Cousins & Bridenbaugh's

NEURAL BLOCKADE
IN CLINICAL ANESTHESIA AND PAIN MEDICINE

Cousins & Bridenbaugh's

NEURAL BLOCKADE
IN CLINICAL ANESTHESIA AND PAIN MEDICINE

Editors

Michael J. Cousins, AM, MB, BS, MD, DSc, FANZCA, FRCA, FFPMANZCA, FAChPM (RACP)
Professor and Head
Department of Anaesthesia and Pain Management
Royal North Shore Hospital
University of Sydney
Professor and Director
Pain Management Research Institute
University of Sydney at Royal North Shore Hospital
St. Leonards, New South Wales
Australia

Daniel B. Carr, MD, DABPM, FFPMANZCA (Hon)
Adjunct Professor
Department of Anesthesiology
Tufts University School of Medicine
Saltonstall Professor of Pain Research
Department of Anesthesiology
Tufts Medical Center
Boston, Massachusetts
Chief Medical Officer
Javelin Pharmaceuticals Inc.
Cambridge, Massachusetts

Terese T. Horlocker, MD
Professor of Anesthesiology and Orthopedics
Department of Anesthesiology
Mayo Clinic College of Medicine
Rochester, Minnesota

Phillip O. Bridenbaugh, MD
Emeritus Professor and Chairman
Department of Anesthesia
University of Cincinnati College of Medicine
Cincinnati, Ohio

 Wolters Kluwer | Lippincott Williams & Wilkins
Health
Philadelphia • Baltimore • New York • London
Buenos Aires • Hong Kong • Sydney • Tokyo

Acquisitions Editor: Brian Brown
Managing Editor: Nicole T. Dernoski
Project Manager: Nicole Walz
Senior Manufacturing Manager: Benjamin Rivera
Senior Marketing Manager: Angela Panetta
Design Coordinator: Teresa Mallon
Cover Designer: Larry Didona
Production Services: Aptara, Inc.

Fourth Edition

© 2009 by Lippincott Williams & Wilkins, a Wolters Kluwer business
© 1998 by Lippincott-Raven Publishers
© 1988 and 1980 by JB Lippincott

Printed in China

Library of Congress Cataloging-in-Publication Data

Cousins and Bridenbaugh's neural blockade in clinical anesthesia and pain medicine / [edited by] Michael J. Cousins, Phillip O. Bridenbaugh – 4th ed.
    p. ; cm.
    Rev. ed. of: Neural blockade in clinical anesthesia and management of pain / editors, Michael J. Cousins, Phillip O. Bridenbaugh. 3rd. ed. c1998.
    Includes bibliographical references and index.
    ISBN-13: 978-0-7817-7388-1
    ISBN-10: 0-7817-7388-1
    1. Nerve block. 2. Anesthesia. 3. Analgesia. I. Cousins, Michael J. II. Bridenbaugh, Phillip O., 1932– III. Neural blockade in clinical anesthesia and management of pain. IV. Title: Neural blockade in clinical anesthesia and pain medicine.
    [DNLM: 1. Nerve Block. 2. Anesthesia, Local. 3. Pain–therapy. WO 300 C867 2009]
    RD84.N48 2009
    617.9′6–dc22   2008029782

10 9 8 7 6 5 4 3 2 1

■ CONTENTS

PART I ■ PHARMACOLOGY AND NEUROPHYSIOLOGY

PART II ■ TECHNIQUES OF NEURAL BLOCKADE IN CLINICAL ANESTHESIA

SECTION A ■ NEURAXIAL BLOCKADE

PART III ▪ APPLICATIONS OF NEURAL BLOCKADE IN CLINICAL ANESTHESIA

PART IV ■ NEURAL BLOCKADE AND THE MANAGEMENT OF PAIN

SECTION A ■ PHYSIOLOGY, PHARMACOLOGY, AND BEHAVIORAL ASPECTS

SECTION B ■ CLINICAL ASSESSMENT OF PERSISTENT PAIN

SECTION C ■ TECHNIQUES OF NEURAL BLOCKADE AND NEUROSTIMULATION

SECTION D ■ APPLICATIONS, COMPLICATIONS, AND THE FUTURE

CONTRIBUTING AUTHORS

Stephen E. Abram, MD
Professor
Department of Anesthesiology
Medical College of Wisconsin
Department of Anesthesiology
Froedtert Memorial Lutheran Hospital
Milwaukee, Wisconsin

Shihab Ahmed, MBBS, MPH
Assistant Professor
Deaprtment of Anesthesia
Harvard Medical School
Assistant in Anesthesia
Department of Anesthesia
Massachusetts General Hospital
Boston, Massachusetts

K. J. S. Anand, MBSS, DPhil
Morris and Hettie Oakley Endowed Chair
    of Critical Care Medicine
Professor of Pediatrics, Anesthesiology, Pharmacology,
    Neurobiology and Developmental Sciences
Director
Pain Neurobiology Laboratory
Arkansas Children's Hospital Research Institute
Little Rock, Arkansas

Francisco Asenjo, MD
Assistant Professor
Department of Anesthesia
McGill University
Staff Anesthesiologist
Department of Anesthesia
McGill University Health Centre
Montreal, Canada

Michael A. Ashburn, MD, MBA, MPH
Professor of Anesthesiology
Director of Pain Medicine and Palliative Care
Penn Pain Medicine Center
University of Pennsylvania
Philadelphia, Pennsylvania

Ralf Baron, Dr. Med
Head, Division of Neurological Pain Research
Department of Neurology
Universitatsklinikum Schleswig-Holstein
Kiel, Germany

Allan L. Basbaum, PhD, FRS
Professor and Chair
Department of Anatomy
University of California San Francisco
San Francisco, California

Fabrizio Benedetti, MD
Professor
Department of Neuroscience
Clinical and Applied Physiology Program
University of Turin Medical School
Turin, Italy

Daniel Benhamou, MD
Professor of Anesthesia and Intensive Care
Department of Anesthesia and Intensive Care
Universite Paris Sud
Chairman
Department of Anesthesia and
    Intensive Care
Hopital Bicetre
Le Kremlin-Bicetre, France

Andreas Binder, DrMed
Division of Neurological Pain Research and
    Therapy
Department of Neurology
Universitatsklinikum Schleswig-Holstein
Kiel, Germany

David J. Birnbach, MD, MPH
Professor and Executive Vice Chair
Department of Anesthesiology
University of Miami
Director
University of Miami–Jackson Memorial
    Hospital Center for Patient Safety
University of Miami Miller School of
    Medicine
Miami, Florida

Hervé Bouaziz, MD
Professor
Department of Anesthesiology
University of Nancy
Praticien Hospitalier
Department of Anesthesiology
University Hospital
Nancy, France

Harald Breivik, MD, DMSc, FRCA (elected)
Professor
Medical Faculty
University of Oslo
Consultant
Department of Anesthesiology and Intensive
    Care
Rikshospitalet Medical Center
Oslo, Norway

David L. Brown, MD
Professor of Anesthesiology and Chair
Institute of Anesthesiology
Cleveland Clinic Foundation
Cleveland, Ohio

Allen W. Burton, MD
Professor
Department of Anesthesiology and Pain Medicine
University of Texas
Chief of Cancer Pain Medicine
Clinical Medical Director
Pain Center
University of Texas–MD Anderson Cancer Center
Houston, Texas

Michael J. Butler, FRCP, FRACP
Senior Lecturer in Medicine
Department of Medicine
University of Auckland
Rheumatologist and Pain Medicine Specialist
Rheumatology Department
The Auckland Regional District Health Board
Auckland, New Zealand

John F. Butterworth, IV, MD
Robert K Stoelting Professor and Chairman
Department of Anesthesia
Indiana University School of Medicine
Co-Chief of Service
Anesthesia Service
Clarian Health Partners–Indiana University Hospital
Indianapolis, Indiana

Xavier Capdevila, MD, PhD
Professor of Anesthesiology and Critical Care Medicine
Montpellier School of Medicine and University
Head of Department
Department of Anesthesia and Critical Care Medicine
Lapeyronie University Hospital
Montpellier, France

Francesco Carli, MD, MPHIL
Professor
Department of Anesthesia
McGill University
Staff Anesthesiologist
Department of Anesthesia
McGill University Health Centre
Montreal, Cananda

Daniel B. Carr, MD, FABPM, FFPMANZCA(Hon)
Adjunct Professor of Anesthesiology
Adjunct Professor of Pharmacology and Experimental
   Therapeutics
Department of Anesthesiology
Tufts University School of Medicine
Saltonstall Professor of Pain Research
Department of Anesthesiology
Tufts Medical Center
Boston, Massachusetts
Chief Medical Officer
Javelin Pharmaceuticals Inc.
Cambridge, Massachusetts

Vincent W.S. Chan, MD, FRCPC
Professor
Department of Anesthesia
University of Toronto
Staff Anesthesiologist
Department of Anesthesiology
Toronto Western Hospital
Toronto, Ontario, Canada

Mark A. Chaney, MD
Associate Professor
Director of Cardiac Anesthesia
Department of Anesthesia and Critical Care
University of Chicago
Chicago, Illinois

Michael J. Cousins, AM, MB, BS, MD, DSc, FANZCA, FRCA, FFPMANZCA, FAChPM (RACP)
Professor and Head
Department of Anaesthesia and Pain Management
Royal North Shore Hospital
University of Sydney
Professor and Director
Pain Management Research Institute
University of Sydney at Royal North Shore Hospital
St. Leonards, New South Wales
Australia

James C. Crews, MD
Associate Professor
Department of Anesthesiology
Wake Forest University
Director, Acute Pain Service
Department of Anesthesiology
Wake Forest University Baptist Medical Center
Winston-Salem, North Carolina

Bernard J. Dalens, MD, PhD
Clinical Professor
Department of Anesthesiology
Université Laval
Anesthesiologist
Department of Anesthesiology
CCHUL-CHUQ
Quebec, Canada

Anthony H. Dickenson, PhD, FMedSci
Professor of Neuropharmacology
Department of Pharmacology
University College London
London, United Kingdom

Dereck Dillane, MB, BCh, BAO, MMedSci, FFARCSI
Assistant Professor
Department of Anesthesiology and Pain Medicine
University of Alberta
University of Alberta Hospital
Edmonton, Canada

F. Kayser Enneking, MD
Professor and Chair
Department of Anesthesiology
College of Medicine
University of Florida
Shands Healthcare System
Gainesville, Florida

Marianne E. Feitl, MD
Arbor Centers for Eye Care
Homewood, Illinois

Perry G. Fine, MD
Professor
Department of Anesthesiology
University of Utah
Salt Lake City, Utah
Vice President for Medical Affairs
National Hospice & Palliative Care Organization
Alexandria, Virginia

B. Raymond Fink, MD (deceased)
Professor Emeritus
Department of Anesthesiology
University of Washington School of Medicine
Seattle, Washington

Damien G. Finniss, MScMed, Bphty, BExSC
Clinical Lecturer
Pain Management and Research Institute
University of Sydney and Royal North Shore Hospital
Sydney, Australia

Brendan T. Finucane, MD, BCh, FRCA, FRCPC
Professor Emeritus
Department of Anesthesiology and Pain Medicine
University of Alberta
Staff Anesthesiologist/Director of Anesthesia Services CCI
Department of Anesthesiology
Leduc Community Hospital and Cross Cancer Institute
Edmonton, Canada

Scott M. Fishman, MD
Professor
Chief, Division of Pain Medicine
Department of Anesthesiology and Pain Medicine
University of California, Davis School of Medicine
Sacramento, California

Julia A. Fleming, MBBS, PhD, FANZCA, FFPMANZCA
Anaesthetist, Head Acute Pain Service
Department of Anaesthetics
Department of Palliative Care
Peter MacCallum Cancer Centre
Victoria, Australia

Rollin M. Gallagher, MD, MPH
Clinical Professor and Director for Pain
    Policy Research and Primary Care
Departments of Psychiatry and
    Anesthesiology and Critical Care
University of Pennsylvania School of Medicine
Director of Pain Medicine
Department of Anesthesia
Philadelphia VA Medical Center
Philadelphia, Pennsylvania

Joseph A. Giovannitti, Jr., DMD
Associate Professor
Department of Anesthesiology
University of Pittsburgh, School of Dental Medicine
Pittsburgh, Pennsylvania

Michael Gofeld, MD
Assistant Professor
Faculty of Medicine
University of Toronto
Staff Physician
Department of Anesthesiology and Pain Medicine
Sunnybrook Health Sciences Centre
Toronto, Canada

David O. Gorman, MD, FFARCSI, DPM
Clinical Lecturer
National University of Ireland
Division of Pain Medicine
Department of Anesthesia
University College Hospital
Galway, Ireland

Dominic C. Harmon, MD
Professor
Department of Medicine
University of Limerick Medical School
Consultant
Department of Anaesthesia and Pain Medicine
Mid-Western Regional Hospital
Limerick, Ireland

Robert D. Helme, MB, BS, PhD, FRACP, FFPMANZCA
Honary Professorial Associate
Department of Medicine
University of Melbourne
Parkville, Australia
Director
Department of Neurology
Western Hospital
Footscray, Australia

Quinn H. Hogan, MD
Professor
Department of Anesthesiology
Medical College of Wisconsin
Milwaukee, Wisconsin

Terese T. Horlocker, MD
Professor of Anesthesiology and Orthopedics
Department of Anesthesiology
Mayo Clinic College of Medicine
Rochester, Minnesota

Constance S. Houck, MD
Assistant Professor
Department of Anaesthesia
Harvard Medical School
Senior Associate in Perioperative Anesthesia
Department of Anesthesiology,
    Perioperative and Pain Medicine
Children's Hospital Boston
Boston, Massachusetts

Narasimhan Jagannathan, MD
Attending Anesthesiologist
Assistant Professor of Anesthesia
Feinberg School of Medicine
Northwestern University
Chicago, Illinois

Joel Katz, PhD
Professor and Canada Research Chair in Health Psychology
Department of Psychology
York University
Senior Scientist
Department of Anesthesia and Pain Management
Toronto General Hospital University Health Network
Toronto, Ontario, Canada

Spencer S. Liu, MD
Clinical Professor of Anesthesiology
Department of Anesthesiology
Weill Cornell Medical Center
Director of Acute Pain Service
Department of Anesthesiology
Hospital for Special Surgery
New York, New York

John D. Loeser, MD
Professor
Departments of Neurological Surgery and Anesthesiology
University of Washington
University of Washington Medical Center
Seattle, Washington

Pamela E. Macintyre, MBBS, MHA, FANZCA, FFPMANZCA
Clinical Lecturer
Discipline of Anaesthesia
University of Adelaide
Director, Acute Pain Service
Department of Anaesthesia, Pain Medicine and Hyperbaric Medicine
Royal Adelaide Hospital
Adelaide, South Australia

Stephen Mannion, MD, MB, MRCPI
Consultant Anaesthetist
Department of Anaesthesia
South Infirmary-Victoria University Hospital
Cork, Ireland

Laurence E. Mather, FANZCA, FRCA
Emeritus Professor of Anesthesia
Department of Anesthesia and Pain Management
University of Sydney at Royal North Shore Hospital
Sydney, Australia

Kathryn E. McGoldrick, MD
Professor and Chair
Department of Anesthesiology
New York Medical College
Director
Department of Anesthesiology
Westchester Medical Center
Valhalla, New York

Graeme A. McLeod, MD, MRCGP, FRCA
Honorary Senior Lecturer
Department of Anaesthesia
University of Dundee
Consultant
Department of Anaesthesia
Ninewells Hospital and Medical School
Dundee, United Kingdom

Ronald Melzack, OC, FRSC, PhD
Emeritus E.P. Taylor Professor of Psychology
McGill University
Montreal, Canada

Michael F. Mulroy, MD
Clinical Professor
Department of Anesthesiology
University of Washington
Anesthesiology Faculty
Department of Anesthesiology
Virginia Mason Medical Center
Seattle, Washington

Joseph M. Neal, MD
Anesthesiology Faculty
Department of Anesthesiology
Virginia Mason Medical Center
Clinical Professor of Anesthesiology
Department of Anesthesiology
University of Washington
Seattle, Washington

David Niv, MD (deceased)
Director Center for Pain Medicine
Tel-Aviv Sourasky Medical Center
Israel

Els Pastijn, MD
Anesthesiology
Université Libre de Bruxelles
Anesthesia Resident
Department of Anesthesiology
Le Centre Hospitalièr Universitairè St. Pierre
Brussels, Belgium

Phillip C. Phan, MD
Assistant Professor
Department of Anesthesiology and Pain Medicine
University of Texas
Director of Interventional Pair Management
Cancer Pain Management MD Anderson Cancer Center
Houston, Texas

James C. Phero, DMD
Professor of Clinical Anesthesia
Professor of Surgery
Professor Pediatrics
Department of Anesthesiology
University of Cincinnati College of Medicine
Faculty Anesthesiologist
Department of Anesthesiology
University Hospitals
University of Cincinnati Medical Center
Cincinnati, Ohio

Carlos A. Pino, MD
Assistant Professor
Department of Anesthesiology
University of Vermont
Director, Center for Pain Medicine
Department of Anesthesiology
Fletcher Allen Health Care
Burlington, Vermont

Mikko Pitkänen, MD, PhD
Associate Professor
Department of Anesthesiology
Helsinki University
Chief Anesthesiologist
Department of Anesthesiology
Orton Orthopaedic Hospital, Invalid Foundation
Helsinki, Finland

Joshua P. Prager, MD, MS
Director
Center for the Rehabilitation of Pain Syndromes (CRPS)
    at UCLA Medical Plaza
Clinical Assistand Professor
Department of Anesthesiology and Internal Medicine
David Geffen School of Medicine at UCLA
Los Angeles. California

James P. Rathmell, MD
Associate Professor of Anaesthesia
Harvard Medical School
Director, Center for Pain Medicine
Department of Anesthesia and Critical Care
Massachusetts General Hospital
Boston, Massachusetts

Per H. Rosenberg, MD, PhD
Professor of Anesthesiology
Department of Anesthesiology and Intensive Care Medicine
University of Helsinki
Chief Anesthesiologist
Department of Anesthesiology and Intensive
    Care Medicine
Helsinki University Hospital
Helsinki, Finland

Morton B. Rosenberg, DMD
Professor of Oral and Maxillofacial Surgery
Head Division of Anesthesia and Pain Control
Tufts University School of Dental Medicine
Associate Professor of Anesthesia
Tufts University School of Medicine
Senior Anesthetist
Department of Anesthesiology
Tufts-New England Medical Center Hospitals
Boston, Massachusetts

William S. Schechter, MD, MS, FAAP
Clinical Professor of Anesthesiology and Pediatrics
Columbia University College of Physicians and Surgeons
Director, Pediatric Pain Medicine Program
Division of Pediatric Anesthesia and Intensive Care
Morgan Stanley Children's Hospital of New York
    Presbyterian
Columbia University Medical Center
New York, New York

Thomas Schricker, MD, MPhD
Associate Professor
Department of Anesthesia
McGill University
Chief
Department of Anesthesia
McGill University Health Centre
Montreal, Canada

David A. Scott, MB, BS, PhD, FANZCA, FFPMANZCA
Associate Professor
Department of Surgery
University of Melbourne
Parkville, Australia
Deputy Director
Department of Anaesthesia
St. Vincent's Hospital, Melbourne
Melbourne, Australia

Lucinda C. Seagrove, MD
Department of Pharmacology
University College London
London, United Kingdom

George D. Shorten, FRCA(RCSI), MD, PhD
Professor and Head
Department of Anaesthesia
National University of Ireland, Cork
Consultant Anaesthetist
Department of Anaesthesia and Intensive Care Medicine
Cork University Hospital
Cork, Ireland

Philip J. Siddall, MBBS, MM (Pain Mgmt), PhD, FFPMANZCA
Clinical Associate Professor
Pain Management Research Institute
University of Sydney
Senior Principal Research Fellow
Department of Anaesthesia and Pain Management
Royal North Shore Hospital
Sydney, Australia

Michael Stanton-Hicks, DrMed, FRCA, ABPM
Professor
Department of Anesthesia
Case Lerner School of Medicine
Vice Chairman
Department of Anesthesia
Cleveland Clinic
Cleveland, Ohio

Gary R. Strichartz, PhD
Professor
Department of Anesthesiology and Pharmacology
Harvard Medical School
Vice-Chairman for Research
Department of Anesthesiology, Perioperative
    and Pain Medicine
Brigham & Women's Hospital
Boston, Massachusetts

Kenji Sugimoto, MD, PhD
Anesthetist
Department of Anesthesiology
Nagoya University Graduate School of Medicine
Nagoya, Japan

Santhanam Suresh, MD, FAAP
Associate Professor of Anesthesiology and Pediatrics
Department of Anesthesia
Feinberg School of Medicine
Northwestern University
Director of Research
Department of Pediatric Anesthesiology
Children's Memorial Hospital
Chicago, Illinois

Joseph D. Tobias, MD
Vice-Chairman, Department of Anesthesiology
Chief, Division of Pediatric Anesthesiology
Russell and Mary Shelden Chair in Pediatric
    Intensive Care Medicine
Professor Anesthesiology and Child Health
University of Missouri
Columbia, Missouri

Mary Ellen Tresgallo, DNP, MS, MPH
Assistant Clinical Professor of Nursing
Columbia University School of Nursing
Attending Nurse Practitioner
Department of Anesthesiology
Pediatric Pain Medicine Program
Morgan Stanley Children's Hospital of
    New York Presbyterian
Columbia University Medical Center
New York, New York

René Truchon, MD, FRCP
Clinical Professor
Department of Anesthesiology
Université Laval
Anesthesiologist
Department of Anesthesiology
CHUL-CHUQ
Québec, Canada

Geoffrey T. Tucker, PhD
Professor and Head of Academic Unit
Academic Unit of Clinical Pharmacology
University of Sheffield
Floor M. Royal Hallamshire Hospital
Sheffield, United Kingdom

Ban C.H. Tsui, MSC, MD, FRCP (C)
Associate Professor
Department of Anesthesiology and Pain Medicine
University of Alberta
Director, Regional Anesthesia and Acute Pain Service
Department of Anesthesiology and Pain Medicine
University of Alberta Hospital
Edmonton, Alberta, Canada

Bernadette T. Veering, MD, PhD
Senior Lecturer
Staff Anesthesiologist
Department of Anesthesiology
Leiden University Medical Center
Leiden, The Netherlands

Christopher D. Vije, MD
Resident Physician
Department of Anesthesiology and Critical Care
Hospital of the University of Pennsylvania
Philadelphia, PA

**Suellen M. Walker, MBBS MM(Pain Management),
MSc, PhD, FANZCA, FEPMANZCA**
Clinical Senior Lecturer in Paediatric
    Anesthesia and Pain Medicine
Portex Anaesthesia Unit
UCL Institute of Child Health
Honorary Consultant
Department of Anaesthesia
Great Ormond Street Hospital for
    Children NHS Trust
London, United Kingdom

Denise J. Wedel, MD
Professor
Department of Anesthesiology
Mayo Clinic College of Medicine
Rochester, Minnesota

J. A. W. Wildsmith, MD, FRCA
Professor Emeritus
Department of Anaesthesia
University of Dundee
Ninewells Hospital and Medical School
Dundee, United Kingdom

Christopher L. Wu, MD
Associate Professor
Department of Anesthesiology
The Johns Hopkins University
Associate Professor
Department of Anesthesiology
The Johns Hopkins Hospital
Baltimore, Maryland

Tony L. Yaksh, PhD
Professor and Vice Chairman for Research
Department of Anesthesiology
University of San Diego
La Jolla, California

Paul Zetlaoui, MD
Staff Anesthesiologist
Department of Anesthesiology and Intensive Care Medicine
Le Kremlin Bicêtre University Hospital
Le Kremlin Bicêtre, France

FOREWORD TO THE FOURTH EDITION

The field of pain research and therapy has made major advances in the past decade. The editors of this excellent, up-to-date fourth edition of *Neural Blockade in Clinical Anesthesia and Pain Medicine* present the science and practice of neural blockade in every setting in which it can be used. It covers analgesia for acute pain relief, as well as regional anesthesia for surgery, obstetrics, posttrauma and postprocedural pain, and includes the management of cancer and chronic noncancer pain.

During the 10 years since the third edition, new evidence has highlighted the importance of effective treatment of acute pain in preventing neural "memory" changes in the nervous system that may lead to the development of persistent pain. This new edition focuses on the important overlap of science and practice in neural blockade, and introduces recent knowledge of genetic and other risk factors that predispose patients to experience higher levels of pain in association with surgery, trauma, and disease states. As these risk factors are increasingly being identified, it becomes possible to identify patients and situations in which the risk is high for the progression from acute to persistent pain. As a result, the anesthesiologist is able to play a crucial "preventive" role. Indeed, future anesthesiologists may routinely practice preventative pain control through their skilled endeavors pre-, intra-, and postoperatively.

Among the major research themes of the past two decades—and now reaching clinical trials—is the role of sodium channel subtype dysregulation in persistent pain. Concurrently, recognition of the role of psychological factors in pain experience has given rise to a major new component of the rapidly growing specialty of pain medicine. Thanks to scientific advances ranging from ion channel molecular biology to the imaging of the brain in a conscious person experiencing pain, we now stand at the threshold of the ability to trace links between tissue injury and the experience of pain. Consequently, multimodal pain relief has emerged as a key concept, aiming to improve pain relief and minimize side effects. Although traditional local anesthetics still play a dominant role, this fourth edition describes the use of many other drugs aiming at targets in addition to the sodium channel. This multimodal approach extends to targeting receptors in diverse anatomic locations in nerve axons, spinal cord, and brain, and is aimed at pain relief during surgery, postoperatively, and posttrauma, as well as for cancer and chronic noncancer pain.

Neural blockade is an option for the relief of severe pain, and much emphasis is given in this edition to its place in the wide spectrum of pain problems that encompass the whole field of pain medicine. Importantly, the use of psychological and environmental manipulation is also elucidated. Neural blockade is undoubtedly the most potent method of relief for acute pain, and thus should be available to severely affected patients. It should likewise be available to patients suffering the many other pain problems described in this text. Finally, it is clear that the use of neural blockade sits firmly within the increasing recognition that "pain management is a fundamental human right," as has been strongly advocated by two of the editors (MC and DC).

Ronald Melzack, O.C., F.R.S.C., Ph.D.
Emeritus E.P. Taylor Professor of Psychology
McGill University
Montreal, Canada

■ FOREWORD TO THE SECOND EDITION

Neural Blockade in Clinical Anesthesia and Management of Pain must be the most ambitious project of its kind ever undertaken. This book ranges from a consideration of the physiology, pharmacology, and toxicology of the local analgesic agents in common use to a number of the less orthodox methods of relieving suffering of various origins. The book is indeed encyclopedic in its coverage, and, like encyclopedias in other sciences, each section has been entrusted to a recognized world authority in his own special field. No book on local analgesia could have a sounder pedigree.

There are situations in which, manifestly, local anesthesia is preferable to general. Apart from these, improved sedation and longer-acting analgesic drugs have improved patient acceptance, but the practitioner still has to acquire the necessary "know-how" to deposit the solution with reasonable accuracy for it to be effective. Both editors are renowned for their practical teaching, which should be a sound guarantee that both the expert and the tyro can turn to this book for guidance and profit.

Neural blockade offers far more to the patient than merely analgesia during surgery. Rapid growth in application of neural blockade to postoperative, posttraumatic, and obstetric pain management is extensively covered in this textbook. Even more extensive is the breadth and depth of scientific information and clinical application of neural blockade in chronic pain; this is presented as completely and concisely as possible.

Sir Robert Macintosh, D.M., F.R.C.S. (EDIN), HON F.E.A.R.C.S.
Emeritus Nuffield Professor of Anaesthetics,
University of Oxford

PREFACE

The decade since publication of the third edition of *Neural Blockade* has been one of vigorous progress in the specialties of anesthesiology and pain medicine, including recognition of the latter as a medical specialty per se. Advances in preclinical knowledge of the anatomy, physiology, and pharmacology of regionally applied drugs have been translated into improved or entirely novel techniques. Progress in molecular biology has improved the understanding of individual differences in response to pain or its treatment, leading to calls for a new era of personalized medical care. Optimal assessment and treatment of pain have always been and will always remain individualized. At the same time, assessments of the evidence for, and outcomes of medical practice are also increasing in an era of economic pressure and concern for efficiency in health care systems worldwide (1).

Many objective economic and physiologic outcomes are improved by early or "preventive" pain control. Yet, even if that were not the case, from the patient's point of view, avoidance of unnecessary pain and suffering are key to improving quality of life (1). As health care systems become increasingly patient-centered, society at large has come to view the appropriate management of pain as a fundamental human right (2). Respecting this right is not only ethical and humane, but also may decrease the likelihood of transition from acute to chronic pain and hence reduce the enormous societal and economic costs of the latter (3). In Australia (population 20 million), a comprehensive 2007 study calculated the annual cost of chronic pain as $34.3 billion Australian, with an associated economic burden of 36.5 million lost workdays annually (4). Substantial savings, both in economic and human terms, can likewise result from shortening the length of stay and postoperative morbidity by improving the management of acute pain (5). Optimal management of cancer pain can increase quality of life, including self-care and independence, decrease caregiver burden, and may extend survival. To fully realize these benefits and savings requires pain control within a multidimensional framework that includes behavioral support, physical conditioning, and (particularly in perioperative care) attention to nutrition, temperature control, and fluid management (6). Maintenance of this infrastructure requires never-ending investment in education for those who provide, as well as those who pay for care.

Because neural blockade and pain medicine are practical skills, no text or syllabus alone can substitute for the hands-on experience required to absorb the many subtleties (including tactile cues) needed to learn and apply these skills safely and effectively. Texts offer the best of all possible means to understand, at one's own pace, the benefits and risks in advance of any proposed intervention. They also allow one to visualize the techniques needed to perform the intervention, and to reflect upon and integrate such knowledge afterward. The process of reading is now known to activate many areas of the brain such as those associated with motor activity, associative memory, and even speech. The editors have not only addressed the text of each contributed chapter, but we have also been most fortunate to enlist as a medical illustrator a protégé of Alan Bentley, a medical illustrator of extraordinary talent whose clear, authoritative figures were so important to prior editions. Marcus Cremonese, the illustrator who has worked on this fourth edition, was able to adhere to Mr. Bentley's signature visual style to continue his tradition of lucid, meticulously prepared illustrations.

Four major trends of importance for regional anesthesia and pain medicine were identified in the Preface to the third edition. They were: (a) the increased use of same-day and short-stay surgery, in part due to wide use of minimally invasive surgical techniques and multimodal analgesia (6); (b) emphasis on rapid rehabilitation even after major surgery; (c) development of acute postoperative pain services and specialized obstetric analgesia services; and (d) a gradual move toward recognition of pain relief as "a basic human right." These trends are very much alive and well. They have been supplemented by an increasing emphasis upon the risks of therapy as well the benefits. To address these ongoing trends, we have added chapters to this fourth edition and expanded prior chapters that describe risks related to techniques of neural blockade, electrical or mechanical failure (e.g., of pump devices or spinal catheters), and co-administered drugs (including anticoagulants). Chapters have also been added on outcomes assessment, the use of newer modalities for regional anesthesia such as microcatheters, socioeconomic factors in pain and disability (including disparities in pain care), the physiologic effects of needle insertion, the placebo response, care of older persons, and palliative care.

A major new theme is that persistent or chronic pain is a disease in its own right. This conclusion follows from extensive research documenting a constellation of physiologic, psychological, and neurochemical responses in persistent pain distinct from those seen in acute pain (7). This new theme underpins current efforts to identify novel targets and develop "target-specific treatments" that directly attack processes that cause and maintain this disease. In the physiologic domain, molecular biology has made major contributions in identifying targets such as the NaV1.7 and NaV1.8 channels as well as the α_2-δ subunit of neuronal calcium channels, and the α_2-adrenoceptor. Other targets also play significant roles in the pathophysiology of persistent pain. Exciting new evidence implicates microglia, partly via tumor necrosis factor (TNF)-α and other inflammatory cytokines, as well as neurotrophic factors in triggering and sustaining persistent pain. These developments represent a major shift in direction and have already led to clinical trials of disease-specific treatments. In contrast, prior efforts aimed solely at relieving pain as a symptom by using morphine, aspirin, and even peripheral nerve blocks. Parallel progress has been made in correlating regional microenvironmental brain and spinal cord neurochemical responses, including metabolic activation, with behavioral and psychological changes during effective treatments. Many new chapters and markedly revised existing chapters in the present edition address this major new theme. Anesthesiologists should note that this theme is equally important to them as well as specialists in pain medicine. The translation of analgesic research into improved clinical outcomes is a major part of the new role of the anesthesiologist as a specialist in perioperative medicine (6). Anesthesiologists are strategically situated to play a crucial role in translating new knowledge about genetic and other risk factors for persistent pain into improved clinical outcomes. In so doing, they will provide enormous humanitarian and economic benefit, and gain profound personal satisfaction.

The third edition concluded with an essay on "new horizons" by the late Professor Patrick Wall, a topic that has been revisited in the final chapter of the current edition by Professor Allan Basbaum. As Professor Basbaum emphasizes, peripheral nociceptive activity plays a pivotal role in all types of acute and persistent pain, thereby ensuring the relevance of this text well into the future. All told, the present edition has expanded the third edition by 17 chapters, from 34 to 51, and the total number of authors from 52 representing 9 countries, to 90 (including 68 new ones) representing 15 countries. The very existence of such an extensive group of international experts—nearly all with their own clinical practices, students, trainees, and junior colleagues—bodes well for the continued mutual strength of regional anesthesia and pain medicine.

References

1. Wittink H, Carr DB, eds. *Pain Management: Evidence, Outcomes and Quality of Life.* New York: Elsevier, 2008.
2. Brennan F, Carr DB, Cousins MJ. Pain management: a fundamental human right. *Anesth Analg* 2007;105:205–221.
3. Van Leeuwen MT, Blyth FM, March LM, et al. Chronic pain and reduced work effectiveness: the hidden cost to Australian employers. *Eur J Pain* 2006; 2:161–166.
4. Blyth FM, Cousins M, Arnold C, et al., for the Pain Epidemiology Research Group, University of Sydney Pain Management Research Institute, Royal North Shore Hospital, Sydney. The high price of persistent pain: the economic impact of persistent pain in Australia. Sydney: Access Economics Pty Limited, 2007. Accessed Sept. 15, 2008 at http://www.anzca.edu.au/fpm/news-and-reports/Thehighpriceofpainfinal-185.pdf.
5. Australian and New Zealand College of Anaesthetists, Faculty of Pain Medicine. *Acute Pain Management: Scientific Evidence,* 2nd ed. Melbourne: Australian and New Zealand College of Anaesthetists, 2005. Accessed Sept. 15, 2008 at http://www.anzca.edu.au/publications/acutepain.htm.
6. White PF, Kehlet H, Neal JM, et al., and the Fast-track Surgery Study Group. The role of the anesthesiologist in fast-track surgery: from multimodal analgesia to perioperative medical care. *Anesth Analg* 2007;104:1380–1396.
7. Siddall PJ. Cousins MJ. Persistent pain as a disease entity: implications for clinical management. *Anesth Analg* 2004;99:510–520.

■ ACKNOWLEDGMENTS

Professor Michael J. Cousins

I thank my mentors, who shaped my now more than 40-year interest and commitment to neural blockade and to pain medicine: Philip Bromage at McGill University Montreal, Canada (1969–1970); Richard I. Mazze at Stanford University, California (1971–1975); Patrick Wall as editor-in-chief of the journal *Pain* while I served as associate editor; Nicholas M. Greene and Ronald Miller as successive editors-in-chief, while I served two separate terms on the editorial board of *Anesthesia & Analgesia*, acting as foundation editor for a new section on pain medicine during my second tour of duty; John J. Bonica, Ronald Melzack, John Loeser, and many other councillors during my more than 20 years on the council of the International Association for the Study of Pain (IASP), serving as IASP President from 1987–1990.

During the years 1975–1990 and 1990–2008, I developed foundation academic departments of anesthesiology and pain medicine at Flinders University, South Australia and Sydney University, respectively. The main academic focus in both cases was the scientific basis of neural blockade and pain medicine. The numerous basic and clinical scientists that I recruited, the research and clinical fellows who trained with me, and our research collaborations all contributed in some way to this text. Many of these colleagues enriched my professional and personal life very greatly. The rigor of the text has been influenced by my experience on the Council of the National Health & Medical Research Council (NHMRC) of Australia; I also served as chair of the NHMRC Clinical Practice Guideline "Acute Pain Management: Scientific Evidence." I continue to gain insight into evolving standards and methodology in medical education as a councillor on the Australian Medical Council and recently as chair of the Presidents of Medical Specialist Colleges of Australia.

Phillip Bridenbaugh and I have worked jointly on this book from 1973 to 2008; this 35-year collaboration has been rewarding, productive, and harmonious at all times—a partnership based on shared interests and friendship akin to family. Sadly, since the third edition, two giants in this field have died: John J. Bonica, the founding father of pain medicine, and Patrick Wall, preeminent basic scientist and founding editor of the journal *Pain*. Both are deeply missed as enormous contributors to this field and as good friends.

The addition of two new editors has recognized the need for a transition to the "next generation." Thus, Phillip Bridenbaugh and I had no hesitation in choosing Terese Horlocker of the Mayo Clinic for her prominence in neural blockade in clinical anesthesia and Dan Carr for his extensive and outstanding role in pain medicine. Numerous very rewarding publication projects have previously been shared with Dan Carr, and our interaction as joint editors of the pain medicine section of the book has been similarly productive and memorable. I thank my personal assistant in Sydney, Helen Johnston, for help beyond the call of duty, which made my contribution to this text possible. I again acknowledge the enormous value of the artwork of Alan Bentley in the first three editions and the excellent work of his protégé Marcus Cremonese for this fourth edition.

On behalf of all of the editors, I thank the staff of Lippincott Williams & Wilkins (Brian Brown, senior acquisitions editor, and Nicole Dernoski, senior managing editor) for their commitment to the high standard set by this text and for their efforts and forbearance, and Max Leckrone for management of its production.

Professor Daniel B. Carr

I thank my countless patients and colleagues for my education in anesthesiology and pain medicine. Michael Rosenblatt, John Potts, and Joseph B. Martin guided me at the start of my academic career in the endocrine unit of the Massachusetts General Hospital, assaying β-endorphin levels alongside Mike Arnold. Richard Kitz, chairman of the MGH Department of Anesthesia and an exceptional mentor and warm friend to many, oversaw the broadening of my research focus to pain and analgesia. Dr. Kitz introduced me to Professor Cousins in the 1980s, and also arranged my apprenticeship to the late Donald Todd in an era before formal pain fellowships. A protégé of Henry Beecher, Don was a pioneer in clinical pain medicine. To be the junior colleague of this remarkably caring clinician of vast knowledge, experience, and humility was a unique privilege. Other close MGH colleagues included Drs. Dementrios Lappas, Ed Lowenstein, Patricia Osgood, Carl Rosow, John Ryan, and Stan Szyfelbein. A long-term collaboration with Professor Lipkowski of Warsaw also began in the 1980s, as did fruitful interactions with colleagues at other Harvard hospitals (Drs. Covino, Ostheimer, Datta, Concepcion, Steinbrook, Ferrante, and Lema).

In the 1990s, Heinrich Wurm, a respected colleague with shared interests in regional anesthesia and pain medicine, invited me to become the Saltonstall Professor of Pain Research at Tufts Medical Center. The Salstontall Fund, led by its principal trustee Dudley Willis, has supported an efficient infrastructure for ongoing research and education within which Evelyn Hall has played a uniquely important role. Her editorial skills and work ethic benefited this volume in many ways. Colleagues at Tufts have shared their insights into pharmacology and analgesic drug development (Drs. Greenblatt and Lasagna), evidence and outcomes (Drs. Lau, Rogers, Wittink, and Chalmers), and professional education (Drs. Lasch, Harrington, Sackler, and Berman; Ms. Connolly, and again, Mike

Rosenblatt). Former fellows at Harvard and Tufts (e.g., Drs. Ballantyne, Cepeda, Eisenberg, Fishman, Goudas, Langlade, McNicol, Silbert, and Strassels), co-editors (e.g., Drs. Addison, Dubois, Gallagher, Gebhart, Loeser, and Morris), colleagues from the American Academy of Pain Medicine, American Pain Society, American Society of Regional Anesthesia and Pain Medicine, Cochrane Collaboration (Phil Wiffen), IASP, and U.S. Agency for Healthcare Research and Quality have all shaped my perspective on pain medicine. The support of Professors Horlocker and Bridenbaugh—and, of course, my family, along with colleagues at Javelin Pharmaceuticals—during completion of this volume amidst other daily responsibilities was indispensable. I especially thank Michael Cousins, whose vast knowledge, tenacity in persisting toward the goal, and commitment to optimizing every detail of the present volume provided a years-long lesson in inspiring leadership. It is an honor and privilege to be a steward of the very same text that, for decades, I have recommended to trainees and colleagues as the single best "desert island" book on neural blockade and pain medicine.

Professor Terese T. Horlocker
I gratefully recognize the many friends, colleagues and teachers who have so generously shared their knowledge of medicine and regional anesthesia. In particular, I look to Professor Denise J. Wedel, who not only put a needle in my hand, but also guided it (as well as my career). Contributing to the fourth edition of *Neural Blockade in Clinical Anesthesia and Management of Pain* has been a humbling experience for me. For over a quarter of a century, this text has defined the specialty; conceptualized, edited, and composed as it was by the patriarchs of regional anesthesia and pain medicine. For the opportunity to collaborate on this volume and also for their mentoring and friendship, I am grateful to my co-editors Professors Cousins, Bridenbaugh, and Carr. Likewise, this edition would not have been possible without the dedication of the contributing authors who selflessly shared their expertise in order to better understand and treat pain and suffering. Finally, I acknowledge the contributions of my family: Randy, Mark, and Caterina, who have steadfastly directed my efforts towards the final goal—in this and so many other endeavors—with their faith, hope, and love.

Professor Phillip O. Bridenbaugh
This fourth edition will conclude my 35 years of editorship. It is impossible to express the relationships—personal, collegial, professional, familial, and memorable—that have developed between myself and Professor Cousins over this time. The nurturing of four editions of *Neural Blockade in Clinical Anesthesia and Management of Pain* has been a life-changing experience for both of us. I owe a debt of gratitude to my wife, Dr. Diann Bridenbaugh, and family, who have been involved directly and indirectly with all four editions. It is impossible to appropriately acknowledge the contributions of all the past authors. I especially thank Professors Carr and Horlocker, who have worked so diligently and efficiently as editors to assure the high quality of science and practical knowledge in this fourth edition. I share their appreciation and gratitude to all contributors to the fourth edition for the quality and timeliness of their offerings. We have also been blessed with the continued support of the same publishers since the first edition of the book—an unusual accomplishment and a key factor accounting for the stellar reputation of this book internationally across multiple medical disciplines. I expect that future editions of *Neural Blockade in Clinical Anesthesia and Management of Pain* will continue to serve the scientific and clinical needs of those in medical practice for generations to come. Thanks to all, past and present, for being part of the *Neural Blockade in Clinical Anesthesia and Management of Pain* legacy. I wish you continued success in future editions.

CHAPTER 1 ■ THE HISTORY OF REGIONAL ANESTHESIA

DAVID L. BROWN AND B. RAYMOND FINK

The popularization of regional anesthesia was not possible until two events occurred. First, a local anesthetic was required, and second, advanced understanding of infectious agents was needed. In 1886, the introduction of cocaine by Koller provided the answer to the first required event, and the increased understanding of infectious complications was made possible by the introduction of the theories of Lister in the 1870s (1). The sequence of these requirements was essential in allowing regional anesthesia to progress since, had physicians progressed to spinal or other regional anesthetics prior to introduction of asepsis to the practice of medicine, it seems likely that regional anesthesia would have been significantly delayed or even prevented from progressing into surgical practices. To most completely understand whence our regional practices have developed, it is helpful to examine a number of issues, including the physiology of neural transmission; the development of local anesthetics (especially cocaine); the use of infiltration anesthesia, intravenous (IV) regional anesthesia, spinal anesthesia, obstetric, and epidural anesthesia; paravertebral anesthesia; and the maturation of the specialty of regional anesthesia within the larger specialty of anesthesiology.

PHYSIOLOGY OF NEURAL TRANSMISSION

Fundamental to modern neural blockade and regional anesthesia is the concept that sensory block is accomplished by pharmacologically interrupting specific nerve fibers, amenable, in principle, to modulation or interruption along the nerve's pathway. This outlook may be traced back to developments in the study of physiology that finally supplanted the view first expressed by Plato and Aristotle that pain, like pleasure, is a passion of the soul—that is, an emotion and not one of the senses (Table 1-1). Philosophical changes from the great scientific revolutions of the 18th century and the birth of biology gradually, although not entirely, effaced the religious connotations of pain in Western civilization (2). These philosophical revolutions of the 18th century were in part based on the mechanistic concepts of biologic function that Descartes developed during the 17th century. Descartes matured the concept of a neural connection from the periphery to the brain (Fig. 1-1). James Moore (1762–1860), a London surgeon (Fig. 1-2), used these mechanistic concepts to promote neural compression as a useful technique for the provision of surgical anesthesia (Table 1-2). As illustrated in Figure 1-3, Moore developed techniques for both upper and lower extremity nerve compression and wrote his monograph, "A Method of Preventing or Di-

minishing Pain in Several Operations of Surgery," only after experimenting upon himself (2a,2b).

The doctrine of specific energies of the senses was first promulgated by Johannes P. Müller (1801–1858) in 1826 (3). This doctrine, although it did not posit specificity for the conduction of pain, initiated the movement of scientific thought toward analysis and classification of the specific characters of different nerves. Earlier, in 1803, Charles Bell defined important functions of the dorsal roots of the spinal nerves as distinct from those of the ventral roots, and he initiated a rigorous search for a more complete understanding of the sensory phenomena. Bell highlighted that dorsal root function is sensory and ventral root function is motor (4). In 1851, von Helmholtz succeeded in measuring the velocity with which the nerve impulse travels and opened the way for the development of modern electrophysiology (5).

The theory that pain was a separate and distinct sense was first definitely formulated by Moritz S. Schiff (1823–1896) in 1858, following experiments on animals (6). A rival theory, the intensity theory, was stated explicitly by Erb in 1874, but had been anticipated by Erasmus Darwin (1731–1802), who said that pain results "whenever the sensorial motions are stronger than usual (6)." Attempts to influence neuralgic pain by applying a drug to the transmitting nerve appear to have been published first by Francis Rynd (1801–1861) (7). Rynd's idea may be said to have foreshadowed both nerve block and, more remotely, opioid regional analgesia.

According to some accounts of the 1850s, Pravaz in Lyon and Wood in Edinburgh invented the syringe and hypodermic hollow needle, respectively (Table 1-2). A thorough sifting of the historical evidence (8) and independent reexamination of the sources support the following outline of the facts. In 1845, Rynd described the idea of introducing a solution of morphine hypodermically in the neighborhood of a peripheral nerve (7), with the intention of allaying neuralgic pain in that nerve. However, he introduced the solution not by syringe but by means of gravity, allowing it to enter passively through a cannula after removal of the trocar. The invention of the syringe is lost in the mists of several centuries preceding Alexander Wood (1817–1884). Wood's contribution was his procedure of subcutaneous injection, which he performed in 1855 using a graduated glass syringe and hollow needle supplied by Ferguson (9). This equipment had been manufactured by Ferguson for a different purpose, namely the injection of ferric perchloride into an aneurysm to produce a coagulum, as proposed by Charles-Gabriel Pravaz (1791–1853) in 1853, following experiments in animals (10). Pravaz himself had used a syringe and trocar (*trois-carre*). Wood thus originated the practice of percutaneous subcutaneous injection to medicate locally a peripheral

TABLE 1-1

CHRONOLOGY OF IDEAS CONCERNING PAIN AND NEURAL BLOCKADE[a]

ca. 500 B.C.	**Alcmaeon (Croton)** The brain is associated with the organs of sense.
ca. 375 B. C.	**Plato (Athens)** Pain is an emotion that dwells in the brain.
ca. 200	**Galen (Pergamon)** Recognized the functional unity of the brain, spinal cord, and peripheral nerves
1752	**Haller (Germany)** Only certain specific parts of the body react to pain, disclosing sensibility.
1826	**Müeller (Germany)** Asserted the doctrine of specific sensory energies; that no direct correlation exists between the external stimulation and the impression received
1855	**Wood (UK)** Neuralgic pain can be treated by circumneural injections of pain-relieving drugs.
1885	**Corning (USA)** Pain can be treated by "medication of the spinal cord."
1900	**Cushing (USA)** Nerve block to prevent pain and "shock" of amputation
1908	**Crile (USA)** "Anociassociation"—neural blockade to prevent noxious stimulation
1929	**Gasser and Erlanger** Nerve fiber size and function
1933	**Brouwer (Netherlands)** Proposed centrifugal influence on centripetal systems in the brain
1934	**O'Shaughnessy and Slome (UK)** Spinal anesthesia decreased mortality in dogs with limb trauma.
1953	**Bonica (USA)** Publication of an encyclopedic treatise on the management of acute pain and chronic pain
1957	**Hagbarth and Kerr (Australia)** Evidence of descending control of sensory input
1958	**Bromage (Canada)** Epidural block restored respiratory function after abdominal surgery.
1963	**Hume and Egdahl** Spinal lesions or spinal anesthesia modified the stress response to surgery in man.
1965	**Melzack and Wall (Canada and UK)** A spinal gate in the dorsal horn controls the transmission of nociceptive messages.
1969	**Reynolds (USA)** Pain-inhibitory impulses descend from the midbrain to the spinal cord. The pathway is activated by electrical stimulation and morphine.
1971	**Bromage (Canada)** Epidural block in humans modifies stress response during and after surgery.
1976	**Yaksh and Rudy (USA)** Spinal application of morphine inhibits nociceptive transmission.
1979	**Cousins and colleagues (Australia)** Epidural administration of opioids in humans results in "selective spinal analgesia" on the basis of studies of pharmacokinetics and neural effects.
1981	**Duggan (Australia)** More than one population of opioid receptors exist in spinal cord.
1983	**Yaksh (USA)** Several different spinal receptor systems mediate antinociception.
1996	**Akopian, Sivilotti and Wood** Noriceptor neuron specific neural blockade via Na V1.8.

[a]See also Chapter 33, Table 33-4.

nerve. His technique was adopted by C. Hunter and renamed *hypodermic injection*, ostensibly because Hunter had in view a different purpose, namely, systemic absorption of the drug.

Carl Koller (1857–1944) (Fig. 1-4) searched for a surgical local surface anesthetic and hit upon cocaine in 1884, and immediately demonstrated its startling effectiveness on the cornea (11). This opened the vast new world of local and regional analgesic therapy. James Leonard Corning (1855–1923) (12) conceived and attempted the direct application of an analgesic to the spinal cord, but a defective rationale and unserviceable technique stultified his approach to the management of chronic pain (Fig. 1-5). A deeper knowledge of the underlying

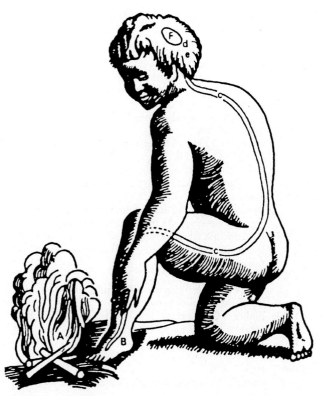

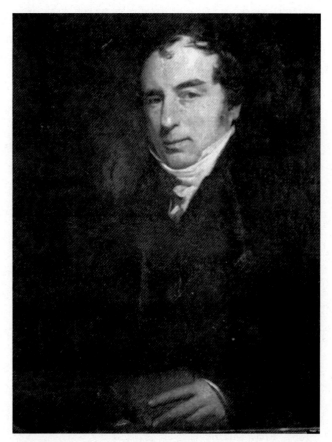

FIGURE 1-1. The path of sensation according to Descartes. He wrote: "If for example fire (A) comes near the foot (B), the minute particles of this fire, which as you know move with great velocity, have the power to set in motion the spot on the skin of the foot which they touch, and by this means pulling upon the delicate thread CC, which is attached to the spot of the skin, they open up at the same instant the pore, d, e, against which the delicate thread ends, just as by pulling at one end of a rope one makes to strike at the same instant a bell which hangs at the other end." From Procacci P, Maresca M. Evolution of the concept of pain. In: Sicuteri F, Terenius L, Veccheit L, Maggi CA, eds. *Pain versus man.* New York: Raven Press, 1992, with permission.

FIGURE 1-2. James Moore (1762–1860).

mechanisms was requisite. Understanding of these mechanisms remained relatively superficial until the era of electrophysiologic and neuropharmacologic microexploration following World War II.

Melzack and Wall's hypothesis that a spinal "gate" controls the cephalad transmission of nociception (13) was based on evidence suggesting that the intensity and quality of pain perceived do not bear a push-button, straight-through, one-to-one relationship to the intensity of the stimulus, but are instead determined by a multiplicity of physiologic and psychologic variables (Figs. 1-6 and 1-7). This led directly to the reintroduction of electrical stimulation as a method of treating chronic pain. Although their gate control theory has been shown to be conceptually incomplete in light of today's understanding, it did provide the framework for most of the advances in understanding spinal cord nociceptive processing.

The search for the mechanism of opioid analgesia and opioid addiction resulted in Reynolds' spectacular demonstration, in 1969, of the analgesic effect of electrical stimulation of the periaqueductal gray matter (14). This seminal discovery gave enormous impetus to pain research and led to the uncovering of a system of descending neurons that inhibit pain and are activated by opiate drugs acting at endorphinergic synapses. Brilliant experimental work by many researchers conceptualized analgesia via a direct spinal action of narcotics, a landmark ad-

vance from which important clinical developments have sprung (15–17). Further experimental studies have now been extended to define, using isolated nerve techniques, the concept of "neuroplasticity" and how multiple spinal cord receptors may be modulated by preemptive analgesia techniques (18). The progression of clinical applications sharply illustrates the process and value of basic medical research.

In the last century, World War II was a stimulus for regional anesthesia development; secondary to two factors: the many injured needing medical care and the introduction of lidocaine to regional techniques. The Seattle personalities Daniel C. Moore and John J. Bonica (Fig. 1-8) led the effort in the United States to grow both regional anesthesia and pain medicine care, with Moore primarily focused on regional anesthesia and Bonica on pain medicine. Both of these men were consummate physicians, and neither lacked confidence or compassion. Further, Moore's interest was primarily clinical research on techniques. He was the primary encourager of the development of the American Society of Regional Anesthesia (ASRA), although not a founding member of the society. Bonica's interest was to better understand matching regional techniques to patients experiencing chronic pain, and his interest ultimately led to the development and leadership of the International Association for the Study of Pain (IASP). Both of these men surrounded themselves with outstanding colleagues.

COCAINE

The mid 19th century was a period of growth in Western science and technology. In 1865, 6 years after the publication of

TABLE 1-2

CHRONOLOGY OF EARLY HISTORY OF LOCAL ANESTHESIA

1564 Paré (France) Local anesthesia by nerve compression	**1897 Braun (Germany)** Cocaine toxicity related to absorption; advocated use of epinephrine
1600 Valverdi (Italy) Regional anesthesia by compression of nerves and blood vessels supplying operative area	**1898 Bier (Germany)** First planned spinal anesthetic
1646 Severino (Italy) Refrigeration anesthesia by use of freezing mixtures of snow and ice	**1899 Tuffier (France)** Report of 125 spinal anesthetics **Tait and Caglieri (USA)** First use of spinal anesthesia in USA (". . . never . . . inject . . . until CSF . . . recognized")
1656 Wren (England) First experiments with intravenous injection	**1900 Tait and Caglieri (USA)** Detailed studies of subarachnoid space and spinal anesthesia in animals and humans
1784 Moore (England) Local anesthesia of extremity by compression of nerve trunks	**1901 Cathelin and Sicard (France)** Independently discovered caudal epidural block using cocaine
1839 Taylor and Washington (USA) Hypodermic injection	**1902 Braun (Germany)** Use of epinephrine in nerve blocking; term *conduction anesthesia* coined
1843 Wood (Scotland) Morphine injection (published 1855)	**1904 Einhorn (Germany)** Synthesis of procaine (Novocaine)
1845 Rynd (Dublin) Hypodermic needle	**1905 Braun (Germany)** Published report: "Local Anesthesia"
1853 Pravaz (France) Hypodermic syringe	**1907 Barker (UK)** Introduction of hyperbaric spinal anesthetic solutions
1855 Gaedcke (Germany) Isolation of alkaloid from leaves of coca plant	**1908 Crile (USA)** Anociassociation: regional block plus light general anesthesia
1860 Niemann (Germany) Purification and naming of cocaine	**1912 Gray and Parsons (UK)** **1915 Smith and Porter (USA)** Blood pressure changes during spinal anesthesia
1873 Bennett (Scotland) Anesthetic properties of cocaine	**1922 Labat (USA)** Published report: "Regional Anesthesia: Its Technique and Clinical Application" Founded American Society of Regional Anesthesia (1923)
1878 von Anrep (Germany) Pharmacologic effects of cocaine (published 1879–1880)	**1942 Allen (USA)** Refrigeration anesthesia for amputation **Edwards and Hingson (USA)** Continuous caudal anesthesia in obstetrics
1884 Koller (Austria) First topical use of cocaine (eye surgery) **Halsted and Hall (USA)** Neural blockade with cocaine (in each other) **Burke (USA)** Removal of bullet from finger under nerve block with cocaine	
1885 Corning (USA) "Spinal anesthesia" (actually injected epidurally)	
1890 Reclus (France) Early use of infiltration anesthesia	
1891 Quincke (Germany) Lumbar puncture technique	
1892 Schleich (Germany) Introduced infiltration anesthesia **François-Franck** Coined term *nerve blocking*	

Charles Darwin's epochal book, Lister opened a new era in surgery by applying Pasteur's proof of nonspontaneous generation to the elimination of sepsis. Pflüger showed that the seat of respiration was in the tissues and not in the blood and, in 1882, the same year that produced the world's first electrical power station (in New York), Ringer demonstrated the need for calcium and potassium salts to maintain the excitability of the heart. The establishment of the coal tar industry in Germany led to large-scale production of pharmaceuticals, of which the marketing of cocaine by Merck was one result. The year 1886 saw the introduction of steam sterilization of dressings by von Bergmann, and the year 1890, the use of surgical rubber gloves, initially for the purpose of protecting the hands of Halsted's instrument nurse from disinfectant.

Koller's demonstration of ocular surface anesthesia with cocaine (11) had antecedents almost as numerous as those of

general anesthesia 40 years earlier. Dr. Scherzer, an Austrian explorer and a member of an expedition to South America, returned with coca leaves to Vienna. Some were sent to Friedrich Wohler for analysis, and subsequently to his pupil, Albert Niemann. Niemann (1834–1861) was successful in isolating and naming the alkaloid from the leaves of *Erythroxylon coca,* as first recorded in 1860 in a report signed W. (for H. Wofler 1800–1882), which also related the passionate chewing of the leaves by the *coqueros* of Peru and the deleterious mental effects this had on them (19,20). Nobody paid a great deal of attention to the benumbing effects of cocaine on the tongue and the lips until the Peruvian army surgeon Moreno y Mayz remarked in 1868 that the sensory paralyzing effects of cocaine might be put to use in medicine (21).

A thorough pharmacologic investigation of the properties of the alkaloid in frogs was presented by von Anrep, a Baltic

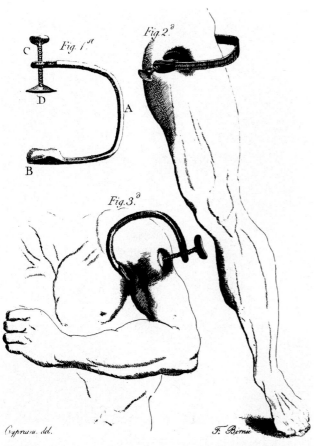

FIGURE 1-3. James Moore's compression instruments for upper and lower extremities. From Moore J. *A method of preventing or diminishing pain in several operations of surgery.* London: T. Cadell, 1784.

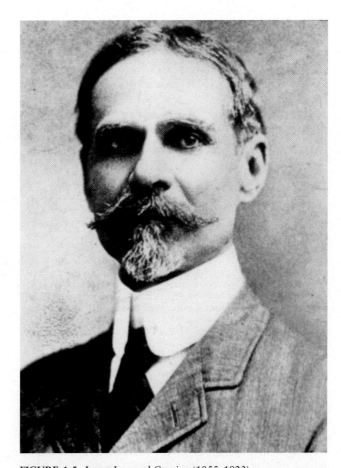

FIGURE 1-5. James Leonard Corning (1855–1923).

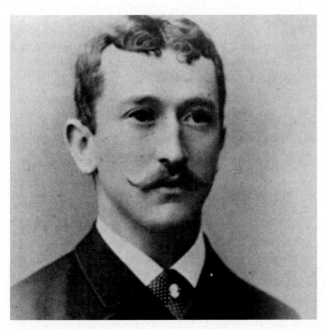

FIGURE 1-4. Carl Koller (1857–1944).

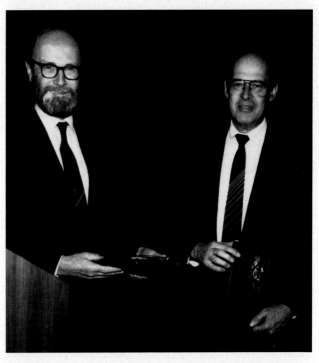

FIGURE 1-6. Patrick Wall *(left)* and Ronald Melzack *(right)* receiving awards at 1989 annual meeting of the American Society of Regional Anesthesia.

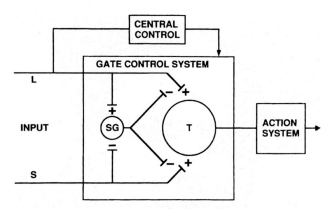

FIGURE 1-7. Schematic representation of the gate control theory of pain mechanisms: *L*, large diameter fibers; *S*, small diameter fibers. The fibers project to the substantia gelatinosa *(SG)* and first central transmission *(T)* cells. The inhibitory effect exerted by SG on the afferent fiber terminals is increased activity in L fibers and decreased activity in S fibers. The central control trigger is represented by a line running from the large-fiber system to the central control mechanisms. These mechanisms, in turn, project back to the gate control system. The T cells project to the entry cells of the action system. +, excitation; −, inhibition. From Melzack R, Wall PD. Pain mechanisms. Science 1965;150:971, with permission. Copyright by the AAAS.

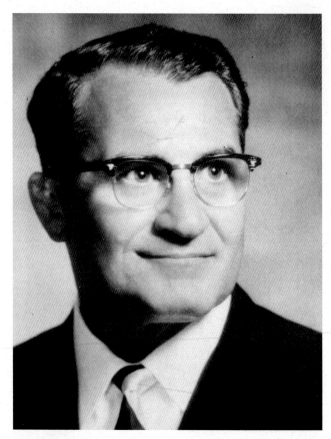

FIGURE 1-8. John J. Bonica (1917–1994).

surgeon. In 1880, von Anrep published an extensive article on the physiologic and pharmacologic effects of cocaine. It is clear that he understood that cocaine had a locally numbing effect on the tongue and that it dilated the pupil upon local application, and he did suggest that this drug might some day become of medical importance (22). He ended the report as follows: "The animal experiments have no practical application; nevertheless I would recommend trying cocaine as a local anesthetic in persons of melancholy disposition (22)." Plainly, von Anrep was most impressed by the stimulating properties of cocaine, and these seem also to have been uppermost in the mind of Sigmund Freud (1856–1939) when he suggested a study of the drug to Koller (23).

Freud wanted to know more about the analeptic action of cocaine, which, he hoped, because of reports from the United States, might be useful in curing one of his great friends of addiction to morphine. This friend was a pathologist who had developed an unbearably painful thenar neuroma after accidentally cutting himself while performing an autopsy. Freud obtained a supply of cocaine from the manufacturing firm of Merck and shared it with Koller, who was to help him investigate its effects on the nervous system. Koller was a junior intern in the Ophthalmological Clinic at the University of Vienna and longed to obtain the coveted appointment of assistant in the clinic, on the strength of a worthy piece of research. In 1884, Koller met Dr. Joseph Gartner at Stricker's Institute for Pathological Anatomy. They dissolved a trace of the white coca powder in distilled water and instilled it in the conjunctival sac of a frog, which allowed its cornea to be touched with no evidence of reflex action or defense. Identical tests were performed on a rabbit and a dog, and the results were equally favorable. Koller wrote: "One more step had now to be taken. We trickled the solution under each other's lifted eyelids, then placed a mirror before us, took pins, and with the head tried to touch the cornea. Almost simultaneously we were able to state jubilantly 'I can't feel anything (20,23).'" After these experiments, he then performed an operation for glaucoma using topical cocaine anesthesia on September 11, 1884, just 4 days before the Congress of Ophthalmology was due to meet in Heidelberg.

Koller immediately wrote a paper for the Congress, but, being an impecunious intern, he could not afford the train fare to Heidelberg, so he gave the paper to a visiting ophthalmologist from Trieste, Dr. Brettauer, who had stopped in Vienna on his way to the Congress. Brettauer's news from Heidelberg reached New York in a letter from H. D. Noyes, an American ophthalmologist who had attended the Heidelberg Congress (24).

Noyes's letter to the *New York Medical Record* excited numerous readers to test the new wonder drug, and many of them rushed into print with astounding experiences. One of the most striking, published within 5 weeks of Noyes's communication, was that of N. J. Hepburn, a New York ophthalmologist (25). There were no standards for drug trials in those days, and the tradition of self-experimentation was inviolate. If a researcher or physician wanted to know whether a drug was safe, he tried it on himself. Hepburn describes how, on October 16, 1884, he experimented with a 2% solution of cocaine, giving himself a series of subcutaneous injections of 0.4 mL (8 mg) at intervals of 5 minutes. He noted that, by the time of the eighth injection, the agreeable stimulating effects of the drug—rapid respiration and pulse, a feeling of warmth, pleasant hallucinations—had reached such a point that he felt it best to stop. For reasons that Hepburn does not state, he repeated the performance 2 days later, and then found it possible to carry the number of 0.4 mL injections to 16 before the general disturbance persuaded him to cease. He records that 4 days later, he was at it again, and this time he tried a larger unit volume and amount (10 mg), and was able to tolerate 16 of these doses. It seems likely that Hepburn was already in the grip of addiction.

By November 29, 1884, the ophthalmologist Bull was able to report that he had used the drug to produce anesthesia of the cornea and conjunctiva in more than 150 cases (26). He gave sound reasons for his enthusiasm: He saved the time required for complete etherization and avoided the enormous engorgement of the ocular blood vessels produced by the ether, the danger of vomiting, and the disadvantage that almost any apparatus for producing anesthesia by inhalation was a physical interference for the operator.

One evening in January 1885, while he was on duty in the emergency room, a workman with an injured finger was brought in. Koller noticed there was a tourniquet applied to the base of the finger. Zinner, Billroth's intern, asked Koller to admit the man to Billroth's service and Koller did so, but he himself urgently removed the tourniquet in order to save the finger. This act aroused Zinner's ire. Zinner called Koller an impudent Jew. Koller in return slapped Zinner's face. Zinner thereupon challenged Koller to a duel. Billroth specified that all duels were strictly prohibited, but both parties were officers in the reserve and members of the Patriotic German Student Society, whose unwritten code dictated that honor must be avenged. The duel was fought with swords the next day, and Koller wounded his opponent. The law impartially charged both parties with the crime. Koller received an official pardon a few months later, but his prospects for advancement in German-speaking Europe were wrecked, destroyed by the first and last duel known to have been fought over a tourniquet. Soon, he immigrated to The Netherlands, and, with Freud's and others' advice, in 1885, to the United States (27). This series of events seems to be in character for Koller, whose own daughter said he was "a difficult tempestuous young man, one who could never be compelled to speak diplomatically even for his own good (28)." Following these earlier events, Koller immigrated to the United States, and he established an ophthalmology practice in New York City.

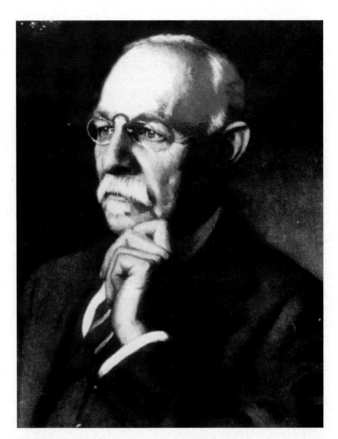

FIGURE 1-9. William Stewart Halsted (1852–1922).

CONDUCTION ANESTHESIA

After the publication of Noyes's 1884 letter, the idea of injecting cocaine directly into tissues to render them insensible occurred simultaneously to several American surgeons. William C. Burke injected 5 minims (drops) of 2% solution close to a metacarpal branch of the ulnar nerve and painlessly extracted a 22-caliber bullet from the base of his patient's little finger (29). But it was William Stewart Halsted (1852–1922) and Richard John Hall (1856–1897) and their associates who most clearly saw the great possibilities of conduction block (Fig. 1-9) (30–32). The term was introduced by François-Franck in 1892 (33), although he may well have borrowed part of it from Corning, for in 1886, Corning was writing that "the thought of producing anaesthesia by abolishing conduction in sensory nerves, by suitable means, should have been rife in the minds of progressive physicians (12)." Corning himself quite possibly got the idea from Halsted, for Halsted later attested that Corning was a frequent observer at the Roosevelt Hospital in New York, where Halsted, assisted by Hall, performed his teaching. In 1884, Hall described how he blocked a cutaneous branch of the ulnar nerve in his own forearm (34). He and Halsted made injections into the musculocutaneous nerve of the leg and the ulnar nerve. Hall noted the appearance of marked constitutional symptoms, giddiness, severe nausea, cold perspiration, and dilated pupils, but this did not daunt these bold pioneers, and that same evening Halsted blocked Hall's supratrochlear nerve and removed an adjoining congenital cystic tumor. He also induced Nash, a dental surgeon, to tend to Hall's own upper incisor tooth after injection of cocaine into the infraorbital nerve at the infraorbital foramen, and Halsted thereafter

performed an inferior dental nerve block on a medical student volunteer and later did the same to Hall. Hall's report was quite explicit in predicting that, once the limits of safety had been determined, this mode of administration would find very wide application in the outpatient department.

The daring experimenters at the Roosevelt Hospital unfortunately became addicted to the new drug, and no more was heard from them about its use in surgery. It appears that Dr. Halsted, with the help of his friend, Dr. William H. Welch, was the only one of the group able to overcome the addiction. In 1886, Halsted, upon an invitation from Dr. Welch, moved to Baltimore. In 1889, after his final recovery from cocaine addiction, he was appointed acting surgeon and head of the outpatient department of the newly established Johns Hopkins Hospital and, in 1890, he became professor of surgery at the new Johns Hopkins Medical School (35). But that Hall and Halsted were the true progenitors of conduction anesthesia can hardly be doubted (34,36).

The great advantage of local anesthesia with cocaine was, of course, that it anesthetized only the part of the body on which the operation was to be performed. However, a price was paid in toxicity and time. Rapid absorption limited the safe quantity of cocaine to 30 mg and the useful duration of anesthesia to 10 to 15 minutes. In 1885, Corning sought a means of prolonging the local anesthetic effects for surgical and other purposes, although he was primarily interested in the application of the drug to the therapeutics of neurologic disease (37). His notion of pharmacokinetics was that, after the introduction of cocaine beneath the skin, a certain period of time elapsed during which the anesthetic agent was diffused throughout the surrounding tissue, with the capillary circulation having a dual effect, first as a distributor and afterward as a dilutor and rapid remover of the anesthetic substance. In his first article of 1885, Corning described how he experimentally injected 0.3 mL of a 4% solution of cocaine into the lateral antebrachial nerve and obtained immediate anesthesia of the skin supplied by this nerve as far as the wrist. He found that simple arrest of the circulation in the involved part by compression or constriction proximal to the point of injection intensified the anesthesia and prolonged it indefinitely. He used an Esmarch bandage for this purpose and pointed out that the method was readily applicable to surgery of all the extremities. The Riva-Rocci cuff tourniquet had not yet been invented. Esmarch had introduced his elastic bandage in 1874, for the purpose of producing a bloodless field in major amputations (38).

As has briefly been mentioned, François-Franck was the first to apply the term *nerve blocking* to the infiltration of a nerve trunk in any part (33,36). He found that the effect of the blocking drug was not limited to the purely sensory fibers because it paralyzed all nerves, whether motor or sensory, and that the sensory anesthesia was manifested much more promptly than was the motor paralysis, a confirmation of von Anrep's observations of 1879 to 1880. François-Franck spoke of the action of cocaine as a "physiological section," transitory and noninjurious.

Corning's principle of prolonging the local anesthetic action of cocaine by arresting the circulation in the anesthetized area inspired Heinrich F. W. Braun (1862–1934) to dispense with the elastic tourniquet and substitute epinephrine, a "chemical tourniquet" as he called it (39). Epinephrine had become available in pure form after Abel isolated it from the suprarenal medulla in 1897 (40).

The suggestion for this use of epinephrine came from ophthalmologic practice, in which it had been introduced to limit hemorrhage and to render the conjunctiva bloodless, as well as to treat certain diseases, notably glaucoma, in which it was found to prolong the local effect of other drugs in general and of cocaine in particular. This observation had been confirmed by rhinologists and had enabled them to reduce the concentration and dose of cocaine and correspondingly to limit the hazard of toxicity (41). Initially, in Braun's solution, the epinephrine was present in concentrations from 1:10,000 to 1:100,000. The first experiments to determine the dosage to be injected subcutaneously were made by Braun on himself. He found his limit of tolerance was 0.5 mg (0.5 mL of 1:1000 solution), after which general symptoms occurred, and he had to lie down.

Braun introduced the term *conduction anesthesia*, and he felt that the use of epinephrine rendered conduction anesthesia in other parts of the body as effective as that in an extremity. In 1905, Braun published a textbook on local anesthesia, giving detailed descriptions of the technique for every region (Table 1-2).

INFILTRATION ANESTHESIA

Some 10 years earlier, a different approach, termed *infiltration anesthesia*, had been advocated by Karl Ludwig Schleich (1859–1922) (42). Schleich's interest in infiltration anesthesia appeared to stem from the poor effects that often followed general anesthesia in that era. Schleich stated: "For however great the improvement that our methods in the treatment of narcosis may undergo in the course of time, it will always remain a dangerous and uncertain interference with the brain mechanism, the working of which we are unable to fathom ... What a blessing, then, if narcosis can be avoided in so great a proportion of cases (35,42)!" Schleich applied the principle that pure water has a weak anesthetic effect but is painful on in-

jection, whereas physiologic saline is not. Although Schleich's initial report on infiltration anesthesia before the Congress of Surgeons in Mainz, Germany, was unfavorably received, by the early 20th century, this technique of anesthesia was widely used. It is reported that Schleich was a meticulous technician who gave great attention to detail, and this likely explains his success over time (35).

The observation that subcutaneous injection of water produced local anesthesia was apparently first made by Potain in 1869. Halsted, in a short letter to the editor of the *New York Medical Journal*, dated September 19, 1885 (31), baldly asserted that "the skin can be completely anesthetized to any extent by cutaneous injections of water;" he had of late used water instead of cocaine in skin incisions, and the anesthesia did not always vanish just as soon as hyperemia supervened.

Schleich believed that there must be a solution of such a concentration between "normal" (0.6% salt solution) and pure water that would not provoke pain on injection and yet be usefully anesthetic, and he thought a 0.2% solution of sodium chloride was ideal. To this, he added cocaine to a concentration of 0.02% and employed the mixture to produce a field of cutaneous anesthesia in the surgery of hydrocele, sebaceous cyst, hemorrhoids, and small abscesses.

The reason why Schleich's hypotonic solutions containing a minuscule amount of cocaine produced impairment of sensation does not appear to have been explained. In the light of later work, it seems possible that loss of electrolyte from nerve fibers may have been involved. Braun dismissed Schleich's solutions as nonphysiologic and insisted that injections into the tissues for whatever purpose must be composed of fluids of the same osmotic tension as the body fluids. Inasmuch as most local anesthetic solutions are hypotonic, a corresponding amount of an indifferent salt, such as sodium chloride, must be added to prevent any injurious action upon the tissue.

Nevertheless, Schleich's infiltration technique was an important advance in that it extended the field of usefulness of a small quantity of anesthetic. Schleich was probably indebted to Paul Reclus for the idea of using a weak solution of cocaine to avoid toxic reactions and fatalities. Enthusiasm for local anesthesia had diminished owing to casualties, but Reclus clearly understood that the basic cause of accidental deaths was overdose from the use of unnecessarily high concentrations (43). He realized that undue absorption could be avoided by using lower concentrations, and he eventually reduced the strength of his cocaine solutions to 0.5%.

LOCAL ANESTHETICS

The toxicity of cocaine, coupled with its vast potential for usefulness in surgery, led to an intensive search for less toxic substitutes. However, decreased toxicity without increased irritancy—or impractically brief effectiveness—proved elusive until the synthesis of procaine (Novocaine) by Einhorn in 1904. No specific report to that effect appears in the literature, so it fell to the lot of the surgeon Heinrich Braun to make the report in 1905, along with descriptions of two other agents, stovaine and alypin (44). Procaine's short duration of activity limited clinical utility; thus, research focused on dibucaine (1925). Meischer synthesized dibucaine, a quinoline derivative, which Uhlmann introduced clinically. In 1928, Eisleb synthesized tetracaine, which was then introduced into clinical practice in 1932. Although dibucaine and tetracaine proved to be potent, long-acting local anesthetics, their increased systemic toxicity limited the usefulness of these agents for many of the regional anesthetic techniques in which large volumes of drugs

TABLE 1-3

CHRONOLOGY OF LOCAL ANESTHETIC AGENTS

Cocaine
1860　Purification and naming by Niemann (Germany)
1884　First clinical use, topical, by Koller (Germany)
　　　First clinical use, nerve block, by Halsted (USA)

Procaine
1904　Synthesis by Einhorn (Germany)
1905　Clinical introduction by Braun (Germany)

Stovaine
1904　Synthesis by Fourneau (France)

Cinchocaine (Nupercaine, dibucaine)
1925　Synthesis by Meischer
1930　Clinical introduction by Uhlmann

Amethocaine (Pontocaine, Tetracaine)
1928　Synthesis by Eisleb
1932　Clinical introduction

Lignocaine (Lidocaine)
1943　Synthesis by Löfgren and Lundqvist
1947　Clinical introduction (Gordh)

Mepivacaine
1956　Synthesis by Ekenstam and Egner
1957　Clinical introduction (Dhunér)

Prilocaine
1959　Synthesis by Lofgren and Tegner
1960　Clinical introduction by Wielding

Bupivacaine
1957　Synthesis by Ekenstam
1963　Clinical introduction by Widman and Telivuo

Etidocaine
1971　Synthesis by Takman
1972　Clinical introduction by Lund

Ropivacaine
1957　Synthesis by Ekenstam
1997　Clinical introduction

Levobupivacaine
Early　First commercial preparation by chiroscience in
　1990s　　collaboration with Mather (Australia) and
　　　　　　Tucker (UK)
1995–　First clinical use
　1998

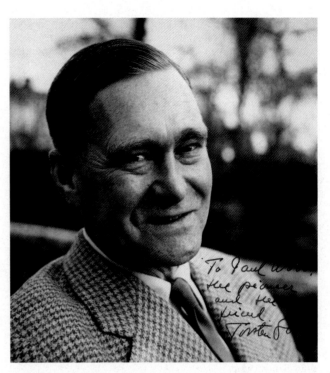

FIGURE 1-10. Torsten Gordh (1907–).

were required. Thus, these agents found their primary use in the field of spinal anesthesia, and they continue to be used today. Most of the chemical compounds synthesized during this first pharmaceutical period were amino ester derivatives, similar in most respects to cocaine. Most of these amino ester agents were relatively unstable and could not be subjected to repeated autoclaving for sterilization. In addition, the hydrolysis of amino esters by the enzyme plasma pseudocholinesterase resulted in the formation of para-aminobenzoic acid, which was responsible for reported allergic reactions (45). Additional crucial properties for wider use of local anesthetics—namely, chemical stability and absence of sensitization—were achieved with lidocaine, which was introduced in 1947 (Table 1-3) (46).

Lidocaine, synthesized in 1943 by Löfgren and Lundqvist, was a stable compound that was not influenced by repeated exposures to high temperatures and thus could be resterilized often. In addition, the metabolites of lidocaine did not include para-aminobenzoic acid; thus, allergic reactions were avoided.

Lundqvist, like many early investigators, started using lidocaine on his own toes and fingers and even for spinal anesthesia. In August 1943, Lundqvist called another friend—Lagergreen—and said that a friend of his had synthesized a new local anesthetic. They arranged a meeting with representatives of the drug company Pharmacia and asked if Lagergreen would come as their medical expert and demonstrate finger blocks on volunteers. This he did, performing five to ten of the blocks, and the results were demonstrated for the executives of Pharmacia. They were to be given a decision within 2 weeks, but Löfgren and Lundqvist never heard from them. Since there had been no response after the respite time, Lundqvist called Lagergreen and said that a Mr. Jordan, science attaché at the U.S. embassy, wanted to meet them. Lagergreen went with them more as an interpreter. Mr. Jordan made an immediate offer of $15,000 for the rights to the discovery, but nothing was decided. The gossip spread like wild fire, and soon Ciba, Roche, and Bayer were out to get this new wonder drug. Also, ICI was interested, and it is said that Löfgren went to London in the tail of a Mustang, a plane flying ball bearings from Sweden to England, by night during the war. However, again no decision was made. This happened between August 23 and September 10, 1943, when Astra laboratories bought the method and patent (47). At this point, the clinical testing of lidocaine was conducted by Gordh (Fig. 1-10) with the assistance of his wife, Ulla, also a physician. Volunteer patients were given 5 crowns (60 cents) for their help. Students were given a copy of Gordh's thesis (1945) or a package of American cigarettes, which were very difficult to obtain during the war. Most of them chose the cigarettes. Gordh made his first presentation of clinical results in 1947, at a meeting of the Swedish Anesthesia Club, the predecessor of the Swedish Society of Anesthesiologists. In the same year, his paper was also presented at the Scandinavian Surgical Society's first meeting after the war. The results were published in *Svenskja Lakartidningen* in 1948 (47).

Subsequent to lidocaine's release, a number of amino amide compounds were synthesized, and four eventually found their way into clinical practice. In 1956, Ekenstam in Sweden synthesized mepivacaine, whose anesthetic properties were similar to lidocaine. In 1959, Löfgren and co-workers synthesized prilocaine in an attempt to produce a local anesthetic whose clinical potency was similar to that of lidocaine, but which was less toxic. Lidocaine and mepivacaine were tertiary amide compounds, whereas prilocaine was a secondary amide. Bupivacaine had been synthesized by Ekenstam at approximately the same time as mepivacaine. However, bupivacaine was not introduced into clinical practice until 1963, by Telivuo. Following the initial reports by Widman concerning the prolonged duration of action of bupivacaine, it gained wide acceptance because of its potency and ability to provide significantly longer anesthesia than was possible with either lidocaine or mepivacaine. In 1971, Takman synthesized etidocaine, which was another amino amide compound similar in structure to lidocaine but with a duration of action comparable to bupivacaine. Unlike bupivacaine, which provided only partial blockade of motor fibers, etidocaine provided profound motor blockade. The most recent amide local anesthetic to be introduced is ropivacaine. The drug was synthesized by Ekenstam in 1957, and is structurally related to bupivacaine and mepivacaine. It is a chiral drug and exists as two stereoisomers (*S* or *R* form). It is manufactured as a single enantiomer, rather than a racemic mixture. Interest in the drug stems from experimental work suggesting that it has less potential for cardiotoxicity than bupivacaine.

INTRAVENOUS REGIONAL ANESTHESIA

In 1908, August K. G. Bier (1851–1949), a surgeon and physiatrist, and first assistant to Johann Friedrich August von Esmarch, devised a very effective method of bringing about complete anesthesia and motor paralysis of a limb (Fig. 1-11) (48). He injected a solution of procaine into one of the subcutaneous veins that were exposed between two constricting bands in a space that had previously been rendered bloodless by an elastic rubber (Esmarch) bandage extending from the fingers or toes. The injected solution permeated the entire section of the limb very quickly, producing what Bier called *direct vein anesthesia* in 5 to 15 minutes. The anesthesia lasted as long as the upper constricting band was kept in place. After it was removed, sensation returned in a few minutes. Heinrich Braun reports that Bier suggested limiting this "vein anesthesia" to those cases in which local anesthesia was not possible (49). Direct vein anesthesia (intravenous regional anesthesia) was not widely used until Holmes reintroduced the technique with lidocaine in 1963 (Table 1-4) (50,51).

SPINAL ANESTHESIA

Somewhat paradoxically, the first spinal anesthesia occurred 5 years before the first lumbar puncture. The term *spinal anesthesia* was introduced by Corning in his famous second paper of 1885 (12). It was the fruit of a brilliant yet erroneous idea, because what he had in mind was neither spinal nor epidural anesthesia as it is currently understood. Corning was under the mistaken impression that the interspinal blood vessels communicated with those of the spinal cord, and his intention was to inject cocaine into the minute interspinal vessels and have it carried by communicating vessels into the spinal cord. He made no mention of the cerebrospinal fluid, nor of how far he introduced the needle into the spinal space.

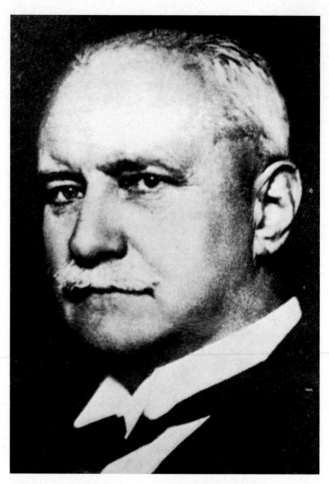

FIGURE 1-11. August K. G. Bier (1851–1949).

Corning's objective was clearly expressed by the title of his article, "Spinal Anaesthesia and Local Medication of the Cord with Cocaine (12)." There is no doubt that Corning was quite literally aiming directly at the spinal cord, as he introduced a hypodermic needle—he does not say of what size—between the spinous processes of the T11 and T12 vertebrae. He wrote:

> I reasoned that it was highly probable that, if the anesthetic was placed between the spinous processes of the vertebrae, it would be rapidly transported by the blood to the substance of the cord and would give rise to anaesthesia of the sensory and perhaps also of the motor tracts of the same. To be more explicit, I hoped to produce artificially a temporary condition of things analogous in its physiological consequences to the effects observed in transverse myelitis or after total section of the cord.

Corning's report was based on a series of two: one dog and one man. In the case of the man, he injected a total of 120 mg of cocaine, about four times the potentially lethal dose, in a period of 8 minutes. Corning implies that he was using the procedure partly as a treatment for masturbation. What he achieved in the man was probably what is now called *epidural* or *extradural anesthesia*, and, in the dog, which received 13 mg, *spinal anesthesia*, as judged by the rates of onset. Corning certainly did have an original idea, as he was at no small pains to indicate, but the results were a lucky accident because the experiment could easily have been fatal and was conceived on the basis of an entirely erroneous notion of the local circulation.

TABLE 1-4

CHRONOLOGY OF EARLY USE OF INDIVIDUAL NEURAL BLOCKADE TECHNIQUES

Spinal analgesia
1898   Bier (Germany)
       First use for surgery in humans
1940   Lemmon (USA)
       Continuous spinal anesthesia
1946   Adriani and Roman-Vega (USA)
       Saddle block spinal

Lumbar epidural analgesia
1921   Pagés (Spain)
       First use for surgery
1931   Dogliotti (Italy)
       Popularized surgical use
1949   Curbelo
       Used Tuohy equipment for continuous blockade

Caudal epidural analgesia
1901   Sicard, Cathelin (France)
       First use for surgery
1909   Stoeckel
       Use in obstetric pain
1910   Läwen (Germany)
       Popularized surgical use
1913   Danis (Belgium)
       Trans-sacral approach
1942   Edwards and Hingson (USA), Manalan
       Continuous caudal

"Continuous" regional techniques
1931   Aburel (Romania)
       Continuous paravertebral lumbosacral plexus block

Paravertebral somatic block
1906   Sellheim
       Thoracic paravertebral block
1912   Kappis
       Paravertebral block for surgery and also for pain relief
1922   Läwen
       Use in diagnosis of abdominal disease

Celiac block
1906   Braun
       Anterior surgical approach
1914   Kappis
       Posterior approach

Paravertebral lumbar sympathetic block
1926   Mandl

Stellate ganglion (cervicothoracic sympathetic) **block**
1930   Labat
       Posterior approach
1934   Leriche and Fontaine
       Anterior approach (used for cerebrovascular accidents)
1948   Apgar
       Anterior approach
1954   Moore
       Paratracheal approach

Brachial plexus block
1884   Halsted
       Injection under direct vision
1897   Crile
1911   Hirschel
       "Blind" axillary injection
       Kulenkampff
       Supraclavicular technique
1940   Patrick
       Basis of current supraclavicular technique
1958   Burnham
       Axillary perivascular technique
1964   Winnie and Collins
       Subclavian
1970   Winnie
       Interscalene

Cervical plexus block
1939   Rovenstine and Wertheim

Intravenous regional analgesia
1908   Bier
       Injection between two cuffs
1963   Holmes
       Injection below a single cuff after exsanguination

Intra-arterial regional anesthesia
1912   Goyanes (Spain)
       Arterial injection below a cuff

Diagnostic blockade in pain management
1924   von Gaza
       Procaine blockade in investigation of pain pathways
1930   Mandl
       Paravertebral procaine block in diagnosis of angina pectoris
1930   White
       Blockade of sensory and sympathetic nerves in pain
         diagnosis

Therapeutic nerve block in pain management
1899   Tuffier
       Spinal cocaine for pain of sarcoma of leg
1901   Cushing
       Regional anesthesia used to describe pain relief by nerve
         block
1903   Schloesser
       Trigeminal alcohol block
1924   von Gaza, Braun, Mandl
       Local anesthetic neural blockade for management of
         visceral pain
1924   Royle
       Surgical sympathectomy for pain of spastic paralysis
1926   Swetlow
       Neurolytic sympathetic block with alcohol for angina
         pectoris and abdominal pain
1930   Dogliotti
       Neurolytic subarachnoid alcohol block
1941   Wertheim and Rovenstine
       Suprascapular local anesthetic nerve block for shoulder pain

There is, of course, no direct communication between the extradural capillaries and those of the spinal cord, so it is rather difficult to understand on what Corning based his expectations. At least as early as 1870, *Gray's Anatomy* (52) had a section on the meninges, including the subarachnoid space and cerebrospinal fluid (53), but Corning apparently was unaware of its existence. He kept the syringe connected to the needle with rubber tubing and thus would not have seen cerebrospinal fluid drip from the needle. Although English-language anatomy books clearly delineated the spinal meninges and cerebrospinal fluid, the contemporary German- and French-language textbooks did not. Corning had a long line of New England ancestors, but he received his medical education in Europe at the University of Wurtzburg (54), and so possibly never learned the basic facts of meningeal anatomy. In any case, how he got the idea that vascular channels existed between the spinous processes of the vertebrae that served as a direct avenue into the spinal cord remains unclear.

Lumbar Puncture

Corning was a neurologist, not a surgeon, and he thought of his spinal use of cocaine as a new means of managing neurologic disorders. He did foresee that it would probably find application as a substitute for etherization in genitourinary or other branches of surgery. However, nothing came of his suggestion until 14 years later, perhaps because conceptual errors flawed his technique at a time when the procedure of lumbar puncture had not yet been invented, let alone standardized. It fell to Heinrich Irenaeus Quincke (1842–1922) to do this, by basing his approach on the anatomic ground that the subarachnoid spaces of the brain and spinal cord were continuous and ended in the adult at the level of S2, whereas the spinal cord extended only to L2 (55). Thus, a puncture effected in the third or fourth lumbar intervertebral space would not damage the spinal cord. Quincke's principal claim to fame was his introduction and popularization of lumbar puncture, first as a method of treatment for tubercular meningitis in children, then as a simple, safe, and necessary clinical development in the investigation of diseases of the nervous system (51).

Lumbar puncture, as the title of Quincke's article indicated (56), was invented as a treatment for hydrocephalus. Quincke acknowledged in his communication that he followed in the steps of Essex Wynter, who, 6 months earlier had described the use of a Southey's tube and trocar for a similar purpose (57). This device was originally designed to drain edema fluid in cases of dropsy. Wynter introduced the tube between the lumbar vertebrae, after making a small incision in the skin, for the purpose of instituting drainage of the fluid in two cases of tuberculous meningitis. Quincke's method was a vast improvement and became the standard technique, thanks to a detailed description that has stood the test of time. Quincke prescribed bed rest for the 24 hours following the puncture. Quincke's needles had an internal diameter of 0.5 to 1.2 mm, and only the larger ones were equipped with a stylet. It is interesting to note that he entered the skin 5 to 10 mm from the midline. Thus, the paramedian approach is and has always been the classic one, and not the median (midline) approach as is sometimes taught.

It took 8 years for Quincke's technique to be applied to the production of what is now called *spinal anesthesia*. No doubt, great courage was required to introduce a drug as toxic as cocaine directly into the nervous system, as Corning had attempted in 1885. Unfortunately, Corning's audacity had no direct sequel unless the title of Bier's paper is taken as an implied tribute to Corning. (Bier does not mention him by name.) August Bier published his celebrated paper on spinal anesthesia in 1899, under the title "Versuche über Cocainisirung des Rückenmarkes" (Research on Cocainization of the Spinal Cord) (58). Apparently Bier also assumed that intrathecal injection of cocaine produced anesthesia by a direct action on the spinal cord. Bier had a certain amount of luck on his side; he worked at the same institution as Quincke and would have been familiar with his technique and might even have borrowed his needles.

Bier, of course, was a surgeon, and it is notable that, for many years, virtually all the extensions of technique in the use of local anesthetics were developed by surgeons. They first performed the block and then performed the operation. This makes Corning's interest in cocaine all the more remarkable, because he was genuinely an outsider in the field and may well have been viewed as such. He seems to have eluded the hazard to which several of the American surgical pioneers of regional anesthesia fell victim when their conscientious zeal led them to experiment on themselves before trying their ideas on patients. Apparently, the first surgeons in the United States to use spinal anesthesia were Tait and Caglieri of San Francisco. On October 26, 1899, they performed an osteotomy of the tibia after the patient received spinal anesthesia (Tables 1-2 and 1-4) (59).

Bier wanted to apply cocaine anesthesia for major operations and saw spinal anesthesia as a way to safely produce a maximum area of anesthesia with a minimum amount of drug. It was his opinion that the spectacular insensitivity to pain evoked by small amounts of cocaine injected into the dural sac resulted from its spread in the cerebrospinal fluid and that it acted not only on the surface of the spinal cord but especially on the unsheathed nerves that traverse the intramembranous space. However, this understanding was not conclusive. The extent of the anesthesia produced was somewhat unpredictable, so Bier decided to obtain an improved insight by experimenting on himself. His assistant, Hildebrandt, performed the lumbar puncture on Bier, but when the time came to attach the syringe to the needle, a crisis developed; the needle did not fit. A considerable amount of cerebrospinal fluid and most of the cocaine dripped onto the floor. To salvage the experiment, Hildebrandt volunteered his own body. This time, there was a good fit and complete success. However, the success was not without sequel. The experimenters celebrated with wine and cigars, and the next day Bier suffered an oppressive headache that lasted for 9 days. Hildebrandt's "hangover" developed even before the night ended. Moreover, while he was anesthetized, Hildebrandt had been scientifically kicked in the shins to demonstrate the depth of the analgesia, and in the aftermath, he duly developed painful bruises in places where no pain had been. As Bier emphasized in his paper, his experiences proved that by the injection of extraordinarily small amounts of cocaine (5 mg) into the dural sac, about two-thirds of the entire body could be made insensible enough for the painless performance of major operations. Complete loss of sensation lasted about 45 minutes. Bier decided that the escape of a considerable amount of cerebrospinal fluid was probably responsible for the after effects. He believed that, in his own case, some type of circulatory disturbance was present, because he felt absolutely well in a supine position but had a sensation of very strong pressure in the head and felt dizzy only if he sat up. Bier concluded that the escape of cerebrospinal fluid should be avoided if possible, and strict bed rest should be observed. Bier said that the size of the needle should be very fine and that, after the dural sac had been entered, the stylet should be withdrawn and the opening immediately closed with a finger so that as little cerebrospinal fluid as possible escaped.

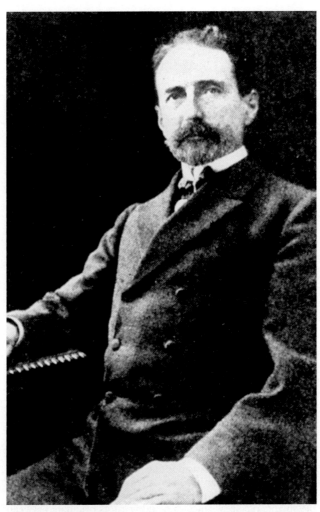

FIGURE 1-12. Theodore Tuffier (1857–1929).

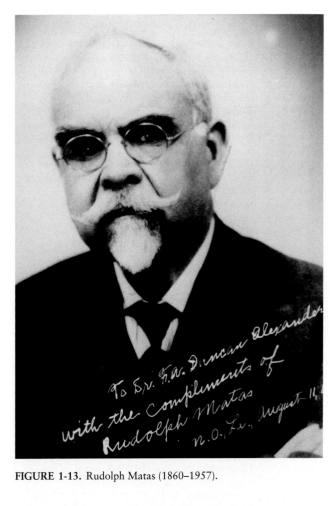

FIGURE 1-13. Rudolph Matas (1860–1957).

Halsted had introduced the use of rubber gloves at operations in the winter of 1889 to 1890, as noted earlier in this chapter, but not with the intention of avoiding wound infection. That consequence was actually serendipitous. His motive was to spare the hands of his operating room nurse (whom he later married), who had developed a dermatitis from exposure to mercurous chloride. Soon the operators took to wearing them as well, but only out of convenience. It was not until 1894 that the wearing of gloves was recommended as part of aseptic technique (32). It surely is a fortunate coincidence that Bier did not start his work on spinal anesthesia until after this important prophylactic measure had become generally available.

The news of Bier's work, published in April 1899, spread quickly, and, although he abandoned it himself, his method of subarachnoid spinal anesthesia was soon brought into prominence by Théodore Tuffier (1857–1929) (Fig. 1-12) (60). In the spring of 1900, in a report on 63 operations, Tuffier enunciated the rule: "Never inject the cocaine solution until the cerebrospinal fluid is distinctly recognized (61,62)." The sensation caused by Tuffier's demonstrations is well conveyed by Hopkins, who wrote: "To be able to converse with a patient during the performance of a hysterectomy, the patient all the while evincing not the slightest indication of pain (and even being unable to tell where the knife was being applied) was

certainly a marvel, and was well worth crossing the Atlantic to see (63)."

In the United States, spinal anesthesia was adopted for obstetrics by Marx and for general surgery by a number of surgeons, most prominently Rudolph Matas (1860–1957) (Fig. 1-13) (64). Matas's article begins with a critical historical review of older methods of local and regional anesthesia. In his description of spinal anesthesia, cocaine hydrochloride, in the amount of 10 to 20 mg, was dissolved in distilled water. The solution instilled was therefore clearly hypotonic. Fowler preferred to have his patients in the sitting position for the injection and, not surprisingly, was often astonished by the rapidity and completeness of the anesthesia (65). Gravity methods were not yet understood.

Aseptic precautions were strictly observed, and E. W. Lee mentions that the injection he used consisted of 12 to 20 minims of a 2% sterilized solution prepared in hermetically sealed tubes by Truax, Green, and Company of Chicago (61). This appears to be the earliest published reference to this method of packaging, an important advance because previously it was necessary for the surgeon to prepare his own solution from tablets and sterilize it.

In 1912, Gray and Parsons of Birmingham, England, undertook an extensive study of variations in blood pressure associated with the induction of spinal anesthesia (66). They concluded that the bulk of the fall in arterial blood pressure during high spinal anesthesia is attributable to the diminished negative intrathoracic pressure during inspiration, which is dependent

TABLE 1-5

CHRONOLOGY OF PIONEERING STUDIES OF COMPLICATIONS OF NEURAL BLOCKADE

1884	**Halsted and associates (USA)**
	Cocaine addiction
1889	**Reclus (France)**
	Toxicity due to systemic absorption defined
	Bier and colleagues (Germany)
	Severe postlumbar puncture headache
1900	**Goldan (USA)**
	Development of anesthetic record of "intraspinal" cocainization
1901	**Dandois (Belgium)**
	Paraplegia after subarachnoid cocaine
1906	**Koenig (USA)**
	Permanent neurologic sequelae in several patients following spinal cocaine
1907	**Barker (UK)**
	Recognition of need to control level of block
1912	**Gray and Parsons (UK)**
	Recognition of vascular pooling due to sympathetic blockade
1927–1928	**Labat (USA)**
	Emphasis on maintenance of cerebral perfusion
1952	**Sancetta and colleagues**
	Cardiovascular effects of "low and high" spinal anesthesia
1953	**Gillies (UK)**
	Studies of cardiovascular effects
	Green (USA)
	Studies of physiologic effects of spinal anesthesia
1954	**Dripps and Vandam (USA)**
	Long-term follow-up of 10,098 spinal anesthetics; failure to discover major neurologic sequelae
	Importance of meticulous technique and safe handling of drugs stressed
1960	**Bromage and colleagues (Canada)**
	Studies of physiology and pharmacology of epidural blockade
1965	**Braid and Scott (UK); Tucker and Mather (USA); Boyes and Covino (USA); Harrison and colleagues (USA); De Jong and colleagues (USA)**
	Studies of pharmacokinetics and toxicity of local anesthetics
1970	**Bonica and colleagues (USA)**
	Studies of cardiovascular effects of central neural blockade

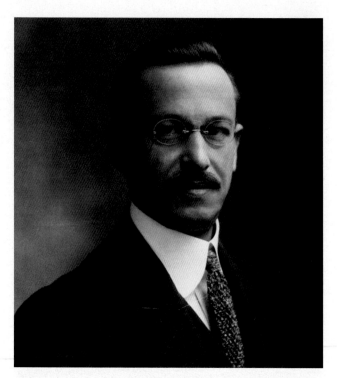

FIGURE 1-14. Gaston Labat (1876–1934).

the splanchnic nerves arise caused as profound a fall in blood pressure as was caused by complete resection of the cord in the upper thoracic region. This, they thought, proved that the fall in blood pressure was not due to toxicity of the drug or to paralysis of the bulbar vasomotor center but to paralysis of the vasomotor fibers that regulate the tonus of the blood vessels in the splanchnic area. Since these nerve roots originate between T2 and T7, Smith and Porter believed that the main clinical objective was to prevent cephalad diffusion of the drug from reaching this height and paralyzing these nerve roots.

Gaston Labat (1877–1934) (68) emphasized that the danger of spinal anesthesia was not the fall in blood pressure per se, but rather the associated cerebral anemia, both being attributable to the increased volume of blood in the viscera caused by splanchnic vascular paralysis and vasomotor collapse (Fig. 1-14). He expressed the belief that this cerebral anemia could be avoided by placing the patient in the Trendelenburg position immediately following the intraspinal injection and that, by this procedure, the brain would be kept amply supplied with blood and irremediable respiratory failure would be avoided. To ensure that the blood pressure would not drop during spinal anesthesia, the practice of administering ephedrine subcutaneously was introduced. The idea of making the injected solution hyperbaric with glucose, to obtain control over the intrathecal spread of the solution, originated with Arthur E. Barker (69). Barker employed stovaine, euphoniously so called from the English translation of its inventor's name, Fourneau (70). Stovaine was less toxic than cocaine but was very slightly irritating and was eventually superseded by procaine. Barker's stovaine came directly from the laboratory of Billon, in Paris, where it was made up in 5% glucose especially for Barker and packaged in sterile ampules. Barker was a professor of surgery at the University of London, and his article is exceedingly thoughtful, based on some 80 cases. He describes experiments with a glass model of the spinal canal, conforming to the shape seen in a mesial

on abdominal and lower thoracic paralysis. They noted that when the negative pressure in the thorax is increased, the arterial blood pressure rises (Tables 1-2 and 1-5).

It was by then quite clear that one of the principal dangers of spinal anesthesia is the lowering of the blood pressure. Believing this to be the primary hindrance to its more universal adoption among urologists, Smith, working with Porter, reported in 1915 the results of 50 experiments on cats (67). They found that the quantity of anesthetic solution was more important for diffusion than its concentration, with dilute solutions usually spreading farther than concentrated ones. The introduction of procaine beneath the dura in the region in which section of a cadaver and bearing a T-junction in the lumbar region to simulate the injection site.

Years later, Pitkin, in 1928, and Etherington-Wilson, in 1934, experimented with a similar apparatus but without acknowledging any debt to Barker (71). Their goal was the opposite of Barker's: to obtain control over the rate of ascent of the drug by making the injected solution hypobaric. Control was achieved by varying the time the patient was kept sitting upright after the injection. Pitkin did this by mixing alcohol with the procaine solutions, a mixture he called *spinocaine*, but he categorically warned against having the patient in the sitting position during injection. He controlled level of blockade by tilting the table and illustrated this with a figure showing an "altimeter" attachment.

Barker stressed such points of technique as raising the head on pillows: Whenever he injected a heavy fluid intradurally, he kept the level of analgesia below the transverse nipple line. At times, he seated the patient on the edge of the table with the feet on a low chair to make the fluid run into the sacral end of the dural sac, where it quickly affected the roots of the nerves supplying the anus and the perineum.

Barker advocated puncture in the midline as being easier and allowing for a more even spread of the injected fluid than the paramedian approach. He, too, emphasized that in no case should the analgesic solution be injected unless the cerebrospinal fluid ran satisfactorily. Above all else, perfect asepsis throughout the entire procedure was absolutely necessary. Moreover, no trace of germicides should be left on the skin, because they could be conveyed by the needle into the spinal canal, where their irritating qualities were particularly undesirable. Barker enjoined that all needles, syringes, and other instruments for the procedure were to be kept apart for this sole use, including the little sterilizer in which they were boiled. Billon's sterilized, sealed ampules were to be opened only a moment before use.

Barker's rational approach to the use of a hyperbaric solution for spinal anesthesia was apparently forgotten when stovaine was replaced by improved drugs, and his technique had to be rediscovered after trials of quasi-isobaric solutions of several new drugs led to unsatisfactory control of spinal level. The lessons of the past were ignored or forgotten by surgeons and not yet learned by anesthesiologists. Indeed, at that time there were few anesthesiologists to learn. In 1920, W. G. Hepburn (69) revived Barker's technique with stovaine, and Sise, an anesthesiologist at the Lahey Clinic, applied it to procaine in 1928 and to tetracaine in 1935 (Fig. 1-15) (72,73).

Tetracaine's great advantage as a spinal anesthetic was its relatively prolonged duration of action without undue toxic effects, but this advantage was partially negated by the vagaries of its segmental spread, which resulted from its being used in an approximately isobaric solution. Therefore, Sise mixed the solution with an equal or greater volume of 10% glucose and injected it while the patient lay on his side on a table tilted head down by 10 degrees. The patient was then turned on his back and a good-sized pillow inserted under his head and shoulders to flex the cervical spine forward as much as possible; the slope of the table was adjusted during the next few minutes as dictated by the level of analgesia needed.

A refinement of this technique was the "saddle-block," described in detail by Adriani and Roman-Vega (53). Anesthesia deliberately confined to the perineal area was obtained by performing the lumbar puncture and injection of hyperbaric solution with the patient sitting on the operating table and remaining so for 35 to 40 seconds after the injection.

An article that announced a hypobaric solution and the associated modifications in the technique of spinal anesthesia was

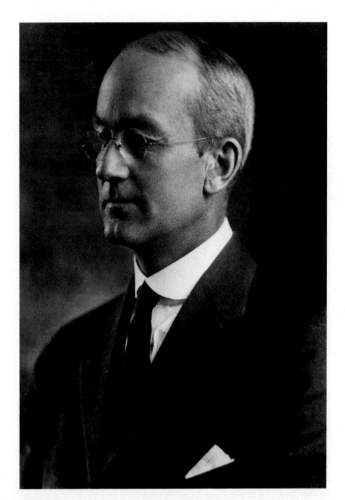

FIGURE 1-15. Lincoln F. Sise (1874–1942).

published by W. W. Babcock in 1912 (74). He dissolved 80 mg of stovaine in 2 mL of 10% alcohol, thus obtaining a solution whose specific gravity was less than 1.000, well below that of the cerebrospinal fluid, which he took to be 1.0065. He believed that the anesthesia that resulted was chiefly a nerve root anesthesia and not the "true spinal cord anesthesia" obtained with the standard solutions. Babcock said that the lightness of this particular anesthetic solution caused it to rise rapidly within the cavity of the arachnoid. He stressed that the patient should promptly have the head and shoulders lowered after the injection, but he rather perversely insisted that, during the injection, the patient should be sitting on the operating table, with his legs hanging over the side of the table. He further remarked: "In most cases spinal anesthesia enables me to operate entirely free from the worry and watchfulness associated with etherization by an untrained assistant ... I have thus been able to operate successfully upon the neck, face, and even the cranium. ... " But let us not fail to note that Babcock also promulgated the following dictum: "*Death from spinal anesthesia usually indicates inefficient or insufficiently prolonged methods of resuscitation.*" The emphasis is his. Further, Babcock's dictum must be considered in light of the report that he was so depressed over the death rate (1 per 500) associated with general anesthetics administered by interns at his Philadelphia institution (Temple University) that spinal anesthesia was preferred over general anesthesia for almost all patients (75).

One of the first lumbar puncture needles was that devised by James Corning, and it was fashioned of either gold or platinum alloy to prevent rusting and fracture. It was by necessity very expensive, and came with an introducer, rather like the introducer described by Sise of Boston in 1928. Other early spinal needles were manufactured from carbon steel "nickeled over," but this stained and rusted on repeated boiling, and occasionally fractures occurred in these needles. Stainless steel, which was really rust-resistant steel, made its appearance in about 1928, following the work of Brearley of Sheffield in England, and it was known as hard-type or martensitic steel. In the 1930s, the German firm of Krupp and Essen produced a truly stainless alloy steel that was given the name austenitic steel of V2A, but it was not until the 1940s that this material was used in the production of spinal needles. By 1945, nearly all needles used for spinal analgesia were made from rust-proof or true stainless steel. Fine-bore needles were employed by Hoit in 1922 and by Green of the University of Oregon in 1923, in attempts to prevent post–lumbar puncture headache. Green's needle also included a pencil-point smooth needle tip that he hoped would reduce dural trauma and thus development of post–dural puncture headaches.

A method for continuous spinal anesthesia was described by W. T. Lemmon in 1940 (76). It was performed with the aid of a special mattress, a malleable needle, and special tubing, and was proposed for long operations that required abdominal relaxation. The equipment was original but not the main idea. In 1907, H. P. Dean wrote of having so arranged the exploring needle that it could be left in situ during the operation and another dose injected without moving the patient beyond a slight degree (77). He proposed that additional injections be made postoperatively to treat pain or abdominal distention. Whether anything ever came of his proposal, he did not say. Lemmon's ponderous technique was quickly simplified by E. B. Tuohy (78). He performed continuous spinal anesthesia by means of a ureteral catheter introduced in the subarachnoid space through a needle with a Huber point.

Other surgeons purposely attempted to achieve widespread regional block via the spinal route to perform a wide variety of surgical procedures. In 1928, Koster detailed the types of procedures he was carrying out during spinal anesthesia (79). Koster reported:

> The purpose of this paper is to describe a technique for safely producing surgical anesthesia of the entire body by the injection of an anesthetic solution into the spinal subarachnoid space. In my clinic, in a general surgical service, spinal anesthesia has been used almost exclusively for the past 3½ years in all cases needing operation on structures below the diaphragm. The only exceptions have been where the anesthesia was needed for such a short period as to make not worth while, e.g., ambulatory cases needing incision, drainage of fingers, abscesses, etc.

Koster went on to include a section on mortality in this report.

> Is the anesthesia safe? We have not as yet had a fatality directly attributable to the anesthesia. Nevertheless: another death occurred in a highly toxic diabetic patient of 62 with a rapid spreading gangrene of the foot and leg. During the course of the guillotine operation at the middle third of the thigh, his pulse suddenly became imperceptible, and stimulation failed to restore his circulation.

One must wonder if this may have been one of the predictable bradycardias that have accompanied spinal anesthesia since its introduction. The variety of procedures carried out under spinal anesthesia in Koster's clinic is indicated in Table 1-6. Koster's work followed an earlier work by Jonnesco, who was an early proponent of the wide use of spinal anesthesia for surgical procedures.

TABLE 1-6

LISTING OF SURGICAL PROCEDURES PROMOTED BY KOSTER AS SUITABLE FOR SPINAL ANESTHESIA, CIRCA 1928

Amputation of lower extremity up to hip
Embolectomy of external iliac artery
Herniotomy
Reduction of fractures and dislocations
Operation for osteomyelitis, lower and upper extremity
Appendectomy
Excision of rectum for carcinoma
Colectomy
Enterectomy
Hemorrhoidectomy
Anterior and posterior colporrhaphy
Tracheoplasty
Interposition operation
Repair of vesicovaginal and rectovaginal fistulae
Salpingo-oophorectomy
Hysterectomy
Hysteropexy
Nephropexy
Nephrectomy
Nephrolithotomy and pyelotomy
Uretotomy
Prostatectomy
Cholecystectomy, choledochotomy, and cholecystenterostomy
Splenectomy
Gastrectomy, pylorectomy, pyloroplasty, and gastroenterostomy
Costectomy and thoracotomy
Radical mastectomy
Embolectomy of the axillary artery
Thyroidectomy
Resection of cervical glands
Excision of tumors of the tongue, face, and scalp
Craniectomy
Mastoidectomy
Nasal plastic
Cesarean section

As with many new ideas, proponents are often characterized as zealots, and such is the case with Thomas Jonnesco of Bucharest (80):

> At a meeting of the German Society of Surgery in Berlin in April, 1909, Professor Beir of Berlin is reported to have said that the method of general spinal analgesia described by me at the Congress of the International Society of Surgery in Brussels, in September, 1908, must be rejected, and Professor Rehn of Frankfurt is reported to have said that experiments on animals showed that considerable danger attended such injections if made higher than the lumbar region as recommended by me. These pronouncements, which seem to be without appeal, prove once more that the method described by myself and my assistant, Dr. Amza Jiano was too novel and too hearty to be accepted without opposition.... During the eight months subsequent to October, 1908, I used spinal analgesia in all my operations, whether performed in the University Clinic, in the Cultza Hospital, or in my private practice; I have never once had recourse to anesthesia by inhalation. There are two essential points of novelty in the method: (1) The puncture is made at the level of the spinal column appropriate to the region to be operated upon; (2) An anesthetic solution is used which, thanks to the addition of strychnine, is tolerated by the higher nervous centers.

OBSTETRIC AND EPIDURAL ANESTHESIA

Tuffier's favorable experience with spinal anesthesia for operative interventions on the lower limbs and urogenital organs led O. Kreis of Basel to give the method a trial in childbirth (81). He injected 10 mg of cocaine at the L4–L5 level, in five parturients, and claimed that this alleviated pain with little impairment of muscular power or uterine motility; however, he recommended the method particularly for forceps delivery. S. Marx (82) in the United States quickly followed with several reports praising the ability of lumbar cocainization to still "the agonizing and maniacal shrieks of these poor women" for 1 to 5 hours, without cessation of uterine contractions; spontaneous bearing down was eliminated, although when told to do so the patient was capable of bringing her abdominal muscles into play as powerfully as under normal conditions. All of this occurred in 1900, but the enthusiasm soon waned.

Interest in obstetric regional anesthesia was revived when W. Stoeckel (83) developed what he termed *sacral anesthesia* using procaine. The feasibility of injecting a local anesthetic by the caudal route was demonstrated by Fernand Cathelin (1873–1945) in 1901. Cathelin based his approach on a thorough anatomic study of the sacral canal and its contents (84). He found that fluids injected into the extradural space through the sacral hiatus rose to a height proportional to the amount and speed of injection. His objective was to develop a method that would be less dangerous but just as effective as subarachnoid lumbar anesthesia. He was successful in reducing the danger, but his efforts to demonstrate the efficiency of the caudal injection for surgical operations were disappointing, and indeed Cathelin himself thought its principal sphere of usefulness lay in the treatment of bladder incontinence and of enuresis in children. Of further interest is that Cathelin's promotion of epidural anesthesia via the sacral route came only a week after Sicard had presented a paper on extradural injections at the Society of Biology meeting in Paris (Fig. 1-16). It seems clear from Cathelin's remarks that competition for priority of publication was well established even at the turn of the century. Quoting Dr. Cathelin, "We believe we should present our results now, remarking only that setting aside all questions or priority, Dr. Sicard and I carried out our experiments simultaneously and independently, one from another." Despite Dr. Cathelin's position that priority was not an issue, in his brief report dates that preempted Dr. Sicard's paper were presented five times (84).

Reflecting on the similarities in the innervation of the bladder and uterus, the gynecologist W. Stoeckel thought that if the pain of childbirth was largely uterine in origin, as seemed probable, the caudal epidural method of the urologist Cathelin offered an ideal approach to painless obstetrics. Cathelin himself had considered pregnancy a contraindication to epidural injection because of the hazard of toxic absorption of cocaine. Stoeckel, however, had begun to use procaine and considered the reduced toxicity of the new drug acceptable. Stoeckel gave the method careful study. He injected colored fluid into the sacral canal of cadavers and noted its extensive spread upward and, contrary to Cathelin's observations, also through the sacral foramina. In 1909, Stoeckel described his experience with caudal anesthesia in the management of labor. He wrote that various concentrations of procaine and epinephrine produced predictably varying degrees of success after a single injection. Pain relief averaged 1 to 1.5 hours in duration, but, warned Stoeckel, the greater the analgesic effect, the greater the hazard of impairing the forces of labor. These reservations, of

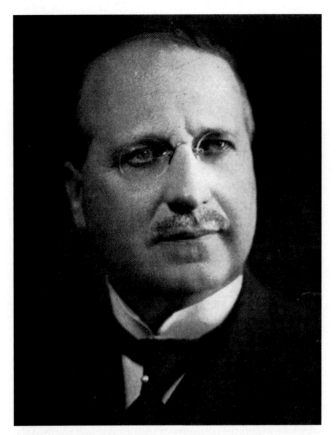

FIGURE 1-16. John Sicard (1872–1929).

course, would not apply to the use of caudal anesthesia for surgical operations, and Läwen, in 1910, described how he used Stoeckel's experience and Cathelin's ideas to perform a variety of interventions in the vicinity of the perineum (85).

Läwen had tested the effectiveness of various concentrations and volumes of procaine–sodium chloride solutions with indifferent success, until he took to preparing and using the bicarbonate salt, as recommended by O. Gros (86). Gros, in the pharmacology laboratory, had established that bicarbonate salts penetrated the nerve sheaths more rapidly than the hydrochloride salts. Läwen exploited this discovery by using increased volumes and stronger concentrations (20 to 25 mL of a 1.5% to 2% solution) to produce anesthesia in the gluteal region, rectum, anus, skin of the scrotum, penis, upper and inner parts of the thigh, and the vulva and vagina. The anesthesia developed after a delay of 20 minutes and lasted for 1.5 to 2 hours. He performed all the common operations on these parts and, hence, was the first to employ sacral anesthesia for operative work, reporting 47 cases with an incidence of failure of 15%.

Pauchet, in 1914, prior to becoming Labat's mentor, was credited with overcoming this incidence of failure by injecting the sacral nerves individually through the posterior sacral foramina, a method that has become known as *transsacral anesthesia* (Fig. 1-17).

The duration of satisfactory anesthesia from a single peridural injection was limited to a few hours. After Lemmon's demonstration of continuous spinal anesthesia in 1940 (76), it was not long before the "continuous" technique (actually replenishments at half-hour intervals) was transferred by Edwards and Hingson to obstetric delivery, in which it had an

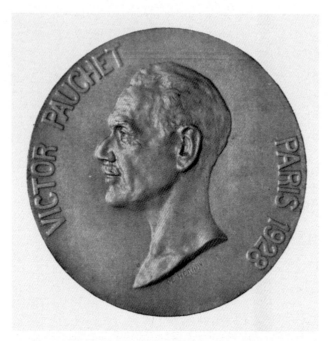

FIGURE 1-17. Likeness of Victor Pauchet, imprinted in Paris in 1928 upon his death.

important sphere of usefulness (Fig. 1-18) (87). This was a rational development, following on the seminal work of Cleland, which identified the pathways of uterine pain and clarified the sources of failure and success of regional obstetric block (55). Cleland had determined that all the sensory fibers that supply the fallopian tubes and uterus enter the spinal cord through T11 and T12, and he blocked them paravertebrally, whereas

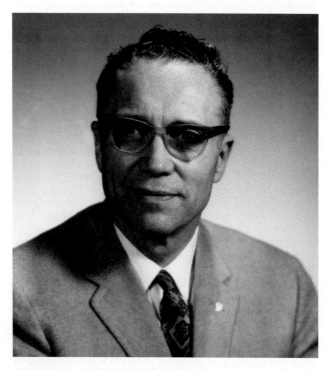

FIGURE 1-18. Robert A. Hingson (1913–).

those from the cervix and perineum were interrupted by caudal block (55). Edwards and Hingson realized that the continuous method enabled them to start the anesthesia early and to continue it for as long as necessary, 5 or 6 hours on the average, to the completion of labor and repair of an episiotomy or laceration. An initial dose of 30 mL of 1.5% Metycaine in physiologic saline produced freedom from pain within 5 minutes.

Caudal block by catheter in obstetrics was announced by Manalan in 1942 (88), independently of Hingson's group, but his described technique of injection was not "continuous." He introduced a No. 4 ureteral silk catheter through the lumen of a 14-gauge needle, advanced the catheter until stopped by the dura, and then withdrew the needle, leaving the catheter in place. The injection, 30 mL of 1% procaine with epinephrine, was withheld until required. Later, he substituted a nylon catheter for the silk catheter because the nylon one could be sterilized more easily. Block and Rochberg devised a continuous gravity drip of procaine and instituted it from the outset, so as to detect any untoward symptoms before a large amount of the drug had been introduced (89). However, the earliest intimation of continuous regional anesthesia in the practice of obstetrics came from Eugene Aburel of Romania (90). For the first stage of labor, he used a specially made combination of catheter and needle: He introduced the needle paravertebrally into the lumbosacral plexus, injected 30 mL of 0.05% dibucaine solution, and then introduced an elastic silk catheter similar to a ureteral catheter through the needle, before withdrawing the needle and fixing the catheter with adhesive tape. Repeated paravertebral injections were given through the catheter, which was "tolerated well, during a rather long period of time." For the second stage, he administered a single (caudal) injection of 30 to 35 mL or infiltrated the perineum. He declared that continuous local anesthesia for obstetrics was henceforth a proven practical procedure, but this claim apparently failed to persuade contemporary obstetricians (Table 1-4).

PARAVERTEBRAL CONDUCTION ANESTHESIA

Matas, the eminent American pioneer and historian of regional anesthesia, recorded that Sellheim, injecting close to the posterior roots of T8 to T12, in addition to the ilioinguinal and iliohypogastric nerves, was able to perform abdominal operations successfully (36). Sellheim was, therefore, credited by Matas as being the originator of the paravertebral method of anesthesia. It was 6 years later, Kappis having in the meantime greatly improved on Sellheim's technique, that the method was first used in urologic surgery. According to Kappis, success with conduction anesthesia of the trigeminal nerve led him to seek an anatomically reliable approach to conduction anesthesia of the spinal nerves at their exit from between the vertebrae (91). In his paper, he described posterior approaches to the lower seven cervical nerves for the purposes of cervical and brachial plexus block. He cautioned against blocking C4 bilaterally at the same time. He made up his own solution of procaine–epinephrine and let it stand for an hour because he believed this improved its effectiveness. The method for paravertebral block of the thoracic nerves and the first four lumbar nerves was given in this same paper, and was used in a great many upper abdominal operations. Finally, Kappis pointed out that these techniques could also be used to treat acute and chronic pain with procaine, or even with alcohol if motor function could be disregarded. Two years later, Kappis described his posterior approach to the splanchnic plexus (92). In 1922, Läwen

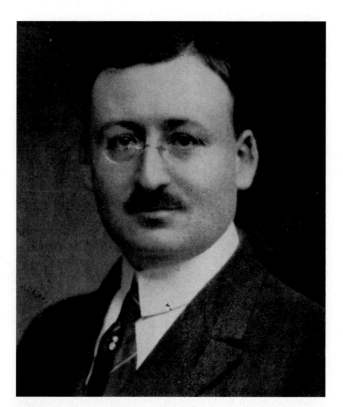

FIGURE 1-19. Fidel Pagés (1886–1923).

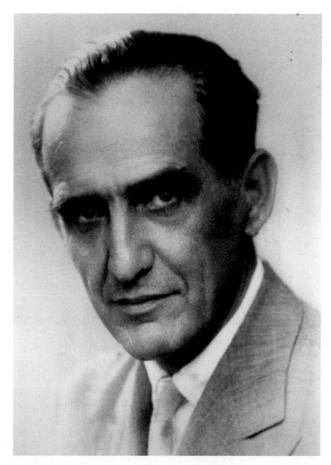

FIGURE 1-20. Achile Mario Dogliotti (1897–1966).

found unilateral paravertebral block of selected spinal nerves useful in the differential diagnosis of intra-abdominal disease (93). For example, he observed that a 10-mL injection of 2% procaine at T10 could completely relieve the pain of a severe biliary colic for 3 hours. The use of segmental paravertebral block for the differential diagnosis of painful conditions was an original idea of Läwen's. At the suggestion of Pal, it was then tried by Brunn and Mandl in 1924 (94), as a therapeutic measure in the hopes of obtaining pain relief in acute cholecystitis, but without significant success. Kappis had treated a case of angina pectoris in this manner in 1923, and von Gaza used 0.5% procaine diagnostically prior to resection of the affected paravertebral nerves (95). In 1925, Mandl reported 16 cases of angina pectoris in which he injected procaine, 0.5%, paravertebrally with excellent results (96).

Segmental peridural anesthesia, under the name of *metameric anesthesia*, was used for the first time in 1921, by Fidel Pagés, a Spanish military surgeon (Fig. 1-19) (97). It is of note that Pagés, reported in his original metameric anesthesia manuscript that the epidural space diameter varies at different levels of the spinal column: "These dimensions are not fixed, and in part, depend on movement of the body." Thus, another early report contains an issue that continues to be highlighted by researchers today (98). To Dogliotti, however, belongs the credit for systematizing and popularizing the peridural principle to produce what he termed *segmental peridural spinal anesthesia* (Fig. 1-20) (99–101). In the light of later theory, which requires that three consecutive internodes be blocked to prevent saltatory conduction, it is interesting to note Dogliotti's iteration of the need to bathe a sufficient length of the spinal nerves. He emphasized that if the anesthetic solution is injected in sufficient quantity (50 to 60 mL) and under adequate pressure, it will be quite easy to subject the spinal nerves to the action of the injected fluid throughout their length in the spinal canal

and the intervertebral foramina, and even beyond. Dogliotti's method was easier and, without question, simpler than paravertebral regional block, since only one puncture was needed. He stressed the sudden loss of resistance when the point of the needle, having pierced the ligamentum flavum, entered the epidural space. The usefulness of this technique was extended further when Curbelo decided to apply the Tuohy armamentarium for continuous spinal anesthesia to continuous segmental peridural anesthesia (102). In one case, he left the catheter in place for as long as 4 days and administered a total of 10 injections of 15 mL each of 2% procaine solution for the production of a continuous sympathetic lumbar block.

ANESTHESIOLOGY AS A SPECIALTY PRACTICE

One of the more noticeable and surprising features in the history of the first 50 years of neural blockade is the almost total lack of involvement by anesthesiologists. Virtually all the developments were devised by surgeons and basic scientists. Also surprising is the miniscule nature of the contribution from Britain, the country of Snow and Lister and pioneering investigation in general. This was not a case of noncommunication, since the very first notice of Koller's discovery in the foreign press had appeared in the London *Lancet*. There is no easy explanation. In most of the medical world, the practice of anesthesia was considered a poor relation, comparatively unhonored

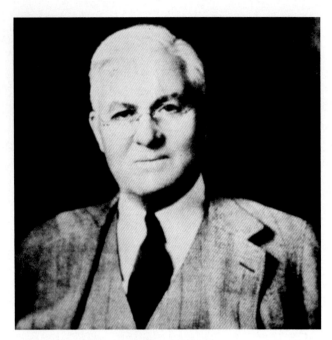

FIGURE 1-21. George W. Crile (1864–1943).

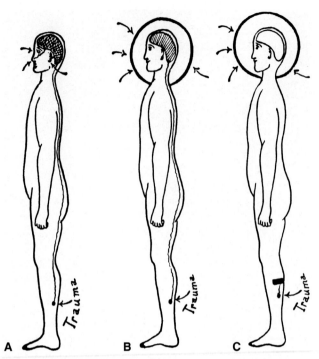

FIGURE 1-22. A: Crile's concept of anociassociation. Schematic drawing illustrating protective effect of anociassociation. **B:** Patient under inhalational anesthesia in whom traumatic noci-impulses only reach the brain. **C:** Patient under complete anociassociation. Auditory, visual, and olfactory impulses are excluded from the brain by inhalational anesthesia. Traumatic impulses from the seat of injury are blocked by Novocaine.

and unskilled, seemingly offering little opportunity or incentive for innovative work. In the British quarter of the globe, general anesthesia was administered by physicians and perhaps generated a certain sense of security and a tendency to leave well enough alone. Everywhere, if local anesthesia was the choice, the surgeon did both the choosing and the injecting. It was not until nerve block began to be perceived as an independent diagnostic and therapeutic tool that a demand arose for regional anesthetic skill independent of surgical operation. One must wonder whether the "choosing and injecting" by the surgeon allowed a more complete view of the perioperative period. The concepts of preemptive analgesia, receiving considerable research attention, have many of their foundations in work by George W. Crile (Fig. 1-21) (103). Crile advanced the thesis that general anesthesia alone was insufficient for shielding patients from the harmful stress of major operations, and he proposed the term *anociassociation* to describe an ideal combination of sedation, local and regional anesthesia, and general anesthetic techniques that protected patients from surgical stress (Fig. 1-22). He subsequently showed that anesthetic prescription affected physiologic variables not only intraoperatively and immediately postoperatively, but also for several days thereafter. In the United States, this period saw the beginnings of anesthesiology as an individual specialty, welcomed by forward-looking surgeons such as William Mayo, who established Labat, one of the first regional anesthesiologists, as a lecturer at the renowned Mayo Clinic in Minnesota.

Not least of the services rendered by the development of regional anesthesia was the stimulation of a higher level of vigilance and physiologic awareness in anesthetic practice as a whole. No better proof of this trend could be desired than that provided by anesthesia records. Charted records of the vital signs during an operation were apparently being kept by Dr. Codman at the Massachusetts General Hospital at the close of the 19th century, stimulated by the recommendations of Cushing. It must be remembered that a convenient method of measuring the blood pressure of a patient was not available until Riva-Rocci invented the arm cuff in 1896, and that 10 years

were to elapse before Korotkoff, a Russian army surgeon, discovered the auscultatory method. Thus, the analgesia charts of Codman at first showed only the pulse rate and, when blood pressure was added, only the systolic pressure. Cushing's insistence on charted records demonstrated his greatness as a medical scientist and surgeon (104). Following the lead of Crile, he sought to combat shock in major amputations by cocainizing the large nerve trunks before dividing them, and he kept graphic track of the patient's condition by having the vital signs measured every 5 minutes (105). The first publication, however, of a chart for recording the progress of a patient during anesthesia should be credited to Sydney Ormond Goldan (1869–1944), who presented a facsimile of one in the *Philadelphia Medical Journal,* November 3, 1900 (106). It was designed specifically for registering the course of "intraspinal cocainization" and provided for the recording of three vital signs—pupil, pulse, and respiration—every 10 minutes (Fig. 1-23). Goldan's paper has a further claim to scholarly distinction; it seems to have been the earliest article in the literature of local anesthesia to include a list of bibliographic citations. Historically, Goldan's contribution is also of interest for his concluding remark: "a remedy for the headache may be found not in simple analgesics, but drugs exerting their influences upon the circulation. . . . Increasing the blood pressure favors an increased tension in the veins retarding absorption."

Goldan gave full details of 16 cases of spinal anesthesia, a large series for that time, and explicitly described himself as an anesthetist. Thus, the practice of careful record-keeping in the operating room, an indispensable foundation to the progress of anesthesiology, was initiated publicly by the first physician

November 3, 1900]

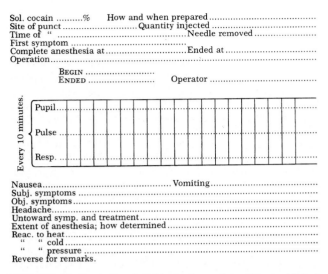

Sol. cocain ....% How and when prepared ....
Site of punct ....Quantity injected ....
Time of " ....Needle removed ....
First symptom ....
Complete anesthesia at ....Ended at ....
Operation ....

BEGIN ....
ENDED ....　　Operator ....

Every 10 minutes.	Pupil										
Pulse										
Resp.										

Nausea...................................Vomiting...................................
Subj. symptoms ....
Obj. symptoms ....
Headache...
Untoward symp. and treatment ....
Extent of anesthesia; how determined ....
Reac. to heat...
　" 　" cold ....
　" 　" pressure ....
Reverse for remarks.

FIGURE 1-23. Facsimile of Goldan's chart, the earliest published anesthesia chart. From Goldan SO. Intraspinal cocainization for surgical anesthesia. *Philadelphia Med J* 1900;6:850, with permission.

to describe himself as an anesthetist in the United States. It is worth noting that Goldan, a much forgotten trailblazer, was also incontrovertibly the first anesthetist to practice regional block anywhere in the world. Goldan disagreed with the approach to anesthetic care that was prevalent in the early 20th century. He objected to the philosophy of one individual performing both the anesthetic and operative procedures. Goldan's beliefs may have contributed to the brevity of his tenure (1896–1903) as a full-time anesthetist. He was an outspoken man, as evidenced by his comments on the question of who should be responsible for the consequences of anesthesia: "There can be but one correct way of viewing this subject, and that is the administrator, whether experienced or not, is responsible for narcosis.... The surgeon should divest himself of the idea that he is doing the anesthetist a favor by having him administer the anesthetic, as he (the anesthetist) is far more important to the patient and the success of the operation (107)."

The interest in regional anesthesia stimulated the formation of the first American Society of Regional Anesthesia (ASRA) on August 2, 1923. The ASRA was founded (a) to develop the methods of local and regional and spinal anesthesia, (b) to promote and further research work along these lines, and (c) to encourage clinical investigations and spread the use of these methods (108). The Society had been a direct outgrowth of a postgraduate course of surgery given at the New York University in Bellevue Hospital Medical College, and, according to notes kept by Dr. Paul Wood, the founders had intended to name this society The Labat Regional Anesthesia Society, but Dr. Labat refused. During the first 10 years of the society's existence, regional anesthesia for surgery made great strides and, toward the end of the decade, regional anesthesia had even extended beyond the scope of surgical anesthesia. It was utilized effectively for diagnostic and prognostic blocks and, with the advent of neurolytic agents, for therapeutic blocks as well. However, as the ASRA (original version) entered its second decade, the role of the physician-anesthetist as a specialist was evolving more rapidly, so that surgeons became less interested and less involved in anesthesia. In the late 1930s, as the specialty of anesthesiology gained momentum, the New

York Society became the American Society of Anesthesiologists (ASA), the American Board of Anesthesiology was founded, and the section on anesthesia of the American Medical Association (AMA) became a separate entity. Indicative of the stature of the ASRA at the time when the American Board of Anesthesiology was founded is the fact that the Board consisted of two representatives from the ASA, two representatives from the section on surgery of the AMA, and two representatives from the ASRA. To this day, the first paragraph of the *Booklet of Information* of the American Board of Anesthesiology and the logo of the Board contain the letters ASRA along with ASA and AMA Board of Specialties. Unfortunately, with the increasing scope of the role of the ASA and the decreasing size of the membership of the ASRA (due to the withdrawal of most of the surgeons), ASRA decided to merge with the ASA and ceased to exist, that is, until its reintroduction in 1976 (109). As Winnie detailed in his 1981 Labat address (108):

But when we anesthesiologists accepted the regional block needle from the surgeon-anesthetist, we did not take with it the body of knowledge that the surgeon-anesthetist had developed to render the use of the needle simple, safe, and effective. We ignored it, or forgot it, or perhaps, even refused to accept it, and, as a result, again and again we have rediscovered and reintroduced techniques which were described accurately and succinctly 50, 60, or 70 years ago.

As of this writing, societies of regional anesthesia, and likely other national societies, have been formed in Europe, Latin America, and Asian and Pacific countries. The ASRA further evolved by changing its name to the American Society of Regional Anesthesia and Pain Medicine. This name change returns the specialty of regional anesthesia to its roots, by linking regional blocks to pain medicine care, much as Moore and Bonica did in the 1940s and 1950s. Another linkage that developed during the last two decades of the 20th century was a return of focus on regional anesthetic techniques to control postoperative surgical pain, thus recalling the subspecialty to one of its primary reasons for growth during the early 20th century. This resurgence of interest resulted from the recognition that many patients could be helped by matching continuous regional techniques to the requirements of individual patients in the early postoperative period (110), for example, through the incorporation of opioids in the local anesthetic solutions used postoperatively (17). The early years of introducing continuous epidural anesthetics into postoperative care resulted in dramatically improved analgesia, yet was accompanied by complications of respiratory depression, occasionally leading to death. These deaths and complications resulted in anesthesiologists organizing acute pain services to optimize this new form of care (111).

The early years of acute pain services were spent in developing the process of how and where these patients should receive advanced analgesia techniques, as well as in undertaking repeated studies focused on the best ways of matching drugs, techniques, and surgical patients. One of the leaders of this effort was Henrik Kehlet, a surgeon from Denmark, who promoted the concept of *multimodal analgesia* (112). This concept utilizes multiple drugs acting on different targets, as well as nondrug strategies to optimize pain amelioration. The concept of "acute rehabilitation" was first raised as a key objective of acute pain management in the 1986 monograph by Michael Cousins in the series *Clinics in Critical Care Medicine* (113). This concept was also a major theme in the first John J. Bonica Lecture of ASRA, delivered by Michael Cousins in 1988 and published in 1989 (114, see particularly page 166 and table 6). Henrik Kehlet and his research group subsequently led a research program that underpinned this important new emphasis for acute pain management. Almost simultaneous with the focus on surgical rehabilitation was promotion of the concept of *preemptive analgesia*. The concept suggested that if regional blockade was introduced prior to surgical pain, the central nervous system (CNS) was prevented from being bombarded with these painful impulses, thereby preventing the development of wind-up and adverse neuroplasticity changes (115). Although preemptive analgesia is a reassuring concept, it has not been proven directly transferrable to clinical practice (116,117). It seems likely that one of the reasons why this concept was so quickly embraced was because it harkened back to the concept of anociassociation promoted by George Crile in the early 20th century. Anociassociation was promoted in an era when general anesthesia was significantly riskier than it is today. Crile suggested that the ideal anesthetic was a combination of regional block along with general anesthesia (103). Many believe we should return to this wise counsel, nearly a century after it was first heralded, but with a different focus.

The modern concept of preemptive analgesia was tested in clinical studies of analgesic regimens given at or before the start of surgery, compared with the same regimens given at the end of surgery. This approach was flawed in that it neglected the large magnitude and lengthy time course of hyperalgesia generated by the postsurgical injury inflammatory response, which has as its basis neuroplastic changes in the nervous system, including the CNS. Thus, existing local anaesthetic and opioid drugs have proven to be suboptimal—particularly if only given in the immediate pre- and/or perioperative period. More recently, a more logical "preventive approach" has been described in which multimodal analgesia is carried over from the preoperative period, through surgery, and well into the postoperative phase. New emphasis is placed on drugs that have powerful effects on neuroplastic changes, such as ketamine, gabapentin, and pregabalin. (The term "preventive analgesia" was first used in the first Bonica Lecture delivered by Michael Cousins in 1988 under the heading "Preventive Treatment of the Injury Response and Acute Pain," which aimed at providing more effective treatment of acute pain and prevention of persistent pain syndromes [114, particularly pages 169–170].)

Hopefully, new drugs and strategies will soon be available to more effectively target the neuroplastic changes associated with the acute injury response, thus allowing a highly effective preventive approach with resulting benefits of more effective acute perioperative pain relief and the prevention of development of persistent pain.

References

1. Brown DL. Anesthesia risk: A historical perspective. In: Brown DL, ed. *Risk and outcome in anesthesia*. Philadelphia: W.B. Saunders Co., 1–29.
2. Caton D. The secularization of pain. *Anesthesiology* 1985;62:493.
2a. Bergman NA. James Morre (1762–1860). An 18th Century advocate of mitigation of pain during surgery. *Anesthesiology* 1994;80:657–662.
2b. Moore J. A method of preventing or diminishing pain in several operations of surgery. London, T. Cadell, 1784.
3. Riese W, Arrington GE Jr. The history of Johannes Müller's doctrine of the specific energies of the senses: Original and later versions. *Bull Hist Med* 1963;37:179.
4. Bell C. *Anatomy of the human body*, 3rd ed. London: T.N. Longman & O. Rees, 1803:224.
5. von Hemholtz H. Ueber di Dauer, und, den Verlauf der durch-stonesschwankungen induzierten elektrischen Strome. *Poggendorf's Annalen Physik Chemie* 1851;83:505.
6. Dallenbach KM. Pain: History and present status. *Am J Psychol* 1939; 52:331.
7. Rynd F. Neuralgia: Introduction of fluid to the nerve. *Dublin Med Press* 1845;13:167.
8. Howard-Jones N. A critical study of the origins and early development of hypodermic medication. *J Hist Med* 1947;2:201.
9. Wood A. New method of treating neuralgia by the direct application of opiates to the painful points. *Edinburgh Med Surg J* 1855;82:265.
10. Pravaz CG. Sur un nouveau moyen d'opérer la coagulation du sang dans les artères, applicable à la guérison des anéurismes. *CR Acad Sci (Paris)* 1853;36:88.
11. Koller C. On the use of cocaine for producing anaesthesia on the eye. *Lancet* 1884;2:990.
12. Corning JL. Spinal anaesthesia and local medication of the cord with cocaine. *NY Med J* 1885;42:483.
13. Melzack R, Wall PD. Pain mechanisms: A new theory. *Science* 1965; 150:971.
14. Reynolds DV. Surgery in the rat during electrical analgesia induced by focal brain stimulation. *Science* 1969;164:444.
15. Kitahata LM, Kosaka Y, Taub A, et al. Lamina-specific suppression of dorsal-horn unit activity by morphine sulfate. *Anesthesiology* 1974;41: 39.
16. Le Bars D, Guilbaud G, Jurna I, Besson JM. Differential effects of morphine on response of dorsal horn lamina V type cells elicited by A and C fibre stimulation in the spinal cat. *Brain Res* 1976;115:518.
17. Yaksh TL, Rudy TA. Analgesia mediated by a direct spinal action of narcotics. *Science* 1976;192:1357.
18. Dickinson AH, Sullivan AF. Subcutaneous formalin-induced activity of dorsal horn neurons in the rate: differential response to an intrathecal opiate administered pre- or postformaline. *Pain* 1987;30:349–360.
19. Niemann A. Ueber eine organische Base in der Coca. *Ann Chem* 1860;114: 213.
20. Vandam LD. Some aspects of the history of local anesthesia. In: Strichartz GR, ed. *Local anesthetics*. Berlin: Springer-Verlag, 1987:1–19.
21. Seelig MG. History of cocaine as a local anesthetic. *JAMA* 1941;117:128.
22. von Anrep B. Ueber die physiologische Wirkung des Cocain. *Pflugers Arch* 1880;21:38.
23. Becker HK. Carl Koller and cocaine. *Psychoanal Quart* 1963;32:309.
24. Noyes HD. The ophthalmological congress in Heidelberg. *Med Record* 1884;26:417.
25. Hepburn WG. Some notes on hydrochlorate of cocaine. *Med Record* 1884;26:534.
26. Bull CS. The hydrochlorate of cocaine as a local anaesthetic in ophthalmic surgery. *NY Med J* 1884;40:609.
27. Fink BR. Leaves and needles: the introduction of surgical local anesthesia. *Anesthesiology* 1985;63:77.
28. Wildsmith JAW. Carl Koller (1857–1944) and the introduction of cocaine into anesthetic practice. *Reg Anesth* 1984;9:161.
29. Burke WC Jr. Hydrochlorate of cocaine in minor surgery. *NY Med J* 1884;40:616.
30. Halsted WS. Practical comments on the use and abuse of cocaine; suggested by its invariably successful employment in more than a thousand minor surgical operations. *NY Med J* 1885;42:294.
31. Halsted WS. Water as a local anesthetic. *NY Med J* 1885;42:327.
32. Halsted WS. *Surgical papers*, Vol. 1. Baltimore: Johns Hopkins Press, 1924: 37–39.
33. Francois-Franck CA. Action paralysant locale de la cocaïne sur les nerfs et les centres nerveux. Applications à la technique expérimentale. *Arch Physiol Norm Pathol* 1892;24:562.
34. Hall RJ. Hydrochlorate of cocaine. *NY Med J* 1884;40:643.
35. Faulconer A Jr., Keys TE. *Foundations of anesthesiology*, Vol. II. Springfield, IL: Charles C. Thomas, 1963.
36. Matas R. Local and regional anesthesia: A retrospect and prospect. *Am J Surg* 1934;25:189.
37. Corning JL. On the prolongation of the anesthetic effect of the hydrochlorate of cocaine, when subcutaneously injected. An experimental study. *NY Med J* 1885;42:317.
38. Esmarch F. Ueber künstliche Blutleere. *Arch Klin Chir* 1874;17:292.
39. Braun H. Ueber den Einfluss der Vitalität der Gewebe auf die örtlichen und allgemeinen Giftwirkungen localanästhesirender Mittel und über die Bedeutung des Adrenalins für die Localanästhesie. *Arch Klin Chir* 1903; 69:541.
40. Abel JJ. On the blood-pressure-raising constituent of the suprarenal capsule. *Johns Hopkins Hosp Bull* 1897;8:151.
41. Mayer E. Clinical experience with adrenaline. *Philadelphia Med J* 1901; 7:819.
42. Schleich CL. Zur Infiltrationsanästhesie. *Therapeutisch Monathefte* 1894;8: 429.

43. Reclus P. Analgésie locale par la cocaïne. *Rev Chir* 1889;9:913.
44. Covino B. One hundred years plus two of regional anesthesia. *Reg Anesth* 1986;11:105.
45. Braun H. Ueber einige neuer örtliche Anaesthetica (Stovain, Alypin, Novocain). *Dtsch Klin Wochenschr* 1905;31:1667.
46. Löfgren N. Studies on local anesthetics. Xylocaine: A new synthetic drug. Inaugural dissertation. Stockholm: Hoeggstroms, 1948.
47. Gordh T. Anesthesiology Topics/January-February. Stockholm, Sweden: Karolinska Hospital, 1986:7.
48. Bier A. Ueber einen neuen Weg Localanästhesie an den Gliedmassen zu erzeugen. *Arch Klin Chir* 1908;86:1007.
49. Braun H. *Local anesthesia: Its scientific basis and practical use,* 3rd ed. Philadelphia: Lea & Febiger, 1914.
50. Holmes GM. Intravenous regional anesthesia: A useful method of producing analgesia of the limbs. *Lancet* 1963;1:245.
51. Lee JA. Labat Lecture: Some foundations on which we have built. *Reg Anesth* 1985;10:99.
52. Gray H. *Anatomy: Descriptive and surgical,* 5th ed. Philadelphia: Henry C. Lea, 1870:572–574.
53. Adriani J, Roman-Vega D. Saddle block anesthesia. *Am J Surg* 1946;71:12.
54. Biographical sketch of Doctor James Leonard Corning of New York City, and his recent remarkable discoveries in local anesthesia. *VA Med Mon* 1886;12:713.
55. Cleland JG. Paravertebral anesthesia in obstetrics. *Surg Gynecol Obstet* 1938;57:57.
56. Quincke H. Die Lumbalpunction des Hydrocephalus. *Ber Klin Wochenschr* 1891;28:929.
57. Wynter WE. Four cases of tuberculosis meningitis in which paracentesis of the theca vertebralis was performed for the relief of fluid pressure. *Lancet* 1891;1:981.
58. Bier A. Versuche über Cocainisirung des Rückenmarkes. *Dtsch Z Chir* 1899;5151:361.
59. Tait D, Caglieri G. Experimental and clinical notes on the subarachnoid space. Transactions Medical Society of California, Abstracted. *JAMA* 1900;35:6.
60. Tuffier T. Analgésie chirurgicale par l'injection sous-arachnoïdienne lombaire de cocaïne. *CR Soc Biol* 1899;1:882.
61. Lee EW. Subarachnoidean injections of cocaine as a substitute for general anesthesia in operations below the diaphragm, with report of seven cases. *Philadelphia Med J* 1900;6:865.
62. Tuffier T. Anesthésie medullaire chirurgicale par injection sous-arachnoidienne lombaire de cocaïne; technique et resultats. *Semaine Medicale* 1900;20:167.
63. Hopkins GS. Anesthesia by cocainization of the spinal cord. *Philadelphia Med J* 1900;6:864.
64. Matas R. Local and regional anesthesia with cocaine and other analgesic drugs, including the subarachnoid method, as applied in general surgical practice. *Philadelphia Med J* 1900;6:820.
65. Fowler RG. Cocaine analgesia from subarachnoid injection, with a report of forty-four cases together with a report of a case in which antipyrine was used. *Philadelphia Med J* 1900;6:843.
66. Gray HT, Parsons L. Blood pressure variations associated with lumbar puncture and the induction of spinal anesthesia. *Quart J Med* 1912;5:339.
67. Smith GS, Porter WT. Spinal anesthesia in the cat. *Am J Physiol* 1915;38:108.
68. Labat G. Circulatory disturbances associated with subarachnoid nerve block. *Long Island Med J* 1927;21:573.
69. Barker AE. Clinical experiences with spinal analgesia in 100 cases and some reflections on the procedure. *Br Med J* 1907;1:665.
70. De Lapersonne F. Un nouvel anesthésique local, la stovaïne. *Presse Med* 1904;12:233.
71. Pitkin G Controllable spinal anesthesia. *Am J Surg* 1928;5:537.
72. Sise LF. Spinal anesthesia for upper and lower abdominal operations. *N Engl J Med* 1928;199:61.
73. Sise LF. Pontocainglucose for spinal anesthesia. *Surg Clin North Am* 1935;15:1501.
74. Babcock WW. Spinal anesthesia; with report of surgical clinics. *Surg Gynecol Obstet* 1912;15:606.
75. Eckenhoff JE. A wide angle view of anesthesiology: Emory A. Rovenstein Memorial Lecture. *Anesthesiology* 1978;48:272.
76. Lemmon WT. A method for continuous spinal anesthesia. *Ann Surg* 1940;111:141.
77. Dean HP. Relative value of inhalation and injection methods of inducing anaesthesia. *Br Med J* 1907;2:869.
78. Tuohy EB. Continuous spinal anesthesia: Its usefulness and technic involved. *Anesthesiology* 1944;5:142.
79. Koster H. Spinal anaesthesia, with special reference to its use in surgery of the head, neck, and thorax. *Am J Surg* 1928;5:554.
80. Jonnesco T. Remarks on general spinal anesthesia. *Br Med J* 1909;2:1396.
81. Kreis O. Ueber Medullarnarkose bei Gebärenden. *Zentralbl Gynakol* 1900;24:724.
82. Marx S. Analgesia in obstetrics produced by medullary injections of cocaine. *Philadelphia Med J* 1900;6:857.
83. Stoeckel W. Ueber sakrale Anästhesie. *Zentralbl Gynaekol* 1909;33:1.
84. Cathelin F. Une nouvelle voie d'injection rachidienne. Méthodes des injections épidurales par le procédé du canal sacré. Applications à l'homme. *CR Soc Biol (Paris)* 1901;53:452.
85. Läwen A. Ueber die Verwertung der Sakralanästhesie fur chirurgische Operationen. *Zentralbl Chir* 1910;37:708.
86. Gros O. Ueber die Narkotika und Localanästhetika. *Arch Exp Pathol Pharmakol* 1910;63:80.
87. Edwards WB, Hingson RA. Continuous caudal anesthesia in obstetrics. *Am J Surg* 1942;57:459.
88. Manalan SA. Caudal block anesthesia in obstetrics. *J Indiana State Med Assoc* 1942;35:564.
89. Block N, Rochberg S. Continuous caudal anesthesia in obstetrics. *Am J Obstet Gynecol* 1943;45:645.
90. Aburel E. L'anesthésie locale continue (prolongée) en obstétrique. *Bull Soc Obstét Gynecol* 1931;20:35.
91. Kappis M. Ueber Leitungsanästhesie an Bauch, Burst, Arm und Hals durch Injektion ans Foramen intervertebrale. *Münch Med Wochenschr* 1912;1:794.
92. Kappis M. Erfahrungen mit Lokalanästhesie bei Bauchoperationen. *Verh Dtsch Ges Chir* 1914;43:87.
93. Läwen A. Ueber segmentäre Schmerzaufhebung durch papavertebrale Novokaininjektionen zur Differentialdiagnose intra-abdominaler. *Erkrankungen Med Wochenschr* 1922;69:1423.
94. Brunn F, Mandl F. Die paravertebral Injektion zur Bekämpfung visceraler Schmerzen. *Wien Klin Wochenschr* 1924;37:511.
95. von Gaza W. Die Resektion der paravertebralen Nerven und die isolierte Durchschneidung des Ramus communicans. *Arch Klin Chir* 1924;133:479.
96. Mandl F. Die Wirkung der paravertebralen Injektion bei "Angina pectoris." *Arch Klin Chir* 1925;136:495.
97. Pagés F. Anestesia metamerica. *Rev Sanid Milit Argen* 1921;11:351–356.
98. Hogan QH. Lumbar epidural anatomy. *Anesthesiology* 1991;75:767–775.
99. Dogliotti AM. Eine neue Methode der regionaren Anästhesie. *Zentralbl Chir* 1931;58:3141.
100. Dogliotti AM. Proposta di un nuovo metodo di cura delle algie periferiche. L'alcoolizzazione sottomeningea delle radici posteriori. Considerazioni sulle prime 30 osservazione cliniche. *Minerva Med* 1931;1:536.
101. Dogliotti AM. A new method of block anesthesia. Segmental peridural spinal anesthesia. *Am J Surg* 1933;20:107.
102. Curbelo MM. Continuous peridural segmental anesthesia by means of a ureteral catheter. *Anesth Analg (Cleve)* 1949;28:13.
103. Crile GW. Nitrous oxide anesthesia and a note on anoci association, a new principle in operative surgery. *Surg Gynecol Obstet* 1911;13:170.
104. Beecher HK. The first anesthesia records (Codman, Cushing). *Surg Gynecol Obstet* 1940;71:789.
105. Cushing H. On the avoidance of shock in major amputations by cocainization of large nerve-trunks preliminary to their division. *Ann Surg* 1902;36:321.
106. Goldan SO. Intraspinal cocainization for surgical anesthesia. *Philadelphia Med J* 1900;6:850.
107. Goldan SO. Anesthetization as a specialty: Its present and future. *Am Med* 1901;2:101.
108. Winne AP. Nothing new under the sun—Labat address. *Reg Anesth* 1982;7:95.
109. Bacon DR, deLeon-Casasola OA, Myers DP, et al. Minutes of the American Society of Regional Anesthesia: 1924–1939. *Anesthesiology* 1993;79:A1028.
110. Yaeger MP, Glass DD, Neff RK, Brinck-Johnsen T. Epidural anesthesia and analgesia in high risk surgical patients. *Anesthesiology* 1987;66:729–736.
111. Ready LB, Oden R, Chadwick HE, et al. Development of an anesthesiology-based postoperative pain management service. *Anesthesiology* 1988;68:100–106.
112. Kehlet H. Postoperative pain relief—a look from the other side. *Reg Anesth* 1994;19:369–377.
113. Cousins MJ, Phillips GD. *Acute pain management clinics in critical care medicine.* New York: Churchill Livingstone, 1986.
114. Cousins MJ. JJ Bonica Lecture: Acute pain and the injury response: immediate and prolonged effects. *Reg Anesth Pain Med* 1989;14:162–179.
115. Katz J, Kavanagh BP, Sandler AN, et al. Preemptive analgesia: Clinical evidence of neuroplasticity contributing to postoperative pain. *Anesthesiology* 1992;77:439–446.
116. Brennan TJ, Kehlet H. Preventive analgesia to reduce wound hyperalgesia and persistent postsurgical pain: Not an easy path. *Anesthesiology* 2005;103:681–683.
117. Brennan TJ. Frontiers in translational research: The etiology of incisional and postoperative pain. *Anesthesiology* 2002;97:535–537.

PART I ■ PHARMACOLOGY AND NEUROPHYSIOLOGY

CHAPTER 2 ■ NEURAL PHYSIOLOGY AND LOCAL ANESTHETIC ACTION

GARY R. STRICHARTZ, ELS PASTIJN, AND KENJI SUGIMOTO

BASIC PHYSIOLOGY AND PHARMACOLOGY

Overview of the Neuron

Local anesthetic drugs reversibly block conduction of nerve impulses at the level of the axonal membrane. In this overview, we review briefly the structure and function of neurons, the impulse generating and conducting cells of the nervous system (1). A typical neuron is composed of a cell body (or soma); dendrites, with multiple small branches close to the cell bodies; and a single long axon for each neuron (Fig. 2-1).

Sensory neurons have their cell bodies in dorsal root ganglia. Only one axon is attached, with its longer branch extending to the periphery and a shorter branch to the spinal cord. Impulses are generated in the small peripheral axon branches at the receptor component of the neuron. The distal nerve endings reside in skin, joints, muscles, viscera, or connective tissue. Impulses may be selectively initiated by mild mechanical, thermal (hot or cold changes in skin temperature), or intense tissue-damaging (noxious) stimuli at the nerve endings, whose anatomic spread determines the receptive field for that particular neuron. Intense mechanical and thermal stimuli that can cause pain lead directly to the opening of ion channels selectively responsive to large mechanical distortions or high temperatures. A widespread example of the latter type is the receptor TRPV1, a member of the transient receptor potential (trp) class of channels that exists in many pain fibers. Tissue damage and inflammation also can result in the release of *sensitizing* chemicals (e.g., bradykinin, prostaglandins) from tissues closely surrounding the endings of nociceptive afferent axons. Such sensitization results in a larger response of nociceptors to specifically noxious stimuli (hyperalgesia) and also to the sensation of pain from stimuli that normally do not cause pain (allodynia). The resulting local depolarization of the nociceptor nerve endings by noxious stimuli leads to trains of impulses with average discharge frequencies that are proportional to the stimulus intensity above the threshold level for impulse generation. Axons then conduct these impulses to the spinal cord, although impulses also invade the soma.

Several axons usually innervate a particular receptive field. As these axons have branches with receptive fields overlapping those of neighboring axons, and each branch alone generates trains of impulses, a convergence occurs in the spinal cord that results in both spatial and temporal summation of afferent impulses. However, the dorsal horn, where primary afferent fibers synapse on second-order neurons, is not merely a relay for transmitting sensory signals. Complex interactions between incoming tactile and nociceptive fibers, as well as modulation by axons descending from the brain, impress sophisticated processing on pain-related activity; in general, these descending pathways have the effect of diminishing pain. As a result, many specifically acting drugs are targeted to receptors for descending axons in the spinal cord to exert a selective analgesia (see Chapters 32 and 33).

Motor neurons have their cell bodies in the ventral horn of the spinal cord gray matter (Fig. 2-1). They are multipolar, in that they have many dendrites in addition to one axon that follows a long course to the periphery. The dendrites and cell body of the motor neuron are specially developed for integrating postsynaptic currents in order to determine the output activity, which occurs as impulse generation. The axon conducts these impulses to its branched, distal terminal enlargements, which contain neurotransmitters to activate effector organs. Skeletal muscles contract rapidly in response to impulses in the large, Aα-fibers that excite them, but their contraction is also strongly dependent on small, myelinated Aγ-fibers that adjust the length threshold for the muscle's response. We will see later, in the section on Fiber Size and Function, how drug effects on Aγ-fibers can account for much of the motor blockade during peripheral nerve block.

Axons and Peripheral Nerves

Axons are cylinders of axoplasm encased in the axonal membrane, which is similar to other plasma membranes (Fig. 2-2). Axons are always enveloped by a Schwann cell. Many unmyelinated axons lie within invaginations of a single Schwann cell (Fig. 2-2C), in contrast to the thick myelin sheath of a myelinated axon, which is formed by a single Schwann cell wrapped many times around the axon (Fig. 2-2B). This myelin sheath is interrupted periodically at the nodes of Ranvier, where the extracellular medium has access to the axolemma (Fig. 2-2A).

Nerve impulses travel along nonmyelinated axons as a uniform wave, similar to the way a flame progressively ignites the fuse of a firecracker. The nerve impulse, or action potential, is a change in the electrical voltage across the membrane that is due to changes in the permeability of ionic channels in the axon membrane (2,3). In nonmyelinated axons, these permeability changes occur relatively uniformly along the axon, supporting a wave of inward ion current that underlies the depolarization of the nerve impulse. In myelinated axons, however, changes in the axon's membrane permeability and the associated inward currents occur only at the nodes of Ranvier; the myelinated internode of the axon is depolarized by the *passive* spread of current from the nodes (4). Thus, impulse conduction in these axons is continuous but not homogeneous.

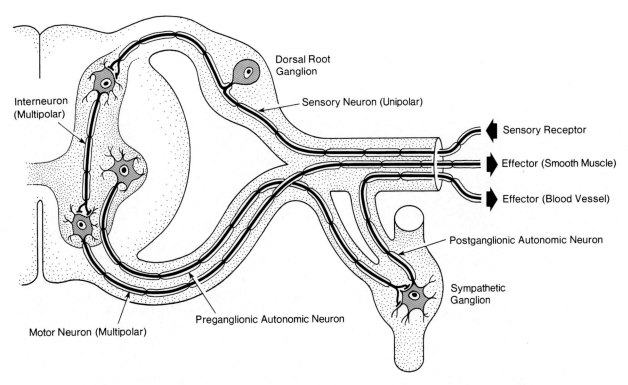

FIGURE 2-1. The neuron. *Sensory neuron*, with a cell body (perikaryon) and an axon with long peripheral and short central branches (unipolar neuron). *Interneuron* with numerous dendrites, a cell body, and one short axon (multipolar neuron). *Motor* neuron with a great many dendrites, a cell body, and a long peripheral axon (multipolar neuron). Two *sympathetic neurons*, one with a cell body in the spinal cord and the other with its cell body in the sympathetic chain, are also shown. Each has several dendrites and a medium-length axon.

Nerve Membranes

The *modern fluid mosaic model* depicts the plasma membrane as a bilayer of phospholipid molecules with their fatty acyl chains facing each other, thus making the inner portion of the membrane hydrophobic (Fig. 2-3). The surfaces of the membrane facing the cytoplasm and extracellular fluid are formed by the charged and polar hydrophilic groups of the phospholipid molecules. Globular proteins are also present, and some of these penetrate through the entire thickness of the membrane. Ionic channels are composed of such transmembrane proteins, as are various transporters and receptors for peptide and nonpeptide transmitters and hormones. Such proteins are heavily glycosylated by carbohydrate groups attached covalently to their extracellular surface and often are covalently bound to lipophilic fatty acids that stabilize their transmembrane domains in the hydrocarbon core of the membrane bilayer (5). An intracellular matrix of cytoskeleton is frequently linked to membrane proteins by other specific proteins. All these attachments secure active proteins within the membrane and also can respond dynamically to cellular activity and metabolism to change the protein populations on the cell membrane. As described later (in Basic Pharmacology), local anesthetic molecules are distributed primarily near the interface of membranes, with aqueous solutions that surround them, and also at protein–membrane interfaces and, sometimes, in the ion-conducting pores of membrane channels. Figure 2-3 shows lidocaine's membrane and protein distribution at the density of drug that occurs for the critical blocking content, which corresponds to one lidocaine molecule for about 100 phospholipid molecules.

Organization of a Peripheral Nerve

In clinical practice, local anesthetics must diffuse across a number of structures before reaching their site of action in the axonal membrane (6). Peripheral nerves contain both afferent and efferent axons (Figs. 2-1 and 2-4). These individual axons and their Schwann cells are linked loosely together by a delicate layer of fine connective tissue (endoneurium) that allows the easy diffusion of most local anesthetics.

Bundles of axons are enclosed in a squamous epithelial cellular "sheath," the perineurium, which comprises several layers of cells and acts as a semipermeable barrier to local anesthetics (7–9). One or more perineurial bundles are covered by an outermost, easily permeable, connective tissue layer, the epineurium. This layer also carries the nutritional blood vessels of larger nerves. Factors that have an important influence on local anesthetic diffusion to the axons include the thickness of the perineurium, the presence or absence of myelin, the size of the axons, and the anatomic position of the axons, either closer to the outer, more superficial mantle layers of the nerve or deeper within the inner "core" sections of the nerve.

Nerve Membranes and Impulses

The generation and propagation of impulses in excitable nerve and muscle cells depend on the flow of specific ionic currents through channels that span the plasma membrane (2). These channels open and close in response to the electrical potential of the cell membrane and are the targets for local anesthetics as they block impulse propagation. This chapter describes the

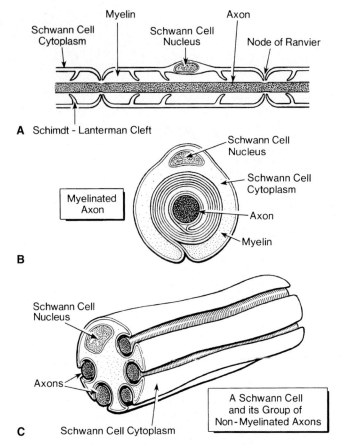

FIGURE 2-2. Diagram of axon. *Myelinated axon.* **A:** Longitudinal section shows the relation of the myelin sheath to the nodes of Ranvier where myelin is absent, but one overlying Schwann cell and a thin layer of "gap substance" are present. The extranodal area is highly specialized and, because of anionic charges bound within it, tends to attract cationic substances such as local anesthetics. **B:** Transverse section of a myelinated fiber shows how the Schwann cell wraps around one axon many times to form the multiple layers of the myelin sheath. **C:** In transverse section, many nonmyelinated axons can be seen embedded in the folds of a single Schwann cell. The Schwann cell surrounds the axon loosely, thus allowing uniform spread of depolarization directly along the axon.

role of ion channels in impulse behavior that account for many of the physiologic effects of local anesthetics.

Most ion channels appear to be very similar in the peripheral nervous system (PNS) and central nervous system (CNS), and in cell bodies as well as axons. Thus, a single description will serve to characterize the essential actions of local anesthetics associated with blockade of impulses anywhere in the nervous system.

Ionic Currents of the Nerve Impulse

Two factors combine to create electric potentials in cells: (a) concentration gradients of ions across membranes and (b) selective permeation of ions through membranes. The gradients are diffusional forces that tend to move the ions; the selective changes in permeability permit that tendency to be manifested as ionic current. Energy from the cell's metabolism is used to create and maintain the gradients.

The concentration of potassium ions (K^+) inside a cell is about 10 times greater than the extracellular K^+ concentration, and vice versa for sodium ions (Na^+). A special protein in the membrane (the Na/K pump) actively transports K^+ into the cell and Na^+ out of the cell, using adenosine triphosphate (ATP) as the source of energy (10). In the resting cell membrane, a selective permeability to K^+ ions exists, permitting the net efflux of a small number of K^+ ions, thus leaving the axoplasm electrically negative (polarized) while making the outside electrically positive. This accounts, for the most part, for the cell's "resting potential," which typically equals -60 to -70 mV (Fig. 2-5).

At rest Na^+ ions tend to flow into the axon, both because the resting axon is electrically negative inside and because the Na^+ ions are more concentrated outside. During a nerve impulse, a selective permeability to Na^+ arises when specific Na channels in the axon membrane are opened (2,3). Figure 2-5 shows the contributions of ionic currents during a conducted nerve impulse. The large inward Na current (I_{Na}^+) accounts for the *depolarizing phase* of the impulse. Opening of Na^+ channels occurs as the membrane is initially depolarized from the resting potential; that is, as the potential becomes less negative. This opening, a result of complex channel activation, is an intrinsic behavior of Na^+ channels, due to charged amino acids that are part of the channel molecule's structure (11). As the membrane depolarizes and the potential becomes less negative, more Na^+ channels open, and they open more rapidly. As more channels open, more Na^+ ions enter the cell, and the resulting depolarization is accelerated (Fig. 2-6). This positive feedback cycle accounts for the "regenerative" behavior of nerve impulses (2).

Action potentials are brief, transient events. Repolarization of the membrane to the negative resting value occurs because of three factors: (a) The driving force moving Na^+ into the cell diminishes as the axoplasmic potential becomes less negative and approaches the Nernst potential for $Na^+ (\sim +50$ mV), (b) the sodium channels eventually close (inactivate) during a depolarization, and (c) voltage-dependent K channels open and permit a large, outward K^+ current that returns the axoplasmic potential to or beyond, its resting value (Fig. 2-5). In simple terms, impulses have a depolarization phase and a repolarization phase. Inward currents, carried by Na^+ ions, depolarize the cell, whereas outward currents, carried by K^+ ions, repolarize the cell. The integrated result of all these factors is diagrammed in Figure 2-6, which summarizes the ionic contribution to the nerve impulse.

With each action potential, a pulse of Na^+ ions enters the cell and a pulse of K^+ leaves it. Small changes in the concentrations of these ions can build up during repeated discharge and thus lessen the ion gradients. However, the Na^+/K^+-ATPase (Na^+/K^+ pump), which is activated by elevation of intracellular Na^+, will return this Na^+ to the extracellular space and, reciprocally, lower the extracellular K^+, removing it to the intracellular compartment, using the energy of ATP. This "electrogenic" pump generates an outward current during this process and thereby hyperpolarizes the cell, contributing to an after-potential (10) and shaping the patterns of impulses that occur in constant or intermittent trains of discharge.

Impulse Propagation

Inward current entering the axon during the depolarizing phase of an impulse flows within the conducting medium of the axoplasm and thereby spreads to adjacent, inactive regions. These adjacent regions are depolarized by this "local circuit" current, usually to levels far in excess of those for threshold conditions,

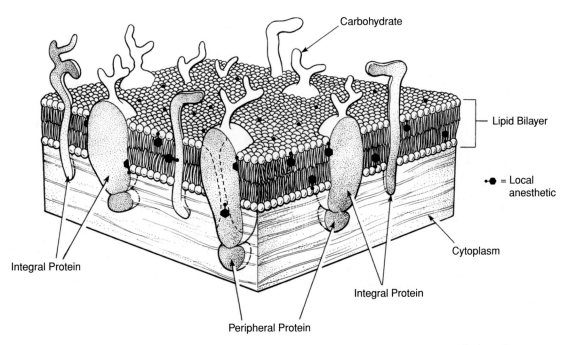

Carbohydrate

Lipid Bilayer

•● = Local anesthetic

Cytoplasm

Integral Protein

Integral Protein

Peripheral Protein

FIGURE 2-3. Axonal membrane. The axonal membrane is similar to the plasma membrane of other cells. Carbohydrate molecules attached to proteins and lipids on the extracellular surface of the membrane form a "cell coat." The lipid bilayer comprises densely packed phospholipids which, nevertheless, freely diffuse laterally in the plane of the membrane. Integral proteins of varying shapes and peripheral protein only on the cytoplasmic surface are associated with enzymatic and receptor functions.

and the regenerative impulse then extends to this region, generating its own inward current. The propagating wave of potential spreads far along axons during any one instant, over distances that are much larger than the fiber's diameter. For example, if an impulse lasts for 1 msec, from the beginning of its depolarizing phase to the time of initial repolarization, and is conducted at a velocity of 1 m/sec, as in the small, nonmyelinated C fibers (of diameter less than 1 μm), then the action potential extends over 1 mm along the axon, 1,000 times the axon's diameter. For large myelinated axons, 20 μm in diameter, impulses travel at 60 to 100 m/sec and thus extend over distances of 60 to 100 mm. Inward currents from all the active nodes add together as they spread toward inactive regions, ensuring that impulse propagation will continue. Therefore, complete block of impulses in about three to five nodes in sequence is necessary for the total prevention of impulse propagation in myelinated fibers (4,12,13). Furthermore, the "action current" flowing into the nerve under the impulse is five to ten times that required to depolarize the next segment to threshold; this ratio is referred to as the *margin of safety* for impulse conduction. Due to this large margin of safety, about 80% of the Na channels in an axon membrane must be inhibited in order to fully block a propagated impulse.

In the face of reduced membrane excitability due to disease, altered metabolism, or drug action, impulses may still occur but will be conducted more slowly. When the net inward current is decreased, the action potential amplitude will be smaller, the rate of impulse depolarization slower, and the velocity of conduction lower. This condition often worsens as an impulse attempts to propagate through a diseased or drugged axon, a situation termed *decremental impulse conduction*. If the decrement is sufficiently great, conduction failure occurs;

if not, then only conduction slowing along the affected axonal region occurs, and normal impulse conduction resumes if the decremented action potential is able to excite the contiguous normal region of the axon. This situation certainly occurs for nerve conduction during the onset and regression of a local anesthetic block. Even in an effectively, fully blocked axon, conduction fails decrementally as an impulse enters the anesthetic-exposed region of the nerve rather than stopping abruptly in a very short distance.

Mechanisms of Anesthetic Action

Local anesthetics block impulses by interfering with the function of Na channels (14,15). In the presence of local anesthetics, Na channels are less likely to open in response to a stimulating depolarization (16–18), the resulting Na$^+$ current is decreased, and, at sufficiently high anesthetic concentrations, enough channels are impaired to prevent impulse generation. When a local anesthetic–containing solution is applied to a *desheathed* peripheral nerve in vitro, inhibition is detected in a minute and a steady-state level of block is usually achieved in 10 minutes or less. At low frequencies of impulse firing, 1 Hz (1/sec) or less, this "tonic block" has a constant value (Fig. 2-7A). Higher-frequency impulses increase the degree of block, a phenomenon called *phasic* or *use-dependent block* (22), which quickly reaches a new steady state (Fig. 2-7B) and quickly reverses to the tonic block level when the stimulation frequency returns to a very low level.

These changes in impulse behavior are caused by reciprocal drug-induced changes in the opening and closing of Na$^+$ channels. Both tonic and phasic block can be accounted for by

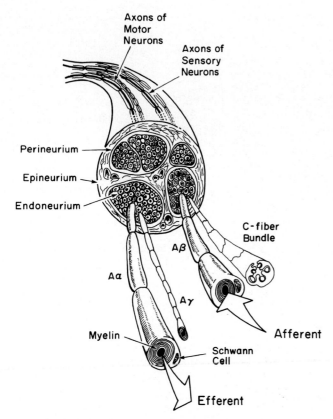

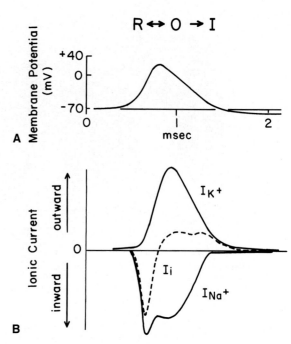

FIGURE 2-5. A propagating action potential and the membrane currents that produce it. **A:** The membrane potential rises from its resting value, about −70 mV in this squid axon, to reverse its sign, becoming positive inside, and then repolarizes. A hyperpolarization actually follows the impulse in this, but not in all, axons. **B:** Inward sodium current (I_{Na}) and outward potassium current (I_K) together yield the net ionic current across the membrane (I_i). The maximum rate of depolarization corresponds to the peak of net inward current, that of repolarization to the largest net outward current. The letters at the top of the figure describe the dominant state of the Na^+ channel during the underwritten phase of the impulse.

FIGURE 2-4. Diagram of a peripheral nerve. The *epineurium,* with its easily permeable collagen fibers, is oriented along the long axis of the nerve. The *perineurium* is a discrete layer of cells, whereas the *endoneurium* is a delicate matrix of connective tissue embedding bundles of axons. Both afferent (sensory) and efferent (motor) axons are shown. Sympathetic efferent axons (not shown) are also present in mixed peripheral nerves.

the modulated receptor hypothesis (MRH) (19,20) (Fig. 2-8). This hypothesis rests on the accepted notion that Na^+ channels normally respond to membrane depolarizations by passing through defined conformational "states," beginning at rest (R), activating through closed intermediate forms (C) to reach an open (O) form—the "activation" response—and then clos-

ing to an inactivated (I) state. According to the MRH, local anesthetics have a higher affinity for open and, especially, inactivated Na^+ channels than they do for resting channels (21,22). During stimulation, some of the channels that are opened and then become inactivated bind local anesthetics more tightly than the resting channels did. This additional binding thus stabilizes the channels in a nonconducting state, and the fraction of channels so bound increases with each stimulating pulse.

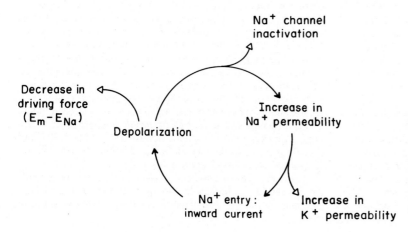

FIGURE 2-6. The positive feedback cycle that underlies the depolarization phase of regenerative action potentials. Each of the three components in the cycle (*filled arrowhead*) is increased by the preceding one and, in turn, increases the subsequent one. Each outlying element (*open arrowhead*) reduces membrane excitability and terminates the action potential. The cycle is initiated by a source of current "external" to the membrane area being studied, for example, an adjacent excited region, a sensory ending depolarized by a physiologic stimulus, or a dendritic arbor that collects postsynaptic currents.

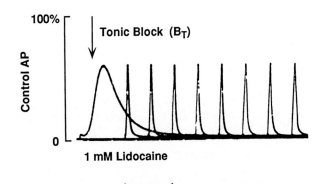

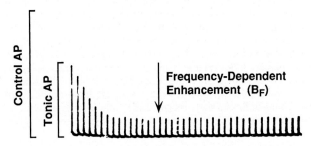

FIGURE 2-7. Tonic (B_T) and use-dependent (B_F) inhibition of action potentials by local anesthetic. **A:** Tonic inhibition is the relative decrease in amplitude of the compound action potential (CAP) in the presence of drug with the nerve stimulated at low frequency (0.016 Hz = 1/min). **B:** Frequency-dependent block (B_F) is the further decrease in amplitude of the action potential during a high-frequency pulse train (40 Hz here), which is completely reversible to the level of B_T when stimulation is slowed. The horizontal bar calibrates the time scale: 2 and 20 msec for the broad and narrow action potentials, respectively, in **A** and 200 msec in **B**. From Bokesch PM, Post C, Strichartz GR. Structure activity relationship of lidocaine homologues on tonic and frequency-dependent impulse blockade in nerve. *J Pharmacol Exp Ther* 1986;237:773, with permission.

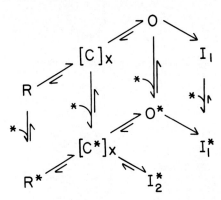

FIGURE 2-8. The revised modulated receptor model. Each letter represents a state of the sodium channel: R, resting; C_x, any one of several intermediate, closed states between R and O, which is the open, ion-conducting state; I_1, an inactivated (non-openable) state that is formed from O; and I_2, a different inactivated state that is formed from the anesthetic-bound C^* states, without going through O. The *vertical arrows* indicate binding reactions of a local anesthetic molecule (*asterisk*). States C and O and I have higher affinities for anesthetics than does R. The $[C^*]_X \rightarrow I_2^*$ reaction may account for much of the resting, tonic blocking activity of local anesthetics, and thus favor the neutral, more hydrophobic drugs. Anesthetic binding reactions of O and I conformations are activated by rapid depolarizations (e.g., action potentials), with the former being faster than the latter. Charged drugs bound to O^* and I_1 and I_2^* dissociate slowly, accounting for much of the phasic blocking behavior.

Some anesthetic-bound channels will return to the resting, unbound state, but much more slowly than inactivated, drug-free channels recover, so that eventually a steady-state level of phasic block will be reached wherein increased drug binding during a depolarization is exactly reversed by drug dissociation in the time between pulses.

The normal inactivated state is not essential for tonic or use-dependent block (23,24). It appears that both open and activated channels react most rapidly with anesthetic molecules and that inactivated channels react more slowly but still have a greater equilibrium drug affinity than resting channels (21). (Clinically, during one, relatively brief nerve impulse [0.5–1 msec], the presence of inactivated channels is limited and drug binding to this state probably contributes little to the observed inhibition. In contrast, cardiotoxicity will arise from this slow binding to cardiac Na^+ channels that remain inactivated during the 200 msec of the action potential's plateau) (25,26). The concept of selective, state-dependent binding of anesthetics lies at the core of the MRH.

Since they lessen the probability that channels will open, local anesthetics have an effect like that of slow depolarization. They shift channels toward an "inactivated-like" state that cannot be directly opened by stimulation (16,19,20). The major difference is that recovery from normal, depolarization-dependent inactivation is fast (a few milliseconds), whereas recovery that depends on local anesthetic unbinding is slow (0.1–1 seconds). In this way, local anesthetics dramatically increase the effective refractory period and thus limit the frequency with which a nerve can fire.

Basic Pharmacology

Exploration of the mechanism of local anesthetic action raises three fundamental questions: Which species of the drug, neutral or protonated, is the active form? Where does the anesthetic molecule act? What is the molecular mechanism of Na^+ channel interference?

Active Species: The Role of Ionization

Under physiologic conditions, most local anesthetics exist in rapid equilibrium between the neutral and protonated, charged species (Fig. 2-9). The ratio of ionized (LH^+) to nonionized (L) molecules is given by the Henderson-Hasselbalch equation:

$$\frac{[LH^+]}{[L]} = 10^{pK_a - pH} \qquad (1)$$

where the pK_a is the value of pH at which the concentrations of the unionized and ionized species are equal. The pK_a values of clinically used local anesthetics range from about 7.7 to 9.5 (27), so that in solution all these drugs are charged more often than they are uncharged. Protonation and deprotonation in solution are very rapid processes, occurring about 10^3 times per second. When the drug is buried in a membrane or bound to a protein molecule, however, these reactions can be much slower.

Both ionized and nonionized drug species can inhibit Na^+ channels. Quaternary derivatives of local anesthetics, which are permanently charged, when placed inside a neuron are potent blockers of impulses and of Na^+ currents (28,29). Interestingly, these drugs have very slowly developing effects when present outside of the axon; their constant charge and low hydrophobicity greatly restrict their passage into and through the membrane.

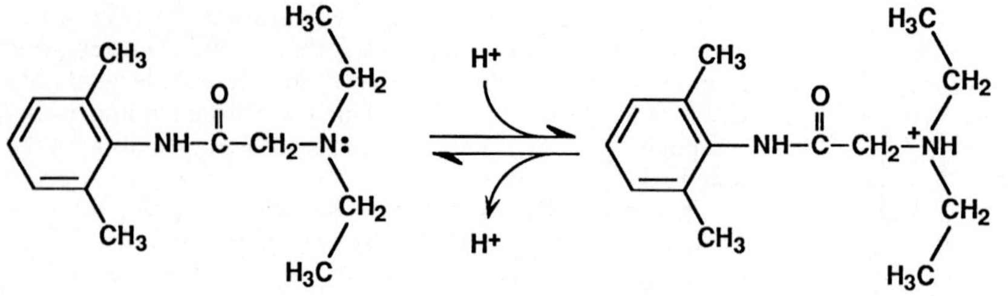

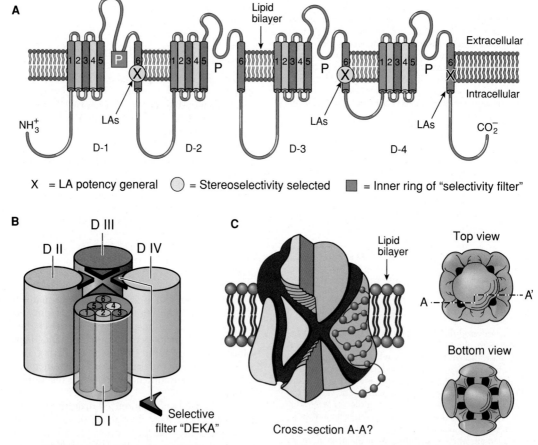

FIGURE 2-9. The ionization (protonation and deprotonation) of lidocaine.

Perpetually uncharged local anesthetics also effectively block impulses and Na^+ channels (30–32), demonstrating that ionization is not essential for pharmacologic activity. The ability of tertiary amine local anesthetics to block Na^+ channels in single cells is faster and greater when the drug is applied externally at alkaline external pH (33–35), or when it is applied by direct internal perfusion at neutral or slightly acidic internal pH (36). Both of these observations are consistent with a model in which the neutral form of the anesthetic dissolves in and passes through the axon membrane and, having reached a cytoplasmic region, becomes protonated.

Changes in the binding and dissociation of local anesthetics by direct mutation of certain amino acids of the large, α-subunit of the channel demonstrate that the drug binds in the inner "pore" of the Na channel (37–40) (Fig. 2-10). One intriguing finding is that dissociation of anesthetic molecules from the closed channel is clearly sensitive to the pH outside the nerve, but relatively insensitive to the intracellular pH (34). Thus, when it is bound in the Na^+ channel, a local anesthetic molecule can interact with extracellular protons. Since the changes in channel structure that underlie its gating also contribute to changes in local anesthetic affinity (see the earlier

FIGURE 2-10. A: Primary sequence of the α-subunit of the Na^+ channel. The locations of amino acid residues that are important for local anesthetic binding are shown by the Xs, circles, and squares. **B:** Arrangement of the domains I to IV of the Na^+ channel to form the central, ion-conducting pore, whose outer region contains the ion selectivity filter. **C:** A three-dimensional rendering of the Na^+ channel showing a possible ion conducting pore and the position of a local anesthetic in the pore-blocking mode.

section, Mechanisms of Anesthetic Action), other factors that influence gating can modify drug blockade. Among these are the concentration of calcium (Ca^{2+}) ions outside the cell (19) and the identity of the smaller β-subunits that are associated with the large α-subunit (41).

Hydrophobicity and Potency

Drug hydrophobicity is also a determinant of potency. The more hydrophobic drugs are more potent blockers of action potentials (42,43) and of Na currents (44–46). This increased potency results from a faster apparent association rate, as well as from a slower dissociation rate, for the binding of the local anesthetics to their channel sites (21,44). In other words, the more hydrophobic local anesthetics can reach the site more easily and appear to leave the site more slowly than the less hydrophobic drugs. Molecular mass of the anesthetics, however, also affects the dissociation of the charged local anesthetics, but not of the neutral ones (45). These results support the concept of two pathways to and from the anesthetic site (19). One pathway may be through the channel's pore (the hydrophilic route, more favorable to charged molecules) and the other may be through the membrane (the hydrophobic route, accessible primarily to uncharged drug molecules). Whether these separate routes eventually lead to a single or several sites of action is unclear at this time.

From this discussion, it appears that pH affects anesthetic potency on isolated neurons by two opposing actions. An alkaline extracellular pH favors the neutral, membrane-permeant form of the drug, facilitating the rise of drug concentration in the membrane and thus inside the cell, whereas an acidic extracellular pH favors the more potent protonated blocking species when drug is present at the site of action. Both neutral and charged forms of anesthetics participate in impulse blockade. Of course, during most clinical procedures, the functional potency of local anesthetics is determined largely by the fraction of injected drug that actually passes into the nerve bundle, and conditions that favor the penetrating, neutral species are desirable (6,47). Other local anesthetics probably have about the same unfavorable distribution properties.

Molecular Mechanisms of Sodium Channel Blockade

Exactly how do local anesthetics interfere with the operation of Na^+ channels? Such questions are addressed by a combination of physiologic and structural studies. Much of this study is anchored on the observation that anesthetics inhibit open and inactivated channels more potently than resting closed channels, and that intentional mutation of specific amino acid residues believed to line the inner region of the pore (37,39) (along the transmembrane helices labelled S6 in Fig. 2-10), leads to changes in the affinities of local anesthetics for different states of the channel (48–50).

Does a local anesthetic molecule inhibit the channel by "plugging" the pore and preventing ions from passing, or by interfering with the conformational changes that underlie channel opening? Both possibilities may occur during the blockade of impulses by tertiary amine drugs, because the channel regions that bind the drug are coupled to those regions that sense the changes in membrane potential and that initially move in order to activate the channel. Other substances that pass through the channel as well as binding within it, such as hydrogen (H^+) and certain cations, also change the gating, providing precedents for the coupled interaction between the pore-forming and the gating domains. Some local anesthetics interfere with the conformational restriction of gating regions (i.e., the molecular equivalent of inactivation), inducing an "inactivation-like"

state by a drug-dependent mechanism rather than stabilizing the normal conformational changes that occur during inactivation.

Susceptibility of Sodium Channels to Local Anesthetics

A differential susceptibility to a local anesthetic of certain Na^+ channel subtypes, for example, those that are selectively expressed in nociceptors more than in motor neurons, would enable a selective analgesia without paralysis, one of the yet-to-be-attained goals for regional anesthesia. Is there experimental evidence to support such channel selectivity?

Voltage-gated Na^+ channels are composed of one large α-subunit and one or two β-subunits. The α-subunit, of which nine have been functionally identified, conducts all the essential activity on Na^+ channels; it contains the "voltage sensor" that moves in response to depolarization, the "ion selectivity filter" that permits the selective permeation of Na^+, and the "gating" structures that respond to voltage sensor movement by opening or closing the channel (Fig. 2-10). β-subunits, four identified so far, are covalently or noncovalently attached to the α-subunits, have immunoglobin-like structures, and chaperone the larger subunits to the membrane, anchoring them to cytoskeletal and extracellular structures. β-subunits also modify the gating of Na^+ channels, which is an important determinant of local anesthetic binding. The various α-subunits are differentially distributed among different tissues and cell types. For example, the $Na_v1.8$ α-subunit occurs only in certain nociceptor neurons, and $Na_v1.5$ is the major channel protein in cardiac muscle (see Chapter 33).

Selective expression is sometimes changed after tissue injury or inflammation (51,52). For example, $Na_v1.8$ in small diameter dorsal root ganglia (DRG) neurons increases after inflammation but decreases after nerve injury. Expression of the $Na_v1.3$ α-subunit is very low in intact adult DRG but is elevated after nerve injury or inflammation (53) and contributes importantly to late Na^+ currents in nociceptors (54,55). β-subunits are also changed by nerve injury, with protein levels of $\beta2$ increasing in both injured and neighboring, noninjured sensory neurons (56). Since β-subunits alter both the density of functional Na^+ channels as well as their gating properties, they would be expected to contribute to local anesthetic action. Indeed, evidence exists of differential effects on local anesthetic blockade by different β-subunits (41,57,58), some of which may arise from altered gating of the α-subunit, whereas others might depend on direct interactions of part of the β-subunit with the local anesthetic binding site (59).

The differential distribution of Na^+ channel subtypes provides the possibility that subtype-selective drugs may modify the target tissue function with fewer side effects on other tissues. In this context, a selective action on pain might be expected from a drug that targets those Na^+ channels whose expression is confined to small-diameter sensory afferents (e.g., $Na_v1.8$ or $Na_v1.9$) (44,60,61). Indeed, the limited clinical use of available Na^+ channel blocking drugs is due to their lack of specificity for neuronal Na^+ channel subtypes (e.g., in comparison to cardiac Na^+ channel subtypes). The overall potency of local anesthetics for the Na^+ channels is relatively low (19,21,22), and the accompanying stereoselectivity for chiral drugs is weak, rarely exceeding 5 (62–64).

Comparison of the amino acid residues believed to bind the Na^+ channels in their different states shows little difference among the known channels, consistent with the similar blocking affinities. Although the amino acid sequence of the α-subunit in homologous domains is quite similar among the different subtypes, particularly for the S6 transmembrane segments that form the cytoplasmic opening of the channel (Fig. 2-10), there may be subtle differences in their spatial orientation in different conformational states of the channel. Furthermore, the contribution of specific residues to local anesthetic binding affinity among the different channel states depends on the local anesthetic molecule, even varying between stereoisomers, for example, *R*- and *S*-bupivacaine (64), such that channel structures that can influence S6 positions (e.g., those on S5), or even cytoplasmic or extracellular connecting peptides, may be able to allosterically alter local anesthetic affinities. Changes in the structure of the selectivity filter, closer to the extracellular pore opening, also modify local anesthetic binding affinity and access to the site, implying that ion flow through the channel also regulates local anesthetic binding (16,65,66).

Importantly, since state-dependent affinities are a strong feature of local anesthetic inhibition, channels that have different gating behaviors may be blocked differently under the same conditions. For example, the mammalian cardiac Na^+ currents, carried by channel $Na_v1.5$, were reported to be more susceptible to lidocaine than are the currents in skeletal muscle (carried by $Na_v1.4$), based on voltage-clamp measurements using the same patterns of membrane potential. Further examination, however, showed that the cardiac channels were more inactivated at the same resting potential, and the apparently higher affinity was actually due to the preferred binding to inactivated channels (67).

When comparing the effect of local anesthetics among different Na^+ channel subtypes in sensory neurons, previous reports suggest that local anesthetics are more potent on tetrodotoxin (TTX)-sensitive Na^+ current (e.g., carried by $Na_v1.7$) than on TTX-resistant current (carried by $Na_v1.8$, $Na_v1.9$) (68). However, the TTX-sensitive Na^+ channels tend to be more inactivated at resting potentials than are the TTX-resistant Na^+ channels (69,70). Thus, the difference in local anesthetic sensitivity between TTX-sensitive and TTX-resistant Na^+ channels might again be defined primarily by gating differences and should be interpreted with caution.

Ropivacaine's actions may present an exception to this concern. This local anesthetic is reported to provide clinically relevant differential block, producing analgesia with less intense motor block (71). Unlike other local anesthetics, ropivacaine is more potent in blocking TTX-resistant Na^+ currents, such as occur in nociceptors, than TTX-sensitive Na^+ channel in DRGs, when the resting membrane potential is set at −80 mV, close to the physiologic condition and at which some of the channels will be in the inactivated state (72). Thus, factors other than gating must account for ropivacaine's preferential inhibition of the TTX-resistant subtype of channel that occurs in nociceptors.

Direct pharmacologic assays for local anesthetics on Na^+ channels determine the potency at the primary target site. However, because the intensity of pain is encoded by the frequency of action potentials in a train of impulses, it is important to note that the local anesthetic concentration for half-maximal blockade of ion currents does not predict the relevant concentration required for a functional blockade of neuronal signal transmission (61). Sensitivity to local anesthetic was higher for reducing the firing frequency than for reducing the peak amplitude of a single TTX-resistant action potential. Thus, an effective dose for pain management might be much lower than the dose for blockade of ion currents. For differential functional blockade, it is essential to realize that the opening and

inactivation kinetics of the same subtype of Na^+ channel may vary substantially among different cell types that have differently shaped action potentials. For example, local anesthetics might selectively block impulses in one type of cell, which has long-lasting action potentials that allow time for the blockade of prolonged open and inactivated states, while sparing those in another cell type that has very brief action potentials. Since excitability properties such as the duration of action potentials, postimpulse de- or hyperpolarization, and even the resting potential are highly sensitive to K^+ channels, which also vary widely in their tissue distribution (73,74), a selective blockade of impulses in one cell type could result from its K^+ channel expression profile, independently of any differences in Na^+ channel expression.

Finally, Na^+ channel gating is modified by enzymes, including protein kinases (75,76), that are activated or suppressed by pathways ordained by G protein-coupled receptors (GPCRs), and/or are influenced by changes in intracellular $[Ca^{+2}]$ influenced strongly by flux through Ca channels. Because local anesthetics also act to inhibit both GPCRs and Ca^{+2} channels (73,77–81), they may thus have an indirect as well as a direct effect on voltage-gated Na^+ channels and cellular excitability.

CLINICAL APPLICATIONS FOR PERIPHERAL AND REGIONAL NERVE BLOCKS

Peripheral Nerve Anatomy and Function

Both anatomical and chemical factors determine the susceptibility of nerve fibers to block by local anesthetics. The particular nerve being blocked and the nature of the agent used and its formulation are important for the rate of onset, maximum degree and duration of nerve block, and differential blockade of different functions by local anesthetics.

Fiber Size and Function

The diameter and myelination of a nerve fiber are correlated with its impulse physiology as well as its message-carrying function (82,83). Nerve fibers are categorized into three major anatomic classes (Table 2-1): myelinated somatic nerves (A-fibers), myelinated preganglionic autonomic nerves (B-fibers), and nonmyelinated axons (C-fibers). The B- and C-fibers are small, ranging in diameter from about 2 μm to less than 1 μm, respectively, whereas the A-fibers vary in diameter from about 4 to 20 μm.

The A-fibers are divided further into four groups according to decreasing impulse conduction velocity and diameter. Largest are the α-fibers, efferent neurons that directly innervate skeletal muscle. Aβ-fibers are afferent, sensory neurons coming from muscle, joints, and skin and transmitting sensations of touch and pressure (as well as unconsciously registered information about body position and force), Aγ-fibers are still smaller efferents that control muscle spindle tone, whereas the thinnest A-fibers—the afferent Aδ group—subserve pain and cold temperature sensations.

The thinly myelinated B-fibers are preganglionic axons of the autonomic system that ultimately control vascular smooth muscle, among others; B-fibers thus assume cardinal importance during spinal or peridural anesthesia. The nonmyelinated C-fibers, like the myelinated Aδ-delta fibers, subserve pain and

TABLE 2-1

CLASSIFICATION AND PHYSIOLOGIC CHARACTERISTICS OF PERIPHERAL NERVE FIBERS

Class	Aα	Aβ	Aγ	Aδ	B	C
Function	Motor	Touch/Pressure	Proprioception/ Motor Tone	Pain/Temperature	Preganglionic autonomic	Pain/temperature
Myelin*	+++	+++	++	++	+	–
Diameter (μm)	12–20	5–12	1–4	1–4	1–3	0.5–1
Conduction speed (m/sec)	70–120	30–70	10–30	12–30	10–15	0.5–1.2
Local anesthetic Sensitivity**	++	++	+++	+++	++	+[†]

* +++, heavily myelinated; ++, moderately myelinated; +, lightly myelinated; –, nonmyelinated;
** +++, most susceptible to impulse blockade; and [†] least susceptible.

temperature transmission, as well as postganglionic autonomic functions. C-fibers are thinner than myelinated fibers (less than 1 μm in diameter) and have a much lower conduction velocity than even Aδ-fibers, less than 1 m/sec.

It is evident from this summary that humans are equipped with two separate conducting systems that convey pain-related messages. One system (fast pain) conducts signals rapidly and is composed of myelinated Aδ-fibers; the other system (slow pain) is composed of slowly conducting, nonmyelinated C-fibers.

Both sensory perception and normal motor activity depend on the integrated actions of afferent and efferent impulses. Sensation is the result of patterns of impulses coding for several different modalities in different primary afferent fiber types, and sensation is tonically modulated by activity in efferent sympathetic nerve fibers (84). Similarly, coordinated gross and deft motor activity depends on efferent impulses in the axons of α motoneurons that are being *tuned* constantly by proprioceptive and muscle spindle afferent input (via Aβ-fibers) to the spinal cord. Recognizing this inherent requirement for integrated afferent and efferent activity in the conduct of normal behavior leads to a realization of the complex pharmacology of peripheral nerve block that underlies clinical anesthesia. Therefore, equating small-fiber inhibition with "sensory" (nociceptive) block and large-fiber inhibition with "motor" block is nonsensical (85).

Impulse Inhibition and Functional Impairment

Clinical local and regional anesthesia is almost always assessed through some behavioral function. Anesthesia of motor function is determined from the patient's ability to perform a requested movement (such as leg lifting) to generate a force (by hand squeeze or resistance to arm movement). Sensory anesthesia is typically assayed by verbal report of perception to weak noxious stimuli (pin prick), light stroking of skin, or rapid cooling (caused by evaporation of alcohol). Quantitative sensory testing is used only rarely to provide a more consistent, objective measure of sensory loss.

Although the neurologic functions of peripheral nerve are dependent on impulse conduction in the nerve's axon, functional loss is not necessarily proportional to impulse blockade. A modest failure of impulses, occurring as a reduction in the number of active fibers or, more likely, as a partial suppression of impulses in many different fibers (e.g., as from frequency-dependent blockade, discussed earlier), may cause no detectable functional deficits, since compensatory mechanisms exist throughout the PNS and CNS to counter such losses as may occur naturally through aging or disease. At the other extreme, total functional loss may occur when some fibers are still conducting impulses, albeit too weakly to support perception of a stimulus or to enable intentional motor activity. Total blockade of impulses, obviously, results in a complete absence of function.

To appreciate how the administration of local anesthetics clinically leads to the observed functional losses, one must know the type as well as the extent of impulse blockade that occurs during a functional block. Since we cannot record peripheral nerve impulses in patients, experimental animals have been used, both to simulate the functional losses in humans during neural blockade and for the invasive measures of impulse activity and measurement of the neuronal content of local anesthetic. The findings from such studies provide an integrated picture of the physiologic changes that underlie neural blockade.

Minimum Blocking Concentration

The minimum blocking concentration (C_m) is the lowest *concentration* of local anesthetic in vivo that blocks all impulse activity in a given nerve within a reasonable period of time (commonly 10–15 minutes). For blockade of mixed somatic nerve function an *administered concentration* of 1% (40 mM) lidocaine in vivo appears to be necessary to achieve the measured C_m of approximately 0.5 to 1.0 mM lidocaine at all the axons (86–89). The concept is important clinically, for only drug concentrations greater than C_m will reliably anesthetize a nerve. Because the pharmacologic potency among different local anesthetics varies greatly (see preceding section), each agent has its own C_m. Drug behavior also depends on the environment, so C_m must be further defined by the prevailing solution conditions, such as pH and temperature (47,88,90).

Because impulse blockade results from the binding of local anesthetic molecules to Na^+ channels in the nerve membrane, the membrane content of drug is most closely related to the primary pharmacologic event. For lidocaine, antinociceptive effects are present when this drug is present at 3 to 5 mM per gram of nerve (91,92). This neural content can be achieved by different dosing procedures, but studies of the dependence of effective functional blockade on the mass of drug injected

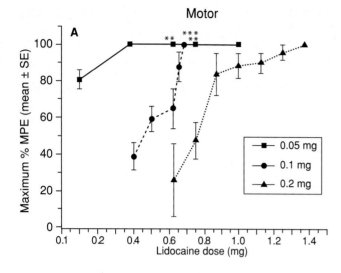

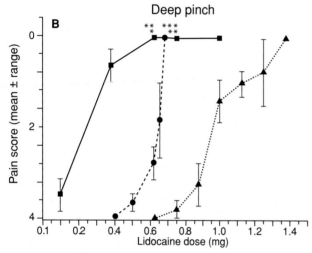

FIGURE 2-11. Dose-response curves for rat sciatic nerve blockade of (**A**) motor function (extensor postural thrust) and (**B**) nocifensive responses to pinch of the lateral-most toes. As the volume of injectate is increased, the dose to achieve equivalent block increases proportionately, showing that lidocaine concentration, rather than total dose, is the important determinant of effectiveness of block. From Rosenberg PH, Heavner JE. Temperature-dependent nerve-blocking action of lidocaine and halothane. *Acta Anaesth Scand* 1980;24:314–332, with permission.

at different volumes show that it is the *concentration* of local anesthetic in the injectate that most determines potency for analgesia (Fig. 2-11). Increasing total drug mass by using larger volumes of the same concentrations does not increase the functional potency, although it does lengthen the duration of blockade (87).

The C_m of an axon may be greater for the peripheral nerve than for the spinal root (93), suggesting that impulse blockade for projections near the neuraxis, such as spiral roots, as occurs in intrathecal and epidural anesthesia, may exceed blockade for peripheral nerve. The local anesthetic pool in vivo, however, is subject to numerous influences that act to reduce the final anesthetic concentration reaching the nerve membrane, so that the same local anesthetic concentration given for peripheral nerve block may result in a different dug concentration over time at

the nerve than one given in the epidural space or intrathecally. Dilution by interstitial fluid, fibrous tissue barriers to diffusion, absorption by fat, and uptake into the vasculature, as well as the local biotransformation, of ester-linked molecules, are all factors that determine the clinical potency. The final concentration of drug eventually arriving at the axon depends on the relative magnitude of these factors and on the length of nerve exposed to drug solution. For example, much less local anesthetic need be applied for subarachnoid than for peridural block, not because the C_m changes when an axon traverses the vertebral canal, but because spinal roots are weakly protected in the subarachnoid space (94). Pharmacokinetic factors clearly are major determinants of the clinical potency of local anesthetics because only a small fraction of the applied dose actually reaches the nerve tissue. In this regard, it is instructive to compare the effective concentrations of lidocaine required for inhibition of Na^+ currents and action potentials with the delivered doses. Lidocaine's half-maximal inhibitory concentration (IC_{50}) for tonic inhibition of Na^+ currents is about 0.2 mM, but for inhibition of the action potential amplitude it is about 0.8 to 1.0 mM. (These numbers are in the ratio predicted by the 80% channel blockade needed for impulse failure.) By comparison, the molar concentration of 1% lidocaine, often used for clinical peripheral nerve blocks, is about 40 mM, about 50 times that needed for impulse blockade of a deshcathed nerve. From laboratory experiments, we know that 0.1 mL of 1% lidocaine injected around the sciatic nerve gives complete motor block and analgesia, but that 0.75% (30 mM) of the same volume (0.1 mL) yields an incomplete functional block of much briefer duration (87,95,96). Why is so much more drug needed for impulse blockade in vivo than in isolated nerve? It is because the perineurial sheath is such an effective barrier against the diffusion of local anesthetics that, under clinical conditions, only about 5% of the lidocaine dose injected actually penetrates into the nerve (91).

Differential Nerve Block

During a peripheral nerve block, it is sometimes observed that pain can be obtunded completely while motor function and touch are less affected (82,97). This situation is one example of functional "differential block." Depending on the perioperative circumstances, differential blockade may or may not be desirable. The presence of motor activity might be disconcerting to a surgeon accustomed to equating anesthesia with flaccid muscles, but total paralysis is not always necessary. On the other hand, as touch and light pressure sensations are conveyed by large fibers, an anxious patient might misinterpret the mechanical perception of pressure from an incision and tissue manipulation as pain.

Differential blockade, observed clinically, has its basis in several possible sources (98). First, it may be a temporal rather than equilibrium phenomenon, with impulses in small fibers being blocked *faster* than those of large ones because of the time course of drug diffusion into the nerve. Differential block can also result from the different *length-dependence* for the susceptibility of impulse blockade, where smaller diameter axons, with shorter length constants, can be blocked by anesthetic spread over lengths of nerve that might not block impulse propagation in larger fibers (12,13,91). Second, some fibers may be slightly more subject to impulse blockade by anesthetics than others because of anatomic features, such as the presence of myelin, which can effectively pool anesthetic molecules near the axon membrane during the dynamics of nerve block. Third, axons per se may be differentially sensitive to block because, for example, some have voltage-gated K^+ channels and some

A
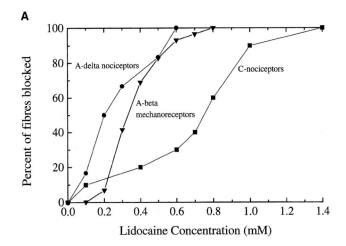

B
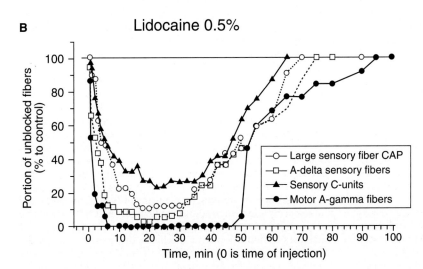

FIGURE 2-12. A: Impulse blockade by lidocaine of individual axons of rat sciatic nerve in vivo. The percentage of fibers conducting at different concentrations of lidocaine for C-fibers (CV <2.0 m/sec, $n = 8$), Aδ-fibers (CV 2.1–30 m/sec, $n = 15$), and Aβ-fibers (CV >30 m/sec, $n = 18$) shows that fibers in all categories are blocked over a range of concentrations from 0.2 to 0.8 mM but that nociceptive C-fibers are significantly less susceptible. From Palade PT, Almers W. Slow calcium and potassium currents in frog skeletal muscle: their relationship and pharmacological properties. *Pflugers Arch* 1985;405:91–101, with permission. **B:** Impulse blockade in the nonequilibrium response to percutaneous bolus injection of 0.5% lidocaine around the rat sciatic nerve. Recordings from spinal roots in these anesthetized rats shows a differential rate and maximum degree of block that is consistent with the results of equilibrium blockade. From Fink BR, Cairns AM. Differential slowing and block of conduction by lidocaine in individual afferent myelinated and unmyelinated axons. *Anesthesiology* 1984;60:111–120, with permission.

do not (99,100), or the Na$^+$ channel types differ (but see earlier discussion) (70), or the membrane lipids differ (101) and thus also the membrane concentration of anesthetics.

However, using these categories to explain differential block presumes speculations about a complex behavior observed clinically. The situation is not much clarified by experimental studies. The relationship between C_m and fiber diameter is far more complex than usually appreciated. Despite widespread belief and persistent mythology, C_m does not increase simply as a function of larger fiber diameter, the so-called "size principle (98)." In many earlier studies of local anesthetics on conduction, the effect was measured as a drop in height of the compound action potential, a signal that results from the summed actions of the hundreds or thousands of axons in a nerve. The amplitude falls because of an overall effect of abolition of impulses in some fibers and slowed but still conducted impulses in others, effectively dispersing the individual action potentials over time. The consequences are unknown for the perception of such differential slowing of conduction, resulting in a reduction of temporal integration in synaptic transmission of afferent information in the spinal cord (86), but are likely to be more difficult to interpret than the numbness that attends the total absence of impulses during a complete physiologic block.

When the ability of individual axons to propagate single action potentials is directly titrated by local anesthetics, the results are clear and consistent. A good example is seen in Figure 2-12A, where the in vivo susceptibility of the smaller Aδ-fibers to equilibrium block during exposure to a constant concentration of lidocaine in rat sciatic nerve is slightly greater than that of the larger Aβ-fibers (102). The susceptibility of impulses in C fibers is significantly less either of the other fiber types. This order of block has been observed by many investigators, in vitro as well as in vivo (103–105).

However, clinical nerve block never achieves the equilibrium drug–nerve interactions that apply for these artificial situations. So, how do the different fiber types respond to local anesthetics during clinical procedures? In rats, percutaneous sciatic nerve blocks using lidocaine produce transient anesthesia (105) with the same order of fiber block as that seen for equilibrium block (Fig. 2-12B), albeit requiring much higher concentrations, as would be expected from the inefficient delivery (see earlier discussion). Aγ efferents are blocked first, resulting in a relaxation of muscle spindles that accounts for the initial phase of flaccid paralysis. The next fibers blocked are the Aδ sensory afferents, and the individual C-fibers are blocked last, even before the impulses in the largest myelinated fibers (Fig. 2-12B). By this accounting, fast pain, transmitted by Aδ-fibers, would disappear earlier and to a greater degree than would the slow pain transmitted by C-fibers. The blocks of these fiber types recover in the reverse order, consistent with a greater individual sensitivity to failure than with any selective diffusion barrier to drug.

A preferred block of Aδ-fibers might mislead an anesthesiologist about the extent of total blockade. If the classic pin-prick method is used to demarcate an "anesthetized" region of the body, but actually only tests sensations conducted by Aδ-fibers (e.g., fast pain), then some C-fibers could still be conducting, and the residual afferent input, although not adequate to realize sensation (106), might still be able to sensitize the CNS and thereby elevate postoperative pain.

Pharmacokinetics of Nerve Block

Delivery Phase

Because local anesthetic solution is usually injected into the space surrounding a nerve, the drug molecules must diffuse through layers of fibrous and other tissue barriers before they ultimately reach individual axons (Fig. 2-4). The density of non-neural tissue components in a peripheral nerve varies. For example, the proximal region of sciatic nerve contains more fibrous tissue, and the sheath is thicker than at its more distal branches. The situation at the brachial plexus versus the radial nerve is another example of this tapering. This pattern changes at the spinal rootlets, however, where nerve fibers are separated from the cerebral spinal fluid of the subarachnoid space by only a thin perineurium (9); drug diffusion and penetration into these nerves after intrathecal injection is accordingly rapid (94), so that just a small dose of local anesthetic produces blockade quickly and fully.

The first step in moving the anesthetic to its neural target site is mass movement (spread) of the injected solution. A large injected volume spreads farther and exposes more nerves to the anesthetic (but, of course, also increases the vascular absorption surface) than does a smaller volume. Mass movement is particularly important in subarachnoid (spinal) anesthesia (107), with the drug spreading upward and downward in the spinal fluid according to the specific gravity of the fluid that contains the local anesthetic and the patient's posture.

Diffusion, the movement of drug molecules out from the volume filled by injection, is governed by concentration gradients and the viscosity of the surrounding liquid. Molecules move from an area of high concentration to one of low concentration, the rate of diffusion increasing with slope of the concentration gradient. Diffusion through solution also depends on the drug's molecular mass, varying with the square root of molecular weight. All local anesthetics are of similar mass, however (e.g., m.w. procaine = 236; m.w. bupivacaine = 288), and thus diffuse in solution at about the same rate. Since diffusion is a relatively slow process, the local anesthetic solution is continually being diluted with tissue fluid, even as it enters the nerve. At the same time, drug is continuously absorbed by vascular and lymphatic channels. In addition, a substantial portion of the supply of available anesthetic is bound to tissue elements encountered along the diffusion path. Since this uptake into membranes and perineural fat depends primarily on hydrophobic absorption (43), the more lipophilic the agent, the more it is bound and the slower is its effective diffusion. Since more potent drugs are generally more hydrophobic (e.g., etidocaine versus lidocaine) and are used at lower concentrations, block from these agents is generally slower to develop.

The most important factor in onset, however, is penetration through the perineurial sheath.

Permeation of the Nerve Sheath

The encasing perineurial sheath presents the major diffusion barrier to local anesthetics reaching the nerve axons (Fig. 2-4) (6,108). In the spinal cord, this structure correlates with the arachnoid membrane. The major route of passage through this network of squamous cells connected by tight junctions (8) is via the cells' plasma membranes. Because the lipid bilayer character of plasma membranes is common to almost all mammalian cells, drug penetration through the sheath is similar to penetration of nerve membranes.

Protonated anesthetic molecules have about 1/1,000 the membrane permeability of the neutral anesthetic species, not because the charged molecules do not bind to the outer surface of the membrane, but because the bound molecules penetrate very slowly across to the inner surface. The electrostatic forces that prevent this transport are largely absent in the unprotonated drug forms, and neutral anesthetic molecules pass across the membrane much more easily (19,32,36).

Pharmaceutic formulations of local anesthetics are always at acid pH. Not only are the anesthetic molecules more chemically stable at low pH, the antioxidants often added to protect the included epinephrine are often themselves weak acids. Since the neutral species of local anesthetics provide a block with faster onset, it seems logical to raise the pH of local anesthetic solutions before injection. This is usually accomplished through the addition of sterile sodium bicarbonate just before injecting. Laboratory studies, however, show that bicarbonate addition, although it speeds the onset, also shortens the duration of the block by plain lidocaine, an effect that does not occur in lidocaine solutions containing epinephrine (47). Alkalinizing plain lidocaine by addition of sodium hydroxide (NaOH) to the same pH as reached with bicarbonate both shortens the onset and increases the duration over the block by acidic lidocaine, delivering advantage at both ends of the block procedure. There are two provisos to alkalinizing procedures: (a) The volume of solution used to raise the pH should not be so large as to reduce its effective potency (e.g., diluting 1% lidocaine to 0.5%), and (b) the pH should not be increased so much that the base form of the local anesthetic, which is considerably less soluble than the protonated form, precipitates from solution (109). Within these confines, valid clinical reasons exist to raise the pH: Onset is briefer, and drug requirements are less.

Hydrophobic adsorption accounts for much of the membrane binding of local anesthetics. But the membrane *permeability* of local anesthetic bases (the neutral, more permeant species) is not directly proportional to their measured hydrophobicity (octanol-to-buffer distribution coefficients) (110). Some hydrophobic quality is necessary for the drug to adsorb to the membrane, but excessive hydrophobicity actually sticks the molecules too tightly at one membrane surface and markedly slows their transport to the other side. For example, lidocaine has only one-tenth the hydrophobicity of bupivacaine (by octanol-to-buffer partition coefficients) (27), but is 2.5 times as permeant through the peridural sheath (108).

Pharmacokinetic considerations for block should focus on those conditions that achieve an adequate neural content of local anesthetic for clinical block, while achieving the lowest plasma, potentially cardiotoxic, concentration. When the amount of lidocaine in a peripheral nerve in vivo is measured at times that correspond to observed behavioral end-points, three noteworthy facts emerge (Fig. 2-13) (87,91,92). First,

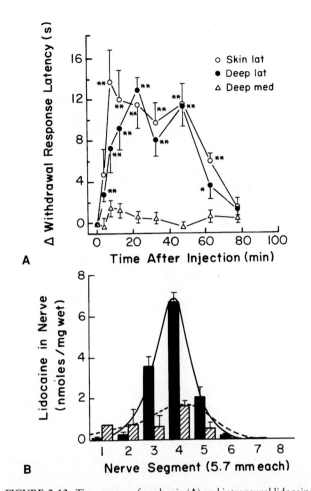

A

B

FIGURE 2-13. Time course of analgesia (**A**) and intraneural lidocaine distribution (**B**) corresponding to blockade of rat sciatic nerve by 0.1 mL of 1% radiolabeled lidocaine injected near the pelvic notch. **A:** Time course of changes in withdrawal response latency (WRL) to pinch of a skin fold on the lateral foot ("skin lat") and deep pinch at the first ("deep med") and fifth toe ("deep lat") during nerve block. Plotted values represent mean values ± standard errors; * $p < 0.05$, ** $p < 0.01$, relative to baseline (pre-drug) values ($n = 12$). From Wong K, Strichartz GR, Raymond SA. On the mechanism of potentiation of local anesthetics by bicarbonate buffer: Drug structure-activity studied on isolated peripheral nerve. *Anesth Anal* 1993;76(1):131–143, with permission. **B:** Distribution of lidocaine along the sciatic nerve removed from rats at two different behavioral end-points: during profound block (15–20 min after injections; *solid bars*) and when movement response to deep pain (toe pinch) had returned (45–55 min; *striped bars*). At full block, the total of all lidocaine in the nerve, exclusive of the sheath, is less than 5% of the injected dose. From Popitz-Bergez FA, Lee-Son S, Strichartz GR, et al. Relation between functional deficit and intraneural local anesthetic during peripheral nerve block: A study in the rat sciatic nerve. *Anesthesiology* 1995;83:583–592, with permission.

the total amount of lidocaine in the nerve is less than 5% of the total dose of anesthetic injected (0.1 mL, 1% lidocaine, pH 6.5). Second, the peak neural concentration (~8 nmol/mg wet nerve) equals only one fifth of the value that would be reached if the nerve had been *equilibrated* with 1% lidocaine. Third, the longitudinal spread of drug along the nerve changes little during the course of the block. These results show how effective a barrier the sheath is, and yet, most movement of drug from its deposition locus is across the sheath and not along the length of the nerve. Interestingly, the amount of lidocaine in the most concentrated segment of the nerve at a time when

"deep pain" sensation returns (45–50 min) corresponds to the amount that would be present at equilibrium in a desheathed nerve bathed by lidocaine just at the marginal blocking concentration (~0.4 mM; Fig. 2-12A). Injection of less lidocaine. (e.g., 0.1 mL, 0.75%) gives an incomplete functional block; injection of more lidocaine prolongs the block.

Although proximity to the nerve is important, blockade can be further enhanced by limiting local vascular drug absorption, usually by incorporating a vasoconstrictor into the local anesthetic solution. The vasoconstrictor (e.g., epinephrine) temporarily lowers the local circulation, so that the rate of vascular absorption of anesthetic is reduced (111). We might suspect that these vasoconstrictive actions endure for the duration of an extended nerve block, slowing the blood flow and associated drug resorption throughout this period. But laboratory studies show that an initial period of vasoconstriction, during the onset of block, allows more drug to enter the nerve, rather than being removed by the local circulation, and it is the longer time required to clear this additional neural content that accounts for the increased block duration (Fig. 2-14) (92,108,112). This "initial loading" mechanism also explains why drug injected into highly perfused tissue (e.g., peridural space), from where it is absorbed much faster than drug injected into a marginally perfused region such as the lumbar subarachnoid space, gives a much briefer block (45).

Highly hydrophobic, fat-soluble local anesthetics, such as etidocaine and bupivacaine, are extensively bound to local tissue depots as well as to plasma proteins. The distribution of such anesthetics between the targeted nerve and vascular uptake appears to be relatively less affected by the addition of epinephrine than is lidocaine, for example. Therefore, epinephrine is less of an influence on the duration of action of more hydrophobic local anesthetics.

Induction Phase

After the local anesthetic has been deposited near a nerve trunk, it diffuses from the nerve's outer surface toward the center (112,114). Accordingly, axons that reside in the outer layers of the nerve (mantle fibers) are anesthetized well before axons that course through the nerve's inner layers (core fibers) (115). Topographically, the fibers in a nerve trunk are arrayed in concentric layers. Fibers that innervate a limb's distal parts assume a central position in the nerve's core, whereas those that innervate the limb's proximal parts lie in the nerve's mantle.

As the local anesthetic diffuses through a nerve trunk from mantle to core, functional anesthesia tends to spread along the limb in a proximal to distal direction (Fig. 2-15). This can easily be observed during axillary block: The subject first notes that the upper arm becomes numb, with anesthesia and analgesia spreading from there down the arm to reach the fingers last. Furthermore, motor block, corresponding to blockade of motor axons residing in the mantle, precedes sensory blockade arising from core fibers that innervate the distal receptive field (112,115).

The rapidity of onset of nerve block is approximately proportional to the logarithm of the concentration of the drug. Thus, doubling the drug concentration will only modestly hasten the onset of block, although, of course, the more concentrated solution also will block the nerve fibers more effectively. Thus, concentrated anesthetic solutions increase the maximum extent of nerve penetration, have a lesser effect on the speed of onset of block, and certainly increase the duration of block. It must be remembered, however, that increasing the concentration also increases the total dose of the drug being given and, therefore, the risk of both systemic and local neural toxicity.

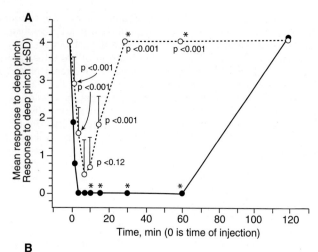

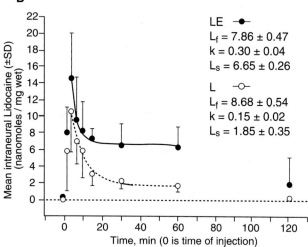

FIGURE 2-14. Effects of vasoconstriction by epinephrine on (A) the time-course of analgesia, as suppression of the nocifensive response to deep pinch of the toe, and (B) the time course of lidocaine content in the nerve, after rat sciatic nerve block by 0.5% lidocaine with (*solid lines, filled circles*) or without epinephrine (*broken lines, open circles*). From Sinnott CJ, Cogswell III LP, Johnson A, et al. On the mechanism by which epinephrine potentiates lidocaine's peripheral nerve block. *Anesthesiology* 2003;98:181–188, with permission.

Recovery from Nerve Block

Diffusion of anesthetic molecules out from the nerve and absorption into the vascular bed mainly account for termination of blockade. It has been found empirically that the duration of the block is proportional to the logarithm of the anesthetic concentration. Thus, repeated doubling of the anesthetic concentration will have progressively less effect on duration. This is probably because, with repeated injections, steady-state distributions of drug are achieved from which the duration of block is completely dependent on the saturation of local tissue depots. More important is the lipophilic solubility of the individual local anesthetic agents; for example, agents with high lipid solubility, such as bupivacaine and etidocaine, are highly concentrated in local tissue, such as cells around the nerve trunk as well as myelin sheaths around individual axons, and dislodge slowly from neural tissue. Blockade therefore persists for a long time.

Dissociation times of local anesthetics from Na^+ channels are on the order of seconds (91) and do not contribute to the

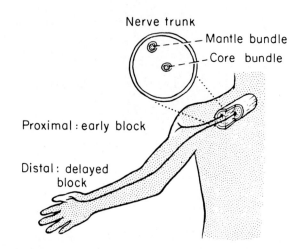

FIGURE 2-15. Somatotopic distribution in peripheral nerve. Axons in large nerve trunks (e.g., axillary terminus of brachial plexus) are arranged so that the outer (*mantle*) fibers innervate the more proximal structures, and the inner (*core*) fibers, the more distal parts of a limb. With the local anesthetic diffusing inward down the mantle-to-core gradient, the analgesia salient sweeps down the limb in proximal-to-distal fashion. From de Jong RH. *Physiology and Pharmacology of Local Anesthesia.* Springfield, IL: Charles C. Thomas, 1970.

kinetics of recovery from clinical block. The oft-mentioned notion that duration of block correlates with degree of protein binding has no mechanistic basis and should not be used to explain clinical pharmacokinetic phenomena.

Although plasma proteins, particularly α_1-acid glycoprotein, can bind local anesthetics at equilibrium to a measurable degree, the bound drug dissociates in seconds from these proteins. As a consequence of this rapidly equilibrating reaction, free anesthetic molecules that pass through the capillary of a perfused tissue are rapidly replaced by drug molecules that dissociate from the plasma proteins. The rate at which blood circulates through an organ is often comparable to the rate of drug dissociation, allowing initially protein-bound drug to be released and to diffuse into the organ. Therefore, the importance of binding to plasma proteins for controlling drug availability, and thus limiting toxicity and metabolism, is far less than would be determined from equilibrium values (116,117).

Lipophilic uptake and release by local tissues is also slower than association with the targeted channels, accounting for the fact that maintenance of block by repeated drug injections does increase the time for recovery, albeit to a limited extent. In addition, more lipophilic drugs have a lower sheath permeability (110) and are thus retained longer within the nerve.

Vascular removal of local anesthetics is an important determinant of block duration. Not only is block duration enhanced by the addition of vasoconstrictors (see the earlier section, Permeation of the Nerve Sheath) but the dynamics of peripheral nerve block recovery can be explained through uptake by the intraneural vasculature (112,115). Thus, in a subclavian block in man, the sensory fibers at the core of the nerve recover function before the motor fibers located in the mantle, apparently because of the rapid vascular removal of drug from the nerve core (115).

Tachyphylaxis with Local Anesthetic

Tachyphylaxis, a drug's declining effectiveness when it is given repeatedly or delivered constantly over a long time, is often

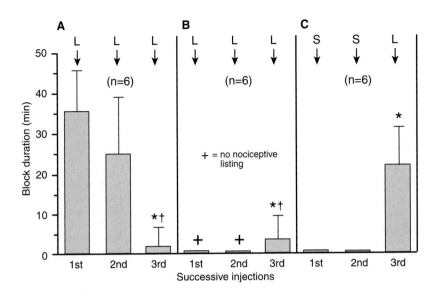

FIGURE 2-16. Tachyphylaxis for lidocaine block of rat sciatic nerve is characterized by decreasing duration of block with repeated administration of the same dose. **A:** Withholding nociceptive testing during the period of the first and second blocks does not alter the abbreviation of the third block (**B**), although injecting saline instead of lidocaine for the first two injections gives only a mildly decreased block duration for the third injection (**C**). From Lee KC, Wilder RT, Smith RL, et al. Thermal hyperalgesia accelerates and MK-801 prevents the development of tachyphylaxis to rat sciatic nerve blockade. *Anesthesiology* 1993;81:1284–1293, with permission.

observed when a long duration of nerve block is attempted. Hallmarks of tachyphylaxis are an ever-shorter duration of action with repeated administration, fading anesthetic potency, and shrinking analgesic field. Tachyphylaxis is less liable to occur if a blocking agent is reinjected soon after the first signs of returning sensation; in fact, the aforementioned augmentation of blockade is more likely to occur than not under these conditions (118). When the block is allowed to lapse, however (as sometimes occurs during attempted postoperative pain relief), tachyphylaxis frequently occurs. Timing, evidently, is a prime consideration that determines whether augmentation or tachyphylaxis follows reinjection.

Tachyphylaxis of local anesthetic blocks may be the result of several independent or related factors. In the laboratory, in vivo nerve block also becomes less effective with repeated reapplication. Both sciatic nerve block and infiltration anesthesia of the hairy skin in the rat are briefer and less profound with repeated administration of 1% lidocaine (Fig. 2-16A). One potential explanation for the reduced efficacy of identical doses is that nociceptive stimulation, from the needle injections that deliver the drug and from the noxious stimuli that are used to test its effect, sensitizes the CNS (by known mechanisms of spinal cord and, probably, brain) and amplifies pain perception, which then requires a higher anesthetic dose for equivalent analgesia. This mechanism may explain why tachyphylaxis occurs clinically when less frequent injections are made, at intervals that allow pain to recur (119). However, in laboratory animals, the injection of saline instead of lidocaine, at the same dosing times, does not induce tachyphylaxis for lidocaine (Fig. 2-16C), and the withholding of mild nociceptive testing (pin prick) during the earlier dosing does not prevent it (Fig. 2-16B), making central sensitization a less complete explanation (120). Nevertheless, in studies in which the blockade was tested electrophysiologically rather than behaviorally, and intense stimuli were used, reduction in the degree of block was dependent on the applied stimulation, consistent with the involvement of central sensitization. The discrepancy between these two findings may reside in the nature of the stimulus and in the elevated peri- and postoperative afferent discharges during and after surgery, which are transmitted by certain classes of C-nociceptors. These nociceptors may be particularly capable of recruiting sensitization pathways and may be important, although not essential, for eliciting tachyphylaxis.

Pharmacokinetic changes also appear to be involved in tachyphylaxis of local anesthesia. The lidocaine content of injected tissues was substantially lower during a third block that was shortened and attenuated by tachyphylaxis compared to the content during a single block using the same dose (120). This reduction is almost certainly due to an enhanced vascular clearance of the drug. But whether the local blood flow was enhanced as a result of altered sympathetic output, driven by central sensitization, or from local responses, such as the reactive hyperemia that would occur after lidocaine-induced vasoconstriction, is not yet known.

Regional Anesthesia: Epidural and Intrathecal Mechanisms

Blockade of large regions of the body by epidural and intrathecal administration of local anesthetics shares many of the characteristics of peripheral nerve blocks. Drugs applied epidurally reach their target tissues by crossing the arachnoid barrier, which is anatomically homologous with the perineurial sheath. These anesthetic molecules not only surround the nerve roots but penetrate deeply into the spinal cord tissue (121), as do intrathecally administered drugs (122) (see also Chapters 10 and 11). The same features of drug molecules and formulations that govern the potency and kinetics of peripheral nerve block are also determinants of epidural block, with the additional aspect that larger injected volumes spread further along the rostrocaudal axis and thus effect a more extensive block of adjacent dermatomes.

Delivery of anesthetics by the epidural or spinal route also distributes them well into the sympathetic paravertebral ganglia and thus can have profound effects on autonomic tone and reflexia (123). (Sympathetic nerve block also occurs during peripheral nerve procedures, of course, but there the consequences are more anatomically restricted.)

The locus and mechanism(s) of spinal/epidural anesthesia are not known with certainty (107). Clearly, local anesthetics in the cerebrospinal fluid (CSF) can block impulses in spinal roots (124). Evidence also suggests that other loci are involved and, indeed, that the site of functionally effective block may shift during the course of a procedure (125). More diverse targets are available to local anesthetics in the spinal cord than in peripheral nerve, because local anesthetics, at the concentrations that occur in during spinal (122) and epidural (121) procedures, are able to inhibit not only Na^+ channels but also various K^+ channels (30,81,126–129), Ca^{+2} channels (83,129,130), and ligand-gated ion channels as well as certain GPCRs (79,80), such as substance P receptors (131). Neurotransmission in the spinal cord is such a complex, integrated result of afferent and supraspinal inputs (86,132), usually involving spinal interneurons (Fig. 2-1), that the possible influences of the relatively nonselective and ubiquitously distributed local anesthetics are intriguing. Future pharmacologic and physiologic analysis should begin to reveal which of the many possible actions are important for regional anesthesia.

Therapeutic Actions of Systemic Local Anesthetics

Persistent pain is often induced by injury and disease of peripheral nerves. These changes induce membrane remodeling in injured afferents and possibly also in the adjacent, uninjured nerves. This gives rise to abnormal expression and trafficking of Na^+ channels, as well as changes in other ion channels (53,54,133,134), that result in increased cellular excitability. Consequently, ectopic impulses, arrhythmogenesis, and enhanced membrane oscillations appear after injury. For many of these cases, immediate and prolonged relief can be provided by the intravenous (IV) infusion of very low concentrations of local anesthetic agents such as lidocaine (135,136).

The mechanism by which such low plasma concentrations may act is not fully known. At these levels (e.g., ~2–5 μg/mL or ~5–10 μM), no resting block of normal nerve impulses occurs and normal physiologic functions are intact. It is not known if lidocaine's actions occur in the PNS or in the CNS, or even if they are primarily on neurons or on some other cell type, such as microglia or astrocytes (137,138), that actively contribute to neuropathic pain. Injured peripheral neurons will be susceptible to these lidocaine levels due to the higher affinity of inactivated channels that are abundant in injured, depolarized but still functional neurons (1,54,134). In addition, the margin of safety for action potential generation and propagation in a depolarized nerve per se is lowered because of the reduction in available channels due to inactivation, the tendency of which is emphasized by local anesthetics (19,35). With respect to the CNS, neuropathic pain needs descending facilitation from the rostral ventromedial medulla (RVM) to be maintained (139,140), so that blockade of such efferent activity would also mute this pain, and very small doses microinjected into the brain are able to reverse injury-related pain in animal models (141).

It is possible to treat these separate regions selectively with quaternary derivatives of local anesthetics, such as the QX314 homologue of lidocaine, that do not easily penetrate the blood–brain barrier and whose IV administration is thus restricted to the peripheral nerves. Systemic administration of this agent resulted in a full reversal of thermal, but not tactile, hypersensitivity caused by peripheral nerve injury. When QX314 was injected into the RVM, a reversal of identically induced tactile hypersensitivity was seen. Thus, we can conclude that thermal and tactile hypersensitivity are mediated through different mechanisms (140). This suggests that lidocaine's acute antihyperalgesic action is both centrally and peripherally mediated in a neuropathic pain state.

Prolonged relief of neuropathic pain has been described after lidocaine administration in animal models and in some patients (142). These actions can sometimes last for weeks following a single 30-minute lidocaine infusion (143,144), despite the

brief serum half-life of lidocaine in the rat (120 minutes); lidocaine's less potent metabolites are present for just a few hours longer. Persistent relief does not occur after intrathecal or regional administration of lidocaine, suggesting that blockade of afferent impulses and neurotransmitter release in the spinal cord is not its complete mechanism (144).

Lidocaine and mexiletine are the clinical drugs of choice for this treatment of neuropathic pain. One regimen is an infusion of 500 mg lidocaine in 250 mL of saline delivered IV over 60 minutes (145), achieving a plasma concentration of 2 to 5 μg/mL. In neuropathic pain treatment, substantial increases in acute analgesic responses are achieved for minimal increases in dosage (146). The difference between the effective dose (ED)50 (372 mg) and the ED90 (416.5 mg) was 44.5 mg of lidocaine, although the resulting plasma lidocaine levels are not known. Mexiletine oral doses range from 400 to 1,200 mg/d with a mean plasma level ranging from 0.36 μg/mL to 0.76 μg/mL (142,147). Mexiletine also relieves experimental tactile allodynia at low plasma levels after nerve injury in rats, but the persistent reversal of neuropathic pain caused by lidocaine does not seem to occur after mexiletine (148). Mexiletine is an orally active class 1B antiarrhythmic agents and a structural analogue of lidocaine. It has a 90% oral bioavailability and is mainly metabolized in the liver, with an elimination half-life of 6 to 17 hours. Mexiletine's benefit over placebo has been shown in diabetic neuropathy and peripheral nerve injury, but no significant benefit occurs after spinal cord injury. In other, broadly classified persistent pain situations, no benefit over placebo is reported, but some benefit is seen in subgroup analyses (149–152). No significant pain relief is observed for patients suffering from HIV-associated neuropathy. Due to the inconsistency of outcomes, side effects, and drug–drug interactions, mexiletine is not widely used (153).

Patients who can benefit from Na^+ channel blockers are those who present with spontaneous pain in combination with allodynia (154,155). This has led some to conclude that Na^+ channel abnormalities are the primary cause for these conditions, but this is erroneous logic. Hyperexcitability of neurons, often corresponding to experimental neuropathic pain in animals, can arise from changes in K^+ and Ca^{2+} as well as Na^+ channels, and from abnormal modulation of these channels by second-messenger systems that modulate channel function, independent of changes in channel density or subunit expression (54,75,107). Regardless of the primary etiology of the hyperexcitability, however, it results in ectopic impulses with a relatively low margin of safety and will be similarly responsive to drugs that block Na^+ channels.

Systemic local anesthetics have also proved effective in reducing postoperative pain scores and the use of opiate analgesics for relieving postoperative pain. Interestingly, through the use of peripherally restricted quaternary local anesthetic derivatives (discussed earlier), it appears that peripheral, rather than central sensitization, plays the critical initial role in postincisional mechanical allodynia and hyperalgesia (156). Whether the same mechanisms that account for persistent pain after nerve injury also cause postoperative pain is not known, but prolonged postoperative pain, which most often follows amputation or skin and nerve compression during prolonged application of retractors, may engage cellular pathways that contribute minimally to the type of postoperative pain that almost always disappears after 2 to 3 days (154).

When lidocaine administration has been used preincisionally (about 1 hour, on average, before surgery), less postoperative pain during movement and less morphine consumption is reported when compared to saline. These effects are most prominent 36 hours after surgery. The preemptive actions of

TABLE 2-2

COMPARISON OF SYSTEMIC LIDOCAINE AND MEXILETINE FOR RELIEF OF
CHRONIC PAIN OF VARIOUS ETIOLOGIES

Pain origin	Lidocaine	Mexiletine
Peripheral, metabolic	Pain relief (156)	Modest analgesic effect (152,188,189)
Peripheral, infectious	Reduction of allodynia (136)	–
Peripheral, CRPS	Reduction of cold-induced pain in CRPS (146)	–
Peripheral, cancer	Reduction of tactile allodynia (190)	–
Central/mixed, vascular or posttraumatic	Reduction of spontaneous pain intensity, brush-induced allodynia, mechanical hyperalgesia (135). Reduction of pain from herniated discs (191) Reduction of post-amputation stump but not phantom pain (192)	(149)
Perioperative	Reduction of movement-induced pain; less morphine consumption, reduced hyperalgesia (157)	Reduction of movement-induced and resting pain (193)

Referenced citation in parentheses.

this treatment are obvious, since administering the same dose of lidocaine in the postoperative period has no analgesic effect (Table 2-2) (157).

Adverse events from systemic lidocaine are nausea, vomiting, abdominal pain, diarrhea, dizziness, tinnitus, and perioral numbness. Less common reported side effects are metallic taste, tremor, dry mouth, insomnia, allergic reactions, and tachycardia. With mexiletine, the most common adverse events are nausea and vomiting. Neurologic (CNS) symptoms are more frequent in patients receiving lidocaine than in those on mexiletine (158). In comparison with the classical drugs given to treat neuropathic pain (carbamazepine, morphine, gabapentin, and amitriptyline), there is a slight, nonsignificant increase in adverse events (151).

The long-term use of lidocaine is limited by the requirement for a subcutaneous or IV delivery system. For patients with second- and third-degree heart blocks, mexiletine is contraindicated. It is also not recommended for patients in uncompensated congestive heart failure. Giving IV lidocaine to test whether patients will respond to subsequent oral mexiletine shows only a moderate correlation. Some patients report better pain relief with mexiletine than with IV lidocaine (159). The inconsistency in reports about the efficacy of oral mexiletine might be due to the inability to achieve sufficiently high plasma levels.

For a better usage of local anesthetics in the treatment of neuropathic pain, further understanding is needed in establishing which patients will benefit from treatment and under what circumstances treatment should be initiated. For its perioperative usage, high-risk surgeries should be recognized and IV lidocaine started when necessary.

In conclusion, for long-term therapy of persistent pain states there remains a need for orally available, well-tolerated drugs.

Toxicity of Local Anesthetics

Local anesthetic toxicity may occur systemically or locally. Allergic or inflammatory reactions have been reported but these are probably due to a component of the vehicle solution or to a local metabolite of ester-linked local anesthetics, for example, para-aminobenzoate (160). Myonecrosis is a well-documented sequel of intramuscular injection of local anesthetic (161), but muscle is an actively restored tissue and, aside from minor pain, no problems arise from this procedure (see also Chapters 3, 5, 12, and 20).

Toxicity from systemic local anesthetics has major manifestations in the CNS and in the cardiovascular system (162). The CNS effects, including tinnitus, dizziness, fainting and, sometimes, convulsions, can be reversed by postural adjustment, waiting until a bolus dose is diluted, or the IV delivery of benzodiazepines. Central nervous system actions for most local anesthetics occur at lower IV concentrations than the cardiovascular complications (140,149), so that the nervous system effects are useful alarms of toxic IV local anesthesia. Injection of small volumes of epinephrine-containing solutions provides a useful indicator of IV needle locations before massive doses of local anesthetic are injected.

Cardiovascular collapse has been reported when certain local anesthetics, most notoriously bupivacaine, are accidentally injected intravenously. The collapse appears to result from direct actions of the drug on the myocardial impulse-conducting tissue (165,166), on the heart's E-C coupling (167) and contractile apparatus (168), and on structures in the CNS (169), as well as actions on vascular tissue. Prompt resuscitation can often prevent death (93,170), but the normal stimulatory actions of adrenergic agents may be blocked by the local anesthetics themselves (93,171), and direct cardiac massage may be required (172).

Systemic concentrations of "free" local anesthetics and their delivery to perfused tissues are affected by several factors. Although a substantial fraction of local anesthetic in the blood is bound to plasma proteins (e.g., α1-acid glycoprotein), this will vary in amount with inflammation and during pregnancy. In the more hydrophobic local anesthetics (particularly those that are "highly bound" [173]), this binding is rapidly reversible and will do little to reduce the bioavailable pool of systemic local anesthetic. Recent studies report that cardiovascular toxicity, in vivo as well as in isolated hearts, can be significantly ameliorated by the IV infusion of lipid emulsions (174–176). Removal of bupivacaine from hearts is accelerated by perfusion with this emulsion after cardiac arrest has occurred (177), showing one mechanism for recovery from toxicity; other means, however, such as reversal of metabolic block or pharmacologic stimulation of ion channel function by free fatty acids, for example, may also contribute.

Local anesthetics also have direct neuropathologic effects. One notorious action is that nerves of the spinal roots may be irreversibly distressed by high concentrations of lidocaine. The delivery of 5% lidocaine in hyperbaric dextrose solutions through continuous spinal catheters has spawned several reports of cauda equina syndrome, as the drug appears to pool around the sacral roots due to inadequate mixing (178). Similar neurologic sequelae have also been reported after multiple (179) and even single (180) intrathecal bolus injections of concentrated local anesthetics. Direct exposure of a desheathed peripheral nerve to 5% lidocaine, a "model" of spinal nerve roots, leads to rapid, complete, and irreversible ablation of the nerve impulse (181–183). Irreversible block has been observed in both A- and C-fibers in mammalian nerve in vitro (184), and some clinical deficits of cauda equina syndrome have been simulated by intrathecal infusion of lidocaine in the rat in vivo (185,186).

The mechanism of this neurotoxic effect may involve several cellular pathways. Local anesthetics are known to disrupt mitochondrial energetics; they are weak bases and thus can short-circuit the proton gradient that composes part of the electromotive force required to synthesize ATP. As a consequence, mitochondria release the Ca^{+2} they have stored into the cytoplasm and also disengage their cytochrome c. The first action can cause a rapid, metabolically induced cell death; the latter action leads, predictably, to apoptosis, the programmed cell death that follows after a day or two. Key intracellular pathways for these processes of death appear to involve some mitogen-activated protein kinases (MAPKs) (169), since inhibitors of the p38 MAPK can greatly reduce neurotoxicity from local anesthetics (187). It is not known whether high concentrations of lidocaine around the nerve roots have a direct effect on neurons per se, either by local actions at the injection site or through diffusion of toxic materials from affected axons to cell bodies, or if the primary cytotoxicity is on glia and Schwann cells, with neuronal effects being a secondary response, such as Wallerian degeneration. Both effects might occur, with glial cell responses inducing a reversible, inflammation-like response, which has been termed "transient radicular irritation," and direct neuronal responses leading to axonal die-back attended by a persistent loss of conduction and of function.

References

1. Kandel ER, Schwartz JH, Jessell T, eds. *Principles of Neural Science*, 4th ed. New York: Elsevier/North-Holland, 2000:105–297.
2. Hille B. *Ionic Channels of Excitable Membranes*, 3rd ed. Sunderland, MA: Sinauer Associates, 2001.
3. Hodgkin AL, Huxley AF. A quantitative description of membrane current and its application to conduction and excitation in nerve. *J Physiol* 1952;117:500–544.
4. Ritchie JM. Physiological basis for conduction in myelinated nerve fibers. In: Morell, P, ed. *Myelin*, 2nd ed. New York: Plenum Press, 1984:117–114.
5. Agnew WS, Levinson SR, Raftery MA. Purification of the tetrodotoxin-binding component associated with the voltage-sensitive sodium channel from electrophorus electroplax membranes. *Proc Natl Acad Sci USA* 1978;75:2606–2610.
6. Ritchie JM, Ritchie B, Greengard P. The effect of the nerve sheath on the action of local anesthetics. *J Pharmacol Exp Ther* 1965;150:160.
7. Akert K, Sandri C, Weibel R, et al. The fine structure of the perineural endothelium. *Cell Tissue Res* 1976;165:281–295.
8. Feng T, Liu YM. The connective tissue sheath of the nerve as effective diffusion barrier. *J Cell Comp Physiol* 1949;34:1–16.
9. Shanthaveerappa TR, Bourne GH. The 'perineural epithelium,' a metabolically active, continuous, protoplasmic cell barrier surrounding peripheral nerve fasciculi. *J Anat London* 1962;96:527.
10. Rang HP, Ritchie JM. On the electrogenic sodium pump in mammalian non-myelinated nerve fibers and its activation by various cations. *J Physiol* 1968;196:183–221.
11. Stühmer W, Conti F, Harukazu S, et al. Structural parts involved in activation and inactivation of the sodium channel. *Nature* 1989;339:597–603.
12. Condouris G, Goebel RH, Brady T. Computer simulation of local anesthetic effects using a mathematical model of myelinated nerve. *J Pharmacol Exp Ther* 1976;196:737–745.
13. Raymond SA, Steffensen S, Gugino LD, et al. The role of length of nerve exposed to local anesthetics in impulse blocking action. *Anesth Anal* 1989;68:563–570.
14. Butterworth JF, Strichartz GR. Molecular mechanism of local anesthesia: A review. *Anesthesiology* 1990;72:711–734.
15. Taylor RE. Effect of procaine on electrical properties of squid axon membrane. *Am J Physiol* 1959;196:1071–1078.
16. Cahalan M, Shapiro BI, Almers W. Relationship between inactivation of sodium channels and block by quaternary derivatives of local anesthetics and other compounds. In: Fink BR, ed. *Molecular Mechanisms of Anesthesia (Progress in Anesthesiology)*, Vol. 2. New York: Raven Press, 1980:17–32.
17. Keynes RD, Rojas E. Kinetics and steady-state properties of the charged system controlling sodium conductance in the squid giant axon. *J Physiol* 1974;239:393–434.
18. Neumcke B, Schwarz W, Stampfli R. Block of Na channels in the membrane of myelinated nerve by benzocaine. *Pflugers Arch* 1981;390:230–236.
19. Hille B. Local anesthetics: Hydrophilic and hydrophobic pathways for the drug-receptor reaction. *J Gen Physiol* 1977;69:497–551.
20. Hille B. Local anesthetic action on inactivation of the Na channel in nerve and skeletal muscle: Possible mechanisms for antiarrhythmic agents. In: Morad M, ed. *Biophysical Aspects of Cardiac Muscle*. New York: Academic Press, 1978:55–74.
21. Chernoff DM. Kinetic analysis of phasic inhibition of neuronal sodium currents by lidocaine and bupivacaine. *Biophys J* 1990;58:53–68.
22. Courtney KR. Mechanism of frequency-dependent inhibition of sodium currents in frog myelinated nerve by the lidocaine derivative GEA-968. *J Pharmacol Exp Ther* 1975;195:225–236.
23. Cahalan M. Local anesthetic block of sodium channels in normal and pronase-treated squid giant axons. *Biophys J* 1978;23:285–311.
24. Strichartz G, Wang K. The kinetic basis for phasic local anesthetic blockade of neuronal sodium channels. In: Miller KW, Roth S, eds. *Molecular and Cellular Mechanisms of Anesthetics*. New York: Plenum Publishing, 1986:217–226.
25. Carmeliet E, Vereecke J, Chaplan S, et al. Electrogenesis of the action potential and atomaticity. In: Berne RM, Sperelakis N, Geiger S, eds. *Handbook of Physiology*, Vol. I. Bethesda, MD: American Physiology Society, 1979:269–334.
26. Noble D. *The Initiation of the Heartbeat*. Oxford: Oxford University Press, 1975.
27. Strichartz GR, Sanchez V, Arthur GR, et al. Fundamental properties of local anesthetics. II. Measured octanol:buffer partition coefficients and pK_a values of clinically-used drugs. *Anesth Anal* 1990;71:158–170.
28. Frazier DT, Narahashi T, Yamada M. The site of action and active form of local anesthetics. II. Experiments with quaternary compounds. *J Pharmacol Exp Ther* 1970;171:45–51.
29. Strichartz GR. The inhibition of sodium currents in myelinated nerve by quaternary derivatives of lidocaine. *J Gen Physiol* 1973;62:37–57.
30. Arhem P, Frankenhaeuser B. Local anesthetics: Effects on permeability properties of nodal membrane in myelinated nerve fibres from Xenopus. Potential clamp experiments. *Acta Physiol Scand* 1974;91:11–21.
31. Chernoff DM, Strichartz GR. Tonic and phasic block of neuronal sodium currents by 5-hydroxyhexano-2',6',-xylidide, a neutral lidocaine homologue. *J Gen Physiol* 1989;93:1075–1090.
32. Ritchie JM, Ritchie BR. Local anaesthetics: Effect of pH on activity. *Science* 1968;162:1394–1395.
33. Hille B. The pH-dependent rate of action of local anesthetics on the node of Ranvier. *J Gen Physiol* 1977;69:475–496.

34. Schwarz W, Palade PT, Hille B. Local anesthetics: Effect of pH on use-dependent block of sodium channels in frog muscle. *Biophys J* 1977;20:343–358.

35. Strichartz G. Interactions of local anesthetics with neuronal sodium channels. In: Covino BG, Fozzard H, Rehder K, Strichartz G, eds. *Effects of Anesthesia. Clinical Physiology Series.* Bethesda, MD: American Physiological Society, 1985:39–52.

36. Narahashi T, Frazier D, Yamada M. The site of action and active form of local anesthetics, I. Theory and pH experiments with tertiary compounds. *J Pharm Exp Ther* 1970;171:132–144.

37. Nau C, Wang SY, Wang GK. Methanethiosulfonate-modification alters local anesthetic block in rNav1.4 cysteine-substituted mutants S1276C and L1280C. *J Membr Biol* 2003;193:47–55.

38. O'Reilly JP, Wang SY, Wang GK. Methanethiosulfonate-modification alters local anesthetic block in rNav1.4 cysteine-substituted mutants S1276C and L1280C. *J Membr Biol* 2003;193:47–55.

39. Ragsdale DS, McPhee JC, Scheuer T, Catterall WA. Molecular determinants of state-dependent block of Na$^+$ channels by local anesthetics. *Science* 1994;265:1724–1728.

40. Wang SY, Mitchell J, Moczydlowski E, Wang G. Block of inactivation-deficient Na+ channels by local anesthetics in stably transfected mammalian cells: Evidence for drug binding along the activation pathway. *J Gen Physiol* 2004;124:691–701.

41. Lenkowski PW, Shah BS, Dinn AEE, et al. Lidocaine block of neonatal Nav1.3 is differentially modulated by co-expression of beta1 and beta3 subunits. *Eur J Pharmacol* 2003;467:23–30.

42. Bokesch PM, Post C, Strichartz GR. Structure activity relationship of lidocaine homologues on tonic and frequency-dependent impulse blockade in nerve. *J Pharmacol Exp Ther* 1986;237:773–781.

43. Skou JC. Local anesthetics: VI. Relation between blocking potency and penetration of a monomolecular layer of lipoids from nerves. *Acta Pharmacol Toxicol* 1954;10:325–337.

44. Chernoff DM, Strichartz GR. Kinetics of local anesthetic inhibition of neuronal sodium channels: pH- and hydrophobicity-dependence. *Biophys J* 1990;58:69–81.

45. Courtney KR. Structure-activity relations for frequency-dependent sodium channel block in nerve by local anesthetics. *J Pharmacol Exp Ther* 1980;213:114–115.

46. Courtney KR, Strichartz GR. Structural elements which determine local anesthetic activity. In: Strichartz GR, ed. *Handbook of Experimental Pharmacology: Local Anesthetics.* New York: Springer-Verlag; 1985:51–94.

47. Sinnott CJ, Garfield JM, Thalhammer JG, et al. Addition of sodium bicarbonate to lidocaine decreases the duration of peripheral nerve block in the rat. *Anesthesiology* 2000;93:1045–1052.

48. Kondratiev A, Tomaselli GF. Altered gating and local anesthetic block mediated by residues in the I-S6 and II-S6 transmembrane segments of voltage-dependent Na$^+$ channels. *Mol Pharmacol* 2003;64:741–752.

49. Lipkind GM, Fozzard HA. Molecular modeling of local anesthetic drug binding by voltage-gated sodium channels. *Mol Pharmacol* 2005;68:1611–1622.

50. Scheib H, McLay I, Guex N, et al. Modeling the pore structure of voltage-gated sodium channels in closed, open, and fast-inactivated conformation reveals details of site 1 toxin and local anesthetic binding. *J Molec Model* 2006;2:813–822.

51. Kim CH, Oh Y, Chung J M, et al. The changes in expression of three subtypes of TTX sensitive sodium channels in sensory neurons after spinal nerve ligation. *Mol Brain Res* 2001;95:153–161.

52. Sleeper AA, Cummins TR, Dib-Hajj SD, et al. Changes in expression of two tetrodotoxin-resistant sodium channels and their currents in dorsal root ganglion neurons after sciatic nerve injury but not rhizotomy. *J Neurosci* 2000;20:7279–7289.

53. Black JA, Liu S, Tanaka M, et al. Changes in the expression of tetrodotoxin-sensitive sodium channels within dorsal root ganglia neurons in inflammatory pain. *Pain* 2004;108:237–247.

54. Amir R, Argoff C, Bennett G, et al. The role of sodium channels in chronic inflammatory and neuropathic pain. *J Pain* 2006;7[Suppl 3]:S1–S29.

55. Lopez-Santiago LF, Pertin M, Morisod X, et al. Sodium channel β2 subunits regulate tetrodotoxin-sensitive sodium channels in small dorsal root ganglion neurons and modulate the response to pain. *J Neurosci* 2006;260:7984–7994.

56. Pertin M, Ji R-R, Berta T. Upregulation of the voltage-gated sodium channel β2 subunit in neuropathic pain models: Characterization of expression in injured and non-injured primary sensory neurons. *J Neurosci* 2005;25:10970–10980.

57. Makielski JC, Limberis J, Fan Z, et al. Intrinsic lidocaine affinity for Na channels expressed in xenopus oocytes depends on alpha (hH1 vs. rSkM1) and beta 1 subunits. *Cardiovasc Res* 1999;42:503–509.

58. Yu EJ, Ko SH, Lenkowski PW. Distinct domains of the sodium channel beta3-subunit modulate channel-gating kinetics and subcellular location. *Biochem J* 2005;392:519–526.

59. Wang GK, Edrich T, Wang SY. Time dependent block and resurgent tail currents induced by mouse $\beta4_{154-167}$ peptide in cardiac Na$^+$ channels. *J Gen Physiol* 2006;27:277–289.

60. Leffler A, Herzog R, Dib-Hajj D, et al. Pharmacological properties of neuronal TTX-resistant sodium channels and the role of a critical serine pore residue. *Pfluugers Arch-Eur J Physiol* 2005;451:454–463.

61. Scholz A, Vogel W. Tetrodotoxin-resistant action potentials in dorsal root ganglion neurons are blocked by local anesthetics. *Pain* 2000;89:47–52.

62. Akerman SB, Camougis G, Sandberg RV. Stereoisomerism and differential activity in excitation block by local anesthetics. *Eur J Pharm* 1969;8:337–347.

63. LeeSon S, Wang GK, Concus A, et al. Stereoselective inhibition of neuronal sodium channels by local anesthetics: Evidence for two sites of action? *Anesthesiology* 1992;77:324–335.

64. Nau C, Wang S-Y, Strichartz GR, et al. Point mutations at N434 in D1-S6 of $\mu1$ Na$^+$ channels modulate binding affinity and stereoselectivity of local anesthetic enantiomers. *Mol Pharm* 1999;56:404–413.

65. Nau C, Wang GK. Topical Review: Interactions of local anesthetics with voltage-gated Na$^+$ channels. *J Membr Biol* 2004;201:1–8.

66. Wang GK. Cocaine-induced closures of single batrachotoxin-activated Na$^+$ channels in planar lipid bilayers. *J Gen Physiol* 1988;92:747–765.

67. Wright SN, Wang SY, Kallen RG, et al. Differences in steady-state inactivation between Na channel isoforms affect local anesthetic binding affinity. *Biophys J* 1997;73: 779–788.

68. Roy ML, Narahashi T. Differential properties of tetrodotoxin-sensitive and tetrodotoxin-resistant sodium channels in rat dorsal root ganglion neurons. *J Neurosci* 1992;12:2104–2111.

69. Chevrier P, Vijayaragavan K, Chahine M. Differential modulation of Nav1.7 and Nav1.8 peripheral nerve sodium channels by the local anesthetic lidocaine. *Br J Pharmacol* 2004;142:576–584.

70. Elliott AA, Elliott JR. Characterization of TTX-sensitive and TTX-resistant sodium currents in small cells from adult rat dorsal root ganglia. *J Physiol* 1993;463:39–56.

71. Van de Velde M, Dreelinck R, Dubois J, et al. Determination of the full dose-response relation of intrathecal bupivacaine, levobupivacaine, and ropivacaine, combined with sufentanil, for labor analgesia. *Anesthesiology* 2007;106:149–156.

72. Oda A, Ohashi H, Komori S, et al. Characteristics of ropivacaine block of Na$^+$ channels in rat dorsal root ganglion neurons. *Anesth Anal* 2000;91:1213–1220.

73. Gold MS, Levine JD, Correa AM. Modulation of TTX-R I$_{Na}$ by PKC and PKA and their role in PGE2-induced sensitization of rat sensory neurons in vitro. *J Neurosci* 1998;18:1045–1055.

74. Rasband MN, Park EW, Vanderah TW, et al. Distinct potassium channels on pain–sensing neurons. *Proc Natl Acad Sci USA* 2001;98:13373–13378.

75. Cardenas LM, Carenas CG, Scroggs RS. 5HT increases excitability of nociceptor-like rat dorsal root ganglion neurons via cAMP-coupled TTX-resistant Na(+) channels. *J Neurophysiol* 2001;86:241–248.

76. Gold MS, Shuster MJ, Levine JD. Characterization of six voltage-gated currents in adult rat sensory neurons. *J Neurophysiol* 1996;75:2629–2646.

77. Hollman MW, Difazio CA, Durieux ME. Ca-signaling G-protein-coupled receptors: A new site of local anesthetic action? *Reg Anesth Pain Med* 2001;26:565–571.

78. Hollman MW, Wieczorek KS, Berger A, et al. Local anesthetic inhibition of G protein-coupled receptor signaling by interference with Galpha(q) protein function. *Mol Pharmacol* 2001;59:294–301.

79. Nietgen GW, Chan CK, Durieux ME. Inhibition of lysophosphatidate signaling by lidocaine and bupivacaine. *Anesthesiology* 1997;86:1112–1119.

80. Oyama Y, Sadoshima J-I, Tokutomi N. Some properties of inhibitory action of lidocaine on the Ca^{2+} current of single isolated frog sensory neurons. *Brain Res* 1988;442:223–228.

81. Palade PT, Almers W. Slow calcium and potassium currents in frog skeletal muscle: their relationship and pharmacological properties. *Pflugers Arch* 1985;405:91–101.

82. Heinbecker P, Bishop GH, O'Leary J. Pain and touch fibers in peripheral nerves. *Arch Neurol Psychiatr* 1933;20:771.

83. Valbo AB, Hagbarth KE, Torebjörk HE, Hallin BG. Somatosensory, proprioceptive and sympathetic activity in human peripheral nerves. *Physiol Rev* 1975;59:919–957.

84. Sato J, Perl ER. Adrenergic excitation of cutaneous pain receptors induced by peripheral nerve injury. *Science* 1991;251:1608–1610.

85. Gissen AJ, Covino BG, Gregus J. Differential sensitivity of mammalian nerves to local anesthetic drugs. *Anesthesiology* 1980;53:467–474.

86. Gardner EP, Martin JH. Coding of sensory information. In: Kandal ER, Schwartz JH, Jessell TH, eds. *Principles of Neural Science*, 4th ed. New York: McGraw Hill, 2000:411–429.

87. Nakamura T, Popitz-Bergez F, Birknes J, et al. The critical role of concentration for lidocaine block of peripheral nerve in vivo. *Anesthesiology* 2003;99:189–197.

88. Rosenberg PH, Heavner JE. Temperature-dependent nerve-blocking action of lidocaine and halothane. *Acta Anaesth Scand* 1980;24:314–332.

89. Thalhammer JG, Vladimirova M, Bershadsky B, et al. Neurological evaluation of the rat during sciatic nerve block with lidocaine. *Anesthesiology* 1995;82:1013–1025.

90. Wong K, Strichartz GR, Raymond SA. On the mechanism of potentiation of local anesthetics by bicarbonate buffer: Drug structure-activity studied on isolated peripheral nerve. *Anesth Anal* 1993;76(1):131–143.

91. Popitz-Bergez FA, Lee-Son S, Strichartz GR, et al. Relation between functional deficit and intraneural local anesthetic during peripheral nerve block: A study in the rat sciatic nerve. *Anesthesiology* 1995;83:583–592.

92. Sinnott CJ, Cogswell III LP, Johnson A, et al. On the mechanism by which epinephrine potentiates lidocaine's peripheral nerve block. *Anesthesiology* 2003;98:181–188.

93. Hurley RJ, Feldman HS, Latch C, Arthur GR. The effects of epinephrine on the anesthetic and hemodynamic properties of ropivacaine and bupivacaine after epidural administration in the dog. *Reg Anaesth* 1991;16: 303–308.

94. Bernards CM, Sorkin LS. Radicular artery blood flow does not redistribute fentanyl from the epidural space to the spinal cord. *Anesthesiology* 1994;80:872–878.

95. Jaffe RA, Rowe MA. Subanesthetic concentrations of lidocaine selectively inhibit a nociceptive response in the isolated rat spinal cord. *Pain* 1995;60:167–174.

96. Thalhammer JG, Raymond S, Strichartz GR. Changes of response pattern of sensory afferent in rats exposed to sub-blocking concentrations of lidocaine. *Abstr Soc Neurosci* 1991;17:440.

97. Jaffe RA, Rowe MA. Differential nerve block. Direct measurements on individual myelinated and unmyelinated dorsal root axons. *Anesthesiology* 1996;84:1455–1464.

98. Raymond SA, Gissen AJ. Mechanisms of differential block. In: Strichartz GR, ed. *Handbook of Experimental Pharmacology*, Vol. 81. Berlin, Heidelberg: Springer-Verlag; 1987:95–164.

99. Bostock H, Sears TA, Sherratt RM. The effects of 4-amino pyridine and tetraethylammonium ions on normal and demyelinated mammalian nerve fibres. *J Physiol* 1981;313:301–313.

100. Drachman D, Strichartz GR. Potassium channel blockers potentiate impulse inhibition by local anesthetics. *Anesthesiology* 1991;75:1051–1061.

101. Strichartz GR. The composition and structure of excitable nerve membrane. In: Jamieson GA, Robinson DM, eds. *Mammalian Cell Membranes*, Vol. 3. London: Butterworths, 1977:173–205.

102. Huang JH, Thalhammer JG, Raymond SA, Strichartz GR. Susceptibility to lidocaine of impulses in different somatosensory afferent fibers of rat sciatic nerve. *J Pharmacol Exp Ther* 1997;292:802–811.

103. Fink BR, Cairns AM. Differential peripheral axon block with lidocaine: Unit Studies in the cervical vagus nerve. *Anesthesiology* 1983;59:182–186.

104. Fink BR, Cairns AM. Differential slowing and block of conduction by lidocaine in individual afferent myelinated and unmyelinated axons. *Anesthesiology* 1984;60:111–120.

105. Gokin AP, Philip B, Strichartz GR. Preferential block of small myelinated sensory and motor fibers by lidocaine: In vivo electrophysiology in the rat sciatic nerve. *Anesthesiology* 2001;95:1441–1454.

106. Benzon HT, Toleikis JR, Dixit P, et al. Onset, intensity of blockade and somatosensory evoked potential changes of the lumbosacral dermatomes after epidural anesthesia with alkanized lidocaine. *Anesth Anal* 1993;76:328–332.

107. Gokin A, Strichartz GR. Local anesthetics acting on the spinal cord. Access, Distribution, Pharmacology and Toxicology. In: Yaksh TL, ed. *Spinal Drug Delivery: Anatomy, Kinetics and Toxicology*. Philadelphia: Elsevier, 1999:477–501.

108. Rosenberg PH, Heavner JE, Kovach K, et al. Dural permeability to epinephrine, bupivacaine, lidocaine and phenol. In: Wüst HJ, Stanton-Hicks MD, eds. *New Aspects in Regional Anaesthesia*, 5th ed. Heidelberg: Springer-Verlag, 1986.

109. Peterfreund RA, Datta S, Ostheimer GW. pH adjustment of local anesthetic solutions with sodium bicarbonate: Laboratory evaluation of alkalinization and precipitation. *Reg Anesth* 1989;14:265–270.

110. Bernards CM, Hill HF. Physical and chemical properties of drug molecules governing their diffusion through the spinal meninges. *Anesthesiology* 1992;77:750–756.

111. Wildsmith JAW, Tucker GT, Cooper S, et al. Plasma concentrations of local anaesthetics after interscalene brachial plexus block. *Br J Anaesth* 1977;49:461–466.

112. Winnie AP, LaVallee DA, Sosa BP, et al. Clinical pharmacokinetics of local anaesthetics. *Can Anaesth Soc J* 1977;24:252–262.

113. Covino BG. Pharmacokinetics of local anesthetic drugs. In: Prys-Roberts C, Hug C Jr., eds. *Pharmacokinetics of Anesthesia*. Oxford: Blackwell Scientific Publications, 1984:202–216.

114. Kristerson L, Nordenram Å, Nordqvist P. Penetration of radioactive local anaesthetic into peripheral nerve. *Arch Int Pharmacodyn Ther* 1965; 157:148–152.

115. Winnie AP, Tay C-H, Patel KP, et al. Pharmacokinetics of local anesthetics during plexus blocks. *Anesth Anal* 1977;56:852–861.

116. Denson D, Coyle D, Thompson G, et al. Alpha I-acid glycoprotein and albumin in human serum bupivacaine binding. *Clin Pharmacol Ther* 1984;35:409–415.

117. Wood M. Plasma drug binding: implications for anesthesiologists. *Anesth Anal* 1986;65:786–804.

118. Bromage PR, Pettigrew RT, Crowell DE. Tachyphylaxis in epidural analgesia. I. Augmentation and decay of local anesthesia. *J Clin Pharmacol* 1969;9:30–38.

119. Lee KC, Wilder RT, Smith RL, et al. Thermal hyperalgesia accelerates and MK-801 prevents the development of tachyphylaxis to rat sciatic nerve blockade. *Anesthesiology* 1993;81:1284–1293.

120. Choi RH, Birknes JK, Popitz-Bergez FA, et al. Pharmacokinetic nature of tachyphylaxis to lidocaine in peripheral nerve blocks and infiltration anesthesia in rats. *Life Sci* 1997;61:177–184.

121. Bromage PR, Joyal AC, Binney JC. Local anesthetics drugs: Penetration from the spinal extradural space into the neuraxis. *Science* 1963;140: 392–398.

122. Cohen EN. Distribution of local anesthetic agents in the neuraxis of the dog. *Anesthesiology* 1968;29:1002–1005.

123. Löfström JB, Cousins MJ. Sympathetic neural blockade of upper and lower extremity. In: Cousins MJ, Bridenbough PO, eds. *Neural Blockade*, 2nd ed. Philadelphia: J.B. Lippincott, 1987:461–500.

124. Frumin MJ, Schwartz H, Burns JJ, et al. Sites of sensory blockade during segmental spinal and segmental peridural anesthesia in man. *Anesthesiology* 1953;14:576–583.

125. Urban BJ. Clinical observations suggesting a changing site of action during induction and recession of spinal and epidural anesthesia. *Anesthesiology* 1973;39:496.

126. Courtney KR, Kendig JJ. Bupivacaine is an effective potassium channel blocker in heart. *Biochim Biophys Acta* 1988;939:163–166.

127. Elliott AA, Harrold JA, Newman JP, Elliott JR. Open channel block and open channel destabilization: contrasting effects of phenol, TEA+ and local anaesthetics on Kv1.1 K+ channels. *Toxicol Lett* 1998;100–101: 277–285.

128. Guo X, Castle N, Chernoff DM, Strichartz GR. Comparative inhibition of voltage-gated cation channels by local anesthetics. In: Miller K, Roth SE, Rubin E, eds. *Molecular and Cellular Mechanisms of Alcohol and Anesthetics. Annals of the New York Academy of Sciences*, Vol. 625. New York: Academy of Sciences, 1991:181–199.

129. Komai H, McDowell TS. Local anesthetic inhibition of voltage-activated potassium currents in rat dorsal root ganglion neurons. *Anesthesiology* 2001;94:1089–1095.

130. Olschewski A, Hemplemann G, Vogel W, et al. Blockade of Na^+ and K^+ currents by local anesthetics in the dorsal horn neurons of the spina cord. *Anesthesiology* 1988;88:172–179.

131. Li Y-M, Wingrove D, Too HP, et al. Local anesthetics inhibit substance P binding and evoked increases in cell Ca^2+. *Anesthesiology* 1995;82:166–173.

132. Basbaum AI. Functional analysis of the cytochemistry of the spinal dorsal horn. In: Fields HL, et al., eds. *Advances in Pain Research and Therapy*, Vol. 9. New York: Raven Press, 1985.

133. Devor M. Sodium channels and mechanisms of neuropathic pain. *J Pain* 2006;7:S3–S12.

134. Waxman SG. The molecular pathophysiology of pain: Abnormal expression of sodium channel genes and its contributions to hyperexcitability of primary sensory neurons. *Pain* 1999;6:S133–S140.

135. Attal N, Gaude V, Brasseur L, et al. Intravenous lidocaine in central pain. *Neurology* 2000;54;564–574.

136. Baranowski A, De Courcey J, Bonello E. A trial of intravenous lidocaine on the pain and allodynia of postherpetic neuralgia. *J Pain Symptom Manage* 1992;7:138–141.

137. Zhuang ZY, Gerner P, Woolf CJ, Ji RR. ERK is sequentially activated in neurons, microglia, and astrocytes by spinal nerve ligation and contributes to mechanical allodynia in this neuropathic pain model. *Pain* 2005;114:149–159.

138. Zhuang ZY, Wen YR, Zhang DR, et al. A peptide c-Jun N-terminal kinase (JNK) inhibitor blocks mechanical allodynia after spinal nerve ligation: Respective roles of JNK activation in primary sensory neurons and spinal astrocytes for neuropathic pain development and maintenance. *J Neurosci* 2006;26:3551–3560.

139. Burgess S, Gardell L, Ossipov M, et al. Time-dependent descending facilitation from the rostral ventromedial medulla maintains, but does not initiate, neuropathic pain. *J Neurosci* 2002;2:5129–5136.

140. Chen Q, King T, Vanderah, T, et al. Differential blockade of nerve injury-induced thermal and tactile hypersensitivity by systemically administered brain-penetrating and peripherally restricted local anesthetics. *J Pain* 2004;5:281–289.

141. Pertovaara A, Wei H, Hamalainen MM. Lidocaine in the rostroventromedial medulla and the periaqueductal gray attenuates allodynia in neuropathic rats. *Neurosci Lett* 1996;218:127–130.

142. Mao J, Chen L. Systemic lidocaine for neuropathic pain relief. *Pain* 2000; 87:7–17.

143. Araujo M, Sinnott C, Strichartz G. Multiple phases of relief from experimental mechanical allodynia by systemic lidocaine: Responses to early and late infusions. *Pain* 2003;103:21–29.

144. Chaplan S, Bach F, Shafer S, et al. Prolonged alleviation of tactile allodynia by intravenous lidocaine in neuropathic rats. *Anesthesiology* 1995;83:775–785.

145. Ferrante M, Paggioli J, Cherukuri S, et al. The analgesic response to intravenous lidocaine in the treatment of neuropathic pain. *Anesth Anal* 1996;82:91–97.

146. Wallace M, Ridgeway B, Leung A, et al. Concentration–effect relationship of intravenous lidocaine on the allodynia of complex regional pain syndrome types I and II. *Anesthesiology* 2000;92:75–83.

147. Chabal C, Russell L, Burchiel K. The effect of intravenous lidocaine, tocainide, and mexiletine on spontaneously active fibers originating in rat sciatic neuromas. *Pain* 1989;38:333–338.

148. Sinnott CJ, Garfield JM, Zeitlin A, et al. Enantioselective relief of neuropathic pain by systemic mexiletine in the rat. *J Pain* 2000;1:128–137.

149. Chiou-Tan FY, Tuel SM, Johnson JC. Effect of mexiletine on spinal cord injury dysesthetic pain. *Am J Phys Med Rehabil* 1996;75:84–87.

150. Dejgard A, Petersen NP, Kastrup J. Mexiletine for treatment of chronic painful diabetic neuropathy. *Lancet* 1988;1:9–11.

151. Kalso E. How strong is the evidence for the efficacies of different drug treatments for neuropathic pain? *Nat Clin Pract Neurol* 2006;2:186–187.

152. Oskarsson P, Ljunggren J, Lins P. Efficacy and safety of mexiletine in the treatment of painful diabetic neuropathy. *Diabetes Care* 1997;20:1594–1597.

153. Markman J, Dworkin R. Ion channel targets and treatment efficacy in neuropathic pain. *J Pain* 2006;7:S38–S47.

154. Ando K, Wallace M, Braun J, Schulteis G. Effect of oral mexiletine on capsaicin-induced allodynia and hyperalgesia: a double-blind, placebo-controlled crossover study. *Reg Anesth Pain Med* 2000;25:468–474.

155. Attal N, Bouhassira D. Translating basic research on sodium channels in human neuropathic pain. *J Pain* 2006;7:S31–S37.

156. Kastrup J, Petersen P, Dejgard A, et al. Intravenous lidocaine infusion-a new treatment of chronic painful diabetic neuropathy. *Pain* 1987;28:69–75.

157. Koppert W, Weigand M, Neuman F, et al. Perioperative intravenous lidocaine has preventive effects on postoperative pain and morphine consumption after major abdominal surgery. *Anesth Anal* 2004;98:1050–1055.

158. Tremont-Lukats I, Challapalli V, McNocol, et al. Administration of local anesthetics to relieve neuropathic pain: A systematic review and meta-analysis. *Anesth Anal* 2005;101:1738–1749.

159. Galer B, Harle J, Rowbotham M. Response to intravenous lidocaine infusion predicts subsequent response to oral mexiletine: a prospective study. *J Pain Symptom Manage* 1996;12:161–167.

160. Aldrete JA, Johnson DA. Evaluation of intracutaneous testing for investigation of allergy to local anesthetic agents. *Anesth Anal* 1970;49:173–183.

161. Benoit PW, Belt WD. Some effects of local anesthetic agents on skeletal muscle. *Exp Neurol* 1972;34:264–278.

162. Scott DB. Evaluation of the toxicity of local anaesthesia agents in man. *Br J Anaesth* 1975;47:56–61.

163. Reiz S, Häggmark S, Johansson G, et al. Cardiotoxicity of ropivacaine—a new amide local anaesthetic agent. *Acta Anaesth Scand* 1989;33:93.

164. Sage D, Feldman H, Arthur GA, et al. The cardiovascular effects of convulsant doses of lidocaine and bupivacaine in the conscious dog. *Reg Anaesth* 1985;10:175–183.

165. Coyle DE, Speralakis N. Bupivacaine and lidocaine blockade of calcium mediated slow action potentials in guinea pig ventricular muscle. *J Pharmacol Exp Ther* 1987;242:1001–1005.

166. Komai H, Rusy BF. Effects of bupivacaine and lidocaine on AV conduction in the isolated rat heart: modification by hyperkalemia. *Anesthesiology* 1981;55:281–285.

167. Lynch C. Local anesthetic effects upon myocardial excitation-contraction (E-C) coupling. *Reg Anaesth* 1985;10:38–43.

168. Wojtczak JA, LaVallee DA, Pesosa B, et al. Bupivacaine cardiotoxicity: "Power failure" and its mechanisms. *Reg Anaesth* 10:43–45.

169. Haller I, Hausott B, Tomaselli B, et al. Neurotoxicity of lidocaine involves specific activation of the p38 mitogen-activated protein kinase, but not extracellular signal-regulated or c-jun N-terminal kinases, and is mediated by arachidonic acid metabolites. *Anesthesiology* 2006;105:1024–1033.

170. Kasten GW, Martin ST. Bupivacaine cardiovascular toxicity: Comparison of treatment with bretylium and lidocaine. *Anesth Anal* 1985;64:491–497.

171. Butterworth IV JF, Brownlow RC, Lieth JP. Bupivacaine inhibits cyclic 3′,5′-adenosine monophosphate production. A possible contributing factor to cardiovascular toxicity. *Anesthesiology* 1993;79:88–95.

172. Feldman HS, Arthur GR, Pitkanen M, et al. Treatment of acute systemic toxicity after the rapid intravenous injection of ropivacaine and bupivacaine in the conscious dog. *Anesth Anal* 1991;73:373–384.

173. Taheri S, Cogswell III LP, Gent A, et al. Hydrophobic and ionic factors in the binding of local anesthetics to the major variant of human α_1-acid glycoprotein. *J Pharmacol Exp Ther* 2003;71:71–80.

174. Litz RJ, Popp S, Stehr N, et al. Successful resuscitation of a patient with ropivacaine-induced asystole after axillary plexus block using lipid infusion. *Anaesthesia* 2006;61:800–801.

175. Weinberg G, Ripper R, Feinstein DL, et al. Lipid emulsion infusion rescues dogs from bupivacaine-induced cardiac toxicity. *Reg Anesth Pain Med* 2003;28:198–202.

176. Weinberg GL, Vadeboncouer T, Ramaraj GA, et al. Pretreatment or resuscitation with a lipid infusion shifts te dose-response to bupivacaine-induced asystole in rats. *Anesthesiology* 1988;88:1071–1075.

177. Weinberg GL, Ripper R, Murphy P, et al. Lipid infusion accelerates removal of bupivacaine and recovery from bupivacaine toxicity in the isolated heart. *Reg Anesth Pain Med* 2006;31:296–303.

178. Rigler ML, Drasner K, Krejcie TC, et al. Cauda equina syndrome after continuous spinal anesthesia. *Anesth Anal* 1991;72:275–281.

179. Rosen MA, Baysinger C, Shnider SM, et al. Evaluation of neurotoxicity after subarachnoid injection of large volumes of local anesthetic solutions. *Anesth Anal* 1983;62:802–808.

180. Schneider M, Ettlin T, Kaufmann M, et al. Transient neurologic toxicity after hyperbaric subarachnoid anesthesia with 5% lidocaine. *Anesth Anal* 1993;76:1154–1157.

181. Bainton CR, Strichartz GR. Concentration dependence of lidocaine-induced irreversible conduction loss in frog nerve. *Anesthesiology* 1994;81:657–667.

182. Lambert LA, Lambert DH, Strichartz GR. Irreversible conduction block in isolated nerve by high concentrations of local anesthetics. *Anesthesiology* 1994;80:1082–1093.

183. Skou JC. The toxic potencies of some local anaesthetics and of butyl alcohol, determined on peripheral nerves. *Acta Pharmacol Toxicol* 1954;10:292–296.

184. Strichartz GR, Manning T, Datta S. Irreversible conduction block in mammalian nerves by direct application of 2% and 5% lidocaine. *Reg Anesth* 1994;19:21.

185. Drasner K, Sakura S, Chan VWS, et al. Persistent sacral sensory deficit induced by intrathecal local anesthetic infusion in rat. *Anesthesiology* 1994;80:847–852.

186. Li DF, Bahar M, Cole G, et al. Neurological toxicity of the subarachnoid infusion of bupivacaine, lignocaine or 2-chloroprocaine in the rat. *Br J Anaesth* 1985;57:424–429.

187. Lirk P, Haller I, Myers RR, et al. Mitigation of direct neurotoxic effects of lidocaine and amitriptyline by inhibition of p38 mitogen-activated protein kinase in vitro and in vivo. *Anesthesiology* 2006;104:206–273.

188. Jarvis B, Coukell A. Mexiletine. A review of its therapeutic use in painful diabetic neuropathy. *Drugs* 1998;56:691–707.

189. Stracke H, Meyer UE, Schumacher HE, et al. Mexiletine in the treatment of diabetic neuropathy. *Diabetes Care* 1992;15:1550.

190. Elleman K, Sjogren P, Banning AM, et al. Trial of intravenous lidocaine on painful neuropathy in cancer patients. *Clin J Pain* 1989;5:291–294.

191. Medrik-Goldberg T, Lifschitz D, Pud D, et al. Intravenous lidocaine, amantadine, and placebo in the treatment of sciatica: A double-blind, randomized, controlled study. *Reg Anesth Pain Med* 1999;24:534–540.

192. Wu C, Tella P, Staats P, et al. Analgesic effects of intravenous lidocaine and morphine on postamputation pain. *Anesthesiology* 2002;96:841–848.

193. Fassoulaki A, Patris K, Sarantopoulos C, Hogan Q. The analgesic effect of gabapentin and mexiletine after breast surgery for cancer. *Anesth Anal* 2002;95:985–991.

CHAPTER 3 ■ PROPERTIES, ABSORPTION, AND DISPOSITION OF LOCAL ANESTHETIC AGENTS

LAURENCE E. MATHER AND GEOFFREY T. TUCKER

It is now more than three decades since the drafting of this chapter for the first edition of this book. In previous editions, the chemical evolution of local anesthetic agents from the ester caines of a century ago into the amide caines and chiral caines commonly used today was outlined as a significant part of anesthesia history. Throughout this evolution, the principle of promoting greater safety in regional anesthesia has not changed—and our dictum from previous editions thus remains unchanged:

> The ideal use of regional anesthesia requires administration of sufficient local anesthetic agent to be effective but not so much so that toxicity develops. The anesthesiologist must have a thorough knowledge of the anatomic and physical landmarks to perform neural blockade in addition to a thorough knowledge of the pharmacology of the individual agents to be used. This includes familiarization with the disposition in the body of local anesthetic agents and, in particular, knowledge of their systemic absorption after the various methods of neural blockade.

The original evolution from prototypic cocaine to the myriad ester caines was driven by the clinical need to have an agent without the toxic and addictive potential of cocaine; the further evolution from ester caines to amide caines was driven by the pharmaceutical need for greater molecular stability. The need for safer, long-acting local anesthetic agents led to the more recent evolution to chiral caines, but it seems likely that continued evolution along the lines of existing chemical entities has now waned. It is, however, still important to examine relationships between the chemical and physicochemical properties of the agents and their fate in the body, and to delineate the role of pharmacokinetics in the overall response to regional anesthesia. Rather than provide a catalog of new and old data, we have continued to concentrate on the underlying principles of safe, effective anesthesia.

STRUCTURE OF LOCAL ANESTHETICS

Many chemically and pharmacologically diverse substances have local anesthetic activity, but remarkably few are used for clinical anesthesia. Conversely, the contemporary clinically useful local anesthetic agents (Table 3-1) have a variety of pharmacologic actions—some of which are exploited therapeutically, and others of which are avoided assiduously. These agents come from a small number of chemical families that still retain the clear ancestral line of cocaine, the original local anesthetic agent; however, paradoxically, cocaine can no longer be regarded as a typical local anesthetic agent, and it is rarely used as such.

Local anesthetic agents can be classified with respect to their chemical structures in two principal, interrelated, ways: by their functional groups and by their physicochemical properties. A comprehensive review of this interrelationship has been provided by Büchi and Perlia (1), albeit with many agents that are unknown except to those with a penchant for anesthetic history.

The functional group requirements for classical local anesthetic agents were established over 100 years ago with the discovery of the local anesthetic anesthesiophore (i.e., the smallest part of the cocaine molecule that retained local anesthetic activity) (2). It was soon realized that the anesthesiophoric part of cocaine was relatively simple and could be reduced to an aromatic (i.e., benzene ring–derived) head that conveys lipophilicity, an amino group that conveys hydrophilicity by way of its ability to form a charged species (or conjugate acid), and a linking chain that joins the two. The amino group was found to be optional, as demonstrated by the preparation of ethyl p-aminobenzoate (benzocaine) in 1890. The need for an injectable substance also required water solubility, and this was achieved and retained through an ionizable amino group, as in cocaine. Cocaine has an ester group in the linking chain, and this group was used in other agents until Löfgren's research showed that it could be replaced with an isosteric (i.e., having similar spatial characteristics) amide group (3). By the late 1960s, local anesthetics were usually classified by their linking chain groups as *ester* or *amide* agents (4). As once-common ester-type local anesthetic agents are now used relatively rarely, this division has more historical significance than pharmacologic importance for contemporary anesthesiologists. A third classification, based upon stereochemistry, is now germane.

The predominant physicochemical properties are *lipophilicity* and the *ionization constant* (pK$_a$)[a] of the amino group. Most other properties, such as affinity for macromolecules and water

---

We dedicate this essay to the memory of our late friends and colleagues who contributed much to our knowledge of local anesthetic agents: Ray Fink (1914–2000), John Bonica (1917–1994), Bruce Scott (1925–1998), Ben Covino (1930–1991), Terry Murphy (1937–1996), and Anton Burm (1949–2005).

---

[a]The dissociation constant of the conjugate acid (K$_a$) expressed as its negative logarithm.

48

TABLE 3-1

PHYSICOCHEMICAL PROPERTIES OF LOCAL ANESTHETICS

Agent	Chemical configuration — Aromatic lipophilic	Intermediate chain	Amine hydrophilic	Molecular weight (Base) (Da)	pK_a (25°C)	Distribution coefficient[b]	Aqueous solubility[c]	Percent protein binding	Equieffective[d] anesthetic concentration	Approximate anesthetic duration (min)[d]	Site of metabolism
Esters											
Benzocaine	H_2N—(ring)—	$COOCH_2CH_3$		165	2.5	81	very low	?	?	?	widely
Butamben	H_2N—(ring)—	$COO(CH_2)_3CH_3$		193	2.3	1028	0.1	?	?	?	?
Procaine	H_2N—(ring)—	$COOCH_2CH_2$—N	C_2H_5 / C_2H_5	236	9.05	1.7	?	6	2	50	Plasma, liver
Chloroprocaine	H_2N—(ring, Cl)—	$COOCH_2CH_2$—N	C_2H_5 / C_2H_5	271	8.97	9.0	?	?	2	45	Plasma, liver
Tetracaine	H_9C_4N—(ring)—, H	$COOCH_2CH_2$—N	CH_3 / CH_3	264	8.46	221	1.4	75.6[e]	0.25	175	Plasma, liver
Amides											
Prilocaine	(ring, CH_3)	$NHCOCH$—N, CH_3	H / C_3H_7	220	7.9	25	?	55 approx.	1	100	Liver, extra-hepatic tissues
Lidocaine		$NHCOCH_2$—N	C_2H_5 / C_2H_5	234	7.91	2.4	24	64[f]	1	100	Liver
Etidocaine		$NHCOCH_2$—N	C_2H_5 / C_3H_7, C_2H_5	276	7.7	800	?	94[f]	0.25	200	Liver
Mepivacaine	(ring, CH_3, CH_3)	NHCO	(piperidine) N—CH_3	246	7.76	21	15	77[f]	1	100	Liver
Ropivacaine		NHCO	(piperidine) N—C_3H_7	262	8.2	115	?	95	0.5	150	Liver
Bupivacaine (and levobupivaine)		NHCO	(piperidine) N—C_4H_9	288	8.16	346	0.83	96[f]	0.25	175	Liver
Articaine	(thiophene ring, CH_3, $COOCH_3$, S)	$NHCO$—CH—N, CH_3	H / C_3H_7	284	7.8	?	?	94	2	?	Plasma, liver

[a] pH corresponds to 50% ionization.
[b] n-octanol/pH 7.4 buffer
[c] Aqueous solubility (mg HCl salt/mL at pH 7.37 and 37°C).
[d] Data derived from rat sciatic nerve blocking procedure.
[e] Nerve homogenate binding.
[f] Plasma protein binding—2 mg/mL.

[Data from Ekenstam, B.: The effect of the structural variation on the local analgetic properties of the most commonly used groups of substances. *Acta Anaesthesiol. Scand.*, 25 (Suppl.): 10, 1966; Truant, A. P., and Takman, B.: Differential physical-chemical and neuropharmacologic properties of local anesthetic agents. *Anesth. Analg. (Cleve.)*, 38:478, 1959; Tucker, G. T.: Biotransformation and toxicity of local anaesthetics. *Int. Anesthesiol. Clin.*, 13:33, 1975; L. E. Mather, Unpublished data; Kamaya, H., Hayes, J. J., and Ueda, I.: Dissociation constants of local anesthetics and their temperature dependence. *Anesth. Analg. (Cleve.)*, 62:1025, 1983; Dudziak, R., and Uihlein, M.: Loslichkeit von Lokalanaesthetika im Liquor cerebrospinalis und ihre Abhangigkeit von der Wasserstoffion-enkonzentration. *Anaesthesist*, 27:32, 1978; Strichartz, G. R., Sanchez, V., Arthur, G. R., Chafetz, R., and Martin, D.: Fundamental properties of local anesthetics. II. Measured octanol: buffer partition coefficients and pK_a values of clinically used drugs. *Anesth. Analg. (Cleve.)*71:158, 1990; Grouls, R. J. E., Ackerman, E. W., Machielsen, E. J. A., and Korsten, H. H. M.: Butyl-p-aminobenzoate. Preparation, characterization and quality control of a suspension injection for epidural analgesia. *Pharm. Wkbl.*, 13:13, 1991; and Malamed SF, Gagnon S, LeBlanc D. Efficacy of articaine: A new amide local anesthetic. *J Amer Dent Assoc.* 2000; 131:635–642.

solubility surface activity, as well as pharmacologic potency for both neural blockade and systemic toxicity, derive from these. Lipophilicity for both esters and amides alike is increased by alkyl and aryl substitution into the carbon framework of the molecule and/or on the amino functional group. The ionization constant determines the relationship between the fractions of local anesthetic agent molecules in the ionized (more water soluble, but more local anesthetically active) and nonionized (more lipophilic) states for any given environmental pH. Amine salts are used to produce water-soluble forms for injection: These are mostly hydrochloride salts (i.e., readily dissociating conjugate acids formed by the interaction of the amine with hydrogen chloride [HCl]), but sometimes other salts such as sulfates from sulfuric acid, acetates from acetic acid, and other compounds are used to achieve the required *water solubility* to produce the necessary local anesthetic concentration. On the premise that nonionized molecules are better able to cross (lipoidal) membranes, these properties determine much of the local and systemic pharmacokinetics and pharmacodynamics of the local anesthetic agents. Together, lipophilicity and hydrophilicity determine *surface activity* and the related *tissue irritancy* (5,6). Not surprisingly, tissue irritancy is used to screen out substances from further development as local anesthetic agents.

Ester Caines

Cocaine was the first local anesthetic to be introduced into modern clinical medicine. Cocaine is an amine extracted from the leaves of the plant *Erythroxylon coca* and other plants of the same genus, native to Peru and Bolivia. During the 1850s, the plant was discovered in South America by German scientists and its principal active ingredient, the (tertiary) amine cocaine ("coca-ine"), was subsequently extracted, purified, and introduced into clinical medicine in the latter part of the 19th century. Final elucidation of the chemical structure of cocaine did not occur until 1924 but, by then, many hundreds of synthetic substitutes had already been prepared and trialed based upon the anesthesiophore of the cocaine molecule. The introduction of procaine (Novocaine)[b] in 1905 heralded a generation of a large family of ester caine local anesthetics having greater safety than cocaine and, most importantly, lacking its addictive/psychostimulant properties. Of these, chloroprocaine (Nesacaine) and tetracaine (amethocaine, Pontocaine) still remain popular with some anesthesiologists—the former for spinal anesthesia and the latter for topical anesthesia—along with some other ester caines, such as oxybuprocaine (Novesine) and proparacaine (Proxymetacaine), that are still used by some ophthalmologists.

As a class, ester caines in solution are subject to degradation by chemical hydrolysis, notably upon heat sterilization. This led to their replacement by amide caines that, as a class, resist chemical hydrolysis. The main pharmacologic benefit of ester caines, however, is that they are readily hydrolyzed metabolically by plasma and tissue esterases. Butamben, a benzocaine derivative of bygone years, received attention again in the late 1990s for its newly discovered ability to provide long-lasting and somewhat selective neural blockade after epidural administration of a suspension, but difficulties with its formulation appear to have precluded its continued development.

[b]The use of individual trade names does not imply that they are only trade names for these substances.

Amide Caines

The early 1930s saw the introduction of dibucaine (cinchocaine, Nupercaine), a quinoline derivative with the ester linkage replaced by a carbamoyl group. This agent is rather toxic, and its use was confined mainly to spinal anesthesia. It still provides the basis of a laboratory test of serum cholinesterase activity. The next major development occurred in two rival Swedish companies, AB Astra and AB Bofors, where some significant variations resulted in a new generation of amide caines. In these, the labile ester linkage was replaced by the chemically sturdier amide group, and this is further protected from chemical, but not enzymic, hydrolysis by steric hindrance from the 2,6-dimethyl groups on the aromatic (xylidine) ring. Lidocaine (lignocaine, Xylocaine, 1940s) was first, followed by mepivacaine (Carbocaine, 1950s), bupivacaine (Marcaine, 1960s), prilocaine (Citanest, 1960s), etidocaine (Duranest, 1970s), articaine (Carticaine, 1970s), ropivacaine (Naropin, 1980s) and levobupivacaine (Chirocaine, 1990s). In etidocaine, the carbon of the amide linking chain is ethyl substituted. In prilocaine, the 2,6-xylidine ring has been replaced by an *o*-toluidine moiety, and the amide linking chain is methyl substituted, thereby protecting the amide link from chemical hydrolysis; prilocaine also has a secondary rather than tertiary amino group, as in its near relatives. Articaine, which was originally introduced for dental anesthesia and relatively recently into mainstream anesthesiology, differs from the other commonly used agents in that the aromatic head is a thiophene ring; it has an amide linking chain to the amino group, but it also has an ester group.

By the late 1970s, routine use of the ester caines had waned, and lidocaine and bupivacaine had become the de facto standards of shorter- and longer-acting agents, mepivacaine and prilocaine continued to have a smaller following among some anesthesiologists and dentists for selected procedures, and etidocaine had developed an unfortunate reputation for producing motor block that outlasted sensory block. At about the same time, concern over the safety of etidocaine and bupivacaine was becoming prominent (7,8).

As safety issues in regional anesthesia have continued to come to the fore, the future place of bupivacaine has now become questionable (9,10), especially with the introduction of ropivacaine and levobupivacaine, which have similar anesthetic activities but greater margins of safety (10,11). Articaine is now finding a wider place among anesthesiologists due to recognition of its relatively greater margin of safety (12).

Chiral Caines

The next major development came in the 1980s, with the development of ropivacaine—the first *synthetic* chiral caine—followed, a decade later, by the development of levobupivacaine.

Many substances, including a wide variety of anesthetic drugs (e.g., halothane, enflurane, isoflurane, desflurane, ketamine, thiopental, mepivacaine, bupivacaine, prilocaine, etidocaine, ropivacaine, and articaine) have a (single) *chiral center* (from the Greek, *cheir*, meaning "hand"). This center, also referred to as an *asymmetric carbon atom* or *center of asymmetry*, has four different functional groups bonded to it. This structure imparts a particular type of *stereoisomerism* known as *enantiomerism*. Where it is required to distinguish between them, substances lacking a chiral center (e.g., lidocaine, procaine, tetracaine and sevoflurane) may be referred to as *achiral*.

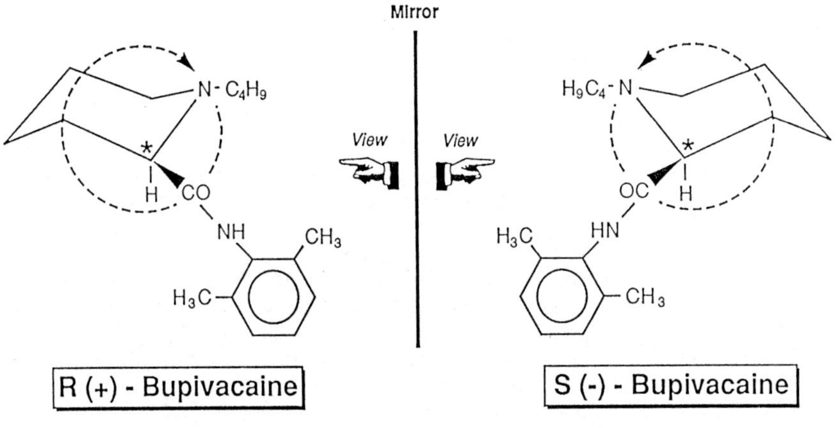

FIGURE 3-1. Application of the sequence rules of Cahn, Ingold, and Prelog to the enantiomers of bupivacaine. The chiral carbon is marked *. The smallest attached group, hydrogen, is projected away from the viewer; the other groups nitrogen (of *n*-N-butyl), carbon (of carbonyl), and carbon (of piperidine ring methylene) are arranged in clockwise order of decreasing size to give *R*-bupivacaine, which is *dextro*-rotatory; its enantiomer, *S*-bupivacaine, has the opposite order and is *levo*-rotatory.

Enantiomers (also referred to as *enantiomorphs*) are *stereoisomers* having nonsuperimposable mirror image relationships (i.e., one enantiomer cannot be superimposed upon the other without chemical bonds being broken and remade differently).

Enantiomers have identical physical and chemical properties, but differ in optical activity—the direction with which they rotate plane polarized light—a distinguishing property for which they became known as *optical isomers*, a now-obsolete term in the context of stereopharmacology. A single stereoisomer, free from its enantiomer, is referred to as *enantiopure*. A *racemate* (*racemic mixture*) consists of equal amounts of both enantiomers (and, therefore, has null rotation of plane polarized light); *nonracemic mixtures* consist of unequal mixtures of enantiomers. *Racemization* is the irreversible production of a racemic mixture from a nonracemic chiral starting material. *Inversion* is conversion of a chiral substance to its enantiomer. *Enantioselectivity* refers to a preference for one enantiomer over the other, whereas *enantiospecificity* refers to marked distinctiveness or exclusivity of that enantiomer. *Diastereoisomers* (or *diastereomers*) have multiple centers of chirality, and they can have multiple pairs of enantiomers (a pair for each chiral center), and normally differ in their chemical and pharmacologic properties (e.g., ephedrine and pseudoephedrine are diastereomers), and each consists of a pair of enantiomers.

Chiral drugs found in nature are usually single enantiomers because they are synthesized enzymically, and such reactions are usually stereospecific. Most synthetic chiral drugs are racemates, unless special synthesis is used to preserve the stereochemistry of a chiral center, or a chiral asymmetric synthesis is used to introduce a chiral center. Racemates are normally produced because there is an equal chance that both stereoisomers around a chiral center will be formed unless there is an energetic advantage for either one. Enantiomers behave essentially identically in an achiral environment, but in the chiral (amino acids, sugars, etc.) environment of the body, they behave as separate entities with potentially different pharmacokinetic and pharmacodynamic properties due to differences in their binding to macromolecules such as receptors (thus effect), membranes (thus distribution), and enzymes (thus metabolism) (13).

Three notations are used to describe chirality and associated optical activity, and all three appear in various publications about local anesthetic agents. First, (+) and (−), or *dextro* and *levo* (or *d* and *l*, now obsolete terminology) are associated with the pairs of enantiomers that rotate plane polarized light, respectively, to the right and left; that is, they are based upon optical properties (first noted in the 1830s). However, the direction of rotation is a phenomenologic feature only. A molecule may rotate plane polarized light in one direction when dissolved in one solvent but in the opposite direction in another solvent. Second, a systematic method of associating the stereochemistry with the direction of optical rotation was developed in 1919 by Emile Fischer and indirectly based upon structure. The Fischer-Rosanoff convention is based upon a molecule's configuration relative to that of (+)-glyceraldehyde (now known to be (*R*)-2,3-dihydropropanal, see below), which was arbitrarily assigned a D configuration (its enantiomer, (−)-glyceraldehyde being designated L-glyceraldehyde), or relative to (−)-serine (L configuration). The configuration of a molecule would be assigned the D configuration if it (or a chemical degradation product that retained the chiral center) had the same direction of optical rotation as the model substance (+)-glyceraldehyde, and the L configuration if the direction of rotation was the reverse. The direction of rotation, as in D-(+)-bupivacaine, also may be added. The D and L notations are still used in sugar and amino acid chemistry. Third, in 1955, the sequence rules of Cahn, Ingold, and Prelog introduced a method for the unequivocal designation of molecular configuration by giving a sequence of priority to the four atoms or groups attached to a tetrahedral chiral center. With the smallest atom or group extending away from the viewer, the arrangement of the largest to smallest groups proceeding clockwise is designated as *R*−(for *rectus*); its enantiomer is designated *S*− (for *sinister*) (Fig. 3-1). If more than one chiral center is present, they must be designated by their configuration at each position. As examples, levobupivacaine, which has one chiral center, is (*S*)-1-butyl-2-piperidylformo-2′,6′-xylidide; natural (−)-cocaine, which has two chiral centers, the position of each being specified, is 3(*S*)-benzoyloxy-2(*R*)-methoxycarbonyl tropane.[c]

Contemporary literature still contains all three notations, depending upon the amount of information available and when the information was acquired, but only the Cahn-Ingold-Prelog notation denotes the absolute configuration. Racemates are designated (±)-, *dl*-, DL-, *rac*-, or *RS*-; nonracemic mixtures are designated by their *enantiomeric excess* (or *ee*), a measure for how much of one enantiomer is present compared to the other; for example, a sample with 40% *ee* in the *R*-enantiomer, would have the remaining 60% as racemic (with 30% of *R*-enantiomer and 30% of *S*-enantiomer), thus having a total of 70% *R*-enantiomer. The naming confusion is preserved by the

---

[c] Further information about chemical nomenclature can be found on sites hosting books and reports of the International Union of Pure and Applied Chemistry (IUPAC). www.iupac.org. Accessed 14 May, 2008.

TABLE 3-2

APPLICATIONS OF STEREOCHEMICAL NOMENCLATURE TO MEPIVACAINE AND BUPIVACAINE

Fischer	Cahn-Ingold-Prelog	$[\alpha]_{25D}$
*Mepivacaine**		
D-(−)-mepivacaine	R-(−)- mepivacaine	−18.6
L-(+)-mepivacaine	S-(+)-mepivacaine	+18.9
DL-(±)-mepivacaine	RS or *rac*-mepivacaine	0
*Bupivacaine**		
D-(+)-bupivacaine	R-(+)-bupivacaine	+12.7
L-(−)-bupivacaine	S-(−)-bupivacaine	−12.0
DL-(±)-bupivacaine	RS or *rac*-bupivacaine	0

$[\alpha]_{25D}$ = rotation of sodium spectrum D-line at 25°C; *racemic clinically used forms of these agents.
Data compiled from Friberger P, Aberg G. Some physicochemical properties of the racemates and the optically active isomers of two local anaesthetic compounds. *Acta Pharm Suec* 1971;8:361–364.

use of international nonproprietary names such as levobupivacaine, which designates optical rotation rather than absolute configuration. The direction of optical rotation is only rarely of pharmacologic significance, so that it is often omitted from the name: (−)-(*S*)-bupivacaine is adequately designated *S*-bupivacaine (or by the nonproprietary name levobupivacaine). Application of the various forms of stereochemical notation is given in Table 3-2 using mepivacaine and bupivacaine as examples (522).

Despite our modern attention to chirality, much was known about the chiral pharmacology of local anesthetics from work performed during the 1960s and 1970s, mainly at the Swedish companies AB Astra and AB Bofors. Prilocaine, mepivacaine, bupivacaine, etidocaine, and articaine were introduced into clinical use as racemates before it was appreciated how important these agents might turn out to be. (Bupivacaine, and the other racemic local anesthetics discussed here, were named originally to designate the racemate, so that there is no need to specify that the particular agent is a racemate unless required by the context. Once in the body, enantioselectivity in pharmacokinetics makes a racemic agent into a nonracemic mixture, so that a measured plasma concentration of bupivacaine, for example, will normally comprise an unequal mixture of *R*- and *S*-bupivacaine.) After the concern was raised about the disproportionate cardiotoxicity of bupivacaine, ropivacaine (which is alone among the synthetic local anesthetic agents to be produced as a single enantiomer from its inception) was announced (14), and levobupivacaine (enantiopure *S*-bupivacaine) was later introduced based upon findings of its lesser toxicity than either bupivacaine or its enantiomer dextrobupivacaine (*R*-bupivacaine) (15,16). Nonracemic mixtures also have been trialed, for example, with bupivacaine (17,18) but have not been developed commercially.

Although pharmacologic enantioselectivity was first recognized by Louis Pasteur in 1858, it is only relatively recently that the pharmacologic consequences of enantiomerism in the context of anesthesiology has been rediscovered (19–24). A variety of studies, mainly using bupivacaine enantiomers in different models and bioassays has, not surprisingly, shown that enantioselectivity at voltage-gated ion channel and other receptors

mediating different neurogenic effects ranges from negligible to considerable (25–38). Presently, drug regulatory authorities are attuned to new chemical entity racemic drugs; these must be demonstrated as being no less safe than their enantiopure counterparts (39).

Analytical separation of local anesthetic (and many other) pairs of enantiomers for pharmacokinetic and other purposes is based on their different affinities for chiral macromolecular stationary phases, typically α_1-acid glycoprotein (also known as orosomucoid), or cyclodextrin, packed into a chromatographic column (40–42). On a manufacturing scale, a racemate such as bupivacaine, an organic base, can be separated into its component *R*- and *S*-enantiomers by combination with a suitable enantiomer of an organic acid, such as tartaric acid, to form two diastereomer salts that have different solubilities and thus unique propensity for selective precipitation; this is a common laboratory process called *resolution*, and commercial methods have been patented for this process (43). Alternatively, *chiral synthesis* to preserve the stereochemistry at the chiral center of the reagents used can be used to produce the required enantiomer selectively (44). For any drug, the commercial method used ultimately depends on cost-effectiveness of the process and the chemistry of the particular drug.

Potency

An agent's potency derives from its structural, stereochemical, and physicochemical properties: These properties govern the fraction of a dose reaching and residing at the relevant receptor, the agent's affinity for the receptor, and its (biochemical and biophysical) efficacy once it has bound to the receptor.

The potency of local anesthetic agents is determined early in drug development by blockade of isolated nerve electrophysiologic studies and/or neural blockade procedures in intact laboratory rodents. Their relative potency is often specified in terms of their *equi-effective anesthetic concentrations*, and some well-known relationships between agents are given in Table 3-1. Equi-effectiveness is sometimes judged by clinical bioassay, for example, by subjects having similar characteristics of neural blockade (e.g., dermatomal–time diagrams) (45), and/or in amount of supplemental analgesic used by patients after surgery when the local anesthetic agent is used for some neural blockade procedure (46). Equal clinical effectiveness is, of course, a desirable standard of judgment, but it is a fairly imprecise standard in that, with reasonably similar agents being tested in typically small cohorts, most studies are more likely to fail to detect a difference between agents rather than show no difference between agents (type II error). More stringently, potency can be specified in terms of the (molar) dose and/or concentration of local anesthetic agent found in preclinical studies that is required to produce a defined extent and/or degree of neural blockade in a particular model or preparation, or the frequency of its occurrence in a certain population.

By-and-large, the same chemical and physicochemical changes that influence anesthetic potency among the various agents also influence potency for toxicity, whether the agents be ester- or amide-type, with some adjustments for differences introduced by also considering chirality. Among these agents, the more potent substances are more lipophilic and less hydrophilic, and this could engender situations in which the physical presentation of the local anesthetic agent is limited by the soluble amount of dose. Greater potency is also usually associated with a longer duration of neural blockade; for example, intrathecal doses of bupivacaine 4- and 8-mg have approximately the same time courses of neural blockade as ropivacaine 8- and 12-mg (47).

Various nerve blocks are now being used to provide a means for assessing the relative potency of local anesthetic agents for producing relevant effects (e.g., sensory or motor block) in a particular population (e.g., primiparous patients in first-stage labor). From studies using the "up-down" sequential single-dose technique, the median effective dose $(ED_{50})^d$ has been determined as a primary measure for comparing potency between agents or for assessing the usefulness of drug combinations (48–50). It has been found, for example, that the mean (and 95% confidence intervals) of the relative analgesic potency ratios in intrathecal labor analgesia were 0.65 (0.56–0.76) for ropivacaine-to-bupivacaine, 0.80 (0.70–0.92) for ropivacaine-to-levobupivacaine, and 0.81 (0.69–0.94) for levobupivacaine-to-bupivacaine, suggesting a potency hierarchy of spinal bupivacaine >levobupivacaine >ropivacaine (51). Similarly, in separate studies, the relative ropivacaine-to-bupivacaine analgesic potency ratio for epidural labor analgesia was found to be 0.6 (0.49–0.74), and that for ropivacaine-to-levobupivacaine potency, the ratio was 0.98 (0.80–1.20) (52,53). The different ratios for ropivacaine-to-levobupivacaine between intrathecal and epidural dosing presumably reflect the more complex milieu of epidural analgesia, as described later.

Some have criticized the use of ED_{50} as the appropriate measure of relative potency, because it represents only the 50th centile; that is, the mid-point of the dose-response curve, and that the ED_{95} would be a more useful measure for extrapolation to clinical practice (48,54,55). Some of the criticism is based on claims that the observed relative potencies of local anesthetics in clinical use do not fit with the observed ED_{50}'s. The ED_{95} is beyond the linearized (ED_{20} to ED_{80}) portion of the slope of the (presumed sigmoidal) dose-response curve, so that the relationship between the ED_{50} and the ED_{95} need not bear the same dose proportionality relationship, which arises when comparing drugs with different slopes. Indeed, the slopes of the dose-response curves for different end points (e.g., sensory and motor blockade) may, and probably do, differ both between closely related agents, as well as within agents (56,57).

The up-down sequential dose method has also been used for assessing the effectiveness of treatments under particular conditions. For example, it has been shown that the ED_{50} for bupivacaine in late labor was greater by a factor of 2.9 (95% CI 2.7–3.2) compared with the MLAC in early labor (58). The up-down sequential dose method is also used assessing combination treatments with additives such as epinephrine or opioids (59,60). Others have also used the more formal isobolographic analysis with several combinations of doses for assessing the ED_{50} for combinations of drugs to determine whether a preferred dosage ratio exists (61).

PHYSICOCHEMICAL PROPERTIES OF LOCAL ANESTHETICS

Basically, three mechanisms are involved in the movement of local anesthetic molecules within the body: bulk flow of the injected solution at the site of administration, diffusion into

---

^{d}Various studies also refer to the minimum local analgesic dose (MLAD) or the minimum local analgesic concentration (MLAC), as appropriate to their study design—the principle is the same. ED_{95} is the 95th percentile, etc.

TABLE 3-3

FEATURES COMMON TO MOST LOCAL ANESTHETICS

Weak bases with pK_a >7.4. (Free base poorly water-soluble)
Thus dispensed as acidic solution of hydrochloride salts (pH 4–7), which are more highly ionized and thus water-soluble
Exist in solution as equilibrium mixture of nonionized, lipid-soluble (free base) and ionized, water-soluble (cationic) forms
Body buffers raised pH and therefore increase amount of free base present
Lipid-soluble (free base) form crosses axonal membrane
Water-soluble (cationic) form is active blocker for most agents

---

and through aqueous and lipoprotein barriers, and vascular transport from the site of administration. Of these, diffusion is most directly dependent on the physicochemical properties of the agent.

According to Fick's Law, the rate of passive diffusion (dQ/dt) of a drug through a biologic membrane at steady state may be approximated by Equation 1, in which D is the diffusion coefficient of the drug in the membrane; A and δ are, respectively, the area and the thickness of the membrane; K is the partition coefficient of drug between the aqueous and membrane phases; and ΔC is the concentration gradient.

$$dQ/dt = D.A.K.\Delta C/\delta \qquad (1)$$

Inasmuch as they determine D, K, and C, physicochemical properties will influence the rate of transport of local anesthetic agent at the membrane level, and potentially, therefore, the time course of anesthetic and pharmacologic effects. By influencing the equilibrium distribution of drugs between fluids and tissues, physicochemical properties also modulate activity and overall drug movement in the bloodstream.

Equation 1 can be simplified to Equation 2, in which the term comprising the constants D, A, K, and δ is combined into a permeability constant P; this equation indicates that the concentration difference across a membrane, ΔC, is the driving force for drug movement.

$$dQ/dt = P.\Delta C \qquad (2)$$

Some physicochemical properties of the clinically used local anesthetics are shown in Tables 3-1 and 3-3. As Table 3-1 shows, structural changes in the aromatic portion of the esters and in the amine group of the amides markedly alter physical properties such as oil or lipid/aqueous partition coefficients and affinity for proteins. These, in turn, have effects on potency, onset time, and duration of anesthesia. For example, with mepivacaine, substitution of a four-carbon n-butyl group for the one-carbon methyl group on the amine function gives bupivacaine a 35-fold increase in distribution coefficient^e, increased protein binding, and increased potency. Lipophilicity is commonly estimated by the distribution coefficient with a suitable organic solvent and an aqueous buffer, typically at pH 7.4, with reference to the pK_a (63). More polar solvents (e.g.,

---

^{e}Whereas *partition coefficient* refers to the equilibrium distribution ratio of concentrations between immiscible phases of the nonionized (neutral, base) form of the drug, *distribution coefficient* refers to the equilibrium concentration ratio of the combined nonionized and ionized (charged, conjugate acid) forms at any specified pH.

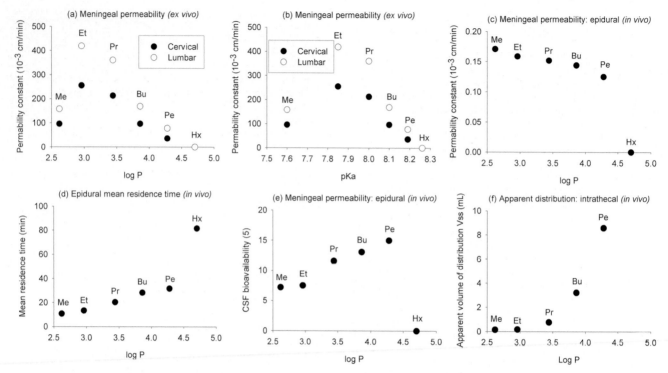

FIGURE 3-2. Composite figure showing the relationships between some physicochemical properties (lipophilicity given by octanol log P, and ionizability given by pK$_a$) of *n*-N-alkyl homolog members of the mepivacaine family and some pharmacokinetic properties in models of spinal anesthesia. In an ex vivo model, **A** and **B:** Meningeal permeabilities. In an in vivo rabbit epidural model. **C:** Meningeal permeabilities. **D:** Epidural mean residence time as a measure of rate of drug dissipation. In an *in vivo* rabbit subarachnoid model, **E:** Bioavailability to CSF. **F:** Distribution within the subdural compartment. Me, methyl (mepivacaine); Et, ethyl; Pr, propyl (ropivacaine); Bu, butyl (bupivacaine); Pe, pentyl; Hx, hexyl. Compiled and redrawn from data in Clément R, Malinovsky JM, Hildgen P, et al. Spinal disposition and meningeal permeability of local anesthetics. *Pharm Res* 2004;21(4):706–716.

chloroform) produce larger values than do less polar solvents (e.g., heptane); *n*-octanol, an amphiphilic solvent that is now commonly used to represent biologic barriers, will dissolve nearly 5% water, thus offering a medium of appreciable solubility of the conjugate acid form of the local anesthetic bases (63–65). The pH–pK$_a$ relationship is relevant because it governs the ratio of concentrations of drug in the ionized (more water soluble) and nonionized (less water soluble) forms. The coefficients also may be calculated from chromatographic retention data (66). Differences in molecular weight among drugs from homologous series are usually also associated with parallel differences in lipophilicity and pK$_a$ making it difficult to isolate the effects of individual variables. Under these circumstances, differences in diffusibility and permeability occur as second-order effects.

Molecular Weight

Molecular weights of the commonly used local anesthetic agent bases vary from 220 to 288 Da (Table 3-1). These agents have essentially the same skeleton with the increases in molecular weight being due to alkyl substitution; hence, lipophilicity and pK$_a$ also change with molecular weight. Because the diffusion coefficient is inversely proportional to the square root of the molecular weight, and differences in molecular weight among related local anesthetic agents are relatively small, the diffusion coefficient does not contribute significantly to differences

in their rates of diffusion. Changes in molecular weight produced by alkyl substitution, however, for example in pK$_a$, are accompanied by changes in other physicochemical properties, and these potentially lead to other related effects (Fig. 3-2).

Ex vivo studies of the dural permeability of drugs have been performed with cadaveric tissues, and these demonstrate a relatively minor influence of molecular weight. Although a relatively simple model, cadaveric membrane-diffusion cell preparations are themselves subject to experimental vagaries of tissue choice (species, site and thickness, etc.) and preparation (notably fresh versus frozen) that probably explain some of the inconsistencies seen in data from different laboratories (67,68). Despite the simplicity, it is still difficult to identify the impact of the various factors and covariates (molecular weight and lipophilicity, for example, because these run together when a homologous series of drugs is used), and corrections need to be made for nonionized (c.f., total) concentration of drug (69). In vivo studies are even more difficult to interpret because of the competing influences of vascular activity, systemic absorption, and uptake into fixed spinal tissues, as well as cardiovascular sequelae of concurrent general anesthesia in the preparation of living subjects. These factors have not yet been investigated systematically, and it is only recently that microdialysis has provided a method for beginning to study in vivo dural permeability and to estimate the bioavailability to cerebrospinal fluid (CSF) of intrathecal and epidural local anesthetics (67,70–72).

When tested with an ex vivo preparation of monkey or rabbit spinal meninges, the permeability coefficients of a heterogeneous series of drugs including lidocaine and bupivacaine were found to be independent of molecular weight (and molecular axis and molecular volume); however, a bell-shaped relationship was found with lipophilicity (as measured by the octanol-to-pH 7.4 buffer distribution coefficient) (73). When tested ex vivo with a series of homologous mepivacaine-like local anesthetics (i.e., progressively increasing molecular weight and lipophilicity), a parabolic relationship between permeability in lumbar and cervical meninges of the rabbit and lipophilicity was found. The permeability of human dura mater ex vivo to a variety of opioids and local anesthetic agents was found to depend on simple diffusion, independent of molecular weight, driven by the concentration gradient, and was not enantioselective (69,74,75). There is, however, some evidence to suggest that molecular weight might be relevant to the diffusion of local anesthetics in the sodium (Na$^+$) channel of the nerve membrane (76).

Recent correspondence in the literature has also drawn attention to the relationship between molar and mass label quantities of some local anesthetic agents that could have implications for differences in dose requirements and the relative potency of similar agents (77–79). It is worth reiterating here some elements of that discussion because it also involves international differences that can occur in labeling requirements.

Local anesthetic agents are normally prepared as %weight/volume solutions of the hydrochloride "salts" of the relevant base, such that the molecular weight is equal to the base + HCl (= 36.5 Da) if anhydrous, additionally + H$_2$O (= 18 Da) if monohydrate, etc. An aqueous solution for injection will be made of the salt, but the concentration of active ingredient may be specified either as that of the salt or the base; the water of crystallization is normally allowed for and adjustments are made. The relative concentrations of bupivacaine and levobupivacaine have the same molecular weight (= 288 Da), but whereas the concentration of bupivacaine is specified as the HCl salt (= 324.5 Da anhydrous), that of levobupivacaine is specified as the base (= 288 Da), at least for the European regulatory authorities. Thereby, the mass concentration of levobupivacaine HCl to make the solution has to be greater by 12.6% to achieve the same molar concentration of base as in a solution of bupivacaine HCl. Levobupivacaine could, therefore, appear to be more potent than bupivacaine if this difference in concentration were to be ignored. The message is plain: *check the locally issued product label/information as to how the concentration of local anesthetic agent is specified!*

Ionization

The inclusion of an amino group in the structure of most local anesthetics confers upon them the "split personality" of a weak base, meaning that they exist in solution partly as the nonionized free base and partly as the ionized cation (conjugate acid) (Equation 3):

Accepts proton (association):

$$\underset{\displaystyle \wedge}{\overset{\displaystyle |}{N:}} + H^+ \; \underset{\displaystyle K_a}{\overset{\longrightarrow}{\longleftarrow}} \; \underset{\displaystyle \wedge}{\overset{\displaystyle |}{N:^+H}} \qquad (3)$$

Donates proton (dissociation):

| nonionized base | hydrogen ion | → ionized ← cation (conjugate acid) |

The position of equilibrium depends on the dissociation constant (K$_a$) of the conjugate acid and on the local hydrogen ion concentration (Equation 4). Thus,

$$K_a = \frac{[H^+][base]}{[conjugate\ acid]} \qquad (4)$$

where the square brackets indicate concentration or, more properly, activity. By rearranging Equation 4 and taking logarithms, the Henderson-Hasselbalch equation (Equation 5) is obtained:

$$pK_a = \frac{pH \log [base]}{[conjugate\ acid]} \qquad (5)$$

where pK$_a$ is defined, by analogy to pH, as the negative logarithm of the dissociation constant of the conjugate acid under particular conditions of solvent and temperature (82–84).

Equation 5 shows that the pK$_a$ is equal to the pH at which the local anesthetic is 50% ionized, that is, when

$$\frac{[base]}{[conjugate\ acid]} = 1, \text{ and } \log 1 = 0.$$

The greater the pK$_a$ of a base, the stronger is that base—that is, it has a greater ability to attract a proton, and the smaller is the proportion of nonionized form at any pH. The ester-type agents have higher pK$_a$ values (8.5–9.1) than the amide types (7.6–8.2) (Table 3-1), which accounts, in part, for relatively poor penetrance and the need to inject these agents close to neural tissue. The effect on pK$_a$ values of differences in structure within the two main types of agents is complex, involving steric factors as well as the inductive effects of alkyl substituents on the amine nitrogen. For example, the greater pK$_a$ of bupivacaine compared with mepivacaine is explained by the effect of greater alkyl substitution, making the nitrogen atom relatively more negative (and able to attract a proton). In contrast, the lower pK$_a$ of etidocaine and of prilocaine reflects the effect of alkyl substituents on the bridging carbon atom in sterically hindering the approach of hydrogen ions to form the conjugate acid and in decreasing stabilization of the resultant cation by hydration.

Ionization is relevant to the solubility and activity of local anesthetics (Table 3-1) and their equilibrium distribution in various body compartments. Because the ionized forms are much more water-soluble than the free bases, the drugs are dispensed as their HCl salts, producing acidic solutions. This also helps to stabilize the esters since they are more readily hydrolyzed in alkaline conditions. The drugs are much more lipid-soluble in their free-base forms than in their conjugate acid forms. Thus, the nonionized fraction becomes essential for passage through lipoprotein diffusion barriers to the site of action on the nerve membrane. The balance between ionized and nonionized forms is shifted in favor of nonionized by the addition of bicarbonate (or other base), at the expense of decreased water solubility and the risk of reducing the effective drug concentration by drug precipitation (85).

Grouls et al. determined the effect of pH on the net flux across human meninges in vitro of lidocaine and bupivacaine. They found that the values at pH 4.0 were less than 20% that of the values measured at pH 7.4 (86). Decreasing ionization by alkalinization of the solution for injection will effectively raise the initial concentration gradient and flux (mass transferred per unit time) of diffusible drug (87,88) thereby increasing the rate of drug transfer. This maneuver has been successful in decreasing the latent period of a peripheral nerve block (89–91) but has not been universally successful for central neural blockade (92–95). Once at the nerve membrane, ionization is again necessary for complete anesthetic activity (96). Increasing the pH of aqueous local anesthetic solution also increases the surface tension (97), and this has been shown to decrease the drop rate when lidocaine solution was being delivered under gravity feed.

The aqueous phases on either side of many body membranes differ in their pH values. Consequently, although nonionized drug concentrations in these phases will be the same at equilibrium, different concentrations of ionized and, therefore, of total drug will exist on either side of the membrane if a pH gradient exists. For a weak base, the equilibrium ratio (R) of total drug concentration across a membrane is given by Equation 6. Thus,

$$R = \frac{1 + 10^{pK_a - pH_1}}{1 + 10^{pK_a - pH_2}} \qquad (6)$$

where the subscripts 1 and 2 refer to the two aqueous compartments. Total drug concentration will be greater in the compartment having the lower pH because a greater proportion will be in the ionized form. Thus, for example, lowered pH owing to infection in tissues surrounding a nerve results in less nonionized drug, which is the form that can cross the axonal membrane. Similarly, local anesthetics will diffuse from blood to acidic gastric contents, thereby maintaining a concentration gradient due to "ion trapping."

Aqueous Solubility

The aqueous solubility of a local anesthetic is related directly to its extent of ionization and inversely to its lipid solubility (Table 3-1; Fig. 3-3). Despite quite large differences in the lipid solubility of the amide local anesthetic bases, the differences in aqueous solubility of the conjugate acids are smaller. Benzocaine and butamben, which lack an (ionizable) amino group, are almost insoluble in water. For this reason, their use is essentially confined to topical anesthesia, or injection for prolonged neural blockade after solubilization with agents such as dextran or suspension in polyethylene glycols. Mixtures of local anesthetic agents with excess bicarbonate will lead to precipitation of the local anesthetic base after the solubilizing acid (normally hydrochloric acid) has been neutralized by the inorganic base.

A low aqueous solubility was thought to be a limiting factor when selecting an agent for subarachnoid block, principally due to the risk of the agent precipitating in CSF and causing

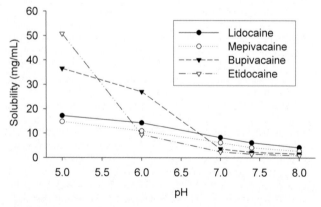

FIGURE 3-3. Aqueous solubility of some selected local anesthetics as a function of pH (Sorensen's phosphate buffer). (Unpublished data from Mather LE.)

neural irritation. It is known that the aqueous solubility is less with more lipophilic agents, and solubility decreases with increasing pH. Transient neurologic disturbances after spinal local anesthetic administration has been reported sporadically for many decades. However, the problem has not vanished by substituting more dilute lidocaine or mepivacaine solutions, suggesting that water solubility of the local anesthetic is not the most critical factor (98,99). Determination of the roles of a particular local anesthetic agent, the particular method of pharmaceutical preparation, and/or any additives have been the subject of much research, but relatively little sound science has emerged (100). How much is due to the local anesthetic, its concentration, and its properties such as surface activity, or the procedure itself, remains controversial (101,102).

Various experiments have been performed with local anesthetics to improve their water solubility, some with pharmaceutical manipulation to affect their local disposition, and some with alterations to the chemical structure. Whether these become useful clinically remains for future studies.

Lipid Solubility

The distribution coefficients of drugs measured in organic solvent/aqueous buffer systems in vitro are commonly used to reflect their relative in vivo distribution characteristics or lipophilicity (83,525). The values obtained normally differ quantitatively between systems due to both the polarity of the solvent and the extent of drug ionization at the chosen pH, such that their best use is in making comparisons between drugs within the same system (522). Net lipid solubility is independent of ester or amide grouping. Tetracaine (amino ester) is regarded as being highly lipid-soluble, as are ropivacaine, bupivacaine, levobupivacaine, and etidocaine (amino amides). Rosenberg et al. (103) have shown good rank order correlation between the *n*-heptane/buffer distribution coefficients of bupivacaine, etidocaine, ropivacaine, and lidocaine and their in vitro distribution into rat sciatic nerve and human epidural and subcutaneous fat. The intrinsic potencies (reciprocals of ED_{50}) of amino ester, amino amide, and piperidine amide local anesthetics have been found to be proportional to their calculated solubility in nerve fibers as determined from their lipid solubility (104). However, the order breaks down when a substance has too great a lipid solubility, and it is suggested that a limiting octanol distribution coefficient of about 5 pertains to useful membrane penetration. This is shown in Figure 3-2, where the *n*-hexyl derivative of mepivacaine fails to significantly penetrate the meninges after epidural administration in rabbits. After lipid solubility reaches this critical level, the apparent anesthetic potency, along with the intrinsic systemic toxicity, decreases (producing bell-shaped curves). This is caused by the drug so favorably distributing into lipoidal barrier membranes that insufficient partitions move into axoplasm (to produce neural blockade) as well as vital organs (producing lethal effects). Nevertheless, local tissue toxicity (cell leakiness) increases continuously with increasing lipid solubility throughout the test series of drugs (79,105).

The relationships for the three classes of agent are essentially parallel but, for the same degree of calculated solubility of the local anesthetic base, the intrinsic potencies were found to be in the order amino ester >amino amide >piperidine amide (106). However, the relationship between potency and physicochemical properties is complex. The distribution coefficients are the result of the composite chemical group effects. Different relationships might apply in vivo, especially for chiral agents. The relative proportions of base and conjugate acid of the individual agents depends on their pK_a. Most relationships are developed in terms of base concentrations only when it is known that both forms are required for membrane stabilizing effect. Overall, a high lipid solubility would be expected to promote drug entry into membranes by increasing the diffusion rate, but this has to be balanced with a high fraction of drug in the nonionized state (106–108). The net effect on onset of maximum anesthetic action is difficult to predict, however, because a faster rate of diffusion is offset by a greater capacity for uptake into a membrane.

It has been found that high lipophilicity alone also does not predict the relative rate of transfer of local anesthetics and chemically similar drugs through meninges in ex vivo models (73). The ex vivo apparent permeability coefficients of homologous N-alkyl piperidine amides and a series of heterologous amide and ester caines follow a bell-shaped curve with increasing lipophilicity; their in vivo rate of absorption from site of administration in the epidural space to CSF constantly decreases with increasing lipophilicity, but their fractional availability to CSF increases (64,67). This apparent paradox reflects the relative balance in competing routes of local distribution into local fixed structures and clearance by local vasculature. Further complexities pertain even within homologous series. Because pK_a values also increase with increasing alkyl substitution, the nonionized fraction increases significantly. Moreover, even when lipid solubility and nonionized fraction are taken into account, the intrinsic potency of the agents is subject to differences in preferred molecular geometry for fit to the local anesthetic receptor site (108). However, it is generally found that by promoting interaction with the hydrophobic components of receptors, a high lipid solubility will increase potency and duration of effect.

Protein Binding

Most drugs *reversibly* bind to/associate with proteins (and various other macromolecules) to some extent. This association, when it occurs within the body, can provide a transport medium and/or a temporary repository for the drug. Drug binding to proteins is a secondary property originating from physicochemical and stereochemical properties that has received much attention with local anesthetic agents.

Thermodynamic characterization of drug binding treats it as an adsorption process and involves the molar concentration of binding protein(s), the molar concentration of binding sites (or number per molecule of protein), and the association/dissociation constants of the interaction. *Pharmacologic characterization*, however, is more concerned with determining which protein(s) are involved, and the extent of binding at various drug and protein concentrations. If more than one drug and/or protein is involved, as typically occurs with drug binding in plasma, the relative extent(s) of binding will be governed by the (competitive) relative affinity constants of the separate drug–protein interactions.

Besides being more lipophilic, the longer-acting local anesthetics also exhibit higher degrees of binding to plasma and tissue proteins (Table 3-1), with greater plasma binding of the agent in its base form at higher pH values (109–114). This suggests that the binding forces are predominantly hydrophobic. Steric factors also apply, so that the enantiomers of chiral local anesthetics usually exhibit differences in degree of binding to proteins, although the differences are usually smaller than those between agents where differences in lipophilicity predominate. Differences between the enantiomers of some drugs may

be large enough to account for differences in some receptor-related effects (e.g., for toxicity) or in pharmacokinetics (e.g., for distribution and/or metabolism).

Adsorption of local anesthetics to binding sites, or solubility within membranes or tissues, although producing relatively high apparent partition coefficients, may result in slower net penetration rates. This may be considered either as a lowering of diffusion coefficient or as a decrease in ΔC, the effective concentration gradient of diffusible drug (Equation 2). Binding of the drugs to proteins associated with the aqueous phases on either side of a membrane will affect the transfer and equilibrium distribution of total drug, analogously to ionization. Only the unbound drug will diffuse readily and, again, this will modify net drug transfer rate by an influence on ΔC.

DRUG ABSORPTION AND DISPOSITION

On the basis of an appreciation of the different structures and physicochemical properties of local anesthetics and the expected consequences of these differences, it is possible to inquire more specifically into their absorption and disposition in various parts of the body. In doing so, the fate of the agents is conveniently divided into consideration of their local disposition, systemic absorption, and systemic disposition and regional disposition (Fig. 3-4). The term *disposition* has a special meaning; it refers collectively to the processes of *drug distribution* into and out of tissues, and *drug elimination* by excretion and/or metabolism, while specifically excluding the process of absorption into the bloodstream.

Local Disposition

In contrast to many drugs, the primary effects of local anesthetics at both the pharmacologic level (neural blockade) and clinical level (analgesia and anesthesia) can be measured fairly objectively. The anesthesiologist is concerned particularly with the onset, spread, quality, and duration of block of one or many nerves with differing morphology. Ultimately, however, these variables depend on the drug's concurrent distribution at, and dissipation from, the site of injection. Therefore, it would be valuable to have chemical measurements of the agents at these sites as a function of time in order to establish pharmacodynamic relationships. Regrettably, such data remain sparse, even from animals. Therefore, knowledge of the local disposition, or neurokinetics, of local anesthetics remains largely theoretical and is deduced from observation of the spatiotemporal changes in anesthetic effect, rather than from direct measurements of intraneural and perineural drug concentrations. Most data have been obtained from studying a particular agent under particular conditions. Despite these limitations, it is possible to draw some general conclusions.

Competing factors that affect local disposition of local anesthetics include dispersion by *bulk flow* of the injected solution, *diffusion*, and *binding* and *vascular uptake* of the agent (or relevant solute). Local blood supply is critical, as this is responsible for local clearance/systemic absorption of drug; metabolic breakdown seems less important, and is probably negligible with amide-type local anesthetic agents. It has been suggested that the local blood supply is responsible for delivery of drug to deeper structures of the spinal cord via the radicular arteries (115,116) but this is now considered unlikely (117). In addition to these factors, the pharmaceutic presentation of the agent can

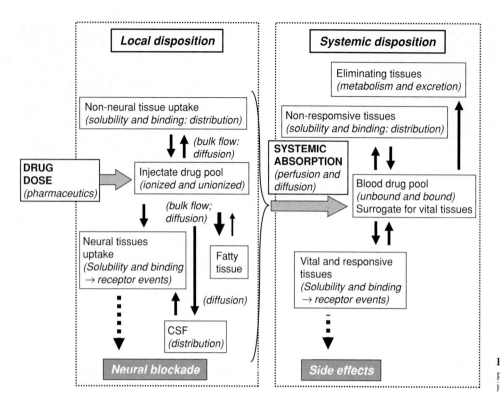

FIGURE 3-4. A conceptual model depicting the fate of local anesthetics injected perineurally.

be manipulated so that the rate of release of agent controls the balance between local and systemic uptake of the agent.

Although lipophilicity is an intrinsic physicochemical property of a drug resulting from its molecular structure, the effective lipophilicity can be altered by pharmaceutic presentation. A variety of drugs have been formulated with innovative methods to increase their local concentrations and/or residence times. Some examples include cyclodextrins to increase the local concentration of local anesthetics by making them more hydrophilic, and liposomes to make them more lipophilic. Both formulations have been found to be longer-acting after subarachnoid administration in laboratory animals than the simple aqueous solutions of the same drugs. The mechanisms of prolongation of action are presumed to differ but have in common the alteration of the rate of drug diffusion. Drugs combined with cyclodextrins are believed to have a slower rate of vascular absorption than aqueous solutions. Liposome or polylactide microsphere encapsulation provides a depot from which drug is released slowly. Liposomal preparations of local anesthetic agents have both a longer duration of action and a lower propensity for systemic toxicity than equivalent doses in aqueous media injected perivascularly, epidurally, or intrathecally in experimental animals (118–121) and in epidural, intercostal, or subcutaneous anesthesia in humans (122–124). Moreover, liposomal preparations of local anesthetic agents have a higher rate of penetration of the dermis than equivalent aqueous solutions (125).

Bulk Flow

The extent of spread of the injected solution might be expected to depend on its volume, the force (rate) with which it is injected, the turbulence generated, the size of the injected space, the physical resistance offered by tissues and fluids, gravity, the position of the patient during and after injection, and the resultant pressure gradients exerted by these factors. Bulk flow

of local anesthetic solutions has been assessed by the use of marker dyes, radiographic contrast media, external counting techniques, and spinal canal models (126–129). Although the spread of analgesia may also indicate the extent of bulk flow, these are not necessarily equivalent because spread of effect is also determined by solute diffusion and local perfusion. For example, the observation that the epidural injection of bupivacaine in glycerol produced longer duration of analgesia than when injected in normal saline was interpreted as being due to a bupivacaine depot (130). Although this may be so, it also may be that the higher viscosity of the glycerol solution reduced the rate of bulk flow, thereby increasing the concentration of bupivacaine diffusing into the nerve structures. Indeed, the presence of fibrous septa within the injected spaces may create compartmentalization of perivascular spaces, thereby becoming the ultimate determinants of the observed effect by affecting the balance between bulk flow of local anesthetic solution and diffusion of local anesthetic agent (131).

Diffusion

Once the local anesthetic has been deposited and has spread physically in the extraneural fluids, it finds its way to sites of action in and on the nerve membrane largely by the process of diffusion (see Chapter 2).

The pattern of drug distribution within the cord is a complex function of accessibility by diffusion from the CSF, the relative myelin (lipoidal) content of various tracts, and the rate of drug removal by local perfusion. Recent studies in pigs, using opioids and microdialysis to sample the epidural space and CSF to perform a kinetic analysis, indicated complexity of the spinal pharmacokinetics of these drugs. The results with a series of opioids that have similar physicochemical properties to local anesthetic revealed that the bioavailability to the CSF and epidural space is determined primarily by their hydrophobicity, with less-hydrophobic drugs having greater bioavailability

(132). Other studies in animals using radiolabeled local anesthetics have shown their accumulation along the posterior and lateral aspects of the spinal cord as well as in the spinal nerve roots, but not to such a degree in the dorsal root ganglion or in the more central parts of the cord. Uptake of drug is higher in the gray matter than in the white matter of the cord, and posterior nerve roots had higher concentrations than anterior roots. Overall, the working model (Fig. 3-4) may be viewed as a reasonable representation of the central neuraxial fate of local anesthetics. By altering the ratio of base and conjugate acid, diffusion of local anesthetic agents can be influenced by a pH gradient, and differences in diffusion of local anesthetics can cause differences in neural penetration, thereby affecting differential block.

Although stereochemical interactions between drugs and biomembranes may occur, the rates of diffusion of bupivacaine enantiomers across isolated meningeal membrane were found not to be enantioselective (69,75). Others have produced evidence for a pharmacokinetic explanation for tachyphylaxis after peripheral intra- or extraneural sciatic or subcutaneous administration of (pH 7.0 adjusted) lidocaine in rats. They found that progressive tachyphylaxis to nociceptive stimuli was associated with diminished respective neural or skin concentrations of lidocaine and claimed a pharmacokinetic (diffusion) basis for tachyphylaxis (133), but local tissue pH, unfortunately, was not measured as a variable.

pH Effects. Any factor that creates local extracellular acidosis should retard net diffusion of local anesthetic to the nerve by increasing and sustaining drug ionization (see Equation 5), and this was demonstrated by Ibusuki, et al. (134), using procaine and crayfish giant axons. A low pH may be preexisting, for example, as a result of infection, or may be induced by injection of the anesthetic solution. A number of studies have indicated that raising the pH of local anesthetic solutions to near neutral often hastens the onset of effects, sometimes prolongs the duration of effects, and usually decreases the local irritation or pain on injection. Capongna et al. (93) found that alkalinization produced the best results with lidocaine and bupivacaine for epidural block, with lidocaine for brachial plexus block, and with mepivacaine for sciatic and femoral nerve blocks. Such effects are not inevitable, however, and shortened onset was not demonstrated with local anesthetic mixtures used for ophthalmic sub-Tenon block or lidocaine for brachial plexus anesthesia (135–137).

Differential Block. The propensity to produce a marked differential blockade is a characteristic of some long-acting local anesthetic agents, particularly tetracaine and etidocaine, which produce profound motor blockade; bupivacaine provides a balance of analgesia and motor loss, whereas ropivacaine and levobupivacaine can provide analgesia with a minimum of motor loss (46,138,139). In the case of epidural block, Bromage (140) suggested that this phenomenon may be due to deeper penetration of the spinal cord by more lipid-soluble agents causing interference with long descending motor pathways. Bupivacaine, however, is more lipid-soluble than tetracaine and lidocaine, which produce less differential sensory loss, and the differences in sensory–motor dissociation seen with the various agents are also apparent after peripheral nerve block procedures, in which penetration of the cord is not a factor (141). To accommodate the latter, differences in the ability of the agents to diffuse into individual sensory and motor fibers have been postulated (106). Thus, from electrophysiologic studies with isolated rabbit vagus nerve, Gissen et al. (142) concluded that, compared to etidocaine, less lipid-soluble bupivacaine diffuses relatively slowly into fast-conducting A (motor) fibers at low concentrations. This is supported by other electrophysiologic studies (143), although Fink and Cairns (144) discount diffusion within a nerve as a contributory factor to differential block. Nevertheless, when comparisons were made between a wide variety of agents, it was found that in vitro blockade of A-fibers occurred before that of C-fibers with procaine, ropivacaine, and bupivacaine and vice versa with tetracaine, etidocaine, and mepivacaine; blockade occurred at the same time with lidocaine. In summarizing the results of their studies, Wildsmith et al. (106) noted that equipotent concentrations of the various drugs blocked C-fibers at the same rate but that blockade of A-fibers was more dependent, as expected, on the physicochemical properties (see Chapter 2).

Metabolism

Local metabolism, if it occurs, has a negligible influence on the neurokinetics of local anesthetics and the time course of conduction blockade.

SYSTEMIC ABSORPTION

Local anesthetics produce their intended effects at or near their site of deposition, without requiring transit through the blood to a blood-perfused "effect site." Indeed, their presence in the circulation is normally undesirable, being associated with lessened intended actions and an increased risk of systemic toxicity. Used in combination with information about putatively "toxic" blood (or plasma or serum) concentrations of local anesthetic agents, knowledge of their systemic absorption helps to set confidence limits on the *likelihood of a systemic toxic reaction* after various block procedures. This, apart from curiosity or regulatory requirement, is the main reason for measuring their blood concentrations. Indirectly, appreciation of rates of systemic absorption can suggest also the relationship between block and the amount of drug remaining at the site of injection, and this information can be useful in assessing other relevant phenomena, such as the relative potency of the drugs.

In humans, measurement of drug concentration–time profiles in the peripheral circulation has been widely used to assess systemic uptake of the different agents after virtually every neural blockade procedure. Tables of these data have been published in many reviews (145,178). *Because these profiles are the net result of both systemic absorption and disposition, they are of value mainly to determine relative changes or differences in drug uptake after different agents, conditions or procedures.* The maximum plasma drug concentration (C_{max}) and the time of its occurrence (T_{max}) are, therefore, not absolute indicators of the absorption kinetics of local anesthetics administered perineurally. Nevertheless, C_{max} and T_{max}, when measured under comparable conditions, are useful in making clinically relevant (but superficial) comparisons between drugs, procedures, and/or subjects, but they must be qualified as to whether they were derived from arterial or venous blood samples, and if venous, which venous. Arterial blood drug concentrations are essentially the same at all sampling points. Venous blood drug concentrations normally differ according to local tissue morphology, venous tone, perfusion, and neural blockade, because the net rate of drug equilibration within the tissues is affected by these factors. Central venous blood drug concentrations resemble arterial concentrations, but are subject to modulation by drug uptake in the lungs.

In general, C_{max} in arterial blood for a particular local anesthetic and block procedure will primarily depend on the total

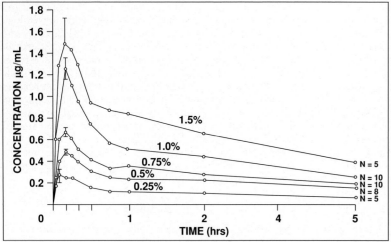
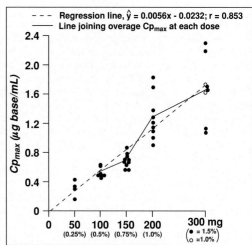

FIGURE 3-5. **A:** Plasma etidocaine concentration–time relationships after intercostal block in surgical patients with different concentrations (achiral assay). **B:** Maximum plasma etidocaine concentrations from the study in **A** showing the relationship of C_{max} to dose. Compiled from Van de Velde M, Dreelinck R, Dubois J, et al. Determination of the full dose–response relation of intrathecal bupivacaine, levobupivacaine, and ropivacaine, combined with sufentanil, for labor analgesia. Data from Bridenbaugh PO, Tucker GT, Moore DC, et al. Preliminary clinical evaluation of etidocaine (Duranest): A new long-acting local anesthetic agent. *Acta Anaesthesiol Scand* 1974;18:165.

dose (Figs. 3-5 and 3-6). As a rule, a larger C_{max} and a shorter T_{max} will occur from drug administration into regions of higher perfusion. In general, the time of greatest risk of systemic toxicity coincides with T_{max} in arterial blood, and this will vary from about 5 to 45 minutes; T_{max} for peripheral venous blood will lag somewhat and vary from about 15 to 90 minutes (Fig. 3-7), with the values being mainly related to the speed of injection (147), drug and site of injection (148,149), and often with

inexplicable variability between subjects for a given treatment (150). Note that T_{max} can be a fairly imprecise variable for comparing between studies as it also depends to some extent on the frequency of blood sampling.

Local Anesthetic Blood Concentrations and Toxicity

Commonly accepted thresholds for "CNS toxic" plasma concentrations from local anesthetic absorbed after uncomplicated

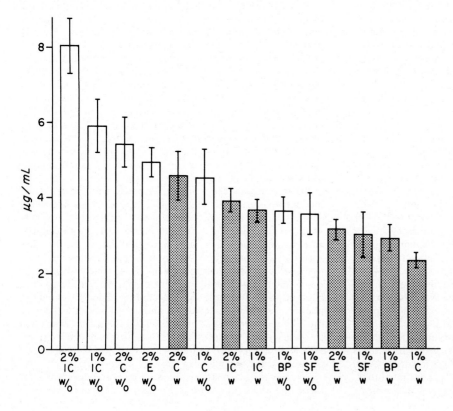

FIGURE 3-6. Systemic absorption of mepivacaine (achiral assay) in surgical patients after various regional block procedures, as indicated by the mean $C_{max} \pm$ SEM of the values. IC, intercostal block; C, caudal block; E, epidural block; BP, brachial plexus block; SF, sciatic/femoral block; w/o, plain solution; w, solution with epinephrine (1:200,000) *stippled bars.* Compiled from Tucker GT, Moore DC, Bridenbaugh PO, et al. Systemic absorption of mepivacaine in commonly used regional block procedures. *Anesthesiology* 1972;37:277.

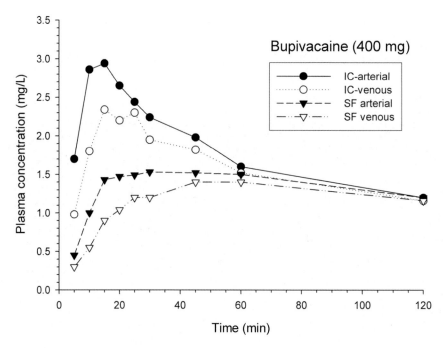

FIGURE 3-7. Arterial and venous mean plasma concentrations of bupivacaine (achiral assay) in surgical patients after intercostal or sciatic/femoral block procedures showing the magnitude and time course of the arteriovenous difference when sampled across the forearm. Compiled and redrawn from Moore DC, Mather LE, Bridenbaugh LD, et al. Arterial and venous plasma levels of bupivacaine (Marcaine) following epidural and intercostal nerve blocks. *Anessthesiology* 1976;45:39; and Moore DC, Mather LE, Bridenbaugh PO, et al. Arterial and venous plasma levels of bupivacaaine following peripheral nerve blocks. *Anesth Analg* 1976;55:763.

perineural administration range from 5 to 10 μg/mL for lidocaine, mepivacaine, and prilocaine, and from 2 to 4 μg/mL for bupivacaine, ropivacaine, and levobupivacaine. Higher values have a higher probability of associated toxic effects, and vice versa.

It is intuitive that a greater circulating blood concentration of any local anesthetic agent is more likely to be associated with a greater risk of systemic toxicity than a lesser one. However, a deterministic relationship between blood drug concentration and toxicity is tenuous for several reasons. First, the rate of change of plasma drug concentrations is an important, but often neglected, element in the relationship because it relates to the degree of equilibration between tissue and blood drug concentrations—that is, how well the blood drug concentrations provide a reliable surrogate for the relevant tissue drug concentrations. Second, toxicity normally occurs concomitantly in different regions, and there can be both direct and indirect effects, for example, with cardiac effects deriving from direct myocardial effects *and* from CNS cardiac control mechanisms. Third, the concurrent physiologic and pharmacologic condition of the subject (e.g., blood gas/electrolyte/acid–base status, state of consciousness, etc.) can have marked influence on the outcome (148,151,152,166,167).

Several scenarios need to be distinguished pharmacokinetically: unusually rapid or normal persistent drug absorption from successful perineural administration, or unintended intravascular (usually IV, but occasionally intra-arterial) administration. Systemic toxicity from rapid absorption is usually acute, but relatively short-lived, whereas that from persistent absorption develops more slowly and recedes more slowly because the greater mass of drug deposited in the vital tissues takes longer to dissipate. Intravenous administration of sufficient dose usually produces sudden-onset, serious, acute generalized (whole body) effects that are usually rapidly receding, with a duration and severity related to the administered dose. Although reported relatively rarely, severely toxic effects can result from unintended intra-arterial injection of very small doses of local anesthetic agent into the afferent vasculature

of vital organs (153,154), and this has been exploited with intended and appropriate doses as a useful research technique for studying regionally selective toxicity (155,156). Thus, it is important to remember that direct toxic effects in one region (notably, the brain) can have profound effects in another region (notably, the heart) via neural and cardiovascular system (CVS) mechanisms. Crucially, both the toxic effects and the associated blood drug concentrations depend on the state of consciousness, so that extrapolation of data between anesthetized and conscious subjects is especially hazardous (473,473a).

Most data documenting local anesthetic toxicity in humans are gathered, essentially opportunistically and retrospectively, from acute incidents in patients undergoing neural blockade, or from prospective studies in a small cohort of healthy volunteers undergoing administration of the drugs for experimental purposes. For ethical reasons, human subjects can be given only mildly toxic doses when local anesthetics are administered intravenously for research, typically to the threshold of CNS subjective symptoms (152,157–162). Information about more serious toxicity must, therefore, be derived either from clinical circumstances in which the objectives are preservation of life and well-being, rather than acquisition of scientific data, or from laboratory animal models. Laboratory rodent and isolated-tissue models are widely used and are especially useful for elucidating mechanisms and for comparisons between drugs (163–165); however, these are generally limited by the restricted data that can be obtained, or because of their destructive nature, or because of the isolation of tissues from their normal milieu. On the other hand, large experimental animals (dogs, pigs, sheep) can be prepared to allow pharmacokinetics and pharmacodynamics to be observed concurrently in a context rather similar to patient treatment. The ultimate goals of such experiments are normally to set "fail-safe" guidelines for human drug use on the grounds that responses among mammalian species are fundamentally the same, and to elucidate principles that can be expected to apply to humans using methods, techniques, and drug doses that are not normally offered in humans.

TABLE 3-4

STUDIES OF THRESHOLD CENTRAL NERVOUS SYSTEM TOXICITY IN HEALTHY YOUNG ADULT VOLUNTEER SUBJECTS PERFORMED WITH INTRAVENOUS INFUSION OF LOCAL ANESTHETIC TO A MAXIMUM DOSE OR ONSET OF SUBJECTIVE SYMPTOMS

Agent	Reference	Number of subjects	Dose rate (mg/min)	Infusion time (min)	Number with subjective symptoms	Number with objective symptoms	Drug conc. (mg/L) Mean ($\pm$SD) or range	Sample site
Lidocaine	159, 160	5	20	12.5	5	2	~ 2.2	Ven
Bupivacaine	152	8	7.5	10	7	0	2.2–4.2	Art
Etidocaine	152	8	7.5	10	6	0	2.1–5.3	Art
Bupivacaine	161	12	15	To 15	Most	0	1.5 ($\pm$0.6)	Ven
Ropivacaine	161	12	15	To 15	Some	0	1.9 ($\pm$0.5)	Ven
Bupivacaine	158	12	10	To 25	All	Most	4.0 ($\pm$1.4)	Art
							2.1 ($\pm$1.2)	Ven
Ropivacaine	158	12	10	To 25	All	Some	4.3 ($\pm$0.6)	Art
							2.2 ($\pm$0.8)	Ven
Bupivacaine	157	14	10	To 15	All T	Some	2.25	Ven
Levobupivacaine	157	14	10	To 15	All T	Some	2.62	Ven

All T: all subjects infused to onset of subjective symptoms; Ven, peripheral venous blood sampling; Art: arterial blood sampling.

Although reported values such as those in Table 3-4 provide some useful guidelines, they refer to the mythic "average subject" and have to be interpreted in the light of many factors. These include whether measurements are made of plasma, serum, or blood drug concentrations; total or unbound (free) drug concentrations; relative enantiomer concentrations (if a racemic local anesthetic); active drug metabolite concentrations, as well as how the drug got into the plasma (intravenously or by vascular absorption), the rate of drug administration, the site of blood sampling (arterial or venous), how soon after drug administration the measured samples were drawn, and, most importantly, the physiologic status of the patient and, in particular, whether the patient was conscious and/or premedicated at the time (473a). In a previous era, the specificity and sensitivity of the drug assay procedure also could have been a factor, but this is rarely a concern with contemporary techniques. Thus, the values in Table 3-4 are more useful when circulating concentrations are not changing rapidly and there is time for equilibration between drug concentrations in plasma and vital tissues. Some individual subjects demonstrate toxic symptoms at lower drug concentrations than the commonly accepted values, whereas others do not demonstrate toxic symptoms despite having values within, or even greater than, those values (473b). In some cases, this is because of the development of locally high drug blood concentration. For example, local anesthetic drugs injected into patients with intracardiac right-left shunts (169) or injected inadvertently into the carotid or vertebral artery during attempted stellate ganglion block, bypass the lung, resulting in a high probability of CNS toxicity (153,154).

Extent and Rate of Absorption

In the absence of local metabolism, all of a dose deposited perineurally will eventually become absorbed into the systemic circulation. The concentration gradient is the main driving force for dissipation of drug both from its (heterogeneous) perineural site of administration into local tissues and uptake into the blood. The net resulting rate of systemic drug absorption will, therefore, be approximated by the sum of exponentials[f] representing different rates of absorption from different local tissues, with the overall rate being governed by the agent's distribution coefficient into, and the local perfusion of, the dominant tissue(s). A similar pattern pertains to drugs in the systemic circulation. Concentration gradients drive the exchange of drug between blood (strictly, plasma water) and tissues (strictly, extracellular fluids), including regions that excrete and metabolize drug. This pattern can also usually be represented by the sum of exponentials, in which the drug concentration approaches zero as time increases because of its excretion and/or metabolism lumped together as elimination (see systemic disposition, which is discussed later in the text).

If blood drug concentration–time profiles are available after perineural and IV administration, then it becomes possible to calculate the rate(s) of drug absorption. The underlying principle of this is that an IV injection reflects the whole-body (systemic) disposition of the drug; that is, distribution and elimination after it has arrived in the systemic circulation. Conversely, a perineural administration reflects the concurrent whole-body disposition of drug while arriving and once in the systemic circulation. The mathematical procedure of *numerical deconvolution* is used to determine the rate of leaving the (perineural) site of administration; this is depicted in Figure 3-8, where "pools" are shown to represent functional regions of drug deposition (rather than precise anatomic spaces). These calculations were originally performed for local anesthetics after IV regional anesthesia (170); subsequently, the method was extended to epidural anesthesia, with determination of the IV pharmacokinetics on a separate occasion (171). More recent technical developments have allowed application to a variety of subjects undergoing epidural and subarachnoid blocks, in which a concurrent small dose of deuterium-labeled agent is administered intravenously (172–177). The two forms of the

---

[f]In which drug concentration in some form is related to time in an exponential product, so that the rate of change of concentration is proportional to how much drug is present at any nominated time (referred to as *first-order kinetics*).

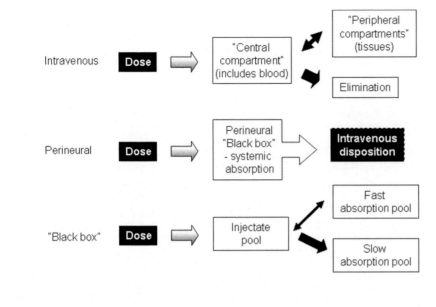

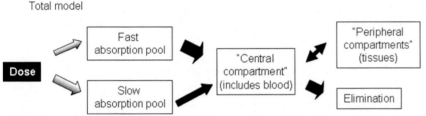

FIGURE 3-8. Conceptual model of local anesthetics injected perineurally used to calculate the rate of systemic absorption using the numerical deconvolution technique. The important assumption is that the systemic disposition of the drug, as revealed by intravenous administration, remains the same when the drug is administered perineurally. With the stable isotope method, the intravenous disposition is determined concurrently with the neural blockade.

agent (native and labeled) are then separated analytically by mass spectrometry, and the rate of absorption of the native form used for the block is again determined by numerical deconvolution.

Such pharmacokinetic calculations provide a mathematical-statistical description of a functional process whereby the drug acts a tracer; nevertheless, the description has physical elements. Because local anesthetics are relatively lipophilic compounds they will partition into tissues around their site of administration. Thus, their vascular absorption rates will be directly related to blood flow and inversely to local tissue binding (distribution coefficient). Important local determinants of systemic absorption include those affecting the tissue distribution, including the site of injection, the lipophilicity and vasoactivity of the agent, the presence of additives such as vasoconstrictors, other formulation factors intended to modify local drug residence and release, the influence of nerve block, and (patho)physiologic features of the patient.

It has been found that systemic absorption after epidural administration can be described, in its simplest form, by a bi-exponential function; that is, the drug behaves as if it has been deposited into two portions with different absorption rate constants, roughly reflecting regions with identifiably different low-affinity/high-perfusion and high-affinity/low-perfusion characteristics. Although a mathematical construct, this can be likened to the drug physically partitioning between aqueous (faster absorption) and fatty (slower absorption) pools; the fraction of the dose going to the slower absorption pool increases with the more lipophilic agents (Table 3-5; Fig. 3-9) and/or when a vasoconstrictor is used (171,172,178). T_{max} for a particular type of nerve block tends to occur at about the same time because the early absorption is dominated by the faster absorption rate constant, which is similar for all agents. However, the half-life of the drug in plasma is dominated by the slower absorption rate constant, and this is normally slower than the elimination rate constant. The real anatomic situation is, however, much more complex than a simple two-pool model.

Overall, for a given blood sampling site, C_{max} and T_{max} are inversely related in that the greater the T_{max} then the lower the value of C_{max}. Extensive data on C_{max} and T_{max} of the amide local anesthetics after various routes of injection have been tabulated elsewhere (145,178). So too have data on (poly)exponential equation exponents and coefficients describing the rate(s) of systemic absorption after epidural administration (171–178). Such data are mainly useful for comparison between drugs, or recipients of drugs.

Agent

Differences between agents need to be assessed under comparable conditions regarding drug administration, subject choice, and subject preparation. Inspection of C_{max} and T_{max} after epidural injection of plain solutions of the amide local anesthetics, and allowing for differences in sampling regimens, shows that the increment in peak whole blood drug concentration per 100 mg of dose is about 0.9 to 1.0 μg/mL for lidocaine and mepivacaine, slightly less for prilocaine, and approximately 50% to 60% as much for bupivacaine, etidocaine, ropivacaine, and levobupivacaine (167,172,178–180). Although differences in disposition kinetics contribute to this order, it appears that, despite similar times of peak concentrations, net absorption of the longer-acting, more lipophilic agents is slower. This is consistent with experimental data on residual concentrations of

TABLE 3-5

MEAN (±SD) FRACTIONS AND HALF-LIVES CHARACTERIZING THE ABSORPTION OF LIDOCAINE, BUPIVACAINE, LEVOBUPIVACAINE, AND ROPIVACAINE AFTER EPIDURAL AND LIDOCAINE AND BUPIVACAINE AFTER SUBARACHNOID ADMINISTRATIONS

	Epidural				Subarachnoid	
	Lidocaine**	Bupivacaine**	Levobupivacaine**	Ropivacaine**	Lidocaine*	Bupivacaine**
FASTER ABSORPTION PROCESS						
F_1	0.38 ± 0.12	0.29 ± 0.08	0.21 ± 0.06	0.27 ± 0.08	–	0.35 ± 0.17
$T_{1/2}$ fast (min)	9.3 ± 3.8	8.1 ± 3.9	6.6 ± 2.9	10.7 ± 5.2	–	50 ± 27
SLOWER ABSORPTION PROCESS						
F_2	0.58 ± 0.07	0.67 ± 0.11	0.83 ± 0.13	0.77 ± 0.12	1.01 ± 0.11	0.96 ± 0.16
$T_{1/2}$ slow (min)	82 ± 19	335 ± 97	426 ± 135	248 ± 64	71 ± 17	408 ± 275

Fraction of dose absorbed (F_{abs}) at time (t) = $F_1 + F_2$ is an exponential function of time. $F_1 + F_2 \approx 1.0$.
*Mono-exponential equation: $F_{abs} = F_2 . e^{-f2.t}$
**Bi-exponential equation: $F_{abs} = F_1 . e^{-f1.t} + F_2 . e^{-f2.t}$
Data were derived using perineural block with each agent in comparable groups of surgical patients. Each patient also had a concurrent intravenous dose of stable isotope-labeled local anesthetic to determine the systemic disposition. From the combined data, the rates of systemic absorption of the agent was determined by numerical deconvolution. Compiled from Burm, AG. Clinical pharmacokinetics of epidural and spinal anaesthesia. *Clin Pharmacokinet* 1989; 16:283–311; Burm, AGL, Vermeulen NPE, Van Kleef JW, et al. Pharmacokinetics of lidocaine and bupivacaine in surgical patients following epidural administration. Simultaneous investigation of absorption and disposition kinetics using stable isotopes. *Clin Pharmacokinet* 1987;13:191; Simon MJ, Veering BT, Stienstra R, et al. Effect of age on the clinical profile and systemic absorption and disposition of levobupivacaine after epidural administration. *Br J Anaesth* 2004;93(4):512–520; Simon MJ, Veering BT, Vletter AA, et al. The effect of age on the systemic absorption and systemic disposition of ropivacaine after epidural administration. *Anesth Analg* 2006;102:276–282; Veering BT, Burm AG, Vletter AA, et al. The effect of age on the systemic absorption, disposition and pharmacodynamics of bupivacaine after epidural administration. *Clin Pharmacokinet* 1992;22:75; Veering BT, Burm, AGL, Vletter AA, et al. The effect of age on systemic absorption and systemic disposition of bupivacaine after subarachnoid administration. *Anesthesiology* 1991;74:250; Simon MJ, Veering BT, Stienstra R, et al. The systemic absorption and disposition of levobupivacaine 0.5% after epidural administration in surgical patients: A stable-isotope study. *Eur J Anaesth* 2004;21:460–470; Veering BT, Burm AG, Feyen HM et al. Pharmacokinetica of bupivacaine during postoperative epidural infusion: Enantioselectivity and role of protein binding. *Anesthesiology* 2002;96(5): 1062–1069; and Veering BT, Burm AGL, Van Kleef JW, et al. Epidural anesthesia with bupivacaine: Effects of age on neural blockade and pharmacokinetics. *Anesth Analg* 1987;66:589.

the agents in epidural fat after injection into sheep (178) and is confirmed by deconvolution calculations of the time course of drug absorption in humans (173–175,178,180).

Differences in the net absorption rates of the various agents have implications for their accumulation during repeated and continuous administration. Whereas systemic accumulation is more marked with the short-acting amides, extensive local accumulation is predicted for the longer-acting compounds, despite their longer dosage intervals (171,181,182). Observations of relatively low blood concentrations of prilocaine with respect to the toxic threshold, particularly after brachial plexus block (Fig. 3-10) and IV regional anesthesia, support the claim that this compound should be the agent of choice for such single-dose procedures (183). For prilocaine and for articaine, a high systemic clearance, rather than slow absorption, is responsible mainly for the relatively low blood drug concentrations (12,183).

Although the rate of systemic absorption of local anesthetics is controlled largely by the extent of local binding, their relative intrinsic vasoactive properties could also modulate local perfusion and hence uptake. However, the effects are a complex function of drug, dose, enantiomer, and type and tone of blood vessel, and their relevance to the overall relative absorption of drugs after peripheral and central nerve blocks is difficult to evaluate (172). Nevertheless, it has been suggested, for example, that an increase in epidural blood flow (whether mediated locally or by change in cardiac output or both), with assumed increase in the systemic absorption rate of bupivacaine, is an important factor leading to regression of anal-

gesia during the continuous epidural infusion of bupivacaine (184). Furthermore, the vasodilatory effect of bupivacaine on cerebral pial, cutaneous, and epidural blood vessels contrasts strikingly with the relative net vasoconstrictor effect of ropivacaine and levobupivacaine, a difference that may contribute to their relative anesthetic profiles (185–187a). Others, however, have found the effects on cutaneous blood vessels to be biphasic: vasodilatory at high concentrations and vasoconstrictive at low concentrations—clearly, the choice of exploratory model and conditions is critical in evaluating the net effects (188,189). Although *R*-bupivacaine was found to be two to three times more potent than *S*-bupivacaine in blocking nerve fibers in vitro (190), this intrinsic difference in action may be modulated in vivo by the dominant stereoselective effects on blood vessels. Thus, the *S*-enantiomer amide local anesthetics are longer acting than the *R*-enantiomers after separate subcutaneous injection, apparently reflecting a greater vasoconstrictor activity and, therefore, a presumed slower systemic absorption (14,191). Similar logic about the greater vasoconstrictor activity of ropivacaine than bupivacaine has been used to rationalize the slower apparent rate of ropivacaine absorption. For example, after caudal administration of 2 mg/kg doses of 0.2% solutions in children undergoing hypospadias repair, there was no significant difference in mean C_{max} of the two agents, but the mean T_{max} of ropivacaine occurred significantly later (65 minutes, c.f. 20 minutes). As the plasma concentrations were measured in peripheral venous blood, it is not possible to confirm this explanation because the C_{max} T_{max} values depended upon the rate of equilibration of drug between blood and

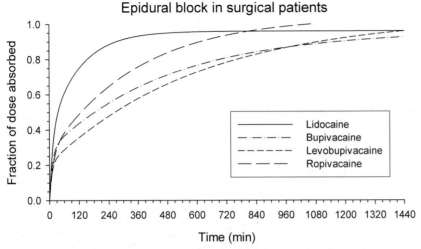

Epidural block in surgical patients

Lidocaine
Bupivacaine
Levobupivacaine
Ropivacaine

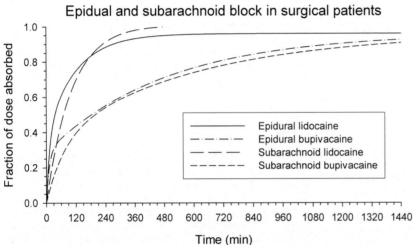

Epidual and subarachnoid block in surgical patients

Epidural lidocaine
Epidural bupivacaine
Subarachnoid lidocaine
Subarachnoid bupivacaine

FIGURE 3-9. Display of fraction of dose absorbed into the systemic circulation plotted as a function of time after epidural injection of selected amide local anesthetics, as determined by the stable isotope method in comparable patient populations. The curves represent bi-exponential functions fitted to the rate of systemic absorption. Compiled and redrawn from Burm, AGL, Vermeulen NPE, Van Kleef JW, et al. Pharmacokinetics of lidocaine and bupivacaine in surgical patients following epidural administration. Simultaneous investigation of absorption and disposition kinetics using stable isotopes. *Clin Pharmacokinet* 1987;13:191; Simon MJ, Veering BT, Stienstra R, et al. Effect of age on the clinical profile and systemic absorption and disposition of levobupivacaine after epidural administration. *Br J Anaesth* 2004;93(4):512–520; Simon MJ, Veering BT, Vletter AA, et al. The effect of age on the systemic absorption and systemic disposition of ropivacaine after epidural administration. *Anesth Analg* 2006;102:276–282; Veering BT, Burm AG, Vletter AA, et al. The effect of age on the systemic absorption, disposition and pharmacodynamics of bupivacaine after epidural administration. *Clin Pharmacokinet* 1992;22:75; Veering BT, Burm, AGL, Vletter AA, et al. The effect of age on systemic absorption and systemic disposition of bupivacaine after subarachnoid administration. *Anesthesiology* 1991;74:250; and Simon MJ, Veering BT, Stienstra R, et al. The systemic absorption and disposition of levobupivacaine 0.5% after epidural administration in surgical patients: A stable-isotope study. *Eur J Anaesth* 2004;24:460–470.

forearm tissues, and was complicated further by the patients being under isoflurane anesthesia (192).

Site of Administration

Anatomic features, such as vascularity and the presence of tissue and fat that can bind local anesthetics, are primary influences on their rate of distribution within, and removal from, specific sites of injection. As revealed by imaging or dyes at various sites of local anesthetic injection, other features, such as the presence of septa or other fibrous tissues (and any resultant pressure gradients), also contribute to distribution of solution and thus spread of anesthesia (131,193–196). This is pertinent to all procedures of neural blockade, but particularly so for the central neuraxis, where the detailed anatomy is complex and obscured from the anesthesiologist, variable between individuals, and still largely unresolved with respect to the resultant block (197,198).

On the whole, and under comparable circumstances, as judged by C_{max} values with regard for the effective dose, the net absorption rate decreases independently of the local anesthetic agent used, in the order intercostal block >caudal block >epidural block >brachial plexus block >sciatic and femoral nerve block (Fig. 3-6) (148,149,199,200). As indicated earlier, arterial plasma drug concentrations precede and exceed

those in peripheral venous plasma, regardless of the agent. A study with epidural ropivacaine found that the forearm arteriovenous gradient diminished exponentially, with the difference essentially extinguished about 1 hour after administration (201), as would be expected from the time needed for drug concentration in the tissues to equilibrate with that in the venous blood. However, different conclusions might have been reached had the same study been performed by determining the drug arteriovenous concentration gradient in a lower limb because the block itself would have influenced the venous tone of the upper and lower limbs differently (171). Concurrent administration of general anesthetics and some medications can alter the time courses of arterial and venous plasma drug concentrations through local and systemic cardiovascular effects, and this may be observed when data from surgical patients and nonsurgical patients or healthy volunteers are compared.

Studies of epidural administration, as discussed earlier, found that the systemic absorption of several local anesthetics could be described as a bi-exponential process, differing only in the net rates; a similar description was proposed for paravertebral ropivacaine (192), and a mono-exponential process was described for subarachnoid lidocaine (172). These descriptions are consistent with anatomic findings, as demonstrated in sheep, of prolonged sequestration of more lipid-soluble local

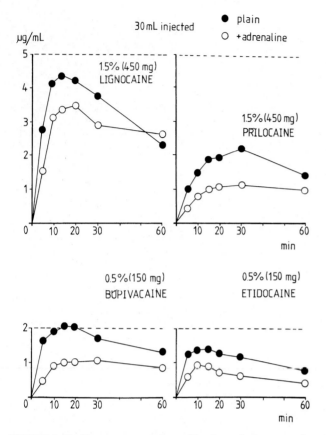

FIGURE 3-10. Plasma concentrations of local anesthetic agents after interscalene brachial plexus block (30 mL volume) with or without added epinephrine. Data from Wildsmith JAW, Tucker GT, Cooper S, et al. Plasma concentrations of local anaesthetics after interscalene brachial plexus block. *Br J Anaesth* 1977;49:237.

anesthetic drugs in epidural fat. Thus, it is clear that the net rates of absorption are mainly sensitive to the lipophilicity of the agent and the fattiness of the region where the agents are deposited.

Intercostal and Interpleural Blocks. The distribution of marker substances after injection into the costal grooves of cadavers has been investigated. It has been pointed out that variations in the anatomy of this region are far more common than has been commonly believed (202) and that information about the spread of solutions derived from cadaver studies may be misleading because of changes occurring postmortem (128). From studies of bupivacaine mixed with methylene blue dye in patients undergoing thoracotomy, Moorthy, et al. (128) concluded that the spread of anesthesia depends on the volume injected: a 5-mL injection spread through one intercostal space, but a 10-mL injection was more likely to spread to two or more intercostal spaces. Maximum absorbed concentrations of the agents after intercostal blocks using plain solutions are usually obtained rapidly, between 5 and 20 minutes, and may exceed individually toxic thresholds, but adverse systemic effects in patients, presumably, may be obtunded by the light general anesthesia/sedative premedication frequently used in patients undergoing these procedures. Since sustained high plasma drug concentrations are achieved during continuous intercostal infu-

sions, supplementary bolus injections are likely to be dangerous (203).

Wide spreading of injectate occurs following interpleural space injection, with pooling in the paravertebral space (204,205). Exposure of drug to a relatively large surface area of tissue, resulting in rapid systemic absorption, emphasizes the potentially small safety margin of the interpleural block technique. Maximum plasma concentrations of bupivacaine are higher but occur later than when the same dose is injected for intercostal block (206). Dosage and plasma drug concentrations measured after interpleural injection of bupivacaine vary widely among studies. However, in patients undergoing cholecystectomy or laparotomy, van Kleef et al. (207) advocate the use of an initial bolus dose of 100 mg followed by continuous infusion of 5 mL/h of 0.25% bupivacaine with epinephrine. This has been shown to be safe, with no further gain in analgesic effect occurring with increased dose. Although Laurito et al. (208) observed that plasma bupivacaine concentrations often increased above the putative toxic threshold of 2 μg/mL using the same infusion rate as van Kleef et al. (206), no adverse effects were observed; this may reflect the postoperative rise in plasma drug binding. In contrast to van Kleef et al. (207) and Laurito et al. (208), who measured continually rising plasma drug concentrations throughout prolonged infusion, Kastrissios et al. (209) observed a steady state.

Epidural and Caudal Blocks. Local anesthetic solution injected epidurally spreads cephalad and caudad as if in a distensible, but leaky, sleeve in which the local anesthetic solution concurrently leaks from foraminae and the local anesthetic agent diffuses into tissues, including dorsal root ganglion cells, and into the CSF (67,71,72,197,198). Although the relationship between injected volume (discrete dose) and number of anesthetized dermatomes has been described mathematically by a cubic polynomial equation (210), this has no physical significance. Not surprisingly, individual variability in the surface area and composition of the epidural space are primary determinants of epidural anesthesia (211,212).

The results of studies on the spread of analgesia indicate a minor influence of injection speed (213–215). It has been suggested that, for comparisons, the dose/segment is a more useful outcome variable than spread alone (216,217). Confounding factors include the drug used, the age and size of the patient, the range of injection pressures, and the approach and direction of the needle bevel (175,196,218,219,219a). It has been claimed that the presence or absence of epinephrine is not a significant factor (216). Insofar as epidural opioids can provide analogies for local anesthetics with similar physicochemical properties, the effects of epinephrine on spinal pharmacokinetics has been found to be more complex than can be explained by simple "greater local retention," and is not predictable from simple observation of plasma drug concentrations (132).

Overall, after epidural administration, the extent of local anesthesia results from cephalad–caudad spread of solution and diffusion of local anesthetic to the spinal cord and nerve roots, as well as transport within the CSF. The apparent rates of systemic absorption and fractions of the dose transferred into CSF of the local anesthetics are inversely proportional to lipophilicity (67). This suggests that competition for drug between the various distribution and clearance processes after epidural administration favors vascular uptake (irreversible local clearance) over transmeningeal distribution. Nevertheless, local anesthetics appear rapidly in the CSF after epidural injection (72,220). Peak drug concentrations in the CSF occur within 10 to 20 minutes and are sufficient to produce blockade of spinal nerve roots. By 30 minutes, high drug concentrations are also achieved in the peripheral cord and in the spinal nerves in the paravertebral space (126). Apart from direct diffusion of drug across the dura, access to the cord, particularly the dorsal horn region, may be mediated (a) by diffusion; (b) by uptake into the posterior radicular branch of spinal segmental arteries, although subsequent work has suggested that this might be more a source of clearance from the cord rather than uptake (70,117); (c) by centripetal subneural and subpial spread from the remote paravertebral nerve trunks (126); and (d) by bulk flow through the arachnoid via the dural root sleeves, although the latter has not been supported by studies using dura ex vivo (70). These suggestions are consistent with clinical observations of the distribution of analgesia during induction and regression of epidural block. A segmental pattern of analgesia during onset may be related to the initial drug diffusion into spinal nerves and roots, with subsequent nonsegmental regression resulting from ultimate diffusion to structures within the cord (221). It is also clear that even a very small hole made during the introduction of an epidural needle can give rise to spuriously high "rates of diffusion" of drugs injected epidurally into the subarachnoid space (222).

Most studies have found no relationship between the various indices of body size and plasma concentrations of local anesthetic agents, but Sharrock et al. suggested that 20% to 40% of the variance in arterial plasma concentrations of bupivacaine could be explained by correlation with body surface in elderly surgical patients (223). The effect of fat deposits within the epidural space in delaying the absorption of local anesthetics has been discussed earlier, and this is the likely explanation for these observations. Local anesthetic will be taken up into the extradural veins and pass from there to the azygos vein. In the presence of raised intrathoracic pressure, absorbed drug could also be redirected up the internal vertebral venous system to cerebral sinuses. Vascular absorption of local anesthetic from different regions of the epidural space (cervical, lumbar, thoracic) appears to be similar (224), although the cardiovascular sequelae may differ markedly and thereby affect the systemic disposition of the agent.

Epidural infusions of local anesthetics are now in widespread use (225). When administered by infusion, the plasma concentrations will increase if the administration rate exceeds the total body clearance. Bupivacaine and ropivacaine both produce good pain relief in obstetric patients, but the plasma concentrations of ropivacaine were found to be greater than those of bupivacaine when administered at equal rates, despite the former having a greater mean total body clearance; such a discrepancy is, therefore, likely to be the result of the net slower absorption of bupivacaine (226). Others have found that ropivacaine plasma concentrations increased with duration of infusion in patients after surgery and were proportional to dose rate, indicating that the administration rate exceeded the mean total body clearance at that time (225a,225b,225c, 335,342,525,530,533).

Subarachnoid Block. Hydrodynamic considerations are more important after subarachnoid injection than after any other regional anesthetic procedure. Indeed, much of the variability in anesthetic spread from subarachnoid injection of local anesthetic results from the consequences of gravity, as well as of the various qualifying factors such as baricity of drug solution and patient posture acting on the local anesthetic solution (227–231). However, a variety of factors in addition to density have some influence on anesthetic spread; for example, the inclusion of glucose to affect baricity will also influence viscosity, whereas changes in solution volume and local anesthetic concentration both must be considered with respect to changes in total local anesthetic dose.

After subarachnoid injection, the relatively high lipid solubility of local anesthetic bases will promote local cord uptake rather than extensive cephalad spread via CSF flow. Thus, drug concentrations in the CSF decline rapidly in both directions from the point of injection and exponentially at the site of injection as uptake proceeds (229,232). Direct diffusion along the concentration gradient from CSF through the pia mater directly into the cord delivers drug only to the superficial parts of the structure. Access to deeper areas is effected by diffusion in the CSF contained in the spaces of Virchow-Robin, which connect with perineural clefts surrounding the bodies of nerve cells within the cord (233).

Because of the relatively small doses used for subarachnoid blocks, plasma drug concentrations are normally quite small and rarely associated with direct systemic effects. Nonetheless, the cardiovascular sequelae of subarachnoid block can be profound and thereby influence pharmacokinetics of the agent and other drugs used concurrently. Systemic uptake after subarachnoid injection is believed to occur predominantly after passage of drug across the dura into the more vascular epidural space, as well as from blood vessels within the spinal space, in the pia mater, and in the cord itself. Extensive diffusion into the epidural space would be expected to result in sequestration in fat, thereby retarding the absorption of the longer-acting agents to a greater extent than the shorter-acting ones. Deconvolution analysis shows that there is a slower net absorption of bupivacaine than lidocaine (Table 3-5). The slower initial uptake from the subarachnoid space may reflect delay imposed by dural diffusion; the similarity of the slower uptake phase for subarachnoid and epidural bupivacaine suggests that the common rate-limiting removal is that from epidural fat.

Brachial Plexus Block. Progression of blockade from upper arm to hand and then to fingers is explained by more rapid diffusion of local anesthetic into mantle fibers that innervate more proximal regions than do the core fibers. To explain why the onset of motor block often precedes that of sensory loss, Winnie et al. (234) suggested that the effect of the larger diameter of the motor fibers is offset by their more peripheral location in the median nerve compared to sensory fibers. According to the classical view, the sequence of recovery should be the same as that of onset: arm first, then hand and fingers. This follows if the concentration gradient within the nerve now becomes reversed, decreasing from core to mantle. However, this has been challenged by Winnie et al. (235), who observed the reverse order of recovery, with significant motor block that outlasted analgesia. To account for these findings, it was proposed that a more rapid vascular uptake of agent occurs near the more distally innervating sensory fibers located in the core of the nerve. As intraneural blood vessels pass from mantle to core, they become increasingly branched and thus offer a larger surface area for drug absorption.

The various techniques for blocking the brachial plexus are not associated with significant differences in local anesthetic absorption rate (236–238). True differences in rates of systemic absorption between similar drugs are not revealed by simple observation of C_{max} and T_{max}, again presumably reflecting their absorption being rate-limited by their uptake from fatty tissues. For example, when administered in the same doses (2.7 mg/kg) for axillary brachial plexus block, bupivacaine and ropivacaine had the same mean plasma C_{max} (1.5 μg/mL) and

T_{max} (0.9 h); however, the mean plasma half-life of ropivacaine was 7.7 hours whereas that of bupivacaine was 17.1 hours (239). As the mean plasma half-life after IV administration for both drugs is only 2 to 3 hours (see later discussion), the longer values after brachial plexus administration of both agents presumably reflect their mean absorption times, with the greater value for bupivacaine.

Plasma concentrations of prilocaine after multiple injections for brachial plexus block were found to be predictable from first-dose data (240). Efficacious prolongation of interscalene block by continuous infusion of ropivacaine (0.75% 30 mL for the initial block, followed by 0.2% 12 or 18 mL/h for 48 hours) has been demonstrated after shoulder surgery. These regimens produce dose-related plasma ropivacaine concentrations without signs or symptoms of toxicity (241).

Head and Neck Blocks. Superficial or deep block of the cervical plexus can be performed with a single large or several small injections: Spread of the injectate is, therefore, an important factor in anesthetic outcome and systemic absorption of the local anesthetic agent (195). Junca et al. (242) compared ropivacaine (0.75%) and bupivacaine (0.5%) for cervical plexus block and found that the arterial C_{max} of bupivacaine (mean 3.02, range 0.98–5.82 μg/mL) was less than that of ropivacaine (4.25, 2.07–6.59 μg/mL) but equivalent when scaled to these equi-anesthetic doses. Others have found that plasma bupivacaine concentrations were the same when 15 mL of 0.5% solution was injected deeply as a single dose or divided into three equal doses (C_{max} single injection 2.3 ± 1.4 versus multiple injections 2.3 ± 1.1 μg/mL; T_{max} single injection 12 ± 7 versus multiple injections 13 ± 4 min), both being below the putative toxic threshold for bupivacaine; furthermore, there were no significant differences in mean block scores between the single-injection and the multiple-injections groups, evaluated either by the anesthesiologists or the surgeon (243).

Patients undergoing scalp block anesthesia for awake craniotomy with local anesthetic solution injected around the base of the scalp have been studied by measuring arterial plasma drug concentrations after injection of ropivacaine 0.75% (mean dose 260 mg) or levobupivacaine 0.5% (mean dose 177 mg), both with freshly added epinephrine (5 μg/mL). Observed mean C_{max} values were 1.5 μg/mL from ropivacaine and 1.6 μg/mL from levobupivacaine, with a T_{max} of around 10 to 20 minutes for both agents (244,245). The plasma concentrations from both agents were considered to be without consequence in these patients, who were obtunded by propofol/remifentanil sedation.

Endotracheal and Endobronchial Administration. Endotracheal doses of lidocaine up to 400 mg are associated with plasma drug concentrations that are well below the toxic threshold (178). The concentrations are significantly lower in spontaneously breathing patients than in paralyzed patients, since the former are more likely to swallow some of the dose, which then undergoes first-pass hepatic metabolism following absorption from the gut (246). Application only to areas below the vocal cords may result in excessive plasma drug concentrations because of reduced transfer to the gut (247). Plasma concentrations of lidocaine were found to be significantly lower when using an ultrasonic nebulizer compared to a conventional spray (248), possibly because of excretion in breath of the smaller particles delivered by the nebulizer. Systemic absorption of local anesthetic from the respiratory tree is, again, biphasic: An initial very rapid peak is followed by a second one at 5 to 30 minutes. The first phase appears to be less prominent after deep endobronchial administration of lidocaine compared to endotracheal instillation (249).

Subcutaneous Infiltration, Direct Tissue Infusion, and Intra-articular Injection. Subcutaneous infiltration of large doses of lidocaine is an essential component of the liposuction technique. When properly applied, the procedure is associated with unmistakably slow systemic drug absorption due, largely, to preferential lidocaine partitioning into fatty tissues prior to suctioning (250). Klein indicated 35 mg/kg as a conservative estimate of the safe maximum dose, based on the observation of C_{max} values well below the toxic threshold at 10 to 15 hours after injection (251). He emphasized the use of a dilute solution with added epinephrine, injected slowly over 45 minutes, whereas injection of large doses over less than 5 minutes results in dangerously rapid drug absorption. Up to about 90% of the dose of lidocaine is absorbed, and up to 30% of the dose is recovered with the removal of the subcutaneous fat tissue (251,252). It has been confirmed that epinephrine (1:1,000,000) significantly retards the absorption of lidocaine administered by the tumescent technique and may allow time for some lidocaine to be removed from the tissues by suction lipectomy (253). Moreover, the high pressure generated in the subcutaneous tissues during injection of the solution does not affect the absorption of lidocaine (253). Regardless of the rate of absorption, a local anesthetic with a rapid local and systemic metabolism presents a more appealing strategy for avoiding systemic toxicity, and recent studies suggest that articaine may be useful in this role (254).

Direct instillation of longer-acting local anesthetics into wounds is currently receiving attention corresponding to the availability of multiport catheters and elastomeric infusion devices that regulate the rate of infusion through controlled contraction of the reservoir. The local anesthetic agent is thereby placed into a milieu of mixed tissues with a possibility of both rapid absorption and depot formation. Mulroy et al. (255) studied the injection of 30 mL of saline or 0.125%, 0.25%, or 0.5% ropivacaine into wounds in 110 healthy patients following hernia repair under spinal anesthesia and reported respective ropivacaine mean C_{max} values of 0.109, 0.249, and 0.399 μg/mL, peaking between 30 and 60 minutes, and remaining elevated for the entire 2-hour sampling period. Bianconi et al. (256) studied a group of adult patients after spinal fusion surgery who were treated with a local loading of ropivacaine 0.5% 40 mL followed by an infusion of 0.2% 5 mL/h for 55 hours. With this pain management regimen, they found an overall superior response compared to patients who had an IV morphine/ketorolac analgetic regimen. Plasma C_{max} of ropivacaine was found to range between 0.3 and 1.6 μg/mL, occurring typically at around 24 hours after commencement of infusion, and no toxic effects were found. A similar regimen of ropivacaine (loading 0.75%, 30 mL, followed by infusion 0.2%, 5 mL/h for 96 hours) was used in a small group of elderly patients (75-86 years) for 96 hours following bowel resection (257). Venous plasma C_{max} of ropivacaine ranged from 2.3 to 8.8 μg/mL, at a T_{max} of 0.75 to 72 hours, and the patients were reported to not exhibit toxic symptoms. The range of ropivacaine concentrations was quite large, approaching some values of concern for toxicity in these patients; however, the unbound concentrations decreased concurrently, presumably the consequence increases in α_1-acid glycoprotein induced by surgery, and this was seen by the authors to confer a safety factor.

Intra-articular injection of local anesthetic agents for pain management after arthroscopic surgery has been found efficacious in some studies, but not in others: Dose and timing seem

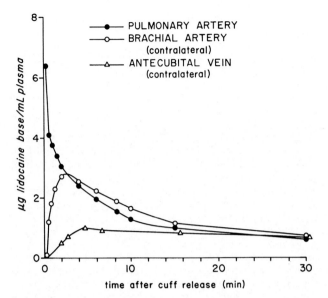

FIGURE 3-11. Plasma lidocaine levels in a subject following cuff release after intravenous regional anesthesia with 3 mg/kg lidocaine (0.5% solution; 45 minutes cuff time). Data from Tucker GT, Boas RA. Pharmacokinetic aspects of intravenous regional anesthesia. *Anesthesiology* 1971;34:538.

to be important factors. A study comparing bupivacaine 0.5% 20 mL with ropivacaine 0.5%, 0.75%, and 1% 20 mL found similar efficacy, with resultant plasma C_{max} values proportional to dose, and with T_{max} values that varied between 20 and 180 minutes (258).

Intravenous Regional Anesthesia. Intravenous regional anesthesia (IVRA) differs pharmacokinetically from other neural blockade procedures because the local anesthetic is deposited within the vascular space—rather than perineurally—whence it must diffuse to its neural target(s). Presentation of the agent to other than local tissues via the systemic circulation is controllable by the anesthesiologist's use of an inflated tourniquet cuff. There is no systemic absorption process as for perineural injections, although there is a systemic resorption process of drug that diffuses into local tissues during cuff inflation.

Analysis of plasma lidocaine concentrations measured after IVRA (170) indicated that, if the cuff is inflated correctly for at least 10 minutes after injection, only about 20% to 30% of the dose enters the systemic circulation during the first minute after cuff release. This is consistent with the observation that only about 12% of the dose can be aspirated from veins shortly after injection. The bulk of the dose remains in arm tissue, with 50% remaining in the limb 30 minutes after cuff release (170). Direct experimental support for this comes from observations of sustained high concentrations of local anesthetic in the venous drainage from the blocked arm after cuff release (Fig. 3-11) (259). Longer application of the cuff delays wash-out of drug from the arm (170). Intermittent deflation of the cuff for 10 to 30 seconds followed by reinflation appears to have little effect on the ultimate maximum plasma drug concentration but does prolong the time to maximum concentration (260).

It is clear that IVRA is preferably performed with a local anesthetic agent with the properties of good and reliable nerve blocking characteristics, the least possible systemic toxicity, and the highest rate of removal from the circulation. Prior logic suggested that prilocaine best filled this role for anesthe-

sia of brief to moderate duration, and that longer duration was not advisable with bupivacaine because of the risks of toxicity associated with cuff leakage or premature deflation. Further future gain for IVRA may come from using an agent that is metabolized locally, such as articaine. Various comparative studies with articaine, prilocaine, and lidocaine indicate that articaine can produce a faster onset with a briefer duration than lidocaine, but its circulating concentrations are much smaller than lidocaine due to extensive local hydrolysis prior to tourniquet release combined with its rapid clearance from the plasma post-tourniquet release (12,261,262).

Dosage Factors

Concentration and Volume

All other things being constant, total dose is the primary determinant of drug plasma concentrations after any route of perineural administration. However, it must be remembered that the drugs are not inert tracers so that their pharmacologic effects, including the neural blockade produced, can also provoke deviations or nonlinearities in their pharmacokinetics, particularly when the local concentration of drug approaches toxic levels or saturation levels for some transport or metabolic binding process.

For example, plasma C_{max} after caudal doses of ropivacaine 1, 2, or 3 mg/kg in children were found to be proportional to dose, but with a tendency toward decreasing T_{max} with increasing dose (263). Similarly, etidocaine intercostal doses of 20 mL in concentrations of 0.25% to 1.5% produced proportionate plasma C_{max} values in surgical patients (Figs. 3-5 and 3-6). Likewise, given up to a 300-mg epidural dose (constant volume) of etidocaine, plasma concentrations increase linearly with dose, but beyond this they become disproportionately higher (264). Some evidence suggests that the absorption rates of local anesthetics after central and peripheral nerve blocks and after IV regional anesthesia are faster from concentrated solutions than from more dilute solutions containing the same dose (Fig, 3-6) (149,170,265). These differences presumably reflect saturation of local binding sites and/or greater vasodilator effects produced by more concentrated solutions. Both of these mechanisms should result in disproportionate increases in plasma drug concentrations when concentration and mass of drug are increased but volume is held constant.

Speed of Injection

It is intuitive that a slower rate of drug administration conveys greater safety than a faster one for a neural blockade procedure. Emphasis on safety improvements in regional anesthesia has led to the practice of *dose fractionation* for avoiding toxicity, whereby the dose is administered slowly or as a series of increments. Although its value seems intuitive, and a predictable relationship exists between C_{max} and the duration of an IV infusion, there has been little systematic investigation into the pharmacokinetic and pharmacodynamic effects of dose fractionation in clinical practice.

Epidural injections given over 1 minute resulted in 16% higher maximum plasma concentrations of lidocaine compared with those injected in 15 seconds (266). Plasma bupivacaine concentrations were not influenced by varying epidural injection speed from 20 to 100 seconds (215). Perivascular axillary injection of mepivacaine as a divided dose with an interval of 20 minutes resulted in slightly lower plasma drug concentrations at up to 90 minutes than did those after a single bolus

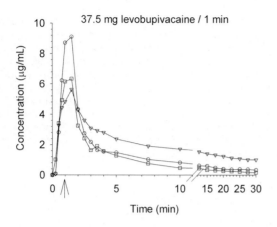

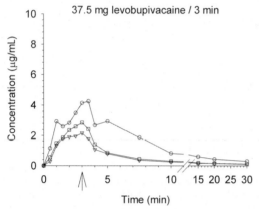

FIGURE 3-12. Comparison of levobupivacaine blood concentrations in three individual sheep when a dose of 37.5 mg was administered intravenously over 1 minute or 3 minutes. The arrow indicates the end of administration. Unpublished data from Mather LE, Copeland SE, Ladd LA.

dose, with no difference in sensory or motor blockade (238). In contrast, the staged administration of an epidural injection of bupivacaine in two aliquots given 15 seconds apart resulted in a prolongation of block, although again there was only a trend for a decrease in the maximum plasma drug concentration (267). Another study performed in sedated surgical patients having epidural anesthesia with plain lidocaine showed that serum lidocaine concentrations were halved if the same dose was administered as an infusion compared to a bolus (147).

The concern of a dose mistakenly being administered intravenously was investigated in sheep, where it was found that prolonging administration of 37.5 mg levobupivacaine from 1 to 3 minutes (as an example) reduced its arterial C_{max} by approximately 40% (Fig. 3-12) (151). Computer simulations of the same dose given variously as a bolus, or by spaced fractionation portions, showed that the agent's C_{max} in arterial blood is definitely attenuated, but a sufficient reduction in drug concentration may not occur to avoid intoxication. The authors suggested that the most important feature of dose fractionation is that it gives the anesthesiologist an early opportunity to cease administering the drug if an adverse effect is detected.

Vasoconstrictors

Vasoconstrictor agents, mainly epinephrine, are often added to local anesthetic solutions to slow the systemic absorption rate, thereby enhancing the local neural uptake and decreasing the

local clearance of local anesthetic agent (74,192,268). Vasoconstrictors enhance the apparent potency of the agent, and this has been demonstrated by the MLAC of epidural bupivacaine being reduced by 29% by epinephrine (59). Although the effects of epinephrine are primarily pharmacokinetic, it can have antinociceptive effects of its own and, when systemically absorbed, may have cardiovascular effects sufficient to modify the systemic pharmacokinetics and effects of other drugs (132,268–270).

The degree to which epinephrine decreases the systemic absorption rate of local anesthetic is a complex function of the type, dose, and concentration of local anesthetic and of the characteristics of the injection site. Although the C_{max} of local anesthetics may be decreased by epinephrine, it does not necessarily prolong the T_{max} (172,271). In general, the greatest effects are seen after intercostal blocks (Fig. 3-10), and more with shorter-acting than longer-acting agents.

In addition to local binding, the inherent vasoactivity of local anesthetics may modulate the vasoconstrictor effect of epinephrine on systemic drug absorption. Thus, vasoconstrictor effects would be expected to augment or override the action of epinephrine at low concentrations of local anesthetic and antagonize it at high concentrations associated with vasodilation. A lack of observed influence of epinephrine on plasma concentrations of ropivacaine after brachial plexus injection (272) might reflect the potent vasoconstrictor effect of this agent overriding that of added epinephrine. Paradoxically, the combined intradermal injection of ropivacaine and epinephrine resulted in less vasoconstriction than injection of epinephrine alone (273). This apparent antiepinephrine effect of ropivacaine would be consistent with a tendency toward longer duration of nerve blockade observed with plain compared with epinephrine-added solutions after brachial plexus injection (274).

Historical studies of lidocaine and prilocaine (266,275) suggest that the use of epinephrine concentrations greater than 5 μg/mL produces only marginally greater decreases in maximum plasma local anesthetic concentration and should, therefore, be avoided in view of side effects associated with excessive systemic levels of epinephrine (276). However, although a concentration of 5 μg/mL epinephrine is commonly employed, the decrease in peak plasma lidocaine concentrations after epidural injection has been shown to be independent of epinephrine concentration between 1.7 and 5 μg/mL (277). The effect of epinephrine on plasma lidocaine concentrations was shown to be attenuated considerably during continuous epidural infusion compared with that observed after the initial loading injection (278). A more recent study found no significant difference between the effectiveness of 5 and 2.5 μg/mL epinephrine used with epidural levobupivacaine (45).

Alternative vasopressor agents to epinephrine include octapressin (279) and phenylephrine (280). Addition of the latter, at a concentration of 50 μg/mL, to lidocaine for epidural block was found to be less effective than epinephrine (5 μg/mL) in lowering blood concentrations of the local anesthetic (281). Phenylephrine had no effect on lidocaine absorption after subarachnoid injection in monkeys, yet it prolonged neural blockade (282). Like epinephrine, phenylephrine prolongs useful clinical blockade after spinal tetracaine (280), possibly because of α-adrenoceptor agonist activity at spinal regions involved in antinociception. Clonidine, which has been used to prolong the duration of sensory anesthesia without significant cardiovascular system effects of its own (283), has been found to exert effects equivalent to epinephrine in reducing C_{max} after epidural lidocaine (284) and blockade of the superficial peroneal nerve (285).

Alkalinization

Alkalinization of ropivacaine solution was found to not cause a reduction of sensory–motor onset, but did provide a significant increase in the duration of the epidural block, with no significant differences between plain solutions and those with epinephrine (286). Alkalinization of lidocaine solutions for epidural anesthesia was found to have no effect on plasma concentrations of the local anesthetic (287). However, studies of IVRA in dogs have shown that the release of bupivacaine into the circulation after deflation of the tourniquet is slowed significantly by prior IV injection of sodium bicarbonate into the occluded limb (288). The effect of the latter is presumably to correct the acidosis caused by ischemia, thereby facilitating tissue uptake of the lidocaine.

Depot Formulations

Several delivery systems based upon local anesthetic-loaded liposomes, polylactide microspheres, or cyclodextrin inclusion complexes have been shown to prolong epidural and subarachnoid block in animals by providing a depot from which local anesthetic is slowly released. This slow local release should also be accompanied by a decrease in the rate of systemic drug absorption. Thus, lower and more prolonged plasma concentrations of lidocaine and bupivacaine have been measured in animals after injection of liposomal and other formulations compared to aqueous solutions (125,289–293). Furthermore, Boogaerts et al. (122) demonstrated that this is accompanied by less risk of systemic toxicity. In humans, dextran (6%–10%) has been shown to attenuate markedly the systemic absorption rate of lidocaine and epinephrine after injection into the scalp (81,295).

Factors Related to Neural Blockade

The neural blockade produced by a local anesthetic agent may, at least theoretically, influence the disposition of the agent through interference with autonomic control mechanisms; for example, hypotension accompanying epidural anesthesia might prolong the duration of blockade owing to decreased perfusion of the epidural space, or it might decrease hepato-splanchnic blood flow and clearance of local anesthetic. In support, prophylactic subcutaneous or IV injection of ephedrine results in shorter durations of anesthesia and elevated blood concentrations of some local anesthetic agents (296). However, no convincing evidence showed that neuraxial blockade to T6–T7 with tetracaine influenced the overall disposition of etidocaine administered intravenously (171). Direct actions of local anesthetic agents on vascular smooth muscle are complex, being both drug- and concentration-dependent (188). Although these effects may contribute to spread, absorption, and effects from certain routes of administration, it is not possible to determine the extent and significance of changes resulting from neural blockade from the existing data.

Physical and Pathophysiological Factors

An overview of the influence of patient-related variables on the disposition of the principal local anesthetic agents was considered as a basis for revision of the maximum recommended doses of local anesthetics (166,167,297). Interpretation of results of studies, however, is somewhat hampered by inconsistency in experimental design, particularly in blood sampling and processing.

Weight and Height

In adults, plasma concentrations of local anesthetics after epidural and other nerve blocks are correlated poorly with body weight and height (149,199,266,298–300). Despite this, and acknowledging that dosage adjustments must be made for the extremes of body weight, various dosage recommendations continue to include total body weight as a primary factor (167).

Age

The effects of aging on the various components of neural blockade and their mechanisms are complex because of concurrent age-related anatomic and physiologic changes that lead to associated local and systemic pharmacokinetic and pharmacodynamic changes. These occur at both ends of the age spectrum.

Veering et al. (176,177) observed increased cephalad spread and faster onset of analgesia in caudad segments in elderly compared to young adult patients after epidural and subarachnoid hyperbaric bupivacaine, but not after subarachnoid glucose-free bupivacaine; they also reported equivocal effects of aging on motor blockade from both epidural and subarachnoid bupivacaine. Whereas Nydahl et al. (301) confirmed a greater cephalad spread in elderly patients compared to young adult volunteers after epidural bupivacaine, they also observed a briefer period of analgesia and motor blockade in the elderly patients. Subsequent studies by Veering et al. with epidural ropivacaine and levobupivacaine again found that cephalad spread increased with age, and that the intensity of motor blockade increased with age for ropivacaine (but not for levobupivacaine) (174,175). The fraction of dose absorbed rapidly was smaller with increased age with ropivacaine and levobupivacaine (but was unaffected with bupivacaine) (174–177). This was probably related to the differences in local disposition and systemic uptake mediated through age-related changes in epidural blood flow and the effective vasoactivity of the local anesthetic agents. Veering et al. (176,177) also found that the total body clearance of bupivacaine decreased with increasing age, presumably because of decreased activity of hepatic enzyme activity.

The introduction of ropivacaine and levobupivacaine appears to have coincided with a resurgence of interest of neural blockade in infants and children (302). Many studies were recently reviewed by Mazoit and Dahlens (145). They noted that two of the main factors producing differences between younger immature and older pediatric patients derive from the relatively lower resting levels of α_1-acid glycoprotein (the major binding protein) during the first 6 to 9 months of life, and the maturation of the hepatic metabolizing enzyme system responsible for drug clearance (303,303a,304). Observed T_{max} data in infants and children are subject to the previously mentioned caveat about blood sampling. Interpretation of C_{max} data in neonatal and infant patients is further complicated by dose-scaling, which is commonly referenced to total body mass, but this is not entirely satisfactory due to age-related differences in body composition. Moreover, it is still not known whether there are age-related changes in the systemic disposition of local anesthetic agents because the appropriate studies with IV administration have not, unsurprisingly, been performed. Nevertheless, the available data suggest a somewhat faster systemic absorption of most local anesthetics than in adults (303,305,306). However, it has been suggested that epidural ropivacaine demonstrates delayed T_{max} in children compared to adults (145), and a delayed T_{max} after caudal block compared to bupivacaine in comparable patients (303a), but this apparently anomalous behavior of ropivacaine is not yet explained.

Pregnancy

Although engorgement of vertebral veins and a hyperkinetic circulation might be expected to enhance absorption of local anesthetics after epidural block, plasma drug concentration–time profiles appear to be similar in pregnant and nonpregnant women (307).

Disease and Surgery

Changes in local perfusion associated with altered hemodynamics as a result of disease or surgery may modify the absorption of local anesthetics and hence duration of anesthesia. For example, acute hypovolemia slows lidocaine absorption after epidural injection in dogs (308) and prolongs anesthesia in patients undergoing thoracotomy with regional block (309). Conversely, a decreased duration of brachial plexus block in patients with chronic renal failure was suggested to reflect a hyperkinetic circulation and enhanced systemic uptake of local anesthetic (310) but this hypothesis has not been substantiated by the results of subsequent studies (311–313). It seems that the main effects of renal and hepatic disease are on the systemic disposition of the agents.

SYSTEMIC DISPOSITION

After absorption from the site of administration, local anesthetics, like other drugs, are distributed by the bloodstream to the organs and tissues of the body and cleared, mostly by hepatic metabolism and to a small extent by renal excretion. In pregnant women, a small proportion of the dose also crosses the placenta into the fetus. However, systemic disposition, free from the complications of absorption, can be studied systematically only with IV administration, ideally in concert with information about cardiovascular and related systems (patho)physiology and concurrent pharmacotherapy (167,314). In humans, such studies with local anesthetics are normally performed with low enough doses to avoid toxicity, and with peripheral blood sampling techniques. The information gathered is, therefore, necessarily limited. More invasive studies to characterize toxic doses, as well as to study the regional pharmacokinetics of the agents and relevant regional physiology, are primarily performed in large animals, usually dogs, pigs, and sheep.

Some pharmacokinetic data describing the systemic disposition of some common local anesthetics in healthy human subjects are given in Table 3-6; these have been derived from compartment model analysis. In some studies, the systemic disposition of a stable (nonradioactive) isotopically labelled local anesthetic has been used to compute the systemic absorption rate (see the earlier section Agents), and these have been found experimentally to not differ to concurrently determined values with native agent (173,180). Such data can be analyzed by several methods. Compartment models—in which the drug is identified as being in one of three places: in a "central compartment" containing sampled blood (along with highly perfused regions), in other regions that have identifiably lower perfusion and drug tissue-to-plasma distribution coefficients (and are lumped together as "peripheral compartments"), or already eliminated—are one, perhaps more readily visualized, method. However, there are a variety of possible compartment models, and a failing of this methodology is that it may not be possible to support one such model unequivocally, or even to determine the "correct" model, from the data obtained. It should be remembered that the model is, after all, a gross oversimplification of a very complex biologic system; hence, it is emphasized that these models are meant to be the simplest mathematical–statistical representations useful for estimating the extent of distribution and the rate of elimination required to balance a known dose with measured drug concentrations (usually blood). Other ways of analyzing such data include noncompartment analysis, in which a compartment structure is not required to be defined, and more or less complex anatomic–physiologic models based on regional blood flow, transit times,

---

TABLE 3-6

MEAN PHARMACOKINETIC VARIABLES DESCRIBING THE SYSTEMIC DISPOSITION OF AMIDE-TYPE LOCAL ANESTHETIC IN ADULT MALE SUBJECTS

Variable	Prilocaine	Lidocaine	Mepivacaine	Ropivacaine	Bupivacaine	Levobupivacaine	Etidocaine
λ	1.1	0.8	0.9	0.7	0.6	~ 0.7	0.6
F_u	0.45	0.30	0.20	0.05	0.05	0.05	0.06
V_{ss} (L)*	191	91	84	61	73	~ 90	134
Vu_{ss} (L)*	~ 445	253	382	742	1,028	$\sim 1,250$	1,478
Cl (L/min)*	2.37	0.95	0.78	0.73	0.58	0.47	1.11
E_H	~ 0.95	0.65	0.52	0.49	0.38	~ 0.67	0.74
$T_{1/2,z}$ (h)	1.6	1.6	1.9	1.9	2.7	1.8	2.7
MBRT (h)	1.3	1.6	1.8	1.4	2.1	2.2	2.0

*specified with respect to arterial blood concentrations except for prilocaine. Approximate average values for λ blood-to-plasma concentration ratio; F_u = fraction unbound in plasma; V_{ss} steady-state apparent volume of distribution; Vu_{ss} steady-state apparent volume of distribution of unbound drug in plasma water; Cl mean total body clearance; E_H estimated hepatic extraction ratio; $T_{1/2,z}$ terminal ("elimination") half-life; MBRT mean body retention time.
Data from Tucker GT, Mather LE. Clinical *pharmacokinetics* of local anaesthetic agents. *Clin Pharmacokinet* 1979;4:241; Simon MJ, Veering BT, Stienstra R, et al. The systemic absorption and disposition of levobupivacaine 0.5% after epidural administration in surgical patients: A stable-isotope study. *Eur J Anaesth* 2004;21:460–470; Arthur GR, Scott DH, Boyes RN, et al. Pharmacokinetic and clinical pharmacological studies with mepivacaine and prilocaine. *Br J Anaesth* 1979;51(6):481–485; and Lee A, Fagan D, Lamont M, et al. Disposition kinetics of ropivacaine in humans. *Anesth Analg* 1989;69(6):736–738.

and like factors, or by simply using a sums-of-exponentials approach that gives no particular structure to the (purely mathematical) model (315–318).

Distribution

The Role of the Lung

The first capillary bed to be exposed to local anesthetic once it has entered the systemic circulation is that in the lungs. This highly perfused maze-like structure acts to (temporarily) sequester an appreciable quantity of drug because of its large surface area for drug uptake and favorable tissue-to-blood distribution coefficient. Hence, after (rapid) IV input, the arterial blood drug concentration that hits the target organs for toxicity—the brain and the heart— is attenuated considerably compared with the drug concentration in the pulmonary artery due to the combined effects of pulmonary capillary transit delay and tissue uptake (Fig. 3-11) (151,170,317,319). The fraction of dose apparently lost into the lungs during first passage (influx) is essentially independent of dose; however, this is soon regained to the circulation by wash-out (efflux), in an exponentially decreasing manner (Fig. 3-13). After slower IV input or normal vascular absorption, the blood-to-tissue drug concentration gradient is small, and lung uptake occurs concurrently with whole body distribution, consequently the pulmonary arterial–arterial blood drug concentration gradient is minimal (200). Several methods have been used to study lung uptake of local anesthetic agents; most are adaptable to other tissues as well.

As indicated, a pulmonary arterial–arterial (i.e., inflow–outflow) drug concentration gradient provides evidence of lung (or other tissue) uptake, but it does not differentiate between drug distribution (reversible) and clearance (irreversible). A concentration gradient at steady state, or an area under the plasma drug concentration–time curve difference at non-steady state, provides evidence of clearance. After an IV dose, the concentration gradient is positive when net influx occurs (blood to tissue mass transfer), zero when blood and tissue concentrations are equal, and negative when net efflux occurs (tissue to blood mass transfer) (320). Studies in humans and sheep readily demonstrate the pulmonary arterial–arterial gradient after IV administration (Fig. 3-11; Fig. 3-13), but there is no good evidence that the lungs extract local anesthetic agents at steady state (200,321,322).

Direct measurement of drug concentrations in lung tissue samples taken serially either repeatedly or discretely in different subjects have been used to demonstrate lung uptake (323,324). Isotopically labeled agents also have been used with appropriate imaging techniques to demonstrate the time course of lung (and other tissue) uptake (325). Comparison of the arterial blood time course of a dye used as a marker of intravascular fluid movement with that of an admixed local anesthetic agent after an IV dose has been used to estimate the transit delay/retention of the agent in the lungs (326–328). Direct determination of uptake and metabolism has been assessed by perfusion of the agent in a medium applied to isolated laboratory rodent lungs either by single-pass or recirculation, or by incubation of agent in preparations of lung tissue. Others have also found a greater uptake of prilocaine than of mepivacaine and bupivacaine in the isolated perfused rat lung, with little evidence of pulmonary metabolism (329). The rank order of uptake in rat lung slices was found to be bupivacaine >etidocaine >lidocaine (330). Other studies using the dye comparison method found that the lung extraction in rabbits is levobupivacaine >ropivacaine (328). There is also evidence for modest enantioselectivity of distribution: Rutten et al. (323) found that the steady-state lung-to-blood distribution coefficients of R-bupivacaine were on average about 40% greater than those of S-bupivacaine in sheep.

The extravascular pH of the lung is low relative to plasma pH, and this encourages ion trapping of local anesthetic (331). Conversely, a relative decrease in plasma pH impairs uptake (332). Other basic drugs, such as propranolol, may compete with local anesthetics for pulmonary binding sites, thereby decreasing their first-pass extraction.

Blood and Plasma Binding

As indicated above, the binding of local anesthetics to macromolecules is a secondary property related to the chemical and physicochemical properties of the agent. Drug binding in blood or plasma is mainly determined ex vivo using equilibrium dialysis or ultrafiltration (114,333). At equilibrium, the concentration of unbound, nonionized drug will be the same on either side of the membrane, but total drug concentrations will differ depending on the relative capacities of the binding sites associated with the two aqueous phases and any pH gradient. The in vitro models are used to infer the relationships between bound and unbound drug concentrations existent in vivo; the mechanism has been used to explain, for example, the unequal distribution of local anesthetic agents across the placenta (333,334). However, both models produce results that depend to some extent upon methodological variables, so that data are better used for comparative than absolute purposes.

Most importantly, the fractional binding of a drug in plasma normally decreases as drug concentrations increase—an indication of saturability of binding sites. For local anesthetics, a

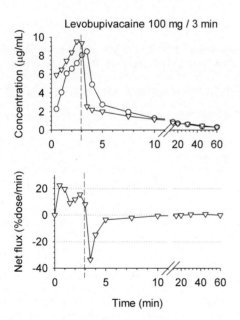

FIGURE 3-13. Lung pharmacokinetics of levobupivacaine infused over 3 minutes in a sheep. Pulmonary aerial and aortic concentrations were measured (*upper panel*). The net flux of levobupivacaine across the lungs was measured from the product of the pulmonary arterial–aortic levobupivacaine concentration gradient and the cardiac output. The net flux is positive (net influx blood to lungs) when the gradient is positive, the lung and blood concentrations are equal when the gradient is zero, and negative (net efflux from lung to blood) when the gradient is negative. Unpublished data from Mather LE, Copeland SE, Ladd LA.

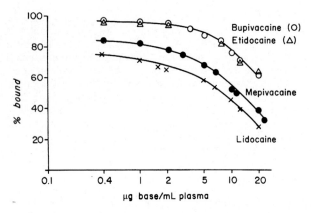

FIGURE 3-14. Plasma binding of amide-type local anesthetics. Data from Tucker GT, Mather LE. Pharmacokinetic of local anaesthetic agents. *Br J Anaesth* 1975;47(Suppl):213–214.

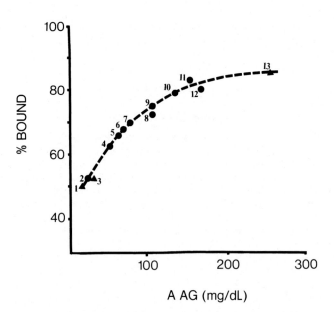

FIGURE 3-15. Relation between the mean percentage of lidocaine bound and the concentration of α_1-acid glycoprotein in plasma in various clinical conditions. ●, patient group data; ▲, individual patient data; 1, patient with nephrotic syndrome; 2, neonates; 3, patient with carcinoma of prostate receiving high-dose estrogens; 4, females on oral conceptives; 5, women under 40 years; 6, men under 40 years; 7, adults over 70 years; 8, subjects with epilepsy; 9, renal transplantation patients; 10, chronic renal failure patients; 11, cancer patients; 12, myocardial infarction patients; 13, patient with myocardial infarction. Data from Jackson PR, Tucker GT, Woods HF. Altered plasma binding in cancer. Role of alpha₁-acid glycoprotein and albumin. *Clin Pharmacol Ther* 1982;32:295; and Tucker GT. Pharmacokinetics of local anaesthetics. *Br J Anaesth* 1986;58:717.

marked change in the fraction bound occurs at total plasma concentrations of around 2 to 4 μg/mL, a concentration range often reached after normal systemic absorption (Fig. 3-14). Thus, it is important to remember that the fraction bound is not a constant, so that binding data need to be collected at relevant drug concentrations. A variety of proteins bind local anesthetic agents to various extents, but their binding can be adequately described by considering that two main classes of binding sites exist: a high-affinity, low-capacity site on α_1-acid glycoprotein, and a low-affinity, high-capacity site on albumin (3,114,335–341). The rank order of binding of local anesthetics to sites in or on erythrocytes is similar to that for plasma binding (171). However, in blood, plasma protein binding competes with blood cell binding, so that harvested plasma drug concentrations increasingly diverge from collected blood drug concentrations with increasing lipophilicity of the agent. Sometimes the value of the average blood-to-plasma drug concentration ratio (λ) is used to provide a numerical factor for converting between equivalent blood and plasma drug concentrations (Table 3-6). A potential hazard of this approach is that λ will normally be dependent on protein and/or drug concentration, hematocrit, acid–base balance, and similar factors.

Human α_1-acid glycoprotein (AAG) is coded by three genes, AGP-A, AGP-B, and AGP-B', and exists as a heterogeneous population of three genetic variants[g], ORM1 F1 and ORM1 S derived from the AGP-A gene, and ORM2 derived from the AGP-B/B' genes, which are involved in plasma binding of local anesthetics and many other drugs (113,342). Individual and disease state–induced differences in the expression of these genes are a source of variation in plasma binding of drugs, including ropivacaine. Binding to the three main AGP phenotypes, F_1S/A, F_1/A, and S/A, is somewhat selective and is competitive among drugs. Ropivacaine binds selectively to the F_1S variants and lidocaine to the F_1S and A variants, so that individual variability in binding may be partly explained, even at similar total AGP plasma concentrations, by these variants (342).

The extent of binding varies with the plasma concentration of α_1-acid glycoprotein (340–342), which becomes elevated considerably in patients with cancer (343), chronic pain (344), trauma (345), inflammatory disease (346), and uremia (346a), and in postoperative (257,348) patients, and after myo-

cardial infarction (349) (Fig. 3-15). Progression through pregnancy, on the other hand, has been found to be associated with progressive decreases in plasma α_1-acid glycoprotein and albumin, along with bupivacaine binding capacity (350). Low plasma concentrations of α_1-acid glycoprotein in neonates are associated with much lower binding of local anesthetics compared with adult plasma (145,333,334,351). The plasma concentration of α_1-acid glycoprotein increases, whereas the free fraction of bupivacaine decreases throughout early infancy (145) and that of lidocaine decreases from early infancy to adolescence (352). In healthy adults, increasing age is not associated with a change in α_1-acid glycoprotein levels (352a,352b) or in the extent of plasma binding of local anesthetic (177). Most studies indicate lower plasma binding of local anesthetics during pregnancy and at term (353,354). Decreases in binding may also occur acutely during and shortly after surgery (342,355). This may be due to competition for binding sites by temporarily increased plasma concentrations of free fatty acids or perturbed acid–base or electrolyte status. Increases in the concentration of α_1-acid glycoprotein after surgery have been found to stabilize the unbound local anesthetic concentrations in the presence of increasing total concentration from continuous epidural infusion (335,356).

Binding also shows modest but significant enantioselectivity. The plasma protein binding of R-bupivacaine was found to be greater than that of S-bupivacaine in sheep plasma, but less than that of S-bupivacaine in plasma from healthy human subjects and postoperative patients (341,355,357,358) (Table 3-7). The binding of R-prilocaine is greater than that of S-prilocaine (359), but that of S-mepivacaine was greater than that of

---

[g] These designations reflect the alternative name for α_1-acid glycoprotein: orosomucoid.

TABLE 3-7

PHARMACOKINETIC PROPERTIES (MEAN [SD]) OF THE SEPARATE ENANTIOMERS OF LOCAL ANESTHETIC AGENTS ADMINISTERED INTRAVENOUSLY OVER 10 MIN AS RACEMATES IN HEALTHY NONSMOKING MALE VOLUNTEERS

Drug [data reference source]	R-pri [500]	S-pri [500]	R/S-pri [500]	R-mep [67]	S-mep [67]	R/S-mep [67]	R-bup [69]	S-bup [69]	R/S-bup [69]
Fu (%)	70 $ [8]	73$ [6]	0.95* [0.05]	36$ [5]	25$ [5]	1.43* [0.10]	6.6# [3.0]	4.5# [2.1]	1.50* [0.09]
CL (L/min)	2.6 [0.5]	1.9 [0.3]	1.36* [0.14]	0.79 [0.12]	0.35 [0.06]	2.25* [0.18]	0.40 [0.08]	0.32 [0.07]	1.25* [0.10]
CLu (L/min)	3.7 [0.6]	3.5 [0.6]	1.05* [0.06]	2.2 [0.3]	1.4 [0.2]	1.58* [0.12]	7.3 [3.6]	8.7 [4.3]	0.84* [0.11]
V_{ss} (L)	279 [94]	291 [93]	0.96 [0.10]	103 [14]	57 [7]	1.79* [0.14]	84 [29]	54 [20]	1.56* [0.27]
V_{ssu} (L)	402 [131]	405 [146]	1.00 [0.10]	290 [32]	232 [30]	1.25* [0.08]	1,576 [934]	1,498 [892]	1.04 [0.17]
$T_{1/2}$ (min)	87 [27]	124 [64]	0.74* [0.12]	113 [17]	123 [20]	0.92* [0.08]	210 [95]	157 [77]	1.36* [0.20]
MRT (min)	108 [30]	155 [59]	0.72* [0.10]	131 [15]	165 [24]	0.80* [0.07]	215 [74]	172 [55]	1.26* [0.31]

Pri = prilocaine; mep = mepivacaine; bup = bupivacaine; R/S = ratio of values for R- and S-enantiomers; Fu = unbound fraction in plasma; CL and CLu = total body clearance based on total plasma and unbound drug concentrations; V_{ss} and V_{ssu} = apparent volume of distribution based on total plasma and unbound drug concentrations; $T_{1/2z}$ = terminal half life; MRT = mean residence time; * = significantly different to unity, thereby denoting enantioselectivity; $ = determined by equilibrium dialysis; # = determined by ultrafiltration.

Group size = 10 for each; doses: prilocaine = 200 mg; mepivacaine = 60 mg; bupivacaine = 30 mg. Peripheral venous blood was sampled and measurements were performed on separated plasma.

Data from Burm AGL, Van der Meer AD, Van Kleef JW, et al. Pharmacokinetics of the enantiomers of bupivacaine following intravenous administration of the racemate. Br J Clin Pharmacol 1994;38:125; van der Meer AD, Burm AG, Stienstra R, et al. Pharmacokinetics of prilocaine after intravenous administration in volunteers: Enantioselectivity. Anesthesiology 1999;90(4):988–992; and Burm AG, Cohen IM, van Kleef JW, et al. Pharmacokinetics of the enantiomers of mepivacaine after intravenous administration of the racemate in volunteers. Anesth Analg 1997;84(1):85–89.

R-mepivacaine (360). Such differences affect secondary pharmacokinetic parameters derived from unbound drug concentrations, where they may offset (or augment) differences in clearance and distribution parameters based upon total drug concentrations, as shown in Tables 3-6 and 3-7.

The role of plasma binding in local anesthetic toxicity has been discussed by Tucker (316). It is important to allow for this phenomenon when interpreting measurements of plasma drug concentrations. For example, accumulation of total plasma drug concentrations postoperatively may not signify a risk of toxicity if this change reflects the postoperative increase in α_1-acid glycoprotein and, therefore, plasma drug binding. Unbound (active) drug concentrations, which are likely to be a

better index of effect, are similar before and after surgery (Fig. 3-16). When systemic drug input is gradual, as after perineural injection, distribution of the dose is spread over time and a large extravascular distribution space and extensive tissue binding ensures that only a small percentage remains in the blood. Under these conditions, any changes in plasma binding are buffered effectively by a high volume of distribution.

Theoretically, plasma binding could limit the first-pass uptake of local anesthetic into the brain and myocardium following inadvertent IV injection, thereby modulating toxicity. However, a toxic dose, especially if delivered rapidly, would overwhelm the binding capacity on first pass through the brain and heart. Studies in sheep have found the myocardial and

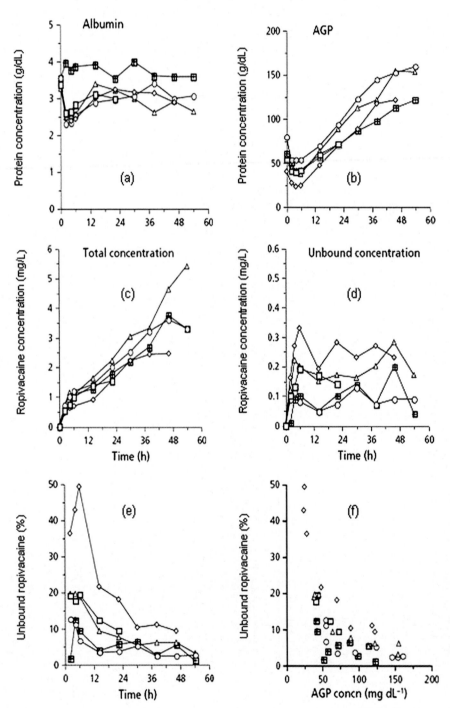

FIGURE 3-16. Binding of ropivacaine in plasma from surgical patients: **A** and **B** show the relationship between change in protein concentrations and time after surgery; **C** and **D** show total and unbound ropivacaine concentrations and time after surgery. Compiled from data in Clément R, Malinovsky JM, Hildgen P, et al. Spinal disposition and meningeal permeability of local anesthetics. *Pharm Res* 2004;21(4):706–716.

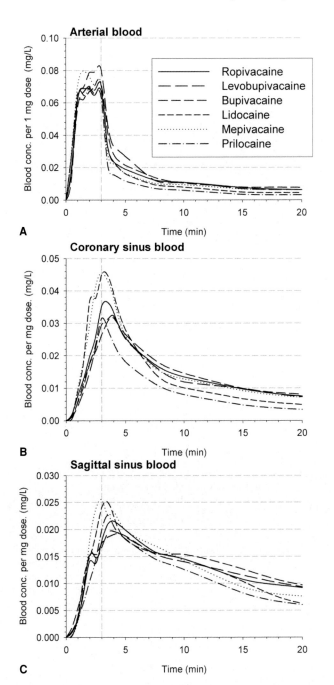

FIGURE 3-17. Comparative normalized (per 1 mg of dose) mean blood concentrations of local anesthetic agents after intravenous administration in sheep. **A:** Arterial concentrations. **B:** Coronary sinus concentrations indicating the drug time course in the heart. **C:** Sagittal sinus concentrations indicating the drug time course in the brain. Local anesthetic doses [bupivacaine (100 mg), levobupivacaine (125 mg), ropivacaine (150 mg), mepivacaine (350 mg), lidocaine (350 mg) and prilocaine (350 mg)) were infused intravenously over 3 minutes in an individual adult female sheep (ca. 50 Kg)]. Compiled from data obtained in a series published as Copeland SE, Ladd LA, Gu X-Q, Mather LE. Effects of general anesthesia on whole body and regional pharmacokinetics of local anesthetics at toxic doses. *Anesth Analg* 2008;106:1440–1449.

brain influxes of all the commonly used local anesthetic agents to be similar, despite differences in their binding (Fig. 3-17) (473a). Furthermore, studies of the initial brain uptake of local anesthetics in rats indicate that there is a facile dissociation from plasma binding sites in the microcirculation (361). The latter observation contrasts with findings in the dog showing that, at a few minutes after rapid IV injection of lidocaine, the extent of drug distribution into brain tissue and CSF was entirely governed by the equilibrium free concentration of drug in plasma (362). Therefore, it appears important to distinguish events after even a few recirculations from those during first pass through an organ. In either case, it should not be assumed that plasma binding modulates the extent of tissue drug uptake, and, therefore, protects against toxicity. A careful distinction should be made between the consequences of changes in unbound or free *fraction* and changes in free drug *concentration* (316,363).

Binding of drugs to specialized transporter proteins can be a regulator of their distribution into, or more importantly out of, various tissues. Binding to transporter proteins appears to plays a part in the active efflux of many drugs, including some used in anesthesia and pain management, from the brain, jejunal cells, testes, and placenta (364,365). The most studied of these transporter proteins is the epithelial cell, membrane-bound P-glycoprotein. P-glycoprotein binding can be inhibited by quinidine, and use is made of this in experimental models. In one such example, the brain-to-plasma concentration ratio of bupivacaine, but not lidocaine, was increased in the presence of quinidine, suggesting that bupivacaine, but not lidocaine, is a substrate for P-glycoprotein transport at the blood–brain barrier (366). Others have failed to find a significant effect attributable to this transporter with ropivacaine, lidocaine, and bupivacaine in intestinal mucosal cells (367).

Tissue Distribution

Tissue affinity or distribution of drugs is normally represented in pharmacokinetic analysis by the steady-state apparent volume of distribution (V_{ss}); this gives, in effect, a numerical value for the equilibrium whole body tissue-to-plasma distribution coefficient under conditions of changing blood drug concentrations. In the amide series of local anesthetics, a greater extent of plasma binding is accompanied by a parallel increase in affinity for tissue components. Thus, steady-state volumes of distribution based on unbound drug in plasma (Vu_{ss}), which reflect net tissue binding, vary over a fivefold range, being greatest for the more lipid-soluble agents (Tables 3-6 and 3-7). Distribution volumes based on total drug concentration in blood vary only twofold, reflecting the balance between blood and tissue binding. Differences in tissue-to-blood distribution coefficients of the enantiomers of local anesthetics, and hence volumes of distribution based on total drug concentration, may be explained by greater stereoselectivity in plasma binding than in tissue binding because the differences in V_{ss} between enantiomers are diminished when Vu_{ss} is considered (323,357).

The rate of uptake of local anesthetic into any particular tissue depends on delivery (perfusion) and capacity (tissue-to-blood distribution coefficient), as well as distribution and clearance elsewhere in the body. In general, tissue concentration is better reflected in the tissue regional venous blood drug concentrations than in arterial blood, a consequence of the transit delay and uptake in that region (320,368). This may or may not correspond to the concentrations in peripheral venous blood samples that are commonly and conveniently obtained in human subjects. The extent of disparity between the various sites of blood sampling depends on the rate and extent of attaining distribution equilibrium of drug concentrations in the relevant tissues.

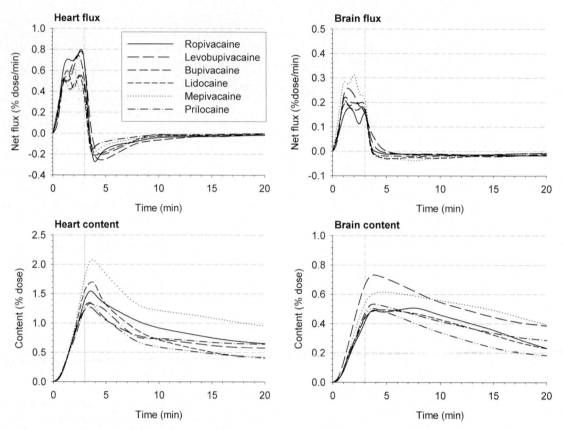

FIGURE 3-18. Comparative normalized (per 1 mg of dose) regional pharmacokinetics of local anesthetic agents after intravenous administration in sheep from the data shown in Figure 3-17. Heart net flux and content of local anesthetic (*left panels*). Brain net flux and content of local anesthetic (*right panels*). The net flux of the agents across membranes was measured from the respective product of the regional blood flow and arteriovenous local anesthetic concentration gradient. Compiled from data obtained in a series published as Copeland SE, Ladd LA, Gu X-Q, Mather LE. Effects of general anesthesia on whole body and regional pharmacokinetics of local anesthetics at toxic doses. *Anesth Analg* 2008;106:1440–1449.

After brief infusions in sheep, the calculated time course of mean myocardial uptake and myocardial concentration of a series of amide local anesthetics was found to correspond more to coronary sinus blood than to arterial, and was not limited to unbound drug (Figs. 3-17 and 3-18). Similarly, the time course of myocardial depressant effects are better correlated with those of the calculated myocardial drug concentrations than with those of arterial or coronary sinus blood drug concentrations (369–371). After prolonged infusions, a greater extent of blood-to-tissue equilibrium is reached, so that arteriovenous concentration gradients diminish until finally a steady state is achieved in which the gradients across non-clearing tissues vanish (321,322). The greater cardiotoxicity of bupivacaine and ropivacaine compared to lidocaine is not explained by a greater fraction of the dose distributing into the myocardium (372); similarly the greater toxicity of R(+)-bupivacaine compared to S(−)-bupivacaine is not adequately explained by stereoselectivity in myocardial drug uptake in the isolated perfused rabbit heart (373).

Treatment of local anesthetic cardiotoxicity, especially when due to bupivacaine, remains a clinical problem (see Chapter 4). Experiments in laboratory animals suggest that lipid infusion (typically with 20% Intralipid) may reduce the cardiotoxic potency of bupivacaine and provide a means of preventing and/or arresting these effects. There are still many unanswered questions about the mechanisms of action, and it is not yet clear whether the lipid formulation achieves its desired effect phar-macodynamically by direct inotropic support or pharmacokinetically by acting as a "sequestering sink" for absorbing bupivacaine from the circulation and/or tissues, or by a combination of effects (374). The applicability to cardiotoxicity from other local anesthetics is not yet established.

CLEARANCE

Drugs are eliminated from the body by concurrent metabolism and excretion, mostly in specialist organs such as liver for metabolism and kidneys for excretion. Some metabolism and/or excretion may also occur outside the liver (all tissues have some metabolic capability; kidneys and lungs are particularly active toward some drugs), and excretion takes place outside the kidneys (e.g. into breath, sweat, milk, etc.).

Excretion

The renal excretion of unchanged local anesthetics is a minor route of elimination, accounting for less than 10% of the dose under normal conditions. Depending on the agent, acidification of the urine increases this proportion to 5% to 20%, which is consistent with less tubular reabsorption as a result of greater ionization (178). However, this increase is insufficient to warrant the use of a forced acid diuresis in treating toxicity.

One study examining the stereoselectivity of bupivacaine urinary excretion reported 14.3% to 39.1% for R-bupivacaine, and 9.2% to 14.0% for S-bupivacaine in five patients having epidural infusions for 60 to 120 hours (40). A possible explanation for these unusually large values is that the $T_{1/2}$ of urinary excretion was greater than 10 hours, presumably reflecting the continued absorption of the agent and the probability that the absorbed dose available for excretion was, therefore, much less than the infused dose as used in the calculations.

Transfer of unchanged local anesthetics down the pH gradient between blood and gastric juice is also a potential route of excretion. However, most of the drug that appears in the stomach contents is subsequently reabsorbed from the intestine and undergoes first-pass metabolism in the liver. Although evacuation of stomach contents has been advocated for treatment of local anesthetic toxicity, especially in neonates (375), it is unlikely that this is of value. Gastric juice-to-blood drug concentration ratios may be high, but the proportion of the dose recycled by way of the stomach is unlikely to be significant.

Although the amide local anesthetic agents are measurable in breast milk, this route of excretion is considered to present a pharmacologically negligible portion of the dose to the nursing infant (376,377).

Metabolism

Enzymatic biotransformation is under strict genetic control; its purpose is to limit the duration of activity of endogenous hormones and autocoids, as well as to preclude/remove exogenous potentially toxic substances from the body. Metabolism generally produces metabolites that are more water-soluble, and thus more readily excreted, than their parent drugs. Primary metabolites may undergo further metabolism before elimination, typically by conjugation with glucuronic acid. Metabolites may have pharmacologic activity profiles similar to or different from the drug from which they were produced; however, the activity of local anesthetic metabolites is relevant essentially only to their potential for systemic toxicity. Moreover, metabolism can be quite complex with racemic drugs because in some, one enantiomer may be metabolically inverted to the other, but there is no evidence that this occurs with local anesthetic agents. Metabolism is often assessed by measurement of metabolites in biofluids and tissues in vivo. In vitro studies using human and other liver microsomes and recombinant cytochromes P450 are being increasingly used to help identify potential metabolic drug interactions, as well as sources of physiologic modification and variation such as gender, maturation, and smoker status (378,379).

Esters

Ester caines are cleared in both the blood and the liver. In vitro half-lives in plasma reflect the action of pseudocholinesterase and, in normal adults, these vary from 10 to 20 seconds for chloroprocaine to 40 seconds for procaine, to several minutes for tetracaine (380–383). In vivo half-lives are longer than those measured in vitro (e.g., that of chloroprocaine after epidural injection is about 3 minutes) (381). However, this value probably reflects rate-limiting redistribution from tissue to plasma rather than metabolic clearance. After high IV doses of procaine, clearances of 0.04 to 0.08 l/min/kg and elimination half-lives of 7 to 8 minutes have been observed, probably reflecting some saturation of the enzyme systems (384). The clinical implication of the rapid clearance of the esters is that, if

a toxic concentration is attained after inadvertent IV injection, the ensuing reaction should be relatively short-lived. Values of the mean plasma elimination half-life of cocaine in humans vary from 40 to 150 minutes (385,386).

The hydrolysis products of procaine, chloroprocaine, and tetracaine have been measured in human plasma but appear to be inactive pharmacologically (382,387), although the aminobenzoic acids may contribute to the rare allergic reaction. The main routes of metabolism of cocaine in humans are ester hydrolysis and N-demethylation (388). The former involves loss of the methyl group to give benzoylecgonine; enzymatic loss of the benzoyl group in plasma and liver, yielding ecgonine methyl ester; and further hydrolysis of both of these compounds to ecgonine. Norcocaine, the product of N-demethylation, undergoes an analogous series of hydrolysis steps (389). Of these metabolites, only norcocaine is believed to have significant pharmacologic activity, but it is not a major product.

Amides

The amide linkage is stable in blood, and most of the clearance of these agents occurs in the liver (526). Mean blood clearance values increase in the order bupivacaine <ropivacaine <mepivacaine (reflecting the size of the n-N-alkyl substituent in this homologous series) <lidocaine <etidocaine <prilocaine (Tables 3-6 and 3-7). Over the whole series, there is no clear relationship to anesthetic potency, lipid solubility, or protein binding. Etidocaine clearance is dependent mostly on liver perfusion, whereas that of bupivacaine and ropivacaine should be more sensitive to changes in intrinsic hepatic enzyme function (357,523,526). The clearance of lidocaine, which has an intermediate extraction ratio, should be dependent on both hepatic perfusion and enzyme activity (390). The blood clearance of prilocaine exceeds liver blood flow, indicating that extrahepatic metabolism of this drug occurs, but the sites of extrahepatic clearance are not yet identified (359,521). There is also evidence from studies in anhepatic patients that some of the N-deethylation of lidocaine may occur at extrahepatic sites (391). There is also evidence that N-deethylation of lidocaine can take place in microsomes from rat lung and, to a lesser extent, from kidney (392). Studies in sheep, in vivo, have found that lidocaine, mepivacaine, bupivacaine, and ropivacaine clearance is essentially confined to the liver (321,322,393,394).

After IV administration, both the mean terminal elimination half-lives and mean body residence times are between 1.5 and 3 hours for all of the agents in humans, reflecting a balance between their distribution and clearance characteristics (Tables 3-6 and 3-7). In humans, the total plasma clearance of R-bupivacaine, the intrinsically more toxic enantiomer, is about 20% to 30% greater than that of S-bupivacaine (357,395). Estimates of the relative unbound clearances of the enantiomers differ, possibly reflecting methodological differences in binding determinations. Whereas Burm et al. (357) reported less extensive plasma binding of R-bupivacaine compared to S-bupivacaine and a lower clearance of unbound drug, Blake et al. (396) found that both the total and unbound clearances of R-bupivacaine exceeded those of S-bupivacaine. However, because of enantiomeric differences in plasma binding, the order of unbound clearances of the isomers is reversed (357). R-mepivacaine is cleared twice as fast as S-mepivacaine in humans but is cleared at the same rate in sheep (360,393,397). Although the clearance of R-prilocaine is greater than that of S-prilocaine (359), they have similar blood concentration–time profiles after perineural injection, with comparable anesthetic activity and acute toxicity in animals; a higher margin for systemic CNS toxicity is not likely to be achieved by substituting racemic prilocaine with one of its enantiomers (42).

With the increasing use of techniques involving the prolonged administration of local anesthetics, it is important to assess any dose or time dependence in their systemic clearance. Under these conditions, the site of injection and drug absorption rate per se have no effect on the eventual steady-state plasma drug concentration. No deleterious effect on clearance has been found with doses of ropivacaine when administered by prolonged epidural infusion over a threefold range, nor when administered intravenously over a fourfold range (150,398). Following short-term intermittent epidural injections of lidocaine and etidocaine given over 5 to 10 hours, increases in plasma drug concentration were consistent with single-dose data (182). As discussed previously, following more prolonged administration in postoperative patients, a time-dependent decrease in systemic clearance (based upon measurement of total bound plus free plasma drug concentration) is expected, as levels of α_1-acid glycoprotein and plasma binding increase (Fig. 3-16). In addition, there is evidence, mostly from animal studies, for a progressive decrease in the intrinsic ability of hepatic enzymes to clear lidocaine, mepivacaine, and bupivacaine (294,393), presumably due to product inhibition by metabolite(s). However, other evidence that bupivacaine showed no time-dependent decrease in clearance when infused intravenously for 24 hours in sheep (321) is consistent with observations that the plasma concentrations of bupivacaine, measured during prolonged interpleural infusion, indicated no decrease in clearance with time. Such evidence is not consistent with either a time-dependent increase in plasma binding or a decrease in intrinsic hepatic clearance (209).

Identification of the biotransformation products of the amides in human urine indicates three major sites of metabolic attack, namely aromatic hydroxylation, N-dealkylation, and amide hydrolysis (399–402). Various metabolites have been measured in human biofluids; these include monoethylglycinexylidide (MEGX), glycinexylidide (GX), and the 4-hydroxy products formed from lidocaine; the 3- and 4-hydroxy products and the N-dealkylated pipecolylxylidide (PPX) from mepivacaine, ropivacaine, and bupivacaine. Of these products, it is likely that MEGX contributes to the systemic effects of the parent drug. On continuous infusion, unbound plasma concentrations of MEGX are 70% of those of lidocaine (403), and studies in rodents indicate that it is about 70% as toxic (404). Plasma concentrations of PPX of about one-third those of parent bupivacaine have been observed on continuous infusion of the latter (405). This metabolite has about half the cardiotoxic potency of bupivacaine in the rat (406). Additional biotransformation products of the chiral piperidine amides include isomeric piperidine ring hydroxylation products and their possible conjugates (400).

Studies using human liver microsomes and recombinant cytochromes P450 indicate that the N-dealkylation of lidocaine to MEGX and of ropivacaine and bupivacaine to PPX is mediated by the CYP3A4 isoform and that the 3'- and 4'-hydroxylation of ropivacaine by human liver microsomes appears to be mediated principally by CYP1A2 (145,407–410). Tanaka et al. (411) reported that five potential co- or premedications (diazepam, lidocaine, cimetidine, vecuronium, and clonidine) did not inhibit ropivacaine metabolism in human liver microsomes at concentrations within the therapeutic range, but that midazolam and thiamylal weakly inhibited its metabolism in a competitive manner. Others have reported dose-dependent competitive inhibitory effects of propofol on ropivacaine metabolism (i.e., PPX production mediated by CYP3A4) in human CYP systems in vitro (412).

Metabolism of prilocaine to o-toluidine and the subsequent N-hydroxylation of this product is responsible for methemoglobinemia which is sometimes discovered in adults after doses above 300 to 400 mg for peripheral or central neural blockade (413). Many case reports also suggest concern about this side effect in children and especially in infants younger than 3 months of age receiving continuous applications of a topical cream containing a eutectic mixture of prilocaine and lidocaine bases (414). Although cases of methemoglobinemia have also been reported with lidocaine, its 2,6-xylidine metabolic product is less potent in this respect than o-toluidine from prilocaine or aniline from benzocaine (414a,415). Both of these aromatic amines are known to be genotoxic in rats, and 2,6-xylidine–hemoglobin adducts have been detected in human blood after low doses of lidocaine (416).

EFFECTS OF PATIENT VARIABLES AND OTHER DRUGS

Much of the information on likely effects of patient variables and other drug therapy on the disposition kinetics of local anesthetics has been obtained from studies with IV lidocaine for cardiotherapy, and it may not always be possible to extrapolate these findings to patients receiving regional anesthesia. This is a problem especially when hemodynamic factors are involved, since the cardiovascular effects of sympathetic nerve block may complicate the issue, and changes in drug elimination may be offset by opposing changes in drug absorption (171). For example, although hypovolemia decreases lidocaine clearance (417), plasma drug concentrations are lower following epidural block in the presence of blood loss as a result of an impaired systemic absorption rate (308). Of the variables considered here, the evidence suggests that cardiovascular disease and liver cirrhosis are associated with clinically more significant alterations in kinetics.

Weight

Limited data on the amide-type agents indicate poor correlations between body weight, surface area, or lean body mass and parameters of drug disposition kinetics in young male subjects with normal height-to-weight ratios (171,178). Weight is an important determinant of systemic clearance in children (418), but is a covariate of other physiologic conditions. A linear relationship of drug dosage with body weight is often used but rarely supported by scientific evidence (167). In obese subjects of either gender with no evidence of cardiac dysfunction, a 50% increase in the terminal elimination half-life of lidocaine was noted. This was explained by an expanded volume of distribution rather than a decreased clearance (80).

Age

Evidence suggests that the clearance of local anesthetics decreases with increasing age in healthy adult subjects. A weak to moderate correlation was seen with bupivacaine and ropivacaine but, surprisingly, not levobupivacaine, the explanation being that hepatic mass is reduced with aging (174–177, 180,219,419). Earlier studies had found no change in lidocaine clearance in geriatric patients, but longer half-lives associated with increased volumes of distribution (420).

Before birth and during the first 3 to 6 months of life, CYP3A4 is deficient, but most of its biotransformation activities are achieved by CYP3A7, which is a major enzyme in the fetus (145). Accordingly, the clearances of bupivacaine and ropivacaine are relatively low at birth and increase through the first year of life (145,421). Elimination half-lives of the amide-type agents are prolonged two- to threefold in neonates, reflecting increased volumes of distribution, decreased clearance, or both (145,303,418,421–424). The renal clearance of lidocaine and mepivacaine was found to be relatively greater in neonates than adults, whereas the hepatic clearance of mepivacaine, but not of lidocaine, was considerably decreased. The first observation may be due to decreased protein binding in neonatal blood and decreased tubular reabsorption owing to higher urine flow rates and lower urine pH in newborns. Less impairment of hepatic lidocaine clearance might be explained by a greater dependence on hepatic perfusion compared to mepivacaine, the elimination of which should be affected more by the function of immature liver enzymes.

Along with suggestions that absorption is faster in children than in adults, the unbound clearance (corrected for body weight) appears to be similar (lidocaine) or greater (bupivacaine and ropivacaine). Corresponding volumes of distribution seem to be similar or higher, such that half-lives are comparable with those in adults (145,421,423,424).

Posture

Prolonged bed rest is associated with increases in plasma and extracellular fluid volumes, and hepatic blood flow is less when standing. Thus, posture might be expected to alter drug disposition. However, although the clearance of lidocaine was observed to decrease on standing (425), no influence of prolonged recumbency on its disposition and plasma binding was found (426).

Pregnancy

Pregnancy is associated with decreases in the plasma half-lives of 2-chloroprocaine and procaine (381–383). Pihlajamaki et al. (307) noted a trend toward lower clearance of bupivacaine in healthy parturients at term compared with controls. They also observed higher plasma concentrations of the N-desbutyl metabolite of bupivacaine (PPX) in the pregnant patients. The clearance of lidocaine was decreased, with no change in plasma binding, in preeclamptic relative to normal parturients (427).

Pregnant ewes were found to clear lidocaine more rapidly, and ropivacaine and bupivacaine less rapidly, than nonpregnant ewes (428–431). This apparent inconsistency may be explained by differences in the determinants of the kinetics of the agents. Thus, clearance of lidocaine is more dependent on hepatic blood flow, which may be raised during pregnancy, whereas that of bupivacaine and ropivacaine is more dependent on the activity of hepatic enzymes, which may be inhibited during pregnancy. Moreover, pregnant ewes had a smaller apparent volume of distribution and a greater plasma binding of both bupivacaine and ropivacaine than nonpregnant ewes, perhaps mediated by competitive tissue binding of pregnancy hormones (428). Pregnant ewes were found to be more susceptible to CNS toxicity at lower doses of bupivacaine, ropivacaine, and levobupivacaine than nonpregnant ewes, although there were no differences in the doses of each agent required to produce more serious cardiovascular system toxicity between

the groups. However, for all three local anesthetics, there were no significant differences between pregnant and nonpregnant ewes in total and free serum drug concentrations when infused at the same dosage rates to the point of circulatory collapse (429).

Cardiovascular Disease

Cardiovascular functioning, and cardiac output in particular, is a determinant of mass balance of solutes in the blood (432); not surprisingly, cardiac output has been found to be a correlate of local anesthetic pharmacokinetics (433).

Plasma concentrations of lidocaine after IV injection in patients with congestive heart failure were found to be about twice as high as those in control subjects receiving the same dose (434). These findings reflect significant decreases in the volume of distribution and clearance of the compounds (Table 3-8). Changes in the rate of drug distribution are a consequence of autoregulatory redistribution of blood from the periphery to vital organs. However, an increase in the extent of distribution, as measured by volume of distribution at steady state (V_{ss}), presumably reflects an altered tissue-to-blood partition or vascular shunting. The impaired clearance appears to be associated with diminished hepatic blood flow secondary to a low cardiac output or impaired hepatic extraction secondary to hepatocellular dysfunction or intrahepatic shunting (417,435). Hypovolemia (417), hypotension (436), and cardiopulmonary resuscitation (437) are associated with changes in the disposition of lidocaine similar to those seen in heart failure. Nonetheless, only minor decreases in the clearance and volume of distribution of lidocaine were observed in patients studied immediately after cardiopulmonary bypass surgery (438). More marked changes seen in the postoperative period were explained, in part, by an increase in plasma binding accompanying the rise in α_1-acid glycoprotein levels.

Liver Disease

Although the plasma half-life of procaine is longer in patients with liver disease, presumably owing to decreased synthesis of pseudocholinesterase, normal esterase activity is preserved in their erythrocytes (383,439).

The clinical significance of altered disposition of the amide local anesthetics in liver disease is greater than that of the esters

TABLE 3-8

LIDOCAINE DISPOSITION IN VARIOUS GROUPS OF PATIENTS

	$t_{1/2,z}$ (h)	V_{ss} (liters/kg)	CL (mL/min/kg)
Normal	1.8	1.32	10.0
Heart failure	1.9	0.88[a]	6.3[a]
Liver cirrhosis	4.9[a]	2.31[a]	6.0[a]
Renal disease	1.3	1.2	13.7

[a]Values differ significantly in comparison to normal subjects. From Thompson P, Melmon KL, Richardson JA, Rowland M. Lidocaine pharmacokinetics in advanced heart failure, liver disease and renal failure in humans. *Ann Intern Med* 1973;78:499.

and depends on the type of liver disease. Assuming that the liver disease does not affect systemic absorption, normal doses can be reasonably considered for single-dose neural blockade, but caution needs to be observed for repeated or continuous dosing because of prolongation of the body residence time of the various agents.

Compared with healthy volunteers, patients with chronic end-stage liver disease had a much lower clearance, a greatly prolonged half-life of intravenously administered ropivacaine, and a decreased urinary excretion of the fraction of the dose metabolized to 3′-OH-ropivacaine (440). In severe cirrhosis, considerable increases occur in the half-life and volume of distribution, and a decrease occurs in the clearance of lidocaine (Table 3-8). The mechanism of the change in distribution may be related to altered plasma or tissue binding, or both (441). The lowered clearance reflects decreased enzyme activity and hepatic blood flow (442). Clearly, systemic accumulation of the amides will be more extensive and prolonged in patients with cirrhosis, and the regression of systemic effects will be slower. In contrast, chronic hepatitis appears to be associated with a higher lidocaine clearance than normal (443), although V_{ss} is also increased secondary to a decreased plasma drug binding (444). The acute phase of viral hepatitis is accompanied by increases in lidocaine half-life and volume of distribution and a trend toward lower clearance. No differences in the plasma binding of the drug were seen in the acute and recovery phases of the disease (445).

Renal Disease

Procaine hydrolysis in sera from patients with impaired renal function is slowed (383). A decreased synthesis of pseudocholinesterase, rather than inhibition or inactivation of the enzyme by other components of uremic serum, appears to be responsible for this effect (446). As in patients with liver disease, red cell esterase is preserved in renal disease (439), and the change in plasma hydrolysis rate may be of little clinical significance.

As might be expected of drugs that are eliminated mostly by the liver, the disposition kinetics of the amides are largely unaffected by renal disease (311) (Table 3-8) but, in patients with severe renal insufficiency, total body clearance was about half that of control subjects (447). However, in contrast to the parent drugs, more polar metabolites will tend to accumulate in patients with renal insufficiency. This is true of GX, formed from lidocaine, although the evidence suggests that the plasma concentrations reached are not likely to cause major toxicity (448).

Diabetes

Patients with non–insulin-dependent diabetes were found to have a significantly lower clearance (60%) of lidocaine after epidural injection compared with controls (449). Although the plasma binding of lidocaine was observed to be less in patients with insulin-dependent diabetes, it was unchanged from normal in type II patients (450). However, in studies with streptozocin-induced diabetes, rats were found to have a significantly higher clearance and decreased apparent volume of distribution compared to control animals that was accompanied by higher plasma concentrations of MEGX (451). The discrepancies are so-far unexplained.

Acidosis and Hypoxia

The toxicity of local anesthetics is believed to be increased significantly by acidosis and hypoxia (452–454). In theory, an increased brain and myocardial concentration of free ionized drug could contribute to this through hemodynamic changes and ion-trapping.

Despite the known effect of arterial CO_2 tension on hepatic blood flow, studies have shown that hypercarbia or hypocarbia does not materially alter the clearance of lidocaine or bupivacaine based on total plasma concentrations (112,455). However, a decrease in plasma binding accompanying acidosis indicates an elevation of free drug concentration under this condition, with the implication of increased toxicity. Nevertheless, deliberate alkalemia produced by IV bicarbonate infusion was associated with greater apparent volume of distribution and concomitant increased half-life of bupivacaine in sheep, whereas deliberate acidemia produced by IV lactic acid infusion produced no significant changes in disposition; neither condition caused significant exacerbation of cardiovascular effects of a sub-convulsant dose of bupivacaine (456).

During metabolic acidosis induced by convulsions, an increase in free drug concentration does not appear to be augmented by an increase in ion trapping within the tissue. Thus, the distribution coefficients of local anesthetics between whole brain or myocardial tissue and blood have been found to be similar (457) or even reduced (112) compared with normal. This is because the lowering of blood pH is similar to, or greater than, the lowering of tissue pH. On the other hand, treatment of convulsions by paralysis and artificial ventilation will tend to exacerbate entry of local anesthetic into the brain, because prevention of the systemic acidosis, but not the cerebral acidosis, promotes ion trapping of drug in the organ (457) (Fig. 3-19). This does not imply that ventilation with oxygen is deleterious, but it may require the use of anticonvulsants during ventilation until the drug is cleared from the brain.

Although the hepatic clearance of lidocaine has been shown to be sensitive to hypoxia in the isolated perfused organ (458), in vivo studies in dogs and sheep with both acute and chronic moderate hypoxia and without hypocapnia indicated no effect

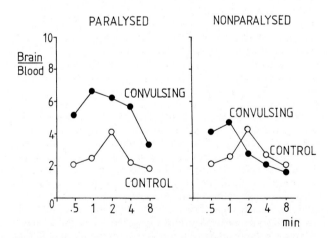

FIGURE 3-19. Brain tissue-to-femoral artery blood partition ratios of lidocaine after intravenous injection into convulsing and nonconvulsing rats. The left panel shows data for animals that were paralyzed with gallamine and ventilated with nitrous oxide/oxygen; the right panel shows data for nonparalyzed animals. Data from Simon RP, Benowitz NL, Culala S. Motor paralysis increases brain uptake of lidocaine during status epilepticas. *Neurology* 1984;34:384, with permission.

on lidocaine clearance or liver blood flow (459,460). However, acute moderate hypoxia was shown to increase the plasma concentrations of the lidocaine metabolites MEGX and GX (459), and hypocapnia was shown to increase the brain concentration of MEGX (461). No effect of hyperbaric hyperoxia was found on the disposition of lidocaine in healthy volunteers (462).

Drug–Drug Interactions

Ideally, interpretation of pharmacokinetic data on drug–drug interactions should be based on measurement of unbound plasma drug concentrations, because these are believed to relate more closely to drug effects than are total concentrations. It becomes especially important in this context to stress the following point. Although the unbound *fraction* of local anesthetic in plasma may be increased by a second drug, this does not necessarily mean that its unbound plasma *concentration* will be significantly greater in vivo, and, therefore, that the risk of toxicity will be increased (316). Failure to appreciate this point has led to confusion in the literature.

Local Anesthetics

There is in vitro evidence that plasma concentrations of etidocaine and bupivacaine in the clinical range can inhibit the hydrolysis of chloroprocaine by 10% to 40% (463,464). Clinically relevant concentrations of bupivacaine may also increase the free *fractions* of lidocaine and mepivacaine (465) in plasma. However, a toxic reaction to a combined block with bupivacaine and mepivacaine due to such a displacement reaction increasing the free concentration of mepivacaine is unlikely.

No differences in plasma concentration–time profiles of etidocaine were observed when intercostal block was performed with etidocaine alone and when it was given with bupivacaine for bilateral block (264,466). Similarly, the plasma concentration–time profiles of lidocaine and bupivacaine were independent of whether they were used alone or in combinations for epidural block (467). However, there are indications of significant enantiomer–enantiomer interactions of the chiral caines. In healthy volunteers, the mean plasma clearance, mean residence time, and (terminal) half-life of levobupivacaine was found to be 465 ± 65 mL/min, 136 ± 20 min, and 115 ± 19 min, respectively, when administered alone, and 317 ± 67 mL/min, 172 ± 55 min, and 157 ± 77 min, when administered as (part of racemic) bupivacaine. Similarly, evidence obtained from sheep also suggests that there may be enantiomer–enantiomer interactions, since the mean total body clearance of R-bupivacaine was 65% greater than that of S-bupivacaine when both enantiomers were administered separately, but only 20% greater when they were administered together as rac-bupivacaine (321,393,468). Moreover, a bolus injection of bupivacaine has been shown to displace lidocaine from binding sites in rabbit lung (469), with possible implications for transient toxicity.

General Anesthetics

Many studies have shown that the disposition of amide local anesthetics, among other drugs, can be altered by volatile anesthetics (470–472). This, to some extent, would appear to be a general effect of all general anesthetics, derived from energy-dependent mechanisms associated with drug transport, processing, and biotransformation.

It has been found that blood concentrations of intravenously infused bupivacaine, levobupivacaine, ropivacaine, lidocaine, mepivacaine, or prilocaine were doubled under halothane anesthesia in sheep; this was the combined result of the drug clearances being decreased by approximately 40%, and apparent volumes of distribution being decreased by approximately 60%. For example, the arterial blood concentrations were doubled and the (calculated) concentrations of these local anesthetics in the myocardium and brain was also increased (473, 473a). Others have shown that the rate of elimination of lidocaine in dogs was slower under halothane anesthesia than while breathing nitrous oxide (474) or air (475). These results are consistent with the effects of halothane in decreasing hepatic blood flow and mixed-function oxidase activity (471,472,476,477). However, the effects of general anesthesia affect more than pharmacokinetics. As described earlier, local anesthetics depress the myocardium in proportion to their local anesthetic potency, but the CNS excitotoxicity they produce heightens sympathetic tone which, inter alia, opposes (reverses) the local anesthetic-induced myocardial depression and alters their pharmacokinetics (Fig. 3-20) (151,478). General anesthesia ablates the CNS response to local anesthetics such that the myocardial depressant effects of the local anesthetics add to the depression induced by the general anesthetic. Figure 3-20 shows, with the example of ropivacaine, a comparison of the pharmacokinetic and pharmacodynamic consequences of the interaction of local anesthetic and general anesthetic in a sheep. Blood and myocardial ropivacaine concentrations are doubled under general anesthesia. When conscious, left ventricular dP/dT_{max} initially decreases, then increases with increased sympathetic tone. Sharp increases occur at the onset of seizure activity, returning to baseline after the CNS response subsides. Under general anesthesia, the depression increases; it too returns to baseline approximately 30 to 60 minutes after cessation of anesthesia.

Adrenoceptor Agonists and Antagonists

Benowitz et al. (417) documented the effects of norepinephrine (α-adrenoceptor stimulation) and of isoproterenol (β-adrenoceptor stimulation) on the disposition kinetics of lidocaine in monkeys. The former decreased initial volume of distribution, decreased clearance by lowering hepatic blood flow, and increased half-life; the latter had the opposite effects.

Inclusion of epinephrine in solutions for epidural block often results in a significant increase in cardiac output and decrease in peripheral resistance and arterial blood pressure over a period of about an hour (479). These effects, together with an increase in liver blood flow (mediated partly through the increase in cardiac output and also by direct action on intrahepatic β_2-receptors), could influence the systemic disposition of local anesthetics. Studies in monkeys (480) and in healthy humans (481) showed that epinephrine absorbed from the epidural space offsets temporarily the lowering of hepatic blood flow caused by sympathetic blockade. In patients receiving epidural injections of bupivacaine, Sharrock et al. (267) observed significantly lower plasma drug concentrations during concomitant IV infusion of epinephrine (maintained cardiac output) compared to phenylephrine (decreased cardiac output). Thus, epinephrine may protect against high systemic exposure to local anesthetic both by decreasing absorption rate and by maintaining or increasing clearance. Intravenous injection of ephedrine (20 mg) was also found to increase the clearance of lidocaine by stimulating hepatic blood flow (482).

Alteration of lidocaine disposition by epinephrine, which increased its brain concentration, was associated with a lower dose threshold for convulsions (483). An increasing number

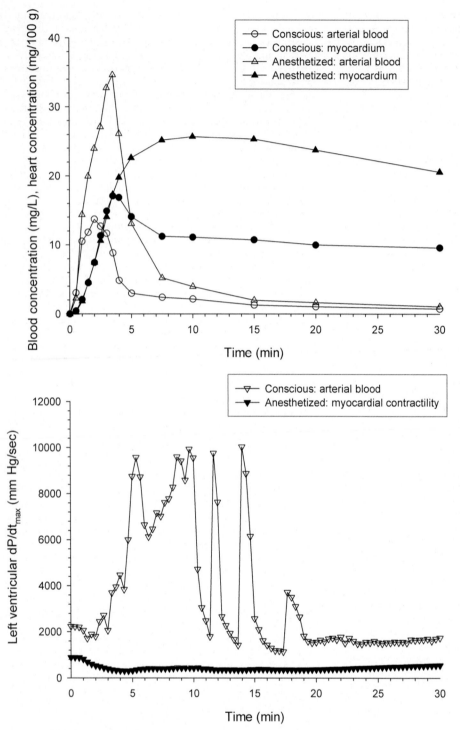

FIGURE 3-20. Interaction between the toxic effects of a local anesthetic and general anesthesia. Ropivacaine (150 mg) was infused intravenously over 3 minutes in an individual adult female sheep (ca. 50 Kg) while the animal was conscious and, on another day, while the sheep was anesthetized with halothane. The dose has produced bouts of excitotoxicity when conscious, corresponding to the increases in LV-dP/dt$_{max}$, but no CNS effects were observed when anesthetized when LV-dP/dt$_{max}$ was already depressed by the halothane anesthesia. These results were similar to the findings also made with other local anesthetics [bupivacaine (100 mg), levobupivacaine (125 mg), mepivacaine (350 mg), lidocaine (350 mg) and prilocaine (350 mg)] in this series. *Upper panels* show arterial and coronary sinus blood ropivacaine concentrations. *Lower panel* shows left ventricular dP/dt$_{max}$. The data were obtained during a series published as Copeland SE, Ladd LA, Gu X-Q, Mather LE. Effects of general anesthesia on whole body and regional pharmacokinetics of local anesthetics at toxic doses. *Anesth Analg* 2008;106:440–449; Copeland SE, Ladd LA, Gu X-Q, Mather LE. Effects of general anesthesia on the central nervous and cardiovascular system toxicity of local anesthetics. *Anesth Analg* 2008;106:1429–1439.

of drugs, mainly well-known CYP inhibitors (484–489), have been shown to alter the disposition kinetics of local anesthetics, but the clinical significance of the changes is largely unknown.

The preanesthetic use of oral clonidine does not impair the clearance of lidocaine (490). In therapeutic doses, propranolol lowers the clearance of lidocaine in humans by about 40%, mainly by direct inhibition of mixed-function oxidase activity and partly by decreasing liver blood flow, through its effect on cardiac output and by intrahepatic β_2 blockade. Other

β-adrenoceptor antagonists have less marked effects, depending on their lipid solubility, cardioselectivity, and intrinsic sympathomimetic activity (491,492). Propranolol also impairs the clearance of bupivacaine (492a).

H$_2$ Antagonists and Proton-pump Inhibitors

Many studies of the potential effect of H$_2$ antagonists on the pharmacokinetics of local anesthetics have been reported, with

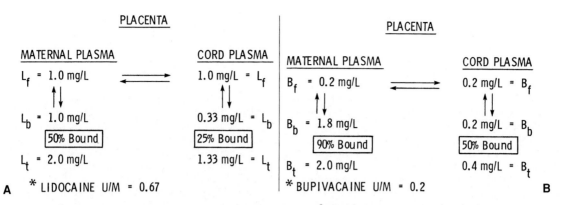

FIGURE 3-21. Schematic showing how transplacental distribution of local anesthetics may be predicted from differences in binding of the drugs in materna. and cord plasma. **A:** Lidocaine. **B:** Bupivacaine; *f, b,* and *t* represent free, bound, and total drug concentrations, respectively.

various permutations of agents, dosage, routes of administration, and duration of treatment (493–498). In isolation, all of these studies suffer from low statistical power owing to the use of few subjects. However, in general, it seems that in single doses for premedication, ranitidine has no effect and cimetidine has little or no effect on the kinetics of either epidural lidocaine or bupivacaine. Used continuously, cimetidine lowers the clearance of lidocaine significantly, but ranitidine has little effect. The effects of multiple doses of cimetidine and ranitidine on bupivacaine clearance have not been determined.

Enzyme-inducing Agents

The systemic clearance of unbound lidocaine was found to be about 25% greater in patients with epilepsy than in controls (499,500). This is presumed to be a consequence of the enzyme-inducing properties of the anticonvulsant. Long-term therapy with phenytoin also induces the synthesis of α_1-glycoprotein, leading to increased plasma binding of lidocaine (500). In contrast, the enzyme inducer rifampicin appears not to influence α_1-acid glycoprotein levels and plasma lidocaine binding in humans (501) but was found to markedly increase the clearance of ropivacaine in both smokers and nonsmokers (485a).

Other Drugs

Administration of inhibitors of plasma pseudocholinesterase, for example, neostigmine and echothiophate, should be avoided in patients receiving ester-type local anesthetics, as should acetazolamide, which blocks hydrolysis by the red cell esterase (439). Nitroprusside in hypotensive doses was shown to have no effect on lidocaine clearance in dogs (146).

Many basic drugs have been shown to displace lidocaine from plasma binding sites, but only when added at supratherapeutic concentrations.

Placental Transfer

Esters

After maternal injection, 2-chloroprocaine appears in both maternal and cord plasma in very low concentrations (62,502). Thus, even though elimination half-lives of chloroprocaine and procaine are twice as long in cord plasma as in maternal plasma, and pregnancy is associated with a decrease in pseudocholinesterase activity (382,383,502), the absolute rate of hydrolysis in the mother remains steady and helps to reduce placental transfer and the risk of fetal intoxication. Cocaine is transferred rapidly and passively across the isolated perfused human placenta (503).

Amides

At delivery, mean values of cord-to-maternal plasma concentration ratios of the amides decrease in the order prilocaine (1.0–1.1), lidocaine (0.5–0.7), mepivacaine (0.7), bupivacaine (0.2–0.4), and etidocaine (0.2–0.3) (178). Comparable values have subsequently been found with bupivacaine, ropivacaine, and levobupivacaine (504–509). These differences broadly reflect differential maternal and fetal plasma binding of the drugs owing to relatively low fetal concentrations of α_1-acid glycoprotein (Fig. 3-21). Equilibrium cord-to-maternal total plasma ratios of the agents are predicted in humans and sheep (admitting species differences in placental morphology) from plasma binding data, with allowance for ion trapping due to fetal acidosis (510–512). As such, therefore, these ratios are not direct predictors of relative fetal toxicity, as corresponding equilibrium ratios of unbound (active) drug across the placenta ought to be close to unity irrespective of the drug; values differing from unity have been found with ropivacaine (509) and mepivacaine (513), and probably reflect disequilibrium values related to the vagaries of labor. (Negative followed by positive deviations from unity are expected with time as the transplacental concentration gradient reverses during the rise and fall of maternal drug concentrations.) Nevertheless, a high maternal-to-fetal binding ratio should delay equilibration of drug in fetal tissues, despite rapid equilibration across the placenta (514). On the other hand, similar umbilical artery-to-umbilical vein concentration ratios observed for the various agents argue against large differences in their equilibration rates in the fetus. As a result of ion trapping, fetal acidosis increases both the cord-to-maternal ratio of unbound drug and the rate of placental transfer of local anesthetic (334,510, 515–519).

Systematic studies performed in sheep at term have found similar placental transmission, along with fetal tissue concentrations of bupivacaine, levobupivacaine, and ropivacaine (324). Papini et al. (520) reported that cord-to-maternal ratios of the bupivacaine enantiomers did not differ when bupivacaine with epinephrine was administered epidurally, but that the ratio for *S*-bupivacaine was slightly greater and exceeded that for *R*-bupivacaine when plain bupivacaine was used. Some degree of enantioselectivity is conceivable and would be consistent with enantioselective disposition in the mother, but the ratio would seem unlikely to be subject to modification by epinephrine.

In the event of inadvertent maternal intravascular injection of local anesthetic, it is advisable to effect the delivery immediately before maximum fetal uptake occurs. Alternatively, providing that clinical conditions allow, there is a theoretical advantage in delaying delivery until significant back-transfer of drug to and clearance by the mother has taken place. An intermediate window will exist in which the body burden to the newborn, whose capacity to eliminate the drug may be impaired, is relatively high. Net back-transfer of bupivacaine, but not of lidocaine, from fetus to mother was observed after a short IV infusion of the agents into ewes (511). The interpretation of this difference with respect to relative rates of equilibration of the drugs in fetal tissues is complicated by the possibility of differential extraction on first pass through the fetal liver. Thus, a higher extraction ratio of lidocaine would amplify its transplacental gradient during infusion, thereby accelerating drug transfer to the fetal circulation. If these findings can be extrapolated to humans, they suggest that back-transfer, which was observed with bupivacaine, might be exploited after an inadvertent injection in the mother by delaying delivery to reduce the burden of drug in the neonate. In contrast, a significant fetal clearance of lidocaine might help to protect against toxicity, and the lack of net back-transfer of this agent would suggest no benefit in delaying delivery.

EPILOGUE

Three decades ago in this essay, we examined relationships between the physicochemical properties of the local anesthetic agents and their fate in the body in order to delineate the role of pharmacokinetics in the overall response to regional anesthesia. This response was then shown to be a complex function of chemistry, pharmacokinetics, pharmacodynamics, the physiologic consequences of neural blockade, and the (patho)physiologic status of the patient. With each revision, some agents have waned in use and new agents have been introduced—and the emphasis has shifted to safer regional anesthesia. Although the maximum tolerated doses may differ, all local anesthetic agents are potentially toxic, regardless of claims, and this is clearly evident by the continual publication of case reports of incidents even with the "safer" chiral caines. The real issue is the separation between the maximum tolerated dose and the minimum effective dose needed for the procedure, and here the agents differ little—but enough to help make choices. Knowledge of the chemical and physicochemical properties provides rationale for these choices.

References

1. Büchi J, Perlia X. Structure-activity relations and physicochemical properties of local anesthetics. In: Lechat P, ed. *Local Anesthetics. International Encyclopedia of Pharmacology and Therapeutics*, Vol. 1. Oxford: Pergamon Press; 1971:39.
2. Calatayud J, González Á. History of the development and evolution of local anesthesia since the coca leaf. *Anesthesiology* 2003;98:1503–1508.
3. Löfgren N. Studies on Local Anesthetics. Xylocaine: A New Synthetic Drug, Inaugural Dissertation for the Degree of Doctor of Philosophy. Stockholm, Faculty of Mathematics and Natural Sciences of the University of Stockholm, 1948. Reprinted, Worcester, Mass, 1958.
4. Lloyd B. The chemical structure and nomenclature of the local anaesthetics. *Br J Anaesth* 1955;27:286–290.
5. Luduena FP. Duration of local anesthesia. *Annu Rev Pharmacol* 1969;9:503–520.
6. Luduena FP. Toxicity and irritancy of local anesthetics. In: Lechat P, ed. *Local Anesthetics, International Encyclopedia of Pharmacology and Therapeutics,* Vol. 1. Oxford: Pergamon Press; 1971:319.
7. Albright GA. Cardiac arrest following regional anesthesia with etidocaine or bupivacaine. *Anesthesiology* 1979;51:285–287.
8. Prentiss JE. Cardiac arrest following caudal anesthesia. *Anesthesiology* 1979;50:51–53.
9. Buckenmaier CC, 3rd, Bleckner LL. Anaesthetic agents for advanced regional anaesthesia: A North American perspective. *Drugs* 2005;65:745–759.
10. Van de Velde M, Dresner M. There is no place in modern obstetrics for racemic bupivacaine. *Int J Obstet Anesth* 2006;15:38–43.
11. Mather LE, Chang DH-T. Cardiotoxicity with modern local anaesthetics: Is there a safer choice? *Drugs* 2001;61:333–342.
12. Vree TB, Gielen MJ. Clinical pharmacology and the use of articaine for local and regional anaesthesia. *Best Pract Res Clin Anaesthesiol* 2005;19(2):293–308.
13. Tucker GT, Lennard MS. Enantiomer specific pharmacokinetics. *Pharmacol Ther* 1989;49:305.
14. Åkerman B, Hellberg I-B, Trossvik C. Primary evaluation of the local anaesthetic properties of the amino amide agent ropivacaine (LEA 103). *Acta Anaesthesiol Scand* 1988;32:571.
15. Åberg G. Toxicological and local anaesthetic effects of optically active isomers of two local anaesthetic compounds. *Acta Pharmacol Toxicol (Copenh)* 1972;31:273–286.
16. Luduena FP, Bogado EF, Tullar BF. Optical isomers of mepivacaine and bupivacaine. *Arch Int Pharmacodyn* 1972;200:359–369.
17. Simonetti MPB, Bird RA. Evaluation of new local anesthetics obtained through the manipulation of the enantiomeric ratio of bupivacaine on the central nervous system of the rat. *The International Monitor, ESRA,* 2000;12:129.
18. Tanaka PP, Tanaka MA, Ogleari MO, Valmorbida PE. Levobupivacaine 0.5% versus 0.5% bupivacaine enantiomeric mixture (S75-R25) versus racemic bupivacaine 0.5% in epidural anesthesia for lower abdominal surgery. *Anesthesiology* 2004;101:A908.
19. Burke D, Henderson DJ. Chirality: A blueprint for the future. *Br J Anaesth* 2002;88:563–576.
20. Calvey TN. Chirality and the mode of action of anaesthetics. *Eur J Anaesth* 1999;16:275–277.
21. Mather LE, Edwards SR. Chirality in anaesthesia: Ropivacaine, ketamine and thiopentone. *Curr Opin Anaesth* 1998;11:383–390.
22. Mather LE, Rutten AJ. Stereochemistry and its relevance in anaesthesiology. *Curr Opin Anaesthesiol* 1991;4:473.
23. Nau C, Strichartz GR. Drug chirality in anesthesia. *Anesthesiology* 2002;97:497–502.
24. Thomas JM, Schug SA. Recent advances in the pharmacokinetics of local anaesthetics. Long-acting amide enantiomers and continuous infusions. *Clin Pharmacokin* 1999;36:67–83.
25. Burmester MD, Schluter KD, Daut J, Hanley PJ. Enantioselective actions of bupivacaine and ropivacaine on coronary vascular resistance at cardiotoxic concentrations. *Anesth Analg* 2005;100(3):707–712.
26. Butterworth J, James RL, Grimes J. Structure-affinity relationships and stereospecificity of several homologous series of local anesthetics for the beta2-adrenergic receptor. *Anesth Analg* 1997;85:336–342.
27. Franqueza L, Longobardo M, Vicente J, et al. Molecular determinants of stereoselective bupivacaine block of hkv1.5 channels. *Circ Res* 1997;81:1053–1064.
28. Graf BM, Abraham I, Eberbach N, et al. Differences in cardiotoxicity of bupivacaine and ropivacaine are the result of physicochemical and stereoselective properties. *Anesthesiology* 2002;96:1427–1434.
29. Kanai Y, Tateyama S, Nakamura T, et al. Effects of levobupivacaine, bupivacaine, and ropivacaine on tail-flick response and motor function in rats following epidural or intrathecal administration. *Reg Anesth Pain Med* 1999;24:444–452.
30. Longobardo M, Delpon E, Caballero R, et al. Structural determinants of potency and stereoselective block of hKv1.5 channels induced by local anesthetics. *Mol Pharmacol* 1998;54:162–169.
31. Mazoit JX, Decaux A, Bouaziz H, Edouard A. Comparative ventricular electrophysiologic effect of racemic bupivacaine, levobupivacaine, and ropivacaine on the isolated rabbit heart. *Anesthesiology* 2000;93:784–792.
32. Muguruma T, Sakura S, Kirihara Y, Saito Y. Comparative somatic and visceral antinociception and neurotoxicity of intrathecal bupivacaine,

levobupivacaine, and dextrobupivacaine in rats. *Anesthesiology* 2006; 104(6):1249–1256.
33. Nau C, Vogel W, Hempelmann G, Brau ME. Stereoselectivity of bupivacaine in local anesthetic-sensitive ion channels of peripheral nerve. *Anesthesiology* 1999;91(3):786–795.
34. Ueta K, Sugimoto M, Suzuki T, et al. In vitro antagonism of recombinant ligand-gated ion-channel receptors by stereospecific enantiomers of bupivacaine. *Reg Anesth Pain Med* 2006;31(1):19–25.
35. Valenzuela C, Delpon E, Tamkun MM, et al. Stereoselective block of a human cardiac potassium channel (Kv1.5) by bupivacaine enantiomers. *Biophys J* 1995;69:418–427.
36. Valenzuela C, Snyders DJ, Bennett PB, et al. Stereoselective block of cardiac sodium channels by bupivacaine in guinea pig ventricular myocytes. *Circulation* 1995;92(10):3014–3024.
37. Vladimirov M, Nau C, Mok WM, Strichartz G. Potency of bupivacaine stereoisomers tested in vitro and in vivo: Biochemical, electrophysiological, and neurobehavioral studies. *Anesthesiology* 2000;93(3):744–755.
38. Zapata-Sudo G, Trachez MM, Sudo RT, Nelson TE. Is comparative cardiotoxicity of S(–) and R(+) bupivacaine related to enantiomer-selective inhibition of L-type Ca(2+) channels? *Anesth Analg* 2001;92(2):496–501.
39. Strong M. FDA policy and regulation of stereoisomers: Paradigm shift and the future of safer, more effective drugs. *Food Drug Law J* 1999;54:463–487.
40. Fawcett JP, Kennedy J, Kumar A, et al. Stereoselective urinary excretion of bupivacaine and its metabolites during epidural infusion. *Chirality* 1999;11(1):50–55.
41. Gu XQ, Fryirs B, Mather LE. High-performance liquid chromatographic separation and nanogram quantitation of bupivacaine enantiomers in blood. *J Chromatography B* 1998;719(1–2):135–140.
42. Tucker GT, Mather LE, Lennard MS, Gregory A. Plasma concentrations of the stereoisomers of prilocaine after administration of the racemate—implications for toxicity? *Br J Anaesth* 1990;65:333–336.
43. Langston M, Dyer UC, Frampton GAC, et al. Racemisation of R-bupivacaine: A key factor in the integrated and economic process for the production of levobupivacaine. *Org Proc Res Dev* 2000;4:530–533.
44. Adger B, Dyer U, Hutton G, Woods M. Stereospecific synthesis of the anaesthetic levobupivacaine. *Tetrahedron Lett* 1996;37:6399.
45. Kopacz DJ, Helman JD, Nussbaum CE, et al. A comparison of epidural levobupivacaine 0.5% with or without epinephrine for lumbar spine surgery. *Anesth Analg* 2001;93:755–760.
46. Dernedde M, Stadler M, Bardiau F, et al. Low vs. high concentration of levobupivacaine for post-operative epidural analgesia: Influence of mode of delivery. *Acta Anaesthesiol Scand* 2003;50(5):613–621.
47. McDonald SB. Hyperbaric spinal ropivacaine: A comparison to bupivacaine in volunteers. *Anesthesiology* 1999;90:971–977.
48. Columb MO, D'Angelo R. Up-down studies: Responding to dosing! *Int J Obstet Anesth* 2006;15:129–136.
49. Columb MO, Lyons G. Determination of the minimum local analgesic concentrations of epidural bupivacaine and lidocaine in labor. *Anesth Analg* 1995;81:833–837.
50. Parpaglioni R, Frigo MG, Lemma A, et al. Minimum local analgesic dose: Effect of different volumes of intrathecal levobupivacaine in early labor. *Anesthesiology* 2005;103(6):1233–1237.
51. Camorcia M, Capogna G, Columb MO. Minimum local analgesic doses of ropivacaine, levobupivacaine, and bupivacaine for intrathecal labor analgesia. *Anesthesiology* 2005;102:646–650.
52. Polley LS, Columb MO, Naughton NN, et al. Relative analgesic potencies of ropivacaine and bupivacaine for epidural analgesia in labor: Implications for therapeutic indexes. *Anesthesiology* 1999;90:944–950.
53. Polley LS, Columb MO, Naughton NN, et al. Relative analgesic potencies of levobupivacaine and ropivacaine for epidural analgesia in labor. *Anesthesiology* 2003;99:1354–1358.
54. Lacassie HJ, Lacassie HP, Muir HA. Is the minimum local analgesic concentration method robust enough? *Anesthesiology* 2004;101(2):550.
55. Van de Velde M, Dreelinck R, Dubois J, et al. Determination of the full dose-response relation of intrathecal bupivacaine, levobupivacaine, and ropivacaine, combined with sufentanil, for labor analgesia. *Anesthesiology* 2007;106(1):149–156.
56. Carvalho B, Durbin M, Drover DR, et al. The ED50 and ED95 of intrathecal isobaric bupivacaine with opioids for cesarean delivery. *Anesthesiology* 2005;103:606–612.
57. Sell A, Olkkola KT, Jalonen J, Aantaa R. Isobaric bupivacaine via spinal catheter for hip replacement surgery: ED50 and ED95 dose determination. *Acta Anaesthesiol Scand* 2006;50:217–221.
58. Capogna G, Celleno D, Lyons G, et al. Minimum local analgesic concentration of extradural bupivacaine increases with progression of labour. *Br J Anaesth* 1998;80:11–13.
59. Polley LS, Columb MO, Naughton NN, et al. Effect of epidural epinephrine on the minimum local analgesic concentration of epidural bupivacaine in labor. *Anesthesiology* 2002;96:1123–1128.

60. Stocks GM, Hallworth SP, Fernando R, et al. Minimum local analgesic dose of intrathecal bupivacaine in labor and the effect of intrathecal fentanyl. *Anesthesiology* 2001;94(4):593–598.
61. Camann W, Abouleish A, Eisenach J, et al. Intrathecal sufentanil and epidural bupivacaine for labor analgesia: Dose-response of individual agents and in combination. *Reg Anesth Pain Med* 1998;23:457–462.
62. Abboud TK, Afrasiabi A, Sarkis F, et al. Continuous infusion epidural analgesia in parturients receiving bupivacaine, chloroprocaine, or lidocaine: Maternal, fetal, and neonatal effects. *Anesth Analg* 1984;63:421.
63. Scott DC, Clymer JW. Estimation of distribution coefficients from the partition coefficient and pKa. *Pharmaceutical Technology* 2002; November: 30–40, at www.pharmtech.com.
64. Grouls RJ, Ackerman EW, Korsten HH, et al. Partition coefficients (n-octanol/water) of N-butyl-p-aminobenzoate and other local anesthetics measured by reversed-phase high-performance liquid chromatography. *J Chromatogr B Biomed Sci Appl* 1997;694:421–425.
65. Schrader W, Andersson JT. Fast and direct method for measuring 1-octanol-water partition coefficients exemplified for six local anesthetics. *J Pharm Sci* 2001;90(12):1948–1954.
66. Meng QC, Zou H, Johansson JS, Eckenhoff RG. Determination of the hydrophobicity of local anesthetic agents. *Anal Biochem* 2001;292:102–106.
67. Clément R, Malinovsky JM, Hildgen P, et al. Spinal disposition and meningeal permeability of local anesthetics. *Pharm Res* 2004;21(4):706–716.
68. Thompson S, Bernards M. Barrier properties of the spinal meninges are markedly decreased by freezing meningeal tissues. *Anesthesiology* 1998;89(5):1276–1278.
69. Grouls RJ, Korsten EH, Hellebrekers LJ, et al. Calculation of the permeability coefficient should take into account the fact that most drugs are weak electrolytes. *Anesthesiology* 2001;95(5):1300–1301.
70. Ratajczak-Enselme M, Estebe JP, Rose FX, et al. Effect of epinephrine on epidural, intrathecal, and plasma pharmacokinetics of ropivacaine and bupivacaine in sheep. *Br J Anaesth* 2007;99(6):881–890.
70a. Rose FX, Estebe JP, Ratajczak M, et al. Epidural, intrathecal, pharmacokinetics, and intrathecal bioavailability of ropivacaine. *Anesth Analg* 2007; 105(3):859–867.
71. Clément R, Malinovsky J, Le Corre P, et al. Spinal biopharmaceutics of bupivacaine and lidocaine by microdialysis after their simultaneous administration in rabbits. *Int J Pharm* 2000;203(1–2):227–234.
72. Clément R, Malinovsky JM, Le Corre P, et al. Cerebrospinal fluid bioavailability and pharmacokinetics of bupivacaine and lidocaine after intrathecal and epidural administrations in rabbits using microdialysis. *J Pharmacol Exp Ther* 1999;289(2):1015–1021.
73. Bernards CM, Hill HF. Physical and chemical properties of drug molecules governing their diffusion through the spinal meninges. *Anesthesiology* 1992;77:750.
74. Bernards CM, Kopacz DJ. Effect of epinephrine on lidocaine clearance in vivo: A microdialysis study in humans. *Anesthesiology* 1999;91(4):962–968.
75. Bernards CM, Ulma GA Jr., Kopacz DJ. The meningeal permeability of R- and S-bupivacaine are not different: Evidence that pharmacodynamic differences between the enantiomers are not the result of differences in bioavailability. *Anesthesiology* 2000;93(3):896–897.
76. Courtney KR. Structure-activity relations for frequency-dependent sodium channel block in nerve by local anesthetics. *J Pharmacol Exp Ther* 1980;213:114.
77. McLeod GA, Columb MO. Moles, weights and potencies: Freedom of expression! *Br J Anaesth* 2005;95:110–111.
78. Rosenberg PH, Schug SA. Levobupivacaine base and levobupivacaine hydrochloride. *Br J Anaesth* 2005;94:544.
79. Åberg G, Dhuner KG, Sydnes G. Studies on the duration of local anaesthesia: Structure/activity relationships in a series of homologous local anesthetics. *Acta Pharmacol Toxicol (Copenh)* 1977;41:432–443.
80. Abernethy DR, Greenblatt DJ. Lidocaine disposition in obesity. *Am J Cardiol* 1984;53:1183.
81. Adams HA, Biscoping J, Kafurke H, et al. Influence of dextran on the absorption of adrenaline-containing lignocaine solutions: A protective mechanism in local anaesthesia. *Br J Anaesth* 1988;60:645.
82. Sanchez V, Arthur GR, Strichartz GR. Fundamental properties of local anesthetics. I. The dependance of lidocaine's ionization and octanol:buffer partitioning on solvent and temperature. *Anesth Analg* 1987;66:159.
83. Strichartz GR, Sanchez V, Arthur GR, et al. Fundamental properties of local anesthetics. II. Measured octanol:buffer partition coefficients and pKa values of clinically used drugs. *Anesth Analg* 1990;71:158–170.
84. Ueda J, Katsuji O, Arakawa K. True oil/water partition coefficients of procaine and lidocaine and estimation of their dissociation constants in organic solvents. *Anesth Analg* 1982;61:56.
85. Fulling PD, Peterfreund RA. Alkalinization and precipitation characteristics of 0.2% ropivacaine. *Reg Anesth Pain Med* 2000;25:518–521.
86. Grouls R, Korsten E, Ackerman E, et al. Diffusion of n-butyl-p-aminobenzoate (BAB), lidocaine and bupivacaine through the human dura-arachnoid mater in vitro. *Eur J Pharm Sci* 2000;12(2):125–131.

87. Fuchsjager-Mayrl G, Zehermayer M, Plass H, Turnheim K. Alkalinization increases penetration of lidocaine across the human cornea. *J Cataract Refract Surg* 2002;28:692–696.
88. Turner D, Williams S, Heavner J. Pleural permeability to local anesthetics: The influence of concentration, pH, and local anesthetic combinations. *Reg Anesth* 1989;14:128.
89. Coventry DM, Todd JG. Alkalinization of bupivacaine for sciatic nerve blockade. *Anaesthesia* 1989;44:467.
90. Quinlan JJ, Oleksey K, Murphy FL. Alkalinization of mepivacaine for axillary block. *Anesth Analg* 1992;74:371.
91. Tetzlaff JE, Yoon HJ, O'Hara J, et al. Alkalinization of mepivacaine accelerates onset of interscalene block for shoulder surgery. *Reg Anesth* 1990;15:242.
92. Ali Z, Chandola HC, Misra MN, Chatterjee S. Effect of pH adjustment on onset and duration of epidural anaesthesia. *J Indian Med Assoc* 1993;91:204–205.
93. Capogna G, Celleno D, Laudano D, Giunta F. Alkalinization of local anesthetics. Which block, which local anesthetic? *Reg Anesth* 1995;20(5):369–377.
94. Candido KD, Winnie AP, Covino BG, et al. Addition of bicarbonate to plain bupivacaine does not significantly alter the onset or duration of plexus anesthesia. *Reg Anesth* 1995;20(2):133–138.
95. Tetzlaff JE, Rothstein L. Alkalinization of mepivacaine does not alter onset of caudal anesthesia. *J Clin Anesth* 1992;4:301.
96. Takman B. The chemistry of local anaesthetic agents. *Br J Anaesth* 1975;47:183.
97. Leor R, Feinstein M, Hod H, et al. The influence of pH on the intravenous delivery of lidocaine solutions. *Eur J Clin Pharmacol* 1990;39:521.
98. Salazar F, Bogdanovich A, Adalia R, et al. Transient neurologic symptoms after spinal anaesthesia using isobaric 2% mepivacaine and isobaric 2% lidocaine. *Acta Anaesthesiol Scand* 2001;45:240–245.
99. Tong D, Wong J, Chung F, et al. Prospective study on incidence and functional impact of transient neurologic symptoms associated with 1% versus 5% hyperbaric lidocaine in short urologic procedures. *Anesthesiology* 2003;98:485–494.
100. Winnie AP, Nader AM. Santayana's prophecy fulfilled. *Reg Anesth Pain Med* 2001;26:6.
101. Kitagawa N, Oda M, Totoki T. Possible mechanism of irreversible nerve injury caused by local anesthetics: Detergent properties of local anesthetics and membrane disruption. *Anesthesiology* 2004;100(4):962–967.
102. Schneider MC, Birnbach DJ. Lidocaine neurotoxicity in the obstetric patient: Is the water safe? *Anesth Analg* 2001;92(2):287–290.
103. Rosenberg PH, Kytta J, Alila A. Uptake of bupivacaine, etidocaine, lignocaine and ropivacaine in n-heptane, rat sciatic nerve and human epidural and subcutaneous fat. *Br J Anaesth* 1986;58:310.
104. Langerman L, Basinath M, Grant GJ. The partition coefficient as a predictor of local anesthetic potency for spinal anesthesia: Evaluation of five local anesthetics in a mouse model. *Anesth Analg* 1994;79:490–494.
105. af Ekenstam B. The effect of the structural variation on the local analgetic properties of the most commonly used groups of substances. *Acta Anaesthesiol Scand* 1966;25[Suppl]:10–18.
106. Wildsmith JAW, Brown PD, Johnson S. Structure activity relationships in differential nerve block at high and low frequency stimulation. *Br J Anaesth* 1989;63:444.
107. Wildsmith JAW, Gissen AJ, Gregus J, Covino BG. Differential nerve blocking ability of amino-ester local anaesthetics. *Br J Anaesth* 1985;57:612.
108. Wildsmith JAW, Gissen AJ, Takman B, Covino BG. Differential nerve block: Esters v amides and the influence of pKa. *Br J Anaesth* 1987;59:379.
109. Bachmann B, Biscoping J, Sinning E, Hempelmann G. Protein binding of prilocaine in human plasma: Influence of concentration, pH and temperature. *Acta Anaesthesiol Scand* 1990;34:311.
110. Coyle DE, Denson DD, Thompson GA, et al. The influence of lactic acid on the serum protein binding of bupivacaine: Species differences. *Anesthesiology* 1984;61:127.
111. Denson DD, Myers JA, Thompson GA, Coyle DE. The influence of diazepam on the serum protein binding of bupivacaine at normal and acidic pH. *Anesth Analg* 1984;63:980.
112. Nancarrow C, Runciman WB, Mather LE, et al. The influence of acidosis on the distribution of lidocaine and bupivacaine into the myocardium and brain of the sheep. *Anesth Analg* 1987;66:925–935.
113. Taheri S, Cogswell, LP, 3rd, Gent A, Strichartz GR. Hydrophobic and ionic factors in the binding of local anesthetics to the major variant of human α1-acid glycoprotein. *J Pharmacol Exp Ther* 2003;304:71–80.
114. Tucker GT, Boyes RN, Bridenbaugh PO, Moore DC. Binding of anilide-type local anesthetics in human plasma. I: Relationships between binding, physicochemical properties and anesthetic activity. *Anesthesiology* 1970;33:287.
115. Bernards CM. Cerebrospinal fluid and spinal cord distribution of baclofen and bupivacaine during slow intrathecal infusion in pigs. *Anesthesiology* 2006;105(1):169–178.
116. Cousins MJ, Mather LE. Intrathecal and epidural administration of opioids. *Anesthesiology* 1984;61:276.
117. Bernards CM, Hill HF. The spinal nerve root sleeve is not a preferred route for redistribution of drugs from the epidural space to the spinal cord. *Anesthesiology* 1991;75:827.
117a. Bernards CM, Sorkin LS. Radicular artery blood flow does not redistribute fentanyl from the epidural space to the spinal cord. *Anesthesiology* 1994;80:872.
118. Grant GJ, Piskoun B, Bansinath M. Analgesic duration and kinetics of liposomal bupivacaine after subcutaneous injection in mice. *Clin Exp Pharmacol Physiol* 2003;30:966–968.
119. Langerman L, Grant GJ, Zakowski M, et al. Prolongation of spinal anesthesia. Spinal action of a lipid drug carrier on tetracaine, lidocaine and procaine. *Anesthesiology* 1992;77:475.
120. McDonald S, Faibushevich AA, Garnick S, et al. Determination of local tissue concentrations of bupivacaine released from biodegradable microspheres and the effect of vasoactive compounds on bupivacaine tissue clearance studied by microdialysis sampling. *Pharm Res* 2002;19(11):1745–1752.
121. Sato S, Baba Y, Tajima K, et al. Prolongation of epidural anesthesia in the rabbit with the use of a biodegradable copolymer paste containing lidocaine. *Anesth Analg* 1995;80:97.
122. Boogaerts JG, Lafont ND, Declercq AG, et al. Epidural administration of liposome-associated bupivacaine for the management of postsurgical pain: A first study. *J Clin Anesth* 1994;6:315.
123. Kopacz DJ, Bernards CM, Allen HW, et al. A model to evaluate the pharmacokinetic and pharmacodynamic variables of extended-release products using in vivo tissue microdialysis in humans: Bupivacaine-loaded microcapsules. *Anesth Analg* 2003;97(1):124–131.
124. Kopacz DJ, Lacouture PG, Wu D, et al. The dose response and effects of dexamethasone on bupivacaine microcapsules for intercostal blockade (T9 to T11) in healthy volunteers. *Anesth Analg* 2003;96(2):576–582.
125. Planas ME, Gonzalez P, Rodriguez L, et al. Noninvasive percutaneous induction of topical analgesia by a new type of drug carrier, and prolongation of local pain insensitivity by anesthetic liposomes. *Anesth Analg* 1992;75:615.
126. Bromage PR. Mechanisms of action of extradural analgesia. *Br J Anaesth* 1975;47[Suppl]:199.
127. Moore DC, Bush WH, Burnett LL. Celiac plexus block: A roentgenographic, anatomic study of technique and spread of solution in patients and corpses. *Anesth Analg* 1981;60:369.
128. Moorthy SS, Dierdorf SF, Yaw PB. Influence of volume on the spread of local anesthetic-methylene blue solution after injection for intercostal block. *Anesth Analg* 1992;75:389.
129. Ross BK, Coda B, Heath CH. Local anesthetic distribution in a spinal model: A possible mechanism of neurologic injury after continuous spinal anesthesia. *Reg Anesth* 1992;17:69+.
130. King HK, Xiao CS, Wooten DJ. Prolongation of epidural bupivacaine analgesia with glycerine. *Can J Anaesth* 1993;40:431.
131. Pippa P, Cuomo P, Panchetti A, et al. High volume and low concentration of anaesthetic solution in the perivascular interscalene sheath determines quality of block and incidence of complications. *Eur J Anaesth* 2006;23(10):855–860.
132. Bernards CM, Shen DD, Sterling ES, et al. Epidural, cerebrospinal fluid, and plasma pharmacokinetics of epidural opioids (part 2): Effect of epinephrine. *Anesthesiology* 2003;99(2):466–475.
133. Choi R, Birknes JK, Popitz-Bergez FA, et al. Pharmacokinetic nature of tachyphylaxis to lidocaine: Peripheral nerve blocks and infiltration anesthesia in rats. *Life Sci* 1997;PL61:177–184.
134. Ibusuki S, Katsuki H, Takasaki M. The effects of extracellular pH with and without bicarbonate on intracellular procaine concentrations and anesthetic effects in crayfish giant axons. *Anesthesiology* 1998;88(6):1549–1557.
135. Chow MY, Sia AT, Koay CK, Chan YW. Alkalinization of lidocaine does not hasten the onset of axillary brachial plexus block. *Anesth Analg* 1998;86(3):566–568.
136. Moharib MM, Mitra S. Alkalinized lidocaine and bupivacaine with hyaluronidase for sub-tenon's ophthalmic block. *Reg Anesth Pain Med* 2000;25(5):514–517.
137. Moharib MM, Mitra S, Rizvi SG. Effect of alkalinization and/or hyaluronidase adjuvancy on a local anesthetic mixture for sub-Tenon's ophthalmic block. *Acta Anaesthesiol Scand* 2002;46(5):599–602.
138. Morrison LMM, Emanuelsson BM, McClure JH, et al. Efficacy and kinetics of extradural ropivacaine: Comparison with bupivacaine. *Br J Anaesth* 1994;72:164.
139. Palmer SK, Bosnjak ZJ, Hopp F, et al. Lidocaine and bupivacaine differential blockade of isolated canine nerves. *Anesth Analg* 1983;62:754.
140. Bromage PR. Lower limb reflex changes in segmental epidural analgesia. *Br J Anaesth* 1974;46:504.
141. Rosenberg PH, Heinonen E. Differential sensitivity of A and C nerve fibres to long-acting amide local anaesthetics. *Br J Anaesth* 1983;55:143.
142. Gissen AJ, Covino BG, Gregus J. Differential sensitivity of fast and slow fibers in mammalian nerve: III. Effect of etidocaine and bupivacaine on fast/slow fibers. *Anesth Analg* 1982;61:570.

143. Ford DJ, Raj PP, Regan KM, Ohlweiler D. Differential peripheral nerve block by local anesthetics in the cat. *Anesthesiology* 1984;60:28.

144. Fink BR, Cairns AM. Diffusional delay in local anesthetic block in vitro. *Anesthesiology* 1984;61:555.

145. Mazoit JX, Dahlens BJ. Pharmacokinetics of local anaesthetics in infants and children. *Clin Pharmacokinet* 2004;43:17–32.

146. Shiroff RA, Schneck DW, Pritchard JF, et al. Effects of acute blood pressure reduction by sodium nitroprusside on serum lidocaine levels. *Fed Proc* 1977;36:958.

147. Xuecheng J, Xiaobin W, Bo G, et al. The plasma concentrations of lidocaine after slow versus rapid administration of an initial dose of epidural anesthesia. *Anesth Analg* 1997;84:570–573.

148. Moore DC, Mather LE, Bridenbaugh LD, et al. Bupivacaine (Marcaine): An evaluation of its tissue and systemic toxicity in humans. *Acta Anaesthesiol Scand* 1977;21:109–121.

149. Tucker GT, Moore DC, Bridenbaugh PO, et al. Systemic absorption of mepivacaine in commonly used regional block procedures. *Anesthesiology* 1972;37:277.

150. Emanuelsson BM, Persson J, Sandin S, et al. Intraindividual and interindividual variability in the disposition of the local anesthetic ropivacaine in healthy subjects. *Ther Drug Monit* 1997;19(2):126–131.

151. Mather LE, Copeland SE, Ladd LA. Acute toxicity of local anesthetics: Underlying pharmacokinetic and pharmacodynamic concepts. *Reg Anesth Pain Med* 2005;30:553–566.

152. Mather LE, Tucker GT, Murphy TM, et al. Cardiovascular, central nervous system effect of long acting local anaesthetics in man. *Anaesth Intensive Care* 1979;7:215–221.

153. Kozody R, Ready LB, Barsa JE, Murphy TM. Dose requirement of local anaesthetic to produce grand mal seizure during stellate ganglion block. *Can J Anaesth* 1982;29:489–491.

154. Perkins WJ, Lanier WL, Sharborough FW. Cerebral and hemodynamic effects of lidocaine accidentally injected into the carotid arteries of patients having carotid endarterectomy. *Anesthesiology* 1988;69:787–790.

155. Chang DHT, Ladd LA, Copeland S, et al. Direct cardiac effects of intracoronary bupivacaine, levobupivacaine and ropivacaine in the sheep. *Br J Pharmacol* 2001;132:649–658.

156. Ladd LA, Chang DH-T, Wilson K, et al. Effects of CNS site-directed carotid arterial infusions of bupivacaine, levobupivacaine and ropivacaine in sheep. *Anesthesiology* 2002;97:418–428.

157. Bardsley H, Gristwood R, Baker H, et al. A comparison of the cardiovascular effects of levobupivacaine and rac-bupivacaine following intravenous administration to healthy volunteers. *Br J Clin Pharmacol* 1998;46:245–249.

158. Knudsen K, Beckman Suurkula M, Blomberg S, et al. Central nervous and cardiovascular effects of i.v. infusions of ropivacaine, bupivacaine and placebo in volunteers. *Br J Anaesth* 1997;78:507–514.

159. Scott DB. Evaluation of the toxicity of local anaesthetic agents in man. *Br J Anaesth* 1975;47[Suppl]:56–61.

160. Scott DB. Toxic effects of local anaesthetic agents on the central nervous system. *Br J Anaesth* 1986;58:732–735.

161. Scott DB, Lee A, Fagan D, et al. Acute toxicity of ropivacaine compared with that of bupivacaine. *Anesth Analg* 1989;69:563–569.

162. Stewart J, Kellett N, Castro D. The central nervous system and cardiovascular effects of levobupivacaine and ropivacaine in healthy volunteers. *Anesth Analg* 2003;97:412–416.

163. Groban L. Central nervous system and cardiac effects from long-acting amide local anesthetic toxicity in the intact animal model. *Reg Anesth Pain Med* 2003;28:3–11.

164. Groban L, Deal DD, Vernon JC, Et al. Does local anesthetic stereoselectivity or structure predict myocardial depression in anesthetized canines? *Reg Anesth Pain Med* 2002;27:460–468.

165. Heavner JE. Cardiac toxicity of local anesthetics in the intact isolated heart model: A review. *Reg Anesth Pain Med* 2002;27:545–555.

166. Reynolds F. Maximum recommended doses of local anesthetics: A constant cause of confusion. *Reg Anesth Pain Med* 2005;30:314–316.

167. Rosenberg PH, Veering BT, Urmey WF. Maximum recommended doses of local anesthetics: A multifactorial concept. *Reg Anesth Pain Med* 2004;29(6):564–575.

168. Munson ES, Tucker WK, Ausinsch B, Malagodi H. Etidocaine, bupivacaine, and lidocaine seizure thresholds in monkey. *Anesthesiology* 1975;42:471–478.

169. Bokesch PM, Castaneda AR, Ziemer G, Wilson JM. The influence of right-to-left cardiac shunt on lidocaine pharmacokinetics. *Anesthesiology* 1987;67:739.

170. Tucker GT, Boas RA. Pharmacokinetic aspects of intravenous regional anesthesia. *Anesthesiology* 1971;34:538.

171. Tucker GT, Mather LE. Pharmacokinetics of local anaesthetic agents. *Br J Anaesth* 1975;47[Suppl]:213–224.

172. Burm AG. Clinical pharmacokinetics of epidural and spinal anaesthesia. *Clin Pharmacokinet* 1989;16:283–311.

173. Burm AGL, Vermeulen NPE, Van Kleef JW, et al. Pharmacokinetics of lidocaine and bupivacaine in surgical patients following epidural adminis-

tration. Simultaneous investigation of absorption and disposition kinetics using stable isotopes. *Clin Pharmacokinet* 1987;13:191.

174. Simon MJ, Veering BT, Stienstra R, et al. Effect of age on the clinical profile and systemic absorption and disposition of levobupivacaine after epidural administration. *Br J Anaesth* 2004;93(4):512–520.

175. Simon MJ, Veering BT, Vletter AA, et al. The effect of age on the systemic absorption and systemic disposition of ropivacaine after epidural administration. *Anesth Analg* 2006;102:276–282.

176. Veering BT, Burm AG, Vletter AA, et al. The effect of age on the systemic absorption, disposition and pharmacodynamics of bupivacaine after epidural administration. *Clin Pharmacokinet* 1992;22:75.

177. Veering BT, Burm AGL, Vletter AA, et al. The effect of age on systemic absorption and systemic disposition of bupivacaine after subarachnoid administration. *Anesthesiology* 1991;74:250.

178. Tucker GT, Mather LE. Clinical pharmacokinetics of local anaesthetic agents. *Clin Pharmacokinet* 1979;4:241.

179. Katz JA, Bridenbaugh PO, Knarr DC, et al. Pharmacodynamics and pharmacokinetics of epidural ropivacaine in humans. *Anesth Analg* 1990;70:16–21.

180. Simon MJ, Veering BT, Stienstra R, et al. The systemic absorption and disposition of levobupivacaine 0.5% after epidural administration in surgical patients: A stable-isotope study. *Eur J Anaesth* 2004;21:460–470.

181. Inoue R, Suganuma T, Echizen H, et al. Plasma concentrations of lidocaine and its principal metabolites during intermittent epidural anesthesia. *Anesthesiology* 1985;63:304.

182. Tucker GT, Cooper S, Littlewood D, et al. Observed and predicted accumulation of local anaesthetic agent during continuous extradural analgesia. *Br J Anaesth* 1977;49:237.

183. Wildsmith JAW, Tucker GT, Cooper S, et al. Plasma concentrations of local anaesthetics after interscalene brachial plexus block. *Br J Anaesth* 1977;49:461.

184. Mogensen T, Hojgaard L, Scott NB, et al. Epidural blood flow and regression of sensory analgesia during continuous postoperative epidural infusion of bupivacaine. *Anesth Analg* 1988;67:809.

185. Dahl JB, Simonsen L, Mogensen T, et al. The effect of 0.5% ropivacaine on epidural blood flow. *Acta Anaesthesiol Scand* 1990;34:308.

186. Iida H, Ohata H, Iida M, et al. The differential effects of stereoisomers of ropivacaine and bupivacaine on cerebral pial arterioles in dogs. *Anesth Analg* 2001;93(6):1552–1556.

187. Kopacz DJ, Carpenter RL, Mackey DC. Effect of ropivacaine on cutaneous capillary blood flow in pigs. *Anesthesiology* 1989;71:69.

188. Newton DJ, Burke D, Khan F, et al. Skin blood flow changes in response to intradermal injection of bupivacaine and levobupivacaine, assessed by laser Doppler imaging. *Reg Anesth Pain Med* 2000;25(6):626–631.

189. Newton DJ, McLeod GA, Khan F, Belch JJ. Vasoactive characteristics of bupivacaine and levobupivacaine with and without adjuvant epinephrine in peripheral human skin. *Br J Anaesth* 2005;94(5):662–667.

189a. Newton DJ, McLeod GA, Khan F, Belch JJ. Mechanisms influencing the vasoactive effects of lidocaine in human skin. *Anaesthesia* 2007;62(2):146–150.

190. Lee-Son S, Wang GK, Concus A, et al. Stereoselective inhibition of neuronal sodium channels by local anesthetics. Evidence for two sites of action? *Anesthesiology* 1992;77:324–335.

191. Åkerman B, Persson H, Tegner C. Local anaesthetic properties of the optically active isomers of prilocaine (Citanest). *Acta Pharmacol Toxicol (Copenh)* 1967;25:233.

192. Karmakar MK, Ho AM, Law BK, et al. Arterial and venous pharmacokinetics of ropivacaine with and without epinephrine after thoracic paravertebral block. *Anesthesiology* 2005;103704–103711.

193. Cardoso MM, Carvalho JC. Epidural pressures and spread of 2% lidocaine in the epidural space: Influence of volume and speed of injection of the local anesthetic solution. *Reg Anesth Pain Med* 1998;23(1):14–19.

194. Cheema S, Richardson J, McGurgan P. Factors affecting the spread of bupivacaine in the adult thoracic paravertebral space. *Anaesthesia* 2003;58(7):684–687.

195. Pandit JJ, Dutta D, Morris JF. Spread of injectate with superficial cervical plexus block in humans: An anatomical study. *Br J Anaesth* 2003;91:733–735.

196. Visser WA, Gielen MJ, Giele JL. Continuous positive airway pressure breathing increases the spread of sensory blockade after low-thoracic epidural injection of lidocaine. *Anesth Analg* 2006;102(1):268–271.

197. Hogan Q. Distribution of solution in the epidural space: Examination by cryomicrotome section. *Reg Anesth Pain Med* 2002;27(2):150–156.

198. Hogan Q, Toth J. Anatomy of soft tissues of the spinal canal. *Reg Anesth Pain Med* 1999;24(4):303–310.

199. Moore DC, Mather LE, Bridenbaugh LD, et al. Arterial and venous plasma levels of bupivacaine (Marcaine) following epidural and intercostal nerve blocks. *Anesthesiology* 1976;45:39.

200. Sharrock NE, Mather LE, Go G, Sculco TP. Arterial and pulmonary arterial concentrations of the enantiomers of bupivacaine after epidural injection in elderly patients. *Anesth Analg* 1998;86(4):812–817.

201. Lee BB, Ngan Kee WD, Plummer JL, et al. The effect of the addition of epinephrine on early systemic absorption of epidural ropivacaine in humans. *Anesth Analg* 2002;95(5):1402–1407.

202. Murphy D. Interpleural analgesia. *Br J Anaesth* 1993;71:426–434.

203. Safran D, Kuhlman G, Orhant EE, et al. Continuous intercostal blockade with lidocaine after thoracic surgery. Clinical and pharmacokinetic study. *Anesth Analg* 1990;70:345.

204. McKenzie AG, Mathe S. Interpleural local anaesthesia: Anatomical basis for mechanism of action. *Br J Anaesth* 1996;76(2):297–299.

205. Skrømstag KE, Minor B, Steen PA. Side effects and complications related to interpleural analgesia: An update. *Acta Anesthesiol Scand* 1990;34:473.

206. Van Kleef JW, Burm AGL, Vletter AA. Single-dose interpleural versus intercostal blockade: Nerve block characteristics and plasma concentration profiles after administration of 0.5% bupivacaine with epinephrine. *Anesth Analg* 1990;70:484.

207. Van Kleef JW, Logeman EA, Burm AGL, et al. Continuous interpleural infusion of bupivacaine for postoperative analgesia after surgery with flank incisions: A double-blind comparison of 0.25% and 0.5% solutions. *Anesth Analg* 1992;75:268.

208. Laurito CE, Kirz LJ, VadeBoncouer TR, et al. Continuous infusion of interpleural bupivacaine maintains effective analgesia after cholecystectomy. *Anesth Analg* 1991;72:516.

209. Kastrissios H, Triggs EJ, Mogg GAG, Higbie JW. The disposition of bupivacaine following a 72h interpleural infusion in cholecystectomy patients. *Br J Clin Pharmacol* 1991;32:251.

210. Kaneko T, Iwama H. The association between injected volume of local anesthetic and spread of epidural anesthesia: A hypothesis. *Reg Anesth Pain Med* 1999;24(2):153–157.

211. Higuchi H, Adachi Y, Kazama T. Factors affecting the spread and duration of epidural anesthesia with ropivacaine. *Anesthesiology* 2004;101(2):451–460.

212. Okutomi T, Minakawa M, Hoka S. Saline volume and local anesthetic concentration modify the spread of epidural anesthesia. *Can J Anaesth* 1999;46(10):930–934.

213. Husemeyer RP, White DC. Lumbar extradural injection pressures in pregnant women. An investigation of relationships between rate of injection, injection pressures and extent of analgesia. *Br J Anaesth* 1980;52:55.

214. Kanai A, Suzuki A, Hoka S. Rapid injection of epidural mepivacaine speeds the onset of nerve blockade. *Can J Anaesth* 2005;52(3):281–284.

215. Rosenberg PH, Saramies L, Alila A. Lumbar epidural anaesthesia with bupivacaine in old patients: Effect of speed and direction of injection. *Acta Anaesthesiol Scand* 1981;25:270.

216. Curatolo M, Orlando A, Zbinden AM, et al. A mutifactorial analysis of the spread of epidural analgesia. *Acta Anaesth Scand* 1994;38:625.

217. Dernedde M, Stadler M, Bardiau F, Boogaerts J. Comparison of different concentrations of levobupivacaine for post-operative epidural analgesia. *Acta Anaesthesiol Scand* 2003;47(7):884–890.

218. Leeda M, Stienstra R, Arbous MS, et al. Lumbar epidural catheter insertion: The midline vs. the paramedian approach. *Eur J Anaesth* 2005;22(11):839–842.

219. Simon MJ, Veering BT, Stienstra R, et al. The effects of age on neural blockade and hemodynamic changes after epidural anesthesia with ropivacaine. *Anesth Analg* 2002;94(5):1325–1330.

219a. Bernards CM, Shen DD, Sterling ES, et al. Epidural, cerebrospinal fluid, and plasma pharmacokinetics of epidural opioids (part 1): Differences among opioids. *Anesthesiology* 2003;99(2):455–465.

220. Wilkinson GR, Lund PC. Bupivacaine levels in plasma and cerebrospinal fluid following peridural administration. *Anesthesiology* 1970;33:482.

221. Urban BJ. Clinical observations suggesting a changing site of action during induction and recession of spinal and epidural anesthesia. *Anesthesiology* 1973;39:496.

222. Bernards CM, Kopacz DJ, Michel MZ. Effect of needle puncture on morphine and lidocaine flux through the spinal meninges of the monkey in vitro. Implications for combined spinal-epidural anesthesia. *Anesthesiology* 1994;80:853.

223. Sharrock NE, Go G, Mineo R, et al. Relationship between body surface area and arterial concentrations of bupivacaine following lumbar epidural anesthesia. *Reg Anesth* 1995;20(2):139–144.

224. Mayumi T, Dohi S, Takahashi T. Plasma concentrations of lidocaine associated with cervical, thoracic, and lumbar epidural anesthesia. *Anesth Analg* 1983;62:578.

225. Schug SA, Saunders D, Kurowski I, Paech MJ. Neuraxial drug administration: A review of treatment options for anaesthesia and analgesia. *CNS Drugs* 2006;20(11):917–933.

225a. Erichsen CJ, Sjovall J, Kehlet H, et al. Pharmacokinetics and analgesic effect of ropivacaine during continuous epidural infusion for postoperative pain relief. *Anesthesiology* 1996;84(4):834–842.

225b. Scott DA, Emanuelsson BM, Mooney PH, et al. Pharmacokinetics and efficacy of long-term epidural ropivacaine infusion for postoperative analgesia. *Anesth Analg* 1997;85(6):1322–1330.

225c. Wiedemann D, Muhlnickel B, Staroske E, et al. Ropivacaine plasma concentrations during 120-hour epidural infusion. *Br J Anaesth* 2000;85(6):830–835.

226. Irestedt L, Ekblom A, Olofsson C, et al. Pharmacokinetics and clinical effect during continuous epidural infusion with ropivacaine 2.5 mg/ml or bupivacaine 2.5 mg/ml for labour pain relief. *Acta Anaesthesiol Scand* 1998;42(8):890–896.

227. Hallworth SP, Fernando R, Columb MO, Stocks GM. The effect of posture and baricity on the spread of intrathecal bupivacaine for elective cesarean delivery. *Anesth Analg* 2005;100(4):1159–1165.

228. Heller AR, Zimmermann K, Seele K, et al. Modifying the baricity of local anesthetics for spinal anesthesia by temperature adjustment: Model calculations. *Anesthesiology* 2006;105(2):346–353.

229. Hocking G, Wildsmith JAW. Intrathecal drug spread. *Br J Anaesth* 2004;93(4):568–578.

230. Nicol ME, Holdcroft A. Density of intrathecal agents. *Br J Anaesth* 1992;68:60.

231. Sinclair CJ, Scott DB, Edstrom HH. Effect of the Trendelenburg position on spinal anaesthesia with hyperbaric bupivacaine. *Br J Anaesth* 1982;54:497.

232. Post C, Freedman J. A new method for studying the distribution of drugs in spinal cord after intrathecal injection. *Acta Pharmacol Toxicol (Copenh)* 1984;54:253.

233. Greene NM. Uptake and elimination of local anesthetics during spinal anesthesia. *Anesth Analg* 1983;62:1013.

234. Winnie AP, Lavallee DA, Sosa BP, Masud KZ. Clinical pharmacokinetics of local anaesthetics. *Can Anaesth Soc J* 1977;24:252.

235. Winnie AP, Tay C-H, Patel KP, et al. Pharmacokinetics of local anesthetics during plexus blocks. *Anesth Analg* 1977;56:852.

236. Maclean D, Chambers WA, Tucker GT, Wildsmith JAW. Plasma prilocaine concentrations after three techniques of brachial plexus blockade. *Br J Anaesth* 1988;60:136.

237. Selander D. Axillary plexus block: Paresthetic or perivascular. *Anesthesiology* 1987;66:726.

238. Vester-Andersen T, Husum B, Lindeburg T, et al. Perivascular axillary block. V: Blockade following 60 ml of mepivacaine 1% injected as a bolus or as 30 + 30 ml with a 20-min interval. *Acta Anaesthesiol Scand* 1984;28:612.

239. Vainionpaa VA, Haavisto ET, Huha TM, et al. A clinical and pharmacokinetic comparison of ropivacaine and bupivacaine in axillary plexus block. *Anesth Analg* 1995;81(3):534–538.

240. Lauven PM, Witow R, Lussi C, Luhr HG. Blutspiegel und pharmakokinetisches modell von prilocain bei der kontinuerlichen plexus-brachialis-blockade. *Reg Anesth* 1990;13:189.

241. Ekatodramis G, Borgeat A, Huledal G, et al. Continuous interscalene analgesia with ropivacaine 2 mg/mL after major shoulder surgery. *Anesthesiology* 2003;98(1):143–150.

242. Junca A, Marret E, Goursot G, et al. A comparison of ropivacaine and bupivacaine for cervical plexus block. *Anesth Analg* 2001;92(3):720–724.

243. Gratz I, Deal E, Larijani GE, et al. The number of injections does not influence absorption of bupivacaine after cervical plexus block for carotid endarterectomy. *J Clin Anesth* 2005;17(4):263–266.

244. Costello TG, Cormack JR, Hoy C, et al. Plasma ropivacaine levels following scalp block for awake craniotomy. *J Neurosurg Anesthesiol* 2004;16(2):147–150.

245. Costello TG, Cormack JR, Mather LE, et al. Plasma levobupivacaine concentrations following scalp block in patients undergoing awake craniotomy. *Br J Anaesth* 2005;94(6):848–851.

246. Scott DB, Littlewood DG, Covino BG, Drum GB. Plasma lignocaine concentrations following endotracheal spraying with an aerosol. *Br J Anaesth* 1976;48:899.

247. Curran J, Hamilton C, Taylor T. Topical analgesia before tracheal intubation. *Anaesthesia* 1975;30:765.

248. Labedzki L, Scavone JM, Ochs HR, Greenblatt DJ. Reduced systemic absorption of intrabronchial lidocaine by high frequency nebulization. *J Clin Pharmacol* 1990;30:795.

249. Prengel AW, Lindner KH, Hahnel JH, Georgieff M. Pharmacokinetics and technique of endotracheal and deep endobronchial lidocaine administration. *Anesth Analg* 1993;77:985.

250. Hagerty P, Klein P. Fat partitioning of lidocaine in tumescent liposuction. *Ann Plast Surg* 1999;42(4):372–375.

251. Klein JA. Tumescent technique for regional anesthesia permits lidocaine doses of 35 mg/kg for liposuction. *J Dermatol Surg Oncol* 1990;16:248.

252. Kenkel JM, Lipschitz AH, Shepherd G, et al. Pharmacokinetics and safety of lidocaine and monoethylglycinexylidide in liposuction: A microdialysis study. *Plast Reconstr Surg* 2004;114(2):516–524.

253. Rubin JP, Bierman C, Rosow CE, et al. The tumescent technique: The effect of high tissue pressure and dilute epinephrine on absorption of lidocaine. *Plast Reconstr Surg* 1999;103(3):990–996.

254. Grossmann M, Sattler G, Pistner H, et al. Pharmacokinetics of articaine hydrochloride in tumescent local anesthesia for liposuction. *J Clin Pharmacol* 2004;44(11):1282–1289.

255. Mulroy MF, Burgess FW, Emanuelsson BM. Ropivacaine 0.25% and 0.5%, but not 0.125%, provide effective wound infiltration analgesia after outpatient hernia repair, but with sustained plasma drug levels. *Reg Anesth Pain Med* 1999;24(2):136–141.

256. Bianconi M, Ferraro L, Ricci R, et al. The pharmacokinetics and efficacy of ropivacaine continuous wound instillation after spine fusion surgery. *Anesth Analg* 2004;98(1):166–172.

257. Corso OH, Morris RG, Hewett PJ, Karatassas A. Safety of 96-hour incision-site continuous infusion of ropivacaine for postoperative analgesia after bowel cancer resection. *Ther Drug Monit* 2007;29(1):57–63.

258. Convery PN, Milligan KR, Quinn P, et al. Efficacy and uptake of ropivacaine and bupivacaine after single intra-articular injection in the knee joint. *Br J Anaesth* 2001;87(4):570–576.

259. Evans CJ, Dewar JA, Boyes RN, Scott DB. Residual nerve block following intravenous regional anaesthesia. *Br J Anaesth* 1974;46:668–670.

260. Sukhani R, Garcia CJ, Munhall RJ, et al. Lidocaine disposition following intravenous regional anesthesia with different tourniquet deflation technics. *Anesth Analg* 1989;68:633.

261. Simon MA, Vree TB, Gielen MJ, Booij LH. Comparison of the effects and disposition kinetics of articaine and lidocaine in 20 patients undergoing intravenous regional anaesthesia during day case surgery. *Pharm World Sci* 1998;20(2):88–92.

262. Vree TB, Simon MA, Gielen MJ, Booij LH. Regional metabolism of articaine in 10 patients undergoing intravenous regional anaesthesia during day case surgery. *Br J Clin Pharmacol* 1997;44(1):29–34.

263. Bosenberg AT, Thomas J, Lopez T, et al. Plasma concentrations of ropivacaine following a single-shot caudal block of 1, 2 or 3 mg/kg in children. *Acta Anaesthesiol Scand* 2001;45(10):1276–1280.

264. Bridenbaugh PO, Tucker GT, Moore DC, et al. Preliminary clinical evaluation of etidocaine (Duranest): A new long-acting local anesthetic agent. *Acta Anaesthesiol Scand* 1974;18:165.

265. Wulf H, Worthmann F, Behnke H, Bohle AS. Pharmacokinetics and pharmacodynamics of ropivacaine 2 mg/mL, 5 mg/mL, or 7.5 mg/mL after ilioinguinal blockade for inguinal hernia repair in adults. *Anesth Analg* 1999;89(6):1471–1474.

266. Scott DB, Jebson PJR, Braid DP, et al. Factors affecting plasma levels of lignocaine and prilocaine. *Br J Anaesth* 1972;44:1040.

267. Sharrock NE, Mineo R, Stanton J, et al. Single versus staged epidural injections of 0.75% bupivacaine: Pharmacokinetic and pharmacodynamic effects. *Anesth Analg* 1994;79:307.

268. Sinnott CJ, Cogswell LP, 3rd, Johnson A, Strichartz GR. On the mechanism by which epinephrine potentiates lidocaine's peripheral nerve block. *Anesthesiology* 2003;98(1):181–188.

269. Brown SA, Lipschitz AH, Kenkel JM, et al. Pharmacokinetics and safety of epinephrine use in liposuction. *Plast Reconstr Surg* 2004;114(3):756–763.

270. Hersh EV, Giannakopoulos H, Levin LM, et al. The pharmacokinetics and cardiovascular effects of high-dose articaine with 1:100,000 and 1:200,000 epinephrine. *J Am Dent Assoc* 2006;137(11):1562–1571.

271. Axelsson K, Widman B. Blood concentration of lidocaine after spinal anaesthesia using lidocaine and lidocaine with adrenaline. *Acta Anaesthesiol Scand* 1981;25:240.

272. Hickey R, Candido KD, Ramamurthy S, et al. Brachial plexus block with a new local anesthetic: 0.5% ropivacaine. *Can J Anaesth* 1990;37:732.

273. Cederholm I, Evers H, Lofstrom JB. Skin blood flow after interdermal injection of ropivacaine in various concentrations with and without epinephrine evaluated by laser Doppler flowmetry. *Reg Anaesth* 1992;17:322.

274. Hickey R, Blanchard J, Hoffman J, et al. Plasma concentrations of ropivacaine given with or without epinephrine for brachial plexus block. *Can J Anaesth* 1990;37:878.

275. Braid DP, Scott DB. The effect of adrenaline on the systemic absorption of local anaesthetic drugs. *Acta Anaesthesiol Scand* 1966;23:334.

276. Dhuner KG. Frequency of general side reactions after regional anaesthesia with mepivacaine with and without vasoconstrictors. *Acta Anaesthesiol Scand* 1972;48:23.

277. Ohno H, Watanabe M, Saitoh JY, et al. Effect of epinephrine concentration on lidocaine disposition during epidural anesthesia. *Anesthesiology* 1988;68:625.

278. Takasaki M, Kajitani H. Plasma lidocaine concentrations during continuous epidural infusion of lidocaine with and without epinephrine. *Can J Anaesth* 1990;37:166.

279. Klingenstrom P, Nylen B, Westermark L. A clinical comparison between adrenaline and octapressin as vasoconstrictors in local anaesthesia. *Acta Anaesthesiol Scand* 1967;11:35.

280. Concepcion M, Maddi R, Francis D, et al. Vasoconstrictors in spinal anesthesia with tetracaine: A comparison of epinephrine and phenylephrine. *Anesth Analg* 1984;63:134.

281. Stanton-Hicks, MD Berges PU, Bonica JJ. Circulatory effects of peridural block: IV. Comparison of the effects of epinephrine and phenylephrine. *Anesthesiology* 1973;39:308.

282. Denson DD, Tumer PA, Bridenbaugh PO, Thompson GA. Pharmacokinetics and neural blockade after subarachnoid lidocaine in the rhesus monkey: III. Effects of phenylephrine. *Anesth Analg* 1984;63:129.

283. Culebras X, Van Gessel E, Hoffmeyer P, Gamulin Z. Clonidine combined with a long acting local anesthetic does not prolong postoperative analgesia after brachial plexus block but does induce hemodynamic changes. *Anesth Analg* 2001;92(1):199–204.

284. Mazoit JX, Benhamou D, Veillette Y, Samii K. Clonidine and or adrenaline decrease lignocaine plasma peak concentration after epidural injection. *Br J Clin Pharmacol* 1996;42(2):242–245.

285. Kopacz DJ, Bernards CM. Effect of clonidine on lidocaine clearance in vivo: A microdialysis study in humans. *Anesthesiology* 2001;95(6):1371–1376.

286. Ramos G, Pereira E, Simonetti MP. Does alkalinization of 0.75% ropivacaine promote a lumbar peridural block of higher quality? *Reg Anesth Pain Med* 2001;26(4):357–362.

287. DiFazio CA, Carron H, Grosslight KR, et al. Comparison of pH-adjusted lidocaine solutions for epidural anesthesia. *Anesth Analg* 1986;65:760.

288. Donchin Y, Ramu A, Olshwang D, et al. Effect of sodium bicarbonate on the kinetics of bupivacaine in i.v. regional anaesthesia in dogs. *Br J Anaesth* 1980;52:969.

289. Estèbe JP, Le Corre P, Chevanne F, Leverge R. Prolongation of spinal anesthesia with bupivacaine-loaded (DL-lactide) microspheres. *Anesth Analg* 1995;81:99.

290. Estèbe JP, Le Corre P, Du Plessis L, et al. The pharmacokinetics and pharmacodynamics of bupivacaine-loaded microspheres on a brachial plexus block model in sheep *Anesth Analg* 2001;93(2):447–455.

291. Estèbe P, Ecoffey C, Dollo G, et al. Bupivacaine pharmacokinetics and motor blockade following epidural administration of the bupivacaine-sulphobutylether 7-β-cyclodextrin complex in sheep. *Eur J Anaesthesiol* 2002;19:308–310.

292. Grant GJ, Vermeulen K, Langerman L, et al. Prolonged analgesia with liposomal bupivacaine in a mouse model. *Reg Anesth* 1994;19:264.

293. Le Corre P, Estèbe JP, Chevanne Y, et al. Spinal controlled delivery of bupivacaine from DL-lactic acid oligomer microspheres. *J Pharm Sci* 1995;84:75.

294. Mazoit JX, Lambert C, Berdeaux A, et al. Pharmacokinetics of bupivacaine after short and prolonged infusions in conscious dogs. *Anesth Analg* 1988;67:961.

295. Ueda W, Hirakawa M, Mon K. Inhibition of epinephrine absorption by dextran. *Anesthesiology* 1985;62:72.

296. Mather LE, Tucker GT, Murphy TM, et al. Haemodynamic drug interactions: Peridural lignocaine and intravenous ephedrine. *Acta Anaesthesiol Scand* 1976;20:207.

297. Heavner JE. Let's abandon blanket maximum recommended doses of local anesthetics. *Reg Anesth Pain Med* 2004;29:524.

298. Hodgkinson R, Husain FJ. Obesity, gravity and spread of epidural anesthesia. *Anesth Analg* 1981;60:421.

299. Moore DC, Mather LE, Bridenbaugh PO, et al. Arterial and venous plasma levels of bupivacaine following peripheral nerve blocks. *Anesth Analg* 1976;55:763.

300. Pihlajamaki KK. Inverse correlation between the peak venous serum concentration of bupivacaine and the weight of the patient during interscalene brachial plexus block. *Br J Anaesth* 1991;67:621.

301. Nydahl P-A, Philipson L, Axelsson K, Johansson J-E. Epidural anesthesia with 0.5% bupivacaine: Influence of age on sensory and motor blockade. *Anesth Analg* 1991;73:780.

302. Ivani G, Conio A, Papurel G, et al. 1,000 consecutive blocks in a children's hospital: How to manage them safely. *Reg Anesth Pain Med* 2001;26(1):93–94.

303. Chalkiadis GA, Anderson BJ, Tay M, et al. Pharmacokinetics of levobupivacaine after caudal epidural administration in infants less than 3 months of age. *Br J Anaesth* 2005;95(4):524–529.

303a. Ala-Kokka TI, Raiha E, Karinen J, et al. Pharmacokinetics of 0.5% levobupivacaine following ilioinguinal-iliohypogastric nerve blockade in children. *Acta Anaesthesiol Scand* 2005;49(3):397–400.

304. Mazoit JX. Pharmacokinetic/pharmacodynamic modeling of anesthetics in children: Therapeutic implications. *Paediatr Drugs* 2006;8(3):139–150.

305. Bricker SRW, Telford RJ, Booker PD. Pharmacokinetics of bupivacaine following intraoperative intercostal nerve block in neonates and in infants aged less than 6 months. *Anesthesiology* 1989;70:942.

306. Rothstein P, Arthur GR, Feldman H, et al. Bupivacaine for intercostal nerve blocks in children: Blood concentrations and pharmacokinetics. *Anesth Analg* 1986;65:625.

307. Pihlajamaki KK, Kanto J, Lindberg R, et al. Extradural administration of bupivacaine: Pharmacokinetics and metabolism in pregnant and nonpregnant women. *Br J Anaesth* 1990;64:556.

308. Morikawa KI, Bonica JJ, Tucker GT, Murphy TM. Effect of acute hypovolaemia on lignocaine absorption and cardiovascular response following epidural block in dogs. *Br J Anaesth* 1974;46:631.

309. Quimby CW. Influence of blood loss on the duration of regional anesthesia. *Anesth Analg* 1965;44:387.

310. Bromage PR, Gertel M. Brachial plexus anesthesia in chronic renal failure. *Anesthesiology* 1972;36:488.

311. Crews JC, Weller RS, Moss J, James RL. Levobupivacaine for axillary brachial plexus block: A pharmacokinetic and clinical comparison

in patients with normal renal function or renal disease. *Anesth Analg* 2002;95(1):219–223.

312. Pere P, Salonen M, Jokinen M, et al. Pharmacokinetics of ropivacaine in uremic and nonuremic patients after axillary brachial plexus block. *Anesth Analg* 2003;96(2):563–569.

313. Rice ASC, Pither CE, Tucker GT. Plasma concentrations of bupivacaine after supraclavicular brachial plexus blockade in patients with chronic renal failure. *Anaesthesia* 1991;46:354.

314. El Desoky ES, Derendorf H, Klotz U. Variability in response to cardiovascular drugs. *Curr Clin Pharmacol* 2006;1:35–46.

315. Mather LE. Anatomical-physiological approaches in pharmacokinetics and pharmacodynamics. *Clin Pharmacokinet* 2001;40:707–722.

316. Tucker GT. Safety in numbers: The role of pharmacokinetics in local anesthetic toxicity. *Reg Anesth* 1994;19:155.

317. Upton RN. A model of the first pass passage of drugs from i.v. injection site to the heart–parameter estimates for lignocaine in the sheep. *Br J Anaesth* 1996;77:764–772.

318. Upton RN, Zheng DA, Grant C, Martinez AM. Development and validation of a recirculatory physiological model of the myocardial concentrations of lignocaine after intravenous administration in sheep. *J Pharm Pharmacol* 2000;52(2):181–189.

319. Upton RN, Doolette DJ. Kinetic aspects of drug disposition in the lungs. *Clin Exp Pharmacol Physiol* 1999;26(5–6):381–391.

320. Mather LE, Huang YF, Pryor ME, Veering BT. Systemic and regional pharmacokinetics of bupivacaine and levobupivacaine in sheep. *Anesth Analg* 1998;86:805–811.

321. Rutten AJ, Mather LE, McLean CF. Cardiovascular effects and regional clearances of i.v. bupivacaine in sheep: Enantiomeric analysis. *Br J Anaesth* 1991;67:247.

322. Rutten AJ, Mather LE, Nancarrow C, et al. Cardiovascular effects and regional clearances of intravenous ropivacaine in sheep. *Anesth Analg* 1990;70:577.

323. Rutten AJ, Mather LE, McLean CF. Tissue distribution of bupivacaine enantiomers in sheep. *Chirality* 1993;5:485–491.

324. Santos AC, Karpel B, Noble G. The placental transfer and fetal effects of levobupivacaine, racemic bupivacaine, and ropivacaine. *Anesthesiology* 1999;90:1698–1703.

325. Feldman HS, Hartvig P, Wiklund L, et al. Regional distribution of 11C-labeled lidocaine, bupivacaine, and ropivacaine in the heart, lungs, and skeletal muscle of pigs studied with positron emission tomography. *Biopharm Drug Dispos* 1997;18(2):151–164.

326. Hasegawa K, Yukioka H, Hayashi M, et al. Lung uptake of lidocaine during hyperoxia and hypoxia in the dog. *Acta Anaesthesiol Scand* 1996;40(4):489–495.

327. Krejcie TC, Avram MJ, Gentry WB, et al. A recirculatory model of the pulmonary uptake and pharmacokinetics of lidocaine based on analysis of arterial and mixed venous data from dogs. *J Pharmacokinet Biopharm* 1997;25(2):169–190.

328. Ohmura S, Sugano A, Kawada M, Yamamoto K. Pulmonary uptake of ropivacaine and levobupivacaine in rabbits. *Anesth Analg* 2003;97(3):893–897.

329. Geng WP, Ebke M, Foth H. Prilocaine elimination by isolated perfused rat lung and liver. *Naunyn Schmiedebergs Arch Pharmakol* 1995;351:93.

330. Post C, Andersson RGG, Ryrfeldt A, Nilsson E. Physicochemical modification of lidocaine uptake in rat lung tissue. *Acta Pharmacol Toxicol (Copenh)* 1979;44:103.

331. Post C, Eriksdotter-Behm K. Dependence of lung uptake of lidocaine in vivo on blood pH. *Acta Pharmacol Toxicol (Copenh)* 1982;51:136.

332. Palazzo MGA, Kalso EA, Argiras E, et al. First-pass lung uptake of bupivacaine: Effect of acidosis in an intact rabbit lung model. *Br J Anaesth* 1991;67:759.

333. Mather LE, Long GJ, Thomas J. The binding of bupivacaine to maternal and foetal plasma proteins. *J Pharm Pharmacol* 1971;23:359–366.

334. Tucker GT, Boyes RN, Bridenbaugh PO, Moore DC. Binding of anilide-type local anesthetics in human plasma. II: Implications in vivo with special reference to transplacental distribution. *Anesthesiology* 1970;33:304.

335. Burm AG, Stienstra R, Brouwer RP, et al. Epidural infusion of ropivacaine for postoperative analgesia after major orthopedic surgery: Pharmacokinetic evaluation. *Anesthesiology* 2000;93(2):395–403.

336. Denson DD, Coyle DE, Thompson G, Myers JA. Alpha₁-acid glycoprotein and albumin in human serum bupivacaine binding. *Clin Pharmacol Ther* 1984;35:409.

337. Kraus E, Polnaszek CF, Scheeler DA, et al. Interaction between human serum albumin and alpha₁-acid glycoprotein in the binding of lidocaine to purified protein fractions and sera. *J Pharmacol Exp Ther* 1986;239:754.

338. Mather LE, Thomas J. Bupivacaine binding to plasma protein fractions. *J Pharm Pharmacol* 1978;30:653.

339. Mazoit JX, Cao LS, Samii K. Binding of bupivacaine to human serum proteins, isolated albumin and isolated alpha-1-acid glycoprotein: Differences between the two enantiomers are partly due to cooperativity. *J Pharmacol Exp Ther* 1996;276(1):109–115.

340. Meunier JF, Goujard E, Dubousset AM, et al. Pharmacokinetics of bupivacaine after continuous epidural infusion in infants with and without biliary atresia. *Anesthesiology* 2001;95(1):87–95.

341. Veering BT, Burm AG, Feyen HM, et al. Pharmacokinetics of bupivacaine during postoperative epidural infusion: Enantioselectivity and role of protein binding. *Anesthesiology* 2002;96(5):1062–1069.

342. Yokogawa K, Shimomura S, Ishizaki J, et al. Involvement of α1-acid glycoprotein in inter-individual variation of disposition kinetics of ropivacaine following epidural infusion in off-pump coronary artery bypass grafting. *J Pharm Pharmacol* 2007;59:67–73.

343. Jackson PR, Tucker GT, Woods HF. Altered plasma binding in cancer: Role of alpha₁-acid glycoprotein and albumin. *Clin Pharmacol Ther* 1982;32:295.

344. Fukui T, Hameroff SR, Gandolfi AJ. Alpha₁-acid glycoprotein and beta-endorphin alterations in chronic pain patients. *Anesthesiology* 1984;60:494.

345. Edwards DJ, Lalka D, Cerra F, Slaughter RL. Alpha₁-acid glycoprotein concentration and protein binding in trauma. *Clin Pharmacol Ther* 1982;31:62.

346. Bruguerolle B, Philip-Joet F, Arnaud C, Arnaud A. Consequences of inflammatory processes on lignocaine protein binding during anaesthesia in fibreoptic bronchoscopy. *Br J Clin Pharmacol* 1985;20:180.

347. Grossman SH, Davis D, Kitchell BB, et al. Diazepam and lidocaine plasma protein binding in renal disease. *Clin Pharmacol Ther* 1982;31(3):350–357.

348. Hasselstrom L, Nortved-Sorensen J, Kehlet H, et al. The influence of systemically administered bupivacaine on cardiovascular function in cholecystectomised patients. *Acta Anaesthesiol Scand* 1985;29:A76.

349. Barchowsky A, Shand DG, Stargel WW, et al. On the role of alpha-l-acid glycoprotein in lignocaine accumulation following myocardial infarction. *Br J Clin Pharmacol* 1981;13:411.

350. Tsen LC, Tarshis J, Denson DD, et al. Measurements of maternal protein binding of bupivacaine throughout pregnancy. *Anesth Analg* 1999;89(4):965–968.

351. Petersen MC, Moore RG, Nation RL, McMeniman W. Relationship between the transplacental gradients of bupivacaine and alpha₁-acid glycoprotein. *Br J Clin Pharmacol* 1981;12:859.

352. Lerman J, Strong A, LeDez KM, et al. Effects of age on the serum concentration of α₁-acid glycoprotein and the binding of lidocaine in pediatric patients. *Clin Pharmacol Ther* 1989;46:219.

352a. Veering BT, Burm AG, Souverijn JH, Serree JM, Spierdijk J. The effect of age on serum concentrations of albumin and alpha 1-acid glycoprotein. *Br J Clinical Pharmacol* 1990;29(2):201–206.

352b. Veering BT, Burm AG, Gladines MP, Spierdijk J. Age does not influence the serum protein binding of bupivacaine. *Br J Clinical Pharmacol* 1991;32(4):501–503.

353. Fragneto RY, Bader AM, Rosinia F, et al. Measurements of protein binding of lidocaine throughout pregnancy. *Anesth Analg* 1994;79:295.

354. Wulf H, Munstedt P, Maier C.H. Plasma protein binding of bupivacaine in pregnant women at term. *Acta Anaesthesiol Scand* 1991;35:129.

355. Rutten AJ, Mather LE, Plummer JL, Henning EC. Postoperative course of plasma protein binding of lignocaine, ropivacaine and bupivacaine in sheep. *J Pharm Pharmacol* 1992;44:355–358.

356. Kakiuchi Y, Kohda Y, Miyabe M, Momose Y. Effect of plasma alpha1-acid glycoprotein concentration on the accumulation of lidocaine metabolites during continuous epidural anesthesia in infants and children. *Int J Clin Pharmacol Ther* 1999;37(10):493–498.

357. Burm AGL, Van der Meer AD, Van Kleef JW, et al. Pharmacokinetics of the enantiomers of bupivacaine following intravenous administration of the racemate. *Br J Clin Pharmacol* 1994;38:125.

358. Groen K, Mantel M, Zeijlmans PW, et al. Pharmacokinetics of the enantiomers of bupivacaine and mepivacaine after epidural administration of the racemates. *Anesth Analg* 1998;86(2):361–366.

359. van der Meer AD, Burm AG, Stienstra R, et al. Pharmacokinetics of prilocaine after intravenous administration in volunteers: Enantioselectivity. *Anesthesiology* 1999;90(4):988–992.

360. Burm AG, Cohen IM, van Kleef JW, et al. Pharmacokinetics of the enantiomers of mepivacaine after intravenous administration of the racemate in volunteers. *Anesth Analg* 1997;84(1):85–89.

361. Terasaki T, Pardridge WM, Denson DD. Differential effect of plasma protein binding of bupivacaine on its in vivo transfer into the brain and salivary gland of rats. *J Pharmacol Exp Ther* 1986;239:724.

362. Marathe PH, Shen DD, Artru AA, Bowdle A. Effect of serum protein binding on the entry of lidocaine into brain and cerebrospinal fluid in dogs. *Anesthesiology* 1991;75:804.

363. Toutain PL, Bousquet-Melou A. Free drug fraction vs. free drug concentration: A matter of frequent confusion. *J Vet Pharmacol Ther* 2002;25:460–463.

364. Upton RN. Theoretical aspects of P-glycoprotein mediated drug efflux on the distribution volume of anaesthetic-related drugs in the brain. *Anaesth Intensive Care* 2002;30(2):183–191.

365. Wandel C, Kim R, Wood M Wood A. Interaction of morphine, fentanyl, sufentanil, alfentanil, and loperamide with the efflux drug transporter P-glycoprotein. *Anesthesiology* 2002;96:913–920.

366. Funao T, Oda Y, Tanaka K, Asada A. The P-glycoprotein inhibitor quinidine decreases the threshold for bupivacaine-induced, but not lidocaine-induced, convulsions in rats. *Can J Anaesth* 2003;50(8):805–811.

367. Berggren S, Hoogstraate J, Fagerholm U, Lennernas H. Characterization of jejunal absorption and apical efflux of ropivacaine, lidocaine and bupivacaine in the rat using in situ and in vitro absorption models. *Eur J Pharm Sci* 2004;21(4):553–560.

368. Chang DHT, Ladd, LA, Wilson KA, et al. Intravenous tolerability of large doses of levobupivacaine in sheep. *Anesth Analg* 2000;91:671–679.

369. Huang YF, Upton RN, Runciman WB. I.V. bolus administration of subconvulsive doses of lignocaine to conscious sheep: Myocardial pharmacokinetics. *Br J Anaesth* 1993;70:326.

370. Huang YF, Upton RN, Runciman WB. I.V. bolus administration of subconvulsive doses of lignocaine to conscious sheep: Myocardial pharmacokinetics. *Br J Anaesth* 1993;70:326–332.

371. Huang YF, Upton RN, Runciman WB. Relationships between myocardial pharmacokinetics and pharmacodynamics. *Br J Anaesth* 1993;70:556.

372. Nancarrow C, Rutten AJ, Runciman WB, et al. Myocardial and cerebral drug concentrations and the mechanisms of death after fatal intravenous doses of lidocaine, bupivacaine, and ropivacaine in the sheep. *Anesth Analg* 1989;69:276–283.

373. Mazoit JX, Boico O, Samii K. Myocardial uptake of bupivacaine: II. Pharmacokinetics and pharmacodynamics of bupivacaine enantiomers in the isolated perfused rabbit heart. *Anesth Analg* 1993;77:477.

374. Weinberg GL, Ripper R, Murphy P, et al. Lipid infusion accelerates removal of bupivacaine and recovery from bupivacaine toxicity in the isolated rat heart. *Reg Anesth Pain Med* 2006;31:296–303.

375. Datta S, Houle GL, Fox GS. Concentration of lidocaine hydrochloride in newborn gastric fluid after elective Caesarian section and vaginal section and vaginal delivery with epidural analgesia. *Can Anaesth Soc J* 1975;22:79.

376. Giuliani M, Grossi GB, Pileri M, et al. Could local anesthesia while breast-feeding be harmful to infants? *J Pediatr Gastroenterol Nutr* 2001;32(2):142–144.

377. Ortega D, Viviand X, Lorec AM, et al. Excretion of lidocaine and bupivacaine in breast milk following epidural anesthesia for cesarean delivery. *Acta Anaesthesiol Scand* 1999;43(4):394–397.

378. Nebert DW, Russell DW. Clinical importance of the cytochromes P450. *Lancet* 2002;360:1155–1162.

379. Palmer SN, Giesecke NM, Body SC, et al. Pharmacogenetics of anesthetic and analgesic agents. *Anesthesiology* 2005;102(3):663–671.

380. Foldes FF, Davidson GN, Duncalf D, Kuwabarra S. The intravenous toxicity of local anesthetic agents in man. *Clin Pharmacol Ther* 1965;6:328.

381. Kuhnert BR, Kuhnert PM, Philipson EH, et al. The half-life of 2-chloroprocaine. *Anesth Analg* 1986;65:273.

382. O'Brien JE, Abbey V, Hinsvark O, et al. Metabolism and measurement of chloroprocaine, an ester-type local anesthetic. *J Pharm Sci* 1979;68:75.

383. Reidenberg MM, James M, Dring LG. The rate of procaine hydrolysis in serum of normal subjects and diseased patients. *Clin Pharmacol Ther* 1972;13:279.

384. Seifen AB, Ferrari AA, Seifen AA, et al. Pharmacokinetics of intravenous procaine infusion in humans. *Anesth Analg* 1979;58:382.

385. Barnett G, Hawks R, Resnick R. Cocaine pharmacokinetics in humans. *J Ethnopharamacol* 1981;3:353.

386. Javaid JI, Musa MN, Fischman M, et al. Kinetics of cocaine in humans after intravenous and intranasal administration. *Biopharm Drug Dispos* 1983;4:9.

387. Krogh K, Jellum E. Urinary metabolites of chloroprocaine. *Anesthesiology* 1982;56:483.

388. Cone EJ, Tsadik A, Oyler J, Darwin WD. Cocaine metabolism and urinary excretion after different routes of administration. *Ther Drug Monit* 1998;20(5):556–560.

389. Stewart DJ, Inaba T, Lucassen M, Kalow W. Cocaine metabolism: Cocaine and norcocaine hydrolysis by liver and serum esterases. *Clin Pharmacol Ther* 1979;25:464.

390. Tucker GT. Pharmacokinetics of local anaesthetics. *Br J Anaesth* 1986;58:717.

391. Sallie RW, Tredger JM, Williams R. Extrahepatic production of the lignocaine metabolite monoethylglycinexylidide (MEGX). *Biopharm Drug Dispos* 1992;13:555.

392. Tanaka K, Oda Y, Asada A, et al. Metabolism of lidocaine by rat pulmonary cytochrome P450. *Biochem Pharmacol* 1994;47:1061.

393. Mather LE. Disposition of mepivacaine and bupivacaine enantiomers in sheep. *Br J Anaesth* 1991;67:239.

394. Morishima HO, Finster M, Pedersen H, et al. Pharmacokinetics of lidocaine in fetal and neonatal lambs and adult sheep. *Anesthesiology* 1979;50(5):431–436.

395. Mather LE, McCall P, McNicol PL. Bupivacaine enantiomer pharmacokinetics after intercostal neural blockade in liver transplant patients. *Anesth Analg* 1995;80:328.

396. Blake DW, Bjorksen A, Dawson P, Hiscock R. Pharmacokinetics of bupivacaine enantiomers during interpleural infusions. *Anaesth Intensive Care* 1994;22:521.

397. Vree TB, Beurner EMC, Lagerwerf AJ, et al. Clinical pharmacokinetics of R(+)- and S(−)-mepivacaine after high doses of racemic mepivacaine with epinephrine in the combined psoas compartment/sciatic nerve block. *Anesth Analg* 1992;75:75.

398. Emanuelsson BM, Zaric D, Nydahl PA, Axelsson KH. Pharmacokinetics of ropivacaine and bupivacaine during 21 hours of continuous epidural infusion in healthy male volunteers. *Anesth Analg* 1995;81(6):1163–1168.

399. Falany CN, Falany JL, Wang J, et al. Studies on sulfation of synthesized metabolites from the local anesthetics ropivacaine and lidocaine using human cloned sulfotransferases. *Drug Metab Dispos* 1999;27(9):1057–1063.

400. Ledger R. Nonaromatic hydroxylation of bupivacaine during continuous epidural infusion in man. *J Biochem Biophys Meth* 2003;57(2):105–114.

401. Pere P, Tuominen M, Rosenberg PH. Cumulation of bupivacaine, desbutyl-bupivacaine and 4-hydroxybupivacaine during and after continuous interscalene brachial plexus block. *Acta Anaesthesiol Scand* 1991;35:647.

402. Tam YK, Ke J, Coutts RT, et al. Quantification of three lidocaine metabolites and their conjugates. *Pharm Res* 1990;7:504.

403. Drayer DE, Lorenzo B, Werns S, Reidenberg MM. Plasma levels, protein binding, and elimination data of lidocaine and active metabolites in cardiac patients of various ages. *Clin Pharmacol Ther* 1983;34:14.

404. Blumer J, Strong JM, Atkinson AJ. The convulsant potency of lidocaine and its N-dealkylated metabolites. *J Pharmacol Exp Ther* 1973;186:31.

405. Rosenberg PH, Pere P, Hekali R, Tuominen M. Plasma concentrations of bupivacaine and two of its metabolites during continuous interscalene brachial plexus block. *Br J Anaesth* 1991;66:25.

406. Rosenberg PH, Heavner JE. Acute cardiovascular and central nervous system toxicity of bupivacaine and desbutylbupivacaine in the rat. *Acta Anaesthesiol Scand* 1992;36:138.

407. Arlander E, Ekstrom G, Alm C, et al. Metabolism of ropivacaine in humans is mediated by CYP1A2 and to a minor extent by CYP3A4: An interaction study with fluvoxamine and ketoconazole as in vivo inhibitors. *Clin Pharmacol Ther* 1998;64(5):484–491.

408. Bargetzi MJ, Aoyama T, Gonzalez FJ, Meyer UA. Lidocaine metabolism in human liver microsomes by cytochrome P450IIIA4. *Clin Pharmacol Ther* 1989;46:521.

409. Gantenbein M, Attolini L, Bruguerolle B, et al. Oxidative metabolism of bupivacaine into pipecolylxylidine in humans is mainly catalyzed by CYP3A. *Drug Metab Dispos* 2000;28(4):383–385.

410. Oda Y, Furuichi K, Tanaka K, et al. Metabolism of a new local anesthetic, ropivacaine, by human hepatic cytochrome P450. *Anesthesiology* 1995;82:214.

411. Tanaka E, Nakamura T, Inomata S, Honda K. Effects of premedication medicines on the formation of the CYP3A4-dependent metabolite of ropivacaine, 2′, 6′-Pipecoloxylidide, on human liver microsomes in vitro. *Basic Clin Pharmacol Toxicol* 2006;98(2):181–183.

412. Osaka Y, Inomata S, Tanaka E, et al. Effect of propofol on ropivacaine metabolism in human liver microsomes. *J Anesth* 2006;20(1):60–63.

413. Vasters FG, Eberhart LH, Koch T. Kranke P, Wulf H, Morin AM. Risk factors for prilocaine-induced methaemoglobinaemia following peripheral regional anaesthesia. *Eur J Anaesthesiol* 2006;23(9):760–765.

414. Gunter JB. Benefit and risks of local anesthetics in infants and children. *Paed Drugs* 2002;4(10):649–672.

414a. McLean S, Starmer GA, Thomas J. Methaemoglobin formation by aromatic amines. *J Pharm Pharmac* 1969;21(7):441–450.

415. Kern K, Langevin PB, Dunn BM. Methemoglobinemia after topical anesthesia with lidocaine and benzocaine for a difficult intubation. *J Clin Anesth* 2000;12:167–172.

416. Bryant MS, Simmons HF, Harrell RE, Hinson JA. 2,6-dimethylaniline-hemoglobin adducts from lidocaine in humans. *Carcinogenicity* 1994;15:2287.

417. Benowitz N, Forsyth RP, Melmon KL, Rowland M. Lidocaine disposition kinetics in monkey and man: II. Effects of hemorrhage and sympathomimetic drug administration. *Clin Pharmacol Ther* 1974;16:99.

418. Chalkiadis GA, Anderson BJ. Age and size are the major covariates for prediction of levobupivacaine clearance in children. *Paediatr Anaesth* 2006;16(3):275–282.

419. Veering BT, Burm AGL, Van Kleef JW, et al. Epidural anesthesia with bupivacaine: Effects of age on neural blockade and pharmacokinetics. *Anesth Analg* 1987;66:589.

420. Nation RL, Triggs EJ, Selig M. Lignocaine kinetics in cardiac patients and aged subjects. *Br J Clin Pharmacol* 1977;4:439.

421. Rapp HJ, Molnar V, Austin S, et al. Ropivacaine in neonates and infants: A population pharmacokinetic evaluation following single caudal block. *Paediatr Anaesth* 2004;14(9):724–732.

422. Ecoffey C, Desparmet J, Maury M, et al. Bupivacaine in children: Pharmacokinetics following caudal anesthesia. *Anesthesiology* 1985;63:447.

423. Hansen TG, Ilett KF, Lim SI, et al. Pharmacokinetics and clinical efficacy of long-term epidural ropivacaine infusion in children. *Br J Anaesth* 2000;85(3):347–353.

424. Van Obbergh LJ, Roelants FA, Veyckemans F, Verbeeck RK. In children, the addition of epinephrine modifies the pharmacokinetics of ropivacaine injected caudally. *Can J Anaesth* 2003;50(6):593–598.

425. Bennett PN, Aarons LJ, Bending MR, et al. Pharmacokinetics of lidocaine and its deethylated metabolite: Dose and time dependency studies in man. *J Pharmacokinet Biopharm* 1982;10:265.

426. Kates RE, Harapat SR, Keefe DLD, et al. Influence of prolonged recumbency on drug disposition. *Clin Pharmacol Ther* 1980;27:624.

427. Ramanathan J, Bottorf M, Jeter JN, et al. The pharmacokinetics and maternal and neonatal effects of epidural lidocaine in preeclampsia. *Anesth Analg* 1986;65:120.

428. Santos AC, Arthur GR, Lehning EJ, Finster M. Comparative pharmacokinetics of ropivacaine and bupivacaine in nonpregnant and pregnant ewes. *Anesth Analg* 1997;85:87–93.

429. Santos A, DeArmas PI. Systemic toxicity of levobupivacaine, bupivacaine, and ropivacaine during continuous intravenous infusion to nonpregnant and pregnant ewes. *Anesthesiology* 2001;95:1256–1264.

430. Santos AC, Pedersen H, Morishima HO, et al. Pharmacokinetics of lidocaine in nonpregnant and pregnant ewes. *Anesth Analg* 1988;67:1154.

431. Santos AC, Pedersen H, Sallusto JA, et al. Pharmacokinetics of ropivacaine in nonpregnant and pregnant ewes. *Anesth Analg* 1990;70:262.

432. Upton RN. Relationships between steady state blood concentrations and cardiac output during intravenous infusions. *Biopharm Drug Dispos* 2000;21(2):69–76.

433. Kuipers JA, Boer F, de Roode A, et al. Modeling population pharmacokinetics of lidocaine: Should cardiac output be included as a patient factor? *Anesthesiology* 2001;94(4):566–573.

434. Benowitz NL, Meister W. Clinical pharmacokinetics of lignocaine. *Clin Pharmacokinet* 1978;3:177.

435. Thompson P, Melmon KL, Richardson JA, Rowland M. Lidocaine pharmacokinetics in advanced heart failure, liver disease and renal failure in humans. *Ann Intern Med* 1973;78:499.

436. Feely J, Wade D, McAllister CB, et al. Effect of hypotension on liver blood flow and lidocaine disposition. *N Engl J Med* 1982;307:866.

437. Chow MSS, Ronfeld RA, Hamilton RA, et al. Effect of external cardiopulmonary resuscitation on lidocaine pharmacokinetics in dogs. *J Pharmacol Exp Ther* 1983;224:531.

438. Holley FO, Ponganis KV, Stanski DR. Effects of cardiac surgery with cardiopulmonary bypass on lidocaine disposition. *Clin Pharmacol Ther* 1984;35:617.

439. Calvo R, Carlos R, Erill S. Effects of disease and acetazolamide on procaine hydrolysis by red cell enzymes. *Clin Pharmacol Ther* 1980;27:175.

440. Jokinen MJ, Neuvonen PJ, Lindgren L, et al. Pharmacokinetics of ropivacaine in patients with chronic end-stage liver disease. *Anesthesiology* 2007;106(1):43–55.

441. Barry M, Keeling PWN, Weir D, Feely J. Severity of cirrhosis and the relationship of α_1-acid glycoprotein concentration to plasma protein binding of lidocaine. *Clin Pharmacol Ther* 1990;47:366.

442. Huet PM, Villeneuve J-P. Determinants of drug disposition in patients with cirrhosis. *Hepatology* 1983;3:913.

443. Huet P-M, LeLorier J. Effects of smoking and chronic hepatitis B on lidocaine and indocyanine green kinetics. *Clin Pharmacol Ther* 1980;28:208.

444. Huet P-M, Arsene D, Richer D. The volume of distribution of lidocaine in chronic hepatitis: Relationship with serum alpha$_1$-acid glycoprotein and serum protein binding. *Clin Pharmacol Ther* 1981;29:252.

445. Williams R, Blaschke TF, Meffin PJ, et al. Influence of viral hepatitis on the disposition of two compounds with high hepatic clearance: Lidocaine and indocyanine green. *Clin Pharmacol Ther* 1976;20:290.

446. Calvo R, Carlos R, Erill S. Procaine hydrolysis defect in uraemia does not appear to be due to carbamylation of plasma esterases. *Eur J Clin Pharmacol* 1983;24:533.

447. De Martin S, Orlando R, Bertoli M, et al. Differential effect of chronic renal failure on the pharmacokinetics of lidocaine in patients receiving and not receiving hemodialysis. *Clin Pharmacol Ther* 2006;80(6):597–606.

448. Collinsworth KA, Strong JM, Atkinson AJ, et al. Pharmacokinetics and metabolism of lidocaine in patients with renal failure. *Clin Pharmacol Ther* 1975;18:59.

449. Peeyush M, Ravishankar M, Adithan C, Sashindran CH. Altered pharmacokinetics of lignocaine after epidural injection in Type II diabetics. *Eur J Clin Pharmacol* 1992;43:269.

450. O'Bryan S, Barry MG, Collins WCJ, et al. Plasma protein binding of lidocaine and warfarin in insulin-dependent and non-insulin-dependent diabetes mellitus. *Clin Pharmacokinet* 1993;24:183.

451. Gawroska-Szklarz B, Musial DH, Pawlik A, Paprota B. Effect of experimental diabetes on pharmacokinetic parameters of lidocaine and MEGX in rats. *Pol J Pharmacol* 2003;55(4):619–624.

452. Englesson S, Matousek M. CNS effects of local anaesthetic agents. *Br J Anaesth* 1975;47[Suppl]:241–246.

453. Heavner JE, Dryden CF, Sanghani V, et al. Severe hypoxia enhances central nervous system and cardiovascular toxicity of bupivacaine in lightly anesthetized pigs. *Anesthesiology* 1992;77:142.

454. Rosen MA, Thigpen JW, Shnider SM, et al. Bupivacaine-induced cardiotoxicity in hypoxic and acidotic sheep. *Anesth Analg* 1985;64:1089.

455. Alexander CM, Berko RS, Gross JB, et al. The effect of changes in arterial CO_2 tension on plasma lidocaine concentration. *Can J Anaesth* 1987;34:343–345.

456. Mather LE, Ladd LA, Chang DHT, Copeland SE. The effects of imposed acid-base derangement on the cardio-activity and pharmacokinetics of bupivacaine and thiopental. *Anesthesiology* 2004;100:1447–1457.

457. Simon RP, Benowitz NL, Culala S. Motor paralysis increases brain uptake of lidocaine during status epilepticus. *Neurology* 1984;34:384.

458. Mets B, Hickman R, Allin R, et al. Effect of hypoxia on the hepatic metabolism of lidocaine in the isolated perfused pig liver. *Hepatology* 1993;17:668.

459. DuSouich P, Saunier C, Hartemann D, Allam M. Effect of acute and chronic moderate hypoxia on the kinetics of lidocaine and its metabolites and on regional blood flow. *Pulm Pharmacol* 1992;5:9–16.

460. Huang YF, Upton RN. The effect of hypoxic hypoxia on the systemic and myocardial pharmacokinetics and dynamics of lidocaine in sheep. *J Pharm Sci* 2003;92(1):180–189.

461. Momota Y, Artru AA, Powers KM, et al. Concentrations of lidocaine and monoethylglycine xylidide in brain, cerebrospinal fluid, and plasma during lidocaine-induced epileptiform electroencephalogram activity in rabbits: The effects of epinephrine and hypocapnia. *Anesth Analg* 2000;91(2):362–368.

462. Rump AF, Siekmann U, Fischer DC, Kalff G. Lidocaine pharmacokinetics during hyperbaric hyperoxia in humans. *Aviat Space Environ Med* 1999;70(8):769–772.

463. Lalka D, Vicuna N, Burrow SR, et al. Bupivacaine and other amide local anesthetics inhibit hydrolysis of chloroprocaine by human serum. *Anesth Analg* 1978;57:534.

464. Raj PP, Ohlweiler D, Hitt BA, Denson DD. Kinetics of local anesthetic esters and effects of adjuvant drugs on 2-chloroprocaine hydrolysis. *Anesthesiology* 1980;53:307.

465. Hartrick CT, Dirkes WE, Coyle DE, et al. Influence of bupivacaine on mepivacaine protein binding. *Clin Pharmacol Ther* 1984;36:546.

466. Bridenbaugh PO. Intercostal nerve blockade for evaluation of local anaesthetic agents. *Br J Anaesth* 1975;47:306.

467. Seow LT, Lips FJ, Cousins MJ, Mather LE. Lidocaine and bupivacaine mixtures for epidural blockade. *Anesthesiology* 1982;56:177.

468. Mather LE, Rutten AJ, Plummer JL. Pharmacokinetics of bupivacaine enantiomers in sheep: Influence of dosage regimen and study design. *J Pharmacokinet Biopharm* 1994;22:481.

469. Ohmura S, Yamamoto K, Kobayashi T, Murakami S. Displacement of lidocaine from the lung after bolus injection of bupivacaine. *Can J Anaesth* 1993;40:676.

470. Nishikawa T, Inomata S, Igarishi M, et al. Plasma lidocaine concentrations during epidural blockade with isoflurane or halothane anesthesia. *Anesth Analg* 1992;75:885.

471. Runciman WB, Myburgh JA, Upton RN, Mather LE. Effects of anaesthesia on drug disposition. In: Feldman SA, Scurr CF, Paton W, eds. *Mechanisms of Action of Drugs in Anaesthetic Practice*, 2nd ed. London: Edward Arnold; 1994:93–128.

472. Wood M. Pharmacokinetic drug interactions in anaesthetic practice. *Clin Pharmacokinet* 1991;21:285–307.

473. Copeland SE, Ladd LA, Gu X-Q, Mather LE. Effects of general anesthesia on the central nervous and cardiovascular system toxicity of local anesthetics. *Anesth Analg* 2008;106:1429–1439.

473a. Copeland SE, Ladd LA, Gu X-Q, Mather LE. Effects of general anesthesia on whole body and regional pharmacokinetics of local anesthetics at toxic doses. *Anesth Analg* 2008;106:1440–1449.

474. Burney RG, DiFazio CA. Hepatic clearance of lidocaine during N_2O anesthesia in dogs. *Anesth Analg* 1976;55:322.

475. Boyce JR, Cervenko FW, Wright FJ. Effects of halothane on the pharmacokinetics of lidocaine in digitalis-toxic dogs. *Can J Anaesth* 1978;25:323.

476. Mather LE, Runciman WB, Carapetis RJ, et al. Hepatic and renal clearances of lidocaine in conscious and anesthetized sheep. *Anesth Analg* 1986;65:943.

477. Runciman WB, Mather LE, Ilsley AH, et al. A sheep preparation for studying interactions between blood flow and drug disposition. III: Effects of general and spinal anaesthesia on regional blood flow and oxygen tensions. *Br J Anaesth* 1984;56:247.

478. Arthur GR, Feldman HS, Covino BG. Alterations in the pharmacokinetic properties of amide local anaesthetics following local anaesthetic induced convulsions. *Acta Anaesthesiol Scand* 1988;32(7):522–529.

479. Bonica JJ, Akamatsu TJ, Berges PU, et al. Circulatory effects of peridural block: II. Effects of epinephrine. *Anesthesiology* 1971;34:514.

480. Amory DW, Sivarajan M, Lindbloom LE. Systemic and regional blood flow during epidural anesthesia with epinephrine in the rhesus monkey. *Acta Anaesthesiol Scand* 1977;21:423.

481. Kennedy WF, Everett GB, Cobb LA, Allen GD. Simultaneous systemic and hepatic hemodynamic measurements during high peridural anesthesia in normal men. *Anesth Analg* 1971;50:1069.

482. Wiklund L, Tucker GT, Engberg G. Influence of intravenously administered epinephrine on splanchnic haemodynamics and clearance of lidocaine. *Acta Anaesthesiol Scand* 1977;21:275.

483. Takahashi R, Oda Y, Tanaka K, et al. Epinephrine increases the extracellular lidocaine concentration in the brain: A possible mechanism for increased central nervous system toxicity. *Anesthesiology* 2006;105(5):984–989.

484. Isohanni MH, Ahonen J, Neuvonen PJ, Olkkola KT. Effect of ciprofloxin on the pharmacokinetics of intravenous lidocaine. *Eur J Anaesthesiol* 2005;22(10):795–799.

485. Jokinen MJ, Ahonen J, Neuvonen PJ, Olkkola KT. The effect of erythromycin, fluvoxamine, and their combination on the pharmacokinetics of ropivacaine. *Anesth Analg* 2000;91(5):1207–1212.

485a. Jokinen MJ, Olkkola KT, Ahonen J, Neuvonen PJ. Effect of rifampin and tobacco smoking on the pharmacokinetics of ropivacaine. *Clin Pharmacol Ther* 2001;70(4):344–350.

486. Jokinen MJ, Ahonen J, Neuvonen PJ, Olkkola KT. Effect of clarithromycin and itraconazole on the pharmacokinetics of ropivacaine. *Pharmacol Toxicol* 2001;88(4):187–191.

487. Jokinen MJ, Olkkola KT, Ahonen J, Neuvonen PJ. Effect of ciprofloxacin on the pharmacokinetics of ropivacaine. *Eur J Clin Pharmacol* 2003; 58(10):653–657.

488. Olkkola KT, Isohanni MH, Hamunen K, Neuvonen PJ. The effect of erythromycin and fluvoxamine on the pharmacokinetics of intravenous lidocaine. *Anesth Analg* 2005;100(5):1352–1356.

489. Orlando R, Piccoli P, De Martin S, et al Effect of the CYP3A4 inhibitor erythromycin on the pharmacokinetics of lignocaine and its pharmacologically active metabolites in subjects with normal and impaired liver function. *Br J Clin Pharmacol* 2003;55(1):86–93.

490. Nishikawa T, Goyagi T, Kimura T, et al. Oral clonidine preanesthetic medication does not alter plasma lidocaine elimination during epidural anesthesia in lightly anesthetized patients. *Can J Anaesth* 1992;39:521.

491. Bax NDS, Tucker GT, Lennard MS, Woods HF. The impairment of lignocaine clearance by propranolol: Major contribution from enzyme inhibition. *Br J Clin Pharmacol* 1985;19:597.

492. Tucker GT, Bax NDS, Lennard MS, et al. Effects of beta-adrenoceptor antagonists on the pharmacokinetics of lignocaine. *Br J Clin Pharmacol* 1984;17:S21.

492a. Bowdle TA, Freund PR, Slattery JT. Propranolol reduces bupivacaine clearance. *Anesthesiology* 1987;66:36.

493. Brashear WT, Zuspan KJ, Lazebnik N, et al. Effect of ranitidine on bupivacaine disposition. *Anesth Analg* 1991;72:369.

494. Feely J, Guy E. Lack of effect of ranitidine on the disposition of lignocaine. *Br J Clin Pharmacol* 1983;15:378.

495. Flynn RJ, Moore J, Collier PS, McClean E. Does pretreatment with cimetidine and ranitidine affect the disposition of bupivacaine? *Br J Anaesth* 1989;62:87.

496. Kishikawa K, Namiki I, Miyashita K, Saitoh K. Effects of famotidine and cimetidine on plasma levels of epidurally administered lignocaine. *Anaesthesia* 1990;45:719.

497. Kuhnert BR, Zuspan KJ, Kuhnert PM, et al. Lack of influence of cimetidine on bupivacaine levels during parturition. *Anesth Analg* 1987;66:986.

498. O'Sullivan GM, Smith M, Morgan B, et al. H2-antagonists and bupivacaine clearance. *Anaesthesia* 1988;43:93.

499. Perucca E, Richens A. Reduction of oral bioavailability of lignocaine by induction of first-pass metabolism in epileptic patients. *Br J Clin Pharmacol* 1979;8:21.

500. Routledge PA, Stargel WW, Finn AL, et al. Lignocaine disposition in blood in epilepsy. *Br J Clin Pharmacol* 1981;12:663.

501. Feely J, Clee M, Pereira L, Guy E. Enzyme inhibition with rifampicin: Lipoproteins and drug binding to alpha1-acid glycoprotein. *Br J Clin Pharmacol* 1983;16:195.

502. Kuhnert BR, Kuhnert PM, Prochaska AL, Gross TL. Plasma levels of 2-chloroprocaine in obstetric patients and their neonates after epidural anesthesia. *Anesthesiology* 1980;53:21.

503. Schenker S, Yang Y, Johnson RF, et al. The transfer of cocaine and its metabolites across the term human placenta. *Clin Pharmacol Ther* 1993;53:329.

504. Bader AM, Tsen LC, Camann WR, et al. Clinical effects and maternal and fetal plasma concentrations of 0.5% epidural levobupivacaine versus bupivacaine for cesarean delivery. *Anesthesiology* 1999;90(6):1596–1601.

505. Decocq G, Brazier M, Hary L, et al. Serum bupivacaine concentrations and transplacental transfer following repeated epidural administrations in term parturients during labour. *Fundam Clin Pharmacol* 1997;11(4):365–370.

506. Downing JW, Johnson HV, Gonzalez HF, et al. The pharmacokinetics of epidural lidocaine and bupivacaine during cesarean section. *Anesth Analg* 1997;84(3):527–532.

507. Johnson RF, Cahana A, Olenick M, et al. A comparison of the placental transfer of ropivacaine versus bupivacaine. *Anesth Analg* 1999;89(3):703–708.

508. Morton CPJ, Bloomfield S, Magnusson A, Jozwiak McClure JH. Ropivacaine 0.75% for extradural anaesthesia in elective Caesarean section: An open clinical and pharmacokinetic study in mother and neonate. *Br J Anaesth* 1997;79:3–8.

509. Porter JM, Kelleher N, Flynn R, Shorten GD. Epidural ropivacaine hydrochloride during labour: Protein binding, placental transfer and neonatal outcome. *Anaesthesia* 2001;56(5):418–423.

510. Kennedy RL, Erenberg A, Robilliard JE, et al. Effects of the changes in maternal-fetal pH on the transplacental equilibrium of bupivacaine. *Anesthesiology* 1979;51:50.

511. Kennedy RL, Miller RP, Bell JU, et al. Uptake and distribution of bupivacaine in fetal lambs. *Anesthesiology* 1986;65:247.

512. Thomas J, Long G, Moore G, Morgan D. Plasma protein binding and placental transfer of bupivacaine. *Clin Pharmacol Ther* 1976;19:426.

513. Bremerich DH, Schlosser RL, L'Allemand N, et al. Mepivacaine for spinal anesthesia in parturients undergoing elective cesarean delivery: Maternal and neonatal plasma concentrations and neonatal outcome. *Zentralbl Gynakol* 2003;125(12):518–521.

514. Hamshaw-Thomas A, Rogerson N, Reynolds F. Transfer of bupivacaine, lignocaine and pethidine across the rabbit placenta: Influence of maternal protein binding and fetal flow. *Placenta* 1984;5:61.

515. Biehl D, Shnider SM, Levinson G, Callender K. Placental transfer of lidocaine: Effects of acidosis. *Anesthesiology* 1978;48:409.

516. Brown WU, Bell GC, Alper MH. Acidosis, local anesthetics and the newborn. *Obstet Gynecol* 1976;48:27.

517. Datta S, Brown WU, Ostheimer GW, et al. Epidural anesthesia for Cesarian section in diabetic parturients: Maternal and neonatal acid-base status and bupivacaine concentration. *Anesthesiology* 1981;60:574.

518. Gaylard DG, Carson RJ, Reynolds F. Effect of umbilical perfusate pH and controlled maternal hypotension on placental drug transfer in the rabbit. *Anesth Analg* 1990;71:42.

519. Johnson RF, Herman NL, Johnson HV, et al. Effects of fetal pH on local anesthetic transfer across the human placenta. *Anesthesiology* 1996;85(3):608–615.

520. Papini O, Mathes AC, Cunha SP, Lanchote VL. Stereoselectivity in the placental transfer and kinetic disposition of racemic bupivacaine administered to parturients with or without a vasoconstrictor. *Chirality* 2004;16(2):65–71.

521. Arthur GR, Scott DH, Boyes RN, Scott DB. Pharmacokinetic and clinical pharmacological studies with mepivacaine and prilocaine. *Br J Anaesth* 1979;51(6):481–485.

522. Friberger P, Åberg G. Some physicochemical properties of the racemates and the optically active isomers of two local anaesthetic compounds. *Acta Pharm Suec* 1971;8:361–364.

523. Lee A, Fagan D, Lamont M, et al. Disposition kinetics of ropivacaine in humans. *Anesth Analg* 1989;69(6):736–738.

524. Malamed SF, Gagnon S, LeBlanc D. Efficacy of articaine: A new amide local anesthetic. *J Amer Dent Assoc* 2000;131:635–642.

525. Truant AP, Takman B. Differential physical-chemical and neuropharmacologic properties of local anesthetic agents. *Anesth Analg* 1959;38:478.

526. Tucker GT, Wiklund L, Berlin-Wahlen A, Mather LE. Hepatic clearance of local anesthetics in man. *J Pharmacokinet Biopharm* 1977;5:111–122.

CHAPTER 4 ■ CLINICAL PHARMACOLOGY OF LOCAL ANESTHETICS

JOHN F. BUTTERWORTH, IV

A review of the clinical pharmacology of local anesthetics must consider those factors that influence the usefulness and toxicity of the drugs as a group, as well as those factors specific to each compound. The various local anesthetics available commercially differ markedly in their clinical applications and potential for toxicity. In clinical practice, not every local anesthetic is suitable for every regional block procedure. Thus, an astute clinician will select among a restricted set of compounds for that one with the onset and duration of action most consistent with surgical needs. The chemical structures of the various agents and the basic pharmacological differences between the ester and amide compounds have been presented in the preceding two chapters and will not be reported herein. This information will not be repeated here. The clinical profiles of the commonly available agents are summarized in Table 4-1.

Local anesthetic toxicity may take the form of central nervous system (CNS) activation (or depression), cardiac arrhythmias or depressed cardiac inotropy, local irritant actions including neurotoxicity and myotoxicity, allergy, or miscellaneous agent-specific reactions such as methemoglobinemia (more common with benzocaine and prilocaine) and addiction (cocaine). Cardiovascular and CNS toxicity is considered in Chapter 5. The remaining forms of toxicity (save for addiction) will be considered in this chapter.

FACTORS THAT INFLUENCE LOCAL ANESTHETIC ACTIVITY

In humans, the potency, onset, and duration of anesthesia have strong statistical associations with the physicochemical properties and inherent vasodilator activites of the various agents. With most agents, onset, duration, and adequacy of anesthesia may be altered by drug dosage and/or addition of vasoconstrictors. The site of injection has a profound influence on the potency, onset, duration and adequacy of anesthesia of a specific local anesthetic dose. Attempts have been made to alter the onset and duration of anesthesia by using mixtures of local anesthetics, carbonation (adding carbon dioxide), or addition of bicarbonate ($NaHCO_3$) or any of a long list of other additives to local anesthetic solutions.

Physicochemical Properties

Important physicochemical properties that associate with measures of local anesthetic activity include lipid solubility, protein binding, and pKa. Measurements of these properties

for the various local anesthetic compounds are provided in Table 3-1.

Lipid solubility has a strong association with the potency of local anesthetic compounds (Fig. 4-1), particularly when chemically similar compounds are compared. Procaine and chloroprocaine, agents of low lipid solubility, have octanol-to-buffer partition coefficients for their free-base neutral form of 100 and 810, respectively, at 36°C. These drugs are typically administered at concentrations of 2% to 3% to attain effective conduction anesthesia in humans. On the other hand, tetracaine, bupivacaine, and etidocaine, compounds of increased lipid solubility, have octanol-to-water partition coefficients for their free-base forms of 5,822; 3,420; and 7,317, respectively, at 37°C (1). Reflecting greater potency, these agents produce effective anesthesia at concentrations between 0.25% to 1.5%. Note, however, that the agent with the greatest free base octanol-to-buffer concentration ratio (etidocaine) is typically applied in greater concentrations than either tetracaine or bupivacaine. Lidocaine and mepivacaine are intermediate both in terms of lipid solubility (partition coefficients of about 366 and 130, respectively) and of their anesthetic potency *in vivo* (typical anesthetic concentration of 1%–2%).

A consistent correlation exists between lipid solubility and anesthetic potency when similar compounds are applied to an isolated nerve *in vitro*. Thus, there is good correlation among potency and solubility when mepivacaine, ropivacaine, and bupivacaine are compared or when procaine and tetracaine are compared. However, the correlation between lipid solubility and anesthetic potency is less consistent in humans owing to other biologic considerations that exist *in vivo* but not in an *in vitro* preparation (Fig. 4-1) (2).

Lipid solubility also associates with duration of action. For unknown reasons, many books and review articles overlook this association. Among certain pairs of related anesthetics—etidocaine and lidocaine, mepivacaine and bupivacaine, and procaine and tetracaine—in every case, the agent with greater lipid solubility will have the more prolonged duration of action. We will consider this association when we discuss protein binding. Increased lipid solubility also associates with increased delay of onset for every drug comparison just cited, save that of etidocaine versus lidocaine, in which etidocaine has at least as fast an onset as lidocaine. Etidocaine's anomalously rapid onset remains poorly understood.

All clinically useful compounds must have at least some minimal lipid solubility. The protonated (charged) forms of local anesthetics have much lower octanol-to-buffer partition coefficients than the neutral (uncharged) forms (1). At 36°C, for bupivacaine, the charged local anesthetic has a coefficient of 2, whereas the uncharged base local anesthetic has a coefficient of

TABLE 4-1

COMMONLY USED LOCAL ANESTHETICS

Agent	Concentration %	Clinical use	Onset	Usual duration (h)	pH of plain solutions	Comments
Amides						
Lidocaine	0.5–1.0	Infiltration	Fast	1.0–2.0	6.5	Most versatile agent
	0.5	IV regional				
	1.0–1.5	Peripheral nerve blocks	Fast	1.0–3.0		
	1.5–2.0	Epidural	Fast	1.0–2.0		
	4	Topical	Moderate	0.5–1.0		
	2–5	Spinal	Fast	0.5–1.5		
Prilocaine	0.5–1.0	Infiltration	Fast	1.0–2.0	4.5	Least toxic amide agent
	0.5	IV regional				
	1.5–2.0	Peripheral nerve blocks	Fast	1.5–3.0		Methemoglobinemia
	2.0–3.0	Epidural	Fast	1.0–3.0		
Mepivacaine	0.5–1.0	Infiltration	Fast	1.5–3.0	4.5	Duration of plain longer than plain lidocaine. Useful when epinephrine is contraindicated.
	1.0–1.5	Peripheral nerve blocks	Fast	2.0–3.0		
	1.5–2.0	Epidural	Fast	1.5–3.0		
	2–4.0	Spinal	Fast	1.0–1.5		
Bupivacaine	0.25	Infiltration	Fast	2.0–4.0	4.5–6	Lower concentrations provide differential sensory/motor block. Ventricular arrhythmias and sudden cardiovascular collapse reported following rapid IV injection.
	0.25–0.5	Peripheral nerve blocks	Slow	4.0–12.0		
	.06–0.25	Obstetrical analgesia	Moderate	2.0–4.0		
	0.5–0.75	Surgical epidural	Moderate	2.0–5.0		
	0.5–0.75	Spinal	Fast	2.0–4.0		
Levobupi-vacaine	0.25	Infiltration	Fast	2.0–4.0		S-Isomer of bupivacaine. Probably less cardiac toxicity than bupivacaine.
	0.25–0.5	Peripheral nerve blocks	Slow	4.0–12.0		
	.06–0.25	Obstetrical analgesia	Moderate	2.0–4.0		
	0.5–0.75	Surgical epidural	Moderate	2.0–5.0		
	0.5–0.75	Spinal	Fast	2.0–4.0		"Plain" solution approved for spinal anesthetic us in USA
Ropivacaine	0.2	Infiltration	Fast	2.0–4.0		
	0.375–0.75	Peripheral nerve blocks	Slow	4.0–12.0		S-Isomer enantiomer of bupivacaine homologue. Probably less cardiac toxicity than bupivacaine.
	0.2	Postoperative analgesia (epidural)	–	–		
	0.2	Obstetrical epidural analgesia	–	–		
	0.75–1.0	Surgical epidural	Moderate	2.0–4.0		
Etidocaine	0.5	Infiltration	Fast	2.0–4.0	4.5	Profound motor block useful for surgical anesthesia but not for obstetrical analgesia.
	0.5–1.0	Peripheral nerve blocks	Fast	3.0–12.0		
	1.0–1.5	Surgical epidural	Fast	2.0–4.0		
Esters						
Procaine	1.0	Infiltration	Fast	30–60	5–6.5	Used mainly for infiltration and spinal anesthesia. Allergic potential.
	1.0–2.0	Peripheral nerve blocks	Slow	30–60		
	2.0	Epidural	Slow	30–60		
	10.0	Spinal	Fast	30–60		

(Continued)

TABLE 4-1

(CONTINUED)

Agent	Concentration %	Clinical use	Onset	Usual duration (h)	pH of plain solutions	Comments
Esters						
Chloroprocaine	1.0	Infiltration	Fast	30–60	2.7–4	Lowest systemic toxicity of all local anesthetics. Fastest onset of spinal anesthetics.
	2.0	Peripheral nerve block	Fast	30–60		
	2.0–3.0	Epidural	Fast	30–60		
	2.0	Spinal	Fast	30–45		
Tetracaine	0.5	Spinal	Fast	2.0–4.0	4.5–6.5	Use is primarily limited to spinal and topical anesthesia
	2.0	Topical	Moderate	30–60		
Cocaine	4.0–10.0	Topical	Moderate	30–60		Topical use only. Addictive, causes vasoconstriction. CNS toxicity initially features marked excitation. May cause cardiac arrhythmias.
Benzocaine	Up to 20	Topical	Moderate	30–60		Useful only for topical anesthesia. Risk of methemoglobinemia.

3,420. Compounds that do not readily permeate membranes (e.g., QX314, an obligatorily charged quaternary analog of lidocaine) will produce nerve block only after a prolonged delay when applied on the extracellular side of a nerve, as would take place during clinical regional anesthesia. Obligatorily charged local anesthetics will potently block sodium (Na) currents when applied within cytoplasm (3).

The pKa of a chemical compound identifies the pH at which the ionized and nonionized forms are present in equal concentrations. In the case of local anesthetics, pKa has a much-discussed, putative association with the speed of onset of anesthesia (4,5). For any local anesthetic that must permeate membrane barriers, rapid onset of action is favored by increasing amounts of drug in the base (uncharged or neutral) form. The percentage of a specific local anesthetic that is present in the base form when injected into tissue is inversely proportional to the pKa of that agent. As a consequence, many reviewers assert that one can predict the relative speed of onset among differing local anesthetics by comparing their pKas (5). This rule is *not valid*, despite the large number of examination questions that have been written on this topic! Mepivacaine, lidocaine, and etidocaine, for example, possess pKas of 7.7, 7.8, and 7.9, respectively, at 36°C (1). When these agents are injected into tissue at a pH of 7.4, roughly 65% of these drugs exist in the ionized form and 35% in the nonionized base form. Yet, the onset of block with etidocaine is at least as fast as with the other two agents. In a similar way, tetracaine possesses a pKa of 8.4 at 36°C. Thus, roughly 5% is present in the nonionized form and 95% exists in the charged cationic form at a tissue pH of 7.4. At the same temperature, chloroprocaine has a pKa of 9.1, meaning that only 2% will be in the free-base form and 98% will be protonated. Nevertheless, the onset of block with chloroprocaine for all forms of regional anesthesia is considerably faster than with tetracaine (and this holds true even when adjustments are made for their relative potencies). The pKas of the various local anesthetic agents are provided in Table 3-1. Those who wish to preserve the pKa "rule" often argue that chloroprocaine is used at greater concentrations and dosages than other local anesthetics, and that the more rapid onset of action could be related simply to the larger number of molecules of this agent that can be safely administered compared to other agents. This explanation collapses when 1% chloroprocaine and 1% lidocaine are compared for spinal anesthesia (Fig. 4-2) (6). Chloroprocaine has a faster

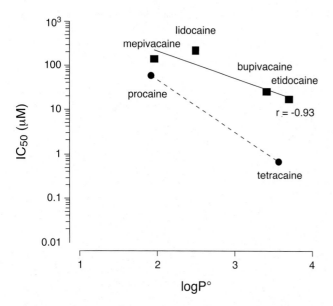

FIGURE 4-1. Strong correlations between local anesthetic potency (at inhibiting sodium currents) with solubility. Local anesthetics lipid solubilities measured as octanol-to-buffer partition coefficient ($\log P^0$). Linear regression gives a correlation coefficient of –0.71 for all local anesthetics (regression line not shown) and –0.93 for only amide-linked structures (mepivacaine, lidocaine, bupivacaine, etidocaine). The slope of the line is –0.6 for amides and –.2 for esters. From Brau M, Vogel W, Hempelmann G. Fundamental properties of local anesthetics: Half-maximal blocking concentrations for tonic block of Na^+ and K^+ channels in peripheral nerve. *Anesth Analg* 1998;87:885–889, with permission.

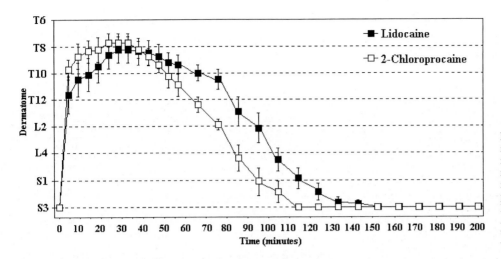

FIGURE 4-2. Faster onset and faster resolution of sensory block determined by pin-prick anesthesia after 2 mL 2% 2-chloroprocaine than after 2 mL 2% lidocaine given as spinal injection. Data derived from Kouri ME, Kopacz DJ. Spinal 2-chloroprocaine: A comparison with lidocaine in volunteers. *Anesth Analg* 2004;98:75–80, with permission.

onset time than lidocaine. Thus, pKa is not nearly as predictive of rate of onset as generations of anesthesiologists have been led to believe.

Many authors have opined that the relative protein binding of various local anesthetics has an influence on their duration of anesthesia. Various unwieldy, logically inconsistent, and almost certainly incorrect explanations have been offered for this association. *Nevertheless, despite the correllation, no direct relationship exists between local anesthetic protein binding and local anesthetic binding to Na channels.* Would any credible pharmacologist argue that a relationship exists between the greater (nonspecific) protein binding of sufentanil versus fentanyl and (specific) binding of these agents to μ-receptors in brain and spinal cord? Certainly not! For all classes of drugs, the less water-soluble the compound the greater fraction of the drug will be protein bound in blood. The only conceivable connection between protein binding and duration of local anesthetic action lies in the fact that local anesthetics of increased lipid solubility (by definition) are protein bound to greater extent when they reach the bloodstream. For thermodynamic reasons, more lipid-soluble agents will have a greater tendency than less lipid-soluble agents to remain in a lipid-rich environment (e.g., the plasma membrane) than diffuse into the blood. The longer that the local anesthetic molecule remains within the membrane (rather than diffusing away from the nerve toward the bloodstream), the longer that the molecule has the potential to bind Na channels and produce nerve block. Once the local anesthetic enters the bloodstream, it is highly unlikely to reenter the nerve membrane and contribute to conduction block.

Bupivacaine is about 95% protein bound (and has an octanol-to-buffer partition coefficient for the free-base form of 3,420) and is a very potent anesthetic with a long duration of action (1). On the other hand, procaine, which is only 6% protein bound (and has an octanol-to-buffer partition coefficient for the free-base form of 100), is less potent and has a relatively short duration of action. Mepivacaine and lidocaine, which are intermediate in terms of protein binding (55%–75%), are also intermediate in terms of lipid solubility (partition coefficients for the free-base forms of 130 and 366, respectively), potency, and anesthetic duration. As should be obvious, it is erroneous to consider the nonspecific binding of a drug to α_1-acid glycoprotein and albumin as having any direct relationship to the binding of that drug to its specific binding site in membrane-spanning region S6 of domains III and IV on the Na channel (7).

Vasodilator Properties

The clinical activity of local anesthetics is also modified by other factors. Faster vascular absorption reduces the number of local anesthetic molecules available for binding to Na channels. Faster absorption into the bloodstream may also reduce the apparent local anesthetic *in vivo* potency and duration of action. All local anesthetics except cocaine exhibit a biphasic effect on vascular smooth muscle (8,9). At extremely low concentrations, they inhibit nitric oxide release in vascular smooth muscle, leading to vasoconstriction. This action is of unknown clinical importance because at the much greater concentrations generally used for regional anesthesia local anesthetics tend to be vasodilators (10). Differences in the relative degree of vasodilation produced by local anesthetics may influence their anesthetic profile. For example, some *in vitro* studies have shown that lidocaine is significantly more potent than mepivacaine on an isolated nerve (consistent with their octanol-to-water partition coefficients) (4). Human studies, however, show little difference in the relative anesthetic potency of these two agents and sometimes find that the duration of action of mepivacaine is longer than that of lidocaine (11). Perhaps these differences relate to greater vasodilation by lidocaine: Addition of epinephrine to lidocaine and mepivacaine reduces both the difference in vasodilator activity and the duration of action (11).

In summary, the clinically important properties of local anesthetics include potency, delay of onset, and duration of action. Associations exist between the clinical profiles of the various agents and their physicochemical properties. *In vivo*, the clinical activity of these drugs may be altered by other actions, such as their relative tendency to produce vasodilation. On the basis of their anesthetic profile in humans, the local anesthetics may be classified as follows:

- Agents of low potency and short duration of action, including procaine and chloroprocaine
- Agents of intermediate potency and duration of action, including lidocaine, mepivacaine, and prilocaine
- Agents of high potency and prolonged duration of action, including tetracaine, bupivacaine, ropivacaine, and etidocaine

In terms of onset, chloroprocaine, lidocaine, mepivacaine, prilocaine, and etidocaine possess a relatively rapid onset of action. Tetracaine, bupivacaine, and ropivacaine have longer latencies of onset (except during spinal anesthesia, during which all anesthetics produce a relatively fast onset of block). *In general, increasing potency associates with increasing lipid solubility, protein binding, delay of onset, and duration of action.*

In addition to these properties, one other important clinical consideration is the ability of local anesthetic agents to differentially inhibit sensory versus motor fibers. Physicians have long known that nerve fibers of differing sizes have differing susceptibility to local anesthetics (as well as to pressure, lack of oxygen, and lack of glucose). In general, among fibers of similar types, the larger the fiber, the more resistant it is to local anesthetic block (12). Smaller myelinated fibers (e.g., Aδ-fibers) are more susceptible to local anesthetics than are larger myelinated fibers (e.g., Aα- or Aβ-fibers). And, larger unmyelinated fibers are less susceptible to block than are smaller unmyelinated fibers. The "size principle" fails when unmyelinated fibers are compared with myelinated fibers. A "pure" differential block of smaller pain fibers cannot be achieved, however, because the unmyelinated fibers (e.g., C-fibers) as a group are *less* susceptible to local anesthetics than are the myelinated fibers (13). Thus, using conventional local anesthetic techniques, one cannot completely block all pain-transmitting Aδ- and C-fibers without also producing some inhibition of motor fibers. Although differential spinal blockade has been produced with reduced intrathecal doses of procaine and used to identify sympathetically mediated pain states of the lower extremities, local anesthetics will not produce surgical analgesia for incision without motor block. Physicians can also use mixtures of local anesthetic and other agents to produce postoperative analgesia via epidural and peripheral neural infusions. Again, these techniques cannot produce analgesia sufficient for surgical incision without motor block.

Bupivacaine and etidocaine, two potent, long-acting local anesthetics introduced into clinical practice at about the same time, provide an interesting contrast in terms of their differential sensory/motor blocking activity. Bupivacaine is widely used in epidural solutions for surgical anesthesia, for obstetric analgesia, and for relief of postoperative pain owing to its ability to provide adequate sensory analgesia while preserving motor function, particularly at concentrations ≤0.25%. Thus, a laboring parturient can be rendered pain-free yet still be able to move her legs (or even walk) (4). Etidocaine, on the other hand, shows little separation between sensory and motor blockade. To achieve adequate epidural sensory anesthesia, 1.5% concentrations of etidocaine are usually required. At these concentrations, etidocaine has an extremely rapid onset of action and a prolonged duration of anesthesia; however, sensory anesthesia is associated with a profound degree of motor blockade, and the motor block can sometimes outlast the sensory block during offset of anesthesia. Thus, etidocaine was useful for surgical epidural anesthesia in which optimum muscle relaxation is desirable, whereas its marked inhibition of motor function rendered it useless for obstetric or postoperative epidural analgesia.

As previously noted, bupivacaine was the first agent that showed some relative specificity for sensory fibers, such that sensory analgesia without profound inhibition of motor fibers often could be observed (14). Unfortunately, the success was incomplete. When the sensory block was adequate for skin incision, there was almost always a significant degree of motor block. Differences among local anesthetics are sometimes apparent during the onset or offset of peripheral nerve block. For example, during the onset of median nerve block with mepivacaine, there is almost no difference in the relative inhibition

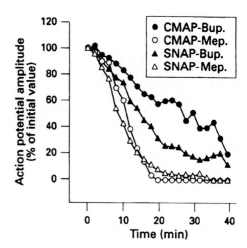

FIGURE 4-3. Differential onset of block with bupivacaine vs. mepivacaine. The median of 10 measurments is plotted in every case. Note that mepivacaine inhibits both compound motor action potentials (CMAPs) and sensory nerve action potentials (SNAPs) faster than bupivacaine. Bupivacaine, unlike mepivacaine, inhibits SNAPs faster than CMAPs. Data derived from Butterworth JF, Ririe DG, Thompson RB, et al. Differential onset of median nerve block: randomized, double-blind comparison of mepivacaine and bupivacaine in healthy volunteers. *Br J Anaesth* 1998;81:515–521, with permission.

of sensory nerve function as assessed by the amplitude of sensory nerve action potentials (SNAPs) recorded from volunteer subjects versus inhibition of motor nerve function as assessed by compound motor action potential (CMAP) amplitude (15). With bupivacaine, the inhibition of SNAP amplitude occurred earlier and was more profound than CMAP. At steady state, both agents inhibited SNAPs and CMAPs comparably and profoundly (Fig. 4-3) (15).

OTHER FACTORS INFLUENCING ANESTHETIC ACTIVITY

Although the inherent pharmacologic properties of the various local anesthetic agents largely determine their anesthetic profile, other factors may influence the quality of regional anesthesia, including (a) dosage of local anesthetic administered, (b) addition of a vasoconstrictors and other additives to the local anesthetic solution, (c) site of administration, (d) the temperature of the local anesthetic solution, (e) pregnancy, and (f) mixtures of local anesthetic solutions.

Dosage of Local Anesthetic Solutions

The mass of drug (the total number of local anesthetic molecules) administered will influence the onset, quality, and duration of anesthesia (Table 4-2) (4). For any agent, as the dose is increased, the likelihood of satisfactory anesthesia and the duration of anesthesia will increase, and the latency of onset of anesthesia will decrease. In general, the dosage of local anesthetic administered can be increased by administering a larger volume of a less concentrated solution or a smaller volume of a more concentrated solution. For example, a dose-response study of bupivacaine for epidural analgesia in laboring women showed that increasing the concentration from

TABLE 4-2

EFFECTS OF DOSE AND EPINEPHRINE ON LOCAL ANESTHETIC PROCEDURES

	Increased dose	Addition of epinephrine
Onset time	↓	↓
Degree of motor block	↑	↑
Degree of sensory block	↑	↑
Likelihood of adequate duration of block	↑	↑
Area (extent) of block	↑	↑
Peak plasma concentration	↑	↓

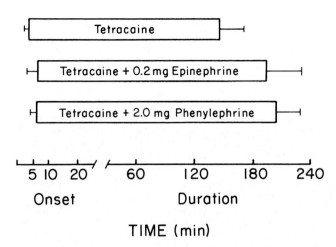

FIGURE 4-4. Comparative effect of epinephrine and phenylephrine on the duration of spinal anesthesia produced by tetracaine. Data derived from Concepcion M, Maddi R, Francis D, et al. Vasoconstrictors in spinal anesthesia with tetracaine. A comparison of epinephrine and phenylephrine. *Anesth Analg* 1984;63:134, with permission.

0.125% to 0.5% while maintaining the same injectate volume (10 mL) decreased latency, improved the incidence of satisfactory analgesia, and increased the duration of sensory analgesia (16). A study of bupivacaine in surgical anesthesia showed that increasing the concentration from 0.5% to 0.75% (increasing the dose from about 100 mg to 150 mg) produced a faster onset and longer duration of sensory anesthesia (17). In addition, the likelihood of satisfactory sensory anesthesia and the degree of motor blockade was increased. When prilocaine (600 mg) was administered in the epidural space either as 30 mL of a 2% solution or 20 mL of 3% solution, there was no difference in onset, adequacy, or duration of anesthesia and onset, depth, and duration of motor blockade (18). In some blocks, the volume of anesthetic solution administered may influence the "spread" of anesthesia; for example, 30 mL of 1% lidocaine administered in the epidural space anesthetized four more dermatomes than did 10 mL of 3% lidocaine (19). On the other hand, some animal studies suggest that a smaller volume of a more concentrated local anesthetic solution produces a denser, more persistant block than a larger volume of a less conventional solution (20). Nevertheless, the consensus from clinical studies suggests that, except for the possible effect on the dermatomal spread of epidural anesthesia, the primary qualities of regional anesthesia, namely, onset, depth, and duration of blockade, are related to the mass of drug injected; that is, the product of volume times concentration, and the proximity of the local anesthetic molecules to the intended target.

Use of Additives with Local Anesthetic Solutions

Vasoconstrictors, typically epinephrine, are frequently added to local anesthetic solutions. Vasoconstrictors decrease the rate of vascular absorption, allowing more anesthetic molecules to reach the nerve membrane, improving depth and prolonging duration of anesthesia (Table 4-2). In clinical anesthesia, local anesthetic solutions usually contain a 1:200,000 (5 μg/mL) concentration of epinephrine, based on studies of lidocaine in epidural and intercostal blocks (4,21). Only limited information is available regarding the optimum concentration of epinephrine with other local anesthetic agents or other block procedures. Other α-agonists, such as clonidine and phenylephrine, have been used as additives to solutions of local anesthetics.

In some studies, phenylephrine produced greater prolongation of spinal anesthesia when combined with tetracaine; however, more recent studies conducted under double-blind conditions found no difference between epinephrine and phenylephrine in prolonging tetracaine spinal anesthesia (Fig. 4-4) (22). Epinephrine has differing effects on specific local anesthetics. Procaine, lidocaine, and mepivacaine are significantly prolonged by epinephrine during infiltration anesthesia, peripheral nerve blocks, or epidural anesthesia (11,23–26). Bupivacaine and etidocaine local infiltration blocks are prolonged by epinephrine (27). The durations of epidural blocks with these agents are not, however, markedly prolonged by epinephrine (24,27,28). It is generally assumed that with bupivacaine and etidocaine the increased lipid solubility and delayed uptake of these agents by the bloodstream may underlie the diminished effect of epinephrine.

The interaction of epinephrine with the long-acting agents, such as bupivacaine, is dependent on the setting, block technique, and concentration of drug used. In epidural analgesia for labor, for example, the frequency and the duration of adequate analgesia were improved when epinephrine 1:200,000 was added to 0.125% and 0.25% bupivacaine (16); however, the addition of epinephrine to 0.5% and 0.75% bupivacaine did not significantly improve epidural blocks in either obstetric or surgical patients (16,29). Epinephrine appears to improve the quality of analgesia provided by dilute intrathecal solutions of bupivacaine plus opioid (30). The degree of motor blockade is increased following the epidural administration of epinephrine-containing solutions of bupivacaine and etidocaine (29). The differing effects of epinephrine in prolonging the duration of differing local anesthetics is most apparent during spinal anesthesia (see Chapter 10). Epinephrine greatly increases the duration of tetracaine spinal anesthesia, but prolongs lidocaine and bupivacaine spinal anesthesia to a lesser extent (22,31–34).

Attempts have been made to modify local anesthetic solutions to shorten their delay of onset and/or to prolong their duration of anesthesia. Carbonation of local anesthetic solutions was thought to speed the onset of action of various local anesthetics (14,35). In isolated nerves, carbon dioxide enhances diffusion of local anesthetics through nerve sheaths and hastens inhibition of action potentials (36,37). Double-blind studies, however, failed to demonstrate a significantly more rapid onset of action when lidocaine carbonate was compared with lidocaine hydrochloride for epidural blockade (38). In fact, addition of $NaHCO_3$ to lidocaine (which would be expected to reduce the fraction of the protonated local anesthetic form) reduced the onset delay relative to the carbonated prepration (39). Other double-blind studies failed to show benefit from carbonation of bupivacaine (40,41). Thus, at present, there appears to be no benefit to carbonation of local anesthetic solutions in terms of onset of block under clinical conditions.

As mentioned, attempts have been made to speed the onset of conduction blockade by adding $NaCHO_3$ to local anesthetic solutions immediately before injection (39,42–44). Sodium bicarbonate will increase the pH of the local anesthetic solution, which in turn will increase the amount of drug in the uncharged base form. Thus, the rate of diffusion across the nerve sheath and nerve membrane could be increased, speeding the onset of anesthesia. *In vitro* studies of pH adjustment suggest that the apparent potency of local anesthetics increases at more basic pH (Fig. 4-5) (45). Addition of $NaCHO_3$ to lidocaine prior to median nerve block decreased the latency of onset of block of compound motor action potentials, but had no effect on the latency of block of sensory nerve action potentials or on inhibition of pin-prick sensibility (46). Numerous clinical studies have been performed in which the addition of $NaCHO_3$ to local anesthetic solutions has had a variable effect on the latency, duration, or effectiveness of blockade (Fig. 4-6) (5,44). Overall, it appears that $NaCHO_3$ has its greatest benefit when added to local anesthetic solutions mixed with epinephrine by the manufacturer. These solutions tend to have a reduced pH (relative to "plain" solutions of local anesthetics) that increases the shelf life of the epinephrine. Bicarbonate would be expected to have a lesser effect on solutions that are less acidic to begin with, and most studies of this topic bear this out (44). Addition

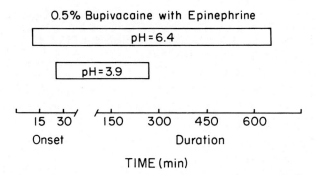

FIGURE 4-6. Faster onset and longer duration of brachial plexus blockade by bupivacaine at more alkaline pH. Data derived from Hilgier M. Alkalinization of bupivacaine for brachial plexus block. *Reg Anesth* 1985;10:59, with permission.

of $NaCHO_3$ consistently reduces the pain of injection of local anethetics (47).

Potassium occasionally has been added to local anesthetic solutions in unsuccessful attempts to improve local anesthesia (48,49). Various attempts have been made to prolong the duration of anesthesia by incorporating dextran into local anesthetic solutions (50,51). In one clinical study, prolonged durations of anesthesia were observed in occasional patients, but the mean duration of intercostal nerve blockade was not significantly altered when solutions of bupivacaine with and without dextran were compared (52). Rosenblatt and Fung have suggested that the difference in results obtained by various investigators may be related to the pH of the dextran solution used with more alkaline dextran solutions producing prolongation and less alkaline dextrans being ineffective (53). Perhaps alkalinization of the anesthetic solution may be responsible for prolonged conduction blockade rather than the dextran itself.

There has been much recent interest in addition of the α_2-agonist clonidine to local anesthetic solutions. Clonidine has local anesthetic properties *in vitro*: Clonidine and other similar agents will block both $A\alpha$- and C-fibers (Fig. 4-7) (54). Thus, it remains unclear whether prolongation of local anesthesia by clonidine is the result of pharmacodynamic prolongation of local anesthetic effects, a direct action of clonidine on nerves, a central action of clonidine, or some combination of effects (55). When added to intermediate-duration agents such as mepivcaine and lidocaine, clonidine markedly prolongs the duration of brachial plexus or femoral nerve blocks. Clonidine prolongs the duration of spinal anesthesia when it is included with mepivacaine. Clonidine even prolongs the duration of tetracaine when clonidine is taken as an oral agent (56,57). Clonidine, like epinephrine, appears to be less useful at prolonging the duration of such agents as bupivacaine or ropivacaine (58).

In the case of spinal anesthesia, probably the most useful additives have been dextrose and opioids (see Chapter 10). Numerous studies have shown that addition of 20 to 25 μg of fentanyl will improve the quality of spinal anesthesia produced by bupivacaine, markedly reduce the likelihood of an inadequate block, and increase the duration of analgesia (without prolonging motor block) (59). In obstetric anesthesia practice, both sufentanil and fentanyl have been popular subarachnoid agents to initiate analgesia during labor (analgesia that will generally be maintained by an epidural local anesthetic infusion) (60).

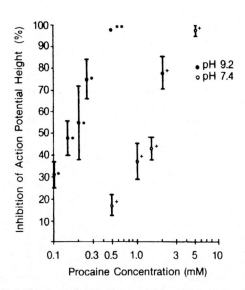

FIGURE 4-5. Increased pH renders procaine more potent at inhibiting action potentials in the isolated frog sciatic nerve. From Butterworth JF, 4th, Lief PA, Strichartz GR. The pH-dependent local anesthetic activity of diethylaminoethanol, a procaine metabolite. *Anesthesiology* 1988;68:501–506, with permission.

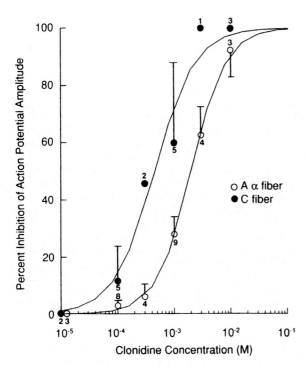

FIGURE 4-7. Concentration-dependant inhibition by clonidine of action potentials in Aα- and C-fibers in rat sciatic nerve. From Butterworth J, Strichartz GR. The alpha 2-adrenergic agonists clonidine and guanfacine produe tonic and phasic block of conduction in rat sciatic nerve fibers. *Anesth Analg* 1993;76:295–301, with permission.

Site of Injection

The site of administration of local anesthetics will influence their pharmacodynamic profile. Although local anesthetics are typically classified as agents of short, moderate, or long duration with a corresponding rapid or slow onset of action, these general properties are influenced by the specific anesthetic procedure performed. Tetracaine, for example, is usually considered an agent of slow onset and long duration, but when administered intrathecally, its onset of action is quite rapid (about 3 minutes) and its duration of spinal anesthesia is only 3 to 4 hours (4,22). In fact, all local anesthetics have a faster onset and shorter duration when used for spinal anesthesia than for other nerve block procedures. In terms of latency, the most rapid onset of action occurs after subcutaneous, intravenous (IV) regional, or spinal administration of local anesthetics, whereas the slowest onset times are observed during the performance of plexus blocks (4). Duration of anesthesia also varies by site. Bupivacaine provides a duration of surgical anesthesia of 3 to 4 hours when administered into the epidural space, but when it is administered for brachial plexus blockade, the anesthesia persists for at least 6 and sometimes 24 hours. Differences in the onset and the duration of anesthesia depending on the site of injection are mainly due to the particular anatomy of the area of injection and differences in the rate of vascular absorption. In the case of spinal anesthesia, the lack of a nerve sheath barrier and the deposition of the local anesthetic solution into a solution that bathes the spinal cord and spinal nerves result in a rapid onset of action. The relatively small amount of drug used for spinal anesthesia almost certainly contributes to the relatively short duration of action

associated with this technique. With brachial plexus blockade, despite large doses of local anesthetic, the onset of anesthesia is slow because the anesthetic agent needs time to diffuse across tissue barriers and the nerve membrane. The longer duration of brachial plexus blockade observed with bupivacaine and ropivacaine is probably related to the slower rate of vascular absorption from that site, and also the absorption of relative larger amounts of drug by the nerve membranes as a consequence of the large doses that are commonly used for plexus blocks.

Mixtures of Local Anesthetics

Mixtures of local anesthetics have long been popular in regional anesthesia despite limited evidence that they are superior to single agents. The theoretical basis for mixing is to compensate for the short duration of action of agents, such as chloroprocaine or lidocaine, and the long latency of other agents, such as tetracaine and bupivacaine. The combination of lidocaine and tetracaine was commonly used before bupivacaine became available. Because the slow onset of tetracaine was often inconvenient, the addition of lidocaine provided a local anesthetic solution with a relatively rapid onset of action and a prolonged duration. In a similar way, mixtures of chloroprocaine and bupivacaine have been used, but with inconsistent results. In some clinicians' hands a mixture of chloroprocaine and bupivacaine produced brachial plexus block with a short latency and a prolonged duration (61). However, others found that a mixture of chloroprocaine and bupivacaine produced epidural anesthesia with a significantly shorter duration than that produced by solutions of pure bupivacaine (62). A variety of complicated explanations have been provided for this reduced duration; however, clinical experience suggests that whenever two agents are mixed in comparable amounts, the onset and duration will always be intermediate between the two (63). In a prospective study of mixtures of lidocaine and bupivacaine, no difference in onset of epidural block was observed among the solutions tested. Duration of blockade with a 50:50 mixture of lidocaine/bupivacaine was only marginally longer than that for lidocaine alone (64). Keckeis and Hofmockel compared onset and duration of brachial plexus block using 30 mL 0.5% bupivacaine or using 15 mL 0.5% bupivacaine to which 15 mL of either 1% lidocaine, 1% mepivacane, 1% prilocaine, or 1% etidocaine was added (65). The mixtures using intermediate-duration local anesthetics all had faster onset but shorter duration than pure bupivacaine. The etidocaine-bupivacaine mixture had a faster onset and a longer duration than pure bupivacaine. In sum, the available data offer vanishingly small evidence for any major advantage to using mixtures of shorter- and longer-acting amide local anesthetics (65). In addition, the use of catheter techniques for epidural anesthesia and plexus blocks makes it possible to provide an anesthetic (and postoperative analgesia) of sufficient duration for almost any appropriate surgical procedure.

Systemic Toxicity

Local anesthetics vary considerably in their potency at causing systemic CNS or cardiovascular toxic reactions. In general, their potency as local anesthetics follows the same rank order as their potency at producing toxic reactions. The relative toxicity of some commonly used agents is depicted in

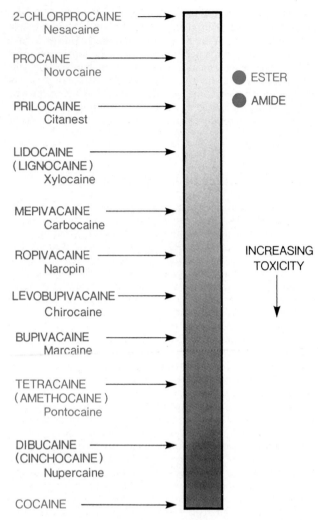

2-CHLORPROCAINE
Nesacaine

PROCAINE
Novocaine

⬤ ESTER
⬤ AMIDE

PRILOCAINE
Citanest

LIDOCAINE
(LIGNOCAINE)
Xylocaine

MEPIVACAINE
Carbocaine

ROPIVACAINE
Naropin

INCREASING
TOXICITY

LEVOBUPIVACAINE
Chirocaine

BUPIVACAINE
Marcaine

TETRACAINE
(AMETHOCAINE)
Pontocaine

DIBUCAINE
(CINCHOCAINE)
Nupercaine

COCAINE

FIGURE 4-8. Local anesthetics are arranged in aproximate order of increasing toxicity. Note that comparisons of all of the agents at "equally effective" concentrations and under the same conditions have not been made in humans.

Figure 4-8. Systemic CNS and cardiovascular toxicity represent large and important topics, and will be covered in Chapter 5.

Peripheral Vascular Effects

Local anesthetics exert a biphasic action on smooth muscle of peripheral blood vessels related to inhibition of nitric oxide mechanisms and vasoconstriction at very reduced concentrations and vasodilation at clinical concentrations (8,9). For example, exposure of arterioles in the cremaster muscle of rats to concentrations of lidocaine of 10 to 1,000 μg/mL produced a dose-related state of vasoconstriction varying from 88% to 60% of the control vascular diameter (9). An increase in the concentration of lidocaine to 10,000 μg/mL produced approximately a 27% increase in arteriolar diameter, indicating a significant degree of vasodilation. Other studies using an isolated rat portal vein preparation have also demonstrated that local anesthetic drugs vasoconstrict at reduced concentrations and inhibit myogenic activity at increased concentrations (8).

In vivo studies have also confirmed the biphasic effect of local anesthetic on the peripheral vasculature (66). Intra-arterial administration of mepivacaine to human volunteers decreases forearm blood flow without changing arterial pressure, which suggests that mepivacaine causes regional vasoconstriction (67). Similar studies with lidocaine also showed an increased tone in capacitance vessels, with less consistent effect on resistance vessels (67). As the dose of local anesthetic agent is increased, the stimulatory or vasoconstrictor action of these agents changes to one of inhibition and vasodilation.

Cocaine is the only local anesthetic that consistently produces vasoconstriction at most doses. Direct blood flow studies in animals have shown that the initial effect of cocaine is one of vasodilation, but this is followed by a long period of vasoconstriction regardless of the dose of cocaine administered (68,69). This unique property of cocaine is related to a direct action of cocaine on inhibition of nitric oxide and to inhibition of reuptake of norepinephrine by tissue (70). No other local anesthetic inhibits the reuptake of norepinephrine. This effect of cocaine is of course related to its actions within the CNS, where it is the only local anesthetic that can produce drug-craving behavior in both animals and humans.

Miscellaneous Systemic Effects

A wide variety of systemic actions have been ascribed to local anesthetic drugs. For example, local anesthetics have neuromuscular blocking, ganglionic blocking, and anticholinergic activity. Local anesthetics have actions on coagulation, inflammation, immune responses, and inhibit a wide variety of enzymes and receptors (71). There is even provocative new evidence that systemically administered lidocaine shortens length of stay and improves outcomes after surgery (72).

A nearly unique systemic side effect of prilocaine is its dose-related ability to initiate methemoglobinemia (73,74). The historic "dogma" was that doses of prilocaine must exceed 600 mg before clinically important fractions (>5%) of methemoglobinemia would appear in adults (4,5). Recent studies suggest that clinically important concentrations (>10%) may occur with prilocaine doses as small as 400 mg in otherwise healthy young adults (75). The formation of methemoglobin is believed to be related to the degradation of prilocaine in the liver to o-toluidine, which converts hemoglobin to methemoglobin (73). Although mild degrees of methemoglobinemia are of little clinical importance in most patients with normal oxygen-carrying capacity, this complication has limited the use of this otherwise potentially valuable drug. Nevertheless, a focus on prilocaine may be inappropriate. Dangerous degrees of methemoglobinemia are more commonly associated with benzocaine than prilocaine, at least in American hospitals (76). In surgical patients, one should be cognizant that dangerous levels of methemoglobin may result from treatment with dapsone (used for opportunistic infections in the immunosuppressed), dehydration, and 20% benzocaine spray used for topical anesthesia (Table 4-3). The methemoglobinemia associated with the use of prilocaine or benzocaines may be treated by the IV administration of methylene blue (1 mg/kg intravenously) over several minutes. Methylene blue treatment may need to be repeated.

Allergic Effects

Many patients report histories suggestive of allergic or hypersensitivity reactions to local anesthetics. There is no question

TABLE 4-3

ETIOLOGIES OF ACQUIRED METHEMOGLOBINEMIA IN 138 PATIENTS

Etiologic agent or context	Total cases	Mean peak methemoglobin % ± standard deviation (range)
Dapsone	58	8 ± 6
Diagnosed intraoperatively	32	3 ± 2
Unknown etiology	24	4 ± 3
Dehydration in children	6	28 ± 21
20% benzocaine	5	44 ± 15
Primaquine	5	6 ± 4
Both dapsone and primaquine	4	17 ± 9
Other etiologies (sepsis, sickle cell crisis, insecticides, or fume inhalation)	4	7 ± 6

From Ash-Bernal R, Wise R, Wright SM. Acquired methemoglobinemia: A retrospective series of 138 cases at 2 teaching hospitals. *Medicine (Baltimore)* 2004;83:265–273.

that an occasional patient may have a local anesthetic allergy, and both anaphylactic and anaphylactoid responses to local anesthetic are possible (77,78). However, systemic toxic reactions to local anesthetic agents are frequently misdiagnosed as allergic or hypersensitivity reactions (72,79). The ester local anesthetics, especially procaine and benzocaine, have long been assumed to have a greater propensity for allergic reactions based on the fact that they are derivatives of p-aminobenzoic acid. According to many textbooks, the advent of the amide local anesthetics, none of which is a derivative of para-aminobenzoic acid, appears to have markedly reduced the incidence of allergic reactions to local anesthetic drugs (4). Nevertheless, good data to support this widely (and strongly) held opinion are sparse indeed. Allergic reactions to the amide local anesthetics are rare (72,77–79). In two studies, none of 149 patients who exhibited hives, wheal and flare, or even an anaphylactoid reaction (requiring resuscitation) actually demonstrated

intradermal test responses to the purported local anesthetic allergen (80). Multiple-dose containers of amide local anesthetics may contain a preservative, methylparaben, the chemical structure of which resembles that of p-aminobenzoic acid. Some patients in whom methylparaben was administered intradermally demonstrate a positive skin reaction (81). Some patients may be allergic to metabisulfite, present in epinephrine-containing local anesthetic solutions. Cross-sensitivity reactions are possible because many other drugs, foods, and beverages contain preservatives such as metabisulfite and hydroxybenzoate.

Progressive challenge with dilute (1:1,000) intradermal local anesthetic injections is often obtained to diagnose immune-based adverse responses to local anesthetics. Given the rarity of true, antibody-related, allergic reactions in patients, it is unclear whether skin testing provides cost-effective information for patients who have experienced an apparent allergic reaction. Skin testing by the anesthesiologist may be useful when local anesthetics are needed acutely (82). Clearly, local anesthetic solutions without additives must be used in such testing, and also used for regional anesthesia in patients with a history of allergy to preservatives in foods or drugs (72).

Local Tissue Toxicity

Local anesthetics rarely produce localized nerve damage in clinical practice (83). In 1980, controversy arose regarding the potential neurotoxicity of chloroprocaine. Prolonged sensory and motor deficits were reported in patients after the epidural or subarachnoid injection of large doses of this agent (84–86).

Initially, animal studies proved contradictory regarding the potential neurotoxicity of chloroprocaine (Table 4-4). In an isolated rabbit vagus nerve preparation, chloroprocaine, but not lidocaine, was associated with signs of neural irritation (87). Rabbit sciatic nerves exposed to chloroprocaine for 6 hours showed no signs of nerve damage (88). Doses of chloroprocaine sufficient to cause total spinal anesthesia in dogs produced paralysis in about 30% of the animals, whereas comparable doses of bupivacaine produced no evidence of permanent neurologic sequelae (89). On the other hand, similar studies in sheep and monkeys failed to show a difference in neurotoxicity between chloroprocaine and other local anesthetics (90).

TABLE 4-4

SUMMARY OF NEUROTOXICITY STUDIES INVOLVING CHLOROPROCAINE AND OTHER AGENTS

Reference	Type of study	Signs of neurotoxicity			
		2-CP	Lidocaine	Bupivacaine	NaHSO$_3$
87	Isolated rabbit vagus nerve	+++	0	−	+++
92	Isolated rabbit vagus nerve	+++	−	0	+++
89	Dog: Total spinal	+++	−	0	−
91	Rabbit: Spinal	+++	−	−	+++
90	Sheep: Total spinal	+	+	0	−
90	Monkey: Total spinal	+	−	+	−
93	Rat: Spinal infusion	+++	−	−	0
148	Rat: Spinal infusion	−	+++	+	−
149	Rat: Spinal infusion	−	+++	+	−

0, no effect; +, mild toxicity; + + +, severe toxicity; − not studied; 2-CP, commercial 2-chloroprocaine solution; NaHSO$_3$, sodium bisulfate.

Later studies in rabbits suggested that the toxicity might be related to sodium bisulfite, which is used as an antioxidant in chloroprocaine solutions (91). Gissen et al. conducted a series of studies on the isolated rabbit vagus nerve to investigate the neurotoxicity of the various components of commercial chloroprocaine solutions (Table 4-4) (92). The results of these studies suggested that the combination of a low pH and the presence of sodium bisulfite may be responsible for the neurotoxic reactions observed following the use of large amounts of chloroprocaine solution. Chloroprocaine, itself, did not appear to be neurotoxic. More recently, Drasner et al. have used a chronic infusion to demonstrate that 2-chloroprocaine caused persisting deficits and the presence of bisulfite reduced the severity of nerve damage after 2-chloroprocaine (93). To make the issue even more confusing, Kopacz and colleagues have performed a detailed series of clinical experiments that document the safety (after several thousand administrations) of preservative-free chloroprocaine as a spinal anesthetic (Fig. 4-2) (6). So, despite more than 20 years of investigation, there remains no consensus regarding the underlying cause (whether it be the drug per se or some combination of drug, pH, and preservative) of cauda equina syndrome following large doses of chloroprocaine.

There has been a raging debate about whether lidocaine remains a suitable local anesthetic for spinal anesthesia. Despite a half-century of use, recent studies suggest that lidocaine may be more likely than other spinal anesthetics to cause transient neurologic symptoms or occasional spinal nerve damage (94,95). When the various spinal anesthetics were applied to desheathed nerves *in vitro*, only 5% lidocaine caused irreversible loss of conduction (96). Clearly lidocaine is now much less popular for spinal anesthesia than a decade ago. Unfortunately, a consensus choice for the "lidocaine substitute" has not yet emerged.

Skeletal muscle appears to be more sensitive to the local irritant properties of local anesthetic agents than other tissues, and skeletal muscle changes have been observed with most currently used local anesthetics (4,97,98). These effects on skeletal muscle tend to be reversible: Muscle regeneration is complete within 2 weeks after injection of local anesthetic agents. These localized changes in skeletal muscle have not been associated with any overt clinical problem other than the possibility that muscle irritation could contribute to back pain following neuraxial techniques.

CLINICAL USE OF LOCAL ANESTHETICS

Ester Agents

Benzocaine

Benzocaine is used exclusively for topical anesthesia. The widespread use of 20% benzocaine spray has led to an apparent increased risk of methemoglobinemia (76). Many hospitals have chosen to remove this product from their formularies.

Procaine

Procaine is rarely used for peripheral nerve or extradural blocks because of its short duration of action. Due to procaine's rapid hydrolysis in blood, the potential for systemic toxic reactions is small. On the other hand, this agent can cause allergic reactions. Currently, procaine is used mainly for local infiltration anesthesia and occasionally for short-duration spinal anesthesias.

Chloroprocaine

Chloroprocaine became very popular for obstetric anesthesia in the United States because of its rapid onset of action and limited systemic toxicity. Chloroprocaine is used for epidural anesthesia in a 3% solution, with a duration of action between 30 and 60 minutes. Injections at 30-minute intervals are needed to maintain adequate anesthesia during longer cases.

In the 1980s, chloroprocaine's popularity declined after reports of prolonged neurologic deficit following accidental subarachnoid injection. As noted previously, this toxicity was attributed to the combination of bisulfite (then included in the commercial preparation as a preservative) and the acidity of the formulation. Because of this, the formulation was changed to one in which disodium ethylenediaminetetraacetic acid (EDTA) was substituted for bisulfite. EDTA may be the explanation for reports (99–102) of chloroprocaine-related back pain (sometimes severe enough to require opioid analgesia). A comparative study found that the use of very large volumes (greater than 40 mL) of chloroprocaine resulted in a significant incidence of the problem, but that 25 mL or less produced no greater incidence of back pain than did other anesthetic agents (103,104).

Chloroprocaine is also useful for peripheral nerve blocks when the duration of surgery is not expected to exceed 30 to 60 minutes. Thus, this drug is well-suited for ambulatory surgery. There is a long history of mixing chloroprocaine with agents such as bupivacaine or tetracaine, seeking a rapid onset and prolonged duration of anesthesia; however, sparse evidence supports this practice. Finally, as previously noted, preservative-free chloroprocaine is gaining ground as a possible replacement for lidocaine for spinal anesthesias of brief duration (6).

Tetracaine

Tetracaine (or amethocaine) remains popular for spinal anesthesia. Although tetracaine may be used as an isobaric or hypobaric solution, the hyperbaric solutions are by far most common. As is true for all local anesthetics during spinal anesthesia, tetracaine provides a relatively rapid onset of anesthesia—within 3 to 5 minutes—and a profound depth of anesthesia. The duration ranges from 2 to 3 hours. Addition of vasoconstrictors can markedly extend the duration of anesthesia to 4 to 6 hours (Fig. 4-4).

Tetracaine is rarely used for other forms of regional anesthesia because of its extremely slow onset of action and its potential for systemic toxic reactions. Tetracaine possesses excellent topical anesthetic properties, and solutions of this agent were commonly used for endotracheal and surface anesthesia. The absorption of tetracaine from mucosa is extremely rapid, and multiple fatalities have been reported following the use of topical tetracaine for endoscopy (105). Recent studies have shown that both tetracaine gel and liposomal tetracaine topical preparations provide faster and better dermal anesthesia than EMLA cream (106–108).

Recent studies have shown a Cochrane systematic review has reached the same conclusions for the use of these products to prevent needle-stick pain in children (109).

Cocaine

Cocaine, the only naturally occuring local anesthetic, is still used clinically for its topical anesthetic and vasoconstrictor properties. Cocaine solutions are frequently used to anesthetize the nasal mucosa before nasotracheal intubation. Cocaine is also one of the most common drugs of abuse, and concerns about drug diversion now limit its use in medical settings.

Amide Agents

Lidocaine

Lidocaine remains the most versatile and most commonly used local anesthetic because of its rapid onset, moderate duration of action, moderate toxicity, and potent topical anesthetic activity. Lidocaine in 0.5%, 1.0%, 1.5%, and 2.0% solutions are available for infiltration, peripheral nerve blocks, and epidural anesthesia. Lidocaine 5% with 7.5% glucose has been widely used for spinal anesthesias of 30 to 60 minutes' duration, but is now less popular due to concerns about the transient neurologic symptoms (in the form of persisting paresthesias in the legs) that seem associated with surgical procedures performed under lidocaine spinal anesthesia in the lithotomy position, and also due to concerns that the 5% solution might be more neurotoxic than other spinal anesthetics. Lidocaine remains commonly used in ointments, jellies, and viscous and aerosol preparations for a variety of topical anesthetic procedures.

The duration of "plain" lidocaine ranges from 1 to 3 hours in various regional anesthetic procedures; addition of epinephrine significantly prolongs its duration. Epinephrine decreases the rate of absorption of lidocaine, significantly decreasing peak blood concentrations and the potential for systemic toxic reactions (see Chapter 3).

Lidocaine possesses a number of nonanesthetic uses. It is administered intravenously to treat patients with ventricular arrhythmias. Lidocaine has been used as IV analgesic agent for chronic pain syndromes, and in combination with CNS depressants such as barbiturates and nitrous oxide to provide a state of balanced anesthesia. This systemic analgesic activity of lidocaine is apparently due to an action within the CNS and not to any effect on peripheral nerves (110).

Lidocaine is also available in the form of Lidoderm patches indicated for topical treatment of postherpetic neuralgia and in eutectic mix of local anesthetic (EMLA) cream (to be discussed in a subsequent section, in liposomal formulation for topical anesthesia, and in combination with tetracaine for topical anesthesia) (108,111,112).

Mepivacaine

Mepivacaine is similar to lidocaine in terms of its anesthetic profile, having a relatively rapid onset and a moderate duration of action. Mepivacaine may be used for infiltration, peripheral nerve blocks, or epidural anesthesia in concentrations varying from 0.5% to 2.0%. In some countries, 4% hyperbaric solutions of mepivacaine are also available for spinal anesthesia, and this agent is undergoing clinical investigation in the United States as a possible replacement for lidocaine (113).

Unlike lidocaine, mepivacaine is not an effective topical anesthetic. The metabolism of mepivacaine is markedly prolonged in the fetus and newborn, such that this agent is usually avoided in obstetric anesthesia. Mepivacaine appears less of a vasodilator (with clinical concentrations) than lidocaine, and this difference may explain why equivalent doses of "plain" mepivacaine provide a somewhat longer duration of anesthesia than "plain" lidocaine. The duration of action of mepivacaine can be significantly prolonged by the addition of a vasoconstrictor such as epinephrine (see Chapter 3). Mepivacaine is widely used in dental anesthesia.

Prilocaine

The clinical nerve-blocking profile of prilocaine resembles that of lidocaine. Prilocaine has a relatively rapid onset of action while providing a moderate duration of anesthesia. This agent causes less vasodilation than lidocaine, permitting its use without epinephrine. In general, the duration of prilocaine without epinephrine is similar to that of lidocaine with epinephrine (see Chapter 3). Prilocaine has been used for infiltration, peripheral nerve blockade, IV regional, and epidural anesthesia. Prilocaine is included in topical anesthetic EMLA cream, which is a eutectic mixture of liodcaine and prilocaine bases.

Prilocaine can induce spinal anesthesia of short duration, and has been used for this purpose (as a lidocaine substitute) in Europe. Prilocaine is no longer available for peripheral nerve block or epidural procedures in the United States, but it remains available and is used in Europe.

The primary advantage of prilocaine compared to lidocaine is its significantly decreased potential for systemic toxic reactions. Studies in animals and human volunteers indicate that prilocaine is approximately 40% less toxic than lidocaine, and is the least toxic of the amide local anesthetics. Thus, this agent has found particular utility for IV regional anesthesia. CNS toxic effects are rarely seen, even with early accidental release of the tourniquet. Forty milliliters of 0.5% prilocaine (200 mg) provides effective anesthesia for hand surgery using the IV regional anesthetic technique (see Chapter 15).

The major deterrent to the use of prilocaine is its dose-related, predictable formation of methemoglobinemia. The classic teaching is that clinically apparent cyanosis will appear when an adult patient receives 600 mg or more of this agent. More recent studies support that methemoglobin concentrations may exceed 10% with doses of 400 mg, particularly in younger patients (75). Fear of methemoglobinemia has virtually eliminated the use of this drug in obstetrics, where the cyanotic appearance of newborns delivered of mothers who have received prilocaine for epidural anesthesia during labor resulted in unnecessary confusion.

Eutectic Mixtures of Local Anesthetics

Oily EMLA cream is used for topical anesthesia. "Eutectic" means equal proportions of solid crystals of prilocaine and lidocaine, and this mixture remains a liquid at room temperature. In comparison, the melting points of lidocaine and prilocaine are 67°C and 37°C, respectively. The eutectic mixture (oil) requires only the addition of an emulsifier (arlatone) and a thickener (carbopol) to give it good consistency as a paste for application (114,115). There is a high concentration of drug in contact with the skin. The base forms of lidocaine and prilocaine more readily passes across the diffusion barrier of the epidermis (116,117).

In typical use, the doses of both drugs are small, and plasma concentrations remain well below toxic levels; methemoglobinemia generally has not been a problem. However, in children younger than 3 years of age, a remote potential for systemic toxicity exists (114,115). Methemoglobinemia may also occur when excessive doses are given to adults (118).

After application of EMLA, at least 60 to 90 minutes is required for a full effect. The analgesia may remain present 1 hour after the cream has been removed (114). EMLA is effective when applied prior to painful superficial procedures such as venipuncture and arterial cannulation, skin graft harvesting, arteriovenous shunt procedures, lumbar puncture, and prior to local anesthetic blocks for dentistry (114,119,120). However, a recent systematic review has concluded that EMLA is inferior to topical tetracaine (amethocaine) prior to venipuncture in children (121).

Synera is a eutectic mixture of lidocaine and tetracaine contained in a patch with a warming element. This product is intended for anesthesia of intact skin in the same manner as EMLA. The advantages of this product include that it produces an adequate clinical effect within 20 to 30 minutes, and that it carries essentially no risk of methemoglobinemia. Most clinical studies have measured tetracaine concentrations in the "barely detectable" range after application of one to four Synera patches (111).

Bupivacaine

Bupivacaine was the first local anesthetic that combined the properties of an acceptable onset, long duration of action, and a tendency for greater sensory anesthesia than motor blockade. This agent is used in concentrations of 0.125%, 0.25%, 0.5%, and 0.75% for various regional anesthetic procedures, including infiltration, peripheral nerve blocks, and epidural and spinal anesthesia. Bupivacaine is not used for topical anesthesia. The typical duration of surgical anesthesia with bupivacaine varies from 3 to 10 hours. Its longest duration of action occurs when major peripheral nerve blocks (such as brachial plexus block) are performed. In these situations, average durations of effective surgical anesthesia of 10 to 12 hours have been reported, and an occasional patient may have analgesia for 18 hours or more followed by complete recovery of sensation. The rate of vascular absorption of bupivacaine is reduced by epinephrine, but less so than for lidocaine.

Bupivacaine achieved its initial widespread use for obstetric analgesia in labor, and it continues to be the standard agent for this application. Typically, bupivacaine is administered epidurally in concentrations varying from 0.06% to 0.25%, often in combination with epidural or intrathecal fentanyl or sufentanil. Under these conditions and doses, adequate analgesia can be achieved without significant motor block. A comparable degree of differential blockade of sensory and motor fibers can also be obtained with bupivacaine in postoperative epidural analgesia (see Chapters 11 and 43).

The obstetric use of bupivacaine has declined in recent years (see also Chapter 24). First, there are continuing concerns about cardiovascular collapse following the accidental rapid IV administration of this agent. Second, competing agents with a reduced propensity for cardiovascular toxicity (ropivacaine and levobupivacaine) were introduced into clinical practice.

Bupivacaine in isobaric and hyperbaric solutions of 0.5% to 0.75% has been used extensively for spinal anesthesia. Onset of bupivacaine spinal anesthesia usually occurs within 5 minutes. Surgical anesthesia usually persists for at least 3 to 4 hours (see Chapter 10).

Ropivacaine

Concerns about the potential of bupivacaine to produce cardiotoxicity after accidental IV injection led to a search for alternative long-acting local anesthetic drugs. Ropivacaine belongs to the same 2′,6′-pipecoloxylidide chemical series as mepivacaine and bupivacaine, being the propyl derivative as opposed to methyl (mepivacaine) or butyl (bupivacaine) (Chapter 3). All three of these local anesthetics contain an asymmetric carbon atom; bupivacaine and mepivacaine are marketed as racemic

mixtures of two optical isomers (enantiomers) (122). However, ropivacaine was marketed as an almost pure solution of the S(−) isomer. Multiple animal studies have shown that the S(−) isomer is less toxic to the heart than the R(+) isomer (123) (see also Chapter 3). Intravenous infusion studies in man have shown that ropivacaine can be administered in larger doses than bupivacaine before early features of either cardiovascular or CNS toxicity are seen (see Chapter 5) (124). The assumption is that the increased concentrations of ropivacaine (e.g., 0.75% or 1.0%) may be used with less risk of severe toxicity than with bupivacaine (122).

Clinical studies suggest that ropivacaine has a block profile very similar to that of bupivacaine (but with a marginally shorter duration) when used for major peripheral (125,126) and epidural block (127–130). In addition, the epidural studies also suggest that the degree of motor block produced by ropivacaine is less than that produced by bupivacaine when similar concentrations are compared, so that it may be possible to achieve a more consistent separation between sensory and motor block when the agent is used for pain relief (see also Chapter 11) (122).

Ropivacaine is commonly used in a dilute formulation for continuous infusion via epidural or peripheral nerve block catheters. As is true with other local anesthetics, ropivacaine has a biphasic effect on blood flow (66,131).

Levobupivacaine

Levobupivacaine is the s(−)-enantiomer of bupivacaine. Preclinical studies suggest that levobupivacaine has less propensity for cardiac toxicity than bupivacaine while having a similar potency at nerve block. Levobupivacaine has been used for the same clinical indications as bupivacaine (36,132).

Etidocaine

Etidocaine, a close chemical relative of lidocaine, is characterized by very rapid onset and prolonged duration of action. Etidocaine has been used for peripheral nerve blockade or epidural anesthesia. Etidocaine may have the fastest onset of anesthesia of any current local anesthetic, and is significantly faster than bupivacaine. In common with lidocaine, concentrations of etidocaine that produce adequate sensory analgesia also produce profound motor blockade. As a result, etidocaine is useful for surgical procedures in which muscle relaxation is required, but not for obstetric or postoperative epidural analgesia.

Other Less Commonly Used Agents

Articaine

Articaine has been used in European dental practices for nearly 20 years and is considered the drug of choice by many (133). It differs from most other local anesthetics in having a thiophene ring rather than a benzene ring (134). Some have claimed that articaine has a faster onset and provides more complete anesthesia than lidocaine when used in dental blocks. On the other hand, comparison with prilocaine for dental blocks showed no significant difference (135). There was no significant difference between articaine and lidocaine in epidural use (136).

Butamben

Butyl aminobenzoate (BAB) is an ester of para-aminobenzoic acid and butyl alcohol patented in 1923 and originally used as a topical preparation, Butesin Picrate. An extraordinarily low pKa of 2.3 results in minimal concentrations of the hydrophilic cation: Thus, BAB has very low water solubility (135). Butyl aminobenzoate also has poor dural permeability, and these properties, together with its rapid hydrolysis, were previously thought to make it unattractive for epidural use. Subsequently, Abbott Laboratories prepared an aqueous suspension of 5% butamben with a pH of 6. Since 1 g of BAB dissolves in about 7 liters of water, very little of the BAB in the suspension is dissolved: The majority of BAB is present in a solid form that acts as a depot for very slow dissolution. These suspension preparations of BAB were found to produce long-lasting sensory blockade when given epidurally to cancer patients (137,138). In this respect, the BAB suspension resembles slow-release morphine preparations (e.g., DepoDur), in which a persisting effect results not from the drug per se, but from the slow and continuous release of the drug. This explains the extraordinarily long duration (weeks to months) of analgesia following epidural administiration of butamben suspension in patients with cancer pain (137,138). In contrast, BAB administered as an aqueous solution epidurally to rats had a shorter duration of action than bupivacaine (139).

Butyl aminobenzoate suspension administered epidurally demonstrates an apparent selectivity for Aδ- and C-fibers: In cancer patients, there is a lack of motor blockade and a sparing of bladder and bowel function (137,138). Aqueous BAB solutions administered epidurally (in rats) do not demonstrate this selectivity. These differences in differential blocking characterists appear to be a result of the physicochemical properties of the suspension, rather than the BAB compound per se (139,140). Necropsy studies in dogs (141) and autopsy in humans (137) revealed semisolid BAB suspension material in the posterior epidural space near the dorsal roots in a metameric pattern. On the other hand, butamben has the unusual (for a local anesthetic) effect of both inhibiting and accelerating low-voltage activated currents in T-type calcium channels in small sensory neurons (142). These tantalizing pilot data on BAB in animals and in cancer patients should prompt further studies with this agent. There is no commercially available preparation of BAB.

DRUGS USED WITH LOCAL ANESTHETICS

Vasoconstrictors

Epinephrine (adrenaline) is, of course, the active agent of the adrenal medulla. It is a powerful vasoconstrictor and has effects on both α- and β-adrenergic receptors.

On exposure to air or light, epinephrine may rapidly lose potency as a result of decomposition. For this reason, stabilizing agents, such as sodium metabisulfite, are used to prolong the epinephrine shelf life by slowing the breakdown of the drug to as little as 2% per year. These agents also permit epinephrine-containing solutions to be autoclaved once without loss of clinical activity. Epinephrine-containing solutions should not, however, be autoclaved more than once. Epinephrine-containing solutions have a reduced pH (3–4.5) compared to plain solutions because of the added antioxidant.

When epinephrine is used with local anesthetic solutions, it must be in a concentration and dose to produce the desired vasoconstriction without leading to epinephrine overdose. Although the optimal concentration untested for most blocks re-

mains controversial, a 1:200,000 (5 μg/mL) concentration is most often used for regional nerve blocks and epidural anesthesia. More dilute solutions have been shown to be useful for some blocks (e.g., cervical plexus); increasing the epinephrine concentration does not provide a significantly reduced peak local anesthetic concentration in blood (relative to 1:200,000) although it does increase the likelihood of toxicity from absorbed epinephrine.

The principal systemic side effects of epinephrine are hypertension, tachycardia (or bradycardia in the presence of β-adrenergic blockers), and arrhythmias, in some cases accompanied by myocardial ischemia. Such reactions are most likely to occur when the local anesthetic solution is accidentally injected intravenously.

Epinephrine also has local side effects, the most important being vasoconstriction of terminal arteries, potentially leading to gangrene. There has been much recent discussion regarding whether epinephrine can be safely used in digital nerve blocks. Although generations of physicians have been warned about epinephrine in digital blocks, there is little published evidence that digital blocks with lidocaine (or any other modern local anesthetic) and epinephrine have ever caused digitial gangrene. Moreover, some studies have shown that the alternative to epinephrine-containing local anesthetic is for the surgeon to use a tourniquet (which can be assumed to reduce digital blood flow as least as much as epinephrine) (143).

Other vasoconstrictors include:

- Phenylephrine (Neosynephrine) is a sympathomimetic drug with selective α-receptor activity. It has been extensively used in spinal anesthesia (Fig. 4-4).
- Felypressin (Octapressin) is a synthetic drug similar to the naturally occurring vasopressin but without the antidiuretic and coronary vasoconstrictor effects of vasopressin. It increases the intensity and duration of dental nerve blocks, and it is used in a concentration of 0.03 U/mL. It is a useful alternative in patients who are sensitive to catecholamines.
- Ornipressin (POR-8) is octapeptide related to vasopressin. A dose of 5 IU in 50 mL of 2% lidocaine has been used for plastic surgery. It is claimed to have a direct effect on the peripheral vasculature with minimal or no direct cardiac effects. Animal studies have revealed teratogenicity in high, subcutaneous doses considerably in excess of the maximum clinical level.
- Levonordefrin (NeoCobefrin) is an α-adrenergic receptor stimulator used with mepivacaine in dental blocks in a 1:20,000 concentration.

α_2 Agonists

Clonidine has achieved wide popularity as a local anesthetic additive and in some instances as a substitute for local anesthetics for postoperative analgesia. When added to local anesthetic solutions, clonidine may increase peak local anesthetic concentration in blood, relative to those measured when epinephrine is added to the local anesthetic (117). Clonidine has been used to improve or prolong spinal anesthesia, epidural anesthesia, caudal analgesia in children, and virtually all common regional nerve block procedures (119,144).

Bicarbonate

Sodium bicarbonate has been added to local anesthetic solutions to increase pH and increase the fraction of local anesthetic molecules that are not protonated. In general, addition of NaCHO$_3$ either speeds the onset and/or improves the "density" of anesthesia, or has no effect, provided that the pH is not increased to the point at which local anesthetic precipates from solution (42,145,146).

Antioxidants

Most of the commonly used local anesthetics, especially the amides, are extremely stable compounds and will remain unchanged in solution indefinitely. Thus ampoules of "plain" local anesthetic solutions do not require additives. If epinephrine is included with the local anesthetic, antioxidants must be added to prevent breakdown of the vasoconstrictor (147). The agent most often used for this purpose is sodium metabisulfite in a concentration of 0.1%. Epinephrine-containing solutions will retain their potency for 2 years with this agent and will withstand single autoclaving. The significance of sodium metabisulfite in producing neurotoxicity with chloroprocaine was addressed in a preceding section.

Antimicrobials

Local anesthetic solutions containing antimicrobials should not be used for any purpose other than local infiltration. The ideal packaging is in a single-use, rubber-capped vial or in an ampoule. Vials are preferred for operator safety and convenience, and because glass fragments may contaminate solutions when ampules are opened (147). In multiple-dose vials for local infiltration, the antimicrobial methylparaben (1%) is often included in the solution.

Methylparaben is effective against gram-positive bacteria and fungi but less so against gram-negative bacteria. It has long been speculated that methylparaben may be responsible for some allergic reactions attributed to local anesthetics—in theory, it should be considerably more antigenic than the local anesthetics.

Chlorocresol has been used as an antibacterial agent and is more effective than methylparaben, but, like phenol, it is neurotoxic and should not be used in spinal, IV, or plexus blocks or extradural injections.

SUMMARY

The clinical pharmacologic properties of local anesthetics affect both their clinical applications and potential toxicities. The most important anesthetic properties are potency, onset, duration of action, and relative blockade of sensory and motor fibers. These qualities are related to the physicochemical properties of the various compounds. The toxicity of local anesthetics involves the CNS and the cardiovascular system. The toxicity of the different drugs is generally correlated with their inherent anesthetic potency but can be modified by the pharmacokinetic and metabolic properties of the specific agents. In general, the local anesthetics for infiltration, peripheral nerve blockade, and epidural anesthesia can be divided into three groups: (a) agents of short duration, such as procaine and chloroprocaine; (b) agents of moderate duration, such as lidocaine, mepivacaine, and prilocaine; and (c) agents of long duration, such as tetracaine, bupivacaine, levobupivacaine, ropivacaine, and etidocaine. These local anesthetics also vary in terms of onset: Chloroprocaine, etidocaine, lidocaine, mepivacaine, and prilocaine have a rapid onset, whereas tetracaine, ropivacaine, levobupivacaine, and bupivacaine are characterized by a longer latency period.

The agents specifically formulated for intrathecal use (the product labeling varies by country) include lidocaine, mepivacaine, levobupivacaine, ropivacaine, and procaine, which have a short duration of action, and tetracaine, dibucaine, and bupivacaine, which provide a prolonged duration of spinal anesthesia. Agents used in topical anesthetic preparations include lidocaine, EMLA, tetracaine, and cocaine.

With regard to the relative systemic toxicity of the various agents, chloroprocaine is the least toxic of the esters, and tetracaine is the most toxic. Among the amides, prilocaine is least toxic, followed in order of increasing toxicity by mepivacaine, lidocaine, etidocaine, ropivacaine, levobupivacaine, and bupivacaine.

An appreciation of the pharmacologic and toxicologic profiles of the various local anesthetics should make it possible to safely match a specific agent to a particular clinical situation.

References

1. Strichartz G, Sanchez V, Arthur GR, et al. Fundamental properties of local anesthetics. II. Measured octanol: Buffer partition coefficients and pKa values of clinically used drugs. *Anesth Analg* 1990;71:158–170.
2. Brau ME, Vogel W, Hempelmann G. Fundamental properties of local anesthetics: Half-maximal blocking concentrations for tonic block of Na+ and K+ channels in peripheral nerve. *Anesth Analg* 1998;87:885–889.
3. Butterworth JF 4th, Strichartz GR. Molecular mechanisms of local anesthesia: A review. *Anesthesiology* 1990;72:711–734.
4. Covino BG, Vassallo HG. *Local Anesthetics. Mechanisms of Action and Clinical Use*. New York: Grune & Stratton, 1976.
5. Tetzlaff J. *Clinical Pharmacology of Local Anesthetics*. Burlington MA: Butterworth-Heinemann, 2000.
6. Kouri ME, Kopacz DJ. Spinal 2-chloroprocaine: A comparison with lidocaine in volunteers. *Anesth Analg* 2004;98:75–80.
7. Lipkind GM, Fozzard HA. Molecular modeling of local anesthetic drug binding by voltage-gated sodium channels. *Mol Pharmacol* 2005;68:1611–1622.
8. Blair MR. Cardiovascular pharmacology of local anaesthetics. *Br J Anaesth* 1975;47:247.
9. Johns RA, DiFazio CA, Longnecker DE. Lidocaine constricts or dilates rat arterioles in a dose dependent manner. *Anesthesiology* 1985;62:141–144.
10. Hogan QH, Stadnicka A, Bosnjak ZJ, et al. Effects of lidocaine and bupivacaine on isolated rabbit mesenteric capacitance veins. *Reg Anesth Pain Med* 1998;23:409–417.
11. Lofstrom JB. Ulnar nerve blockade for the evaluation of local anaesthetic agents. *Br J Anaesth* 1975;47:297.
12. Raymond SA, Gissen AJ. Mechanisms of differential nerve block. In: Strichartz GR, ed. *Local Anesthetics. (Handbook of Experimental Pharmacology)*, Vol. 81. New York: Springer-Verlag, 1987.
13. Huang JH, Thalhammer JG, Raymond SA, et al. Susceptibility to lidocaine of impulses in different somatosensory afferent fibers of rat sciatic nerve. *J Pharmacol Exp Ther* 1997;292:802–811.
14. Bromage PR. An evaluation of two new local anesthetics for major conduction blockade. *Can Anaesth Soc J* 1970;17:557.
15. Butterworth J, Ririe DG, Thompson RB, et al. Differential onset of median nerve block: Randomized, double-blind comparison of mepivacaine and bupivacaine in healthy volunteers. *Br J Anaesth* 1998;81:515–521.
16. Littlewood DG, Buckley P, Covino BG, et al. Comparative study of various local anesthetic solutions in extradural block in labour. *Br J Anaesth* 1979;51:47.
17. Scott DB, McClure JH, Giasi RM, et al. Effects of concentration of local anaesthetic drugs in extradural block. *Br J Anaesth* 1980;52:1033.

18. Crawford OB. Comparative evaluation in peridural anesthesia of lidocaine, mepivacaine, and L-67, a new local anesthetic agent. *Anesthesiology* 1964;25:321.

19. Erdimir HA, Soper LE, Sweet RB. Studies of factors affecting peridural anesthesia. *Anesth Analg* 1965;44:400.

20. Nakamura T, Popitz-Berger F, Birknes J, Strichartz GR. The critical role of concentration for lidocaine block of peripheral nerve *in vivo*: Studies of function and drug uptake in the rat. *Anesthesiology* 2003;99:1189–1197.

21. Braid DP, Scott DB. The systemic absorption of local analgesic drugs. *Br J Anaesth* 1965;37:394.

22. Concepcion M, Maddi R, Francis D, et al. Vasoconstrictors in spinal anesthesia with tetracaine. A comparison of epinephrine and phenylephrine. *Anesth Analg* 1984;63:134.

23. Albert J, Lofstrom B. Bilateral ulnar nerve blocks for the evaluation of local anaesthetic agents. *Acta Anaesthesiol Scand* 1965;9:203.

24. Bromage PR. A comparison of the hydrochloride salts of lignocaine and prilocaine for epidural analgesia. *Br J Anaesth* 1965;37:753.

25. Grambling ZW, Ellis RG, Volpitto PP. Clinical experiences with mepivacaine (Carbocaine). *J Med Assoc Ga* 1964;53:16.

26. Swerdlow M, Jones R. The duration of action of bupivacaine, prilocaine, and lignocaine. *Br J Anaesth* 1970;42:335.

27. Buckley FP, Littlewood DG, Covino BG, Scott DB. Effects of adrenaline and the concentration of solution on extradural block with etidocaine. *Br J Anaesth* 1978;50:171.

28. Keir L. Continuous epidural analgesia in prostatectomy: Comparison of bupivacaine with and without adrenaline. *Acta Anaesthesiol Scand* 1974;18:1.

29. Sinclair CJ, Scott DB. Comparison of bupivacaine and etidocaine in extradural blockade. *Br J Anaesth* 1984;56:147.

30. Soetens FM. Levobupivacaine-sufentanil with or without epinephrine during epidural labor analgesia. *Anesth Analg* 2006;103:182–186.

31. Armstrong IR, Littlewood DG, Chambers WA. Spinal anesthesia with tetracaine: Effect of added vasoconstrictor. *Anesth Analg* 1983;62:793.

32. Chambers WA, Littlewood DG, Logan MR, Scott DB. Effect of added epinephrine on spinal anesthesia with lidocaine. *Anesth Analg* 1981;60:417.

33. Chambers WA, Littlewood DG, Scott DB. Spinal anesthesia with hyperbaric bupivacaine: Effect of added vasoconstrictors. *Anesth Analg* 1982;61:49.

34. Moore JM, Liu SS, Pollock JE, et al. The effect of epinephrine on small-dose hyperbaric bupivacaine spinal anesthesia: Clinical implications for ambulatory surgery. *Anesth Analg* 1998;86:973–977.

35. Bromage PR. A comparison of the hydrochloride and carbon dioxide salts of lidocaine and prilocaine in epidural analgesia. *Acta Anaesthesiol Scand Suppl* 1965;16:55.

36. Catchlove RFH. The influence of CO_2 and pH on local anesthetic action. *J Pharmacol Exp Ther* 1972;181:298–309.

37. Gissen AJ, Covino BG, Gregus J. Differential sensitivity of fast and slow fibers in mammalian nerve. IV. Effect of carbonation of local anesthetics. *Reg Anaesth* 1985;10:68.

38. Morrison DH. A double-blind comparison of carbonated lidocaine and lidocaine hydrochloride in epidural anaesthesia. *Can Anaesth Soc J* 1981;28:387.

39. Curatolo M, Petersen-Felix S, Arendt-Nielse L, et al. Adding sodium bicarbonate to lidocaine enhances the depth of epidural blockade. *Anesth Analg* 1998;86:341–347.

40. Brown DT, Morrison DH, Covino BG, Scott DB. Comparison of carbonated bupivacaine and bupivacaine hydrochloride for extradural anaesthesia. *Br J Anaesth* 1980;52:419.

41. McClure JH, Scott DB. Comparison of bupivicaine hydrochloride and carbonated bupivacaine in brachial plexus block by the inter-scalene technique. *Br J Anaesth* 1981;53:523.

42. Arakawa M, Aoyama Y, Ohe Y. Block of the sacral segments in lumbar epidural anaesthesia. *Br J Anaesth* 2003;90:173–178.

43. Candido KD, Winnie AP, Covino BG, et al. Addition of bicarbonate to plain bupivacaine does not significantly alter the onset or duration of plexus anesthesia. *Reg Anesth* 1995;20:133–138.

44. Hilgier M. Alkalinization of bupivacaine for brachial plexus block. *Reg Anaesth* 1985;10:59.

45. Butterworth JF 4th, Lief PA, Strichartz GR. The pH-dependent local anesthetic activity of diethylaminoethanol, a procaine metabolite. *Anesthesiology* 1988;68:501–506.

46. Ririe DG, Walker FO, James RL, Butterworth J. Effect of alkalinization of lidocaine on median nerve block. *Br J Anaesth* 2000;84:163–168.

47. Davies RJ. Buffering the pain of local anesthetics: A systematic review. *Emerg Med (Fremantle)* 2003;15:81–88.

48. Aldrete JA, Barnes DR, Sidon MA, McMullen RB. Studies on effects of addition of potassium chloride to lidocaine. *Anesth Analg* 1969;48:269.

49. Bromage PR, Burfort MD. Quality of epidural blockade. II. Influence of physico-chemical factors: Hyaluronidase and potassium. *Br J Anaesth* 1966;38:857.

50. Loder RE. A local anesthetic solution with longer action. *Lancet* 1960;2:346.

51. Rosenblatt RM, Fung DL. Optimal ratio of bupivacaine and dextran for regional anaesthesia. *Reg Anaesth* 1979;4:2.

52. Bridenbaugh LD. Does the addition of low molecular weight dextran prolong the duration of action of bupivacaine? *Reg Anaesth* 1978;3:6.

53. Rosenblatt RM, Fung DL. Mechanism of action of dextran prolonging regional anesthesia. *Reg Anaesth* 1980;5:3.

54. Butterworth JF, Strichartz G. The alpha 2-adrenergic agonists clonidine and guanfacine produe tonic and phasic block of conduction in rat sciatic nerve fibers. *Anesth Analg* 1993;76(2):295–301.

55. Gaumann DM, Brunet PC, Jirounek P. Clonidine enhances the effects of lidocaine on C-fiber action potential. *Anesth Analg* 1992;74:719–725.

56. Larsen B, Dorscheid E, Macher-Hanselmann F, Buch U. Does intrathecal clonidine prolong the effect of spinal anesthesia with hyperbaric mepivacaine? A randomized double-blind study. *Anaesthesist* 1998;47:741–746.

57. Ota K, Namiki A, Iwasaki H, Takahashi I. Dose-related prolongation of tetracaine spinal anesthesia by oral clonidine in humans. *Anesth Analg* 1994;79:1121–1125.

58. Ilfeld BM, Morey TE, Thannikary LJ, et al. Clonidine added to a continuous interscalene ropivacaine perineural infusion to improve postoperative analgesia: A randomized, double-blind, controlled study. *Anesth Analg* 2005;100:1172–1178.

59. Kuusniemi KS, Pihlajamaki KK, Pitkanen MT, Helenius HY. The use of bupivacaine and fentanyl for spinal anesthesia for urologic surgery. *Anesth Analg* 2000;91:1452–1456.

60. Wong CA, Scavone BM, Peaceman AM, et al. The risk of cesarean delivery with neuraxial analgesia given early versus late in labor. *N Engl J Med* 2005;352:655–665.

61. Cunningham NL, Kaplan JA. A rapid onset long acting regional anesthetic technique. *Anesthesiology* 1974;41:509.

62. Cohen SE, Thurlow A. Comparison of a chloroprocaine-bupivacaine mixture with chloroprocaine and bupivacaine used individually for obstetric epidural analgesia. *Anesthesiology* 1979;51:288.

63. Galindo A, Witcher T. Mixtures of local anesthetics: Bupivacaine-chloroprocaine. *Anesth Analg* 1980;59:683.

64. Seow LT, Lips FJ, Cousins MJ, Mather LE. Lidocaine and bupivacaine mixtures for epidural blockade. *Anesthesiology* 1982;56:177.

65. Keckeis A, Hofmockel R. Mixtures of diferent local anesthetics for subaxillary plexus anesthesia. *Anaesthesiol Reanim* 1994;19:32–36.

66. Cederholme I, Evers H, Lofstrom JB. Skin blood flow after intradermal injection of ropivacaine in various concentrations with and without epinephrine evaluated by laser doppler flowmetry. *Reg Anesth* 1992;17:322.

67. Jorfeldt L, Lofstrom B, Pernow B, Wahren J. The effect of mepivacaine and lidocaine on forearm resistance and capacitance vessels in man. *Acta Anaesthesiol Scand* 1970;14:183.

68. Benzaquen BS, Cohen V, Eisenberg MJ. Effects of cocaine on the coronary arteries. *Am Heart J* 2001;142:402–410.

69. Nishimura N, Morioka T, Sato S, Kuba T. Effects of local anesthetic agents on the peripheral vascular system. *Anesth Analg* 1965;44:135.

70. He J, Yang S, Zhang L. Effects of cocaine on nitric oxide production in bovine coronary artery endothelial cells. *J Pharmacol Exp Ther* 2005;314:980–986.

71. Butterworth J, Brownlow RC, Leith JP, et al. Bupivacaine inhibits cyclic-$3',5'$-adenosine monophosphate production. *Anesthesiology* 1993;79:88–95.

72. Herroeder S, Pecher S, Schönherr ME, et al. Systemic lidocaine shortens length of hospital stay after colorectal surgery: a double-blind, randomized, placebo-controlled trial. *Ann Surg* 2007;246:192–200.

73. Hjelm M, Holmdahl MH. Biochemical effects of aromatic amines II. Cyanosis, methemoglobinemia and Heinz-body formation induced by a local anaesthetic agent (prilocaine). *Acta Anaesthesiol Scand* 1965;2:99.

74. Lund PC, Cwik JC. Propitocaine (Citanest) and methemoglobinemia. *Anesthesiology* 1965;26:569–571.

75. Vasters FG, Eberhart LH, Koch T, et al. Risk factors for prilocaine-induced metheaemoglobinaemia following peripheral regional anaesthesia. *Eur J Anaesthesiol* 2006;23:760–765.

76. Ash-Bernal R, Wise R, Wright SM. Acquired methemoglobinemia: A retrospective series of 138 cases at 2 teaching hospitals. *Medicine* 2004;83:265–273.

77. Brown DT, Beamish D, Wildsmith JAW. Allergic reaction to an amide local anaesthetic. *Br J Anaesth* 1981;53:435.

78. Reynolds F. Allergy reaction to an amide local anaesthetic. *Br J Anaesth* 1981;53:901.

79. Jacobsen RB, Borch JE, Bindslev-Jensen C. Hypersensitivity to local anaesthetics. *Allergy* 2005;60:261–264.

80. deShazo RD, Nelson HS. An approach to the patient with a history of local anesthetic hypersensitivity: Experience with 90 patients. *Allergy Clin Immunol* 1979;63:387–394.

81. Aldrete JA, Johnson DA. Evaluation of intracutaneous testing for investigation of allergy to local anesthetic agents. *Anesth Analg* 1970;49:173.

82. Finucane BT. Allergies to local anesthetics – the real truth. *Can J Anesth* 2003;50:869–874.

83. Skou JC. Local anesthetics. II. The toxic potencies of some local anesthetics and of butyl alcohol, determined on peripheral nerve. *Acta Pharmacol Toxicol* 1954;10:292.

84. Moore DC, Spierdijk J, VanKleef JD, et al. Chloroprocaine neurotoxicity: Four additional cases. *Anesth Analg* 1982;61:155.

85. Ravindran RS, Bond VK, Tasch MD, et al. Prolonged neural blockade following regional analgesia with 2-chloroprocaine. *Anesth Analg* 1980;58:447.

86. Reisner LS, Hochman BN, Plumer MH. Persistent neurological deficit and adhesive arachnoiditis following intrathecal 2-chloroprocaine injection. *Anesth Analg* 1980;58:452.

87. Barsa JE, Batra M, Fink BR, Sumi SM. Prolonged neural blockade following regional analgesia with 2-chloroprocaine. *Anesth Analg* 1982;61:961.

88. Pizzalato D, Reneger OJ. Histopathologic effects of long exposure to local anesthetics on peripheral nerves. *Anesth Analg* 1959;38:138.

89. Ravindran RS, Turner MS, Muller T. Neurological effects of subarachnoid administration of 2-chloroprocaine-CE, bupivacaine and low pH normal saline in dogs. *Anesth Analg* 1982;61:279.

90. Rosen MA, Baysinger CL, Shnider SM, et al. Evaluation of neurotoxicity after subarachnoid injection of large volumes of local anesthetic solutions. *Anesth Analg* 1983;62:802–808.

91. Wang BC, Hillman DE, Spiedholz NI, Turndorf H. Chronic neurological deficits and Nesacaine-CE: An effect of the anesthetic, 2-chloroprocaine, or the antioxidant, sodium bisulfite? *Anesth Analg* 1984;63:445.

92. Gissen AJ, Datta S, Lambert D. The chloroprocaine controversy II. Is chloroprocaine neurotoxic? *Reg Anaesth* 1984;9:135.

93. Taniguchi M, Bollen AW, Drasner K. Sodium bisulfite: Scapegoat for chloroprocaine neurotoxicity? *Anesthesiology* 2004;100:85–91.

94. Freedman JM, Li D, Drasner K, et al. Transient neurologic symptoms after spinal anesthesia: An epidemiologic study of 1,863 patients. *Anesthesiology* 1998;89:633–641.

95. Rigler ML, Drasner K, Krejcie TC, et al. Cauda equina syndrome after continuous spinal anesthesia. *Anesth Analg* 1991;72:275–281.

96. Lambert LA, Lambert DH, Strichartz GR. Irreversible conduction block in isolated nerve by high concentrations of local anesthetics. *Anesthesiology* 1994;80:1082–1093.

97. Benoit PW, Belt WD. Some effects of local anesthetic agents on skeletal muscle. *Exp Neurol* 1972;34:264.

98. Libelius R, Sonesson B, Stamenovic BA, Thesleff S. Denervation-like changes in skeletal muscle after treatment with a local anesthetic (Marcaine). *J Anat* 1970;106:297.

99. Ackerman WE. Correspondence: Back pain after epidural Nesacaine MPF. *Anesth Analg* 1990;70:224.

100. Hynson JM, Sessler DI, Glosten B. Back pain in volunteers after epidural anesthesia with chloroprocaine. *Anesth Analg* 1991;72:253.

101. Levy L, Randel GI, Pandit SK. Correspondence: Does chloroprocaine (Nesacaine MPF) for epidural anesthesia increase the incidence of backache? *Anesthesiology* 1989;71:476.

102. Stevens RA, Chester WL, Artuso JD, et al. Back pain after epidural anesthesia in volunteers: A preliminary report. *Reg Anaesth* 1991;16:199.

103. Munnur U, Suresh MS. Backache, headache, and neurologic deficit after regional anesthesia. *Anesthesiol Clin North America* 2003;21:71–86.

104. Stevens RA, Urmey WF, Urquhart BL, Kao TC. Back pain after epidural anesthesia with chloroprocaine. *Anesthesiology* 1993;78:492.

105. Palmer ED, Deutsch DL. Sudden death during preparation for esophagoscopy with tetracaine gargle. *Am J Dig Dis* 1955;22:95–96.

106. Fisher R, Hung O, Mezei M, et al. Topical anaesthesia of intact skin: Liposome-encapsulated tetracaine vs EMLA. *Br J Anaesth* 1998;81:972–973.

107. O'Brien L, Taddio A, Lyszkiewicz DA, et al. A critical review of the topical local anesthetic amethocaine (Ametop) for pediatric pain. *Paediatr Drugs* 2005;7:41–54.

108. Schecter AK, Pariser DM, Pariser RJ, et al. Randomized, double-blind, placebo-controlled study evaluating the lidocaine/tetracaine patch for induction of local anesthesia prior to minor dermatologic procedures in geriatric patients. *Dermatol Surg* 2005;31:287–291.

109. Lander JA, Weltman BJ, So SS. EMLA and amethocaine for reduction of children's pain associated with needle insertion. *Cochrane Database Syst Rev* 2006;19:3:CD004236.

110. Butterworth J, Cole L, Marlow G. Inhibition of brain cell excitability by lidocaine, QX314, and tetrodotoxin: A mechanism for analgesia from infused local anesthetics. *Acta Anaesthesiol Scand* 1993;37:516–523.

111. Sethna NF, Verghese ST, Hannallah RS, et al. A randomized controlled trial to evaluate S-Caine patch for reducing pain associated with vascular access in children. *Anesthesiology* 2005;102:403–408.

112. Taddio A, Soin HK, Schuh S, et al. Liposomal lidocaine to improve procedural success rates and reduce procedural pain among children: A randomized controlled trial. *CMAJ* 2005;172:1691–1695.

113. YaDeau JT, Liguori GA, Zayas VM. The incidence of transient neurologic symptoms after spinal anesthesia with mepivacaine. *Anesth Analg* 2005;101:661–665.

114. Buckley MM, Benfield P. Eutectic lidocaine/prilocaine cream: A review of the topical anesthetic/analgesic efficacy of a eutectic mixture of local anesthetics (EMLA). *Drugs* 1993;46:126.

115. Freeman JA, Doyle E, Ng TI, Morton NS. Topical anaesthesia of the skin: A review. *Paediatr Anaesth* 1993;3:129.

116. Bjerring P, Arendt-Nielsen L. Depth and duration of skin analgesia to needle insertion after topical application of EMLA cream. *Br J Anaesth* 1990;64:173.

117. Dalens B. Some current controversies in paediatric regional anaesthesia. *Curr Opin Anaesthesiol* 2006;19:301–308.

118. Hahn IH, Hoffman RS, Nelson LS. EMLA-induced methemoglobinemia and systemic topical anesthetic toxicity. *J Emerg Med* 2004;26:85–88.

119. Chang PC, Goresky GV, O'Connor G, et al. A multicentre randomised study of single-unit dose package of EMLA patch vs EMLA 5% cream for venipuncture in children. *Can J Anaesth* 1994;41:59.

120. Eidelman A, Weiss JM, Lau J, et al. Topical anesthetics for dermal instrumentation: A systematic review of randomized, controlled trials. *Ann Emerg Med* 2005;46:343–351.

121. Taddio A, Gurguis MG, Koren G. Lidocaine-prilocaine cream versus tetracaine gel for procedural pain in children. *Ann Pharmacother* 2002;36:687–692.

122. McClure JH. Ropivacaine [Review]. *Br J Anaesth* 1996;76:300.

123. Vanhoutte F, Vereecke J, Verbeke N, Carmeliet E. Stereoselective effects of the enantiomers of bupivacaine on the electrophysiological properties of the guinea-pig papillary muscle. *Br J Pharmacol* 1991;103:1275.

124. Scott DB, Lee A, Fagin D, et al. Acute toxicity of ropivacaine compared with that of bupivacaine. *Anesth Analg* 1989;69:563.

125. Hickey R, Hoffman J, Ramamurthy S. A comparison of ropivacaine 0.5% and bupivacaine 0.5% for brachial plexus block. *Anesthesiology* 1991;74:639.

126. Hickey R, Rowley CL, Candido KD, et al. A comparative study of 0.25% ropivacaine and 0.25% bupivacaine for brachial plexus block. *Anesth Analg* 1992;75:602.

127. Brockway MS, Bannister J, McClure JH, et al. Comparison of extradural ropivacaine and bupivacaine. *Br J Anaesth* 1991;66:31.

128. Brown DL, Carpenter RL, Thompson GE. Comparison of 0.5% ropivacaine and 0.5% bupivacaine for epidural anesthesia in patients undergoing lower-extremity surgery. *Anesthesiology* 1990;72:633.

129. Concepcion M, Arthur GR, Steele SM, et al. A new local anesthetic, ropivacaine: Its epidural effects in humans. *Anesth Analg* 1990;70:80.

130. Katz JA, Knarr D, Bridenbaugh PO. A double-blind comparison of 0.5% bupivacaine and 0.75% ropivacaine administered epidurally in humans. *Reg Anesth* 1990;15:250.

131. Dahl JB, Simonsen L, Morgensen T, et al. The effect of 0.5% ropivacaine on epidural blood flow. *Acta Anaesth Scand* 1990;34:308.

132. Casati A, Putzu M. Bupivacaine, levobupivacaine and ropivacaine: Are they clinically different? *Best Pract Res Clin Anaesthesiol* 2005;19:247–268.

133. Vree TB, Gielen MJ. Clinical pharmacology and the use of articaine for local and regional anaesthesia. *Best Pract Res Clin Anaesthesiol* 2005;19:293–308.

134. Winther J, Patirupanusara B. Evaluation of carticaine: A new local analgesic. *Int J Oral Surg* 1974;3:422.

135. Haas D, Harper D, Saso M, Young E. Comparison of articaine and prilocaine anesthesia by infiltration in maxillary and mandibular arches. *Anesth Prog* 1990;37:230.

136. Brinklov M. Clinical effects of Carticaine, a new local anaesthetic. *Acta Anaesth Scand* 1977;21:5.

137. Korsten HHM, Ackerman EW, Grouls RJE, et al. Long-lasting epidural sensory blockade by n-butyl-p-aminobenzoate in the terminally ill intractable cancer pain patient. *Anesthesiology* 1991;75:950.

138. Shulman, M.: Treatment of cancer pain with epidural butyl-amino-benzoate suspension. Reg. Anesth., 12:1, 1987.

139. Grouls RJE, Meert TF, Korsten HHM, et al. Epidural and intrathecal n-butyl-p-aminobenzoate solution in the rat: Comparison with bupivacaine. *Anesthesiology* 1997;86:181.

140. Van den Berg RJ, van Soest PF, Wang Z, et al. The local anaesthetic n-butyl-p-aminobenzoate selectively affects inactivation of fast sodium currents in cultured rat sensory neurons. *Anesthesiology* 1995;82:1463.

141. Korsten HHM, Hellebrekers LJ, Grouls RJE, et al. Long-lasting sensory blockade by n-butyl-p-aminobenzoate in the dog. Neurotoxic or local anaesthetic effect? *Anesthesiology* 1990;73:491.

142. Beekwilder JP, van Kempen GT, van den Berg RJ, et al. The local anesthetic butamben inhibits and accelerates low-voltage activated T-type currents in small sensory neurons. *Anesth Analg* 2006;102:141–145.

143. Denkler K. A comprehensive review of epinephrine in the finger: To do or not to do. *Plast Reconstr Surg* 2001;108:114–124.

144. Molnar RR, Davies MJ, Scott DA, et al. Comparison of clonidine and epinephrine in lidocaine for cervical plexus block. *Reg Anesth* 1997;22:137–142.

145. Moharib MM, Mitra S, Rizvi SG. Effect of alkalinization and/or hyaluronidase adjuvancy on a local anesthetic mixture for sub-Tenon's ophthalmic block. *Acta Anaesthesiol Scand* 2002;46:599–602.

146. Ramos G, Pereira E, Simonetti MP. Does alkalinization of 0.75% ropivacaine promote a lumbar peridural block of higher quality? *Reg Anesth Pain Med* 2001;26:357–362.

147. Reichert MG, Butterworth J. Local anesthetic additives to increase stability and prevent organism growth. *Tech Reg Anesth Pain Manag* 2004;8:106–109.

148. Sakura S, Kirihara Y, Muguruma T, et al. The comparative neurotoxicity of intrathecal lidocaine and bupivacaine in rats. *Anesth Analg* 2005;101:541–547.

149. Takenami T, Yagishita S, Murase S, et al. Neurotoxicity of intrathecally administered bupivacaine involves the posterior roots/posterior white matter and is milder than lidocaine in rats. *Reg Anesth Pain Med.* 2005;30:464–472.

PART I: PHARMACOLOGY

CHAPTER 5 ■ LOCAL ANESTHETIC SYSTEMIC TOXICITY

GRAEME A. McLEOD, JOHN F. BUTTERWORTH, IV, AND J. A. W. WILDSMITH

Systemic toxicity is the term used to describe the clinical symptoms associated with extreme plasma concentrations of local anesthetics. Most reactions involve the central nervous system (CNS) first, with cardiovascular collapse being secondary to hypoxia consequent upon central respiratory depression. However, primary cardiovascular complications can occur under certain circumstances, most commonly the rapid, but accidental, intravascular injection of a large dose of drug, particularly one of the longer-acting agents. The drugs vary in their potential for causing systemic toxicity; the general view of the relative risk of this complication is shown in Figure 4-8 and clearly relates to local anesthetic potency. Although some variation in early symptoms exists between individuals, the actual features of a toxic reaction are drug nonspecific and generally demonstrate the consequences of progressive CNS depression, as noted in Figure 5-1. Classically, the initial features include perioral numbness or paresthesia, light-headedness, tinnitus, dysarthria, visual disturbances, and muscular twitching. This may be followed by convulsions, coma, respiratory arrest and, finally, cardiovascular depression. Cardiovascular features may include heart block, hypotension, bradycardia, ventricular arrhythmia (such as torsade de pointes), and cardiac arrest. Resuscitation from local anesthetic–induced cardiac arrest is extremely difficult, and has often been unsuccessful.

Such a major, life-threatening reaction can occur as the result of a simple, but very significant, overdose with a correctly placed injection. Excessive dosing during a continuous block is a more likely cause, although the many factors that can affect systemic absorption (Chapter 3) may interact to cause occasional problems with otherwise appropriate doses. However, most severe reactions are the result of unusually rapid increases in plasma concentration. Inflammation at the site of injection may contribute to this by speeding absorption, but the accidental intravascular injection of significant amounts of drug is the more likely cause, with sudden cuff deflation during intravenous (IV) regional anesthesia being a block-specific variation. It will not escape notice that all of these factors are subject to some degree of operator control and, given that the reactions are extremely difficult to treat, the overall message must be that prevention is better than cure (see Fig. 4-8).

HISTORICAL BACKGROUND

Systemic toxicity secondary to local anesthetics was recognized historically, but only as the stereotypical progression from prodromal symptoms to convulsions to circulatory collapse illustrated in Figure 4-8. However, in 1979, an editorial by Albright (1) described six cases of cardiac arrest without preceding CNS symptoms and made the claim that these were due to inadvertent intravascular injection of bupivacaine or etidocaine. Four years later, at a meeting of the U.S. Food and Drug Administration (FDA), Albright presented a total of 53 cases of prolonged and difficult resuscitation after inadvertent intravascular injection of bupivacaine or etidocaine, with death being the outcome in 31. An important feature was that 24 out of 35 pregnant women died (69%) of systemic reactions following an epidural block, whereas only seven out of 18 nonpregnant patients (39%) died (the latter group had received a variety of regional techniques). The outcome from the FDA meeting was that 0.75% bupivacaine was no longer recommended for obstetric anesthesia, despite having being used in only 27 (51%) of the reported patients, another eight (15%) having received the 0.5% preparation.

Ironically, the introduction of bupivacaine into anesthetic practice in the 1960s had done much to develop the subspecialty of obstetric anesthesia. Compared to lidocaine, bupivacaine caused less cumulative toxicity because of a more convenient duration of action and did not require epinephrine to limit systemic absorption or prolong its effect. Further clinical benefits of epidural bupivacaine include a greater degree of differential sensory block (that is, analgesia with relative sparing of motor function) and limited transfer of local anesthetic to the fetus. In these circumstances, it was not surprising that anesthesiologists did not wish to dispense with bupivacaine, but sought to alter anesthetic practice. Greater attention to the use of test doses (both of local anesthetics and other markers of intravascular injection), careful aspiration (especially of the epidural catheter) before injection, and incremental injection (dividing the total dose into 4- to 5-mL aliquots and injecting these at 45- to 60-second intervals) were partially successful in reducing the incidence of systemic toxicity. However, not even the use of all these techniques seems to be able to prevent the occasional accidental intravascular injection, and cases of systemic toxicity have continued to occur in different clinical settings.

The incidence of systemic toxicity reported in several observational studies performed during the last quarter of a century or so is summarized in Table 5-1. The most obvious feature is that the overall incidence of convulsions from all types of regional block has reduced dramatically—from 1 in 518 in 1978 to 1 in 4,510 in 1997, and to 1 in 17,564 in 2002. However, analysis of these data according to the site of injection (either neuraxial or major limb block) reveals a rather more disturbing picture. The incidence of convulsions secondary to limb block varied from 1 in 502 to 1 in 8,371, between four and sixteen times greater than the incidence of convulsions associated with epidural block. In one series, for example, Brown

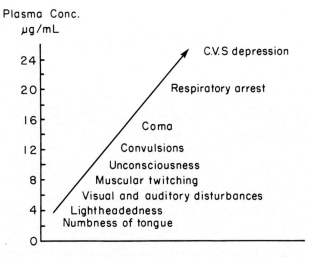

FIGURE 5-1. Relationship of signs and symptoms of local anesthetic toxicity to plasma concentrations of lidocaine.

et al. (2) recorded eight convulsions in 6,620 axillary blocks (1 in 827) and seven convulsions in 912 interscalene/supraclavicular blocks (1 in 130), suggesting that nerve block above the clavicle is particularly hazardous, even when compared with other types of brachial plexus block, let alone epidural anesthesia (1 in 8,435). Fortunately, none of the 58 patients suffering a convulsion in the combined series of Brown (2) and Auroy (3,4) progressed to cardiac collapse.

It might be argued that such reactions are the consequence of poor clinical practice, but this position is confounded by considering the results from controlled clinical trials conducted for approval of newer, safer local anesthetics. One of the consequences of cardiac toxicity following bupivacaine was the search for safer long-acting agents. Two such agents, ropivacaine (Astra-Zeneca, Sweden) and levobupivacaine (Abbott, Chicago), underwent a rigorous series of phase III studies for the FDA and the European regulatory authorities before being licensed for clinical practice. Data gathered in regulatory studies such as these provide detailed descriptions of the clinical management of the patients and any adverse events, particularly their relationship to systemic toxicity (5,6). All of the prospective, randomized, ethically approved

studies were undertaken in hospitals noted for their expertise in regional anesthesia, and the blocks were performed by experienced staff, such as consultants or dedicated research fellows.

In spite of that high level of care, nine adults out of approximately 4,500 patients were identified as experiencing systemic toxicity secondary to accidental IV administration of local anesthetic (seven women, two men). Three patients were pregnant and scheduled for Cesarean section. Six patients received ropivacaine, two bupivacaine, and one patient levobupivacaine. Seizures occurred in the two patients undergoing upper limb block (one ropivacaine, one bupivacaine), but not in any of the seven patients having epidural anesthesia, with incremental dosing probably preventing a major reaction. The proximity of the brachial plexus to large blood vessels, the use of large volumes/doses of local anesthetics, and the use of transarterial techniques probably explains the higher rate of serious complications with upper limb blocks and corroborates the findings of Brown (2) and Auroy (3,4). Most importantly, the conclusion must be that even experts must recognize that accidental intravascular injections are nearly always possible.

More recently, tumescent anesthesia (the extensive subcutaneous infiltration of local anesthetics administered by plastic surgeons for liposuction) has been associated with death secondary to systemic toxicity. Many of these operations were performed in private offices, without an anesthesiologist or any regulatory requirement to report adverse events (even deaths). A typical combination of drugs for tumescent anesthesia is lidocaine 1,000 mg, epinephrine 0.25 to 1.0 mg, and sodium bicarbonate 12.5 mmol/L of crystalloid solution. The injection of doses as great as 55 mg/kg of lidocaine is not uncommon during liposuction. Practitioners claim that most of it is aspirated with the subcutaneous fat that is being removed. However, the dangers of the technique came to prominence with a report (7) to the Chief Medical Examiner of New York City of five deaths after 47,000 procedures, and a survey (8) of U.S. plastic surgeons that estimated that the mortality rate was 1 in 5,224 procedures. As well as excessive plasma lidocaine concentration, death after tumescent anesthesia and liposuction (9) has been attributed to pulmonary embolism, pulmonary edema, epinephrine-induced side effects, excessive sedation, and reduction in venous return due to tight abdominal compression.

In the United Kingdom, death from inadvertent intravascular injection has occurred during continuous epidural

TABLE 5-1

INCIDENCE OF CONVULSIONS IN LARGE-SCALE STUDIES OF REGIONAL ANESTHESIA: EPIDURAL AND PERIPHERAL BLOCK

	Epidural			Peripheral block			All regional blocks		
	Total (n)	ST (n)	Incidence	Total (n)	ST (n)	Incidence	Total (n)	ST (n)	Incidence
Moore, 1978	6,729	13	1 in 518				6,729	13	1 in 518
Tanaka	17,439	20	1 in 872				17,439	20	1 in 872
Brown, 1995	16,870	2	1 in 8,435	7,532	15	1 in 502	25,697	26	1 in 988
Auroy, 1997	30,413	4	1 in 7,603	21,278	16	1 in 1,329	103,730	23	1 in 4,510
Auroy, 2002	35,379	3	1 in 11,793	50,223	6	1 in 8,371	158,083	9	1 in 17,564
Borgeat Single isomers 1995–1999				521	1	1 in 521	521	1	1 in 521
							4,500	2	1 in 2,250

ST, systemic toxicity

administration using electromechanical infusion devices (10). On two occasions, epidural infusions were connected to IV lines by mistake and, in another, the epidural infusion was connected to the central venous line. The local anesthetic infusion resulted in cardiac arrest and the death of the patient on the operating table. However, these appear not to be isolated events. Between January 2005 and May 2006, the National Patient Safety Agency's (NPSA) National Reporting and Learning System identified more than 346 incidents involving problems with epidural infusions that resulted in moderate, low, or no harm to patients (10). Reports such as these illustrate how the increased complexity of modern anesthesia, involving multiple monitoring modalities and drug infusions, produces new problems that must be overcome. The risks of regional anesthesia identified by the NPSA concerned the appropriate labeling of solutions and ready discrimination between the electronic pumps and lines used for epidural and other routes of parenteral administration. In considering both these problems, and the complications of tumescent anesthesia described in the previous paragraph, the point must be repeated that operators have a major role in prevention.

At the outset, some assumed that the simple substitution of the new drugs (ropivacaine and levobupivacaine) for bupivacaine would eradicate the problem of systemic toxicity. However, overwhelming evidence (as just summarized) from national surveys, FDA and European regulatory bodies, and patient safety groups suggests that local anesthetic systemic toxicity still occurs and remains a source of patient mortality. Part of the problem may be an overly simplistic view of local anesthetic pharmacology, especially among nonanesthesiologists, but another reason is that the nature of regional anesthesia has changed. The increased popularity of major limb blocks, a tendency to inject greater doses of the allegedly "safer" local anesthetics, and wider use of electronic infusion devices have all created a new milieu within which systemic toxicity may occur. Unfortunately, its very nature makes systemic toxicity very difficult to study formally in the clinical setting. To understand the basis of systemic toxicity and develop strategies for its management, most of the studies, in vitro and in vivo, have been in a range of animal models, albeit supplemented with some evidence from human volunteer studies and the clinical arena. Proper understanding of the problem requires that all levels of evidence, from ion channels to man, need to be reviewed, starting with the physicochemical and chiral properties of the drugs themselves.

INDIVIDUAL DRUG CHARACTERISTICS

Detailed consideration of the pharmacology of individual agents has been provided in Chapters 2 and 3, with physicochemical drug characteristics (pKa, lipid solubility, protein binding, vasoactivity, and stereoisomerism) to illustrate important determinants of the differences between drugs. Generally, systemic toxicity is regarded, as noted already, as relating primarily to lipid solubility, just as is local anesthetic potency, but a few other factors are important. Vasoactivity (11,12) has some relevance, with most drugs causing a degree of vasodilatation that will increase the rate of absorption. Some, however, such as prilocaine and ropivacaine, are less vasoactive. Prilocaine is also sequestered in lung tissue and is metabolized in the liver more rapidly than other amide drugs, making it a preferred agent for blocks with a relatively high risk of toxicity, the classic example being IV regional anesthesia. The degree of binding to plasma proteins is often taken as an indicator of the risk of toxicity, the erroneous argument being that drugs that are highly protein-bound (such as bupivacaine) are "retained" in the plasma, and do not cross into the tissues to exert a toxic effect. In fact, simply relating the data (Table 5-2) for protein binding to the known clinical risk (see Fig. 4-8) will show that the least protein-bound of the amides (prilocaine) is actually the least toxic, and the most protein-bound (bupivacaine) the most toxic. The final factor to be mentioned comes as consequences of more than 20 years' of investigation into the basis of bupivacaine cardiotoxicity: namely, extensive consideration of the role of stereoisomerism and drug chirality in its generation.

Chirality, the existence of structural stereoisomers, is a characteristic of many chemicals, and it may influence both the potency and toxicity of local anesthetics (see Table 5-3 for definitions).

One of the drugs introduced as a long-acting alternative to bupivacaine, levobupivacaine, is simply a single isomer derivative of the original drug. They are both potent, lipid-soluble local anesthetics, and have exactly the same physicochemical characteristics; the only difference between them is the number of isomers in solution. Their identical high lipid solubility (partition coefficient 346) and pKa (8.1) imply that the two drugs will cross physiologic membranes equally readily, whether at the cell wall or at intracellular structures such as mitochondria.

TABLE 5-2

PHYSICOCHEMICAL CHARACTERISTICS OF LOCAL ANESTHETICS

	MW	pKa[†]	Protein binding	Partition coefficient[*]	Onset	Duration	Relative toxicity
Procaine	236	8.9	6	1.7	Slow	Short	Low
Chloroprocaine	271	9.1	?	9.0	Fast	Short	Low
Tetracaine	264	8.5	75	4.1	Slow	Long	High
Etidocaine	276	7.7	94	800	Moderate	Long	High
Lidocaine	234	7.9	65	2.4	Fast	Medium	Medium
Prilocaine	220	7.7	55	25	Fast	Medium	Medium
Mepivacaine	246	7.6	78	21	Fast	Medium	Medium
Bupivacaine	288	8.1	95	346	Moderate	Long	High
Ropivacaine	274	8.1	94	115	Moderate	Long	High
L-Bupivacaine	288	8.1	95	346	Moderate	Long	High

[*]Octanol-to-buffer partition coefficient presented as a measure of lipid
[†]pKa measured at 37°C. solubility.

TABLE 5-3

CHIRAL TERMINOLOGY

Chiralit	Spatial arrangement of atoms, nonsuperimposable on each other
Isomer	A molecular entity with the same atomic composition but different stereochemical formulas and hence different physical or chemical properties
Stereoisomers	Isomers that possess identical constitution but which differ in the arrangement of their atoms in space
Enantiomers	One of a pair of molecular entities that are mirror images of each other and non-superimposable
Racemate	An equimolar mixture of a pair of enantiomers

The other newer drug, ropivacaine, is also a single *S* isomer, and comes from the same homologous series as bupivacaine, but the butyl side chain is replaced by a propyl group. This results in a lower partition coefficient (115), which implies that the drug will be less potent as well as less toxic. However, ropivacaine may produce less vasodilatation, and this might compensate for a lower inherent potency by increasing uptake into tissues (14). The underlying principle in the development of both ropivacaine and levobupivacaine was that if a significant difference in cardiotoxicity between the new agents and bupivacaine was coupled with equivalent potency for nerve block, then the gain in therapeutic index warranted their clinical use.

MECHANISMS OF TOXICITY

Early Investigations

Before the public exposure of bupivacaine toxicity in 1979, researchers had already conducted in vitro studies of the *dextro* (D) and *levo* (L) isomers of bupivacaine. Both Aberg (15) and Luduena (16), identified (in a variety of small animal studies) a difference in toxicity between enantiomers, showing that levobupivacaine had a 66% to 76% higher median lethal dose (LD50) than D-bupivacaine, and a 41% to 45% higher LD50 than bupivacaine. Studies after Albright's disclosure sought to determine further the dose and concentration relationships between convulsions and lethality. Intriguingly, a study in mice (17) showed a consistent ratio between the median convulsant (CD50) and lethal doses of local anesthetics. The CD50-to-LD50 ratio was 1.0 for bupivacaine and 1.2 for lidocaine, indicating a very narrow margin between convulsive and cardiotoxic effect, but no obvious difference in the "margin of safety" between these two systemic toxic effects. However, further studies with dog (18–20) and sheep (21,22) models in the mid 1980s demonstrated that bupivacaine was associated with the early onset of severe arrhythmias, these often occurring before the onset of convulsions, and that pregnancy increased susceptibility to systemic toxicity (23). Thus, accumulating evidence showed that bupivacaine was much more toxic than previously believed, and that its toxicity was substantially out of proportion to its clinical potency relative to lidocaine. These early studies were the basis for further investigation of the differential effects of local anesthetics on sodium (Na^+),

potassium (K^+), and calcium (Ca^{2+}) channels; mitochondrial function; myocardial electrical conduction; contractility; and the genesis of arrhythmias.

Sodium Channel Block

Local anesthetics preferentially block Na^+ channels when they are in the open (conducting) or inactivated (nonconducting) states, as opposed to the resting (nonconducting) state (24). Opportunities for binding to open or inactivated Na^+ channels are enhanced by increased frequency of nerve depolarization; this phenomenon is described as *phasic* or *use-dependent block*. However, recovery from block during repolarization (the onset of diastole in cardiac muscle) is slow, the dissociation time constant for bupivacaine being some tenfold slower than that for lidocaine. Bupivacaine block of cardiac Na^+ channels can be described as being "fast-in, slow-out," and allowing substantial block to accumulate in the physiologic heart rate range, prolonging conduction, and inducing reentry-type arrhythmias. Metabolic changes, such as hypoxia, acidosis, and hyperkalemia, further enhance systemic toxicity by increasing the proportion of Na^+ channels in the inactivated state during diastole.

Cardiac Na^+ channels arise from a specific gene, and may have important electrophysiologic differences from Na^+ channels in nerve cells. Moreover, the action potential in axons consists of a very brief depolarization due to rapid influx of Na^+ ions followed immediately by an equally rapid repolarization due to channel inactivation and termination of Na^+ ion flux. In contrast, the action potential of cardiac cells is prolonged, repolarization being delayed by Ca influx during the "plateau" phase, when local anesthetic binding is favored because most Na^+ channels are in the inactivated state. Experimentally, Na^+ channel block by local anesthetics may be measured in electrophysiologic studies by measuring the maximum upstroke velocity of the action potential (V_{max}) and the action potential duration (APD), studies that are often performed in guinea pig papillary muscle. Translated to the clinical EKG, reductions in V_{max} correlate with QRS widening, and changes in APD are associated with ventricular arrhythmias related to lengthening of the QT interval.

Data from several studies using the whole-cell voltage clamp technique in isolated cardiac muscle showed that both bupivacaine (25,26) and dextrobupivacaine (27,28) suppressed V_{max} more than lidocaine, ropivacaine (25,26), or levobupivacaine (26–28) (Table 5-4). Furthermore, recovery from block was faster with levobupivacaine and ropivacaine, implying that systemic toxicity due to these drugs may be easier to overcome. In addition, Vanhoutte et al. (27) and Valenzuela et al. (28) demonstrated, also in isolated guinea pig papillary muscle, that the enantiomers of bupivacaine possess marked stereoselectivity in their effects on the inactivated Na^+ channel. The D-enantiomer reduced V_{max}, between 65% and 72% more than the L, and shortened the action potential duration more (Table 5-4). Phasic (or frequency-dependent) block may also exhibit stereospecific features (29). Although no differences were seen in V_{max} when D-bupivacaine, L-bupivacaine, and ropivacaine were applied to crayfish giant axons stimulated at a frequency of 0.1 Hz, a significant decrease in V_{max} occurred (in the order L-bupivacaine >D-bupivacaine >ropivacaine) when the stimulation rate was 5 Hz, suggesting a greater frequency dependent effect of L-bupivacaine.

One reason for the development of cardiac arrhythmias is a concentration and use-dependent slowing of ventricular conduction, progressing to a degree that might allow

IN VITRO AND ISOLATED ORGAN STUDIES

Author/year	Measurement	Model	Bup >Lido	Dex >Levo	Bup >Levo	Bup >Rop	Levo >Rop
Vanhoutte (27), 1991	Na^+ channel block	Guinea pig papillary muscle		28%			
Valenzuela (28), 1995	Na^+ channel block	Guinea pig papillary muscle		65%	54%	60%	4%
Harding (26), 1998	Na^+ channel	Guinea pig papillary muscle		47%			
Nau (133), 2000	Na^+ channel	Cloned human cardiac		566%		1,850%	193%
Valenzuela (31), 1995 and (41), 1997	K^+ channel hKv1.5	Cloned human cardiac muscle					
Kindler (43), 2003	K^+ channel TASK 2	Oocyte			152%	1,288%	449%
Zapata-Sudo (46), 2001	L-type Ca^{2+} channel	Rat, ventricular myocytes					
Butterworth (50), 1993	$\beta2$-receptor	Human lymphocytes basal cAMP			23%	74%	
Butterworth (134), 1997	First pass pulmonary uptake	Rabbit lungs	14%	14%	−5%	−5%	0%
Ohmura (135), 2003	Mitochondrial ATP	Rat, isolated heart mitochondria					37%
Sztark (55), 1998	Mitochondrial ATP	Rat, isolated heart mitochondria				150%	
Sztark (57), 2000	Mitochondrial complex 1 inhibition	Rat, isolated heart mitochondria		18%			
Aya (30), 2002	Myocardial conduction velocity	Rabbit heart			37%	70%	
Graf (59), 1997	AV conduction	Guinea pig		54%	30%		
Mazoit (136), 1993	QRS duration	Rabbit	1,400%				
Mazoit (137), 2000	QRS duration	Rabbit			150%	307%	
Denson (63), 1992	Arrhythmogenesis	Rat		200%			
Denson (63)	Time to peak decrease in firing rate in NTS	Rat		100%			63%

>, more potent than; Bup, bupivacaine; dex, dextrobupivacaine; levo, levobupivacaine; lido, lidocaine; rop, ropivacaine.

electrical reentry. Isolated frozen rabbit hearts, but with a thin layer of surviving epicardial muscle, were stimulated using 256 unipolar minielectrodes, attached to a programmable constant-current stimulator, in the presence of 0.1, 1.0, and 10 μM concentrations of bupivacaine, L-bupivacaine, or ropivacaine (30). Use-dependency was determined by pacing cycle length (PCL), longitudinal ventricular conduction velocity (θL), transverse ventricular conduction velocity (θT), conduction velocities, and the maximal decrease in conduction velocity (E_{max}) at a PCL of 600 ms. In addition, the ventricular effective refractory period was calculated. Each local anesthetic induced a use-dependent slowing in θL (bupivacaine = L-bupivacaine), and θT (ratio of bupivacaine to L-bupivacaine/ropivacaine of 1:0.74 at 600 ms), and a concentration-dependent prolongation in ventricular effective refractory period (bupivacaine = L-bupivacaine >ropivacaine). The results suggest that equimolar concentrations of ropivacaine are less cardiotoxic than bupivacaine because of less use-dependent conduction block, and that L-bupivacaine cardiotoxicity is intermediate.

Potassium Channel Block

Potassium channels (all of which may interact with local anesthetics) are a relatively heterogeneous group compared to Na^+ channels. Three basic forms exist, with the following nomenclature:

- Six transmembrane segments, single-pore, voltage-gated channel (31–33). Examples include Kv1 to Kv9, and human *ether-a-go-go*-related potassium (HERG) channels (34,35).
- Two transmembrane segments, single-pore, inward rectifier channel. Examples include Kir 1,1, 1.2, 3.1, 6.2, and others (36,37), which are important in setting the resting membrane potential.
- Four transmembrane segments, two-pore channel (38,39), representing perhaps the most abundant class of K^+ channels (e.g., TWIK, TREK, TASK, or TRAAK channels).

During the cardiac action potential, K^+ channels are responsible for repolarization and stabilization of the cell membrane resting potential. Potassium channel block contributes to the systemic toxicity of local anesthetics by lengthening the cardiac action potential, predisposing the heart to ventricular arrhythmias such as torsade de pointes. Evidence of K^+ ion involvement in systemic toxicity and a propensity for cardiac arrhythmias is suggested by prolongation of the Q-Tc interval on a 12-lead EKG (40). Further evidence for the effects of ropivacaine, L-bupivacaine, and D-bupivacaine was obtained by studies on cloned human cardiac delayed- rectifier K^+ channels expressed in a mouse fibroblast cell line, using a patch clamp technique. Apparent dissociation constant (K_D) values of 27.3 μM and 4.1 μM were calculated for L-bupivacaine and D-bupivacaine, respectively, indicating that the latter has sevenfold greater affinity for the K^+ channel (31). Using the same model, the same research group found that ropivacaine had an apparent K_D of 80 μM (41), suggesting that the relative potency of local anesthetic K^+ channel block is in the order bupivacaine >L-bupivacaine >ropivacaine. In contrast, the optical isomers of mepivacaine showed no stereospecific effect (42).

Bupivacaine, L-bupivacaine, and ropivacaine were also shown to block both the open and inactivated states of HERG channels in a time- and concentration-dependent manner. However, the evidence for stereoselective block is conflicting. Gonzalez et al. (33) found that L-bupivacaine was twice as potent as D-bupivacaine in blocking HERG channels, whereas Friederich et al. (34) showed no stereospecific effect at HERG and HERG/MiRP1 channels. Studies on tandem-pore domain K^+ channels (2P K^+) also produced some controversy (39). These channels are widely expressed in the CNS, and are involved in the control of the resting membrane potential and the firing pattern of excitable cells. Thus, their inhibition results in membrane depolarization, increasing the affinity of both open and inactivated Na^+ channels for local anesthetics. TASK-2, but not TASK-1, K^+ channels showed agent-specific, dose-dependent, and stereoselective responses (43), with half maximal inhibitory concentration (IC50) values of 17 μM and 43 μM for D-bupivacaine and L-bupivacaine, and 85 μM and 236 μM for D-ropivacaine and ropivacaine, respectively (Table 5-4).

Calcium Channel Block

Calcium ions stimulate myocardial contractility by passing through long-lasting (L)-type Ca^{2+} channels, binding to ryanodine receptors in the sarcoplasmic reticulum, and triggering Ca-induced Ca release (44). Relaxation of the myocardium is an energy-dependent process, and is reliant on the removal of Ca from troponin binding sites and active return of Ca to the sarcoplasmic reticulum by an adenosine triphosphate (ATP)-dependent regulatory protein called SERCA2.

Rossner (45) showed that bupivacaine inhibited cardiac Ca^{2+} channels tonically in a concentration-dependent manner. Zapata-Sudo et al. (46) subsequently investigated the effect of D-bupivacaine and L-bupivacaine on L-type calcium channels in isolated perfused rat ventricular myocytes. At a concentration of 10 μM, significant differences occurred between the isomers (D >L) in the incidence of ventricular arrhythmias, and lengthening of the PR and QRS intervals of the EKG. In addition to these global stereospecific differences, specific inhibitory effects on Ca^{2+} channels were investigated using the whole-cell clamp technique. Maximal reduction of inward Ca currents (I_{Ca}) was 57% for D-bupivacaine 20 μM and 51% for L-bupivacaine 10 μM, indicating that differences between the isomers could be attributed to stereoscopic effects at Na^+ and K^+ channels, but not Ca channels.

Thus, the propensity of local anesthetics to produce systemic toxicity, in the forms of myocardial depression and poor response to traditional resuscitation, may be only partially explained by stereoselective ion channel block; local anesthetics also have intracellular actions linked to the bioenergetics of the mitochondria (47–49).

Effects on Mitochondrial Function

Much recent work on local anesthetic toxicity relates to effects on mitochondrial function, an important area, because 70% of myocardial energy needs are supplied by the oxidation of fatty acids. Discussion of the cellular mechanisms of actions of local anesthetics requires first a description of the pathways involved in fatty acid breakdown.

Long-chain fatty acids react with coenzyme A (CoA) in an ATP-dependent process catalyzed by long-chain acyl-CoA synthetase (LCAS) located in the outer mitochondrial membrane (Fig. 5-2). To cross the inner mitochondrial membrane, Acyl-CoA is transformed into acylcarnitine by carnitine palmitoyltransferase I (CPT I), located in the outer membrane. After crossing the inner membrane, acylcarnitine is then regenerated to acyl-CoA by carnitine palmitoyltransferase II (CPT II) within the matrix compartment, and acyl-CoA is metabolized to H_2O

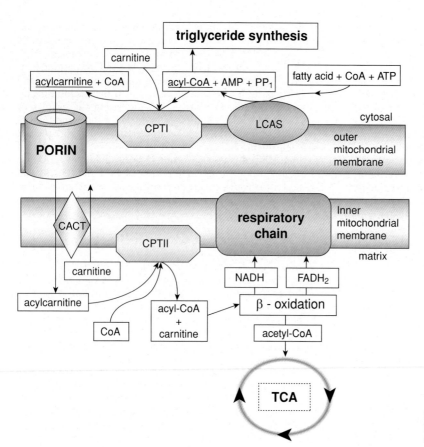

FIGURE 5-2. An ATP-dependent process catalyzed by long-chain acyl-CoA synthetase (LCAS) located in the outer mitochondrial membrane.

and CO_2 in the tricarboxylic acid cycle. In tissues, almost 90% of ATP is formed by a mitochondrial process termed *oxidative phosphorylation*. Located within the inner mitochondrial membrane is a chain of "respiratory" enzymes and coenzymes that transport hydrogen or electrons, developing enough energy to transport protons from the mitochondrial inner compartment or matrix into the intermembrane space.

It has been known for several years that lipophilic local anesthetics interfere with mitochondrial energy-linked processes by uncoupling oxidative phosphorylation on complex I of the intracellular mitochondrial respiratory chain (50,51) and inhibiting respiratory chain enzymes (52,53). In addition, local anesthetics inhibit state 3, active respiration (oxygen consumed in converting ADP to ATP), and state 4 respiration (oxygen consumed in the resting state to maintain the chemiosmotic gradient) (54). Furthermore, less disturbance of mitochondrial energy metabolism by ropivacaine (55), hence less reduction of cAMP, indicated that this effect correlates with lipid solubility (56), but not stereoisomerism (57).

Whole-Organ Studies

The results of ion channel studies have been extended by work on isolated whole guinea pig or rabbit hearts, in which such effects as conduction defects and ventricular arrhythmias may be observed independent of any systemic effects of the drugs on other organs (e.g., brain).

In a study by Mazoit et al. (58), a two-step infusion of L-bupivacaine, D-bupivacaine, or bupivacaine was administered to isolated perfused rabbit hearts and the effects mon-

itored continuously using a surface EKG. Although myocardial pharmacokinetics were similar for all three local anesthetics, QRS widening, as well as the occurrence of severe arrhythmias, was much less pronounced in the hearts receiving L-bupivacaine than in those receiving D-bupivacaine or bupivacaine. All but one heart infused with D-bupivacaine or bupivacaine developed ventricular fibrillation or asystole. In contrast, four out of six hearts receiving L-bupivacaine developed atrioventricular block, but none progressed to cardiac arrest. A similar study (59) of isolated perfused guinea pig heart was designed to measure the effect of increasing concentrations of L-bupivacaine, bupivacaine, and D-bupivacaine on atrioventricular (AV) conduction time and second-degree heart block. At 10 μM concentration, AV conduction time was 54% longer with D-bupivacaine and 30% longer with bupivacaine compared to L-bupivacaine. Second degree heart block occurred in 83% of D-bupivacaine, 33% of bupivacaine, and 8% of L-bupivacaine hearts. Using an identical model, AV conduction time was increased by 84 seconds with ropivacaine 10 μM, compared to 105 seconds with levobupivacaine 10 μM (60).

Thus, L-bupivacaine and ropivacaine have been shown to cause less QRS widening and fewer episodes of ventricular tachycardia, fibrillation, or asystole, than bupivacaine.

Central Nervous System Studies

Classically, during progressive local anesthetic intoxication, CNS toxicity precedes cardiovascular system toxicity. An initial, apparently excitatory phase, characterized by muscle twitching, tremors, and convulsions, precedes overt CNS depression, which results in hypoventilation and then respiratory arrest, with hypoxia (and probably other systemic actions of local anesthetics) leading to cardiac arrest.

A primary role of the CNS in cardiovascular toxicity was proposed in early studies that observed arrhythmias after direct application of local anesthetics to the brain. After injection of bupivacaine into the lateral cerebral ventricle of 10 cats (61), all developed tachycardia and ventricular arrhythmias at doses of five to 11 times less than needed by the IV route. In a study in rats by Thomas et al. (62), bupivacaine and lidocaine injected into the nucleus tractus solitarius produced a significant decrease in neuronal firing rate, associated with marked bradycardia and hypotension. The effect on arrhythmias was dependent on the local anesthetic injected; animals given lidocaine reverted to sinus rhythm, whereas half of the animals given bupivacaine died. The same team investigated the differential effects of an IV dose of D-bupivacaine and L-bupivacaine 2 mg/kg in 24 rats (63). Cell firing rate (CFR) was recorded continuously, along with EKG and arterial blood pressure. The time to maximum decrease in CFR was twice as long with L-bupivacaine as D-bupivacaine. Moreover, D-bupivacaine produced severe bradycardia, progressive hypotension, apnea, and death in all animals, whereas L-bupivacaine produced only a mild bradycardia in one-third. Malignant ventricular arrhythmias occurred in one-third of D-bupivacaine treated rats, but in none of those given L-bupivacaine.

To further investigate the influence of CNS toxicity on cardiac arrhythmogenesis, equimolar doses of L-bupivacaine, bupivacaine, and ropivacaine were infused bilaterally into the carotid arteries of sheep over 3 minutes (64), thus targeting local anesthetic to the brain, not the heart. Convulsions and signs of sympathetic stimulation were seen in the order bupivacaine >L-bupivacaine >ropivacaine. However, no difference was seen between the local anesthetics in the incidence or severity of CNS-associated arrhythmias. The conclusion from the study was that fatal arrhythmias did not result from direct CNS excitation or convulsions caused by CNS site-directed supraconvulsant doses of local anesthetic agents. Thus, conflict remains regarding the relative importance of CNS contributions to local anesthetic cardiovascular toxicity.

Large-Animal Models

The use of in vitro and in vivo studies using small animal models has improved understanding of local anesthetic toxicity, but does not simulate accurately the accidental intravascular administration of local anesthetic during neural block. Injection into the systemic and coronary circulation of large animals and direct intravascular infusion of local anesthetics into human volunteers replicates more closely clinical toxicity, and provides a controlled environment in which CNS and cardiovascular system side effects can be observed. The nature of the large-animal experiments used has varied according to the nature of the scientific question being asked. Undoubtedly, IV bolus administration of local anesthetic into a conscious animal best replicates accidental intravascular injection, although early cerebral excitation may confound cardiovascular changes. In contrast, injection in anesthetized, mechanically ventilated dogs limits seizure effects and allows observation of the progressive signs of toxicity by allowing relative control of Po_2, Pco_2, and pH. Continuous infusion in a pregnant sheep model allows measurement of drug concentrations in fetal tissue, whereas injection into carotid or coronary arteries minimizes recirculation and allows site-specific assessment of toxicity.

Conscious Sheep Model

A series of studies has been performed investigating the CNS and cardiovascular toxicity of graded doses of IV lidocaine, bupivacaine, ropivacaine, and L-bupivacaine in a chronically instrumented, conscious sheep preparation. Preparation involves prior surgical instrumentation to allow direct measurement of blood pressure, EKG, EEG, left ventricular contractility (dP/dt_{max}), and pulmonary artery and myocardial blood flows.

Common to all experiments is an initial decrease in myocardial contractility then, coincidental with the onset of CNS stimulation, a sudden increase in myocardial contractility, blood pressure, and heart rate. The appearance of convulsions is often associated with widened QRS complexes and ventricular arrhythmias. The amount of local anesthetic required to induce convulsions varied with the drug. Relative to bupivacaine (65), mean requirements were 144%, 33%, and 21% greater with lidocaine, ropivacaine, and L-bupivacaine (66) respectively (Table 5-5). In addition, fewer and less deleterious arrhythmias were induced by ropivacaine and L-bupivacaine, and these arrhythmias were more likely to revert to sinus rhythm.

When the dose of local anesthetic was increased further, the mean fatal doses of lidocaine (67), ropivacaine (67), and L-bupivacaine (68) were 829%, 108%, and 78% greater than bupivacaine (67), respectively, with the cause of death varying with the local anesthetic (Table 5-6). Bupivacaine was associated with the sudden onset of ventricular tachycardia-fibrillation, but without hypoxia or acidosis. Lidocaine overdose led to respiratory depression, bradycardia, and hypotension, but without arrhythmias, and death was attributed to "pump failure." Interestingly, the animals given ropivacaine and L-bupivacaine experienced a variety of modes of death; some died of ventricular fibrillation, but others died of electromechanical dissociation or pump failure.

Conscious Pregnant Sheep Model

The high proportion of fatalities in pregnant women suffering bupivacaine toxicity has stimulated much research into whether pregnancy is associated with any increased sensitivity to local anesthetic toxicity, with in vitro studies of rabbit myocardium suggesting that progesterone enhances the arrhythmogenicity of bupivacaine (69).

The model described in the previous section has been used to evaluate the effects of equimolar concentrations of L-bupivacaine, bupivacaine, and ropivacaine in pregnant sheep, with two methods of injection being used: bolus to mimic inadvertent intravascular injection, and constant rate infusion to mimic cumulative toxicity. Nonpregnant and pregnant ewes were randomized to receive lidocaine (70), bupivacaine (71), ropivacaine (71,72), or L-bupivacaine at a constant rate of 0.5 mg/kg$^-$/min until circulatory collapse. In pregnant sheep, the dose threshold for convulsions was lower than in nonpregnant animals, but no difference existed for the onset of cardiac arrhythmias. There were no significant differences between pregnant and nonpregnant ewes in plasma drug concentrations, except in pregnant animals at the time of circulatory collapse (73). The rank order for toxicity was defined according to convulsive dose and plasma concentration and was found to be in the sequence bupivacaine >L-bupivacaine >ropivacaine. Furthermore, there was no significant difference between the three drugs in uterine blood flow or fetal plasma and tissue concentrations.

TABLE 5-5

SYSTEMIC TOXICITY IN VARIOUS SPECIES

	Symptom	Species	Bup >Lido	Rop >Lido	Dex >Levo	Bup >Levo	Bup >Rop	Levo >Rop
de Jong (17), 1980	Convulsions	Mouse	91%					
Aberg (15), 1972	Convulsions	Mouse/rat			74%	42%		
Ohmura (138), 2001	Convulsions	Rat				38%	42%	3%
Liu, 1982	Convulsions	Dog	171%					
Liu (20), 1983	Convulsions	Dog	344%					
Feldman (139), 1989	Convulsions	Dog	382%	326%			13%	
Feldman (100), 1991	Convulsions	Dog					14%	
Rutten (65), 1989	Convulsions	Sheep	144%	33%			83%	
Huang (66), 1998	Convulsions	Sheep				21%		
Santos (73), 2001	Convulsions	Pregnant sheep				15%	46%	27%
Santos (73), 2001	Convulsions	Nonpregnant Sheep				29%	50%	17%
Dony (140), 2000	First CNS or CVS sign	Rat					61%	
Ohmura (138), 2001	Dysrhythmias	Rat	1,400%	570%		231%	595%	110%
Reiz (74), 1989	VF	Pig					138%	
Morrisson (75), 2000	VF	Pig				87%	113%	14%
Chang (76), 2001	VF	Sheep				29%	29%	0%
Groban (99), 2001	CVS collapse	Dog	486%			24%	92%	52%
Ohmura (138), 2001	Asystole	Rat				45%	172%	88%
de Jong (17), 1980	Lethality	Mouse	127%					
Aberg (15), 1972	Lethality	Mouse/rat			76%	41%		
Luduena (16), 1972	Lethality	Mouse/rat/rabbit			66%	45%		
Nancarrow (67), 1989	Lethality	Sheep	829%	346%			108%	

>, more potent than; Bup, bupivacaine; dex, dextrobupivacaine; levo, levobupivacaine; lido, lidocaine; rop, ropivacaine.

TABLE 5-6

MEAN DOSE OF LOCAL ANESTHETIC FOR ONSET OF CONVULSIONS AND DEATH AND THE RATIO OF CONVULSIVE TO LETHAL DOSE

			$Dose_{convulsion}$ (*mg, mg/kg, or $^\phi$mmol/kg)	$Dose_{fatal}$ (mg,*mg/kg, or $^\phi$mmol/kg)	Dose ratio (convulsion/fatal)
De Jong (17), 1980	Mouse (intra- peritoneal)	Lido	111.0	133.1	1.2
		Bup	57.7	58.7	1.0
Aberg (15), 1972	Mouse, rat	Levo	4.7	9.7	2.1
		Bup	3.3	6.9	2.1
		Dex	2.7	5.5	2.0
Ohmura (138), 2001	Rat	Bup	9.3	39.6	4.3
		Levo	12.8	57.4	4.5
		Rop	13.2	107.8	8.2
Santos (71), 1995	Pregnant sheep	Bup	5.0	8.5	1.7
		Rop	7.5	12.9	1.7
Santos (71), 1995	Nonpregnant sheep	Bup	4.7	8.9	1.9
		Rop	6.0	11.6	1.9
Santos (73), 2001	Pregnant sheep	Bup	0.013^ϕ	0.026^ϕ	2.0
		Levo	0.015^ϕ	0.031^ϕ	2.1
		Rop	0.19^ϕ	0.038^ϕ	2.0
Santos (73), 2001	Nonpregnant sheep	Bup	0.014^ϕ	0.024^ϕ	1.7
		Levo	0.018^ϕ	0.031^ϕ	1.7
		Rop	0.021^ϕ	0.038^ϕ	1.8
Nancarrow (67), 1989	Sheep	Lido	320*	1450*	14
		Bup	69*	156*	2.2
		Rop	155*	325*	2.1
Chang (68), 2000	Sheep	Levo	127*	277*	2.2

Bup, bupivacaine; dex, dextrobupivacaine; levo, levobupivacaine; lido, lidocaine; rop, ropivacaine.

Direct Coronary Injection Model

The in vivo cardiotoxicities of lidocaine (74), bupivacaine (74,75), L-bupivacaine (75), and ropivacaine (74,75) were evaluated by their direct injection into the coronary arteries of pigs at doses sufficient to mimic (but only in cardiac blood vessels) the plasma concentrations found following IV injection. A catheter was inserted into the left anterior descending coronary artery in anesthetized pigs and increasing doses of drug were injected. Systemic hemodynamics, left ventricular pressures, and 12-lead EKG were recorded continuously, and prolongation of the QRS interval was regarded as an electrophysiologic measure of toxicity. Early studies consistently demonstrated a toxicity ratio of >15:1 for bupivacaine and lidocaine, 2.5 to 4 times greater than calculated potency differences between the two drugs. Compared with bupivacaine, significantly higher doses of L-bupivacaine and ropivacaine had to be administered to achieve the same degree of QRS prolongation, giving relative toxicity ratios of 2.1:1.2:1. Death was due to ventricular fibrillation in all cases. A similar direct intracoronary injection study was performed in sheep (76) using incremental equimolar doses. Bupivacaine, L-bupivacaine, and ropivacaine suppressed myocardial contractility and increased QRS duration. Although two-thirds of the sheep died of ventricular fibrillation, no differences were detected between drugs, in contrast to the studies in the pig model.

Human Volunteer Studies

Despite animal studies implying that both ropivacaine and L-bupivacaine have a lower level of toxicity than bupivacaine,

the ideal study would demonstrate similar effects in man. The difficulties are obvious, but a useful model was derived: acute tolerance to constant IV infusion. Volunteers were first given an infusion of lidocaine to acquaint them with the CNS effects of local anesthetics. They then received, on separate days, 10 mg/min of bupivacaine, ropivacaine, or L-bupivacaine in crossover, randomized, double-blind studies. Each drug was infused to a maximum dose of 150 mg or until the volunteers reported early CNS effects such as paresthesias, visual changes, light-headedness, or tinnitus. Changes in conductivity and myocardial contractility were monitored using EKG parameters (PR interval, QRS duration, QTc, QTd), echocardiography, or thoracic bioimpedance. QTc dispersion is a validated predictor of arrhythmogenesis, is obtained by measuring the difference between the shortest and longest QT interval, and is corrected for time.

Overall, human volunteer studies have shown that bupivacaine is more likely to impair myocardial contractility, extend QRS duration, and produce more symptoms and signs of toxicity than L-bupivacaine or ropivacaine. The first two studies both showed that a larger dose of ropivacaine (124 mg [77] and 115 mg [78]) was tolerated better than that of bupivacaine (99 mg [77] and 103 mg [78]). Both drugs impaired left ventricular systolic and diastolic function compared with placebo, but the effect was greater with bupivacaine. Symptoms of CNS toxicity were similar with both drugs, but tended to occur earlier, with a lower dose and at a lower plasma concentration with bupivacaine. Side effects were similar except for an increased incidence of muscle twitching in the volunteers given bupivacaine.

In subsequent studies, the volunteers were able to tolerate only much lower local anesthetic doses, possibly because of greater anxiety about their effects. Bardsley et al. (79) compared bupivacaine and L-bupivacaine, with the doses tolerated being 47 mg and 56 mg, respectively. The subjects receiving bupivacaine had greater decreases in stroke index, acceleration index, and ejection fraction as measured by thoracic bioimpedance. A similar comparison of L-bupivacaine and ropivacaine (80) in volunteers did not detect any difference in myocardial function or symptoms of systemic toxicity, but the mean tolerated doses were even lower: 39 mg for L-bupivacaine and 37 mg for ropivacaine. Mean time to the first onset of CNS symptoms was similar for L-bupivacaine and ropivacaine (3.7 min versus 3.9 min), although L-bupivacaine had fewer symptoms recorded than ropivacaine. The symptoms that occurred exclusively during the ropivacaine infusion were chest pain, circumoral paresthesia, pain, taste perversion, and vasodilatation, whereas only a feeling of detachment and hyperventilation occurred exclusively with L-bupivacaine. Changes in stroke index, cardiac index, acceleration index, and all measured ECG parameters were similar with both drugs.

Only one study (81) has been conducted to investigate the effect of local anesthetics on EEG signals. L-bupivacaine or bupivacaine 40 mg was infused over 35 minutes in 12 subjects, both drugs producing a slowing of the EEG consistent with CNS depression. Levobupivacaine had less excitatory characteristics, judged in terms of their magnitude and the extent of the brain involved, and the volunteers suffered more adverse events, such as tinnitus and dizziness, with bupivacaine.

Overview

In vitro studies suggest that L-bupivacaine and ropivacaine are less potent than D-bupivacaine and bupivacaine in multiple models of cardiotoxicity, and have less affinity for cardiac Na^+ and K^+ channels. Moreover, local anesthetics would appear to have important nonstereo-specific effects on Ca channels and mitochondrial function, although the evidence is not totally consistent. Large-animal and human volunteer studies have demonstrated that both L-bupivacaine and ropivacaine show a reduced propensity toward Ca arrhythmias, require greater doses for a lethal effect in animal models, and have less effect on cardiac mechanical function in human volunteers.

Treatment

As indicated earlier, prevention is better than a cure, thus adequate patient evaluation and preparatory steps are essential. Prior knowledge of the differential diagnosis of local anesthetic reactions is also vital. In the event of a systemic toxic reaction to any local anesthetic occurring as a result of inadvertent intravascular injection or any other cause, full life support measures should be instigated immediately. In general terms, management should follow established guidelines such as those of the American Heart Association (82) or U.K. Resuscitation Council (83) and, although some specific aspects must be considered further, the general principles of a prioritized approach based on the standard sequence of airway, breathing, circulation (ABC) is required. A full-blown toxic reaction, even with a drug such as lidocaine, is life-threatening and requires skilled management if the patient is to recover unharmed. Few will have to deal with more than one or two such events in a career, so adherence to standard resuscitation protocols is important because the training given for other settings should mean that the routines are well ingrained (see Tables 5-7 to 5-9). Regrettably, recent surveys (84) indicate that, in North American

TABLE 5-7

DIFFERENTIAL DIAGNOSIS OF LOCAL ANESTHETIC REACTIONS

Etiology	Major clinical features	Comments
Local anesthetic toxicity		
Intravascular injection	Immediate convulsion and/or cardiac toxicity	Injection into vertebral or a carotid artery may cause convulsion after administration of small dose.
Relative overdose	Onset in 5 to 15 minutes of irritability, progressing to convulsions	
Reaction to vasoconstrictor	Tachycardia, hypertension, headache, apprehension	May vary with vasopressor used
Vasovagal reaction	Rapid onset Bradycardia Hypotension Pallor, faintness	Rapidly reversible with elevation of legs
Allergy		
Immediate	Anaphylaxis ($\downarrow$ BP, bronchospasm, edema)	Allergy to amides extremely rare
Delayed	Urticaria	Cross-allergy possible, for example, with preservatives in local anesthetics and food
High spinal or epidural block	Gradual onset Bradycardia[a] Hypotension Possible respiratory arrest	May lose consciousness with total spinal block and onset of cardiorespiratory effects more rapid than with high epidural or with subdural block.
Concurrent medical episode (e.g., asthma attack, myocardial infarct)	May mimic local anesthetic reaction	Medical history important

[a]Sympathetic block above T4 adds cardioaccelerator nerve blockade to the vasodilation seen with blockade below T4; total spinal block may have rapid onset.
BP, blood pressure.

TABLE 5-8

MEASURES TO MINIMIZE RISK OF TOXICITY FROM NEURAL BLOCKADE[a]

PATIENT EVALUATION
Identification of significant systemic disease, age, and other factors, to permit individualization of local anesthetic dose

PREMEDICATION
Diazepam or other appropriate CNS depressant in moderate dosage

PREPARATION
Resuscitative drugs
   Midazolam or thiopental, succinylcholine, atropine, vasopressor

Equipment
   Oxygen administration and suction equipment
   Airway (oropharyngeal airway, laryngoscope, endotracheal tube)
Ensure adequate IV available
Discard any cloudy solutions or those containing crystals
Physically separate neural blockade tray from any other drugs

PREVENTION
Personally check dose of local anesthetic and vasoconstrictor
Use effective test dose and incremental injection with repeated aspiration thereafter
Aspirate frequently and discard solution colored by blood
Monitor cardiovascular signs (rapid ↑ heart rate if epinephrine injected intravenously)
Constant verbal contact with patient past time of peak plasma concentration

[a]Local anesthetic toxicity may result in convulsions; however, with rapid and appropriate treatment, these should never be fatal in themselves. See also cardiac effects of bupivacaine in text
   CNS, central nervous system; IV, intravenous.

TABLE 5-9

TREATMENT OF ACUTE LOCAL ANESTHETIC TOXICITY

AIRWAY
Establish clear airway; suction, if required

BREATHING
Oxygen with face mask
Encourage adequate ventilation (avoid ↑ CO_2 ↓ O_2) acidosis which potentiate cardiotoxicity.
Artificial ventilation, if required

CIRCULATION
Elevate legs
Increase IV fluids if ↓ blood pressure
CVS support drug if ↓ blood pressure persists (see below) or ↓ heart rate

DRUGS
Anticonvulsant
Diazepam 0.15–3 mg/kg IV, Midazopam 0.075–0.15mg/kg IV
Thiopental 1.4 mg/kg IV, Propofol 1–2mg/kg IV
Muscle relaxant
   Succinylcholine 1 mg/kg, if inadequate control of ventilation with above measures (requires artificial ventilation and may necessitate intubation)
CVS support
Treat arrhythmias using standard life support protocols and consider lipid infusion (see text)

CNS, central nervous system; CVS, cardiovascular system; IV, intravenous.

centers at least, there is much confusion about the best drugs to use in the event of a local anesthetic toxic reaction. Some clinicians even designated a drug that had not been available for several years as their preferred, first-line agent for use in the event of local anesthetic–induced ventricular arrhythmias.

Clearly, the clinician's first actions must be immediate and clear to all: call for further help and assistance, secure and maintain a clear airway, and administer 100% oxygen, by artificial ventilation if breathing is inadequate or absent. The maintenance of full oxygenation will be an ongoing requirement needing constant attention. If the onset of the reaction has not, perforce, resulted in the cessation of local anesthetic administration, then the clinician must ensure that this is the case. Particularly if apnea has occurred, or one of the longer-acting drugs is involved, an early check of the pulse rate and rhythm is vital—remember that the EKG will, almost certainly, be distorted by extensive electrical activity due to the muscle contraction associated with seizures. Simple, basic management may be all that is required in the event of a seizure following drugs such as lidocaine and mepivacaine, and may even suffice for the longer-acting ones, but some further points need to be made.

Acidosis and Hypoxia

It is impossible to overstress the importance of avoiding hypoxia and acidosis. Studies on isolated atrial tissue have shown that hypercarbia, acidosis, and hypoxia tend to potentiate the negative chronotropic and inotropic effects of both lidocaine

and bupivacaine (85,86), with the combination of hypoxia and acidosis having a marked effect on the toxicity of bupivacaine. This finding was confirmed by studies in intact sheep (22). Interestingly, this enhanced toxicity may not be related to greater myocardial uptake of drug because rabbit studies have shown a decrease in the uptake of bupivacaine in the presence of acidosis (87). Thus, the extreme cardiovascular effects of the more potent drugs such as bupivacaine may be due, in part at least, to an interaction with severe acid–base changes. Hypercarbia, acidosis, and hypoxia, as can occur in some patients because of the metabolic consequences of vigorous muscle activity during seizures, may be reduced by adequate lung ventilation with oxygen, but they may not be overcome. This is the rationale for taking a more active approach to the management of convulsions.

Controlling Seizure Activity

It has long been taught that convulsions due to an accidental IV bolus of local anaesthetic are brief, and that persisting seizures should raise the possibility that hypoxia is not being controlled adequately. There is probably more than a modicum of truth in this, and it is important to check that the lungs are being ventilated adequately with 100% oxygen. This does not negate the need to consider what further treatment is needed to stop the convulsions; convulsions may be the cause of inadequate lung ventilation. Two schools of thought exist on management:

■ *Anticonvulsant drugs.* Almost any drug with an anticonvulsant action might be used, but, with speed being of the essence, the clinician is advised to use familiar and immediately available agents. Intravenous thiopental (1–4 mg/kg), propofol (1–2 mg/kg), diazepam (0.15–0.3 mg/kg), or midazolam (0.075–0.15 mg/kg) are all suitable, and at least one is likely to be close to hand. The important point is to note the low doses advocated: These drugs are much more potent as anticonvulsants than as anesthetics, and use of anesthetic doses will add to the cardiovascular depression caused by local anesthetic toxicity.[a] A side issue is that benzodiazepines, such as diazepam and clonazepam, can completely protect rats against local anesthetic-induced convulsions (88,89). However, patients who are heavily medicated with these agents may not show any of the earlier signs of local anesthetic toxicity, with cardiac arrest being the presenting feature.

■ *Suxamethonium.* Because of concerns about the cardiovascular effects of sedative drugs, some advocate the use of this short-acting neuromuscular blocking drug in a dose of about 50 mg. The patient will become, if not already, totally apneic and thus dependent on the clinician's ability to intubate the trachea and ventilate the lungs. Suxamethonium will only stop the manifestations of seizure activity; it will not stop the seizures, and evidence exists (see earlier discussion) that seizures may contribute to the arrhythmogenesis. Thus, other drug treatment may be needed anyway.

Sparse evidence exists, despite firmly held opinions, as to the best method of controlling convulsions. Each method has its positive and negative features, and the clinician is advised to think the matter through *before* the clinical need arises, so that treatment is prompt and appropriate at the time.

Treatment of Arrhythmias

In the absence of evidence to the contrary, any arrhythmia that occurs should be treated according to the standard life support protocols mentioned earlier. However, evidence suggests that some drugs are better avoided in the setting of local anesthetic toxicity. These include Ca channel blockers, sodium valproate, phenytoin, and bretylium (89). Phosphodiesterase inhibitors, such as amrinone and milrinone, have generally failed to show benefit. That bretylium is now advised against is an indicator of the difficulties that can arise in drawing up recommendations for treating rare events; for many years, bretylium was the drug of choice for treating ventricular arrhythmias in this setting. Such difficulties also explain the considerable amount of research done in treatment of reactions.

Early Resuscitation Studies

Cats (90), dogs (91), sheep (91), and pigs (92,93) have all been used for studies of resuscitation from bupivacaine overdose, but it is important to note that mode of death (to say nothing of the doses of bupivacaine, L-bupivacaine, and ropivacaine required to cause cardiovascular collapse) tends to vary according to the experimental animal model used. One of the most striking differences is that animals given intracoronary local anesthetic die only from ventricular fibrillation, whereas after intravascular injection they die from either ventricular fibrillation or pump failure. If nothing else, this emphasizes the importance of viewing the evidence on treatment regimens with some caution before applying them to man.

In an early study by Kasten et al. (91), resuscitation of sheep and dogs was attempted after aliquots of bupivacaine 3 mg/kg were injected into the right atrium at 1-minute inter-

vals. The nature of the cardiovascular collapse was different in the two species: electromechanical dissociation and asystole occurred in the dogs, whereas ventricular fibrillation and asystole were more likely in sheep. Furthermore, the initial dose of bupivacaine used to cause cardiovascular collapse was sevenfold greater in dogs (24.6 mg/kg) compared to sheep (3.5 mg/kg). Resuscitation was performed using open chest heart massage, bretylium for treatment of ventricular arrhythmias, and epinephrine and atropine for treatment of electromechanical dissociation or asystole. Despite the larger dose needed for cardiovascular collapse, dogs were resuscitated after 2.1 min compared to 36.9 min for sheep. Dogs, unlike sheep, showed a resistance to further cardiovascular collapse.

Alternative Drugs for Resuscitation

Resuscitation of bupivacaine toxicity is often protracted, difficult, and associated with a poor outcome. Thus, drugs such as vasopressin (92,93), insulin (94,95), and amiodarone (96) have all been proposed to supplement the traditional advanced life support algorithms, with amiodarone being the only one of these to become a standard treatment for advanced life support.

Two studies were undertaken in pigs to investigate the efficacy of vasopressin during bupivacaine-induced cardiac arrest. In the first, epinephrine and vasopressin were compared (92). After 1 minute of untreated ventricular fibrillation, and 3 minutes of basic life support, the animals were randomized to receive either epinephrine (45, 45, and 200 μg/kg) or vasopressin (0.4, 0.4, and 0.8 U/kg) every 5 minutes. Vasopressin increased coronary perfusion pressure more than epinephrine, but only in those animals without concomitant epidural block. Animals were more likely to develop bradycardia with vasopressin, but metabolic acidosis was increased in animals receiving epinephrine. In the second pig study (93), the effects of saline, epinephrine, vasopressin, and the combination of epinephrine with vasopressin, were assessed after bupivacaine-induced cardiac arrest. Ventilation was interrupted for 3 minutes until asystole occurred, then cardiopulmonary resuscitation was started 1 minute later. After 2 minutes of cardiopulmonary resuscitation, each of the 28 animals was randomized to a study group. Resuscitation drugs and electroshock were administered every 5 minutes. In the combination group, all of the pigs survived; in the vasopressin group, five of seven survived; in the epinephrine group, four of seven; and in the placebo group, none of seven. Thus, both studies suggest that vasopressin may be an effective drug for resuscitation from bupivacaine toxicity, particularly when combined with epinephrine. Indeed, the Advanced Cardiac Life Support (ACLS) (82) guidelines state that one dose of vasopressin 40 U may replace the first or second dose of epinephrine during pulseless arrest.

Insulin has been proposed as a treatment for systemic local anesthetic toxicity, with the aim of improving myocardial energetics and performance. To test this hypothesis, 24 anesthetized dogs (94) were infused with bupivacaine until the mixed venous oxygen saturation decreased to 60% and then randomly assigned to one of four treatment groups: normal saline; glucose; glucose and insulin; and glucose, insulin and potassium. Mean arterial pressure (MAP), cardiac output, heart rate, and mixed venous oxygen saturation recovered toward baseline level more rapidly in the glucose-insulin and glucose-insulin-potassium groups, suggesting a beneficial effect on cardiac depression due to bupivacaine. In a similar experiment, also in anesthetized dogs, glucose-insulin-potassium reversed cardiovascular collapse (defined as a mean blood pressure of 40 mm Hg) induced by bupivacaine (95). The benefits of a glucose-insulin-potassium regimen may be attributed to enhanced

---

[a] See *Anesth Analg.* 2008;106:1429–1449.

repolarization of the myocyte action potential and increased delivery of glucose and pyruvate to the myocardial cells as metabolic substitutes for lipid. As noted earlier, the heart relies predominantly on long-chain fatty acid metabolism, but bupivacaine reduces ATP production by that route. However, excessive glucose is known to worsen CNS outcome after an ischemic insult, and the decision to use a glucose-insulin-potassium infusion should be balanced between overall benefits and side effects.

Amiodarone is recommended for treatment of arrhythmias in the ACLS guidelines, although its use may be associated with hypotension. One study (96) has investigated the efficacy of amiodarone therapy in a pig model of bupivacaine toxicity, exacerbated by hypoxia and hypercarbia. Although outcome was 50% better in pigs treated with amiodarone, more experience is needed before amiodarone can be promoted as the standard treatment of arrhythmias in the setting of local anesthetic systemic toxicity.

Advanced Life Support

The majority of animal studies have shown that resuscitation using sympathomimetics, particularly norepinephrine and epinephrine, improves outcome by increasing myocardial contractility. In addition, rapid elevations in blood pressure increase coronary perfusion pressure during resuscitation and facilitate local anesthetic cardiac washout (97). However, sympathomimetic drugs may have adverse effects. Epinephrine exacerbates arrhythmias without improving cardiac output or cardiac relaxation, especially in the setting of local anesthetic overdose (98,99).

A study by Feldman et al. (100) investigated whether modern advanced life support procedures improved survival from cardiac arrest after local anesthetic overdose. Twelve beagles received IV ropivacaine or bupivacaine, in a dose just sufficient to precipitate convulsions, followed 48 hours later by IV injection of twice the convulsive dose. Two dogs in the bupivacaine group developed ventricular fibrillation that was resistant to full advanced cardiopulmonary resuscitation, whereas all the beagles receiving ropivacaine survived.

More recent experimental resuscitation of dogs after incremental injection of lidocaine, bupivacaine, L-bupivacaine, and ropivacaine has used epinephrine, open-chest massage, and advanced cardiac life support protocols to treat hypotension and arrhythmias (99,101) when MAP was 45 mm Hg or lower. Mortality was significantly greater after bupivacaine (50%) and L-bupivacaine (30%) than after ropivacaine (10%) and lidocaine (0%), although, interestingly, six out of seven dogs that received lidocaine required a continuing epinephrine infusion to counteract myocardial depression, compared with two out of seven dogs receiving any of the longer-acting local anesthetics. As with the sheep model, epinephrine-induced ventricular fibrillation occurred more frequently after administration of bupivacaine.

These resuscitation studies, if they can be extrapolated to man, suggest that patients with ropivacaine-induced systemic toxicity are more responsive to epinephrine resuscitation than those with bupivacaine-induced toxicity. Further, improved survival from cardiac arrest induced by ropivacaine (versus bupivacaine) may be attributable to its smaller molecular size and not to its stereospecificity, because the results with L-bupivacaine were less strikingly different (101,102).

Lipid Infusion

Interference of local anesthetics with mitochondrial energy-linked processes by the uncoupling of oxidative phosphory-lation (50,51) and inhibition of respiratory chain enzymes was well recognized in the 1990s. However, translation of the relevance of this observation to the clinical setting of bupivacaine toxicity was not made until a 16-year-old with isovaleric acidemia, an autosomal recessive disease of leucine catabolism characterized by intermittent episodes of metabolic acidosis, presented for bilateral axillary liposuction (103). After infiltration of only 22 mg of bupivacaine under general anesthesia, her EKG showed a junctional bradycardia then a wide complex ventricular dysrhythmia. Hypotension was treated with 100% oxygen, immediate cessation of inhalational anesthesia, and IV ephedrine 15 mg.

A subsequent study of rat ventricular myocyte mitochondria (104) showed that bupivacaine inhibited carnitine-acylcarnitine translocase, the enzyme necessary for transport of fatty acids into the mitochondrial matrix, reducing the primary supply of energy for the heart. Inhibition of carnitine-acylcarnitine translocase (Fig. 5-2) is consistent with the reductions in intracellular ATP levels, inhibition of myocardial contractility, and the poor recovery from resuscitation often seen in systemic toxicity. Furthermore, it is consistent with the exacerbation of bupivacaine-induced cardiotoxicity by hypoxia and the relatively narrow window between convulsions and cardiovascular collapse.

A chance finding (105) that lipid pretreatment increased the dose of bupivacaine required to produce asystole in rats stimulated research into the use of IV lipid for resuscitation. Infusion of lipid was tested initially in rats (106) and dogs (107) to investigate survival from bupivacaine-induced cardiac arrests. In the first study, 24 rats were randomized to receive the same volume of saline or three (10%, 20%, or 30%) concentrations of Intralipid, then were given 0.75% bupivacaine until asystole occurred (106). The results showed a clear correlation between the dose of bupivacaine needed to produce asystole and the amount of lipid infused, the dose of bupivacaine increasing by 56%, 181%, and 363% above control (saline) with each dose of lipid, and signifying marked protection against bupivacaine toxicity. In the dog study, 12 animals were given IV bupivacaine 10 mg/kg. After cardiac arrest, the dogs received internal cardiac massage for 10 minutes to replicate clinical practice. They were then randomized to receive saline (placebo) or intravenous lipid 20%, each administered as a bolus of 4 mL/kg followed by a continuous infusion of 0.5 mL/kg/min (107). All of the dogs treated with Intralipid were resuscitated successfully, whereas none of the animals treated with saline survived.

In addition to this animal work, two case reports have been published (108,109) documenting successful resuscitation, including the use of lipid infusion, after cardiac arrest due to inadvertent IV injection of large doses of local anesthetic.

In one report, a 58-year-old man with coronary artery disease and presenting for arthroscopic repair of a torn shoulder rotator cuff developed a tonic–clonic seizure shortly after the interscalene injection of bupivacaine (100 mg) and mepivacaine (300 mg). The seizure was stopped briefly by the administration of propofol, but recurred 90 seconds later, so more propofol was administered. However, the patient developed asystole, and advanced life support was initiated. Despite a total of 3 mg epinephrine, 2 mg atropine, 300 mg amiodarone, 40 U arginine vasopressin, and cardioversion for ventricular tachycardia/fibrillation, resuscitation was initially unsuccessful. After 20 minutes, 100 mL of IV 20% Intralipid was given, followed by an infusion of 0.5 mL/kg/min over 2 hours. Resuscitation was successful, and the patient made a full recovery.

In the second report, 40 mL of ropivacaine 1% was injected mistakenly (0.5% was intended) for axillary plexus block in an

84-year-old woman. After 15 minutes, she complained of dizziness and drowsiness, and developed a generalized tonic–clonic seizure followed by an asystolic cardiac arrest of 10 minutes' duration. A 100 mL bolus of Intralipid 20% was administered, followed by a continuous infusion of 10 mL/min. After a total 200 mL had been given, spontaneous electrical activity and cardiac output were restored, and the patient recovered completely.

In view of these reports of successful resuscitation in both experimental animals and human patients, recommendations for the use of Intralipid in local anesthetic-induced cardiac arrest unresponsive to standard resuscitation procedures have been issued (105):

- Bolus of Intralipid 20% 1.5 mL/kg over 1 minute
- Infusion of Intralipid at a rate of 0.25 mL/kg/min
- Chest compressions (lipid must circulate)
- Repeated bolus of Intralipid 20% every 3 to 5 minutes, up to 3 mL/kg total dose until circulation is restored
- Intralipid infusion continued until hemodynamic stability is restored and infusion rate increased to 0.5 mL/kg/min if the blood pressure declines
- A maximum total dose of 8 mL/kg is recommended

However, it must be recognized that these recommendations represent no more than a "best guess" in humans, interesting though the work is. Intralipid has only been reported twice in the medical literature for this purpose in humans. Its side effects in this setting remain unknown, and much more research is needed to define the optimum regimen and its relationship to other components of the resuscitation regimen. In addition, the immediate relevance of the animal work to man is unclear, and both case reports are open to criticism: the adequacy of basic resuscitation has been questioned in the first (110), and the second was clearly due to a failure to check the labels of the ampoules from which the injection was drawn. Nevertheless, additional case reports of lipid resuscitation used in local anesthetic intoxication should be reported to, and reviewed on, the web site maintained by Weinberg (104).

Two hypotheses have been proposed to explain the mechanism of the lipid effect in local anesthetic–induced systemic toxicity. The indirect hypothesis proposes that lipid acts as "sink" for the lipid-soluble local anesthetic, drawing it from tissues, especially those of the myocardium, and back into the circulation. However, reversal of toxicity occurs very quickly and at a rate incompatible with bulk extraction of drug from myocardial tissue. The alternative "direct" hypothesis proposes a metabolic benefit of lipid therapy, the suggestion being that high plasma triglyceride concentrations override the inhibition of mitochondrial carnitine-acylcarnitine translocase by local anesthetics. Using an isolated rat heart model, Stehr et al. (111) and Weinberg et al. (112) have shown faster restoration of cardiac contractility and rate pressure product and accelerated removal of bupivacaine from heart tissue, but neither the direct nor the indirect hypothesis remains proven.[b]

Prevention

Despite translational advances in cell biology and case reports of apparently effective resuscitation with lipid, the best means for dealing with systemic toxicity remains its prevention. Regional anesthesia should always be performed in an environment equipped to manage anesthesia and cardiac arrest: an

anesthetic machine, a reliable oxygen supply, full noninvasive monitoring (EKG, NIBP, SPo_2, Fio_2, and $ETCo_2$), suction, a full range of anesthetic and resuscitative drugs, and trained assistance. Recourse to resuscitation efforts still means, however, a failure of prevention.

The prevention of systemic toxicity requires a careful, almost obsessive, approach to safety. Both the selection of local anesthetic and its dose should be appropriate for the planned block and the individual patient. The suitability of different drugs for the various block procedures is dealt with in relevant chapters of this book. Dose selection requires a consideration of a range of patient-related factors, in addition to the requirements and risks (especially rate of absorption) of a particular block. Age, weight, pregnancy, and preexisting medical conditions such as cardiac, hepatic, and renal disease all influence the plasma concentrations of local anesthetics (113,114) (see Chapter 3), and each may suggest a reduction in dose. Elderly patients are particularly sensitive to local anesthetic effect, and patients with chronic liver disease and other causes of reduced drug clearance are particularly prone to toxicity from repeated injection or continuous infusion. Taking these factors into consideration, it is evident that a "one safe maximum dose fits all approach" (in either absolute or weight-related terms) is inappropriate. It makes no sense to consider that the same dose may be used safely in an 80-year-old with significant intercurrent disease as in a healthy 20-year-old just because they are of the same weight and are having the same block performed.

Ampoules and other containers must be checked carefully before, during, and after the solution is drawn up, with syringes or infusion systems clearly labelled immediately, and infusion lines equally clearly identified when continuous blocks are being used. If drugs are being mixed with others or diluted for infusion, it makes sense to have the solution prepared (in a sterile environment apart from anything else) by the hospital pharmacy.

All possible care must be taken to minimize the possibility of intravascular injection. Usually IV injection is the concern, but blocks in the head and neck raise the possibility of arterial injection, in which only a small dose can produce a major CNS reaction. As some epidemiologic data presented earlier suggest, it may be that exists a certain minimal incidence that cannot be reduced, but that does not mean that every effort should not be made to avoid a life-threatening complication.

Prevention is the sole responsibility of the anesthesiologist and requires constant vigilance during *and after* injection. Whatever local anaesthetic drug or concentration is used, the clinician must keep communicating with the patient and observing standard monitors. Before injection, the syringe or catheter must be aspirated gently to detect any vascular placement, although a negative aspiration test does not guarantee that this has not occurred: Gentle aspiration must be used to prevent a negative pressure that causes the vessel to collapse and no blood to run out. If a catheter has been inserted, it may be better to hold the operator's end below the level of the heart to see if blood simply siphons out.

Recognition that the aspiration test can produce false-negative responses led to the introduction of the test dose: the initial injection of a small aliquot of solution with the aim of demonstrating a systemic effect. The usual constituents of a test dose are either a local anesthetic and/or epinephrine, with systemic placement resulting in the prodromal features of toxicity or tachycardia, respectively. However, neither approach is ideal. Patients may not understand what is expected of them when questioned about subtle symptoms such as paresthesias and tinnitus, and many factors can cause an increase in heart rate and blood pressure (or obscure such changes) in the

---

[b]See *Anesth Analy.* 2008;106:1333–1342.

preoperative or laboring patient (115). Furthermore, any test dose must contain enough agent to have a high probability of producing a systemic effect without causing harm. If a local anesthetic test dose is to be used, 5 mL lidocaine 2% (or its equivalent) is required; if epinephrine is used, then up to 15 μg may be needed, but neither is definitive. Thus, even after negative aspiration and test dose, slow incremental injection of the anesthetic dose in 5-mL aliquots at 60-second intervals is recommended. The benefits are a reduction in plasma concentration of local anesthetic if the injection is accidentally intravascular (116) and an opportunity for the anesthesiologist to note the early clinical signs and symptoms of developing toxicity. Currently, no practical method exists for physically demonstrating with absolute certainty that an epidural catheter does or does not lie within a vessel.

CURRENT POSITION

Sadly, the introduction of the potentially safer local anesthetics, such as L-bupivacaine and ropivacaine, has not eliminated systemic toxicity. Accumulating case reports have described agitation and convulsions with L-bupivacaine (117–120) and ropivacaine (121–128). Of greater concern are three publications describing cardiac arrest with ropivacaine. In the first, a 76-year-old woman received a femoral block with 20 mL of 1.5% mepivacaine and 1:400,000 epinephrine and an anterior sciatic block with 32 mL of 0.5% ropivacaine and 1:400,000 epinephrine (129). Despite negative aspiration and incremental injection, she had a convulsion followed by ventricular fibrillation. In the second report, a patient experienced cardiac arrest after injection of ropivacaine for posterior lumbar plexus blockade (130). In the third case (131), a patient with severe myocardial disease and renal failure underwent brachial plexus block for formation of an arteriovenous fistula when accidental intravascular injection of ropivacaine resulted in ventricular fibrillation. All patients made a full recovery after resuscitation, but it is clear that use of an allegedly "safer" drug alone is not enough to ensure that adverse events will not occur.

Curiously, local anesthetic–induced cardiac arrest was not described by Brown (2) or Auroy (3,4) in their studies of local anesthetic complications; convulsions were the most serious manifestation of systemic toxicity that they reported. It is imperative that introduction of new local anesthetics does not lead to changes in practice that offset the margin of safety that these drugs offer. For example, if a new local anesthetic offers a 30% to 40% improvement in toxicity compared to bupivacaine, then giving a 50% larger dose of the new agent not only negates any safety advantage, but actually increases the risk of toxicity. So too does the assumption that, at lower doses, this "safer" drug can be injected quickly.

Judicious alterations in practice have the potential to reduce further the incidence of systemic toxicity. The change from the rapid injection of large volumes of bupivacaine to incremental injection through a catheter quickly resulted in a reduction in the problems seen with this anesthetic during epidural block.

Perhaps the more routine use of perineural catheters for major limb blocks will have a similar effect in reducing the present concerning incidence of adverse effects.

Recently, enthusiastic claims have been made (103) for the potential of ultrasound imaging to improve the success and minimize the complications of regional anesthesia. Ultrasound does allow the clinician to visualize the position of the needle or catheter, their relationship to other structures such as nerves and large blood vessels, and the spread of local anesthetic solution. A retrospective study of 1,146 infraclavicular blocks for hand surgery conducted by Sandhu et al. (132) reported a 99.3% block success rate and no cases of nerve injury, pneumothorax, or local anesthetic toxicity. This is a good start, but the total number of cases is small relative to the predicted incidence of accidental intravascular injections. Ultrasound is a technique that requires careful training and informed use if it is to deliver its potential benefits, to say nothing of justifying its cost. As with new and safer drugs, it is not a substitute for careful practice; it is another adjunct to it. No reports have been published of complications associated with ultrasound use, but anecdotal reports of problems have surfaced, usually in connection with the fact that the responsible clinician had not received appropriate training—which remains the source of all safe practice.

APPENDIX

In light of several recent editorials and publications on the subject of lipid emulsion for the treatment of local anesthetic toxicity, the authors encourage readers to review the following articles of interest:

Rowlingson J. Lipid Rescue: A Step Forward in Patient Safety? Likely So! *Anesth Analg.* 2008;106:1333–1336.

Brull SJ. Lipid Emulsion for the Treatment of Local Anesthetic Toxicity: Patient Safety Implications. *Anesth Analg.* 2008;106:1337–1339.

Weinberg GL. Lipid Infusion Therapy: Translation to Clinical Practice. *Anesth Analg.* 2008;106:1340–1342.

Litz RJ, Roessel T, Heller AR, et al. Reversal of central nervous system and cardiac toxicity after local anesthetic intoxication by lipid emulsion injection. *Anesth Analg.* 2008;106:1575–1577.

Ludot H, Tharin J-Y, Belooudah M, et al. Successful resuscitation after ropivacaine and lidocaine-induced ventricular arrhythmia following posterior lumbar plexus block in a child. *Anesth Analg.* 2008;106:1572–1574.

Mayr VD, Mitterschiffthaler L, Neurauter A, et al. A comparison of the combination of epinephrine and vasopressin with lipid emulsion in a porcine model of asphyxial cardiac arrest after intravenous injection of bupivacaine. *Anesth Analg.* 2008;106:1566–1571.

Warren J, Brian T, Georgescu A, et al. Intravenous lipid infusion in the successful resuscitation of local anesthetic-induced cardiovascular collapse after supraclavicular brachial plexus block. *Anesth Analg.* 2008;106:1578–1580.

References

1. Albright G. Cardiac arrest following regional anesthesia with etidocaine or bupivacaine. *Anesthesiology* 1979;51:285–287.
2. Brown DL, Ransom DM, Hall JA, et al. Regional anesthesia and local anesthetic-induced systemic toxicity: Seizure frequency and accompanying cardiovascular changes. *Anesth Analg* 1995;81(2):321–328.
3. Auroy Y, Narchi P, Messiah A, et al. Serious complications related to regional anesthesia: Results of a prospective survey in France. *Anesthesiology* 1997;87(3):479–486.
4. Auroy Y, Benhamou D, Bargues L, et al. Major complications of regional anesthesia in France: The SOS Regional Anesthesia Hotline Service. *Anesthesiology* 2002;97(5):1274–1280.

5. McClure JH. Ropivacaine. *Br J Anaesth* 1996;76:300–307.
6. McLeod GA, Burke D. Levobupivacaine. *Anaesthesia* 2001;56(4):331–341.
7. Rao RB, Ely SF, Hoffman RS. Deaths related to liposuction. *N Engl J Med* 1999;340(19):1471–1475.
8. Grazer FM, de Jong RH. Fatal outcomes from liposuction: Census survey of cosmetic surgeons. *Plast Reconstr Surg* 2000;105:436–448.
9. Toledo LS, Mauad R. Complications of body sculpture: Prevention and treatment. *Clin Plast Surg* 2006;33(1):1–11, v.
10. NPS Agency. Patient Safety Alert No 21. At www.npsa.nhs.uk/site/media/documents/2462_Epidural_alert_FINAL.pdf. Accessed 08 April 2008.
11. Newton DJ, Amyes AK, Khan F, et al. Vasoactive properties of lignocaine administered by iontophoresis in human skin. *Clin Sci (Lond)* 2003;104(1):87–92.
12. Newton DJ, McLeod GA, Khan F, Belch JJ. Vasoactive characteristics of bupivacaine and laevo-bupivacaine with and without adjuvant epinephrine in peripheral human skin. *Br J Anaesth* 2005;94(5):662–667.
13. Moss GP. Basic Terminology of Stereochemistry. International Union of Pure and Applied Chemistry and (IUPAC), 1996.
14. Vladimirov M, Nau C, Mok WM, Strichartz G. Potency of bupivacaine stereoisomers tested in vitro and in vivo: Biochemical, electrophysiological, and neurobehavioral studies. *Anesthesiology* 2000;93(3):744–755.
15. Aberg G. Toxicological and local anaesthetic effects of optically active isomers of two local anaesthetic compounds. *Acta Pharmacol Toxicol (Copenh)* 1972;31(4):273–286.
16. Luduena FP, Bogado EF, Tullar BF. Optical isomers of mepivacaine and bupivacaine. *Arch Int Pharmacodyn Ther* 1972;200(2):359–369.
17. de Jong RH, Bonin JD. Deaths from local anesthetic-induced convulsions in mice. *Anesth Analg* 1980;59(6):401–405.
18. Liu P, Feldman HS, Covino BM, et al. Acute cardiovascular toxicity of intravenous amide local anesthetics in anesthetized ventilated dogs. *Anesth Analg* 1982;61:317–322.
19. Hotvedt R, Refsum H, Helgesen KG. Cardiac electrophysiologic and hemodynamic effects related to plasma levels of bupivacaine in the dog. *Anesth Analg* 1985;64:388–394.
20. Liu PL, Feldman HS, Giasi R, et al. Comparative CNS toxicity of lidocaine, etidocaine, bupivacaine, and tetracaine in awake dogs following rapid intravenous administration. *Anesth Analg* 1983;62(4):375–379.
21. Kotelko DM, Shnider SM, Dailey PA, et al. Bupivacaine-induced cardiac arrhythmias in sheep. *Anesthesiology* 1984;60(1):10–18.
22. Rosen MA, Thigpen JW, Shnider SM, et al. Bupivacaine-induced cardiotoxicity in hypoxic and acidotic sheep. *Anesth Analg* 1985;64(11):1089–1096.
23. Morishima HO, Pedersen H, Finster M, et al. Bupivacaine toxicity in pregnant and nonpregnant ewes. *Anesthesiology* 1985;63(2):134–139.
24. Clarkson CW, Hondeghem LM. Mechanisms for bupivacaine depression of cardiac conduction: Fast block of sodium channels during the action potential with slow recovery from block during diastole. *Anesthesiology* 1985;62:396–405.
25. Arlock P. Actions of three local anaesthetics: Lidocaine, bupivacaine and ropivacaine on guinea pig papillary muscle sodium channels (Vmax). *Pharmacol Toxicol* 1988:96–104.
26. Harding DP, Collier PA, Huckle R. Cardiotoxic effects of laevo-bupivacaine, bupivacaine and ropivacaine: An in vitro study in guinea-pig and human cardiac muscle. *Br J Pharmacol* 1998;125[Suppl]:P127.
27. Vanhoutte F, Vereecke J, Verbeke N, Carmeliet E. Stereoselective effects of the enantiomers of bupivacaine on the electrophysiological properties of the guinea-pig papillary muscle. *Br J Pharmacol* 1991;103(1):1275–1281.
28. Valenzuela C, Snyders DJ, Bennett PB, et al. Stereoselective block of cardiac sodium channels by bupivacaine in guinea pig ventricular myocytes. *Circulation* 1995;92(10):3014–3024.
29. Kanai Y, Katsuki H, Takasaki M. Comparisons of the anesthetic potency and intracellular concentrations of S(−) and R(+) bupivacaine and ropivacaine in giant crayfish giant white axon. *Anesth Analg* 2000;90:415–420.
30. Aya AG, de la Coussaye JE, Robert E, et al. Comparison of the effects of racemic bupivacaine, laevo-bupivacaine, and ropivacaine on ventricular conduction, refractoriness, and wavelength: An epicardial mapping study. *Anesthesiology* 2002;96(3):641–650.
31. Valenzuela C, Delpon E, Tamkun MM, et al. Stereoselective block of a human cardiac potassium channel (Kv1.5) by bupivacaine enantiomers. *Biophys J* 1995;69(2):418–427.
32. Longobardo M, Gonzalez T, Navarro-Polanco R, et al. Effects of a quaternary bupivacaine derivative on delayed rectifier K(+) currents. *Br J Pharmacol* 2000;130(2):391–401.
33. Gonzalez T, Arias C, Caballero R, et al. Effects of laevo-bupivacaine, ropivacaine and bupivacaine on HERG channels: Stereoselective bupivacaine block. *Br J Pharmacol* 2002;137:1269–1279.
34. Friederich P, Solth A, Schillemeit S, Isbrandt D. Local anaesthetic sensitivities of cloned HERG channels from human heart: Comparison with HERG/MiRP1 and HERG/MiRP1T8A. *Br J Anaesth* 2004;92:93–101.
35. Siebrands CC, Schmitt N, Friederich P. Local anesthetic interaction with human ether-a-go-go-related gene (HERG) channels: Role of aromatic amino acids Y652 and F656. *Anesthesiology* 2005;103(1):102–112.

36. Zhou W, Arrabit C, Choe S, Slesinger PA. Mechanism underlying bupivacaine inhibition of G protein-gated inwardly rectifying K+ channels. *Proc Natl Acad Sci USA* 2001;98(11):6482–6487.
37. Kawano T, Oshita S, Takahashi A, et al. Molecular mechanisms of the inhibitory effects of bupivacaine, laevo-bupivacaine, and ropivacaine on sarcolemmal adenosine triphosphate-sensitive potassium channels in the cardiovascular system. *Anesthesiology* 2004;101(2):390–398.
38. Punke MA, Licher T, Pongs O, Friederich P. Inhibition of human TREK-1 channels by bupivacaine. *Anesth Analg* 2003;96(6):1665–1673.
39. Kindler CH, Yost CS. Two-pore domain potassium channels: New sites of local anesthetic action and toxicity. *Reg Anesth Pain Med* 2005;30(3):260–274.
40. Barr CS, Naas A, Freeman M, et al. QT dispersion and sudden unexpected death in chronic heart failure. *Lancet* 1994;343(8893):327–329.
41. Valenzuela C, Delpon E, Franqueza L, et al. Effects of ropivacaine on a potassium channel (hKv1.5) cloned from human ventricle. *Anesthesiology* 1997;86(3):718–728.
42. Longobardo M, Gonzalez T, Caballero R, et al. Bupivacaine effects on hKv1.5 channels are dependent on extracellular pH. *Br J Pharmacol* 2001;134(2):359–369.
43. Kindler CH, Paul M, Zou H, et al. Amide local anesthetics potently inhibit the human tandem pore domain background K+ Channel TASK-2 (KCNK5). *J Pharmacol Exp Ther* 2003;306:84–92.
44. Komai H, Lokuta AJ. Interaction of bupivacaine and tetracaine with the sarcoplasmic reticulum Ca2+ release channel of skeletal and cardiac muscle. *Anesthesiology* 1999;90(3):835–843.
45. Rossner KL, Freese KJ. Bupivacaine inhibition of L-type calcium current in ventricular cardiomyocytes of hamster. *Anesthesiology* 1997;87(4):926–934.
46. Zapata-Sudo G, Trachez MM, Sudo RT, Nelson TE. Is comparative cardiotoxicity of S(−) and R(+) bupivacaine related to enantiomer-selective inhibition of L-type Ca(2+) channels? *Anesth Analg* 2001;92(2):496–501.
47. Dabadie P, Bendriss P, Erny P, Mazat JP. Uncoupling effects of local anesthetics on rat liver mitochondria. *FEBS Lett* 1987;226(1):77–82.
48. Terada H, Shima O, Yoshida K, Shinohara Y. Effects of the local anesthetic bupivacaine on oxidative phosphorylation in mitochondria. Change from decoupling to uncoupling by formation of a leakage type ion pathway specific for H+ in cooperation with hydrophobic anions. *J Biol Chem* 1990;265(14):7837–7842.
49. Schonfeld P, Sztark F, Slimani M, et al. Is bupivacaine a decoupler, a protonophore or a proton-leak-inducer? *FEBS Lett* 1992;304(2–3):273–276.
50. Butterworth JF 4th, Brownlow RC, Leith JP, et al. Bupivacaine inhibits cyclic-3′,5′-adenosine monophosphate production. A possible contributing factor to cardiovascular toxicity. *Anesthesiology* 1993;79(1):88–95.
51. Sztark F, Tueux O, Erny P, et al. Effects of bupivacaine on cellular oxygen consumption and adenine nucleotide metabolism. *Anesth Analg* 1994;78(2):335–339.
52. Floridi A, Barbieri R, Pulselli R, et al. Effect of the local anesthetic bupivacaine on the energy metabolism of Ehrlich ascites tumor cells. *Oncol Res* 1994;6(12):593–601.
53. Pulselli R, Arcuri E, Paggi MG, Floridi A. Changes in membrane potential induced by local anesthetic bupivacaine on mitochondria within Ehrlich ascites tumor cells. *Oncol Res* 1996;8(7–8):267–271.
54. Sztark F, Ouhabi R, Dabadie P, Mazat JP. Effects of the local anesthetic bupivacaine on mitochondrial energy metabolism: Change from uncoupling to decoupling depending on the respiration state. *Biochem Mol Biol Int* 1997;43(5):997–1003.
55. Sztark F, Malgat M, Dabadie P, Mazat JP. Comparison of the effects of bupivacaine and ropivacaine on heart cell mitochondrial bioenergetics. *Anesthesiology* 1998;88(5):1340–1349.
56. Nava-Ocampo AA, Bello-Ramirez AM. Lipophilicity affects the pharmacokinetics and toxicity of local anaesthetic agents administered by caudal block. *Clin Exp Pharmacol Physiol* 2004;31(1–2):116–118.
57. Sztark F, Nouette-Gaulain K, Malgat M, et al. Absence of stereospecific effects of bupivacaine isomers on heart mitochondrial bioenergetics. *Anesthesiology* 2000;93(2):456–462.
58. Mazoit JX, Boico O, Samii K. Myocardial uptake of bupivacaine: II. Pharmacokinetics and pharmacodynamics of bupivacaine enantiomers in the isolated perfused rabbit heart. *Anesth Analg* 1993;77(3):477–482.
59. Graf BM, Martin E, Bosnjak ZJ, Stowe DF. Stereospecific effect of bupivacaine isomers on atrioventricular conduction in the isolated perfused guinea pig heart. *Anesthesiology* 1997;86(2):410–419.
60. Graf BM, Eberl S, Abraham I, et al. *Anesthesiology* 1998;89:A–76.
61. Heavner JE. Cardiac dysrhythmias induced by infusion of local anesthetics into the lateral cerebral ventricle of cats. *Anesth Analg* 1986;65:133–138.
62. Thomas RD, Behbehani MM, Coyle ED, Denson DD. Cardiovascular toxicity of local anesthetics. *Anesth Analg* 1986;65:444–450.
63. Denson DD, Behbehani MM, Gregg RV. Enantiomer-specific effects of an intravenously administered arrhythmogenic dose of bupivacaine on neurons of the nucleus tractus solitarius and the cardiovascular system in the anesthetized rat. *Reg Anesth* 1992;17(6):311–316.

64. Ladd LA, Chang DH, Wilson KA, et al. Effects of CNS site-directed carotid arterial infusions of bupivacaine, laevo-bupivacaine, and ropivacaine in sheep. *Anesthesiology* 2002;97(2):418–428.

65. Rutten AJ, Nancarrow C, Mather LE, et al. Hemodynamic and central nervous system effects of intravenous bolus doses of lidocaine, bupivacaine, and ropivacaine in sheep. *Anesth Analg* 1989;69(3):291–299.

66. Huang YF, Pryor ME, Mather LE, Veering BT. Cardiovascular and central nervous system effects of intravenous laevo-bupivacaine and bupivacaine in sheep. *Anesth Analg* 1998;86(4):797–804.

67. Nancarrow C, Rutten AJ, Runciman WB, et al. Myocardial and cerebral drug concentrations and the mechanisms of death after fatal intravenous doses of lidocaine, bupivacaine, and ropivacaine in the sheep. *Anesth Analg* 1989;69(3):276–283.

68. Chang DH, Ladd LA, Wilson KA, et al. Tolerability of large-dose intravenous laevo-bupivacaine in sheep. *Anesth Analg* 2000;91(3):671–679.

69. Moller RA, Datta S, Fox J, et al. Effects of progesterone on the cardiac electrophysiologic action of bupivacaine and lidocaine. *Anesthesiology* 1992;76(4):604–608.

70. Morishima HO, Finster M, Arthur GR, Covino BG. Pregnancy does not alter lidocaine toxicity. *Am J Obstet Gynecol* 1990;162(5):1320–1324.

71. Santos AC, Arthur GR, Wlody D, et al. Comparative systemic toxicity of ropivacaine and bupivacaine in nonpregnant and pregnant ewes. *Anesthesiology* 1995;82(3):734–740; [Discussion, 27A].

72. Santos AC, Arthur GR, Pedersen H, et al. Systemic toxicity of ropivacaine during ovine pregnancy. *Anesthesiology* 1991;75(1):137–141.

73. Santos AC, DeArmas PI. Systemic toxicity of laevo-bupivacaine, bupivacaine, and ropivacaine during continuous intravenous infusion to nonpregnant and pregnant ewes. *Anesthesiology* 2001;95(5):1256–1264.

74. Reiz S, Haggmark S, Johansson G, Nath S. Cardiotoxicity of ropivacaine–a new amide local anaesthetic agent. *Acta Anaesthesiol Scand* 1989;33(2):93–98.

75. Morrison SG, Dominguez JJ, Frascarolo P, Reiz S. A comparison of the electrocardiographic cardiotoxic effects of racemic bupivacaine, laevo-bupivacaine, and ropivacaine in anesthetized swine. *Anesth Analg* 2000;90(6):1308–1314.

76. Chang DH, Ladd LA, Copeland S, et al. Direct cardiac effects of intracoronary bupivacaine, laevo-bupivacaine and ropivacaine in the sheep. *Br J Pharmacol* 2001;132(3):649–658.

77. Scott DB, Lee A, Fagan D, et al. Acute toxicity of ropivacaine compared with that of bupivacaine. *Anesth Analg* 1989;69(5):563–569.

78. Knudsen K, Beckman Suurkula M, et al. Central nervous and cardiovascular effects of i.v. infusions of ropivacaine, bupivacaine and placebo in volunteers. *Br J Anaesth* 1997;78(5):507–514.

79. Bardsley H, Gristwood R, Baker Hea. A comparison of the cardiovascular effects of laevo-bupivacaine and rac-bupivacaine following intravenous administration to administration to healthy volunteers. *Br J Clin Pharmacol* 1998;46:245–249.

80. Stewart J, Kellett N, Castro D. The central nervous system and cardiovascular effects of laevo-bupivacaine and ropivacaine in healthy volunteers. *Anesth Analg* 2003;97(2):412–416.

81. Van F, Rolan PA, Brennan N. Differential effects of laevo-bupivacaine and racemic bupivacaine on the EEG in volunteers. *Reg Anesth Pain Med* 1998;23:48.

82. American Heart Association Guidelines For Cardiopulmonary Resuscitation and Emergency Cardiovascular Care. *Circulation* 2005:58–66.

83. *Advanced Life Support*, 5th ed. London: Resuscitation Council (UK) Trading Ltd, 2006.

84. Corcoran W, Butterworth J, Weller RS, et al. Local anesthetic-induced cardiac toxicity: A survey of contemporary practice strategies among academic anesthesiology departments. *Anesth Analg* 2006;103(5):1322–1326.

85. Sage DJ, Feldman HS, Arthur GR, et al. Influence of lidocaine and bupivacaine on isolated guinea pig atria in the presence of acidosis and hypoxia. *Anesth Analg* 1984;63(1):1–7.

86. Heavner JE, Dryden CF Jr., Sanghani V, et al. Severe hypoxia enhances central nervous system and cardiovascular toxicity of bupivacaine in lightly anaesthetized pigs. *Anesthesiology* 1992;77:142–147.

87. Halpern SH, Eisler EA, Shnider SM. Myocardial tissue uptake of bupivacaine and lidocaine after intravenous injection in normal and acidotic rabbits. *Anesthesiology* 1984;61:A208.

88. De Jong RH, Heavner JE. Diazepam prevents local anesthetic seizures. *Anesthesiology* 1971;34(6):523–531.

89. Sawaki K, Ohno K, Miyamoto K, et al. Effects of anticonvulsants on local anaesthetic-induced neurotoxicity in rats. *Pharmacol Toxicol* 2000;86(2):59–62.

90. Chadwick HS. Toxicity and resuscitation in lidocaine- or bupivacaine-infused cats. *Anesthesiology* 1985;63(4):385–390.

91. Kasten GW, Martin ST. Comparison of resuscitation of sheep and dogs after bupivacaine-induced cardiovascular collapse. *Anesth Analg* 1986;65(10):1029–1032.

92. Krismer AC, Hogan QH, Wenzel V, et al. The efficacy of epinephrine or vasopressin for resuscitation during epidural anesthesia. *Anesth Analg* 2001;93(3):734–742.

93. Mayr VD, Raedler C, Wenzel V, et al. A comparison of epinephrine and vasopressin in a porcine model of cardiac arrest after rapid intravenous injection of bupivacaine. *Anesth Analg* 2004;98(5):1426–1431.

94. Cho HS, Lee JJ, Chung IS, et al. Insulin reverses bupivacaine-induced cardiac depression in dogs. *Anesth Analg* 2000;91(5):1096–1102.

95. Kim JT, Jung CW, Lee KH. The effect of insulin on the resuscitation of bupivacaine-induced severe cardiovascular toxicity in dogs. *Anesth Analg* 2004;99(3):728–733.

96. Haasio J, Pitkanen MT, Rosenberg PH. Treatment of bupivacaine-induced cardiac arrhythmias in hypoxic and hypercarbic pigs with amio. *Reg Anesth* 1991;15:174–179.

97. Igarashi T, Hirabayashi Y, Saitoh K, et al. Dose-related cardiovascular effects of amrinone and epinephrine in reversing bupivacaine-induced cardiovascular depression. *Acta Anaesthesiol Scand* 1998;42(6):698–706.

98. Bernards CM, Carpenter RL, Kenter ME, et al. Effect of epinephrine on central nervous system and cardiovascular system toxicity of bupivacaine in pigs. *Anesthesiology* 1989;71(5):711–717.

99. Groban L, Deal DD, Vernon JC, et al. Cardiac resuscitation after incremental overdosage with lidocaine, bupivacaine, laevo-bupivacaine, and ropivacaine in anesthetized dogs. *Anesth Analg* 2001;92(1):37–43.

100. Feldman HS, Arthur GR, Pitkanen M, et al. Treatment of acute systemic toxicity after the rapid intravenous injection of ropivacaine and bupivacaine in the conscious dog. *Anesth Analg* 1991;73(4):373–384.

101. Groban L, Deal DD, Vernon JC, et al. Does local anesthetic stereoselectivity or structure predict myocardial depression in anesthetized canines? *Reg Anesth Pain Med* 2002;27(5):460–468.

102. Graf BM, Abraham I, Eberbach N, et al. Differences in cardiotoxicity of bupivacaine and ropivacaine are the result of physicochemical and stereoselective properties. *Anesthesiology* 2002;96(6):1427–1434.

103. Weinberg GL, Laurito CE, Geldner P, et al. Malignant ventricular dysrhythmias in a patient with isovaleric acidemia receiving general and local anesthesia for suction lipectomy. *J Clin Anesth* 1997;9(8):668–670.

104. Weinberg GL, Palmer JW, VadeBoncouer TR, et al. Bupivacaine inhibits acylcarnitine exchange in cardiac mitochondria. *Anesthesiology* 2000;92(2):523–528.

105. Weinberg GL. LipidRescue: Resuscitation for local anesthetic toxicity. At www.lipidrescue.org. Accessed 01 Jan 1997.

106. Weinberg GL, VadeBoncouer T, Ramaraju GA, et al. Pretreatment or resuscitation with a lipid infusion shifts the dose-response to bupivacaine-induced asystole in rats. *Anesthesiology* 1998;8(4):1071–1075.

107. Weinberg G, Ripper R, Feinstein DL, Hoffman W. Lipid emulsion infusion rescues dogs from bupivacaine-induced cardiac toxicity. *Reg Anesth Pain Med* 2003;28(3):198–202.

108. Rosenblatt MA, Abel M, Fischer GW, et al. Successful use of a 20% lipid emulsion to resuscitate a patient after a presumed bupivacaine-related cardiac arrest. *Anesthesiology* 2006;105(1):217–218.

109. Litz RJ, Popp M, Stehr SN, Koch T. Successful resuscitation of a patient with ropivacaine-induced asystole after axillary plexus block using lipid infusion. *Anaesthesia* 2006;61(8):800–801.

110. de Jong R. Lipid infusion for cardiotoxicity: Promise? Yes-Panacea? Not. *Anesthesiology* 2007;106(3):635–636.

111. Stehr SN, Ziegeler JC, Pexa A, et al. The effects of lipid infusion on myocardial function and bioenergetics in l-bupivacaine toxicity in the isolated rat heart. *Anesth Analg* 2007;104(1):186–192.

112. Weinberg GL, Ripper R, Murphy P, et al. Lipid infusion accelerates removal of bupivacaine and recovery from bupivacaine toxicity in the isolated rat heart. *Reg Anesth Pain Med* 2006;31(4):296–303.

113. Heavner JE. Let's abandon blanket maximum recommended doses of local anesthetics. *Reg Anesth Pain Med* 2004;29(6):524.

114. Rosenberg PH, Veering BT, Urmey WF. Maximum recommended doses of local anesthetics: A multifactorial concept. *Reg Anesth Pain Med* 2004;29(6):564–575; [Discussion, 524].

115. Mulroy MF. Systemic toxicity and cardiotoxicity from local anesthetics: Incidence and preventive measures. *Reg Anesth Pain Med* 2002;27(6):556–561.

116. Mather LE, Copeland SE, Ladd LA. Acute toxicity of local anesthetics: Underlying pharmacokinetic and pharmacodynamic concepts. *Reg Anesth Pain Med* 2005;30(6):553–66.

117. Kopacz DJ, Allen HW. Accidental intravenous laevo-bupivacaine. *Anesth Analg* 1999;89(4):1027–1029.

118. Pirotta D, Sprigge J. Convulsions following axillary brachial plexus blockade with laevo-bupivacaine. *Anaesthesia* 2002;57(12):1187–1189.

119. Crews JC, Rothman TE. Seizure after laevo-bupivacaine for interscalene brachial plexus block. *Anesth Analg* 2003;96(4):1188–1190.

120. Breslin DS, Martin G, Macleod DB, et al. Central nervous system toxicity following the administration of laevo-bupivacaine for lumbar plexus block: A report of two cases. *Reg Anesth Pain Med* 2003;28(2):144–147.

121. Abouleish EI, Elias M, Nelson C. Ropivacaine-induced seizure after extradural anaesthesia. *Br J Anaesth* 1998;80(6):843–844.

122. Plowman AN, Bolsin S, Mather LE. Central nervous system toxicity attributable to epidural ropivacaine hydrochloride. *Anaesth Intensive Care* 1998;26(2):204–206.

123. Ruetsch YA, Fattinger KE, Borgeat A. Ropivacaine-induced convulsions and severe cardiac dysrhythmia after sciatic block. *Anesthesiology* 1999;90(6):1784–1786.

124. Klein SM, Benveniste H. Anxiety, vocalization, and agitation following peripheral nerve block with ropivacaine. *Reg Anesth Pain Med* 1999;24(2):175–178.

125. Ala-Kokko TI, Lopponen A, Alahuhta S. Two instances of central nervous system toxicity in the same patient following repeated ropivacaine-induced brachial plexus block. *Acta Anaesthesiol Scand* 2000;44(5):623–626.

126. Muller M, Litz RJ, Huler M, Albrecht DM. Grand mal convulsion and plasma concentrations after intravascular injection of ropivacaine for axillary brachial plexus blockade. *Br J Anaesth* 2001;87(5):784–787.

127. Bisschop DY, Alardo JP, Razgallah B, et al. Seizure induced by ropivacaine. *Ann Pharmacother* 2001;35(3):311–313.

128. Dernedde M, Furlan D, Verbesselt R, et al. Grand mal convulsion after an accidental intravenous injection of ropivacaine. *Anesth Analg* 2004;98(2):521–523.

129. Klein SM, Pierce T, Rubin Y, et al. Successful resuscitation after ropivacaine-induced ventricular fibrillation. *Anesth Analg* 2003;97(3):901–903.

130. Huet O, Eyrolle LJ, Mazoit JX, Ozier YM. Cardiac arrest after injection of ropivacaine for posterior lumbar plexus blockade. *Anesthesiology* 2003;99(6):1451–1453.

131. Khoo LP, Corbett AR. Successful resuscitation of an ASA 3 patient following ropivacaine-induced cardiac arrest. *Anaesth Intensive Care* 2006;34(6):804–807.

132. Sandhu N, Joseph S, Manne MD, et al. Sonographically guided infraclavicular brachial plexus block in adults a retrospective analysis of 1146 cases. *J Ultrasound Med* 2006;25:1555–1561.

133. Nau C, Wang SY, Strichartz GR, Wang GK. Block of human heart hH1 sodium channels by the enantiomers of bupivacaine. *Anesthesiology* 2000;93:1022–33.

134. Butterworth J, James RL, Grimes J. Structure-affinity relationships and stereospecificity of several homologous series of local anesthetics for the beta2-adrenergic receptor. *Anesth Analg* 1997;85(2):336–342.

135. Ohmura S, Sugano A, Kawada M, Yamamoto K. Pulmonary uptake of ropivacaine and laevo-bupivacaine in rabbits. *Anesth Analg* 2003;97(3):893–897.

136. Mazoit JX, Orhant EE, Boico O, et al. Myocardial uptake of bupivacaine: I. Pharmacokinetics and pharmacodynamics of lidocaine and bupivacaine in the isolated perfused rabbit heart. *Anesth Analg* 1993;77(3):469–476.

137. Mazoit JX, Decaux A, Bouaziz H, Edouard A. Comparative ventricular electrophysiologic effect of racemic bupivacaine, laevo-bupivacaine, and ropivacaine on the isolated rabbit heart. *Anesthesiology* 2000;93(3):784–792.

138. Ohmura S, Kawada M, Ohta T, et al. Systemic toxicity and resuscitation in bupivacaine-, laevo-bupivacaine-, or ropivacaine-infused rats. *Anesth Analg* 2001;93(3):743–748.

139. Feldman HS, Arthur GR, Covino BG. Comparative systemic toxicity of convulsant and supraconvulsant doses of intravenous ropivacaine, bupivacaine, and lidocaine in the conscious dog. *Anesth Analg* 1989;69(6):794–801.

140. Dony P, Dewinde V, Vanderick B, et al. The comparative toxicity of ropivacaine and bupivacaine at equipotent doses in rats. *Anesth Analg* 2000;91(6):1489–1492.

CHAPTER 6 ■ MODIFICATION OF METABOLIC RESPONSES TO SURGERY BY NEURAL BLOCKADE

FRANCESCO CARLI AND THOMAS SCHRICKER

CATABOLIC CHANGES INDUCED BY SURGICAL STRESS

The endocrine, metabolic, and inflammatory response to surgery make up the constellation of physiologic changes termed the *catabolic response to surgery*. Accumulated evidence suggests that this phenomenon, if untreated, is accompanied by undesirable effects leading to morbidity and mortality. Pharmacologic, nutritional, and physical interventions have been used to prevent or attenuate catabolic illness. Regional anesthesia and, in particular, neuraxial blockade has been found to modulate some aspects, with potential implication for the anesthetic practice. Nevertheless, the realization that the pathophysiology of surgical stress is multifactorial requires a global perspective in the use of interventional strategies.

Although previous publications have covered in great detail all various aspects of the neuroendocrine and inflammatory response to surgery and the changes produced by regional anesthesia, the purpose of this chapter is to focus on clinically relevant alterations, with emphasis on the effectiveness of some of the most common regional anesthesia procedures.

METABOLIC AND FUNCTIONAL CONSEQUENCES OF SURGERY

Hyperglycemia

The human body's circulating concentration of glucose, contrary to other metabolic substrates such as ketone bodies, fatty acids, or amino acids, is controlled within a narrow range (Fig. 6-1). Metabolically healthy subjects maintain glycemia between 3.6 and 7.8 mmol/L irrespective of their physiologic state (fasting, feeding, exercise). Blood glucose levels increase during periods of stress, including sepsis, injury, and surgery (1).

The degree of intraoperative hyperglycemia depends on the type, severity, and extent of surgical tissue trauma (Fig. 6-2). In fasting patients undergoing elective intraperitoneal procedures, blood glucose levels typically increase to values between 7 and 10 mmol/L (2). During cardiac surgery the disturbance of glucose homeostasis is impressive, with blood glucose values frequently exceeding 15 mmol/L in nondiabetic (3,4) and 20 mmol/L in diabetic subjects (5).

The occurrence of hyperglycemia is related to stereotypical metabolic and endocrine alterations induced by the surgical insult: stimulated glucose production (6), decreased glucose utilization (7), enhanced renal absorption of filtered glucose (8), inadequate insulin secretion, and decreased insulin activity (9,10). Although hyperglycemia per se is usually restricted to the immediate perioperative period, metabolic derangements are severe enough to produce insulin resistance up to 2 weeks after abdominal surgery (9,10).

Glucose is toxic under certain conditions such as surgical stress, which triggers the release of mediators. These mediators serve two roles: on one hand, they inhibit the expression of the insulin-dependent membrane glucose transporter glut-4, which is mainly located in the myocardium and the skeletal muscle (Fig. 6-3). On the other hand, they stimulate the expression of the insulin-independent membrane glucose transporters glut-1, -2, and -3, which are located in the brain, endothelium, liver, and some blood cells. Although insulin-dependent cells are protected by insulin resistance, most of the circulating glucose enters cells that do not require insulin for uptake, resulting in a cellular glucose overload: once inside the cell, glucose either nonenzymatically glycosylates proteins such as immunoglobins and renders them dysfunctional or enters glycolysis and oxidative phosphorylation. That pathway generates excess superoxide molecules that bind to nitric oxide (NO), lead to the formation of peroxynitrate, and ultimately result in mitochondrial dysfunction and cell death (Fig. 6-3) (13).

Evidence has mounted that even moderate increases in blood glucose are associated with poor outcome. Patients with fasting glucose levels of over 7 mmol/L or random blood glucose levels of more than 11.1 mmol/L on general surgical wards showed an 18-fold increased in-hospital mortality, a longer length of stay, and a greater risk of infection (11). In a heterogenous group of critically ill patients, mortality was directly correlated with increasing glucose levels above 5 mmol/L (12). The lowest hospital mortality occurred in patients with a mean blood glucose of 4.5 to 5.5 mmol/L. Patients with cardiovascular disease appear to be particularly sensitive to changes in glycemia.

Overall studies in both the basic and clinical sciences are compelling in demonstrating that acute hyperglycemia is detrimental to patient outcome.

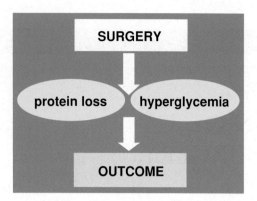

FIGURE 6-1. Major metabolic changes occurring with surgery.

Loss of Protein

The cumulative net nitrogen losses after elective abdominal operations range between 40 and 80 g of nitrogen; complications that delay the use of the gastrointestinal tract may result in nitrogen losses of up to 150 g (Fig. 6-4) (14). Patients suffering from multiple injury and septic shock lose more than 200 g of nitrogen, whereas nitrogen losses after severe burns can exceed 300 g. The principal underlying defect appears to be an accelerated rate of protein breakdown and amino acid oxidation, along with an insufficient increase in protein synthesis (15–17). Endogenous amino acid oxidation and amino acid release from the muscle after abdominal surgery have been shown to increase by 90% and 30%, respectively, whereas whole body protein synthesis increases by 10% only (17). The magnitude of this alteration is substantial considering the fact that muscle tissue represents approximately 45% of body weight and contributes as much as 20% to total body protein synthesis. The clinical importance of this catabolic pattern can be appreciated more readily when one remembers that 1 g of nitrogen is the equivalent of 30 g of hydrated lean tissue. Therefore, a loss of 50 g of nitrogen, as seen after uncomplicated chole-

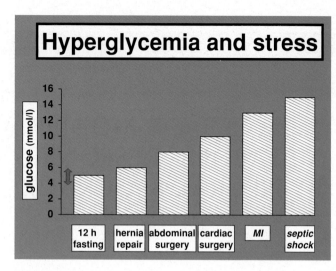

FIGURE 6-2. Intensity of stress and levels of hyperglycemia.

cystectomy, would be the equivalent of 1,500 g of lean tissue. The latter point is of utmost clinical relevance, as the length of time for return of normal physiologic function after discharge from the hospital is related to the extent of loss of lean body mass during hospitalization (18). Because protein represents both structural and functional body components, erosion of lean tissue also may lead to devastating consequences such as delayed wound healing (19), compromised immune function, and diminished muscle strength that result in prolonged convalescence and increased morbidity (20,21).

Lipotoxicity

Free fatty acid (FFA) levels during and after surgery are increased as a result of prolonged preoperative fasting, sympathoadrenergic responses to surgical injury, and the lipolytic

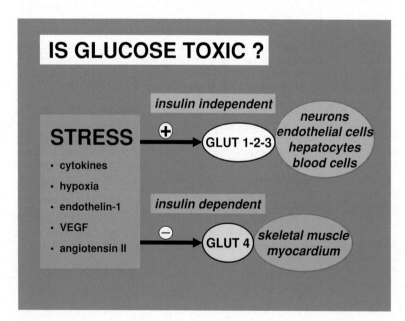

FIGURE 6-3. Pathways of glucose potential toxicity.

TABLE 6-1

HORMONAL EFFECTS ON PROTEIN LOSS AND BLOOD GLUCOSE

Hormone	Protein loss (%)	Blood glucose
Thyroid hormone	⌂ (+ 20)	↑
Growth hormone	↑	↑
Cortisol	↑ (+20)	↑
Glucagon	↑ (+30)	↑
Epinephrine	→	↑
Insulin	↓	↓

↑ increase, → no change, ↓ decrease.

TABLE 6-2

FUNCTIONAL CHANGES AFTER SURGERY

Study	Type of surgery	Days after surgery	% of Preop capacity
Christensen et al.	Abdominal	20	65
Wood	Abdominal	10	77
Zeidermann	Abdominal	3	60

action of heparin administered for the prevention of thrombosis (22). High levels of FFA have been shown to depress myocardial contractility (23), inhibit glycolytic flux, and increase myocardial oxygen consumption without a concomitant increase in myocardial work (24–25). Furthermore, fatty acids may impair calcium homeostasis and increase the production of free radicals, leading to electrical instability and ventricular arrhythmias. Elevated fatty acids also have been found to cause endothelial dysfunction and impair endothelium-dependent vasodilatation through the inhibition of endothelial nitric oxide synthase (eNOS) (26).

Functional Impairment

Muscle fatigue is characterized by a decreased ability to carry out activities of daily living together with an element of depression and muscle weakness (Table 6-2) (27). After major surgery, fatigue and tiredness can last for 4 to 6 weeks. Although the mechanism for muscle weakness has not been elucidated, it appears to be a combination of impaired nutritional intake, the inflammatory-metabolic response, immobilization, and a subjective feeling of fatigue (28). A decrease in handgrip strength has been found to be related to the magnitude of surgical stimulus, and can last up to 3 to 4 weeks. A decrease in vital capacity

has also been reported to be particularly relevant after upper abdominal surgery (29,30). Assessment of energy expenditure after surgery shows a marked decrease in adaptability to exercise manifested as increased heart rate and circulating levels of lactate (Table 6-1).

CATABOLIC RESPONSE TO ACUTE PAIN

Severe acute surgical pain results in an abnormal response characterized by sympathetic over-reactivity and increased heart rate, systemic vascular resistance, cardiac output, and coronary vasoconstriction. An isolated painful stimulus response cannot be entirely separated from that associated with surgical injury, and attempts have been made to identify the neuroendocrine and metabolic changes associated with experimental pain in the absence of surgery. Following electrical stimulation of the abdominal wall, a painful response (visual analogue scale 8 out of 10) elicits a stress response with significant increase in cortisol, catecholamines, and glucagon, and a decrease in insulin sensitivity and glucose uptake (31). This response continues for a certain period of time that is directly related to the time and extent of injury. As it is difficult to dissociate the inflammatory component from the nociceptive stimulus, it is assumed that endocrine and humoral responses are directly integrated.

Although these metabolic changes occur after surgery in all patients undergoing major surgery and experiencing pain, there are certain patient populations in whom the catabolic response is exaggerated.

METABOLICALLY CHALLENGED PATIENTS

Diabetes Mellitus

Depending on the type of the procedure, the prevalence of type 2 diabetes in surgical patients ranges from 12% to 28% (Fig. 6-5) (32). Type 2 diabetic patients experience a higher mortality and morbidity in response to surgical treatment and have a more prolonged convalescence than those who are nondiabetic (33). Insulin resistance is associated with catabolic changes in protein and glucose metabolism (34,35). Poorly controlled type 2 diabetic subjects show increased protein loss (36), although protein homeostasis in the presence of good glucose control appears to be preserved (Figs. 6-6 and 6-7) (37).

Because the metabolic and endocrine alterations observed in patients with type 2 diabetes are similar to those induced by surgical tissue trauma per se ("diabetes of the injury"), it was

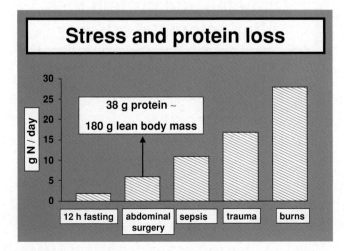

FIGURE 6-4. Intensity of stress and protein loss.

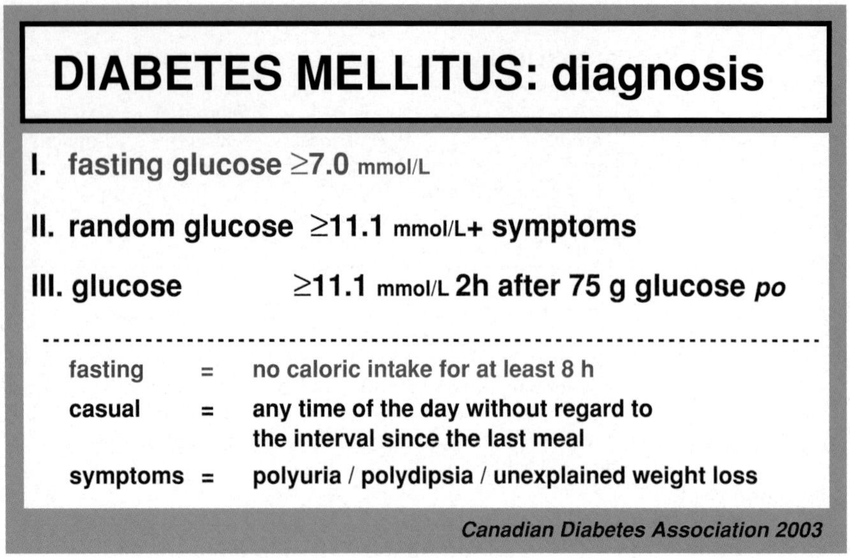

DIABETES MELLITUS: diagnosis

I. **fasting glucose ≥7.0** mmol/L

II. **random glucose ≥11.1** mmol/L **+ symptoms**

III. **glucose ≥11.1** mmol/L **2h after 75 g glucose** *po*

- -

fasting	=	no caloric intake for at least 8 h
casual	=	any time of the day without regard to the interval since the last meal
symptoms	=	polyuria / polydipsia / unexplained weight loss

Canadian Diabetes Association 2003

FIGURE 6-5. Definition of diabetes and levels of blood glucose.

previously held that the metabolic abnormalities after surgery are accentuated in diabetic patients (38,39). Recently, evidence was provided that the catabolic response to colorectal surgery is indeed increased in patients with type 2 diabetes mellitus as reflected by a 50% greater protein loss, glucose production, and glucose plasma concentration (40). Feeding is poorly tolerated by the diabetic patient, because it is followed by an exaggerated hyperglycemic response (Table 6-3).

Cancer

Malnutrition and depletion of lean body mass are characteristic of patients with cancer. Many clinical and biochemical indices have been used to characterize the nutritional status of surgical patients, but all techniques have limitations (41); anthropometric and body composition measurements must be treated with caution in subjects who are dehydrated and who have edema or ascites (42). Serum proteins are pathophysiologic markers and not specific for the nutritional state (43), because they are affected by influences other than malnutrition or catabolism, including inflammation with redistribution and dilution.

Quantitative assessment of preoperative protein catabolism in surgical patients becomes relevant because the frequency of extreme forms of undernutrition seems to decline. Contrary to earlier studies reporting incidences of up to 40% on hospital admission (44), more recent reports indicate that severe malnutrition occurs in only 6% to 20% of hospitalized patients (45). Less than 5% of patients undergoing surgery for colorectal cancer are malnourished. The development of malnutrition represents a systemic response to the tumor. Anorexia and reduced intake, rather than changes in energy expenditure, result in negative energy balance (46).

Evidence suggests a link between the occurrence of weight loss and alterations in whole body protein catabolism. Protein loss in well-nourished, weight-stable cancer patients was

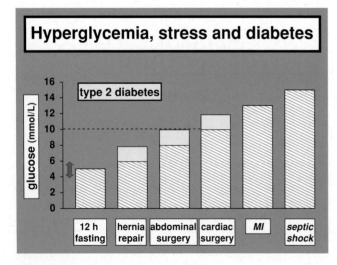

FIGURE 6-6. Circulating levels of blood glucose in diabetic and non-diabetic patients with surgical and medical pathologies.

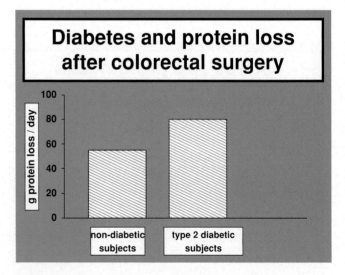

FIGURE 6-7. Postoperative loss of body protein in diabetic and non-diabetic patients.

TABLE 6-3

BLOOD GLUCOSE AND PROTEIN LOSS DURING FASTED AND IV INFUSION OF DEXTROSE

	Diabetic		Nondiabetic	
	Fast	Dextrose	Fast	Dextrose
Blood glucose (mmol/L)	7 ± 1	14 ± 5	5 ± 1	10 ± 1
Protein loss (μmol/kg/h)	112 ± 9	152 ± 16	105 ± 8	98 ± 7

Data from Schricker T, Gougeon R, Eberhart L, et al. Type 2 diabetes mellitus and the catabolic response to surgery. *Anesthesiology* 2002;97:943–951.

normal, whereas it was significantly increased in malnourished, weight-losing subjects suffering from gastrointestinal malignancy (47). These results confirm earlier observations that, in cancer cachexia, a maladaptation to the starved state occurs, with a continued mobilization of protein and calorie reserves in the face of a decreased intake (48).

Aging

In animals, experiments have shown that the acute stress response becomes blunted with age (49). Elderly critically ill patients have been found to possess a higher baseline cortisolemia but a lower response to adrenocorticotropic hormone (ACTH) stimulation than younger patients, implying that adrenal glands in this population function close to maximal levels and have a decreased ability to cope with injury and trauma (50,51). This relative adrenal insufficiency undoubtedly contributes to the increased morbidity and mortality observed in older patients. In the past, it was expected that elderly patients, because of a decrease in skeletal lean tissue mass and a proportional increase in visceral lean tissue mass would need an increased stress response and plasma glucose to provide glycemic fuel to their viscera. However, most studies have concluded that, compared with young patients, hyperglycemia is not increased in elderly patients (52–54). Therefore, the prevailing data points to an attenuation of the acute stress response in the elderly.

Regarding protein metabolism, aging is associated with sarcopenia (loss of skeletal muscles). Although incompletely understood, the etiology of sarcopenia is multifactorial: An increased first-pass hepatic extraction of dietary amino acids occurs that decreases substrate availability for protein synthesis (55). Furthermore, the synthesis of myofibrillar, mitochondrial, and myosin heavy chain proteins declines with age (56).

In geriatric patients with trauma, protein breakdown is attenuated, suggesting that the elderly cannot respond to injury as readily as their younger counterparts (57) and have a worse prognosis (58). They suffer from more cardiorespiratory complications, have less postoperative strength, and are slower to recuperate. The malnourished elderly fare the worst (59).

PREOPERATIVE FASTING

Elective surgery is routinely performed after an overnight fast to minimize the risk of aspiration when general anesthesia is induced. Fasting periods before abdominal surgery usually amount to a longer time (up to 40 h) because bowel preparation on the preoperative day impedes oral food intake. This period of fasting is long enough to substantially deplete hepatic glycogen stores, thereby increasing the demand for amino acids for gluconeogenesis rather than tissue repair (60). Animal studies showed that coping with stress is much improved if the animals enter the trauma under fed rather than fasted conditions (61,62). The effect of changing the metabolic setting from an overnight fasted to a fed state before surgical trauma on the development of the catabolic response has only recently been tested in humans. Overnight treatment with glucose infusions prevented the postoperative decrease in insulin sensitivity (63), inhibited urinary urea excretion (64), and reduced fatigue, as reflected by improved voluntary muscle function (65). Clinical studies demonstrating better outcome with preoperative nutrition, particularly in malnourished patients (66,67), further emphasize that the avoidance of fasting before surgery could make patients less vulnerable to postoperative complications that result in a decreased length of hospital stay.

NEURAXIAL BLOCKADE AND THE CATABOLIC RESPONSE TO SURGERY

Ample evidence has accumulated to identify the peripheral and central nervous systems as common pathways for triggering the catabolic responses to surgery (68). Stimulation of afferent sensory and sympathetic fibers by tissue trauma and activation of efferent hypothalamopituitary pathways has been considered to be one of the main release mechanisms (69). Blockade of these pathways by local anesthetics prevents the increase in circulating counterregulatory hormones, thereby improving insulin sensitivity (Fig. 6-8).

The effect of neuraxial blockade on the endocrine and metabolic response has been extensively investigated previously (68), and a consensus exists on the importance of the nature of the blockade and the adequacy of analgesia. High doses of local anesthetics provide an adequate somatic and autonomic blockade that prevents stimulation of the hypothalamic-pituitary-adrenal axis and is capable of attenuating the cortisol and catecholamine response. However, this depends upon the type and concentration of local anesthetic (68), as well as the extent of the block. There is still an active search for the ideal local anesthetic agent able to provide an adequate block of afferent and efferent nervous fibers with minimal side effects. Evidence shows that a symmetrical block extended from T4 to S5 dermatomes effectively suppresses the sympathetic-hypothalamic response, if initiated before surgery and continued for a reasonable period of time, which seems to be 48 hours (70). Although injection of local anesthetics in the subarachnoid space provides a dense block with significant attenuation of catabolic hormones and gluconeogenic metabolites (71), this technique is time limited. The epidural block, in contrast, can be maintained beyond surgery and as these local anesthetics can be injected and an adequate sensory block monitored. Studies on epidural blockade and stress response can be divided in two groups. The first group includes surgery below the umbilicus, in which local anesthetics have been injected into the epidural space to provide different levels of sensory block and the endocrine response has been measured. If the sensory block is below T10, the neuroendocrine response is not inhibited, whereas it remains suppressed when the block is above T6. The catecholamine response is totally inhibited only when the block is above T4.

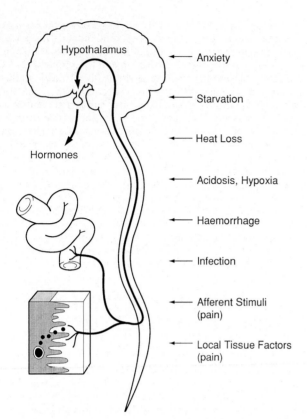

FIGURE 6-8. Release mechanisms of the endocrine metabolic response to surgery. The principal mechanisms are afferent neural stimuli (*arrows on right*) due to noxious surgical/trauma stimuli and local tissue factors released at the trauma site; both of these categories of stimuli may be associated with pain. Interleukin-1 is released from circulating macrophages and forms part of the "inflammatory soup" that sensitizes nociceptors. Secondary amplifiers of the response are psychological factors (e.g., anxiety), starvation, heat loss, acidosis, hypoxia, hemorrhage, and infection. Noxious stimuli from viscera (e.g., gut) travel via visceral nociceptive afferents (via sympathetic ganglia) and contribute to the trauma stimuli, and local tissue factors are also involved. Central responses to afferent stimuli involve hypothalamus and other central nervous system areas mediating the efferent humoral and neural components of the endocrine-metabolic response.

The second group includes upper abdominal surgery, in which it appears that epidural block (T4–S5) with local anesthetics can only partly blunt the cortisol response, probably due to the unblocked afferent vagal stimulation and diaphragmatic and peritoneal nerve terminals (Fig. 6-9) (72). Despite this partial inhibition, some studies have reported significant decrease in circulating gluconeogenic metabolites, indicating that cortisol might be only partially involved in modulating the metabolic stress response (73).

Studies on the effect of small and moderate doses of spinal opioids on the catabolic response to surgery indicate that the modifying effect of opioids are modest compared with those induced by local anesthetics (74). Although a significant reduction of circulating levels of cortisol occurs, circulating concentrations of catecholamine and metabolites are not modified. In contrast, large doses of lipophilic opioids cause segmentary neural block, with consequent inhibition of sympathetic activity (75). This technique has several limitations, and therefore it is restricted to major surgery, in which postoperative ventilation and surveillance are required. No metabolic advantages of neuraxial opioids have been found (76).

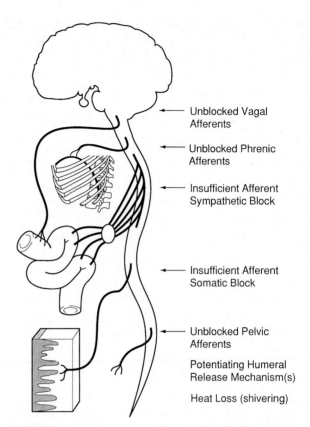

FIGURE 6-9. Factors that may explain the demonstrated reduced inhibition of the surgical stress response by epidural analgesia during major (upper) abdominal procedures compared to procedures in the lower abdomen and lower extremities. Existent data suggest that the main cause is an insufficient afferent somatic and sympathetic block, whereas unblocked parasympathetic afferents probably are of minor importance. The role of potentiating humoral release mechanisms (local tissue factors and interleukin-1) and increased metabolism by shivering due to heat loss have not been fully evaluated.

Hyperglycemia

The hyperglycemic response to surgery is reduced or blocked by neural blockade through inhibition of hepatic glycogenolytic response to surgical injury (Fig. 6-8) (77). With the block of sympathetic hyperactivity, epinephrine response is abolished and the efferent sympathetic neural pathways to the liver are inhibited. Insulin sensitivity is preserved by neural blockade through inhibition of the catabolic hormones, both of which are responsible for inhibiting peripheral glucose clearance. Postoperative impaired glucose tolerance is reversed by epidural blockade, therefore facilitating glucose utilization by peripheral tissues (Fig. 6-10). Recent studies using normoglycemic hyperinsulinemic clamp and labeled tracers have shown the positive effect of epidural anesthetics in reversing postoperative insulin resistance (78). The production of gluconeogenic substrates is also inhibited, and oxygen consumption is reduced.

Protein Catabolism

Based on the early studies on hysterectomy and limb surgery, there has been a realization that neuraxial blockade could

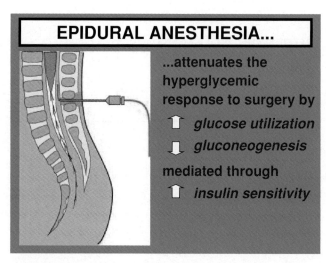

EPIDURAL ANESTHESIA...

...attenuates the hyperglycemic response to surgery by

⇧ *glucose utilization*

⇩ *gluconeogenesis*

mediated through

⇧ *insulin sensitivity*

FIGURE 6-10. Effects of epidural analgesia on aspects of glucose metabolism.

reduce protein catabolism in patients undergoing major abdominal surgery and therefore influence outcome. The magnitude and duration of the deafferentation and the extent of the sensory block influence the degree of protein loss. The provision of continuous epidural blockade for 48 hours improves postoperative protein balance by decreasing the loss of nitrogen and attenuating the fall in synthesis of new lean tissue (70).

Lipid Metabolism

Injured patients have raised lipolysis and utilize fat as major source of energy. Early studies on the effect of intraoperative epidural anesthesia on fat metabolism reported decreased circulating levels of plasma glycerol and FFAs (79). More recently, labeled tracers were used to assess the effect of dextrose supplementation and epidural analgesia on postoperative lipid turnover and oxidation in patients undergoing upper abdominal surgery. The elevated rates of lipolysis were not suppressed by epidural analgesia, probably due to the limited extent of sensory blockade and the inability to modulate the persistent postoperative state of insulin resistance (80). In contrast, a reduction in fat metabolism and circulating levels of ketones was reported in patients receiving epidural local anesthetics for lower body surgery.

Integration Epidural Analgesia and Nutrition

The majority of earlier reports documenting the protein-sparing effects of epidural analgesia were conducted in patients receiving alimentary support (81,70), making it impossible to differentiate between the impact of epidural analgesia and changes resulting from nutritional factors (Table 6-4) (82,83). Studies in patients with controlled feeding status enabled researchers to conclude that, under fasting conditions, when energy intake is absent, epidural analgesia has no effect on protein catabolism (84,85). However, epidural analgesia, in contrast to intravenous (IV) analgesia with morphine, facilitates the oxidative utilization of exogenous glucose (85), thereby preventing the postoperative amino acid loss and sav-

ing almost 100 g of lean body mass per day (86). The extent of protein sparing was found to be greater than that previously achieved with pharmacologic and nutritional interventions after elective abdominal surgery. Although epidural analgesia has anticatabolic effects in the presence of energy supply, patients could not be rendered anabolic. Whole body protein balance remained negative, most likely due to the lack of anabolic substrate provision. The validity of this assumption was confirmed by the demonstration of the anabolic effects of epidural analgesia during the administration of glucose and amino acids (87). Epidural, not IV analgesia, was associated with a protein gain during a 3-hour infusion of glucose and amino acids 2 days after colorectal surgery. In patients receiving epidural analgesia, a perioperative *hypo*caloric feeding regimen providing glucose and amino acids or amino acids alone induced an anabolic state on the second postoperative day (88). The advantage of infusing amino acids alone is the absence of hyperglycemia and a positive protein balance in the postoperative period. It appears that the effect of high doses of amino acids on protein metabolism is stronger than the modulatory effect of epidural blockade in the sense that the former attenuates protein breakdown and enhances protein gain (Table 6-5) (89,90).

Neuraxial Blockade and Functional Impairment

An epidural mixture of local anesthetic and opioids provides superior analgesia, facilitates mobilization, and accelerates food intake (Fig. 6-11). Within an accelerated recovery program that included epidural analgesia, postoperative

TABLE 6-4

INTERACTION BETWEEN EPIDURAL ANALGESIA AND NUTRITION

Substrate infused	Protein loss	Protein gain	Blood glucose
Fasting	→	→	→
Low-dose glucose	↓	→	↑
Low-dose glucose + amino acids	↓↓	↑	↑
Amino acids	↓↓	↑	→

Glucose infused: 200 g /day; Amino acids: 1 g protein/kg/day
↑ increase, → no change, ↓ decrease.

TABLE 6-5

PROTEIN SAVING AFTER COLORECTAL SURGERY

Intervention	LBM (g/day)
Growth hormone and hypocaloric glucose	50
Growth hormone and hypocaloric glucose and amino acids	71
Glutamine and hypercaloric nutrition	60
Epidural analgesia and hypocaloric glucose	150

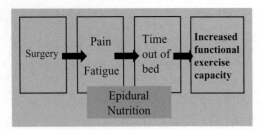

FIGURE 6-11. Model of interaction of surgical stress, pain intervention, and functional recovery.

TABLE 6-6

PROTEIN METABOLISM AND CIRCULATING BLOOD GLUCOSE IN DIABETIC AND NONDIABETIC PATIENTS

		Protein loss	Protein gain	Blood glucose
Diabetic	Glucose infusion	↓	→	+ +
	AA infusion	↓↓	↑↑	−
Nondiabetics	Glucose infusion	→	→	+
	AA infusion	↓	↑	−

↑ increase, → no change, ↓ decrease; AA = amino acids.

cardiopulmonary response to treadmill exercise has been shown to return to normal levels more quickly (91). In addition, out-of-bed activity immediately after surgery is enhanced, thus facilitating the recuperation of functional exercise capacity during the first 6 weeks after surgery (92). This might be explained by the positive influence of a combination of epidural analgesia and nutritional substrate on protein and glucose metabolism leading to preservation of muscle protein and a decrease in whole body protein catabolism through the amelioration of insulin sensitivity (Fig. 6-11).

PERIPHERAL NERVE BLOCK AND CATABOLIC RESPONSE TO SURGERY

It is logical to suppose that interruption of peripheral neural pathways by infiltration anesthesia or peripheral neural blockade might decrease the stress response by reducing afferent nociceptive stimuli. Application of local anesthetics at the site of the surgical incision provides pain relief, but does not inhibit the neuroendocrine response after abdominal and gynecologic surgery. Other techniques, such as interpleural administration of bupivacaine, also did not reduce the stress response to surgery despite decreased opioid requirement and satisfactory degree of analgesia (93). Nerve blocks with local anesthetics have been shown to be effective in attenuating the catecholamine and hyperglycemic response following cataract surgery (94) and thoracic surgery (95). In particular, retrobulbar block in diabetic patients was associated with better postoperative glycemic control (94).

In contrast, continuous femoral and sciatic block did not attenuate the endocrine stress response to knee arthroplasty, and the endogenous glucose production was reduced independently of the anesthesia technique used (96). It is possible that, for the deafferentation of the knee area, other nerve fibres, such as the obturator and the lateral musculotaneous, need to be blocked.

DIABETES AND REGIONAL ANESTHESIA

As patients with type 2 diabetes mellitus tend to become more catabolic after surgery than nondiabetic patients (97), it would make sense to establish an epidural block in order to attenuate the loss of proteins from the body while avoiding hyperglycemia. Infusion of amino acids after surgery blunts protein breakdown and stimulates protein synthesis, resulting in a pos-

itive protein balance with a greater significant effect in patients with epidural blockade compared to patient-controlled analgesia (PCA) (98). In addition, the infusion of amino acids is preferable to that of dextrose to maintain blood glucose within physiologic limits (Table 6-6).

ROLE OF MINIMALLY INVASIVE SURGERY AND REGIONAL ANESTHESIA AND ANALGESIA

Endoscopic surgical techniques have been shown to cause less tissue damage than open procedures, and therefore the rise in markers of inflammation is significantly attenuated (99). The clinical implications of attenuated inflammatory response result in decreased incidence of wound infection and postoperative complications. In contrast, the neuroendocrine and metabolic response to endoscopic surgery is similar to that caused by open surgery. The creation of pneumoperitoneum mounts a significant sympathetic response, with changes in cortisol and metabolites. The rise persists in the immediate postoperative period, although the magnitude is less than one would see with open procedure. With regard to the metabolic changes associated with laparoscopic surgery, the administration of dextrose after colon surgery promoted a significant suppression of endogenous glucose production, an index of gluconeogenesis, with no protein-sparing capacity (100). This implies an enhanced whole body glucose uptake, utilization, and oxidation of exogenous glucose.

Attempts to attenuate the metabolic and inflammatory response to endoscopic techniques with regional anesthesia have failed, and this might be due to the inability of neuraxial blockade to ablate some of the autonomic fibers innervating the splanchnic area and the little effect the neural blockade has on modulating tissue trauma (Fig. 6-9). Nevertheless, the beneficial effect of epidural anesthesia and analgesia for laparoscopic colon resection on gut motility has been shown recently, implying that this technique attenuates the sympathetic hyperactivity associated with surgery and facilitates earlier restoration of gut motility (101). Similar results were found when IV lidocaine was infused during laparoscopic colon resection. Early bowel function was promoted, probably by lidocaine modulating the inflammatory response and preventing the spinal hypersensitivity (102).

REGIONAL ANESTHESIA/ANALGESIA TO MODULATE THE METABOLIC STRESS RESPONSE WITHIN THE FRAMEWORK OF MULTI-INTERVENTIONAL STRATEGY

Sufficient published data confirms that regional anesthesia modulates some aspects of the stress response and attenuates the rise of catabolic hormones and gluconeogenic substrates. Most of the studies have focused on neuraxial blockade, with particular interest in the use of local anesthetics. Although the mechanism of stress modulation is not well known, it appears that neural blockade inhibits the establishment of an insulin-resistant state that, on its own, contributes to loss of body mass and decreased glucose utilization. Although it is evident that neural blockade could play a main role in attenuating some of the metabolic responses, it is rather presumptuous to expect that this intervention alone would be able to suppress the constellation of responses that are part of surgical stress (Figs. 6.8 and 6.9). It is for this reason that an attempt to determine the effect of epidural blockade on postoperative outcome failed. In addition, there is evidence that the inflammatory, rather than the endocrine, response to surgical stress is to some extent linked to postoperative morbidity, and neural blockade does not inhibit the former response. It is therefore necessary that, to optimize and enhance the effectiveness of neural blockade, a multimodal intervention be put in place in

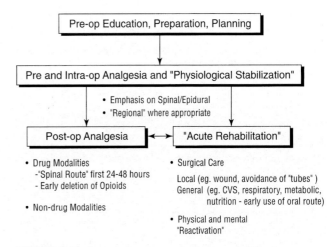

FIGURE 6-12. Acute pain treatment and acute rehabilitation.

which pharmacologic, physical, psychological, and nutritional strategies are part of the therapy modulating organ dysfunction and facilitating the recovery process (103). It is evident that every effort made in providing epidural analgesia should be with the intention of optimizing pain relief, which in turn facilitates early mobilization and oral nutrition. An integrated surgical care that would actively control the perioperative period would contribute to a reduction in postoperative organ dysfunction and enhance rehabilitation (Fig. 6-12).

References

1. Schricker T, Lattermann R, Schreiber M, et al. The hyperglycemic response to surgery: Pathophysiology, clinical implications and modification by the anaesthetic technique. *Clin Intensive Care* 1998;9:118–128.
2. Lattermann R, Carli F, Wykes L, Schricker T. Epidural blockade modifies perioperative glucose production without affecting protein catabolism. *Anesthesiology* 2002;97:374–381.
3. Chaney MA, Nikolov MP, Blakeman BP, Bakhos M. Attempting to maintain normoglycemia during cardiopulmonary bypass with insulin may initiate postoperative hypoglycemia. *Anesth Analg* 1999;89:1091–1095.
4. Carvalho G, Moore A, Qizilbash B, et al. Maintenance of normoglycemia during open cardiac surgery. *Anesth Analg* 2004;99:319–324.
5. Schricker T, Carvalho G. An ounce of prevention worth a pound of cure. *Can J Anesth* 2004;51:948–949.
6. Thorell A, Rooyackers O, Myrenfors P, et al. Intensive insulin treatment in critically ill trauma patients normalizes glucose by reducing endogenous glucose production. *J Clin Endocrinol Metab* 2004;89:5382–5386.
7. Tsubo T, Kudo T, Matsuki A, Oyama T. Decreased glucose utilization during prolonged anaesthesia and surgery. *Can J Anesth* 1990;37:645–649.
8. Braden H, Cheema-Dhadli S, Mazer D, et al. Hyperglycemia during normothermic cardiopulmonary bypass: The role of the kidney. *Ann Thorac Surg* 1998;65:1588–1593.
9. Thorell A, Nygren J, Ljungqvist O. Insulin resistance: A marker of surgical stress. *Curr Opin Clin Nutr Metab Care* 1999;2:69–78.
10. Ljungqvist O, Nygren J, Thorell A. Insulin resistance and elective surgery. *Surgery* 2000;128:757–760.
11. Van den Berghe G. How does blood glucose control with insulin save lives in intensive care? *J Clin Invest* 2004;114(9):1187–1195.
12. Umpierrez GE, Isaacs SD, Bazargan H, et al. Hyperglycemia: An independent marker of in-hospital mortality in patients with undiagnosed diabetes. *J Clin Endocrinol Metab* 2002;87:978–982.
13. Krinsley JS. Association between hyperglycemia and increased hospital mortality in a heterogenous population of critically ill patients. *Mayo Clin Proc* 2003;78:1471–1478.
14. Kinney J, Elwyn D. Protein metabolism and injury. *Ann Rev Nutr* 1983; 3:433–466.
15. Carli F, Webster J, Ramachandra V, et al. Aspects of protein metabolism after elective surgery in patients receiving constant nutritional support. *Clin Sci* 1990;78:621.
16. Shaw J, Wolfe R. An integrated analysis of glucose, fat, and protein metabolism in severely traumatized patients. *Ann Surg* 1989;209:63–72.
17. Harrison R, Lewin M, Halliday D, Clark C. Leucine kinetics in surgical patients I: A study of the effect of surgical stress. *Br J Surg* 1989;76:505–508.
18. Chandra R. Nutrition, immunity and infection: Present knowledge and future directions. *Lancet* 1983;1(8326):688–691.
19. Windsor J, Hill G. Weight loss with physiologic impairment. *Ann Surg* 1988; 207:290–296.
20. Watters J, Clancey S, Moulton S, et al. Impaired recovery of strength in older patients after major abdominal surgery. *Ann Surg* 1993;218:380–393.
21. Christensen T, Bendix T, Kehlet H. Fatigue and cardiorespiratory function following abdominal surgery. *Br J Surg* 1982;69:417–421.
22. Lazar HH, Chipkinn SR, Fiztgerald CA, et al. Tight glycemic control in diabetic coronary artery bypass graft patients improves perioperative outcomes and decreases recurrent ischemic events. *Circulation* 2004;109:1497–502.
23. Korvald C, Elvenes OP, Myrmel T. Myocardial substrate metabolism influences left ventricular energetics in vivo. *Am J Physiol Heart Circ Physiol* 2000;279:H1345–H1351.
24. Liu Q, Docherty JC, Rendell JCT, et al. High levels of fatty acids delay the recovery of intracellular pH and cardiac efficiency in post-ischemic hearts by inhibiting glucose oxidation. *J Am Coll Cardiol* 2002;39:718–725.
25. Olivier MF, Opie LH. Effects of glucose and fatty acids on myocardial ischaemia and arrhythmias. *Lancet* 1994;343:155–158.
26. Steinberg HO, Tarshoby M, Monestel M, et al. Elevated circulating free fatty acid levels impair endothelium-dependent vasodilatation. *J Clin Invest* 1997;100:1230–1239.
27. Schroeder D, Hill GL. Predicting postoperative fatigue: Importance of preoperative factors. *World J Surg* 1993;17:226–231.
28. Christensen T, Nygaard F, Stage JG, Kehlet H. Skeletal muscle enzyme activities and metabolic substrates during exercise in patients with postoperative fatigue. *Br J Surg* 1990;77:312–317.
29. Wood CD. Postoperative exercise capacity following nutritional support with hypotonic glucose. *Surg Gynecol Obstet* 1981;152:39–47.

30. Zeidermann MR, Welchew EA, Clark RG. Changes in cardiorespiratory and muscle function associated with the development of postoperative fatigue. *Br J Surg* 1990;77:576–585.

31. Greisen J, Juhl CB, Grofte T, et al. Acute pain induces insulin resistance in humans. *Anesthesiology* 2001;95:578–584.

32. Nashef SA, Roques F, Michael P, et al. Coronary surgery in Europe: Comparison of the national subsets of the European system for cardiac operative risk evaluation database. *Eur J Cardiothorac Surg* 2000;17:396–399.

33. Leurs LJ, Laheij RJ, Buth J, Eurostar Collaborators. Influence of diabetes mellitus on the endovascular treatment of abdominal aortic aneurysms. *J Endovasc Ther* 2005;12(3):288–296.

34. Charlton MR, Nair KS. Role of hyperglucagonemia in catabolism associated with type 1 diabetes: Effects on leucine metabolism and the resting metabolic rate. *Diabetes* 1998;47:1748–1756.

35. Inchiostro S, Biolo G, Bruttomesso D, et al. Effects of insulin and amino acid infusion on leucine and phenylalanine kinetics in type 1 diabetes. *Am J Physiol* 1992;262:E203–E210.

36. Umpleby AM, Scobie IN, Boroujerdi MA, et al. Diurnal variation in glucose and leucine metabolism in non-insulin-dependent diabetes. *Diabetes Res Clin Pract* 1990;9:89–96.

37. Halvatsiotis P, Short KR, Bigelow M, Nair SK. Synthesis rate of muscle proteins, muscle functions, and amino acid kinetics in type 2 diabetes. *Diabetes* 2002;51:2395–2404.

38. Shamoon M, Hendler R, Sherwin R. Altered responsiveness to cortisol, epinephrine, and glucagon in insulin-infused juvenile-onset diabetes. A mechanism for diabetic instability. *Diabetes* 1980;29:284–291.

39. Barker JP, Robinson PN, Vafidis GC, et al. Metabolic control of non-insulin-dependent diabetic patients undergoing cataract surgery: Comparison of local and general anesthesia. *Br J Anaesth* 1995;74:500–505.

40. Schricker T, Gougeon R, Eberhart L, et al. Type 2 diabetes mellitus and the catabolic response to surgery. *Anesthesiology* 2002;97:943–951.

41. Allison S. Malnutrition, disease, and outcome. *Nutrition* 2000;16:590–593.

42. Downs J, Haffejee A. Nutritional assessment in the critically ill. *Curr Opin Clin Nutr Met Care* 1998;1:275–279.

43. Allison S, Lobo D, Stanga Z. The treatment of hypoalbuminemia. *Clin Nutr* 2001;20:275–279.

44. McWhirter J, Pennington C. Incidence and recognition of malnutrition in hospital. *Br Med J* 1994;308:945–948.

45. Fettes S, Davidson H, Richardson R, Pennington C. Nutritional status of elective gastrointestinal surgery patients pre- and postoperatively. *Clin Nutr* 2002;21:249–254.

46. Douglas R, Shaw J. Metabolic effects of cancer. *Br J Surg* 1990;77:246–254.

47. Jeevanandam M, Horowitz G, Lowry S, Brennan M. Cancer cachexia and protein metabolism. *Lancet* 1984;1(8392):1423–1426.

48. Brennan M. Uncomplicated starvation versus cancer cachexia. *Cancer Res* 1977;37:2359–2236.

49. Oclio MR, Brodish A. Effects of age on metabolic responses to acute and chronic stress. *Am J Physiol* 1988;254(5 pt 1);E617–E624.

50. Seals DR, Esler MD. Human ageing and the sympathoadrenal system. *J Physiol* 2000;528(3):407–417.

51. Beale E, Zhu J, Belzberg H. Changes in serum cortisol with age in critically in patients. *Gerontology* 2002;48:84–92.

52. Walters JM, Narris SB, Kirkpatrick SM. Endogenous glucose production following injury increases with age. *J Clin Endocrinol Metab* 1997;82:3005–3010.

53. Walters JM, Moulton SB, Claucey SM, et al. Aging exaggerates glucose intolerance following injury. *J Trauma* 1994;37(5):786–791.

54. Cregerman RI, Bierman EL. Aging and hormones. In: Williams RH, ed. *Textbook of Endocrinology*, 6th ed. Philadelphia: Saunders, 1981.

55. Boirie Y, Gachon P, Beaufrere B. Splanchnic and whole-body leucine kinetics in young and elderly men. *Am J Clin Nutr* 1997;65:489–495.

56. Short KR, Nari KS. The effect of age on protein metabolism. *Am Opin Clin Nutr Metab Care* 2000;3(1):39–44.

57. Jeevanandam M, Petersen SR, Shamos RF. Protein and glucose fuel kinetics and hormonal changes in elderly trauma patients. *Metabolism* 1993;42(10):1255–1262.

58. Burdge JJ, Katz B, Edwards R, et al. Surgical treatment of burns in elderly patients. *J Trauma* 1988;28:219–227.

59. Linn BS, Robinson AS, Klismas NG. Effects of age and nutritional status on surgical outcomes. *Ann Surg* 1988;207(3):267–273.

60. Dahn M, Mitchell R, Lange P, et al. Hepatic metabolic response to injury and sepsis. *Surgery* 1995;117:520–530.

61. Eshali A, Boija P, Ljungqvist O, et al. Twenty-four-hour food deprivation increases endotoxin lethality in the rat. *Eur J Surg* 1991;157:85–89.

62. Ljungqvist O, Boija P, Eshali A, et al. Food deprivation alters glycogen metabolism and endocrine responses to hemorrhage. *Am J Physiol* 1990;259:E692–E698.

63. Nygren J, Thorell A, Soop M, et al. Perioperative insulin and glucose infusion maintains normal insulin sensitivity after surgery. *Am J Physiol* 1998;275:E140–E148.

64. Ljungqvist O, Thorell A, Gutniak M, et al. Glucose infusion instead of preoperative fasting reduces postoperative insulin resistance. *J Am Coll Surg* 1994;178:329–336.

65. Crowe P, Dennison A, Royle G. The effect of preoperative glucose loading on postoperative nitrogen metabolism. *Br J Surg* 1984;71:635–637.

66. Veterans Affairs Total Parenteral Nutrition Study Group. Perioperative parenteral nutrition in surgical patients. *N Engl J Med* 1991;325:525–529.

67. Bozzetti F, Gavazzi C, Miceli R, et al. Perioperative total parenteral nutrition in malnourished gastrointestinal cancer patients: A randomized clinical trial. *J Parent Enteral Nutr* 2000;24:7–14.

68. Kehlet H. Modification of responses to surgery by neural blockade: Clinical implications. In: Cousins MJ, Bridenbaugh PO, eds. *Neural Blockade in Clinical Anesthesia and Management of Pain*, 3rd ed. Philadelphia: Lippincott; 1998:129–175.

69. Kehlet H. The stress response to surgery: Release mechanisms and the modifying effects of pain relief. *Acta Chir Scand* [Suppl] 1989;55[Suppl]:22–33.

70. Carli F, Halliday D. Modulation of protein metabolism in the surgical patient: Effect of 48-h continuous epidural blockade with local anesthetics on leucine kinetics. *Reg Anesth* 1996;21:430.

71. Carli F, Barnard M, Webster J. Metabolic response to colonic surgery: Spinal versus extradural anaesthesia. *Br J Anaesth* 1991;67:567.

72. Segawa H, Mori K, Kasai K, et al. The role of the phrenic nerves in stress response in upper abdominal surgery. *Anesth Analg* 1996;82:1215–1220.

73. Tsuji H, Shirasaka C, Asoh T, Uchida I. Effects of epidural administration of local anaesthetics and morphine on postoperative nitrogen loss and catabolic hormones. *Br J Surg* 1987;74:421–427.

74. Ruthberg H, Havanson E, Anderberg L, et al. Effects of extradural administration of morphine or bupivacaine on the endocrine response to upper abdominal surgery. *Br J Anaesth* 1984;56:233–241.

75. Goodarzi M, Narasimhan RR. The effect of large-dose intrathecal opioids on the autonomic nervous system. *Anesth Analg* 2001;93:456–459.

76. Schricker T, Wykes L, Eberhardt L, et al. Epidural ropivacaine vs. epidural morphine and the catabolic response to colonic surgery: Stable isotope kinetic studies in the fasted state and during the infusion of glucose. *Anesthesiology* 2004;100(4):973–978.

77. Lattermann R, Carli F, Wykes L, Schricker T. Epidural blockade modifies perioperative glucose production without affecting protein catabolism. *Anesthesiology* 2002;97:374–381.

78. Uchida I, Asoh T, Shirasaka C, Tsuji H. Effect of epidural analgesia on postoperative insulin resistance as evaluated by insulin clamp technique. *Br J Surg* 1988;75:557–562.

79. Lattermann R, Carli F, Schricker T. Epidural blockade suppresses lipolysis during major abdominal surgery. *Reg Anesth Pain Med* 2002;27:469–475.

80. Carli F, Lattermann R, Schricker T. Epidural analgesia and postoperative lipid metabolism: Stable isotope studies during a fasted/fed state. *Reg Anesth Pain Med* 2002;27:132–138.

81. Vedrinne C, Vedrinne J, Giraud M, et al. Nitrogen-sparing effect of epidural administration of local anesthetics in colon surgery. *Anesth Analg* 1989;69:354–359.

82. Lariviere F, Wagner D, Kupranycz D, Hoffer L. Prolonged fasting as conditioned by prior protein depletion: Effect on urinary nitrogen excretion and whole-body protein turnover. *Metabolism* 1990;39:1270–1277.

83. Nolte K, Kehlet H. Epidural anaesthesia and analgesia—effects on surgical stress responses and implications for postoperative nutrition. *Clin Nutr* 2002;21:199–206.

84. Schricker T, Wykes L, Carli F. Epidural blockade improves substrate utilization after surgery. *Am J Physiol* 2000;279:E646–E653.

85. Hjortso R, Lewin M, Halliday D, Clark C. Effects of extradural administration of local anesthetic agents and morphine on the urinary excretion of cortisol, catecholamines and nitrogen following abdominal surgery. *Br J Anaesth* 1985;57:400–406.

86. Schricker T, Meterissian S, Lattermann R, Carli F. Postoperative protein sparing with epidural analgesia and hypocaloric glucose. *Ann Surg* 2004;240:916–921.

87. Schricker T, Wykes L, Eberhart L, et al. The anabolic effect of epidural blockade requires energy and substrate supply. *Anesthesiology* 2002;97:943–951.

88. Schricker T, Wykes L, Eberhart L, et al. Randomized clinical trial of the anabolic effect of hypocaloric parenteral nutrition after abdominal surgery. *Br J Surg* 2005;92:947–953.

89. Donatelli F, Schricker T, Asenjo JF, et al. Intraoperative infusion of amino acids induces anabolism independently of the type of anesthesia. *Anesth Analg* 2006;103:1549–1556.

90. Donatelli F, Schricker T, Mistraletti G, et al. Postoperative infusion of amino acids induces a positive protein balance independently of the type of analgesia used. *Anesthesiology* 2006;105:253–259.

91. Basse L, Raskov HH, Hjort Jakobsen D, et al. Accelerated postoperative recovery programme after colonic resection improves physical performance, pulmonary function and body composition. *Br J Surg* 2002;89:446–453.

92. Carli F, Mayo N, Klubien K, et al. Epidural analgesia enhances functional exercise capacity and health-related quality of life. Results of a randomized trial. *Anesthesiology* 2002;97:540–549.

93. Rademaker BM, Shir L, Kalkman CJ, et al. Effects of interpleurally administered bupivacaine 0.5% on opioid analgesic requirements and endocrine

response during and after cholecystectomy: A randomized double blind study. *Acta Anaesthesiol Scand* 1991;35:108–115.

94. Barker JP, Robinson PN, Vafidis GC, et al. Metabolic control of non-insulin dependent diabetic patients undergoing cataract surgery: Comparison of local and general anesthesia. *Br J Anaesth* 1995;74:500–505.

95. Richardson J, Sabanathan S, Jones J, et al. A prospective, randomized comparison of preoperative and continuous balanced epidural or paravertebral bupivacaine on post-thoracotomy pain, pulmonary function and stress responses. *Br J Anaesth* 1999;83:387–392.

96. Mistraletti G, DeLaQuadra JC, Asenjo JF, et al. Comparison of analgesic methods for total knee arthroplasty: Metabolic effect of exogenous glucose. *Reg Anesth Pain Med* 2006;31:260–269.

97. Schricker T, Gougeon R, Eberhart L, et al. Type 2 diabetes mellitus and the catabolic response to surgery. *Anesthesiology* 2005;102:320–326.

98. Kopp LA, Donatelli F, Chricker T, et al. Epidural analgesia enhances the postoperative anabolic effect of amino acids in diabetes mellitus type 2 patients undergoing colon surgery. *Anesthesiology* 2008;108: in press.

99. Buunen M, Gholghesaei M, Veldkamp R, et al. Stress response to laparoscopic surgery. *Surg Endosc* 2004;18:1022–1028.

100. Carli F, Galeone M, Gzodzic B, et al. Effect of laparoscopic colon resection on postoperative glucose utilization and the protein sparing effect. *Arch Surg* 2005;140:593–597.

101. Taqi A, Hong X, Mistraletti G, et al. Thoracic epidural analgesia facilitates the restoration of bowel function and dietary intake in patients undergoing laparoscopic colon resection with a traditional, non-accelerated, perioperative care program. *Surg Endosc* 2007;21:247–252.

102. Kaba A, Laurent SR, Detroz BJ, et al. Intravenous lidocaine infusion facilitates acute rehabilitation after laparoscopic colectomy. *Anesthesiology* 2007;106:11–18.

103. Kehlet H, Wilmore DW. Multimodal strategies to improve surgical outcome. *Am J Surg* 2002;183:630–641.

CHAPTER 7 ■ NEURAL BLOCKADE: IMPACT ON OUTCOME

CHRISTOPHER L. WU AND SPENCER S. LIU

The importance of effective management of acute pain is clear from multiple studies documenting the undertreatment of pain and introducing guidelines and regulatory standards for the assessment and treatment of acute pain. The presence of uncontrolled acute pain may potentially result in widespread adverse responses that may contribute to a number of perioperative complications. As described in the preceding chapter by Drs. Schricker and Carli, the effective management of acute pain may attenuate several of these adverse responses and, in turn, improve patient outcomes. Many different classes of analgesic agents and different analgesic techniques exist, each of which has a unique profile (e.g., quality of analgesia, presence of side effects, attenuation of adverse physiologic responses, and impact on outcomes). However, regional anesthesia and analgesic techniques, including neuraxial and peripheral regional analgesia, are especially effective in the provision of postoperative analgesia and attenuation of perioperative pathophysiology. In this chapter, we review the evidence, focusing on available systematic review and meta-analyses, for the effects of regional anesthetic and analgesia techniques (both peripheral and neuraxial) on patient outcomes.

PATHOPHYSIOLOGY OF ACUTE PAIN

The noxious stimuli from iatrogenic surgical injury or accidental trauma set a cascade of events into motion, cumulating in the perception of "pain." Many interrelated components contribute to the processing of nociceptive stimuli. These pathways are generally divided into peripheral and central (i.e., spinal and supratentorial) processes. Clinicians should recognize that the neurobiology of nociception is extremely complex, with multiple levels of redundancy such that no "hardwired" or "final common" pathway exists for the process of nociception. Comprehensive discussions of the neuroanatomy and pharmacology of nociception are provided in Chapters 31 through 33. For the purposes of the present chapter, we will concisely survey these processes and limit our description of central nociceptive processing to that taking place in the spinal cord.

Peripheral Nociceptive Processing

Surgical incision initiates a variety of noxious stimuli (mechanical or chemical) that ultimately are processed, conveyed to higher brain centers, and perceived as "pain." In the periphery, information from the noxious stimulus is processed by receptors and neurons whose primary function is the processing of nociceptive information. Primary afferent nociceptors, which are distinct from those that carry innocuous somatic sensory information, convert a wide range of environmental noxious stimuli into electrochemical signals. Activation of primary afferent nociceptors may also initiate the process of neurogenic inflammation and the release of neurotransmitters, particularly substance P and calcitonin gene-related peptide (CGRP), that may cause vasodilation and plasma extravasation (1). Release of these neurotransmitters, along with inflammatory mediators (e.g., bradykinin, prostaglandins, serotonin, neurotrophins) released at the site of injury, may initiate the process of peripheral sensitization (1). The electrochemical signals processed by the primary afferent nociceptors are transmitted toward the spinal cord in the small diameter Aδ- and C-fibers that primarily transmit nociceptive information.

Primary sensory afferent nociceptors synapse with neurons in the dorsal horn of the spinal cord. Neurotransmission across the synapse, originating from peripheral afferent Aδ- and C-fibers, is mediated by a number of peptides and amino acids that interact with specific receptors postsynaptically. For example, substance P, which is specific to the small-diameter primary afferents and released by noxious thermal, mechanical, and chemical stimuli in the periphery, will interact with the neurokinin (NK)-1 receptor postsynaptically.

In addition, the excitatory amino acid glutamate is also present within small-diameter primary afferents, released by noxious stimulation, and may interact with one of three receptor classes: α-amino-3-hydroxy-5-methyl-4-isoxazolepropionic acid (AMPA)/kainate, N-methyl-D-aspartate (NMDA), and metabotropic glutamate receptors (mGluR). Although postsynaptic interaction occurs with the AMPA, NK-1, mGluR, and NMDA receptors, as described in Chapters 31 through 33, presynaptic interactions may also exist (e.g., mGluR, voltage-gated calcium channels) that may affect neurotransmitter release (2).

Central (Spinal) Nociceptive Processing and Descending Modulation

Although the primary afferents release neurotransmitters to activate the second-order neurons in the spinal cord, the specific actions depend on the particular receptor activated, since the second-order neurons in the dorsal horn contain a wide variety of neurotransmitter receptors. Activation of certain receptors, such as the NMDA, AMPA/kainate, mGluR, and NK-1, results in depolarization and increased nociceptive pain transmission. Activation of other receptors, such as the opioid γ-aminobutyric acid-A (GABA$_A$) and serotonin, results in hyperpolarization and a decrease or inhibition of nociceptive pain transmission. Actual transmission of nociceptive information may also be modified by descending inhibitory systems including serotonin, enkephalin, and noradrenergic neurons (see Chapters 31 and 32).

Although not all nociceptive input results in a pathologic process, a certain percentage of patients who undergo surgical procedures will exhibit prolonged central sensitization and chronic pain. Pathologic nociceptive input may cause a central sensitization that is marked by hyperexcitable spinal neurons that exhibit a decreased threshold for activation, increased and prolonged response to noxious input, expansion of receptive fields, possible spontaneous activity, and activation by normally non-noxious stimuli (33). Induction and maintenance of central sensitization emphasizes different receptor–neurotransmitter combinations, including NMDA receptors, prostaglandins, and neuropeptides (substance P, CGRP, neurokinin A) (3). Ultimately, transcriptional changes (including induction of genes), structural changes in synaptic connections (e.g., contact between low-threshold afferent and nociceptive neurons), and loss of inhibitory interneurons may result in a persistent state of central sensitization (4).

Effects on Individual Organ Systems

The noxious stimuli and resultant pathophysiology associated with surgery may affect many organ systems and result in postoperative complications, particularly in patients in certain subgroups (e.g., older patients, those with decreased physiologic reserve, and those undergoing specific procedures such as lung resection or coronary artery bypass [CAB]).

Cardiovascular

It has traditionally been thought that an imbalance of myocardial oxygen supply and demand, such as an increase in demand (e.g., increase in heart rate or blood pressure) or decrease in supply (e.g., decreased coronary blood flow to the vulnerable subendocardial areas), may contribute to perioperative cardiac events particularly in patients with decreased cardiac reserve (5). Although many factors may contribute to an imbalance of myocardial oxygen supply and demand, uncontrolled postoperative pain may be especially detrimental and contribute to cardiac morbidity through activation of the sympathetic nervous system, other surgical stress responses, and the coagulation cascade. Increased sympathetic nervous system activity can increase myocardial oxygen demand by increasing heart rate, blood pressure, and contractility or even decrease myocardial oxygen supply, which in turn may lead to angina, dysrhythmias, and areas of myocardial infarction (5). In addition, sympathetic activation may enhance perioperative hypercoagulability, which may contribute to perioperative coronary thrombosis or vasospasm, thus reducing myocardial oxygen supply (7,8).

Pulmonary

The pathophysiology of pulmonary dysfunction after surgery is multifactorial. Relevant factors include disruption of normal respiratory muscle activity that may result from either surgery or anesthesia, reflex inhibition of phrenic nerve activity with subsequent decrease in diaphragmatic function, and uncontrolled postoperative pain, which may contribute to volun-

tary inhibition of respiratory activity or splinting (9). Although the pathophysiology of breathing and respiratory muscle function following surgery is complex, it is clear that anesthetic or analgesic agents administered in the perioperative period affect the central regulation of breathing and activities of respiratory muscles. This incoordination of respiratory muscle function (which may last well into the postoperative period) will impair lung mechanics (9), increasing the risk of hypoventilation, atelectasis, and pneumonia. Visceral stimulation may decrease phrenic motoneuron output, which results in a decrease in diaphragmatic descent and lung volumes (9).

Gastrointestinal

Although decreased gastrointestinal (GI) motility is expected after abdominal surgery, return of GI function usually occurs within several days postoperatively. However, some patients will develop paralytic ileus, a protracted and more severe state of GI immotility. Although the pathophysiology of postoperative ileus and decreased GI motility is multifactorial, the primary mechanisms include neurogenic (spinal, supraspinal adrenergic pathways), inflammatory (i.e., local inflammatory responses initiate neurogenic inhibitory pathways), and iatrogenic pharmacologic (e.g., opioids) mechanisms (10). In the acute postoperative phase, neurogenic (spinal and supraspinal) mechanisms are primary mediators of decreased GI motility (10). Activation of splanchnic afferents and increased sympathetic outflow, along with the possible use of opioids, are the predominant mechanisms for decreased GI motility immediately following surgery (10). However, over the subsequent postoperative days, a prolonged phase of postoperative ileus occurs. The presumed etiology of the latter is distinct, and involves an enteric molecular inflammatory response that impairs local neuromuscular function and activates neurogenic inhibitory pathways (10). Our understanding of the mechanisms of postoperative ileus is not complete, and it is likely that these three mechanisms are not discrete phenomena but interrelated (10).

Coagulation

It is recognized that hypercoagulability occurs in association with surgical procedures. Although the pathophysiology of coagulation-related events (e.g., formation of deep venous thrombosis [DVT]) has essentially been unchanged since Virchow's initial description of the triad of stasis, blood vessel injury, and hypercoagulability (11), our current understanding of the coagulation system is that it is a complex system with many other functions including tissue repair, autoimmune regulation, arteriosclerosis, and tumor growth and metastasis (12). Nevertheless, the primary components of the coagulation systems comprise cellular (e.g., platelets, endothelial cells, monocytes, and erythrocytes) and molecular (e.g., coagulation factors and inhibitors, fibrinolysis factors and inhibitors, adhesive and intercellular proteins, acute-phase proteins, immunoglobulins, phospholipids, prostaglandins, and cytokines) components (12). The normal process of coagulation involves several steps including initiation (damaged vascular endothelium expresses tissue factor, which ultimately leads to generation of thrombin), amplification (augmentation of the effects of thrombin), propagation (formation of clot), and stabilization (formation of a stable fibrin meshwork that protects the clot from fibrinolytic attack) (12). However, following surgery, the normal process of coagulation may become unbalanced, which may result in a tendency toward thrombosis. Immediately after surgical incision, there are increases in levels of tissue factor, tissue plasminogen activator, plasminogen activator inhibitor-1, and von Willebrand factor, which contribute to a hypercoagulable and hypofibrinolytic state postoperatively (12).

Cognitive Function

The etiology of postoperative cognitive dysfunction (PCD) is uncertain but most likely involves the combination of many factors, including dysregulation of cerebral neurotransmitters, patient factors (e.g., age, comorbidities, preoperative cognitive function and general health), surgical procedure undertaken (certain procedures such as CAB may have a higher incidence), and perioperative drug therapy. It is believed that a perioperative imbalance of neurotransmitter systems, especially acetylcholine and serotonin, or increase in inflammatory mediators, such as cytokines, may contribute to the development of PCD, especially in the elderly, who may have a decreased neurophysiologic reserve at baseline (13,14). Central cholinergic deficiency through anticholinergic mechanisms or impaired acetylcholine production may be an important factor in the development of PCD, with a possible dose-response relationship between the degree of pharmacologic anticholinergic activity and severity of delirium (15). In addition, an excessive amount or enhanced transmission of serotonin, which is important for mediating mood, sleep, and cognition, can result in confusion and restlessness (15). Surgery will result in the release of cytokines, which may ultimately influence neurotransmitter activity and contribute to PCD, since administration of interleukin (IL)-2 has been associated with cognitive dysfunction and delirium (14). Finally, some surgical procedures may be specific etiologies of PCD, especially in patients undergoing cardiac surgery. Besides the possible etiologies of PCD discussed earlier, PCD after cardiac surgery may reflect additional factors including cerebral microembolization, global cerebral hypoperfusion, cerebral temperature perturbations, cerebral edema, and possible blood–brain barrier dysfunction (16).

Immunologic Function

It is clear that patients experience an alteration in immune status following surgery. Following major surgical procedures, an early hyperinflammatory response occurs, with release of proinflammatory tumor necrosis factor (TNF)-α, IL-1 and IL-6 cytokine, neutrophil activation and microvascular adherence, and uncontrolled polymorphonuclear (PMN) and macrophage oxidative activity (17). This hyperinflammatory response is followed by significant cell-mediated immunosuppression marked by monocyte deactivation, decreased microbicidal activity of phagocytes, and an overall imbalance between proinflammatory and anti-inflammatory cytokines and immunocompetent cells (17,18). Surgery in the abdominal cavity may also elicit an enhanced immunologic response, as manipulation of the GI tract initiates an inflammatory cascade within the intestinal wall muscularis that results in a decrease in GI motility (18). Cytokines released into the peritoneal fluid during abdominal surgery may decrease organ function and increase the risk of anastomotic leakage, particularly during sepsis (18). The resultant immunosuppression may lead to an increased risk of postoperative infection and could in theory influence outcomes in oncologic patients. However, it is possible that laparoscopic surgery, which results in less trauma than conventional open surgery, might be associated with a reduced inflammatory response and subsequent immunosuppression due to a decrease in the production of cytokines and in activation of cellular and humoral immune responses (18).

EFFECTS AND EFFICACY OF ACUTE PAIN MANAGEMENT ON POSTOPERATIVE OUTCOME

Epidural and Spinal Neural Blockade

Mortality

Despite controversy (due in part to some of the methodologic issues present in studies, such as underpowered trials) as to the overall benefits of perioperative neuraxial anesthesia and analgesia on mortality, some credible data suggest that the use of both intraoperative neuraxial anesthesia and postoperative epidural analgesia may significantly lower mortality. A systematic review of randomized controlled trials (RCTs) comparing patients who received intraoperative neuraxial blockade or not included 141 trials (prior to January 1997) with 9,559 patients (19). The risk of mortality within 30 days of the surgical procedure was reduced by about a third in patients who received neuraxial anesthesia (103 deaths per 4,871 patients versus 144 deaths per 4,688 patients, odds ratio (OR) = 0.70, 95% confidence interval (CI): 0.54–0.90, $p = 0.006$) (Fig. 7-1) (19). A subsequent meta-analysis (20) indicated that the 30-day mortality after mixed orthopedic procedures was significantly lower with use of neuraxial anesthesia (versus general anesthesia) although many methodologic issues are present when interpreting the evidence. Despite the findings of some larger recent RCTs (21,22) that found no differences in mortality between neuraxial and general anesthesia, a meta-analysis suggested that high-risk patients may benefit from regional anesthesia (22).

Large-scale observational data also suggest that postoperative epidural analgesia may be associated with a significantly lower odds of death (23). A 5% random sample of the Medicare claims database from 1997 through 2001 was analyzed. Patients undergoing a variety of surgical procedures (colectomy, esophagectomy, gastrectomy, hysterectomy, liver resection, nephrectomy, pulmonary resection, radical retropubic prostatectomy, and total knee replacement) were stratified according to the presence ($n = 12,780$ subjects) or absence ($n = 55,943$) of a bill for postoperative epidural analgesia. After adjusting for comorbidities, age, gender, and hospital size, regression analysis revealed that the presence of postoperative epidural analgesia was associated with a significantly lower odds ratio for both 7-day (OR = 0.52; 95% CI: 0.38–0.73, $p = 0.0001$) and 30-day (OR = 0.74; 95% CI: 0.63–0.89, $p = 0.0005$) mortality (23). Not unexpectedly, there was a significantly lower mortality in patients who received postoperative epidural analgesia for higher-risk procedures (e.g., lung resection, colectomy) but no difference in mortality between patients who did or did not receive postoperative epidural analgesia in lower-risk procedures (e.g., total knee replacement, hysterectomy) undergone by patients with lower comorbidity indices.

Morbidity

Cardiovascular. Given that 8 million of the 27 million patients in the United States who have surgery every year have coronary artery disease or risk factors for cardiovascular disease, cardiac-related events are one of the most common causes of perioperative mortality (24). Within the United States alone, 1 million patients annually have perioperative cardiac complications (at an estimated cost of $20 billion) (25) and worldwide, approximately 5% of the surgical population will develop some type of perioperative cardiac complication (26).

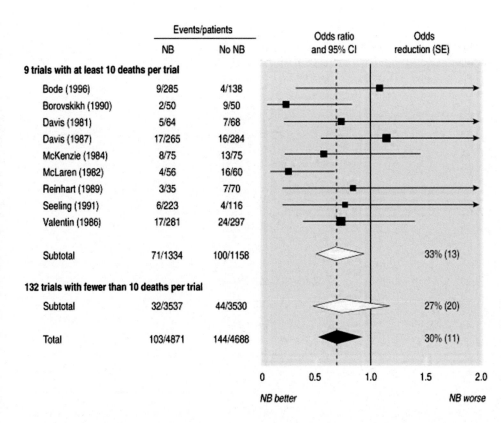

| | Events/patients | | Odds ratio | Odds |
| | NB | No NB | and 95% CI | reduction (SE) |

9 trials with at least 10 deaths per trial

	NB	No NB	
Bode (1996)	9/285	4/138	
Borovskikh (1990)	2/50	9/50	
Davis (1981)	5/64	7/68	
Davis (1987)	17/265	16/284	
McKenzie (1984)	8/75	13/75	
McLaren (1982)	4/56	16/60	
Reinhart (1989)	3/35	7/70	
Seeling (1991)	6/223	4/116	
Valentin (1986)	17/281	24/297	
Subtotal	71/1334	100/1158	33% (13)

132 trials with fewer than 10 deaths per trial

	NB	No NB	
Subtotal	32/3537	44/3530	27% (20)
Total	103/4871	144/4688	30% (11)

0   0.5   1.0   1.5   2.0
NB better   *NB worse*

FIGURE 7-1. Pooled estimate of randomized controlled trials indicating that use of perioperative neuraxial anesthesia (compared to general anesthesia) is associated with a significantly lower odds (30%) of 30-day mortality after a variety of surgical procedures. From Rogers et al. *BMJ* 2000;321: 1493–1497, with permission.

Experimental data from animal studies suggest that thoracic epidural analgesia with local anesthetics (thoracic epidural analgesia; TEA) will provide a favorable balance of myocardial oxygen supply and demand particularly in patients with decreased cardiac reserve. Thoracic epidural analgesia may increase the diameter of stenotic epicardial coronary arteries in patients with coronary artery disease without changing the diameter of nonstenotic segments, and it does not induce any changes in coronary perfusion pressure, total myocardial blood flow, coronary venous oxygen content, or regional myocardial oxygen consumption (27). During myocardial ischemia, TEA may also attenuate an ischemia-induced decrease in myocardial pH (28), and it lessens the degree of regional ischemia induced by intracoronary injection of endothelin, a potent vasoconstrictor (29). Other animal studies indicate that TEA improves functional recovery from myocardial stunning and reduces infarct size after myocardial ischemia and reperfusion injury (30,31). In part through its favorable physiologic effects (blockade of sympathetic outflow, attenuation of stress response, increased coronary flow in stenotic segments) on the myocardium, TEA has been shown in animal studies to decrease the incidence of malignant ventricular arrhythmias and may actually protect against the generation of ventricular arrhythmias (32,33). It is important to remember that these physiologic benefits are provided only by TEA (a "catheter-incision congruent" technique) and not lumbar epidural analgesia (LEA; a "catheter-incision *in*congruent" technique) as there may be a compensatory *increase* in sympathetic activity above the level of blockade during lumbar epidural analgesia, which may not be particularly physiologically beneficial to the heart (34). Finally, in patients with multivessel ischemic heart disease, TEA increased myocardial blood flow in all vascular territories (35).

Several systematic reviews and meta-analyses examine the effects of neuraxial anesthesia and analgesia on cardiovascu-

lar events. Although the results of these meta-analyses might seem equivocal, they in fact are consistent when one asks whether a catheter-incision congruent technique was employed and whether the neuraxial technique persisted into the postoperative period, thus maximizing the physiologic benefits of neuraxial analgesia. One of the largest meta-analyses examined 141 RCTs describing 9,559 patients who were randomized to receive intraoperative neuraxial or general anesthesia (19). Although the patients who were randomized to receive neuraxial anesthesia had a significantly lower risk of 30-day mortality, there was no significant decrease in the risk of myocardial infarction (Fig. 7-2). It should be noted that the vast majority of patients received LEA or spinal anesthesia, which, as previously mentioned, may not provide the physiologic benefit of TEA.

Two meta-analyses examining the efficacy of postoperative epidural analgesia and cardiovascular events suggest a benefit for epidural analgesia. The first meta-analysis examined 11 RCTs comprising 1,173 patients undergoing a variety of surgical procedures in whom epidural analgesia was extended at least 24 hours into the postoperative period (36). There was no difference in the in-hospital death rate; however, the rate of myocardial infarction was significantly lower in those who received epidural analgesia (rate difference = −3.8%; 95% CI: −7.4%, −0.2%; p = 0.049). Subgroup analysis revealed that TEA but not LEA provided a significant reduction in the rate of myocardial infarction (rate difference = −5.3%; 95% CI: −9.9%, −0.7%; p = 0.04) (36), again supporting experimental data demonstrating physiologic cardiac benefits of TEA but not necessarily of LEA. The second meta-analysis examined 15 RCTs with 1,178 patients undergoing CAB surgery (37). There were no differences in the incidences of mortality or myocardial infarction; however, the use of TEA (versus systemic opioids) was associated with a significant reduction in the risk of dysrhythmias (24.8% versus 29.1%) (Table 7-1).

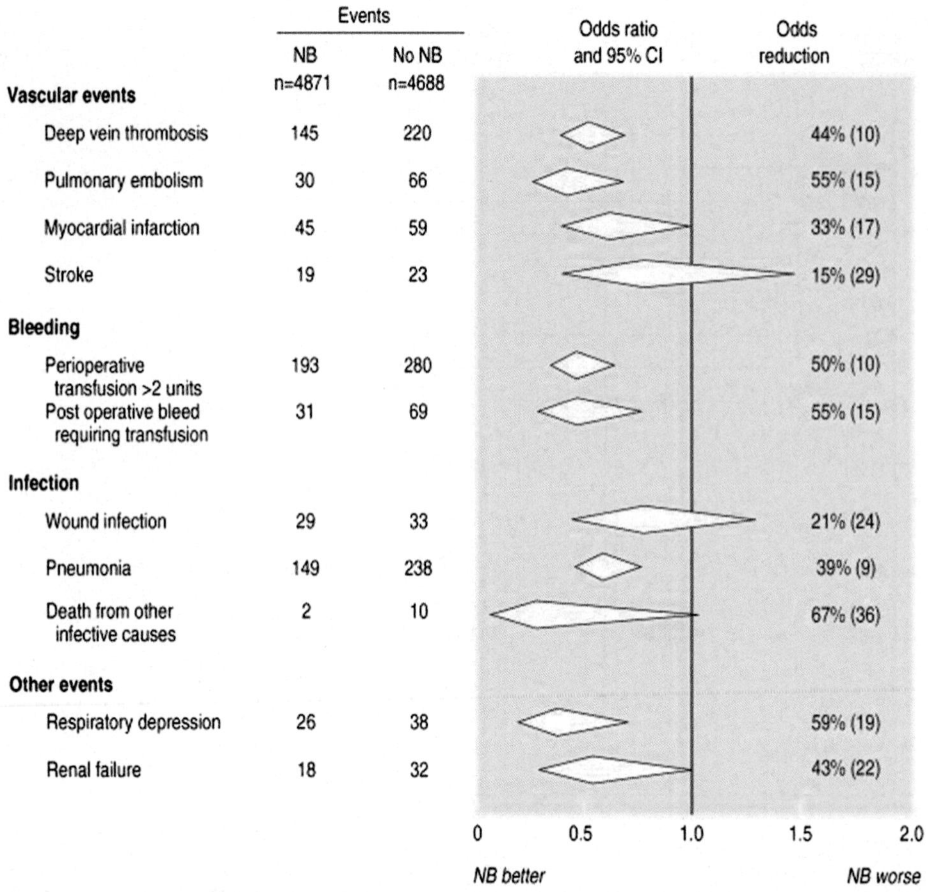

FIGURE 7-2. Subgroup analysis of Figure 7-1. Pooled estimates suggest that use of perioperative neuraxial anesthesia (compared to general anesthesia) is associated with a significantly lower odds of deep venous thrombosis, pulmonary embolism, bleeding complications, pneumonia, and respiratory depression. From Rogers et al. *BMJ* 2000;321:1493–1497, with permission.

Pulmonary. Postoperative pulmonary complications (PPC) are a significant problem affecting approximately 10% of patients undergoing elective abdominal surgery (9) and are as common as cardiac complications in those undergoing noncardiac procedures (38,39). Compared to postoperative cardiac complications, PPC may be a better predictor of long-term postoperative

mortality (39). Many factors, including uncontrolled postoperative pain, may result in decreased lung volumes, which in turn may contribute to the development of atelectasis and PPC.

Epidural analgesia, particularly that using a local anesthetic–based solution, will confer superior analgesia compared to systemic opioids, including IV PCA (40,41). Segmental block from TEA may result in increased tidal volume and vital capacity related in part to improved pain control and interruption of the reflex inhibition of phrenic nerve activity, thus improving diaphragmatic activity (9). Thoracic epidural analgesia using bupivacaine 0.25% did not impair ventilatory mechanics and inspiratory respiratory muscle strength in patients with severe chronic obstructive pulmonary disease (42). Despite the presence of sympathetic blockade, TEA does not worsen airway obstruction in patients with severe chronic obstructive pulmonary disease (43). Although there are apparent benefits, the physiologic effects of TEA on respiratory muscle function are complex, with TEA possibly paralyzing other respiratory muscles such as the intercostals or abdominals (9).

Several meta-analyses indicate that the use of regional anesthesia and analgesia (versus general anesthesia and systemic opioids) may be associated with a significant decrease in the risk of PPC (19,37,44). An earlier meta-analysis of 48 RCTs demonstrated that the use of epidural analgesia using a local anesthetic-based regimen (versus systemic opioids) was associated with a significant decrease in PPC (44). These benefits were not seen with epidural opioids, intercostal blocks, or intrapleural analgesia (44). The subgroup analysis of a previously described meta-analysis (19) noted neuraxial anesthesia-analgesia reduce the odds of developing pneumonia by 39%,

TABLE 7-1

EFFECTS OF SINGLE-SHOT PERIPHERAL NERVE BLOCKS VERSUS GENERAL ANESTHESIA FOR AMBULATORY SURGERY

Outcome	N	PNB (mean)	GA (mean)	p
VAS pain (mm)	359	10	36	0.0001
Nausea (%)	319	7	30	0.0001
Need for rescue analgesics (%)	259	6	42	0.001
Excellent patient satisfaction (%)	158	88	72	0.001

A total of seven randomized controlled trials with 359 patients were included. Data from Liu SS, Strodtbeck WM, Richman JM, Wu CL. A comparison of regional versus general anesthesia for ambulatory anesthesia: A meta-analysis of randomized controlled trials. *Anesth Analg* 2005;101:1634–1642, with permission.

compared to general anesthesia and systemic opioids. In addition, a more recent meta-analysis examining the perioperative use of TEA in patients undergoing CAB revealed that TEA was associated with a significant decrease in PPC (OR = 0.41; 95% CI: 0.28–0.61) (37). However, PPC might not be decreased with use of regional anesthesia-analgesia in all procedures: A meta-analysis of general versus regional anesthesia in patients undergoing hip fracture repair noted no difference in the risk of developing pneumonia (45). Finally, one systematic review suggested that IV PCA with opioids versus as-needed (PRN) systemic opioids was associated with a statistically significant decrease in PPC (OR = 0.93; 95% CI: 0.86–0.99) (46); however, two other meta-analyses examining the same topic (i.e., IV PCA versus PRN opioids) did not reveal any benefit of IV PCA in decreasing the incidence of PPC (47,48). Many methodologic issues contribute to the controversy of whether neuraxial anesthesia-analgesia decreases PPC, including the fact that there is no universally accepted definition of what constitutes a PPC.

Gastrointestinal. Postoperative ileus and decreased GI motility may cost the U.S. health care system several billions dollars annually (49). The pathophysiology of postoperative ileus and decreased GI motility is multifactorial and includes neurogenic (spinal, supraspinal adrenergic pathways), inflammatory (i.e., local inflammatory responses initiate neurogenic inhibitory pathways), and pharmacologic (e.g., opioids) mechanisms (10). Analgesic agents differ in their effects on GI motility and, as such, it is not unreasonable to expect a difference in rate of return of GI function with different analgesic regimens.

Experimental data consistently indicate that epidural analgesia shortens the duration of intestinal paralysis (50,51). Other experimental data indicate that epidural analgesia may actually increase the strength of colonic contractions without impairing anastomotic healing or increasing the risk of anastomotic leakage (52). Epidural analgesia has been shown to hasten recovery from postischemic paralytic ileus in a rat model (53) and to prevent endotoxin-induced gut mucosal injury in rabbits (54). In addition, there is also data suggesting that TEA may improve gastric microcirculation and minimize intestinal acidosis (55,56).

A systematic review of RCTs published in the Cochrane Library indicates consistently quicker return of GI function in subjects receiving epidural local anesthetic compared with those receiving systemic or epidural opioid (37 hours and 24 hours, respectively) (57). Other reviews also confirm that epidural analgesia enhances recovery after GI surgery (58,59). This benefit, however, was seen only in RCTs in which there was proper placement of the epidural catheter (i.e., "catheter-incision congruent analgesia," in which the catheter tip placement corresponds with the incisional dermatome). In such studies, there was consistent benefit from (thoracic) epidural analgesia with regard to return of GI function (59). Use of a catheter-incision *in*congruent analgesia technique (e.g., LEA for upper abdominal surgery), even with local anesthetic, will obscure any possible benefit of epidural analgesia in providing an earlier return of GI function (59). It should be noted that the advantages of epidural analgesia with respect to return of GI function are greatest when used as part of a multimodal, accelerated rehabilitation care pathway (60) and that other factors, such as fluid therapy, may also influence postoperative GI motility (61).

Coagulation. In general, approximately 600,000 patients annually develop pulmonary embolism (PE), with 60,000 deaths resulting from this complication (11). During the perioperative period, coagulation-related complications may be an important cause of morbidity. It is widely recognized that DVT is a major complication following orthopedic procedures. In addition, PE is the most frequent cause of death associated with childbirth (11). In the absence of thromboembolic prophylaxis, the incidence of *fatal* PE ranges from 0.1% to 0.8% after general surgery, 0.3% to 1.7% after elective hip surgery, and 4% to 7% after emergency hip surgery (11).

Spinal and epidural anesthesia using local anesthetic regimens will attenuate perioperative hypercoagulability and may provide physiologic benefits (e.g., increased blood flow) to prevent perioperative coagulation-related complications (49). Following surgical incision, there is an increase in coagulation factors and platelet activity and a decrease in fibrinolytic activity (49). Intraoperative neuraxial anesthesia has been shown to attenuate perioperative increases in coagulation proteins (62) and platelet activity (63), to preserve fibrinolytic activity (7), and to increase arterial and venous blood flow. Local anesthetics administered for epidural anesthesia and analgesia may be absorbed systemically and thereby exert systemic antithrombotic effects, including reduction in platelet aggregation, inhibition of thrombus formation, and reduction in blood viscosity (64).

Several meta-analyses have demonstrated that intraoperative use of neuraxial anesthesia (versus general anesthesia) is associated with significant decreases in the odds of DVT and PE (19,45,65,66). Subgroup analysis of a large meta-analysis revealed that intraoperative neuraxial anesthesia (versus general anesthesia) was associated with a significant decrease in the odds of developing DVT by 44% and PE by 55% (Fig. 7-2) (19). A more recent meta-analysis also found that neuraxial anesthesia compared to general anesthesia for hip fracture surgery significantly decreased the risk of developing DVT. Regional anesthesia was associated with a reduced risk of DVT (relative risk [RR] = 0.64; 95% CI: 0.48–0.86) (66). Another meta-analysis in patients undergoing hip fracture repair revealed that regional anesthesia lowered the odds of DVT (OR = 0.41; 95% CI: 0.23–0.72) (45).

In addition, some RCTs suggest that use of epidural anesthesia and analgesia may decrease coagulation-related events in patients undergoing abdominal and lower extremity vascular grafts procedures. In one RCT, patients undergoing vascular surgery received either general anesthesia followed by systemic opioids or a combined general-epidural anesthesia followed by epidural analgesia (63). Patients who were randomized to receive epidural anesthesia-analgesia had one-ninth the incidence of vascular graft occlusion (63). In another RCT in patients undergoing lower extremity revascularization, patients were randomized to receive either general anesthesia followed by systemic opioids, or epidural anesthesia followed by epidural analgesia (67). Patients who were randomized to receive epidural anesthesia and analgesia had one-fifth the incidence of reoperation (67).

Despite the benefits for regional anesthesia shown in these trials and meta-analyses, it is unclear if the physiologic benefits conferred by intraoperative neuraxial anesthesia continue into the postoperative period. Further, the effect of epidural analgesia per se on coagulation-related events is not straightforward: Some experimental data suggest that postoperative epidural analgesia using common local analgesic concentrations (≤0.125% bupivacaine) does not provide any significant increase in whole-limb, venous, or cutaneous blood flow nor decrease in postoperative hypercoagulability (68,69). Another methodologic issue in trials of the effect of regional analgesia is the fact that many older studies in this area did not use concurrent prophylactic anticoagulation.

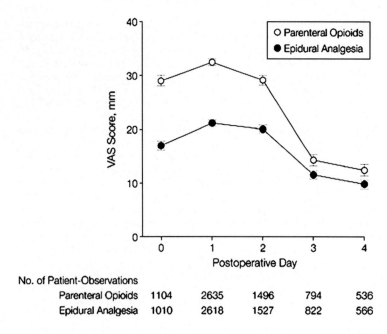

FIGURE 7-3. Compared to systemic parenteral opioids, epidural analgesia provides statistically lower pain scores for up to 4 days after a variety of surgical procedures. From Block BM, Liu SS, Rowlingson AJ, et al. Efficacy of postoperative epidural analgesia: A meta-analysis. *JAMA* 2003;290:2455–2463, with permission.

Chronic Pain. Chronic pain following surgery has only recently been considered as a significant postoperative complication (see Chapter 43). The incidence of chronic pain after surgery varies by procedure but may be quite high, with reported incidences of 30% to 81% after limb amputation, 22% to 67% after thoracotomy, 17% to 57% after breast surgery, 6% to 56% after cholecystectomy, and 4% to 37% after hernia repair (70). Persistent pain has also recently been reported after cesarean section in approximately 12% of patients at 10 months after surgery (71). As mentioned earlier in this chapter and discussed at length in Chapters 31 through 33, peripheral and central sensitization may occur following surgery, ultimately leading to chronic pain with hyperalgesia and allodynia. It is important to recognize that, although many risk factors are possible (e.g., psychological factors, whether the surgical incision has a nerve-sparing orientation, preexisting pain intensity), the severity of acute postoperative pain appears to be an important risk factor for the development of chronic postsurgical pain (70). Theoretically, the use of epidural analgesia could confer superior analgesia (compared to systemic opioids) (Fig. 7-3) and thereby reduce the incidence of chronic postsurgical pain. Epidural anesthesia-analgesia that is initiated prior to incision might confer a "preemptive" effect and may be more efficacious in decreasing or even preventing chronic postsurgical pain. Although there are few trials in this area, some RCTs have suggested that use of preincisional epidural analgesia might decrease the incidence of chronic postsurgical pain (72,73). Patients undergoing thoracic surgery under general anesthesia were randomized to receive either continuous epidural block before surgical incision or at completion of surgery. Postoperative pain was less in the group that received continuous epidural block prior to surgical incision. This group also had lower postoperative pain scores and a higher percentage of pain-free patients at 3 and 6 months after surgery (73). In another RCT in patients undergoing thoracic procedures, patients who received TEA pre- and intraoperatively (compared to those who received general anesthesia with IV PCA morphine for postoperative analgesia) had a lower incidence and intensity of pain at 6 months (72).

Confusion and Cognitive Function. Postoperative central nervous system disorders are generally marked by deficits in cognition and memory. These disorders encompass a wide range of postoperative states including delirium or dementia (impairment in cognitive function), amnesia (impairment in memory), and sedation (impairment of consciousness). The etiologies of these disorders are complex and may be distinct for specific disorders. However, mental function typically reaches a nadir in the early postoperative period, with a recovery to preoperative levels by 1 week following surgery in most patients (74,75). Certain subgroups, especially those undergoing certain types of surgery (e.g., CAB), and those with coexisting medical diseases, preexisting cognitive dysfunction, or advanced age (76), are at higher risk for developing postoperative cognitive dysfunction. Delirium is a particularly problematic subset of postoperative cognitive dysfunction as it may contribute to at least an additional 17.5 million inpatient days and $4 billion in health care expenditures annually (77). Delirium may occur in 9% to 11% of elderly patients undergoing elective noncardiac surgery (78,79) and as many as 36.8% of patients undergoing hip fracture repair (80).

A systematic review examining the effect of intraoperative anesthetic technique upon postoperative cognitive dysfunction noted that, of the 19 RCTs (24 total) obtained from the literature search, 18 did not demonstrate a difference in cognitive function after *intra*operative general versus regional anesthesia (81). Although the effect of *post*operative regional analgesia on cognitive dysfunction is uncertain, it is plausible that it may have a greater impact than intraoperative regional anesthesia. Higher degrees of postoperative pain severity are associated with a higher incidence of postoperative cognitive dysfunction (especially delirium) (82,83). Since postoperative regional analgesia provides superior analgesia (40,84), it is theoretically possible that postoperative regional analgesia (versus systemic opioids) might result in a lower incidence of postoperative cognitive dysfunction, including delirium. However, the effect of postoperative analgesia on mental function has not been rigorously investigated as trials in this area generally lack control of the postoperative analgesic regimen.

Patient-oriented Outcomes

Patient-oriented ("nontraditional") outcomes, such as patient satisfaction, quality of life, and quality of recovery, are important, valid outcomes that have been widely used in other areas of medicine and are becoming more important in the field of anesthesiology and perioperative care. Although many diverse patient-oriented outcomes exist, several aspects of regional anesthesia and analgesia (e.g., quality of analgesia, presence of side effects) might theoretically influence patient-oriented outcomes. For example, it is recognized that different analgesic regimens provide different degrees of postoperative analgesia, with postoperative regional analgesic techniques (e.g., continuous epidural and peripheral) providing superior analgesia compared to systemic opioids including IV PCA (40,82). There may be differences even when comparing the same regional analgesic technique to different systemic analgesic control groups, as IV PCA opioids in general appear to provide superior analgesia compared to PRN systemic opioids (46–48).

Nausea, Vomiting, and Pruritus. Although provision of analgesia is a commonly recognized goal for postoperative pain control, the presence of analgesic agent–related side effects, typically from opioids or local anesthetics, differ among analgesic techniques and may be an important influence on patient-oriented outcomes. For example, although continuous epidural analgesia (CEA) may provide superior analgesia compared to patient-controlled epidural analgesia (PCEA), patients who were randomized to CEA had a higher incidence of some side effects such as motor block (41). In addition, PCEA (when compared to IV PCA with opioids) is associated with a lower incidence of postoperative nausea and vomiting (PONV) and sedation but a higher incidence of pruritus and motor block (41). Compared to systemic opioids, CEA is associated with a lower incidence of PONV, sedation, and pruritus but a higher incidence of motor block (84).

Patient Satisfaction. Patient satisfaction has become an important outcome measurement and indicator of quality of medical care. Although assessing patient satisfaction might seem intuitively easy, the concept of patient satisfaction incorporates many dimensions and domains and is quite complex, embracing various theories, definitions, and ideas regarding patient satisfaction still not clearly codified by consensus. Appropriate methods to assess patient satisfaction must utilize validated survey instruments that have been psychometrically constructed (85). Many assessments of satisfaction with regional anesthesia have not relied upon validated instruments; however, it is possible that regional analgesia may result in superior satisfaction compared to other techniques due in part to the superior analgesia provided. A systematic review examining the effect of regional anesthesia and analgesia on patient satisfaction revealed that, of the 10 RCTs that assessed satisfaction, seven trials showed greater satisfaction with regional analgesic techniques compared to systemic opioids (86). It is not clear whether there may be differences in patient satisfaction among different regional analgesic techniques; however, different techniques appear to be associated with differences in the frequency and severity of analgesic-related side effects such as nausea, pruritus, sedation, and motor block. For example, patients who received epidural anesthesia for elective cesarean section had higher maternal satisfaction (using a validated instrument) compared with those who were randomized to receive spinal anesthesia, due in part to the increased side effects (i.e., pruritus) associated with intrathecal morphine (87).

Further research is necessary to elucidate the effect of different analgesic techniques on patient satisfaction.

Health-related Quality of Life. Health-related quality of life (HRQL) is a comprehensive assessment of the medical care received by a patient and conceptually assesses the domains of physical functioning, mental health, cognitive functioning, symptoms (e.g., pain), role and social functioning, general health perceptions, sleep, and energy. Typically, HRQL is best measured using validated instruments, either generic or specific. As with other patient-oriented outcomes, HRQL is widely recognized as a valid end-point and important outcome in research, particularly in the assessment of chronic diseases and the long-term effects of surgery. Although HRQL may be assessed in the postoperative period, the time frame for assessment of HRQL is typically over a period of months, not days, which might be more relevant to assessment of the immediate postoperative period.

Theoretically, many factors such as fatigue, physical functioning, mental health, degree of analgesia, and presence of analgesic agent–related side effects may influence HRQL; however, few studies examine the effect of postoperative analgesic regimens on HRQL as a primary end-point. An RCT in patients undergoing colectomy randomized patients to either IV PCA opioid or epidural analgesia and assessed HRQL using a validated generic HRQL instrument, the SF-36 (88). Patients who were randomized to receive epidural analgesia had lower pain and fatigue scores, increased mobilization, and significantly better preservation of HRQL scores compared with those who received IV PCA (88).

Complications

A variety of complications may occur with neuraxial anesthesia and analgesia. These are discussed in detail in the context of perioperative care in Chapters 12 and 20, and in relation to pain management in Chapter 50. For the purposes of the present chapter, we will mention these. The vast majority of adverse events are limited and not life-threatening (e.g., nausea, vomiting, pruritus) and are generally related to the medications used in the anesthetic technique. Some of the more serious complications are discussed here. In light of these serious adverse effects, clinicians must carefully weigh the risks and benefits of contemplated neuraxial techniques on an individual basis.

Respiratory. Neuraxial opioids may produce severe respiratory depression. The incidence of neuraxial opioid-induced respiratory depression is dose-dependent and is reported to occur in approximately 0.1% of patients, a rate significantly lower than that from IV PCA using opioids (1.9%) (90). Although neuraxial administration of both lipophilic (e.g., fentanyl, sufentanil) and hydrophilic (e.g., morphine, hydromorphone) opioids may cause respiratory depression, "delayed" respiratory depression with neuraxial administration attributed to hydrophilic opioids typically occurs within 12 hours following injection (91). Risk factors for the development of respiratory depression after administration of neuraxial opioids include increasing dose, increasing age, concomitant use of systemic opioids or sedatives, and possibly prolonged or extensive surgery, presence of comorbidities, and thoracic surgery (91).

Neurologic, Including Hematoma. Neurologic injury after neuraxial techniques may be either transient or permanent; it is uncommon, with an estimated incidence of between 0.002% and 0.16% (92–95). Although the cross-sectional area of the epidural space is smaller at the thoracic than at the lumbar level, the risk of neurologic injury does not appear to be greater with placement of thoracic epidural catheters. A prospective series of 4,185 patients with thoracic epidural catheters reported a 0.7% incidence of neurologic injury, with none of these injuries resulting in paraplegia (95).

Epidural hematoma is one of the most feared complications of neuraxial techniques. Although epidural vessel puncture may occur in up to 12% of epidural catheter placements (96), the development of symptomatic epidural hematomas is rare, with an estimated incidence of approximately 1:150,000 after epidural anesthesia/analgesia (97). However, the introduction of low-molecular-weight heparin (LMWH) in North America may have increased the risk of epidural hematoma, notwithstanding the extensive prior safety experience in Europe with LMWH (approximately 100,000 patients with spinal or epidural anesthesia in combination with LMWH, with six reported cases of epidural hematoma) (98). A consensus statement for the administration of neuraxial techniques in patients receiving anticoagulants has been published by the American Society of Regional Anesthesia and Pain Medicine (www.asra.com).

Infectious. Epidural abscess formation is fortunately relatively uncommon, with a reported incidence of 0.02% to 0.05% with epidural analgesia (92,99). Although an epidural catheter offers a route of entry into the epidural space, epidural abscesses are more likely to result from hematogenous rather than direct spread (100) and are rare with routine postoperative use (101). Patients who develop an epidural abscess are more likely to have a prolonged epidural catheterization time and be immunocompromised, although the level of catheter insertion does not appear to be related to the risk of abscess formation (99).

Peripheral Nerve Analgesia and Outcomes

Peripheral nerve blocks and catheter placement for continuous local anesthetic infusion have become increasingly popular in acute postoperative pain management. Peripheral techniques offer potential advantages over systemic analgesic regimens in terms of better analgesia with fewer side effects than opioid-based regimens (Fig. 7-4, Tables 7-2 and 7-3). Peripheral techniques offer more targeted and limited sensory and motor block than central neuraxial analgesia and offer reduced risk of catastrophic complications such as spinal hematomas

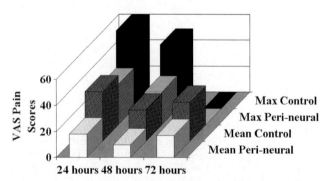

FIGURE 7-4. Mean and maximum pain scores for continuous perineural versus systemic opioid analgesia after a variety of surgical procedures. Pain scores were significantly lower for perineural analgesia for all time points. From Richman JM, Liu SS, Courpas G, et al. Does continuous peripheral nerve block provide superior pain control to opioids? A meta-analysis. *Anesth Analg* 2006;102:248–257, with permission.

TABLE 7-2

EFFECTS OF SINGLE-SHOT PERIPHERAL NERVE BLOCKS VERSUS GENERAL ANESTHESIA FOR AMBULATORY SURGERY

Outcome	N	PNB (mean)	GA (mean)	p
VAS pain (mm)	359	10	36	0.0001
Nausea (%)	319	7	30	0.0001
Need for rescue analgesics (%)	259	6	42	0.001
Excellent patient satisfaction (%)	158	88	72	0.001

A total of seven randomized controlled trials with 359 patients were included.
Data from Liu SS, Strodtbeck WM, Richman JM, Wu CL. A comparison of regional versus general anesthesia for ambulatory anesthesia: A meta-analysis of randomized controlled trials. *Anesth Analg* 2005;101:1634–1642, with permission.

and abscesses. The amount of residency training devoted to regional anesthesia and peripheral nerve blocks has steadily increased in the United States as a reflection of this increased interest and the potential benefits. A survey of American anesthesiology residency program directors in 2002 indicated that nearly 60% of programs now offer a specific peripheral nerve block rotation (102). A review of clinical case logs submitted from residents to the Residency Review Committee for Anesthesiology demonstrated a growth in use of regional anesthesia techniques from 21% of cases in 1980 to 30% of cases in 2000 (103).

Single-shot Peripheral Nerve Blocks

Although excellent evidence exists for increased interest and training in peripheral nerve blocks, there remains little evidence that these techniques affect clinical outcomes. Conceptually, single-shot peripheral nerve blocks would offer limited means to reduce the mechanisms of major perioperative complications described thus far. Duration of analgesia after a single injection of long-acting local anesthetic is at most about 12 hours (104), whereas maximal postoperative pain after major surgery has an average duration of 3 days (40). Thus, single-shot peripheral

TABLE 7-3

COMPARISON OF INCIDENCES OF SIDE EFFECTS BETWEEN CONTINUOUS PERINEURAL ANALGESIA VERSUS SYSTEMIC OPIOIDS

Side effects	Perineural analgesia	Opioids	Odds ratio	NNT
Nausea/Vomiting (%)	21	49	0.28	4
Sedation	27	52	0.33	4
Pruritus	10	27	0.3	6

All differences are statistically significant (p <0.01).
Data from Richman JM, Liu SS, Courpas G, et al. Does continuous peripheral nerve block provide superior pain control to opioids? A meta-analysis. *Anesth Analg* 2006;102:248–257, with permission.

nerve blocks are temporally inadequate to affect ongoing pain and subsequent outcomes. As discussed earlier, cardiopulmonary complications are the most frequent source of major morbidity (23) and often occur later than 12 hours into the postoperative period. Postoperative myocardial infarction remains the leading cause of major postoperative morbidity, and patients remain at risk for at least 24 hours after surgery (36). Although less severe but more common than cardiac complications, postoperative pulmonary complications may be associated with significantly longer increments of hospital stay (9). The most important postoperative ventilatory change is the delayed decrease in functional residual capacity. Because this decrease is maximal at 24 to 48 hours after surgery, single-shot peripheral nerve blocks are temporally insufficient to affect pulmonary outcome. In addition, the limited spatial targeting of conduction block with peripheral neural blockade, although generally an attractive feature, may also restrict potentially beneficial effects on postoperative pathophysiology. For example, blocks limited to the periphery have minimal direct effects on sympathetic activation, which is an important contributor to cardiovascular (105) and gastrointestinal (106) morbidity, as well as limited effects on phrenic afferent stimulation, which may be detrimental to pulmonary function (9). Finally, the ability of peripheral nerve blocks per se to affect outcome may be diluted by the frequent use of adjunct analgesics. Due to a block's relatively brief duration, limited anatomic spread, and inherent sensory and motor block, peripheral nerve blocks are frequently supplemented with systemic analgesics such as nonsteroidal anti-inflammatory drugs (NSAIDs) or opioids. This multimodal approach may benefit the patient but lessens potential contribution of peripheral nerve blocks per se upon outcome.

Mortality and Morbidity. Perhaps reflecting their limited effect upon underlying pathophysiologic mechanisms, the published evidence that single-shot peripheral nerve blocks may affect postoperative outcomes is sparse. A 2006 search of Medline for clinical trials in the last decade examining single-shot peripheral nerve blocks and postoperative complications (with search terms "nerve block" and "postoperative complications" and limited to Clinical trial, Adult, and English) returned 271 abstracts. The largest single RCT enrolled only 100 patients and was designed to evaluate analgesia and minor, immediate complications after ambulatory surgery (107). The largest meta-analysis of RCTs included a total of 359 patients randomized to single-shot peripheral nerve block versus general anesthesia for ambulatory anesthesia (107). The largest prospective clinical series examined lumbar plexus blocks for outpatient anterior cruciate ligament (ACL) repair in 948 patients and was again designed to evaluate analgesia and minor, immediate complications (108). As previously discussed, reasonably designed outcome studies examining mortality and major morbidity (e.g., myocardial infarction) would require enrollment of 1.2 million low-risk patients (mostly undergoing ambulatory procedures) or 5,000 high-risk patients (23,37). Thus, no conclusions can be drawn from the current literature regarding the effects of single-shot peripheral nerve blocks on major outcomes. Given the limited mechanistic effects and the typically less-invasive, lower-risk procedures in which single-shot peripheral nerve blocks are applied, it seems unlikely that such evidence will be forthcoming or even detectable.

Patient-oriented Outcomes. In contrast, there is considerable and growing evidence for patient-oriented benefits, such as analgesia, from single-shot peripheral nerve blocks. In general,

RCTs studying peripheral nerve blocks are very heterogeneous with widely varying surgical procedures, types and techniques of nerve block, types of control group, and agents for nerve blocks. Although this diversity makes summary statements difficult, two recent systematic reviews provide insight for hospitalized and outpatient procedures. A Cochrane Review of nerve blocks for analgesia after hip fracture repair examined effects of subcostal, lateral femoral cutaneous, femoral, three-in-one, and psoas blocks from eight RCTs enrolling 328 patients (109). Analgesia after hip fracture is an important topic, as hip fracture repair is a worldwide health issue due to an increasing elderly population. The World Health Organization has estimated that 6.3 million individuals per annum will suffer a hip fracture by 2050 (110). In aggregate, RCTs of single-shot peripheral nerve blocks showed decreases in pain intensity scores and opioid consumption, but clinical trial heterogeneity precluded an assessment of clinical impact or discernment of differences between different types of nerve block. Another recent systematic review assessed the effect of single-shot peripheral nerve blocks for ambulatory surgery (107). A total of seven RCTs reporting 359 patients were included. Again, a variety of surgical procedures, nerve blocks, and agents were used. Overall, use of single-shot nerve blocks resulted in better analgesia, reduced need for rescue medications, reduced risk of nausea, and increased patient satisfaction (Table 7-1). Finally, single-shot nerve blocks may also provide improvement in economic outcomes for ambulatory surgery. Although time until discharge from the Ambulatory Surgery Unit has been previously measured as a cost surrogate, other studies suggest that this parameter has little direct impact (111). Indeed, the just-reviewed meta-analysis did not detect a statistically significant reduction in time spent in the Ambulatory Surgical Unit in patients who received nerve blocks, despite improved analgesia and reduced side effects. On the other hand, the ability to prevent hospitalization after an outpatient procedure is another outcome that may better reflect gains from nerve blocks. An observational study of 948 ambulatory patients undergoing ACL repair reported a reduction in unplanned hospitalization rates from 17% to 4% with use of nerve blocks. Cost savings is institution-dependent but were modeled to be approximately $100,000 per annum for this single procedure (108).

Continuous Perineural Analgesia

In contrast to the limited duration of single-shot peripheral nerve blocks, continuous perineural analgesia offers prolonged duration of postoperative analgesia and has grown in reported popularity. Duration of analgesia with perineural analgesia can be more easily matched to duration of maximal postoperative pain. However, the potential for perineural analgesia to affect postoperative physiology remains limited by the restricted extent of the conduction block, and it is further diluted by the frequent use of multimodal analgesia.

Mortality and Morbidity. A meta-analysis published in 2006 of all available RCTs comparing perineural analgesia to systemic opioids included 19 RCTs with a total of 603 patients (84). This number is clearly insufficient to evaluate the effects on mortality or major morbidity. For example, as described in detail in several chapters in the second half of this volume, the development of chronic postoperative pain is increasingly recognized as a major postoperative morbidity (70). As noted earlier, consistent evidence suggests that the severity of acute postoperative pain is a risk factor for development of chronic pain, and that single-shot nerve blocks and continuous

TABLE 7-4

A SUMMARY OF DURATION OF HOSPITAL STAY, PHYSICAL THERAPY, ANALGESIA, AND SIDE EFFECTS IN RANDOMIZED CONTROLLED TRIALS COMPARING CONTINUOUS PERINEURAL ANALGESIA TO SYSTEMIC OR EPIDURAL ANALGESIA

Outcome	Singelyn 1998	Capdevila 1999	Barrington 2005	Salinas ** 2006	Zaric 2006
Hospital stay (days)					
Perineural	17	40	5.3	3.8	8
Epidural	16	37	5.4		7
Systemic opioid	21*	50*		3.9	
Discharge knee flexion (°)					
Perineural	94	90	81		88
Epidural	97	90	82		90
Systemic opioid	88*	80*			
3-month knee flexion (°)					
Perineural	124	125		117	
Epidural	121	130			
Systemic opioid	116	125		113	
24-hr active VAS (mm)					
Perineural	36	28	18	17	40
Epidural	33	22	15		27
Systemic opioid	52*	55*		33*	
48-hr active VAS (mm)					
Perineural	25	22	10	9	
Epidural	30	30	10		37
Systemic opioid	42	49*		32*	40
Nausea (%)					
Perineural	33	5	N/A	N/A	8
Epidural	27	12	N/A		13
Systemic opioid	40	21*		N/A	

*, statistically significant (versus other groups); **systemic opioid group also received single-shot femoral nerve block.
Data from Zaric D, Boysen K, Christiansen C, et al. A comparison of epidural analgesia with combined continuous femoral-sciatic nerve blocks after total knee replacement. *Anesth Analg* 2006;102:1240–1246; Singelyn FJ, Deyaert M, Joris D, et al. Effects of intravenous patient-controlled analgesia with morphine, continuous epidural analgesia, and continuous three-in-one block on postoperative pain and knee rehabilitation after unilateral total knee arthroplasty. *Anesth Analg* 1998;87:88–92; Barrington MJ, Olive D, Low K, et al. Continuous femoral nerve blockade or epidural analgesia after total knee replacement: A prospective randomized controlled trial. *Anesth Analg* 2005;101:1824–1829; Capdevila X, Barthelet Y, Biboulet P, et al. Effects of perioperative analgesic technique on the surgical outcome and duration of rehabilitation after major knee surgery. *Anesthesiology* 1999; 91:8–15; and Salinas FV, Liu SS, Mulroy MF. The effect of single-injection femoral nerve block versus continuous femoral nerve block after total knee arthroplasty on hospital length of stay and long-term functional recovery within an established clinical pathway. *Anesth Analg* 2006;102: 1234–1239, with permission.

perineural analgesia offer superior pain control. The combination of these two factors suggests the hypothesis that these peripheral analgesic techniques may decrease the risk of chronic postoperative pain. Unfortunately, evidence for this hypothesis is still lacking. Evidence reviews in 2000 and 2004 did not identify any RCTs that specifically evaluated these techniques as a method to reduce the risk of chronic postoperative pain and complex regional pain syndrome (70,112). A recent (2006) search of Medline (using the search terms "postoperative analgesia" or "nerve blocks" or "regional anesthesia" and "chronic pain," limited to human, English, and clinical trials) yielded 177 abstracts but no RCTs that specifically studied this question. Currently, the question of the impact of nerve blocks and continuous perineural techniques on the development of chronic postsurgical pain remains unaddressed, yet potentially fruitful.

Patient-oriented Outcomes. Excellent evidence exists for the analgesic efficacy of perineural analgesia in both hospitalized and ambulatory patients (84,113). The previously mentioned meta-analysis (84) pooled data from both hospitalized and ambulatory patients to create summary comparisons. Overall, patients who received perineural analgesia had lower pain scores, decreased opioid use, and fewer opioid-related side effects (Fig. 7-1, Table 7-2).

Two other short-term outcomes related to perineural analgesia are worth noting. Earlier RCTs examining perineural analgesia for total knee replacement observed improved analgesia compared to systemic analgesic regimens, as well as faster physical rehabilitation and shortened hospital stays (Table 7-4) (114,115). However, physical function was similar in both groups by 3 months, and the durations of hospitalizations were quite long compared to current standards (Table 7-3). Recent RCTs have revisited this question in the context of present-day clinical pathways structured to accelerate postoperative physical rehabilitation and hospital discharge after knee replacement (116–118). These newer studies have noted much briefer durations of hospital stay than the previously published studies, and these durations are similar to those reported in current large orthopedic surgery patient registries (119). These recent

TABLE 7-5

SUMMARY OF LARGER SURVEILLANCE STUDIES EXAMINING COMPLICATIONS AFTER SINGLE-SHOT AND CONTINUOUS PERIPHERAL NERVE BLOCKS

	N	Types of block (hours of catheter)	Neurologic injury incidence (%)	Local infection incidence (%)	Bacteremia incidence (%)
Single shot					
Auroy, 2002	21,278	Mixed		N/A	N/A
2-day			0.04		
3-month			0.02		
Auroy, 1997	43,946	Mixed		N/A	N/A
8-day			0.03		
3-month			0.02		
Continuous perineural					
Capdevila, 2005	1,416	Mixed (56)	0.21	0.07	0
Bergman, 2003	405	Axillary (55)	0.5	0	1.5
Borgeat, 2003; 2001	934	Interscalene (72)		0.8*	N/A
10-day			8.7		
1-month			3.3		
3-month			0.9		
6-month			0.3		
Cuvillon, 2001	211	Femoral (48)	0.5	0	1.5%

*, only reported for 2003 study.
Data from Auroy Y, Narchi P, Messiah A, et al. Serious complications related to regional anesthesia. *Anesthesiology* 1997;87:479–486; Auroy Y, Benhamou D, Bargues L, et al. Major complications of regional anesthesia in France: The SOS Regional Anesthesia Hotline Service. *Anesthesiology* 2002;97:1274–1280; Borgeat A, Ekatodramis G, Kalberer F, Benz C. Acute and nonacute complications associated with interscalene block and shoulder surgery: A prospective study. *Anesthesiology* 2001;95:875–880; Capdevila X, Pirat P, Bringuier S, et al. Continuous peripheral nerve blocks in hospital wards after orthopedic surgery: A multicenter prospective analysis of the quality of postoperative analgesia and complications in 1,416 patients. *Anesthesiology* 2005;103:1035–1045; Cuvillon P, Ripart J, Lalourcey L, et al. The continuous femoral nerve block catheter for postoperative analgesia: Bacterial colonization, infectious rate and adverse effects. *Anesth Analg* 2001;93:1045–1049; Bergman BD, Hebl JR, Kent J, Horlocker TT. Neurologic complications of 405 consecutive continuous axillary catheters. *Anesth Analg* 2003;96:247–252; and Borgeat A, Dullenkopf A, Ekatodramis G, Nagy L. Evaluation of the lateral modified approach for continuous interscalene block after shoulder surgery. *Anesthesiology* 2003;99:436–442, with permission.

RCTs did not observe any current benefit upon physical rehabilitation or duration of hospitalization with perineural analgesia compared to single-shot nerve blocks or epidural analgesia (Table 7-4). Thus, in current practice, the ability of perineural analgesia to affect physical rehabilitation and length of stay for inpatients after knee replacement surgery appears limited. On the other hand, reports are beginning to appear describing perineural analgesia as a means to facilitate the conversion of major orthopedic procedures (total shoulder, elbow, hip, and knee replacements) to short-stay or ambulatory procedures (120–123). If this trend continues, reduced use of hospital resources through the application of perineural analgesia may produce substantial economic benefit.

Complications

Neurologic and Infectious. Detailed discussions of neurologic and other complications related to peripheral and neuraxial regional anesthesia and pain management are provided in Chapters 12, 20, and 50. Because these adverse outcomes of regional anesthesia must be weighed against beneficial ones, a mention of the former is appropriate here. Permanent injuries from single-shot and continuous nerve blocks appear to be clinically uncommon, and thus risks are difficult to estimate. The two largest prospective surveillance studies on regional anesthesia are limited by reliance on voluntary reporting and were both conducted only in France (Table 7-5). In these studies (in 1997 and 1999), initial incidences were eight neurologic injuries in 21,278 nerve blocks (0.038%) and

12 in 43,946 nerve blocks (0.027%). At 3-month follow-up, both incidences declined to 0.02%, reflecting patient recovery from injury (94,124). Use of continuous perineural analgesia is a recent development, with even less data available to address risk. The largest prospective study was performed in eight participating French institutions that utilized a variety of perineural catheters (femoral most common, followed in descending order by interscalene, popliteal, and axillary) for diverse surgical procedures (Table 7-5) (125). This study enrolled 1,416 patients and reported 394 (28%) minor adverse events (n = 253, 18%). Bacterial colonization of the catheters was common (30%), but only one abscess was reported. Neurologic injury occurred in three patients (0.21%), all with femoral catheters. The largest surveys to specify individual perineural techniques include 934 patients with interscalene catheters, 405 patients with axillary catheters, and 211 patients with femoral catheters (126–129). Information from these surveys is summarized in Table 7-5; all reported similar incidences of neurologic injury at 6 months (0.3%–0.5%). Some incidences were quite high early in the postoperative period. For example, there was a 9% incidence of neurologic injury with interscalene catheters at the 10-day examination period; this subsequently declined to 0.3% at 6 months (126,127). Although risk estimates from current data are imprecise, long-term neurologic injury is clearly uncommon after perineural catheter use. Nonetheless, current data is consistent with a potential five- to tenfold increase in risk for continuous peripheral nerve blocks compared to single-shot blocks. Further large-scale survey studies are needed to confirm this possibility.

SUMMARY

Effective acute pain management using both neuraxial and peripheral regional analgesia may benefit patient outcomes in a number of areas. Improvements in mortality, major morbidity, and patient-oriented outcomes have been identified in a literature that has for the most part focused upon the effects of epidural analgesia. Echoing the conclusions of the prior chapter by Drs. Carli and Schricker, placement and maintenance of peripheral and neuraxial regional analgesic techniques can provide superior analgesia and attenuate perioperative pathophysiologies that contribute to perioperative complications. Although epidural analgesic techniques seem to be associated with decreases in perioperative mortality and major morbidity and improvement in patient-oriented outcomes, methodologic issues in the relevant literature preclude definitive statements on this matter. Despite the potential analgesic and other benefits of peripheral and neuraxial regional analgesic techniques, risks are associated with these techniques, and an individualized risk–benefit assessment needs to be undertaken for each patient for whom these techniques are being considered.

References

1. Julius D, Basbaum AI. Molecular mechanisms of nociception. *Nature* 2001; 413:203–210.
2. Scholz J, Woolf CJ. Can we conquer pain? *Nat Neurosci* 2002;5[Suppl]: 1062–1067.
3. Schaible HG, Richter F. Pathophysiology of pain. *Langenbecks Arch Surg* 2004;389:237–243.
4. Wu CL, Garry MG, Zollo RA, Yang J. Gene therapy for the management of pain: Part I: Methods and strategies. *Anesthesiology* 2001;94:1119–1132.
5. Warltier DC, Pagel PS, Kersten JR. Approaches to the prevention of perioperative myocardial ischemia. *Anesthesiology* 2000;92:253–259.
6. Wu CL, Fleisher LA. Outcomes research in regional anesthesia and analgesia. *Anesth Analg* 2000;91.1232–1242.
7. Rosenfeld BA, Beattie C, Christopherson R, et al. The effects of different anesthetic regimens on fibrinolysis and the development of postoperative arterial thrombosis. *Anesthesiology* 1993;79:435–443.
8. Parker SD, Breslow MJ, Frank SM, et al. Catecholamine and cortisol responses to lower extremity revascularization: Correlation with outcome variables. *Crit Care Med* 1995;23:1954–1961.
9. Warner DO. Preventing postoperative pulmonary complications: The role of the anesthesiologist. *Anesthesiology* 2000;92:1467–1472.
10. Bauer AJ, Boeckxstaens GE. Mechanisms of postoperative ileus. *Neurogastroenterol Motil* 2004;16[Suppl 2]:54–60.
11. Hirsh J, Hoak J. Management of deep vein thrombosis and pulmonary embolism. A statement for healthcare professionals. Council on Thrombosis (in consultation with the Council on Cardiovascular Radiology), American Heart Association. *Circulation* 1996;93:2212–2245.
12. Bombeli T, Spahn DR. Updates in perioperative coagulation: Physiology and management of thromboembolism and haemorrhage. *Br J Anaesth* 2004;93:275–287.
13. Flacker JM, Lipsitz LA. Neural mechanisms of delirium: Current hypothesis and evolving concepts. *J Gerontol* 1999;54:B239–B246.
14. van der Mast RC. Pathophysiology of delirium. *J Geriat Psych Neurol* 1998;11:138–145.
15. Flacker JM, Lipsitz LA. Serum anticholinergic activity changes with acute illness in elderly medical patients. *J Gerontol* 1999;54A:M12–M16.
16. Grocott HP, Homi HM, Puskas F. Cognitive dysfunction after cardiac surgery: Revisiting etiology. *Semin Cardiothorac Vasc Anesth* 2005;9:123–129.
17. Menger MD, Vollmar B. Surgical trauma: Hyperinflammation versus immunosuppression? *Langenbecks Arch Surg* 2004;389:475–484.
18. Sido B, Teklote JR, Hartel M, et al. Inflammatory response after abdominal surgery. *Best Pract Res Clin Anaesthesiol* 2004;18:439–454.
19. Rodgers A, Walker N, Schug S, et al. Reduction of postoperative mortality and morbidity with epidural or spinal anaesthesia: Results from overview of randomised trials. *Br Med J* 2000;321:1493.
20. Ballantyne JC, Kupelnick B, McPeek B, Lau J. Does the evidence support the use of spinal and epidural anesthesia for surgery? *J Clin Anesth* 2005; 17:382–391.
21. Park WY, Thompson JS, Lee KK. Effect of epidural anesthesia and analgesia on perioperative outcome: A randomized, controlled Veterans Affairs cooperative study. *Ann Surg* 2001;234:560–569.
22. Rigg JR, Jamrozik K, Myles PS, et al. Epidural anaesthesia and analgesia and outcome of major surgery: A randomised trial. *Lancet* 2002;359:1276–1282.
23. Wu CL, Hurley RW, Anderson GF, et al. Effect of postoperative epidural analgesia on morbidity and mortality following surgery in Medicare patients. *Reg Anesth Pain Med* 2004;29:525–533.
24. Mangano DT. Perioperative cardiac morbidity. *Anesthesiology* 1990;72: 153–184.
25. Mangano DT, Goldman L. Preoperative assessment of patients with known or suspected coronary disease. *N Engl J Med* 1995;333:1750–1756.
26. Mangano DT. Assessment of the patient with cardiac disease: An anesthesiologist's paradigm. *Anesthesiology* 1999;91:1521–1526.
27. Blomberg S, Emanuelsson H, Kvist H, et al. Effects of thoracic epidural anesthesia on coronary arteries and arterioles in patients with coronary artery disease. *Anesthesiology* 1990;73:840–847.
28. Tsuchida H, Omote T, Miyamoto M, et al. Effects of thoracic epidural anesthesia on myocardial pH and metabolism during ischemia. *Acta Anaesthesiol Scand* 1991;35:508–512.
29. Fujita S, Tsuchida H, Kanaya N, et al. Effects of thoracic epidural anesthesia on changes in ischemic myocardial metabolism induced by intracoronary injection of endothelin in dogs. *J Cardiothorac Vasc Anesth* 1996;10:903–908.
30. Rolf N, Van de Velde M, Wouters PF, et al. Thoracic epidural anesthesia improves functional recovery from myocardial stunning in conscious dogs. *Anesth Analg* 1996;83:935–940.
31. Groban L, Zvara DA, Deal DD, et al. Thoracic epidural anesthesia reduces infarct size in a canine model of myocardial ischemia and reperfusion injury. *J Cardiothorac Vasc Anesth* 1999;13:579–585.
32. Blomberg S, Ricksten SE. Thoracic epidural anaesthesia decreases the incidence of ventricular arrhythmias during acute myocardial ischaemia in the anaesthetized rat. *Acta Anaesthesiol Scand* 1988;32:173–178.
33. Meissner A, Eckardt L, Kirchhof P, et al. Effects of thoracic epidural anesthesia with and without autonomic nervous system blockade on cardiac monophasic action potentials and effective refractoriness in awake dogs. *Anesthesiology* 2001;95:132–138.
34. Taniguchi M, Kasaba T, Takasaki M. Epidural anesthesia enhances sympathetic nerve activity in the unanesthetized segments in cats. *Anesth Analg* 1997;84:391–397.
35. Nygard E, Kofoed KF, Freiberg J, et al. Effects of high thoracic epidural analgesia on myocardial blood flow in patients with ischemic heart disease. *Circulation* 2005;111:2165–2170.
36. Beattie WS, Badner NH, Choi P. Epidural analgesia reduces postoperative myocardial infarction: A meta-analysis. *Anesth Analg* 2001;93:853–858.
37. Liu SS, Block BM, Wu CL. Effects of perioperative central neuraxial analgesia on outcome after coronary artery bypass surgery: A meta-analysis. *Anesthesiology* 2004;101:153–161.
38. Lawrence VA, Cornell JE, Smetana GW, American College of Physicians. Strategies to reduce postoperative pulmonary complications after noncardiothoracic surgery: Systematic review for the American College of Physicians. *Ann Intern Med* 2006;144:596–608.
39. Smetana GW, Lawrence VA, Cornell JE, American College of Physicians. Preoperative pulmonary risk stratification for noncardiothoracic surgery: Systematic review for the American College of Physicians. *Ann Intern Med* 2006;144:581–595.
40. Block BM, Liu SS, Rowlingson AJ, et al. Efficacy of postoperative epidural analgesia: A meta-analysis. *JAMA* 2003;290:2455–2463.
41. Wu CL, Cohen SR, Richman JM, et al. Efficacy of postoperative patient-controlled and continuous infusion epidural analgesia versus intravenous patient-controlled analgesia with opioids: A meta-analysis. *Anesthesiology* 2005;103:1079–1088.
42. Gruber EM, Tschernko EM, Kritzinger M, et al. The effects of thoracic epidural analgesia with bupivacaine 0.25% on ventilatory mechanics in patients with severe chronic obstructive pulmonary disease. *Anesth Analg* 2001;92:1015–1019.
43. Groeben H, Schafer B, Pavlakovic G, et al. Lung function under high thoracic segmental epidural anesthesia with ropivacaine or bupivacaine in patients with severe obstructive pulmonary disease undergoing breast surgery. *Anesthesiology* 2002;96:536–541.
44. Ballantyne JC, Carr DB, deFerranti S, et al. The comparative effects of postoperative analgesic therapies on pulmonary outcome: Cumulative meta-analyses of randomized, controlled trials. *Anesth Analg* 1998;86:598–612.

45. Urwin SC, Parker MJ, Griffiths R. General versus regional anaesthesia for hip fracture surgery: A meta-analysis of randomized trials. *Br J Anaesth* 2000;84:450–455.

46. Walder B, Schafer M, Henzi I, Tramer MR. Efficacy and safety of patient-controlled opioid analgesia for acute postoperative pain. A quantitative systematic review. *Acta Anaesthesiol Scand* 2001;45:795–804.

47. Ballantyne JC, Carr DB, Chalmers TC, et al. Postoperative patient-controlled analgesia: Meta-analyses of initial randomized control trials. *J Clin Anesth* 1993;5:182–193.

48. Hudcova J, McNicol E, Quah C, et al. Patient controlled intravenous opioid analgesia versus conventional opioid analgesia for postoperative pain: A quantitative systematic review. *Acute Pain* 2005;7:115–132.

49. Liu SS, Carpenter RL, Neal JM. Epidural anesthesia and analgesia: Their role in postoperative outcome. *Anesthesiology* 1995;82:1474–1506.

50. Jansen M, Fass J, Tittel A, et al. Influence of postoperative epidural analgesia with bupivacaine on intestinal motility, transit time, and anastomotic healing. *World J Surg* 2002;26:303–306.

51. Thorn SE, Wickbom G, Philipson L, et al. Myoelectric activity in the stomach and duodenum after epidural administration of morphine or bupivacaine. *Acta Anaesthesiol Scand* 1996;40:773–778.

52. Jansen M, Lynen Jansen P, Junge K, et al. Postoperative peridural analgesia increases the strength of colonic contractions without impairing anastomotic healing in rats. *Int J Colorectal Dis* 2003;18:50–54.

53. Udassin R, Eimerl D, Schiffman J, Haskel Y. Epidural anesthesia accelerates the recovery of postischemic bowel motility in the rat. *Anesthesiology* 1994;80:832–836.

54. Kosugi S, Morisaki H, Satoh T, et al. Epidural analgesia prevents endotoxin-induced gut mucosal injury in rabbits. *Anesth Analg* 2005;101:265–272.

55. Ai K, Kotake Y, Satoh T, et al. Epidural anesthesia retards intestinal acidosis and reduces portal vein endotoxin concentrations during progressive hypoxia in rabbits. *Anesthesiology* 2001;94:263–269.

56. Lazar G, Kaszaki J, Abraham S, et al. Thoracic epidural anesthesia improves the gastric microcirculation during experimental gastric tube formation. *Surgery* 2003;134:799–805.

57. Jorgensen H, Wetterslev J, Moiniche S, Dahl JB. Epidural local anaesthetics versus opioid-based analgesic regimens on postoperative gastrointestinal paralysis, PONV and pain after abdominal surgery. *Cochrane Database Syst Rev* 2000;4:CD001893.

58. Fotiadis RJ, Badvie S, Weston MD, Allen-Mersh TG. Epidural analgesia in gastrointestinal surgery. *Br J Surg* 2004;91:828–841.

59. Hodgson PS, Liu SS. Thoracic epidural anaesthesia and analgesia for abdominal surgery: Effects on gastrointestinal function and perfusion. *Balliere's Clinical Anesthesiology* 1999;13:9–22.

60. Basse L, Thorbol JE, Lossl K, Kehlet H. Colonic surgery with accelerated rehabilitation or conventional care. *Dis Colon Rectum* 2004;47:271–277.

61. Joshi GP. Intraoperative fluid restriction improves outcome after major elective gastrointestinal surgery. *Anesth Analg* 2005;101:601–605.

62. Donadoni R, Baele G, Devulder J, et al. Coagulation and fibrinolytic parameters in patients undergoing total hip replacement: Influence of anaesthesia technique. *Acta Anaesthesiol Scand* 1989;33:588–592.

63. Tuman KJ, McCarthy RJ, March RJ, et al. Effects of epidural anesthesia and analgesia on coagulation and outcome after major vascular surgery. *Anesth Analg* 1991;73:696–704.

64. Hollmann MW, Wieczorek KS, Smart M, Durieux ME. Epidural anesthesia prevents hypercoagulation in patients undergoing major orthopedic surgery. *Reg Anesth Pain Med* 2001;26:215–222.

65. Sorenson RM, Pace NL. Anesthetic techniques during surgical repair of femoral neck fractures. A meta-analysis. *Anesthesiology* 1992;77:1095–1104.

66. Parker MJ, Handoll HH, Griffiths R. Anaesthesia for hip fracture surgery in adults. *Cochrane Database Syst Rev* 2004;4:CD000521.

67. Christopherson R, Beattie C, Frank SM, et al. Perioperative morbidity in patients randomized to epidural or general anesthesia for lower extremity vascular surgery. *Anesthesiology* 1993;79:422–434.

68. Bew SA, Bryant AE, Desborough JP, Hall GM. Epidural analgesia and arterial reconstructive surgery to the leg: Effects on fibrinolysis and platelet degranulation. *Br J Anaesth* 2001;86:230–235.

69. Markel DC, Urquhart B, Derkowska I, et al. Effect of epidural analgesia on venous blood flow after hip arthroplasty. *Clin Orthop Relat Res* 1997;334:168–174.

70. Perkins FM, Kehlet H. Chronic pain as an outcome of surgery. A review of predictive factors. *Anesthesiology* 2000;93:1123–1133.

71. Nikolajsen L, Sorensen HC, Jensen TS, Kehlet H. Chronic pain following Caesarean section. *Acta Anaesthesiol Scand* 2004;48:111–116.

72. Senturk M, Ozcan PE, Talu GK, et al. The effects of three different analgesia techniques on long-term postthoracotomy pain. *Anesth Analg* 2002;94:11–15.

73. Obata H, Saito S, Fujita N, et al. Epidural block with mepivacaine before surgery reduces long-term post-thoracotomy pain. *Can J Anaesth* 1999;46:1127–1132.

74. Riis J, Lomholt B, Haxholdt O, et al. Immediate and long-term mental recovery from general versus epidural anesthesia in elderly patients. *Acta Anaesthesiol Scand* 1983;27:44–49.

75. Edwards H, Rose EA, Schorow M, King TC. Postoperative deterioration in psychomotor function. *JAMA* 1981;245:1342–1343.

76. Dyer CB, Ashton CM, Teasdale TA. Postoperative delirium: A review of 80 primary data-collection studies. *Arch Intern Med* 1995;155:461–465.

77. Inouye SK, Schlesinger MJ, Lydon TJ. Delirium: A symptom of how hospital care is failing older persons and a window to improve quality of hospital care. *Am J Med* 1999;106:565–573.

78. Marcantonio ER, Lee G, Orav JE, et al. The association of intraoperative factors with the development of postoperative delirium. *Am J Med* 1998;105:380–384.

79. Litaker D, Locala J, Franco K, et al. Preoperative risk factors for postoperative delirium. *Gen Hosp Psychiatry* 2001;23:84–89.

80. Zakriya KJ, Christmas C, Wenz JF, Sr., et al. Preoperative factors associated with postoperative change in confusion assessment method score in hip fracture patients. *Anesth Analg* 2002;94:1628–1632.

81. Wu CL, Hsu W, Richman JM, Raja SN. Postoperative cognitive function as an outcome of regional anesthesia and analgesia. *Reg Anesth Pain Med* 2004;29:257–268.

82. Lynch EP, Lazor MA, Gellis JE, et al. The impact of postoperative pain on the development of postoperative delirium. *Anesth Analg* 1998;86:781–785.

83. Vaurio LE, Sands LP, Wang Y, et al. Postoperative delirium: The importance of pain and pain management. *Anesth Analg* 2006;102:1267–1273.

84. Richman JM, Liu SS, Courpas G, et al. Does continuous peripheral nerve block provide superior pain control to opioids? A meta-analysis. *Anesth Analg* 2006;102:248–257.

85. Fung D, Cohen MM. Measuring patient satisfaction with anesthesia care: A review of current methodology. *Anesth Analg* 1998;87:1089–1098.

86. Wu CL, Naqibuddin M, Fleisher LA. Measurement of patient satisfaction as an outcome of regional anesthesia and analgesia: A systematic review. *Reg Anesth Pain Med* 2001;26:196–208.

87. Morgan PJ, Halpern S, Lam-McCulloch J. Comparison of maternal satisfaction between epidural and spinal anesthesia for elective Cesarean section. *Can J Anaesth* 2000;47:956–961.

89. Carli F, Mayo N, Klubien K, et al. Epidural analgesia enhances functional exercise capacity and health-related quality of life after colonic surgery: Results of a randomized trial. *Anesthesiology* 2002;97:540–549.

90. Cashman JN, Dolin SJ. Respiratory and haemodynamic effects of acute postoperative pain management: Evidence from published data. *Br J Anaesth* 2004;93:212–223.

91. Mulroy MF. Monitoring opioids. *Reg Anesth* 1996;21(6S):89.

92. de Leon-Casasola OA, Parker B, Lema MJ. Postoperative epidural bupivacaine-morphine therapy. Experience with 4,227 surgical cancer patients. *Anesthesiology* 1994;81:368–375.

93. Moen V, Dahlgren N, Irestedt L. Severe neurological complications after central neuraxial blockades in Sweden 1990–1999. *Anesthesiology* 2004;101:950–959.

94. Auroy Y, Narchi P, Messiah A, et al. Serious complications related to regional anesthesia. *Anesthesiology* 1997;87:479–486.

95. Giebler RM, Scherer RU, Peters J. Incidence of neurologic complications related to thoracic epidural catheterization. *Anesthesiology* 1997;86:55–63.

96. Mulroy MF, Norris MC, Liu SS. Safety steps in epidural injection of local anesthetics: Review of the literature and safety recommendations. *Anesth Analg* 1997;85:1346–1356.

97. Vandermeulen EP, Aken V, Vermylen J. Anticoagulants and spinal-epidural anesthesia. *Anesth Analg* 1994;79:1165–1169.

98. Horlocker TT, Wedel DJ, Benzon H, et al. Regional anesthesia in the anticoagulated patient: Defining the risks. *Reg Anesth Pain Med* 2003;28:172–197.

99. Wang LP, Hauerberg J, Schmidt JF. Incidence of spinal epidural abscess after epidural analgesia: A national 1-year survey. *Anesthesiology* 1999;91:1928–1936.

100. Baker AS, Ojemann RG. Spinal epidural abscess. *N Engl J Med* 1975;293:463–468.

101. Darchy B, Forceville X, Bavoux E, et al. Clinical and bacteriologic survey of epidural analgesia in patients in the intensive care unit. *Anesthesiology* 1996;85:988–998.

102. Chelly JE, Greger J, Gebhard R, et al. Training of residents in peripheral nerve blocks during anesthesiology residency. *J Clin Anesth* 2002;14:584–588.

103. Kopacz DJ, Neal JM. Regional anesthesia and pain medicine: Residency training–the year 2000. *Reg Anesth Pain Med* 2002;27:9–14.

104. Weber A, Fournier R, Riand N, Gamulin Z. Duration of analgesia is similar when 15, 20, 25 and 30 mL of ropivacaine 0.5% are administered via a femoral catheter. *Can J Anaesth* 2005;52:390–396.

105. London MJ, Zaugg M, Schaub MC, Spahn DR. Perioperative beta-adrenergic receptor blockade: Physiologic foundations and clinical controversies. *Anesthesiology* 2004;100:170–175.

106. Mythen MG. Postoperative gastrointestinal tract dysfunction. *Anesth Analg* 2005;100:196–204.

107. Liu SS, Strodtbeck WM, Richman JM, Wu CL. A comparison of regional versus general anesthesia for ambulatory anesthesia: A meta-analysis of randomized controlled trials. *Anesth Analg* 2005;101:1634–1642.

108. Williams BA, Kentor ML, Vogt MT, et al. Economics of nerve block pain management after anterior cruciate ligament reconstruction: Potential hospital cost savings via associated postanesthesia care unit bypass and same-day discharge. *Anesthesiology* 2004;100:697–706.

109. Parker MJ, Griffiths R, Appadu BN. Nerve blocks (subcostal, lateral cutaneous, femoral, triple, psoas) for hip fractures. *Cochrane Database Syst Rev* 2002;CD001159.

110. Urwin SC, Parker MJ, Griffiths R. General versus regional anaesthesia for hip fracture surgery: A meta-analysis of randomized trials. *Br J Anaesth* 2000;84:450–455.

111. Macario A, Glenn D, Dexter F. What can the postanesthesia care unit manager do to decrease costs in the postanesthesia care unit? *J Perianesth Nurs* 1999;14:284–293.

112. Reuben SS. Preventing the development of complex regional pain syndrome after surgery. *Anesthesiology* 2004;101:1215–1224.

113. Ilfeld BM, Enneking FK. Continuous peripheral nerve blocks at home: A review. *Anesth Analg* 2005;100:1822–1833.

114. Capdevila X, Barthelet Y, Biboulet P, et al. Effects of perioperative analgesic technique on the surgical outcome and duration of rehabilitation after major knee surgery. *Anesthesiology* 1999;91:8–15.

115. Singelyn FJ, Deyaert M, Joris D, et al. Effects of intravenous patient-controlled analgesia with morphine, continuous epidural analgesia, and continuous three-in-one block on postoperative pain and knee rehabilitation after unilateral total knee arthroplasty. *Anesth Analg* 1998;87:88–92.

116. Zaric D, Boysen K, Christiansen C, et al. A comparison of epidural analgesia with combined continuous femoral-sciatic nerve blocks after total knee replacement. *Anesth Analg* 2006;102:1240–1246.

117. Salinas FV, Liu SS, Mulroy MF. The effect of single-injection femoral nerve block versus continuous femoral nerve block after total knee arthroplasty on hospital length of stay and long-term functional recovery within an established clinical pathway. *Anesth Analg* 2006;102:1234–1239.

118. Barrington MJ, Olive D, Low K, et al. Continuous femoral nerve blockade or epidural analgesia after total knee replacement: A prospective randomized controlled trial. *Anesth Analg* 2005;101:1824–1829.

119. Anderson FA Jr., Hirsh J, White K, Fitzgerald RH Jr. Temporal trends in prevention of venous thromboembolism following primary total hip or knee arthroplasty 1996–2001: Findings from the Hip and Knee Registry. *Chest* 2003;124:S349–S356.

120. Ilfeld BM, Wright TW, Enneking FK, et al. Total shoulder arthroplasty as an outpatient procedure using ambulatory perineural local anesthetic infusion: A pilot feasibility study. *Anesth Analg* 2005;101:1319–1322.

121. Ilfeld BM, Wright TW, Enneking FK, Vandenborne K. Total elbow arthroplasty as an outpatient procedure using a continuous infraclavicular nerve block at home: A prospective case report. *Reg Anesth Pain Med* 2006; 31:172–176.

122. Ilfeld BM, Gearen PF, Enneking FK, et al. Total hip arthroplasty as an overnight-stay procedure using an ambulatory continuous psoas compartment nerve block: A prospective feasibility study. *Reg Anesth Pain Med* 2006;31:113–118.

123. Ilfeld BM, Gearen PF, Enneking FK, et al. Total knee arthroplasty as an overnight-stay procedure using continuous femoral nerve blocks at home: A prospective feasibility study. *Anesth Analg* 2006;102:87–90.

124. Auroy Y, Benhamou D, Bargues L, et al. Major complications of regional anesthesia in France: The SOS Regional Anesthesia Hotline Service. *Anesthesiology* 2002;97:1274–1280.

125. Capdevila X, Pirat P, Bringuier S, et al. Continuous peripheral nerve blocks in hospital wards after orthopedic surgery: A multicenter prospective analysis of the quality of postoperative analgesia and complications in 1,416 patients. *Anesthesiology* 2005;103:1035–1045.

126. Borgeat A, Ekatodramis G, Kalberer F, Benz C. Acute and nonacute complications associated with interscalene block and shoulder surgery: A prospective study. *Anesthesiology* 2001;95:875–880.

127. Borgeat A, Dullenkopf A, Ekatodramis G, Nagy L. Evaluation of the lateral modified approach for continuous interscalene block after shoulder surgery. *Anesthesiology* 2003;99:436–442.

128. Bergman BD, Hebl JR, Kent J, Horlocker TT. Neurologic complications of 405 consecutive continuous axillary catheters. *Anesth Analg* 2003;96:247–252.

129. Cuvillon P, Ripart J, Lalourcey L, et al. The continuous femoral nerve block catheter for postoperative analgesia: Bacterial colonization, infectious rate and adverse effects. *Anesth Analg* 2001;93:1045–1049.

CHAPTER 8 ■ PERIOPERATIVE MANAGEMENT OF PATIENTS AND EQUIPMENT SELECTION FOR NEURAL BLOCKADE

JAMES C. CREWS AND VINCENT W. S. CHAN

The essential elements for optimal perioperative management of patients for neural blockade include a physician, well-trained in the principles and techniques of regional anesthesia, working in a well-equipped, well-staffed anesthetizing location designed for safe and efficient patient care. The anesthesiologist must be skilled, not only in the technical aspects of how to accomplish a selected neural blockade technique, but also in its indications and contraindications, as well as appropriate intraoperative patient management. Ideally, these skills and knowledge are taught beginning early in the anesthesia training period by experts in the subspecialty. From this beginning, the anesthesiologist who has a sincere interest in neural blockade, and who is convinced of its efficacy, will continue to apply and refine her technical skills until they become an essential part of the anesthetic armamentarium.

A thorough knowledge of the pertinent anatomy, obtained from textbooks and atlases, should be reinforced through the study of cadavers and surgical specimens. In addition, one should be familiar with the physiology of neural blockade, the pharmacology of the local anesthetic agents themselves, and the physiologic effects and potential complications associated with the various regional anesthetic techniques. One can, therefore, anticipate changes in the patient's status and not only determine the suitability of a given technique for a specific patient and procedure, but also be prepared to institute appropriate therapy if and when these changes occur.

Finally, this thorough knowledge of the requirements for successful neural blockade also requires that the anesthesiologist undertake these activities in a location well equipped with not only suitable neural blockade equipment, but also with all other appropriate monitors, resuscitation drugs, and equipment. This equipment should be located in such a way as to allow easy access to commonly used monitors and supplies, and allow ample room for the patient, the anesthesiologist, and an assistant. The anesthesiologist and the assistant must have ample room to move about without feeling confined. The area should also allow the patient adequate privacy from other nearby patients or visitors.

PATIENT SELECTION

The most important determinant in the selection of a regional anesthetic technique is the suitability of that technique to that specific patient for that specific procedure. Unless thorough and careful consideration is given to the patient, all else will likely fail. Specific patient factors to be considered include the patient's anatomy, coexisting medical conditions, and neuropsychological state.

Because nearly all regional anesthetic techniques are based on the identification and utilization of anatomic landmarks, both surface and bony, it is useful that the patient display those landmarks to a sufficient degree. Examples of anatomic impediments to the conduct of a successful neural blockade technique include morbid obesity, arthritis, and other physical deformities that would limit patient positioning or palpation of local landmarks at the site of the block. The use of ultrasound imaging may be helpful in some situations in which anatomic surface landmarks are difficult to determine.

Complicating coexisting medical conditions may be either local or systemic. Local conditions such as infection, anatomic abnormalities, trauma, burns, or dressings could all preclude the opportunity to perform a satisfactory block technique. More subtle, and often more important, are the systemic problems of the patient. Clearly, a severely hypovolemic patient should not be considered for a technique that involves major sympathetic neural blockade unless appropriate fluid resuscitation is accomplished beforehand. Patients with neurologic disease, coagulopathies, or severe cardiovascular disease require a thorough preanesthetic medical and laboratory evaluation of their pathology. In some circumstances, one type of block technique will be contraindicated whereas another might be perfectly acceptable. It must be remembered that the anesthetic choice involves not only the selection of a block technique but also consideration of the risks and benefits of all anesthetic options tailored to the individual patient for the best possible outcome. Coincident with the assessment of the patient's pathophysiology is the consideration of the patient's preoperative medications. Special management considerations may be required for some neural blockade techniques in patients receiving antihypertensive agents, β-adrenergic receptor blockers, anticoagulant medications, antiplatelet agents, or high-dose opioid analgesics. The use of certain neural blockade techniques for patients with various preexisting medical conditions (e.g., patients with coagulopathies or history of anticoagulant/antiplatelet therapy, patients with preexisting neurologic disease or deficits, and patients with localized or systemic infections) is a controversial and highly subjective issue. The literature does not contain absolute documentation of when it is safe or unsafe, indicated or contraindicated, preferable or optional to apply a given anesthetic technique or agent. The decision is multifactorial but ultimately becomes the responsibility of the attending anesthesiologist (1). The risks versus benefit of any given technique must be viewed in the context of the individual patient.

Finally, the patient's attitude or preconceptions regarding regional anesthesia may play a role in determining patient acceptance of a specific neural blockade technique. For example, an individual patient may accept a peripheral nerve block for open fixation of an ankle fracture yet might be completely opposed to consideration of a spinal anesthetic for the same procedure. A study by Matthey in 2004 demonstrated that the general public is not very well informed about the matters related to regional anesthesia, and that people's fears and conceptions about regional anesthesia are greatly distorted (2). Preoperative discussion of reasonable anesthetic options for a surgical procedure may require some degree of patient education regarding regional anesthesia versus general anesthesia or the selection of an individual block technique. Tetzlaff and colleagues found in patients undergoing reconstructive shoulder surgery that interscalene block was found to be highly acceptable to those who had undergone previous shoulder surgery with general anesthesia. These authors supported the belief that the key to patient acceptance of regional anesthesia involves patient education and preparation (3).

The anesthesiologist must also undertake all the other common elements of a preanesthetic evaluation, including a complete history and physical examination. The usual elements of systemic disease, current medications, past operations and anesthetics, allergies, airway and dentition, and family history of anesthetic problems must be recorded. Laboratory studies essential for the conduct of a general anesthetic must also be recorded. Patients must first be evaluated as candidates for general anesthesia and then evaluated for suitability for regional anesthesia.

PATIENT INTERVIEW

Once the anesthesiologist has determined an anesthetic plan, it is discussed with the patient and informed consent is obtained. A broad but useful definition of informed consent is the obligation to explain to the patient the risks and benefits of the selected anesthetic plan, as opposed to the risks and benefits of an alternate plan. A significant number of patients refuse a regional anesthetic because "they don't want to be awake during the operation." It is essential, therefore, that the anesthesiologist describe in chronological detail the events that will occur from arrival in the surgical/anesthesia area through admission to the recovery area. Patients should be assured that as soon as an intravenous (IV) infusion is established, systemic sedatives will be given to make the patient comfortable prior to the anesthetic. Patients also need to be told, early in the interview, that they will be provided with additional systemic

drugs throughout the operation to produce a state of sedation (with possible progression to general anesthesia) as needed for their comfort. When available, the use of headphones with music, visual screens, and other distracting techniques should be discussed.

The anesthesiologist should describe in detail the performance of the block and the patient's role in that process. This description should include the need for starting of an IV infusion, and the requirement for patient positioning. The neural blockade procedure should be described, including the possibility of producing paresthesias, neuromuscular stimulation, or the use of ultrasound guidance, as well as the signs and symptoms of normal onset of neural blockade, and the possibility of systemic effects and adverse events.

Informing the patient about the rationale for neural blockade will further motivate patients toward acceptance. Factors such as a reduced likelihood of side effects from inhalational general anesthetics, muscle relaxants, and endotracheal intubation should be noted. The increased public awareness of postoperative pain relief facilitates patient acceptance of regional anesthesia. The painless emergence from operative sedation in the recovery unit with a plan for earlier discharge with fewer risks of inhaled anesthetic- or opioid analgesic-related side effects, and the possibility of extending neural blockade into the postoperative period with continuous catheter techniques should also be discussed. The amount of information given will vary for each patient; however, such discussions invariably increase the confidence of the patient and may positively affect the recovery. Figure 8-1 shows an informed consent document developed at Wake Forest University that outlines the risks of various selected regional anesthesia and general anesthesia techniques separately to allow the patient a clearer understanding of the risks associated with individual procedures and techniques.

PREMEDICATION OF PATIENTS FOR NEURAL BLOCKADE TECHNIQUE

Just as the principles applied to preoperative preparation of a patient for a regional anesthetic technique are primarily those used for general anesthesia, so too are the basic tenets similar in the administration of the preanesthetic medications.

Preanesthetic Fasting

In the past, *all* patients scheduled to receive any type of anesthetic were restricted from all oral intake for a minimum of 6 hours and preferably from midnight the day before surgery. The efficacy of this practice was reexamined in the early 1990s. Because unconsciousness may be a required or desired part of any surgical procedure performed with a regional anesthetic, the rationale for preanesthetic fasting should be the same as that for a surgical procedure performed with a general anesthetic. There are many individual circumstances, especially in pediatric procedures, where these practices will be modified, but some general guidelines are helpful.

Phillips et al. (4) prospectively compared the effect of allowing unrestricted clear fluids until the time of oral medication (2 hours prior to surgery). Patients otherwise underwent conventional fasting. The residual volume and pH of gastric contents after induction of anesthesia were measured in 100 elective surgical patients allocated randomly to a group

	Patient Name	
ANESTHESIA REQUEST RISK DISCLOSURE FORM	Medical Record #	
	Age	
	Race Sex	
	(Patient name plate stamp)	

You have requested anesthesia for your surgery, for pain relief, or both. The type of anesthesia will be determined by what you want, but also by what we normally use for the planned surgery, your medical condition, and your surgeon's preferences. Sometimes a type of anesthesia technique may not work well for the surgery planned and another type may have to be used. **All types of anesthesia carry some risk.** Although rare, severe complications could occur including infection, drug reactions, blood clots, paralysis, stroke, heart attack, brain damage, and death. **Anesthesia could injure a fetus: tell your anesthesiologist if you think you may be pregnant.** Some of the risks for specific types of anesthesia, monitoring, and blood transfusion are listed below.

Consent for Anesthesia and Pain Relief

☐ **General Anesthesia**	Technique	Medicines injected into the bloodstream and breathed into the lungs using a tube placed in the windpipe or throat after unconsciousness.
	Expected Result	Total unconsciousness during surgery
	Specific Risks	Breathing stomach contents into the lungs, pneumonia, nausea and vomiting, mouth or throat pain, hoarseness, injury to mouth or teeth, awareness under anesthesia, nerve injury.
☐ **Spinal or Epidural Anesthesia**	Technique	Medicines injected through a needle or tube placed between the bones of the back.
	Expected Result	Temporary loss of feeling and/or movement to the lower part of the body or to the chest and belly.
	Specific Risks	Convulsions, headache, backache, nausea and vomiting, nerve injury- permanent weakness, numbness, or pain.
☐ **Peripheral Nerve Block**	Technique	Numbing medicines injected through a needle or tube placed near nerves of a limb, part of a limb, chest wall, or belly.
	Expected Result	Temporary loss of feeling and movement of a limb or part of a limb, chest wall, or belly.
	Specific Risks	Convulsions, injury to blood vessel, nerve injury – permanent weakness, numbness, or pain. ☐ Lung collapse
☐ **Intravenous Regional Anesthesia**	Technique	Numbing medicine injected into a vein of an arm while using a tourniquet.
	Expected Result	Loss of feeling and movement of arm during surgery.
	Specific Risks	Convulsions, nerve injury, injury to blood vessels.
☐ **Sedation with constant monitoring**	Technique	Medicines injected into the bloodstream, producing a semi-conscious or unconscious state.
	Expected Result	Reduced anxiety and pain, partial or total unconsciousness, amnesia.
	Specific Risks	slowed breathing, nausea and vomiting, injury to blood vessels.

FIGURE 8-1. Anesthesia risk disclosure form developed at Wake Forest University Baptist Medical Center describing specific anesthetic, pain management, and special monitoring procedures, expected results, and associated risks associated with each different type of anesthetic technique. Developed by Gerancher JC, 2006. Used with permission.

allowed unrestricted fluids or to a control group who fasted for 6 hours (mean = 388 mL versus 0 mL). There was no significant difference in mean residual gastric volume (22 mL versus 19 mL) or pH (2.64 versus 2.26) between the study group and the control group. Problems with aspiration were not encountered. The authors concluded that elective surgical patients could be allowed to drink clear fluids until 2 hours before anesthesia to enhance patient comfort without compromising safety. An accompanying editorial in the *British Journal of Anaesthesia* (5) also stated: "Returning to elective operations which concern the vast majority of patients requiring an anaesthetic, it is clear that 'nil by mouth after midnight' should be abandoned. In its place, there should be agreement by anesthetists, surgeons, and nurses on guidelines that both day-case and inpatients may take, if they wish, clear fluids by mouth up to 3 hours before surgery." The list of clear fluids excluded alcoholic drinks and those containing milk or sugar but it did include orange juice and apple juice.

In 2002, the American Society of Anesthesiologists released its *Practice Guidelines for Preoperative Fasting and the Use of Pharmacologic Agents to Reduce the Risk of Pulmonary Aspiration: Application to Healthy Patients Undergoing Elective*

Consent for Special Monitoring

☐ **Arterial Line** ☐ **Central Line** ☐ **Pulmonary Artery Line** ☐ **TEE** ☐ **Lumbar Drain**	Technique	Placing a tube in an artery of the arm or leg to monitor pressures. Placing a tube in the neck to monitor pressures in the vein. Placing a tube in the neck to monitor pressures within the heart. Placing a ultrasound probe into the throat to monitor the heart. Placing a tube between the bones of the back to remove spinal fluid and measure spinal pressures.	
	Expected Result	Monitoring during anesthesia , frequent blood sampling, injecting medicines into veins	
	Specific Risks	Injury to blood vessels. Lung collapse. Irregular heart rhythm. Mouth or throat pain, hoarseness, injury to mouth or teeth. Headache, backache, nausea and vomiting, nerve injury ñ permanent weakness, numbness, or pain.	

Consent for Blood or Blood Component Transfusion

☐ **I give consent for blood transfusion** ☐ **I will not accept blood transfusion even as a life saving measure**	In order to maintain your health and provide proper medical care while you are anesthetized during surgery, transfusion of blood or one of its components may become necessary. Such a transfusion would only be begun if it is absolutely necessary and all other measures are first used. Although blood is carefully tested, transfusion has the small risk of unexpected reactions or the transmission of hepatitis, HIV, and other infectious agents.

I have read this form or had read to me. I understand what it says. I have been given a chance to ask questions. The types of anesthesia, monitoring and blood transfusion have been explained to me. I believe I have enough information to give my permission for you to use these as needed.

_____

Signature of the patient or person authorized to sign for the patient

I have discussed the contents of this form with the patient (or person authorized to sign).

_____   _____   ___/___/___   (___:___)

Person obtaining the signature   Physician discussing the form   Date and time

FIGURE 8-1. (*Continued*)

Procedures (6), and made the following recommendations for preanesthesia fasting:

> It is appropriate to fast from intake of clear liquids for 2 or more hours before procedures involving general anesthesia, regional anesthesia, or sedation/analgesia. . . . Examples of clear liquids include but are not limited to water, fruit juices without pulp, carbonated beverages, clear tea, and black coffee.

These guidelines are not intended to include patients with coexisting diseases or conditions that might affect gastric emptying or fluid volume (e.g., pregnancy, obesity, diabetes, hiatal hernia, gastroesophageal reflux disease, ileus or bowel obstruction, emergency care, or enteral tube feeding) or patients in whom airway management might be difficult. In urgent, emergent, or other situations in which gastric emptying is impaired, the fasting status of the patient and the risk potential for pulmonary aspiration of gastric contents must be considered in determining the timing of the intervention and the degree of sedation/analgesia.

Preanesthetic Medications

The advent of ambulatory surgery and the current practice that most patients are seen for the first time by their anesthesiologist a few hours before surgery has changed the rationale and types of drugs used for premedication. Even the former practice of writing preanesthetic medication orders for inpatients "on-call to the OR" has generally been abandoned in favor of receiving unmedicated patients into the preanesthesia holding area and then providing preanesthetic sedation after a final opportunity for discussing the anesthetic and answering patient's questions immediately prior to the surgical procedure.

Timing of Administration

Premedication has as its goals the rapid onset of anxiolysis, amnesia, and analgesia with a relatively short duration of action. It is essential that all preanesthetic and presurgical discussions and consents be obtained and documented prior to

TABLE 8-1

OBSERVER'S ASSESSMENT OF ALERTNESS/SEDATION (OAA/S) SCALE

Response	Speech	Facial expression	Eyes	Composite score
Responds readily to name spoken in normal tone	Normal	Normal	Clear, no ptosis	5
Lethargic response to name spoken in normal tone	Mild slowing or thickening	Mild relaxation	Glazed or mild ptosis (less than half the eye)	4
Responds only after name is called loudly or repeatedly	Slurring or prominent slowing	Marked relaxation (slack jaw)	Glazed and marked ptosis (half the eye or more)	3
Responds only after mild prodding or shaking	Few recognizable words			2
Does not respond to mild prodding or shaking				1
Does not respond to noxious stimulus				0

From Chernick DA, Gillings D, Laine H, et al. Validity and reliability of the Observer's Assessment of Alertness/Sedation Scale: Study with intravenous midazolam. *J Clin Psychopharmcol* 1990;10:244–251, with permission.

administration of any premedication. Not infrequently, changes in the surgical or anesthetic plan may be required for a variety of reasons. Patients may fail to arrive on time for the procedure, they may have eaten prior to arrival, they may have previously unknown (or missing) abnormal laboratory values, electrocardiogram (ECG) changes, or chest radiographic results, there may have been an interim illness since the last office visit requiring reevaluation with the potential for surgical postponement or cancellation. Thus, the anesthesiologist must be sure that a scheduled procedure will take place, and that the surgeon and patient have had an opportunity to resolve all relevant issues that may require an addition, deletion, or revision of the surgical consent before administering sedative premedications to the patient.

Before administration of sedatives or analgesics, it should be verified and confirmed that the patient is the correct patient, for the correct procedure, to be performed on the correct side of the body, and that these parameters are clearly outlined in the patient's consent for surgery and anesthesia. This interaction may occur as a "time-out" session, during which these issues are verified by the patient and confirmed by a member of the anesthesia or surgical team and a witness. After this confirmation of correct patient and procedure, and attention to any last-minute patient question's or concerns, the anesthesiologist may proceed with premedication and positioning of the patient for the neural blockade procedure.

Monitoring During Sedation

Any time supplemental IV agents are being used, it is especially important that the anesthesiologist have an assistant to monitor the patient's vital signs and level of consciousness and ensure maintenance of proper patient positioning for the procedure. Minimum monitoring standards for patients undergoing neural blockade procedures should include pulse oximetry monitoring of pulse rate and oxygen saturation (7). ECG and blood pressure should monitored or monitoring equipment should be immediately available. For patients receiving supplemental sedative-hypnotic or opioid analgesic drugs, supplemental oxygen administration should be considered, and supplemental oxygen administration is recommended for all patients re-

ceiving moderate or deeper levels of sedation, or for patients receiving combinations of drugs or dose titrations (Table 8-1). Following the administration of supplemental sedative or analgesic drugs or performance of the neural blockade procedure, the patient should be intermittently monitored and should not be left alone until adequate recovery of consciousness and respiratory function has been established. Regular verbal contact should be maintained to ensure consciousness and comfort until the patient has recovered from the effects and the potential side effects of all drugs administered and until delayed systemic toxicity from the local anesthetics is ruled out.

Selection of Sedative/Analgesic Medications

The goal of the anesthesiologist is to provide the patient with a pleasant anesthetic experience throughout the entire perioperative period. The amount of additional supplemental sedative or analgesic medication required for the nerve block procedure depends not only on the specific requirements of the patient, but also on the degree of painful stimulation associated with the performance of the selected block technique. Most patients require little additional supplementation for the simple, single-injection procedures such as spinal, epidural, and axillary block. In fact, patients often are more easily positioned and responsive to paresthesias or nerve stimulation if they are not heavily medicated. Conversely, procedures such as deep paravertebral blocks (psoas compartment, celiac plexus, and sympathetic blocks) or multiple intercostal nerve blocks are quite painful and will likely require additional parenteral sedation and/or analgesics. Nervous or hypersensitive patients may also benefit from additional parenteral supplementation.

As discussed earlier, the selection of sedative or analgesic drugs for administration prior to and during performance of a neural blockade procedure is as individual as the choice of premedication. The common goal, however, is to produce adequate sedation, analgesia, and anxiolysis while maintaining meaningful contact with the patient throughout the procedure. If deeper levels of sedation are required for brief periods during the procedure, very short-acting medications that will allow a rapid return of consciousness are preferable. Excessive sedation incurs the risks of airway obstruction or circulatory collapse and will also mask the early warnings of complications of the block, such as an unintentional high spinal or epidural block, a painful intraneural injection, or an intravascular injection. Excessive doses of some of the psychotropic or dissociative drugs may also render a previously cooperative patient excitable or unmanageable. Short-acting IV drugs given in small doses or by a continuous infusion can be carefully titrated to produce the desired level of sedation and analgesia and still ensure a rapid recovery at the conclusion of the block.

Anticholinergics

Most practitioners of regional anesthesia have abandoned the routine use of anticholinergic drugs unless they plan to combine their technique with an inhalation anesthetic. Those abandoning the preoperative use of these drugs considered their action as primarily antisialagogue. Anticholinergic drugs in adult, premedication doses do not alter gastric fluid pH or volume (8). A published review of postoperative nausea and vomiting states that "the incidence of nausea and vomiting during spinal anesthesia is decreased by the intravenous administration of atropine." However, the quoted references date to the late 1950s and raise the question of whether such conclusions are still valid (9).

In summary, the preanesthetic use of this class of drugs is limited to a knowledge of their various clinical actions and the application of that action to the specific needs of a select patient. Routine use of anticholinergics as premedications for regional anesthesia is not recommended.

Antiemetics

One of the inducements anesthesiologists offer to patients when comparing regional and general anesthesia is the reduced likelihood of postoperative nausea and/or vomiting (PONV) with regional anesthesia, especially as compared to general anesthesia using volatile anesthetic agents. Postoperative nausea and vomiting remains as a significant perioperative occurrence despite recent advances and treatment. Patients generally consider PONV to be among the most undesirable perioperative anesthesia-related concerns (10). PONV continues to be among the most common factors delaying inpatient discharge from the post anesthesia care unit (PACU), outpatient discharge to home, and unanticipated hospital admission for ambulatory surgery patients (11). Volatile anesthetics, nitrous oxide, large-dose neostigmine, and intra- or postoperative opioids are well established anesthesia-related risk factors for PONV (12), and regional anesthesia techniques generally avoid or minimize the exposure of the patient to these agents. Although some randomized, controlled clinical studies have confirmed that general anesthesia may cause a greater frequency or severity of PONV than regional anesthetic techniques, the results are far from conclusive (13–16). Although regional anesthesia may be considered as an attractive alternative to general anesthesia, the confusion arises from the practice of using concomitant IV sedatives and opioids during regional anesthesia to provide anxiolysis and analgesia. Thus, it is difficult to separate the emetic effects of the sedative/analgesic medications from those associated with neural blockade.

The incidence of emesis associated with central neuraxial block is greater than with peripheral nerve block because of the side effects of the resultant sympathetic nervous system blockade (i.e., hypotension and perhaps central hypoxemia). Studies of the actual benefit of central neuraxial block in reducing emesis are conflicting. Even studies with local anesthesia and monitored anesthesia care fail to document conclusively that neural blockade is better. Clearly, the multifactorial causes of perioperative nausea and vomiting are influenced more by total patient management than by the use of any single drug or technique. Reviews of PONV confirm this point (12,17). Therefore, for patients undergoing surgical procedures with regional anesthesia, as for those with general anesthesia, routine prophylactic treatment of PONV with antiemetic agents such as ondansetron, droperidol, dexamethasone, or promethazine should be limited to at-risk patients. With respect to reducing the risk for PONV in patients undergoing surgical procedures with regional anesthesia, attention to maintenance of adequate hydration, administration of supplemental oxygen, and judicious use of oral or IV analgesic adjuvants while minimizing perioperative opioid exposure may be the best strategies to allow the benefits of regional anesthesia to be most clearly demonstrated.

Analgesics

A popular belief among many anesthesiologists is that induction of anesthesia is not painful and thus does not require administration of an analgesic agent in the preanesthetic period. However, practitioners of regional anesthesia or other potentially painful invasive procedures should give strong consideration to their use. Furthermore, the regional anesthetic renders only portions of the patient's anatomy analgesic. An analgesic will enhance total body comfort and likely reduce the dosage of supplementary sedation.

Two major determinants for the inclusion of an opioid preanesthetic are the type of nerve block and the mental attitude of the patient. Nerve blocks that require paresthesias or multiple insertions, especially paravertebral, are painful and analgesia is beneficial. Similarly, the more apprehensive or excitable the patient, the greater the need for both analgesia and sedation. Excitable patients heavily medicated with sedatives may tend to be drowsy and relaxed until painfully stimulated, when they are likely to overreact or react inappropriately and uncooperatively during an invasive procedure.

Selection of a specific opioid as a preanesthetic analgesic must be made with a consideration of the patient's analgesic requirements during the ensuing procedure and recovery period. For a brief period of painful stimulus associated with positioning or placement of a nerve block, a short-acting opioid with a fast onset is best. Fentanyl is probably the preanesthetic opioid of choice for analgesia during nerve block procedures because its analgesic effects at 50- to 150-μg doses produce few side effects and provide a cooperative patient with a relatively clear sensorium.

Sedatives

Early practitioners of regional anesthesia combined short-acting barbiturates with opioids as their premedication of choice. Usually, atropine or scopolamine accompanied that combination. As noted earlier, most anesthesia practices today are for same-day patients, many of whom will leave the hospital or surgical facility 1 to 3 hours after their procedure. In addition to the desirable analgesia prior to regional anesthesia, most patients prefer to be sedated and usually amnestic during presurgical procedures. Just as the selection of an analgesic considers the needs and duration of the procedure, so too does the selection of a sedative. The chosen drug may be continued into the operative management of the patient as well.

The benzodiazepines, principally midazolam, are commonly used as sedative agents because of their wide spectrum of central nervous system (CNS) depressant activity, low incidence of side effects, and wide margin of safety. All

TABLE 8-2

COMMONLY USED IV AND INHALATION SEDATIVE AND ANALGESIC DRUGS AND DOSES RECOMMENDATIONS

Drug	Dose	Infusion	Clinical effect	Reference
Midazolam	1–3 mg	0.5–2.5 μg/kg/min	Anxiolysis, mild to moderate sedation	2–1
Fentanyl	50–150 μg	25–100 μg/kg/h	Analgesia	–
Propofol	10–30 mg over 1 min	25–75 μg/kg/min	Sedation, amnesia	2–2
Ketamine	10–20 mg		Analgesia, sedation	–
Propofol–Ketamine infusion (9.4 mg/mL–0.94 mg/mL)		25–75 μg/kg/min P 2.5–7.5 μg/kg/min K	Sedation, analgesia, amnesia	2–2
Dexmedetomidine	0.5–1.0 μg/kg	0.2–0.8 μg/kg/h	Sedation, mild analgesia, amnesia	2–3,4
Sevoflurane		0.2–1.2%	Sedation, amnesia	2–5

1. White PF, Negus JB. *J Clin Anesth* 1991;3:32–39. Nishiyama T, Yokoyama T, Hanaoka K. Sedation guidelines for midazolam infusion during combined spinal and epidural anesthesia. *J Clin Anesth* 2004;16:568–572.
2. Badrinath S, Avramov MN, Shadrick M, et al. The use of ketamine-propofol combination during monitored anesthesia care. *Anesth Analg* 2000;90:858–862.
3. Hall JE, Ulrich TD, Barney JA, et al. Sedative, amnestic, and analgesic properties of small-dose dexmedetomidine infusions. *Anesth Analg* 2000;90:699–705.
4. McCutcheon CA, Orme RM, Scott DA, et al. A comparison of dexmedetomidine versus conventional therapy for sedation and hemodynamic control during carotid endarterectomy performed under regional anesthesia. *Anesth Analg* 2006;102:668–675.
5. Ibrahim AE, Taraday JK, Kharasch ED. Bispectral index monitoring during sedation with sevoflurane, midazolam, and propofol. *Anesthesiology* 2001;95:1151–1159.

benzodiazepines possess the same properties of anxiolysis, amnesia, and sedation to varying degrees. A secondary benefit of using benzodiazepines as premedication for regional anesthesia techniques is their anticonvulsant properties. De Jong (18) first reported the superiority of diazepam over barbiturates in preventing seizures from local anesthesia overdose in animals. As a result of those studies, diazepam enjoyed widespread use as a prophylactic against local anesthetic seizures as well as for its sedative properties. A serious criticism must be given, however, against the use of benzodiazepines as a prophylactic to permit the use of larger than recommended safe doses of local anesthetic. Many factors contribute to a given patient's toxicity threshold to local anesthetics. It is important, therefore, that the selected dose of a local anesthetic be at or below that recommended dose. Currently, midazolam is the most frequently used benzodiazepine for preanesthetic sedation. Because it is water-soluble, it causes significantly less pain on injection than diazepam (19). Midazolam has a rapid onset of action and a short elimination half-life (2–4 hours) and is significantly more potent than diazepam. Refer to Table 8-2 for commonly used sedative agents and dose recommendations. The other benzodiazepines, lorazepam and oxazepam, are potent amnestic agents but have such a prolonged duration of action that they are less suitable as premedication or supplements to most regional anesthesia procedures (20,21).

Other drugs have been used as preanesthetic adjuvants prior to administration of regional anesthesia. The tranquilizing drugs (phenothiazines and butyrophenones) were popular earlier, but their hypotensive effects in conjunction with sympathetic blocks resulting from regional anesthesia led to some major complications. The perceived advantage of the butyrophenones is their ability to produce a state of mental calm and indifference with little hypnotic effect. It was discovered, however, that larger doses, especially without analgesic or sedative drugs already present, could produce hallucinations, restlessness, and even extrapyramidal dyskinesia (22). Droperidol is still useful, however, in low doses (0.625 mg), as a potent antiemetic. Excess sedation and delayed discharge time are likely only after doses of droperidol greater than 2.5 mg (23).

Although not truly in the category of preanesthetic medication, the need for a rapid-acting sedative or analgesic to alleviate the anxiety or pain during the positioning for or the performance of a regional block technique can be effectively met with thiopental, methohexital, propofol, or ketamine. (These agents are discussed later in this chapter.) During a regional blockade procedure, small IV bolus doses may be given with close monitoring of the patient's airway, vital signs, and level of consciousness. The advantage of the use of low doses of these drugs is the rapid recovery of sensorium soon after the block technique is completed. This allows for accurate patient response to onset and level of sensory and motor blockade. The disadvantage of using these drugs lies primarily in their extreme potency and potential for relative overdose, resulting in significant respiratory depression (or apnea) that may require ventilatory support. It must be kept in mind that neither the barbiturates or propofol are analgesic, and may perhaps be even hyperalgesic, so supplemental analgesia may be required with opioid analgesics if these drugs are used for producing brief, moderate or deep levels of sedation.

For patients with painful medical conditions or associated injuries requiring extensive repositioning for an indicated neural blockade procedure, IV ketamine titrated in small, intermittent doses should be considered as an additional adjuvant to the benzodiazepines and opioids. It is our practice for patients in whom we are anticipating significant discomfort associated with positioning for neural blockade (e.g., patient's with multiple extremity fractures, rib fractures, burn injury, etc.) to titrate doses of midazolam 2 to 3 mg and fentanyl 100 to 200 μg, followed by small IV doses of ketamine (10–20 mg, in 5- to 10-mg increments) to a level of sedation and analgesia that allows positioning without pain.

Perioperative Adjuvant Analgesics

In addition to the administration of sedatives and analgesics to provide sedation, anxiolysis, and analgesia for the performance of neural blockade techniques, it is common to administer adjuvant analgesic agents in the preoperative period to help manage pain in the intra- and postoperative period. Commonly administered adjuvant analgesics include acetaminophen, non-steroidal anti-inflammatory drugs (NSAIDs), cyclo-oxygenase inhibitors (COXIBs), and, more recently, gabapentin. Acetaminophen, NSAIDs (such as ibuprofen, naproxen, or ketorolac), and COXIBs (such as celecoxib), with administration starting preoperatively or immediately postoperatively and continued during the postoperative period, have demonstrated a 15% to 55% reduction in postoperative opioid requirement (24–26). Meta-analysis of clinical trials with the use of perioperative NSAID administration have also demonstrated significant reductions in opioid-related side effects such as nausea, vomiting, and sedation (26). Recent studies have demonstrated that gabapentin in preoperative oral doses of 600 to 1,200 mg can improve analgesia and reduce postoperative opioid requirement as well (27,28). Although the use of local anesthetics in neural blockade for infiltration, peripheral nerve block, or neuraxial block remains the most potent of the nonopioid analgesic techniques, these other nonopioid analgesics are important adjuvants in the multimodal approach to postoperative pain management. A more thorough discussion of multimodal analgesia in postoperative pain management can be found in Chapter 43.

EQUIPMENT, SUPPLIES, LOCATION, AND PATIENT POSITIONING

Equipment and Supplies

Prior to performing any neural blockade procedure, the anesthesiologist should locate and ensure the proper functioning of the necessary monitoring and resuscitation equipment and drugs. Minimal basic resuscitation drugs and equipment for airway management (airways, suction equipment, laryngoscope, endotracheal tubes, muscle relaxants), support of cardiorespiratory function (oxygen, mask and reservoir bag, epinephrine, anticholinergic drugs, inotropic and/or vasopressor drugs), and sedative/induction agents (benzodiazepines, barbiturates) should be immediately available in case of adverse patient reaction associated with the procedure or the anesthetic agents administered. The Regional Anesthesia Section at Wake Forest University have developed a special "Local Anesthetic Toxicity" box, with special equipment and supplies to treat patients in the event of an unintentional intravascular injection of local anesthetic, in addition to routine resuscitation drugs and equipment.

Monitoring should include, at a minimum, the application of a pulse oximeter to monitor pulse rate, peripheral perfusion, and oxygen saturation (7). For all but the least invasive, least complicated procedures, one should consider electrocardiograph and blood pressure monitoring as well. Peripheral temperature monitoring may be helpful if monitoring for effects of sympathetic blockade.

Location

The location most appropriate for performance of neural blockade procedures will vary according to the type of procedure and practice setting. Local anesthetic infiltration and minor neural blockade procedures may be safely performed in outpatient locations such as physicians' offices and emer-

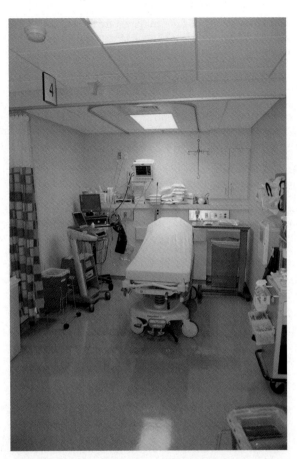

FIGURE 8-2. Regional anesthesia preoperative procedure and holding room. One of four patient care areas with full monitoring and resuscitation equipment, where all patients undergoing surgical procedures with regional anesthesia are brought for placement of their neural blockade prior to going to the operating room.

gency departments. More complex neural blockade procedures should be carried out in an otherwise suitable anesthetizing location such as the preinduction area, operating room, PACU, or an appropriately equipped special procedure area (radiologic procedure area, pain management unit, etc.). Regardless of the location, an area of sufficient size, with proper lighting and equipment to safely and efficiently perform the procedure, is required. Neural blockade procedures for surgical patients may be more conveniently and efficiently performed in a dedicated regional anesthesia holding area, similar to induction areas, where the block can be performed while a preceding operative procedure is being completed or while the operating room is being prepared for the patient. This system has been used in several centers and provides a significant efficiency advantage in terms of improving operating room turnover times, improving the success rate of neural blockade procedures, and improving overall acceptance of regional anesthesia techniques (Fig. 8-2).

Patient Positioning and Documentation

Considerations for patient positioning for neural blockade procedures should ensure patient safety and comfort and optimize the successful performance of the anesthetic procedure. Some neural blockade procedures may require the enlistment of an assistant to help maintain patient safety and comfort. Special care should be taken with patients placed in the sitting position following or during the administration of sedative medications.

Appropriate documentation of neural blockade procedures is important for continuity of patient care, medicolegal considerations, and billing and compliance issues. Simple neural blockade procedures may only require a brief note on the anesthetic record or in the progress notes of the patient's chart. More extensive procedures may require more extensive documentation including the patient's consent, patient positioning, sedative agents administered, skin preparation, block technique, needle or catheter used, local anesthetic used and total dose administered, patient response, and documentation of any problems or complications. Because of the amount of space required on the anesthetic record for this level of documentation, and to standardize and improve efficiency of documentation of regional anesthesia procedures, a standardized neural blockade procedure note may be helpful (Figs. 8-3 and 8-4).

Equipment Specific to Neural Blockade

The necessary equipment for a neural blockade procedure will again vary according to the anesthetic procedure being performed. Nonetheless, suggestions regarding basic equipment may be useful to most and can be modified to the needs of the specific procedure, patient, and practitioner.

Block Trays

Three types of neural blockade procedures are most frequently performed by the anesthesiologist: (a) spinal (subarachnoid) neural blockade, (b) epidural or caudal neural blockade, and (c) peripheral neural blockade. Because the specific equipment required for each of these three types of blockade procedures is sufficiently different, most anesthesia departments find it most efficient to have separate block trays for each procedure. However, with the popularity of the combined spinal-epidural technique, it may be more cost-effective to have a single spinal-epidural tray that can be used for either procedure or the combination. The specific requirements for needles, syringes, and ancillary equipment are discussed in the chapters that describe the various neural blockade techniques.

Apart from the needles, syringes, local anesthetic agents, adjuvant drugs, and ancillary equipment specific to the procedure, some basic supplies are required for all neural blockade procedures including (a) a container for a skin preparation solution, (b) sponges or other applicators for skin preparation solution application, (c) sterile drapes, and (d) gauze sponges for wiping the skin during the procedure. These supplies may be assembled from individual sterile packages at the time of the procedure or be supplied as components of either a preassembled nerve block pack or a commercially prepared, disposable nerve block tray.

Anesthesiologists have witnessed a progressive improvement in the quality and reliability of disposable, commercially prepared nerve block trays. In many high-volume centers, commercially produced "custom trays" tailored to the specific needs and preferences of the department are frequently used. The convenience of the prepackaged tray, improvements in the quality of disposable needles and other equipment components, and the desirability of single-use equipment from the standpoint of sterility and patient safety have virtually eliminated the use of internally prepared nerve block trays in most centers. Convenience, efficiency, and flexibility in the practice of regional anesthesia may be further enhanced through the use of a specially equipped regional anesthesia cart (Fig. 8-5).

Syringes, Needles, and Drugs

The major variation in what otherwise might be an "all purpose" block tray is the numbers and kinds of syringes, needles, and drugs that would be included. Other than the personal preferences for size, glass versus plastic, or three-ringed versus plain syringes, there is little to choose among syringes.

Interest in needles has focused primarily on patient safety and comfort, speed of injection, angle of bevel, and the role of needle size in nerve trauma and association with the incidence of postdural puncture headache. Commensurate with the ability to aspirate blood as an indication of possible intravascular injection, generally one should consider using the smallest needle possible. Because most practitioners must do multiple needle insertions to accomplish a successful block, all patients deserve skin and subcutaneous infiltration with a 25-gauge or smaller needle. The use of a needle with a security bead at its proximal shaft has been advocated to preclude loss of broken needles (29). The use of high-quality disposable needles makes this practice unnecessary and expensive. The role of the needle, its size, and angle of bevel (i.e., sharp point) in producing nerve injury has been studied (30,31) and is discussed in Chapter 20.

A word of caution must be given concerning the use of long-bevel disposable needles. The metal with which these needles are made is relatively soft. After such a needle point strikes a bony surface (rib or spine), it may develop a hook or barb at its tip. This barb can cause significant damage as it passes through nerves, vessels, and tissue. Frequent observation for development of deformities at the needle tip or wiping of the tip of the needle across sterile cotton or gauze will allow recognition of this problem. Needles that are bent or otherwise deformed during the performance of a neural blockade procedure should be discarded and a new needle should be used.

Drugs packaged in commercially prepared, disposable trays have been sterilized, usually with ethylene oxide. In an effort to determine the safety of subjecting these drugs to gas autoclaving with ethylene oxide, Abram (32) studied both ampules and vials of local anesthetic agents, some of which had intentionally been "pre-cracked." There was no evidence of ethylene oxide metabolites—that is, ethylene glycol—in any of the intact ampules. However, some of the drugs in vials with rubber stoppers or in pre-cracked ampules had detectable ethylene glycol. In a separate animal study of the neurologic effect of ethylene glycol, Abram found no effect in doses several times greater than that found in the "cracked ampules." His conclusion was that it was safe to sterilize local anesthetic agents with ethylene oxide, especially those in snap-top ampules. It is important, however, that 24 to 72 hours be allowed for the extrusion of ethylene oxide if it is used to sterilize the entire block tray. Without regard to how trays are sterilized, there should be indicator tape or tags to assure the anesthesiologist that the equipment has, in fact, been sterilized.

Special Equipment and Techniques

To improve the success rate of neural blockade or to make it possible in very difficult cases or extreme circumstances, special devices, needles, and pieces of equipment have been advocated or introduced. Various needles and modifications of the technique of identification of the epidural space have been described (see Chapter 11). Radiologic localization of needle placement

Anesthesiology Procedure Note

PERIPHERAL NERVE BLOCKADE

Peripheral Nerve Block(s) performed

Patient Name

Medical Record #

Age   Sex

(Patient name plate stamp)

Approach: _____ ☐ **Left** ☐ **Right** side confirmed

Indication: ☐ Analgesia ☐ Surgical anesthesia   Dx/pain location:_____

☐ Specifically requested for management of pain by Dr. _____

Date: _____/_____/20_____ **Start time** (:) **End time** (:)

Pt Condition: **Initial BP:**____/____ **HR:** ____ **VAS Pain score:** 0 1 2 3 4 5 6 7 8 9 10

☐ awake   ☐ sedate with meaningful contact maintained

☐ PNB performed under spinal / epidural / general anesthesia. Indication: _____

Preparation: ☐ povidone-iodine ☐ chlorhexidine ☐ iodophor/isopropyl ☐ alcohol ☐ drape

Position: ☐ supine   ☐ prone   ☐ LLD   ☐ RLD ☐ sitting

Needle(s): ☐ short-bevel   ☐ Tuohy   ☐ long-bevel   ☐ pencil-tipped

Manufacturer, length, gauges: _____

Technique: ☐ injection through needle   ☐ catheter placement **(depth at skin_____cm).**

☐ nerve stimulation   ☐ infiltration   ☐ ultrasound

☐ paresthesia. describe quality of paresthesia :_____

Motor response or paresthesia obtained	mA	mS	depth (cm)	Sedation Given	mg/mcg
				Midazolam	
				Fentanyl	

Injectate: ☐ **bupivacaine** ☐ **ropivacaine** ☐ **mepivacaine** ☐ **lidocaine** ☐ **2-CP**

Concentration (%)	Volume (mL)	Adjunct	Epinephrine
			☐ 1/____00,000
			☐ not used

Narrative: Injection was made incrementally with constant monitoring and aspiration every _____ ml's.

		Action Taken
Blood aspirated:	☐ no	☐ yes
Intravenous test using epinephrine:	☐ negative	☐ positive
Pain on injection noted:	☐ no	☐ yes
Resistance on injection	☐ normal	☐ high

Events: ☐ none: easy and well tolerated   ☐ difficult:

Success: ☐ complete ☐ partial ☐ failed ☐ aborted ☐ full evaluation pending

Pt Condition: **Post BP:**____/____ **HR:** ____ **VAS Pain score:** 0 1 2 3 4 5 6 7 8 9 10

☐ The procedure was performed by _____(sign). I was present and medically directed.

☐ I performed the procedure myself. **ATTENDING MD SIGNATURE:** _____

FIGURE 8-3. A peripheral neural blockade procedure note for standardized documentation of regional anesthetic procedures for the patient's record. The document has a second copy that goes to the billing department for charge documentation. From Gerancher JC, Viscusi ER, Liguori GA, et al. Development of a standardized peripheral nerve block procedure note form. *Reg Anesth Pain Med* 2005;30:67–71, with permission

Anesthesiology Procedure Note
NEURAXIAL BLOCKADE

Block(s) performed	Surgical site confirmed:

□ **Left** □ **Right** □ **Midline**

□ **Anticoagulation/antithrombosis status was reviewed**

Patient Name

Medical Record #

Age   Sex

(Patient name plate stamp)

Indication: □ Analgesia □ Anesthesia   □ Specifically requested for management
Dx/pain location: of pain by Dr. _____

Date: _____/_____/20_____   **Start time** (:)   **End time** (:)

Pt Condition: Initial BP:_____/_____ HR:_____O2 Sat:_____ VAS Pain: 0 1 2 3 4 5 6 7 8 9 10

□ awake   □ sedate with meaningful contact maintained

□ Performed under general anesthesia with the indication: _____

Preparation: □ drape   □ povidone-iodine □ chlorhexidine □ alcohol   □ iodophor/isopropyl

Position: □ LLD   □ RLD   □ sitting   □ prone

Technique: □ mid-line □ paramedian   □ loss of resistance to saline □ loss of resistance to air

Approximate interspace: □ Thoracic: **T -T**   □ Lumbar: **L -L .**

□ injection given through needle □ **Loss of resistance at depth:** _____cm.

□ **Catheter insertion, mark at skin:** _____cm.

Needle(s):   □ Epidural needle gauge: _____   □ Needle length if not 3.5 inches:_____

□ Spinal needle gauge: _____   □ Pencil-tip   □ Quincke □ introducer

Manufacturer of neuraxial needle/catheter/ tray:

Injectate:

Spinal Local Anesthetic	Dose (mg)	Baricity	Adjuncts	Epinephrine

Epidural Local Anesthetic	Volume (ml)		Adjuncts	Epinephrine
				□ 1/__00,000
				□ not used

Narrative: **The test dose given was:**   **Action Taken**

Paresthesia encountered	□ no	□ yes	
CSF via catheter or epidural	□ no	□ yes	
Blood aspirated:	□ no	□ yes	
Intravenous/Spinal test:	□ negative	□ positive	
Pain on injection noted:	□ no	□ yes	

Injection was made incrementally with constant monitoring and aspiration every _____ml's.

Events: □ none: easy/ well tolerated □ difficult:

Success: **Block Level(s):** _____ □ failed   □ aborted   □ a full evaluation is pending

Pt Condition: Post BP:_____/_____ HR:_____O2 Sat:_____ VAS Pain: 0 1 2 3 4 5 6 7 8 9 10

Sedation Given	Dose (mcg /mg)

□ The procedure was performed by _____(sign). I was present and medically directed.

□ I performed the procedure myself. **ATTENDING MD SIGNATURE:** _____

FIGURE 8-4. A central neural blockade procedure note for standardized documentation of regional anesthetic procedures for inclusion in the patient's medical record. The document has a second copy that goes to the billing department for charge documentation. From Viscusi ER, Gerancher JC, Weller R, et al. "Not Documented? Not Done!: A proposed procedure note for neuraxial blockade. [Abstract] American Society of Regional Anesthesia and Pain Medicine 2005 Annual Spring Meeting April 21–24, 2005, Toronto, Canada, with permission

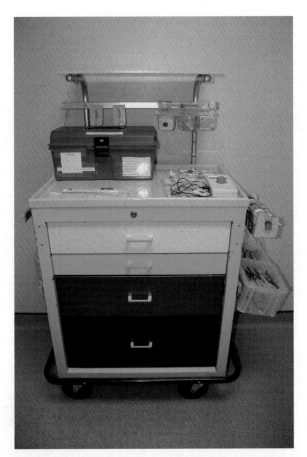

FIGURE 8-5. Regional anesthesia procedure cart. The top shelf is the work surface for resuscitation drugs and equipment or block tray. The drawers contain syringes, needles, skin preparation solutions, dressing supplies, peripheral nerve stimulator. and insulated needles.

using fluoroscopy or computed tomography guidance may be indicated for certain more difficult neural blockade procedures (e.g., placement of neurolytic solutions for celiac plexus block), but they may be too expensive and time-consuming to become routine daily practice. The use of Doppler and most recently ultrasound guidance to locate nerves or associated vascular structures has attracted a great deal of attention, and ultrasound may become the standard of future practice.

Peripheral Nerve Stimulators

The use of a nerve stimulator to assist in the location of peripheral nerves with motor fiber components has been advocated for peripheral neural blockade procedures on the basis of efficacy, efficiency, and patient safety (33–39). The peripheral nerve stimulator allows for localization of a peripheral nerve without the need for elicitation of a paresthesia; thus, peripheral neural blockade can be performed in patients who are sedated, unconscious, or otherwise unable to understand or cooperate, or in circumstances in which the nerve is difficult to localize due to anatomic variability.

The technique of peripheral nerve stimulation was originally described in 1912 (40). The stimulating current was transmitted to the nerve using a pure nickel needle insulated with lacquer down to the tip. Needle localization of nerves with motor responses using electrical stimulation with an insulated needle

was described in 1955 (41). In 1962, the construction and use of a portable needle nerve stimulator–locator as an instrument to assist in the locating of nerves for neural blockade procedures was reported (42).

In 1973, the use of a nerve stimulator with standard, unsheathed (uninsulated) needles commonly used for neural blockade procedures was described (42). The reported advantages of the use of uninsulated needles included superior detection of the tissue planes, fewer complications resulting from problems with the insulating materials, and less dependence on special equipment. Although the use of uninsulated needles may result in stimulation of the nerve because of proximity of the nerve to segments of the needle other than the tip, experimental investigation demonstrated greater current density at the tip of unsheathed hypodermic needles than at the shaft.

In a comparative investigation of sheathed and unsheathed needles in the cat, sheathed (insulated) needles were reported to be more precise in locating the peripheral nerve (43). In this study, it was reported that unsheathed (uninsulated) needles were capable of displaying the "least stimulating current" when the tip of the needle was beyond the nerve by as much as 0.8 cm. In a study of the electrical characteristics of peripheral nerve stimulators that contributed to the localization of peripheral nerves (44), the following characteristics were found to be important:

- A *linear output*; that is, a plot of percent output versus percentage of meter scale gives a straight line passing through zero and with 100% of the meter scale corresponding to 100% output.
- *High and low output ranges* that allow the use of higher output when the needle is distant from the nerve and a wide range of low-output control when the needle is close to the nerve. Stimulators developed for monitoring neuromuscular blockade may not have the required control in the low-output range, making them unsuitable for use in the location of peripheral nerves for neural blockade.
- *Clearly marked polarity of the output* extending to the ends of the connecting cables. It is important to attach the cathode (−) to the stimulating needle and the anode (+) to the surface of the patient. On some stimulators, it is difficult to determine which is the cathode (−) by color, but by convention the cathode (−) is usually black and the anode (+) is usually red.
- *Constant-current output*; that is, current output remains the same regardless of different resistance applied to the output. In contrast, a constant-voltage output instrument will decrease current output as resistance increases.
- A *short stimulation pulse*. The shorter the stimulation pulse, the greater the ratio of the current required to stimulate the nerve when the needle is 1 cm away from the nerve, compared to when the needle is on the nerve. For example, for a pulse width of 40 μsec, this ratio is 11, whereas for a pulse width of 1,000 μsec the ratio is only 5. Newer nerve stimulators now offer stimulation of variable pulse durations (0.1 ms, 0.3 ms, and 1 ms) for sensory and motor nerve stimulation.
- *Design features*, including a large, easily turned current-output dial, a digital current-output meter, and a battery check.

Several sophisticated peripheral nerve stimulators and a variety of prepackaged, sterile, single-use, insulated needle systems are currently commercially available that incorporate the design features outlined above (Fig. 8-6).

Polarity of the stimulating needle when using a peripheral nerve stimulator affects the current required for nerve

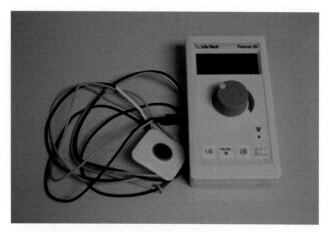

FIGURE 8-6. Peripheral nerve stimulator with low-output, variable-intensity control with connecting cable and ground electrode.

stimulation during neural blockade procedures (45). In a study of patients undergoing axillary brachial plexus blockade, as much as two to three times the current output of the nerve stimulator was required to obtain nerve stimulation when the stimulating needle was attached to the positive terminal (anode) compared to when the stimulating needle was attached to the negative terminal (cathode). For this reason, it is imperative that the stimulating needle be connected to the negative output terminal (cathode) of the nerve stimulator and the patient be connected via the positive terminal (anode) to allow nerve stimulation detection at the lowest possible current output.

Technical Considerations

1. The anode (+) terminal of the stimulator (usually red) is connected to an electrode on the patient's skin clear of the prepped site of the block.
2. The cathode (−) terminal of the stimulator (usually black) is connected to the stimulating needle. The needle is inserted and advanced near the nerve. The stimulator is set to an output of 1 to 2 mA. Local muscle contraction should be minimal at this setting.
3. Stimulation of the nerve to be blocked should be measured by observing or feeling for muscle contractions within the motor distribution of the nerve. When using an insulated (sheathed) needle, stimulation will increase as the needle tip approaches the nerve and then decrease as the needle tip passes the nerve. The current output of the stimulator is decreased, as the needle approaches the nerve, to the lowest output that results in nerve stimulation and muscle contraction (usually less than 0.5 mA). At the point of maximum stimulation with the minimum stimulator output, the needle tip should be proximate to the nerve and the local anesthetic solution may be injected.
4. Injection of 1 to 2 mL of local anesthetic will immediately abolish nerve stimulation and muscle contraction if the tip of the needle is at the site of the nerve. If this does not occur, the needle should be withdrawn slightly and the process repeated. A further test is to increase the output of the stimulator after the test dose. It should still be possible to elicit some muscle response at the higher output. After a successful test dose, the full dose of local anesthetic required for the nerve block may be injected.
5. Injection of dextrose 5% solution (D5W), a nonconducting medium, can reliably confirm needle-to-nerve contact.

Electrophysiologic studies in humans (46) and animals (47) have demonstrated that D5W can increase current density at the needle tip with the same delivered current intensity, thus intensifying an existing motor response (the Tsui test). Injection of D5W can also bring about the return of a motor response that has disappeared after initial saline injection.

Newer Developments. The peripheral nerve stimulator has traditionally been used to locate nerves with motor fiber components, as just described. However, the use of a peripheral nerve stimulator to determine the location of a peripheral nerve with purely sensory fiber components also has been described recently (48). Peripheral surface stimulation of peripheral nerves and proximal location of nerve trunks using detection of mixed nerve action potentials has also been reported as a method to facilitate peripheral neural blockade (49). A percutaneous electrode guidance (PEG) system (50) was recently developed to identify target nerve location prior to actual needle puncture, thus minimizing the number of random searches and painful needle attempts. The PEG system uses a cylindrical, smooth-tipped metallic electrode probe to indent the skin and subcutaneous tissue and bring the cutaneous electrode tip close to the underlying nerve for transcutaneous stimulation. Once obtaining a satisfactory motor response with the surface electrode (often requiring 2 to −5 mA and a 0.3 to 1 msec pulse duration), an insulated needle is then advanced inside the PEG device to reach the target nerve underneath the skin. Needle-to-nerve contact is further confirmed by electrical stimulation through the needle, with a lower threshold current (e.g., 0.2–0.7 mA and 0.1 msec). A modified and improved PEG system has been reported recently (51), but commercialization of this product is pending. In the meantime, successful transcutaneous electrical stimulation through an insulated needle has been reported to prelocate individual terminal branches of the brachial plexus in the axilla (52). Conceivably, it may be challenging for transcutaneous electrical stimulation to reach nerves that are located deep (e.g., sciatic nerve in the gluteal region or brachial plexus in the infraclavicular region), and this may pose a possible limitation to this technique.

Another new method of nerve localization under investigation is called sequential electrical nerve stimulation (SENS) (53). In the prototype, the nerve stimulator is set to deliver repeating sequenced electrical nerve stimuli through an insulated needle at 3 Hz, with increasing pulse duration of 0.1 msec, 0.3 msec, and 1 msec. Because SENS can trigger a motor response with a stronger stimulus (0.3 msec and 1 msec) when the needle is still far away from the nerve, this method of nerve localization is potentially more sensitive than the conventional 0.1-msec pulsed stimulation. The final end-point is the elicitation of three sustainable motor responses at 0.5 mA or less.

Stimulating catheters have been developed to improve the accuracy of perineural catheter placement and to reduce secondary block failure (i.e., inadequate analgesia during local anesthetic infusion) associated with non−stimulating catheters (54) (Fig. 8-7). Similar to the stimulating needle concept, a nerve stimulated motor response observed during catheter advancement indicates proper catheter placement along the course of the target nerve, guides the direction and depth of insertion, and confirms final catheter position. Disappearance of the motor response during catheter advancement, on the other hand, indicates migration of the catheter away from the target nerve and requires adjustment. The aim is to advance 3 to 5 cm of indwelling catheter segment while maintaining a low current-stimulated motor response (less than 0.5 mA). Clinical outcome data associated with stimulating catheters are mixed. Although anesthesia and analgesia was noted to be superior

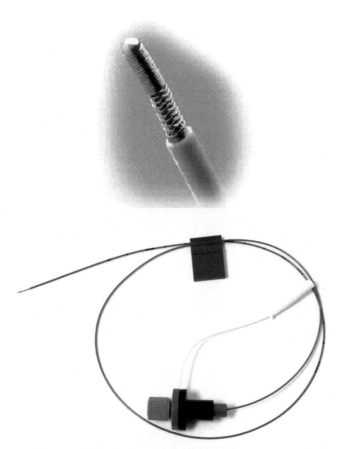

FIGURE 8-7. An example of a stimulating catheter with a metal bullet tip. (Arrow's StimuCath system.)

with stimulating catheters in a volunteer study (55) and clinical studies involving foot surgery (56,57), similar favorable outcome was not found in patients who received continuous femoral nerve blocks for total knee arthroplasty (58–60).

Electrical stimulation through a metal-reinforced epidural catheter primed with saline (a conducting medium) can confirm proper catheter placement in the epidural space. This forms the basis of the electrical nerve stimulation test (Tsui test) (61). A positive test is indicated by a segmental motor response, unilateral or bilateral, in a dermatome congruent with the epidural insertion level induced by a stimulating current between 1 and 10 mA (1 Hz and 0.2 msec pulse width). Depending on the catheter tip location, electrical stimulation may cause anal sphincter contraction (S2–S4) with a caudal catheter, leg contraction with a lumbar catheter, intercostal or abdominal muscle contraction with a thoracic catheter, and upper limb contraction with a cervical catheter. It is important to connect the cathode lead of the stimulator to the metal hub of an adapter connected to the epidural catheter and the anode (ground) lead on the body. Local twitching commonly observed under the grounding electrode should not be confused with the segmental motor response. This test is reportedly 80% sensitive but the positive predictive value is around 100% (no false-positive) (62). It is important to note that a higher current (10 to 15 mA) may be required for catheter stimulation (63), although a current of greater than 15 mA is generally not recommended. Conversely, a motor response occurring at less than 1 mA likely indicates intrathecal or subdural catheter placement or the catheter in close proximity to a nerve root.

A nonelectrical stimulation technique to confirm epidural catheter placement is epidural pressure waveform guidance (62).

In addition to position confirmation, electrical stimulation can also guide catheter advancement in the epidural space. For example, a styleted, saline-primed, 20-gauge epidural catheter (FlexTip Plus) can be reliably advanced from the caudal to lumbar or thoracic epidural space in children, and guided by electrical stimulation (1 to 10 mA) and the corresponding segmental motor responses (64). Similarly, in adults, the catheter has been successfully placed at the thoracic level (e.g., T4) and advanced to the cervical space (e.g., C5) using the same catheter assembly and stimulation technique for upper limb surgery (65). A nonelectrical stimulation technique to assist with epidural catheter advancement is electrocardiographic guidance (66).

Ultrasound Imaging

In recent years, ultrasound imaging has been recognized as a noninvasive, practical method for localizing peripheral nerve that may improve block success and safety (Fig. 8-8) (67–69). Contrary to conventional approaches that rely on surface anatomic landmarks, ultrasound provides visualization of target nerve structures and surrounding bony, muscular, and vascular structures underneath the skin. Nerves in cross-section often appear round or oval on ultrasound and demonstrate different echogenicity-hypoechoic (dark, showing the neural component) or hyperechoic (bright, showing the connective tissue component). Pre-block scanning helps to define the best

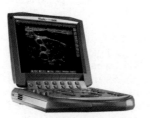

SonoSite MicroMaxx

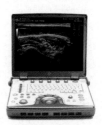

GE LOGIQ E

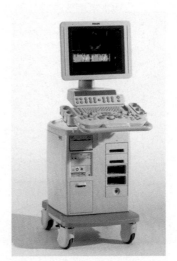

Philips HD 11 XE

FIGURE 8-8. State-of-the-art ultrasound machines, compact-sized (SonoSite MicroMaxx and GE LOGIQe) and cart-based (Philips HD 11XE), for regional anesthesia.

PART II: TECHNIQUES

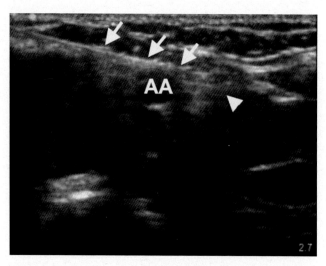

FIGURE 8-9. A transverse sonogram showing a block needle (*arrows*) in contact with the ulnar nerve (*arrowhead*) in the axilla; needle is advanced using the in-plane needle approach. AA, axillary artery.

possible site for needle insertion. Needle imaging during advancement provides real-time visual guidance to minimize random needle movement as the block needle is advanced toward the target nerves. Needle-to-nerve contact is further confirmed by nerve movement with or without concomitant electrical stimulation. Most important of all, accurate needle placement is confirmed when circumferential local anesthetic spread is observed around the nerves at the time of injection (Figs. 8-9 and 8-10).

Those ultrasound probes most useful for superficial scanning (within 3 to 4 cm deep; e.g., brachial plexus and femoral nerve) are in the range of 10 to 15 MHz, which provides high-resolution images. Ultrasound scanning for the brachial plexus in the interscalene, supraclavicular, infraclavicular, and axillary regions and its peripheral branches and that for the femoral

nerve and popliteal sciatic nerve is technically straightforward. Preliminary outcome data showing benefits of ultrasound-guided brachial plexus blocks include shortened procedure time, quicker block onset, improvement in block quality, prolonged block duration, and a decrease in block-related complications (e.g., vascular puncture) (70–72).

Scanning the sciatic nerve in the gluteal region and lumbar plexus in the psoas compartment in adults and older children can be challenging because of the deep locations of these nerves. Lower-frequency probes (5 to 7 MHz) are required for deep beam penetration at the expense of image clarity. Innovative advanced techniques for imaging nerves of small caliber (e.g., ilioinguinal and iliohypogastric nerves, infrapatellar nerve, and occipital nerve) have also been reported. It is important to realize that the success of ultrasound-guided nerve block demands: (a) proper nerve imaging technique, (b) proficiency in tracking needle advancement in real time, (c) recognition of needle-to-nerve contact, and (d) a sufficient amount of local anesthetic deposit around the target nerve.

Although ultrasound technology for nerve imaging is advancing rapidly, a number of technical limitations remain. Nerve localization is highly dependent on the proficiency of the operator's scanning skill. Image clarity and the depth of penetration are inversely related, thus it is technically challenging to visualize deep structures with clarity. Anatomic structures deep to bones (e.g., neuraxial structures and intercostal nerves) are often shadowed by bone, and imaging accessibility is highly restricted. Accurate needle tracking during advancement can be difficult in the absence of an echogenic needle tip design.

INTRAOPERATIVE MANAGEMENT OF PATIENTS FOR NEURAL BLOCKADE

An important, and often the most challenging aspect of the successful practice of regional anesthesia, is the intraoperative management of the patient. A major concern of patients when discussing regional anesthesia for their surgery is that they will have to remain awake. This approach to the management of patients with nerve blockade may be traced back to the earliest days of surgery when there were no, or too few, anesthesiologists. Surgeons performed the nerve blocks first, then they proceeded with the surgical procedure. It is not surprising, then, that early anesthesiologists were expected only to provide general anesthesia to those patients and/or procedures not suitable for a nerve block administered by the surgeon.

Gaston Labat (73), a surgeon and the "Father of Regional Anesthesia," acknowledged in his early writings the importance of sedative supplementation of regional anesthesia. Even more important are his comments relating to excessive noise in the operating room, unnecessary conversation that might be misinterpreted by the patient, and avoidance of the surgeon querying the patient about his level of sedation or comfort. Many patients would be content with little or no sedation if the operating room environment were quiet and nonthreatening.

Patient Considerations

Often, the compelling indication for a regional block technique rather than a general anesthetic is the patient who should *not* be rendered unconscious. This may be due to a full stomach, difficult airway, or high risk (poor physical status), all factors that

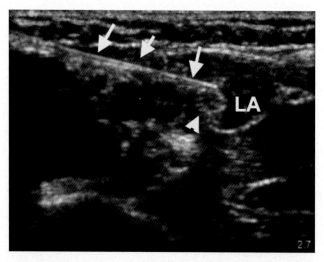

FIGURE 8-10. A transverse sonogram showing a needle (*arrows*) and local anesthetic (*LA*) injection around the ulnar nerve (*arrowhead*); local anesthetic spread is indicated by a hypoechoic fluid collection (*LA*).

impose serious risks under general anesthesia. Clearly, these patients should be awake or sedated just enough to provide anxiolysis and a cooperative attitude. Specific pharmacologic agents will be discussed later, but this is a situation in which "vocal anesthesia" (reassuring conversation) or music via headphones can be very helpful.

The antithesis of the high-risk, slightly sedated patient is the pediatric or otherwise overly anxious patient who will likely become uncooperative or agitated intraoperatively. Although these patients may need to be asleep during surgery, it does not preclude their receiving a regional anesthetic for surgical anesthesia prior to induction of unconscious sedation. Supplementation of regional anesthesia thus covers the extremes of patient needs. It is a rare patient, however, who must be denied any kind of supplementation just as a matter of principle. Our armamentarium of drugs and techniques no longer makes this argument valid.

Surgical Considerations

Frequently, the determinant of supplemental drugs and techniques is the location or anticipated duration of the surgical procedure, or both. In general, the closer the surgical procedure is to the head and neck, the more complex the anesthetic management. Patients tend to be more apprehensive about operations in these areas. The proximity of darkening and smothering surgical drapes, retractors, and surgical manipulation around the eyes and the airway may further add to the patient's apprehension and feelings of claustrophobia. For these reasons, one may tend toward heavy sedation. Unfortunately, as the surgical team occupies the area at the head of the patient, the anesthesiologist is likely dislocated to areas more distant, requiring vigilance and caution in balancing sedation with airway management and safety. In these surgical procedures, the anesthesiologist must never render patients unconscious without first securing the airway. Anesthesiologists who work with otolaryngologists, ophthalmologists, oral surgeons, and plastic surgeons providing monitored anesthesia care (MAC) are especially vulnerable to the aforementioned balance of "conscious airways" in comfortable and cooperative patients.

One must also review if and what drugs were given in the pre-block period because many are of short duration. A continuum of necessary sedation and analgesia must be maintained throughout the perioperative period.

Anesthetic Considerations

At least three features of regional anesthesia are primary indications for supplementation. First is a thorough knowledge of the neural elements involved in the surgical procedure and of the regional block to be performed. For example, the use of an intercostal nerve block is extremely beneficial as the anesthetic technique for placement of a gastrostomy feeding tube. One must appreciate, however, that the intercostal nerve block provides only somatic sensory blockade of that portion of the abdominal wall. When the surgeon enters the abdomen, visceral pain will be noted by the patient since the viscera are innervated via the unblocked autonomic fibers. As a result, some degree of supplemental analgesia will be required.

Second is the possibility that the block is inadequate due to missed or partially blocked neural elements. This could result from poor technique or improper choice of local anesthetic drug, concentration, or volume. On occasion, the operation extends beyond the area of neural blockade. In these cases, sup-

plementary analgesia and sedation in the amount and duration necessary to provide completely satisfactory anesthesia must be rapidly instituted. However, one should supplement only to the degree and duration necessary to restore the contribution of the regional technique to overall anesthetic satisfaction.

A final factor overlooked by anesthesiologists and surgeons alike is total comfort for the patient. The duration of the surgical procedure affects the complete range of supplemental pharmacology. Extremely short procedures may require no supplemental drugs, whereas lengthy procedures will likely require both sedation and analgesia. Depending on surgical position, most patients will become progressively more uncomfortable from lying still on an operating table. Although high sensory levels of spinal or epidural anesthesia supply their own analgesia, low levels of block and peripheral nerve blocks have limited areas of analgesia. Remember, "all of the body wants to be comfortable." The patient may have a totally numb and paralyzed extremity only to subsequently suffer progressive back and body aches and pains from lying immobilized on a hard operating surface. A ready solution to this problem for healthy patients receiving epidural or spinal anesthesia is to produce a higher level of sensory blockade. For example, a T11 spinal anesthetic would be sufficient for lower extremity surgery. However, if no significant adverse physiologic effects are anticipated, then a T6 level would provide patient comfort up to the mid-thorax without use of large doses of systemic analgesics. Too many "perfect blocks" have been abandoned because of poor management of the patient's total anesthetic needs.

Drugs and Techniques

Specific agents or techniques for intraoperative supplementation of regional anesthesia include the entire gamut of anesthesia practice. For a variety of surgical, anesthetic, and patient factors, every regional anesthetic could potentially require induction of a general anesthetic at a moment's notice, and the anesthetic preparations should be made accordingly. With that in mind, supplementation methods will be discussed from the least to the most intrusive since that is actually the recommended practice—that is, to give no more or do no more than is required to provide a satisfactory anesthetic.

Nonpharmacologic Techniques

A surprising number of patients will request a regional anesthetic because they are actually afraid of being rendered unconscious. Other patients are ambivalent about the need for or desirability of sedation and defer to the anesthesiologist. Among the most common reasons for patients' reluctance to have a regional anesthetic is the desire that they do not "hear what is going on" even if they are convinced they will not "feel anything" during the surgical procedure. A thorough explanation to the patient of the anesthetic and surgical happenings will be helpful in their decision. Reassurance that the anesthesiologist will be in constant attendance and able to increase levels of supplementation as required or desired is essential. It is important that patients be unaware of the actual events of the procedure—that they are psychologically or pharmacologically distracted from the operative procedures.

Techniques for distraction vary, but are designed to prevent anticipation of pain and fear by the patient. Office practitioners of local or nerve block anesthesia become adept at these techniques of "vocal anesthesia." It is equally important that all operating room personnel project the same professional reassurance to the patient. Minimization of extraneous conversation, especially that which is not patient-related, should be encouraged for all the operating room staff.

Music has been a part of the surgical experience for nearly a century, beginning with live performances in dental and operating theaters (74). Music exerts a calming or distracting influence on patients both in the preoperative holding area and during the surgical procedure. Portable CD or MP3 players with headphones and a sufficient music library may provide music of the patient's choice. Patients may even be encouraged to bring their own music or appropriate devices with them for their use during the perioperative period. Studies have demonstrated that listening to music throughout the perioperative period is associated with decreased supplemental sedation and analgesic medication requirement in patients undergoing surgical procedures with regional anesthesia (75,76). Many recovery units now provide closed-circuit or commercial television viewing for patients awaiting discharge home.

Pharmacologic Techniques

All practitioners of local and regional anesthesia must know the fundamentals of administering and monitoring sedation, whether it is done by anesthesiologists or other operating room personnel. For the nonanesthesiologist, the practice guidelines for sedation and analgesia as outlined by the American Society of Anesthesiologists are excellent basic principles that all should follow (77).

The most common method of administering sedative and analgesic drugs intraoperatively is intravenously. With development of more sophisticated levels of technology, the single or combined uses of bolus, continuous drip, continuous infusion, and even patient-controlled administration are now available. The selection of methods should be tailored to the circumstances of patient and procedure. For relatively shorter procedures or for patients who request that very minimal sedation be administered intraoperatively, small doses of sedative medications titrated in intermittent doses to achieve the desired effect may be most appropriate. However, although the technique of intermittent dosing throughout the perioperative period is possible, intraoperative administration of ongoing sedation in a stable surgical procedure can be easily accomplished using any of a variety of continuous infusion devices.

Nonopioids. A variety of nonopioid drugs have been commonly used for intraoperative sedation for patients undergoing surgical procedures with regional anesthesia, including barbiturates (methohexital, pentobarbital) and benzodiazepines (diazepam, midazolam). Midazolam, propofol (alone or in combination with ketamine), and dexmedetomidine are currently the most commonly used intraoperative sedative agents for patients with neural blockade.

Midazolam. Midazolam, being the most commonly used benzodiazepine for preoperative sedation and anxiolysis, is commonly used to produce intraoperative sedation as well. Effective dosing regimens for midazolam may be accomplished by either initial dosing of 1 to 2 mg, followed by subsequent intermittent doses of 0.5 to 1.0 mg, or by continuous infusion at a dose of 1.0 to 2.5 μg/kg/min to produce mild to moderate sedation (78,79).

In 1991, sedative infusions of midazolam were compared to propofol during local and regional anesthesia. This early study demonstrated that, although the overall quality of sedation was similar in the two groups, the use of propofol was associated with less postoperative sedation, drowsiness, and confusion,

and a more rapid recovery of cognitive function. Midazolam was associated with less pain on injection and more effective intraoperative amnesia (78).

Propofol. Propofol in combination with ketamine was initially used to attempt to minimize the hemodynamic effects sometimes seen with propofol infusion alone (80). Later studies looked at the analgesic effect of propofol–ketamine infusion and demonstrated that the combination was associated with a reduced requirement for "rescue" opioid doses, as compared to propofol alone, in patients undergoing breast biopsy procedures. This study suggested that ketamine was a useful adjuvant to propofol sedation at an optimal propofol–ketamine dose ratio of 10:1 (81). It is our common clinical practice to add 20 mg of ketamine to 20 mL of propofol (10 mg/mL) to produce a final concentration of approximately 9 mg/mL propofol to 0.9 mg/mL administered in combination as a continuous infusion for intraoperative sedation and supplemental analgesia for patients with neural blockade. Adverse psychotomimetic responses to ketamine are reduced with this low-dose ketamine–propofol combination and premedication with a small dose of IV midazolam (2 mg).

Ketamine. The analgesic activity of ketamine has been linked primarily to its noncompetitive antagonist effect at the N-methyl-D-aspartate (NMDA) receptor (82,83), although it also interacts at non-NMDA glutamate receptors, nicotinic and muscarinic cholinergic receptors, and monoaminergic and opioid receptors (84). NMDA receptor antagonists have been demonstrated to modify peripheral afferent noxious stimulation and reduce the activation of spinal sensory neurons (85). Intraoperative low-dose ketamine has also been demonstrated to significantly reduce postoperative opioid requirements (86–88). Therefore, in addition to its preoperative and intraoperative benefits as a potent sedative and analgesic, intraoperative infusion of low-dose ketamine (0.5 mg/kg/h) can provide significant adjuvant analgesic effects for postoperative pain management as well.

Clonidine. The α_2-adrenergic receptor agonist clonidine, has been used as an anesthetic premedication, as well as for perioperative sedation and intraoperative and postoperative analgesia. In regional anesthesia, clonidine is more widely used as an additive to local anesthetics to prolong and intensify the analgesic effects of neural blockade and as an analgesic/anesthetic adjuvant for neuraxial blockade (89). Dexmedetomidine, a more highly selective α_2-adrenergic receptor agonist with a shorter half-life than clonidine, has been demonstrated to be useful as an IV sedative agent (90). The other potential benefits of dexmedetomidine as an IV sedative agent include easily arousable sedation, minimal respiratory depression, mild analgesic effects, and rapid recovery. Dexmedetomidine doses of 0.2 to 0.8 μg/kg/min following a loading dose of 0.5 to 1.0 μg/kg over 10 minutes have been used in volunteers and in patients undergoing surgical procedures with regional anesthesia (90,91).

Opioids. The use of low-dose opioids alone to supplement regional anesthesia is of limited value. Although their use will address the additional analgesic needs of the patient, most opioids at low doses have little effect on levels of consciousness and do not produce amnesia. The combination of an opioid analgesic and a benzodiazepine for sedation has been shown to reduce the requirements of both agents. Combinations of midazolam–alfentanil and propofol–fentanyl provided highly satisfactory intraoperative conditions during extracorporeal shock wave lithotripsy compared with a purely epidural technique (92). Caution and careful monitoring are important when combining opioid and benzodiazepine sedation for long procedures and/or in poor-risk patients. Respiratory depression is clearly the most dangerous of the opioid side effects. In a study of volunteers receiving fentanyl 2 μg/kg, 50% developed hypoxemia as defined by oxygen saturation (SaO$_2$) of less than 90% (93). Although midazolam alone (0.05 mg/kg) produced no adverse respiratory events, the combination of those doses of fentanyl and midazolam produced hypoxemia in 92% of the patients and apnea lasting more than 15 seconds in 50%. The use of supplemental oxygen and adequate monitoring of respiratory function and hemoglobin oxygen saturation are essential for all regional anesthesia techniques in which sedation and analgesia, alone or in combination, are used.

Remifentanil. The implementation of continuous infusion techniques for intraoperative supplementation has led to the use of very potent, short-acting agents. In the opioid class of drugs, remifentanil, a fentanyl derivative, has attracted interest. It is rapidly metabolized by tissue esterases, with a short, context-sensitive half-time of 3.2 minutes even following an infusion for 8 hours or more. Its brief duration of action avoids the issue of postoperative respiratory depression but also provides no postoperative analgesia. In a study of the use of remifentanil (0.05 μg/kg/min) versus propofol (16 μg/kg/min) for sedation during carotid endarterectomy under cervical plexus block, although both groups of patients experienced similar sedative effects, remifentanil was associated with a higher incidence of significant respiratory depression (94). Studies of low-dose remifentanil infusion (0.05 μg/kg/min) in combination with small doses of midazolam (2 mg) have demonstrated fewer opioid-related side effects including nausea, vomiting, and hypoventilation as compared to remifentanil (0.1 μg/kg/min) alone (95). The combination of midazolam with remifentanil potentiates the sedative and respiratory depressant effects of remifentanil (96). For patients requiring additional analgesia in addition to sedation for painful procedures, such as retrobulbar block, the use of remifentanil (0.03 μg/kg/min) in combination with propofol (12 μg/kg/min) has demonstrated adequate levels of sedation, better analgesia, and less respiratory depression for patients as compared to either fentanyl or propofol alone (97).

Inhalation Techniques. Three major reasons exist for combining inhalation techniques with a regional anesthetic technique. First, there are operative positions and procedures about the head, neck, thorax, and upper abdomen that require endotracheal tube protection of the airway against obstruction or aspiration. Although patients in critical care units tolerate indwelling endotracheal tubes with little or no sedation, most surgical patients need to be anesthetized if the endotracheal tube is to be tolerated during surgical manipulation. Second, procedures of very long duration can be performed with regional anesthesia using continuous catheter techniques or long-acting local anesthetics such as bupivacaine or ropivacaine. However, the cumulative doses of the parenteral sedatives and opioids can become very high over several hours of administration, leading to a prolonged postoperative recovery time. In these instances, once significant basal sedation is achieved with sedatives and opioids, it may be desirable to switch to low concentrations of inhaled agents. Third, there is always the possibility that the regional anesthetic technique, even with significant sedative supplementation, will not meet all of the needs of the patient or the surgeon. At that point, it is essential to proceed to an inhalation anesthetic technique. In some cases, the limitation of

the regional anesthetic may be anticipated, as in the use of thoracic epidural anesthesia for thoracotomy or upper abdominal surgery, where the use of a general anesthetic in combination with the epidural anesthetic is the planned technique. Anesthesiologists must always remember that the goal is to provide the patient with the very best anesthetic possible throughout the surgical procedure.

For situations in which an endotracheal tube is not required for protection of the airway, there is greater opportunity of using very low concentrations of inhaled drugs as another means of continuously administered sedation or analgesia in a spontaneously breathing patient. This can be administered by mask, nasal airway, or laryngeal mask airway (LMA). For patients who dislike or resist the claustrophobic feeling of head straps and face mask, a nasal airway connected to the circle breathing circuit of an anesthetic machine may be a satisfactory alternative. After gentle insertion of the lubricated airway into the anesthetized nasal passage, an endotracheal tube connector is inserted into the proximal end of the airway and the breathing circuit of the anesthesia machine is attached (Fig. 8-11).

The use of inhaled agents for supplemental sedation is very common in dental practice. Because IV injections are not required, this technique is of benefit to pediatric patients. More importantly, inhalation agents are rapidly eliminated through the lungs, so that recovery may be faster than that following administration of IV drugs. Nitrous oxide was traditionally the most popular of the supplemental inhalation agents because of its significant analgesic properties and its low potency, which provide a wide margin of safety. Recommended concentrations of nitrous oxide for "inhalation sedation" are 25% to 50%. An early study (98) involved 394 patients who received 1,005 outpatient dental treatments with the usual local anesthetic techniques plus a fixed concentration of 25% nitrous oxide via a nasal mask. Ninety-nine percent of these patients received adequate analgesia without loss of consciousness. More important, the change in anxiety level on subsequent treatments declined from the initial 86% who were "very anxious" to less than 10% on the fourth visit. Generally, these results apply to the proper management of most regional anesthetic procedures. The patient who is pain-free and sedated will be less anxious and more compliant toward future regional anesthetics.

Low concentrations of potent volatile anesthetics may also be used to provide intraoperative sedation and analgesia. In a crossover study of patients in labor, inhalation of 0.75% isoflurane provided analgesia superior to 50% nitrous oxide. Patients receiving isoflurane also had more drowsiness (99). Another study in dental patients compared inhalation of 0.5% isoflurane with 33% nitrous oxide. Patients breathing isoflurane were more relaxed, had marginally more rapid recovery and, in spite of a slightly unpleasant odor, would prefer isoflurane again (100). Sevoflurane is attractive as an inhalation agent for sedation in patients with regional anesthesia because of its characteristics of nonpungency, rapid onset, and quick elimination. A comparison of patients receiving sedation with IV midazolam versus inhaled sevoflurane demonstrated that sevoflurane was associated with faster recovery of post-administration memory and cognitive function. However, sedation with sevoflurane was associated with a high incidence of intraoperative excitement, resulting in conversion to general anesthesia (101). Because of the potency of the inhalation anesthetics, especially if administered in conjunction with other sedatives and opioids, extreme vigilance and careful monitoring of SaO$_2$ and other vital signs must be used. Supplemental oxygen should be administered to all patients receiving significant doses of sedative and analgesic drugs without regard to route of administration.

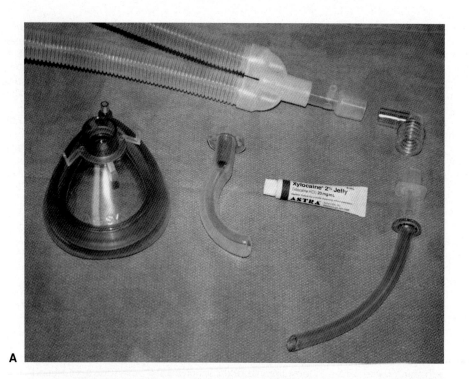

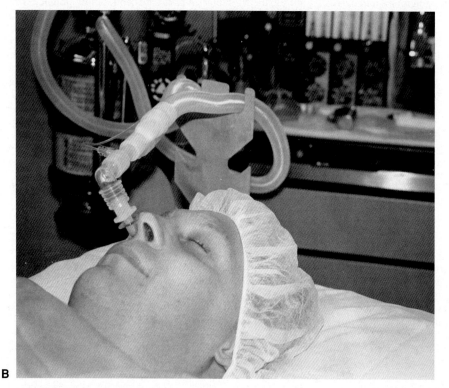

FIGURE 8-11. A: Equipment used for inhalation supplement of neural blockade using the anesthesia system. The plastic mask with or without oral airway may be used. Alternatively, the plastic nasal airway plus a standard 15-mm fitting may be adapted to the circle system. B: Demonstration of the use of the plastic nasal airway and circle system used for inhalation anesthesia supplement of neural blockade.

It is important to remember when using any potent sedative agents that sedation is a continuum that can range from a mild depression of consciousness to general anesthesia. The titration of "adequate" sedation for an individual patient may require a depth of sedation anywhere along this continuum, and the anesthesiologist must be prepared to move seamlessly through the required levels of sedation to maintain patient comfort.

SUMMARY

The use of sedative and analgesic adjuncts during local and regional anesthesia can enhance patient comfort and improve operative conditions. In turn, this can expand the range of procedures that can safely and comfortably be performed without a major general anesthetic.

Two basic principles may be derived from the preceding discussion of perioperative management of patients undergoing neural blockade. First, neural blockade is just one technique in the total armamentarium of the anesthesiologist. The anesthesiologist must be intellectually, psychologically, and technically prepared to perform inhalation or IV anesthesia techniques, as well as regional anesthesia techniques. The successful outcome of regional as well as general anesthesia practices requires provision of adequate space, equipment, and assistance. Finally, and most important, regional anesthesia techniques should not be considered failures if additional drugs and techniques are required for complete patient or surgical satisfaction. To exploit each drug and technique, alone or in combination, to the maximum benefit is the ultimate consultant practice of anesthesiology.

Second, the use of regional anesthesia techniques is only a part of the total anesthetic care of the patient. The anesthesiologist must deal with the whole patient, from the preanesthetic visit through discharge from the facility. The goal of correct premedication and supplementation of regional anesthesia is to maximize the benefits of what was, presumably, the appropriately selected and well-administered regional anesthetic technique. Empirical or premature overmedication carries the risk of respiratory and cardiovascular complications. Conversely, refusing to supplement when and to the degree necessary will only incur the ill will of the patient and surgeon. The appropriate use of analgesics and sedatives as premedication and for intraoperative supplementation is the key to an ever-increasing acceptance of the practice of regional anesthesia.

References

1. Horlocker TT, Wedel DJ, Benzon H, et al. Regional anesthesia in the anticoagulated patient: Defining the risks: The second ASRA consensus conference on neuraxial anesthesia and anticoagulation. *Reg Anesth Pain Med* 2003;28:172–197.
2. Matthey PW, Finegan BA, Finucane BT. The public's fears about and perceptions of regional anesthesia. *Reg Anesth Pain Med* 2004;29:86–89.
3. Tetzlaff JE, Yoon HJ, Brems J. Patient acceptance of interscalene block for shoulder surgery. *Reg Anesth* 1993;18:30–33.
4. Phillips S, Hutchinson S, Davidson T. Preoperative drinking does not affect gastric contents. *Br J Anaesth* 1993;70:6.
5. Strunin L. How long should patients fast before surgery? Time for new guidelines [Editorial]. *Br J Anaesth* 1993;70.
6. Practice Guidelines for sedation and analgesia by non-Anesthesiologists: An updated report by the American Society of Anesthesiologists task force on sedation and analgesia by non-anesthesiologists. *Anesthesiology* 2002;96:1004–1017.
7. American Society of Anesthesiologists, House of Delegates. Standards for Basic Intraoperative Monitoring. Park Ridge, IL: ASA, October 21, 1986, amended October 13, 1993.
8. Stoelting RK. Responses to atropine, glycopyrrolate, and Riopan of gastric fluid pH and volume in adult patients. *Anesthesiology* 1978;48:367.
9. Watcha MF, White PF. Postoperative nausea and vomiting, its etiology, treatment and prevention. *Anesthesiology* 1992;77:162.
10. Macario A, Weinger M, Carney S, Kim A. Which clinical anesthesia outcomes are important to avoid? The perspective of patients. *Anesth Analg* 1999;89:652–658.
11. Borgeat A, Ekatodramis G, Schenker CA. Postoperative nausea and vomiting in regional anesthesia. *Anesthesiology* 2003;98:530–547.
12. Gan TJ. Risk factors for postoperative nausea and vomiting. *Anesth Analg* 2006;102:1884–1898.
13. Richardson MG, Dooley JW. The effects of general versus epidural anesthesia for outpatient extracorporeal shock wave lithotripsy. *Anesth Analg* 1998;86:1214–1218.
14. Pusch F, Freitag H, Weinstabl C, et al. Single-injection paravertebral block compared with general anesthesia in breast surgery. *Acta Anaesthesiol Scand* 1999;43:770–774.
15. Wulf H, Biscoping J, Beland B, et al. Ropivacaine epidural anesthesia and analgesia versus general anesthesia and intravenous patient-controlled analgesia with morphine in the perioperative management of hip replacement. *Anesth Analg* 1999;89:111–116.
16. Standl T, Eckert S, Esch ISA. Postoperative complaints after spinal thiopentone-isoflurane anaesthesia in patients undergoing orthopaedic surgery: Spinal versus general anaesthesia. *Anaesthesiol Scan* 1996;40:222–226.
17. Carpenter RL, Caplan RA, Brown DL, et al. Incidence and risk factors for side effects of spinal anesthesia. *Anesthesiology* 1992;76:909–916.
18. deJong RH, Heavner JE. Diazepam prevents local anesthetic seizures. *Anesthesiology* 1971;34:523.
19. Dundee JW, Wilson B. Amnesic action of midazolam. *Anaesthesia* 1980;35:459.
20. Dundee JW, Lilburn JK, Toner W, Howard PJ. Plasma lorazepam levels. A study following single dose administration of 2 and 4 mg by different routes. *Anaesthesia* 1978;33:15.
21. McKay AC, Dundee JW. Effect of oral benzodiazepines on memory. *Br J Anaesth* 1980;52:1247.
22. Vickers MD, Wood-Smith FG, Stewart HC. Central nervous system depressants. In: *Drugs in Anaesthetic Practice*, 5th ed. London: Butterworth & Co.; 1978:66.
23. Stoelting RK. Responses to atropine, glycopyrrolate, and Riopan of gastric fluid pH and volume in adult patients. *Anesthesiology* 1978;48:367.
24. Mason L, Edwards JE, Moore RA, McQuay HJ. Single dose oral naproxen and naproxen sodium for acute postoperative pain. *Cochrane Database Syst Rev* 2004(4):CD004234.
25. Straube S, Derry S, McQuay HJ, Moore RA. Effect of preoperative COX-II-selective NSAIDs (COXIBs) on postoperative outcomes: A systematic review of randomized studies. *Acta Anaesthesiol Scand* 2005;49:601–613.
26. Elia N, Lysakowski C, Tramer MR. Does multimodal analgesia with acetaminophen, nonsteroidal antiinflammatory drugs, or selective cyclooxygenase-2 inhibitors and patient-controlled analgesia morphine offer advantages over morphine alone? Meta-analyses of randomized trials. *Anesthesiology* 2005;103:1296–1304.
27. Ho KY, Gan TJ, Habib As. Gabapentin and postoperative pain: Systematic review of randomized controlled trials. *Pain* 2006;126:91–101.
28. Seib RK, Paul JE. Preoperative gabapentin for postoperative analgesia: A meta-analysis. *Can J Anaesth* 2006;53:461–469.
29. Moore DC. *Regional Block*, 4th ed. Springfield, IL: Charles C. Thomas Publishers, 1965.
30. Selander D, Edshage S, Wolff T. Paresthesiae or no paresthesiae? *Acta Anaesthesiol Scand* 1979;23:27.
31. Selander D, Dhuner KG, Lundborg G. Peripheral nerve injury due to injection needles used for regional anesthesia. *Acta Anaesthesiol Scand* 1977;21:182.
32. Abram SE, Ho KC, Doumas BT. Ethylene oxide sterilization of local anesthetics a potential hazard? *Reg Anesth* 1979;4:2.
33. Baranowski AP, Pither CE. A comparison of three methods of axillary brachial plexus anaesthesia. *Anaesthesia* 1990;45:362.
34. Bosenberg AT. Lower limb nerve blocks in children using unsheathed needles and a nerve stimulator. *Anaesthesia* 1995;50:206.
35. Davies MJ, McGlade DP. One hundred sciatic nerve blocks: A comparison of localisation techniques. *Anaesth Intensive Care* 1993;21:76.
36. Lavoie J, Martin R, Tetrault J-P, et al. Axillary plexus block using a peripheral nerve stimulator: Single or multiple injections. *Can J Anaesth* 1992;39:538.
37. Riegler FX. Brachial plexus block with the nerve stimulator: Motor response characteristics at three sites. *Reg Anaesth* 1992;17:295.
38. Smith BL. Efficacy of a nerve stimulator in regional analgesia; experience in a resident training program. *Anaesthesia* 1976;31:778.
39. Zahari DT, Englund K, Girolamo M. Peripheral nerve block with use of nerve stimulator. *J Foot Surg* 1990;29:162.
40. vonPerthes G. Uker leitungsanasthesie unter zuhilfenahme elektrischer reizung. *Med Wschr* 1912;47:2545.
41. Pearson B. Nerve block in rehabilitation: A technique of needle localization. *Arch Phys Med Rehab* 1955;36:631.
42. Montgomery SJ, Raj PP, Nettles D, Jenkins MT. The use of the nerve stimulator with standard unsheathed needles in nerve blockade. *Anesth Analg* 1973;52:827.
43. Ford DJ, Pither C, Raj PP. Comparison of insulated and uninsulated needles for locating peripheral nerves with a peripheral nerve stimulator. *Anesth Analg* 1984;63:925.
44. Ford DJ, Pither CE, Raj PP. Electrical characteristics of peripheral nerve stimulators: Implications for nerve localization. *Reg Anaesth* 1984;9:73.

45. Tulchinsky A, Weller RW, Rosenblum M, Gross JB. Nerve stimulator polarity and brachial plexus block. *Anesth Analg* 1993;77:100.
46. Tsui BC, Kropelin B. The electrophysiological effect of dextrose 5% in water on single-shot peripheral nerve stimulation. *Anesth Analg* 2005;100:1837–1839.
47. Tsui BC, Wagner A, Finucane B. Electrophysiologic effect of injectates on peripheral nerve stimulation. *Reg Anesth Pain Med* 2004;29:189–193.
48. Selander D, Dhuner KG, Lundborg G. Peripheral nerve injury due to injection needles used for regional anesthesia. *Acta Anaesthesiol Scand* 1977;21:182.
49. Wee MYK, Geeurickx A, Wimalaratna S. A method to facilitate regional anaesthesia by detection of mixed nerve action potentials. *Br J Anaesth* 1992;69:411.
50. Urmey WF, Grossi P. Percutaneous electrode guidance: A noninvasive technique for prelocation of peripheral nerves to facilitate peripheral plexus or nerve block. *Reg Anesth Pain Med* 2002;27:261–267.
51. Urmey WF, Grossi P. Percutaneous electrode guidance and subcutaneous stimulating electrode guidance: Modifications of the original technique. *Reg Anesth Pain Med* 2003;28:253–255.
52. Capdevila X, Lopez S, Bernard N, et al. Percutaneous electrode guidance using the insulated needle for prelocation of peripheral nerves during axillary plexus blocks. *Reg Anesth Pain Med* 2004;29:206–211.
53. Urmey WF, Grossi P. Use of sequential electrical nerve stimuli (SENS) for location of the sciatic nerve and lumbar plexus. *Reg Anesth Pain Med* 2006;31:463–469.
54. Pham-Dang C, Kick O, Collet T, et al. Continuous peripheral nerve blocks with stimulating catheters. *Reg Anesth Pain Med* 2003;28:83–88.
55. Salinas FV, Neal JM, Sueda LA, et al. Prospective comparison of continuous femoral nerve block with nonstimulating catheter placement versus stimulating catheter-guided perineural placement in volunteers. *Reg Anesth Pain Med* 2004;29:212–220.
56. Rodriguez J, Taboada M, Carceller J, et al. Stimulating popliteal catheters for postoperative analgesia after hallux valgus repair. *Anesth Analg* 2006;102:258–262.
57. Casati A, Fanelli G, Koscielniak-Nielsen Z, et al. Using stimulating catheters for continuous sciatic nerve block shortens onset time of surgical block and minimizes postoperative consumption of pain medication after hallux valgus repair as compared with conventional nonstimulating catheters. *Anesth Analg* 2005;101:1192–1197.
58. Morin AM, Eberhart LH, Behnke HK, et al. Does femoral nerve catheter placement with stimulating catheters improve effective placement? A randomized, controlled, and observer-blinded trial. *Anesth Analg* 2005;100:1503–1510.
59. Jack NT, Liem EB, Vonhogen LH. Use of a stimulating catheter for total knee replacement surgery: Preliminary results. *Br J Anaesth* 2005;95:250–254.
60. Hayek SM, Ritchey RM, Sessler D, et al. Continuous femoral nerve analgesia after unilateral total knee arthroplasty: Stimulating versus nonstimulating catheters. *Anesth Analg* 2006;103:1565–1570.
61. Tsui BC, Finucane B. Verifying accurate placement of an epidural catheter tip using electrical stimulation. *Anesth Analg* 2002;94:1670–1671.
62. de Medicis E, Tetrault JP, Martin R, et al. A prospective comparative study of two indirect methods for confirming the localization of an epidural catheter for postoperative analgesia. *Anesth Analg* 2005;101:1830–1833.
63. Tsui BC. Epidural stimulation test criteria. *Anesth Analg* 2006;103:775–776.
64. Tsui BC, Wagner A, Cave D, Kearney R. Thoracic and lumbar epidural analgesia via the caudal approach using electrical stimulation guidance in pediatric patients: A review of 289 patients. *Anesthesiology* 2004;100:683–689.
65. Tsui BC, Bateman K, Bouliane M, Finucane B. Cervical epidural analgesia via a thoracic approach using nerve stimulation guidance in an adult patient undergoing elbow surgery. *Reg Anesth Pain Med* 2004;29:355–360.
66. Tsui BC. Thoracic epidural catheter placement in infants via the caudal approach under electrocardiographic guidance: Simplification of the original technique. *Anesth Analg* 2004;98:273.
67. Marhofer P, Greher M, Kapral S. Ultrasound guidance in regional anaesthesia. *Br J Anaesth* 2005;94:7–17.
68. Gray AT. Ultrasound-guided regional anesthesia: Current state of the art. *Anesthesiology* 2006;104:368–373.
69. Grau T. Ultrasonography in the current practice of regional anaesthesia. *Best Pract Res Clin Anaesthesiol* 2005;19:175–200.
70. Williams SR, Chouinard P, Arcand G, et al. Ultrasound guidance speeds execution and improves the quality of supraclavicular block. *Anesth Analg* 2003;97:1518–1523.
71. Marhofer P, Sitzwohl C, Greher M, Kapral S. Ultrasound guidance for infraclavicular brachial plexus anaesthesia in children. *Anaesthesia* 2004;59:642–646.
72. Soeding PE, Sha S, Royse CE, et al. A randomized trial of ultrasound-guided brachial plexus anaesthesia in upper limb surgery. *Anaesth Intensive Care* 2005;33:719–725.
73. Labat G. *Regional Anesthesia*. Philadelphia: W.B. Saunders, 1922.
74. Neal JJ, McMahon DJ. Equipment. In: Brown DB, ed. *Regional Anesthesia and Analgesia*, 1st ed. Philadelphia: Saunders; 1996:162.
75. Koch ME, Kain ZN, Ayoub C, Rosenbaum SH. The sedative and analgesic sparing effect of music. *Anesthesiology* 1998;89:300–306.
76. Lepage C, Drolet P, Girard M, et al. Music decreases sedative requirements during spinal anesthesia. *Anesth Analg* 2001;93:912–916.
77. Practice Guidelines for sedation and analgesia by non-anesthesiologists: An updated report by the American Society of Anesthesiologists task force on sedation and analgesia by non-anesthesiologists. *Anesthesiology* 2002;96:1004–1017.
78. White PF, Negus JB. Sedative infusions during local and regional anesthesia: A comparison of midazolam and propofol. *J Clin Anesth* 1991;3:32–39.
79. Nishiyama T, Yokoyama T, Hanaoka K. Sedation guidelines for midazolam infusion during combined spinal and epidural anesthesia. *J Clin Anesth* 2004;16:568–572.
80. Frizelle HP, Duranteau J, Samil K. A comparison of propofol with a propofol-ketamine combination for sedation during spinal anesthesia. *Anesth Analg* 1997;84:1318–1322.
81. Badrinath S, Avramov MN, Shadrick M, et al. The use of ketamine-propofol combination during monitored anesthesia care. *Anesth Analg* 2000;90:858–862.
82. Thomson AM. Comparison of responses to transmitter candidates at an N-methylaspartate receptor mediated synapse, in slices of rat cerebral cortex. *Neuroscience* 1986;17:37–47.
83. Gordh T, Karlsten R, Kristensen J. Intervention with spinal NMDA, adenosine, and NO systems for pain modulation. *Ann Med* 1995;27:229–234.
84. Kohrs R, Durieux ME. Ketamine: Teaching an old drug new tricks. *Anesth Analg* 1998;87:1186–1193.
85. Honore P, Chapman V, Buritova J, Besson JM. Concomitant administration of morphine and an N-methyl-D-aspartate receptor antagonist profoundly reduces inflammatory evoked spinal c-Fos expression. *Anesthesiology* 1996;85:150–160.
86. Menigaux C, Fletcher D, Dupont X, et al. The benefits of intraoperative small-dose ketamine on postoperative pain after anterior cruciate ligament repair. *Anesth Analg* 2000;90:129–135.
87. Aida S, Yamakura T, Baba H, et al. Preemptive analgesia by intravenous low-dose ketamine and epidural morphine in gastrectomy: A randomized double-blind study. *Anesthesiology* 2000;92:1624–1630.
88. Kararmaz A, Kaya S, Karaman H, et al. Intraoperative ketamine in combination with epidural analgesia: Postoperative analgesia after renal surgery. *Anesth Analg* 2003;97:1092–1096.
89. Eisenach JC, De Kock M, Klimscha W. Alpha-2-adrenergic agonists for regional anesthesia. *Anesthesiology* 1996;85:655–674.
90. Hall JE, Uhrich TD, Barney JA, et al. Sedative, amnestic, and analgesic properties of small-dose dexmedetomidine infusions. *Anesth Analg* 2000;90:699–705.
91. McCutcheon CA, Orme RM, Scott DA, et al. A comparison of dexmedetomidine versus conventional therapy for sedation and hemodynamic control during carotid endarterectomy performed under regional anesthesia. *Anesth Analg* 2006;102:668–675.
92. Monk TG, Boure B, White PF, et al. Comparison of intravenous sedative-analgesic techniques for outpatient immersion lithotripsy. *Anesth Analg.* 1991;72:616.
93. Bailey PL, Pace NL, Ashburn MA, et al. Frequent hypoxemia and apnea after sedation with midazolam and fentanyl. *Anesthesiology* 1990;73:826.
94. Krenn H, Deusch E, Jellinek H, et al. Remifentanil or propofol for sedation during carotid endarterectomy under cervical plexus block. *Br J Anaesth* 2002;89:637–640.
95. Gold MI, Watkins WD, Sung YF, et al. Remifentanil versus remifentanil/midazolam for ambulatory surgery during monitored anaesthesia care. *Anesthesiology* 1997;87:51–57.
96. Avramov MN, Smith I, White PF. Interactions between midazolam and remifentanil during monitored anesthesia care. *Anesthesiology* 1996;85:1283–1289.
97. Holas A, Krafft P, Marcovoc M, Quehenberger F. Remifentanil, propofol or both for conscious sedation during eye surgery under regional anaesthesia. *Eur J Anaesthesiol* 1999;16:741–748.
98. Edmunds DH, Rosen M. Inhalation sedation with 25% nitrous oxide. *Anaesthesia* 1984;39:183.
99. McLead DD, Ramayya GP, Tunstall ME. Self-administered isoflurane in labour. A comparative study with Entonox. *Anaesthesia* 1985;40:424.
100. Rodrigo MR, Rosenquist JB. Isoflurane for conscious sedation. *Anaesthesia* 1988;43:369.
101. Ibrahim AE, Ghoneim MM, Kharasch ED. Speed of recovery and side-effect profile of sevoflurane sedation compared with midazolam. *Anesthesiology* 2001;94:87–94.

CHAPTER 9 ■ ANATOMY OF THE NEURAXIS

QUINN H. HOGAN

Anatomy, the oldest of medical sciences, holds a central position in regional anesthesia because of the obvious necessity of correctly delivering the therapeutic solution to the target neural structures. Beyond this, anatomic understanding is required to avoid complications due to needle damage or incorrectly placed injection, to understand the physiologic events resulting from neural blockade, and to develop new techniques for anesthesia and pain treatment. The spinal column, and the soft tissues and neuraxial elements contained within it, have been the subject of examination for hundreds of years, but we do not yet fully understand important aspects of their structure. This is in part due to the special interests of anesthesiologists in such matters as the organization of tissue planes and the permeability of various barriers that regulate distribution of fluids, interests shared by few other physicians and scientists. An additional challenge is the difficulty of observing the contents of the spinal canal, which are enclosed by sturdy bones and ligaments. Removal of these structures disrupts the natural arrangement of the soft tissues within the canal. Only recently have techniques become available for analyzing these features. This chapter anatomically tours the neuraxis, generally from outer to inner structures, and includes new observations wherever possible.

VERTEBRAL BONES

The stacked vertebral bones reveal a segmentation that is otherwise minimally evident in human anatomy. This metameric arrangement into individual vertebrae also dictates that communication of the peripheral nervous system with the spinal cord must be likewise segmented, despite the lack of any organization into subunits within the spinal cord. Typically, there are 7 cervical vertebrae, 12 thoracic, 5 lumbar, 5 sacral, and 4 coccygeal (Fig. 9-1). Common palpable landmarks (Fig. 9-2) may locate particular levels, including the most prominent spinous process (vertebra prominens), which usually indicates the seventh cervical. The seventh thoracic spine is usually opposite the inferior angle of the scapula, and the line connecting the iliac crests (Tuffier line) crosses the vertebral column most often at the L4–L5 disc. However, clinical ability to estimate segmental level from palpable landmarks is often overestimated, and these indices are subject to natural variability in anatomic parameters (Fig. 9-3) (1). For instance, the first thoracic vertebral spine may be more prominent than the seventh cervical. Also, the Tuffier line may cross the vertebral column as high as the L3–L4 disc or as low as the L5–S1 disc (2–5). For this reason, and because of a variable amount of subcutaneous fat, the accuracy of predicting the vertebral level of needle insertion is about 50% at best when unaided by radiologic imaging. Most often, the error occurs when the clinician selects a level one or two segments higher than the intended level in the lower tho-

racic and lumbar regions, or selects a space too low in the upper thoracic and cervical region (6–9). Errors are comparable in the sitting and lying positions, are greater with obese subjects, and are greater using the vertebra prominens as a reference point compared to the Tuffier line (10,11).

The numerical designations of the vertebra may differ between individuals because of anomalous patterns of vertebral segmentation, which are predominantly found in the lumbosacral spine (12). This parallels the phylogenetic stability of mammalian cervical and thoracic segmentation and the marked variability in the number of lumbar vertebrae, even among primates (13). The last lumbar or first sacral vertebrae is often indeterminate in configuration, with fusion of L5 to S1 in 6.2% (sacralization of L5, bilateral in 1.5%), or incomplete fusion of S1 to S2 in 5.3% (lumbarization of S1, bilateral in 4.1%) (12).

Although the vertebrae differ in design at the various levels of the vertebral column, common elements can be defined. Each consists of posterior elements forming a vertebral arch and the body (or soma) anteriorly (Fig. 9-4A). The lumbar vertebral bodies are distinctly narrowed into an hourglass shape, with a diameter 15% less at the middle than at the endplates (14). Stout pedicles arise on the posterolateral aspects of the body and fuse with the platelike laminae to encircle the vertebral foramen. Together, the vertebral foramina of the adjacent vertebrae in sequence form the vertebral (or spinal) canal. In the cervical and lumbar regions (Fig. 9-4B), the canal approaches a triangular shape, but it is circular and smaller in the thoracic vertebrae. The width of the canal measured between the pedicles is narrowest in the thoracic region (about 17 mm), but widens in both the cervical (25 mm) and lumbar regions (about 22 mm at L1 to about 27 mm at L5) (15–20). In contrast, the anterior/posterior diameter of the vertebral canal is fairly constant (about 16 mm) throughout the vertebral column (21).

Between the pedicles of each adjacent pair of vertebrae, there remains a gap called the *intervertebral foramen* (or *nerve root canal*; Fig. 9-5) that provides a passage between the paravertebral space and the vertebral canal, and conveys the segmental nerves as well as other neural and vascular structures. The transverse process is based at the junction of the pedicle and lamina and passes laterally. The spinous process projects posteriorly from the midline junction of the laminae, is often bifid in the cervical column, and may not lie in the midline at other levels.

The pattern described here varies somewhat in different regions of the vertebral column. Vertebral bodies are relatively massive at the lumbar levels, but less so in the thoracic column and especially in the cervical region. Whereas the transverse processes are attached to the pedicles and laminae in the lumbar and thoracic zones, they take their origin from the vertebral body in the cervical vertebrae. The spinous processes are steeply angled caudally in the thoracic region, but are nearly

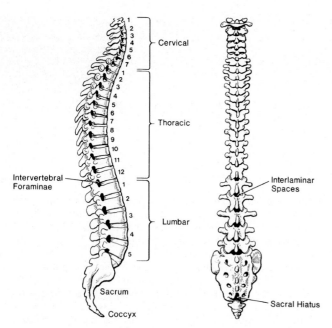

FIGURE 9-1. Vertebral column, in lateral view (*left*) and posterior view (*right*), illustrating curvatures, lumbar interlaminar spaces, and the sacral hiatus.

perpendicular to the axis of the column in cervical and lumbar vertebrae.

The sacral vertebral column is a special case. In childhood, the sacral vertebrae are connected by cartilage, but progressively fuse into a single structure after puberty. In the adult, only a narrow residue of the sacral discs persists. The fusion of adjacent vertebrae eliminates the intervertebral foramina. Instead, the concave anterior surface of the sacrum features four pairs of large anterior sacral foramina that provide passage from the midline sacral canal for the anterior rami of the upper four sacral nerves. In contrast with their posterior counterparts, which provide an exit for the posterior primary rami at each level, the anterior foramina are unsealed and provide a ready passage for escape of local anesthetic solution injected into the sacral canal. On the posterior surface of the sacrum, there is a median crest with three or more, but commonly four, variably prominent tubercles, representing the sacral spinous processes. Lateral to this crest and medial to the four posterior sacral foramina is the intermediate sacral crest with a row of four tubercles, representing the upper four sacral articular processes. The remnants of the S5 inferior articular processes are free and prominent, and flank the sacral hiatus, constituting the sacral cornua.

The sacrum is the least predictable portion of vertebral anatomy. Specifically, the volume of the adult sacral canal may vary from 12 mL to 65 mL (22). Typically, fusion of the posterior roof of the sacral vertebral canal is complete down to the S5 level, where the sacral hiatus persists as an opening bordered by the sacral cornua on either side and is covered by the thick, fibrous posterior sacrococcygeal ligament (Fig. 9-6). However, either an entire lack of any posterior bony roof or virtually complete closure of the sacral vertebral canal are found in about 8% of subjects (Fig. 9-7) (23). In 5% of adult sacral bones, the anterior–posterior diameter of the canal at the hiatus is 2 mm or less (22), making access by needle placement very difficult or impossible in some subjects. In children, however, the sacral hiatus is predictably open and access is readily performed.

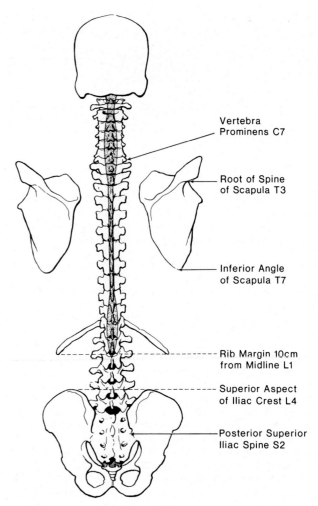

FIGURE 9-2. Surface anatomy and landmarks for epidural blockade. The spinous process (vertebra prominens) at C7 is the most prominent spinous process when the neck is flexed. The spinous process at T3 lies opposite the root of the spine of the scapula (arm by side). The spinous process at T7 lies opposite the inferior angle of the scapula (arm by side). The spinous process at L1 (*lower border*) is noted by a line meeting the costal margin 10 cm from the midline. The spinous process at L4 (*center*) lies at the top of the iliac crests. S2 is noted by the posterior superior iliac spines. Despite these guidelines, natural variability occurs between subjects, and it is common to be at least one segment off when using these landmarks to determine vertebral level.

The coccyx is a small triangular bone consisting of three to five fused rudimentary vertebrae; it attaches by means of its upper articular surface to the lower articular surface of the sacrum. It has two prominent coccygeal cornua that abut their sacral counterparts. The bone tends to be angulated forward from the sacrococcygeal junction, with its pelvic surface facing anteriorly and upward.

JOINTS OF THE VERTEBRAL COLUMN

The ligamentous system of the vertebral column must bond the adjacent segments adequately while allowing for a degree of bending motion. The joints between the successive vertebral bones (Fig. 9-8) control this motion.

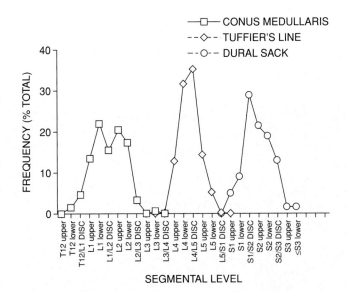

FIGURE 9-3. Natural distribution of three anatomic features: the conus medullaris, where the Tuffier line (between the iliac crests) intersects the vertebral column, and the terminus of the dural sac. Because of natural variability between subjects, these and other anatomic features form a normal distribution. The peak incidence for the conus medullaris is at approximately the L1–L2 disc, for the Tuffier line at the L4–L5 disc, and for the dural sac at the S1–S2 disc.

The adjacent vertebral bodies are joined at their endplates by the discs, which are composed of fibrocartilaginous joints with an avascular gelatinous core—the nucleus pulposus—surrounded by a reinforcing annular ligament made of collagenous lamellae. These serve the purposes of bearing weight while permitting flexibility. In the cervical region, the lateral upper edge of the vertebral bodies extends as the uncinate process, which articulates with the body of the next cephalad vertebra as the uncovertebral joint (of Luschka). Arthritic degeneration and expansion of this joint may encroach upon the cervical nerve root canals.

The posterior elements of adjacent vertebrae articulate by true diarthrodial joints, the zygapophyseal (or facet) joints. The inferior articular process projecting caudally overlaps the superior articular process from the next most caudal vertebra. In the cervical and lumbar column, the facet joints are posterior to the transverse processes, whereas the thoracic facets are anterior to the transverse processes. Joint surfaces are angled midway between the axial and coronal planes in the cervical region, but are much more vertically deployed at thoracic levels, and are almost in a coronal plan (24). At lumbar levels, the facet joints are distinctly curved, such that the posterior portion is in the sagittal plane whereas the anterior portion is almost in the coronal plane. The transition from the characteristic thoracic to lumbar type articulation is gradual in half of subjects, with intermediate articular orientation at T11–T12 (25). In others, the change is abrupt, with a coronal superior facet and a curved/sagittal inferior facet on a single vertebra at T12 (29%), T11 (16%), or L1 (0.5%), with frequent asymmetry.

The orientation of the facets guides and constrains movements between the two vertebrae. Specifically, minimal rotation is allowed at lumbar levels because of the sagittally opposing

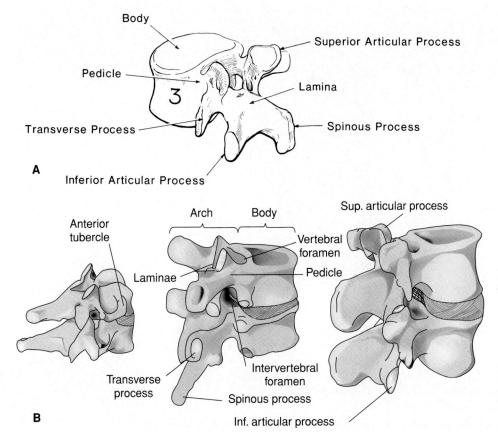

FIGURE 9-4. A: Components of a lumbar vertebra. **B:** Distinctions between vertebra at different levels. Spinous processes are relatively straight posteriorly directed at cervical and lumbar levels, but caudally inclined at thoracic levels. Vertebral bodies become progressively larger going from cervical to lumbar. The point of origin of the transverse processes is from the vertebral body at cervical levels, but from the pedicle and lamina at thoracic and lumbar levels. The angle of the articular surfaces for the facet joints differs at each level.

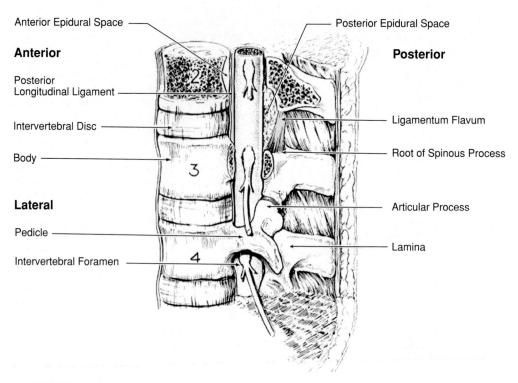

FIGURE 9-5. Boundaries of the epidural space. Note that the posterior epidural space at each level has its greatest anterior–posterior dimension at its most superior portion.

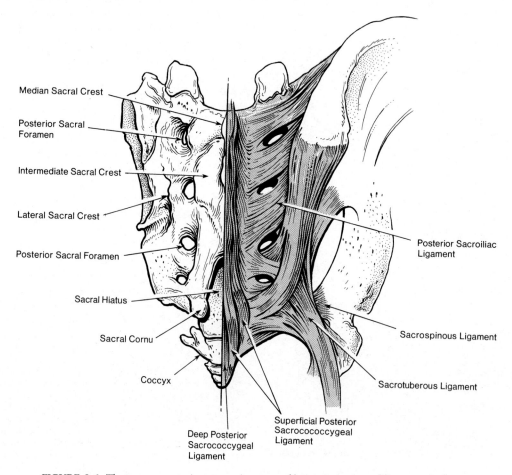

FIGURE 9-6. The sacrum, posterior aspect. Anatomy of bone structures and ligaments is shown.

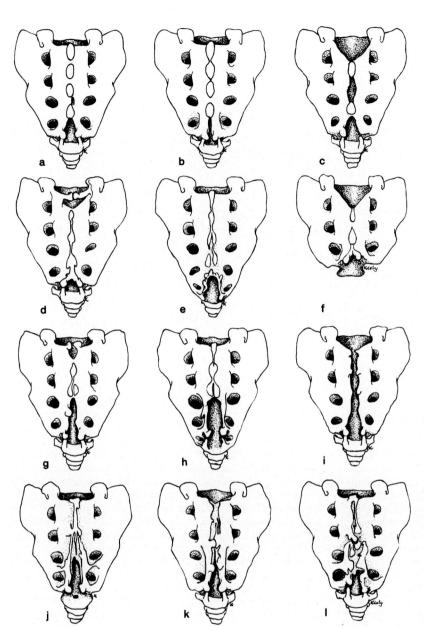

FIGURE 9-7. Anatomic variants of dorsal wall of sacrum and sacral hiatus. Dorsal wall: Despite its many structural variations, the sacral canal is open at the lower half of S5, and the hiatus is invariably in line with the median sacral crest (where present and palpable). Sacral hiatus: (*a*) most common pattern; (*b*) longitudinal, slit-like hiatus; (*c*) second midline hiatus; (*d*) transverse hiatus; (*e*) large hiatus with absent cornua; (*f*) transverse hiatus with absent coccyx and two prominent cornua, with two proximal "decoy" hiatuses lateral to the cornua; (*g, h, i*) large midline defects in posterior sacral wall continuous with sacral hiatus; (*j, k, l*) enlarged longitudinal hiatuses, each with an overlying "decoy hiatus." In (*l*), the "decoy hiatus" is large and is surrounded by "cornua-like" structures, which could lead to needle insertion through posterior sacral ligaments but not into the sacral canal. Also in (*l*), the sacral cornu is absent on the left side; this could lead to identification of the right S4 posterior sacral foramen as the sacral hiatus.

portions, whereas thoracic facets permit rotation but limit flexion. In the cervical column, movement in all planes is less restricted and includes translation (anterior/posterior sliding) between adjacent vertebrae controlled by the uncinate processes as lateral guide rails (24). Movement in the sagittal plane (flexion and extension) is maximal in the cervical region and at L5–S1. In addition to restricting motion, the facets bear weight in the cervical region (26) and at the lumbosacral joint (27). Lumbar posterior joints may transmit load in part through contact of the tip of the inferior articular process with the lamina of the vertebra below (28).

The capsule of the facets is loose and redundant at the inferior and superior ends of the joint, and injection of the joints is often accompanied by leakage of the solution into the epidural space from medial disruption of the capsule (29–31). Rudimentary fibroadipose menisci and synovial folds cushion the superior and inferior poles of the lumbar zygapophyseal joints

(32), but these typically disappear with age and the cartilage on the joint surfaces thins (33). Although small myelinated nerves innervate the facet menisci (34), no clear evidence implicates them in chronic back pain.

Facet arthritis with periarticular exostoses is another etiology of cord and nerve compression (35), and pathologic medial expansion of facets may interfere with epidural or spinal needle placement as well.

LIGAMENTS OF THE VERTEBRAL COLUMN

The supraspinous ligament joins the tips of the spinous processes as a heavy band (Fig. 9-8), but thins and vanishes in the lower lumbar region (36), which allows greater flexion

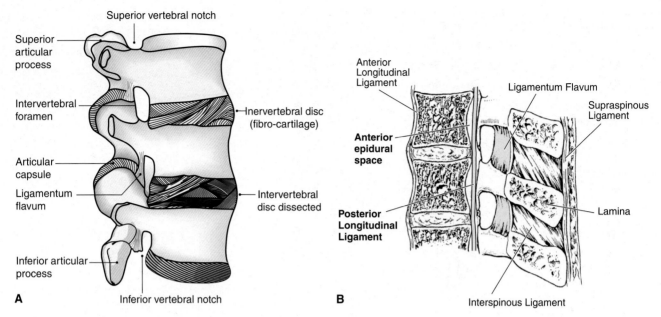

FIGURE 9-8. Ligaments of the lumbar vertebral column, shown in lateral view (**A**) and sagittal section (**B**).

at the L5–S1 joint. Between the spinous processes, the interspinous ligament forms a narrow web. It may have a slit-like midline cavity filled with fat (36), which may mistakenly give a positive loss-of-resistance sign during epidural needle insertion. The supraspinous and intraspinous ligaments are largely composed of collagen so that a needle passing through them generates a characteristic snapping sensation as the fibers are parted. In contrast, the ligamentum flavum is 80% elastin, with a dense and homogenous texture that is readily appreciated as a needle passes through it. In normal posture, the ligamentum flavum is under tension, so that it retracts to half its length when cut. It spans from the anterior surface of the upper lamina of an adjacent pair of vertebrae to the posterior aspect of the lower lamina. The right and left halves meet at an angle of less than 90 degrees, and a gap may be present in the midline (37). Its lateral edges wrap anteriorly around the medial margin of the facet joints, reinforcing the joint capsule. Bone may grow into the margins of the ligamentum flavum even in young individuals, especially at mid and lower thoracic levels (38–41), which may result from the increased rotatory strains at these levels (40). These fine bone spurs in the ligamentum flavum may impede the progress of a spinal or epidural needle and may be mistaken for fracture fragments on x-ray images.

With age, the intervertebral discs become desiccated and lose height, which in turn causes increased overlap of the facets. This decreases the longitudinal dimensions of the intervertebral foramen and foreshortens the ligamentum flavum, causing it to buckle into the foramen, further contributing to foraminal narrowing.

The broad anterior longitudinal ligament reinforces the anterior aspect of the discs and binds the vertebral bodies together. Posterior to the vertebral bodies, the posterior longitudinal ligament likewise constrains the relative motion of the vertebral bodies. It runs along the anterior surface of the dural sac as a tight band, but broadens and merges tightly with the discs at each level (Fig. 9-9). This reinforcement typically prevents herniations of the disc in the midline. At cervical and thoracic levels, ossification may result in spinal stenosis (41).

EPIDURAL SPACE

Everything outside the dural sac but within the vertebral canal can be considered to constitute the epidural space. Its outer boundaries are thus the walls of the vertebral canal, including the vertebral bodies and discs anteriorly, pedicles laterally, and laminae and ligamenta flava posteriorly. It is commonly said that the epidural space is a "potential space," but it naturally has contents, specifically fat, vessels, and nerves. There is no clear physiologic purpose in having fat within the spinal canal. Indeed, the cranial epidural space is entirely empty. Whereas the brain is protected by a rigid case, the spinal cord must exist within the flexible vertebral column. Perhaps the epidural fat, which is nearly fluid in texture and which has nonadherent surfaces to permit gliding movement of the neural structures, provides a padding effect.

The distance from the skin to the lumbar epidural space in the midline is on average about 5 cm, but may be as small as 3 cm and rarely greater than 8 cm. Distance loosely correlates with weight, and it is somewhat greater at L3–L4 than at other lumbar levels (42–47). A practitioner must be cautious when using these dimensions clinically, however, since substantial variability makes it unreliable to expect the actual depth to be close to the published mean.

The distribution of epidural contents is highly nonuniform. Investigations by cryomicrotome sectioning (Figs. 9-10 through 9-14) (37) and in vivo imaging avoid the dissection artifact. These methods show that the undisturbed lumbar vertebral canal is nearly filled by the dural sac. Thus, the epidural space is empty in large areas, where the dura contacts bone and ligament. It is important to recognize, however, that the dura is not adherent to the canal wall in these empty areas, and solutions and catheters may pass through them. Separated by these empty areas, the epidural contents occur as a series of metamerically and circumferentially discontinuous compartments (Fig. 9-15). In contrast to this general pattern, the dural sac inferior to the L4–L5 disc and in the sacral canal tapers to a smaller diameter and does not fill the canal as completely,

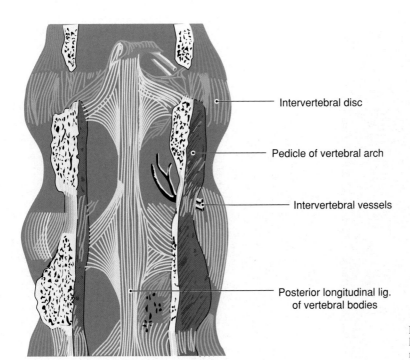

Intervertebral disc

Pedicle of vertebral arch

Intervertebral vessels

Posterior longitudinal lig.
of vertebral bodies

FIGURE 9-9. Posterior view of the posterior longitudinal ligament, viewed with the posterior vertebral structures removed.

resulting in a proportionate increase in epidural fat. This may contribute to difficulty in delivering local anesthetic to the L5 and sacral nerve roots during epidural anesthesia, since solution is not confined in close proximity with neural structures at these levels.

Because of their distinct designs, the various epidural compartments are considered separately in detail.

Posterior Epidural Compartment

The portion of the epidural space posterior to the dura is filled by a fat pad that is triangular in axial section (Figs. 9-13 and 9-14). (In epidurograms and epiduroscopy, the stretched posterior epidural fat is often mistakenly identified as an epidural fibrous band.) It is enclosed by the ligamenta flava, but also extends slightly under the caudal-most portion of the lamina above (Fig. 9-16). The largest posterior epidural compart-

ment is at the mid-lumbar level, with progressive decrease in anterior–posterior dimension at thoracic levels (Fig. 9-17) (48). Rostral to the C7 level, the posterior epidural space vanishes and the posterior dura lies entirely in contact with the ligamentum flavum and laminar bone (Fig. 9-18). Movement of the dura within the canal during spinal flexion (49–52) is facilitated by the nonadherent gliding surface of the posterior fat pad.

The cleft-like space between the epidural fat and canal wall (Fig. 9-19) allows passage of catheters and injected fluids, with only a minor impediment in the posterior midline, where the dura may adhere to the lamina or fat (53). This arrangement of apposing nonadherent tissue planes is ideally designed to demonstrate the normal subatmospheric pressure within tissues (54), generated by the usual action of lymphatics and the balance of osmotic and hydrostatic forces across the capillary endothelium (Starling forces). This produces the force that aspirates a hanging drop into the needle hub as the tip enters the compartment. Alternatively, pressurized air or saline enters readily into the plane between the nonadherent posterior fat pad and canal wall at the moment the advancing needle tip passes anterior to the ligamentum flavum, thus signaling entry into the spinal canal by the loss-of-resistance method. Rarely, the needle might pass directly into the substance of the posterior fat pad, allowing a loss of resistance to injection but making catheter passage difficult.

The geometry of the posterior epidural space dictates the distance that a needle must travel after entering the epidural space within the ligamentum flavum before contacting the dura. This dimension is a maximum of about 8 mm at the cephalad extent of the interlaminar space and in the midline (55). However, if the needle enters the spinal canal away from the midline, it may encounter the dura with no further advancement since the posterior epidural fat pad thins laterally and the dura contacts the ligamentum flavum there.

The only point of attachment for this fat is to the posterior midline by a vascular pedicle that enters through the gap between the right and left ligamenta flava (Fig. 9-20).

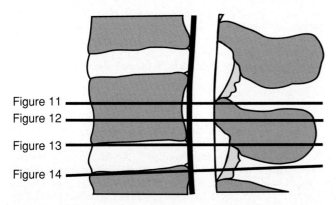

Figure 11

Figure 12

Figure 13

Figure 14

FIGURE 9-10. Schematic sagittal section of lumbar vertebrae, indicating the levels of the subsequent figures. Yellow indicates ligamentum flavum, brown indicates bone.

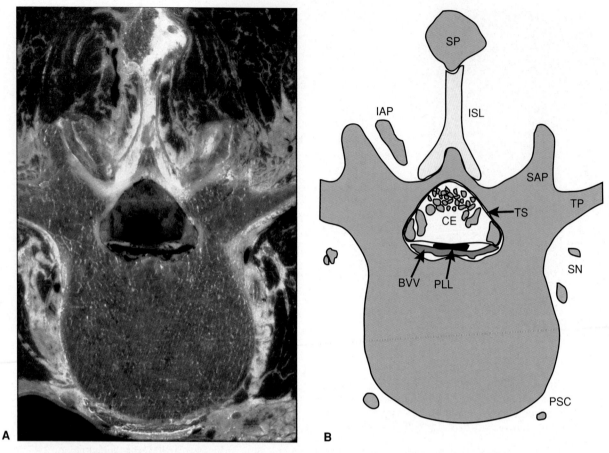

FIGURE 9-11. Axial cryomicrotome section (**A**) and index diagram (**B**) of a third lumbar vertebra. *BVV*, basivertebral vein; *CE*, cauda equina; *IAP*, inferior articular process; *ISL*, interspinous ligament; *PLL*, posterior longitudinal ligament; *PSC*, perivertebral sympathetic chain; *SAP*, superior articular process; *SN*, spinal nerve branches; *SP*, spinous process; *TP*, transverse process; *TS*, thecal sac. Bone is brown, nerves are pink, and veins are blue.

This mesentery-like attachment and the accompanying fat pad may be seen as a midline filling defect in radiologic contrast studies (56–58), and as an incomplete "membrane" during epiduroscopy (59,60). The native posterior epidural compartment is entirely without fibrous tissue (61–63), although fibrous proliferation takes place after laminectomy.

Epidural lipomatosis, in which the posterior epidural fat expands and compresses the dural sac (Fig. 9-21), is well recognized during systemic steroid therapy or endogenous Cushing syndrome and may produce neurologic compromise (64,65). Additionally, symptomatic epidural lipomatosis may occur after epidural steroid treatments (66), associated with morbid obesity (67), or in a normal individual (68). Even the normal posterior epidural fat may contribute to pathology when its displacement by facet arthropathy contributes to central vertebral canal stenosis (69).

Lateral Epidural Compartment

No epidural contents exist lateral to the dural sac where it is in contact with the vertebral pedicles. Between the pedicles, however, the lateral epidural compartment forms just medial to each intervertebral foramen and is filled with segmental nerves, vessels, and fat (Fig. 9-22). Except in extreme cases of degen-

erative disease, the intervertebral foramina are wide open (Fig. 9-23) and allow the free egress of solution injected within the vertebral canal (53,70). Early observations of a "fibrous operculum" occluding the foramen probably represented an artifact of specimen desiccation. Because of the flexibility of the tissues occupying the lateral epidural space and the lack of a rigid barrier in the intervertebral foramina, the pressure in the epidural space closely reflects abdominal pressure. Increased abdominal pressure, such as happens during a cough or pregnancy, is therefore readily transmitted to the epidural space (71). There is no reason to believe that veins passing through the intervertebral foramina in some way play a special role in conducting pressure changes from the abdomen to the vertebral canal.

Anterior Epidural Space

A fine membrane, sometimes called the *fascia of the posterior longitudinal ligament*, stretches laterally from the posterior longitudinal ligament and completely separates the anterior epidural compartment from the rest of the vertebral canal (Fig. 9-22). This membrane effectively blocks spread of injected solution from passing anterior to the plane of the posterior longitudinal ligament, and funnels solution toward the spinal nerves

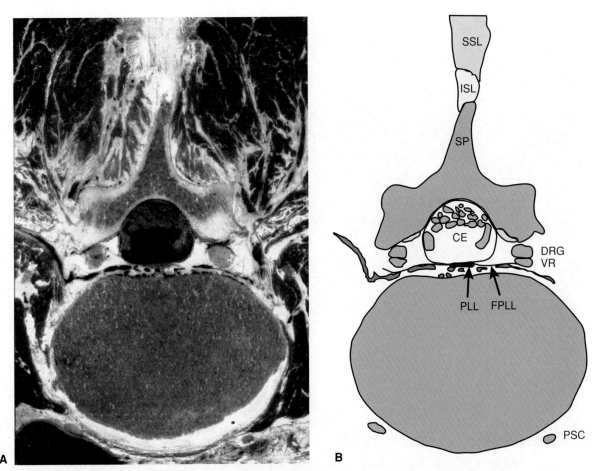

FIGURE 9-12. Axial cryomicrotome section (**A**) and index diagram (**B**) of a third lumbar vertebra, caudal to the image in Figure 9-11. *CE,* cauda equina; *DRG,* dorsal root ganglion; *FPLL,* fascia of the poster longitudinal ligament; *ISL,* interspinous ligament; *PLL,* posterior longitudinal ligament; *PSC,* perivertebral sympathetic chain; *SN,* spinal nerve branches; *SP,* spinous process; *SSL,* supraspinous ligament; *VR,* ventral root. Bone is brown, nerves are pink, and veins are blue.

(Fig. 9-24) (70). At the longitudinal level of the narrow midportion of the vertebral body, this anterior space is almost entirely occupied by a nearly confluent internal vertebral plexus, from which the midline basivertebral vein originates as it penetrates into the vertebral body (Figs. 9-25 and 9-26). Catheters that transgress into the anterior epidural space through the fascia of the posterior longitudinal ligament are likely to enter the venous plexus. At the level of each disc, the anterior epidural compartment is obliterated by attachment of the posterior longitudinal ligament to the disc.

Functional Implications

Few attachments exist between various structures in the spinal canal. Although dura, fat, nerves, and spinal canal wall are in contact, these tissues are not bound to one another. Therefore, solution injected into the epidural space readily spreads circumferentially at a given level and passes out of the intervertebral foramina (Fig. 9-27), and likewise freely passes longitudinally within the vertebral canal (Fig. 9-28).

As a catheter is advanced through the needle, there may be a brief resistance to advancement as the tip encounters the dura. Computed tomography (CT) shows that catheter tips inserted

3 cm into the vertebral canal most commonly travel laterally to the internal aspect of an intervertebral foramen (Fig. 9-29), because of the stiffness of the fairly short segment of catheter that has emerged from the needle. Nonetheless, injected solutions still surround the dura circumferentially (Fig. 9-30). Even when the catheter tip lies exterior to the intervertebral foramen in the paravertebral space, distribution of the injectate is preferentially back into the vertebral canal. This is explained by high pressures that develop with injection into the muscular confines of the perivertebral space. In contrast, the adjacent spinal canal has a maximum pressure set by the cerebrospinal fluid (CSF) pressure of approximately 15 cm H_2O, and therefore accepts flow by displacing CSF. Thus, fluid may arrive in the epidural space during any block around the vertebral column, including brachial plexus blocks (72–74), stellate ganglion and lumbar sympathetic chain blocks (75,76), and especially intercostal (77) and paravertebral spinal nerve blocks (78).

MENINGES

The spinal cord, nerve roots, and CSF are enclosed in membranes termed *meninges* (Fig. 9-31).

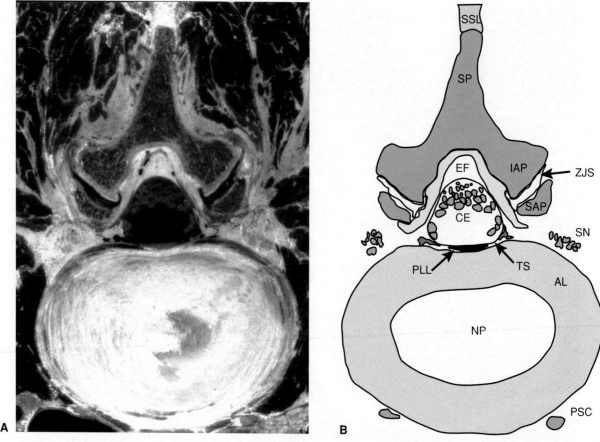

FIGURE 9-13. Axial cryomicrotome section (**A**) and index diagram (**B**) through the L3–L4 interverte-bral disc, caudal to the image in Figure 12. *AL*, annular ligament; *CE*, cauda equina; *EF*, epidural fat; *IAP*, inferior articular process; *NP*, nucleus pulposus; *PLL*, posterior longitudinal ligament; *PSC*, periver-tebral sympathetic chain; *SAP*, superior articular process; *SN*, spinal nerve; *SP*, spinous process; *SSL*, supraspinous ligament; *TS*, thecal sac; *ZJS*, zygapophyseal joint space. Ligamentum flavum is yellow, bone is brown, nerves are pink, and veins are blue.

Dura

The outermost meningeal layer is the dura mater, a connective tissue sack that extends from the skull, where its fusion with the foramen magnum terminates the epidural space. The cau-dal tip of the spinal dura is at about the S2 level (Fig. 9-3). The dural sac is attached to the posterior longitudinal ligament, particularly in the lumbar region (79), and is also anchored by the attachment of the anterior aspect of dural nerve root sleeves to the epineural tissue in the intervertebral foramen. The dura develops a posterior midline fold, termed a *plica me-diana dorsalis*, when foreign matter such as injected air or fluid compresses the dural sac (Fig. 9-30B). Under these conditions, scattered attachments of the dura to the posterior epidural fat and lamina produce a tethering effect that tents the dura poste-riorly. This is not seen, however, in the undisturbed dura, which is oval in axial section (Figs. 9-12 and 9-13) (37), except where it assumes a triangular shape where the nerve root sheaths diverge laterally (Figs. 9-11 and 9-14). The dura is thickest in the posterior midline and thinner in the lumbar area than more rostral (80). Still, lumbar dura is impenetrable by epidural catheters (81).

The structure of the dura is composed of collagenous lamel-lae and some elastin elements, separated by clefts filled with ground substance (82), which account for dural permeability (83). Although the fibrous strands run in both circumferen-tial and longitudinal fashion (82), the predominant direction is lengthwise (84). Dura is somewhat elastic, especially in the circumferential dimension (84). Because the dura is freely com-pressible, shifts in CSF from the intracranial space or between different sections of the vertebral dural sac are reflected as dy-namic changes in shape and volume of the sac. For instance, the Valsalva maneuver dramatically and immediately collapses the lumbar and thoracic dural sac, displacing CSF rostrally (85–88). The displaced CSF distends the cervical dural sac, but does not enter the skull, which is a fixed space and is pressur-ized comparable to the thoracoabdominal cavity. Tensing of the dura with flexion of the vertebral column, especially at cer-vical levels, causes an increased CSF pressure (89) and a rostral shift of the dural sac within the vertebral canal of close to 2 cm (49–52).

Arachnoid and Pia

Immediately within the dura is the arachnoid mater, a thin membrane that encloses the subarachnoid space and the CSF. Delicate trabeculae span the subarachnoid space from the

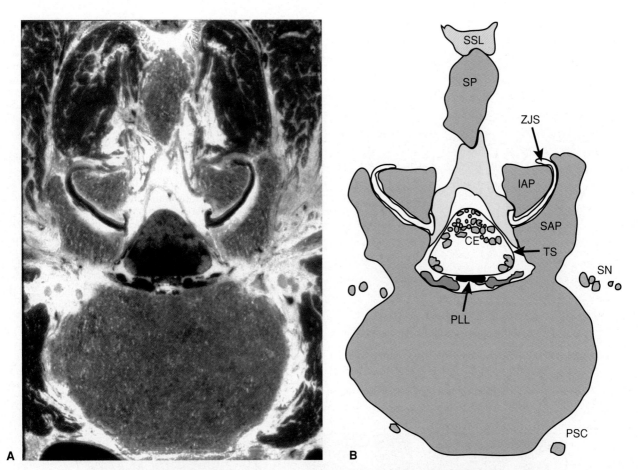

FIGURE 9-14. Axial cryomicrotome section (**A**) and index diagram (**B**) of a fourth lumbar vertebra, caudal to the image in Figure 13. *CE*, cauda equina; *IAP*, inferior articular process; *PLL*, posterior longitudinal ligament; *PSC*, perivertebral sympathetic chain; *SAP*, superior articular process; *SN*, spinal nerve branches; *SP*, spinous process; *SSL*, supraspinous ligament; *TS*, thecal sac; *ZJS*, zygapophyseal joint space. Bone is brown, nerves are pink, and veins are blue.

PART II: TECHNIQUES

thecal sac to the pia mater that envelops the surface of the cord and nerve roots (Fig. 9-32). (Because of the intimate relationship, common embryologic origin, and similar microscopic structure of the inner two meninges, they are often designated jointly as pia-arachnoid or *leptomeninges*.) The basal lamina and tight intracellular junctions of the arachnoid cells, together with those of the pia mater, constitute a physiologically active barrier (20). Whereas the substantia dura can be cleanly punctured, the arachnoid is velamentous and filmy in texture and withdraws from an advancing needle. In doing so, it may delaminate between its component layers (90), forming the commonly termed *subdural space*. This is probably a misnomer, since the cleft that most easily forms when arachnoid is pulled away from dura is not between the dura and arachnoid membranes, but more properly between layers of arachnoid (91). Conventional radiographic imaging is not adequate to distinguish between fluid layering inside or outside the dura. Secondary indicators have been used, such as lack of flow of contrast along exiting spinal nerves and a cylindrical pattern of uniform layering. However, these have not been suitably validated. For instance, a study of intentional subdural injection shows that solution preferentially passes out along the nerve roots (92), and routine epidural injections may also layer cylindrically outside the dura. A dural-based loculation on CT does, however, prove a subdural injection.

Cerebrospinal Fluid

About 500 mL of CSF is formed each day (93,94) principally by the choroid plexuses of the cerebral ventricles (95,96). Bulk flow distributes the fluid into the cisterns at the base of the brain, from which most CSF flows along the convexities of the brain (Fig. 9-32). Along the sagittal sinus, macroscopic defects in the dura accommodate outward herniations of arachnoid membrane, termed *arachnoid granulations* or *Pacchionian bodies*. These permit passage of CSF, and probably account for much of the CSF absorption back into the venous circulation, although other mechanisms participate (94). Particulate matter as large as 7 μm may pass through the granulations from CSF into venous blood (97) and electron microscopy has confirmed widened intracellular spaces (98) and transcellular fenestrations (99) in arachnoid granulations. A one-way valve mechanism, by which these passages open only when exposed to a CSF pressure in excess of the venous pressure, assures that flow will only be from CSF to veins. The pressure-sensing feature of arachnoid granulations regulates CSF pressure to about 10 to 20 cm H_2O in the lateral position (100).

The bulk of the CSF remains in the skull, whereas a minority of CSF produced leaves the cranial cavity and enters the spinal subarachnoid space to pass downward posterior to the cord

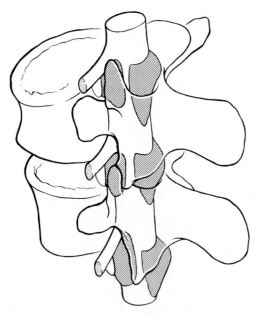

FIGURE 9-15. Drawing of the compartments of the epidural space (*stippled*). The epidural contents are discontinuous circumferentially and repeat metamerically. Where no contents are represented, the dura is in contact with the spinal canal wall. The pedicles are concealed behind the transverse processes. From Hogan QH. Lumbar epidural anatomy. A new look by cryomicrotome section. *Anesthesiology* 1991;75:767, with permission

and return upward anterior to the cord (Fig. 9-33). Superimposed upon this bulk flow is a longitudinal oscillation of the CSF column in synchrony with the pulsations of the arteries in the skull (101). The amplitude of this movement is substantial, about 9 mm per cycle in the cervical CSF and about 4 mm at the thoracolumbar junction. It is likely that this oscillatory CSF pulsation facilitates anesthetic distribution after subarachnoid injection. This could in part explain how material injected into the lumbar CSF ascends to the basal cisterns within an hour (102).

Despite its key role as the diluting volume for subarachnoid anesthetic solutions, the volume of the spinal CSF has only recently been explored. Of the approximately 100 mL of CSF in the vertebral canal, approximately half resides in the distal thecal sac. However, there is a dramatic interindividual variability, ranging from 30 to 80 mL in the zone distal to the T11–T12 disc (103,104). At least part of the interindividual variability is attributable to differences in body habitus, since subjects with high body mass index (BMI) have less CSF, probably due an elevated intraabdominal pressure (103,104). A small CSF volume may account for the higher anesthetic levels following subarachnoid local anesthetic administration in high-BMI subjects (105,106).

The composition of CSF (107) is similar to serum but with lower pH (7.32), potassium (2.9 mEq/L), and glucose (about two-thirds concurrent serum concentration) levels, and higher pCO_2 (47 mm Hg), magnesium (2.2 mEq/L), sodium (145 mEq/L), and chloride (125 mEq/mL) levels. Protein concentrations are much less than in serum, with greater

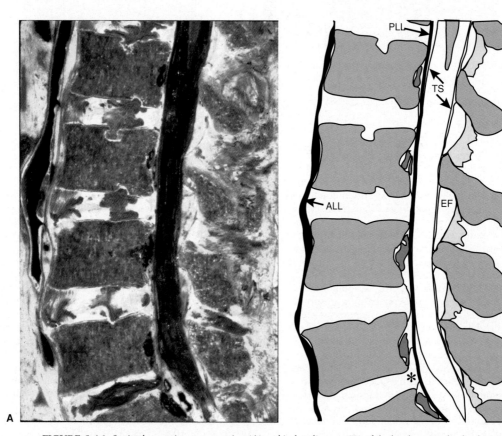

FIGURE 9-16. Sagittal cryomicrotome section (**A**) and index diagram (**B**) of the lumbar vertebral column, including vertebrae one through four and parts of the twelfth thoracic and fifth lumbar vertebrae. *ALL*, anterior longitudinal ligament; *EF*, epidural fat; *PLL*, posterior longitudinal ligament; *TS*, thecal sac; ∗ indicates a herniated nucleus pulposus. Ligamentum flavum is yellow, bone is brown, the spinal cord is pink, and veins are blue.

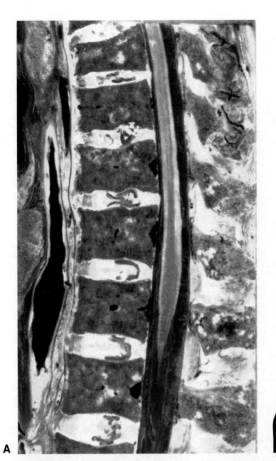
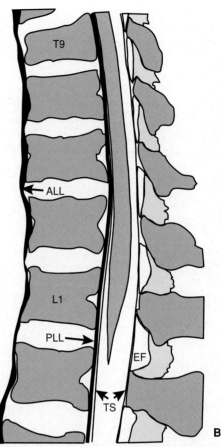

FIGURE 9-17. Sagittal cryomicrotome section (**A**) and index diagram (**B**) of the lower thoracic and upper lumbar vertebral column, including vertebrae T9 through L2 and parts of the eighth thoracic and third lumbar vertebrae. *ALL,* anterior longitudinal ligament; *EF,* epidural fat; *PLL,* posterior longitudinal ligament; *TS,* thecal sac. Ligamentum flavum is yellow, bone is brown, the spinal cord is pink, and veins are blue.

concentrations in lumbar CSF (300 mg/L) than in ventricular CSF (170 mg/L). The specific gravity of lumbar CSF is about 1.006.

Subarachnoid Space

Although the anterior subarachnoid space is empty of structures, the posterior subarachnoid space is crowded with membranous elements (Fig. 9-34) (108–110). Remnants of embryologic connective tissue persist as the mesh of arachnoid trabeculae (111). Denticulate ligaments, which are more substantial than trabeculae, extend laterally from the sides of the cord to suspend it within the dural sac and stabilize the position of the cord, particularly in the cervical zone (112).

The main subarachnoid structure is a variably fenestrated partition, the subarachnoid septum or septum posticum, which extends from the posterior midline of the cord to the inner aspect of the arachnoid. A continuous membrane is present at upper lumbar levels in 28% of cadavers and virtually always at thoracic and cervical levels (109). Other membranes extend from each posterior nerve root to the septum posticum and dorsolateral arachnoid, forming a lateral oblique cul-de-sac (108).

Particularly relevant to the anesthesiologist is the occurrence of cysts within the subarachnoid space, formed as saccular dilatations of the septum posticum. In normal subjects, these collections of loculated CSF occur in 45% (113) to 84% (114) of upright films in which adequately large amounts of oily radiographic contrast have been employed. Injection into them is a potential cause of inadequate spinal anesthesia.

Nerve Root Sheath

As nerve roots exit the dural sac, they are initially surrounded by their pial membrane, CSF, and the arachnoid membrane lining the dural cuff (Fig. 9-27). These extensions of the main neuraxial elements project laterally only as far as the proximal pole of the posterior root ganglion, which averages about 6 mm at L1 to about 15 mm long at S1 and S2 (115,116). At the lateral end of this nerve root sheath, the subarachnoid space is a closed off cul-de-sac in which the arachnoid reflects back along the nerve root. The dural sleeve in this area may also exhibit macroscopic arachnoid granulations similar to those in the intracranial dural sinuses, especially with advanced age (117–119), but they are not plentiful and lack the surrounding connective tissue cleft and accompanying venous confluence evident with cerebral granulations.

The pial layer of the nerve root is in continuity with the perineurium of the peripheral nerve (120,121) that defines a

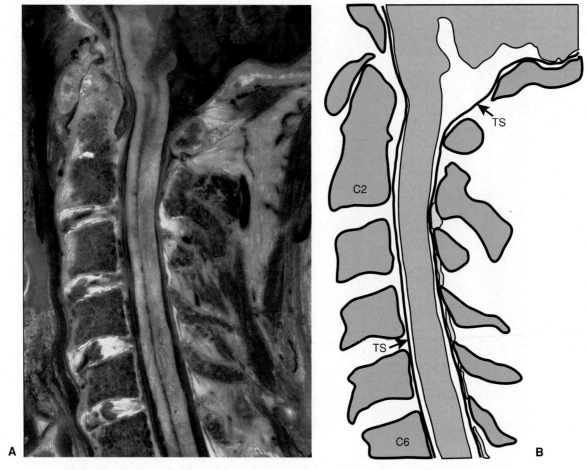

FIGURE 9-18. Sagittal cryomicrotome section (**A**) and index diagram (**B**) of the cervical vertebral column, down to the sixth cervical vertebra. *TS*, thecal sac. Ligamentum flavum is yellow, bone is brown, and the spinal cord and brain are pink.

fascicle. It is recognized that injection within a peripheral nerve fascicle may transmit injected solution longitudinally through the fascicle (122–124). By this route, intrafascicular peripheral injections travel in minutes to hours into the subpial space of the roots and then into the CSF or spinal cord (125,126). Damage to the cord or delayed spill into the CSF have been demonstrated (123,124).

Particulate ink injected into the CSF collects as a cuff at the furthest lateral extent of the CSF space along the posterior root ganglion and nerve roots, indicating egress of CSF and trapping of particulate matter at these sites (127). The arachnoid granulations are too few to account for this, so other imperfections in the meninges at the nerve root sleeve must account for the passage of material out of the CSF at this "ink cuff" (128). Accordingly, the lateral recess of the subarachnoid space terminates as a maze of lacunae filled with cellular debris and macrophages (129), and probably provides an important drainage and cleansing site. Root sleeves may also be a portal for the entry of local anesthetic from the epidural space into the CSF, however not because of increased permeability (130), but rather because of their particular geometry. Specifically, the nerve roots are close to the epidural space in this region, and the surface area of the dural root sleeve is large in comparison to the minimal CSF available at this site to dilute the entering anesthetic.

Degeneration and distention of root sheath arachnoid granulations can lead to saccular herniation of a subarachnoid diverticulum outside the dural sac proper (131). They usually occupy the intervertebral foramina and are referred to as *perineural cysts*. However, they occasionally expand into the vertebral canal, especially at lower thoracic levels (132), where they are termed *arachnoid cysts*. Saccular diverticula of thoracic, lumbar, and sacral nerve root sheaths are found in between 9% and 18% of asymptomatic subjects (133–135). They are usually multiple and symmetrical in a given subject, and often erode adjacent bone. At the sacral level, perineural cysts are termed *Tarlov cysts*. These are the largest and most common cysts, and may destroy sacral bone and even expand into the pelvic cavity (136,137). Cystic lesions of the nerve root sheath are also observed at lower cervical vertebral levels in 30% of aged normal subjects, but these do not exceed 7 mm diameter (138). At other than sacral levels, it is exceptional for either the normal nerve root sheath (139) or sheath diverticula (134) to extend laterally to the dorsal root ganglion and intervertebral foramen. Because of this, injection into such a sheath or cyst after a paravertebral needle insertion is likely only if the needle is mistakenly advanced into the intervertebral foramen.

Synovial cysts and *ganglion cysts*, which differ only histologically, are an uncommon form of fluid-filled vertebral canal mass. They originate as a dilatation of the capsule of a degenerating facet joint on its anterior and medial aspect. They may compress the dural sac from its posterolateral aspect (140,141), and may produce radiculopathy. Facet joint arthrography might demonstrate a connection to the joint space. Other uncommon types of ganglion cysts arise from the posterior or anterior longitudinal ligaments, dura mater, or ligamentum flavum. Injection into such ganglion cysts could be the rare cause of failed spinal or epidural anesthesia.

SPINAL CORD

The adult spinal cord measures approximately 41 to 48 cm in length and weighs between 24 and 36 g (142). It is about 1 cm in diameter, with cervical and lumbosacral expansions in the lateral dimension to accommodate the greater gray matter for the limbs at these levels. The tapered end of the cord is called the *conus medullaris* (Fig. 9-31) and usually lies at about the level of the L1–L2 intervertebral disc, although this is variable and may be as low as L3 (5,143–145). Continuing from the tip of the conus medullaris is a fibrous extension, the filum terminale (Fig. 9-31 and Fig. 9-35), which travels internally in the subarachnoid space with the nerve roots of the cauda equina. It penetrates the caudal terminus of the thecal sac and continues externally as a fine filament that inserts on the dorsum of the first sacral vertebral soma.

Flexion of the vertebral column stretches parts of the spinal cord by as much as 18 to 24% (49,50). The cervical cord moves anteriorly within the thecal sac with flexion and moves posteriorly during extension (146). There is no longitudinal movement of the conus medullaris with flexion (147). Both the cord and roots assume a dependent position ("sink") within the thecal sac (148,149).

PART II: TECHNIQUES

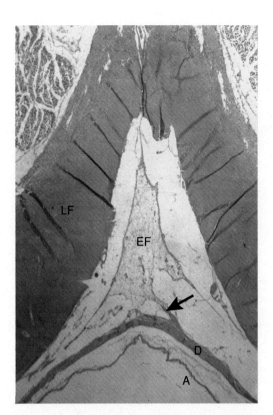

FIGURE 9-19. Histologic preparation of the contents of the human posterior vertebral canal in axial section. The arrow indicates an attachment of the epidural fat (*EF*) to the dura (*D*), and the fat is also attached at its apex to the ligamentum flavum (*LF*). These attachments are longitudinally incomplete, and thus are present only in some sections. *A*, arachnoid membrane. Lines across the LF are wrinkles created during preparation.

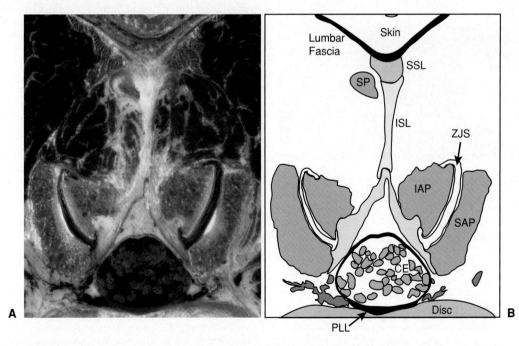

FIGURE 9-20. Axial cryomicrotome section (**A**) and index diagram (**B**) through the L4–L5 intervertebral disc. *CE*, cauda equina; *IAP*, inferior articular process; *ISL*, interspinous ligament; *PLL*, posterior longitudinal ligament; *SAP*, superior articular process; *SP*, spinous process; *SSL*, supraspinous ligament; *ZJS*, zygapophyseal joint space. Ligamentum flavum is yellow, bone is brown, nerves are pink, and veins are blue.

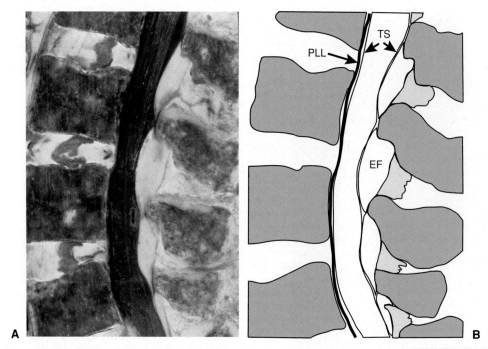

FIGURE 9-21. Epidural lipomatosis, in a subject having received systemic corticosteroids. A sagittal cryomicrotome section (**A**) and index diagram (**B**) show expanded posterior epidural fat (*EF*) that displaces the thecal sac (*TS*) anteriorly. *PLL,* posterior longitudinal ligament. Ligamentum flavum is yellow and bone is brown.

NERVE ROOTS

Rootlets that emerge from the spinal cord fuse into anterior nerve roots that carry afferent sensory fibers, and posterior

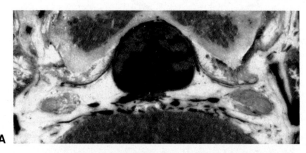

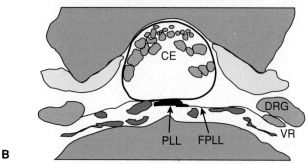

FIGURE 9-22. Axial cryomicrotome section (**A**) and index diagram (**B**) of a lumbar vertebra. *CE,* cauda equina; *DRG,* dorsal root ganglion; *FPLL,* fascia of the poster longitudinal ligament; *PLL,* posterior longitudinal ligament; *VR,* ventral root. Ligamentum flavum is yellow, bone is brown, the spinal cord is pink, and veins are blue.

spinal roots that carry efferent motor fibers. As rootlets emerge from the cord and join together as a root, each takes along a thin layer of pia, which continues along the entire length of the root, separating the root into fascicles. These meningeal coverings of the roots and their basement membrane are notably mesh-like and porous. The axons in the nerve roots are therefore freely bathed by the surrounding CSF, which gives ready access to drugs and particulate matter from the subarachnoid space.

Segments that contribute to a plexus innervating the upper or lower extremity have roots considerably larger in diameter than at other levels (Fig. 9-36). The L5 through S2 roots are largest, with a fair degree of interindividual variation (150). Large roots may be the most resistant to local anesthetic, contributing to delayed or absent blockade at L5 through S2 and variable results among individuals.

Since the human cord is much shorter than the entire vertebral canal, lumbar and sacral roots acquire a long oblique course within the dural sac and together compose the cauda equina (Fig. 9-31). These nerve roots, which vary in length from 7 cm at L1 to 27 cm at S5 (151), settle toward the most dependent part of the dural sac, regardless of posture (152).

Within the dural sac, multiple connections between adjacent roots are found in all specimens (153,154). Because the nerve roots pivot tightly around the inner and caudal aspect of the pedicle as they exit the vertebral canal, flexion of the vertebral column, especially of the neck, tenses the lumbosacral roots compared to their relaxed and redundant condition during spinal extension (51). Anomalous patterns of distribution at the foramina are discovered in dissections of 14% of normal subjects (155) and include two root pairs exiting at one level with an adjacent empty foramen (156–158). These occasionally aberrant arrangements may result in an unexpected distribution of anesthesia following foraminal injection for intended spinal nerve blockade (157).

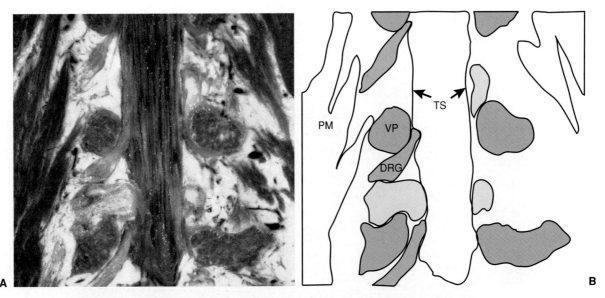

FIGURE 9-23. Coronal cryomicrotome section (**A**) and index diagram (**B**) of the vertebral column, spanning from the second to fourth lumbar vertebrae. *DRG,* dorsal root ganglion; *PM,* psoas muscle; *TS,* thecal sac; *VP,* vertebral pedicle. Ligamentum flavum is yellow, bone is brown, the spinal cord is pink, and veins are blue.

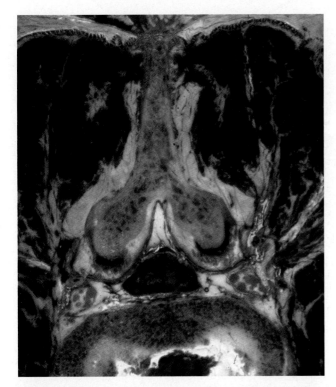

FIGURE 9-24. Axial cryomicrotome section at the fifth lumbar level, showing the distribution of green ink injected into the epidural space post mortem. Flow patterns include out the intervertebral foramina, accumulation around the spinal nerves in the perivertebral space, and into the posterior musculature.

SEGMENTATION

The anterior and posterior roots diverge toward the lateral thecal sac just rostral to the point at which they perforate the dural sac through a common aperture. Also at this point, the posterior root swells into the posterior root ganglion, which holds the somata of the sensory neurons. The anterior root lies in immediate apposition to the ganglion, and the two fuse at the distal pole of the ganglion to form the spinal nerve. The ganglion resides in the foramen directly inferior to the pedicle in the lumbar region (115), but lies further into or beyond the foramen in the cervical region, and within the vertebral canal in the sacrum. No simple relationship exists between the layers of the meninges and the layers of the peripheral nerves where they meet at the origin of the spinal nerve. Whereas both the peripheral nerve and meninges form a functional barrier to penetration by chemical agents, the capsule of the posterior root ganglion uniquely lacks such a function (159).

There is no evident segmentation in the spinal cord. However, the clumping of rootlets into nerve root fascicles and their exit through a common intervertebral foramen to form a spinal nerve defines a neuronal segment in the periphery. Although there are only seven cervical vertebrae, there are eight cervical neural segments. The eighth spinal nerve emerges between the seventh cervical and first thoracic vertebrae, whereas the other cervical nerves emerge *above* their same numbered vertebral bones, and the thoracic, lumbar, and sacral nerves exit the vertebral column *below* their same numbered bony segment.

A single spinal nerve projects its sensory axons to an innervated cutaneous surface. Each vertebral segment is associated with a dermatome, defined as the cutaneous area supplied by that spinal nerve. The first cervical spinal nerve is an exception. No sensory area has been identified for this segment, although mechanical or electrical stimulation of the posterior root at this level produces orbital and forehead pain (160). Rootlets that contribute to a root innervate serially overlapping portions of the greater root dermatome, ordered in sequence

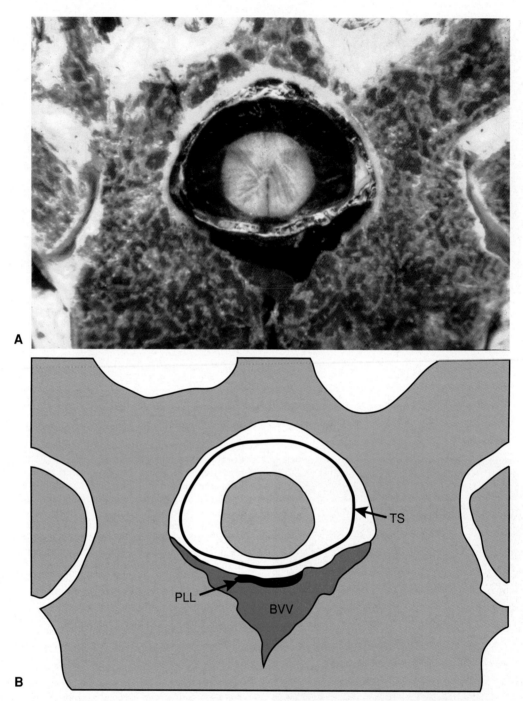

FIGURE 9-25. Axial cryomicrotome section (**A**) and index diagram (**B**) of a midthoracic vertebrae after epidural injection of green ink. Epidural accumulation surrounding the thecal sac (*TS*) is shown, as well as the barrier provided by the posterior longitudinal ligament (*PLL*) and the fascia that extends laterally from it, such that the injectate is excluded from the basivertebral vein (*BVV*). Bone is brown, the spinal cord is pink, and veins are blue.

from the cephalad to caudal end of the dermatome according to their order along the cord (161). Although simple diagrams are often presented showing highly specific areas for each segmental dermatome, the neuroanatomic reality is much more complex. Extensive overlap clearly occurs between consecutive peripheral dermatomes, since the division of an individual root rarely produces an appreciable loss of sensibility (162). This is

in large part attributable to divergence of afferent fibers immediately upon entry into the spinal cord in the tract of Lissauer. After transection of the ascending and descending fibers of the Lissauer tract above and below the entry of a given root into the cord, sensory responses can be elicited from skin two segments away. Thus, each cutaneous point is innervated by fibers from as many as five different roots (163).

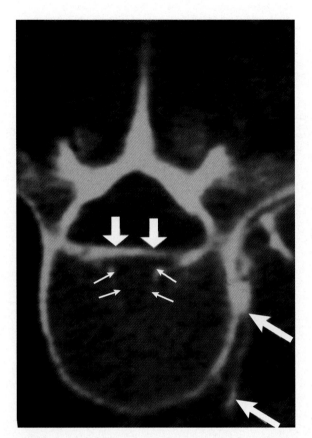

FIGURE 9-26. Axial computed tomographic scan of a patient with a functioning lumbar epidural catheter. Radiographic contrast injected through the catheter appears in the anterior epidural space (*wide arrows*), in contact with the basivertebral vein (*small arrows*). These spaces are separated by the posterior longitudinal ligament and its fascia, which are not visible per se. The injected contrast also tracks perivertebrally to the area of the sympathetic chain (*long arrows*).

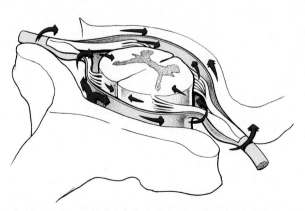

FIGURE 9-27. Schematic representation of circumferential distribution of local anesthetic injected into the epidural space. After initially spreading by bulk flow in the posterior and anterior epidural space, anesthetic and other drugs then enter the subarachnoid space, including through the dural cuff (root sleeve) region. Drug effects evolve after subsequent uptake into the nerve roots and spinal cord.

Various techniques have been employed to identify the segmental distribution of fibers to the skin, including mapping zoster eruptions, identifying areas of residual sensation after sectioning the roots on either side of an intact segment, defining regions of absent sensation after root section or anesthesia, observing vasodilatation during stimulation of roots, or delineating the radiation of pain with nerve root compression and visceral disease (164). The resulting diagrams, however, show considerable disagreement (Fig. 9-37) (165), and substantial variability between subjects has been noted (166). Thus, there is no way to be certain that a particular spinal nerve conveys sensation from a given skin area. Also, the dermatome for pain and temperature sensibility usually exceeds the dimensions of the dermatome for touch for the same root (162).

Similar to the definition of dermatomes, maps may be made of the spinal nerve levels contributing motor innervation to various muscles. As with dermatome maps, there is a degree of inconsistency in the segmental innervation of extremity muscles (166). For instance, marked departure from the usual distribution of L5 and S1 motor fibers is found in 16% of subjects (167), in whom stimulation of L5 produces movement typical of S1 and the reverse.

NEURAL SUPPLY OF THE VERTEBRAL COLUMN

Various portions of the vertebral column are provided with sensory innervation (168–172).

Posterior Structures

Immediately after its formation from the merging of the anterior root and posterior root ganglion, the spinal nerve splits into a dominant anterior primary ramus and a much smaller posterior primary ramus. The median branch of the posterior primary ramus supplies the posterior vertebral structures, including the supraspinous and intraspinous ligaments, periosteum, and fibrous capsule of the facet joint (Fig. 9-38). Of these, the facet joint is consistently found to be most thoroughly innervated, including nociceptive fibers penetrating the capsule as well as into the synovial folds (173). Recent work has also identified nerve fibers in the intraspinous and supraspinous ligaments, with specialized nerve endings indicative of a role in sensing motion and mechanical load (174). Few pain fibers are observed in these ligaments, explaining their general insensitivity to needle insertion. The few nerve endings of the ligamentum flavum are found only on its surface.

Sensory divergence in the tract of Lissauer is particularly extensive for afferent fibers from deep somatic structures such as vertebral joints and ligaments. Sensory fibers from a single facet joint terminate in the cord bilaterally as far rostral as the thoracolumbar junction and as far caudal as S1 (175), making somatotopic localization of pain originating in these deep structures especially difficult. It is possible that all fibers innervating these posterior skeletal structures pass through the sympathetic chain on their afferent course to the cord (172).

Few nerve fibers are seen in the posterior spinal canal or dura (173,176), accounting for the lack of sensations from these tissues during anesthetic procedures.

Anterior Structures

The innervation of the anterior longitudinal ligament, vertebral bodies, discs, and structures within the spinal canal are

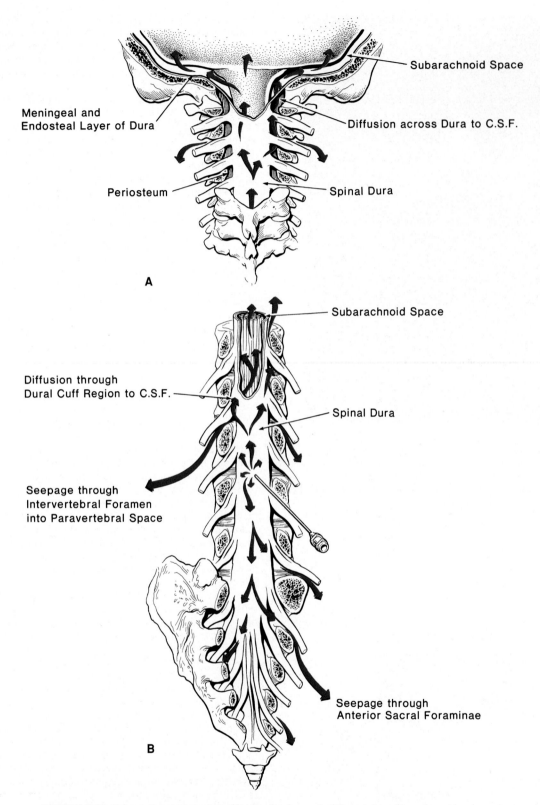

FIGURE 9-28. Schematic representation of longitudinal spread of drugs injected into the epidural space. **A:** Spread superiorly to base of skull, with diffusion into the cerebrospinal fluid by diffusion across dura, including in the region of the dural cuffs at the origins of the spinal nerves. **B:** Spread inferiorly to caudal canal with seepage by way of anterior sacral foramina. Seepage also occurs through the intervertebral foramina into the paravertebral space.

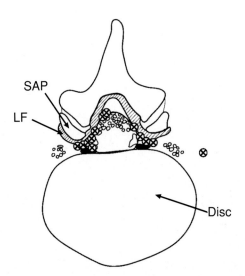

FIGURE 9-29. Location of the tips of lumbar epidural catheters (⊗) after placement by a midline approach. Following advancement of catheters 3 to 4 cm into the epidural space, the tips typically lie anteriorly in the area of the intervertebral foramen. Functioning catheters may also lie well outside the spinal canal (*far right* in the image). Data from Hogan Q. Epidural catheter tip position and distribution of injectate evaluated by computerized tomography. *Anesthesiology* 1999;90:964–970, with permission.

derived from cells with their somas in dorsal root ganglia at that level (177) through sympathetic pathways, including perivascular nerve plexuses and the sympathetic chain (Fig. 9-39) (172). Up to five sinuvertebral nerves (also called the *recurrent nerves, meningeal rami,* or the *nerves of Luschka*) travel through each intervertebral foramen anterior to the dorsal root ganglion on their passage into the vertebral canal (172,178). They originate from the rami communicantes and the anterior primary ramus of the spinal nerve. They contribute to an extensive plexus that follows the posterior longitudinal ligament and passes fibers to the anterior dura. Other filaments supply the outer annulus of the posterior aspect of the disc (171,172,179,180). The inner annulus, center of the disc, and vertebral endplates have no nerves, although free nerve endings may invade the interior of a degenerating disc (181,182). Ascending and descending branches from the sinuvertebral nerve span as many as eight vertebral segments and cross the midline (171,172,177,178,183), accounting for a wide distribution of pain from stimulation of these structures at a single level.

Functional Significance

It is highly likely that the fibers innervating certain vertebral structures produce pain. Substance P, a polypeptide neurotransmitter characteristic of small nociceptive fibers, is found in nerves of the posterior longitudinal ligament (184,185), dura (186), pia on the anterior aspect of the cord and on the ventral roots (187), supraspinous ligament (188), annular ligament of the disc (185), and facet joint capsule (188,189). Little is found in facet menisci (190), the central disc, and ligamentum flavum (184,185,189). Consistent with these anatomic findings, physiologic recordings in laboratory animals have documented mechanoreceptive sensory fields in facet joints (191,192), disc, dura, ligaments, periosteum, paraspinous muscles (191,193,194), and the pial surface of the ventral roots (195). The receptive field of central nervous system sensory

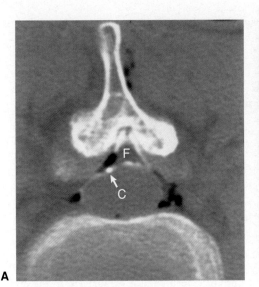

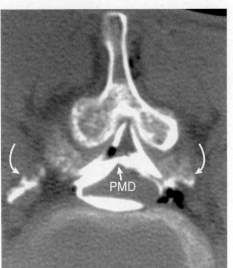

FIGURE 9-30. Computed axial tomograph of mid-lumbar level of an epidural injection. The epidural catheter (*C*) is in the posterior epidural space, which is not typical (see Fig. 9-29). After injection of 0.4 mL of radiologic contrast through the catheter (**A**), the posterior epidural fat (*F*) is outlined by contrast, which appears white. Black areas represent air, which is found in the track of the epidural needle along the spinous process and in the epidural space posteriorly and bilaterally in the intervertebral foramina. After injection of an additional 14 mL of contrast (**B**), the dura is collapsed by the pressure of the injected contrast, except where it is tethered by the posterior epidural fat, producing a plica mediana dorsalis (*PMD*). Injectate in the anterior epidural space further compresses the thecal sac. The posterior epidural fat is seen as a triangle well surrounded by contrast, except where it is suspended from the posterior laminar bone. Air bubbles do not impede distribution of injected solution, and solution passes out each intervertebral foramen (*curved arrows*).

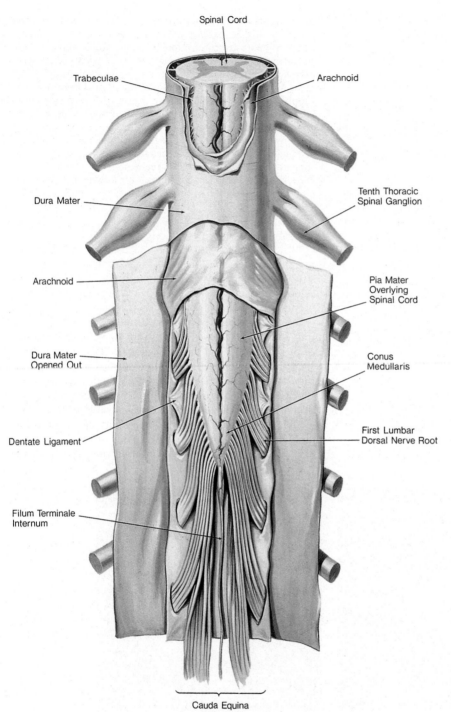

Spinal Cord

Trabeculae

Arachnoid

Dura Mater

Tenth Thoracic
Spinal Ganglion

Arachnoid

Pia Mater
Overlying
Spinal Cord

Dura Mater
Opened Out

Conus
Medullaris

Dentate Ligament

First Lumbar
Dorsal Nerve Root

Filum Terminale
Internum

Cauda Equina

FIGURE 9-31. Terminal spinal cord and cauda equina, showing relationship of overlying structures.

cells typically is very large and always includes multiple tissues.

Anatomic exploration in human subjects has immediate relevance to clinical conditions. Various methods have been used to test the sensitivity of vertebral structures in humans, such stimulation with needles or hypertonic saline during surgery under local anesthesia (169,196–208). Stimulation has also been performed using threads attached to various tissues during surgery (209). Consistent findings are particular sensitivity of the posterior longitudinal ligament and anterior dura, which

produce deep pain at or adjacent to the midline of the back and into the buttock. At cervical levels, manipulation of these structures can induce chest pain. Irritation of the surface of the disc or the inner portion of a degenerated disc produces typical deep back pain with radiation to the pelvis and abdomen, and only rarely radiation into the lower extremity. Mechanical stimulation of the posterior root produces an electric sensation, whereas manipulation of the anterior root evokes a deep ache. Inflamed roots produce particularly intense pain even with minimal manipulation. Facet joint stimulation creates low back

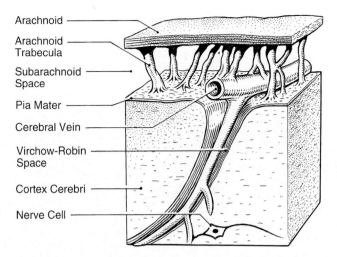

Arachnoid
Arachnoid Trabecula
Subarachnoid Space
Pia Mater
Cerebral Vein
Virchow-Robin Space
Cortex Cerebri
Nerve Cell

FIGURE 9-32. Diagram of the subarachnoid space, showing blood vessels and arachnoid trabecula. Redrawn after Strong OS, Elwyn A. *Human Neuroanatomy.* Baltimore: Williams & Wilkins, 1959, with permission.

pain that radiates into the thigh, with extensive overlap of referral areas from the various joints even when L1–L2 and L4–L5 joints are compared. Interspinous and supraspinous ligaments produce only minimal local and sometimes referred pain, and the ligamentum flavum, posterior dura, lamina, vertebral body, and the spinous process are essentially insensitive.

Sympathetic Pathways

Afferent fibers carrying deep somatic sensation of midline structures pass predominantly through sympathetic rami and trunks. This is evident from the pattern of nerve connections noted above (172), from retrograde neural labeling (210), and from induction of activity in the sympathetic rami and trunks by stimulation of vertebral structures (193,211). In human subjects, electrical stimulation of the sympathetic chain or rami provokes localized back pain (212,213) or extremity pain (214). These observations would indicate that blocks or ablation of the chain might have therapeutic potential in back pain.

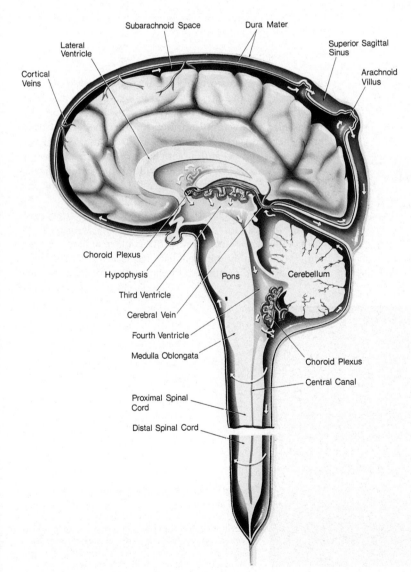

Lateral Ventricle
Subarachnoid Space
Dura Mater
Superior Sagittal Sinus
Cortical Veins
Arachnoid Villus
Choroid Plexus
Hypophysis
Third Ventricle
Cerebral Vein
Fourth Ventricle
Medulla Oblongata
Pons
Cerebellum
Choroid Plexus
Central Canal
Proximal Spinal Cord
Distal Spinal Cord

FIGURE 9-33. Production, circulation, and resorption of cerebrospinal fluid.

PART II: TECHNIQUES

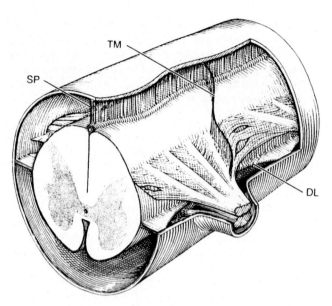

FIGURE 9-34. Diagram of subarachnoid membranes at the thoracic level, including the septum posticum (*SP*), transverse membranes (*TM*), and the dentate ligaments (*DL*).

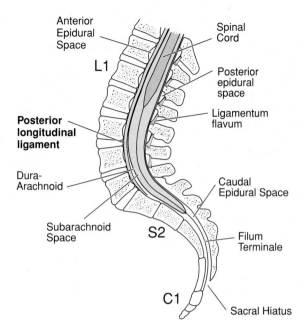

FIGURE 9-35. Lumbosacral portion of vertebral column, showing terminal spinal cord and its coverings.

Roots and Cord

The investing pial membrane of the anterior and posterior roots has sensory innervation (215), as does the pia of the cord (216), and injury to the root leads to increased small-fiber innervation of the pia (217). However, the contribution of these pathways to clinical pain conditions is unknown.

VASCULAR SUPPLY OF THE VERTEBRAL COLUMN

Arteries

The arterial supply of the vertebral structures originates from segmental spinal arteries, which in turn are branches of the thyrocervical and costocervical trunks and the vertebral artery in the neck, and the intercostal and lumbar arteries more caudally (Fig. 9-40). The nucleus pulposus of the intervertebral disc is avascular, receiving its nutrition through the flow of tissue fluid generated through a pumping mechanism of alternating compression and expansion with flexion and extension of the vertebral column (218). The extent of this process is indicated by the loss of enough fluid during axial loading to result in a loss of about 2 cm height through the day (219).

At every intervertebral foramen, the segmental artery gives off radicular arteries that enter the spinal canal with each posterior and anterior root and provide nutrient flow to them (Fig. 9-41). In addition, medullary feeder arteries that deliver blood flow to the intrinsic system of the cord travel along

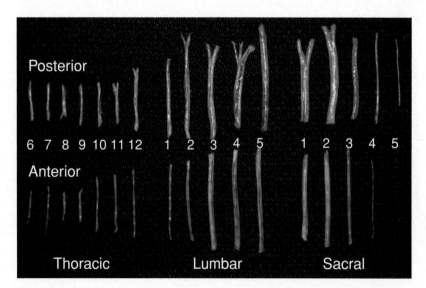

FIGURE 9-36. Spinal nerve roots harvested at autopsy. The segmental levels are indicated by number. The diameter of the roots is largest for those that contribute to the lumbosacral plexus, and posterior roots are generally larger than anterior roots. Note that many roots are multifascicular and readily separate into components without dissection.

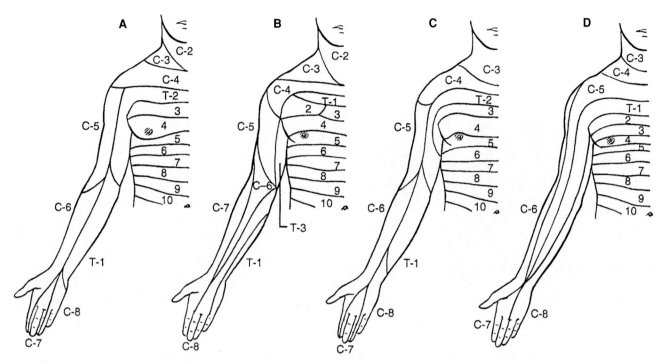

FIGURE 9-37. Spinal nerve dermatome charts. Disagreement exists about the exact dermatome specifications, depending on the method for determination. **A:** Foerster's chart was devised by sectioning roots and observing vasodilatation during stimulation of nerve stumps. **B:** Head determined dermatomes using distribution of herpes zoster lesions. **C:** Bonica mapped dermatomes by observation of effects of nerve blocks and radiation of mechanical paresthesias during needle placement. **D:** Keegan identified patterns of hyperalgesia observed in cases of clinical radiculopathy and following rhizotomy and local anesthetic injection.

approximately eight of the anterior and 12 of the posterior roots (220). The anterior feeders split at the anterior median fissure of the cord into ascending and descending divisions, which link to make an anastomotic chain (221), the anterior median longitudinal arterial trunk of the spinal cord (or anterior spinal artery). Similar linking of posterior medullary feeders produces right and left postero-lateral longitudinal arterial trunks (or posterior spinal arteries) just posterior to the ori-

gin of the posterior nerve roots. Penetrating midline branches (sulcal arteries) from the anterior spinal artery ramify in the anterior two-thirds of the spinal cord, whereas the posterior arteries supply the posterior one-third, with negligible overlap between the fields. A circumferential pial network contributes minimal nutrient flow to the cord (222).

The longitudinal arteries of the cord, which are the sole source of medullary perfusion, are not substantial or

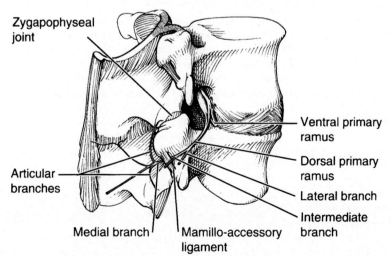

Zygapophyseal joint

Articular branches

Medial branch

Mamillo-accessory ligament

Ventral primary ramus

Dorsal primary ramus

Lateral branch

Intermediate branch

FIGURE 9-38. Innervation of posterior structures by the posterior primary ramus of the segmental spinal nerve.

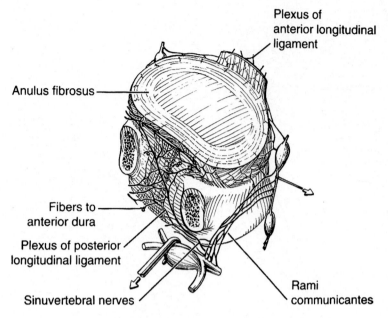

FIGURE 9-39. Innervation of the vertebral body, intervertebral disc, and the posterior and anterior longitudinal ligaments. A plexus along the posterior longitudinal ligament distributes fibers to the anterior epidural space and dural sac. There originate from the sinuvertebral nerves the rami communicantes. This highly complex pattern is revealed using acetylcholinesterase histochemical staining. After Groen GJ, Baljet B, Drukker J. Nerves and nerve plexuses of the human vertebral column. *Am J Anat* 1990;188:282–296, with permission.

continuous throughout the length of the cord (223,224). Along the length of these arteries, which are the longest in the body, blood flow is not uniformly in one direction, but rather depends on the proximity of the nearest contributing feeder (225), and flow direction at any point may change in response to physiologic and pathologic influences (226). Therefore, although the anterior arterial system of the cord is usually anatomically continuous, it is functionally a longitudinal series of independent vascular beds centered upon the regional medullary feeder (227), with linkage to the adjacent bed to assure redundancy of supply to this critical tissue. For this reason, the term anastomotic "trunk" may be preferable to "artery" for the longitudinal channels.

Numerous descriptions of the pattern of medullary feeders have identified dominant vessels at certain levels, but without much consistency. Typically, a major contribution is made by a single anterior medullary feeder, known as the artery of Adamkiewicz, which may enter at a level between T7 and L4 on the left (Fig. 9-40). Often, however, a uniquely conspicuous artery is not apparent. Rather, the site and size of a dominant feeder to the lumbosacral cord is so unpredictable that the concept cannot be applied in a clinically useful manner (228). Each segmental artery must be considered critical (229), although specific anatomic details about an individual may aid surgical planning (230).

The anterior and deep portions of the cord supplied by the anterior spinal artery are most prone to damage during ischemia, systemic hypotension, or hypoxia without vascular damage (231–233), due in part to an inherent sensitivity of the anterior horn motor neurons (232–235). Vascular anatomy also contributes to making the anterior cord prone to ischemic injury, since anterior medullary feeders are larger but fewer than their posterior counterparts (229). Anatomic definition of anterior cord damage is usually overstated, and clinical and experimental ischemic injuries are rarely limited to the anterior two-thirds of the cord that is considered the classical zone of anterior spinal cord infarction (236). Rather, injury is greatest

in the deep gray matter, with progressively less damage in concentrically surrounding zones. Consequently, at least some of the superficial dorsal columns survive with accompanying distal nonpainful sensation, giving rise to the inexact diagnosis of anterior spinal artery syndrome, despite the infrequent confirmation of the anatomic lesion of anterior spinal cord infarction by autopsy (237).

Vulnerable watershed areas of the anterior arterial supply of the cord occur especially in the mid-thoracic zone (238), where feeders are most rare. Furthermore, this zone has the lowest density of penetrating branches from the anterior trunk (223,224), and the intercostal arteries providing feeder vessel in the thorax lack the extensive interconnections that provide alternative supply to the extraspinal arteries in the neck and lumbosacral region (237). As a result, the most common levels for nonsurgical spinal stroke are T3 to T9 (233), and cord infarction after thoracolumbar aortic surgery is typically at a thoracic segmental level (239). Disruption of spinal arteries during abdominal aortic surgery usually cause conus and lumbosacral ischemic injuries.

The arterial supply of the nerve roots has been intensively studied (240,241). Like the anterior spinal trunk, the radicular arteries appear as a single continuous vessel from the intervertebral foramen to the cord but are in fact functionally two vessels, with flow originating both at the cord end and in the intervertebral foramen (221,241). Thus, an obstruction will not block flow to either side but only in the compressed area. No collateral arterial inflow occurs along the course of the roots, which may be 20 cm long, but nutrients and oxygen can be absorbed from the ambient CSF (241,242). This alternative path provides a greater share of nutrient exchange than the vascular route.

Veins

Veins of the epidural space form a primitive, valveless plexus (243) composed of high-capacitance and thin-walled vessels

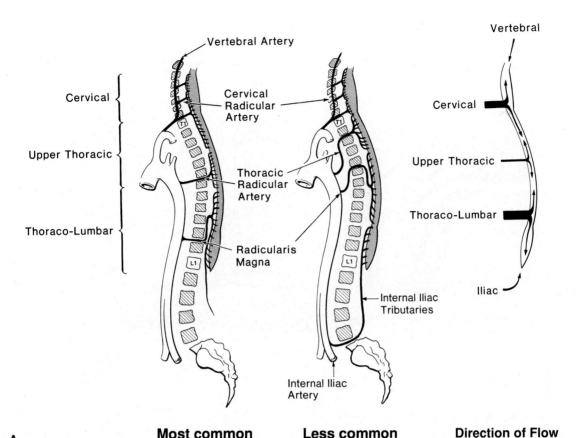

Most common   **Less common**   **Direction of Flow**

A

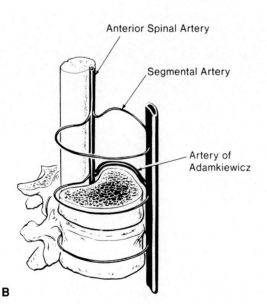

B

FIGURE 9-40. **A:** Blood supply of spinal cord, vertical distribution; functional concept. In the most common case, note the relatively discrete vertical areas with little anastomosis. In less common situations (high take-off), the iliac artery branch may supply the lower thoracolumbar region of cord, entering by way of the intervertebral foramen in the vicinity of L4–L5. Direction of flow is dependent on the proximity of a major feeder artery. A large proportion of flow originates from the radicularis magna artery (artery of Adamkiewicz) in the thoracolumbar region. **B:** Blood supply of spinal cord; anatomic description. This highlights the segmental anatomic distribution of spinal arteries. However, note that, although all spinal arteries reach the spinal cord, many are extremely small and offer only a minimal contribution to nutritive blood flow. Modified from data of Crock HV, Yoshizawa H. *The Blood Supply of the Vertebral Column and Spinal Cord in Man.* New York: Springer-Verlag, 1977, with permission.

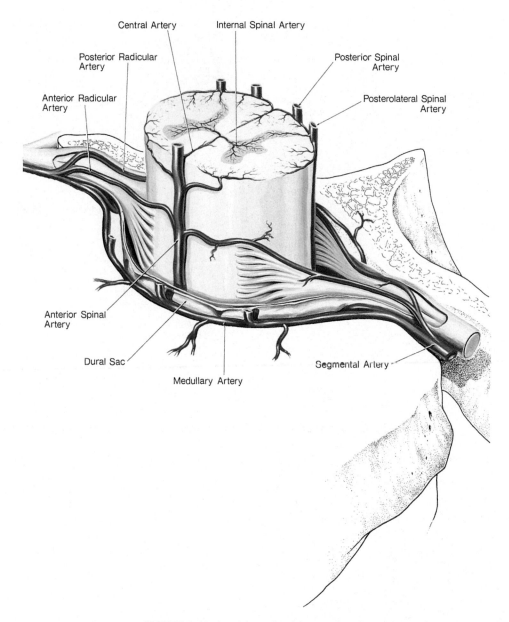

FIGURE 9-41. Arterial supply of the spinal cord.

that are easily punctured (244,245). This system conducts flow in any direction, dictated by the relative pressures in the pelvis, abdomen, chest, and head (246). Batson (244) and others (247) proposed that venous metastasis might be distributed via this route during caval occlusion. Increased intra-abdominal pressure is unlikely to divert systemic venous flow into the vertebral canal since epidural pressure rises in tandem with intra-abdominal pressure. Selective occlusion of the vena cava, however, does encourage venous flow into the alternative pathway of the epidural system by increasing venous pressures distal to the blockage (248,249), and flow reversal during caval occlusion by external abdominal compression has been observed (250–252).

The internal vertebral veins of the anterior epidural space are usually depicted as a double system, with a medial and lateral component, but dissection (253), venography (254), and cryomicrotome section (37) show a virtually confluent pool between disc levels (Fig. 9-11). There are essentially no veins in the posterior epidural space (252), except caudal to the L5–S1 disc, where the veins are widely distributed (254).

Large, tortuous venous trunks, found on the anterior and posterior midline of the cord surface, drain to medullary veins that exit through the intervertebral foramina. Whereas arteries of roots are tolerant to chronic compression and maintain patency (255), venous obliteration and nerve root edema follow even a brief interval of root compression (256), and may produce radicular pain (257). Crowding of the intervertebral foramen by disc or facet disease produces venous obstruction before impinging upon the nerve and leads to fibrosis of the roots (258).

Lymphatics

Little is known about the lymphatic system of the vertebral column. Lymphatics begin draining particulate matter from the epidural space within 5 minutes after epidural ink injection in rabbits (259), and they play a minor role in the uptake of epidural drugs (260). Dissipation of extruded disc material (261,262) and of blood injected for the treatment of post-lumbar puncture headache (263) indicates an active lymphatic system in the vertebral canal.

SUMMARY

A thorough knowledge of the spinal column and the soft tissues and neuraxial elements contained within it is required to accurately place local anesthetic solutions, avoid complications due to needle damage or incorrectly placed injection, predict the physiologic events resulting from neural blockade, and develop new approaches for intraoperative anesthesia and acute and chronic pain management.

References

1. Hogan, Q. Tuffier's line: The normal distribution of anatomic parameters. *Anesth Analg* 1993;78:194–195.
2. Edwards E. Operative anatomy of the lumbar sympathetic chain. *Angiology* 1951;2:184–198.
3. MacGibbon B, Farfan HF. A radiologic survey of various configurations of the lumbar spine. *Spine* 1979;4:258–266.
4. Quinnell RC, Stockdale HR. The use of in vivo lumbar discography to assess the clinical significance of the position of the intercrestal line. *Spine* 1983;8:305–307.
5. Kim JT, Bahk JH, Sung J. Influence of age and sex on the position of the conus medullaris and Tuffier's line in adults. *Anesthesiology* 2003;99:1359.
6. Lirk P, Messner H, Deibl M, et al. Accuracy in estimating the correct intervertebral space level during lumbar, thoracic and cervical epidural anaesthesia. *Acta Anaesthesiol Scand* 2004;48:347–349.
7. Sjögren P, Gefke K, Banning A, et al. Lumbar epidurography and epidural analgesia in cancer patients. *Pain* 1989;36:305–309.
8. Gielen MJ, Slappendel R, Merx JL. Asymmetric onset of sympathetic blockade in epidural anesthesia shows no relation to epidural catheter position. *Acta Anaesthesiol Scand* 1991;35:81–84.
9. Van Gessel EF, Forster A, Gamulin Z. Continuous spinal anesthesia: Where do spinal catheters go? *Anesth Analg* 1993;76:1004–1007.
10. Broadbent CR, Maxwell WB, Ferrie R, et al. Ability of anaesthetists to identify a marked lumbar interspace. *Anaesthesia* 2000;55:1122–1126.
11. Holmaas G, Frederiksen D, Ulvik A, et al. Identification of thoracic intervertebral spaces by means of surface anatomy: A magnetic resonance imaging study. *Acta Anaesthesiol Scand* 2006;50:368–373.
12. Willis TA. An analysis of vertebral anomalies. *Am J Surg* 1929;6:163–168.
13. Todd TW. Numerical significance in the thoracolumbar vertebrae of the mammilia. *Anat Rec* 1922;24:261–286.
14. Ericksen MF. Some aspects of aging in the lumbar spine. *Am J Phys Anthrop* 1976;45:575–580.
15. Amonoo-Kuofi HS. Maximum and minimum lumbar interpedicular distances in normal adult Nigerians. *J Anat* 1982;135:225–233.
16. Berry JL, Moran JM, Berg WS, Steffee AD. A morphometric study of human lumbar and selected thoracic vertebrae. *Spine* 1987;12:362–367.
17. Scoles PV, Linton AE, Latimer B, et al. Vertebral body and posterior element morphology: The normal spine in middle life. *Spine* 1988;10:1082–1086.
18. Hurme M, Alaranta H, Aalto T, et al. Lumbar spinal canal size of sciatica patients. *Acta Radiol* 1989;30:353–357.
19. Panjabi MM, Takata K, Goel V, et al. Thoracic human vertebrae: Quantitative three-dimensional anatomy. *Spine* 1991;16:889–901.
20. Panjabi MM, Duranceau J, Goel V, et al. Cervical human vertebrae: Quantitative three-dimensional anatomy of the middle and lower regions. *Spine* 1991;16:861–869.
21. Amonoo-Kuofi HS. The sagittal diameter of the lumbar vertebral canal in normal adult Nigerians. *J Anat* 1985;140:69–78.
22. Trotter M. Variations of the sacral canal: Their significance in the administration of caudal analgesia. *Anesth Analg* 1947;26:192–202.
23. Norenberg A, Johanson DC, Gravenstein JS. Racial differences in sacral structure in caudal anesthesia. *Anesthesiology* 1979;50:549–551.
24. Milne N. The role of zygapophysial joint orientation and uncinate processes in controlling motion in the cervical spine. *J Anat* 1991;178:189–201.
25. Singer KP, Breidahl PD, Day RE. Variations in zygapophyseal joint orientation and level of transition at the thoracolumbar junction. *Surg Radiol Anat* 1988;10:291–295.
26. Pal GP, Routal RV. A study of weight transmission through the cervical and upper thoracic regions of the vertebral column in man. *J Anat* 1986;148:245–261.
27. Davis PR. Human lower lumbar vertebrae: Some mechanical and osteological considerations. *J Anat* 1961;95:337–344.
28. Yang KH, King AI. Mechanism of facet load transmission as a hypothesis for low-back pain. *Spine* 1984;9:557–565.
29. Dory MA. Arthrography of the lumbar facet joints. *Radiology* 1981;140:23–27.
30. Raymond J, Dumas J-M. Intraarticular facet block: Diagnostic test of therapeutic procedure? *Radiology* 1984;151:333–336.
31. Moran R, O'Connell D, Walsh MG. The diagnostic value of facet injections. *Spine* 1988;13:1407.
32. Bogduk N, Engel R. The menisci of the lumbar zygapophyseal joints. *Spine* 1984;9:454–460.
33. Wang ZL, Yu S, Haughton VM. Age-related changes in the lumbar facet joints. *Clin Anatomy* 1989;2:55–62.
34. Giles LGF, Taylor JR, Cockson A. Human zygapophyseal joint synovial folds. *Acta Anat* 1986;126:110–114.
35. Epstein JA, Epstein BS, Lavine LS, et al. Lumbar nerve root compression at the intervertebral foramina caused by arthritis of the posterior facets. *J Neurosurg* 1973;39:362–369.
36. Heylings JA. Supraspinous and intraspinous ligaments of the human lumbar spine. *J Anat* 1978;125:127–131.
37. Hogan Q. Lumbar epidural anatomy: A new look by cryomicrotome section. *Anesthesiology* 1991;75:767–775.
38. Williams DM, Gabrielsen TO, Latack JT. Ossification in the caudal attachments of the ligamentum flavum. *Radiology* 1982;145:693–697.
39. Williams DM, Gabrielsen TO, Latack JT, et al. Ossification in the cephalic attachment of the ligamentum flavum. *Radiology* 1984;150:423–436.
40. Maigne JY, Ayral X, Guerin-Surville H. Frequency and size of ossifications in the caudal attachments of the ligamentum flavum of the thoracic spine. Role of rotatory strains in their development. *Surg Radiol Anat* 1992;14:119–124.
41. Miyasaka K, Kaneda K, Ito T, et al. Ossification of spinal ligaments causing thoracic radiculomyelopathy. *Radiology* 1982;143:463–468.
42. Cork RC, Kryc JJ, Vaughan RW. Ultrasonic localization of the lumbar epidural space. *Anesthesiology* 1980;52:513–516.
43. Palmer SK, Abram SE, Maitra AM, von Colditz JH. Distance from the skin to the lumbar epidural space in an obstetric population. *Anesth Analg* 1983;62:944–946.
44. Rosenberg H, Keykhah MM. Distance to the epidural space in nonobstetric patients. *Anesth Analg* 1984;63:538–546.
45. Currie JM. Measuring of the depth to the extradural space using ultrasound. *Br J Anaesth* 1984;56:345–347.
46. Harrison GR, Clowes NWB. The depth of the lumbar epidural space from the skin. *Anaesthesia* 1985;40:685–687.
47. Sutton DN, Linter SPK. Depth of extradural space and dural puncture. *Anaesthesia* 1991;46:97–98.
48. Hogan QH. Epidural anatomy examined by cryomicrotome section: Influence of age, level and disease. *Reg Anesth* 1996;21:395–406.
49. Smith CG. Changes of length and position of the segments of the spinal cord with changes in posture in the monkey. *Radiology* 1956;66:259–265.
50. Reid JD. Effects of flexion-extension movements of the head and spine upon the spinal cord and nerve roots. *J Neurol Neurosurg Psychiat* 1960;23:214–221.
51. Brieg A, Marions O. Biomechanics of the lumbosacral nerve roots. *Acta Radiol [Diagn]* 1962;1:1141–1160.
52. Kubik S, Muntener M. Zur topographie der spinalen Nervenwurzeln. *Acta Anat* 1969;74:149–168.
53. Hogan Q. Epidural catheter tip position and distribution of injectate evaluated by computerized tomography. *Anesthesiology* 1999;90:964–970.
54. Guyton AC, Granger HJ, Taylor AE. Interstitial fluid pressure. *Physiol Rev* 1971;51:527–563.
55. Nickalls RWD, Kokri MS. The width of the epidural space in obstetric patients. *Anaesthesia* 1986;41:432–433.
56. Luyendijk W, van Voorthuisen AE. Contrast examination of the spinal epidural space. *Acta Radiol [Diagn]* 1966; 5:1051.

57. Hatten HP. Lumbar epidurography with metrizamide. *Radiology* 1980;137:129–136.
58. Savolaine ER, Pandya JB, Greenblatt SH, Conover SR. Anatomy of the human lumbar epidural space: New insights using CT-epidurography. *Anesthesiology* 1988;68:217–220.
59. Blomberg R. The dorsomedian connective tissue band in the lumbar epidural space of humans: An anatomical study using epiduroscopy in autopsy cases. *Anesth Analg* 1986;65:747–752.
60. Blomberg R, Olsson SS. The lumbar epidural space in patients examined with epiduroscopy. *Anesth Analg* 1989;68:157–160.
61. Hogan Q, Toth J. Anatomy of soft tissues of the spinal canal. *Reg Anesth Pain Med* 1999;24:303–10.
62. Ramsey HJ. Fat in the epidural space of young and adult cats. *Am J Anat* 1959;104:345–380.
63. Ramsey HJ. Comparative morphology of fat in the epidural space. *Am J Anat* 1959;105:219–232.
64. George WE, Wilmot M, Greenhouse A, Hammeke M. Medical management of steroid-induced epidural lipomatosis. *N Engl J Med* 1983;308:316–319.
65. Quint DJ, Boulos RS, Sanders WP, et al. Epidural lipomatosis. *Radiology* 1988;169:485–490.
66. Sandberg DI, Lavyne MH. Symptomatic spinal epidural lipomatosis after local epidural corticosteroid injections: Case report. *Neurosurgery* 1999;45:162–165.
67. Badami JP, Hinck VC. Symptomatic deposition of epidural fat in a morbidly obese woman. *AJNR* 1982;3:664–665.
68. Bednar DA, Esses SI, Kucharczuk W. Symptomatic lumbar epidural lipomatosis in a normal male. *Spine* 1990;15:52–53.
69. Herzog RJ, Kaiser JA, Saal JA, Saal JS. The importance of posterior epidural fat pad in lumbar central canal stenosis. *Spine* 1991;16:S227–S233.
70. Hogan QH. Distribution of solution in the epidural space: Examination by cryomicrotome section. *Reg Anesth Pain Med* 2002;27:150–156.
71. Shah JL. Influence of cerebrospinal fluid on epidural pressure. *Anaesthesia* 1981;36:627–631.
72. Kumar A, Battit GE, Froese AB, Long MC. Bilateral cervical and thoracic epidural blockade complicating interscalene brachial plexus block: A case report of two cases. *Anesthesiology* 1971;35:650–652.
73. Scammell SJ. Inadvertent epidural anaesthesia as a complication of interscalene brachial plexus block. *Anaesth Intensive Care* 1979;7:56–57.
74. Lombard TP, Couper JL. Bilateral spread of analgesia following interscalene brachial plexus block. *Anesthesiology* 1983;58:472–473.
75. Evans JA, Dobben GD, Gay GR. Peridural effusion of drugs following sympathetic blockade. *JAMA* 1967;200:93–98.
76. Moore DC. *Complications of Regional Anesthesia.* Springfield IL: Charles C. Thomas, 1955:53–54.
77. Middaugh RE, Menk EJ, Reynolds WJ, et al. Epidural block using large volumes of local anesthetic solution for intercostal nerve block. *Anesthesiology* 1985;63:214–216.
78. Krempen JS, Smith B, DeFreest LJ. Selective nerve root infiltration for the evaluation of sciatica. *Orthop Clin North Am* 1975;6:311–315.
79. Blikra G. Intradural herniated lumbar disc. *J Neurosurg* 1969; 31:676–679.
80. Cheng PA. The anatomical and clinical aspects of epidural anesthesia. *Anesth Analg* 1963;42:398–415.
81. Hardy PAJ. Can epidural catheters penetrate dura mater? An anatomic study. *Anaesthesia* 1986;41:1145–1147.
82. Fink BR, Walker S. Orientation of fibers in human dorsal lumbar dura mater in relation to lumbar puncture. *Anesth Analg* 1989;69:768–772.
83. Bernards C, Hill H. Morphine and alfentanil permeability through the spinal dura, arachnoid and pia mater of dogs and monkeys. *Anesthesiology* 1990;73:1214–1219.
84. Patin DJ, Eckstein EC, Harum K, Pallares VS. Anatomic and biochemical properties of human lumbar dura mater. *Anesth Analg* 1993;76:535–540.
85. Reitan H. On movements of fluid inside the cerebrospinal space. *Acta Radiol* 1941;22:762–779.
86. Scott WG, Furlow LT. Myelography with Pantopaque and a new technique for its removal. *Radiology* 1944;43:241–249.
87. Epstein BS. The effect of increased interspinal pressure on the movement of iodized oil within the spinal canal. *Am J Roentgen* 1944;52:196–199.
88. Martins BS, Wiley JK, Myers PW. Dynamics of the cerebrospinal fluid and the spinal dura mater. *J Neurol Neurosurg Psychiat* 1972;35:468–473.
89. Watanabe S, Yamaguchi H, Ishizawa Y. Level of spinal anesthesia can be predicted by the cerebrospinal fluid pressure difference between full-flexed and non-full-flexed lateral position. *Anesth Analg* 1991;73:391–393.
90. Reina MA, de Leon Casasola O, Lopez A, et al. The origin of the spinal subdural space: Ultrastructure findings. *Anesth Analg* 2002;94:991–995.
91. Shantha TR. Subdural space: What is it? Does it exist? *Reg Anesth* 17, S 1992;5.
92. Mehta M, Maher R. Injection into the extra-arachnoid subdural space. *Anaesthesia* 1977;32:760–766.
93. Rubin RC, Henderson ES, Ommaya A, et al. The production of cerebrospinal fluid in man and its modification by acetazolamide. *J Neurosurg* 1966;25:430–436.
94. Cuttler RWP, Page L, Galicich PJ, Watters GV. Formation and absorption of cerebrospinal fluid in man. *Brain* 1968;91:707–720.
95. Milhorat TH. The third circulation revisited. *J Neurosurg* 1975;42:628–645.
96. Oreskovic D, Whitton PS, Lupret V. Effect of intracranial pressure on cerebrospinal fluid formation in isolated brain ventricles. *Neuroscience* 1991;41:773–777.
97. Welch K, Pollay M. Perfusion of particles through arachnoid villi of monkey. *Am J Physiol* 1961;201:651–654.
98. Gomez DG, Potts DG. The surface characteristics of arachnoid granulations. *Arch Neurol* 1974;31:88–93.
99. Levine JE, Povlishock JT, Becker DP. The morphological correlates of primate cerebrospinal fluid absorption. *Brain Res* 1982;241:31–41.
100. Gilland O. Normal cerebrospinal pressure. *N Engl J Med* 1969;280:904–905.
101. Enzmann DR, Pelc NJ. Normal flow patterns of intracranial and spinal cerebrospinal fluid defined with phase-contrast cine MR imaging. *Radiology* 1991;178:467–474.
102. DiChiro G. Observations on the circulation of the cerebrospinal fluid. *Acta Radiol* 1966;5:988–1002.
103. Hogan QH, Prost R, Kulier A, et al. Magnetic resonance imaging of cerebrospinal fluid volume and the influence of body habitus and abdominal pressure. *Anesthesiology* 1996;84:1341–1349.
104. Sullivan JT, Grouper S, Walker MT, et al. Lumbosacral cerebrospinal fluid volume in humans using three-dimensional magnetic resonance imaging. *Anesth Analg* 2006;103:1306–1310.
105. Carpenter RL, Liu S, Hogan Q, Crane B. Lumbosacral CSF volume is the primary determinate of sensory block height and duration of spinal anesthesia. *Anesthesiology* 1998;89:24–29.
106. Higuchi H, Adachi Y, Kazama T. The influence of lumbosacral cerebrospinal fluid volume on extent and duration of hyperbaric bupivacaine spinal anesthesia: A comparison between seated and lateral decubitus injection positions. *Anesth Analg* 2005;101:555–560.
107. Lentner C. *Geigy Scientific Tables*, Vol. 1, 8th ed. Basle: Ciba-Geigy Limited, 1981:165–177.
108. Jirout J. *Pneumomyelography*, 2nd ed. Springfield IL: Charles C. Thomas, 1969:27–41.
109. DiChiro G, Timins EL. Supine myelography and the septum posticum. *Radiology* 1974;111:319–327.
110. Nauta HJW, Dolan E, Yasaargil MG. Microsurgical anatomy of spinal subarachnoid space. *Surg Neurol* 1983;19:431–437.
111. Osaka K, Hanada H. Matsumoto S, Yasuda M. Development of the cerebrospinal fluid pathway in the normal and abnormal human embryos. *Child's Brain* 1980;6:26–38.
112. Tubbs RS, Salter G, Grabb PA, Oakes WJ. The denticulate ligament: Anatomy and functional significance. *J Neurosurg* 2001;94:271–275.
113. Teng P, Papatheodorou C. Spinal arachnoid diverticula. *Br J Radiol* 1966;39:249–254.
114. Teng P, Rudner N. Multiple arachnoid diverticula. *AMA Arch Neurol* 1960;2:348–356.
115. Cohen MK, Wall EJ, Brown RA, et al. Cauda equina anatomy II; extrathecal nerve roots and dorsal root ganglia. *Spine* 1990;15:1248–1251.
116. Brierley JB. The penetration of particulate matter form the cerebrospinal fluid into the spinal ganglia, peripheral nerves, and perivascular spaces of the central nervous system. *J Neurol Neursurg Psychiat* 1950;13:203–215.
117. Basmajian JV. The depressions for the arachnoid granulations as a criterion of age. *Anat Rec* 1952;112:843–846.
118. Grossman CB, Potts DG. Arachnoid granulations: Radiology and anatomy. *Radiology* 1974;113:95–100.
119. Shanatha TR, Evans JA. The relationship of epidural anesthesia to neural membranes and arachnoid villi. *Anesthesiology* 1972;37:543–557.
120. McCabe JS, Low FN. The subarachnoid angle: An area of transition in peripheral nerve. *Anat Rec* 1969;164:15–34.
121. Haller FB, Haller AC, Low FN. The fine structure of cellular layers and connective tissue space at spinal nerve root attachments in the rat. *Anat Rec* 1972;133:109–124.
122. Brierley JB, Field EJ. The fate of intraneural injection as demonstrated by the use of radio-active phosphorus. *J Neurol Neurosurg Psychiat* 1949;12:86–99.
123. Moore DC, Hain RF, Ward A, Bridenbaugh LD. Importance of the perineural spaces in nerve blocking. *JAMA* 1954;156:1050–1053.
124. Sullivan WE, Mortensen OA. Visualization of the movement of a brominized oil along peripheral nerves. *Anat Rec* 1934;59:493–501.
125. French JD, Strain WH, Jones GE. Mode of extension of contrast substances injected into peripheral nerves. *J Neuropath Exp Neurol* 1948;7:47–58.
126. Selander D, Sjostrand J. Longitudinal spread of intraneurally injected local anesthetics. *Acta Anaesthesiol Scand* 1978;22:622–634.
127. Brierley JB, Field EJ. The connections of the spinal sub-arachnoid space with the lymphatic system. *J Anat* 1948;82:153–166.
128. Hassin GB. Villi (Pacchionian bodies) of the spinal arachnoid. *Arch Neurol Psychiat* 1930;23:65–78.

129. Himango WA, Low FN. The fine structure of a lateral recess of the subarachnoid space in the rat. *Anat Rec* 1971;171:1–20.

130. Bernards CM, Hill HF. The spinal nerve root sleeve is not a preferred route for redistribution of drugs from the epidural space to the spinal cord. *Anesthesiology* 1991;75:827–832.

131. Nabors M, Pait TG, Byrd EB, et al. Updated assessment and current classification of spinal meningeal cysts. *J Neurosurg* 1988;68:366–377.

132. Gortvai P. Extradural cysts of the spinal canal. *J Neurol Neurosurg Psychiat* 1963;26:223–230.

133. Tarlov IM. *Sacral Nerve Root Cysts: Another Cause of the Sciatic or Cauda Equina Syndrome.* Springfield IL: Charles C. Thomas, 1953.

134. Smith DT. Cystic formations associated with human spinal nerve roots. *J Neurosurg* 1961;18:654–660.

135. Larsen JL, Smith D, Fossan G. Arachnoid diverticula and cystlike dilatations of the nerve-root sheaths in lumbar myelography. *Acta Radiol [Diag]* 1980; 21:141–145.

136. North RB, Kidd DH, Wang H. Occult, bilateral anterior sacral and intrasacral meningeal and perineural cysts: Case report and review of the literature. *Neurosurgery* 1990;27:981–986.

137. Thomas M, Halaby FA, Hirschauer JS. Hereditary occurrence of anterior sacral meningocele: Report of ten cases. *Spine* 1987;12:351–354.

138. Holt S, Yates PO. Cervical nerve root "cysts." *Brain* 1964;87:481–490.

139. Lindblom K. The subarachnoid spaces of the root sheaths in the lumbar region. *Acta Radiol* 1948;30:419–426.

140. Hemminghytt S, Daniels DL, Williams AL, Haughton VM. Intraspinal synovial cysts: Natural history and diagnosis by CT. *Radiology* 1982;145:375–376.

141. Knox AM, Fon GT. The appearances of lumbar intraspinal synovial cysts. *Clin Radiol* 1991;44:397–401.

142. Barson AJ, Sands J. Regional and segmental characteristics of the human adult spinal cord. *J Anat* 1977;123:797–803.

143. McCotter RE. Regarding the length and extent of the human medulla spinalis. *Anat Rec* 1916;26:559–564.

144. Needles JH. The caudal level of termination of the spinal cord in whites and Negroes. *Anat Rec* 1935;63:417–425.

145. Reimann AF, Anson BJ. Vertebral level of termination of the spinal cord with report of a case of sacral cord. *Anat Rec* 1944;88:127–138.

146. Muhle C, Wiskirchen J, Weinert D, et al. Biomechanical aspects of the subarachnoid space and cervical cord in healthy individuals examined with kinematic magnetic resonance imaging. *Spine* 1998;23:556–567.

147. Fettes PDW, Leslie K, McNabb S, Smith PJ. Effect of spinal flexion on the conus medullaris. *Anaesthesia* 2006;61:521–523.

148. Takiguchi T, Yamaguchi S, Okuda Y, Kitajima T. Deviation of the cauda equina by changing position. *Anesthesiology* 100:754–755.

149. Witkamp TD, Vandertop WP, Beek FJA, et al. Medullary cone motion in subjects with a normal spinal cord and in patients with a tethered cord. *Radiology* 2001;220:208–212.

150. Hogan QH. Size of human lower thoracic and lumbosacral nerve roots. *Anesthesiology* 1996;85:37–42.

151. Sunderland S. Avulsion of nerve roots. In: *Handbook of Clinical Neurology*, Vol. 25. Vinken PJ, Bruyn GW, eds. New York: Elsevier, 1975:393–435.

152. Fink BR, Gerlach R, Maravilla KR, Richards T. Postural mobility of cauda equina: Evidence from fast sequence magnetic resonance imaging (MRI). *Anesthesiology* 1993;79:28.

153. Pallie W. The intersegmental anastomoses of posterior spinal rootlets and their significance. *J Neurosurg* 1959;16:188–196.

154. Pallie W, Manuel JK. Intersegmental anastomoses between dorsal spinal rootlets in some vertebrates. *Acta Anat* 1968;70:341–351.

155. Kadish LJ, Simmons EH. Anomalies of the lumbosacral nerve roots. *J Bone Jnt Surg* 1984;66B:411–416.

156. Kikuchi S, Hasue M, Nishiyama K, Ito T. Anatomic and clinical studies of radicular symptoms. *Spine* 1984;9:23–30.

157. Nitta H, Tajima T, Sugiyama H, Moriyama A. Study of dermatomes by means of selective lumbar spinal nerve block. *Spine* 1993;13:1782–1786.

158. Neidre A, MacNab I. Anomalies of the lumbosacral nerve roots: Review of 16 cases and classification. *Spine* 1983;8:294–299.

159. Abram SE, Yi J, Fuchs A, Hogan QH. Permeability of injured and intact peripheral nerves and dorsal root ganglia. *Anesthesiology* 2006;105:146–153.

160. Kerr FWL. A mechanism to account for frontal headache in cases of posterior-fossa tumors. *J Neurosurg* 1961;18:605–609.

161. Kuhn RA. Organization of tactile dermatomes in cat and monkey. *J Neurophysiol* 1953;16:169–182.

162. Foerster O. The dermatomes in man. *Brain* 1933;56:1–39.

163. Denny-Brown D, Kirk EJ, Yanagisawa N. The tract of Lissauer in relation to sensory transmission in the dorsal horn of spinal cord in the macaque monkey. *J Comp Neurol* 1973;151:157–199.

164. Bonica JJ. *The Management of Pain*, 2nd ed. Philadelphia: Lea and Febiger, 1990:133–146.

165. Keegan JJ, Garrett FD. The segmental distribution of the cutaneous nerves in the limbs of man. *Anat Rec* 1948;102:409–437.

166. Liguori R, Drarup C, Trojaborg W. Determination of the segmental sensory and motor innervation of the lumbosacral spinal nerves. *Brain* 1992;115:915–935.

167. Young A, Getty J, Jackson A, et al. Variations in the pattern of muscle innervation by the L5 and S1 nerve roots. *Spine* 1983;6:616–624.

168. Stilwell DL. The nerve supply of the vertebral column and its associated structures in the monkey. *Anat Rec* 1956;125:139–162.

169. Edgar MA, Ghadially JA. Innervation of the lumbar spine. *Clin Orthop Related Res* 1976;115:35–41.

170. Bogduk N. The innervation of the lumbar spine. *Spine* 1983;8:286–293.

171. Forsythe WB, Ghoshal NG. Innervation of the canine thoracolumbar vertebral column. *Anat Rec* 1984;208:57–63.

172. Groen GJ, Baljet B, Drukker J. Nerves and nerve plexuses of the human vertebral column. *Am J Anat* 1990;188:282–296.

173. Giles LGF, Taylor JR. Human zygapophyseal joint capsule and synovial fold innervation. *Br J Rheumatol* 1987;26:93–98.

174. Jiang H, Russell G, Raso J, et al. The nature and distribution of the innervation of human supraspinal and interspinal ligaments. *Spine* 1995;20:869–876.

175. Gillette RG, Kramis RC, Roberts WJ. Spinal projections of cat primary fibers innervating lumbar facet joints and multifidus muscle. *Neurosci Lett* 1993;157:67–71.

176. Edgar MA, Nundy S. Innervation of the spinal dura mater. *J Neurol Neurosurg Psychiat* 1966;29:530–534.

177. Kojima Y, Maeda T, Arai R, Shichicawa K. Nerve supply to the posterior longitudinal ligament and the intervertebral disc of the rat vertebral column as studied by acetylcholinesterase histochemistry. II. Regional differences in the distribution of the nerve fibers and their origins. *A Anat* 1990;169:247–255.

178. Kimmel DL. Innervation of spinal dura mater and dura mater of the posterior cranial fossa. *Neurology* 1961;11:800–809.

179. Bogduk N, Tynan W, Wilson AS. The nerve supply to the human lumbar intervertebral discs. *A Anat* 1981;132:39–56.

180. Kojima Y, Maeda T, Arai R, Shichicawa K. Nerve supply to the posterior longitudinal ligament and the intervertebral disc of the rat vertebral column as studied by acetylcholinesterase histochemistry. I Distribution in the lumbar region. *A Anat* 1990;169:237–246.

181. Sinohara H. Lumbar disc lesion with special reference to the histological significance of nerve endings of the lumbar discs. *J Jap Orthop Assoc* 1970;44:553–570.

182. Coppes MH, Marini E, Thomeer RTWM, et al. Innervation of annulus fibrosis in low back pain. *Lancet* 1990;336:189–190.

183. Groen GJ, Baljet B, Drukker J. The innervation of the spinal dura mater: Anatomy and clinical implications. *Acta Neurochir* 1988;92:39–46.

184. Korkala O, Gronblad M, Liesi P, Karaharju E. Immunohistochemical demonstration of nociceptors in the ligamentous structures of the lumbar spine. *Spine* 1985;10:156–157.

185. Konttinen Y, Gronblad M, Antti-Poika I, et al. Neuroimmunohistochemical analysis of peridiscal nociceptive neural elements. *Spine* 1990;15:383–386.

186. Edvinsson L, Rosedal-Helgesen S, Uddman R. Substance P: Localization, concentration and release in cerebral arteries, choroid plexus and dura mater. *Cell Tissue Res* 1983;234:1–7.

187. Dalsgaard CJ, Risling M, Cuello C. Immunohistochemical localization of substance P in the lumbosacral spinal pia mater and ventral roots of the cat. *Brain Res* 1982;246:168–171.

188. El-Bohy A, Cavanaugh JM, Getchell ML, et al. Localization of substance P and neurofilament immunoreactive fibers in the lumbar facet joint capsule and supraspinous ligament of the rabbit. *Brain Res* 1988;460:379–382.

189. Ashton IK, Ashton BA, Gibson SJ, et al. Morphological basis for back pain: The demonstration of nerve fibers and neuropeptides in the lumbar facet joint capsule but not in ligamentum flavum. *J Orthop Res* 1992;10:72–78.

190. Gronblad M, Korkala O, Konttinen YT, et al. Silver impregnation and immunohistochemical study of nerves in lumbar facet joint plical tissue. *Spine* 1991;16:34–38.

191. Cavanaugh JM, El-Bohy A, Hardy WN, et al. Sensory innervation of soft tissues of the lumbar spine in the rat. *J Ortho Res* 1989;7:378–388.

192. Yamashita T, Cavanaugh JM, El-Bohy AA, et al. Mechanosensitive afferent units in the lumbar facet joint. *J Bone Jnt Surg* 1990;72A:865–870.

193. Bahns E, Ernsberger U, Janig W, Nelke A. Discharge properties of mechanosensitive afferents supplying the retroperitoneal space. *Pfluggers Arch* 1986;407:519–525.

194. Gillette RG, Kramis RC, Roberts WJ. Characterization of spinal somatosensory neurons having receptive fields in lumbar tissues of cats. *Pain* 1993;54:85–98.

195. Habler HJ, Janig W, Klotzenberg M, McMahon SB. A quantitative study of the central projection patterns of unmyelinated ventral root afferents in the cat. *J Physiol* 1990;422:265–287.

196. Edgar MA, Ghadially JA. Innervation of the lumbar spine. *Clin Orthop Related Res* 1976;115:35–41.

197. Kellgren JH. On the distribution of pain arising from deep somatic structures with charts of segmental pain areas. *Clin Sci* 1939;4:35–46.

198. Sinclair DC, Feindel WH, Weddell G, Falconer MA. The intervertebral ligaments as a source of segmental pain. *J Bone Jnt Surg* 1948;30B:515–521.
199. Hockaday JM, Whitty CWM. Patterns of referred pain in the normal subject. *Brain* 1967;90:481–496.
200. Mooney V, Robertson J. The facet syndrome. *Clin Orthop Rel Res* 1976;115:149–156.
201. McCall IW, Park WM, O'Brien JP. Induced pain referral from posterior lumbar elements in normal subjects. *Spine* 1979;4:441–446.
202. El-Mahdi MA, Latif FYA, Janko M. The spinal nerve root "innervation", and a new concept of the clinicopathological interrelations in back pain and sciatica. *Neurochirurgia* 1981;24:137–141.
203. Falconer MA, McGeorge M, Begg AC. Observations on the cause and mechanism of symptom-production in sciatica and low-back pain. *J Neurol Neurosurg Psychiatr* 1948;11:13–26.
204. Wiberg G. Back pain in relation to the nerve supply of the intervertebral disc. *Acta Orthop* 1949;19:211–221.
205. Frykholm R, Hyde J, Norlen G, Skoglund CR. On pain sensations produced by stimulation of ventral roots in man. *Acta Physiol Scand* S 1953;06:455–467.
206. Fernstrom U. A discographical study of ruptured lumbar intervertebral discs. *Acta Chir Scand* S 1960;58:10–60.
207. Murphey F. Sources and patterns of pain in disc disease. *Clin Neurosurg* 1968;15:343–351.
208. Kuslich SD, Ulstrom CL. The tissue origin of low back pain and sciatica: A report of pain response to tissue stimulation during operations on the lumbar spine using local anesthesia. *Orthop Clin N Am* 1991;22:181–187.
209. Smyth MJ, Wright V. Sciatica and the intervertebral disc. *J Bone Jnt Surg* 40 1958;40A:1401–1418.
210. Janig W, McLachlan EM. Identification of distinct topographical distribution of lumbar sympathetic and sensory neurons projecting to end organs with different functions in the cat. *J Comp Neurol* 1986;246:104–112.
211. Gillette RG, Kramis RC, Roberts WJ. Sympathetic activation of cat spinal neurons responsive to noxious stimulation of deep tissues in the low back. *Pain* 1994;56:31–42.
212. Walker AE, Nulson F. Electrical stimulation of the upper thoracic portion of the sympathetic chain in man. *Arch Neurol Psychiatry* 1948;59:559–560.
213. Sluijter ME. The use of radiofrequency lesions for pain relief in failed back patients. *Int Disabil Studies* 1988;10:37–43.
214. Echlin F. Pain responses on stimulation of the lumbar sympathetic chain under local anesthesia. *J Neurosurg* 1949;6:530–533.
215. Hromada J. On the nerve supply of the connective tissue of some peripheral nervous system components. *Acta Anat* 1963;55:343–351.
216. Clark SL. Innervation of the pia mater of the spinal cord and medulla. *J Comp Neurol* 1931;53:129–141.
217. Raine CS, Brown AM, McFarlin DE. Heterotopic regeneration of peripheral nerve fibers into the subarachnoid space. *J Neurocytol* 1982;11:109–118.
218. Holm S, Nachemson A. Variations in the nutrition of the canine intervertebral disc induced by motion. *Spine* 1983;8:866–874.
219. Tyrrell AR, Reilly T, Troup JDG. Circadian variation in stature and the effects of spinal loading. *Spine* 1985;10:161–164.
220. Dommisse GF. The arteries, arterioles, and capillaries of the spinal cord. *Ann Royal Coll Surg* 1980;62:369–376.
221. Parke WW, Gammell K, Rothman RH. Arterial vascularization of the cauda equina. *J Bone Jnt Surg* 1981;63A:53–62.
222. Koyanagi I, Tator CH, Lea PJ. Three-dimensional analysis of the vascular system in the rat spinal cord with scanning electron microscopy of vascular corrosion casts. Part 1: Normal spinal cord. *Neurosurgery* 1993;33:277–284.
223. Woollam DHM, Millen JW. The arterial supply of the spinal cord and its significance. *J Neurol Neurosurg Psychiat* 1955;18:97–102.
224. Lazorthes G, Gouaze A, Zadeh JO, et al. Arterial vascularization of the spinal cord: Recent studies of the anastomotic substitution pathways. *J Neurosurg* 1971;35:253–262.
225. Fried LC, Doppman JL, DiChiro G. Direction of blood flow in the primate cervical spinal cord. *J Neurosurg* 1970;33:325–330.
226. DiChiro G, Fried LC. Blood flow currents in spinal cord arteries. *Neurology* 1971;21:1088–1096.
227. Suh TH, Alexander L. Vascular system of the human spinal cord. *Arch Neurol Psychiatry* 1939;41:660–676.
228. Dommisse GF. *The Arteries and Veins of the Human Spinal Cord from Birth.* New York: Livingstone, 1975.
229. Ross RT. Spinal cord infarction in disease and surgery of the aorta. *Can J Neurol Sci* 1985;12:289–295.
230. Savander SJ, Williams GM, Trerotola SO, et al. Preoperative spinal artery localization and its relationship to postoperative neurologic complications. *Radiology* 1993;189:165–171.
231. Krogh E. The effect of acute hypoxia on the motor cells of the spinal cord. *Acta Physiol Scand* 1950;20:263–292.
232. Giles FH, Nag D. Vulnerability of human spinal cord in transient cardiac arrest. *Neurology* 1971;21:833–839.
233. Silver JR, Buxton PH. Spinal stroke. *Brain* 1974;97:539–550.
234. Gelfan S, Tarlov IM. Differential vulnerability of spinal cord structures to anoxia. *J Neurophysiol* 1955;18:170–188.
235. Harreveld AV, Schade JP. Nerve cell destruction by asphyxiation of the spinal cord. *J Neuropath Exp Neurol* 1962;21:410–423.
236. Fried LC, Aparicio O. Experimental ischemia of the spinal cord. *Neurology* 1973;23:289–293.
237. Turnbull IM. Blood supply of the spinal cord: Normal and pathological considerations. *Clin Neurosurg* 1972;20:56–84.
238. Dommisse GF. *The Arteries and Veins of the Human Spinal Cord from Birth.* New York: Livingstone, 1975:19.
239. Mawad ME, Rivera V, Crawford S, et al. Spinal cord ischemia after resection of thoracoabdominal aortic aneurysms: MR findings in 24 patients. *Am J Roentgen* 1990;155:1303–1307.
240. Rydevik B, Brown MD, Lundborg F. Pathoanatomy and pathophysiology of nerve root compression. *Spine* 1984;9:7–15.
241. Yoshizawa H, Kobayashi S, Hachiya Y. Blood supply of nerve roots and dorsal root ganglia. *Ortho Clin N Am* 1991;22:195–211.
242. Rydevik B, Holm S, Brown MD, Lundborg G. Diffusion from the cerebrospinal fluid as a nutritional pathway for spinal nerve roots. *Acta Physiol Scand* 1990;138:247–248.
243. Abrams HL. The vertebral and azygos venous systems, and some variations in systemic venous return. *Radiology* 1957;69:508–526.
244. Batson OV. The function of the vertebral veins and their role in the spread of metastases. *Ann Surg* 1940;112:138–149.
245. Dommisse GF. *The Arteries and Veins of the Human Spinal Cord from Birth.* New York: Livingstone, 1975:90–92.
246. Herlihy WF. Revision of the venous system: The role of the vertebral veins. *Med J Australia* 1947;1:661–672.
247. Coman DR, DeLong RP. The role of the vertebral venous system in the metastasis of cancer to the spinal column. *Cancer* 1951;4:610–618.
248. Anderson R. Diodrast studies of the vertebral and cranial venous systems. *J Neurosurg* 1951;8:411–422.
249. Nordenstrom B. A method of angiography of the azygos vein and the anterior internal venous plexus of the spine. *Acta Radiol* 1955;44:201–298.
250. Helander CG, Lindbom A. Sacrolumbar venography. *Acta Radiol* 1955;44:410–416.
251. Schobinger RA, Krueger EG, Sobel GL. Comparison of intraosseous vertebral venography and Pantopaque myelography in the diagnosis of surgical conditions of the lumbar spine and nerve roots. *Radiology* 1961;77:376–397.
252. Gershater R, St. Louis EL. Lumbar epidural venography. *Radiology* 1979;131:409–421.
253. Crock HV, Yoshizawa H. *The Blood Supply of the Vertebral Column and Spinal Cord in Man.* New York: Springer-Verlag, 1977; 51.
254. Meijenhorst GCH. Computed tomography of the lumbar epidural veins. *Radiology* 1982;145:687–691.
255. Watanabe R, Parke WW. Vascular and neural pathology of lumbosacral spinal stenosis. *J Neurosurg* 1986;64:64–70.
256. Olmarker K, Rydevik B, Holm S. Edema formation in spinal nerve roots induced by experimental graded compression. *Spine* 1989;14:569–573.
257. Parke WW. The significance of venous return impairment in ischemic radiculopathy and myelopathy. *Ortho Clin N Am* 1991;22:213–221.
258. Hoyland JA, Freemont AJ, Jayson MIV. Intervertebral foramen venous obstruction: A cause of periradicular fibrosis? *Spine* 1989;15:558–569.
259. Nohara Y, Brown MD, Eurell JC. Lymphatic drainage of epidural space in rabbits. *Ortho Clin N Am* 1991;22:189–194.
260. Durant PAC, Yaksh TL. Distribution in spinal fluid, blood, and lymph of epidurally injected morphine and inulin in dogs. *Anesth Analg* 1986;65:583–592.
261. Saal JA, Saal JS, Herzog RJ. The natural history of lumbar intervertebral disc extrusions treated nonoperatively. *Spine* 1990;15:683–686.
262. Bush K, Cowen N, Katz DE, Gishen P. The natural history of sciatica associated with disc pathology. *Spine* 1991;17, 1205–1212.
263. DiGiovanni AL, Galbert MW, Wahle WM. Epidural injection of autologous blood for post lumbar-puncture headache. II. Additional clinical experiences and laboratory investigation. *Anesth Analg* 1972;51:276–232.

CHAPTER 10 ■ SPINAL (SUBARACHNOID) BLOCKADE

MIKKO PITKÄNEN

HISTORY

Spinal anesthesia creates an intense sensory and motor block that can effectively be achieved with a small amount of local anesthetic. In the late nineteenth century, soon after the discovery of the local anesthetic properties of cocaine, spinal anesthesia was introduced into clinical practice. In the first experiments and clinical use, the local anesthetic used was cocaine (Table 10-1) (1). The use of spinal cocaine caused a high frequency of central nervous system (CNS) side effects, muscle spasms, and pain. Therefore, the use of spinal anesthesia was limited to a few enthusiasts until safer local anesthetics—procaine (2) and later tetracaine (3)—caused a widespread interest in its use. In the ensuing years, the popularity of spinal blockade has waxed and waned. The development of modern general anesthesia using muscle relaxants and an endotracheal tube, together with the fear of neurologic complications, decreased the interest in spinal anesthesia in 1940s and 1950s (6). As operations became more radical, their duration and extensiveness were often incompatible with spinal anesthesia. Dedicated enthusiasts, however, continued to use the method and believe in its safety (7), and, about 40 years ago, spinal anesthesia started to regain its place in anesthesia care. Since the 1980s, modern disposable needles and especially the use of bupivacaine has greatly increased the interest in spinal anesthesia in many countries (8,9). The fact that general anesthesia also has its risks and problems has made spinal anesthesia a valuable option for surgery of the lower abdomen and extremities. It is used in short ambulatory procedures as a restricted saddle block or as unilateral anesthesia to provide a fast, limited, short-lasting, and reliable anesthesia with good-quality postoperative pain relief (10). Combined spinal anesthesia with epidural catheter (CSE) is widely used for anesthesia in obstetrics and vascular and orthopedic surgery (11). Continuous spinal anesthesia (CSA) using a spinal catheter can be used in hemodynamically unstable patients, for complicated operations lasting for several hours, and may be continued for postoperative pain relief (12).

INDICATIONS

All operations in the lower abdomen, perineum, and lower extremities can be performed under spinal anesthesia. The spinal anesthesia technique and dose, and the properties of the local anesthetic can be adapted to obtain optimal spread and duration of the anesthesia for the planned surgery.

Specifically, spinal anesthesia is appropriate in patients who choose to remain conscious or whose medical condition requires consciousness during the surgery, but who still need high-quality anesthesia. Patients with respiratory problems or difficult airways may not need an endotracheal tube if spinal anaesthesia is employed. The risk of vomiting and aspiration is diminished (but not eliminated) during spinal anesthesia. A full stomach is not as great a risk as with general anesthesia because the conscious patient may be able to protect the airway, but because of the possibility of untoward reactions or inadequate block needing deep sedation or conversion to general anesthesia with endotracheal intubation, the same guidelines for preoperative fasting should be used as with general anesthesia. In cesarean section, the benefits of spinal anesthesia or the CSE technique are well verified. Endoscopic urologic procedures have a risk of hypervolemia secondary to absorption of irrigating fluid causing transurethral resection (TUR) syndrome; the changes in mental status caused by TUR syndrome can be better observed during spinal anesthesia.

Cholecystectomies and gastrectomies have successfully been performed under spinal anesthesia. However, upper abdominal operations require a T4 level of sensory anesthesia. As a safety margin, the upper level should be still higher, and some unwanted reflexes may appear; thus, spinal anesthesia as a sole anesthetic technique for these operations. It can and has been used as an adjunct that enables lighter general anesthesia. In cardiac surgery, the use of intrathecal narcotics enables faster recovery (13). High spinal anesthesia (37.5 mg of bupivacaine) with general anesthesia has caused less β-receptor dysfunction and a lower stress response during coronary artery bypass graft surgery (14). For renal transplant surgery, combined spinal–epidural anesthesia has been as safe and as well tolerated as general anesthesia (15). An extreme example of the use of spinal anesthesia is a patient with severe lung disease who successfully underwent a laparoscopic cholecystectomy under segmental subarachnoid (spinal) anaesthesia performed at the low thoracic level (16).

In lower extremity surgery, peripheral blocks are used with increasing frequency for surgical anesthesia. Spinal anesthesia has the advantage of being simpler and more rapidly induced, the tolerance of a tourniquet is better, and it is also suitable for bilateral procedures. The number and complexity of nerve blocks needed for good anesthesia for operations on the knees, thigh, and hip are so great that spinal anesthesia is often the preferred technique.

CONTRAINDICATIONS

Contraindications for spinal anesthesia are classified usually as absolute or relative. Absolute contraindications are:

TABLE 10-1

MILESTONES OF SPINAL ANESTHESIA

1899	Bier (Germany) Cocaine spinal anesthesia (1)
1905	Braun (Germany) Procaine spinal anesthesia (2)
1935	Sise (USA) Tetracaine spinal anesthesia (3)
1940	Lemmon (USA) Continuous spinal anesthesia (4)
1949	Gordh (Sweden) Lidocaine spinal anesthesia (5)
1954	Woolley and Roe case (United Kingdom) Report of paraplegia in association with spinal anesthesia (6)
1954	Dripps and Vandam (USA) Absence of neurologic sequelae (7)
1966	Ekblom (Sweden) Bupivacaine spinal anesthesia (8)

■ Patient's refusal despite adequate information. There are several indications for which spinal anesthesia would be a better choice than general anesthesia, but rarely is general anesthesia absolutely contraindicated and, in those cases, the patient usually understands the need for regional anesthesia and accepts the choice.
■ Infections at the site of injection. No needle should pass through an infected area before entering into the subarachnoid space.
■ Dermatologic conditions (e.g., psoriasis) that preclude aseptic preparation of the skin at the site of injection.
■ Septicemia or bacteremia. In these circumstances, the infection may spread to the CNS. Central neuronal block is not recommended in patients with untreated systemic infection; however, if appropriate antibiotic therapy has been initiated, patients who have shown a response to therapy may safely undergo single-dose spinal anesthesia (17).
■ Shock or severe hypovolemia. Since spinal anesthesia causes sympathetic block and vasodilatation, the hypotension in a hypovolemic patient may cause severe problems.
■ Abnormality in blood clotting mechanism (see Chapter 12).
■ Increased intracranial pressure. Because of lumbar puncture, the pressure of cerebrospinal fluid (CSF) in the spine may be lowered; therefore, the high intracranial pressure may cause herniation of the medullary vasomotor and respiratory centers.
■ Lack of skill in spinal anesthesia.
■ Allergy to local anesthetics. This is extremely rare, and usually another choice of local anesthetic is available.

Relative contraindications include:

■ Deformities of the spinal column (spinal stenosis, severe arthritis, severe kyphoscoliosis, ankylosing spondylitis). These may cause difficulties in finding the subarachnoid space. Multiple punctures increase the risk of bleeding in the epidural space and, indeed, spinal stenosis was found to be a risk factor for spinal hematoma (18).
■ Preexisting disease of the spinal cord. The hypothesis is that abnormal nervous tissue is more susceptible to the neurotoxicity of local anesthetics than normal nervous tissue. There are no objective data, but common sense and medicolegal considerations make it prudent to avoid spinal anesthesia in patients with progressive disease involving the cord. Otherwise, the progression of the disease may be blamed on the spinal anesthetic. However, if the neurologic status is stable and there is a common agreement with the patient about the risks and benefits of regional anesthesia, no contraindication exists to proceeding with spinal anesthesia. There are several

case reports on the safe use of spinal anesthesia in patients with postpolio syndrome or multiple sclerosis (19,20).
■ Chronic headache or backache. These can sometimes be aggravated by spinal anesthesia; however, if sufficient information is provided and agreement about the procedure is obtained from the patient, spinal anesthesia can be safely used.
■ Inability to achieve a spinal tap in three attempts. One should either abandon spinal anesthesia or obtain the help of a more experienced anesthesiologist.
■ Certain cardiac diseases. Marked aortic stenosis is considered a contraindication to spinal anesthesia. The sympathetic block and vasodilatation causes a sudden decrease in systemic vascular resistance that may lead to a profound decrease in coronary perfusion. However, if only a limited block or continuous techniques with the possibility to titrate the dose carefully are used, spinal anesthesia can safely be used even in patients with aortic stenosis (21).
■ Tattoo on the back. The recent trend of having tattoos in the lumbar area can cause a concern if the needle has to pass through pigmented tissue. It is possible that the needle may transfer pieces of the pigment into the subarachnoid space. This could theoretically cause inflammation or a granulomatous response. Naturally, the tattoo should not be punctured, and usually there is pigment-free skin in another interspace or paramedially where the needle can be passed. Use of an introducer needle does not abolish this risk. If the pigmented skin must be punctured, a small superficial skin incision before introducing the needle has been suggested (22). A good practice may also be to allow some drops of CSF to drip from the needle before injecting the anesthetic.

PHARMACOLOGY

Local Anesthetics

Almost all local anesthetics have also been used at some point in spinal anesthesia. This chapter concentrates on their special properties in the subarachnoid space and on possible factors that influence the spread and duration of spinal anesthesia (Table 10-2).

The spinal nerves in the subarachnoid are without the protection of dura mater and arachnoid membranes, since only a thin layer of pia mater covers them. Thus they are more vulnerable to damage than are the peripheral nerves, which have extensions of dura and arachnoid with layers of connective tissues, fat cells, and blood vessels to protect them. The lack of this protection makes fast and intense block with a small amount of local anesthetic possible. On the other hand, it is also possible to produce irreversible injury by administering high concentrations of local anesthetic in a small area. This was observed when relative overdoses of hyperbaric lidocaine, 50 mg/mL, were used for continuous spinal anesthesia through microcatheters. The tip of the catheter was probably located caudally, and the local anesthetic accumulated in a small area and caused permanent neurologic damage (23). This happened even though lidocaine had been safely used for spinal anesthesia for almost 50 years.

Procaine

Procaine is a fast and short-acting local anesthetic. It was the first relatively safe and widely used spinal anesthetic. When the appearance of transient neurologic symptoms was associated

TABLE 10-2

DRUGS USED FOR SPINAL ANESTHESIA AND APPROXIMATE DURATIONS OF BLOCKS

Drug	Concentrations	Doses	Duration Th12	Ambulation
Bupivacaine	5–7.5 mg/mL	4 mg	60 min	2–3 h
		20 mg	3–4 h	7–8 h
Ropivacaine	5–10 mg/mL	7.5 mg	60 min	3 h
		15–20 mg	2–3 h	5–6 h
Levobupivacaine	5–7.5 mg/mL	5 mg	60 min	3 h
		20 mg	4 h	7–8 h
Lidocaine	20 mg/mL	60 mg	60 min	2–3 h
Tetracaine	5–10 mg/mL	6 mg	60 min	3 h
		16 mg	3 h	4–6 h
Procaine	5 mg/mL	75–200 mg	40–70 min	2–3 h
2–Chloroprocaine	10–20 mg/mL	40 mg	60 min	2 h
Prilocaine	20 mg/mL	50–80 mg	100 min	3–4 h
Articaine	30–40 mg/mL	60–80 mg	80 min	2–3 h

with lidocaine, procaine was again studied to see if it could replace lidocaine as a spinal anesthetic for ambulatory surgery. The transient neurologic symptoms (TNS) frequency with procaine is small, but unfortunately it causes a high frequency of nausea and the quality of the block is not adequate (24,25). The frequency of pruritus when it is used with fentanyl is high (26).

Lidocaine

Lidocaine, 50 mg/mL, as a hyperbaric solution was widely used for spinal anesthesia since the 1950s. In the early 1990s, however, came reports of cauda equina syndrome when overdoses of anesthetic mixtures containing lidocaine were used for continuous spinal anesthesia through microcatheters (23). Soon thereafter, reports of transient radicular irritation (TRI), later called TNS, were published (27). In a prospective survey from France, 75% of the neurologic deficits after nontraumatic spinal anesthesia occurred in patients who had received hyperbaric lidocaine, 50 mg/mL, at a frequency of 14.4 per 10,000 (28). Plain lidocaine with a reduced concentration (20 mg/mL) and dose is still used. However, the incidence of TNS does not decrease even though the concentration of lidocaine is decreased to 5 mg/mL (29,30).

Tetracaine

Tetracaine was a popular and widely used spinal anesthetic but the amide local anesthetics have replaced it in many places. Tetracaine is long-acting, and epinephrine further increases its duration of action. It is perhaps not as reliable as bupivacaine (31). It does not prevent tourniquet pain as well as bupivacaine, and it seems to cause more hypotension than bupivacaine (32,33). The mechanism for these differences is unknown.

Bupivacaine

Bupivacaine is probably the most widely used spinal anesthetic (9). It is used as a 2.5 to 7.5 mg/mL concentration with and without glucose. Plain solution is often called *isobaric* but at body temperature it is *hypobaric*. Therefore the term *plain bupivacaine* instead of *isobaric bupivacaine* should be used for additive-free bupivacaine solutions. The duration and extent of anesthesia depend on the dose and baricity. Using a 4 mg hyperbaric solution, an ambulatory arthroscopy of the knee with

duration less than 1 hour and with rapid home discharge can be performed (34). On the other hand, using 20 mg plain solution provides anesthesia for bilateral knee arthroplasty with duration of 3 to 4 hours. The spread of plain bupivacaine solution is unpredictable (35). The later discussion of factors affecting the spread of spinal anesthesia is based mostly on studies with plain bupivacaine.

Levobupivacaine

Levobupivacaine is less cardiotoxic than bupivacaine. However, the doses used for spinal anesthesia (maximum of 25 mg) do not cause cardiotoxicity even if accidentally injected intravenously, thus this issue is not a concern in spinal anesthesia. In several experiments in which the spinal anesthetic properties of levobupivacaine and bupivacaine have been compared, they appear identical (36,37). Therefore, there should be no benefit in using levobupivacaine for spinal anesthesia. On the other hand, if bupivacaine is not available, it can be replaced by levobupivacaine (38).

Ropivacaine

Ropivacaine, another levo- isomer of the amide local anesthetics, is less potent and of shorter duration than bupivacaine. In a volunteer study, the potency of ropivacaine for spinal anesthesia appeared to be only half that of bupivacaine (39). When relatively large doses (17.5 mg) of spinal bupivacaine or ropivacaine were compared in patients scheduled for hip arthroplasty, little difference was noted in the duration of the sensory block (median duration at T10, 3 versus 3.5 hours) but the median duration of motor block (Bromage score 3) was shorter after ropivacaine than bupivacaine (2.1 versus 3.9 hours) (40). When ropivacaine doses of 15 and 20 mg were compared to a bupivacaine dose of 10 mg, the conclusion was that the duration of sensory block from ropivacaine was two-thirds and the duration of motor block one-half when compared with bupivacaine, with calculations based on the duration-per-milligram of the local anesthetic (41). When smaller doses were compared, the effective dose of ropivacaine was 1.5 times higher than that for levobupivacaine or bupivacaine (42,43). In herniorrhaphy, 8 mg of hyperbaric levobupivacaine and 12 mg of hyperbaric ropivacaine provided similar unilateral anesthesia (42). Likewise, for arthroscopy of the knee, 5 mg of hyperbaric levobupivacaine and 7.5 mg of hyperbaric ropivacaine provided

TABLE 10-3

ADDITIVES TO SPINAL ANESTHETICS AND USUAL DOSES

α_2–Adrenergic agonists	Opioids	Vasoconstrictors
Clonidine 15–45 μg	Morphine 0.1–0.4 mg	Epinephrine 0.2–0.3 mg
Dexmedetomidine 3 μg	Fentanyl 10–25 μg	Phenylephrine 2–5 mg
	Sufentanil 2.5–10 μg	

adequate blockade. The home discharge criteria were fulfilled faster with ropivacaine (43). In two studies in which hyperbaric and plain spinal ropivacaine (15 mg) were compared, the hyperbaric solution produced a faster onset and recovery as well as better reliability (44,45). For ambulatory surgery, hyperbaric ropivacaine may be a good option, allowing fast recovery of motor function. Unfortunately, hyperbaric solutions are not yet available, and they must be mixed at the bedside, which may pose the risk of possible miscalculations or wrong ingredients being used.

2-Chloroprocaine

Recently 2-chloroprocaine has gained interest in spinal anesthesia for ambulatory surgery. The neurotoxicity of 2-chloroprocaine or its additives has been the center of a controversy for several years. When preservative-containing preparations were used for epidural anesthesia, permanent neurologic injury after unintentional subarachnoid injection was reported. The additive sodium bisulfite and low pH were claimed to be the reason for neurotoxicity (46,47).

Preservative-free preparations of 2-chloroprocaine have been tested for spinal anesthesia; 40 mg of 2-chloroprocaine, 10 or 20 mg/mL, produces a reliable block for 60 minutes, with a fast onset and rapid recovery (48,49). No TNS has been reported in the preliminary studies. The safety of this preparation needs to be confirmed, since in a neurotoxicity study in rats 2-chloroprocaine caused significant functional impairment and histologic damage and, surprisingly, the additive bisulfite seemed to actually protect the rats from histologic damage (50). On the other hand, in a similar earlier experimental study from the same group, comparable changes in histology were observed with lidocaine and prilocaine (51). In these studies, the 2-chloroprocaine concentration was 30 mg/mL and that for lidocaine and prilocaine 25 mg/mL. Even though no neurologic damage has been observed in these clinical studies, more studies are needed before 2-chloroprocaine can be recommended for widespread use.

Articaine

The need for safe, short-acting agents has caused renewed interest in another old spinal anesthetic, articaine. It has been found comparable to lidocaine, and it has been used in some parts of Europe (52). When it was used for ambulatory surgery, an 84-mg dose of hyperbaric articaine provided anesthesia for 70 minutes and no TNS was observed (53).

Prilocaine

In some countries, prilocaine is used for short-lasting spinal anesthesia. Its properties are similar to those of lidocaine, although it may have a slightly longer duration of action. Transient neurologic symptom frequency is less than with lidocaine (54).

Additives

Different additives (Table 10-3) have been used with local anesthetics for spinal anesthesia, mostly in order to prolong or intensify the block. For example, the duration of tetracaine spinal anesthesia can be prolonged by 25% to 50% with the addition of epinephrine 0.2 to 0.5 mg (31,55). Additives have also been used with the aim of intensifying anesthesia without prolonging recovery. One indication is also the prevention of postoperative pain.

The safety of drugs injected into the subarachnoid space must be affirmed by animal research before they are used clinically (56).

Opioids

The local anesthetics and opioids have synergistic analgesic properties in the intrathecal space (57). This synergism does not affect the motor block. The major effect of intrathecally administered opioids is achieved through binding to μ-opioid receptors (58). Opioids selectively modulate nociceptive afferent input from A- and C-fibers; in addition, other receptors (κ) have analgesic effects (59).

Morphine

Morphine is a hydrophilic opioid with a long duration of action in the intrathecal space because of its low spinal cord distribution volume and slow clearance into plasma (60).

It is used as a 0.1- to 0.5-mg dose in combination with local anesthetic, and it provides good postoperative pain relief for up to 24 hours. Because of its hydrophilicity, morphine spreads in the intrathecal space; therefore, even after lumbar injection it can relieve pain after thoracic surgery. However, there is a delay in onset of analgesia of several hours. It is also carried rostrally to the level of the brainstem, and delayed respiratory depression can occur. Fortunately, this complication is rare but can occur even 24 hours after the injection.

The needed dose depends on the surgery. For example, for cesarean section, 0.1 mg provides good analgesia; 0.2 mg is adequate for hip arthroplasty, but even a dose of 0.3 mg did not relieve the pain after knee arthroplasty (61).

With increasing dose, the risk of side effects, nausea, vomiting, pruritus, and respiratory depression increases.

Morphine has also been used combined with bupivacaine for continuous intrathecal analgesia after orthopedic surgery (62). Intrathecal morphine cannot be recommended for ambulatory surgery. With a small dose (0.05 mg), the pain relief was enhanced but nausea, pruritus, and delay in voiding prevent the use of intrathecal morphine in ambulatory surgery (63).

Lipophilic Opioids

Fentanyl and sufentanil are lipophilic opioids which, after intrathecal injection, rapidly penetrate to the spinal cord and also through the dura to the epidural fat. Late respiratory depression is not a risk, but fast rostral spread may cause respiratory depression immediately (20–30 minutes) after the injection. Because of the high lipophilicity, the main effect of these opioids is on those dermatomes close to the injection (64,65).

Fentanyl. Fentanyl is typically used for ambulatory surgery. Small doses (10–25 μg) intensify the block without markedly prolonging it. With the use of fentanyl, the dose of local anesthetic can be diminished; the recovery of sensory and motor block is fast, without risking an excessive level of analgesia during surgery. When 4 mg intrathecal bupivacaine was compared to 3 mg intrathecal bupivacaine plus 10 μg fentanyl for arthroscopic surgery of the knee (66), the level of analgesia was equal but recovery of motor block was faster and time in the post anesthesia care unit shorter in the fentanyl group. In another study, the addition of 10 μg fentanyl to 5 mg of hyperbaric bupivacaine increased the success rate of spinal anesthesia from 75% to 100% (67). In ambulatory surgery, intrathecal fentanyl causes a high frequency of pruritus, which sometimes can be disturbing (68).

Sufentanil. Sufentanil is mostly used in the relief of labor pain and in cesarean sections. Doses of 2.5 to 7.5 μg have been used for the relief of labor pain and 2.5 to 10 μg with a low dose of bupivacaine for cesarean section. Its properties are very similar to those of fentanyl (64,65).

Side Effects of Intrathecally Administered Opioids

Respiratory Depression. Respiratory depression is the most feared complication of the use of intrathecal opioids. As already discussed, the risk differs depending on the properties of the opioid (hydro- versus lipophilic).

Pruritus. The pathophysiology and possibilities for treatment of this sometimes troublesome side effect are summarized in an extensive review by Szarvas and co-workers (68). This side effect is most commonly observed in obstetric and ambulatory patients. The incidence has been reported to be between 30% and 100%, and it seems to be equally common after fentanyl, sufentanil, and morphine. Different treatments and prevention modes have been tried, but it seems that naloxone is the best treatment. 5-HT3 receptor antagonists have been tested with variable success (69).

Antihistamines provide relief from the itching but do not prevent pruritus (70).

Nausea. Regardless of the path of administration—perorally, intravenously, or intrathecally—opioids may cause nausea and vomiting. Nausea is common after intrathecal morphine (35%–75%), and it seems to be dose dependent. In a volunteer study, intrathecal morphine caused a dose-related increase in emesis (71). Similarly, in clinical studies, the frequency of nausea increased with the dose of morphine used (72). If small doses of intrathecal morphine (<100 μg) have been used, the frequency of nausea is smaller. When small doses of sufentanil or fentanyl have been used in ambulatory surgery, nausea and vomiting is not a significant problem. Similar results have been reported when these lipophilic opioids have been used for labor pain or during cesarean delivery.

Vasoconstrictors

The mechanism of the vasoconstrictors in prolonging the effect of local anesthetics is reduction of the blood flow, which decreases the absorption of local anesthetics into the systemic circulation. Thus, the local anesthetics remain longer in the spinal space and their action is prolonged. There has been concern that the vasoconstrictors produce ischemia of the spinal cord and may lead to neurologic complications. This has been observed in animal experiments (73). On the other hand, in several controlled clinical studies in which spinal anesthesia with or without vasoconstrictives have been compared, no neurologic complications were attributed to the use of vasoconstrictors.

The recommended dose for epinephrine is 0.2 to 0.3 mg, and for phenylephrine 2 to 5 mg (74). They both prolong the duration of tetracaine spinal anesthesia and, in rigidly controlled studies, even a dose-response effect can be seen (75). When equipotent doses of epinephrine and phenylephrine are used, the prolongation is equal. When epinephrine has been used with lidocaine or bupivacaine, the duration of the block has not markedly changed (76,77). The reason for this difference is likely the different intrinsic vasodilatation/constriction properties of the local anesthetics. On the other hand, with hyperbaric lidocaine, epinephrine prolonged surgical anesthesia but also, significantly, prolonged the time required to regain the ability to void (78). When epinephrine was added to 2-chloroprocaine, it increased the duration of the block, but the use of epinephrine and 2-chloroprocaine caused vague, nonspecific flu-like symptoms and therefore is not recommended (79).

The use of vasoconstrictors is not advisable in ambulatory surgery. Vasoconstrictors may be used to prolong tetracaine spinal anesthesia in major operations, but they do not prolong the effect of bupivacaine (80).

α_2-Adrenergic Agonists

Clonidine was initially introduced as an antihypertensive drug. Now its main indication is in pain therapy. Its action is mediated by α_2-adrenergic receptors. These receptors are found in the substantia gelatinosa (81) of the dorsal horn of the spinal cord and also in primary afferent terminals and within several brainstem nuclei implicated in analgesia (82), thus explaining clonidine's analgesic effect after systemic, intrathecal, and local administration. In spinal anesthesia, clonidine intensifies and prolongs both sensory and motor block. Clonidine also potentiates the effects of intrathecal opioids in a synergistic way. Because clonidine is an antihypertensive drug, hypotension, bradycardia, and sedation are common side effects.

Even a small dose of clonidine (15 μg) prolongs markedly the sensory block if a large dose of local anesthetic is used (bupivacaine 17.5 mg) (83). The same dose has also improved analgesia for inguinal herniorrhaphy (84). Doses of up to 300 μg have been used intrathecally; however, these doses have caused marked hemodynamic changes and sedation (85). Interestingly, oral doses of 150 to 300 μg as premedication also have intensified spinal anesthesia, although, unfortunately hypotension is more common than after intrathecal use (86,87). If 3 μg/kg of clonidine is given intravenously after the spinal injection of bupivacaine (10 to 50 minutes), it may increase the duration of spinal anesthesia by 60 to 80 minutes (88).

Dexmedetomidine, another α_2-adrenergic receptor agonist, has also been studied in spinal anesthesia with bupivacaine. Dexmedetomidine at a dose of 3 μg had a similar effect in prolonging the block as 30 μg of clonidine when injected with 12 mg of bupivacaine (89).

MECHANISM OF SPINAL ANESTHESIA

Uptake

The nerves of the subarachnoid space do not have the protection of dura or arachnoid. Therefore even a small amount of local anesthetic in the CSF will cause a profound block of nerve transmission. Local anesthetic for spinal anesthesia is usually injected into the subarachnoid space between the spinous processes of the third and fourth lumbar vertebra. The needle will enter the dura in the area of the cauda equina, where the nerve roots cross the subarachnoid space from the spinal cord to their points of exit through the dura. The surface area of the nerve roots is considerable, thus making them vulnerable to the effects of local anesthetic (90). The nerve roots differ markedly in their size. The smallest roots have the relatively largest surface area, and local anesthetic penetrates them rapidly. Large individual variability exists among the properties of spinal anesthesia (Table 10-4). One reason for this may be the size of nerve roots, which differ greatly among individuals (e.g., the area for posterior L5, the most variable root, ranges from 2.2 mm^2 to 7.4 mm^2) (91).

The spinal cord itself also takes up local anesthetic, mostly by diffusion through the pia mater. This is a slow process and affects only the superficial portions of the cord. Local anesthetics can also penetrate to the deeper structures of the cord through the extensions of the subarachnoid space, which exist around those blood vessels that make their way through the pia mater. Because of the easy accessibility of local anesthetic to the nerve roots, it would be logical to assume that concentrations of local anesthetics are higher in nerve roots than in the cord. However, in experiments of the neuraxis of the dog, it seems that the opposite is true (90), because local anesthetics are lipid soluble, and highly myelinated fibers in the spinal cord will take up high concentrations.

Differential Sensitivity of Nerve Fibers

The major anesthetizing effect is caused by the local anesthetic in spinal nerve roots and dorsal root ganglia. The spread of local anesthetic in the spinal space is determined by diffusion, movement of CSF and, most importantly, baricity (relationship of the density of the local anesthetic and CSF). When the distance from the injection site increases, the amount of local anesthetic decreases and fewer molecules are available to produce

TABLE 10-4

UPTAKE AND ELIMINATION OF LOCAL ANESTHETICS FROM CEREBROSPINAL FLUID

Factors affecting uptake of local anesthetic (LA) into neural tissue:
Concentration of LA in cerebrospinal fluid (CSF)
Surface area of neural tissue exposed to CSF
Lipid content of nerve
Blood flow of nerve
Elimination of LA from CSF:
Through the arachnoidea and dura to epidural space
Vascular absorption via subarachnoid and epidural blood vessels

a block of nerve transmission. This, together with the fact that the nerve fibers differ in their sensitivity to the blocking agents, provides the explanation for the zones of differential blockade seen in spinal anesthesia. Traditionally, the extent of the spinal block has been differentiated between sympathetic block, sensory block, and motor block. Several reports note that the measured loss of cold-temperature discrimination (sensitive C-fibers and comparatively sympathetic fibers) occurs two to four spinal segments above the level of pin-prick sensory blockade (Aδ-fibers), which again is one or two segments higher than the level of anesthesia to light touch (Aβ-fibers) (92,93). The correlation of different modalities of sensation and fiber size appears accurate. Sensation of touch correlates with Aβ-fiber function, sensation of pin-prick with Aδ-fibers, and sensation of cold with C-fiber function. This correlation of fiber function and sensation during recovery was reported by Liu and co-workers after lidocaine spinal anesthesia in volunteers (94). They determined cutaneous current-perception thresholds at different frequencies and found a good correlation between recovery of the different nerve fibers and touch, pin-prick, and cold, respectively. Return of Aβ current-perception threshold (touch) correlated with duration of surgical anesthesia as assessed using an electrical stimulation model.

The block and recovery of sensory fibers occurs in this order: The most sensitive sensory fibers—C-fibers (sensation to cold)—are blocked first and remain blocked longest; Aδ-fibers (pin-prick) are the second to be blocked and recover; and Aβ-fibers (touch) are the last to block and first to recover (Fig. 10-1).

The preganglionic sympathetic fibers (B-fibers) are most sensitive to the local anesthetics. Traditionally, the spread of

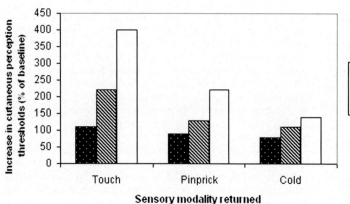

FIGURE 10-1. Sequential return of nerve function by class of nerve fiber correlates with sequential return of different sensation modalities at the L2–L3 dermatome after lidocaine spinal anesthesia (100% = baseline). Redrawn from Brull SJ, Greene NM. Time courses of zones of differential spinal anesthesia with hyperbaric tetracaine or bupivacaine. *Anesth Analg* 1989;69:342–347, with permission.

sympathetic block during spinal anesthesia was supposed to extend as high as the block of cold sensation (C-fibers). However, the sympathetic block during spinal anesthesia is more complex, because sympathetic fibers are not necessarily blocked when the sense to cold is blocked. In studies in which sympathetic function during spinal anesthesia has been measured by thermography, laser Doppler flowmetry, or skin conductance responses (95–97), an inconsistency is noted in the extent of the sympathetic block compared to the block of pin-prick or touch. In another, more recent study, a high-level spinal anesthesia with hyperbaric lidocaine, bupivacaine, or tetracaine attenuated sympathetic function but did not produce complete sympathectomy when tested by cold pressor test (98).

The motor fibers (Aα, the largest fibers) are less sensitive to local anesthetics than are sensory fibers. The level of motor block is supposed to be two to four dermatomes lower than the level of sensory anesthesia.

This difference between sensory and motor block seems inconsistent. Motor function is better preserved because more local anesthetic is needed to anesthetize the thick motor fibers. This is well observed in ambulatory surgery, when very small doses of local anesthetics are used. Despite adequate sensory block, the amount of local anesthetic is too small to cause significant motor blockade (99).

These zones of differing reaction to spinal anesthesia remain constant also during the emergence from spinal anesthesia.

Elimination

As local anesthetic molecules are absorbed by neuronal tissues, the concentration in the CSF decreases. This is a time-consuming procedure, since free local anesthetic can be detected in the CSF over 60 minutes after the injection. (The level of anesthesia changes after the repositioning of the patient when plain or hyperbaric bupivacaine is used [100,101].) However, even a small amount of free local anesthetic in the CSF can cause block—an important consideration since increase in the level of anesthesia can also increase the risk of hypotension.

The duration of spinal anesthesia is dependent on the rate of elimination of the local anesthetic. Elimination occurs entirely by vascular absorption (102,103). No intrathecal metabolism occurs. The duration of the block and rate of elimination depend on the extent of spinal anesthesia. Because of large individual variability, a dose of 15 mg of bupivacaine can cause a block to a level of T2 or L2. If the block is at the T2 level, a much larger area of absorption is present and therefore faster elimination and shorter duration of the block occurs in the upper dermatomes. The vascular absorption happens within the subarachnoid space, principally through vessels in the pia mater. The free local anesthetic in the CSF passes also through the dura outward to the epidural space, where the rich vasculature rapidly eliminates the local anesthetic to the systemic circulation (104). A difference exists in the absorption kinetics of lidocaine and bupivacaine. Lidocaine is absorbed through a single first-order absorption process (half-life, 71 minutes), whereas the more lipophilic bupivacaine binds to the epidural fat and its absorption can be characterized by two parallel first-order absorption processes (half-lives of 50 and 408 minutes). The first absorption equals that of lidocaine; the second, slower one is caused by the slow absorption from epidural fat (105). The plasma concentrations after spinal anesthesia are small: When 15 mg of plain or hyperbaric bupivacaine (5 mg/mL) was used, mean peak plasma concentrations of 63 ng/mL were observed (103). Interestingly, the times to peak concentration were shorter when hyperbaric bupivacaine was used (103,106).

This reflects the shorter duration of the block with hyperbaric solutions, in which the *baricity* or glucose concentration interferes with the absorption.

Increasing age affects the pharmacokinetics of intrathecally injected local anesthetics. The total plasma clearance of intrathecally administered bupivacaine is decreased and the elimination half-life increased with increasing age (107,108). The most probable reason for this is a decrease in hepatic enzyme activity. With local anesthetic doses used for spinal anesthesia, the plasma concentrations will not increase to systemic toxic levels.

Factors Affecting Intrathecal Spread

The spread of spinal anesthesia, especially with plain local anesthetic solutions (local anesthetic solutions without additives), is unpredictable (35). Fortunately, several things can help the anesthesiologist to decide the required technique, dose, and characteristics of the local anesthetic solution to anesthetize the area for a planned surgery for sufficient duration. Unnecessarily high or low blocks can be avoided by choosing the appropriate technique.

Greene, in his classical review from 1985, listed several factors that may influence the distribution of local anesthetic solution in the subarachnoid space (109). Some of these factors are controllable and others (e.g., patient characteristics) cannot be controlled. Thus, when we know the characteristics of the patient, we can modify our technique in order to get a good and safe spinal anesthesia. Some important factors are presented in Table 10-5.

Patient Characteristics

Age. It seems that, with advancing age, the nerves become more vulnerable to local anesthetics. The number of myelinated nerves decreases (110) and conduction velocity, especially in motor nerves, slows (111). There is sensory neuron loss, distal axonal degeneration, axonal atrophy, and an accumulation of multiple mitochondrial DNA mutations in muscle, and physical inactivity and deconditioning occur (112). With increasing age, the volume of CSF decreases, and its specific gravity increases (113). The results of different studies are not uniform but it seems that there is a tendency for spinal anesthesia, administered using the same technique and dose, to cause a faster onset, higher level of blockade, and longer lasting anesthesia with increasing age (108,114,115).

Height. In normal-sized adults, height does not influence the spread of anesthetics, but when extremes are compared, height plays a role. For example, when an identical dose of local anesthetic is injected into the spinal space of an individual 210 cm tall, the spread cannot be expected to be the same as in an individual 130 cm tall. Theoretically, the length of vertebral column would be even more important than height, but, within the limits of normal-sized adults, this parameter does not seem to affect the spread of anesthesia (116).

Weight. No linear correlation exists between obesity and spread of spinal anesthesia. If body mass index (BMI; an index of relative weight [kg/m²]) instead of weight is used, some effect on anesthetic spread can be observed. When the spread of spinal anesthesia using 15 mg plain bupivacaine in thin (BMI <21 kg/m²) versus obese (BMI >30 kg/m²) patients was compared, the spread was higher in obese patients (mean T5 versus T10). However, a large individual variability was also observed (T9–C7 versus L2–T4) (117).

TABLE 10-5

FACTORS AFFECTING DISTRIBUTION OF LOCAL ANESTHETIC IN CEREBROSPINAL FLUID

Factors with no proven effects	Factors with some effect	Factors with major effect
CSF composition	Age	Needle (directional needles)*
Circulation of CSF	Weight	Volume of CSF
Barbotage	Extremes of height	Density of LA solution (baricity)*
Gender	Rate of injection*	Dose of LA*
Volume or concentration of the local anesthetic	Site of injection*	Position of patient during and after injection*
	Anatomical configuration of spinal column	
	Temperature of the LA solution*	

*Factors that are not patient-related and can be manipulated.
CSF, cerebrospinal fluid; LA, local anesthetic.

It is possible that the abdominal mass in obese patients decreases the CSF volume and thus leads to a larger spread of spinal anesthesia (see the section on Cerebrospinal Fluid Properties) (118,119).

The influence of these patient characteristics (age, weight, height) is not uniform. Some correlation can be observed, as shown in a study by Pargger and co-workers (116), who performed spinal anesthesia using 18 mg plain bupivacaine in 100 patients over 49 years of age. In a multiple regression analysis age, weight, and height were found to significantly correlate with sensory level. However, the predictive value was low.

Cerebrospinal Fluid Properties

According to the traditional literature, the volume of CSF in the spinal subarachnoid space varies between 25 and 35 mL. Modern technology has allowed us to accurately measure the volume of CSF. In 25 healthy volunteers, the volume of CSF was measured using magnetic resonance images (MRI) (118). The mean volume from the T11–T12 disc to the sacral terminus of the dural sac was 49.9 ± 12.1 mL. Large individual variability occurs, with a range of 28.0 to 81.1 mL. Interestingly, this volume was significantly less in relatively obese subjects (42.9 ± 9.5 mL) than in nonobese subjects (53.5 ± 12.9 mL). In another MRI study, slightly smaller values of CSF volume (10–61 mL) were observed (119). A correlation was again noted with obesity; patients with spinal stenosis also had smaller CSF volumes. In a volunteer study, an inverse correlation between CSF volume measured by MRI and peak sensory height of hyperbaric lidocaine spinal anesthesia was observed (Fig. 10-2) (120). The same observations were recently repeated in a clinical study using plain bupivacaine (121). Lumbosacral CSF volume inversely correlated with peak sensory block level ($p = 0.65$, $P < 0.0001$).

These studies confirm that, if the volume of CSF is small, there will be more extensive spread of the local anesthetic in the intrathecal space, and maximum spread of anesthesia will be higher.

It is speculated that the decreased CSF volume is caused by abdominal pressure, which compresses the epidural space and displaces the CSF. Abdominal compression does diminish the CSF volume (118,122). As mentioned earlier, a correlation does exist between the volume of CSF and BMI. The CSF volume is also diminished in the elderly. Thus, it seems that at least part of the reason for the larger spread of spinal anesthesia in obesity or pregnancy is the compression of the epidural space, which diminishes the CSF volume.

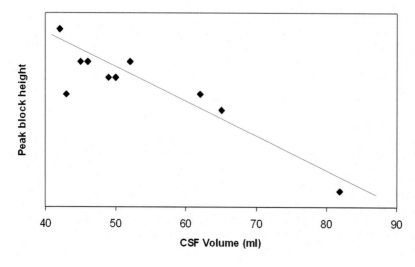

FIGURE 10-2. Correlation between cerebrospinal fluid volume measured by magnetic resonance imaging and peak sensory block height after lidocaine spinal anesthesia in volunteers ($r = 0.91$, by linear regression analysis). Redrawn from Hogan QH, Prost R, Kulier A, et al. Magnetic resonance imaging of cerebrospinal fluid volume and the influence of body habitus and abdominal pressure. *Anesthesiology* 1996;84:1341–1349, with permission.

Density of CSF has a minor effect on the maximum spread of plain bupivacaine (121,123). When 15 mg of plain bupivacaine was used for spinal anesthesia, a correlation was noted between the maximum extent of the block and CSF density (123). Different components of CSF (glucose, proteins) affect its density, but the effect of these components on the spread of the block has not been verified (123,124).

Site of Injection

When spinal anesthesia is performed at the L4–L5 level compared to L2–L3 level, the spread after the former injection is lower, but the variation is large (125). However, the routine use of L2–L3 or higher levels for spinal anesthesia is not recommended. This difference in the spread of anesthesia is therefore theoretical. When injections to L3–L4 and L4–L5 have been compared, little difference in the properties of the block have been noted (126).

If the needle is inserted through the L2–L3 interspace into the subarachnoid space, it should not reach the conus in most adults. Unfortunately, the ability to accurately identify the lumbar interspaces is not good. In 100 patients scheduled for lumbar MRI, anesthesiologists were asked to identify and mark the lumbar interspace. The marker was one space higher than assumed in 51% of cases and the interspace was identified correctly in only 29%. Obesity made it more difficult to place the markers accurately. In 19% of patients, the spinal cord extended lower than L1 (127).

In another MRI study, the margin between the conus medullaris and the Tuffier line was measured. The conus medullaris was at the L1 (median; range of T12–L2) level in men and L1–L2 (median; range of T12–L3) in women. The Tuffier line was at L4–L5 (L3–S1) and L4–L5 (L4–5), respectively (128).

Thus, there should be a two- to four-segment difference between the Tuffier line and the conus medullaris but, because of the difficulty in correctly identifying this line and considerable differences in the extent of the conus medullaris, spinal puncture above L3 is not recommended. Indeed, seven patients with neurologic damage were reported after introducing the spinal needle at a level that was believed to be the L2–L3 level. All experienced pain during insertion of the needle. On MRI, conus damage, fluid collection, and hemorrhage were observed (129).

Previous Spinal Anesthesia

If adequate information is available about the properties (spread, duration) of a previous spinal anesthesia, this knowledge can be used to obtain a second successful spinal anesthesia. It has been observed that a subsequent spinal anesthesia using exactly the same technique and dose of local anesthetic (plain bupivacaine) in an individual behaves in manner similar to a previous one (130,131). This observation supports the fact that the properties of the patient (height, weight, CSF volume, etc.) play a role in the spread of spinal anesthetic.

If one knows that the spread of previous anesthesia was unnecessarily high or low, technique can be adjusted to obtain a satisfactory spread.

Needle

It is possible to influence the spread of anesthesia by using directional needles. The extreme example is unilateral anesthesia with hyperbaric or clearly hypobaric local anesthetic solution, in which the direction of the needle aperture is important (132). Placing the opening of the Whitacre needle in the cranial direction has caused a higher sensory level and longer duration of lidocaine spinal anesthesia compared to the caudal direction when patients were in the horizontal side position during the injection (133).

Speed of Injection

Theoretically, fast injection through a small needle causes turbulence and perhaps faster mixing of the local anesthetic within the CSF, hence a larger spread of anesthesia. However, the results are not uniform. When plain bupivacaine was used, minor differences in the spread have been observed between 10- and 180-second injection times (slower injection caused larger spread) (134). However, in another study, in which injection times of 10 and 250 seconds were compared, the results were opposite (135). When 6 and 60 seconds were compared, no difference of effect was observed (136). For unilateral anaesthesia, reduced speed did not effect spread (137). When extremely slow injection speed (0.5 mL/min to 3 min) and fast injection speed (7.5 mL/min to 10 seconds) were compared, unilaterality was better with the slow injection (138). When clinically applicable injection speeds are used, the effect on spread seems to be limited.

Barbotage

The term *barbotage* has several definitions; here, the word is used to describe the technique of aspirating a certain volume of CSF either before or after injecting the local anesthetic, then reinjecting the CSF, sometimes repeating the process. Usually the volume of CSF is equal to the volume of the local anesthetic. With hyperbaric solutions, this method may shorten the time to full development of analgesia (139); however, this has not been observed with plain solutions (140). With modern thin needles, barbotage is difficult because of the very slow flow rate through the needle and difficulties in aspirating large volumes.

Volume, Concentration and Dose of the Local Anesthetic

Several studies have compared the parameters (volume and concentration) influencing the dose of the local anesthetic injected intrathecally. With these comparisons, one has to remember that if the volume of the solution is changed, either the concentration or dose also will change. Thus, only one parameter at a time can be standardized. The changes in volume or concentration do not seem to have a major effect on the spread or duration of anesthesia. Instead, increase in dose (in milligrams), especially with plain solutions, causes higher spread and longer duration of anesthesia. A comparison of bupivacaine doses of 10, 15, or 20 mg as 5-mg/mL or 7.5-mg/mL solutions indicated that the total dose is more important than volume or concentration (141). When dose was increased from 10 to 20 mg, both the level of anesthesia and the duration of the block increased. On the other hand, if the volume or concentration was changed, but the dose remained constant, there were no major differences in the properties of the block. Similar observations were reported with plain lidocaine at a 70-mg dose, using a 5- to 100-mg/mL solution (142). It produced the same level of analgesia, motor block, and duration of anesthesia regardless of the broad range of concentrations and volumes (0.7–14 mL). With hyperbaric solutions, the spread is more influenced by baricity, and differences are not as easily observed. However, the duration of the block also increases with the increased dose when hyperbaric solutions are used (143,144). When a hyperbaric bupivacaine dose was decreased from 15 to 5 mg, without changing the volume (it was diluted with saline to 3 mL), the duration of the block decreased with the decrease in dose (145). In this study, baricity might have had some effect also, since the addition of saline decreased the baricity of the solutions.

Density of Local Anesthetics and Baricity

Density is a physical characteristic expressed as weight in grams of 1 mL of a solution (g/mL) at a specified temperature. The density of a local anesthetic has an important role in spread within the intrathecal space. The relationship between the density of the local anesthetic and the density of the CSF is called *baricity*. Anesthetic substances that have a greater density than CSF are *hyperbaric*; likewise, those with a lower density are *hypobaric*. Local anesthetics with a density close to that of the CSF are called *isobaric*. By definition, the baricity of an isobaric solution is 1. *Specific gravity* is another expression used for comparison of densities of substances. Specific gravity is the relationship of the density of a substance to the density of water. The following discussion concentrates on both density and baricity.

The density of CSF in humans varies. Certain factors, such as gender and hormonal status in women (menopause, pregnancy), affect on CSF density. The densities vary from 1.00033 g/mL in pregnant women to 1.00067 g/mL in men (146).

Therefore, an isobaric local anesthetic may be hypobaric in some and hyperbaric in others. Since it is impractical to measure the density of CSF before each spinal anesthesia procedure, certain assumptions must be made. By definition, the local anesthetic behaves as an isobaric solution (the position of the patient does not have marked effect on the spread) if the density of the solution is within a mean of ± 3 SD of the density of CSF (representing 99.73% of the population) (109,147). Using this definition (results of Lui and co-workers from 131 patients [146]), the range of isobaricity is 0.9999 to 1.00119 g/mL.

What makes this more complicated is that CSF density changes with temperature. Increasing temperature decreases the density of a solution. Usually, local anesthetics are injected intrathecally at room temperature. The temperature equilibrates rapidly to that of the CSF and the physical characteristics change likewise (density decreases). When densities are expressed, they should be at normal human body temperature. Plain bupivacaine, 5 mg/mL solution, has a density of 1.00376 at 23°C but of 0.99944 at 37°C (148). The effect of temperature was studied in patients when plain bupivacaine 5 mg/mL solutions equilibrated at 20°C or 37°C were compared for spinal anesthesia in the sitting position. After injection of 3 mL (15 mg), as can be expected, the warmer solution (lower density; hypobaric solution) caused a significantly higher maximum level. Of note, the variability of the spread also was clearly less than with the solution at room temperature (149).

Heller and co-workers (150), using sophisticated measurement and mathematic models, calculated *isobaric temperatures* (temperature at which the local anesthetic is isobaric) for different local anesthetics of different concentrations. Their calculations revealed that at normal body temperature plain solutions of the usual concentrations of prilocaine, lidocaine, articaine, ropivacaine, bupivacaine, and levobupivacaine all were hypobaric (density less than that of CSF, i.e., −3 SD). In Heller's study, the true isobaric local anesthetics at 37°C were mepivacaine 10 and 15 mg/mL and articaine 15 mg/mL. Mepivacaine and articaine 20 mg/mL were hyperbaric (density at 37°C >CSF + 3 SD). The isobaric temperature for plain bupivacaine 5 mg/mL is 34.3°C to 35.8°C. To get the advantages of isobaric solution, the temperature of the local anesthetic must be at this isobaric temperature. The clinical relevance of this finding must be verified. The effect of temperature is, however, of short duration, because when room-temperature local anesthetic is injected into the CSF, the temperature increases rapidly to that of CSF (151).

The baricity of the local anesthetic solution can be changed by adding either glucose (hyperbaric) or distilled water (hypobaric) to it. There are several commercially available hyperbaric solutions that contain glucose 50 to 80 mg/mL. Their densities at room temperature are 1.02 to 1.03 mg/mL, thus they are clearly hyperbaric. The position of the patient after the injection is important when hyper- or hypobaric solutions are used. In the supine horizontal position, there is a tendency for anesthesia to spread to the level of thoracic kyphosis, which approximates the T4 level. The spread can be limited or extended by positioning the patient. If the hyperbaricity of the bupivacaine solution is decreased (glucose concentration of only 8 mg/mL; baricity of 1.0045 at 23°C), the extent of the block is not as high as with the more hyperbaric (glucose concentration 80 mg/mL; baricity 1.02) solution. These two baricities of bupivacaine 15 mg were compared in spinal anesthesia. The injection was made at the L3–L4 interspace with patients in the sitting position. The range in the spread of anesthesia after the less hyperbaric solution was more limited (T5–T9 versus T2–T9) and was useful in predicting the spread of the block (152).

Hyperbaric solutions are especially practical in small doses for saddle block and unilateral anesthesia. Hypobaric solutions have traditionally been used for rectal and perineal surgery when injected in the lateral decubitus or jack-knife position. There are no commercially available hypobaric solutions, and they must be mixed bedside. Hypobaricity can be used to produce unilateral anesthesia (153,154). This is especially useful in patients who cannot lie on their side due to fractures (155). The hypobaric solutions must be used carefully, because when hypobaric bupivacaine (8 mL; 1.9 mg/mL) was injected in the sitting position, undesirably extensive block followed up to the cervical dermatomes (even to C1 and C2) in three out of 14 patients (156). Hyperbaric solutions have a shorter duration of action than plain solutions (Table 10-6; Fig. 10-3) (45,157–158).

PHYSIOLOGIC RESPONSES

Cardiovascular

The most important physiologic responses to spinal anesthesia involve the cardiovascular system (159). These responses are mediated by the combined effects of autonomic denervation and, with higher levels of neural blockade, the added effects of vagal nerve innervation. Spinal anesthesia always causes some degree of hypotension and reflex bradycardia because of reduction in cardiac output and systemic vascular resistance. Usually, these can be considered as the normal effects of spinal anesthesia. Depending on the definition, the frequency of hypotension or bradycardia needing treatment varies; frequencies of hypotension of 8% to 30% and bradycardia of 10% to 15% have been reported. Unfortunately, sometimes these effects may lead to severe hypotension and asystole, leading to morbidity and even mortality in previously asymptomatic patients. In 1988, Caplan and co-workers searched through the insurance claims for major anesthetic mishaps and found 14 cardiac arrests—six of these fatal—occurring after normal spinal anesthesia in healthy patients (160). They emphasized

TABLE 10-6

DENSITIES OF LOCAL ANESTHETICS AT 37°C

Solution	Density at 37°C mg/mL mean ± 3 SD
CSF	1.00059 ± 0.00060
Bupivacaine 5 mg/mL	0.99944 ± 0.00012
Bupivacaine 7.5 mg/mL	0.99938 ± 0.00017
Levobupivacaine 5 mg/mL	1.00024 ± 0.00009
Levobupivacaine 7.5 mg/mL	1.00056 ± 0.00010
Ropivacaine 5 mg/mL	0.99953 ± 0.00013
Ropivacaine 7.5 mg/mL	0.99953 ± 0.00014
Ropivacaine 10 mg/mL	0.99950 ± 0.00010
2-chloroprocaine 20 mg/mL	1.00123 ± 0.00009
2-chloroprocaine 30 mg/mL	1.00257 ± 0.00009
Lidocaine 20 mg/mL	0.99890 ± 0.00042
Bupivacaine 1.8 mg/mL; sterile water	0.997 (25°C)
Bupivacaine 5 mg/mL glucose 80 mg/mL	1.02890 ± 0.00051
Levobupivacaine 5 mg/mL glucose 80 mg/mL	1.03042 ± 0.00026
Ropivacaine 5 mg/mL glucose 80 mg/mL	1.02980 ± 0.00060

CSF, cerebrospinal fluid; SD, standard deviation.

that vigilance and careful monitoring are essential during spinal anesthesia, even in low-risk patients and situations. In a large survey from France from 1997, the incidence of cardiac arrest after spinal anesthesia was 26 in 40,640 cases (6.4 per 10,000); six of these were fatal (161). Later, in another survey from the same group, the incidence was slightly less at 2.7 per 10,000 cases (28). A similar frequency was reported in a 20-year report from the Mayo Clinic, where the risk of cardiac arrest during spinal anesthesia was 2.9 per 10,000 cases (162).

Plasma levels of local anesthetics during spinal anesthesia are below those required to produce direct effects on the myocardium or on peripheral vascular smooth muscles (163), and the generalization that local anesthetics and vasoactive substances administered in small doses intrathecally lack direct cardiovascular effect remains accurate. Sympathetic denervation has great influence in the genesis of cardiovascular changes during spinal anesthesia.

Sympathetic Denervation

Because the level of sympathetic denervation determines the magnitude of cardiovascular responses to spinal anesthesia, it might be anticipated that the higher the level of neural blockade, the greater the change in cardio-circulatory parameters. This seems to be accurate, at least in high levels of anesthesia. However, the relationship is more complicated since, in the presence of partial sympathetic blockade, a reflex increase in sympathetic activity occurs in sympathetically intact areas. The result is vasoconstriction that tends to compensate for the peripheral vasodilation taking place in the sympathetically denervated areas. This can be seen in the changes in arterial pulse wave contours and in cutaneous blood flow in the upper extremities in the presence of low or midthoracic sensory levels of spinal anesthesia (164). The risk of hypotension and bradycardia is increased if the level of anesthesia is T5 or higher;

Hypobaric

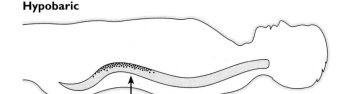

Injection

Isobaric

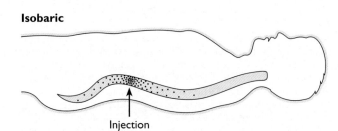

Injection

Hyperbaric

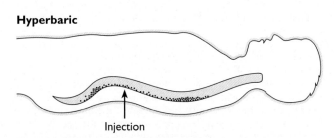

Injection

FIGURE 10-3. The spread of local anesthetic in the intrathecal space depends on the baricity (see chapter 11, Tables 11-2, 11-3).

however, with proper intraoperative management, vascular hypotension may be modest or even absent even with sensory anesthesia up to T2 (see chapter 11, Tables 11-2, 11-3).

Arterial Circulation

Sympathetic denervation produces arterial and, physiologically more important, arteriolar vasodilation, although vasodilation is not maximal. Vascular smooth muscle on the arterial side of the circulation retains a significant degree of autonomous tone following acute, pharmacologically induced sympathetic denervation. As a result, total peripheral vascular resistance (TPVR) decreases only modestly, about 15% to 18% in normal subjects, even in the presence of total sympathetic denervation, provided cardiac output, the other determinant of blood pressure, is kept normal (159). Because TPVR decreases only 15% to 18%, mean arterial pressure decreases only 15% to 18% in the presence of a normal cardiac output (see Fig. 11-3).

Venous Circulation. Veins and venules, with only a few smooth muscles in their walls, retain no significant residual tone following acute pharmacologic denervation, and so they can vasodilate maximally. Whether they do so or not is determined by intraluminal hydrostatic pressure. Intraluminal hydrostatic pressure on the venous side of the circulation depends on gravity. If denervated veins lie below the level of the right atrium, gravity causes peripheral pooling of blood in these capacitance vessels. If the denervated veins lie above the level of the right atrium, gravity causes the blood to flow back to the heart.

Preload—that is, venous return to the heart—therefore depends on the position of the patient during spinal anesthesia, especially during high spinal anesthesia.

Cardiac Output. Preload is an important determinant of cardiac output. During levels of spinal anesthesia high enough to produce total sympathetic denervation, cardiac output remains unchanged in normovolemic subjects as long as they are positioned with the legs elevated above the level of the heart. The head-up (legs-down) position, on the other hand, leads to severe decreases in venous return to the heart, and thus to significant decreases in cardiac output (see Fig. 11-3).

Heart Rate. Heart rate characteristically decreases during spinal anesthesia in the absence of autonomically active drugs and medications. The bradycardia is due in part to blockade of preganglionic cardiac accelerator fibers arising from T1 to T4 during high (i.e., T3–T4) levels of anesthesia (165). Indeed, in prospective studies, the incidence of episodes of bradycardia is increased if the sensory block level is T5 or higher (166,167). The bradycardia is also mediated by significant decreases in right atrial pressure and pressure in the great veins as they enter the right atrium. This can be seen during fixed levels of high spinal anesthesia. Placing the patient in the modest head-down position (or with legs elevated) increases venous return, which in turn increases right atrial pressure and thus heart rate at a time when blockade of cardiac accelerator fibers remains constant. The slight head-up position, on the other hand, further decreases venous return, right atrial pressure, and heart rate. The direct relationship between right atrial pressure and heart rate during high spinal anesthesia is mediated by intrinsic chronotropic stretch receptors located in the right atrium and adjacent great veins. Severe bradycardia may develop even without complete sympathetic blockade (168). Several factors and reflexes affect the heart rate. They are complex, and their effects may antagonize each other. It seems that the sudden severe bradycardia with spinal anesthesia is very similar to that in vasovagal syncope, with a decrease in venous return (169). It may be that the cardiovascular response described as the Bezold-Jarisch reflex is the mechanism for these changes. This reflex is triggered by reduced cardiac venous return as well as through affective mechanisms such as pain or fear. It is probably mediated in part via afferent nerves from the heart, but also by various noncardiac baroreceptors that may become paradoxically active (170,171) (see also Chapter 11, Fig. 11-4).

Hypotension

As discussed, slight decreases in arterial pressure in the range of 15% or so during high spinal anesthesia in normovolemic patients can be ascribed to decreases in afterload, that is, decreases in TPVR. Severe hypotension, however, can be due only to decreases in cardiac output secondary to decreases in preload associated with peripheral pooling of blood in vasodilated capacitance vessels or to hypovolemia, or both.

The indications for treatment of arterial hypotension during spinal anesthesia and the methods to be used are best considered in light of what arterial hypotension caused by sympathetic denervation means in terms of oxygenation of the myocardium and the CNS (the organs most susceptible to hypoxia). Hypovolemic subjects are highly susceptible to the hypotensive effects of spinal anesthesia because, in the presence of hypovolemia, maintenance of cardiovascular function depends on compensatory reflex increases in sympathetic activity. Elimination of these compensatory reflexes by sympathetic denervation during spinal anesthesia can result in such catastrophic hypotension (due to decreases in TPVR and venous return to the heart) that spinal anesthesia is contraindicated in the presence of hypovolemia. (See also Chapter 11.)

Myocardial Oxygenation

A major determinant of coronary blood flow, and thus myocardial oxygen supply, is the perfusion pressure in the coronary vasculature. A decrease in mean arterial pressure during spinal anesthesia is therefore associated with a decrease in coronary blood flow (172). Myocardial oxygen demands decrease during hypotension associated with spinal anesthesia for three reasons: (a) afterload decreases—the resistance against which the left ventricle ejects blood during systole is diminished, and therefore left ventricular work decreases; (b) preload decreases—as venous return and cardiac output decrease, so too does the work load of both ventricles because the amount of blood to be ejected per unit of time is lessened; and (c) heart rate decreases—the ventricular work load is diminished as the frequency of contraction diminishes. Myocardial work and oxygen requirements diminish to essentially the same extent as does myocardial oxygen supply during moderate levels of arterial hypotension caused by spinal anesthesia in normal subjects.

Cerebral Blood Flow

Cerebrovascular autoregulatory mechanisms maintain cerebral blood flow in humans at constant levels, even in the presence of wide fluctuations in mean arterial pressure. Not until mean arterial pressure decreases below 50 to 55 mm Hg does cerebral blood flow become pressure dependent. Cerebrovascular autoregulation is independent of the sympathetic nervous system.

The level of blood pressure during spinal anesthesia that requires initiation of corrective measures is higher in hypertensive than in normotensive patients, both in absolute terms and in terms of percent decrease in pressure from preanesthetic control levels. Neither normotensive nor hypertensive patients need arterial pressure to be maintained at preoperative levels during spinal anesthesia in order to ensure maintenance of adequate cerebral perfusion.

Regional Blood Flow

In addition to the effects of spinal anesthesia on cardiac and cerebral blood flow, it is of interest to know whether blood flow to other organs, such as kidney and liver, is affected and whether the changes are of clinical importance. In awake, unrestrained sheep, the effects of five drugs with flow-limited characteristics on regional blood flow and organ oxygen tensions were compared with the effects induced by spinal anesthesia (173). Aside from a 10% decrease in hepatic blood flow, there were no significant changes in any hemodynamic variable or in any of the arterial or venous oxygen tensions induced by spinal anesthesia. The intravenous (IV) infusion of adequate volumes of saline at the time of the spinal blockade probably contributed to the maintenance of the normal variables.

Management of Hypotension

Oxygenation of the two most critical organs, the brain and the myocardium, is recognized as being maintained in normal subjects in the presence of moderate levels of hypotension during spinal anesthesia. It is thus no longer considered necessary or desirable to maintain blood pressure at "normal" levels during spinal anesthesia. There comes a point, nevertheless, at which hypotension becomes so great that decreases in cerebrovascular resistance and decreases in myocardial oxygen requirements are no longer able to compensate for decreases in cerebral and coronary artery perfusing pressures. Exactly what this critical pressure is has not yet been defined. Pragmatically, however, decreases in systolic blood pressure to levels 33% below resting control levels (preferably as measured before the patient gets out of bed in the morning) need not be treated during spinal anesthesia in healthy, asymptomatic patients. Although also not quantitated, similar levels of hypotension may be tolerated in patients with coronary arterial disease. Such statements are based on equivalent decreases in arterial blood pressure being deliberately induced in coronary care units by use of nitroprusside or nitroglycerin as a means of favorably affecting the ratio between myocardial oxygen supply and demand, even in patients with demonstrable myocardial ischemia. Physiologic responses to nitroprusside or nitroglycerin are quite similar to those associated with spinal anesthesia. Pragmatically, in patients with essential hypertension, it would appear prudent to initiate corrective measures when systolic blood pressure decreases to more than 25% below the resting control levels. Clearly, appropriate monitors to detect significant blood pressure and ST segment changes, as well as delivery of supplemental oxygen, are to be recommended (Table 10-7).

Vasopressors in the management of hypotension during spinal anesthesia must be used carefully. If extreme bradycardia or cardiac arrest is present, epinephrine is the primary drug of choice and there should be no hesitation in using it (160). On the other hand, with milder hypotension certain conservatism in using vasoactive agents is needed. α-Adrenoceptor agonists, such as methoxamine and phenylephrine, may so increase afterload that increases in left ventricular oxygen demand, because of increased work load, may exceed the increase in myocardial oxygen supply brought about by the increase in coronary perfusion pressure. Also, of course, a hypotension significant enough to require treatment during spinal anesthesia is not caused by a decrease in TPVR, which α-adrenoceptor agonists would correct, but rather by decreases in preload and cardiac output, neither of which is favorably affected by α-adrenoceptor agonists. Proportionately greater increases in myocardial oxygen requirements than in myocardial oxygen supply may also result when positive chronotropic drugs, including atropine, are used to elevate blood pressure by increasing heart rate and thus cardiac output.

Positive inotropic agents that increase cardiac output by increasing myocardial contractility may not be effective either. Myocardial contractility is not impaired by spinal anesthesia. Increasing ventricular contractility when end diastolic filling volumes are decreased because of decreased preload may be misguided. The ideal vasopressor for treatment of hypotension during spinal anesthesia would be one that acts selectively to produce venoconstriction without affecting afterload, heart rate, or myocardial contractility. Such an ideal vasopressor would selectively remedy the cause of severe hypotension—decreased preload—during spinal anesthesia. Such an ideal vasopressor, however, is not available. The best means for treating hypotension during spinal anesthesia is thus physiologic, not pharmacologic. In instances in which physiologic measures (discussed next) need to be supplemented by vasopressors, the most useful are ephedrine and mephentermine. Both have at least some venoconstrictive properties without major undesirable effects on the ratio between myocardial oxygen supply and demand.

Physiologic treatment of hypotension during spinal anesthesia consists of restoration of preload by increasing venous return to the heart, thus restoring cardiac output. This is most simply and effectively done by providing the patient with an *internal autotransfusion*: Merely place the patient in the slight head-down or legs-up position. By doing so, the venous return and cardiac output improve and, in normovolemic patients, blood pressure returns to near normal levels (174). The remaining minor decrease in blood pressure represents a decrease in afterload secondary to arterial and arteriolar vasodilatation. The head-down position need not, and should not, exceed about 20 degrees. An extreme Trendelenburg position may be counterproductive by increasing internal jugular venous pressure to such an extent that effective cerebral perfusion pressure and cerebral blood flow are diminished. Use of the head-down position to maintain blood pressure or to correct hypotension during hyperbaric spinal anesthesia may result in unnecessarily high levels of anesthesia. This can be avoided by elevating the lower body above the level of the heart at the same time the upper thorax and cervical area are elevated at about the T4 level by placing a pillow or other support under the patient's shoulders. This arrests the rising spinal anesthesia at the T4 level at the same time that venous return is being maximized. This technique also reduces the chance of producing significant respiratory depression.

Another means for restoring venous return, preload, and cardiac output during spinal anesthesia consists of the rapid IV infusion of large volumes of electrolyte solutions. Restoration of blood pressure alone, however, is not the sole objective in treating hypotension during spinal anesthesia. The objective is restoration of tissue oxygenation, especially myocardial oxygenation. Vasoconstrictors also restore blood pressure, as discussed earlier, but their adverse effects on the balance between myocardial oxygen supply and demand are so well recognized that they should be used infrequently today. The rapid IV infusion of a relatively large volume of fluids (1.0–1.5 L/70 kg) within 10 to 15 minutes for treatment of arterial hypotension

TABLE 10-7

TREATMENT OF HYPOTENSION ASSOCIATED WITH SPINAL ANESTHESIA

Treat hypotension only if systolic arterial pressure decreases 30% from baseline
  However, monitor cardiovascular system (ST-segment, arrhythmias) and central nervous system (alertness) and begin treatment earlier if necessary
Treatment steps
  1. Elevate legs or Trendelenburg position
    Be careful if hyperbaric anesthetics are used
  2. Oxygen
  3. IV fluids: Not effective if normovolemic
  4. Ephedrine
Principles of use of vasopressors
  Ephedrine: Indirect action, stimulation of α, β_1, and β_2 receptors, IV dose 5–15 mg
  Phenylephrine: Direct action, only α stimulation, IV dose 50–100 μg
  Epinephrine: Direct action, more β than α stimulation; potent drug—do not hesitate to use in extreme bradycardia; dose 5 μg

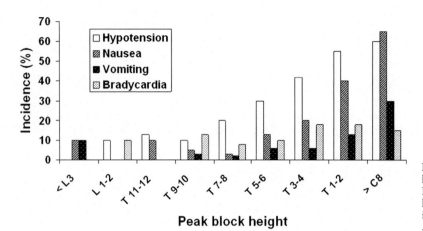

FIGURE 10-4. Incidence of side effects related to the height of spinal anesthesia. Redrawn from Tarkkila P, Isola J. A regression model for identifying patients at high risk of hypotension, bradycardia and nausea during spinal anesthesia. *Acta Anaesthesiol Scand* 1992;36: 554–558, with permission.

during spinal anesthesia has been reported (175,176). In one such study, Venn and colleagues (176) concluded that the fluid preload was only of benefit in reducing the extent of the hypotension induced by spinal anesthesia, and even then, only in those patients in whom the sympathetic block extended above the T6 dermatome. By contrast, a vasopressor such as ephedrine was much more effective in treating hypotension, even when fluid administration (1 L or more) was ineffective. In another study, Coe and Revanas compared the incidence of hypotension induced by spinal anesthesia in patients who received no intravascular volume preload, with the incidence of hypotension in patients given 8 mL or 16 mL of intravascular fluid (Ringer's acetate solution) per kg body weight. The authors found that the incidence of hypotension was a function of the level of sympathetic denervation, occurring in 60% of patients with a T7 sympathectomy, and in 100% of patients with a T4 or higher level of sympathectomy. However, the overall incidence of hypotension (27%) was similar in the three groups of patients, regardless of the IV fluid preload. Even when the IV fluid administration was guided by objective criteria such as central venous pressure monitoring, fluid preloading failed to prevent significant blood pressure decreases in 35% of patients (174). It is apparent, then, that IV fluid preloading is relatively ineffective in the prophylaxis or treatment of hypotension induced by clinical spinal anesthesia in patients with normal circulating blood volume.

In addition to being relatively ineffective, other considerations are to be borne in mind when large amounts of IV fluids are administered to patients undergoing spinal anesthesia. Although IV crystalloids may increase peripheral blood flow by decreasing viscosity and improving blood rheology, the oxygen content is decreased because of hemodilution. Thus, the decreased oxygen delivery to the tissues may exceed the benefits of increased tissue perfusion. Relatively large amounts of IV fluids also may be poorly tolerated by patients with myocardial dysfunction or those with valvular heart disease. Excess IV fluids also increase the need for postoperative urinary bladder catheterization, because the duration of parasympathetic nervous system denervation induced by spinal anesthesia far outlasts the duration of sensory denervation. These patients (and especially elderly males with some degree of prostate hyperplasia) are much more likely to develop urinary retention and some of the complications associated with catheterization, such as urinary bladder infection. Finally, IV crystalloid administration may counteract the salutary effects of spinal anesthesia on the coagulatory system; according to one study, IV crystalloids increased coagulability and the incidence of deep venous thrombosis (177).

Prophylaxis. The prophylactic use of colloids instead of crystalloids decreases the incidence of hypotension, especially in patients with possible relative hypovolemia (178).

Also, the prophylactic use of vasopressors decreases episodes of hypotension after spinal anesthesia. On the other hand, increased frequency of tachycardia and overcorrection of hypotension has also been reported after the use of vasopressors (179).

Certain patient-related and anesthesia-related factors are predictive for developing hypotension or bradycardia during spinal anesthesia. Patients with these factors must be treated with special caution in order to be able to observe and treat these side effects. Prospective studies agree that sensory block to T5 or higher is highly predictive for developing hypotension (Fig. 10-4). Other factors increasing the risk of hypotension are age older than 40 to 50 years and a BMI of more than 30 kg/m², baseline systolic blood pressure less than 120 mm Hg, spinal puncture at or above L2–L3 (this should be avoided), urgency of surgery, history of hypertension, and chronic alcohol consumption (166,167,180). Another interesting approach to predicting hypotension after spinal anesthesia has been reported by Hanss and co-workers (181,182): They analyzed the heart rate variability, especially the low-to-high frequency ratio (LF/HF) from the echocardiogram (ECG). Heart rate variability reflects the activity of the autonomic nervous system (183) and therefore could predict the reaction of the sympathetic nervous system to spinal anesthesia. Indeed, in patients scheduled for prostate brachytherapy, high LF/HF predicted systolic blood pressure decrease after spinal anesthesia (181). Use of LF/HF-guided vasopressor therapy prevented hypotension after spinal anesthesia for cesarean section (182).

Ventilatory

Arterial blood gas tensions are unaffected during high spinal anesthesia in patients spontaneously breathing room air (159). Resting tidal volume, maximum inspiratory volume, and negative intrapleural pressure during maximal inhalation are similarly unaffected (184). These parameters remain unaltered despite intercostal paralysis associated with high thoracic sensory levels of spinal anesthesia because diaphragmatic activity is unimpaired. Maximum breathing capacity and maximum expiratory volumes, on the other hand, are significantly diminished during high thoracic levels of anesthesia, as are maximum intrapleural pressures during forced exhalation, including coughing. Pulmonary mechanics during exhalation are impaired because the muscles involved in forced exhalation, especially the anterior abdominal muscles, are denervated by high thoracic levels of spinal anesthesia. The effects of high spinal anesthesia on forced exhalation are of clinical importance in patients with tracheal or bronchial secretions in whom the ability to maintain clear airways depends on their ability to cough. In obese patients, the use of the Trendelenburg position or legs- and head-up position for correcting hypotension because of high block may cause difficulties in ventilation. The abdomen may compress the diaphragm and, if the intercostal muscles are blocked, adequate ventilation is not possible.

The phrenic nerves are unaffected by even midcervical levels of sensory anesthesia because the level of motor blockade is usually below the level of sensory anesthesia, as discussed previously. Respiratory arrest owing to phrenic paralysis secondary to an excessively high or "total" spinal is relatively rare. Even the concentration of local anesthetic in cisternal CSF during high spinal anesthesia, greater than that in ventricular CSF, is below the threshold concentration of local anesthetic required to produce depression of the central respiratory neurons when applied directly to the medulla. The most likely cause of transient respiratory arrest during high spinal anesthesia is ischemia of medullary respiratory neurons secondary to decreases in blood pressure and cardiac output severe enough to impair cerebral blood flow. Medullary ischemia as the cause of apnea during high spinal anesthesia is evidenced by the fact that respiratory arrest rarely occurs in the absence of hypotension severe enough to be associated with impending loss of consciousness. Further, restoration of blood pressure and cardiac output in cases of respiratory arrest during spinal anesthesia, if done promptly, is associated with immediate return of spontaneous respiration. This would not happen if the respiratory arrest were caused by pharmacologic block of the phrenic nerves or central respiratory neurons.

The character of spontaneous respiration serves as a valuable indication of the adequacy of medullary blood flow during high spinal anesthesia. It is therefore advisable to let patients breathe spontaneously during high spinal anesthesia rather than to control ventilation. Elimination of the negative intrapleural pressure of spontaneous inhalation by positive pressure ventilation not only removes a valuable indication of the adequacy of cerebral blood flow, but also may further decrease venous return, cardiac output, and arterial blood pressure.

The frequency and the type of postoperative respiratory complications have been reported to be similar after spinal anesthesia, local infiltration anesthesia, and general anesthesia in healthy patients, as well as in patients with preexisting respiratory disease, provided all other factors involved in determining the incidence of postoperative respiratory complications are kept constant. These other factors include the site and type of operation; age, sex, obesity, and smoking history of the patient; and frequency with which narcotics are administered for relief of postoperative pain. In studies of spinal anesthesia, no special advantage has been reported in the respiratory cripple. There may be an advantage, however, in using saddle block or low spinal anesthesia for perineal, urologic, and other surgery in order to avoid general anesthesia and possible artificial ventilation in patients on the brink of respiratory failure, with severe bronchospasm, excessive amounts of sputum, or a difficult airway. Data are lacking to document these theoretic advantages.

Sedation

It is a common observation that spinal anesthesia causes sedation and decreases requirements for sedative medication. One

reason is probably the profound block of afferent stimulation caused by spinal anesthesia. Experimental studies support this. In goats, lidocaine spinal anesthesia causes depression of excitability of reticulo-thalamo-cortical arousal mechanisms by blocking ascending somatosensory transmission (185).

In rats, subarachnoid bupivacaine decreases anesthetic requirements for thiopental (186). Spinal anesthesia with 50 mg of bupivacaine has caused significant sedation in unmedicated volunteers, with the sedative effect dependent on the level of sensory block (187). Similar observations have been reported also from clinical studies (188). The need for propofol during high spinal anesthesia was less than during low spinal anesthesia when the administration of propofol was guided by bispectral index (BIS) monitoring (189).

Thermoregulation

Shivering is commonly observed during or after spinal anesthesia. It is usually caused by a decrease in core temperature. Hypothermia does not always lead to shivering, especially in elderly patients (190).

Hypothermia during neuraxial anesthesia is nearly as severe as with general anesthesia. Extensive spinal blockade impairs central thermoregulatory control more than less extensive blockade (191). The main cause of hypothermia during spinal anesthesia is the redistribution of blood flow and heat to the periphery because of vasodilation. This can cause shivering, which is limited to unblocked segments. If the block is high, the area available for compensating the heat loss is smaller and the expected heat loss is larger. Usually, shivering is treated pharmacologically, thus abolishing physiologic mechanism to prevent heat loss.

The core temperature returns to normal levels by active heating faster after spinal than general anesthesia probably because the residual peripheral vasodilation during spinal anesthesia enables faster periphery-to-core heat transfer (192).

To prevent hypothermia, active warming through warm infusions, warm air, and coverings are essential during the operation and in the recovery room. Monitoring of central body temperature is indicated, especially in elderly patients.

TECHNIQUE OF LUMBAR PUNCTURE FOR SPINAL ANESTHESIA

A thorough knowledge of the anatomy of the lumbar spine (see Chapter 9) is an essential prerequisite to successful spinal anesthesia.

Preparation and Monitoring of the Patient

Inasmuch as all regional anesthesia may potentially become general anesthesia, the preparation for spinal anesthesia should be the same as that for general anesthesia. This includes a functional IV line, blood pressure and heart rate monitor, pulse oximeter, and appropriate equipment for airway management, suction, and oxygen administration. Emergency drugs must also be prepared. Because bradycardia and hypotension may appear rapidly, it is a good practice to have anticholinergic (atropine) and vasopressor (ephedrine) ready in the syringes. As in the management of any technique, the spinal anesthesia should be administered to a cooperative patient who is lying on a table that can be tipped upward or downward. One advantage of spinal over epidural anesthesia is the ability to control the spread of the anesthetic by manipulation of the baricity of the solution and the position of the patient. Similarly, the anesthesiologist must be able to assess the spread of anesthesia for limited procedures. The spread in overly sedated or anesthetized patients is virtually impossible to assess and can lead to a greater degree of failure or complications (see Chapter 8).

Position of the Patient

Lateral decubitus position (Fig. 10-5) is undoubtedly the most popular position for the performance of spinal anesthesia because of the comparative comfort it affords the patient. The patient should be placed on the very edge of the table closest to the anesthesiologist. The vertebral column is then flexed to widen the interlaminar spaces; this is accomplished by drawing the knees up to the chest and putting the chin down on the chest, the head supported by a pillow. (Care must be taken so that the vertebral column remains parallel with the edge of the table and the iliac crest and shoulders perpendicular to the table.) An assistant must stand in front of the patient to help the patient maintain the correct position. If the patient is to be positioned prone or supine at the conclusion of administering the spinal anesthetic, the location of the operative site is irrelevant. If, on the other hand, unilateral or hypobaric techniques

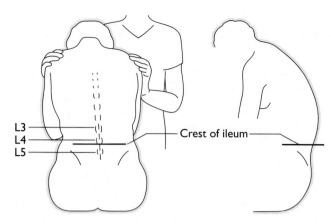

FIGURE 10-6. Sitting position of patient for spinal anesthesia.

are being used, then position of the operative site appropriate to the baricity of solution is essential.

Sitting position (Fig. 10-6) is used less frequently than lateral decubitus, with the exceptions of low spinal anesthesia in obstetrics, certain gynecologic and urologic procedures, and certain hypobaric and hyperbaric techniques. The sitting position also facilitates identification of the midline and the performance of lumbar puncture in obese patients. Precautions should be taken to prevent hypotension when patients who have received moderate to heavy premedication or who are subject to fainting are in the sitting position. The patient sits on the table as close to the anesthesiologist as possible, the feet supported by a stool. The patient's neck and back are flexed to provide maximum opening of the interspinous spaces. An assistant must stand in front of the patient at all times both to provide support and to maintain the correct position of the patient.

The prone position is used primarily for the hypobaric technique for procedures on rectum or sacrum. Preferably, the patient is placed prone on the operating table to avoid repositioning after induction of spinal anesthesia. The technique is most easily accomplished if the lumbar curve is extended by flexion of the table or by placing a pillow under the patient's abdomen. The CSF pressure is low in this position, and therefore aspiration may be necessary to obtain a free flow of CSF. Flow of CSF may be facilitated by elevating the head of the table. If this is to be done with a hypobaric technique, it is critical that the table be repositioned before injection of the anesthetic, so that the highest portion of the vertebral column is at the desired level of anesthesia. For operations of the lumbar spine, spinal anesthesia can be performed with the patient positioned for the surgery (knee-chest or similar position). The lumbar spine is already flexed, and the subarachnoid space is easier to find than in the prone position. The same precautions for the free flow of CSF and position of the table must be taken.

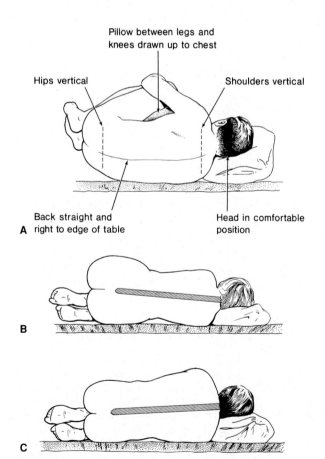

FIGURE 10-5. Lateral decubitus position for spinal anesthesia. Note skeletal differences of female (B) and male (C) on level of subarachnoid space.

Aseptic Technique

Before the spinal anesthesia, the anesthesiologist must perform a thorough surgical scrub using alcohol-based antiseptic solutions. All jewelry (rings, watches) must be removed, and sterile surgical gloves must be used. The use of surgical masks reduces the likelihood of contamination from the microorganisms in the upper airway of clinicians. In one study, the use of surgical gowns did not reduce the infection rates beyond that achieved with gloves alone (193). However, the use of a sterile gown may prevent contamination of the procedure site from nonsterile clothing.

The patient's back is widely prepared with an alcohol-based antiseptic solution and sterile drapes are applied. The antiseptic solution must be allowed to dry before proceeding. The anesthetic is drawn into the syringe and the equipment is checked, with constant vigilance against contamination of drugs or equipment. It is best to avoid combining different ingredients at the bedside; the local anesthetic to be should be premixed to the right concentration with needed additives to reduce the risk for large differences in the composition of spinal anesthetic mixtures when they are made at the bedside (194). If glass ampoules are used, the aspiration of the local anesthetic into the syringe should be done through a filter needle to prevent small pieces of glass being injected into the subarachnoid space.

The insertion site for lumbar puncture should be identified by the line between the upper border of the iliac crests, which passes through either the spinous process of L4 or the interspace between L4 and L5. The anesthesiologist should be positioned with the tray on the right (if right-handed) and the patient as nearly at eye level as possible. One may sit or stand as desired. Before any injection, the spinal needle should be inspected to ascertain that the stylet fits properly and that there are no barbs or foreign material on the tip of the needle. Care is taken to avoid handling the plunger of the syringe, which contains the spinal anesthetic solution, or touching the shaft of the spinal needle, which will subsequently be introduced into the subarachnoid space.

Depending on the interspace and approach selected (see Site of Injection, above), an intracutaneous skin wheal is made at the puncture site with a 25- to 27-gauge, 1-cm needle attached to a 2- to 5-mL syringe. One to 2 mL of lidocaine 10 mg/mL is the usual dosage and drug for skin wheals. After this, subcutaneous infiltration of additional local anesthetic may be accomplished with a 2- to 3-cm, 22-gauge needle. The patient is then ready for the spinal needle to be introduced.

Midline Approach

The midline approach, with the patient in the lateral position, is the most popular approach. First, an introducer needle is inserted through the skin wheal firmly into the interspinous ligament. Then, the spinal needle is introduced through the introducer. If Quincke-type needles are used, the bevel of the spinal needle should be directed laterally, so that the dural fibers that run longitudinally are spread rather than transected, thus diminishing the risk of posture-dependent postdural puncture headache (PDPPH). With these needles, a risk of deviation of the needle from the midline is possible, and it is suggested to start with the bevel oriented transversely, then turn the bevel 90° degrees longitudinally when the tip is close to the dura. After traversing the skin and subcutaneous tissues, the needle is advanced in a slightly cephalad direction (100–105 degrees on the cephalad side) with the long axis of the vertebral column, care again being taken to stay absolutely in the midline. (Even in the lumbar area, where the spinous processes of the lumbar vertebrae are relatively straight, the interlaminar space is slightly cephalad to the interspinous space.) A characteristic change in resistance occurs as the needle traverses the ligamentum flavum and dura arachnoid, a change that becomes quite recognizable as experience is gained with this technique. Especially when a noncutting needle is used, a characteristic "click" sensation can be observed when the dura is pierced. The stylet is removed and CSF allowed to appear at the hub of the needle. If proper flow of CSF does not occur, the needle is rotated in 90-degree increments until good flow is achieved. Occasionally, with patients in the prone position or if a small-bore spinal needle is being used, free flow of CSF will not be apparent. Gentle aspiration with a small, sterile syringe may then be used to obtain fluid.

With the hub of the spinal needle held firmly between the thumb and index finger of the left hand—the back of the left hand against the patient's back to prevent either withdrawal or advance of the spinal needle—the syringe containing the local anesthetic solution is firmly attached to the needle. Aspiration of CSF is then performed, and if there is free flow, the local anesthetic solution is injected. If a hyperbaric solution (with glucose) is used a typical turbulence is observed in the syringe when CSF mixes with the local anesthetic. Before removing the spinal needle, one again performs aspiration and reinjection of a small amount of fluid to reconfirm that the tip of the needle is still in the subarachnoid space. The patient is then placed in the desired position; cardiovascular and respiratory functions are monitored frequently, and the analgesic level to pin-prick or temperature level is checked at 5-minute intervals until the desired level is achieved. The patient should be repositioned as necessary, according to the baricity of the injected solution, to achieve this desired level.

Paramedian (Lateral) Approach

Many variations of the paramedian (lateral) approach (Fig. 10-7) avoid traversing the sometimes narrowed or calcified interspinous space. This approach is especially useful when degenerative changes are encountered in the interspinous structures (e.g., in elderly patients) and when ideal positioning of the patient cannot be achieved, owing to pain (e.g., fractures or dislocations involving the hips and lower extremities).

The patient is placed in the flexed lateral decubitus position, and a skin wheal is raised 1.5 cm lateral to the midline directly opposite the cephalad edge of the spinous process below the selected interspace. The direction of the spinal needle is at an angle of about 15 to 20 degrees with the midline and slightly cephalad, 100 to 105 degrees on the cephalad side. As with the midline approach, a characteristic "click" is encountered as the needle passes through the ligamentum flavum and dura arachnoid. At this point, the advance is stopped and the stylet withdrawn to allow CSF to appear in the hub of the needle. If periosteum rather than the subarachnoid space is encountered, the needle should be redirected slightly cephalad, thus walked off the laminae into the interspace. Anesthesiologists should remember that the interlaminar space is created by the failure of the laminae to unite in the midline. If the needle is walked off the laminae, it should enter the interlaminar space and go into the subarachnoid space. Once the tip of the needle lies within the subarachnoid space, the remainder of the technique for administering spinal anesthesia is identical to that described previously for the midline approach.

Problems

■ *The spinal needle is already deeply inserted, and it feels as if it is in the right place but there is no CSF.* Rotate the needle 90 degrees and wait for 10 to 15 seconds; repeat if necessary. Insert the stylet and remove it. Try to aspirate at different rotating angles. If no CSF can be aspirated, you

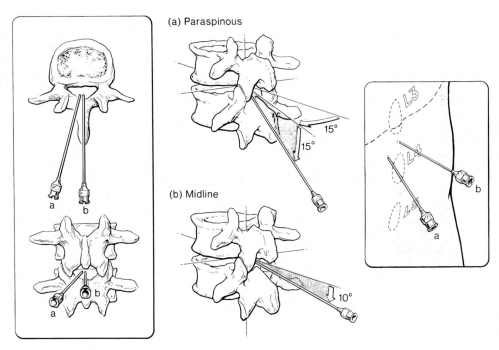

FIGURE 10-7. Two common techniques of lumbar puncture for spinal anesthesia. **A:** Paraspinous, para-median, or lateral approach. **B:** Midline.

have directed the needle too laterally. Withdraw the needle, check the position of the patient, and try again.

■ *There is blood in the needle.* There may be some blood from the epidural space; usually, it clears when a few drops of CSF are allowed to drip. However, if the blood continues to drip, the position of the needle must be changed. Most probably it is in an epidural vein.

■ *The needle causes pain in the leg.* Do not inject anything. Withdraw the needle and redirect it more medially.

■ *The needle hits bone all the time.* Reposition the patient. Change the needle—the tip of the needle is damaged from contact with bone. Try a different interspace or paramedian technique. Remember that the risk of spinal hematoma is increased in patients with spinal stenosis. Therefore, if you are not able to find the subarachnoid space, change the anesthesia method and do not stubbornly persist with further attempts at lumbar puncture.

Unilateral Spinal Anaesthesia

In 1961, Tanasichuk and colleagues published a paper in which a technique called *spinal hemianalgesia* was described (195). To achieve spinal hemianalgesia, they injected a hyperbaric solution through a Whitacre needle into a patient in the lateral decubitus position, the basic procedure used to produce unilateral spinal anesthesia. The technique did not garner much interest until the 1990s, when rapid ambulation and home discharge after surgery became important. Several groups have published papers on this technique, using terms such as *restricted, asymmetric, selective,* and *unilateral spinal anesthesia* to describe spinal anesthesia that achieves motor and sensory block limited to one side of the body (34,138,153,154,196) (although, usually, after turning the patient supine, some spread to the other side appears).

With a limited block, the surgery—most often arthroscopy of the knee—can be successfully performed and the recovery is

fast. Because the block is unilateral, the sympathetic block is also mostly unilateral, and hypotension and bradycardia risks are less. It seems also that bladder function is partly preserved, and thus problems with urinary retention preventing ambulation do not appear. However, bladder function after unilateral spinal anesthesia has not been adequately studied. It is questionable if voiding before discharge is needed after ambulatory surgery of the extremities; with the help of bladder ultrasound and proper patient information, most patients can be successfully discharged without mandatory voiding (197). Both hypo- and hyperbaric techniques have been used, but unilaterality is better achieved if hyperbaric anesthetic is used (153,154). The hypobaric techniques are used only in cases when the patient cannot be positioned on the side to be operated, for instance because of a fracture or if the operation is to be performed in the side-lying position (155). For unilateral block, the patient must be in a side-lying position. The best unilaterality is achieved with directional needles, where the injection can be directed to the appropriate side (132). Some dispute surrounds the role of injection speed in the spread of the block, because fast injection through a thin needle may cause turbulence and bilateral spread. Thus, suggestions for a low-flow technique (0.5 mL/min) have been made (138), but in clinical practice these extremely slow injections are difficult to achieve. The dose of the local anesthetic has to be small, otherwise it will spread bilaterally. After the injection, the patient must remain in the lateral position for at least 15 to 20 minutes. Usually, after turning the patient to the supine position some spread of the anesthesia to the other side will appear (99).

This technique is practical especially in lower extremity surgery with a duration of less than 1 hour. Tourniquet pain is also adequately blocked. It is used also in patients undergoing inguinal herniorrhaphy, but higher doses of local anesthetic are needed to ensure the spread of the block.

Hyperbaric bupivacaine, 5 mg/mL, 4 to 8 mg, injected through a directional needle with a lateral opening, and with the patient kept in the lateral position for 15 minutes following injection will result in a unilateral block in 80% of patients. For a hypobaric block, 6 to 8 mg of bupivacaine 1.8 to 2 mg/mL, diluted with water (1.8–2 mL of plain bupivacaine 5 mg/mL mixed with sterile water, 3–3.2 mL) has been used, but the unilaterality is not as good as with a hyperbaric technique (153,154).

Spinal Anesthesia for Lumbar Spine Surgery

Spinal anesthesia can also be used for lumbar spine surgery. The technique has certain benefits. The patient can move himself into the desired position and, because he is awake, the risk of pressure to the arms or eyes is avoided. Intubation is not needed. Spinal block has been performed with the patient placed for the surgery in the knee-chest position, but in that position aspiration of CSF is necessary to identify the subarachnoid space because the CSF will not freely come up through the thin needle. Alternatively, the subarachnoid injection can be performed with the patient in the lateral position and immediately thereafter he can move himself into the prone position for surgery. When this position is used, deep sedation must be avoided since securing the airway could be a problem. Plain bupivacaine doses of 10 to 15 mg will provide good anesthesia for herniated lumbar disk surgery (198,199). If the surgery lasts longer than the anesthesia, another dose of local anesthetic can be injected into the subarachnoid space through the operation wound.

Continuous Spinal Anesthesia

To produce continuous spinal anesthesia, a catheter may be inserted into the subarachnoid space and small, repeated doses of local anesthetic given. The benefits of this technique are that it could prevent the hypotension due to excessive sympathetic block caused by the large spread of anesthesia, and it would allow adequate anesthesia to be continued for as long as needed. Because the relatively large needle needed to insert a regular catheter causes the risk of headache, small microcatheters (32-gauge) that could be inserted through 25-gauge needles were introduced early in the 1990s (200). Unfortunately, the use of these microcatheters, together with overdoses of hyperbaric local anesthetics, caused several permanent cauda equina syndromes (23) and U.S. Food and Drug Administration (FDA) prohibited their use (244–245).

Continuous spinal anesthesia is, however, still quite commonly used. Either epidural catheters in the subarachnoid space, inserted through 18- to 20-gauge Tuohy needles, special catheters (CoSpan, Kendall; 28-gauge catheter through a 22-gauge needle), or a specially designed catheter-over-the-needle design (Spinocath; BBraun) are used. In the latter, an 18-gauge Crawford-type epidural needle is first inserted in the epidural space and then a special 22-gauge catheter over a 27-gauge needle is advanced through the Crawford needle and the dura is punctured. After ascertaining CSF flow through the catheter, it is kept immobile while the needle is withdrawn (201).

For continuous spinal anesthesia, the catheter should point cranially, and this is best achieved by using directional needles. If the needle has a Quincke-type tip, the catheter is easily directed caudally or curled (202). With a caudally directed catheter, the spread of anesthesia is limited and an increase in dose causes the local anesthetic to accumulate in a small area, thus increasing the risk of neurotoxicity. The catheter should be introduced only 2 to 3 cm, otherwise the tip may be too cranial or turn to the side and anesthesia may become seg-

mental. Plain (close to isobaric) solutions are preferred (203). The spread is easier to predict with plain solutions, and all the known cauda equina cases happened after the use of hyperbaric solutions. So far, the most experience is with bupivacaine (12,204). Levobupivacaine or ropivacaine may be as good and safe alternatives (205). Even though it would be logical to use fast and short-acting lidocaine, it is not recommended because of the potential for neurotoxicity. If the anesthesia has not spread after a reasonable dose (10–15 mg of bupivacaine) and time (20 minutes), one must assume that the catheter is pointing caudally and extreme caution should accompany any extra doses. If onset of spinal block occurs, but the spread is not adequate, a small dose of local anesthetic with different baricity (bupivacaine and sterile water; hypobaric) is worth a try. If the spread is still not adequate, the technique must be abandoned (204).

This technique is used mostly in elderly and hemodynamically unstable (the small dose lessens the risk of hypotension) and long operations (to continue the anesthesia for as long as needed). These patients are not in the highest-risk groups of PDPPH (206). It is also assumed that, because the catheter remains through the dura, it causes an inflammatory reaction that promotes the closure of the hole and diminishes the leak of CSF. The risk of headache is higher in younger, active populations. In a study (207) of 18- to 30-year-old healthy volunteers, in which through-catheter or catheter-over-needle techniques were used, 78% experienced PDPPH. The catheters were used for collecting of CSF samples (17 × 0.5 mL) for 4 hours. This situation is different from that in the surgical setting, and the clinical relevance may be questionable.

Continuous spinal anesthesia has also been used also for treatment of postoperative pain (62,208).

EQUIPMENT

Only disposable needles should be used, since reusable needles carry a small risk of infection and contamination by disinfectants. The thin spinal needles are especially difficult to clean (209).

Needles for Spinal Anesthesia

A needle with a close-fitting, removable stylet is essential. This will prevent coring of the skin and the rare, though possible, occurrence of epidermoid spinal cord tumors from the introduction of pieces of epidermis into the subarachnoid space. Over the years, a large number of spinal needles of various diameters with numerous types of points have been developed (Fig. 10-8). In general, in order to keep the incidence of postpuncture headache to a minimum, needles either of small bore or with a rounded, noncutting bevel (Whitacre or Sprotte) should be used.

The Quincke-Babcock spinal needle, the so-called standard spinal needle, has a sharp point with a medium-length cutting bevel.

The Whitacre needle, originally introduced in 1951 (210), and the Sprotte needle introduced in 1987 (211), have a completely rounded, noncutting bevels with solid tips. The needles' openings are on the side, 2 to 4 mm proximal to the tip. The Huber point Tuohy needle has a curved tip for introducing catheters into the subarachnoid space. Many other designs of spinal needles have been introduced, but their use is limited. Atraucan spinal needles have a tip designed to make a small linear cut (as opposed to a V-shaped cut) in the dura mater. The cut

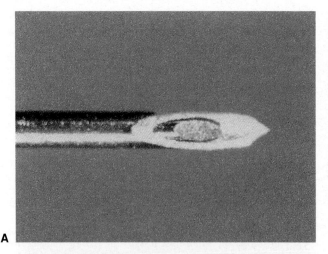

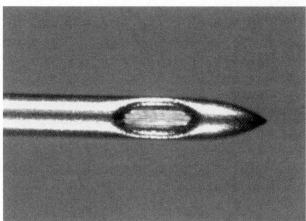

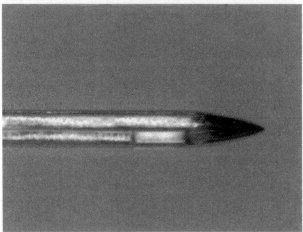

FIGURE 10-8. Tips of commonly used 27-gauge spinal needles. A: Quincke. B: Sprotte. C: Whitacre.

is shorter than the outside diameter of the needle and is dilated as the needle passes through the dura (212). A pencil-point needle with two holes (two circular holes opposing each other) has been used with the aim of enhancing symmetrical spread of anesthesia (213,214). Another spinal needle (Ballpen), with a pencil-like tip formed by a stylet that is withdrawn after penetration of the dura, has also been used (215).

Historically, the diameter of needles has been measured in *gauges*. Gauges are described in fractions of an inch; therefore, when the needle becomes thinner, the gauge number increases. There may be small differences among various manufacturers in the outer diameters of same gauge-size needles (Table 10-8) (216).

For the inexperienced, the use of a 25-gauge Whitacre or Sprotte needle is recommended. These slightly thicker needles allow the operator to become familiar with the characteristic "feel" of the various structures, especially the characteristic "click" sensation when the needle pierces the dura. The 25-gauge needles simultaneously keep the incidence of PDPPH low (2%–7%).

Combined spinal–epidural sets are becoming increasingly popular. Although slight modifications exist among manufacturers, all sets provide a Tuohy needle for introduction of an epidural catheter and a slightly longer spinal needle for subarachnoid injection of local anesthetics or narcotics. Some Tuohy needles have two holes: the usual one at the end of the tip for the passage of the catheter and a smaller one on the

outer curve (back-eye) to enable the passage of the spinal needle without needle bending (see Chapter 11, Fig. 11-13).

Regardless of the size of the needle used, care must be taken so that the dural fibers that run longitudinally are separated rather than transected. With that in mind, the opening bevel is always on the side of the notch on the hub of the needle; the notch is then arranged so that the needle bevel is parallel to the longitudinal dural fibers.

TABLE 10-8

NEEDLE SELECTION

The diameters of the needles used for anesthesia are expressed as gauge units. There are small differences in these diameters (in millimeters) among different manufacturers.

Gauge	Outer diameter (mm)
16	1.6
18	1.3
22	0.7
25	0.5
27	0.41
29	0.34

Introducers

Various introducers have been developed both to facilitate the introduction of small-bore spinal needles, which are difficult to direct alone, and to prevent contact of the spinal needle with the skin. The introducer needle usually does not have a stylet and thus does not seem to reduce tissue coring. As an alternative, a disposable 18-gauge needle may be used. The use of an introducer is particularly helpful with 25- or 27-gauge needles.

In order to limit the risk of PDPPH, small needles with non-cutting tips should be used (217). There does not seem to be a major difference between Sprotte and Whitacre needles. In scanning electron microscopy studies, Whitacre-type needles produce a more traumatic dural lesion than Quincke-type needles (218). It is suggested that the lower incidence of PDPPH after the use of noncutting needles might be caused by the inflammatory reaction produced by the tearing of the collagen fibers after dural penetration. This inflammatory reaction may result in a significant edema, which may act as a plug to limit the leakage of CSF.

Needle Deflection

Quincke-type needles tend to deviate toward the leading point of the tip and, in experimental models (219), the largest amount of deviation was seen with beveled spinal needles (Quincke, Atraucan; range 4.42–5.90 mm/50 mm tissue). The thicker needles have a larger tendency toward deviation (220). This can lead to difficulties finding the spinal space and perhaps more readily cause bone contacts. This deflection has not been observed with noncutting needles. The use of an introducer needle diminishes this problem.

Needle Deformation

The tip of thin Quincke-type needles is easily damaged when contacting bone. This happens mainly with thin 25- to 27-gauge needles. The clinical significance seems to be limited since when untoward postanesthetic signs (headache, back pain, numbness) were compared, there was no difference between the needles that had not been damaged (no bone contact prior the spinal puncture) and those that were damaged (bone contact before the puncture) (221).

Tissue Coring

It is possible for tissue particles (skin, fat) or disinfectant solution to be carried intrathecally with the needle (222). The role of these tissue particles in causing spinal epidermoid tumors has been suggested; thus, all precautions to prevent this must be used. The use of an introducer does not necessarily prevent the introduction of debris intrathecally, but tissue coring appears to be less with the use of noncutting needles. To reduce the risk of introducing foreign matter, the stylet of the needle should fit well, and it has been suggested that several drops of CSF be allowed to escape from the needle to clear it of tissue particles before injecting local anesthetic (223).

Spread of Local Anesthetic. The conventional Quincke-type needle has an opening at the tip causing injectate to flow in an almost straight direction (Fig. 10-9). In a pencil-point needle with the hole in the side, the flow is directed approximately 45 degree from the longitudinal axis (133). Thus, it is possible to limit the spread of anesthesia (saddle block, unilateral block) with pencil-point needles and a hypo- or hyperbaric local anesthetic solution.

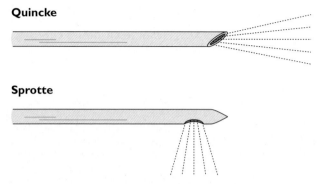

FIGURE 10-9. The direction of flow is different from Quincke and Sprotte needles.

INTRAOPERATIVE AND POSTOPERATIVE MANAGEMENT

Clinically, the extent of the sensory block can be tested with cold (acetone drops, ice, iced tubes, alcohol swabs, ethyl chloride spray), pin-prick (short-bevel 18-gauge needle), pinch, or touch. Several recent studies have reported on the use of tolerance to transcutaneous electrical stimulation (TES) with a peripheral nerve stimulator as a test for the spread of sensory anesthesia. A 60-mA current at 50-Hz for 5 seconds is considered equivalent to surgical stimulation (to test for analgesia), but smaller currents have been used to predict surgical anesthesia (224).

A bed-side test for the extent of motor block for epidural anesthesia was described 40 years ago by Bromage (225), and modifications of this test are still in use. The Bromage score does not always predict recovery but, during the induction phase of the block, it is practical for everyday clinical use. More sophisticated methods for motor block testing have been evaluated, but their correlation to the Bromage score is not always good (226). An electromyelographic (EMG)-based method for testing motor block during surgery has been used to guide the administration of "top-up doses" of bupivacaine during continuous spinal anesthesia (227).

In clinical practice, a method that is easy to use at the bedside and that has a reasonable predictive value is needed to test the spread of a block. If one uses loss of sensation to cold, there must be a safety margin of two to four dermatomes over the planned incision. It is practical first to touch an area where sensation is normal; thus, the patient is able to differentiate between normal and abnormal sensation. For sensory analgesia testing, TES might be a good alternative. The Bromage test is easily used at bedside, and a score of 2 to 3 predicts good muscle relaxation (see Table 11-5).

The first 5 to 10 minutes after administration of the spinal anesthetic are the most critical in adjusting the level of anesthesia when hyperbaric or hypobaric solutions are used. Levels of spinal anesthesia required for common surgical procedures are shown in Table 10-9. The first 10 to 20 minutes are also the most critical in assessing the cardiovascular responses to spinal anesthesia. Frequent measurements of blood pressure and heart rate will allow early recognition of any degree of hypotension. Patient monitoring should include blood pressure (noninvasive or invasive depending on the patient and surgery), pulse oximetry, and electrocardiogram.

If after 10 minutes there are no signs of spinal anesthesia—that is, motor function and sensation are still normal—it is

TABLE 10-9

LEVEL OF SPINAL ANESTHESIA REQUIRED FOR COMMON SURGICAL PROCEDURES

Level	Surgical procedure
T4–T5 (nipple)	Upper abdominal surgery
T6–T8 (xiphoid)	Intestinal surgery including appendectomy, gynecologic pelvic surgery, renal surgery
T10 (umbilicus)	Transurethral resection, hip surgery, hernia surgery
T12	Thigh tourniquet
L1 (inguinal ligament)	Knee surgery, lower limb amputation
L2–L3 (below knee)	Foot surgery
S2–S5	Perineal surgery, hemorrhoidectomy

apparent that the injection was not intrathecal. Depending on the patient, another spinal injection or other methods of anesthesia must be used. If the block is not high enough, the baricity of the local anesthetic can be altered and the position of the patient can be changed in order to increase the level. If the block is too high, one must prepare for treatment of hypotension or bradycardia and assure and comfort the patient. During the first 20 minutes, and if the level of the block is high, changes to the position of the patient must be made with caution. A legs-down position with hyperbaric anesthetic will eliminate the upward movement of the local anesthetic but also limit the circulatory volume, thus increasing risk of hypotension. Usually, hyperbaric solution does not spread higher than the thoracic kyphosis (T4).

After surgical anesthesia levels and cardiovascular stability have been achieved, the anesthesiologist may determine whether supplemental drugs should be administered to make the patient comfortable. Not all patients will need IV medications during the course of surgery under spinal anesthesia. Many need only reassurance by a caring, empathetic anesthesiologist. The opportunity to follow the surgery from the monitor during arthroscopic procedures is appreciated by most of the patients. The possibility to listen one's own music is another way to distract attention away from the procedure. When drugs are required to attenuate apprehension or discomfort arising from the unanesthetized upper extremities and trunk, benzodiazepines, which have both sedative and anxiolytic properties, are most useful. The object of intraoperative medication during spinal anesthesia is to render the patient free of fear, anxiety, and discomfort. The object is not to induce light general anesthesia unless the patient or surgical circumstances require it. Benzodiazepines, for example, should be administered in low doses, and their effects should be assessed frequently, especially in the elderly; once the desired effect is achieved, maintenance of sedation should be accomplished with additional low doses at increasingly longer intervals. Opioids during spinal anesthesia are best reserved for management of discomfort or slight pain from the operative site and for discomfort that occurs in the unanesthetized upper part of the body when patients lie immobile on the operating table for long periods. The low doses of opioids required for this type of analgesia will have minimal depressant effects on respiration. If pain is severe because the level of spinal anesthesia is inadequate, induction of light general anesthesia is preferred instead of reliance upon large doses of opioids.

Although supplemental oxygen by mask or by nasopharyngeal insufflation is usually not necessary in normal patients with low levels of spinal anesthesia, it is often used in patients with high thoracic levels or if the patient's respirations are depressed by hypnotics, tranquilizers, or opioids. The anesthesiologist should bear in mind that supplemental oxygen given to a hypoventilating patient may improve arterial oxygenation, but it will not relieve the accompanying increase in arterial carbon dioxide tension and may even aggravate it. If the sedation is too deep and the airway needs to be secured, the laryngeal mask airway is usually well tolerated and enables smooth recovery.

The anesthesiologist's role postoperatively can be divided into two periods. The first is a continued monitoring of the anesthetized patient in the recovery unit until complete cessation of the spinal anesthesia has occurred. Concerns during this period start with the careful movement and transport of the patient from the operating room to the unit. The level of anesthesia can change even more than 60 minutes after the block, indicating that free anesthetic is present in the CSF (101). Therefore, sudden movements too soon after the anesthesia may increase the spread of anesthesia and lead to hypotension in the recovery room. Movements may also cause some degree of hypotension owing to redistribution of blood volume with movement; thus careful monitoring of the blood pressure is essential. If blood loss has occurred during surgery and there is relative hypovolemia, the risk of hypotension is increased. If the patient does not have an indwelling urinary catheter, recovery room personnel should be alert for a distended bladder. The voiding mechanism is mediated through sacral autonomic fibers, which are the last to regain function after spinal anesthesia. Even after patients are able to move their extremities and respond to sensory stimuli, they may have some residual autonomic blockade, and thus may not only be unable to void but may also become hypotensive in the sitting or standing position. Unilateral spinal anesthesia seems to diminish this problem. Ultrasound devices help in deciding the volume of urine in the bladder and thus unnecessary catheterizations are avoided (197,228). Posture-dependent postdural puncture headache is not related, either in severity or in incidence, to the patient's position while spinal anesthesia is wearing off and during the immediate postoperative period. Patients are kept flat in bed after spinal anesthesia only if necessary to avoid hypotension, not postoperative headaches. The role of the anesthesiologist in the postoperative period becomes one of surveillance, with special attention to the possible development of postanesthetic complications. Equally as important as the detection of bona fide complications is good rapport with the patient, which will permit the explanation of postsurgical aches and pains and the appropriate dismissal of them when clearly not caused by spinal anesthesia.

POSTURE-DEPENDENT POSTDURAL PUNCTURE HEADACHE

Headache used to be a very common postoperative side effect of spinal anesthesia, a condition more appropriately called *postdural puncture headache* rather than *spinal headache*. Because the headache usually appears in the erect position and is relieved by recumbency, the term *posture-dependent postdural puncture headache* is most accurate.

The incidence of PDPPH over the years has varied from 0.2% to 24% (210,217,229,230). Posture-dependent postdural puncture headache is more frequent in women and in younger patients. The highest incidence is in obstetric patients. Also, the larger the size of the needle, the more frequent and severe are the PDPPHs. Although headaches after spinal anesthesia can be a post spinal-anesthetic problem, diagnostic lumbar punctures and myelography are associated with an even higher incidence of headaches. Further, postoperative headaches occur after general anesthesia. Not all headaches after spinal anesthesia are due to the dural puncture. It is important, therefore, to be conversant with the diagnostic features that are unique to this complication.

Clinical Features

Although a history of dural puncture is helpful, the clinical features of PDPPH are still diagnostic. First, the onset of headache occurs a minimum of several hours after the puncture but usually within the first or second day post puncture. A controlled study showed that bed rest did not prevent, but merely postponed, the onset of headache (231). The headache has been described as invariably bifrontal and occipital, frequently involving the neck and upper shoulders (232). Severity varies from mild to incapacitating and may be aggravated, especially by the upright position and also by coughing and straining. The headache usually subsides completely when the patient is lying down. Associated symptoms are related to the severity of the headache and may include nausea and loss of appetite, photophobia, and changes in hearing acuity and tinnitus, and depression. Patients whose headache persists for any period of time feel miserable, tearful, bedridden, and dependent. In more severe cases, diplopia and cranial nerve palsies have been attributed to traction on corresponding nerves.

The most probable reason for headache is the loss of CSF through the dural tear. The larger hole in the dura, the more probable is the headache. In an MRI study in patients suffering from PDPPH, extrathecal CSF and hemosiderosis indicating the site of dural puncture was observed. In another MRI study, clear reductions of intracranial CSF volume were observed in patients with PDPPH (233,234).

Once the diagnosis of PDPPH has been established, prompt treatment is essential. When considering the treatment options, one must remember that the process is self-limiting. The earliest measure was prophylactic in the form of enforced flat bed rest for 24 to 48 hours. This, of course, became therapeutic once the headache had occurred. Symptomatic treatment with analgesics or sedatives is just that, and probably has no beneficial effect in reversing the process.

Because the reason for the symptoms is probably the loss of CSF through the dural tear and decreased pressure in the CSF, therapeutic modalities have been directed at restoring the pressure relationships in the epidural and subarachnoid spaces. This has included measures such as abdominal binders to force more venous blood through the epidural plexus; injection of saline in large volumes into the epidural space; overhydration of the patient, orally or intravenously, to stimulate production of CSF; and antidiuresis. In practical terms, many mild headaches may be resolved with forced fluid intake of 3 L/day or more, plus the use of a tight abdominal binder when the patient is sitting or standing. Cerebral vasoconstrictors have been used with the aim to decrease the cerebral blood volume. Caffeine perorally or intravenously has been used with variable success (235). (It seems that part of the headaches is due to withdrawal of caffeine during the perioperative period and therefore an extra dose of caffeine relieves headache.)

The most efficient treatment relies on the assumption that the hole in the dura and leak of the CSF is the reason for headache. Therefore, sealing the hole would resolve the headache (Table 10-10).

TABLE 10-10

POSTURE-DEPENDENT POSTDURAL PUNCTURE HEADACHE

Prevention:
Noncutting thin spinal needles
If dural tap with epidural needle, consider inserting catheter into the intrathecal space for 24 hours

Diagnosis:
Headache 12–72 hours after dural puncture
Posture-dependent
May involve nausea, vomiting, double vision, tinnitus

Differential diagnosis:
Migraine
Caffeine, tobacco withdrawal, fasting
Meningitis
Intracranial bleeding

Treatment:
Bed rest, hydration, caffeine, mild analgesics

If >24 hours and prevents ambulation, perform epidural blood patch:
Aseptic technique; max 20 mL blood from cubital vein
Epidural puncture same level or below
Stop epidural injection if pain or paresthesia: 30–60 min bedrest

Indeed, in 1960, Gormley (229) reported injecting 2 to 3 mL of a patient's own blood into the epidural space in seven patients with good results. Probably because of the small number studied, this technique did not become popular before the 1970s, when DiGiovanni (230) reported on 50 patients who received epidural injections of 20 mL autologous blood as successful treatment for post–lumbar puncture headache. Subsequently, and despite fears of infection and neurologic sequelae, the procedure has become an important therapy, employed progressively earlier. Abouleish summarized 524 cases reported by 11 centers. He also reported a prospective study of an additional 118 patients (236). In another large study of 504 patients, 75% achieved complete pain relief and 18% experienced some relief (237).

The technique of autologous blood patch is simply the insertion of a needle into the epidural space by the usual methods, followed by the injection of 20 mL of blood drawn aseptically from the patient's own antecubital vein. If the patient expresses backache or pain, the injection must be stopped. In MRI, after epidural blood patch (EBP), a large extradural hematoma extending over four spinal segments, extending out through the neural outlet foramina, and tamponading the site of dural puncture can be seen (238).

If patients are at all volume-depleted, it is desirable to simultaneously infuse 1,000 mL of IV fluid. Subsequent to the injection, the patient remains supine for 30 to 60 minutes. The success rate after the first injection varies from 89% to 95%. The procedure may be repeated 24 hours later and will provide equivalent success. Reported complications are few and mild but include backache (35%), neck ache (0.9%), and transient temperature elevation (5%) of 24 to 48 hours' duration. It appears, then, that this is a worthwhile procedure with known minor risk that should be considered if early conservative measures fail.

There are different opinions on the right timing and indication of EBP. Since the symptom is self-limiting and the epidural puncture and handling of blood carry certain risks, it is reasonable to be conservative. The success rate of EBP is smaller if it is performed during the first 24 hours. On the other hand, waiting longer increases the suffering of the patient and limits ambulation. Therefore, in a patient with PDPPH limiting ambulation, optimal time to place EBP is 24 hours after the dural puncture (239).

Prevention

Especially in young females, a thin (27-gauge) noncutting spinal needle must be used. If a dural tap with an epidural needle is used, the risk of PDPPH in the obstetric population

can be as high as 90%. Different options are possible after an accidental dural tap with an epidural needle. Immediate infusion of saline epidurally may delay PDPPH but does not prevent it. Immediate blood patch does not relieve the headache, either (240,241).

If the catheter is introduced intrathecally through the hole and left to remain 24 hours, the frequency of PDPPH decreases to 6% (242,243).

As mentioned earlier, an intrathecal catheter seems to cause an inflammatory reaction that seals the hole and prevents leakage. If the catheter is removed after the delivery, the frequency of PDPPH is increased; the same phenomenon occurs after spinal needle removals. Quincke-type needles cause a neat hole compared to Whitacre needles (218), but the risk of headache is smaller if Whitacre needles are used.

References

1. Bier A. Versuche über Kokainisierung des Rückenmarks. *Langenbecks Arch Klin Chir Ver Dtsch Z Chir* 1899;51:361–369.
2. Braun H. Über einige neue örtliche Anästhetica (Stovain, Alypine, Novokain). *Dtsch Med Wochenschr* 1903;31:1667–1671.
3. Sise LF. Pontocaine-glucose solution for spinal anesthesia. *Surg Clin North Am* 1935;124:1501–1511.
4. Lemmon WT, Paschal GW. Continuous—serial, fractional, controllable, intermittent—spinal anesthesia. *Surg Gynecol Obst* 1942;74:948–956.
5. Gordh T. Xylocain: A new local analgesic. *Anaesthesia* 1949;4:4–9.
6. Cope RW. The Woolley and Roe Case. *Anaesthesia* 1954;9:249–270.
7. Dripps RD, Vandam LD. Long-term follow-up of patients who received 10,098 spinal anesthetics: Failure to discover major neurological sequelae. *J Am Med Assoc* 1954;156:1486–1491.
8. Ekblom L, Widman B. LAC-43 and tetracaine in spinal anaesthesia. *Acta Anaesthesiol Scand* 1966;[Suppl 23]:419–425.
9. Tuominen M. Bupivacaine spinal anaesthesia. *Acta Anaesthesiol Scand* 1991;35:1–10.
10. Urmey WF. Spinal anaesthesia for outpatient surgery. *Best Pract Res Clin Anaesthesiol* 2003;17:335–346.
11. Rawal N. Combined spinal-epidural anaesthesia. *Curr Opin Anaesthesiol* 2005;18:518–521.
12. Bevacqua BK. Continuous spinal anaesthesia: What's new and what's not. *Best Pract Res Clin Anaesthesiol* 2003;17:393–406.
13. Liu SS, Block BM, Wu CL. Effects of perioperative central neuraxial analgesia on outcome after coronary artery bypass surgery: A meta-analysis. *Anesthesiology* 2004;101:153–161.
14. Lee TW, Grocott HP, Schwinn D, Jacobsohn E. High spinal anesthesia for cardiac surgery: Effects on beta-adrenergic receptor function, stress response, and hemodynamics. *Anesthesiology* 2003;98:499–510.
15. Hadimioglu N, Ertug Z, Bigat Z, et al. A randomized study comparing combined spinal epidural or general anesthesia for renal transplant surgery. *Transplant Proc* 2005;37:2020–2022.
16. van Zundert AA, Stultiens G, Jakimowicz JJ, et al. Segmental spinal anaesthesia for cholecystectomy in a patient with severe lung disease. *Br J Anaesth* 2006;96:464–466.
17. Wedel DJ, Horlocker TT. Regional anesthesia in the febrile or infected patient. *Reg Anesth Pain Med* 2006;31:324–333.
18. Moen V, Dahlgren N, Irestedt L. Severe neurological complications after central neuraxial blockades in Sweden 1990–1999. *Anesthesiology* 2004;101:950–959.
19. Drake E, Drake M, Bird J, Russell R. Obstetric regional blocks for women with multiple sclerosis: A survey of UK experience. *Int J Obstet Anesth* 2006;15:115–123.
20. Lambert DA, Giannouli E, Schmidt BJ. Postpolio syndrome and anesthesia. *Anesthesiology* 2005;103:638–644.
21. McDonald SB. Is neuraxial blockade contraindicated in the patient with aortic stenosis? *Reg Anesth Pain Med* 2004;29:496–502.
22. Raynaud L, Mercier FJ, Auroy Y, Benhamou D. SOS ALR—Epidural anaesthesia and lumbar tattoo: What to do? *Ann Fr Anesth Reanim* 2006;25:71–73.
23. Rigler ML, Drasner K, Krejcie TC, et al. Cauda equina syndrome after continuous spinal anesthesia. *Anesth Analg* 1991;72:275–281.
24. Hodgson PS, Liu SS, Batra MS, et al. Procaine compared with lidocaine for incidence of transient neurologic symptoms. *Reg Anesth Pain Med* 2000;25:218–222.
25. Le Truong HH, Girard M, Drolet P, et al. Spinal anesthesia: A comparison of procaine and lidocaine. *Can J Anaesth* 2001;48:470–473.
26. Mulroy MF, Larkin KL, Siddiqui A. Intrathecal fentanyl-induced pruritus is more severe in combination with procaine than with lidocaine or bupivacaine. *Reg Anesth Pain Med* 2001;26:252–256.
27. Schneider M, Ettlin T, Kaufmann M, et al. Transient neurologic toxicity after hyperbaric subarachnoid anesthesia with 5% lidocaine. *Anesth Analg* 1993;76:1154–1157.
28. Auroy Y, Benhamou D, Bargues L, et al. Major complications of regional anesthesia in France: The SOS Regional Anesthesia Hotline Service. *Anesthesiology* 2002;97:1274–1280.
29. Eberhart LH, Morin AM, Kranke P, et al. Transiente neurologische symptome nach spinal anästhesie. *Anaesthesist* 2002;51:539–546.
30. Pollock JE, Liu SS, Neal JM, Stephenson CA. Dilution of spinal lidocaine does not alter the incidence of transient neurologic symptoms. *Anesthesiology* 1999;90:445–450.
31. Moore DC. Spinal anesthesia: Bupivacaine compared with tetracaine. *Anesth Analg* 1980;59:743–750.
32. Concepcion MA, Lambert DH, Welch KA, Covino BG. Tourniquet pain during spinal anesthesia: A comparison of plain solutions of tetracaine and bupivacaine. *Anesth Analg* 1988;67:828–832.
33. Tuominen M, Pitkanen M, Doepel M, Rosenberg PH. Spinal anaesthesia with hyperbaric tetracaine: Effect of age and body mass. *Acta Anaesthesiol Scand* 1987;31:474–478.
34. Valanne JV, Korhonen AM, Jokela RM, et al. Selective spinal anesthesia: A comparison of hyperbaric bupivacaine 4 mg versus 6 mg for outpatient knee arthroscopy. *Anesth Analg* 2001;93:1377–1379.
35. Logan MR, McClure JH, Wildsmith JA. Plain bupivacaine: An unpredictable spinal anaesthetic agent. *Br J Anaesth* 1986;58:292–296.
36. Glaser C, Marhofer P, Zimpfer G, et al. Levobupivacaine versus racemic bupivacaine for spinal anesthesia. *Anesth Analg* 2002;94:194–198.
37. Alley EA, Kopacz DJ, McDonald SB, Liu SS. Hyperbaric spinal levobupivacaine: A comparison to racemic bupivacaine in volunteers. *Anesth Analg* 2002;94:188–193.
38. Milligan KR. Recent advances in local anaesthetics for spinal anaesthesia. *Eur J Anaesthesiol* 2004;21:837–847.
39. McDonald SB, Liu SS, Kopacz DJ, Stephenson CA. Hyperbaric spinal ropivacaine: A comparison to bupivacaine in volunteers. *Anesthesiology* 1999;90:971–977.
40. McNamee DA, McClelland AM, Scott S, et al. Spinal anaesthesia: Comparison of plain ropivacaine 5 mg ml(-1) with bupivacaine 5 mg ml(-1) for major orthopaedic surgery. *Br J Anaesth* 2002;89:702–706.
41. Kallio H, Snall EV, Kero MP, Rosenberg PH. A comparison of intrathecal plain solutions containing ropivacaine 20 or 15 mg versus bupivacaine 10 mg.*Anesth Analg* 2004;99:713–717.
42. Casati A, Moizo E, Marchetti C, Vinciguerra F. A prospective, randomized, double-blind comparison of unilateral spinal anesthesia with hyperbaric bupivacaine, ropivacaine, or levobupivacaine for inguinal herniorrhaphy. *Anesth Analg* 2004;99:1387–1392.
43. Cappelleri G, Aldegheri G, Danelli G, et al. Spinal anesthesia with hyperbaric levobupivacaine and ropivacaine for outpatient knee arthroscopy: A prospective, randomized, double-blind study. *Anesth Analg* 2005;101:77–82.
44. Kallio H, Snall EV, Tuomas CA, Rosenberg PH. Comparison of hyperbaric and plain ropivacaine 15 mg in spinal anaesthesia for lower limb surgery. *Br J Anaesth* 2004;93:664–669.
45. Fettes PD, Hocking G, Peterson MK, et al. Comparison of plain and hyperbaric solutions of ropivacaine for spinal anaesthesia. *Br J Anaesth* 2005;94:107–111.

46. Wang BC, Hillman DE, Spielholz NI, Turndorf H. Chronic neurological deficits and Nesacaine-CE: An effect of the anesthetic, 2-chloroprocaine, or the antioxidant, sodium bisulfite? *Anesth Analg* 1984;63:445–447.

47. Gissen A, Datta S, Lambert D. The chloroprocaine controversy. *Reg Anesth Pain Med* 1984;9:124–145.

48. Yoos JR, Kopacz DJ. Spinal 2-chloroprocaine for surgery: An initial 10-month experience. *Anesth Analg* 2005;100:553–558.

49. Casati A, Danelli G, Berti M, et al. Intrathecal 2-chloroprocaine for lower limb outpatient surgery: A prospective, randomized, double-blind, clinical evaluation. *Anesth Analg* 2006;103:234–238.

50. Taniguchi M, Bollen AW, Drasner K. Sodium bisulfite: Scapegoat for chloroprocaine neurotoxicity? *Anesthesiology* 2004;100:85–91.

51. Kishimoto T, Bollen AW, Drasner K. Comparative spinal neurotoxicity of prilocaine and lidocaine. *Anesthesiology* 2002;97:1250–1253.

52. Kaukinen S, Eerola R, Eerola M, Kaukinen L. A comparison of carticaine and lidocaine in spinal anaesthesia. *Ann Clin Res* 1978;10:191–194.

53. Kallio H, Snall EV, Luode T, Rosenberg PH. Hyperbaric articaine for daycase spinal anaesthesia. *Br J Anaesth* 2006;97:704–709.

54. Ostgaard G, Hallaraker O, Ulveseth OK, Flaatten H. A randomised study of lidocaine and prilocaine for spinal anaesthesia. *Acta Anaesthesiol Scand* 2000;44:436–440.

55. Park WY, Balingot PE, McNamara TE. Effects of patient age, pH of cerebrospinal fluid and vasopressor on onset and duration of spinal anesthesia. *Anesth Analg* 1975;54:455–458.

56. Eisenach J. Safety in numbers: How do we study toxicity of spinal analgesics? *Anesthesiology* 2002;97:1047–1049.

57. Walker SM, Goudas LC, Cousins MJ, Carr DB. Combination spinal analgesic chemotherapy: A systematic review. *Anesth Analg* 2002;95:674–715.

58. Tejwani GA, Rattan AK, McDonald JS. Role of spinal opioid receptors in the antinociceptive interactions between intrathecal morphine and bupivacaine. *Anesth Analg* 1992;74:726–734.

59. Yamada H, Shimoyama N, Sora I, et al. Morphine can produce analgesia via spinal kappa opioid receptors in the absence of mu opioid receptors. *Brain Res* 2006;1083:61–69.

60. Ummenhofer WC, Arends RH, Shen DD, Bernards CM. Comparative spinal distribution and clearance kinetics of intrathecally administered morphine, fentanyl, alfentanil, and sufentanil. *Anesthesiology* 2000;92:739–753.

61. Rathmell JP, Pino CA, Taylor R, et al. Intrathecal morphine for postoperative analgesia: A randomized, controlled, dose-ranging study after hip and knee arthroplasty. *Anesth Analg* 2003;97:1452–1457.

62. Bachmann M, Laakso E, Niemi L, et al. Intrathecal infusion of bupivacaine with or without morphine for postoperative analgesia after hip and knee arthroplasty. *Br J Anaesth* 1997;78:666–670.

63. Gürkan Y, Canatay H, Özdamar D, et al. Spinal anesthesia for arthroscopic knee surgery. *Acta Anaesthesiol Scand* 2004;48:513–517.

64. Rathmell JP, Lair TR, Nauman B. The role of intrathecal drugs in the treatment of acute pain. *Anesth Analg* 2005;101:S30–S43.

65. Hamber EA, Viscomi CM. Intrathecal lipophilic opioids as adjuncts to surgical spinal anesthesia. *Reg Anesth Pain Med* 1999;24:255–263.

66. Korhonen AM, Valanne JV, Jokela RM, et al. Intrathecal hyperbaric bupivacaine 3 mg + fentanyl 10 μg for outpatient knee arthroscopy with tourniquet. *Acta Anaesthesiol Scand* 2003;47:342–346.

67. Ben-David B, Solomon E, Levin H, et al. Intrathecal fentanyl with small-dose dilute bupivacaine: Better anesthesia without prolonging recovery. *Anesth Analg* 1997;85:560–565.

68. Szarvas S, Harmon D, Murphy D. Neuraxial opioid-induced pruritus: A review. *J Clin Anesth* 2003;15:234–239.

69. Sarvela PJ, Halonen PM, Soikkeli AI, et al. Ondansetron and tropisetron do not prevent intraspinal morphine- and fentanyl-induced pruritus in elective cesarean delivery. *Acta Anaesthesiol Scand* 2006;50:239–244.

70. Horta ML, Morejon LC, da Cruz AW, et al. Study of the prophylactic effect of droperidol, alizapride, propofol and promethazine on spinal morphine-induced pruritus. *Br J Anaesth* 2006;96:796–800.

71. Bailey PL, Rhondeau S, Schafer PG, et al. Dose-response pharmacology of intrathecal morphine in human volunteers. *Anesthesiology* 1993;79:49–59.

72. Yamaguchi H, Watanabe S, Fukuda T, et al. Minimal effective dose of intrathecal morphine for pain relief following transabdominal hysterectomy. *Anesth Analg* 1989;68:537–540.

73. Dohi S, Matsumiya N, Takeshima R, Naito H. The effects of subarachnoid lidocaine and phenylephrine on spinal cord and cerebral blood flow in dogs. *Anesthesiology* 1984;61:238–244.

74. Covino BG, Scott DB, Lambert DH. *Handbook of Spinal Anaesthesia and Analgesia.* Philadelphia: Mediglobe, 1994.

75. Concepcion M, Maddi R, Francis D, et al. Vasoconstrictors in spinal anesthesia with tetracaine: A comparison of epinephrine and phenylephrine. *Anesth Analg* 1984;63:134–138.

76. Chambers WA, Littlewood DG, Logan MR, Scott DB. Effect of added epinephrine on spinal anesthesia with lidocaine. *Anesth Analg* 1981;60:417–420.

77. Chambers WA, Littlewood DG, Scott DB. Spinal anesthesia with hyperbaric bupivacaine: Effect of added vasoconstrictors. *Anesth Analg* 1982;61:49–52.

78. Chiu AA, Liu S, Carpenter RL, et al. The effects of epinephrine on lidocaine spinal anesthesia: A cross-over study. *Anesth Analg* 1995;80:735–739.

79. Smith KN, Kopacz DJ, McDonald SB. Spinal 2-chloroprocaine: A dose-ranging study and the effect of added epinephrine. *Anesth Analg* 2004;98:81–88.

80. Liu SS, McDonald SB. Current issues in spinal anesthesia. *Anesthesiology* 2001;94:888–906.

81. Khan ZP, Ferguson CN, Jones RM. Alpha-2 and imidazoline receptor agonists. Their pharmacology and therapeutic role. *Anaesthesia* 1999;54:146–165.

82. Unnerstall JR, Kopajtic TA, Kuhar MJ. Distribution of alpha 2 agonist binding sites in the rat and human central nervous system: Analysis of some functional, anatomic correlates of the pharmacologic effects of clonidine and related adrenergic agents. *Brain Res* 1984;319:69–101.

83. Dobrydnjov I, Axelsson K, Gupta A, et al. Improved analgesia with clonidine when added to local anesthetic during combined spinal-epidural anesthesia for hip arthroplasty: A double-blind, randomized and placebo-controlled study. *Acta Anaesthesiol Scand* 2005;49:538–545.

84. Dobrydnjov I, Axelsson K, Thorn SE, et al. Clonidine combined with small-dose bupivacaine during spinal anesthesia for inguinal herniorrhaphy: A randomized double-blinded study. *Anesth Analg* 2003;96:1496–1503.

85. Niemi L. Effects of intrathecal clonidine on duration of bupivacaine spinal anaesthesia, haemodynamics, and postoperative analgesia in patients undergoing knee arthroscopy. *Acta Anaesthesiol Scand* 1994;38:724–728.

86. Liu S, Chiu AA, Neal JM, et al. Oral clonidine prolongs lidocaine spinal anesthesia in human volunteers. *Anesthesiology* 1995;82:1353–1359.

87. Dobrydnjov I, Axelsson K, Samarutel J, Holmstrom B. Postoperative pain relief following intrathecal bupivacaine combined with intrathecal or oral clonidine. *Acta Anaesthesiol Scand* 2002;46:806–814.

88. Rhee K, Kang K, Kim J, Jeon Y. Intravenous clonidine prolongs bupivacaine spinal anesthesia. *Acta Anaesthesiol Scand* 2003;47:1001–1005.

89. Kanazi GE, Aouad MT, Jabbour-Khoury SI, et al. Effect of low-dose dexmedetomidine or clonidine on the characteristics of bupivacaine spinal block. *Acta Anaesthesiol Scand* 2006;50:222–227.

90. Cohen EN. Distribution of local anesthetic agents in the neuraxis of the dog. *Anesthesiology* 1968;29:1002–1005.

91. Hogan Q. Size of human lower thoracic and lumbosacral nerve roots. *Anesthesiology* 1996;85:37–42.

92. Brull SJ, Greene NM. Time courses of zones of differential spinal anesthesia with hyperbaric tetracaine or bupivacaine. *Anesth Analg* 1989;69:342–347.

93. Wildsmith JA, McClure JH, Brown DT, Scott DB. Effects of posture on the spread of isobaric and hyperbaric amethocaine. *Br J Anaesth* 1981;53:273–278.

94. Liu S, Kopacz DJ, Carpenter RL. Quantitative assessment of differential sensory nerve block after lidocaine spinal anesthesia. *Anesthesiology* 1995;82:60–63.

95. Bengtsson M, Nilsson GE, Lofstrom JB. The effect of spinal analgesia on skin blood flow, evaluated by laser Doppler flowmetry. *Acta Anaesthesiol Scand* 1983;27:206–210.

96. Bengtsson M, Lofstrom JB, Malmqvist LA. Skin conductance responses during spinal analgesia. *Acta Anaesthesiol Scand* 1985;29:67–71.

97. Chamberlain DP, Chamberlain BD. Changes in the skin temperature of the trunk and their relationship to sympathetic blockade during spinal anesthesia. *Anesthesiology* 1986;65:139–143.

98. Stevens RA, Frey K, Liu SS, et al. Sympathetic block during spinal anesthesia in volunteers using lidocaine, tetracaine, and bupivacaine. *Reg Anesth* 1997;22:325–331.

99. Kuusniemi KS, Pihlajamaki KK, Pitkanen MT, Korkeila JE. A low-dose hypobaric bupivacaine spinal anesthesia for knee arthroscopies. *Reg Anesth* 1997;22:534–538.

100. Povey HM, Jacobsen J, Westergaard-Nielsen J. Subarachnoid analgesia with hyperbaric 0.5% bupivacaine: Effect of a 60-min period of sitting. *Acta Anaesthesiol Scand* 1989;33(4):295–297.

101. Niemi L, Tuominen M, Pitkanen M, Rosenberg PH. Effect of late posture change on the level of spinal anaesthesia with plain bupivacaine. *Br J Anaesth* 1993;71:807–809.

102. Denson DD, Bridenbaugh PO, Turner PA, Phero JC. Comparison of neural blockade and pharmacokinetics after subarachnoid lidocaine in the rhesus monkey. II: Effects of volume, osmolality, and baricity. *Anesth Analg* 1983;62:995–1001.

103. Burm AG, van Kleef JW, Gladines MP, et al. Plasma concentrations of lidocaine and bupivacaine after subarachnoid administration. *Anesthesiology* 1983;59:191–195.

104. Greene NM. Uptake and elimination of local anesthetics during spinal anesthesia. *Anesth Analg* 1983;62:1013–1024.

105. Burm AG, Van Kleef JW, Vermeulen NP, et al. Pharmacokinetics of lidocaine and bupivacaine following subarachnoid administration in surgical patients: Simultaneous investigation of absorption and disposition kinetics using stable isotopes. *Anesthesiology* 1988;69:584–592.

106. Axelsson KH, Sundberg AE, Edstrom HH, et al. Venous blood concentrations after subarachnoid administration of bupivacaine. *Anesth Analg* 1986;65:753–759.

PART II: TECHNIQUES

107. Veering BT, Burm AG, van Kleef JW, et al. Spinal anesthesia with glucose-free bupivacaine: Effects of age on neural blockade and pharmacokinetics. *Anesth Analg* 1987;66:965–970.

108. Veering BT, Burm AG, Spierdijk J. Spinal anaesthesia with hyperbaric bupivacaine. Effects of age on neural blockade and pharmacokinetics. *Br J Anaesth* 1988;60:187–194.

109. Greene NM. Distribution of local anesthetic solutions within the subarachnoid space. *Anesth Analg* 1985;64:715–730.

110. Corbin KB, Gardner ED. Decrease in number of myelinated fibers in human spinal roots with age. *Anat Rec* 1937;68:63–74.

111. Dorfman LJ, Bosley TM. Age related changes in peripheral and central nerve conduction in man. *Neurology* 1979;29:38–44.

112. Flanigan KM, Lauria G, Griffin JW, Kuncl RW. Age-related biology and diseases of muscle and nerve. *Neurol Clin* 1998;16:659–669.

113. May C, Kaye JA, Atack JR, et al. Cerebrospinal fluid production is reduced in healthy aging. *Neurology* 1990;40:500–503.

114. Cameron AE, Arnold RW, Ghoris MW, Jamieson V. Spinal analgesia using bupivacaine 0.5% plain. *Anaetshesia* 1981;36:318–322.

115. Pitkanen M, Haapaniemi L, Tuominen M, Rosenberg PH. Influence of age on spinal anaesthesia with isobaric 0.5% bupivacaine. *Br J Anaesth* 1984;56:279–284.

116. Pargger H, Hampl KF, Aeschbach A, et al. Combined effect of patient variables on sensory level after spinal 0.5% plain bupivacaine. *Acta Anaesthesiol Scand* 1998;42:430–434.

117. Pitkanen MT. Body mass and spread of spinal anesthesia with bupivacaine. *Anesth Analg* 1987;66:127–131.

118. Hogan QH, Prost R, Kulier A, et al. Magnetic resonance imaging of cerebrospinal fluid volume and the influence of body habitus and abdominal pressure. *Anesthesiology* 1996;84:1341–1349.

119. Sullivan JT, Grouper S, Walker MT, et al. Lumbosacral cerebrospinal fluid volume in humans using three-dimensional magnetic resonance imaging. *Anesth Analg* 2006;103:1306–1310.

120. Carpenter RL, Hogan QH, Liu SS, et al. Lumbosacral cerebrospinal fluid volume is the primary determinant of sensory block extent and duration during spinal anesthesia. *Anesthesiology* 1998;89:24–29.

121. Higuchi H, Hirata J, Adachi Y, Kazama T. Influence of lumbosacral cerebrospinal fluid density, velocity, and volume on extent and duration of plain bupivacaine spinal anesthesia. *Anesthesiology* 2004;100:106–114.

122. Barclay DL, Renegar OJ, Nelson EW, Jr. The influence of inferior vena cava compression on the level of spinal anesthesia. *Am J Obstet Gynecol* 1968;101:792–800.

123. Schiffer E, Van Gessel E, Fournier R, et al. Cerebrospinal fluid density influences extent of plain bupivacaine spinal anesthesia. *Anesthesiology* 2002;96:1325–1330.

124. Kalso E, Tuominen M, Rosenberg PH. Effect of posture and some c.s.f. characteristics on spinal anaesthesia with isobaric 0.5% bupivacaine. *Br J Anaesth* 1982;54:1179–1184.

125. Tuominen M, Taivainen T, Rosenberg PH. Spread of spinal anaesthesia with plain 0.5% bupivacaine: Influence of the vertebral interspace used for injection. *Br J Anaesth* 1989;62:358–361.

126. Veering BT, Ter Riet PM, Burm AG, et al. Spinal anaesthesia with 0.5% hyperbaric bupivacaine in elderly patients: Effect of site of injection on spread of analgesia. *Br J Anaesth* 1996;77:343–346.

127. Broadbent CR, Maxwell WB, Ferrie R, et al. Ability of anaesthetists to identify a marked lumbar interspace. *Anaesthesia* 2000;55:1122–1126.

128. Kim JT, Bahk JH, Sung J. Influence of age and sex on the position of the conus medullaris and Tuffier's line in adults. *Anesthesiology* 2003;99:1359–1363.

129. Reynolds F. Damage to the conus medullaris following spinal anaesthesia. *Anaesthesia* 2001;56:238–247.

130. Tuominen M, Kuulasmaa K, Taivainen T, Rosenberg PH. Individual predictability of repeated spinal anaesthesia with isobaric bupivacaine. *Acta Anaesthesiol Scand* 1989;33:13–14.

131. Taivainen TR, Tuominen MK, Kuulasmaa KA, Rosenberg PH. A prospective study on reproducibility of the spread of spinal anesthesia using plain 0.5% bupivacaine. *Reg Anesth* 1990;15:12–14.

132. Casati A, Fanelli G, Cappelleri G, et al. Effects of spinal needle type on lateral distribution of 0.5% hyperbaric bupivacaine. *Anesth Analg* 1998;87:355–359.

133. Urmey WF, Stanton J, Bassin P, Sharrock N. The direction of the Whitacre needle aperture affects the extent and duration of isobaric spinal anesthesia. *Anesth Analg* 1997;84:337–341.

134. Tuominen M, Pitkanen M, Rosenberg PH. Effect of speed of injection of 0.5% plain bupivacaine on the spread of spinal anaesthesia. *Br J Anaesth* 1992;69:148–149.

135. Horlocker TT, Wedel DJ, Wilson PR. Effect of injection rate on sensory level and duration of hypobaric bupivacaine spinal anesthesia for total hip arthroplasty. *Anesth Analg* 1994;79:773–777.

136. Stienstra R, Van Poorten F. Speed of injection does not affect subarachnoid distribution of plain bupivacaine 0.5%. *Reg Anesth* 1990;15:208–210.

137. Casati A, Fanelli G, Cappelleri G, et al. Does speed of intrathecal injection affect the distribution of 0.5% hyperbaric bupivacaine? *Br J Anaesth* 1998;81:355–357.

138. Enk D, Prien T, Van Aken H, et al. Success rate of unilateral spinal anesthesia is dependent on injection flow. *Reg Anesth Pain Med* 2001;26:420–427.

139. Janik R, Dick W, Stanton-Hicks MD. Influence of barbotage on block characteristics during spinal anesthesia with hyperbaric tetracaine and bupivacaine. *Reg Anesth* 1989;14:26–30.

140. Nightingale PJ. Barbotage and spinal anaesthesia. The effect of barbotage on the spread of analgesia during isobaric spinal anaesthesia. *Anaesthesia* 1983;38:7–9.

141. Sheskey MC, Rocco AG, Bizzarri-Schmid M, et al. A dose-response study of bupivacaine for spinal anesthesia. *Anesth Analg* 1983;62:931–935.

142. Van Zundert AA, Grouls RJ, Korsten HH, Lambert DH. Spinal anesthesia. Volume or concentration–what matters? *Reg Anesth* 1996;21:112–118.

143. Axelsson KH, Edstrom HH, Sundberg AE, Widman GB. Spinal anaesthesia with hyperbaric 0.5% bupivacaine: Effects of volume. *Acta Anaesthesiol Scand* 1982;26:439–445.

144. Chambers WA, Littlewood DG, Edstrom HH, Scott DB. Spinal anaesthesia with hyperbaric bupivacaine: Effects of concentration and volume administered. *Br J Anaesth* 1982;54:75–80.

145. Ben-David B, Levin H, Solomon E, et al. Spinal bupivacaine in ambulatory surgery: The effect of saline dilution. *Anesth Analg* 1996;83:716–720.

146. Lui AC, Polis TZ, Cicutti NJ. Densities of cerebrospinal fluid and spinal anaesthetic solutions in surgical patients at body temperature. *Can J Anaesth* 1998;45:297–303.

147. Horlocker TT, Wedel DJ. Density, specific gravity, and baricity of spinal anesthetic solutions at body temperature. *Anesth Analg* 1993;76:1015–1018.

148. McLeod GA. Density of spinal anaesthetic solutions of bupivacaine, levobupivacaine, and ropivacaine with and without dextrose. *Br J Anaesth* 2004;92:547–551.

149. Stienstra R, van Poorten JF. The temperature of bupivacaine 0.5% affects the sensory level of spinal anesthesia. *Anesth Analg* 1988;67:272–276.

150. Heller AR, Zimmermann K, Seele K, et al. Modifying the baricity of local anesthetics for spinal anesthesia by temperature adjustment: Model calculations. *Anesthesiology* 2006;105:346–353.

151. Ernst EA. In vitro changes of osmolality and density of spinal anesthetic solutions. *Anesthesiology* 1968;29:104–109.

152. Sanderson P, Read J, Littlewood DG, et al. Interaction between baricity (glucose concentration) and other factors influencing intrathecal drug spread. *Br J Anaesth* 1994;73:744–746.

153. Kuusniemi KS, Pihlajamaki KK, Pitkanen MT. A low dose of plain or hyperbaric bupivacaine for unilateral spinal anesthesia. *Reg Anesth Pain Med* 2000;25:605–610.

154. Kaya M, Oguz S, Aslan K, Kadiogullari N. A low-dose bupivacaine: A comparison of hyperbaric and hypobaric solutions for unilateral spinal anesthesia. *Reg Anesth Pain Med* 2004;29:17–22.

155. Faust A, Fournier R, Van Gessel E, et al. Isobaric versus hypobaric spinal bupivacaine for total hip arthroplasty in the lateral position. *Anesth Analg* 2003;97:589–594.

156. Taivainen T, Tuominen M, Rosenberg PH. Spinal anaesthesia with hypobaric 0.19% or plain 0.5% bupivacaine. *Br J Anaesth* 1990;65:234–236.

157. Stienstra R, van Poorten JF. Plain or hyperbaric bupivacaine for spinal anesthesia. *Anesth Analg* 1987;66:171–176.

158. Na KB, Kopacz DJ. Spinal chloroprocaine solutions: Density at 37 degrees C and pH titration. *Anesth Analg* 2004;98:70–74.

159. Greene NM, Brull SJ. *Physiology of Spinal Anesthesia*, 4th ed. Baltimore: Williams & Wilkins, 1993.

160. Caplan RA, Ward RJ, Posner K, Cheney FW. Unexpected cardiac arrest during spinal anesthesia. A closed claims analysis of predisposing factors. *Anesthesiology* 1988;68:5–11.

161. Auroy Y, Narchi P, Messiah A, et al. Serious complications related to regional anesthesia: Results of a prospective survey in France. *Anesthesiology* 1997;87:479–486.

162. Kopp SL, Horlocker TT, Warner ME, et al. Cardiac arrest during neuraxial anesthesia: Frequency and predisposing factors associated with survival. *Anesth Analg* 2005;100:855–865.

163. Giasi RM, D'Agostino E, Covino BG. Absorption of lidocaine following subarachnoid and epidural administration. *Anesth Analg* 1979;58:360–363.

164. Bridenbaugh PO, Moore DC, Bridenbaugh L. Capillary Po₂ as a measure of sympathetic blockade. *Anesth Analg* 1971;50:26–30.

165. Ward RJ, Bonica JJ, Freud FG, et al. Epidural and subarachnoid anesthesia: Cardiovascular and respiratory effects. *JAMA* 1965;191:275–278.

166. Tarkkila P, Isola J. A regression model for identifying patients at high risk of hypotension, bradycardia and nausea during spinal anesthesia. *Acta Anaesthesiol Scand* 1992;36:554–558.

167. Carpenter RL, Caplan RA, Brown DL, et al. Incidence and risk factors for side effects of spinal anesthesia. *Anesthesiology* 1992;76:906–916.

168. Stienstra R. Mechanisms behind and treatment of sudden unexpected circulatory collapse during central neuraxis blockade. *Acta Anaesthesiol Scand* 2000;44:965–971.

169. Salinas FV, Sueda LA, Liu SS. Physiology of spinal anaesthesia and practical suggestions for successful spinal anaesthesia. *Best Pract Res Clin Anaesthesiol* 2003;17:289–303.

170. Campagna JA, Carter C. Clinical relevance of the Bezold-Jarisch reflex. *Anesthesiology* 2003;98:1250–1260.

171. Kinsella SM, Tuckey JP. Perioperative bradycardia and asystole: Relationship to vasovagal syncope and the Bezold-Jarisch reflex. *Br J Anaesth* 2001; 86:859–868.

172. Hackel DB, Sancetta SM, Kleinerman J. Effect of hypotension due to spinal anesthesia on coronary blood flow and myocardial metabolism in man. *Circulation* 1956;13:92–97.

173. Runciman WB, Mather LE, Ilsley AH, et al. A sheep preparation for studying interactions between blood flow and drug disposition. III: Effects of general and spinal anaesthesia on regional blood flow and oxygen tensions. *Br J Anaesth* 1984;56:1247–1258.

174. Sidi A, Pollak D, Floman Y, Davidson JT. Hypobaric spinal anesthesia in the operative management of orthopedic emergencies in geriatric patients. *Isr J Med Sci* 1984;20:589–592.

175. Coe AJ, Revanäs B. Is crystalloid preloading useful in spinal anaesthesia in the elderly? *Anaesthesia* 1990;45:241–243.

176. Venn PJH, Simpson DA, Rubin AP, Edstrom HH. Effect of fluid preloading on cardiovascular variables after spinal anaesthesia with glucose-free 0.75% bupivacaine. *Br J Anaesth* 1989;63:682–687.

177. Janvrin SB, Davies G, Greenhalgh RM. Postoperative deep vein thrombosis caused by intravenous fluids during surgery. *Br J Surg* 1980;67:690–693.

178. Dahlgren G, Granath F, Pregner K, et al. Colloid vs. crystalloid preloading to prevent maternal hypotension during spinal anesthesia for elective cesarean section. *Acta Anaesthesiol Scand* 2005;49:1200–1206.

179. Yap JC, Critchley LA, Yu SC, et al. A comparison of three fluid-vasopressor regimens used to prevent hypotension during subarachnoid anaesthesia in the elderly. *Anaesth Intensive Care* 1998;26:497–502.

180. Hartmann B, Junger A, Klasen J, et al. The incidence and risk factors for hypotension after spinal anesthesia induction: An analysis with automated data collection. *Anesth Analg* 2002;94:1521–1529.

181. Hanss R, Bein B, Weseloh H, et al. Heart rate variability predicts severe hypotension after spinal anaesthesia. *Anesthesiology* 2006;104:537–545.

182. Hanss R, Bein B, Francksen H, et al. Heart rate variability-guided prophylactic treatment of severe hypotension after subarachnoid block for elective cesarean delivery. *Anesthesiology* 2006;104:635–643.

183. Pomeranz B, Macaulay RJ, Caudill MA, et al. Assessment of autonomic function in humans by heart rate spectral analysis. *Am J Physiol* 1985; 248:H151–H153.

184. Freund FG, Bonica JJ, Ward RJ, et al. Ventilatory reserve and level of motor block during high spinal and epidural anesthesia. *Anesthesiology* 1967;28:834–837.

185. Antognini JF, Jinks SL, Atherley R, et al. Spinal anaesthesia indirectly depresses cortical activity associated with electrical stimulation of the reticular formation. *Br J Anaesth* 2003;91:233–238.

186. Eappen S, Kissin I. Effect of subarachnoid bupivacaine block on anesthetic requirements for thiopental in rats. *Anesthesiology* 1998;88:1036–1042.

187. Gentili M, Huu PC, Enel D, et al. Sedation depends on the level of sensory block induced by spinal anaesthesia. *Br J Anaesth* 1998;81:970–971.

188. Ben-David B, Vaida S, Gaitini L. The influence of high spinal anesthesia on sensitivity to midazolam sedation. *Anesth Analg* 1995;81:525–528.

189. Ozkan-Seyhan T, Sungur MO, Senturk E, et al. BIS guided sedation with propofol during spinal anaesthesia: Influence of anaesthetic level on sedation requirement. *Br J Anaesth* 2006;96:645–649.

190. Vassilieff N, Rosencher N, Sessler DI, Conseiller C. Shivering threshold during spinal anesthesia is reduced in elderly patients. *Anesthesiology* 1995;83:1162–1166.

191. Leslie K, Sessler DI. Reduction in the shivering threshold is proportional to spinal block height. *Anesthesiology* 1996;84:1327–1331.

192. Szmuk P, Ezri T, Sessler DI, et al. Spinal anesthesia speeds active postoperative rewarming. *Anesthesiology* 1997;87:1050–1054.

193. Hebl JR. The importance and implications of aseptic techniques during regional anesthesia. *Reg Anesth Pain Med* 2006;31:311–323.

194. Dull RO, Peterfreund RA. Variations in the composition of spinal anesthetic solutions: The effects of drug addition order and preparation methods. *Anesth Analg* 1998;87:1326–1330.

195. Tanasichuk MA, Schultz EA, Matthews JH, Van Bergen FH. Spinal hemianalgesia: An evaluation of a method, its applicability, and influence on the incidence of hypotension. *Anesthesiology* 1961;22:74–85.

196. Fanelli G, Borghi B, Casati A, et al. Unilateral bupivacaine spinal anesthesia for outpatient knee arthroscopy. Italian Study Group on Unilateral Spinal Anesthesia. *Can J Anaesth* 2000;47:746–751.

197. Mulroy MF, Salinas FV, Larkin KL, Polissar NL. Ambulatory surgery patients may be discharged before voiding after short-acting spinal and epidural anesthesia. *Anesthesiology* 2002;97:315–319.

198. Laakso E, Pitkanen M, Kytta J, Rosenberg PH. Knee-chest vs horizontal side position during induction of spinal anaesthesia in patients undergoing lumbar disc surgery. *Br J Anaesth* 1997;79:609–611.

199. Jellish WS, Shea JF. Spinal anaesthesia for spinal surgery. *Best Pract Res Clin Anaesthesiol* 2003;17:323–334.

200. Hurley RJ, Lambert DH. Continuous spinal anesthesia with a microcatheter technique: Preliminary experience. *Anesth Analg* 1990;70:97–102.

201. Puolakka R, Pitkanen MT, Rosenberg PH. Comparison of three catheter sets for continuous spinal anesthesia in patients undergoing total hip or knee arthroplasty. *Reg Anesth Pain Med* 2000;25:584–590.

202. Standl T, Eckert S, Straub U. The effect of puncture needle on the subarachnoid catheter position in continuous spinal anesthesia. *Anaesthesist* 1995;44:826–830.

203. Van Gessel EF, Forster A, Schweizer A, Gamulin Z. Comparison of hypobaric, hyperbaric, and isobaric solutions of bupivacaine during continuous spinal anesthesia. *Anesth Analg* 1991;72:779–784.

204. Pitkanen M. Continuous spinal anesthesia and analgesia. *Tech Reg Anesth Pain Manag* 1998;2:96–102.

205. Sell A, Olkkola KT, Jalonen J, Aantaa R. Minimum effective local anesthetic dose of isobaric levobupivacaine and ropivacaine administered via a spinal catheter for hip replacement surgery. *Br J Anaesth* 2005;94:239–242.

206. Denny N, Masters R, Pearson D, et al. Postdural puncture headache after continuous spinal anesthesia. *Anesth Analg* 1987;66:791–794.

207. Gosch UW, Hueppe M, Hallschmid M, et al. Post-dural puncture headache in young adults: Comparison of two small-gauge spinal catheters with different needle design. *Br J Anaesth* 2005;94:657–661.

208. Mollmann M, Cord S, Holst D, Auf der Landwehr U. Continuous spinal anaesthesia or continuous epidural anaesthesia for post-operative pain control after hip replacement? *Eur J Anaesthesiol* 1999;16:454–461.

209. Tuominen MK, Keskinen K, Rosenberg PH. Scanning electron microscopic examination of resterilized 29-gauge spinal needles. *Anesthesiology* 1988;69:123–125.

210. Hart JR, Whitacre RG. Pencil-point needle in prevention of post spinal headache. *JAMA* 1951;147:657–658.

211. Sprotte G, Schedel R, Pajunk H, Pajunk H. Eine "atraumatische" Universakanüle für einzeitige Regionalanaesthesien. *Reg Anaesth* 1987;10:104–108.

212. Scott DB, Dittmann M, Clough DG, et al. Atraucan: A new needle for spinal anesthesia. *Reg Anesth* 1993;18:213–217.

213. Eldor J. Double-hole pencil-point spinal needle. *Reg Anesth* 1996;21:74–75.

214. Puolakka R, Haasio J, Rosenberg PH, Tuominen M. Comparison of double-hole and single-hole pencil-point needles for spinal anesthesia with hyperbaric bupivacaine. *Reg Anesth Pain Med* 1998;23:271–277.

215. Standl T, Stanek A, Burmeister MA, et al. Spinal anesthesia performance conditions and side effects are comparable between the newly designed Ballpen and the Sprotte needle: Results of a prospective comparative randomized multicenter study. *Anesth Analg* 2004;98:512–517.

216. Poll JS. The story of the gauge. *Anaesthesia* 1999;54:575–581.

217. Santanen U, Rautoma P, Luurila H, et al. Comparison of 27-gauge (0.41-mm) Whitacre and Quincke spinal needles with respect to post-dural puncture headache and non-dural puncture headache. *Acta Anaesthesiol Scand* 2004;48:474–479.

218. Reina MA, de Leon-Casasola OA, Lopez A, et al. An in vitro study of dural lesions produced by 25-gauge Quincke and Whitacre needles evaluated by scanning electron microscopy. *Reg Anesth Pain Med* 2000;25:393–402.

219. Kopacz DJ, Allen HW. Comparison of needle deviation during regional anesthetic techniques in a laboratory model. *Anesth Analg* 1995;81:630–633.

220. Sitzman BT, Uncles DR. The effects of needle type, gauge, and tip bend on spinal needle deflection. *Anesth Analg* 1996;82:297–301.

221. Puolakka R, Jokinen M, Pitkanen MT, Rosenberg PH. Comparison of postanesthetic sequelae after clinical use of 27-gauge cutting and noncutting spinal needles. *Reg Anesth* 1997;22:521–526.

222. Puolakka R, Andersson LC, Rosenberg PH. Microscopic analysis of three different spinal needle tips after experimental subarachnoid puncture. *Reg Anesth Pain Med* 2000;25:163–169.

223. Campbell DC, Douglas MJ, Taylor G. Incidence of tissue coring with the 25-gauge Quincke and Whitacre spinal needles. *Reg Anesth* 1996;21:582–585.

224. Moore JM, Liu SS, Pollock JE, et al. The effect of epinephrine on small-dose hyperbaric bupivacaine spinal anesthesia: Clinical implications for ambulatory surgery. *Anesth Analg* 1998;86:973–977.

225. Bromage PR. A comparison of hydrochloride and carbon dioxide salts of lidocaine and prilocaine in epidural analgesia. *Acta Anaesthesiol Scand* 1965;[Suppl 16]:55–69.

226. Axelsson K, Hallgren S, Widman B, et al. A new method for measuring motor block in the lower extremities. *Acta Anaesthesiol Scand* 1985;29:72–78.

227. Niemi-Murola L, Paloheimo M. Feasibility of electromyography (sEMG) in measuring muscular activity during spinal anaesthesia in patients undergoing knee arthroplasty. *Acta Anaesthesiol Scand* 2005;49:558–562.

228. Pavlin DJ, Pavlin EG, Gunn HC, et al. Voiding in patients managed with or without ultrasound monitoring of bladder volume after outpatient surgery. *Anesth Analg* 1999;89:90–97.

229. Gormley JB. Treatment of postspinal headache. *Anesthesiology* 1960;21: 565–566.
230. DiGiovanni AJ, Dunbar BS. Epidural injections of autologous blood for postlumbar-puncture headache. *Anesth Analg* 1970;49:268–271.
231. Carbaat PAT, Van Crevel H. Lumbar puncture headache: Controlled study of the preventive effect of 24 hours bedrest. *Lancet* 1981;21;2:1133–1135.
232. Brownridge P. Management of headache following dural puncture in obstetric patients. *Anaesth Intensive Care* 1983;11:4–15.
233. Vakharia SB, Thomas PS, Rosenbaum AE, et al. Magnetic resonance imaging of cerebrospinal fluid leak and tamponade effect of blood patch in postdural puncture headache. *Anesth Analg* 1997;84:585–590.
234. Grant R, Condon B, Hart I, Teasdale GM. Changes in intracranial CSF volume after lumbar puncture and their relationship to post-LP headache. *J Neurol Neurosurg Psychiatry* 1991;54:440–442.
235. Camann WR, Murray RS, Mushlin PS, Lambert DH. Effects of oral caffeine on postdural puncture headache. A double-blind, placebo-controlled trial. *Anesth Analg* 1990;70:181–184.
236. Abouleish E, Vega S, Blendinger I, Tio TO. Long-term follow-up of epidural blood patch. *Anesth Analg* 1975;54:459–463.
237. Safa-Tisseront V, Thormann F, Malassine P, et al. Effectiveness of epidural blood patch in the management of post-dural puncture headache. *Anesthesiology* 2001;95: 334–339.

238. Griffiths AG, Beards SC, Jackson A, Horsman EL. Visualization of extradural blood patch for post lumbar puncture headache by magnetic resonance imaging. *Br J Anaesth* 1993;70:223–225.
239. Vilming ST, Kloster R, Sandvik L. When should an epidural blood patch be performed in postlumbar puncture headache? A theoretical approach based on a cohort of 79 patients. *Cephalalgia* 2005;25:523–527.
240. Charsley MM, Abram SE. The injection of intrathecal normal saline reduces the severity of postdural puncture headache. *Reg Anesth Pain Med* 2001;26:301–305.
241. Scavone BM, Wong CA, Sullivan JT, et al. Efficacy of a prophylactic epidural blood patch in preventing post dural puncture headache in parturients after inadvertent dural puncture. *Anesthesiology* 2004;101:1422–1427.
242. Ayad S, Demian Y, Narouze SN, Tetzlaff JE. Subarachnoid catheter placement after wet tap for analgesia in labor: Influence on the risk of headache in obstetric patients. *Reg Anesth Pain Med* 2003;28:512–515.
243. Kuczkowski KM, Benumof JL. Decrease in the incidence of post-dural puncture headache: Maintaining CSF volume. *Acta Anaesthesiol Scand* 2003;47:98–100.
244. Drasner K, Smiley R. Continuous spinal analgesia for labor and delivery: A born-again technique? *Anesthesiology*. 2008;108:184–186.
245. Arkoosh VA, Palmer CM, Yunem et al. A randomized double-masked, multicenter comparison of the safety of continuous intrathecal labor analgesia using a 28-guage catheter versus continuous epidural labor analgesia. *Anesthesiology*. 2008;108:286–298.

CHAPTER 11 ■ EPIDURAL NEURAL BLOCKADE

BERNADETTE T. VEERING AND MICHAEL J. COUSINS

Although techniques of epidural anesthesia do not offer the economy of drug dosage or degrees of blockade of spinal anesthesia, they are currently more versatile and better studied. No other neural blockade techniques are used as extensively in each of the fields of surgical anesthesia, obstetric anesthesia, and diagnosis and management of acute and chronic pain. Epidural blockade is also unique because of special features of the anatomic site of injection and the resultant diverse sites of action of the local anesthetic solution.

The most practical and widely used continuous method of neural blockade is spinal epidural blockade; pharmacokinetic data have helped to increase the efficacy and safety of epidural infusion techniques (see Chapter 40). Continuous caudal blockade has useful but limited applications, and continuous spinal anesthesia is beginning to be used more frequently. As indicated in Chapters 32 and 40, new developments in the understanding of pain conduction have extended the use of continuous epidural blockade to the administration of drugs that selectively block pain conduction, while leaving sensation, motor power, and sympathetic function essentially unchanged. The safety and reliability of spinal epidural catheter techniques, with the addition of bacterial filters, have permitted relief of acute pain (see Chapters 24, 40, and 43) and chronic pain (see Chapters 44 and 45) for many days, often with patients remaining ambulatory. This has heralded an even more vigorous and fruitful era of investigation and clinical application of epidural blockade than did the unprecedented development of the past 20 years.

ANATOMY OF EPIDURAL NEURAL BLOCKADE

Key anatomic features of the epidural space and of approaches to needle/catheter insertion are described in Chapter 9.

Epidural Pressures

The epidural space is identified traditionally by a sensation of negative pressure when entering the space. This negative pressure is believed to be created by tenting of the dura by the advancing needle, especially by blunt needles with side openings (1,2).

By using a closed measurement system that permitted continuous measurement of positive and negative pressure, lumbar epidural space pressures seem to be always positive with the needle stationary in the epidural space, except when the subarachnoid space was to be entered (Fig. 11-1) (3) At thoracic level, high negative epidural pressures up to −60 mm Hg were only observed at the moment of epidural puncture, equilibrating to a positive value within 90 seconds in both expiratory and inspiratory phases (4). This suggests that subsequent adaptation of the surrounding tissue results in restoration of the normal positive epidural pressure.

The lumbar epidural pressure increased with stimuli known to increase cerebrospinal fluid (CSF) pressure such as jugular venous compression, ventilation with carbon dioxide, and positive end expiratory pressure (5). This suggests that the lumbar epidural pressure is in equilibrium with the prevailing spinal CSF pressure (6).

Epidural injection of two different volumes of bupivacaine resulted in the same plateau pressure in both groups at the upper limit of normal for CSF pressure, suggesting a pressure-limiting feature in the epidural space (7).

Successful entry into the epidural space is sometimes followed by "drip back" when local anesthetic is subsequently injected, especially in elderly patients (8). This is probably due to a lower compliance of the epidural space, compared to that in younger patients.

In severe lung diseases such as emphysema, epidural negative pressure may be abolished, particularly if the patient is lying down (9). Any factor that increases abdominal pressure and/or occlusion of the inferior vena cava may distend the epidural veins and increase pressure in the lumbar epidural space. This results in only slight changes in the thoracic epidural space, particularly if the patient is sitting (6).

During labor, baseline lumbar epidural pressures are higher in women in the supine position compared with those in the lateral position. As labor progresses, baseline pressures increase with peaks of epidural pressure during each uterine contraction (10,11).

Coughing or a Valsalva maneuver increases both intrathoracic and intra-abdominal pressure, so that pressure in thoracic and lumbar epidural space increases (6), resulting in high positive pressures being recorded throughout the epidural space.

Comparison of patients having prior lumbar surgery to those who did not revealed a higher baseline lumbar epidural pressure in patients with previous lumbar surgery (12). However, additional pressure from epidural injections decays at a rate similar to that in patients who did not undergo operations. This suggests that the alteration induced by surgery is one of different *initial* condition, rather than a change in distensibility. On the other hand, the resistance to fluid injection in the epidural space was higher in patients with a diseased space, as the result of epidural arachnoiditis, compared with that of the normal space (13). Therefore, one should be careful with the

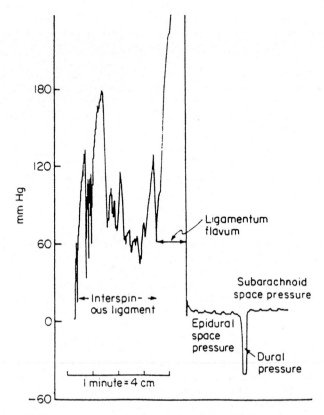

FIGURE 11-1. A typical pressure-compared-with-time recording. Note the increasing pressure during passage through the interspinous ligaments, the high pressure generated during passage through the ligamentum flavum, and the precipitous decrease in pressure on entering the epidural space. The pressure is only negative on entry into the subarachnoid space. From Telford RJ, Holbway TE. Observations on deliberate dural puncture with a Tuohy needle: Pressure measurement. *Anaesthesia* 1991;46:725, 1991, with permission.

injection of fluid into parts of the epidural space that do not communicate freely with their surroundings.

PHYSIOLOGIC EFFECTS OF EPIDURAL BLOCKADE

With currently available local anesthetic agents, spinal epidural neural blockade implies sympathetic blockade accompanied by somatic blockade, in the form of sensory and motor blockade alone or in combination. Although it is possible to avoid blockade of "peripheral" lumbar sympathetic fibers if only sacral segments are blocked by a caudal approach to the epidural space, spinal epidural blockade almost invariably results in some degree of sympathetic blockade. Some of the most important (but not all) of the physiologic effects of epidural blockade can be discussed in relation to either sympathetic blockade only of vasoconstrictor fibers (below T4) and/or of cardiac sympathetic fibers (T1–T4; Fig. 11-2). Many clinicians prefer to have a wide margin of safety if they are intent on avoiding major sympathetic blockade. Thus, they aim to restrict the level of analgesia to T10. Studies discussed in Chapter 38, however, indicate that the level of sympathetic block with epidural anesthesia may be lower than the level of sensory block and more incomplete in terms of the quality of block (14). This concept of sympathetic blockade is still a practical approach in considering the physiologic effects of epidural blockade because inguinal, perineal, urologic, and lower limb surgical procedures can be carried out with blockade to T10 or lower, which at most will produce only a "peripheral" sympathetic blockade. However, lower abdominal surgery (such as appendectomy, gynecologic surgery, and cesarean section) necessitates blockade to T4. Thus, the most frequent use of epidural block will be to either the T4 or T10 level. Occasionally, a T1 level is needed for chest injury or thoracotomy. We will consider the cardiovascular

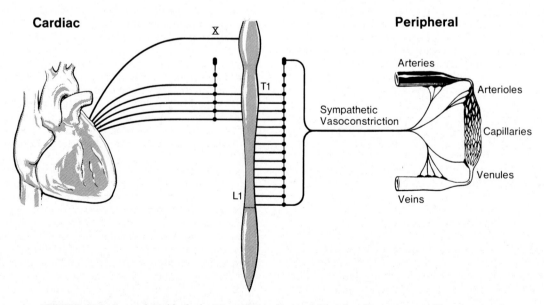

FIGURE 11-2. Sympathetic blockade: "Central" (cardiac) and "peripheral" components. These consist of T1–T4 cardiac sympathetic fibers and T1–L2 "peripheral" sympathetic fibers. Note important innervation of veins and venules. Vagal cardiac fibers are also shown. Level of sympathetic block is the same as (or lower than) sensory with epidural blockade. In comparison, sympathetic block is two to three segments higher than sensory level with subarachnoid block.

effects of epidural block with respect to the degree of sympathetic block (and its effects) with sensory blockade to T1, T4, or T10.

Subtler and somewhat more indirect is the reduced input to the central nervous system (CNS), which accompanies various levels of sensory blockade. This "deafferentation" has long been thought capable of exerting a "protective" effect that reduces the efferent neurohumoral response to surgical stimulation or trauma. Objective data have now become available to support this hypothesis (see Chapters 6 and 7).

Finally, it is important to remember that extensive epidural blockade often requires large doses of local anesthetic (with or without epinephrine) (Fig. 11-3). Large doses themselves may cause physiologic changes as a result of the direct pharmacologic effects of circulating blood concentrations. These are an inevitable outcome of vascular absorption from the epidural space. Because of the unique epidural venous system (see Chapter 9), direct intravascular injection may result in the rapid attainment of high concentrations of local anesthetic in the brain and/or heart, with the potential for convulsions and/or sudden depression of cardiac output (see Chapters 3 to 5). Also, important changes in vagal tone accompany sympathetic block (Fig. 11-4). The various mechanisms for physiologic effects of epidural block are summarized in Table 11-1.

Cardiovascular Effects of Epidural Blockade

Block of sympathetic innervation accounts for the cardiovascular responses to epidural anesthesia. The preganglionic sympathetic innervation plays an important role in regulating regional blood flow. Blockade of sympathetic nerve fibers and resulting loss of vasomotor tone will therefore cause considerable changes in blood flow to various organs, depending on the level achieved (Fig. 11-2) (15). Postganglionic sympathetic nerves are important in controlling cardiac function and vascular tone. High thoracic epidural anesthesia (TEA), from the first to fifth thoracic segments, blocks the cardiac afferent and efferent sympathetic fibers, with loss of chronotropic and inotropic drive to the myocardium (16). Epidural anesthesia that is restricted to the level of the low thoracic and lumbar region (T5–L4) results in a peripheral sympathetic blockade with vascular dilatation in the pelvis and lower limbs.

Cardiovascular depression may occur with both epidural and subarachnoid blockade (Fig. 11-3) and is at least partly related to the level of sympathetic blockade (Fig. 11-2, see also Chapter 10) (17,18).

Also, vascular absorption of local anesthetic and vasoconstrictor may result in significant hemodynamic changes after epidural but not after subarachnoid blockade; the reason for this lies predominantly in the much larger doses of drugs used in epidural blockade and in the proximity of the large epidural veins, which, owing to their anatomy, have considerable potential for rapid transport of drug to the heart (Table 11-2) and CNS.

When comparing the physiologic effects of spinal and epidural anesthesia, it is relevant to consider if spinal anesthesia does result in a more complete sympathetic blockade than does epidural anesthesia. A possible approach to investigate the intensity of sympathetic block is to measure catecholamine response to immersion of a limb in cold water (cold pressor test). Plasma catecholamines and hemodynamic responses were similar following both techniques, indicating that spinal anesthesia did not result in a more profound attenuation of the sympathetic response than did epidural anesthesia (19).[a]

High Thoracic Segmental Epidural Anesthesia (T1–T5)

Epidural blockade of T1–T5 segments has the following effects on cardiac sympathetic activity: (a) blockade of segmental cardiac reflexes in segments T1–T4, (b) blockade of outflow from vasomotor center to cardiac sympathetic fibers (T1–T4), and (c) vasoconstrictor nerve blockade in head, neck, and upper limbs. Denervation of preganglionic cardiac accelerator fibers leaving the cord at T1–T5 results in minimal vasodilatory consequences.

However, changes in heart rate, LV function, and myocardial oxygen demand may occur because of high thoracic epidural blockade and are discussed next.

Heart Rate. During cardiac sympathetic denervation, parasympathetic cardiovascular responses, including those involved in baroreflexes may dominate.

A high TEA covering the cardiac segments (T1–T4) produces small but significant reductions in heart rate (20,21,22). Because changes in cardiac rate are known to be controlled chiefly by the balance of sympathetic and parasympathetic tone at any moment, it must be assumed that parasympathetic tone is reduced to almost the same degree as sympathetic tone to maintain heart rate at a normal or near normal level (21,22) (Table 11-3). Whether the sympathetic nervous system functions as a direct cardioaccelerator or indirectly by modifying the parasympathetic tone needs to be clarified.

Left Ventricular Function and Myocardial Oxygen Demand. Blockade from T1 to T5 influences the contractility of the LV. However, discrepancies exist among studies that have evaluated the influence of high TEA on the LV contractility. Some studies demonstrated that blockade from T1 to T5 is associated with a negative inotropic effect on the LV (23,24). The LV contractility decreased with an approximate 15% reduction of stroke volume in patients with TEA from C5 to T5. On the other hand, high segmental TEA did not produce a reduction in LV function, as measured by the suprasternal Doppler method (25) or by echocardiography (26) in patients scheduled for elective noncardiac surgery. Both studies documented a small but statistically significant decrease in heart rate, a minor decrease in mean arterial pressure, and essentially no change in cardiac index. A study in healthy volunteers receiving thoracic epidural blockade from C7 to T6 produced only a minor decrease in systolic blood pressure and no significant change in cardiac output (27).

In contrast in patients with coronary artery disease (CAD) subjected to physical stress, high TEA improves global and regional LV function while diminishing associated changes in ST segments (28). The most likely explanation for the improvements in LV global and regional function during TEA and exercise is that TEA beneficially affects the oxygen supply-to-demand ratio in the ischemic area mainly by reducing myocardial oxygen demand. The LV diastolic function appears to improve in resting patients with CAD after high TEA (29).

---

[a]Level of sympathetic block is the same as (or lower than) sensory with epidural blockade. In comparison, sympathetic block is two to three segments higher than sensory level with subarachnoid block.

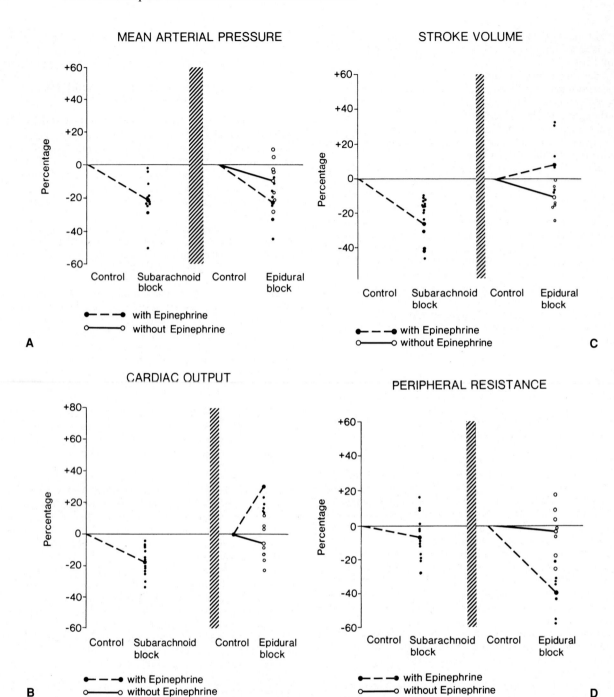

FIGURE 11-3. Cardiovascular effects of epidural block to T5 level, with and without epinephrine. **A:** Mean arterial pressure. **B:** Cardiac output. **C:** Stroke volume. **D:** Peripheral resistance. Percentage changes for each variable are shown after epidural block, with a comparison given for a similar level of subarachnoid block. From Ward RJ, et al. Epidural and subarachnoid anesthesia. Cardiovascular and respiratory effects. *JAMA* 1965;25:275, with permission.

Effects of Thoracic Epidural Blockade on the Ischemic Heart[a]

With a high TEA, the cardiac sympathetic nerves are blocked and this will have an impact on the myocardium (30).

Following high TEA in an animal model the size of experimentally induced myocardial infarcts was reduced after experimental coronary occlusion (31). In another animal study, it was demonstrated that the endocardial-to-epicardial blood flow ratio increased, and this may have decreased ischemic injury in association with TEA (32). In addition, the incidence of ischemia-induced malignant arrhythmias in anesthetized rats was reduced by high TEA (33). Thus, high TEA exerts a cardioprotective effect during experimental myocardial ischemia by improving the myocardial oxygen supply-to-demand ratio.

TABLE 11-1

MECHANISMS FOR PHYSIOLOGIC EFFECTS OF EPIDURAL ANALGESIA

By way of vascular absorption of local anesthetic (L.A.) or Epinephrine (EPI)	By way of direct neural blocking effects or indirect results of blockade

Receptor
  β-stimulation by EPI
  α-stimulation by EPI or phenylephrine
Smooth muscle
  Blood vessels, L.A. or EPI
  Heart, L.A. or EPI
  Other organs, L.A. or EPI
Cardiac muscle
  By L.A. or EPI
Neural tissue
  CNS, by L.A.
  Conducting system of heart, by L.A.
Miscellaneous
  Neuromuscular junction by L.A.
	Spinal nerves (roots and trunks) by axonal blockade
	  Sympathetic
	    Efferent blockade
	      Peripheral (T1–L2) vasoconstrictor
	      "Adrenal" (T6–L1)
	      "Central" (T1–T4) cardiac sympathetic
	  Sensory
	    Afferent blockade
	      Reduced peripheral sensation
	      Blockade of visceral pain fibers
	      Reduced efferent neurohumoral response to surgical or other stimulus within the blocked area
	  Motor
	    Efferent blockade
	      Varying degrees of motor paralysis
	      Reflex muscle relaxation without paralysis (deafferentation)
	  Spinal cord
	    Axons
	      Superficial, sensory tracts blocked (e.g., bupivacaine, lidocaine, and etidocaine)
	      Deep motor paths blocked (e.g., etidocaine)
	        Dorsal horn modulation of pain transmission (? axons, ?cells)
	        Possibility of "antianalgesic" effect owing to block of inhibitors paths
	    Cell Bodies: "selective" blockade, by opioids (see Chapter 40)
	  Secondary changes in parasympathetic activity
	    Sympathetic block to T5 + ↓ venous return may → ↑↑ vagus
	    Sympathetic block to T1 → unopposed vagus (see Fig. 11.5)
	  Secondary changes in vasoactive hormones
	    Sympathetic block to T1 → blockade of ↑ renin but not ↑ vasopressin, that usually helps maintain BP in response to ↓ BP challenge (see Fig. 11-6)

BP, blood pressure; CNS, central nervous system

High TEA in humans improves an ischemia-induced LV dysfunction; reduces electrocardiographic, echocardiographic, and angiographic signs of coronary insufficiency; decreases the incidence of arrhythmias; and provides relief of ischemic chest pain (34–36). Furthermore, it has been reported that high TEA improves ischemia-induced LV global and regional wall motion abnormalities while diminishing associated changes in ST segments in patients with CAD under physical stress (28). This is probably related to the decrease in LV afterload per se improving regional wall motion (see also Chapter 7).

High TEA has probably no influence upon the autoregulation of coronary resistance vessels; it should therefore not adversely affect regional blood flow distribution in patients with CAD with a pattern that provides a basis for coronary steal (i.e., maldistribution of coronary blood flow) (37,38). In addition, in patients with multivessel ischemic heart disease, TEA partly normalizes the myocardial blood flow response to sympathetic stimulation (39).

Thoracic Epidural Anesthesia (T1–T12). An epidural block from T1 to T12 (using a mid to high thoracic catheter) or even involving the upper lumbar segments is associated with extensive sympathetic block. Consequently, hypotension will occur, partly by the block's cardio depressant action and consequent reduction in systemic vascular resistance. Such block decreases

preload and afterload as a result of increased venous capacitance and redistribution of blood volume in the affected dilated splanchnic vascular beds (T6–L1). Denervation of the splanchnic fibers leads to vasodilatation of the visceral (splanchnic) venous bed, resulting in pooling of blood in the gut and abdominal viscera. The splanchnic veins produce the majority of the total systemic reflex capacitance changes and account for almost all of the reflex venoconstriction that buffers the systemic circulatory volume changes (40).

The depressant effects are partly counteracted by vasoconstriction in the diminished remaining innervated body regions (41). This increased efferent sympathetic activity is mediated predominantly (by means of the baroreceptors) by those sympathetic vasoconstrictor nerves (T1–T5) that remain unblocked and by circulating catecholamines released from the adrenal medulla, owing to increased activity in any unblocked fibers in the splanchnic nerves (T6–L1). Although blood vessels in some viscera, such as the kidney, appear to be more responsive to direct neural stimuli in other vascular beds, both neural and hormonal influences have major effects, although at different levels of the vasculature. Major arterioles respond mostly to neural stimuli, whereas small arterioles and venules near the capillary bed respond predominantly to circulating catecholamines. Thus, while any splanchnic fibers remain unblocked, there is a potential for vasoconstrictor activity below (as well as above)

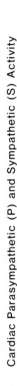

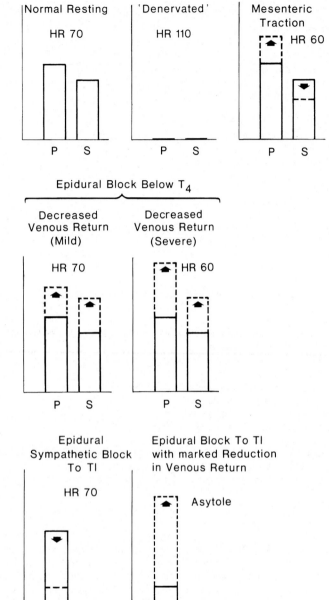

FIGURE 11-4. Vagal effects of epidural block. **Top, left:** The balance of cardiac parasympathetic (P) activity and sympathetic (S) activity is shown with a normal resting heart rate of 70. **Top, middle:** The presence of a heart rate of 110 following complete "denervation" of the heart emphasizes the dominant action of the vagus. **Top, right:** Autonomic reflexes such as mesenteric traction usually result in bradycardia by an opposite change in P and S. **Center:** Epidural block to T4. **Center, left:** A mild reduction in venous return results in increased vagal tone, which may offset the increase in sympathetic tone (arterial baroreceptors), so that heart rate is unchanged or slightly decreased. **Center, right:** Marked reduction in venous return stimulates a marked increase in P, and S increases in an attempt to minimize the bradycardia. **Bottom:** Epidural block to T1. **Bottom, left:** Usual situation, in which P has diminished to compensate for a blocked S. A heart rate of 70 is the result of the same dominance of P over S that exists at rest; however, P is now completely unopposed. **Bottom, right:** Marked reduction in venous return (or other stimulus to P) results in unopposed increase in P, which may lead to asystole. Such responses are much more likely in the conscious patient.

the level of blockade, through release of catecholamines from the adrenal medulla. Finally, the ability of precapillary sphincters to achieve autoregulation within a short time of cessation of neural activity (42) provides a further mechanism for regaining vascular tone and minimizing vascular pooling below the level of blockade.

Catecholamine response to immersion of a limb in cold water (cold pressor test) revealed that epidural anesthesia with a sensory level to T1 did not produce complete sympathectomy regardless of the local anesthetic used, since plasma concentrations of catecholamines were nearly unchanged (43). Blockade of preganglionic sympathetic fibers innervating the adrenal medulla and innervating peripheral sympathetic fibers appeared to be incomplete, even during quite extensive epidural anesthesia to C8 (44).

Epidural anesthesia is probably associated with a reduction in sympathetic neural transmission rather than a complete blockade of sympathetic fibers.

The potential magnitude of cardiovascular changes has been documented in unmedicated volunteers with a blockade of C5–S5; that is, complete blockade of cardio-accelerator fibers and adrenal medullary catecholamine secretion (17,45). The mean arterial blood pressure was reduced approximately 20%, with a similar reduction in total peripheral resistance, minimal changes in heart rate, and a rise central venous pressure (26%). This small change in heart rate gives a deceptive picture of cardiac sympathetic activity, since Otton and Wilson have shown that blockade of T1–T4 alone produced an increase in central venous pressure (CVP) without an increase in stroke volume output of the heart (27).

TABLE 11-2

CARDIOVASCULAR EFFECTS OF EPIDURAL BLOCKADE

Mechanism	Effect
Neural effects	
"Peripheral" sympathetic block (T10–L2)	
Blockade of vasoconstrictor fibers to lower limbs	Arteriolar dilatation. Increased venous capacitance and pooling of blood in lower limbs → decreased venous return → ↓ CO
Reflex increase in vasoconstrictor fiber activity in upper limbs via baroreceptors	Increased vasomotor tone in upper limbs → ↑ venous return → ↑ CO
Reflex increase in cardioaccelerator nerve activity	↑ HR ↑ CO
Reduced right atrial pressure, due to ↓ venous return[a]	? ↓ HR (Note ↓↓ RA pressure → ↓ HR[a]; see Fig. 11-15)
Adrenal medullary sympathetic block (T6–L1)	
(Blockade of splanchnic nerves)	
Vasoconstrictor fibers to abdominal viscera	Pooling of blood in gut → decreased venous return
Adrenal medullary catecholamine secretion	Decreased levels of circulating catecholamines → ↓ HR ↓ CO
"Central" sympathetic block (T1–T4)	
Blockade of	
Cardiac sympathetic outflow from vasomotor center	↓ HR ↓ CO
Cardiac sympathetic reflexes at segmental level	
Vasoconstrictor fibers to head, neck, and arms	Vasodilatation in upper limbs. Blockade of compensatory lower limb vasoconstriction if T5–L1 is also blocked
Vagal predominance	"Inappropriate bradycardia"; "sudden bradycardia"; vagal arrest (see Fig. 11-5 and Table 11-4)
Effects of drug absorption	
Absorbed local anesthetic	Usually no measurable effects on HR, CO, MAP, or TPR even in patients with vascular disease
Moderate blood levels	
Antiarrhythmic	Lidocaine may → ↑ CO, which is balanced ↓ TPR, so that MAP is unchanged
Maintenance of normal CO	
Minimal reduction in vascular tone	
High blood levels (toxic)	↓ CO ↓ HR
Decreased contractility	↓ MAP
If convulsions occur hypoxia results in further reduction in CO	
Cardiac conducting tissue, ? unidirectional blockade	Bupivacaine (very high levels) may → VT, VF, and cardiac arrest
Vascular dilatation	↓ TPR
Absorbed epinephrine	↑ CO ↑ HR ↓ TPR
β-stimulation	MAP may be unchanged or slightly reduced
	Antagonism of reflex vasoconstriction above level of blockade because of β-effects on muscle vasculature (→ ↓ TPR)

CO, Cardiac output; HR, heart rate; MAP, mean arterial pressure; TPR, total peripheral resistance; VT, ventricular tachycardia; VF, ventricular fibrillation.

[a]Decreased venous return was associated with increased vagal activity in one study. This may offset any increases in sympathetic activity.[48]

Mid Thoracic to Lumbar Epidural Anesthesia (T5–S5). Epidural blockade that is restricted to the level of the low thoracic and lumbar region (T5–L4) results in a "peripheral" sympathetic blockade with vascular dilatation in the pelvis and lower limbs; if all splanchnic fibers are blocked (T6–L1), then pooling of blood in the gut and abdominal viscera also may occur (Table 11-2). This peripheral blockade has been demonstrated by measurements of large increases in lower limb blood flow owing to arteriolar vasodilation (46) and pooling of blood in the venous capacitance vessels (47). Because the latter contain 80% of blood volume, venodilatation has a potential for dramatic changes in venous return, reduction in right atrial pres-

sure, and reduced cardiac output. The decrease in venous return has been shown to result in increased cardiac vagal tone. This explains why heart rate remains unchanged or decreased despite hypotension and activation of cardiac sympathetic accelerator fibers (48).

While any splanchnic fibers remain unblocked, there is a potential for vasoconstrictor activity below (as well as above) the level of blockade, through release of catecholamines from the adrenal medulla. Increased activity in cardiac sympathetic fibers (T1–T4) may result in increased cardiac contractility and increased heart rate; similar effects are produced by increased levels of circulating catecholamines. Evidence that the latter

TABLE 11-3

DANGER SIGNALS: CARDIOVASCULAR EFFECTS OF EPIDURAL BLOCK

Signal	Mechanisms and potential sequelae	Treatment
↑ HR ↓ BP in supine parturient with sensory level T11–L4 or ↓ HR ↓ BP—a more dangerous sign	Inferior vena caval occlusion venodilatation in lower limbs → ↓ Venous return, ↓ CO, ↓ organ perfusion (incl. fetus) → Epidural vein engorgement → ↓ spinal cord perfusion → "spinal stroke" → ↑ Sympathetic → ↑ HR (baroreceptors) vasoconstriction activity (above level of block) in upper limbs → ↓ RA pressure → ↓ HR (↑ vagal tone) (Note ↓↓ RV pressure may → ↓↓ HR; see Table 11-4 and Fig. 11-5)	Lateral position IV fluids, oxygen until MAP normal May require atropine and/or ephedrine if above measures fail
Gradual ↓ HR ↓ BP with level above T4	Venodilatation (as above) ↓ cardiac sympathetic activity → ↓ CO ↓ HR ↓ MAP → ↓ Cardiac sympathetic activity initially accompanied by ↓ parasympathetic (see also Fig. 11-5). → However, ↓↓ venous return → ↑ vagal activity Therefore, ↓↓ HR may occur before blockade of all T1-T4	IV fluids. Elevate legs. Atropine. Oxygen until MAP normal. Vasopressor (ephedrine) if required
"Sudden bradycardia" in either condition above	↓↓ Venous return may result in sudden ↑ parasympathetic tone ("faint response"); see Table 11-4; Fig. 11-5) ↓↓ HR → cardiac arrest	As above, but emphasis on sequence: elevate legs, oxygen, IV atropine, IV fluids—ephedrine rapidly if no response to above. May need epinephrine[a]
"Inappropriate" bradycardia (i.e., "normal" HR inface of ↓ MAP with sensory level T3–T4)	Peripheral vasodilatation should evoke an ↑ HR. But ↓ venous return → ↑ vagal tone, so HR remains at preblock rate but is "inappropriately" slow	IV atropine if MAP does not respond to fluids and elevation of legs, and relief of venous obstruction
Reduced blood volume or known obstruction of inferior vena cava ↓ HR with visceral traction in presence of blockade to T1	Hemorrhage Increased intra-abdominal pressure Total sympathetic block Unopposed vagus Changes in vagal tone → profound changes in HR; may → transient asystole (see Table 11-4 and Fig. 11-5)	Restore blood volume ⎫ Before epidural Relieve vena caval ⎬ block obstruction ⎭ IV atropine (?) Local infiltration to block vagal stimulus Ensure venous return adequate + arterial Po₂ adequate since ↑ HR (atropine) → ↑ myocardial oxygen demand

[a]Sudden bradycardia and hypotension may also result from cardiac toxicity of local anesthetics. This may require rapid resuscitative measures. Including large doses of epinephrine.
BP, blood pressure; CO, cardiac output; HR, heart rate; IV, intravenous; MAP, mean arterial pressure; RA, right atrial; RV, right ventricular.

are important in maintaining homeostasis in some clinical situations is provided by the surprisingly small changes in heart rate and cardiac output (−16%) with blockade of C5–T4, but with splanchnic fibers to the adrenal medulla (T6–L1) intact (27).

Distribution of blood to the splanchnic area was studied by Arndt et al. in healthy young volunteers after injection of 20 mL of plain 2% lidocaine into the lumbar region. Splanchnic

blood volume decreased as assessed by distribution of radio-labeled red cells. Radioactivity also decreased in thorax and upper limbs, indicating compensatory vasoconstriction (49).

Low Thoracic to Lumbar Epidural Anesthesia (T10–S5). Lumbar epidural anesthesia (LEA) with a sympathetic blockade below T10 results in minimal vasodilatory consequences because fewer vasoconstrictor fibers are included, and neither the splanchnic nerves nor the nerve supply to the adrenal medulla are affected. Since muscle veins lack sympathetic innervation, venodilatation of the extremities is limited to the skin, and so minimal capacitance increase results from blocks of the lower extremities (50). A block below L3 does not affect the sympathetic system, and the hemodynamic upset is minimal.

Lumbar epidural anesthesia with a sympathetic blockade extending to the lower segments may occasionally be associated with profound bradycardia and circulatory collapse without any obvious precipitating event. This issue is discussed in the section on central volume depletion.

Absorbed Local Anesthetics

Relatively large amounts of local anesthetic solutions are required to achieve satisfactory epidural anesthesia. Local anesthetics exhibit a direct biphasic action on vascular smooth muscle, depending upon the local anesthetic agent, its concentration and stereochemical configuration, the type of blood vessel (capacitance or resistance), and preexisting vascular tone (see Chapter 3). At low concentrations, local anesthetics cause vasoconstriction. At concentrations used for epidural anesthesia, vessels tend to vasodilatate (51). At high concentrations of lidocaine, Bonica observed stimulatory effects on the circulation (17). Such stimulation was thought to be caused by a central effect of lidocaine enhancing sympathetic activity by means of remaining cardiac sympathetic fibers. Generally, the systemic effects produced by concentrations of local anesthetics in blood that are associated with correctly performed epidural block have little, if any, clinical significance (Table 11-2).

Epinephrine-Containing Solutions. Epinephrine injected alone into the epidural space (i.e., 100 μg; 20 mL of 5 μg/mL) will be absorbed slowly because of its local vasoconstrictor effect. The systemic effects of achieved epinephrine blood levels are β-adrenergic; that is, a moderate increase in heart rate, increased cardiac output, decreased peripheral resistance, and unchanged mean arterial pressure. The vasodilatation results in augmentation of the vasodilatation induced by the sympathetic denervation associated with epidural anesthesia, so that the total effect in epidural block is likely to be a larger decrease in mean arterial pressure than if solutions of plain local anesthetic are used. The early cardiovascular changes observed with absorbed epinephrine are, however, transient. Therefore, the prolonged cardiovascular changes seen with local anesthetics containing epinephrine probably relate to sympathetic blockade. The most likely explanations for the more pronounced cardiovascular effects of epinephrine-containing local anesthetic solutions appear to be as follows:

▨ Systemic absorption of epinephrine. β-Adrenergic effects on the heart, resulting in increased heart rate and cardiac output; peripheral vascular β-adrenergic effects, resulting in further vasodilatation within the area of sympathetic block; and antagonism of compensatory vasoconstrictor responses outside the area of blockade. Thus, total peripheral resistance falls, and mean arterial blood pressure is reduced to a degree comparable to that seen with equivalent levels of subarachnoid blockade (Fig. 11-3).

▨ More intense neural penetration or more extensive spread of neural blockade, resulting in more reliable sympathetic block.

Hypovolemia and Epidural Block

Bonica demonstrated in healthy volunteers that epidural block to T5 was associated with major reductions in heart rate, car-

diac output, and mean arterial pressure in the presence of hypovolemia in comparison to mild cardiovascular changes at normovolemia (17,45,52). Cardiovascular homeostasis was better maintained with epinephrine–lidocaine blockade. However, marked reductions in mean arterial blood pressure still occurred (Fig. 11-5). Because cardiac sympathetic fibers were thought not to be blocked in these patients, an explanation was sought for the large reductions in heart rate and cardiac output. The abrupt bradycardia resulting in cardiovascular collapse in human subjects is probably a sudden vagal response to marked reductions in venous return (53–56) (Tables 11-3 and 11-4). The mechanism is discussed in detail in the next section, on central volume depletion.

The less pronounced cardiovascular depression in hypovolemic subjects receiving epidural block with lidocaine–epinephrine is probably due to an increase in heart rate due to absorption of epinephrine. This may have protected the heart from increases in vagal activity although it has been noted that a high level of sympathetic activity may accentuate cholinergic effects in patients with poor venous return (56). It is also possible that peak arterial blood concentrations of lidocaine were higher after plain lidocaine in patients with hypovolemia, owing to decreased cardiac output and thus a smaller volume of distribution (see Chapter 3). In this situation, the myocardium receives a larger percentage of cardiac output and thus is potentially exposed to higher concentrations of local anesthetics (see Chapter 5). Any coexistent hypercapnia or acidosis would tend to accentuate the depressant effects of local anesthetic on the myocardium (see Chapter 3). The moral of Bonica's study is clear (18): Epidural block should be avoided or used with great care in patients with uncorrected hypovolemia or in any other patient in whom venous return is markedly impaired (e.g., patients with large intra-abdominal masses in whom the pressure of the mass on the vena cava cannot be relieved before blockade).

Central Volume Depletion

Epidural anesthesia with and without involvement of cardiac segments may be associated with profound bradycardia and, in some patients, with transient cardiac arrest without any obvious precipitating event (57) (Tables 11-3 and 11-4). Apparently, responses by vagal reflex predominate, associated with echocardiographic evidence of smaller LV chamber size (58). This bradycardia seems to be mediated via the LV mechanoreceptors, activated by a reduction in end-systolic volume, occurring as a result of decrease in venous return. A vago-vagal reflex (the Bezold-Jarisch reflex) elicited from and returning to the heart is thereby activated and is likely a protective reflex (59,60). This reflex slowing should allow time for more complete filling of the heart. So, hypovolemia can precipitate not only classic vagal symptoms, but also full cardiac arrest in healthy patients. Vagal activation with bradycardia is thus a protective reflex that prevents the heart from contracting when relatively empty. Possible CNS hypoperfusion and an obtunded response to hypoxia from epidural block may intensify the bradycardic response to volume depletion (61).

Recent animal research demonstrated the cardiodepressor response to be mediated from regions in the brainstem triggering the sympathoinhibitory reflex to central hypovolemia (62).

Epidural Anesthesia and General Anesthesia

Thoracic epidural anesthesia associated with light general anesthesia is increasingly used for upper abdominal surgery and for

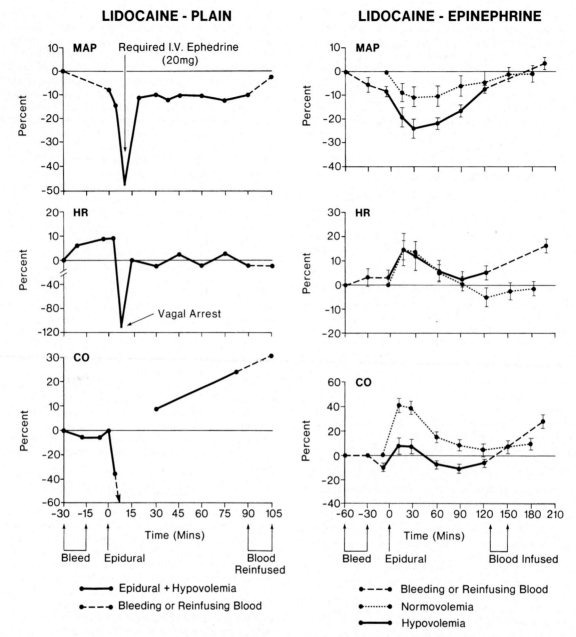

FIGURE 11-5. Cardiovascular effects of epidural block, effect of hypovolemia in conscious volunteers; epidural block to T5 with plain and epinephrine-containing solutions. The mean percentage of change is shown for each variable. **Right:** Lidocaine–epinephrine. The cardiovascular changes after lidocaine-epinephrine in the presence of normovolemia are compared with hypovolemia (−13%). During normovolemia, note the marked increase in heart rate and cardiac output, lasting about 60 minutes. During hypovolemia, mean arterial pressure is significantly lower (−23%), but cardiac output remains close to control levels as a result of an elevated heart rate. **Left:** Lidocaine plain. A representation of a typical response is shown. Severe bradycardia is associated with extreme hypotension, and in two subjects, vagal arrest occurred that required rapid resuscitation with ephedrine and oxygen. In only one subject was hypotension associated with increased heart rate, and this prevented the extreme hypotension seen in the other five subjects. Modified from data of Bonica JJ. Berges PU, Morikawa K. Circulatory effects of epidural block: I. Effects of levels of analgesia and dose of lidocaine. *Anesthesiology* 1970;33:1619; Bonica JJ, Akamatsu TJ, Berges PU, et al. Circulatory effects of epidural block: II. Effects of epinephrine. *Anesthesiology* 1971;34:514; and Bonica JJ, Kennedy WF, Akamatsu TJ, Gerbershagen HU. Circulatory effects of peridural block. III. Effects of acute blood loss. *Anesthesiology* 1972;36:219, with permission.

TABLE 11-4

VAGAL AND SYMPATHETIC ACTIVITY: EFFECTS ON HEART RATE

	Venous return "sensors" in great veins, atria, ventricles	Arterial pressure "sensors" in carotid sinus and aortic arch
Afferent path	Vagus	Vagus, glossopharyngeal
Efferent path	Vagus	Sympathetic
Effect of increased venous return + ↑ BP	↑ Venous return	↑ BP
	↘ ↓ Vagal activity → ↑ HR	↘ ↓ sympathetic activity → ↓ HR
Effect of decreased venous return + ↓ BP		
Mild ↓:	↑ Vagal activity → ↓ HR	↑ sympathetic activity → ↑ HR
(? ↓ atrial volume)	↓ HR (vagus) balanced by ↑ HR (sympathetic).: HR unchanged	
Severe ↓↓: (? ↓ ventricular pressure)	↑↑ Vagal activity → ↓↓ HR	↑↑ Sympathetic activity
	If cardiac sympathetics blocked, vagus is unopposed, and with sensitized vagal receptors (serum catecholamines) → ↓↓ HR and possible cardiac arrest	? Accentuates activation of vagal receptors in ventricle[a]

[a] ↓↓ BP also → ↓ carotid body oxygen supply. This initiates a "hypoxic" response and further increases vagal efferent activity.
BP, blood pressure; HR, heart rate

major vascular surgery. Lumbar epidural anesthesia combined with general anesthesia is commonly used for prolonged major lower abdominal and pelvic surgery. Combined epidural and general anesthesia offers the advantage of a rapid and less painful recovery. This combination technique may result in a greater degree of hypotension than with each technique alone (63,64).

Such hypotension arises mainly from a decrease in venous return and is also due to attenuation of the compensatory vasoconstriction of nonanesthetized sympathetic tone via central depressant effects on vasomotor center (65,66). Obviously, the greatest concern for the consequences of hypotension is in patients with CAD. Thoracic epidural anesthesia plus light general anesthesia did not worsen (or improve) ventricular wall motion or induce myocardial ischemia, suggesting that myocardial oxygen balance was maintained (67). On the other hand, LEA with general anesthesia may cause impairment of segmental ventricular wall motion (SWM), indicating myocardial ischemia (68). In comparing these two studies, it would seem that the block of efferent sympathetic innervation to the heart that occurs with TEA but not with lumbar epidural blockade has beneficial effects.

In clinical practice, ephedrine and phenylephrine are the two agents that are commonly recommended to treat hypotension during epidural anesthesia associated with general anesthesia (69). Ephedrine appears to be the drug of choice to restore blood pressure under TEA associated with general anesthesia (70,71), since LV function was not compromised.

Phenylephrine seems to be the drug of choice to restore mean arterial pressure in patients who were moderately hypotensive during LEA combined with general anesthesia (71).

In summary, it appears that light general anesthesia can be safely combined with epidural block to the level of T5 in healthy patients. Use of a slight head-down tilt to maintain venous return and small incremental doses of atropine to maintain heart rate at approximately 90 beats per minute are recommended to treat moderate hypotension during combined lumbar epidural and general anesthesia. If additional cardio-

vascular support is required, ephedrine should be used depending on each patient's cardiovascular status.

Important Aspects of Venous Return and Epidural Blockade

As indicated in Tables 11-3 and 11-4 and in Figures 11-4 and 11-5, reduced venous return may play a dominant role in initiating sudden reductions in cardiac rate, which should be viewed as a danger signal that venous return is markedly reduced and oxygenation of the myocardium is at risk. Obstruction to venous return, by whatever means, must be avoided in patients being given epidural block. If postural changes are added to obstruction in the presence of the increased venous capacitance of epidural block, serious impairment of venous return will follow. In addition, pressure in epidural veins will rise owing to channeling of blood from the pelvis by way of the alternative route of the vertebral venous plexus and azygos vein to the right atrium; this has important consequences for increased spread of segmental analgesia and may impair arterial blood flow to the spinal cord (72).

Situations in which venous return may be compromised may be summarized as follows:

■ *Supine hypotensive syndrome* in pregnancy resulting from uterine compression of the vena cava is accentuated by increased venous capacitance owing to sympathetic block of epidural analgesia and postural changes favoring pooling of blood in the lower limbs (73,74).

■ *Uterine contraction* during labor in supine position may cause compression. Mean brachial arterial pressure may be maintained at deceptively normal levels because of simultaneous compression of vena cava and aorta (Poiseiro effect). However, mean femoral arterial pressure drops precipitously, as does uterine blood flow (75). These effects are accentuated by epidural block if the patient is allowed to remain supine.

■ *Intestinal obstruction, ascites, and large intra-abdominal tumors* may compress the vena cava at three main sites: (a) *below the liver*, owing to abdominal distention, by intestinal obstruction (76), or by ascites (77) (this site is also commonly occluded by overenthusiastic retraction or by abdominal packs during upper abdominal surgery); (b) *in the upper lumbar region*, by large intra-abdominal tumors (including within the uterus); and (c) *at the pelvic brim*, by stretching of the iliac vessels owing to extreme backward tilting of the pelvis. This is sometimes an accompaniment of later pregnancy and may also result from extreme lordotic posturing on the operating table. The "extended lordotic posture" may occlude the vena cava below the liver as well—with potential for venous congestion in the kidney and resultant proteinuria (78).

The most common causes of vena caval obstruction in surgical applications of epidural block are poor positioning, heavy-handed retraction, and incorrect use of abdominal packs. Extreme positions, such as the jackknife prone, lateral "kidney," and hyperflexed lithotomy, should be avoided in association with any anesthetic technique and with epidural block in particular (73,79). Whenever possible, caval obstruction should be relieved before epidural block or carefully avoided after epidural block. If it occurs and cannot be corrected for a period of time, venous return may be assisted by restoring venous capacitance to normal levels by using carefully titrated doses of ephedrine (5–10 mg) intravenously. In some patients with large abdominal tumors, both the aorta and vena cava may be partially obstructed, but with maintenance of sufficient venous return to keep mean arterial pressure normal, with a partly occluded aorta. Sudden relief of the aortic obstruction as the tumor is removed may cause a precipitous fall in blood pressure owing to the reactive hyperemia below the level of obstruction. This situation may be avoided by ensuring adequate hydration and perhaps by using appropriate amounts of colloid before tumor removal. Also, one should be prepared to use small doses of ephedrine until reactive hyperemia subsides.

Epidural Blockade and Reduction of Blood Loss

Although initial emphasis on methods to reduce operative blood loss focused on reduction of arterial blood pressure, it was also well known that position played an important part (80). There has been a gradual recognition of the importance of avoidance of venous obstruction and the use of position in combination with sympathetic blockade to aid venous pooling away from the operative site. Thus, although epidural blockade has been used to produce hypotension and, in turn, control operative blood loss (81,82), others have found that blood loss can be reduced without the levels of hypotension commonly required if general anesthesia and hypotensive drugs are used (83,84). Keith deliberately avoided arterial hypotension in a randomized prospective study of blood loss using epidural or general anesthesia for surgery for total hip replacement (83). Blood loss was determined intraoperatively by a colorimetric technique and postoperatively by closed suction drains. Patients receiving epidural block had operative blood losses that were half those associated with general anesthesia. In contrast, there was no difference in postoperative blood losses between the two groups. Other studies reported a reduction in blood loss by 30% to 40% if epidural block is used for hip surgery (85,86). Thus, it appears that epidural block may reduce oper-

ative blood loss by factors other than a mild reduction in arterial blood pressure, increased venous capacitance (47), and the use of appropriate position. Additional factors may include the prevention of high venous pressure in response to sympathetic activity resulting from pain (87), avoidance of "reactive arterial hypertension," and avoidance of increased airway pressure with resultant effects on venous pressure.

Function of Hollow Viscera After Epidural Blockade

The Bladder

One of the most commonly observed sequels of lumbar epidural block is temporary atonia of the bladder owing to blockade of sacral segments S2–S4. This is similar to lower motor neuron lesions in which bladder sensation is lost. Fortunately, this type of effect after epidural blockade is usually short-lived and causes no or minimal increases in postblock bladder dysfunction (88). However, careful postepidural monitoring of bladder function is advised (e.g., by postvoid bladder scans).

When continuous epidural techniques are used, however, catheterization of the bladder may be necessary (89). On the other hand, segmental thoracic epidural block (e.g., T5–L1) may spare the sacral segments and thus leave bladder sensation intact. In addition, relief of severe abdominal pain by epidural block from T5 to L1 may prevent reflex sympathetic activity (via T12–L1 spinal segments), which increases bladder sphincter tone and may predispose to acute retention.

The Gut

Epidural block extending from T6 to L1 effectively denervates the splanchnic sympathetic supply to the abdominal viscera (see Chapter 39, Fig. 39-1). The sympathetic blockade results in a small contracted gut owing to parasympathetic dominance.

Colorectal surgery is associated with postoperative ileus, which contributes to delayed discharges. Blockade of nociceptive afferent and sympathetic efferent nerves are believed to be key initiators of ileus. Thoracic epidural anesthesia with postoperative thoracic epidural analgesia has been shown to shorten the time to first bowel movement (90). The duration of postoperative colonic ileus is shortened with TEA using local anesthetics (91,92), compared with parental and epidural opioids (93). The main mechanism appears to be a block of the nociceptive afferent fibres and the thoracolumbar nociceptive efferent fibres with unopposed parasympathetic efferent fibers (90).

Lumbar epidural blockade appears to be not effective in inhibiting bowel motility (94). Perioperative intestinal hypoperfusion is a major contributing factor leading to organ dysfunction. Thoracic epidural anesthesia during and after major surgery has been shown to protect the gut from decreased microvascular perfusion and to improve the mucosal blood flow, even under conditions of decreased perfusion pressure (95,96).

Blood flow in the intestine, as assessed by laser Doppler flowmetry, has been shown to increase in patients undergoing colon surgery (97) and during experimental gastric tube formation (98) under epidural anesthesia. This increase may be beneficial and may contribute to the healing of the gut anastomoses if epidural local anesthetic agents are used for postoperative analgesia (see also Chapters 6 and 7).

Thus, epidural anesthesia with local anesthetics seems to be the best method for relieving pain after gastrointestinal surgery because of its minimal effects on gastric emptying, stimulating effects on bowel motility, and possibly beneficial effects on the integrity of bowel anastomoses.

Thermoregulation and Shivering

Hypothermia (a decrease in core temperature) is common in patients undergoing surgery with epidural anesthesia and is thought to result from heat loss to the cold environment due to sympathectomy-induced vasodilatation. The normal process by which thermoregulation usually minimizes intraoperative core temperature is prevented, since epidural anesthesia directly inhibits vasoconstriction in the analgesic dermatomes.

Hypothermia following epidural injection of local anesthetic solution may result in part from redistribution of heat from central to peripheral regions (99–101). Warming the body via the skin for 2 hours before inducing epidural anesthesia raised the skin temperature (but not the core temperature) and helped prevent hypothermia during the induction of epidural anesthesia (99).

With epidural anesthesia, shivering-like tremors occur in approximately 30% of patients (102). The decrease in core temperature triggers thermoregulatory vasoconstriction and shivering above the level of epidural anesthesia (100,101).

Cold solutions injected into the epidural space may directly affect thermosensitive structures within the spinal cord to cause shivering during epidural anesthesia in pregnant subjects (103,104) but not in nonpregnant subjects (101). This suggests that pregnancy may enhance the contribution of spinal thermoregulatory input.

Injection of either epidural meperidine (25 mg) or epidural fentanyl (50 μg) has been reported to abolish shivering during epidural local analgesia in a high percentage of patients in labor (105,106) and during cesarean section (107).

In summary, tremor during epidural anesthesia is due to normal thermoregulatory shivering, which results largely from central hypothermia and is preceded by peripheral vasoconstriction above the level of sympathetic blockade.

Neuroendocrine Effects of Epidural Blockade

Surgical stress is associated with a variety of changes in endocrine and metabolic function, including protein metabolism, leading to a state of negative nitrogen balance in the postoperative period. Most of the surgically induced endocrine and metabolic changes are abolished by an appropriate level of sensory blockade produced by regional anesthesia. If the level of anesthesia extends from T4 to S5, and if the epidural blockade is initiated before the onset of surgery, epidural anesthesia for lower abdominal procedures and operations on the lower extremities may completely abolish the hormonal and metabolic response. However, epidural anesthesia is less efficient in decreasing the surgical stress response to major upper abdominal and thoracic procedures (108). This is probably due to the inability of the epidural anesthetic to completely block all nociceptive afferent pathways (109). Also, evidence suggests that the afferent neural impulses as well as humoral factors, such as cytokines, which are released from the site of injury, may initiate the stress response in the hypothalamus during upper

abdominal surgery (110). Combinations of local anesthetics and opioids administered epidurally in the postoperative period provide more complete blunting of the neuroendocrine response than do opioids alone (111).

The metabolic alterations observed during surgery and the modifying effect of intra- and postoperative epidural anesthesia–analgesia on the metabolic stress response to surgery are discussed in detail in Chapter 6.

Vasoactive Hormones

The arginine-vasopressin (AVP) system and the renin-angiotensin system (RAS) play an important role in maintaining arterial blood pressure under conditions in which the sympathetic system is impaired (112,113). In an animal model, vasopressin concentrations increased during high TEA, most likely to compensate for decreased cardiac filling and/or arterial blood pressure when sympathoadrenal responses are impaired (114).

However, in humans, both renin and vasopressin support blood pressure and prevent severe hypotension following epidural anesthesia (115).

In nonpremedicated patients, active renin and vasopressin concentrations were measured in response to sodium nitroprusside (SNP)-induced arterial hypotension both before and during sympathetic blockade by epidural anesthesia (116). Sodium nitroprusside-induced hypotension was associated with increased plasma renin concentrations with the sympathetic system intact, but not during sympathetic blockade by TEA. Vasopressin plasma concentrations increased during SNP-induced hypotension in the presence of widespread epidural sympathetic blockade by segmental thoracic epidural blockade from T1 to T11, but not with the sympathetic system intact (Fig. 11-6B). During sympathetic blockade by epidural anesthesia, the responses to the second hypotensive challenge were significantly different from the first: Heart rate increased by less than half of the increase following the first challenge (Fig. 11-6A).

In summary, sympathetic blockade by TEA abolished the increase in renin activity in response to arterial hypotension. This indicates that, in humans, the renal sympathetic system probably plays a key role in mediating renin release in response to hypotension. In addition, TEA activates the vasopressin system in response to hypotension.

Understanding the role of these endogenous vasopressor systems in maintaining blood pressure after epidural blockade in healthy subjects may help to explain why certain high-risk patients become hypotensive during high TEA.

Effects of Epidural Blockade on Respiration

Two important questions concerning respiration and epidural blockade require an answer: Does epidural block interfere with respiration? Is the ability to cough impaired?

The following aspects of epidural blockade may influence respiration:

- Sensory ("afferent") neural blockade reduces nociceptive afferent drive to respiratory center
- Motor ("efferent") neural blockade of intercostal muscles, abdominal muscles, and diaphragm (rarely)
- Sympathetic neural blockade with resultant changes in cardiac output and pulmonary blood flow
- Vagal dominance in the presence of complete sympathetic blockade

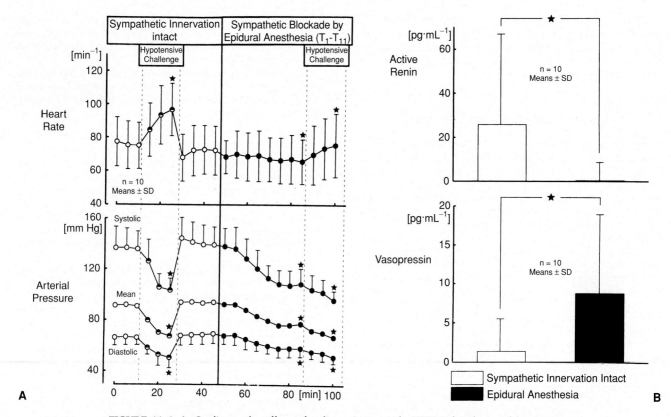

FIGURE 11-6. A: Cardiovascular effects of sodium nitroprusside (SNP)-induced arterial hypotension (hypotensive challenge; *vertical stippled lines*) in awake, nonsedated patients. Data points are mean values with standard deviations. **Left:** With the sympathetic innervation intact (o-o). Note the marked increase in heart rate and decrease in arterial blood pressure. **Right:** With sympathetic blockade by thoracic epidural blockade from T1 to T11 with plain bupivacaine (•—•). Heart rate increased albeit to a much smaller extent, whereas blood pressure decreased significantly. Sympathetic blockade by thoracic epidural anesthesia is usually (and here) associated with a decrease of both heart rate and blood pressure. **B:** Changes in plasma renin and vasopressin concentrations evoked by hypotensive challenge. SNP-induced hypotension was associated with increased renin plasma concentrations with the sympathetic system intact, but not during sympathetic block by epidural anesthesia. In contrast, vasopressin plasma concentrations remained unchanged with SNP-induced hypotension, but increased significantly during epidural anesthesia. From Hopf HB, Schlaghecke R, Peters J. Sympathetic neural blockade by thoracic epidural anesthesia suppresses renin release in response to arterial hypotension. *Anesthesiology* 1994;80:992, with permission.

Systematically absorbed epinephrine and local anesthetic have effects upon:

- Respiratory control center in midbrain and chemoreceptors in medulla and carotid bodies
- Myoneural junction
- Metabolism of succinylcholine in serum

The potential for phrenic (C3–C5) palsy is extremely low with epidural block, since even blockade to T1 produces motor blockade to only the T4–T5 level. The only exception may be intentional epidural block at the cervical level or inadvertent epidural block during interscalene brachial plexus block (see Chapter 13).

Respiratory arrest during high epidural blockade is not usually the result of the effects of sensory or motor blockade, nor is it due to depressant effects of local anesthetic in the CSF; the concentrations attained in the brain by means of this route are insufficient to depress neuronal activity unless gross overdosage is administered (117). The most common causes of the rare instances of respiratory arrest associated with epidural block are extensive sympathetic blockade, reduced cardiac output, and

reduced oxygen delivery to the CNS. It cannot be overemphasized that meticulous attention to maintenance of organ perfusion, by means of the clinical measures described earlier, should ensure that respiratory arrest in association with epidural block occurs extremely seldom and that such an occurrence should be rapidly reversible, with proper management.

It has been claimed that extensive sensory blockade may result in loss of consciousness owing to lack of input to the reticular activating system. However, epidural block to T1 does not cause loss of consciousness. This requires complete afferent blockade, including blockade of cervical nerve roots and the cranial nerves (87).

Many factors may contribute to the respiratory effects of epidural block. At present, our knowledge in this area is meager. However, the documented changes produced by epidural block per se appear to be mild. For example, a sensory level of T3, associated with a motor level of T8, may be expected to result in essentially no change in vital capacity (VC) and functional residual capacity (FRC) in normal patients, so that respiration and the ability to cough are not impaired (118,119). In patients with severe pain, epidural block probably improves

VC and FRC as well as Pa$_{O_2}$, at least in the early postoperative period (see also Chapter 39); this may result in improved respiratory exchange and more effective coughing (87,120–123).

Effect of Thoracic Epidural Anesthesia on Respiration

Since epidural anesthesia induces segmental block of spinal nerves, an adequate extension of the block of motor nerves can selectively affect respiratory muscles in the rib cage. Therefore the effect of TEA on the performance of the parasternal intercostal muscles was investigated by measuring electromyographic activity and length changes of the parasternal muscles in anesthetized, spontaneously breathing dogs (124). Thoracic epidural anesthesia caused rib cage distortion by impaired contraction of the parasternals and conceivably other respiratory muscles in the rib cage as well. Extrapolation to the clinical situation is difficult. However, in healthy awake volunteers, TEA caused a reduction of ventilatory response to CO_2 during spontaneous respiration principally because of decreased contribution of the rib cage to tidal breathing (125). Mechanical impairment of rib cage movement can produce decreased ventilatory response to carbon dioxide, probably reflecting blockade of the efferent or afferent pathway (or both) of the intercostal nerve roots. These changes, however, are of an order unlikely to be of clinical relevance. Prevention of respiratory failure by blocking pain-related effects on ability to cough and breathe deeply usually outweighs any consideration of ventilatory impairment from the block itself, especially as diaphragmatic function may be improved.

Furthermore TEA does not impair the hypoxic drive; for example, the ventilatory response to progressive isocapnic hypoxemia as has been shown in non-premedicated patients (126). There appears to be no reason to avoid TEA in patients who are reliant on hypoxic drive, such as those with chronic airway disease.

Diaphragmatic dysfunction is a major determinant of the impaired respiratory function observed after upper abdominal and thoracic surgery. Mankikian et al. (1988) showed that TEA increased postoperative esophageal and gastric pressure and diaphragmatic motion indices of diaphragmatic function after upper abdominal surgery in humans, suggesting a partial reversal of the diaphragmatic dysfunction (127). These results, however, were based upon indirect measurements and may also reflect changes in abdominal muscle activity. Pansard et al. (1993) obtained direct diaphragmatic electromyogram recording from intramuscular electrodes that had been inserted into the costal and crural parts of the muscle during elective abdominal aorta surgery (128). The electrical diaphragmatic activity was increased but was not associated with improved diaphragmatic contractility. It seems unlikely that diaphragmatic activity increased during TEA as a compensation for reduction in parasternal muscle inspiratory activity produced by motor blockade, since rib cage motion did not change after thoracic epidural blockade. In an awake sheep model 24 hours after thoracotomy, there was a significant decrease of both costal and crural diaphragmatic shortening; following TEA using lidocaine, tidal volume increases were recorded, but there was markedly reduced rib cage expansion (129). This finding may be due to a shift of the work load of breathing from the chest wall to the diaphragm, thus explaining the unexpected observation that rib cage function decreased in this animal model. By using the same study design in humans undergoing thoracic

surgery, this group observed a marked impairment of active diaphragmatic shortening, which was not reversed by TEA, despite improvement of other indices of respiratory function (130). This probably suggests that diaphragmatic contraction could not overcome the increased external forces placed upon it by other respiratory muscles (see also Chapter 7).

In summary, the effects of epidural anesthesia on diaphragmatic function after upper abdominal and thoracic surgery are complex. The most likely explanation for the TEA-related increase in diaphragmatic activity seems to be the interruption of an inhibitory reflex of phrenic nerve motor drive, either related to direct deafferentation of visceral sensory pathways or related to a diaphragmatic load reduction due to increased abdominal compliance.

Segmental high TEA can be used in patients with severe chronic obstructive pulmonary disease (COPD) and asthma undergoing chest wall surgery (131). In patients with bronchial hyperactivity, high TEA does not alter airway resistance, suggesting that reported cases of severe bronchospasm during epidural anesthesia are unrelated to sympathetic blockade and may be caused by mechanisms other than pulmonary sympathetic denervation (132).

Epidural Block and Motor Function

Clinical Applications of Deliberate Preservation of Motor Function

With respect to respiratory function, it is clear from the previous section that the aim is to use the appropriate drug and regimen to preserve motor function, and thus to permit deep breathing and coughing. In postoperative patients, continuous infusion of bupivacaine has proved to be an attractive method of achieving this goal. This method is described in detail in Chapter 43. Preservation of motor function also permits ultra-early ambulation, since patients who are pain-free are able to ambulate soon after surgery (87). It may be necessary to use vasopressors if epidural block is continued with only local anesthetic. Alternatives are to use dilute bupivacaine plus opioid (some risk of hypotension) or opioid alone (no risk of hypotension), as described in Chapter 43. Ultra-early ambulation probably decreases the risk of venous thrombosis and may decrease the hospitalization time (87). More controlled data are required (see also Chapter 7).

Clinical Applications of Motor Function Depression

In abdominal and hip surgery, depression of motor function is necessary during surgery. In this situation, the powerful motor blockade of etidocaine or lidocaine may be used (Fig. 11-7). Some of the motor effects are obtained by "deafferentation," preventing reflex muscle contraction by blocking nociception before it reaches the spinal cord.

Factors determining motor effects of epidural block are as follows (see pharmacology section):

- *The local anesthetic drug:* Ropivacaine has the least motor effects; etidocaine has the most potent effects.
- *Dose of drug:* Degree of motor blockade is increased as dose of drug increases.
- *Repeated doses of drug:* With "top-up" techniques, both motor and sensory blockade tend to become more intense with repeated doses; however, if dilute solutions of ropivacaine, levobupivacaine, or bupivacaine are used by

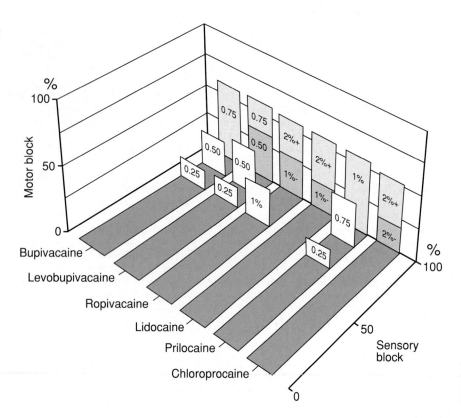

FIGURE 11-7. Motor and sensory block percentage success rate. Comparison of agents, concentrations, and addition of epinephrine is based on subjective data, so that only approximate comparisons can be made.

controlled continuous infusion, motor blockade can be kept to a minimum.

■ *Epinephrine as an adjuvant* increases the degree of motor blockade.

Epidural Blockade and Pregnancy

The known and potential physiologic effects of epidural block on mother, placenta, and fetus must be viewed in the light of contemporary knowledge of the physiology and pathophysiology of pregnancy, fetal physiology, and pharmacology. The detailed implications for regional anesthesia are discussed further in Chapter 24. By recognizing the modifications in management that are predicted by the impact of the physiologic changes of pregnancy, one can administer epidural anesthesia to gravid women with efficacy and safety.

PHARMACOLOGY OF EPIDURAL BLOCKADE

The essence of the clinical pharmacology of epidural block is the provision of safe and effective neural blockade. To safely institute an epidural block, a knowledge of the physiology of epidural block is necessary, as well as a revision of the pharmacokinetics of local anesthetics as related to their administration by means of the epidural route. The efficacy of epidural block depends on this and on the clinical effects of the local anesthetics used (see Chapters 2–5).

In considering the pharmacokinetics of local anesthetics, both the systemic absorption and systemic disposition are of importance. Systemic absorption of local anesthetics limits the duration of nerve blocks and is of concern in view of systemic toxicity. The general absorption and disposition characteristics of local anesthetics are discussed in detail in Chapter 3. The potential for systemic toxicity should also be considered when choosing a local anesthetic agent for epidural use. The pharmacokinetic characteristics of the local anesthetics currently used for epidural analgesia and the implications for the time course of neural blockade and systemic toxicity have been reviewed in detail by Burm (133,134). Toxic effects of local anesthetics mainly involve the CNS and the cardiovascular system, depending on the rapidity of absorption from the epidural space and the total dose of the drug administered. This topic is covered in detail in Chapters 3, 4, and 5.

Thus, a thorough knowledge of the pharmacokinetics and toxicity of local anesthetics is a prerequisite to the safe use of epidural analgesia.

Sites of Action

Local anesthetics may act on the periphery of the spinal cord, the spinal roots, the dorsal root ganglia, and the extradural nerves (87). However, the spinal nerve roots, at the location where they leave the subarachnoid space and enter the nerve root sheath, are suggested to be the primary sites of action during spinal and epidural anaesthesia (87,135). This is substantiated by significantly higher tissue concentrations in the intradural spinal roots than in the spinal cord (136,137) and the close proximity of the epidural space and the nerve roots (135). Both dura and arachnoid-mater appear to be thinner in this region (138,139). In addition, the diffusion surface is increased by the dispersion of the bundles into individual fascicles (135). Subsequently, diffusion of local anesthetics from the epidural space through the dura mater into the CSF occurs to the periphery of the spinal cord (136,140).

Likewise, opioids rapidly gain access to CSF (see also Chapter 40) (141,142).

Furthermore, extensions of the subarachnoid space provide a large area for penetration of the local anesthetic into the nerve structures and also possibly provide retaining pockets of high concentration of local anesthetics, limiting dilution into a greater pool of CSF (135). Despite lower tissue penetration of local anesthetics in the spinal cord (with concentration being highest in the lateral and posterior column and lowest in the gray matter) (137), involvement of the spinal cord in nerve blocking during epidural anesthesia has been demonstrated (143–145). Even lower tissue concentrations have been demonstrated in the dorsal root ganglia after epidural administration of local anesthetics (137). Nevertheless, this site has also been proposed as the primary site of action (138).

Longitudinal Spread of Solutions in the Epidural Space

The longitudinal spread of local anesthetics in the epidural space accounts primarily for the extent of epidural neural blockade, although they do not necessarily correspond exactly. This is because diffusion and vascular transport possibly influence the ultimate spread of analgesia (see Chapter 3). Longitudinal spread has shown to be more in a cephalad than caudad direction (146,147), and it depends largely on bulk flow during and after administration and on those structures in the epidural space that resist flow (148). In this context, the epidural space can be regarded as a reservoir that is collapsible, distensible, and leaky. The spread of analgesia may be modified by outflow of local anesthetics through the intervertebral foramina. Continuous positive airway pressure increased the spread of sensory blockade in TEA, primarily by a more caudad extension of sensory blockade (149).

Changes in the anatomy of the intervertebral foramina by disease or advancing age may alter the spread of analgesia by this mechanism (see Chapter 9).

Clinical Considerations for the Efficacy of Epidural Blockade

There is no question now that epidural block can be effective in nearly all cases if attention is paid to the anatomy, physiology, and pharmacology of the technique. Yet there are still many major medical centers throughout the world that hold the belief that epidural blockade has a high failure rate compared with subarachnoid blockade. This merely serves to underline the relatively recent acquisition of relevant data on which to base the effective use of epidural block.

Assessment of Epidural Blockade

In defining important factors in effective epidural block, the development of standardized methods of assessment of epidural block has been essential.

Sensory Block. Sensory block is graphed by testing for loss and return of pin-prick sensation (*partial sensory block*) in each dermatome on both sides of the body. An alternative method of testing initial onset is to use an alcohol swab to assess loss of temperature sensation, which is the most sensitive indicator of initial onset of sensory block (see Chapter 2, Table 2-1). Complete loss of touch sensation may also be charted (150,151).

From a "time-segment" graph can be obtained (a) time to initial onset and complete spread of analgesia, (b) time to regression of two segments and complete regression of analgesia, (c) total number of segments blocked on both sides of the body, (d) milliliters of local anesthetic per mean segmental spread (total segments R + L divided by two), and (e) area of the segment–time diagram (segment minutes), which can be related to the dose of local anesthetic, in segment minutes per dose. The latter expression is used to assess the development of tachyphylaxis (see later discussion).

Somatosensory Evoked Potentials. Cortical-derived somatosensory evoked potentials (SEPs) have been used in the qualitative assessment of the intensity of peripheral and central neural blockade (152–158).

Somatosensory evoked potentials reflect the net results of neuronal activities coming from peripheral nerves through the spinal cord to the brain. Somatosensory evoked potentials are generated by repetitive stimulation of peripheral nerves and can be monitored at several points along the sensory pathway, including over the spinal cord, subcortical structures, and cerebral cortex. Intraoperative monitoring of SEPs is an accepted technique to assess the functional integrity of the sensory pathways, particularly during spinal and scoliosis surgery (159).

Despite a clinically adequate block as assessed by pin-prick, afferent impulses generating SEPs still passed through an expected blocked area following epidural administration of bupivacaine, mepivacaine, or etidocaine. This probably indicates that total afferent blockade often is not obtained. Abolishment of SEP has only been accomplished using 1.5% etidocaine (154). This is possibly due to the ability of etidocaine to penetrate the white matter of the spinal cord more readily (144).

Sympathetic Block. Sympathetic block is assessed by measuring skin temperature with a telethermometer thermography, or temperature-sensitive papers. Alternatively, a digital plethysmogram may be used. Skin conductance can be measured in the clinical setting by use of the psychogalvanic response; reliable measurements are much more difficult than usually acknowledged. More precise, but of research application only, are the use of various sweat tests, such as cobalt blue and starch iodine, or the response of skin plethysmography to ice during venous occlusion plethysmography. A full discussion of the clinical and laboratory tests of sympathetic block is given in Chapter 39.

Motor Block. Motor block is usually assessed by use of the Bromage scale for motor blockade in the lower limbs (87) (Table 11-5).

TABLE 11-5

BROMAGE SCALE

No block (0%)	Full flexion of knees and feet possible
Partial (33%)	Just able to flex knees, still full flexion of feet possible
Almost complete (66%)	Unable to flex knees. Still flexion of feet
Complete (100%)	Unable to move legs or feet

Motor blockade in the lower limbs can be assessed with reference to specific myotomes (e.g., L2, hip flexion) (151). A score of 0 is assigned for no block and 1 for complete block (no movement) at each joint on each side. Thus, maximal motor block is present bilaterally with a score of 10:

	Right	Left
Hip flexion (L2)	1	1
Knee extension (L3)	1	1
Ankle dorsiflexion (L4)	1	1
Great toe dorsiflexion (L5)	1	1
Ankle plantar flexion (S1)	1	1

5 + 5 = 10 (complete motor block)

This test removes some observer error because only a "move" (0) or "no move" (1) decision needs to be made at each joint.

An onset profile for motor blockade can be presented as a "myotome score–time" diagram. For research purposes, Axelsson reported an apparatus that measures maximal isometric strength by a force transducer at ankle, knee, and hip. This provides objective, reproducible measurements of muscle power (160).

Abdominal muscle power may be assessed by the rectus abdominis muscle (RAM) test (Table 11-6) (161). This is useful in abdominal surgery, when abdominal muscle blockade is required rather than lower limb muscle blockade. On the other hand, the Bromage scale is useful for lower limb surgery. Both scales may be used when a comprehensive picture is required: RAM-test (T5–T12) and Bromage scale (L1–S2).

Testing of 100% and 80% power has limitations in patients with vasodilation; blood pressure and pulse rate must be carefully monitored if these tests are to be used.

A broad comparison of agents used for epidural block can be compiled based on their success rate in producing motor and sensory block. Because different methods of testing have been used in many studies, the comparisons are only qualitative (Fig. 11-7).

Electromyography. Few studies have used the more quantitative method of electromyography (EMG), although this would provide more sensitive assessment.

Reflex Response. Under general anesthesia without muscle relaxation, sensation can still be crudely assessed by use of reflex response to pinch by a forceps at appropriate segmental levels. Alternatively, the tendon reflexes in the lower limbs give a gross index of both motor and sensory block, while reflexes such as those of the cremaster, anal, and abdominal muscles may also be useful as a gross guide to adequacy of blockade.

Factors Affecting Epidural Blockade

Many factors may affect the efficacy, spread of blockade, fiber types blocked, and other aspects of epidural blockade: site of injection and nerve root size; age; position; speed of injection;

TABLE 11-6

RAM TEST OF ABDOMINAL MUSCLES

100%	Able to rise from supine to sitting position with hands behind head
80% power	Can sit only with arms extended
60% power	Can lift only head and scapulae off bed
40% power	Can lift only shoulders off bed
20% power	An increase in abdominal muscle tension can be felt during effort; no other response

dose and choice of local anesthetic; adjuvants; number and frequency of injections.

Site of Injection and Nerve Root Size

Blockade tends to be most intense and has the most rapid onset close to the site of injection. The subsequent spread of analgesia depends to some extent on whether the injection is made in thoracic or lumbar regions.

After *lumbar epidural* injection, a somewhat greater cranial than caudal spread of analgesia occurs and there may be a delay in the L5 and S1 segments. The delay in onset at these segments appears to be due to the large size of these nerve roots (162).

After *midthoracic epidural* injection, analgesia spreads quite evenly from the site of injection. However, the upper thoracic and lower cervical segments are resistant to blockade because of the large size of the nerve roots and the large number of nerve fibers within them. Repeated doses by the mid thoracic route eventually may cause analgesia to spread into lumbar and sacral segments, with the expected lag in onset at L5–S1. Careful control of dose in the thoracic region permits sparing of the lumbar segments and thus avoidance of sympathetic block in the lower limbs and maintenance of normal bladder function—that is, a true segmental block. Similarly, a small dose injected at L2–L3 for labor pain may block only T11 and L3–L4 segments, while it spares the sacral segments.

The profile of onset of caudal epidural block spreads upward from S5, and the S1 segment is the last to be blocked, as expected.

Age

Over the past several years, the anesthesiologist has been faced with a growing number of elderly patients presenting for surgery. Epidural anesthesia has enjoyed a resurgence of popularity for elderly patients undergoing surgery in areas amenable to conduction anesthesia. With advancing age, anatomic changes do occur in the epidural space (136). In the young individual, the areolar tissue around the intervertebral foramina is soft and loose. In the elderly, this areolar tissue becomes dense and firm, partially sealing the intervertebral foramina (87). With aging, the dura becomes more permeable to local anesthetic because of significant increase in the size of the arachnoid villi (138). Discrepancies exist among studies in which the influence of age on epidural anesthesia has been assessed. The classic study of Bromage regarding the influence of age on epidural spread reported a strong relationship between age and the epidural segmental dose requirement (ESDR); that is, the amount (dose) of local anesthetic required to block one spinal segment (163). Assuming a linear dose-relationship, Bromage demonstrated that, with age, the ESDR decreased in a linear way. In contrast to Bromage's assumption, others have found no direct linear relationship between volume and anesthetic spread (164–166). The greater the total amount used, the greater the ESDR calculated. From this it can be concluded that the results of Bromage's study concerning the linear decrease of ESDR with age are questionable because he assumed a direct linear relationship between the amount (dose) of local anesthetic and extent of anesthesia and because he used variable total anesthetic amounts (163). Using a given dose (fixed volume and concentration), other investigators have found a significantly greater number of spinal segments blocked in older patients. However, the magnitude of this effect was small: only one to three segments more in the elderly patients compared to younger adult patients (Fig. 11-8) (164,165,167–171). When using different volumes, the dose-effect relationships varied with these volumes (166,172).

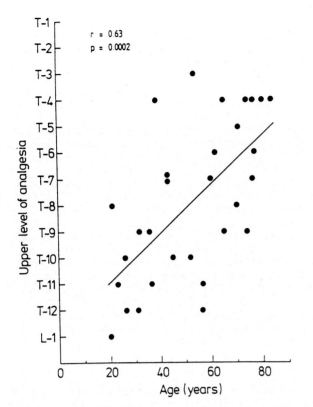

FIGURE 11-8. Relationship between the upper level of analgesia and age after epidural administration of 0.5% bupivacaine. Segmental spread is increased with age. From Veering BT, Burm AGL, Van Kleef JW, et al. Epidural anesthesia with bupivacaine: Effects of age on neural blockade and pharmacokinetics. *Anesth Analg* 1987;66:589, with permission.

The spread was also greater in the elderly patients than in younger ones after epidural anesthesia with the relatively new long-acting local anesthetics ropivacaine (173) and levobupivacaine (174). The higher spread with ropivacaine in elderly patients was accompanied with a high incidence of hypotension and bradycardia (Fig. 11-9). This problem is a particularly important issue in elderly patients with cardiovascular disease such as hypertension, because the risk for ischemia secondary to hypotension is increased (175,176).

Since aging is associated with reduced β-adrenergic responsiveness, a small dose of epinephrine added to a local anesthetic does not appear to be a reliable detector of unintentional intravascular injection of local anesthetic solution (177).

Age has also been shown to be associated with a higher upper level of analgesia following TEA of a fixed dose; increased levels of analgesia with increasing age have been attributed to reduced leakage of local anesthetic solution because of progressive sclerotic closure of intervertebral foramina (87,136). Also, the cephalad spread of radioactivity after epidural injection of ^{131}I mixed in 2% lidocaine was higher in patients older than 50 years than in those younger (147). Radiologic studies, however, have failed to show a relationship between age and spread in the epidural space (146). It is possible that radiopaque material and local anesthetic do not spread in an identical manner. On the other hand, the increased permeability of the dura with aging, as described by Shantha and Evans (138), may contribute to the higher levels of analgesic spread in the elderly. Usubiaga reported that older patients have a higher residual pressure and that a positive relationship exists between residual epidural pressure and the extent of analgesic spread. Also, increased epidural compliance and decreased epidural resistance with advancing age may contribute to this enhanced spread in the elderly (178).

The onset time to maximal caudad spread has been reported to decrease with advancing age following epidural administration of bupivacaine, thus allowing surgery in areas innervated

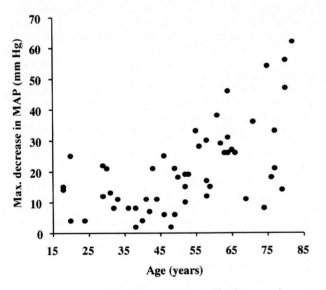

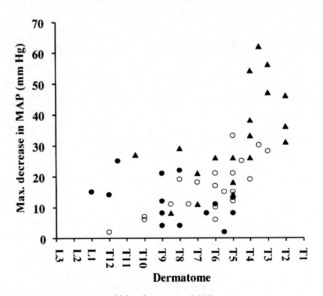

FIGURE 11-9. Relationship between the maximum decrease of the mean arterial blood pressure (MAP; mm Hg) during the first hour after the induction of epidural anesthesia and age. **Right:** Relationship between the maximum decrease of the mean arterial blood pressure (MAP; mm Hg) during the first hour after the induction of epidural anesthesia and the highest level of analgesia for the three age groups (●: Group 1: 19–40 yr, o: Group 2: 41–60 yr; ▲: Group 3: >61 yr). Adapted from Simon, Veering BT, Stienstra R, et al. The effects of age on the neural blockade and hemodynamic changes following epidural anesthesia with ropivacaine. *Anesth Analg* 2002;94:1325, with permission.

by these segments to be started sooner in older patients than in younger (170,171). In addition, a more rapid onset and enhanced intensity of motor blockade has been shown in older patients (171). With aging, the neural population declines steadily within the spinal cord, and peripheral nerves show a linear reduction in conduction velocity, especially in motor nerves (179). This could make older patients more sensitive to local anesthetics, which is probably (partially) the cause of the shorter onset time of analgesia in the caudad segments and the altered motor block profile. Nydahl (167) reported a shorter duration of motor blockade, as assessed by EMG recordings, following epidural administration of epinephrine-containing bupivacaine solutions. This may be attributed to a stronger reaction in younger subjects to epinephrine (180).

Epidural anesthesia carries some problems in elderly patients. The technique is technically more difficult, and so a chance of a failure is always present. This is partially attributed to the fact that the ligamentum flavum probably changes into a form that is easily ossified (181). The more extensive spread of analgesia is likely to be accompanied by more extensive sympathetic blockade. Therefore, prevention of hypotension by intravenous (IV) administration of crystalloid fluids will be important in older patients. It should be emphasized, however, that rapid volume preloading constitutes a potential risk in elderly patients with poor cardiac function, in whom there is a risk of pulmonary edema and cardiac failure.

With epidural anesthesia, a decline in the thermoregulatory response occurs with age, as has been shown by the decrease in core temperature (182). Consequently, the postoperative rewarming process will occur more slowly in older patients. Lumbar epidural anesthesia (LEA) using lidocaine did not affect the resting ventilation parameters, such as minute ventilation and tidal volume, in older patients, and it stimulated the ventilatory response to hypercapnia to the same degree as in young patients (126). Therefore, LEA appears to be a safe technique in elderly patients.

Important considerations for the use of epidural anesthesia in pediatric patients is covered in Chapter 27.

Position

Comparison of sitting and lateral positions for epidural block reveals no significant differences in cephalad spread (183). An exception is the obese patient, who achieves a lower level of block when seated (184). Caudad spread of block in seated patients is slightly favored by the sitting position (185). From these studies, it seems that the differences between sitting and lateral positions are small. The lateral position favors spread of analgesia to the dependent side in both pregnant and nonpregnant patients (186–188), but the differences are small. In surgical patients, however, Seow and associates found that onset of sensory and motor block was significantly more rapid on the dependent side and had a longer duration. In addition to being more rapid in onset, motor blockade was greater on the dependent side at all time intervals tested out to 40 minutes after injection. Onset time for sympathetic block was not faster on the dependent side, but duration of maximum elevation of skin temperature was greater on the dependent side (188). The differences in sensory and motor block are great enough to indicate an advantage in placing patients on the operative side during epidural block before lower limb surgery (188). There appears to be no correlation between spread of analgesia and weight and height in adults (87).

Speed of Injection

Increasing the speed of injection has no effect on the bulk flow of solutions in the epidural space (146,147). Also, spread of analgesia is only minimally influenced. However, rapid injection of large volumes of solution may increase CSF pressure (189), decrease spinal cord blood flow, increase intracranial pressure, and pose a risk of spinal or cerebral complications. In susceptible patients, sudden increases in CSF pressure may compromise spinal cord blood flow (see Chapter 12), and this may increase susceptibility to neurotoxicity (189) or, in patients with atherosclerosis, may possibly cause "spinal stroke." Evidence exists that nutritive vessels crossing the perineurium of nerves are subject to a pathologic "valve" mechanism initiated by perineurial edema (190). This edema could be initiated by sudden increases in CSF pressure. Subsequent hypotension owing to sympathetic block may decrease spinal cord flow if CSF pressure and perineurial pressure remain high. A combination of these effects could result in neural damage (see also Chapter 12).

Sudden increases in intracerebral pressure may cause headache, cerebral hemorrhage, or isolated hemorrhage in a small vessel, such as a retinal vessel. Headache is commonly reported if epidural solutions are injected rapidly. Intraocular hemorrhage has been described after rapid epidural injection of 30 mL of local anesthetic solution (191). Thus, rapid injection is not only ineffective in "forcing solution up the epidural space," but also potentially dangerous. Local anesthetics should be injected into the epidural space slowly and preferably in incremental doses.

Volume, Concentration, and Dose of Local Anesthetic

Extensive studies by Bromage indicated that the dose of drug (concentration × volume) determined the spread of analgesia (136), at least between the concentrations of 2% and 5% lidocaine and 0.2% and 0.5% tetracaine. However, data were not obtained to compare 0.5% lidocaine with a range of 1% to 2%, which is a typical clinical range of concentrations. It did appear from Bromage's data that dose requirements diminished from about 30 mg per segment to 20 mg per segment when concentration was reduced from 2% to 1% lidocaine. Erdemir et al. have shown that 30 mL of 1% lidocaine produced a higher sensory level than 10 mL of a 3% solution (192). Burn et al. showed that large volumes of contrast media (40 mL) were more likely to spread into cervical regions compared with higher concentrations and smaller volumes (20 mL) (146). With regard to motor blockade, dosage becomes less important when dilute solutions are used. Below concentrations of 1% lidocaine, motor block is minimal regardless of dose, unless injections are repeated at intervals. Then, intensity of sensory and motor block increases with each successive injection. This mechanism is important in obstetric analgesia when dilute solutions of 0.125% or 0.065% bupivacaine are used.

Increasing dosage results in a linear increase in degree of sensory block and duration of epidural block, whereas increasing concentration results in a reduction in onset time and intensity of motor blockade (Fig. 11-7). A general summary of the effects of local anesthetic dose and added epinephrine is given in Chapter 4. However, it should be recognized that choice of drug influences these effects.

Choice of Local Anesthetic

The concept of a "spectrum" of local anesthetics, as depicted in Chapter 4, relates significantly to epidural block. The great flexibility of sensory and motor block that can be obtained by careful choice of drug is seen in Figure 11-7. For example, 0.25% bupivacaine, 0.5% ropivacaine, or 0.25% levobupivacaine may provide satisfactory analgesia for acute pain with

TABLE 11-7

CLINICAL EFFECTS OF LOCAL ANESTHETIC SOLUTIONS COMMONLY USED FOR EPIDURAL BLOCKADE

Drug	Time spread to ± four segments ±1 SD (min)	Approximate time to two-segment regression ±2 SD[a] (min)	Recommended "top-up" time from initial dose[a] (min)
Lidocaine, 2%	15 ± 5	100 ± 40	60
Prilocaine, 2%–3%	15 ± 4	100 ± 40	60
Chloroprocaine, 2%–3%	12 ± 5	60 ± 15	45
Mepivacaine, 2%	15 ± 5	120 ± 150	60
Bupivacaine, 0.5%–0.75%	18 ± 10	200 ± 80	120
Ropivacaine, 0.75%–1%	20.5 ± 7.9	177 ± 49	120
Levobupivacaine, 0.5%–0.75%	19.5 ± 9	200 ± 80	120

[a]Note "top-up" time is based on duration minus 2 SD, which encompasses the likely duration in 95% of the population. In a conscious, cooperative patient, an alternative is to use frequent checks of segmental level to indicate need to top-up. All solutions contain 1:200,000 epinephrine, except ropivacaine and levobupivacaine. Data from Bromage PR. *Epidural Analgesia*. Philadelphia: W.B. Saunders, 1978; Brockway MS, Bannister JP, McClure JH, et al. Comparison of extradural ropivacaine and bupivacaine. *Br J Anaesth* 1991;66:31; Casati A, Putzu M. Bupivacaine, levobupivacaine and ropivacaine: are they clinically different? *Best Pract Res Clin Anaesthesiol* 2005;19:247; Cederholm J, Anskar S, Bengtsson M. Sensory, motor, and sympathetic lock during epidural analgesia with 0.5% and 0.75% ropivacaine with and without epinephrine. *Reg Anesth* 1994;19:18; Cohen SE, Thurlow A. Comparison of a chloroprocaine-bupivacaine mixture with chloroprocaine and bupivacaine used individually for obstetric epidural analgesia. *Anesthesiology* 1979;51:288; Seow LT, Lips FJ, Cousins MJ, Mather LE. Lidocaine and bupivacaine mixtures for epidural blockade. *Anesthesiology* 1982;56:177; and Simon MJG, Veering BT, Burm AGL, et al. The effect of age on the clinical profile and the systemic absorption and disposition of levobupivacaine following epidural anaesthesia. *Br J Anaesth* 2004;93:512, with permission.

close to zero motor block, whereas 0.25% etidocaine results in close to 50% motor block, but variable analgesia.

If more potent analgesia with minimal motor block is required, 0.5% bupivacaine, 0.5% ropivacaine, 0.5% levobupivacaine, or 2% plain lidocaine may be chosen, although the former is the best choice for continuous techniques. The requirements of profound sensory block and excellent muscle relaxation (e.g., for surgery or operative obstetrics) are best met by 2% lidocaine with epinephrine or 1.5% etidocaine (193) or 0.75% to 1.0% ropivacaine (if long duration is required).

Chloroprocaine has become an attractive alternative for short procedures and for obstetric analgesia; it is a safe drug because of its high rate of metabolism (however, see Chapter 4).

Use of prilocaine for epidural block is worthy of consideration. It is still the safest amide agent when used in a dose of less than 600 mg and should be considered for single-shot epidural block, except in obstetrics. Of practical use, the 2% plain solution provides intense sensory block and minimal motor block; with 2% plain solutions, levels are similar to those of the 2% epinephrine-containing solution, provided the dose is below 400 mg. This solution has appeal for outpatient caudal blocks or for single-shot epidural blocks for brief procedures. Alternatively, the 3% solution may be used if rapid onset is required, although a 20-mL dose produces some degree of motor block even with the plain solution.

Ropivacaine is the first enantiomerically pure local anesthetic and exists as the *S*-enantiomer (194,195). Its lipid-solubility is lower and this may contribute to a greater differential block of sensory and motor function than bupivacaine (196).

Both in animals and healthy human volunteers, ropivacaine has less cardiovascular and CNS toxicity than racemic bupivacaine (197–200).

In general, with epidural anesthesia, the onset, potency, and duration of anesthesia and analgesia of ropivacaine is comparable to that of bupivacaine (196) (Table 11-7). Ropivacaine shows, like bupivacaine, a dose-dependent duration of sensory (196,201,202) and motor block (203), but the duration of motor blockade seems to be shorter than with bupivacaine (201). Addition of epinephrine to ropivacaine did not result in prolongation of sensory or motor blockade (202). The use of more highly concentrated solutions of ropivacaine (0.75% and 1.0%) increases the clinical efficacy for lower limb surgery (204).

Ropivacaine has been shown to be effective in treating postoperative pain (see Chapter 43).

Levobupivacaine is the pure *S*(−)-enantiomer of racemic bupivacaine and is the most recently developed agent. Animal studies have demonstrated that levobupivacaine had less potential for CNS and cardiac system toxicity than does bupivacaine (205,206). This is consistent with findings of greater subjective tolerability of levobupivacaine than bupivacaine by human volunteers (207). Levobupivacaine infused intravenously appeared to be less arrhythmogenic than the same dose range of bupivacaine in healthy volunteers (208).

Levobupivacaine and bupivacaine after epidural administration show similarity in their clinical profiles (Table 11-8). Levobupivacaine 0.5% and 0.75%, used for lower limb surgery and lower abdominal surgery, had a very similar sensory and motor blockade as bupivacaine 0.5% and 0.75% (209–211). The addition of epinephrine to levobupivacaine led to an

increased rate of satisfaction of neural blockade (212). However, variables of sensory and motor blockade did not differ between the plain solution and the solutions containing
epinephrine. Levobupivacaine has been shown to be effective
in treating postoperative pain.

Differential Block. The differential capabilities of local anesthetics to block sensory and motor fibers has been referred to
as "sensory-motor dissociation" (Fig. 11-7). The basis for this
phenomenon is discussed in Chapters 2 and 3.

Local Anesthetic Mixtures. The basis of mixing (compounding) of local anesthetic agents is to obtain a rapid onset as well
as a long duration of blockade. 2-Chloroprocaine was used
in combination with bupivacaine to produce a faster onset as
well as prolonged sensory block following epidural anesthesia
in the obstetric setting (213). Unfortunately, 2-chloroprocaine
shortened the duration of bupivacaine's block. Isolated nerve
studies suggest that a metabolite of chloroprocaine may inhibit the binding of bupivacaine to the membrane site of action
(214).

Currently, no clinically significant advantage appears to ac-
crue to the use of mixtures of local anesthetic agents if a catheter
technique is to be used. The use of continuous techniques of
administration of the shorter-acting agents has considerable
advantages in that duration is not a problem and a rapid effect
can be obtained with a single drug. Only when a single-dose
(through-the-needle) technique is used does the 1:1 mixture of
lidocaine–bupivacaine have some merit in achieving rapid onset of profound motor blockade, followed by some increases in
duration of analgesia compared with lidocaine alone; however,
the gains are small (215).

Adjuvants

Epinephrine. Epinephrine reduces vascular absorption to a
variable extent (see Chapter 3, and Fig. 3-9) and enhances
the efficacy of epidural blockade. Enhancement of blockade
is much less marked with the longer-acting agents bupivacaine
and etidocaine; addition of fresh epinephrine in a concentration of 1:200,000 may enhance the intensity of motor block,
quality of sensory blockade, and duration of blockade, at least
for lidocaine and prilocaine (216).

Commercial preparations of local anesthetics containing
epinephrine are quite acidic. As a consequence, very little local
anesthetic is available in the nonionized base form that more
easily penetrates neural tissue. This will result in an increased
latency to onset of sensory blockade (216).

However, the addition of fresh epinephrine to local anesthetic, *at the time of injection*, does not prolong the onset of
clinical epidural or subarachnoid neural blockade with lidocaine or bupivacaine. In fact, with lidocaine or etidocaine, the
opposite has been reported (217,218) (Fig. 11-10).

Epinephrine has a hypalgesic effect when given alone
epidurally (219,220). enhancement of analgesia seen with
epinephrine is due to activation of dorsal horn inhibitory systems via α_2-adrenoceptors (221). For more detailed information on α-agonists, the reader is referred to Chapter 40.

Clonidine

Clonidine is a selective α_2-adrenergic agonist with some α_1-
agonist property. Clonidine acts synergistically with local anesthetics because of its action of opening potassium channels.
Thus, the duration of both sensory and motor blockade from
epidural block with local anesthetics is prolonged (222).

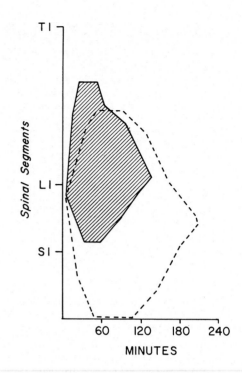

- - - - - Lidocaine with adrenaline 5 μg/ml

——— Lidocaine without adrenaline

FIGURE 11-10. Effect of epinephrine; segmental spread and duration
of sensory blockade for lidocaine. Segmental spread and duration of
analgesia are enhanced by addition of epinephrine. Caudad spread of
analgesia is also markedly improved with epinephrine-containing solutions. *Broken line,* + epinephrine (5 μg/ml); *solid line,* plain solution.
From Murphy TM, Mather LE, Stanton-Hicks MDA, et al. Effects of
adding adrenaline to etidocaine and Lignocaine in extradural anaesthesia: I. Block characteristics and cardiovascular effects. *Br J Anaesth*
1976;48:893, with permission.

Arterial hypotension is the most commonly reported side effect of neuraxial use of clonidine (223). Hypotension is mostly
due to direct inhibition of sympathetic outflow of preganglionic
neurons in the spinal cord. Other side effects include sedation
and a reduction of the heart rate (see also Chapter 40).

Ketamine

Ketamine is a noncompetitive antagonist of the N-methyl-D-
aspartate (NMDA) receptor calcium channel. Ketamine blocks
the open calcium channel on the NMDA receptor complex.
Thus, ketamine inhibits excitatory transmission by decreasing
depolarization. S(+)-ketamine, the left-handed optical isomer
of racemic ketamine, has a fourfold higher affinity for NMDA
receptors than right-handed R(−)-ketamine (224).

In clinical practice, conflicting results have been reported
when epidural administration of ketamine was used for pain
management. One study found a reduction in the onset time
of sensory block following epidural administration of 25 mg
ketamine with bupivacaine compared to epidural bupivacaine
(225). However, postoperative analgesic duration was comparable between the groups. Others found that the combination of S(+)-ketamine and ropivacaine following epidural administration increased postoperative pain relief when
compared with ropivacaine (226). Potential complementary

antinociceptive action of the two drugs used may play a role (see Chapters 40 and 43).

Neostigmine

The cholinergic system is thought to modulate pain perception and transmission by a spinal mechanism (227) (Chapter 40). Acetylcholine is one of more than 25 neurotransmitters that participate in the spinal cord's modulation of pain processing. Mainly muscarinic receptors play a part in producing analgesia. Analgesia by neostigmine is not associated with respiratory depression, but a significant incidence of nausea, vomiting, and more rarely anxiety has been noted to occur.

Epidural neostigmine 1 to 4 μg added to a local anesthetic solution produced a dose-independent analgesic effect in patients after minor orthopedic procedures (228).

Number and Frequency of Local Anesthetic Injections

Whether augmentation or diminution of neural blockade occurs after repeated epidural injection of local anesthetics depends on the local anesthetic agent, the number of injections, and the timing between injections (Fig. 11-11).

A single "repeat" dose (20% of total dose) given approximately 20 minutes after the main dose of local anesthetic has been said to consolidate blockade within the level of blockade already established. Thus, "missed segments" may be "filled in," but the level of blockade may not be extended (229).

A second dose of approximately 50% of initial dosage will maintain the initial segmental level of analgesia if given when the upper level of segmental analgesia has receded one to two dermatomes. On the other hand, administration of the same dose as given for induction of block will result in augmentation of blockade level at this time. Clinical practice relies on either mean duration times (Table 11-7) or careful monitoring for signs of regression of blockade to determine the need for a second or refill dose.

A "refill" dose given more than 10 minutes outside regression of analgesia (the "interanalgesic interval") may result in *tachyphylaxis*; that is, an *increase* in dosage is required to maintain a constant level of blockade. Tachyphylaxis increases with the length of interanalgesic interval up to 60 minutes, but then it remains constant; at 60 minutes there is a 30% to 40% decrease in effect of a repeated dose (Fig. 11-11) (230).

In addition, tachyphylaxis increases with the number of injections especially when short-acting amides—lidocaine, prilocaine, or mepivacaine—are used. It appears the tachyphylaxis can be attenuated when small amounts of local anesthetics are used as compared to high-dose regimen (Fig. 11-11). This again indicates the desirability of using long-acting agents.

TECHNIQUE OF EPIDURAL BLOCKADE

Epidural Trays

A large number of commercially prepared, disposable epidural trays are available that contain a variable number of the ideal components for epidural blockade. Individual preference plays a considerable part in choice of a tray. However, there are several desirable features to be considered.

Separation of a preparation section from the equipment section of the tray is desirable. Glass syringes for testing loss of resistance should be of highest quality, with freely moving, snug-fitting plungers. High-quality plastic "loss-of-resistance" syringes are also available. Disposable epidural needles should not have the "chisel" tip of the original Tuohy needle, since this increases the risk of dural puncture. Some disposable epidural needles are dangerously sharp (Fig. 11-12A).

Epidural needle stylets should fit the needle precisely, particularly at the needle tip. Epidural catheters should be made of clear material, so that aspirated blood can be clearly seen in the catheter. Also, catheters should be strong and flexible, should be inert, and should not have sharp tips capable of tearing blood vessels or puncturing dura. They should also be marked for roentgenographic detection.

Local anesthetics to be used in disposable trays should be packed in sterile protective coverings on the tray or in individual sterile containers. Single-use vials are available with a "top hat"–shaped cap that can easily be grasped and pulled off without contaminating the solution with particles of glass or rubber, as may occur with ampules and some types of vials.

Mixing cups should be free of any particulate matter. Unfortunately, many disposable trays fall short of these ideals.

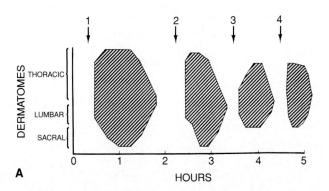

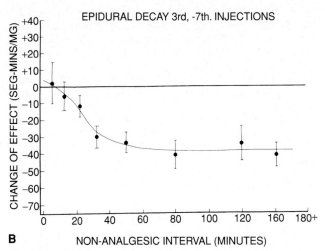

EPIDURAL DECAY 3rd, -7th. INJECTIONS

FIGURE 11-11. Tachyphylaxis. **A:** Diminished segmental spread and duration of action of repeated epidural injections of the same dose of local anesthetic, injected at each arrow. Note reinjection has been made at least 30 minutes after analgesia has regressed two segments. **B:** "Nonanalgesic interval." As the time lag from loss of analgesia to reinjection exceeds 10 to 15 minutes, a progressive reduction in analgesic effect occurs that reaches a maximum reduction of about 35% to 40% at 60 minutes. From Bromage PR, Pettigrew RT, Crowell DE. Tachyphylaxis in epidural analgesia: I. Augmentation and decay of local anesthesia. *J Clin Pharmacol* 1969;9:30, with permission.

PART II: TECHNIQUES

However, sterility is guaranteed by the manufacturer, and needles and syringes should be free of imperfections.

Many anesthesiologists still prefer department-prepared trays, which contain all items decided on by that particular group. This works well in a practice in which all can agree on a standard tray, and a dedicated and skilled staff prepare the trays to ensure sterility and exclusion of chemical materials that may be neurolytic. In smaller hospitals that use epidural trays infrequently, commercial trays may be a valuable insurance against chemical and bacterial contamination. Larger units may prefer to design their own trays and use carefully maintained, reusable, high-quality needles and syringes. The following pitfalls should be avoided.

Syringe barrels and plungers should be kept together, since "odds" may not fit with the precision required for loss-of-resistance testing. Powder or other material on syringe plungers may result in sticking, which can be dangerous if entry into the epidural space is missed, particularly above the level of L1; plastic epidural loss-of-resistance syringes have special plungers that prevent this problem.

Epidural needles should be skillfully machined and maintained, so that rough and sharp edges are avoided. Stylets must fit perfectly to avoid tissue damage or plugs in the end of the needle.

Epidural local anesthetics must be carefully sterilized, using a technique approved by a trained pharmacist, so that sterility, potency, and freedom from chemical contamination are ensured.

Hospital-prepared anesthetic trays should have the date of sterilization marked on the outside of the pack and a sterilization indicator included inside the pack.

Epidural Needles

As for spinal analgesia, a close-fitting removable stylet is essential for epidural anesthesia, to prevent plugging of the needle tip with skin and failure to recognize loss of resistance. The possibility of a large epidermal plug being carried into the epidural or subarachnoid space must also be avoided. The epidural space can also be identified by compression of a 10- to 20 mL air-filled syringe attached to a 22-gauge Greene or Whitacre spinal needle; this is a useful teaching aid while performing lumbar puncture and may also be an alternative technique for single-shot epidural block. The standard Tuohy needle has a gentle curve of the Huber tip, but with a rather sharp point at the end, and this is favored by some experienced epiduralists. For the novice, a rounded blunt needle end to the Huber tip is less likely to puncture the dura (231) (Fig. 11-12A). This type of needle end also permits easier identification of the ligamentum flavum, sometimes requiring considerable force to penetrate the ligament. Some authorities like to teach with a 16-gauge needle and then let the novice graduate to an 18-gauge needle.

A useful refinement is the Scott needle, which has the shaft protruding from the hub (110). This permits easier threading and advancement of epidural catheters, particularly with 18-gauge catheters, which sometimes kink and curl within the standard hub. Calibrated needles with centimeter markings also are available (232,233).

The 18-gauge Crawford thin-walled needle is often used for the paramedian, "paraspinous" (Fig. 11-12B) approach, since a catheter threads directly up the epidural space if the needle is angled at 45 to 60 degrees upward. With a Tuohy needle, the catheter is sometimes difficult to thread using this approach, since the recurved needle tip is angled back against the ligamentum flavum or lamina. However, the Crawford needle with its

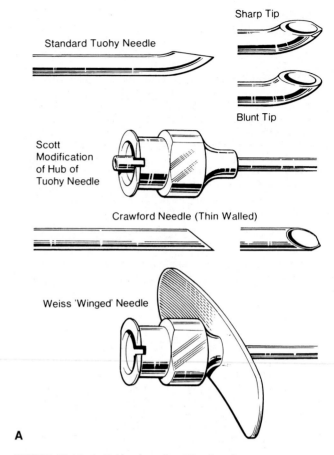

FIGURE 11-12. A: Epidural needles. (*Continued*)

front-end orifice is more likely to penetrate the tissues, rather like an apple corer, and to become plugged with tissue fragments than is the Tuohy needle with its recurved orifice. Other needles, such as the large Cheng (234) and Crawley needles (235) and the fine 22-gauge Wagner needle, are less commonly used, since they have little advantage over standard needles.

Winged needles are ideal for "hanging-drop" (Gutierrez) techniques, since the grip on the needle should be well away from the fluid drop on the hub of the needle. Many variants of the original Labat winged needle are available, and detachable wings made of plastic have also been designed (236) for use with standard Tuohy needles. Some anesthesiologists prefer more versatile and more solid spool-type needles with a Barker style of hub (e.g., the Bromage needle).

Epidural Catheters

Plastic epidural catheters have replaced those made of other materials. Various plastic materials are used, and no systematic study has been made of the requirements for epidural catheters and the features of different plastic materials. Only sporadic information is available. For example, some Teflon catheters were found to kink, and this led to breakages in the wall. Bromage has summarized ideal characteristics: biochemical inertness, low coefficient of friction, high tensile strength, maneuverable rigidity, kink resistance, atraumatic tip, depth indicators, and radiopacity. A stylet is not recommended, since it increases the risk of trauma to blood vessels, nerve roots, and so on. One

LUMBAR EPIDURAL

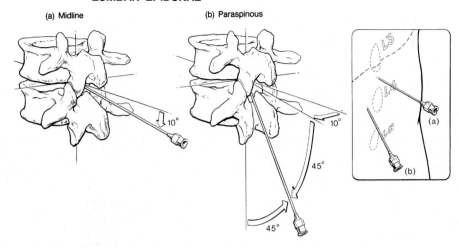

(a) Midline   (b) Paraspinous

THORACIC EPIDURAL

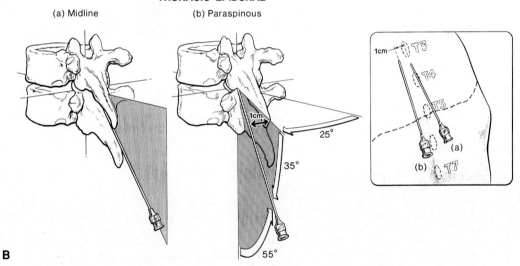

(a) Midline   (b) Paraspinous

B

FIGURE 11-12. (*Continued*) **B:** Epidural block: Sites of needle insertion. **Upper panel:** Lumbar epidural: (*a*) midline; note insertion closer to the superior spinous process and with a slight upward angulation; (*b*) paraspinous (paramedian). Note insertion beside caudad edge of "inferior" spinous process, with 45-degree angulation to long axis of spine below. **Lower panel:** Thoracic epidural: (*a*) midline; note extreme upward angulation required in midthoracic region, therefore, a paraspinous approach may be easier; (*b*) paraspinous. Note needle insertion next to caudad tip of the spinous process above interspace of intended level of entry through ligamentum flavum. Upward angulation is 55 degrees to long axis of spine below, and inward angulation is 10 to 15 degrees.

catheter (the Racz catheter) has a stainless steel coil at the tip that makes the tip flexible.

Epidural Cannulas

In an attempt to overcome the risk of pulling a catheter back through a Tuohy needle and shearing it off, epidural "cannula-over-needle" equipment was developed, analogous to intravascular equipment. This includes the Winnie-Jelco cannula, the Henkin-Bard cannula, and others (87). They all suffer from the need to connect the cannula to a catheter after it is advanced over the straight epidural needle. In our view, this equipment is not an advantage over standard equipment.

Epidural equipment should be simple (Table 11-8). A steady pair of hands with a highly trained feel for loss of resistance, a

freely running glass syringe, and a high-quality epidural needle are far superior to the multitude of mechanical devices offered as aids to identify the epidural space (237).

Some practitioners prefer to have sterilized vials of local anesthetic on the tray and to draw them up into 10-mL glass or plastic syringes, rather than using a mixing container and exposing the solution to possible contamination. Although Millipore filters have not been conclusively shown to reduce the incidence of epidural infection, they may have other advantages. Particulate matter has been reported from mixing containers and "snap-neck" glass ampules (238). The Millipore filter offers some protection against this material reaching the epidural space. (See Chapter 8 for general information regarding equipment for neural blockade and preparation of the patient.)

REQUIRED EQUIPMENT FOR EPIDURAL BLOCKADE

A satisfactory preparation section of tray (sterilizing fluid cup, swabs, swab holder, sterile towels)
1 × 2.5 cm, 25-gauge needle for skin analgesia
1 × 4 cm, 22-gauge needle for deep infiltration
1 × 18 gauge needle for drawing up epidural solutions and then piercing skin[a] before inserting the epidural needle
Epidural needle (Tuohy, Crawford)
Epidural catheter
1 × 2 mL, plastic syringe for infiltration, syringe mount
2 × 10 mL, all-glass syringes for loss of resistance tests[b] and drawing up local anesthetic
Local anesthetic mixing cup
Normal saline
Local anesthetics
Filters and caps for epidural catheter
Sterility indicator

[a]Alternatively a small scalpel blade is used.
[b]Excellent plastic "testing syringes" are available.

Combined Spinal-Epidural Anesthesia

A combined spinal-epidural technique (CSE) can be used to reduce or eliminate some of the disadvantages of spinal and epidural anesthesia while preserving advantages of both. Spinal anesthesia offers rapid onset of action, reliable surgical anesthesia, and full muscle relaxation. On the other hand, an indwelling epidural catheter offers the advantage of adding local anesthetic top-up doses to extend the duration of the block, improve inadequate spinal block, and provide postoperative pain relief. This sequential technique has been shown to be particularly useful in patients undergoing cesarean section and major hip and knee surgery (239). Controlled studies comparing a regular or epidural block with sequential CSE block for cesarean section showed that CSE technique proved to be as safe and effective as spinal and epidural anesthesia for cesarean section (312). Initially, an epidural needle was introduced at one lumbar interspace followed by a subarachnoid puncture at another interspace (240). Brownridge (241) advocated this double-interspace technique for cesarean section (see Chapter 24).

The most commonly used technique is the single-interspace spinal needle through the epidural needle method, as first described by Coates in 1982 (Fig. 11-13A) (242). A 16- or 18-gauge Tuohy needle is used to identify the epidural space, after which a long spinal needle is inserted through it to perforate the dura mater. Correct placement of the spinal needle in the subarachnoid space is confirmed by aspiration of CSF. After the subarachnoid injection of a local anesthetic solution, the spinal needle is removed, and the epidural catheter is introduced into the epidural space in the usual manner.

Specially designed needle sets for CSE have been produced. For example, a modified Tuohy needle with a hole (back eye) in its curve has been manufactured, so that the spinal needle passes through the back eye directly into the subarachnoid space, instead of exiting from the end of the Tuohy needle (Fig. 11-13B). This back eye is only of importance in those Tuohy needles with a long distal curve, and it has been developed to eliminate the need to thread the spinal needle through the distal opening of the Tuohy needle with all the supposed disadvan-

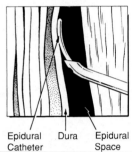

FIGURE 11-13. A: Combined spinal and epidural needle, showing a needle-through-needle technique. **B:** Tuohy needle with back eye. *Left panel* shows subarachnoid needle protruding through back eye of Tuohy needle into subarachnoid space, while the Tuohy needle remains in the epidural space. *Right panel* shows an epidural catheter subsequently threaded into the epidural space for continuous epidural analgesia.

tages. Very recently, Joshi et al. (1994) evaluated the CSE technique using the standard 16-gauge Tuohy needle or the modified Tuohy needle with the back eye (243). It was concluded that an improved needle set for the "needle-through-needle" technique would be one with a modified Tuohy needle having the back eye and a spinal needle protruding more than 13 mm beyond the Tuohy needle.

Concerns regarding the CSE technique include an accidental passage of the epidural catheter through the hole in the dura mater, the possibility of extensive subarachnoid effects from epidurally injected local anesthetics by passage through the hole in the dura, and failure to thread the epidural catheter after the intrathecal injection has been given. Routine precautions to avoid intravascular or intrathecal injection should be carried out, including aspiration and test dose administration. Spinal-epidural needle-through-needle technique may cause metallic fragments by friction between the spinal needle and the epidural bent-tip inner surface (244). Theoretically, the particles produced by the friction between the two needles can be pushed forward by the force extended into the epidural space. It is clear that this technique requires technical skills and therefore should be performed only by substantially experienced anesthesiologists.

Patient Evaluation and Preparation

As in any preanesthetic evaluation, certain essential information should be obtained. Its implications must be considered before epidural blockade is selected as part of the anesthetic

TABLE 11-9

CHECKLIST: A SAFETY PROCEDURE BEFORE SPINAL EPIDURAL BLOCKADE

Patient evaluation
Psychological suitability
Physical suitability with emphasis on the following:
Obesity and/or bony spine abnormalities
Pre-existing neurologic disease
Cardiorespiratory function (e.g., ability to withstand
sympathetic blockade)
Blood volume
Drug factors:
Anticoagulants, aspirin, and other antiplatelet drugs,
sensitivity to local anesthetics, antihypertensive agents,
monoamine oxidase inhibitors (and other drugs
interferring with sympathetic function)
History of previous anesthetic and other drug administration
Family history of adverse drug effects

Patient preparation
Explanation of blockade procedure and its benefits
(intraoperative and postoperative)
Inquiry as to patient's desire for sedation or full
unconsciousness
Baseline information
Spine imaging for undefined pathology, blood sugar level
for diabetics
Correction of reversible abnormalities (e.g., dehydration)
Informed consent is obtained.
Record history and management plan in notes
Order
Changes (if any) in current medication
Premedication

Preoperative discussion
Operative details with surgeon to determine the following:
Level of blockade required
Appropriate supplementation
Necessity for intubation
Management plan with surgical staff: equipment and drug
requirements
Timing for patient transport to operating room
Assistance from nursing staff

regimen. If epidural block seems appropriate, the necessary preoperative steps should be taken: The minimum entails adequate psychological preparation, adequate baseline data (e.g., blood sugar levels in a patient with diabetes), and correction of reversible abnormalities, such as dehydration (Table 11-9). Informed consent is obtained.

Preoperative Discussion with Medical Staff

A discussion with the medical staff should not be omitted just because the choice of anesthesia is considered the province of the anesthesiologist. Consultation with the surgeon is necessary to help determine the precise nature of operative approach and therefore the level of blockade required, the need for sup-

plementation, and the necessity for intubation if exploration will markedly impinge on upper abdominal areas. Preoperative communication with nursing staff can be accomplished by a telephone call, to inform them beforehand of requirements for special equipment, timing of transportation of the patient to the operating room, and the need for assistance during positioning of the patient for a block (Table 11-9).

Planning for Technique of Block and Drug Dose

Choice of patient position for puncture follows the same principles outlined in Chapter 10; although the effect of gravity may be debatable, reliability of blockade of S1 is probably increased with the patient in the sitting position.

The key anatomy for safe placement of a needle in the epidural space is summarized in Tables 11-10–11-12.

Also, it is easier to enter the epidural space in obese patients if the sitting position is used. On the other hand, patients who have a history of fainting or who are heavily premedicated should have their block induced while in the lateral position. Site of puncture is usually at L2–L3 or L3–L4, unless the anesthesiologist is an experienced epiduralist; puncture at L5–S1 aids in ensuring blockade of the resistant S1 segment for ankle or knee surgery. At higher levels, experienced epiduralists may choose an interspace close to the center of the dermatomal segments required (245). However, the degree of difficulty of needle insertion should also be considered. Thus, one may choose T9–T10 for a thoracic operation, even though the more difficult T5–T6 level may be closer to the center of the required dermatomes. Similarly, C7–T1 level may be chosen for an upper thoracic procedure rather than the more difficult T3–T4 level. We believe that the midline approach should be learned thoroughly before using the paraspinous (lateral) approach, since the chance of needle entry into the lateral aspects of the ligamentum flavum may be greater if inexperienced attempts are made to "angle" the needle toward the midline. However, careful use of the spinous process to guide the needle for a paraspinous approach to a midline entry through the ligamentum flavum can be extremely reliable and easy in the hands of an experienced epiduralist (Table 11-11), and this feature is helpful in the midthoracic region (Table 11-10). In the cervical region, midline puncture becomes more reliable again, and it is best to choose the C7–T1 level, since the epidural space is wider than at higher cervical levels, and access between the spinous processes is easy if the neck if flexed (Table 11-10).

The *technique chosen for identification of epidural space* depends largely on personal preference and familiarity with technique (246). We prefer the loss-of-resistance technique, using an air-filled syringe at all levels, provided the firm "Bromage" grip is used (87). Certainly, the two-handed grip of the hanging-drop (Gutierrez) technique ensures excellent control; however, the slight risk that there may be a plug in the needle tip and the occurrence of low or no negative pressure tends to outweigh the benefits of the hanging-drop technique. We prefer to use the midline approach (Fig. 11-12) with an air-filled syringe (Figs. 11-14 and 11-15) at lumbar, low-thoracic, and C7–T1 levels, unless midline entry proves difficult; then a paraspinous approach is used. In the midthoracic region, the paramedian, paraspinous (lateral) approach (Fig. 11-12) is routinely used with an air-filled syringe.

A case for avoiding air-filled syringes could be made in patients presenting for ablation of renal stones by extracorporeal shock wave lithotripsy (247). The focused shock waves set up

TABLE 11-10A

KEY ANATOMIC FEATURES FOR ADMINISTRATION OF LUMBAR EPIDURAL ANESTHESIA

Spine and ligaments	Relationships of epidural space

Spinous process
    Widest in midlumbar region
    Only slight downward angulation
    Inferior border opposite widest point of interlaminar space
    Superior border over upward-sloping lamina
    Narrower superiorly. Needle Inserted beside spinous process guided into midline by lateral aspect of spinous process
Interspinous ligament
    Well defined above L4. Below L4 narrower and loose—may offer less resistance
Lamina
    Posterior surface slopes down and back
    Needle may strike lamina superficially at inferior aspect of slope or deep at superior aspect of slope
Interlaminar space
    Increased by flexing lumbar spine
    Larger "target" area in midline and in midlumbar region
    Smaller target laterally
Articular facets
    Needle directed past lateral aspect of interlaminar space may impinge on articular facets, causing severe radiating pain and muscle spasm
Ligamentum flavum
    Thickest in midlumbar region in midline
    Attached to anteroinferior aspects of lamina above and posterosuperior aspects of lamina below; thus, needle entering at inferior aspect may be held up by lamina
	Epidural space
	    Widest in midlumbar region in midline (5–6 mm), narrower next to articular processes where ligamentum flavum and dura almost touch
	    Widens laterally where spinal nerve surrounded by dural cuff
	    Communicates with paravertebral space by way of intervertebral foramen therefore, epidural catheter may stimulate spinal nerve—unisegmental paresthesia
	Spinal nerve
	    Needle inserted past depth of lamina with lateral angulation on same side may penetrate past spinous process to spinal nerve
	    Needle angled across midline to *opposite side* may run in substance of ligamentum flavum laterally to reach spinal nerve and/or dural cuff
	Arterial supply of spinal cord (see Chapter 9)
	    Only one anterior spinal artery
	    In thoracolumbar region fed mainly by "radicularis magna," which usually enters by way of an intervertebral foramen on left side at T11–T12 (may be at other interspaces T8–L3)
	    Supply to anterior thoracolumbar cord is discontinuous with higher levels
	    Sharp demarcation between anterior and posterior spinal artery territory
	Epidural veins
	    Prominent in lateral portion of epidural space
	    Drain to azygos vein and connect to pelvic veins, providing an alternative route from pelvis to right heart. Therefore, they become distended when inferior vena cava is obstructed
	    Also connect to cerebral venous sinuses by way of basivertebral veins

TABLE 11-10B

KEY ANATOMIC FEATURES FOR ADMINISTRATION OF MIDTHORACIC EPIDURAL ANESTHESIA

Spinous process
    Extreme downward slope, inferior border opposite midpoint of lamina below
    Small posterior surface, processes close together and difficult to identify
    Therefore, the paraspinous (paramedian) technique is easier (see Fig. 11-12B)
Interspinous ligament
    Difficult to identify because spinous processes close to one another
Lamina
    Broader than lumbar laminae, but shorter in vertical dimension
    Large area available for location of depth of ligamentum flavum with less fear of accidental puncture of dura
Ligamentum flavum
    Thick but less so than midlumbar
Epidural space
    In midline 3–5 mm, narrow laterally

TABLE 11-10C

KEY ANATOMIC FEATURES FOR ADMINISTRATION OF CERVICOTHORACIC EPIDURAL ANESTHESIA

Spinous process
    At C7 (vertebra prominens) and T1, direction is almost horizontal
    Inferior border C7 opposite widest point of C7–T1 interlaminar space
Lamina
    Shaped like narrow rectangle
Interlaminar space
    Accessible with midline puncture if neck flexed
Ligamentum flavum
    Thinner than at any other level
Epidural space
    Width at first thoracic interspace is 3 to 4 mm (note width at C3–C6 is 2 mm)
    Increased width if neck flexed
    Usually marked negative pressure (increased if sitting)

TABLE 11-11

STRUCTURES ENCOUNTERED DURING EPIDURAL BLOCK*

Structure	Comment
With Correct Procedure (Midline Technique)	
Skin	Prior puncture with 19-gauge needle should ensure no "drag" on epidural needle
Supraspinous ligament	Needle sits *firmly* in midline
Interspinous ligament	Clear-cut resistance to syringe plunger (above L4)
	? Poorly defined resistance (below L4, or sometimes at other levels, ? choose another interspace)
Ligamentum flavum	Increase in resistance to syringe plunger, with marked "elastic" quality
	Increased resistance to advancing needle
Epidural space	*Controlled* and well-defined loss of resistance
	No resistance to injected solution
	No, or minimal, "drip back" of injected solution
	Catheter passes easily
Incorrect Procedure or Unintentional Misplacement of Needle	
Skin	Lack of prior puncture causes marked "drag" on epidural needle
Supraspinous ligament	Entered to one side, causes needle to angle laterally
	Missed completely, causes needle to flop to one side and appear to have no support
Interspinous ligament	Entered obliquely, results in transient resistance, then loss of resistance, which is interpreted as entrance to epidural space; however, there is marked run back of injected solution, and catheter will not thread
	Missed completely, results in low resistance—needle in paravertebral muscles
Spinous process	Very superficial contact: interspace not marked ?; spine flexed?
	Deep contact: needle angled much too acutely?
Lamina	Posterior end of slope: superficial obstruction to needle advancement
	Anterior end of slope: deep obstruction
Articular processes	Sudden pain in back
	Muscle spasm on one side of back
Ligamentum flavum (LF)	
LF pierced midline but with poor control of entry	Needle "overshoots" through epidural space and punctures dura (see Table 11-12)
LF pierced to side of midline where dura close and veins prominent	Dural puncture ± CSF flow; or cannulation of epidural vein, +/− bleeding
Failure to identify LF with subsequent entry into subdural space	No CSF aspirated
	Some resistance to injected solution and "drip back," which is local anesthetic
	Catheter passes with difficulty
	Small dose of local anesthetic results in widespread block with bizarre distribution
Needle enters lateral aspect from opposite side and continues within ligament to region of spinal nerve	Continued "elastic resistance" for several millimeters and then sudden unisegmental paresthesia
	May be followed by CSF flow if dural cuff entered
Epidural space	
Entry uncontrolled, needle against dura, no solution injected to expand epidural space	Catheter threads with difficulty or sudden loss of resistance—CSF in catheter
Entry to side of midline into epidural vein or CSF	Blood or CSF via needle or bleeding as catheter threaded—clot in catheter unless flushed with saline
Entry at extreme inferior aspect of ligamentum flavum at attachment to lamina of lower vertebra	Loss of resistance to syringe plunger but needle progress halted by upper edge of lamina and catheter will not thread
Entry at extreme superior aspect with only tip of needle piercing ligament	Loss of resistance to syringe plunger but some resistance to injected solution and catheter will not thread
	Further progress of needle easy
Entry at lateral aspect	Catheter may impinge on spinal nerve

CSF, cerebrospinal fluid.
*See Figures in Chapter 9.

TABLE 11-12

SUSPECTED DURAL PUNCTURE

Sign	Cause	Management
Second loss of resistance and fluid flows from needle	Dural puncture	Convert to spinal anesthetic or move to higher interspace for epidural
Second loss of resistance after identifying ligamentum flavum and no fluid flows from needle, but injected solution → some "drip back"	? Entry into subdural space ? Dural puncture	Test "drip back" on arm: Cold = L.A.; warm = CSF Drip into container[a] With glucose test tape: CSF → color change If drip back only L.A. withdraw needle and reidentify epidural space If drip back = CSF ± L.A., move to a rostrad[b] interspace or convert to spinal anesthetic
One loss of resistance only; however, "drip back" at: A shallow level	Interspinous ligament pierced and needle in paravertebral muscle	Reinsert needle in midline
A deeper level	Low compliance of epidural fat Needle only partially through ligamentum flavum Needle in CSF	Test as above, if drip back only L.A.: Attempt to pass catheter → easy passage Attempt to pass catheter → does not pass Superiorly needle can be advanced and then catheter threaded Inferiorly needle will not advance Test for CSF, if positive move to rostrad interspace or convert to spinal

[a]Few drops of CSF in thiopental will form a precipitate; however local anesthetic will also form a precipitate with thiopental.[255] Positive identification of CSF can be made by measuring a special protein, beta-transferrin, only present in CSF. This is *not* an acute test since it will take 48 hrs to obtain a result but may be valuable if a chronic epidural or intrathecal catheter has been placed and definitive diagnosis of ongoing CSF leak is important.
[b]Do not attempt to withdraw needle into epidural space at the same level, as this may result in subdural cannulation.[265]
L.A. local anesthetic; CSF, cerebrospinal fluid.

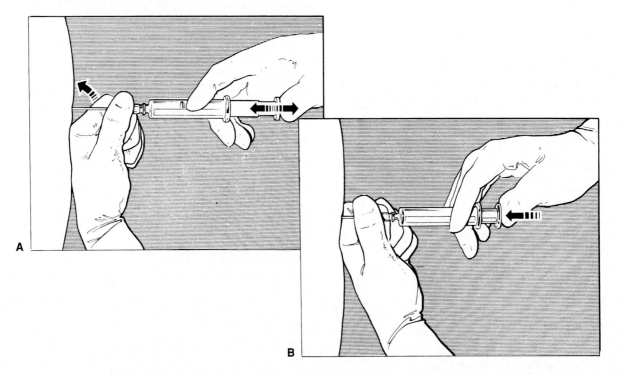

FIGURE 11-14. "Bromage" grip for loss-of-resistance technique. **A:** Note the vise-like grip of needle between thumb and entire fist. Metacarpal heads are braced against the back. The needle is advanced by rotation of the entire hand around the metacarpal heads; only a small, highly controlled movement is possible without repositioning the hand on the needle. Continual compression of syringe plunger is present, with a "bouncing" movement. **B:** As soon as the ligamentum flavum is pierced, resistance to syringe plunger is lost, and the needle is immediately halted. (This sequence is seen from above.)

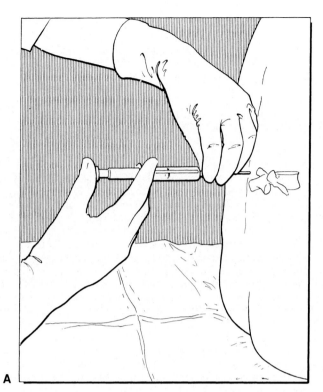
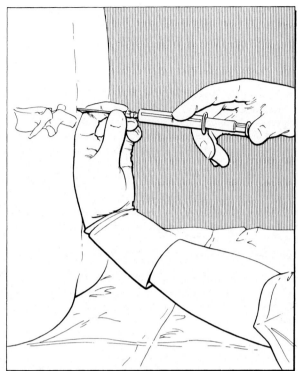

FIGURE 11-15. Alternative, less-controlled grips. **A:** Hand gripping needle from above. **B:** Hand gripping needle from below. Note that in both **A** and **B**, the hand holding the needle is braced against the patient's back at all times, and the needle is advanced by forward movement of the forefinger and thumb. **B:** It may be helpful to leave the infiltration needle in situ and to use this as a guide to the location of the spinous process when the epidural needle is inserted by means of a separate "track."

turbulence and tissue damage at air–water or air–tissue interfaces, and so epidural or paravertebral bubbles of air might conceivably predispose to local neural damage if traversed by the shock beam. Thus, theoretic grounds exist for using saline-filled syringes for loss of resistance in such cases (247). The chances of problems arising from epidural bubbles would seem to be extremely remote if puncture is made in the thoracic region and above the path of the shock beam.

It is desirable when puncture is made above the L2 level to routinely infiltrate down beside the spinous process and check the depth of the lamina as a guide to the depth of the interlaminar space. This avoids the danger of continuing to advance a needle with a plug in the end. Experience with the use of the Bromage grip develops a keen sense of resistance in the hand advancing the needle and the hand compressing the syringe plunger. Unfortunately, the hanging-drop is not under the anesthesiologist's control; it may impart a visual sign only on entry into the epidural space without premonitory sign of increased plunger resistance, which becomes highly developed during routine use of lumbar epidural block. Nevertheless, many anesthesiologists find that the two-handed grip of the hanging-drop technique gives them greater control. If this technique is used, the stylet must not be withdrawn until the needle is close to the ligamentum flavum. It should be reinserted if the needle contacts periosteum and requires repositioning. Also, it is preferable to advance the needle only during inspiration, so that negative pressure in the epidural space is maximal.

Incorrect procedure (Tables 11-11 and 11-12), or sometimes inadvertent aberrant needle placement owing to anatomic difficulties, may result in quite a different sequence of events than that described earlier and contact with different anatomic structures.

The *choice of single-shot or catheter technique* depends on the patient and the type of operation. Catheter techniques are useful in debilitated and aged patients, since level of blockade can be gradually extended to the required level; this is also a wise approach in operative obstetrics. Prolonged surgery requires catheter techniques. Healthy patients undergoing brief procedures can be adequately managed with a single shot via the needle, even if it is planned to thread a catheter for "insurance." In this situation, we prefer to inject the dose by way of the needle, since catheters may malfunction owing to transforaminal escape or superficial placement (248), "curling up (249)," or sometimes passage into the anterior epidural space. Threading catheters only 3 to 4 cm into the epidural space reduces, but does not eliminate, malfunction (250).

Dosage calculation and choice of agent depend on the factors discussed earlier. Single-shot techniques depend on a generous calculation of dose requirements, so that catheter techniques are preferable if it is essential to restrict dose and level of blockade. Needle insertion under general anesthesia is certainly more comfortable for the patient. However, comfort is bought at the price of safety, since valuable signs of contact with neural tissue and of intravascular or subarachnoid injection may be lost, so that considerable experience or supervision by an experienced epiduralist is required.

Conduct of Epidural Blockade

Epidural neural blockade should be viewed as part of a complete anesthetic procedure, which includes preparative steps, continuous surveillance, and appropriate responses (e.g., supplementation if indicated). It should be stressed that technical expertise in inserting an epidural needle is insufficient, by itself, to safely manage epidural block. Reports of anesthetic mortality committees (251) have drawn attention to:

- Deficiencies in knowledge of physiology and pharmacology of epidural blockade and treatment of altered physiology and of pharmacologic side effects
- Inadequate preparation (e.g., failure to restore blood volume)
- Inadequate monitoring before, during, and after surgery
- Inadequate supplementation and general management (e.g., failure to use artificial ventilation in situations where it is required)
- Slowness and inappropriate responses to sudden changes in physiology
- Lack of appropriate resuscitative skills

All of these issues have parallels in the safe administration of *general* anesthesia. Somehow, some individuals attempting to use epidural block have failed to realize that the same level of knowledge, surveillance, and technical skill is required for epidural block and its management.

Once the patient arrives in the operating room, all equipment and drugs should be ready, and activity should then concentrate on aspects relating directly to the patient. For example, adequacy of sedation before needle insertion should be assessed. Any recent untoward events, such as severe angina during the night, should be elicited. The medical record should be checked. In particular, drug therapy should be scrutinized to determine whether prescribed drugs (e.g., insulin) have been given and undesired drugs (e.g., heparin) have been discontinued. The steps of the procedure should be reassuringly outlined for the patient, and any changes in patient requirements determined (e.g., a desire to be completely asleep rather than lightly sedated).

Although there are many approaches to *locating the desired interspace*, we prefer to make an indentation with the thumb nail in the chosen interspace, leave a mark at the level of the anterior superior iliac crest with the skin preparation solution, and then finally palpate the rib margin as a guide to location of L1. Using this approach, the landmarks can be identified immediately before needle insertion. In contrast, marking with a skin pen is carried out before skin preparation, and the patient may move in the interim. Baseline blood pressure and heart rate should always be recorded on the anesthetic record before blockade.

Skin preparation and preparation of the neural block tray should require two separate steps. Also, it should be stressed that the neural block tray must be kept separate from all other drugs, since human error may result in injection of inappropriate agents into the epidural space with potentially disastrous sequelae (252). It is preferable to complete the skin preparation before uncovering the epidural needles and drugs. In any event, splashing of preparatory solutions on neural block equipment must be avoided.

Except for skin infiltration, complete preparation of neural block equipment should take place before the block is begun. The remaining steps are completed while skin analgesia ensues. It should be noted that the local anesthetic to be used for epidural block is drawn up and ready to inject and the catheter (if used) has been checked and is ready to thread. Care should be taken that glove powder or other material does not soil the barrel of the loss-of-resistance syringe, since this may result in dangerous sticking of the barrel.

Midline Technique

The essential anatomy of needle insertion in the midline is described in detail in Chapter 9 (see also Figs. 11-14 and 11-15). The anesthesiologist should constantly think of the structures the needle encounters. If the Bromage grip shown in Figure 11-14 is used, it is possible to readily identify changes in resistance, transmitted by the hand holding the needle and the syringe plunger, as the needle enters supraspinous ligament, interspinous ligament, and ligamentum flavum. Constant pressure on the syringe plunger permits immediate recognition of loss of resistance as the needle tip enters the epidural space, and the vice-like grip on the needle permits immediate halting of needle progress. Gentle aspiration or, preferably, mere disconnection of the syringe is carried out to check for flow of CSF or blood. If neither is present, 4 mL of solution is immediately injected to push the dura away from the needle tip. Two points require emphasis: The injected solution should meet no resistance, and the hand holding the needle must remain braced against the patient's back; otherwise, the needle may be advanced as the solution is injected. The syringe is disconnected again and any drip back is tested as in Table 11-15 while the patient is questioned about warmth and numbness in lower limbs; a subarachnoid injection results in almost immediate onset of blockade of β-fibers (Chapter 2, Table 2-1). If no evidence of onset of a subarachnoid block is present, one may proceed to inject the calculated epidural dose as follows:

Single-shot Techniques. After gentle aspiration, a *test dose* of 5 mL (preferably epinephrine-containing) local anesthetic solution is injected at 10 mL/min. The syringe is disconnected, and any drip back is tested (Table 11-12). The patient is observed for increased heart rate owing to intravascular injection of epinephrine and is questioned about sudden onset of warmth or numbness in the legs. If the response to these is negative, further 5-mL increments are injected until the full dose has been given. It should be noted that a negative response to a test dose does not provide absolute proof of correct placement.

Catheter Techniques. The catheter is inserted 3 to 4 cm while the hand holding the needle is braced against the patient's back to ensure that the needle does not move. After removal of the needle and careful aspiration, a 5-mL test dose (see previous section) is then injected through the catheter. After 5 to 10 minutes, the level of blockade, heart rate, and blood pressure are checked; if satisfactory, a careful aspiration test is carried out, and the remainder of the dose is injected. Alternatively, the remainder of the dose can be injected slowly in 5-mL increments. Needle or catheter insertion should be halted if undue force is required or if paresthesias or muscle twitches are elicited. If blood flows freely from an epidural needle, it may be necessary to move to an adjacent interspace and ensure that the subsequent entry through the ligamentum flavum is in the midline. If clear solution drips back or is aspirated from needle or catheter, the steps outlined in Table 11-12 must be taken to determine whether the fluid is local anesthetic or CSF (253,254).

A few drops of CSF in thiopental will form a precipitate; however, local anesthetic will also form a precipitate with pentothal (255). Aspiration of blood from the epidural catheter may be overcome by withdrawing the catheter (*provided the catheter is not still in the epidural needle*) or by injecting some saline. The catheter must not be left with blood in it, since it may rapidly become occluded. If blood aspiration does not cease, the catheter should be reinserted at another level. Two further indications to reposition needles or catheters are important: If resistance is poorly defined at any level, it is helpful to either try another interspace or choose the paraspinous (lateral) approach, which permits checking laminar depth through use of an exploring needle; if onset of analgesia is excessively prolonged, it is likely that injection has not been made into the epidural space.

Paraspinous Techniques (Paramedian)

Paraspinous, paramedian (lateral) insertion is a useful alternative technique. The term *paraspinous* is favored for the following reasons:

- The needle should be inserted close to the spinous process because in both lumbar and thoracic regions, the spinous process narrows superiorly and thus guides the needle to a midline entry through the ligamentum flavum.
- Extreme lateral angulation of the needle should be avoided, since it may result in oblique penetration of the ligamentum flavum and vascular or neural damage. In most instances, the needle need not be angulated—because merely follows the spinous process, "paraspinous" describes the essence of the technique.

Techniques with extreme angulation of the needle should be disregarded in favor of the safer paraspinous approach (Fig. 11-12B).

In the lumbar region, infiltration is made 1 cm lateral to the caudad tip of the inferior spinous process of the chosen interspace. A 9- to 10-cm, 22-gauge spinal needle is then used to infiltrate perpendicular to the skin beside the spinous process; this permits the depth of the lamina to be determined before the epidural needle is inserted. It is worth noting that the epidural space can be identified, for single-shot techniques, if an air-filled syringe is attached to the 22-gauge needle and constant pressure is applied to the plunger. However, in most patients, an 18-gauge epidural needle is next inserted beside the spinous process and angled upward at 45 degrees to the skin (Fig. 11-12B); often, the spinous process carries the needle slightly inward 10 to 15 degrees to the sagittal plane. This may not always be so, and the needle may pass directly to the ligamentum flavum without any necessity for inward angulation. With this technique, resistance to the advancing needle and syringe plunger is encountered only when the needle tip enters the ligamentum flavum. Thus, careful location of the depth of ligamentum flavum is essential; from this point, the technique is identical to that at the midline.

In the thoracic region, skin infiltration is made 1 cm lateral to the caudad tip of the spinous process, *cephalad to* the intended level of needle insertion (Fig. 11-12B). Infiltration down to the level of the lamina is carried out as described earlier. The epidural needle is inserted beside the spinous process and 55 to 60 degrees to the skin (sagittal plane); this angulation should permit the needle to reach ligamentum flavum *caudad to* the chosen spinous process (Fig. 11-12B). For both thoracic and lumbar paraspinous approaches, the Crawford 18-gauge thin-wall needle is an option for single-shot and catheter techniques. The angulation of the needle may permit easier threading of a catheter if a straight-tip Crawford needle is used rather than the Huber tip of the Tuohy needle.

Technique for Obese Subjects and Those with Impalpable Spinous Processes

If preoperative evaluation determines that the patient is obese or of a very "squat" stature, or if bony landmarks are impalpable for other reasons, additional maneuvers may be required. In this situation it may be helpful to plan to carry out the epidural block with the patient in the sitting position, since landmarks may be more readily palpable and epidural puncture is often easier than in the lateral position.

At the time of epidural block, absence of bony landmarks need not cause dismay, since they can be identified during gentle infiltration with local anesthetic. A 5-cm, 22-gauge needle is used to infiltrate the deeper tissues in the region where the spinous processes are judged to lie. The needle is used to probe gently for the underlying spine (87). Each time the needle touches bone, the depth is noted and the needle is systematically redirected medially or laterally until bone is located at the most superficial depth (i.e., the spinous process). At this stage, it may be necessary to infiltrate a new "track" directly toward the spinous process. The epidural needle is then inserted as for the midline technique described earlier. Alternatively, the lamina may also be located and the paramedian approach used, as already described. An additional strategy is to ask the patient to indicate whether a pin-point stimulus is to left or right or exactly midline. Many patients can be extremely accurate.

Continuing Management

Monitoring and response to altered physiology are important aspects of the conduct of epidural block. The management of sudden reactions to the injection of local anesthetic requires a sound knowledge of the differential diagnosis of local anesthetic reactions (Chapter 5, Tables 5-7–5-9) and their treatment, as well as detailed knowledge of the cardiovascular effects of epidural block (Tables 11-1–11-4). Only with constant monitoring can the appropriate responses to physiologic changes be made (Table 11-13). Atropine is often used for situations of vagal dominance (Table 11-3). Ephedrine is useful for cardiovascular support if it is desired to use bolus injections of a medium-duration drug. Ephedrine is not useful in patients with depleted norepinephrine in sympathetic nerve endings, such as some elderly and debilitated patients and those under treatment with drugs that chronically deplete norepinephrine stores. In this situation, direct-acting drugs, such as epinephrine and norepinephrine, are required (Table 11-13). Both of these drugs have a brief duration of action, and thus it is more rational to use them by IV infusion, with careful titration against response.

Vasopressin (40 U IV, once) has been recommend in place of, or in addition to, epinephrine. This appears logical in the setting of bupivacaine toxicity because epinephrine may exacerbate local anesthetic-induced arrhythmias (256,257).

The induction of 20% lipid infusion has been used in successful treatment of local anesthetic-induced cardiovascular collapse both in animals (258) and in human patients who were unresponsive to standard therapy (259–261). The exact mechanism by which lipid reverses local anesthetic toxicity is not yet known.

Surveillance also permits appropriate supplementation with sedative opioid or anesthetic agents and also appropriately timed top-up doses for the epidural block.

TABLE 11-13

CARDIOVASCULAR SUPPORT, EPIDURAL BLOCK: CARDIOACTIVE DRUGS (70-kg ADULT)

Drugs of choice	
Atropine	0.3 mg IV increments
Ephedrine	5–10 mg IV increments
Epinephrine	1 mg in 500 mL solution (2 μg/mL)
	Infuse at rate 2–4 μg/min
	Titrate against heart rate, mean arterial blood pressure, improved tissue perfusion
	At low rates of infusion mainly β-effects; at higher rates, increasing α-effects
Norepinephrine	1 mg in 500 mL solution (2 μg/mL)
	Infuse at rate 2–4 μg/min
	Titrate as above
	At <6 μg/min β- as well as α-effects, and thus perfusion (e.g., urine flow) not reduced
	2–4 μg/min usually sufficient to maintain blood pressure in presence of total sympathetic block
Other drugs	
Dopamine and dobutamine are alternatives to epinephrine; however, dopaminergic receptors are blocked by butyrophenones and phenothiazines.	
Vasopressin	40 U IV, once
Amiodarone	300 mg over 20–60 min, followed by an infusion of 900 mg in 24 h.

Maintenance of effective epidural block may entail overcoming common deficiencies in blockade and problems in the management of epidural catheters.

Problems in Epidural Blockade

Blockade Too Low at Upper Level or Inadequate Blockade at Lower Level. Approximately half the initial dose is administered 30 minutes after the first dose. However, if the initial dose was small (e.g., 4–8 mL), it may be necessary to repeat the initial dose. This is particularly so in the region of L5–S1, which is difficult to block. If not already done, it may be helpful to add opioid to the local anesthetic solution, since this will speed onset of block and will also extend the number of segments blocked; rapid-acting opioids such as fentanyl and hydromorphone may be the best choices (see Chapter 43).

Missed Segments. "Missed segments" are managed in the same way as too-low or inadequate blockade (described in the previous section), depending on the size of initial dose and size of nerve root of the missed segment(s). If a segment is missed on one side, it is worthwhile turning the patient onto that side before injection (188). Epinephrine-containing solutions are the most effective, particularly 2% lidocaine with 1:200,000 epinephrine, in dealing with missed segments or inadequate block. This is a useful practice even if another agent has been used for the initial injection. If available, 2% lidocaine–carbon dioxide is a good choice for such problems.

Inadequate Motor Block Within the Segmental Area Blocked. This requires further injection, 30 minutes after the initial dose,

of approximately half this dose, preferably as 2% lidocaine with epinephrine.

Level Too High but Inadequate Sacral Analgesia. Careful monitoring of the physiologic effects of the high block and appropriate treatment are essential. Approximately 30 to 60 minutes after the initial dose, a small dose of 8 to 10 mL may be injected by a separate single-shot caudal needle. Such a dose will reliably block sacral segments without extending the upper level of lumbar epidural block. If access to the sacral hiatus is impossible, it is preferable to wait as long as possible (approximately 60 minutes) and inject a small increment (e.g., 5–8 mL by the epidural catheter), since blockade tends to spread progressively into the sacral segments with each repeat injection. Careful monitoring is required for signs of total epidural block. Another alternative is a single-shot subarachnoid saddle block (see Chapter 10); the spinal needle can be inserted without discomfort since the lumbar segments are already blocked, also there is no need for time delay since the additional dose of local anesthetic is small.

"Visceral" Pain During Lower Abdominal Surgery. It is not commonly recognized that peritoneal stimulation during appendectomy and sometimes during a difficult herniorrhaphy may require blockade to the level of T5–T6. Thus, adequate provision should be made to block to this level or, alternatively, to top-up to this level if required. If there is a delay in onset of T5 block, IV or epidural opioid or light general anesthesia may be required.

Inability to Thread Epidural Catheter. This is often a confirmatory sign that a false loss of resistance has been encountered in a tissue space dorsal to the ligamentum flavum and that the needle has been halted superficial to the ligamentum flavum. Clearly, injection of local anesthetic at this point will be ineffectual. The most prudent course is to withdraw the needle and catheter together, after noting the depth of the needle. The needle is then redirected in the midline and maintained in resistant ligamentous tissues until a convincing loss of resistance is achieved.

On the other hand, if the anesthetist is firmly convinced, by all the evidence available, that the needle is properly sited and if the planned operative procedure is likely to be accomplished within the duration of a long-acting local anesthetic, it may be reasonable to proceed with a single-shot injection through the needle, using bupivacaine or etidocaine. However, the latter course of action involves two assumptions: that the needle is properly sited and that the operation will not extend longer than expected. One or both of these assumptions may be wrong; thus this course is not recommended because of the unpredictability of outcome.

Dural Puncture. Often it is feasible to convert to a subarachnoid block merely by maintaining the needle in position and injecting the appropriate intrathecal dose of tetracaine, dibucaine, or bupivacaine. If the anesthesiologist wants to persevere with epidural block, another interspace should be chosen (preferably above) and a catheter should be threaded upward. Injection should be made entirely by the catheter and should be slow. A test dose (described earlier) is essential.

Subarachnoid Cannulation. This may occur at the time of initial insertion of the needle or epidural catheter (262). It has an incidence of 0.2% to 0.7% (262). Failure to recognize malplacement of needle or catheter and injection of the usual epidural dose would result in a total spinal anesthesia.

Epidural catheters have also been found to penetrate the dura at the time of a top-up dose, having initially functioned as if normally placed in the epidural space (263). Thus, a small test dose administered by an epidural catheter is always advisable.

Subdural Cannulation. This results from perforation of the dura without penetration of the underlying arachnoid membrane (see Chapter 12). This is a rare result of intended epidural cannulation (264,265). It occurs frequently during myelography (266) and in spinal anesthesia, with an incidence of up to one in 100. Spread of analgesia is patchy, markedly asymmetric, and sometimes extensive (264,265). Replacement of the epidural catheter to a more rostrad interspace level is required (see also Chapter 10).

Cannulation of an Epidural Vein. This is a greater hazard, especially in pregnant women, because of epidural venous distention during labor, particularly if the needle or catheter enters the epidural space other than in the midline. Usually the risk of epidural venous cannulation is small (267). The best treatment is *prevention*, which depends on gentle insertion of catheters that do not have sharp ends and avoidance of use of stylets, insertion of only 3 to 4 cm of the catheter length, aspiration before injection by way of an epidural catheter, and use of a test dose, preferably with epinephrine (injected into an epidural vein, this results in a rapid increase in heart rate and blood pressure).

Injection of a small amount of saline and withdrawal of the catheter by 1 to 2 cm usually permits retrieval of the catheter from the vein; if not, the catheter should be reinserted at another level. Delayed entry of a catheter into a vein may occur at the time of a top-up dose, with resulting CNS toxicity (268). Once again, the catheter must be withdrawn, or if it is inaccessible, epidural block must be discontinued.

Venous cannulation is less likely to occur if the catheter is inserted into a "wet" epidural space, expanded by prior injection of local anesthetic, rather than into a "dry" one (269). The practice of injecting a priming dose of local anesthetic through the needle is therefore a logical precaution against venous cannulation. Expansion of the epidural space can be accomplished by using a test dose of 4 mL via the needle, before inserting the catheter.

Epidural Hematoma. Needle or catheter trauma to epidural veins may result in bleeding, but this is usually minimal and stops rapidly; it is rare for an epidural hematoma and neurologic symptoms to arise if coagulation is normal. Only one case is currently recorded (270). However, patients on anticoagulant therapy may develop large epidural hematomas and, possibly, paraplegia if either an epidural needle or catheter is inserted (271,272) (see Chapter 12).

In the majority of cases, alternative means of providing most of the beneficial effects of epidural block are now available if anticoagulation is believed to be essential. For example, epidural block increases graft blood flow in association with vascular procedures on the lower limb (46). However, limb blood flow may also be increased by prior sympathetic blockade using long-acting local anesthetics or intravascular reserpine injected into the affected limb, or even surgical sympathectomy (see Chapter 39). It is also important to note that surgical procedures involving the abdominal aorta may cause paraplegia. This may be the result of prolonged clamping of the aorta (273) or sectioning of nutrient arteries to nerve plexuses and the spinal cord (252). Thus, whereas, in lower limb vascular surgery, anticoagulation or epidural block, or both, may lead to epidural hematoma and paraplegia, in aortic surgery, direct

cord ischemia must be added to the differential diagnosis of postoperative paraplegia (however, see Chapter 12).

It is important to assess any sensory or motor deficits, by decreasing a continuous epidural block as soon as possible after the surgery. The use of low-dose bupivacaine and opioid infusion usually does not result in significant motor or sensory loss; upon monitoring of neurologic function, it is usually readily apparent when sudden onset of new symptoms and signs occur in the form of sensorimotor disturbances and/or back pain. Failure to recover function fully and, in some cases, severe lumbar pain indicate the possibility of epidural hematoma. Anticoagulants should then be stopped and myelography and/or CT scan carried out immediately because most patients who have recovered from epidural hematoma have been decompressed within 12 hours of the onset of symptoms (274). The variability in individual response to low-dose heparin therapy means that some patients may still develop epidural hematomas, and this risk will continue until rapid methods are available to measure plasma levels of heparin and to assess the effect of heparin therapy on coagulation (275). Patients with potential interference with normal hemostatic mechanisms include those with disease (e.g., severe preeclampsia, intrauterine death) or medication (e.g., heparinization or oral warfarin, aspirin and other nonsteroidal anti-inflammatory drugs). Epidural puncture should be avoided if the platelet count falls below 100,000/mm^3. However, aspirin-like drugs do not change platelet *count;* they alter platelet *function.* In patients with preeclampsia and other conditions likely to alter the coagulation cascade, a full range of clotting studies should be performed in consultation with a hematologist.

The consequences of the wide use of anticlotting drugs by patients scheduled for surgery when considering a regional technique are discussed in detail in Chapter 12.

Management of Epidural Catheters

Accurate placement of a minimal length of catheter is described in the foregoing discussion as an essential aid to successful continuous catheter epidural blockade. The problems of patchy blockade, missed segments, intravascular cannulation, and subarachnoid and subdural cannulation can usually be effectively managed if the correct procedure is carefully followed and close monitoring is carried out. The long-term complications of catheter placement, owing to damage to neural tissue, should be avoidable if catheters are withdrawn at the first sign of pain or paraesthesias on insertion or on reinjection. The complications of epidural hematoma are mostly (but not always) avoidable.

Prevention of Infection

Perhaps the most important aspect of epidural catheter management is the avoidance of infections:

- A strict antiseptic routine should always be carried out during catheter insertion. Adequate time should be allowed for the skin preparation to exert its antibacterial effect, and great care should be taken not to contaminate the epidural catheter before insertion.
- Multidose local anesthetic vials should not be used: Preservative-free, single-use local anesthetic solutions should be used, and any residuum should be discarded after injection.
- Local anesthetics should not be aspirated through rubber bungs in tops of local anesthetic vials; the top should be removed and the vial discarded after single use.

▨ Glass syringes should be used only once and then resterilized, since the outside of the plunger may be contaminated during use. Many hospitals now use plastic single-use syringes.

▨ During top-up, the syringe nozzle and epidural catheter connection must not be contaminated, and if they are touched directly, the appropriate components should be changed. Wiping with alcohol swabs is not advised, since it is possible that neurolytic alcohol solution may then be carried into the epidural space.

▨ The use of micropore (Millipore) filters has been shown in one study to reduce catheter contamination (276). Although other studies have not substantiated this finding (277), it seems reasonable to recommend the use of such filters; they provide at least some protection against infection and reduce the chance of contamination with particulate matter (278).

If reasonable precautions are taken, the risk of infection from contamination of epidural catheters or local anesthetic solution should be small (e.g., 30,000 epidurals without a single infection) (87). However, endogenous infection owing to blood-borne spread from a preexisting focus of infection may be a hazard (279). Also, patients with septicemia clearly pose a considerable risk of metastatic epidural infection, and insertion of an epidural catheter is best avoided in such patients. Infection in the pelvic region could possibly spread to the epidural space by way of the venous connections to epidural veins; thus, the use of epidural catheters should be avoided unless the pelvic infection has been treated adequately with antibiotics. The risk of metastatic infection is even further increased in patients with diabetes and in patients with suppressed immune responses (280). The diabetic patient has proved to be a problem with long-term epidural catheters in treatment of cancer pain. However, immunosuppressed patients with cancer have been safely managed with long-term totally implanted epidural systems (see Chapter 40).

More complex measures to combat contamination at reinjection include the enclosure of large-volume syringes in a sterile bag (87) and the use of continuous drips and syringe pumps (281).

Procedure for Top-up and Catheter Removal

In conscious and cooperative patients, careful monitoring for signs of segmental regression will indicate the need for "top-up." In other situations, it is most convenient to top-up at the approximate time of regression of analgesia (−2 SD) as determined in clinical studies (Table 11-7), provided that this timing coincides with safe blood concentrations of local anesthetic (see Chapters 3 and 4). The mean −2 SD predicts the duration in 95% of patients. In practice, injection of half the initial dose of lidocaine approximately every hour results in maintenance of blockade associated with a small but significant gradual increase in blood lidocaine concentration (see Chapter 3). This is usually not of importance during surgery, when one to two top-ups are often sufficient. In contrast, for the long-acting agents bupivacaine and ropivacaine, topping up with half the initial dose every 2 hours maintains level of blockade without appreciable increase in blood concentration over many successive top-ups. Thus, for long-term catheter techniques, bupivacaine, ropivacaine, or levobupivacaine are preferable with respect to toxicity and because the generous margin between top-up and two-segment regression lessens the chance that tachyphylaxis may occur. It should be clearly understood that we are interested in duration of blockade from time of complete spread to regression of two segments, provided an appropriate level of blockade is achieved with the initial dose; duration to two-segment regression is considerably shorter than complete duration. If the initial level of blockade is much too high, initial top-up should be appropriately delayed, and size of top-up dose should be reduced in proportion to the level of "overshoot." A routine for topping-up is important:

1. *Check level if possible.* Pin-prick or ice in conscious patients to test reflexes, and presence or absence of bradycardia (? level above T2) in anesthetized patients. Do not top-up if a high level is suspected.
2. *Aspirate for CSF or blood.* Inject a small test dose (3–4 mL) of epinephrine-containing solution and check heart rate and blood pressure: Intravascular injection results in rapid increase in heart rate and blood pressure; subarachnoid injection results in extensive blockade with hypotension and sometimes bradycardia.
3. *Inject remainder of top-up dose slowly* with frequent aspiration, only if no complications ensue after the step 2.
4. *Monitor closely for one-half hour after top-up.* If the patient is conscious and mobile, he should lie flat during top-up and for one-half hour afterward. In any patient, be prepared to increase rate of IV infusion or to manage local anesthetic reactions or extensive sympathetic blockade (see Chapter 5, Tables 5-7 to 5-9).

Routine for Catheter Removal

Epidural catheters left in place for more than 2 weeks have been reported. Bromage advocated replacement of catheters at a different site every 72 hours (87), and this is supported on the grounds that epidural catheters become walled off by fibrous tissue reaction after about 72 hours (282). However, if a catheter is functioning satisfactorily with no sequela, it is reasonable for it to remain in situ for approximately 1 week (see also Chapter 40). Catheters should be removed gently, and the end of the catheter should be carefully checked for completeness. If difficulty is experienced in withdrawing the catheter, the spine should be flexed and gentle continuous traction exerted. There is a remote possibility that a knot may form in the catheter if excessively long lengths have been inserted; this is impossible if only 3 to 4 cm of catheter is inserted into the epidural space. An even more remote possibility exists that a catheter may loop around a spinal nerve if excess lengths are inserted; pain on removal of catheter should alert the anesthesiologist to this possibility. If subsequent radiographs, after injection of 0.3 mL of contrast media into the catheter, show that it is located in the region of a spinal nerve, removal by laminectomy may have to be considered. Sequestration of a small amount of catheter in the epidural space should be noted, and the patient must be carefully assessed over the ensuing weeks. However, it is usually not necessary to remove this foreign body, nor is it technically easy to locate it at laminectomy. Thus, in general, laminectomy is reserved for situations associated with symptoms or signs.

APPLICATIONS OF EPIDURAL BLOCKADE

A discussion of the indications and contraindications of epidural block is not within the scope of this chapter. The preceding material in this chapter has provided a broad anatomic, technical, pharmacologic, and physiologic basis on which to answer two important questions: Does epidural blockade offer significant benefits to the *individual* patient under consideration for the proposed operative or other application? Do the benefits outweigh the risks, owing to factors peculiar to the patient and/or procedure?

When viewed in this context, lists of indications and contraindications can be misleading and dangerous, since they cannot take into consideration factors that vary in individual patients. The only absolute *contraindications* to epidural blockade are patient refusal, major coagulation defects, uncorrected hypovolemia, infection in the area of proposed needle insertion, or severe systemic infection. As with spinal anesthesia, the benefits of epidural blockade in patients with neurologic disease should be carefully weighed; it appears wise, although there is no clear supportive evidence, to avoid blockade in patients with unstable neurologic disease, particularly if the spinal cord is involved. However, if epidural block offers significant benefits in patients with stable peripheral neurologic disease, such as diabetic neuropathy, its use may be considered in light of individual patients and procedures. The use of epidural block in many thousands of patients with back pain and neurologic deficit after back surgery (see Chapter 44) attests to its safety in carefully selected patients with stable neurologic signs. Abnormalities of the bony spine may increase the difficulty of epidural block, although by no means do they make it impossible; this difficulty must be weighed against the skill of the anesthesiologist and the risk–benefit ratio for the patient and procedure; both anteroposterior and lateral radiographs of the lumbar spine may be useful in making such a decision.

These considerations enable the anesthesiologists to determine which benefits epidural blockade offers to each patient in each clinical setting. The potential applications may include operative surgery; postoperative pain management; post-trauma pain management (see also Chapter 43); obstetric analgesia and operative obstetrics (see also Chapter 24); chronic and cancer pain diagnosis and management (see also Chapters 38, 40, and 45); and special applications in the management of particular medical and surgical conditions (Table 11-14).

COMPLICATIONS OF EPIDURAL BLOCKADE

The issues detailed in the earlier Problems in Epidural Blockade section may be considered minor complications. Any complication should be viewed in the light of a sound knowledge of the anatomy, pharmacology, and physiology of epidural block.

Complications Relating to Anatomic or Technical Problems

Several problems have been discussed elsewhere: inadvertent dural puncture and total spinal blockade, massive subdural spread, total epidural blockade, epidural venous injection, epidural hematoma, epidural abscess, anterior spinal artery syndrome, ligation of spinal cord blood supply during major vascular surgery, injection of local anesthetics contaminated with neurolytic agents, injection of the "wrong drug" (e.g., thiopental), broken epidural catheters, and local anesthetic toxicity.

Rigid adherence to a "therapeutic procedure" greatly reduces the risks of major complications.

■ *The occurrence and management of postdural puncture headache* is discussed in Chapter 10.

TABLE 11-14

SOME APPLICATIONS OF EPIDURAL BLOCKADE

1. Surgery
   Upper and lower abdominal surgery, urologic surgery, pelvic surgery, hip surgery, vascular surgery, surgery in the obese patient, thoracic surgery, surgery of the neck and upper limb, radical mastectomy
2. Postoperative and post-trauma pain relief See Chapter 43.
3. Obstetrics (see also Chapter 24)
   For patient comfort, to avoid incoordinate uterine action, to minimize fetal acidosis, to reduce use of "urgent" instrumental delivery or "painful delivery" needing general anesthesia, to relieve pain during labor for medical indications, preeclampsia, for cesarean section
4. Diagnosis and management of chronic pain
   "Differential" epidural block (see Chapter 38)
   "Diagnostic epidural opioid blockade" (see Chapter 38)
   Epidurography with metrizamide
   Neurolytic epidural block (see Chapter 45)
   Pain due to vasospasm due to ergot poisoning, cold injuries of extremities, Raynaud disease or phenomenon and other vasospastic problems, phantom limb pain and causalgia, postherpetic neuralgia, pancreatitis, renal colic, acute priapism
5. Epidural techniques
   Epidural electrical stimulation of spinal cord (see Chapter 41)
   Epidural opioids (see Chapter 40)

■ *Backache* is supposed to be more severe when large epidural needles (compared with spinal needles) are used. However, no data support this contention.

■ *Bladder dysfunction* is a distinct possibility if blockade of the sacral segments continues into the postoperative period. As discussed in more detail in Chapter 43, it is important to attempt to restrict epidural block to the required segments, which often do not include S2–S5. Also, it is vital to ensure that the bladder does not become overdistended if epidural block extends into the sacral segments during surgery; this is particularly important in aged men with incipient prostatic obstruction. Careful management of blockade level in obstetric patients results in a similar incidence of catheterization, whether or not epidural block is used (283). Urinary bladder volumes can be measured by portable ultrasound imaging (bladder scan).

■ *Major neurologic sequelae* of epidural block are potentially the same as for spinal anesthesia (see Chapter 10) and are discussed in Chapter 12. By determining the segments involved, it is possible to attempt to anatomically localize the lesion (Fig. 11-16).

Complications Relating to Altered Physiology

The potential for complications owing to alteration in oxygen delivery to vital organs is outlined in detail in Tables 11-3 and 11-4. Thus, like general anesthesia, it is possible for epidural block to result in compromise of oxygen delivery to heart, brain, liver, or kidney, with sequelae that depend on the degree and duration of compromise. Full knowledge of preexisting physical status and careful monitoring throughout the use of epidural block are essential to avoid such complications.

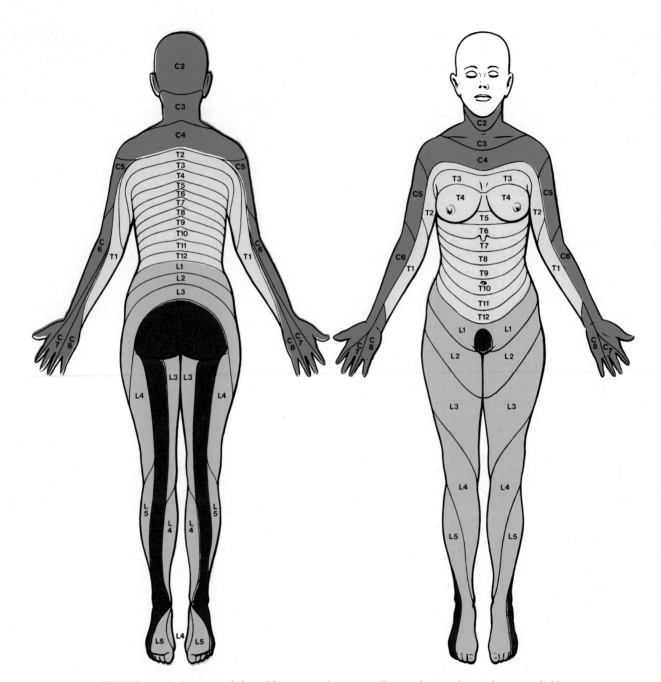

FIGURE 11-16. Dermatomal chart. The segmental areas are illustrated to emphasize the most reliable cutaneous area to test for blockade of individual spinal cord segments.

Complications of epidural block are given further consideration in Chapter 12.

CONCLUSION

Epidural neural blockade is capable of great diversity in terms of its range of neural blocking effects and the clinical applications of these effects. It is undoubtedly a most complex technique in terms of the anatomy involved, site of action, physiology, and pharmacology. Because of this, it is a technique for the specialist—the anesthesiologist. However, if used with due attention to the data presented in this chapter, it can be used with a high degree of safety and efficacy.

CAUDAL EPIDURAL BLOCKADE

Local anesthetic injection into the sacral canal by way of the sacral hiatus, or caudal anesthesia as it is now known, was first introduced in 1901 (284) and was used as the only available form of epidural anesthesia until the lumbar approach was described by Pages, in Spain, in 1921. Since that time, caudal epidural blockade has consistently suffered from comparison with central neural blockade induced at a higher level by both lumbar epidural and subarachnoid spinal techniques.

The reasons for these unfavorable comparisons are clear. First, there is considerable variation in the anatomy of the tissues near the sacral hiatus, in particular, in the bony sacrum. Frequently, the bony landmarks are obscured to a greater or lesser extent both by asymmetric bony overgrowth and by the overlying fibrous or fatty soft tissues. Attempts have been made to assess the incidence of sacral bony features that would make caudal blockade "impossible." One old study quoted an incidence of 7.7% of "absent hiatus" (285). This pessimistic figure takes no account of differences with advancing age, it being well accepted that distorted anatomy is less common in younger patients and quite rare in children. It is difficult to correlate this figure with some modern success rates of 94% and greater (286,287). It remains conjectural whether this represents a difference in the age distribution of the population studied, or whether a modern study of bony abnormalities would reveal a lesser incidence of "impossible" anatomy. There is certainly no doubt that the failure rate with caudal blockade decreases markedly with greater experience. Another reason for the unfavorable comparison of caudal with lumbar block is also anatomic, relating to the dermatomal distribution of the nerve roots, the site of the entry hiatus at the exit of the most terminal roots, and the frequency of minor bony obstructions in the sacral canal. In the lumbar region, spread of anesthetic solution can occur both cephalad and caudad, giving rise to a wide dermatomal distribution of anesthesia. Clearly, with caudal entry to the epidural space, spread can only be cephalad and may be limited by minor bony obstructions, with the result that the total number of segments blocked is bound to be less. To achieve a wide distribution of anesthesia predictably, with marked cephalad spread of solution, a large dose of local anesthetic drug must be used, with its inherent risk of drug toxicity and occasional excessive spread. Although single-dose caudal anesthesia has been and still is used to block thoracic segments, it seems an inappropriate use of the technique and partly to blame for the block's poor reputation. When an indwelling catheter is inserted via the sacral hiatus and is freely introduced in the line of the canal, so that the tip of the catheter lies closer to the lumbosacral junction, there is a greater likelihood of cephalad spread with a moderate dose. This is a worthwhile technique as long as the primary requirement for anesthesia is still in the lumbosacral distribution.

If one viewed the caudal approach merely as the lowest of segmental approaches to the epidural space, and restricted the block to the dermatomes supplied by lumbosacral roots, the technique would have a much lower failure rate, a lower incidence of complications, and, hence, a much greater popularity.

PHARMACOLOGY

Various studies have attested to safety of caudal anesthesia in terms of the local anesthetic blood levels attained. As would be expected, such wide variations occur between the doses, concentrations, and drugs used in the different studies that comparisons are difficult to make. In addition, some of these studies have measured the time of onset of the block and the duration. This information has been tabulated in Tables 11-15 and 11-16. The following generalizations can be made from this information:

- Plasma levels for all local anesthetic drugs tend to be low after caudal administration (288–295). Even very large doses in children have given plasma levels well below the accepted adult toxic levels (296). Higher peak serum concentrations in infants under 12 kg, and the presence of a greater free fraction, suggest that greater caution should be exercised with dose in this age group (290,297). The addition of epinephrine 1:200,000 to bupivacaine solutions injected in children under 5 years of age provides a significantly longer duration of action than in adults, in whom epinephrine is of questionable value (298).
- Onset time or latent interval seems to be longer with caudal than with lumbar epidural anesthetic when similar drugs and doses are administered (299).
- The time to attainment of maximum spread is variable and takes longer than for lumbar epidural block. Ranges from 10 to 60 minutes have been reported with a mean of about 30 minutes (290,297,300).
- Block of the large-diameter S1 root is less predictable than it is after lumbar epidural block when moderate doses are used (299).
- Concentrations of solution adequate to block sensory fibers are bupivacaine, ropivacaine, and levobupivacaine 0.2%; etidocaine, 1%; mepivacaine, 1%; lidocaine, 1%; prilocaine, 1%; and chloroprocaine, 2%. Increased concentration will increase the degree of motor block and, possibly, will improve speed of onset. The addition of epinephrine will increase the degree of motor block, decrease the plasma levels and increase the duration of the shorter-acting drugs (see also Chapter 3) (301,302).

Dose and Spread

Through the years, many factors have been implicated in influencing the spread of a standard dose of local anesthetic solution injected into the caudal canal. Such factors as age, weight, height, dose (both volume and concentration of drug), speed of injection, and patient position, will be known or controllable. Their influences have been studied by a number of investigators. There are, however, a number of other factors in which the influences remain both unknown and uncontrollable, and which must inevitably give rise to the significant unpredictability of all epidural spread, but particularly in the sacral canal. These factors are (303):

- The size of the caudal epidural space
- The size and patency of the sacral canal and the anterior sacral foramina
- The amount of bony distortion of the sacral canal
- The presence of septa in the epidural space
- The amount and nature of the soft tissues in the epidural space, especially fatty tissues
- The permeability of the neural tissue and dural cuffs to the drug

Adults. The only factors that have been shown to affect caudal spread in adults are volume, speed of injection (303), and patient posture (304).

In another study, 30 mL of 1.5% lidocaine with epinephrine 1:200,000 injected over 1 minute gave a mean upper level of T6–T7 (L3–T1), whereas a similar volume injected over 2 minutes gave a mean upper level of T11 (S2–T2) (303). There was an 8% incidence of transient acute hypertension and tachycardia in the more rapid injection group. The lack of influence of age in adults is well shown in a study in which the dose of

TABLE 11-15

PHARMACOKINETICS AND CAUDAL BLOCK

Study (Ref.)	Drug	Dose	Mean peak blood concentration and range	Mean time to peak blood concentration	Comments
Mazze et al., 1966 (292) Young adults	1.5% lidocaine with epinephrine 1:200,000	5.8–7.5 mg/kg Mean 428 mg = 28.5 mL	1.4 μg/mL (0.5–2.9)	30 min	Lower blood levels with caudal than with lumbar epidural on IV regional
Moore et al., 1968 (310) Obstetric patients with caudal catheter	1.5% mepivacaine	300–450 mg = 20–30 mL	About 3.0 μg/mL	Not stated; 40 min for one patient	Blood levels rose after equivalent top-up doses to reach 7–9 μg/mL in four of five patients at delivery
Freund et al., 1984 (291) Young males <40 years compared with older males >55 years; caudal catheters inserted to 10 cm	2% lidocaine or 0.75% bupivacaine, both with epinephrine 1:200,000	Lidocaine 6 mg/kg, bupivacaine 2.2 mg/kg	Lidocaine <40 y 2.47 μg/mL ± 0.23 Lidocaine >55 y 2.61 μg/mL ±1.45 bupivacaine <40 y 0.86 μg/mL ±0.22 Bupivacaine >50 y 0.69 μg/mL ±0.25	Lidocaine <40, 45 min, lidocaine >55 y, 25 min, bupivacaine <40 y, 30 min, bupivacaine >55 y, 20 min	No significant difference between peak plasma lidocaine or bupivacaine levels with age; no significant difference in dermatomal levels for the four groups
Ecoffey et al., 1984 (289) Children	1% lidocaine	5 mg/kg	2.05 ± 0.08 μg/mL	28.2 ± 2.9 min	Long terminal half-life in children attributed to large volume of distribution
Takasaki 1984 (302) Children Lönnqvist et al., 2000 (293) Chalkiadis et al., 2004 (294) Children Chalkiadis et al., 2005 (295) Infants	1.5% lidocaine, 1.5% mepivacaine, 0.5% bupivacaine, all with epinephrine 0.2% ropivacaine 0.25% levobupivacaine 0.25% levobupivacaine	Lidocaine 11 mg/kg, Mepivacaine 11 mg/kg, bupivacaine 3.7 mg/kg 2 mL/kg 2 mg/kg 2 mg/kg	Lidocaine 2.2 μg/mL, mepivacaine 2.53 μg/mL, bupivacaine 0.67 μg/mL 0.47 ± 0.16 μg/mL 0.91 ±0 .4 μg/mL 0.72 ± 0.23 μg/mL	45 min 45 min 45 min 30 min (5–60) 49.5 min 12–249 min	Low blood concentrations with slow decrease in concentrations

IV, intravenous; y = years of age.

anesthetic per spinal segment is plotted against age for both lidocaine HCl and carbonated lidocaine (286) (Fig. 11-17). In the same study, there was also no correlation with height or weight. In another study, comparing spread with both lidocaine and bupivacaine in a group of older and a group of younger adult males, there was no significant difference between any of the four groups (291).

The effect of posture on the spread of caudal solutions was studied in patients in the horizontal position, 15 degrees head-up, and 15 degrees head-down. Higher levels of analgesia were obtained in the head-up position (304).

Children. In children, the situation is different: Schulte-Steinberg and Rahlfs (1970) established a high correlation between dose and age (305). There were lesser degrees of correlation between dose and weight and dose and height in children. In 1977, the same authors produced a single regression line for three drugs (1% lidocaine, 1% mepivacaine, and 0.25% bupivacaine, all with epinephrine) showing in children the linear relation between age and spread (measured in mL/spinal segment) (306). Reference to this study shows that an adequate dosing schedule would be 0.1 mL/segment/yr + 0.1 mL/segment (see Chapter 27).

TABLE 11-16

ONSET AND DURATION OF CAUDAL BLOCK

Study (Ref.)	Drug	Onset (min)	Spread (segments)	Two-segment regression (min)	Total regression (min)	Comments
Seow et al., 1976 (301) Adults	1% etidocaine with epinephrine 1:200,000, 25 mL	7.06 SD = 4.54	11.7 SD = 3.9	Not measured	Not measured	Rapid onset but persisting motor block noted with etidocaine
	1.5% lidocaine with epinephrine 1:200,000, 25 mL	12.44 SD = 6.14	12.7 SD = 5.8	Not measured	Not measured	
Park et al., 1979 (303)	30 mL 1.5% lidocaine with 1:200,000 epinephrine					Several instances of acute hypertension >200/100 in 1 min injection group
	Injection over 1 min	3.9 (2–15)	17 (8–22)		203 ± 5.3	
	Injection over 2 min	3.6 (2–12)	12 (3–21)	Not measured	192 ± 11	

| | | Block of S1 Root | | | | |
Study (Ref.)	Drug	Delay (min)	Failure (%)	Spread	Total regression	Comments
Galindo et al., 1978 (299)	1.5% chloroprocaine	4.8 (SD = 1.5)	20	20 (8.6)		All onset times are similar and very fast. The delay in the block of the large S1 root is very variable.
	3% chloroprocaine		25	24.3 (6.7)		
	2% mepivacaine	5.5 (0.7)	23	27 (8.4)		
Breschan et al., 2005 (361) Children	0.75% bupivacaine	5.9 (2.6)	13	17.9 (5.6)		
	1% etidocaine	4.9 (2.0)	0	17.8 (3.5)		
	1.5% etidocaine	4.9 (1.4)	0	15 (3.8)		
	All with epinephrine 1:200,000 – dose range, 10–20 mL	4.2 (2.5) 10 (SD = 2.2)		T7.6 (SD = 1.1) T8 (1.4)	Not measured	Because individual doses range from 10–20 mL, it is difficult to assess the significance of these data
	0.2% ropivacaine 1 mL/kg	11.4 (3.3) 10 (1.8)		T7.7 (1.2)		
	0.2% levobupivacaine 1 mL/kg					342 (SEMe = 48)
	0.1% bupivacaine 1 mL/kg					345 (39) 321 (78)

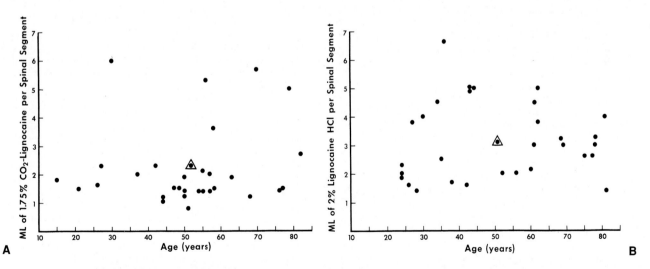

FIGURE 11-17. Caudal blockade in adults: Segmental spread analgesia with advancing age. **A:** 1.75% lidocaine carbonate. **B:** 2% lidocaine hydrochloride. Dose requirements in milliliter per spinal segment are plotted against age, with the mean dose indicated by a dot in a triangle. There is no consistency in spread of analgesia at any age or any correlation between age and segmental spread. From Cousins MJ, Bromage PR. A comparison of the hydrochloride and carbonated salts of lignocaine for caudal analgesia in outpatients. *Br J Anaesth* 1971;43:1149, with permission.

Strong agreement exists between this work and that done by Bromage with lumbar epidural anesthesia (307).

Despite the academic appeal of the dosing schedule cited above, it has been challenged by a number of authors. This has given rise to a bewildering collection of formulae, some for specific purposes, and some for such vague indications as "routine surgical procedures." Three dosing schedules are worthy of further mention. The Armitage formula of 0.5 mL of 0.25% bupivacaine/kg for circumcision and anal surgery (low sacral) is easy to use, reliable, and safe, but requires much larger doses of drug (308). The same author recommends 1 mL/kg of 0.25% bupivacaine to block the lower thoracic nerves and 1.25 mL/kg to block the midthoracic nerves (e.g., for orchidectomy or umbilical herniorrhaphy). This latter dose is high, but seems to have proven safe in children.

In the second study, Busoni and Andreuccetti (309) analyzed 763 caudal blocks in children and produced two graphs. The first related spread of analgesia to dose and age, while the second related spread of analgesia to dose and weight. Knowing the age and/or weight, the dose required for a given degree of spread can be determined. Weight proved to be a better predictor in infants, whereas age was better for older children (see also Chapter 27).

The third study (287) is notable for the extent of the detail presented. It states that with at least 97% confidence, 0.55 mL of 1% to 2% lidocaine/kg will produce a block to S3 or higher, 1.1 mL/kg will produce a block to L3 or higher, and 1.7 mL/kg will produce a block to T11 or higher. These doses gave rise to some excessively high blocks, and there was an alarmingly high incidence of respiratory or cardiac arrest (2.8%), or both, which one must deduce was at least contributed to by the very high doses of drug given. Such large doses should not be administered.

The detailed implications for caudal anesthesia in pediatrics are further discussed in Chapter 27.

Dose by Means of Caudal Catheter. As previously stated, the tip of a caudal catheter may readily reach the L5–S1 level. The block then tends to behave more like a lumbar epidural. Estimation of dose can be done using the criteria that one uses for this latter block. Top-up doses should be scaled down, as with lumbar epidural top-ups. Accumulation of 1.5% mepivacaine during labor, with steadily rising blood levels and toxicity, has occurred, in which caudal top-up doses have been the same as the initial dose (310).

Onset and Duration

To understand and use rationally any regional anesthetic technique, it is important to know the following time intervals: (a) the time to achieve maximum spread of block and (b) the duration (usually measured for a central block as the time from onset to regression of two spinal segments). It is also useful to know the onset interval (latency) and the time to total regression of the block. Only limited data are available on this subject, the most notable feature of which is the great variability, particularly with regard to onset interval (Table 11-19). This is probably due to the use of different methods as criteria for onset. In most studies, time of onset is the period from injection until the patient first notices loss of sensation to pin-prick or other stimulus.

Physiologic Effects

A limited sacral block from a caudal epidural would be expected to cause minimal physiologic trespass. Besides the sen-

sory and motor block of the sacral roots, one could expect a degree of autonomic block. The sacral component of the parasympathetic craniosacral outflow (the pelvic splanchnic nerves) will be blocked, causing loss of visceromotor function in the bladder and bowel distally from the splenic flexure of the colon. There should, in theory, also be an increase in anal and bladder sphincter tone, but this is seldom seen in practice because of a coexistent sympathetic block, which is outlined below. Since the sympathetic outflow from the spinal cord ends at L1 level, a limited caudal block should theoretically avoid any sympathetic block. It would seem in practice, however, that this is not necessarily so. Vascular dilatation in the lower limb is often seen with a low level of caudal block. There seems no doubt that the level of sympathetic block is higher than that of sensory block, although there is very little hard evidence in the literature to confirm this. An often-quoted study (311) has shown evidence of sympathetic block of the eye in 17 of 20 consecutive obstetric patients having caudal analgesia. Although in this study the dose of drug and supine positioning of the patient have been rightly criticized, nevertheless the upper level of sensory block was significantly lower than T1 in all patients. It would seem, therefore, that the potential exists for a degree of unwanted sympathetic block. Pooling of blood in the denervated lower extremities, and reflex vasoconstriction in the innervated upper limbs, has been shown to occur (312). Carotid flow was unchanged. Of course, if an extensive sensory block occurs (intentional or otherwise), inevitably a similarly extensive sympathetic block will occur, with all the consequences outlined in this chapter. Likewise, similar respiratory and neuroendocrine effects of high epidural anesthesia would be expected with an extensive caudal block.

Changes in adrenocorticotropic hormone (ACTH), immunoreactive β-endorphin, antidiuretic hormone (ADH), cortisol, catecholamines, insulin, and growth hormone levels were measured in children undergoing surgery with either halothane anesthesia or caudal anesthesia. The normal rises in these hormone levels associated with general anesthesia and surgery in the perioperative period were blocked by caudal anesthesia (313,314).

Technique of Caudal Block

As in the preparation for any major regional anesthetic technique, all equipment must be assembled and checked, including block tray, resuscitation equipment, monitors, and suction. Secure IV access must be obtained (see Chapter 8).

The needles used for this procedure will depend to some extent on the clinical circumstances. For single-injection caudal block in a child, a 2- to 3-cm disposable 23- to 25-gauge needle should be used. In an adult, the slightly greater rigidity of a 22-gauge needle may make the procedure easier. The needles should be short-bevelled, because they give a better feel when different tissues are penetrated, they have less tendency to form barbs if bone is struck, the bevel is more likely to fully enter the canal when it is very shallow, and they may cause less trauma to blood vessels. If a catheter is to be inserted, a short 5- to 7-cm 18T-gauge Crawford-tip needle and a standard epidural catheter are recommended. Some operators prefer to use a plastic IV cannula of small caliber (315). Although this has some advantages, it has a tendency to kink and is less reliable. A large-gauge IV needle can be used to insert a standard epidural catheter. The use of a Tuohy needle to insert a catheter is not recommended because the needle will lie in the long axis of the canal and the Tuohy tip will direct the catheter toward the wall, rather than into the axis of the canal, as would happen with a Crawford or an IV needle.

The patient can be positioned in one of three ways: The preferred position is the lateral Sims position (left-side down for a right-handed operator), with the lower leg only slightly flexed at the hip and the upper leg more flexed so that it lies over and above the lower leg and is also in contact with the bed. This maneuver tends to separate the buttocks. In contrast to lumbar epidural block, excess hip flexion is unnecessary and may on occasion stretch the skin to such an extent that palpation of the landmarks may become more difficult. This position has the advantages of comfort for the patient, a familiar working position for the anesthesiologist, and easy access to the airway if the patient is sedated, or in the event of an adverse reaction. Sagging of the gluteal cleft occasionally may cause some confusion in confirming landmarks in inexperienced hands, but can be readily corrected by an assistant, who holds the upper buttock to reposition the gluteal cleft in the median plane of the sacrum. This is in accordance with the general principle that skin creases are poor landmarks for regional anesthesia (Fig. 11-18A).

The prone position, with a pillow under the pelvis, is still popular with some anesthesiologists. Both legs are rotated so that the toes of both feet are facing medially. This again separates the buttocks. In this position, there is no distortion from movement of the gluteal cleft, but access to the mouth and airway is compromised.

The less popular knee-chest position may still be useful, particularly for the pregnant patient.

Skin preparation should be done over a large area, so that all the landmarks can be palpated aseptically. If alcoholic solutions are used, a swab should be placed deep in the gluteal cleft, to prevent pain in the exposed sensitive perineal area.

Confirmation of bony landmarks is the key to success. In a thin, young patient, the protrusions of the sacral cornua can be seen without palpation, and the shallow depression over the sacral hiatus can be seen between them. Successful needle placement in these circumstances is exceedingly easy; however, the majority of patients have less obvious surface anatomy and require very careful palpation of all the bony landmarks. Needle penetration of a posterior sacral foramen may mimic the feel of entering the sacral hiatus. Often, closed bony depressions covered by fibrous ligament can also mimic the sacral hiatus, although injection is impossible (Fig. 11-19B). Only the most meticulous attention to the landmarks can prevent needle entry into these "decoy hiatuses."

It is important, initially, to identify the midline positively. This can be achieved by palpating the tip of the coccyx with the finger and moving cephalad, about 4 to 5 cm in an adult, until the fingertip lies over the sacral hiatus with the prominent sacral cornua palpable on each side by moving the fingertip from side to side (Fig. 11-18B). The use of excessive pressure while moving the finger in this latter manner can be painful. Considerable variability occurs in the prominence of the cornua, causing problems for the unwary. If one cornu is much less obvious than the other, there may be a tendency to palpate further laterally until a prominent tubercle of the lateral sacral crest at the inferior lateral sacral angle is felt. The importance of establishing the midline of the sacrum cannot be overemphasized. Palpation of the median sacral crest in a caudad direction can also lead to the sacral hiatus, but it is a less reliable method. The posterior superior iliac spines form an equilateral triangle with the sacral hiatus; this should be used as a confirmatory landmark for correct needle placement. Unfortunately, these spines are not always readily palpable. It is useful to remember that the line joining these spines is an approximate indication of the level of termination of the dural sac (S2 level). In patients in whom landmark palpation is difficult, digital examination, with one finger inserted into the rectum, may be performed to help select a point of needle entry. A useful alternative method of palpating the cornua and hiatus, using the thumb of each hand has been described (316).

Once the area of the suspected hiatus has been found, one should keep the palpating hand in position until after the needle insertion, because the landmarks can be quickly obscured, especially in an obese patient. Because the canal has a tendency to become deeper as one progresses cephalad, canal entry is facilitated if a point of needle entry is chosen toward the upper end of the hiatus. The initial angle of needle insertion should be about 120 degrees to the back (Fig. 11-18C). Penetration of the sacrococcygeal ligament has a characteristic feel to it. This "pop" can be learned only by practice. There is a feeling of nonresistance after penetration of the ligament, until the anterior sacral wall is contacted. This contact should not be sought deliberately. The needle, both hub and shank, should be depressed toward the skin to align the needle approximately in the long axis of the canal. It may then be inserted a further centimeter (Fig. 11-18C). On occasion, further needle insertion is not possible because of obstruction of some kind. This should be accepted. After both aspiration and a test of the local anesthetic drug are safely accomplished, the full dose of local anesthetic may be injected in 3 to 5 mL increments.

Signs of Correct Needle Placement

The following are the objective and subjective signs of accurate needle positioning, and those that appear appropriate should be elicited before completion of injection; the first four should be regarded as essential (modified from McCaul [316]):

■ Presence of sacral bone on each side of, in front of, and behind the needle at its point of insertion does not exclude the possibility of entry into a decoy hiatus, but does protect against injection lateral to the sacral or coccygeal margins or into the presacral tissues or rectum.

■ The lack of CSF, air, or blood on aspiration is important. Light blood staining is not uncommon and may indicate that entry into the sacral canal has been achieved and that repeat aspiration should be attempted during the injection of solution.

■ There should be no subcutaneous bulge or superficial crepitus after rapid injection of 2 or 3 mL of anesthetic solution or air.

■ There should be no tissue resistance to injection; the force required to inject should not exceed that necessary to overcome syringe and needle resistances and should be constant throughout. Injection should feel like any other injection into the epidural space.

■ The so-called "whoosh" test can be used to predict successful needle placement (317,318). This involves listening with a stethoscope over the midline lumbar spine for a characteristic "whoosh" sound on injection of 2 to 3 mL of air via the caudal needle. This test is more reliable than the "pop" of sacrococcygeal ligament penetration or loss-of-resistance tests (319). Venous air embolism in an 11-kg child has been suggested following the use of 2.5 mL of air for this test (320).

■ When correctly positioned, the needle should be able to move in the canal, pivoting at the point of penetration of the sacrococcygeal ligament. Eliciting the sign may, however, cause trauma to the tissues in the canal, particularly blood vessels, and usually is not necessary.

■ There should be no local pain during injection of solution; pain indicates misplacement of the needle, and injection should stop.

A

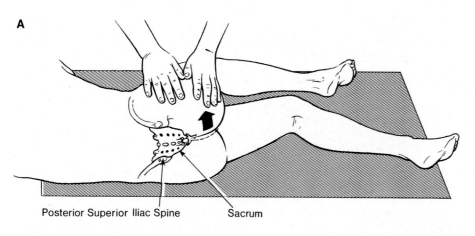

Posterior Superior Iliac Spine   Sacrum

B

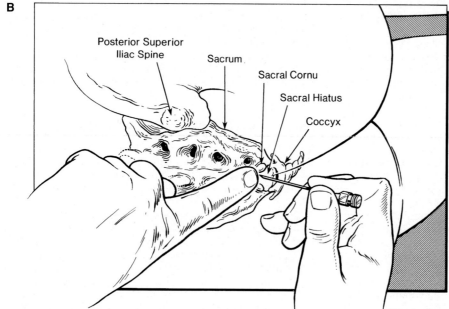

Posterior Superior
Iliac Spine   Sacrum   Sacral Cornu

Sacral Hiatus

Coccyx

C

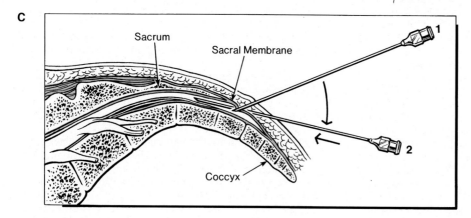

Sacrum   Sacral Membrane

1

2

Coccyx

FIGURE 11-18. Technique of caudal block. **A:** Positioning for caudal block. **B:** Palpation of landmarks and needle insertion. **C:** Needle insertion through sacrococcygeal (sacral) membrane.

■ Paresthesia or a feeling of fullness that extends from the sacrum to the soles of the feet is common during injection, but ceases on completion and portends successful blockade.

■ The feeling of grating as the needle moves along the anterior wall of the sacral canal indicates accurate positioning but should not be purposefully elicited lest the sacral venous plexus be damaged.

■ An epidural catheter or other plastic cannula should enter the canal freely with the same or greater ease than in the lumbar epidural space.

It is recommended that one use a test dose containing epinephrine before the full dose is given. Because of the proximity of needle and catheter to venous plexuses, there is a risk of intravascular injection and a toxic reaction. Slow injection

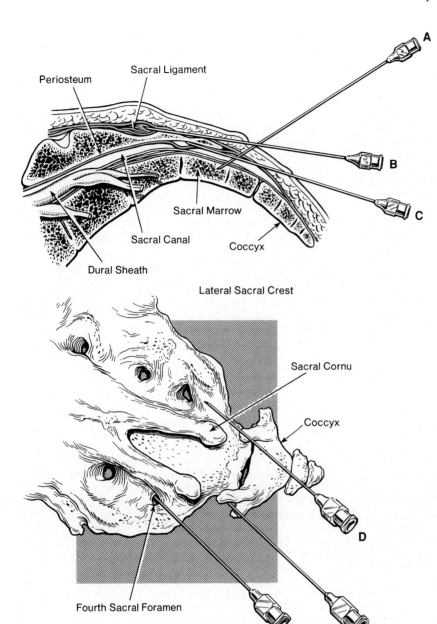

Periosteum
Sacral Ligament
Dural Sheath
Sacral Canal
Sacral Marrow
Coccyx

A
B
C

Lateral Sacral Crest

Sacral Cornu
Coccyx

Fourth Sacral Foramen

D
E
F

FIGURE 11-19. Misplacement of needle during attempted caudal block. Note injection into posterior sacral ligaments (**B**); subperiosteal injection (**C**); and injection into marrow (**A**); lateral injection into a "decoy hiatus" (**D**); injection lateral to coccyx and toward anterior sacral wall (**E**), with a risk of damaging intrapelvic structures (including a fetus); injection into fourth sacral foramen (**F**), perhaps one of the most common causes of a unilateral limited block.

PART II: TECHNIQUES

is also recommended in order to avoid rapid increases in spinal and intraepidural pressure.

Catheter Techniques

The epidural catheter should enter the canal without difficulty. Because of the angle of insertion, it will progress cephalad more predictably in all age groups (321–324) than will lumbar epidural catheters.

Fixation of the epidural catheter to prevent soiling is important. One secure method is to spray the area lightly with an adhesive, such as tincture of benzoin compound, and then apply a sterile adhesive plastic dressing initially into the previously separated gluteal cleft, and then directly over the site of insertion of the catheter. Because many of these patients will have surgery in the lithotomy position, the aim is to have a very adherent dressing in the gluteal cleft that will *not* form a pocket to collect fluids from the operative site, which may run down directly over the anus.

Monitoring

Despite the limited extent of block anticipated with caudal anesthesia, it is still mandatory to monitor the patient, including blood pressure, electrocardiogram (ECG), and pulse oximetry. Intravenous or intraosseous misplacement of the caudal needle or excessive spread of block may give rise to unwanted effects. Maintaining verbal communication with the patient is the simplest, and in some ways the most reliable method of detecting adverse side effects. However, blood pressure and pulse should be measured frequently, and the progress of the block should be plotted.

Indications

Obstetric Anesthesia and Analgesia

The widespread and safe use of epidural analgesia to control the pain of labor has been a major factor in increasing the popularity of regional anesthesia for elective and emergency surgery (see also Chapter 24). Although the lumbar approach is now used as the technique of choice in most obstetric units, it should be remembered that it was the 1943 report by Hingson and Edwards (325) that first popularized the method. The advantages were immediately obvious: high-quality analgesia with a low incidence of complications and a low failure rate for that time of only 7%.

In later years, clinical studies confirmed some of the advantages (326,327). Most, but not all (328), studies showed that caudal analgesia had essentially no effect on uterine activity during labor. Local anesthetic blood levels did not correlate with any measured changes in uterine activity (329). Cardiac output increases during labor were decreased, and the tachycardia of the second stage and the early postpartum period was prevented by caudal analgesia (330,331). One study demonstrated the prolongation of analgesia achieved by adding epinephrine to the caudal local anesthetic solution (332). It also reported that epinephrine, 25 mL of 1:200,000 dilution, significantly prolonged labor; however, top-up doses of 15 to 20 mL were given in this study, and patients were supine; thus the epinephrine dose was large and some supine hypotension may have occurred.

As regional anesthetic techniques became more refined, it became apparent that there were significant objections to the use of the caudal route for routine analgesia in labor. The pathways for the pain of first-stage labor are by way of T10–L1 (see Chapter 24). Thus, a technique that initially and predominantly blocked sacral roots was less effective for early labor. Large doses of local anesthetic drug needed to be given. Admittedly, the caudal approach offered superb management of the sacrally mediated pain of second stage, but it did so for what could be a lengthy period of first stage, when it was not required. What was previously a tolerable failure rate of 7% became no longer acceptable. An unfortunate objection was the report of four cases in which local anesthetic drugs were injected into the fetus during attempted caudal injection (333,334). For these reasons, continuous caudal analgesia in labor fell into disuse in most obstetric units, to an extent that facility in performing the technique has now been largely lost. There is still a place for continuous caudal analgesia in labor in those cases in which lumbar epidural analgesia is contraindicated because of anatomic abnormalities or localized infection. On occasions, sacral analgesia is required either early in labor or cannot be obtained via a lumbar catheter.

A two-catheter technique, one lumbar and one caudal, has been used in an effort to lower the total dose of local anesthetic drug (335,336). This would seem to compound the likelihood of complications without a sufficiently significant positive advantage. The technique of using a lumbar catheter for first-stage analgesia, supplemented late in labor by single-injection caudal block, is popular in some centers (316,317). Single-injection caudal anesthesia is useful as an alternative to saddle-block spinal anesthesia for forceps delivery. In these circumstances, the proximity of the needle to the presenting part of the fetus must be remembered. The procedure is safe if bone of the sacrum and coccyx is palpable on all sides of the needle. Rectal examination is advised when there is any doubt. It has been stated that caudal block should not be performed if the presenting part is at the perineum (316).

An excellent review of the use of caudal anesthesia in obstetrics is provided by Paull in a symposium on obstetric anesthesia (337).

Pediatric Anesthesia

Caudal block has been used successfully for anesthesia in children since about 1960, with many studies attesting to its success (see also Chapter 27). It is in this group of patients that the caudal technique has found its greatest application. In children, the sacral hiatus is usually very easy to palpate, making the procedure very simple, quick, and reliable (287,339,340). Because of the ease of its performance in children, the block has been recommended for a wide variety of surgical procedures, both as the sole anesthetic and in combination with light general anesthesia. In summary, the surgical indications for the block divide into three groups: sacral block (e.g., circumcision, anal surgery), lower thoracic block (e.g., inguinal herniotomy), and upper thoracic block.

The significance of these three groups relates to the doses of local anesthetic drug required to consistently achieve the desired spread. This subject has been discussed at length in a previous section, but it should be reemphasized here that no justification exists for the use of doses of lidocaine in excess of 5 to 7 mg/kg, despite the allegations of safety by some authors. Mid abdominal or upper abdominal surgery is not an indication for conventional caudal block. Thoracic epidural anesthesia in children has been achieved via a 24-gauge epidural catheter inserted through the sacral hiatus. The radiographically determined epidural catheter tip position was within two segments of the target position in 17 of 20 patients (323).

For subumbilical surgery, caudal anesthesia is excellent. Since young children do not tolerate the frightening environment of the operating room, light general anesthesia seems to be the preferred technique for both induction of the caudal block and throughout the surgery. In those patients in whom sedation or general anesthesia is not desired or is contraindicated (341,342,387), eutectic mixture of local anesthetics (EMLA) cream under adhesive plastic can be applied to the skin over the sacral hiatus an hour or so prior to the procedure (343).

A modification of the standard caudal technique has been described by Busoni and Sarti for use in children (300). This sacral intervertebral epidural block is based on the fact that fusion of the sacral segments is not complete until after the 25th year. The caudal needle is inserted into the S2–S3 space in the midline just below a line drawn between the posterior superior iliac spines. The epidural space was identified by loss of resistance to air. Successful block was achieved in 100% of 74 children aged between 2 months and 13 years.

Low-birth-weight and preterm or former preterm neonates constitute a high risk group of patients for whom the appropriate use of regional anesthesia can obviate the need for general anesthesia and minimize the associated serious respiratory complications common to this group (344). The author's personal series, as well as several published studies, attest to the success and safety of single-shot or continuous caudal anesthesia for lower abdominal and perineal surgery in this challenging group of patients (340,345–350).

A specific indication for caudal anesthesia in children is surgery in patients with congenital dystrophia myotonica. Regional anesthesia enables the anesthesiologist to avoid the respiratory depression associated with general anesthesia in these patients (351,352).

Relief of pain in the early postoperative period is probably the major advantage of caudal anesthesia in children. Several studies have confirmed the benefit of caudal anesthesia for control of postoperative pain following circumcision (353–357). It would seem to be better than intramuscular (IM) morphine, IM buprenorphine (356), and IM dihydrocodeine (358), and at least equivalent to penile block (357), wound infiltration (359), and ilioinguinal/iliohypogastric block, when appropriate (307) (see also Caudal Opioids). The subsequent coexistent motor block has, however, been considered a disadvantage by some authors (357,360). For postoperative pain management, bupivacaine 0.125% with epinephrine 1:200,000 is equianalgesic but has less motor block than 0.25% bupivacaine with epinephrine. The newer long-acting local anesthetic agents ropivacaine 0.2% and levobupivacaine 0.2% have been associated with less motor weakness compared to bupivacaine 0.2% administered caudally (361,362). Suggested safe infusion rates for caudal bupivacaine are 0.2 to 0.3 mg/kg/hr in infants and 0.2 to 0.5 mg/kg/hr in older children, with a limit of 48 hours. Higher infusion rates have given rise to toxicity (363). Safe guidelines have been described by Berde (364).

The duration of postoperative analgesia with caudal bupivacaine was significantly increased by the addition of 1 μg/kg of clonidine (365). Caudal ketamine 0.5 mg/kg is equianalgesic with 0.25% bupivacaine (366). S-ketamine 0.5 mg/kg when added to 0.2% caudal ropivacaine provides better postoperative analgesia than clonidine 2 μg/kg without any clinically significant side-effect (367).

Adult Anesthesia

Caudal blockade can be used whenever the area of surgery is primarily innervated by the sacral and lumbar nerve roots. When the area is innervated from a higher level, lumbar epidural blockade and spinal subarachnoid block are preferable techniques. The following procedures are appropriate indications: anal surgery, especially hemorrhoidectomy and anal dilatation; surgery on the vulva and vagina; surgery on the scrotal skin and penis; and surgery of the lower limb. If a caudal catheter is used with its tip positioned higher in the canal, a higher level of anesthesia can be assured and more extensive surgery accommodated. Such procedures could include vaginal hysterectomy and inguinal herniorrhaphy. The use of caudal blockade for relief of postoperative pain following hemorrhoidectomy is well documented (368) and has been recommended for pain relief following lower limb surgery (369).

Chronic Pain Management

The caudal approach to the epidural space has been used for many years by pain physicians both to diagnose and to treat a variety of largely unspecified low back pain syndromes. In the main, the therapeutic techniques have involved injecting large volumes (up to 64 mL) of diluted procaine, lidocaine, or bupivacaine, with or without steroid, often at a fairly rapid rate (370–373). Cure or improvement rates of more than 50% have been claimed (371,374) (see Chapter 44). Rapid injection of large volumes of any solution into the epidural space is not recommended. Such practice can result in a large increase in spinal CSF pressure, with a risk of cerebral hemorrhage, visual disturbances, headache, or compromised spinal cord blood flow (spinal stroke). Central nervous system vascular catastrophes are particular hazards in patients with atherosclerosis.

Caudal Opioids. The caudal epidural route has been used for the administration of opioids, with varying claims of success (375–378). With the exception of analgesia following hemorrhoidectomy, there is a paucity of studies of the use of caudal opioids in adults. However, in children, numerous clinical studies compare the postoperative pain relief obtained from cau-

dal opioids with that obtained from a wide variety of regional anesthetic techniques and drugs given by other routes. From this large amount of literature, the following statements can be made:

- Caudal morphine is effective and safe and has a prolonged duration of action for postoperative analgesia (379–382).
- An effective caudal analgesic dose of morphine is 50μg/kg, which gives rise to plasma levels lower than those generally required for systemic analgesia (381).
- Caudal morphine gives a significantly longer duration of analgesia than IM/IV morphine or caudal bupivacaine (377,379,381), but is approximately equivalent to caudal buprenorphine (383).
- The addition of fentanyl to caudal solutions of bupivacaine (384) or ropivacaine (386) does not prolong the duration of analgesia.
- Single-shot caudal morphine can provide adequate postoperative analgesia following thoracic surgery (380).
- Despite the alleged safety of caudal opioids, respiratory depression is still possible (387,388), particularly in infants (389). All the usual precautionary measures must be taken.

In general, the side effects of caudal epidural opioids are similar to those from the more common lumbar epidural route. Certainly, itching has been reported and claimed in a single report to be dose-related (390).

Complications

The range of complications seen with caudal anesthesia is predictable and, in common with most other regional anesthetic procedures, decreases markedly with experience and with meticulous attention to technique (see Chapter 12) (391).

Improper Needle Placement

It is to be expected that in this region of renowned variability of anatomy, malpositioning of the caudal needle, particularly by novices, is not uncommon. There is no substitute for practical experience coupled with a sound knowledge of the possible anatomic variants. The possible consequences of improper needle placement follow.

Absent or Patchy Block. Particularly in an obese patient, the needle may come to lie in the soft tissues superficial to the sacrum. The experienced hand can often detect the absence of firm needle fixation that is present when the needle has correctly penetrated the sacrococcygeal ligament. Palpation over the needle tip during rapid injection of air or fluid will detect the appearance of a subcutaneous lump (Fig. 11-19B). With malplacement of the needle under periosteum, either outside the canal or inside the canal anteriorly or posteriorly, the needle will be fixed, but there will be considerable resistance to injection (Fig. 11-19C).

If the needle is misplaced laterally, it may penetrate a posterior sacral foramen, or it may miss any hiatus and lie in the presacral soft tissues (Figs. 11-19E, F). In either case, injection may be easy, but absent or patchy block will result. Penetration of a ligament-covered sealed depression (decoy hiatus) may sometimes give the correct feel, but injection will be impossible (Fig. 11-19D). With any malplacement in which periosteum is needled or stretched, the awake patient will feel pain that can be severe. This pain may continue into the postoperative period and give rise to patient complaints. There is no place for persistent clumsy attempts to locate the correct hiatus.

Intravenous or Intraosseous Placement. Claims for a high incidence of local anesthetic toxic reactions during caudal anesthesia are not substantiated by studies (392). Nevertheless, the potential exists for producing early-onset high blood levels of local anesthetic due either to IV or intraosseous injection (393). When a fine needle is used, free aspiration of blood on entering an epidural vein may not be obvious.

Several cases have been reported of cardiac arrhythmias associated with hemodynamic changes following caudal injection of bupivacaine with adrenaline in children (287,339,394,395). Of particular interest were case reports of five infants who developed ST segment elevation and increased T-wave amplitude in association with a significant *decrease* in heart rate, but without seizures (394). The importance of the test dose is again emphasized.

Of at least equal importance in toxicity potential is the possibility of intraosseous injection, produced by penetrating the thin layer of cortical bone of the sacral canal's anterior wall, in those circumstances when the ligament penetration has not been felt (Fig. 11-19A). The feeling of bone penetration may be confused with that of ligament penetration, and then it is possible that the local anesthetic drug will be injected into the marrow. The result is similar to an IV injection—rapid attainment of a high blood level of local anesthetic; this, again, supports the use of a test dose. This complication was reported initially following aspiration of marrow cells during clinical caudal anesthesia (397,396) and was reproduced in animal studies (397). A further, more recent, case has been reported (398). Any suggestion of a feeling of "granularity" during needle insertion or during attempted aspiration should alert one to the possibility of this hazard; the test dose provides the only practical protection against this complication.

Dural Puncture. With the dural sac ending at the S2 level, or approximately on a line joining the posterior-superior iliac spines, dural puncture should be exceedingly rare. An incidence of more than 1% has been quoted (392), although the rate of consequent accidental spinal block was much lower, at 0.1%. Total spinal anesthesia has been reported following attempted caudal block in infants (399). A knowledge of the variable distance from the tip of the sac to the apex of the sacral hiatus should warn of the possibility of dural puncture. Advancement of the needle, in adults, by more than 1 to 2 cm in the sacral canal should be avoided, whereas in children it should be correspondingly less.

Subdural Injection. As with epidural injection at any level, subdural injection is possible, although less likely, when the needle is inserted via the sacral hiatus. A slow onset but extensive block is highly suggestive of subdural injection (400).

Injection into Fetus. There have been reports of fetal intoxication by local anesthetic drug injected into the fetal scalp during attempted caudal injection (333,334). Two babies died. Unfortunately, these isolated reports have done much to discourage the use of caudal anesthesia during labor, despite the fact that the risk exists only when the presenting part has descended to the perineum and questionable techniques are used.

Excessive Spread

Unpredictability of spread of the local anesthetic solution, especially in adults (286), has already been mentioned. Although *limited* cephalad spread is a more common problem with caudal, on rare occasions *excessive* spread may occur to a high thoracic level, even in the absence of a subarachnoid or subdural injection (392). This extensive region of blockade is of itself no particular problem. After all, such levels are deliberately sought with lumbar epidural anesthesia for a variety of surgical procedures, and the physiologic changes that result are well controlled by simple standard measures. There is, however, a difference in the degree of expectation of these changes, often resulting in a lesser degree of vigilance by the anesthesiologist. One must not forget that the potential exists for a caudal to give rise to a somatic and sympathetic block at least as extensive as a lumbar epidural block, although it is less common. Secure IV access, adequate monitoring, and normal resuscitation equipment must be assured (see Chapter 5, Tables 5-7 to 5-9 for details of management of extensive epidural or total spinal block).

Catheter Problems

Problems from caudal epidural catheters are no different from those that occur with lumbar insertion. Catheter insertion when the needle is correctly placed is generally very easy, occurring more readily than with lumbar insertion. Early resistance to insertion is usually an indication that the needle is incorrectly placed. The catheter should never be withdrawn through the needle because of the risk of shearing it off. Shearing has also been reported when a properly placed needle was being withdrawn over the catheter in the accepted fashion (401). This was caused by a barb directed toward the lumen, which had developed during a difficult insertion. Dural or venous puncture by the catheter is possible, particularly with older, more rigid catheters with sharper tips. There has also been a case report of a catheter knotting in the caudal canal, requiring neurosurgical exploration for its removal (401).

Postoperative Problems

Pain. Pain at the injection site is the most common postoperative complaint. Ligament penetration without periosteal trauma will give rise to only minimal pain both during insertion and postoperatively. On the other hand, a periosteal hematoma may cause pain that lasts several weeks. There is no substitute for careful technique, using the information from all landmarks before needle insertion. It is worth remembering that coccygodynia resulting from the stress of childbirth may be erroneously blamed on the caudal block.

Urinary Retention. There seems little doubt that some increased risk of urinary retention occurs after epidural block of the sacral segments, especially when a long-acting local anesthetic drug is used (402). The likelihood of retention may be greater in those patients who would normally be considered at risk, that is, elderly men, puerperal women, and those who will undergo ano-perineal surgery. These groups, of course, make up the bulk of the indications for adult caudal blockade. A single bladder catheterization should not cause significantly increased morbidity if proper technique is followed (402).

Infection. Intuitively, one would think that the infection rate would be significantly higher with caudal block than with lumbar epidural block. In a bacteriologic comparison between simultaneous caudal and lumbar epidural catheters (two-catheter technique) during childbirth, cultures were taken from skin at the puncture site, catheter tip, catheter fluid, and catheter subcutaneously (403). Specimens from the skin surface in the caudal area produced a significantly larger number of positive cultures than did those from the epidural area. This result was repeated when a more extensive skin preparation, including povidone-iodine ointment, was used in the caudal area; however, no clinical infections occurred, and in fact all cultures in both areas taken from sites deep into the skin were negative. The study indicates that the risk of infection, although remote, does exist. Compromises in sterile technique have no place in regional anesthesia.

Neurologic Complications. In common with lumbar epidural and subarachnoid anesthesia, caudal epidural anesthesia is inevitably associated with some slight risk of neurologic damage. In his analysis of complications, Dawkins mentions one permanent lesion in nearly 23,000 cases, but the details are not specified (392). Whatever the true incidence, it must be very small. Of greater significance is the likelihood that a coexistent neurologic lesion will be blamed on the block. Neurologic sequelae of traumatic vaginal delivery notoriously fall into this group. As anesthesiologists, we need to ensure that our medical colleagues maintain a balanced view of regional anesthetic techniques and that any neurologic lesions be thoroughly examined and investigated. In almost all cases, such investigations will reveal the coincident nature of the lesion (see Chapter 12).

Conclusion

Objective data obtained from randomized, prospective, controlled studies are still needed for many aspects of caudal blockade. Such data as are available indicate that caudal block can provide safe, effective analgesia of lumbosacral spinal segments.

The caudal route to the epidural space is particularly attractive in children (see Chapter 27) and in adults who require sacral block. In children, the technique is reliable, easy to perform, and has a consistent dose-spinal segment response relationship. In adults, there is an inevitable failure rate that is higher than that for lumbar epidural block, but with a knowledge of pertinent anatomy and with practical experience, this failure rate can be reduced to an acceptable level.

References

1. Bromage PR. The "hanging-drop" sign. *Anaesthesia* 1953;8:237.
2. Usubiaga JE, Dos Reis A, Usubiaga LE. Epidural misplacement of catheters and mechanisms of unilateral blockade. *Anesthesiology* 1970;32:158.
3. Telford RJ, Hollway TE. Observations on deliberate dural puncture with a Tuohy needle: Pressure measurement. *Anaesthesia* 1991;46:725.
4. Okutomi T, Watanable S, Goto F. Time course in thoracic epidural pressure measurement. *Can J Anaesth* 1993;40:1044.
5. Shah JL. Positive lumbar extradural space pressure. *Br J Anaesth* 1994;73:309.
6. Usubiaga JE, Moya F, Usubiaga LE. Effect of thoracic and abdominal pressure changes on the epidural space pressure. *Br J Anaesth* 1967;39:612.
7. Paul DL, Wildsmith JAW. Extradural pressure following the injection of two volumes of bupivacaine. *Br J Anaesth* 1989;62:368.
8. Usubiaga JE, Wikinski JA, Usubiaga LE. Epidural pressure and its relation to spread of anesthetic solutions in epidural space. *Anesth Analg* 1967;46:440.
9. Frank NR, Mead J, Ferris BG. The mechanical behaviour of the lungs in healthy elderly persons. *J Clin Invest* 1957;36:1680.
10. Galbert MW, Marx GF. Extradural pressures in the parturient patient. *Anesthesiology* 1974;40:499.
11. Bromage PR. Epidural needle. *Anesthesiology* 1961;22:1018.
12. Thomas PS, Gerson JI, Strong G. Analysis of human epidural pressures. *Reg Anesth* 1992;17:212.
13. Rocco AG, Scott DA, Boas RA, Philip JH. Epidural space behaves as a Starling resistor and inflow resistance is higher in spinal stenosis than in disc disease. *Anesthesiology* 1990;73:A816.
14. Bengtsson M. Changes in skin blood flow and temperature during spinal analgesia evaluated by laser Doppler flowmetry and infra-red thermography. *Acta Anaesthesiol Scand* 1984;28:625.
15. Bromage PR. Physiology and pharmacology of epidural analgesia. *Anesthesiology* 1967;28:592–622.
16. Bonica JL. Autonomic innervation of the viscera in relation to nerve block. *Anesthesiology* 1968;29:793–813.
17. Bonica JJ, Berges PU, Morikawa K. Circulatory effects of peridural block. I. Effects of levels of analgesia and dose of lidocaine. *Anesthesiology* 1970;33:619.
18. Bonica JJ, Kennedy WF, Ward RJ, Tolas AG. A comparison of the effects of high subarachnoid and epidural anesthesia. *Acta Anaesthesiol Scand* 1966;23[Suppl]:429.
19. Stevens RA, Beardsley D, White JL, et al. Does the choice of local anesthetic affect the catecholamine response to stress during epidural anesthesia. *Anesthesiology* 1993;79:1219–1226.
20. Tanaka K, Harada T, Dan K. Low-dose thoracic epidural anesthesia induces discrete thoracic analgesia without reduction in cardiac output. *Reg Anesth* 1991;16:318.
21. Goertz A, Heinrich H, Seeling W. Baroreflex control of heart rate during high thoracic epidural anaesthesia. *Anaesthesia* 1992;47:984–987.
22. Dohi S, Tsuchida H, Mayumi T. Baroreflex control of heart rate during cardiac sympathectomy by epidural anesthesia in lightly anesthetized humans. *Anesth Analg* 1991;62:815.
23. Reiz S. Circulatory effects of epidural anesthesia in patients with cardiac disease. *Acta Anaesthesiol Belg* 1968;39[Suppl 2]:21.
24. Goertz AW, Seeling W, Heinrich H, et al. Influence of high thoracic epidural anesthesia on left ventricular contractility assessed using end-systolic-pressure-length relationship. *Acta Anaesthesiol Scan* 1993;37:38.
25. Niimi Y, Ichinose F, Saegusa H, et al. Echocardiographic evaluation of global left ventricular function during high thoracic epidural anesthesia. *J Clin Anesth* 1997;9:118–124.
26. Ottesen S. The influence of thoracic epidural analgesia on the circulation at rest and during physical exercise in man. *Acta Anaesthesiol Scand* 1978;22:537–547.
27. Otton PE, Wilson EJ. The cardiocirculatory effects of upper thoracic epidural analgesia. *Can Anaesth Soc J* 1966;13:541.
28. Koch M, Blomberg S, Emanuelsson H, et al. Thoracic epidural anesthesia improves global and regional left ventricular function during stress induced myocardial ischemia in patients with coronary artery disease. *Anesth Analg* 1990;71:625.
29. Schmidt C, Hinder F, van Aken H. The effect of high thoracic epidural anesthesia on systolic and diastolic left ventricular function in patients with coronary artery disease. *Anesth Analg* 2005;100:1561–1569.
30. Veering BT, Cousins MJ. Cardiovascular and pulmonary effects of epidural anaesthesia. *Anaesth Intensive Care* 2000;28:620–635.
31. Davis RF, DeBoer WV, Maroko PR. Thoracic epidural anesthesia reduces myocardial infarct size after coronary artery occlusion in dogs. *Anesth Analg* 1986;65:711.
32. Klassen GA, Bramwell RS, Bromage PR, Zborowska-Sluis DT. The effect of acute sympathectomy by epidural anesthesia on the canine coronary circulation. *Anesthesiology* 1980;52:8.
33. Blomberg S, Ricksten SE. Thoracic epidural anesthesia decreases the incidence of ventricular arrhythmias during acute myocardial ischemia in anaesthetised rats. *Acta Anaesthesiol Scand* 1988;32:173.
34. Blomberg S, Curelaru J, Emanuelsson H, et al. Thoracic epidural anaesthesia in patients with unstable angina pectoris. *Eur Heart J* 1989;10:437.
35. Blomberg S, Emanuelsson H, Ricksten SE. Thoracic epidural anesthesia and central hemodynamics in patients with unstable angina pectoris. *Anesth Analg* 1989;69:558.
36. Olausson K, Magnusdottir H, Lurje L, et al. Anti-ischemic and anti-anginal effects of thoracic epidural anesthesia versus those of conventional medical therapy in the treatment of severe refractory unstable angina pectoris. *Circulation* 1997;96:2178.
37. Buffington CW, Davis KB, Gillispie S. The prevalence of steal prone-coronary anatomy in patients with coronary artery disease: An analysis of the coronary artery surgery study registry. *Anesthesiology* 1988;69:721.
38. Heusch G, Deussen A, Thamer V. Cardiac sympathetic nerve activity and progressive vasoconstriction distal to coronary stenosis: Feedback aggravation of myocardial ischemia. *J Auton Nerve Syst* 1985;13:311.
39. Nygard E, Kofoes KF, Freiberg J. Effects of high thoracic epidural analgesia on myocardial blood flow in patients with ischemic heart disease. *Circulation* 2005;111:2165.

PART II: TECHNIQUES

40. Hainsworth R. Vascular capacitance: Its control and importance. *Rev Physiol Biochem Pharmacol* 1986;105:101.

41. Baron J-F, Payon D, Coriat P, et al. Forearm vascular tone and reactivity during lumbar epidural anesthesia. *Anesth Analg* 1988;67:1065.

42. Granger HJ, Guyton AC. Autoregulation of the total systemic circulation following destruction of the central nervous system in the dog. *Circ Res* 1969;25:379.

43. Stevens RA, Beardsley D, White JL, et al. Does the choice of local anesthetic affect the catecholamine response to stress during epidural anesthesia. *Anesthesiology* 1993;79:1219.

44. Stevens RA, Artuso JD, Kao T-Z, et al. Changes in human plasma catecholamine concentrations during epidural anesthesia depend on the level of the block. *Anesthesiology* 1991;74:1029.

45. Bonica JJ, Akamatsu TJ, Berges PU, et al. Circulatory effects of peridural block. II. Effects of epinephrine. *Anesthesiology* 1971;34:514.

46. Cousins MJ, Wright CJ. Graft, muscle, skin blood flow after epidural block in vascular surgical procedures. *Surg Gynecol Obstet* 1971;133:59.

47. Shimosato S, Etsten BE. The role of the venous system in cardiocirculatory dynamics during spinal and epidural anesthesia in man. *Anesthesiology* 1969;30:619.

48. Baron JF, Decaux-Jacolot A, Edouard A, et al. Influence of venous return on baroreflex control of heart rate during lumbar epidural anesthesia in humans. *Anesthesiology* 1986;64:188.

49. Arndt J, Hock A, Stanton-Hicks M, Stuhmeier KD. Peridural anesthesia and the distribution of blood in supine humans. *Anesthesiology* 1985;63:616.

50. Fluxe K, Sedvall G. The distribution of adrenergic nerve fibers to the blood vessels in skeletal muscle. *Acta Physiol Scand* 1965;64:75.

51. Salevsky FC, Whalley DG, Kalant D, Crawhall J. Epidural epinephrine and the systemic circulation during peripheral vascular surgery. *Can J Anaesth* 1990;37:16.

52. Bonica JJ, Kennedy WF, Akamatsu TJ, Gerbershagen HU. Circulatory effects of peridural block. III. Effects of acute blood loss. *Anesthesiology* 1972;36:219.

53. Oberg B, Thoren P. Studies on left ventricular receptors signalling in non-medullated vagal afferents. *Acta Physiol Scand* 1972;85:145.

54. Oberg B, Thoren P. Increased activity in left ventricular receptors during hemorrhage or occlusion of caval veins in the cat. A possible cause of vasovagal reaction. *Acta Physiol Scand* 1972;85:164.

55. Oberg B, White S. Circulatory effects of interruption and stimulation of cardiac vagal afferents. *Acta Physiol Scand* 1970;80:383.

56. Oberg B, White S. The role of vagal cardiac nerves and arterial baroreceptors in the circulatory adjustments to hemorrhage in the cat. *Acta Physiol Scand* 1970;80:395.

57. Kopp SL, Horlocker TT, Warner ME, et al. Cardiac arrest during neuraxial anesthesia: Frequency and predisposing factors associated with survival. *Anesth Analg* 2005;100:855.

58. Jacobsen J, Sofelt S, Brocks V, et al. Reduced left ventricular diameters at onset of bradycardia during epidural anesthesia. *Acta Anaesthesiol Scand* 1992;36:831.

59. Campagna JP, Carter C. Clinical relevance of the Bezold-Jarisch reflex. *Anesthesiology* 2003;98:1250.

60. Mark AL. The Bezold-Jarisch reflex revisited: Clinical implications of inhibitory reflexes originating in the heart. *J Am Coll Cardiol* 1983;1:90.

61. Schadt JC, Ludbrook J. Hemodynamic and neurohumoral responses to acute hypovolemia in conscious mammals. *Am J Physiol* 1991;260:H305.

62. Sander-Jensen K, Marving J, Secher N, et al. Does the decrease in heart rate prevent a decremental decrease of the end-systolic volume during central hypovolemia in man? *Angiology* 1990;41:687.

63. Stephen GW, Lees MM, Scott DB. Cardiovascular effects of epidural block combined with general anaesthesia. *Br J Anaesth* 1969;41:933.

64. Nancarrow C, Plummer JL, Ilsley AH, et al. Effects of combined extradural blockade and general anaesthesia on indocyanine green clearance and halothane metabolism. *Br J Anaesth* 1986;58:29.

65. Reiz S, Balfors E, Sorensen MB, et al. Coronary hemodynamic effects of general anesthesia and surgery: Modification by epidural analgesia in patients with ischemic heart disease. *Reg Anesth* 1982;7[Suppl]:8–18.

66. Wattwil M, Sundberg A, Arvill A, Lennquist C. Circulatory changes during high thoracic epidural anaesthesia: Influence of sympathetic block and of systemic effect of the local anaesthetic. *Acta Anaesthesiol Scand* 1985;29:849.

67. Saada M, Catoire P, Bonnet F, et al. Effects of thoracic epidural anesthesia with general anesthesia on segmental wall motion assessed by transesophageal echocardiography. *Anesth Analg* 1992;75:329.

68. Saada M, Duval AM, Bonnet F, et al. Abnormalities in myocardial segmental wall motion during lumbar epidural anesthesia. *Anesthesiology* 1989;71:26.

69. Wright PMC, Fee JPH. Cardiovascular support during combined extradural and general anaesthesia. *Br J Anaesth* 1992;68:585.

70. Samain E, Coriat P, Le Bret F, et al. Ephedrine vs phenylephrine for hypotension due to thoracic epidural anesthesia associated with general anesthesia: Effects on left ventricular function. *Anesthesiology* 1989;73:A82.

71. Goertz AW, Seeling W, Heinriech H, et al. Effect of phenylephrine bolus administration on left ventricular function during high thoracic and lumbar epidural anesthesia combined with general anesthesia. *Anesth Analg* 1993;76:541.

72. Silver JR, Buxton PH. Spinal stroke. *Brain* 1974;97:539.

73. Scott DB. Inferior vena caval pressure. Changes occurring during anaesthesia. *Anaesthesia* 1963;18:135.

74. Scott DB. Inferior vena caval occlusion in late pregnancy. *Clin Anesth* 1973;10:37.

75. Bieniarz J, Branda LA, Maqueda E, et al. Aortocaval compression by the uterus in late human pregnancy. II: An arteriographic study. *Am J Obstet Gynecol* 1968;100:203.

76. Bellis CJ, Wangensteen OH. Venous circulatory change in the abdomen and lower extremities attending intestinal distention. *Proc Soc Exp Biol Med* 1939;41:490.

77. Ranninger K, Switz DM. Local obstruction of the inferior vena cava by massive ascites. *AJR Am J Roentgenol* 1965;93:935.

78. Bull GM. Postural proteinuria. *Clin Sci Mol Med* 1948;7:77.

79. Malatinsky J, Kadlic T. Inferior vena caval occlusion in the left lateral position. *Br J Anaesth* 1974;46:165.

80. Enderby GEH. Controlled circulation with hypotensive drugs and posture to reduce bleeding in surgery. Preliminary results with pentamethonium iodide. *Lancet* 1950;1:1145.

81. Urquhat-Hay D, Marshall NG, Marsland JM. Comparison of epidural and hypotensive anaesthesia in open prostatectomy. Series 1. *N Z Med J* 1969;69:280.

82. Urquhat-Hay D, Marshall NG, Marsland JM. Comparison of epidural and hypotensive anaesthesia in open prostatectomy. Series 2. *N Z Med J* 1969;70:223.

83. Keith I. Anaesthesia and blood loss in total hip replacement. *Anaesthesia* 1977;32:444.

84. Thorud T, Lund I, Holme I. The effect of anesthesia on intraoperative and postoperative bleeding during abdominal prostatectomies: A comparison of neurolept anesthesia, halothane anesthesia and epidural anesthesia. *Acta Anaesthesiol Scand* 1975;57[Suppl]:83.

85. Modig J, Borg T, Karlstrom G, et al. Thromboembolism after total hip replacement: Role of epidural and general anesthesia. *Anesth Analg* 1933;62:174.

86. Stanton-Hicks, MD. A study using bupivacaine for continuous peridural analgesia in patients undergoing surgery of the hip. *Acta Anaesthesiol Scand* 1971;15:97.

87. Bromage PR. *Epidural Analgesia*. Philadelphia: W.B. Saunders, 1978.

88. Crawford JS. *Principles and Practice of Obstetric Anaesthesia*, 4th ed. Oxford: Blackwell Scientific Publications, 1978.

89. Holmdahl MH, Sjögren S, Strom G, Wright B. Clinical aspects of continuous epidural infusion for postoperative pain relief. *Ups J Med Sci* 1972;77:47.

90. Steinbrook RA. Epidural anesthesia and gastrointestinal motility. *Anesth Analg* 1998;86:837.

91. Carli F, Trudel JL, Belliveau P. The effect of intraoperative thoracic epidural anesthesia and postoperative analgesia on bowel function after colorectal surgery: A prospective, randomized trial. *Dis Colon Rectum* 2001;44:1083.

92. Zugel N, Bruer C, Breitschaft K, Angster R. Effect of thoracic epidural analgesia on the early postoperative phase after interventions on the gastrointestinal tract. *Chirurgia* 2002;73:262.

93. Scheinin B, Asantila R, Orko R. The effect of bupivacaine and morphine on pain and bowel function after colonic surgery. *Acta Anaesthesiol Scand* 1987;31:161.

94. Scott AM, Starling JR, Ruscher AE. Thoracic versus lumbar epidural anesthesia's effect on pain control and ileus resolution after restorative proctocolectomy. *Surgery* 1996;120:688.

95. Sielenkamper AW, Eicker K, Van Aken H. Thoracic epidural anesthesia increases mucosal perfusion in ileum of rats. *Anesthesiology* 2000;93:844.

96. Adolphs J, Schmidt DK, Mousa SA, et al. Thoracic epidural anesthesia attenuates hemorrhage-induced impairment of intestinal perfusion in rats. *Anesthesiology* 2003;99:685.

97. Johansson K, Ahn H, Lindhagen J, Tryselius U. Effect of epidural anaesthesia on intestinal blood flow. *Br J Surg* 1988;75:73.

98. Lazar G, Kaszaki J, Abraham S, et al. Thoracic epidural anesthesia improves the gastric microcirculation during experimental gastric tube formation. *Surgery* 2003;134:799.

99. Glosten B, Hynson J, Sessler DI, McGuire J. Preanesthetic skin-surface warming reduces redistribution hypothermia caused by epidural block. *Anesth Analg* 1993;77:488.

100. Hynson JM, Sessler DI, Glosten B, McGuire J. Thermal balance and tremor patterns during epidural anesthesia. *Anesthesiology* 1991;74:680.

101. Sessler DI, Ponte J. Shivering during epidural anesthesia. *Anesthesiology* 1990;72:816.

102. Glosten B, Sessler DI, Faure AM, et al. Central temperature changes are poorly perceived during epidural anesthesia. *Anesthesiology* 1992;77:10.

103. Ponte J, Sessler DI. Extradurals and shivering: Effects of cold and warm extradural saline injections in volunteers. *Br J Anaesth* 1990;64:731.

104. Walmsley AJ, Giesecke AH, Lipton JM. Epidural temperature: A cause of shivering during epidural anesthesia. *Anesth Analg* 1986;65:S1.

105. Brownridge P. Shivering related to epidural blockade in labor, and the influence of epidural pethidine. *Anaesth Intensive Care* 1986;14:412.

106. Shehabi Y, Gatt S, Buckman T, Isert P. Effect of adrenaline, fentanyl and warming of injectate on shivering following extradural analgesia in labour. *Anaesth Intensive Care* 1990;18:31.

107. Sutherland J, Seaton H, Lowry C. The influence of epidural pethidine on shivering during lower segment caesarean section under epidural anaesthesia. *Anaesth Intensive Care* 1991;19:282.

108. Hjorts NC, Neumann P, Frsig F, et al. A controlled study on the effect of epidural analgesia with local anesthetics and morphine on morbidity after abdominal surgery. *Acta Anaesthesiol Scand* 1985;29:790.

109. Kehlet H. Surgical stress: The role of pain and analgesia. *Br J Anaesth* 1989;63:189.

110. Naito Y, Tamai S, Shingu K. Responses of plasma adrenocorticotropic hormone, cortisol and cytokines during and after upper abdominal surgery. *Anesthesiology* 1992;77:426.

111. Cousins MJ. Acute pain and the injury response: Immediate and prolonged effects. *Reg Anesth* 1989;14:162.

112. Brand PH, Metting PJ, Britton SL. Support of arterial blood pressure by major pressor systems in conscious dogs. *Am J Physiol* 1988;255:H483.

113. Quail AW, Woods RL, Korner PJ. Cardiac and arterial baroreceptor influences in release of vasopressin and renin during hemorrhage. *Am J Physiol* 1987;252:H1120.

114. Peters J, Schlaghecke R, Thouet H, Arndt JO. Endogenous vasopressin supports blood pressure and prevents severe hypotension during epidural anesthesia in conscious dogs. *Anesthesiology* 1990;72:694.

115. Carp H, Vadherra R, Jayaram A, Garvey D. Endogenous vasopressin and renin-angiotensin systems support blood pressure after epidural block in humans. *Anesthesiology* 1994;80:1000.

116. Hopf HB, Schlaghecke R, Peters J. Sympathetic neural blockade by thoracic epidural anesthesia suppresses renin release in response to arterial hypotension. *Anesthesiology* 1994;80:992.

117. Bromage PR, Joyal AC, Binney JC. Local anesthetic drugs: Penetration from the spinal extradural space into the neuraxis. *Science* 1963;140:392.

118. McCarthy GS. The effect of thoracic extradural analgesia on pulmonary gas distribution. Functional residual capacity and airway closure. *Br J Anaesth* 1976;48:243.

119. Wahba WM, Craig DB, Don HF, Becklake MR. The cardio-respiratory effects of thoracic epidural anaesthesia. *Can Anaesth Soc J* 1972;19:8.

120. Holmdahl MH, Sjögren S, Strom G, Wright B. Clinical aspects of continuous epidural blockade for postoperative pain relief. *Ups J Med Sci* 1972;77:47.

121. Miller L, Gertel M, Fox GS, MacLean LD. Comparison of effect of narcotic and epidural analgesia on postoperative respiratory function. *Am J Surg* 1976;131:291.

122. Sjögren S, Wright B. Circulation, respiration and lidocaine concentration during continuous epidural blockade. *Acta Anaesthesiol Scand* 1972;16[Suppl]:5.

123. Wahba WM, Don HF, Craig DB. Post-operative epidural analgesia: Effects on lung volumes. *Can Anaesth Soc J* 1975;22:519.

124. Sugimori K, Kochi T, Nishiro T, et al. Thoracic epidural anesthesia causes rib cage distortion in anesthetised, spontaneously breathing dogs. *Anesth Analg* 1993;77:494.

125. Kochi T, Sako S, Nishino T, Mizuguchi T. Effect of high thoracic extradural anaesthesia on ventilatory response to hypercapnia in normal volunteers. *Br J Anaesth* 1989;62:362.

126. Sakura S, Saito Y, Kosaka Y. Effect of lumbar epidural anesthesia on ventilatory response to hypercapnia in young and elderly patients. *J Clin Anesth* 1993;5:109.

127. Mankikian B, Cantineau JP, Bertrand M, et al. Improvement of diaphragmatic function by a thoracic extradural block after upper abdominal surgery. *Anesthesiology* 1988;68:379.

128. Pansard JL, Mankikian B, Bertrand M, et al. Effects of thoracic extradural block on diaphragmatic electrical activity and contractility after upper abdominal surgery. *Anesthesiology* 1993;78:63.

129. Polaner DM, Kimball WR, Fratacci M, et al. Thoracic epidural anesthesia increases diaphragmatic shortening after thoracotomy in the awake lamb. *Anesthesiology* 1993;79:808.

130. Fratacelli M, Kimball WR, Wain JL, et al. Diaphragmatic shortening after thoracic surgery in humans. Effects of mechanical ventilation and thoracic epidural anesthesia. *Anesthesiology* 1993;79:654.

131. Groeben H. Lung function under high thoracic segmental epidural anesthesia with ropivacaine or bupivacaine in patients with severe chronic obstructive pulmonary disease undergoing breast surgery. *Anesthesiology* 2002;96:536.

132. Gruber EM, Tschernko EM, Kritzinger M, et al. The effects of thoracic epidural analgesia with bupivacaine 0.25% on ventilatory mechanics in patients with severe chronic obstructive pulmonary disease. *Anesth Analg* 2001;92:1015.

133. Burm AGL. Clinical pharmacokinetics of epidural and spinal anaesthesia. *Clin Pharmacokinet* 1989;16:283.

134. Veering BT, Burm AGL. Pharmacokinetics and pharmacodynamics of medullar agents. *Baillieres Clin Anaesthesiol* 1993;7:557.

135. Hogan Q, Toth J. Anatomy of soft tissues of the spinal canal. *Reg Anaesth Pain Med* 1999;24:303–310.

136. Bromage PR. Mechanism of action of extradural analgesia. *Br J Anaesth* 1975;47:199.

137. Cohen EN. Distribution of local anesthetic agents in the neuraxis of the dog. *Anesthesiology* 1968;29:1002–1005.

138. Shantha TR, Evans JA. The relationship of epidural anesthesia to neural membranes and arachnoid villi. *Anesthesiology* 1972;37:543–557.

139. Zenker W, Bankoul S, Braun JS. Morphological indications for considerable diffuse reabsorption of cerebrospinal fluid in spinal meninges particularly in the areas of meningeal funnels. An electron microscopical study including tracing experiments in rats. *Anat Embryol (Berl)* 1994;189:243–258.

140. Covino BG, Scott DB. *Handbook of Epidural Anaesthesia and Analgesia.* Orlando: Grune & Stratton, 1985.

141. Cousins MJ, Mather LE. Intrathecal and epidural administration of opioids. *Anesthesiology* 1984;61:276.

142. Cousins MJ, Mather LE, Glynn CJ, et al. Selective spinal analgesia. *Lancet* 1979;1:1141.

143. Bromage PR. Lower limb reflexes changes in segmental epidural analgesia. *Br J Anaesth* 1974;46:504–508.

144. Cusick JF, Myklebust JB, Abram SE. Differential neural effects of epidural anesthetics. *Anesthesiology* 1980;53:299–306.

145. Cusick JF, Myklebust JB, Abram SE, Davidson A. Altered neural conduction with epidural bupivacaine. *Anesthesiology* 1982;57:31–36.

146. Burn JM, Guyer PB, Langdon L. The spread of solutions injected into the epidural space: A study using epidurograms in patients with the lumbosciatic syndrome. *Br J Anaesth* 1973;45:338.

147. Nishimura N, Kitahara T, Kusakabe T. The spread of lidocaine and 1–131 solution in the epidural space. *Anesthesiology* 1959;20:785.

148. Rocco AC, Philip JH, Boas RA, Scott D. Epidural space as a Starling resistor and elevation of flow resistance in a diseased epidural space. *Reg Anesth* 1997;22:167–177.

149. Visser WA, Gielen MJM, Gielen JLP. Continuous positive airway pressure breathing increases the spread of sensory blockade after low-thoracic epidural injection of lidocaine. *Anesth Analg* 2006;102:268.

150. Cousins MJ, Augustus JA, Gleason M, et al. Epidural block for abdominal surgery: Aspects of clinical pharmacology of etidocaine. *Anaesth Intensive Care* 1978;6:105.

151. Seow LT, Lips FJ, Cousins MJ, Mather LE. Lidocaine and bupivacaine mixtures for epidural blockade. *Anesthesiology* 1982;56:177.

152. Benzon HT, Toleikis JR, Shanks C, et al. Somatosensory evoked potential quantification of ulnar nerve blockade. *Anesth Analg* 1986;65:843.

153. Dahl JB, Rosenberg J, Lund C, Kehlet H. Effect of thoracic epidural bupivacaine 0.75% on somatosensory evoked potentials after dermatomal stimulation. *Reg Anesth* 1990;15:73.

154. Dirkes WE, Rosenberg J, Lund C, Kehlet H. The effect of subarachnoid lidocaine and combined subarachnoid lidocaine and epidural bupivacaine on electrical sensory thresholds. *Reg Anesth* 1991;16:262.

155. Lund C, Hansen OB, Kehlet H, et al. Effects of etidocaine administered epidurally on changes in somatosensory evoked potentials after dermatomal stimulation. *Reg Anesth* 1991;16:38.

156. Lund C, Hansen OB, Mogensen T, et al. Effect of thoracic epidural bupivacaine on somatosensory evoked potentials after dermatomal stimulation. *Anesth Analg* 1987;66:731.

157. Lund C, Selmar P, Hansen OB, et al. Effect of epidural bupivacaine on somatosensory evoked potentials after dermatomal stimulation. *Anesth Analg* 1987;66:34.

158. Malmquist EL-A, Berg S, Holmgren H. Effects of epidural bupivacaine or mepivacaine on somatosensory evoked potentials and skin resistance responses. *Reg Anesth* 1992;17:205.

159. Grundy BL, Heros RC, Tung AS, Doyle E. Intraoperative loss of somatosensory evoked potentials predicts loss of spinal cord function. *Anesthesiology* 1982;57:321.

160. Axelsson KH. A double-blind study of motor blockade in the lower limbs. Studies during spinal anaesthesia with hyperbaric and glucose-free 0.5% bupivacaine. *Br J Anaesth* 1985;57:960.

161. Van Zundert A, Vaes L, Van Der AP, et al. Motor blockade during epidural anesthesia. *Anesth Analg* 1986;65:333.

162. Galindo A, Hernandez J, Benavides O, et al. Quality of spinal extradural anaesthesia: The influence of spinal nerve root diameter. *Br J Anaesth* 1975;47:41.

163. Bromage PR. Ageing and epidural dose requirements. Segmental spread and predictability of epidural analgesia in youth and extreme age. *Br J Anaesth* 1969;41:1016.

164. Grundy EM, et al. Extradural analgesia revisited. A statistical study. *Br J Anaesth* 1978;50:805.

165. Park WY, Massengale M, Kin SI, et al. Age and the spread of local anesthetic solutions in the epidural space. *Anesth Analg* 1980;59:768.

166. Sharrock NE. Epidural anesthetic dose responses in patients 20 to 80 years old. *Anesthesiology* 1978;49:425.

167. Nydahl PA, Philipson L, Axelsson K, Johansson JE. Epidural anesthesia with 0.5% bupivacaine: Influence of age on sensory and motor blockade. *Anesth Analg* 1991;73:780.

168. Park WY, Hagins FM, Rivat EL, MacNamara TE. Age and epidural dose response in adult men. *Anesthesiology* 1982;56:318.

169. Rosenberg PH, Saramies L, Alila A. Lumbar epidural anaesthetic with bupivacaine in old patients: Effect of speed and direction of injection. *Acta Anaesth Scand* 1981;25:270.

170. Veering BT, Burm AGL, Van Kleef JW, et al. Epidural anesthesia with bupivacaine: Effects of age on neural blockade and pharmacokinetics. *Anesth Analg* 1987;66:589.

171. Veering BT, Burm AGL, Vletter AA, et al. The effect of age on the systemic absorption and systemic disposition of bupivacaine after epidural administration. *Clin Pharmacokinet* 1992;22:75.

172. Anderson S, Cold GE. Dose response studies in elderly patients subjected to epidural analgesia. *Acta Anaesthesiol Scand* 1981;25:279.

173. Simon MJG, Veering BT, Stienstra R, et al. The effects of age on the neural blockade and hemodynamic changes following epidural anesthesia with ropivacaine. *Anesth Analg* 2002;94:1325.

174. Simon MJG, Veering BT, Burm AGL, et al. The effect of age on the clinical profile and the systemic absorption and disposition of levobupivacaine following epidural anaesthesia. *Br J Anaesth* 2004;93:512.

175. Juelsgaard P, Sand NP, Felsby S, et al. Perioperative myocardial ischaemia in patients undergoing surgery for fractured hip randomized to incremental spinal, single-dose spinal or general anaesthesia. *Eur J Anaesthesiol* 1998;15:656.

176. Racle JP, Poy JY, Haberer JP, Benkhadra AA. comparison of cardiovascular responses of normotensive and hypertensive elderly patients following bupivacaine spinal anesthesia. *Reg Anesth* 1989;14:66.

177. Tanaka M, Nishikawa T. Aging reduces the efficacy of the simulated epidural test dose in anesthetized adults. *Anesth Analg* 2000;91:657.

178. Hirabayashi Y, Shimizu R, Matsuda I, Inoue S. Effect of extradural compliance and resistance on spread of extradural analgesia. *Br J Anaesth* 1990;65:508.

179. Dorfman LJ, Bosley TM. Age-related changes in peripheral and central nerve conduction in man. *Neurology* 1979;29:38.

180. Vestal RE, Wood AJJ, Shand DG. Reduced beta-adrenoceptor sensitivity in the elderly. *Clin Pharmacol Ther* 1979;26:181.

181. Okada A, Harata S, Takeda Y, et al. Age-related changes in proteoglycans of human ligamentum flavum. *Spine* 1993;18:2261.

182. Frank SM, Shir Y, Raja SN, et al. Core hypothermia and skin surface temperature gradients. Epidural versus general anesthesia and the effects of age. *Anesthesiology* 1994;80:502.

183. Park WY, Hagins FM, Massengale MD, MacNamara Y. The sitting positions and anesthetic spread in the epidural space. *Anesth Analg* 1984;63:863.

184. Hodgkinson R, Husain FJ. Obesity gravity and spread of epidural anesthesia. *Anesth Analg* 1981;60:421.

185. Bromage PR. Spread of analgesic solutions in the epidural space and their site of action: A statistical study. *Br J Anaesth* 1962;34:161.

186. Apostolou GA, Zarmakoupis PK, Mastrokostopoulos GT. Spread of epidural anesthesia and the lateral position. *Anesth Analg* 1981;60:584.

187. Grundy EM, Rao LN, Winnie AP. Epidural anesthesia and the lateral position. *Anesth Analg* 1978;57:95.

188. Seow LT, Lips FJ, Cousins MJ. Effect of lateral posture on epidural blockade for surgery. *Anaesth Intensive Care* 1983;11:97.

189. Gissen AJ, Datta S, Lambert D. The chloroprocaine controversy. *Reg Anesth* 1984;9:124.

190. Low PA. Endoneural fluid pressure and microenvironment of nerve. In: Dyck PJ, Thomas PK, Lambert EH, Bunge R, eds. *Peripheral Neuropathy.* Philadelphia: W. B. Saunders; 1984:599.

191. Clarke CJ, Whitewell J. Intradural haemorrhage after epidural injection. *Br Med J* 1961;2:1612.

192. Erdemir HA, Soper LE, Sweet RB. Studies of factors affecting peridural anesthesia. *Anesth Analg* 1965;44:400.

193. Löfström B. Blocking characteristics of etidocaine (Duranest). *Acta Anaesthesiol Scand* 1975;60[Suppl]:21.

194. Casati A, Putzu M. Bupivacaine, levobupivacaine and ropivacaine: Are they clinically different? *Best Pract Res Clin Anaesthesiol* 2005;19:247.

195. McClellan KJ, Faulds D. Ropivacaine: An update of its use in regional anaesthesia. *Drugs* 2000;60:1065.

196. Whiteside JB, Wildsmith JAW. Developments in local anaesthetics drugs. *Br J Anaesth* 2001;87:27.

197. Ohmura S, Kawada M, Ohta T, et al. Systemic toxicity and resuscitation in bupivacaine-, levobupivacaine-, or ropivacaine-infused rats. *Anesth Analg* 2001;93:743.

198. Nancarrow C, Rutten AJ, Runciman WB, et al. Myocardial and cerebral drug concentrations and the mechanisms of death after intravenous doses of lignocaine, bupivacaine, and ropivacaine in the sheep. *Anesth Analg* 1989;69:276–283.

199. Scott DB, Lee A, Fagan D, et al. Acute toxicity of ropivacaine compared with that of bupivacaine. *Anesth Analg* 1989;69:563.

200. Knudsen K, Beckman Suurküla M, Blomberg S., et al. Central nervous and cardiovascular effects of i.v. infusions of ropivacaine, bupivacaine and placebo in volunteers. *Br J Anaesth* 1997;78:507.

201. Brockway MS, Bannister JP, McClure JH, et al. Comparison of extradural ropivacaine and bupivacaine. *Br J Anaesth* 1991;66:31.

202. Cederholm J, Anskar S, Bengtsson M. Sensory, motor, and sympathetic lock during epidural analgesia with 0.5% and 0.75% ropivacaine with and without epinephrine. *Reg Anesth* 1994;19:18.

203. Zaric D, Axelsson K, Nydahl PA, et al. Sensory and motor blockade during epidural analgesia with 1%, 0.75% and 0.5% ropivacaine: A double-blind study. *Anesth Analg* 1991;72:509.

204. Wolff AP, Hasselstrom L, Kerkkamp HE, Gielen MJ. Extradural ropivacaine and bupivacaine in hip surgery. *Br J Anaesth* 1995;74:458.

205. Mazoit JX, Decaux A, Bouaziz H, Edouard A. Comparative ventricular electrophysiologic effect of racemic bupivacaine, levobupivacaine and ropivacaine on the isolated rabbit heart. *Anesthesiology* 2000;93:784.

206. Huang YF, Pryor ME, Mather LE, et al. Cardiovascular and central nervous system effects of intravenous levobupivacaine and bupivacaine in sheep. *Anesth Analg* 1998;86:797.

207. Gristwood RW, Greaves JL. Levobupivacaine: A new safer long acting local anaesthetic agent. *Expert Opin Invest Drug* 1999;8:861–876.

208. Bardsley H, Gristwood R, Baker H, et al. A comparison of the cardiovascular effects of levobupivacaine and rac-bupivacaine following intravenous administration to healthy volunteers. *Br J Clin Pharmacol* 1998;46:245.

209. Cox CR, Faccenda KA, Gilhooly C, et al. Extradural S(-)-bupivacaine: Comparison with racemic RS-bupivacaine. *Br J Anaesth* 1998;80:289.

210. Peduto VA, Baroncini S, Montanini S, et al. A prospective, randomized, double-blind comparison of epidural levobupivacaine 0.5% with epidural ropivacaine 0.75% for lower limb procedures. *Eur J Anaesthesiol* 2003;20:979.

211. Casati A, Santorsola R, Aldegheri G, et al. Intraoperative epidural anesthesia and postoperative analgesia with levobupivacaine for major orthopedic surgery: A double-blind, randomized comparison of racemic bupivacaine and levobupivacaine. *J Clin Anesth* 2003;15:126.

212. Kopacz DJ, Helman JD, Nussbaum CE, et al. A comparison of epidural levobupivacaine 0.5% with or without epinephrine for lumbar spine surgery. *Anesth Analg* 2001;93:755.

213. Cohen SE, Thurlow A. Comparison of a chloroprocaine-bupivacaine mixture with chloroprocaine and bupivacaine used individually for obstetric epidural analgesia. *Anesthesiology* 1979;51:288.

214. Corke BG, Carlson CG, Dettbarn WD. The influence of 2-chloroprocaine on the subsequent analgesic potency of bupivacaine. *Anesthesiology* 1984;60:25.

215. Seow LT, Lips FJ, Cousins MJ, Mather LE. Lidocaine and bupivacaine mixtures for epidural blockade. *Anesthesiology* 1982;56:177.

216. Bromage PR, Burfoot MF, Crowell DF, Pettigrew RT. Quality of epidural blockade. I. Influence of physical factors. *Br J Anaesth* 1964;36:342.

217. Bridenbaugh PO, Tucker GT, Moore DC, et al. Role of epinephrine in regional block anesthesia with etidocaine: A double-blind study. *Anesth Analg* 1974;53:430.

218. Murphy TM, Mather LE, Stanton-Hicks MD, et al. Effects of adding adrenaline to etidocaine and lignocaine in extradural anaesthesia. I. Block characteristics and cardiovascular effects. *Br J Anaesth* 1976;48:893.

219. Bromage PR, Camporesi EM, Durant PA, et al. Influence of epinephrine as an adjuvant to epidural morphine. *Anesthesiology* 1983;58:257–262.

220. Curatolo M, Petersen-Felix S, Arendt-Nielsen L, et al. Epidural epinephrine and clonidine: Segmental analgesia and effects on different pain modalities. *Anesthesiology* 1997;87:785–794.

221. Reddy SVR, Yaksh TL. Spinal noradrenergic terminal system mediates antinociception. *Brain Res* 1980;189:391.

222. Carabine UA, Milligan K, Moore J. Extradural clonidine and bupivacaine for postoperative analgesia. *Br J Anaesth* 1992;68:132.

223. Dobrydnjov I, Axelsson K, Gupta A, et al. Improved analgesia with clonidine when added to local anesthetic during combined spinal-epidural anesthesia for hip arthroplasty: A double-blind, randomized and placebo-controlled study. *Acta Anaesthesiol Scand* 2005;49:538.

224. Zeilhofer HU, Swandulla D, Geisslinger G, Brune K. Differential effects of ketamine enantiomers on NMDA receptor currents in cultures neurons. *Eur J Pharmacol* 1992;213:155.

225. Yanli Y. The effect of extradural ketamine on onset time and sensory block in extradural anesthesia with bupivacaine. *Anesthesia* 1996;51:84.

226. Himmelseher S, Ziegler-Pithamitsis D, Argiriadou H, et al. Small-dose S(+)-ketamine reduces postoperative pain when applied with ropivacaine in epidural anesthesia for total knee arthroplasty. *Anesth Analg* 2001;92:1290.

227. Gordh T Jr., Jansson I, Hartvig P, et al. Interactions between noradrenergic and cholinergic mechanisms involved in spinal nociceptive processing. *Acta Anaesthesiol Scand* 1989;33:39.

228. Lauretti GR, de Oliveira R, Reis MP, et al. Study of three different doses of epidural neostigmine coadministered with lidocaine for postoperative analgesia. *Anesthesiology* 1999;90:534.

229. Bromage PR. *Spinal Epidural Analgesia*. Edinburgh: E&S Livingstone, 1954.
230. Bromage PR, Pettigrew RT, Crowell DE. Tachyphylaxis in epidural analgesia. I. Augmentation and decay of local anesthesia. *J Clin Pharmacol* 1969; 9:30.
231. Tuohy EB. Continuous spinal anesthesia: A new method of utilising a ureteral catheter. *Surg Clin North Am* 1945;25:834.
232. Doughty A. A precise method of cannulating the lumbar epidural space. *Anaesthesia* 1974;29:63.
233. Lee JA. Specially marked needle to facilitate extradural block. *Anaesthesia* 1960;15:186.
234. Cheng PA. Blunt-tip needle for epidural anesthesia. *Anesthesiology* 1958; 19:556.
235. Corning JL. Spinal anaesthesia and local medication of the cord. *NY Med J* 1885;42:483.
236. Winnie AP. A grip to facilitate the insertion of epidural needles. *Anesth Analg* 1971;50:23.
237. Dawkins CJM. The identification of the epidural space. A critical analysis of the various methods employed. *Anaesthesia* 1963;18:66.
238. Katz H, Borden H, Hirscher D. Glass-particle contamination of color-break ampules. *Anesthesiology* 1973;39:354.
239. Vandermeersch E. Combined spinal-epidural anaesthesia. In: Van Aken H, ed. *New Developments in Epidural and Spinal Drugs Administration*. London: Bailliere Tindall; 1993:691.
240. Rawal N, Schollin J, Wesstrom G. Epidural versus combined spinal epidural block for caesarean section. *Acta Anaesthesiol Scand* 1988;32:61.
241. Brownridge P. Epidural and subarachnoid analgesia for elective cesarean section. *Anaesthesia* 1981;36:70.
242. Coates MB. Combined subarachnoid and epidural techniques. *Anaesthesia* 1982;37:89.
243. Joshi GP, McCarroll SM. Evaluation of combined spinal-epidural anesthesia using two different techniques. *Reg Anesth* 1994;19:169.
244. Eldor J. Metallic particles in the spinal-epidural needle technique. Letter to the Editor. *Reg Anesth* 1994;19:219.
245. Holmdahl MH, Sjögren S, Strom G, Wright B. Clinical aspects of continuous epidural blockade for postoperative pain relief. *Ups J Med Sci* 1972;77:47.
246. Moore DC. *Regional Block*, 4th ed. Springfield: Charles C Thomas, 1976.
247. Abbott MA, Samuel JR, Webb DR. Anaesthesia for extracorporeal shock wave lithotripsy. *Anaesthesia* 1985;40:1065.
248. Bridenbaugh LD, Moore DC, Bagdi P, Bridenbaugh PO. The position of plastic tubing in continuous block techniques: An x-ray study of 552 patients. *Anesthesiology* 1968;29:1047.
249. Sanchez R, Acuna L, Rocha F. An analysis of the radiological visualization of the catheters placed in the epidural space. *Br J Anaesth* 1967;39:485.
250. Shanks CA. Four cases of unilateral analgesia. *Br J Anaesth* 1968;40:999.
251. South Australian Health Commission, 1985. Report of the Anaesthetics Mortality Committee. Anaesthetic Deaths in South Australia, 1974–1983.
252. Usubiaga JE. Neurological complications following epidural anesthesia. *Int Anaesthesiol Clin* 1975;13:2.
253. Catterberg J. Local anesthetic vs. spinal fluid. *Anesthesiology* 1977;46:309.
254. Gavin R. Continuous epidural analgesia, an unusual case of dural perforation during catheterisation of the epidural space. *N Z Med J* 1965;64:280.
255. Ackerman WE, Mustaque Juneja MM, Kaczorowski DO. The accuracy of using thiopental or test strips to detect dural puncture during continuous epidural analgesia. *Reg Anesth* 1988;13:169.
256. Groban L, Deal DD, Vernon JC, et al. Cardiac resuscitation after incremental overdosage with lidocaine, bupivacaine, levobupivacaine, and ropivacaine in anesthetized dogs. *Anesth Analg* 2001;92:37–43.
257. Heavner JE, Pitkanen MT, Shi B, Rosenberg PH. Resuscitation from bupivacaine-induced asystole in rats: Comparison of different cardioactive drugs. *Anesth Analg* 1995;80:1134–1139.
258. Weinberg G, Ripper R, Feinstein DL, et al. Lipid emulsion infusion rescues dogs from bupivacaine-induced cardiac toxicity. *Reg Anesth Pain Med* 2003;28:198–202.
259. Rosenblatt MA, Abel M, Fischer GW, et al. Successful use of a 20% lipid emulsion to resuscitate a patient after a presumed bupivacaine-related cardiac arrest. *Anesthesiology* 2006;105:217–218.
260. Litz RJ, Popp M, Stehr SN, Koch T. Successful resuscitation of a patient with ropivacaine-induced asystole after axillary plexus block. *Anaesthesia* 2006;61:800–801.
261. Foxal G, McCahon R, Lamb J, et al. Levobupivacaine-induced seizures and cardiovascular collapse treated with Intralipid. *Anaesthesia* 2007;62:516–518.
262. Kalas DB, Hehre EW. Continuous lumbar peridural anesthesia in obstetrics. VIII. Further observations on inadvertent lumbar puncture. *Anesth Analg* 1972;51:192.
263. Philip JH, Brown WU. Total spinal anesthesia late in the course of obstetric bupivacaine epidural block. *Anesthesiology* 1976;44:340.
264. Boys JE, Norman PF. Accidental subdural analgesia. *Br J Anaesth* 1975;47:1111.
265. Stevens RA, Stanton-Hicks MD. Subdural injection of local anesthetic: A complication of epidural anesthesia. *Anesthesiology* 1985;63:323.
266. Cohen CA, Kallos T. Failure of spinal anesthesia due to subdural catheter placement. *Anesthesiology* 1972;37:352.
267. Hylton RR, Eger EI, Rovno SH. Intravascular placement of epidural catheters. *Anesth Analg* 1964;43:379.
268. Ryan DW. Accidental intravenous injection of bupivacaine: A complication of obstetrical epidural anaesthesia. *Br J Anaesth* 1973;45:907.
269. Verniquet AJW. Vessel puncture with epidural catheters. Experience in obstetric patients. *Anaesthesia* 1980;35:660.
270. Lerner SM, Gutterman P, Jenkins F. Epidural hematoma and paraplegia after numerous lumbar punctures. *Anesthesiology* 1973;39:550.
271. De Angelis J. Hazards of subdural and epidural anesthesia during anticoagulant therapy: A case report and review. *Anesth Analg* 1972;51:676.
272. Gingrich TF. Spinal epidural hematoma following continuous epidural anesthesia. *Anesthesiology* 1968;29:162.
273. Coupland GAE, Reeve TS. Paraplegia: A complication of excision of abdominal aortic aneurysm. *Surgery* 1968;64:878.
274. Blomberg RG, Olsson SS. The lumbar epidural space in patients examined with epiduroscopy. *Anesth Analg* 1989;68:157.
275. Yin EI, Wessler S, Butler JV. Plasma heparin: A unique, practical, submicrogram sensitive assay. *J Lab Clin Med* 1973;81:298.
276. James FM, George RH, Haiem H, White GJ. Bacteriologic aspects of epidural analgesia. *Anesth Analg* 1976;55:187.
277. Abouleish E, Amortegui AJ, Taylor FH. Are bacterial filters needed in continuous epidural analgesia for obstetrics? *Anesthesiology* 1977;46:351.
278. Katz H, Borden H, Hirscher D. Glass-particle contamination of color-break ampules. *Anesthesiology* 1973;39:354.
279. Baker AS, Ojemann RG, Swartz MN, Richardson EP. Spinal epidural abscess. *N Engl J Med* 1975;293:463.
280. Schreiner EJ, Lipson SF, Bromage PR, Camporesi EM. Neurological complications following general anaesthesia. *Anaesthesia* 1983;38:226.
281. Scott DB, Walker LR. Administration of continuous epidural analgesia. *Anaesthesia* 1963;18:82.
282. Durant PA, Yaksh TL. Epidural injections of bupivacaine, morphine, fentanyl, lofentanil, and DADL in chronically implanted rats: A pharmacologic and pathologic study. *Anesthesiology* 1986;64:43.
283. Crawford JS. The prevention of headache consequent upon dural puncture. *Br J Anaesth* 1972;44:598.
284. Cathelin MF. Une nouvelle voie d'injection rachidienne: Methôde des injections épidurales pas le procède du canal sacré. *CR Soc Biol (Paris)* 1901;53:452.
285. Black MG. Anatomic reasons for caudal anesthesia failure. *Anesth Analg* 1949;28:33.
286. Cousins MJ, Bromage PR. A comparison of the hydrochloride and carbonated salts of lignocaine for caudal analgesia in outpatients. *Br J Anaesth* 1971;43:1149.
287. McGown RG. Caudal analgesia in children. *Anaesthesia* 1982;37:806.
288. Camboulives J, Couvely JP, Alphonsi R, Unal D. Plasma determination of lidocaine and bupivacaine after caudal anesthesia in children. *Ann Fr Anesth Reanim* 1986;5:115.
289. Ecoffey C, Desparmet J, Berdeaux A, et al. Pharmacokinetics of lignocaine in children following caudal anaesthesia. *Br J Anaesth* 1984;56:1399.
290. Ecoffey C, Desparmet J, Maury M, et al. Bupivacaine in children: Pharmacokinetics following caudal anesthesia. *Anesthesiology* 1985;63:447.
291. Freund PR, Bowdle TA, Slattery JT, Bell LE. Caudal anesthesia with lidocaine or bupivacaine: Plasma local anesthetic concentration and extent of sensory spread in old and young patients. *Anesth Analg* 1984;63:1017.
292. Mazze RI, Dunbar RW. Plasma lidocaine concentrations after caudal, lumbar epidural, axillary block, and intravenous regional anesthesia. *Anesthesiology* 1966;27:574.
293. Lönnqvist PA, Westrin P, Larsson BA, et al. Ropivacaine pharmacokinetics after caudal block in 1–8 year old children. *Br J Anaesth* 2000;85:506–511.
294. Chalkiadis GA, Eyres RL, Cranswick N, et al. Pharmacokinetics of levobupivacaine 0.25% following caudal administration in children under 2 years of age. *Br J Anaesth* 2004;92:218–222.
295. Chalkiadis GA, Anderson BJ, Tay M, et al. Pharmacokinetics of levobupivacaine after caudal epidural administration in infants less than 3 months of age. *Br J Anaesth* 2005;95:524–529.
296. Takasaki M, Dohi S, Kawabata Y, Takahashi T. Dosage of lidocaine for caudal anesthesia in infants and children. *Anesthesiology* 1977;47:527.
297. Mazoit JX, Denson DD, Samii K. Pharmacokinetics of bupivacaine following caudal anesthesia in infants. *Anesthesiology* 1988;68:387.
298. Warner MA, Kunkel SE, Offord KO. The effects of age, epinephrine, and operative site on duration of caudal analgesia in pediatric patients. *Anesth Analg* 1987;66:995.
299. Galindo A, Benavides O, Ortega De Munos S, et al. Comparison of anesthetic solutions used in lumbar and caudal peridural anesthesia. *Anesth Analg* 1978;57:175.
300. Busoni P, Sarti A. Sacral intervertebral epidural block. *Anesthesiology* 1987;67:993.
301. Seow LT, Chiu HH, Tye CY. Clinical evaluation of etidocaine in continuous caudal analgesia for pelvic floor repair and postoperative pain relief. *Anaesth Intensive Care* 1976;4:239.

302. Takasaki M. Blood concentrations of lidocaine, mepivacaine and bupivacaine during caudal analgesia in children. *Acta Anaesthesiol Scand* 1984; 28:211.
303. Park WY, Massengale M, MacNamara TE. Age, height, and speed of injection as factors determining caudal anesthetic level, and occurrence of severe hypertension. *Anesthesiology* 1979;51:81.
304. Williams NE, Hardy PA, Evans AF. Spread of local anaesthetic solutions following sacral extradural (caudal) block: Influence of posture. *J Spinal Disord* 1989;2:249.
305. Schulte-Steinberg O, Rahlfs VW. Caudal anaesthesia in children and spread of 1 percent lignocaine: A statistical study. *Br J Anaesth* 1970;42:1093.
306. Schulte-Steinberg O, Rahlfs VW. Spread of extradural analgesia following caudal injection in children: A statistical study. *Br J Anaesth* 1977;49:1027.
307. Bromage PR. *Epidural Analgesia*. Philadelphia, W. B. Saunders, 1978.
308. Armitage EN. Caudal block in children. *Anaesthesia* 1979;34:396.
309. Busoni P, Andreuccetti T. The spread of caudal analgesia in children: A mathematical model. *Anaesth Intensive Care* 1986;14:140.
310. Moore DC, Bridenbaugh LD, Bagdi PA, Bridenbaugh PO. Accumulation of mepivacaine hydrochloride during caudal block. *Anesthesiology* 1968;29:585.
311. Mohan J, Potter JM. Pupillary constriction and ptosis following caudal epidural analgesia. *Anaesthesia* 1975;30:769.
312. Payen D, Ecoffey C, Carli P, Dubousset AM. Pulsed Doppler ascending aortic, carotid, brachial and femoral artery blood flows during caudal anesthesia in infants. *Anesthesiology* 1987;67:681.
313. Giaufre E, Conte-Devolx B, Morrison-Lacombe G, et al. Caudal epidural anesthesia in children: Study of endocrine changes. *Presse Med* 1985;14:201.
314. Nakamura T, Takasaki M. Metabolic and endocrine responses to surgery during caudal analgesia in children. *Can J Anaesth* 1991;38:969.
315. Owens WD, Slater EM, Battit GE. A new technique of caudal anesthesia. *Anesthesiology* 1973;39:451.
316. McCaul K. Caudal blockade. In: Cousins MJ, Bridenbaugh PO, eds. *Neural Blockade in Clinical Anesthesia and Management of Pain*, 1st ed. Philadelphia: J. B. Lippincott; 1980:275–293.
317. Bollinger D, Mayne P. The "whoosh" test in children (letter). *Anaesthesia* 1992;47:1002.
318. Lewis MP, Thomas P, Wilson LF, Mulholland RC. The "whoosh" test: A clinical test to confirm correct needle placement in caudal epidural injections. *Anaesthesia* 1992;47:57.
319. Chan SY, Tay HB, Thomas E. "Whoosh" test as a teaching aid in caudal block. *Anaesth Intensive Care* 1993;21:414.
320. Guinard JP, Borboen M. Probable venous air embolism during caudal anesthesia in a child. *Anesth Analg* 1993;76:1134.
321. Bonica JJ. *Principles and Practice of Obstetric Analgesia and Anesthesia*. Philadelphia: F. A. Davis, 1967.
322. Bosenberg AT, Bland BA, Schulte-Steinberg O, Downing JW. Thoracic epidural anesthesia via caudal route in infants. *Anesthesiology* 1988;69:265.
323. Gunter JB, Eng C. Thoracic epidural anesthesia via the caudal approach in children. *Anesthesiology* 1992;76:935.
324. Zaaijman JD, Slabber CF. The position of epidural catheters in obstetric regional anaesthesia. *S Afr Med J* 1979;55:915.
325. Hingson RA, Edwards WB. Continuous caudal analgesia: An analysis of the first ten thousand confinements thus managed with the report of the authors' first thousand cases. *JAMA* 1943;123:538.
326. Fernandez-Sepulveda R, Gomez-Rogers C. Single dose caudal anesthesia: Its effect on uterine contractility. *Am J Obstet Gynecol* 1967;98:847.
327. Hingson RA, Cull WA, Benzinger M. Continuous caudal analgesia in obstetrics: Combined experience of a quarter of a century in clinics in New York, Philadelphia, Memphis, Baltimore, and Cleveland. *Anesth Analg* 1961;40:119.
328. Alexander JA, Franklin RR. Effects of caudal anesthesia on uterine activity. *Obstet Gynecol* 1966;27:436.
329. Tyack AG, Parsons RJ, Millar DR, Nicholas ADG. Uterine activity and plasma bupivacaine levels after caudal epidural analgesia. *J Obstet Gynaecol Br Common W* 1973;80:896.
330. Hansen JM, Ueland K. The influence of caudal analgesia on cardiovascular dynamics during normal labour and delivery. *Acta Anaesthesiol Scand* 1966;23[Suppl]:449.
331. Ueland K, Hansen JM. Maternal cardiovascular dynamics III: Labour and delivery under local and caudal analgesia. *Am J Obstet Gynecol* 1969;103:8.
332. Gunther RE, Bellville JW. Obstetrical caudal anesthesia: II. A randomized study comparing 1 percent mepivacaine with 1 percent mepivacaine plus epinephrine. *Anesthesiology* 1972;37:288.
333. Finster M, Poppers PJ, Sinclair JC, et al. Accidental intoxication of the fetus with local anesthetic drug during caudal anesthesia. *Am J Obstet Gynecol* 1965;92:922.
334. Sinclair JC, Fox HA, Lentz JF, et al. Intoxication of the fetus by a local anesthetic: A newly recognized complication of maternal caudal anesthesia. *N Engl J Med* 1965;273:1173.
335. Abouleish E. *Pain Control in Obstetrics*. Philadelphia: J. B. Lippincott; 1977:285.
336. Cleland JGP. Continuous peridural and caudal analgesia in obstetrics. *Anesth Analg* 1949;28:61.
337. Paull JD. The place of caudal anaesthesia in obstetrics. *Anaesth Intensive Care* 1990;18:313.
338. Spiegel P. Caudal anesthesia in pediatric surgery: A preliminary report. *Anesth Analg* 1962;41:218.
339. Dalens B, Hasnaoui A. Caudal anesthesia in pediatric surgery: Success rate and adverse effects in 750 consecutive patients. *Anesth Analg* 1989;68:83.
340. Veyckemans F, Van Obbergh LJ, Gouverneur JM. Lessons from 1,100 pediatric caudal blocks in a teaching hospital. *Reg Anesth* 1992;17:119.
341. Fortuna A. Caudal analgesia: A simple and safe technique in paediatric surgery. *Br J Anaesth* 1967;39:165.
342. Hassan SZ. Caudal anesthesia in infants. *Anesth Analg* 1977;56:686.
343. Giaufre E, Le Gal M, Trinquet F. Clinical study of EMLA analgesic cream in pediatric regional anesthesia. *Ann Fr Anesth Reanim* 1992;11:384.
344. Watcha MF, Thach BT, Gunter JB. Postoperative apnea after caudal anesthesia in an ex-premature infant. *Anesthesiology* 1989;71:613.
345. Gunter JB, Watcha MF, Forestner JB, et al. Caudal epidural anesthesia in conscious premature and high-risk infants. *J Pediatr Surg* 1991;26:9.
346. Henderson K, Sethna NF, Berde CB. Continuous caudal anesthesia for inguinal hernia repair in former preterm infants. *J Clin Anesth* 1993;5:129.
347. Peutrell JM, Hughes DG. Epidural anaesthesia through caudal catheters for inguinal herniotomies in awake ex-premature babies. *Anaesthesia* 1993;48:128.
348. Spear RM, Deshpande JKM, Maxwell LG. Caudal anesthesia in the awake high-risk infant. *Anesthesiology* 1988;69:407.
349. Tobias JD, Flannagan J, Brock J, Brin E. Neonatal regional anesthesia: Alternative to general anesthesia for urologic surgery. *Urology* 1993;41:362.
350. Touloukian RJ, Wugmeister M, Pickett LK, Hehre FW. Caudal anesthesia for neonatal anoperineal and rectal operations. *Anesth Analg* 1971;50:565.
351. Alexander C, Wolf S, Ghia JN. Caudal anesthesia for early onset myotonic dystrophy. *Anesthesiology* 1981;55:597.
352. Bray RJ, Inkster JS. Anaesthesia in babies with congenital dystrophia myotonica. *Anaesthesia* 1984;39:1007.
353. Kay B. Caudal block for postoperative pain relief in children. *Anaesthesia* 1974;29:610.
354. Lunn JN. Postoperative analgesia after circumcision: A randomized comparison between caudal analgesia and intramuscular morphine in boys. *Anaesthesia* 1979;34:552.
355. Martin LV. Postoperative analgesia after circumcision in children. *Br J Anaesth* 1982;54:1263.
356. May AE, Wandless J, James RH. Analgesia for circumcision in children. A comparison of caudal bupivacaine and intramuscular buprenorphine. *Acta Anaesthesiol Scand* 1982;26:331.
357. Yeoman PM, Cooke R, Hain WR. Penile block for circumcision: A comparison with caudal blockade. *Anaesthesia* 1983;38:862.
358. Bramwell RG, Bullen C, Radford P. Caudal block for postoperative analgesia in children. *Anaesthesia* 1982;37:1024.
359. Schindler M, Swann M, Crawford M. A comparison of postoperative analgesia provided by wound infiltration or caudal anaesthesia. *Anaesth Intensive Care* 1991;19:46.
360. White J, Harrison B, Richmond P, et al. Postoperative analgesia for circumcision. *Br Med J* 1983;286:1934.
361. Breschan C, Jost R, Krumpholz R, et al. A prospective study comparing the analgesic efficacy of levobupivacaine, ropivacaine and bupivacaine in pediatric patients undergoing caudal blockade. *Paediatr Anaesth* 2005;15:301–306.
362. Ivani G, De Negri P, Lonnqvist PA, et al. A comparison of three concentrations of levobupivacaine for caudal block in children. *Anesth Analg* 2003;97:368–371.
363. McCloskey JJ, Haun SE, Deshpande JK. Bupivacaine toxicity secondary to continuous caudal epidural infusion in children. *Anesth Analg* 1992;75:287.
364. Berde CB. Convulsions associated with pediatric regional anesthesia. *Anesth Analg* 1992;75:164.
365. Jamali S, Monin S, Begon C, et al. Clonidine in pediatric caudal anesthesia. *Anesth Analg* 1994;786:633.
366. Naguib M, Sharif AM, Seraj M, et al. Ketamine for caudal analgesia in children: Comparison with caudal bupivacaine. *Br J Anaesth* 1991;67:559.
367. De Negri P, Ivani G, Visconti C, et al. How long to prolong postoperative analgesia after caudal anaesthesia with ropivacaine in children. S-ketamine versus clonidine. *Paediatr Anaesth* 2001;11:679–683.
368. Berstock DA. Haemorrhoidectomy without tears. *Ann R Coll Surg Engl* 1979;61:51.
369. McCrirrick A, Ramage DT. Caudal blockade for postoperative analgesia: A useful adjunct to intramuscular opiates following emergency lower leg orthopaedic surgery. *Anaesth Intensive Care* 1991;19:551.
370. Cyriax JH. *Textbook of Orthopaedic Medicine. Diagnosis of Soft Tissue Lesions*, Vol. 1. London: Bailliere Tindall, 1978.
371. Gordon J. Caudal extradural injection for the treatment of low back pain. *Anaesthesia* 1980;35:515.

372. Natelson SE, Gibson CE, Gillespie RA. Caudal block: Cost-effective primary treatment for back pain. *South Med J* 1980;73:286.

373. Sharma PK. Indications, technique and results of caudal epidural injection for lumbar disc retropulsion. *Postgrad Med J* 1977;53:1.

374. Hauswirth R, Michot F. Sacral epidural anesthesia in the treatment of lumbosacral backache. *Schweiz Med Wochenschr* 1982;112:222.

375. Boskovski N, Lewinski A, Xuereb J, Mercieca V. Caudal epidural morphine for postoperative pain relief. *Anesthesia* 1981;36:67.

376. Jensen BH. Caudal block for post-operative pain relief in children after genital operations: A comparison between bupivacaine and morphine. *Acta Anaesthesiol Scand* 1981;25:373.

377. Jensen PJ, Siem-Jorgensen P, Nielsen TB, Wichmand-Nielson H. Epidural morphine by the caudal route for postoperative pain relief. *Acta Anaesthesiol Scand* 1982;26:511.

378. Pybus DA, Dubras BE, Goulding G, et al. Post-operative analgesia for haemorrhoid surgery. *Anaesth Intensive Care* 1983;11:27.

379. Krane EJ, Jacobsen LE, Lynn AM, et al. Caudal morphine for postoperative analgesia in children: A comparison with caudal bupivacaine and intravenous morphine. *Anesth Analg* 1987;66:647.

380. Rosen KR, Rosen DA. Caudal epidural morphine for control of pain following open heart surgery in children. *Anesthesiology* 1989;70:418.

381. Wolf AR, Hughes D, Hobbs AJ, Prys-Roberts C. Combined morphine–bupivacaine caudals for reconstructive penile surgery in children: Systemic absorption of morphine and postoperative analgesia. *Anaesth Intensive Care* 1991;19:17.

382. Vetter T, Carvallo D, Johnson JL, et al. A comparison of single-dose caudal clonidine, morphine, or hydromorphone combined with ropivacaine in pediatric patients undergoing urethral reimplantation. *Anesth Analg* 2007;104:1356–1363.

383. Girotra S, Kumar S, Rajendran KM. Comparison of caudal morphine and buprenorphine for postoperative analgesia in children. *Eur J Anaesthesiol* 1993;10:309.

384. Campbell FA, Yentis SM, Fear DW, Bissonnette B. Analgesic efficacy and safety of a caudal bupivacaine–fentanyl mixture in children. *Can J Anaesth* 1992;39:661.

385. Jones RD, Gunawardene WM, Yeung CK. A comparison of lignocaine 2% with adrenaline 1:200,000 and lignocaine 2% with adrenaline 1:200,000 plus fentanyl as agents for caudal anaesthesia in children undergoing circumcision. *Anaesth Intensive Care* 1990;18:194.

386. Kawaraguchi Y, Otomo T, Uchida N, et al. A prospective, double-blind, randomized trial of caudal block using ropivacaine 0.2% with or without fentanyl 1 μg kg in children. *Br J Anaesth* 2006;97:858–861.

387. Krane EJ. Delayed respiratory depression in a child after caudal epidural morphine. *Anesth Analg* 1988;67:79.

388. Stienstra R, Van Poorten F. Immediate respiratory arrest after caudal epidural sufentanil. *Anesthesiology* 1989;71:993.

389. Valley RD, Bailey RG. Caudal morphine for postoperative analgesia in infants: A report of 138 cases. *Anesth Analg* 1991;72:120.

390. Hirlekar G. Is itching after caudal epidural morphine dose related? *Anaesthesia* 1981;36:68.

391. DeJong RH. Anesthetic complications during continuous caudal analgesia for obstetrics: Analysis of 826 cases. *Anesth Analg* 1961;40:384.

392. Dawkins CJM. An analysis of the complications of extradural and caudal block. *Anaesthesia* 1969;24:554.

393. Prentiss JE. Cardiac arrest following caudal anesthesia. *Anesthesiology* 1979;50:51.

394. Freid EB, Bailey AG, Valley RD. Electrocardiographic and haemodynamic changes associated with unintentional intravascular injection of bupivacaine with adrenaline in infants. *Anesthesiology* 1993;79:394.

395. Ved SA, Pinosky M, Nicodemus H. Ventricular tachycardia and brief cardiovascular collapse in two infants after caudal anesthesia using a bupivacaine–epinephrine solution. *Anesthesiology* 1993;79:1121.

396. McGown RG. Accidental marrow sampling during caudal anaesthesia. *Br J Anaesth* 1972;44:613.

397. DiGiovanni AJ. Inadvertent intraosseous injection: A hazard of caudal anesthesia. *Anesthesiology* 1971;34:92.

398. Weber S. Caudal anesthesia complicated by intraosseous injection in a patient with ankylosing spondylitis. *Anesthesiology* 1985;63:716.

399. Desparmet JF. Total spinal anesthesia after caudal anesthesia in an infant. *Anesth Analg* 1990;70:665.

400. Calder TM, Harris AP. Subdural block during attempted caudal epidural analgesia for labor. *Anesthesiology* 1992;76:316.

401. Chun L, Karp M. Unusual complications from placement of catheters in caudal canal in obstetrical anesthesia. *Anesthesiology* 1966;27:96.

402. Bridenbaugh LD. Catheterization after long- and short-acting local anesthetics for continuous caudal block for vaginal delivery. *Anesthesiology* 1977;46:357.

403. Abouleish E, Orig T, Amortegui AJ. Bacteriologic comparison between epidural and caudal techniques. *Anesthesiology* 1980;53:511.

CHAPTER 12 ■ NEUROLOGIC COMPLICATIONS OF NEURAXIAL BLOCK

TERESE T. HORLOCKER AND DENISE J. WEDEL

Perioperative nerve injuries have long been recognized as a complication of spinal and epidural anesthesia. Neurologic complications associated with neuraxial anesthesia may be divided into two categories: those which are unrelated to the spinal or epidural anesthetic but coincide temporally, and those which are a direct result of the regional technique. Postoperative neurologic injury due to pressure from improper patient positioning or from tightly applied casts or surgical dressings, as well as surgical trauma, are often attributed to the neuraxial anesthetic. For example, Marinacci (1) evaluated 542 patients with postoperative neurologic deficits allegedly caused by spinal anesthesia. In only four cases were the findings related to the spinal anesthetic (cauda equina syndrome, arachnoiditis, and chronic radiculitis). In the remaining 538 patients, the neurologic deficits exhibited an apparent, but not causal relationship to the spinal anesthetic. Marinacci's study demonstrates the difficulty in reporting the actual incidence, pathogenesis, and prognosis of neurologic dysfunction that occurs as a result of spinal or epidural anesthesia.

The etiologies of neurologic complications following neuraxial anesthesia include spinal cord ischemia (hypothesized to be related to the use of vasoconstrictors or prolonged hypotension, as well as expanding spinal hematoma), traumatic injury to the spinal cord or nerve roots during needle or catheter placement, infection (meningitis and epidural abscess), and choice of local anesthetic solution (2–7). Patient factors such as body habitus or a preexisting neurologic dysfunction may also contribute (8,9). The safe conduct of neuraxial anesthesia involves knowledge of the large patient surveys, as well as individual case reports of neurologic deficits following central neural blockade. Prevention of complications, along with early diagnosis and treatment, are important factors in the management of neuraxial anesthetic risks.

Complications of long-term neuraxial analgesia, via intrathecal or epidural infusion of various drugs, are discussed in Chapter 50 (see Figs. 50-1, 50-19, 50-21, 50-22).

INCIDENCE OF NEUROLOGIC COMPLICATIONS

Although severe or disabling neurologic complications are rare, recent epidemiologic series suggest the frequency of some serious complications, including spinal hematoma and central nervous system (CNS) infections, is increasing. A prospective survey in France recently evaluated the incidence and characteristics of serious complications related to regional anesthesia (2). Participating anesthesiologists kept a log of all cases and detailed information of serious complications occurring during or after regional anesthetics. All patients with a neurologic deficit lasting more than 2 days were examined by a neurologist; patients with cauda equina syndrome were evaluated with a computed tomography (CT) scan to rule out compressive etiology. A total of 103,730 regional anesthetics, including 40,640 spinal and 30,413 epidural anesthetics, were performed over a 5–month period. The incidence of cardiac arrest and neurologic complications was significantly higher after spinal anesthesia than other types of regional procedures (Table 12-1). Neurologic recovery was complete within 3 months in 29 of 34 patients with deficits. In 12 of 19 cases of radiculopathy after spinal anesthesia, and in all cases of radiculopathy after epidural or peripheral block, needle placement was associated with either paresthesia during needle insertion or pain with injection. In all cases, the radiculopathy had the same topography as the associated paresthesia. The authors concluded that needle trauma and local anesthetic neurotoxicity were the etiologies of most neurologic complications. In a follow-up investigation performed with similar methodology 5 years later, the investigators reported a slight decrease of neurologic complications related to regional anesthetic technique (10).

An epidemiologic study evaluating severe neurologic complications after neuraxial block conducted in Sweden between 1990 and 1999 reported some disturbing trends (8). During the 10–year study period, approximately 1,260,000 spinal and 450,000 epidural (including 200,000 epidural blocks for labor analgesia) were performed. A total of 127 serious complications were noted, including spinal hematoma (33), cauda equina (32), meningitis (29), and epidural abscess (13) (Table 12-2). The nerve damage was permanent in 85 patients. Complications occurred more often after epidural than spinal blockade, and were different in character: cauda equina syndrome, spinal hematoma, and epidural abscess were more likely to occur after epidural block, whereas meningitis was more often associated with a spinal technique. Undiagnosed spinal stenosis (detected during evaluation of the new neurologic deficits) was a risk factor for cauda equina syndrome and paraparesis with both techniques. In the 18 cases of cauda equina syndrome following spinal anesthesia, 5% hyperbaric lidocaine was administered in eight cases, whereas bupivacaine (hyperbaric or isobaric) was the local anesthetic in 11 cases. This large series suggests that the incidence of severe anesthesia-related complications is not as low as previously reported. Moreover, since serious complications were noted to occur even in the presence of experienced anesthesiologists, continued vigilance in patients undergoing neuraxial anesthesia is warranted.

For example, Cheney and colleagues (11) examined the American Society of Anesthesiologists (ASA) Closed Claims

TABLE 12-1

NUMBER AND INCIDENCE OF SEVERE COMPLICATIONS RELATED TO SPINAL AND EPIDURAL ANESTHESIA

Neuraxial technique	Cardiac arrest	Death	Seizure	Neurologic injury	Radiculopathy	Cauda equina syndrome	Paraplegia
Spinal N = 40,640	26* (3.9–8.9)	6 (0.3–2.7)	0 (0–0.9)	24* (3.5–8.3)	19* (2.6–6.8)	5 (0.1–2.3)	0 (0–0.9)
Epidural N = 30,413	3 (0.2–2.9)	0 (0–1.2)	4 (0.4–3.4)	6 (0.4–3.6)	5 (0.5–3.8)	0 (0–1.2)	1 (0–1.8)

Data presented are number and (95% confidence interval).
*Spinal versus epidural (p <0.05). Adapted from Auroy Y, Narchi P, Messiah A, et al. Serious complications related to regional anesthesia. *Anesthesiology* 1997;87:479–486, with permission.

database to determine the role of nerve damage following regional/pain block or general anesthesia in malpractice claims filed against anesthesia care providers. Of the 4,183 claims reviewed, 670 (16%) were for anesthesia-related nerve injury, including 189 claims involving the lumbosacral roots (105 claims) or spinal cord (84 claims); spinal cord injuries were the leading cause of claims for nerve injury that occurred in the 1990s, whereas previously, injuries to the ulnar nerve or brachial plexus were more common. In addition, lumbosacral nerve root injuries having identifiable etiology were associated predominantly with a regional (compared to general) anesthetic technique (92%), and were related to paresthesias during needle or catheter placement or pain during injection of local anesthetic. Major factors associated with spinal cord injury were blocks for chronic pain management and systemic anticoagulation in the presence of neuraxial block (see also Chapter 50). A more recent Closed Claims analysis of the 1,005 cases of regional anesthesia claims from 1980–1999, reported that the majority of neuraxial complications associated with regional anesthesia claims resulted in permanent neurologic deficits (12). Hematoma was the most common cause of neuraxial injuries, and the majority of these cases were associated with either an intrinsic or iatrogenic coagulopathy; 89% of patients had a permanent deficit. Conversely, complications caused by meningitis or abscess were more likely to be temporary. In a subset comparison of obstetric versus nonobstetric

neuraxial anesthesia claims, obstetrics had a higher proportion of claims with low-severity and temporary injuries.

NERVE INJURY FROM NEEDLE AND CATHETER PLACEMENT

Direct needle- or catheter-induced trauma rarely results in permanent or severe neurologic injury. A recent retrospective study of 4,767 spinal anesthetics noted the presence of a paresthesia during needle placement in 298 (6.3%) of patients. Importantly, four of the six patients with a persistent paresthesia postoperatively complained of a paresthesia during needle placement, identifying elicitation of a paresthesia as a risk factor for a persistent paresthesia (13). In the series by Auroy and colleagues (2), two-thirds of the patients with neurologic complications experienced pain during needle placement or injection of local anesthetic. In all cases, the neurologic deficit had the same distribution as the elicited paresthesia. In addition, the neurologic injury occurred even though the investigators did not continue to inject in the presence of pain. It is unknown whether clinicians should abandon the procedure if a paresthesia is elicited (rather than replacing the needle) in an effort to decrease the risk of nerve injury. This decision is complicated by the series of conus medullaris injuries following spinal (three

TABLE 12-2

COMPLICATIONS ACCORDING TO TYPE OF CENTRAL NEURAXIAL BLOCKADE

	Epidural blockade	Combined spinal epidural blockade	Spinal blockade	Continuous spinal blockade	Total
Spinal hematoma	21	4	7	1	33
Cauda equina syndrome	8	4	18	2	32
Purulent meningitis	5	1	20	3	29
Epidural abscess	12	–	1	–	13
Traumatic cord lesion	8	–	1	–	9
Cranial subdural hematoma	3	–	2	–	5
Paraparesis	3	–	1	–	4
Other	2	–	–	–	2
Total	62	9	50	6	127

Spinal hematoma followed thoracic epidural blockade in eight cases and lumbar epidural blockade in 17 cases. From Moen V, Dahlgren N, Irestedt L. Severe neurological complications after central neuraxial blockades in Sweden 1990–1999. *Anesthesiology* 2004;101:950–959, with permission.

cases) or combined spinal-epidural (four cases) anesthesia using a pencil-point needle reported by Reynolds (14). All seven cases complained of pain on needle insertion (only one noted pain on injection) and suffered damage to more than a single nerve root. In all patients, the anesthesiologist believed needle placement to have occurred at or below L2–L3. A syrinx was noted on magnetic resonance imaging (MRI) in six cases, suggesting intracord injection was the etiology of the deficits. Cases of cord damage from needle insertion were also reported in the series by Auroy and colleagues (10) and Moen and colleagues (8). Importantly, in all cases, the proceduralist had presumed the level of insertion to be below L1. These cases support the recommendation to insert needles below L3 to reduce the risk of direct needle trauma (14,15).

The passage and presence of an indwelling catheter into the subarachnoid or epidural space presents an additional source of direct trauma. However, a lower frequency of persistent paresthesia/radiculopathy occurs following epidural techniques, which are typically associated with catheter placement, compared to single-injection spinal anesthesia (2,10). Although the incidence of neurologic complications associated with thoracic epidural techniques has historically been judged to be higher than that of lumbar placement, Giebler and colleagues (16) noted only a 0.2% incidence of postoperative radicular pain in 4,185 patients undergoing thoracic epidural catheterization; all cases were responsive to catheter removal. Placement of a subarachnoid catheter most likely further increases the risk of neurologic dysfunction. In one study, the incidence of paresthesias was 13% with a single-dose and 30% with a continuous catheter spinal anesthetic (CSA) technique (17). The incidence of postoperative neurologic deficits was also significantly increased following CSA (0.66%) compared to single-dose techniques (0.13%). Laboratory studies have demonstrated demyelination and inflammation adjacent to the catheter tract in both the spinal root and cord of rats following placement of indwelling subarachnoid catheters (18). The use of a catheter may indirectly contribute to neurologic injury. Poor mixing resulting from very slow injection rates through spinal microcatheters may increase the risk of developing high concentrations of hyperbaric local anesthetics in dependent areas of the spinal canal. This is the presumed mechanism of cauda equina syndrome following continuous spinal anesthesia (19–22) (see also the discussion in the section Local Anesthetic Toxicity). In a series of 603 consecutive CSAs, including 127 delivered through a 28-gauge microcatheter, three patients reported pain (persistent paresthesia) postoperatively. In two patients, the symptoms resolved in 4 days; the other patient was discharged 8 days postoperatively with residual foot pain. One patient with aseptic meningitis and one patient with a sensory cauda equina syndrome (still present after 15 months) were also reported (23). A recent multicenter study compared the efficacy and safety of continuous spinal (329 patients) with continuous epidural (100 patients) anesthesia for labor analgesia (24). In the CSA group, sufentanil was continuously infused and bupivacaine administered as a bolus (0.25 mg isobaric bolus, with 1 hour maximum = 7.5 mg). No neurologic complications occurred; however, in 15% of cases, the intrathecal catheters were moderately difficult/difficult to remove and one catheter broke during extraction, leaving a 4-cm remnant in the patient. The catheter was left in situ with no apparent complication. Overall, the initial analgesia was superior in the CSA group, but there were also more technical difficulties and catheter failures, compared to continuous epidural analgesia. Although this study is the largest study to date evaluating spinal microcatheter techniques, the use of an infusion (which potentiates maldistribution) and administration of small (labor analgesia)

doses of local anesthetic does not allow for extrapolation to other patient populations. In addition, the lack of a clear superiority with CSA also suggests that application of this technique may be limited.

LOCAL ANESTHETIC TOXICITY

Neurologic complications after neuraxial anesthesia may be a direct result of local anesthetic toxicity. Both laboratory and clinical evidence suggests that local anesthetic solutions are potentially neurotoxic and that the neurotoxicity varies among local anesthetic solutions (5,18,20,25). Neurotoxicity is dependent on pKa, lipid solubility, protein binding, and potency. In histopathologic, electrophysiologic, and neuronal cell models, lidocaine and tetracaine appear to have a greater potential for neurotoxicity than bupivacaine at clinically relevant concentrations (26). Additives such as epinephrine and bicarbonate may also affect neurotoxicity. The presence of a preexisting neurologic condition may predispose the nerve to the neurotoxic effects of local anesthetics (25).

Although most local anesthetics administered in clinical concentrations and doses do not cause nerve damage (27), prolonged exposure, high dose, and/or high concentrations of local anesthetic solutions at the spinal roots may result in permanent neurologic deficits (22). For example, cauda equina syndrome has been reported after single-dose and continuous spinal anesthesia, intrathecal injection during intended epidural anesthesia, and repeated intrathecal injection after failed spinal block with lidocaine (2,20,28). In the late 1980s, three manufacturers introduced 27- to 32-gauge "microcatheters" capable of passage through standard 22- to 26-gauge needles. Experience with these devices was just gaining popularity when the occurrence of eleven cases of cauda equina syndrome led to their withdrawal from the U.S. market by the U.S. Food and Drug Administration (FDA) in 1992 (29). Presumably, injection (and/or reinjection) results in high concentrations of local anesthetic within a restricted area of the intrathecal space and causes neurotoxic injury. In the study by Auroy and co-workers, (2) 75% of the neurologic complications after uneventful (atraumatic) spinal anesthesia occurred in patients who received hyperbaric lidocaine, including one patient who received 350 mg over 5 hours with a 5% lidocaine infusion. Drasner (30) has recommended a maximum dose of 60 mg of lidocaine and the avoidance of epinephrine to prolong lidocaine spinal anesthesia. In addition, many clinicians recommend the use of isobaric solutions to reduce the risk of nonuniform distribution within the intrathecal space. Attention to patient positioning, total local anesthetic dose, and careful neurologic examination (evaluating for preferential sacral block) will assist in the decision to inject additional local anesthetic in the face of a patchy or failed block (31) (Tables 12-3 and 12-4).

2-Chloroprocaine was introduced nearly 50 years ago as a local anesthetic for epidural administration. However, concern for neurotoxicity emerged two decades ago, with a series of eight cases of neurologic injury associated with the use of Nesacaine-CE, a chloroprocaine solution containing the antioxidant sodium bisulfite. In all cases, the injury occurred after a large volume of anesthetic solution intended for the epidural space was accidentally administered intrathecally. Subsequent laboratory investigations evaluating the toxic contributions of 2-chloroprocaine, bisulfite, epinephrine, and pH reported that the commercial solution of 3% chloroprocaine (containing 0.2% sodium bisulfite, pH 3) produced irreversible block, but exposure to the same solution buffered to pH 7.3 resulted in complete recovery (32). It was assumed that bisulfite was the

TABLE 12-3

RECOMMENDATIONS FOR ANESTHETIC ADMINISTRATION WITH CONTINUOUS SPINAL ANESTHESIA

1. Insert catheter 2–4 cm, which should be adequate to confirm and maintain placement.
2. Use the lowest effective anesthetic concentration.
3. Place a limit on the amount of anesthetic to be used.
4. Administer a test dose and assess the extent of block.
5. If maldistribution is suspected, use maneuvers to increase the spread of local anesthetic (e.g., change the patient's position, alter the lumbosacral curvature, switch to a solution with a different baricity).
6. If well-distributed sensory anesthesia is not achieved before the dose limit is reached, abandon the technique.

From Drasner K. Local anesthetic neurotoxicity: Clinical injury and strategies that may minimize risk. *Reg Anesth Pain Med* 2002;27: 576–580, with permission.

source of neurotoxicity and that solutions that were bisulfite-free were safe for intrathecal use. More recently, these experiments were repeated with a more appropriate animal model and yielded different results: nerve injury scores were greater after administration of plain chloroprocaine compared to those of chloroprocaine containing bisulfite. These findings suggest clinical deficits associated with unintentional intrathecal injection of chloroprocaine likely resulted from a direct effect of the anesthetic, not the preservative. In addition, the data suggest that bisulfite can actually reduce neurotoxic damage induced by intrathecal local anesthetic (33). Although recent clinical and volunteer studies (34) have not reported neurologic symptoms following spinal anesthesia with low-dose 2-chloroprocaine

TABLE 12-4

RECOMMENDATIONS FOR ANESTHETIC ADMINISTRATION AFTER A "FAILED SPINAL"

1. Aspiration of cerebrospinal fluid (CSF) should be attempted before and after injection of anesthetic.
2. Sacral dermatomes should always be included in an evaluation of the presence of a spinal block.
3. If CSF is aspirated after anesthetic injection, it should be assumed that the local anesthetic has been delivered into the subarachnoid space; total anesthetic dosage should be limited to the maximum dose a clinician would consider reasonable to administer in a single injection.
4. If an injection is repeated, the technique should be modified to avoid reinforcing the same restricted distribution (e.g., alter patient position or switch to a local anesthetic of different baricity).
5. If CSF cannot be aspirated after injection, repeat injection of a full dose of local anesthetic should not be considered unless careful sensory examination (conducted after sufficient time for development of sensory anesthesia) reveals no evidence of block.

From Drasner K. Local anesthetic neurotoxicity: Clinical injury and strategies that may minimize risk. *Reg Anesth Pain Med* 2002;27: 576–580, with permission.

(30–40 mg), the laboratory evidence for toxicity warrants a cautious approach until additional toxicity data are available.

TRANSIENT NEUROLOGIC SYMPTOMS

Transient neurologic symptoms (TNS) were first formally described in 1993. Schneider and colleagues (3) reported four cases of severe radicular back pain occurring after resolution of hyperbaric lidocaine spinal anesthesia. All four patients had undergone surgery in the lithotomy position. No sensory or motor deficits were detected on examination, and the symptoms resolved spontaneously within several days. Multiple laboratory and clinical studies have been performed in an attempt to define the etiology, clinical significance, and risk factors associated with TNS. However, our understanding remains incomplete.

The incidence of TNS has ranged between 0% and 37% (35,36), and is dependent on anesthetic, surgical, and probably undefined patient factors. A prospective randomized study reported a 16% incidence of TNS in patients receiving either hyperbaric 5% lidocaine with epinephrine or 2% isobaric lidocaine. However, no patient receiving 0.75% hyperbaric bupivacaine developed TNS (35). In addition, the incidence was higher among patients positioned with knees or hips flexed (genitourinary, arthroscopy) than in patients positioned supine (herniorrhaphy), presumably because the flexion results in additional stretch on the nerve roots. A subsequent study comparing the incidence of TNS in knee arthroscopy patients undergoing spinal anesthesia with 50 mg of lidocaine in 2%, 1%, and 0.5% concentrations also failed to note a concentration effect; the incidence was similar in all groups (37). The lack of concentration (37) or dose effect (38) suggests that neurotoxicity is not the etiology of TNS, but does not rule out an alternative intrathecal source. Neurophysiologic evaluation in volunteers during TNS did not reveal abnormalities in somatosensory evoked potentials, electromyography, or nerve conduction studies (39).

A large multicenter epidemiologic study involving 1,863 patients was recently performed to identify potential risk factors for TNS (38). The incidence of TNS with lidocaine (11.9%) was significantly higher than that with tetracaine (1.6%) or bupivacaine (1.3%). The pain was described as severe in 30% of patients and resolved within a week in over 90% of cases. Outpatient status, obesity, and lithotomy position also increase the risk of TNS for patients who receive lidocaine. This suggests that the risk of TNS is high among outpatients in the lithotomy position (24.3%) and low for inpatients having surgery in positions other than lithotomy (3.1%). However, these variables were not risk factors with tetracaine or bupivacaine. The authors also reported that neither gender, age, history of back pain or neurologic disorder, lidocaine dose/concentration, spinal needle/size, aperture direction, nor addition of epinephrine increased the risk of TNS (Table 12-5). A previous study has identified the addition of phenylephrine as a risk factor for TNS with tetracaine spinal anesthesia (40). These findings were confirmed in a systematic review of TNS. The analysis included 14 trials reporting 1,347 patients (117 of whom developed TNS). The relative risk for developing TNS after spinal anesthesia with lidocaine was higher (4.35 [95% confidence interval (CI), 1.98–9.54]) than with other local anesthetics (bupivacaine, prilocaine, procaine, and mepivacaine) (41). There was no evidence of neurologic deficits; in all patients, the symptoms disappeared spontaneously by the 10th postoperative day.

TABLE 12-5

FACTORS THAT DID NOT INCREASE THE RISK OF DEVELOPING TRANSIENT NEUROLOGIC SYMPTOMS AFTER LIDOCAINE SPINAL ANESTHESIA

Gender
Age (<60 vs. 60+ years)
Preexisting neurologic disorder or back pain
Needle type (Quincke vs. Pencil point)
Needle size (22-gauge vs. 24–25 gauge vs. 26–27 gauge)
Bevel direction during injection (caudad vs. cephalad vs. lateral)
Lidocaine dose (<50 mg vs. 51–74 mg vs. >75 mg)
Intrathecal epinephrine
Intrathecal opioid
Intrathecal dextrose
Paresthesia during needle placement

Adapted from Freedman JM, Li D, Drasner K, Jaskela MC, et al. Transient neurologic symptoms after spinal anesthesia. An epidemiologic study of 1,863 patients. *Anesthesiology* 1998;89: 633–641, with permission.

The high frequency of TNS with lidocaine spinal anesthesia has resulted in a search for a safe and effective alternative. The intrathecal administration of 2-chloroprocaine is under reconsideration due to the concern regarding toxicity, as previously mentioned. Mepivacaine may be a suitable substitute; in a series of 1,273 patients undergoing spinal or combined spinal-epidural anesthesia, TNS occurred in only 78 (6.4%; 95% CI, 5.1%–8%) (42).

The etiology and clinical significance of TNS are unknown. Recent studies suggest a local anesthetic toxicity, although the mechanism may not be identical to that of cauda equina syndrome (43). Although many anesthesiologists believe that the reversible radicular pain is on one side of a continuum leading to irreversible cauda equina syndrome, no data support this concept. It is important to distinguish between factors associated with serious neurologic complications, such as cauda equina syndrome, and transient symptoms when making recommendations for the clinical management of patients. For example, increasing the concentration/dose of lidocaine and adding epinephrine increases the risk of irreversible neurotoxicity, but has little effect on the risk of TNS. Therefore, the clinician must determine the appropriate intrathecal solution, including adjuvants, given the surgical duration and intraoperative position for each individual patient.

ANTERIOR SPINAL ARTERY SYNDROME

The blood supply to the spinal cord is precarious due to the relatively large distances between the radicular vessels. Systemic hypotension or localized vascular insufficiency with or without a spinal anesthetic may produce spinal cord ischemia resulting in flaccid paralysis of the lower extremities (including sphincter dysfunction) or anterior spinal artery syndrome (44). Classically, proprioception and sensation are spared or preserved, relative to motor loss. Characteristics of anterior spinal artery syndrome, spinal abscess, and spinal hematoma are reported in (45) (Table 12-6). Local anesthetic solutions have a varied effect on spinal cord blood flow. For example, lidocaine and tetracaine either maintain or increase blood flow, whereas bupivacaine and levobupivacaine result in a decrease (46–48). The addition of epinephrine or phenylephrine results in a further decrease. However, in laboratory investigations, the alterations in blood flow are not accompanied by changes in histology or behavior. Likewise, large clinical studies have failed to identify the use of vasoconstrictors as a risk factor for temporary or permanent deficits. Most presumed cases of vasoconstrictor-induced neurologic deficits have been reported as single case reports, often with several other risk factors present (2,49).

Finally, the addition of vasoconstrictors may potentiate the neurotoxic effects of local anesthetics. In a laboratory model, it was determined that the neurotoxicity of intrathecally administered lidocaine was increased by the addition of epinephrine (50). A recent investigation by Sakura and colleagues (40) noted that the addition of phenylephrine increased the risk of TNS in patients undergoing tetracaine spinal anesthesia (although no patient had sensory or motor deficits). The actual risk of significant neurologic ischemia causing neurologic compromise in patients administered local anesthetic solutions

TABLE 12-6

DIFFERENTIAL DIAGNOSIS OF SPINAL ABSCESS, SPINAL HEMATOMA, AND ANTERIOR SPINAL ARTERY SYNDROME

	Spinal abscess	Spinal hematoma	Anterior spinal artery syndrome
Age of patient	Any age	50% over 50 years	Elderly
Previous history	Infection*	Anticoagulants	Arteriosclerosis/Hypotension
Onset	1–3 days	Sudden	Sudden
Generalized symptoms	Fever, malaise, back pain	Sharp, transient back and leg pain	None
Sensory involvement	None or paresthesias	Variable, late	Minor, patchy
Motor involvement	Flaccid paralysis, later spastic	Flaccid paralysis	Flaccid paralysis
Segmental reflexes	Exacerbated*, later obtunded	Abolished	Abolished
Myelogram/CT scan	Signs of extradural compression	Signs of extradural compression	Normal
Cerebrospinal fluid	Increased cell count	Normal	Normal
Laboratory data	Rise in sedimentation rate	Prolonged coagulation time*	Normal

*Infrequent findings.
From Wedel DJ, Horlocker TT. Risks of regional anesthesia-infectious, septic. *Reg Anesth* 1996;21:57–61, with permission.

containing vasoconstrictors appears to be very low. Clinicians should be aware of other surgical and patient factors predisposing to spinal cord ischemia, including major aortic vascular or spinal column procedures, arthrosclerosis, sustained hypotension, and anemia. The decision to perform a neuraxial block in these patients is based on risk–benefit evaluation and the ability to diagnosis/intervene should a reversible etiology of ischemia occur.

SPINAL HEMATOMA

The actual incidence of neurologic dysfunction resulting from hemorrhagic complications associated with neuraxial blockade is unknown; however, the incidence cited in the literature is estimated to be less than one in 150,000 epidural and less than one in 220,000 spinal anesthetics (51). In a review of the literature between 1906 and 1994, Vandermeulen and colleagues (52) reported 61 cases of spinal hematoma associated with epidural or spinal anesthesia. In 87% of patients, a hemostatic abnormality or traumatic/difficult needle placement was present. More than one risk factor was present in 20 of 61 cases. Importantly, although only 38% of patients had partial or good neurologic recovery, spinal cord ischemia tended to be reversible in patients who underwent laminectomy within 8 hours of onset of neurologic dysfunction.

The need for prompt diagnosis and intervention in the event of a spinal hematoma was also demonstrated in a review of the ASA Closed Claims project, which noted that spinal cord injuries were the leading cause of claims in the 1990s (11). Spinal hematomas accounted for nearly half of the spinal cord injuries. Risk factors for spinal hematoma included epidural anesthesia in the presence of intravenous (IV) heparin during a vascular surgical or diagnostic procedure. Importantly, the presence of postoperative numbness or weakness was typically attributed to local anesthetic effect rather than spinal cord ischemia, which delayed the diagnosis. Patient care was rarely judged to have met standards (1 of 13 cases), and the median payment was very high.

It is impossible to conclusively determine risk factors for the development of spinal hematoma in patients undergoing neuraxial blockade solely through review of the case series, which represent only patients with the complication and do not define those who underwent uneventful neuraxial analgesia. However, large inclusive surveys that evaluate the frequencies of complications (including spinal hematoma), as well as identify subgroups of patients with higher or lower risk, enhance risk stratification. In the series by Moen and co-workers (8) involving nearly 2 million neuraxial blocks, 33 spinal hematomas occurred. The methodology allowed for the calculation of frequency of spinal hematoma among patient populations. For example, the risk associated with epidural analgesia in women undergoing childbirth was significantly less (one in 200,000) than that in elderly women undergoing knee arthroplasty (one in 3,600, $p < 0.0001$). Likewise, women undergoing hip fracture surgery under spinal anesthesia had an increased risk of spinal hematoma (one in 22,000) compared to all patients undergoing spinal anesthesia (one in 480,000).

Overall, these series suggest that the risk of clinically significant bleeding varies with age (and associated abnormalities of the spinal cord or vertebral column), the presence of an underlying coagulopathy, difficulty during needle placement, and an indwelling neuraxial catheter during sustained anticoagulation (particularly with standard or low-molecular-weight heparin [LMWH]). They also consistently demonstrate the need for prompt diagnosis and intervention.

CURRENT RECOMMENDATIONS FOR THE PREVENTION AND TREATMENT OF VENOUS THROMBOEMBOLISM

Prevention of venous thromboembolism remains a crucial component of patient care following major surgery. Although neuraxial anesthesia and analgesia reduce the risk of venous thrombosis, a significant risk remains, even in the presence of a continuous epidural infusion containing a local anesthetic (53). As a result, pharmacologic (and/or mechanical) prophylaxis is warranted. Thromboprophylaxis is based upon identification of risk factors. The risk factors for thromboembolism include trauma, immobility/paresis, malignancy, previous thromboembolism, increasing age (over 40 years), pregnancy, estrogen therapy, obesity, smoking history, varicose veins, and inherited or congenital thrombophilia. Not surprisingly, only the healthiest patients undergoing minor surgery are not considered candidates for thromboprophylaxis postoperatively.

Guidelines for antithrombotic therapy including appropriate pharmacologic agent, degree of anticoagulation desired, and duration of therapy continue to evolve. There is a trend toward initiating thromboprophylaxis in close proximity to surgery. However, early postoperative (and intraoperative) dosing of LMWH was associated with an increased risk of neuraxial bleeding. Likewise, the duration of prophylaxis has been extended to a minimum of 10 days following total joint replacement or hip fracture surgery, whereas the recommended duration for hip procedures is 28 to 35 days. It has been demonstrated that the risk of bleeding complications is increased with the duration of anticoagulant therapy. The interaction of prolonged thromboprophylaxis and previous neuraxial instrumentation, including difficult or traumatic needle insertion, is unknown.

Recommendations from the Seventh American College of Chest Physicians (ACCP) in 2004 are based upon prospective randomized studies that assess the efficacy of therapy using contrast venography or fibrinogen leg scanning to diagnose asymptomatic thrombi (54) (Table 12-7). Clinical outcomes, such as fatal pulmonary embolism and symptomatic deep venous thrombosis are not primary endpoints. Despite the successful reduction of asymptomatic thromboembolic events with routine use of antithrombotic therapy, an actual reduction of clinically relevant events has been more difficult to demonstrate.

Neuraxial Anesthesia and Anticoagulation

Practice guidelines or recommendations summarize evidence-based reviews. However, the rarity of spinal hematoma defies a prospective-randomized study, and no current laboratory model exist. As a result, the consensus statements developed by the American Society of Regional Anesthesia and Pain Medicine represent the collective experience of recognized experts in the field of neuraxial anesthesia and anticoagulation. They are based on case reports, clinical series, pharmacology, hematology, and risk factors for surgical bleeding. An understanding of the complexity of this issue is essential to patient management.

Oral Anticoagulants

Few data exist regarding the risk of spinal hematoma in patients with indwelling epidural catheters who are anticoagulated with

TABLE 12-7

PHARMACOLOGIC VENOUS THROMBOEMBOLISM PROPHYLAXIS AND TREATMENT REGIMENS

Minor general surgery, spine, vascular, and arthroscopic procedures (with NO additional risk factors present)*

Early mobilization

No pharmacologic thromboprophylaxis

Minor general surgery, vascular or spine surgery (with additional risk factors present) and major general or gynecologic surgery (with NO additional risk factors present)

Unfractionated heparin	5,000 U SC q12h, started 2 hours before surgery
LMWH	≤3,400 U SC qd, started 1–2 hours before surgery

Major general or gynecologic surgery, and open urologic procedures (with additional risk factors present)

Unfractionated heparin	5,000 U SC q8h, started 2 hours before surgery
LMWH	>3400 U SC qd, started 1–2 hours before surgery

Total hip or knee arthroplasty and hip fracture surgery

Fondaparinux	2.5 mg SC qd started 6–8 hours after surgery
LMWH*	5,000 U SC qd started 12 hours before surgery, or
	2500 U SC 4–6 given hours after surgery, then 5,000 U SC daily
Warfarin	Started the night before or immediately after surgery and adjusted to prolong the INR = 2.0–3.0

SC, subcutaneous; LMWH, low-molecular-weight heparin; INR, international normalized ratio.
*The risk factors for thromboembolism and include trauma, immobility/paresis, malignancy, previous thromboembolism, increasing age (over 40 years), pregnancy, estrogen therapy, obesity, smoking history, varicose veins, and inherited or congenital thrombophilia
Based on recommendations from Geerts WH, Pineo GF, Heit JA, et al. Prevention of venous thromboembolism: The Seventh ACCP Conference on Antithrombotic and Thrombolytic Therapy. *Chest* 2004;126:338S–400S.

warfarin. The optimal duration of an indwelling catheter and the timing of its removal also remain controversial. To date, only three studies have evaluated the risk of spinal hematoma in patients with indwelling spinal or epidural catheters who receive oral anticoagulants perioperatively. Odoom and Sih (55) performed 1,000 continuous lumbar epidural anesthetics in vascular surgical patients who were receiving oral anticoagulants preoperatively. The thrombotest (a test measuring factor IX activity) was decreased (but not below 10% activity) in all patients prior to needle placement. Heparin was also administered intraoperatively. Epidural catheters remained in place for 48 hours postoperatively. No neurologic complications occurred. Although these results are reassuring, the obsolescence of the thrombotest as a measure of anticoagulation, combined with the unknown coagulation status of the patients at the time of catheter removal limit the usefulness of these results. Therefore, except in extraordinary circumstances, spinal or epidural needle/catheter placement and removal should not be performed in fully anticoagulated patients.

No symptomatic spinal hematomas were reported in two smaller series with a total of nearly 700 patients undergoing neuraxial block in combination with warfarin anticoagulation perioperatively (56,57). In both studies, epidural catheters were left indwelling approximately for 2 days. The mean international normalized ratio (INR) at the time of catheter removal was 1.4, although in a small number of patients, the INR was therapeutic (2.0–3.0). A large variability in patient response to warfarin was also noted, demonstrating the need for close monitoring of the coagulation status (56). A large series of patients is required to confirm these results. However, the small number of hematomas reported and widespread use of warfarin thromboprophylaxis (at least in the United States) in patients administered neuraxial block suggests that patients receiving oral anticoagulants may safely undergo re-

gional techniques with appropriate monitoring of the level of anticoagulation.

Intravenous and Subcutaneous Standard Heparin

The safety of neuraxial techniques in combination with intraoperative heparinization is well documented, providing no other coagulopathy is present. In a study involving over 4,000 patients, Rao and El-Etr (58) demonstrated the safety of indwelling spinal and epidural catheters during systemic heparinization during vascular surgery. However, the heparin was administered at least 60 minutes after catheter placement, level of anticoagulation was closely monitored, and the indwelling catheters were removed at a time when circulating heparin levels were relatively low. A subsequent study in the neurologic literature by Ruff and Dougherty (59) reported spinal hematomas in seven of 342 patients (2%) who underwent a diagnostic lumbar puncture and subsequent heparinization. Traumatic needle placement, initiation of anticoagulation within 1 hour of lumbar puncture, and concomitant aspirin therapy were identified as risk factors in the development of spinal hematoma in anticoagulated patients. Subsequent studies using similar methodology have verified the safety of this practice, provided the monitoring of anticoagulant effect and the time intervals between heparinization and catheter placement/removal are maintained.

There have been continued discussions regarding the relative risk (and benefit) of neuraxial anesthesia and analgesia in the patient undergoing complete heparinization for cardiopulmonary bypass. A review has recommended certain precautions to be taken, including delay of surgery for 24 hours in case of traumatic needle/catheter placement (60). Although no spinal hematomas were reported in the small series of patients who have undergone epidural block for cardiac surgery, investigators repeatedly observe that this technique remains controversial because of the degree of anticoagulation required and the associated risk of permanent spinal cord damage from an epidural hematoma. Such a risk must be balanced by important clinical advantages if the technique is to be justified (6).

Low-dose subcutaneous standard (unfractionated) heparin is administered for thromboprophylaxis in patients undergoing major thoracoabdominal surgery and in patients at increased risk of hemorrhage using oral anticoagulant or LMWH therapy. A review of the literature by Schwander and Bachmann (61) noted no spinal hematomas in over 5,000 patients who received subcutaneous heparin in combination with spinal or epidural anesthesia. Only three cases of spinal hematoma are associated with neuraxial blockade in the presence of low-dose heparin, two of which involved a continuous epidural anesthetic technique (52). It is important to note that while the ACCP guidelines are more often recommending thrice daily dosing of subcutaneous heparin (due to patient comorbidities and increased risk of thromboembolism), the safety of neuraxial block in these patients is unknown.

Low-molecular-weight Heparin

Extensive clinical testing and utilization of LMWH in Europe over the last 10 years suggested that there was not an increased risk of spinal hematoma in patients undergoing neuraxial anesthesia while receiving LMWH thromboprophylaxis perioperatively (52,62). However, in the 5 years since the release of LMWH for general use in the United States in May 1993, over 60 cases of spinal hematoma associated with neuraxial anesthesia administered in the presence of perioperative LMWH prophylaxis were reported to the manufacturer (6,63). Many of these events occurred when LMWH was administered intraoperatively or early postoperatively to patients undergoing continuous epidural anesthesia and analgesia. Concomitant antiplatelet therapy was present in several cases. The apparent difference in incidence in Europe compared to the United States may be a result of a difference in dose and dosage schedule. For example, in Europe, the recommended dose of enoxaparin is 40 mg once daily (with LMWH therapy initiated 12 hours preoperatively), rather than 30 mg every 12 hours. However, timing of catheter removal may also have an impact. It is likely that the lack of a trough in anticoagulant activity associated with twice daily dosing resulted in catheter removal occurring during significant anticoagulant activity. Importantly, no data suggest that the risk of spinal hematoma is increased with certain LMWH formulations (63). The incidence of spinal hematoma in patients undergoing neuraxial block in combination with LMWH has been estimated at one in 40,800 spinal anesthetics and one in 3,100 continuous epidural anesthetics (64). It is interesting in that the frequency of spinal hematoma in this series is similar to that reported by Moen and colleagues (8) for women undergoing total knee replacement with epidural analgesia.

The indications and labeled uses for LMWH continue to evolve. Indications for thromboprophylaxis as well as treatment of thromboembolism or myocardial infarction (MI) have been introduced. These new applications and corresponding regional anesthetic management warrant discussion (54). Several off-label applications of LMWH are of special interest to the anesthesiologist. LMWH has been demonstrated to be efficacious as a "bridge therapy" for patients chronically anticoagulated with warfarin, including parturients, and patients with prosthetic cardiac valves, a history of atrial fibrillation, or preexisting hypercoagulable condition. The doses of LMWH are those associated with deep venous thrombosis (DVT) treatment, not prophylaxis, and are much higher. An interval of at least 24 hours is required for the anticoagulant activity to resolve.

Antiplatelet Medications

Antiplatelet medications are seldom used as primary agents of thromboprophylaxis. However, many orthopedic patients report chronic use of one or more antiplatelet drugs. Although Vandermeulen and colleagues (52) implicated antiplatelet therapy in three of the 61 cases of spinal hematoma occurring after spinal or epidural anesthesia, several large studies have demonstrated the relative safety of neuraxial blockade in both obstetric, surgical, and pain clinic patients receiving these medications (65–67). In a prospective study involving 1,000 patients, Horlocker and co-workers (65) reported that preoperative antiplatelet therapy did not increase the incidence of blood present at the time of needle/catheter placement or removal, suggesting that trauma incurred during needle or catheter placement is neither increased nor sustained by these medications. The clinician should be aware of the possible increased risk of spinal hematoma in patients receiving antiplatelet medications who undergo subsequent heparinization (59).

Ticlopidine and clopidogrel are also platelet aggregation inhibitors. These agents interfere with platelet–fibrinogen binding and subsequent platelet–platelet interactions. The effect is irreversible for the life of the platelet. Ticlopidine and clopidogrel have no effect on platelet cyclooxygenase, acting independently of aspirin. However, these medications have not been tested in combination. Platelet dysfunction is present for 5 to 7 days after discontinuation of clopidogrel and 10 to 14 days with ticlopidine. Platelet glycoprotein IIb/IIIa receptor antagonists, including abciximab (ReoPro), eptifibatide (Integrilin), and tirofiban (Aggrastat), inhibit platelet aggregation by interfering with platelet–fibrinogen binding and subsequent platelet–platelet interactions. Time to normal platelet aggregation following discontinuation of therapy ranges from 8 hours (eptifibatide, tirofiban) to 48 hours (abciximab). Increased perioperative bleeding in patients undergoing cardiac and vascular surgery after receiving ticlopidine, clopidogrel, and glycoprotein IIb/IIIa antagonists warrants concern regarding the risk of anesthesia-related hemorrhagic complications.

Herbal Medications

Herbal medications are widely used in surgical patients. Morbidity and mortality associated with herbal use may be more likely in the perioperative period because of the polypharmacy and physiologic alterations that occur. Such complications include bleeding from garlic, ginkgo, and ginseng, and potential interaction between ginseng–warfarin. Because the current regulatory mechanism for commercial herbal preparations sold in the United States does not adequately protect against unpredictable or undesirable pharmacologic effects, it is especially important for anesthesiologists to be familiar with related literature on herbal medications when caring for patients in the perioperative period. It appears that herbal drugs, by themselves, appear to represent no added significant risk for the development of spinal hematoma in patients having epidural or spinal anesthesia. This is an important observation, since it is likely that a significant number of these surgical patients utilize alternative medications preoperatively and perhaps during their postoperative course. There is no wholly accepted test to assess adequacy of hemostasis in the patient reporting preoperative herbal medications. Careful preoperative assessment of the patient to identify alterations in health that might contribute to bleeding is crucial. Data on the combination of herbal therapy with other forms of anticoagulation are lacking. However, the concurrent use of other medications affecting clotting mechanisms may increase the risk of bleeding complications in these patients (6).

Anesthetic Management of the Anticoagulated Patient

The decision to perform spinal or epidural anesthesia/analgesia and the timing of catheter removal in a patient receiving thromboprophylaxis should be made on an individual basis, weighing the small, although definite risk of spinal hematoma with the benefits of regional anesthesia for a specific patient. Alternative anesthetic and analgesic techniques exist for patients considered to be at an unacceptable risk. The patient's coagulation status should be optimized at the time of spinal or epidural needle/catheter placement, and the level of anticoagulation must be carefully monitored during the period of epidural catheterization (Table 12-8). It is important to note that patients respond with variable sensitivities to anticoagulant medications. Indwelling catheters should not be removed in the presence of a significant coagulopathy, as this appears to significantly increase the risk of spinal hematoma (8,52). In addition, communication between clinicians involved in the perioperative management of patients receiving anticoagulants for thromboprophylaxis is essential to decrease the risk of serious hemorrhagic complications. The patient should be closely monitored in the perioperative period for signs of cord ischemia. If spinal hematoma is suspected, the treatment of choice is immediate decompressive laminectomy. Recovery is unlikely if surgery is postponed for more than 10 to 12 hours; less than 40% of the patients in the series by Vandermeulen and colleagues (52) had partial or good recovery of neurologic function.

MENINGITIS AND EPIDURAL ABSCESS

Bacterial infection of the central neuraxis may present as meningitis or cord compression secondary to abscess formation. Possible risk factors include underlying sepsis, diabetes, depressed immune status, steroid therapy, localized bacterial colonization or infection, and chronic catheter maintenance. Bacterial infection of the central neural axis may present as meningitis or cord compression secondary to abscess formation. The infectious source for meningitis and epidural abscess may result from distant colonization or localized infection with subsequent hematogenous spread and CNS invasion. The anesthetist may also transmit microorganisms directly into the CNS by needle/catheter contamination through a break in aseptic technique or passage through a contiguous infection. An indwelling neuraxial catheter, although aseptically sited, may be colonized with skin flora and consequently serve as a source for ascending infection to the epidural or intrathecal space.

Historically, the frequency of serious CNS infections such as arachnoiditis, meningitis, and abscess following spinal or epidural anesthesia was considered to be extremely low, with cases were reported individually or in small series (68,69). However, recent epidemiologic series from Europe suggest that the frequency of infectious complications associated with neuraxial techniques is increasing (8,70). In a national study conducted from 1997 to 1998 in Denmark, Wang and colleagues (70) reported the incidence of epidural abscess after epidural analgesia was 1:1,930 catheters. Patients with epidural

---

TABLE 12-8

RECOMMENDED GUIDELINES FOR PERFORMING SPINAL PROCEDURES IN ANTICOAGULATED PATIENTS

Warfarin	Discontinue chronic warfarin therapy 4–5 days before spinal procedure and evaluate INR. INR should be within the normal range at time of procedure to ensure adequate levels of all vitamin K-dependent factors. Postoperatively, daily INR assessment with catheter removal occurring with INR <1.5
Antiplatelet medications	No contraindications with aspirin or other NSAIDs. Thienopyridine derivatives (clopidogrel and ticlopidine) should be discontinued 7 days and 14 days, respectively, prior to procedure. GP IIb/IIIa inhibitors should be discontinued to allow recovery of platelet function prior to procedure (8 hours for tirofiban and eptifibatide, 24–48 hours for abciximab).
Thrombolytics/fibrinolytics	No available data suggest a safe interval between procedure and initiation or discontinuation of these medications. Follow fibrinogen level and observe for signs of neural compression.
LMWH	Delay procedure at least 12 hours from the last dose of thromboprophylaxis LMWH dose. For "treatment" dosing of LMWH, at least 24 hours should elapse prior to procedure. LMWH should not be administered within 24 hours after the procedure. Indwelling epidural catheters should be maintained with caution and only with once-daily dosing of LMWH and strict avoidance of additional hemostasis-altering medications, including ketorolac.
Unfractionated SQ heparin	There are no contraindications to neuraxial procedure if total daily dose is less than 10,000 units. For higher dosing regimens, manage according to intravenous heparin guidelines.
Unfractionated IV heparin	Delay needle/catheter placement 2–4 hours after last dose, document normal aPTT. Heparin may be restarted 1 hour following procedure. Sustained heparinization with an indwelling neuraxial catheter associated with increased risk; monitor neurologic status aggressively.

NSAIDs, nonsteroidal antiinflammatory drugs; GP IIb/IIIa, platelet glycoprotein receptor IIb/IIIa inhibitors; INR, international normalized ratio; LMWH, low-molecular-weight heparin; aPTT, activated partial thromboplastin time. Adapted from Horlocker TT, Wedel DJ, Benzon H, et al. Regional anesthesia in the anticoagulated patient: Defining the risks (the second ASRA Consensus Conference on Neuraxial Anesthesia and Anticoagulation). *Reg Anesth Pain Med* 2003;28:172–197.

abscess had an extended duration of epidural catheterization (median 6 days, range 3–31 days). In addition, the majority of the patients with epidural abscess were immunocompromised. Often the diagnosis was delayed; the time to first symptom to confirmation of the diagnosis was a median of 5 days. *Staphylococcus aureus* was isolated in 67% of patients. Patients without neurologic deficits were successfully treated with antibiotics, whereas those with deficits underwent surgical decompression, typically with only moderate neurologic recovery. It is difficult to determine why the frequency of symptomatic epidural abscess was so high in this series. Since perioperative antithrombotic therapy was involved in most cases, it is possible that the epidural abscesses were infected "micro" epidural hematomas, but this is not strongly supported by the diagnostic imaging studies and neurosurgical findings (see Fig. 50-22).

In the series by Moen and colleagues (8), 42 serious infectious complications were reported. Epidural abscess occurred in 13 patients; nine (70%) were considered immunocompromised as a result of diabetes, steroid therapy, cancer, or alcoholism. Six patients underwent epidural block for analgesia following trauma. The time from placement of the epidural catheter to first symptoms ranged from 2 days to 5 weeks (median 5 days). Although prevailing symptoms were fever and sever backache, five developed neurologic deficits. All seven positive cultures isolated *S. aureus*. Overall neurologic recovery was complete in seven of 12 patients. However, four of the five patients with neurologic symptoms did not recover. Meningitis was reported in 29 patients, for an overall incidence of 1:53,000. A documented perforation of the dura (intentional or accidental) occurred in 25 of 29 cases. In the 12 patients in whom positive cultures were obtained, α-hemolytic streptococci were isolated in 11 patients and *S. aureus* in one.

These large epidemiologic studies represent new and unexpected findings regarding the demographics, frequency, etiology, and prognosis of infectious complications following neuraxial anesthesia. Epidural abscess is most likely to occur in immunocompromised patients with prolonged durations of epidural catheterization. The most common causative organism is *S. aureus*, which suggests the colonization and subsequent infection from normal skin flora as the pathogenesis. Delays in diagnosis and treatment result in poor neurologic recovery, despite surgical decompression. Conversely, patients who develop meningitis following neuraxial blockade typically are healthy and have undergone uneventful spinal anesthesia. Furthermore, the series by Moen and colleagues (8) validates the findings of individual case reports of meningitis after spinal anesthesia—the source of the pathogen is mostly likely to be the upper airway of the proceduralist. Although the frequency of serious infectious complications is much higher than reported previously, the results may be due to differences in reporting and/or clinical practice (asepsis, perioperative antibiotic therapy, duration of epidural catheterization).

Meningitis after Dural Puncture and Neuraxial Anesthesia

Dural puncture has long been considered a risk factor in the pathogenesis of meningitis. Exactly how bacteria cross from the blood stream into the spinal fluid is unknown. The presumed mechanisms include introduction of blood into the intrathecal space during needle placement and disruption of the protection provided by the blood–brain barrier. However, lumbar puncture is often performed in patients with fever or infection of unknown origin. If dural puncture during bacteremia results

in meningitis, definite clinical data should exist. In fact, clinical studies are few, and often antiquated (71–75) (Table 12-9).

Initial investigations were performed over 80 years ago. In 1919, Weed and colleagues (76) demonstrated that lumbar or cisternal puncture performed during septicemia (produced by lethal doses of an intravenously administered gram-negative bacillus) invariably resulted in a fatal meningitis. In the same year, Wegeforth and Latham (71) reported their clinical observations on 93 patients suspected of having meningitis who received a diagnostic lumbar puncture. Blood cultures were taken simultaneously. The diagnosis was confirmed in 38 patients. The remaining 55 patients had normal cerebrospinal fluid (CSF). However, six of these 55 patients were bacteremic at the time of lumbar puncture. Five of the six bacteremic patients subsequently developed meningitis. It was implied, but not stated, that patients with both sterile blood and CSF cultures did not develop meningitis. Unfortunately, these lumbar punctures were performed during two epidemics of meningitis occurring at a military installation, and it is possible that some (or all) of these patients may have developed meningitis without lumbar puncture. These two historical studies provided support for the claim that lumbar puncture during bacteremia was a possible risk factor for meningitis.

Subsequent clinical studies reported conflicting results regarding the causal relationship between dural puncture during bacteremia and meningitis (Table 12-9). However, the protective effect of antibiotic administration prior to lumbar puncture was suggested (74).

Prevention of lumbar puncture–induced meningitis with antibiotic therapy was also supported by a more recent animal study. Carp and Bailey (77) investigated the association between meningitis and dural puncture in bacteremic rats. Twelve of 40 rats subjected to cisternal puncture with a 26-gauge needle during *Escherichia coli* bacteremia subsequently developed meningitis. In addition, bacteremic animals not undergoing dural puncture, as well as animals undergoing dural puncture in the absence of bacteremia, did not develop meningitis. Meningitis occurred only in animals with a blood culture result of more than 50 colony forming units/mL at the time of dural puncture. Treatment of a group of bacteremic rats with a single dose of gentamicin immediately prior to cisternal puncture apparently eliminated the risk of meningitis, as none of these animals developed infection. This study demonstrates that dural puncture in the presence of bacteremia is associated with the development of meningitis in rats, and that antibiotic treatment before dural puncture reduces this risk. Unfortunately, this study did not include a group of animals that were treated with antibiotics after dural puncture. Since many surgeons defer antibiotic therapy until after cultures are obtained, the actual clinical scenario remains unstudied. There are several other limitations to this study. Although *E. coli* is a common cause of bacteremia, it is an uncommon cause of meningitis. In addition, the authors knew the sensitivity to the bacteria injected, allowing for appropriate antibiotic coverage. The authors also performed a cisternal puncture (rather than lumbar puncture) and utilized a 26-gauge needle, producing a relatively large dural defect in the rat compared to dural puncture with spinal needles in humans. Finally, no local anesthetic was injected. Local anesthetic solutions are typically bacteriostatic, which may reduce the risk of meningitis in normal clinical settings. These results do not apply to administration of epidural anesthesia in the febrile patient (which involves placement of an indwelling catheter).

Prior to large surveys, meningitis after spinal anesthesia was rarely reported, with cases occurring as a single event or small series (Table 12-10) (78–85). In a study evaluating the

TABLE 12-9

MENINGITIS AFTER DURAL PUNCTURE

Author, year	Number of patients	Population	Microorganism(s)	Patients with spontaneous meningitis	Patients with lumbar puncture–induced meningitis	Comments
Wegeforth, 1919 (71)	93	Military personnel	Neisseria meningitidis Streptococcus pneumonia	38 of 93 (41%)	5 of 93, including 5 of 6 bacteremic patients	Lumbar punctures performed during meningitis epidemics
Pray, 1941 (72)	416	Pediatric with bacteremia	Streptococcus pneumonia	86 of 386 (22%)	8 of 30 (27%)	80% of patients with meningitis <2 yrs of age
Eng, 1981 (73)	1089	Adults with bacteremia	Atypical and typical bacteria	30 of 919 (3.3%)	3 of 170 (1.8%)	Atypical organisms responsible for lumbar puncture induced meningitis
Teele, 1981 (74)	271	Pediatric with bacteremia	Streptococcus pneumonia Neisseria meningitidis Haemophilus influenza	2 of 31 (8.7%)	7 of 46 (15%)*	All cases of meningitis occurred in children <1 yr of age. Antibiotic therapy reduced risk
Smith, 1986 (75)	11	Preterm with neonatal sepsis	NA (No cases of meningitis)	0%	0%	

*Significant association (*p* <0.001). Spontaneous meningitis = concurrent bacteremia and meningitis (without a preceding lumbar puncture). Lumbar puncture-induced meningitis = positive blood culture with sterile CSF on initial exam; subsequent positive CSF culture (same organism present in blood). From Wedel DJ, Horlocker TT. Risks of regional anesthesia-infectious, septic. *Reg Anesth* 1996;21:57–61, with permission.

frequency of meningitis in patients undergoing spinal anesthesia, Kilpatrick and Girgis (86) retrospectively reviewed records of all patients admitted to the meningitis ward in Cairo, Egypt. During a 5-year period from 1975 to 1980, 17 of 1,429 patients admitted with a diagnosis of meningitis had a history of recent spinal anesthesia. The patients developed meningeal symptoms 2 to 30 days (mean 9 days) after spinal anesthesia and were symptomatic for 1 to 83 days (mean 15 days) prior to hospital admission. Ten of the 17 had positive CSF cultures: eight were *Pseudomonas aeruginosa*, one was *S. aureus*, and one was *Streptococcus mitis*. These organisms were not cultured from patients who had not had spinal anesthesia. Two additional patients with a history of recent spinal anesthesia demonstrated evidence of tuberculous meningitis. The lack of positive CSF cultures was presumed to be a result of oral antibiotic therapy, which was present in over half of patients at the time of admission. However, all patients, including those with negative CSF cultures, were treated with antibiotic therapy. Four of the 17 patients died. These results suggest that meningitis occurring in patients with a history of recent spinal anesthesia is often due to unusual or nosocomial organisms and that aggressive bacteriologic evaluation and antibiotic coverage is warranted.

The risk of meningitis in parturients undergoing spinal or combined spinal-epidural blockade deserves special discussion. In a review of published reports of meningitis following neuraxial blockade in obstetric patients, Reynolds (87) reports that, in the majority of parturients, meningitis is "surprisingly rare when spinals are used for elective caesarean section." Reasons cited for the relative risk in laboring patients includes the location of block performance (operating room versus delivery

suite), antibiotic pretreatment, decreased likelihood of streptococcal bacteremia, and the patient is not lying in an "amniotic fluid–soaked bed." As a result, it was recommended that "the dura should not be punctured during labor if an epidural would do instead" (87).

EPIDURAL ABSCESS AFTER EPIDURAL ANESTHESIA

Several relevant studies have specifically examined the risk of epidural abscess in patients receiving epidural anesthesia and/or analgesia. Bader and colleagues (80) investigated the use of regional anesthesia in women with chorioamnionitis; 319 women were identified from a total of 10,047 deliveries. Of the 319 women, 100 had blood cultures taken on the day of delivery. Eight of these had blood cultures consistent with bacteremia. Two-hundred ninety-three of the 319 patients received a regional anesthetic; in 43 patients antibiotics were administered prior to needle or catheter placement. No patient in the study, including those with documented bacteremias, had infectious complications. In addition, mean temperatures and leukocyte counts in patients who received blood cultures showed no significant differences between bacteremic and nonbacteremic groups. These authors continue to administer spinal and epidural anesthesia in patients with suspected chorioamnionitis because the potential benefits of regional anesthesia outweigh the theoretical risk of infectious complications.

The safety of epidural analgesia in 75 patients admitted to the intensive care unit was prospectively evaluated by Darchy

TABLE 12-10

INFECTIOUS COMPLICATIONS FOLLOWING REGIONAL ANESTHESIA

Author, year	No of patients	Population	Neuraxial techniques	Antibiotic prophylaxis	Duration of indwelling catheter	Complications
Kane, 1981 (44)	115,000	Surgical and obstetric	65,000 spinal 50,000 epidural	Unknown	Unknown	3 Meningitis (all after spinal anesthesia)
DuPen, 1990 (78)	350	Cancer and AIDS patients	Permanent (tunneled) epidural analgesia	No	4–1,460 days	30 Insertion site infections, 19 deep track or epidural space infections; treated with catheter removal and antibiotics, 15 uneventfully replaced
Scott, 1990 (79)	505,000	Obstetrical	Epidural	Unknown	Unknown	1 Epidural abscess; laminectomy with partial recovery
Bader, 1992 (80)	319	Parturients with chorioamnionitis	General (26), epidural (224), spinal (29), local (50) anesthesia	Yes (13%)	Surgical	None
Strafford, 1993 (81)	1,620	Pediatric surgical	Epidural analgesia	No	2.4 days median	3 Positive epidural catheter tip cultures 1 Candida colonization of epidural space (along with necrotic tumor)
Goodman, 1996 (82)	531	Parturients with chorioamnionitis	Spinal (14), epidural (517) anesthesia and analgesia	Yes (23%)	>24 h in (64 patients)	None
Dahlgren, 1995 (49)	18,000	All indications and ages of patients	Spinal (8,768) and Epidural (9,232)	Unknown	Unknown	None
Kindler, 1996 (83)	13,000	4000 Obstetrical 9000 Surgical	Epidural	Unknown	Unknown	2 Epidural abscess, both requiring laminectomy
Auroy, 1997 (2)	71,053	Surgical	Spinal (40,640) Epidural (30,413)	Unknown	Unknown	None
Aromaa, 1997 (84)	720,000	Surgical	Epidural (170,000) Spinals (550,000)	Unknown	Unknown	4 Meningitis 2 Epidural abscess 2 Discitis 2 Superficial skin infections
Albright, 1999 (85)	6,002	Surgical and obstetric	CSE	Unknown	Unknown	None
Wang, 1999 (70)	17,372	Surgical, cancer & trauma	Epidural	Unknown	11 days mean 6 days median	9 Epidural abscess; 7 required laminectomy; complete recovery in 6 of 10 patients 2 Subcutaneous infections
Auroy, 2002 (10)	78,104	Surgical and obstetrical	Spinal (41,251) Epidural (35,379) CSE (1474)	Unknown	Unknown	1 Meningitis
Moen, 2004 (8)	1,710,000	Pain, surgical and obstetrical	Spinal (1,260,000) Epidural (450,000)	Unknown	2d-5wk	29 Meningitis; partial sequelae in 6 patients 13 Epidural abscess, laminectomy performed in six patients; 4 of 5 patients with deficits did not recover

Modified from Wedel DJ, Horlocker TT. Regional anesthesia in the febrile or infected patient. *Reg Anesth Pain Med* 2006;31:324–333, with permission.

and co-workers (88). No epidural abscesses occurred. However, five of nine patients with positive cultures of the catheter insertion site also had positive catheter tip cultures (epidural catheter infection); *Staphylococcus epidermidis* was the most commonly cultured microorganism. Local infection of the catheter site was treated with catheter removal, but antibiotic therapy was not specifically prescribed. Concomitant infection at other sites, antibiotic prophylaxis, and duration of epidural analgesia were not risk factors for epidural-analgesia related infections. The authors noted that the presence of both erythema and local discharge is a strong predictor of local and epidural catheter infection.

Epidural anesthesia and analgesia in a patient with a known systemic or localized infection remains controversial. Jakobsen and colleagues (89) retrospectively reviewed the records of 69 patients with abscesses or wound infections who underwent epidural catheter placement for surgical debridement over a 7-year period. Several patients had more than one catheter inserted. Catheters were left indwelling for a mean of 9 days. On 12 occasions (eight patients), the catheter was removed because of local infection. None of the patients demonstrated signs or symptoms of neuraxial infection. The authors concluded that epidural anesthesia is relatively safe for patients requiring repeated surgical treatment of localized infection. In contrast, Bengtsson and colleagues (90) reported three epidural catheter–related infections in patients with cutaneous wounds over a 4-year period. All patients were treated with antibiotic therapy; one patient underwent transcutaneous drainage of an epidural abscess. However, no neurologic deficits occurred. It is difficult to determine the actual risk of epidural abscess in patients with chronic localized infections who undergo epidural catheter placement due to the small number of patients studied and the rarity of this complication. Therefore, the clinician must maintain vigilance in neurologic monitoring to assure early recognition and treatment.

NEURAXIAL BLOCKADE IN THE IMMUNOCOMPROMISED PATIENT

Large series have demonstrated that patients with immunodeficiencies are at increased risk for infectious complications compared to those with intact immune function. However, few investigations have evaluated the frequency of meningitis or epidural abscess within a specific immunodeficient population (8,70,91) (Table 12-11). Strafford and colleagues (81) reviewed 1,620 pediatric patients who received epidural analgesia for postoperative pain relief. Epidural catheters were left indwelling for a median of 2 days (range, 0–8 days). No patient developed an epidural abscess. One patient with osteosarcoma metastatic to spine, chest wall, and lungs became febrile after 10 days of epidural catheterization. When the catheter was removed, culture demonstrated candidal contamination. A second thoracic epidural catheter was placed 4 days later to provide analgesia. Two weeks later, she developed an acute sensory and motor block at T2. Magnetic resonance imaging showed an epidural fluid collection; an emergent laminectomy was performed. A large amount of necrotic tumor, as well as fluid containing *C. tropicalis*, was present in the epidural space. Her neurologic deficits resolved postoperatively. Three additional patients with chronic pain syndromes were evaluated for epidural infection; all workups were negative. The authors concluded that, for terminally ill patients, the risk of infection with long-term epidural catheterization is acceptable, but

TABLE 12-11

INFECTIOUS COMPLICATIONS FOLLOWING NEURAXIAL ANESTHESIA IN THE IMMUNOCOMPROMISED PATIENT

- The attenuated inflammatory response within the immunocompromised patient may diminish the clinical signs and symptoms often associated with infection and result in a delay in diagnosis and treatment.
- The range of microorganisms causing invasive infection in the immunocompromised host is much broader than that affecting the general population and includes atypical and opportunistic pathogens.
- Initiation of early and effective therapy is paramount in optimizing neurologic outcome; consultation with an infectious disease specialist is advised.
- Prolonged antibiotic therapy (weeks–months) is often required because of persistent and immunologic deficiencies.
- Since eradication of infection is difficult once established, prevention of infection is paramount in caring for immunocompromised patients.

From Horlocker TT, Wedel DJ. Regional anesthesia in the immunocompromised patient. *Reg Anesth Pain Med* 2006;31: 334–345, with permission.

recommended careful monitoring to avoid serious neurologic sequelae.

Chronic epidural catheterization in cancer patients is also a potential risk for epidural infection. Du Pen and co-workers (78) studied 350 patients in whom permanent (tunneled) epidural catheters were placed. The authors examined three areas of the catheter track for evidence of infection: exit site, superficial catheter track, and epidural space. The rate of epidural and deep-track catheter-related infections was one in every 1,702 days of catheter use in the 19 patients who developed deep-track or epidural infections. (Four of the 19 patients had both deep track and epidural involvement.) Bacteria cultured were most frequently skin flora. All 19 patients with deep infections were treated with catheter removal and antibiotics; none required surgical decompression or debridement. Catheters were replaced in 15 of the 19 patients who requested them after treatment with no recurrent infections. The authors state recommendations similar to Strafford and colleagues (81); long-term epidural catheterization is safe when patients are carefully monitored for signs of infection and receive prompt treatment when the diagnosis is established.

HERPES SIMPLEX VIRUS

Herpes simplex virus type 2 (HSV-2) infection is an incurable, recurrent disease characterized by asymptomatic periods alternating with recrudescence of genital lesions. The primary infection is associated with viremia and can be accompanied by a variety of symptoms, including fever, headache, and rarely aseptic meningitis. In contrast, recurrent or secondary infections present as genital lesions without evidence of viremia. When obstetric patients present for delivery with evidence of active HSV-2 infection, cesarean section is recommended to avoid exposing the neonate to the virus during vaginal delivery. Neuraxial block in these patients is controversial because of the theoretical potential of introducing the virus into the CNS. However, little data support these concerns.

Bader and colleagues (92) reviewed the management of 169 parturients with HSV-2 infections, five of which were primary infections. Although general anesthesia was administered to 59 patients, the remaining 110 patients received spinal or epidural techniques. One patient with primary HSV-2 infection developed transient unilateral leg weakness after bupivacaine spinal anesthesia. The authors concluded that neuraxial block was safe in cases of secondary infection. Additional investigations support these recommendations, although the total number of patients studied is too limited to make a definitive assessment (93,94). In addition, since the risk of neurologic complications in patients undergoing neuraxial block in the presence of primary infection remains unknown, a conservative approach is recommended.

Herpes simplex virus type 1 (HSV-1), the infectious agent of oral herpes, rarely causes genital lesions. However, recurrent HSV-1 infection has been described in parturients receiving intrathecal and epidural opioids (95). The postnatal association is controversial, since other factors including emotional or physical stress, have been implicated as causes of recurrent HSV-1 infection.

HUMAN IMMUNODEFICIENCY VIRUS

The risk of performing neuraxial block in patients infected with human immunodeficiency virus (HIV) is largely undetermined. Approximately 40% of patients with the diagnosis of acquired immune deficiency syndrome (AIDS) have clinical signs of neuropathy, and 70% to 80% have neuropathic changes present at autopsy. Since the virus infects the CNS early in the disease, it is unlikely that neuraxial block would result in new CNS transmission. However, the neurologic symptoms associated with HIV infection such as aseptic meningitis, headache, and polyneuropathy would be indistinguishable from those related to regional technique. Hughes and colleagues (96) reported safe administration of neuraxial block to 18 HIV-infected parturients. The patients studied showed no postpartum change in immune, infectious, or neurologic status. Avidan and colleagues (97) and Bremerich and colleagues (98) also reported a low complication rate for parturients with HIV infection on antiretroviral therapy who underwent spinal anesthesia. However, in all three series (with a combined total of 117 patients), the patients were relatively healthy and in the early stage of their disease. The effects of anesthesia on patients with more advanced disease are unreported.

Uncomplicated placement of an epidural blood patch for treatment of postdural puncture headache in nine HIV-positive patients has also been described (99). A clear understanding of the association of CNS symptoms with HIV infection is important to interpret postblock (or post blood patch) neurologic findings.

ASEPTIC TECHNIQUE

Although previous publications have repeatedly recommended meticulous aseptic technique, only recently have standards for asepsis during the performance of regional anesthetic procedures been defined (100) (Table 12-12). Hand-washing remains the most crucial component of asepsis; gloves should be regarded as a supplement to—not a replacement for—hand-

TABLE 12-12

VARIABLES THAT MAY INFLUENCE INFECTIOUS COMPLICATIONS

Site of catheter placement (thoracic vs. lumbar vs. caudal)
Choice of antiseptic and technique of application
Choice of barrier protection (masks, gloves, gowns)
Timing and selection of perioperative antibiotics
Duration of neuraxial or peripheral catheterization
Use of bacterial filters
Dressing type(s) (transparent vs. dry gauze dressing; use of antiseptic dressings)

From Hebl JR. The importance and implications of aseptic techniques. *Reg Anesth Pain Med* 2006;31:311–323, with permission.

washing (101). The use of an antimicrobial soap reduces bacterial growth and reduces the risk of bacteria being released into the operative field should gloves become torn or punctured during the procedure. An alcohol-based antiseptic provides the maximum degree of antimicrobial activity and duration. Prior to washing, all jewelry (rings, watches, etc.) should be removed; higher microbial counts have been noted in health care workers who do not routinely remove these items before hand-washing. Sterile gloves protect not only patients from contamination, but also health care workers from blood-borne pathogens and are required by the Occupational Safety and Health Administration (OSHA) (100). Glove leaks are more likely to occur with vinyl compared to latex gloves (24% versus 2%), with contamination of the health care workers' hands noted following the leaks in 23% of cases (102). Conversely, the use of gowns does not further reduce the likelihood of cross-contamination in an intensive care unit setting compared to gloves alone. At this time, there are insufficient data to make recommendations regarding routine use for single-injection or temporary neuraxial/peripheral catheter placement. However, placement of an indwelling permanent device, such as a spinal cord stimulator, warrants the same asepsis as a surgical procedure, including gowns, hats, and antibiotic pretreatment (100,103).

Surgical masks, initially considered a barrier to protect the proceduralist from patient secretions and blood, are now required by the Center for Disease Control (104) due to the increasing number of cases of post spinal meningitis, many of which result from contamination of the epidural or intrathecal space with pathogens from the operator's buccal mucosa (8,105–108). Interestingly, similar reports have been noted among patients undergoing pain procedures. Masks are also recommended as a crucial protective measure against blood-borne pathogen exposure by OSHA (100).

Antiseptic Solutions

Controversy still exists regarding the most appropriate and safe antiseptic solution for patients undergoing neuraxial and peripheral techniques. Povidone iodine and chlorhexidine gluconate (with or without the addition of isopropyl alcohol) have been most extensively studied (109,110). In nearly all clinical investigations, the bactericidal effect of chlorhexidine was more rapid and more effective (extending its effect hours following its application) than povidone iodine. The addition of isopropyl alcohol accelerates these effects. Chlorhexidine is effective against nearly all nosocomial yeasts and bacteria (gram-positive and gram-negative); resistance is extremely rare. It also remains effective in the presence of organic compounds, such as blood. It must be noted that chlorhexidine-alcohol labeling contains a warning against use as a skin preparation prior to lumbar puncture. The FDA has not formally approved chlorhexidine for skin preparation prior to lumbar puncture because of the lack of animal and clinical studies examining the neurotoxic potential of chlorhexidine, not due to a number of reported cases of nerve injury. Indeed, it is important to note that there are no cases of neurotoxicity with either chlorhexidine or alcohol (100). Therefore, as a result of its superior effect, alcohol-based chlorhexidine solutions are considered the antiseptic of choice for skin preparation before any regional anesthetic procedure (100).

Anesthetic Management of the Infected or Febrile Patient

In summary, several clinical and laboratory studies have suggested an association between dural puncture during bacteremia and meningitis. The data are not equivocal, however. The clinical studies are limited to pediatric patients who are historically at high risk for meningitis. Many of the original animal studies utilized bacterial counts that were far in excess of those noted in humans in early sepsis, making CNS contamination more likely. Despite these conflicting results, it is generally recommended that, except in the most extraordinary circumstances, central neuronal block should not be performed in patients with untreated bacteremia (7).

Patients with evidence of systemic infection may safely undergo spinal anesthesia, if antibiotic therapy is initiated prior to dural puncture and the patient has demonstrated a response to therapy, such as a decrease in fever. Placement of an indwelling epidural (or intrathecal) catheter in this group of patients remains controversial; patients should be carefully selected and monitored for evidence of epidural infection. Spinal anesthesia may be safely performed in patients at risk for low-grade transient bacteremia after dural puncture. Once again, little information exists concerning the risk of epidural anesthesia in patients suspected of developing an intraoperative transient bacteremia (such as during a urologic procedure). However, short-term epidural catheterization is most likely safe (7).

The attenuated inflammatory response within the immunocompromised patient, including patients with HSV and HIV, may diminish the clinical signs and symptoms often associated with infection. Likewise, the range of microorganisms causing invasive infection in the immunocompromised host is much broader than that affecting the general population and includes atypical and opportunistic pathogens. Consultation with an infectious disease specialist is advised to facilitate initiation of early and effective therapy (91).

Meticulous aseptic technique, including hand-washing with chlorhexidine, wearing of mask and sterile gloves by the proceduralist, skin asepsis with chlorhexidine, and antibiotic pretreatment for the placement of permanent devices, is critical to the prevention of infectious complications related to regional anesthesia (100).

All patients with an established local or systemic infection should be considered at risk for developing CNS infection. A delay in diagnosis and treatment of even a few hours significantly worsens neurologic outcome. Bacterial meningitis is a medical emergency. Mortality is approximately 30%, even with antibiotic therapy. Meningitis presents most often with fever, severe headache, altered level of consciousness, and meningis-

mus. The diagnosis is confirmed with a lumbar puncture. Lumbar puncture should not be performed if spinal abscess is suspected, as contamination of the intrathecal space may result. The CSF examination in the patient with meningitis reveals leukocytosis, a glucose level of less than 30 mg/dL, and a protein level greater than 150 mg/dL.

The clinical course of epidural abscess progresses from spinal ache and root pain, to weakness (including bowel and bladder symptoms), and eventually paralysis. The initial back pain and radicular symptoms may remain stable for hours to weeks. However, the onset of weakness often progresses to complete paralysis within 24 hours. Although the diagnosis was historically made with myelogram, radiologic examination such as CT scan, or more preferably MRI, is currently recommended. A combination of antibiotics and surgical drainage remains the treatment of choice. As with spinal hematoma, neurologic recovery is dependent on the duration of the deficit and the severity of neurologic impairment before treatment.

NEURAXIAL BLOCK IN PATIENTS WITH PREEXISTING NEUROLOGIC DISORDERS

Patients with preexisting neurologic disease present a unique challenge to the anesthesiologist. The cause of postoperative deficits is difficult to evaluate, because neural injury may occur as a result of surgical trauma, tourniquet pressure, prolonged labor, improper patient positioning, or anesthetic technique. Progressive neurologic diseases such as multiple sclerosis may coincidentally worsen perioperatively, independent of the anesthetic method. The most conservative legal approach is to avoid regional anesthesia in these patients. However, high-risk patients, including those with significant cardiopulmonary disease, may benefit medically from regional anesthesia and analgesia. The decision to proceed with a regional anesthesia in these patients should be made on a case-by-case basis.

Patients with preexisting neurologic disorders of the CNS, such as multiple sclerosis or amyotrophic lateral sclerosis (ALS), lumbar radiculopathy, and ancient poliomyelitis present potential management dilemmas for anesthesiologists. The presence of preexisting deficits, signifying chronic neural compromise, theoretically places these patients at increased risk for further neurologic injury. The presumed mechanism is a "double crush" of the nerve at two locations, resulting in a nerve injury of clinical significance. The double-crush concept suggests that nerve damage caused by traumatic needle placement/local anesthetic toxicity during the performance of a regional anesthetic may worsen neurologic outcome in the presence of an additional patient factor or surgical injury. Progressive neurologic diseases may also coincidentally worsen perioperatively, independent of the anesthetic method. If a neuraxial anesthetic is indicated or requested, the patient's preoperative neurologic examination should be formally documented, and the patient must be made aware of the possible progression of the underlying disease process.

It is difficult to define the actual risk of neurologic complications in patients with preexisting neurologic disorders who receive regional anesthesia; no controlled studies have been performed, and accounts of complications have appeared in the literature only as individual case reports. The decision to use regional anesthesia in these patients is determined on a case-by-case basis and involves understanding the pathophysiology of neurologic disorders, the mechanisms of neural injury associated with regional anesthesia, and the overall incidence of neurologic complications after regional techniques. Although laboratory studies have identified multiple risk factors for the development of neurologic injury after regional anesthesia, clinical studies are lacking. Even less information is available on the variables affecting neurologic damage in patients with preexisting neurologic disease. Several neurologic conditions warrant a more comprehensive discussion.

Multiple Sclerosis

Multiple sclerosis is a degenerative disease of the CNS, characterized by multiple sites of demyelination in the brain and spinal cord. The peripheral nerves are not involved. The course of the disease consists of exacerbations and remissions of symptoms, and the unpredictability in the patient's changing neurologic status must be appreciated when selecting an anesthetic technique. Stress, surgery, and fatigue have been implicated in the exacerbation of multiple sclerosis. Epidural and, more often, spinal anesthesia have been associated with relapse of multiple sclerosis, although the evidence is not strong (111). The mechanism by which spinal anesthesia may exacerbate multiple sclerosis is unknown, but it may be direct local anesthetic toxicity. Epidural anesthesia has been recommended over spinal anesthesia because the concentration of local anesthetic in the white matter of the spinal cord is one-fourth the level after epidural administration (112). The largest series of neuraxial anesthesia in the patient with a preexisting CNS condition involved 139 patients (9). Postpolio syndrome and multiple sclerosis were the most common CNS disorders. Twenty-five patients had a coexisting radiculopathy, peripheral sensorimotor neuropathy, or spinal stenosis. The CNS diagnoses were present a mean of 23 ± 23 years. The majority of patients had sensorimotor deficits at the time of block placement. There were no patients with new or worsening postoperative neurologic deficits when compared to preoperative findings (0.0%; 95% CI, 0.0%–0.3%). The investigators concluded that the risks commonly associated with neuraxial block in patients with preexisting CNS disorders may not be as high as thought and that these conditions should not be an absolute contraindication to spinal or epidural techniques. Because multiple sclerosis is a disorder of the CNS, peripheral nerve blocks do not affect neurologic function and are considered appropriate anesthetic techniques.

Diabetes Mellitus

A substantial proportion of diabetic patients report clinical symptoms of a neuropathy. However, a subclinical neuropathy may be present before the onset of pain, paresthesia, or sensory loss, and may remain undetected without electrophysiologic testing showing typical slowing of nerve conduction velocity. The presence of underlying nerve dysfunction suggests that patients with diabetes may have a decreased requirement for local anesthetic. The diabetes-associated microangiopathy of nerve blood vessels decreases the rate of absorption, resulting in prolonged exposure to local anesthetic solutions. The combination of these two mechanisms may cause nerve injury with an otherwise safe dose of local anesthetic in diabetic patients. In a study examining the effect of local anesthetics on nerve conduction block and injury in diabetic rats, Kalichman and Calcutt (25) reported that the local anesthetic requirement is decreased and the risk of local anesthetic–induced nerve injury is increased in diabetes. These findings suggest that di-

abetic patients may require less local anesthetic to produce anesthesia and that a reduction in dose may be necessary to reduce the risk of neural injury by doses considered safe in non-diabetic patients. However, confirmatory human studies are lacking.

A recent retrospective review of 567 patients with a sensorimotor neuropathy or diabetic polyneuropathy who underwent neuraxial block evaluated the risk of neurologic complications. All patients had a single neurologic diagnosis; there were no coexisting spinal canal or CNS disorder (113). The majority of patients had sensorimotor deficits at the time of surgery. Two (0.4%; 95% CI, 0.1%–1.3%) patients experienced new or worsening postoperative neurologic deficits in the setting of uneventful neuraxial block and without surgical/positioning risk factors. In these patients, who had severe sensorimotor neuropathy preoperatively, it is likely the neuraxial technique contributed to the injury. The investigators concluded that clinicians should be aware of this potentially high-risk subgroup of patients.

Spinal Stenosis and Lumbar Root Disease

Moen and colleagues (8) identified spinal stenosis as a risk factor for postoperative cauda equina syndrome and paraparesis. Importantly, deficits would often occur after uneventful neuraxial technique. These findings agree with those of a recent investigation that examined the overall success and neurologic complication rates among 937 patients with spinal stenosis or lumbar disc disease undergoing neuraxial block between 1988 and 2000 (114). Of these, 210 patients had a coexisting peripheral neuropathy in addition to their spinal cord pathology. Neurologic diagnoses were present a mean of 5 ± 6 years; half of patients had active symptoms at the time of block. In addition, 207 patients had a history of prior spinal surgery before undergoing neuraxial block, although the majority were simple laminectomies or discectomies. Success rates did not differ between patients who had previous surgery and those who had undergone a spine procedure. Ten (1.1%; 95% CI, 0.5%–2.0%) patients experienced new or progressive neurologic deficits when compared to preoperative findings. Although the majority of the deficits were related to surgical trauma or tourniquet ischemia, the neuraxial block was the primary etiology in four patients. The preliminary nature of these data warrants care in their interpretation. However, overall, patients with spinal stenosis or lumbar disc disease may undergo successful neuraxial block without a significant increase in neurologic complications. Importantly, this includes patients who have undergone prior (minor) spine surgery.

In summary, patients with preexisting neurologic disorders such as multiple sclerosis, polio, or ALS may develop new neurologic deficits perioperatively. It is often difficult to differentiate between surgical or anesthetic causes (1). The medicolegal issue, however, remains, and if a regional anesthetic is indicated (or requested), the patient's preoperative neurologic examination should be formally documented, and the patient must be made aware of the possible progression of the underlying disease process. Although stable preexisting neurologic conditions, such as an inactive lumbosacral radiculopathy or hemiparesis associated with an ancient cerebrovascular accident, are not contraindications to neuraxial anesthesia, the underlying etiology of such neurologic deficits requires careful evaluation.

Patients with preoperative neurologic deficits may undergo further nerve damage more readily from needle or catheter placement, local anesthetic systemic toxicity, and vasopressor-induced neural ischemia. Dilute or less potent local anesthetic solutions should be used when feasible to decrease the risk of local anesthetic toxicity. Because epinephrine and phenylephrine also prolong the block and therefore neural exposure to local anesthetics, the appropriate concentration and dose of local anesthetic solutions must be thoughtfully considered.

PERFORMANCE OF NEURAXIAL BLOCKADE IN PATIENTS UNDER ANESTHESIA

The performance of neuraxial blockade on anesthetized patients theoretically increases the risk of perioperative neurologic complications, since these patients are unable to respond to the pain associated with needle- or catheter-induced paresthesias or intraneuronal injections. Case reports of spinal cord and root damage have been reported following thoracic and lumbar neuraxial techniques (115). However, with such a rare (albeit catastrophic) event, a comparative study is unlikely due to the large number of patients required. Hence, the relative risk of neurologic complications in patients undergoing neuraxial techniques while anesthetized or heavily sedated has been difficult to establish.

Regional Anesthesia in Anesthetized Children

The majority of children who undergo regional anesthetic techniques are either heavily sedated or under general anesthesia (116–118). Although this is considered "acceptable" anesthetic management, it could also be argued that, except in cases where there is a documented improvement in perioperative morbidity and mortality (not just superior analgesia), the patient is placed at an "unacceptable" increased risk. Nevertheless, studies involving regional anesthesia in the pediatric population are perhaps the best source of evaluating the risk of neurologic complications in anesthetized patients.

The largest prospective study evaluating the morbidity of regional anesthesia in children was performed by Giaufre and colleagues (119). There were 24,409 regional blocks; 89% were performed under general anesthesia, 6% were performed in the presence of sedation. Approximately half of the blocks were performed in patients between 3 and 12 years of age. Neuraxial blocks, the majority of which were caudal blocks, accounted for 15,013 (>60%) of all regional anesthetics. However, there were 506 spinals (75% of which were performed in premature infants), and 135 thoracic epidural anesthetics. Catheters were placed in only 1,026 of 2,396 (43%) epidural patients. All 23 complications occurred after neuraxial block, for an overall incidence of 1.5 per 1,000 cases. None resulted in long-term sequelae or medicolegal action.

This study is significant for several reasons. Firstly, it documents the safety of regional anesthesia in children. Although it is possible that not all neurologic complications were discovered, it is doubtful that major morbidity went unreported. The etiology of complications is also important. Half of the 23 reported complications, four total spinals, six intravascular injections, and two transient paresthesias, may have been influenced by the patient's alertness during the performance of the neural blockade. These data also support meticulous regional anesthetic technique, including careful calculation of total local anesthetic dose, the use of a test dose, intermittent injection/aspiration, and continuous electrocardiographic monitoring.

Neuraxial Anesthesia in Anesthetized Adults

No prospective studies evaluate the performance of neuraxial techniques in anesthetized adults. However, several retrospective reviews have suggested that, under certain circumstances, neuraxial block may be safe. Horlocker and co-workers (120) reviewed the records of 4,392 consecutive epidural catheters placed in anesthetized adult patients undergoing upper abdominal or thoracic surgery. Epidural catheters were placed either immediately after induction and tracheal intubation or upon completion of the surgical procedure, prior to emergence. Epidural catheterization occurred at the lumbar level in all but four patients who underwent thoracic epidural placement. Nearly all infusions (98.4%) contained an opioid only. There were no documented neurologic complications including spinal hematoma, epidural abscess or catheter site infections, or radicular symptoms (95% CI, 0.0%–0.08%). In one patient, the epidural catheter broke during removal and a portion was retained; no long-term sequelae were noted.

Neurosurgical patients frequently undergo needle/catheter placement (without administration of local anesthetics) under general anesthesia. Grady and colleagues (121) assessed the frequency of neurologic complications in 478 patients undergoing transsphenoidal surgery in conjunction with intraoperative spinal drainage. Malleable needles or spinal drainage catheters were placed after tracheal intubation. Although the drains were used intraoperatively for air injection or CSF removal in 54% and 41% of patients, respectively, no potentially neurotoxic agent was administered. No neurologic deficits were attributable to spinal drainage (95% CI, 0.0–0.8%). Although it is possible that minor neurologic sequelae were missed due to the retrospective nature of these two reviews, it is doubtful that any significant complications were undiscovered.

Although these results are reassuring, they must be carefully interpreted. Although the safety of regional blockade performed on anesthetized pediatric patients is well documented, the decision to perform a regional anesthetic on a heavily sedated or anesthetized patient should not be made indiscriminately. Experts repeatedly question the need to perform epidurals under general anesthesia, noting that more than a million lumbar epidurals are performed on laboring women annually without sedation or anesthesia (115,122).

DIAGNOSIS AND EVALUATION OF NEUROLOGIC COMPLICATIONS

It is imperative that all preoperative neurologic deficits are documented to allow early diagnosis of new or worsening neurologic dysfunction postoperatively. A comprehensive discussion of perioperative neuralgic deficits is beyond the scope of this chapter. However, the clinician is referred to previous reviews of the topic (123). Postoperative sensory or motor deficits must also be distinguished from residual (prolonged) local anesthetic effect. Imaging techniques, such as CT and MRI are useful in identifying infectious and inflammatory processes, as well as expanding hematomas. Although most neurologic complications resolve completely within several days or weeks, significant neural injuries necessitate neurologic consultation to document the degree of involvement and coordinate further workup. Neurophysiologic testing, such as nerve conduction studies, evoked potentials, and EMG are often useful in establishing a diagnosis and prognosis. A reduced amplitude in evoked responses indicates axonal loss, whereas increased latency occurs in the presence of demyelination. Fibrillation

TABLE 12-13

ELECTROMYOGRAPHIC ABNORMALITIES AFTER AXONAL INJURY

Time after injury	Insertional activity	Fibrillation	Recruitment	Amplitude
Acute (<14 days)	Normal	Absent	Reduced	Normal
Subacute (14–21 days)	Increased	Present	Reduced	Normal
1–3 months	Increased	Present	Reduced	May be increased
>6 months	May be increased	Present, but decreased	Reduced	Increased

Adapted from Hogan Q, Hendrix L, Safwan J. Evaluation of neurologic injury after regional anesthesia. In: Finucane BT (Ed). *Complications of Regional Anesthesia*, 2nd ed. New York: Springer, 2007:386–409.

potentials are present during active axonal degeneration. They appear 2 to 3 weeks after injury and are maximal at 1 to 3 months (123) (Table 12-13). Because of the decreased number of axons present in patients with neurologic conditions, a reduction in neuron recruitment occurs during voluntary effort. The degree of reduction parallels the severity of the disorder. Despite many applications, nerve conduction studies have several limitations. Typically, only the large sensory and motor nerve fibers are evaluated; dysfunction of small unmyelinated fibers would not be detected. In addition, abnormalities will not be noted on EMG immediately after injury, but rather require several weeks to evolve. Although it is often recommended to wait until evidence of denervation has appeared before performing neurophysiologic testing, a baseline study (including evaluation of the contralateral extremity, where subclinical symptoms may exist) would be helpful in ruling out underlying pathology or a preexisting condition.

ARACHNOIDITIS AND SPINAL DRUG ADMINISTRATION

It is very unlikely that arachnoidits results from spinal administration of approved spinal drugs. However the inadvertent injection of the wrong drug has the potential to cause inflammation of the meninges and development of arachnoiditis (see Chapter 50, Table 50-2). Unfortunately wrong drug injection continues to occur, albeit rarely, both epidurally and intrathecally. It must be scrupulously guarded against.

Arachnoiditis can lead to the formation of extensive sclerosis of arachnoid membranes (see Fig. 50-21), with constriction of the vascular supply to neural tissue, and potentially to causa equina syndrome (see Chapter 50). It is important to note that arachnoiditis can be caused by intraspinal bleeding associated with occult or overt spinal trauma or by spinal surgery. Such events could result in the delayed development of arachnoiditis.

There are many other potential causes of arachnoiditis such as tuberculosis, syphilis, intrathecal injection of radiological contrast medium (see Chapter 50 and Fig. 50-21).

Thus a patient receiving spinal anesthesia years after spinal surgery or trauma, who subsequently develops arachnoiditis could be inappropriately labelled as "post spinal anesthesia arachnoidits". Careful review of history prior to spinal anesthesia may reveal pre-existing symptoms or signs of arachnoiditis (see Table 50-2).

SUMMARY

In conclusion, major complications after neuraxial techniques are rare, but can be devastating to the patient and the anesthesiologist. Prevention and management begin during the preoperative visit with a careful evaluation of the patient's medical history and appropriate preoperative discussion of the risks and benefits of the available anesthetic techniques. Alternative anesthetic techniques, such as peripheral regional techniques or general anesthesia, should be considered for patients at increased risk for neurologic complications following neuraxial block. The decision to perform a regional anesthetic technique on an anesthetized patient must be made with care, since these patients are unable to report pain on needle placement or injection of local anesthetic. Efforts should also be made to decrease neural injury in the operating room through careful patient positioning. Postoperatively, patients must be followed closely to detect potentially treatable sources of neurologic injury, including expanding spinal hematoma or epidural abscess, constrictive dressings, improperly applied casts, and increased pressure on neurologically vulnerable sites. New neurologic deficits should be evaluated promptly by a neurologist or neurosurgeon to document formally the patient's evolving neurologic status, arrange further testing or intervention, and provide long-term follow-up.

PART II: TECHNIQUES

References

1. Marinacci AA. Neurological aspects of complications of spinal anesthesia with medico-legal implications. *Bull Los Angeles Neurol Soc* 1960;25:170–192.
2. Auroy Y, Narchi P, Messiah A, et al. Serious complications related to regional anesthesia. *Anesthesiology* 1997;87:479–486.
3. Schneider M, Ettlin T, Kaufmann M, et al. Transient neurologic toxicity after hyperbaric subarachnoid anesthesia with 5% lidocaine. *Anesth Analg* 1993;76:1154–1157.
4. Myers RR, Heckman HM. Effects of local anesthesia on nerve blood flow: Studies using lidocaine with and without epinephrine. *Anesthesiology* 1989;71:757–762.
5. Ready LB, Plumer MH, Haschke RH, et al. Neurotoxicity of intrathecal local anesthetics in rabbits. *Anesthesiology* 1985;63:364–370.
6. Horlocker TT, Wedel DJ, Benzon H, et al. Regional anesthesia in the anticoagulated patient: Defining the risks (the second ASRA Consensus Conference on Neuraxial Anesthesia and Anticoagulation). *Reg Anesth Pain Med* 2003;28:172–197.
7. Wedel DJ, Horlocker TT. Regional anesthesia in the febrile or infected patient. *Reg Anesth Pain Med* 2006;31:324–333.
8. Moen V, Dahlgren N, Irestedt L. Severe neurological complications after central neuraxial blockades in Sweden 1990–1999. *Anesthesiology* 2004;101:950–959.

9. Hebl JR, Horlocker TT, Schroeder DR. Neuraxial anesthesia and analgesia in patients with preexisting central nervous system disorders. *Anesth Analg* 2006;103:223–228.

10. Auroy Y, Benhamou D, Bargues L, et al. Major complications of regional anesthesia in France: The SOS Regional Anesthesia Hotline Service. *Anesthesiology* 2002;97:1274–1280.

11. Cheney FW, Domino KB, Caplan RA, Posner K. Nerve injury associated with anesthesia. A closed claims analysis. *Anesthesiology* 1999;90:1062–1069.

12. Lee LA, Posner KL, Domino KB, et al. Injuries associated with regional anesthesia in the 1980s and 1990s: A closed claims analysis. *Anesthesiology* 2004;101:143–152.

13. Horlocker TT, McGregor DG, Matsushige DK, et al. A retrospective review of 4767 consecutive spinal anesthetics: Central nervous system complications. *Anesth Analg* 1997;84:578–584.

14. Reynolds F. Damage to the conus medullaris following spinal anaesthesia. *Anaesthesia* 2001;56:238–247.

15. Reynolds F. Logic in the safe practice of spinal anaesthesia. *Anaesthesia* 2000;55:1045–1046.

16. Giebler RM, Scherer RU, Peters J. Incidence of neurologic complications related to thoracic epidural catheterization. *Anesthesiology* 1997;86:55–63.

17. Dripps RD. A comparison of the malleable needle and catheter techniques for continuous spinal anesthesia. *NY State J Med* 1950;50:1595–1599.

18. Myers RR, Sommer C. Methodology for spinal neurotoxicity studies. *Reg Anesth* 1993;18:439–447.

19. Ross BK, Coda B, Heath CH. Local anesthetic distribution in a spinal model: A possible mechanism of neurologic injury after continuous spinal anesthesia. *Reg Anesth* 1992;17:69–77.

20. Rigler ML, Drasner K, Krejcie TC, et al. Cauda equina syndrome after continuous spinal anesthesia. *Anesth Analg* 1991;72:275–281.

21. Lambert DH, Hurley RJ. Cauda equina syndrome and continuous spinal anesthesia. *Anesth Analg* 1991;72:817–819.

22. Drasner K, Sakura S, Chan VW, et al. Persistent sacral sensory deficit induced by intrathecal local anesthetic infusion in the rat. *Anesthesiology* 1994;80:847–852.

23. Horlocker TT, McGregor DG, Matsushige DK, et al. Neurologic complications of 603 consecutive continuous spinal anesthetics using macrocatheter and microcatheter techniques. Perioperative Outcomes Group. *Anesth Analg* 1997;84:1063–1070.

24. Arkoosh VA, Palmer CM, Yun EM, et al. A randomized, double-masked, multicenter comparison of the safety of continuous intrathecal labor analgesia using a 28-gauge catheter versus continuous epidural labor analgesia. *Anesthesiology* 2008;108:286–298.

25. Kalichman MW, Calcutt NA. Local anesthetic-induced conduction block and nerve fiber injury in streptozotocin-diabetic rats. *Anesthesiology* 1992;77:941–947.

26. Hodgson PS, Neal JM, Pollock JE, Liu SS. The neurotoxicity of drugs given intrathecally (spinal). *Anesth Analg* 1999;88:797–809.

27. Selander D. Neurotoxicity of local anesthetics: Animal data. *Reg Anesth* 1993;18:461–468.

28. Drasner K, Rigler MA, Sessler DI, Stoller ML. Cauda equina syndrome following intended epidural anesthesia. *Anesthesiology* 1992;77:582–585.

29. U.S. Food and Drug Administration. FDA safety alert: Cauda equina syndrome associated with use of small-bore catheters in continuous spinal anesthesia. May 29, 1992.

30. Drasner K. Lidocaine spinal anesthesia. A vanishing therapeutic index. *Anesthesiology* 1997;87:469–472.

31. Drasner K. Local anesthetic neurotoxicity: Clinical injury and strategies that may minimize risk. *Reg Anesth Pain Med* 2002;27:576–580.

32. Gissen A, Datta S, Lambert D. The chloroprocaine controversy. II. Is chloroprocaine neurotoxic? *Reg Anesth* 1984;9:135–144.

33. Taniguchi M, Bollen AW, Drasner K. Sodium bisulfite: Scapegoat for chloroprocaine neurotoxicity? *Anesthesiology* 2004;100:85–91.

34. Yoos JR, Kopacz DJ. Spinal 2-chloroprocaine for surgery: An initial 10-month experience. *Anesth Analg* 2005;100:553–558.

35. Pollock JE, Neal JM, Stephenson CA, Wiley CE. Prospective study of the incidence of transient radicular irritation in patients undergoing spinal anesthesia. *Anesthesiology* 1996;84:1361–1367.

36. Hampl KF, Schneider MC, Ummenhofer W, Drewe J. Transient neurologic symptoms after spinal anesthesia. *Anesth Analg* 1995;81:1148–1153.

37. Pollock JE, Liu SS, Neal JM, Stephenson CA. Dilution of spinal lidocaine does not alter the incidence of transient neurologic symptoms. *Anesthesiology* 1999;90:445–450.

38. Freedman JM, Li D, Drasner K, et al. Transient neurologic symptoms after spinal anesthesia. An epidemiologic study of 1863 patients. *Anesthesiology* 1998;89:633–641.

39. Pollock JE, Burkhead D, Neal JM, et al. Spinal nerve function in five volunteers experiencing transient neurologic symptoms after lidocaine subarachnoid anesthesia. *Anesth Analg* 2000;90:658–665.

40. Sakura S, Sumi M, Sakaguchi Y, et al. The addition of phenylephrine contributes to the development of transient neurologic symptoms after spinal anesthesia with 0.5% tetracaine. *Anesthesiology* 1997;87:771–778.

41. Zaric D, Christiansen C, Pace NL, Punjasawadwong Y. Transient neurologic symptoms after spinal anesthesia with lidocaine versus other local anesthetics: A systematic review of randomized, controlled trials. *Anesth Analg* 2005;100:1811–1816.

42. YaDeau JT, Liguori GA, Zayas VM. The incidence of transient neurologic symptoms after spinal anesthesia with mepivacaine. *Anesth Analg* 2005;101:661–665.

43. Johnson ME, Uhl CB, Spittler KH, et al. Mitochondrial injury and caspase activation by the local anesthetic lidocaine. *Anesthesiology* 2004;101:1184–1194.

44. Kane RE. Neurologic deficits following epidural or spinal anesthesia. *Anesth Analg* 1981;60:150–161.

45. Wedel DJ, Horlocker TT. Risks of regional anesthesia-infectious, septic. *Reg Anesth* 1996;21:57–61.

46. Kristensen JD, Karlsten R, Gordh T. Spinal cord blood flow after intrathecal injection of ropivacaine: A screening for neurotoxic effects. *Anesth Analg* 1996;82:636–640.

47. Kozody R, Swartz J, Palahniuk RJ, et al. Spinal cord blood flow following sub-arachnoid lidocaine. *Can Anaesth Soc J* 1985;32:472–478.

48. Kozody R, Palahniuk RJ, Cumming MO. Spinal cord blood flow following subarachnoid tetracaine. *Can Anaesth Soc J* 1985; 32:23–29.

49. Dahlgren N, Tornebrandt K. Neurologic complications after anaesthesia. A follow-up of 18,000 spinal and epidural anaesthetics performed over three years. *Acta Anaesthesiol Scand* 1995;39:872–880.

50. Hashimoto K, Hampl KF, Nakamura Y, et al. Epinephrine increases the neurotoxic potential of intrathecally administered lidocaine in the rat. *Anesthesiology* 2001;94:876–881.

51. Tryba M. Epidural regional anesthesia and low molecular heparin: Pro (German). *Anästh Intensivmed Notfallmed Schmerzther* 1993;28:179–181.

52. Vandermeulen EP, Van Aken H, Vermylen J. Anticoagulants and spinal-epidural anesthesia. *Anesth Analg* 1994;79:1165–1177.

53. Liu S, Carpenter RL, Neal JM. Epidural anesthesia and analgesia. Their role in postoperative outcome. *Anesthesiology* 1995;82:1474–1506.

54. Geerts WH, Pineo GF, Heit JA, et al. Prevention of venous thromboembolism: The Seventh ACCP Conference on Antithrombotic and Thrombolytic Therapy. *Chest* 2004;126:S338–S400.

55. Odoom JA, Sih IL. Epidural analgesia and anticoagulant therapy. *Anaesthesia* 1983;38:254–259.

56. Horlocker TT, Wedel DJ, Schlichting JL. Postoperative epidural analgesia and oral anticoagulant therapy. *Anesth Analg* 1994;79:89–93.

57. Wu CL, Perkins FM. Oral anticoagulant prophylaxis and epidural catheter removal. *Reg Anesth* 1996;21:517–524.

58. Rao TLK, El-Etr AA. Anticoagulation following placement of epidural and subarachnoid catheters: An evaluation of neurologic sequelae. *Anesthesiology* 1981;55:618–620.

59. Ruff RL, Dougherty JH. Complications of lumbar puncture followed by anticoagulation. *Stroke* 1981;12:879–881.

60. Chaney MA. Intrathecal and epidural anesthesia and analgesia for cardiac surgery. *Anesth Analg* 1997;84:1211–1221.

61. Schwander D, Bachmann F. Heparin and spinal or epidural anesthesia: Decision analysis. *Ann Fr Anesth Reanim* 1991;10:284–296.

62. Bergqvist D, Lindblad B, Matzsch T. Low molecular weight heparin for thromboprophylaxis and epidural/spinal anaesthesia: Is there a risk? *Acta Anaesthesiol Scand* 1992;36:605–609.

63. Horlocker TT, Wedel DJ. Neuraxial block and low molecular weight heparin: Balancing perioperative analgesia and thromboprophylaxis. *Reg Anesth Pain Med* 1998;23:164–177.

64. Schroeder DR. Statistics: Detecting a rare adverse drug reaction using spontaneous reports. *Reg Anesth Pain Med* 1998;23:183–189.

65. Horlocker TT, Wedel DJ, Offord KP, et al. Preoperative antiplatelet therapy does not increase the risk of spinal hematoma associated with regional anesthesia. *Anesth Analg* 1995;80:303–309.

66. CLASP (Collaborative Low-Dose Aspirin Study in Pregnancy): CLASP: A randomized trial of low-dose aspirin for the prevention and treatment of pre-eclampsia among 9364 pregnant women. *Lancet* 1994;343:619–629.

67. Horlocker TT, Bajwa ZH, Ashraf Z, et al. Risk assessment of hemorrhagic complications associated with nonsteroidal antiinflammatory medications in ambulatory pain clinic patients undergoing epidural steroid injection. *Anesth Analg* 2002;95:1691–1697.

68. Ready LB, Helfer D. Bacterial meningitis in parturients after epidural anesthesia. *Anesthesiology* 1989;71:988–990.

69. Baker AS, Ojemann RG, Swartz MN, Richardson EP. Spinal epidural abscess. *New Engl J Med* 1975;293:463–468.

70. Ericsson M, Algers G, Schliamser SE. Spinal epidural abscesses in adults: Review and report of iatrogenic cases. *Scand J Infect Dis* 1990;22:249–257.

71. Wegeforth P, Latham JR. Lumbar puncture as a factor in the causation of meningitis. *Am J Med Sci* 1919;158:183–202.

72. Pray LG. Lumbar puncture as a factor in the pathogenesis of meningitis. *Am J Dis Child* 1941;295:62–68.

73. Eng RHK, Seligman SJ. Lumbar puncture-induced meningitis. *JAMA* 1981; 245:1456–1459.

74. Teele DW, Dashefsky B, Rakusan T, Klein JO. Meningitis after lumbar puncture in children with bacteremia. *N Engl J Med* 1981;304:1079–1081.

75. Smith KM, Deddish RB, Ogata ES. Meningitis associated with serial lumbar punctures and post-hemorrhagic hydrocephalus. *J Pediatr* 1986;109:1057–1060.

76. Weed LH, Wegeforth P, Ayer JB, Felton LD. The production of meningitis by release of cerebrospinal fluid during an experimental septicemia. *JAMA* 1919;72:190–193.

77. Carp H, Bailey S. The association between meningitis and dural puncture in bacteremic rats. *Anesthesiology* 1992;76:739–742.

78. Du Pen SL, Peterson DG, Williams A, Bogosian AJ. Infection during chronic epidural catheterization: Diagnosis and treatment. *Anesthesiology* 1990;73:905–909.

79. Scott DB, Hibbard BM. Serious non-fatal complications associated with extradural block in obstetric practice. *Br J Anaesth* 1990;64:537–541.

80. Bader AM, Datta S, Gilbertson L, Kirz L. Regional anesthesia in women with chorioamnionitis. *Reg Anesth* 1992;17:84–86.

81. Strafford MA, Wilder RT, Berde CB. The risk of infection from epidural analgesia in children: A review of 1,620 cases. *Anesth Analg* 1995;80:234–238.

82. Goodman EJ, DeHorta E, Taguiam JM. Safety of spinal and epidural anesthesia in parturients with chorioamnionitis. *Reg Anesth* 1996;21:436–441.

83. Kindler C, Seeberger M, Siegemund M, Schneider M. Extradural abscess complicating lumbar extradural anaesthesia and analgesia in an obstetric patient. *Acta Anaesthesiol Scand* 1996;40:858–861.

84. Aromaa U, Lahdensuu M, Cozanitis DA. Severe complications associated with epidural and spinal anaesthetics in Finland 1987–1993. A study based on patient insurance claims. *Acta Anaesthesiol Scand* 1997;41:445–452.

85. Albright GA, Forster RM. The safety and efficacy of combined spinal and epidural analgesia/anesthesia (6,002 blocks) in a community hospital. *Reg Anesth Pain Med* 1999;24:117–125.

86. Kilpatrick ME, Girgis NI. Meningitis: A complication of spinal anesthesia. *Anesth Analg* 1983;62:513–515.

87. Reynolds F. Neurological infections after neuraxial anesthesia. *Anesthesiol Clin* 2008;26:23–52.

88. Darchy B, Forceville X, Bavoux E, et al. Clinical and bacteriologic survey of epidural analgesia in patients in the intensive care unit. *Anesthesiology* 1996;85:988–998.

89. Jakobsen KB, Christensne MK, Carlsson PS. Extradural anaesthesia for repeated surgical treatment in the presence of infection. *Br J Anaesth* 1995;75:536–540.

90. Bengtsson M, Nettelblad H, Sjoberg F. Extradural catheter-related infections in patients with infected cutaneous wounds. *Br J Anaesth* 1997;79:668–670.

91. Horlocker TT, Wedel DJ. Regional anesthesia in the immunocompromised patient. *Reg Anesth Pain Med* 2006;31:334–345.

92. Bader AM, Camann WR, Datta S. Anesthesia for cesarean delivery in patients with herpes simplex type-2 infections. *Reg Anesth* 1990;15:261–263.

93. Crosby ET, Halpern SH, Rolbin SH. Epidural anaesthesia for cesarean section in patients with active recurrent genital herpes simplex infections: A retrospective review. *Can J Anaesth* 1989;36:701–704.

94. Ramanathan S, Sheth R, Turndorf H. Anesthesia for cesarean section in patients with genital herpes infections. A retrospective study. *Anesthesiology* 1986;64:807–809.

95. Crone LL, Conly JM, Storgard C, et al. Herpes labialis in parturients receiving morphine after cesarean section. *Anesthesiology* 1990;73:208–213.

96. Hughes SC, Dailey PA, Landers D, et al. Parturients infected with human immunodeficiency virus and regional anesthesia. *Anesthesiology* 1995;82:32–37.

97. Bremerich DH, Ahr A, Buchner S, et al. Anesthetic regimen for HIV positive parturients undergoing elective cesarean section. [German]. *Anaesthesist* 2003;52:1124–1131.

98. Avidan MS, Groves P, Blott M, et al. Low complication rate associated with cesarean section under spinal anesthesia for HIV-1-infected women on antiretroviral therapy. *Anesthesiology* 2002;97:320–324.

99. Tom DJ, Gulevich SJ, Shapiro HM, et al. Epidural blood patch in the HIV-positive patient. *Anesthesiology* 1992;76:943–947.

100. Hebl JR. The importance and implications of aseptic techniques. *Reg Anesth Pain Med* 2006;31:311–323.

101. Saloojee H, Steenhoff A. The health professional's role in preventing nosocomial infections. *Postgrad Med J* 2001;77:16–19.

102. Olsen RJ, Lynch P, Coyle MB, et al. Examination gloves are barriers to hand contamination in clinical practice. *JAMA* 1993;270:350–353.

103. Rathmell JP, Lake T, Ramundo MB. Infectious risks of chronic pain treatments. *Reg Anesth Pain Med* 2006;31:346–352.

104. Centers for Disease Control and Prevention. Isolation guidelines. Retrieved July 31, 2008 from http://www.cdc.gov/ncidod/dhqp/pdf/guidelines/Isolation2007.pdf.

105. Schneeberger PM, Janssen M, Voss A. Alpha-hemolytic streptococci: A major pathogen of iatrogenic meningitis following lumbar puncture. Case reports and a review of the literature. *Infection* 1996;24:29–35.

106. Trautmann M, Lepper PM, Schmitz FJ. Three cases of bacterial meningitis after spinal and epidural anesthesia. *Eur J Clin Microbiol Infect Dis* 2002;21:43–45.

107. Couzigou C, Vuong TK, Botherel AH, et al. Iatrogenic Streptococcus salivarius meningitis after spinal anaesthesia: Need for strict application of standard precautions. *J Hosp Infect* 2003;53:313–314.

108. Molinier S, Paris JF, Brisou P, et al. Two cases of iatrogenic oral streptococcal infection: Meningitis and spondylodiscitis. [French]. *Rev Med Interne* 1998;19:568–570.

109. Kinirons B, Mimoz O, Lafendi L, et al. Chlorhexidine versus povidone iodine in preventing colonization of continuous epidural catheters in children: A randomized, controlled trial. *Anesthesiology* 2001;94:239–244.

110. Birnbach DJ, Stein DJ, Murray O, et al. Povidone iodine and skin disinfection before initiation of epidural anesthesia. *Anesthesiology* 1998;88:668–672.

111. Crawford J, James FM, Nolte H, et al. Regional analgesia for patients with chronic neurologic disease and similar conditions. *Anaesthesia* 1981;36:821.

112. Warren TM, Datta S, Ostheimer GW. Lumbar epidural anesthesia in a patient with multiple sclerosis. *Anesth Analg* 1982;61:1022–1023.

113. Hebl JR, Kopp SL, Schroeder DR, Horlocker TT. Neurologic complications after neuraxial anesthesia or analgesia in patients with preexisting peripheral sensorimotor neuropathy or diabetic polyneuropathy. *Anesth Analg* 2006;103:1294–1299.

114. Hebl JR, Horlocker TT, Schroeder DR. Neurologic complications after neuraxial anesthesia or analgesia in patients with pre-existing spinal stenosis or lumbar disc disease. *Reg Anesth Pain Med* 2005;29:A89.

115. Drasner K. Thoracic epidural anesthesia: Asleep at the wheal? *Anesth Analg* 2004;99:578–579.

116. Berde C. Epidural analgesia in children. *Can J Anaesth* 1994;41:555–560.

117. Berde C. Regional anesthesia in children: What have we learned? *Anesth Analg* 1996;83:897–900.

118. Wood C, Goresky GV, Klassen KA, Neil SG. Complications of continuous epidural infusions for postoperative analgesia in children. *Can J Anaesth* 1994;41:613–620.

119. Giaufre E, Dalens B, Gombert A. Epidemiology and morbidity of regional anesthesia in children: A one-year prospective survey of the French-Language Society of Pediatric Anesthesiologists. *Anesth Analg* 1996;83:904–912.

120. Horlocker TT, Abel MD, Messick JM, Schroeder DR. Small risk of serious complications related to lumbar epidural catheter placement in anesthetized patients. *Anesth Analg* 2003;96:1547–1552.

121. Grady RE, Horlocker TT, Brown RD, et al. Neurologic complications of spinal drainage. *Anesth Analg* 1999;88:388–392.

122. Rosenquist RW, Birnbach DJ. Epidural insertion in anesthetized adults: Will your patients thank you? *Anesth Analg* 2003;96:1545–1546.

123. Hogan Q, Hendrix L, Safwan J. Evaluation of neurologic injury after regional anesthesia. In: Finucane BT, ed. *Complications of Regional Anesthesia*, 2nd ed. New York: Springer; 2007:386–409.

PART II: TECHNIQUES

CHAPTER 13 ▪ THE UPPER EXTREMITY: SOMATIC BLOCK

JOSEPH M. NEAL

Upper extremity regional anesthesia is the most common form of peripheral nerve block performed by anesthesiologists, even when intravenous (IV) regional anesthesia techniques are excluded. Fellowship-trained regional anesthesiologists also perform more upper than lower extremity regional anesthesia (1). This chapter provides a comprehensive review of brachial plexus regional anesthesia, including its affect on patient outcome, the anatomy and pharmacology of the brachial plexus, complications specific to these techniques, and practical advice on performing regional anesthesia at the various approaches to the brachial plexus.

HYPERTENSION AND BRADYCARDIA

Nonanesthesiologists may surmise that regional anesthesia of the brachial plexus is safer for patients than is general anesthesia. No evidence supports this belief. Indeed, the prudent anesthesiologist recognizes that in certain patient subsets, regional anesthesia may be riskier than general anesthesia despite an intuitive sense to the contrary. For example, upper extremity regional anesthesia may be presumed safer than general anesthesia in patients with severe pulmonary disease, when in fact above-the-clavicle approaches place these patients at risk for further pulmonary compromise from transient hemidiaphragmatic paresis. The absence of evidence that upper extremity block reduces major morbidity should not be surprising, since upper extremity surgery itself does not adversely impact cardiac or pulmonary pathophysiology. However, upper extremity regional anesthesia can positively impact lesser outcomes during the first 24 hours after surgery. Randomized clinical trials have consistently shown that the use of a regional anesthetic technique for shoulder (2), hand, or wrist (3,4) surgery improves analgesia; reduces opioid requirement, with consequent reduction of opioid-related side effects; lessens time to discharge; and lessens the need for hospital admission as compared to fast-track general anesthesia techniques. Furthermore, benefits such as superior analgesia and improved sleep can be prolonged if regional analgesia is extended into the postoperative period with the use of a continuous perineural catheter (5,6). Limited evidence suggests that continuous brachial plexus analgesia improves hard outcomes, such as better rehabilitation or earlier return to work (7). Preliminary studies suggest that continuous perineural techniques can aid early hospital discharge and facilitate rehabilitation on an outpatient basis, provide superior analgesia, and reduced opioid-related side effects after major procedures such as total shoulder arthroplasty (8,9). Importantly, the use of continuous perineural techniques does not appear to increase the risk of major neurologic or infectious complications, as compared to single-injection techniques. (10,11).

BRACHIAL PLEXUS ANATOMY

The Brachial Plexus

Brachial plexus anatomy can be daunting to skilled anatomists, and is even more so to the occasional practitioner of regional anesthesia. The brachial plexus forms from the ventral primary rami of the fifth through eighth cervical (C5–C8) and the first thoracic (T1) nerves. The C4 and T2 nerve roots may also contribute to the brachial plexus. From these separate nerve roots, the brachial plexus undergoes a complex series of convergences and divergences (Fig. 13-1). As the nerve roots traverse the space between the anterior and middle scalene muscles, they converge into three vertically arranged trunks (upper, middle, and lower), which shortly thereafter diverge into anterior and posterior divisions as they cross over the lateral border of the first rib. From this point forward, the posterior division innervates the posterior arm, primarily as the radial and axillary nerves. As the divisions proceed distally, they wrap around the second part of the axillary artery and form three distinct cords. The posterior cord is simply a continuation of the posterior division and lies posterior to the artery. The anterior division splits into the medial and lateral cords, which are defined by their relationship to the axillary artery. Both of these cords usually contain portions of what will eventually become the median nerve, while the musculocutaneous nerve is derived from the lateral cord and the ulnar nerve is derived from the medial cord. By the time the neurovascular bundle reaches the axilla, the four terminal nerves remain separate and distinct for the remainder of their distal travel, with the musculocutaneous nerve typically coursing within the belly or fascia of the coracobrachialis muscle (12).

Structurally, the brachial plexus exhibits marked variation in its configuration; at least 29 known variations exist (13), and two–thirds of humans will have a different brachial plexus configuration on their right as compared to their left side (14). This variation in anatomic configuration is ultimately mirrored in upper extremity cutaneous sensory innervation. Schematic depictions of the arm's sensory innervation seldom represent clinical reality (Fig. 13-2). Innervation of the arm is characterized by significant overlap of cutaneous distribution, especially in the volar forearm and hand, where the sensory fields blend and thus impair the anesthesiologist's ability to assess which terminal nerves are adequately anesthetized or may require anesthetic

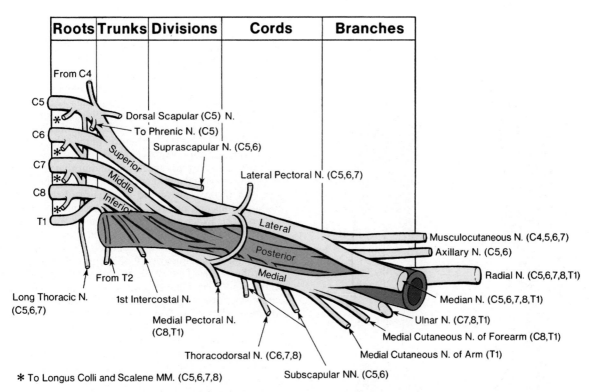

FIGURE 13-1. Schematic illustration of the left brachial plexus. Note how intermediary branches diverge from various portions of the brachial plexus to innervate progressively distal portions of the shoulder and arm. Anesthesiologists should be aware that this idealized version of the brachial plexus is unlikely to represent the actual configuration in any individual and indeed, right- and left-sided configurations differ in up to two-thirds of patients.

supplementation. A frequently used technique for assessing upper extremity anesthetic distribution isolates sensory or motor characteristics specific to each terminal nerve, rather than attempting to use and then potentially misinterpret traditional sensory or motor tests such as loss of pin-prick or grip strength. The practitioner can thereby more accurately link inadequate block to a specific nerve. This assessment technique—*Push—Pull—Pinch—Pinch*—isolates the four terminal nerves in the following manner. Inability to *push* by extending the forearm against resistance confirms anesthesia of the radial nerve. Loss of the ability to *pull* the forearm by flexing it against resistance signifies anesthesia of the musculocutaneous nerve. Inability to recognize *pinches* at the palmar bases of the index finger or the little finger indicates anesthesia of the median nerve and ulnar nerve, respectively (15).

Basic understanding of upper extremity motor innervation is essential for correctly interpreting motor responses to peripheral nerve electrical stimulation. Shoulder elevation and/or biceps contraction signifies stimulation of the upper trunk and correct needle placement during the interscalene approach, whereas posterior shoulder movement is unacceptable because it indicates dorsal scapular nerve stimulation and needle placement that is too posterior. Triceps movement indicates radial nerve stimulation, but is a less desirable end-point than extension of the wrist or fingers during axillary block (16). Musculocutaneous nerve stimulation results in forearm flexion. Median nerve stimulation causes forearm pronation, wrist flexion, and thumb/index finger opposition. Ulnar nerve stimulation is identified by ulnar deviation of the wrist, thumb adduction, and little finger flexion (Fig. 13-3).

Important Brachial Plexus Branches and Non-brachial Plexus Nerves

Knowledge of certain important branches of the brachial plexus, together with select nerves that are not part of the brachial plexus, is crucial for intelligently providing upper extremity anesthesia (Fig. 13-1). The *supraclavicular nerve* (C3–C4) innervates the "cape of the shoulder." Although it is frequently blocked from cephalad local anesthetic spread during the interscalene approach, adequate anesthesia is often absent after the supraclavicular brachial plexus approach. The *suprascapular nerve* (C5–C6) branches from the upper trunk. Depending on how proximally this branching occurs in relationship to where the block needle is placed, the suprascapular nerve may require a separate anesthetizing procedure for surgery involving the shoulder joint. The *intercostobrachial nerve* (T2) is not part of the brachial plexus and therefore requires separate anesthesia when surgery involves the upper posterior medial arm. The *medial antebrachial cutaneous nerve* innervates the medial volar forearm and may remain unanesthetized when an axillary or midhumeral block is placed distal to where it branches from the medial cord.

Important Anatomic Relationships

The brachial plexus maintains relatively consistent anatomic relationships with surrounding structures that aid in the provision of upper extremity regional anesthesia (Fig. 13-4). As the

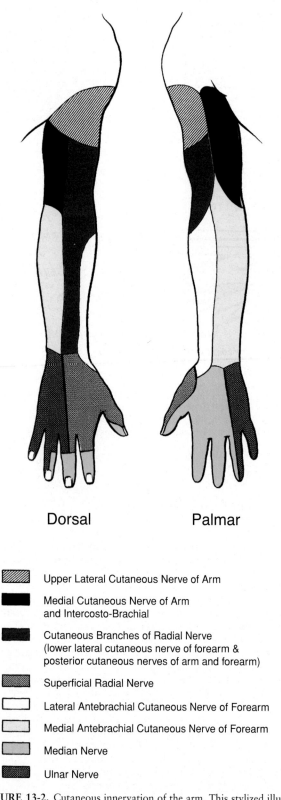

Dorsal   Palmar

▨	Upper Lateral Cutaneous Nerve of Arm
■	Medial Cutaneous Nerve of Arm and Intercosto-Brachial
▦	Cutaneous Branches of Radial Nerve (lower lateral cutaneous nerve of forearm & posterior cutaneous nerves of arm and forearm)
▨	Superficial Radial Nerve
▢	Lateral Antebrachial Cutaneous Nerve of Forearm
▢	Medial Antebrachial Cutaneous Nerve of Forearm
▨	Median Nerve
■	Ulnar Nerve

FIGURE 13-2. Cutaneous innervation of the arm. This stylized illustration may not reflect reality, because significant overlapping of sensory fields occur within the arm, particularly on the volar forearm and hand.

cervical nerve roots exit their respective intervertebral foramina, they invaginate the prevertebral fascia, which purportedly forms the brachial plexus sheath, the clinical significance of which is controversial (14,17–21). Early descriptions of the brachial plexus sheath described it as a tubular structure containing the various components of the brachial plexus—from the roots extending to beyond the axilla (21). Newer imaging methodologies place this concept into question and instead describe the brachial plexus as being contained within a tissue plane defined by the rigid structures of the chest wall, humerus, pectoral fascia, and scapula (17). This tissue plane, rather than a sheath, provides the structural conduit that facilitates tracking of injected local anesthetic solutions along the plexus. Proximally, the convergence and divergence of the trunks, roots, and divisions are mirrored by their accompanying connective tissues (22), which likely facilitates the even spread of anesthesia associated with blocks placed at these approaches (17). At the level of the first rib, cryomicrotome evidence suggests that the structural integrity of these connective tissues becomes less robust (14) (Fig. 13-5). Farther distally, as the terminal nerves and their connective tissue coverings become separate and distinct, the tubular integrity of the sheath and/or the rigid anatomy of the tissue plane become less apparent and less clinically relevant (18–20). The distal incongruity of tissue planes and connective tissues can be correlated with clinical evidence that multiple-injection techniques at these levels are generally more successful than single-injection techniques (14).

Muscular and vascular structures help to further guide and refine upper extremity block. The brachial plexus typically passes between the anterior and middle scalene muscles as it traverses from the neck to the arm in a lateral, 45-degree anterior, and caudad trajectory. Portions of the nerve roots occasionally pass directly through the anterior scalene muscle. The relationship of brachial plexus to scalene muscles defines the interscalene groove and provides surface landmarks used for the interscalene and some supraclavicular approaches (Fig. 13-4). Key vascular relationships include the vertebral arteries, which lie anterior to the nerve roots as they exit the intervertebral foramina, a position that makes them susceptible to intravascular injection from needles placed too medially and deeply (Fig. 13-6). The brachial plexus consistently resides posterior, lateral, and cephalad to the subclavian artery at the level of the first rib (Fig. 13-5). This relationship provides valuable information if blood is aspirated during the supraclavicular approach. The second part of the axillary artery defines the anatomic positioning of the three cords. More distally at the axilla, the four terminal nerves maintain a variably predictable relationship to the axillary artery (14) (Fig. 13-1). The dome of the pleura resides anterior and medial to the lower trunk (Fig. 13-5).

BRACHIAL PLEXUS PHARMACOLOGY

Local Anesthetics

Local Anesthetic Selection

Selection of local anesthetic for upper extremity regional anesthesia is predicated primarily on the desired duration of surgical anesthesia and/or postoperative analgesia. Despite some favorable preliminary reports, no extended-release local anesthetic preparation is commercially available (23). Extended block duration may be unwise for surgeries that are expected to generate

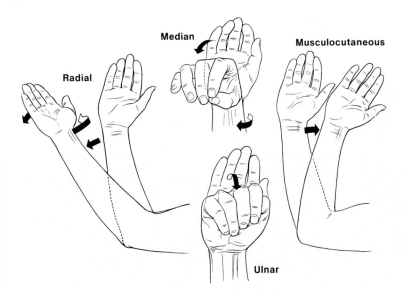

FIGURE 13-3. Typical motor responses to electrical neurostimulation. Radial nerve stimulation results in elbow, wrist, and/or finger extension. Median nerve stimulation causes forearm pronation, wrist flexion, and thumb/index finger opposition. Musculocutaneous nerve stimulation is indicated by elbow flexion. Ulnar nerve stimulation results in wrist ulnar deviation, little finger flexion, and thumb adduction.

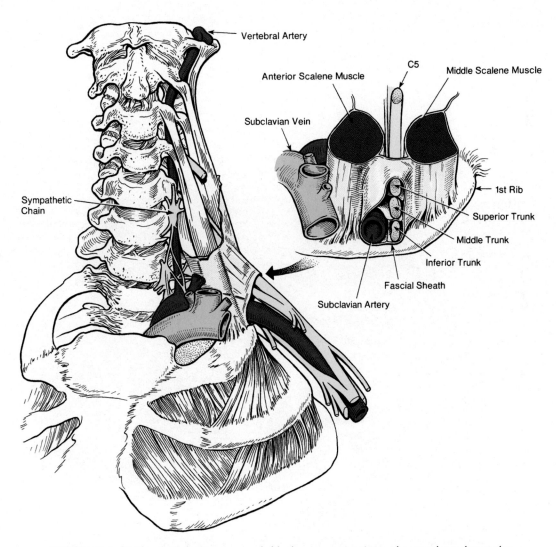

FIGURE 13-4. The brachial plexus is surrounded by key connective tissue, plus vascular and muscular structures that play important roles in upper extremity regional anesthesia. The concept of a substantial fascial sheath derived from the prevertebral fascia has become less relevant as information from modern imaging techniques question its importance. The anterior and middle scalene muscles define the interscalene groove. The vertebral artery is accessible to deeply placed needles. The brachial plexus takes an anterolateral and caudad path toward the shoulder. The trunks stack vertically and continue along a path that takes them posterior and lateral to the subclavian artery.

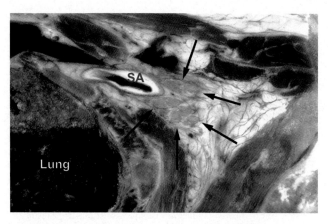

FIGURE 13-5. Cryomicrotome section at the base of the neck (top is anterior). Arrows denote the brachial plexus without an obvious surrounding sheath structure. The subclavian artery (*SA*) is posterior and lateral to the plexus. Note the proximity of the lung. Cryomicrotome by Quinn H. Hogan, MD. Used with permission of the American Society of Regional Anesthesia and Pain Medicine (14).

mild to moderate pain, because some patients are distressed by the numbness and heaviness that accompany long-acting local anesthetic blockade. The possibility of compartment syndrome should be determined in consultation with the surgeon, since even analgesic blocks can mask early signs of impaired circulation. Prolonged sensory and especially motor block demand that patients are provided with protective slings and counseled to avoid sources of heat, cold, or trauma that could injure their insensate arm Using proper precautions, patients with anesthetized arms and/or continuous perineural infusions can be discharged home with minimal risk of injury (5,6,24).

Most upper extremity surgery is amenable to anesthesia using the intermediate-acting local anesthetics lidocaine and mepivacaine. When prolonged analgesia is desired, bupivacaine generally results in 8 to 14 additional hours of analgesia than mepivacaine, or 2 to 6 more hours as compared with ropivacaine. Plain bupivacaine applied to the brachial plexus for surgical anesthesia is approximately 33% more potent than plain ropivacaine (bupivacaine 0.5% = ropivacaine 0.75%) (25,26). Thus, the reduction in cardiotoxicity inherent to ropivacaine can be compromised if larger doses of ropivacaine are used in an attempt to mimic the characteristics of a bupivacaine

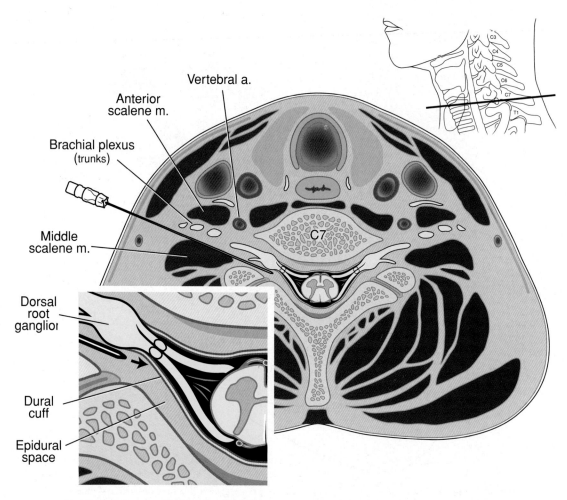

FIGURE 13-6. Unintended neuraxial anesthesia can be associated with interscalene block. Needles placed too deeply can gain access to the subarachnoid, subdural, or epidural spaces. Local anesthetic can also enter the epidural space in a retrograde manner or enter the subarachnoid space via long dural root sleeves. From Neal JM, Rathmell JP. *Complications in Regional Anesthesia and Pain Medicine.* New York: Elsevier Saunders, 2007, with permission.

block. Levobupivacaine and racemic bupivacaine share similar anesthetic characteristics when applied to the brachial plexus (27).

Local Anesthetic Dosing

For neuraxial local anesthetic blockade, total drug mass delivered to the target nerve is the most important factor in determining block effectiveness (28), yet its role is relatively inconsequential for brachial plexus blockade. Based on the studies of Vester-Andersen and colleagues (29–32), there is little evidence that brachial plexus block characteristics can be improved by manipulating local anesthetic dosing regimens. Specifically, block onset, quality, and duration are unaffected by increasing the volume, concentration, and/or total dose of local anesthetic. These data imply that many brachial plexus blocks are performed with more local anesthetic than necessary. Because systemic local anesthetic toxicity is related to the total dose delivered (33), and local anesthetic neurotoxicity in animal models is concentration-dependent (34), logic dictates that attempts to enhance brachial plexus block by using a high volume of concentrated local anesthetic not only fails to significantly improve block quality, but conceivably places the patient at increased risk should an unintended intravascular injection or nerve injury occur. Drug mass should be especially reduced in patients with altered local anesthetic metabolism, such as the elderly and those with congestive heart failure or liver disease (33).

Adjuvants

A myriad of adjuvants have been proposed to improve block quality in terms of faster onset, denser block, and/or longer analgesia. Clinical evidence suggests that only two adjuvants unequivocally accomplish these goals–epinephrine and clonidine—and that their most dramatic effects occur only in conjunction with the intermediate-acting local anesthetics lidocaine and mepivacaine. This phenomenon is explained by the inherent analgesic duration of long–acting local anesthetics being longer than the pharmacokinetic effects of the adjuvant.

Epinephrine intensifies block quality, prolongs block duration, decreases systemic uptake of local anesthetic (and thus the rapid rise of plasma levels that is most associated with systemic toxicity), and acts as a marker of intravascular injection. Epinephrine's availability and low cost argue for its being the adjuvant of choice for brachial plexus blockade. When used in a 1:400,000 concentration (2.5 μg/mL), epinephrine extends local anesthetic blockade to almost the same degree as a 1:200,000 (5 μg/mL) concentration, but without concurrent tachycardia (35). Despite warnings to the contrary, there is no evidence that epinephrine significantly affects blood flow to end arteries, such as those in the fingers (36).

Clonidine prolongs anesthesia and analgesia of intermediate-acting local anesthetics by approximately 50%. When used in 0.5 μg/kg doses (<150 μg), clonidine does not cause significant hypotension, bradycardia, or sedation (37,38). In the United States, the use of clonidine is somewhat restricted by its expense relative to epinephrine and its inability to act as an intravascular marker. There is no benefit to adding clonidine to perineural infusions (39,40).

One other adjuvant—buprenorphine 0.3 mg—has been shown in a single study to increase the duration of mepivacaine upper extremity blocks. All other adjuvants, including opioids, neostigmine, hyaluronidase, tramadol, and calcium channel blockers (14), and most recently dexamethasone (41)

and magnesium (42), have not been consistently shown to improve local anesthetic blockade of the brachial plexus and/or have unresolved toxicity issues.

The practice of alkalinizing local anesthetics to hasten block onset is beneficial in some neuraxial models, but not so for brachial plexus blocks. The addition of sodium bicarbonate ($NaHCO_3$) to plain local anesthetic or to local anesthetic freshly admixed with epinephrine (43) does not result in significantly faster block onset at the brachial plexus; indeed, animal studies suggest that alkalinization of plain lidocaine reduces block quality and duration (44). The addition of $NaHCO_3$ to local anesthetic premixed with epinephrine results in statistically, but perhaps not clinically, significant faster block onset. There is no evidence that alkalinizing local anesthetics improves other measures of block quality (14).

COMPLICATIONS UNIQUE TO BRACHIAL PLEXUS ANESTHESIA

Neurologic and Infectious Complications

Neurologic and infectious complications associated with upper extremity regional anesthesia are exceedingly rare. Details of these complications are presented in Chapters 12 and 20.

Unintended Local Anesthetic Destinations

Intravascular Injection

As compared to epidural anesthesia, unintentional intravascular injection during peripheral nerve block is five times more likely to result in seizures (45). This observation is particularly important in brachial plexus anesthesia, because injection into the nearby vertebral, carotid, or subclavian arteries transports local anesthetic directly to the brain. Predictably, seizure is approximately five times more likely to be associated with the interscalene or supraclavicular approaches than with the axillary approach (46). Intraarterial injections are characterized by immediate seizure activity that resolves quickly if the injection is promptly stopped, which emphasizes the importance of using a 1-mL local anesthetic test dose. Subsequent fractionated 5-mL aliquots of local anesthetic (preferably with epinephrine as an intravascular marker) allow time to develop signs of local anesthetic systemic toxicity and/or epinephrine-induced tachycardia before systemic toxicity occurs from IV injection (47).

Neuraxial Anesthesia

Unintended neuraxial anesthesia can result from a malpositioned needle during the interscalene approach, although the frequency of this complication may be decreased with technique modification (48,49). The distance from the skin overlying the interscalene groove to the intervertebral foramen can be as little as 25 mm (49), and as little as 35 mm to the neuraxis (50). A needle placed too deeply can thus enter the epidural, subdural, or subarachnoid space. Because some nerve root dural sleeves extend far laterally, even properly placed needles can gain access to cerebrospinal fluid and cause unexpected high spinal anesthesia (14) (Fig. 13-6). The use of shorter (25-mm) needles and fractionated dosing regimens may decrease the incidence of this rare complication, but no studies support these recommendations (51).

The presentation of unintended neuraxial anesthetic is determined by where the local anesthetic is injected. Subarachnoid injection results in rapid, bilateral anesthesia that extends from the cervical levels to the lower extremities and may result in immediate unconsciousness and/or apnea. Epidural anesthesia is delayed for 5 to 15 minutes and is more segmental and perhaps unilateral in presentation. In either case, bradycardia and hypotension are common signs (14). Similar to spinal anesthesia-induced hypotension and bradycardia, anesthetic blockade of the cardioaccelerator fibers and sympathetic vasomotor fibers require that resuscitation is rapid and aggressive, including the early use of epinephrine if hemodynamic perturbations fail to immediately respond to atropine and/or ephedrine. Needles can also be unintentionally placed through the intervertebral foramen and into the spinal cord (52).

Cervicothoracic Sympathectomy

The cervicothoracic sympathetic trunk lies in close proximity to the lower brachial plexus (Fig. 13-7). It is therefore not

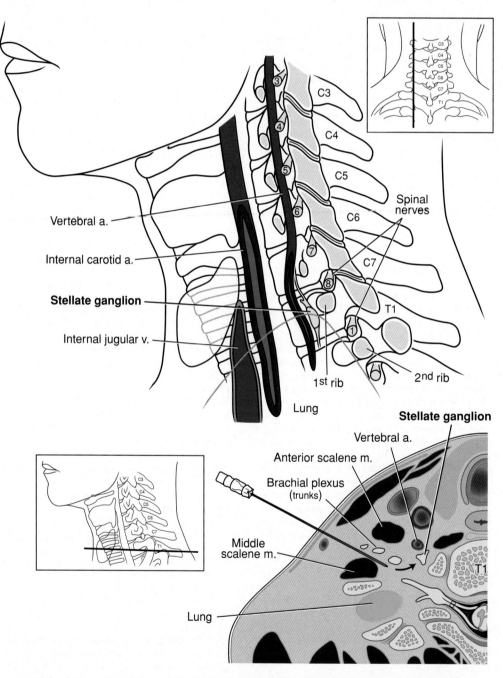

FIGURE 13-7. Unintended anesthesia of the cervicothoracic sympathetic chain/stellate ganglion is a frequent side effect of supraclavicular and interscalene blocks. Even properly placed local anesthetics intended for brachial plexus targets can track through tissue planes toward the stellate ganglion. From Neal JM, Rathmell JP. *Complications in Regional Anesthesia and Pain Medicine.* New York: Elsevier Saunders, 2007, with permission.

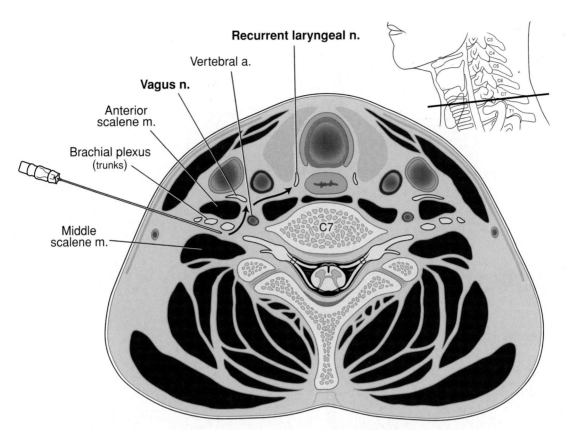

FIGURE 13-8. Unintended anesthesia of the recurrent laryngeal nerve is a frequent side effect of interscalene, and occasionally, supraclavicular blocks. Even properly placed local anesthetics intended for brachial plexus targets can track through tissue planes toward the recurrent laryngeal or the vagus nerves. From Neal JM, Rathmell JP. *Complications in Regional Anesthesia and Pain Medicine.* New York: Elsevier Saunders, 2007, with permission.

surprising that 20% to 90% of supraclavicular (53), 60% of cervical paravertebral (54), 7% of infraclavicular (55), and some interscalene blocks are associated with the development of ipsilateral Horner syndrome (miosis, ptosis, anhydrosis). This nuisance side effect resolves in concert with local anesthetic block resolution.

Recurrent Laryngeal Nerve Anesthesia

Local anesthetic injected into the neck during proximal approaches to the brachial plexus can also diffuse through tissue planes and affect the recurrent laryngeal and/or the vagus nerve (Fig. 13-8). When this occurs, hoarseness results. The reported incidence is higher with the interscalene approach (6% to 12%) (56) than it is with the supraclavicular approach (<2%) (53). This nuisance side effect will resolve along with dissipation of the local anesthetic block (51).

Hemidiaphragmatic Paresis

Ipsilateral hemidiaphragmatic paresis occurs when local anesthetic deposited around the brachial plexus unintentionally blocks the phrenic or accessory phrenic nerve. Although this can take place from direct local anesthetic contact with the phrenic nerve as it crosses the anterior scalene muscle, it most typically results from cephalad spread of local anesthetic to the C3-C5 nerve roots (57) (Fig. 13-9). The incidence and sever-

ity of hemidiaphragmatic paresis varies with the approach to the brachial plexus; the more cephalad the approach, the more likely the diaphragm is affected. Hemidiaphragmatic paresis is associated with 100% of interscalene blocks and can reduce spirometric measures of pulmonary function by 25% to 33% (57,58). The incidence of hemidiaphragmatic paresis is much lower with the supraclavicular approach (~50%) and has no effect on pulmonary function in healthy volunteers (59). The sternocleidomastoid approach is associated with up to 60% incidence of hemidiaphragmatic paresis (60). The vertical infraclavicular approach has a 26% incidence of hemidiaphragmatic impairment with accompanying, but clinically unapparent, diminution in pulmonary function (61), whereas the more distal coracoid approach rarely affects diaphragmatic function (62).

Diaphragm impairment mirrors the onset and waning of local anesthetic effects. Because hemidiaphragmatic paresis with associated diminution in pulmonary function is both prevalent and unpredictable when using proximal approaches to the brachial plexus, these blocks are contraindicated in patients with contralateral diaphragm or phrenic nerve dysfunction, contralateral pneumonectomy, or in patients who may not withstand a 25% reduction in pulmonary function and/or those with a forced vital capacity of less than 1 L (63). Neither digital pressure proximal to the injection site and/or lowering injected volume to 20 mL (14,64), nor the infusion of motor-sparing local anesthetics such as bupivacaine or ropivacaine appreciably and predictably reduces the incidence of hemidiaphragmatic

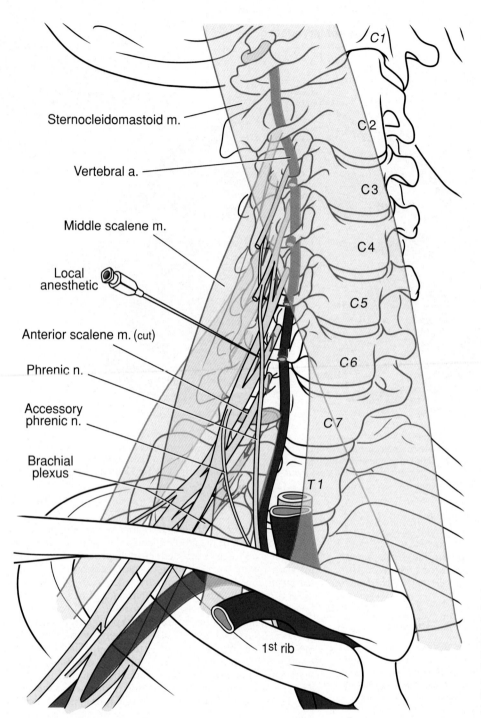

Sternocleidomastoid m.

Vertebral a.

Middle scalene m.

Local anesthetic

Anterior scalene m. (cut)

Phrenic n.

Accessory phrenic n.

Brachial plexus

C1

C2

C3

C4

C5

C6

C7

T1

1st rib

FIGURE 13-9. Unintended anesthesia of the phrenic nerve occurs most frequently from cephalad spread and direct local anesthesia of the C3–C5 nerve roots. Local anesthesia can also affect the phrenic nerve as it courses along the anterior scalene muscle. From Neal JM, Rathmell JP. *Complications in Regional Anesthesia and Pain Medicine.* New York: Elsevier Saunders, 2007, with permission.

paresis (65–67). Single-injection ropivacaine 0.5% has been associated with diaphragm impairment (68), whereas interscalene analgesic infusion of ropivacaine appears to result in a similar incidence of hemidiaphragmatic paresis to that seen with IV opioid analgesia (69). Although most studies suggest that manipulation of local anesthetic type, dose, concentration, or volume have insignificant effect on pulmonary function after interscalene block, one study has shown that reducing the volume and concentration of bupivacaine can minimize adverse respiratory effects (70).

Pneumothorax

Pneumothorax is an especially feared complication of the supraclavicular approach and is rarely possible from wayward needles placed using the interscalene or sternocleidomastoid approaches. Although the supraclavicular approach has been associated with a 0.6% to 6% incidence of pneumothorax, these data refer to the classic, but rarely used, Kulenkampff technique (71). The more contemporary "plumb-bob" (72) and

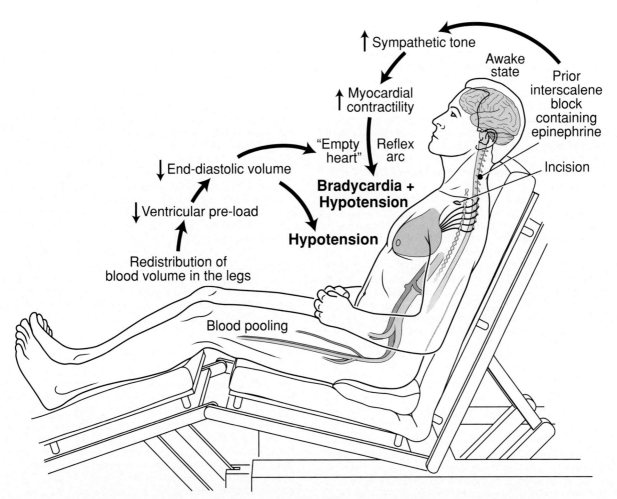

FIGURE 13-10. Mechanisms of hypotension/bradycardia associated with interscalene block in awake shoulder surgery patients in the beach chair position. Hypovolemia and increased sympathetic tone lead to a vigorously contracting, empty heart, which activates reflexes that cause hypotension and bradycardia. From Neal JM, Rathmell JP. *Complications in Regional Anesthesia and Pain Medicine.* New York: Elsevier Saunders, 2007, with permission.

subclavian perivascular (21) techniques were designed in part to reduce the risk of pneumothorax. Although there are no sufficiently powered studies to confirm this impression, no pneumothoraces were reported in separate studies of 1,001 (73) and 2,020 (74) subclavian perivascular blocks. The more medially placed vertical infraclavicular approach theoretically carries a small risk of pneumothorax; risk should be exceedingly low using the more lateral coracoid approach (75–77). Since the pleura is easily identifiable using ultrasound, it is speculated that this technology might further reduce the incidence of pneumothorax.

Symptoms of pneumothorax are frequently delayed 10 to 12 hours after block placement, particularly in the absence of mechanical ventilation. This delay has obvious implications for performing these blocks in outpatients. The most common presenting symptom of pneumothorax in these patients is pleuritic chest pain, not dyspnea (63).

Hypotension Bradycardia

Interscalene block has been linked to the occurrence of hypotension and bradycardia in 13% to 24% of awake patients who undergo shoulder surgery in the beach chair position (78,79). The sudden onset of these hemodynamic alterations occurs about 60 minutes after block placement (78). The presumptive mechanism involves a hyperdynamic myocardium (associated with epinephrine used as block or irrigating solution additives, and/or from patient anxiety) that vigorously contracts against an empty ventricle (decreased preload from the beach chair position). These conditions combine to activate mechanoreceptors in the ventricular wall and reflexively cause bradycardia (Bezold-Jarish reflex) (Fig. 13-10). The frequency of this complication can be reduced by titrating metoprolol or similar β-blocker to a heart rate of less than 60 beats/min, but is unaffected by prophylactic glycopyrrolate (80).

TECHNIQUES TO OPTIMIZE BLOCK SUCCESS

Nerve Localization

The essence of regional anesthesia technique is safely placing the block needle sufficiently close to the target plexus or nerve to ensure optimal local anesthetic effect. For upper extremity block, multiple options exist for localizing the target nerve, including paresthesia-seeking, peripheral nerve stimulation, ultrasound, and transarterial and perivascular techniques. Existing data suggest that no technique is clearly superior to another in terms of block success rates or safety (14,81,82). A growing body of knowledge and experience demonstrates that ultrasonic localization of target nerves is associated with highly successful and safe brachial plexus regional anesthesia (83). Yet, minimal evidence to date shows that ultrasound guidance improves success or safety as compared to other techniques. However, one must acknowledge that early investigators' relative inexperience with ultrasound techniques, as compared to standard localization techniques, may potentially bias favorable outcomes toward the latter (84).

Of at least equal importance to localization technique is how many stimulations or injections should be carried out at each block approach. For above-the-clavicle blocks, a single localization end-point and subsequent injection is sufficient for successful block (14,81). However, as one proceeds distally along the course of the brachial plexus, multiple nerve localizations and injections clearly improve block success (82,85). Two injections are generally superior to a single injection for the infraclavicular (86) and transarterial axillary approaches (14), whereas three or more injections improve axillary block success when using a paresthesia, nerve stimulation, or perivascular technique (14,82).

Mechanical Maneuvers

A number of creative mechanical maneuvers have been proposed to improve brachial plexus block characteristics. These include applying digital pressure proximal or distal to the injection site in an attempt to direct local anesthetic flow in a desirous path, adduction of the arm during and/or after local anesthetic injection, cooling local anesthetic solutions, mixing short- and long-acting local anesthetics, or exercising the arm as the block sets up. None of these maneuvers have unequivocally proven beneficial in well-designed studies (14).

APPROACHES TO THE BRACHIAL PLEXUS

The following section provides technical details of commonly used approaches to the brachial plexus. Each subsection discusses the indications for, technique of, and complications of the given approach. Even though several techniques are often described for each approach, this chapter focuses on only a single technique unless an alterative exists that offers a unique advantage. The choice of technique reflects the author's experience and bias. Indeed, a significant deficit in regional anesthesia literature is that, although multiple techniques have been described for nearly every approach to the brachial plexus, exceedingly few comparative studies assess the superiority or equivalency of one over another (14).

Interscalene Approach

Indications

The interscalene approach is ideally suited for shoulder surgery since it consistently anesthetizes the upper trunk. The approach is unsuitable for most forearm and hand surgeries because inferior trunk anesthesia can be incomplete in up to 50% of blocks (87). Using interscalene block for ambulatory shoulder surgery results in better analgesia, more postanesthesia care unit (PACU) bypass, and patients ready for discharge sooner than if fast-track general anesthesia is used (2). A continuous interscalene technique provides superior analgesia when compared to a subacromial catheter for arthroscopic rotator cuff surgery (88). Continuous techniques also provide excellent analgesia and may improve rehabilitation and functional recovery after major shoulder surgery (7–9,89).

Because interscalene block is placed relatively high along the nerve roots, cephalad spread of local anesthetic usually involves the non-brachial plexus supraclavicular nerve, thereby ensuring anesthesia of the shoulder cape. Separate blockade of the suprascapular nerve is unnecessary when an interscalene block is used for anterior, open shoulder surgery (90), but may be a valuable adjunct for surgery that involves the posterior shoulder joint, such as total shoulder arthroplasty or shoulder arthroscopy. The interscalene approach occasionally fails to anesthetize the anterior axilla for anterior arthroscopic port placement, which then requires supplementation of the intercostobrachial nerve.

Technique

The classic Winnie technique (91) for interscalene block begins with identification of the interscalene groove in a supine patient whose head is turned to the side, 45 degrees away from the operative side (Fig. 13-11). If the groove is difficult to palpate, the patient is asked to lift his head off the bed while the practitioner places a finger on the contracting sternocleidomastoid muscle. The patient then relaxes his head, and the anesthesiologist's finger moves laterally, off the muscle and into the interscalene groove. At the level of the cricoid cartilage, the needle is directed into the interscalene groove using a trajectory that is perpendicular to all planes of the skin, with a slightly caudad angulation. The needle is advanced until a paresthesia to the arm or anterior shoulder (92) occurs, or a motor response that involves the deltoid muscles is obtained (93). If the desired end-point is not found, the needle is moved systematically and perpendicularly across the interscalene groove (Fig. 13-12). Block success and technical qualities are similar whether a paresthesia technique or electrical stimulation is chosen to localize the nerves (81). When seeking a motor response, careful attention should be paid to movement of the diaphragm, which indicates stimulation of the phrenic nerve and the need to reposition the needle more posteriorly (Fig. 13-9). Trapezius muscle/posterior shoulder movement indicates the need to redirect the needle slightly more anteriorly. Once the desired end-point is attained, 1 mL of local anesthetic is injected slowly to rule out intra-arterial injection. This is followed by fractionated injection of 20 to 30 mL of local anesthetic. Pain on injection may indicate intraneural injection and should prompt immediate cessation of injection and repositioning of the needle.

Despite being the interscalene approach of choice for over three decades, the safety of the Winnie technique and its suitability for continuous catheter techniques have been questioned (49,94). In response to these concerns, several modifications of the interscalene approach have been proposed (48,49,95). These modifications advocate entering the interscalene groove at a slightly more caudad level and/or angling the needle more acutely and laterally in an attempt to avoid needle entry into the intervertebral foramen, with its inherent risk of entry into the neuraxis. Although no randomized studies prove the

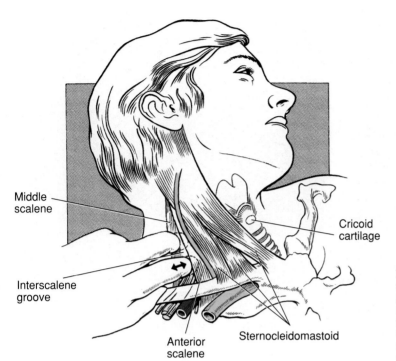

Middle scalene

Cricoid cartilage

Interscalene groove

Anterior scalene

Sternocleidomastoid

FIGURE 13-11. Identifying the interscalene groove is essential for any interscalene technique. The anesthesiologist's fingers are placed into the groove between the anterior and middle scalene muscles. If the groove is difficult to palpate, have the patient lift his head from the bed. Place the fingers on the contracted sternocleidomastoid muscle. As the neck is relaxed, sweep the fingers slowly and laterally, off the sternocleidomastoid and into the interscalene groove.

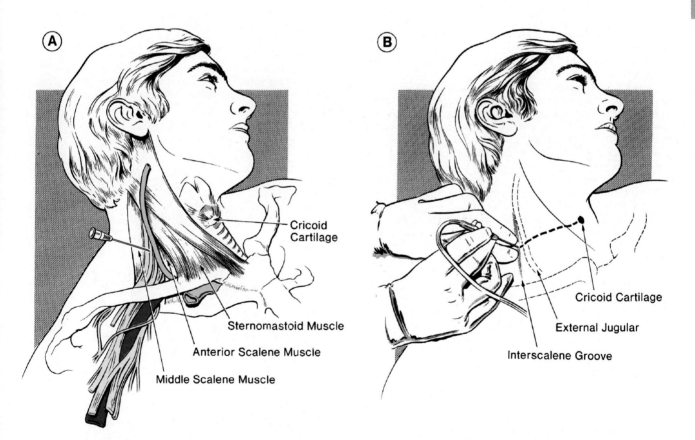

Ⓐ

Cricoid Cartilage

Sternomastoid Muscle

Anterior Scalene Muscle

Middle Scalene Muscle

Ⓑ

Cricoid Cartilage

External Jugular

Interscalene Groove

FIGURE 13-12. Modified Winnie technique for the interscalene approach. A line is drawn laterally about 0.5 cm caudad to the cricoid cartilage (C6 level). The needle entry point is at this level, into the interscalene groove. The needle is angulated 50 to 70 degrees from the skin and advanced along the line of the interscalene groove. If an appropriate paresthesia or motor response is not obtained, the needle is systematically fanned over the groove until the desired end-point is identified (*note insert*).

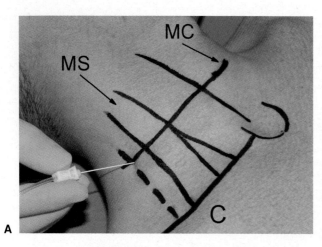
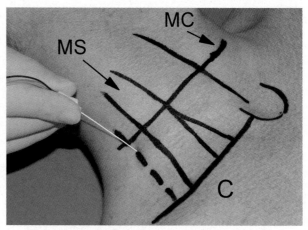

FIGURE 13-13. Comparison of Winnie's technique (**A**) and the modified lateral approach (**B**). Note that the modified approach places the needle 0.5 cm more caudad. The angulation of the needle is more acute and thus away from the midline. The modified lateral approach directs the needle along the line of the interscalene groove. From Neal JM, Rathmell JP. *Complications in Regional Anesthesia and Pain Medicine*. New York: Elsevier Saunders, 2007, with permission.

superiority of these techniques to the classic Winnie technique, reasonable experience with the block (51) and small published studies (10,48) have been devoid of neuraxial complications. Furthermore, imaging studies suggest that caudad angulation of the needle to 50 degrees or more (as compared to a median 7 degrees at C6 and a median 29 degrees at C7 using the Winnie approach) may reduce the likelihood of needle entry into the intervertebral foramen (49).

If one accepts that the theoretical arguments and noncomparative clinical experience are reasonable, then the Borgeat modified lateral approach (48,96) for interscalene block is a good alternative to the Winnie approach (Fig. 13-13). For this technique, the interscalene groove is traced out. The needle is inserted 0.5 cm below the level of the cricoid cartilage and angled at 50 to 60 degrees to the neck (96). The needle is ultimately angled laterally or slightly medially, matching the plane of the interscalene groove. Motor response end-points are identical to those used for the Winnie technique.

Continuous perineural catheter placement from the interscalene approach can be problematic using the Winnie technique, because the catheter must exit the needle at a 75-to-90-degree angle. This impediment can be overcome by reducing the needle angle after obtaining the desired motor response but before threading the catheter. Alternatively, the modified lateral technique facilitates catheter threading into the interscalene space at a straighter and more direct angle. A stimulating or nonstimulating catheter is threaded 2 to 3 cm along the plexus and then secured by tunneling it subcutaneously (48,97).

If the brachial plexus is localized using ultrasound, a high-frequency probe is situated with its axis perpendicular to the underlying brachial plexus (Fig. 13-14). It is easiest to first identify the pulsating carotid artery and internal jugular vein, and then slowly sweep the probe laterally to identify the anterior scalene muscle. The plexus is seen as hypoechoic structures that reside between the anterior and middle scalene muscles, averaging only 1 cm in skin-to-nerve distance (Fig. 13-15). Although an out-of-plane needle approach is possible, most North American experts suggest approaching the brachial plexus with the needle in plane with the ultrasound probe. Under direct vision, a ring of local anesthetic is injected around the nerves (98).

Complications

Several significant complications can occur with the interscalene approach. Because the brachial plexus is proximate to the vertebral and carotid arteries (Fig. 13-6), intraarterial injection with immediate seizure is possible. Furthermore, the vascularity of the neck lends itself to IV needle placement and systemic local anesthetic toxicity that is slightly delayed in onset from intra-arterial injection and therefore may result in more significant toxicity because higher volumes of local anesthetic are

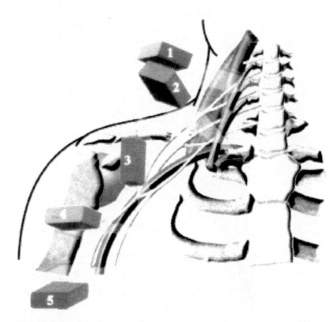

FIGURE 13-14. Ultrasound probe positions for the interscalene (*1*), supraclavicular (*2*), infraclavicular (*3*), axillary (*4*), and midhumeral (*5*) approaches. From Perlas A, Chan VWS, Simons M. Brachial plexus examination and localization using ultrasound and electrical stimulation. *Anesthesiology* 2003;99:429–435, with permission.

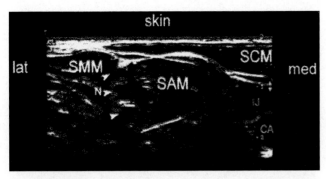

FIGURE 13-15. Transverse ultrasound image of the interscalene region. Arrows delineate the hypoechoic brachial plexus as it resides between the anterior (*SAM*) and middle (*SMM*) scalene muscles. SCM, sternocleidomastoid muscle; IJ, internal jugular vein; CA, carotid artery. From Perlas A, Chan VWS, Simons M. Brachial plexus examination and localization using ultrasound and electrical stimulation. *Anesthesiology* 2003;99:429–435, with permission.

injected prior to discovery. The relatively short distance (25–35 mm) from the skin to the neuraxis (49) makes the interscalene approach risky for unintended high spinal or epidural anesthesia. Reports of intramedullary needle placement, subsequent local anesthetic injection, and cervical spinal cord injury in patients who were under general anesthesia during block placement strongly warns that interscalene block should not be performed in anesthetized or heavily sedated patients (52,99).

Less consequential than unintended intravascular or neuraxial injection, hemidiaphragmatic paresis occurs in all patients undergoing interscalene block and is therefore contraindicated in any patient who cannot withstand a 25% re-

duction in pulmonary function (63). Anesthesia of the cervicothoracic sympathetic chain and/or the recurrent laryngeal nerve is a relatively common nuisance side effects associated with the interscalene approach.

Cervical Paravertebral Approach

Indications

The cervical paravertebral approach (originally described by Kappis in 1923, modified by Pippa in 1990 [100], and repopularized by Boezaart [54,101]) is a posterior approach to the brachial plexus block that is especially useful for placement of continuous perineural catheters. The block is primarily indicated for shoulder and upper arm surgeries. When compared to Winnie's lateral approach, the (Pippa) posterior cervical paravertebral approach resulted in similarly effective anesthesia for shoulder and upper arm surgery (102).

Technique

The patient is positioned lateral decubitus. At the level of the C6 spinous process, a stimulating Tuohy needle is placed at the apex of a "V" formed by the levator scapulae and trapezius muscles and directed medially and 30 degrees caudad (aiming towards the suprasternal notch). The needle is expected to contact the pars intervertebralis or transverse process of C6 in about 4 to 6 cm. Once this bony landmark is encountered, the needle is directed laterally off the bone and, using loss-of-resistance to air for confirmation, advanced another 0.5 to 1 cm until a motor response is observed in the shoulder (Fig. 13-16). A stimulating catheter is then manipulated to pass 3 to 5 cm beyond the needle tip while maintaining the motor

PART II: TECHNIQUES

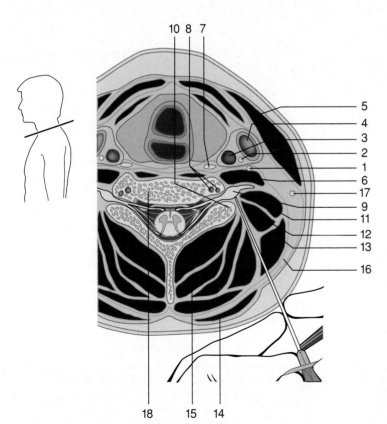

FIGURE 13-16. Posterior cervical paravertebral approach. Axial section of the neck at the C6 spinous process. A needle is placed at the apex of a "V" formed by the levator scapulae and trapezius muscles and directed medially and 30 degrees caudad (aiming toward the suprasternal notch). The needle is expected to contact the pars intervertebralis or the transverse process of C6 in approximately 4 to 6 cm. Once this bony landmark is encountered, the needle is directed laterally off the bone toward the brachial plexus. Top is anterior. 1, anterior scalene muscle; 2, middle scalene muscle; 3, brachial plexus; 4, phrenic nerve; 5, superior cervical ganglion; 6, vertebral artery; 7, pars intervertebralis of C6; 8, extensor muscles of neck; 9, trapezius muscle; 10, levator scapulae muscle. From Boezaart A, Koorn R, Rosenquist RW. Paravertebral approach to the brachial plexus: An anatomic improvement in technique. *Reg Anesth Pain Med* 2003;28:241–244; with permission of The American Society of Regional Anesthesia and Pain Medicine.

response at approximately 0.5 mA. A bolus of 20 to 30 mL local anesthetic is followed by infusion at 5 mL/h (101).

Complications

The Boezaart approach is less painful than previously described posterior approaches, yet 22% of patients note neck discomfort. Horner syndrome is common (40%). Although 8% of patients report dyspnea, no direct studies assess the effect of this approach on diaphragmatic function. As with other paravertebral approaches, epidural spread is possible (4%). Similar to the modified lateral interscalene techniques, the cervical paravertebral approach should have minimal chance of entering the neuraxis. In a series of 256 continuous blocks using a stimulating catheter, no nerve injuries were noted (54).

Supraclavicular Approach

Indications

The supraclavicular approach consistently provides anesthesia for the upper arm, elbow, and forearm. It is also a reasonable choice for shoulder surgery if supplementation of the supraclavicular nerve is provided to ensure anesthesia of the cape of the shoulder. Ultrasound-guided supraclavicular block is more reliable for anesthesia of the radial nerve than is ultrasound-guided infraclavicular block, although these results may be biased by the single-injection technique chosen for the infraclavicular block (103). Because the inferior trunk is the furthest away from the block needle and may reside behind the subclavian artery, the supraclavicular approach may rarely fail to provide adequate anesthesia in the ulnar nerve distribution. Even in obese patients, the supraclavicular block can be performed with high success (~94%) and low complication rates (74).

Technique

Supraclavicular block approaches the brachial plexus where the relatively compact trunks/divisions track under the clavicle and over the first rib, residing posterior, lateral, and cephalad to the subclavian artery (Fig. 13-17). Several techniques have been described for the supraclavicular approach (21,72,104). One of the most straightforward is Brown and Bridenbaugh's plumb-bob technique (72) (Fig. 13-18). The patient is placed supine, without a pillow, with the head turned slightly away from the operated side and the arm at the side. The patient is asked to raise his head off the bed to identify the lateral border of the sternocleidomastoid muscle. The needle entry point is at the posterior border of the muscle, just above the clavicle. The needle is directed toward the floor, just as a brick mason's plumb-bob would hang. Based on studies using the subclavian perivascular technique, elicitation of a motor response to the fingers at 0.9 mA is just as effective as eliciting the same motor response at 0.5 mA (105). Evidence suggests that more distal surgeries are associated with higher success rates if the middle or lower trunks are stimulated (106,107). If an appropriate paresthesia or motor response to the arm or shoulder is not obtained during the plumb-bob technique, the needle is incrementally fanned cephalad by several degrees until it has traveled 20 degrees. It is then fanned caudally until it reaches 20 degrees caudad. During all needle movements, it is essential to keep the needle in the parasagittal plane, because unintentional medial deflection increases the likelihood of pleural puncture (Fig. 13-18). If the subclavian artery is encountered, the needle is directed slightly posterior and lateral to identify the brachial

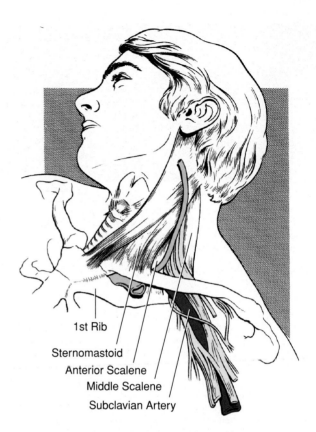

1st Rib
Sternomastoid
Anterior Scalene
Middle Scalene
Subclavian Artery

FIGURE 13-17. Supraclavicular approach. The compacted brachial plexus moves under the clavicle and over the first rib as it courses anterolateral and caudad. The plexus lies posterior and lateral to the subclavian artery.

plexus (Figs. 13-5 and 13-17). Once the plexus is identified, a 1-mL test dose to rule out intraneural and intra-arterial injection (retrograde flow into the carotid or innominate arteries can cause seizures) is followed by fractionated delivery of 20 to 30 mL of local anesthetic. Especially for tall, asthenic individuals whose pleural dome can be more cephalad, Klaastad and co-workers (108) have suggested initial needle angulation at 45 degrees cephalad and then incrementally moving the needle more caudad. If a continuous perineural technique is planned, the catheter is simply threaded 2 or 3 cm beyond the needle tip and then tunneled or otherwise secured near the supraclavicular fossa.

For ultrasonic localization, a high-frequency probe is placed obliquely at the base of the neck, just above the clavicle (Fig. 13-14). The plexus is identified lateral to the pulsating subclavian artery. Local anesthetic is injected to form a ring around the plexus, taking care to identify and avoid the pleura (Fig. 13-19). A study by experienced practitioners has shown that ultrasound can speed block execution and provide a more complete ulnar nerve block, as compared to using a peripheral nerve stimulator (109).

Complications

The most feared complication of the supraclavicular approach is pneumothorax. This complication appears to occur less frequently with the newer plumb-bob or subclavian perivascular (73,74,105) techniques, as compared to the classic Kulenkampff technique, although no adequately powered

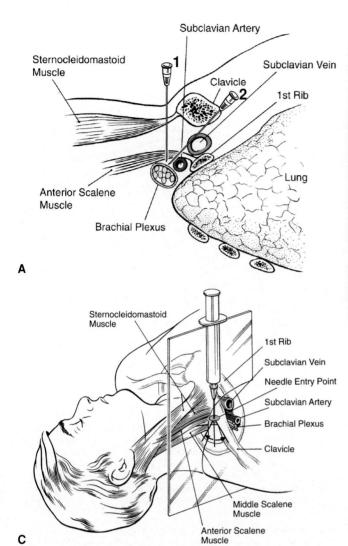

A

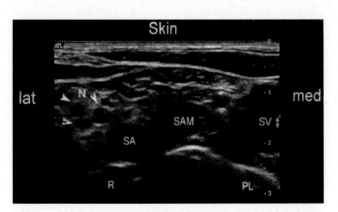

C

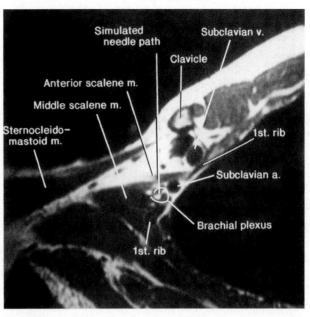

B

FIGURE 13-18. The plumb-bob technique for the supraclavicular approach. A: The relevant parasagittal anatomy. Note that the brachial plexus is below the clavicle and slightly cephalad to the brachial plexus. Needle 1 follows the classic plumb-bob trajectory, while Needle 2 begins with a cephalad direction that may avoid the pleural dome in taller individuals. B: Magnetic resonance image of the parasagittal anatomy. C: Needle movement within the parasagittal plane.

studies confirm this impression. No comparative data demonstrate that ultrasound guidance, with its inherent ability to visualize the pleura, reduces the incidence of pneumothorax, although limited reports have not listed pneumothorax as a complication (103,109). Supraclavicular block is associated with less hemidiaphragmatic paresis (95% confidence interval, 14%–86%) (59) as compared to the interscalene approach, but is still contraindicated for patients unable to withstand a significant reduction in pulmonary function. Minor side effects associated with the supraclavicular approach include unintended anesthesia of the cervicothoracic sympathetic chain and the recurrent laryngeal nerve. Subclavian artery hematoma is rare, but the inability to compress this vessel argues against performing supraclavicular block in anticoagulated patients (110).

Infraclavicular Approach

Indications

The infraclavicular approach to the brachial plexus is ideal for surgeries distal to the shoulder. For outpatient hand and wrist surgery, the infraclavicular approach offers better analgesia, more PACU bypass, faster times to discharge readiness, and less nausea and vomiting when compared to fast-track general

FIGURE 13-19. Transverse ultrasound image of the supraclavicular region. Arrows delineate the hypoechoic brachial plexus as it resides lateral to the subclavian artery (*SA*). Note the pleura (*PL*) deep to the plexus. R, first rib; SAM, anterior scalene muscle; SV, subclavian vein. From Perlas A, Chan VWS, Simons M. Brachial plexus examination and localization using ultrasound and electrical stimulation. *Anesthesiology* 2003;99:429–435, with permission.

anesthesia (4). This approach more reliably anesthetizes the axillary and musculocutaneous nerves compared to the axillary approach (111,112); therefore, it is an excellent choice for surgeries within the distribution of these nerves. Conversely, ultrasound-guided single-injection infraclavicular block is less likely to anesthetize the radial nerve, as compared to the supraclavicular approach (103). For arm and hand surgery, the infraclavicular approach has similar anesthetic qualities as the midhumeral approach in terms of success and anesthesia time, and is more comfortable to perform in trauma patients (113,114). The infraclavicular approach is also more comfortable for patients than is the axillary approach. Whether the decreased number of painful paresthesias with the infraclavicular approach also reduces the risk for postoperative nerve injury is unknown (115). When used for continuous perineural techniques, the infraclavicular approach improves analgesia and patient satisfaction while decreasing opioid-related side effects (116).

Technique

Several different techniques for placing infraclavicular block have been described (76,77,113,117–119). Although each has its advantages, the coracoid approach (as modified by Wilson [77]) is straightforward in its surface landmarks and subsequent needle movements: The patient is placed supine, with the arm to be blocked ideally at his side, although an advantage of this approach is that the arm can be placed in any comfortable position. The neural target are the cords as they wrap around the second part of the axillary artery (Figs. 13-1 and 13-17). Magnetic resonance imaging (MRI) studies demonstrate that the three cords lie within 2 cm of the artery and are grouped between the 3 o'clock and 11 o'clock positions (12 o'clock anterior) (120).

The needle entry point is identified 2 cm medial and 2 cm caudad to the lateral border of the coracoid process (Fig. 13-20). Based on magnetic resonance neurography, the medial and caudad distances should be increased by 0.5 to 1 cm in tall, broad-shouldered patients (121). The needle is advanced in a posterior direction toward the floor and in the parasagittal plane until an initial stimulation is observed and maintained at approximately 0.5 mA, followed by injection of 15 to 20 mL of local anesthetic. The needle is then redirected to obtain a second stimulation pattern, as dictated by the originally observed stimulation. For example, if the first stimulation involves the lateral cord, then the needle is redirected further caudad and deeper to identify the posterior cord. Although controversial, the preponderance of studies (55,86,122,123) suggests that a double-injection technique results in a more effective block than a single-injection technique. For a single-injection coracoid (124) or vertical lateral (125) technique, success is enhanced by injecting on a posterior cord stimulation.

When linking the observed motor response to which cord is being stimulated, the mnemonic tool "at the cords, the pinkie towards" is useful. The operator observes the patient's little finger movement in response to stimulation: *posterior movement* is associated with stimulation of the posterior cord, *lateral movement* (little finger moving away from the body when the arm is in anatomic position) indicates stimulation of the lateral cord, and *medial movement* (little finger toward the body) is linked with stimulation of the medial cord (126).

Because the infraclavicular approach is a deep block near a vascular structure, it is particularly amenable to ultrasound guidance. A low-frequency ultrasound probe is placed above the needle entry point for the coracoid technique, with the long axis oriented in the parasagittal plane (Fig. 13-14). The axillary

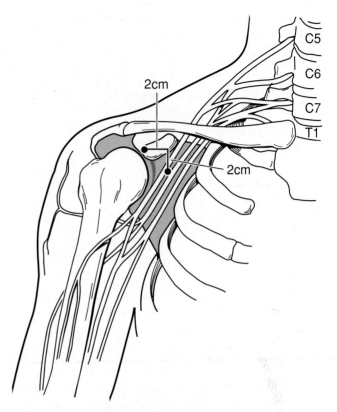

FIGURE 13-20. Coracoid technique for the infraclavicular block. The brachial plexus is located by plotting a point 2 cm medial from the lateral border of the coracoid process and 2 cm caudad. The cords of the brachial plexus reside lateral (cephalad), posterior, and medial (caudad) to the second part of the axillary artery. Redrawn from Mulroy MF. *Regional Anesthesia: A Procedural Guide.* Philadelphia: Lippincott, Williams, and Wilkins, 2002, with permission.

artery is identified by its pulsation. The posterior cord is usually visualized posterior lateral to the artery, whereas the medial cord usually resides in a triangular groove between the axillary artery and vein, but is the most variable in its relationship to the artery. The lateral cord is lateral (cephalad) to the artery and most superficial (Fig. 13-21). The needle is manipulated

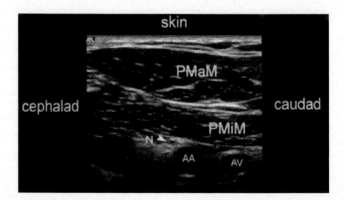

FIGURE 13-21. Transverse ultrasound image of the infraclavicular region. Arrows delineate the hypoechoic brachial plexus as it resides below the fascial layers of the pectoralis major (*PMaM*) and pectoralis minor (*PMiM*) muscles. AA, axillary artery; AV, axillary vein. From Perlas A, Chan VWS, Simons M. Brachial plexus examination and localization using ultrasound and electrical stimulation. *Anesthesiology* 2003;99:429–435, with permission.

to deposit local anesthetic around the posterior cord and one of the other cords. Alternatively, MRI suggests that, for single-injection, the ideal midpoint between the three cords is next to the artery at the 8 o'clock position (120).

The infraclavicular approach is an excellent choice for continuous perineural catheter techniques (5,39,116). Operators may encounter technical difficulty maneuvering the catheter, which exits the needle tip at a right angle to travel along the path of the brachial plexus. However, once this is accomplished, the catheter easily maintains its position during subsequent infusion.

Complications

As long as the stimulating needle remains in the parasagittal plane, there is little risk of pneumothorax with the infraclavicular approach, especially when using the (most lateral) coracoid technique. Hemidiaphragmatic paresis is extremely rare using the coracoid technique, probably because local anesthetic spread with this approach is restricted to below the clavicle (127). However, the frequency of phrenic nerve involvement begins to increase as needle placement becomes more medial, such as with the vertical technique. The presence of the deep and noncompressible axillary artery argues against performing infraclavicular block in anticoagulated patients (110).

Axillary Approach

Indications

The axillary approach is the workhorse block for upper extremity regional anesthesia. It is suitable for surgeries involving the hand and forearm, and is a reliable alternative for elbow surgery (128). For ambulatory hand surgery, axillary block offers short-term (<24 hours) benefits as compared to general anesthesia—earlier fast-track eligibility, less pain, and fewer opioid-related side effects (3). Single-stimulation infraclavicular and axillary blocks appear to be equally effective for hand surgery (111). However, a four-stimulation axillary block has been shown to be more effective than a two-stimulation infraclavicular block, although comparison of unequal stimulation techniques is problematic (112). The disadvantages of this approach are that it requires the arm be abducted 90 degrees at the shoulder, which can be problematic in some patients, and that the musculocutaneous nerve has usually split away from the other terminal nerves and therefore requires a separate blocking procedure to ensure adequate forearm anesthesia.

Technique

Several techniques are described for the axillary approach. Common to these techniques is that multiple injection/stimulation techniques result in superior block quality, as compared to single- or double-injection techniques (82,85). Comparative studies are limited, but existing data suggest that overall effectiveness and safety of the various techniques of axillary block are equivalent (14).

A key to successful axillary block is visualizing the relationship of the terminal nerves to the axillary artery (Fig. 13-22). Although these relationships can vary among individual patients, the median and ulnar nerves are typically more superficial, and are found superior and inferior to the axillary artery, respectively (when the arm is abducted 90 degrees at the shoulder and flexed 90 degrees at the elbow). The musculocutaneous nerve is superior to the artery, deeper, and usually within the belly or fascia of the coracobrachialis muscle. The radial nerve is inferior and posterior to the artery. At the axillary level, little anatomic or clinical evidence exists of a functional sheath, but rather a more compartmentalized configuration of connective tissue (18–20,85) (Fig. 13-22). Importantly, the median and ulnar nerves, and the triceps branches of the radial nerve all lie in a superficial compartment. Conversely, the main branch of the radial nerve lies in a deeper compartment that must be accessed if successful radial anesthesia is to be ensured (18,85,129).

Generally, five different techniques may be used for axillary brachial plexus block. All depend on identification of the axillary artery as the primary surface landmark. This is best accomplished by pressing the long finger into the axilla to palpate the artery, keeping the finger's axis in continuity with the artery's long axis. By slightly pressing the fingertip into the pulsation, the operator gains a sense of the side-to-side dimensions of the artery. The *transarterial* technique relies on identification of the axillary artery and subsequent fractionation of 30 to 40 mL of local anesthetic posterior and anterior to the artery (130–132). The *perivascular* technique relies on fanning small amounts of local anesthetic immediately inferior and superior to the axillary artery, injecting through a constantly moving needle. This technique does not rely on further localization of the individual nerves (133) (Fig. 13-23). Successful blocks from the next two axillary techniques, which use either peripheral nerve stimulation (134) or paresthesia (135) to localize individual terminal nerves, are particularly amenable to multiple stimulations and injections. Determination of which nerve is most essential to anesthetize is somewhat dependent on surgical requirements. For complete anesthesia of the arm, it is most important to localize the radial nerve and least important to localize the ulnar nerve (136,137). Three stimulations/injections are clearly superior to a single or double end-point, (82,85,138), whereas localization of all four nerves does not significantly improve block success, but does increase performance time (136). The final technique for axillary block is ultrasound guidance (Figs. 13-14 and 13-24). Although ultrasound-guided techniques for axillary block have been described (129), no comparative evidence suggests that they are superior to more traditional techniques. Axillary catheter techniques have been described, but offer little advantage over catheter placement at more proximal approaches, and suffer from a high frequency of catheter dislodgment.

At the axilla, the musculocutaneous nerve has usually diverged from the other terminal nerves and lies within the belly or fascia of the coracobrachialis muscle (Fig. 13-22). Because axillary techniques frequently fail to anesthetize the musculocutaneous nerve, it is best blocked by infiltrating 5 mL of local anesthetic into the muscle belly. Alternatively, the nerve can be more precisely localized with peripheral nerve stimulation or ultrasound.

Complications

Unintended intravascular injection can result in systemic local anesthetic toxicity, although seizures are about five times less likely to occur with the axillary approach (1–2 per 1,000 patients) as compared to either the interscalene or supraclavicular approaches (46). Pulmonary complications are not associated with axillary brachial plexus block. Half of patients undergoing axillary block report at least one minor side effect, including soreness, bruising, or transient numbness (139). Whether multiple stimulation techniques for axillary block increase the risk of nerve injury is unknown (82), although limited data

PART II: TECHNIQUES

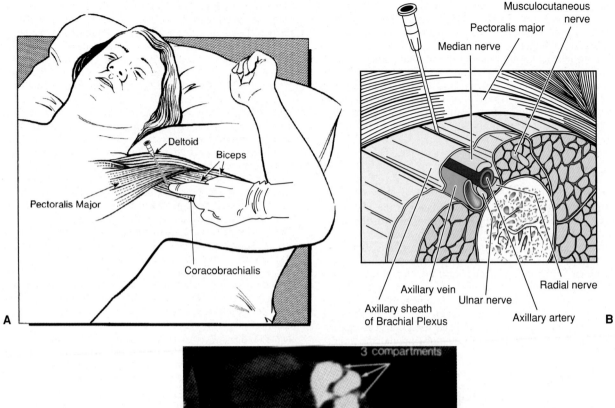

FIGURE 13-22. Axillary block. The axillary artery is palpated and fixed along its long axis by the middle finger of the operator's hand. The needle is directed toward the target, as dictated by the technique chosen—transarterial, perivascular, paresthesia, or peripheral nerve stimulation. C: The compartmentalized nature of the connective tissue as it surrounds the terminal nerves.

suggest that the practice may be safe if the block is performed expeditiously (140).

Midhumeral Approach

Indications

The midhumeral approach is appropriate for surgeries from the distal one-third of the arm to the hand. Compared to a two-stimulation axillary block, a four-stimulation midhumeral block was more successful in blocking all nerves of the upper extremity (54% versus 88%, respectively), but required a longer onset time (mean difference of 10 minutes) (134). Because the terminal nerves are relatively separate and distinct at this level, the midhumeral approach offers the unique oppor-

tunity to tailor desired anesthetic action to specific nerve distributions. Such specificity is most useful for minimizing motor block while maximizing sensory block. To this end, the midhumeral approach can selectively deliver shorter-duration local anesthetics to the radial and musculocutaneous nerves and longer-duration local anesthetic (141) and/or an adjuvant such as clonidine (142) to the ulnar and median nerves.

Technique

The midhumeral approach was described by Dupre (143) and popularized by Bouaziz and Narchi (134) in the mid 1990s (Fig. 13-25). The upper arm is abducted 80 degrees in a supine patient. The brachial artery is palpated at the junction of the upper and middle thirds of the arm. The median nerve is approached tangentially just superior to the artery; it is identified

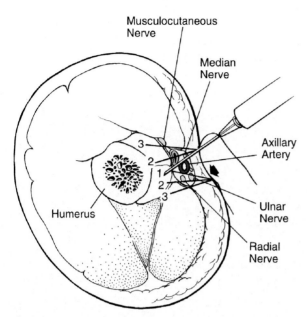

FIGURE 13-23. Perivascular technique of axillary block. The axillary artery is identified by its pulsation. The anesthesiologist then makes several fanning passes of the needle both superior and inferior to the artery. The local anesthetic is constantly injected through the constantly moving needle. Note also the configuration of the terminal nerves around the axillary artery, including the musculocutaneous nerve as it lies within the coracobrachialis muscle.

by wrist and finger flexion in response to nerve stimulation. Directing the needle deeper toward the coracobrachialis muscle while seeking forearm flexion identifies the musculocutaneous nerve. The needle is redirected tangentially and inferior to the artery to localize the ulnar nerve (ulnar deviation of the wrist, flexion of the little finger). The needle is finally advanced deep to the artery, alongside the humerus, to identify the radial nerve (wrist and finger extension) (Fig. 13-3). Only 5 to 7 mL of local anesthetic is injected after satisfactory stimulation at 0.5 mA or less. Ultrasound can also be used to localize the terminal nerves at the midhumeral approach (Fig. 13-14).

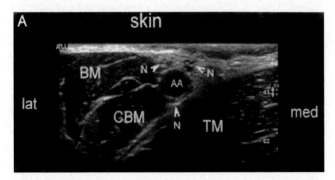

FIGURE 13-24. Transverse ultrasound image of the axillary region. Arrows delineate the hypoechoic reflections of the median, and ulnar nerves. AA, axillary artery; TM, triceps muscle; CBM, coracobrachiolis muscle; BM, biceps muscle. From Perlas A, Chan VWS, Simons M. Brachial plexus examination and localization using ultrasound and electrical stimulation. *Anesthesiology* 2003;99:429–435, with permission.

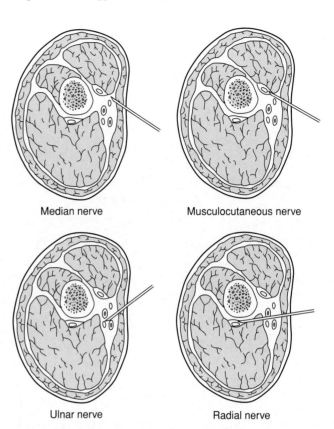

FIGURE 13-25. Midhumeral block showing the sequential needle movements required to anesthetize the four terminal nerves. Redrawn from Neal JM. Upper Extremity Blocks. In: Rathmell JP, Neal JM, Viscomi CM, eds. *Requisites in Anesthesiology: Regional Anesthesia.* Philadelphia: Elsevier Mosby, 2004; and Mulroy MF. *Regional Anesthesia: A Procedural Guide.* Philadelphia: Lippincott, Williams, and Wilkins, 2002, with permission.

Complications

The complication profile of the midhumeral approach essentially mirrors that of the axillary approach—intravascular injection, bruising, soreness, and rare nerve injury.

Selective Nerve Blocks

The previously described techniques are intended to anesthetize the entire brachial plexus by approaching it at various points along its course from the cervical nerve roots to the terminal nerves. On occasion, one finds it necessary to selectively anesthetize individual nerves that are either separate from the brachial plexus itself or are branches of the plexus that require supplementation anesthesia. Individual nerves can be selectively anesthetized as the primary block for surgery of the forearm or hand, but realistically, the variability and overlap of sensory innervation necessitates anesthesia of two or more nerves. Selective block can also be performed secondarily as a supplement to an incomplete or failed proximal brachial plexus block, although this practice can be associated with an increased risk of nerve injury (144).

Supraclavicular Nerve Block

The supraclavicular nerve (C3–C4) provides sensory innervation to the cape of the shoulder, which covers the area from

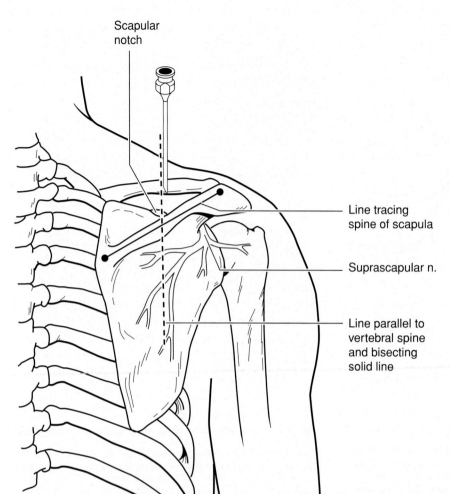

Scapular
notch

Line tracing
spine of scapula

Suprascapular n.

Line parallel to
vertebral spine
and bisecting
solid line

FIGURE 13-26. Suprascapular nerve block. The needle is directed toward the suprascapular notch to block the suprascapular nerve as it exits toward the shoulder. Redrawn from Rathmell JP, Neal JM, Viscomi CM, eds. *Requisites in Anesthesiology: Regional Anesthesia.* Philadelphia: Elsevier Mosby, 2004, with permission.

the neck to the deltoids and from the second rib anteriorly to the top of the scapula posteriorly. Because the supraclavicular nerve is not part of the brachial plexus, it can remain unanesthetized using the supraclavicular brachial plexus approach and thus require supplementation for full anesthesia of the shoulder. Supplementation is less likely to be required when the interscalene approach is used, probably because local anesthetic tracks cephalad to involve the C3 and C4 nerve roots.

The supraclavicular nerve block (also referred to as the superficial cervical plexus block) is accomplished by simply injecting 5 to 10 mL of local anesthetic subcutaneously along the posterior border of the sternocleidomastoid muscle. The external jugular vein should be identified so as to avoid hematoma and bruising. The block has no significant complications (144).

Suprascapular Nerve Block

The suprascapular nerve (C5–C6) branches from the superior trunk to innervate the posterior two-thirds of the shoulder joint, the acromioclavicular joint, and the anterior axilla in approximately 10% of patients. As a supplement to general anesthesia, suprascapular nerve block improves analgesia and reduces opioid-related side effects in patients undergoing shoulder arthroscopy (145). It provides superior analgesia to intraarticular local anesthesia, but not to interscalene block for shoulder arthroscopy (146). Because it is part of the brachial

plexus, separate suprascapular nerve anesthesia is seldom necessary when an interscalene block is used (90), but may add value for total shoulder arthroplasty or as a supplement when an interscalene block does not fully anesthetize the anterior axilla during arthroscopic surgery.

The suprascapular nerve is approached as it exits the suprascapular notch just above the scapular spine. With the patient seated, a line is drawn along the scapular spine and then bisected by a second line drawn parallel to the vertebral spine. Needle entry is 2 cm along a third line that bisects the upper outer quadrant. The needle is directed parallel to the vertebral spine until it contacts the scapular spine near the suprascapular notch (Fig. 13-26). Ten milliliters of local anesthetic is injected as a field block, or alternatively, after shoulder external rotation is obtained with nerve stimulation. Keeping the needle parallel to the vertebral spine avoids traversing the suprascapular notch and entering the pleural space (147).

Intercostobrachial Nerve Block

The intercostobrachial nerve is a terminal sensory branch of T2 and occasionally T1. Along with the medial cutaneous nerve, it innervates the medial/posterior upper arm and the anterior axilla. Not a part of the brachial plexus, the intercostobrachial nerve requires separate anesthesia when surgery involves areas within its sensory field, including anterior arthroscopic ports when that area is not fully anesthetized by an interscalene block. A common misperception is that anesthesia of the intercostobrachial nerve blocks tourniquet pain. Although the nerve transmits tourniquet sensation, it is not the sole messenger of ischemic/compressive tourniquet pain. The intercostobrachial nerve is blocked by simple subcutaneous injection of local anesthetic along the axillary crease. The block is virtually devoid of complications.

Medial and Lateral Antebrachial Cutaneous Nerve Blocks

The medial antebrachial cutaneous nerve (MAC; an intermediary branch of the medial cord) and the lateral antebrachial cutaneous nerve (LAC; the terminal cutaneous portion of the musculocutaneous nerve) provide cutaneous innervation to the volar forearm. Primary block of these nerves is a useful alternative for superficial surgeries such as arteriovenous fistula creation or revision (148). Because sensory innervation of the volar forearm is notoriously overlapping, combined MAC and LAC blocks are recommended.

The MAC is anesthetized by placing a 5-mL subcutaneous half-ring of local anesthetic along the medial upper arm, about one-fourth of the distance from the epicondyles to the shoulder. Anesthesia of the LAC requires two 5-mL local anesthetic injections. The first is deposited just lateral to the biceps tendon at the level of the antecubital crease. The second injection is deposited subcutaneously and lateral from the initial needle entry site (Figs. 13-27 and 13-28). Because the MAC and LAC are superficial, there is little chance of nerve injury. This suggests that these blocks are safer alternatives to selective musculocutaneous nerve or medial cord blocks, especially for supplementation after failed or incomplete proximal plexus blocks.

Selective Nerve Blocks at the Elbow

Few indications exist for selective nerve block at the elbow. When one considers that multiple nerves must be blocked to overcome the inherent overlap of the arm's sensory distribution pattern, that upper arm tourniquet sensation is not blocked, and that these nerves are relatively deep in the arm, the benefits of selective elbow block seems rather low. The only advantage of blocking individual nerves at the elbow rather than the wrist is that doing so blocks forearm extensor and flexor muscles. The theoretical risk of nerve injury from placing needles near terminal nerves that have been fully or partially anesthetized by a failed proximal block is indirectly supported by reports of injury when supplemental elbow blocks were used in these scenarios (14,149). If supplemental elbow blocks are performed, the risk of injury may be reduced by performing the block within 5 minutes after placement of the more proximal block and by accepting a higher electrical current end-point (≥ 1 mA) (140), but this recommendation lacks confirmatory data.

The *musculocutaneous nerve* is best anesthetized using the axillary or midhumeral approaches, as previously described. There are no indications to block the *ulnar nerve* at the elbow unless motor blockade of the hand is required. A common misperception is that sensory innervation of the medial forearm is from the ulnar nerve when indeed it is from the MAC. Placing a needle 2 cm proximal to the ulnar groove and directing it toward the groove until a paresthesia or motor response is elicited blocks the ulnar nerve; 2 to 3 mL of local anesthetic is then injected.

For radial and median nerve blocks at the elbow, the arm is abducted with the elbow extended and the forearm supinated. The *radial nerve* is approached at the intercondylar level with

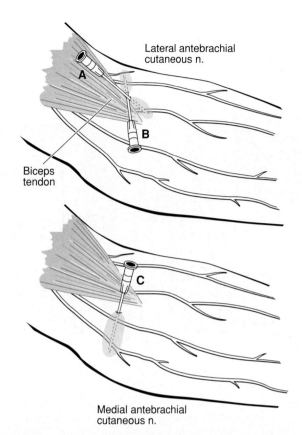

FIGURE 13-27. Lateral and medial antebrachial cutaneous blocks. For the lateral antebrachial cutaneous block, 3 mL of local anesthetic is first injected deep on the lateral side of the biceps tendon. Then, a subcutaneous local anesthetic wheal is deposited laterally. The medial antebrachial cutaneous block is a simple subcutaneous injection of local anesthetic around the medial arm. Redrawn from Viscomi CM, Reese J, Rathmell JP. Medial and lateral antebrachial cutaneous nerve blocks: An easily learned regional anesthetic for forearm arteriovenous fistula surgery. *Reg Anesth* 1996;21:2–5, with permission of the American Society of Regional Anesthesia and Pain Medicine.

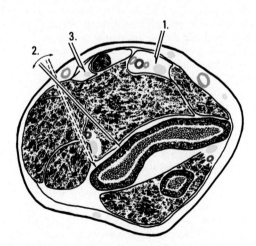

FIGURE 13-28. Cross-section of the arm at the elbow. Needle 1 is approaching the median nerve, medial to the brachial artery. Needle 2 illustrates the radial nerve block, as it resides deep and close to the humerus. Needle 3 shows the first injection for the lateral antebrachial cutaneous nerve, which is lateral to the biceps tendon and deep to the fascia.

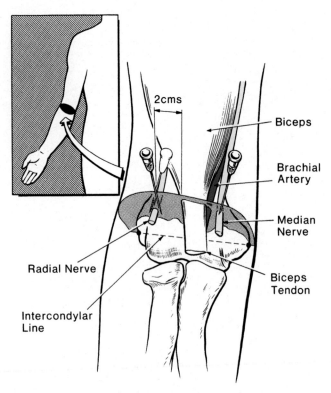

FIGURE 13-29. Landmarks for selective radial and median nerve blocks at the elbow. For radial nerve block, the needle is inserted approximately 2 cm lateral to the biceps tendon, placed against the lateral epicondyle, then redirected medially. The median nerve is approached just medial to the brachial artery pulsation.

a needle placed approximately 2 cm lateral to the biceps tendon and directed straight toward the lateral epicondyle and subsequently redirected medially. An injection of 5 mL of local anesthetic is placed near the humerus at the conclusion of each needle fan, or alternatively after confirmatory paresthesia, ultrasound visualization, or finger extension from peripheral nerve stimulation. The *median nerve* is approached at the intercondylar level by placing a needle just medial to the brachial artery pulsation and directing it perpendicular to the skin; 5 to 10 mL of local anesthetic is injected after confirmatory paresthesia, wrist flexion and/or thumb opposition, or ultrasound guidance (144) (Figs. 13-28 and 13-29).

Selective Nerve Blocks at the Wrist

Selective nerve blocks at the wrist can be placed primarily for carpal tunnel release or hand operations. When used for the former indication, selective wrist blocks result in stable intraoperative hemodynamics and faster discharge from the hospital (150).

For wrist blocks, the patient is supine with the arm abducted. All wrist blocks require only 3 to 5 mL of local anesthetic. The *ulnar nerve* can be blocked at the proximal flexion crease of the wrist by placing a needle just radial to the flexor ulnaris tendon and advancing downward. However, it is often easier to use a lateral approach to the nerve from the ulnar side by directing the needle just posterior to the flexor ulnaris tendon and advancing it 1 to 2 cm. The end-point can be a paresthesia, a motor response to the little finger, or the block can be performed with ultrasound guidance. An additional subcuta-

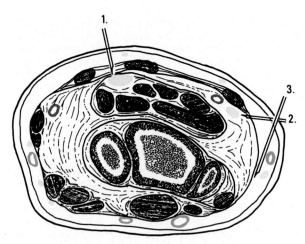

FIGURE 13-30. Cross-section of the forearm at the wrist. Needle 1 is placed next to the radial border of the palmaris longus tendon and pierces the fascia prior to contacting the median nerve. Needles 2 and 3 depict blocking the ulnar nerve from the ulnar side and directing the needle posterior to the flexor carpi ulnaris tendon; they are then redirected laterally to anesthetize the superficial branch of the nerve.

neous injection along the ulnar border of the wrist will ensure anesthesia of the superficial branches of the ulnar nerve. The *median nerve* is blocked at the level of the proximal flexion crease by a needle placed just radial to the palmaris longus tendon. If the tendon is absent, the needle is placed approximately 1 cm to the ulnar side of the flexor carpi radialis tendon. Within 1 cm of advancement, the needle should penetrate fascia. The median nerve at this level is primarily a sensory nerve, so a paresthesia or sensory stimulation is more likely than a motor response (151) (Figs. 13-30 and 13-31). The *radial nerve* block at the wrist requires two subcutaneous injections to ensure that both branches are anesthetized. The first injection of local anesthetic is placed proximally along the course of the extensor pollicis longus tendon from the base of the first metacarpal to the radial styloid. The needle is then withdrawn to the starting point and directed at right angles across the anatomic "snuffbox" to the extensor pollicis brevis tendon (144) (Fig. 13-32).

SUMMARY

Regional anesthesia of the upper extremity is the most common form of peripheral nerve block. Its use can improve patient outcomes, such as providing better analgesia during the first 24 hours and allowing more efficient discharge from the hospital. Continuous perineural techniques can extend these benefits, and they have the potential to positively impact functional rehabilitation. Fundamental knowledge of brachial plexus anatomy and pharmacology can greatly enhance one's ability to provide outstanding patient care. Brachial plexus regional anesthesia is associated with common, but generally benign, side effects. Serious complications such as nerve injury, systemic local anesthetic toxicity, and pneumothorax are rare; furthermore, there is evidence that knowledge and technique modifications can reduce their incidence. Each approach along the brachial plexus offers advantages and disadvantages, therefore each should be tailored to surgical and patient needs.

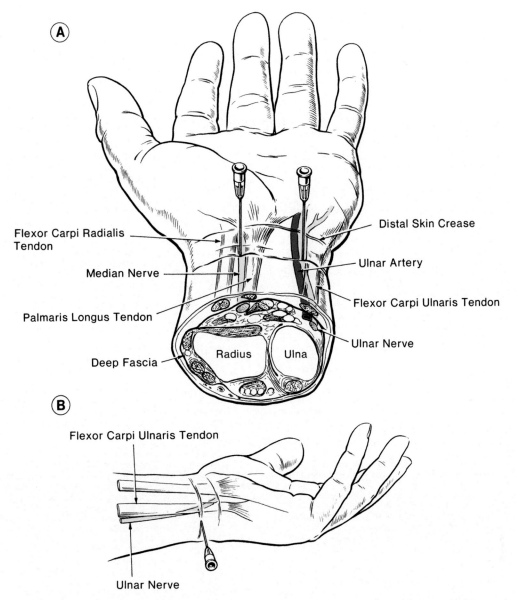

(A)

(B)

Flexor Carpi Radialis Tendon

Median Nerve

Palmaris Longus Tendon

Deep Fascia

Distal Skin Crease

Ulnar Artery

Flexor Carpi Ulnaris Tendon

Ulnar Nerve

Radius   Ulna

Flexor Carpi Ulnaris Tendon

Ulnar Nerve

FIGURE 13-31. Surface landmarks for wrist blocks. The median nerve is approached between the flexor carpi radialis and palmaris longus tendons. The ulnar nerve can be approached either from the volar forearm, just radial to the flexor carpi ulnaris tendon or from the ulnar side of the forearm.

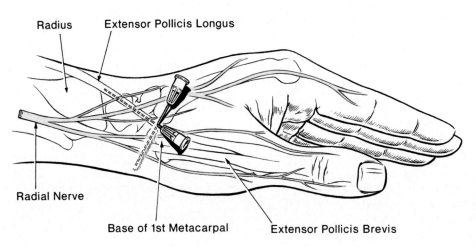

Radius   Extensor Pollicis Longus

Radial Nerve

Base of 1st Metacarpal   Extensor Pollicis Brevis

FIGURE 13-32. Surface landmarks and needle paths for radial nerve block at the wrist.

ACKNOWLEDGMENT

The author wishes to recognize the American Society of Regional Anesthesia and Pain Medicine's (ASRA) intensive workshops initiative. From this project comes much of the information summarized in this chapter (14). The following physicians have made significant scholarly contributions to the upper extremity regional anesthesia project: Drs. Carlo D. Franco, J. C. Gerancher, James R. Hebl, Quinn H. Hogan, Brian M. Ilfeld, Colin J. L. McCartney, and Joseph M. Neal.

References

1. Neal JM, Kopacz DJ, Liguori GA, et al. The training and careers of regional anesthesia fellows: 1983–2002. *Reg Anesth Pain Med* 2005;30:226–232.
2. Hadzic A, Williams BA, Karaca PE, et al. For outpatient rotator cuff surgery, nerve block anesthesia provides superior same-day recovery after general anesthesia. *Anesthesiology* 2005;102:1001–1007.
3. McCartney CJ, Brull R, Chan VW, et al. Early but no long-term benefit of regional compared with general anesthesia for ambulatory hand surgery. *Anesthesiology* 2004;101:461–467.
4. Hadzic A, Arliss J, Kerimoglu B, et al. A comparison of infraclavicular nerve block versus general anesthesia for hand and wrist day-case surgeries. *Anesthesiology* 2004;101:127–132.
5. Ilfeld BM, Enneking FK. Continuous peripheral nerve blocks at home: A review. *Anesth Analg* 2005;100:1822–1833.
6. Ilfeld BM, Esener DE, Morey TE, et al. Ambulatory perineural infusion: The patients' perspective. *Reg Anesth Pain Med* 2003;28:418–423.
7. Capdevila X, Dadure C, Bringuier S, et al. Effect of patient-controlled perineural analgesia on rehabilitation and pain after ambulatory orthopedic surgery. A multicenter randomized trial. *Anesthesiology* 2006;105:566–573.
8. Ilfeld BM, Vandenborne K, Duncan PW, et al. Ambulatory continuous interscalene nerve blocks decrease the time to discharge readiness after total shoulder arthroplasty. A randomized, triple-masked, placebo-controlled study. *Anesthesiology* 2006;105:999–1007.
9. Ilfeld BM, Wright TW, Enneking FK, et al. Joint range of motion after total shoulder arthroplasty with and without a continuous interscalene nerve block: A retrospective, case-control study. *Reg Anesth Pain Med* 2005;30:429–433.
10. Borgeat A, Ekatodramis G, Kalberer F, et al. Acute and nonacute complications associated with interscalene block and shoulder surgery. A prospective study. *Anesth Analg* 2001;95:875–880.
11. Capdevila X, Pirat P, Bringuier S, et al. Continuous peripheral nerve blocks in hospital wards after orthopedic surgery. *Anesthesiology* 2005;103:1035–1045.
12. Williams PL, Warwick R, Dyson M, et al. *Gray's Anatomy*. London: Churchill Livingstone, 1989.
13. Bergman RA, Thompson SA, Afifi AK, et al. *Compendium of Human Anatomic Variation*. Baltimore: Urban and Schwarzenberg, 1988.
14. Neal JM, Gerancher JC, Ilfeld BM, et al. Brachial plexus anesthesia: Essentials of our current understanding. *Reg Anesth Pain Med* 2008;33: in press.
15. Thompson GE, Brown DL. The common nerve blocks. In: Nunn JF, Utting JE, Brown BR, eds. *General Anaesthesia*. London: Butterworths; 1989:1068–1069.
16. Sia S, Lepri A, Magherini M, et al. A comparison of proximal and distal radial nerve motor responses in axillary block using triple stimulation. *Reg Anesth Pain Med* 2005;30:458–463.
17. Cornish PB, Leaper C. The sheath of the brachial plexus. Fact or fiction? *Anesthesiology* 2006;105:563–565.
18. Klaastad O, Smedby O, Thompson GE, et al. Distribution of local anesthetic in axillary brachial plexus block: A clinical and magnetic resonance imaging study. *Anesthesiology* 2002;96:1315–1324.
19. Partridge BL, Benirschke K. Functional anatomy of the brachial plexus sheath: Implications for anesthesia. *Anesthesiology* 1987;66:743–747.
20. Thompson GE, Rorie DK. Functional anatomy of the brachial plexus sheaths. *Anesthesiology* 1983;59:117–122.
21. Winnie AP, Collins VJ. The subclavian perivascular approach of brachial plexus anesthesia. *Anesthesiology* 1964;25:353–363.
22. Cornish PB, Greenfield LJ. Brachial plexus anatomy. *Reg Anesth* 1997;22:106–107.
23. Rose JS, Neal JM, Kopacz DJ. Extended-duration analgesia: Update on microspheres and liposomes. *Reg Anesth Pain Med* 2005;30:275–285.
24. Klein SM, Nielsen KC, Greengrass RA, et al. Ambulatory discharge after long-acting peripheral nerve blockade: 2382 blocks with ropivacaine. *Anesth Analg* 2002;94:65–70.
25. Raeder JC, Drosdahl S, Klaastad O, et al. Axillary brachial plexus block with ropivacaine 7.5 mg/ml. A comparative study with bupivacaine 5 mg/ml. *Acta Anaesthesiol Scand* 1999;43:794–798.
26. Vaghadia H, Chan V, Ganapathy S, et al. A multicentre trial of ropivacaine 7.5 mg × ml(−1) vs bupivacaine 5 mg × ml(−1) for supraclavicular brachial plexus anaesthesia. *Can J Anaesth* 1999;46:946–951.
27. Cox CR, Checketts MR, Mackenzie N, et al. Comparison of S(-)-bupivacaine with racemic (RS)-bupivacaine in supraclavicular brachial plexus block. *Br J Anaesth* 1998;80:594–598.
28. Covino BG, Wildsmith JAW. Clinical pharmacology of local anesthetic agents. In: Cousins MJ, Bridenbaugh PO, eds. *Neural Blockade in Clinical Anesthesia and Management of Pain*. Philadelphia: Lippincott-Raven Publishers; 1998:97–128.
29. Vester-Andersen T, Christiansen C, Sorensen M, et al. Perivascular axillary block I: blockade following 40 mL 1% mepivacaine with adrenaline. *Acta Anaesthesiol Scand* 1982;26:519–523.
30. Vester-Andersen T, Christiansen C, Sorensen M, et al. Perivascular axillary block II: influence of injected volume of local anesthetic on neural blockade. *Acta Anaesthesiol Scand* 1983;27:95–98.
31. Vester-Andersen T, Eriksen C, Christiansen C. Perivascular axillary block III: blockade following 40 ml of 0.5%, 1% or 1.5% mepivacaine with adrenaline. *Acta Anaesthesiol Scand* 1984;28:95–98.
32. Vester-Andersen T, Husum B, Lindeburg T, et al. Perivascular axillary block IV: Blockade following 40, 50 or 60 ml of mepivacaine 1% with adrenaline. *Acta Anaesthesiol Scand* 1984;28:99–105.
33. Rosenberg P, Veering BT, Urmey WT. Maximum recommended doses of local anesthetics: A multifactorial concept. *Reg Anesth Pain Med* 2004;29:564–575.
34. Lambert LA, Lambert DH, Strichartz GR. Irreversible conduction block in isolated nerve by high concentrations of local anesthetics. *Anesthesiology* 1994;80:1082–1093.
35. Kennedy WF, Bonica JJ, Ward RJ, et al. Cardiorespiratory effects of epinephrine when used in regional anesthesia. *Acta Anaesthesiol Scand* 1966;23:320–333.
36. Denkler K. A comprehensive review of epinephrine in the finger: To do or not to do. *Plast Reconstr Surg* 2001;108:114–124.
37. Singelyn FJ, Dangoisse M, Bartholomee S, et al. Adding clonidine to mepivacaine prolongs the duration of anesthesia and analgesia after axillary brachial plexus block. *Reg Anesth* 1992;17:148–150.
38. Singelyn FJ, Gouverneur J-M, Robert A. A minimum dose of clonidine added to mepivacaine prolongs the duration of anesthesia and analgesia after axillary brachial plexus block. *Anesth Analg* 1996;83:1046–1050.
39. Ilfeld BM, Morey TE, Enneking FK. Continuous infraclavicular perineural infusion with clonidine and ropivacaine compared with ropivacaine alone: A randomized, double-blind, controlled study. *Anesth Analg* 2003;97:706–712.
40. Ilfeld BM, Morey TE, Thannikary LJ, et al. Clonidine added to a continuous interscalene ropivacaine perineural infusion to improve postoperative analgesia: A randomized, double-blind, controlled study. *Anesth Analg* 2005;100:1172–1178.
41. Movafegh A, Razazian M, Hajimaohamadi F, et al. Dexamethasone added to lidocaine prolongs axillary brachial plexus block. *Anesth Analg* 2006;102:263–267.
42. Gunduz A, Bilir A, Gulec S. Magnesium added to prilocaine prolongs the duration of axillary plexus block. *Reg Anesth Pain Med* 2006;31:233–236.
43. Chow MYH, Sia ATH, Koay CK, et al. Alkalinization of lidocaine does not hasten the onset of axillary brachial plexus block. *Anesth Analg* 1998;86:566–568.
44. Sinnott CJ, Garfield JM, Thalhammer JG, et al. Addition of sodium bicarbonate to lidocaine decreases the duration of peripheral nerve block in the rat. *Anesthesiology* 2000;93:1045–1052.
45. Auroy Y, Narchi P, Messiah A, et al. Serious complications related to regional anesthesia. Results of a prospective survey in France. *Anesthesiology* 1997;87:479–486.
46. Brown DL, Ransom DM, Hall JA, et al. Regional anesthesia and local anesthetic-induced systemic toxicity: Seizure frequency and accompanying cardiovascular changes. *Anesth Analg* 1995;81:321–328.
47. Groban L, Butterworth J. Local anesthetic systemic toxicity. In: Neal JM, Rathmell JP, eds. *Complications in Regional Anesthesia and Pain Medicine*. Philadelphia: Saunders Elsevier; 2007:55–66.
48. Borgeat A, Dullenkopf A, Ekatodramis G, et al. Evaluation of the lateral modified approach for continuous interscalene block after shoulder surgery. *Anesthesiology* 2003;99:436–442.

49. Sardesai AM, Patel R, Denny NM, et al. Interscalene brachial plexus block: Can the risk of entering the spinal cord by reduced? A study of needle angles in volunteers undergoing magnetic resonance imaging. *Anesthesiology* 2006;105:9–13.

50. Lombard TP, Couper JL. Bilateral spread of analgesia following interscalene brachial plexus block. *Anesthesiology* 1983;58:472–473.

51. Borgeat A, Blumenthal S. Unintended destinations of local anesthetics. In: Neal JM, Rathmell JP, eds. *Complications in Regional Anesthesia and Pain Medicine*. Philadelphia: Saunders Elsevier; 2007:157–163.

52. Benumof JL. Permanent loss of cervical spinal cord function associated with interscalene block performed under general anesthesia. *Anesthesiology* 2000;93:1541–1544.

53. Hickey R, Garland TA, Ramamurthy S. Subclavian perivascular block: Influence of location of paresthesia. *Anesth Analg* 1989;68:767–771.

54. Boezaart AP, de Beer JF, Nell ML. Early experience with continuous cervical paravertebral block using a stimulating catheter. *Reg Anesth Pain Med* 2003;28:406–413.

55. Kilka HG, Geiger P, Mehrkens HH. Infraclavicular vertical brachial plexus blockade: A new technique of regional anaesthesia. *Anaesthetist* 1995; 44:339–344.

56. Seltzer JL. Hoarseness and Horner's Syndrome after interscalene brachial plexus block. *Anesth Analg* 1977;56:585–586.

57. Urmey W, McDonald M. Hemidiaphragmatic paresis during interscalene brachial plexus block: Effects on pulmonary function and chest wall mechanics. *Anesth Analg* 1992;74:352–357.

58. Urmey WF, Talts KH, Sharrock NE. One hundred percent incidence of hemidiaphragmatic paresis associated with interscalene brachial plexus anesthesia as diagnosed by ultrasonography. *Anesth Analg* 1991;72:498–503.

59. Neal JM, Moore JM, Kopacz DJ, et al. Quantitative analysis of respiratory, motor, and sensory function after supraclavicular block. *Anesth Analg* 1998;86:1239–1244.

60. Pham-Dang C, Gunst JP, Gouin F, et al. A novel supraclavicular approach to brachial plexus block. *Anesth Analg* 1997;85:111–116.

61. Rettig HC, Gielen MJM, Boersma E, et al. Vertical infraclavicular block of the brachial plexus: Effects on hemidiaphragmatic movement and ventilatory function. *Reg Anesth Pain Med* 2005;30:529–535.

62. Rodriguez J, Barcena M, Rodriguez V, et al. Infraclavicular brachial plexus block effects on respiratory function and extent of block. *Reg Anesth Pain Med* 1998;23:564–568.

63. Urmey WF. Pulmonary complications. In: Neal JM, Rathmell JP, eds. *Complications in Regional Anesthesia and Pain Medicine*. Philadelphia: Saunders Elsevier; 2007:147–156.

64. Urmey WF, Grossi P, Sharrock NE, et al. Digital pressure during interscalene block is clinically ineffective in preventing anesthetic spread to the cervical plexus. *Anesth Analg* 1996;83:366–370.

65. Pere P. The effect of continuous interscalene brachial plexus block with 0.125% bupivacaine plus fentanyl on diaphragmatic motility and ventilatory function. *Reg Anesth* 1993;18:93–97.

66. Pere P, Pitkanen M, Rosenberg PH, et al. Effect of continuous interscalene brachial plexus block on diaphragm motion and on ventilatory function. *Acta Anaesthesiol Scand* 1992;36:53–57.

67. Altintas F, Gumus F, Kaya G, et al. Interscalene brachial plexus block with bupivacaine and ropivacaine in patients with chronic renal failure: Diaphragmatic excursion and pulmonary function changes. *Anesth Analg* 2005;100:1166–1171.

68. Casati A, Fanelli G, Cedrati V, et al. Pulmonary function changes after interscalene brachial plexus anesthesia with 0.5% and 0.75% ropivacaine: A double blind comparison with 2% mepivacaine. *Anesth Analg* 1999;88:587–592.

69. Borgeat A, Perschak H, Bird P, et al. Patient-controlled interscalene analgesia with ropivacaine 0.2% versus patient-controlled intravenous analgesia after major shoulder surgery. Effects on diaphragmatic and respiratory function. *Anesthesiology* 2000;92:102–108.

70. al-Kaisy AA, Chan VW, Perlas A. Respiratory effects of low-dose bupivacaine interscalene block. *Br J Anaesth* 1999;82:217–220.

71. Winnie AP. *Plexus Anesthesia: Perivascular Techniques of Brachial Plexus Block*. Philadelphia: W B Saunders, 1990.

72. Brown DL, Cahill DR, Bridenbaugh LD. Supraclavicular nerve block: Anatomic analysis of a method to prevent pneumothorax. *Anesth Analg* 1993;76:530–534.

73. Franco CD, Vieira ZE. 1,001 subclavian perivascular brachial plexus blocks: Success with a nerve stimulator. *Reg Anesth Pain Med* 2000;25:41–46.

74. Franco CD, Gloss FJ, Voronov G, et al. Supraclavicular block in the obese population: An analysis of 2020 blocks. *Anesth Analg* 2006;102:1252–1254.

75. Desroches J. The infraclavicular brachial plexus block by the coracoid approach is clinically effective. *Can J Anaesth* 2003;50:253–257.

76. Whiffler K. Coracoid block-a safe and easy technique. *Br J Anaesth* 1981; 53:845–848.

77. Wilson JL, Brown DL, Wong GY. Infraclavicular brachial plexus block: Parasagittal anatomy important to the coracoid technique. *Anesth Analg* 1998;87:870–873.

78. D'Alessio JG, Weller RS, Rosenblum M. Activation of the Bezold-Jarisch reflex in the sitting position for shoulder arthroscopy using interscalene block. *Anesth Analg* 1995;80:1158–1162.

79. Kahn RL, Hargett MJ. Beta-adrenergic blockers and vasovagal episodes during shoulder surgery in the sitting position under interscalene block. *Anesth Analg* 1999;88:378–381.

80. Liguori GA, Kahn RL, Gordon J, et al. The use of metoprolol and glycopyrrolate to prevent hypotension/bradycardic events during shoulder arthroscopy in the sitting position under interscalene block. *Anesth Analg* 1998;87:1320–1325.

81. Liguori GA, Zayas VM, YaDeau JT, et al. Nerve localization techniques for interscalene brachial plexus blockade: A prospective, randomized comparison of mechanical paresthesia versus electrical stimulation. *Anesth Analg* 2006;103:761–777.

82. Handoll HHG, Koscielniak-Nielsen ZJ. Single, double or multiple injection techniques for axillary brachial plexus block for hand, wrist or forearm surgery. *Cochrane Database Syst Rev* 2006;CD003842, CD14003842.

83. Marhofer P, Greher M, Kapral S. Ultrasound guidance in regional anesthesia. *Br J Anaesth* 2004;94:7–17.

84. Gray AT. Ultrasound-guided regional anesthesia. Current state of the art. *Anesthesiology* 2006;104:368–373.

85. Koscielniak-Nielsen ZJ. Multiple injections in axillary block: Where and how many? [Editorial]. *Reg Anesth Pain Med* 2006;31:192–195.

86. Rodriguez J, Barcena M, Taboada-Muniz M, et al. A comparison of single versus multiple injections on the extent of anesthesia with coracoid infraclavicular brachial plexus block. *Anesth Analg* 2004;99:1225–1230.

87. Lanz E, Theiss D, Jankovic D. The extent of blockade following various techniques of brachial plexus block. *Anesth Analg* 1983;62:55–58.

88. Delaunay L, Souron V, Lafosse L, et al. Analgesia after arthroscopic rotator cuff repair: Subacromial versus interscalene continuous infusion of ropivacaine. *Reg Anesth Pain Med* 2005;30:117–122.

89. Ilfeld BM, Wright TW, Enneking FK, et al. Total shoulder arthroplasty as an outpatient procedure using ambulatory perineural local anesthetic infusion: A pilot feasibility study. *Anesth Analg* 2005;101:1319–1322.

90. Neal JM, McDonald SB, Larkin KL, et al. Suprascapular nerve block prolongs analgesia after nonarthroscopic shoulder surgery, but does not improve outcome. *Anesth Analg* 2003;96:982–986.

91. Winnie AP. Interscalene brachial plexus block. *Anesth Analg* 1970;49:455–466.

92. Roch JJ, Sharrock NE, Neudachin L. Interscalene brachial plexus block for shoulder surgery: A proximal paresthesia is effective. *Anesth Analg* 1992;75:386–388.

93. Silverstein WB, Saiyed MU, Brown AR. Interscalene block with a nerve stimulator: A deltoid motor response is a satisfactory endpoint for successful block. *Reg Anesth Pain Med* 2000;25:356–359.

94. Borgeat A. All roads do not lead to Rome [Editorial]. *Anesthesiology* 2006;105:1–2.

95. Meier G, Bauereis C, Heinrich C. Interscalene brachial plexus catheter for anesthesia and postoperative pain therapy: Experience with a modified technique. *Anaesthetist* 1997;46:715–719.

96. Borgeat A, Ekatodramis G. Anesthesia for shoulder surgery. *Best Pract Res Clin Anaesthesiol* 2002;16:211–225.

97. Ilfeld BM, Morey TE, Wright TW, et al. Continuous interscalene brachial plexus block for postoperative pain control at home: A randomized, double-blinded, placebo-controlled study. *Anesth Analg* 2003;96:1089–1095.

98. Perlas A, Chan VWS, Simons M. Brachial plexus examination and localization using ultrasound and electrical stimulation. *Anesthesiology* 2003;99:429–435.

99. Neal JM. Anatomy and pathophysiology of spinal cord injuries associated with regional anesthesia and pain medicine. *Reg Anesth Pain Med*. 2008;33: in press.

100. Pippa P, Cominelli E, Marinelli C, et al. Brachial plexus block using the posterior approach. *Eur J Anaesth* 1990;7:411–420.

101. Boezaart A, Koorn R, Rosenquist RW. Paravertebral approach to the brachial plexus: An anatomic improvement in technique. *Reg Anesth Pain Med* 2003;28:241–244.

102. Rettig HC, Gielen MJM, Jack NTM, et al. A comparison of the lateral and posterior approach for brachial plexus block. *Reg Anesth Pain Med* 2006;1:119–126.

103. Arcand G, Williams SR, Chouinard P, et al. Ultrasound-guided infraclavicular block versus supraclavicular block. *Anesth Analg* 2005;101:886–890.

104. Kulenkampff D, Persky MA. Brachial plexus anesthesia: Its indications, technic, and dangers. *Ann Surg* 1928;87:883.

105. Franco CD, Domashevich V, Voronov G, et al. The supraclavicular block with a nerve stimulator: To decrease or not to decrease, that is the question. *Anesth Analg* 2004;98:1167–1171.

106. Hickey R, Blanchard J, Hoffman J, et al. Plasma concentrations of ropivacaine given with or without epinephrine for brachial plexus block. *Can J Anaesth* 1990;37:878–882.

107. Smith BE. Distribution of evoked paraesthesiae and effectiveness of brachial plexus block. *Anaesthesia* 1986;41:1112–1115.
108. Klaastad O, VadeBoncouer TR, Tillung T, et al. An evaluation of the supra-clavicular plumb-bob technique for brachial plexus block by magnetic resonance imaging. *Anesth Analg* 2003;96:862–867.
109. Williams SR, Chouinard P, Arcand G, et al. Ultrasound guidance speeds execution and improves the quality of supraclavicular block. *Anesth Analg* 2003;97:1518–1523.
110. Horlocker TT, Wedel DJ, Benzon H, et al. Regional anesthesia in the anti-coagulated patient: Defining the risks (The second ASRA consensus conference on neuraxial anesthesia and anticoagulation). *Reg Anesth Pain Med* 2003;28:172–197.
111. Kapral S, Jandrasits O, Schabernig C, et al. Lateral infraclavicular plexus block vs. axillary block for hand and forearm surgery. *Acta Anaesthesiol Scand* 1999;43:1047–1052.
112. Koscielniak-Nielsen ZJ, Rotboll Nielsen P, Risby Mortensen C. A comparison of coracoid and axillary approaches to the brachial plexus. *Acta Anaesthesiol Scand* 2000;44:274–279.
113. Minville V, Fourcade O, Idabouk L, et al. Infraclavicular brachial plexus block versus humeral block in trauma patients: A comparison of patient comfort. *Anesth Analg* 2006;102:912–916.
114. Minville V, Amathieu R, Luc N, et al. Infraclavicular brachial plexus block versus humeral approach: Comparison of anesthetic time and efficacy. *Anesth Analg* 2005;101:1198–1201.
115. Koscielniak-Nielsen ZJ, Rasmussen H, Hesselbjerg L, et al. Infraclavicular block causes less discomfort than axillary block in ambulatory patients. *Acta Anaesthesiol Scand* 2005;49:1030–1034.
116. Ilfeld BM, Morey TE, Enneking FK. Continuous infraclavicular brachial plexus lock for postoperative pain control at home: A randomized, double-blinded, placebo-controlled study. *Anesthesiology* 2002;96:1297–1304.
117. Klaastad O, Smith H-J, Smedby O, et al. A novel infraclavicular brachial plexus block: The lateral and sagittal technique, developed by magnetic resonance imaging studies. *Anesth Analg* 2004;98:252–256.
118. Raj PP, Montgomery SJ, Nettles Dea. Infraclavicular brachial plexus block: A new approach. *Anesth Analg* 1973;52:897–904.
119. Sims JK. A modification of landmarks for infraclavicular approach to brachial plexus block. *Anesth Analg* 1977;56:554–555.
120. Sauter AR, Smith H-J, Stubhaug A, et al. Use of magnetic resonance imaging to define the anatomical location closest to all three cords of the infraclavicular brachial plexus. *Anesth Analg* 2006;103:1574–1576.
121. Raphael DT, McIntee D, Tsuruda JS, et al. Frontal slab composite magnetic resonance neurography of the brachial plexus. *Anesthesiology* 2005;103:1218–1224.
122. Gaertner E, Estebe JP, Cuby C, et al. Triple-injection method using peripheral nerve stimulator is superior to single injection in infraclavicular plexus block: A preliminary study. *Reg Anesth Pain Med* 2001;26S:A30.
123. Jandard C, Gentilli ME, Girard F, et al. Infraclavicular block with lateral approach and nerve stimulation: Extent of anesthesia and adverse effects. *Reg Anesth Pain Med* 2002;27:590–594.
124. Lecamwasam H, Mayfield J, Rosow L, et al. Stimulation of the posterior cord predicts successful infraclavicular block. *Anesth Analg* 2006;102:1564–1568.
125. Bloc S, Garnier T, Komly B, et al. Single-stimulation, low-volume infraclavicular plexus block: Influence of the evoked distal motor response on success rate. *Reg Anesth Pain Med* 2006;31:433–437.
126. Borene SC, Edwards JN, Boezaart AP. At the cords, the pinkie towards: Interpreting infraclavicular motor responses to neurostimulation. *Reg Anesth Pain Med* 2004;29:125–129.
127. Rodriguez J, Barcena M, Alvarez J. Restricted infraclavicular distribution of the local anesthetic solution after infraclavicular brachial plexus block. *Reg Anesth Pain Med* 2003;28:33–36.
128. Schroeder LE, Horlocker TT, Schroeder DR. The efficacy of axillary block for surgical procedures about the elbow. *Anesth Analg* 1996;83:747–751.

129. Retzl G, Kapral S, Greher M, et al. Ultrasonographic findings in the axillary part of the brachial plexus. *Anesth Analg* 2001;92:1271–1275.
130. Cockings E, Moore PL, Lewis RC. Transarterial brachial plexus blockade using high doses of 1.5% mepivacaine. *Reg Anesth* 1987;12:159–164.
131. Hickey R, Hoffman J, Tingle LJ, et al. Comparison of the clinical efficacy of three perivascular techniques for axillary brachial plexus block. *Reg Anesth* 1993;18:335–338.
132. Youssef MS, Desgrand DA. Comparison of two methods of axillary brachial plexus anaesthesia. *Br J Anaesth* 2001;60:841–844.
133. Thompson G. The multiple compartment approach to brachial plexus anesthesia. *Tech Reg Anesth Pain Manag* 1997;1:163–168.
134. Bouaziz H, Narchi P, Mercier FJ, et al. Comparison between conventional axillary block and a new approach at the midhumeral level. *Anesth Analg* 1997;84:1058–1062.
135. Yamamoto K, Tsubokawa T, Shibata K, et al. Area of paresthesia as determinant of sensory block in axillary brachial plexus block. *Reg Anesth* 1995;20:493–497.
136. Sia S, Bartoli M. Selective ulnar nerve localization is not essential for axillary brachial plexus block using a multiple nerve stimulation technique. *Reg Anesth Pain Med* 2001;26:12–16.
137. Sia S. A comparison of injection at the ulnar and the radial nerve in axillary block using triple stimulation. *Reg Anesth Pain Med* 2006;31:514–518.
138. Rodriguez J, Taboada M, Valino C, et al. A comparison of stimulation patterns in axillary block: Part 2. *Reg Anesth Pain Med* 2006;31:202–205.
139. Cooper K, Kelley H, Carrithers J. Perceptions of side effects following axillary block used for outpatient surgery. *Reg Anesth* 1995;20:212–216.
140. Fanelli G, Casati A, Garancini P, et al. Nerve stimulator and multiple injection technique for upper and lower limb blockade: Failure rate, patient acceptance, and neurologic complications. Study Group on Regional Anesthesia. *Anesth Analg* 1999;88:847–852.
141. Bouaziz H, Narchi P, Mercier FJ, et al. The use of selective axillary nerve block for outpatient hand surgery. *Anesth Analg* 1998;86:746–748.
142. Iskandar H, Guillaume E, Dixmerias F, et al. The enhancement of sensory blockade by clonidine selectively added to mepivacaine after midhumeral block. *Anesth Analg* 2001;93:771–775.
143. Dupre LJ. Bloc du plexus brachial au canal humeral. *Cah Anesthesiol* 1994;42:767–769.
144. Neal JM. Cutaneous blocks for the upper extremity. In: Hadzic A, ed. *Modern Regional Anesthesia*. New York: McGraw Hill, 2006.
145. Ritchie E, Tong D, Chung F, et al. Suprascapular nerve block for postoperative pain relief in arthroscopic shoulder surgery: A new modality? *Anesth Analg* 1997;84:1306–1312.
146. Singelyn FJ, Lhotel L, Fabre B. Pain relief after arthroscopic shoulder surgery: A comparison of intraarticular analgesia, suprascapular nerve block, and interscalene brachial plexus block. *Anesth Analg* 2004;99:589–592.
147. Neal JM. Upper extremity blocks. In: Rathmell JP, Neal JM, Viscomi CM, eds. *Requisites in Anesthesiology: Regional Anesthesia*. Philadelphia: Elsevier Mosby, 2004.
148. Viscomi CM, Reese J, Rathmell JP. Medial and lateral antebrachial cutaneous nerve blocks: An easily learned regional anesthetic for forearm arteriovenous fistula surgery. *Reg Anesth* 1996;21:2–5.
149. Selander D, Edshage S, Wolff T. Paresthesiae or no paresthesiae? Nerve lesions after axillary blocks. *Acta Anaesthesiol Scand* 1979;23:27–33.
150. Gebhard RE, Al–Samsam T, Greger J, et al. Distal nerve blocks at the wrist for outpatient carpal tunnel surgery offer intraoperative cardiovascular stability and reduce discharge time. *Anesth Analg* 2002;95:351–355.
151. Macaire P, Choquet O, Jochum D, et al. Nerve blocks at the wrist for carpal tunnel release revisited: The use of sensory–nerve and motor-nerve stimulation techniques. *Reg Anesth Pain Med* 2005;30:536–540.
152. Neal JM, Rathmell JP. *Complications in Regional Anesthesia and Pain Medicine*. New York: Elsevier Saunders, 2007.

CHAPTER 14 ■ THE LOWER EXTREMITY: SOMATIC BLOCKADE

F. KAYSER ENNEKING, DENISE J. WEDEL, AND TERESE T. HORLOCKER

Lower extremity peripheral nerve blocks (PNBs) have traditionally been less popular and less utilized compared to other forms of regional anesthesia. Epidural and subarachnoid anesthesia, which provide rapid, reliable, and safe anesthesia of the lower extremities, are more widely taught to anesthesiologists than lower extremity peripheral neural blockade techniques. Unlike the upper extremity, the entire lower extremity cannot be anesthetized with a single injection, and injections are generally deeper than those required for upper extremity block. Over the past decade, several developments have led to an increased interest in lower extremity PNBs, including transient neurologic symptoms associated with spinal anesthesia, increased risk of epidural hematoma associated with more aggressive antithromboembolic prophylaxis regimens, and evidence of improved rehabilitation outcome with lower extremity single-injection and continuous PNBs (1).

Like other forms of neural blockade, lower extremity techniques are not new. As early as 1887, Crile performed amputations by exposing the sciatic nerve in the gluteal fold and the femoral nerve in the inguinal fold, and injecting cocaine intraneurally. Braun mentions that blockade of the lateral cutaneous femoral nerve was described by Nystrom in 1909 (2). Laewen expanded on this by describing the additional blockade of the anterior crural nerve, and Keppler improved both techniques by advocating the elicitation of paresthesias. Subsequently, no fewer than six others advocated percutaneous approaches to the sciatic nerve alone. Many of these same authors described blockade of other nerves of the lower extremity as well (Chapter 1). Importantly, many of the techniques currently utilized are nearly identical to the original descriptions. This emphasizes remarks made by Labat that: "Anatomy is the foundation upon which the entire concept of regional anesthesia is built"; and that "The anesthetist should attempt to visualize the anatomic structures traversed by the needle and utilize the tactile senses to determine the impulses transmitted by the point of the needle as it approaches a deep landmark (e.g., bone)" (3). Labat localized neural structures using fascial "pops" and the elicitation of one or more paresthesias, as well as field infiltration. Advances in needles, catheters, and nerve stimulator technology have facilitated localization of neural structures and improved success rates. Even more recently, direct imaging using ultrasound, fluoroscopy, computer tomography (CT), and magnetic resonance imaging (MRI) has been utilized.

ANATOMY

Anatomically, the lumbosacral plexus consists of two distinct entities: the lumbar plexus and the sacral plexus. Some communication exists between these plexus via the lumbosacral trunk, but for functional purposes these are distinct entities (4). The lumbosacral plexus arises from at least eight spinal nerve roots, each of which contains anterior and posterior divisions that innervate the embryologic ventral or dorsal portions of the limb. With the exception of a small cutaneous portion of the buttock (which is supplied by upper lumbar and sacral segmental nerves), the innervation of the lower extremity is entirely through branches of the lumbosacral plexus (Tables 14-1 and 14-2; Figs. 14-1 and 14-2). The nerves to the muscles of the anterior and medial thigh are from the lumbar plexus. The muscles of the buttocks, the posterior muscles in the thigh, and all the muscles below the knee are supplied by the sacral plexus.

Lumbar Plexus Anatomy

The lumbar plexus is formed within the psoas muscle from the anterior rami of T12–L4 (4–7) (Fig. 14-1). Although the lumbosacral plexus as a whole contributes to the nerve supply of the lower extremities, the upper part of the lumbar division supplies the iliohypogastric and ilioinguinal nerves, which are in series with the thoracic nerves and innervate the trunk above the level of the extremity (Chapter 16). Specifically, the *iliohypogastric nerve* provides cutaneous innervation to the skin of the buttock and the muscles of the abdominal wall. The *ilioinguinal nerve* supplies the skin of the perineum and adjoining portion of the inner thigh (see Chapter 16). A third nerve, the *genitofemoral nerve*, arises from the first and second lumbar nerves. It supplies filaments to the genital area and adjacent parts of the thigh. It also gives off a lumboinguinal branch, which supplies the skin over the area of the femoral artery and femoral triangle (Table 14-1). The branches of the lumbar plexus and the iliohypogastric, ilioinguinal, genitofemoral, lateral femoral cutaneous, femoral, and obturator nerves, emerge from the psoas laterally, medially, and anteriorly. Of these, the *femoral nerve* (sometimes called the anterior crural nerve), *lateral femoral cutaneous nerve*, and *obturator nerve* are most important for lower extremity surgery (Figs. 14-1 and 14-2).

Sacral Plexus Anatomy

The sacral plexus gives off two nerves important for lower extremity surgery, the *posterior cutaneous nerve of the thigh* and the *sciatic nerve* (Fig. 14-2). The posterior cutaneous nerve has sometimes been referred to as the "lesser sciatic" nerve. It derives from the first, second, and third sacral nerves, as does the larger sciatic nerve, which also receives branches of the anterior

TABLE 14-1

LUMBAR PLEXUS ANATOMY

Nerve	Spinal segment	Motor innervation	Motion observed*	Sensory innervation	Articular branches
Iliohypogastric	T12–L1	Int/ext oblique Transverse abdominis	Ant abdominal wall	Inferior abd wall Upper lat quadrant of buttock	None
Ilioinguinal	L1	Int oblique	Ant abdominal wall	Inferior to medial aspect of inguinal ligament Portion of genitalia	None
Genitofemoral	L1–L2	Cremaster	Testicular	Inferior to mid portion of inguinal ligament Spermatic cord	None
Lateral Femoral Cutaneous	L2–L3	None		Anterior lateral and posterior aspects of thigh terminating in prepatellar plexus	
Femoral Anterior division	L2–L4	Sartorious	Medial aspect of the lower thigh	Anterior medial skin of the thigh	None
		Pectineus	Adductor of thigh	None	
Posterior division		Quadriceps Saphenous	Knee extension, patellar ascension	Ant thigh Medial leg from the tibia to the medial aspect of the foot	Hip and knee
Obturator Anterior division	L2–L4	Gracilis, adductor brevis and longus pectineus	Thigh adduction	Variable, posterior medial thigh, medial knee	Hip
Posterior division		Obturator externus, adductor magnus	Thigh adduction with lateral hip rotation		Knee

*Motion observed refers to the observed motor response with electrical stimulation of that nerve. Int, internal; Ext, external; Ant, anterior; Abd, abdominal; Lat, lateral. From Enneking FK, Chan V, Greger J, et al. Lower extremity peripheral nerve blocks: Essentials of our current understanding. *Reg Anesth Pain Med* 2005;30:4–35, with permission.

TABLE 14-2

SACRAL PLEXUS ANATOMY

Nerve	Spinal segment	Motor innervation	Motion observed*	Sensory innervation	Articular branches
Gluteal nerves	L4–S2	Piriformis, sup/inf gemellus obturator internus, quadratus femoris	Buttocks with lat hip rotation	Upper medial aspect of buttock	Hip
Sciatic, Tibial	L4–S3	Biceps femoris, semitendinosus, adductor magnus Popliteus Gastrocnemius, soleus, flexors of foot	Hamstrings with knee extension Knee flexion Plantar flexion Toe flexion	Medial and lat heel Sole of foot	Hip and Knee and Ankle
Sciatic, Peroneal Superficial Deep	L4–S3	Short head of biceps femoris peroneus longus, brevis Extensors of foot, toes	Knee flexion Foot inversion Dorsiflexion of foot, ankle	Distal anterior leg, dorsum of foot Web space of first toe	Knee and ankle Ankle
Sural Components from peroneal and tibial		None	None	None Post calf, lat border of foot and fifth toe	None
Post cut nerve of thigh	S1–S3	None	None	Distal medial quadrant of buttock perineum, post thigh including popliteal fossa	None

*Motion observed refers to the observed motor response with electrical stimulation of that nerve. Abbreviations: Sup, superior; Inf, inferior; Lat, lateral; Post, posterior; Cut, cutaneous.
From Enneking FK, Chan V, Greger J, et al. Lower extremity peripheral nerve blocks: Essentials of our current understanding. *Reg Anesth Pain Med* 2005;30:4–35, with permission.

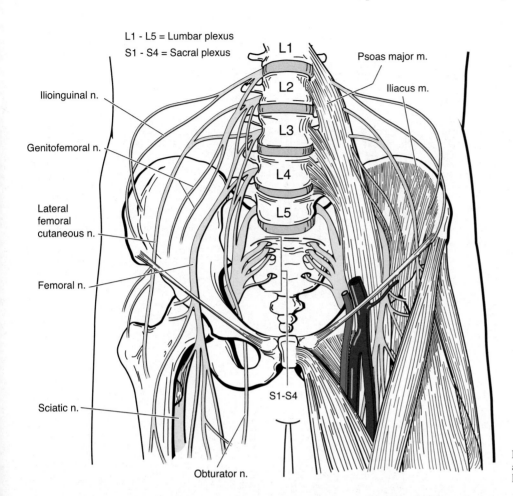

L1 - L5 = Lumbar plexus
S1 - S4 = Sacral plexus

L1
L2
L3
L4
L5

Psoas major m.

Iliacus m.

Ilioinguinal n.

Genitofemoral n.

Lateral
femoral
cutaneous n.

Femoral n.

Sciatic n.

S1-S4

Obturator n.

FIGURE 14-1. Lumbosacral plexus and major peripheral nerves of the lower extremity.

rami of the fourth and fifth lumbar nerves. Inasmuch as the two nerves course through the pelvis together and out through the greater sciatic foramen, they are considered together when techniques for blocking the sciatic nerve above the gluteal fold are discussed.

The sciatic nerve is really an association of two major nerve trunks. The first is the tibial, derived from the ventral branches of the anterior rami of the fourth and fifth lumbar and first, second, and third sacral nerves. The second is the common peroneal, derived from the dorsal branches of the anterior rami of the same five nerves. These two major nerve trunks pass as the sciatic to the proximal angle of the popliteal fossa, where they separate, with the tibial portion passing medially and the common peroneal (lateral popliteal) laterally. This division can occur more cephalad or caudad to the popliteal fossa. The smaller branches of these nerves, which provide distal innervation of the lower extremity, are discussed in detail in conjunction with techniques for nerve block at the knee and ankle.

PARAVERTEBRAL APPROACHES TO BLOCKADE OF THE LUMBAR PLEXUS

The lumbar plexus, as previously noted, is formed by the anterior (ventral) divisions of the first, second, third, and fourth lumbar nerves, with about 50% inclusion of a branch from the twelfth thoracic nerve and occasionally from the fifth lum-

bar nerve. The spinal nerve that leaves the spinal cord at each level is formed by the union of a ventral motor root with a dorsal sensory root. This mixed spinal nerve gives off a dorsal ramus, a ventral ramus, and a ramus communicans; the latter contributes to the formation of the sympathetic ganglion and trunk. The lumbar plexus is formed in front of the transverse processes of the lumbar vertebrae into a series of oblique loops that lie deep in the substance of the psoas major muscle and at the medial border of the quadratus lumborum muscle (Fig. 14-3). From here, the individual nerves form and course in the direction of their terminal innervation.

The relationship of the lumbar plexus to the sympathetic chain is important, since each may be blocked separately, but with a similar approach. The first and second lumbar spinal nerves, frequently the third, and sometimes the fourth, send communicating rami to form the lumbar portion of the sympathetic trunk. The sympathetic trunk lies on the ventrolateral surface of the lumbar and sacral bodies medial to the anterior foramina. It is apparent, therefore, that although these two nerve systems are separated by distance, muscle, and tissue planes, they have considerable intercommunication (Fig. 14-3).

Indications

The lumbar plexus supplies the cutaneous nerves not only to the upper thigh but also to the lower abdominal area. (Analgesia for the abdomen is covered more completely in Chapter 16.)

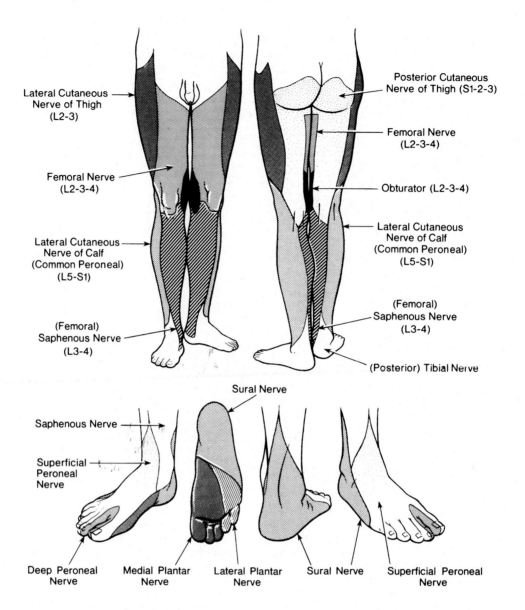

FIGURE 14-2. Cutaneous nerve distribution of the lower limb.

Branches of the first three lumbar nerves provide cutaneous distribution to the inner and outer aspects of the thigh and the posterior gluteal region, along with adjacent perineal and suprapubic areas. Complete lumbar plexus blockade may be accomplished by discretely blocking the five individual lumbar somatic nerves (assuring blockade of the iliohypogastric, ilioinguinal, genitofemoral nerves, if needed for the anticipated procedure) or with a single large injection (psoas compartment block). Recent applications have typically utilized the psoas compartment approach. Sacral blockade must also be performed to achieve complete blockade of the lower extremity.

The psoas compartment block was first described by Chayen in 1976 (8). It can be performed as a single-injection technique or with a catheter placed for prolonged analgesia. It has been used to provide anesthesia for thigh surgery. In combination with parasacral nerve block, it has been used for hip fracture repair (9), to provide analgesia following total hip arthroplasty (THA) or total knee arthroplasty (TKA) (5,6,10,11), and also in the treatment of chronic hip pain (12).

Continuous psoas techniques have been described to provide analgesia following a variety of operations including THA, TKA, open reduction and internal fixation (ORIF) of acetabular fractures, ORIF of femur fractures, and anterior cruciate ligament reconstruction (5,10,11,13–15). Interest in this block developed as practitioners sought alternatives to neuraxial techniques that could provide consistent analgesia following hip, femur, and knee surgery.

Technique: Lumbar Paravertebral Nerve Block

The classic approach to blockade of the lumbar somatic nerves is paravertebral. The original block description of Labat advocates having the patient lie on the side opposite the one to be blocked (3). A soft roll placed between the iliac crest and the costal margin will minimize the lateral spinal curvature. A

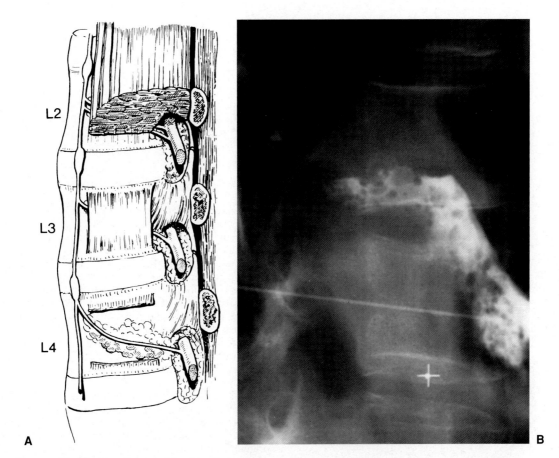

FIGURE 14-3. Relationship of lumbar somatic nerve roots to sympathetic chain. Note the separation of somatic and sympathetic nerves by the psoas major muscle; however, there is also a potential path of communication via the fibrous arch illustrated at the L4 level (see also Chapter 39).

preferred position, is that of having the patient lie prone over a soft pillow, which will flatten/minimize the lordotic curve. Regardless of patient position, the landmarks used are the spinous processes of the lumbar vertebrae. Skin wheals are raised opposite the cephalad aspect of the spinous processes, on a line 3 to 4 cm laterally from, and parallel to, the midline of the back (Fig. 14-4). Depending on the size of the patient, a 10- or 15-cm insulated needle is inserted through each of the skin wheals and advanced perpendicular to the surface of the skin until its tip comes into contact with the transverse process of the vertebral body, usually at a depth of 4 to 5 cm. The needle is then partially withdrawn and reintroduced slightly more cephalad and medially, making an angle of about 25 degrees with the sagittal plane of the body. This should allow the needle to pass just tangential to the superior aspect of the transverse process and to be advanced an additional 2 to 3 cm. Following elicitation of the appropriate motor response (abdominal wall versus lower extremity), 8 to 10 mL of the selected local anesthetic solution is injected.

Importantly, the spinous processes of the lumbar vertebrae, unlike those of the thoracic vertebrae, do not slope downward, their upper and lower borders being more nearly horizontal. Their average thickness is from 0.5 to 1 cm. The distance between the tip of the lumbar spinous process and its attachment to the vertebral lamina is approximately 3 to 4 cm. A horizontal line drawn tangentially to the superior aspect of the spinous process will overlie the transverse process of that ver-

tebrae. The transverse processes of the lumbar vertebrae are short, accounting for the paravertebral skin wheal being only 2 to 3 cm from the midline. The average depth of the transverse process to the skin is 5 cm, which varies with the size of the patient and the paraspinous musculature. The transverse processes of L4 and L5 are more deeply situated than are those of the vertebrae above. When the needle passes superior to the transverse process, it is in proximity to the somatic nerve of the preceding segment (the needle passing over the transverse process of L1 injects the T12 nerve root). The L5 root is blocked through the same skin wheal as L4, by redirecting the needle in a caudad direction until it passes from the lower border of the L4 transverse process and by injecting the nerve root in a manner similar to the technique used in other roots (Fig. 14-4, *lower panel*).

Technique: Psoas Compartment Block

Several descriptions of the needle entry site for the psoas compartment blocks have been described (5,7,16–19). All rely on bony contact with the transverse process as a guide to depth of needle placement. The patient is placed in the lateral position, hips flexed and operative extremity uppermost. A line is drawn to connect the iliac crests (intercristal line) identifying the fourth lumbar spine. After skin preparation, a skin wheal is raised 3 cm caudad and 5 cm lateral to the midline

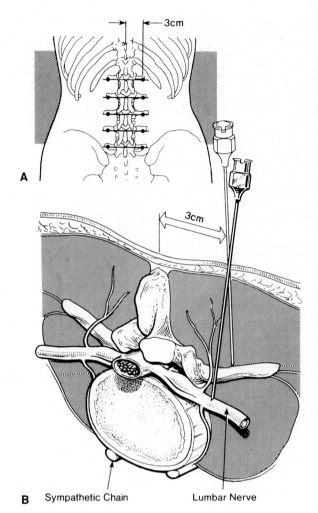

FIGURE 14-4. Paravertebral lumbar somatic nerve block. **A:** Skin markings are made by drawing lines across the cephalad aspect of spinous processes and then drawing vertical lines 3 cm from the midline. **B:** A needle inserted perpendicular to the skin will contact the cephalad edge of a spinous process. The lumbar plexus is identified approximately 2 cm deep to the transverse process, between the quadratus lumborum and the psoas muscles.

on the side to be blocked. A 21-gauge, 10-cm stimulating needle is then advanced perpendicular to the skin entry site until it contacts the fifth lumbar transverse process. The needle is redirected cephalad until it passes the transverse process (Fig. 14-4, *lower panel*). Traversing from posterior to anterior at the level of L4–L5, the following structures would be encountered: posterior lumbar fascia, paraspinous muscles, anterior lumbar fascia, quadratus lumborum, and the psoas muscle (20). The common iliac artery and vein are situated anterior to the psoas muscle. The lumbar plexus is identified by elicitation of a quadriceps motor response, and 30 mL of solution is injected.

Based on anatomic imaging studies, Capdevila et al. (5) modified the classic psoas technique. Needle insertion site is the junction of the lateral third and medial two thirds of a line between the spinous process of L4 and a line parallel to the spinal column passing through the posterior superior iliac spine (PSIS). (The spinous process of L4 was estimated to be approximately 1 cm cephalad to the upper edge of the iliac crests.) The needle is advanced perpendicularly to the skin un-

til contact with the transverse process of L4 is obtained and advanced caudad off the transverse process until quadriceps femoris muscle twitches are elicited (Fig. 14-5). Despite a difference between men and women in the depth of the lumbar plexus (median values, 8.5 and 7.0 cm, respectively), the distance from the L4 transverse process to the lumbar plexus was comparable (median value, 2 cm) in both sexes. Thus, the authors stressed the importance of achieving contact with the L4 transverse process to establish appropriate needle depth and position.

Complications

The deep needle placement with the lumbar paravertebral and psoas compartment approaches increases the risk of possible renal hematoma, retroperitoneal hematoma, pneumocele, and unintended intra-abdominal and intervertebral disk catheter placement (5,21–24). Seizures have been reported following negative aspiration and intermittent injection (25). To ensure the proper position of the needle during these deep techniques and to avoid excessive needle insertion, it is recommended that the transverse process be intentionally sought. Peripheral nerve damage is also a potential risk with this technique. A side effect of the paravertebral approach to the lumbar plexus is the development of a sympathetic block secondary to spread of local anesthetic. This unilateral sympathectomy is usually of little consequence.

Epidural spread of local anesthetic is another common side effect of psoas compartment block, occurring in 9% to 16% of adult patients (7,26). In children, Dalens et al. reported a greater than 90% incidence of epidural spread when using the original landmarks of Chayen, compared to no epidural spread when using the landmarks as modified by Winnie (27). This side effect is usually attributed to retrograde diffusion of the local anesthetic to the epidural space when large volumes of local anesthetic are used (greater than 20 mL). In most cases, residual lumbar plexus blockade is apparent after the resolution of the contralateral block. However, there are case reports of total spinal anesthesia occurring during lumbar plexus blockade, and vigilance must be maintained during the management of this block (22,28,29).

BLOCKADE OF BRANCHES OF THE LUMBAR PLEXUS

Femoral Nerve Block

The femoral nerve is formed by the dorsal divisions of the anterior rami of the second, third, and fourth lumbar nerves. The femoral nerve emerges from the psoas muscle in a fascial compartment between the psoas and iliacus muscles, where it gives off articular branches to the hip. It enters the thigh posterior to the inguinal ligament. There it lies lateral and posterior to the femoral artery. This relationship to the femoral artery exists near the inguinal ligament, but not after the nerve enters the thigh. As the nerve passes into the thigh, it divides into an anterior and a posterior division and quickly arborizes. At the level of the inguinal ligament, dense fascial planes are present: the fascia lata and fascia iliaca (Fig. 14-6). The femoral nerve is situated deep to these fascial planes. The femoral artery, vein, and lymphatics reside in a separate fascial compartment medial to the nerve.

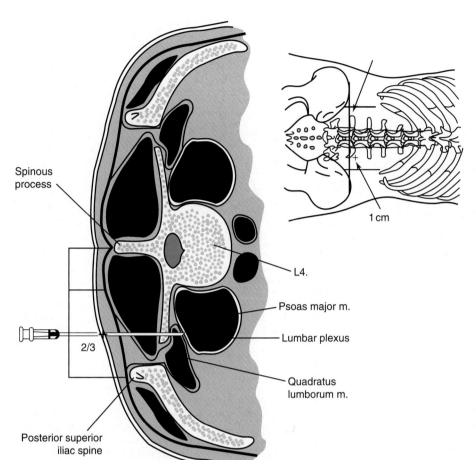

Spinous
process

L4.

Psoas major m.

Lumbar plexus

2/3

Quadratus
lumborum m.

Posterior superior
iliac spine

1 cm

FIGURE 14-5. Psoas compartment block. Needle entry is marked 1 cm cephalad to the intercristal line, two-thirds the distance from the midline to the posterior superior iliac spine line. The lumbar plexus is identified between the transverse processes of L4 and L5. Dural sleeves extend 3 to 5 cm laterally. The cross indicates the site of needle insertion.

The anterior division of the femoral nerve gives off the medial and intermediate cutaneous nerves that supply the skin of the medial and anterior surfaces of the thigh. The muscular branches of the anterior division of the femoral nerve supply the sartorius muscle and the pectineus muscle and articular branches to the hip. The posterior division of the femoral nerve gives off the saphenous nerve, which is the largest cutaneous branch of the femoral nerve, and the muscular branches to the quadriceps muscle and articular branches to the knee.

The terminal nerves of the posterior division of the femoral nerve, the saphenous and the vastus medialis nerves, continue distally through the adductor canal. The saphenous nerve exits from the lower part of the canal, emerging between the sartorius and gracilis muscles, where is gives off an infrapatellar branch. The nerve becomes subcutaneous below the sartorius at the medial side of the knee. It descends down the medial border of the tibia immediately behind the long saphenous vein, although its course can be quite variable. The nerve crosses with the vein in front of the medial malleolus and extends as far as the base of the great toe. The saphenous nerve supplies an extensive cutaneous area over the medial side of the knee, leg, ankle, and foot (Fig. 14-2).

Indications

Indications for single-injection femoral nerve block include anesthesia for knee arthroscopy in combination with intra-articular local anesthesia, and analgesia for femoral shaft frac-

tures, anterior cruciate ligament reconstruction (ACL), and TKA as a part of multimodal regimes (30–35). Their use in complex knee operations is associated with lower pain scores and fewer hospital admissions following same-day surgery (36).

Technique: Femoral Nerve Block

The patient lies supine with the anesthesiologist standing next to the side that is to be blocked. After careful palpation, a skin wheal is raised just lateral to the femoral artery, where it emerges distal to the inguinal ligament (Fig. 14-6). A 22-gauge 5-cm insulated needle is inserted just over the tip of the palpating finger in a cephalad direction. Commonly, the anterior branch of the femoral nerve will be identified first. Vloka et al. reported this to be the first motor response elicited 97% of the time (37). Stimulation of this branch leads to contraction of the sartorius muscle on the medial aspect of the thigh and should not be accepted, as the articular and muscular branches derive from the posterior branch of the femoral nerve. The needle should be redirected slightly laterally and with a deeper direction to encounter the posterior branch of the femoral nerve. Stimulation of this branch is identified by *patellar ascension* as the quadriceps contract. The needle is then fixed and a volume of 25 to 30 mL of local anesthetic is injected.

Three-in-One Block versus Femoral Block

During femoral nerve block, it has been advocated to use a higher volume of local anesthetic and apply firm pressure just

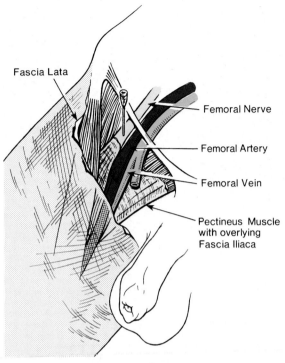

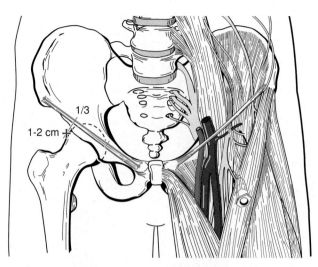

FIGURE 14-7. Fascia iliacus block. Needle entry is marked 1 to 2 cm below the junction between the outer one third and the inner two thirds of the line connecting the anterior superior iliac spine and the pubic tubercle. Two discernible fascial "pops" are noted as the needle traverses the fascia lata and then the fascia iliaca. Since the needle insertion site overlies the hip joint capsule, a third pop may signify insertions into the joint space.

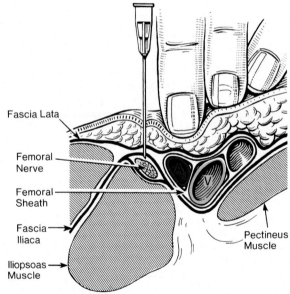

FIGURE 14-6. Femoral triangle. Inguinal structures showing fascial envelope around femoral nerve and relationships for inguinal paravascular femoral nerve block techniques. Note that the femoral nerve is under the fascia iliaca; both the fascia lata and fascia iliaca must be penetrated.

distal to the needle during and a few minutes after injection to block the femoral, lateral femoral cutaneous, and obturator nerves, the so named "three-in-one block" (38). However, despite many efforts to consistently produce a three-in-one block, the effectiveness of these maneuvers has not been demonstrated. In most reports, the femoral nerve is the only nerve consistently blocked with this approach (39–42). Blockade of the lateral femoral cutaneous nerve occurs through lateral diffusion of local anesthetic and not through proximal

spread to the lumbar plexus (41). The obturator nerve is less frequently anesthetized during three-in-one block than the lateral femoral cutaneous nerve, which is not surprising given the number of fascial barriers between these structures at the level of the inguinal ligament. As a result of the lack of scientific support for the term "three-in-one," the perivascular or three-in-one approach is now most often referred to as a *femoral nerve block*.

Technique: Modified Femoral (Fascia Iliacus) Block

Dalens originally described the fascia iliacus block in children (43). The indications for its use are the same as those for single-injection femoral nerve block (44). Advocates believe its utility lies in the "double-pop" technique for applying this block. The double-pop refers to the sensation felt as the needle traverses the fascia lata then the fascia iliaca. Penetration of both layers of fascia is important for successful fascia iliacus blockade. To facilitate the appreciation of the "clicks" or "pops," the use of a short bevel- or pencil-tipped needle has been advocated to provide more tactile feedback than cutting needles. This technique does not require a nerve stimulator; however, confirmatory motor responses may be sought. The needle entry site for the fascia iliacus block is determined by drawing a line between the pubic tubercle and the anterior superior iliac crest and dividing this line into thirds. The needle entry point is 1 cm caudal to the intersection of the medial two-thirds and lateral one-third along this line. This site is well away from the femoral artery, making this useful for patients in whom femoral artery puncture is contraindicated (Fig. 14-7).

Continuous Femoral and Fascia Iliacus Blockade

Continuous femoral and fascia iliacus block have been shown to improve outcome following major knee and vascular surgery of the lower extremity compared to intravenous (IV) narcotic therapy or continuous infusion or injection of analgesics (45–53).

However, both continuous techniques have been associated with a high rate of inaccurate catheter placement. In a prospective study, Capdevila et al. showed that continuous femoral nerve block using a standard approach led to unpredictable catheter placement, with only 25% of the catheters lying near the lumbar plexus (54). Most often the catheters tended to course medially in the direction of the psoas muscle or laterally in the direction of the iliacus muscle. The accuracy of final catheter placement correlated with the degree of analgesia following proximal lower limb surgery (54). Ganapathy et al. (52) reported similar results with final placement of fascia iliaca catheters; CT scans noted only 40% of catheters placed were ideally positioned (superior to the upper third of the sacroiliac joint in the psoas sheath). Comparing a stimulating catheter to a nonstimulating catheter, Salinas et al. were able to increase the success rate of continuous femoral nerve block in volunteers from 85% to 100% (55).

Technique: Saphenous Nerve Block

Saphenous nerve blocks are commonly performed as a component of knee and ankle blocks. Supplemental block of the saphenous nerve is required for surgical procedures to the medial aspect of the leg, ankle, and foot, or when a tourniquet or Esmarch bandage is applied. Patients with thigh tourniquet placement require a more proximal block near the saphenous nerve origin in the femoral triangle. Various nerve block approaches are described, from its origin in the femoral triangle to the medial malleolus.

Saphenous Nerve Block at the Level of the Femoral Triangle

The patient is positioned supine with the leg extended at the knee and the long axis of the foot at a 90-degree angle to the table. The anesthesiologist stands at the side to be blocked. The femoral artery pulse is palpated and marked. Needle insertion site is 1 to 2 cm lateral to the artery and medial to the upper border of the sartorius muscle. A 22-gauge 5-cm insulated needle is introduced perpendicular to the skin at the needle insertion site and advanced until an evoked vastus medialis muscle response is elicited at 0.5 mA or less. A total of 5 to 10 mL of solution is injected incrementally after negative aspiration. Alternatively, a more proximal block of the femoral nerve may be performed as described earlier if total volume of anesthetic solution is not of concern (see Fig. 14-6).

Saphenous Nerve Block at the Level of the Knee

Saphenous nerve blocks at the level of the knee are based on the relationship of the nerves to the superior pole of the patella, tibial tuberosity, medial head of gastrocnemius muscle, sartorius muscle, and saphenous vein. No motor response is sought with distal saphenous approaches, since the saphenous nerve is purely sensory, distal to the femoral triangle. However, the nerve may be localized using a nerve stimulator and eliciting sensory "electrical" pulsations (56,57).

Field Block Technique. The patient is positioned supine with the leg extended at the knee. A 25-gauge 5-cm needle is inserted above the medial surface of the tibia and 5 to 7 mL of solution is infiltrated subcutaneously in a fan-like pattern. Classically, this saphenous nerve block was performed as a blind subcuta-

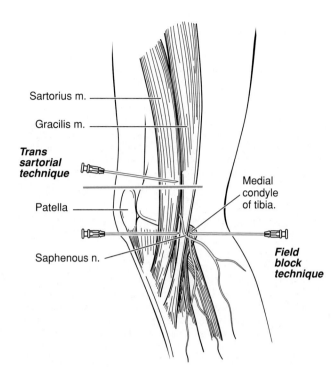

FIGURE 14-8. Saphenous nerve block at the knee joint. Transsartorial technique (*upper needle*): At the upper pole of the patella, the sartorius muscle is palpated and a needle is advanced through the muscle belly, at an angle of 45 degrees from the coronal plane, until a "pop" is noted when the needle penetrates the deep aspect of the sartorius fascia (at a depth of 1.5–3 cm). Field block technique (*lower needles*): A needle is inserted just superior to the medial condyle of the tibia. Local anesthetic is injected subcutaneously in a fan-like pattern.

neous infiltration over the medial surface of the tibia (between the tibial tuberosity and the medial head of the gastrocnemius muscle) (Fig. 14-8). However, success rates with this technique ranged between 33% and 65%.

Transsartorial Technique. The patient is positioned supine with the leg extended at the knee. The sartorius muscle is palpated on the medial side, just above the knee joint. At the level of the upper pole of the patella, a 22-gauge 5-cm needle is advanced 45 degrees from the coronal plane, through the muscle belly of the sartorius, until a fascial pop or click is noted (1.5–3 cm) (Fig. 14-8). After negative aspiration, 10 mL of local anesthetic is injected. Success rates for the transsartorial approach are 70% to 80% (58).

Paravenous Technique. The patient is placed supine with the leg extended at the knee. Below the knee, the saphenous nerve is immediately adjacent to the saphenous vein. The saphenous vein is identified by placing a thigh tourniquet and allowing the leg to dangle for at least 60 seconds. Ultrasound guidance also may be helpful. A subcutaneous paravascular injection is performed using a 25-gauge 5 cm needle with 5 mL of local anesthetic on each side of the vein, taking care to avoid IV injection. The success rate is approximately 100%. However, painless hematomas often occur with this approach (59).

Complications

Intravascular injection and hematoma are possible because of the close proximity of vascular structures throughout the course of the nerve. However, anatomically, the nerve and femoral artery are located in separate sheaths approximately 1 cm apart (Fig. 14-6). In most patients with normal anatomy, the femoral artery can be easily palpated, allowing correct, safe needle positioning lateral to the pulsation. The presence of femoral vascular grafts is a relative contraindication to femoral block; however, the fascia iliacus approach may be utilized in these patients because of the lateral needle insertion site. Nerve damage is rare with this technique (60). Both local inflammation and proximal abscess have been reported with indwelling catheters (1). Finally, the presence of femoral or combined femoral–sciatic block may lead to lateral gait instability, resulting in difficulty with pivoting maneuvers and patient falls (61).

OBTURATOR NERVE BLOCK

The obturator nerve (L2–L4) derives its major source from L3–L4—the portion coming from L2 is very small and sometimes even lacking. The nerve appears at the medial border of the psoas muscle, covered anteriorly by the external iliac vessels, and passes downward in the pelvis. It continues with the obturator vessels along the obturator groove and passes through the obturator foramen into the thigh. As the nerve passes through the obturator canal, it divides into posterior and anterior branches. The anterior branch supplies an articular branch to the hip joint, the anterior adductor muscles, and cutaneous branches to the lower inner thigh (Fig. 14-2). The size or existence of this cutaneous innervation is small and variable depending on which anatomic reference material is quoted; recent investigations suggest that the only way to effectively evaluate obturator nerve function is to assess adductor strength (62,63). The posterior branch innervates the deep adductor muscles and frequently sends an articular branch to the knee joint, which may be important in providing analgesia for knee surgery.

Some anatomic descriptions include an accessory obturator nerve that leaves the medial border of the psoas muscle in company with the obturator nerve. It has been said to be incorrectly named, having much more in common with the femoral nerve (64). Like the femoral nerve, it passes over, not under, the pubic ramus where it supplies the pectineus muscle. It is present in about one third of individuals.

Indications

Indications for a single-injection obturator nerve block are generally limited to diagnostic applications or therapeutic relaxation of the adductor muscles of the thigh (65). Despite the significant amount of literature that has been devoted to anesthetic sparing of this nerve with many approaches to the lumbar plexus, only two studies have examined the effect of the addition of an obturator nerve block to improve analgesia after major knee surgery (66,67). Both studies reported a decrease in opioid consumption and pain scores in patients undergoing TKA receiving obturator nerve block in addition to a femoral or femoral and sciatic nerve block.

Technique: Obturator Nerve Block

The patient is placed supine with the leg to be blocked in slight abduction. Caution should be taken to protect the skin of the genitalia from irritating antiseptic solutions used in preparing the area. It is not necessary to shave the pubic area. A skin wheal is raised at a point 1 to 2 cm lateral and 1 to 2 cm caudad to the pubic tubercle, and a 22-gauge, 8- to 10-cm needle is advanced perpendicular to the skin entry site with a slight medial direction. The inferior pubic ramus is encountered at a depth of 2 to 4 cm, and the needle is walked in a lateral and caudad direction, until it passes into the obturator canal. Identification of the bony wall verifies that the needle has passed into the canal rather than into the soft tissues (e.g., bladder or vagina) medially or superiorly (Fig. 14-9A). The obturator nerve is located 2 to 3 cm past the initial point of contact with the pubic ramus. After negative aspiration, 10 to 15 mL of local anesthetic is injected. A nerve stimulator is helpful in locating the obturator nerve; correct needle position is evidenced by contraction of the adductor muscles of the medial thigh. The presence of successful obturator nerve block is determined by demonstrating paresis of the adductor muscles, since the cutaneous distribution is small and inconstant.

The classic approach to obturator nerve block involves painful periosteal contact and multiple needle redirection. An alternate interadductor approach was described by Wasseff (65). In this technique, the needle is inserted behind the adductor tendon, near its pubic insertion, and is directed laterally toward a mark on the skin 1 to 2 cm medial to the femoral artery and immediately below the inguinal ligament, representing the obturator canal. The nerve is identified by a motor response to peripheral nerve stimulation in the adductor muscle (Fig. 14-9B).

A modification of this technique advocates searching for paresthesias to the area of the inner thigh (68). If paresthesias are not elicited, then it is suggested that a fan-like wall of anesthesia be deposited. The major difference in the two techniques lies in a greater attempt to palpate the tendon on the adductor longus muscle, which constitutes the upper medial aspect of the obturator foramen. With gentle, deep palpation, one may be able to palpate the entire foramen and, placing the skin wheal inferior to the midpoint of the superior pubic ramus, gain a more precise location of the obturator nerve.

Complications

Obturator nerve block has vascular and neural complications and side effects nearly identical to those of the femoral nerve.

LATERAL FEMORAL CUTANEOUS NERVE BLOCK

The lateral femoral cutaneous nerve (L2–L3) emerges at the lateral border of the psoas muscle at a level lower than the ilioinguinal nerve. It passes obliquely under the fascia iliaca and across the iliac muscle to enter the thigh deep to the inguinal ligament, at a point approximately 1 to 2 cm medial to the anterior superior iliac spine (Fig. 14-10). It then crosses or passes through the tendinous origin of the sartorius muscle, and courses downward beneath the fascia lata. It emerges from the fascia lata at a point 7 to 10 cm below the anterior superior iliac spine, where it branches into anterior and posterior branches. The anterior branch supplies the skin over the anterolateral aspect of the thigh as low as the knee. The posterior branch pierces the fascia lata and passes backward to supply the skin on the lateral side of the thigh from just below the greater trochanter to about the middle of the thigh (Fig. 14-10).

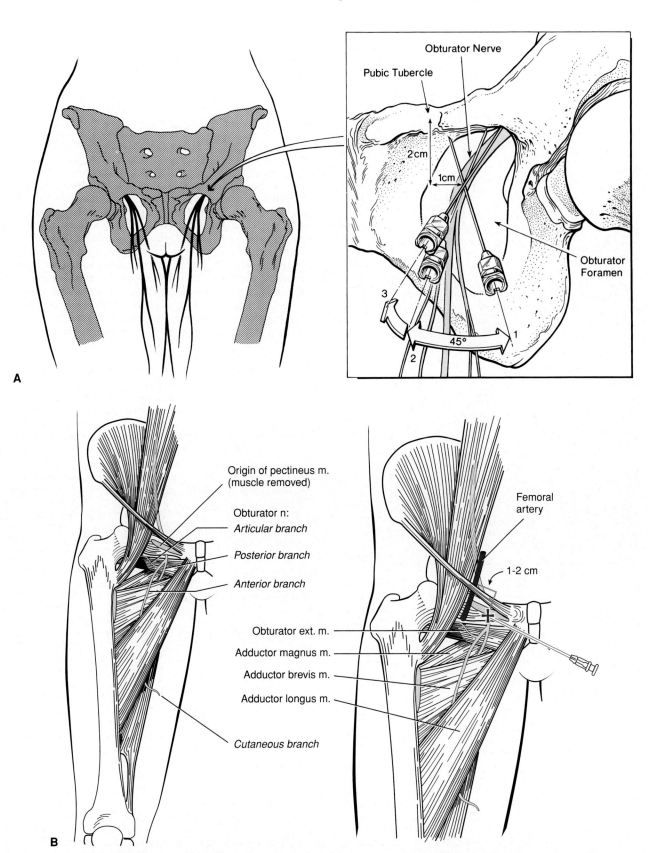

PART II: TECHNIQUES

FIGURE 14-9. A: Obturator nerve block. The needle entry site is 1 to 2 cm lateral and 1 to 2 cm caudad to the pubic tubercle. The obturator nerve is blocked in the obturator canal. **B:** Interadductor approach to obturator nerve block. A needle is inserted superolaterally adjacent to the pubic tubercle insertion of the adductor longus tendon. The needle traverses the adductor longus, aiming posteriorly to a point 1 to 2 cm lateral to the femoral artery to reach the obturator canal.

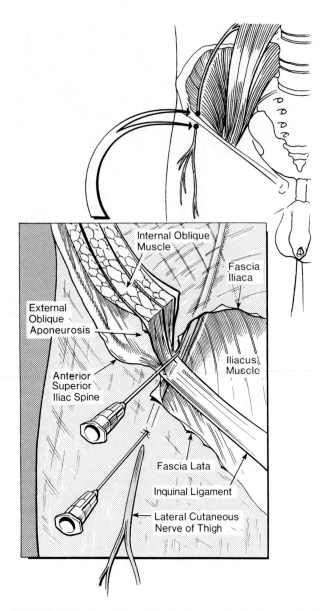

FIGURE 14-10. Lateral femoral cutaneous nerve block. The lateral cutaneous nerve of the thigh passes inferiorly on iliacus muscle covered by iliacus fascia. Just medial to the anterior superior iliac spine, it turns anteriorly to pass just below the inguinal ligament and runs deep to the fascia lata until it emerges subcutaneously. The lateral cutaneous nerve can be blocked just medially to the anterior superior iliac spine or 1 to 2 cm below it.

Indications

The lateral femoral cutaneous nerve of the thigh is a purely sensory nerve that supplies a large but variable area from the inguinal ligament to the knee on the lateral aspect of the thigh (69). Lateral femoral cutaneous nerve block is most commonly used as the sole anesthetic during diagnostic muscle biopsy and harvesting of split thickness skin grafts (70,71). It has also been used to provide analgesia in elderly patients undergoing hip fracture repair (72). However, in a study comparing lateral femoral cutaneous nerve block, femoral nerve block, and patients receiving no block following femoral neck repair, lateral

femoral cutaneous nerve block was not as effective at controlling postoperative pain as femoral nerve block (73). Femoral nerve block has been reported following lateral femoral cutaneous block (74). This is not surprising given the bulk of data reporting spread to the lateral femoral cutaneous nerve during femoral nerve block (Fig. 14-2).

Technique: Lateral Femoral Cutaneous Nerve Block

The patient is placed in the supine position. After palpation of the anterior superior iliac spine, a skin wheal is placed 2 to 3 cm inferior and 2 to 3 cm medial to it. A 3- to 4-cm needle with syringe attached is then inserted through the wheal and perpendicular to the skin surface. Soon after passing through the skin, the firm fascia lata is felt and then a sudden release as the needle passes through. Then, 10 mL of a local anesthetic solution should be deposited fanwise as the needle is moved superiorly and inferiorly, depositing solution both above and below the fascia; most of it should be deposited below (Fig. 14-10).

An alternate technique is to direct the needle through the skin wheal in a slightly lateral and cephalad direction to strike the iliac bone, just medially and below the anterior superior iliac spine. Since the nerve emerges here, the deposition of 10 mL of local anesthetic solution in a medial fanwise fashion will also accomplish satisfactory blockade of the nerve.

Although blockade of this sensory nerve is accomplished using a fan technique with variable success, Shannon et al. compared the traditional fan technique for lateral femoral cutaneous nerve block to the use of a nerve stimulator technique seeking tingling in the distribution of the nerve (75). They reported a 40% success rate with the fanning technique compared to 100% with the nerve stimulating technique. There was no difference in the extent of the blockade in successful blocks.

Complications

With the exception of a remotely possible dysesthesia or hypoesthesia, there are no serious complications associated with this nerve block technique.

COMPARISON OF APPROACHES TO THE LUMBAR PLEXUS

Psoas Compartment Block Versus Femoral Nerve Block

Parkinson et al. were the first to compare the extent of blockade following single-injection femoral nerve block and psoas compartment block (26) (Table 14-3). They compared the extent of blockade of the lumbar plexus with five different methods: posterior approach at L3 and L4–L5 with a nerve stimulator using noninsulated needles, and anterior femoral nerve block approaches with a paresthesia technique and nerve stimulating technique (26). They reported a 100% success rate of femoral nerve blockade with all techniques. The lateral femoral cutaneous nerve success rate was 85% to 95%. The obturator nerve, as assessed by thigh adduction, was blocked 100% of the time with the posterior approaches and never with the anterior approaches. Limitations of this report include lack of details

TABLE 14-3

SUCCESS RATE OF LUMBAR PLEXUS BLOCK WITH VARIOUS NEURAL LOCALIZATION TECHNIQUES*

Reference	N	Technique	Sensory Block			Motor Block		Number of failures (Number of epidural spread)
			Fem	Lateral Femoral Cutaneous	OBT	Fem	OBT	
Parkinson et al., 1989 (26)[†]	27	Psoas at L3, NS		95%		100%	100%	7 (4 epidural)
	23	Psoas at L4–L5		95%		100%	100%	3 (1 epidural)
	20	Femoral, paresthesia		95%		100%	0%	None reported
	20	Femoral, NS[‡]		85%		100%	0%	None reported
Seeberger et al., 1995 (42)	39	Femoral, NS 20 mL		41%		92%	62%	4
	41	Femoral, NS 40 mL		44%		93%	78%	3
Lang et al., 1993 (40)	32	Femoral, Paresthesia 30 mL		96%		81%	4%	6
Farny et al., 1994 (7)	45	Psoas, NS 1.0–0.5 mA		100%		100%	100%	5 (4 epidural)
Morau et al., 2003 (78)	20	Femoral, NS at 0.5 mA bolus via catheter	100%	70%	88%			2
	20	Fascia iliaca bolus via catheter	86%	92%	55%			2
Tokat et al., 2002 (76)	30	Psoas, NS	100%	97%	77%	80%	63%	0 (2 epidural)
	30	Femoral, NS	93%	63%	47%	73%	30%	3
Pandin et al., 1998 (96)	132	Psoas, NS at 0.3 mA bolus via catheter	100%	93%	91%	80%	63%	4 (2 epidural)
Capdevila et al., 1998 (79)	50	Femoral, NS at 0.5 mA 30 mL	90%	62%	52%	76%	32%	5
	50	Fascia iliaca, 30 mL	88%	90%	38%	80%	20%	6
Kaloul et al., 2004 (77)	20	Femoral, NS at 0.5 mA bolus via catheter				95%	47%	Not reported
	20	Psoas, NS at 0.5 mA bolus via catheter				90%	93%	Not reported

[†]Use of uninsulated needles, no mA given.
[‡]These studies reported rate of success for blocking the components of the lumbar plexus using a variety of nerve localization techniques and approaches to the nerves. Fem, femoral; LFC, lateral femoral cutaneous; OBT, obturator; NS, nerve stimulator. From Enneking FK, Chan V, Greger J, et al. Lower extremity peripheral nerve blocks: Essentials of our current understanding. *Reg Anesth Pain Med* 2005;30:4–35, with permission.

regarding the type of nerve stimulation, the small sample size, and exclusion of patients in whom femoral nerve block failed to develop. A more recent comparison has been made between psoas compartment blocks and femoral nerve blocks (76). In this study, patients receiving a psoas compartment block developed a sensory block of the femoral, lateral femoral cutaneous, and obturator nerves in 100%, 97%, and 77% of patients versus 93%, 63%, and 47% of the patients receiving a femoral nerve block. Kaloul et al. (77) noted that psoas block was associated with a greater likelihood of obturator block than the femoral approach, but there was no difference in pain scores or morphine consumption in patients undergoing TKA.

Femoral Nerve Block Versus Fascia Iliacus Block

Direct comparisons of the extent of blockade between the fascia iliaca block and femoral nerve block has been done in both adults and children. In adults, the fascia iliaca block, performed with the double-pop technique, provided faster onset and a higher rate of blockade of the lateral femoral cutaneous nerve compared to femoral nerve blocks performed with a nerve stim-

ulator (78). Both techniques provide adequate postoperative analgesia (79). In children, the fascia iliaca block is more likely to block the lateral femoral cutaneous nerve compared to a femoral nerve block (43). However, the duration of analgesia from these single-injection techniques was somewhat shorter in the fascia iliaca group. The authors speculated this was related to greater spread of the local anesthetic.

A single study directly comparing continuous fascia iliacus blocks to continuous femoral nerve blocks has been reported (78). Again, the degree of analgesia was highly correlated with catheter positioning. Overall, there was a greater degree of blockade of the lateral femoral cutaneous nerve in the fascia iliacus group and a greater likelihood of blocking the obturator nerve in the femoral group.

APPROACHES TO BLOCKADE OF THE SACRAL PLEXUS

Since the derivation of the sciatic nerve comes in part from spinal roots S1–S3, blockade of these roots must be combined with lumbar somatic block if complete anesthesia of the lower extremity is to be obtained.

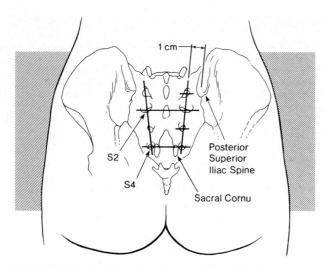

FIGURE 14-11. Landmarks for transsacral plexus block.

The sacral plexus is formed by the union of the first three sacral nerves and the fourth and fifth lumbar nerves. It also connects with the ascending division of the fourth sacral nerve. The sacral plexus is located on the anterior surface of the sacrum and is separated from the sacrum by the piriformis muscle. It is covered by the parietal portion of the pelvic fascia. In front of it lie the ureter, the pelvic colon, part of the rectum, and the iliac artery and vein. The plexus gives off two sets of branches: the collateral and the terminal. The collateral branches (anterior and posterior) supply the pudendal plexus, the hip joint, the gluteal structures, and the adductor and hamstring muscles. More pertinent to this discussion is that the terminal branches supply the greater and lesser sciatic nerves.

The sacrum consists of the fused, lower five sacral vertebrae, attached by joints and ligaments to the iliac bones. On its posterior surface are two rows of openings—the posterior sacral foramina, present on each side of the fused spinous processes (Chapter 9). The posterior divisions of the sacral nerves pass through these foramina to the soft tissues of the sacral region at the back. Although these rows of foramina are not exactly parallel, angling toward the midline, they are not as steeply angulated as the edges of the sacrum. This is an important point to remember when surface landmarks are plotted (Fig. 14-11).

Another important anatomic relationship is that of the anterior sacral foramina to the posterior foramina, which constitute the transsacral canal. The depth of the canal varies from 2.5 cm at the level of S1 to 0.5 cm at S4. Knowledge of these anatomic relationships are important during transsacral block to avoid introducing the needle into the pelvis.

Indications

Sacral block provides anesthesia over the upper thigh, hip, and perineum; complete sacral plexus block is not achieved with more peripheral sciatic approaches. Obturator blockade is not reliably attained (80). This technique is utilized to provide anesthesia for high amputations and for the relief of sciatic pain. It is also useful when immediate access to the individual nerves is not possible; for example, owing to trauma or infection.

Technique: Transsacral Nerve Block

The patient is prone over a pillow placed under the hips (Fig. 14-11). The posterior superior iliac spine and the sacral cornu

are palpated and marked bilaterally. A skin wheal is raised immediately lateral to and above the sacral cornu, and another placed 1 cm medial to and 1 cm below the posterior superior iliac spine of the side to be blocked. The distance between the wheals is bisected, and an additional wheal is raised at this site. Those three wheals thus identify the second, third, and fourth sacral foramina. The first sacral foramen is found by placing a wheal 1 to 2 cm above the second and on the same line as the others. There is no fifth sacral foramen. The fifth sacral nerves lie 1 to 2 cm caudad to the fourth foramen on the lines marked. The thickness of the soft tissues overlying the sacrum is greater superiorly—and, therefore, requires longer needles—than the lower segments. A 10-cm, 21-gauge insulated needle is adequate for S1 and S2, and a 5-cm needle for the lower segments. The second foramen is often easiest to locate and thus usually attempted first. The needle is inserted toward the posterior aspect of the sacrum, inclined slightly medially until striking bone. The needle is then withdrawn and reintroduced until it enters the respective transsacral canal. The needle is advanced approximately 2 to 2.5 cm into the first sacral canal and in 0.5-cm decrements for each succeeding canal, moving caudally. Similarly, 5 to 7 mL of solution should be injected into the first sacral foramen, the volume being reduced by 1 to 1.5 mL for each subsequent injection. Elicitation of proximal or distal lower extremity musculature stimulation is sufficient. Access to sacral foramina can be greatly enhanced by the use of an image intensifier (see Chapter 42).

Technique: Parasacral Block

The parasacral nerve block has been described as more than an isolated sciatic nerve block (81). It has been used to provide analgesia following major foot and ankle reconstruction. Parasacral block will consistently block both components of the sciatic nerve and the posterior cutaneous nerve of the thigh. Spread of local anesthetic may also anesthetize other branches of the sacral plexus including the superior and inferior gluteal, and pudendal nerves. The pelvic splanchnic nerves (S2–S4), the terminal portion of the sympathetic trunk, the inferior hypogastric plexus, and the obturator nerve all lie in close proximity to the elements of the sacral plexus and may all be anesthetized with this approach. For procedures about the knee, this may provide an advantage over more distal approaches to the sciatic nerve (81,82). For procedures below the knee, the adductor weakness from the obturator and superior gluteal nerve block may actually be disadvantageous for mobilization of the patient. The sympathetic nerve supply to the bladder is also in close proximity but problems with voiding and the need for bladder catheterization after parasacral block have not been reported (81). A notable difference from other approaches to the sciatic nerve is the type of muscle response deemed acceptable as an end-point for injection. Contraction of the hamstring muscles (biceps femoris, semitendinous) above the knee is associated with the motor response most consistent with success (81).

This approach is based on the bony relationship of the posterior superior iliac spine and the ischial tuberosity. The patient is positioned laterally with the side to be blocked uppermost. The most prominent aspects of the posterior superior iliac spine and the ischial tuberosity are identified, and a line is drawn joining these two points. Along the line, a mark is made at 6 cm inferior to the posterior superior iliac spine, defining the needle insertion site (Fig. 14-12). A 21-gauge 10-cm insulated needle is advanced in a sagittal plane until an evoked motor response is elicited, typically at a depth 5 to 7 cm from the skin. Plantar flexion of the foot (tibial nerve component) or dorsiflexion

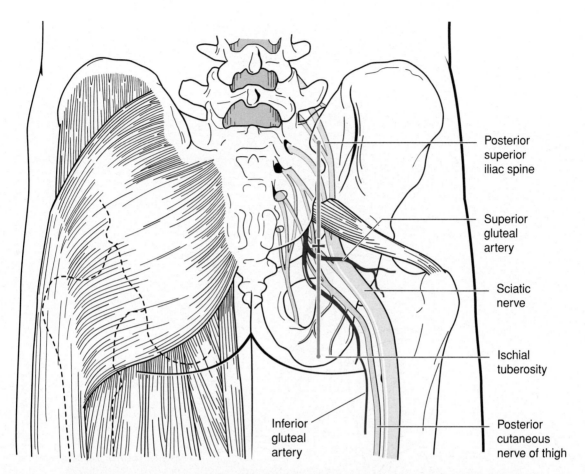

FIGURE 14-12. Parasacral block. This is the most proximal approach to the sciatic nerve and also results in block of the posterior femoral cutaneous nerve. The most prominent aspects of the posterior superior iliac spine and the ischial tuberosity are identified, and a line is drawn joining these two points. Needle insertion site is along the line, 6 cm inferior to the posterior superior iliac spine.

(common peroneal nerve) is an acceptable motor response. Because of the proximal nature of the block, a hamstring motor response also is acceptable. If the needle is too cephalad, it may contact bone (ilium above the upper margin of the sciatic notch). The needle should be reinserted caudally 2 to 3 cm along the posterior superior iliac spine–ischial tuberosity marked line. If the needle is directed too medially, the sacrum is encountered. Once the needle is properly placed, 20 to 30 mL of solution is slowly and incrementally injected.

Complications

Since the sacral nerves represent the parasympathetic portion of the autonomic nervous system, sympathetic blockade and its potential for hypotension are not seen with transsacral block unless excessive volumes of solution spread proximally to the lumbar sympathetic fibers. Loss of parasympathetic function to bowel, bladder, and sphincters may occur (83), however. Injection of local anesthetic through misdirected needles into the subarachnoid or vascular compartments is a remote risk. Classically, the dural sac terminates at the lower border of S2; however, there are clinical reports of subarachnoid puncture with a 6- to 7-cm caudal needle, thus suggesting individual variations below this "classic" location (see Chapter 9). Finally, an appreciation of the pelvic contents, especially colon, rectum, and bladder, is important; should a deeply inserted needle enter

the colon or rectum and not be noticed, it could result in seeding fecal material into the sacral canals.

SCIATIC NERVE BLOCK

The sciatic (L4–L5, S1–S3) is the largest of the four major nerves supplying the leg. The sciatic nerve, as previously noted, arises from the sacral plexus, where it is nearly 2 cm in width as it leaves the pelvis in company with the posterior cutaneous nerve of the thigh. It passes from the pelvis through the sacrosciatic foramen beneath the lower margin of the piriformis muscle, and between the tuberosity of the ischium and the greater trochanter of the femur. After the sciatic nerve passes between the ischial tuberosity and the greater trochanter, it lies just anterior to the gluteus maximus muscle. The nerve is accompanied at this point by the sciatic artery and the inferior gluteal veins, but they are relatively small vessels. The nerve becomes superficial at the lower border of the gluteus maximus muscle. From there, it courses down the posterior aspect of the thigh to the popliteal fossa, where it divides into the tibial and common peroneal nerves. Branches supplying the posterior thigh are given off during the descent of the nerve to the popliteal fossa. The sciatic nerve supplies sensory innervation to the posterior thigh and entire leg and foot from just below the knee (Fig. 14-2).

Labels on figure:
- Posterior superior iliac spine
- Superior gluteal artery
- Sciatic nerve
- Ischial tuberosity
- Posterior cutaneous nerve of thigh
- Inferior gluteal artery

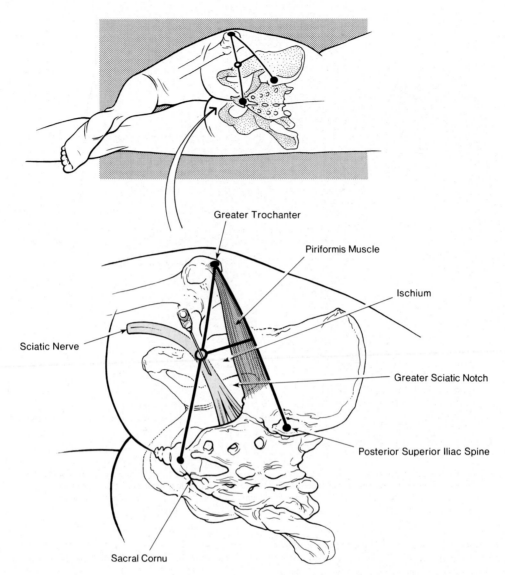

Greater Trochanter

Piriformis Muscle

Ischium

Sciatic Nerve

Greater Sciatic Notch

Posterior Superior Iliac Spine

Sacral Cornu

FIGURE 14-13. Sciatic nerve block (posterior approach of Labat). Needle insertion is 3 cm caudad along the perpendicular line that bisects a line connecting the posterior superior iliac spine and the greater trochanter. The superior gluteal artery is immediately medial to the sciatic nerve at this level.

Indications

The most common indications for sciatic nerve block are anesthesia and analgesia for foot and ankle surgery. Frequently, it is combined with blockade of one or more components of the lumbar plexus to provide a significantly larger field of surgical anesthesia, including complete unilateral lower extremity block. The use of sciatic block, either single-injection or with the continuous infusion technique, for treatment of long-term pain, acute or chronic, secondary to ischemia, or sympathetically mediated pain, has also been reported (84,85).

A variety of approaches to the sciatic nerve block are possible, and their success rate is widely variable, ranging from 33% to 95% (84,86–88). Gaston Labat first described, at the beginning of the 20th century, the sciatic nerve block that is now referred to as the Classic Approach of Labat (3). This approach is based on the bony relationship of the PSIS and the greater trochanter with the patient positioned in a modi-

fied Sims position. Winnie was the first to modify the original description by adding an additional landmark, the sacral hiatus to greater trochanter distance, to more precisely account for varying body habitus (88). Several alternate approaches to blockade of the sciatic nerve have been proposed, primarily to avoid positioning problems that are difficult for trauma patients and the elderly.

Technique: Classic Approach of Labat

The classic approach to the sciatic nerve block is with the patient lying on the side opposite the one to be blocked, rolled forward onto the flexed knee, with the heel in opposition to the knee of the outstretched, dependent leg (Fig. 14-13). A line is drawn between points made over the upper aspect of the greater trochanter of the femur and the posterior superior iliac spine. This line should coincide with the upper border of the piriformis muscle and also the upper border of the sacrosciatic foramen (sciatic notch). A line perpendicular and bisecting this is then drawn downward 3 cm and represents the needle insertion point. Verification of this point may be made by projecting a line from the greater trochanter to a point 1 to 2 cm below the sacral cornua. This line crosses the perpendicular at about 3 cm and also represents a point overlying the sciatic nerve where it exits from the pelvis (88).

A 10- to 15-cm needle is inserted through a wheal made at this point in a direction perpendicular to the skin. The needle may enter the sciatic notch and localize the nerve on the first needle advance. If bone is encountered, the needle is redirected medially. If blood is aspirated (superior gluteal artery), the needle is redirected laterally. Motor responses must be elicited in the leg *below* the level of the thigh to assure complete sciatic blockade. Plantar flexion and inversion produce a more reliable (complete) block compared to dorsiflexion and eversion (89, 90). The sciatic is a large nerve, and it is often helpful to seek a second motor response in the previously unstimulated sciatic branch and inject a total volume of 20 to 30 mL of solution. The double-injection technique had a faster onset of blockade and higher efficacy with no increase in complications (91).

Surface landmarks can be difficult to identify accurately in sciatic nerve blockade, because of the variable amount of subcutaneous tissue overlying the bony landmarks. The use of vacular imaging guides may provide a more consistent landmark, the superior gluteal artery. The superior gluteal artery, the largest branch of the internal iliac artery, passes between L5 and S1 and emerges from the upper border of the piriformis muscle at the upper aspect of the sciatic notch. A pencil-probe Doppler study was used to locate this structure in 20 patients, followed by localization of the sciatic nerve with a stimulator. The artery was located 1 to 2 cm medial to the Labat line and usually slightly cephalad to Labat's point, with the nerve slightly inferior and lateral to the artery. The authors reported a 70% success rate with one or two needle passes, and only one failure, in a diabetic patient (92).

Technique: Subgluteal Sciatic Nerve Block (Posterior Approach)

A posterior subgluteal approach to the sciatic nerve was first described by Ichiyanagi in 1959 (93). Other investigators have described a high success rate using this high lateral approach with a slightly more caudal entry point (84). When using this approach, the success rate of the blockade of the posterior cutaneous nerve of the thigh was 83%. This may have implications for patients undergoing knee surgery or procedures requiring the use of a thigh tourniquet.

With this approach, the patient is positioned laterally in a modified Sims position: The leg to be blocked is rolled forward onto the flexed knee as the heel rests on the knee of the dependent (nonoperative) leg. This approach is based on the bony relationship to the greater trochanter and the ischial tuberosity. The most prominent aspects of the greater trochanter and the ischial tuberosity are identified by palpation, and a line is drawn joining these two points. A perpendicular line is drawn bisecting this line and extending 4 to 6 cm caudad. The second line approximates the location of the sciatic nerve. The site of the needle insertion may be at the intersection of the two lines or as far as 6 cm distally along the second line. A 21-gauge 10-cm insulated needle is inserted perpendicularly until a tibial or peroneal evoked motor response in the ankle or foot is elicited, then 20 to 30 mL of solution is injected incrementally (Fig.

14-14). The target response is an evoked muscle contraction below the knee; stimulation of the tibial nerve component produces plantar flexion and inversion of the foot, and common peroneal nerve stimulation produces dorsiflexion and eversion. If no motor response is elicited, the needle may be redirected 1 to 2 cm medially or laterally to the original direction of the needle. It may be helpful to palpate or visualize the groove that can be seen or palpated on the posterior aspect of the thigh. If bony contact is made, the needle is withdrawn and redirected medially.

Technique: Sciatic Nerve Block Anterior Approach

The anterior approach to the sciatic nerve has the appeal of supine positioning and a single prep of the patient for combined femoral and sciatic nerve blocks. Its popularity had long been limited by its low success rate and relatively painful use of the femur as a deep landmark (94,95). The patient is placed supine with the lower extremity in a neutral position. A line that represents the inguinal ligament is trisected, and a perpendicular line from the junction of the middle and medial thirds of this line is extended downward and laterally on the anterior aspect of the thigh. The greater trochanter is located by palpation and a line extended from its tuberosity medially across the anterior surface of the thigh, parallel to the inguinal ligament. The point of intersection of this line and the perpendicular line from the inguinal ligament represents the point of injection (Fig. 14-15). A 10- to 15-cm needle is inserted through a wheal at this point and directed slightly laterally from a plane perpendicular to the skin. The needle is advanced until bone is contacted, then withdrawn and redirected medially and more perpendicularly to pass 5 cm beyond the femur, where it should be resting slightly posterior and medial to the femur within the neurovascular compartment (containing the sciatic nerve).

Technique: Subgluteal Sciatic Nerve Block (Lithotomy Approach)

Raj described a supine approach to the sciatic nerve in the flexed hip (lithotomy) position, initiating the block at the midpoint between the greater trochanter of the femur and the ischial tuberosity (87).

The patient is placed supine, and the extremity to be blocked is flexed at the hip (90–120 degrees). The extremity may be supported by stirrups, mechanical devices, or by an assistant. In this position, the gluteus maximus muscle is flattened and the sciatic nerve relatively more superficial, lying in the readily palpable hollow between the semitendinosus and biceps femoris muscles. A line is drawn between the ischial tuberosity and the greater trochanter, and a wheal is raised at its midpoint. A 10- to 15-cm insulated needle is inserted perpendicular to the skin and advanced until a motor response involving the foot or ankle is elicited. Twenty to 25 mL of a local anesthetic solution is then injected (Fig. 14-16).

Technique: Sciatic Nerve Block (Lateral Approach)

A lateral approach to the sciatic nerve has also been described (84). The sciatic nerve is approached from the lateral thigh

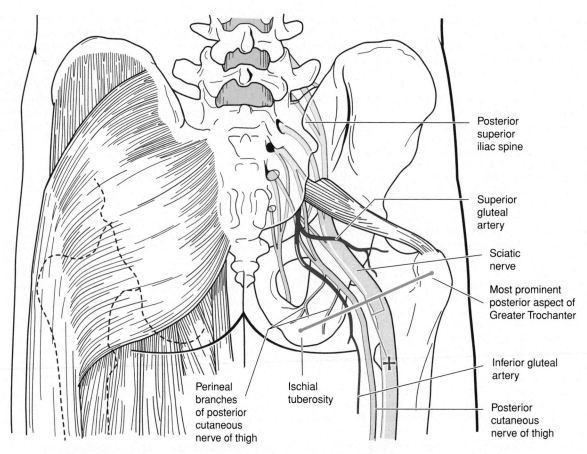

FIGURE 14-14. Sciatic nerve block (subgluteal approach). The sciatic nerve is relatively superficial at this level. Needle insertion is near the gluteal crease, between the hamstring muscles.

with the patient lying supine. The earliest report of a lateral approach was by Ichiyanagi in 1959; it was thought by many to be "extremely difficult" (93). The quadratus femoris is the lowermost of the short rotators of the hip, crossed by the sciatic nerve on its way to the posterior compartment of the thigh. The subgluteal space, within which the sciatic nerve lies as it crosses this muscle, can be identified in relation to the femur and the ischial tuberosity. The posterior cutaneous nerve is not reliably blocked with this more distal approach to the sciatic nerve (96).

The block is performed with a 15-cm insulated needle. The patient lies supine with the whole limb exposed and with the hip held in the natural position. After appropriate skin preparation and drape, the needle is inserted through a skin wheal made 3 cm distal to the point of maximum lateral prominence of the trochanter, along the posterior profile of the femur (Fig. 14-17). Upon striking the bone of the femoral shaft, the needle is redirected to slide under the femur and is advanced to a total depth of 8 to 12 cm to reach the sciatic nerve. The nerve stimulator may elicit responses from either of the motor components of the sciatic. After localization of the nerve, 20 to 30 mL of local anesthetic is injected.

Complications

Serious complications of sciatic nerve block are rare. However, theoretical concerns regarding muscle trauma and puncture of a variety of vascular structures, must be considered.

Sciatic nerve block is primarily a somatic nerve block. It does carry some sympathetic fibers to the extremity, however, and may, therefore, allow pooling of small quantities of blood—usually insufficient to cause significant hypotension. On some occasions, such as limb reimplantations and sympathetically mediated pain conditions, this sympathetic block may be advantageous. The effect of compensatory vasoconstriction on the opposite extremity should, however, be considered. There is some evidence that tissue oxygenation may be further reduced during this period of compensation, although it is unlikely that this is of clinical significance (97). Residual dysesthesias for periods of 1 to 3 days are not uncommon, but usually resolve within several months (98,99). Importantly, many orthopedic surgical procedures (including TKA and THA) are associated with neurapraxia to one or both components of the sciatic nerve. Thus, thoughtful application of this technique is required to optimize neurologic outcome for patients considered to be at high risk of perioperative nerve injury from surgery or preexisting neurologic dysfunction.

SCIATIC NERVE BLOCK AT THE LEVEL OF THE POPLITEAL FOSSA

The posterior muscles of the thigh are the biceps femoris, the semimembranosus, semitendonosus, and the posterior portion of the adductor magnus. As these muscles are traced distally from their origin on the ischial tuberosity, they separate into medial (semimembranosus, semitendonosus) and lateral (biceps) musculature, and form the upper border of the popliteal fossa. The lower border of the popliteal fossa is defined by the two heads of the gastrocnemius. In the upper part of the popliteal fossa, the sciatic nerve lies posterolateral to the popliteal vessels. Specifically, the popliteal vein is medial to the nerve, while the popliteal artery is most anterior, lying on the popliteal surface of the femur. Near the upper border of the popliteal fossa, the two components of the sciatic nerve separate. The peroneal nerve diverges laterally and the larger tibial branch descends almost straight down through the fossa. The tibial nerve and popliteal vessels then disappear deep to the converging heads of the gastrocnemius muscle (Fig. 14-18A).

Importantly, to provide complete anesthesia/analgesia at the level of the popliteal fossa (e.g., medial surgical procedure or use of a calf tourniquet/Esmarch), the sciatic block must be supplemented with a saphenous technique.

Indications

Popliteal fossa block is chiefly used for foot and ankle surgery (100–102). Short saphenous vein stripping may also be performed under combined popliteal and posterior cutaneous nerve block (103). The block has also been successfully utilized in the pediatric population. Popliteal fossa block anesthetizes the entire leg below the tibial plateau except the skin of the medial aspect of the calf and foot; that is, the saphenous nerve distribution (Fig. 14-2). Potential advantages of popliteal block over ankle block are improved calf tourniquet tolerance and an immobile foot. The components of the sciatic nerve may be blocked at the level of the popliteal fossa via posterior or lateral approaches. Patient positioning—prone, lateral (operative side nondependent), or supine (with leg flexed at the hip and knee)—may determine the optimal approach for an individual patient (104). Continuous techniques have been described using both posterior (105–107) and lateral (108) approaches.

Technique: Popliteal Fossa Block (Posterior Approach)

The classic approach to the posterior popliteal fossa block is with the patient positioned prone. However, access may also occur with the patient in the lateral (operative side nondependent), or supine (with leg flexed at the hip and knee) positions. The borders of the popliteal fossa are identified by flexing the knee joint. A triangle is constructed, with the base consisting of the skin crease behind the knee, and the two sides composed of the semimembranosus (medially) and the biceps (laterally). A bisecting line is drawn from the apex to the base of the triangle, and a 5-cm needle is inserted at a site 5 to 10 cm above the skin fold and 0.5 to 1 cm lateral to the bisecting line (Fig. 14-18A). Classically, the 5-cm distance was described (102). However, in an attempt to block the sciatic nerve prior to its division, a 7 to 10 cm distance has been recommended (109).

The needle is advanced at a 45-degree angle toward the apex of the triangle until a nerve stimulator response is elicited; inversion of the foot is the motor response most predictive of complete neural block of the foot (110). The distance from skin to nerve in the average adult is 1.5 to 2.0 cm (102). Injection of approximately 30 mL of local anesthetic solution is sufficient. Success rate is typically 90% to 95% (102,110). No formal comparison between paresthesia and nerve stimulator

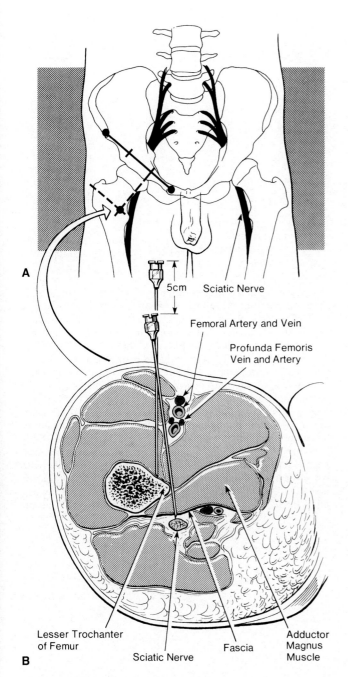

FIGURE 14-15. Sciatic nerve block (anterior approach) **A:** The inguinal ligament is trisected, and a perpendicular line from the junction of the middle third and medial third of this line is extended downward and laterally on the anterior aspect of the thigh. The greater trochanter is located by palpation, and a line is extended from its tuberosity medially across the anterior surface of the thigh, parallel to the inguinal ligament. Needle insertion is the point of intersection of this line and the perpendicular line from the inguinal ligament. **B:** Cross-section of the leg at the level of the lesser trochanter demonstrating the relationship between the sciatic nerve and the femur, and the fascia separating it from adductor magnus.

Labels in figure:
A
5cm   Sciatic Nerve
Femoral Artery and Vein
Profunda Femoris Vein and Artery
Lesser Trochanter of Femur
Sciatic Nerve
Fascia
Adductor Magnus Muscle
B

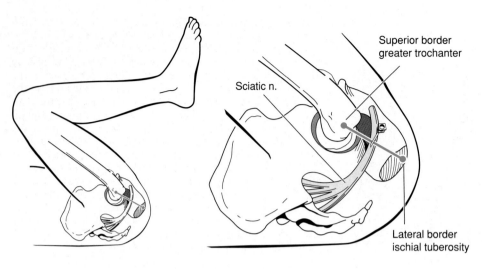

FIGURE 14-16. Sciatic nerve block (lithotomy position-subgluteal approach).

techniques has been performed to assess efficacy and complications. It is believed that incomplete block is the result of poor diffusion (due to the size of the sciatic nerve), the separate fascial coverings of the tibial and peroneal nerves, or to blockade of only a single component of the sciatic nerve. Identification of both tibial and peroneal components decreases onset time and improves success rate (111).

Technique: Popliteal Fossa Block (Lateral Approach)

A lateral approach to blockade of the sciatic nerve in the popliteal fossa has been described (112). Onset and quality of block are similar to the posterior approach (113). However, time to complete the block was slightly longer with the lateral

approach (mean 8 minutes; range 1–17 minutes) compared to the posterior approach (mean 6 minutes; range 1–16 minutes).

The lateral approach allows the patient to be positioned supine and eliminates the need for repositioning. The patient's leg is extended, with the long axis of the foot at a 90-degree angle to the table. A horizontal line is drawn across the upper edge of the patella. The site of insertion is the intersection of the vertical line drawn across the upper edge of the patella and the groove between the lateral border of the biceps femoris and vastus lateralis (Fig. 14-18B). A 10-cm needle is advanced at a 30-degree angle posterior to the horizontal plane. Since the common peroneal nerve is located lateral to the tibial nerve, the stimulating needle encounters the common peroneal nerve first with the lateral approach (Fig. 14-18C). As with the posterior approach, an elicited tibial (inversion) response is sought (110,114). If a response associated with common peroneal nerve stimulation (such as eversion) is elicited, the needle

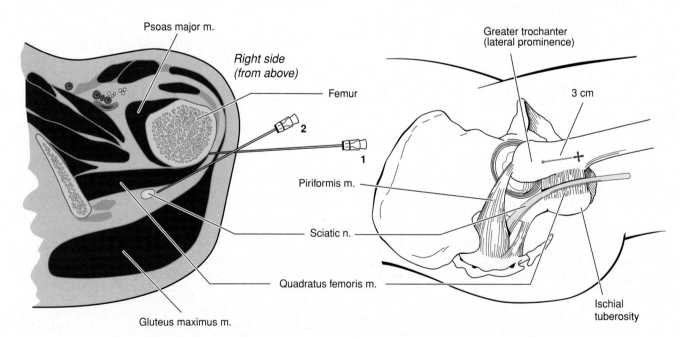

FIGURE 14-17. Sciatic nerve block (lateral approach). Needle insertion is 3 cm distal to the point of maximum lateral prominence of the greater trochanter. Upon striking the femoral shaft, the needle is redirected to slide posterior to the femur and is advanced to a total depth of 8 to 12 cm to reach the sciatic nerve.

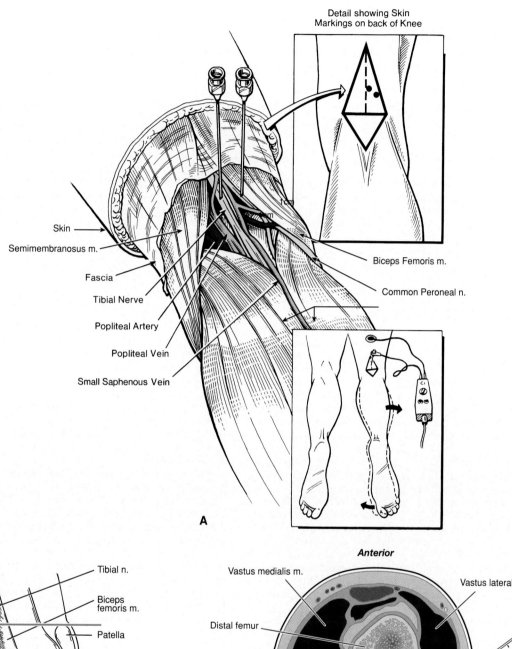

Detail showing Skin
Markings on back of Knee

Skin

Semimembranosus m.

Fascia

Tibial Nerve

Popliteal Artery

Popliteal Vein

Small Saphenous Vein

Biceps Femoris m.

Common Peroneal n.

A

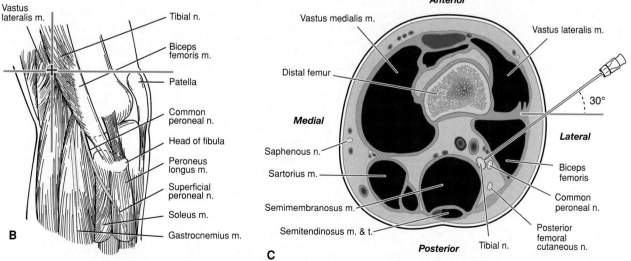

Vastus
lateralis m.

Tibial n.

Biceps
femoris m.

Patella

Common
peroneal n.

Head of fibula

Peroneus
longus m.

Superficial
peroneal n.

Soleus m.

Gastrocnemius m.

B

Anterior

Vastus medialis m.

Vastus lateralis m.

Distal femur

30°

Medial

Lateral

Saphenous n.

Biceps
femoris

Sartorius m.

Common
peroneal n.

Semimembranosus m.

Posterior
femoral
cutaneous n.

Semitendinosus m. & t.

Tibial n.

Posterior

C

FIGURE 14-18. A: Popliteal fossa block. The tibial and common peroneal (lateral popliteal) nerves diverge in the popliteal fossa, which is bounded by biceps femoris muscle laterally and semimembranosus muscle medially. A perpendicular line is drawn bisecting the popliteal crease line and extending 7 to 8 cm cephalad. The needle entry site is just lateral (0.5–1 cm) to the perpendicular line. **B:** Popliteal fossa: lateral approach. Surface markings. **C:** Popliteal fossa block. Lateral approach. Cross-section with needle in place.

is redirected more posteriorly. After neural localization, 30 mL of local anesthetic is injected.

A comparison of classic Labat, subgluteal, and lateral popliteal approaches to the sciatic nerve showed similar success rates (96%, 92%, and 96%, respectively) but slower onset time for the lateral popliteal group compared to the more proximal approaches (115). This difference was attributed to the greater distance separating the components of the sciatic nerve as it traverses through the popliteal fossa.

Complications

As with other PNBs, neuropathy is the most common complication. Intravascular injection may occur as a result of the presence of vascular structures within the popliteal fossa. Performance of popliteal fossa block in patients with previous total knee arthroplasty or vascular bypass (femoral–popliteal) should be done with care. However, to date, there are no cases of graft disruption or joint infections relating to needle placement in these patients.

ANKLE BLOCK

Five branches of the principal nerve trunks supply the ankle and foot: posterior tibial, sural, superficial peroneal (musculocutaneous), saphenous, and deep peroneal (anterior tibial) (116). These nerves are relatively easy to block at the ankle (Fig. 14-19). There are no important variants in the innervation of the distal musculature. However, considerable variation does occur in the branching and distribution of the sensory nerves of the foot. For this reason, blockade of all five nerves has been advocated (117). Neural blockade of the posterior tibial nerve has been described at the supramalleolar (117–119), midmalleolar (120), subcalcaneal (121,122), and midtarsal (123) levels with no evidence of superiority for any technique.

All five nerve blocks at the ankle, undertaken simultaneously, would produce a ring of infiltration around the ankle at the level of the malleoli. However, with circular infiltration, there is the hazard of vascular occlusion if large volumes of anesthetic solutions are injected, especially if they contain epinephrine. In general, block of a specific nerve, with smaller quantities of non-epinephrine–containing solutions of local anesthetic agents has the highest success rate with less risk.

A technique for a "midtarsal" approach to nerve block of the forefoot has also been described (123). Injections are made immediately distal to the ankle joint where the nerves are accessible without having to reposition the patient.

Indications

Indications for blockade of the terminal nerves of the lumbosacral plexus distally, at the ankle and midtarsal levels, include anesthesia for surgery to the foot, including Morton neuroma; operations on the great toe, including bunionectomy and amputation; amputation of midfoot and toes for peripheral vascular disease; metatarsal osteotomy; and incision, drainage, and debridement procedures (120,124). Diagnostic block has also been described (125). Few studies evaluating perioperative outcomes with ankle block exist (126) although the technique has been performed for decades (3). Rather, most publications describe variations to improve success rate. Peak blood levels of

local anesthetic occur around 90 minutes after blockade and are very low even after bilateral ankle block (127). Chronic edema may obscure landmarks, but in the absence of draining infected lesions, needle insertion is not contraindicated.

A prospective evaluation compared popliteal fossa block using the lateral approach with ankle block in patients undergoing ambulatory foot surgery (128). In both groups, the local anesthetic consisted of 20 mL of 0.5% bupivacaine. There was no difference in the pain scores in the recovery room or at the time of hospital discharge. However, during the first 24 hours postoperatively, only 14% of patients in the popliteal fossa block rated their pain as severe, whereas 60% of patients with ankle block complained of severe pain. The duration of analgesia was also significantly longer in the popliteal fossa group, 18 hours compared to 6 hours. The authors concluded that popliteal fossa block provided effective analgesia and was associated with a high level of patient satisfaction. A recent review also recommended popliteal fossa block as the technique of choice in patients undergoing major foot or ankle surgery (129).

Technique: Tibial Block

The tibial nerve (L4–L5, S1–S3) reaches the distal part of the leg from the medial side of the Achilles tendon, where it lies behind the posterior tibial artery. The nerve then gives off the medial calcaneal branch to the inside of the heel, after which it divides at the back of the medial malleolus into the medial and lateral plantar nerves, both under the abductor hallucis running to the sole of the foot. The medial branch supplies the medial two thirds of the sole and plantar portion of the medial three and a half toes up to the nail. The lateral branch supplies the lateral one third of the sole and plantar portion of the lateral one and a half toes (Fig. 14-2).

The patient lies prone or supine with the ankle supported by a pillow or foot rest. A skin wheal is raised lateral to the posterior tibial artery, if the artery is palpable. If the artery is not palpable, then the wheal is placed to the medial side of the Achilles tendon, level with the upper border of the medial malleolus. A 1- to 3-cm needle is advanced through the wheal at a right angle to the posterior aspect of the tibia, lateral to the artery. Shifting the needle in a mediolateral position may elicit a paresthesia, and then 3 to 5 mL of local anesthetic solution should be injected. If paresthesias are not obtained, 5 to 7 mL of local anesthetic solution is injected against the posterior aspect of the tibia, while the needle is withdrawn 1 cm (Fig. 14-19).

Technique: Sural Nerve Block

The sural nerve is a cutaneous nerve that arises through the union of a branch from the tibial nerve and one from the common peroneal nerve. It becomes subcutaneous distal to the middle of the leg and proceeds along with the short saphenous vein behind and below the lateral malleolus to supply the lower posterolateral surface of the leg, the lateral side of the foot, and the lateral part of the fifth toe (Fig. 14-2).

With the patient in the same position as for tibial nerve block, a skin wheal is raised lateral to the Achilles tendon at the level of the lateral malleolus. A 1- to 3-cm needle is inserted through the wheal approximately 1 cm and angled toward the fibula, where paresthesias may be sought. If no paresthesias occur, subcutaneous infiltration is accomplished from the Achilles

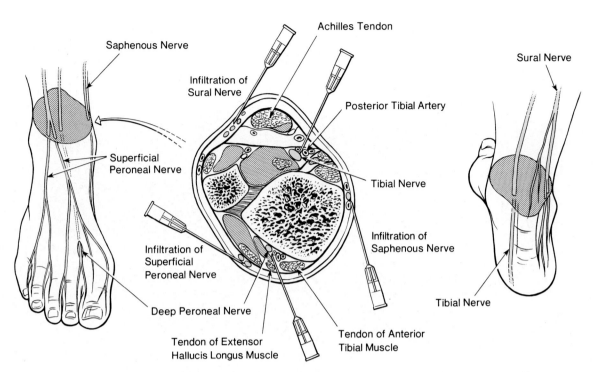

FIGURE 14-19. Anatomic relationships and needle placement for ankle block.

tendon to the outer border of the lateral malleolus. Three to 5 mL of local anesthetic solution, injected fanwise, are usually sufficient to produce analgesia (Fig. 14-19).

Technique: Superficial Peroneal Nerve Block

The superficial peroneal nerve (L4–L5, S1–S2) perforates the deep fascia on the anterior aspect of the distal two thirds of the leg and runs subcutaneously to supply the dorsum of the foot and toes, except for the contiguous surfaces of the great and second toes, which are supplied by the deep peroneal nerve (Fig. 14-2).

The superficial peroneal nerve is blocked immediately above and medial to the lateral malleolus. A subcutaneous infiltration of 5 to 10 mL of local anesthetic solution is injected from the anterior border of the tibia to the superior aspect of the lateral malleolus (Fig. 14-19).

Technique: Deep Peroneal Nerve Block

The deep peroneal nerve (L4–L5, S1–S2) courses down the anterior aspect of the interosseus membrane of the leg and continues midway between the malleoli onto the dorsum of the foot. Here, it innervates the short extensors of the toes, as well as the skin on the adjacent areas of the first and second toes (Fig. 14-2). At the level of the foot, the anterior tibial artery lies medial to the nerve, as does the tendon of the extensor hallucis longus muscle.

The deep peroneal nerve is blocked in the lower portion of the leg by placing a wheal between the tendons of the anterior tibial and extensor hallucis longus muscles, at a level just su-

perior to the malleoli. Often the anterior tibial artery may be palpated. If this is possible, the skin wheal and nerve should be just lateral to the artery. The needle is advanced toward the tibia, and 3 to 5 mL of local anesthetic solution is injected (Fig. 14-19).

Technique: Saphenous Nerve Block

The saphenous nerve, the sensory terminal branch of the femoral nerve, becomes subcutaneous at the lateral side of the knee joint. It then follows the great saphenous vein to the medial malleolus and supplies the cutaneous area over the medial side of the lower leg, anterior to the medial malleolus and the medial part of the foot, as far forward as the midportion (Fig. 14-2). Occasionally, its innervation extends to the metatarsophalangeal joint.

To block the saphenous nerve, a skin wheal is raised immediately above and anterior to the medial malleolus, and 3 to 5 mL of local anesthetic solution is infiltrated subcutaneously around the great saphenous vein (Fig. 14-19).

Complications

No major complications have been reported. In one major series, only one patient complained of dysesthesias for 3 to 4 weeks (123). A simple alternative to a calf or upper leg tourniquet is the midfoot Esmarch bandage tourniquet. Following routine exsanguination of the foot, the elastic bandage is left tightly wound around the midfoot, serving as a sterile tourniquet within the anesthetized area.

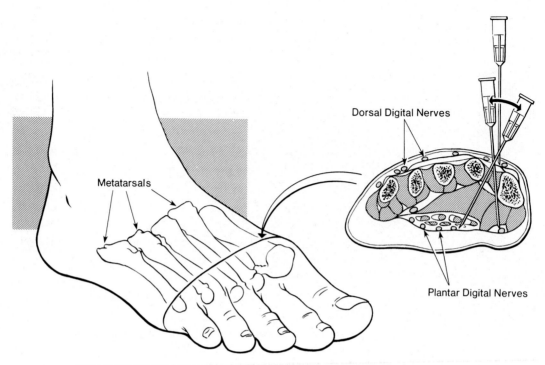

FIGURE 14-20. Anatomic relationships and needle placement for metatarsal nerve block.

METATARSAL AND DIGITAL NERVE BLOCK

The relationship of the terminal nerves to the metatarsal bones and the toes is very similar to that of the structures of the hand, with the nerve fibers passing through the intermetatarsal space and alongside each toe, where they become the digital nerves.

Nerve block in the intermetatarsal space is very similar to the metacarpal block. Skin wheals are raised on the dorsum of the foot just proximal to the metatarsal heads of the toes to be blocked. Local anesthetic solutions are then infiltrated in a fanwise direction between the two wheals, taking care not to pierce the sole of the foot. Solution should be injected carefully around the plantar surface of the metatarsal bone as well. Digital block alone can be accomplished by injecting through the wheals at the webs of the toes, depositing 2 to 3 mL of local anesthetic solution along either side of the toes to be blocked. Use of epinephrine in the anesthetic solutions and excessive volumes should be avoided in these blocks (Fig. 14-20).

INTRAVENOUS REGIONAL ANESTHESIA

Although IV regional anesthesia in the upper extremity is a widely used technique (130), it has not been reported extensively for use in the lower limbs (see Chapter 15). When a tourniquet is applied to the thigh, a large dose of local anesthetic agent is required, with resultant failures and occasional reports of toxicity. The tourniquet may be placed either prox-

imally on the thigh or above the ankle. With the tourniquet placed at the thigh, larger volumes of more dilute solutions are advocated. Lidocaine 0.25% to a total dose of 3.3 mg/kg is recommended (131). This will provide the 75 to 100 mL of solution desired.

Use of the lower limb tourniquet just above the ankle has also been reported (132). A double-cuff tourniquet was used and arterial occlusion pressures measured before the start of anesthesia. Cuffs were inflated 100 mm Hg above occlusion pressure. A maximum volume of 40 to 50 mL of a dilute solution of local anesthetic agent was used (0.25%–0.5% lidocaine or mepivacaine). No major complications were noted (131,132), but occasional cases of tinnitus or signs of transient vascular absorption were noted.

INTRA-ARTICULAR BLOCKS

Intra-articular injections of local anesthetics, opioids, or combinations have become routine for perioperative pain management following arthroscopic knee surgery (133,134). In an early comparison of femoral nerve block, intra-articular injection, or nothing, there was no difference in pain relief between intra-articular bupivacaine and the control, whereas only one of 10 patients receiving a femoral nerve block had any pain (135). A number of recent reports enthusiastically recommend the use of this technique; however, the results are conflicting. Comparison of reports is difficult because of variability in underlying anesthetic techniques, different dosages and concentrations of local anesthetic, and frequent lack of control groups. Multivariate analysis in one study showed that gender, preoperative pain scores, and the type and length of surgical procedure were all significant in predicting postoperative pain, whereas the use of bupivacaine dropped out as a significant factor (136). Two reports of intra-articular morphine or bupivacaine in patients undergoing arthroscopy under regional anesthesia indicated minimal efficacy (137,138). In patients having general anesthesia, conflicting reports recommend intra-articular morphine alone (139,140) or conclude that intra-articular morphine and bupivacaine are equally efficacious, but both provide less analgesia than continuous lumbar plexus block for 24 hours postoperatively (141). The safety of injecting large volumes of intra-articular bupivacaine has been ascertained (142), and side effects are rare following intra-articular doses of morphine. Since these techniques are simple and low-risk and afford pain relief under some conditions, they will likely be continued to be utilized.

COMPARISON OF NERVE LOCALIZATION TECHNIQUES

Nerve Stimulation Versus Paresthesia for Lower Extremity Peripheral Nerve Block

Few studies directly compare success rate with paresthesia techniques versus peripheral nerve stimulation techniques in lower extremity PNB. However, nerve stimulation provides a success rate comparable to earlier reports of paresthesia techniques (26,143–148). In addition, it may improve patient comfort during block performance. However, its biggest advantage may be the redirection cues that are provided to the operator. For example, when performing a sciatic nerve block in the gluteal region, one may observe knee flexion as a result of stimulation of the superior gluteal nerve. This likely indicates that the needle is posterior, lateral, and cephalad to the sciatic nerve and should be repositioned appropriately.

Multistimulation Versus Single-stimulation Techniques

Multiple stimulation techniques by definition require individual stimulation of each component of a peripheral nerve, with deposition of a small volume of local anesthetic at each site. For instance, during performance of a sciatic block, a peroneal motor response is elicited first and a small volume of local anesthetic is deposited. The needle is then redirected medially to obtain a tibial nerve motor response with subsequent deposition of additional local anesthetic. Advocates of multiple-stimulation techniques believe the technique increases the success rate, decreases onset time, and allows the injection of a smaller volume of local anesthetic (111,149–151). Advocates of single-injection techniques believe multistimulation and -injection techniques may add risk of nerve injury during redirection of the needle through partially anesthetized nerves. However, no neurologic complications have been reported in any of these studies (111,149,150). This is in agreement with the large cohort of patients (more than 2,000) studied by Fanelli using multistimulation techniques, who found no nerve injury attributed to nerve block (98). However, nerve injury is a rare event after PNB, and even a study of this size may not provide a large enough sample to deter-

mine the relative risk of multiple- versus single-injection techniques.

Ultrasound-guided Lower Extremity Block

In recent years, the number of prospective randomized studies comparing ultrasound-guided and electrical stimulation techniques have steadily increased. In general, onset times and number of needle passes required to obtain a motor response are reduced with the use of ultrasound guidance (152–154). Ultrasound guidance increases success rate provided that (a) the needle is redirected (as necessary) to achieve uniform spread around the neural structure and (b) blocks in the control group are performed using a single injection (1). To date, no studies have compared multistimulation lower extremity block to ultrasound-guided block, perhaps a more appropriate comparison group. Ultrasound images of local anesthetic distribution have provided clinicians with a visualization of successful block (154,156,157) and documented *why* single-injection techniques are less reliable. Although it has been theorized that visualization of needle advancement would decrease the frequency (or severity) of needle misadventures, the small patient numbers reported precludes determination of either the absolute or relative frequency of neurologic complications. Both intraneural needle placement and injection have been reported during ultrasound (154,158). However, the risk of large-volume intravascular injection of local anesthetic may be reduced in experienced ultrasonographers' hands.

LOCAL ANESTHETIC AGENTS

The choice of local anesthetic and the addition of adjuvants for lower extremity PNB are dependent on the anticipated duration of surgery, the need for prolonged analgesia, and the timing of ambulation/weight-bearing postoperatively (1). Prolonged blockade for 24 hours (or greater) may occur with long-acting agents such as bupivacaine, levobupivacaine, or ropivacaine. Although this feature may result in excellent postoperative pain relief for the inpatient, it may be undesirable or a cause for concern in the ambulatory patient because of the potential for falls with a partially insensate/weak lower extremity. A medium-acting agent may be more appropriate in the outpatient setting for orthopedic procedures with minimal to moderate postoperative pain. In general, equipotent concentrations of the long-acting amides have a similar onset and quality of block. However, bupivacaine may have a slightly longer duration than levobupivacaine or ropivacaine. Likewise, higher concentrations are more likely to be associated with profound sensory *and* motor block, whereas infusions of 0.1% to 0.2% bupivacaine or ropivacaine often allow complete weight bearing without notable motor deficits. Recent investigations have suggested that increasing the local anesthetic concentration will alter the character (i.e., degree of sensory and/or motor block), but not the duration of anesthesia (see Chapter 4).

The lowest effective dose and concentration should be utilized to minimize local anesthetic systemic and neural toxicity (Chapter 5). Essentially, the safe dose of a local anesthetic should be individualized based on site of injection, patient age, and the presence of medical conditions that affect local anesthetic pharmacology and toxicity (Chapters 4 and 5). These considerations are believed to be most critical when large doses of local anesthetics are injected or in association with repeated blocks/continuous infusions because of the potential for local anesthetic accumulation.

Adjuvants

Epinephrine

Epinephrine decreases local anesthetic uptake and plasma levels, improves the quality of block, and increases the duration of postoperative analgesia during lower extremity peripheral blockade. Epinephrine also allows for the early detection of intravascular injection. Importantly, concentrations of epinephrine ranging from 1.7 to 5 μg/mL (1:600,000 to 1:200,000 dilution) reduce the uptake and prolong the blockade of medium-duration local anesthetics to a similar extent. However, concentrations of 1.7 to 2.5 μg/mL have little effect on nerve blood flow, which theoretically may reduce the risk of nerve injury for patients with a preexisting angiopathy or neuropathy (159). In addition, larger doses of epinephrine injected systemically may cause undesirable side effects in patients with known cardiac disease. Concerns regarding neural or cardiac ischemia must be balanced with the need to detect intravascular injection. In general, because of the high doses of local anesthetics administered during lower extremity peripheral block, the benefits of adding epinephrine outweigh the risks (see Chapters 3, 4, and 5).

Commercially prepared solutions with epinephrine have a lower pH than those in which it is freshly added, resulting in a higher percentage of ionized drug molecules. These ionized molecules do not readily cross the neural membrane, thus delaying the onset of local anesthetic action after injection (see Chapter 3). Epinephrine should not be added for ankle block. The addition of epinephrine to local anesthetics with intrinsic vasoconstrictive properties, such as ropivacaine, may not increase block duration, but would still facilitate detection of intravascular injection.

Clonidine

Clonidine consistently prolongs the time to first analgesia when added to intermediate-acting agents during brachial plexus block. The effect is most likely peripherally mediated and dose-dependent. Side effects such as hypotension, bradycardia, and sedation do not occur with a dose less than 1.5 μg/kg or a maximum dose of 150 μg. Conversely, the efficacy of clonidine as an adjuvant for lower extremity single-injection and continuous techniques is less defined; at most, a modest (20%) prolongation with the addition of clonidine to long-acting local anesthetic solutions can be expected (160,161).

Opioids

Although opioids, including morphine, sufentanil, and fentanyl, are often added to lumbar plexus infusions, no convincing data suggest that block onset, quality, or duration is improved when opioids are added to the local anesthetic solution.

Systemic Local Anesthetic Toxicity

The potential for systemic local anesthetic toxicity would seem to be very high for lower extremity PNBs due to the relatively large doses of local anesthetic injected and the proximity of needle/catheter insertion to vascular structures and highly vascularized muscle beds. Clinical investigations have consistently reported levels below toxic values, however, even with combined lumbar plexus–sciatic techniques (77,162,163). The few cases of systemic toxicity requiring resuscitation occurred shortly after injection, suggesting accidental intravascular injection or vascular channeling, rather than systemic absorption, as the mechanism (99). Prevention and treatment of local anesthetic toxicity is dependent on the injection of an appropriate volume and concentration of local anesthetic, the use of a vasoconstrictor adjuvant, slow injection with frequent aspiration, and increased vigilance for the early detection of toxic reactions (see Chapters 3, 4, and 5). It is notable that local anesthetic levels may not peak for 60 minutes or more following deposition in lower extremity peripheral block (162). Furthermore, large variations in plasma concentrations may occur (164). Thus, patients should be appropriately monitored for signs and symptoms of rising blood levels during this duration. Resuscitation equipment and medications should also be readily available (Chapter 5).

SUMMARY

The role of plexus and peripheral blockade of the lower extremity has expanded from the operating suite into the arena of postoperative and chronic pain management. With appropriate selection and sedation, these techniques can be used in all age groups. Skillful application of lower extremity somatic block broadens the anesthesiologist's range of options in providing optimal anesthetic care.

References

1. Enneking FK, Chan V, Greger J, et al. Lower extremity peripheral nerve blocks: Essentials of our current understanding. *Reg Anesth Pain Med* 2005; 30:4–35.
2. Braun H. *Anesthesia—Its Scientific Basis and Practical Use*, 2nd ed. Philadelphia: Lea & Febiger, 1924.
3. Labat G. *Regional Anesthesia: Its Technic and Clinical Application.* Philadelphia: W. B. Saunders Co, 1922.
4. Gray H. *Anatomy of the Human Body.* Philadelphia, PA: Lea & Fibiger, 1918.
5. Capdevila X, Macaire P, Dadure C, et al. Continuous psoas compartment block for postoperative analgesia after total hip arthroplasty: New landmarks, technical guidelines and clinical evaluation. *Anesth Analg* 2002;94: 1606–1613.
6. Chudinov A, Berkenstadt H, Salai M, et al. Continuous psoas compartment block for anesthesia and perioperative analgesia in patients with hip fractures. *Reg Anesth Pain Med* 1999;24:563–568.
7. Farny J, Girard M, Drolet P. Posterior approach to the lumbar plexus combined with a sciatic nerve block using lidocaine. *Can J Anaesth* 1994; 41:486–491.
8. Chayen D, Nathan H, Chayen M. The psoas compartment block. *Anesthesiology* 1976;45:95–99.
9. Ho AM, Karmakar MK. Combined paravertebral lumbar plexus and parasacral sciatic nerve block for reduction of hip fracture in a patient with severe aortic stenosis. *Can J Anaesth* 2002;49:946–950.
10. Luber MJ, Greengrass R, Parker T. Patient satisfaction and effectiveness of lumbar plexus and sciatic nerve block for total knee arthroplasty. *J Arthroplasty* 2001;16:17–21.
11. Turker G, Uckunkaya N, Yavascaoglu B, et al. Comparison of the catheter-technique psoas compartment block and the epidural block for analgesia in partial hip replacement surgery. *Acta Anaesthesiol Scand* 2003;47: 30–36.
12. Goroszeniuk T, di Vadi PP. Repeated psoas compartment blocks for the management of long-standing hip pain. *Reg Anesth Pain Med* 2001;26:376–378.

13. Matheny JM, Hanks GA, Rung GW, et al. A comparison of patient-controlled analgesia and continuous lumbar plexus block after anterior cruciate ligament reconstruction. *Arthroscopy* 1993;9:87–90.

14. Pandin PC, Vandesteene A, d'Hollander AA. Lumbar plexus posterior approach: A catheter placement description using electrical stimulation. *Anesth Analg* 2002;95:1428–1431.

15. Pagnano MW, Hebl J, Horlocker T. Assuring a painless total hip arthroplasty: A multimodal approach emphasizing peripheral nerve blocks. *J Arthroplasty* 2006;21:80–84.

16. Bridenbaugh PO, Wedel DJ. The lower extremity: Somatic blockade. In: Cousins MJ, Bridenbaugh PO, eds. Neural Blockade: Clinical Anesthesia and Management of Pain. Philadelphia, PA: Lippincott-Raven; 1998:374–376.

17. Brown DL. Psoas compartment block. In: Brown DL, ed. *Atlas of Regional Anesthesia*, 2nd ed. Philadelphia: W. B. Saunders; 1999:88–91.

18. Solanski D. Posterior lumbar plexus (psoas) block. In: Chelly JE, ed. *Peripheral Nerve Blocks: A Color Atlas*. Philadelphia: Lippincott, Williams & Wilkins; 1999:90–92.

19. Winnie AP, Ramamurthy S, Durrani Z, Radonjic R. Plexus blocks for lower extremity surgery. *Anesthesiol Rev* 1974;1:11–16.

20. Gray H. *Anatomy of the Human Body*. Philadelphia, PA: Lea & Fibiger; 1918:416.

21. Aida S, Takahashi H, Shimoji K. Renal subcapsular hematoma after lumbar plexus block. *Anesthesiology* 1996;84:452–455.

22. Pousman RM, Mansoor Z, Sciard D. Total spinal anesthetic after continuous posterior lumbar plexus block. *Anesthesiology* 2003;98:1281–1282.

23. Reddy MB. Pneumocoele following psoas compartment block. *Anaesthesia* 2002;57:938–939.

24. Aveline C, Bonnet F. Delayed retroperitoneal haematoma after failed lumbar plexus block. *Br J Anaesth* 2004;93:589–591.

25. Breslin DS, Martin G, Macleod DB, et al. Central nervous system toxicity following the administration of levobupivacaine for lumbar plexus block: A report of two cases. *Reg Anesth Pain Med* 2003;28:144–147.

26. Parkinson S, Mueller J, Little W, Bailey SL. Extent of blockade with various approaches to the lumbar plexus. *Anesth Analg* 1989;68:243–248.

27. Dalens B, Tanguy A, Vanneuville G. Lumbar plexus block in children: A comparison of two procedures in 50 patients. *Anesth Analg* 1988;67:750–758.

28. Muravchick S, Owens WD. An unusual complication of lumbar plexus block: A case report. *Anesth Analg* 1976;55:350–352.

29. McLitz RJ, Vicent O, Wiessner D, Heller AR. Misplacement of a psoas compartment catheter in the subarachnoid space. *Reg Anesth Pain Med* 2004;29:60–64.

30. Fletcher AK, Rigby AS, Heyes FL. Three-in-one femoral nerve block as analgesia for fractured neck of femur in the emergency department: A randomized, controlled trial. *Ann Emerg Med* 2003;41:227–233.

31. Frost S, Grossfeld S, Kirkley A, et al. The efficacy of femoral nerve block in pain reduction for outpatient hamstring anterior cruciate ligament reconstruction: A double-blind, prospective, randomized trial. *Arthroscopy* 2000;16:243–248.

32. Goranson BD, Lang S, Cassidy JD, et al. A comparison of three regional anaesthesia techniques for outpatient arthroscopy. *Can J Anaesth* 1997;44:371–376.

33. McCarty EC, Spindler KP, Tingstad E, et al. Does intraarticular morphine improve pain control with femoral nerve block after anterior cruciate ligament reconstruction? *Am J Sports Med* 2001;29:327–332.

34. Mulroy MF, Larkin KL, Batra MS, et al. Femoral nerve block with 0.25% or 0.5% bupivacaine improves postoperative analgesia following outpatient arthroscopic anterior cruciate ligament repair. *Reg Anesth Pain Med* 2001;26:24–29.

35. Wang H, Boctor B, Verner J. The effect of single-injection femoral nerve block on rehabilitation and length of hospital stay after total knee replacement. *Reg Anesth Pain Med* 2002;27:139–144.

36. Williams BA, Kentor ML, Vogt MT, et al. Femoral-sciatic nerve blocks for complex outpatient knee surgery are associated with less postoperative pain before same-day discharge. *Anesthesiology* 2003;98:1206–1213.

37. Vloka JD, Hadžić A, Drobnik L, et al. Anatomic landmarks for femoral nerve block: A comparison of four needle insertion sites. *Anesth Analg* 1999;89:1467–1470.

38. Winnie AP, Ramamurthy S, Durrani Z. The inguinal paravascular technic of lumbar plexus anesthesia: The "3-in-1 block." *Anesth Analg* 1973;52:989–996.

39. Cauhepe C, Oliver M, Colombani R, Railhac N. The "3-in-1" block: Myth or reality. *Ann Fr Anesth Reanim* 1989;8:376–378.

40. Lang SA, Yip RW, Chang P, Gerard M. The femoral 3-in-1 block revisited. *J Clin Anesth* 1993;5:292–296.

41. Marhofer P, Nasel C, Sitzwohl C, Kapral S. Magnetic resonance imaging of the distribution of local anesthetic during the three-in-one block. *Anesth Analg* 2000;90:119–124.

42. Seeberger M, Urwyler A. Paravascular lumbar plexus block: Block extension after femoral nerve stimulation and injection of 20 vs. 40 ml mepivacaine 10 mg/ml. *Acta Anaesthesiol Scand* 1995;39:769–773.

43. Dalens B, Vanneuville G, Tanguy A. Comparison of the fascia iliaca compartment with "3-in-1" block in children. *Anesth Analg* 1989;69:705–713.

44. Lopez S, Gros T, Bernard N, et al. Fascia iliaca compartment block for femoral bone fractures in prehospital care. *Reg Anesth Pain Med* 2003;28:203–207.

45. Capdevila X, Barthelet Y, Biboulet P, et al. Effects of perioperative analgesic technique on the surgical outcome and duration of rehabilitation after major knee surgery. *Anesthesiology* 1999;91:8–15.

46. Chelly JE, Greger J, Gebhard R, et al. Continuous femoral blocks improve recovery and outcome of patients undergoing total knee arthroplasty. *J Arthroplasty* 2001;16:436–445.

47. Dauri M, Polzoni M, Fabbi E, et al. Comparison of epidural, continuous femoral block and intraarticular analgesia after anterior cruciate ligament reconstruction. *Acta Anaesthesiol Scand* 2003;47:20–25.

48. Griffith JP, Whiteley S, Gough MJ. Prospective randomized study of a new method of providing postoperative pain relief following femoropopliteal bypass. *Br J Surg* 1996;83:1735–1738.

49. Singelyn FJ, Deyaert M, Joris D, et al. Effects of intravenous patient-controlled analgesia with morphine, continuous epidural analgesia, and continuous "3-in-1" block on postoperative pain and knee rehabilitation after unilateral total knee arthroplasty. *Anesth Analg* 1998;87:88–92.

50. Singelyn FJ, Gouverneur JM. Extended "3-in-1" block after total knee arthroplasty: Continuous versus patient-controlled techniques. *Anesth Analg* 2000;91:176–180.

51. Singelyn FJ, Vanderelst P, Gouverneur JM. Extended femoral nerve sheath block after total hip arthroplasty: Continuous versus patient-controlled techniques. *Anesth Analg* 2001;92:455–459.

52. Ganapathy S, Wasserman RA, Watson JT, et al. Modified continuous femoral three-in-one block for postoperative pain after total knee arthroplasty. *Anesth Analg* 1999;89:1197–1202.

53. Paut O, Sallabery M, Schreiber-Deturmeny E, et al. Continuous fascia iliaca compartment block in children: A prospective evaluation of plasma bupivacaine concentrations, pain scores, and side effects. *Anesth Analg* 2001; 92:1159–1163.

54. Capdevila X, Biboulet P, Morau D, et al. Continuous three-in-one block for postoperative pain after lower limb orthopedic surgery: Where do the catheters go? *Anesth Analg* 2002;94:1001–1006.

55. Salinas FV, Neal JM, Sueda LA, et al. Prospective comparison of continuous femoral nerve block with nonstimulating catheter placement versus stimulating catheter-guided perineural placement in volunteers. *Reg Anesth Pain Med* 2004;29:212–220.

56. Comfort VK, Lang SA, Yip RW. Saphenous nerve anesthesia: A nerve stimulator technique. *Can J Anaesth* 1996;43:852–857.

57. Mansour NY. Sub-sartorial saphenous nerve block with the aid of a nerve stimulator. *Reg Anesth* 1993;18:266–268.

58. van der Wal M, Lang SA, Yip RW. Trans-sartorial approach for saphenous nerve block. *Can J Anaesth* 1993;40:542–546.

59. De Mey JC, Deruyck LJ, Cammu G, et al. A paravenous approach for the saphenous nerve block. *Reg Anesth Pain Med* 2001;26:504–506.

60. Atchabahian A, Brown AR. Postoperative neuropathy following fascia iliaca compartment blockade. *Anesthesiology* 2001;94:534–536.

61. Muraskin SI, Conrad B, Zheng N, et al. Falls associated with lower-extremity-nerve blocks: A pilot investigation of mechanisms. *Reg Anesth Pain Med* 2007;32:67–72.

62. Bouaziz H, Vial F, Jochum D, et al. An evaluation of the cutaneous distribution after obturator nerve block. *Anesth Analg* 2002;94:445–449.

63. Atanassoff PG, Weiss BM, Brull SJ, et al. Electromyographic comparison of obturator nerve block to three-in-one block. *Anesth Analg* 1995;81:529–533.

64. Last RJ. *Anatomy: Regional and Applied*, Section 5. New York: Churchill Livingstone, 1978.

65. Wassef MR. Interadductor approach to obturator nerve blockade for spastic conditions of adductor thigh muscles. *Reg Anesth* 1993;18:13–17.

66. Macalou D, Trueck S, Meuret P, et al. Postoperative analgesia after total knee replacement: The effect of an obturator nerve block added to the femoral 3-in-1 nerve block. *Anesth Analg* 2004;99:251–254.

67. McNamee DA, Parks L, Milligan KR. Post-operative analgesia following total knee replacement: An evaluation of the addition of an obturator nerve block to combined femoral and sciatic nerve block. *Acta Anaesthesiol Scand* 2002;46:95–99.

68. Parks CR, Kennedy WF. Obturator nerve block: A simplified approach. *Anesthesiology* 1967;28:775–778.

69. Hopkins PM, Ellis FR, Halsall PJ. Evaluation of local anaesthetic blockade of the lateral femoral cutaneous nerve. *Anaesthesia* 1991;46:95–96.

70. Karacalar A, Karacalar S, Uckunkaya N, et al. Combined use of axillary block and lateral femoral cutaneous nerve block in upper-extremity injuries requiring large skin grafts. *J Hand Surg [Am]* 1998;23:1100–1105.

71. Maccani RM, Wedel DJ, Melton A, Gronert GA. Femoral and lateral femoral cutaneous nerve block for muscle biopsies in children. *Paediatr Anaesth* 1995;5:223–227.

PART II: TECHNIQUES

72. Jones SF, White A. Analgesia following femoral neck surgery. Lateral cutaneous nerve block as an alternative to narcotics in the elderly. *Anaesthesia* 1985;40:682–685.

73. Coad NR. Postoperative analgesia following femoral-neck surgery: A comparison between 3 in 1 femoral nerve block and lateral cutaneous nerve block. *Eur J Anaesthesiol* 1991;8:287–290.

74. Sharrock NE. Inadvertent "3-in-1 block" following injection of the lateral cutaneous nerve of the thigh. *Anesth Analg* 1980;59:887–888.

75. Shannon J, Lang SA, Yip RW, Gerard M. Lateral femoral cutaneous nerve block revisited. A nerve stimulator technique. *Reg Anesth* 1995;20:100–104.

76. Tokat O, Turker YG, Uckunkaya N, Yilmazlar A. A clinical comparison of psoas compartment and inguinal paravascular blocks combined with sciatic nerve block. *J Int Med Res* 2002;30:161–167.

77. Kaloul I, Guay J, Cote C, Fallaha M. The posterior lumbar plexus (psoas compartment) block and the three-in-one femoral nerve block provide similar postoperative analgesia after total knee replacement. *Can J Anaesth* 2004;51:45–51.

78. Morau D, Lopez S, Biboulet P, et al. Comparison of continuous 3-in-1 and fascia iliaca compartment blocks for postoperative analgesia: Feasibility, catheter migration, distribution of sensory block, and analgesic efficacy. *Reg Anesth Pain Med* 2003;28:309–314.

79. Capdevila X, Biboulet P, Bouregba M, et al. Comparison of the three-in-one and fascia iliaca compartment blocks in adults: Clinical and radiographic analysis. *Anesth Analg* 1998;86:1039–1044.

80. Jochum D, Iohom G, Choquet O, et al. Adding a selective obturator nerve block to the parasacral sciatic nerve block: An evaluation. *Anesth Analg* 2004;99:1544–1549.

81. Morris GF, Lang SA, Dust WN, Van der Wal M. The parasacral sciatic nerve block. *Reg Anesth* 1997;22:223–228.

82. Gaertner E, Lascurain P, Venet C, et al. Continuous parasacral sciatic block: A radiographic study. *Anesth Analg* 2004;98:831–834.

83. Helayel PE, Ceccon MS, Knaesel JA, et al. Urinary incontinence after bilateral parasacral sciatic-nerve block: Report of two cases. *Reg Anesth Pain Med* 2006;31:368–371.

84. Guardini R, Waldron BA, Wallace WA. Sciatic nerve block: A new lateral approach. *Acta Anaesthesiol Scand* 1985;29:515–519.

85. Smith BE, Fischer ABJ, Scott PU. Continuous sciatic nerve block. *Anaesthesia* 1984;39:155–157.

86. McNichol LR. Sciatic nerve block for children: Sciatic nerve block by anterior approach for postoperative pain relief. *Anaesthesia* 1985;40:410–414.

87. Raj PP, Parks RI, Watson TD, Jenkins MT. A new single-posterior supine approach to sciatic-femoral nerve block. *Anesth Analg* 1975;54:489–494.

88. Winnie AP. Regional anesthesia. *Surg Clin North Am* 1975;55:861–892.

89. Taboada M, Atanassoff PG, Rodriguez J, et al. Plantar flexion seems more reliable than dorsiflexion with Labat's sciatic nerve block: A prospective, randomized comparison. *Anesth Analg* 2005;100:250–254.

90. Sukhani R, Nader A, Candido KD, et al. Nerve stimulator-assisted evoked motor response predicts the latency and success of a single-injection sciatic block. *Anesth Analg* 2004;99:584–588.

91. Bailey SL, Parkinson SK, Little WL, Simmerman SR. Sciatic nerve block: A comparison of single versus double injection technique. *Reg Anesth* 1994;19:9–13.

92. Hullander M, Spillane W, Leivers D, Balsara Z. The use of Doppler ultrasound to assist with sciatic nerve blocks. *Reg Anesth* 1991;16:282–284.

93. Ichiyanagi K. Sciatic nerve block: Lateral approach with patient supine. *Anesthesiology* 1959;20:601–604.

94. Beck GP. Anterior sciatic nerve block. *Anesthesiology* 1963;24:222–224.

95. Magora F, Pessachovitch B, Shoham I. Sciatic nerve block by the anterior approach for operations on the lower extremity. *Br J Anaesth* 1974;46:121–123.

96. Pandin P, Vandesteene A, D'Hollander A. Sciatic nerve blockade in the supine position: A novel approach. *Can J Anaesth* 2003;50:52–56.

97. Bridenbaugh PO, Moore DC, Bridenbaugh LD. Capillary PO$_2$ as a measure of sympathetic blockade. *Anesth Analg* 1972;50:26–30.

98. Fanelli G, Casati A, Garancini P, Torri G. Nerve stimulator and multiple injection technique for upper and lower limb blockade: Failure rate, patient acceptance, and neurologic complications. Study Group on Regional Anesthesia. *Anesth Analg* 1999;88:847–852.

99. Auroy Y, Benhamou D, Bargues L, et al. Major complications of regional anesthesia in France: The SOS regional anesthesia hotline service. *Anesthesiology* 2002;97:1274–1280.

100. Hansen E, Eshelman MR, Cracchiolo A. Popliteal fossa neural blockade as the sole anesthetic technique for outpatient foot and ankle surgery. *Foot Ankle Int* 2000;21:38–44.

101. Rongstad K, Mann RA, Prieskorn D, et al. Popliteal sciatic nerve block for postoperative analgesia. *Foot Ankle Int* 1996;17:378–382.

102. Rorie DK, Byer DE, Nelson DO, et al. Assessment of block of the sciatic nerve in the popliteal fossa. *Anesth Analg* 1980;59:371–376.

103. Vloka JD, Hadžić A, Mulcare R, et al. Combined popliteal and posterior cutaneous nerve of the thigh blocks for short saphenous vein stripping in

104. Vloka JD, Hadžić A, Koorn R, Thys D. Supine approach to the sciatic nerve in the popliteal fossa. *Can J Anaesth* 1996;43:964–967.

105. Ilfeld BM, Morey TE, Wang RD, Enneking FK. Continuous popliteal sciatic nerve block for postoperative pain control at home: A randomized, double-blinded, placebo-controlled study. *Anesthesiology* 2002;97:959–965.

106. Schimek F, Deusch H. New technique of sciatic nerve block in the popliteal fossa. *Eur J Anaesth* 1995;12:163–169.

107. Singelyn FJ, Aye F, Gouverneur JM. Continuous popliteal sciatic nerve block: An original technique to provide postoperative analgesia after foot surgery. *Anesth Analg* 1997;84:383–386.

108. Levecque JP, Borne M, Saissy JM. Analgesia with continuous lateral posterior tibial nerve block (letter). *Reg Anesth Pain Med* 1999;24:191–192.

109. Volka JD, Hadžić A, April E, Thys DM. The division of the sciatic nerve in the popliteal fossa: Anatomical implications for popliteal nerve blockade. *Anesth Analg* 2001;92:215–217.

110. Benzon HT, Kim C, Benzon HP, et al. Correlation between evoked motor response of the sciatic nerve and sensory blockade. *Anesthesiology* 1997;87:547–552.

111. Paqueron X, Bouaziz H, Macalou D, et al. The lateral approach to the sciatic nerve at the popliteal fossa: One or two injections? *Anesth Analg* 1999;89:1221–1225.

112. Zetlaoui PJ, Bouaziz H. Lateral approach to the sciatic nerve in the popliteal fossa. *Anesth Analg* 1998;87:79–82.

113. Hadžić A, Vloka JD. A comparison of the posterior versus lateral approaches to the block of the sciatic nerve in the popliteal fossa. *Anesthesiology* 1998;88:1480–1486.

114. Arcioni R, Palmisani S, Della Rocca M, et al. Lateral popliteal sciatic nerve block: A single injection targeting the tibial branch of the sciatic nerve is as effective as a double-injection technique. *Acta Anaesthesiol Scand* 2007;51:115–121.

115. Taboada M, Alvarez J, Cortes J, et al. The effects of three different approaches on the onset time of sciatic nerve blocks with 0.75% ropivacaine. *Anesth Analg* 2004;98:242–247.

116. McCutcheon R. Regional anesthesia for the foot. *Can Anaesth Soc J* 1965;12:465–474.

117. Delgado-Martinez AD, Marchal-Escalona JM. Supramalleolar ankle block anesthesia and ankle tourniquet for foot surgery. *Foot Ankle Int* 2001;22:836–838.

118. Gerbert J. The location of the terminal branching of the posterior tibial nerve and its effect on administering a posterior tibial nerve block. *J Am Podiatry Assoc* 1971;61:8–11.

119. Lichtenfeld NS. The pneumatic ankle tourniquet with ankle block anesthesia for foot surgery. *Foot Ankle* 1992;13:344–349.

120. Schurman DJ. Ankle-block anesthesia for foot surgery. *Anesthesiology* 1976;44:348–352.

121. Colgrove RC. Posterior tibial nerve block. *Foot Ankle Int* 2001;22:839–840.

122. Wassef MR. Posterior tibial nerve block. A new approach using the bony landmark of the sustentaculum tali. *Anaesthesia* 1991;46:841–844.

123. Sharrock NE, Waller JF, Fierro LE. Midtarsal block for surgery of the forefoot. *Br J Anaesth* 1986;58:37–40.

124. Pinzur MS, Morrison C, Sage R, et al. Syme's two-stage amputation in insulin-requiring diabetics with gangrene of the forefoot. *Foot Ankle* 1991;11:394–396.

125. Harvey CK. Dilute lidocaine ankle blocks in the diagnosis of sympathetically maintained pain. *J Am Podiatr Med Assoc* 1997;87:473–477.

126. Needoff M, Radford P, Costigan P. Local anesthesia for postoperative pain relief after foot surgery: A prospective clinical trial. *Foot Ankle Int* 1995;6:11–13.

127. Mineo R, Sharrock NE. Venous levels of lidocaine and bupivacaine after midtarsal ankle block. *Reg Anesth* 1992;17:47–49.

128. McLeod DH, Wong DH, Claridge RJ, Merrick PM. Lateral popliteal sciatic nerve block compared with subcutaneous infiltration for analgesia following foot surgery. *Can J Anaesth* 1994;41:673–676.

129. Singelyn FJ. Single-injection applications for foot and ankle surgery. *Best Pract Res Clin Anaesthesiol* 2002;16:247–254.

130. Hilgenhurst G. The bier block after 80 years: A historical review. *Reg Anesth* 1990;15:2–5.

131. Lehman WL, Jones WW. Intravenous lidocaine for anesthesia in the lower extremity. *J Bone Joint Surg Am* 1984;66:1056–1060.

132. Davies JAH, Walford AJ. Intravenous regional anaesthesia for foot surgery. *Acta Anaesthesiol Scand* 1986;30:145–147.

133. Chirwa SS, MacLeod BA, Day B. Intra-articular bupivacaine (Marcaine) after arthroscopic meniscectomy: A randomized double-blind controlled study. *Arthroscopy* 1989;5:33–35.

134. Stein C, Comisel K, Haimerl E, et al. Analgesic effect of intra-articular morphine after arthroscopic knee surgery. *N Engl J Med* 1991;325:1123–1126.

135. Hughes DG. Intra-articular bupivacaine for pain relief in arthroscopic surgery. *Anaesthesia* 1985;40:821.

outpatients: An alternative to spinal anesthesia. *J Clin Anesth* 1997;9:618–622.

136. Osborne D, Keene G. Pain relief after arthroscopic surgery of the knee: A prospective, randomized, and blinded assessment of bupivacaine and bupivacaine with adrenaline. *Arthroscopy* 1993;9:177–180.
137. Niemi L, Pitkanen M, Tuominen M, et al. Intra-articular morphine for pain relief after knee arthroscopy performed under regional anaesthesia. *Acta Anaesthesiol Scand* 1994;38:402–405.
138. Raja SN, Dickstein RE, Johnson CA. Comparison of postoperative analgesic effects of intra-articular bupivacaine and morphine following arthroscopic knee surgery. *Anesthesiology* 1992;77:1143–1147.
139. Joshi GP, McCarroll SM, O'Brien TM, Lenane P. Intra-articular analgesia following knee arthroscopy. *Anesth Analg* 1993;76:333–336.
140. Khoury GF, Chen AC, Garland DE, Stein C. Intra-articular morphine, bupivacaine, and morphine/bupivacaine for pain control after knee video arthroscopy. *Anesthesiology* 1992;77:263–266.
141. De Andres J, Bellver J, Barrera L, et al. A comparative study of analgesia after knee surgery with intra-articular bupivacaine, intra-articular morphine and lumbar plexus block. *Anesth Analg* 1993;77:727–730.
142. Katz JA, Kaeding CS, Hill JR, Henthorn TK. The pharmacokinetics of bupivacaine when injected intra-articularly after knee arthroscopy. *Anesth Analg* 1988;67:872–875.
143. Davies MJ, McGlade DP. One hundred sciatic nerve blocks: A comparison of localization techniques. *Anaesth Intensive Care* 1993;21:76–78.
144. Hirst GC, Lang SA, Dust WN, et al. Femoral nerve block. Single injection versus continuous infusion for total knee arthroplasty. *Reg Anesth* 1996;21:292–297.
145. Kaiser H, Niesel HC, Klimpel L. Influence of minimum current for peripheral nerve stimulation on the latency and success rate of sciatic blockade. *Reg Anesth* 1988;11:92–97.
146. Rosenblatt R. Continuous femoral anesthesia for lower extremity surgery. *Anesth Analg* 1980;59:631–632.
147. Singelyn FJ, Gouverneur JM. Postoperative analgesia after total hip arthroplasty: IV PCA with morphine, patient-controlled epidural analgesia, or continuous "3-in-1" block: A prospective evaluation by our acute pain service in more than 1300 patients. *J Clin Anesth* 1999;11:550–554.
148. Tetzlaff JE, Andrish J, O'Hara J Jr., et al. Effectiveness of bupivacaine administered via femoral nerve catheter for pain control after anterior cruciate ligament repair. *J Clin Anesth* 1997;9:542–545.
149. Bailey SL, Parkinson SK, Little WL, Simmerman SR. Sciatic nerve block: A comparison of single vs double injection technique. *Reg Anesth* 1994;19:9–13.
150. Cuvillon P, Ripart J, Jeannes P, et al. Comparison of the parasacral approach and the posterior approach, with single- and double-injection techniques, to block the sciatic nerve. *Anesthesiology* 2003;98:1436–1441.
151. Casati A, Fanelli G, Beccaria P, et al. The effects of single or multiple injections on the volume of 0.5 % ropivacaine required for femoral nerve blockade. *Anesth Analg* 2001;93:83–86.
152. Dingemans E, Williams SR, Arcand G, et al. Neurostimulation in ultrasound-guided block: A prospective randomized trial. *Anesth Analg* 2007;104:1275–1280.
153. Domingo-Triado V, Selfa S, Martinez F, et al. Ultrasound guidance for lateral midfemoral sciatic nerve block: A prospective randomized study. *Anesth Analg* 2007;104:1270–1274.
154. Gray AT. Ultrasound-guided regional anesthesia: Current state of the art. Review. *Anesthesiology* 2006;104:368–373.
155. Neal JM, Hebl JR, Gerancher JC, Hogan QH. Brachial plexus anesthesia: Essentials of our current understanding. *Reg Anesth Pain Med* 2002;27:402–428.
156. Marhofer P, Greher M, Kapral S. Ultrasound guidance in regional anaesthesia. *Br J Anaesth* 2005;94:7–17.
157. Marhofer P, Chan VWS. Ultrasound-guided regional anesthesia: Current concepts and future trends. *Anesth Analg* 2007;104:1265–1269.
158. Chan VWS, Brull R, McCartney CJL, et al. An ultrasonographic and histological study of intraneuronal injection and electrical stimulation in pigs. *Anesth Analg* 2007;104:1281–1284.
159. Neal JM. Effects of epinephrine in local anesthetics on the central and peripheral nervous systems: Neurotoxicity and neural blood flow. *Reg Anesth Pain Med* 2003;28:124–134.
160. Casati A, Magistris L, Fanelli G, et al. Small-dose clonidine prolongs postoperative analgesia after sciatic-femoral nerve block with 0.75% ropivacaine for foot surgery. *Anesth Analg* 2000;91:388–392.
161. Casati A, Vinciguerra F, Cappelleri G, et al. Adding clonidine to the induction bolus and postoperative infusion during continuous femoral nerve block delays recovery of motor function after total knee arthroplasty. *Anesth Analg* 2005;100:866–872.
162. Vanterpool S, Steele SM, Nielsen KC, et al. Combined lumbar-plexus and sciatic-nerve blocks: An analysis of plasma ropivacaine concentrations. *Reg Anesth Pain Med* 2006;31:417–421.
163. Simon MA, Gielen MJ, Lagerwerf AJ, Vree TB. Plasma concentrations after high doses of mepivacaine with epinephrine in the combined psoas compartment/sciatic nerve block. *Reg Anesth* 1990;15:256–260.
164. Snoeck MM, Vree TB, Gielen MJ, Lagerwert AJ. Steady state bupivacaine plasma concentrations and safety of a femoral "3-in-1" nerve block with bupivacaine in patients over 80 years of age. *Int J Clin Pharmacol Ther* 2003;41:107–113.

PART II: TECHNIQUES

CHAPTER 15 ■ INTRAVENOUS REGIONAL NEURAL BLOCKADE

PER H. ROSENBERG

Intravenous (IV) regional neural blockade, or IV regional anesthesia (IVRA) is mainly used for short surgical procedures of the upper extremity. It can also be used for analgesia or anesthesia of the lower extremity, but certain toxicologic risks and methodologic circumstances make the use of IVRA of the lower extremity less attractive. In the last 10 years there has been very little change in this anesthetic technique itself (1–3); instead, in recent years, clinical research has focused on pharmacokinetics, toxicity, and benefits of additives in the local anesthetic solutions used.

HISTORY

Intravenous regional neural blockade was first described by the German surgeon August Bier in 1908 (4). The technique initially consisted of exsanguination of the arm by winding an Esmarch bandage from the fingers to above the elbow, application of two pneumatic tourniquets on the arm, one above the elbow and the other on the antebrachium, and then performing a surgical cutdown under local anesthesia in the cubital or antebrachial region to locate a superficial vein. A slit was made in the vein and a cannula was inserted in the peripheral direction and secured with a tie. The vein was ligated centrally to the slit.

After injection of procaine (0.25% or 0.5%), Bier noted a rapid initial analgesia in the region between the tourniquets, sufficient for starting the surgical procedure. A slower developing sensory block was noted in the region distal to the peripheral tourniquet.

Harvey Cushing introduced the pneumatic tourniquet, an adaptation of the original sphygmomanometer, in 1904. This device contained a hand pump, similar in design to that of bicycle pumps. Later, a manometer was added and the pump replaced with compressed pipeline air.

MECHANISMS OF ACTION

The mechanisms of action in intravenous regional neural blockade are multiple and depend primarily on ischemia and on the transport of local anesthetic solution through a venous network into veins inside nerve trunks.

The nerve trunks of the extremities are composed of bundles covered with a connective tissue layer called *epineurium,* which also contain the blood vessels that supply the nerves. The *endoneurium* encloses the individual nerve fibers and contains capillary plexuses that extend interneurally as *vasae nervorum.*

Nerve fibers at the center of the fascicle are more distant from the lipoprotein-containing epineurium, and they are not protected by a strong diffusion barrier between the vessels and the nerve axons. Therefore, this is likely the reason for the commonly noted centripetal progression of the sensory block in IVRA.

Nerve endings in the skin are easily reached by the local anesthetic solution through valveless venules. The intercostobrachial nerves are not near a rich vessel network; that is, they cannot be rapidly reached by intravenously injected local anesthetic solution, therefore, their innervation region may sometimes be insufficiently blocked.

Surgical anesthesia in IVRA is produced by multiple and complementary mechanisms of action (Table 15-1). Initially, sensory block of the skin occurs along the veins (venules) filled with local anesthetic, a result of nerve conduction blockade of small nerves and nerve endings (peripheral mechanism of action). In the radiographic study by Fleming and co-workers (5), the development of skin analgesia followed the distribution of the injected mixture of local anesthetic and contrast medium. On the other hand, others have demonstrated an accumulation of injected contrast medium (6,7) or radioactive lidocaine (8) in the vicinity of the major nerves near the elbow in IVRA of the arm. When distal flow of a solution of local anesthetic and contrast medium was prevented by a tourniquet, anesthesia developed also in those parts peripheral to the distal tourniquet (7). This phenomenon was described by August Bier in 1908.

The uptake of lidocaine into the main nerves occurs rapidly (2–4 minutes), as shown by positron emission tomography, after the injection of [^{11}C]lidocaine for IVRA (8). After tourniquet release, positron emission in the nerves decreased rapidly. More lipid-soluble and strongly protein-bound local anesthetics, such as bupivacaine and etidocaine, stay in the nerves longer, which in IVRA has resulted in prolonged analgesia after the deflation of the tourniquet cuff (9,10).

As long as the pressure in the tourniquet cuff stays low, nerve conduction block in IVRA through direct nerve damage probably plays a minor role (11). Ischemia, on the other hand, plays a major role, and total conduction block of the arm ensues after 15 to 45 minutes of ischemia (12–14). In conditions similar to those in a clinical IVRA of the arm, injection of saline instead of local anesthetic in volunteers resulted in complete sensory block of the skin with paralysis of the arm in 20 to 25 minutes (15).

EQUIPMENT

Equipment needed for IVRA are a pneumatic tourniquet, a pressure regulator with pressure gauges, an elastic bandage for exsanguination, an IV cannula in the extremity to be anesthetized, and syringes containing local anesthetic solution.

TABLE 15-1

MULTIPLE MECHANISMS OF ACTION OF INTRAVENOUS REGIONAL ANESTHESIA

Block of peripheral small nerves and nerve endings (initial effect)

Block of large nerves at a proximal site (e.g., cubital region in intravenous regional nerve block of the arm), as well as via intraneural venous distribution of the local anesthetic solution

Ischemia (blocks nerve conduction and motor end-plate function)

Compression of nerves under the tourniquet cuff (slow component)

Tourniquets

Soft padding on the extremity under the tourniquet is required. This is usually accomplished by applying either cast padding or tubular cotton stockinette, placing it as wrinkle-free as possible against the skin.

Tourniquets of different length and width are available for IVRA of the arm, with specially designed dual-bladder cylindrical or contour cuffs and with Velcro fasteners. Currently, the newest models are latex-free. The contour cuffs are particularly suitable in muscular or very obese adults. Two separate tourniquet cuffs may be used on the upper arms of very large patients, providing that enough room remains between the elbow and the axilla for two 7- or 9-cm wide cuffs. For IVRA of the whole lower extremity, two separate tourniquet cuffs fit well on the thigh. On the other hand, for IVRA of the leg below the knee, a single-cuff tourniquet is often applied on the calf, clearly below the head of the fibula (Fig. 15-1), with an un-

pressurized safety tourniquet in place on the thigh. In athletic patients, the calf tourniquet should be of the contour design and as wide as possible to diminish discomfort and tourniquet pain.

To prevent nerve injuries from the tourniquet, is important to minimize the destructive effect of the cuff pressure, especially the shear stress under the cuff edges. The pressure should be kept as low as possible; the wider the cuff, the lower the minimal limb blood flow occlusion pressure. For IVRA of the arm, with the tourniquet on the upper arm, a cuff pressure of 50 to 100 mm Hg above the systolic arterial blood pressure (i.e., 200–275 mm Hg in adults) is needed (16). For a thigh tourniquet cuff in adults, at least 100 mm Hg above the systolic arterial blood pressure (i.e., 250–300 mm Hg) is needed.

When the tourniquet cuff is inflated, several destructive mechanical and metabolic events are initiated (11). The tourniquet cuff itself, and in particular its edges, compresses the underlying nerves, disturbing both their structure and perfusion. Prolonged nerve conduction times at this region can be detected in 5 to 10 minutes (17,18). After about 30 minutes of compression at 300 mm Hg, a conduction block develops distal to the cuff. Tourniquet release resulted in recovery in about 5 minutes, but the conduction time at the level of the tourniquet, particularly across the proximal border region, was the last to recover (17). Interestingly, only 75% recovery of nerve conduction velocity was observed across the tourniquet zone 1 hour after the release of the cuff.

The metabolic changes include hypoxia, hypercapnia, metabolic acidosis, lacticemia, and loss of muscle cell membrane integrity. As a result, a local (isolated limb) and systemic inflammatory response (19) involving fibrinolysis (20) ensues.

When the tourniquet is inflated for a long time, a risk arises for the development of a reperfusion syndrome. In fact, the muscle tissue is quite vulnerable, with a critical tissue ischemic time of 4 hours (21). It may be of note that reversible histologic, ultrastructural, and neuromuscular deteriorating changes can

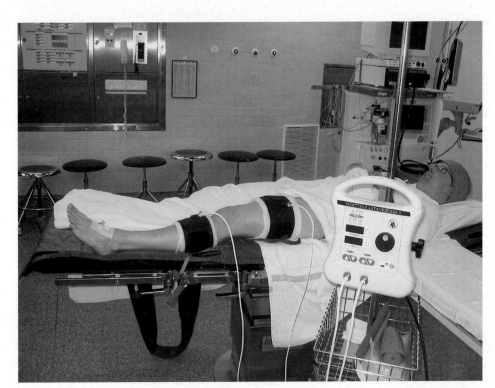

FIGURE 15-1. Tourniquet cuff placement for intravenous regional anesthesia (IVRA) below the knee. The distal cuff is around the calf, the upper edge clearly below the head of the fibula. Only the distal cuff is inflated for IVRA below the knee. The proximal cuff around the thigh is kept prepared to be immediately inflated if the proximal cuff fails during the procedure.

PART II: TECHNIQUES

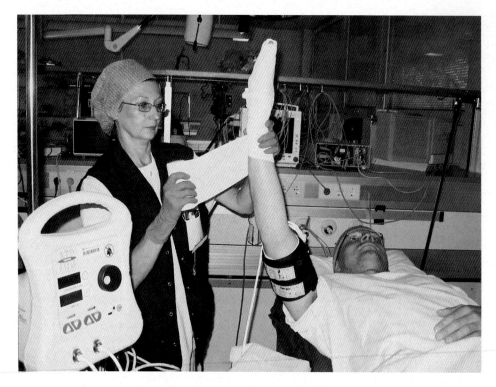

FIGURE 15-2. Intravenous regional anesthesia of upper limb. Exsanguination of the extremity is performed by winding an elastic bandage tightly from the fingertips down onto the distal tourniquet cuff. The double-cuff tourniquet has been applied over soft cotton fabric.

be observed after 1.5 to 2 hours of ischemia (22,23), and irreversible muscle cell damage starts after 3 hours of ischemia (24). Such studies have been guides to the determination of the safe duration of the application of an inflated tourniquet in clinical patients (i.e., 1.5–2 hours). In an awake patient (e.g., in IVRA), tourniquet pain usually limits the time to 1 hour.

Exsanguination

The extremity is best exsanguinated by winding an elastic rubber Esmarch, Martin, or other elastic bandage tightly from the periphery to the tourniquet (Fig. 15-2). August Bier was the first to apply this bandage in IVRA, but initially, both Johannes von Esmarch and Henry A. Martin used their elastic rubber bandages as a method of applying diffuse pressure on the entire lower extremity for the treatment of stasis ulcers and to prevent reoccurrence of effusion after aspiration of the knee joint.

In comparison of various techniques of exsanguination of the arm in volunteers, the Esmarch bandage reduces blood volume of the arm on average by 69% (25), whereas the reduction was only about 45% by elevation of the arm (Table 15-2). In patients with a traumatized arm, an elevation/arterial compression (brachial artery) exsanguination technique results in sufficient emptying of the veins for IVRA (26). The degree of emptiness of the veins is probably related to the evenness and efficacy of the distribution of the injected local anesthetic but this does not seem to affect the development and success of anesthesia of the arm (27). Overfilling and distention of the veins may result in swelling of the tissue structures and oozing of blood during surgery, which may be so disturbing that some hand surgeons do not allow anesthesiologists to use IVRA in their patients. This problem may be overcome by using exsanguination with an Esmarch bandage and injecting only moderate volumes of anesthetic solution (20–30 mL) for IVRA

of the arm, or by using the so-called "second-wrap" technique (described later).

Today, other types of elastic bands (e.g., bands using elasthane or crepe), 6 to 12 cm wide, have replaced the classic rubber bandage. However, their efficacy in emptying the limb of blood without damaging the skin must still be confirmed.

Pressure Gauge

Tourniquet-induced muscle and nerve damage (tourniquet paralysis) was a great problem when the rubber bandage itself

TABLE 15-2

EFFICACY OF EXSANGUINATION OF THE UPPER EXTREMITY BY VARIOUS METHODS, AS STUDIED WITH A SCINTIGRAPHIC TECHNIQUE

Method of exsanguination	Reduction of blood volume
Elevation of the upper extremity	
5 s	44%
60 s	46%
240 s	42%
Esmarch bandage	69%
Gauze bandage	63%
Pomidor roll-cuff*	66%
Inflatable arm splint (Urias)	57%

*An annular tube of elastic material, which contains pressurized air, to be rolled onto a limb. The tube has a valve member to which a pressure-regulating unit can be connected. Modified from Blond L, Madsen JL. Exsanguination of the upper limb in healthy young volunteers. *J Bone Joint Surg* 2002;84B:489–491, with permission.

was used as a tourniquet (11,28). Uncontrolled very high pressures were created under the bandage. Thus, the development of pneumatic tourniquets with pressure gauges connected were of great significance, perhaps more so for the safe conductance of extremity surgery.

Modern pressure-control devices (tourniquet control units; Fig. 15-1) contain two different regulators and gauges, one for either of two tourniquet cuffs. In addition, these units contain alarms for time limits and self-regulation systems for maintaining either a set pressure or the limb occlusion pressure (LOP). In the IVRA technique, pressures slightly higher than LOP should be used, as recommended earlier, because of the risk of IV leakage of local anesthetic during and immediately after injection.

DRUGS FOR INTRAVENOUS REGIONAL ANESTHESIA

Lidocaine and Prilocaine

All available local anesthetics have been used for IVRA (Table 15-3). In principle, the least toxic local anesthetic should be chosen because the dose initially injected intravenously either in the upper or lower extremity is large enough to cause severe systemic intoxication if the dose mistakenly enters the circulation directly. Thus, the amide-linked local anesthetics lidocaine and prilocaine have been popular and safe drugs in IVRA. In countries in which prilocaine has not been available, lidocaine has been the first choice. Because of practical reasons determined by the use of a tourniquet, the onset of the IV neural blockade should be rapid; therefore, solutions of 5 mg/mL (0.5%) are commonly used. A few minutes may be won by using higher concentrations, but with the expense of causing toxic damage to the endothelium of the veins (39). In adults, the volume injected should, in principle, replace the volume removed by exsanguination; that is, 32 mL in women and 63 mL in men, on average (26). In an earlier study of adults, it was shown that 20 to 50 mL would suffice to fill the venous channels of an exsanguinated arm (40). The commonly used volumes for IVRA of the upper extremity in adults are 40 to 50 mL. The volume to fill the veins in an exsanguinated whole

lower limb would probably be at least double these amounts, and in clinical practice, volumes of 100 to 120 mL have been applied (41). In the comparative study of the use of 6 mg/kg of either lidocaine or prilocaine, the plasma concentrations after cuff deflation (Fig. 15-3), as well as the incidence of central nervous system (CNS) toxicity symptoms were clearly lower when prilocaine was used, again emphasizing the advantage regarding the safety of prilocaine when large doses are applied. In a clinical situation, such a high dose of lidocaine is not recommended. As the concentration of the local anesthetic in the injected solution for IVRA of the whole lower extremity needs to be kept low, the onset of anesthesia is sometimes disturbingly long. The high pressure in the thigh tourniquet (often as high as 300 mm Hg) and the relatively slow onset of analgesia make the IVRA technique of the whole lower extremity less attractive in comparison with spinal anesthesia or peripheral nerve blocks. However, IVRA below the knee, or IVRA around the knee (discussed later) are interesting alternatives, lacking some of the problems linked to whole lower extremity IVRA.

With prilocaine 6 mg/kg, a moderate rise in methemoglobin (met-Hb) levels was noted after IVRA of the whole lower extremity (Fig. 15-4), albeit without clinical signs of cyanosis or hypoxemia (41). It has been shown that two metabolites of prilocaine, o-toluidine and nitrosotoluidine oxidize ferrous iron in the hemoglobin molecule to the ferric state (42). The interindividual variation in met-Hb concentrations after prilocaine anaesthesia are huge (41,42). The maximum dose recommendation of 600 mg prilocaine in adults for the avoidance of clinically serious methemoglobinemia is more circumstantial than evidence-based (43). The prediction of the occurrence of this side effect/complication is hampered also by the fact that exposure to several other drugs and chemicals (e.g., chloroquine, primaquine, glyceryl trinitrate, sulfonamides, phenacetin) may induce met-Hb of varying degree (44).

More concentrated prilocaine solutions (7.5–20 mg/mL) have been used for IVRA of both the upper and lower extremity (45,46). The onset of the neural blockade is shorter, but otherwise the blocking profile is very similar to that of IVRA with prilocaine 5 mg/mL. The occurrence of mild symptoms of CNS toxicity is more frequent with the more concentrated solutions if the dose is not reduced.

Mepivacaine

Mepivacaine 5 mg/mL for IVRA produces blocks equivalent to lidocaine 5 mg/mL and prilocaine 5 mg/mL (47,48).

Bupivacaine and Analogues

Bupivacaine was popular for IVRA in the early 1980s (10,49). Concentrations from 2 to 5 mg/mL were used until severe intoxications (50) and deaths (51) were reported associated with bupivacaine-induced IVRA. Although bupivacaine is no longer recommended for IVRA, a questionnaire in North America taken during the mid 1990s showed that 1.2% of respondents still used bupivacaine (16). (See also Chapter 5.)

The less toxic enantiomer, levobupivacaine, at 1.25 mg/mL concentration has been tested for upper extremity IVRA in volunteers (35). Loss of sensation occurred at a similar rate as with lidocaine 5 mg/mL, but recovery after tourniquet cuff deflation was at least twice as long with levobupivacaine as with lidocaine. With ropivacaine 2 mg/mL for upper extremity IVRA, the block develops slightly more slowly compared with either lidocaine 5 mg/mL (52,53) or prilocaine 5 mg/mL (54). Although

TABLE 15-3

LOCAL ANESTHETICS USED IN INTRAVENOUS REGIONAL ANESTHESIA

Local anesthetic	Concentration (%)	Study (Ref.)
Articaine	0.5	Eerola, 1974 (32)
Bupivacaine	0.2–0.5	Ware, 1975 (33)
2-Chloroprocaine	0.5–1	Dickler et al., 1965 (29)
Cocaine	0.5	Hitzrot, 1909 (30)
Etidocaine	0.25	Evans et al., 1974 (34)
Levobupivacaine	0.125	Atanassoff et al., 2002 (35)
Lidocaine	0.15–1	Holmes, 1963 (1)
Mepivacaine	0.5	Cox, 1964 (36)
Prilocaine	0.25–2	Hooper, 1964 (37)
Procaine	0.25–0.5	Bier, 1908 (4)
Tetracaine	0.1–0.25	Durrani et al., 1982 (31)
Ropivacaine	0.2–0.36	Chan et al., 1999 (38)

PART II: TECHNIQUES

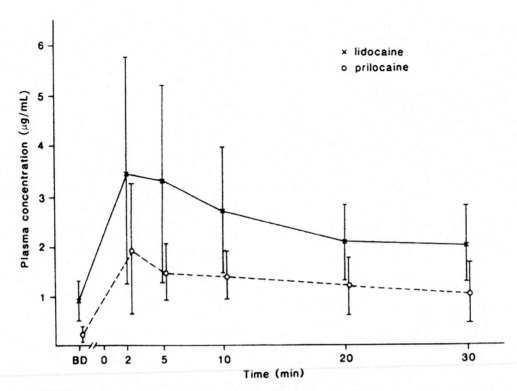

FIGURE 15-3. Mean plasma concentrations (±SD) of lidocaine and prilocaine in patients after intravenous regional anesthesia of the whole lower extremity using 6 mg/kg of the drugs. Statistically significant difference occurred only at the 5-minute time point. Modified from Valli HK, Rosenberg PH, Hekali R. Comparison of lidocaine and prilocaine for intravenous regional anesthesia of the whole lower extremity. *Reg Anesth* 1987;12:128–134, with permission.

the sensation of the hand and arm recovers slightly more slowly after both levobupivacaine 1.25 mg/mL or ropivacaine 2 mg/mL, the prolongation of the sensory block has only a limited clinical (surgical) significance.

Articaine

Another amide-type local anesthetic, articaine (4-methyl-3-[2-propylamino-propionamido]-thiophene-2-carboxylic acid hydrochloride), with properties similar to those of lidocaine, but less toxic (55) has also been used in IVRA and found to be more rapidly acting than lidocaine 5 mg/mL or prilocaine 5 mg/mL in patients (56)and similar to prilocaine 5 mg/mL in volunteers (57). In some of the volunteers, articaine caused an anaphylactoid-type reaction in the exposed arm, along the veins, suggesting a direct irritation of the endothelium by the acidic solution (57). In spite of the fact that articaine belongs to the amide-type local anesthetics, the breaking of an ester bond in the molecule in tissues and plasma inactivates the molecule (55). After the release of the tourniquet following IVRA, $t_{1/2\alpha}$ was 5 minutes and $t_{1/2\beta}$ was 59 minutes (56).

Procaine and Analogues

Ester-type local anesthetics have also been used in IVRA. In fact, procaine was the first such anesthetic used (4), followed by cocaine. Tetracaine has been studied (31). The North American questionnaire on IVRA (16) indicated that tetracaine was reported to be mixed with lidocaine by some anesthesiologists.

2-Chloroprocaine is an ester-type local anesthetic used in IVRA during the 1960s, initially in a solution containing both preservative and antioxidant (29,58). This formulation was soon abandoned because of the development of thrombophlebitis in the exposed veins. More recently, 40 mL of an additive-free 2-chloroprocaine 5 mg/mL solution has been found less irritating to the veins, but otherwise quite similar in effect as prilocaine 5 mg/mL (59,60). The fast breakdown of 2-chloroprocaine in plasma (half-life of approximately 22 seconds) is the basis for its low degree of systemic toxicity. However, by increasing the concentration of 2-chloroprocaine to 10 mg/mL (1%), CNS toxicity symptoms occur quite frequently after the release of the tourniquet cuff (61).

Conclusion

To summarize, the general experience with different local anesthetics in IVRA clearly shows no evidence base or clinically practical reason to use any drugs other than preservative-free lidocaine 5 mg/mL and preservative-free prilocaine 5 mg/mL. Both have been proved safe and effective in 50 years of use in IVRA.

Adjuncts to Local Anesthetics for Intravenous Regional Anesthesia

The general reasons for the addition of various kinds of drugs to local anesthetics for IVRA include certain more or less important drawbacks of IVRA, such as relatively slow onset, poor

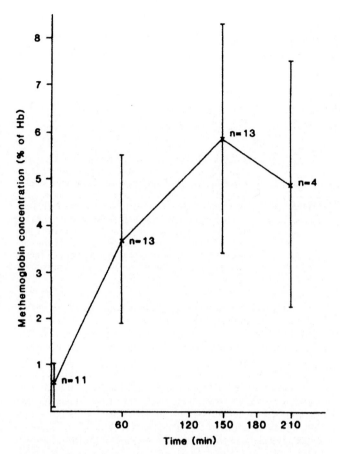

FIGURE 15-4. Mean methemoglobin concentrations (percentage of hemoglobin concentration, ± SD) after intravenous regional anesthesia of the whole lower extremity with prilocaine 6 mg/kg. Modified from Valli HK, Rosenberg PR, Hekali R. Comparison of lidocaine and prilocaine for intravenous regional anesthesia of the whole lower extremity. *Reg Anesth* 1987;12:128–134, with permission.

muscle relaxation, tourniquet pain, and short duration of postoperative analgesia.

Studies on opioids (fentanyl, sufentanil, morphine, meperidine, tramadol), nonsteroidal anti-inflammatories (NSAID; lysine acetylsalicylate, ketorolac, tenoxicam), α_2-adrenergic ag-

onists (clonidine), and muscle relaxants (atracurium, mivacurium, pancuronium) as adjuncts have been analyzed in a systematic review in 2002 (62). In addition to drugs, the influence of alkalinization of the solution and hypothermia of the extremity was also included in the analysis.

The only group of drugs showing clinical benefit was the NSAID group, providing prolonged postoperative analgesia and less need for supplemental analgesics; this prolonged analgesia extended for up to 24 hours when ketorolac was used (63,64).

Chronic Pain and Intravenous Regional Anesthesia

No convincing evidence in the literature suggests that any drug with analgesic potential is clinically beneficial for the treatment of complex regional pain syndromes (CRPS) (65,66).

No evidence suggests any benefit to the use of the commonly administered guanethidine, a sympatholytic drug earlier used for arterial hypertension (67). On the contrary, adverse effects, such as prolonged arterial hypotension, may hamper this therapy. Some support of analgesic effectiveness in the treatment of CRPS using the IVRA technique has been obtained with bretylium, an antiarrhythmic drug that blocks the release of norepinephrine from sympathetic nerve endings, added to lidocaine (68), and with ketanserin, a blocker of serotonin vasoconstrictor receptors ($5HT_2$), earlier tested for treatment of arterial hypertension (69). (See also Chapter 46.)

Clinical Pharmacology of Intravenous Regional Anesthesia

The peak blood or plasma concentrations of lidocaine are much higher after immediate IV bolus administration of a certain dose than after the release of the upper extremity tourniquet cuff in IVRA with the same dose (70). Prolongation of the tourniquet inflation time allows more local anesthetic to be bound to tissues and, thus, peak plasma concentrations decrease proportionally with duration of the tourniquet time (Fig. 15-5).

After a tourniquet time of 10 minutes, about 30% of the lidocaine dose is released immediately in the first flush of blood

PART II: TECHNIQUES

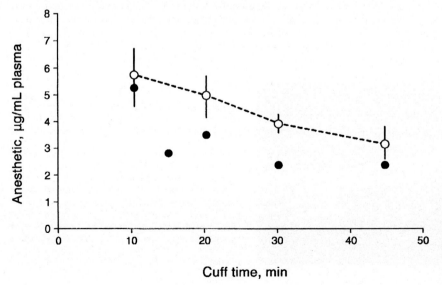

FIGURE 15-5. The longer the tourniquet time, the lower the arterial plasma concentrations of lidocaine at 1 minute after tourniquet cuff deflation in intravenous regional anesthesia. *Open circles* represent the mean of lidocaine concentrations after the use of a 1% solution; *closed circles* are individual values when a 0.5% solution of lidocaine was used. Modified from Tucker GT, Boas RA. Pharmacokinetic aspects of intravenous regional anesthesia. *Anesthesiology* 1971;34:538–549, with permission.

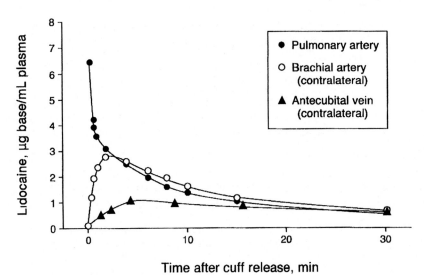

Time after cuff release, min

FIGURE 15-6. Plasma concentrations of lidocaine in a subject following tourniquet cuff release after intravenous regional anesthesia with lidocaine 3 mg/kg; tourniquet time was 45 minutes. The difference in concentrations in pulmonary artery and peripheral artery indicates immediate elimination of lidocaine into the lung tissue during its first pulmonary circulatory passage(s). Modified from Tucker GT, Boas RA. Pharmacokinetic aspects of intravenous regional anesthesia. *Anesthesiology* 1971;34:538–549, with permission.

after the deflation of the cuff; after 30 minutes, about 45% of the dose still remains in the arm (70). Prolonging the tourniquet time to 45 minutes, the release of a 30% portion takes about 4 minutes. In such circumstances, about 55% of the dose is still in the arm after 30 minutes. It is probable that such differences in peak plasma concentrations cannot be detected when tourniquet time exceeds 40 minutes (Fig. 15-6), in particular when the characteristics of local anesthetic include both great lipid solubility and extensive protein binding (71).

Occasionally observed secondary plasma concentration peaks (48,72) may result from exercise of the limb and extreme vasodilatation in the immediate postinflation period. By administering the same dose as a larger volume of more dilute solution, plasma concentrations after tourniquet cuff deflation seem to decrease slightly (70), but in IVRA with prilocaine of the lower extremity below the knee, no difference was seen when the same dose had been administered in a more dilute solution (73).

Drugs released from the blocked extremity first pass through the lungs before entering the systemic arterial circulation (Fig. 15-5). The lungs, therefore, are in a highly strategic position, clearing the blood of a substantial amount of local anesthetic and thus protecting the CNS and heart from the toxic effect of high concentrations of drug. One reason for the clinical popularity of prilocaine in IVRA is its low degree of toxicity, which is due, in part, to the rapid uptake into the lungs, to a greater extent than that of lidocaine, during the first pulmonary passage (74). The pH of lung tissue is low in comparison with the

pH of plasma, thus enhancing uptake of local anesthetic by ion trapping mechanisms (75).

Mild CNS toxicity sometimes occurs soon after the deflation of the tourniquet cuff, even when prilocaine is used (41,60). Such symptoms have included numbness of the tongue, tinnitus, and visual disturbances. Convulsions and loss of consciousness associated with recommended doses of lidocaine or prilocaine in IVRA are rare. However, severe intoxications have been reported when bupivacaine has been used for IVRA, either due to leakage under the tourniquet cuff (Fig. 15-7) or due to sudden release into the circulation because of faulty equipment (51).

As mentioned earlier, low doses of ropivacaine (80 mg) (52–54) and levobupivacaine (50 mg) (35) have been safely used in IVRA of the upper extremity. Higher doses of ropivacaine (1.2 and 1.8 mg/kg) have also been tested in volunteers in a feasibility study (38). Total plasma concentrations of ropivacaine after cuff deflation in the studies using the fixed low dose (80 mg) vary considerably and reach mean peak levels of 0.6 μg/mL (54) and 1.2 μg/mL in 3 to 5 minutes (53). Mild CNS symptoms after tourniquet cuff deflation occurred in one of five volunteers who received 1.8 mg/kg, and in six of the ten volunteers who received 80 mg (53), whereas none of the 30 patients in the clinical study (54) who received 80 mg experienced any symptoms. Peak total plasma concentrations of local anesthetic after tourniquet cuff release do not seem to correlate with occurrence and severity of toxic CNS symptoms (38,73). This may be due, in part, to the fact that it is the unbound

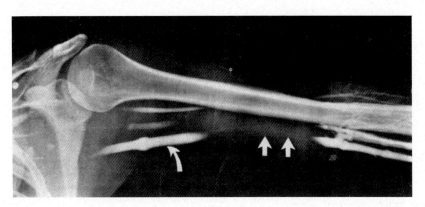

FIGURE 15-7. Phlebography performed in a female volunteer in a similar fashion as an intravenous regional anesthesia. The tourniquet cuff pressure was 250 mm Hg. Instead of local anesthetic, 50 mL of contrast medium was injected into a vein on the dorsum of the hand at a speed of 1 mL/sec. After 15 seconds, contrast medium was noticed in the axillary vein (*curved arrow*), and there were streaks of contrast medium under the inflated cuff (*straight arrows*). From Rosenberg PH, Kalso EA, Tuominen MK, et al. Acute bupivacaine toxicity as a result of venous leakage under the tourniquet cuff during a Bier block. *Anesthesiology* 1983;58:95–98, with permission.

drug concentration in plasma, not the total concentration, that causes toxic effects (76), and the unbound concentration was not measured in any of the above-mentioned ropivacaine IVRA studies. Toxic symptoms in the volunteers receiving 40 mL of levobupivacaine 1.25 mg/mL for upper extremity IVRA were not encountered (35).

As mentioned earlier, an increase occurs in met-Hb concentration in blood formed after IVRA with prilocaine (41,77). After IVRA of the whole lower extremity with prilocaine 6 mg/kg, the rise in met-Hb was found to be quite modest, and maximum mean percentage of hemoglobin was approximately 6% (41). It has been estimated that cyanosis becomes visible when methemoglobin concentrations exceed 10% to 15%, and symptoms of hypoxemia may occur when the percentage rises to 30% (78).

Allergy to amide-type local anesthetics is very rare (79). There are a few case reports of hypersensitivity reactions to plain prilocaine 5 mg/mL in IVRA (80), as well as reports on occasional skin reactions and venous irritation in the exposed area associated with the use of articaine (57), 2-chloroprocaine, and prilocaine (59). The risk of hypersensitivity-type skin reactions is increased when the local anesthetic solution contains the antimicrobial preservative methylparaben (80,81). As a rule, only preservative-free local anesthetic solutions should be used in IVRA, in order to avoid irritation and the anaphylaxis occasionally caused by preservatives such as methylparaben or bisulfites.

CLINICAL ASPECTS OF INTRAVENOUS REGIONAL ANESTHESIA

Intravenous Regional Anesthesia of Upper Limb

Indications for IVRA of the upper extremity are surgery of the hand, wrist, forearm, or elbow that normally will last less than 1 hour. The surgical diagnoses include carpal tunnel syndrome, ganglion of the wrist and hand region, tendon ruptures of the fingers, and Colles fracture.

General contraindications are obviously patient refusal, and in addition, severe arterial hypertension, athletic build (large, strong muscles), skeletal muscle disorder, increased intracranial pressure (ICP) in a traumatized patient (risk of additional increase in ICP when tourniquet cuff is deflated), and known hypersensitivity to local anesthetics.

When surgery is performed as a day-case, usually no premedication is given, but when prolonged surgery is expected, a small dose of oral or IV diazepam or midazolam may be administered before the start. Presently, it is common to premedicate day-case patients with an oral NSAID or cyclooxygenase (COX) inhibitor with the aim of reducing postoperative pain (82,83), but whether this reduces or prevents tourniquet-induced pain during surgery has remained a matter of controversy.

Patients must be monitored in the same way as any other anesthetized patients in the operating room, using electrocardiogram (ECG), automatic noninvasive arterial blood pressure measurement, and pulse oximetry. Since a large dose of a local anesthetic will be given IV, preparedness for immediate cardiopulmonary resuscitation by the advanced life support principle and for treatment of convulsions with propofol or thiopental and succinylcholine is required. Propofol is equally effective as thiopental in aborting grand mal seizures due to toxic doses of local anesthetics (84,85). It is possible that propofol should be preferred in cases of severe local anesthetic toxicity because the local anesthetic will partition into the lipid phase of propofol and a portion of at least the more lipid soluble local anesthetics is thus temporarily eliminated (86,87).

A small plastic IV cannula (20–22-gauge) is placed as peripherally as possible on the arm to be blocked and another is placed in the opposite extremity for supplemental drug administration. Sometimes an IV infusion of Ringer's solution or physiologic saline may be needed, especially if there is a change in operation schedules that causes a prolonged latency between past fluid intake and start of surgery, or if the patient is nauseated.

A suitable piece of a cotton stockinette is placed on the arm, or alternatively, a thin, soft, unwrinkled cast padding fabric is wrapped around the limb. A contoured double-bladder tourniquet or two separate tourniquets (each approximately 7 cm wide) is fitted around the padding, so that the tourniquet edges are not in direct contact with the skin (Fig. 15-2). The Velcro straps are fastened, and the security ribbons are thoroughly tied around the cuffs, over the straps.

For exsanguination, the arm is first kept elevated for 1 to 2 minute, then an Esmarch rubber bandage (or equivalent elastic bandage) is wrapped tightly around the arm, from the fingertips all the way to and partly over the distal of the two brachial tourniquet cuffs. Then the distal cuff is inflated to a pressure approximately 100 mm Hg above the current systolic arterial pressure, normally to 200 to 275 mm Hg in adults. The pressure reading and lack of peripheral arterial pulsation, by hand or by pulse oximeter, must be verified. Thereafter the proximal cuff is inflated to the same pressure and the distal cuff is deflated. Again, the pressure reading and lack of pulsation are verified. The elastic bandage is removed. Before the start of injection of local anesthetic, it is advisable to visually observe the veins of the exsanguinated arm for 1 to 2 minutes to note any undesired venous filling. If refilling is clearly visible, the exsanguination process and tourniquet inflation procedures must be repeated, and the tourniquet cuff pressure may be raised by 30 to 50 mm Hg. If venous refilling still occurs, the IVRA technique should be abandoned and another technique chosen.

In case of trauma or infection, exsanguination by the wrapping method may not be feasible, and adequate exsanguination using another technique, although not as efficacious as that using an elastic bandage (Table 15-2), can be obtained for IVRA.

The local anesthetic solution (approximately 3 mg/kg of preservative- and antioxidant-free lidocaine 5 mg/mL or prilocaine 5 mg/mL) is injected slowly (e.g., at a rate of 20 mL/min). Faster rates may raise the venous pressure to near that of tourniquet cuff pressure (27,88,89). The onset of analgesia of the skin normally occurs in a few minutes, but surgical anesthesia by lidocaine or prilocaine 5 mg/mL may not develop until 15 to 20 minutes. With the use of more concentrated solutions of local anesthetic (e.g., prilocaine 7.5 mg/mL), the onset of surgical anesthesia may occur slightly faster. Since ischemia is a major part of the mechanism of action of IVRA, a partly incomplete block often develops further to completeness merely through patiently waiting for a few more minutes.

When the extremity is prepared and scrubbed for surgery, it is important to prevent the flow of disinfectant solution under the tourniquet cuff because it may easily damage the ischemic skin.

Tourniquet pain may sometimes be problematic, especially if surgery unexpectedly will become prolonged. Pain is often eased substantially by switching the pressurization to the distal cuff, and deflating the proximal cuff. This procedure is critical and should be performed in the presence of the attending anesthesiologist because a mistake may lead to severe local anesthetic intoxication. In order to guarantee the tissue binding of a substantial amount of the local anesthetic, cuff pressure switching should not be performed until about 20 minutes after injection of the local anesthetic. If the tourniquet pain continues or escalates, small doses of short-acting opioids, fentanyl, or alfentanil, may be administered intravenously.

MODIFICATIONS OF INTRAVENOUS REGIONAL ANESTHESIA OF THE ARM

Second Wrap

Sometimes oozing at the site of surgery may become a problem in spite of the initial exsanguination with an elastic bandage and adequate tourniquet pressure. A second wrap with a sterile elastic bandage from the fingers all the way up over the distal cuff will dry up the surgical field (90). It has been shown that a second wrap performed 15 to 20 minutes after the local anesthetic injection does not influence the quality of the sensory and motor block, but the tolerance of the tourniquet cuff seems to be improved (91). As the second-wrap technique includes the release of both tourniquet cuffs for a very short time, a small amount of local anesthetic will inevitably escape into the circulation when the wrap is completed. Therefore the technique is suitable only when local anesthetics with low degrees of toxic potential (such as prilocaine, lidocaine, articaine, or 2-chloroprocaine) are used; even then, the second wrap should not be performed until about 20 minutes after the injection of the local anesthetic dose, usually immediately before surgery (Fig. 15-7).

Additional Tourniquets

Peripherally injected local anesthetic solution may be forced to distribute as peripherally as possible by applying a tight temporary tourniquet (e.g., a Penrose drain) around the forearm before the injection and keeping it in place for 5 to 10 minutes after the injection. Nerve endings in the periphery will be rapidly blocked, allowing start of surgery in this region a few minutes earlier than usual (92).

INTRAVENOUS REGIONAL ANESTHESIA OF THE LOWER EXTREMITY

Aspects of Application

Although the technique of IVRA of the lower extremity is, in principle, similar to that of the upper extremity, certain important differences must be kept in mind. First, as the volume of the solution for the block of the whole lower extremity must be large (approximately double in comparison with that for the arm), also the dose of local anesthetic is large. The risk of local anesthetic intoxication is great if there is leakage past the tourniquet cuff, and also when the cuff is deflated at the end of a short surgical case. Second, the cuff pressure in the thigh tourniquet must be relatively high—300 mm Hg (sometimes

even higher) in adults—which results in a high incidence of tourniquet pain (41).

In adults, two separate 9-cm wide tourniquets are placed upon a cotton stockinette around the thigh. The tourniquet must not be in direct contact with the skin, and the pneumatic bladder must surround the thigh by more than one and a half turns.

A venous cannula for local anesthetic injection is placed as peripherally as possible. Exsanguination is performed by winding an Esmarch bandage, or another type of elastic bandage tightly from toes to thigh. Exsanguination by bandage should not be performed in patients suspected of having developed deep vein thrombosis (e.g., in elderly patients with a traumatized leg).

The preferred local anesthetic is plain prilocaine, 6 mg/kg, diluted so that the total volume is approximately 100 mL for a 70-kg patient. Lidocaine, 4 mg/kg, may also be used. In short-lasting surgery of the foot or ankle, the distal cuff may be applied on the calf, clearly below the head of the fibula (away from the peroneal nerve), and the proximal cuff on the thigh (Fig. 15-1). The leg is exsanguinated with a bandage up to the tourniquet on the calf, which is inflated. The local anesthetic volume and dose can be the same as for an upper extremity IVRA (i.e., 35–50 mL of lidocaine 5 mg/mL or prilocaine 5 mg/mL). The proximal tourniquet on the thigh is not inflated, but is kept ready as a back-up, if the distal cuff fails.

Surgery indications for lower extremity IVRA are short-lasting orthopedic procedures (30–45 min) on the foot, removal of plates and screws from the bones below the knee, and foreign-body removal from the foot.

Two Tourniquet Technique for Intravenous Regional Anesthesia of the Knee

A similar principle as that initially described by Bier in 1908 (4), providing IVRA between two tourniquet cuffs, has recently been rediscovered for anesthesia of the knee (93). After exsanguination with an Esmarch bandage on the leg, first a double-cuff tourniquet is inflated on the thigh and 40 mL of lidocaine 5 mg/mL is injected. Immediately thereafter, another single-cuffed tourniquet is placed on the calf, followed by re-exsanguinated with the bandage, from toes to the distal cuff, and the cuff is inflated. Complete anesthesia develops between the two cuffs, with patchy anesthesia distal to the calf tourniquet cuff. Both cuffs are kept inflated during surgery (knee arthroscopy). The principal advantage of this modification is the use of a relatively small dose (volume) of the local anesthetic.

TOURNIQUET CUFF DEFLATION

Severe local anesthetic intoxication after the release of the tourniquet cuff is rare when 40 mL of 5 mg/mL concentrations of lidocaine, prilocaine, articaine, or 2-chloroprocaine have been used for upper extremity IVRA. As a rule, the tourniquet cuff should not be released before 20 minutes have passed from the injection of the local anesthetic. Such precaution guarantees that a substantial amount of the drug has been taken up by the tissues, and the bolus-type release of the local anesthetic remaining in the veins will not induce severe toxicity. Occasionally, mild CNS toxicity symptoms (dizziness, tinnitus, lightheadedness) occur, more often after lidocaine than after prilocaine (41). The patient may experience such symptoms even when relatively heavily sedated (94).

After the use of the above-mentioned doses, the tourniquet cuff may normally be released in one step, and the tourniquet is immediately removed to allow unobstructed circulation to the skin. However, if for some reason the cuff must be deflated earlier than 20 minutes after local anesthetic injection, or if the patients has a disease that may increase the risk of cardiotoxicity, the cuff may be deflated and reinflated in cycles until confirmation of no complications is made. The reinflation should not be longer that 30 seconds, in order to avoid stasis of blood and tissue swelling.

INTRAVENOUS REGIONAL ANESTHESIA IN CHILDREN

The IVRA technique is applicable in children, although usually not in children under 3 years of age, for operations of short duration (less than 20 minutes) (95,96). Indications include, for example, repositioning of painful fractures of the elbow and forearm and minor operations of the hand or foot. There are case reports of successful treatment of complex regional pain syndrome in children (11 and 15 years old) with the IVRA technique using lidocaine and ketorolac (97).

In small children, local anesthetic cream or ointment is useful for pain-free IV cannulation; rarely, exsanguination with an Esmarch bandage is needed. Elevation of the extremity for 1 to 2 minutes may suffice.

For IVRA of the upper extremity in small children, a single tourniquet is used, but in older children with room on the arm, specially designed double-cuff pediatric tourniquets are applied. The cuffs are pressurized to 50 to 75 mm Hg above the systolic arterial pressure, and the switching-between-cuff principle is practiced, as in adults.

Whole lower extremity IVRA can be provided only to older children, because of need for cooperation and the patient's acceptance of a tourniquet cuff pressure of 200 to 250 mm Hg.

The local anesthetic dose has to be modified according to the size of the extremity and the child, starting from 10 to 15 mL (lidocaine or prilocaine 5 mg/mL) in a 3- to 4-year-old child to 25 to 30 mL in a 11- to 12-year-old child. For the whole lower extremity, volumes (doses) are approximately double.

References

1. Holmes C. Intravenous regional analgesia: A useful method of producing analgesia of the limb. *Lancet* 1963;1:245–247.
2. Rosenberg PH. Intravenous regional anesthesia. In: Brown DL, ed. *Regional Anesthesia and Analgesia*. Philadelphia: W. B. Saunders; 1996:385–394.
3. Holmes C. Intravenous regional nerve block. In: Cousins MJ, Bridenbaugh PO, eds. *Neural Blockade in Clinical Anesthesia and Management of Pain*, 3rd ed. Philadelphia: Lippincott-Raven Publishers; 1998:385–409.
4. Bier A. Ueber einen neuen Weg Localanästhesie an den Gliedmassen zu erzeugen. *Arch Klin Chir* 1908;86:1007–1016.
5. Fleming SA, Veiga-Pires JA, McCutcheon RM, et al. A demonstration of the site of action of intravenous lignocaine. *Can Anaesth Soc J* 1966;13:21–27.
6. Sorbie C, Chancha P. Regional anaesthesia by the intravenous route. *Br Med J* 1965;1:957–960.
7. Raj PP, Garcia CE, Burleson JW, et al. The site of action of intravenous regional anesthesia. *Anesth Analg* 1972;51:776–786.
8. Hallén J, Rawal N, Hartwig P, et al. Pharmacokinetic and pharmacodynamic studies of 11C-lidocaine following intravenous regional anaesthesia (IVRA) using positron emission tomography (abstract). *Acta Anaesthesiol Scand* 1991;35[Suppl 96]:214.
9. Finucane BT, McClain DA, Smith SR. A double-blind comparison of etidocaine and lidocaine for IV regional anesthesia. *Reg Anesth* 1980;5[Suppl]:17–18.
10. Magora F, Stern L, Zylber-Katz E, et al. Prolonged effect of bupivacaine hydrochloride after cuff release in i.v. regional anaesthesia. *Br J Anaesth* 1980;52:1131–1136.
11. Lundborg G, ed. *Nerve Injury and Repair*, 2nd ed. Philadelphia: Churchill Livingstone, 2005.
12. Lewis T, Pickering GW, Rothschild P. Centripetal paralysis arising out of arrested blood-flow to the limb, including notes on a form of tingling. *Heart* 1931;16:1–32.
13. Lundborg G. Ischemic nerve injury. Experimental studies on intraneural microvascular pathophysiology and nerve function in a limb, subjected to temporary circulatory arrest. *Scand J Plast Reconstr Surg* 1970;[Suppl]:1–113.
14. Iizuka T. Effect of ischemia on peripheral nerve-evoked potential: Experimental and clinical study. *J Jap Orthop Ass* 1984;58:307–322.
15. Heavner JE, Leinonen L, Haasio J, et al. Interaction of lidocaine and hypothermia in Bier blocks in volunteers. *Anesth Analg* 1989;69:53–59.
16. Henderson C, Warriner B, McEwen JA, Merrick PM. A North American survey of intravenous regional anesthesia. *Anesth Analg* 1997;85:858–863.
17. Hurst LN, Weiglein O, Brown WF, et al. The pneumatic tourniquet: A biomechanical and electrophysiological study. *Plast Reconstr Surg* 1981;67:648–652.
18. Yates SK, Hurst LN, Brown WF. The pathogenesis of pneumatic tourniquet paralysis in man. *J Neurol Neurosurg Psychiatr* 1981;44:759–767.
19. Wakai A, Wang JH, Winter DC, et al. Tourniquet-induced systemic inflammatory response in extremity surgery. *J Trauma* 2001;51:922–926.
20. Niemi TT, Kuitunen AH, Vahtera EM, Rosenberg PH. Haemostatic changes caused by i.v. regional anaesthesia with lignocaine. *Br J Anaesth* 1996;76:822–828.
21. Steinau H-U, ed. *Major Limb Replantation and Postischemia Syndrome: Investigation of Acute Ischemia-induced Myopathy and Reperfusion Injury*. New York: Springer Verlag, 1988.
22. Solonen KA, Hjelt L. Morphological changes in striated muscle during ischaemia. A clinical and histological study in man. *Acta Orthop Scand* 1968;39:13–19.
23. Patterson S, Kleinerman L. The effect of pneumatic tourniquets on the ultrastructure of skeletal muscle. *J Bone Joint Surg* 1979;61:178–183.
24. Blaisdell FW. The pathophysiology of skeletal muscle ischemia and the reperfusion syndrome: A review. *Cardiovasc Surg* 2002;10:620–630.
25. Blond L, Madsen JL. Exsanguination of the upper limb in healthy young volunteers. *J Bone Joint Surg* 2002;84B:489–491.
26. Mabee J, Orlinsky M. Bier block exsanguination: A volumetric comparison and venous pressure. *Acad Emerg Med* 2000;7:105–113.
27. Haasio J, Hiippala S, Rosenberg PH. Intravenous regional anaesthesia of the arm. Effect of the technique of exsanguination on the quality of anaesthesia and prilocaine plasma concentrations. *Anaesthesia* 1989;44:19–21.
28. Eckhoff NL. Tourniquet paralysis: Plea for extended use of pneumatic tourniquet. *Lancet* 1931;2:243–245.
29. Eerola R. A comparative study of carticaine and prilocaine in regional intravenous analgesia (German). *Prakt Anästh* 1974;9:171–175.
30. Ware RJ. Intravenous regional analgesia using bupivacaine. *Anaesthesia* 1975;30:817–822.
31. Dickler DJ, Friedman PL, Susman IC. Intravenous regional anesthesia with chloroprocaine (abstract). *Anesthesiology* 1965;26:244–245.
32. Hitzrot JM. Intravenous local anaesthesia. *Ann Surg* 1909:1:782–785.
33. Evans CJ, Dewar JA, Boyes RN, et al. Residual nerve block following intravenous regional anaesthesia. *Br J Anaesth* 1974:46:668–670.
34. Atanassoff PG, Aouad R, Hartmannsgruber MW, et al. Levobupivacaine 0.125% and lidocaine 0.5% for intravenous regional anesthesia in volunteers. *Anesthesiology* 2002;97:325–328.
35. Cox JMR. Intravenous regional anaesthesia. *Can Anaesth Soc J* 1964;11:503–508.
36. Hooper RL. Intravenous regional analgesia: A report on a new local anaesthetic agent. *Can Anaesth Soc J* 1964;11:247–251.
37. Durrani Z, Russell J, Zsigmond EK, et al. Tetracaine for intravenous regional anesthesia (abstract). *Reg Anesth* 1982;7:81–82.
38. Chan VWS, Weisbrod MJ, Kaszas Z, Dragomir C. Comparison of ropivacaine and lidocaine for intravenous regional anesthesia in volunteers: A preliminary study on anesthetic efficacy and blood level. *Anesthesiology* 1999;90:1602–1608.
39. Suzuki N, Pitkänen M. Sariola H, et al. The effect of plain 0.5% 2-chloroprocaine on venous endothelium after intravenous regional anaesthesia in the rabbit. *Acta Anaesthesiol Scand* 1994;38:653–656.
40. Adams JP, Dealy EJ, Kenmore PI. Intravenous regional anesthesia in hand surgery. *J Bone Joint Surg* 1964;46A:811–816.
41. Valli HK, Rosenberg PH, Hekali R. Comparison of lidocaine and prilocaine for intravenous regional anesthesia of the whole lower extremity. *Reg Anesth* 1987;12:128–134.

42. Vasters FG, Eberhart LH, Koch T, et al. Risk factors for prilocaine-induced methaemoglobinaemia following peripheral regional anaesthesia. *Eur J Anaesthesiol* 2006;23:760–765.

43. Hjelm M, Holmdahl MH. Clinical chemistry of prilocaine and clinical evaluation of methaemoglobinaemia induced by this agent. *Acta Anaesthesiol Scand* 1965;16[Suppl]:161–170.

44. Hall AH, Kulig KW, Rumack BH. Drug- and chemical-induced methaemoglobinaemia. Clinical features and management. *Med Toxicol* 1986;1:253–260.

45. Tryba M, Zenz M, Hausmann E. Controlled study on intravenous regional anesthesia using high and low concentration prilocaine (German). *Regional-Anästhesie* 1983;6:27–29.

46. Prien T, Goeters C. Intravenous regional anesthesia of the arm and foot using 0.5, 0.75 and 1.0 percent prilocaine (German). *Anaesth Intensivther Notf Med* 1990;25:59–63.

47. Solonen KA, Tarkkanen L. Intravenous anaesthesia in surgery of the hand. *Arch Orthop Unfallchir* 1966;60:115–121.

48. Thorn-Alquist AM. Intravenous regional anaesthesia. *Acta Anaesthesiol Scand* 1971;[Suppl 40]:1–35.

49. Gooding JM, Tavakoli MM, Fitzpatrick WO, et al. Bupivacaine: Preferred agent for intravenous regional anesthesia? *South Med J* 1981;74:1282–1283.

50. Rosenberg PH, Kalso EA, Tuominen MK, et al. Acute bupivacaine toxicity as a result of venous leakage under the tourniquet cuff during a Bier block. *Anesthesiology* 1983;58:95–98.

51. Heath NL. Deaths after intravenous regional anaesthesia (editorial). *Br Med J* 1982;285:913–914.

52. Haartmannsgruber MW, Silverman DG, Halaszynski TM, et al. Comparison of ropivacaine 0.2% and lidocaine 0.5% for intravenous regional anesthesia in volunteers. *Anesth Analg* 1999;89:727–731.

53. Atanassoff PG, Ocampo CA, Bande MC, et al. Ropivacaine 0.2% and lidocaine 0.5% for intravenous regional anesthesia in outpatient surgery. *Anesthesiology* 2001;95:627–631.

54. Niemi TT, Neuvonen PJ, Rosenberg PH. Comparison of ropivacaine 2 mg ml⁻¹ and prilocaine 5 mg ml⁻¹ for i.v. regional anaesthesia in outpatient surgery. *Br J Anaesth* 2006;96:640–644.

55. Vree TB, Gielen MJM. Clinical pharmacology and the use of articaine for local and regional anaesthesia. *Best Pract Res Clin Anaesthesiol* 2005;19:293–308.

56. Simon MA, Gielen MJ, Alberink N, et al. Intravenous regional anesthesia (IVRA) with 0.5% articaine, 0.5% lidocaine, or 0.5% prilocaine. A double-blind randomized clinical study. *Reg Anesth* 1997;22:29–34.

57. Pitkänen MT, Xu M, Haasio J, Rosenberg PH. Comparison of 0.5% articaine and 0.5% prilocaine in intravenous regional anesthesia of the arm: A cross-over study in volunteers. *Reg Anesth Pain Med* 1999;24:131–135.

58. Harris WH. Choice of anesthetic agent for intravenous regional anesthesia. *Acta Anaesthesiol Scand* 1969;[Suppl 36]:47–52.

59. Pitkänen MT, Suzuki N, Rosenberg PH. Intravenous regional anaesthesia with 0.5% prilocaine or 0.5% chloroprocaine. A double-blind comparison in volunteers. *Anaesthesia* 1992;47:618–619.

60. Pitkänen M, Kyttä J, Rosenberg PH. Comparison of 2-chloroprocaine and prilocaine for intravenous regional anaesthesia of the arm: A clinical study. *Anaesthesia* 1993;48:1091–1093.

61. Marsch SC, Sluga M, Studer W, et al. 0.5% versus 1.0% 2-chloroprocaine for intravenous regional anesthesia: A prospective, randomized, double-blind trial. *Anesth Analg* 2004;98:1789–1793.

62. Choyce A, Peng P. A systematic review of adjuncts for intravenous regional anesthesia for surgical procedures. *Can J Anesth* 2002;49:32–45.

63. Reuben SS, Steinberg RB, Kreitzer JM, et al. Intravenous regional anesthesia using lidocaine and ketorolac. *Anesth Analg* 1995;81:110–113.

64. Reuben SS, Duprat KM. Comparison of wound infiltration with ketorolac versus intravenous regional anesthesia with ketorolac for postoperative analgesia following ambulatory hand surgery. *Reg Anesth* 1996;21:565–568.

65. Kingrey WS. A critical review of controlled clinical trials for peripheral neuropathic pain and complex regional pain syndromes. *Pain* 1997;73:123–139.

66. Rowbotham MC. Pharmacologic management of complex regional pain syndrome. *Clin J Pain* 2006;22:425–429.

67. Jadad AR, Carroll D, Glynn CJ, et al. Intravenous regional sympathetic blockade for pain relief in reflex sympathetic dystrophy: A systematic review and a randomized, double-blind crossover study. *J Pain Sympt Manag* 1995;10:13–20.

68. Hord AH, Rooks MD, Stephens BO, et al. Intravenous regional bretylium and lidocaine for treatment of reflex sympathetic dystrophy: A randomized, double-blind study. *Anesth Analg* 11992;74:818–821.

69. Hanna MH, Peat SJ. Ketanserin in reflex sympathetic dystrophy. A double-blind placebo controlled cross-over trial. *Pain* 1989;38:145–150.

70. Tucker GT, Boas RA. Pharmacokinetic aspects of intravenous regional anesthesia. *Anesthesiology* 1971;34:538–549.

71. Kalso A, Tuominen M, Rosenberg PH, et al. Bupivacaine blood levels after intravenous regional anaesthesia of the arm. *Regional-Anästhesie* 1982;5:81–84.

72. Cotev S, Robin GC. Experimental studies on intravenous regional anaesthesia using radioactive lignocaine. *Br J Anaesth* 1966;38:936–940.

73. Valli H, Rosenberg PH. Intravenous regional anaesthesia below the knee. A cross-over study with prilocaine in volunteers. *Anaesthesia* 1986;41:1196–1201.

74. Arthur GR. Distribution and elimination of local anaesthetic agents: The role of lung, liver and kidney. Ph.D. Thesis. University of Edinburgh, Scotland, 1981.

75. Post C, Eriksdotter-Behm K. Dependence of lung uptake of lidocaine in vivo on blood pH. *Acta Pharmacol Toxicol (Copenh)* 1982;51:136–140.

76. Tucker GT. Pharmacokinetics of local anaesthetic. *Br J Anaesth* 1986;58:717–731.

77. Harris WH, Cole DW, Mital M, et al. Methemoglobin formation and oxygen transport following intravenous regional anesthesia using prilocaine. *Anesthesiology* 1968;29:65–69.

78. Adriani I, Naraghi M. Drug induced methemoglobinemia: Local anesthetics. *Anesthesiol Rev* 1985;12:54–59.

79. Sindel LJ, deShazo RD. Accident resulting from local anesthetics. True or false allergy? *Clin Rev Allergy* 1991;9:379–395.

80. Ruiz K, Stevens JD, Train JJ, et al. Anaphylactoid reactions to prilocaine. *Anaesthesia* 1987;42:1078–1080.

81. Kajimoto Y, Rosenberg ME, Kyttä J, et al. Anaphylactoid skin reactions after intravenous regional anaesthesia using 0.5% prilocaine with or without preservative: A double-blind study. *Acta Anaesthesiol Scand* 1995;39:782–784.

82. Watcha MF, Issioui T, Klein KW, White PF. Costs and effectiveness of rofecoxib, celecoxib, and acetaminophen for preventing pain after ambulatory otolaryngologic surgery. *Anesth Analg* 2003;96:987–994.

83. Kim JT, Sherman O, Cuff G, et al. A double-blind prospective comparison of rofecoxib vs ketorolac in reducing postoperative pain after arthroscopic knee surgery. *J Clin Anesth* 2005;17:439–443.

84. Heavner JE, Arthur J, Zou J, et al. Comparison of propofol with thiopentone for treatment of bupivacaine-induced seizures in rats. *Br J Anaesth* 1003;71:715–719.

85. Ohmura S, Ohta T, Yamamoto K, et al. A comparison of the effects of propofol and sevoflurane on the systemic toxicity of intravenous bupivacaine in rats. *Anesth Analg* 1999;88:155–159.

86. Weinberg G, Ripper R, Feinstein DL, et al. Lipid emulsion infusion rescues dogs from bupivacaine-induced cardiac toxicity. *Reg Anesth Pain Med* 2003;28:198–202.

87. Litz RJ, Popp M, Stehr SN, et al. Successful resuscitation of a patient with ropivacaine-induced asystole after axillary plexus block using lipid infusion. *Anaesthesia* 2006;61:800–801.

88. Duggan J, McKeown DW, Scott DB. Venous pressure in intravenous regional anaesthesia. *Reg Anesth* 1984;9:70–72.

89. Lawes EG, Johnson T, Pritchard P, et al. Venous pressure during simulated Bier's block. *Anaesthesia* 1984;39:147–149.

90. Haas LM, Lendeen FH. Improved intravenous regional anesthesia for surgery of the hand, wrist, and forearm. The second wrap. *J Hand Surg* 1978;3:194–195.

91. Rawal N, Hallén J, Amilon A, et al. Improvement in i.v. regional anaesthesia by re-exsanguination before surgery. *Br J Anaesth* 1993;70:280–285.

92. Eastwood D, Griffiths S, Jack J, et al. Bier's block: An improved technique. *Injury* 1986;17:187–188.

93. Al-Metwall R, Mowafi HA. A modification of the inter-cuff technique of IVRA for the use in knee arthroscopy. *Can J Anesth* 2002;49:687–689.

94. Haasio J, Hekali R, Rosenberg PH. Influence of premedication on lignocaine-induced acute toxicity and plasma concentrations of lignocaine. *Br J Anaesth* 1988;61:131–134.

95. FitzGerald B. Intravenous regional anaesthesia in children. *Br J Anaesth* 1976;48:485–486.

96. Rudzinski JP, Ampel LL. Pediatric application of intravenous regional anesthesia. *Reg Anesth* 1983;8:69–72.

97. Suresh S, Wheeler M, Patel A. Case series: IV regional anesthesia with ketorolac and lidocaine: Is it effective for the management of complex regional pain syndrome 1 in children and adolescents? *Anesth Analg* 2003;96:694–695.

CHAPTER 16 ■ INTERCOSTAL, INTRAPLEURAL, AND PERIPHERAL BLOCKADE OF THE THORAX AND ABDOMEN

DOMINIC C. HARMON AND GEORGE D. SHORTEN

Peripheral nerve blocks (PNBs) are applicable to virtually every thoracic and abdominal surgical procedure. Regional anesthesia and, in particular, PNBs can provide the basic foundation to allow a considerably less stressful operation, less deterioration in many physiologic functions, and improved postoperative analgesia.

For the purposes of this chapter, the thorax and abdomen will be considered separately. The thoracic component will concentrate on intercostal and paravertebral blocks, whereas the abdominal component will deal with ilioinguinal/iliohypogastric nerve block, rectus sheath block, and the recently described transversus abdominis plane (TAP) block. Intrapleural blockade applies to both regions. Ultrasound-guided techniques will be discussed where relevant.

The trunk is divided into thorax and abdomen. The nerve supply to the thorax is derived from the anterior primary rami of T1 to T6. The nerve supply of the abdominal wall is derived from the anterior primary rami of T6 to L1. The sensory components of these nerves branch in the mid-axillary line. Important surface anatomic landmarks are (Fig. 16-1):

■ Manubriosternal joint	T2
■ Nipple line	T4
■ Xiphoid process	T6
■ Umbilicus	T10
■ Symphysis pubis	T12

ANALGESIA IN THE POSTOPERATIVE PERIOD

Assessment of the impact of anesthetic and analgesic techniques commonly focuses on the incidence of mortality and major complications after major surgical procedures. Nevertheless, other postoperative adverse events such as pain, nausea and vomiting, and urinary retention may also impair patient comfort, recovery, and rehabilitation after minor and major surgical procedures. In addition, growing evidence suggests that acute postoperative events may lead to long-term consequences. For example, uncontrolled postoperative pain is related to the development of chronic pain syndromes (1); to postoperative myocardial ischaemia and infarction, which are risk factors for death from cardiac causes in the following months (2); and to postoperative cognitive decline, which can be persistent (3). As postoperative pain is often the predominant symptom, it can be considered an important outcome of surgery.

Pain is a key component in the alteration of lung function after thoracic and upper abdominal surgery. This highlights the importance of providing effective postoperative analgesia to reduce pulmonary complications and attenuate the stress response. Minor surgeries, such chest and abdominal wall procedures, are often performed on an outpatient basis. Postoperative analgesia in this setting is often not optimum (4), with associated adverse patient outcomes (4).

Peripheral nerve blockade has particular advantages over other analgesic techniques such as neuroaxial blocks and systemic opioids (5). This is also true in the setting of thoracic and abdominal surgery. Studies have examined the effects of intercostal blocks on lung volumes and gas flow rates following either abdominal or thoracic surgery. Most authors have used peak expiratory flow as a measure of the maximal expiratory effort that can be generated by a patient. When compared with opioid analgesia, intercostal block results in higher peak expiratory flows (6). This is true whether measured immediately after surgery or on the following day. In healthy volunteers, Jakobson found that bilateral intercostal nerve blocks with 0.25% bupivacaine or 0.5% etidocaine caused no change in the normal pattern of breathing (7). Minor changes were noted in several of the lung capacities and flows. Total lung capacity, forced vital capacity, and peak expiratory flow, all decreased by 4%. Functional residual capacity decreased by 8%, and peak expiratory airway pressure decreased by 7%.

Epidural analgesia is considered by many to be the best method of pain relief after major surgery. Although effective, side effects include hypotension, urinary retention, incomplete (or failed) block, and, in rare cases, paraplegia. Paravertebral block (PVB) is an alternative technique that may offer comparable analgesic effectiveness and a better side-effect profile. Davies and colleagues (8) performed a meta-analysis of all relevant randomized trials comparing PVB with epidural analgesia in thoracic surgery. Ten trials that had enrolled 520 thoracic surgery patients were identified. All of the trials were small ($n < 130$), and none were blinded. There was no significant difference between PVB and epidural groups for pain scores. Pulmonary complications occurred less often with PVB (odds ratio [OR] 0.36; 0.14, 0.92). Urinary retention (OR 0.23; 0.10, 0.51), nausea and vomiting (OR 0.47; 0.24, 0.53), and hypotension (OR 0.23; 0.11, 0.48), were less common with PVB. Rates of failed block were lower in the PVB group, OR 0.28 (0.2,

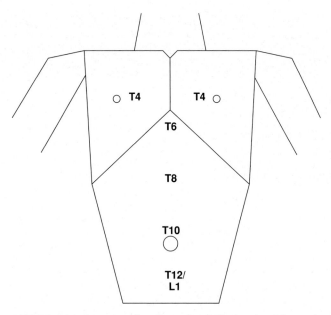

FIGURE 16-1. Dermatomal surface anatomic landmarks of the trunk and abdomen.

0.6). The authors (8) concluded that PVB and epidural analgesia provide comparable pain relief after thoracic surgery, but PVB has a better side-effect profile and is associated with a reduction in pulmonary complications.

PATIENT COMFORT

Patient comfort during regional anesthesia relates to comfort during needle insertion, peripheral nerve stimulation if applicable, duration of surgery, and the postoperative period. Patient comfort during regional anesthesia is also an important teaching point for trainees (9). In ensuring patient comfort during regional anesthesia, several steps are involved. Some of these are outlined below.

Preoperative Preparation, Psychology and Communication

Psychology and communication play an important part in the success of any anesthetic technique (10). Patients' previous experiences of regional anesthesia should be sought. Simple and precise language should be used.

Premedication

Pharmacologic premedication facilitates patient comfort during regional anesthesia performance (11). Advantages of premedication include improved patient satisfaction, acceptance, and cooperation. Disadvantages include unpredictable response, side effects, and interference with cooperation (12). In some cases, particularly with elderly patients and in ambulatory surgery, premedication is omitted.

When possible, premedication with nonopioid analgesics is optimum.

Sedation

Certain aspects of the regional technique often require both sedation and analgesia. Sedation alone in the presence of pain may cause confusion and restlessness. Conscious sedation is defined as a state of depressed consciousness that allows protective reflexes to be maintained, and the patient to respond appropriately to physical and verbal stimulation (13) (see also Chapter 8).

Regional Anesthetic Technique

In the performance of regional anesthesia, factors that impact on patient comfort should be optimized. The use of analgesics immediately prior to patient positioning can help increase patient comfort (14). Skilled, gentle digital palpation of surface anatomic landmarks is required. The pain on skin puncture is the most negative aspect of the patients' experience of regional anesthesia (15). The smallest gauge needle (25–30 gauge) should be used for infiltration of skin and subcutaneous tissues.

Regional anesthesia can be a stressful patient experience, and all measures to establish and maintain patient comfort should be considered. The aim is to produce a relaxed patient who is comfortable and cooperative. In practice, achieving this ideal may be the most challenging part of regional anesthetic practice. Multiple techniques and drug regimes exist. No single algorithm or guideline can address the management challenges for a heterogenous patient population. A patient-centered approach, with individualized regimes, including procedures and drugs, will ensure a high standard of patient comfort without compromising safety.

ULTRASOUND-GUIDED NERVE BLOCK TECHNIQUES

Ultrasound imaging is an attractive tool for regional anesthesia because of the many potential clinical benefits. Both cart-based and portable, compact ultrasound machines are now available and suited for nerve imaging. In theory, visual guidance can impart confidence to anesthesiologists, improve safety of patients, and enhance efficient time utilization in the operating room. Outcomes data to demonstrate convincingly that the clinical benefits of ultrasound are pending. There is no doubt that this imaging technology will be a valuable and enduring part of practice in regional anesthesia. In this chapter, where relevant, ultrasound-guided block techniques and available literature will be discussed.

General Principles of Ultrasound-guided Nerve Block Techniques

Certain general principles apply to the successful use of ultrasound to guide nerve block techniques:

■ The quality of ultrasonographic nerve images is dependent on the quality of the ultrasound machine and transducers, proper transducer selection (e.g., frequency) for each nerve location, the anesthesiologist's familiarity and interpretation of sonographic anatomy pertinent to the block, and good eye-hand coordination to track needle movement during needle advancement.

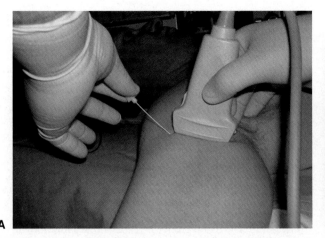
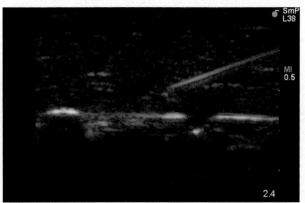

FIGURE 16-2. A: Long-axis needle approach with block needle parallel to the ultrasound beam. **B:** Ultrasound image of long-axis needle approach. The needle shaft and tip are visible.

- Optimal patient positioning and sterile technique are required. This is particularly important for continuous catheter techniques. Sterile conducting gel and a sterile plastic sheath to fully cover the entire transducer should be used especially for catheter techniques.
- Nerve localization by ultrasound can be combined with nerve stimulation. Ultrasonography provides anatomic information, while a motor response to nerve stimulation provides functional information about the nerve in question.
- Observing local anesthetic spread is a valuable feature of ultrasound in addition to real-time visual guidance to navigate the needle toward the target nerve. Correct spread pattern predicts block success.

Two approaches are generally used to block peripheral nerves. The first approach aims to align and move the block needle parallel to the ultrasound beam (Fig. 16-2). The needle shaft and tip can thus be clearly visualized. This approach is preferred when it is important to track the needle tip at all times. The second approach aims to align and move the block needle perpendicular to the ultrasound beam (Fig. 16-3).

In this case, the ultrasound image captures a transverse view of the needle, which is shown as a hyperechoic "dot" on the screen. Accurate moment-to-moment tracking of the needle tip location can be difficult, and needle tip position is often inferred indirectly by tissue movement and local anesthetic spread. This approach, however, is particularly useful for continuous catheter placement along the long axis of the nerve.

BLOCK PREPARATION

The topic of equipment selection for neural blockade has been reviewed in detail, together with the general topic of perioperative management of patients undergoing neural blockade by Crews and Chan in Chapter 8. As for all regional anesthetic procedures, after checking that the emergency equipment is complete and in working order, intravenous (IV) access, electrocardiogram (ECG), pulse oximetry, and blood pressure monitoring are established. Asepsis is observed.

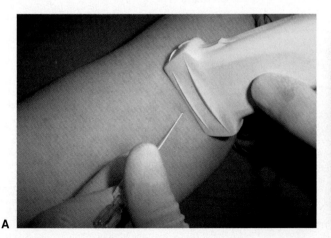

FIGURE 16-3. A: Short-axis needle approach with block needle perpendicular to the ultrasound beam. **B:** Ultrasound image of short-axis needle approach. The needle is seen as a hyperechoic dot with loss of image beneath.

INTERCOSTAL NERVE BLOCK

Anatomy

The intercostal nerves are the anterior primary rami of T1 through T11. T12 is not an intercostal nerve because it does not run a course between two ribs; it is more appropriately termed a subcostal nerve. Some of its fibers unite with fibers from the first lumbar nerve and are terminally represented as the iliohypogastric and ilioinguinal nerves.

A typical intercostal nerve has four significant branches (Fig. 16-4). The first are the paired gray and white rami communicantes, which pass anteriorly to and from the sympathetic ganglion and chain. The second branch arises as the posterior cutaneous branch and supplies the skin and muscles in the paravertebral region. The third branch is the lateral cutaneous division, which arises just anterior to the midaxillary line. This branch is of most concern to the anesthesiologist because it immediately sends subcutaneous fibers coursing both posteriorly and anteriorly to supply skin of much of the chest and abdominal wall. The final branch of an intercostal nerve is the anterior cutaneous branch. In the upper five nerves, this branch terminates after penetrating the external intercostal and pectoralis major muscles to innervate the breast and front of the thorax. The lower six anterior cutaneous nerves terminate after piercing the sheath of the rectus abdominis muscle, to which they supply motor branches. Some final branches continue an-

teriorly and become superficial near the linea alba, to provide cutaneous innervation to the midline of the abdomen.

Medial to the posterior angles of the ribs, the intercostal nerves lie between the pleura and the fascia of the internal intercostal muscle. This fascial layer is also known as the *posterior intercostal membrane*. In the paravertebral region, there is only fatty connective tissue between nerve and pleura. At the angle of the rib (6 to 8 cm from the spinous processes), the nerve comes to lie between the internal intercostal muscle and the intercostalis intimus muscle. At this position, the costal groove is broadest and deepest. Cadaver studies have shown that the nerve itself remains subcostal only 17% of the time, has most frequently (73%) moved inferiorly into the midzone between ribs, and is often branching at this point (16). The nerve is accompanied by intercostal veins and an artery, which lie superior to the nerve in the inferior groove of each rib (Fig. 16-5). The costal groove becomes a sharp inferior edge of the rib, about 5 to 8 cm anterolateral to the angle of the rib. At this point, the intercostal groove ceases to exist, the lateral cutaneous branch is given off (Fig. 16-4), and the intercostal nerve lies more inferiorly and moves toward the center of the intercostal space.

Technique

For technical ease of performance and for an optimal teaching or learning experience, the patient is best placed in a prone

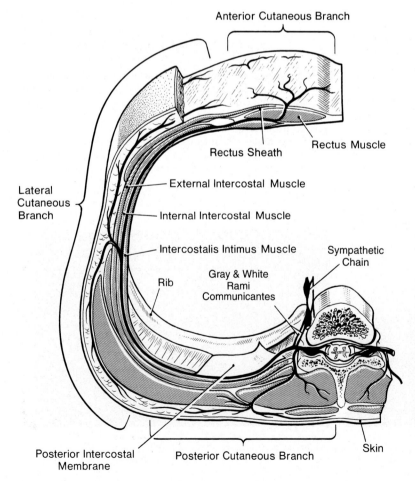

FIGURE 16-4. An intercostal nerve and its branches. Approximate area of skin supplied by branches is also shown. There is evidence, however, that local anesthetic injected near the lateral cutaneous branch diffuses posteriorly to reach the posterior cutaneous branch (see also Figure 16-9). Note also (a) the spinal nerves and dorsal root ganglia in the region of intervertebral foramen, with risk of perineurial spread into spinal fluid after intraneural injection in this region; (b) direct injection into an intervertebral foramen may reach spinal fluid by means of a dural cuff; (c) local anesthetic may gain access to epidural space by diffusing into an intervertebral foramen; (d) close to the midline, the intercostal nerve lies directly on the posterior intercostal membrane and pleura; and (e) paravertebrally, solution may diffuse to rami communicantes and sympathetic chain.

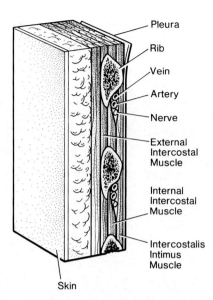

FIGURE 16-5. Cross-section of rib and intercostal space. Section is shown in region of costal groove, which extends from near the head of the rib to 5 to 8 cm anterior to the angle of the rib. At the level of the angle of the rib, the intercostal nerve (one or more) lies inferior to vein and artery in the intercostal groove.

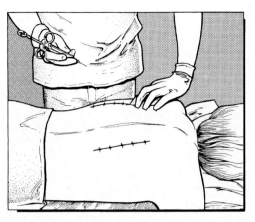

FIGURE 16-6. Technique for intercostal block and corresponding deep anatomy. Skin markings at lateral edge of sacrospinalis muscle (6–8 cm from midline). Note the medial curve of the line superiorly to avoid the scapulae. Ribs and interspaces are palpated. The lowest (most inferior) intercostal nerve is blocked first because the lower ribs are easy to palpate.

position. The prone position is particularly favored if bilateral blocks are to be performed. A pillow is placed under the abdomen to decrease the lumbar lordosis and to accentuate the intercostal spaces posteriorly. The arms should be allowed to hang down from the edge of the block table to permit the scapula to rotate as far laterally as possible. If multiple levels are to be blocked then sedation is mandatory.

The next step is the process of using skin markings (Fig. 16-6). First, a vertical line should be drawn along the posterior vertebral spines. The next step is to palpate laterally to the edge of the sacrospinalis group of muscles, where the ribs are most superficial. This distance is somewhat variable, depending on body size, muscle mass, and physique, but is usually 6 to

8 cm from the midline. Subsequent lines are drawn somewhat parallel to the first one, but with a trend to angle medially at the upper levels as the sacrospinalis muscles taper, so as to avoid the scapulae. The caudal end of the line should cross near the end of the shortened twelfth rib, which is generally easy to palpate. Then, by successively palpating and marking the inferior edge of each rib (or interspaces between ribs) a diagram is completed along these two vertical lines (Fig. 16-7). For abdominal surgery, six or seven (T5–T11 or T12) pairs of ribs are marked. For thoracic or other unilateral chest wall surgery, only the appropriate side and ribs are marked.

The anesthesiologist stands beside and behind the patient. The needle insertion point is infiltrated with local anesthetic using a 25-gauge needle. The needle insertion point is at the angle of the ribs. The ribs and intercostal spaces are thicker at the angle of the rib, allowing a larger margin of safety before pleura is contacted.

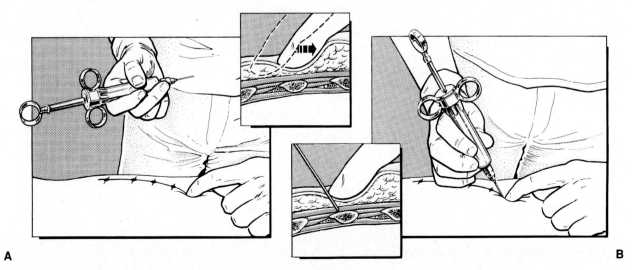

FIGURE 16-7. A: Skin at lower edge of rib retracted superiorly onto rib. B: Needle inserted onto rib (see also inset). Note finger palpating rib still in place and hand holding syringe firmly braced against back.

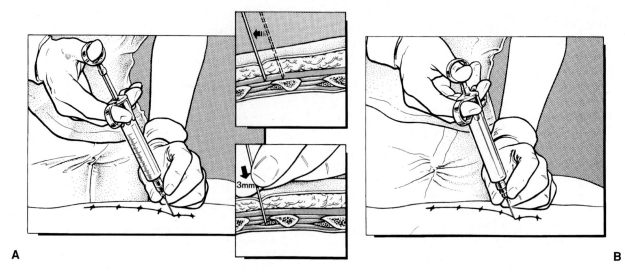

FIGURE 16-8. A: The position of the hands now change. Note left hand now rests against the back and holds the needle as it is walked off the inferior edge of the rib and advanced 3 mm. Right hand is free to aspirate and inject. **B:** Injection completed with left hand still firmly against patient's back and controlling the needle.

The index and third finger of left hand retract skin up and over rib. A 25-gauge 15-mm or a 23-gauge 25-mm needle is introduced in 20-degree cephalad orientation through the skin between the tip of the retracting fingers and advanced until it contacts rib. The left hand now holds needle hub and shaft between the thumb, index, and the middle fingers (Fig. 16-8). The left hand hypothenar eminence is firmly placed against the patient's back. The needle and syringe move as a whole. This allows maximal control of the needle depth as the left hand walks the needle off the inferior margin of the rib and into the intercostal groove at a distance of 2 to 4 mm past the edge of the rib, where 3 to 5 mL of local anesthetic is injected after aspiration (Fig. 16-9). The average distance from posterior rib to pleura averages 8 mm (17), so advancing a small distance (2–3 mm) after walking off the rib is safe.

Intercostal nerve blocks can also be placed at the midaxillary line while the patient is lying supine. This position is considerably more convenient in many situations (e.g., after induction of general anesthesia), but there is less margin of safety, the costal groove no longer exists, the nerve has often split into several main branches, and the lateral cutaneous branch of the nerve could be missed by the injected solution. Computed tomographic studies show, however, that solutions spread readily along the subcostal groove for several centimeters and can come in contact with the origin or takeoff of this large branch (Figs. 16-4 and 16-9).

Continuous intercostal techniques have been described. Percutaneous techniques are associated with a failure rate of 10% to 30% (18,19). Catheters can also be placed under direct vision at the time of thoracotomy (20). A systematic review of randomized trials indicates that intercostal infusion provides analgesia that is at least as effective as an epidural and significantly better than systemic opioids alone (21).

Sonoanatomy of the Intercostal Block

Only one report of ultrasound-guided intercostal nerve block appears in the literature (22). The authors report poor inter-

costal nerve visibility due to its proximity to the bony channel within which the nerve lies. The chest wall is best imaged in a coronal (vertical) plane (Fig. 16-10). Using a high-frequency transducer, the intercostal space can be visualized (Fig. 16-11). The ribs appear as dense, dark oval structures with a bright surface (periosteum). A dark shadow is cast deep to the rib on ultrasound, illustrating the phenomenon of echo shadowing. The pleura and lungs may also be visualized deep to the intercostal space between the echo shadows.

Ultrasound-guided Intercostal Block

The intercostal space is generally found at a depth of 2 to 3 cm from the skin. The uppermost rib is kept in the center of the field of view. The needle entry site is at the caudad edge of the linear transducer (Fig. 16-12). A 23-gauge needle is advanced under real-time ultrasound guidance, and local anesthetic is deposited along the needle entry path. A free-hand technique rather than the use of a needle guide is preferred. A 21-gauge needle is inserted parallel to the axis of the beam of the ultrasound transducer. The needle is attached to sterile extension tubing, which is connected to a 20-mL syringe and flushed with local anesthetic solution to remove all air from the system. It is then introduced at the caudad edge of the transducer and visualized along its entire path to the intercostal space. It is important not to advance the needle without proper visualization, achieving which may require needle or transducer adjustment.

The needle is advanced toward the inferior border of the rib. On contacting the rib, the needle is redirected inferiorly to pass no more than 0.5 cm beyond the inferior rib margin. Following a negative test aspiration, 2 to 5 mL of local anesthetic solution is injected.

Surgical Indications

Surgical intercostal block indications include upper abdominal and thoracic superficial procedures, such as insertion of

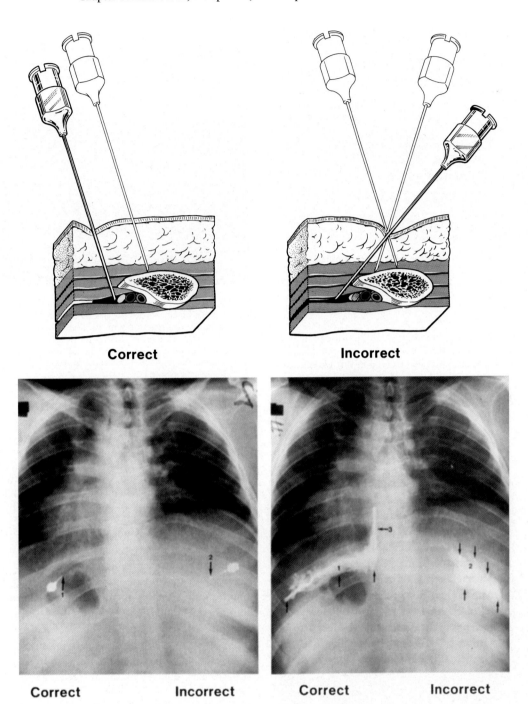

FIGURE 16-9. A: Comparison of correct (*left*) and incorrect (*right*) technique. **A:** Radiograph showing correct needle insertion (*1*) compared to incorrect position (*2*). Radiograph showing injection of x-ray contrast medium. **B:** Injection from correctly placed needle results in spread along intercostal groove (*1*) and also into paravertebral space (*3*). Injection from incorrectly placed needle results in a localized "blob" in intercostal muscles (*2*). Arrows indicate extent of spread of solution.

thoracotomy and gastrostomy tubes. Minor breast surgery (23,24), extracorporeal lithotripsy (25), and cardiac pacemaker insertion (26) have been described using intercostal blockade. Relatively few surgical procedures can be performed under intercostal nerve block alone; for major abdominal surgery, celiac plexus or splanchnic nerve block is required (see Chapters 42 and 45).

Nonsurgical Applications

Intercostal nerve block is extremely effective in providing pain relief for fractured ribs. Because vigorous palpation of broken ribs can be quite painful in the obese or in the patient with excessive local swelling, localization of the ribs and performance

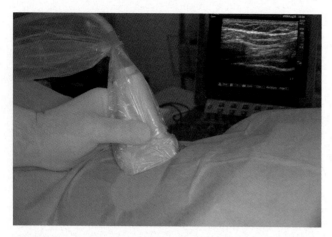

FIGURE 16-10. Ultrasound transducer orientation (coronal) for the intercostal block. From Harmon D, Frizelle HP, Sandhu NS, et al. *Perioperative Diagnostic and Interventional Ultrasound.* New York: Saunders, 2007, with permission.

of the block can be aided by ultrasound (22). Pleuritic pain and pain from flail chest also can be relieved in this manner. Herpes zoster pain may be relieved and even treated in this way. Intercostal nerve block can be helpful in the differential diagnosis of visceral versus abdominal wall pain. Chronic pain conditions such as intercostal neuralgia and tumor-related pain may also be treated.

Complications

Preoperative and postoperative chest films in 200 consecutive patients resulted in a pneumothorax incidence of 0.42% (1/2,610 intercostal nerve blocks) (27). Treatment of pneumothorax, by needle aspiration or merely by careful observation, is usually all that is needed.

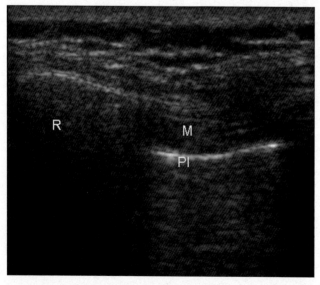

FIGURE 16-11. Ultrasound appearance of the intercostal space. *R,* rib; *M,* intercostal muscle; *Pl,* pleura. From Harmon D, Frizelle HP, Sandhu NS, et al. *Perioperative Diagnostic and Interventional Ultrasound.* New York: Saunders, 2007, with permission.

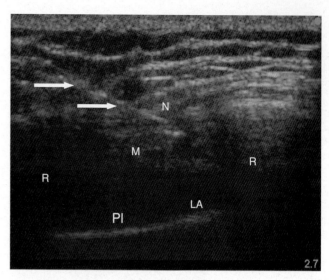

FIGURE 16-12. Real-time imaging of needle insertion for the intercostal nerve block. Notice the needle shaft marked with arrows and the needle tip (N) position with local anesthetic injected into the intercostal space. *R,* Rib; *M,* Intercostal Muscle; *Pl,* Pleura; *LA,* Local Anesthetic. From Harmon D, Frizelle HP, Sandhu NS, et al. *Perioperative Diagnostic and Interventional Ultrasound.* New York: Saunders, 2007, with permission.

A second complication relates to the toxic effects of absorbed local anesthetic and epinephrine following intercostal block. Blood levels of the anesthetic drug after intercostal and interpleural blockade are higher than after any other regional anesthetic procedure. Systemic toxic reactions rarely occur in patients having diagnostic or therapeutic blocks, because smaller volumes of more dilute solution of drug are used. Greater amounts of more concentrated drug are injected to provide complete motor and sensory block in the surgical patient.

Performance of intraoperative intrathoracic intercostal injection appears to be associated with a higher incidence of complications. Multiple cases of total spinal anesthesia have been reported after intrathoracic intercostal blockade conducted during surgery under general anesthesia (28,29). In most of these instances, the blocks were performed under direct vision at a site more medial than would likely be chosen for the percutaneous approach. Injection of local anesthetic into a dural root cuff or directly into nerve tissue itself, with extensive intrafascicular followed by spinal spread, has been proposed as the mechanism for the resultant widespread blockade, which manifests as hypotension and bradycardia, dilated pupils, and prolonged anesthesia and paralysis.

INTERPLEURAL BLOCKADE

Anatomy

Interpleural block can provide analgesia over the chest wall and upper abdomen. Anesthesia is attained by diffusion of local anesthetic solution to nerves that run in proximity to the pleural surfaces. Anteriorly, laterally, and posteriorly, the parietal pleura is in close approximation to the intercostal nerves. Superiorly, the inferior roots of the brachial plexus pass a short distance over the cupola before reaching the first rib. Medially, the sympathetic chain, splanchnic, phrenic, and vagus nerves are also adjacent. The epidural and subarachnoid spaces are at a greater distance and are generally not felt to be a site of local anesthetic action during interpleural anesthesia.

Technique

Spread of local anesthetic solution within the interpleural space is governed by gravity, the amount of volume injected, and the location of the catheter itself (30). The hallmark of this technique is detection of the negative interpleural pressure, so that placement should be performed either pre- or postoperatively in the awake patient, or during general anesthesia with the patient breathing spontaneously. Placement should be avoided during positive pressure ventilation, as the interpleural pressure is no longer negative, and the risk of pneumothorax and its evolution to tension pneumothorax is greatly increased (31).

The patient is placed in either the sitting, lateral, or prone position. After sterile prepping and draping, the skin is anesthetized at a point 8 to 10 cm lateral from the midline, overlying the top edge of a rib. Infiltration is carried deeper until the rib is contacted (Fig. 16-13). After recontacting the rib with a 16- or 18-gauge Tuohy needle, the needle is gently walked cephalad until it is felt to slide off the superior edge of the rib.

A loss-of-resistance technique to positive pressure is used (32) (Fig. 16-13). Once in the interpleural space, the syringe is removed, and the interpleural catheter is gently passed 5 to 6 cm. The needle is removed, then an occlusive dressing is applied. If this technique is employed preoperatively, nitrous oxide should not be used during subsequent general anesthesia, because of the risk of significant expansion of the small pneumothorax that inevitably arises during even a brief interval of communication between the interpleural space and the atmosphere.

Prior to local anesthetic injection, the patient should be placed in a position to maximize the desired effect. As the movement of injected solution is governed by gravity, blockade will localize at the dependent point (33). Positioning the patient with the operative side up causes solution to pool medially, which maximizes the amount of subsequent sympathetic blockade (Fig. 16-13, lateral), while the supine and operative-side-down positions cause solution to accumulate near the intercostal nerves (Fig. 16-13, supine), minimizing the degree of sympathetic blockade. A head-down positioning can increase the amount of cervical and upper thoracic sympathetic blockade and, in some instances, can produce anesthesia of the inferior roots of the brachial plexus.

The total dose (e.g., 20–30 mL of 0.5% bupivacaine) should be given intermittently in divided doses over 2 to 3 minutes, and the position maintained for 20 to 30 minutes. The duration

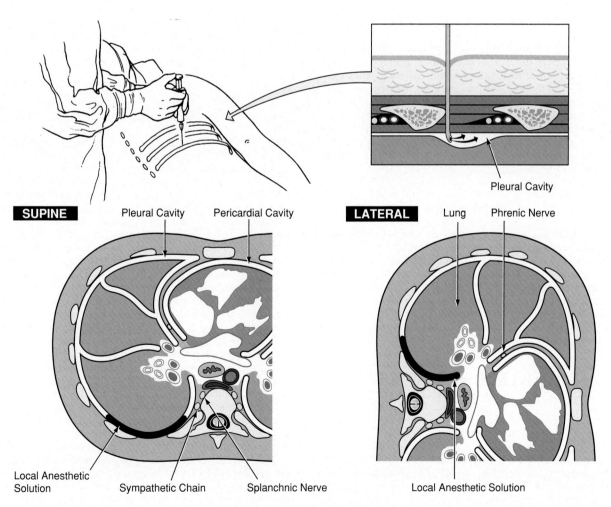

FIGURE 16-13. Interpleural block.

of action appears to be proportional to the milligram amount of drug given, rather than to its concentration or volume (34). Continuous infusion is at a rate of 0.125 mL/kg/hour (35).

Surgical Applications

Interpleural analgesia is an established technique for providing hemithoracic analgesia and sympathetic block and offers some advantage in the management of widespread chest wall pain by minimizing the number of injections required compared with intercostal block. Interpleural analgesia is best utilized for open cholecystectomy, renal surgery, and unilateral breast procedures. After cholecystectomy, opioid requirements and visual analog scale (VAS) pain scores are decreased, and pulmonary parameters are improved when interpleural analgesia is used (36,37).

Its usefulness during thoracotomy is controversial, because the duration of blockade appears to be significantly reduced when the parietal pleura is interrupted and a thoracostomy drainage tube is present (38,39). Compared to paravertebral analgesia for thoracic surgery, VAS scores are similar but interpleural block is associated with decreased preservation of lung function and a greater number of side effects (40).

Nonsurgical Applications

Treatment of pain associated with multiple rib fractures improves pulmonary function as assessed by several parameters (41). Case reports of treating upper limb ischemia, reflex sympathetic dystrophy, and the pain of acute and chronic pancreatitis have been described (42–45). Pain relief associated with tumor invasion of the brachial plexus, vertebral metastases, and severe postherpetic neuralgia has also been reported (46,47). Catheters can be tunneled subcutaneously for the long-term management of thoracic pain in patients with pain due to cancer (48).

Complications

Pneumothorax occurs in approximately 2% (49). The analgesia also tends to be less intense and of shorter duration compared to that produced by intercostal block (50). Phrenic nerve paresis occurs in some instances (51,52). Ipsilateral bronchospasm has been reported in one patient (53). Horner syndrome occurs frequently. Cholestasis, documented by clinical and laboratory findings, has been described in three patients with right interpleural catheters used to treat upper extremity reflex sympathetic dystrophy (54).

PARAVERTEBRAL THORACIC SOMATIC NERVE BLOCK

Anatomy

The paravertebral space is a wedged-shaped area on either side of the vertebral column (Fig. 16-14). The boundaries of the space are: posteriorly, the superior costotransverse ligament; laterally, the posterior intercostal membrane; anteriorly, the parietal pleura; and base of triangle (medially), the posterolat-

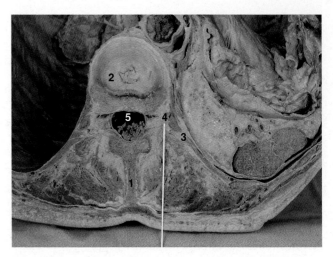

FIGURE 16-14. Cadaveric illustration of thoracic paravertebral space. Needle tip is positioned in the paravertebral space.

eral aspect of the vertebral body, disc, and intervertebral foramen (Fig. 16-15). The contents of the paravertebral space include fatty tissue, intercostal vessels, spinal (intercostal) nerve, dorsal ramus, rami communicantes, and the sympathetic chain (anteriorly). The paravertebral space is contiguous medially with the epidural space and laterally with the intercostal space. The inferior limit of this space occurs at the origins of the psoas major muscle. The superior limit extends into the cervical region.

Technique

The patient is placed in the sitting or lateral position, with the head in the flexed position and the back bent forward. After the anesthesiologist chooses the dermatomes involved in the operative field, the corresponding spinal processes are palpated and marked with a skin marker. A point 2.5 cm lateral to the spinous processes is marked. Single- and multi-injection techniques have been described (55). The needle insertion site is first infiltrated with local anesthetic using a 25-gauge needle. For a single-injection technique, an 18-gauge Tuohy needle is inserted perpendicular to the skin until contact is made with the transverse process (Fig. 16-16). This usually occurs between 2 and 4 cm deep to the skin. At this point, further local anesthetic is injected, as contact with periosteum is painful. Locating the transverse process is critical to the proper performance of this block. If this contact is not made, it is likely that the needle lies between the transverse processes and should be withdrawn and redirected in a caudal or cephalad direction (Fig. 16-17). Once the transverse process is identified, the needle is withdrawn and redirected in a cephalad or caudad direction to walk over the transverse process. There are advantages to both directions. A greater distance exists between the superior aspect of the transverse process and the pleura, which may decrease the incidence of pneumothorax because the spinal nerve and vessels lie closer to the inferior aspect of the transverse process.

The paravertebral space is usually reached by advancing the needle tip 1 to 1.5 cm beyond the transverse process, while maintaining its cephalad or caudad orientation. It is imperative that the needle should not be advanced further once its tip has entered the paravertebral space, as a risk of pleural puncture

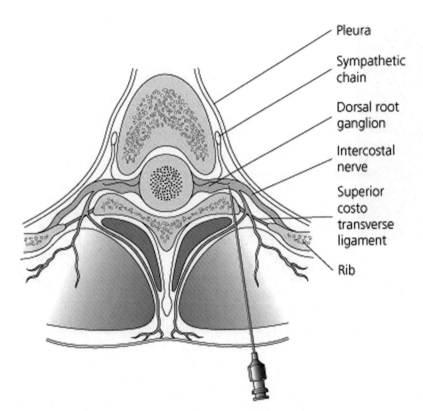

FIGURE 16-15. Anatomy of the paravertabral space.

exists. A subtle "click" or loss of resistance is usually felt as the needle passes through the costotransverse membrane. Incremental injection of local anesthetic (e.g., 5 mL of 0.5% bupivacaine) is made with repeated aspiration. For a single-injection multisegment block, the total volume used should be 15 to 25 mL. Although the onset of analgesia occurs within minutes after injection of local anesthetic, up to 20 minutes is typically required for surgical anesthesia. If a catheter is required, it may be advanced into the paravertebral space through the needle, 3 to 4 cm beyond the needle tip, after completion of the bolus injection.

Recently, a nerve stimulation-based technique has been described to identify the thoracic paravertebral space (56). Ultrasound can identify the transverse process and the pleura (57). An ultrasound-guided technique has not been described.

Local anesthetic solution injected into the paravertebral space may remain localized, spread to the ipsilateral paravertebral spaces above and below the injection site, pass laterally through the intercostal space (Fig. 16-4), or spread medially through the epidural space or across the vertebral bodies. Thermographic studies have demonstrated that 15 mL of 0.5% bupivacaine produces a somatic block of five dermatomes and

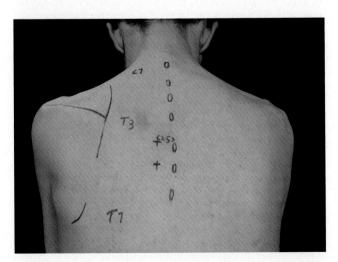

FIGURE 16-16. Paravertebral block technique. The epidural needle is directed perpendicular to the skin until contact is made with the transverse process.

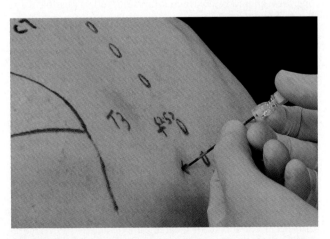

FIGURE 16-17. Paravertebral block technique. The epidural needle is then directed cephalad to the transverse process and advanced until the loss of resistance is felt.

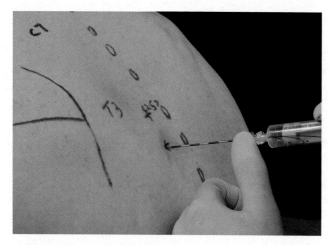

FIGURE 16-18. Paravertebral block technique. Use of syringe to detect loss of resistance as needle passes through costotransverse membrane.

a sympathetic block over eight dermatomes. Little is known regarding the factors that influence spread.

Surgical Applications

Paravertebral thoracic somatic nerve block can be used to provide anesthesia for thoracic surgery, breast surgery, cholecystectomy, renal and ureteric surgery, herniorrhaphy, and appendicectomy, as well as for video-assisted thoracoscopic surgery and minimally invasive cardiac surgery.

Nonsurgical Applications

Paravertebral thoracic somatic nerve block may be used to reduce the risk of chronic pain after breast surgery (58). Acute pain management for fractured ribs and flail chest; intercostal neuralgia associated with osteoporotic vertebral fractures; and liver capsular pain after blunt abdominal trauma are additional indications, as are relief of acute herpes zoster pain (59), acute postamputation pain, and tumor-related pain. Prolonged postoperative analgesia (continuous infusion) (60) is possible using this technique.

Complications

Because of the proximity of the sympathetic chain and splanchnic nerves, ipsilateral sympathetic blockade is to be expected. If bilateral blockade is performed, sympathetic blockade equivalent to thoracic spinal or epidural anesthesia, with accompanying hypotension, should be anticipated. Intravascular, epidural, and subarachnoid injections are possible. The incidence of solution tracking into the ipsilateral epidural space is as high as 70% in some reports, with bilateral epidural spread occurring in 7% (61). Bilateral anesthesia suggests an epidural or intrathecal injection, the likelihood of which is decreased by avoiding any medial orientation of the needle. Bilateral anaesthesia may also occur via spread of local anesthetic across the vertebral bodies.

Pneumothorax has an incidence of 0.5% (62). As with all unguided peripheral blocks, an incidence of block failure is

possible (62). Postdural puncture headache has been reported (63).

PARAVERTEBRAL LUMBAR SOMATIC NERVE BLOCK

Anatomy

The lumbar nerves exit their respective intervertebral foramina just inferior to the caudad edge of each transverse process. These nerves divide immediately into anterior and posterior branches. The small posterior branches supply the skin of the lower back and the paravertebral muscles. Of primary interest, however, are the anterior branches of the first four lumbar nerves. These nerves, together with a small branch from the twelfth thoracic nerve, form the lumbar plexus. This plexus is formed largely within the substance of the psoas major muscle, and most of the peripheral branches exit laterally in a plane between the psoas and quadratus lumborum muscles.

The major branches of the lumbar plexus (i.e., the iliohypogastric, ilioinguinal, and lateral femoral cutaneous nerves) continue laterally around the rim of the pelvis. Their terminal branches approach and pass near the anterior superior iliac spine. The femoral nerve passes almost directly caudad after emerging from the lateral edge of the psoas major. The obturator nerve emerges from the medial edge of the psoas major, descends under the common iliac vessels, and finally emerges from the pelvis through the obturator foramen. The ultimate cutaneous distribution of each of these nerves in the groin, inguinal crease, and anterolateral leg is quite variable. Considerable overlap also occurs of the cutaneous branches of individual nerves. The primary peripheral branches of the lumbar plexus are listed in Table 16-1 and illustrated in Figure 16-19. It is apparent that paravertebral nerve block of L1–L4 will result in sensory and motor block of the groin and much of the leg. For intra-abdominal, pelvic, or groin operations, only the upper two lumbar segments need to be blocked. In general, the lumbar nerves tend to slope sharply caudad as they emerge from the intervertebral foramina. In doing so, they tend to course anterior to the tips of the transverse processes of the next lower lumbar vertebral bodies. A needle placed at the inferior edge of a transverse process will be close to nerves from two lumbar segments. Medially, it will be close to the nerve exiting the vertebral foramen; laterally, it will be near the nerve from the next more cephalad vertebral level. Hence, local anesthetic solution injected at the proper depth inferior to one lumbar vertebral process actually can result in nerve block of two or more root segments.

TABLE 16-1	

ORIGINS AND DISTRIBUTION OF THE LUMBAR PLEXUS

Peripheral Nerve	Root Segments
Iliohypogastric	T12, L1
Ilioinguinal	L1
Genitofemoral	L1, L2
Lateral femoral cutaneous	L2, L3
Femoral	L2, L3, L4
Obturator	L2, L3, L4

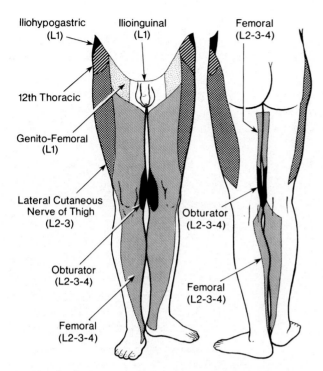

FIGURE 16-19. Cutaneous branches of lumbar plexus and the areas of skin that they supply.

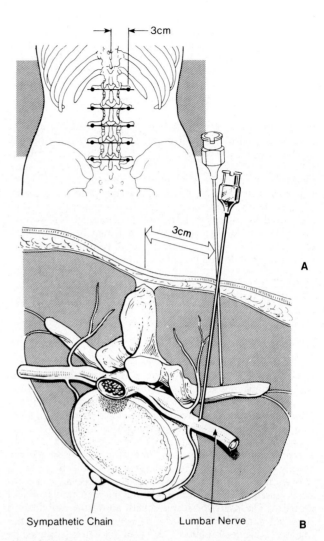

FIGURE 16-20. Paravertebral lumbar somatic nerve block. **A:** Skin markings are made by drawing lines across the cephalad aspect of spinous processes and then drawing vertical lines 3 cm from the midline. **B:** A needle inserted perpendicular to the skin will contact the caudad edge of a transverse process. Angulation of the needle in a caudad direction to slide caudad to the transverse process will reach the spinal nerve 1 to 2 cm deeper than the transverse process.

Technique

The patient is placed in the prone or lateral position. The injection sites are marked while keeping in mind that the cephalad edge of a lumbar posterior spinous process lies opposite the caudad edge of its homologous transverse process. Visualizing and then locating the transverse process is fundamental to a successful block. After palpating and marking each of the lumbar vertebral spinous processes, the anesthesiologist draws horizontal lines at the cephalad edge of each one and projects them laterally. Two vertical lines should then be drawn parallel to, and 3 to 5 cm lateral from, the midline. The points of intersection of the vertical and horizontal lines mark the sites where skin wheals are raised (Fig. 16-20). An 8-cm, 22-gauge needle is inserted perpendicularly to the skin until it contacts the transverse process at a depth of 3 to 5 cm. The needle then should be withdrawn to a subcutaneous level, and redirected to slide off the caudad edge of the transverse process. The needle is advanced another 2 to 3 cm beyond the point where it previously made contact with bone, and 6 to 10 mL of local anesthetic solution is injected. Paresthesiae are not sought. This process is repeated at each of the lumbar levels at which anesthesia is desired. The useful concentrations of local anesthetic are the same as those used for intercostal block.

Surgical Applications

Although most widely used to facilitate thoracic and breast procedures, paravertebral blocks have proven to be effective in providing analgesia for both upper and lower abdominal procedures. Such procedures include major abdominal vascular surgery (64), transcutaneous hepatic biliary drainage (65), thoracoabdominal esophagectomy (66), and inguinal hernior-

rhaphy (with the block performed at T10–L2) (67). Saito and colleagues (68) have provided an anatomic explanation for the efficacy of paravertebral blocks performed at thoracic levels in producing analgesia for incisions of the abdominal wall. In a cadaver study, dye injected into the paravertebral space at T11 entered the abdominal cavity through the lateral and medial arcuate ligaments and in the transversalis fascia to stain subcostal, ilioinguinal, iliohypogastric, genitofemoral, lateral femoral cutaneous, and femoral nerves (68).

Nonsurgical Applications

When the block is used for diagnostic purposes, only small volumes of local anesthetic solution should be injected, so as to limit spread centrally or to adjacent lumbar nerves. Some physicians use fluoroscopy or a nerve stimulator to position the needle precisely and then inject only 0.5 to 1 mL of drug.

A diagnostic use of paravertebral lumbar somatic block is in evaluating groin or genital pain, such as the nerve entrapment syndromes that sometimes follow inguinal herniorrhaphy.

Complications

It is possible to inject into intravascular, epidural, or subarachnoid spaces during performance of this block. Should the needle be inserted too far medially, it could enter a vertebral foramen or penetrate a dural sleeve to produce spinal anesthesia. Perineural spread of solution into the epidural space may also occur, with a consequent variable degree of anesthesia over the lower extremities. Intravascular injection can be minimized by aspiration tests, and by avoiding large-volume injections. The lumbar sympathetic chain may be anesthetized. Intraperitoneal injection, or puncture of retroperitoneal (kidney) or intra-abdominal organs, is possible.

RECTUS SHEATH BLOCK

Anatomy

As the lower five intercostal nerves course anteriorly, they become more superficial and terminate after penetrating the rectus abdominis muscle. These nerves enter the rectus sheath at the posterolateral border of the body of that muscle. The tendinous intersections of the rectus tend to create segmental distributions of individual intercostal nerves, but some overlap of adjacent fibers occurs. Anteriorly, the rectus sheath is tough and fibrous from pubis to xiphoid. Posteriorly, it is strong and readily identifiable down to the level of the umbilicus, but then it fades into a thin sheath of transversalis fascia, which adheres closely to the peritoneum below the semicircular line of Douglas. The posterior rectus sheath above the umbilicus is quite substantial and can serve as a "backboard" for injecting local anesthetic solution. This solution will be confined by the tendinous intersections, but within those limits will spread up and down to anesthetize the peripheral motor and sensory branches of the intercostal nerves.

Technique

The patient lies supine, and the anesthesiologist may stand at either side. Two to six sites are chosen for injections, the number depending on the location and size of surgical incision (Fig. 16-21). If performed while the patient is awake, skin wheals are raised at the middle of each segment of the rectus muscle body that can be palpated between tendinous intersections. A reusable or short-bevel 5-cm, 22-gauge needle is passed through skin and subcutaneous tissue until it meets the firm resistance of the anterior rectus sheath. The block should be discontinued unless this sheath can be convincingly demonstrated upon advancing the needle. With controlled, steady pressure, the needle is pushed to penetrate this sheath with a definite snap. Advancing further passes the needle through the softer belly of the muscle, and as the needle approaches the posterior rectus sheath, the anesthesiologist will feel firm resistance again. Using this posterior sheath as a backboard, 10 mL of local anesthetic solution is injected. The process is repeated at each injection site. Blocks above the umbilicus should be performed first, and needle depth noted, before attempting any additional blocks below the umbilicus, where injection just after

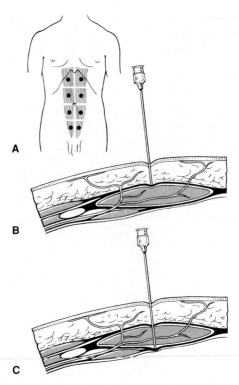

FIGURE 16-21. Rectus block. **A:** Skin wheals are raised in the center of rectus segments. These are delineated by a vertical line through umbilicus and horizontal lines at umbilical level, and midway between umbilicus and xiphisternum, and umbilicus and pubis, respectively. **B:** Short bevel needle contacts resistance of anterior rectus sheath. **C:** Needle penetrates rectus muscle and is halted by resistance of posterior rectus sheath. Note the latter structure is absent below the line midway between umbilicus and pubis. Thus, these two rectus injections are made last.

the loss-of-resistance of the anterior sheath may be safer and sufficient.

Sonoanatomy of Rectus Sheath Block

The rectus abdominis muscle is readily visualized in a transverse ultrasound plane, with the sheath highlighted as a bright hyperechoic structure surrounding the muscle (Fig. 16-22). Willschke and colleagues (69) have described the performance of ultrasound-guided rectus sheath block in children undergoing umbilical hernia repair. They report satisfactory analgesia using 0.1 mL/kg of 0.25% levobupivacaine. The use of ultrasound may help the anesthesiologist decrease the incidence of complications and improve the success rate of the block. Whether it actually does so has yet to be studied.

Ultrasound-guided Rectus Sheath Block Technique

Using ultrasonic guidance, the target is kept in the center of the field of view, and the needle entry site is at the lateral-most end of the linear transducer. A 21-gauge needle is inserted parallel to the axis of the beam of the ultrasound transducer (Fig. 16-23). The needle is visualized along its entire path to the posterior rectus sheath (Fig. 16-24). It is important not to advance the

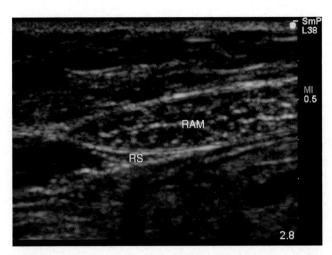

FIGURE 16-22. Ultrasound appearance of the rectus abdominis muscle (*RAM*) and rectus sheath (*RS*). From Harmon D, Frizelle HP, Sandhu NS, et al. *Perioperative Diagnostic and Interventional Ultrasound.* New York: Saunders, 2007, with permission.

needle without good visualization. This may require transducer adjustment.

Surgical Applications

The rectus sheath block can provide good intra- and postoperative analgesia for abdominal surgery requiring a midline incision. The block has proven useful in the management of surgical pain after incisional and umbilical hernia repair, postpartum and laparoscopic tubal ligation, cesarean section when a midline incision is used (70), and outpatient laparoscopy (71). It is widely used for pediatric patients, particularly in the ambulatory surgical setting.

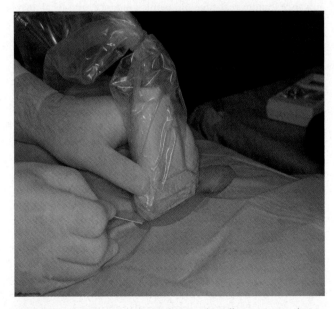

FIGURE 16-23. Ultrasound transducer and needle positioning during ultrasound-guided rectus sheath block. From Harmon D, Frizelle HP, Sandhu NS, et al. *Perioperative Diagnostic and Interventional Ultrasound.* New York: Saunders, 2007, with permission.

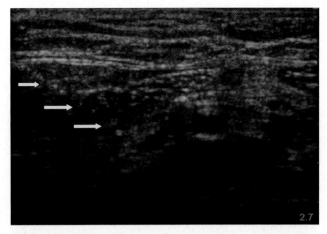

FIGURE 16-24. Real-time imaging of needle insertion (arrows) for rectus sheath block.

Nonsurgical Applications

Rectus block may be useful in diagnosing abdominal nerve entrapment syndromes or localized myofascial problems.

Complications

It is difficult to identify the posterior rectus sheath where it lies near the xiphoid and pubis. Attempting this block at these levels may result in penetration of peritoneum and underlying organs such as liver, intestine, bladder, or uterus. In the patient with a distended abdomen, the thinly stretched rectus may prevent clear identification of anterior and posterior sheaths. A visible bulge in the abdominal wall upon injection indicates that the needle is too superficial, and a poor block will result. The block is more difficult in the obese, cachectic, or elderly patient with poor abdominal muscle tone.

Once the needle has been placed in the posterior sheath, 2 to 3 mL of local anaesthetic solution is injected to confirm correct needle placement; 10 mL of solution may then be injected and observed to fill the posterior aspect of the sheath (Fig. 16-25). The procedure is repeated on either side of the midline, as blockade of the contralateral sensory afferents is necessary to obtain midline analgesia.

ILIOINGUINAL/ ILIOHYPOGASTRIC NERVE BLOCKS

Anatomy

The ilioinguinal, iliohypogastric, and twelfth thoracic nerves pass near the anterior superior iliac spine. At or near the level of the anterior superior iliac spine, the twelfth thoracic and iliohypogastric nerves lie between the internal and external oblique muscles. The ilioinguinal nerve lies between the transversus abdominis and internal oblique muscles initially and then penetrates the internal oblique at a variable distance medial to the anterior superior iliac spine (Fig. 16-26). These three nerves continue anteromedially and become superficial as they terminate in branches to skin and muscles of the inguinal region.

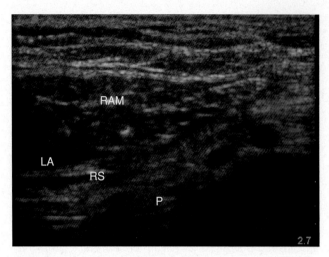

FIGURE 16-25. Ultrasound appearance of anesthetic solution injected into the posterior rectus sheath. *LA*, local anesthetic; *RAM*, rectus abdominus muscle; *RS*, rectus sheath; *P*, peritoneum.

Using the anterior superior iliac spine as a primary point of orientation, the anesthesiologist can block these nerves. Success depends on spreading a large volume of anesthetic solution between abdominal wall muscle layers. The block is inadequate to provide total anesthesia for inguinal herniorrhaphy, because structures that enter the inguinal canal through the internal inguinal ring will not be anesthetized, but the surgeon can block the latter adequately with direct local infiltration of the spermatic cord during the procedure.

Technique

The procedure can be performed with the patient lying in the supine position, awake or anesthetized. The skin puncture point is 1 cm medial and 1 cm inferior to the anterior superior iliac spine. A 35-mm 21-gauge needle is advanced at right angles to the skin in all planes (Fig. 16-27). A characteristic "click" may be felt on penetrating the external oblique, at which point 6 to 8 mL of local anaesthetic is injected, following aspiration, in increments of 2.5 mL, to anesthetize the iliohypogastric nerve. Advancing the needle further will result in a second characteristic "click" as the needle penetrates the internal oblique. A further 6 to 8 mL is injected at this point (with the usual precautions) to anesthetize the ilioinguinal nerve.

Without withdrawing the needle through the skin, redirection laterally toward the ilium will permit subcutaneous injection of local anesthetic (3–5 mL) to block the lateral cutaneous branch of the subcostal nerve. A similar subcutaneous injection can be made toward the midline to block other branches of the subcostal nerve.

If herniorrhaphy is to be performed, a second skin wheal may be raised 2 to 3 cm above the midinguinal point. A 5-cm needle is inserted, perpendicular to the skin, to a depth of 3 to 5 cm. Infiltration of 10 to 15 mL of local anesthetic solution in fan-wise fashion will anesthetize the genitofemoral nerve, sympathetic fibers, and peritoneal sac. However, there is a risk of hematoma owing to trauma to the femoral artery. Thus, it may be preferable for the surgeon to inject 2 to 3 mL of local anesthetic circumferentially into the spermatic cord as soon as it is exposed.

Sonoanatomy of Ilioinguinal/Iliohypogastric Nerve Blocks

The nerves are visualized by placing the ultrasound transducer medial to the anterior superior iliac spine in an oblique axial orientation (Fig. 16-28). The nerves appear as hypoechoic fascicular structures with hyperechoic rims sandwiched between the two layers of muscle (Fig. 16-29). As already reported, the use of ilioinguinal and iliohypogastric nerve blocks is popular, yet clinical experience with this technique indicates block failure rates of 10% to 25% (72). Willschke and co-workers (73) have reported that the use of ultrasound in locating the ilioinguinal and iliohypogastric nerves yields a higher success rate than the classic landmark technique. Four percent of patients in the ultrasound group required supplemental intraoperative analgesia compared to 26% in the landmark group. They also reported a significant reduction in the volume of anesthetic agent required for successful block in the ultrasound group. Thus, ultrasonic guidance would appear to improve the quality and success rate of ilioinguinal and iliohypogastric nerve block when compared to traditional landmark techniques. Visualization of the needle, nerve, and peritoneum should help prevent nerve injury and also visceral injury associated with traditional, blind techniques.

Ultrasound-guided Ilioinguinal/Iliohypogastric Nerve Block Technique

The image of the abdominal wall at this level reveals the internal oblique and transversus abdominis muscles, with the peritoneum and intestine deep to these (Fig. 16-28). The nerves are kept in the center of the field of view, and the needle entry site is at the medial border of the linear transducer (Fig. 16-29).

A free-hand technique, rather than the use of a needle guide, is preferred. A 21-gauge needle is inserted parallel to the axis of the beam of the ultrasound transducer. A 23-gauge needle is advanced under real-time ultrasonic guidance, and local anesthetic is deposited along the needle entry path. The needle is attached to sterile extension tubing, which is connected to a 20-mL syringe and preflushed with local anesthetic solution to clear all air from the system. The needle is then introduced at the medial edge of the transducer and visualized along its entire path to the ilioinguinal nerve (Fig. 16-30). It is important not to advance the needle without good visualization, which may require transducer adjustment.

Surgical Applications

Ilioinguinal/iliohypogastric nerve blocks can provide adequate anesthesia for field block for groin surgery (in combination with genitofemoral nerve block/surgical infiltration at deep and superficial inguinal rings) and postoperative analgesia. Bilateral ilioinguinal nerve block, using 10 mL plain 0.5% bupivacaine per side, during general anesthesia for cesarean section has also been shown to significantly reduce pain scores and opiate requirements in the first 24 hours after surgery (17).

Nonsurgical Applications

Ilioinguinal/iliohypogastric nerve blocks can aid in the diagnosis of nerve entrapment syndromes following herniorrhaphy.

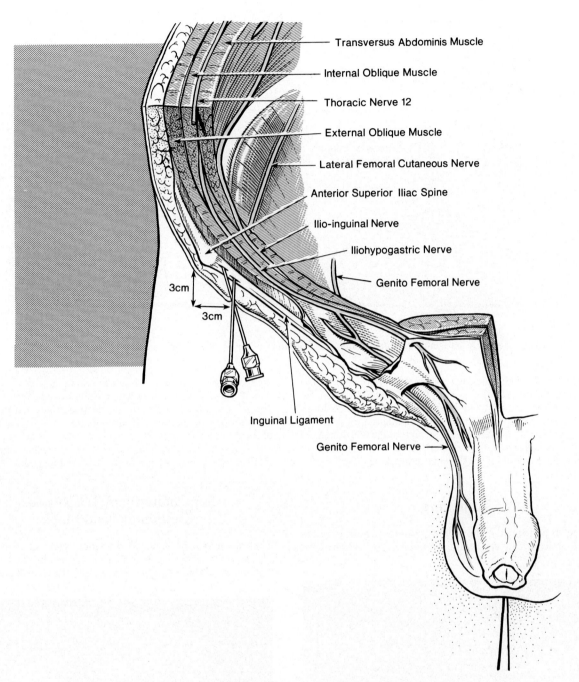

- Transversus Abdominis Muscle
- Internal Oblique Muscle
- Thoracic Nerve 12
- External Oblique Muscle
- Lateral Femoral Cutaneous Nerve
- Anterior Superior Iliac Spine
- Ilio-inguinal Nerve
- Iliohypogastric Nerve
- Genito Femoral Nerve

3cm

3cm

Inguinal Ligament

Genito Femoral Nerve

FIGURE 16-26. Iliac crest block. Note point of needle insertion 3 cm caudad to and 3 cm medial to anterior superior iliac spine. Initial direction of needle is superolateral to reach the inner aspect of iliac bone. Then, the needle is redirected approximately perpendicular to the long axis of the body (see also Fig. 14–13). Note the locations of nerves in relation to muscles of the abdominal wall. An alternative technique is to insert the needle 3 cm along a line from anterior superior iliac spine to umbilicus.

Complications

Hematoma (both subcutaneous and pelvic) (74) is possible with this technique, as is local anaesthetic toxicity (particularly if performed in combination with surgical infiltration during inguinal hernia repair). A femoral nerve block may occur if the needle tip is too deep (75); bowel perforation is a rare complication (76).

TRANSVERSUS ABDOMINIS FIELD BLOCK

Anatomy

The transversus abdominis plane is traversed by all the nerves that provide sensory innervation of the anterolateral

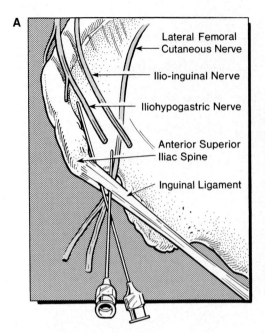

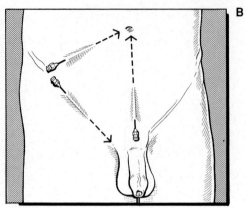

FIGURE 16-27. A: Bone and ligamentous landmarks in relation to nerves. **B:** Superficial infiltration for herniorrhaphy.

abdominal wall. This muscular plane lies between internal oblique and transversus abdominus muscles in the mid-axillary line between the iliac crest and the subcostal region. Deposition of local anesthetic in this plane produces analgesia for patients undergoing surgical procedures via an abdominal incision. McDonnell and colleagues have demonstrated the feasibility of delivering local anesthetic to this anatomic plane (77).

Technique

The block is performed in the supine position in awake or anesthetized patients. The needle insertion point is just superior to

the iliac crest and posterior to the midaxillary line. After the skin is anesthetized, an 18-gauge Tuohy needle is used. Two "pops" are appreciated as the needle penetrates first the external oblique and then the internal oblique muscle. Twenty mL of local anesthetic (e.g., 0.25% plain bupivacaine) is injected. For a midline incision, bilateral blocks are necessary to ensure that sensory afferents from both sides are blocked.

Sonoanatomy of Transversus Abdominis Field Block

The muscles of the anterior abdominal wall are readily visible as three distinct layers (external oblique, internal oblique, transversus abdominis) (Fig. 16-31) with the transducer placed

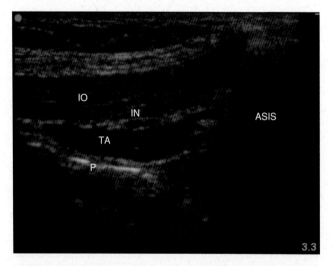

FIGURE 16-28. Ultrasound appearance of ilioinguinal nerve. *IO*, internal oblique; *TA*, transversus abdominis; *IN*, ilioinguinal nerve; *P*, peritoneum; *ASIS*, anterior superior iliac spine. From Harmon D, Frizelle HP, Sandhu NS, et al. *Perioperative Diagnostic and Interventional Ultrasound.* New York: Saunders, 2007, with permission.

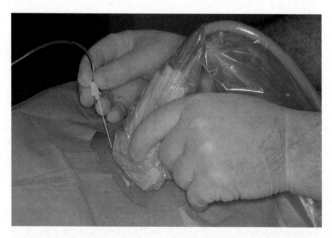

FIGURE 16-29. Ilioinguinal nerve block. Ultrasound transducer is placed medial to the anterior superior iliac spine in an oblique axial orientation. Needle orientation is parallel to the ultrasound beam. From Harmon D, Frizelle HP, Sandhu NS, et al. *Perioperative Diagnostic and Interventional Ultrasound.* New York: Saunders, 2007, with permission.

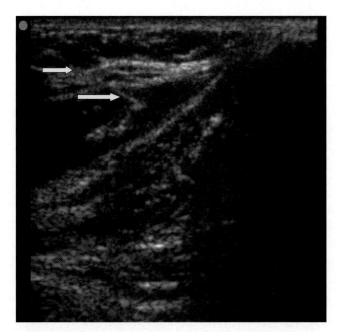

FIGURE 16-30. Real-time imaging of needle insertion (arrows) for ilioinguinal nerve block. From Harmon D, Frizelle HP, Sandhu NS, et al. *Perioperative Diagnostic and Interventional Ultrasound.* New York: Saunders, 2007, with permission.

in a longitudinal orientation in the flank. The muscle layers are seen as marbled transverse structures surrounded by bright hyperechoic fascial coverings. The muscles have different echogenicity patterns due to their differing orientation. The peritoneum and intestine are seen deep to the muscles (Fig. 16-31). No published data are available on ultrasound-guided transversus abdominis block. The use of ultrasound may decrease the incidence of complications and improve the success rate of the block, but this benefit has yet to be studied.

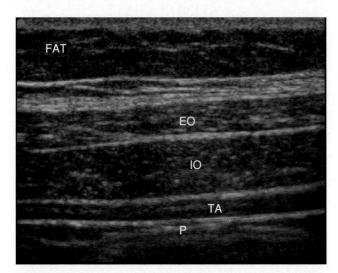

FIGURE 16-31. Ultrasound appearance of the lateral abdominal wall. *EO*, external oblique muscle; *IO*, internal oblique muscle; *TA*, transversus abdominis muscle; *P*, peritoneum. From Harmon D, Frizelle HP, Sandhu NS, et al. *Perioperative Diagnostic and Interventional Ultrasound.* New York: Saunders, 2007, with permission.

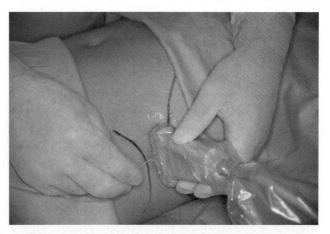

FIGURE 16-32. Ultrasound transducer and needle positioning during the ultrasound-guided transversus abdominis plane block.

Ultrasound-guided Transversus Abdominus Field Block Technique

The needle insertion point on the lateral abdominal wall is just cephalad to the iliac crest, behind the midaxillary line (Fig. 16-32). The target is kept in the center of the field of view, and the needle entry site is at the inferior border of the linear transducer. After skin infiltration, a 21-gauge needle is introduced at the inferior border of the transducer and visualized along its entire path to the transversus abdominis muscle (Fig. 16-33).

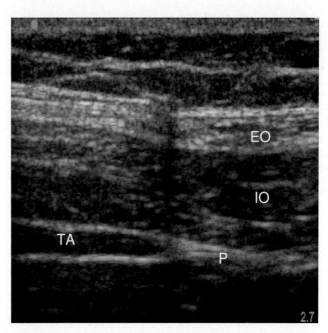

FIGURE 16-33. Real-time imaging of needle insertion for the transabdominis plane block. *EO*, external oblique; *IO*, internal oblique muscle; *TA*, transversus abdominis muscle; *P*, peritoneum. From Harmon D, Frizelle HP, Sandhu NS, et al. *Perioperative Diagnostic and Interventional Ultrasound.* New York: Saunders, 2007, with permission.

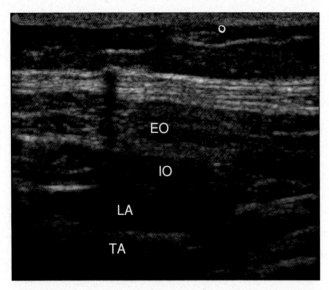

FIGURE 16-34. Ultrasound appearance of 20 mL of local anesthetic solution filling the transversus abdominis plane. *LA*, local anesthetic; *EO*, external oblique muscle; *IO* internal oblique muscle; *TA* transversus abdominis muscle. From Harmon D, Frizelle HP, Sandhu NS, et al. *Perioperative Diagnostic and Interventional Ultrasound.* New York: Saunders, 2007, with permission.

It is important not to advance the needle without good visualization, which may require transducer adjustment.

Injection in the correct plane can be confirmed by injecting 3 to 5 mL of solution and observing the spread in the desired plane. Following confirmation of correct needle placement, 20 mL of solution may then be injected and observed to fill the plane (Fig. 16-34).

Surgical Applications

Analgesic efficacy of the transverses abdominus block has been demonstrated for retropubic prostatectomy (78,79). The authors have also used this block successfully in combination with general anesthesia for inguinal hernia and appendectomy surgery.

Nonsurgical Applications

These blocks are useful in diagnosing nerve entrapment syndromes following herniorrhaphy.

Complications

Hematoma may occur following femoral nerve block, if local anaesthetic reaches the plane between the transversus abdominis and transversalis fascia, and tracks deep to the iliacus fascia to anesthetize the femoral nerve (80).

PERITONEAL LAVAGE

Once the peritoneal cavity has been entered, additional nociceptive pathways are recruited: These are the afferent pain fibers of the sympathetic and parasympathetic nervous systems. Lavage of the peritoneal cavity with large volumes of local anesthetic solution will result in analgesia; however, it is difficult to lavage all peritoneal surfaces, and the solution must be left in the abdomen for 10 minutes. One hundred to 300 mL of solution (e.g., 0.15% lidocaine or 0.10% bupivacaine) are instilled into the peritoneal cavity after entrance into the cavity. Slight jostling of the abdomen may aid distribution. The Trendelenburg position aids the flow of the solution over the celiac area and the inferior surface of the diaphragm; this often improves analgesia. Although local anesthetic solutions are absorbed readily from mucosal surfaces, serum local anesthetic levels are surprisingly low (highest level, 2.2 μg/mL after 500 mg of 0.5% lidocaine) (81). The laparoscope may also be used to deliver lavage solution. Peritoneal instillation of either lidocaine or bupivacaine has been shown to reduce markedly the incidence and severity of referred shoulder pain after laparoscopy (82), and is adequate as a sole anesthetic for laparoscopic tubal ligation (81), if surgical manipulation is deliberately gentle and overdistention of the pneumoperitoneum is avoided. Combined with wound infiltration (or rectus sheath block), peritoneal lavage can often provide a prolonged pain-free period for patients after laparoscopic surgery (83).

In contrast to its value for laparoscopic procedures, the benefit of intraperitoneal local anesthetic after open laparotomy is controversial. Although some studies have demonstrated improvements in analgesia, a decreased hyperglycemic (stress) response, and improved colonic motility (84), others have not shown these benefits (85), even when local anesthetic is infused continuously through an intraperitoneal catheter (86).

SUMMARY

Peripheral nerve blocks and other regional anesthetic techniques such as intrapleural or intraperitoneal instillation of local anesthetic are readily taught and learned, and have a high success rate, particularly when sonographic techniques are used to supplement traditional palpation of landmarks. These methods may be used to supplement or substitute for epidural anesthesia and analgesia (described in Chapters 11 and 23 by Veering and Cousins, and Carli and Asenjo, respectively). These straightforward methods are broadly applicable to most thoracic and abdominal surgical procedures, and have proven themselves generally effective in providing postoperative analgesia and, in certain cases, blunting associated stress responses.

References

1. Macrae WA. Chronic pain after surgery. *Br J Anaesth* 2001;87:88–98.
2. Filipovic M, Jeger R, Probst C, et al. Heart rate variability and cardiac troponin I are incremental and independent predictors of one-year all cause mortality after major noncardiac surgery in patients at risk of coronary artery disease. *J Am Coll Cardiol* 2003;42:1767–1776.
3. Duggleby W, Lander J. Cognitive status and postoperative pain: Older adults. *J Pain Symptom Manage* 1994;9(1):19–27.
4. Kamming D, Chung F, Williams D, McGrath BM, Curti B. Pain management in ambulatory surgery. *J Perianesth Nurs* 2004;19(3):174–182.
5. Klein SM, Evans H, Nielsen KC, Tucker MS, Warner DS, Steele SM.

Peripheral nerve block techniques for ambulatory surgery. *Anesth Analg* 2005;101(6):1663–1676.

6. Rawal N, Sjostrand U, Dahlstrom B, et al. Epidural morphine for postoperative pain relief: A comparative study with intramuscular narcotic and intercostal block. *Anesth Analg* 1982;61:93.

7. Jakobson S, Fridriksson H, Hedenstrom H, Ivarsson I. Effects of intercostal nerve blocks on pulmonary mechanics in healthy men. *Acta Anaesthesiol Scand* 1980;24:482.

8. Davies RG, Myles PS, Graham JM. A comparison of the analgesic efficacy and side-effects of paravertebral vs epidural blockade for thoracotomy—a systematic review and meta-analysis of randomized trials. *Br J Anaesth* 2006;96(4):418–426.

9. Hargett MJ, Beckman JD, Liguori GA, et al. Education Committee in the Department of *Anesthesiology* at Hospital for Special Surgery. Guidelines for regional anesthesia fellowship training. *Reg Anesth Pain Med* 2005;30(3):218–225.

10. Kopp VJ, Shafer A. Anesthesiologists and perioperative communication. *Anesthesiology* 2000;93(2):548–555.

11. Tryba M. Choices in sedation. *Eur J Anaesthesiol Suppl* 1996;13:22–25.

12. Kenny GN. Patient sedation: Technical problems and developments. *Eur J Anaesthesiol* 1996;13[Supp 13]:18–21.

13. Practice guidelines for sedation and analgesia by non-anesthesiologists: A Report by the American Society of Anesthesiologists Task Force on Sedation and Analgesia by Non-Anesthesiologists. *Anesthesiology* 1996;84:459–471.

14. Bailey PL, Egan TD, Stanley TH. Intravenous opioids anesthetics. In: Miller RD, ed. *Anesthesia*, 5th ed. New York: Churchill-Livingstone, 2000:273–376.

15. Gairaj NM, Sharma SK, Souter AJ, et al. A survey of obstetric patients who refuse regional anaesthesia. *Anaesthesia* 1995;50(8):740–741.

16. Hardy PA. Anatomical variation in the position of the proximal intercostal nerve. *Br J Anaesth* 1988;61:338.

17. Nunn J, Slavin C. Posterior intercostal nerve block for pain relief after cholecystectomy. *Br J Anaesth* 1980;52:253.

18. Conacher ID, Kokri M. Postoperative paravertebral blocks for thoracic surgery. A radiological appraisal. *Br J Anaesth* 1987;59:155–161.

19. Lönnqvist PA, MacKenzie J, Soni AK, Conacher ID. Paravertebral blockade. Failure rate and complications. *Anaesthesia* 1995;50:813–815.

20. Detterbeck FC. Subpleural catheter placement for pain relief after thoracoscopic resection. *Ann Thorac Surg* 2006;81:1522–1523.

21. Detterbeck FC. Efficacy of methods of intercostal nerve blockade for pain relief after thoracotomy. *Ann Thorac Surg* 2005;80:1550–1559.

22. Eichenberger U, Greher M, Curatolo M. Ultrasound in interventional pain management. *Tech Reg Anesth Pain Manage* 2004;8:171–178.

23. Atanassoff PG, Alon E, Pasch T, et al. Intercostal nerve block for minor breast surgery. *Reg Anesth* 1991;16:23.

24. Atanassoff PG, Alon E, Weiss BM. Intercostal nerve block for lumpectomy: Superior postoperative pain relief with bupivacaine. *J Clin Anesth* 1994;6(1):47–51.

25. Malhotra V, Long CW, Meister MJ. Intercostal blocks with local infiltration anesthesia for extracorporeal shock wave lithotripsy. *Anesth Analg* 1987;66:85.

26. Raza SM, Vasireddy AR, Candido KD, et al. A complete regional anesthesia technique for cardiac pacemaker insertion. *J Cardiothorac Vasc Anesth* 1991;5:54.

27. Moore D, Bridenbaugh L. Pneumothorax: Its incidence following intercostal nerve block. *JAMA* 1962;182:1005.

28. Gauntlett IS. Total spinal anesthesia following intercostal nerve block. *Anesthesiology* 1986;65:82.

29. Sury M, Bingham R. Accidental spinal anaesthesia following intrathoracic intercostal nerve block. *Anaesthesia* 1986;41:401.

30. Iwama H, Tase C, Kawamae K, et al. Catheter location and patient position affect spread of interpleural regional analgesia. *Anesthesiology* 1993;79:1153.

31. Symreng T, Gomez MN, Johnson B, et al. Intrapleural bupivacaine—technical considerations and intraoperative use. *J Cardiothorac Anesth* 1989;3:139.

32. Reiestad F, Stromskag K. Interpleural catheter in the management of postoperative pain: A preliminary report. *Reg Anesth* 1986;11:89.

33. Riegler FX, Vade BT, Pelligrino DA. Interpleural anesthetics in the dog: Differential somatic neural blockade. *Anesthesiology* 1989;71:744.

34. Stromskag KE, Reiestad F, Holmqvist EL, Ogenstad S. Intrapleural administration of 0.25%, 0.375%, and 0.5% bupivacaine with epinephrine after cholecystectomy. *Anesth Analg* 1988;67:430.

35. Seltzer JL, Larijani GE, Goldberg ME, Marr AT. Intrapleural bupivacaine-a kinetic and dynamic evaluation. *Anesthesiology* 1987;67:798–800.

36. Frenette L, Boudreault D, Guay J. Interpleural analgesia improves pulmonary function after cholecystectomy. *Can J Anaesth* 1991;38:71.

37. Rademaker BM, Sih IL, Kalkman CJ, et al. Effects of interpleurally administered bupivacaine 0.5% on opioid analgesic requirements and endocrine response during and after cholecystectomy: A randomized, double-blind, controlled study. *Acta Anaesthesiol Scand* 1991;35:108.

38. Ferrante FM, Chan VW, Arthur GR, Rocco AG. Interpleural analgesia after thoracotomy. *Anesth Analg* 1991;72:105.

39. Symreng T, Gomez MN, Rossi N. Intrapleural bupivacaine vs. saline after thoracotomy: Effects on pain and lung function—A double-blind study. *J Cardiothorac Anesth* 1989;3:144, 1989.

40. Richardson J, Sabanathan S, Mearns AJ, Shah RD, Goulden C. A prospective, randomized comparison of interpleural and paravertebral analgesia in thoracic surgery. *Br J Anaesth* 1995;75:405–408.

41. Rocco A, Reiestad F, Gudman J, McKay W. Intrapleural administration of local anesthetics for pain relief in patients with multiple rib fractures. *Reg Anesth* 1987;12:10.

42. Ahlburg P, Noreng M, Molgaard J, Egebo K. Treatment of pancreatic pain with interpleural bupivacaine: An open trial. *Acta Anaesthesiol Scand* 1990;34:156.

43. Perkins G. Interpleural anaesthesia in the management of upper limb ischaemia: A report of three cases. *Anaesth Intensive Care* 1991;19:575.

44. Reiestad F, McIlvaine WB, Kvalheim L, et al. Successful treatment of chronic pancreatitis pain with interpleural analgesia. *Can J Anaesth* 1989;36:713.

45. Reiestad F, McIlvaine WB, Kvalheim L, et al. Interpleural analgesia in treatment of upper extremity reflex sympathetic dystrophy. *Anesth Analg* 1989;69:671.

46. Dionne C. Tumour invasion of the brachial plexus: Management of pain with intrapleural analgesia. *Can J Anaesth* 1992;39:520.

47. Reiestad F, McIlvaine WB, Barnes M, et al. Interpleural analgesia in the treatment of severe thoracic postherpetic neuralgia. *Reg Anesth* 1990;15:113.

48. Vaghadia H, Jenkins LC. Use of a Doppler ultrasound stethoscope for intercostal nerve block. *Can J Anaesth* 1988;35:86.

49. Stromskag KE, Minor B, Steen PA. Side effects and complications related to interpleural analgesia: An update. *Acta Anaesthesiol Scand* 1990;34:473.

50. van Kleef J, Burm A, Vletter AA. Single-dose interpleural vs. intercostal blockade: Nerve block characteristics and plasma concentration profiles after administration of 0.5% bupivacaine with epinephrine. *Anesth Analg* 1990;70(5):484–488.

51. Kowalski SE, Bradley BD, Greengrass RA, et al. Effects of interpleural bupivacaine (0.5%) on canine diaphragmatic function. *Anesth Analg* 1992;75:400.

52. Lauder GR. Interpleural analgesia and phrenic nerve paralysis. *Anaesthesia* 1993;48:315.

53. Shantha TR. Unilateral bronchospasm after interpleural analgesia. *Anesth Analg* 1992;74:291.

54. Billstrom R, Blomberg HM. Cholestasis after interpleural bupivacaine for chronic upper limb pain. *Anesth Analg* 1993;76:1158.

55. Naja ZM, El-Rajab M, Al-Tannir MA, et al. Thoracic paravertebral block: Influence of the number of injections. *Reg Anesth Pain Med* 2006;31(3):196–201.

56. Lang SA, Saito T. Thoracic paravertebral nerve block, nerve stimulator guidance and the endothoracic fascia. *Anaesthesia* 2005;60(9):930–931.

57. Pusch F, Wildling E, Klimscha W, Weinstabl C. Sonographic measurement of needle insertion depth in paravertebral blocks in women. *Br J Anaesth* 2000;85(6):841–843.

58. Kairaluoma PM, Bachmann MS, Rosenberg PH, Pere PJ. Preincisional paravertebral block reduces the prevalence of chronic pain after breast surgery. *Anesth Analg* 2006;103(3):703–708.

59. Naja ZM, Maaliki H, Al-Tannir MA, et al. Repetitive paravertebral nerve block using a catheter technique for pain relief in post-herpetic neuralgia. *Br J Anaesth* 2006;96(3):381–383.

60. Boezaart AP, Raw RM. Continuous thoracic paravertebral block for major breast surgery. *Reg Anesth Pain Med* 2006;31(5):470–476.

61. Purcell-Jones G, Pither C, Justins D. Paravertebral somatic nerve block: A clinical, radiographic, and computed tomography study in chronic pain patients. *Anesth Analg* 1989;68:32.

62. Naja Z, Lönnqvist P-A. Somatic paravertebral nerve blockade Incidence of failed block and complications. *Anaesthesia* 2001;56(12):1181–1201.

63. Lin HM, Chelly JE. Post-dural headache associated with thoracic paravertebral blocks. *J Clin Anesth* 2006;18(5):376–378.

64. Richardson J, Vowden P, Sabanathan S. Bilateral paravertebral analgesia for major abdominal vascular surgery: A preliminary report. *Anaesthesia*. 1995;50(11):995–998.

65. Culp WC Jr., Culp WC. Thoracic paravertebral block for percutaneous transhepatic biliary drainage. *J Vasc Interv Radiol* 2005;16(10):1397–1400.

66. Kelly FE, Murdoch JA, Sanders DJ, Berrisford RG. Continuous paravertebral block for thoraco-abdominal oesophageal surgery. *Anaesthesia* 2005;60(1):98–99.

67. Klein SM, Pietrobon R, Nielsen KC, et al. Paravertebral somatic nerve block compared with peripheral nerve blocks for outpatient inguinal herniorrhaphy. *Reg Anesth Pain Med* 2002;27(5):476–480.

68. Saito T, Den S, Tanuma K, et al. Anatomical bases for anaesthetic paravertebral block: Fluid communication between the thoracic and lumbar paravertebral regions. *Surg Radiol Anat* 1999;21:359–363.

PART II: TECHNIQUES

69. Willschke H, Bosenberg A, Marhofer P, et al. Ultrasonography-guided rectus sheath block in paediatric anaesthesia—a new approach to an old technique. *Br J Anaesth* 2006;97(2):244–249.

70. Templeton T. Rectus block for postoperative pain relief. *Reg Anesth* 1993; 18:258.

71. Bunting P, McConachie I. Ilioinguinal nerve blockade for analgesia after caesarean section. *Br J Anaesth* 1988;61:773.

72. Van Schoor AN, Boon JM, Bosenberg AT, et al. Anatomical considerations of the pediatric ilioinguinal/iliohypogastric nerve block. *Paediatr Anaesth* 2005;15(5):371–377.

73. Willschke H, Marhofer P, Bosenberg A, et al. Ultrasonography for ilioinguinal/iliohypogastric nerve blocks in children. *Br J Anaesth* 2005;95(2):226–230.

74. Vaisman J. Pelvic haematoma after an ilio-inguinal nerve block for orchialgia. *Anesth Analg* 2001;92:1048–1049.

75. Ghani KR, McMillan R, Peterson-Brown S. Transient femoral nerve palsy following ilio-inguinal nerve blockade for day case inguinal hernia repair. J R Coll Surg Edinburgh 2002;47:626–639.

76. Amory C, Mariscal A, Guyot E, et al. Is ilio-inguinal/ilio-hypogastric nerve block always totally safe in children? *Paed Anesth* 2003;13:164–166.

77. McDonnell JG, O'Donnell B, Tuite D, et al. Tomographic and Anatomical identification of a novel approach to the transversus abdominis neurovascular fascial plane. *Anesthesiology* 2004;101:A899.

78. O'Donnell BD, McDonnell JG, McShane AJ. The transversus abdominis plane block in open retropubic prostatectomy. *Reg Anesth Pain Med* 2006;31:91.

79. McDonnell JG, O'Donnell BD, Heffernan A, et al. The analgesic efficacy of transversus abdominis plane block after abdominal surgery: A prospective randomized controlled trial. *Anesth Analg* 2007;104(1):193–197.

80. Rosario DJ, Jacob S, Luntley K, et al. Mechanism of femoral nerve palsy complicating ilio-inguinal field block. *Br J Anaesth* 1997;78:314–316.

81. Deeb R, Viechnicki M. Laparoscopic tubal ligation under peritoneal lavage anesthesia. *Reg Anesth* 1985;10:24.

82. Narchi P, Benhamou D, Fernandez H. Intraperitoneal local anaesthetic for shoulder pain after day-case laparoscopy. *Lancet* 1991;338:1569.

83. Helvacioglu A, Weis R. Operative laparoscopy and postoperative pain relief. *Fertil Steril* 1992;57:548.

84. Rimback G, Cassuto J, Faxen A, et al. Effect of intra-abdominal bupivacaine instillation on postoperative colonic motility. *Gut* 1986;27:170.

85. Wallin G, Cassuto J, Hogstrom S, Hedner T. Influence of intraperitoneal anesthesia on pain and the sympathoadrenal response to abdominal surgery. *Acta Anaesthesiol Scand* 1988;32:553.

86. Scott N, Mogensen T, Greulich A, et al. No effect of continuous IP infusion of bupivacaine on postoperative analgesia, pulmonary function, and the stress response to surgery. *Br J Anaesth* 1988;61:165.

CHAPTER 17 ■ SOMATIC BLOCKADE OF THE HEAD AND NECK

SANTHANAM SURESH AND NARASIMHAN JAGANNATHAN

Regional anesthesia for head and neck procedures have a long and successful history of use and application in dental surgery and otolaryngology. The application of these blocks has now extended into the breadth of plastic surgery (1), neurosurgical procedures (2), and, in addition, to outside the operating room, such as in treatment of chronic pain states. Important advantages of regional techniques include decrease in intraoperative and postoperative opioids use (3) as well as a less stressful perioperative experience. Regional anesthesia for procedures involving the head and neck can potentially provide excellent postoperative analgesia without the adverse effects of opioids (4).

Regional anesthetic techniques involving the head and neck are predominantly sensory nerve blocks, and adverse effects such as nerve damage are rarely reported. Because of the anatomy of the area, and the close relationship of cranial and cervical nerves to many vital structures, meticulous placement of the needle and smaller volumes of the anesthetic agent are required. The landmarks for regional anesthesia in the head and neck are relatively constant, easily located, and mostly predictable. Despite these advantages, nerve blocks to the head and neck remain underutilized in routine clinical practice.

Applied anatomic knowledge is of vital importance for the success of regional anesthesia in general and particularly so in providing regional anesthesia of the head and neck. Cadaveric dissections, reviewing the anatomy with a regional anesthesia atlas, and frequent reference to a model skull is advisable, both while learning how to perform these blocks and prior to such procedures. The availability of these techniques on dedicated regional anesthesia web sites, with video-assisted demonstrations of these blocks, has increased their usage in anesthesia practice.

As more prospective studies are performed and peer-reviewed literature of regional anesthesia for head and neck procedures are made available, the demand and popularity of these techniques may increase. This chapter will elucidate the anatomy, technique, and potential advantages and adverse effects of commonly used peripheral nerve blocks of the head and neck. Regional blockade of the mouth and circumoral structures, as well as the eye, are described in detail in Chapters 18 and 19, respectively. These techniques will be only briefly discussed in the current chapter.

APPLIED ANATOMY

The trigeminal nerve and the cervical plexus primarily provide the cutaneous sensory innervation to the face, head, and neck. In addition, the glossopharyngeal and vagus nerves supply the pharynx and larynx.

Embryology

The anatomy and complexity of the nerve supply of the head, neck, and face in the adult is perhaps best understood in light of its development in the embryo, as the face forms around the primitive mouth (the stomodeum). Initially, the stomodeum is surrounded caudally by the mandibular arch (which is supplied by the mandibular nerve), laterally on each side by the maxillary processes (which are supplied by the maxillary division of the trigeminal nerve), and rostrally by the forebrain capsule, from which develops the frontonasal process (which is supplied by the first division of the trigeminal nerve, the ophthalmic nerve). The frontonasal process grows down into the primitive stomodeum from the forebrain capsule, and eventually this will form the nose of the mature embryo (Fig. 17-1). The two maxillary processes grow inward from either side and join together below the primitive nose, as shown, and they then form the rostral margin of the primitive mouth. Thus, in the mature face, the forehead, eyebrows, upper eyelids, and nose are supplied by the first ophthalmic division of the trigeminal nerve. The lower eyelid, cheek, and upper lip are supplied by the second division (i.e., the maxillary nerve), and the lower lip, chin, mandibular, and temporal regions are supplied by the third division, mandibular nerve. Because of the disproportionate growth of the cranial cavity in humans, these dermatomal distributions are distorted cranially, with the result that some skin innervated by the cervical plexus is drawn up over the angle of the mandible onto the face and posteriorly over the occipital area and the scalp as far forward as the vertex (Fig. 17-2).

The Trigeminal Nerve

The trigeminal nerve is the predominant sensory nerve of the head and face, and is also the motor supply for the muscles of mastication. It originates from the pons. The sensory fibers derive from the cells of the semilunar temporal bone. As it enters the pons, it divides into upper and lower roots. Three branches arise, the ophthalmic V1, maxillary V2, and the mandibular V3 divisions. Both the ophthalmic and maxillary divisions consist exclusively of sensory fibers, whereas the mandibular nerve also has a motor component (Table 17-1).

The semilunar ganglion, also known as the Gasserian ganglion, lies posteromedially in the middle cranial fossa at the junction of its floor and the cavernous sinus just anterior to the ridge of the petrous temporal bone. The ganglion invaginates the dura and therefore lies in a dural pouch—Meckel's cave—which contains cerebrospinal fluid (CSF).

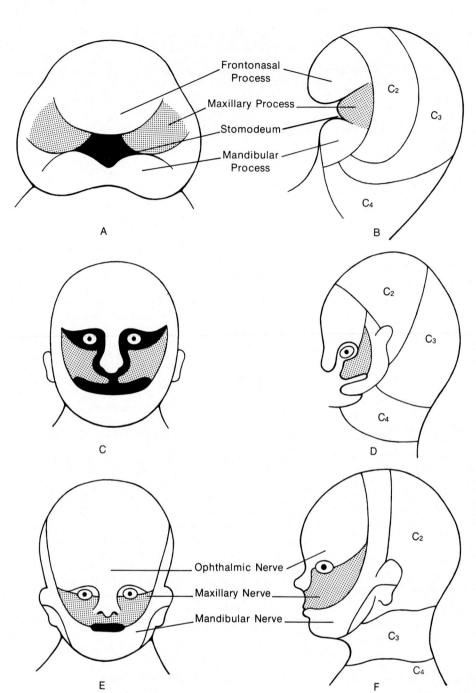

FIGURE 17-1. Frontal and lateral views of development of dermatomes of the head and neck. **A, B:** The primitive stomodeum (mouth) is surrounded by the three parts of the developing face. **C, D:** The frontonasal process (supplied by the ophthalmic nerve) grows in from above, the maxillary processes (maxillary nerve) grow in from each side, and the mandibular process (mandibular nerve) forms the caudal margin. **E, F:** The frontonasal process forms the brow, eyebrows, upper eyelid, and nose in the fully developed face. The maxillary process forms both cheeks, lower eyelid, and upper lip. The mandibular process gives rise to the lower lip, the chin, and a strip of skin extending up the side of the face, often to the vertex, including the superior anterior two-thirds of the anterior surface of the ear. The cervical plexus derivatives of the second, third, and fourth cervical nerves supply the posterior part of the head and neck from the vertex down. Note in **F** that the skin over the angle of the jaw and the lower part of the auricle on the anterior surface and all of its posterior surface are supplied by cervical plexus dermatomes (C2).

Ophthalmic (V1) Division Trigeminal Nerve

In its intracranial course, the trunk of the ophthalmic nerve does not lend itself to regional anesthesia. The intraorbital branches of the nasociliary nerve are blocked by retrobulbar block. The intraorbital branches, anterior ethmoidal and infratrochlear, can also be blocked in the orbit. The terminal divisions in the forehead and nose are suitable for peripheral nerve blocks of the scalp and face (6).

The ophthalmic nerve is the smallest division of the trigeminal nerve. It supplies the cornea, conjunctiva, ciliary body, and the iris. The lacrimal gland; mucous membranes of the nasal cavity; the skin of the eyebrow, eyelids, and forehead; and the nose are also supplied by this division. The frontal nerve is the largest branch and may be regarded as the continuation of the first division of the trigeminal nerve. As it enters the orbit through the superior orbital fissure, it proceeds forward between the levator palpebrae superioris and the periosteum. The two branches, the supraorbital and the supratrochlear nerve supply sensory innervation to the forehead and anterior scalp (Fig. 17-3). The supraorbital nerve and vessels emerge from the supraorbital foramen and continue superiorly on the anterior portion of the forehead and scalp. The supraorbital nerve trunk divides into a deep and a superficial branch. The deep branch courses superiorly and laterally, running parallel to

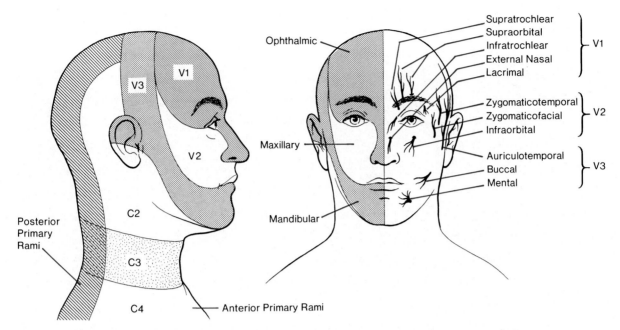

FIGURE 17-2. Dermatomes and cutaneous nerves of head, neck, and face. Note that the supraorbital, infraorbital, and mental nerves all lie in the same vertical plane as the pupil, with the eye looking straight forward. The external nasal area is innervated by infratrochlear and external nasal (from anterior ethmoidal *n.*) branches of V1 and the infraorbital branch of V2. The internal nasal cavity is shown in Figure 17-6.

the superior temporal line of the skull in the loose areolar tissue between the galea and the pericranium. The terminal branches of the deep supraorbital nerve branch pierces the galea near the coronal suture to supply scalp sensation. The superficial division lies medially at its origin and quickly divides into multiple branches that pierce the frontalis muscle. These smaller branches pass cephalad to supply the forehead and up to 3.5 cm of the frontal scalp.

The supratrochlear nerves exit the orbit at the superior orbital rim through a notch, above the trochlea and medial to the supraorbital notch. At the supraorbital rim, the nerves penetrate the corrugator muscle and the frontalis muscle. The nerves supply cutaneous sensation to a central vertical strip of forehead and to the medial upper eyelid (7).

TABLE 17-1

TRIGEMINAL NERVE DISTRIBUTION

Trigeminal nerve and its branches
Ophthalmic V1
Supraorbital nerve
Supratrochlear nerve
Maxillary V2
Maxillary division of the trigeminal nerve (Infraorbital nerve)
Greater palatine nerve
Mandibular V3
Mental nerve
Mandibular nerve
Auriculotemporal nerve

Maxillary Division (V2) of the Trigeminal Nerve

The maxillary nerve is purely sensory and is called the *infraorbital nerve* when it reaches the infraorbital fossa. It divides into four branches: the external nasal, the internal nasal, the inferior palpebral, and the superior labial. The nerve can be easily accessed superficially. The posterior superior alveolar branch arises from the trunk of the nerve just before it enters the infraorbital groove. It enters the infratemporal surface of the maxilla communicating with the middle superior alveolar branch, giving off branches to the lining membrane of the maxillary sinus and branches to the molar teeth. The middle superior alveolar branch arises from the nerve in the posterior part of the infraorbital canal and runs downward and forward in a canal along the lateral wall of the maxillary sinus. The anterior superior alveolar nerve branches off just as it exits the infraorbital foramen and descends in a canal in the anterior wall of the maxillary sinus. It communicates with the middle superior alveolar branch, which supplies the mucous membrane of the anterior part of the inferior meatus and the floor of the nasal cavity, communicating with the branches from the sphenopalatine ganglia. The external nasal branches supply the skin of the nose and of the septum mobile nasi and joins with the terminal branches of the nasociliary nerve. The superior labial branches, the largest, descend behind the quadratus labii superioris and are distributed to the skin of the upper lip, the mucous membrane of the mouth, and the labial glands. They are joined, immediately below the orbit by filaments from the facial nerve, forming with them the infraorbital plexus (7). A computed tomography (CT)-guided imaging study demonstrated that the infraorbital foramen is located approximately 2 cm lateral to the midline in most children at the level of the inferior rim of the orbit (8). The superior anterior part of both

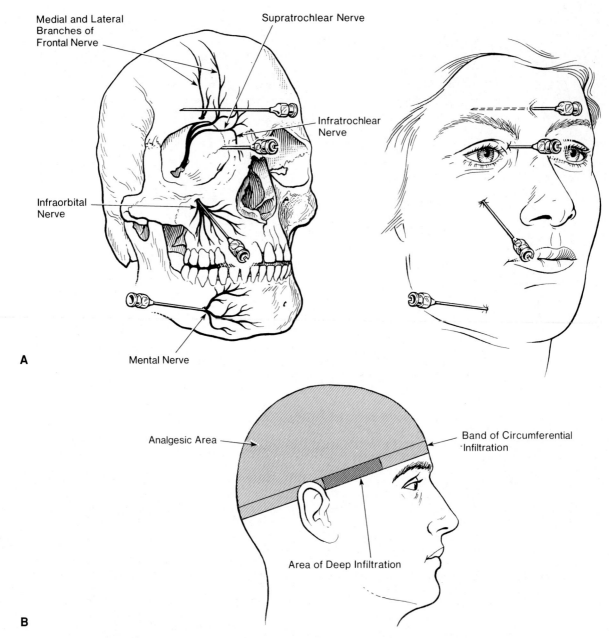

FIGURE 17-3. A: Nerve block of the superficial branches of the trigeminal nerve. The supraorbital and supratrochlear branches of the first division (ophthalmic) can be blocked as they emerge above the orbit. A single-needle insertion in the mid brow above the root of the nose can anesthetize the forehead bilaterally by infiltrations on either side through the same insertion. Note that this injection needs to be undertaken above the level of the eyebrow to prevent periorbital hematoma. The infratrochlear nerve (and also anterior ethmoidal nerve) is blocked by inserting a needle 1 cm above the inner canthus and just lateral to the medial wall of the orbit. The needle is directed posteriorly and slightly medially to a depth of about 2.5 cm. The infraorbital nerve is located one finger's breadth below the orbital rim in the same vertical position as the pupil with the eye looking forward. To enter the infraorbital foramen, advance the needle cephalad and laterally. It is not necessary, however, to enter the foramen, but just to infiltrate the nerve as it emerges at the foramen. The mental nerve is anesthetized again in the same vertical line as the pupil; to enter the mental foramen, direct the needle medially as shown in the diagram. The mental foramen lies at a different vertical level in the mandible at different ages. **B:** Circumferential infiltration of scalp. Note that infiltration is superficial except in the temporal region, where infiltration deep to deep fascia is useful to help prevent movement of the temporalis muscle during surgery. If periosteum will be stimulated, injection must be made deep to deep fascia.

septum and lateral wall of the nose receive contributions from the anterior ethmoidal branch of the ophthalmic nerve. The entire hard palate is supplied by the maxillary nerve via the sphenopalatine ganglion.

Palatine Nerve

The palatine nerves are distributed to the roof of the mouth, soft palate, tonsil, and lining membrane of the nasal cavity. Most of their branches are derived from the sphenopalatine branches of the maxillary nerve. There are three main branches: the anterior, middle, and posterior branches.

The *anterior palatine nerve* descends through the pterygopalatine canal and emerges in the hard palate through the greater palatine foramen. It passes in a groove in the hard palate as far as the incisor teeth. It supplies the gums, and the mucous membrane and glands of the hard palate.

The *middle palatine nerve* emerges through one of the minor palatine foramen and provides the sensory supply to the uvula, tonsils, and the soft palate.

The *posterior palatine nerve* descends through the pterygopalatine canal and emerges through a special opening behind the greater palatine foramen. It supplies the sensory branches to the soft palate, tonsils, and uvula. The middle and posterior palatine branches join the tonsillar branch of the glossopharyngeal to form a plexus (cirrus tonsillaris) around the tonsils (7).

Mandibular Division (V3) of the Trigeminal Nerve

The mandibular nerve emerges from the cranial cavity through the floor of the middle cranial fossa, via the foramen ovale, to enter the infratemporal fossa. This fossa is a rectangular compartment bounded anteriorly by the posterior wall of the maxilla and posteriorly by the styloid apparatus and carotid sheath. The lateral wall is the ramus of the mandible, and the medial wall is composed anteriorly of the lateral pterygoid plate of the sphenoid bone and posteriorly by the constrictor muscles of the pharynx. It has no floor, but its roof is the floor of the middle cranial fossa. In the infratemporal fossa, the mandibular nerve divides into its terminal branches.

Glossopharyngeal Nerve

The glossopharyngeal nerve supplies the posterior third of the tongue and the oropharynx from its junction with the nasopharynx at the level of the hard palate. It supplies the pharyngeal surfaces of the soft palate and the epiglottis, and the pharyngeal wall, as far down as the pharyngoesophageal junction at the level of the cricoid cartilage (C6).

Vagus Nerve

The vagus nerve supplies sensation to the larynx. The undersurface of the epiglottis and the laryngeal inlet down to the vocal folds are supplied by the internal laryngeal branch of the vagus. This nerve reaches the larynx by piercing the thyrohyoid membrane, which joins the thyroid to the hyoid cartilages. Below the cords, the larynx and trachea are supplied by the recurrent branch of the vagus that ascends in the neck, in the groove between the trachea and esophagus. The recurrent laryngeal nerve also supplies motor function to all the intrinsic muscles of the larynx (except the cricothyroid muscle), and bilateral motor block produces loss of phonation and loss of ability to close the glottis.

Cervical Plexus

The cervical plexus contributes to the supply of both the deep and the superficial structures of the neck. The first cervical nerve, C1, is a motor nerve to the muscles of the suboccipital triangle and has no sensory distribution to skin. The skin of the neck is supplied in a sequential dermatomal pattern (like the trunk) by the cutaneous branches of C2–C4 by both anterior and posterior primary rami. The cervical plexus is formed by the ventral rami of the upper four cervical nerves. Their dorsal and ventral roots combine to form spinal nerves as they exit through the intervertebral foramen. The anterior rami of C2 through C4 form the cervical plexus. The cervical plexus lies behind the clavicular head of the sternocleidomastoid, giving out both the superficial and deep branches. The superficial cervical plexus wraps around the belly of the clavicular head of the sternocleidomastoid to form four branches: (a) the lesser occipital, (b) the great auricular, (c) the transverse cervical, and (d) the supraclavicular nerves. The great auricular nerve is the largest of the ascending branches. It arises from the second and third cervical nerve roots, winds around the posterior border of the sternocleidomastoid and, after perforating the deep fascia, ascends behind the clavicular head of the sternocleidomastoid beneath the platysma to the parotid gland, where it divides into an anterior and posterior branch. The anterior branch (ramus anterior; facial branch) is distributed to the skin of the face over the parotid gland and communicates in the substance of the gland with the facial nerve. The posterior branch (ramus posterior; mastoid branch) supplies the skin over the mastoid process and on the back of the auricle, except at its upper part; a filament pierces the auricle to reach its lateral surface, where it is distributed to the lobule and the lower part of the concha. The posterior branch communicates with the smaller lesser occipital, the auricular branch of the vagus, and the posterior auricular branch of the facial nerve (7).

In the region of the scalp, the nerves of supply have long superficial upward courses. Four sensory nerves pass in front of the ear to the scalp (supratrochlear and supraorbital from V1, zygomaticotemporal from V2, auriculotemporal from V3), and four pass behind the ear (great auricular and greater, lesser, and least occipital nerves from cervical plexus) (Figs. 17-2 and 17-3).

TRIGEMINAL NERVE BLOCK

Gasserian Ganglion Block

Indications

Gasserian ganglion block results in extensive anesthesia of the ipsilateral face, over the area shown in Figure 17-4. It was once used solely for surgery of the head and neck. With the advent of endotracheal intubation and more sophisticated techniques for general anesthesia, its appeal as a primary surgical anesthetic declined. However, it is still used diagnostically and therapeutically for neuralgias of the trigeminal system. It has merit as a diagnostic block, a permanent neurolytic block, and as a means

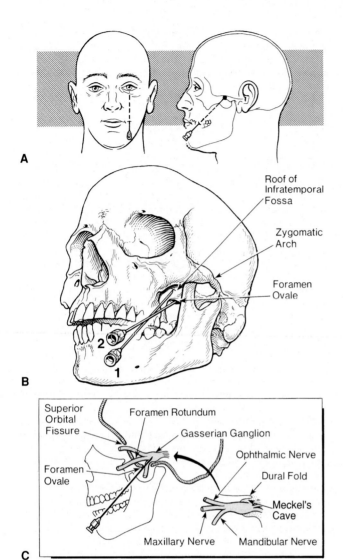

tains the carotid artery, and the third, fourth, and sixth cranial nerves. Superiorly, it is the inferior surface of the temporal lobe of the brain, and posterior to the ganglion lies the brainstem. Any of these structures might be damaged by the introduction of the needle through the foramen ovale. The ganglion is partially bathed in CSF, hence injections into the area might spread into the spinal fluid (Fig. 17-4).

Technique

An 8- to 10-cm, 22-gauge needle is required for Gasserian ganglion block. The point of introduction of the needle is approximately one finger's breadth posterior to the lateral margin of the mouth, next to the medial border of the masseter muscle (Table 17-2). In edentulous patients, this landmark may not permit a sufficient angle of approach to enter the foramen ovale, and therefore a point of insertion more caudad is needed. The direction of the needle is both rostral and medial, to a point that coincides with the midpoint of the zygomatic arch when viewed from the lateral aspect, and the pupil from the anterior view (with the eyes looking straight forward), as in Figure 17-4. It is important to keep a guiding finger in the oral cavity, palpating the cheek to ensure that the needle does not enter the mouth, which might, potentially, introduce contaminating bacteria into deeper structures. Such an approach usually causes the needle to impinge on the roof of the infratemporal fossa (i.e., the base of the skull, which is also the floor of the middle cranial fossa). The needle is then adjusted until it slips through the foramen ovale; usually, just prior to this, a mandibular nerve paresthesia is obtained in the lower jaw or lip. This maneuver is optimally (but not necessarily) performed under radiographic control, so that the needle and its path through the foramen ovale can be visualized (5). After the foramen ovale is entered, the needle should not be advanced more than 1 cm, and usually its advance is guided by the appropriate paresthesia.

Initially, there will be a third-division mandibular paresthesia, but this can occur while the needle is still in the infratemporal fossa. A second-division maxillary paresthesia must be obtained, or a first-division paresthesia to the upper jaw or frontal area of the face, respectively, to confirm that the needle

FIGURE 17-4. Gasserian ganglion block. **A:** Note that the needle is inserted in the cheek about 1 cm posterior to the angle of the mouth, as shown, and directed toward the pupil in the anterior view and the midpoint of the zygoma in the lateral view. In patients with teeth, needle insertion in the cheek is superficial to the teeth of the upper jaw. In edentulous patients, this may lie a variable distance between the angle of the mouth and a line midway between upper lip and nose. A palpating finger in the mouth helps to prevent needle penetration into the mouth. **B:** As the needle is advanced into the infratemporal fossa, it will usually strike the roof of the infratemporal fossa initially (*1*); this is the correct depth to seek the foramen ovale. The needle is then directed slightly posteriorly (*2*) to obtain a mandibular nerve (V3) paresthesia. **C:** The needle can then be advanced through the foramen ovale into the middle cranial fossa, where it will be adjacent to the Gasserian ganglion, as shown. Note the relationships of the dural fold and Meckel cave, containing cerebrospinal fluid (CSF). A needle advanced too far through the foramen ovale can enter the Meckel cave, and subsequent injections could enter the cranial CSF and produce total spinal anesthesia.

of introducing heated probes for the newer techniques of thermogangliolysis (11) (Chapters 42 and 45).

The Gasserian ganglion is reached with a needle by traversing the infratemporal fossa and entering the middle cranial fossa by way of the foramen ovale. Medially, the Gasserian ganglion is bounded by the cavernous venous sinus, which con-

TABLE 17-2	
GASSERIAN GANGLION BLOCK	
Indications:	Diagnostic and therapeutic blocks for trigeminal neuralgia
Technique:	One finger breadth posterior to the lateral margin of the mouth, close to the medial border of the masseter muscle
	Needle direction is rostral and medial to the midpoint of the zygomatic arch
	Keep finger in mouth to prevent needle entering the oral cavity
	Needle is adjusted until it slips through the foramen ovale
	Needle should not be advanced more than 1 cm
Confirmation:	Fluoroscopy, paresthesia of third division of mandibular nerve
Caution:	Aspirate for blood or cerebrospinal fluid (CSF) (if Meckel cave is entered)
Complication:	Intrathecal injection, unconsciousness

is in fact in the immediate vicinity of the Gasserian ganglion. A stimulating device may be used to confirm the position of the needle in patients who are unable to locate the paresthesia accurately. This, being a painful procedure, would require some intravenous (IV) analgesics or sedation prior to performance of the block. For diagnostic blocks, however, it is better not to alter the sensorium with any analgesics in order to obtain a more accurate assessment of the block.

Prior to injection, aspiration tests are mandatory to ensure that the needle has not entered a blood vessel or, in a more likely outcome, the Meckel cave, with its CSF contents. If these aspiration tests are negative, then the anesthetizing agent, either a local anesthetic (1% lidocaine or the equivalent) or a neurolytic agent, is injected in small aliquots (e.g., 0.25 mL at a time) until the desired analgesic effect is obtained. If injection affords evidence of analgesia in only one of the divisions, then adjustment of the needle sometimes can affect spread to the other divisions—in patients in whom the needle is in the same vertical axis as the ganglion. However, there appear to be some patients in whom the ganglion lies at a more horizontal axis, and in these patients it is sometimes difficult, if not impossible, to obtain a first-division paresthesia.

Complications

Depending upon the manipulations needed to produce satisfactory block, the patient's face quite frequently will be painful for few days following the block, and there is often bruising at the injection site. This usually responds well to treatment with mild oral analgesics. Probably the most serious side effect is injection of local anesthetic or neurolytic agent into the CSF contained within the Meckel cave and its resulting spread into the circulating CSF of the cranial cavity. Injections of as little as 0.25 mL of 1% lidocaine have resulted in unconsciousness and profound paralysis of the ipsilateral cranial nerve system, albeit temporary, with the patient needing cardiorespiratory support for a brief period (10 minutes). If a hyperbaric solution is used (e.g., lidocaine with epinephrine or phenol in glycerine), then the drug that emerges from the Meckel cavity will tend to flow over the free margin of the tentorium cerebelli to affect, immediately, cranial nerves VI, VIII, IX, X, XI, and XII, and usually the patient loses consciousness. If hypobaric solutions are used (e.g., lidocaine without epinephrine, or alcohol), then the flow will tend to be cephalad, probably involving the trochlear and oculomotor nerves initially, and almost certainly affecting consciousness to a variable extent.

Clinical Application of Gasserian Ganglion Blockade in Pain States

Local anesthetics injected into the ganglion can produce profound analgesia in certain pain states, such as tic douloureux (but only for short periods), and neurolytic blocks with alcohol were used in the past by some therapists for this condition (5,12,13). The pain relief is obtained at the price of hemifacial and corneal analgesia, with saliva often dribbling out of the ipsilateral, numb side of the mouth. Such blocks, for long-term pain relief, are rarely performed by pain specialists today (Chapters 42 and 45).

Gangliolysis, or thermogangliolysis, has great therapeutic implications because of its proven results (14). For gangliolysis, an insulated needle is placed through the foramen ovale. Electrical stimuli are delivered, and the needle tip is adjusted until paresthesias are elicited in the area of pain and a radiofrequency lesion is made, using a thermistor. This appears to be a suc-

cessful maneuver in those 30% of tic douloureux patients who do not benefit from carbamazepine or other medication therapy, and approximately 80% will get at least 1 year's relief of pain. An alternative to thermal coagulation for tic douloureux is provided by "bathing" the trigeminal ganglion in glycerol (0.1–0.3 mL) (15). Proponents of this technique claim the relief is as satisfactory as thermal coagulation, with a greater degree of safety with regard to the production of excessive neural damage. However, it is claimed that glycerol gangliolysis is less likely to produce corneal anesthesia than are radiofrequency lesions of the first division, and so it may have some advantages (16). Gangliolysis has improved success over neurolytic block, surgical neurectomy, and rhizotomy therapies. However, which of the gangliolysis methods is superior is still debated among the proponents of the different techniques.

Blockade of Ophthalmic Nerve Branches: Supraorbital, Supratrochlear, Anterior Ethmoidal Nerves

Indications

Supraorbital and supratrochlear nerve analgesia is a simple block that can produce excellent analgesia of the forehead and scalp back from eyebrows to the vertex (6).

These techniques can be utilized for surgery performed on the scalp, repair to lacerations, removal of cysts, frontal craniotomies, midline dermoid excisions, frontal ventriculoperitoneal shunts, Omaya reservoir placement in neonates (2), and nevus excisions on the anterior portion of the scalp (6) (Table 17-3).

Technique (Supraorbital Block)

The supraorbital foramen is palpated at the roof of the orbital rim, approximately at the level of the pupil in most patients. A 30-gauge needle is utilized. The insertion of the needle is at the level of the eyebrow, at the mid-pupillary line (Fig. 17-3). A subcutaneous wheal of local anesthetic solution is injected with the needle directed parallel to the eyebrow at the site of the needle insertion in a subcutaneous plane. Care should be exercised to avoid placing the needle directly into the foramen. One to 1.5 mL of volume is sufficient for analgesia. Firm pressure should be applied to the area after the needle is withdrawn, preventing the formation of a hematoma.

TABLE 17-3

SUPRAORBITAL/SUPRATROCHLEAR BLOCKS

Indications:	Scalp surgery, supplement for craniotomies, midline dermoid surgery
Technique:	Supraorbital foramen, located at the upper orbital rim
	Midpoint of pupil coincides with supraorbital foramen
	Insert 27-gauge needle subcutaneous at the level of the supraorbital foramen
	For supratrochlear injection, insert needle medially
Confirmation:	Sensory nerve; in an awake patient, paresthesia can be demonstrated
Complication:	Ecchymosis, hematoma formation

Complications

Hematoma formation, intravascular injection, intraneural injection may occur.

Technique (Combined Infratrochlear and Anterior Ethmoidal Block)

Anterior ethmoidal and infratrochlear nerve blocks accompanied with an infraorbital nerve block can be very effective when they are performed bilaterally for plastic surgical procedures and fracture reduction operations on the nose (9).

The nasociliary nerve divides into its terminal branches—anterior ethmoidal and infratrochlear—on the medial wall of the orbit 2.5 cm from the orbital margin. Both branches are blocked by inserting a 5-cm, 25-gauge needle 1 cm above the inner canthus. The needle is directed backward and slightly medially to pass just lateral to the inner wall of the orbit and medial to the eyeball and medial rectus muscle. Depth of insertion is 2.5 cm, and at this point 1 mL of 2% lidocaine, or equivalent, is injected, while the needle is slowly withdrawn. Orbital veins may be easily damaged, resulting in proptosis; thus, small-gauge needles (27-gauge) should be used, and repeated insertion should be avoided (Fig. 17-3).

The infratrochlear nerve can be blocked separately by infiltrating at the superomedial border of the orbit and along its medial wall with 2 to 4 mL of local anesthetic. The external nasal branch of the anterior ethmoidal nerve can also be blocked separately, by infiltration at the junction of nasal bone with cartilage.

If the mucous membrane of the nose is likely to be stimulated, as it would be in reduction of a fractured nose, then branches of the anterior ethmoidal nerve and sphenopalatine ganglion that supply the septum and lateral wall of the nose should be blocked by topical application (pledgets soaked) of local anesthetic (Figs. 17-5 and 17-6).

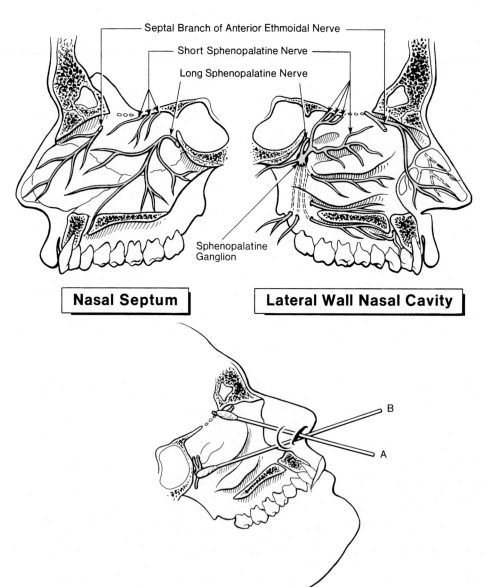

Septal Branch of Anterior Ethmoidal Nerve

Short Sphenopalatine Nerve

Long Sphenopalatine Nerve

Sphenopalatine Ganglion

Nasal Septum

Lateral Wall Nasal Cavity

FIGURE 17-5. Nerve supply of nasal septum and lateral wall of nasal cavity. Pledgets of cotton wool soaked in local anesthetic and inserted as shown to contact branches of the anterior ethmoidal nerve (A) and the sphenopalatine ganglion and nerves (B). Note pledget A is inserted parallel with the line of the external nose until it reaches the superior extent of the nasal cavity. Pledget B is inserted about 20 to 30 degrees with the horizontal line through the floor of the nose, to reach the region sphenopalatine foramen.

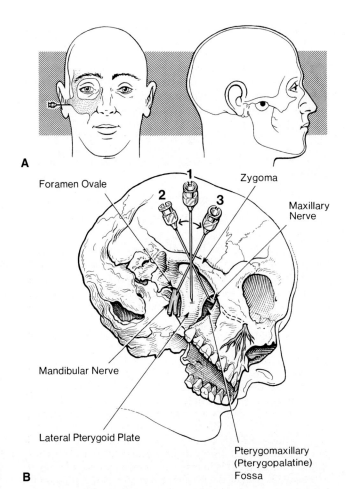

FIGURE 17-6. A. The coronoid notch is located below the midpoint of the zygoma. A finger is placed at this point and the patient asked to open his mouth. The condyle of the mandible should be palpable immediately, deep to the fingertip, as the mouth opens. The fingertip should then sink into the coronoid notch as the mouth is closed. **B:** The maxillary and mandibular nerves are approached by way of the coronoid notch below the midpoint of zygoma. (*1*) The needle passes through the infratemporal fossa to reach the lateral pterygoid plate. Initial direction of the needle should be medial and slightly anterior. (*2*) The needle is then walked anteriorly until it passes into the pterygomaxillary (pterygopalatine) fossa, where the maxillary nerve is blocked. (*3*) The needle is then walked from position (*1*) posteriorly until it passes just posterior to the lateral pterygoid plate to block the mandibular nerve as it emerges from the foramen ovale. The needle point is kept at the same depth as the lateral pterygoid plate to prevent accidental introduction of the needle into the posterior pharynx.

Topical Analgesia of Nasal Cavities

As noted in the description of nerve supply, only two main sites require blockade, the sphenopalatine ganglion and the anterior ethmoidal nerve, both located in the region of the sphenoethmoidal recess (Fig. 17-5).

Pledget Technique

Prior spraying of the nasal cavities with 0.5 mL of 5% cocaine solution on each side provides analgesia and some shrinking

TABLE 17-4

TOPICAL ANALGESIA OF THE NASAL CAVITIES

Indications:	For nasal surgery
Nerve supply:	Sphenopalatine ganglion, anterior ethmoidal nerve
Technique:	Cotton applicators to nasal cavities Use pledget to pass cephalad about 5 cm (close to the cribriform plate)
Complications:	Overdose if cocaine is used

of the mucous membrane, making the insertion of applicators more comfortable for the patient. The anesthesiologist then employs a headlight and nasal speculum and gradually applies cocaine paste upward and backward in the nasal cavity (Table 17-4). Initially, insertion should be close to the septum to avoid injuring the lateral wall. Finally, one applicator is inserted parallel to the anterior border of the nasal cavity until it reaches the anterior end of the cribriform plate at a depth of approximately 5 cm. A second applicator is inserted at an angle of about 20 degrees to the floor of the nose, until bone is felt at a depth of approximately 6 to 7 cm. The end of the applicator should now lie close to the sphenopalatine foramen. The two applicators are left in place for 10 to 15 minutes, and the patient is asked to breathe through the mouth. Cocaine pastes of 10% are also available and are preferable if bilateral blocks are to be performed. It should be noted that the total administered dose of solution and paste should not exceed 200 mg (e.g., 1 mL 5% solution [50 mg] + 1.5 mL 10% paste [150 mg]). Because of the danger of cocaine overdose, some now prefer to use a 10% lidocaine spray for initial anesthesia (20 mg/puff) and then 5% to 10% lidocaine solution up to a maximum dose of 500 mg. Oxymetazoline hydrochloride has replaced the use of cocaine for vasoconstriction. This does not provide analgesia and hence an additional blockade may be necessary.

Instillation Technique

Instillation into sphenoethmoidal recess is unsatisfactory if the mucous membrane is grossly thickened, or if other pathology exists. This procedure requires the patient to lie with the head upside down, which is distressing to many patients.

The mucous membrane is initially sprayed with local anesthetic solution, as previously described. The patient is then placed supine with a pillow under the shoulders, and the neck is extended so that the skull is upside down. The patient is told to breathe through the mouth. A blunt-nosed 10-cm cannula with a 120-degree angle at its midpoint is inserted through the nares until the angle lies at the external nares. The cannula is now swiveled, keeping close to the septum, until the end reaches the roof of the nose. Local anesthetic (e.g., 2 mL 10% lidocaine) is instilled. The procedure is repeated on the other side, and the position maintained for 10 minutes. Then the patient rolls supine, while holding the nares pinched, and lets the solution run out of the external nares. Injections into the nasal cavity do have significant potential for spread beyond the cavity. Attempts to anesthetize the anterior ethmoidal nerve close to the cribriform plate have resulted in total spinal anesthesia (19).

MAXILLARY NERVE BLOCK

Block of Main Trunk in Pterygopalatine (Pterygomaxillary) Fossa

Indications

As it crosses the pterygopalatine fossa, the maxillary nerve is usually blocked by a lateral approach. The resulting block will produce profound anesthesia of the upper jaw and its teeth on the ipsilateral side of the face (Fig. 17-6).

Technique

The nerve is approached by way of the infratemporal fossa, and the needle is inserted in the skin at a point below the midpoint of the zygomatic arch overlying the coronoid notch of the mandible. Location of the point of needle insertion is aided by asking the patient to open the mouth wide and palpating the condyle of the mandible as it moves anteriorly to the midpoint of the zygoma. When the mouth is closed, the condyle leaves a clear entry path through the coronoid notch. An 8-cm, 22-gauge needle is inserted through the skin and subcutaneous tissues, which contain the parotid gland and possibly some of the rostral portions of the pes anserinus branches of the facial nerve destined for the orbicularis oculi muscles (Table 17-5). An extensive subcutaneous infiltration of local anesthetic at this site may result in some temporary weakness of these muscles. Having traversed the coronoid notch of the mandible, the needle is directed medially until it reaches the medial wall of the infratemporal fossa, where it will strike the lateral surface of the lateral pterygoid plate, usually at a depth of about 5 cm. The needle is now walked anteriorly from the lateral pterygoid plate until it enters the pterygopalatine fossa, where it is advanced a further centimeter into the fossa. Usually, a paresthesia is not obtained or sought, and 5 mL of local anesthetic is injected into this fossa to produce anesthesia of the maxillary nerve. It has been suggested that the sphenopalatine ganglion can be selectively blocked at this site and used for treatment of refractory headaches (20). It is almost impossible to block selectively this ganglion without involving the second division of the trigeminal nerve. This more or less precludes the use of permanent blockade in this area, even if such headaches could be shown conclusively to be relieved by such blockade.

Complications

Because of the highly vascular nature of the contents of the infratemporal fossa (containing as it does the five terminal branches of the maxillary artery with all their venae comitantes, plus the veins that drain the orbit by way of the inferior orbital fissure), a hematoma is frequently a sequel to this block. Such a hematoma can spread into the orbit and produce a profound black eye, which usually resolves in a few days. Spread of local anesthetic to the optic nerve may occur, producing temporary blindness. The patient should be forewarned of these potential complications. This approach is not favored for neurolytic blockade because of proximity to the orbit. If maxillary division neurolytic blockade is required, it is common practice to employ the approach described under Gasserian ganglion block.

Block of the Infraorbital Nerve

Indications

Cleft lip repair (21,22), endoscopic sinus surgery (23), nasal septal repair (9), and transsphenoidal hypophysectomy are applications of infraorbital nerve block (24). There are two common approaches. These are discussed in depth in Chapter 18.

Extraoral Approach. The location of the infraorbital foramen is approximately 25 mm from the midline at the floor of the orbital rim (directly inferior to the pupils) (25). The foramen is located by palpation of the floor of the orbit, and a 27-gauge needle is inserted through the skin (transcutaneously) toward the foramen. The needle need not be placed into the foramen since the nerve arborizes outside the foramen to provide the sensory supply to the midface. This will also prevent intraneural injections with the potential for dysesthesia and chronic pain. About 0.5 mL (for cleft lip repairs) to 2 mL (for endoscopic sinus surgery) is injected on each side. Careful pressure to the area is provided with gentle massage of the area to provide adequate spread of the local anesthetic solution.

Intraoral Approach. The infraorbital foramen is located at the floor of the orbital rim at about the level of the pupil. The external landmarks include the incisor and the first premolar. A needle is inserted in the buccal mucosa in the subsulcal groove at about the level of the canine or the first premolar. The needle is inserted until it reaches proximal to the infraorbital foramen. A finger is placed externally at the level of the infraorbital foramen to prevent the needle from cephalad insertion into the globe of the eye. Bending the needle about 70 degrees prior to injection facilitates passage of the needle on the maxillary process toward the infraorbital foramen. After careful aspiration, 2 mL of local anesthetic solution is injected (see Chapter 18, Figs. 18-10 through 18-12) (Table 17-6).

TABLE 17-5

MAXILLARY NERVE BLOCK: PTERYGOPALATINE FOSSA BLOCK

Indications:	Refractory headaches
Technique:	Pterygopalatine fossa; nerve approach is by the infratemporal fossa
	Needle is inserted below the midpoint of the zygomatic arch overlying the coronoid notch of the mandible
	8-cm, 22-gauge needle is advanced through the skin, subcutaneous tissue, and the rostral portion of the facial nerve
	After the needle traverses the coronoid notch of the mandible, direct needle medially until it reaches the medial wall of the infratemporal fossa
	Needle will strike the lateral pterygoid plate and enter the pterygopalatine fossa
	5 mL local anesthetic injected
Complications:	Hematoma, ecchymosis, and black eye; spread to optic nerve causing temporary blindness

TABLE 17-6

MAXILLARY NERVE BLOCK: PERIPHERAL BRANCH BLOCK

Indications:	Cleft lip repair, nasal septal repair
Technique:	Infraorbital route; lower margin of the orbit at midpoint of the pupil
	Evert lip and advance 27-gauge needle at the level of the premolars and toward the infraorbital foramen.
Complications:	Hematoma, ecchymosis

Complications

Intravascular injection and hematoma formation are possible. It is important to stress the potential for numbness of the upper lip in older patients since this can lead to significant concern after the block is performed.

Alternate Approaches to the Maxillary Nerve

Blockade by Way of the Orbit

An alternative approach for blocking the maxillary nerve involves traversing the inferolateral borders of the orbit and depositing the local anesthetic in the pterygopalatine fossa superolaterally. A 6-cm, 22-gauge needle is inserted at the junction of the inferior and lateral borders of the orbit, and, keeping close to the bone, is advanced for a distance of 4 cm. It will then have entered the inferior orbital fissure, and its tip lies in the pterygopalatine fossa. No attempts are made to seek a paresthesia, and 5 mL of local anesthetic is injected at this site. This approach also may be complicated by hematoma production or spread of local anesthetic to the optic nerve, producing temporary blindness. The eye itself does not encroach directly upon the path of the needle in this block, being held off the floor of the orbit by the suspensory ligament of Lockwood.

Although this is not recommended as a first choice for second-division trigeminal block, it is an alternative when local conditions (e.g., trauma or infection) may preclude the conventional approach by the infratemporal fossa.

Alternate Approach by Way of the Infratemporal Fossa

Yet another alternative approach to the maxillary nerve is by way of the anterior aspect of the infratemporal fossa. Here, the needle is introduced anterior to the coronoid process of the mandible at a point below the anterior aspect of the zygomatic arch. This permits a medial approach toward the pupil of the eye, passing posterior to the posterior surface of the maxilla, directly into the pterygopalatine fossa. The needle should not be inserted to a depth greater than 5 cm, because this approach can lead unchecked into the optic nerve and by way of its foramen into the cranial cavity (7). Although the bony landmarks for this block are usually constant, sometimes the zygomatic arch is relatively low in position, and if this is the case, then the second division of the trigeminal can actually be reached in the pterygomandibular fossa by advancing the needle superior to the zygoma (26). In contrast, the approach by way of the coronoid notch involves an anterior direction, so that if the needle is advanced too deeply it will impinge on the posterior surface of the maxillary or palatine bones, and thereby, hopefully, be prevented from damaging deeper structures.

MANDIBULAR NERVE BLOCK

Block of Main Trunk in the Infratemporal Fossa

Indications

Third-division block (V3) here produces analgesia of the skin over the lower jaw (except at the angle) of the superior two-thirds of the anterior surface of the auricle, and of a strip of skin that often extends up to the temporal area. If sufficient concentration of local anesthetic is injected to result in motor blockade (1% lidocaine or equivalent), then the muscles of mastication will also be anesthetized, resulting in some incoordination of ipsilateral movements of the jaw. This is well-tolerated after temporary blocks, but could be a long-term distressing complication of permanent blockade. The otic ganglion, lying in such intimate connection posterior to the mandibular division just below the foramen ovale, is inevitably blocked. This nerve supplies secretomotor fibers to the parotid gland, which pursue a peripatetic course from the inferior salivary nucleus; thus, permanent impairment of secretion by this gland is a possible sequel of neurolytic blockade of the mandibular nerve.

Technique

The approach for blocking the main division of the mandibular branch in the infratemporal fossa is the same, initially, as that described for the maxillary nerve; that is, a 6-cm, 22-gauge needle is introduced below the midpoint of the zygomatic arch and passes through the coronoid notch of the mandible, directed medially across the infratemporal fossa until it impinges upon the bony medial wall (i.e., the lateral aspect of the lateral pterygoid plate) (Fig. 17-6). At this stage, the directions differ from those for a maxillary nerve block; for here the needle is walked posteriorly from the lateral pterygoid plate until a third-division paresthesia is obtained. If a paresthesia is not obtained, the needle, once it leaves the posterior aspect of the lateral pterygoid plate, can pierce the attached superior constrictor muscle and enter the pharynx. It should not, therefore, be inserted to a depth greater than the lateral pterygoid plate (Table 17-7).

Mental Nerve Block

Indications

Mental nerve block is performed for surgery to the mandible and lower lip surgery. Similar to the infraorbital nerve block, an intraoral or an extraoral route can be utilized.

Technique: Intraoral Block of Mental Nerve

After eversion of the lip, the lower canine or the first premolar is identified. The needle is then gently passed into the buccal mucosa until it approximates the mental foramen. A dose of 2 mL of local anesthetic solution is injected after careful aspiration to prevent intravascular placement (Table 17-8).

TABLE 17-7

MANDIBULAR NERVE: MAIN TRUNK IN THE INFRATEMPORAL FOSSA

Indications:	Mandibular fractures
Technique:	Insert 22-gauge needle below the midpoint of the zygomatic arch and pass it through the coronoid notch of the mandible directed medially until it impinges on the lateral plate of the lateral pterygoid plate
	The needle is walked posterior from the lateral pterygoid plate until a third-division paresthesia is obtained
Complications:	Intravascular injection

Technique: Extraoral Block of Mental Nerve

The mental foramen, as mentioned, lies in the same vertical line as the supraorbital and infraorbital foramen and the pupil, with the pupil in the midposition (Fig. 17-3). The position of the mental foramen varies with age and dentition, being more caudal on the mandibular ramus in youth and closer to the alveolar margin of the mandible in the edentulous aged person. To enter the mental foramen, the needle must be directed anterior and caudad. However, it is not necessary actually to enter the foramen, and an infiltration over the midpoint of the mandible in the vertical line of the pupil is usually ample to produce analgesia of the lower lip and chin, and is effective anesthesia for operative procedures there.

Auriculotemporal Nerve Block

This nerve can be blocked as it ascends over the posterior root of the zygoma (Fig. 17-2) behind the superficial temporal artery, and infiltration of 3 to 5 mL 1% lidocaine, or the equivalent, produces anesthesia of the upper two-thirds of the temporal fossa. This also provides analgesia for the temporal portion of the scalp and is used in combination with other blocks of the trigeminal ganglion including the supraorbital nerve block.

Glossopharyngeal Nerve Block

Indications

The ninth cranial nerve emerges via the jugular foramen in very close relationship to the vagus and accessory nerves, along with

TABLE 17-8

MANDIBULAR NERVE: BLOCKADE OF BRANCHES

Indications:	Mandible and lower lip surgery
Technique:	Evert the lip; needle insertion is at the level of the canine or first premolar
	Needle is inserted a few mm, inject after aspiration
Complications:	Hematoma formation

the internal jugular vein. It is blocked just below this point, and therefore both temporary and permanent blocks usually involve these other two cranial nerves, all three of which lie in the groove between the internal jugular vein and the internal carotid artery. Glossopharyngeal nerve block is most frequently used for inoperable carcinomas that invade the distribution of the nerve in either the posterior third of the tongue or the pharyngeal trapezius muscles, and with numbness of the laryngeal inlet and trachea, and paralysis of the ipsilateral vocal cords (with resulting hoarseness).

Technique

The landmarks for this block involve locating the styloid process of the temporal bone. This osseous process represents the calcification of the cephalic end of the stylohyoid ligament. This fibrous band, which passes from the base of the skull to the lesser cornu of the hyoid bone, ossifies to a different extent in different patients. Although it is relatively easy to identify in people with a large styloid process, if ossification has been limited, then the styloid process sometimes cannot be located with the exploring needle. The styloid process may be anatomically absent in certain individuals.

A 5-cm, 22-gauge needle is inserted at a point midway on a line joining the angle of the mandible to the tip of the mastoid process of the occipital bone (Fig. 17-7). The needle is advanced directly medially, until it locates the styloid process. In the event that the styloid process is not located, the needle is inserted to a depth of 3 cm. In patients who have had a radical neck dissection (and therefore are often candidates for this kind of block), the removal of the sternocleidomastoid muscle places the styloid process, and its adjacent nerves and vessels, in a much more superficial plane. In fact, in these patients, the styloid process can often be palpated in the interval between mastoid process and the posterior border of the mandible. The needle will then need to be inserted only 1 to 2 cm. Ideally, the styloid process is located as a bony end-point and the needle adjusted posterior to this at the same depth as the process. An injection of 1 to 2 mL of 1% lidocaine or the equivalent will produce anesthesia of the glossopharyngeal, and the vagus and accessory nerves as well. At this site, it is not usually possible to block one of these three nerves selectively.

Complications

The carotid artery and jugular vein may be punctured during attempts to block these nerves at this site, resulting in either intravascular injection or hematoma. Even very small amounts (e.g., 0.25 mL) of local anesthetic injected into the carotid artery at this point can produce quite profound effects of convulsion and loss of consciousness. Therefore, as always, aspiration tests must be meticulous. Likewise, injection of neurolytic agents at this site, so close to the large vascular conduits, is cause for concern because of the possibility of damage to the walls of these vessels, which might result in slough and necrosis, with potentially disastrous sequelae. However, such a complication has not yet been reported.

VAGUS NERVE BLOCK (MAIN TRUNK AND BRANCHES)

The main trunk of the vagus nerve is rarely, if ever, blocked intentionally as a primary procedure. However, the branches of sensory distribution to the larynx can be blocked simply and efficiently, thereby rendering the laryngeal inlet and trachea

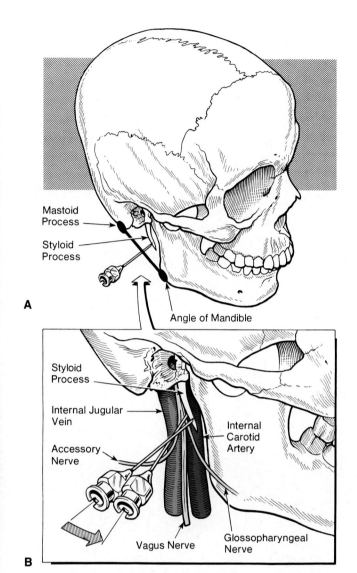

FIGURE 17-7. Glossopharyngeal nerve block. **A:** The needle is inserted at a point midway between the mastoid process and the angle of the mandible. **B:** The needle is inserted at a right angle to the skin. At a depth of 2 to 3 cm, the styloid process will be contacted (if present). The needle is then walked posteriorly off the styloid process. Local anesthetic deposited at this point will block glossopharyngeal, accessory, and vagus nerves. Note the proximity of the internal carotid artery and the internal jugular vein.

insensitive to pain. This is very useful for intubations performed on conscious patients and for other endoscopic procedures. These branches can also be blocked permanently, for pain relief in terminal neoplastic disease in the area.

Superior Laryngeal Nerve Block

This branch of the vagus nerve is easily blocked as it sweeps around the inferior border of the greater cornu of the hyoid bone, which is readily palpable, even in the most obese patients. By pressing on the opposite greater cornu of the hyoid bone, the laryngeal structures can be displaced toward the side to be blocked (Fig. 17-8). A small 2.5-cm, 25-gauge needle is usually all that is required. It is walked from the inferior border

of the greater cornu of the hyoid near its tip, and 3 mL of local anesthetic is infiltrated both superficially and deep to the thyrohyoid membrane. Penetration of this membrane is felt as a slight loss of resistance. The procedure is repeated on the other side. This will produce anesthesia over the inferior aspect of the epiglottis and the laryngeal inlet, as far down as the vocal cords. It will also produce motor blockade (if the concentration of lidocaine exceeds 1%, or the equivalent for other drugs) of the cricothyroid muscles.

Recurrent Laryngeal Nerve Block

The recurrent laryngeal nerve supplies the wall of the trachea below that of the vocal cords. It is possible to block this nerve specifically (and, in fact, blockade of this nerve frequently occurs while performing a stellate ganglion block).

In the event blockade of the recurrent laryngeal nerve is required (e.g., for a possible neurolytic block for cancers of the vocal cords or below), then the nerve, which lies in the groove between esophagus and trachea, can be blocked at any cervical level below the cricoid cartilage. Attempts at this block would, of course, demand meticulous technique to avoid involvement of brachial plexus with deep insertion of the needle.

To produce anesthesia below the cords, the simplest and most useful method is transtracheal puncture. Here, a relatively wide-bore needle (i.e., 20- or 22-gauge) is used, so that air can be aspirated and rapid injection performed. The needle is introduced in the midline through the cricothyroid membrane. Entry of the needle into the trachea is identified by aspiration of air, and the patient will usually cough slightly at this stage. Rapid injection of 3 to 5 mL of local anesthetic will produce a dramatic cough in all but the most obtunded patients, and this spreads the local anesthetic up and down the trachea, yielding satisfactory topical anesthesia. It is usually necessary to use a higher concentration for this topical anesthesia than it is for nerve block, and 4% lidocaine is frequently chosen, although 2% lidocaine will produce adequate blockade but will take a little longer (Fig. 17-8).

Auricular Nerve Block

Block of the auricular branch of the vagus has even been used for resolving bronchial asthma (27), where the nerve exits from the base of the skull between the mastoid process and the external tympanic plate of the temporal bone. Recently, our group has used this to provide analgesia for children undergoing myringotomy and tube placement.

Accessory Nerve (11th Cranial Nerve) Block

Indications

There are very few indications for blocking the accessory nerve. It is useful for trapezius muscle paralysis, or as an adjunct to interscalene nerve blocks of the brachial plexus for surgery on the shoulder. With interscalene block alone, the patient has adequate analgesia of the operative site, but motor power is maintained in the trapezius muscle. They can, by shrugging their shoulders, accidentally interfere with the surgical procedure; by blocking the accessory nerve in the posterior triangle of the neck, the trapezius muscle is paralyzed and surgery often facilitated.

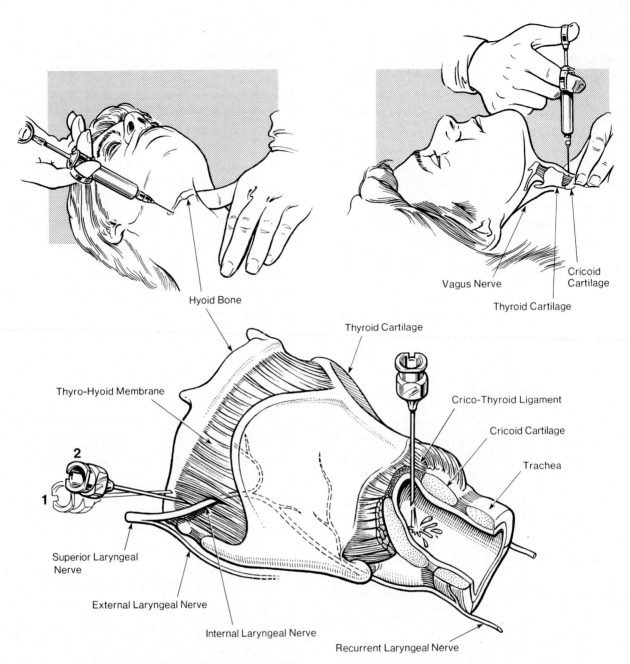

FIGURE 17-8. Superior and recurrent laryngeal nerve block. The superior laryngeal nerve and its internal and external branches are blocked inferior to the lateral limits of the greater cornu of the hyoid bone. This landmark is brought into prominence by pressing medially on the contralateral cornu of the hyoid bone. (*1*) A needle is inserted onto the greater cornu of the hyoid bone and then walked off the inferior edge of the hyoid (*2*). Needle depth is not increased beyond the depth of the hyoid to avoid the needle's piercing the larynx. Local anesthetic injected at (*2*) blocks the internal laryngeal nerve and produces anesthesia of the laryngeal inlet, down to the level of the vocal cords. The recurrent laryngeal nerve is blocked by introducing a needle through the cricothyroid membrane. Note one hand grasping the cricoid cartilage. The other hand is steadied against the patient's chin. Injection is made after aspirating for air. It is important that the local anesthetic be injected rapidly, and the needle immediately removed, since the patient will cough vigorously. Anesthesia is produced over the inferior surface of the vocal cords and the trachea.

Technique

The posterior triangle of the neck is a compartment bounded anteriorly by the posterior border of sternomastoid muscle, laterally by the anterior border of the trapezius, and inferiorly by the middle third of the clavicle. The accessory nerve traverses this triangle in a very superficial location (Fig. 17-9). It emerges from the substance of the sternomastoid muscle at the junction of the superior and middle thirds of the posterior border of the muscle, and proceeds in a downward and lateral course across the triangle, to enter the trapezius muscle at the junction of the middle and inferior third of its anterior border. Anywhere along

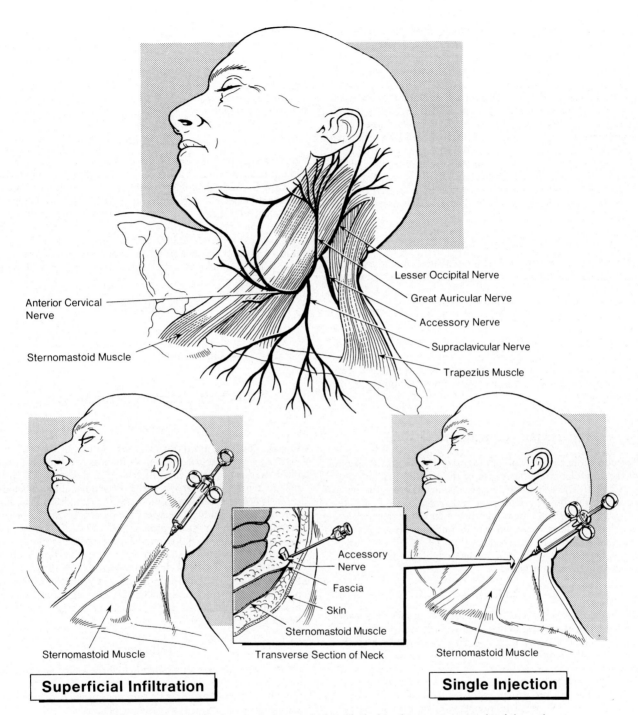

Lesser Occipital Nerve

Great Auricular Nerve

Accessory Nerve

Supraclavicular Nerve

Trapezius Muscle

Anterior Cervical Nerve

Sternomastoid Muscle

Accessory Nerve

Fascia

Skin

Sternomastoid Muscle

Transverse Section of Neck

Sternomastoid Muscle

Sternomastoid Muscle

Superficial Infiltration

Single Injection

FIGURE 17-9. The superficial cervical plexus, which is blocked in the posterior triangle of the neck as it emerges adjacent to the midpoint of the posterior border of the sternomastoid muscle. Superficial infiltration is extended along the middle third of the posterior border of the sternomastoid muscle. Note the close relationship of the accessory nerve as it emerges from the posterior border of the sternomastoid muscle at the junction of its middle and upper third; that is, just above the emerging superficial cervical plexus. *Single injection technique for accessory nerve block*. Note that the accessory nerve lies deep to the deep fascia of the neck and that this needs to be pierced as shown in the "*single injection*," which is sometimes used as an adjunct to produce muscle paralysis of the trapezius muscle in shoulder operations. Successful block of the superficial cervical plexus results in analgesia corresponding to the C2, C3, and C4 dermatomes shown in Figure 17-2.

this course, it can successfully be blocked (28). The accessory nerve lies superficial to the prevertebral fascia and therefore is lying deep only to skin, platysma, and deep cervical fascia. Therefore, if a needle is introduced at the junction of the middle and superior thirds of the sternomastoid muscle at its lateral border, and an infiltration of 10 mL of local anesthetic is used, blockade of the nerve can be accomplished. Accuracy can be increased if a stimulating device is used to locate the nerve. Ramamurthy and co-workers (29) have described a technique for blocking this nerve as it lies within the sternomastoid muscle. This is accomplished by infiltrating the substance of the muscle with 10 to 20 mL of local anesthetic below its attachment to the mastoid process. It can be used for the therapy of spasms and painful conditions of the sternomastoid muscle itself.

Complications

This nerve, not infrequently, is blocked inadvertently when a superficial cervical plexus block is performed, and vice versa.

CERVICAL PLEXUS BLOCK

The cervical plexus is formed by loops between the anterior primary rami of the upper four cervical nerves. Its muscular branches are distributed to the prevertebral muscles, strap muscles of the neck, and provide a minor contribution to the phrenic nerve.

Superficial Cervical Plexus Block

The cutaneous distribution of the cervical plexus is to the skin of the anterolateral neck by way of the anterior primary rami of C2–C4. These emerge as four distinct nerves (the lesser occipital, the great auricular, the transverse cervical, and the supraclavicular) from the posterior border of the sternocleidomastoid muscle at approximately its midpoint, just below the emergence of the accessory nerve (Fig. 17-9). All four nerves can be blocked by infiltration at the midpoint of the posterior border of the sternomastoid.

Indications

Blockade of the superficial cervical plexus can provide sensory analgesia for the postauricular area of the scalp (lesser occipital), the external pinna (30), and the posterior auricular area as well as the temporoparietal area of the scalp (greater auricular), the anterior portion of the neck (transverse cervical) (31), and supply to the supraclavicular area (supraclavicular branch). The greater auricular nerve block has been successfully used for pain relief following tympanomastoid surgery (4) and otoplasty (30). Children who undergo tympanomastoid surgery may have a greater predisposition to nausea and

vomiting, which can be decreased by performing a great auricular nerve block and avoiding or reducing the need for opioids in the perioperative period. Blockade of the superficial cervical plexus bilaterally can provide analgesia for surgery on the anterior part of the neck. This can be used for thyroid surgery (32) as well as for anterior neck procedures including medialization thyroplasty (31).

Technique

After sterile preparation of the neck, the cricoid cartilage is identified. The posterior border of the sternocleidomastoid is identified. With a 60-degree bend to the needle, a 27-gauge needle is placed superficially along the posterior border of the clavicular head of the sternocleidomastoid at the level of C6 (Fig. 17-9). A wheal is raised with 2 mL of 0.25% bupivacaine with 1:200,000 epinephrine after careful aspiration to prevent intravascular injection. Recently, ultrasonography has been used to localize the superficial cervical plexus (Table 17-9).

Complications

Intravascular injection, potential for deep cervical plexus block with associated Horner syndrome, unilateral phrenic nerve paralysis (19), and hematoma formation have been reported.

Block of Greater Occipital Nerve

Indications

The skin over the posterior extensor muscles of the neck and extending up over the occiput as high as the vertex, is supplied by the posterior rami of the cervical nerves. Of these, the greater occipital nerve is perhaps the most clinically significant. It is easily blocked as it crosses the superior nuchal line, approximately midway between the external occipital protuberance and the mastoid process (Fig. 17-10). The nerve is located at this site by palpating the occipital artery that lies adjacent to it. Blockade of the occipital nerve will result in a band of anesthesia from the occiput to the vertex. This can be used for providing pain relief for posterior craniotomies as well for pain secondary to occipital neuralgia (33). It is also a useful block in both diagnosis and treatment of occipital "tension" headaches (Table 17-10).

Technique

The occipital artery is palpated below the occipital protuberance. A 27-gauge needle is placed next to the artery and in the subcutaneous plane while fanning laterally. After careful aspiration to rule out intravascular placement, 2 to 3 mL of local anesthetic solution is injected. Gentle massage of the area allows easy spread of the local anesthetic solution.

TABLE 17-9	
SUPERFICIAL CERVICAL PLEXUS	
Indications:	Mastoid surgery, anterior neck surgery, thyroidectomy, parietal craniotomy
Technique:	Palpate the posterior border of the sternal border of the sternocleidomastoid; insert needle in a subcutaneous plane at the level of the cricoid and posterior border of the sternocleidomastoid
Complications:	Deep cervical plexus block, intravascular injection

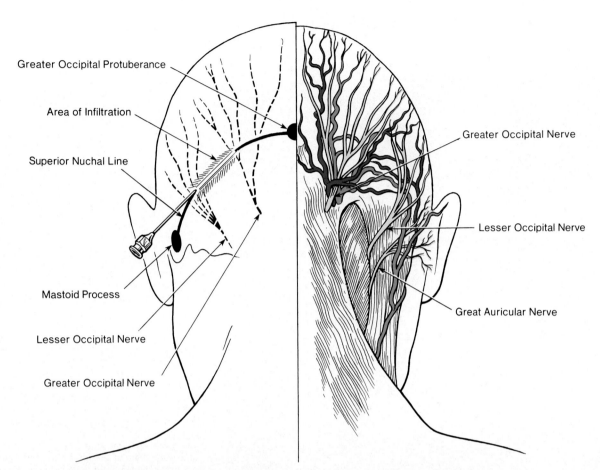

FIGURE 17-10. Greater and lesser occipital nerve block. Note the greater and lesser occipital nerve branches crossing the superior nuchal line approximately halfway between the greater occipital protuberance and the mastoid process. Superficial infiltration along this line will produce analgesia of the posterior scalp. The greater occipital nerve can be located by identifying the pulsations of the posterior occipital artery, which crosses the nuchal line in company with the nerve.

Complications

Complications are very rarely seen. Intravascular injection should be avoided by careful aspiration. This block is used along with blocks of the supraorbital, supratrochlear, auriculotemporal, and lesser occipital nerves to render the scalp anesthetized for surgery (2).

TABLE 17-10

OCCIPITAL NERVE BLOCKS

Indications:	Occipital neuralgia, occipital craniotomy
Technique:	Palpate occipital protuberance, lateral to the midline and inferior to the occipital protuberance
	2 mL of local anesthetic is injected in a fan-like manner in the subcutaneous plane
Complications:	Intravascular injection

Deep Cervical Plexus Block

Indications

This block is sometimes useful for such procedures as thyroidectomy and tracheostomy under local anesthesia (although rarely, see later discussion), and is also used effectively for unilateral carotid endarterectomy or for unilateral removal of cervical lymph nodes.

Technique

Deep cervical plexus block is, in effect, a paravertebral nerve block of C2–C4 spinal nerves as they emerge from the foramina in the cervical vertebrae. Each nerve lies in the sulcus in the transverse process of these vertebrae (Fig. 17-11). Three needles are traditionally used, being inserted at the levels of C2, C3, and C4. The sites of insertion are located by reference to a line that joins the tip of the mastoid process with the Chassaignac tubercle of C6, which is readily palpated at the level of the cricoid cartilage. The C2 transverse process is commonly located approximately one finger's breadth caudad to the mastoid process on this line, and C3 and C4 are at similar intervals

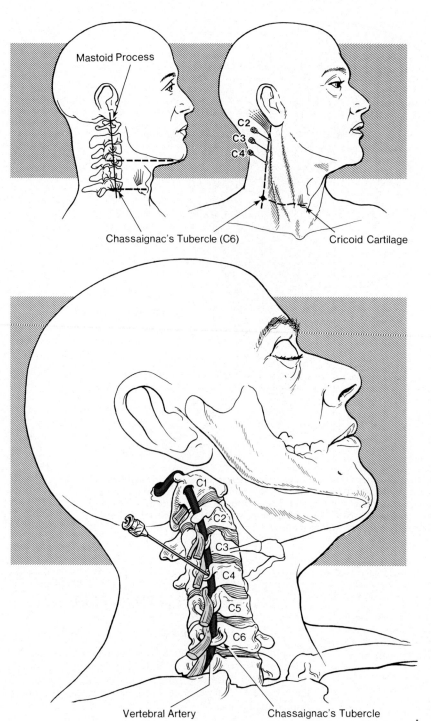

FIGURE 17-11. Deep cervical plexus block. A line is drawn from mastoid process to the Chassaignac tubercle (C6). The latter lies on a line extended laterally from the cricoid cartilage. This line lies over the "gutters" in the superior surface of the transverse processes, upon which the cervical nerve roots pass laterally. The C4 nerve root is located at the junction of the vertical line and a line horizontally drawn to the lower border of the mandible, with the head in a neutral position. The C3 and C2 nerve roots can be located by dividing the distance between the mastoid and horizontal line into thirds (see *right upper panel*). The C5 nerve root lies midway between the "C6 line" and the line above. Individual cervical nerve roots may be blocked by injecting small volumes of local anesthetics, as shown in the upper right. Single-injection block of cervical plexus can be obtained by a technique similar to interscalene brachial plexus block, since the cervical nerve roots are contained in a continuous space between the scalene muscles. A single needle is inserted on the vertical line at the C4 level and directed medially and slightly caudad to contact the "gutter" of the transverse process (*lower panel*). Note that caudad direction is essential to avoid penetration of an intervertebral foramen, with possible injection into epidural space or dural sleeve (and thus direct entry to cerebrospinal fluid). Note also the proximity of the vertebral artery passing through the foramina transversaria of the transverse processes.

caudally on the same line. A horizontal line through the lower border of the ramus of the mandible intersects this line at C4; 5-cm, 22-gauge needles are directed medially and caudad. The reason for the caudad direction is to avoid entering the intervertebral foramen and producing a peridural or spinal block. The end-point is the bony landmark of the transverse process, and paresthesias are obtained. Injection of 3 to 4 mL of 1% lidocaine or the equivalent on each nerve is generally adequate for anesthesia. The paravertebral space communicates freely in the cervical region, and hence the anesthetic solution spreads easily to adjacent levels. Deep cervical plexus block therefore can quite often be obtained with injections at just one level, with a larger volume of 6 to 8 mL. Deep cervical plexus block is a frequent adverse effect following a single-needle interscalene approach for brachial plexus block. If digital pressure is maintained distally over the interscalene groove and the patient placed in a horizontal (or even head-down posture), cervical plexus block can be predictably produced using the same needle insertion technique as for the interscalene brachial plexus block (Table 17-11).

TABLE 17-11

DEEP CERVICAL PLEXUS BLOCK

Indication:	Carotid endarterectomy, cervical lymph node biopsy
Technique:	A line is drawn between C6 and the mastoid process. Three needles are inserted. C2 transverse process is one finger breadth below the mastoid process on this line, and C3 and C4 are similar distances caudad. Needles are inserted medially and caudad until they reach the transverse process and paresthesias are obtained. 3 to 4 mL of local anesthetic solution is injected at each level.
Complications:	Intravascular injection, brachial plexus blockade

Complications

A significant complication of the block is due to the proximity of the vertebral artery, because accidental direct intra-arterial injection may produce profound and very rapid toxic side effects of convulsions, unconsciousness, and blindness; therefore, aspiration tests are of great importance. Extension of the anesthetic into the epidural or subdural spaces is theoretically possible by either dural sleeves or leakage through intervertebral foramen; thus, patients who undergo such procedures must be observed very carefully. When the block is performed bilaterally, bilateral phrenic nerve block is a potentially serious hazard. The deep cervical plexus lies deep to the deep cervical fascia, and hence spread to the cervical sympathetic chain should not occur. If, however, infiltration has spread anterior to the prevertebral fascia, then the cervical sympathetic chain will be involved, with resultant Horner syndrome, and will spread also to the recurrent laryngeal nerve, resulting in hoarseness (34). Both of these complications in a failed block will indicate that, in fact, the anesthetic has been injected at a site superficial to the deep cervical fascia.

Regional Anesthesia of the Ear

The pinnae of the ear are supplied by both cervical plexus and trigeminal nerves. The cervical plexus branch of the great auricular nerve (and maybe the lesser occipital) supplies the posterior surface of the ear and the lower third of the anterior surface. The superior two-thirds of the anterior surface is supplied by the auriculotemporal branch of the mandibular division of the trigeminal (Fig. 17-2).

The cervical plexus supply to the ear can be anesthetized by infiltration along the posterior aspect of the auricle over the mastoid process, where 5 to 8 mL of local anesthetic is infiltrated (Fig. 17-12). The auriculotemporal contribution to the anterior surface of the ear can be anesthetized by infiltration over the posterior aspect of the zygoma. A branch of the auriculotemporal nerve supplies the interior of the auditory canal over its superior aspect, and is injected at the junction between the bony and cartilaginous parts of the anterior wall of the auditory canal, where it can be reached with a 5- to 6-cm needle. Subcutaneous infiltration at this osseous cartilaginous junction is usually done with 2 mL of 1% lidocaine with 1:200,000 epinephrine. The external pinna can be anesthetized using a superficial cervical plexus approach and by blocking the great auricular nerve (30).

The floor of the external auditory canal and the lower part of the tympanum are supplied by a branch of the vagus nerve. This can be anesthetized by infiltrating the osseous cartilaginous junction of the external auditory canal over its lower aspect with 2 mL of 1% lidocaine with 1:200,000 epinephrine. The tympanum can also be anesthetized by direct application of a 4 to 10% lidocaine spray, directing the spray at the roof of the auditory canal and permitting the solution to drain passively over the tympanum rather than directing the spray at the tympanum itself.

CERVICAL EPIDURAL ANESTHESIA

In addition to the discrete regional blocks described for head and neck surgical procedures, it must be remembered that it is quite feasible to produce epidural blockade in the cervical regional, which can facilitate extensive head and neck surgery (35). This might be particularly appropriate, because many patients who are candidates for head and neck surgery belong to the older age group and have coexisting chronic obstructive pulmonary and arteriosclerotic cardiovascular disease. Despite significant preoperative attempts to improve their cardiopulmonary conditions, these patients frequently pose significant operative risks. Since the surgical procedures often are very lengthy, the opportunity for administering continuous local anesthetics is enhanced by an epidural catheter (36).

Because of the poor health of many elderly patients, invasive hemodynamic monitoring may be required. Resting ventilation following cervical epidural block is similar to that following thoracic epidural block and, although there may be some statistically significant changes in both CO_2 accumulation and oxygenation, Takasaki and co-workers (37) deemed these not clinically significant in a group of surgical patients studied on whom this technique was used. Thus, it may provide a useful form of analgesia for patients with compromised cardiorespiratory reserve who need major prolonged head and neck reconstructive surgery (38).

ADVERSE EFFECTS OF REGIONAL ANESTHESIA OF HEAD AND NECK

Regional anesthesia to the head and neck is a relatively safe procedure. However, like all other forms of therapy and intervention, adverse effects including postinjection infection, local tissue trauma, and hematoma; allergic reactions may be seen with head and neck blocks (Table 17-12). There are also some specific complications peculiar to regional anesthetics in this area. These usually involve damage to adjacent structures or spread to the central nervous system via direct or vascular

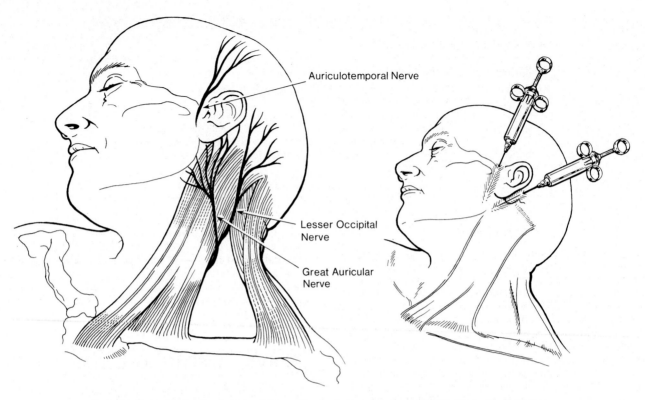

FIGURE 17-12. Regional anesthesia of the ear. The auriculotemporal nerve (V3) is blocked by infiltration over the posterior aspect of zygoma. The great auricular nerve and lesser occipital nerve (branches of the cervical plexus) are blocked by infiltration over the mastoid process posterior to the ear.

spread, which can produce convulsions or extensive neuraxial anesthesia, requiring cardiopulmonary resuscitation.

Accidental injection into one of the vascular conduits carrying blood directly to the brain (e.g., carotid or vertebral artery, or one of their branches) can produce significant transient losses of consciousness and/or convulsion, following accidental injection of small (0.5 mL or less) volumes of local anesthetic into the vertebral artery. Total, reversible, blindness has also been described following similar accidental injections of small amounts (1 mL) of local anesthetic into a vertebral artery. It is also possible for local anesthetic procedures to result in spread of local anesthetic into the neuraxis, either through direct penetration of the foramina of the skull or of the intervertebral

foramen in the cervical spine, producing total brainstem anesthesia (32).

Infection is a rare complication of regional anesthesia in the head and neck, despite many of the injections being placed through the mucous membranes of the mouth. There is scant reference in the literature to infectious complications, although two surprising cases of atlantoaxial subluxation were deemed to be caused by infection of the anterior transverse ligament following local anesthesia for tonsillectomy (41).

Systemic toxic reactions to local anesthetic uptake can be produced by application of such agents to mucous membranes in the nose, oropharynx, and larynx, and attention to dose administered is critically important here, as in other forms of regional anesthesia. The use of benzocaine and prilocaine has been associated with episodes of methemoglobinemia induced following their application to mucous membranes in the throat and trachea.

TABLE 17-12

ADVERSE EFFECTS OF REGIONAL ANESTHESIA OF THE HEAD AND NECK

Minor:
    Syncope
    Infection
    Local tissue trauma
    Hematoma
    Allergic reactions to local anesthetic

Major:
    Intravascular injection
    Temporary blindness
    Convulsions
    Neuraxial spread

SUMMARY

Skill in regional anesthesia of this area of the body is a challenging and technically satisfying addition to the anesthesiologist's repertoire. Regional anesthesia of the head and neck also provides optimal anesthesia for certain kinds of surgical procedures, and it can provide long-lasting postoperative pain relief while reducing the incidence of postoperative morbidity, including postoperative nausea and vomiting (4).

Understanding the anatomy of the region is of prime importance in executing any regional anesthetic, but especially so around the complex anatomic structures in the head and neck. Other innovative techniques have been devised by applying similar basic anatomic knowledge of this area for lateral chest wall pain by blocking the long thoracic nerve of Bell (nerve of supply to the serratus anterior muscle), another branch (C5, C6, and C7) of the brachial plexus roots, which can be located and blocked in the posterior triangle of the neck.

Successful blockade permits reduction, or deletion, of doses of supplemental analgesia. If long-acting local anesthetics, such as bupivacaine or ropivacaine, are employed, then the patient also receives the benefit of excellent postoperative analgesia in situations where analgesic doses of narcotics are relatively contraindicated (e.g., surgery in close proximity to the airway).

Most operations of the head and neck area can be performed with some form of supplementary neural blockade. We have consistently used head and neck blocks routinely in our practice for children coming in for head and neck procedures for over a decade with very good results. It should be recognized that selection of the appropriate peripheral nerves for blockade can permit very effective and efficient analgesia for a wide range of plastic surgery procedures. Volumes of local anesthetic as small as 1 mL can be employed for individual nerves and then supplemented by minimal infiltration of the incision line. As a result, almost all plastic surgical cases, as well as otolaryngology cases in our institution, are provided with peripheral nerve blocks of the head and neck for perioperative pain relief.

References

1. Bosenberg AT, Kimble FW. Infraorbital nerve block in neonates for cleft lip repair: Anatomical study and clinical application. *Br J Anaesth* 1995;74:506–508.
2. Suresh S, Bellig G. Regional anesthesia in a very low-birth-weight neonate for a neurosurgical procedure. *Reg Anesth Pain Med* 2004;29:58–59.
3. Allen BT, Anderson CB, Rubin BG, et al. The influence of anesthetic technique on perioperative complications after carotid endarterectomy. *J Vasc Surg* 1994;19:834–842.
4. Suresh S, Barcelona SL, Young NM, et al. Postoperative pain relief in children undergoing tympanomastoid surgery: Is a regional block better than opioids? *Anesth Analg* 2002;94:859–862, table.
5. Waldman S. *Blockade of the Gasserian Ganglion and the Distal Trigeminal Nerve, Interventional Pain Management*, 1st ed. Waldman S, Winnie A, eds. Philadelphia: W. B. Saunders; 1996:230–246.
6. Suresh S, Wagner AM. Scalp excisions: Getting "ahead" of pain. *Pediatr Dermatol* 2001;18:74–76.
7. Gray H. *Anatomy of the Human Body: Gray's Anatomy*, 30th ed. Baltimore, MD: Williams & Wilkins, 1985.
8. Suresh S, Heffner CL, Voronov P, Curran J. Infraorbital nerve block in children: A computerized tomographic measurement of the location of the infraorbital foramen. (Abstract). *Am Soc Anesthesiol* 2004.
9. Molliex S, Navez M, Baylot D, et al. Regional anesthesia for outpatient nasal surgery. *Br J Anaesth* 1996;76:151–153.
10. Kountakis SE. Effectiveness of perioperative bupivacaine infiltration in tonsillectomy patients. *Am J Otolaryngol* 2002;23:76–80.
11. Onofrio BM. Radiofrequency percutaneous Gasserian ganglion lesions. Results in 140 patients with trigeminal pain. *J Neurosurg* 1975;42:132–139.
12. Rosenberg M, Phero JC. Regional anesthesia and invasive techniques to manage head and neck pain. *Otolaryngol Clin North Am* 2003;36:1201–1219.
13. Peterson JN, Schames J, Schames M, King E. Sphenopalatine ganglion block: A safe and easy method for the management of orofacial pain. *Cranio* 1995;13:177–181.
14. Pradel W, Hlawitschka M, Eckelt U, et al. Cryosurgical treatment of genuine trigeminal neuralgia. *Br J Oral Maxillofac Surg* 2002;40:244–247.
15. Wilkinson HA. Trigeminal nerve peripheral branch phenol/glycerol injections for tic douloureux. *J Neurosurg* 1999;90:828–832.
16. Sweet WH. Percutaneous methods for the treatment of trigeminal neuralgia and other faciocephalic pain: Comparison with microvascular decompression. *Semin Neurol* 1988;8:272–279.
17. Mullan S, Lichtor T. Percutaneous microcompression of the trigeminal ganglion for trigeminal neuralgia. *J Neurosurg* 1983;59:1007–1012.
18. Lichtor T, Mullan JF. A 10-year follow-up review of percutaneous microcompression of the trigeminal ganglion. *J Neurosurg* 1990;72:49–54.
19. Hill JN, Gershon NI, Gargiulo PO. Total spinal blockade during local anesthesia of the nasal passages. *Anesthesiology* 1983;59:144–146.
20. Lebovits AH, Alfred H, Lefkowitz M. Sphenopalatine ganglion block: Clinical use in the pain management clinic. *Clin J Pain* 1990;6:131–136.
21. Prabhu KP, Wig J, Grewal S. Bilateral infraorbital nerve block is superior to peri-incisional infiltration for analgesia after repair of cleft lip. *Scand J Plastic Reconst Surg & Hand Surg* 1999;33:83–87.
22. Bosenberg AT, Kimble FW. Infraorbital nerve block in neonates for cleft lip repair: Anatomical study and clinical application. *Br J Anaesth* 1995;74:506–508.
23. Suresh S, Patel AS, Dunham ME, et al. A randomized double-blind controlled trial of infraorbital nerve block versus intravenous morphine sulfate for children undergoing endoscopic sinus surgery: Are postoperative outcomes different? *Anesthesiology* 2002;97:10–11.
24. McAdam D, Muro K, Suresh S. The use of infraorbital nerve block for postoperative pain control after transsphenoidal hypophysectomy. *Reg Anesth Pain Med* 2005;30:572–573.
25. Suresh S, Voronov P, Curran J. Infraorbital nerve block in children: A computerized tomographic measurement of the location of the infraorbital foramen. *Reg Anesth Pain Med* 2006;31:211–214.
26. Priman J, Eterr LE. Significance of variations of the skull in blocking the maxillary nerve: An anatomical and radiological study. *Anesthesiology* 1961;22:42–48.
27. Goel AC. Auricular nerve block in bronchial asthma. *J Indian Med Assoc* 1981;76:132–134.
28. Krause HR, Kornhuber A, Dempf R. A technique for diagnosing the individual patterns of innervation of the trapezius muscle prior to neck dissection. *J Craniomaxillofac Surg* 1993;21:102–106.
29. Ramamurthy S, Akkineni SR, Winnie AP. A simple technic for block of the spinal accessory nerve. *Anesth Analg* 1978;57:591–593.
30. Cregg N, Conway F, Casey W. Analgesia after otoplasty: Regional nerve blockade vs local anaesthetic infiltration of the ear. *Can J Anaesth* 1996;43(2):141–147.
31. Suresh S, Templeton L. Superficial cervical plexus block for vocal cord surgery in an awake pediatric patient. *Anesth Analg* 2004;98:1656–1657, table.
32. Dieudonne N, Gomola A, Bonnichon P, Ozier YM. Prevention of postoperative pain after thyroid surgery: A double-blind randomized study of bilateral superficial cervical plexus blocks. *Anesth Analg* 2001;92:1538–1542.
33. Ward JB. Greater occipital nerve block. *Semin Neurol* 2003;23:59–62.
34. Hogan QH, Taylor ML, Goldstein M, et al. Success rates in producing sympathetic blockade by paratracheal injection. *Clin J Pain* 1994;10:139–145.
35. Wittich DJ Jr., Berny JJ, Davis RK. Cervical epidural anesthesia for head and neck surgery. *Laryngoscope* 1984;94:615–619.
36. Catchlove RF, Braha R. The use of cervical epidural nerve blocks in the management of chronic head and neck pain. *Can Anaesth Soc J* 1984;31:188–191.
37. Takasaki M, Yao K, Kosaka Y, Takahashi T. [Respiratory effects of cervical epidural analgesia (author's transl)]. *Masui* 1978;27:397–401.
38. Catchlove RF, Braha R. The use of cervical epidural nerve blocks in the management of chronic head and neck pain. *Can Anaesth Soc J* 1984;31:188–191.
39. Sakawi Y, Groudine S, Roberts K, et al. Carotid endarterectomy surgery and ICU admissions: A regional anesthesia perspective. *J Neurosurg Anesthesiol* 1998;10:211–217.
40. Harbaugh RE, Pikus HJ. Carotid endarterectomy with regional anesthesia. *Neurosurgery* 2001;49:642–645.
41. Bowyer MW, Zierold D, Loftus JP, et al. Carotid endarterectomy: A comparison of regional versus general anesthesia in 500 operations. *Ann Vasc Surg* 2000;14:145–151.
42. Stoneham MD, Knighton JD. Regional anaesthesia for carotid endarterectomy. *Br J Anaesth* 1999;82:910–919.
43. Prough DS, Scuderi PE, Stullken E, Davis CH Jr. Myocardial infarction following regional anaesthesia for carotid endarterectomy. *Can Anaesth Soc J* 1984;31:192–196.

PART II: TECHNIQUES

CHAPTER 18 ■ NEURAL BLOCKADE OF ORAL AND CIRCUMORAL STRUCTURES

MORTON B. ROSENBERG, JOSEPH A. GIOVANNITTI, JR., AND JAMES C. PHERO

The ability to provide safe, effective local anesthesia is the foundation of clinical dentistry. Neural blockade of oral and circumoral structures can be achieved via *extraoral or intraoral* techniques. With their in-depth knowledge of intraoral anatomy and familiarity with the oral cavity, most dentists use the intraoral approaches. However, there may be specific indications in which one method is preferred over the other. The presence of anatomic anomalies, infection, the nature of an injury and the extent of the procedure, or the use of local anesthetic techniques for diagnosis or management for acute and/or chronic pain syndromes, for example, may mitigate for or against a particular technique, drug, or approach. Generally, the extraoral approach is designed to provide anesthesia of a major nerve trunk (e.g., V2, V3). The effect of this type of blockade is to block neural conduction to a wide area of the face, head, or neck.

This chapter discusses the most common intraoral techniques used by dentists to anesthetize soft and hard tissues of the oral cavity. Local anesthetic techniques involving both intraoral and extraoral approaches to the trigeminal nerve are reviewed. In addition, the armamentarium unique to dentistry and the pharmacology of the local anesthetics routinely employed are presented.

Intraoral local anesthesia, as well as dental therapy, is often complicated by the existence of multifactorial psychological considerations associated with the delivery of dental care. Anticipation of pain is the most common cause of anxiety associated with a dental visit and accounts for the avoidance behavior of 6% to 9% of the U.S. population who neglect needed dental care (1), and it is responsible for the large number of dental phobics who find dental treatment highly stressful. It is imperative for health care professionals to understand and appreciate these issues and employ perioperative behavioral management strategies such as progressive relaxation, hypnosis, biofeedback, systematic desensitization, or the use of sedative drugs to reduce anxiety, fear, and apprehension to acceptable levels. Like any regional anesthetic technique, the effectiveness and utility of any intraoral injection depends upon patient considerations, the extent and duration of the procedure, and the skill and experience of the clinician. Every clinician should be aware of her skill limitations, as well as the limitations of the contemplated technique and agents. These factors must be clearly understood, as they will directly impact on successful outcomes and the potential for severe complications. The management of the apprehensive dental patient remains one of the most challenging problems in health care.

PREPARATION

As with any anesthetic, medical, dental, or surgical procedure, a careful and thorough preoperative evaluation including, but not limited to, a review of the medical history with special emphasis on past anesthetic experiences, focused physical examination, and determination of physical status and the potential of drug interactions must be conducted prior to selection of technique and agents. Based on this information and practitioner knowledge base, a reasonable and rational anesthesia plan, taking into account the risk–benefit balance, may be successfully formulated.

Special Injection Considerations

Patient Position

Intraoral injections are best achieved with the patient seated comfortably in a semireclining position (Fig. 18-1). This position offers at least two distinct advantages over the conventional upright or horizontal position. First, the oral cavity can be easily accessed and landmarks identified to provide optimal working conditions for the dentist. Second, this position provides a physiologically sound cardiovascular and respiratory position. Venous return is facilitated from both upper and lower extremities, and diaphragmatic movement is unrestricted. Vasodepressor syncope remains the most common medical emergency in dentistry and is often associated with the administration of local anesthesia. This may be due to the high incidence of phobia and stress or the anticipated (and sometime actual) pain that is often associated with intraoral injections.

Tissue Preparation

Tissue preparation for regional anesthesia at extraoral sites involves disinfection of the area with a suitable preparatory solutions and the use of appropriate aseptic technique. For local anesthetic injections within the oral cavity, true "asepsis" is neither necessary nor attainable. Nevertheless, certain basic principles may be adhered to, to reduce the risk of infection, particularly into deep structures. Prior to injection, the hands of the operator should be scrupulously cleansed and gloved. A surgical mask and eye protection is worn to protect the operator from inadvertent exposure to blood, saliva, or mucus. Prior to inserting a needle into the tissues of the oral cavity, the operator should dry the area with a sterile cotton-tipped

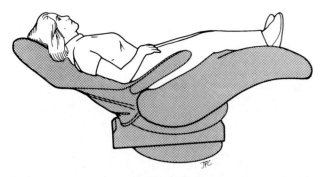

FIGURE 18-1. Patient should be placed in semi-reclining position with legs and thorax slightly elevated.

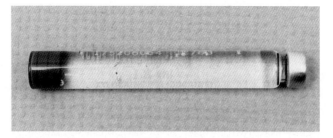

FIGURE 18-2. Needle end (*right*) of the cartridge is sealed with a metal cap. A rubber plunger at the other end is used to expel the contents.

applicator or a 2 × 2 gauze sponge. A suitable topical antiseptic may then be applied to the site of injection, and the antiseptic wiped from the tissue to prevent its introduction into the tissues during needle penetration.

Topical Anesthesia

The topical application of a local anesthetic can play an important role in reducing the pain of needle insertion. It also provides psychological reinforcement to the patient that everything is being done to reduce pain. Topical anesthesia usually only reaches a depth of 2 to 3 mm and is usually achieved using high concentrations of benzocaine or lidocaine. A new addition to the dental topical local anesthesia armamentarium is the introduction of a periodontal topical eutectic local anesthetic gel consisting of 2.5% lidocaine and 2.5% prilocaine that is expressed as a liquid onto the gingiva and becomes an adherent gel at body temperature (2).

SUPPLIES AND EQUIPMENT

Although in theory similar to the armamentarium used for other types of neural blockade, the equipment used in dentistry for intraoral anesthesia is sufficiently different enough to warrant description. Traditional plastic syringes and needles with Luer-Lok hubs can be substituted for this specialized equipment, but are unwieldy in the dental environment. The equipment used in dentistry intraoral neural blockade (3) includes:

- Glass cartridges containing the anesthetic solution
- Aspirating syringes
- Needles
- Auxiliary equipment and supplies

Cartridge

The introduction of the single-use local anesthetic cartridge for dentistry was a major advance because it ensured sterility, uniformity of solution composition, reduced cost, and integration into the dental aspirating syringe system. The cartridge is a glass tube sealed at one end by a movable rubber stopper that can be forced into the tube by the plunger of the cartridge-type syringe (Fig. 18-2). The other end of the tube is sealed by an aluminum cap over a rubber or latex-free diaphragm that is punctured by the cartridge end of the needle (Fig. 18-3).

Cartridges are hermetically sealed and contain approximately 1.8 mL of local anesthetic solution.

Cartridges are supplied by the manufacturer in either vacuum-packed cans or sealed cartons. Local anesthetic cartridges are color-coded as to their contents. After the package containing the cartridges has been opened, it is recommended that cartridges be stored in their original container at room temperature. Cartridges should not be placed or submerged in any germicide, since germicides may corrode the metal caps or penetrate the rubber stopper, and the potentially neurolytic germicidal agent may eventually seep into the cartridge. The contents of a dental local anesthetic cartridge include the local anesthetic drug, sodium chloride, and sterile distilled water. A vasoconstrictor, such as epinephrine or levonordefrin, may often be present, as well as sodium bisulfite, which acts as a preservative for the vasoconstrictor. Local anesthetic cartridges should never be heat-sterilized as this will cause deterioration of the vasoconstrictive agent. The internal contents of the local anesthetic cartridges are sterile. If the cartridges are to be used in a sterile system, they should be disinfected with an appropriate agent prior to handling. The shelf life of a plain local anesthetic solution (no vasoconstrictor) in a dental cartridge is approximately 48 months. Local anesthetic solutions containing epinephrine and levonordefrin have shelf lives of 18 months and 12 months, respectively.

Problems with Cartridges

Despite quality control in the manufacturing of local anesthetic cartridges, several minor problems may develop:

- *Bubbles.* Small bubbles (1–2 mm) may be visible within the cartridge. These bubbles are usually nitrogen gas, which has been introduced into the cartridge during the manufacturing

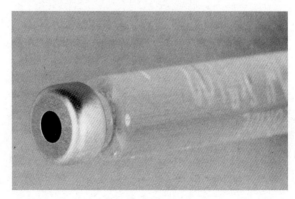

FIGURE 18-3. Cartridge with aluminum cap over rubber diaphragm.

process to prevent oxygen from entering the cartridge, the presence of which would cause deterioration of the vasoconstrictor. Although these small bubbles are harmless, large bubbles in cartridges, with or without plungers extruded beyond the end of the cartridge, may be caused by freezing during transit and should be discarded.

■ *Extruded plungers.* Extruded plungers in cartridges that contain no bubbles usually indicate that the cartridge has been stored in disinfecting solution and that some of the solution has passed through the rubber stopper or diaphragm and contaminated the anesthetic solution. These should be discarded.

■ *Corrosion of aluminum cap.* Corrosion of the cap is usually caused by immersing the cartridge in chemical disinfecting solutions that contain nitrate antirust materials; these cartridges should not be used.

Syringes

The most commonly used syringe in dentistry for intraoral injections is the metal, side-loading metal cartridge aspirating syringe (Fig. 18-4). These syringes are extremely durable, autoclavable, accept a wide variety of cartridge and needles, and can produce negative pressure during the injection process.

To load, the piston is retracted and the cartridge inserted, plunger end first, into the syringe (Fig. 18-5A). Next, the piston is pushed forward with moderate pressure until the harpoon on the plunger (Fig. 18-5B) is firmly engaged into the rubber stopper. This will allow the stopper to be advanced and withdrawn when negative or positive pressure is applied to the piston to facilitate aspiration. The needle is then affixed to the threaded end of the syringe and pierces the diaphragm of the cartridge (Fig. 18-5C). A few drops of solution are expressed to ensure that the unit is properly assembled and ready for use (Fig. 18-5D).

Several other types of cartridge syringe systems may be used for intraoral injections. One of these is the self-aspirating, cartridge-type syringe, which is a variation of the conventional side-loading syringe previously described. This syringe has no barbed or harpoon plunger, but instead allows aspiration to occur by depression of a thumb disk at its base. This action causes distortion of the cartridge diaphragm, which then rebounds as the thumb disk is released, producing negative pressure. Subsequently, during the injection process, any release of forward plunger pressure will result in negative pressure in the syringe, resulting in aspiration.

Needles

Needles designed for use in the standard dental syringe are divided into five parts: the bevel, shank, hub, syringe adapter, and syringe end of the needle (Fig. 18-6). Needles for intraoral injection range from 30 to 25 gauge and from 1.5 to 5 cm in length and are for one-time use. For deep intraoral injections, the 25-gauge, 5 cm needle is preferred by most practitioners. This needle may be inserted painlessly and directed to the

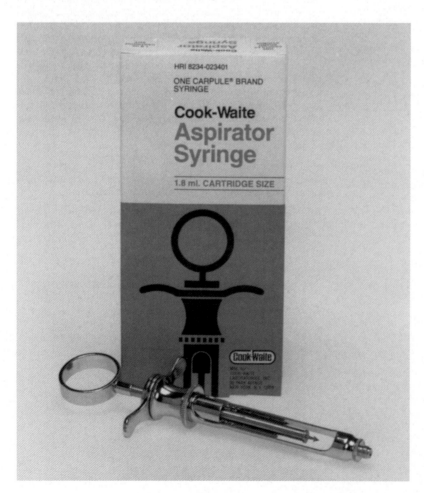

FIGURE 18-4. Metal aspirating syringe that can be resterilized. (Courtesy of Cook-Waite Laboratories, Inc., New York.)

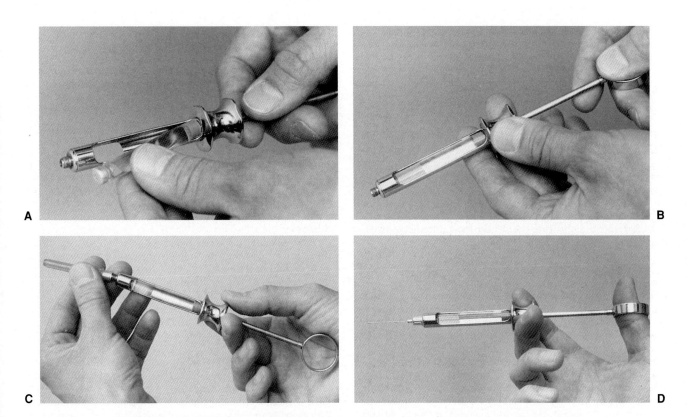

FIGURE 18-5. A: Plunger is retracted and cartridge inserted into syringe. **B:** Piston is pushed forward until harpoon engages plunger. **C:** Needle is affixed to syringe top. **D:** Prepared syringe is ready for use.

desired site with minimal deflection, yet is of sufficient gauge to allow reliable aspiration.

Emergency (Resuscitation) Equipment

Because complications and emergencies can occur during the administration of any local anesthetic, it is imperative that medical emergency equipment and supplies be immediately available and that practitioners who use these drugs be proficient in resuscitation (see Chapter 5).

Although local anesthesia within the oral cavity generally uses relatively small doses and volumes of local anesthetic drugs, the head and neck is a very vascular area, with direct and immediate connection to the central nervous system (CNS). Unintentional intra-arterial or intravenous (IV) injection or the rapid absorption of even relatively small amounts of local anesthetic doses may result in immediate and severe toxic manifestations of local anesthetic toxicity. Indeed, it is estimated that 90% of all medical emergencies occurring in dental offices occur in conjunction with, but are not necessarily directly attributable to, the administration of local anesthesia. Acute medical emergencies such as angina, syncope, hyperventilation

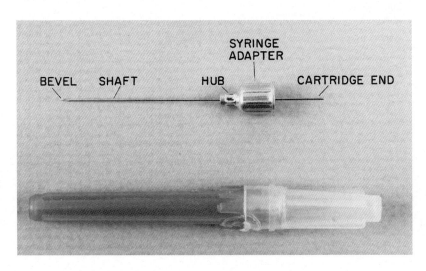

FIGURE 18-6. Segments of dental needle.

syndrome, acute-onset seizure activity, bronchospasm, and myocardial infarction have all been reported to have been precipitated by anticipatory fear, pain, and accidental intravascular injections (4) (see also Chapter 5).

LOCAL ANESTHETIC SOLUTIONS

Although any available local anesthetic solution acceptable for neural blockade in other parts of the body may be used for regional anesthesia of the head and neck, only eight agents are currently available in cartridge form for dentistry (Table 18-1). It is important to note that procaine (Novocaine), the first local anesthetic with true dental utility, is no longer available in North America in dental cartridges. Therefore, only amide local anesthetics constitute the dental local anesthetic armamentarium.

As in other types of neural blockade, the choice of anesthetic agent and amount, type, and concentration of vasoconstrictor is based on many factors such as physical status, age, and weight of the patient, duration of the procedure, and the need for hemostasis. Local anesthesia toxicity is a concern whenever large volumes of concentrated local anesthetic are used. Clinicians must to avoid injecting more milligrams per kilogram than is recommended to avoid a toxic response with the potential of leading to CNS, respiratory, and cardiac depression. When a large volume of local anesthetic must be administered, the incidence of toxicity can be avoided by using the lowest concentration of local anesthetic that will produce the required block and calculating the maximum volume of this solution that each patient may receive in advance of starting the injection. This is especially true in pediatric, severely compromised, and geriatric patients, in whom drug toxicity can become a life-threatening complication if maximum doses are not strictly followed (Table 18-2).

In the past, dental local anesthetic cartridges also contained methylparaben as a bacteristatic agent. Since the dental anesthetic cartridge is designed for one-time use, methylparaben has been eliminated. On the other hand, sodium (meta) bisulfite as an antioxidant is present in any dental cartridge containing a vasopressor (epinephrine or levonordefrin) to prevent oxidation and a decrease in potency.

Since 1948, lidocaine, the first amino-amide local anesthetic, became the "gold standard" against which all other dental local anesthetics are compared. Lidocaine, mepivacaine, and prilocaine combined with a vasoconstrictor provide reliable and profound pulpal anesthesia for approximately 60 minutes with a duration of soft tissue anesthesia ranging from 3 to 5 hours (5).

The increase in longer and more invasive surgical procedures with significant postoperative pain led to the introduction of longer-acting local anesthetics available in the dental cartridge. Currently, bupivacaine, 0.5% with 1:200,000 epinephrine is the only long-lasting local anesthetic available in dental cartridges in North America. Despite its relatively long onset (6 to 10 minutes), injections of bupivacaine with up to 12 hours of soft tissue anesthesia play an important role in reducing pain in the postoperative period.

Articaine, the newest local anesthetic available in dental cartridges, was introduced in 1976 in Europe and in 2000 in the United States. Articaine with epinephrine appears to have a similar clinical profile as lidocaine, mepivacaine, and prilocaine with vasoconstrictors (6). Despite the anecdotal reports of greater success and efficacy with articaine than with other local anesthetics, at this time, a lack of evidence supports these claims. Controversy also exists concerning reports

---

TABLE 18-1

LOCAL ANESTHETICS IN CARTRIDGE FORM

Generic name	Trade name(s)	Vasoconstrictor
Bupivacaine 0.5%	Marcaine	1:200,000 epinephrine
Lidocaine 2%	Octocaine	Without vasoconstrictor
	Xylocaine	1:50,000 epinephrine
	Alphacaine	1:100,000 epinephrine
	Lignospan	
	Lignospan Forte	
Mepivacaine 2%	Carbocaine	1:20,000 Levonordefrin
Mepivacaine 3%	Carbocaine	Without vasoconstrictor
Mepivacaine	Isocaine	
Mepivacaine	Polocaine	
	Arestocaine	
	Scandanest	
Prilocaine 4%	Citanest Plain	Without vasoconstrictor
Prilocaine 4%	Citanest Forte	1:200,000 epinephrine
Articaine 4%	Ultracaine D-S Forte	1:100,000 epinephrine
Articaine 4%	Ultracaine D-S	1:200,000 epinephrine
Procaine 2%		

[a]Propoxycaine 0.4% and procaine 2% are combined in the same cartridge. Both compounds are ester-type anesthetic drugs. They are the only esters currently marketed in cartridge form. All other agents are amides.

TABLE 18-2

DURATION AND MAXIMUM SAFE DOSAGE OF AGENTS USED IN DENTISTRY

Drug	Duration pulpal/soft tissue	Maximum dose
Bupivacaine 0.4% 1:200,000 epinephrine	1–2 h/>10 h	1.3 mg/kg 90 mg max (10 cart)
Lidocaine 2% (without vasoconstrictor)	5–10 min/60–120 min	4.4 mg/kg 300 mg max (8.3 cart)
Lidocaine 2% 1:50,000 epinephrine	60–90 min/3–4 h	7.0 mg/kg 500 mg max (13.8 cart)[a]
Lidocaine 2% 1:100,000 epinephrine	60–90 min/3–4 h	7.0 mg/kg 500 mg max (13.8 cart)[a]
Mepivacaine 3%	20–40 min/2–3 h	6.6 mg/kg 400 mg max (7.4 cart)
Mepivacaine 2% 1:20,000 Levonordefrin	40–60 min/2–4 h	6.6 mg/kg 400 mg max (11.1 cart)[b]
Prilocaine 4%	10–15 min/2–4 h	7.9 mg/kg 600 mg max (8.3 cart)
Prilocaine 4% 1:200,000 epinephrine	60–90 min/2–4 h	7.9 mg/kg 600 mg max (8.3 cart)
Articaine 4% 1:100,000 epinephrine	75 min/2–4 h	7.0 mg/kg 500 mg max (7 cart)
Articaine 4% 1:200,000 epinephrine	45 min/2–4 h	7.0 mg/kg 500 mg max (7 cart)

[a]Exceeds maximum recommended epinephrine dose
[b]Exceeds maximum recommended levonordefrin dose

that the 4% local anesthetic solutions (articaine and prilocaine) may be implicated in a slightly higher rate of prolonged paresthesia following inferior alveolar block than other agents (7).

VASOCONSTRICTORS

Vasoconstrictors are used to prolong the duration of anesthetic effect, decrease the rate of absorption of local anesthetics, and decrease localized bleeding at the site of administration. The most pronounced effect on duration is achieved by adding a vasoconstrictor to lidocaine and mepivacaine. By contrast, addition of a vasoconstrictor to bupivacaine does little to prolong its duration, as this drug produces prolonged duration of anesthesia following mandibular block, primarily because of bupivacaine's high degree of lipid solubility. The two most commonly used vasoconstrictors in dentistry are epinephrine and levonordefrin. In dental cartridges, epinephrine is available in three concentrations, 5 μg/mL (1:200,000), 10 μg/mL (1:100,000), and 20 μg/mL (1:50,000). A standard dental cartridge with 1:100,000 epinephrine contains 18 μg of epinephrine. Levonordefrin is found only in dental cartridges containing mepivacaine, in a concentration of 50 μg/mL (1:20,000). A standard dental cartridge with 1:20,000 levonordefrin contains 90 μg of levonordefrin. Al-

though levonordefrin is a relatively weaker adrenergic agonist than epinephrine, consideration should be given to the fact that the 1:20,000 concentration is five times greater than the standard concentration of epinephrine. Therefore, fewer cartridges containing levonordefrin may be safely used in comparison with cartridges containing epinephrine. Table 18-3 gives generally accepted dosages for vasoconstrictors in healthy patients, as well as in those with cardiovascular compromise.

The mucosa of the oral cavity is highly vascularized, and the systemic uptake of vasoconstrictors following intraoral injection may be rapid. A single dental cartridge of lidocaine 2% with 1:100,000 epinephrine can double the resting epinephrine titer within minutes (8,9). Furthermore, the intraoral administration of eight dental cartridges of a 1:100,000 epinephrine solution may produce plasma epinephrine concentrations equivalent to those present during heavy exercise (10). It is important to limit the amount of vasoconstrictor-containing local anesthetic solutions to patients with severe anxiety and/or cardiovascular disease. As a general rule, the minimum possible amount of vasoconstrictor should be used. One cartridge (1.8 mL) of a 1:100,000 epinephrine-containing solution should be well-tolerated even in patients with significant cardiovascular disease. Caution should also be exercised in patients taking nonspecific β-adrenergic blockers, adrenergic neuron blockers, tricyclic antidepressants, and phenothiazine derivatives.

TABLE 18-3

MAXIMUM RECOMMENDED DOSE OF VASOCONSTRICTORS (70 kg)

	Healthy	ASA II	ASA III
Epinephrine 1:100,000	3 μg/kg 200 μg max (11.1 cart)	1.5 μg/kg 100 μg/kg (5.5 cart)	0.75 μg/kg 40 μg/kg (2.22 cart)
Levonordefrin 1:20,000	7 μg/kg (5.4 cart)	3.5 μg/kg (2.7 cart)	1.5 μg/kg (1.2 cart)

Vasoconstrictive agents should be used intraorally when a plain local anesthetic solution fails to provide profound anesthesia, when the length of the planned procedure is longer than the expected duration of anesthesia with a plain solution, and when local hemostasis is required.

EXTRAORAL AND INTRAORAL INJECTION TECHNIQUES

Anatomy

Innervation of the head and neck is by the trigeminal and cervical nerves (Fig. 18-7). The trigeminal nerve is the largest of the

cranial nerves. It contains both sensory and motor fibers. General somatic afferent nerve fibers carry sensory impulses from the face. Somatic impulses, including thermal, touch, and pain, are transmitted from the skin of the face and forehead, mucous membranes of the nasal surfaces and oral cavity, the teeth, the anterior two-thirds of the tongue, and anterior portions of the cranial dura. Proprioceptive impulses are carried from the teeth, periodontium, hard palate, and temporomandibular joint. The trigeminal nerve carries afferent impulses from stretch receptors in the muscles of mastication. Additionally, visceral efferent fibers innervate the muscles of mastication, the tensor tympani and tensor veli palatine muscles, muscles of the eye, and facial muscles.

The trigeminal nerve is divided into the ophthalmic (V1), maxillary (V2), and mandibular (V3) divisions. Areas of the oral cavity are innervated by either V2 or V3.

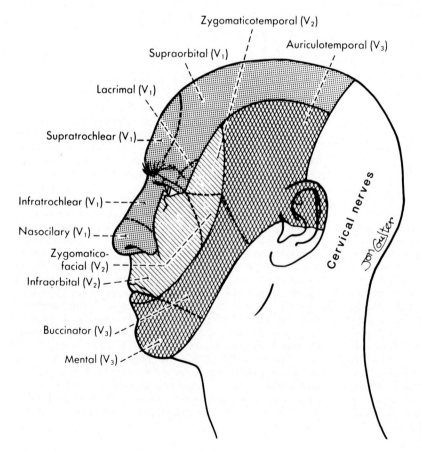

FIGURE 18-7. Superficial sensory nerves of the head and neck.

Anatomy of the Ophthalmic Division (V1)

The ophthalmic division is entirely sensory, and is the smallest of the three trigeminal divisions. It exits the cranium and enters the orbit via the superior orbital fissure, where it divides into its three main branches: the frontal, nasociliary, and lacrimal nerves. These nerves supply the eyeball, conjunctiva, lacrimal gland, portions of the mucous membranes of the nose and sinuses, and the skin of the forehead, eyelids, and nose. Blockade of these nerves is rarely used for oral and circumoral surgery and is discussed in detail in Chapter 17.

Techniques of Neural Blockade for the Maxillary Nerve and Its Subdivisions

Anatomy of the Maxillary Division (V2)

The maxillary nerve is entirely sensory (Fig. 18-8). It exits the skull through the foramen rotundum and enters the pterygopalatine fossa, whence it progresses forward into the inferior orbital fissure and passes into the orbital cavity. Here, it turns slightly laterally in the infraorbital groove on the orbital surface of the maxilla. As it continues forward, it passes through the infraorbital canal and exits onto the front of the maxilla through the infraorbital foramen.

The branches of the maxillary nerve (V2) and associated areas of sensory innervation occur (a) within the pterygopalatine fossa, (b) within the infraorbital groove and canal, and (c) as terminal branches to the face.

The branches within the pterygopalatine fossa are:

- Pharyngeal branch: Mucosa of pharynx
- Middle and posterior palatine: Tonsil and soft palate
- Greater palatine: Mucosa of posterior palate
- Nasopalatine branch: Septal mucosa through incisive canal to the anterior hard palate
- Posterior and superior lateral nasal branch: Lateral walls of nasal cavity
- Posterior superior alveolar branch: Second and third maxillary molars, as well as palatal and distobuccal root of first molar, alveolus, and overlying buccal soft tissue. (The mesiobuccal root of the maxillary first molar is innervated by the middle superior alveolar nerve)
- Zygomatic branch: Skin of the temple and over the zygomatic bone. At this point, the maxillary division becomes known as the *infraorbital nerve.*

Branches within the infraorbital groove and canal are:

- Middle superior alveolar nerve: Anterior walls of the maxillary sinus, bicuspid teeth, buccal gingiva, and mucosa
- Anterior superior alveolar nerve: Incisor and cuspid teeth and labial soft tissue

The terminal branches to the face are:

- Inferior palpebral: Lower eyelid
- Lateral nasal: Skin of the side of the nose
- Superior labial: Cheek, skin, and mucosa of the upper lid

In order to provide the necessary anesthesia for procedures on maxillary hard and soft tissue, it may be necessary

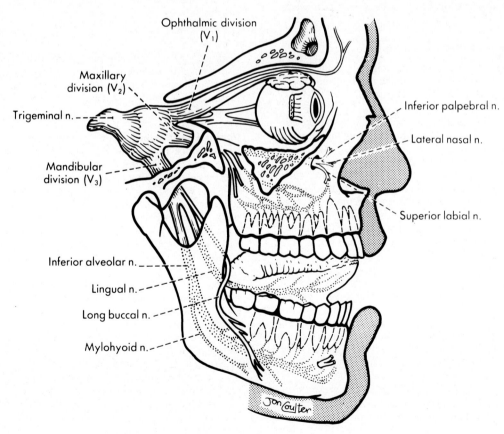

FIGURE 18-8. Distribution of the trigeminal nerve.

TABLE 18-4

REGIONAL ANALGESIA OF THE MAXILLA

Nerves anesthetized	Areas anesthetized
Posterior superior alveolar nerve	Maxillary molars (except mesiobuccal root of first molar); buccal alveolar bone and soft tissues; lining of maxillary sinus corresponding to the molar teeth
Middle superior alveolar nerve	Mesiobuccal root of first molar; premolars; corresponding buccal alveolar bone and soft tissues; lining of maxillary sinus
Anterior superior alveolar nerve	Canines, lateral incisors, central incisors; corresponding buccal alveolar bone and soft tissues
Greater palatine nerve	Hard palate and overlying mucosa from molars to first bicuspids
Nasopalatine nerve	Hard and soft tissues of the entire anterior hard palate to the canines bilaterally
Infraorbital nerve	Lower eyelid, side of nose, upper lip; areas supplied by the middle and anterior superior alveolar nerves

to block either one or a combination of the these nerves or nerve branches which are listed in Table 18-4. Although most dental professionals access the maxillary nerve via intraoral techniques, extraoral techniques are also possible in selected cases.

Intraoral Techniques

Local Infiltration. Soft tissues of the oral cavity may be satisfactorily anesthetized with local infiltration (i.e., injection of local anesthesia directly into the soft tissues).

Technique. After the application of a topical anesthetic, a 2.5-cm, 25-gauge needle is inserted beneath the mucous membrane into the connective tissue in the area to be anesthetized and the solution is slowly infiltrated. Because in many areas of the oral cavity the mucosa is adherent to the underlying periosteum, care must be taken to avoid depositing large volumes of solution. Large volumes may strip the periosteum from the underlying bone or result in pressure-induced soft tissue ischemia and resultant tissue slough; this injection into tightly adherent tissues can be extremely painful.

Block of Terminal Branches. Terminal branch block is indicated for anesthetizing a single maxillary tooth. The maxilla is better suited for this type of injection because of the porosity of the maxillary bone, which allows diffusion of the anesthetic solution. The technique is rarely successful in the mandible because of the density of the cortical plate, except in the anterior region where most children and some adults have a thin cortical plate.

Technique. After the application of topical anesthesia, a 2.5-cm, 25-gauge needle is inserted through the mucous membrane and underlying connective tissue until it contacts the periosteum over the apex of the tooth (or teeth) (Fig. 18-9). A dose of 1 to 2 mL of anesthetic solution should be injected slowly, al-

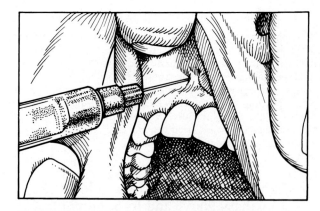
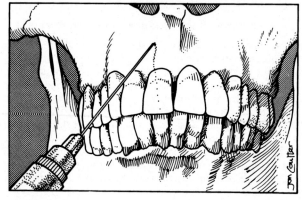

FIGURE 18-9. Field block or infiltration. The needle is inserted through mucous membrane in the area of the tooth or teeth to be anesthetized.

lowing about 5 minutes for maximum effect. The maxillary incisors, cuspids, and bicuspids may be anesthetized in this manner. Maxillary molars may require other techniques, because these teeth are multirooted and divergent, and the overlying bone is dense.

Intraoral and Extraoral Approaches for the Infraorbital Nerve Block (Block of the Anterior and Middle Superior Alveolar Nerves). The infraorbital nerve block is useful for providing anesthesia of the lower eyelid, lateral inferior portion of the nose and vestibule, and the upper lid and mucosa. The anterior superior alveolar nerve branches from the infraorbital nerve in the anterior part of the infraorbital canal and innervates the maxillary incisors, cuspid teeth (including their bony support), and surrounding labial soft tissue. Block of these areas can be accomplished via intraoral and extraoral approaches.

Intraoral technique. The patient is instructed to look directly forward while the operator palpates the supraorbital and infraorbital notches. An imaginary straight line drawn vertically through these landmarks will pass through the pupil of the eye, infraorbital foramen, the bicuspid teeth, and the mental foramen (Fig. 18-10). When the infraorbital notch is identified, the palpating finger should follow the vertical line inferiorly about 0.5 cm, at which point a shallow depression is felt. The infraorbital foramen is located within the depression.

For a block on the right side, the thumb of the operator's left hand is placed over the previously located foramen and the index finger is used to retract the lip (Fig. 18-11). A 4-cm, 25-gauge needle is then inserted along the imaginary vertical line

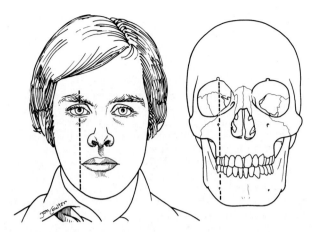

FIGURE 18-10. Supraorbital notch, pupil of the eye, infraorbital notch, infraorbital frame, bicuspid teeth, and mental foramen lie on a straight vertical line.

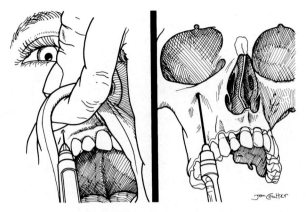

FIGURE 18-11. Infraorbital block. The thumb is maintained in place over the infraorbital foramen.

until the foramen is reached. The needle should be inserted a sufficient distance (about 0.5 cm) from the labial plate to bridge the canine fossa. The thumb in place over the foramen should be used to maneuver the needle into position, so that it contacts the bone at the entrance to the foramen. The needle should not penetrate soft tissue for more than 2 cm. About 2 mL of solution is deposited. The skin over the infraorbital foramen should be massaged to promote the spread of the anesthetic solution into the foramen.

Tingling and numbness of the lower eyelid, side of the nose, and upper lip will ensue, but is not necessarily an indication of a successful block. To anesthetize the anterior and middle superior alveolar nerves that supply the teeth, the solution must enter the infraorbital foramen and flow proximally through the infraorbital canal. Instrumentation of the teeth in question will demonstrate success or failure of the block.

Figure 18-12 depicts the anatomic relationships involved when performing the infraorbital nerve block.

Extraoral approach. The extraoral approach to the infraorbital nerve is accomplished by first identifying the infraorbital ridge of the maxillary bone and palpating the infraorbital

foramen, located approximately 2 cm from the lateral surface of the nose. The anterior portion of the canal in the orbit is typically covered with a thin plate of bone, so that needle insertion should occur 0.5 cm below and slightly medial to the foramen to allow for the backward and upward slant of the infraorbital canal. The needle must be advanced past the opening of the infraorbital canal, or the anterior superior alveolar nerve will not be blocked. However, the needle should not be advanced more than 0.5 cm past the entry into the infraorbital foramen. A volume of 1 to 3 mL of local anesthetic is sufficient for nerve blockade.

Posterior Superior Alveolar Nerve Block. This nerve block provides anesthesia of the third and second maxillary molars, and two-thirds of the first maxillary molar, as well as supporting hard and buccal soft tissues.

Since the first maxillary molar has dual innervation via the middle superior alveolar nerve, the posterior superior alveolar nerve block must often be coupled with infiltration over the mesiobuccal root to provide total pulpal anesthesia. The posterior superior alveolar nerve arises from the maxillary nerve before it enters the body of the maxilla. It is located distal to the maxillary tuberosity.

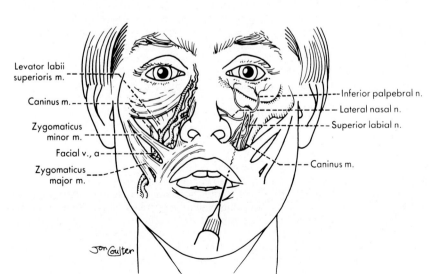

Levator labii
superioris m.

Caninus m.

Zygomaticus
minor m.

Facial v., a

Zygomaticus
major m.

Inferior palpebral n.

Lateral nasal n.

Superior labial n.

Caninus m.

FIGURE 18-12. Anatomic relationships relative to the infraorbital nerve block.

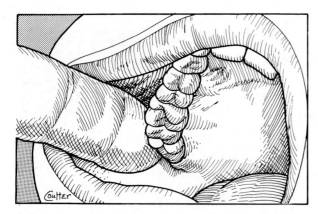

FIGURE 18-13. Posterior superior alveolar nerve block. The operator moves the left index finger posteriorly over the buccal surface of the maxillary molars until the zygomatic process of the maxilla is reached.

Technique. For a block on the right side, the operator places the left forefinger on the buccal surface of the maxillary molars parallel to the occlusal plane. The finger is moved posteriorly until the zygomatic process of the maxilla is reached (Fig. 18-13). At this point, the finger is rotated (Fig. 18-14). The index finger is now pointing in the exact direction the needle is to follow. The mouth should be opened only partially, because excessive opening may cause the coronoid process of the mandible to impinge upon the target area and/or impair visualization. A 4-cm, 25-gauge needle is inserted into the mucosa slightly posterior to the zygomatic arch, at a 45-degree angle to all three planes of orientation. The insertion is made for a distance of 1.5 to 2 cm, going upward, inward, and behind the tuberosity.

To avoid hematoma caused by unintentional trauma to the pterygoid venous plexus, the needle should be kept in contact with the posterior surface of the maxilla throughout the injection. Hematoma caused by a rent in an artery in this area will be rapidly manifest as swelling to the side of the face. Venous hematomas will develop more slowly. Either may produce swelling of surprising proportion. Cold compresses should be applied immediately if a hematoma is detected.

The patient should not experience subjective signs of anesthesia, such as numbness or tingling, following this injection.

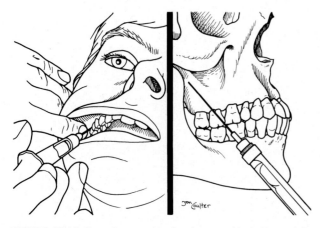

FIGURE 18-14. Posterior superior alveolar nerve block. Rotated finger points to path of needle insertion.

Adequacy of the nerve block must be ascertained prior to surgery by careful probing of the involved area.

Maxillary Nerve Block

Intraoral high tuberosity and greater palatine canal approaches and extraoral approach. The entire second division of the trigeminal nerve producing total anesthesia of the hemimaxilla may be accomplished by two intraoral approaches or an extraoral approach. The high tuberosity approach closely mimics the posterior superior alveolar nerve block, except that the needle is slightly bent to bypass the maxillary tuberosity. The needle is inserted to a depth of 30 mm, and an entire cartridge of local anesthesia is injected. The greater palatine canal approach to the maxillary nerve relies on first identifying the greater palatine foramen, which is located at the level of the maxillary molar near the junction of the maxillary alveolar process and the hard palate. After ensuring topical anesthesia, either by direct pressure over the foramen or the use of topical agents, the needle is carefully and slowly advanced up the canal with the bevel directed downward. When the canal has been traversed to a depth of 30 mm after aspiration, the cartridge of local anesthetic solution is injected. Any resistance encountered should not be overcome with force, but the needle should be withdrawn and again advanced slowly. If continued resistance is met, regardless of how slight, the attempt should be discontinued.

The *extraoral* approach to the maxillary nerve can be achieved via a lateral approach. The needle enters the skin at the point of intersection of the lower border of the zygoma and the anterior border of the mandibular ramus through the coronoid notch. For blockade of the maxillary nerve, the needle is directed slightly upward, forward, and medially until it meets the greater wing of the sphenoid. The local anesthetic is then slowly injected.

Nasopalatine Nerve Block. Anesthesia of the nasopalatine nerve will provide palatal hard and soft tissue anesthesia bilaterally from the bicuspids forward and can also supplement anesthesia of the nasal passages. The procedure for anesthetizing the nasopalatine nerve is relatively simple, but because of the inelastic nature of the palatal tissue in this area, it can be painful if the injection is not performed slowly.

Technique. A 2.5-cm, 25-gauge needle is inserted into the incisive papilla just behind the maxillary central incisors (Fig. 18-15). The needle need not be introduced directly into the nasopalatine canal for successful anesthesia. Because the soft tissue (particularly submucosal connective tissue) is sparse in this area, only a drop or two of solution can be injected. Care must be taken to avoid injecting too large a quantity of solution, to avoid postinjection pain and tissue slough.

Greater (Anterior) Palatine Nerve Block. The greater palatine nerve innervates the posterior portion of the hard palate medially to the midline and anteriorly as far as the first premolar.

Technique. The greater palatine nerve enters the palate via the greater palatine foramen and courses forward in a groove parallel to the molar teeth. The foramen is usually located between the second and third maxillary molars, about 1 cm from the teeth, at the junction of the maxillary alveolar processes and palatine bone.

The foramen is approached from the opposite side with a 2.5-cm, 25-gauge needle that is kept as near to a right angle as possible to the curvature of the palatal bone (Fig. 18-16). A

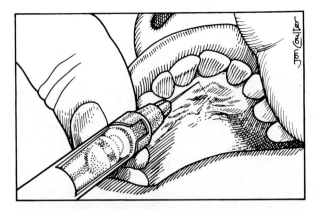

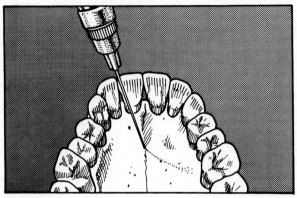

FIGURE 18-15. Naso palative nerve block. Needle is inserted into the incisive papilla behind the maxillary central incisors.

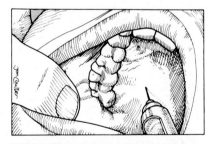

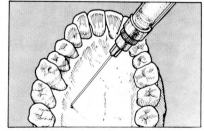

FIGURE 18-16. Block of anterior palatine nerve. Needle is inserted from the opposite side, keeping it as near to a right angle as possible with the curvature of the palate.

volume of 0.25 to 0.5 mL is injected. For satisfactory palatal anesthesia, the greater palatine foramen and canal need not be entered.

Techniques of Neural Blockade for the Mandibular Nerve and Its Subdivisions

Anatomy of the Mandibular Division (V3)

The mandibular division of the trigeminal nerve is both sensory and motor. The motor division does not emerge from the Gasserian ganglion, but joins the sensory branch after it leaves the anteroinferior part of the gasserian ganglion. For a short distance, they travel side by side, then form a single trunk to exit the skull through the foramen ovale. From this trunk, a motor branch passes to the internal pterygoid and two tensor muscles. The trunk then divides into anterior and posterior divisions.

The branches of the anterior division and associated areas of innervation are:

- External pterygoid nerve: Motor
- Masseter nerve: Motor
- Temporal muscle nerve: Motor
- Long buccal nerve: Sensory

The long buccal nerve passes between the two heads of the pterygoid muscle, crosses the anterior border of the ramus at the level of the occlusal plane of the teeth, and supplies the skin and mucous membranes of the cheek and buccal gingiva, from the retromolar triangle to the bicuspid teeth.

The branches of the posterior division and associated areas of innervation are:

- Auriculotemporal nerve: Sensory to the parotid gland, temporomandibular joint, external auditory meatus, and scalp in the temporal region
- Lingual nerve: Sensory to the lingual mucous membranes, anterior two-thirds of the tongue, and floor of the mouth. (The chorda tympani nerve from the seventh cranial nerve joins the lingual nerve shortly after its origin and supplies fibers of special sense to taste buds of the anterior two-thirds of the tongue.)
- Inferior alveolar nerve: Sensory to the mandibular teeth, body of the mandible, and labial gingiva anterior to the bicuspid teeth. This nerve passes downward on the medial side of the external pterygoid muscle and the medial side of the mandibular ramus. On the medial side of the ramus, in the pterygomandibular space, it enters the mandibular foramen. It then travels anteriorly within the body of the mandible. In the region of the mental foramen, the inferior alveolar nerve divides into two terminal branches:
  - Mental nerve: Exits the body of the mandible through the mental foramen and is sensory to the skin of the chin and lower lip and mucous membrane lining the lower lip.
  - Incisive nerve: Continues anteriorly within the body of the mandible to supply anterior teeth and their supporting hard tissues.

It may be necessary to block one or more of the nerves or nerve branches for successful mandibular anesthesia (Table 18-5). Three intraoral approaches to the inferior alveolar nerve are possible: the standard, Halstead, or classic; the closed mouth; and the Gow-Gates.

TABLE 18-5
REGIONAL ANALGESIA OF THE MANDIBLE

Nerves anesthetized	Areas anesthetized
Inferior alveolar nerve	Mandibular teeth; surrounding hard and soft tissues unilaterally to the midline (does not innervate buccal soft tissue in the molar area)
Lingual nerve	Mucosa of floor of mouth, anterior 2/3 of tongue; lingual gingiva
Long buccal nerve	Mucosa of cheek; buccal mucosa and mucoperiosteum of molar region
Mental nerve	Buccal gingiva; mucoperiosteum from bicuspids to midline; skin of chin and lower lip (does not innervate teeth)
Incisive nerve	First bicuspid, canine, incisor unilaterally to the midline; areas innervated by the mental nerve

Intraoral Techniques

Classic Inferior Alveolar Nerve Block (Standard or Halstead Approach). This commonly used nerve block provides anesthesia for the hemimandible from the mandibular teeth to the midline, the body of the mandible and inferior portion of the ramus, buccal mucoperiosteum, and mucous membrane from the bicuspid teeth to the midline, anterior two-third of the tongue and floor of the mouth, and lingual soft tissues. The large distribution of anesthesia is due to the fact that, in addition to blockade of the inferior alveolar nerve, which is a branch of the posterior division of the mandibular nerve, the incisive, mental, and often, the lingual nerves are also anesthetized with this single injection. Occasionally, it may be necessary to perform a separate lingual nerve block. For anesthesia of the buccal soft tissues and periosteum adjacent to the second and third molars, an additional buccal nerve block is necessary.

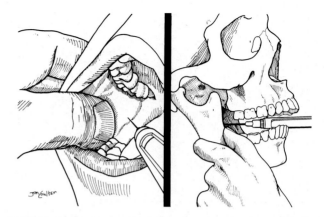

FIGURE 18-18. Inferior alveolar nerve block. The ramus is grasped between an intraorally placed thumb and an extraorally positioned index finger.

Technique. The patient is instructed to open the mouth as widely as possible. For a block on the right side, the operator palpates the mucobuccal fold in the area of the molar teeth with the left thumb. The thumb is moved posteriorly until contact is made with the external oblique ridge on the anterior border of the ramus of the mandible. The deepest concavity on the anterior border of the ramus, the coronoid notch, is then identified. The apex of the coronoid notch is in a direct line with the lingula, the point at which the inferior alveolar nerve enters the ramus of the mandible (Fig. 18-17).

The palpating thumb is then moved medially onto the internal oblique ridge, the inner "edge" of the ramus. This maneuver helps estimate the width of the ramus. The thumb is once again moved to the lateral side of the ramus, retracting soft tissues of the cheek while doing so. At this point, the left index finger grasps the posterior border of the mandible from the extraoral approach (Fig. 18-18). In this manner, the operator is holding the ramus of the mandible between the thumb and index

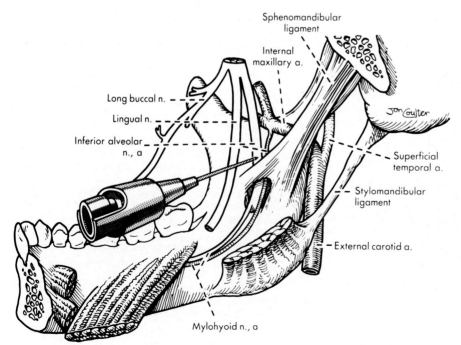

FIGURE 18-17. Inferior alveolar nerve block. Coronoid notch is in a direct line with the point at which the inferior alveolar nerve enters the ramus of the mandible.

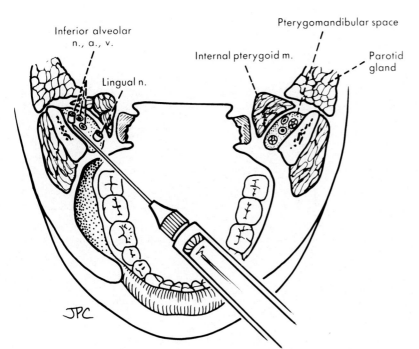

FIGURE 18-19. Inferior alveolar nerve block. Needle is inserted parallel to the medial surface of the ramus.

finger, thus allowing the operator to estimate the anteroposterior width of the ramus.

After application of a topical anesthetic, a 4-cm, 25-gauge needle is inserted parallel to the occlusal plane, lateral to the pterygomandibular raphe, at a height indicated by the coronoid notch just medial to the internal oblique ridge. The needle should approach the ramus at an angle that is parallel to the inner surface of the ramus from the contralateral side (Fig. 18-19). Depth of insertion may be determined by estimating when the needle tip has been advanced half the distance between the thumb and index finger. For proper position for deposition of solution, the needle tip will be close to the inferior alveolar nerve, artery, and vein. Bony contact should occur at a depth of 20 to 25 mm. If bone is not contacted at this depth or is contacted much earlier, then the needles should be withdrawn and redirected. The target area for this block is slightly above the lingula, where the inferior alveolar nerve enters the body of the ramus. After careful aspiration, about two-thirds of a dental cartridge is injected and the needle withdrawn about half of its inserted depth; the remainder of the cartridge is injected to anesthetize the lingual nerve.

Closed-mouth (Vazirani-Akinosi) Approach to Mandibular Nerve Block. In clinical situations in which limited mouth opening is encountered, the closed-mouth technique may be a reasonable alternative to the standard alveolar approach. Since the height of needle insertion and deposition of anesthetic solution is considerably superior to the target area for the standard inferior alveolar nerve block, more of the mandibular nerves (inferior alveolar, incisive, mental, lingual, and mylohyoid nerves) may be anesthetized with this single injection (11).

Technique. With the teeth in occlusion, the lips are retracted and the needle and syringe are aligned parallel to the occlusal plane at the level of the mucogingival junction of the maxillary molar teeth. The needle penetrates mucosa (Fig. 18-20) just medial to the ramus and is inserted to a depth of about 30 mm.

Following negative aspiration, the entire contents of the cartridge is slowly deposited.

Since this technique relies on few bony landmarks, determining the depth of needle insertion is difficult. In addition, improper angulation in a superior direction may result in partial or complete anesthesia of the maxilla, particularly if improper medial angulation occurs simultaneously. The needle must be inserted parallel to the medial surface of the ramus or the target zone will not be accessed.

The Gow-Gates Block. The Gow-Gates approach is a unique technique for mandibular nerve anesthesia using both intra- and extraoral landmarks and is the closest intraoral approach to a true mandibular block anesthetizing the inferior alveolar, mental, incisive, lingual, mylohyoid, auriculotemporal, and often the buccal nerve. The target area is on the lateral side of the neck of the mandibular condyle (see Fig. 21-2).

Technique. The extraoral landmarks for this block are established by visualizing a line drawn from the corner of the widely

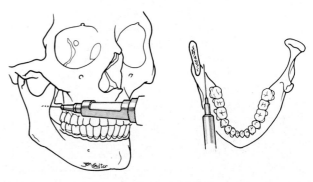

FIGURE 18-20. Inferior alveolar nerve block. With the teeth in occlusion, the needle is aligned parallel to the occlusal plane and positioned at the level just superior to the maxillary molars.

opened mouth to the intertragic notch. The intraoral height of injection is accomplished by the placement of the needle tip below the mesiolingual cusp of the second maxillary molar, with penetration of the mucosa just distal to the maxillary second molar. The needle is advanced until bone is contacted, typically at a depth of approximately 25 mm. After negative aspiration, a full dental cartridge is slowly injected. Once again, bone must be contacted prior to injection (see Fig. 21-2).

Extraoral Approach. For the extraoral approach to the mandibular nerve, as with the extraoral approach to the maxillary nerve, the needle enters the skin at the point of intersection of the lower border of the zygoma and the anterior border of the mandibular ramus through the coronoid notch. After the needle contacts the lateral pterygoid plate, it is withdrawn and reinserted upward and slightly posterior until a paresthesia is noted or the needle has reached a depth of 5 cm (Fig. 17-6).

Long Buccal Nerve Block. To provide anesthesia of the soft tissue buccal to mandibular posterior molars, the long buccal nerve block is often performed to supplement the inferior alveolar and lingual nerve blocks. The long buccal nerve branches from the mandibular nerve at a point superior to the site for an inferior alveolar nerve block (Fig. 18-17).

Technique. The coronoid notch and external oblique ridge are identified. The cheek is retracted and the needle inserted through the soft tissue at the height of the occlusal plane. The needle is directed to the external oblique ridge and inserted until bony contact is made (Fig. 18-21) (9,11); 0.25 to 0.5 mL of solution is sufficient to anesthetize the long buccal nerve.

Mental Nerve Block. The mental nerve exits the body of the mandible through the mental foramen located between the bicuspid teeth, near their apices. A block of this nerve provides soft tissue anesthesia of the chin, lower lip, and its underlying mucosa and gingiva.

Technique. A syringe with 2.5-cm needle attached is inserted through the mucosa and directed to a point approximating the apices of the bicuspid teeth (Fig. 18-22); 0.5 to 1 mL of solution is deposited (see also Fig. 17-3).

Incisive Nerve Block. The incisive nerve is the continuation of the inferior alveolar nerve within the anterior body of the

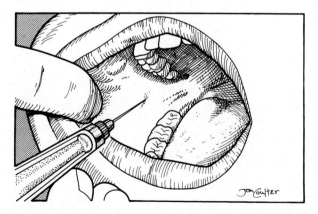

FIGURE 18-21. Long buccal nerve block. The needle is inserted through the mucosa and directed toward the external oblique line at the level of the occlusal plane.

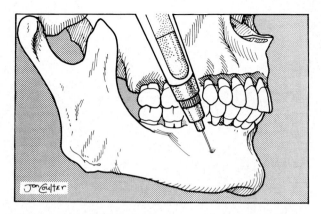

FIGURE 18-22. To block the incisive nerve, direct the needle into the mental foramen and canal. The mental nerve will be blocked simultaneously.

mandible. It innervates the anterior mandibular teeth and their supporting hard tissues.

Technique. Access to the incisive nerve is gained through the mental foramen and canal. The mental foramen and canal are located, and its downward, forward direction ascertained and gently probed by the needle tip. The needle must be directed into the canal at an angle parallel to its long axis.

After deposition of 0.25 to 0.5 mL of solution, anesthesia of the lower anterior teeth and their supporting structures will be produced. Because the mental nerve will be simultaneously anesthetized, anesthesia of the chin and lower lip will ensue.

ANCILLARY TECHNIQUES

Electronic Dental Anesthesia

Transcutaneous electrical nerve stimulation (TENS) has been used successfully since the early 1970s for the management of chronic pain syndromes and acute postsurgical pain. Similar technology has been applied in dentistry to control the pain of intraoral instrumentation without use of local anesthetics. Transcutaneous electrical nerve stimulation may be an alternative mode of anesthesia in patients with needle phobias, and in those patients for whom local anesthetics or vasoconstrictors might be contraindicated, due to cardiac disease, intolerance, or allergy. Additional uses may be in the relief of muscle trismus or in the management of temporomandibular joint pain.

Two basic devices have been studied for electronic dental anesthesia: the classic high-current (100 to 150 mA), low-frequency (55 to 150 Hz) TENS unit with an H-wave generator, and a low-current (4 mA), high-frequency (15,000 Hz) device (12).

Technique

A TENS unit with either extraoral or intraoral electrodes may be used. Extraoral electrodes should be placed bilaterally on the affected jaw, over the infraorbital foramina in the maxilla, and over the mental foramina in the mandible. Intraoral electrodes consisting of conducting filaments embedded in cotton rolls are placed in the mucobuccal fold, directly adjacent to the affected teeth. The unit is activated and the wave amplitude is set to a level predetermined by the manufacturer. The frequency is slowly increased until mild muscle contractions occur. Instrumentation or manipulation may begin at this point.

Electronic dental anesthesia has been claimed to provide clinically successful anesthesia in 80% to 90% of patients undergoing restorative dentistry (13). However, the success rate decreases with the depth of restoration, for crown preparations, tooth extractions, or for molar teeth. It is not reliable for endodontic therapy. The efficacy of electronic dental anesthesia can be increased by the addition of nitrous oxide and aspirin-like drugs (14,15). In order for electronic dental anesthesia to gain more widespread acceptance, further research is needed to determine the optimum frequency of stimulation and waveform. Attempts are under way to improve the quality and adherent properties of intraoral electrodes. This local anesthetic technique still has not been embraced by the majority of dentists.

COMPLICATIONS OF NEURAL BLOCKADE AND REASONS FOR FAILURE

Local Complications

Paresthesia

One of the most devastating localized complications following any intraoral injection is the occurrence of a *paresthesia* in any of the trigeminal nerve distributions. It may result from direct mechanical needle trauma to the nerve; hemorrhage, either extraneural or intraneural; edema, either extraneural or intraneural; contaminated anesthetic; or from chemical neurotoxicity of the local anesthetic drug itself or adjuvants in the local anesthetic cartridge. Although relatively uncommon, paresthesia most likely is associated with blocks of the inferior alveolar nerve and result in lingual nerve paresthesia. The altered sensation is usually transient and usually resolves spontaneously within days, weeks, or months. In rare instances, the damage can, however, be permanent.

Muscle Trismus

Muscles trismus can also be a sequelae of mandibular blocks. Limitation of muscular function after an intraoral injection may be caused by hematoma formation, direct muscle injury secondary to needle trauma, localized muscle necrosis secondary to the anesthetic drug or vasoconstrictor, infection in a fascial space, or the introduction of a foreign body. The treatment of intraoral trismus may include nonsteroidal anti-inflammatory agents, saline mouth rinses, antibiotics, and physical therapy.

Hematoma

Bleeding complications are the result of direct needle trauma to a blood vessel, and most likely to occur following a posterior superior alveolar nerve block, and after greater palatine canal and high tuberosity approaches to the maxillary nerve. Signs and symptoms of hematoma include rapid swelling, a sensation of fullness in the area, facial asymmetry, and mild trismus. Management of a hematoma includes reassurance for the patient and application of ice to the affected area on the day of injury, followed in 24 hours by application of heat. When indicated, posttreatment antibiotics may also be necessary.

Mucosal Irritation

Local irritation may be produced by a number of different causes. For example, topical anesthetics, when applied to the mucosa for extended periods, may compromise the capillary integrity of the underlying tissue and produce irritation. The injection of excessive volumes of local anesthetics with vasoconstrictors under pressure into tightly attached tissue may produce localized tissue ischemia and ulceration. The tissue overlying the hard palate is most frequently damaged in this manner. High-pressure injection techniques, such as the periodontal ligament injection, have been reported to produce irritation and even necrosis of the interdental papilla, with exposure of the underlying bone. Self-inflicted injuries, such as cheek-, lip-, and tongue-biting, are common causes of mucosal irritation following local anesthesia in children and occasionally in adults.

Infection

Although infection is an extremely rare complication of local anesthesia, it may result from injection into or through an infected area, the use of the same cartridge or needle in more than one patient, and multiple uses of the same needle in the same patient. Preparing the injection site with an antiseptic agent prior to injection may reduce the amount of bacteria at the site, but it is inconclusive as to whether this action prevents infection from intraoral needle injections.

Needle Breakage

Needle breakage is a an uncommon complication during intraoral anesthetic techniques. The advent of the single-use, disposable needles coupled with high-quality manufacturing techniques have minimized this problem. However, unexpected patient movement, excessive lateral force by the operator, manufacturing defects, intentional repeated bending of the needle, and use of higher-gauge needles have been implicated in needle breakage. Needles are most susceptible to breakage at the hub and therefore should never be inserted to this distance, as the needle will not be easily retrieved and will require surgical consultation.

Clinical Anesthesia Difficulties

Accidental blockade of other nerves other than those expected may result from local anesthetic administration. This may result from misdirection of the needle, or from an extensive pattern of anesthetic distribution or anatomic considerations. For example, injection into the parotid capsule will result in anesthesia of the facial nerve and will cause a transient hemifacial paralysis, whereas anesthesia of the recurrent laryngeal nerve will cause hoarseness and difficulty with speech.

Failure to Achieve Anesthesia

With an understanding of the anatomic foundations of clinical techniques, the use of properly sized needles, and the correct choice of a local anesthetic agent, the success rate for neural blockade of the dentition and soft tissue of the oral cavity is very high. The most common cause of a failed injection is improper identification of appropriate anatomic landmarks or a patient exhibiting anatomic variations. Inappropriate needle selection may also contribute to failure. For example, a needle that is too long or too short, coupled with uncertainty about the required depth of penetration, will lead to failure and may lead to breakage. In addition, the selection of a thin needle for certain injections may result in deflection away from the intended path of insertion as it passes through mucosa, muscle, and soft tissue. For this reason, a 25-gauge needle is preferable to a 27- or 30-gauge needle for intraoral injections, and this size needle also results in less false-negatives during aspiration.

Occasionally, patients may experience some subjective signs of anesthesia but may not be able to withstand instrumentation without pain. This may be due in part to injection of an inadequate volume of anesthetic solution or not waiting long enough for the action of the local anesthetic to penetrate the neural sheath. Increasing the volume of injected solution will often remedy this problem.

Cross-innervation from the contralateral side, especially in procedures in and around the midline or from other less common neural elements, must always be considered. In the mandible, variant branches of the inferior alveolar nerve may leave the nerve before it enters the mandibular foramen. These branches are not blocked by the conventional inferior alveolar nerve block. A more superiorly oriented injection may be necessary for success in a case such as this. The mylohyoid nerve, which supplies sensory and motor function to the mylohyoid muscle and anterior belly of the digastric, may enter the mandible on the lingual side via a foramen in the bicuspid region. This occurs in about 10% of patients and may provide sensory innervation to the incisor teeth. Again, an apparently successful inferior alveolar block will not affect this nerve; however, a higher injection or lingual infiltration may result in success.

Finally, when the just-mentioned causes for failed anesthesia have been ruled out, the possibility of alternative innervation should be considered. Variant nerves may exist that supply structures not usually associated with them. This can occur in patients with an extremely high palate and long alveolar process. The nasopalatine nerve may exchange fibers with the anterior superior alveolar nerve and contribute to the innervation of the incisor teeth. The long buccal nerve, although a branch of the third division of the trigeminal nerve, may innervate the buccal soft tissue in the maxillary molar area.

Occasionally, the pharyngeal plexus of nerves, which normally supply the pharynx, may supply impacted mandibular third molars. Very rarely, the cutaneous coli nerve, a branch of the cervical plexus, may enter the mandible on the inner surface of the lingual cortical plate and provide accessory innervation to the mandibular teeth.

Another possible causes for failed local anesthesia is the presence of tissue inflammation. Most significantly, inflammation lowers the tissue pH and creates an acidic environment in which the anesthetic solution must work. Lowered tissue pH significantly reduces the ability of local anesthetic drugs to block nervous tissue and may render them ineffective. Injecting through areas of active inflammation is to be avoided, and blocks more proximal to the lesion are advised.

SUMMARY

The performance of neural blockade for the majority of hard and soft tissue dental procedures are the hallmark of clinical dental care. Topical and infiltrative blockade of specific terminal nerve techniques have been described. The safety, efficacy, and patient acceptance of these intra- and extraoral techniques are extremely high and continue to be refined. The introduction of newer local anesthetic agents gives the practitioner choice as to duration and presence, type and quantity of vasoconstrictors.

References

1. Quarnstrom FC, Milgrom P. Clinical experience with TENS and TENS combined with nitrous oxide-oxygen. Report of 371 patients. *Anesth Prog* 1989;36(2):66–69.
2. van Steenberghe D, Bercy P, De Boever J, et al. Patient evaluation of a novel non-injectable anesthetic gel: A multicenter crossover study comparing the gel to infiltration anesthesia during scaling and root planing. *J Periodontol* 2004;75(11):1471–1478.
3. Bennett CR. *Conscious-sedation in Dental Practice*, 2nd ed. St. Louis: Mosby, 1978.
4. Kajander KC. Evaluation of low-intensity transcutaneous electrical nerve stimulation in combination with aspirin for reduction of controlled thermal sensation. *Anesth Prog* 1988;35(5):195–198.
5. American Dental Association. 2002 Survey of Dental Practice—Characteristics of Dentists in Private Practice & Their Patients. Chicago: American Dental Association; 2002.
6. Malamed SF, Gagnon S, Leblanc D. Efficacy of articaine: A new amide local anesthetic. *J Am Dent Assoc* 2000;131(5):635–642.
7. Haas DA, Lennon D. A 21-year retrospective study of reports of paresthesia following local anesthetic administration. *J Can Dent Assoc* 1995;61(4):319–330.
8. Cryer PE. Physiology and pathophysiology of the human sympathoadrenal neuroendocrine system. *N Engl J Med* 1980;303(8):436–444.
9. Monheim LM, Bennett CR. *Monheim's Local Anesthesia and Pain Control in Dental Practice*, 7th ed. St. Louis: Mosby, 1984.
10. Cioffi GA, Chernow B, Glahn RP, et al. The hemodynamic and plasma catecholamine responses to routine restorative dental care. *J Am Dent Assoc* 1985;111(1):67–70.
11. Akinosi JO. A new approach to the mandibular nerve block. *Br J Oral Surg* 1977;15(1):83–87.
12. Cooke-Waite Laboratories. Marcaine Package Insert, 1985.
13. Malamed SF. *Handbook of Medical Emergencies in the Dental Office*, 6th ed. St. Louis: Mosby, 2007.
14. Dionne RA, Goldstein DS, Wirdzek PR. Effects of diazepam premedication and epinephrine-containing local anesthetic on cardiovascular and plasma catecholamine responses to oral surgery. *Anesth Analg* 1984;63(7):640–646.
15. Quarnstrom F. Electronic dental anesthesia. *Anesth Prog* 1992;39(4–5):162–177.

CHAPTER 19 ■ NEURAL BLOCKADE OF THE EYE

KATHRYN E. MCGOLDRICK AND MARIANNE E. FEITL

Orbital injection of local anesthetic was first performed in 1884, with cocaine, for enucleation of the globe (1). However, it was not until the 1930s, when the less toxic procaine and, later, the amide anesthetics became available, that orbital block was commonly used for ophthalmic surgery. Atkinson's 1936 paper (2) popularized a technique that became firmly entrenched as the traditional retrobulbar block. Over the next five decades, anesthesiologists and ophthalmologists reported serious complications of retrobulbar blockade that were vision-threatening or life-threatening. Attempts to circumvent these complications led to the development in the mid-1980s of peribulbar block. However, peribulbar block is also associated with serious adverse sequelae. Advances in cataract surgery have enabled faster surgery with greater control and less trauma and allowed ophthalmologists to reexamine the use of topical anesthesia for this procedure, obviating, in many cases, the need for injection techniques.

Clearly, the requirements and complications of local anesthesia for intraocular and specialized extraocular surgical procedures are unique. A thorough understanding of the mechanism of neural blockade in ophthalmologic surgery is inextricably linked to detailed knowledge of the relevant anatomy. This chapter outlines the anatomy and techniques germane to the successful administration of local anesthesia for ophthalmic surgery. Moreover, in-depth discussion is presented of associated potential complications and their prevention.

TOPICAL ANESTHESIA

Agents and Complications

Topical anesthesia frequently is used to eliminate corneal and conjunctival reflexes, in order to obtain ocular measurements. In addition, these agents are used for removal of superficial foreign bodies, suture removal, and irrigation of the lacrimal system. Cocaine is frequently administered during dacryocystorhinostomy to provide analgesia, vasoconstriction, and shrinkage of the nasal mucous membranes.

Although many agents that cause surface analgesia are available for topical use (Table 19-1), the most widely used agents are proparacaine and tetracaine. All agents have a rapid onset of action, within 30 to 60 seconds, and a duration of action from 10 to 20 minutes.

Ocular or serious systemic reactions to topical anesthetic agents are almost nonexistent, with the exception of cocaine. Cocaine penetrates the eye, where it blocks the reuptake of catecholamines at the nerve terminal and has a sympathetic potentiating effect. Pupillary dilation occurs.

Although 1 g of cocaine is considered to be the usual lethal dose for an adult, considerable variation occurs. The usual maximum dose of cocaine employed in clinical practice is 200 mg for a 70-kg adult, or 3 mg/kg. However, systemic reactions may occur with as little as 20 mg. Meticulous attention must be paid to the volume and concentration used because a narrow range spans safety to toxicity to death. Meyers (3) described two cases of cocaine toxicity during dacryocystorhinostomy, emphasizing that cocaine is contraindicated in hypertensive patients or in patients receiving adrenergic-modifying drugs such as guanethidine, tricyclic antidepressants, or monoamine oxidase inhibitors. Additionally, sympathomimetics, such as epinephrine hydrochloride or phenylephrine hydrochloride, should not be administered with cocaine.

Signs of cocaine toxicity can be evident in the respiratory, cardiovascular, and central nervous systems (CNS). Cocaine's effect on the CNS is biphasic: Initial stimulation is followed by depression as inhibitory synapses are stimulated (4). The patient rapidly becomes excited, anxious, garrulous, and confused. Initially, reflexes are augmented. Headache is common. The pulse becomes rapid, and hypertension develops. Respiration becomes erratic. A chill may herald the sudden onset of hyperthermia. The pupils become dilated, and exophthalmos occurs. Nausea, vomiting, and abdominal pain are common. The patient may complain of something crawling on his or her skin. Delirium, Cheyne-Stokes breathing, convulsions, and, finally, unconsciousness ensues. Indeed, death may be very rapid following acute cocaine overdosage, and resuscitative maneuvers must be initiated quickly.

Before administering cocaine, the physician should thoroughly evaluate for possible contraindications, including the use of concurrent medications. To avoid toxic levels, dosages of dilute solutions should be calculated meticulously and administered carefully. Intravenous (IV) labetalol may be administered to treat serious cardiovascular complications (5). Initially, propranolol had been used to control cocaine-induced hypertension (6). However, a lethal hypertensive exacerbation has been ascribed to unopposed α-adrenergic stimulation (7). Thus, labetalol offers the advantage of both α- and β-blockade. To combat the CNS symptoms of cocaine toxicity, IV barbiturates should be given. Cooling measures may be required to treat hyperthermia, including a cooling blanket and ice water or alcohol sponging. In the event of cardiopulmonary arrest, the usual resuscitative measures must be attempted.

All of the topical agents can be toxic to the corneal epithelium with frequent repeated administrations and may delay the healing of corneal epithelial defects by inhibiting cell division

TOPICAL OPHTHALMOLOGIC ANESTHETIC AGENTS

Agent	Concentration %
Proparacaine HCl (Ophthaine, Ophthetic)	0.5
Tetracaine HCl (Pontocaine)	0.5
Benoxinate (Dorsacaine)	0.4
Dibucaine HCl (Nupercaine)	0.1
Phenacaine HCl (Holocaine, Tanicaine)	1.0
Piperocaine HCl (Metycaine)	2.0 solution
	4.0 ointment
Cocaine	1.0–4.0

and migration (8). Therefore, topical anesthetics should be used for surgery or diagnostic tests and not for repeated symptomatic relief. Cocaine has the added disadvantage of causing loosening of the epithelium, which can result in large corneal erosions. Thus, cocaine has been replaced in many clinics by one of the alternatives shown in Table 19-1.

Topical Anesthesia for Cataract Surgery

Recent refinements in cataract surgery have been extremely impressive and have enabled the use of topical analgesia for these procedures. During the last few decades, the transition from intracapsular surgery to planned extracapsular and then phacoemulsification has enabled surgeons to have greater control of the intraocular environment. Small incisions, scleral tunnel incisions, sutureless wounds, and now clear corneal incisions have minimized surgical trauma and accelerated healing and visual recovery. Moreover, the implantation of intraocular lenses through small incisions became possible with the development of continuous circular capsulorrhexis and foldable implants.

Although Tomas Morena y Maiz of Peru first suggested the medical use of cocaine as a topical anesthetic in 1868, it was in 1884 that Koller and Freud in Vienna first instilled cocaine into the conjunctival sac for local ophthalmic analgesia. Then, in 1910, Julius Hirschberg reported on his extensive, favorable experience administering 2% cocaine chloride for topical anesthesia in cataract surgery (9). The advances in cataract surgery previously mentioned have allowed ophthalmologists to reexamine the use of topical anesthesia for this procedure. Phacoemulsification, with its small incisions, is the procedure of choice in using topical anesthesia. Although planned extracapsular procedures may be performed under topical anesthesia alone, it is frequently advisable to supplement with 1 to 2 mL of subconjunctival 1% lidocaine superiorly. If surgery is prolonged, topical analgesia may need to be supplemented with sub-Tenon's lidocaine. This may be administered via a cannula for greater safety.

Topical anesthesia circumvents potential complications of peribulbar or retrobulbar block that can result in blindness or death. It also allows the patient to see well almost immediately after the surgery. Potential disadvantages of topical anesthesia include eye movement during surgery, patient anxiety, and (rarely) allergic reactions. Immediate allergic reactions are manifested by hyperemia, stinging, itching, and chemosis of the conjunctiva. Delayed hypersensitivity can occur as well. Proparacaine and especially cocaine have the greatest toxicity to the epithelium. Tetracaine, although less toxic, purportedly does not produce adequate deep anesthesia. Lidocaine has minimal epithelial toxicity and produces satisfactory deep analgesia of sufficient duration (8).

Patient selection is critical and should be restricted to individuals who are alert, able to follow instructions, and can control their eye movements. Patients who are demented, photophobic, or are unable to communicate are inappropriate candidates. Similarly, patients with small pupils, which may require significant iris manipulation, those requiring large scleral incisions, or those with an inflamed eye may be contraindicated for topical anesthesia.

In 1992, Charles Williamson developed a technique using topical 4% lidocaine for phacoemulsification surgery through a stepped clear corneal wound. Williamson described his technique, beginning with the instillation of two drops of 0.5% tetracaine into the operative eye prior to the application of dilating drops (10). (Tetracaine prevents the stinging associated with mydriatics.) Then, before the patient is brought to the operating room, two sets of topical 4% lidocaine, four drops every 5 to 10 minutes, are administered. After the patient is positioned on the operating room table, four more drops of topical 4% lidocaine are instilled. A well-dilated pupil is necessary to provide adequate visualization of the lens and to prevent the need for excessive iris manipulation. Orbital decompression devices are not used because they are uncomfortable and unnecessary; there is no solution in the orbit to cause external pressure. Minimal, if any, sedation is given because it is crucial that the patient be able to cooperate with the surgeon's instructions. Some analgesic supplementation, however, is often required because topical application of local anesthetic in this setting does not provide the dense and profound analgesia associated with retrobulbar blockade (11,12). Moreover, supplementation of topical anesthesia with preservative free intraocular lidocaine may help to improve the comfort of both the patient and surgeon during cataract surgery using topical analgesia. After preoperative instillation of topical local anesthetic, preservative-free 1% lidocaine (0.3 mL) is injected into the anterior chamber after a corneal stab incision is performed. Viscoelastic is then instilled to fill the anterior chamber, and the remainder of the surgery is conducted using the standard technique.

LOCAL ANESTHETICS AND ADJUVANTS FOR OPHTHALMOLOGIC NEURAL BLOCKADE

Agents injected for regional anesthesia in ophthalmic surgery (Table 19-2) are the same as those used in other peripheral nerve blocks (see Chapter 4). Lidocaine was traditionally the commonly used agent. In the last two decades, however, there has been a tendency to use local anesthetics of longer duration, such as bupivacaine, that reduce the need for postoperative analgesics and minimize eye movements immediately after surgery. These agents can be used alone or in combination with lidocaine, to take advantage of the rapid onset of lidocaine and the long duration of bupivacaine. In addition, the longer-duration agents can provide adequate anesthesia for the more lengthy and complex procedures such as combined vitrectomy and retinal reattachment surgery.

Epinephrine frequently is added to the injection solution for ophthalmologic neural blockade to counteract the vasodilator action of the anesthetic agent and to reduce bleeding. Epinephrine can also serve as a marker of accidental IV

TABLE 19-2

LOCAL ANESTHETIC AGENTS USED IN OPHTHALMOLOGY

Agent	Concentration %	Maximum dose (mg)	Onset of action (min)	Duration of action
Procaine (Novocaine)	1–4	500	6–8	30–45 min
Mepivacaine (Carbocaine)	1–2	400	3–5	90–120 min
Lidocaine (Xylocaine)	1–2	400	4–6	30–60 min
Prilocaine (Citanest)	1–2	600	3–5	60–90 min
Bupivacaine (Marcaine)	0.25–0.75	175	3–5	4–12 h

injection and to facilitate augmentation and longer duration of action of lidocaine, mepivacaine, or bupivacaine. Dilute concentrations of 1:200,000 (1 mg/200 mL) should be used to avoid tissue injury secondary to ischemia. The use in the orbit of premixed anesthetic solutions with epinephrine is discouraged, because of their high concentration of metabisulfite, an allergenic and neurotoxic substance. Rather, the addition of 0.1 mL of 1:1,000 epinephrine at time of use to 20 mL ampules or vials, or 0.15 mL of 1:1,000 to 30 mL vials, to produce 1:200,000 solutions is recommended. Importantly, retrobulbar epinephrine may reduce blood flow to the optic nerve and is best avoided in patients with glaucomatous optic nerve damage.

The enzyme hyaluronidase is often added to the anesthetic solution to enhance solution diffusion through the tissues; this action is accomplished by hydrolysis of extracellular hyaluronic acid. For ophthalmic solutions, 7.5 to 15 turbidity-reducing units (TRU) per mL are used. The addition of hyaluronidase allows a more complete, reliable block with the use of less anesthetic solution, and thus less tissue distortion. Additionally, improved dispersal of the anesthetic agent may reduce the incidence of myotoxicity and subsequent postoperative diplopia.

The myotoxic effects of local anesthetics on muscle fibers of humans and animals have been well-established (13–15). Rainin and Carlson (16) reported three cases of permanent and one case of temporary vertical muscle paresis after injection of 0.75% bupivacaine directly into the extraocular muscles of four patients. Subsequently, Carlson and associates (17) showed that only 1 mL of 0.75% bupivacaine, 2% lidocaine, or 2% mepivacaine, injected retrobulbarly into rhesus monkeys, led to damage of the extraocular muscles closest to the site of injection, usually the inferior recti and oblique muscles. The same substances injected into human extraocular muscles caused massive lesions, which often occupied the bulk of the cross-section of the muscle. Within such lesions, all of the muscle fibers were uniformly destroyed (17). Lidocaine appears preferentially to destroy white fibers, whereas bupivacaine is more toxic to red fibers. However, at higher concentrations of local anesthetics, this specificity is abolished, and all striated muscle is injured. Interestingly, other tissues such as smooth muscle, neurons, and connective tissue are unaffected by the same concentration of local anesthetic.

Clearly, intramuscular injection of local anesthetics above a threshold concentration (18) causes myonecrosis with loss of myotubules. Damaged fibers become hyalinized and are invaded by macrophages. However, cell nuclei appear to be spared. Regeneration (16,19) can begin after several days and is often complete in 6 weeks if the microcirculation of the nerve and muscle is intact. In addition to being concentration-dependent, myotoxicity is also dependent on the volume of

muscle into which the local anesthetic is injected and on limited epimysial or perimysial spread. Because damage is more likely to be irreversible if the blood supply to the muscle is damaged, injection into the extraocular muscles in the area of the hilum should be assiduously avoided. Early recognition of myotoxicity and selective patching of the eye during regeneration are important.

Ptosis following cataract surgery is not uncommon, and multiple factors have been implicated in its etiology (20,21). These include the presence of a preexisting ptosis, injection of anesthetic solution into the upper lid when performing facial nerve block, retrobulbar injection, injection of peribulbar anesthesia through the upper eyelid at the 12-o'clock position, ocular compression or massage, the eyelid speculum, placement of a superior rectus bridle suture with traction on the superior rectus-levator complex, creation of a large conjunctival flap, prolonged or tight patching in the postoperative period, and postoperative eyelid edema. Direct intramuscular injection of local anesthetics may also account for many cases of transient and permanent ptosis (16). A recent magnetic resonance imaging (MRI) study performed immediately after the diagnosis of diplopia in four patients who received peribulbar blockade disclosed inflammatory edema of the paralyzed extraocular muscle consistent with direct local anesthetic–induced myotoxicity after presumed inadvertent intramuscular injection (22).

Feibel and colleagues (20) believe that the development of postcataract ptosis is multifaceted and that no single aspect of cataract surgery is the sole contributor. That the local anesthetic injection cannot be isolated as a primary factor is underscored by the observation that postsurgical ptosis is seen in patients undergoing surgery with general anesthesia.

ANATOMY OF THE ORBIT AND THE EYE

A thorough knowledge of the anatomy of the orbit and eye (23), especially of the innervation of the orbital structures, is essential to obtain effective neural blockade. Anatomy related to specific anesthetic blocks is detailed under the description of the regional block.

Orbit

The bony orbit has the shape of a pear with the stem directed toward the optic canal (Fig. 19-1). The orbit is covered by the outer periosteal layer of the dura mater (periorbita). The orbit contains the muscles, nerves, and vessels that enable the eye to function properly. A number of blood vessels and nerves

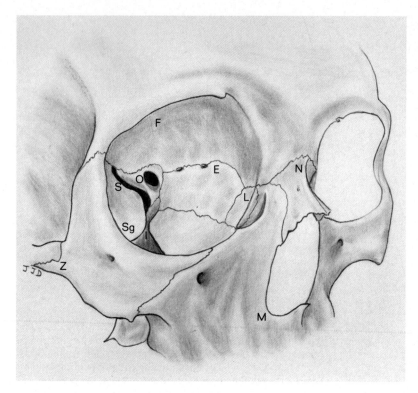

FIGURE 19-1. Bony orbit showing the medial wall and floor. N, nasal bone; M, maxilla; L, lacrimal bone; E, ethmoid bone; F, frontal bone; O, optic foramen; S, superior orbital fissure; Sg, orbit plate of greater wing of sphenoid; I, inferior orbital fissure; Z, zygomatic bone. From Krupin T, Waltman SR, eds. *Complications in Ophthalmic Surgery*. Philadelphia: JB Lippincott, 1984, with permission.

supplying areas of the face around the orbital aperture pass through the orbit. Important surrounding anatomic structures include the anterior cranial fossa above, the maxillary sinus below, and the nasal cavity and ethmoidal air cells medially. There are nine canals and fissures in the orbit, the most important being the optic foramen, the superior and inferior orbital fissures, and the supraorbital and infraorbital foramina (Fig. 19-2).

Eye

The normal globe is about 24 mm in the anteroposterior diameter. This dimension is increased in myopic (nearsighted) eyes. The eyeball has three concentric layers: an outer fibrous layer (the cornea and sclera), a middle vascular layer (the iris, ciliary body, and choroid), and an inner neural layer (the retina). Intraocular contents are: aqueous humor in the anterior chamber

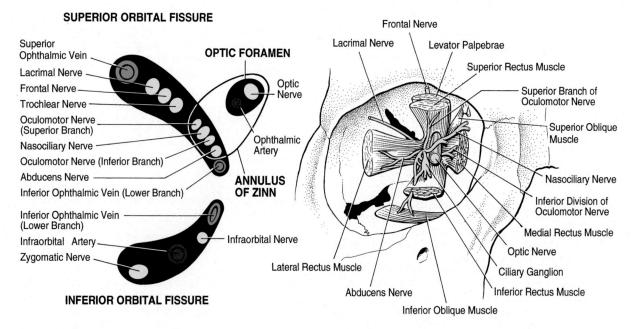

FIGURE 19-2. Bony orbit with the superior and inferior orbital fissures and optic canal at the apex of the muscle cone.

(space lined by the cornea, iris, and pupil) and in the posterior chamber (space behind the iris and in front of the vitreous), the crystalline lens, and the vitreous humor (space behind the lens and in front of the retina).

The optic nerve (cranial nerve II) pierces the globe just above and 3 mm medial to the posterior pole. The nerve has a diameter of 1.5 mm and an intraorbital length of about 30 mm. The nerve exits the orbit by way of the optic foramen. The traditional upward and inward position of the globe during retrobulbar anesthesia (see following) results in stretching, as well as a downward and outward displacement of the optic nerve. This position places the nerve in a vulnerable position for direct traumatization (24,25). Thus, having the patient look in primary gaze should reduce the risk of direct injury.

Six extraocular striated muscles control the movements of the globe. The four rectus muscles (superior, medial, inferior, and lateral) originate from a common tendon ring that encircles the optic foramen (annulus of Zinn) with their tendinous insertion 5.5 to 7.5 mm from the limbus of the cornea. The superior oblique muscle originates above and medial to the optic foramen, runs medially to the trochlea, then bends backward to insert on the globe beneath the superior rectus muscle. The inferior oblique muscle originates medially from the periosteum of the lacrimal bone, runs beneath the inferior rectus muscle, and inserts on the posterolateral aspect of the globe. The seventh striated muscle in the orbit is the levator of the upper eyelid, which originates from the periosteum of the apex of the orbit above the superior oblique muscle. The levator runs forward between the roof of the orbit and superior rectus

muscle and spreads out into an aponeurosis that inserts into the skin and tarsal plate of the upper eyelid. Cranial nerves III, IV, and VI innervate these striated muscles (Table 19-3 and Fig. 19-3A,B).

Innervation of the Eye and Orbital Contents

The sensory supply to the eye and its adnexa is derived from the trigeminal nerve (cranial nerve V). This is a mixed nerve

TABLE 19-3

MOTOR INNERVATION TO OCULAR ADNEXAL MUSCLES

Nerve (cranial nerve)	Muscle innervation
Oculomotor (III)	Superior rectus
	Medial rectus
	Inferior rectus
	Inferior oblique
	Levator palpebrae superioris
Trochlear (IV)	Superior oblique
Abducens (VI)	Lateral rectus
Facial (VII)	
Upper zygomatic branch	Frontalis
	Orbicularis oculi upper lid
Lower zygomatic branch	Orbicularis oculi lower lid

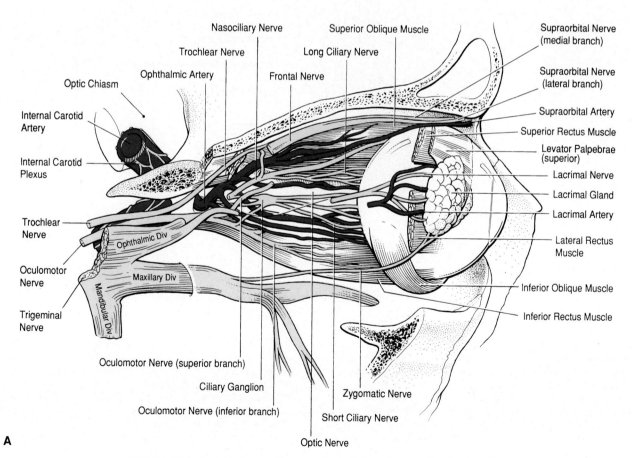

FIGURE 19-3. A: Orbital anatomy as seen from the lateral approach. (*Continued*)

PART II: TECHNIQUES

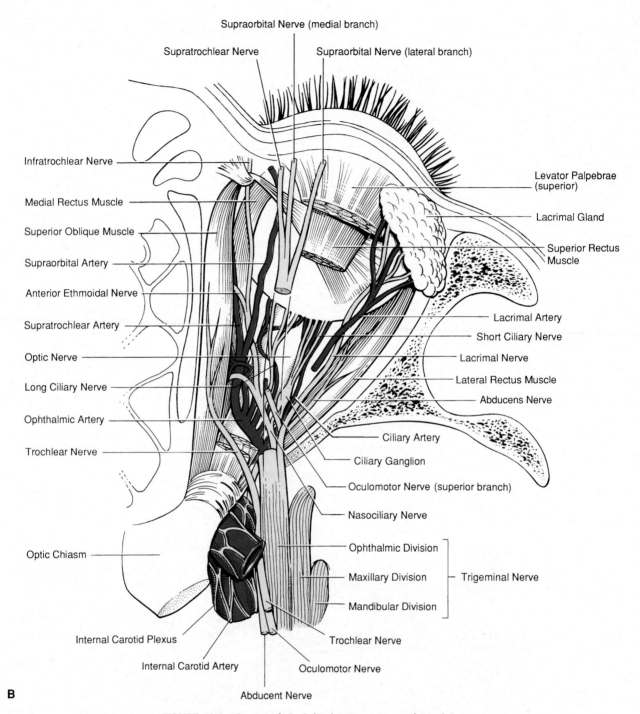

Supraorbital Nerve (medial branch)

Supratrochlear Nerve

Supraorbital Nerve (lateral branch)

Infratrochlear Nerve

Medial Rectus Muscle

Superior Oblique Muscle

Supraorbital Artery

Anterior Ethmoidal Nerve

Supratrochlear Artery

Optic Nerve

Long Ciliary Nerve

Ophthalmic Artery

Trochlear Nerve

Optic Chiasm

Internal Carotid Plexus

Internal Carotid Artery

Levator Palpebrae (superior)

Lacrimal Gland

Superior Rectus Muscle

Lacrimal Artery

Short Ciliary Nerve

Lacrimal Nerve

Lateral Rectus Muscle

Abducens Nerve

Ciliary Artery

Ciliary Ganglion

Oculomotor Nerve (superior branch)

Nasociliary Nerve

Ophthalmic Division

Maxillary Division   Trigeminal Nerve

Mandibular Division

Trochlear Nerve

Oculomotor Nerve

Abducent Nerve

B

FIGURE 19-3. (*Continued*) B: Orbital anatomy as seen from above.

that comprises a large sensory part and a small motor part. The sensory portion of the nerve divides at the trigeminal ganglion into three branches: ophthalmic, maxillary, and mandibular (Table 19-4, Figs. 19-3 and 19-4).

The motor supply to the extraocular muscles and levator palpebrae muscle of the upper eyelid is provided by cranial nerves III, IV, and VI (Table 19-3). The facial nerve (cranial nerve VII) supplies all the muscles of expression, including the orbicularis oculi in the eyelids. The nerve emerges through the stylomastoid foramen, just below the osseous part of the outer ear. The facial nerve then turns forward and enters the parotid gland superficial to the neck of the mandible, where it divides into five branches: temporal, zygomatic, buccal, mandibular, and cervical. The temporal division supplies the upper part of the orbicularis oculi, the corrugator supercilii, and the frontalis muscle. The zygomatic branch supplies the lower part of the orbicularis oculi muscle (Fig. 19-5).

The autonomic nervous system supplies the eye through the sympathetic and parasympathetic systems (Table 19-5, Fig. 19-4).

TABLE 19-4

TRIGEMINAL (V CRANIAL NERVE) SENSORY INNERVATION OF THE EYE AND ADNEXAL STRUCTURES

Trigeminal nerve division	Branch	Sub-branch	Innervation
Ophthalmic	Frontal	Supratrochlear	Skin of lower forehead, skin root of nose, skin and conjunctiva of medial part of upper eyelid
		Supraorbital	Scalp and skin of forehead, skin and conjunctiva of upper eyelid
		Long ciliary	Cornea, iris, ciliary muscle
	Nasociliary	Infratrochlear	Medial upper and lower eyelid, skin and conjunctiva of inner canthus, caruncle, skin root of nose, lacrimal sac
		Long sensory root	Ciliary ganglion (cornea, iris, ciliary body via short ciliary nerves to the ganglion)
		Anterior ethmoid	Tip of nose
	Lacrimal		Outer upper and lower eyelid skin and conjunctiva, lateral canthus, and lacrimal gland
Maxillary	Infraorbital		Entire lower lid, medial and lateral parts of upper and lower lid, lacrimal sac, nasolacrimal duct, upper lip, skin over temple and lateral orbital wall
	Zygomatic		Skin of temporal area and lateral wall of the orbit

PART II: TECHNIQUES

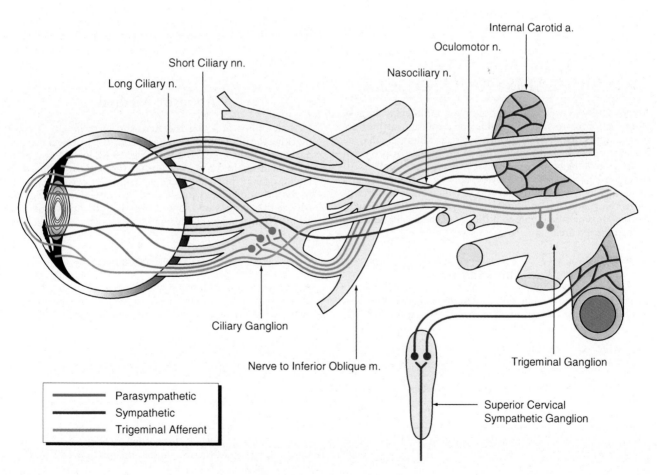

FIGURE 19-4. Innervation of the eye.

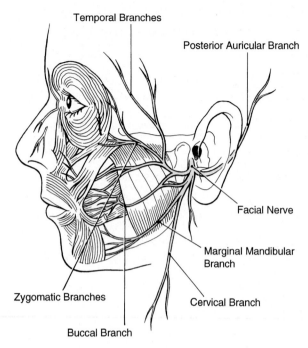

FIGURE 19-5. *Facial nerve* and distribution of its branches.

AKINESIA OF THE ORBICULARIS OCULI MUSCLE

Akinesia of the eyelids is important for intraocular surgery to prevent compression of the lids and expulsion of intraocular contents. Paralysis of the orbicularis oculi muscle may be achieved either by local infiltration of the muscle or proximal infiltration of the branches of the facial nerve that supply it. Although a separate block to provide akinesia of the orbicularis oculi muscle is typically performed in conjunction with *retrobulbar* blockade, this additional maneuver is unnecessary with *peribulbar* blockade owing to diffusion of the local anesthetic to the targeted area.

Van Lint Method

In 1914, van Lint was the first to describe akinesia of the orbicularis oculi for cataract extraction (26). The classic van Lint technique involves inserting the needle at the lateral orbital rim and making a small intradermal wheal. The needle is advanced into the deep tissues along the inferolateral orbital margin. As the needle is withdrawn, 2 to 4 mL of anesthetic is injected. The needle is then redirected along the supertemporal orbital margin. Again, anesthetic is injected as the needle is withdrawn. Pressure is applied to the eye to promote diffusion of the anesthetic. This method has the side effect of producing lid edema. Therefore, the technique has been modified by placing the injections more laterally to block the facial nerve as it crosses the periosteum of the orbital rim, and is followed by inferior and superior injections (Fig. 19-6).

O'Brien Method

In 1927, O'Brien described a facial nerve block over the mandibular condyle, inferior to the posterior zygomatic process (27). The condyle can be palpated as the patient moves his jaw. The needle is inserted approximately 1 cm to the level of the periosteum (Fig. 19-7). Anesthetic solution (2 to 3 mL) is injected as the needle is withdrawn. Because of the variable course of the facial nerve, the block may be incomplete. Hence, the following modifications have been recommended: After injecting over the condyle, partially withdraw the needle and redirect it inferiorly along the posterior edge of the ramus of the mandible. Then, inject the anesthetic solution while withdrawing the needle; reposition the needle anteriorly along the zygomatic arch, and inject the anesthetic while withdrawing the needle.

Atkinson Method

First described in 1953, the Atkinson method (28) involves blocking the branches of the facial nerve to the orbicularis oculi as they cross the zygomatic arch (Fig. 19-8). First, a skin wheal is made at the lower margin of the zygomatic arch below the lateral orbital rim. The needle is then directed superiorly and posteriorly along the zygoma (aimed just lateral to the midpoint between the tragus and lateral orbital rim). Anesthetic (5 to 10 mL) is injected as the needle is withdrawn.

Combined Methods

A number of injection techniques are described that combine the classic with the modified van Lint, O'Brien, and Atkinson methods. Inconsistencies of the resultant facial nerve blockade

---

TABLE 19-5

AUTONOMIC NERVOUS SYSTEM INNERVATION TO THE EYE

System	Source	Nerves	Supply
Sympathetic	Superior cervical ganglion	Long ciliary nerve, (2) short ciliary nerves	Vascular system of choroid, ciliary body, iris (vasoconstrictors); motor impulses to iris dilator muscle
Parasympathetic	Oculomotor nerve (preganglionic fibers) to ciliary ganglion	Short ciliary nerves (postganglionic)	Ciliary body, motor impulse to the iris sphincter muscle and to the ciliary muscle

See also Fig. 19-4.

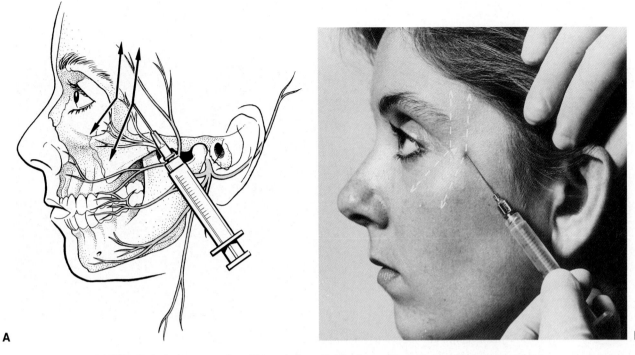

FIGURE 19-6. A: Anatomy of van Lint technique. **B:** Classic van Lint technique blocks the facial nerve at the lateral orbital rim. The modified technique (needle site) places the injection more lateral to avoid lid edema.

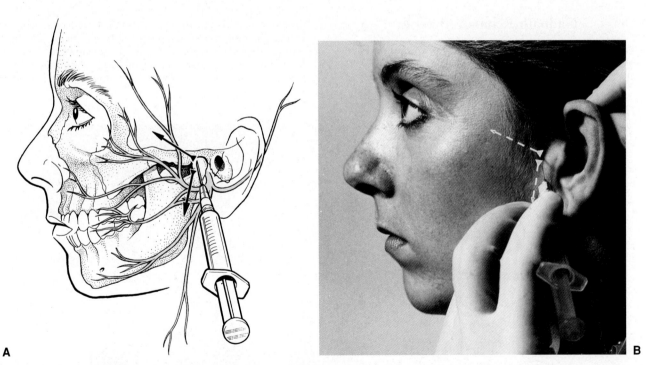

FIGURE 19-7. A: Anatomy of O'Brien technique for facial nerve block. **B:** O'Brien technique for facial nerve block. Injection is performed over the mandibular condyle (tip of the needle). A modified technique (*dotted lines*) adds injections along the posterior edge of the mandible and anteriorly along the zygomatic arch.

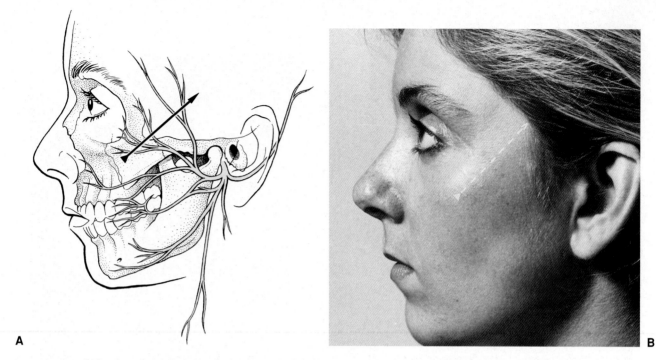

FIGURE 19-8. A: Anatomy of Atkinson method for facial nerve block. **B:** Atkinson method for facial nerve block.

relate to individual variability in the course of the nerve after it enters the parotid gland and subsequently divides into the five facial branches.

Nadbath-Rehman Method

Complete akinesia of the muscles innervated by the facial nerve may be achieved with the Nadbath-Rehman block (29), initially described in 1963. The main trunk of the facial nerve is blocked at the concavity just below the external auditory meatus between the anterosuperior border of the mastoid process and the posterior border of the mandibular ramus (Fig. 19-9). The site can be identified by palpation, and confirmed by having the patient open and close his jaw. A 25-gauge, 12-mm needle is inserted into the skin, and an intradermal wheal is made. The needle is advanced its full length, perpendicularly, into the tissue. The stylet is withdrawn to assure that the needle is not intravascular, and about 3 mL of anesthetic solution is injected as the needle is withdrawn. Gentle massage

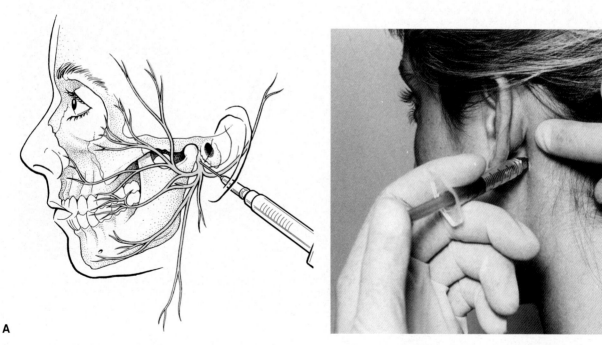

FIGURE 19-9. A: Anatomy of Nadbath-Rehman facial nerve block. **B:** Nadbath-Rehman facial nerve block.

is applied to the injection site to diffuse the anesthetic. This technique produces complete facial nerve akinesia. The major advantage of this technique is the consistent course of the facial nerve from the stylomastoid foramen to the posteromedial surface of the parotid gland, before branching of the nerve. Akinesia of the lower facial musculature also occurs; the patient must be informed of this associated occurrence preoperatively and be reassured that the effect is transient. Patients may also develop sudden dysphagia, hoarseness, respiratory distress, pooling of secretions, or laryngospasm (30,31). Presumably these symptoms result from ipsilateral paralysis of the glossopharyngeal, vagus, and spinal accessory nerves, which exit the skull via the jugular foramen located a mere 10 mm medial to the stylomastoid foramen. Complete facial hemiparesis can be undesirable in the outpatient setting, because family members may misinterpret its effects as a stroke. Moreover, profound facial hemiparesis interferes with liquid and solid intake.

RETROBULBAR BLOCK

Technique

Retrobulbar injection of local anesthetic provides akinesia of the extraocular muscles by blocking cranial nerves III, IV, and VI, and anesthesia of the cornea and uvea by blocking the ciliary nerves. Retrobulbar anesthesia, combined with a separate block to provide akinesia of the orbicularis oculi muscle, permits intraocular surgery under local anesthesia. Topical anesthetic applied to the conjunctiva is helpful in providing total comfort for the patient.

Appropriate patient preparation, including monitoring, sedation, and positioning, is discussed elsewhere in this volume. Traditionally, patients had been instructed to look upward and inward during the retrobulbar injection, in order to place the inferior oblique muscle out of the trajectory of the retrobulbar needle and the patient's gaze away from the needle and the site of puncture. In 1981, however, Unsöld and colleagues (24), using computed tomography (CT) scanning of a cadaver orbit as the retrobulbar needle is inserted, exposed the hazards of the traditional Atkinson position of superonasal gaze during inferotemporal needle placement for retrobulbar block. They discovered that in this position, the optic nerve, ophthalmic artery and its branches, superior orbital vein, and the posterior pole of the globe rotated *into* the path of the retrobulbar needle. The chance of perforating the optic nerve or of piercing the meningeal sheath surrounding the optic nerve, thereby allowing local anesthesia to spread throughout the CNS, is also increased, because the nerve is put on stretch in this position. Hence, the current recommendation is to have the patient look in *primary gaze*, or *inferonasally* (32,33).

Conventional wisdom in ophthalmology had long maintained that the force required to perforate an eye during retrobulbar injection is noticeably greater with a specially designed blunt needle than with a standard hypodermic needle (Fig. 19-10). In 1993, Waller and colleagues (34) measured scleral perforation pressure with specific needle tips in preserved and unpreserved human cadaver eyes. These investigators confirmed that the noncutting edge, blunt-tipped needles do indeed have higher scleral perforation pressures than those with cutting edges (Table 19-6). Conversely, there is, also a possibility that a perforating blunt needle tip does more serious retinal damage than its sharper counterpart (32). Moreover, large caliber (23-gauge) needles require more force to perfo-

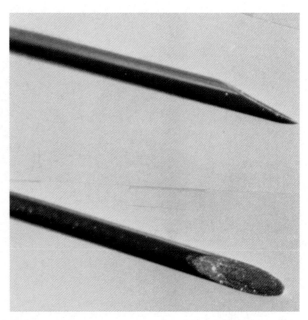

FIGURE 19-10. Frontal and lateral views of the Atkinson needle for retrobulbar injection.

rate the globe than do 25-gauge needles of the same tip design (34). Thus, some clinicians prefer to use fine disposable needles and small-volume syringes to detect subtle changes in resistance (35).

A "painless injection" may be achieved by first instilling local anesthetic eyedrops to afford conjunctival analgesia and then making an injection in the inferotemporal quadrant: The lower eyelid is retracted and a 30-gauge, 12-mm needle is inserted, tangentially to the globe, through the conjunctiva to a depth of 1 cm. The needle will have pierced the capsulopalpebral ligament, and 1 mL of local anesthetic inserted here

TABLE 19-6

SCLERAL PERFORATION PRESSURES

	Scleral perforation pressure (mm Hg) mean ± SD
Preserved Eyes	
30-gauge hypodermic	2 ± 0.5
27-gauge hypodermic	2 ± 0.5
18-gauge hypodermic	3 ± 1.3
23-gauge Atkinson	12 ± 2.6
Fresh Cadaver Eyes	
30-gauge hypodermic	1 ± 1
25-gauge hypodermic	2 ± 1
23-gauge Atkinson	10 ± 1
25-gauge Straus	12 ± 3.8
23-gauge Straus	12 ± 1
23-Gauge Thornton	29 ± 4.5
SD, standard deviation	35 ± 5

Reprinted Waller SG, Taboado J, O'Connor P. Retrobulbar anesthesia risk: Do sharp needles really perforate the eyes more easily than blunt needles? *Ophthalmology* 1993;100:506, with permission.

PART II: TECHNIQUES

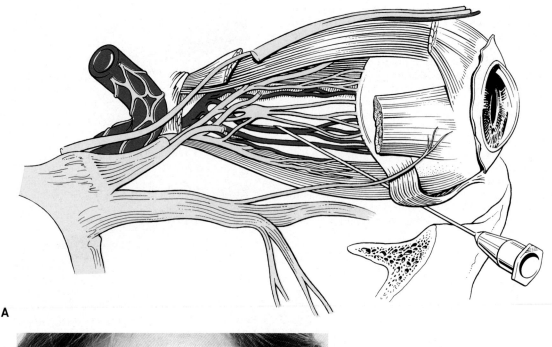

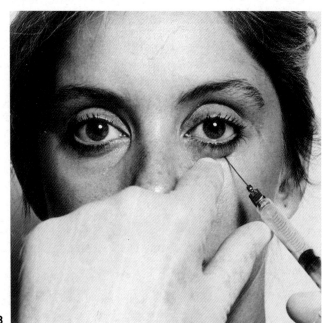

FIGURE 19-11. A: Anatomy of retrobulbar injection. **B:** Retrobulbar injection with the eye in primary gaze. The index finger is palpating the orbital rim. The needle is directed slightly below the apex of the orbit.

will eliminate any pain from subsequent needle insertion for peribulbar or retrobulbar block, using the inferotemporal site of needle insertion. The retrobulbar needle is inserted through the lower lid in the inferotemporal quadrant, at the junction of the lateral and middle thirds of the margin (Fig. 19-11). The needle (no longer than 31 mm [36]) is then directed perpendicular to the skin surface, with the bevel facing the globe to reduce the risk of perforation. After the needle passes the equator of the globe, it should be directed slightly lower than the orbital apex, toward the inferior part of the superior orbital fissure. The syringe should be aspirated before injection to be

certain that the needle is not inside a vessel. Satisfactory retrobulbar block is achieved using injections of 1.5 to 2.0 mL of anesthetic solution into the muscle cone. Many clinicians will inject larger volumes (4.0 to 5.0 mL) and use hyaluronidase to enhance diffusion through the orbit. These larger volumes may produce additional pressure on the globe and chemosis of the conjunctiva. After the injection, firm intermittent digital pressure is applied for about 5 minutes to help distribute the anesthetic and lower intraocular pressure (IOP); some clinicians prefer pressure devices that apply measurable pressure. If complete akinesia and adequate analgesia have not been achieved, it may be necessary to perform a supplemental retrobulbar injection, or a transconjunctival quadrant block, adjacent to the functioning extraocular muscle. The superior oblique muscle, located outside the annulus of Zinn, will not be paralyzed following retrobulbar blockade. Thus, the eye may intort when the patient is instructed to look down.

Although many clinicians perform the retrobulbar injection through the lower eyelid, a transconjunctival approach may be used also. The lower lid is pulled down and the needle inserted through the inferior cul-de-sac. Otherwise, the direction and technique are as described previously.

Complications

Retrobulbar injection is associated with both local and systemic complications (37) (Table 19-7). Perforation of the globe can occur during retrobulbar injection, despite the use of a blunted retrobulbar needle. Published studies from two retinal surgery practices show an approximate incidence of 1 in 1,000 (38,39). More recently, Waller and co-workers (34), in a review of more than 4,000 charts, found no incidence of scleral perforation during retrobulbar or peribulbar injection. Risk factors for globe perforation include an anteroposterior (AP) length of greater than 26 mm by ultrasound, commonly noted in high myopes, severe enophthalmos, previous scleral buckle, repeated surgeries, posterior staphyloma, repeated injections, and an uncooperative patient who moves. The patient typically has intense and immediate ocular pain with sudden loss of vision following perforation of the globe (40). Approximately 50% of the time, the clinician will not recognize unintentional ocular perforation on administering the block, because the scleral perforation pressure may be so low as to be imperceptible, especially with sharp needles. In 30% of cases, the eye may feel hypotonic, possibly owing to loss of vitreous. In 10% of cases, the eye may feel very hard because of elevated IOP, following injection of local anesthetic into the globe. In this case, the scheduled surgical procedure must be postponed and appropriate retinal treatment undertaken.

Retrobulbar Hemorrhage

Retrobulbar hemorrhage is the most common complication, occurring as often as 1% to 3% of the time after retrobulbar injection (41). Vascular or hematologic disease may predispose a patient to develop a retrobulbar hemorrhage. In addition, systemic therapy with aspirin or anticoagulation therapy may be associated with this complication. Many ophthalmologists prefer that patients avoid aspirin for at least 10 days before intraocular surgery, with or without retrobulbar injection. If the patient is taking systemic anticoagulants, his internist should be consulted regarding cessation of, or lowering the dose of, anticoagulation treatment. Discontinuing anticoagulation can have serious medical consequences, including cerebrovascular accident and deep venous thrombosis, and several studies suggest that cataract surgery can be safely performed under regional anesthesia without discontinuing anticoagulants (42–44), especially if the prothrombin time is approximately 1.5 times control (45). A recent multicenter study of almost 20,000 cataract patients older than 50 years of age attempted to establish the risks and benefits of continuing aspirin or Coumadin therapy (46). The investigators found that the rate of complications was so low that absolute differences in risk were minimal. Patients who continued therapy did not have more ocular hemorrhage; those who discontinued treatment did not have a greater incidence of medical events.

Signs and symptoms of retrobulbar hemorrhage include pain, increasing proptosis, and frequently subconjunctival or eyelid ecchymoses. The patient's IOP and central retinal artery pulsations should be monitored carefully by an ophthalmologist for signs of an impending retinal arterial occlusion. Because the oculocardiac reflex may be triggered several hours after the initial retrobulbar hemorrhage, electrocardiographic monitoring of the patient should be performed accordingly. If external pressure on the globe is sufficient to produce compression of the retinal arteries, then a deep lateral canthotomy should be performed to decompress the orbit rapidly. If this does not reestablish normal retinal blood flow, an anterior chamber paracentesis should be done to decompress the globe.

TABLE 19-7

COMPLICATIONS OF RETROBULBAR ANESTHESIA

Complications	Signs and symptoms	Mechanism
Ocular		
Perforation of the globe	Ocular pain, intraocular hemorrhage, restlessness	Direct trauma: myopic eye, posterior staphyloma, repeated injections
Retrobulbar hemorrhage	Subconjunctival or eyelid ecchymosis, increasing proptosis, pain, ± increased IOP	Direct trauma (artery or vein)
Optic nerve damage	Visual loss, optic disc pallor	Direct injury to nerve or blood vessels, vascular occlusion
Systemic		
Intra-arterial injection	Cardiopulmonary arrest, convulsions	Retrograde flow to internal carotid and access to midbrain structures
Optic nerve sheath injection	Agitation, confusion, ptosis, mydriasis, dysphagia, dizziness, confusion, contralateral ophthalmoplegia, respiratory depression or arrest	Subdural or subarachnoid injection
Oculocardiac reflex	Bradycardia, other arrhythmias, asystole	Trigeminal nerve (afferent arc) to floor of fourth ventricle with efferent arc via vagus nerve

Reprinted from Feitl ME, Krupin T. Retrobulbar anesthesia. *Ophthalmol Clin North Am* 1990;3:83, with permission.

Inadequate or delayed treatment of this complication may result in total loss of vision unilaterally. Some retrobulbar hemorrhages may be minimal, even subclinical, and on rare occasions the surgeon may consider continuing surgery. There is, however, significant risk of repeat hemorrhage intraoperatively, with devastating sequelae. Therefore, the recommended course following a recognized retrobulbar hemorrhage is to postpone surgery until all signs of the hemorrhage have resolved. Moreover, it may be prudent to plan general anesthesia for the rescheduled surgery.

Optic atrophy and permanent loss of vision may occur, even in the absence of retrobulbar hemorrhage (47). Postulated mechanisms include direct injury to the nerve, injection into the nerve sheath with subsequent compressive ischemia, and intraneural sheath hemorrhage (47,48). In addition, retinal vascular occlusion has been observed after retrobulbar injection, without evidence of a retrobulbar hemorrhage (47,49). Each of these patients experiencing vascular occlusion without concomitant hemorrhage had a severe hematologic or vascular disorder. Another apparent risk factor is a previous episode. Therefore, it seems prudent to avoid future retrobulbar injection (and perhaps peribulbar injection) in a patient who has developed this rare complication (49).

Systemic Complications

Systemic complications associated with retrobulbar blocks are rare, but potentially fatal. A partial list of these sequelae includes stimulation of the oculocardiac reflex arc, producing associated dysrhythmias, including asystole; intravascular injection of local anesthetic triggering initial CNS excitation (50), which can be followed by obtundation and cardiovascular collapse; and unintentional injection of local anesthetic into the CNS, which can result in respiratory arrest.

Although the amount of local anesthetic administered during retrobulbar blockade is not usually sufficient to produce toxicity if unintentionally injected into a vein, this is not true for inadvertent intra-arterial injection. Indeed, only 1.8 mL of 2% lidocaine unintentionally injected into an artery of the head or neck region can produce profound toxicity (51). These complications include virtually instantaneous seizures secondary to ophthalmic artery injection, with retrograde flow into the cerebral circulation.

From 1980 onward, several reports appeared in the literature documenting serious CNS depression after retrobulbar block. Although an incidence rate of 0.79% was reported in one paper (52), other investigators suggest that the occurrence is more unusual, typically appearing once in 350 to 500 cases (53–55). A continuum of sequelae exists, depending on the amount of drug that gains entrance to the CNS and the specific area to which the drug spreads. Onset of symptoms is variable, ranging from 2 to 40 minutes (56). The protean CNS signs may include violent shivering (57), contralateral amaurosis, eventual loss of consciousness, apnea, and hemiplegia, paraplegia, quadriplegia, or hyperreflexia. Blockade of the eighth to twelfth cranial nerves will result in deafness, vertigo, vagolysis, dysphagia, aphasia, and loss of neck muscle power. Although these signs may be present in various combinations, once it is apparent that the local anesthetic has spread to the CNS, the anesthesiologist must be prepared to provide immediate cardiopulmonary resuscitation. When properly treated, these patients recover quickly and completely. However, delay in diagnosing and treating respiratory arrest, secondary to brainstem anesthesia, can result in death.

Much is now known about prevention of brainstem anesthesia. Attention has focused on ocular position when retrobulbar block is performed, and on the length of the needle selected. The traditional Atkinson position of superonasal gaze places the optic nerve in closer proximity to the advancing needle, where the needle tip can pierce the meningeal sheath surrounding the optic nerve, allowing local anesthesia to spread throughout the CNS. With the globe in primary gaze, or looking inferonasally (58), the optic nerve is less vulnerable. Moreover, avoidance of deep penetration of the orbit is important to prevent this and other serious complications, including perforation of the globe. Even in the absence of penetration of the optic nerve sheath, central spread of local anesthetic from deep orbital injection *may* be a rare possibility (59). Hence, the maximum needle length currently recommended for retrobulbar block is 31 mm (1.25 inches) (33).

PERIBULBAR BLOCK

Technique

Since the late 1980s, peribulbar block has gained increasing popularity. Peribulbar block is considered by many to be easier, safer, and less painful than retrobulbar block, because the muscle cone is not entered (Fig. 19-12), and the need for separate facial nerve block is eliminated because the relatively large volume (8 to 10 mL) of injected local anesthetic usually diffuses into the eyelids. It is important to understand that cadaveric dissections have demonstrated the fallacy of the classic concept of the cone. There is no truly complete intermuscular septum encircling the rectus muscles, linking them together to form an impermeable compartment behind the globe, akin to the brachial plexus sheath in the axilla. Ripart and colleagues (60) recently demonstrated that extraconal injections of dye into cadaveric specimens diffused into the intraconal space, and solutions placed within the cone distributed to the extraconal space.

Davis and Mandel (61) advocated a peribulbar or periconal technique in 1986, and several modifications of their original protocol have since developed. In the most common technique, two injections are required; these are placed inferotemporally and superonasally, just below and medial to the supraorbital notch. There are differing views as to which injection should be made first; the lower lid puncture may be safer (25). A 25-gauge, 1.25-inch needle is used and directed just beyond the equator of the globe. Following careful aspiration, 4 to 5 mL of anesthetic solution is injected in each site. Onset is usually slower than with retrobulbar blockade and may be delayed for as long as 15 to 20 minutes. Zahl and colleagues (62) reported that onset is accelerated by adding sodium bicarbonate to bupivacaine and hyaluronidase. However, others believe that pH adjustment of local anesthetic bottled at pH 6.0 or above to reach 7.4 has minimal effect (63). In an area of rapid blood flow, such as in orbital connective tissue, transcapillary extraction is also facilitated when a concentration of base form predominates.

Ortiz and colleagues (25) confirmed, by a CT scan study, that superior midline and supertemporal puncture may cause perforation of the globe. Thus, these approaches are not used.

One approach is to use a single inferotemporal injection, and to supplement only if needed. Others use inferotemporal *or* superonasal injection first, and then, routinely, supplement with the other.

A further approach is to give a medial injection transconjunctivally, on the medial side of the caruncle, at the extreme medial side of the palpebral fissure. The bevel of the needle

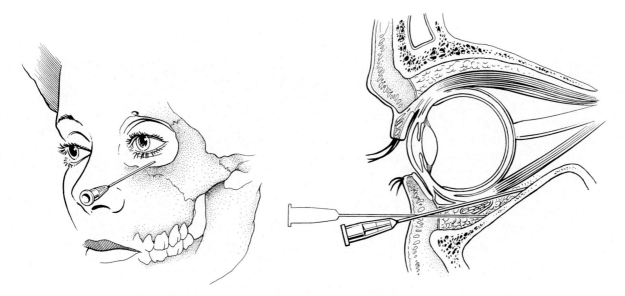

FIGURE 19-12. Peribulbar block. With peribulbar block, the muscle cone is not entered. At both the superonasal injection site, and the inferotemporal site (shown here), anesthetic solution is deposited just past the equator.

faces the medial orbital wall, and the needle passes posteriorly, in the transverse plane, directed at a 5-degree angle away from the sagittal plane and toward the medial orbital wall. It is recommended that a 27-gauge, 20- to 25-mm disposable needle be used, and inserted until the hub reaches the plane of the iris (33).

Some authors recommend the combination of inferotemporal retrobulbar block and complementary peribulbar injection, with the medial caruncle technique favored (35).

Complications

Peribulbar block typically has a higher failure rate than retrobulbar block. Additionally, the larger volume of anesthetic solution deposited in the orbit produces increased forward pressure on the globe, which some surgeons find objectionable. Eyelid ecchymoses occasionally appear. More serious complications have included peribulbar hemorrhage and perforation of the globe.

Feibel and colleagues (20) conducted a randomized, double-blinded study of 317 patients and demonstrated that the incidence of postcataract ptosis is the same in both two-injection peribulbar or retrobulbar anesthesia. However, Esswein and von Noorden (64) retrospectively studied nine patients with a permanent paresis of a vertical rectus muscle after cataract extraction. Peribulbar anesthesia was the most consistent feature in seven of the nine cases, and the authors postulated that permanent paresis of a vertical rectus muscle may be caused by a myotoxic effect of the local anesthetic. As typically performed, the peribulbar needle lies directly under the inferior rectus muscle and directly over the superior rectus muscle. To decrease the incidence of myotoxic complications when performing peribulbar injections, Esswein and von Noorden recommend avoiding the muscle belly (by injecting slightly medially and laterally to a vertical rectus muscle); using the lowest concentration and smallest quantity of local anesthetic needed to obtain analgesia and akinesia; injecting with a short, blunt-tipped needle;

and waiting at least 30 minutes for effect before repeating injections (64).

CRANIAL NERVE BLOCKADE FOR OPHTHALMOLOGIC SURGERY

Frontal Nerve

The frontal nerve, while still within the orbit, divides into the supraorbital and supratrochlear nerves. A sensory frontal nerve block is very useful in adults undergoing frontalis suspensory surgery for ptosis repair. The block retains motility to the upper eyelid and globe, while providing sensory anesthesia to the upper eyelid and eyebrow. A local block can be performed on the frontal nerve within the orbit, or on its two branches near the orbital rim.

Frontal Nerve Block

A rigid 22-gauge, 4-cm needle is passed through the center of the eyelid just below the eyebrow and orbital margin. The needle is directed posteriorly, in a step-like fashion, along the roof of the orbit, until the entire 4-cm length of the needle has been passed (Fig. 19-13). At this location, the frontal and lacrimal nerves enter the orbit. The needle is kept near the roof of the orbit to avoid penetration of the intermuscular septum, which would result in motor anesthesia of the levator and superior rectus muscles, as well as in sensory anesthesia. Not more than 0.5 mL of local anesthetic solution, with epinephrine but without hyaluronidase, is injected. Complications include penetration of the muscle cone and retrobulbar hemorrhage.

Supraorbital Nerve Block

The supraorbital nerve supplies the upper eyelid, upper conjunctiva, upper portion of the lacrimal fossa, upper lacrimal duct, and supraorbital portion of the forehead. The nerve runs

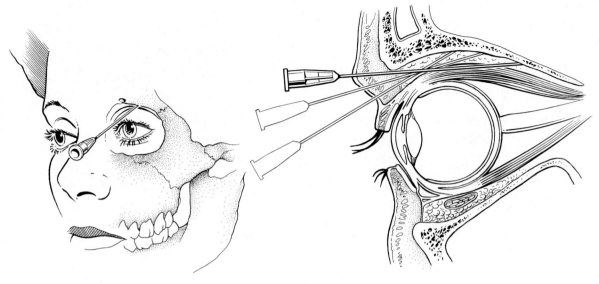

FIGURE 19-13. Frontal nerve block.

from the superior orbital fissure immediately beneath the peri-orbita, along the orbital roof, to emerge from the orbit through the supraorbital foramen or notch. The notch is a separation in the superior orbital rim at the junction of its lateral two-thirds and medial one-third, and is easily palpated. This landmark is on a line with the pupil when the eye is in the primary position. The nerve is blocked by inserting a needle through a skin wheal at the notch and injecting 2 to 3 mL of anesthetic solution (Fig. 19-14). Bleeding can occur from the accompanying supraorbital artery.

Supratrochlear Nerve Block

The supratrochlear nerve supplies the medial part of the upper eyelid, conjunctiva, and forehead. After branching from the frontal nerve, it runs medially to the supraorbital nerve just beneath the periorbita of the orbital roof. The nerve emerges from the orbit between the pulley (trochlea) of the superior

oblique muscles and the supraorbital foramen or notch. The supratrochlear nerve can be blocked by inserting a needle 1 to 1.5 cm along the superomedial wall, just above the trochlea (Fig. 19-15); 1 to 1.5 mL of anesthetic is injected.

Nasociliary Nerve

The nasociliary branch of the ophthalmic nerve divides within the orbit into the anterior and posterior ethmoidal nerves and the infratrochlear nerve. The anterior ethmoidal nerve supplies the lateral wall of the nose in the area of the lacrimal fossa and the skin covering the ala nasi. The infratrochlear nerve runs just beneath the periorbita, along the medial orbital wall, and just above the medial rectus muscle. This nerve innervates the skin of the nose, the skin and the conjunctiva of the inner canthus, and the lacrimal sac. Infiltrative anesthesia of the

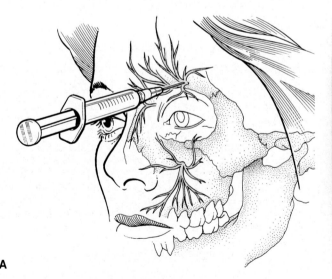

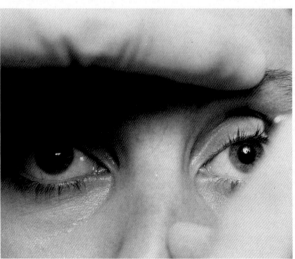

A   B

FIGURE 19-14. A: Anatomy of supraorbital nerve block. B: Supraorbital nerve block. The needle is inserted at the supraorbital notch.

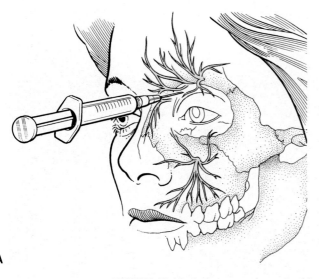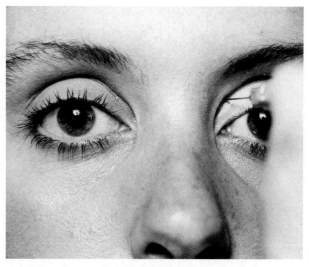

A

B

FIGURE 19-15. A: Anatomy of supratrochlear nerve block. **B:** Supratrochlear nerve block.

infratrochlear and infraorbital nerves is used for surgery on the lacrimal sac (dacryocystorhinostomy).

Infratrochlear Nerve Block

The infratrochlear nerve is blocked by inserting a 25-gauge needle below the trochlea and just above the medial canthal ligament, along the medial orbital wall (Fig. 19-16). The needle is inserted to a depth of 2 to 2.5 cm, and 1.5 to 2.0 mL of anesthetic is injected. Introduction of the needle to a depth of 2.5 to 3.5 cm will also anesthetize the anterior ethmoidal nerve.

Terminal branches of the ophthalmic artery and small tributaries of the superior ophthalmic vein can be encountered during an infratrochlear nerve block. Retrobulbar hemorrhage can occur in approximately 2% of blocks. If the hemorrhage is severe, the operation must be postponed.

Lacrimal Nerve

The lacrimal nerve is located at the superior part of the lateral orbital wall. The nerve supplies the lacrimal gland and the skin and conjunctiva of the lateral part of the upper eyelid. The nerve is anesthetized by introducing a 25-gauge needle through an intradermal wheal in the upper eyelid at the lateral wall of the orbit (Fig. 19-17). The needle is inserted along the lateral wall to a depth of 2.5 cm, and 2 mL of anesthetic solution is injected.

Maxillary Nerve

The maxillary nerve, the second division of the trigeminal nerve, runs through the orbit in the infraorbital groove. The nerve divides into the zygomatic and infraorbital nerves.

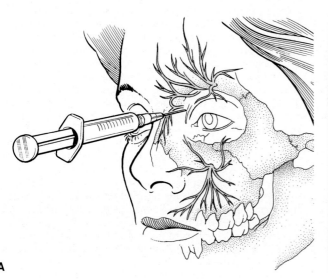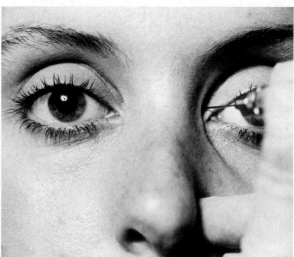

A

B

FIGURE 19-16. A: Anatomy of infratrochlear nerve block. **B:** Infratrochlear nerve block.

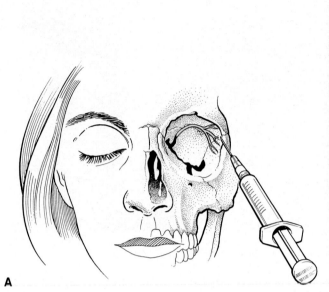
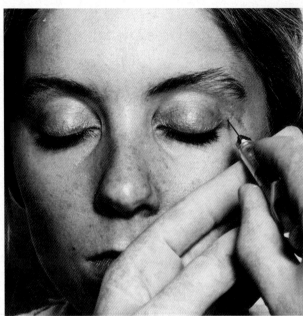

A   B

FIGURE 19-17. **A:** Anatomy of lacrimal nerve block. **B:** Lacrimal nerve block.

Zygomatic Nerve Block

The zygomatic nerve innervates the skin of the temporal area and the lateral wall of the orbit. Zygomaticotemporal and zygomaticofacial branches exit through small foramen in the zygomatic bone at the junction of the lateral and inferior orbital rims. Infiltrative anesthesia at these sites will block these nerves.

Infraorbital Nerve Block

The infraorbital nerve, within its canal, gives off alveolar nerves to the upper teeth, maxillary sinus, and nasal cavity. The infraorbital groove in the central orbital floor is bridged-over at its midportion to continue forward as the infraorbital canal. The nerve emerges on the face from the infraorbital foramen on the maxilla. The foramen is palpable as a small depression 1.5 cm below the inferior orbital rim. The foramen is on a line with the supraorbital notch and pupil. The nerve supplies the lower eyelid and cheek, inner canthus, and part of the lacrimal sac. Infraorbital combined with infratrochlear nerve block are used for dacryocystorhinostomy.

The infraorbital nerve can be blocked where it enters the canal on the orbital floor. A 2-mL injection of anesthetic is given along the floor, 1.0 to 1.5 cm behind the orbital rim. A block can also be done at the infraorbital foramen. The foramen is palpated on the maxilla, 1.5 cm below the orbital rim, on a line with the supraorbital notch and pupil (Fig. 19-18). Anesthetic solution of 1.5 to 2.0 mL is injected at the external opening of the foramen or just within the canal.

SUB-TENON BLOCK

In 1992, Stevens described a technique that delivers a direct infiltration of local anesthetic to the posterior sub-Tenon space via a blunt, curved cannula (65). Satisfactory analgesia and akinesia for cataract and anterior segment surgery is obtained with fewer risks than those associated with the use of sharp-needle injection methods. The conjunctiva is infiltrated with anesthetic, and the sub-Tenon space is opened with a pair of microscissors; then a blunt cannula is inserted and advanced about 1.7 cm, curving round the globe of the eye (Fig. 19-19). Onset of analgesia is rapid. The degree of abolition of extraocular muscle movement is proportional to the volume and depth of injectate.

The anatomic basis of the sub-Tenon block is the fascial plane called the Tenon capsule. The extraocular muscles are connected by a sheet of condensed fascial tissue, and, external to this incomplete intermuscular septum, is a fascial plane—the Tenon capsule. This capsule is a dense fascial layer that surrounds the globe and extraocular muscles from the limbus to the optic nerve. A potential space exists between the sclera of the eye and Tenon capsule. A small incision in conjunctiva 5 mm posterior to the limbus will pass through conjunctiva, the Tenon capsule, and the intermuscular septum. This gains access to the area known as the sub-Tenon space.

One large prospective study by Guise (66) of 6,000 sub-Tenon blocks noted the technique to be highly effective. Advantages, particularly for very myopic patients who have elongated axial lengths, include reduced risk of posterior pole perforation because needles are not placed into the posterior orbit. It is common, however, for local anesthetics to leak retrograde out of the incision site where the cannula is introduced. Conjunctival bleeding (especially if diathermy is not used), chemosis, and ballooning up of the conjunctiva and Tenon capsule are common. Fortunately, these are cosmetic issues that seldom affect outcome. Guise (66) estimated that the incidence of minor hemorrhage is less than 10%. Thus, the sub-Tenon block may be a prudent ocular anesthesia technique for the anticoagulated patient at risk for retrobulbar hemorrhage. A study comparing topical and sub-Tenon anesthesia in routine cataract surgery reported that patients receiving sub-Tenon anesthesia reported less pain than those receiving only topical anesthesia (67). Nonetheless, topical anesthesia was found to be well tolerated by patients.

Major complications of sub-Tenon anesthesia (performed via either episcleral needle or catheter techniques) include

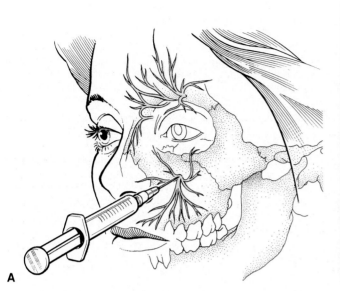
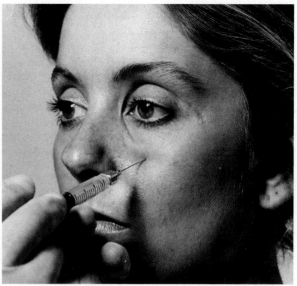

FIGURE 19-18. **A:** Anatomy of infra-orbital nerve block. **B:** Infra-orbital nerve block.

globe perforation (68), major orbital hemorrhage, rectus muscle trauma, postoperative strabismus, orbital cellulitis, and inadvertent brainstem anesthesia (69). A greater proportion of complications seem to be associated with longer (18 to 25 mm), more rigid, metallic cannulae. Shorter (12 mm), more flexible, plastic cannulae may be preferable. However, shorter cannulae are associated with a higher incidence of conjunctival hemorrhage and chemosis. Recently, an ultrashort cannula (6 mm) was introduced.

Technique

Topical local anesthetic (Table 19-1) is applied to the cornea and conjunctiva, followed by one drop of epinephrine 0.1%

(to reduce bleeding). The patient is asked to look outward and upward with the eye to be blocked; this helps with access to the conjunctiva in the inferonasal quadrant, 5 mm from the limbus. At this point, a blunt ophthalmologic (Wescott) scissors is used to make a small nick in the conjunctiva. A blunt Southampton curved cannula is then used to deliver a small bleb of local anesthetic; this helps to elevate the Tenon fascia. Moorfield forceps are used to grip the incised conjunctival edge, and the curved cannula is inserted onto bare sclera. The cannula is then glided along a path following the contour of the globe, until posterior to the equator, at a depth of about 1.7 cm from the limbus. Passage posterior to the equator may be aided by injecting 1 mL of local anesthetic at the level of the equator. An additional 3 to 3.5 mL is slowly injected

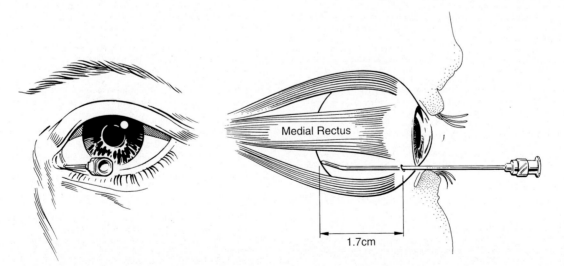

FIGURE 19-19. Sub-Tenon's space block. Blunt Cannula (Southampton) is shown entering the conjunctiva at the inferonasal quadrant, approximately 5 mm from the limbus. An initial nick in the conjunctiva is made to aid cannula insertion. To aid access to the inferonasal conjunctiva, the patient is asked to look upwards and laterally with the eye to be blocked: This also aids passage of the blunt cannula. The final position of the cannula is shown in this figure with the eye in the anatomic position, to facilitate visualization of relationship of cannula to orbit.

posteriorly, depending on the size of the globe. Solution diffuses to cover the nerve supply of the cornea and conjunctiva, with variable cover of the nerve supply of the extraocular muscles. Hyaluronidase may be added to the solution to enhance diffusion. Since there is no true separation of compartments in the orbit, solution may also diffuse into the intracone (retrobulbar) area.

SUMMARY

Surgery to the eye may be achieved with topical anesthesia or discrete neural blockade of orbital structures with retrobulbar, peribulbar and sub-Tenon blockade. Advances in cataract surgery have enabled faster surgery with greater control and less trauma and allowed ophthalmologists to perform addi-

tional procedures under topical anesthesia, thus reducing the overall need for injection techniques. A thorough understanding of the relevant anatomy and the various techniques of ophthalmologic neural blockade is necessary for the successful administration of local anesthesia for surgery to the eye, as well as the prevention and treatment of associated potential complications.

ACKNOWLEDGMENT

The authors wish to acknowledge the valuable assistance of Cheryl Silver, Head of Information Processing and Assistant Director of the New York Medical College Health Sciences Library, in the preparation of this manuscript.

References

1. Knapp H. On cocaine and its use in ophthalmic and general surgery. *Arch Ophthalmol* 1884;13:402–448.
2. Atkinson WS. Retrobulbar injection of anesthetic within the muscle cone. *Arch Ophthalmol* 1936;16:494–503.
3. Meyers EF. Cocaine toxicity during dacryocystorhinostomy. *Arch Ophthalmol* 1980;98:842–843.
4. Schenck NL. Cocaine: Its use and misuse in otolaryngology. *Trans Am Acad Ophthalmol Otolaryngol* 1975;80:343–351.
5. Gay GR, Loper KA. Control of cocaine-induced hypertension with labetalol. *Anesth Analg* 1988;67:92.
6. Rappolt RT, Gray GR, Inaba DS. Propranolol in the treatment of cardiopressor effects of cocaine (letter). *N Engl J Med* 1976;448.
7. Ramoska E, Sacchetti AD. Propranolol-induced hypertension in treatment of cocaine intoxication. *Ann Emerg Med* 1985;14:1112–1113.
8. Marr WG, Wood R, Senterfit L, Sigelman S. Effect of topical anesthetics on regeneration of the corneal epithelium. *Am J Ophthalmol* 1957;43:606–610.
9. Hirschberg J. *History of Ophthalmology.* Amsterdam: Kugler, 1910:234.
10. Williamson CH. Clear corneal incision with topical anesthesia. In: Gills JP, Hustead RF, Sanders DR, eds. *Ophthalmic Anesthesia.* Thorofare, New Jersey: Slack, Inc.; 1993:176.
11. Fung D, Cohen M, Stewart S, et al. What determines patient satisfaction with cataract care under topical local anesthesia and monitored sedation in a community hospital setting? *Anesth Analg* 2005;100:1644–1650.
12. Jonas JB, Pakdaman B, Sauder G, et al. Is intraoperative monitoring necessary in cataract surgery under topical anesthesia? *J Cataract Refract Surg* 2004;30:2645–2646.
13. Libelius R, Sonesson B, Stamenovic BA, et al. Denervation-like changes in skeletal muscle after treatment with a local anesthetic (Marcaine). *J Anat* 1970;106[Pt 2]:297–309.
14. Steer JH, Mastaglia FL, Papadimitriou, et al. Bupivacaine-induced muscle injury: The role of extracellular calcium. *J Neurol Sci* 1986;75:205–217.
15. Foster AH, Carlson MB. Myotoxicity of local anesthetics and regeneration of damaged muscle fibers. *Anesth Analg* 1980;58:727–736.
16. Rainin EA, Carlson BM. Postoperative diplopia and ptosis: A clinical hypothesis based on the myotoxicity of local anesthetics. *Arch Ophthalmol* 1985;103:1337–1339.
17. Carlson BM, Emerich S, Komorowski TE, et al. Extraocular muscle regeneration in primates: Local anesthetic-induced lesions. *Ophthalmology* 1992;99:582–589.
18. Yagiela JA, Benoit PW, Buoncristiani RD, et al. Comparison of myotoxic effects of lidocaine with epinephrine in rats and humans. *Anesth Analg* 1981; 60:471–480.
19. Rao VA, Kawatra VK. Ocular myotoxic effects of local anesthetics. *Can J Ophthalmol* 1988;23:171–173.
20. Feibel RM, Custer PL, Gordon MO. Postcataract ptosis: A randomized, double-masked comparison of peribulbar and retrobulbar anesthesia. *Ophthalmology* 1993;100:660–665.
21. Kaplan LJ, Jaffee NS, Clayman HM. Ptosis and cataract surgery. *Ophthalmology* 1985;92:237–242.
22. Taylor G, Devys JM, Heran F, et al. Early exploration of diplopia with magnetic resonance imaging after peribulbar anaesthesia. *Br J Anaesth* 2004; 92:899–901.
23. Johnson RW. Anatomy for ophthalmic anesthesia. *Br J Anaesth* 1995;75:80–87.
24. Unsöld R, Stanley JA, DeGroot J. The CT-topography of retrobulbar anesthesia: Anatomic-clinical correlation of complications and suggestions of a modified technique. *Albrecht von Graefes Arch Klin Exp Ophthalmol* 1981; 217:125–136.
25. Ortiz M, Vallis R, Vallés J, et al. Topography of peribulbar anesthesia. *Reg Anesth* 1995;20:337–342.
26. van Lint A. Paralysie palpebrale temporaire provoquée par l'opération de la câtaracte. *Ann Ocul (Paris)* 1914;151:420–424.
27. O'Brien CS. Akinesia during cataract extraction. *Arch Ophthalmol* 1929;1: 447–449.
28. Atkinson WS. Akinesia of the orbicularis. *Am J Ophthalmol* 1953;36:1255–1258.
29. Nadbath RP, Rehman I. Facial nerve block. *Am J Ophthalmol* 1963;55:143–146.
30. Wilson CA, Ruiz RS. Respiratory obstruction following the Nadbath facial nerve block. *Arch Ophthalmol* 1985;103:1454–1456.
31. Cofer HF. Cord paralysis after Nadbath facial nerve block (letter). *Arch Ophthalmol* 1986;104:337.
32. Grizzard WS, Kirk NM, Pavan PR, et al. Perforating ocular injuries caused by anesthesia personnel. *Ophthalmology* 1991;98:1011–1016.
33. Katsev DA, Drews RC, Rose BT. An anatomic study of retrobulbar needle path length. *Ophthalmology* 1989;96:1221–1224.
34. Waller SG, Taboada J, O'Connor P. Retrobulbar anesthesia risk: Do sharp needles really perforate the eye more easily than blunt needles? *Ophthalmology* 1993;100:506–510.
35. Hamilton RC. Techniques of orbital regional anaesthesia. *Br J Anaesth* 1995;75:88–92.
36. Petruscak J, Smith RB, Breslin PP. Mortality related to ophthalmological surgery. *Arch Ophthalmol* 1973;89:106–109.
37. Rubin AP. Complications of local anesthesia for ophthalmic surgery. *Br J Anaesth* 1995;75:93–96.
38. Cibis PA. General discussion. In: Schepens CL, Regan CDJ, eds. *Controversial Aspects in the Management of Retinal Detachment.* Boston: Little, Brown;1965:222–233.
39. Ramsay RC, Knobloch WH. Ocular perforation following retrobulbar anesthesia for retinal detachment surgery. *Am J Ophthalmol* 1978;86:61–64.
40. Duker JS, Belmont JB, Benson WE, et al. Inadvertent globe perforation during retrobulbar and peribulbar anesthesia: patient characteristics, surgical management, and visual outcome. *Ophthalmology* 1991;98:519–526.
41. Morgan CM, Schatz H, Vine AKM, et al. Ocular complications associated with retrobulbar injections. *Ophthalmology* 1988;95:660–665.
42. McMahan LB. Anticoagulants and cataract surgery. *J Cataract Refract Surg* 1988;14:569–571.
43. Hall DL, Steen WH Jr., Drummond JW, et al. Anticoagulants and cataract surgery. *Ophthalmic Surg* 1988;19:221–223.
44. Robinson GA, Nylander A. Warfarin and cataract extraction. *Br J Ophthalmol* 1989;73:702–703.
45. Feitl ME, Krupin T. Retrobulbar anesthesia. *Ophthalmol Clin North Am* 1990;3(1):83–91.
46. Katz J, Feldman MA, Bass EB, et al. Risks and benefits of anticoagulant and antiplatelet medication use before cataract surgery. *Ophthalmology* 2003; 110:1784–1788.
47. Klein MI, Jampol LM, Condon PI, et al. Central retinal artery occlusion without retrobulbar hemorrhage after retrobulbar anesthesia. *Am J Ophthalmol* 1982;93:573–577.

48. Sullivan KL, Brown GC, Forman AR, et al. Retrobulbar anesthesia and retinal vascular obstruction. *Ophthalmology* 1983;90:373–377.

49. Cowley M, Campochiaro PA, Newman SA, et al. Retinal vascular occlusion without retrobulbar or optic nerve sheath hemorrhage after retrobulbar injection of lidocaine. *Ophthalmic Surg* 1988;19:859–861.

50. Meyers EF, Ramirez RC, Boniu KI. Grand mal seizures after retrobulbar block. *Arch Ophthalmol* 1978;847–848.

51. Aldrete JA, Roma-Salas F, Arora S, et al. Reverse arterial blood flow as a pathway for central nervous system toxic responses following injection of local anesthetics. *Anesth Analg* 1978;57:428–433.

52. Wittpenn JR, Rapoza P, Sternberg P, et al. Respiratory arrest following retrobulbar anesthesia. *Ophthalmology* 1986;93:867–870.

53. Nicoll JMV, Acharya PA, Ahlen K, et al. Central nervous system complications after 6,000 retrobulbar blocks. *Anesth Analg* 1987;66:1298–1302.

54. Hamilton RC, Gimbel HV, Strunin L. Regional anesthesia for 12,000 cataract extraction and intraocular lens implantation procedures. *Can J Anaesth* 1988;35:615–623.

55. Ahn JC, Stanley JA. Subarachnoid injection as a complication of retrobulbar anesthesia. *Am J Ophthalmol* 1987;103:225–230.

56. Hamilton RC. Brain stem anesthesia as a complication of regional anesthesia for ophthalmic surgery. *Can J Ophthalmol* 1992;27:323–325.

57. Nicoll JMV, Acharya PA, Edge KR, et al. Shivering following retrobulbar block. *Can J Anaesth* 1988;35:671.

58. Liu C, Youl B, Moseley I. Magnetic resonance imaging of the optic nerve in extremes of gaze: Implications for the positioning of the globe for retrobulbar anaesthesia. *Br J Ophthalmol* 1992;76:728–733.

59. Shantha TR. The relationship of retrobulbar local anesthetic spread to the neural membranes of the eyeball, optic nerve, and arachnoid villi in the optic nerve (abstract). *Anesthesiology* 1990;73[Suppl]:A850.

60. Ripart J, Lefrant JY, de la Coussaye JE, et al. Peribulbar versus retrobulbar anesthesia for ophthalmic surgery: An anatomical comparison of extraconal and intraconal injections. *Anesthesiology* 2001;94:56–62.

61. Davis DB, Mandel MR. Posterior peribulbar anesthesia: An alternative to retrobulbar anesthesia. *J Cataract Refract Surg* 1986;12:182–184.

62. Zahl K, Jordan A, McGroarty J, et al. pH-adjusted bupivacaine and hyaluronidase for peribulbar block. *Anesthesiology* 1990;72:230–232.

63. Hustead RF, Hamilton RC. Pharmacology. In: Gills JP, Husteaf RF, Sanders DR, eds. *Ophthalmic Anesthesia*. Thorofare, New Jersey: Slack, Inc.; 1993: 69.

64. Esswein MB, von Noorden GK. Paresis of a vertical rectus muscle after cataract extraction. *Am J Ophthalmol* 1993;116:424–430.

65. Stevens JD. A new local anaesthesia technique for cataract extraction by one quadrant sub-Tenon's infiltration. *Br J Ophthalmol* 1992;76:670–674.

66. Guise PA. Sub-Tenon's anesthesia: A prospective study of 6000 blocks. *Anesthesiology* 2003;98:964–968.

67. Srinivasan S, Fern AT, Selvaraj S, Hasan S. Randomized double-blind clinical trial comparing topical and sub-Tenon's anaesthesia in routine cataract surgery. *Br J Anaesth* 2004;93:683–686.

68. Frieman BJ, Friedberg MA. Globe perforation associated with sub Tenon's anesthesia. *Am J Ophthalmol* 2001;131:520–521.

69. Ruschen H, Bremner FD, Carr C. Complications after sub-Tenon's eye block. *Anesth Analg* 2003;96:273–277.

CHAPTER 20 ■ NEUROLOGIC COMPLICATIONS OF PERIPHERAL NEURAL BLOCKADE

HERVÉ BOUAZIZ AND DAN BENHAMOU

The exponential increase in the utilization of peripheral nerve blocks (PNBs) began in the 1990s. This increase has been more marked (and earlier to occur) in Europe than in the United States (1). In France, a 1996 national survey showed that regional anesthesia was used in more than 20% of surgical procedures, a 14-fold increase in use when compared with data obtained in 1980 (2). Epidural and spinal anesthesia, which are associated with well-defined benefits in several patient populations, gained widespread acceptance during this interval. However, PNBs also were used more often, despite lack of definite and proven benefits. Conversely, the American Society of Anesthesiologists Closed Claims project confirmed the limited utilization of PNB in North America during this same period (3). For example, when claims between 1980 and 1999 were reviewed, PNBs accounted for 13% of all regional anesthesia claims and 21% of nonobstetric regional anesthesia claims. Axillary plexus blocks were used in the majority of cases followed by intravenous (IV) regional blocks and interscalene blocks (44%, 21%, and 19% respectively). Although the number of claims cannot be directly related to the frequency of use of each technique because denominators are not known, these data provide indirect evidence that a major evolution has occurred in the type of blocks used during the last decade.

With increasing utilization, case reports describing major morbidity or even death related to the use of PNB were reported. New technical developments, including stimulating peripheral catheters, ultrasound guidance, and portable infusion devices, were perceived to improve safety. However, safety is difficult to assess in the absence of large series of patients (4), and the real risk associated with these techniques remains unknown. Although most data are reassuring (5), others are less so (6), and the overall incidence of PNB-related severe morbidity and mortality remains unknown.

INCIDENCE OF NEUROLOGIC COMPLICATIONS AND IDENTIFICATION OF ETIOLOGY

Although PNBs have been practiced for years, large series of consecutive cases have only been gathered recently. This is in stark contrast to neuraxial blocks, for which several large series were published more than 50 years ago (7). As previously mentioned, this difference reflects the limited use of peripheral techniques compared to neuraxial blocks. However, with the increasing use of PNB during the last 15 years, investigators have started compiling total case numbers and their associated complications.

Incidence of Complications

Although the information provided by these series is invaluable, several limits should be acknowledged. Most series that have been reported are dominated by groups (or individuals) highly trained in regional anesthesia; intuitively, it may be suspected that complications are less frequently encountered in these practices. However, few data support this hypothesis. In a series of 1,000 consecutive axillary brachial plexus blocks (8) performed over a 12-year period, there was a 0.2% overall incidence of persistent paresthesia that fully recovered within 8 months. The occurrence of these complications did not decrease with increasing experience *in contrast* to the success rate, which increased significantly over the years. Other published reports come from university teaching hospitals and reflect the dynamics of learning, with subtle changes in the incidence of complications (and a likely reduction in the level of risk) over time. Numbers are often low, and conclusions drawn from rare complications should be treated with caution.

From the cases included in the closed-claims study (9), it is apparent that peripheral nerve injury may be associated with either regional or general anesthesia, since factors common to both—such as positioning, preexisting medical conditions, tourniquet use, and surgically induced complications—can be the cause of postoperative neurologic complications (10).

Etiology of Complications

Peripheral nerve techniques, even more than neuraxial blocks, are performed in the context of limb orthopedic surgery, which can itself produce complications. An example is hip replacement, which can lead to sciatic and/or femoral nerve lesion. When surgery is performed with the use of combined femoral and sciatic nerve block, controversy over which technique is at fault may arise when a postoperative neurologic injury occurs (11). Furthermore, neurophysiologic evaluation (electromyography, evoked potentials, nerve conduction studies) may not definitively differentiate the cause of the nerve trauma, as anesthetic and surgical injury are situated in the same site (12). By contrast, if sciatic nerve injury occurs after knee replacement performed under combined sciatic–femoral nerve block, the site at which the nerve has been injured is often easier to recognize (site of needle insertion for regional anesthesia–related injury and level of the peroneal nerve for surgery-related injury). Separating the mechanisms of injury can also be made more difficult in orthopedic surgery because, during limb surgery, tourniquet use may lead to nerve/muscle trauma. In this context of difficult differential diagnosis to separate anesthetic and surgical technique as the cause of nerve injury, it is important to consider the respective incidence of lesions caused by each technique. For example, hip replacement (performed under general anesthesia) is associated with a 0.5% to 2% incidence of sciatic nerve lesion (13), and this high incidence has led several experts to use evoked potentials during surgery to facilitate early detection of nerve trauma (14). Sciatic and/or femoral nerve blocks are associated with nerve injury in one to two of 1,000 anesthetic procedures—an incidence much lower than that for surgery-induced nerve trauma. This comparison should lead one to consider that, in difficult-to-diagnose cases, a surgery-induced lesion should be considered first. A sciatic nerve lesion is more often encountered after revision/reoperation or acetabular reconstruction for dysplasia in females and with an inexperienced surgeon (13,15). When one or several of these risk factors exist, then a surgical etiology is more likely the cause of nerve injury than is the sciatic nerve block. By contrast, femoral nerve lesion can occur but has been very rarely described after hip replacement (16), leaving more uncertainty as to the cause of the injury.

Similar risk ratios of surgery- and anesthesia-related nerve injury can be found in other situations. Lynch and co-workers observed an incidence of severe neurologic injuries of 4.3% after 417 total shoulder arthroplasty procedures (17). Of patients with a neurologic complication, only 17% had an interscalene block. In a study of 693 patients receiving an interscalene block, the incidence, distribution, and resolution of neurologic sequelae were determined using a standardized assessment that was performed repeatedly until the fourth postoperative week (18). In all but one case, symptoms were reported within the first 2 weeks and were only sensory. Neurologic symptoms were noticed in 4.2% of patients during the first month, but all had resolved within 4 to 6 weeks, except one case of brachial plexopathy that resolved in 12 weeks (1.4/1,000). A retrospective study of a total of 1,614 axillary blocks performed on 607 patients also reported that of the 62 nerve injuries, seven (11%) were related to the anesthetic technique whereas the remaining 55 (89%) were a result of the surgical procedure (19). These comparative data again show that surgically induced nerve injuries are generally much more common than those related to PNB.

Even minor surgery may lead to neurologic symptoms, as shown by a study that analyzed the postoperative course of 100 patients who had undergone ambulatory hand surgery after randomized use of either general anesthesia or axillary block using a transarterial technique (20). On postoperative day 1, 60% of patients of either group had paresthesia; the incidence declined to 12% at 1-year follow-up, still with no difference between the two groups. This reports also highlights the role surgery itself can play in obscuring the analysis of postoperative complications due to regional anesthesia.

Duration of Neurologic Dysfunction

An additional difficulty when counting PNB-induced neurologic complications relates to the fact that most lesions observed immediately after surgery resolve rapidly and do not lead to long-term sequelae. Sufficient patient numbers must thus be large enough to separate time-limited and long-lasting complications. Lesions are indeed most often caused by neurapraxia or axonotmesis than by neurotmesis, the prognosis for which is much more severe (12). Axonotmesis results from nerve disruption with endoneurium and other supportive tissue preserved. Complete recovery is expected more or less rapidly for these two lesions. Neurotmesis by contrast, reflects complete disruption of nerve and supporting connective tissue and its prognosis is poor. In contrast, neurapraxia results from a mild degree of injury with impulse conduction failure. Electromyography demonstrates an unaltered pattern combined with decreased conduction and increased latency. Assessment of neurologic complications therefore requires calculating both early and late incidences of events. In a prospective survey, 521 patients scheduled for elective shoulder surgery performed with an interscalene block (6) were assessed at regular intervals, with the final evaluation at 9 months. Although 14% reported some neurologic abnormality unrelated to surgery on the tenth day, only one patient (0.2%) had symptoms remaining at 9 months. The high incidence of early symptoms (i.e., 14%) is only an approximation, as neurologic symptoms evolved as a dynamic condition. Spontaneous resolution was rapid in most patients, leaving an incidence of only 7.9% at 1 month. By contrast, in 0.2% of patients, symptoms became apparent only 2 to 3 weeks after the procedure, depending on the formation of perineural edema, inflammation, and microhematoma (6).

The extreme situation (i.e., high initial incidence of neurologic symptoms and extremely rare late complications) is found with the risk of diaphragm dysfunction after interscalene block. Diaphragmatic paresis is present in 100% of patients in the first hours after the block (21), explaining why this technique is contraindicated in patients with limited respiratory reserve. It was traditionally thought that no long-term sequelae exist. There are, however, a few recent reports describing permanent diaphragmatic paralysis after an apparently uneventful interscalene block (22,23).

In 1997, the first prospective large series of regional anesthetic procedures was reported (24). In this series, 21,278 PNBs were performed by experienced anesthesiologists over a 6-month period. All peripheral blockade–related neurologic complications were present on the second postoperative day. With an incidence of 1.9 per 10,000 cases, peripheral techniques were less likely associated with a neurologic complication than spinal anesthesia (5.9/1,000) and were complicated by neurologic injury at a rate similar to that of epidural anesthesia (2/10,000, NS). The vast majority of these neurologic symptoms had recovered at 3 months. More recently, the same group (25) reiterated their analysis of complications observed after regional anesthesia and surveyed prospectively 50,223 peripheral blocks also performed by highly trained anesthesiologists. Although only 12 patients had a peripheral neuropathy after a peripheral block (2.3/10,000), seven of them had sequelae still present after 6 months. Only serious adverse events were recorded, explaining why the incidences reported were much lower than in smaller series, which reported even mild symptoms (6,18). Patients had their neurologic injury diagnosed through the usual follow-up (usually surgeon-based), and it remains possible that some complications were not reported to anesthesiologists, suggesting that underestimation might exist. This concern may however be unjustified, as shown by a prospective survey of 5,147 patients who had undergone surgery using PNB for anesthesia (26). Patients were evaluated at 24 hours and again at 7 days after surgery. An overall incidence of four per 10,000 neurologic complications was found, consistent with incidences found in previous reports.

TABLE 20-1

COMPARATIVE INCIDENCE OF NEUROLOGIC COMPLICATIONS AFTER CONTINUOUS PERIPHERAL NERVE BLOCK (CPNB) IN PUBLISHED STUDIES

Type of CPNB studied	Number of patients	Incidence, severity and timing of evaluation	Reference
Femoral	$n = 214$	0.5%, partial recovery at 1 year follow-up	111
Interscalene	$n = 700$	Minor = 2.4% at 1 month, 0.3% at 3 months and complete recovery at 6 months	29
		Serious = 0.2%, complete recovery at 19 and 28 weeks follow-up	
Axillary	$n = 405$	0.5%*	28
Mixed	$n = 1,416$	Minor = 0.21%, complete resolution before/at 10 weeks	27
Popliteal	$n = 1,001$	0%	32

*Prognosis of anesthesia-related nerve complications unclear from the article.

Continuous Peripheral Nerve Blocks

In the large series by Auroy and colleagues (25), patients were included in 1998–1999, a time period during which the use of continuous PNBs was still limited. However, several series have evaluated the incidence of neurologic complications following the use of continuous peripheral techniques (Table 20-1). In an important study, 1,416 patients were followed in the postanesthesia care unit and every day for up to 5 days, to examine efficacy and complications related to the use of continuous catheters (27). Twelve patients (0.84%) experienced serious adverse events and three (0.21%) patients had neurologic lesions attributed to the continuous peripheral nerve catheter. All three nerve injuries were seen after a femoral nerve block, perhaps reflecting the fact that this technique was used in half of the surveyed patients. Nerve damage resolved 36 hours to 10 weeks later. A similarly relatively high incidence can be extracted from the report by Bergman and colleagues, who reported a series of 405 axillary catheters (28), two of which were associated with new and anesthesia-related neurologic injury (0.5%). Although the absolute number in these two studies is low, the incidence *may* be ten times greater than after single-injection nerve blocks. These results are refuted by Borgeat and co-workers (6), who reported the incidence of neurologic complications was 30% to 50% less after continuous (compared to single-injection) interscalene block. In both groups, however, a similar pattern of progressive decrease in the number of patients with persistent neurologic symptoms was observed. The same authors noted a similar complication rate in another prospective study that included 700 interscalene catheters (29).

Complications Associated with Selection of Peripheral Technique

It has been suggested that, even more so than the placement of a catheter, the insertion site for interscalene block might be a risk factor for an increased incidence and/or prolonged duration of complications compared to other techniques. For example, no late neurologic complications occurred in a prospective study involving 500 popliteal blocks (263 single-injection and 237 continuous techniques) (30). Likewise, in a large series of 3,396 peripheral blocks, the incidence of postoperative neurologic dysfunction was the lowest after axillary plexus blocks and the largest after interscalene block (4.0%, 2.0%, and 1.0%: interscalene, femoral–sciatic, axillary, respectively) although statistical differences were not significant regarding interscalene block (31). By contrast, Auroy and co-workers

(25) found a greater incidence of neurologic complications following popliteal blocks than after interscalene blocks, whereas Borgeat and colleagues, prospectively studying 1,001 consecutive popliteal blocks, did not record any anomaly at 10 days and again at 3 months' follow-up (32). These data suggest that needle insertion site (specific block) is difficult to associate with a high or low incidence of neurologic complications.

Mechanisms of Neurologic Injury

Neural damage is a possible complication of central and PNB and may significantly impact the quality of life of patients. Injury may be due to ischemic, mechanical, or chemical mechanisms—all of these factors occurring alone or in combination—and may aggravate preexisting nerve lesions (26,33). Trauma may disrupt neural blood vessels or neural barriers, cause extra- or intraneural hematoma or edema, and lead to degenerative changes or discontinuity of fibers. Intrafascicular injection (within the perineurium) (Fig. 20-1) is more likely to be associated with injury than intraneural extraperineural injection (34). Unduly high concentrations or intrafascicular injections of local anesthetics may lead to severe nerve injury. Histopathologic studies have shown that all local

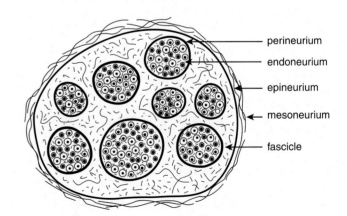

FIGURE 20-1. Cross-section of a peripheral nerve. Reproduced from Bigeleisen PE. Nerve puncture and apparent intraneural injection during ultrasound-guided axillary block does not invariably result in neurologic injury. *Anesthesiology* 2006;105:779–783, with permission.

TABLE 20-2

INTRA- OR EXTRAFASCICULAR INJECTION AS A RISK FACTOR OF NERVE INJURY

	Degree of nerve fiber damage	
Agent	Extrafascicular injection	Intrafascicular injection
Bupivacaine HCl 0.5%	−	+
Mepivacaine HCl 1%	−	+
Lidocaine HCl 1% ± epinephrine	−	++
Lidocaine HCl 2% ± epinephrine	−	++
Bupivacaine HCl 0.5% + epinephrine	−	++
Lidocaine hydrocarbonate 2%	−	+++
Procaine HCl 2%	−	+++
Tetracaine HCl 1%	−	+++

−, no evidence of nerve damage ; +, minimal nerve injury with occasional nerve fiber injury ; ++, moderate nerve injury with focal axonal and myelin damage; +++, severe nerve fiber injury with widespread axonal and myelin degeneration.
Reproduced from Gentili F, Hudson A, Kline DG, Hunter D. Peripheral nerve injection injury: An experimental study. *Neurosurgery* 1979;4:244–253, with permission.

anesthetics induce a concentration-dependent breakdown of the blood–nerve barrier, with concomitant edema and degenerative changes of nerve fibers (35). By contrast, extrafascicular injection results in a low risk, if any, of nerve damage (36) (Table 20-2).

Preexisting Patient Factors

Patients with preexisting peripheral nerve disorders may be at risk of neurologic injury after receiving a PNB, according to the "double-crush" theory described first by Upton and Mc-Comas (37). As postulated by these authors, the presence of a more proximal lesion renders the more distal nerve trunk more vulnerable to compression, with subsequent damage that far exceeds the expected additive injury caused by each isolated insult. Therefore, the performance of PNBs in patients with preexisting peripheral nerve disease may theoretically place them at increased risk of occurrence of a double-crush syndrome. In streptozotocin-diabetic rats, local anesthetic requirement is reduced and the risk of local anesthetic–induced nerve injury is increased during sciatic block (38). Moreover patients with diabetes may be theoretically at greater risk of nerve ischemia after receiving epinephrine due to the underlying microangiopathy. Although, it is not possible to conclude whether or not these patients are at greater risk of developing new or worsening neurologic symptoms after PNB, clinicians should consider lower concentrations of local anesthetic and assess the risks–benefit ratio before adding epinephrine to the anesthetic solution in these patients. In a large retrospective study, a higher success rate after a popliteal sciatic nerve block has been observed in diabetic patients (*n* = 371) versus nondiabetic patients (*n* = 971) (39), suggesting a higher sensitivity of nerve fibers to local anesthetic in diabetic patients. No difference was observed, however, regarding neurologic complications (there were none in either group), in contrast with animal studies discussed earlier (38). Another retrospective study compared patients with preexisting neuropathy who underwent ulnar nerve transposition under regional anesthesia (*n* = 100) or general anesthesia (*n* = 260) and also found a similar incidence (6%) of new or worsening postoperative neuropathy (40). More recently, analysis of a large cohort of 5,147 patients showed that diabetes

mellitus and preexisting peripheral neuropathy were independent risk factors for the occurrence of paresthesia/dysesthesia at 24 hours after a PNB, as well as for prolonged duration of motor and sensory block (26). Furthermore, nerve stimulation does not always provide easy electrolocalization in patients with preexisting nerve disease, even at high current intensity (41,42). It thus seems reasonable to consider the individual risk–benefit ratio when deciding which anesthetic technique should be preferred in a patient with preexisting peripheral nerve disease.

Direct Trauma from the Injection Needle/Catheter

Elicitation of paresthesia may be used intentionally for PNBs and even when other methods are used, unintentional paresthesia may occur in as often as 40% of cases (43). The classic controversy regarding relative safety of elicitation of a paresthesia compared to other methods (mainly nerve stimulation) remains undetermined. Auroy and colleagues reported that all cases of persistent paresthesia after PNBs occurred in the same territory as the associated paresthesia (25). Lee and co-workers, in evaluation of the ASA Closed Claims database, recorded 13 neuropathies associated with a peripheral block (3); a paresthesia occurred before injection in four of these cases and during injection in two additional cases. Candido and colleagues also disclosed that paresthesia at needle insertion was an independent predictor of postoperative interscalene block–related sequelae (18). By contrast, no regional anesthetic technique risk factors, including elicitation of a paresthesia, selection of local anesthetic, or addition of epinephrine, were identified by Horlocker and co-workers; however, similar to Auroy and colleagues (25), the nerve deficit occurred in the distribution of an elicited paresthesia in five of the seven patients (19).

Multiple stimulation techniques (including withdrawal and redirection of the stimulating needle) as well as performance of repeated regional blocks (even within 1 week), which both theoretically may increase the rate of neurologic injury, do not seem to be risk factors for the occurrence of nerve injury (19,31). The deleterious role of paresthesia elicitation is indeed difficult to ascertain even in large series in which paresthesia elicitation is used in every patient, as neurologic complications only occur in a very small percentage of cases.

Interpreting the Role of Paresthesia in Nerve Injury. Elicitation of a paresthesia has been considered to be the surrogate marker of contact between the needle and the nerve. Unfortunately, recent studies demonstrate that the problem is more complex. First, definition of paresthesia is variable among authors, and patients often find it difficult to explain precisely the sensation felt. Second, a recent ultrasound study demonstrated that paresthesia is reported in only 37% of patients, and limb movement is obtained in 78% of patients at the time of direct needle-to-nerve contact (44), suggesting that nerve contact does not necessarily trigger paresthesia. As well, in studies in which paresthesia is the clinical end-point used to perform a brachial plexus block, nerve stimulation does not always produce muscle movement when paresthesia is obtained (45). Paresthesia may also be frequently associated with intraneural injection (observed using ultrasound guidance) but with no postoperative nerve injury, most likely because of extra-perineural injection (46). Likewise, during nerve stimulation at low current intensity (0.2–0.4 mA), patients do not spontaneously report paresthesia, although half of them describe electrical paresthesia on careful questioning (47). Klein and co-workers have recently provided an additional possible explanation as to why elicitation of a paresthesia is not always associated with motor response, and they describe the mechanism of nerve injury that can occur while using a nerve stimulation technique (48). Using a mathematical model of nerve stimulation, it was calculated that an intense stimulation close to the nerve (paresthesia suggesting close proximity) can block propagation. This could explain clinical situations in which the needle is advanced quickly at relatively high current and fails to elicit motor response until gradually withdrawn. In addition, nerve injury might then occur during needle movement with no motor response.

Techniques of Neural Localization. Direct prospective comparisons have also been unable to solve the controversy. In a nonrandomized study, Selander and co-workers enrolled a total of 533 patients—290 in the paresthesia group and 243 in the transarterial group (43). Clinical evidence of nerve damage occurred in 2.8% of the patients in the paresthesia group and in 0.8% in the artery group, the difference being not statistically significant. More recently, a study compared the incidence of complications using electrical stimulation or mechanical paresthesia for nerve localization in 218 patients who underwent interscalene block for shoulder surgery (49). The risk of developing postoperative neurologic symptoms was again comparable between the two methods. It should be stressed, however, that in these clinical studies, statistical power may have been too low to ensure that true differences become significant because of the low rate of complications with either technique, thus maintaining the uncertainty. Nevertheless, it is well documented that the use of a nerve stimulator does not guarantee that such complications will not occur and that nerve injury can occur with either method, even in the hands of experienced anesthesiologists.

Needle Bevel and Design. Bevel design and needle size may also affect the risk of nerve injury. Indeed, it has been found both in vivo and in vitro that a nerve fascicle tends to roll or slide away from an advancing needle point, especially when the needle is short-beveled (45 versus 14 degrees) (50). On the other hand, should a nerve fascicle become impaled, the lesions induced by a short-beveled needle (27 degrees) are more severe and take longer to repair than those induced by a long-beveled

needle (12 degrees); introduction of the needle bevel transverse (compared to parallel) to the nerve fibers further increases the resultant injury (51). Others recommend the use of a tapered injection needle after having shown that this design produced the least damage after nerve puncture (52). Nevertheless, the relatively long distance between the tip of the needle and the side orifice results in local anesthetic solution injection at a site distant from the nerve. To solve this problem, a long-tapered double needle has been developed and compared to the beveled needle (Quincke), short-tapered needle (Whitacre), and long-tapered needle (Sprotte) with encouraging results. However, the ability of different bevels to penetrate the nerve or to push them away in the clinical setting is still not known. It should be noted that, in particular situations, the nerve can be potentially pinned between needle tip and bony structure, such as during block of the ulnar nerve at the elbow and common peroneal nerve at the neck of the fibula (53). Finally, the short-bevel needle may be preferred as it is easier to discern the crossing of fascia, thus enabling the delivery of local anesthetics in the right place.

Intrafascicular Injection. Results of experimental studies clearly showed that the site of injection was the most crucial factor in determining the degree of nerve fiber injury, with the most severe fiber damage following intrafascicular injection (54) (Table 20-2). The intrafascicular injection pressures measured are generally high, exceeding the capillary perfusion pressure, and these remain so longer than the duration of the injection (55). In clinical practice, sharp, lancinating pain during injection has been suggested as a possible sign of impending intraneural injection (56). It is for this reason that blocks are not recommended in anesthetized or heavily sedated patients. However, nerve injury may occur even in the absence of pain on injection, making this symptom difficult to rely on as a definitive warning sign (57). Several recent studies focused on the injection pressure and concluded that this parameter, when high, may indicate intraneural placement leading to severe fascicular injury and persistent neurologic deficit (58,59). If this observation, coming from animal studies, applies to human, avoiding excessive pressures during nerve blockade may reduce the risk of nerve injuries. Unfortunately, it has been also demonstrated that anesthesiologists vary widely in their perception of appropriate force and rate of injection, making the syringe-feel method of assessing injection force difficult to rely on (60). Techniques aimed to standardize block injection pressures have been assessed in order to maintain pressure below the level associated with significant nerve injury, with varying success (61).

Local Neurotoxicity

Cauda equina syndrome after a central block may be the typical clinical expression of permanent neurologic sequelae that results from local anesthetic toxicity (62). However, this relation between clinical symptoms and local anesthetic toxicity is less clear for transient neurologic symptoms after spinal anesthesia, and nerve damage, whatever the severity, after PNB. Electrophysiologic, histopathologic, and behavioral animal studies have been employed to study local anesthetic toxicity (Fig. 20-2). The mechanism of local anesthetic cytotoxicity remains unclear. Inhibition of voltage-gated sodium (Na^+) channels, cytoplasmic calcium (Ca) dysregulation, membrane solubilization, and apoptosis have all been evoked. The neurotoxicity of local anesthetics depends on the agent used, its concentration, and the duration of exposure.

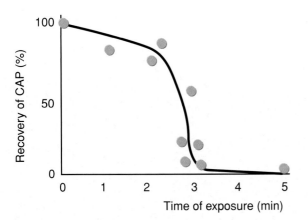

FIGURE 20-2. Lidocaine neurotoxicity. The effect of duration of exposure to 5% lidocaine in 7.5% dextrose. Each point represents a value from a separate nerve exposed to 5% lidocaine for the time shown on the horizontal axis and then washed with Ringer's solution for 3 hours before the measurement of the compound action potential (CAP), which is shown on the vertical axis as a percentage of the initial value. The solid line was drawn by eye. Reproduced from Lambert LA, Lambert DH, Strichartz GR. Irreversible conduction block in isolated nerve by high concentrations of local anesthetics. *Anesthesiology* 1994;80:1082–1093, with permission.

In clinical practice, the incidence of injury resulting from lidocaine toxicity is relatively low. This low incidence may be related to the fact that the concentration of lidocaine at the neuronal membrane rarely reaches levels required to induce injury (63). Dilution of local anesthetic in the cerebrospinal fluid is a factor that minimizes the risk of injury after spinal anesthesia. Exceptionally, a nonhomogeneous mixing and pooling of local anesthetic is responsible for highly concentrated solution to pool around the relatively unprotected nerve fibers of the cauda equina and expose them to a high concentration of local anesthetic. With peripheral routes of administration, even larger barriers to diffusion exist, since axons are surrounded by epineural tissue. As such, intraneuronal lidocaine concentration is only 1.6% of the injected concentration at full block, provided the solution has being extraneurally administered. The relative potency for producing injury varies with the agent used (35,64). Based on electrophysiologic studies, it has been demonstrated that 5% lidocaine and 0.5% tetracaine cause irreversible conduction block in desheathed bullfrog sciatic nerves, whereas 1.5% lidocaine or 0.75% bupivacaine causes 25% to 50% residual block (65). Lidocaine causes a nonreversible block that begins at concentrations as low as 40 mM (~1%), and increases in a graded fashion with increasing concentrations to complete ablation of the compound action potential at 80 mM (~2%). Applied on a crayfish giant axon, 2% lidocaine has a direct neurotoxic effect, with generation of action potentials being more vulnerable than the maintenance of resting membrane potentials (66). Sakura and colleagues showed that local anesthetic–induced neurotoxicity in vivo does not result from blocking voltage-gated Na^+ channels (67). Indeed, concentrations of lidocaine inducing neuronal death are much greater than those required for complete and reversible block of voltage-gated Na^+ channels and action potential generation. Lidocaine, at concentrations that cause neuronal death, also causes rapid depolarization of the neuronal membrane as well as an increase in $[Ca^{2+}]_{intracellular}$ that apparently results from Ca^{2+} influx through the plasma membrane, in addition to Ca^{2+} release from intracellular stores (68). It is

interesting to note that preventing lidocaine-induced increase in $[Ca^{++}]_{intracellular}$ significantly attenuates lidocaine-induced neurotoxicity (69). However, disturbance in Ca^{2+} homeostasis is mostly associated with the use of high concentrations of lidocaine. Work in non-neuronal subcellular particles has suggested that local anesthetics may affect the mitochondrial activities responsible for apoptosis or necrosis (70). As such, using cell culture made of mature neurons, it has been shown that the earliest manifestation of lidocaine toxicity was a complete loss of mitochondrial membrane potential within 5 minutes of exposure at a concentration of 19 mM or greater (71). Lidocaine at a concentration of 37 mM or greater almost completely inhibited oxygen consumption in intact ND7 neurons and was responsible for a dose-dependent release of cytochrome C from mitochondria to cytoplasm. Mitochondrial injury by lidocaine seems to occur upstream of caspase (apoptosis-related proteases) activation. Neuroprotective drugs interacting with apoptotic pathways (as is the case for p38 mitogen-activated protein kinase) may be of considerable benefit (72). The clinical implications for these findings during peripheral techniques remains unclear because of the low concentration of local anesthetic present intraneuronally.

Several experimentations have been conducted on the neurotoxicity of local anesthetics using the growth cone. The *growth cone* is the highly motile structure at the end of growing axons and dendrites. It has a crucial role in pathfinding and cytoarchitecture establishment in the developing nervous system. When the growth cone is surrounded by toxic substances, a new growth cone cannot be formed after growth cone collapse. Using dorsal root ganglia of 7-day-old chick embryos, Saito and colleagues showed that short-term exposure to tetracaine produced irreversible changes in growing neurons (73). Growth cones were quickly affected, and neurites degenerated subsequently. Sensitivity varied with neuronal tissue. Intra–growth cone Ca^{2+} concentration increased simultaneously to the growth cone collapse (74). When neurotrophic factors (brain derived neurotrophic factor [NTF], glial derived NTF, or neurotrophin 3) were added to the replacement medium at a minimum concentration, significantly high reversibility of the lidocaine-induced growth cone collapse was observed (75). It has been proposed that NTFs may protect neurons by reducing the elevation of Ca^{2+} ions. When local anesthetics are compared for their neurotoxicity on growing neurons, the order of neurotoxicity is procaine = mepivacaine <ropivacaine = bupivacaine <lidocaine <tetracaine <dibucaine (76,77) (Fig. 20-3).

Ischemic Nerve Lesions

Peripheral nerves receive a dual blood supply made of intrinsic exchange vessels in the endoneurium and the extrinsic plexus of supply vessels in the epineurial space that cross the perineurium to anastomose with the intrinsic circulation. Persistent reduction of peripheral nerve blood flow can lead to pathologic changes in the structure of nerve fibers and their supporting cells; hence the study of nerve blood flow (NBF) after perineural application of local anesthetics has been used for neurotoxicologic screening. Using a laser Doppler flow probe, it has been shown that lidocaine, levobupivacaine, and ropivacaine are responsible for a significant reduction in rat sciatic NBF, with ropivacaine producing the greatest reduction (78) (Fig. 20-4). The addition of epinephrine (which itself causes a reduction of nerve blood flow) to lidocaine reduces NBF to a greater extent than lidocaine alone (79–81). However, when added to 0.75% ropivacaine, epinephrine does not seem to further reduce NBF compared to 0.75% ropivacaine alone (78).

PART II: TECHNIQUES

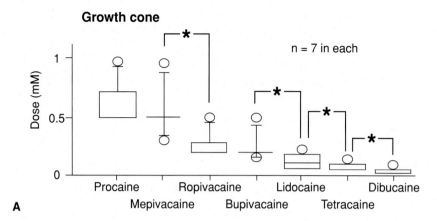

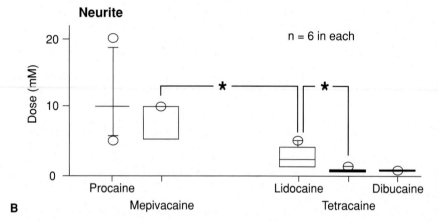

FIGURE 20-3. Compared neurotoxicity of local anesthetics. Comparison of the doses of local anesthetics giving moderate morphologic changes for the growth cones (**A**) and the neurites (**B**) from the freshwater snail *Lymnaea stagnalis*. *Boxes* indicate median and range of 10% to 90%. *Small circles* indicate the cases that were outside of the range between 10% and 90%. *P <0.05. Reproduced from Kasaba T, Onizuka S, Takasaki M. Procaine and mepivacaine have less toxicity in vitro than other clinically used local anesthetics. *Anesth Analg* 2003;97:85–90, with permission.

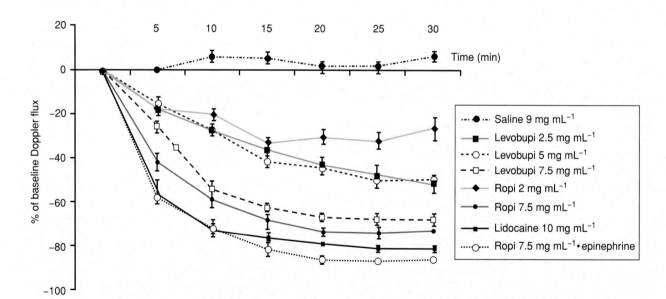

FIGURE 20-4. Effect of different local anesthetics on peripheral nerve blood flow. Data are mean (SEM). Reproduced from Bouaziz H, Iohom G, Estebe JP et al. Effects of levobupivacaine and ropivacaine on rat sciatic nerve blood flow. *Br J Anaesth* 2005;95:696–700, with permission.

TABLE 20-3
NEUROLOGIC COMPLICATIONS OF PERIPHERAL NERVE BLOCKS: RECOMMENDATIONS FOR ADEQUATE PRACTICE
1. Anesthesiologists must consider carefully the choice of local anesthetic agent.
2. Low-concentration local anesthetic solutions should be favored for peripheral nerve blockade.
3. Ultrasound-guided technique may decrease inadvertent intraneural injection and therefore may decrease neurotoxicity.
4. When epinephrine is used as an adjuvant, lower doses should be preferred to obtain a solution at 1:400,000 instead of 1:200,000.
5. High injection pressure may indicate an intrafascicular injection, and should make the anesthesiologist stop immediately.
6. Duration of catheter placement should be as short as possible.

Bupivacaine produces dose-dependent reduction of NBF, with the lowest concentration (0.25%) producing the greatest reduction and the highest concentrations (0.75%) producing the least. Tetracaine (0.5% and 1%) does not produce any significant change in NBF. Table 20-3 finally summarizes recommendations that can diminish the risk of nerve injury during peripheral regional techniques.

Myotoxicity

The myotoxicity of local anesthetics is predictable and intense (82). Intramuscular injections of local anesthetics regularly result in striated muscle damage and myonecrosis, with a drug-specific and dose dependent rate of toxicity (83–86). Compared with local anesthetic application, muscle injury does not occur after the injection of corresponding volumes of normal saline, indicating that fluid volumes are not responsible for tissue alterations (87). Similarly, needle trauma to muscles produces minor and focal lesions and therefore can be eliminated as a relevant mechanism of myotoxicity (88). Finally, the functional muscle denervation following the blockade of neuronal Na^+ channels is not involved in local anesthetic myotoxicity (89). All local anesthetics that have been studied are myotoxic in clinical concentrations, and agent-specific rates of myotoxicity differ in a quantitative but not a qualitative manner. In this respect, tetracaine and procaine have been shown to produce the least, and chloroprocaine and bupivacaine the most severe muscle injury (87,90,91). Furthermore, the extent of muscle damage deteriorates with continuous or serial application. Except after co-injection of steroids and epinephrine, toxic effects are strictly confined to the muscle fiber, and neither vasculature and neural structures nor connective tissue elements appear to be affected (83,92–94).

The histologic pattern and time course of skeletal muscle injury appear uniform and nonspecific, with hypercontracted myofibrils observed several minutes after exposure, then lytic degeneration of striated muscle sarcoplasmic reticulum and mitochondria within the following hours. At that time, a whole spectrum of necrobiotic changes can be encountered, ranging from fiber vacuolation and myocyte edema to a total disinte-

gration of intracellular structures and myonecrosis. Sarcolemmal structures remain morphologically intact for a long period, indicating that fiber degeneration mainly occurs intracellularly. Muscle tissue remains in this state of destruction over the next 24 to 48 hours until it become invaded by phagocytic cells. Muscular regeneration is generally observed within 3 to 4 weeks (95).

Basic pathomechanisms of local anesthetic–induced myotoxicity are still not understood. Local anesthetic agents are known to perturb both internal and external membrane systems of striated myocytes. Benoit and co-workers were the first to propose that local anesthetic–induced muscle necrosis may be the result of an intracellular increase in free Ca^{2+} rather than disturbances of sarcolemmal Na^+ conduction (96). In fact, pathologic Ca^{2+} release from the sarcoplasmic reticulum (SR) seems to be the major mechanism involved in local anesthetic toxicity. In this respect, bupivacaine has been identified to induce Ca^{2+} release from the SR and to inhibit Ca^{2+} reuptake simultaneously (97–100). The increase of myoplasmic Ca^{2+} levels is the result of a direct interaction of local anesthetics with the Ca^{2+} release channel ryanodine receptor at the SR membrane. Beside these disturbances in SR function, other pathways are likely to be involved in local anesthetic myotoxicity. As such, many local anesthetics uncouple oxidative phosphorylation in isolated mitochondria in a dose-dependent fashion. This effect results in intracellular adenosine triphosphate (ATP) depletion, which in turn contributes to intracellular Ca^{2+} dysregulation (101). In addition, bupivacaine may be responsible for mitochondrial depolarization and pyridine nucleotide oxidation, thus inducing the opening of the permeability transition pore supposed to play a role in many forms of cell death (102). Finally, increasing oxidative stress is also supposed to be involved in the pathogenesis of local anesthetic myotoxicity, with hydroxyl radical and superoxide anion formation induced by cytochrome C release (103).

Among long-acting local anesthetics, ropivacaine is characterized by a smaller rate of myotoxicity in comparison to bupivacaine (99). Bupivacaine causes severe tissue damage, whereas ropivacaine induces fiber injury of smaller extent in an acute model of mini pigs in vivo (87) (Fig. 20-5). Moreover, bupivacaine induces apoptosis in striated muscle fibers in vitro and in vivo, conversely to ropivacaine, indicating that the induction of programmed cell death seems to be a unique and specific property to bupivacaine. In addition, long-term myotoxic effects of bupivacaine significantly exceed those of ropivacaine, according to histologic changes observed after 7 and 28 days (104). On the other hand, bupivacaine disturbs heart cell mitochondrial bioenergetics more significantly than does ropivacaine (105).

The clinical impact of local anesthetic neurotoxicity is presently not considered to be a major problem; muscle injury after application of local anesthetics remains subclinical (asymptomatic) in most cases and is reversible within weeks. Indeed, few case reports of myotoxic complications have been published, mainly after continuous PNBs, infiltration of wound margins, trigger point injections, and peri- and retrobulbar blocks, with bupivacaine involved in most of these cases (90,106). The incidence of anesthesia-related diplopia has been documented in 3,587 cataract surgeries after retrobulbar/peribulbar/topical anesthesia (107). In this retrospective review, 26 cases of persistent diplopia were found (0.72% incidence), nine of which (0.25%) were considered to be related to anesthetic factors. Surgery was required to correct the diplopia in two cases; a prism was employed in six; and, in the remaining patient, treatment was not considered necessary. The outcome has been satisfactory in eight patients at the time of the

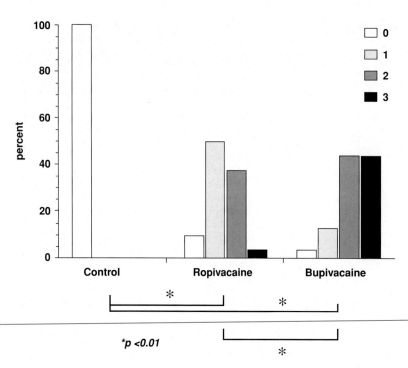

FIGURE 20-5. Myotoxicity of ropivacaine and bupivacaine. Severity score of skeletal muscle damage. Scoring system with 0: no fiber damage; 1: localized and/or sparsely scattered fiber destruction; 2: more extensive necrosis of major connective tissue planes and involving numerous muscle fascicles; 3: destruction of essentially the entire muscle mass in the eye-field. Reproduced from Zink W, Seif C, Bohl JR et al. The acute myotoxic effects of bupivacaine and ropivacaine after continuous peripheral nerve blockade. *Anesth Analg* 2003;97:1173–1179, with permission.

publication. Retrobulbar block was found to be more often involved in such complication than was peribulbar blocks (107). Local anesthetic toxicity should be suspected when localized muscle dysfunction and tenderness follow anesthetic injection into the area. Biopsy aids in differential diagnosis and magnetic resonance imaging (MRI) might be used in noninvasively establishing the diagnostic.

Recommendations that can be formulated to avoid myotoxic complications are overall the same as those to minimize neurotoxic events (Table 20-3).

Infectious Complications

The incidence of infectious complications following PNB appears to be very low. Indeed, according to large prospective epidemiologic studies, no such complication had been reported after more than 70,000 PNBs (25). The only case of severe infection complicating a single-injection PNB is a fatal streptococcal necrotizing fasciitis after an axillary brachial plexus block for carpal tunnel decompression (108). Sporadic cases reported in the literature after continuous peripheral techniques include psoas and thigh abscesses complicating continuous femoral and sciatic nerve block, respectively (109,110). Large recent series describing signs and symptoms of infection (including local pain, redness, induration, systemic sepsis, or abscess requiring removal of the catheter with or without surgical drainage/antibiotic therapy) after continuous peripheral blockade suggest an incidence between one in 100 and one in 10,000 depending on the severity of symptoms required to define infection (27–29,32,111).

Sources of infections may be related to the underlying health of the patients, as is the case for those with diabetes mellitus or in patients admitted to an ICU in whom compromised cellular immunity may contribute to a higher risk. Besides these intrinsic sources, invasion of skin bacteria along the catheter or contamination of the material used for the procedure may oc-

cur. The time during which the catheter has remained in place is a risk factor for infection (112); catheter duration longer than 48 hours is associated with a relative risk of inflammation/infection of 4.6 (27). Admission to an ICU and repeated changing of catheter dressings have also been identified as risk factors for local infection/inflammation (27,113). Antibiotic prophylaxis used to prevent surgical site infection may be associated with a decreased risk of infection (27,113).

The incidence of colonization of a perineural catheter has been evaluated by several studies and varies according to the site of the catheter (Table 20-4). The colonization rate may be greater after continuous femoral nerve block than after axillary blocks (111,113,114) but may be greater after axillary plexus block than after popliteal block (27). Interscalene blocks may also be at increased risk (112), whereas anterior proximal sciatic catheters might be at low risk although the puncture site is close to the femoral area (112). The density of sebaceous glands in the different insertion sites impacts the ability of local disinfectants to reduce the number of microorganisms and may explain this variability. Coagulase-negative *Staphylococcus* is the most frequently isolated bacteria from continuous PNBs (27,112). This microorganism is primarily cultured following interscalene and popliteal catheter placement, whereas *Enterococcus* and gram-negative bacilli may be more often isolated from axillary and femoral catheter sites (27). Two or more organisms are observed in one-third to one-half of cases.

The relatively low incidence of infection following peripheral techniques may be in part related to the time- and concentration-dependent antimicrobial activity of most local anesthetics (115,116). This antibacterial activity has been described in many in vitro studies. Antimicrobial effects of local anesthetics include growth inhibition, reduction of the number of viable cells, lysis of protoplasts, permeability modifications, alteration of ultrastructural characteristics, and inhibition of membrane-bound enzymatic activity. The observed antibacterial effect of local anesthetics may depend not only on drug

TABLE 20-4

CATHETER CULTURE FOR EACH CONTINUOUS PERIPHERAL NERVE BLOCK (CPNB) GROUP

	Interscalene (n = 256)	Axillary (n = 126)	PCB (n = 20)	Femoral (n = 683)	Fascia I (n = 94)	Sciatic (n = 32)	Popliteal (n = 167)	Distal (n = 38)
Catheters with culture, (n)%	(n = 166) 64.9	(n = 77) 61.1	(n = 15) 76.9	(n = 485) 71.1	(n = 65) 69.3	(n = 25) 77.4	(n = 112) 67.5	(n = 24) 63.3
Colonized catheters, %	25.6	36.5	20	28.6	28.6	30.4	18.9	35.5
[95% CI]	[19–32]	[25.5–47.4]	[2.4–37.5]	[14.9–52.2]	[14.9–49.2]	[11.6–49.2]	[11.6–26.2]	[24–47.4]
Organisms, %								
Coagulase-negative staphylococcus	83	56.7	66.7	52.3	35.7	75	77.3	69.6
Staphylococcus aureus	4.3	6.7	0	4.6	7.1	0	0	8.7
Enterococcus	2.1	3.3	0	9.9	14.3	12.5	0	0
Other gram-positive cocci	6.4	3.3	0	1.3	0	0	0	0
Gram-negative bacillus	0	26.7	33.3	27.1	42.7	12.5	18.1	21.7
Others	4.2	6.6	0	4.8	0.2	0	4.6	0

Axillary, axillary catheter; CI, confidence interval; CPNB, continuous peripheral nerve block; Distal, distal nerve block catheter; Femoral, femoral catheter; Interscalene, catheter of the brachial plexus through interscalene approach; PCB, catheter in the lumbar plexus through a posterior approach; Popliteal, popliteal catheter; Sciatic, sciatic catheter through a parasacral approach.
Reproduced from Capdevila X, Pirat P, Bringuier S, et al. Continuous peripheral nerve blocks in hospital wards after orthopedic surgery: A multicenter prospective analysis of the quality of postoperative analgesia and complications in 1,416 patients. *Anesthesiology* 2005;103:1035–1045, with permission.

TABLE 20-5

INFECTIOUS COMPLICATIONS OF PERIPHERAL NERVE BLOCKS: RECOMMENDATIONS FOR ADEQUATE PRACTICE

Protective measure	Comment	Grade*
A new facial mask should be worn for each new case.	The use of surgical masks during regional anesthesia will maximize sterile barrier precautions. In particular, surgical masks have been found to significantly reduce the likelihood of site contamination from microorganisms grown in the upper airway of clinicians. Although the routine use of masks has not been found to reduce infectious complications related to regional anesthesia, they do remain a vital protective measure against blood-borne pathogen exposure	(Grade B)
Wash hands thoroughly with alcohol-based antiseptic solutions.	Thorough hand-washing greatly reduces the risk of cross-contamination and should be done before performing any regional anesthetic technique. The duration and method of washing (standard hand washing vs. full surgical scrub) required to reduce infectious complications is currently unknown. Alcohol-based antiseptic solutions will provide the maximal degree of antimicrobial activity with extended duration when compared with nonalcoholic antimicrobial or non antimicrobial preparations.	Grade A
Apply alcohol-containing chlorhexidine antiseptic solution on the puncture site.	Chlorhexidine antiseptic solutions significantly reduce the likelihood of catheter and site colonization and maximize the rapidity and potency of bactericidal activity when compared to other antiseptic agents. Alcohol-based antiseptics reinforce efficacy and should be considered the antiseptic of choice before regional anesthetic techniques.	Grade A
	At least two disinfections of the puncture site with solution-soaked sterile gauze are necessary. These disinfections must be large, comprehensive, and performed in a centrifuge manner.	Grade D
	Allow time for the antiseptic to dry and to produce its effects between each disinfection (1 minute for alcohol iodine and alcoholic chlorhexidine).	Grade B
Maximize barrier precautions.	Install sterile drapes. Disposable equipment only must be used. The catheter is covered with a transparent sterile dressing (Tegaderm, Opsite).	Grade D
Remove jewelry before hand-washing.	Higher microbial counts have been identified in health care workers who do not remove jewelry before hand-washing. Therefore, it may be prudent to remove all jewelry items (rings, watches, and so on) before hand-washing to reduce the risk of contamination.	Grade B
Wear surgical gloves.	Sterile surgical gloves should be used and considered a supplement to, not a replacement for, hand-washing. The use of surgical gloves is advocated not only to protect patients from cross-contamination but also to protect health care workers from blood-borne pathogen exposure.	Grade A
The decision for catheter placement should be evidence-based, and the duration of catheter placement should be as short as possible.		Grade D
Wear a surgical gown if a catheter is placed for days.	Several intensive care unit investigations have shown that the use of surgical gowns does not reduce patient colonization, infection, or mortality rates beyond that achieved with gloves alone. There is currently insufficient data to make recommendations with regard to routine use during regional techniques within the operating room environment. However, as catheter duration is associated with an increased risk of catheter infection, wearing a gown in these cases can be supported.	Grade D
Insert a bacterial filter if a catheter is used.	Currently, the literature does not support the routine use of bacterial filters with short-term epidural or perineural catheter infusions as their use has not been demonstrated to decrease the risk of infection. However, they are useful for catheter identification and therefore avoiding erroneous injections.	Grade B
Consider using antibiotics before catheter placement.	In the absence of surgical indication for antibiotic prophylaxis, consider using single-shot dosing of antistaphylococcal antibiotics before catheter placement.	Grade C
Use adjuvant only if necessary.	Adjuvant use adds further risk of infection (vial opening), and its use should also be evidence-based.	Grade D
Infuse sterile mixtures.	Sterile infusion (prepared in 250–500 mL bag and which can be transferred into the continuous infusion system through a three-way-stopcock) is preferable to top-up administration, which requires frequent disconnection maneuvers and which may cause hub colonization.	Grade D

*Grade A, evidence obtained from at least one proper meta-analysis or from a properly randomized controlled trial; Grade B, evidence obtained from a well-designed controlled trial without randomization or from other types of quasi-experimental studies; Grade C, evidence obtained from descriptive studies such as comparative studies, correlation studies, and case-control studies; Grade D, opinions of respected authorities or reports of expert committees.
Modified from Benhamou D, Mercier FM, Dounas M. Hospital policy for prevention of infection after neuraxial blocks in obstetrics. *Int J Obstet Anesth* 2002;11:265–269; and Hebl JR. The importance and implications of aseptic techniques during regional anesthesia. *Reg Anesth Pain Med* 2006;31:311–323, with permission.

concentration or time of exposure but also on the local anesthetic tested (bupivacaine has a stronger inhibition on growth of bacteria than ropivacaine) and on methods used to evaluate bacterial growth (direct versus indirect method, room temperature versus 37°C) (117,118). Among additives, clonidine has been shown to exhibit a concentration- and time-dependent bactericidal activity (119). However, anesthesiologists should not rely on such antibacterial properties of local anesthetics to use less rigorous antiseptic protocols. Ultrasound imaging is gaining popularity as a method of peripheral nerve localization. This technique may be associated with an increased incidence of infection, as the presence of the ultrasound probe itself and the increased complexity of the procedure can interfere with aseptic technique. Aids can be used to maintain asepsis, such as sterile gels and sleeve covers (120), but they add to the cost and complexity of the procedure. Simpler and cheaper techniques to maintain asepsis during ultrasound guided block are needed. Furthermore, in the absence of validated guidelines for prevention of infection in regional anesthesia, some groups and societies have implemented their own standards (121,122) (Table 20-5).

SUMMARY

In conclusion, the frequency and mechanism of neurologic complications following PNB is currently the focus of laboratory, clinical, and epidemiologic studies. Ongoing efforts to improve methods of neural localization, avoid intraneural injection of local anesthetics, as well as identify patients at risk for neurologic complications will continue to increase the utilization and safety of PNB.

References

1. Benhamou D, Pequignot F, Auroy Y, et al. Factors associated with use of regional anaesthesia: A multivariate analysis in seven surgical procedures in France. *Eur J Anaesthesiol* 2004;21:576–578.
2. Clergue F, Auroy Y, Pequignot F, et al. French survey of anesthesia in 1996. *Anesthesiology* 1999;91:1509–1520.
3. Lee LA, Posner KL, Domino KB, et al. Injuries associated with regional anesthesia in the 1980s and 1990s: A closed claims analysis. *Anesthesiology* 2004;101:143–152.
4. Pronovost PJ, Miller MR, Wachter RM. Tracking progress in patient safety: An elusive target. *JAMA* 2006;296:696–699.
5. Klein SM. Continuous peripheral nerve blocks: Fewer excuses. *Anesthesiology* 2005;103:921–923.
6. Borgeat A, Ekatodramis G, Kalberer F, Benz C. Acute and nonacute complications associated with interscalene block and shoulder surgery: A prospective study. *Anesthesiology* 2001;95:875–880.
7. Dripps RD, Vandam LD. Long-term follow-up of patients who received 10,098 spinal anesthetics: Failure to discover major neurological sequelae. *JAMA* 1954;156:1486–1491.
8. Perris TM, Watt JM. The road to success: A review of 1000 axillary brachial plexus blocks. *Anaesthesia* 2003;58:1220–1224.
9. Kroll DA, Caplan RA, Posner K, et al. Nerve injury associated with anesthesia. *Anesthesiology* 1990;73:202–207.
10. Horlocker TT, Hebl JR, Gali B, et al. Anesthetic, patient, and surgical risk factors for neurologic complications after prolonged total tourniquet time during total knee arthroplasty. *Anesth Analg* 2006;102:950–955.
11. Ben-David B, Joshi R, Chelly JE. Sciatic nerve palsy after total hip arthroplasty in a patient receiving continuous lumbar plexus block. *Anesth Analg* 2003;97:1180–1182.
12. Aminoff MJ. Electrophysiologic testing for the diagnosis of peripheral nerve injuries. *Anesthesiology* 2004;100:1298–1303.
13. DeHart MM, Riley LH Jr. Nerve injuries in total hip arthroplasty. *J Am Acad Orthop Surg* 1999;7:101–111.
14. Satcher RL, Noss RS, Yingling CD, et al. The use of motor-evoked potentials to monitor sciatic nerve status during revision total hip arthroplasty. *J Arthroplasty* 2003;18:329–332.
15. Nercessian OA, Macaulay W, Stinchfield FE. Peripheral neuropathies following total hip arthroplasty. *J Arthroplasty* 1994;9:645–651.
16. Darmanis S, Pavlakis D, Papanikolaou A, Apergis E. Neurovascular injury during primary total hip arthroplasty caused by a threaded acetabulum cup. *J Arthroplasty* 2004;19:520–524.
17. Lynch NM, Cofield RH, Silbert PL, Hermann RC. Neurologic complications after total shoulder arthroplasty. *J Shoulder Elbow Surg* 1996;5:53–61.
18. Candido KD, Sukhani R, Doty R Jr., et al. Neurologic sequelae after interscalene brachial plexus block for shoulder/upper arm surgery: The association of patient, anesthetic, and surgical factors to the incidence and clinical course. *Anesth Analg* 2005;100:1489–1495.
19. Horlocker TT, Kufner RP, Bishop AT, et al. The risk of persistent paresthesia is not increased with repeated axillary block. *Anesth Analg* 1999;88:382–387.
20. Brull R, McCartney CJ, Chan VW, et al. Effect of transarterial axillary block versus general anesthesia on paresthesiae 1 year after hand surgery. *Anesthesiology* 2005;103:1104–1105.
21. Urmey WF, Talts KH, Sharrock NE. One hundred percent incidence of hemidiaphragmatic paresis associated with interscalene brachial plexus anesthesia as diagnosed by ultrasonography. *Anesth Analg* 1991;72:498–503.
22. Deruddre S, Vidal D, Benhamou D. A case of persistent hemidiaphragmatic paralysis following interscalene brachial plexus block. *J Clin Anesth* 2006;18:238–239.
23. Robaux S, Bouaziz H, Boisseau N, et al. Persistent phrenic nerve paralysis following interscalene brachial plexus block. *Anesthesiology* 2001;95:1519–1521.
24. Auroy Y, Narchi P, Messiah A, et al. Serious complications related to regional anesthesia: Results of a prospective survey in France. *Anesthesiology* 1997;87:479–486.
25. Auroy Y, Benhamou D, Bargues L, et al. Major complications of regional anesthesia in France: The SOS Regional Anesthesia Hotline Service. *Anesthesiology* 2002;97:1274–1280.
26. Capdevila X, Bringuier S, Choquet O, et al. Patient's pre-existing disease interfere with complications after peripheral nerve block. [Abstract] *Anesthesiology* 2006;105:A889.
27. Capdevila X, Pirat P, Bringuier S, et al. Continuous peripheral nerve blocks in hospital wards after orthopedic surgery: A multicenter prospective analysis of the quality of postoperative analgesia and complications in 1,416 patients. *Anesthesiology* 2005;103:1035–1045.
28. Bergman BD, Hebl JR, Kent J, Horlocker TT. Neurologic complications of 405 consecutive continuous axillary catheters. *Anesth Analg* 2003;96:247–252.
29. Borgeat A, Dullenkopf A, Ekatodramis G, Nagy L. Evaluation of the lateral modified approach for continuous interscalene block after shoulder surgery. *Anesthesiology* 2003;99:436–442.
30. Borgeat A, Blumenthal S, Karovic D, et al. Clinical evaluation of a modified posterior anatomical approach to performing the popliteal block. *Reg Anesth Pain Med* 2004;29:290–296.
31. Fanelli G, Casati A, Garancini P, Torri G. Nerve stimulator and multiple injection technique for upper and lower limb blockade: Failure rate, patient acceptance, and neurologic complications. Study Group on Regional Anesthesia. *Anesth Analg* 1999;88:847–852.
32. Borgeat A, Blumenthal S, Lambert M, et al. The feasibility and complications of the continuous popliteal nerve block: A 1001-case survey. *Anesth Analg* 2006;103:229–233.
33. Blumenthal S, Borgeat A, Maurer K, et al. Preexisting subclinical neuropathy as a risk factor for nerve injury after continuous ropivacaine administration through a femoral nerve catheter. *Anesthesiology* 2006;105:1053–1056.
34. Borgeat A. Regional anesthesia, intraneural injection, and nerve injury: Beyond the epineurium. *Anesthesiology* 2006;105:647–648.
35. Kalichman MW, Moorhouse DF, Powell HC, Myers RR. Relative neural toxicity of local anesthetics. *J Neuropathol Exp Neurol* 1993;52:234–240.
36. Gentili F, Hudson A, Kline DG, Hunter D. Peripheral nerve injection injury: An experimental study. *Neurosurgery* 1979;4:244–253.
37. Upton AR, McComas AJ. The double crush in nerve entrapment syndromes. *Lancet* 1973;2:359–362.
38. Kalichman MW, Calcutt NA. Local anesthetic-induced conduction block and nerve fiber injury in streptozotocin-diabetic rats. *Anesthesiology* 1992;77:941–947.
39. Singelyn FJ, Gerard C, Fuzier R. The influence of diabetes mellitus on the success rate of posterior popliteal sciatic nerve blockade [Abstract]. *Anesthesiology* 2004;101:A1125.
40. Hebl JR, Horlocker TT, Sorenson EJ, Schroeder DR. Regional anesthesia does not increase the risk of postoperative neuropathy in patients undergoing ulnar nerve transposition. *Anesth Analg* 2001;93:1606–1611.

41. Sites BD, Gallagher J, Sparks M. Ultrasound-guided popliteal block demonstrates an atypical motor response to nerve stimulation in 2 patients with diabetes mellitus. *Reg Anesth Pain Med* 2003;28:479–482.
42. Minville V, Zetlaoui PJ, Fessenmeyer C, Benhamou D. Ultrasound guidance for difficult lateral popliteal catheter insertion in a patient with peripheral vascular disease. *Reg Anesth Pain Med* 2004;29:368–370.
43. Selander D, Edshage S, Wolff T. Paresthesia or no paresthesia? *Acta Anaesth Scand* 1979;23:27–33.
44. Perlas A, Niazi A, McCartney C, et al. The sensitivity of motor response to nerve stimulation and paresthesia for nerve localization as evaluated by ultrasound. *Reg Anesth Pain Med* 2006;31:445–450.
45. Urmey WF, Stanton J. Inability to consistently elicit a motor response following sensory paresthesia during interscalene block administration. *Anesthesiology* 2002;96:552–554.
46. Bigeleisen PE. Nerve puncture and apparent intraneural injection during ultrasound-guided axillary block does not invariably result in neurologic injury. *Anesthesiology* 2006;105:779–783.
47. Karaca P, Hadzic A, Yufa M, et al. Painful paresthesiae are infrequent during brachial plexus localization using low-current peripheral nerve stimulation. *Reg Anesth Pain Med* 2003;28:380–383.
48. Johnson CR, Barr RC, Klein SM. A computer model of electrical stimulation of peripheral nerves in regional anesthesia. *Anesthesiology* 2007;106(2):323–330.
49. Liguory GA, Zayas VM, YaDeau JT, et al. Nerve localization techniques for interscalene brachial plexus blockade: A prospective, randomized comparison of mechanical paresthesia versus electrical stimulation. *Anesth Analg* 2006;103:761–767.
50. Selander D, Dhuner KG, Lundborg G. Peripheral nerve injury due to injection needles used for regional anesthesia. An experimental study of the acute effects of needle point trauma. *Acta Anaesthesiol Scand* 1977;21:182–188.
51. Rice ASC, McMahon SB. Peripheral nerve injury caused by injection needles used in regional anesthesia: Influence of bevel configuration, studied in a rat model. *Br J Anaesth* 1992;69:433–438.
52. Maruyama M. Long-tapered double needle used to reduce needle stick nerve injury. *Reg Anesth* 1997;22:157–160.
53. McQuillan PM, Hahn MB. Does location matter in ulnar and common peroneal nerve block? [Letter] *Lancet* 1996;348:490–491.
54. Gentili F, Hudson AR, Hunter DA, Kline DG. Nerve injection injury with local anesthetic agents: A light and electron microscopic, fluorescent microscopic, and horseradish peroxidase study. *Neurosurgery* 1980;6:263–272.
55. Selander D, Sjostrand J. Longitudinal spread of intraneurally injected local anesthetics. An experimental study of the initial neural distribution following intraneural injections. *Acta Anaesthesiol Scand* 1978;22:622–634.
56. Kaufman BR, Nystrom E, Nath S, et al. Debilitating chronic pain syndromes after presumed intraneural injections. *Pain* 2000;85:283–286.
57. Bonner SM, Pridie AK. Sciatic nerve palsy following uneventful sciatic nerve block. *Anaesthesia* 1997;52:1205–1207.
58. Hadzic A, Dilberovic F, Shah S, et al. Combination of intraneural injection and high injection pressure leads to fascicular injury and neurologic deficits in dogs. *Reg Anesth Pain Med* 2004;29:417–423.
59. Kapur E, Vuckovic I, Dilberovic F, et al. Neurologic and histologic outcome after intraneural injections of lidocaine in canine sciatic nerves. *Acta Anaesthesiol Scand* 2007;51(1):101–107.
60. Claudio R, Hadzic A, Shih H, et al. Injection pressures by anesthesiologists during simulated peripheral nerve block. *Reg Anesth Pain Med* 2004;29:201–205.
61. Tsui BC, Pillay JJ. Compressed air injection technique to standardize block injection pressures. *Can J Anesth* 2006;53:1098–1102.
62. Rigler ML, Drasner K, Krejcie TC, et al. Cauda equina syndrome after continuous spinal anesthesia. *Anesth Analg* 1991;72:275–281.
63. Popitz-Berger FA, Leeson S, Strichartz GR, Thalhammer JG. Relation between functional deficit and intraneural local anesthetic during peripheral nerve block: A study in the rat sciatic nerve. *Anesthesiology* 1995;83:583–292.
64. Kalichman MW, Powell HC, Myers RR. Quantitative histologic analysis of local anesthetic-induced injury to rat sciatic nerve. *J Pharmacol Exp Ther* 1989;250:406–413.
65. Lambert LA, Lambert DH, Strichartz GR. Irreversible conduction block in isolated nerve by high concentrations of local anesthetics. *Anesthesiology* 1994;80:1082–1093.
66. Kanai Y, Katsuki H, Takasaki M. Graded, irreversible changes in crayfish giant axon as manifestations of lidocaine neurotoxicity in vitro. *Anesth Analg* 1998;86:569–573.
67. Sakura S, Bollen AW, Ciriales R, Drasner K. Local anesthetic neurotoxicity does not result from blockade of voltage-gated sodium channels. *Anesth Komai* 1995;81:338–346.
68. Gold MS, Reichling DB, Hampl KF, et al. Lidocaine toxicity in primary afferent neurons from the rat. *J Pharmacol Exp Ther* 1998;285:413–421.
69. Johnson ME, Saenz JA, DaSilva AD, et al. Effect of local anesthetic on neuronal cytoplasmic calcium and plasma membrane lysis (necrosis) in a cell culture model. *Anesthesiology* 2002;97:1466–1476.
70. Sztark F, Ouhabi R, Dabadie P, Mazat JP. Effects of the local anesthetic bupivacaine on mitochondrial energy metabolism: Change from uncoupling to decoupling depending on the respiration state. *Biochem Mol Biol Int* 1997;43:997–1003.
71. Johnson ME, Uhl CB, Spittler KH, et al. Mitochondrial injury and caspase activation by the local anesthetic lidocaine. *Anesthesiology* 2004;101:1184–1194.
72. Lirk P, Haller I, Myers RR, et al. Mitigation of direct neurotoxic effects of lidocaine and amitriptyline by inhibition of p38 mitogen-activated protein kinase in vitro and in vivo. *Anesthesiology* 2006;104:1266–1273.
73. Saito S, Radwan I, Obata H, et al. Direct neurotoxicity of tetracaine on growth cones and neuritis of growing neurons in vitro. *Anesthesiology* 2001;95:726–733.
74. Saito S, Radwan IAM, Nishikawa K, et al. Intracellular calcium increases in growth cones exposed to tetracaine. *Anesth Analg* 2004;98:841–845.
75. Radwan IAM, Saito S, Goto F. Growth cone collapsing effect of lidocaine on DRG neurons is partially reversed by several neurotrophic factors. *Anesthesiology* 2002;97:630–635.
76. Kasaba T, Onizuka S, Takasaki M. Procaine and mepivacaine have less toxicity in vitro than other clinically used local anesthetics. *Anesth Analg* 2003;97:85–90.
77. Radwan IAM, Saito S, Goto F. The neurotoxicity of local anesthetics on growing neurons: A comparative study of lidocaine, bupivacaine, mepivacaine, and ropivacaine. *Anesth Analg* 2002;94:319–324.
78. Bouaziz H, Iohom G, Estebe JP, et al. Effects of levobupivacaine and ropivacaine on rat sciatic nerve blood flow. *Br J Anaesth* 2005;95:696–700.
79. Myers RR, Heckman HM. Effects of local anesthesia on nerve blood flow: Studies using lidocaine with and without epinephrine. *Anesthesiology* 1989;71:757–762.
80. Partridge BL. The effects of local anesthetics and epinephrine on rat sciatic nerve blood flow. *Anesthesiology* 1991;75:243–251.
81. Selander D, Mansson LG, Karlsson L, Svanvik J. Adrenergic vasoconstriction in peripheral nerves of the rabbit. *Anesthesiology* 1985;62:6–10.
82. Grim M, Rerabkova L, Carlson BM. A test for muscle lesions and their regeneration following intramuscular drug application. *Toxicol Pathol* 1988;16:432–442.
83. Forster AH, Carlson BM. Myotoxicity of local anesthetics and regeneration of the damaged muscle fibers. *Anesth Analg* 1980;59:727–736.
84. Pere P, Watanabe H, Pitkanen M, et al. Local myotoxicity of bupivacaine in rabbits after continuous supraclavicular brachial plexus block. *Reg Anesth* 1993;18:304–307.
85. Kytta J, Heinon E, Rosenberg PH, et al. Effects of repeated bupivacaine administration on sciatic nerve and surrounding muscle tissue in rats. *Acta Anaesthesiol Scand* 1986;30:625–629.
86. Sadeh M, Czyzewski K, Stern L. Chronic myopathy induced by repeated bupivacaine injections. *J Neurol Sci* 1985;67:229–238.
87. Zink W, Seif C, Bohl JR, et al. The acute myotoxic effects of bupivacaine and ropivacaine after continuous peripheral nerve blockade. *Anesth Analg* 2003;97:1173–1179.
88. Benoit PW, Belt WD. Some effects of local anesthetic agents on skeletal muscle. *Exp Neurol* 1972;34:264–278.
89. Schultz E, Lipton BH. The effect of Marcaine on muscle and non-muscle cells in vitro. *Anat Rec* 1978;191:351–369.
90. Hogan Q, Dotson R, Erickson S, et al. Local anesthetic myotoxicity: A case and review. *Anesthesiology* 1994;80:942–947.
91. Yagiela JA, Benoit PW, Buoncristiani RD, et al. Comparison of myotoxic effects of lidocaine with epinephrine in rats and humans. *Anesth Analg* 1981;69:471–480.
92. Benoit PW. Reversible skeletal muscle damage after administration of local anesthetics with and without epinephrine. *J Oral Surg* 1978;36:198–201.
93. Basson MD, Carlson BM. Myotoxicity of single and repeated injections of mepivacaine (Carbocaine) in the rat. *Anesth Analg* 1980;59:275–282.
94. Benoit PW. Microscarring in skeletal muscle after repeated exposures to lidocaine with epinephrine. *J Oral Surg* 1978;36:530–533.
95. Zink W, Graf BM. Local anesthetic myotoxicity. *Reg Anesth Pain Med* 2004;29:333–340.
96. Benoit PW, Yagiela A, Fort NF. Pharmacologic correlation between local anesthetic-induced myotoxicity and disturbances of intracellular calcium distribution. *Toxicol Appl Pharmacol* 1980;52:187–198.
97. Zink W, Graf BM, Sinner B, et al. Differential effects of bupivacaine on intracellular Ca2+ regulation: Potential mechanisms of its myotoxicity. *Anesthesiology* 2002;97:710–716.
98. Komai H, Lokuta AJ. Interaction of bupivacaine and tetracaine with the sarcoplasmic reticulum Ca2+ release channel of skeletal and cardiac muscles. *Anesthesiology* 1999;90:835–843.
99. Zink W, Kunst G, Martin E, Graf BM. Differential effects of S(-)-ropivacaine and bupivacaine on intracellular Ca2+ homeostasis in mammalian skeletal muscle fibers. *Anesthesiology* 2005;102:793–798.

100. Takahashi S. Local anesthetic bupivacaine alters function of sarcoplasmic reticulum and sarcolemmal vesicles from rabbit masseter muscle. *Pharmacol Toxicol* 1994;75:119–128.
101. Sztark F, Nouette-Gaulain K, Malgat M, et al. Absence of stereospecific effects of bupivacaine isomers on heart mitochondrial bioenergetics. *Anesthesiology* 2000;93:456–462.
102. Irwin W, Fontaine E, Agnolucci L, et al. Bupivacaine myotoxicity is mediated by mitochondria. *J Biol Chem* 2002;277:12221–12227.
103. Wakata N, Sugimoto H, Iguchi H, et al. Bupivacaine hydrochloride induces muscle fiber necrosis and hydroxyl radical formation dimethyl sulphoxide reduces hydroxyl radical formation. *Neurochem Res* 2001;26:841–844.
104. Zink W, Bohl JRE, Hacke N, et al. The long term myotoxic effects of bupivacaine and ropivacaine after continuous peripheral nerve blocks. *Anesth Analg* 2005;101:548–554.
105. Sztark F, Malgat M, Dabadie P, Mazat JP. Comparison of the effects of bupivacaine and ropivacaine on heart cell mitochondrial bioenergetics. *Anesthesiology* 1998;88:1340–1349.
106. Parris WC, Dettbarn WD. Muscle atrophy following nerve block therapy [Letter]. *Anesthesiology* 1988;69:289.
107. Gomez-Arnau JI, Yanguela J, Gonzalez A, et al. Anaesthesia-related diplopia after cataract surgery. *Br J Anaesth* 2003;90:189–192.
108. Nseir S, Pronnier P, Soubrier S, et al. Fatal streptococcal necrotizing fasciitis as a complication of axillary brachial plexus block. *Br J Anaesth* 2003; 92:427–429.
109. Adam F, Jaziri S, Chauvin M. Psoas abscess complicating femoral nerve block catheter. *Anesthesiology* 2003;99:230–231.
110. Compère V, Cornet C, Fourdrinier V, et al. Thigh abscess as a complication of continuous popliteal sciatic nerve block. *Br J Anaesth* 2005;95:255–256.
111. Cuvillon P, Ripart J, Lalourcey L, et al. The continuous femoral nerve block catheter for postoperative analgesia: Bacterial colonization, infectious rate and adverse effects. *Anesth Analg* 2001;93:1045–1049.
112. Neuburger M, Buttner J, Blumenthal S, et al. Inflammation and infection complications of 2285 perineural catheters: A prospective study. *Acta Anaesthesiol Scand* 2007;51(1):108–114.
113. Morin AM, Kerwat KM, Klotz M, et al. Risk factors for bacterial catheter colonization in regional anaesthesia. *BMC Anesthesiol* 2005;5:1.
114. Gaumann DM, Lennon RL, Wedel DJ. Continuous axillary block for postoperative pain management. *Reg Anesth* 1988;13:77–82.
115. Sakuragi T, Ishino H, Dan K. Bactericidal activity of preservative-free bupivacaine on microorganisms in the human skin flora. *Acta Anaesthesiol Scand* 1998;42:1096–1099.
116. Feldman JM, Chapin-Robertson K, Turner J. Do agents used for epidural analgesia have antimicrobial properties? *Reg Anesth* 1994;19:43–47.
117. Aydin ON, Eyigor M, Aydin N. Antimicrobial activity of ropivacaine and other local anaesthetics. *Eur J Anaesthesiol* 2001;18:687–694.
118. Pere P, Lindgren L, Vaara M. Poor antibacterial effect of ropivacaine. Comparison with bupivacaine. *Anesthesiology* 1999;91:884–886.
119. Boselli E, Guillier M, Freney J, et al. Antibacterial activity of clonidine and neostigmine in vitro. *Anesth Analg* 2005;101:121–124.
120. Tsui BC, Twomey C, Finucane BT. Visualization of the brachial plexus in the supraclavicular region using a curved ultrasound probe with a sterile transparent dressing. *Reg Anesth Pain Med* 2006;31:182–184.
121. Benhamou D, Mercier FM, Dounas M. Hospital policy for prevention of infection after neuraxial blocks in obstetrics. *Int J Obstet Anesth* 2002; 11:265–269.
122. Hebl JR. The importance and implications of aseptic techniques during regional anesthesia. *Reg Anesth Pain Med* 2006;31:311–323.

PART II: TECHNIQUES

CHAPTER 21 ■ NEURAL BLOCKADE FOR SURGERY TO THE HEAD AND NECK

BAN C. H. TSUI, DEREK DILLANE, AND BRENDAN T. FINUCANE

Regional anesthesia techniques for the head and neck region are diversified. The majority of head and neck surgical procedures are amenable to some form of regional anesthesia, including being used as the sole anesthetic (stand-alone), as a component of a balanced general anesthesia technique, or for effective postoperative pain control. In addition, regional block procedures in this area can serve both in a diagnostic role and for the therapeutic management of acute and chronic pain syndromes. Head and neck regional blockade is effective in the management of somatic pain, and the techniques can range from local infiltration to field blocks to specific nerve blocks. This chapter briefly reviews the major clinical uses of head and neck regional anesthesia with respect to the wide range of relevant surgical disciplines. Specific regional techniques are described in detail in Chapters 17–19, and are discussed in this chapter only where applicable.

OPHTHALMIC SURGERY

Conventional prerequisites for intraocular surgery under regional anesthesia are globe and conjunctival anesthesia; globe, lid, and periorbital akinesia; and intraocular hypotonia (1). Because of the widespread use of phacoemulsification techniques, surgical requests for total akinesia and lowered intraocular pressure have decreased (2). Despite retrobulbar anesthesia being originally regarded as the gold standard in ocular anesthesia, major complications of the technique are well documented (3). These include globe perforation, retinal vascular occlusion, retrobulbar hemorrhage, optic nerve damage, and even cardiac and respiratory arrest (4–6). Greater emphasis is now placed on safety during eye block, and this has led to the evolution of several newer techniques, even at the price of incomplete akinesia. These techniques may be beneficial in anterior segment surgery, in particular cataract surgery, which 2 million patients undergo each year in the United States (7). However, some surgeons may express a wish for more complete anesthesia, especially for posterior segment surgery and for individual patients. Analgesic requirements are highest for evisceration and less so in order from enucleation through to ablation surgery, glaucoma surgery, complicated cataract surgery, and uncomplicated cataract surgery (8).

Eye Surgery

Classically, retrobulbar anesthesia is assumed to be more successful than peribulbar anesthesia. If a sufficient volume of injectate is used however, both techniques appear to have sim-

ilar efficacies (9). The Atkinson "up and in" position of gaze for retrobulbar anesthesia was abandoned when Liu and co-workers (10) and Unsold and co-workers (11) demonstrated that this position placed the optic nerve nearer the path of the needle and increased the risk of nerve injury. Patients are now asked to hold the eye in the primary or neutral position (10,12,13). Some advocate for the addition of a facial nerve block with retrobulbar anesthesia to prevent blinking due to the extraocular course of the superior branch of the facial nerve to the orbicularis oculi muscle (see Figs. 19-6–19-9) (14). However, when hyaluronidase is used with local anesthetics in higher volume, effective spread through the orbital septum occurs, resulting in complete eyelid immobility (15).

Peribulbar anesthesia appears less hazardous by avoiding the risk of injury to the major structures in the intraconal space. This superiority in safety has never been proven because of the very low rate of complications and subsequent lack of power of comparative studies (2). A larger volume is needed with peribulbar anesthesia (6–12 mL) to allow spread into the intraconal space, and to the lids to provide block of the orbicularis muscle and lids immobility. The classical technique for peribulbar anesthesia involves two injections, inferotemporal and supernasal. Comparative studies confirm that a single-injection technique is effective, provided the volume of injection is sufficient (16) (see Fig. 19-12). Some authors recommend avoiding the superior nasal injection site as the distance between the orbital roof and the globe is reduced at this location, thus increasing the risk of perforation (17). The medial canthus is proposed as an alternative puncture site, and a second injection may be performed here for supplementary anesthesia in the case of a failed first injection. Spread of local anesthetic within the corpus adiposum of the orbit is unpredictable, and an additional injection is required in up to 50% of peribulbar blocks in order to achieve akinesia (18,19). This is the main disadvantage of peribulbar anesthesia (20).

Perforation of the globe has an incidence of between one in 350 and seven in 50,000 cases (21,22). The principal risk factors are physician inexperience and a highly myopic eye (22). Edge and Navon demonstrated that myopic staphyloma was the greatest risk factor (21). Vohra and Good, using B-mode ultrasound, observed that the incidence of staphyloma is greater in highly myopic than in slightly myopic eyes (23). Thus an ultrasound measurement of the globe should be performed and if the axial length is greater than 26 mm, then retrobulbar block is contraindicated.

Sub-Tenon or episcleral anesthesia places local anesthetic solution into the episcleral space. One technique that has been described involves a surgical approach using blunt scissors and a curved cannula to infiltrate the sub-Tenon canal through the conjunctiva at the inferonasal quadrant, allowing the local anesthetic to spread circumferentially around the scleral part of the globe (see Fig. 19-19) (24). High-quality analgesia is produced with relatively low volumes (3–5 mL), and the use of higher volumes (8–11 mL) causes spread to the extraocular muscles, producing effective akinesia (25–28). Briggs and co-workers performed a comparative study between peribulbar and sub-Tenon anesthesia for cataract surgery. They conclude that sub-Tenon anesthesia reduces the overall level of discomfort associated with the administration of local anesthetic compared with the peribulbar method, in addition to providing superior intraoperative pain control (29). Several prospective studies have found that sub-Tenon anesthesia is as effective or better than retrobulbar injection for cataract surgery (30–33) or vitreoretinal surgery (34). Roman and co-workers investigated the complications associated with sub-Tenon anesthesia in 109 patients, 76 of whom were having cataract surgery. The investigators reported chemosis involving one quadrant in 39.4% of patients and conjunctival hemorrhages in 56% of patients (35). The occurrence of chemosis is associated with the injection of higher volumes (2). The surgical approach to sub-Tenon anesthesia appears to be the technique of choice as an intraoperative supplemental injection when initial anesthesia is insufficient (2). In a prospective study of 6,000 surgical sub-Tenon blocks, Guise reported no serious complications—7% of patients with subconjunctival hematoma and 6% with subconjunctival edema (36). This approach offers greater safety by avoiding the blind insertion of a needle into the orbit.

In recent years, topical anesthesia has become very popular for cataract surgery, being used in up to 50% of procedures in some series (7). However, intraoperative pain control appears to be more consistent when retrobulbar (37,38) or sub-Tenon anesthesia (39,40) is performed. Conversely, Johnston and colleagues, in a prospective study comparing topical and peribulbar anesthesia, report that topical anesthesia for phacoemulsification was well tolerated, but add that patient cooperation is an important factor in its success (41). In a prospective randomized comparison of peribulbar and topical anesthesia for cataract surgery, Sauder and Jonas (42) found that patient comfort and surgery-related complications did not differ between the two groups, and they recommend the use of topical anesthesia for routine cataract surgery. Ultimately, the use of topical anesthesia should be limited to uncomplicated surgery in cooperative patients. Topical anesthesia is inappropriate whenever phacoemulsification is not possible and total akinesia is required.

Intracameral injection of local anesthetic has been proposed as an adjunct to topical anesthesia but safety issues have been raised about local anesthetic toxicity to the corneal endothelium, which is incapable of regeneration. The American Academy of Ophthalmology in a report on intracameral anesthesia (43) recount the equivocal nature of studies investigating the effectiveness of the technique. It would appear that preservative-free lidocaine 1% is well tolerated by the corneal endothelium but that higher concentrations are toxic. They recommend the use of intracameral anesthesia for supplementary incremental analgesia for patients who cannot tolerate topical anesthesia alone. However, they stress that, although short-term studies seem to indicate safety, the long-term effects of intracameral anesthesia are unknown.

NEUROSURGERY

Neurosurgery under local anesthesia was originally introduced for surgical treatment of epilepsy during the 1930s. Regional anesthesia is performed to facilitate resection of abnormal brain tissue without damaging surrounding normal tissue. With the assistance of cortical mapping and a conscious patient, this goal can be readily achieved through observing the effects of stimulation on speech and movement areas. Another common procedure performed under local anesthesia is carotid endarterectomy (CEA).

Craniotomy

Requirements for craniotomy include sufficient depth of anesthesia during opening and closing of the bone flap, return to full consciousness during brain mapping, smooth transition between anesthesia and consciousness, as well as immobility and comfort throughout surgery (44). An asleep-awake-asleep technique is usually utilized (45,46).

A skull block involves regional anesthesia to the nerves that innervate the scalp, including the greater and lesser occipital nerves, the supraorbital and supratrochlear nerves, the zygomaticotemporal nerves, the auriculotemporal nerves, and the greater auricular nerves (Fig. 21-1; see also Figs. 17-2, 17-3, and 17-10) (47).

Girvin described his experience with local anesthesia for awake craniotomy using 60 mL of 0.33% bupivacaine with epinephrine 1:200,000 infiltrated into the scalp flap, plus an additional 12 mL of 0.5% bupivacaine for individual nerve blocks (48). More recently, a similar regional technique using ropivacaine up to 4.3 mg/kg with added epinephrine 5 μg/mL has been advocated to provide surgical anesthesia for awake craniotomy (49). Extensive blockade of the scalp bilaterally warranted minimal sedation, which the authors (49) suggest

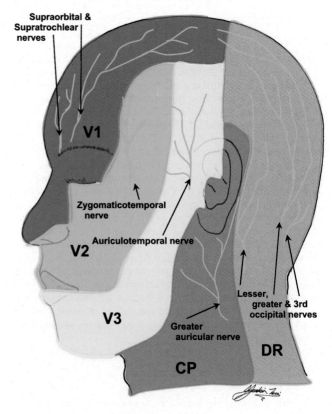

FIGURE 21-1. Skull block. Nerve block sites for regional anesthesia to nerves that innervate the scalp.

contrasts with other recognized awake craniotomy techniques that require a period of general anesthesia prior to the wake-up period.

Blanshard and co-workers reported retrospectively on the feasibility of performing craniotomy in awake patients for removal of intracranial tumors on an ambulatory basis. The investigators provided anesthesia using local infiltration with 2% lidocaine for insertion of the pins for rigid head fixation and 0.25% bupivacaine with epinephrine for the surgical incision. There was only one conversion to general anesthesia out of 241 patients. An overall morbidity rate of 32% was reported including neurologic, systemic, and regional complications. These results are comparable to those of a similar study of craniotomy under general anesthesia (50).

Pinosky advocates the use of a bupivacaine skull block to attenuate the hemodynamic response to craniotomy during general anesthesia (47). Insertion of cranial pins, incision, and periosteal–dural contact can result in tachycardia and hypertension, causing further increases in intracranial pressure (ICP) in patients with intracranial pathology and a higher risk of rupture of intravascular aneurysms. The requirement for additional anesthesia or vasoactive drugs was removed in patients who received a skull block with 0.5% bupivacaine.

The use of scalp nerve blocks has also been recommended to attenuate postoperative pain after craniotomy (51,52). Prospective studies report that 60% to 80% of patients experience moderate to severe pain after craniotomy (53,54). Data on the best analgesic method for this population are scarce. Intramuscular opioids or intravenous (IV) patient-controlled analgesia with morphine is associated with the side effect of sedation, which may be perceived as a neurosurgical complication. Nguyen and co-workers, in a prospective, randomized, and double-blind study reported on the successful use of a ropivacaine scalp block at skin closure, in patients undergoing supratentorial craniotomy (51). The supraorbital and supratrochlear nerves, auriculotemporal and postauricular branches of the greater auricular nerves, and the greater, lesser, and third occipital nerves were blocked using a total of 20 mL 0.75% ropivacaine. The analgesic effect lasted for 48 hours, as demonstrated using visual analog scale scores.

Blockade of the supraorbital and greater occipital nerves can facilitate frame placement during stereotactic neurosurgery (55). Watson and colleagues demonstrated that nerve blocks and subcutaneous infiltration provided comparable anesthesia for frame placement (56). Nerve blocks were less painful than infiltration at both frontal and orbital sites. Supraorbital nerve blocks were associated with more supplementation than either greater occipital nerve blocks or subcutaneous infiltration. Reasons given include straying of the frontal pin of the frame into the region supplied by the zygomaticotemporal nerve in addition to anomalous variation in the anatomy of the supraorbital nerve. The supraorbital nerve may exit the skull undivided, or its lateral and medial branches may exit separately. Failure to block the lateral branch may account for inadequate anesthesia during frame pin placement (57).

Carotid Endarterectomy

Carotid endarterectomy is the one of the most frequent surgical procedure performed to prevent ischemic stroke in patients with severe symptomatic stenosis (>70%–99%) of the extracranial internal carotid artery. A series of large, randomized controlled trials (ECST, NASCET) (58–60) have demonstrated the superiority of the procedure over medical therapy in this cohort, and it is of smaller but definite benefit in symptomatic

patients with 50% to 69% stenosis (American Academy Neurology Therapeutics and Technology Assessment). However, the procedure itself carries an inherent risk of stroke and mortality, estimated at 5% to 7 % within 30 days of surgery. If the perioperative risks could be reduced, the benefits from CEA would be greater. Regional anesthesia for CEA has been favored by some practitioners for over two decades, but whether it reduces the incidence of these risks remains unproven.

A recent body of evidence suggests that morbidity and mortality may be reduced if CEA is performed under regional anesthesia. Cerebral protection during carotid cross-clamping and the signs that herald hypoperfusion are the principal surgical issues of concern. The use of carotid artery stump pressure measurement, electroencephalogram (EEG), and transcranial Doppler of the middle cerebral artery may be used either alone or in combination to determine which patients require insertion of an internal carotid artery shunt to bypass the carotid cross-clamp. However, these measurements are neither sufficiently sensitive nor specific to accurately detect hypoperfusion, and many patients have their blood pressure pharmacologically elevated during carotid cross-clamping in an effort to maintain perfusion.

The conscious patient having the procedure performed under regional block acts as his own monitor of the adequacy of cerebral perfusion throughout. Any change in speech, cerebration, or motor function indicates the need for immediate shunting. This facilitates the use of selective shunting—some surgeons use a shunt in all CEAs under general anesthesia. Studies (61–63) suggest a rate of shunting as low as 10% to 15% in procedures carried out under a regional procedure, which may improve morbidity, as shunting itself carries a risk of stroke (64).

Other advantages of a regional technique include lower cardiovascular morbidity (65), shorter ICU and overall hospital stays, and less expense (66). However, there is insufficient evidence from randomized trials comparing regional and general techniques to prove that one technique is superior to the other. Nonrandomized studies suggest potential benefits as outlined, but these studies may be biased (65).

Regional anesthesia for CEA requires blockade of the second (C2) to the fourth (C4) cervical dermatomes. This may be performed by using a superficial cervical plexus block, a combination of superficial and deep cervical plexus blocks, or, less commonly, by cervical epidural. Most practitioners appear to favor a combination of deep and superficial blocks. The deep block may be performed by single injection at C3 or C4, as described originally by Winnie and co-workers (67), or by the standard three-injection technique (see Fig. 17-11) (68).

Stoneham and colleagues compared the efficacy of superficial block alone with deep block alone (69). No differences were found between the blocks in terms of the amount of supplemental local anesthetic required, although this was influenced by the presence or absence of paresthesia during placement of the deep block. Paresthesiae occurring during deep cervical plexus block placement resulted in a more effective block. In two prospective randomized studies comparing superficial versus combined (superficial and deep) cervical plexus block, no differences were detected in terms of the need for supplemental local anesthesia (70,71). The deep branches of the cervical plexus supplying the neck muscles are not anesthetized with a superficial block. This in theory may lead to difficulty operating on deep structures because of the absence of neuromuscular block. However, there is little evidence to support this (72).

A number of case series support the use of cervical epidural anesthesia (73–76). However, there is a high incidence of associated cardiovascular morbidity, respiratory failure requiring intubation in 1%, dural puncture in 0.5%, and alterations in pulmonary function in all recipients (66). Therefore its use is not widely advocated. A single-injection posterior cervical paravertebral block and interscalene cervical plexus block using a nerve stimulator have been successfully used (77,78).

Several potentially life-threatening complications may arise from deep cervical plexus blockade. These include vertebral artery, subarachnoid, or epidural injection. Phrenic nerve palsy leading to hemidiaphragmatic paresis (79) is a common occurrence and may lead to respiratory embarrassment in patients with underlying pulmonary disease. Other well-described complications include Horner syndrome (80,81), stellate ganglion block (66), and hoarseness due to recurrent laryngeal nerve block. There are a number of reports of complete respiratory obstruction due to preexisting contralateral recurrent laryngeal nerve block (82,83). There is no evidence to suggest that a single-injection technique is safer that a three-injection technique or vice-versa (67).

Common problems encountered during CEA usually relate to sedation or incomplete block. Intravenous sedation may lead to obtundation and hypoventilation or agitation. Small-dose IV clonidine may offer an advantage as an adjunct, as well as decreasing the incidence of postoperative hypertension (84). The most common reason for incomplete block is usually incisional pain near the midline mediated by contralateral fibers. Local anesthetic infiltration by the surgeon usually minimizes this problem. Occasionally, pain is experienced during dissection of the carotid sheath, pain which may be mediated by fibers from the ansa cervicalis or vagus nerves (72,85). Again, this is usually alleviated by local anesthetic supplementation. Pain caused by dissection high in the neck or by metal retractors is not prevented by cervical plexus block but may be ameliorated by performing a mandibular nerve block (86).

SURGERY TO THE ORAL CAVITY AND NASOPHARYNX

Interventional skills and mastery of the airway are crucial for all anesthesiologists, and airway blockade is one of most important regional blocks to perfect to accomplish these goals. Other common procedures in which regional anesthesia is useful include tonsillectomy and endonasal surgery.

Airway

Awake fiberoptic intubation is a well-established technique in the management of the anticipated difficult airway (87,88). Advantages of this technique of airway control include patient cooperation, spontaneous respiration throughout the procedure, and maintenance of airway patency through conscious control of the airway muscles (89). Several techniques for providing airway anesthesia have been described, including direct application of local anesthetics to the respiratory mucosa using sprays and nebulizers, as well as a variety of nerve blocks. Being airway experts and frequently called upon in the management of difficult airways, these techniques are extremely important for all anesthesiologists in their clinical practices.

A good working knowledge of the neuroanatomy of the nasal and oral cavities, the pharynx, larynx, and trachea is important when manipulating the airway in the awake state. The nasal cavity is entirely innervated by branches of the trigeminal nerve (90). The anterior parts of the nasal cavity and septum are supplied by the anterior ethmoidal nerve, which itself is a branch of the ophthalmic nerve. The remainder of the nasal cavity receives its innervation from branches of the maxillary nerve. The glossopharyngeal nerve provides sensation to the posterior third of the tongue, the fauces and tonsils, the epiglottis, and all of the pharynx. The superior laryngeal nerve arises from the vagus nerve before dividing into internal and external branches. The external branch provides motor innervation to the cricothyroid muscle. The internal branch provides visceral sensory and secretomotor innervation to the larynx above the vocal cords. The recurrent laryngeal nerve, also a branch of the vagus nerve, provides sensory innervation to the laryngeal mucous membranes inferior to the vocal cords and to the upper trachea. It provides motor innervation to all of the laryngeal musculature except the cricothyroid (91).

These nerves participate in a number of brainstem-controlled reflex pathways concerning airway protection (89). The gag reflex is initiated by mechanical and chemical stimulation of areas innervated by the glossopharyngeal nerve (92). A selective bilateral block of the glossopharynx can abolish conduction in the afferent limb of the gag reflex and greatly increase the chances of a successful awake intubation (93). The laryngeal closure reflex can be stimulated by irritation of the sensory area innervated by the internal branch of the superior laryngeal nerve. This reflex can be attenuated by either topical anesthesia or direct nerve blocks (93). The cough reflex is relayed by sensory afferents from the trachea and larynx in the internal branch of the superior laryngeal nerve and the recurrent laryngeal nerve. This can also be blocked by both direct nerve blocks and topical anesthesia (93). The cardiovascular reflex response to airway manipulation is hypertension, tachycardia, and bradycardia. Laryngeal and glottic receptors are responsible for increased sympathetic activity with stimulation of the airway mucosa. This is relayed to the brainstem via the corresponding cranial nerve innervating these areas. The cardiovascular response may be blocked by targeting mechanoreceptor stimulation using topical or regional anesthesia (93).

There is considerable debate in the literature about the most effective means of achieving adequate airway anesthesia. Topical anesthesia may be applied indirectly by spraying with a nebulizer or atomizer, or it may applied directly by swabbing, gargling, inhaling, or via the fiberoptic bronchoscope itself (89). The two most common local anesthetic techniques used to provide anesthesia are the superior laryngeal nerve block for the supraglottic larynx and the transtracheal injection for subglottic structures. The glossopharyngeal nerve block is very effective for obtunding the gag reflex but is not often used in clinical practice. Reasoner and co-workers compared topical anesthesia and nerve blocks for awake intubation in neurosurgical patients with cervical spine instability. Topical anesthesia was administered using nebulized 4% lidocaine (20 mL) and transtracheal injection of 4% lidocaine (3 mL). Nerve block patients underwent bilateral glossopharyngeal and superior laryngeal nerve blocks with 2% lidocaine in addition to a transtracheal injection of 4% lidocaine. They found no difference in patient perception of discomfort during the procedure (94). Similarly, Kundra and co-workers compared nebulized 4% lidocaine with combined superior laryngeal and transtracheal nerve blocks and demonstrated better patient comfort and hemodynamic stability with the combined nerve block technique. However, they failed to show a difference between the two groups with respect to intubating conditions (95). Conversely, Graham and colleagues reported better laryngotracheal anesthesia following translaryngeal injection of lidocaine when compared to nebulization.

Many authors recognize the potential for toxic plasma levels of lidocaine with topical application owing to the relatively large amounts of concentrated solutions used (95,96). It is believed, however, that a large amount of the drug is "wasted" (97), with one group working on the assumption that up to 75% of the nebulized drug is lost (98). The toxic plasma concentration of lidocaine is widely accepted as 5 mg/L (96,99–101), and side effects are reported to develop when concentrations reach 4 mg /L. Recent guidelines issued by the British Thoracic Society suggest the total dose of lidocaine applied during bronchoscopy should be limited to 8.2 mg/kg (101).

The glossopharyngeal nerve block can be performed by using either an intraoral or a peristyloid approach (102). If the intraoral approach is used, the patient must have sufficient mouth-opening so that visualization of the posterior tonsillar pillar is possible. Benumof (88) described the use of an anterior tonsillar pillar injection that has been advocated elsewhere because of better exposure to the anterior tonsillar pillar in cases of limited mouth opening and better patient tolerance (103). The peristyloid approach does not rely on reliability of mouth opening but requires access to the lateral neck and the ability to recognize bony landmarks (89) (see Fig. 17-8).

The internal branch of the superior laryngeal nerve may be blocked by either an anterior or a lateral approach (104). Furlan (104), in a study of 50 human cadavers, demonstrated the proximity of the superior laryngeal nerve to the greater cornu of the hyoid bone. The mean distance from internal superior laryngeal nerve to the greater horn of the hyoid bone in a craniocaudal direction was 2.4 mm. The lateral approach uses the greater cornu of the hyoid bone as the target from which the needle is directed inferiorly and advanced 2 to 3 mm, so that the tip rests between the thyrohyoid membrane laterally and the laryngeal mucosa medially (89) (Fig. 17-8). Using an anterior approach, the needle is walked in a cephalad direction off the superior cornu of the thyroid cartilage. Recognized complications include vasovagal response (105,106), which may be explained by spread of local anesthetic to the carotid bulb or the main trunk of the vagus.

Alternative uses for nerve blocks used in providing anesthesia for awake intubation have been described. Sulica and Blitzer reported using bilateral superior laryngeal nerve blocks and transtracheal injection to provide anesthesia for office-based laryngeal surgery including soft tissue biopsy and CO_2 laser ablation of respiratory tract papilloma (105). Superior laryngeal blocks have been used in the treatment and prevention of laryngospasm and stridor (107) and to facilitate placement of transesophageal echocardiography probes (108,109).

Tonsillectomy

Post tonsillectomy pain can be severe and remains a significant obstacle to rapid recovery. The pain in adult patients is maximal in the first 5 days (110) and in children a return to normal activity and diet may take up to 12 days (111).

Reported benefits of local anesthetic techniques include diminished perioperative bleeding, postsurgical pain, and nausea in addition to improved surgical planes of dissection (112–117). However, there are numerous conflicting reports regarding the efficacy of regional anesthesia for post tonsillectomy analgesia.

The tonsillar bed receives innervation from a number of sources known collectively as the circulus tonsillaris (118). The nerves involved are the glossopharyngeal nerve, branches from the lesser palatine nerves, and branches from the lingual nerve.

Since there is no uniform approach for blocking this area, most practitioners describe a variation of the glossopharyngeal nerve block.

In the most comprehensive review to date of several randomized trials Hollis and co-workers (119) concluded that recent studies of injection of local anesthetic were too small and did not show a benefit to the practice. In addition, sites of injection are not well described in most studies, ranging from the somewhat vague peritonsillar injection to glossopharyngeal nerve block.

Regional anesthesia for tonsillectomy has been associated with several adverse events. There are several anecdotal reports of inadvertent vagal nerve blockade (120,121), recurrent laryngeal nerve paralysis (122–124), and hypoglossal nerve paralysis (125) as well as dyspnea of unknown etiology. These complications are more than likely related to using larger doses of local anesthetic solution in the confined space of the lateral pharyngeal fossa (126). This space has no structures to limit the spread of local anesthetic. Therefore, it is not surprising to read reports of partial or complete bilateral recurrent laryngeal nerve paralysis leading to vocal cord adduction and bilateral hypoglossal nerve paralysis leading to loss of motor function of the tongue. It has been suggested that smaller volumes of local anesthetic are appropriate, especially in children (12–25 kg), in whom 1 mL of 0.25% bupivacaine is reported to be safe and effective (126).

Sinonasal Surgery

Advances in minimally invasive nasal surgery techniques have been associated with an increased frequency of endonasal surgery over the past 20 years (127). The use of local anesthesia is well established for most rhinologic procedures (128). In addition, reduction of nasal fractures can be performed under regional or local anesthesia. Many of these procedures are carried out on an ambulatory basis, and evidence suggests that operative times, postanesthesia recovery times, and complications during sinonasal surgery are less when local anesthesia is employed (129).

Most studies investigating nasal fracture manipulation report using local infiltration techniques rather than individual nerve blocks (130–133). This usually consists of a combination of intranasal spray, topical paste, and interalar injection or a so-called *hematoma block*. Evidence in support of external nasal fixation under local anesthesia is anecdotal in nature and hence there is no clear consensus on the issue (133). Available studies suggest a favorable surgical outcome (132–134) in terms of progression to open surgical correction. Patient discomfort has been likened to that of a minor dental procedure, and satisfaction ratings range from 69% (134) to 92% (135).

Evidence comparing local infiltration versus individual nerve blockade is sparse and conflicting. One study comparing combined infraorbital and infratrochlear nerve blocks with external infiltration revealed the internal route to be significantly more painful with no advantage in terms of nasal patency or cosmesis (136). Conversely, a different study investigating combined nasociliary and infraorbital nerve blocks in 24 patients for nasal surgery found that the blocks were technically easy to perform, with high patient satisfaction and minor complications. Because adrenaline is not used to avoid retinal artery spasm, the authors suggest blocking the nasociliary nerve before the infraorbital nerve block. No major complications were reported, and swelling of the eyelid, the more common side effect of nasociliary block can be prevented by local pressure during injection.

It has been suggested that endoscopic sinus surgery is safer in the conscious patient because of the patient's ability to report ocular pain from orbital penetration. Infiltrative local anesthesia has been an accepted surgical technique for sinus surgery in selected patients. It is indicated for surgery of the maxillary sinus, frontoethmoidal recess, and anterior and posterior ethmoid cells (137). Fedok and co-workers report shorter recovery times with less epistaxis, nausea, and emesis using local infiltration (129). Infraorbital nerve block in combination with general anesthesia has been described to reduce blood pressure and alleviate postoperative pain for endoscopic sinus surgery (138). Sphenopalatine nerve block has also been documented for this surgery (139).

PLASTIC SURGERY

Individual nerve blocks have been described for cutaneous laser resurfacing and repairs of facial lacerations and cleft lips. Current trends in cosmetic surgical procedures of the face suggest that local infiltration is still popular, but an organized approach to regional blockade using clear anatomic landmarks can lead to complete facial anesthesia (140). Otoplasty is another common plastic surgery that is amenable to regional anesthesia.

Regional Anesthesia of the Face

The safety profile of dermatologic surgery performed without the need to resort to general anesthesia appeals to both patient and surgeon. A combination of tumescent local infiltration and nerve block anesthesia has been described for full-face laser resurfacing (141). This involves a "horseshoe" subcutaneous infiltration bilaterally beginning at the temporal hairline and extending sequentially to the preauricular area, jawline, and chin. Upper and lower eyelids and nose are also infiltrated with tumescent local anesthesia. Supraorbital, supratrochlear, infratrochlear, and mental nerve blocks are then given (see Figs. 17-3 and 17-12, and Figs. 19–13 to 19–18). A criticism of this technique is the frequent failure to obtain complete facial anesthesia with local infiltration. It has been suggested that anatomically based block methods would increase the probability of full anesthesia being achieved (142,143).

Peripheral blocks of the terminal branches of the trigeminal nerve offer a safe and effective alternative to local infiltration for soft-tissue injury of the face (140,144). There is a paucity of evidence in this regard but one retrospective study of 59 patients investigated the failure rate and side effects associated with blocks of the supraorbital, supratrochlear, nasociliary, infraorbital, and mental nerves (145). In this study, 22% of patients had incomplete anesthesia in the surgical area, which was rectified by additional local infiltration. The failures occurred with the supraorbital and infraorbital nerve blocks. The authors attribute this to a less than full understanding of the sensory innervation of the face. The intraoral route for blockade of the infraorbital nerve is thought to be more reliable than the external percutaneous approach (146,147). However, a comparison of both approaches—the intraoral route on one side of the face and the percutaneous route on the other—failed to demonstrate any difference between the techniques (146).

Infraorbital nerve block can provide analgesia after cleft lip repair (148). This is a common procedure in infants, and it is important to ensure that the child is pain-free in the postoperative period as surgical dehiscence may result from vigorous crying (149). Conversely, profound respiratory depression has been reported after opioid administration (150). Hence, the requirement for a form of adequate analgesia without the risk of respiratory depression (151,152). Peri-incisional infiltration has been used with varied results (153), but it may cause distortion of the repair.

Adult landmarks used to perform infraorbital nerve blocks are absent or difficult to palpate in the neonate and, by the same token, the neonatal facial configuration is different from that in the adult. Concern about correct needle placement is ever present, especially when using an intraoral route. In one cadaveric study, it has been suggested that the infraorbital nerve lies halfway between the midpoint of the palpebral fissure and the angle of the mouth (153). The authors report good clinical correlation. Computerized tomographic evidence suggests a linear relationship between age and distance of the infraorbital foramen from the midline.

Otoplasty

Otoplasty is an elective cosmetic procedure generally performed on healthy pediatric patients. A high incidence of severe pain and vomiting occurs, particularly on the first postoperative day (154–156). Moreover, opioid analgesia exacerbates postoperative nausea and vomiting (PONV) and delays early resumption of diet in addition to causing excessive sedation.

The pinna of the ear is supplied by branches of the cervical plexus and the trigeminal nerve. The posterior surface and the lower third of the anterior surface are supplied by the great auricular and the lesser occipital nerves, branches of the cervical plexus. The upper two-thirds of the anterior surface is innervated by the auriculotemporal nerve, a branch of the mandibular division of the trigeminal nerve (see Fig. 17-12).

Postoperative pain may be controlled by regional anesthesia (157,158) and local infiltration (159,160). By blocking the great auricular and lesser occipital nerves, Burtles and co-workers (154) found a reduction in opioid use with an associated reduction in the incidence of PONV. The block was performed using bupivacaine 0.25% or 0.5% to a maximum of 2 mg/kg. Regional nerve blockade has been compared with an infiltrative technique by Cregg and co-workers (161). The greater auricular and lesser occipital nerves were blocked by injecting 0.4 mL/kg 0.5% bupivacaine subcutaneously from the angle of the mandible to the mastoid process. In addition, the auriculotemporal nerve was blocked by injection over the posterior aspect of the zygoma. When comparing with opioid alone, this study found both regional and infiltrative techniques were comparable forms of analgesia for otoplasty but with a lower requirement for opioids and incidence of PONV. Local infiltration has also been used for surgical anesthesia. In 1985, Atwood and Evans advocated the use of local anesthesia as an acceptable alternative to general anesthesia in selected adult and pediatric cases (162). Lancaster and co-workers (163) reported on a retrospective comparison of general and infiltrative anesthesia. In the local anesthesia group, percutaneous infiltration comprised a circumauricular block followed by infiltration to both surfaces of the pinna. Despite infiltration being well tolerated, there was no demonstrable difference in surgical outcome and there was a highly significant difference in postoperative vomiting in favor of the infiltrative technique.

SURGERY TO THE NECK

Various regional anesthesia techniques can form a basis for superficial surgical anesthesia procedures to the head and neck.

Procedures such as sebaceous cyst excision, scar revision, skin excision, and lymph node biopsy can rely on anesthesia through simple local infiltration or field blocks. Minimally invasive surgical procedures of the neck, involving structures such as the parathyroid and thyroid glands, as well as the previously discussed carotid artery (CEA) have been gaining popularity as more surgeons and anesthesiologists gain related experience.

Parathyroid Surgery

Primary hyperparathyroidism can be attributed to a solitary benign adenoma in 80% of cases (164). To date, bilateral neck exploration under general anesthesia has been the preferred surgical management (165). Technological preoperative imaging advances including sestamibi scintigraphy in addition to intraoperative parathyroid hormone measurement has led to the development of minimally invasive techniques through a small unilateral incision under regional anesthesia (164–168). Patients suitable for minimally invasive surgery should have a nonfamilial form of hyperthyroidism, no previous thyroid or parathyroid surgery, no previous neck irradiation, and no suspicion of malignancy (165).

Not surprisingly, a similar diversity of regional techniques as that described for minimally invasive thyroidectomy has been reported in the literature. This range includes local infiltration, and superficial and deep cervical plexus blocks either alone or in various combinations. Cervical epidural anesthesia has been proposed in one series (169).

The most common approach is that described by Lo Gerfo's group and cited by others (165,166,170,171). According to an initial report from Lo Gerfo's group, this involves a combination of C2–C4 superficial cervical plexus block, infiltration along the incision line, and infiltration of the upper thyroid pedicle (170) (see Fig. 17-11). However, various descriptions of technique, including a modified deep/superficial cervical blockade (e.g., using needle insertion similar to the deep plexus block at each of C2 and C3, yet withdrawing the needle to place anesthetic in the space between the sternocleidomastoid muscle and the transverse processes; Fig. 17–11) have been reported (171,172). It seems as though incorporating both superficial and deep plexus blockade may be needed for successful anesthesia. Of additional importance, Lo Gerfo's group also pointed out that the upper pole of the thyroid was the most important area to extensively infiltrate with local anesthetic (170).

In the largest study of its kind to date, Carling and colleagues reported on 441 patients who underwent minimally invasive parathyroidectomy under superficial cervical plexus and local field block (164); 10.6% of patients required conversion to general anesthesia. The most common reasons for conversion were unrecognized concomitant thyroid pathology. This was followed by multiglandular parathyroid hyperplasia, as heralded by a less than 50% drop in parathyroid hormone levels requiring conversion to general anesthesia and more extensive bilateral exploration. Other reasons for conversion to general anesthesia included difficulty ensuring adequate protection of the recurrent laryngeal nerve, patient discomfort, and intraoperative diagnosis of parathyroid carcinoma requiring bilateral exploration. Bilateral deep cervical plexus block has been described without complication (165) to enable bilateral exploration but is not widely recommended because of the inherent danger of bilateral phrenic nerve block.

Comparisons with bilateral exploration under general anesthesia are favorable with respect to cure rates (166,168). Signif-

icantly shorter anesthetic and operative times leading to early hospital discharge (166,168) have been reported with regional anesthesia techniques regardless of approach. Reduced hospital costs (166) and significantly better postoperative pain relief (165) are also known advantages.

Thyroid Surgery

Thyroid surgery is usually performed under general anesthesia in contemporary practice but historically regional anesthesia played a far greater role. In 1907, Sir Thomas Peel Dunhill reported a series of seven thyroidectomies for toxic goiter under regional anesthesia (173,174), and by 1932, G. W. Crile had performed more than 20,000 thyroidectomies in the conscious patient (175). As the safety profile of general anesthesia improved, the need for regional anesthesia for thyroid surgery became redundant. Over the past 20 years there has been a renewal of interest in regional anesthesia for thyroid surgery. This is related to the development of minimally invasive approaches to thyroid and parathyroid surgery in addition to the refinement of cervical plexus block techniques. Anesthesia may be successfully achieved either by cervical plexus block (C2–C4) in combination with an anterior field block (176) or by anterior field block alone (177). Subsequent success or failure is dependent on adaptation of a minimally invasive surgical technique in conjunction with patient cooperation.

Indications for regional anesthesia for thyroid surgery have evolved with surgical experience with the procedure. Initially deemed unsuitable, patients with moderate substernal goiter, clinical regional thyroid cancer, and previous neck surgery are now being considered in some centers (176). Contraindications include recurrent laryngeal nerve paralysis, retrotracheal or retroesophageal goiter, cervical lymphadenopathy, and locally invasive tumor (176). Minimally invasive thyroid surgery may be indicated in 5% to 35% of patients requiring thyroid surgery, depending on surgical technique and fine needle aspiration cytology (178).

Favorable results have been reported with superficial cervical plexus block alone (179), anterior field block alone (180), or a combination of the two techniques (176). The superficial plexus block is a relatively easy technique to learn and, being a sensory block, it may be performed bilaterally (181). In a prospective randomized study comparing the efficacy of anterior field block alone versus general anesthesia, Snyder and co-workers reported similar operative and clinical results in 58 patients undergoing thyroidectomy (180). In a comparison of superficial cervical block and general anesthesia in 175 patients undergoing thyroidectomy, Specht and co-workers found no difference between the two groups in terms of anesthetic efficacy (179).

Reported complications with the superficial cervical plexus block are usually related to deep supplemental injection in cases of failure of superficial plexus blockade. Phrenic nerve paralysis leading to diaphragmatic dysfunction (69), vagus nerve block with resultant recurrent nerve paralysis (179), and inadvertent intravascular injection have been reported (182).

The most extensive series on thyroid surgery under locoregional anesthesia has been conducted by Lo Gerfo, who reported on 1,025 cases over 16 years (176). A combination of superficial cervical plexus and anterior field block was utilized. Patients with substernal goiter and extensive cancer accounted for two-third of cases converted to general anesthesia; 20% (34 patients) of converted cases were directly related to regional anesthesia. Three patients developed agitation and anxiety, three developed laryngospasm due to laryngeal pressure, and one patient had inadvertent intra-arterial injection of local anesthetic.

Among the benefits of locoregional anesthesia, Lo Gerfo cites avoidance of general anesthesia in high-risk patients. He reports nine patients in his series with amiodarone-induced hyperthyroidism or Graves disease who were successfully managed using a regional technique. Patient satisfaction is positive (183), and reports of the postoperative analgesic efficacy of cervical plexus blockade are for the most part encouraging (184,185). In addition, the potential for early discharge of selected patients after shorter inpatient times has been reported (179,186).

Any reduction in operative and recovery time with any resultant economic benefit must be balanced against the potential for life-threatening complications associated with thyroidectomy. The problems encountered by patients undergoing local thyroid surgery are no different from those occurring after general anesthesia (176,178).

The three principal complications are wound hematoma and airway obstruction, hypocalcemia, and recurrent laryngeal nerve injury. These must be taken into account if a six-hour discharge time is implemented.

CHRONIC PAIN

Regional anesthesia has both diagnostic and therapeutic roles in the management of chronic pain of the head and neck including headache, trigeminal neuralgia, intractable cancer pain, and postherpetic pain.

Occipital Nerve Block

The use of peripheral nerve blockade for the management of primary headache syndromes is well documented (187,188). The greater occipital nerve block is reported with greatest frequency for this purpose, whereas the lesser occipital and supraorbital blocks are used occasionally (189). Patients with chronic headache complain of pain affecting both the trigeminally innervated anterior regions of the head and the posterior region innervated by the greater occipital nerve (190). The bilocational nature of chronic headache may be due to the convergence of trigeminal and cervical sensory fibers upon the trigeminal nucleus caudalis (191) (see also Chapter 41).

Greater occipital nerve block has been used for a variety of headache syndromes including cervicogenic headache, occipital neuralgia, migraine, and cluster headache (192). However, only a small number of studies determine the efficacy of nerve blocks for headache management (187,188,190,193,194). The duration of response exceeded local anesthetic effect, as also reported by Caputi and Firetto (187). The therapeutic effect was maintained for the 6-month period of observation. It has been suggested that this prolonged duration of effect may be due to changes in brain nociceptive pathways (190). Gawel and Rothbart demonstrated the efficacy of greater occipital nerve block in combination with corticosteroid injection for patients with refractory migraine and posttraumatic headache; 72% of the posttraumatic patients and 54% of migraine patients were significantly improved up to 6 months after the block (188). Peres and co-workers, in a study of patients with cervicogenic headache, demonstrated a 64% positive response to greater occipital nerve block combined with corticosteroid injection (194). Occipital nerve block and occipital nerve stimulation and the oncologic applications of occipital nerve block are discussed in Chapters 41, 42 and 44.

Trigeminal Neuralgia

Sporadic case reports are available in the literature of the use of local anesthetic blocks for the treatment of trigeminal neuralgia, while the mainstay of treatment continues to be either pharmacologic or neuroablative (Chapter 42). A standard (single-injection) block that anesthetizes the facial region containing the sensitive trigger zone may result in a reduction in attacks for prolonged periods of time, often outlasting the duration of the anesthetic agent used (195,196). Umino and co-workers describe the use of an indwelling mandibular nerve catheter in a single patient for long-term pain control in trigeminal neuralgia (197). They cite the usefulness of this technique as a temporizing measure in patients scheduled to undergo microvascular decompression. Local anesthetic blockade is reversible and only mildly toxic, in contrast to the potential toxic effects of neurolytic blocks using glycerol and alcohol.

Sphenopalatine Ganglion Block

Sphenopalatine ganglion block can be used to treat headache and facial pain. Transnasal, transoral, and lateral approaches may be used (198). The transnasal application of topical anesthetic is the simplest and best tolerated of the three approaches (see Fig. 17–5) (199–201). It can easily be performed with a cotton-tipped applicator soaked with local anesthetic (202). The potential for sloughing of the nasal mucosa during needle insertion has been reported (203), which led to the development of a transnasal endoscopic technique (204). However, unpredictable diffusion of anesthetic to the ganglion may occur with this approach, and analgesia is not long lasting (205). Varghese and Koshy (206) describe the successful use of endoscopic transnasal neurolytic sphenopalatine ganglion blockade with phenol for head and neck cancer pain. Cohen and colleagues (207) describe using a transnasal approach with eutectic mixture of local anesthetic (EMLA) cream for parturients with tension headache and migraine during the labor and postpartum period. With the transoral approach, the needle may pass beyond the sphenoid to anesthetize other structures (203,208). The lateral infratemporal approach depends on imaging guidance for its success (199,203,209).

DENTAL APPLICATIONS

Neural blockade of oral and circumoral structures is discussed at length in Chapter 18. This section briefly describes nuances in the selection of a specific peripheral block (including reasons for failed block and block supplementation) to provide anesthesia to dental structures.

It is widely believed by convention that innervation of the maxillary teeth comes from three nerves: the anterior, middle, and posterior superior alveolar nerves. However, in many people, the middle superior alveolar nerve, which is associated with premolar innervation, is missing (210,211). In this case, the premolar and canine region is innervated by the posterior superior alveolar nerve, but no anatomic predictors are present for this pattern of innervation (212). A further anatomic irregularity in the premolar area is the zygomaticoalveolar crest. This is a bony prominence that approaches the apices of the premolar teeth and may prevent infiltrative anesthesia. The posterior superior alveolar nerve block can be used to anesthetize the maxillary molar teeth and is usually employed when infiltrative anesthesia is inadequate. Failure of this block may be associated with displaced branches of the posterior superior alveolar nerves entering the lingual aspect of the premolars, the palatal aspect of the molars, or both (213). A greater palatine nerve block may augment the effectiveness of a posterior superior alveolar block.

The mucosa of the hard palate and the palatal gingiva are innervated by the greater palatine nerve and nasopalatine nerves, respectively. It may occasionally be necessary to perform a nasopalatine nerve block to completely anesthetize the central incisors because nerve fibers from the superior alveolar plexus occasionally join the nasopalatine nerve below the nasal floor and travel with the nasopalatine nerve to the central incisor (212–215). The greater palatine foramen, through which a greater palatine nerve block is performed, is traditionally placed palatally opposite the second molar. Recent studies (216–218) have ascribed a more posterior location for this foramen, one study localizing it to an area opposite or slightly distal to the third molar (217). An ineffective posterior superior alveolar nerve block may be supplemented with a greater palatine injection, as mentioned earlier (214,215).

Unlike the maxilla, the mandible consists of dense cortical bone that makes infiltrative anesthesia less effective than that undertaken at corresponding maxillary teeth (219). The inferior alveolar nerve block is the most commonly used block in dentistry (220) but it has a relatively high failure rate of 15% to 30% (221,222). There are a number of reasons for the failure rate of this block (223). Poor block technique due to inadequate mouth opening or incorrect needle placement is the most common reason for failure (224). If mouth opening is inadequate, the inferior alveolar nerve is relaxed and at a distance from the medial wall of the mandibular ramus. When the mouth has opened adequately, the nerve is flush against the medial wall of the ramus and moves into the target area (224). Incorrectly placing the needle in front of or behind the target area is another common mistake (223) (Chapter 18).

Before it enters the mandibular foramen, the inferior alveolar nerve gives rise to the mylohyoid nerve (Fig. 21-2). This is primarily a motor nerve but has been shown to have a sensory component from some mandibular teeth. Because of this dual innervation, a conventional inferior alveolar nerve block may not be solely sufficient in achieving mandibular anesthesia. The mylohyoid nerve has been demonstrated to originate 14.7 mm from the mandibular foramen (225). This distance may be beyond the area of anesthetic spread in a conventional inferior alveolar nerve block. The Gow-Gates high mandibular block may be useful in this situation (Fig. 21-2). It is technically more difficult, but reports suggest a higher overall success rate when compared to conventional mandibular nerve blocks (220). The needle is introduced across the contralateral mandibular canine and directed across the mesiopalatal cusp of the ipsilateral upper second molar until bony contact is achieved. The point of bony contact is the condylar head just below the attachment of the lateral pterygoid muscle (226). The needle is withdrawn slightly before injection. A 20% to 30% increase in efficacy is reported when this technique is used (227) (Fig. 21-2; see also Figs. 18-17–18-19).

The presence of a bifid mandibular nerve has been reported in 0.1% (228) to 0.9% (229) of the population. It is easily detectable on panoramic radiographs due to the presence of an accessory mandibular foramen. An inferior alveolar nerve block may not be sufficient, as the nerve bifurcates before it enters the mandibular foramen. A Gow-Gates block may block the accessory nerve at or above its branch point. The presence of a retromolar foramen containing accessory innervation is thought to occur in a significant proportion of the population (230). This innervation may arise from either the long buccal

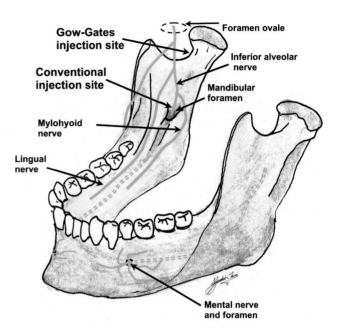

FIGURE 21-2. The Gow-Gates high mandibular block site as compared to the conventional inferior alveolar nerve block site. This site may improve mandibular anesthesia by incorporating the mylohyoid nerve.

nerve or accessory branches of the inferior alveolar nerve (231). Sufficient mandibular anesthesia should be achieved with a Gow-Gates block. Alternatively, a small amount of anesthetic can be injected directly into the tissue of the retromolar area (219).

A number of alternative approaches are possible to successful mandibular anesthesia when the conventional inferior alveolar nerve block fails. The closed-mouth or Akinosi block may be useful when the patient cannot open the mouth completely, for example during trismus (232,233). A separate buccal nerve block may be required to anesthetize the tissues buccal to the mandibular molars, as the buccal nerve may not be blocked in some cases (220) (Chapter 18).

SUMMARY

In summary, regional anesthesia is clinically useful for such broad applications as providing diagnostic and postoperative analgesia, as well as intraoperative anesthesia. Head and neck regional blockade can be of benefit for many situations, including: facilitating and transforming surgery into an outpatient procedure for certain patient groups (dental surgery, cataract, minor plastic procedures), providing optimal solitary anesthetic care for patients with comorbidities, and reducing the amount of opioids administered while maintaining or improving analgesia.

Regional nerve blockade for head and neck surgery may be used as the sole surgical anesthetic agent where indicated or when requested by the patient. Obviously, certain patients may not be suitable subjects for surgery under regional block, but may benefit from its use in combination with general anesthesia. If favorable results are to be ensured, meticulous attention must be paid to preoperative assessment and planning with respect to each particular surgery, careful intraoperative monitoring, and active postoperative care in any clinical situation.

Before each surgical procedure, the appropriate combination of specific nerve block with type, volume, and concentration of local anesthetic drug must be careful determined. Careful attention to titration, with the appropriate sedation, is paramount. Detailed explanation of the procedures involved and any expected complications (e.g., bruising from the injection site particularly on the face) should be provided to the patient or family members before any approach is initiated. Good communication skills are essential for every anesthesiologist attempting regional blockade for surgical anesthesia.

ACKNOWLEDGMENTS

Simplified anatomic drawings for this chapter were produced by and used with permission from Mr. Jenkin Tsui.

References

1. Hamilton RC. Techniques of orbital regional anaesthesia. *Br J Anaesth* 1995;75:88–92.
2. Ripart J, Nouvellon E, Chaumeron A. Regional anesthesia for eye surgery. *Reg Anesth Pain Med* 2005;30:72–82.
3. Ahmad S, Ahmad A. Complications of ophthalmologic nerve blocks: A review. *J Clin Anesth* 2003;15:564–569.
4. Morgan CM, Schatz H, Vine AK, et al. Ocular complications associated with retrobulbar injections. *Ophthalmology* 1988;95:660–665.
5. Capo H, Roth E, Johnson T, et al. Vertical strabismus after cataract surgery. *Ophthalmology* 1996;103:918–921.
6. Nicoll JM, Acharya PA, Ahlen K, et al. Central nervous system complications after 6000 retrobulbar blocks. *Anesth Analg* 1987;66:1298–1302.
7. Leaming DV. Practice styles and preferences of ASCRS members: 2003 survey. *J Cataract Refract Surg* 2004;30:892–900.
8. Kallio H, Rosenberg PH. Advances in ophthalmic regional anaesthesia. *Best Pract Res Clin Anaesthesiol* 2005;19:215–227.
9. Demediuk OM, Dhaliwal RS, Papworth DP, et al. A comparison of peribulbar and retrobulbar anesthesia for vitreoretinal surgical procedures. *Arch Ophthalmol* 1995;113:908–913.
10. Liu C, Youl B, Moseley I. Magnetic resonance imaging of the optic nerve in extremes of gaze. Implications for the positioning of the globe for retrobulbar anaesthesia. *Br J Ophthalmol* 1992;76:728–733.
11. Unsold R, Stanley JA, DeGroot J. The CT-topography of retrobulbar anesthesia. Anatomic-clinical correlation of complications and suggestion of a modified technique. *Albrecht Von Graefes Arch Klin Exp Ophthalmol* 1981;217:125–136.
12. Javitt JC, Addiego R, Friedberg HL, et al. Brain stem anesthesia after retrobulbar block. *Ophthalmology* 1987;94:718–724.
13. Pautler SE, Grizzard WS, Thompson LN, Wing GL. Blindness from retrobulbar injection into the optic nerve. *Ophthalmic Surg* 1986;17:334–337.
14. Allen ED, Elkington AR. Local anaesthesia and the eye. *Br J Anaesth* 1980;52:689–694.
15. Martin SR, Baker SS, Muenzler WS. Retrobulbar anesthesia and orbicularis akinesia. *Ophthalmic Surg* 1986;17:232–233.
16. Demirok A, Simsek S, Cinal A, Yasar T. Peribulbar anesthesia: One versus two injections. *Ophthalmic Surg Lasers* 1997;28:998–1001.
17. Hustead RF, Hamilton RC, Loken RG. Periocular local anesthesia: Medial orbital as an alternative to superior nasal injection. *J Cataract Refract Surg* 1994;20:197–201.
18. Bloomberg LB. Anterior periocular anesthesia: Five years experience. *J Cataract Refract Surg* 1991;17:508–511.
19. Davis DB, Mandel MR. Efficacy and complication rate of 16,224 consecutive peribulbar blocks. A prospective multicenter study. *J Cataract Refract Surg* 1994;20:327–337.
20. Davis DB, Mandel MR. Posterior peribulbar anesthesia: An alternative to retrobulbar anesthesia. *J Cataract Refract Surg* 1986;12:182–184.
21. Edge R, Navon S. Scleral perforation during retrobulbar and peribulbar anesthesia: Risk factors and outcome in 50,000 consecutive injections. *J Cataract Refract Surg* 1999;25:1237–1244.
22. Duker JS, Belmont JB, Benson WE, et al. Inadvertent globe perforation during retrobulbar and peribulbar anesthesia. Patient characteristics, surgical management, and visual outcome. *Ophthalmology* 1991;98:519–526.
23. Vohra SB, Good PA. Altered globe dimensions of axial myopia as risk factors for penetrating ocular injury during peribulbar anaesthesia. *Br J Anaesth* 2000;85:242–245.
24. Stevens JD. A new local anaesthesia technique for cataract extraction by one quadrant sub-Tenon's infiltration. *Br J Ophthalmol* 1992;76:670–674.
25. Ripart J, Prat-Pradal D, Vivien B, et al. Medial canthus episcleral (sub-Tenon) anesthesia imaging. *Clin Anat* 1998;11:390–395.
26. Ripart J, Metge L, Prat-Pradal D, et al. Medial canthus single-injection episcleral (sub-Tenon anesthesia): Computed tomography imaging. *Anesth Analg* 1998;87:42–45.
27. Ripart J, Lefrant JY, Vivien B, et al. Ophthalmic regional anesthesia: Medial canthus episcleral (sub-Tenon) anesthesia is more efficient than peribulbar anesthesia: A double-blind randomized study. *Anesthesiology* 2000;92:1278–1285.
28. Li HK, Abouleish A, Grady J, et al. Sub-Tenon's injection for local anesthesia in posterior segment surgery. *Ophthalmology* 2000;107:41–6.
29. Briggs MC, Beck SA, Esakowitz L. Sub-Tenon's versus peribulbar anaesthesia for cataract surgery. *Eye* 1997;11[Pt 5]:639–643.
30. Kapran Z, Uyar M, Eltutar K, Dincer N. One quadrant sub-Tenon's capsule anesthesia in anterior segment surgery. *Eur J Ophthalmol* 1996;6:131–136.
31. Khoo BK, Lim TH, Yong V. Sub-Tenon's versus retrobulbar anesthesia for cataract surgery. *Ophthalmic Surg Lasers* 1996;27:773–777.
32. Fukasaku H, Marron JA. Pinpoint anesthesia: A new approach to local ocular anesthesia. *J Cataract Refract Surg* 1994;20:468–471.
33. Nielsen PJ, Allerod CW. Evaluation of local anesthesia techniques for small incision cataract surgery. *J Cataract Refract Surg* 1998;24:1136–1144.
34. Lai MM, Lai JC, Lee WH, et al. Comparison of retrobulbar and sub-Tenon's capsule injection of local anesthetic in vitreoretinal surgery. *Ophthalmology* 2005;112:574–579.
35. Roman SJ, Chong Sit DA, Boureau CM, et al. Sub-Tenon's anaesthesia: An efficient and safe technique. *Br J Ophthalmol* 1997;81:673–676.
36. Guise PA. Sub-Tenon anesthesia: A prospective study of 6,000 blocks. *Anesthesiology* 2003;98:964–968.
37. Rebolleda G, Munoz-Negrete FJ, Gutierrez-Ortiz C. Topical plus intracameral lidocaine versus retrobulbar anesthesia in phacotrabeculectomy: Prospective randomized study. *J Cataract Refract Surg* 2001;27:1214–1220.
38. Boezaart A, Berry R, Nell M. Topical anesthesia versus retrobulbar block for cataract surgery: The patients' perspective. *J Clin Anesth* 2000;12:58–60.
39. Sekundo W, Dick HB, Schmidt JC. Lidocaine-assisted Xylocaine jelly anesthesia versus one quadrant sub-Tenon infiltration for self-sealing sclerocorneal incision routine phacoemulsification. *Eur J Ophthalmol* 2004;14:111–1116.
40. Ruschen H, Celaschi D, Bunce C, Carr C. Randomised controlled trial of sub-Tenon's block versus topical anaesthesia for cataract surgery: A comparison of patient satisfaction. *Br J Ophthalmol* 2005;89:291–293.
41. Johnston RL, Whitefield LA, Giralt J, et al. Topical versus peribulbar anesthesia, without sedation, for clear corneal phacoemulsification. *J Cataract Refract Surg* 1998;24:407–410.
42. Sauder G, Jonas JB. Topical versus peribulbar anaesthesia for cataract surgery. *Acta Ophthalmol Scand* 2003;81:596–599.
43. Karp CL, Cox TA, Wagoner MD, et al. Intracameral anesthesia: A report by the American Academy of Ophthalmology. *Ophthalmology* 2001;108:1704–1710.
44. Yamamoto F, Kato R, Sato J, Nishino T. Anaesthesia for awake craniotomy with non-invasive positive pressure ventilation. *Br J Anaesth* 2003;90:382–385.
45. Huncke K, Van de WB, Fried I, Rubinstein EH. The asleep-awake-asleep anesthetic technique for intraoperative language mapping. *Neurosurgery* 1998;42:1312–1316.
46. Tongier WK, Joshi GP, Landers DF, Mickey B. Use of the laryngeal mask airway during awake craniotomy for tumor resection. *J Clin Anesth* 2000;12:592–594.
47. Pinosky ML, Fishman RL, Reeves ST, et al. The effect of bupivacaine skull block on the hemodynamic response to craniotomy. *Anesth Analg* 1996;83:1256–1261.
48. Girvin JP. Resection of intracranial lesions under local anesthesia. *Int Anesthesiol Clin* 1986;24:133–155.
49. Costello TG, Cormack JR, Hoy C, et al. Plasma ropivacaine levels following scalp block for awake craniotomy. *J Neurosurg Anesthesiol* 2004;16:147–150.
50. Sawaya R, Hammoud M, Schoppa D, et al. Neurosurgical outcomes in a modern series of 400 craniotomies for treatment of parenchymal tumors. *Neurosurgery* 1998;42:1044–1055.
51. Nguyen A, Girard F, Boudreault D, et al. Scalp nerve blocks decrease the severity of pain after craniotomy. *Anesth Analg* 2001;93:1272–1276.
52. Law-Koune JD, Szekely B, Fermanian C, et al. Scalp infiltration with bupivacaine plus epinephrine or plain ropivacaine reduces postoperative pain

after supratentorial craniotomy. *J Neurosurg Anesthesiol* 2005;17:139–143.

53. De BG, Lorenzetti A, Migliore M, et al. Postoperative pain in neurosurgery: A pilot study in brain surgery. *Neurosurgery* 1996;38:466–469.

54. Quiney N, Cooper R, Stoneham M, Walters F. Pain after craniotomy. A time for reappraisal? *Br J Neurosurg* 1996;10:295–299.

55. Kocuj F, Epple J, Polarz H, et al. Nerve blocks in stereotactic neurosurgery. *Stereotact Funct Neurosurg* 2002;78:29–38.

56. Watson R, Leslie K. Nerve blocks versus subcutaneous infiltration for stereotactic frame placement. *Anesth Analg* 2001;92:424–427.

57. Knize DM. A study of the supraorbital nerve. *Plast Reconstr Surg* 1995; 96:564–569.

58. Beneficial effect of carotid endarterectomy in symptomatic patients with high-grade carotid stenosis. North American Symptomatic Carotid Endarterectomy Trial Collaborators. *N Engl J Med* 1991;325:445–453.

59. MRC European Carotid Surgery Trial: Interim results for symptomatic patients with severe (70–99%) or with mild (0–29%) carotid stenosis. European Carotid Surgery Trialists' Collaborative Group. *Lancet* 1991;337:1235–1243.

60. Randomised trial of endarterectomy for recently symptomatic carotid stenosis: Final results of the MRC European Carotid Surgery Trial (ECST). *Lancet* 1998;351:1379–1387.

61. Castresana EJ, Shaker IJ, Castresana MR. Incidence of shunting during carotid endarterectomy: Regional versus general anesthesia. *Reg Anesth* 1997;22:S23.

62. Fiorani P, Sbarigia E, Speziale F, et al. General anaesthesia versus cervical block and perioperative complications in carotid artery surgery. *Eur J Vasc Endovasc Surg* 1997;13:37–42.

63. Forssell C, Takolander R, Bergqvist D, et al. Local versus general anaesthesia in carotid surgery. A prospective, randomised study. *Eur J Vasc Surg* 1989;3:503–509.

64. Sundt TM Jr., Houser OW, Sharbrough FW, Messick JM Jr. Carotid endarterectomy: Results, complications, and monitoring techniques. *Adv Neurol* 1977;16:97–119.

65. Rerkasem K, Bond R, Rothwell PM. Local versus general anaesthesia for carotid endarterectomy. *Cochrane Database Syst Rev* 2004;CD000126.

66. Stoneham MD, Knighton JD. Regional anaesthesia for carotid endarterectomy. *Br J Anaesth* 1999;82:910–919.

67. Winnie AP, Ramamurthy S, Durrani Z, Radonjic R. Interscalene cervical plexus block: A single-injection technic. *Anesth Analg* 1975;54:370–375.

68. Moore DC. *Regional Block: A Handbook for Use in the Clinical Practice of Medicine and Surgery,* 4th ed. Springfield, IL: Charles C Thomas, 1978.

69. Stoneham MD, Doyle AR, Knighton JD, et al. Prospective, randomized comparison of deep or superficial cervical plexus block for carotid endarterectomy surgery. *Anesthesiology* 1998;89:907–912.

70. Pandit JJ, Bree S, Dillon P, et al. A comparison of superficial versus combined (superficial and deep) cervical plexus block for carotid endarterectomy: A prospective, randomized study. *Anesth Analg* 2000;91:781–786.

71. de Sousa AA, Filho MA, Faglione W Jr., Carvalho GT. Superficial vs combined cervical plexus block for carotid endarterectomy: A prospective, randomized study. *Surg Neurol* 2005;63[Suppl 1]:S22–S25.

72. Davies MJ, Silbert BS, Scott DA, et al. Superficial and deep cervical plexus block for carotid artery surgery: A prospective study of 1000 blocks. *Reg Anesth* 1997;22:442–446.

73. Bonnet F, Derosier JP, Pluskwa F, et al. Cervical epidural anaesthesia for carotid artery surgery. *Can J Anaesth* 1990;37:353–358.

74. Bonnet F, Szekely B, Abhay K, et al. Baroreceptor control after cervical epidural anesthesia in patients undergoing carotid artery surgery. *J Cardiothorac Anesth* 1989;3:418–424.

75. Campkin TV. Cervical epidural analgesia during carotid artery surgery. *Anaesthesia* 1987;42:437–439.

76. Kainuma M, Shimada Y, Matsuura M. Cervical epidural anaesthesia in carotid artery surgery. *Anaesthesia* 1986;41:1020–1023.

77. Merle JC, Mazoit JX, Desgranges P, et al. A comparison of two techniques for cervical plexus blockade: Evaluation of efficacy and systemic toxicity. *Anesth Analg* 1999;89:1366–1370.

78. Boezaart AP, Nosovitch MA. Carotid endarterectomy using single injection posterior cervical paravertebral block. *Anesth Analg* 2005;101:1885–1886.

79. Castresana MR, Masters RD, Castresana EJ, et al. Incidence and clinical significance of hemidiaphragmatic paresis in patients undergoing carotid endarterectomy during cervical plexus block anesthesia. *J Neurosurg Anesthesiol* 1994;6:21–23.

80. Castresana MR, Brooks AG, Maters RD, et al. Incidence of dysphagia in patients undergoing carotid endarterectomy using deep and superficial cervical plexus block anesthesia. *Anesth Analg* 1994;79:S52.

81. Masters RD, Castresana EJ, Castresana MR. Superficial and deep cervical plexus block: Technical considerations. *AANA J* 1995;63:235–243.

82. Kwok AO, Silbert BS, Allen KJ, et al. Bilateral vocal cord palsy during carotid endarterectomy under cervical plexus block. *Anesth Analg* 2006;102:376–377.

83. Weiss A, Isselhorst C, Gahlen J, et al. Acute respiratory failure after deep cervical plexus block for carotid endarterectomy as a result of bilateral re-

current laryngeal nerve paralysis. *Acta Anaesthesiol Scand* 2005;49:715–719.

84. Schneemilch CE, Bachmann H, Ulrich A, et al. Clonidine decreases stress response in patients undergoing carotid endarterectomy under regional anesthesia: A prospective, randomized, double-blinded, placebo-controlled study. *Anesth Analg* 2006;103:297–302.

85. Einav S, Landesberg G, Prus D, et al. A case of nerves. *Reg Anesth* 1996; 21:168–170.

86. Bourke DL, Thomas P. Mandibular nerve block in addition to cervical plexus block for carotid endarterectomy. *Anesth Analg* 1998;87:1034–1036.

87. Caplan RA, Benumof JL, Berry F, et al. Practice guidelines for management of the difficult airway: A report by the ASA Task Force Management of the Difficult Airway. *Anesthesiology* 1993:597–602.

88. Benumof JL. Management of the difficult adult airway. With special emphasis on awake tracheal intubation. *Anesthesiology* 1991;75:1087–1110.

89. Simmons ST, Schleich AR. Airway regional anesthesia for awake fiberoptic intubation. *Reg Anesth Pain Med* 2002;27:180–192.

90. Netter FH, Mitchell GAG. Cranial Nerves. *Ciba Collection of Medical Illustrations,* Volume I: The Nervous System, Part 1: Anatomy and Physiology. West Caldwell, NJ: Ciba Pharmaceuticals Company, 1983.

91. Snell RS. *Clinical Anatomy for Medical Students,* 4th ed. Boston: Little Brown and Company, 1992.

92. Hermanowicz N, Turong DT. Cranial nerves IX (glossopharyngeal) and X (vagus). In: Goetz C, ed. *Textbook of Clinical Neurology.* Philadelphia: Saunders; 1999:206–207.

93. Fulling PD, Roberts JT. Fiberoptic intubation. *Int Anesthesiol Clin* 2000;38:189–217.

94. Reasoner DK, Warner DS, Todd MM, et al. A comparison of anesthetic techniques for awake intubation in neurosurgical patients. *J Neurosurg Anesthesiol* 1995;7:94–99.

95. Kundra P, Kutralam S, Ravishankar M. Local anaesthesia for awake fibreoptic nasotracheal intubation. *Acta Anaesthesiol Scand* 2000;44:511–516.

96. Mostafa SM, Murthy BV, Hodgson CA, Beese E. Nebulized 10% lignocaine for awake fibreoptic intubation. *Anaesth Intensive Care* 1998;26:222–223.

97. Clay MM, Clarke SW. Wastage of drug from nebulisers: A review. *J R Soc Med* 1987;80:38–39.

98. Williams KA, Barker GL, Harwood RJ, Woodall NM. Combined nebulization and spray-as-you-go topical local anaesthesia of the airway. *Br J Anaesth* 2005;95:549–553.

99. Parkes SB, Butler CS, Muller R. Plasma lignocaine concentration following nebulization for awake intubation. *Anaesth Intensive Care* 1997;25:369–371.

100. Efthimiou J, Higenbottam T, Holt D, Cochrane GM. Plasma concentrations of lignocaine during fibreoptic bronchoscopy. *Thorax* 1982;37:68–71.

101. British Thoracic Society Bronchoscopy Guidelines Committee, a Subcommittee of Standards of Care Committee of British Thoracic Society. British Thoracic Society Guidelines on diagnostic flexible bronchoscopy. *Thorax* 2001;11–21.

102. Glossopharyngeal block. In: Brown D, ed. *Atlas of Regional Anesthesia.* Philadelphia: Saunders; 1999:205–208.

103. Henthorn RW, Amayem A, Ganta R. Which method for intraoral glossopharyngeal nerve block is better? *Anesth Analg* 1995;81:1113–1114.

104. Furlan JC. Anatomical study applied to anesthetic block technique of the superior laryngeal nerve. *Acta Anaesthesiol Scand* 2002;46:199–202.

105. Sulica L, Blitzer A. Anesthesia for laryngeal surgery in the office. *Laryngoscope* 2000;110:1777–1779.

106. Wiles JR, Kelly J, Mostafa SM. Hypotension and bradycardia following superior laryngeal nerve block. *Br J Anaesth* 1989;63:125–127.

107. Monso A, Riudeubas J, Palanques F, Braso JM. A new application for superior laryngeal nerve block: Treatment or prevention of laryngospasm and stridor. *Reg Anesth Pain Med* 1999;24:186–187.

108. Risk C, Fine R, D'Ambra MN, O'Shea JP. A new application for superior laryngeal nerve block: Transesophageal echocardiography. *Anesthesiology* 1990;72:746–747.

109. Reed AP. Successful transesophageal echocardiography in an unsedated critically ill patient with superior laryngeal nerve blocks. *Am Heart J* 1991;122:1472–1474.

110. Murthy P, Laing MR. Dissection tonsillectomy: Pattern of post-operative pain, medication and resumption of normal activity. *J Laryngol Otol* 1998;112:41–44.

111. Nunez DA, Provan J, Crawford M. Postoperative tonsillectomy pain in pediatric patients: Electrocautery (hot) vs cold dissection and snare tonsillectomy: A randomized trial. *Arch Otolaryngol Head Neck Surg* 2000;126:837–841.

112. Ohlms LA. Injection of local anesthetic in tonsillectomy. *Arch Otolaryngol Head Neck Surg* 2001;127:1276–1278.

113. Jebeles JA, Reilly JS, Gutierrez JF, et al. Tonsillectomy and adenoidectomy pain reduction by local bupivacaine infiltration in children. *Int J Pediatr Otorhinolaryngol* 1993;25:149–154.

114. Jebeles JA, Reilly JS, Gutierrez JF, et al. The effect of pre-incisional infiltration of tonsils with bupivacaine on the pain following tonsillectomy under general anesthesia. *Pain* 1991;47:305–308.

PART III: APPLICATIONS

115. Broadman LM, Patel RI, Feldman BA, et al. The effects of peritonsillar infiltration on the reduction of intraoperative blood loss and post-tonsillectomy pain in children. *Laryngoscope* 1989;99:578–581.
116. Goldsher M, Podoshin L, Fradis M, et al. Effects of peritonsillar infiltration on post-tonsillectomy pain. A double-blind study. *Ann Otol Rhinol Laryngol* 1996;105:868–870.
117. McClairen WC Jr., Strauss M. Tonsillectomy: A clinical study comparing the effects of local versus general anesthesia. *Laryngoscope* 1986;96:308–310.
118. El-Hakim H, Nunez DA, Saleh HA, et al. A randomised controlled trial of the effect of regional nerve blocks on immediate post-tonsillectomy pain in adult patients. *Clin Otolaryngol Allied Sci* 2000;25:413–417.
119. Hollis LJ, Burton MJ, Millar JM. Perioperative local anaesthesia for reducing pain following tonsillectomy. *Cochrane Database Syst Rev* 2000;CD001874.
120. Hald F, Godtfredsen E. Transitory occurrence of Horner syndrome. *Acta Otolaryngolog* 1942;30:156–161.
121. Garretson HD, Elvidge AR. Glossopharyngeal neuralgia with cerebral and cardiovascular symptomatology. *Trans Am Neurol Assoc* 1962;87:204–206.
122. Burack SM. Kausuistik der Komplikationen nack Adeno-und Tonsillektomien. *Z Laryngol Rhinol Otol* 1911;21:477–486.
123. Sewell L. Remarks of certain dangers associated with the operation for the removal of tonsils and adenoids. *Med Chron Fourth Ser* 1911;21:212–216.
124. Link R. Eigenartiger Zwischenfall nack Infiltrationsanaesthesie bei Tonsillektomie. *Z Hals Nasen Ohrenerzt* 1941;31:368–372.
125. Urbanitsch E. Tonsillektomie-Komplikationen. *Wien Med Wochenschr* 1931;81:1600–1602.
126. Sher MH, Laing DI, Brands E. Life-threatening upper airway obstruction after glossopharyngeal nerve block: Possibly due to an inappropriately large dose of bupivacaine? *Anesth Analg* 1998;86:678.
127. Manoukian PD, Wyatt JR, Leopold DA, Bass EB. Recent trends in utilization of procedures in otolaryngology-head and neck surgery. *Laryngoscope* 1997;107:472–477.
128. Armstrong M Jr. Office-based procedures in rhinosinusitis. *Otolaryngol Clin North Am* 2005;38:1327–1338.
129. Fedok FG, Ferraro RE, Kingsley CP, Fornadley JA. Operative times, postanesthesia recovery times, and complications during sinonasal surgery using general anesthesia and local anesthesia with sedation. *Otolaryngol Head Neck Surg* 2000;122:560–566.
130. Courtney MJ, Rajapakse Y, Duncan G, Morrissey G. Nasal fracture manipulation: A comparative study of general and local anaesthesia techniques. *Clin Otolaryngol Allied Sci* 2003;28:472–475.
131. Wild DC, El Alami MA, Conboy PJ. Reduction of nasal fractures under local anaesthesia: An acceptable practice? *Surgeon* 2003;1:45–47.
132. Owen GO, Parker AJ, Watson DJ. Fractured-nose reduction under local anaesthesia. Is it acceptable to the patient? *Rhinology* 1992;30:89–96.
133. Houghton DJ, Hanafi Z, Papakostas K, et al. Efficacy of external fixation following nasal manipulation under local anaesthesia. *Clin Otolaryngol Allied Sci* 1998;23:169–171.
134. Rajapakse Y, Courtney M, Bialostocki A, et al. Nasal fractures: A study comparing local and general anaesthesia techniques. *ANZ J Surg* 2003;73:396–399.
135. Waldron J, Mitchell DB, Ford G. Reduction of fractured nasal bones: Local versus general anaesthesia. *Clin Otolaryngol Allied Sci* 1989;14:357–359.
136. Cook JA, Murrant NJ, Evans K, Lavelle RJ. Manipulation of the fractured nose under local anaesthesia. *Clin Otolaryngol Allied Sci* 1992;17:337–340.
137. Keles N, Ilicali OC, Deger K. Objective and subjective assessment of nasal obstruction in patients undergoing endoscopic sinus surgery. *Am J Rhinol* 1998;12:307–309.
138. Higashizawa T, Koga Y. Effect of infraorbital nerve block under general anesthesia on consumption of isoflurane and postoperative pain in endoscopic endonasal maxillary sinus surgery. *J Anesth* 2001;15:136–138.
139. Friedman M, Venkatesan TK, Lang D, Caldarelli DD. Bupivacaine for postoperative analgesia following endoscopic sinus surgery. *Laryngoscope* 1996;106:1382–1385.
140. Eaton JS, Grekin RC. Regional anesthesia of the face. *Dermatol Surg* 2001;27:1006–1009.
141. Hanke CW. The tumescent facial block: Tumescent local anesthesia and nerve block anesthesia for full-face laser resurfacing. *Dermatol Surg* 2001;27:1003–1005.
142. Field LM. Alternative and additional techniques for tumescent facial block anesthesia. *Dermatol Surg* 2002;28:442.
143. Zide BM, Swift R. How to block and tackle the face. *Plast Reconstr Surg* 1998;101:840–851.
144. Kays CR. Local infiltration versus regional anesthesia of the face: Case report and review. *J S C Med Assoc* 1988;84:494–496.
145. Pascal J, Charier D, Perret D, et al. Peripheral blocks of trigeminal nerve for facial soft-tissue surgery: Learning from failures. *Eur J Anaesthesiol* 2005;22:480–482.
146. Lynch MT, Syverud SA, Schwab RA, et al. Comparison of intraoral and percutaneous approaches for infraorbital nerve block. *Acad Emerg Med* 1994;1:514–519.
147. Hanke CW. The tumescent facial block: Tumescent local anesthesia and nerve block anesthesia for full-face laser resurfacing. *Dermatol Surg* 2001;27:1003–1005.
148. Prabhu KP, Wig J, Grewal S. Bilateral infraorbital nerve block is superior to peri-incisional infiltration for analgesia after repair of cleft lip. *Scand J Plast Reconstr Surg Hand Surg* 1999;33:83–87.
149. Bromley GS, Rothaus KO, Goulian D Jr. Cleft lip: Morbidity and mortality in early repair. *Ann Plast Surg* 1983;10:214–217.
150. Doyle E, Hudson I. Anaesthesia for primary repair of cleft lip and cleft palate: A review of 244 procedures. *Paediatr Anaesth* 1992;2:139–145.
151. Hatch DJ. Analgesia in the neonate. *Br Med J (Clin Res Ed)* 1987;294:920.
152. Yaster M. Analgesia and anesthesia in neonates. *J Pediatr* 1987;111:394–396.
153. Bosenberg AT, Kimble FW. Infraorbital nerve block in neonates for cleft lip repair: Anatomical study and clinical application. *Br J Anaesth* 1995;74:506–508.
154. Burtles R. Analgesia for "bat ear" surgery. *Ann R Coll Surg Engl* 1989; 71:332.
155. Roberts RH, Tan ST, Sinclair SW. Lignocaine vs bupivacaine in prominent ear correction: A controlled trial. *Br J Plast Surg* 1992;45:533–535.
156. Sossai R, Johr M, Kistler W, et al. Postoperative vomiting in children. A persisting unsolved problem. *Eur J Pediatr Surg* 1993;3:206–208.
157. Broadman LM. Regional anaesthesia in paediatric practice. *Can J Anaesth* 1987;34:S43–S48.
158. Yaster M, Maxwell LG. Pediatric regional anesthesia. *Anesthesiology* 1989; 70:324–338.
159. Analgesia in children after day-case surgery. *Lancet* 1988;1:1084–1085.
160. Reid MF, Harris R, Phillips PD, et al. Day-case herniotomy in children. A comparison of ilio-inguinal nerve block and wound infiltration for postoperative analgesia. *Anaesthesia* 1987;42:658–661.
161. Cregg N, Conway F, Casey W. Analgesia after otoplasty: Regional nerve blockade vs local anaesthetic infiltration of the ear. *Can J Anaesth* 1996;43:141–147.
162. Attwood AI, Evans DM. Correction of prominent ears using Mustarde's technique: An out-patient procedure under local anaesthetic in children and adults. *Br J Plast Surg* 1985;38:252–258.
163. Lancaster JL, Jones TM, Kay AR, McGeorge DD. Paediatric day-case otoplasty: Local versus general anaesthetic. *Surgeon* 2003;1:96–98.
164. Carling T, Donovan P, Rinder C, Udelsman R. Minimally invasive parathyroidectomy using cervical block: Reasons for conversion to general anesthesia. *Arch Surg* 2006;141:401–404.
165. Miccoli P, Barellini L, Monchik JM, et al. Randomized clinical trial comparing regional and general anaesthesia in minimally invasive video-assisted parathyroidectomy. *Br J Surg* 2005;92:814–818.
166. Chen H, Sokoll LJ, Udelsman R. Outpatient minimally invasive parathyroidectomy: A combination of sestamibi-SPECT localization, cervical block anesthesia, and intraoperative parathyroid hormone assay. *Surgery* 1999;126:1016–1021.
167. Bergenfelz A, Kanngiesser V, Zielke A, et al. Conventional bilateral cervical exploration versus open minimally invasive parathyroidectomy under local anaesthesia for primary hyperparathyroidism. *Br J Surg* 2005;92:190–197.
168. Cohen MS, Finkelstein SE, Brunt LM, et al. Outpatient minimally invasive parathyroidectomy using local/regional anesthesia: A safe and effective operative approach for selected patients. *Surgery* 2005;138:681–687.
169. Michalek P, David I, Adamec M, Janousek L. Cervical epidural anesthesia for combined neck and upper extremity procedure: A pilot study. *Anesth Analg* 2004;99:1833–1836.
170. Ditkoff BA, Chabot J, Feind C, Lo Gerfo P. Parathyroid surgery using monitored anesthesia care as an alternative to general anesthesia. *Am J Surg* 1996;172:698–700.
171. Lo Gerfo P, Kim L. Technique for regional anesthesia: Thyroidectomy and parathyroidectomy. *Operative Techniques in General Surgery* 1999;1:95–102.
172. Brichkov I, Lo Gerfo P. Thyroidectomy under local or regional anesthesia. *Operative techniques in otolaryngology. Head Neck Surg* 2002;13:239–241.
173. Vellar ID. Thomas Peel Dunhill: Pioneer thyroid surgeon. *Aust N Z J Surg* 1999;69:375–387.
174. Taylor S. Sir Thomas Peel Dunhill (1876–1957). *World J Surg* 1997;21:660–662.
175. Crile G Jr. Regional anesthesia for certain patients undergoing thyroid and parathyroid surgery. *Surgery* 1989;105:455.
176. Spanknebel K, Chabot JA, DiGiorgi M, et al. Thyroidectomy using local anesthesia: A report of 1,025 cases over 16 years. *J Am Coll Surg* 2005;201:375–385.
177. Hochman M, Fee WE Jr. Thyroidectomy under local anesthesia. *Arch Otolaryngol Head Neck Surg* 1991;117:405–407.
178. Henry JF. Minimally invasive surgery of the thyroid and parathyroid glands. *Br J Surg* 2006;93:1–2.
179. Specht MC, Romero M, Barden CB, et al. Characteristics of patients having thyroid surgery under regional anesthesia. *J Am Coll Surg* 2001;193:367–372.

180. Snyder SK, Roberson CR, Cummings CC, Rajab MH. Local anesthesia with monitored anesthesia care vs general anesthesia in thyroidectomy: A randomized study. *Arch Surg* 2006;141:167–173.

181. Cousins MJ, Bridenbauch PO. *Neural Blockade*, 2nd ed. Philadelphia: Lippincott-Raven, 1990.

182. Tobias JD. Cervical plexus block in adolescents. *J Clin Anesth* 1999;11:606–608.

183. Schwartz AE, Clark OH, Ituarte P, Lo Gerfo P. Therapeutic controversy: Thyroid surgery: The choice. *J Clin Endocrinol Metab* 1998;83:1097–1105.

184. Aunac S, Carlier M, Singelyn F, De KM. The analgesic efficacy of bilateral combined superficial and deep cervical plexus block administered before thyroid surgery under general anesthesia. *Anesth Analg* 2002;95:746–750.

185. Dieudonne N, Gomola A, Bonnichon P, Ozier YM. Prevention of postoperative pain after thyroid surgery: A double-blind randomized study of bilateral superficial cervical plexus blocks. *Anesth Analg* 2001;92:1538–1542.

186. Hisham AN, Aina EN. A reappraisal of thyroid surgery under local anaesthesia: Back to the future? *ANZ J Surg* 2002;72:287–289.

187. Caputi CA, Firetto V. Therapeutic blockade of greater occipital and supraorbital nerves in migraine patients. *Headache* 1997;37:174–179.

188. Gawel MJ, Rothbart PJ. Occipital nerve block in the management of headache and cervical pain. *Cephalalgia* 1992;12:9–13.

189. Ashkenazi A, Silberstein SD. Headache management for the pain specialist. *Reg Anesth Pain Med* 2004;29:462–475.

190. Afridi SK, Shields KG, Bhola R, Goadsby PJ. Greater occipital nerve injection in primary headache syndromes: Prolonged effects from a single injection. *Pain* 2006;122:126–129.

191. Kerr RW. A mechanism to account for frontal headache in cases of posterior-fossa tumors. *J Neurosurg* 1961;18:605–609.

192. Anthony M. Cervicogenic headache: Prevalence and response to local steroid therapy. *Clin Exp Rheumatol* 2000;18:S59–S64.

193. Bovim G, Sand T. Cervicogenic headache, migraine without aura and tension-type headache. Diagnostic blockade of greater occipital and supraorbital nerves. *Pain* 1992;51:43–48.

194. Peres MF, Stiles MA, Siow HC, et al. Greater occipital nerve blockade for cluster headache. *Cephalalgia* 2002;22:520–522.

195. Naja MZ, Al-Tannir M, Naja H, et al. Repeated nerve blocks with clonidine, fentanyl and bupivacaine for trigeminal neuralgia. *Anaesthesia* 2006;61:70–71.

196. Goto F, Ishizaki K, Yoshikawa D, et al. The long lasting effects of peripheral nerve blocks for trigeminal neuralgia using high concentration of tetracaine dissolved in bupivacaine. *Pain* 1999;79:101–103.

197. Umino M, Kohase H, Ideguchi S, Sakurai N. Long-term pain control in trigeminal neuralgia with local anesthetics using an indwelling catheter in the mandibular nerve. *Clin J Pain* 2002;18:196–199.

198. Yang Y, Oraee S. A novel approach to transnasal sphenopalatine ganglion injection. *Pain Physician* 2006;9:131–134.

199. Peterson JN, Schames J, Schames M, King E. Sphenopalatine ganglion block: A safe and easy method for the management of orofacial pain. *Cranio* 1995;13:177–181.

200. Saberski L, Ahmad M, Wiske P. Sphenopalatine ganglion block for treatment of sinus arrest in postherpetic neuralgia. *Headache* 1999;39:42–44.

201. Shah RV, Racz GB. Long-term relief of posttraumatic headache by sphenopalatine ganglion pulsed radiofrequency lesioning: A case report. *Arch Phys Med Rehabil* 2004;85:1013–1016.

202. Russell AL. Sphenopalatine block: The cheapest technique in the management of chronic pain. *Clin J Pain* 1991;7:256–257.

203. Cambareli J. Sphenopalatine ganglion. In: Thomas PS, ed. *Image Guided Pain Management*. Philadelphia: Lippincott Raven Publishers; 1997:27–33.

204. Prasanna A, Murthy PS. Sphenopalatine ganglion block under vision using rigid nasal sinuscope. *Reg Anesth* 1993;18:139–140.

205. Janzen VD, Scudds R. Sphenopalatine blocks in the treatment of pain in fibromyalgia and myofascial pain syndrome. *Laryngoscope* 1997;107:1420–1422.

206. Varghese BT, Koshy RC. Endoscopic transnasal neurolytic sphenopalatine ganglion block for head and neck cancer pain. *J Laryngol Otol* 2001;115:385–387.

207. Cohen S, Trnovski S, Zada Y. A new interest in an old remedy for headache and backache for our obstetric patients: A sphenopalatine ganglion block. *Anaesthesia* 2001;56:606–607.

208. Sluder G. Injection of the nasal ganglion and comparison methods. *Ann Otol Rhinol Laryngol* 1927;86:648–655.

209. Day M. Sphenopalatine ganglion analgesia. *Curr Rev Pain* 1999;3:342–347.

210. Loetscher CA, Walton RE. Patterns of innervation of the maxillary first molar: A dissection study. *Oral Surg Oral Med Oral Pathol* 1988;65:86–90.

211. Heasman PA. Clinical anatomy of the superior alveolar nerves. *Br J Oral Maxillofac Surg* 1984;22:439–447.

212. Blanton PL, Jeske AH. The key to profound local anesthesia: Neuroanatomy. *J Am Dent Assoc* 2003;134:753–760.

213. DuBrul EL. *Sicher's Oral Anatomy*, 7th ed. St. Louis: Ishiyaku EuroAmerica, 1980.

214. DuBrul EL. *Sicher & DuBrul's Oral Anatomy*, 8th ed. St. Louis: Ishiyaku EuroAmerica, 1988.

215. Phillips WH. Anatomic considerations in local anesthesia. *J Oral Surg* 1943;1:112–121.

216. Slavkin HC, Canter MR, Canter SR. An anatomic study of the pterygomaxillary region in the craniums of infants and children. *Oral Surg Oral Med Oral Pathol* 1966;21:225–235.

217. Westmoreland EE, Blanton PL. An analysis of the variations in position of the greater palatine foramen in the adult human skull. *Anat Rec* 1982;204:383–388.

218. Slavkin HC. Anatomical investigation of the greater palatine foramen and canal. *Alpha Omegan* 1965;58:148–151.

219. DeSantis JL, Liebow C. Four common mandibular nerve anomalies that lead to local anesthesia failures. *J Am Dent Assoc* 1996;127:1081–1086.

220. Malamed SF. Techniques of mandibular anesthesia. *Handbook of Local Anaesthesia*. Noida, India: Harcourt Brace; 1997:193–219.

221. Malamed SF. *Handbook of Local Anesthesia*, 4th ed. St Louis: Mosby, 1997.

222. Kaufman E, Weinstein P, Milgrom P. Difficulties in achieving local anesthesia. *J Am Dent Assoc* 1984;108:205–208.

223. Meechan JG. How to overcome failed local anaesthesia. *Br Dent J* 1999;186:15–20.

224. DuBrul EL. Anatomy of mandibular anesthesia. *Sicher & DuBrul's Oral Anatomy*. St. Louis: Ishiyaku EuroAmerica, 1988.

225. Wilson S, Johns P, Fuller PM. The inferior alveolar and mylohyoid nerves: An anatomic study and relationship to local anesthesia of the anterior mandibular teeth. *J Am Dent Assoc* 1984;108:350–352.

226. Madan GA, Madan SG, Madan AD. Failure of inferior alveolar nerve block: Exploring the alternatives. *J Am Dent Assoc* 2002;133:843–846.

227. Levy TP. An assessment of the Gow-Gates mandibular block for third molar surgery. *J Am Dent Assoc* 1981;103:37–41.

228. Grover PS, Lorton L. Bifid mandibular nerve as a possible cause of inadequate anesthesia in the mandible. *J Oral Maxillofac Surg* 1983;41:177–179.

229. Nortje CJ, Farman AG, Grotepass FW. Variations in the normal anatomy of the inferior dental (mandibular) canal: A retrospective study of panoramic radiographs from 3612 routine dental patients. *Br J Oral Surg* 1977;15:55–63.

230. Sawyer DR, Kiely ML. Retromolar foramen: A mandibular variant important to dentistry. *Ann Dent* 1991;50:16–18.

231. Loizeaux AD, Devos BJ. Inferior alveolar nerve anomaly. *J Hawaii Dent Assoc* 1981;12:10–11.

232. Vazirani SJ. Closed mouth mandibular nerve block: A new technique. *Dent Dig* 1960;66:10–13.

233. Akinosi JO. A new approach to the mandibular nerve block. *Br J Oral Surg* 1977;15:83–87.

CHAPTER 22 ■ NEURAL BLOCKADE FOR CARDIOVASCULAR SURGERY

MARK A. CHANEY

Adequate postoperative analgesia prevents unnecessary patient discomfort, may decrease morbidity, may decrease postoperative hospital length of stay, and may thus decrease cost. Because postoperative pain management has been deemed important, the American Society of Anesthesiologists has published practice guidelines regarding this topic (1). Furthermore, in recognition of the need for improved pain management, the Joint Commission on Accreditation of Healthcare Organizations has recently developed standards for the assessment and management of pain in accredited hospitals and other health care settings (2).

Surgical or traumatic injury initiates changes in the peripheral and central nervous system that must be addressed therapeutically to promote postoperative analgesia and, potentially, improve clinical outcome. The physical processes of incision, traction, and cutting of tissues stimulate free nerve endings and a wide variety of specific nociceptors. Receptor activation and activity is further modified by the local release of chemical mediators of inflammation and sympathetic amines released via the perioperative surgical stress response. The perioperative surgical stress response peaks during the immediate postoperative period following cardiovascular surgery (intraoperative period during cardiac surgery associated with cardiopulmonary bypass) and exerts major effects on many physiologic processes (many detrimental). The potential clinical benefits of attenuating the perioperative surgical stress response has received much attention during the last decade and remains controversial (3). However, it seems clear that inadequate postoperative analgesia and/or an uninhibited perioperative surgical stress response following cardiovascular surgery has the potential to initiate pathophysiologic changes in all major organ systems, including the cardiovascular, pulmonary, gastrointestinal, renal, endocrine, immunologic, and/or central nervous system, all of which may lead to substantial postoperative morbidity.

Achieving optimal pain relief following cardiovascular surgery is often difficult. Furthermore, inadequate analgesia and/or an uninhibited stress response during the immediate postoperative period may increase morbidity by causing adverse hemodynamic, metabolic, immunologic, and hemostatic alterations (4–6). Aggressive control of postoperative pain, associated with an attenuated stress response, may decrease morbidity and mortality not only in high-risk patients following noncardiac surgery (7,8) and may also decrease morbidity and mortality in patients following cardiac surgery (9,10). Adequate postoperative analgesia following cardiovascular surgery may be attained via a wide variety of techniques (Table 22-1). Choice of technique is substantially influenced by type of surgery performed (i.e., cardiac surgery, thoracoabdominal aortic reconstruction, lower extremity revascularization). Traditionally, analgesia following cardiovascular surgery has been obtained mainly with IV (IV) opioids (specifically morphine), and this technique remains quite popular. However, IV opioid use is associated with definite detrimental side effects (nausea/vomiting, pruritus, urinary retention, respiratory depression), and longer-acting opioids such as morphine may delay tracheal extubation during the immediate postoperative period because of excessive sedation and/or respiratory depression. Thus, in the current era of early extubation ("fast-tracking") following all types of surgeries, cardiovascular anesthesiologists are exploring unique options other than traditional IV opioids for control of postoperative pain in patients following all types of cardiovascular surgery (11,12). No single analgesic technique is clearly superior; each possesses distinct advantages and disadvantages. It is becoming increasingly clear that a multimodal approach/combined analgesic regimen (utilizing a variety of techniques) is likely the best way to approach postoperative pain to maximize analgesia and minimize side effects. When addressing postoperative analgesia and appropriateness of neural blockade techniques in cardiovascular surgical patients, choice of technique(s) is made only after a thorough analysis of the risk-benefit ratio of each technique in each specific patient in whom analgesia is desired. This chapter focuses on the clinical applications (advantages and disadvantages) of neural blockade techniques in patients undergoing cardiovascular surgery.

CLINICAL APPLICATIONS FOR CARDIAC SURGERY

Pain following cardiac surgery may be intense and originates from many sources, including the incision (sternotomy, thoracotomy, etc.), intraoperative tissue retraction and dissection, vascular cannulation sites, vein harvesting sites, and chest tubes, among others (13,14). Patients in whom an internal mammary artery is surgically exposed and used as a bypass graft may have substantially more postoperative pain (15). A recently published prospective clinical investigation involving 200 consecutive patients undergoing cardiac surgery via median sternotomy assessed the location, distribution, and intensity of postoperative pain (13). All patients received 25 to 50 μg/kg of intraoperative IV fentanyl, were subjected to routine cardiopulmonary bypass, had their arms positioned along their body on the operating table, had their sternum closed with five peristernal wires, and received mediastinal and thoracic drains passed through the rectus abdominis muscle just below the xiphoid. A subgroup (127 patients) also underwent long

TABLE 22-1

TECHNIQUES AVAILABLE FOR POSTOPERATIVE ANALGESIA

Local anesthetic infiltration
Nerve blocks
Opioids
Nonsteroidal anti-inflammatory agents
α-Adrenergic agents
Intrathecal techniques
Epidural techniques
Multimodal analgesia

saphenous vein harvesting either from the calf (men) or thigh (women). All patients were extubated before the first postoperative morning. Postoperative analgesic management was standardized and included IV morphine, oral paracetamol, oral tramadol, and subcutaneous morphine. The investigators found that maximal pain intensity was highest on the first postoperative day and lowest on the third postoperative day. However, maximal pain intensity was only graded as "moderate" (mean pain score was approximately 3.8 on a 0-10 scale), did not diminish during the first two postoperative days, then started to decline between postoperative day 2 and 3. Pain distribution did not appear to vary throughout the postoperative period, yet location did (more shoulder pain observed on the seventh postoperative day). As time from operation increased, pain usually moved from primarily incisional/epigastric to osteoarticular. Another source of postoperative pain in patients following cardiac surgery is thoracic cage rib fractures, which may be common (16,17). Furthermore, sternal retraction, causing posterior rib fracture, may lead to brachial plexus injury. In these patients, routine chest radiographs may be normal despite the presence of fracture. Thus, bone scans (superior to chest radiographs in detecting rib fractures) are recommended whenever unexplained postoperative nonincisional pain occurs in a patient who has undergone sternal retraction (17). Other studies have indicated that the most common source of pain in patients following cardiac surgery is the chest wall. Age also appears to impact pain intensity; patients younger than 60 often have higher pain intensity than patients older than 60. Although maximal pain intensity following cardiac surgery is usually only moderate, improvement in analgesic control to minimize pain intensity, especially during the first few postoperative days, is warranted.

Persistent pain following cardiac surgery, while rare, can be problematic (18–20). The cause of persistent pain following sternotomy is multifactorial; tissue destruction, intercostal nerve trauma, scar formation, rib fractures, sternal infection, stainless-steel wire sutures, and/or costochondral separation may all play roles. Chronic pain is often localized to the arms, shoulders, or legs. Postoperative brachial plexopathies may also occur and have been attributed to rib fracture fragments, internal mammary artery dissection, suboptimal positioning of patients during surgery, and/or central venous catheter placement. Postoperative neuralgias of the saphenous nerve have also been reported following harvesting of saphenous veins for coronary artery bypass grafts (CABG). Younger patients appear to be at higher risk for developing chronic pain. The correlation of severity of acute postoperative pain and development of chronic pain syndromes has been suggested (patients requiring more postoperative analgesics may be more likely to develop chronic pain), yet the causative relationship is still vague. Ho and associates assessed via survey 244 patients following cardiac surgery and median sternotomy and found that persistent pain (defined as pain still present 2 or more months following surgery) was reported in almost 30% of patients (18). The incidence of persistent pain at any site was 29% (71 patients) and for sternotomy was 25% (61 patients). Other common locations of persistent pain reported to these investigators were the shoulders (17.4%), back (15.9%), and neck (5.8%). However, such persistent pain was usually reported as mild, with only 7% of patients reporting interference with daily living. The most common words used to describe the persistent pain were "annoying" (57%), "nagging" (33%), "dull" (30%), "sharp" (25%), "tiring" (22%), "tender" (22%), and "tight" (22%). The temporal nature of this pain was mostly reported as being brief/transient and periodic/intermittent. Twenty patients (8%) also described symptoms of numbness, burning pain, and tenderness over the internal mammary artery harvesting site, symptoms suggestive of internal mammary artery syndrome. Thus, Ho and associates conclude that mild persistent pain following cardiac surgery and median sternotomy is common, but infrequently interferes substantially with daily life.

Although the most common source of pain in patients following cardiac surgery remains the chest wall, leg pain from vein graft harvesting can be problematic as well. Such pain may not become apparent until the late postoperative period, which may be related to the progression of patient mobilization as well as the decreasing impact of sternotomy pain (unmasking leg incisional pain). The recent utilization of minimally invasive vein graft harvesting techniques (endoscopic vein graft harvesting) decreases postoperative leg pain intensity and duration compared to conventional open techniques (21). Furthermore, leg morbidity (infection, dehiscence, etc.) may be less in patients undergoing endoscopic vein harvest when compared to patients undergoing conventional open techniques, because of different incisional lengths.

Patient satisfaction with quality of postoperative analgesia (following any surgical procedure) is as much related to the comparison between anticipated pain and experienced pain as it is to the actual level of pain experienced. Patients undergoing cardiac surgery remain concerned regarding the adequacy of postoperative pain relief and tend to preoperatively expect a greater amount of postoperative pain than that which is actually experienced (14). Because of these unique preoperative expectations, patients following cardiac surgery who receive only moderate analgesia postoperatively will likely still be satisfied with their pain control. Thus, patients may experience pain of moderate intensity after cardiac surgery yet still express very high satisfaction levels (14,15).

Inadequate analgesia (coupled with an uninhibited stress response) during the postoperative period following cardiac surgery may lead to many adverse hemodynamic (tachycardia, hypertension, vasoconstriction), metabolic (increased catabolism), immunologic (impaired immune response), and hemostatic (platelet activation) alterations. In patients undergoing cardiac surgery, perioperative myocardial ischemia (diagnosed by electrocardiography [ECG] and/or transesophageal echocardiography [TEE]) is most commonly observed during the immediate postoperative period and appears to be related to outcome (22,23). Intraoperatively, initiation of cardiopulmonary bypass causes substantial increases in stress response hormones (norepinephrine, epinephrine, etc.) that persist into the immediate postoperative period and may also contribute to myocardial ischemia observed during this time (24–26). Furthermore, postoperative myocardial ischemia may be aggravated by cardiac sympathetic nerve activation, which disrupts the balance between coronary blood flow and myocardial oxygen demand (27). Thus, during the pivotal immediate postoperative period after cardiac surgery, adequate analgesia (coupled with stress response attenuation) may potentially decrease morbidity and enhance health-related quality of life (27,28).

Evidence exists that aggressive control of postoperative pain in patients following cardiac surgery may beneficially affect outcome (9,10,29). Unfortunately, aggressive control of postoperative pain in patients following cardiac surgery through the use of relatively large amounts of IV opioids does not allow tracheal extubation to occur in the immediate postoperative period (a goal of current practice). Regional techniques may perhaps allow one to obtain intense postoperative analgesia while allowing early postoperative tracheal extubation.

Local Anesthetic Infiltration

Pain following cardiac surgery is often related to median sternotomy (peaking during the first 2 postoperative days). Because of problems associated with traditional IV opioid analgesia (nausea and vomiting, pruritus, urinary retention, respiratory depression) and the more recently introduced nonsteroidal antiinflammatory drugs (NSAIDs) and cyclooxygenase (COX) inhibitors (gastrointestinal bleeding, renal dysfunction), alternative methods of achieving postoperative analgesia in cardiac surgical patients have been sought. One alternative method is continuous infusion of local anesthetic in the sternotomy incision. In a prospective, randomized, placebo-controlled, double-blind clinical trial, White and associates studied 36 patients undergoing cardiac surgery (30). Intraoperative management was standardized. All patients had two indwelling infusion catheters placed at the median sternotomy incision site at the end of surgery (one in the subfascial plane above the sternum, one above the fascia in the subcutaneous tissue). Patients received either 0.25% bupivacaine ($n = 12$), 0.5% bupivacaine ($n = 12$), or normal saline ($n = 12$) via a constant rate infusion through the catheter (4 mL/hr) for 48 hours following surgery. Average times to tracheal extubation were similar in the three groups (approximately 5–6 hours). Compared with the control group (normal saline), there was a statistically significant reduction in verbal rating scale pain scores and IV patient-controlled morphine analgesia use in the 0.5% bupivacaine group. Patient satisfaction with their pain management was also improved in the 0.5% bupivacaine group versus saline control. However, there were no significant differences in patient-controlled morphine analgesia use between the 0.25% bupivacaine and control groups. Although tracheal extubation time and the duration of the intensive care unit stay (30 hours versus 34 hours, respectively) were not significantly altered, time to ambulation (1 day versus 2 days, respectively) and duration of hospital stay (4.2 days versus 5.7 days, respectively) were lower in the 0.5% bupivacaine group than in the control group. Serum bupivacaine concentrations in patients were reasonable. One complication related to the local anesthetic delivery system was encountered when a catheter tip was inadvertently broken off during its removal from the incision site, which required surgical reexploration of the wound under local anesthesia. The authors conclude that continuous infusion of 0.5% bupivacaine at 4 mL/hour is effective for decreasing postoperative pain and the need for postoperative supplemental opioid analgesic medication, as well as for improving patient satisfaction (earlier ambulation, reduced length of hospital stay) with pain management after cardiac surgery.

Another published clinical investigation reveals the potential benefits of using a continuous infusion of local anesthetic

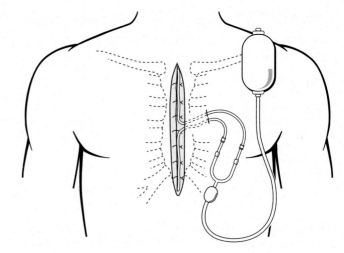

FIGURE 22-1. Intraoperative placement of the pressurized elastomeric pump and catheters.

combined with intercostal nerve blocks in patients following cardiac surgery (31). In this prospective, randomized, placebo-controlled, double-blind clinical trial, Dowling and associates studied 35 healthy patients undergoing cardiac surgery (31). Patients undergoing elective CABG via median sternotomy were randomized to either ropivacaine or placebo groups. At the end of the operation, prior to wound closure, bilateral intercostal nerve injections from T1 to T12 were performed using 20 mL of either 0.2% ropivacaine or normal saline. After sternal reapproximation with wires, two catheters with multiple side openings were placed anterior to the sternum (Fig. 22-1). Infusions of 0.2% ropivacaine or normal saline at approximately 4 mL/hour for 48 hours were delivered through these catheters. Both groups exhibited similar postoperative extubation times (approximately 8 hours). Total mean patient-controlled morphine analgesia consumption during the immediate postoperative period (72 hours) was significantly decreased in the ropivacaine group when compared with the placebo group (47.3 mg versus 78.7 mg, respectively, $p = 0.038$). Mean overall pain scores (0–10 scale) were also significantly decreased in the ropivacaine group when compared with the placebo group (1.6 versus 2.6, respectively, $p = 0.005$). Most interestingly, patients receiving ropivacaine had a significantly shorter length of stay of 5.2 days ± 1.3 days compared with 8.2 days ± 7.9 days for patients receiving normal saline ($p = 0.001$). One patient in the placebo group had an extremely long postoperative hospitalization (39 days). However, the difference between the two groups regarding length of hospital stay remained statistically significant even if this outlier was removed (5.2 days ± 1.3 days versus 6.3 days ± 2.8 days, respectively, $p < 0.01$). Despite differences in postoperative analgesia, postoperative pulmonary function (assessed via forced expiratory volume in 1 second and peak expiratory flow) was similar between the two groups. There was no difference in wound infections or wound healing between the two groups during hospitalization or after hospital discharge. No complications related to placement of the sternal wound catheters or performance of the intercostal nerve blocks were encountered. The significant decrease in hospital length of stay observed by the investigators is intriguing, may result in substantial cost reductions, and deserves further study.

The management of postoperative pain with continuous direct infusion of local anesthetic into the surgical wound has been described following a wide variety of surgeries other than cardiac (inguinal hernia repair, upper abdominal surgery, laparoscopic nephrectomy, cholecystectomy, knee arthroplasty, shoulder surgery, and gynecologic operative laparoscopy) (32). The infusion pump systems used for anesthetic wound perfusion are regulated by the U.S. Food and Drug Administration (FDA) as medical devices. Thus, adverse events reported to the FDA include tissue necrosis, surgical wound infection, and cellulitis following orthopedic, gastrointestinal, podiatric, and other surgeries. None of these reported adverse events as of yet have involved patients undergoing cardiac surgery. The most commonly reported complication is tissue necrosis, an adverse event almost never seen following normal surgical procedures. Furthermore, consequences of these reported adverse events were typically severe and required intervention and additional medical and/or surgical treatment. Although these initial reports may be isolated incidents, they may also represent an early warning that is representative of a widespread problem. Nevertheless, these reports provide a potentially important signal, suggesting the need for further investigation into the relationship between use of these infusion pumps for direct continuous infusion of local anesthetics and other drugs into surgical wounds and the effect on tissue necrosis, serious infections, or cellulitis. Neither of the two clinical investigations involving local anesthetic infusion in patients following cardiac surgery with median sternotomy report such wound complications (30,31). Regardless, these safety issues merit careful consideration because of the importance of sternal wound complications in this setting.

Nerve Blocks

With the increasing popularity of minimally invasive cardiac surgery, which utilizes non sternotomy incisions (minithoracotomy), the use of nerve blocks in cardiac surgical patients has increased as well (33–38). Thoracotomy incisions (transverse anterolateral minithoracotomy, vertical anterolateral minithoracotomy), owing to trauma of the costal cartilage tissue, damage to ribs, tissue damage to muscles, and tissue damage to peripheral nerves, may induce more intense postoperative pain than median sternotomy. Adequate analgesia following thoracotomy is important because pain is a key component in alteration of lung function following thoracic surgery. Uncontrolled pain causes a reduction in respiratory mechanics, reduced mobility, and increases in hormonal and metabolic activity. Perioperative deterioration in respiratory mechanics may lead to pulmonary complications and hypoxemia, which may in turn lead to myocardial ischemia/infarction, cerebrovascular accidents, thromboembolism, and/or delayed wound healing, further leading to increased morbidity and prolonged hospital stay. Various analgesic techniques have been developed to treat postoperative thoracotomy pain. The most commonly utilized techniques include intercostal nerve blocks, intrapleural administration of local anesthetics, and thoracic paravertebral blocks.

Intercostal nerve block has been used extensively for analgesia following thoracic surgery (33,35). Intercostal nerve blocks can be performed either intraoperatively or postoperatively and usually provide sufficient analgesia lasting approximately 6 to 12 hours (depending on amount and type of local anesthetic utilized); these blocks may need to be repeated if additional analgesia is required. Local anesthetics may be administered as a single treatment under direction vision, before chest closure; as a single preoperative percutaneous injection; as multiple percutaneous serial injections; or via an indwelling inter-

costal catheter. Blockade of intercostal nerves interrupts C-fiber afferent transmission of impulses to the spinal cord. A single intercostal injection of a long-acting local anesthetic can provide pain relief and improve pulmonary function in patients following thoracic surgery for up to 6 hours. To achieve longer duration of analgesia, a continuous extrapleural intercostal nerve block technique may be used in which a catheter is placed percutaneously into an extrapleural pocket by the surgeon. A continuous intercostal catheter allows frequent dosing or infusions of local anesthetic agents and avoids multiple needle injections. Various clinical studies have confirmed the analgesic efficacy of this technique, and the technique compares favorably with thoracic epidural analgesic techniques (33). A major concern associated with intercostal nerve block is the potentially high amount of local anesthetic systemic absorption, yet multiple clinical studies involving patients undergoing thoracic surgery have documented safe blood levels with standard techniques. Clinical investigations involving patients undergoing thoracic surgery indicate that intercostal nerve blockade by intermittent or continuous infusion of 0.25% to 0.5% bupivacaine with epinephrine is an effective method for supplementing systemic IV opioid analgesia for postthoracotomy pain. The value of single preclosure injections remains doubtful.

Intrapleural administration of local anesthetics initiates analgesia via mechanisms that remain incompletely understood (33,35). However, the mechanism of action of extrapleural regional anesthesia seems to depend primarily on diffusion of the local anesthetic into the paravertebral region. Local anesthetic agents then affect not only the ventral nerve root but also afferent fibers of the posterior primary ramus. Posterior ligaments of the posterior primary ramus innervate posterior spinal muscles and skin and are traumatized during posterolateral thoracotomy. Intrapleural administration of local anesthetic agent to this region through a catheter inserted in the extrapleural space thus creates an anesthetic region in the skin. The depth and width of the anesthetic region depends on diffusion of the local anesthetic agent in the extrapleural space. With this technique, local anesthetics may be administered via an indwelling intrapleural catheter placed between the parietal and visceral pleura by intermittent or continuous infusion regimens. Systemic absorption of local anesthetic and toxicity are always a concern with this technique, but have not been substantiated in clinical studies that assayed plasma levels (33,35). A handful of clinical investigations involving patients undergoing thoracic surgery via thoracotomy incision suggest that 0.25% to 0.5% bupivacaine may improve analgesia in patients following thoracic surgery, yet its true efficacy as a postoperative analgesic in this patient population remains somewhat controversial (36). The analgesic benefits are of short duration, and there does not appear to be a significant overall opioid-sparing effect. Furthermore, the optimum concentration and duration remains to be defined. However, a recently published prospective, randomized clinical study involving 50 patients undergoing minimally invasive direct CABG (via minithoracotomy) reported that an intrapleural analgesic technique (using 0.25% bupivacaine) is safe and effective and compares favorably to a conventional thoracic epidural technique (37). However, careful catheter positioning, chest tube clamping, and anchoring of the catheter are mandatory for postoperative intrapleural analgesia to be effective. A major factor implicated in lack of efficacy regarding intrapleural techniques is loss of local anesthetic solution through intercostal chest drainage tubes. Although clamping the chest tubes during the postoperative period will increase analgesic efficacy, it may not be safe to clamp chest tubes, as they provide important drainage of hemorrhage and air and allow for enhanced lung patency and expansion.

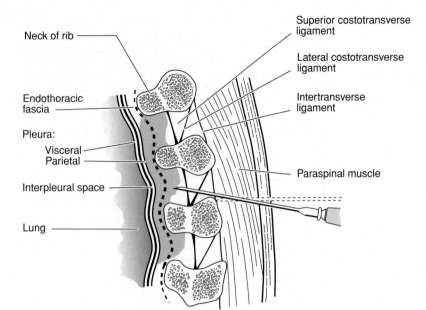

FIGURE 22-2. Sagittal section through the thoracic paravertebral space showing a needle that has been advanced above the transverse process.

Apart from proper catheter positioning (insertion of catheter under direct vision and anchoring catheter to skin is essential), effective analgesia with this technique also appears to depend on whether surgery to the lung was performed or whether the pleural anatomy and physiology are relatively intact.

Thoracic paravertebral block involves injection of local anesthetic adjacent to the thoracic vertebrae, close to where the spinal nerves emerge from the intervertebral foramina (Fig. 22-2 and see Figs. 16-4, and 16-15 to 16-17). Thoracic paravertebral block, when compared to thoracic epidural analgesic techniques, provides equivalent analgesia, is technically easier, and may harbor less risk. Several different techniques exist for successful thoracic paravertebral block, and have recently been extensively reviewed (34) (Chapter 16). These blocks may be effective in alleviating acute and chronic pain of unilateral origin from the chest and/or abdomen. Unilateral paravertebral block is useful for attaining postthoracotomy analgesia, because pain following lateral thoracotomy is essentially always unilateral. The benefits of unilateral paravertebral blockade are a lesser incidence of adverse events (hypotension, urinary retention) and a decreased risk of systemic local anesthetic toxicity because less local anesthetic is used. The clinical investigations involving unilateral paravertebral block in patients undergoing thoracic surgery are few (33,35). Therefore, it is not possible to determine from the available literature whether the technique of paravertebral blockade (single injection) is truly useful in the postoperative analgesic management of patients following thoracotomy. Continuous thoracic paravertebral infusion of local anesthetic, placed under direct vision at thoracotomy or using a loss-of-resistance technique, is an effective method of providing analgesia following thoracotomy. Indeed, continuous thoracic paravertebral block, as part of a balanced analgesic regimen, may provide effective pain relief with very few side effects following thoracotomy and appears to be comparable to thoracic epidural analgesia (34). Bilateral use of thoracic paravertebral block has been described.

In summary, intercostal nerve blocks, intrapleural administration of local anesthetics, and thoracic paravertebral block offer the advantages of simplicity and efficacy in controlling postoperative pain in patients undergoing thoracic incisions for cardiac surgery. However, although the analgesic efficacy of these techniques sometimes is comparable to intrathecal techniques and epidural techniques, these techniques appear to work best as a part of a multimodal analgesic regimen. The patient must be observed for complications associated with infiltrations of large quantities of local anesthetic when utilizing these analgesic techniques.

Intrathecal and Epidural Techniques

Intrathecal and/or epidural techniques, utilizing opioids and/or local anesthetics, initiate reliable postoperative analgesia in patients following cardiac surgery (39). Additional potential advantages of using intrathecal and/or epidural techniques in patients undergoing cardiac surgery include stress response attenuation and thoracic cardiac sympathectomy. Intrathecal or epidural anesthesia and analgesia (with local anesthetics or opioids) can effectively inhibit the stress response associated with surgical procedures (27). Local anesthetics appear to possess greater efficacy than opioids in perioperative stress response attenuation, perhaps because of their unique mechanism of action. Although still a matter of some debate, perioperative stress response attenuation with epidural local anesthetics and/or opioids in high-risk patients after major noncardiac surgery may potentially decrease morbidity and mortality (7,8,27). Unfortunately, to achieve perioperative stress response attenuation in patients undergoing cardiac surgery using IV opioids in this manner does not allow tracheal extubation to occur in the immediate postoperative period. Intrathecal or epidural anesthesia and analgesia techniques (particularly with local anesthetics) are attractive alternatives because of their potential to attenuate the perioperative stress response yet still allow tracheal extubation to occur in the immediate postoperative period.

The myocardium and coronary vasculature are densely innervated by sympathetic nerve fibers that arise from T1 to T5 and profoundly influence total coronary blood flow and distribution (40). Cardiac sympathetic nerve activation initiates coronary artery vasoconstriction (41) and paradoxical coronary vasoconstriction in response to intrinsic vasodilators (42). In patients with coronary artery disease, cardiac sympathetic nerve activation disrupts the normal matching of coronary blood flow and myocardial oxygen demand (43,44). Animal models have revealed an intense poststenotic coronary vasoconstrictive mechanism mediated by cardiac sympathetic nerve activation that attenuates local metabolic coronary vasodilation in response to myocardial ischemia (45,46). Furthermore, myocardial ischemia initiates a cardiocardiac reflex mediated by sympathetic nerve fibers, which augments the ischemic process (47). Cardiac sympathetic nerve activation likely plays a central role in initiating postoperative myocardial ischemia by decreasing myocardial oxygen supply via these mechanisms (27,48).

Thoracic epidural anesthesia with local anesthetics effectively blocks cardiac sympathetic nerve afferent and efferent fibers, whereas epidural opioids are unable to effectively block such cardiac sympathetic nerve activity (27). Patients with symptomatic coronary artery disease benefit clinically from cardiac sympathectomy; the application of thoracic sympathetic blockade in the management of angina pectoris was described as early as 1965 (49). Thoracic epidural anesthesia with local anesthetics increases the diameter of stenotic epicardial coronary artery segments without causing dilation of coronary arterioles (43), decreases determinants of myocardial oxygen demand (44), improves left ventricular function (50), and decreases anginal symptoms (44,51). Furthermore, cardiac sympathectomy increases the endocardial-to-epicardial blood flow ratio (52,53), beneficially affects collateral blood flow during myocardial ischemia (53), decreases poststenotic coronary vasoconstriction (46), and attenuates the myocardial ischemia-induced cardiocardiac reflex (46). In an animal model, thoracic epidural anesthesia with local anesthetics actually decreased myocardial infarct size following coronary artery occlusion (52). Of note, these beneficial effects are not caused by systemic absorption of the local anesthetic (52). In short, thoracic epidural anesthesia with local anesthetics may benefit patients undergoing cardiac surgery by effectively blocking cardiac sympathetic nerve activity and improving the myocardial oxygen supply-demand balance.

Intrathecal Techniques

Application of intrathecal analgesia to patients undergoing cardiac surgery was initially reported by Mathews and Abrams in 1980 (54). They described the administration of intrathecal morphine (1.5–4.0 mg) to 40 adults after the induction of general anesthesia for cardiac surgery. Somewhat remarkably, all 40 patients awakened pain-free at the end of surgery (prior to leaving the operating room) and 36 patients were tracheally extubated prior to transfer to the intensive are unit. Postoperatively, all 40 patients were entirely pain-free for the first 27.5 postoperative hours, and 17 did not require any supplemental analgesics prior to discharge from the hospital. Mathews and Abrams summarize: "The benefits of recovering from surgery free from pain have been impressive. This has been particularly appreciated by patients who have had previous operations with conventional anaesthesia and postoperative analgesic drugs. The patients have been remarkably comfortable, able to move more easily in bed, and more cooperative, thus greatly helping their nursing care" (54). After this impressive clinical display, other investigators have subsequently applied intrathecal anesthesia and analgesia techniques to patients undergoing cardiac surgery (55–83). Most clinical investigators have used intrathecal morphine to provide prolonged postoperative analgesia, although some clinical investigators have used intrathecal fentanyl, sufentanil, and/or local anesthetics. A recently published

anonymous survey of members of the Society of Cardiovascular Anesthesiologists indicates that almost 8% of practicing anesthesiologists incorporate intrathecal techniques into their anesthetic management of adults undergoing cardiac surgery (83). Of these anesthesiologists, 75% practice in the United States, 72% perform the intrathecal injection prior to induction of anesthesia, 97% utilize morphine, 13% utilize fentanyl, 2% utilize sufentanil, 10% utilize lidocaine, and 3% utilize tetracaine (83).

Intrathecal Analgesia and Tracheal Extubation

Two randomized, blinded, placebo-controlled clinical studies revealed the ability of intrathecal morphine to induce significant postoperative analgesia following cardiac surgery (69,76). In 1988, Vanstrum and associates prospectively randomized 30 patients to receive either intrathecal morphine (0.5 mg) or intrathecal placebo prior to induction of anesthesia (76). Intraoperative anesthetic management was standardized, and all patients postoperatively received exclusively IV morphine administered by a nurse who attempted to keep the linear analog pain score at less than four (1–10 scale). Although pain scores between groups were not significantly different at any postoperative time interval tested, patients who received intrathecal morphine required significantly less IV morphine than placebo controls (2.4 mg versus 8.3 mg, respectively, $p <0.02$) during the initial 30 hours following intrathecal injection. Associated with this enhanced analgesia in patients receiving intrathecal morphine was a substantially decreased need for antihypertensive medications (sodium nitroprusside, nitroglycerine, hydralazine) during the immediate postoperative period. Time to tracheal extubation (approximately 20 hours) and postoperative arterial blood gas tensions following anesthesia were not significantly affected by the use of intrathecal morphine. In 1996, Chaney and associates prospectively randomized 60 patients to receive either intrathecal morphine (4.0 mg) or intrathecal placebo prior to induction of anesthesia for elective CABG (69). Intraoperative anesthetic management was standardized and, after tracheal extubation, all patients received exclusively IV morphine via patient-controlled analgesia (PCA). The mean time from intensive care unit arrival to tracheal extubation was similar in all patients (approximately 20 hours). However, patients who received intrathecal morphine required significantly less IV morphine than placebo controls (33.2 mg versus 51.1 mg, respectively, $p <0.05$) during the initial postoperative period. Despite enhanced analgesia, no clinical differences between groups existed regarding postoperative morbidity (pruritus, nausea, vomiting, urinary retention, prolonged somnolence, atrial fibrillation, ventricular tachycardia, myocardial infarction, cerebral infarction), mortality, nor duration of postoperative hospital stay (approximately 9 days in each group).

The mid 1990s saw the emergence of fast-track cardiac surgery, with the goal being tracheal extubation in the immediate postoperative period. Chaney and associates, in 1997, were the first to study the potential clinical benefits of intrathecal morphine when used in patients undergoing cardiac surgery and early tracheal extubation (68). They prospectively randomized 40 patients to receive either intrathecal morphine (10 μg/kg) or intrathecal placebo prior to induction of anesthesia for elective CABG. Intraoperative anesthetic management was standardized (IV fentanyl, 20 μg/kg, and IV midazolam, 10 mg) and all patients postoperatively received exclusively IV morphine via PCA. Of the patients who were tracheally extubated during the immediate postoperative period, the mean time from intensive care unit arrival to tracheal extubation was significantly prolonged in those who received intrathecal morphine (10.9 hours ± 4.4 hours; $p = 0.02$) when compared to placebo controls (7.6 hours ± 2.5 hours). Three patients who received intrathecal morphine had tracheal extubation substantially delayed (12–24 hours) because of prolonged ventilatory depression, likely secondary to intrathecal morphine. No clinical differences existed between groups regarding IV morphine use for 48 hours, postoperative morbidity, mortality, nor duration of postoperative hospital stay (approximately 9 days in each group).

These somewhat discouraging findings (absence of enhanced analgesia, prolongation of tracheal extubation time) stimulated the same group of investigators, in 1999, to repeat the study, but decrease intraoperative IV fentanyl administration to 10 μg/kg (66). Of the patients tracheally extubated during the immediate postoperative period, mean time to tracheal extubation was similar in patients who received intrathecal morphine (6.8 hours ± 2.8 hours) when compared to intrathecal placebo patients (6.5 hours ± 3.2 hours). However, once again, four (10%) patients who received intrathecal morphine had tracheal extubation substantially delayed (14 hours, 14 hours, 18 hours, 19 hours) because of prolonged respiratory depression (likely secondary to intrathecal morphine). No clinical differences existed between groups regarding postoperative morbidity, mortality, nor duration of postoperative hospital stay (approximately 6 days in each group). Based on these three prospective, randomized, double-blind, placebo-controlled clinical investigations, the authors concluded that, although intrathecal morphine certainly can initiate reliable postoperative analgesia, its use in the setting of fast-track cardiac surgery and early tracheal extubation may be detrimental by potentially delaying tracheal extubation in the immediate postoperative period.

Since this time, however, other clinical investigators have revealed that certain combinations of intraoperative anesthetic technique, coupled with appropriate doses of intrathecal morphine, will allow both tracheal extubation following cardiac surgery within the immediate postoperative period along with enhanced analgesia (58). Importantly, limiting the amounts of intraoperative IV opioids and IV sedatives and the application of a postoperative tracheal extubation protocol may be more important in achieving the goal of early tracheal extubation following cardiac surgery than adequate pain control during the immediate postoperative period.

Many other suboptimally designed clinical investigations attest to the ability of intrathecal morphine to induce substantial postoperative analgesia in patients following cardiac surgery (Table 22-2). Intrathecal doses of 0.5 to 10.0 mg administered prior to cardiopulmonary bypass initiate reliable postoperative analgesia, the quality of which depends not only on the intrathecal dose administered but also on the type and amount of IV analgesics and sedatives used for the intraoperative baseline anesthetic. The optimal dose of intrathecal morphine for achieving the maximum postoperative analgesia with minimum undesirable drug effects is uncertain. Naturally, when larger doses of intrathecal morphine are used, more intense and prolonged postoperative analgesia is purchased at the expense of more undesirable side effects, including nausea and vomiting, pruritus, urinary retention, and respiratory depression.

Attenuation of Stress Response

Because of morphine's low lipid solubility, analgesic effects following intrathecal injection are delayed. Thus, even large doses of intrathecal morphine administered to patients prior to cardiac surgery will not initiate reliable intraoperative analgesia (76–78,81) and therefore would not be expected to potentially attenuate the intraoperative stress response associated with cardiopulmonary bypass. Only an extremely large dose of intrathecal morphine (10.0 mg) may initiate reliable intraoperative analgesia (80). A single clinical investigation has examined the ability of intrathecal morphine to potentially attenuate the intraoperative stress response associated with cardiopulmonary bypass as measured by blood catecholamine levels (69). In this clinical investigation by Chaney and associates, patients were prospectively randomized to receive either intrathecal morphine (4.0 mg) or intrathecal placebo prior to induction of anesthesia for elective CABG with cardiopulmonary bypass. Intraoperative anesthetic management was standardized, and multiple arterial blood samples were obtained perioperatively to ascertain norepinephrine and epinephrine levels. Patients who were administered intrathecal morphine experienced similar perioperative increases in blood catecholamine levels when compared with placebo controls. Thus, it appears that intrathecal morphine (even in relatively large doses) is unable to reliably attenuate the perioperative stress response associated with cardiac surgery and cardiopulmonary bypass.

However, although unable to reliably attenuate the perioperative stress response associated with cardiopulmonary bypass, intrathecal morphine (by initiating postoperative analgesia) may potentially attenuate the stress response during the immediate postoperative period (76). Vanstrum and associates revealed that patients who were administered 0.5 mg of intrathecal morphine prior to the induction of anesthesia not only required significantly less IV morphine postoperatively when compared to placebo controls but also required significantly less IV nitroprusside (58.1 mg versus 89.1 mg, respectively, $p < 0.05$) during the initial 24 postoperative hours to control hypertension, suggesting partial postoperative stress response attenuation.

Intrathecal fentanyl, sufentanil, and/or local anesthetics have been used in patients undergoing cardiac surgery, hoping to provide intraoperative anesthesia and analgesia (and stress response attenuation), with mixed results (Table 22-2). Intrathecal sufentanil (50 μg), administered prior to the induction of anesthesia for cardiac surgery can reduce volatile anesthetic requirements during mediastinal dissection but is unable to reliably block intraoperative hemodynamic responses to laryngoscopy and intubation (73).

Hemodynamic Effects of Intrathecal Local Anesthetics

Administration of intrathecal local anesthetics to patients after the induction of anesthesia for cardiac surgery may help promote intraoperative hemodynamic stability (70,72).

In 1994, in a retrospective review, 18 adult patients were administered lumbar intrathecal hyperbaric bupivacaine (23–30 mg) and/or hyperbaric lidocaine (150 mg) mixed with morphine (0.5–1.0 mg) following the induction of anesthesia (72). In an attempt to produce a "total spinal" and, thus, thoracic cardiac sympathectomy, the Trendelenburg position was maintained for at least 10 minutes following intrathecal injection. Heart rate decreased significantly (baseline mean 67 bpm to postinjection mean 52 bpm) after the intrathecal injection (indicating cardiac sympathectomy was obtained) and not a single patient exhibited ECG evidence of myocardial ischemia prior to cardiopulmonary bypass. Although these authors report that

TABLE 22-2

REPORTS OF INTRATHECAL ANESTHESIA AND ANALGESIA FOR CARDIAC SURGERY

First author	Year	Study design	Total patients	Drugs: dose	Intraoperative management	Remarks
Metz	2004	Retrospective	112	Morphine: 0.3–1.6 mg	Not Standardized	May facilitate intraoperative extubation; May increase respiratory depression
Lena	2003	Prospective, randomized	45	Morphine: 4 μg/kg; Clonidine: 1 μg/kg	Not Standardized	Reliable postoperative analgesia; Facilitated early extubation
Lee	2003	Prospective, randomized blind, placebo-controlled	38	Bupivacaine: 37.5 mg	Standardized	Potential stress-response attenuation
Bowler	2002	Prospective, randomized	24	Morphine: 2.0 mg	Not Standardized	No benefit
Bettex	2002	Prospective, randomized	24	Morphine: 0.5 mg; Sufentanil: 50 μg	Not Standardized	Reliable postoperative analgesia; Facilitated early extubation
Alhashemi	2000	Prospective, randomized, blind, placebo-controlled	50	Morphine: 250 μg or 500 μg	Standardized	Significant postoperative analgesia
Latham	2000	Prospective, randomized	40	Morphine: 8 μg/kg	Standardized	No benefit
Zarate	2000	Prospective, randomized	40	Morphine: 8 μg/kg	Standardized	Reliable postoperative analgesia
Peterson	2000	Retrospective	18	Morphine: 5–10 μg/kg; Tetracaine: 1–2 mg/kg	Not Standardized	No benefit
Hammer	2000	Retrospective	25	Morphine: 7–10 μg/kg; Tetracaine: 0.5–2 mg/kg	Not Standardized	No benefit
Chaney	1999	Prospective, randomized, blind, placebo-controlled	40	Morphine: 10 μg/kg	Standardized	No benefit
Shroff	1997	Prospective, randomized	21	Morphine: 10 μg/kg; Fentanyl: 25 μg	Not Standardized	Reliable postoperative analgesia, facilitated early extubation
Chaney	1997	Prospective, randomized, blind, placebo-controlled	40	Morphine: 10 μg/kg	Standardized	Hindered early extubation
Chaney	1996	Prospective, randomized, blind, placebo-controlled	60	Morphine: 4.0 mg	Standardized	Significant postoperative analgesia, no stress-response attenuation
Taylor	1996	Retrospective	152	Morphine: 30 μg/kg	Not Standardized	Reliable postoperative analgesia
Kowalewski	1994	Retrospective	18	Morphine: 0.5–1.0 mg; Bupivacaine: 23–30 mg; Lidocaine: 150 mg	Not Standardized	Reliable postoperative analgesia, possible thoracic cardiac sympathectomy

(continued)

TABLE 22-2

(CONTINUED)

First author	Year	Study design	Total patients	Drugs: dose	Intraoperative management	Remarks
Swenson	1994	Retrospective	10	Morphine: 0.5 mg Sufentanil: 50 μg	Not Standardized	Reliable postoperative analgesia, facilitated early extubation
Fitzpatrick	1988	Prospective, randomized	44	Morphine: 1.0–2.0 mg	Not Standardized	Significant postoperative analgesia
Vanstrum	1988	Prospective, randomized, blind, placebo-controlled	30	Morphine: 0.5 mg	Standardized	Significant postoperative analgesia, possible stress-response attenuation
Casey	1987	Prospective, randomized, blind, placebo-controlled	40	Morphine: 20 μg/kg	Standardized	No benefit
Cheun	1987	Prospective, observational	180	Morphine: 0.1 mg/kg Meperidine: 1.5 mg/kg	Not Standardized	Reliable postoperative analgesia
Aun	1985	Prospective, randomized	60	Morphine: 2.0–4.0 mg	Not Standardized	Significant postoperative analgesia
Jones	1984	Prospective, observational	56	Morphine: 20–30 μg/kg	Not Standardized	Reliable postoperative analgesia
Mathews	1980	Retrospective	40	Morphine: 1.5–4.0 mg	Not Standardized	Reliable postoperative analgesia

the technique provided stable perioperative hemodynamics, 17 of 18 patients required IV phenylephrine at some time intraoperatively to increase blood pressure. In 1996, the same group of investigators reported similar hemodynamic changes in a case report involving a 10-year-old child with Kawasaki disease who underwent CABG and receiving intrathecal hyperbaric bupivacaine mixed with morphine via a lumbar puncture following induction of anesthesia (70).

A recently published, small ($n = 38$ patients), prospective, randomized, blinded clinical investigation reveals that large doses of intrathecal bupivacaine (37.5 mg) administered to patients immediately prior to induction of general anesthesia (19 patients received intrathecal bupivacaine, 19 patients served as controls) for elective CABG may potentially initiate intraoperative stress response attenuation (assessed via serum mediator levels, hemodynamics, and qualitative/quantitative alterations in myocardial β-receptors) (84). However, no effect on real clinical outcome parameters (i.e., tracheal extubation times, respiratory function, perioperative spirometry) was observed. Mean tracheal extubation times (measured from the time of sternotomy dressing application) were extremely short in both groups (11–19 minutes). Postoperative pain scores and morphine use via PCA did not differ between the two groups. Not surprisingly, phenylephrine use was more common in patients who received intrathecal bupivacaine when compared to control patients.

In summary, the many clinical investigations involving the use of intrathecal analgesic techniques in patients undergoing cardiac surgery indicate that the administration of intrathecal morphine to patients prior to cardiopulmonary bypass initiates reliable postoperative analgesia following cardiac surgery. Intrathecal opioids or local anesthetics cannot reliably attenuate the perioperative stress response associated with cardiopulmonary bypass that persists during the immediate postoperative period. Although intrathecal local anesthetics (not opioids) may induce perioperative thoracic cardiac sympathectomy, the hemodynamic changes associated with a "total spinal" makes the technique unsuitable for patients with cardiac disease.

Epidural Techniques

Thoracic epidural anesthesia and analgesia with local anesthetics and/or opioids induces significant postoperative analgesia in patients undergoing cardiac procedures. A recently published anonymous survey of members of the Society of Cardiovascular Anesthesiologists indicates that 7% of practicing anesthesiologists incorporate thoracic epidural techniques into their anesthetic management of adults undergoing cardiac surgery (83). Of these anesthesiologists, 58% practice in the United States. Regarding the timing of epidural instrumentation, 40% perform instrumentation before induction of general anesthesia, 12% perform instrumentation following induction of general anesthesia, 33% perform instrumentation at the end of surgery, and 15% perform instrumentation on the first postoperative day (83).

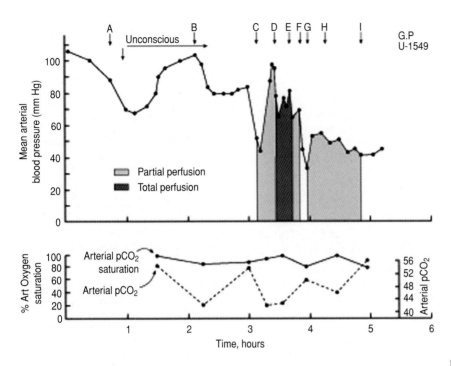

FIGURE 22-3. Graph of clinical course of initial cardiac patient receiving presurgical epidural anesthesia in 1954. From Clowes et al. (85).

A = Epidural Anesthesia started; **B** = Chest open; **C** = Star pump; **D** = Clamp Pulmonary artery; **E** = Unclamp Pulmonary artery; **F** = Pump off; **G** = Pump on; **H** = Chest closed; **I** Pump off

The initial description of thoracic epidural anesthesia and analgesia applied to a cardiac surgical patient occurred in 1954 (85). Clowes and associates describe their presurgical anesthetic technique in a 55-year-old man with severe cardiac failure: "An endotracheal tube was passed with topical anesthesia. Under extradural block of the upper thorax, hypotension developed but responded to the administration of a vasopressor drug. At this time the patient became comatose" (Fig. 22-3) (85). The patient eventually expired. Application of thoracic epidural anesthesia and analgesia to patients undergoing cardiac surgery during the modern surgical era was initially reported by Hoar and associates in 1976 (86). They described the intraoperative insertion of thoracic epidural catheters in 12 patients following CABG (after IV protamine, prior to transfer to intensive care unit). The epidural catheters were injected with lidocaine and bupivacaine during the immediate postoperative period to promote analgesia and effectively control hypertension. Administration of epidural local anesthetics to these patients significantly decreased postoperative blood pressure in hypertensive and normotensive patients; not a single patient required cardiac or peripheral vascular stimulants during the immediate postoperative study period.

The 1987 report by El-Baz and Goldin was the first to describe the insertion of thoracic epidural catheters in patients *prior* to cardiac surgery and also involved epidural opioids, rather than local anesthetics (87). In prospective, randomized fashion, patients undergoing elective CABG received either routine treatment for postoperative pain ($n = 30$ patients, IV morphine) or a continuous infusion of morphine (0.1 mg/hr) via a thoracic epidural catheter ($n = 30$ patients). Thoracic epidural catheters were inserted at T3–T4 immediately prior to induction of anesthesia on the day of surgery. Intraoperative anesthetic technique was standardized; mean postoperative tracheal extubation time was significantly shorter in patients receiving thoracic epidural anesthesia when compared to con-

trol patients (9 ± 3 hours versus 18 ± 5 hours, respectively, $p < 0.01$). Continuous thoracic epidural infusion of morphine also achieved better postoperative pain relief in patients than IV morphine (significantly better pain scores, significantly less supplemental IV morphine). Furthermore, in a subgroup of 20 patients (10 per group), postoperative "stress" was assessed via serum cortisol and β-endorphin levels. Patients receiving thoracic epidural anesthesia had significantly lower postoperative levels of these mediators when compared to control patients, indicating potential postoperative stress response attenuation. Continuous thoracic epidural infusion of morphine (when compared to controls) was also associated with a lower incidence of opioid-related side effects during the immediate postoperative period. The insertion of the thoracic epidural catheter immediately prior to systemic heparin administration was not associated with any neurologic problems.

Since this initial report of potential benefits (reliable postoperative analgesia, stress response attenuation, facilitation of early tracheal extubation), others clinical investigators have subsequently applied thoracic epidural anesthesia and analgesia to patients undergoing cardiac surgery (88–123) (Table 22-3). For example, patients randomized to receive intermittent boluses of thoracic epidural infusion intraoperatively, followed by continuous infusion postoperatively, exhibited significantly decreased blood levels of norepinephrine and epinephrine (98,101) and cortisol (98) perioperatively when compared with patients managed similarly without thoracic epidural catheters (101). Furthermore, increased blood catecholamine levels in these patients were associated with increased systemic vascular resistance (101). Continuous thoracic epidural bupivacaine and sufentanil infusion administered perioperatively significantly decreased blood levels of norepinephrine following sternotomy when compared to conventional analgesic methods (104). Other clinical studies further attest to the ability of thoracic epidural anesthesia with

TABLE 22-3

REPORTS OF EPIDURAL ANESTHESIA AND ANALGESIA FOR CARDIAC SURGERY

First author	Year	Study design	Total patients	Drugs: dose	Intraoperative management	Remarks
Hansdottir	2006	Prospective, randomized	113	Bupivacaine, Fentanyl infusion	Standardized	Facilitated early extubation
Barrington	2005	Prospective, randomized	120	Ropivacaine, Fentanyl infusion	Not standardized	Reliable postoperative analgesia Facilitated early extubation No myocardial protection
Royse	2003	Prospective, randomized	80	Ropivacaine, Fentanyl infusion	Not Standardized	Reliable postoperative analgesia
Pastor	2003	Prospective, observational	714	Bupivacaine or Ropivacaine boluses plus infusion	Not Standardized	No hematoma formation
Priestley	2002	Prospective, randomized	100	Ropivacaine, Fentanyl infusion	Not Standardized	Reliable postoperative analgesia
de Vries	2002	Prospective, randomized	90	Bupivacaine: bolus plus infusion Sufentanil: bolus plus infusion	Standardized	Reliable postoperative analgesia Facilitated early extubation Possible decreased hospital stay
Canto	2002	Prospective, observational	305	Ropivacaine: bolus plus infusion	Not Standardized	No hematoma formation
Fillinger	2002	Prospective, randomized	60	Bupivacaine: bolus plus infusion Morphine: bolus plus infusion	Not Standardized	No benefit
Jideus	2001	Prospective, randomized	41	Bupivacaine: bolus plus infusion Sufentanil: infusion	Not Standardized	Stress response attenuation Thoracic cardiac sympathectomy
Scott	2001	Prospective, randomized	206	Bupivacaine: bolus plus infusion Clonidine: infusion	Standardized	Decreased postoperative arrhythmias Improved postoperative pulmonary function Decreased postoperative renal failure Decreased postoperative confusion
Dhole	2001	Prospective, randomized	41	Bupivacaine: bolus plus infusion	Not Standardized	No benefit
Djaiani	2001	Retrospective	37	Bupivacaine: bolus plus infusion	Not Standardized	Facilitated early extubation
Warters	2000	Retrospective	278	Not specified	Not Standardized	No hematoma formation
Loick	1999	Prospective, randomized	25	Bupivacaine: bolus plus infusion Sufentanil: bolus plus infusion	Standardized	Stress response attenuation Thoracic cardiac sympathectomy Facilitated early extubation
Tenling	1999	Prospective, randomized	14	Bupivacaine: bolus plus infusion	Not Standardized	Reliable postoperative analgesia Facilitated early extubation
Sanchez	1998	Prospective, observational	571	Bupivacaine: boluses	Not Standardized	No hematoma formation

(continued)

TABLE 22-3

(CONTINUED)

First author	Year	Study design	Total patients	Drugs: dose	Intraoperative management	Remarks
Fawcett	1997	Prospective, randomized	16	Bupivacaine: bolus plus infusion	Standardized	Reliable postoperative analgesia Improved pulmonary function Stress response attenuation
Hoar	1976	Prospective, observational	12	Lidocaine: boluses Bupivacaine: boluses	Not Standardized	Reliable postoperative analgesia Possible stress response attenuation
Turfrey	1997	Retrospective	218	Bupivacaine: bolus plus infusion Clonidine: infusion	Not Standardized	Facilitated early extubation Possible thoracic cardiac sympathectomy
Shayevitz	1996	Retrospective	54	Morphine: bolus plus infusion	Not Standardized	Reliable postoperative analgesia Facilitated early extubation
Stenseth	1996	Prospective, randomized	54	Bupivacaine: bolus plus infusion	Not Standardized	Facilitated early extubation Possible thoracic cardiac sympathectomy
Moore	1995	Prospective, randomized	17	Bupivacaine: bolus plus infusion	Standardized	Stress response attenuation Possible thoracic cardiac sympathectomy
Stenseth	1995	Prospective, randomized	30	Bupivacaine: bolus plus infusion	Standardized	Thoracic cardiac sympathectomy
Kirno	1994	Prospective, randomized	20	Mepivacaine: bolus	Standardized	Stress response attenuation Thoracic cardiac sympathectomy
Stenseth	1994	Prospective, randomized	30	Bupivacaine: bolus plus infusion	Standardized	Stress response attenuation Possible thoracic cardiac sympathectomy
Liem	1992	Prospective, randomized	54	Bupivacaine: bolus plus infusion Sufentanil: bolus plus infusion	Not Standardized	Reliable postoperative analgesia Stress response attenuation Possible thoracic cardiac sympathectomy
Rosen	1989	Prospective, randomized	32	Morphine: bolus	Not Standardized	Reliable postoperative analgesia Facilitated early extubation
Joachimsson	1989	Observational	28	Bupivacaine: boluses	Not Standardized	Reliable postoperative analgesia
El-Baz	1987	Prospective, randomized	60	Morphine: infusion	Standardized	Reliable postoperative analgesia Stress response attenuation Facilitated early extubation
Robinson	1986	Prospective, observational	10	Meperidine: bolus	Standardized	Reliable postoperative analgesia
Hoar	1976	Prospective, observational	12	Lidocaine: boluses Bupivacaine: boluses	Not Standardized	Reliable postoperative analgesia Possible stress response attenuation

PART III: APPLICATIONS

local anesthetics to promote perioperative hemodynamic stability in patients undergoing cardiac surgery, which suggests perioperative stress response attenuation (86,100,101,104).

One unique clinical investigation directly compared thoracic epidural anesthesia and IV clonidine in patients undergoing cardiac surgery (91). Loick and associates prospectively randomized 70 patients undergoing elective CABG to receive either thoracic epidural anesthesia supplementation (bupivacaine, sufentanil continuous infusion) perioperatively to general anesthesia ($n = 25$ patients), IV clonidine supplementation (continuous infusion) perioperatively to general anesthesia ($n = 24$ patients), or only general anesthesia ($n = 21$ patients, controls) (91). Both the thoracic epidural anesthesia and IV clonidine groups experienced postoperative decreases in heart rate compared with the control group, without jeopardizing cardiac output or perfusion pressure. The effects on stress response mediators were unpredictable and variable. Electrocardiographic evidence of ischemia (ST-segment elevation, ST-segment depression) occurred in 70% of control patients, 50% of thoracic epidural anesthesia patients, and 40% of IV clonidine patients. The release of troponin T was attenuated when compared with controls in the thoracic epidural anesthesia group only, with no effect in the IV clonidine group. Interestingly, the highest quality of postoperative analgesia was found in the patients receiving IV clonidine; visual analog pain scores were nearly halved when compared with the two other groups. Sedation scores were similar among the three groups, with the exception of the 24-hour value in the IV clonidine group, which was higher than that in the thoracic epidural anesthesia group. The postoperative comfort scores (rated between excellent and good) did not differ among the three groups.

Cardiac Sympathectomy

Two provocative clinical studies demonstrate the ability of thoracic epidural anesthesia to induce significant thoracic cardiac sympathectomy in patients undergoing cardiac surgery (99,100). In the first study, patients undergoing CABG were evaluated with reverse thermodilution catheters that had been inserted into the mid coronary sinus under fluoroscopic guidance prior to the induction of anesthesia (99). Intraoperative anesthetic management was standardized. Coronary sinus blood flow was measured by a constant infusion technique, and coronary vascular resistance was calculated utilizing coronary perfusion pressure (arterial diastolic pressure minus pulmonary capillary wedge pressure) and coronary sinus blood flow. Patients who received intermittent boluses of thoracic epidural bupivacaine intraoperatively followed by a continuous infusion postoperatively exhibited significant decreases in coronary vascular resistance post cardiopulmonary bypass when compared with pre-cardiopulmonary bypass values, whereas patients managed similarly without thoracic epidural catheters exhibited significant increases in coronary vascular resistance post cardiopulmonary bypass. In the second study, patients undergoing CABG were evaluated with catheters that had been inserted into the coronary sinus under fluoroscopic guidance and continuous pressure monitoring prior to the induction of anesthesia (100). Intraoperative anesthetic management was standardized, and all patients received a continuous IV infusion of tritiated norepinephrine (which allowed assessment of cardiac norepinephrine spill-over to plasma via isotope dilution technique). To assess cardiac sympathetic activity, blood samples were obtained from the coronary sinus and radial artery, and the rate of norepinephrine spill-over from the heart was calculated according to the Fick principle. Pa-

tients who received a single bolus of thoracic epidural mepivacaine immediately following induction of anesthesia exhibited significantly decreased cardiac norepinephrine spill-over after sternotomy when compared with patients managed similarly without thoracic epidural catheters. Furthermore, 20% of patients managed without thoracic epidural catheters exhibited ECG evidence of myocardial ischemia following sternotomy, whereas no patient managed with a thoracic epidural catheter exhibited myocardial ischemia during this time.

Perioperative cardiac sympathectomy induced via thoracic epidural anesthesia with local anesthetics may clinically benefit patients undergoing cardiac surgery by increasing myocardial oxygen supply (43,52,53). However, such a cardiac sympathectomy may offer additional benefits to patients undergoing cardiac surgery. For example, thoracic epidural anesthesia with local anesthetics significantly decreases heart rate before (104) and after (98,104) initiation of cardiopulmonary bypass and significantly decreases the need to administer β-blockers following cardiopulmonary bypass (101). Thoracic epidural anesthesia with local anesthetics also significantly decreases systemic vascular resistance before (100,101) and after (104,108) initiation of cardiopulmonary bypass. Furthermore, patients undergoing cardiac surgery who receive thoracic epidural anesthesia with local anesthetics not only exhibit significant decreases in postoperative heart rate and systemic vascular resistance, but also exhibit significant decreases in postoperative ECG evidence of myocardial ischemia when compared with patients managed similarly without thoracic epidural catheters (104).

Potential Benefits of Thoracic Anesthesia and Analgesia

A relatively large clinical investigation published in 2001 highlights the potential benefits of thoracic epidural anesthesia in cardiac surgical patients (89). Scott and associates prospectively randomized (nonblinded) 420 patients undergoing elective CABG to receive either thoracic epidural anesthesia (bupivacaine/clonidine) and general anesthesia or general anesthesia alone (control group) (89). The two groups received similar intraoperative anesthetic techniques. In thoracic epidural anesthesia patients, the thoracic epidural infusion was continued for 96 hours following surgery (titrated according to need). In control patients, target-controlled infusion alfentanil was used for the first 24 postoperative hours, followed by patient-controlled morphine analgesia for the next 48 hours. Postoperatively, striking clinical differences were observed between the two groups (Fig. 22-4). Postoperative incidence of supraventricular arrhythmia, lower respiratory tract infection, renal failure, and acute confusion were all significantly lower in patients receiving thoracic epidural anesthesia when compared with control patients. However, data from this clinical investigation must be viewed with caution. The clinical protocol dictated that β-adrenergic blocker therapy could not be used intraoperatively or postoperatively for the 5 days of the study period (except in those patients who developed a new arrhythmia requiring additional therapy). Since approximately 90% of this study's patients were taking β-adrenergic blockers preoperatively, this unique perioperative management clouds interpretation of postoperative supraventricular arrhythmia data. Also, despite prospective randomization, substantially fewer patients receiving thoracic epidural anesthesia were active smokers preoperatively when compared to controls (5.8% versus 13.4%, respectively), which clouds interpretation of

Outcome	TEA (*n* = 206), *n* (%)	GA (*n* = 202), *n* (%)
Supraventricular arrhythmia	21 (10.2)	45 (22.3)
Lower respiratory tract infection	31 (15.3)	59 (29.2)
Renal failure	4 (2.0)	14 (6.9)
CVA	2 (1.0)	6 (3.0)
Acute confusion	3 (1.5)	11 (5.5)
Significant bleeding	35	23
Any complications	84	108

FIGURE 22-4. Various outcomes of patients. Significant (unadjusted) differences existed between groups regarding supraventricular arrhythmia ($p = 0.0012$), lower respiratory tract infection ($p = 0.0007$), renal failure ($p = 0.016$), acute confusion ($p = 0.031$), and any complications ($p = 0.011$). TEA, thoracic epidural analgesia; GA, general anesthesia; CVA, cerebrovascular accident. Data from Scott et al. (89).

postoperative lower respiratory tract infection data. These investigators also found that postoperative preextubation maximal expiratory lung volumes were increased in thoracic epidural anesthesia patients (when compared to controls) and postoperative tracheal extubation was facilitated via thoracic epidural anesthesia as well (yet thoracic epidural anesthesia patients and control patients were managed somewhat differently during the immediate postoperative period). Although postoperative analgesia was not definitively assessed in this clinical investigation, 11.9% of control patients were converted to thoracic epidural anesthesia during the first 24 postoperative hours because of suboptimal postoperative analgesia, whereas only 2.9% of thoracic epidural anesthesia patients were converted to target-controlled infusion alfentanil or patient-controlled morphine analgesia because of suboptimal postoperative analgesia. Although the results of this clinical investigation are intriguing, definitive conclusions regarding the use of thoracic epidural techniques in patients undergoing cardiac surgery cannot be drawn because of the study's substantial limitations, highlighted by an accompanying editorial (124) and three subsequent letters to the editor (125–127).

In contrast to the encouraging findings of the clinical investigation by Scott and associates, two other prospective, randomized, nonblinded clinical investigations reveal that using thoracic epidural anesthesia techniques in patients undergoing cardiac surgery may not offer substantial clinical benefits (128,129). In 2002, Priestly and associates prospectively randomized 100 patients undergoing elective CABG to receive either thoracic epidural anesthesia (ropivacaine/fentanyl) and general anesthesia or general anesthesia alone (control group) (129). The two groups received quite different (nonstandardized) intraoperative anesthetic techniques. Postoperatively, thoracic epidural anesthesia patients received epidural ropivacaine/fentanyl for 48 hours (supplemental analgesics available if needed), whereas control patients received nurse-administered IV morphine, followed by patient-controlled morphine analgesia. Patients receiving thoracic epidural anesthesia were extubated sooner than controls (3.2 hours versus 6.7 hours, respectively, $p < 0.001$), yet this difference may have been secondary to the different amounts of intraoperative IV opioid administered to the two groups. Postoperative pain scores at rest were significantly lower in patients receiving thoracic epidural anesthesia only on postoperative days 0 and 1 (equivalent on days 2 and 3). Postoperative pain scores during coughing were significantly lower in patients receiving thoracic epidural anesthesia only on postop-

erative day 0 (equivalent on days 1, 2, and 3) (Fig. 22-5). There were no significant differences between the two groups in postoperative oxygen saturation on room air, chest radiograph changes, or spirometry (Fig. 22-6). Furthermore, no clinical differences were detected between the two groups regarding

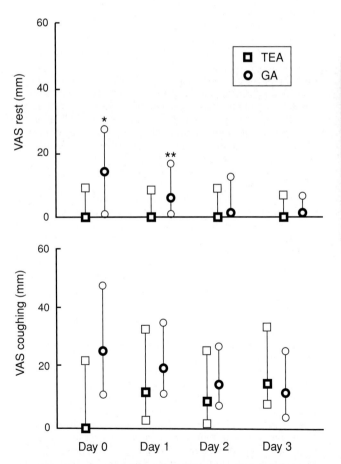

FIGURE 22-5. Visual analog scale (VAS) scores. Visual analog scale scores for pain at rest (*top*) and with coughing (*bottom*) on the day of surgery and the first 3 postoperative days. Significant differences ($p < 0.03$) existed between the two groups only on day 0 (rest and coughing) and on day 1 (rest only). TEA, thoracic epidural analgesia; GA, general anesthesia. Data from Priestley et al. (129).

Outcome	FEV$_1$ (TEA) (L)	FEV$_1$ (GA) (L)	FVC (TEA) (L)	FVC (GA) (L)
Predicted	2.9 (0.4)	2.9 (0.5)	3.9 (0.5)	3.9 (0.6)
Preoperative	2.5 (0.4)	2.6 (0.8)	3.3 (0.8)	3.4 (0.9)
Postoperative Day 1	1.0 (0.3)	1.0 (0.4)	1.2 (0.4)	1.4 (0.5)
Postoperative Day 2	1.1 (0.3)	1.1 (0.4)	1.4 (0.4)	1.5 (0.5)
Postoperative Day 4	1.4 (0.4)	1.3 (0.5)	1.8 (0.6)	1.7 (0.6)

FIGURE 22-6. Spirometry results. No significant differences existed between patients receiving thoracic epidural analgesia (TEA) and control patients (GA). TEA, thoracic epidural analgesia; GA, general anesthesia; FEV$_1$ = forced expiratory volume in 1 second; FVC, forced vital capacity. Values are mean (SD). Data from Priestley et al. (129).

postoperative mobilization goals, atrial fibrillation, postoperative hospital discharge eligibility, or actual postoperative hospital discharge. In short, this clinical investigation revealed that thoracic epidural anesthesia may provide enhanced postoperative analgesia (though brief) and enhance early postoperative tracheal extubation, yet has no effect on important clinical parameters (morbidity, hospital length of stay). In 2003, Royse and associates prospectively randomized 80 patients undergoing elective CABG to receive either thoracic epidural anesthesia (ropivacaine/fentanyl) and general anesthesia or general anesthesia alone (control group) (128). The two groups received quite different intraoperative anesthetic techniques. Postoperatively, thoracic epidural anesthesia patients received epidural ropivacaine/fentanyl until the third postoperative day, whereas control patients received nurse-administered IV morphine followed by patient-controlled morphine analgesia. Patients receiving thoracic epidural anesthesia were tracheally extubated sooner during the immediate postoperative period than controls (2.6 hours versus 5.4 hours, respectively, $p < 0.001$), yet this difference may have been secondary to the different amounts of intraoperative IV anesthetics administered (intraoperative anesthetic technique was not standardized). Postoperative pain scores at rest and with cough were significantly lower in patients receiving thoracic epidural anesthesia on postoperative days 1 and 2 only (equivalent on postoperative day 3) (Fig. 22-7). Much like the Priestley investigation, there were no substantial differences between the two groups regarding important postoperative clinical parameters (respiratory function, renal function, atrial fibrillation, intensive care unit length of stay, hospital length of stay).

Two recently published clinical investigations add to the expanding amount of literature that indicates that thoracic epidural techniques may not offer substantial clinical benefits to patients undergoing cardiac surgery (130,131). Barrington and associates, in 2005, prospectively randomized 120 patients undergoing elective cardiac surgery to receive either general anesthesia (with postoperative IV morphine) or general anesthesia with thoracic epidural infusion of ropivacaine/fentanyl (commenced 1 hour after induction of general anesthesia and continued until the morning of the third postoperative day) (131). Patients receiving thoracic epidurals experienced shorter extubation times and enhanced postoperative analgesia, yet no differences between the groups were detected regarding biochemical (troponin levels, creatine kinase myocardial fraction levels) or electrocardiographic evidence of myocardial ischemia/infarction. In 2006, Hansdottir and associates prospectively randomized 113 patients undergoing elective cardiac

surgery to receive either patient-controlled thoracic epidural analgesia (catheter inserted the day prior to surgery: bupivacaine, fentanyl, and adrenalin utilized) or patient-controlled IV morphine analgesia during the immediate postoperative period (130). Perioperative care was standardized (all patients underwent general anesthesia and received a median sternotomy). When the two groups were compared, the only difference was a shorter time to postoperative tracheal extubation in patients receiving thoracic epidural analgesia (2.3 hours versus 7.3 hours). No differences were observed regarding postoperative analgesia (at rest and during cough), degree of sedation, lung volumes (forced vital capacity, forced vital capacity at 1 second, peak expiratory flow), degree of ambulation, global quality of recovery score (including all five domains), cardiac morbidity, renal morbidity, neurologic outcome, intensive care unit stay, nor hospital length of stay.

Chronic Pain Following Cardiac Surgery

Despite enhanced postoperative analgesia offered via thoracic epidural techniques, such analgesia does not appear to decrease

Pain Score	High Thoracic Epidural Analgesia (Mean ± Standard Deviation)	Control (Mean ± Standard Deviation)
Rest day 1	0.02 ± 0.2	0.8 ± 1.8
Cough day 1	1.0 ± 1.7	4.4 ± 3.1
Rest day 2	1.5 ± 0.4	1.2 ± 2.7
Cough day 2	1.5 ± 2.0	3.6 ± 3.1
Rest day 3	0.2 ± 1.7	0.3 ± 1.1
Cough day 3	1.7 ± 2.3	2.7 ± 3.0

FIGURE 22-7. Visual analog scale scores. Mean pain scores at rest and with cough for days 1, 2, and 3. Significant differences ($p < 0.05$) existed between groups on days 1 and 2 (at rest and with cough), yet not on day 3. Data from Royse et al. (128).

Coronary Artery Bypass Grafting in the Conscious Patient Without Endotracheal General Anesthesia

Haldum Y. Karagoz, MD, Beril Sönmez, MD, Beyhan Bakkaloglu, MD,
Murat Kurtoglu, MD, Melih Erdinc, MD, Aylin Türkeli, MD, and Kemal Bayazit, MD

Department of Cardiovascular Surgery and Department of Cardiovascular Anesthesiology, Guven Hospital, Ankara, Turkey

FIGURE 22-8. Initial report of awake cardiac surgery published in the Annals of Thoracic Surgery in 2000.

the incidence of persistent pain following cardiac surgery. Ho and associates assessed via survey 244 patients following cardiac surgery via median sternotomy (18); 150 patients received perioperative supplementation of general anesthesia with thoracic epidural anesthesia (ropivacaine/fentanyl infusion initiated prior to induction of anesthesia and continued postoperatively for 2 to 3 days) and 94 patients received general anesthesia and routine postoperative nurse-controlled IV morphine infusion for analgesia (along with intraoperative wound infiltration with ropivacaine at chest wall closure). Persistent pain (defined as pain still present 2 or more months following surgery) was similar in the two cohorts (reported in almost 30% of patients). However, persistent pain reported by these patients was mild in most cases, infrequently interfering with daily life.

The quality of analgesia obtained with thoracic epidural anesthetic techniques is sufficient to allow cardiac surgery to be performed in awake patients without general endotracheal anesthesia. The initial report of awake cardiac surgery was published in the *Annals of Thoracic Surgery* in 2000 (Fig. 22-8) (132). Karagoz and associates, in Turkey, described the perioperative course of five patients who underwent elective off-pump single-vessel CABG via minithoracotomy with only thoracic epidural anesthesia (spontaneous ventilation throughout). All five patients did well, and none had to be converted to general endotracheal anesthesia. Soon thereafter, a group of investigators from Germany described the perioperative course of 12 patients who underwent elective off-pump multivessel coronary artery bypass grafting via complete sternotomy with only thoracic epidural anesthesia (133). All patients did well, yet two patients required conversion to general endotracheal anesthesia (one for incomplete analgesia, one for pneumothorax). Also that year (2002), investigators from Brazil revealed that "outpatient" CABG was possible (discharge to home within 24 hours of hospital admission) in a small (*n* = 20) group of patients undergoing cardiac surgery solely via thoracic epidural anesthesia (134). Since these initial small clinical reports appeared, larger series of patients have been published, proving that "awake" cardiac surgery is feasible and safe (135–145). In 2003, the first case report of awake cardiac surgery requiring cardiopulmonary bypass was published (146). In this astonishing case report from Austria, a 70–year-old man with aortic stenosis underwent aortic valve replacement with assist of normothermic cardiopulmonary bypass (total time 123 minutes, cross-clamp time 82 minutes) solely via thoracic epidural anesthesia. Verbal communication with the patient was possible on demand throughout cardiopulmonary bypass. The patient did well and experienced an unremarkable postoperative course.

In summary, the many clinical investigations involving the use of epidural analgesic techniques in patients undergoing cardiac surgery indicate that administration of thoracic epidural opioids or local anesthetics before and/or after cardiopulmonary bypass initiates reliable postoperative analgesia following cardiac surgery. Administration of thoracic epidural local anesthetics (not opioids) can both reliably attenuate the perioperative stress response associated with cardiopulmonary bypass (that persists during the immediate postoperative period) and induce perioperative thoracic cardiac sympathectomy. Enhanced postoperative analgesia likely facilitates early tracheal extubation following cardiac surgery, yet one may tracheally extubate patients following cardiac surgery (with or without cardiopulmonary bypass) in the operating room without assistance of thoracic epidural techniques (147).

Regional Anesthesia for Minimally Invasive Cardiac Surgery

With the increasing popularity of minimally invasive cardiac surgery, the utilization of nonsternotomy (thoracotomy, minithoracotomy, etc.) incisions has increased as well, and thus deserves brief mention here (because many anesthesiologists utilize epidural techniques in patients undergoing thoracotomy incisions). Pain following thoracotomy can be intense, which may produce pulmonary complications following surgery (148). Many factors are involved in the occurrence of pulmonary dysfunction following thoracotomy. Postoperative changes in pulmonary function result from lung resection, atelectasis, and/or volume loss due to pneumothorax and also inspiratory muscle dysfunction. Somewhat surprisingly, patients undergoing a "clamshell" incision (transverse thoracosternotomy) for bilateral lung transplantation do not experience more postoperative pain than patients undergoing a standard thoracotomy for single-lung transplantation. In addition, lung transplant recipients undergoing thoracotomy have a lower incidence of adequate pain relief than patients undergoing thoracotomy for other indications (149). These clinical observations emphasize that the condition of the patient may play a major role (along with type of incision) regarding adequacy of postoperative pain control (149). Clearly, when compared to standard thoracotomy incisions, patients receiving minithoracotomy incisions experience less postoperative pain and consume less supplemental analgesics during the immediate postoperative period. Importantly, up to half of all patients undergoing thoracotomy incision will develop chronic pain related to the surgical site. Evidence exists that indicates adequate postoperative pain control following thoracotomy may help prevent the development of chronic postoperative thoracotomy pain. Therefore, an effective postoperative analgesic plan must be developed for these patients. In contrast to median sternotomy incisions and minithoracotomy incisions, there appears to be some clinical evidence indicating that use of regional anesthetic techniques may decrease postoperative complications following thoracotomy incisions. Specifically, Ballantyne and associates (150) and Licker and associates (151) provide ample evidence that postoperative pain control with epidural techniques following thoracotomy incision may reduce pulmonary morbidity and overall patient

PART III: APPLICATIONS

TABLE 22-4

OUTCOMES FOR TEA AND IT VS. GA FOR CARDIAC SURGERY

Outcome	No.	TEA	GA	OR or WMD (95% Confidence interval)	P value
Death	1,178	0.7%	0.3%	1.56 (0.35–6.91)	0.56
Myocardial infarction	1,026	2.3%	3.4%	0.74 (0.34–1.59)	0.44
Dysryhthmias	913	17.8%	30%	0.52 (0.29–0.93)	0.03
Pulmonary complications	644	17.2%	30.3%	0.41 (0.27–0.60)	<0.00001
Time to tracheal extubation, h	905	6.9*	10.4*	−4.5 (−7 to −2)	0.0005
VAS pain score at rest, mm	392	12.4*	19.6*	−7.8 (−15 to −0.6)	0.03
VAS pain score with activity, mm	222	14*	27.6*	−11.6 (−19.7 to −3.5)	0.005
Death	668	0.3%	0.6%	0.88 (0.13–5.72)	0.89
Myocardial infarction	290	3.9%	5.7%	0.75 (0.24–2.31)	0.61
Dysryhthmias	204	24.8%	29.1%	0.81 (0.42–1.53)	0.51
Time to tracheal extubation, h	588	10.4*	10.9*	−0.85 (−1.83 to 0.12)	0.09
Time to tracheal extubation for small-dose IT, h	189	7.1*	9.3*	−1.2 (−1.8 to −0.7)	<0.0001
Morphine use per day, mg	816	14*	22*	−11 (−15 to −7)	<0.00001
VAS pain score, mm	315	13.4*	23.4*	−16 (−27 to −4.9)	0.005
Pruritus	506	10.1%	2.5%	2.9 (1.2–6.7)	0.01
Nausea/vomiting	490	31.3%	28.5%	1.27 (0.81–2.0)	0.3

Random effects model used for all analyses.
*Weighted by number of subjects.
GA = general anesthesia; IT = intrathecal analgesia; OR = odds ratio; TEA = thoracic epidural analgesia; VAS = visual analog scale; WMD = weighted mean difference (inverse variance method).
From Liu SS, Block B, Wu CLM. Effects of perioperative central neuraxial analgesia on outcome after coronary artery bypass surgery: A meta-analysis. *Anesthesiology* 2004;101(1):153–161.

mortality, respectively. However, although ample evidence exists suggesting that thoracic epidural analgesia offers superior postoperative analgesia, not all clinical studies have shown that such techniques truly improve postoperative pulmonary function and reduce postoperative pulmonary complications (Chapter 23).

Clinical Outcomes

All clinical reports involving utilization of intrathecal and thoracic epidural anesthesia and analgesia techniques for cardiac surgery involve small numbers of patients and few (if any) are well designed (Tables 22-2 and 22-3). Only a handful of clinical studies involving intrathecal analgesia are prospective, randomized, blinded, and placebo-controlled (Table 22-2). There are no blinded, placebo-controlled clinical studies involving thoracic epidural anesthesia and analgesia (Table 22-3). Furthermore, none of the existing clinical studies involving intrathecal and thoracic epidural anesthesia and analgesia techniques for cardiac surgery use clinical outcome as a primary end-point. Thus, clear deficiencies in the literature prohibit definitive analysis of the risk-benefit ratio of intrathecal and thoracic epidural anesthesia and analgesia techniques as applied to patients undergoing cardiac surgery.

A recently published (2004) meta-analysis by Liu and associates assessed effects of perioperative central neuraxial analgesia on outcome after CABG (152). These authors, via MEDLINE and other databases, searched for randomized controlled trials in patients undergoing coronary artery bypass surgery with cardiopulmonary bypass. Fifteen trials enrolling 1,178 patients were included for thoracic epidural anesthesia analysis and 17 trials enrolling 668 patients were included for

intrathecal analysis. Thoracic epidural techniques did not affect incidences of mortality or myocardial infarction, yet did reduce risk of dysrhythmias (atrial fibrillation and tachycardia), risk of pulmonary complications (pneumonia and atelectasis), time to tracheal extubation, and analog pain scores. Intrathecal techniques did not affect incidences of mortality, myocardial infarction, dysrhythmias, or time to tracheal extubation, and only modestly decreased systemic morphine utilization and pain scores (while increasing incidence of pruritus). These authors conclude that central neuraxial analgesia does not affect rates of mortality or myocardial infarction following CABG, yet is associated with improvements in time until tracheal extubation, decreased pulmonary complications and cardiac dysrhythmias, and reduced pain scores (Table 22-4). However, the authors also note that the majority of potential clinical benefits offered by central neuraxial analgesia (earlier extubation, decreased dysrhythmias, enhanced analgesia) may be reduced and/or eliminated with changing cardiac anesthesia practice using fast-track techniques, use of β-adrenergic blockers or amiodarone, and/or use of NSAIDs or COX-2 inhibitors. These authors also note that the risk of spinal hematoma (addressed later in this chapter) due to central neuraxial analgesia in patients undergoing full anticoagulation for cardiopulmonary bypass remains uncertain.

CLINICAL APPLICATIONS FOR VASCULAR SURGERY

Patients undergoing major vascular surgery (like cardiac surgical patients) have a high incidence of coexisting disease (diabetes, hypertension, coronary artery disease, etc.) and are subjected to substantial intraoperative stressors (major arterial cross-clamping and unclamping, large blood losses, etc.). Thus, it is not surprising that perioperative morbidity/morbidity is exceedingly high following vascular surgery relative to that of other surgical procedures (even cardiac surgery). Ongoing controversy continues over proper choice of anesthetic technique and influence on outcome because vascular procedures often lend themselves to a wide variety of local, regional, general, or combined regional/general anesthetic techniques.

Patients having vascular surgery are a unique group, with a high incidence of coexisting disease associated with advanced age, cigarette smoking, diabetes, and hypertension (among others). Coronary artery disease is easily the leading cause of perioperative mortality following vascular surgery, and long-term survival following these procedures is significantly limited by a high incidence of morbid cardiac events. Given the systemic nature of atherosclerotic disease, very few patients who present for vascular surgery have normal coronary arteries, and more than half of the patients have advanced or severe coronary artery disease (153). Needless to say, these patients usually only have borderline function in important organ systems (heart, kidneys, lungs, etc.). Furthermore, assessing perioperative risk in these sick individuals before vascular surgery is a difficult and controversial task.

Most operative procedures on the thoracic and/or abdominal aorta and its major branches require large incisions and extensive dissection, clamping and unclamping of the aorta and its major branches, varying duration of organ ischemia, significant fluid shifts and temperature fluctuations, thus stimulating activation of the neuroendocrine stress response (most importantly during the immediate postoperative period). The pathophysiology of aortic cross-clamping and unclamping is complex and depends on many factors, including the level of the cross-clamp, extent of coronary artery disease and myocardial dysfunction, degree of aortic collateralization, blood volume and distribution, activation of the sympathetic nervous system, and the anesthetic agents/techniques utilized. Of greatest concern to the anesthesiologist managing these patients is changes in blood pressure, systemic vascular resistance, cardiac output, and myocardial function with cross-clamp application and removal.

Inadequate analgesia (coupled with an uninhibited stress response) during the postoperative period following vascular surgery (like cardiac surgery) may lead to many adverse hemodynamic (tachycardia, hypertension, vasoconstriction), metabolic (increased catabolism), immunologic (impaired immune response), and hemostatic (platelet activation) alterations. In patients undergoing vascular surgery, perioperative myocardial ischemia is most commonly observed during the immediate postoperative period and appears to be related to outcome. Furthermore, postoperative myocardial ischemia may be aggravated by cardiac sympathetic nerve activation, which disrupts the balance between coronary blood flow and myocardial oxygen demand (27). Thus, during the immediate postoperative period after vascular surgery, adequate analgesia (coupled with stress response attenuation) may potentially decrease morbidity and enhance health-related quality of life (27,28).

Occasionally, vascular surgical procedures such as embolectomy and femoral pseudoaneurysm repair can be completed with the patient under local anesthesia with IV sedation. Because these procedures may often progress to more invasive arterial reconstruction, a regional or general anesthetic initiated before the procedure begins may avoid an unplanned and unwanted conversion to general anesthesia. In some patients,

a specific anesthetic technique (regional or general) may be preferable to others. For example, patients who are anticoagulated (heparin, thrombolytics) before surgery are usually not candidates for regional techniques.

Because patients undergoing vascular surgery usually have a surgical incision on the lower half of the body, the vast majority of neural blockade techniques in these patients involve intrathecal and/or epidural techniques. As with cardiac surgery, it is clear from numerous clinical investigations that intrathecal and/or epidural techniques (utilizing opioids and/or local anesthetics) initiate reliable postoperative analgesia in patients following vascular surgery. Likewise, additional potential advantages of using intrathecal and/or epidural techniques in patients undergoing vascular surgery include stress response attenuation and thoracic cardiac sympathectomy. However, as with cardiac surgery, whether such enhanced postoperative analgesia, stress response attenuation, and thoracic cardiac sympathectomy via intrathecal and/or epidural techniques truly affects morbidity and mortality in patients undergoing vascular surgery is controversial.

Thoracoabdominal Aortic Reconstruction

Perhaps no surgery is more challenging for the anesthesiologist than thoracoabdominal aortic reconstruction. Management issues include lung separation, extracorporeal circulatory support, hypothermia, spinal cord protection, renal protection, hemodynamic instability, large blood losses, and coagulopathy, among others. Even in centers where numerous such surgeries are performed, morbidity and mortality remains high.

Although the surgical incision is quite large and painful (thoracic and abdominal cavities entered), most clinicians are hesitant to utilize epidural techniques because these patients are at increased risk for epidural hematoma formation due to systemic heparinization (required for extracorporeal circulatory support), coagulopathy from hypothermia, and massive transfusion. Furthermore, most clinicians insert indwelling intrathecal catheters for perioperative cerebrospinal fluid (CSF) drainage in order to hopefully decrease risk of postoperative paraplegia. Thus, we believe that the use of epidural techniques in these patients needlessly (no proven substantial clinical benefits) increases risk of hematoma formation (above and beyond risk associated with CSF drainage catheter insertion) and may complicate postoperative differentiation between lower extremity paralysis from an epidural hematoma versus paralysis from spinal cord ischemia, for which the definitive treatment is much different. Heller and Chaney describe such a case in a patient who underwent uneventful thoracoabdominal aortic aneurysm repair (154). A thoracic epidural catheter was inserted the night before surgery, and a lumbar CSF drainage catheter was inserted immediately after induction of general anesthesia. Tracheal extubation occurred 6 hours after intensive care unit arrival. On the first postoperative day, the patient had full motor strength and function of both lower extremities and was ambulating without difficulty. At this time, pain was well-controlled with thoracic epidural infusion of bupivacaine 1.0% and fentanyl 5 μg/mL at 10 mL/hr. Within 30 minutes of CSF catheter removal on postoperative day one, the patient reported bilateral lower extremity weakness. One hour following catheter removal, he could not move his left lower extremity, and soon thereafter could not move either lower extremity. The epidural infusion was decreased to 7 mL/hr. Seven hours after catheter removal, the patient was unable to move either lower extremity against gravity. The epidural catheter was pulled back and the infusion was decreased to

6 mL/hr. Ten hours after catheter removal, the patient was unable to move either lower extremity. At this time, the epidural infusion was stopped. Emergency magnetic resonance imaging revealed no signs of extradural mass or epidural hematoma, yet demonstrated spinal cord infarction in the anterior spinal artery distribution. By the fifth postoperative day, sensory level to pin-prick had stabilized at T10, and the patient had no motor function in his legs. Posterior cord function (position sense and vibratory sensation) remained intact. The authors note that postoperative management of an epidural (lumbar or thoracic) catheter in a patient after thoracoabdominal aortic surgery is certainly challenging and somewhat controversial. However, in this unique patient population, concern always exists regarding neurologic deficit related to the surgery itself. One could argue that, in this patient, the thoracic epidural infusion should have been immediately discontinued when the neurologic deficit was first noted and that magnetic resonance imaging should have been performed earlier. Perhaps with earlier detection of spinal cord ischemia, prognosis in this patient would have been altered.

At our institution, we utilize CSF drainage catheters in essentially all of our patients; these are inserted in the operating room immediately following induction of general anesthesia. After the large-bore introducer needle is placed in the intrathecal space (prior to insertion of the CSF drainage catheter), we inject a large dose (6–10 mg) of intrathecal morphine for postoperative analgesia (155). In our experience, this technique works well (patients usually are not extubated within the immediate postoperative period, morphine will not mask presentation of postoperative paralysis), providing high-quality postoperative analgesia. However, a study involving aortic occlusion in rats indicates that spinal administration of large doses of morphine after transient aortic occlusion may be associated with a potential risk of paraparesis and the corresponding development of neurologic dysfunction (156). These authors caution against the use of large doses of intrathecal morphine for postoperative analgesia in patients undergoing thoracoabdominal aortic aneurysm repair.

Thus, we believe intrathecal morphine is an excellent way to initiate substantial postoperative analgesia in patients undergoing the large and painful incision required for thoracoabdominal aortic reconstruction. A relatively large dose (6–10 mg), administered immediately prior to or soon after induction of general anesthesia, usually provides substantial postoperative analgesia and will allow tracheal extubation to occur 6 to 8 hours after intensive care unit arrival. The advantage of this technique is its simplicity, reliability, and low risk. Because these surgeries are often quite long (approximately 6 hours) and are associated with substantial hemodynamic alterations, the use of intrathecal local anesthetics cannot be recommended. Although epidural techniques, on one hand, are appealing and allow enhanced analgesic flexibility, we believe they increase complexity and risk (perhaps needlessly). However, if one chooses to use epidural techniques in patients undergoing thoracoabdominal aortic reconstruction, an opioid-based technique is recommended to minimize perioperative hypotension (which may lead to spinal cord ischemia and paralysis) and avoid complicating postoperative differentiation between lower extremity paralysis from an epidural hematoma versus paralysis from spinal cord ischemia.

Abdominal Aortic Reconstruction

A wide variety of anesthetic techniques and drugs may be used safely in patients undergoing abdominal aortic reconstruction.

General anesthesia alone, regional anesthesia alone, and combined techniques have all been used successfully. Because the required surgical incision is usually large, local anesthetic infiltration and nerve blocks are used infrequently, if at all. Thus, the vast majority of neural blockade techniques for patients undergoing abdominal aortic reconstruction involve intrathecal and/or epidural techniques (mostly in supplementation of general anesthesia). A number of possibilities exist regarding the choice of intrathecal/epidural administration of local anesthetic/opioid. Intrathecal opioids initiate reliable intraoperative and postoperative analgesia following surgery, yet will not reliably attenuate the perioperative stress response that persists into the immediate postoperative period. Although intrathecal local anesthetics, but not opioids, may induce perioperative thoracic cardiac sympathectomy, the hemodynamic changes (hypotension) associated with this technique makes it unpalatable in patients with cardiac disease. Epidural techniques with opioids and/or local anesthetics also initiate reliable intraoperative and postoperative analgesia. Administration of thoracic epidural local anesthetics (not opioids) can reliably attenuate the perioperative stress response as well as induce perioperative thoracic cardiac sympathectomy. The ultimate decision regarding anesthetic technique should be made only after thoughtfully considering many factors. One must keep in mind that morbidity and mortality following abdominal aortic reconstruction is likely influenced most by maintenance of perioperative hemodynamic stability. This may be safely achieved in many ways (with or without associated neural blockade).

Intrathecal techniques, as applied to patients undergoing abdominal aortic reconstruction, are primarily limited to use of intrathecal morphine for postoperative analgesia. Use of more lipophilic opioids, such as fentanyl, would only provide short-term analgesia and would not be appropriate for these long surgeries. Use of intrathecal local anesthetics would provide analgesia for a longer period of time, yet the induced sympathectomy is undesirable in these patients, especially during hemodynamic changes associated with aortic clamping and unclamping.

A wide variety of epidural techniques (local anesthetics and/or opioids) without (157,158) or (more commonly) with general anesthesia may be used. Most clinicians use a mixture of epidural local anesthetic and opioid throughout the intraoperative period (along with general anesthesia) and well into the immediate postoperative period following tracheal extubation (159,160). One must be careful not to administer excessive intraoperative epidural local anesthetic, as this can lead to hypotension at the time of aortic cross-clamp removal, increased fluid requirements, and/or increased vasopressor requirements (161–163).

Thus, a wide variety of intrathecal and/or epidural techniques may be safely used in patients undergoing abdominal aortic reconstruction. Although regional anesthesia may be used alone, most clinicians use these techniques to supplement general anesthesia. An enormous amount of possibilities exist that allow one to achieve desired perioperative goals safely and efficaciously.

Lower Extremity Revascularization

A wide variety of anesthetic techniques and drugs may be used safely in patients undergoing lower extremity revascularization. General anesthesia alone, regional anesthesia alone, and combined techniques have all been used successfully. Because the required surgical incisions are smaller and more peripheral than those used during thoracoabdominal and abdominal aortic reconstruction, local anesthetic infiltration and/or nerve blocks may potentially be used. Despite this, the vast majority of neural blockade techniques for patients undergoing lower extremity revascularization involve intrathecal and/or epidural techniques (164). Although most anesthesiologists supplement a general anesthetic, a fair amount of lower extremity revascularizations can be performed solely under intrathecal and/or epidural techniques, in contrast to thoracoabdominal and abdominal aortic reconstruction. Selection of technique is similar to considerations for patients undergoing aortic reconstruction: intrathecal/epidural route and administration of local anesthetic/opioid and the associated changes in the stress response and hemodynamics. This may be safely achieved many ways, with or without associated neural blockade.

Outcome

Two early clinical studies indicated that use of epidural anesthesia and analgesia in patients following noncardiac surgery may beneficially affect outcome (7,8). In 1987, Yeager and associates, in a small ($n = 53$ patients), randomized, controlled clinical trial involving patients undergoing major thoracic/vascular surgery, revealed that patients who were managed to receive epidural anesthesia and analgesia demonstrated decreased postoperative morbidity and improved operative outcome (8). In 1991, Tuman and associates, in another small ($n = 80$ patients), randomized, controlled clinical trial involving patients undergoing lower extremity revascularization, revealed that patients who were managed to receive epidural anesthesia and analgesia demonstrated improved outcome when compared with patients receiving routine on-demand IV narcotic analgesia (7).

Despite an enormous amount of research and published material over the last 20 years, the question of whether general anesthesia, regional anesthesia, or a combination of the two is preferable for patients undergoing vascular surgery remains extremely controversial (165–169). Furthermore, studies assessing outcome cannot determine whether potential benefits result from the intraoperative anesthetic technique, from the postoperative pain regimen, or from a combination of the two. The effects of anesthetic/analgesic technique on the incidence of myocardial ischemia have also received considerable attention as well, and this issue also remains extremely controversial (170–175). Also, there is little evidence from well-designed clinical studies to demonstrate improved pulmonary outcome with regional anesthetic techniques. However, a recent review of the role of epidural anesthesia and analgesia in surgical practice, by Moraca and associates (166), indicates that epidural anesthesia/analgesia may improve postoperative outcome. Specifically, in four large studies they assessed involving high-risk (aortic reconstruction) surgery patients, significant reductions in cardiac morbidity were associated with use of intraoperative and postoperative epidural anesthesia/analgesia using local anesthetics plus opioids (166). In addition, they concluded that intraoperative epidural administration of local anesthetics may blunt the physiologic hypercoagulable surgical stress response and thus modify the perioperative hypercoagulable state, stating "reductions in morbidity due to thrombotic complications in complex vascular operations make epidural anesthesia and analgesia the standard of care in these settings" (166).

Perhaps the only substantial clinical benefit of regional anesthetic techniques in patients undergoing vascular surgery is enhanced postoperative graft patency. Christopherson and co-workers (174) and Tuman and co-workers (7) report an approximately five-fold greater incidence of graft occlusion following general anesthesia alone. Most graft occlusions occurred during the immediate postoperative period (1–3 days following surgery), suggesting that anesthetic technique may play a substantial role. The proposed mechanism that perhaps explains this observation is that general anesthesia alone is associated with a hypercoagulable state in the immediate postoperative period, whereas regional anesthetic techniques may attenuate this effect (176). It appears from several studies that fibrinolysis is decreased after general anesthesia yet is normal following regional anesthesia. These findings may be linked to stress response attenuation with regional anesthesia, thus profoundly affecting postoperative catecholamines, acute phase reactants, and platelets. Another important potential mechanism for increased lower extremity graft patency with regional anesthetic techniques may be increased lower extremity blood flow associated with sympathectomy (177).

Thus, as with cardiac surgery, clear deficiencies in the literature prohibit definitive analysis of the risk-benefit ratio of intrathecal and epidural anesthesia and analgesia techniques as applied to patients undergoing vascular surgery. Although some evidence from meta-analyses suggest that there may be benefits from regional anesthetic techniques on postoperative pulmonary complications, postoperative myocardial infarction, and even mortality, these have mostly not been confirmed by recent randomized controlled clinical trials. In summary, although regional anesthetic techniques certainly provide excellent pain relief following vascular surgery, the supposition that the techniques decrease morbidity and mortality remains unproven.

SIDE EFFECTS OF INTRATHECAL AND EPIDURAL LOCAL ANESTHETICS

Because essentially all patients undergoing cardiovascular surgery have some degree of cardiac disease (coronary artery disease, left ventricular dysfunction, etc.), hypotension is the most troubling and undesirable drug effect of intrathecal and epidural local anesthetics. Spinal anesthesia to upper thoracic dermatomes produces a decrease in mean arterial blood pressure that is accompanied by a parallel decrease in coronary blood flow (178,179). Exactly what percentage of blood pressure decrease is acceptable remains speculative, especially in patients with coronary artery disease. Disturbances in myocardial oxygenation appear to occur in patients with coronary artery disease if coronary perfusion pressure is allowed to decrease by more than 50% during induction of thoracic epidural anesthesia with local anesthetics (180). Furthermore, if α-adrenergic agonists are used to increase blood pressure during this time, detrimental effects (vasoconstriction) may occur on the native coronary arteries and bypass grafts (181,182). Of the 19 patients who received intrathecal local anesthetics to produce a "total spinal" for cardiac surgery, 18 required IV phenylephrine intraoperatively to increase blood pressure, indicating that hypotension is a substantial problem with this technique (70,72). Hypotension also appears to be relatively common when thoracic epidural local anesthetics are used in patients undergoing cardiovascular surgery. Volume replacement, β-adrenergic agonists, and/or α-adrenergic agonists are required in a fair proportion of patients, and coronary perfusion pressure may decrease in susceptible patients.

PART III: APPLICATIONS

Following epidural administration, local anesthetics can produce blood concentrations of drug that may initiate detrimental cardiac electrophysiologic effects and myocardial depression (183). In fact, myocardial depression has been detected in patients receiving thoracic epidural anesthesia with bupivacaine, a clinical effect at least partially caused by increased blood concentrations of the drug (184). Concomitant use of β-adrenergic blockers may further decrease myocardial contractility in this setting (185,186). Patients undergoing cardiac surgery who were randomized to receive intermittent boluses of thoracic epidural bupivacaine intraoperatively followed by continuous infusion postoperatively exhibited significantly increased pulmonary capillary wedge pressures following cardiopulmonary bypass when compared with patients managed similarly without epidural catheters (10.8 versus 6.4 mm Hg, respectively, p <0.001), which suggests myocardial depression (101).

Two case reports also indicate that the use of epidural anesthesia and analgesia may either mask myocardial ischemia or initiate myocardial ischemia (187,188). Oden and Karagianes describe the perioperative course of an elderly patient who had a history of exertional angina and underwent uneventful cholecystectomy (188). Postoperatively, analgesia was achieved with continuous lumbar epidural fentanyl. On the second postoperative day, with continuous lumbar epidural fentanyl being administered, ST-segment depression was noted on the ECG. The patient was awake, alert, and did not experience angina. Initiation of IV nitroglycerin at this time resulted in normalization of ischemic ECG changes. It was believed by these authors that epidural fentanyl-induced analgesia masked the patient's typical anginal pain. Easley and associates describe the perioperative course of a middle-aged patient without cardiovascular symptoms ("borderline" hypertension) who was scheduled for exploratory laparotomy (187). Prior to surgery, a low thoracic epidural catheter was inserted and local anesthetic was administered (sensory level peaked by pin-prick at T2). The patient at this time began complaining of left-sided jaw pain, and substantial (2.7 mm) ST-segment depression was noted on the ECG. Surgery was cancelled, and the patient was treated with aspirin and nitroglycerin. The electrocardiogram normalized, yet, based on ECG changes, troponin levels, and creatine kinase-MB fractions, the patient was diagnosed with a non-Q-wave myocardial infarction. Coronary angiography on the following day was unremarkable, and a presumptive diagnosis of coronary artery spasm was made. It was believed by these authors that low thoracic epidural-induced sympathectomy led to alterations in the sympathetic-parasympathetic balance (i.e., vasoconstriction above level of block) and thus led to coronary artery spasm.

SIDE EFFECTS OF INTRATHECAL AND EPIDURAL OPIOIDS

Although many have been described, the four clinically relevant undesirable drug effects of intrathecal and epidural opioids are pruritus, nausea and vomiting, urinary retention, and respiratory depression (189). Following administration of intrathecal or epidural opioids, the most common side effect is pruritus. The incidence varies widely (from 0% to 100%) and is often identified only after direct questioning of patients. Severe pruritus is rare, occurring in only approximately 1% of patients. The incidence of nausea and vomiting is approximately 30%. The incidence of urinary retention varies widely (from 0% to 80%),

and occurs most frequently in young male patients. When intrathecal or epidural opioids are used in patients undergoing cardiovascular surgery, the incidence of pruritus, nausea and vomiting, and urinary retention is similar to that just described. Of note, if a large dose (4.0 mg) of intrathecal morphine is administered, prolonged postoperative urinary retention may occur (69).

The most important undesirable drug effect of intrathecal and epidural opioids is respiratory depression (which may delay postoperative tracheal extubation). Only 4 months after the initial use of intrathecal (190) and epidural (191) opioids in humans, life-threatening respiratory depression was reported (192–194). The incidence of respiratory depression that requires intervention after conventional doses of intrathecal and epidural opioids is approximately 1%, the same as that after conventional doses of intramuscular and IV opioids. Early respiratory depression occurs within minutes of opioid injection and is associated with administration of intrathecal or epidural fentanyl or sufentanil. Delayed respiratory depression occurs hours after opioid injection and is associated with administration of intrathecal or epidural morphine. Delayed respiratory depression results from cephalad migration of morphine in CSF and the subsequent stimulation of opioid receptors located in the ventral medulla (195). Factors that increase the risk of respiratory depression include large and/or repeated doses of opioids, intrathecal utilization, advanced age, and concomitant use of IV sedatives (189). The magnitude of postoperative respiratory depression is profoundly influenced by the dose of intrathecal or epidural morphine administered and the type and amount of IV analgesics and amnestics used for the intraoperative baseline anesthetic. Prolonged postoperative respiratory depression may delay tracheal extubation, and naloxone may be required in some patients. Children may be more susceptible to developing postoperative respiratory depression when intrathecal morphine is used in this setting. Of 56 children (aged 1–17 years) administered either 20 or 30 μg/kg intrathecal morphine prior to surgical incision for cardiac surgery, three of 29 who received 20 μg/kg and six of 27 receiving 30 μg/kg required naloxone postoperatively for respiratory depression (81) (see Chapter 40).

One clinical study indicates that administration of intrathecal morphine to patients undergoing cardiac surgery may be contraindicated if early extubation is planned (68). Patients were randomized to receive either intrathecal morphine (10 μg/kg) or intrathecal placebo prior to the induction of anesthesia. Intraoperative anesthetic management was standardized and consisted of IV fentanyl (20 μg/kg) and IV midazolam (10 mg total) along with inhaled isoflurane and/or IV nitroglycerin, if required. The mean time from intensive care unit arrival to extubation was significantly increased in those who received intrathecal morphine compared with those who received intrathecal placebo (10.9 versus 7.6 hours, respectively, p = 0.02). However, other clinical studies indicate that intrathecal or epidural morphine may yet prove to be a useful adjunct for cardiac surgery and early extubation. All of the clinical studies involving use of intrathecal or epidural morphine in patients undergoing vascular surgery indicate that if appropriate amounts are used, tracheal extubation may occur in a timely manner. In summary, the optimal dose of intrathecal or epidural morphine in patients undergoing cardiovascular surgery, along with the optimal intraoperative baseline anesthetic that will provide significant postoperative analgesia yet not delay tracheal extubation in the immediate postoperative period, remains to be elucidated. In contrast to intrathecal and epidural opioids, epidural local anesthetics (which initiate no respiratory depression) should not delay tracheal extubation in the immediate postoperative period.

RISK OF HEMATOMA FORMATION

Essentially all patients undergoing cardiovascular surgery are subjected to a certain degree of systemic anticoagulation. Intrathecal or epidural instrumentation entails risk, the most feared complication being epidural hematoma formation (196) (see Chapter 12).

Although spontaneous hematomas can occur in the absence of intrathecal or epidural instrumentation (197), most occur when instrumentation is performed in a patient with a coagulopathy (from any cause) or when instrumentation is difficult or traumatic (196). Although intrathecal or epidural instrumentation has been performed safely in patients with known clinical coagulopathy, major alteration in hemostasis is considered a contraindication to neuraxial block (198,199).

Risk is increased when intrathecal or epidural instrumentation is performed prior to systemic heparinization (essentially all patients undergoing cardiovascular surgery), and hematoma formation has occurred in patients when diagnostic or therapeutic lumbar puncture has been followed by systemic heparinization (200–203). When lumbar puncture is followed by systemic heparinization, concurrent use of aspirin, difficult or traumatic instrumentation, and administration of IV heparin within 1 hour of instrumentation increases the risk of hematoma formation (202). Certainly, by observing certain precautions, intrathecal or epidural instrumentation can be performed safely in patients who will subsequently receive IV heparin (204,205). By delaying surgery 24 hours in the event of a traumatic tap, delaying heparinization 60 minutes after catheter insertion, and maintaining tight perioperative control of anticoagulation, more than 4,000 intrathecal or epidural catheterizations were performed safely in patients undergoing peripheral vascular surgery who received IV heparin following catheter insertion (205). A retrospective review involving 912 patients further indicates that epidural catheterization prior to systemic heparinization for peripheral vascular surgery is safe (204). Certainly, the magnitude of anticoagulation in these two studies (activated partial thromboplastin time approximately 100 seconds [204] and activated clotting time approximately twice the baseline value [205]) involving patients undergoing peripheral vascular surgery was substantially less than the degree of anticoagulation required in patients subjected to cardiopulmonary bypass (activated clotting time usually between 400–500 seconds).

Most clinical studies investigating the use of intrathecal or epidural anesthesia and analgesia techniques in patients undergoing cardiac surgery include precautions to decrease risk of hematoma formation. Some used the technique only after the demonstration of laboratory evidence of normal coagulation parameters, delayed surgery 24 hours in the event of traumatic tap, or required that the time from instrumentation to systemic heparinization exceed 60 minutes. Additionally, systemic heparin effect and reversal should be tightly controlled (smallest amount of heparin used for the shortest duration compatible with therapeutic objectives), and patients should be closely monitored postoperatively for signs and symptoms of hematoma formation (39). Although most studies investigating the use of epidural anesthesia and analgesia techniques in patients undergoing cardiac surgery insert catheters the day before scheduled surgery, recent investigators have performed instrumentation on the same day of surgery (39). Institutional practice (same-day admit surgery) may eliminate the option of epidural catheter insertion on the day before scheduled surgery. An alternative is to perform epidural instrumentation postoperatively (prior to or after tracheal extubation), following the demonstration via laboratory evidence of normal coagulation parameters. An obvious economic disadvantage of intrathecal or epidural instrumentation in patients prior to cardiac surgery is the possible delay in surgery in the event of a traumatic tap. However, one study involving more than 4,000 intrathecal or epidural catheterizations via a 17-gauge Tuohy needle indicates that the incidence of traumatic tap (blood freely aspirated) is rare (less than 0.10%) (205).

Whereas most investigators agree that risk of hematoma is likely increased when intrathecal or epidural instrumentation is performed in patient prior to systemic heparinization required for cardiopulmonary bypass, the absolute degree of increased risk is somewhat controversial; some believe the risk may be as high as 0.35% (200). A recently published extensive mathematical analysis by Ho and associates of the approximately 10,840 intrathecal injections in patients subjected to systemic heparinization required for cardiopulmonary bypass (without a single episode of hematoma formation), estimated that the maximum risk of hematoma formation was 1:3,600 (95% confidence level) or 1:2,400 (99% confidence level) (206). Similarly, of the approximately 4,583 epidural instrumentations in patients subjected to systemic heparinization required for cardiopulmonary bypass (without a single episode of hematoma formation), estimated maximum risk of hematoma formation was calculated to be 1:1,500 (95% confidence level) or 1:1,000 (99% confidence level) (206).

In 2004, the first case report of an epidural hematoma associated with a thoracic epidural catheter inserted in a patient prior to cardiac surgery was published (207). The 18-year-old male patient had a thoracic (T9–T10) epidural catheter uneventfully inserted following induction of general anesthesia (patient had intense fear of needles) immediately prior to initiation of cardiopulmonary bypass for aortic valve replacement surgery. Three hours elapsed from instrumentation to systemic heparinization. The entire intraoperative course and immediate postoperative course were uneventful; the patient was extubated soon after surgery and ambulated without difficulty on the first postoperative day. Forty-nine hours following surgery, IV heparin therapy was initiated (prosthetic valve thromboprophylaxis). Fifty-three hours following surgery, alteplase was used to flush a dysfunctional IV catheter. Within 2 hours of IV alteplase administration, the patient reported intense back pain while ambulating. At this point, the epidural catheter was removed. The activated partial thromboplastin time assessed at the time of catheter removal was 87.4 seconds (normal range 24.8–37.3 seconds). The patient was also thrombocytopenic at this time. Upon catheter removal, the patient experienced sudden onset of numbness and weakness distal to T9. Intravenous heparin was discontinued, a computed tomographic scan was inconclusive, requiring a magnetic resonance imaging scan, which revealed an epidural hematoma. Five hours from the onset of neurologic symptoms, the patient underwent surgical evacuation of the hematoma, which extended from the T8 to T11 levels. Intraoperatively, IV methylprednisolone (30 mg/kg) was administered, followed by an infusion (5.4 mg/kg/hr), which was continued for 72 hours. Twenty-four hours postlaminectomy, the patient demonstrated mild residual lower extremity motor and sensory deficits. Six weeks later, his neurologic examination had returned to normal. The authors note the factors affecting coagulation in this patient (heparin, alteplase, thrombocytopenia) that likely led to hematoma formation and theorize that removing the catheter may have increased bleeding, further compounding the problem. Although this represents the first-ever published case report of an epidural hematoma associated with a thoracic epidural catheter inserted prior to cardiac surgery, this author is aware of at least three additional unpublished cases (in the United States alone) of permanent paralysis secondary to epidural hematoma in patients who had thoracic epidural catheters inserted for elective cardiac surgery.

Thromboembolic complications may occur when coagulation parameters are normalized to allow neuraxial catheter removal. A recent case report describes the perioperative course of a patient who underwent cardiac surgery with thoracic epidural supplementation and experienced a thromboembolic phenomenon during the postoperative period, when normalization of coagulation parameters was achieved to safely remove the thoracic epidural catheter (208). In this patient, a thoracic epidural catheter was inserted 2 days prior to uneventful cardiac surgery. The immediate postoperative period was uneventful, yet required anticoagulation for the patient's mechanical aortic valve. On the seventh postoperative day, coagulation parameters were normalized in order to safely remove the epidural catheter. Following catheter removal, the patient experienced an acute onset of aphasia. Neurologic examination at this time revealed intact cranial nerves and normal sensory and motor function, yet the patient could not name familiar objects or repeat words and spoke in nonsensical sentences. Computed tomographic scanning eventually revealed new ischemic changes in the left temporal lobe consistent with the patient's clinical symptoms. Thus, the increased risk for thromboembolic phenomenon in patients requiring anticoagulation therapy should be considered when assessing the risk-benefit ratio of applying epidural techniques in patients undergoing cardiovascular surgery.

In summary, the performance of regional anesthetic techniques in patients undergoing cardiac surgery, although increasing in popularity, remains extremely controversial because of perceived hematoma risk and lack of clinical benefits, thus prompting numerous editorials by recognized experts in the field of cardiac anesthesia (209–214). One of the main reasons such controversy exists (and likely will continue for some time) is that the numerous clinical investigations regarding this topic are suboptimally designed and utilize a wide array of disparate techniques that prevent clinically useful conclusions all can agree on (215,216). On the other hand, most clinicians believe that the use of regional anesthetic techniques is relatively safe in patients with normal coagulation undergoing vascular surgeries that require a lesser degree of anticoagulation than that required for cardiac surgery.

MULTIMODAL ANALGESIA

The possibility of synergism between analgesic drugs is a concept that is nearly a century old (217,218). Although subsequent research has elucidated the difference between additivity and synergy, the fundamental strategy behind such combinations ("multimodal" or "balanced" analgesia) remains unchanged: enhanced analgesia with minimization of adverse physiologic effects. For decades, the utilization of analgesic combinations during the postoperative period, specifically the combination of traditional IV opioids with other analgesics (NSAIDs, COX-2 inhibitors, ketamine), has been proven clinically effective following cardiovascular surgery. Early clinical investigations simply reported analgesic efficacy, whereas more recent clinical investigations have additionally evaluated and

described specific opioid-sparing effects that should lead to a reduction in side effects (see Chapter 43 on acute pain management).

The American Society of Anesthesiologists Task Force on Acute Pain Management in the Perioperative Setting reports that the literature supports the administration via a single route of two analgesic agents that act by different mechanisms to provide superior analgesic efficacy with equivalent or reduced adverse effects (1). Potential examples include epidural opioids administered in combination with epidural local anesthetics or clonidine, and IV opioids in combination with ketorolac or ketamine. Dose-dependent adverse effects reported with administration of a medication occur whether it is given alone or in combination with other medications (opioids may cause nausea, vomiting, pruritus, or urinary retention, and local anesthetics may produce motor block). The Task Force believes that NSAID, COX-2 inhibitor, or acetaminophen administration has a dose-sparing effect for systemically administered opioids. The literature suggests that two routes of administration, when compared with a single route, may be more effective in providing perioperative analgesia. Examples include intrathecal or epidural opioids combined with IV, intramuscular, oral, transdermal, or subcutaneous analgesics versus intrathecal or epidural opioids alone. Another example is IV opioids combined with oral NSAIDs, COX-2 inhibitors, or acetaminophen versus IV opioids.

SUMMARY

Multiple important factors during the perioperative period potentially affect outcome and quality of life following cardiovascular surgery, including type and quality of surgical intervention and postoperative analgesia and the extent of postoperative neurologic dysfunction, myocardial dysfunction, pulmonary dysfunction, renal dysfunction, coagulation abnormalities, and/or systemic inflammatory response, among others (Table 22-5) (219). The list of factors in Table 22-5 is presented in no particular order; obviously, depending on specific clinical situations (surgical procedure, patient comorbidity), certain factors will be more important than others. One must keep in mind that morbidity and mortality following cardiovascular surgery is profoundly influenced by maintenance of perioperative hemodynamic stability. It is extremely difficult (if not impossible) to determine exactly how important attaining adequate postoperative analgesia truly is in relation to all of these clinical factors surrounding a patient undergoing cardiovascular surgery. A clear link between "adequate" or "high-quality" postoperative analgesia in patients following cardiovascular surgery has yet to be established (220–222).

TABLE 22-5
FACTORS AFFECTING OUTCOME FOLLOWING CARDIOVASCULAR SURGERY
Type and quality of surgical intervention Extent of postoperative neurologic dysfunction Extent of postoperative myocardial dysfunction Extent of postoperative pulmonary dysfunction Extent of postoperative renal dysfunction Extent of postoperative coagulation abnormalities Quality of postoperative analgesia Extent of systemic inflammatory response

However, despite the absence of substantiating scientific evidence, most clinicians intuitively believe that attaining high-quality postoperative analgesia is important because it may prevent adverse hemodynamic, metabolic, immunologic, and hemostatic alterations, all of which may potentially impact postoperative morbidity. Although many analgesic techniques are available, IV systemic opioids form the cornerstone of post-cardiovascular surgery analgesia. Opioids have been used for many years in the treatment of postoperative pain in patients following cardiovascular surgery with good results. Neural blockade techniques (used as part of a multimodal analgesic approach) certainly offer unique benefits to these patients. Although NSAIDs (specifically COX-2 inhibitors) have received much recent attention, very important clinical issues regarding their safety (gastrointestinal, renal, hemostatic, immunologic effects) must be resolved. Although PCA techniques are commonly used, their clear superiority over traditional nurse-controlled analgesic techniques remains unproven. As a general rule, it is likely best to avoid intense, single-modality therapy for the treatment of acute postoperative pain. One should strive for an approach that uses a number of different therapies (mul-timodal therapy), each counteracting pain via different mechanisms. Preemptive analgesia, while intriguing, needs further study to determine its role in affecting postoperative analgesia and outcome (223–226).

Last, the American Society of Anesthesiologists Task Force on Acute Pain Management in the Perioperative Setting offers sound advice (1). It recommends that anesthesiologists who manage perioperative pain should utilize analgesic therapeutic options only after thoughtfully considering the risks and benefits for the individual patient. The therapy (or therapies) selected should reflect the individual anesthesiologist's expertise, as well as the capacity for safe application of the chosen modality in each practice setting. This capacity includes the ability to recognize and treat adverse effects that emerge after initiation of therapy. Whenever possible, anesthesiologists should employ multimodal pain management therapy. Dosing regimens should be administered to optimize efficacy while minimizing the risk of adverse events. The choice of medication, dose, route, and duration of therapy should always be individualized. For the anesthesiologist caring for patients undergoing cardiovascular surgery, sounder advice could not be offered.

References

1. American Society of Anesthesiologists Task Force on Acute Pain Management. Practice guidelines for acute pain management in the perioperative setting: An updated report by the American Society of Anesthesiologist Task Force on Acute Pain Management. *Anesthesiology* 2004;100:1573–1581.
2. Joint Commission on Accreditation of Healthcare Organization. Pain assessment and management: An organizational approach. At http://www.jacho.org. Accessed 15 May 2008.
3. Royston D, Kovesi T, Marczin N. The unwanted response to cardiac surgery: Time for a reappraisal? [Editorial]. *J Thorac Cardiovasc Surg* 2003;125:32–35.
4. Weissman C. The metabolic response to stress: An overview and update [Review article]. *Anesthesiology* 1990;73:308–327.
5. Kehlet H. Surgical stress: The role of pain and analgesia [Review article]. *Br J Anaesth* 1989;63:189–195.
6. Roizen MF. Should we all have a sympathectomy at birth? Or at least pre-operatively? [Editorial]. *Anesthesiology* 1988;68:482–484.
7. Tuman KJ, McCarthy RJ, March RJ, et al. Effects of epidural anesthesia and analgesia on coagulation and outcome after major vascular surgery. *Anesth Analg* 1991;73:696–704.
8. Yeager MP, Glass DD, Neff RK, et al. Epidural anesthesia and analgesia in high-risk surgical patients. *Anesthesiology* 1987;66:729–736.
9. Mangano DT, Siliciano D, Hollenberg M, et al. Postoperative myocardial ischemia: Therapeutic trials using intensive analgesia following surgery. *Anesthesiology* 1992;76:342–353.
10. Anand KJS, Hickey PR. Halothane-morphine compared with high-dose sufentanil for anesthesia and postoperative analgesia in neonatal cardiac surgery. *N Engl J Med* 1992;326:1–9.
11. Wallace AW. Is it time to get on the fast track or stay on the slow track? [Editorial]. *Anesthesiology* 2003;99:774.
12. Myles PS, Daly DJ, Djaiani G, et al. A systematic review of the safety and effectiveness of fast-track cardiac anesthesia [Review article]. *Anesthesiology* 2003;99:982–987.
13. Mueller XM, Tinguely F, Tevaearai HT, et al. Pain location, distribution, and intensity after cardiac surgery. *Chest* 2000;118:391–396.
14. Nay PG, Elliott SM, Harrop-Griffiths AW. Postoperative pain, expectation and experience after coronary artery bypass grafting. *Anaesthesia* 1996;51:741–743.
15. Meehan DA, McRae ME, Rourke DA, et al. Analgesic administration, pain intensity, and patient satisfaction in cardiac surgical patients. *Am J Crit Care* 1995;4:435–442.
16. Moore R, Follette DM, Berkoff HA. Poststernotomy fractures and pain management in open cardiac surgery. *Chest* 1994;106:1339–1342.
17. Greenwald LV, Baisden CE, Symbas PN. Rib fractures in coronary bypass patients: Radionuclide detection. *Radiology* 1983;148:553–554.
18. Ho SC, Royse CF, Royse AG, et al. Persistent pain after cardiac surgery: An audit of high thoracic epidural and primary opioids analgesia therapies. *Anesth Analg* 2002;95:820–823.
19. Kalso E, Mennander S, Tasmuth T, et al. Chronic post-sternotomy pain. *Acta Anaesthesiol Scand* 2001;45:935–939.
20. Chaney MA, Morales M, Bakhos M. Severe incisional pain and long thoracic nerve injury after port-access minimally invasive mitral valve surgery [Case report]. *Anesth Analg* 2000;91:288–290.
21. Davis Z, Jacobs HK, Zhang M, et al. Endoscopic vein harvest for coronary artery bypass grafting: Technique and outcomes. *J Thorac Cardiovasc Surg* 1998;116:228–235.
22. Smith RC, Leung JM, Mangano DT. Postoperative myocardial ischemia in patients undergoing cardiac artery bypass graft surgery. SPI Research Group. *Anesthesiology* 1991;74:464–473.
23. Leung JM, O'Kelly B, Browner WS, et al. Prognostic importance of post-bypass regional wall-motion abnormalities in patients undergoing coronary artery bypass graft surgery. *Anesthesiology* 1989;71:16–25.
24. Philbin DM, Rosow CE, Schneider RC, et al. Fentanyl and sufentanil anesthesia revisited: How much is enough? *Anesthesiology* 1990;73:5–11.
25. Reves JG, Karp RB, Buttner EE, et al. Neuronal and adrenomedullary catecholamine release in response to cardiopulmonary bypass in man. *Circulation* 1982;66:49–55.
26. Roberts AJ, Niarchos AP, Subramanian VA, et al. Systemic hypertension associated with coronary artery bypass surgery: Predisposing factors, hemodynamic characteristics, humoral profile, and treatment. *J Thorac Cardiovasc Surg* 1977;74:846–859.
27. Liu S, Carpenter RL, Neal MJ. Epidural anesthesia and analgesia: Their role in postoperative outcome [Review article]. *Anesthesiology* 1995;82:1474–1506.
28. Wu CL, Naqibuddin M, Rowlingson AJ, et al. The effect of pain on health-related quality of life in the immediate postoperative period. *Anesth Analg* 2003;97:1078–1085.
29. Rogers MC. Do the right thing: Pain relief in infants and children [Editorial]. *N Engl J Med* 1992;326:55–56.
30. White PF, Rawal S, Latham P, et al. Use of a continuous local anesthetic infusion for pain management after median sternotomy. *Anesthesiology* 2003;99:918–923.
31. Dowling R, Thielmeier K, Ghaly A, et al. Improved pain control after cardiac surgery: Results of a randomized, double-blind, clinical trial. *J Thorac Cardiovasc Surg* 2003;126:1271–1278.
32. Brown SL, Morrison AE. Local anesthetic infusion pump systems adverse events reported to the Food and Drug Administration. *Anesthesiology* 2004;100:1305–1306.
33. Soto RG, Fu ES. Acute pain management for patients undergoing thoracotomy. *Ann Thorac Surg* 2003;75:1349–1357.
34. Karmakar MK. Thoracic paravertebral block [Review article]. *Anesthesiology* 2001;95:771–780.
35. Kavanagh BP, Katz J, Sandler AN. Pain control after thoracic surgery, a review of current techniques [Review article]. *Anesthesiology* 1994;81:737–759.

PART III: APPLICATIONS

36. Bilgin M, Akcali Y, Oguzkaya F. Extrapleural regional versus systemic analgesia for relieving postthoracotomy pain: A clinical study of bupivacaine compared with metamizol. *J Thorac Cardiovasc Surg* 2003;126:1580–1583.

37. Mehta Y, Swaminathan M, Mishra Y, et al. A comparative evaluation of intrapleural and thoracic epidural analgesia for postoperative pain relief after minimally invasive direct coronary artery bypass surgery. *J Cardiothorac Vasc Anesth* 1998;12:162–165.

38. Riedel BJCJ. Regional anesthesia for major cardiac and noncardiac surgery: More than just a strategy for effective analgesia? [Editorial]. *J Cardiothorac Vasc Anesth* 2001;15:279–281.

39. Chaney MA. Intrathecal and epidural anesthesia and analgesia for cardiac surgery [Review article]. *Anesth Analg* 2006;102:45–64.

40. Feigl E. Coronary physiology [Review article]. *Physiol Rev* 1983;63:1–205.

41. Lee DDP, Kimura S, DeQuattro V. Noradrenergic activity and silent ischaemic in hypertensive patients with stable angina: Effect of metoprolol. *Lancet* 1989;1:403–406.

42. Vanhoutte PM, Shimokawa H. Endothelium-derived relaxing factor and coronary vasospasm. *Circulation* 1989;80:1–9.

43. Blomberg S, Emanuelsson H, Kvist H, et al. Effects of thoracic epidural anesthesia on coronary arteries and arterioles in patients with coronary artery disease. *Anesthesiology* 1990;73:840–847.

44. Blomberg S, Curelaru I, Emanuelsson H, et al. Thoracic epidural anaesthesia in patients with unstable angina pectoris. *Eur Heart J* 1989;10:437–444.

45. Heusch G, Deussen A, Thamer V. Cardiac sympathetic nerve activity and progressive vasoconstriction distal to coronary stenosis: Feed-back aggravation of myocardial ischemia. *J Auton Nerv Syst* 1985;13:311–326.

46. Heusch G, Deussen A. The effects of cardiac sympathetic nerve stimulation on perfusion of stenotic coronary arteries in the dog. *Circ Res* 1983;53:8–15.

47. Uchida Y, Murao S. Excitation of afferent cardiac sympathetic nerve fibers during coronary occlusion. *Am J Physiol* 1974;226:1094–1099.

48. Mangano DT. Perioperative cardiac morbidity [Review article]. *Anesthesiology* 1990;72:153–184.

49. Birkett DA, Apthorp GH, Chamberlain DA, et al. Bilateral upper thoracic sympathectomy in angina pectoris: Results in 52 cases. *Br Med J* 1965; 2:187–190.

50. Kock M, Blomberg S, Emanuelsson H, et al. Thoracic epidural anesthesia improves global and regional left ventricular function during stress-induced myocardial ischemia in patients with coronary artery disease. *Anesth Analg* 1990;71:625–630.

51. Blomberg SG. Long-term home self-treatment with high thoracic epidural anesthesia in patients with severe coronary artery disease. *Anesth Analg* 1994;79:413–421.

52. Davis RF, DeBoer LWV, Maroko PR. Thoracic epidural anesthesia reduces myocardial infarct size after coronary artery occlusion in dogs. *Anesth Analg* 1986;65:711–717.

53. Klassen GA, Bramwell RS, Bromage PR, et al. Effect of acute sympathectomy by epidural anesthesia on the canine coronary circulation. *Anesthesiology* 1980;52:8–15.

54. Mathews ET, Abrams LD. Intrathecal morphine in open heart surgery (correspondence). *Lancet* 1980;2:543.

55. Metz S, Schwann NM, Hassanein W, et al. Intrathecal morphine for off-pump coronary artery bypass grafting. *J Cardiothorac Vasc Anesth* 2004; 18:451–453.

56. Lena P, Balarac N, Arnulf JJ, et al. Intrathecal morphine and clonidine for coronary artery bypass grafting. *Br J Anaesth* 2003;90:300–303.

57. Bowler I, Djaiani G, Abel R, et al. A combination of intrathecal morphine and remifentanil anesthesia for fast-track cardiac anesthesia and surgery. *J Cardiothorac Vasc Anesth* 2002;16:709–714.

58. Alhashemi JA, Sharpe MD, Harris CL, et al. Effect of subarachnoid morphine administration on extubation time after coronary artery bypass graft surgery. *J Cardiothorac Vasc Anesth* 2000;14:639–644.

59. Latham P, Zarate E, White PF, et al. Fast-track cardiac anesthesia: A comparison of remifentanil plus intrathecal morphine with sufentanil in a desflurane-based anesthetic. *J Cardiothorac Vasc Anesth* 2000;14:645–651.

60. Zarate E, Latham P, White PF, et al. Fast-track cardiac anesthesia: Use of remifentanil combined with intrathecal morphine as an alternative to sufentanil during desflurane anesthesia. *Anesth Analg* 2000;91:283–287.

61. Bowler I, Djaiani G, Hall J, et al. Intravenous remifentanil combined with intrathecal morphine decreases extubation times after elective coronary artery bypass graft (CABG) surgery [Abstract]. *Anesth Analg* 2000;90:S33.

62. Lee TWR, Jacobsohn E, Maniate JM, et al. High spinal anesthesia in cardiac surgery: Effects on hemodynamics, perioperative stress response, and atrial β-receptor function [Abstract]. *Anesth Analg* 2000;90:SCA90.

63. Peterson KL, DeCampli WM, Pike NA, et al. A report of two hundred twenty cases of regional anesthesia in pediatric cardiac surgery. *Anesth Analg* 2000;90:1014–1019.

64. Hammer GB, Ngo K, Macario A. A retrospective examination of regional plus general anesthesia in children undergoing open heart surgery. *Anesth Analg* 2000;90:1020–1024.

65. Djaiani G, Bowler I, Hall J, et al. A combination of remifentanil and intrathecal morphine improves pulmonary function following CABG surgery [Abstract]. *Anesth Analg* 2000;90:SCA64.

66. Chaney MA, Nikolov MP, Blakeman BP, Bakhos M. Intrathecal morphine for coronary artery bypass graft procedure and early extubation revisited. *J Cardiothorac Vasc Anesth* 1999;13:574–578.

67. Shroff A, Rooke GA, Bishop MJ. Effects of intrathecal opioid on extubation time, analgesia, and intensive care unit stay following coronary artery bypass grafting. *J Clin Anesth* 1997;9:415–419.

68. Chaney MA, Furry PA, Fluder EM, et al. Intrathecal morphine for coronary artery bypass grafting and early extubation. *Anesth Analg* 1997;84:241–248.

69. Chaney MA, Smith KR, Barclay JC, et al. Large-dose intrathecal morphine for coronary artery bypass grafting. *Anesth Analg* 1996;83:215–222.

70. Kowalewski R, MacAdams C, Froelich J, et al. Anesthesia supplemented with subarachnoid bupivacaine and morphine for coronary artery bypass surgery in a child with Kawasaki disease [Case report]. *J Cardiothorac Vasc Anesth* 1996;10:243–246.

71. Taylor A, Healy M, McCarroll M, et al. Intrathecal morphine: One year's experience in cardiac surgical patients. *J Cardiothorac Vasc Anesth* 1996;10:225–228.

72. Kowalewski RJ, MacAdams CL, Eagle CJ, et al. Anaesthesia for coronary artery bypass surgery supplemented with subarachnoid bupivacaine and morphine: A report of 18 cases. *Can J Anaesth* 1994;41:1189–1195.

73. Swenson JD, Hullander RM, Wingler K, et al. Early extubation after cardiac surgery using combined intrathecal sufentanil and morphine. *J Cardiothorac Vasc Anesth* 1994;8:509–514.

74. Shroff AB, Bishop MJ. Intrathecal morphine analgesia speeds extubation and shortens ICU stay following coronary artery bypass grafting (CABG) [Abstract]. *Anesthesiology* 1994;81:A129.

75. Fitzpatrick GJ, Moriarty DC. Intrathecal morphine in the management of pain following cardiac surgery, a comparison with morphine i.v. *Br J Anaesth* 1988;60:639–644.

76. Vanstrum GS, Bjornson KM, Ilko R. Postoperative effects of intrathecal morphine in coronary artery bypass surgery. *Anesth Analg* 1988:67:261–167.

77. Casey WF, Wynands JE, Ralley FE, et al. The role of intrathecal morphine in the anesthetic management of patients undergoing coronary artery bypass surgery. *J Cardiothorac Vasc Anesth* 1987;1:510–516.

78. Cheun JK. Intraspinal narcotic anesthesia in open heart surgery. *J Kor Med Sci* 1987;2:225–229.

79. Aun C, Thomas D, St. John-Jones L, et al. Intrathecal morphine in cardiac surgery. *Eur J Anaesth* 1985;2:419–426.

80. Vincenty C, Malone B. Mathru M, et al. Comparison of intrathecal and intravenous morphine in post coronary bypass surgery [Abstract]. *Crit Care Med* 1985;13:308.

81. Jones SEF, Beasley JM, Macfarlane DWR, et al. Intrathecal morphine for postoperative pain relief in children. *Br J Anaesth* 1984;56:137–140.

82. Bettex DA, Schmidlin D, Chassot PG, et al. Intrathecal sufentanil-morphine shortens the duration of intubation and improves analgesia in fast-track cardiac surgery. *Can J Anesth* 2002;49:711–717.

83. Goldstein S, Dean D, Kim SJ, et al. A survey of spinal and epidural techniques in adult cardiac surgery. *J Cardiothorac Vasc Anesth* 2001;15:158–168.

84. Lee TWR, Grocott HP, Schwinn D, et al. High spinal anesthesia for cardiac surgery: Effects on β-adrenergic receptor function, stress response, and hemodynamics. *Anesthesiology* 2003;98:499–510.

85. Clowes GHA, Neville WE, Hopkins A, et al. Factors contributing to success or failure in the use of a pump oxygenator for complete by-pass of the heart and lung, experimental and clinical. *Surgery* 1954;36:557–579.

86. Hoar PF, Hickey RF, Ullyot DJ. Systemic hypertension following myocardial revascularization, a method of treatment using epidural anesthesia. *J Thorac Cardiovasc Surg* 1976;71:859–864.

87. El-Baz N, Goldin M. Continuous epidural infusion of morphine for pain relief after cardiac operations. *J Thorac Cardiovasc Surg* 1987;93:878–883.

88. Jideus L, Joachimsson P, Stridsberg M, et al. Thoracic epidural anesthesia does not influence the occurrence of postoperative sustained atrial fibrillation. *Ann Thorac Surg* 2001;72:65–71.

89. Scott NB, Turfrey DJ, Ray DAA, et al. A prospective randomized study of the potential benefits of thoracic epidural anesthesia and analgesia in patients undergoing coronary artery bypass grafting. *Anesth Analg* 2001;93:528–535.

90. Warters D, Knight W, Koch SM, et al. Thoracic epidurals in coronary artery bypass surgery. *Anesth Analg* 2000;90:767.

91. Loick HM, Schmidt C, Van Aken H, et al. High thoracic epidural anesthesia, but not clonidine, attenuates the perioperative stress response via sympatholysis and reduces the release of troponin T in patients undergoing coronary artery bypass grafting. *Anesth Analg* 1999;88:701–709.

92. Tenling A, Joachimsson PO, Tyden H, et al. Thoracic epidural anesthesia as an adjunct to general anesthesia for cardiac surgery: Effects on ventilation-perfusion relationships. *J Cardiothorac Vasc Anesth* 1999;13:258–264.

93. Sanchez R, Nygard E. Epidural anesthesia in cardiac surgery: Is there an increased risk? *J Cardiothorac Vasc Anesth* 1998;12:170–173.

94. Loick HM, Mollhoff T, Erren M, et al. Thoracic epidural anesthesia lowers catecholamine and TNF α release after CABG in humans [Abstract]. *Anesth Analg* 1998;86:S81.

95. Warters RD, Kroch SM, Luehr SL, et al. Thoracic epidural anesthesia in CABG surgery [Abstract]. *Anesth Analg* 1998;86:S116.
96. Shayevitz JR, Merkel S, O'Kelly SW, et al. Lumbar epidural morphine infusions for children undergoing cardiac surgery. *J Cardiothorac Vasc Anesth* 1996;10:217–224.
97. Frank RS, Bolts MG, Sentivany SK, et al. Combined epidural-general anesthesia for the repair of atrial septal defects in children resulting in shorter ICU stays [Abstract]. *Anesthesiology* 1995;83:A1176.
98. Moore CM, Cross MH, Desborough JP, et al. Hormonal effects of thoracic extradural anesthesia for cardiac surgery. *Br J Anaesth* 1995;75:387–393.
99. Stenseth R, Berg EM, Bjella L, et al. Effects of thoracic epidural analgesia on coronary hemodynamics and myocardial metabolism in coronary artery bypass surgery. *J Cardiothorac Vasc Anesth* 1995;9:503–509.
100. Kirno K, Friberg P, Grzegorczyk A, et al. Thoracic epidural anesthesia during coronary artery bypass surgery: Effects on cardiac sympathetic activity, myocardial blood flow and metabolism, and central hemodynamics. *Anesth Analg* 1994;79:1075–1081.
101. Stenseth R, Bjella L, Berg EM, et al. Thoracic epidural analgesia in aortocoronary bypass surgery I: Haemodynamic effects. *Acta Anaesthesiol Scand* 1994;38:826–833.
102. Stenseth R, Bjella L, Berg EM, et al. Thoracic epidural analgesia in aortocoronary bypass surgery II: Effects on the endocrine metabolic response. *Acta Anaesthesiol Scand* 1994;38:824–839.
103. Shapiro JH, Wolman RL, Lofland GK. Epidural morphine as an adjunct for early extubation following congenital cardiac surgery [Abstract]. *Anesth Analg* 1994;78:S385.
104. Liem TH, Booij LHDJ, Hasenbos MAWN, et al. Coronary artery bypass grafting using two different anesthetic techniques: Part 1: Hemodynamic results. *J Cardiothorac Vasc Anesth* 1992;6:148–155.
105. Liem TH, Hasenbos MAWM, Booij LHDJ, et al. Coronary artery bypass grafting using two different anesthetic techniques: Part 2: Postoperative outcome. *J Cardiothorac Vasc Anesth* 1992;6:156–161.
106. Liem TH, Booij LHDJ, Gielen MJM, et al. Coronary artery bypass grafting using two different anesthetic techniques: Part 3: Adrenergic responses. *J Cardiothorac Vasc Anesth* 1992;6:162–167.
107. Rosen KR, Rosen DA. Caudal epidural morphine for control of pain following open heart surgery in children. *Anesthesiology* 1989;70:418–421.
108. Joachimsson PO, Nystrom SO, Tyden H. Early extubation after coronary artery surgery inefficiently rewarmed patients: A postoperative comparison of opioid anesthesia versus inhalational anesthesia and thoracic epidural anesthesia. *J Cardiothorac Vasc Anesth* 1989;3:444–445.
109. Robinson RJS, Brister S, Jones E, et al. Epidural meperidine analgesia after cardiac surgery. *Can Anaesth Soc J* 1986;33:550–555.
110. Pastor MC, Sanchez MJ, Casas MA, et al. Thoracic epidural analgesia in coronary artery bypass graft surgery: Seven years' experience. *J Cardiothorac Vasc Anesth* 2003;17:154–159.
111. Vlachtsis H, Vohra A. High thoracic epidural with general anesthesia for combined off-pump coronary artery and aortic aneurysm surgery. *J Cardiothorac Vasc Anesth* 2003;17:226–229.
112. Sisillo E, Salvi L, Juliano G, et al. Thoracic epidural anesthesia as a bridge to redo coronary artery bypass graft surgery. *J Cardiothorac Vasc Anesth* 2003;17:629–631.
113. Varadarajan B, Whitaker DK, Vohra A, et al. Case 2–2002. Thoracic epidural anesthesia in patients with ankylosing spondylitis undergoing coronary artery surgery (case conference). *J Cardiothorac Vasc Anesth* 2002;16:240–245.
114. de Vries AJ, Mariani MA, van der Maaten JMAA, et al. To ventilate or not after minimally invasive direct coronary artery bypass surgery: The role of epidural anesthesia. *J Cardiothorac Vasc Anesth* 2002;16:21–26.
115. Canto M, Casas A, Sanchez MJ, et al. Thoracic epidurals in heart valve surgery: Neurologic risks evaluation. *J Cardiothoracic Vasc Anesth* 2002;16:723–726.
116. Fillinger MP, Yeager MP, Dodds TM, et al. Epidural anesthesia and analgesia: Effects on recovery from cardiac surgery. *J Cardiothorac Vasc Anesth* 2002;16:15–20.
117. Dhole S, Mehta Y, Saxena H, et al. Comparison of continuous thoracic epidural and paravertebral blocks for postoperative analgesia after minimally invasive direct coronary artery bypass surgery. *J Cardiothorac Vasc Anesth* 2001;15:288–292.
118. Djaiani GN, Ali M, Heinrich L, et al. Ultra-fast-track anesthetic technique facilitates operating room extubation in patients undergoing off-pump coronary revascularization surgery. *J Cardiothorac Vasc Anesth* 2001;15:152–157.
119. Visser WA, Liem TH, Brouwer RMHJ. High thoracic epidural anesthesia for coronary artery bypass graft surgery in a patient with severe obstructive lung disease. *J Cardiothorac Vasc Anesth* 2001;15:758–760.
120. Liem TH, Williams JP, Hensens AG, et al. Minimally invasive direct coronary artery bypass procedure using a high thoracic epidural plus general anesthetic technique [Case report]. *J Cardiothorac Vasc Anesth* 1998;12:668–672.
121. Fawcett WJ, Edwards RE, Quinn AC, et al. Thoracic epidural analgesia started after cardiopulmonary bypass, adrenergic, cardiovascular and respiratory sequelae. *Anaesthesia* 1997;52:294–299.
122. Turfrey DJ, Ray DAA, Sutcliffe NP, et al. Thoracic epidural anaesthesia for coronary artery bypass graft surgery, effects on postoperative complications. *Anaesthesia* 1997;52:1095–1097.
123. Stenseth R, Bjella L, Berg EM, et al. Effects of thoracic epidural analgesia on pulmonary function after coronary artery bypass surgery. *Eur J Cardiothorac Surg* 1996;10:859–865.
124. O'Connor CJ, Tuman KJ. Epidural anesthesia and analgesia for coronary artery bypass graft surgery: Still forbidden territory? [Editorial]. *Anesth Analg* 2001;93:523–525.
125. Amar D. Beta-adrenergic blocker withdrawal confounds the benefits of epidural analgesia with sympathectomy on supraventricular arrhythmias after cardiac surgery (correspondence). *Anesth Analg* 2002;95:1119.
126. Riedel BJ, Shaw AD. Thoracic epidural anesthesia & analgesia in patients undergoing coronary artery bypass surgery (correspondence). *Anesth Analg* 2002;94:1365.
127. Alston RP. Thoracic epidurals and coronary artery bypass grafting surgery (correspondence). *Anesth Analg* 2002;94:1365.
128. Royse C, Royse A, Soeding P, et al. Prospective randomized trial of high thoracic epidural analgesia for coronary artery bypass surgery. *Ann Thorac Surg* 2003;75:93–100.
129. Priestley MC, Cope L, Halliwell R, et al. Thoracic epidural anesthesia for cardiac surgery: The effects on tracheal intubation time and length of hospital stay. *Anesth Analg* 2002;94:275–282.
130. Hansdottir V, Philip J, Olsen MF, et al. Thoracic epidural versus intravenous patient-controlled analgesia after cardiac surgery: A randomized controlled trial on length of hospital stay and patient-perceived quality of recovery. *Anesthesiology* 2006;101:142–151.
131. Barrington MJ, Kluger R, Watson R, et al. Epidural anesthesia for coronary artery bypass surgery compared with general anesthesia alone does not reduce biochemical markers of myocardial damage. *Anesth Analg* 2005;100:921–928.
132. Karagoz HY, Sonmez B, Bakkaloglu B, et al. Coronary artery bypass grafting in the conscious patient without endotracheal general anesthesia. *Ann Thorac Surg* 2000;70:91–96.
133. Aybek T, Dogan S, Neidhart G, et al. Coronary artery bypass grafting through complete sternotomy in conscious patients. *Heart Surg Forum* 2002;5:17–21.
134. Souto GLL, Junior CSC, de Souza JBS, et al. Coronary artery bypass in the ambulatory patient. *J Thorac Cardiovasc Surg* 2002;123:1008–1009.
135. Aybek T, Kessler P, Dogan S, et al. Awake coronary artery bypass grafting: Utopia or reality? *Ann Thorac Surg* 2003;75:1165–1170.
136. Aybek T, Kessler P, Khan MF, et al. Operative techniques in awake coronary artery bypass grafting. *J Thorac Cardiovasc Surg* 2003;125:1394–1400.
137. Karagoz HY, Kurtoglu M, Bakkaloglu B, et al. Coronary artery bypass grafting in the awake patient: Three years' experience in 137 patients. *J Thorac Cardiovasc Surg* 2003;125:1401–1404.
138. Chakravarthy M, Jawali V, Patil TA, et al. High thoracic epidural anesthesia as the sole anesthetic for redo off-pump coronary artery bypass surgery [Case report]. *J Cardiothorac Vasc Anesth* 2003;17:84–86.
139. Chakravarthy M, Jawali V, Patil TA, et al. High thoracic epidural anesthesia as the sole anaesthetic technique for minimally invasive direct coronary artery bypass in a high-risk patient [Case report]. *Ann Cardiac Anaesth* 2003;6:62–64.
140. Kessler P, Neidhart G, Bremerich DH, et al. High thoracic epidural anesthesia for coronary artery bypass grafting using two different surgical approaches in conscious patients. *Anesth Analg* 2002;95:791–797.
141. Vanek T, Straka Z, Brucek P, et al. Thoracic epidural anesthesia for off-pump coronary artery bypass without intubation. *Eur J Cardiothorac Surg* 2001;20:858–860.
142. Anderson MB, Kwong KF, Furst AJ, et al. Thoracic epidural anesthesia for coronary bypass via left anterior thoracotomy in the conscious patient [Case report]. *Eur J Cardiothorac Surg* 2001;20:415–417.
143. Paiste J, Bjerk RJ, Williams JP, et al. Minimally invasive direct coronary artery bypass surgery under high thoracic epidural [Case report]. *Anesth Analg* 2001;93:1486–1488.
144. Zenati MA, Paiste J, Williams JP, et al. Minimally invasive coronary bypass without general endotracheal anesthesia [Case report]. *Ann Thorac Surg* 2001;72:1380–1382.
145. Chakravarthy M, Jawali V, Patil TA, et al. High thoracic epidural anesthesia as the sole anesthetic for performing multiple grafts in off-pump coronary artery bypass surgery. *J Cardiothorac Vasc Anesth* 2003;17:160–164.
146. Schachner T, Bonatti J, Balogh D, et al. Aortic valve replacement in the conscious patient under regional anesthesia without endotracheal intubation [Case report]. *J Thorac Cardiovasc Surg* 2003;25:1526–1527.
147. Straka Z, Brucek P, Vanek T, et al. Routine immediate extubation for off-pump coronary artery bypass grafting without thoracic epidural analgesia. *Ann Thorac Surg* 2002;74:1544–1547.

PART III: APPLICATIONS

148. Ochroch EA, Gottschalk A, Augostides J, et al. Long-term pain and activity during recovery from major thoracotomy using thoracic epidural analgesia. *Anesthesiology* 2002;97:1234–1244.

149. Richard C, Girard F, Ferraro P, et al. Acute postoperative pain in lung transplant recipients. *Ann Thorac Surg* 2004;77:1951–1955.

150. Ballantyne JC, Carr DB, deFerranti S, et al. The comparative effects of postoperative analgesic therapies on pulmonary outcome: Cumulative meta-analyses of randomized, controlled trials. *Anesth Analg* 1998;86:598–612.

151. Licker M, de Perrot M, Hohn L, et al. Perioperative mortality and major cardiopulmonary complications after lung surgery for non-small cell carcinoma. *Eur J Cardiothorac Surg* 1999;15:314–319.

152. Liu SS, Block BM, Wu CL. Effects of perioperative central neuraxial analgesia on outcome after coronary artery bypass surgery: A meta-analysis. *Anesthesiology* 2004;101:153–161.

153. Norris EJ, Frank SM. Anesthesia for vascular surgery. In: Miller RD, ed. *Anesthesia*, 5th ed. Philadelphia: Churchill Livingstone; 2000:1849–1893.

154. Heller LB, Chaney MA. Paraplegia immediately following removal of a cerebrospinal fluid drainage catheter in a patient after thoracoabdominal aortic aneurysm surgery. *Anesthesiology* 2001;95:1285–1287.

155. Chaney MA. High-dose intrathecal morphine for thoracoabdominal aneurysm repair (correspondence). *J Cardiothorac Vasc Anesth* 1996;10: 306–307.

156. Kakinohana M, Fuchigami T, Nakamura S, et al. Intrathecal administration of morphine, but not small dose, induced spastic paraparesis after a noninjurious interval of aortic occlusion in rats. *Anesth Analg* 2003;96:759–775.

157. Rosenbaum GJ, Arroya PJ, Sivina M. Retroperitoneal approach used exclusively with epidural anesthesia for infrarenal aortic disease. *Am J Surg* 1994;168:136–139.

158. Pecoraro JP, Dardik H, Mauro A, et al. Epidural anesthesia as an adjunct to retroperitoneal aortic surgery. *Am J Surg* 1990;160:187–191.

159. Boylan JF, Katz J, Kavanagh BP, et al. Epidural bupivacaine-morphine analgesia versus patient-controlled analgesia following abdominal aortic surgery: Analgesic, respiratory, and myocardial effects. *Anesthesiology* 1998;89:585–593.

160. Gold MS, DeCrosta D, Rizzuto C, et al. The effect of lumbar epidural and general anesthesia on plasma catecholamines and hemodynamics during abdominal aortic aneurysm repair. *Anesth Analg* 1994;78:225–230.

161. Davies MJ, Silbert BS, Mooney PJ, et al. Combined epidural and general anaesthesia versus general anaesthesia for abdominal aortic surgery: A prospective randomized trial. *Anaesth Intensive Care* 1993;21:790–794.

162. Blunt TJ, Manzuk M, Varley K. Continuous epidural anesthesia for aortic surgery: Thoughts on peer review and safety. *Surgery* 1987;101:706–714.

163. Lunn JK, Dannemiller FJ, Stanley TH. Cardiovascular responses to clamping of the aorta during epidural and general anesthesia. *Anesth Analg* 1979; 58:372–376.

164. Breslow MJ, Parker SD, Frank SM, et al. Determinants of catecholamine and cortisol responses to lower extremity revascularization. *Anesthesiology* 1993;79:1202–1209.

165. Wu CL, Cohen SR, Richman JM, et al. Efficacy of postoperative patient-controlled and continuous infusion epidural analgesia versus intravenous patient-controlled analgesia with opioids: A meta-analysis. *Anesthesiology* 2005;103:1079–1088.

166. Moraca RJ, Sheldon DG, Thirlby RC. The role of epidural anesthesia and analgesia in surgical practice [Review article]. *Ann Surg* 2003;238:663–673.

167. Block BM, Liu SS, Rowlingson AJ, et al. Efficacy of postoperative epidural analgesia: A meta-analysis. *JAMA* 2003;290:2455–2463.

168. Dolin SJ, Cashman JN, Bland JM. Effectiveness of acute postoperative pain management: I. Evidence from published data. *Br J Anaesth* 2002;89:409–423.

169. Young Park W, Thompson JS, Lee KK, et al. Effect of epidural anesthesia and analgesia on perioperative outcome: A randomized, controlled veterans affairs cooperative study. *Ann Surg* 2001;234:560–571.

170. Bois S, Couture P, Boudreault D, et al. Epidural analgesia and intravenous patient-controlled analgesia result in similar rates of postoperative myocardial ischemia after aortic surgery. *Anesth Analg* 1997;85:1233–1239.

171. Dodds TM, Burns AK, DeRoo DB, et al. Effects of anesthetic technique on myocardial wall motion abnormalities during abdominal aortic surgery. *J Cardiothorac Vasc Anesth* 1997;11:129–136.

172. Garnett RL, MacIntyre A, Lindsay P, et al. Perioperative ischemia in aortic surgery: Combined epidural/general anesthesia and epidural analgesia vs general anesthesia and i.v. analgesia. *Can J Anaesth* 1996;43:769–777.

173. Bode RH, Lewis KP, Zarich SW, et al. Cardiac outcome after peripheral vascular surgery: Comparison of general and regional anesthesia. *Anesthesiology* 1996;84:3–13.

174. Christopherson R, Beattie C, Frank SM, et al. Perioperative morbidity in patients randomized to epidural or general anesthesia for lower extremity vascular surgery: Perioperative ischemia randomized anesthesia trial study group. *Anesthesiology* 1993;79:422–434.

175. Baron JF, Bertrand M, Barre E, et al. Combined epidural and general anesthesia versus general anesthesia for abdominal aortic surgery. *Anesthesiology* 1991;75:611–618.

176. Rosenfeld BA, Beattie C, Christopherson R, et al. The effects of different anesthetic regimens on fibrinolysis and the development of postoperative arterial thrombosis. *Anesthesiology* 1993;79:435–443.

177. Haljamae H, Frid I, Holm J, et al. Epidural vs. general anesthesia and leg blood flow in patients with occlusive atherosclerotic disease. *Eur J Vasc Surg* 1988;2:395–400.

178. Sivarajan M, Amory DW, Lindbloom, LE, et al. Systemic and regional blood-flow changes during spinal anesthesia in the rhesus monkey. *Anesthesiology* 1975;43:78–88.

179. Hackel DB, Sancetta SM, Kleinerman J. Effect of hypotension due to spinal anesthesia on coronary blood flow and myocardial metabolism in man. *Circulation* 1956;13:92–97.

180. Reiz S, Nath S, Rais O. Effects of thoracic epidural block and prenalterol on coronary vascular resistance and myocardial metabolism in patients with coronary artery disease. *Acta Anaesthesiol Scand* 1980;24:11–16.

181. DiNardo JA, Bert A, Schwartz MJ, et al. Effects of vasoactive drugs on flows through left internal mammary artery and saphenous vein grafts in man. *J Thorac Cardiovasc Surg* 1991;102:730–735.

182. Heusch G. α-adrenergic mechanisms in myocardial ischemia. *Circulation* 1990;81:1–13.

183. Reiz S, Nath S. Cardiotoxicity of local anaesthetic agents. *Br J Anaesth* 1986; 58:736–746.

184. Wattwil M, Sundberg A, Arvill A, et al. Circulatory changes during high thoracic epidural anaesthesia: Influence of sympathetic block and of systemic effect of the local anaesthetic. *Acta Anaesthesiol Scand* 1985;29:849–855.

185. Blomberg S, Ricksten SE. Effects of thoracic epidural anaesthesia on central haemodynamics compared to cardiac beta adrenoceptor blockade in conscious rats with acute myocardial infarction. *Acta Anaesthesiol Scand* 1990;34:1–7.

186. Hotvedt R, Refsum H, Platou ES. Cardiac electrophysiological and hemodynamic effects of β-adrenoceptor blockade and thoracic epidural analgesia in the dog. *Anesth Analg* 1984;63:817–824.

187. Easley RB, Rosen RE, Linderman KS. Coronary artery spasm during initiation of epidural anesthesia [Case report]. *Anesthesiology* 2003;99:1015–1017.

188. Oden RV, Karagianes TG. Postoperative myocardial ischemia possibly masked by epidural fentanyl analgesia. *Anesthesiology* 1991;74:941–943.

189. Chaney MA. Side effects of intrathecal and epidural opioids [Review article]. *Can J Anaesth* 1995;42:891–903.

190. Wang JK, Nauss LA, Thomas JE. Pain relief by intrathecally applied morphine in man. *Anesthesiology* 1979;50:149–151.

191. Behar M, Magora F, Olshwang D, et al. Epidural morphine in treatment of pain. *Lancet* 1979;1:527–529.

192. Glynn CJ, Mather LE, Cousins MJ, et al. Spinal narcotics and respiratory depression (correspondence). *Lancet* 1979;2:356–357.

193. Liolios A, Andersen FH. Selective spinal analgesia (correspondence). *Lancet* 1979;2:357.

194. Scott DB, McClure J. Selective epidural analgesia (correspondence). *Lancet* 1979;1:1410–1411.

195. Shook JE, Watkins WD, Camporesi EM. Differential roles of opioid receptors in respiration, respiratory disease, and opiate-induced respiratory depression. *Am Rev Respir Dis* 1990;142:895–909.

196. Vandermeulen EP, Van Aken H, Vermylen J. Anticoagulants and spinal-epidural anesthesia. *Anesth Analg* 1994;79:1165–1177.

197. Markham JW, Lynge HN, Stahlman EB. The syndrome of spontaneous spinal epidural hematoma, report of three cases. *J Neurosurg* 1967;26:334–342.

198. Waldman SD, Feldstein GS, Waldman HJ, et al. Caudal administration of morphine sulfate in anticoagulated and thrombocytopenic patients. *Anesth Analg* 1987;66:267–268.

199. Odoom JA, Sih IL. Epidural analgesia and anticoagulant therapy, experience with one thousand cases of continuous epidurals. *Anaesthesia* 1983;38:254–259.

200. Owens EL, Kasten GW, Hessel EA. Spinal subarachnoid hematoma after lumbar puncture and heparinization: A case report, review of the literature and discussion of anesthetic implications. *Anesth Analg* 1986;65:1201–1207.

201. Brem SS, Hafler DA, Van Uitert RL, et al. Spinal subarachnoid hematoma: A hazard of lumbar puncture resulting in reversible paraplegia. *N Engl J Med* 1981;303:1020–1021.

202. Ruff RL, Dougherty JH. Complications of lumbar puncture followed by anticoagulation. *Stroke* 1981;12:879–881.

203. Varkey GP, Brindle GF. Peridural anaesthesia and anti-coagulant therapy. *Can Anaesth Soc J* 1974;21:106–109.

204. Baron HC, LaRaja RD, Rossi G, et al. Continuous epidural analgesia in the heparinized vascular surgical patient: A retrospective review of 912 patients. *J Vasc Surg* 1987;6:144–146.

205. Rao TLK, El-Etr AA. Anticoagulation following placement of epidural and subarachnoid catheters: An evaluation of neurologic sequelae. *Anesthesiology* 1981;55:618–620.

206. Ho AMH, Chung DC, Joynt GM. Neuraxial blockade and hematoma in cardiac surgery: Estimating the risk of a rare adverse event that has not (yet) occurred. *Chest* 2000;117:551–555.
207. Rosen DA, Hawkinberry DW, Rosen KR, et al. An epidural hematoma in an adolescent patient after cardiac surgery [Case report]. *Anesth Analg* 2004;98:966–969.
208. Chaney MA, Labovsky JK. Thoracic epidural anesthesia and cardiac surgery: Balancing postoperative risks associated with hematoma formation and thromboembolic phenomenon. *J Cardiothorac Vasc Anesth* 2005; 19:768–771.
209. Chaney MA. Cardiac surgery and intrathecal/epidural techniques: At the crossroads? [Editorial]. *Can J Anesth* 2005;52:783–788.
210. Chaney MA. How important is postoperative pain after cardiac surgery? [Editorial]. *J Cardiothorac Vasc Anesth* 2005;19:705–707.
211. Mora Mangano CT. Risky business [Editorial]. *J Thorac Cardiovasc Surg* 2003;125:1204–1207.
212. Castellano JM, Durbin CG. Epidural analgesia and cardiac surgery: Worth the risk? [Editorial]. *Chest* 2000;117:305–307.
213. Schwann NM, Chaney MA. No pain, much gain? [Editorial]. *J Thorac Cardiovasc Surg* 2003;126:1261–1264.
214. Gravlee GP. Epidural analgesia and coronary artery bypass grafting: The controversy continues [Editorial]. *J Cardiothorac Vasc Anesth* 2003;17: 151–153.
215. de Leon-Cassasola OA. When it comes to outcome, we need to define what a perioperative epidural technique is [Editorial]. *Anesth Analg* 2003;96:315–318.
216. Rosenquist RW, Birnbach DJ. Epidural insertion in anesthetized adults: Will your patients thank you? [Editorial]. *Anesth Analg* 2003;96:1545–1546.
217. White PF. The role of non-opioid analgesic techniques in the management of pain after ambulatory surgery [Review article]. *Anesth Analg* 2002;94:577–585.
218. Kehlet H, Dahl JB. The value of "multimodal" or "balanced analgesia" in postoperative pain treatment [Review article]. *Anesth Analg* 1993;77:1048–1056.
219. Myles PS, Hunt JO, Fletcher H, et al. Relation between quality of recovery in hospital and quality of life at 3 months after cardiac surgery. *Anesthesiology* 2001;95:862–867.
220. Fleron MH, Weiskopf RB, Bertrand M, et al. A comparison of intrathecal opioid and intravenous analgesia for the incidence of cardiovascular, respiratory, and renal complications after abdominal aortic surgery. *Anesth Analg* 2003;97:2–12.
221. Beattie WS, Badner NH, Choi P. Epidural analgesia reduces postoperative myocardial infarction: A meta-analysis. *Anesth Analg* 2001;93:853–858.
222. Wu CL, Raja SN. Optimizing postoperative analgesia: The use of global outcome measures [Editorial]. *Anesthesiology* 2002;97:533–534.
223. Gottschalk A, Ochroch EA. Preemptive analgesia: What do we do now? (correspondence). *Anesthesiology* 2003;98:280–281.
224. Hogan QH. No preemptive analgesia: Is that so bad? [Editorial]. *Anesthesiology* 2002;96:526–527.
225. Moiniche S, Kehlet H, Dahl JB. A qualitative and quantitative systematic review of preemptive analgesia for postoperative pain relief: The role of timing of analgesia [Review article]. *Anesthesiology* 2002;96:725–741.
226. Katz J, Cohen L, Schmid R, et al. Postoperative morphine use and hyperalgesia are reduced by preoperative but not intraoperative epidural analgesia: Implications for preemptive analgesia and the prevention of central sensitization. *Anesthesiology* 2003;98:1449–1460.

CHAPTER 23 ■ NEURAL BLOCKADE FOR ABDOMINAL AND THORACIC (NON-VASCULAR) SURGERY

FRANCISCO ASENJO AND FRANCESCO CARLI

REGIONAL ANESTHESIA FOR THORACIC (NONCARDIAC) SURGERY

Thoracic surgery has benefited greatly from advances in anesthesia. Sixty years ago, intubation allowed control of the airway and ventilation. Then, the ability to separate the lungs with one-lung ventilation techniques provided better surgical conditions. Lately, regional anesthesia and analgesia have decreased morbidity and improved outcome in the perioperative period (see Chapters 6 and 7).

Neuroanatomy of the Chest and Abdomen

The somatic innervation of the chest and abdominal wall is supplied by the intercostal nerves from T2 to T12. After exiting through the intervertebral foramina, the roots divide into ventral branches, dorsal branches, and sympathetic nerves. The dorsal branches run posteriorly to innervate the dorsal paravertebral muscles as well as the skin from midline to 8 to 10 cm laterally. The ventral branches progress antero-laterally under the ribs accompanied by the intercostal artery and vein to innervate the chest wall and breast. This course of the nerves explains the inconsistency between the more superior segmental innervation found in the posterior paravertebral cutaneous innervation and the lower anterior distribution. The ventral branches give origin to two or three perforating cutaneous nerves that divide to innervate the skin from 8 to 10 cm lateral of the dorsal midline to the ventral midline. The primary sensory nerves conveying pain from skin, ribs, and soft tissues are Aδ- and C-type neurons (see Figs. 16-1 and 16-4).

The shoulder girdle is innervated by the brachial plexus. The brachial plexus supplies the motor nerve component of the chest wall muscles that stabilize the shoulder girdle (i.e., pectoralis, latissimus dorsi). The sensation to the skin below the clavicle is provided by cutaneous branches of the cervical superficial plexus (supraclavicular nerve) (see Chapter 13).

The autonomic nervous system supplies the innervation of the viscera, both in the chest and abdomen. In the chest, sympathetic nerves from T1 to T5 travel bilaterally to the heart, carrying efferent nerves that contribute to increase contractility and frequency of the heartbeat as well as to regulate the coronary circulation. In healthy coronaries, the activation of these nerves produces coronary dilatation; however, the con-

trary occurs in patients with coronary artery disease (CAD). Afferent sensory nerves convey ischemic pain from the heart. Other sympathetic fibers carry the afferent and efferent innervation of the bronchi, pericardium, and other thoracic visceral anatomic structures. Sympathetic nerves from T4–T6 to T10 bilaterally form the greater, lesser, and lowest splanchnic nerves that course adjacent to the spine. These fibers cross under the diaphragmatic crura to the abdominal cavity at the level of T12 or L1 to merge as a group of ganglia in front of the celiac trunk to form the celiac plexus. Fibers from the vagus nerve also course to the abdomen along the esophagus. Similar ganglia are present around the origin of the superior mesenteric artery coming from a lower origin in the spine. These ganglia contain the soma of the postganglionic sympathetic neurons providing vascular tone to the abdominal vascular structures, as well as regulation of hormonal and metabolic functions of the viscera (i.e., catecholamine release from the adrenal glands, renin-angiotensin-kallikrein system). Through these ganglia pass the preganglionic parasympathetic neurons that connect with their terminal synapses in the viscera that they are traveling to. The ganglia also include sensory afferent fibers that carry pain signals from the abdominal viscera and peritoneum. Another important visceral sensory structure is the superior hypogastric plexus located in front of the sacral promontorium. This plexus conveys the afferent and efferent innervation (sympathetic/parasympathetic) of the pelvic visceral structures (see Chapter 39, Figs. 39-1 to 39-10 and Figs. 39-21 to 39-23). The phrenic nerves originate bilaterally from C3–C4/5 and give the motor activity to the diaphragm. However, it has been recognized that the phrenic nerves also provide sensory visceral innervation to the diaphragm from both the thoracic as well as the abdominal directions. In fact, because the phrenic nerves share dermatomes with the somatic innervation of the shoulder, patients who have had intrathoracic procedures frequently complaint about ipsilateral shoulder pain in spite of excellent incisional and chest tube area analgesia. However, this pain can also result from other sources including myocardial ischemia, a chest drain impinging on the apex of the pleura and the brachial plexus, and malposition or compression of the shoulder during the surgery (see also Chapter 45).

The vagus nerve supplies parasympathetic innervation to the mediastinal and upper abdominal viscera, including the stomach, liver, kidneys, small bowel, and the ascending and proximal transverse colon (see Figs. 39-5 and 39-21).

The cervical superficial plexus (C3–C4) innervates the skin, fascia, and most of the musculature of the neck. Consideration should be given to this innervation when esophageal surgery is planned with a neck (as well as thoracic) incision (1).

Physiologic Considerations of Thoracic Epidural Blockade

Cardiovascular Effects

Cardiovascular changes occur when local anesthetics are injected into the thoracic epidural space. The extension and intensity of the changes depend upon the volume/mass of local anesthetic injected, the age of the patient, and the spinal level at which the anesthetic agents are deposited. These factors affect the impact on the sympathetic nervous system produced by the local anesthetics. The nerve roots in the intervertebral foramina contain afferent sympathetic fibers, as well as efferent fibers regulating the "tone" of the vascular structures they innervate. These are small neurons that are easily blocked by small concentrations of local anesthetics, leaving the arteries and veins to regulate their caliber in a "low-resistance state." Therefore, the blood flow toward the regions affected by the decrease in vascular sympathetic tone increases (abdomen). Pooling of venous blood decreases central venous pressure, cardiac output, and subsequently, blood pressure (2). A compensatory vasoconstriction in the vasculature of the unblocked regions may attenuate to certain extent the drop in blood pressure and increase cardiac output in healthy individuals. Thoracic epidural anesthesia leads to compensatory reduction of myocardial work and oxygen demand. In patients with CAD, thoracic epidural anesthesia improves cardiac function through an effect on diastolic function and near normalization in the coronary blood flow (3). As shown by echocardiographic testing, a reduction in mean arterial pressure leads to myocardial wall motion dysfunction only during lumbar epidural anesthesia, not during thoracic epidural anesthesia (4) (see Chapter 11).

The visceral sympathetic innervation reaching the suprarenal gland will also be blocked. As a consequence, the systemic circulation of catecholamines released by the adrenal gland will decrease, thus compounding the drop in peripheral resistance, venous return, cardiac output, and blood pressure.

If the epidural blockade reaches the cardiac sympathetic fibers (T1–T5), in addition to the vasodilatation and systemic catecholamine decrease just mentioned, a drop in chronotropism and inotropism is observed in healthy people. Hypotension can be profound in patients with poor cardiovascular reserve and requires prompt action to correct. Thoracic epidural anesthesia is associated with a significant reduction in the arrhythmias associated with cardiac surgery and thoracic surgery, but not in esophageal cancer resection (5–8).

Respiratory Effects

Epidural blockade in the thoracic spine from T1 to T5 is related to minor physiologic respiratory changes (5% decreases in vital capacity [VC] and forced expiratory volume [FEV] 1.0; 0.16 kPa increases in $PaCo_2$) in healthy patients. Shunt fraction and alveolar-arterial differences in Pao_2 do not change with thoracic epidural anesthesia. To affect the mechanical function of the intercostal muscles, a thoracic epidural blockade would require a highly concentrated local anesthetic covering segments from T2 to T8. Motor blockade is about four to five dermatomes below the sensory level. Epidural blockade with mepivacaine 2% from dermatomes C4 to T7 and from T5 to L4 leads to a decrease of 25% in VC and of 13% in FEV_1 (9). In chronic obstructive pulmonary disease (COPD) patients, epidural block with bupivacaine 0.5% (sensory block

from C4 to T8) leads to a decrease of only 8% from baseline in VC and FEV_1. With extensive epidural block, the sitting position is poorly tolerated. Supine position is often associated with decreases in VC and FEV_1, up to 23%. On the other hand, hypotension and hypoperfusion of the respiratory centers in the brainstem from thoracic blockade can produce severe changes in the respiratory physiology (see Chapter 11).

During the postoperative period Whaba (10) and Mankikian (11) have shown improvements in functional residual capacity (FRC) and VC with the use of thoracic epidural local anesthetics. Mankikian also demonstrated that postoperative thoracic epidural block corrects postoperative diaphragmatic dysfunction. In patients with COPD or increased bronchial reactivity, high thoracic epidural block does not disrupt mechanical and functional respiratory patterns more than in healthy patients. The unopposed bronchial reactivity due to the sympathetic blockade might be attenuated by the systemic effect of the local anesthetics (see Chapter 11).

Regional Anesthesia Techniques for Thoracotomy

Thoracotomy is associated with atelectasis, intrapulmonary shunt, and ventilation–perfusion mismatch. General anesthesia, postoperative immobilization, and systemic administration of opioids and sedative drugs adversely affect ventilation and gas exchange and cause respiratory complications. Open lung surgery is also a cause for intra- and postoperative arrhythmias. An ideal anesthesia and analgesia technique for thoracotomy should be rapid in onset, facilitate recovery, and should provide optimum analgesia for a minimum of 3 postoperative days (as long as chest drains are in situ). Patients should be able to move, take deep breaths, produce effective coughs, and cooperate with physiotherapy. Dietary intake and bowel function should be restored soon after surgery. The most common regional anesthesia techniques for thoracic surgical procedures involving the opening of the chest include thoracic epidural, paravertebral, intercostal, and interpleural blockade.

Thoracic Epidural Blockade

Thoracic epidural anesthesia is achieved by approaching the epidural space with a paramedian or mid-line technique. Thoracic epidural anesthesia has been used for lung, chest wall, esophageal, and plastic/reconstructive surgeries (see Chapter 11).

Epidural local anesthetics increase Pao_2 and decrease the incidence of pulmonary infections and pulmonary complications overall. Gruber and co-workers evaluated the effects of thoracic epidural anesthesia in patients with end-stage COPD (12) and showed better ventilatory mechanics with no changes in either gas exchange or inspiratory muscle force. Effectiveness of the sensory block should be established before induction of general anesthesia with either cold or pin-prick testing and by autonomic response such as a decrease in blood pressure or pupillary reflex dilation in response to noxious stimulation (13). Intraoperative thoracic epidural blockade has been shown to decrease chronic pain after thoracotomy (14,15). One-lung ventilation causes significant increases in shunt fraction associated with a decrease in Pao_2. However, Pao_2 remains significantly increased in patients with thoracic epidural anesthesia and general anesthesia compared with total intravenous anesthesia (TIVA) alone (16). Thoracic epidural anesthesia in combination with general anesthesia does not impair arterial oxygenation to the same extent as TIVA, which might be a result of the changes in cardiac output. It is suggested that patients with cardiopulmonary disease and impaired oxygenation before one-lung ventilation might benefit from thoracic epidural anesthesia combined with general anesthesia. In a meta-analysis of 65 studies, Ballantyne and associates concluded that postoperative epidural pain control may significantly decrease pulmonary morbidity (17). Commonly used opioid–local anesthetic mixtures include fentanyl-bupivacaine, morphine-bupivacaine, and fentanyl-ropivacaine. Very-low-dose ketamine (approximately 3 mg/hr for 72 hours) potentiates morphine–ropivacaine analgesia and reduces post-thoracotomy pain (18) (see Chapter 11).

The Direct Search Procedure technique has been utilized to find proper doses, infusion rates, and combinations of drugs to achieve optimal analgesia with thoracic epidural anesthesia (19,20). A sophisticated mathematical model tested multiple solutions and infusion rates based on bupivacaine, fentanyl, and clonidine. The three best combinations of bupivacaine dose (mg/h), fentanyl dose (μg/h), clonidine dose (μg/h), and infusion rate (mL/h) were: 9-21-5-7, 8-30-0-9, and 13-25-0-9. Mixing an opioid (fentanyl 2–3 μg/mL or sufentanil 0.5–1 μg/mL) with a local anesthetic improves pain control with thoracic epidural anesthesia; side effects may increase, decrease, or remain unchanged. Adding epinephrine to mixtures of opioids with low-concentration solutions of local anesthetics has proven beneficial for thoracic epidural analgesia (20), but the role of clonidine remains undetermined.

A recent well-conducted study of analgesia after thoracotomy showed a minor difference between intercostal block and IV patient-controlled analgesia (PCA) versus epidural analgesia with local anesthetics and fentanyl on pain and lung function (21) (see Chapter 11).

Level of Catheter Insertion. Most robust evidence for the analgesic and functional benefits provided by thoracic epidural anesthesia comes from studies using local anesthetics with or without opioids (2,22–24). Epidural catheters placed in the lumbar area for thoracic/upper abdominal surgery require hydrophilic opioids to produce analgesic effects in the thoracic region. However, no clear functional benefits have been documented with this approach. To achieve maximal analgesia, the epidural catheter should be placed in the dermatome corresponding to the mid-point of the surgical incision. Therefore, it is recommended that the catheter be inserted at the T4–T6 level for thoracic surgery. Epidural catheters placed in the lower thoracic spine do not provide adequate analgesia to incisions in the T4– 6 region during thoracic surgery. Increasing the infusion rate to improve analgesia produces unwanted motor blockade in the lower extremities and impairs mobilization. Likewise, catheters inserted above T4 tend not to cover the insertion site of the chest drains, producing only partial analgesia. Blocking the upper thoracic dermatomes is usually accompanied by hypotension secondary to cardiac sympathetic blockade, decrease in cardiac output, and blockade of the sympathetic innervation of the suprarenal glands. This is more noticeable when patients sit and ambulate after surgery. Compensatory sympathetic activity and vasoconstriction occur in the nonblocked distal territories (25,26). Moderate intravascular volume load and cardiostimulant drugs are recommended to reestablish cardiac output and blood pressure in this scenario. Up to 50% of the patients faint when placed in the sitting position for epidural catheterization (27). Sedation and glycopyrrolate or atropine before the procedure may decrease this side effect.

Assessment of Inadequate Analgesia. Postoperative analgesia may be associated with primary failure (inadequate analgesia immediately postoperatively) or secondary failure (initial adequate analgesia followed by an increase in pain/inadequate analgesia). Techniques to determine the etiology of epidural failure are discussed in Table 23-1.

Duration of Epidural Catheterization. Recommended practice is to remove thoracic epidural catheters 48 to 72 hours after chest operations or once the chest drains have been removed. An exception is the esophagectomy, in which some teams remove the epidural catheter by the fourth or fifth day after the barium test has been performed (28).

Treatment of Thoracic Epidural Anesthesia–induced Hypotension. Holte and co-workers assessed plasma volume before and 90 minutes after thoracic epidural anesthesia in 12 volunteers (29). They then administered 7 mL/kg hydroxyethyl starch or 0.2 mg/kg ephedrine. The authors concluded that epidural anesthesia does not lead to any changes in intravascular volume and, as both ephedrine and fluids have comparable hemodynamic effects, vasopressors might be preferred in the treatment of hypotension associated with epidural anesthesia (in patients who are well hydrated), especially for patients with cardiopulmonary diseases in which perioperative fluid overload is undesirable (see also Chapter 11).

Paravertebral Blockade

Paravertebral analgesia for thoracotomy can be provided by the surgeon once the chest is open or percutaneously by the anesthesiologist; both approach have similar success rate. The technique has been described under several different terms: paravertebral, continuous intercostal nerve block, extrapleural intercostal nerve block, extrapleural paravertebral, and retropleural analgesia (see Chapter 16, Figs. 16-15 to 16-18).

Typically, paravertebral catheters are located posterior to the parietal pleura in close proximity to the paravertebral pleural recess, where they provide analgesia by putting the local anesthetic in contact with the intercostal nerves close to their exit from the spine. This anatomic position explains why, in most cases, unilateral analgesia occurs in the affected side of the chest, but in a variable percentage of the patients, it migrates in part to the epidural space via the intervertebral foramen to produce a partial epidural block as well. The analgesic action may also be attributed to the local anesthetic's action on the nerve roots or intercostal nerves and in part to a blockade of the sympathetic chain (31). Different local anesthetics have been successfully used (bupivacaine 0.25%, 0.5%; ropivacaine 0.5%; lidocaine 1%, 2%). A bolus of lidocaine 0.25 mL/kg provides excellent hemodynamic stability (32), as well as bupivacaine-fentanyl and ropivacaine-fentanyl mixtures (33) at 0.1 mL/kg/hr. Clonidine, when used as an adjunct to bupivacaine for continuous paravertebral block, improves analgesic efficacy. Hypotension occurs more frequently among patients receiving clonidine, but this responds well to treatment with volume (34). Sedation is the major adverse effect of clonidine that interferes with its clinical application.

A number of publications support a superior effect of paravertebral versus systemic opiates associated with the lower use of rescue analgesics and respiratory complication rates (35). FEV_1 is also better preserved with paravertebral anesthesia when compared to systemic opiate administration. Randomized trials have compared paravertebral versus epidural anesthesia for thoracotomy in a recent meta-analysis (36) that included a total of 520 patients from 10 trials. Patients who received paravertebral anesthesia had a quality of analgesia at 4, 8, 24, and 48 postoperative hours similar to that of thoracic epidural anesthesia; however, patients with paravertebral anesthesia had better pulmonary function, lower rates of

TABLE 23-1

MOST COMMON CAUSES OF EPIDURAL FAILURE/PROBLEMS AND CORRECTION

Problem	Assessment	Etiology	Action
No intraoperative or post operative analgesia	Cold test after short acting local anesthesia (SALA) bolus (−)	The catheter is not in the epidural space	Reinsert catheter
Good pain control in PACU but not now	a. Cold test to SALA (+) b. Cold test to SALA (−) c. Cold test to SALA (+)	a. Infusion rate too low or weak b. Catheter displaced c. Pump malfunction	a. Increase infusion rate or concentration b. Reinsert catheter c. Change infusion pump
Chest tube area is hurting	Positive block of higher segments	Catheter is placed too high	Reinsert the catheter two segments below or partially withdraw if it has been advanced excessively
Incision area is hurting, but site of drains comfortable	Cold test to SALA (−) over incision, positive block of lower segments	Catheter is placed too low	Reinsert the catheter two segments higher
Poor analgesia and unilateral block noted	Cold test to SALA (−); catheter is partially withdrawn, positive block noted, then pain returns	a. Catheter in paravertebral area b. Catheter exited epidural space by the foramen	a. Try higher infusion rate or reinsert b. Withdrawing catheter 2–3 cm may bring the catheter back into de epidural space
Analgesia is adequate but patient is hypotensive	Stop infusion for 2 hours and restart at lower rate. Aspirate through catheter and test for CSF glucose	a. Rate of infusion too large b. Catheter is intrathecal c. Rule out surgical bleeding, asymptomatic aortic stenosis, initial sepsis, or other causes of hypotension/hypovolemia	a. Decrease infusion rate b. Consider removing catheter or restarting at lower infusion rate c. Consider: (1) decrease in epidural infusion rate, (2) vasopressors, and/or (3) IV fluids bolus (lactated Ringer's 500 mL challenge)
Adequate thoracic analgesia, but shoulder hurts	Check dynamic shoulder pain	a. If it doesn't change with shoulder movement, possible "referred pain" from diaphragm b. If pain increases with movement, check shoulder	a. Optimize multimodal analgesia and rule out coronary artery disease b. Optimize multimodal analgesia; if pain persists after 48 hours, consult orthopedics
Chest pain complaint in spite of good epidural	Test with SALA (+) Is the patient opioid-tolerant (chronic opioids before surgery)? Have preoperative opioids been continued perioperatively?	a. Patient may require higher doses b. Patient may be in withdrawal	a. Add small regular dose of mild opioid (codeine, tramadol) b. Determine "morphine equivalent" and reestablish previous opioid therapy

CSF, cerebrospinal fluid. Cold test: ice cube or alcohol swab.

pulmonary complications, less morphine consumption, and lower incidences of postoperative nausea and vomiting (PONV), urinary retention, and hypotension (36). Interestingly, the failure rate with paravertebral seems to be lower than with epidural anesthesia (37). The concept that epidural anesthesia is the gold standard for postoperative management of pain after thoracic surgery has been challenged by these publications supporting the paravertebral technique. Plasma levels of bupivacaine are between 3 and 4 μg/mL following a few days of infusion. For ropivacaine 0.2% at rates of infusion of 6 to 10 mL/hr, plasma ropivacaine concentrations remain below the toxic threshold. Paravertebral and multimodal analgesia have been also compared with PCA plus multimodal analgesia. Dy-

namic and static pain scores were lower in the paravertebral group. Side effects (nausea, vomiting, urinary retention) were less frequent in the paravertebral group (30% versus 75%; $p < 0.005$) (35) (see also Chapter 16).

Intercostal Blockade

Intercostal blockade (single-injection or continuous) was more popular for thoracotomy before thoracic epidural anesthesia became widespread. The injections can be done either under direct view by the surgeon from inside the chest or percutaneously. Single-injection intercostal nerve blocks for thoracotomy provide better pain relief than opioids alone, with less total opioid requirement, and they improve briefly the FEV$_1$ (37a). In a large study, an incidence of pneumothorax of 0.07% was reported, and peak plasma levels were reached at 10 minutes (bupivacaine 0.19–1.46 μg/mL) (38–40) with no signs of toxicity. Intercostal nerve blockade can be considered a reasonable alternative to paravertebral and thoracic epidural anesthesia (see Chapter 16 and Figs. 16-4 to 16-12).

Cryoanalgesia

Cryoanalgesia is performed by applying a cryoprobe to the nerve under direct view by the surgeon and freezing the nerve to –60°C to –80°C for 2 minutes. This local cold shock destroys the myelin sheath without damaging the axons, an effect that may last for 3 months. As with intercostal blocks, the technique is applied at the level of the surgical incision and the levels above and below (41,42). Studies comparing cryoanalgesia to systemic opiates showed conflicting results in pain relief as well as pulmonary function with a marginal advantage toward cryoanalgesia. The technique fell into disgrace when a number of studies demonstrated painful neuromas in 20% to 30% of patients after cryoanalgesia for thoracic surgery, occurring at about 6 weeks post surgery and lasting for about 4 weeks (43,44). In one study, a decrease in the post thoracotomy pain syndrome was found with cryoanalgesia versus opioids or epidural or interpleural anesthesia (45).

Interpleural Analgesia

Interpleural analgesia consists of depositing local anesthetics between the parietal and visceral pleura. It plays a minor role in thoracotomy patients since they have chest drains in place that preclude a proper effect of the local anesthetic due to its short "residence time" in the target area. Explanations for the limited analgesic efficacy of interpleural analgesia include (a) loss of local anesthetic through the chest tube, (b) dilution of local anesthetic with blood and exudative fluid present in the pleural cavity, (c) binding of local anesthetic with proteins, and (d) altered diffusion across the parietal pleural following surgical manipulation and inflammation. Studies have shown limited or no improvement in analgesia with interpleural analgesia (46–48) (see Chapter 16 and Fig. 16-14).

Phrenic Nerve Infiltration

Approximately one-third of patients undergoing thoracic surgery with thoracic epidural anesthesia complain of ipsilateral shoulder pain due to diaphragmatic irritation (49). This pain is often not covered with epidural blockade. A recent study evaluated the effect of infiltration of 10 mL of 1% lidocaine into the paraphrenic fat pad at conclusion of surgery at the level of the diaphragm in patients undergoing thoracotomy. Patients receiving lidocaine had a significantly decreased incidence of ipsilateral shoulder pain and an overall reduction in pain score compared with placebo infiltration. This may be a simple and effective technique for optimizing postoperative pain control when used in conjunction with epidural analgesia (50). On the contrary, blocking the suprascapular nerve does not contribute to control of referred pain in the shoulder after thoracotomy (51) unless it is a consequence of malpositioning in the operating table and consequently a true shoulder injury.

Regional Anesthesia for Visually-assisted Thoracoscopic Surgery (VATS)

Most commonly visually-assisted thoracoscopic surgery (VATS) is used for lung biopsy, wedge resection, lobectomy, and volume-reduction surgery. VATS has also been successfully used for pneumonectomy as a "fast-track" 24-hour hospital stay procedure. Pain after VATS varies. In the first 24 hours after surgery, the median morphine consumption is similar for lung biopsy and pleurectomy but significantly lower than for pleural biopsy and sympathectomy (52,53). On the second postoperative day (24–48 hours), PCA requirements are significantly reduced, although morphine consumption remains relatively high in pleurectomy patients.

Intercostal nerve blockade with bupivacaine 0.375% or 0.5% provides good-quality analgesia for a median duration of 16 hours with a significant reduction in morphine requirements (52,53). Intercostal blocks with bupivacaine 0.5% are superior to PCA and interpleural block, but only in the first 24 hours after surgery. Analgesic use at the third and seventh days, as well as lung function test recovery pattern, are unaffected by regional anesthesia (54). Plasma levels of ropivacaine after intercostal block for VATS is dose-dependent and reaches peak between 10 and 15 minutes after injection (55). These levels are twice as high as the same dose given via the epidural route. Ropivacaine 0.5% 3 mL per level seems to be appropriate and safe. Preoperative multiple-injection paravertebral block using bupivacaine 0.5% with epinephrine 5 μg/mL (five levels, 4–5 mL per level) provides effective pain relief and a significant reduction in opioid requirements. This approach may also contribute to earlier postoperative ambulation and to lower intraoperative opioid requirements. In a well-conducted double-blind, randomized clinical trial (RCT) (56), time to first analgesic requirement, visual analog scale (VAS) pain scores at first analgesic request, maximum VAS pain scores during 48-hour study period, PCA rescue morphine requirements in the first 48 hours, patient satisfaction with analgesia, time to first mobilization, and time to hospital discharge were all reduced in the paravertebral group. Another RCT also showed better pain control with paravertebral anesthesia up to 24 hours post procedure (57). In a subsequent study, better pain control was noted only through the sixth postoperative hour by Hill, without the prolonged effect previously reported (58). A major difference between these studies is that, in the first one, all blocks were determined to be successful before inducing general anesthesia, whereas in the Hill study, a number of failed blocks were included. Investigators have reported improved pain control and improved postoperative respiratory function in patients receiving continuous epidural local anesthetic with opioid compared with IV narcotic analgesia for patients undergoing thoracoscopy (59). However, there is no consensus (60). The disadvantages of continuous thoracic epidural infusion for patients undergoing VATS procedures include neuraxial opioid side effects in short-stay surgery patients and more intensive postoperative monitoring requirements.

Regional Anesthesia in Patients with Chest Trauma

The excruciating pain caused by coughing, deep breaths, and movement remains a management issue in patients with chest trauma and rib fractures. An ideal method to control pain in these patients should be safe, provide complete and prolonged analgesia, and facilitate deep breathing and clearance of secretions during chest physiotherapy. The method used should ideally also improve respiratory dynamics, have minimal central nervous and systemic side effects, and permit early mobilization. Systemic opioids may provide good static pain control but cause respiratory depression and hypoxemia. The hypoxemia may be caused also by obstructive apnea, paradoxical breathing, or a diminution in the number of sigh breaths. Opioids also cause sedation, respiratory depression, and cough suppression (61). Various peripheral nerve blocks are available to control pain in these patients.

Intercostal Blocks

Intercostal blocks produce excellent pain relief. It is necessary to perform the blocks proximal to the site of the fracture and to block at least one level above and below the same fractured rib since there is overlap in the innervation of the thoracic dermatomes. The disadvantage is the need for repeated block due to the short action of the local anesthetics. In addition, multiple injections are required, and together with fast absorption from the intercostal area, toxic levels of local anesthetics can easily be reached. The addition of epinephrine 1:200,000 to bupivacaine 0.5% during intercostal blocks results in lower peak blood bupivacaine levels and may reduce the potential for local anesthetic toxicity (62). Multiple intercostal blocks nerve blocks for rib fractures also predispose to a higher incidence of pneumothorax. The reported incidence of pneumothorax after intercostal blocks in patients with multiple rib fractures is 1.4% for each intercostal blocks and 5.6% when multiple intercostal blocks are performed (63). Typically, the effect lasts for 6 to 12 hours (see also Chapter 16).

Thoracic Epidural Anesthesia

The use of thoracic epidural anesthesia in patients with thoracic trauma who are older than 60 years of age is an independent predictor of both decreased mortality and decreased incidence of pulmonary complications (64). Performed in patients with chest wall trauma, thoracic epidural anesthesia produces dramatic pain relief, which results in an increase in FRC, dynamic lung compliance, and vital capacity; a decrease in airway resistance; and a significant increase in PaO_2. Shallow breathing improves to near normal levels and paradoxical chest wall movements are reduced. Epidural analgesia also modifies the immune response in patients with chest trauma, as evidenced by a reduction in the plasma levels of interleukin (IL)-8, a proinflammatory chemoattractant implicated in acute lung injury (65). Patients on a thoracic epidural anesthesia regimen are alert, able to cough adequately and comply with chest physiotherapy, and develop fewer complications (see Chapter 11).

Thoracic epidural anesthesia could be technically demanding, especially in patients distressed with pain. The neural blockade can mask intra-abdominal injuries and may be associated with hypotension during the early phase of treatment, potentially resulting in cardiovascular collapse and cardiac arrest in the inadequately resuscitated patient. Luchette and co-workers evaluated analgesia for 72 hours in 19 blunt trauma patients with unilateral rib fractures (66). They found that thoracic epidural bupivacaine 0.125%, 8 to 10 mL/h, compared to intrapleural bupivacaine 0.5% intermittent boluses of 20 mL every 8 hours, resulted in significantly lower VAS pain scores, less use of rescue opioids, and greater tidal volume and negative inspiratory force. In a comparison of PCA and thoracic epidural anesthesia using a combination of bupivacaine and morphine in 34 patients with thoracic trauma, epidural analgesia provided better pain relief and was associated with superior ventilatory dynamics, as evidenced by greater tidal volumes and maximal inspiratory force on day 3, and lower plasma levels of IL-8 on days 2 and 3. In the PCA group, there was a progressive decline in tidal volume and maximal inspiratory force throughout the 3-day study period. There were no differences in plasma IL-1, IL-2, IL-6, tumor necrosis factor, or urinary catecholamine levels, although there was a trend for lower IL-6 levels in patients receiving epidural analgesia (65).

Interpleural analgesia is less effective than epidural or paravertebral block. It can result in high plasma levels of local anesthetic as a result of high vascularization of the pleural space (66).

Regional Anesthesia for Esophagectomy

Esophagectomy is a major surgical procedure performed in patients with esophageal cancer and is associated with high morbidity (20%–50%) and mortality (0%–30%). The procedure involves large thoraco-abdominal incisions. Thoracic epidural anesthesia is recommended as part of the intraoperative anesthetic management and is continued to provide analgesia for 3 to 5 postoperative days. In addition to a beneficial effect on respiration and gut perfusion, epidural anesthesia facilitates immediate extubation in the operating room, thereby reducing the risks associated with prolonged mechanical ventilation. Neal and co-workers also emphasized the importance of providing optimal analgesia with thoracic epidural anesthesia as part of the fast-track strategy. Thoracic epidural anesthesia facilitates ambulation the same day of the surgery, reduces the incidence of ileus and deep venous thrombosis, and allows early enteral feeding (67). Esophageal anastomotic leak is a potentially life-threatening complication of esophagectomy related to the disastrous consequences of leakage of GI contents with mediastinitis, septic shock, adult respiratory distress syndrome (ARDS), and death. Thoracic epidural anesthesia used during the postoperative course has been shown to decrease the risk for anastomotic leakage (68).

Regional Anesthesia for Breast Surgery

Intercostal, paravertebral, and cervical or thoracic epidural anesthesia have been used for breast surgery. It was recently shown in a retrospective series that the use of continuous paravertebral blockade (placed before induction of anesthesia into the ipsilateral paravertebral space at the level of T2 or T3 and maintained for 48 hours postoperatively), when compared to PCA with morphine, improved recurrence- and metastasis-free survival at 24 and 36 month follow-up (94% versus 82% and 94% versus 77%, respectively, $p < 0.038$) (69). Buggy and co-workers studied the effect of continuous paravertebral anesthesia with levobupivacaine on the oxygen tension in the latissimus dorsi flap after mastectomy (70). The mean PtO_2 over the 20-hour period was significantly higher in patients receiving paravertebral block (75 versus 44 mm Hg; $p < 0.03$). Intraoperative blood loss was also less in paravertebral patients (1.2 ± 0.4 versus 1.7 ± 0.5 l; $p < 0.04$). Dynamic VAS pain scores were significantly lower in the paravertebral group.

Preincisional paravertebral anesthesia has been shown to reduce chronic pain after breast surgery. At 1-month after surgery, patients who received paravertebral anesthesia in the perioperative period had a lower intensity of motion-related pain. At 6 months, the prevalence of any type of pain continued to be lower, and at 12-month follow-up motion as well as pain at rest were significantly lower in the paravertebral group. Segmental high thoracic epidural anesthesia (blockade of C4–T8 with bupivacaine or C5–T9 with ropivacaine) has been successfully used in women with COPD also receiving minimal sedation with propofol or midazolam (12). Similar results were recently observed with cervical epidural anesthesia (71).

REGIONAL ANESTHESIA FOR ABDOMINAL SURGERY

Regional anesthesia was commonly performed for abdominal surgery in the 1920s, when Gaston Labat described surgery under bilateral paravertebral combined with visceral block. Neuraxial blockade became popular later as their safety increased and applications for postoperative analgesia were developed. More recently came the realization that regional anesthesia may influence some of the perioperative factors intrinsically tied with postoperative outcome (see also Chapter 7).

Physiological Considerations and the Influence of Regional Anesthesia

Splanchnic Blood Flow

The splanchnic circulation receives approximately 30% of cardiac output, and it is characterized by high oxygen extraction.

Major decreases in splanchnic blood flow occur during low cardiac output states, and if this persists, the gut mucosal barrier may be disrupted, resulting in generation of inflammatory mediators which, together with ischemia–reperfusion injury, precipitate gastrointestinal organ dysfunction (72). The control of splanchnic blood flow is regulated through a fine balance involving sympathetic and parasympathetic systems. Other local and systemic factors also modulate the tone of the mesenteric vasculature. Neuraxial blockade causes splanchnic vasodilatation, with the mesenteric venules subsequently containing up to 30% of the body's total blood volume (73–75). The resulting decreased venous return and systemic hypotension may compromise gut mucosal integrity. The use of vasopressors is more effective than IV fluids in restoring adequate splanchnic blood flow (see also Chapter 11).

Gastrointestinal Motility

Peristalsis is under the control of sympathetic and parasympathetic systems (Fig. 23-1). The former inhibits motility, whereas the parasympathetic enhances it. Surgery, pain, direct gut

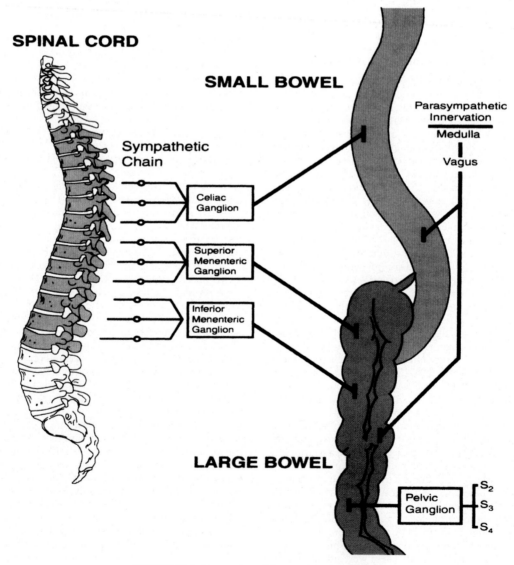

FIGURE 23-1. Innervation of the gastrointestinal tract.

manipulation, circulating inflammatory mediators, or injury to the gut causes an increase in sympathetic activity resulting in ileus. Local anesthetic neuraxial blockade of the sympathetic fibers innervating the gut (T4–L2) inhibits sympathetic hyperactivity and enhances vagal activity with restoration of gut motility (see Chapters 7 and 11).

Surgical Considerations and Regional Anesthesia

Preoperative Fasting

Tradition dictates patients to be fasted the day and night before surgery. In addition, patients undergoing gastrointestinal surgery undergo chemical bowel preparation during the 18 to 24 hours prior to surgery. Recent evidence documents the metabolic benefit of carbohydrate-rich clear liquids continued up until 2 hours preoperatively in reverting gluconeogenesis and attenuating perioperative insulin resistance (76). Clear fluids are rapidly eliminated from the stomach with minimal risk of aspiration. For patients undergoing gastrointestinal surgery with neuraxial blockade, maintenance of hydration may minimize hypotensive episodes associated with sympathetic block (see also Chapter 6 and Fig. 6-8).

Bowel Preparation

The mechanical preparation of the bowel achieved using a large volume of osmotically active fluid is practiced to lower the risk of peritoneal contamination, anastomotic breakdown, and wound infection. On average, patients lose 1 to 2 liters over a period of 24 hours and arrive dehydrated on the morning of surgery (unless they have been encouraged to replenish the fluid loss). Neuraxial blockade can precipitate severe hypotension if rehydration does not occur. Two large randomized studies have not been able to show any advantage of bowel preparation on postoperative anastomotic complications and infection (77–78).

Bowel Anastomosis

Anastomotic healing is very fast, but may be impaired by diabetes, infection, malnutrition, anemia, steroids, and radiation. Anastomotic leakage can lead to severe morbidity and mortality, if not immediately identified and treated. Neuraxial blockade has not been shown to increase the incidence of anastomotic leakage in colorectal surgery (78a).

Postoperative Ileus

Surgery of the small and large intestine is associated with a period of ileus, which, if not treated might be a cause for considerable morbidity. Neuraxial blockade with local anesthetics has been shown to attenuate the sympathetic hyperactivity and facilitate the restoration of peristalsis (79–81).

Postoperative Early Feeding

Considerable fluid shift occurs with major abdominal surgery requiring correction with appropriate fluids (82–84). Although there has been some anxiety regarding oral feeding within the first 24 hours and the integrity of the anastomosis, several studies have demonstrated no difference in rate of anastomotic dehiscence (85). Epidural analgesia facilitates dietary intake as a result of opioid-sparing, increased mobilization/ambulation, and restored active peristalsis. Advantages of early feeding are less infection, better tissue healing, and reduction of hospital length of stay (85) (see also Chapter 7).

Endoscopic Surgery and Regional Anesthesia

Endoscopic surgery, extensively used in gastrointestinal surgery, has been shown to attenuate the inflammatory response and the incidence of wound infections compared with conventional open techniques. In addition, the small incisions cause less postoperative pain and allow patients to be more mobile. However, the endoscopic approach per se has not been shown to accelerate restoration of bowel function, probably because of the lack of direct effect on anastomosis or the inability to reverse postoperative ileus (86). Recently, local anesthetics, administered either intravenously or epidurally, have been shown to accelerate bowel motility after laparoscopic colon surgery (87–88) (see also Chapter 7).

Open Abdominal Surgery and Regional Anesthesia

Spinal

Spinal anesthesia for abdominal surgery is an attractive proposition since it requires small amounts of local anesthetic and provides a reliable and extended sensory blockade with adequate muscle relaxation. Adequate mesenteric blood flow is particularly required for the viability of anastomosis. Hyperbaric local anesthetics are used when a high (T3–T4) sensory block is needed for upper abdominal surgery, whereas hypobaric local anesthetics can also be used for lower abdominal/pelvic surgery. Because of the relatively short duration of spinal anesthesia (2 hours), adjuvants such as epinephrine and morphine have been added to extend the duration of sensory block and enhance analgesia. Lipophilic opioids, fentanyl, and sufentanil have been shown to extend and potentiate the sensory block with decreased likelihood of pruritus and urinary retention (see also Chapter 10).

Although high spinal anesthesia provides excellent operating conditions, the relatively short duration of sensory deafferentation makes this technique of limited use for major and prolonged abdominal surgery. A combined spinal–epidural technique has been successfully used for abdominal surgery, to prolong the duration of anesthesia. Upper abdominal surgery has been performed under high spinal anesthesia in which patients were required to remain either conscious or had airway problems. Spinal catheters have been also used for abdominal surgery, but large concentrated doses of local anesthetic (lidocaine) resulted in major neurologic complications. The reintroduction of spinal catheters in practice for abdominal surgery should be restricted to specific clinical conditions. Presently, spinal anesthesia is used for ambulatory surgery of groin hernia and anorectal surgery.

Epidural Anesthesia

Epidural blockade plays an important role in abdominal surgery because of perioperative optimization of splanchnic blood flow, early restoration of bowel motility, and attenuation of the stress response. As such, epidural block has been adopted as part of the anesthetic technique for the majority of abdominal surgical interventions (see also Chapter 11).

Site of Epidural Needle Insertion. Appropriate needle insertion and catheter placement are dependent on the level of surgical incision; typically, the thoracic route is preferred. The location of the catheter should correspond to the segment of the surgical incision. As a progressive increase occurs in the width of epidural space from C7 down to T12, high thoracic epidural has minimal cephalad and extensive caudal spread. Recommended insertion sites are: for upper abdominal surgery (esophagus, stomach, pancreas, liver, spleen), T4–T6; for small bowel and colon, T8–T9; and for sigmoid colon and rectum, T10–T11. The lumbar approach is discouraged because of insufficient upper sensory block covering the surgical incision, lack of blockade of sympathetic fibers innervating the gut, and presence of lower extremity motor block (limiting ambulation).

Intraoperative Management

There are several advantages in establishing neuraxial blockade with local anesthetic prior to surgical incision: (a) verification that the sensory block is bilateral and extended to cover the surgical incision, (b) reduction in the requirement for volatile anesthetic agents, and (c) a reduction in the need for muscle relaxation. Verification of the sensory block can be achieved by using lidocaine 2%, 3 to 5 mL, and assessing the blocked dermatome distribution with alcohol or ice. Bupivacaine 0.5%, 5 to 10 mL, can be then injected to provide adequate bilateral deafferentation extending from T3 down to L3. A continuous infusion of bupivacaine 0.5%, 3 mL/h or 0.25%, 5 to 8 mL/h may be administered throughout surgery. Hypotension can occur in those subjects who have received bowel preparation and are in a hypovolemic state, or are dehydrated or malnourished. In this case, prompt rehydration with 1 to 2 L of crystalloids is recommended. Blood pressure may be restored by administration of vasopressors ephedrine and neosynephrine sympathetic agents. Animal studies have demonstrated the protective effect of colloids (hydroxyethyl starch) on anastomosis, through a decrease in fluid entrapment and swelling of the mucosa (80a).

Most abdominal interventions also receive general anesthesia, which can be achieved with either inhalational agents or propofol infusion. Patients can continue to breath spontaneously with either an endotracheal tube or a laryngeal airway or be ventilated using a positive pressure ventilator.

Postoperative Analgesia

Epidural

Epidural analgesia is widely used following abdominal surgery when pain relief is required beyond 24 hours. Administration of epidural local anesthetics alone is associated with poor to moderate pain relief and motor block. Although epidural opioids alone adequately relieve postoperative pain at rest (VAS less than 3), with movement, the pain is rated moderate to severe. A combination of opioids and local anesthetics enhances the analgesic effect and reduces the side effects associated with each component (81). A consensus has been reached whereby a combination of low-dose of local anesthetic (0.1%) with a small dose of opioid (morphine 0.06–0.1 mg/mLc, fentanyl 3 μg/mLc, sufentanil is recommended. Morphine is added to the local anesthetic when the surgical incision is extended beyond the limits covered by the epidural local anesthetics. Adjuvants, including clonidine and epinephrine, have been shown to potentiate the quality of analgesia, but side effects (hypotension, bradycardia, sedation, urinary retention) have been reported. The rate of epidural infusion varies between 4 and 15 mL/h and should be titrated according to the patient's assessment of pain at rest, during movements, and on coughing, as well as ability to ambulate. The use of patient-controlled epidural analgesia in abdominal surgery has been associated with

adequate quality of analgesia, a dose-sparing effect, and fewer side effects. Optimization of postoperative epidural analgesia can be achieved if patients are assessed regularly and adjustments are made when needed (see Chapter 43).

Side Effects of Epidural

Motor block (Bromage score >2) can seriously limit patient's mobilization. This can be the result of either insertion of the epidural catheter at lumbar level or of a large dose of local anesthetic. It is advised to correct the motor block initially by decreasing the dose of local anesthetic or by replacing the epidural at a higher level (thoracic).

Postoperative hypotension can occur with either thoracic or lumbar epidural anesthesia. The incidence has been reported between 3% and 10%, during the first 24 to 48 hours (89). Postoperative hypotension is generally treated with either IV fluids, vasopressors, and/or decreasing the rate of epidural infusion. The hypotension induced by the sympathetic block triggers an increase in plasma volume as a result of a movement of plasma from the interstitial to the intravascular space (90–91). Recommendations include caution in the use of crystalloids, and administration of an α/β-sympathomimetic agent, such as ephedrine, or an α-sympathomimetic such as Neo-Synephrine or methoxamine (see Chapter 11).

Abdominal Wall Block

Recently, a transversus abdominis plane block has been reported to be quite effective for abdominal surgery (92). This block of the neural afferent nerves to the anterior abdominal wall is achieved by identifying the lumbar triangle of Petit as an access to the neurofascial plane situated between the internal oblique and the transversus abdominis. A single injection of bupivacaine 0.375% has been shown to provide pain relief for up to 18 hours (see Figs. 16-33, 16-34).

Emergency Abdominal Surgery and Regional Anesthesia

Exploratory laparotomy is one of the most common emergency operations and is associated with considerable morbidity. The risks factors are not only related to the surgical conditions, but also to preoperative comorbidities. As such, there is some reluctance to use regional anesthesia in emergency surgery, in which the potential benefits of regional anesthesia and analgesia must be balanced against the risks of serious events. Hypovolemia and severe cardiac disorders remain a relative contraindication to the use of neuraxial blockade. Absolute contraindications traditionally include severe bleeding, deranged clotting, and systemic sepsis that could lead to devastating complications if neuraxial blockade is used. However, if appropriate fluid resuscitation, correction of clotting abnormalities, and/or antibiotic prophylaxis are established as soon as the patient is referred to the anesthesiologist, it is possible that neuraxial blockade may be safely performed with the intention that epidural catheter placement would minimize the surgical stress response and attenuate sympathetic hyperactivity. Experimental thoracic epidural block administered to ewes in the presence of hyperdynamic endotoxemia did not cause significant hypotension (93). Local anesthetics should be given in small doses, as they are sufficient to cause extensive neural blockade. Hypotension in response to sympathetic blockade must be corrected aggressively to maintain adequate mesenteric blood flow. Hypothermia, another potential consequence of epidural blockade, should be treated by using active warming during surgery to avoid shivering in the immediate postoperative period. Local anesthetics may be beneficial in these circumstances as a result of their anti-inflammatory properties, but, administered in large doses in the presence of sepsis, they can inhibit phagocytosis (94).

Fast-track Colonic Surgery and Epidural Anesthesia and Analgesia

During the last decade, attempts have been made to apply techniques widely used in ambulatory surgery to major upper and lower abdominal surgery with the intent of accelerating the recovery process. Epidural blockade remains a critical intervention, considered necessary for a rapid recovery program following colonic resection, because of the benefits relating to reduced stress response, effective analgesia, and early restoration of bowel function, early food intake, and early mobilization (95–97). These immediate effects translate into a number of late benefits. However, a number of investigations have shown that, despite the excellent analgesia provided by an effective working epidural, postoperative recovery is not accelerated (80); typically because the pathophysiology of surgical stress is made up of a constellation of components that require attenuation possible only with a multimodal approach. This perioperative program requires optimization of preoperative surgical and medical care, pharmacologic and physiologic attenuation of intraoperative stress response, goal-directed fluid balance, maintenance of normothermia, a minimally invasive surgical approach, optimal analgesia, enforced mobilization, and oral feeding. The benefits of epidural analgesia become most apparent when used as part of a multimodal analgesic regimen. Based on this program, some prospective controlled studies have been able to show an accelerated recovery process with minimal morbidity (98–101). The benefits of the anesthesiologist's fast-track techniques can only be fully appreciated if they are incorporated into the comprehensive perioperative care plan and if all parties involved in the care of the surgical patient participate in the organization and monitoring of the clinical progress (102,103) (see also Chapters 6 and 7).

Inguinal Hernia Repair and Regional Anesthesia

Hernia repair is a very common operation performed on an ambulatory basis. Different anesthetic techniques are available, including general anesthesia, spinal anesthesia, inguinal field block, and paravertebral block (104). Inguinal field block is widely used for ambulatory hernia repair. It has the advan-

tage that it does not require particular technical skill, provides excellent anesthesia and postoperative analgesia lasting up to 18 hours, and is associated with minimal side effects, thus allowing early recovery. The inguinal field block has the advantages of faster recovery, minimal urinary retention, and excellent patient satisfaction (see also Figs. 16-26 to 16-29). Spinal anesthesia with bupivacaine is associated with prolonged recovery and a high incidence of postoperative urinary retention compared with general anesthesia and local infiltration (104).

Anorectal Surgery and Regional Anesthesia

Anorectal surgery includes hemorrhoidectomy, biopsy, fistulotomy, sphincterotomy, polyp removal, and excision of rectal tumors. To facilitate the surgical approach, patients are positioned either prone, in lateral decubitus, or lithotomy. Prone position is preferred because of the quality of surgical exposure. Minor procedures may be performed under local infiltration; although the injection is extremely painful, it has the advantage of minimal recovery time, good postoperative pain control, and no urinary retention.

Regional anesthesia for anorectal surgery includes caudal and spinal techniques. Caudal blockade provides selective sensory and motor block in the anorectal area, which facilitates ambulation and early discharge. However, the identification of the caudal space can be difficult in the adult. The addition of adjuvants (morphine, fentanyl, epinephrine, clonidine) provides analgesia for 12 to 18 hours for inpatient procedures. Conversely, spinal anesthesia provides a rapid-onset, reliable block with a great success rate. A saddle block of the S2–S5 dermatomes is achieved with 0.6 to 1.0 mL of 0.75% hyperbaric bupivacaine. Fentanyl 10 to 25 μg can be added to prolong postoperative analgesia. Urinary retention is a recognized complication of both techniques compared with local infiltration and sedation (105).

SUMMARY

In summary, surgery to the thorax and abdomen were initially performed under regional anesthesia—primarily peripheral/plexus combined with visceral blockade. As the safety of general and neuraxial techniques increased, peripheral block was seldom utilized. Outcome studies support the use of neuraxial anesthesia and analgesia to improve pain relief, normalize respiratory function (and reduce respiratory infections), facilitate return of bowel function, and allow early hospital discharge. Recent investigations suggest that plexus (paravertebral) as well as peripheral (intercostal, abdominal wall block, field infiltration) may also be associated with these benefits (see also Chapters 6 and 7).

References

1. Hamilton WJ. *Textbook of Human Anatomy*, 2nd ed. New York: Macmillan, 1976.
2. Waurick R, Van Aken H. Update in thoracic epidural anaesthesia. *Best Pract Res Clin Anaesthesiol* 2005;19(2):201–213.
3. Schmidt C, Hinder F, Van Aken H, et al. The effect of high thoracic epidural anesthesia on systolic and diastolic left ventricular function in patients with coronary artery disease. *Anesth Analg* 2005;100:1561–1569.
4. Nygård E, Kofoed KF, Freiberg J, et al. Effects of high thoracic epidural analgesia on myocardial blood flow in patients with ischemic heart disease. *Circulation* 2005;111:2165–2170.
5. Oka T, Ozawa Y, Ohkubo Y. Thoracic epidural bupivacaine attenuates supraventricular tachyarrhythmias after pulmonary resection. *Anesth Analg* 2001;93:253–259.
6. Turfrey DJ, Ray DA, Sutcliffe NP, et al. Thoracic epidural anaesthesia for coronary artery bypass grafting surgery. Effects of postoperative complications. *Anaesthesia* 1997;52:1090–1095.
7. Scott NB, Turfrey DJ, Ray DA, et al. A prospective randomised study of the potential benefits of thoracic epidural anesthesia and analgesia in patients undergoing coronary artery bypass grafting. *Anesth Analg* 2001;93:528–535.

8. Ahn HJ, Sim WS, Shim YM, Kim JA. Thoracic epidural anesthesia does not improve the incidence of arrhythmia after thoracic esophagectomy. *Eur J Cardiothorac Surg* 2005;28:19–21.

9. Groeben H. Epidural anesthesia and pulmonary function. *J Anesth* 2006;20:290–299.

10. Whaba WM, Craig DB, Don HF, Becklake MR. The cardio-respiratory effects of thoracic epidural anaesthesia. *Can Anaesth Soc J* 1972;19:8–19.

11. Mankikian B, Cantineau JP, Bertrand M, et al. Improvement of diaphragmatic function by a thoracic extradural block after abdominal surgery. *Anesthesiology* 1988;68:379–386.

12. Gruber EM, Tschernko EM, Kritzinger M, et al. The effects of thoracic epidural analgesia with bupivacaine 0.25% on ventilatory mechanics I. Patients with severe chronic obstructive pulmonary disease. *Anesth Analg* 2001;92:1015–1019.

13. Huybrechts I, Barvais L, Ducart A, et al. Assessment of thoracic epidural analgesia during general anesthesia using pupillary reflex dilation: A preliminary study. *J Cardiothorac Vasc Anesth* 2006;20(5):664–667.

14. Senturk M, Ozcan PE, Talu GK, et al. The effects of three different analgesia techniques on long-term postthoracotomy pain. *Anesth Analg* 2002;94:11–15.

15. Tippana E, Nilsson E, Kalso E. Post thoracotomy pain after thoracic epidural analgesia: A prospective follow-up study. *Acta Anesth Scand* 2003;47:433–438.

16. Von Dossow V, Welte M, Zaune U, et al. Thoracic epidural anesthesia combined with general anesthesia: The preferred anesthetic technique for thoracic surgery. *Anesth Analg* 2001;92:848–854.

17. Ballantyne JC, Carr DB, deFerranti S, et al. The comparative effects of postoperative analgesic therapies on pulmonary outcome: Cumulative meta-analyses of randomized, controlled trials. *Anesth Analg* 1998;86:598–612.

18. Suzuki M, Haraguti S, Sugimoto K, et al. Low-dose intravenous ketamine potentiates epidural analgesia after thoracotomy. *Anesthesiology* 2006;105:111–119.

19. Curatolo M, Sveticis G. Drug combination in pain treatment: A review of the published evidence and a method for finding the optimal combination. *Best Pract Res Clin Anesth* 2002;16(4):507–519.

20. Curatolo M, Schnider TW, Petersen-Felix S, et al. A direct search procedure to optimize of epidural bupivacaine, fentanyl: And for postoperative analgesia combinations clonidine. *Anesthesiology* 2000;92:325–337.

21. Concha M, Dagnino J, Cariaga M, et al. Analgesia after thoracotomy: Epidural fentanyl/bupivacaine compared with intercostal nerve block plus intravenous morphine. *J Cardiothorac Vasc Anesth* 2004;18(3):322–326.

22. Kahn L, Baxter FJ, Dauphin A, et al. A comparison of thoracic and lumbar epidural techniques for post-thoracoabdominal esophagectomy analgesia. *Can J Anaesth* 1999;46:415–422.

23. Grant GJ, Zakowski M, Ramanathan S, et al. Thoracic versus lumbar administration of epidural morphine for postoperative analgesia after thoracotomy. *Reg Anesth* 1993;18:351–355.

24. Guinard JP, Mavrocordatos P, Chiolero R, Carpenter RL. A randomized comparison of intravenous versus lumbar and thoracic epidural fentanyl for analgesia after thoracotomy. *Anesthesiology* 1992;77:1108–1115.

25. Arndt JO, Hock A, Stanton-Hicks M, et al. Peridural anesthesia and distribution of blood in supine humans. *Anesthesiology* 1985;63:616–623.

26. Baron JF, Payen D, Choriat P, et al. Forearm vascular tone and reactivity during lumbar epidural anesthesia. *Anesth Analg* 1988;67:1065–1070.

27. Nishi M, Usukaura A, Kidani Y, et al. Which is a better position for insertion of a high thoracic epidural catheter: Sitting or lateral decubitus? *J Cardiothorac Vasc Anesth* 2006;20(5):656–658.

28. Michelet P, D'Journo XB, Roch A, et al. perioperative risk factors for anastomotic leakage after esophagectomy: Influence of thoracic epidural analgesia. *Chest* 2005;128:3461–3466.

29. Holte K, Foss N, Svensen C, et al. Epidural anesthesia, hypotension, and changes in intravascular volume. *Anesthesiology* 2004;100:281–286.

30. Myles PS, Bain C. Underutilization of paravertebral block in thoracic surgery. *J Cardiothorac Vasc Anesth* 2006;20(5):635–638.

31. Naja MZ, Gustafsson AC, Ziade MF, et al. Distance between the skin and the thoracic Paravertebral space. *Anaesthesia* 2005;60:680–684.

32. Garutti L, Olmedilla L, Pérez-Peña JM, et al. Hemodynamic effects of lidocaine in the thoracic paravertebral space during one-lung ventilation for thoracic surgery. *J Cardiothorac Vasc Anesth* 2006;20:648–651.

33. Navlet M, Garutti I, Olmedilla L, et al. Paravertebral ropivacaine, 0.3%, and bupivacaine, 0.25%, provide similar pain relief after thoracotomy. *J Cardiothorac Vasc Anesth* 2006;20(5):644–647.

34. Bhatnagar S, Mishra S, Madhurima S, et al. Clonidine as an analgesic adjuvant to continuous paravertebral bupivacaine for post-thoracotomy pain. *Anaesth Intensive Care* 2006;34(5):586–591.

35. Marret E, Bazelly B, Taylor G, et al. Paravertebral block with ropivacaine 0.5% versus systemic analgesia for pain relief after thoracotomy. *Ann Thorac Surg* 2005;79:2109–2114.

36. Davies RG, Myles PS, Graham JM. A comparison of the analgesic efficacy and side-effects of paravertebral vs epidural blockade for thoracotomy: A systematic review and meta-analysis of randomized trials. *Br J Anaesthesia* 2006;96(4):418–426.

37. Casati A, Alessandrini P, Nuzzi M, et al. A prospective, randomized, blinded comparison between continuous paravertebral and epidural infusion of 0.2% ropivacaine after lung resection surgery. *Eur J Anesth* 2006;23(12):999–1004.

37a. Detterbeck D, Franck C. Efficacy of methods of intercostal nerve blockade for pain relief after thoracotomy. *Ann Thorac Surg* 2005;80:1550–1559.

38. Moore DC. Intercostal nerve block for postoperative somatic pain following surgery of thorax and upper abdomen. *Br J Anaesth* 1975;47[Suppl]:284–286.

39. Toledo-Pereyra LH, DeMeester TR. Prospective randomized evaluation of intrathoracic intercostal nerve block with bupivacaine on postoperative ventilatory function. *Ann Thorac Surg* 1979;27:203–205.

40. Kaplan JA, Miller ED Jr., Gallagher EG Jr. Postoperative analgesia for thoracotomy patients. *Anesth Analg* 1975;54:773–777.

41. Moorjania N, Zhaob F, Tianb Y, et al. Effects of cryoanalgesia on postthoracotomy pain and on the structure of intercostal nerves: A human prospective randomized trial and a histological study. *Eur J Cardiothorac Surg* 2001;20:502–507.

42. Barnard D. The effects of extreme cold on sensory nerves. *Ann R Coll Surg Engl* 1980;62:180–187.

43. Moorjani N, Zhao F, Tian Y, et al. Effects of cryoanalgesia on postthoracotomy pain and on the structure of intercostal nerves: a human prospective randomized trial and a histological study. *Eur J Cardiothorac Surg* 2001;20:502–507.

44. Maiwand MO, Makey AR, Rees A. Cryoanalgesia after thoracotomy. Improvement of technique and review of 600 cases. *J Thorac Cardiovasc Surg* 1986;92:291–295.

45. Miguel R, Hubbell D. Pain management and spirometry following thoracotomy: A prospective, randomized study of four techniques. *J Cardiothorac Vasc Anesth* 1993;7:529–534.

46. Schneider RF, Villamena PC, Harvey J, et al. Lack of efficacy of intrapleural bupivacaine for postoperative analgesia following thoracotomy. *Chest* 1993;103:414–416.

47. Ferrante FM, Chan VW, Arthur GR, Rocco AG. Interpleural analgesia after thoracotomy. *Anesth Analg* 1991;72:105–109.

48. Filomon M, Claus T, Huwer H, et al. Interpleural analgesia does not influence postthoracotomy pain. *Anesth Analg* 2000;91:44–50.

49. Burgess FW, Anderson DM, Colonna D, et al. Ipsilateral shoulder pain following thoracic surgery. *Anesthesiology* 1993;78:365–368.

50. Scawn ND, Pennefather SH, Soorae A, et al. Ipsilateral shoulder pain after thoracotomy with epidural analgesia: The influence of phrenic nerve infiltration with lidocaine. *Anesth Analg* 2001;93:260–264.

51. Tan N, Agnew NM, Scawn ND, et al. Suprascapular nerve block for ipsilateral shoulder pain after thoracotomy with thoracic epidural analgesia: A double-blind comparison of 0.5% bupivacaine and 0.9% saline. *Anesth Analg* 2002;94:199–202.

52. Taylor R, Massey S, Stuart-Smith K. Postoperative analgesia in video-assisted thoracoscopy: The role of intercostal blockade. *J Cardiothorac Vasc Anesth* 2004;18(3):317–321.

53. Bolotin G, Lazarovici H, Uretzky G, et al. The efficacy of intraoperative internal intercostal nerve block during video-assisted thoracic surgery on postoperative pain. *Ann Thorac Surg* 2000;70:1872–1875.

54. Leger R, Ohlmer A, Scheiderer U, et al. Pain relief after thoracoscopy (video-assisted thoracic surgery): Patient-controlled analgesia (PCA) with IV opioids vs. intercostal blocks or interpleural analgesia. *Chirurg* 1999;70:682–689.

55. Benhke H, Wulf H. Plasma concentration of ropivacaine after intercostal block for video-assisted thoracic surgery. *Br J Anaesth* 2002;89(2):251–253.

56. Kaya FN, Turker G, Basagan-Mogol E, et al. Preoperative multiple-injection thoracic paravertebral blocks reduce postoperative pain and analgesic requirements after video-assisted thoracic surgery. *J Cardiothorac Vasc Anesth* 2006;20(5):639–643.

57. Vogt A, Stieger DS, Theurillat C, Curatolo M. Single-injection thoracic paravertebral block for postoperative pain treatment after thoracoscopic surgery. *Br J Anaesth* 2005;95(6):816–821.

58. Hill SE, Keller RA, Stafford-Smith M, et al. Efficacy of single-dose, multilevel paravertebral nerve blockade for analgesia after thoracoscopic procedures. *Anesthesiology* 2006;104:1047–1053.

59. Yoshioka M, Mori T, et al. The efficacy of the epidural analgesia after video-assisted thoracoscopic surgery: A randomized control study. *Ann Thorac Cardiovasc Surg* 2006;12(5):313–318.

60. Fernandez MI, Martin-Ucara AE, Leea HD, et al. Does a thoracic epidural confer any additional benefit following video-assisted thoracoscopic pleurectomy for primary spontaneous pneumothorax? *Eur J Cardiothorac Surg* 2005;27:671–674.

61. Karmakar MK, Ho A. Acute pain management of patients with multiple fractured ribs. *J Trauma* 2003;54:615–625.

62. Johnson MD, Mickler T, Arthur GR, et al. Bupivacaine with and without epinephrine for intercostal nerve block. *J Cardiothorac Anesth* 1990;4:200–203.

63. Shanti CM, Carlin AM, Tyburski JG. Incidence of pneumothorax from intercostal nerve block for analgesia in rib fractures. *J Trauma* 2001;51:536–539.

64. Wisner DH. A stepwise logistic regression analysis of factors affecting morbidity and mortality after thoracic trauma: Effect of epidural analgesia. *J Trauma* 1990;30:799–804.

65. Moon MR, Luchette FA, Gibson SW, et al. Prospective, randomized comparison of epidural versus parenteral opioid analgesia in thoracic trauma. *Ann Surg* 1999;229(5):684–692.

66. Karmakar MJ, Ho AM-H. Acute management of patients with multiple fractured ribs. *The Journal of Trauma* 2003;54:615–625.

67. Neal JM, Wilcox RT, Allen HW, Low DE. Near-total esophagectomy: The influence of standardize multimodal management and Intraoperative fluid restriction. *Reg Anesth Pain Med* 2003;28:328–334.

68. Ragni J, Thomas P, Auffray JP, et al. Perioperative risk factors for anastomotic leakage after esophagectomy: Influence of thoracic epidural analgesia. *Chest* 2005;128:3461–3466.

69. Exadaktylos AK, Buggy DJ, Moriarty DC, et al. Can anesthetic technique for primary breast cancer. Surgery affect recurrence or metastasis? *Anesthesiology* 2006;105:660–664.

70. Buggy DJ, Kerin MJ. Paravertebral analgesia with levobupivacaine increases postoperative flap tissue oxygen tension after immediate latissimus dorsi breast reconstruction compared with intravenous opioid analgesia. *Anesthesiology* 2004;100:375–380.

71. Singh AP, Tewari M, Singh DK, Shukla HS. Cervical epidural anesthesia: A safe alternative to general anesthesia for patients undergoing cancer breast surgery. *World J Surg* 2006;30:2043–2047.

72. Takala J. Determinants of splanchnic blood flow. *Br J Anaesth* 1996;77:50–58.

73. Hogan Q, Stadnicka A, Stekiel T, et al. Region of epidural blockade determines sympathetic and mesenteric capacitance effects in rabbits. *Anesthesiology* 1995;83:604–610.

74. Sielekamper AW, Eicker K, Van Haken H. Thoracic epidural anesthesia increases mucosal perfusion in ileum of rats. *Anesthesiology* 2000;93:844–851.

75. Adolphs J, Schmidt DK, Mousa SA, et al. Thoracic epidural anesthesia attenuates hemorrhage-induced impairment of intestinal perfusion in rats. *Anesthesiology* 2003;99:685–692.

76. Nygren J, Soop M, Thorell A, et al. Preoperative oral carbohydrates and postoperative insulin resistance. *Clin Nutr* 1999;18:117–120.

77. Zmora O, Mahajma A, Bar-Zakai B, et al. Colon and rectal surgery without mechanical bowel preparation: A randomized prospective trial. *Ann Surg* 2003;237:363–367.

78. Ram E, Sherman Y, Weil B, et al. Is mechanical bowel preparation mandatory for elective colon surgery? A prospective randomized study. *Arch Surg* 2005;140:285–288.

78a. Holte K, Kehlet H. Epidural analgesia and the risk of anastomotic leakage. *Regional Anesthesia and Pain Medicine* 2001;26:111–117.

79. Steinbrook RA. Epidural anesthesia and gastrointestinal motility. *Anesth Analg* 1998;86:837–844.

80. Carli F, Trudel JL, Belliveau P. The effect of intraoperative thoracic epidural anesthesia and postoperative analgesia on bowel function after colorectal surgery: A prospective randomized trial. *Dis Colon Rectum* 2001;44:1083–1089.

80a. Boldt J. Fluid management of patients undergoing abdominal surgery. More questions than answers. *European Journal of Anaesthesiology* 2006;23:631–640.

81. Jorgensen H, Wettersley J, Moniche S, et al. Epidural local anesthetics versus opioid-based-analgesic regimens on postoperative gastrointestinal paralysis. PONV and pain after abdominal surgery. *Cochrane Database Syst Rev* 2000:CD001893.

82. Branstrup B, Tonnessen H, Bejer-Holgersen R, et al. Effects of intravenous fluid restriction on postoperative complications: Comparison of two perioperative fluid regimens: A randomized assessor-blinded multicenter trial. *Ann Surg* 2003;238:641–648.

83. Nisanevich V, Felsenstein I, Almogy G, et al. Effects of intraoperative fluid management on outcome after intra-abdominal surgery. *Anesthesiology* 2005;103:25–32.

84. Lobo DN, Bostock KA, Neal KR, et al. Effect of salt and water balance on recovery of gastrointestinal function after elective colonic resection: A randomised controlled trial. *Lancet* 2002;359:1812–1818.

85. Lewis SJ, Egger M, Sylvester PA, Topic ST. Early enteral feeding versus "nil by mouth" after gastrointestinal surgery: Systematic review and meta-analysis of controlled trials. *Br Med J* 2001;323:773–776.

86. Kehlet H, Kennedy RH. Laparoscopic colonic surgery-mission accomplished or work in progress? *Colorectal Dis* 2006;8:514–517.

87. Taqi A, Hong X, Mistraletti G, et al. Thoracic epidural analgesia facilitates the restoration of bowel function and dietary intake in patients undergoing laparoscopic colon resection with a traditional, non-accelerated, perioperative care program. *Surg Endosc* 2007;21:247–252.

88. Kaba A, Laurent SR, Detroz BJ, et al. Intravenous lidocaine infusion facilitates acute rehabilitation after laparoscopic colectomy. *Anesthesiology* 2007;106:11–18.

89. Cashman JN, Dolin SJ. Respiratory and haemodynamic effects of acute postoperative pain management: Evidence from published data. *Br J Anaesth* 2004;93:212–223.

90. Hahn RG. Increased haemodilution in hypotension induced by epidural anaesthesia. *Acta Anaesthesiol Scand* 1993;37:357–360.

91. Hahn RG. Haemoglobin dilution from epidural-induced hypotension with and without fluid loading. *Acat Anaesthesiol Scand* 1992;36:241–244.

92. McDonnell JG, O'Donnell B, Curley G, et al. The analgesic efficacy of transverses abdominis plane block after abdominal surgery: A prospective randomized controlled trial. *Anesth Analg* 2007;104:193–197.

93. Daudel F, Ertmer C, Stubbe HD, et al. The hemodynamic effects of thoracic epidural anesthesia in ovine hyperdynamic endotoxemia. *Reg Anesth Pain Med* 2007;32(4):311–316.

94. Ploppa A, Kiefer RT, Kreuger WA, et al. Local anesthetics time-dependently inhibit *Staphylococcus aureus* phagocytosis, oxidative burst and CD 11b expression in human neutrophils. *Reg Anesth Pain Med* 2007, in press.

95. Cassuto J, Sinclair R, Benderovic M. Anti-inflammatory properties of local anesthetics and their present and potential clinical implications. *Acta Anesthesiol Scand* 2006;50:265–282.

96. Finucane B, Ganapathy S, Carli F S, et al. Prolonged epidural infusions of ropivacaine (2mg/ml) after colonic surgery: The impact of adding fentanyl. *Anesth Analg* 2001;92:1276–1285.

97. Carli F, Mayo N, Klubien K, et al. Epidural analgesia enhances functional exercise capacity and health-related quality of life after colonic surgery: Results of a randomized trial. *Anesthesiology* 2002;97:540–549.

98. Brodner G, Van Aken H, Hertle L, et al. Multimodal perioperative management combining thoracic epidural analgesia, forced mobilization, and oral nutrition reduces hormonal and metabolic stress and improves convalescence after major urological surgery. *Anesth Analg* 2001;92:1594–1600.

99. Fearon KCH, Ljungquist O, Von Meyenfeldt M, et al. Enhanced recovery after surgery: A consensus of clinical care for patients undergoing colonic surgery. *Clin Nutr* 2005;24:466–477.

100. Basse L, Hjorte Jakobsen D, Billesbolle P, et al. A clinical pathway to accelerate recovery after colonic resection. *Ann Surg* 2000;232:51–57.

101. Basse L, Jakobsen RH, Bardram L, et al. Functional recovery after open versus laparoscopic colonic resection: A randomized blinded study. *Ann Surg* 2005;241:416–423.

102. Kehlet H, Wilmore DW. Multimodal strategies to improve surgical outcome. *Am J Surg* 2002;183:630–641.

103. Kehlet H, Wilmore DW. Fast-track surgery. *Br J Surg* 2005;92:3–4.

104. Kehlet H, White PF. Optimizing anesthesia for inguinal herniorrhaphy: General, regional or local anesthesia? *Anesth Analg* 2001;93:1367–1369.

105. Li S, Coloma M, White P, et al. Comparison of the cost and recovery profiles of 3 anesthetic techniques for ambulatory anorectal surgery. *Anesthesiology* 2000;93:1225–1230.

CHAPTER 24 ■ NEURAL BLOCKADE FOR OBSTETRICS AND GYNECOLOGIC SURGERY

DAVID O. GORMAN AND DAVID J. BIRNBACH

Pain management in the parturient is a challenging clinical situation that requires knowledge of maternal and fetal physiology in addition to the technical skills required to achieve rapid, effective analgesia on demand. Because of the dynamic nature of parturition, the ability to rapidly achieve surgical anesthesia to facilitate cesarean delivery is also required. The capacity to work in a multidisciplinary environment is essential, as clinical situations in obstetrics can change instantly and frequently, requiring changes in the plan of anesthetic management.

Gynecologic surgery is ideally suited to the use of regional anesthesia alone or in combination with general anesthesia. For example, developments in the surgical and oncologic management of gynecologic cancer have resulted in an increased incidence of intra-abdominal lymph node sampling, which often requires higher levels of regional anesthesia and even modification of anesthetic technique.

MANAGEMENT OF PAIN IN LABOR

Labor pain is a subjective, multidimensional experience that is unique to each individual (1). The International Association for the Study of Pain (IASP) has defined pain as "an unpleasant sensory and emotional experience, associated with actual or potential tissue damage and described in terms of such damage" (2). Given the sensory and affective component involved in any painful process, pain assessment with appropriate institution of therapy is difficult to perform with precision in the parturient. Demographic, social, and psychological factors have all been shown to predict maximum pain during labor (3). Pain increases as labor advances and is greater when labor is induced or augmented (Fig. 24-1).

Labor pain is real, with subjective and objective manifestations. It has been described as severe, very severe, and intolerable in both parous (46%) and nulliparous women (61%). Use of the McGill Pain questionnaire in labor has shown comparisons between various painful conditions in multiparas and nulliparas (4,5) (Figs. 24-2 and 24-3). Although questionnaires such as the McGill Pain Questionnaire are valid and reliable, their interpretation can be limited by a patient's previous experience of pain, and researchers continue to look for an accurate, reliable, and reproducible tool for pain measurement. The combination of muscle electromyography combined with visual analogue scales (VAS) has been used to assess the adequacy of pain management in labor (6). Attempts to find diagnostic markers in the measurement of pain, such as cerebrospinal levels of the proteinase inhibitor cystatin C, showed no difference between laboring and nonlaboring women (7).

The development of functional magnetic resonance imaging (fMRI), positron emission tomography (PET), and neurophysiologic techniques have allowed researchers to examine cortical representation of painful stimuli and to establish the role of the brainstem, descending pathways, and multiple locations in pain processing (8–10). However, the use of these in the parturient has not been established.

CONSEQUENCES OF LABOR PAIN

Successful management of labor pain is essential to minimize physiologic perturbations that may have a potentially deleterious effect on the fetus. Pregnancy itself is associated with alterations in the maternal physiology due to anatomic and neurohumoral factors. Many of these physiologic changes can be exacerbated by the presence of untreated labor pain and, independently, can have an impact on the technique and effective management of anesthesia and analgesia in the parturient.

Respiratory System

Because of increased metabolism in pregnancy, maternal oxygen consumption can be increased by up to 60% (11) (Table 24-1). Respiratory changes in pregnancy mean that, despite the anatomic changes of increased diaphragmatic and reduced chest wall excursion, vital capacity, total lung capacity, and inspiratory reserve volume remain essentially unchanged. The reduced expiratory reserve volume (−25%) and functional residual capacity (FRC) (−20%) can result in airway closure in 50% of mothers at term (12,13). This situation can be further aggravated by concomitant obesity or in the assumption of a recumbent or lithotomy position. The supine FRC in the parturient has been shown to be only 70% of that in the upright position (14). Pain-associated hyperventilation can be associated with increases in minute ventilation of up to 300% in the second stage of labor (15). This can lead to hypocarbia and alkalosis with hypoventilation between painful contractions, resulting in maternal and fetal hypoxemia and altered maternal neurologic status (16). Studies have shown that administration of effective regional anesthesia is associated with reduced maternal hyperventilation and oxygen consumption (17,18).

Cardiovascular

Increases in stroke volume (25%) and heart rate (25%) can lead to a concomitant increase in cardiac output in early

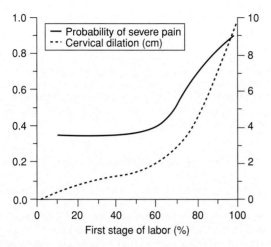

FIGURE 24-1. Likelihood of severe pain during labor. From Hardy JD, Javert CT. Studies on pain: Measurements of pain intensity in childbirth. *J Clin Invest* 1949;28:153–162, with permission.

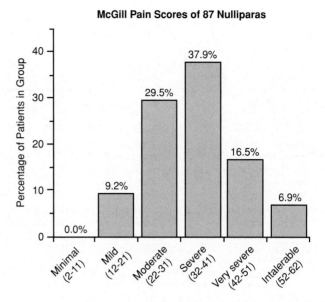

FIGURE 24-3. Variation in severity of labor pain in nulliparous women. From Melzack R, Taezner P, Feldman P, Kinch RA. Labour is still painful after prepared childbirth training. *Can Med Assoc J* 1981;125:357–363, with permission.

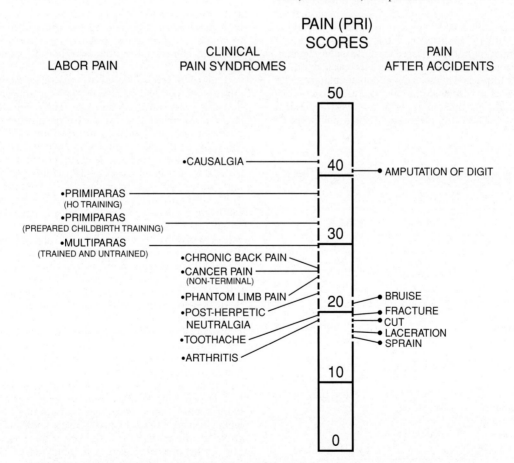

FIGURE 24-2. Comparison of pain scores, using the McGill Pain Questionnaire, obtained from women during labor (5), from patients in the general hospital pain clinic (Melzack R. The short form McGill Pain Questionnaire. *Pain.* 1987;30:191) and an emergency department (Melzack et al. Acute pain in an emergency clinic: latency of onset and descriptor patterns. *Pain.* 1982;14:33).

PART III: APPLICATIONS

TABLE 24-1

CHANGES IN PULMONARY MECHANICS IN PREGNANCY

Parameter	Change	Amount
Tidal volume	Increased	40%
Rate	Unchanged	—
Minute volume	Increased	40%
Alveolar ventilation	Increased	40%
Inspiratory capacity	Increased	15%
Expiratory reserve volume	Decreased	15%
Forced vital capacity	Maintained	—
Total lung capacity	Decreased	5%
Inspiratory capacity	Increased	15%
Vital capacity	Minor increase	1–200 mL
Functional residual capacity	Decreased	20%
Residual volume	Decreased	15%

Values derived from references 5, 177–179.
From Birnbach DJ, Datta S, Gatt SP (eds.). *Textbook of Obstetric Anesthesia*. New York: Churchill Livingstone, 2000, with permission.

pregnancy, resulting in increases of up to 35% to 40% of baseline values, and peaking in the early to mid third trimester (12,19,20) (Table 24-2). Uterine contractions can be associated with increases in both cardiac output (up to 25%) and blood pressure (5%–20%) (21). Effective labor analgesia is associated with attenuation of these related cardiovascular changes, with little detrimental effect on uteroplacental perfusion (22–25). Pregnancy imposes dynamic changes on circulation, with dramatic increases in cardiac output and decreases in systemic resistance. Because uteroplacental perfusion is very dependent on maternal blood pressure, profound hypotension is poorly

TABLE 24-2

CARDIOVASCULAR CHANGES IN PREGNANCY

Parameter	Change	Amount
Heart rate	Increased	20–30%
Stroke volume	Increased	20–50%
Cardiac output	Increased	30–50%
Contractility	Variable	±10%
Central venous pressure	Unchanged	—
Pulmonary capillary wedge pressure	Unchanged	—
Systemic vascular resistance	Decreased	20%
Systemic blood pressure	Slight decrease	Midtrimester 10–15 mm Hg then rises 30%
Pulmonary vascular resistance	Decreased	
Pulmonary artery pressure	Slight decrease	—

Values derived from references 43, 46, 49, and 107.
From Birnbach DJ, Datta S, Gatt SP (eds.). *Textbook of Obstetric Anesthesia*. New York: Churchill Livingstone, 2000, with permission.

tolerated and should be treated rapidly. Aortocaval compression is a common cause of hypotension and should be avoided in the term parturient, especially one who has received a neuraxial block. Although most pregnant women can tolerate the supine position without developing hypotension, some will develop *supine hypotensive syndrome*, which may be associated with profound hypotension, nausea, sweating, and loss of consciousness (Fig. 24-4). Left uterine displacement reduces aortocaval compression (Fig. 24-5).

Neuroendocrine Effects

Interestingly, population-based studies suggest that marked gender variations occur in the reporting of pain. Some suggest that women report symptoms of pain more frequently than do men. In addition, both preclinical and clinical models of acute pain in humans suggest that females are more sensitive to certain noxious stimuli, and report a lower pain threshold than do men (26–29). (Although these data are of scientific interest, it would probably be inappropriate to mention these results in a busy labor and delivery ward.) Pregnancy itself is associated with an endogenous antinociception that is multifactorial in origin. Peripheral processes (ovarian sex steroids), visceral afferent activity, and spinal opioid antinociceptive pathways are all thought to play a role in pain modulation (30). Animal and human studies have demonstrated an increase in pain threshold in pregnancy, possibly due to increased secretion and reduced degradation of endorphins. This mechanism may be a developmentally induced endorphin-mediated response to counteract the pain of parturition, as pain has also been shown to be reduced by administration of opioid antagonists (31–33).

Endorphin levels in labor are related to the frequency and duration of uterine contractions and thus are considered to reflect the stress state of labor (34). The combination of pain, stress, and anxiety associated with parturition lead to an increase in maternal plasma catecholamines. The effect of increased plasma catecholamines on the maternal–placental unit has been demonstrated in animal studies, with reductions of up to 50% in uterine blood flow (35). Human studies have similarly shown increases in plasma catecholamines in pregnancy of between four and seven times that of nonpregnant controls following modest exercise (36). Plasma catecholamine levels are increased in labor by a factor of up to five times normal values, with a higher urinary level of catecholamine excretion. This leads to increases in maternal peripheral vascular resistance and blood pressure. Increased sympathetic activity with release of gastrin leads to gastric hyperacidity, which, combined with pain-related gastric stasis and reduced parasympathetic activity, increases the risk of aspiration should general anesthesia be required.

Pain in labor can have a marked physiologic effect on both mother and fetus. Increased epinephrine release from the adrenal medulla due to pain and anxiety leads to increased glucagon formation and increases in maternal free fatty acids and lactate levels. These hormonal responses to the increases in catecholamine levels, combined with maternal hyperventilation and compensatory metabolic changes during painful labor, lead to a state of maternal catabolism. The resulting stress on the maternal physiologic system leads to stimulation of the hypothalamus, with both adrenergic and pituitary responses. This leads to an increase in systemic cortisol, β-endorphins, and lipotropins and a corresponding increase in serum antidiuretic hormone (ADH) release. Increased sympathetic stimulation leads to increased gluconeogenesis

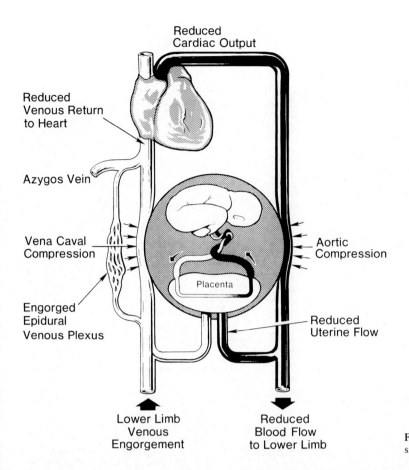

FIGURE 24-4. Circulatory effects of aortocaval compression.

in the medulla and peripheral norepinephrine effects in the periphery.

High maternal concentrations of catecholamines may have a deleterious effect on both mother and fetus in terms of uterine blood flow, and effective analgesia in labor is essential to reduce this effect (Figs. 24-6 and 24-7). Researchers have demonstrated a reduction of more than 50% in maternal plasma epinephrine levels associated with epidural and intrathecal analgesia (37–39). However, studies have shown that epidural analgesia in labor has not been associated with reductions in fetal and neonatal levels of catecholamines and β-endorphins, which are thought to play a central role in the mediation of several adaptive processes in the fetus after delivery, including surfactant synthesis, nonshivering thermogenesis, glucose homeostasis, and water metabolism (40).

Concomitant Illnesses

With improvements in reproductive medicine and increases in the average maternal age in pregnancy, the impact of increased sympathetic activity on cardiac output and maternal blood pressure may be associated with increased morbidity. This is illustrated by the increasing number of high-risk pregnancies in which maternal cardiac disease is a factor.

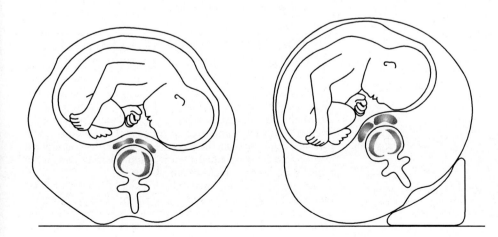

FIGURE 24-5. Aortocaval decompression with left lateral tilt.

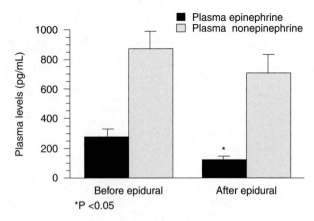

FIGURE 24-6. Maternal plasma catecholamine concentrations before and after initiation of epidural analgesia. From Shnider SM, Abboud TK, Artal R, et al. Maternal catecholamines decrease during labor after lumbar epidural anesthesia. *Am J Obstet Gynecol* 1983;147:13–15, with permission.

Psychological Effects of Pain in Labor

Perception of pain in labor can be modulated by many factors. The psychological effects of painful labor are not clearly understood. Anxiety and fear of pain may occur in the nulliparous patient, possibly in association with other ongoing psychological issues. Multiparous patients may also have a morbid fear of pain, especially if they have had a previously bad experience with medical care (41).

Negative outlook, low levels of education, and neuroendocrine factors all correlate with increased perception of pain. It is likely that these factors could impact on long-term psycho-

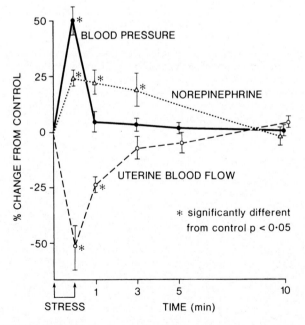

FIGURE 24-7. Effects of norepinephrine concentrations on uterine blood flow. From Snider SM, Wright RG, Levinson G, et al. Uterine blood flow and plasma norepinephrine changes during maternal stress. *Anesthesiology* 1979;50:524, with permission.

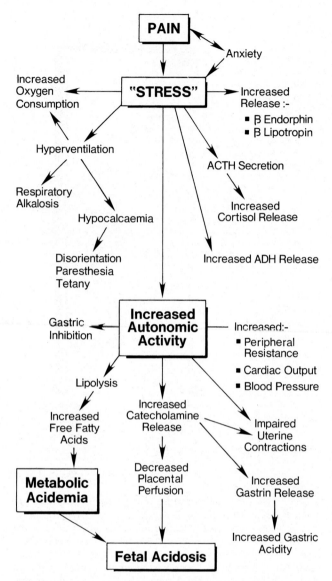

FIGURE 24-8. Physiologic and psychologic changes secondary to pain in labor.

logical issues, including bonding, long-term emotional stress, and postpartum mood dysfunction (Fig. 24-8).

REGIONAL ANALGESIA AND MATERNAL–FETAL CIRCULATION

The circulations of mother and fetus merge in the placenta and allow for the exchange of many physiologic substrates. In addition, the placenta serves a variety of functions, including the ongoing endocrine support of pregnancy. Fetal blood travels from the fetal heart to the placenta by way of two umbilical arteries and returns (nutrient-enriched and waste free) to the fetus by means of a single umbilical vein.

The placenta is composed of both maternal and fetal tissues that form a basal and chorionic plate. Essentially, the placenta is a semipermeable membrane that provides an interface for maternal and fetal circulation. The intervillous space separates the plates and is subdivided by decidual tissue. Chorionic villi and spiral arteries project extensively into the intervillous space. Maternal blood flows into the intervillous space from the spiral artery and, at this site, maternofetal placental transfer occurs. It is estimated that up to 80% of the uterine blood flow passes through the intervillous space.

Between 40% and 50% of the fetal cardiac output goes to the placenta, and a similar amount returns to the heart via the umbilical vein. Fetal blood enters the placenta via the two umbilical arteries, which arise from the internal iliac arteries. These arteries subdivide and eventually form umbilical capillaries that traverse the chorionic villi. The fetal blood flow is approximately 75 mL/kg/min. Although fetal and maternal blood pressures are uneven, placental transfer occurs rapidly for most drugs.

The umbilical–placental circulation is regulated by physiologic reflex changes and is also modified by neuroendocrine effects. Prostaglandins, endorphins, catecholamines, vasopressins, and other systemic factors modulate umbilical–placental perfusion.

Uterine Blood Flow

Uterine blood flow increases progressively throughout pregnancy and reaches a mean value of 500 to 700 mL/min at term. Uterine vessel blood flow is high, with a low vascular resistance (42). Pain may play a significant role, as uterine artery flow is dependent on maternal blood pressure and cardiac output. The uterine vessels are maximally dilated during pregnancy, thus no autoregulation is present. Therefore, any factor that interferes with blood flow through the uterus can potentially adversely affect fetal blood flow. Uterine blood flow is determined by the following relationship:

$$\text{Uterine blood flow} = \frac{(\text{uterine arterial pressure}) - (\text{uterine venous pressure})}{(\text{Uterine vascular resistance})}$$

$$(24\text{-}1)$$

Factors that reduce uterine blood flow include maternal hypotension, hypovolemia, hemorrhage, aortocaval compression, and sympathectomy. Similarly, conditions that increase the frequency or duration of uterine contractions (uterine hypercontractility/tetany) and changes in hypertension-induced increases in uterine vascular tone may also adversely affect blood flow. Both general and regional anesthesia can have a marked influence on uterine blood flow, causing alterations in perfusion pressure and/or changes in uterine vascular resistance. Sympathetic blockade following neuraxial techniques, especially as practiced prior to 1990 using higher concentrations of local anesthetics, can produce maternal hypotension and thus reduce uterine blood flow. This can be marked in a fasting and potentially dehydrated parturient with ongoing insensible fluid losses. Fluid preloading prior to proceeding with regional anesthetic technique may reduce the impact of the local anesthetic–induced sympathectomy and resulting hypotension. This becomes more important as the concentration of local anesthetic increases and neuraxial analgesia progresses to neuraxial anesthesia. Appropriate fluid preloading, with maintenance of maternal cardiac output, has a beneficial effect on uteroplacental blood flow (43). Studies have demonstrated that maternal cardiac output correlates with the uterine artery pulsatility index and umbilical artery pH; therefore, these can be used as a surrogate index of fetal homeostasis (44,45). Volatile agents used in the maintenance of general anesthesia are po-

tent myocardial depressants and can also lead to systemic vasodilatation. Aortocaval compression can further exacerbate this situation, and the parturient should, whenever possible, be positioned with left uterine displacement to optimize fetal oxygenation.

Hypotension as a result of regional anesthesia for labor and cesarean delivery can have a potentially deleterious affect on the fetus. Intravenous (IV) fluid therapy and avoidance of aortocaval compression are essential, but often must be combined with pharmacologic management. Ephedrine is extensively used in obstetric anesthesia for treatment of the effects of sympathectomy, as it has a low incidence of uteroplacental vasoconstriction. However, ephedrine can produce tachycardia and has been shown to produce depression of fetal pH and base excess (46). Ephedrine has mixed α- and β-adrenergic effects that may lead to an increase in blood pressure secondary to increased cardiac output and increased peripheral vascular resistance. Studies in pregnant ewes demonstrated that ephedrine was superior to metaraminol and methoxamine in maintaining uteroplacental blood flow (47).

Phenylephrine is a potent vasoconstrictor that is easy to titrate and has minimal associated fetal acidosis (Fig. 24-9). However, phenylephrine may decrease maternal heart rate and cardiac output and, although safe in the healthy parturient, few data are available on its use in high-risk cases. Vasopressors such as phenylephrine have direct α-adrenergic receptor activity and have been shown in animal studies to increase intrinsic vascular resistance and thus reduce uterine blood flow (48). There has been renewed interest and popularity in the use of phenylephrine as a vasopressor in routine clinical practice; studies have demonstrated that it is as efficacious as ephedrine in maintaining maternal blood pressure and umbilical artery pH values (49–51). Although a recent study has suggested that combination therapy with ephedrine and phenylephrine may be the optimal technique for maintaining normotension, ephedrine is still considered the vasopressor of choice by many anesthesiologists (52,53).

Relative to the high-risk parturient, animal studies of compromised maternal–fetal physiology with maternal hypoxemia and hypotension found that phenylephrine administration was associated with impaired uterine and placental hemodynamics and increased fetal lactate concentrations, when compared to ephedrine (54). Despite the more favorable effects on uterine and placental circulations of ephedrine over phenylephrine, no significant differences in fetal acid–base status or lactate concentrations were observed in other similar investigations (55). At Jackson Memorial Hospital, we have changed our practice so that mild hypotension is still treated with 5 mg of IV ephedrine. If this dose does not correct the hypotension, combinations of ephedrine and phenylephrine are subsequently administered.

Furthermore, in studies to evaluate the impact of both vasopressors in the maintenance of maternal–fetal parameters during ritodrine tocolysis and epidural-induced hypotension, both agents were shown to provide similar restoration of maternal mean arterial pressure. However, ephedrine was shown to be superior to phenylephrine in restoring uterine blood flow and fetal oxygenation (56). Comparison of both agents in the treatment of hypotension following anesthesia for cesarean delivery suggested that, unlike ephedrine, phenylephrine had a greater impact on uterine and placental flow indices as measured using Doppler velocimetry. These findings suggest that, although both agents have been well described in the treatment of maternal hypotension, caution should be exercised with phenylephrine in the presence of a potentially compromised fetus (57).

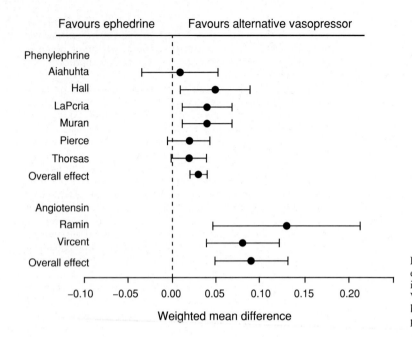

FIGURE 24-9. Meta-analysis of trials comparing phenylephrine and ephedrine for management of hypotension during spinal anesthesia for cesarean section. From Ngan Kee W, Khaw KS. Vasopressors in obstetrics: What should we be using? *Curr Opin Anesthesiol* 2006;19:238–243, with permission.

REGIONAL ANESTHESIA AND THE PLACENTA

The potential transfer of anesthetic agents across the placenta is a concern in the management of pain in the parturient. Drugs cross the placenta by three main processes: simple diffusion, active transport, or pinocytosis. The extent of drug transfer is dependent on numerous factors including lipid solubility, molecular weight, protein binding, concentration gradient, and maternal and fetal pH. The Fick principle governs the rate of transfer of a drug across a membrane:

$$Q/t = \frac{KA(Cm - Cf)}{D} \qquad (24\text{-}2)$$

where Q/t is the rate of diffusion, K is the diffusion coefficient, A is the surface area of membrane available for exchange, Cm-Cf is the concentration gradient between the maternal and fetal circulations, and D is the thickness of the membrane.

The potency and duration of action of local anesthetic agents is determined by their lipid solubility. This leads to the binding of a drug close to its target of action and also to reduced metabolism by liver enzymes and plasma esterases. Local anesthetic agents are weak bases and are poorly water soluble. Structurally, most local anesthetic agents are composed of a benzene ring (lipid-soluble/hydrophobic) and an amine group (water-soluble/hydrophilic), which is ionizable. These components are linked by a chemical chain, the structure of which is either ester (–CO) or amide (–HNC). The uncharged hydrophobic fraction of drug crosses the lipid membrane and initiates blockade of the hydrophobic sodium (Na^+) channel. The extent of hydrophobicity of a drug may also increase its risk of toxicity. Placental transfer is thus more active for lipid-soluble anesthetic agents.

Local anesthetics agents bind systemically to tissue and plasma proteins (albumin and α_1-acid glycoproteins [AAGs]). The protein-bound fraction is pharmacologically inactive, thus increased protein binding leads to reduced transfer of local anesthetic agent across the placenta. High-molecular-weight molecules are less likely to cross the placenta, whereas

molecules with weights under 500 daltons will cross easily. Most drugs administered to the parturient in labor have low molecular weight and therefore transfer easily to the fetus.

Highly ionized substances with low lipid solubility (such as non-depolarizing muscle relaxants) have very limited transfer. In fact, non-depolarizing muscle relaxants have been directly administered to the fetus during fetal surgery, with no impact on the mother. Fetal pH and serum protein binding directly affect drug disposition in the fetal circulation (58).

The degree of ionization greatly influences drug transfer because only nonionized portions of the drug can cross the placenta. The degree of ionization of a drug is determined by the Henderson-Hasselbalch equation:

$$pH = pKa + \log[base]/[acid] \qquad (24\text{-}3)$$

where pKa is the negative logarithm of the acid dissociation constant. The pKa of a drug is the pH at which it is 50% ionized and 50% nonionized.

The pKa of a local anesthetic agent determines the ratio of ionized to uncharged (base) form of the drug. The pKa for local anesthetic agents ranges from 7.6 to 9.2. The pKa generally correlates with the speed of onset of most local anesthetics agents. The closer the pKa is to physiologic pH, the faster its onset of action. Bupivacaine has a pKa of 8.1 and is only 15% nonionized at physiologic pH. Lidocaine has a more rapid onset, with a pKa of 7.7, and with 25% of drug nonionized at physiologic pH. However, 2-chloroprocaine is an exception, exhibiting a rapid onset of action, possibly due to increased tissue penetrability, despite having a pKa of 9.0. Similarly, agents with a pKa closer to physiologic pH have a higher degree of placental transfer. The umbilical vein-to-maternal artery (UV:MA) ratio for mepivacaine (pKa 7.6) is 0.8, compared to 0.3 for bupivacaine (pKa 8.1) (see also Chapters 3 and 4).

Pain thresholds may be increased in pregnancy, with a possible corresponding increased sensitivity to local anesthetic agents (32,59). Therefore, changes in maternal and fetal acid–base status, combined with altered protein binding, can have a major impact on the management and technique of regional anesthesia. Fetal acidosis leads to increased ionization of local anesthetic agents that have crossed the placenta into the fetal circulation. These ionized agents are unable to transfer back (ion trapping) across the placenta into the maternal circulation. Fetal acidosis and systemic insult can lead to increased perfusion of the heart and brain, thus increasing the delivery of drug to these important organs. This can lead to further accumulation of drugs in an already compromised fetus (60). Although this is a major theoretical concern, the clinical significance of this phenomenon is unclear (see Chapter 3).

The fetal circulation can have a major impact on drug distribution within the fetus. As previously described, drugs enter the fetal circulation via the umbilical vein following their passage across the placenta. The liver is perfused by umbilical venous blood, and significant hepatic uptake can occur, which may have a protective effect on the fetus (61). Approximately 40% of the umbilical venous blood bypasses the liver via the ductus venosus (62). Further dilution of umbilical venous blood across the foramen ovale and ductus arteriosus can also occur.

PARTURITION AND STAGES OF LABOR

The delivery of the fetus (parturition) is achieved by the intermittent involuntary contraction of smooth muscle, facilitated by maternal bearing down. When stretched, the uterus has the ability to expel any foreign body within its cavity. The precise mechanism of maintenance of pregnancy and onset of labor is unknown, although numerous hypotheses have been suggested. Declines in serum progesterone, increasing levels of estrogen, increased prostaglandin production, increases in oxytocin receptors, structural changes in the myometrium, and many fetal factors are all thought to play a role in the onset of labor (63).

Labor is divided into three stages, each stage of which has a particular type and nature of pain. The first stage begins with maternal awareness of regular and painful uterine contractions and ends with complete dilatation of the cervix. This discomfort usually reflects a minimal intrauterine pressure of approximately 25 mm Hg and reflects stretching and distension during contraction (64).

During the first stage of labor, the pain experienced is mostly visceral in nature, arising from afferents in the uterus and its adnexa during contractions. The painful afferents pass through the superior hypogastric plexus and lumbar sympathetic chain and enter the spinal cord through the posterior segments of T10–T12 (Fig. 24-10). The intensity of pain is related to the contraction strength and subsequent pressure generated against the cervix and perineum (65). Chemical metabolites resulting from neurohumoral pathways or contraction-induced ischemia may also lead to local stimulation of painful chemoreceptors by several chemical mediators including prostaglandins, serotonin, substance P, and lactic acid (64,66).

The painful afferents from the lower uterine segment and the endocervix have their cell bodies located in the thoracolumbar dorsal root ganglia. However, the upper vagina and vaginal cervix have cell bodies in the sacral dorsal root ganglia that are mostly comprised of C-fibers. These enter the spinal cord through the dorsal root ganglion and develop a loose network of synapses in the ventral and dorsal horn (superficial and deep). Because of the significant convergence of the visceral pain pathways, the pain experienced in this stage of labor is often poorly localized and can be referred to the rectum, lower back, and along the abdominal wall (67). As the fetal head descends along the birth canal and into the pelvis, pressure on the pelvic viscera and stimulation of the lumbosacral plexus can lead to perception of pain from L1–S1. This has implica-

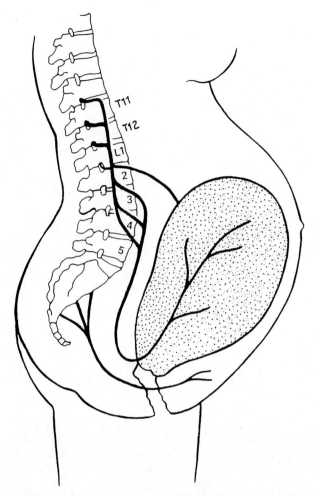

FIGURE 24-10. Peripheral pain pathways during labor (see also Fig. 31-23).

tions in the provision of neuraxial analgesia, because to achieve effective pain management during this stage, the lumbar and upper sacral nerve roots require effective blockade. Neurons at the level of the dorsal horn transmit afferent information to the contralateral spinothalamic tract and other ascending pathways to the higher centers of the brain responsible for the localization and affective component of pain (see Fig. 31-19).

The second stage of labor begins with full dilatation of the cervix and ends with the delivery of the fetus. Ongoing pain stimuli from contractions of the uterine body continue, in addition to pain from distension of the lower uterine segment. The contribution of pain from cervical dilatation slowly diminishes. However, the presenting fetus, as it presses on pelvic structures, leads to stimulation of superficial somatic structures and their afferents via the pudendal nerve (S2–S4); pain arises from tearing of ligaments, and pressure on fascia, muscles, bladder, urethra, and rectum. The pudendal nerve also supplies the motor fibers to the skeletal muscles of the pelvic floor and perineum. The anterior perineum also receives fibers from the genital branch of the genitofemoral nerve (L1–L2) and the ilioinguinal nerve (L1). The lateral aspect of the perineum is also supplied by the posterior femoral cutaneous nerve (S1–S3) (68–70) (Fig. 24-11). Thus, pain in the second stage is often sharply localized. This somatic pain is transmitted via C- and Aδ-fibers that enter the spinal cord through the dorsal

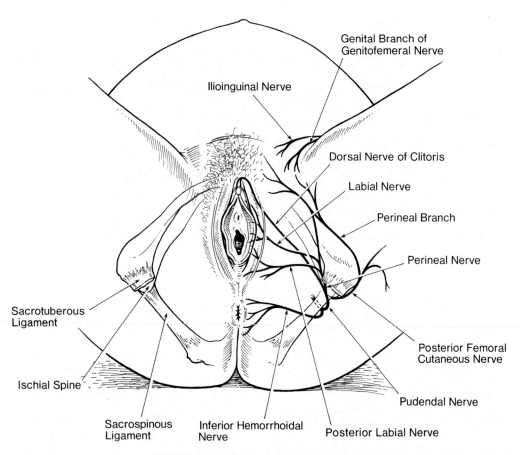

FIGURE 24-11. Nerve supply to the perineum.

roots and terminate in synapses in the ipsilateral superficial laminae of the dorsal horn. Provision of appropriate analgesia during the second stage of labor requires analgesia from a level of T10 extending caudally to include the somatic nerves of the perineum (S2–S4). This may not always be blocked by a continuous epidural using low-dose anesthetic, and increased dosing (top-offs) may be necessary at this stage.

The third stage of labor commences with the completed delivery of the fetus and ends with the completed delivery of the placenta and attached membranes. The analgesia requirements for the third stage of labor are usually less than that of the first and second stages. However, if there is delay in the delivery of the placenta or if manual removal by the obstetrician is required, increased doses of analgesia or anesthesia of the perineum and lower uterus are usually required.

Management of Pain in Labor

Comprehensive patient education programs regarding labor pain and its management options form a key part of antenatal care. Pain management in labor ideally should be multidisciplinary in nature. Appropriate psychological preparation and support is essential whenever possible. This can be accomplished by high levels of antenatal care and patient education prior to onset of labor, thus enabling the patient to make decisions in advance in relation to her pain management and also increasing the likelihood that, despite the pains of labor, the parturient has made an informed decision and gives vital consent.

The use of psychological techniques including positive outlook, relaxation therapies, and diversionary techniques may be considered as adjuncts to neuraxial pain management (71). The role of the patient's partner in this situation cannot be underestimated; relatives and caregivers who provide an appropriately relaxing and supportive environment are clearly beneficial. Use of hypnosis in labor has been limited by refractory patients, whereas the role of nonconventional therapies including aromatherapy and reflexology is unclear. Transcutaneous electrical nerve stimulation (TENS) can be useful in early labor when pain scores are low, but its role in established painful labor has not been supported (72).

Intradermal injections of water have been described in the management of lower back pain in labor. These injections are thought to produce analgesia by counterirritation. Relief of labor back pain has been described for up to 90 minutes following injection (73).

Systemic Analgesia

Systemic analgesia is used when regional techniques are either not available or contraindicated. This may include situations in which no anesthesiologist is available, or in the high-risk parturient in whom neuraxial techniques are contraindicated, such as in a coagulopathic patient. The administration of intramuscular opioids has been a well-established technique that has been widely used historically, despite suggestions that labor pain is insensitive to systemically administered opioids and that the IV route is preferable to intramuscular injection (74). The associated maternal and fetal neurologic depressant effects, combined with risks of accumulation of excitatory metabolites, have limited the use of parenteral opioids. Lack of established efficacy, combined with nausea, vomiting, and sedation all preclude widespread use and have made this option unpopular with parturients (75). Opioid administration in labor has been shown to produce relief of moderate pain in 70% to 80% of patients, but only in 35% to 60% of those experiencing severe pain (64,65). Of note, the majority of women in labor experience severe pain, as illustrated by the classic studies performed more than 50 years ago (76–82).

Insufficient evidence is available to evaluate the comparative efficacy and index of safety among opioids used in labor analgesia. Intramuscular meperidine (Demerol) has been widely used for labor analgesia and is associated with modest analgesia (76), but the potential for maternal, fetal, and neonatal side effects exist. Accumulation of the excitatory metabolite normeperidine has not been widely described in labor. In terms of pain relief, interval to delivery, and instrument/operative delivery, no difference was noted between meperidine and tramadol. However, meperidine was associated with a higher incidence of nausea, vomiting, and drowsiness (77,78).

Use of fentanyl has been considered because of its potency (100 times that of morphine) and rapid onset. Intravenous doses of 50 μg of fentanyl have been reported to be of value in the first stage of labor, although its short duration of action compared to morphine requires frequent administration or use of continuous infusions. In addition, because of its lipid solubility, fentanyl has been shown to cross the placenta easily, and fetal levels of drug can rise rapidly (79). Use of patient-controlled IV remifentanil (0.27–0.93 μg/kg) has been shown to be superior to IV meperidine in terms of pain relief, with a lower incidence of fetal heart rate abnormalities; research is ongoing to find optimal dosing regimens (82). Finally, the potential benefit of combining μ- and κ-receptor agonists has not been borne out by clinical studies (81).

Neural Blockade in Obstetric Anesthesia and Analgesia

Regional blockade provides the least depressant and most effective form of analgesia and anesthesia in obstetrics. Peripheral techniques are commonly used by the surgeon in situations in which regional techniques have not been utilized or to supplement blockade in the presence of sparing of the sacral dermatomes due to an ineffective block.

Infiltration of local anesthetic along the perineum is performed in a fan-shaped pattern along the ischiorectal fossa prior to episiotomy or for suture of same post delivery. Lidocaine 0.5% to 1.0% with epinephrine (1:200,000) can be used, up to a total dose of 7 mg/kg. Local anesthetic infiltration has been described for emergency use for cesarean delivery, although central neuraxial blockade has largely replaced this practice. The technique may still have a place in the situation of profound fetal bradycardia with no anesthesia provider present (83).

Paracervical and Pudendal Blocks

The paracervical block is an alternate technique for the parturient who does not want or cannot receive central neuraxial block for the first stage of labor. It is a relatively simple procedure to perform and provides relief of pain in the first stage of labor without adversely affecting the progress of labor. Local

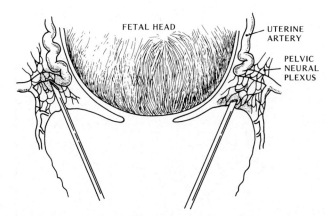

FIGURE 24-12. Neurovascular anatomy associated with a paracervical block in obstetrics. The needle in the right fornix is short-beveled and shows distribution of the local anesthetic. From Bloom SL, Horswill, CW, Curet, LB. Effects of paracervical blocks on the fetus during labor: A prospective study with the use of direct fetal monitoring. *Am J Obstet Gynecol* 1972;114:218, with permission.

anesthetic is injected submucosally into the fornix of the vagina lateral to the cervix. Blockade of neural transmission through the paracervical ganglion is achieved, which lies lateral and posterior to the junction of the cervix and uterus. Paracervical blockade does not affect somatic sensory fibers from the perineum and thus offers no pain relief for the second stage of labor. Currently, this technique is predominantly performed by obstetricians for nonobstetric surgery, such as dilatation and curettage. Its use in obstetric practice has profoundly decreased over the past two decades as neuraxial blockade has become safer, more effective, and increasingly more available. Significant adverse reactions to paracervical blockade have been reported including profound fetal bradycardia, systemic local anesthetic toxicity, postpartum neuropathy, and infection (84). It has been suggested that the etiology of fetal bradycardia is related to reductions in uterine blood flow and elevated local anesthetic levels in fetal blood (85,86) (Fig. 24-12).

The pudendal nerves originate from the lower sacral nerve roots (S2–S4). These nerves transmit sensory innervation for the lower vagina, vulva, and perineum, and provide motor innervation to the perineal muscles. Injection of local anesthetic behind the bilateral sacrospinous ligament transvaginally provides excellent anesthesia of these nerves (87). Pudendal nerve block provides satisfactory analgesia for spontaneous and instrumental vaginal delivery at the level of the vaginal outlet. However, pudendal nerve blocks do not provide sufficient analgesia for mid-forceps delivery, repair of vaginal lacerations, or exploration of the uterine cavity (88). Although complications are rare, failure of block, systemic local anesthetic toxicity, infections, and hematoma formation have been described. The proximity of needle placement to the fetal head may also be an issue of great concern (89) (Fig. 24-13).

Lumbar Sympathetic and Thoracolumbar Paravertebral Blocks

Anatomy and Innervation

The autonomic nervous system is divided into the sympathetic and parasympathetic nervous systems. Preganglionic nerves of the sympathetic nervous system arise from the thoracic and lumbar segments of the spinal cord; in the parasympathetic

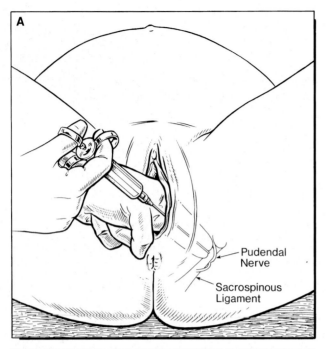

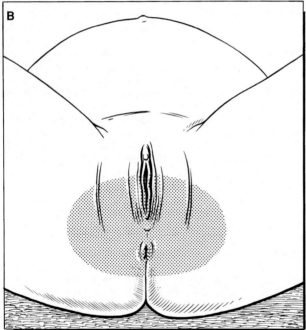

FIGURE 24-13. Pudendal block by the transvaginal approach.

sels pass under the dense fascia toward the epidural space, thus creating a potential passageway to the epidural space (90,91).

White rami communicantes are aggregates of preganglionic fibers that leave the spinal cord from the intermediolateral cell column and lateral horn (T1–L2). They leave the spinal canal with the corresponding anterior spinal nerves and join the sympathetic chain. They are white in color, as they are only slightly myelinated. The postganglionic fibers (gray rami communicantes) leave the sympathetic chain in association with the spinal nerves. They are unmyelinated and appear gray in color. The preganglionic fibers (white rami communicantes) may synapse in the sympathetic chain and then travel with the spinal nerve. Some may ascend or descend to another level of the spinal cord and synapse at this level before traveling with the spinal nerve. Some white rami communicantes transverse the sympathetic chain without synapsing. These preganglionic sympathetic fibers form the greater, lesser, and least splanchnic nerves (T6–T12), which synapse in the celiac and superior mesenteric ganglia within the abdomen. The postganglionic sympathetic fibers from these ganglia are distributed to the abdominal organs. The sympathetic nerves are usually accompanied by afferent fibers conducting sensory information from the appropriate viscera (see Figs. 39-1, 39-2, 39-5).

Lumbar Sympathetic Blockade

Early studies have suggested that the lower uterine and cervical afferent sensory fibers join the sympathetic chain at L2–L3. There were some reports of effective blockade of afferent sensory transmission from these structures to the spinal cord using lumbar sympathetic blocks (92,93). Lumbar sympathetic blocks provided effective analgesia of long duration (94). In addition, lumbar sympathetic blocks in nulliparous parturients with induced labor were associated with effective analgesia and rapid cervical dilatation during the first 2 hours of analgesia, and were also associated with a shorter duration of the second stage when compared to epidural analgesia (95). These findings, however, have not widely convinced clinicians to embrace this technique, which remains unpopular.

Blockade of the paravertebral sympathetic chain interrupts visceral afferents and sympathetic efferent transmission. The specificity and sensitivity of this procedure and the role of the sympathetic nervous system in the pain of parturition is unclear (96). The precise mechanism of action of lumbar sympathetic blocks in labor is also unclear, given the close anatomic relationship between the sensory afferents and the sympathetic chain (see Fig. 39-4).

The lumbar sympathetic nerves at the thoracolumbar level are reasonably amenable to non–image guided regional anesthesia techniques. However, the afferent nerves from the distal one-third of colon and all the pelvic viscera are less so. These fibers travel with the sympathetic fibers of the superior hypogastric plexus, which is located retroperitoneally in the pelvis at the level of L5–S1. Needle placement is technically difficult and thus impractical to use during labor (97,98). In addition, use of fluoroscopic guidance to facilitate needle placement in the parturient would be exceptionally rare because of risks of fetal exposure to radiation (see Figs. 45-15, 45-16).

Lumbar sympathetic blockade requires placement of a 22-gauge 10-cm needle approximately 2 cm deep to the transverse process of L2, bilaterally. Incremental local anesthetic injections can be administered. Bilateral doses of 10 mL of bupivacaine 0.5% with 25 μg of fentanyl and 50 μg epinephrine have been used to good effect (95). Complications include bleeding, infection, hypotension, genitofemoral neuralgia, unintentional epidural/spinal injection, and perforation of viscera

nervous system, they arise from the brainstem and sacral spinal cord. Most visceral structures (except blood vessels and sweat glands) receive both sympathetic and parasympathetic innervation. The sympathetic chain lies along the anterolateral surface of the lumbar vertebral bodies. The psoas muscle and fascia separate the lumbar sympathetic chain from the somatic nerves. Anatomic studies have shown marked variability in the distribution of the ganglia, but suggest optimum blockade of the ganglia will result from sympathetic blocks at the level of the L3 vertebral body (90). However, caution should be exercised at the level of the middle one-third, where the segmental ves-

or blood vessels (91,99). As previously mentioned, these complications, combined with the potential for block failure, have limited the clinical usefulness of these blocks.

Thoracolumbar Paravertebral Blockade

The paravertebral space is a narrow triangular space lateral to the vertebral column. The boundaries of the paravertebral space are formed by the iliopsoas anterolaterally; vertebral body, intervertebral disc, and foramen medially; and by the costotransverse ligament posteriorly. The space contains the sympathetic chain, dorsal and ventral nerve roots, and rami communicantes. Analgesia is achieved by deposition of local anesthesia in the distribution of the lateral aspect of the intervertebral foramen, within the paravertebral space, resulting in blockade of the ventral nerve roots and accompanying sympathetic nerves (see Figs. 16-4 and 16-15 to 16-18).

In the sitting position, the iliac crests (corresponding to L3–L4 ± 1 interspace) and spinous processes (midline) are identified and marked (see Chapter 16, Fig. 16-20). A line is drawn cephalad/caudad 2.5 cm lateral to midline, parallel to the spinous process of the thoracolumbar spine. Needle placement is along this line at the level of those nerve roots requiring blockade (T9–L1). Contact is made with the transverse process at each level required, and the needle is then angled 10 degrees cephalad/caudad and advanced 1 cm beyond the transverse process. Some anesthesiologists use a loss-of-resistance technique to identify the paravertebral space, although this can be quite subjective. This technique results in dermatomal analgesia at the level of the nerve roots blocked. The block is volume-dependent, and 20 mL of local anesthetic administered via a single needle should provide analgesia to approximately five somatic dermatomes and eight sympathetic levels. This volume of anesthetic agent may pose risks to the parturient in the event of accidental intravascular or intrathecal injection. Catheter techniques may be used to facilitate prolonged analgesia through the use of local anesthetic infusions and bolus doses as required. The absorption of local anaesthetic is difficult to predict, with analgesia of between 1 and 10 hours reported following a single injection (100,101) (see also Chapter 16).

The failure rate for paravertebral blocks performed in surgical patients is approximately 10%, with side effects including hypotension (4.6%), vascular puncture (3.8%), pleural puncture (1.1%), and pneumothorax (0.5%). The incidence of urinary complications and hypotension was found to be lower than with epidural analgesia (102,103). Total spinal anesthesia has also been reported as a complication (104). Paravertebral hematoma formation may also occur, although cadaveric studies suggest that fluid spread in the paravertebral space is caudal and lateral, thus away from the central neuraxis (105).

Bilateral lumbar sympathetic and paravertebral blocks have been described as effective techniques that can be used as an alternative to epidural labor analgesia (95,106). These, however, are non–image guided techniques (in the parturient), and the needle entry point is chosen on the basis of anatomic landmarks. The needle end-point is based on varying distances beyond contact with the transverse processes. This presents quite a large margin for error, and the distinction between the benefits of sympathectomy and nerve root block may be difficult to make for either procedure. These techniques have been suggested as suitable alternatives for epidural analgesia when central neuraxial blockade is deemed inappropriate for anatomic or medical reasons, but further investigation in the high-risk parturient is necessary. Use of short-acting IV opioid infusions may prove to be a safer and more flexible option.

Central Neuraxial Blockade

Epidural analgesia resulting in blockade of the lumbosacral plexus has been demonstrated to be a safe and effective technique for the management of labor pain in the parturient (107–109).

Epidural placement should be performed in an area with appropriate staffing, and familiarity with central neuraxial blockade is essential. Appropriate resuscitation equipment must be readily available. In addition, ongoing maternal and fetal monitoring should be maintained, and provision must be made for the placement of the epidural catheter in a sterile environment. Appropriate facilities for ongoing epidural management, including physiologic monitoring and post epidural management protocols, must be in place. There has been much discussion regarding both the proximity and levels of anesthesiology staffing required to provide safe and effective care using epidural analgesia in labor. International practice varies widely and, in the future, it is likely that a combination of quality assurance, financial constraints, and medicolegal issues may ultimately establish a more uniform standard of care.

Full preprocedure evaluation and preparation of the parturient should be performed. In addition, anesthesiologists are obliged to obtain consent and inform their patients of the risks associated with regional anesthesia and analgesia. The timing, effectiveness, and extent of this consent have been the subject of much debate (110). No clear consensus exists as to what the appropriate levels of informed consent are. Some anesthesiologists believe that the forum for obtaining and documenting consent for labor analgesia should be during the antenatal preparation of the parturient, as acute pain might have a marked impact on the understanding and acceptance of clinical risks (111). However, the consensus of opinion is that most women are capable of giving informed consent even during active labor. Theoretically, similar ethical problems may arise should a mother fail to give consent for epidural analgesia in the antenatal period, and then change this decision on experiencing acute pain refractory to parenteral opioids. The previous administration of parenteral opioids does not necessarily preclude subsequent placement of an epidural. However, each case must be decided individually. Anesthesiologists have differing views regarding the extent of inclusiveness of both risks and their associated incidences, and may limit patient discussion regarding rare complications such as epidural hematoma (112).

Patient Position

The technique of epidural insertion in labor differs in some ways from standard epidural placement in the nonpregnant patient. Pregnancy-related anatomic changes can make positioning and identification of landmarks problematic. In addition, ongoing acute pain and associated distress during contractions can lead to difficulty in positioning the patient and can lead to ongoing physical and emotional stress to both patient and medical staff. Epidural insertion can be performed with the patient in the lateral decubitus or sitting position. Some evidence suggests that uteroplacental perfusion may be optimum in the lateral decubitus position (113). Likewise, the potential for the reduction of venous congestion by adopting the lateral recumbent head-down position may be associated with a reduction in the incidence of lumbar epidural venous puncture (114). However, the incidence of successful epidural placement may be higher in the sitting position, especially in the obese parturient. In the management of obese and morbidly obese patients, the sitting position may be associated with easier identification of the midline and possibly improved respiratory parameters (115). To complicate the issue further, a decreased incidence of aortocaval compression during the identification of the epidural space was demonstrated in the sitting position compared to the left lateral decubitus position (116). Taking all these factors into account, we believe that positioning of the patient for epidural placement should be done taking user experience and preference into account. In addition, patient factors and preferences should also be considered. One report even suggested that use of the prone (knee-chest) position had a role in epidural placement (117). There is no doubt that the dynamic nature of acute pain medicine requires that each practitioner should be familiar with a broad range of procedures and positions in the performance of epidural, spinal, and combined spinal–epidural techniques.

Aseptic Technique

Strict asepsis is essential in the performance of neuraxial blocks, especially those involving epidural catheter insertion. Several case reports have identified iatrogenic causes of meningitis during central neuraxial procedures (118–121). The routine use of face masks in the prevention of iatrogenic contamination by anesthesiologists has shown wide user variation. Surveys of United Kingdom obstetric anesthesiologists and of fellows of the Australia and New Zealand College of Anaesthetists with a special interest in obstetric practice showed a marked variation in practice standards. In the United Kingdom, more than 50% of anesthesiologists did not wear face masks for central neuraxial procedures, and this precaution was not seen to be essential in 29% of the latter group (122–123). The infectious disease community however, is united in their view that aseptic techniques, including use of face masks, is essential.

Disinfection of the skin with chlorhexidine, povidone iodine, or similar agent is strongly recommended. Standard aseptic precautions, including use of sealed bottles or single-use packets of povidone iodine, have proved to be more effective than multiuse bottles (124,125). In vitro studies have shown the effectiveness of iodine products for asepsis, although recent clinical evidence suggests that chlorhexidine in alcohol solution is more efficient as an antimicrobial agent (126). This combination agent has been extensively evaluated for use in placing central lines; however, its use in epidural or spinal placement has not been fully established. Although there is some worry about neurotoxicity based on preliminary animal research, clinical evidence in Europe suggests that chlorhexidine is both efficacious and safe for use as a disinfectant for neuraxial blocks (127,128).

Identification of the Epidural Space

Following appropriate antiseptic preparation of the lumbosacral spine, the skin is draped and local anaesthesia is administered to the skin and interspinal ligament. Use of clear plastic drapes offers the advantage of providing a sterile field while allowing better visualization of landmarks. Placement of the epidural needle at the L3–L4 ±1 intervertebral level should provide appropriate coverage of the lumbar and sacral nerve roots required for analgesia during labor and delivery. Use of loss-of-resistance techniques to both saline and air have been extensively described. Studies have assessed the quality of analgesia in women randomized to either technique (129,130): Beilin and co-workers found that patients who had epidural placement using a loss-of-resistance technique to air had a higher requirement for rescue medications following initial analgesia (129). The merits of a saline technique include avoidance of pneumocephalus-induced headache, nonuniform

spread of local anesthetic, and nerve root irritation, all of which have been described following injection of epidural air (131,132) (see Figs. 11-12 to 11-15).

However, the judicious use of air during the loss-of-resistance technique should avoid many of these side effects. In fact, the use of air when performing a combined spinal–epidural (CSE) technique can be advantageous, as it allows clear identification of cerebrospinal fluid (CSF) without introducing any confusion caused by the concomitant use of saline. Because of the unpredictable duration of labor and the ever-present need to facilitate cesarean section delivery should it be necessary, placement of the epidural catheter is performed more commonly than performing a single-injection technique.

Selection of Epidural Catheter

The use of both single-port (uniport) and multiport (multiple-orifice) epidural catheters has been widely described. The proposed advantage of the single-port (open-end) catheter is the delivery of medication to a single anatomic site, which may have safety implications. However, single-port catheters may also be associated with reduced spread of medication, leading to incomplete and/or unilateral blocks. This problem may be reduced through the use of the newly developed flexible-tip single-port catheters, which may also potentially offer the advantage of decreased incidence of paresthesias and intravascular placement (133).

Comparisons between multi- and single-port catheters showed that significantly fewer catheters needed replacement in the multiport group because of inadequate analgesia (defined as unblocked segments or unilateral block) and that paresthesias were less common in this same group (134,135). A comparison of multiport, firm-tipped, close-ended epidural catheters with uniport, open-ended, soft-tipped, wire-reinforced catheters showed the softer uniport to have a lower incidence of paresthesias and vascular puncture (136).

Multiport (closed-end) catheters have the theoretical disadvantage of potentially delivering anesthetic agent to more than one anatomic site, such as to the epidural and subarachnoid spaces at the same time. However, studies have not shown multiport catheters to be associated with multicompartment placement, and the incidence of vascular puncture and dislodgement requiring replacement were similar for both catheter types (single- and multiport). Multiport catheters have consistently been shown to be associated with a reduced incidence of inadequate analgesia and thus require less manipulation, presumably because of a more even distribution of medication (133,135).

A further technique suggested in the prevention of accidental vascular puncture during epidural catheter placement includes injection of 3 to 5 mL of saline through the epidural needle prior to advancing the catheter. This is thought to expand the epidural space, possibly decreasing the likelihood of unintentional IV cannulation (137).

Technical factors may play a major role in determining the effectiveness of labor analgesia. In a study of 100 laboring women, insertion of multiport catheters to a depth of 5 cm was shown to be associated with the highest incidence of satisfactory analgesia and minimal complications, compared to a higher rate of insertion complications at a 7-cm depth (138). Cephalad orientation of the epidural needle at catheter placement has also been shown to be associated with increased effectiveness and reduced complications. Epidural catheters are not fixed in the epidural space however, and their position can vary according to the posture of the parturient. Change of position from sitting to lateral recumbent can be associated with movement of the catheter of between 1 and 2.5 cm, which can lead to inadequate analgesia (139). To minimize the risk of catheter displacement, especially in obese patients, it has been suggested that multiorifice catheters should be inserted to a depth of more than 4 cm into the epidural space and secured only upon assuming the lateral position (140).

Epidural Test Dose

Confirmation of successful catheter placement within the epidural space is often best measured by effective analgesia. Prior to administration of appropriate medications to achieve this degree of analgesia, unanticipated intrathecal or IV catheter placement must be excluded. Although this may not ensure appropriate epidural placement, it does however reduce the cardiorespiratory and neurologic risks associated with administration of a dose intended for epidural use into the CSF or systemic circulation. The use of test doses in labor has also been the subject of much controversy. Use of an appropriate test dose is considered important by some anesthesiologists, especially as many patients may subsequently require larger doses of concentrated local anesthetic administered epidurally in the event of emergency cesarean delivery (141). The sensitivity and specificity of test dosing is critically important in determining the appropriate placement of an epidural catheter. Given the extent of patient movement during labor and the potential for the epidural catheter to move according to patient position, it could be argued that frequent test dosing might be required. In addition, the impact of this epidural test dose on motor function in ambulating patients, and in preeclamptic patients and patients with cardiac disease, should also be considered (142–146). However, in clinical practice, if an epidural catheter has been placed and local anesthesia/opioid solution is infusing uneventfully into a comfortable parturient with minimal motor deficit, the catheter can be considered to be appropriately sited in the epidural space.

Intrathecal injection of 3 mL of lidocaine 1.5% (45 mg) with epinephrine 1:200,000 (5 μg/mL) will result in dense motor blockade within 2 to 4 minutes. Intravascular injection of 15 μg of epinephrine will result in tachycardia. The administration of this dose of local anesthetic systemically can result in lightheadedness and circumoral numbness or tingling within 1 minute of injection (141–143). Administration of the test dose should not be performed immediately before or during a uterine contraction, as labor pain itself is associated with increased heart rate variability. Aspiration of epidural catheters should be performed, but does not adequately identify all cases of intravascular or intrathecal catheter placement, especially if a single-port catheter is used (147,148).

Use of the "air test" combined with epidural catheter aspiration has also been described as a method to out rule accidental intravascular catheter placement (149). Injection of 1 mL of epidural air with concomitant precordial Doppler detection has been used successfully to identify intravascular placement. However, the sensitivity for this test appears to be less with use of the newer multiport epidural catheters (150).

Selection of Local Anesthetic Agent and Adjuvant

Bupivacaine

The use of the amide local anesthetic bupivacaine is well established in obstetric anesthesia. Its prolonged duration of action, differential sensory blockade, and relative lack of tachyphy-laxis make it an ideal agent for use in epidural and spinal anesthesia (151). The degree of drug ionization at physiologic pH and the extent of protein binding determine the degree of placental transfer. Bupivacaine is highly ionized at physiologic pH (pKa of 8.05) and is 95% protein bound, thus placental transfer is limited. The ratio at delivery of the concentration of local anesthetic in blood or plasma from the umbilical vein to the concentration of local anesthetic in maternal blood (UV:MA ratio) for bupivacaine ranges from 0.31 to 0.44 and is much lower than that of lidocaine (152). Bupivacaine has been the subject of concern in relation to its systemic cardiovascular toxicity (153,154), and the use of bupivacaine 0.75% concentration solution in the epidural space has been prohibited in obstetric practice by the U.S. Food and Drug Administration (FDA). Bupivacaine consists of two stereoisomers $S(-)$ and $R(+)$, and is marketed as a racemic mixture of these. The R enantiomer was found to contribute to bupivacaine's unwanted toxicity (155,156). Levobupivacaine and ropivacaine are the pure $S(-)$ enantiomers of N-butyl- and N-propyl-2',6'-pipercoloxylidide, which were developed as less cardiotoxic alternatives to bupivacaine (157) (see also Chapter 3).

Ropivacaine

Ropivacaine is a homologue of bupivacaine and mepivacaine formulated as a single levo rotary enantiomer. The putative advantages of ropivacaine over bupivacaine are the suggested lower risks of cardiovascular depression and neurologic toxicity (158) (see also Chapter 3).

In addition, sheep studies have shown faster clearance associated with ropivacaine compared to bupivacaine following intravascular administration, which suggests a greater margin of safety after unintentional intravascular injection (159).

Use of the minimum local anesthetic concentration (MLAC) in determining local anesthetic potency has shown that ropivacaine is 40% less potent than bupivacaine when used as a bolus for initiation of epidural analgesia in early labor (158,160). However, dilute ropivacaine (0.08%) with fentanyl (2 μg/mL) produced effective labor analgesia with preservation of spontaneous voiding and ambulation in parturients (161). Comparison between bupivacaine 0.075% and ropivacaine 0.075% using a patient-controlled epidural analgesia (PCEA) technique during labor showed both agents to be equally effective (162). Thus, there appears to be no clear clinical advantage of ropivacaine over bupivacaine for epidural labor analgesia in terms of either obstetric or neonatal outcome. However, cost may become a factor in the selection of any anesthetic technique, and ropivacaine is currently more expensive than racemic bupivacaine (163–165).

Levobupivacaine

Levobupivacaine is a long-acting local anesthetic with a similar clinical profile to bupivacaine. Studies have shown that the cardiotoxicity of bupivacaine was more pronounced with the $R(+)$ enantiomer, and use of levobupivacaine—the $S(-)$ enantiomer—has gained acceptance in clinical practice (166). The safety of levobupivacaine has been compared to racemic bupivacaine in both animal and human volunteer studies (167–169). The lethal dose of levobupivacaine was 1.3- to 1.6-fold higher than that of bupivacaine in several animal studies, supporting the added safety of levobupivacaine should inadvertent intravascular injection occur (170) (see also Chapters 3 and 5).

Levobupivacaine crosses the placenta, with UV:MA ratios for levobupivacaine demonstrated to be 0.3 in women undergoing elective cesarean delivery following the epidural administration of 30 mL 0.5% levobupivacaine (171).

PART III: APPLICATIONS

Levobupivacaine has been shown to compare favorably to bupivacaine for epidural use for cesarean delivery (172). Assessment of speed of onset and quality of sensory block between 0.5% bupivacaine and 0.5% levobupivacaine has shown similar results. There appears to be no difference between speed of onset and duration of sensory block when patients received either levobupivacaine 0.5% or bupivacaine 0.5% for cesarean delivery. In addition, the onset and reversal of sensory/motor blockade, quality of anesthesia, and muscle relaxation were comparable between the two groups. Levobupivacaine has also been used extensively to provide epidural analgesia for labor. A recent multicenter study comparing levobupivacaine and bupivacaine reported these drugs as having equivalent analgesic efficacy (173,174). Concomitant use of fentanyl has been shown to have a dose-sparing effect on levobupivacaine requirements. Levobupivacaine is not currently marketed in the United States, but is available in many other countries worldwide.

Lidocaine

Lidocaine has been widely used in obstetric anesthesia. The rapid onset of action associated with lidocaine and its intermediate duration of action are particularly useful for many obstetric procedures. The UV:MA ratios reported are within the range of 0.4 to 0.6 (175). Epidurally administered lidocaine 2% solution combined with epinephrine is widely used for operative delivery; however, its duration of action and degree of motor blockade make it less ideal for use in facilitation of prolonged labor analgesia. Although early reports suggested that lidocaine compromised neonatal neurobehavioral function, this has not been borne out by further investigation or clinical experience (176,177).

Concerns regarding the use of 5% hyperbaric lidocaine for spinal anesthesia developed because of reports of cauda equina syndrome (CES) (178,179). The FDA suggested dilution of lidocaine with saline or CSF prior to intrathecal injection, and these precautions were subsequently incorporated into the package insert for this drug. However, despite dilution of drug, lidocaine concentration of 2.5% and 2% solutions may still cause CES. This has resulted in many anesthesiologists abandoning this once favored drug (Chapter 12).

2-Chloroprocaine

2-Chloroprocaine is an ester local anesthetic with a rapid onset time and short duration of action. Metabolism is rapid via ester hydrolysis ($t_{1/2} = 45$ seconds); thus, since almost no drug crosses the placenta, it is a very safe agent for use in obstetrics (180). By virtue of its safety profile and speed of onset, its predominant role in obstetric anesthesia is in the establishment of anesthesia for emergency cesarean delivery when an epidural catheter is in situ. The short duration of action and its rapid reversal of anesthesia require ongoing vigilance regarding fading levels of intraoperative anesthesia. Another potential disadvantage of 2-chloroprocaine is its anomalous action of decreasing the analgesic effectiveness of subsequently administered neuraxial opioids (181). Although 2-chloroprocaine has binding affinity at the μ and κ opioid receptor sites, it may not act through an opioid receptor in terms of this antagonism (182). In addition, animal studies have shown that pretreatment with chloroprocaine may interfere with the local anesthetic action of subsequently administered bupivacaine (183).

Concerns regarding 2-chloroprocaine neurotoxicity and arachnoiditis following inadvertent intrathecal injections were initially thought to be related to a combination of low pH and contained preservatives (184,185). Replacement of metabisulfite and methylparaben with safer preservatives has presumably decreased the risk of neurotoxicity. Although recent reports advocate the use of spinal chloroprocaine, its use remains controversial (186,187) (see also Chapter 12).

Spinal Analgesia

Intrathecal injection of local anesthesia and/or opioid produces very rapid onset and effective analgesia in labor. This single injection has a limited duration of action and cannot provide the flexibility of a catheter technique. However, intrathecal injection can be a useful method of providing analgesia to facilitate instrumental deliveries in a patient without an epidural catheter in situ. In addition, analgesia can be rapidly achieved with intrathecal injection of medication, which in a very distressed patient may allow more controlled conditions for subsequent epidural catheter placement.

In the situation in which unanticipated dural puncture occurs during attempted epidural placement, intrathecal insertion of the catheter should be considered. This can produce excellent analgesia in labor and may reduce the risk of the development of post–dural puncture headache (PDPH) (188).

Continuous spinal analgesia may be considered in these cases of accidental dural puncture or in the very high-risk parturient in whom an effective regional anesthesia may be required urgently (188). Appropriate safety measures should be put in place to prevent accidental local anesthetic overdosage during administration of top-ups or transfer to the operating room for cesarean delivery. These safety measures should include appropriate labeling, disclosure to the patient and nurses, and use of a closed system for administration of drug.

The use of small-bore intrathecal catheters for administration of local anesthesia has been shown to be associated with rapid onset of analgesia with a potentially reduced risk of PDPH (188). However, these microcatheters were withdrawn from clinical practice because of reports of CES associated with their use. Inadequate mixing of local anesthetic solutions within the CSF and pooling of high concentrations of potentially neurotoxic local anesthetic agents (5% lidocaine) were considered to be responsible for this problem (189,190). A recent study reevaluated spinal catheters and concluded that they were safe (191). The concept of intrathecal catheter use in clinical practice has been well received; however, much work needs to be done prior to their full acceptance into the practice of obstetric anesthesia. Appropriate catheter placement can be technically difficult to achieve, especially with degenerative disease of the lumbar spine. In addition, catheter-over-needle techniques (22-gauge Spinocath, B. Braun) may have several advantages compared to the microcatheter (28-gauge Portex). The larger catheters have been shown to be associated with improved insertion, maintenance, and clinical effects, and with a potentially reduced risk of catheter breakage and neurotoxicity (192–194).

Combined Spinal–Epidural Analgesia

Combined spinal–epidural techniques for labor analgesia offer effective, rapid-onset analgesia with minimal motor block, and with the flexibility of prolonging the duration of analgesia as required via the epidural catheter. In addition, at any time, surgical anesthesia can be readily achieved should operative delivery be required. The near immediate onset of spinal analgesia is ideal for use in the labor suite, and the duration of action (2–3 hours) is often sufficient for delivery. The insertion of the epidural catheter gives added security should emergency

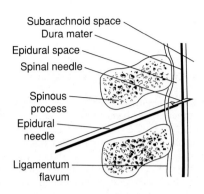
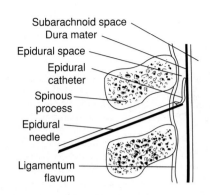

FIGURE 24-14. The needle-through-needle technique. From Birnbach DJ, Datta S, Gatt SP (eds.). *Textbook of Obstetric Anesthesia.* New York: Churchill Livingstone, 2000, with permission.

cesarean delivery become necessary. The duration of spinal analgesia with bupivacaine and sufentanil has been shown to be dependent on the extent of cervical dilatation and stage of labor at time of placement. Shorter durations of analgesia were associated with advanced labor (7–10 cm cervical dilatation) (195). Use of CSE in labor has been associated with a high degree of patient satisfaction compared to standard epidural techniques, possibly because of the rapid onset, reduced motor block, and feeling among patients of having greater self-control (196,197).

Intrathecal labor analgesia was initially described with use of sufentanil or fentanyl; however, the addition of "isobaric" bupivacaine to opioids has been shown to produce excellent and prolonged sensory blockade with minimal motor deficit (198,199). Intrathecal doses of fentanyl 25 μg or sufentanil 10 μg were initially described; however, evidence suggests that lower doses of sufentanil (5 μg) or fentanyl (15 μg) may be sufficient to achieve labor analgesia (169,200). In addition, recent studies have suggested that ropivacaine and levobupivacaine can be substituted for intrathecal bupivacaine to provide labor analgesia (201). Although 2.5 mg bupivacaine was originally described for intrathecal use, many anesthesiologist are now using half that dose (199,200).

The minimal motor blockade associated with the CSE techniques theoretically allows the parturient to ambulate. Other potential advantages over conventional epidural placement include good coverage of the sacral dermatomes with more complete, uniform analgesia and a lack of negative impact on the duration and progress of labor. In healthy nulliparous parturients in early labor, CSE was also associated with more rapid cervical dilation compared to epidural analgesia (202,203).

Combined spinal–epidural analgesia can be accomplished using a variety of techniques: The epidural space can be cannulated using a standard technique, with the spinal analgesia administered one interspace below; a single-level epidural needle can be placed beside the spinal needle, using specially designed needles; and the most common approach uses a single-segment "needle-through-needle" technique (Fig. 24-14). In this technique, a standard epidural needle or specially designed CSE epidural needle (for example, the Espocan needle, B. Braun) is used to identify the epidural space and, through this, entry into the intrathecal space is achieved using a long, finebore, atraumatic pencil-point spinal needle. Once flow of CSF is confirmed, appropriate medication is injected intrathecally and the spinal needle is withdrawn. The epidural catheter is then advanced into the epidural space. Various commercial interlocking/docking systems are available to prevent movement of the spinal needle within the epidural needle during intrathecal injection. Despite the development of the locking needle system, comparison of single-segment needle-through-needle (with interlock), needle-through-needle with epidural needle "back-eye," and two-segment technique in orthopedic surgery showed no time advantage and demonstrated a higher incidence of technical problems, including unsuccessful CSE technique and damaged spinal needles (204). A recent obstetric anesthesia study however, suggested that the back-hole epidural needle may be associated with a decreased incidence of paresthesia during spinal needle placement (205). Occasionally, despite epidural placement of the epidural needle, no CSF can be obtained via the spinal needle, as illustrated in Figure 24-15.

The rapid onset of profound spinal analgesia associated with spinal opioids is ideal in labor, especially when it is advanced. Side effects include pruritus, nausea and vomiting, and urinary retention. Respiratory depression due to cephalad spread of opioid may occur, but is very rare when using lipid-soluble opioids. In addition, in contrast with morphine, if respiratory depression occurs, it is almost immediately after spinal injection (206,207). There is some suggestion of possible increased frequency of nonreassuring fetal heart rate tracing and fetal bradycardia associated with CSE (208–210). The etiology of fetal bradycardia following CSE remains unclear, but it may be related to an acute reduction in systemic maternal catecholamines resulting from rapid onset of analgesia. Also, it has been postulated that an imbalance between epinephrine and norepinephrine levels causes unopposed α-adrenoceptor effects on uterine tone and may decrease uterine blood flow (211,212). However, preliminary reports suggest there may be no alteration in uteroplacental blood flow (213). If it occurs, the resulting short-lived fetal bradycardia is usually self-limiting (208). Therefore, these cases do not generally require an emergency cesarean delivery. A retrospective study of 1,240 patients who received regional labor analgesia (CSE 98%) and 1,140 patient who received parenteral medication or no analgesia demonstrated no significant difference in the rates of cesarean delivery, with rates of 1.3% and 1.4%, respectively. No emergency cesarean deliveries were performed for acute fetal distress in the absence of obstetric indications up to 90 minutes following intrathecal sufentanil administration (214).

Continuous Epidural Infusion

Labor analgesia is commonly initiated by either conventional epidural or intrathecal medication, and is then followed by a continuous epidural infusion technique.

Local anesthetics such as ropivacaine, bupivacaine, and levobupivacaine in concentrations ranging from 0.0625% to 0.125% have been described alone or in combination with

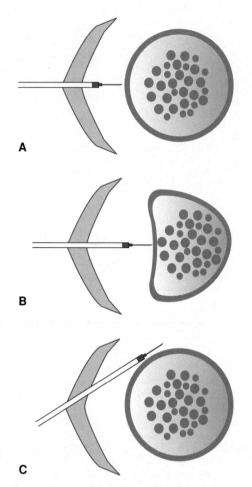

FIGURE 24-15. Reasons for combined spinal–epidural failure. **A:** Length of spinal needle is too short. **B:** Tenting of the dura. **C:** Malposition of the epidural needle off midline. Modified from Birnbach DJ, Datta S, Gatt SP (eds.). *Textbook of Obstetric Anesthesia.* New York: Churchill Livingstone, 2000, with permission.

opioids (215–217). Larger concentrations are seldom required and are invariably associated with motor blockade.

Use of epidural infusions in labor should be associated with smooth maintenance of analgesia and allow titration of dose to effect. Earlier studies suggested that use of infusions was associated with a reduced risk of cesarean delivery in primiparous women (218). A systematic review of epidural analgesia using low concentrations of bupivacaine compared to parenteral opioid analgesia revealed no increase in the rate of cesarean delivery and improved quality of analgesia. It was suggested, however, that the second stage of labor was prolonged using the former and that there was a potentially higher risk of instrumental vaginal delivery (219). This does not appear to be the case with current practice.

Comparison of CSE and low-dose epidural infusion techniques with traditional epidural techniques (intermittent bolus top-ups) revealed that infusion techniques were associated with a lower incidence of instrumental delivery but a higher incidence of Apgar scores of 7 or less at 5 minutes (220). Compared to traditional epidural techniques, continuous infusions were reported to be as effective, and CSE techniques superior in terms of pain relief, with reduced incidence of instrumental delivery (220). When evaluated by the National Institutes

of Health, the consensus was that neuraxial analgesia is not associated with increased risk of cesarean delivery (221,222).

Adjuvant Agents for Neuraxial Analgesia

The use of clonidine, neostigmine, and epinephrine as neuraxial adjuvants in obstetric practice has been shown to enhance analgesia with minimal side effects (223,224). The addition of epinephrine to this infusion has been shown to improve quality of analgesia by possibly reducing vascular uptake and/or systemic absorption of local anesthetic, or by a direct agonist effect on α_2 spinal receptors (225). However, addition of epinephrine (1:800,000) to bupivacaine and sufentanil infusion has been shown to be associated with improved analgesia at the expense of increased incidence of motor block and a potentially prolonged second stage of labor. In one study, lower Apgar scores were also reported at 1 and 5 minutes in the epinephrine group (226).

Patient-controlled Epidural Analgesia

Use of PCEA in labor offers several potential advantages, including improved analgesia, patient satisfaction, reduced dose of local anesthetic, and fewer physician interventions (227,228). This reduction in local anesthetic dose was shown to diminish the risk of side effects, including motor blockade and hypotension. Patient satisfaction was shown to be high, presumably due to independence and self control of analgesia.

Options for PCEA during labor include continuous infusion plus demand-dose, or demand-dose only (229). Comparison of epidural infusion of ropivacaine 0.16% solution with sufentanil 0.5 μg/mL with a PCEA bolus of 4 mL (lockout 20 minutes) or demand alone with PCEA bolus of 4 mL (lock out 15 minutes) found the continuous infusion to be more effective in treating pain in the parturient without any increase in dose requirement (230). Background infusions were not found to be beneficial in another study in terms of patient satisfaction and were shown to be associated with a greater consumption of ropivacaine 0.1%. This study also suggested that demand-only regimens were not associated with a higher incidence of physician/midwife intervention (231).

REGIONAL ANESTHESIA FOR CESAREAN DELIVERY

Cesarean delivery has become the most common hospital-based operative procedure in the United States, accounting for approximately 30% of all live births. The increased incidence of operative delivery has been attributed to the broadening of the definition of *fetal distress.* In addition, the increased incidence of cesarean delivery has had an effect on the incidence of repeat elective cesarean delivery (232). Cesarean delivery can be associated with risks from anesthesia, puerperal infection, and venous thromboembolism. A population-based case control study performed in France estimated the risk of postpartum death to be 3.6 times higher after cesarean section compared to vaginal delivery. The risks associated with postpartum hemorrhage did not differ between vaginal and cesarean delivery (233). However, a study performed in the United States suggested that cesarean delivery might be a marker for the existence of preexisting morbidities associated with increased mortality risk, rather than an independent risk factor for death.

This raises the question of difficulty in separating preexisting mortality risk from delivery method (234). The same difficulty could be considered in relation to preexisting mortality risk, and the impact that risk has on the choice and outcome of anesthetic technique employed by choice or by clinical circumstance. Neonatal mortality rates were also found to be higher among infants delivered by cesarean delivery (1.77 per 1,000 live births) compared with those delivered vaginally (0.62 per 1,000 live births) even after adjustment for deaths secondary to congenital malformations, demographic, and medical factors (235). Despite these data, many consider it a woman's right to choose an elective primary cesarean delivery, and there is much debate regarding nonmedical indications for cesarean delivery (236–238).

The most common indications for cesarean delivery in obstetric practice include nonreassuring fetal status, failure to progress, cephalopelvic disproportion, malpresentation, issues related to prematurity, and prior uterine surgery. Fetal macrosomia is increasing as obesity and diabetes increase, and this may have an impact on caesarean rates. The technique of anesthesia for cesarean delivery depends on the indications for the surgery, degree of urgency of delivery, maternal–fetal status, and the wishes of the patient (239). In addition, the anticipated duration of the procedure must also be considered. For example, a single-injection spinal anesthetic may be insufficient if the routine duration of surgery is in excess of 90 minutes.

Anesthesia-related complications are the sixth most common cause of maternal death in pregnancy in the United States. The anesthesia-related maternal mortality rate decreased from 4.3 per million live births between 1979 and 1981, to 1.7 million in the period between 1988 and 1990. Maternal deaths related to general anaesthesia were higher than those associated with regional anesthesia. The mortality related to regional anesthesia was predominantly related to issues of toxic levels of local anesthetics and excessively high levels of regional block. The evidence suggests that the mortality associated with regional anesthesia is decreasing, possibly because of technical developments in the specialty. The number of deaths involving general anesthesia, however, has remained relatively constant. The relative risk of fatality during general anesthesia was estimated to be more than 16 times that of regional anesthesia (240), although with the development of alternative methods for securing the airway after failed intubation (e.g., laryngeal mask airway [LMA] and Combitube), this statistic may decrease.

General anesthesia has the potential advantages of speed of induction, definitive airway maintenance, and a theoretically greater control over the degree of sympathectomy compared with regional techniques. The institutional frequency of general anesthesia for cesarean delivery can depend on many factors, including the numbers of patients receiving epidural analgesia, the percentage of high-risk parturients within the institute, and the skills of the anesthesiologist. Although no absolute contraindications to general anesthesia exist, previous history of failed intubation, uninvestigated family history of malignant hyperthermia, or anticipated airway difficulties may require modification of anesthetic technique. Potential causes of morbidity or mortality with general anesthesia for cesarean delivery includes failed intubation, aspiration pneumonitis, neonatal depression, and risks of maternal awareness. However, general anesthesia is considered to be the ideal technique for certain conditions, including massive maternal hemorrhage, overt coagulopathy, imminent fetal demise, or in cases in which a patient refuses regional anesthesia despite appropriate risk–benefit discussion during the consent process (111).

Data suggest that the use of general anesthesia for cesarean delivery has been steadily decreasing in the United States. In general, regional anesthetic techniques avoid the need for endotracheal intubation and thus avoid the risks associated with failed intubation and aspiration of gastric contents. The avoidance of the risks of IV and inhalational anesthesia and their associated neurologic and cardiovascular depressant effects is also of benefit to both mother and fetus. Most mothers express a preference for regional anesthesia and enjoy being awake and partaking (with or without an accompanying partner) in the birth experience, despite any accompanying hypotension-induced nausea. In addition, blood loss may be reduced under regional anesthesia for cesarean delivery (241,242).

Spinal Anesthesia

Spinal anesthesia offers many advantages for cesarean delivery. Intrathecal anesthesia has a rapid onset and provides a dense neural block. Small doses of local anesthetic with or without opioid are used, thus there is little risk of local anesthetic toxicity and placental transfer of drug is minimal. In addition, the failure rates for spinal anesthesia, including incomplete or failed blocks, are lower than with epidural blocks (243). Disadvantages of this technique include the finite duration of anesthesia and a higher incidence of hypotension and associated nausea and vomiting (244). Intrathecal hyperbaric bupivacaine is the most commonly used anesthetic agent for cesarean delivery. Its duration of action of up to 2 hours correlates well with the average duration of surgery. Although calculation of the appropriate intrathecal dose can be done using patient height parameters, many physicians use a set dose of hyperbaric bupivacaine because height, weight, and body mass index parameters appear to have little or no correlation with block height (245) (see Chapter 10).

Increased doses of spinal anesthetic are associated with increases in level of block; doses above 15 mg significantly increase the risk of complications of high motor block and longer duration of anesthesia (246). The availability of spinal hyperbaric bupivacaine varies internationally, and it is marketed in concentrations of 0.5%, 0.75%, and 1.0%. The level of spinal anesthesia achieved following intrathecal injection appears to be unrelated to the concentration of the agent; however, the quality of sensory block may be improved with 0.75% bupivacaine compared to the 0.5% concentration in similar doses (247). Studies comparing 0.75% with 1.0% bupivacaine found no difference in onset times or quality of block. There was, however, an increased incidence of backache reported in the bupivacaine 1.0% group (248). Use of a single intrathecal injection of local anesthetic with or without opioid has been shown to provide rapid onset of effective anesthesia at a decreased cost, compared to epidural anesthesia (249).

The optimal position for initiation of central neuraxial block in relation to patient comfort, uteroplacental perfusion, and associated risks of intravascular injection have been discussed previously (113–116). Spinal anesthesia can be initiated with the parturient in the sitting or the lateral position. Plain or hyperbaric solutions can be used, although most clinicians currently favor hyperbaric preparations for cesarean anesthesia. The sitting position has been shown to have advantages in the performance of central neuraxial blockade in obese parturients as it reduces the distance between skin and central neuraxis (250). Hyperbaric solutions exhibit a greater predictability of block height compared to plain solutions, and further adjustment of block height can be achieved safely by adjusting table position (251). Regional anesthesia to the sensory level of

T4–T5 appears to be an appropriate predictive level for a pain-free cesarean delivery (252). Despite achieving this level of anesthesia, many women experience some degree of visceral discomfort during cesarean delivery, especially when exteriorization of the uterus is performed to facilitate repair. Interestingly, exteriorization of the uterus for repair was associated with a decrease in postoperative febrile days, no difference in blood loss, and a nonsignificant trend toward increased nausea and vomiting when performed under a regional anesthetic technique (253). Those adjuvant agents injected intrathecally that have been shown to improve the quality of the spinal anesthesia include epinephrine, morphine, and either fentanyl or sufentanil (254–257).

Epidural Anesthesia

Epidural anesthesia for cesarean delivery is indicated when the flexibility to prolong the duration of anesthesia is required, as when difficult surgery is anticipated. This may be necessary if there is a history of complicated pregnancy, anatomic abnormalities, or multiple previous cesarean deliveries. If the indication for surgery is failure to progress, presumed fetal jeopardy, or problematic labor in a parturient with an existing labor epidural, appropriate dosing of the in situ epidural can provide levels of anesthesia sufficient for cesarean delivery (T4). Occasionally, in high-risk parturients, elective early preemptive placement and appropriate testing of an epidural catheter can ensure effective functioning should emergency cesarean delivery be necessary. This situation highlights the importance of continual assessment of epidural catheter effectiveness during labor analgesia. High-risk cases may also be performed using an elective spinal catheter technique and are discussed later in this chapter.

Administration of an epidural local anesthetic with rapid onset of sensory block and with a reproducible duration of action is ideal for use in cesarean delivery. Commonly used agents include 2-chloroprocaine, lidocaine, levobupivacaine, and bupivacaine. Unlike spinal anesthesia, larger doses of local anesthetic are used to achieve the appropriate levels for cesarean delivery, thus concerns exist regarding systemic toxicity. Epidural catheters may migrate, and therefore consideration must be given to aspiration tests, repeat test dosing, and intermittent injections of local anesthetic to avoid the risks of intrathecal or intravascular injection. Safer drugs (such as chloroprocaine and lidocaine) or the newer amide local anesthetics (such as ropivacaine and levobupivacaine) should be considered when available.

Epidural adjuncts can be used to improve the quality of epidural anesthesia. Since local anesthetics are all weak bases prepared in an acidic solution, they are ionized and do not readily cross lipid membranes. Adding small quantities of sodium bicarbonate ($NaHCO_3$) can increase the pH of the local anesthetic solution and, in so doing, increase the proportion of nonionized local anesthetic. This can result in a faster onset of action (258). The addition of $NaHCO_3$ to solution increases the speed of onset of action of lidocaine and chloroprocaine; however, not all studies have demonstrated this effect with bupivacaine (259). In addition, lower doses of $NaHCO_3$ must be used with bupivacaine (0.1 mEq per 20 mL local anesthetic) to avoid risks of precipitation. Commercially prepared solutions of local anesthetic with epinephrine have a lower pH, therefore have a slower onset time. The addition of epinephrine to the local anesthetic immediately before injection may achieve more rapid anesthesia with lidocaine; however, this may not be the case with bupivacaine (260,261).

The quality of intraoperative epidural analgesia can be improved with use of other adjuvants, including fentanyl (50–100 µg) or sufentanil (10–20 µg) (262,263). Clonidine has also been used as an additive to epidural local anesthetic solutions; however, its use has been associated with side effects including sedation, bradycardia, and hypotension (264).

Combined Spinal–Epidural Technique

Use of CSE was described for cesarean delivery in 1984, and it is widely used for both labor analgesia and cesarean delivery anesthesia (265). The CSE technique has the advantage of producing a rapid onset of surgical anesthesia while allowing for the flexibility of an epidural technique, with the ability to prolong or extend the level of block as required. Placement of an epidural catheter may also have a dose-sparing effect on the initial intrathecal dose, thus potentially reducing the incidence of high spinal block and hypotension (266). In addition, this technique allows decreased (mini-dose) spinal doses, which may be associated with a reduction in side effects. Epidural administration of preservative-free normal saline to extend the level of spinal anesthesia has been described (267).

Disadvantages of CSE include the inability to fully test the catheter in the presence of dense spinal anesthesia. In addition, enhanced spread of intrathecal dosage has been described after early administration of medication through the epidural catheter (268). However, this phenomenon can also be seen as an advantage, and can be exploited as a method of increasing the level of spinal anesthesia if required (269).

Continuous Spinal Anesthesia

Continuous spinal anesthesia has many potential advantages over single-bolus intrathecal injection or continuous epidural techniques. The classic technique required the use of large-bore epidural needles/catheters; as technology evolved, continuous spinal anesthesia could be performed using 32-gauge microcatheters inserted through an intrathecally placed spinal needle (270). The technique gained in popularity in the 1980s, despite technical difficulties, but was abandoned following withdrawal of approval for microcatheters by the FDA. Continuous intrathecal infusions may have an advantage, especially in high-risk parturients, in whom careful titration of incremental subarachnoid dosage is required to maintain hemodynamic stability. To reduce the risk of headache associated with insertion of a "macrocatheter," it has been suggested that the introducer needle be turned, so that it is parallel to the dural fibers at the time of puncture. Further prophylactic measures for headache reduction include leaving the catheter in situ for more than 12 hours and injecting a bolus of preservative-free normal saline prior to removal of the spinal catheter (271).

Central neuraxial anesthesia–induced sympathectomy leads to peripheral vasodilatation, reduced preload, and subsequently decreased cardiac output. The incidence and extent of hypotension depends on the height of the block, the parturient's position, and whether appropriate measures were instituted prophylactically to minimize hypotension (48). Fluid preloading and avoidance of aortocaval compression with left uterine displacement to avoid further mechanical reductions in preload can decrease the risk. Continuous fetal heart rate monitoring allows appropriate intervention should maternal hemodynamic instability have a detrimental effect on fetal status. With early recognition and appropriate prompt treatment, transient maternal hypotension should not be associated with maternal or neonatal morbidity (272,273). Treatment of central neuraxial blockade–induced hypotension includes maternal and fetal resuscitation, including maternal oxygen delivery, optimal lateral uterine displacement, and increased IV fluid administration. Use of ephedrine (initially boluses of 5–10 mg IV) and phenylephrine (50–100 μg) as vasopressors have been extensively described (52,53). The *prophylactic* administration of commonly used doses of ephedrine appears to provide no benefit (53,274,275).

Many methods for preventing hypotension during spinal anesthesia for cesarean delivery have been investigated, but no single technique has proved to be completely effective and reliable. Use of simultaneous rapid crystalloid infusion (cohydration) with titration of high-dose phenylephrine (100 μg/min) immediately following subarachnoid injection to achieve normotension has been described as an effective treatment to reduce the risk of hypotension during cesarean delivery (48).

Complications

Accidental Dural Puncture

A relatively common and problematic complication of epidural placement in the pregnant patient is that of accidental dural puncture. This complication can lead to the development of PDPH in up to 70% of cases (276). Orthostatic positional headache following dural puncture is pathognomonic of PDPH. The parturient may describe bilateral occipital and/or frontal headache, often accompanied by photophobia, nausea, vomiting, visual symptoms, and occasionally mental changes. Auditory symptoms include tinnitus and hearing loss, although vestibular dysfunction has also been reported following spinal anesthesia independent of PDPH (277,278,279).

The incidence of PDPH has been reported at between 10% and 70% of patients following dural puncture. Technical factors related to this relationship include needle size, needle tip characteristics, and the orientation of the tip on dural penetration (280,281). A direct relationship exists between the degree of CSF leakage and the size of the dural puncture. However, increased technical difficulty is associated with use of smaller needles, and potential failure of the technique must be balanced against efforts to avoid PDPH. A lower incidence of PDPH occurs with the use of noncutting atraumatic needles compared to the traditional cutting needle. A comparison of smaller-bore cutting needles (27 gauge) and larger-gauge atraumatic needles (25 gauge) revealed a PDPH incidence of 2.7% with the former and 1.2% with the latter, showing the importance of needle design characteristics over size (280,281). Use of the blunt tip is thought to produce a nonuniform hole in the dura, which may be associated with increased inflammatory response, thus promoting closure of defect. In theory, the relevance of bevel orientation and needle characteristics in relation to separation as opposed to cutting of dural fibers is likely to be of lesser relevance given the complex anatomic structure of the dural fibers on electron microscopy (282,283). The dura has been shown to be comprised of many overlapping layers in multiple planes, thus creation of a defect specifically parallel to theses fibers would be extremely difficult (284).

Independent risk factors for the development of PDPH include female gender, pregnancy, and age 20 to 50 years, thus careful attention to technique in obstetric practice is essential. The incidence of PDPH in obstetric analgesia and analgesia is thought to be between 1.1% and 5.2%, depending on needle size and tip characteristics (285). As previously mentioned, up to 70% of patients will develop PDPH following accidental dural puncture during the course of epidural insertion. However, not all postpartum headaches occur as a result of a dural puncture (286,287,288,289). A review of headaches in the parturient showed symptoms in 15% of parturients who did not receive an epidural, and in 12% of parturients who had an epidural with no evidence of dural puncture (286). Other causes of headache in the postpartum period include nonspecific headache, migraine, hypertension, caffeine withdrawal, pneumocephalus, infection (including sinusitis and meningitis), cortical vein thrombosis, and intracerebral pathology. One report also described neurocysticercosis, which presented initially as positional headache following spinal anesthesia (287). Therefore, a thorough history and physical examination is essential in the assessment of all patients complaining of PDPH to ensure additional pathology is not missed. Changes in quality of headaches, loss of the postural component, or onset of new neurologic signs may indicate additional pathology that requires immediate attention and further workup.

The pathophysiology of PDPH is unclear, although an imbalance is thought exist between CSF production and leakage through a presumed dural puncture. Prevention of PDPH in obstetric anesthesia depends on operator and technical factors. Needle selection is critical, as smaller-gauge atraumatic needles have the lowest incidence of PDPH. In addition, insertion of cutting needles with their orientation parallel to the long axis of the spinal cord also appears to reduce the incidence of PDPH (290,291,292,293,294). Use of a paramedian approach to spinal anesthesia has been suggested to be associated with a lower incidence of PDPH, as the angle of dural puncture may create a self-sealing defect in the dura. However, familiarity with use of the paramedian approach to neuraxial block has been shown to be low in a review of regional anesthesia practice, and it has been suggested that failure rates are higher with this technique. Comparison between paramedian and midline approaches to the epidural space showed speed of catheter insertion to be faster using the paramedian approach. There was also a trend toward a higher incidence of paraesthesias with the midline approach in female patients, although not statistically significant (295).

The traditional management of accidental dural puncture is to resite the epidural at a different interspace. Recently, however, many anesthesiologists have advocated that the epidural catheter should be passed into the subarachnoid space, thus providing intrathecal delivery of local anesthetic as a continuous spinal technique. This establishes rapid and effective pain relief. Analysis of aggregate data from limited retrospective trials demonstrates a significant reduction in the incidence of PDPH and the subsequent need for epidural blood patch (EBP) in those patients who receive continuous spinal analgesia after unintentional dural puncture (188,296). In addition, the catheter provides excellent labor analgesia and a route toward almost instant onset of blockade for cesarean delivery. Some evidence suggests that by maintaining CSF volume, a reduction in PDPH can be observed, and the injection of up to 10 mL of preservative-free normal saline following inadvertent dural puncture has been advocated (271). Insertion of an intrathecal catheter for a period of 24 hours through the dural deficit following inadvertent dural puncture with an 18-gauge Tuohy needle has been shown to reduce the incidence of PDPH (296). Other measures that have been advocated include a combination of reinjection of CSF immediately, insertion of an epidural catheter intrathecally for analgesia/anesthesia, injection of preservative-free normal saline through the intrathecal catheter prior to catheter removal, and administration of continuous intrathecal labor analgesia (271).

Symptoms of PDPH tend to occur as early as 24 hours and as late as 7 days following dural puncture (297). If symptoms occur earlier, one should consider pneumocephalus. The symptoms typically last from 12 hours to 7 days, and occasionally even longer. Therefore, any decision to treat PDPH should be made with a degree of caution. Medical management, interventional treatments, and placement of intrathecal catheters are all associated with their own inherent risks that may outweigh any potential morbidity associated with PDPH. That said, PDPH is often very severe, precluding ambulation, hospital discharge, and maternal care of the newborn.

Generally, PDPH is initially treated conservatively with increased intake of oral or IV fluid, often with supplemental administration of caffeine and regular analgesics. Bed rest gives good symptomatic relief but with little therapeutic benefit. No evidence shows that increasing the fluid intake will cause a greater production of CSF. Aggressive fluid rehydration is common practice, although little evidence suggests that fluid and medical management has any impact on pain scores in PDPH unless the patient is severely dehydrated (298). Conversely, this may lead to more frequent bathroom trips and less periods of recumbency, with the potential to worsen headache symptoms.

Drugs that have been used to treat PDPH include caffeine (methylxanthines), vasopressin, theophylline, sumatriptan, and adrenocorticotrophic hormone. Caffeine is a central nervous stimulant and has cerebral vasoconstrictor activity. The benefits of caffeine in the management of PDPH appear to be transient. Oral doses of 300 mg have been described or IV doses of 500 mg/L of normal saline (repeated after 4 hours) (299). In addition, caffeine is more likely to be successful following a headache caused by a small-gauge spinal needle, rather than one caused following an accidental "wet-tap" during the course of epidural placement. Caffeine may be associated with undesirable side effects such as insomnia and irritability (300). In addition, there also have been reports of grand mal seizures and cardiac arrhythmias following caffeine administration (301,302). Caffeine levels can be detected in breast milk in the postpartum period, although this has not been found to have a deleterious effect on the newborn (303). Use of prophylactic IV caffeine (500 mg/L normal saline) within 90 minutes of spinal anesthesia (unlike oral caffeine) was shown to be an effective preemptive treatment to avoid PDPH in general and orthopedic surgery, but this has not been used in obstetric anesthesia (304). Theophylline can also produce cerebral vasoconstriction and is available in a long-acting formulation. A paucity of information exists regarding its effectiveness, which has not been studied in a randomized, double-blinded fashion. The serotonin agonist sumatriptan (which has cerebral vasoconstriction properties and is routinely used to treat migraine headaches) may have a role to play in management of PDPH (305). Subcutaneous doses of 6 mg of sumatriptan have been described with mixed results (305–308). Adrenocorticotrophic hormone infusion has also been anecdotally reported as an effective treatment for PDPH (309).

The decision to proceed with more invasive treatments in the management of PDPH should be made following careful discussion with the patient in terms of risk–benefit analysis. If the PDPH symptoms are intolerable, limit ambulation, or are associated with neurologic symptoms related to the dural puncture (such as double vision), an EBP is advisable. This administration of autologous blood into the epidural space has become the most effective means of PDPH treatment. Complete success rates have been reported in approximately 75% of patients. The effectiveness of EBP as a treatment of PDPH appears to be related to the size of the needle used during original puncture of the dura (310). Immediate relief has been described in 88% to 96% of patients following EBP for PDPH;

however, postprocedure follow-up has revealed less promising results. Patients reported return of their symptoms to a lesser extent (16%–36%), with symptoms continuing until gradual resolution in all patients. Most important, a high degree of patient satisfaction was reported with this treatment of PDPH (311).

Contraindications for EBP are the same as for all regional anesthetic techniques. Ethical issues related to performance of EBP in patients of Jehovah's Witness faith has led to use of alternative techniques including closed-loop systems of autologous blood collection, although EBP without modification of technique may be accepted by some members (312). Regional anesthesia is not recommended in the presence of systemic sepsis, and administration of autologous blood into the epidural space is therefore relatively contraindicated in a febrile patient (313). As previously mentioned, the precise method by which EBP exerts its benefit is unclear. The success of an EBP is not solely due to a direct blockade of the dural puncture, as the CSF volume replacement is not sufficiently rapid to account for the immediate resolution of headache. Other explanations for the effectiveness of EBP include the increase in CSF pressure and cerebral vasoconstriction (314). There is some controversy regarding the optimal volume of blood to be injected; however, most anesthesiologists use 15 to 25 mL of blood and stop injection if severe pain is experienced. Although the incidence of complications (especially back pain) increases with increased volume, it appears that increased volume also increases the success rate (315).

Epidural blood injectate has been shown to spread both longitudinally and circumferentially over up to four vertebral levels, thus reducing the intradural volume, pushing the cranial contents cephalad, and reducing meningeal traction (315,316). Epidural blood patches have been shown to produce a focal hematoma around the injection site, thus compressing the thecal sac and nerve roots and possibly producing tamponade (317). This effect has been shown to have resolved radiologically by 7 hours; however, widely distributed clots adherent to the thecal sac are still evident at 18 hours (318). Radiologic studies using radiopaque dye while performing EBP have demonstrated that blood inserted into the epidural space will travel one space below the level of insertion of the epidural needle and up to four spaces above the site (316). However, endogenous bridging of the dural defect may be well established by the clot resolution. Failure of EBP has been described in the presence of technical factors, if performed within 24 hours, or if residual local anesthetic is present in the epidural space (319,320).

In view of the cephalad spread of injectate, EBP is commonly performed caudal to the site of dural puncture. Remaining supine following EBP for up to 2 hours has been shown to be associated with greater benefit from treatment compared to 30 minutes in the supine position (321).

Other agents that have been described in the management of PDPH include fibrin glue and epidural Dextran-40 (322–324). Surgical and computed tomography–guided techniques are sometimes considered should severe symptoms persist (323). Complications associated with EBP are few and similar to any central neuraxial regional technique. Transient low back and radicular symptoms have been described that may be related to the presence of blood at a foraminal level, as shown radiologically (315).

Total Spinal Anesthesia

Total spinal anesthesia is a rare and life-threatening complication that occurs following excessive cephalad spread of local anesthetic. It has been reported following spinal anesthesia, the intrathecal spread of epidural medication (for example, following unintentional dural puncture or catheter migration), or subdural injection (325,326). Single-injection spinal anesthesia preformed subsequent to failed spinal anesthesia or partial epidural blockade may also precipitate total spinal anesthesia (327). Several possible mechanisms exist for high spinal blocks in this clinical scenario. Compression of the spinal canal may result from the presence of epidural injectate, with a reduction in intradural volume. This may precipitate excessive cephalad spread of intrathecal drug and rising levels of blockade. Transfer of local anesthetic across the dura from the epidural space through a dural hole may also occur. In addition, dose requirements of local anesthetic may be reduced in the presence of partial epidural blockade (328).

In the case of a nonemergent cesarean delivery with a nonuniform block, several options are available to the obstetric anesthesiologist. An epidural catheter can be resited, and the level of anesthesia titrated using this more effective delivery alternative. Alternatively, CSE can be placed, in which a fraction of the usual intrathecal dose can be administered; again, the catheter can be used to titrate to a desired level. Continuous spinal anesthesia may also be considered. If the procedure is totally elective, the patient can be transferred to the postanesthesia care unit until the partial block resolves, and thereafter a repeat spinal injection can then be performed.

Because of changes in obstetric practice and the changing medicolegal environment in which we now practice, every parturient should be considered a potential candidate for emergency cesarean delivery; therefore, strict attention should be given to the quality of epidural analgesia. Efforts should be made at a departmental level to have policies in place to ensure that poorly functioning epidural catheters are identified and replaced.

NEUROLOGIC COMPLICATIONS

The incidence of permanent neurologic injury following regional anesthesia is exceedingly rare. Central neuraxial techniques account for in excess of 70% of regional blocks, and permanent neurologic injury has been estimated at between 0.02% and 0.07% (329). A comprehensive retrospective Swedish study revealed a risk of 0.004% of permanent neurologic injury following epidural injection (330) (see Chapter 12).

The American Society of Anesthesiologists Closed Claim Project evaluates adverse outcomes in anesthesia collected from closed anesthesia malpractice insurance claims. Analysis of claims between 1980 and 1999 related to regional anesthesia in both obstetric and nonobstetric neuraxial blocks revealed a total of 1,005 claims. Obstetric anesthesia had a higher proportion of neuraxial anesthesia claims with temporary and low-severity injury (71%), compared with the nonobstetric group (38%) (331,332) (see Chapter 12).

Neurologic complications in obstetric patients can occur because of both obstetric- and anesthesia-related factors. Although the presence of existing neurologic disease is not an absolute contraindication for regional anesthesia, careful consideration of both maternal and fetal factors is essential prior to proceeding with central neuraxial anesthesia (333). Specific, guided history taking and clinical evaluation is necessary prior to performing any regional technique. Exacerbation of preexisting neurologic deficits has been reported following central neuraxial blockade in patients who did not volunteer their neurologic history (334) (see Chapter 12).

Paresthesia or pain on injection of medication is a warning sign of the potential for neurologic injury, and adjustment of technique or resiting of the needle/catheter should be considered to avoid further injury (329). Neurologic injury in obstetrics can be independent of anesthesia, directly related to anesthesia, or indirectly related to anesthesia, which can have a contributory effect on the condition (335,336). Neurologic examination of postpartum women may reveal asymptomatic transient postpartum sensory dysfunction in up to 21% of parturients, and these signs are often unrelated to regional anesthesia (337).

Neurologic complications are five times more common after childbirth itself than after regional blockade (338). Many postpartum neurologic injuries can be related to obstetric factors and may occur as a result of instrumentation, nonanatomic positioning during labor, use of stirrups or lithotomy position, and/or compression of sacral nerve roots by the fetal head during delivery (179).

Transient Neurologic Symptoms

Transient neurologic symptom (TNS) injuries following central neuraxial block occur with a frequency of 0.01% to 0.8% and are defined as pain and/or dysesthesia occurring in radicular distribution involving the legs or buttocks (329,339). Typically, symptoms develop within 24 hours following recovery from anesthesia and usually resolve completely at 72 hours (340,341). The role of intrathecal lidocaine in the development of neurologic injury has been discussed previously (178,179). The incidence of TNS following subarachnoid injection of lidocaine is similar to mepivacaine, but higher than with use of bupivacaine, prilocaine, and procaine (341–343) (see Chapter 12).

The treatment of TNS following obstetric regional anesthesia is that of supportive care with nonsteroidal anti-inflammatory drugs (NSAIDs), physical therapy, opioid analgesics, and muscle relaxants as required. Although usually self-limiting in terms of nature and duration, suffering from a transient debilitating injury in the postpartum period is not ideal. Patients may require extended hospital admission, and community nursing and family support should be in place prior to discharge. Telephone and outpatient anesthesia follow-up should also be arranged to ensure appropriate continuation of care and further evaluation if required (332).

Cauda Equina Syndrome

Cauda equina syndrome is a very rare but potentially devastating complication of central neuraxial blockade. It has been reported after use of intrathecal lidocaine, but also with bupivacaine, epidural triamcinolone/bupivacaine, chloroprocaine, and procaine (344–347) and after an uneventful single spinal administration of 0.5% hyperbaric bupivacaine (348). The etiology of CES is thought to include direct or indirect trauma to the nerve roots and/or spinal cord, focal local anesthetic neurotoxicity, or spinal cord ischemia. The functional anatomy of the cauda equina render them very sensitive to injury in the absence of a protective sheath. In conjunction with the use of spinal microcatheter techniques, CES was thought to be related to high volumes and concentrations of local anesthetic in the distribution of the cauda equina, but single injections of local anesthetic have also been implicated (348). There is no formal treatment for CES, and generalized supportive care is advised. Regular urologic review and frequent catheterization is required to avoid bladder distension and detrusor muscle damage (see Chapter 12).

Adhesive Arachnoiditis

Adhesive arachnoiditis occurs when there is acute localized inflammation of the arachnoid layer of the meningeal sac, leading to fibrosis, adhesion, and scarring. The process can occur up to months following spinal anesthesia. The condition presents as gradual, progressive sensory and motor deficits that can progress to paraplegia. Symptoms of transient nerve root irritation, CES, radiculitis, pachymeningitis, pseudomeningocele, and syringomyelia can develop (349–351) (see Chapter 12).

This syndrome has been described in association with pathologic processes in the spinal cord, including epidural abscess, injection of neurolytic solutions, intrathecal corticosteroids, and infection. Local anesthetics, detergents, antiseptic solutions, and radiocontrast material have also been implicated. The initial inflammatory process can lead to a cascade of inflammation and localized ischemia of the spinal cord.

Traumatic spinal needle placement and paresthesias on needle placement may increase the risk of development of arachnoiditis. Supportive care is required in the management of adhesive arachnoiditis, and imaging should be performed to confirm the diagnosis and rule out concomitant pathology. Some evidence suggests that systemic corticosteroids may be of benefit in treatment during the early inflammatory phase. Surgery is generally not recommended. Adhesive arachnoiditis is exceedingly rare in obstetrics, and labor analgesia techniques are considered to be of low risk for its development (352).

Back Pain Following Central Neuraxial Blockade

Localized back pain following regional anesthesia is quite common. The incidence appears to be higher following epidural compared to spinal anesthesia, which is hardly surprising as it correlates with the differences in needle size (329).

Many patients have a perception that their back pain is related to epidural analgesia, regardless of the etiology. Studies of the relationship between labor epidurals and postpartum backache showed no increase in back pain in women who had received epidural analgesia (353). A different group reported an 18% incidence of new-onset postpartum back pain in those women who delivered with an epidural compared with 12% of those who delivered without (354). Other prospective studies evaluating labor epidural analgesia and postpartum back pain failed to find a significant link between epidural administration and back pain (355,356). One study reported that the incidence of postpartum backache in women who received epidural anesthesia was equivalent to those who did not (44% versus 45%) (356). Further data analyses demonstrated an association between new-onset postpartum back pain with greater weight and shorter stature. Postpartum back pain was also associated with a previous history of back pain and younger age. Similarly, another recent study found no difference in the incidence of long-term low back pain in patients receiving epidurals for labor compared with controls (357).

Central Nervous System Infections

In routine anesthesia practice, the reported incidence of central neuraxial infection following regional anesthesia is extremely low. Infections such as arachnoiditis, meningitis, and epidural abscess with cord compression appear as single case reports in the literature. In addition, spontaneous epidural ab-

scess formation has been estimated in 1 of 10,000 hospital admissions in the United States (358). A prospective study of the incidence of epidural abscess following epidural analgesia over a 1-year period estimated the risk of abscess formation to be 1:1,930 (359). Abscess formation can occur at any of the tissue levels breached following subarachnoid injection. Abscess formation at the level of skin, soft tissues, or epidural space with spinal cord compression can occur. Superficial infection generally presents with local signs of fever, hyperemia, drainage, and pain. There are seldom any neurologic issues associated with these. Formation of epidural abscess may present days to weeks following a neuraxial procedure. The patient may present with severe focal back pain, paraplegia, urinary or fecal incontinence, and radicular pain with systemic signs of infection both clinically and hematologically. Typical signs and symptoms include fever, back pain, and localized infection at the level of the epidural site. Infection may be exogenous in origin due to the contamination of equipment or drug, catheter colonization, local spread from a proximal site of infection, lymphatic spread from a paraspinous focus, or—the most common route—hematogenous spread from another site in the body (360,361).

Serious infectious complications following neuraxial analgesia and anesthesia are rare, but they can have devastating consequences. Colonization of minimal clinical significance has been estimated in between 6% and 22% of epidural catheters. The rates of catheter infection as high as 5.3% has been reported. Localized infection is thought to occur in up to 12% of patients. *Staphylococcus aureus* is responsible for more than 60% of all epidural abscesses, however parasitic, fungal, and gram-negative aerobic and anaerobic organisms have also been described. Epidural abscess formation can lead to neurologic sequelae by virtue of the mechanical effect on the spinal cord itself or via ischemic compression of its blood supply. Localized inflammatory processes are also thought to be contributory (361). Meningitis following spinal anesthesia often involves the same phage type of organism; *Streptococcus viridans* was isolated from the patient and the anesthesiologist who performed the procedure. Often, the bacteria come from the nares of the anesthesiologist (362).

Early diagnosis and treatment is essential in the management of epidural abscess formation. Magnetic resonance imaging (MRI) scanning and performance of blood cultures can provide definitive diagnosis and identify causative organism, respectively. Treatment recommendations consist of urgent laminectomy with decompression of the lumbar spine. Evacuation and drainage of pus with ongoing antimicrobial therapy for approximately 3 months is required.

Although no established U.S. national guidelines exist on infection-control precautions for neuraxial techniques, strict attention to aseptic technique should reduce risk of infection (122,123). Use of epidural and drug aspiration filters, protective adhesive sterile dressing, continuous infusions in place of intermittent bolus top-ups, flow-hood drug infusion preparation stations, and inspection protocols should further reduce risks. Particular caution should be exercised in certain patient subgroups: a higher incidence of infectious complications occurs in patients with a history of immunocompromise, alcoholism, diabetes mellitus, chronic corticosteroid consumption, and malignant disease (see Chapter 12).

Spinal and Epidural Hematoma

Bleeding within the central neuraxis following spinal or epidural analgesia is fortunately a very rare complication of neuraxial anesthesia. The incidence of neurologic injury resulting from central hematoma is estimated at less than 1 in 150,000 for spinal anesthesia, and less than 1 in 220,000 for epidural anesthesia respectively and is often related to anticoagulant administration (339,363–367). Use of neuraxial techniques in the patient taking low-molecular-weight heparin (LMWH) is discussed in Chapter 12.

Preeclampsia and HELLP syndrome

Preeclampsia describes the development of proteinuria and hypertension (a sustained systolic blood pressure elevation of ≥140 mm Hg or diastolic ≥90 mm Hg) occurring after 20 weeks of gestation (368) (Fig. 24-16). It occurs in between 6% and 8% of pregnancies, with 85% of cases involving women in their first pregnancy (368,369). Thrombocytopenia can occur in up to 30% of patients with preeclampsia or eclampsia (370). Thrombocytopenia without other coagulation abnormalities, in the presence of hemolysis and liver enzyme abnormalities, is found in the variant of preeclampsia known as *HELLP syndrome* (*h*emolysis, *e*levated *l*iver enzymes, and *l*ow *p*latelets) (371).

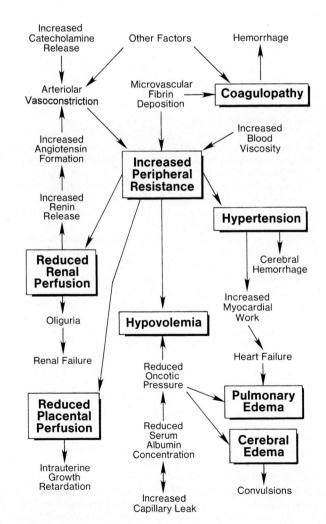

FIGURE 24-16. Pathophysiologic changes in preeclampsia (pregnancy-induced hypertension).

The optimal anesthetic technique in severely preeclamptic women remains controversial, but many anesthesiologists consider subarachnoid block to be safe (372). Although no absolute platelet count is necessary to guarantee the safety of neuraxial block, many anesthesiologists choose 100,000, 75,000, or 50,000 as a cut-off (373). Although some have advocated other methods to determine a safe level, such as thromboelastography, no evidence suggests that these alternatives provide greater safety than the platelet count (374). We place neuraxial block in patients with platelet counts over 75,000. If the platelet count is between 50,000 and 75,000, and there are no other signs of coagulopathy, we proceed. Neuraxial blockade without platelet transfusion is not attempted below 50,000 at our institution.

Antiphospholipid Syndrome and Low-molecular-weight Heparin

Antiphospholipid syndrome (APS) is a disorder characterized by recurrent venous or arterial thrombosis and/or fetal losses associated with typical laboratory abnormalities. These include persistently elevated levels of antibodies directed against membrane anionic phospholipids. Antiphospholipid syndrome can be associated with adverse pregnancy outcomes. Several trials suggest that a combination of heparin and acetylsalicylic acid (aspirin) may improve pregnancy outcomes in APS (375,376). Spontaneous fetal loss can occur at any time in pregnancy; however, it most commonly occurs in the second or third trimester (377,378).

Reports suggest that an association may exist between various thrombophilias and maternal and neonatal morbidity/mortality, including preeclampsia, abruptio placentae, intrauterine growth restriction, recurrent abortions, and fetal death (379–382). Limited evidence definitively recommends use of LMWH for women with previous adverse pregnancy outcomes and thrombophilias, however anticoagulation therapy in pregnancy is increasingly recommended in certain high risk pregnancies (383).

In vitro studies have shown that LMWHs do not cross the placenta (384,385). In retrospective studies, no specific adverse fetal effects or teratogenicity have been detected with LMWH (386,387). It should be noted that LMWHs are classified by the FDA as pregnancy category B (no evidence of adverse effects on humans). The concentration of LMWH in maternal milk was very low, more than 10 times lower than in maternal serum, and thus had no clinical significance. Women treated with LMWHs can safely breast-feed (386). Recent guidelines by the American Society of Regional Anesthesia (ASRA) suggest that neuraxial techniques should be deferred for 10 to 12 hours in the parturient who has received preoperative LMWH or for 24 hours for those parturients on higher doses of LMWH (e.g., enoxaparin 1 mg/kg twice daily) (388).

MORBIDITY AND MORTALITY ISSUES IN OBSTETRIC ANESTHESIA

The worldwide estimated number of maternal deaths in 2000 was 529,000. These deaths were divided almost equally between Asia (253,000) and Africa (251,000). Less that 1% of maternal deaths occurred in the developed world (389). The most widely accepted definition of maternal mortality comes from the Tenth Revision of the International Classification of Diseases (ICD-10), which defines a maternal death as the death of a woman while pregnant or within 42 days of termination of pregnancy, irrespective of the duration and site of the pregnancy, from any cause related to or aggravated by the pregnancy or its management but not from accidental or incidental causes (390). Given that medical intervention can prolong life and delay death, further qualification of maternal mortality in ICD-10 also includes the concept of late maternal death, which is defined as death of a woman from direct or indirect obstetric causes more than 42 days but less than 1 year after termination of pregnancy. The ICD-10 further divides maternal deaths into two groups: (a) direct obstetric deaths, to include deaths due to obstetric complications of the pregnancy itself, in addition to death due to interventions, omission, incorrect treatment, or from a chain of events resulting from any of the above; and (b) indirect obstetric deaths, defined as deaths resulting from previous existing disease or diseases that developed during pregnancy and which was not due to direct obstetric causes, but was aggravated by physiologic effects of pregnancy. Deaths by accidental or incidental means have historically been excluded from maternal mortality statistics, although the ICD-10 further qualifies maternal deaths with *irrespective of the cause of death* in their definition of maternal mortality (390).

Measurement of maternal mortality is difficult and complex, due to under-reporting, misclassification, and difficulties experienced comparing information from multiple sources. Under-reporting is common even in the developed world, where underestimation of incidence by a factor of up to 30% has been suggested (390,391).

In the United Kingdom, analysis of data related to maternal mortality has been the subject of the *Report on Confidential Enquiry in to Maternal Deaths* (392). Similarly, in the United States, a National Pregnancy-Related Mortality Surveillance System was organized in 1987, which analyzes a broad range of statistics to establish a measure of maternal mortality. This analysis has shown that the risk of death from pregnancy-related complications has reduced from approximately 850 maternal deaths per 100,000 live births in 1950 to 7.5 per 100,000 in 1982 (393). This incidence has increased since then, despite advances in patient care, and most likely reflects improved collection of information and increased ascertainment of pregnancy-related deaths. Furthermore, it appears that the risks of pregnancy-related maternal mortality among African Americans is three to four times greater than that of Caucasian women (393). Obstetric complications during labor and delivery were also found to be higher in African-American and Asian women compared to Caucasian women (394).

Anesthesia-related deaths are the sixth leading cause of pregnancy-related death in the United States. Review of the Pregnancy Mortality Surveillance data revealed anesthesia-related mortality to be 1.7 per million live births (1988–1990), down from 4.3 per million as reported in the previous triennium (1979–1981). The number of deaths following general anesthesia has remained stable and that of regional anesthesia has continued to decrease. General anesthesia may be associated with aspiration of gastric contents, failure to secure the airway appropriately, inadequate postoperative care, and misuse of drugs or equipment. Evidence suggests that communication between anesthesiologist and obstetrician is essential to ensure appropriate selection of anesthetic technique for surgery (240). In addition, it is recommended that anesthesia for these patients be planned and carried out by an anesthesiologist with a minimum of 12 months of training in anesthesia.

NEURAL BLOCKADE FOR ASSISTED REPRODUCTIVE TECHNIQUES

With the development of medical management of maternal illnesses, increased maternal age, and societal changes, an increase has occurred in both expectation and outcome in relation to age and difficult pregnancy management. Assisted reproductive techniques include hormonal stimulation, retrieval of oocytes, in vitro fertilization, and transfer of gamete to the uterine cavity or fallopian tubes. Hormonal stimulation is performed to produce oocytes that can be retrieved for assisted reproduction. Initially, ovarian downregulation is performed, followed by hyperstimulation. This results in the release of multiple follicles and oocytes, and is accomplished via manipulation of the pituitary axis through the administration of gonadotrophin-releasing hormone agonists (e.g., leuprolide acetate) and can be confirmed by imaging and low serum levels of estrogen. When maturation of the follicles occurs, ovulation is achieved with human chorionic gonadotrophin (hCG), then oocyte retrieval is performed (395,396).

Oocyte retrieval is commonly performed transvaginally, under ultrasound guidance. The follicles are identified and their contents aspirated and placed in culture media, awaiting the next step in the assisted-fertilization process. The oocyte is processed using in vitro fertilization (IVF) or gamete intrafallopian transfer (GIFT). In vitro fertilization is the process whereby fertilization of the oocyte occurs in a culture medium. Fertilization is confirmed microscopically and the resulting embryo is then transferred into the fallopian tubes or uterine cavity. Various options are available to achieve this transfer, based on the cell stage of the resulting embryo. The IVF process allows identification and confirmation of fertilization prior to transfer. In GIFT procedures, this confirmation is not made, as the oocyte and sperm are both placed in the fallopian tubes directly and the fertilization process occurs in vivo.

Increasing pregnancy success via assisted reproductive technology (ART) has been shown to be at times associated with an increased risk of neonatal morbidity. In addition to the increased incidence of multiple births, ART has also led to an increase in prematurity, low birth weight, and perinatal morbidity and mortality. Therefore, caution in selection of anesthetic technique in the facilitation of this process is imperative to minimize the impact of intervention on maternal–fetal homeostasis. Several studies have examined the causal effect of anesthesia on neonatal well-being. The impact of anesthesia on the oocyte as it progresses to embryonic stage, however, is less clear. In addition, the relationship between the selected ART technique and choice of anesthetic technique is also the subject of much debate.

The impact of serum levels of local anesthesia depends on the route of administration and extent of protein binding of each agent. The toxicity of local anesthetic agents on embryogenesis is unknown. Animal studies suggest a dose-dependent deleterious effect of local anesthetics on in vitro fertilization and embryonic development. Lidocaine was associated with adverse effects to a greater extent than chloroprocaine, whereas bupivacaine was only shown to negatively impact fertilization and embryonic development at the highest dosage studied (397). Human studies showed that, despite use of paracervical nerve blocks with lidocaine to facilitate transvaginal follicle aspiration, there was no difference in fertilization or embryonic cleavage rates compared with patients without local anesthetic exposure (398).

Oocyte retrieval can be done transvaginally or transabdominally. Transabdominal techniques can be done under general anesthesia, neuraxial anesthesia, or with local anesthetic infiltration techniques. A retrospective review of retrieval procedures showed that use of general anesthesia, particularly nitrous oxide, had a potentially adverse effect on IVF outcome, with lower pregnancy and delivery rates. Local anesthesia combined with sedation, and regional anesthesia were shown to have less impact on IVF results. Transvaginal oocyte retrieval is now much more commonly performed and, although the procedure may potentially be performed without anesthesia or analgesia, this may not be tolerated well by patients secondary to discomfort and pain (399). Epidural and spinal anesthesia have been shown to be effective techniques for transvaginal oocyte retrieval, but without apparent improved pregnancy rates compared to general anesthesia. There is however, a reduced incidence of postoperative nausea and vomiting under neuraxial block, which may be associated with improved patient satisfaction and reduced length of hospital stay (400). Specifically, spinal anesthesia results in rapid-onset, uniform anesthesia with low doses of local anesthetic, which has merit in relation to potential oocyte exposure to drug. Intrathecal hyperbaric lidocaine 1.5% to 5% (45 mg) combined with low-dose fentanyl (10 μg) has been described for spinal anesthesia to facilitate oocyte retrieval (401,402).

NONOBSTETRIC PAIN IN PREGNANCY

Nonobstetric pain can occur in pregnancy due to factors directly or indirectly related to pregnancy. These conditions may not be specific to pregnancy but can commonly occur because of a combination of mechanical, hormonal, or physiologic factors. Tension headache can occur in pregnancy, although more sinister causes must be ruled out. Conditions such as preeclampsia, subarachnoid hemorrhage, intracerebral tumor, and other vascular causes must be excluded when a pregnant patient presents with severe headache. This is especially the case when the patient has never had a previous headache or when she states that it is "the worst headache of my life" (403, 404).

Back pain is common during pregnancy and the postpartum period, and occurs in approximately 50% of mothers (405–407). Sacroiliac joint pain is thought to account for up to 15% of all back complaints and is more common in pregnancy because of both mechanical and hormonal factors (408). Symptoms may be difficult to differentiate from radiculopathy, and provocative testing of the joint can be difficult to perform clinically in the pregnant patient. Magnetic resonance imaging of pregnant and nonpregnant women suggests that lumbosacral disk bulges and herniations are common in women of childbearing age, regardless of whether they are pregnant. No evidence, however, suggests an increased prevalence of disk abnormalities in pregnant patients (408). In fact, mechanical factors and traction on the lumbosacral plexus itself may mimic symptoms of radiculopathy (406).

Conservative therapy is the treatment of choice for back pain, including bed rest, physical therapy, heat, massage, and exercise therapy, with use of acetaminophen as required. Opioid therapy can be considered, as can interventional treatments including non–image guided interventional techniques including trigger point, sacroiliac joint, and epidural steroid injection. Computed tomography and fluoroscopy are not typically recommended (407).

The use of radiologic imaging is important in the diagnosis and treatment of many painful syndromes. When possible, imaging should be avoided entirely during pregnancy; however, if essential to diagnosis, postponement until the fetus has reached a gestational age of 15 weeks is recommended (409).

In some circumstances, however, imaging during pregnancy is essential. The stimulatory effects of pregnancy on conditions including meningioma, hemangioblastoma, metastatic tumors, and prolactinoma also suggest that early use of central nervous system imaging may avoid the consequences of delayed diagnosis (410).

Complex regional pain syndrome (previously known as *reflex sympathetic dystrophy*) of the lower extremity has been described in pregnancy. These patients usually present in the third trimester, mostly with pelvic and lower extremity pain, with fractures occurring in 19% of patients. Symptoms were reported to have subsided at varying intervals following delivery of the fetus (411,412).

Nerve entrapment, including carpal tunnel syndrome or meralgia paresthetica, may also occur in pregnancy due to fluid retention or mechanical factors, respectively.

Abdominal pain in pregnancy may be related to obstetric or gynecologic factors including placental abruption, uterine rupture, or amnionitis. Nonobstetric causes including appendicitis, gastritis, and perforated viscus must also be considered. Other significant conditions including sickle cell crises, pulmonary embolism, and trauma must also be considered as nonobstetric causes of pain in the pregnant patient.

Medical Management of Pain in Pregnancy and Lactation

Diagnosis and treatment of painful conditions in the pregnant woman can be complicated by risks to both mother and fetus. Administration of drugs during pregnancy increases the risk of fetal exposure and, in addition, postpartum administration of medication may also have an impact on the neonate if secreted into breast milk. The effect of drug exposure depends on dose, gestational age of the fetus, and pharmacologic factors specific to the drug. The extent of transfer of drug to both fetus and nursing child depends mostly on passive diffusion; thus, lipid solubility, protein binding, concentration gradient, and diffusing capacity of the placental membrane (intrauterine exposure) are all factors of importance when considering intrauterine exposure. Caution must be exercised in the medical management of nonobstetric pain in the pregnant patient, and nonpharmacologic management should be utilized if possible. Should medical management be required, careful consideration of the risk–benefit ratio of each drug should be made, and fetal exposure should be reduced, if possible, by administering the minimal dose for the shortest possible duration.

Maternal, infant, and drug factors determine the quantity of drug to which the nursing child is exposed. The maternal dose, dose schedule, volume of feedings, and elimination half-life of the drug determine the degree of excretion of drug into breast milk. Breast milk is slightly acidic and thus favors the passive diffusion of weakly basic drugs. Passive diffusion is high in drugs that are lipid soluble and have low protein binding. Despite this, infant plasma concentrations are usually less than 2% of the breast milk concentration (409).

Acetaminophen and NSAIDs are considered to be safe for use in nursing mothers and are the current mainstay of pain therapy (413). Inhibition of prostaglandin synthesis with use of NSAIDs has been shown to be effective for the prevention of premature labor and in the treatment of polyhydramnios.

The risks of fetal renal impairment, maternal and fetal hemorrhage, and the potential to produce premature closure of the fetal ductus arteriosus, have limited the use of NSAIDs in pregnancy (414). Similarly, the potential for drug transfer to the neonate via breast milk is also a concern postpartum. Concerns regarding the potential development of Reye syndrome has limited the use of aspirin in breast-feeding mothers. However, low-dose aspirin (up to 100 mg/day) appears to be safe in lactating mothers (414). The propionic acid derivatives and indomethacin cross into the breast milk in small quantities, and the possible effects are considered negligible. Diclofenac has not been detected in breast milk at doses up to 100 mg/day; however, very small amounts have been detected in breast milk at doses of 150 mg/day (414–416). Transfer of between 0.16% and 0.4% of the total daily maternal dose of ketorolac has been reported in maternal milk (417). Thus, caution is recommended with use of ketorolac for postoperative pain.

Opioids pass freely into breast milk, but are considered safe for use in breast-feeding. However, IV PCA in nursing mothers was shown to be associated with neurobehavioral changes in infants (418). Similarly, closer monitoring of those infants whose nursing mothers use oral opioids with active metabolites (especially meperidine) is often required.

The general recommendations for pain management in lactating mothers include administration of the lowest effective maternal dose and avoidance of breast-feeding at times of peak drug concentration in breast milk. Because breast milk confers potential nutritional, immunologic, and other advantages to the infant, the risk–benefit ratio should be assessed on an individual basis. Patients should not be expected to choose between analgesia and breast-feeding (414).

Antiepilepsy drugs, such as phenytoin, carbamazepine, and sodium valproate, are used in the treatment of neuropathic pain and are considered to be safe during lactation (419). Less evidence is available regarding the newer membrane-stabilizing adjuvant drugs, including lamotrigine and topiramate. No large human studies have analyzed the effect of the more recently developed and widely used drugs pregabalin and gabapentin on lactating mothers. However, it has been suggested that gabapentin is safe for the neonate, despite transfer of drug into breast milk (420). Selective serotonin reuptake inhibitors and the tricyclic antidepressants amitriptyline and imipramine, but not doxepin, are thought to be compatible with breast-feeding (421).

NEURAL BLOCKADE FOR GYNECOLOGIC SURGERY

Regional anesthesia, alone or in combination with general anesthesia, is ideal for vaginal and intra-abdominal pelvic surgery. Vaginal procedures with involvement of the ovarian pedicles will require anesthesia to T10. Major intra-abdominal surgery can be performed with regional anesthesia, however, depending on the duration of the surgery, light sedation or general anesthesia could be added with patient comfort in mind. Laparoscopic procedures are mostly performed under general anesthesia. However, local anesthesia and regional techniques have been described (422–424). Recent work suggests that laparoscopically performed myomectomy may be associated with improved postoperative pain scores when compared to open procedures (425).

Tubal ligation is a commonly performed sterilization procedure. Many patients prefer to have this procedure performed during their inpatient stay during the postpartum period. This raises several moral and ethical issues regarding the timing of the procedure and consent. Issues regarding the permanence of the procedure and the potential of sterilization failure (1.85% over 10 years) must be carefully discussed with the patient prior to proceeding with surgery (426). The timing of consent in the postpartum period to a permanent surgical procedure in the presence of pain, emotional lability, hormonal changes, and sleep deprivation is sometimes less than ideal. Performance of an elective procedure, with ongoing airway and aspiration risks, is not without hazard. Regional anesthesia is ideal for postpartum tubal ligation, as the risk of aspiration remains a concern despite relief of the mechanical risk factors with the delivery of the fetus. Spinal or epidural anesthesia also can be used effectively for postpartum tubal ligation. If an epidural catheter is in situ following labor analgesia, this can be used for operative analgesia. A sensory level to T4 is required for patient comfort, as visceral pain can be uncomfortable on manipulation of the fallopian tubes. Failure of epidural reactivation may be a problem (22%–26%) and appears to be time dependent. Reactivation of an epidural catheter was successful in 95% of patients if the epidural catheter was used within 4 hours of delivery. Spinal anesthesia has been found to be very effective for postpartum tubal ligation and has a superior cost analysis (427,428).

References

1. Clark WC, Yang JC, Tsui SL et al. Unidimensional pain rating scales: A multidimensional affect and pain survey (MAPS) analysis of what they really measure. *Pain* 2002;98:241–247.
2. Mersky H, Bogduku P, eds. *Classification of Chronic Pain*, 2nd ed. Seattle: IASP Press, 1994.
3. Lang AJ, Sorrell JT, Rodgers CS, Lebeck MM. Anxiety sensitivity as a predictor of labor pain. *Eur J Pain* 2006;10(3):267–270.
4. Melzack R. The myth of painless childbirth (The John J. Bonica Lecture). *Pain* 1984;19:321–337.
5. Melzack R, Taenzer P, Feldman P, Kinch RA. Labour is still painful after prepared childbirth training. *Can Med Assoc J* 1981;125(4):357–363.
6. Ackerman WE, Andrews PJ, Juneja M, et al. Sensory evoked facial muscle electromyography for the quantification of acute labor pain. *J Ky Med Assoc* 1994;92(1):14–17.
7. Eisenach JC, Thomas JA, Rauck RL, et al. Cystatin C in cerebrospinal fluid is not a diagnostic test of pain in humans. *Pain* 2004;107(3):199–201.
8. Brooks J, Tracey I. From nociception to pain perception: Imaging the spinal and supraspinal pathways. *J Anat* 2005 207(1):19–33.
9. Casey KL, Lorenz J, Minoshima S. Insight into the pathophysiology of neuropathic pain through functional brain imaging. *Exp Neurol* 2003;184:S80–S88.
10. Schweinhardt P, Lee M, Tracey I. Imaging pain in patients: Is it meaningful? *Curr Opin Neurol* 2006;19(4):392–400.
11. Spätling L, Fallenstein F, Huch A, et al. The variability of cardiopulmonary adaptation to pregnancy at rest and during exercise. *Br J Obstet Gynaecol* 1992;99[Suppl 8]:1–40.
12. Conklin KA. Maternal physiological adaptations during gestation, labor and the puerperium. *Semin Anesth* 1991;10:221–234.
13. Baldwin GR, Moorthi DS, Whelton JA, MacDonnell KF. New lung functions and pregnancy. *Am J Obstet Gynecol* 1977;127:235–239.
14. Russell IP, Chamber WA. Closing volume in normal pregnancy. *Br J Anaesth* 1981;53:1043–1047.
15. Cole PV, Nainby-Lumoore RC. Respiratory volumes in labour. *Br Med J* 1962;1:1118.
16. Miller FC, Petrie RHP, Arce JJ, et al. Hyperventilation in labor. *Am J Obstet Gynecol* 1974;120:489–495.
17. Sangoul F, Fox GS, Houle GL. Effect of regional anesthesia on maternal oxygen consumption during the first stage of labor. *Am J Obstet Gynecol* 1975;121:1080–1083.
18. Hagerdal M, Morgan CW, Sumner AE, Gutsche BB. Minute ventilation and oxygen consumption during labor with epidural analgesia. *Anesthesiology* 1983;59:425–427.

19. Robson SC, Hunter S, Boys RJ, Dunlop W. Serial study of factors influencing changes in cardiac output during human pregnancy. *Am J Physiol* 1989;256:H1060–H1065.

20. Desai DK, Moodley J, Naidoo DP. Echocardiographic assessment of cardiovascular hemodynamics in normal pregnancy. *Obstet Gynecol* 2004; 104(1):20–29.

21. Hendricks CH. Hemodynamics of a uterine contraction. *Am J Obstet Gynecol* 1958;76:968–982.

22. Ueland K, Hansen JM. Maternal cardiovascular dynamics. III. Labor and delivery under local and caudal analgesia. *Am J Obstet Gynecol* 1969;103:8–18.

23. Hansen JM, Ueland K. Maternal cardiovascular dynamics during pregnancy and parturition. *Clin Anesth* 1974;10(2):21–36.

24. Patton DE, Lee W, Miller J, Jones M. Maternal, uteroplacental, and fetoplacental hemodynamic and Doppler velocimetric changes during epidural anesthesia in normal labor. *Obstet Gynecol* 1991;77(1):17–19.

25. Alahuhta S, Rasanen J, Jouppila R, et al. Effects of extradural bupivacaine with adrenaline for caesarean section on uteroplacental and fetal circulation. *Br J Anaesth* 1991;67(6):678–682.

26. Unruh AM. Gender variations in clinical pain experience. *Pain* 1996;65:123–167.

27. Aloisi AM, Albonneti ME, Carli G. Sex differences in the behavioural response to persistent pain in rats. *Neurosci Lett* 1994;179:79–84.

28. Mogil JS, Chesler EJ, Wilson SG, et al. Sex difference in thermal nociception and morphine antinociception in rodents depend on the genotype. *Neurosci Behav Rev* 2000;24:375–389.

29. Riley JL, Robinson ME, Wise EA, et al. Sex differences in the perception of noxious experimental stimuli: A meta-analysis. *Pain* 1998;74:181–187.

30. Liu NJ, Gintzler AR. Gestational and ovarian sex steroid antinociception: Relevance of uterine afferent and spinal alpha(2)-noradrenergic activity. *Pain* 1999;83(2):359–368.

31. Cosontos K, Rust M. Halt V, et al. Elevated plasma B-endorphins in pregnant women and neonates. *Life Sci* 1979:25:835–844.

32. Cogan R, Spinnato JA. Pain and discomfort thresholds in late pregnancy. *Pain* 1986;27:63–68.

33. Gintzler AR. Endorphin-mediated increases in pain threshold during pregnancy. *Science* 1980;210:193–195.

34. Pilkington JW, Nemeroff CB, Mason GA, Prange AJ. Increase in plasma B-endorphin like immunoreactivity at parturition in normal women. *Am J Obstet Gynecol* 1983;145:11–13.

35. Shnider SM, Wright RG, Levinson G, et al. Uterine blood flow and plasma norepinephrine changes during maternal stress in the pregnant ewe. *Anesthesiology* 1979;50:524–527.

36. Baron WM, Mujais SK, Zinaman M, et al. Plasma catecholamine responses to physiological stimuli in normal human pregnancy. *Am J Obstet Gynecol* 1986;154:80–84.

37. Shnider SM, Abboud T, Artal R, et al. Maternal catecholamines decrease during labor after lumbar epidural analgesia. *Am J Obstet Gynecol* 1983; 147:13–15.

38. Cascio M, Pygon B, Bernett C, Ramanathan S. Labour analgesia with intrathecal fentanyl decreases maternal stress. *Can Anaesth Soc J* 1997;44:605–609.

39. Vogl SE, Worda C, Egarter C, et al. Mode of delivery is associated with maternal and fetal endocrine stress response. *BJOG* 2006;113(4):441–445.

40. Abboud TK, Artal R, Henriksen EH, et al. Effects of spinal anesthesia on maternal circulating catecholamines. *Am J Obstet Gynecol* 1982;1423:252–254.

41. Saisto T, Halmesmaki E. Fear of childbirth: A neglected dilemma. *Acta Obstet Gynecol Scand* 2003;82:201–208.

42. Trudinger BJ, Giles WB, Cook CM. Uteroplacental blood flow velocity time wave forms in normal and complicated pregnancy. *Br J Obstet Gynaecol* 1985;92:39–45.

43. McKinlay J, Lyons G. Obstetric neuraxial anaesthesia: Which pressor agents should we be using? *Int J Obstet Anesth* 2002;11:77–152.

44. Skjölderbrand A, Eklund J, Johansson H, et al. Uteroplacental blood flow measured by placental scintigraphy during epidural anaesthesia for caeserean section. *Acta Anaesthesiol Scand* 1990;34:79–84.

45. Robson SC, Boys RJ, Rodeck C, et al. Maternal and fetal haemodynamic effects of spinal and extradural anaesthesia for elective caeserean section. *Br J Anaesth* 1992;68:54–59.

46. Reynolds F, Seed PT. Anaesthesia for caesarean section and neonatal acid-base status: A meta-analysis. *Anaesthesia* 2005;60(7):636–653.

47. Ralston DH, Schnider SM, deLorimar AA. Effects of equipotent ephedrine, metaraminol, mephentermine and methoxamine on uterine blood flow in the pregnant ewe. *Anesthesiology* 1974;40:354–370.

48. Ngan Kee WD, Khaw KS. Vasopressors in obstetrics: What should we be using? *Curr Opin Anaesthesiol* 2006;19(3):238–243.

49. Ramanathan S, Grant GJ. Vasopressor therapy for hypotension due to epidural anesthesia for cesarean section. *Acta Anaesthesiol Scand* 1988;32:559–565.

50. Thomas DG, Robson SC, Redfern N, et al. Randomized trial of bolus phenylephrine or ephedrine for maintenance of arterial pressure during spinal anesthesia for cesarean section. *Br J Anaesth* 1996;76:61–65.

51. Moran DH, Perillo M, La Porta RF, et al. Phenylephrine in the prevention of hypotension following spinal anesthesia for cesearean delivery. *J Clin Anesth* 1991;3:301–305.

52. Mercier FJ, Riley ET, Frederickson WL, et al. Phenylephrine added to prophylactic ephedrine infusion during spinal anesthesia for elective Cesarean section. *Anesthesiology* 2001;95:668–674.

53. Burns SM, Cowan CM, Wilkes RG. Prevention and management of hypotension during spinal anaesthesia for elective caeseran section: A survey of practice. *Anaesthesia* 2001;56:794–798.

54. Erkinaro T, Kavasmaa T, Pakkila M, et al. Ephedrine and phenylephrine for the treatment of maternal hypotension in a chronic sheep model of increased placental vascular resistance. *Br J Anaesth* 2006;96(2):231–237.

55. Erkinaro T, Makikallio, Kavasmaa T, et al. Effects of ephedrine and phenylephrine on uterine and placental circulations and fetal outcome following fetal hypoxaemia and epidural-induced hypotension in a sheep model. *Br J Anaesth* 2004;93(6):825–832.

56. McGrath JM, Chestnut DH, Vincent RD, et al. Ephedrine remains the vasopressor of choice for treatment of hypotension during ritodrine infusion and epidural anesthesia. *Anesthesiology* 1994;80(5):1073–1078.

57. Alahuhta S, Rasanen J, Jouppila P, et al. Ephedrine and phenylephrine for avoiding maternal hypotension due to spinal anaesthesia for caesarean section. Effects on uteroplacental and fetal haemodynamics. *Int J Obstet Anesth* 1992;1(3):129–134.

58. Kingston HGG, Kendrick A, Sommer KM, et al. Binding of thiopental in neonatal serum. *Anesthesiology* 1990;72(3):428–431.

59. Rosenberg PH, Veering BT, Urmey WF. Maximum recommended doses of local anesthetics: A multifactorial concept. *Reg Anesth Pain Med* 2004;29 (6):564–575.

60. Brown WU Jr., Bell GC, Alper MH. Acidosis, local anesthetics and the newborn. *Obstet Gynecol* 1976;48:27–30.

61. Finster M, Morishima HO, Mark LC, et al. Tissue thiopental concentrations in the fetus and newborn. *Anesthesiology* 1972;336:155.

62. Pang LM, Mellins RB. Neonatal cardiorespiratory physiology. *Anesthesiology* 1975;43:171.

63. Casey ML, MacDonald PC. Biochemical processes in the initiation of parturition: Decidual activation. *Clin Obstet Gynecol* 1988;31:533–552.

64. Bonica JJ. *Principles and Practice of Obstetric Analgesia and Anesthesia*, Vol. 1. Philadelphia: FA Davis;1967:104.

65. Bonica JJ. The nature of pain in parturition. In: Van Zundert A, Ostheimer GW, eds. *Pain Relief and Anesthesia in Obstetrics*. New York: Livingstone;1996:19–52.

66. Brownridge P. The nature and consequences of childbirth pain. *Eur J Obstet Gynecol Reprod Biol* 1995;59[Suppl]:S9–S15.

67. Bonica JJ. Peripheral mechanisms and pathways of parturition pain. *Br J Anaesth* 1979;51:3S.

68. Reynolds SRM. Innervation of the uterus: Functional features. In: Reynolds SRM, ed. *Physiology of the Uterus*. New York: Harper and Brothers; 1949: 477–490.

69. Berkley KJ, Robbins A, Sato Y. Afferent fibers supplying the uterus in the rat. *J Neurophysiol* 1988;59:142–163.

70. Berkley KJ, Wood E. Responses to varying intensities of vaginal distension in the awake rat. *Abstr Soc Neurosc* 1989;15:979.

71. Simkin P, O'Hara M. Non pharmacological relief of pain during labor: A systematic review of five methods. *Am J Obstet Gynaecol* 2002;186:S131–S159.

72. Carroll D, Tramer M, McQuay H, et al. Transcutaneous electrical nerve stimulation in labour pain: A systematic review. *Br J Obstet Gynaecol* 1997;104:169–175.

73. Ader L, Hansson B, Wallin G. Parturition pain treated by intracutaneous injections of sterile water. *Pain* 1990;41(2):133–138.

74. Olofsson C, Ekblom A, Ekman-Ordeberg G, et al. Lack of analgesic effect of systemically administered morphine or pethidine on labor pain. *Br J Obstet Gynaecol* 1996;103(10):968–972.

75. Erberle RL, Norris MC. Labor analgesia. A risk-benefit analysis. *Drug Saf* 1996;14:239–251.

76. Tsui MH et al. A double blinded randomised placebo-controlled study of intramuscular pethidine for pain relief in the first stage of labour. *BJOG* 2004;111(7):648–655.

77. Bricker L, Lavender T. Parenteral opioids for labor pain relief: A systematic review. *Am J Obstet Gynecol* 2002;186:S94–S109.

78. Elbourne D, Wiseman RA. Types of intramuscular opioids for maternal pain relief in labour. *Cochrane Database Syst Rev* 2000;(2):CD001237.

79. Rosaeg OP, Kitts JB, Koren G, Byford LJ. Maternal and fetal effects of intravenous patient-controlled fentanyl analgesia during labour in a thrombocytopenic parturient. *Can J Anaesth* 1992;39(3):277–281.

80. Hardy JD, Javert CT. Studies on pain: Measurements of pain intensity in childbirth. *J Clin Invest* 1949;28:153–162.

81. Nelson KE, Eisenach JC. Intravenous butorphanol, meperidine, and their combination relieve pain and distress in women in labor. *Anesthesiology* 2005;102(5):1008–1013.

82. Evron S, Glezerman M, Sadan O, et al. Remifentanil: A novel systemic analgesia for labor pain. *Anesth Analg* 2005;100(1):233–238.

83. Ranney B, Stanage WF. Advantages of local anesthesia for cesarean section. *Obstet Gynecol* 1975;45(2):163–167.

84. Baxi LV, Petrie RH, James LS. Human fetal oxygenation following paracervical block. *Am J Obstet Gynecol* 1979;135:1109–1112.

85. Shnider SM, Asling JH, Holl JW, et al. Paracervical block anesthesia in obstetrics: I. Fetal complications and neonatal morbidity. *Am J Obstet Gynecol* 1970;107:619–625.

86. Asling JH, Shnider SM, Margolis AJ, et al. Paracervical block anesthesia in obstetrics: II: Etiology of fetal bradycardia following Paracervical block. *Am J Obstet Gynecol* 1970;107:626–634.

87. Klink EW. Perineal nerve block: An anatomic and clinical study in the female. *Obstet Gynecol* 1953;1:137–146.

88. Hutchins CJ. Spinal anesthesia for instrumental delivery: A comparison with pudendal nerve block. *Anaesthesia* 1980;35:376–377.

89. Scudamore JH, Yates MJ. Pudendal block: A misnomer? *Lancet* 1966;1:23–24.

90. Umeda S, Arai T, Hatano Y, et al. Cadaver anatomic analysis of the best site for chemical lumbar sympathectomy. *Anesth Analg* 1987;66:643–646.

91. Rocco AG, Palombi D, Raeke D. Anatomy of the lumbar sympathetic chain. *Reg Anesth* 1995;20(1):13–19.

92. Cleland JGP. Paravertebral anaesthesia in obstetrics. Experimental and clinical basis. *Surg Gynecol Obstet* 1933;57:51–62.

93. Jarvis SM. Paravertebral sympathetic nerve block: A method for the safe and painless conduct of labor. *Am J Obstet Gynecol* 1944;47:335–342.

94. Meguiar RV, Wheeler AS. Lumbar sympathetic block with bupivacaine: Analgesia for labor. *Anesth Analg* 1978;57(4):486–492.

95. Leighton BL, Halpern SH, Wilson DB. Lumbar sympathetic blocks speed early and second stage induced labor in nulliparous women. *Anesthesiology* 1999;90(4):1039–1046.

96. Hogan QH, Abram SE. Neural blockade for diagnosis and prognosis. A review. *Anesthesiology* 1997;86(1):216–241.

97. De Leon-Casasola OA, Kent E, Lema MJ. Neurolytic superior hypogastric plexus block for chronic pelvic pain associated with cancer. *Pain* 1993;54:145–151.

98. Plancarte R, de Leon Casasola OA, El-Helealy M, et al. Neurolytic superior hypogastric plexus block for chronic pelvic pain associated with cancer. *Reg Anesth* 1997;22:562–568.

99. Cousins MJ, Reeve TS, Glynn CJ, et al. Neurolytic lumbar sympathetic blockade: Duration of denervation and relief of rest pain. *Anaesth Intensive Care* 1979;7:121–135.

100. Eason MJ, Wyatt R. Paravertebral thoracic block: A reappraisal. *Anaesthesia* 1979;34:638–642.

101. Richardson J, Vowden P, Sabanathan S. Bilateral paravertebral analgesia for major abdominal vascular surgery: A preliminary report. *Anaesthesia* 1995;50:995–998.

102. Matthews PJ, Govenden V. Comparison of continuous paravertebral catheters and extradural infusions of bupivacaine for pain relief after thoracotomy. *Br J Anaesth* 1989;62:204–205.

103. Longquist PA, MacKensie J, Soni AK. Paravertebral blockade: Failure rate and complications. *Anaesthesia* 1995;50:813–815.

104. Gay GR, Evans JA. Total spinal anesthesia following lumbar paravertebral block: A potentially lethal complication. *Anesth Analg* 1971;50:344–348.

105. Saito T, Den S, Tanuma K, et al. Anatomical bases for paravertebral anesthetic block: Fluid communication between the thoracic and lumbar paravertebral regions. *Surg Radiol Anat* 1999;21(6):359–363.

106. Nair V, Henry R. Bilateral paravertebral block: A satisfactory alternative for labor analgesia. *Can J Anaesth* 2001;48(2):179–184.

107. MacArthur C, Lewis M, Knox EG. Evaluation of obstetric analgesia and anaesthesia: Long term maternal recollection. *Int J Obstet Anesth* 1993;2:3.

108. Sheiner E, Shohm-Vardi I, Sheiner EK, et al. A comparison between the effectiveness of epidural analgesia and parenteral pethidine during labor. *Arch Gynecol Obstet* 2000;263(3):95–98.

109. Philipsen T, Jensen NH. Maternal opinion about analgesia in labour and delivery. A comparison of epidural blockade and intramuscular pethidine. *Eur J Obstet Gynecol Reprod Biol* 1990;34(3):205–210.

110. Swan HD, Borshoff DC. Informed consent: Recall of risk information following epidural analgesia in labour. *Anaesth Intensive Care* 1994;22(2):139–141.

111. Pattee C, Ballantyne M, Milne B. Epidural analgesia for labour and delivery: Informed consent issues. *Can J Anaesth* 1997;44:918–923.

112. Black JD, Cyna AM. Issues of consent for regional analgesia in labor: A survey of obstetric anaesthetists. *Anaesth Intensive Care* 2006;34(2):254–260.

113. Suonio S, Simpanen AL, Olkkonen H, Haring P. Effect of the left lateral recumbent position compared with the supine and upright positions on placental blood flow in normal late pregnancy. *Ann Clin Res* 1976;8(1):22–26.

114. Bahar M, Chanimov M, Cohen ML, et al. The lateral recumbent head-down position decreases the incidence of epidural venous puncture during catheter insertion in obese parturients. *Can J Anaesth* 2004;51(6):577–580.

115. Vincent RD, Chestnut DH. Which position is more comfortable for the parturient during identification of the epidural space? *Int J Obstet Anesth* 1991;1:9–11.

116. Andrews PJ, Ackerman WE, Juneja MM. Aortocaval compression in the sitting and lateral decubitus positions during extradural catheter placement in the parturient. *Can J Anaesth* 1993;40(4):320–324.

117. Bamberger PD, Birnbach DJ. Lumbar epidural anesthesia initiated in the knee-chest position. *Reg Anesth* 1991;16(4):240–241.

118. Kaiser E, Suppini A, de Jaurequiberry JP, et al. Acute streptococcus salivarius meninigitis after spinal anesthesia. *Ann Fr Anesth Reanim* 1997;16(1):47–49.

119. Trautmann M, Lepper PM, Schmitz FJ. Three cases of bacterial meningitis after spinal and epidural anesthesia. *Eur J Clin Microbiol Infect Dis* 2002;21(1):43–45.

120. Molinier S, Paris JF, Brisou P, et al. Two cases of iatrogenic oral streptococcal infection: Meningitis and spondylodiscitis. *Rev Med Interne* 1998;19(8):568–570.

121. Schneeberger PM, Janssen M, Voss A. Alpha-hemolytic streptococci: A major pathogen of iatrogenic meningitis following lumbar puncture. Case reports and a review of the literature. *Infection* 1996;24:29–35.

122. Panikkar KK, Yentis SM. Wearing of masks for obstetric regional anaesthesia. A postal survey. *Anaesthesia* 1996;51(4):398–400.

123. Sellors JE, Cyna AM, Simmons SW. Aseptic precautions for inserting an epidural catheter: A survey of obstetric anaesthetist. *Anaesthesia* 2002;57(6):593–596.

124. Birnbach DJ, Stein DJ, Murray O, et al. Povidone iodine and skin disinfection before initiation of epidural anesthesia. *Anesthesiology* 1998;88(3):668–672.

125. O'Rourke E, Runyan D, O'Leary J, Stern J. Contaminated iodophor in the operating room. *Am J Infect Control* 2003;31(4):255–256.

126. Clevenot D, Robert S, Debaene B, Mimoz O. Critical review of the literature concerning the comparative use of two antiseptic solutions before intravascular or epidural catheterization. *Ann Fr Anesth Reanim* 2003;22(9):787–797.

127. Henschen A, Olson L. Chlorhexidine-induced degeneration of adrenergic nerves. *Acta Neuropathol* 1984;63(1):18–23.

128. Robins K, Wilson R, Watkins EJ, et al. Chlorhexidine spray versus single use sachets for skin preparation before regional nerve blockade for elective cesarean section: An effectiveness, time and cost study. *Int J Obstet Anesth* 2005;14(3):189–192.

129. Beilin Y, Arnold I, Telfeyan C, et al. Quality of analgesia when air versus saline is used for identification of the epidural space in the parturient. *Reg Anesth Pain Med* 2000;25(6):596–599.

130. Saberski LR, Kondamuri S, Osinubi OY. Identification of the epidural space: Is loss of resistance to air a safe technique? A review of the complications related to the use of air. *Reg Anesth* 1997;22(1):3–15.

131. Dalens B. Gone with the wind: The fate of epidural air. *Reg Anesth* 1990;15(3):150–151.

132. Kennedy TM, Ullman DA, Harte FA, et al. Lumbar root compression secondary to epidural air. *Anesth Analg* 1988;67(12):1184–1186.

133. Dickson MA, Moores C, McClure JH. Comparison of single, end-holed and multi-orifice extradural catheters when used for continuous infusion of local anaesthetic during labour. *Br J Anaesth* 1997;79(3):297–300.

134. Segal S, Eappen S, Datta S. Superiority of multi-orifice over single-orifice epidural catheters for labor analgesia and cesarean delivery. *J Clin Anesth* 1997;9(2):109–112.

135. D'Angelo R, Foss ML, Livesay CH. A comparison of multiport and uniport epidural catheters in laboring patients. *Anesth Analg* 1997;84(6):1276–1279.

136. Jaime F, Mandell GL, Vallejo MC, Ramanathan S. Uniport soft-tip, open-ended catheters versus multiport firm-tipped close-ended catheters for epidural analgesia: A quality assurance study. *J Clin Anesth* 2000;12(2):89–93.

137. Gadalla F, Lee SH, Choi KC, et al. Injecting saline through the epidural needle decreases the iv epidural catheter placement rate during combined spinal-epidural labour analgesia. *Can J Anaesth* 2003;50(4):382–385.

138. Beilin Y, Bernstein HH, Zucker-Pinchoff B. The optimal distance that a multiorifice epidural catheter should be threaded into the epidural space. *Anesth Analg* 1995;81(2):301–304.

139. Richardson MG, Wissler RN. The effects of needle bevel orientation during epidural catheter insertion in laboring parturients. *Anesth Analg* 1999;88(2):352–356.

140. Hamilton CL, Riley ET, Cohen SE. Changes in the position of epidural catheters associated with patient movement. *Anesthesiology* 1997;86(4):778–784.

141. Birnbach DJ, Chestnut DH. The epidural test dose in obstetric patients: Has it outlived its usefulness? *Anesth Analg* 1999;88(5):971–972.

142. Moore DC, Batra MS. The components of an effective test dose prior to epidural block. *Anesthesiology* 1981;55(6):693–696.

143. Gaiser RR. The epidural test dose in obstetric anesthesia: It is not obsolete. *J Clin Anesth* 2003;15(6):474–477.

144. Reynolds F. Epidural catheter migration during labour. *Anaesthesia* 1988;43(1):69.

145. Seidman SF, Marx GF. Epinephrine test dose is not warranted for confirmation of intravascular migration of epidural catheter in a parturient. *Can J Anaesth* 1988;35(1):104–106.

146. Leighton BL, Norris MC, DeSimone CA, Epstein R. The epinephrine test dose revisited again. *Anesthesiology* 1988;68(5):807–809.

147. Norris MC. Ferrenbach D, Dalman H, et al. Does epinephrine improve the diagnostic accuracy of aspiration during labor epidural analgesia? *Anesth Analg* 1999;88(5):1073–1076.

148. Colonna-Romano P, Nagaraj L. Tests to evaluate intravenous placement of epidural catheters in laboring women: A prospective clinical study. *Anesth Analg* 1998;86(5):985–988.

149. Leighton BL, Norris MC, DeSimone CA, et al. The air test as a clinically useful indicator of intravenously placed epidural catheters. *Anesthesiology* 1990;73(4):610–613.

150. Leighton BL, Topkis WG, Gross JB, et al. Multiport epidural catheters: Does the air test work? *Anesthesiology* 2000;92(6):1617–1620.

151. Albaladejo P, Bouaziz H, Benhamou D. Epidural analgesics: How can safety and efficacy be improved? *CNS Drugs* 1998;10:91–104.

152. Poppers PJ. Evaluation of local anesthetic agents for regional anesthesia in obstetrics. *Br J Anaesth* 1975;47S:322–327.

153. Albright G. Cardiac arrest following regional anesthesia with etidocaine or bupivacaine. *Anesthesiology* 1979;51:285–287.

154. Heath ML. Deaths after intravenous regional anaesthesia. *Br Med J* 1982;285:913–994.

155. Aberg G. Toxicological and local anaesthetic effects of optically active isomers of 2 local anaesthetic compounds. *Acta Pharmacologia Toxicologica* 1972;31:273–286.

156. Luduena FP, Bogado EF, Tullar BF. Optical isomers of Mepivacaine and Bupivacaine. *Arch Intern Pharmacodynam* 1972;200:359–369.

157. Thomas JM, Schug SA. Recent advances in the pharmacokinetics of local anaesthetics. Long-acting amide enantiomers and continuous infusions. *Clin Pharmacokinet* 1999;36(1):67–83.

158. Polley LS, Columb MO, Naughton NN, et al. Relative analgesic potencies of ropivacaine and bupivacaine for epidural analgesia in labor: Implications for therapeutic indexes. *Anesthesiology* 1999;90(4):944–950.

159. Santos AC, Arthur GR, Lehning EJ, Finster M. Comparative pharmacokinetics of ropivacaine and bupivacaine in nonpregnant and pregnant ewes. Anesth Analg 1997;85(1):87–93.

160. Capogna G, Celleno D, Fusco P, et al. Relative potencies of bupivacaine and ropivacaine for analgesia in labour. *Br J Anaesth* 1999;82(3):371–373.

161. Campbell DC, Zwack RM, Crone LA, Yip RW. Ambulatory labor epidural analgesia: Bupivacaine versus ropivacaine. *Anesth Analg* 2000;90(6):1384–1389.

162. Owen MD, Thomas JA, Smith T, et al. Ropivacaine 0.075% and bupivacaine 0.075% with fentanyl 2 microg/mL are equivalent for labor epidural analgesia. Anesth Analg 2002;94(1):179–183.

163. Halpern SH, Breen TW, Campbell DC, et al. A multicenter, randomized, controlled trial comparing bupivacaine with ropivacaine for labor analgesia. Anesthesiology 2003;98(6):1431–1435.

164. Pitimana-aree S, Visalyaputra S, Komoltri C, et al. An economic evaluation of bupivacaine plus fentanyl versus ropivacaine alone for patient-controlled epidural analgesia after total-knee replacement procedure: A double-blinded randomized study. Reg Anesth Pain Med 2005;30(5): 446–451.

165. Panni M, Segal S. New local anesthetics. Are they worth the cost? *Anesthesiol Clin North America* 2003;21(1):19–38.

166. Nath S, Haggamrk S, Johansson G, Reiz S. Differential depressant and electrophysiological cardiotoxicity of local anesthetic: An experimental study with special reference to lidocaine and bupivacaine. *Anesth Analg* 1986;65(12):1263–1270.

167. Foster RH, Markham A. Levobupivacaine: A review of its pharmacology and use as a local anesthetic. *Adis Drug Evaluation* 2000;59:3.

168. Gristwood RW, Greaves JL. Levobupivacaine: A new safer long acting local anaesthetic agent. *Expert Opin Invest Drug.* 1999;8:861–876.

169. Vercauteren MP, Hans G, De Decker K, Adriaensen HA. Levobupivacaine combined with sufentanil and epinephrine for intrathecal labor analgesia: A comparison with racemic bupivacaine. *Anesth Analg* 2001;93(4):996–1000.

170. Morrison SG, Dominquez JJ, Frascarolo P, Reiz S. A comparison of the electrocardiographic effects of racemic bupivacaine, levobupivacaine, and ropivacaine in anesthetized swine. *Anesth Analg* 2000;90(6):1308–1314.

171. Bader AM, Tsen LC, Camann WR, et al. Clinical effects and maternal and fetal plasma concentrations of 0.5% epidural levobupivacaine versus bupivacaine for cesarean delivery. *Anesthesiology* 1999;90(6):1596–1601.

172. Cheng CR, Su TH, Hung YC, et al. A comparative study of the safety and efficacy of 0.5% levobupivacaine and 0.5% bupivacaine for epidural anesthesia in subjects undergoing elective caesarean section. *Acta Anaesthesiol Sin* 2002;40:13–20.

173. Burke D, Henderson DJ, Simpson A, et al. Comparison of 0.25% S(-) bupivacaine with 0.25% R-S bupivacaine for epidural analgesia in labour. *Br J Anaesth* 1999;83:750–755.

174. Robinson AP, Lyons GR, Wilson RC, et al. Levobupivacaine for epidural analgesia in labor: The sparing effect of epidural fentanyl. *Anesth Analg* 2001;92;410–414.

175. Brown WU, Bell GC, Lurie AL, et al. Newborn blood levels of lidocaine and mepivacaine in the first postnatal day following maternal epidural anesthesia. *Anesthesiology* 1975;42:698–707.

176. Scanlon JW, Brown WJ Jr., Weiss JB, et al. Neurobehavioral responses of newborn infants after maternal epidural anaesthesia. *Anesthesiology* 1974;40:121.

177. Kunhert BR, Harrison MJ, Linn PL, et al. Effects of maternal epidural anesthesia on neonatal behavior. *Anesth Analg* 1984;63:301.

178. Hampl KF, Schneider MC, Thorin D, et al. Hyperosmolarity does not contribute to transient radicular irritation after spinal anesthesia with hyperbaric 5% lidocaine. *Reg Anesth* 1995;20(5)363–368.

179. Pollock JE, Neal JM, Stephenson CA, et al. Prospective study of the incidence of transient radicular irritation (TRI) in patients undergoing spinal anesthesia. *Anesthesiology* 1996;84:1361–1367.

180. Kuhnert BR, Kuhnert PM, Philipson EH, et al. The half life of 2-chloroprocaine. *Anesth Analg* 1986;65:273.

181. Karambelkar DJ, Ramanathan S. 2 chloroprocaine antagonism of epidural morphine analgesia. *Acta Anaesthesiol Scand* 1997;41:774–778.

182. Coda B, Bausch S, Haas M, et al. The hypothesis that antagonism of fentanyl analgesia by 2 chloroprocaine is mediated by direct action on opioid receptors. *Reg Anesth* 1997;22:43–52.

183. Corke BC, Carlson CG, Dettbarn W. The influence of 2-chloroprocaine on the subsequent analgesic potency of bupivacaine. *Anesthesiology* 1984;60: 25–27.

184. Reisner LS, Hochman BN, Plumer MH. Persistent neurologic deficit and adhesive arachnoiditis following intrathecal 2-chloroprocaine injection. *Anesth Analg* 1980;59:452.

185. Gissen AJ, Datta S, Lambert D. The chloroprocaine controversy. I. A hypothesis to explain the neural complications of chloroprocaine epidural. *Reg Anesth* 1984;9:124.

186. Winnie AP, Nader AM. Santayana's prophecy fulfilled. *Reg Anesth Pain Med* 2001;26:558–564.

187. Kopacz DJ. Spinal 2-chloroprocaine: Minimum effective dose. *Reg Anesth Pain Med* 2005;30(1):36–42.

188. Russell I. In the event of accidental dural puncture by an epidural needle in labour, the catheter should be passed into the subarachnoid space. *Int J Obstet Anesth* 2002;11:23–27.

189. Rigler ML, Drasner K. Distribution of catheter-injected local anesthetic in a model of the subarachnoid space. *Anesthesiology* 1991;75:684–692.

190. Ross BK, Coda B, Heath CH. Local anesthetic distribution in a spinal model: A possible mechanism of neurologic injury after continuous spinal anesthesia. *Reg Anesth* 1992;17:69–77.

191. Arkoosh VA, Palmer CM, Yun E, et al. Continuous spinal labor analgesia: Safety and efficacy. *Anesthesiology* 2003;99:A1561.

192. Arkoosh VA, Palmer CM, Van Maren GA, et al. Continuous intrathecal labor analgesia: Safety and efficacy. *Anesthesiology* 1998;89:A1041.

193. Puolakka R, Pitkanen MT, Rosenberg PH. Comparison of three catheter sets for continuous spinal anesthesia in patients undergoing total hip or knee arthroplasty. *Reg Anesth Pain Med* 2000;25(6):584–90.

194. Muralidhar V, Kaul HL, Mallick P. Over-the-needle versus microcatheter-through-needle technique for continuous spinal anesthesia: A preliminary study. *Reg Anesth Pain Med* 1999;24(5):417–421.

195. Viscomi CM, Rathmell JP, Pace NL. Duration of intrathecal labor analgesia. Early versus advanced labor. *Anesth Analg* 1997;84:1108–1112.

196. Collis RE, Davies DW, Aveling W. Randomised comparison of combined spinal epidural and standard epidural analgesia in labour. *Lancet* 1995;345:1413–1416.

197. Wilson MJ, Cooper G, MacArthur C, Shennan A. Comparative Obstetric Mobile Epidural Trial (COMET) study group UK. Randomized controlled trial comparing traditional with two "mobile" epidural techniques: Anesthetic and analgesic efficacy. *Anesthesiology* 2002;97(6):1567–1575.

198. Palmer CM, Randall CC, Hays R, et al. The dose-response relation of intrathecal fentanyl for labor analgesia. *Anesthesiology* 1998;88:355–361.

199. Campbell DC, Camann WR, Datta S, et al. The addition of bupivacaine to intrathecal sufentanil for labor analgesia. *Anesth Analg* 1995;81:305–309.

200. Sia AT, Chong JL, Chiu JW. Combination of intrathecal sufentanil 10 mcg plus bupivacaine 2.5mg for labor analgesia. Is half the dose enough? *Anesth Analg* 1999;88:362–366.

201. Hughes D, Hill D, Fee JP. Intrathecal ropivacaine or bupivacaine with fentanyl for labour. *Br J Anaesth* 2001;87:733–737.

202. Tsen L, Thue B, Datta S, et al. Is combined spinal-epidural analgesia associated with more rapid cervical dilation in nulliparous patients when compared with conventional epidural analgesia? *Anesthesiology* 1999;91:920–925.

203. Wong C, Scavone, Peaceman A, et al. The risk of cesarean delivery with neuraxial analgesia given early versus late in labor. *N Engl J Med* 2005;352(7):655–656.

204. Puolakka R, Pitkanen MT, Rosenberg PH. Comparison of technical and block characteristics of different combined spinal and epidural anesthesia techniques. *Reg Anesth Pain Med* 2001;26(1):17–23.

205. Browne I, Birnbach DJ, Stein D, et al. A comparison of Espocan and Tuohy needles for the combined spinal-epidural technique for labor analgesia. *Anesth Analg* 2005;101(2):535–540.

206. Wells J, Paech MJ. Evans SF. Intrathecal fentanyl-induced pruritus during labour: The effect of prophylactic ondansetron. *Int J Obstet Anesth* 2004;13(1):35–39.

207. Van de Velde M. Neuraxial opioids for labour analgesia: Analgesic efficiency and effect on labour. *Curr Opin Anaesth* 2002;15(3):299–303.

208. Clarke VT, Smiley RM, Finster M. Uterine hyperactivity after intrathecal injection of fentanyl for analgesia during labor: A cause of fetal bradycardia? *Anesthesiology* 1994;81:1083.

209. D'Angelo R, Eisenach JC. Severe maternal hypotension and fetal bradycardia after a CSE. *Anesthesiology* 1997;81:116–118.

210. Rolfseng OK, Skogvoll E, Borchgrevink PC. Epidural bupivacaine with sufentanil or fentanyl during labour: A randomized, double blind study. *Eur J Anaesthesiol* 2002;19(11):812–818.

211. Van de Velde M, Teunkens A, Hanssens M, et al. Intrathecal sufentanil and fetal heart abnormalities: A double-blind, double placebo-controlled trial comparing two forms of combined spinal epidural analgesia with epidural analgesia in labor. *Anesth Analg* 2004;98(4):1153–1159.

212. Van de Velde M, Vercauteren M, Vandermeersch E. Fetal heart rate abnormalities after regional analgesia for labor: The effect of intrathecal opioids. *Reg Anesth Pain Med* 2001;26(3):257–262.

213. O'Gorman D, Birnbach DJ, Kuczkowski KM, et al. Use of umbilical flow velocimetry in the assessment of the pathogenesis of fetal bradycardia following combined spinal epidural analgesia in parturients (Abs). *Anesthesiology* 2000;92:A2.

214. Albright GA, Forster RM. Does combined spinal-epidural analgesia with subarachnoid sufentanil increase the incidence of emergency cesarean delivery? *Reg Anesthesia and Pain Med* 1997;22:400–405.

215. Debon R, Allaouchiche B, Duflo G, et al. The analgesic effect of sufentanil combined with ropivacaine 0.2% for labor analgesia: A comparison of three sufentanil doses. *Anesth Analg* 2001;92(1):180–183.

216. Buyse I, Stockman W, Columb M, et al. Effect of sufentanil on minimum local analgesic concentrations of epidural bupivacaine, ropivacaine, and levobupivacaine in nullipara in early labour. *Int J Obstet Anesth* 2007;16(1):22–28.

217. Camorcia M, Capogna G. Epidural levobupivacaine, ropivacaine, and bupivacaine in combination with sufentanil in early labour: A randomized trial. *Eur J Anaesthesiol* 2003;20(8):636–639.

218. Driver I, Popham P, Glazebrook C, Palmer C. Epidural bupivacaine/fentanyl infusions vs intermittent top-ups: A retrospective study of the effects on mode of delivery in primiparous women. *Eur J Anaesthesiol* 1996;13(5):515–520.

219. Liu EH, Sia AT. Rates of caesarean section and instrumental delivery in nulliparous women after low concentration epidural infusions or opioid analgesia: A systemic review. *BR MED J* 2004;328(7453):1410.

220. Comparative Obstetric Mobile Epidural Trial (COMET) study group UK. Effect of low-dose mobile versus traditional epidural techniques on mode of delivery: A randomised controlled trial. *Lancet* 2001;358(9275):19–23.

221. Zhang J, Yancey MK, Klebanoff MA, et al. Does epidural analgesia prolong labor and increase risk of cesarean delivery? A natural experiment. *Am J Obstet Gynecol* 2001;185:128–134.

222. Zhang J, Klebanoff M, DerSimonian R. Epidural analgesia in association with duration of labor and mode of delivery: A quantitative review. *Am J Obstet Gynecol* 1999;180(4):970–977.

223. Roelants F, Lavand'homme PM, Mercier-Furzier V. *Anesthesiology* 2005;102(6):1025–1010. Roelants F. The use of neuraxial adjuvant drugs (neostigmine, clonidine) in obstetrics. *Curr Opin Anaesthesiol* 2006;19(3):33–37.

224. Boelants E. The use of neuraxial adjuvant drugs (neostigmine, clonidine) in obstetrics. *Curr Opin Anaesthesiol* 2006;19:33–37.

225. Curatolo M, Petersen-Felix S, Arendt-Nielson L, et al. Epidural epinephrine and clonidine, segmental analgesia and effects on different pain modalities. *Anesthesiology* 1997;87:785–794.

226. Soetens FM, Soeten MA, Vercauten MP. Levobupivacaine-sufentanil with or without epinephrine during epidural labor analgesia. *Anesth Analg* 2006;103(1):182–186.

227. Viscomi C, Eisenach JC. Patient controlled epidural analgesia during labor. *Obstet Gynecol* 1991;77:348.

228. Carvalho B, Wang P, Cohen S. A survey of labor patient-controlled epidural anesthesia practice in California Hospitals. *Int J Obstet Anesth* 2006;15(3):217–222.

229. Paech MJ. Patient controlled epidural analgesia in obstetrics. *Int J Obstet Anesth* 1996;5:115–125.

230. Bremerich DH, Waibel HJ, Meirdl S, et al. Comparison of continuous background infusion plus demand dose and demand-only parturient-controlled epidural analgesia (PCEA) using ropivacaine combined with sufentanil for labor and delivery. *Int J Obstet Anesth* 2005;14(2):114–120.

231. Boselli E, Debon R, Cimino Y, et al. Background infusion is not beneficial during labor patient-controlled analgesia with 0.1% ropivacaine plus 0.5% microg/ml sufentanil. *Anesthesiology* 2004;100(4):968–972.

232. Depp R. Cesarean delivery and other surgical procedures. In: Gabbe SG, Niebyl JR, Simpson JL, eds. *Obstetrics: Normal and Problem Pregnancies*. New York: Church and Livingston; 1991;20:635.

233. Deneux-Tharaux C, Carmona E, Bouvier-Colle MH, Breart G. Postpartum maternal mortality and cesarean delivery. *Obstet Gynecol* 2006;108[3 Pt 1]:541–548.

234. Lydon-Rochelle M, Holt VL, Easterling TR, Martin DP. Cesarean delivery and postpartum mortality among primiparas in Washington State, 1987–1996(1). *Obstet Gynecol* 2001;97(2):169–174.

235. MacDorman MF, Declercq E, Meancker F, Malloy MH. Infant and neonatal mortality for primary caesarean and vaginal births to women with "no indicated risk," United States, 1998–2001 birth cohorts. *Birth* 2006;33(3):175–182.

236. Grisaru S, Samueloff A. Primary non-medically indicated cesarean section (section on request): Evidence based or modern vogue? *Clin Perinatol* 2004;31(3):409–430.

237. National Institutes of Health state-of-the-science conference statement: Cesarean delivery on maternal request March 27–29, 2006. *Obstet Gynecol* 2006;107(6):1386–1397.

238. Bettes B, Coleman V, Zinberg S, et al. Cesarean delivery on maternal request: Obstetrician-gynecologists' knowledge, perception, and practice patterns. *Obstet Gynecol* 2007;109(1):57–66.

239. Brownridge P, Jefferson J. Central neural blockade and caesarean section II: Patient assessment of the procedure. *Anaesth Intensive Care* 1979;7(2):163–168.

240. Hawkins JL, Koonin LM, Palmer SK, et al. Anesthesia-related deaths during obstetric delivery in the United States, 1979–1990. *Anesthesiology* 1999;86:277–284.

241. Andrews WW, Ramin SM, Maberry MC, et al. Effect of type of anesthesia on blood loss at elective repeat cesarean section. *Am J Perinatol* 1992;9:197–200.

242. Afolabi BB, Lesi FE, Merah NA. Regional versus general anesthesia for caesarean section. *Cochrane Database Syst Rev* 2006;18(4):CD004350.

243. Pan PH, Bogard TD, Owen MD. Incidence and characteristics of failures in obstetric neuraxial analgesia and anesthesia: A retrospective analysis of 19,259 deliveries. *Int J Obstet Anesth* 2004;13(4):227–233.

244. Balki M, Carvalho JC. Intraoperative nausea and vomiting during caesarean section under regional anesthesia. *Int J Obstet Anesth* 2005;14(3):230–241.

245. Norris MC. Height, weight and the spread of subarachnoid hyperbaric bupivacaine in the term parturient. *Anesth Analg* 1988;67:555.

246. De Simone CA, Leighton BL, Norris MC. Spinal anesthesia for cesarean delivery: A comparison of two doses of hyperbaric bupivacaine. *Reg Anesth* 1995;20:90.

247. Vucevic M, Russell IF. Spinal anesthesia for caesarean section: 0.125% plain bupivacaine 12mL compared with 0.5% plain bupivacaine 3mL. *Br J Anaesth* 1992;68:590–595.

248. Runza M, Albani A, Tagliabue M, et al. Spinal Anesthesia using 3 ml hyperbaric 0.75% versus hyperbaric 1% bupivacaine for cesarean section. *Anesth Analg* 1998;87:1099–1013.

249. Riley ET, Cohen SE, Macario A, et al. Spinal versus epidural anesthesia for cesarean section: A comparison of time efficiency, costs, charges, and complications. *Anesth Analg* 1995;80:709–712.

250. Hamza J, Mohammed S, Benhamou D, et al. Parturient's posture during epidural puncture affects the distance from the skin to epidural space. *J Clin Anesth* 1995;7:1–4.

251. Russell IF. Spinal anaesthesia for caesarean section: The use of 0.5% bupivacaine. *Br J Anaesth* 1983;55:309–314.

252. Congreve K, Gardner I, Laxton C, Scrutton M. Where is T5? A survey of anaesthetists. *Anaesthesia* 2006;61(5):453–455.

253. Wilkinson C, Enkin MW. Uterine exteriorization versus intraperitoneal repair at caesarean section. *Cochrane Database Syst Rev* 2000;(2):CD000085.

254. Abouleish EL. Epinephrine improves the quality of spinal hyperbaric bupivacaine for cesarean section. *Anesth Analg* 1987;66:395–400.

255. Abouleish E, Rawal N, Fallon K, et al. Combined intrathecal morphine and bupivacaine for cesarean section. *Anesth Analg* 1988;67:370–374.

256. Hunt CO, Naulty J, Bader AM, et al. Perioperative analgesia with subarachnoid fentanyl-bupivacaine for cesarean delivery. *Anesthesiology* 1989;71:535–540.

257. Courtney MA, Bader AM, Hartwell B, et al. Perioperative analgesia with subarachnoid sufentanil administration. *Reg Anesth* 1992;17:274–278.

258. Di Fazio CA, Carron H, Grosslight RR, et al. Comparison of pH-adjusted lidocaine solutions for epidural anesthesia. *Anesth Analg* 1986;65:760–764.

259. Benhamou D, Labaille T, Bonhomme L, et al. Alkalinization of epidural 0.5% bupivacaine for cesarean section. *Reg Anesth* 1980;14:240–243.

260. Lam DT, Ngan Kee WD, Khaw KS. Extension of epidural blockade in labour for emergency Cesarean section using 2% lidocaine with epinephrine and fentanyl, with or without alkalinization. *Anaesthesia* 2001;56:790–794.

261. Laishley RS, Morgan BM. A single dose epidural technique for caesarean section: A comparison between 0.5% bupivacaine plain and 0.5% bupivacaine with adrenaline. *Anaesthesia* 1988;43:100–103.

262. Preston PG, Rosen MA, Hughes SC, et al. Epidural anesthesia with fentanyl and lidocaine for cesarean section: Maternal effects and neonatal outcome. *Anesthesiology* 1988;68:938.

263. Vertommen JD, Van Aken H, Vandermeulen E, et al. Maternal and neonatal effects of adding epidural sufentanil to 0.5% bupivacaine for cesarean delivery. *J Clin Anesth* 1991;3:371–376.

264. Eisenach J, Detweiler D, Hood D. Hemodynamic and analgesic actions of epidurally administered clonidine. *Anesthesiology* 1993;78:277–287.

265. Carrie LES, O'Sullivan GM. Subarachnoid bupivacaine 0.5% for cesarean section. *Eur J Anaesth* 1984;1:275–283.

266. Crowhurst J, Birnbach DJ. Low dose neuraxial block. Heading towards the new millennium. *Anesth Analg* 2000;90:241–242.

267. Stienstra R, Dilrosun-Alhadi B, Dahan A, et al. The epidural "top-up" in combined spinal-epidural anesthesia: The effect of volume versus dose. *Anesth Analg* 1999;88(4):810–814.

268. Blumgart CH, Ryall D, Dennison B, et al. Mechanism of extension of spinal anaesthesia by extradural injection of local anesthetic. *Br J Anaesth* 1992;69:457.

269. Rawal N, Van Zunder A, Holmstrom B, et al. Combined spinal-epidural technique. *Reg Anesth* 1997;22:406–423.

270. Hurley RJ, Lambert DH. Continuous spinal anesthesia with a microcatheter technique. Preliminary experience. *Anesth Analg* 1990;70:97–102.

271. Charsley MM, Abrams SE. The injection of intrathecal normal saline reduces the severity of postdural puncture headache. *Reg Anesth Pain Med* 2001;26(4):301–305.

272. Dick WE. Anaesthesia for caesarean section (epidural and general): Effects on the neonate. *Eur J Obstet Gynecol Reprod Biol* 1995;59:S1–S7.

273. Scherer R, Holzgreve W. Influence of epidural analgesia on fetal and neonatal well-being. *Eur J Obstet Gynecol Reprod Biol* 1995;59:S17–S29.

274. Tsen LC, Boosalis P, Segal S, et al. Hemodynamic effects of simultaneous administration of intravenous ephedrine and spinal anesthesia for cesarean delivery. *J Clin Anesth* 2000;12:378–382.

275. Ngan Kee Wd, Khaw K, Lee BB, et al. A dose-response study of prophylactic intravenous ephedrine for the prevention of hypotension during spinal anesthesia for cesarean delivery. *Anaesth Analg* 2000;90:1390–1395.

276. Reynolds F. Dural puncture and headache. *BR MED J* 1993;306:874–875.

277. Day CJE, Shutt LE. Auditory, ocular and facial complications of central neural blockade: A review of possible mechanisms. *Reg Anesth* 1996;21:97–201.

278. Wong AYC, Irwin MG. Post dural puncture tinnitus. *Br J Anaesth* 2003;91:762–763.

279. Malhotra SK, Iver BR, Gupta AK, et al. Spinal analgesia and auditory functions: Comparison of two size Quincke needle. *Minerva Anestesiol* 2006;12:Epub.

280. Ahmed SV, Jayawarna C, Jude E. Post dural puncture headache: Diagnosis and management. *Postgrad Med J* 2006;82(973):713–716.

281. Richman JM, Joe EM, Cohen SR, et al. Bevel direction and postdural puncture headache: A meta-analysis. *Neurologist* 2006;12(4):224–228.

282. Lambert DH, Hurley RJ, Herrwig L, et al. Role of needle gauge and tip configuration in the production of lumbar puncture headache. *Reg Anesth* 1997;22:66–72.

283. Norris MC, Leighton BL, DeSimone CA. Needle bevel orientation and headache after inadvertent dural puncture. *Anesthesiology* 1989;70:729–731.

284. Reina MS, Dittman M, Garcia AL, et al. New perspectives in the microscopic structure of human dura mater in the dorsolumbar region. *Reg Anesth* 1997;22:161–166.

285. Van De Velde M, Teunkens A, Hannens M, et al. Post dural puncture headache following combined spinal epidural or epidural anaesthesia in obstetric patients. *Anaesth Intensive Care* 2001;29(6):595–599.

286. Benhamou D, Hamza J, Ducot B. Postpartum headache after epidural analgesia without dural puncture. *Int J Obstet Anesth* 1995;4:17–20.

287. Browne I, Birnbach DJ. Neurocysticercosis: A new differential in the diagnosis of postdural puncture headache. *Anesth Analg* 2003;97(2):580–582.

288. Benzon HT, Iqbal M, Tallman MS, et al. Superior sagittal sinus thrombosis in a patient with postdural puncture headache. *Reg Anesth Pain Med* 2003;28:64–67.

289. Mokri B. Headaches caused by decreased intracranial pressure: Diagnosis and management. *Curr Opin Neurol* 2003;16:319–326.

290. Schaller B, Graf R. Different compartments of intracranial pressure and its relationship to cerebral blood flow. *J Trauma* 2005;59(6):1521–1531.

291. Mokri B. The Monroe-Kellie hypothesis: Applications in CSF volume depletion. *Neurology* 2001;56:1746–1748.

292. Halpern S, Preston R. Postdural puncture headache and spinal needle design. Meta analyses. *Anesthesiology* 1994;81:1376–1383.

293. Hatfalvi BI. Postulated mechanisms for post dural puncture headache and review of laboratory models clinical experience. *Reg Anesth* 1995;20:329–336.

294. Wantman A, Hancox N, Howell PR. Techniques for identifying the epidural space: A survey of practice amongst anaesthetists in the UK. *Anaesthesia* 2006;61(4):370–375.

295. Leeda M, Stienstra R, Arbous MS, et al. Lumbar epidural catheter insertion: The midline vs. the paramedian approach. *Eur J Anaesthesiol* 2005;22(11):839–842.

296. Ayad S, Demain Y, Narouze SN, et al. Subarachnoid catheter placement after wet tap for analgesia in labor. Influence on the risk of headache in obstetric patients. *Reg Anaesth Pain Med* 2003;28:512–515.

297. Choi PT, Galinski SE, Takeuchi L, et al. PDPH is a common complication of neuraxial blockade in parturients: A meta-analysis of obstetrical studies. *Can J Anaesth* 2003;50(5):460–469.

298. Sandesc D, Lupei MI, et al. Conventional treatment or epidural blood patch for the treatment of different etiologies of post dural puncture headache. *Acta Anaesthesiol Belg* 2005;56(3):265–269.

299. Camann WR, Murray RS, Mushlin PS, et al. Effects of oral caffeine on postdural puncture headache: A double-blind placebo-controlled trial. *Anesth Analg* 1990;70:181–184.

300. Yucel A, Ozyalcin S, Talu GK, et al. Intravenous administration of caffeine sodium benzoate for postdural puncture headache. *Reg Anesth Pain Med* 1999;24:51–54.

301. Bolton VE, Leicht CH, Scanlon TS. Postpartum seizure after epidural blood patch and intravenous caffeine sodium benzoate. *Anesthesiology* 1989;70:146–149.

302. Cohen SM, Laurito CE, Curran MJ. Grand mal seizure in a post partum patient following intravenous infusion of caffeine benzoate to treat persistent headache. *J Clin Anesth* 1992;4:48–51.

303. Ryu JE. Effect of maternal caffeine consumption on heart rate and sleep time of breast fed infants. *Dev Pharmacol Ther* 1985;8:353–363.

304. Esmaoglu A, Akpinar H, Ugur F. Oral multidose caffeine-paracetamol combination is not effective for the prophylaxis of postdural puncture headache. *J Clin Anesth* 2005;17(1):58–61.

305. Hodgson C, Roitberg-Henry A. The use of sumatriptan in the treatment of postdural puncture headache. *Anaesthesia* 1997;52:808.

306. Carp H, Singh PJ, Vadhera R, et al. Effects of the serotonin-receptor agonist sumatriptan on postdural puncture headache: Report of six cases. *Anesth Analg* 1994;79:180–182.

307. Connolly NR, Parker RK, Rahimi A, et al. Sumatriptan in patients with postdural puncture headache. *Headache* 2000;40:316–319.

308. Lhuissier C, Mercier FJ, Dounas M, Benhamou D. Sumatriptan: An alternative to epidural blood patch. *Anaesthesia* 1996;51(11):1078.

309. Kshatri AM, Foster PA. ACTH infusion as a novel treatment for postdural puncture headache. *Reg Anesth* 1997;22:432–434.

310. Safa-Tisseront V, Thormann F, Malassine P, et al. Effectiveness of epidural blood patch in the management of post-dural puncture headache. *Anesthesiology* 2001;95:334–339.

311. Taivaninen T, Pitkanen M, Touminen M, et al. Efficacy of epidural blood patch for postdural puncture headache. *Acta Anaesthesiol Scand* 1993;37:702–705.

312. Bearb ME, Pennant JH. Epidural blood patch in a Jehovah's Witness. *Anesth Analg* 1987;66:1052.

313. Anwari JS. Epidural blood patch (EBP) and septic complication. *Can J Anaesth* 2000;47(3):289–290.

314. Coombs DW, Hooper D. Subarachnoid pressure with epidural blood patch. *Reg Anesth* 1979;4:3–6.

315. Szeinfeld M, Ihmeidan IH, Moser MM, et al. Epidural blood patch: Evaluation of the volume and spread of blood injected into the epidural space. *Anesthesiology* 1986;64:820–822.

316. Djurhuus H, Rasmussen M, Jensen EH. Epidural blood patch illustrated by CT-epidurography. *Acta Anaesthesiol Scand* 1995;39:613–617.

317. Griffith AG, Beards SC, Jackson A, Horsman EL. Visualization of extradural blood patch for post lumbar puncture headache by magnetic resonance imaging. *Br J Anaesth* 1993;70(2):223–225.

318. Beards SC, Jackson A, Griffiths AG, Horsman EL. Magnetic resonance imaging of extradural blood patches: Appearance from 30 min to 18 h. *Br J Anaesth* 1993;7(12):182–188.

319. Tobias MD, Henry C, Augostides YGT. Lidocaine and bupivacaine exert differential effects on whole blood coagulation. *J Clin Anesth* 1999;11:52–55.

320. Loeser EA, Hill GE, Bennett GM, et al. Time vs. success rate for epidural blood patch. *Anesthesiology* 1978;49:147–148.

321. Martin R, Jourdain S, Clairoux M, et al. Duration of decubitus position after epidural blood patch. *Can J Anaesth* 1994;41:23–25.

322. Kamada M, Fujita Y, Ishii R, et al. Spontaneous intracranial hypotension successfully treated by epidural patching with fibrin glue. *Headache* 2000;40:844–847.

323. Gladstone JP, Nelson K, Patel N, Dodick DW. Spontaneous CSF leak treated with percutaneous CT-guided fibrin glue. *Neurology* 2005;64(10):1818–1819.

324. Souron V, Hamza J. Treatment of post dural puncture headaches with colloid solutions: An alternative to epidural blood patch. *Anesth Analg* 1999;89:1333–1334.

325. Philip JH, Brown WU. Total spinal anesthesia late in the course of obstetric bupivacaine epidural block. *Anesthesiology* 1976;44:340.

326. Lee A, Dodd KW. Accidental subdural catheterisation. *Anaesthesia* 1986;41:847.

PART III: APPLICATIONS

327. Mets B, Broccoli E, Brown AR. Is spinal anesthesia after failed epidural anesthesia contraindicated for cesarean section? *Anesth Analg* 1993;77:629–631.

328. Gupta A, Enhund G, Bengtsson M. Spinal anaesthesia for cesarean section following epidural analgesia in labour. *Int J Obstet Anaesth* 1994;3:153–156.

329. Faccenda KA, Finucane BT. Complications of regional anesthesia: Incidence and prevention. *Drug Saf* 2001;24:413–442.

330. Moen V, Dahlgren N, Irestedt L. Severe neurological complications after central neuraxial blockades in Sweden 1990–1999. *Anesthesiology* 2004;101(4):950–959.

331. Lee LA, Posner KL, Domino KB, et al. Injuries associated with regional anesthesia in the 1980s and 1990s: A closed claim analysis. *Anesthesiology* 2004;101(1):143–152.

332. Ross BK. ASA closed claims in obstetrics: Lessons learned. *Anesthesiol Clin North American* 2003;21(1):183–197.

333. Hebl JR, Horlocker TT, Schroeder DR. Neuraxial anesthesia and analgesia in patients with pre-existing central nervous system disorders. *Anesth Analg* 2006;103(1):223–228.

334. Aldrete JA, Reza-Medina M, Daud O, et al. Exacerbation of preexisting neurological deficits by neuraxial anesthesia: Report of 7 cases. *J Clin Anesth* 2005;17(4):304–313.

335. Bromage PR. Neurological complications of epidural and spinal techniques. In: Van Aken H, ed. *New Developments in Epidural and Spinal Drugs Administration*. London: Balliere's Clinical Anesthesiology; 1992;7:793–815.

336. Hebl JR, Kopp SL, Schroeder DR, Horlocker TT. Neurologic complications after neuraxial anesthesia or analgesia in patients with preexisting peripheral sensorimotor neuropathy or diabetic polyneuropathy. *Anesth Analg* 2006;103(5):1294–1299.

337. O'Donnell D, Rottmann R, Kotelko D, et al. Incidence of maternal postpartum neurologic dysfunction (Abs). *Anesthesiology* 1994;81:A1127.

338. Durbridge J, Holdcroft A. The long-term effects of analgesia in labour. *Baillieres Clin Obstet Gynaecol* 1998;12:485–498.

339. Horlocker TT, McGregor D, Matsushige DK, et al. A retrospective review of 4767 consecutive spinal anesthetics: Central nervous system complications. Perioperative Outcomes Group. *Anesth Analg* 1997;84:578–584.

340. Pollock JE. Transient neurological symptoms: Etiology, risk factors, and management. *Reg Anesth Pain Med* 2002;27:581–586.

341. Hampl KF, Schneider MD, Pargger H, et al. A similar incidence of transient neurological symptoms after spinal anesthesia with 2% and 5% lidocaine. *Anesth Analg* 1996;83:1051–1054.

342. Salmela L, Aromma U. Transient radicular irritation after spinal anesthesia induced with hyperbaric solutions of cerebrospinal fluid-diluted lidocaine 50 mg/ml or mepivacaine 40 mg/ml or bupivacaine 5 mg/ml. *Acta Anaesthesiol Scand* 1998;42:765–769.

343. Ostgaard G, Hallaraker O, Ulveseth OK, et al. A randomised study of lidocaine and prilocaine for spinal anesthesia. *Acta Anaesthesiol Scand* 2000;44:436–440.

344. Chabbouh T, Lentschener C, Zuber M, et al. Persistent cauda equina syndrome with no identifiable facilitation condition after an uneventful single spinal administration of 0.5% hyperbaric bupivacaine. *Anesth Analg* 2005;101(6):1847–1848.

345. Bilir A, Gulec S. Cauda equina syndrome after epidural steroid injection: A case report. *J Manipulative Physiol Ther* 2006;29(6):1–3.

346. Auroy Y, Benhamou D, Bargeus L, et al. Major complications of regional anesthesia in France. *Anesthesiology* 2002;97:1274–1280.

347. Loo CC, Irsted L. Cauda equina syndrome after spinal anesthesia with hyperbaric 5% lidocaine: A review of six cases of cauda equine syndrome reported to the Swedish pharmaceutical insurance 1993–1997. *Acta Anaesthesiol Scand* 1999;43:371–379.

348. Gerancher JC. Cauda equina syndrome following a single spinal administration of 5% hyperbaric lidocaine through a 25-gauge Whitacre needle. *Anesthesiology* 1997;87:687–689.

349. Aldrete JA. Neurological deficits and arachnoiditis following neuroaxial anesthesia. *Acta Anaesthesiol Scand* 2003;47(1):3–12.

350. Petty PG, Hudgson P, Hare WS. Symptomatic lumbar spinal arachnoiditis: Fact or fallacy? *J Clin Neurosci* 2000;7(5):395–399.

351. Dolan RA. Spinal adhesive arachnoiditis. *Surg Neurol* 1993;39(6):479–484.

352. Rice I, Wee MY, Thomson K. Obstetric epidurals and chronic adhesive arachnoiditis. *Br J Anaesth* 2004;92(1):109–120.

353. Macarthur C, Lewis M, Knox FG, et al. Epidural anaesthesia and long-term backache after childbirth. *Br Med J* 1990;301:9–12.

354. Russell R, Groves P, Taub N, et al. Assessing long term backache after childbirth. *Br Med J* 1993;306:1299–1303.

355. Macarthur AJ, Macarthur C, Weeks SK. Is epidural anesthesia in labor associated with chronic lower back pain? A prospective cohort study. *Anesth Analg* 1997;85(5):10066–10070.

356. Breen TW, Ransil BJ, Groves PA, et al. Factors associated with back pain after childbirth. *Anesthesiology* 1994;81:29–34.

357. Howell CJ, Dean T, Lucking L, et al. Randomised study of long-term outcome after epidural versus non-epidural analgesia during labour. *Br Med J* 2002;325:357–361.

358. Hlavin ML, Kaminski HJ, Ross JS, et al. Spinal epidural abscess: A 10 year perspective. *Neurosurgery* 1990;27:177–184.

359. Wang LP, Hauerberg J, Schmidt JF. Incidence of spinal epidural abscess after epidural analgesia. *Anesthesiology* 1999;91:1928–1936.

360. Horlocker TT, Wedel DJ. Neurological complications of spinal and epidural anesthesia. *Reg Anesth Pain Med* 2000;25:83–98.

361. Brookman CA, Rutledge MLC. Epidural abscess. Case report and literature review. *Reg Anesth Pain Med* 2000;25:428–431.

362. Schneeberger PM, Janssen M, Voss A. Alpha-hemolytic streptococci: A major pathogen of iatrogenic meningitis following lumbar puncture: Case reports and a review of the literature. *Infection* 1996;24:29–35.

363. Tryba M. Epidural regional anesthesia and low molecular weight heparin: Pro (German). *Anästh Intensivmed Notfallmed Schmerzther* 1993;28:179–181.

364. Vandermeulen EP, Van Aken H, Vermylen J. Anticoagulants and spinal epidural anesthesia. *Anesth Analg* 1994;79:1165–1177.

365. Greer IA. Anticoagulants in pregnancy. *J Thromb Thrombolysis* 2006;21(1):57–65.

366. Many A. Koren G. Low molecular-weight heparins during pregnancy. *Can Fam Physician* 2005;51:199–201.

367. Huxtable LM, Tafreshi MJ, Ondreyco SM. A protocol for the use of enoxaparin during pregnancy: Results from 85 pregnancy including 13 multiple gestational pregnancies. *Clin Appl Thromb Hemost* 2005;11(2):171–181.

368. Cunningham FG, MacDonald PC, Gant NF, et al. Hypertensive disorders in pregnancy. In: *Williams Obstetrics*, 20th ed. Stamford, Conn: Appleton and Lange; 1997:693–744.

369. Sibai BM, Gordon T, Thom E, et al. Epidemiology of preeclampsia and eclampsia in the United States, 1979–1986. *Am J Obstet Gynecol* 1990;163:460–465.

370. Kam PC, Thompson SA, Liew AC. Thrombocytopenia in the parturient. *Anaesthesia* 2004;59(3):255–264.

371. O'Brien JM, Barton JR. Controversies with the diagnosis and management of HELLP syndrome. *Clin Obstet Gynecol* 2005;48(2):460–477.

372. Santos AC, Birnbach DJ. Spinal anesthesia for cesarean delivery in severely preeclamptic women: Don't throw out the baby with the bathwater! *Anesth Analg* 2005;101:859–861.

373. Schneider MC, Landau R, Mortl MG. New insights in hypertensive disorders of pregnancy. *Curr Opin Anaesthesiol* 2001;14(3):291–297.

374. Davies JR, Fernando R, Hallworth SP. Hemostatic function in healthy pregnant and preeclamptic women: An assessment using the platelet function analyzer (PFA-100) and thromboelastograph. *Anesth Analg* 2007;104(2):416–420.

375. Rai R, Cohen H, Dave M, Regan L. Controlled trial of aspirin and aspirin plus heparin in pregnant women with recurrent miscarriage associated with phospholipid antibodies (or antiphospholipid antibodies). *BR MED J* 1997;314(7076):253–257.

376. Duley L, Henderson-Smart D, Knight M, King J. Antiplatelet drugs for prevention of pre-eclampsia and its consequences: Systematic review. *BR MED J* 2001;322:329–333.

377. Belilos E, Carsons S. Rheumatologic disorders in women. *Med Clin North Am* 1998;82(1):77–101.

378. Gomez-Puerta JA, Cervera R, Espinosa G, et al. Pregnancy and puerperium are high susceptibility periods for the development of catastrophic antiphospholipid syndrome. *Autoimmune Rev* 2006;6(2):85–88.

379. Dekker GA, de Vries JIP, Doelitzsch PM, et al. Underlying disorders associated with severe early-onset preeclampsia. *Am J Obstet Gynecol* 1995;173:1042–1048.

380. Kupferminc MJ, Eldor A, Steinman N, et al. Increased frequency of the genetic thrombophilia in women with complications of pregnancy. *N Engl J Med* 1999;340:9–13.

381. Martinelli I, Taioli E, Cetin I, et al. Mutations in coagulation factors in women with unexplained late fetal loss. *N Engl J Med* 2000;343:1015–1018.

382. Many A, Elad R, Yaron Y, et al. Third-trimester unexplained intrauterine fetal death is associated with inherited thrombophilia. *Obstet Gynecol* 2002;99:684–687.

383. Gris JC, Mercier E, Quere I, et al. Low-molecular-weight heparin versus low-dose aspirin in women with one fetal loss and a constitutional thrombophilic disorder. *Blood* 2004;103:3695–3699.

384. Placental transfer of drugs. In: Yaffe J, Aranda JU, eds. *Neonatal and Pediatric Pharmacology*. Philadelphia, PA: Lippincott Williams and Wilkins; 2005:136.

385. Dimitrakakis C, Papageorgiou P, Papageorgiou I, et al. Absence of transplacental passage of the low molecular weight heparin enoxaparin. *Haemostasis* 2000;30:243–248.

386. Richter C, Sitzmann J, Lang P, et al. Excretion of low molecular weight heparin in human milk. *Br J Clin Pharmacol* 2001;52(6):708–710.

387. Seshadri N, Goldhaer SZ, Elkayam U, et al. The clinical challenge of bridging anticoagulation with low-molecular-weight heparin in patients with mechanical prosthetic heart valves: An evidence-based comparative review focusing on anticoagulation options in pregnant and nonpregnant patients. *Am Heart J* 2005;150(1):27–34.

388. Regional anesthesia in the anti-coagulated patient: Defining the risks. American Society of Regional Anesthesia Consensus Statement. At www.asra.com. Accessed 11 May 2008.

389. Maternal Mortality in 2000. Estimates developed by WHO, UNICEF and UNFPA. Department of Reproductive Health and Research. Geneva: World Health Organization, 2004.

390. International Statistical Classification of Diseases and Related Health Problems. 10th Revision Version for 2006, World Health Organization.

391. Bouvier-Colle MH, Varnoux N, Costes P, Hatton F. Reasons for the under reporting of maternal morbidity in France, as indicated by surveying all deaths in women of childbearing age. *Int J Epidemiol* 1991;20:717–721.

392. UK Health Departments. *Reports on Confidential Enquiries into Maternal Deaths in the UK, 1991–1993.* London: Her Majesty's Stationery Office, 1996.

393. Chang J, Elam-Evans LD, Berg CJ, et al. Pregnancy-related mortality surveillance—United States, 1991–1999. *MMWR Surveill Summ* 2003; 52(2):1–8.

394. Guendelman S, Thornton D, Gould J, Hosang N. Obstetric complications during labor and delivery: Assessing ethnic differences in California. *Womens Health Issues* 2006;16(4):189–197.

395. De Ziegler D, Cedars MI, Randle D, et al. Suppression of the ovary using gonadotrophin-releasing hormone agonist prior to stimulation for oocyte retrieval. *Fertil Steril* 1987;48:807–810.

396. Edwards RG, Steptoe PC, Purdy JM. Establishing full-term human pregnancies using cleaving embryos grown in vitro. *Br J Obstet Gynaecol* 1980; 87:737–756.

397. Schnell VL, Sacco AG, Savoy-Moore RT, et al. Effects of oocyte exposure to local anesthetics on in vitro fertilization and embryo development in the mouse. *Reprod Toxicol* 1992;6(4):323–327.

398. Wikland M, Evers H, Jakobsson AH, et al. The concentration of lidocaine in follicular fluid when used for paracervical block in a human IVF-ET programme. *Hum Reprod* 1990;5(8):920–923.

399. Gonen O, Shulman A, Ghetler Y, et al. The impact of different types of anesthesia on in vitro fertilization-embryo transfer treatment outcome. *J Assist Reprod Genet* 1995;12(10):678–682.

400. Botta G, D'Angelo A, D'Ari G, et al. Epidural anesthesia in an in vitro fertilization and embryo transfer program. *J Assist Reprod Genet* 1995; 12(3):187–190.

401. Endler GC, Magyar DM, Hayes MF, Moghiosi KS. Use of spinal anesthesia in laparoscopy for IVF. *Fertil Steril* 1985;43:809–810.

402. Martin R, Tsen LC, Tzeng G, et al. Anesthesia for in vitro fertilization: The addition of fentanyl to 1.5% lidocaine. *Anesth Analg* 1999;88:523–526.

403. Fox AW, Diamond M, Spierings EL. Migraine during pregnancy: Options for therapy. *CNS Drugs* 2005;19(6):465–481.

404. Maderia LM, Hoffman MK, Shlossman PA. Internal carotid artery dissection as a cause of headache in the second trimester. *Am J Obstet Gynecol* 2007;196:7–8.

405. Ostgard HC, Andersson GB, Karlsson K. Prevalence of back pain in pregnancy. *Spine* 1991;16:549–552.

406. Fast A, Shapiro D, Ducommun EJ, et al. Low back pain in pregnancy. *Spine* 1987;12:368–371.

407. Foley BS, Buschbacher RM. Sacroiliac joint pain: Anatomy, biomechanics, diagnosis and treatment. *Am J Phys Med Rehab* 2006;85(12):997–1006.

408. Weinreb JC, Wolbarsht LB, Cohen JM, et al. Prevalence of lumbosacral intervertebral disk abnormalities on MR images in pregnant and asymptomatic nonpregnant women. *Radiology* 1989;170:125–128.

409. Rathmell JP, Viscomi CM, Ashburn MA. Management of nonobstetric pain during pregnancy and lactation. *Anesth Analg* 1997;85(5):1081–1082.

410. Berlin L. Radiation exposure and the pregnant patient. *Am J Roentgenol* 1996;167(6):1377–1379.

411. Zak IT, Dulai HS, Kish KK. Imaging of neurological disorders associated with pregnancy and the postpartum period. *Radiographics* 2007;27(1):95–108.

412. Poncelet C, Perdu M, Levy-Wall F, et al. Reflex sympathetic dystrophy in pregnancy: Nine cases and a review of the literature. *Eur J Obstet Gynecol Reprod Biol* 1999;86(1):55–63.

413. Lee JJ, Rubin AP. Breast feeding and anaesthesia. *Anaesthesia* 1993;48:616–625.

414. Schoenfeld A, Bar Y, Merlob P, Ovadia Y. NSAIDs: Maternal and fetal considerations. *Am J Reprod Immunol* 1992;28(3–4):141–147.

415. Bar-Oz B, Bulkowstein M, Benyamini L, et al. Use of antibiotics and analgesic drugs during lactation. *Drug Saf* 2003;26(13):925–935.

416. Spigset O, Hagg S. Analgesics and breast-feeding: Safety considerations. *Paediatr Drugs* 2000;2(3):223–238.

417. Wischnik A, Manth SM, Lloyd J, et al. The excretion of ketorolac tromethamine into breast milk after multiple oral dosing. *Eur J Clin Pharmacol* 1989;36(5):521–524.

418. Wittens B, Glosten B, Faure EA, et al. Post cesarean analgesia with both epidural morphine and intravenous patient-controlled analgesia: Neurobehavioral outcomes among nursing neonates. *Anesth Analg* 1997;85:600–606.

419. Bar-Oz B, Nulman I, Koren G, Ito S. Anticonvulsants and breast feeding: A critical review. *Paediatr Drugs* 2000;2(2):113–126.

420. Ohman I, Vitols S, Tomson T. Pharmacokinetics of gabapentin during delivery, in the neonatal period, and lactation: Does a fetal accumulation occur during pregnancy? *Epilepsia* 2005;46(10):1621–1624.

421. Eberhard-Gran M, Eskild A, Opjordsmoen S. Use of psychotropic medications in treating mood disorders during lactation: Practical recommendations. *CNS Drugs* 2006;20(3):187–198.

422. Penfield AJ. Laparoscopic sterilization under local anesthesia: 1200 cases. *Obstet Gynecol* 1977;49(6):725–727.

423. Bridenbaugh LD, Soderstrom RM. Lumbar epidural block anesthesia for outpatient laparoscopy. *J Reprod Med* 1979;23(2):85–86.

424. Gerges FJ, Kanazi GE, Jabbour-Khouri SI. Anesthesia for laparoscopy: A review. *J Clin Anesth* 2006;18(1):67–78.

425. Holzer A, Jirecek ST, Illievich UM, et al. Laparoscopic versus open myomectomy: A double-blind study to evaluate postoperative pain. *Anesth Analg* 2006;102(5):1480–1484.

426. Baill IC, Cullins VE, Pati S. Counseling issues in tubal sterilization. *Am Fam Physician* 2003;67(6):1287–1294.

427. Viscomi CM., Rathmell JP. Labor epidural catheter reactivation or spinal anesthesia for delayed postpartum tubal ligation: A cost comparison. *J Clin Anesth* 1995;7:380–383.

428. Vincent RD, Reid RW. Epidural anesthesia for postpartum tubal ligation using epidural catheters placed during labor. *J Clin Anesth* 1993;5:289–291.

PART III: APPLICATIONS

CHAPTER 25 ■ NEURAL BLOCKADE FOR ORTHOPEDIC SURGERY

XAVIER CAPDEVILA, PAUL ZETLAOUI, AND STEPHEN MANNION

Anesthesia for orthopedic surgery is a significant anesthetic subspecialty. The concurrent use of antithrombotic therapy, risk of significant blood loss, increased difficulties in airway management, and the common use of neural blockade require specialized anesthesiologists. Furthermore, the ability to perform safe and effective regional anesthesia/analgesia is a prerequisite skill for an anesthesiologist working in the field of orthopedic surgery.

RISKS AND CONTRAINDICATIONS OF NEURAL BLOCKADE IN ORTHOPEDIC SURGERY

For every patient and orthopedic procedure, there is invariably a neural block that can be performed, even if general anesthesia is also indicated. The advantages of neural blockade, especially for postoperative analgesia, indicate that most patients presenting for orthopedic surgery should receive neural blockade unless specific contraindications exist.

Sepsis and Neural Blockade

Performing Regional Anesthesia in Septic Patients

Perioperative infection or septic complications are not unusual in orthopedic patients and may result in revision surgical procedures. It is still a matter of debate whether neuraxial blockade can be performed safely in septic patients. Recent recommendations state that (1):

■ Even if the risk of central neuraxial infection is very low after spinal or epidural anesthesia or analgesia, the decision to perform a central blockade must be established on an individual basis, whenever a patent risk of infection is present.
■ Central neural blockade should not be performed in patients with an untreated or uncontrolled septic state.
■ Conversely, a controlled infection is not a contraindication for regional anesthesia, if appropriate antibiotic therapy has been initiated before the block and there is evidence of clinical improvement.

Recommendations are less evident for plexus or peripheral anesthesia. Overall, it appears that, when the puncture is performed distant from the site of infection (axillary block for hand infection), a peripheral block can be performed safely in cases of local infection, after verifying that no infective lymphadenopathy is present at the puncture site. However, case reports suggest that local anesthesia is less efficient if local in-

fection, such as paronychia or acute infection of the fingers or toes, is present. The causes for this are not clearly understood, but the addition of clonidine to local anesthetics can shorten the onset time and enhance the quality of both anesthesia and analgesia (2).

Infectious Complications of Regional Anesthesia and Analgesia

Infective complications may be catastrophic events in patients undergoing orthopedic surgery, especially following arthroplasty, and antibiotic prophylaxis guidelines and aseptic techniques must be respected to prevent these from occurring (3).

The infectious risk of regional anesthesia is very low, particularly after single-injection plexus or peripheral blocks. There are few case reports of infection after single-injection neural techniques in chronic pain patients despite the concurrent use of steroids or nonsteroidal anti-inflammatory drugs (NSAIDs). The use of neuraxial or peripheral catheters does raise concerns regarding infective complications. Several studies have confirmed a risk of bacterial colonization of the catheter (4–7). A large survey by Capdevila and co-workers, involving nearly 1,500 patients, reported that the incidence of bacterial colonization of catheters was about 30% (4). However, only 3% of patients had signs of local inflammation. Risk factors for local inflammation or infection were postoperative monitoring in an intensive care setting, catheter duration greater than 48 hours, male gender, and the absence of antibiotic prophylaxis. Despite these findings, clinical infection is very rare and there are no reports of septic prothesis complications related to a peripheral neural catheter.

The use of an epidural catheter for postoperative analgesia is controversial because of the potential for rare but serious complications from neuraxial infection (6). The incidence of bacterial colonization is also nearly 30%. However, similarly, clinical infection is very rare; the incidence of epidural abscess has been reported as 0.12% in a controlled study involving 800 patients (6). As the bacterial species most frequently found were coagulase-negative staphylococcus (in two-third of cases) proper skin preparation, dressing, and asepsis are required for catheter placement (4,6,7).

Regional Anesthesia and Disorders of Coagulation

Coagulation Disorders

In most cases, inherited coagulation disorders such as hemophilia or von Willebrand disease are traditionally considered

566

TABLE 25-1

NEURAXIAL ANESTHESIA IN THE PATIENT RECEIVING THROMBOPROPHYLAXIS

Antiplatelet medications	No contraindication with NSAIDs; Discontinue ticlopidine 14 days, clopidogrel 7 days, Discontinue GP IIb/IIIa inhibitors 8–48 hours in advance
Subcutaneous unfractionated heparin	No contraindications; consider delaying heparin until after block if technical difficulty anticipated
Intravenous unfractionated heparin	Heparinize 1 hour after neuraxial technique; remove catheter 2–4 hour after last heparin dose; no mandatory delay if traumatic puncture
Low-molecular-weight heparin (LMWH)	Twice daily dosing: Stop LMWH 24 hours before surgery, regardless of technique; remove neuraxial catheter 2 hours before next LMWH dose. Single daily dosing: according to European statements
Pentasaccharide fondaparinux	Single-injection neuraxial technique: Discontinue fondaparinux for 24 hours; begin treatment 6–8 hours after the end of surgery Catheter removal: Discontinue fondaparinux for 36 hours before removal; reintroduce 12 hours after
Warfarin	Document normal INR after discontinuation (prior to neuraxial technique); remove catheter when INR less than 1.5 (initiation of therapy)
Thrombolytics	No data on safety interval for performance of neuraxial technique or catheter removal; follow fibrinogen level
Herbal therapy	No evidence for mandatory discontinuation prior to neuraxial technique; be aware of potential drug interactions

From Horlocker TT, Wedel DJ, Benzon H, et al. Regional anesthesia in the anticoagulated patient: defining the risks (the second ASRA Consensus Conference on Neuraxial Anesthesia and Anticoagulation). *Reg Anesth Pain Med* 2003;28:172–197; this recommendation is that of the EXPERT study; see Singelyn FJ, Felicissimo P, Piovella F, et al. Extended thromboprophylaxis with fondaparinux (Arixtra®) after major orthopedic lower limb surgery: The EXPERT Study. *J Thromb Haemost* 2005;3:[Suppl 1]:1102. NSAIDs, nonsteroidal anti-inflammatory drugs; GP IIb/IIIa, platelet glycoprotein receptor IIb/IIIa inhibitors; INR, international normalized ratio.

absolute contraindications for regional anesthesia. Only intravenous (IV) regional anesthesia is usually recommended for these patients. However, a recent study by Marcou and Zetlaoui reported the safe placement and use of continuous femoral nerve block for total knee arthroplasty in hemophiliac patients (8). After appropriate factor substitution, the use of peripheral neural blockade is possible in these patients if performed by an experienced anesthesiologist using a nerve stimulation or ultrasonographic technique. Neuraxial blockade is contraindicated because of the risk of blind, uncontrolled, and late bleeding.

Antithrombotic Agents

Patients receiving regional anesthesia, especially neuraxial blocks, are at risk of serious hemorrhagic complications if they are treated with thrombolytic or fibrinolytic agents, as a result of the profound effects of these drugs on hemostasis and the risk of bleeding related to regional anesthesia. Furthermore, it is likely that the clinical risk of bleeding is increased when several agents, such as heparin or its derivatives (low-molecular-weight heparin; LMWH), pentasaccharide, warfarin, aspirin, NSAIDs, or other antiplatelet medications (clopidogrel or ticlopidine) are used concurrently in the perioperative period. According to the American Society of Regional Anesthesia and Pain Medicine (ASRAPM) recommendations, regional techniques can be performed in patients treated with antithrombotic agents. The recommendations of the ASRAPM are reported in Table 25-1 (9). The timing of the initial LMWH dose, as well as that of subsequent doses, relative to the neuraxial block is especially challenging if a catheter is placed. According to local practice, each clinical team must propose and respect written guidelines to ensure patient safety (10).

Preexisting Central Nervous System Disorders

The presence of a preexisting central nervous system (CNS) disorder is typically considered a contraindication for neuraxial blockade. The postulated risk of worsening neurologic outcome following a mechanical trauma, a drug-induced toxicity, or neural ischemia is commonly reported as contraindication to neuraxial blockade in patients suffering from these conditions. A retrospective study from the Mayo Clinic involving 139 patients with a CNS disorder who underwent spinal anesthesia or epidural anesthesia/analgesia showed no new postoperative worsening of the preexisting CNS disorder (11). These results suggest that a preexisting CNS disorder is not an absolute contraindication for neuraxial blockade, but support an individualized discussion with the patient regarding the risk–benefit profile. However, two subgroups of patients appear to be at higher risk of neurologic complication after neuraxial blockade: (a) patients presenting with uncontrolled or unstable CNS disorders such as Guillain-Barré syndrome and (b) patients suffering from chronic, stable, neurologic sensorimotor or diabetic polyneuropathies. These patients are at increased risk of new or progressive postoperative neurologic deficits after neuraxial blockade (12). In a retrospective study including 567 stable patients, the risk of worsening or developing a new neurologic dysfunction after neuraxial blockade has been found to be 0.4% (13).

Amputees

Although it has been suggested that in scheduled limb amputation perioperative neuraxial blockade could prevent severe phantom limb pain, the use of spinal anesthesia in amputees has a low (5%) but real risk of phantom pain recurrence (14,15). Rare cases have also been reported after peripheral plexus blocks (16). Accordingly, spinal anesthesia or plexus blocks are relatively contraindicated for patients with previous lower limb amputation, and their use should be made on an individual basis considering the anesthetic alternatives.

Performance of Regional Anesthesia in Anesthetized Patients

In orthopedic surgery, association of general anesthesia with regional anesthesia (or analgesia) is common practice, but the timing of regional anesthesia in relation to general anesthesia remains controversial. Benumof, on the basis of four cases, stated that interscalene block should not be performed in anesthetized patients because of the risk of spinal cord injury (17). Prospective studies do not demonstrate an increased risk of neurologic complications associated with regional anesthesia performed under general anesthesia (18,19). Two studies report that the risk of neural damage after epidural or subdural catheter placement in anesthetized patients is very low and probably not different from the relative risk of neuraxial catheter placement in awake patients (20,21). However, according to Benumof, it should be recommended in current practice to perform regional anesthesia in awake or lightly sedated patients. Regional anesthesia performed under general anesthesia is not contraindicated, but should only be considered as an alternative technique in suitable cases.

ADVANTAGES OF REGIONAL ANESTHESIA IN ORTHOPEDIC SURGERY

Emergencies

The use of regional anesthesia in the management of a patient undergoing emergency surgery is a reasonable choice because of the nonfasted state and often preoperative pain. Plexus or peripheral blocks are suitable for limb surgery in emergency conditions, as they assure preoperative and postoperative analgesia, and intraoperative anesthesia. Depending on the technique and the administered drugs, extensive or long-duration surgery such as finger replantation is possible. The placement of a perineural catheter should be considered early in these patients as the duration of surgery may be unpredictable (operating room time, staff availability), and continuous techniques provide reliable pain relief, especially if repeated procedures are necessary (22).

In civilian or war casualties, large series or cases reports describe the use of regional anesthesia for pain control in femoral shaft fracture, and hand or foot trauma. If regional anesthesia is suitable for a trauma patient, techniques are selected on the basis of surgical site, presence of fractures and associated injuries, and need for prolonged analgesia. For example, for elbow, forearm, and hand surgery, infraclavicular block is perhaps a good choice, as it does not need upper limb mobilization (23). Furthermore, ultrasound-guided infraclavicular block without nerve stimulation may be a better choice, as movement of the limb and hence fracture is avoided. Although often sufficient, IV regional anesthesia (Bier block) may be unsuitable for a Colles fractures, because wrapping the fracture with an Esmarch bandage is a painful procedure and IV regional anesthesia does not provide postoperative pain control after open surgical repair. In case of confirmed or suspected traumatic pneumothorax, interscalene and supraclavicular block should be replaced with distal approaches to the brachial plexus. For lower limb traumatic emergencies, anterior or lateral thigh or lateral popliteal approaches of the sciatic nerve are preferred, as they do not require moving the trauma patient. After hip fracture, early fascia iliaca block provides efficient preoperative analgesia and allows pain-free patient positioning for spinal anesthesia if indicated (24,25). The main disadvantage of spinal and epidural anesthesia in trauma patients is hypovolemia related to hemorrhage, dehydration, and the affects of chronic medication such as angiotensin antagonists on vascular tone.

Finally, although the risk of compartment syndrome must be considered in all limb injuries, high-impact traumatic fractures of the forearm and leg are at highest risk. It is important that the orthopedic and anesthetic teams discuss patient management concerning the use of regional anesthesia and the risk–benefit profile (26). If regional anesthesia is performed, the use of short-acting local anesthetics, compartment pressure monitoring, and increased clinical vigilance are sensible precautions. The use of IV regional anesthesia is best avoided because of tourniquet placement, with subsequent local anesthetic volume injection (27).

Ambulatory Surgery

Regional anesthesia techniques such as spinal anesthesia and peripheral nerve blocks (PNBs) are ideal techniques for ambulatory surgery. There is excellent evidence that these techniques provide effective and rapid-onset anesthesia and, compared with general anesthesia, reduce adverse effects and unanticipated hospital admission and provide improved postoperative analgesia, especially if continuous PNBs are performed.

Spinal anesthesia provides fast, reliable, and profound surgical block with a single injection of small amounts of local anesthetics. Disadvantages of using spinal anesthesia in the outpatient setting relate to the effect of spinal block on the recovery of motor and bladder function after the block and the risk of postdural puncture headaches. A recent study compared clinical markers of motor block resolution (Bromage scale) and objective data of functional balance (ability to safely ambulate). The results of the study suggest that the standard markers of motor function are poor predictors of functional balance following ambulatory spinal anesthesia, and the actual ability to walk was more important for safe patient discharge (28). Mulroy and co-workers recently evaluated the efficacy and safety of applying an accelerated discharge pathway after spinal block by not requiring the patient to void (29). This study suggested that waiting for voiding after short-duration spinal anesthesia for surgical procedures with a low-risk of urinary problems might be not necessary, and could result in prolonged discharge time. Accordingly, the dose and drug used for spinal anesthesia must be balanced to achieve the fastest recovery of unassisted ambulation after the procedure while maintaining adequate efficacy of intraoperative anesthesia. Lidocaine provides intense and short-lasting spinal block. However, in the last 10 years, the occurrence of transient neurologic symptoms (TNS) after spinal lidocaine has increased concerns about its use. Freedman and colleagues, evaluating the epidemiology and risk factors for TNS after spinal anesthesia in more than 1,800 patients, clearly demonstrated that TNS was associated with lidocaine spinal anesthesia (30). Other authors have recommended the use of very low doses of local anesthetics (lidocaine or bupivacaine) that have an incidence of side effects lower than that previously reported with 50 to 60 mg lidocaine and a time to discharge of 145 minutes (31,32). However, this reduction in doses of local anesthetics requires the addition of intrathecal opioids (20–25 μg fentanyl) to improve analgesia. Very good results have been reported with small doses of long-acting agents such as bupivacaine (8 mg of iso- and hyperbaric solutions) and using the concept of unilateral spinal block for orthopedic lower limb surgery (33,34). It has been recently reported that small doses of ropivacaine (10–12 mg) could be an acceptable option for ambulatory surgery, allowing fast recovery of ambulation after the procedure, with discharge times similar to those for small-dose lidocaine anesthesia (35). In some patients, epidural anesthesia may be used with or without general anesthesia. Williams and colleagues demonstrated that combined general and regional anesthesia care is better than general anesthesia alone (36). Patients with the combined technique showed improved recovery profiles, had fewer unanticipated hospital admissions, and required fewer nursing interventions for common postoperative symptoms. Patients receiving epidural anesthesia had discharge outcomes similar to those patients receiving general anesthesia with femoral nerve block. Postanesthesia care unit (PACU) bypass (fast-tracking) was more likely in patients in the regional anesthesia (peripheral or spinal) clinical pathway when compared to the general anesthesia clinical pathway (see also Chapter 26).

Peripheral nerve blocks with long-acting local anesthetics are an attractive alternative for ambulatory surgery (37). These techniques are site-specific, have few side effects, and provide excellent surgical conditions, as well as superior analgesia compared to systemic opioids. Furthermore, despite analgesia with oral and intra-articular drugs, postdischarge pain with systemic opioids is often evaluated as moderate to severe. Mulroy and co-workers evaluated femoral nerve block for postoperative analgesia following outpatient arthroscopic anterior cruciate ligament repair (38). The authors reported that femoral nerve block with 25 mL of 0.25% bupivacaine provided good analgesia for the first 24 hours after surgery. Jankowski and co-workers compared psoas compartment block with low-dose spinal and general anesthesia for outpatient knee arthroscopy (39). Patients undergoing psoas compartment block received 40 mL of 1.5% mepivacaine with epinephrine. For patients receiving spinal anesthesia, 6 mg of isobaric bupivacaine with 15 μg of fentanyl were injected. General anesthesia was induced with propofol and fentanyl, and maintained with propofol and nitrous oxide. All patients received 20 mL of 0.25% bupiva-

caine intra-articularly at the end of the procedure. All patients receiving spinal anesthesia and all except one (inadvertent bilateral psoas compartment blocks performed with subsequent epidural anesthesia) receiving a psoas compartment block bypassed the PACU, whereas only 35% of general anesthesia patients were able to bypass. Discharge time did not differ among the three groups. There was no difference among groups regarding opioid consumption. However, pain scores were highest in general anesthesia patients until 2 hours postoperatively. The authors concluded that spinal anesthesia or psoas compartment block is superior to general anesthesia when considering hospital resource utilization. The advantages of single-injection PNBs may be limited because of the duration of long-acting local anesthetics (10–24 hours) (40). After resolution of PNBs, postoperative pain management is often difficult to manage and inadequate in the ambulatory setting. Continuous PNBs allow prolonged site-specific local anesthetic delivery in the outpatient setting, resulting in profound analgesia, minimal side effects, and avoidance of premature regression of an analgesic block. Klein and colleagues investigated 40 patients undergoing major shoulder surgery who received an interscalene block and perineural catheter preoperatively, and were randomized to receive either perineural ropivacaine 0.2% or normal saline postoperatively (10 mL/h) (41). Patients receiving perineural ropivacaine averaged 10 on a visual analog score (VAS) pain scale of 0–100 mm, compared with a 30 mm for subjects receiving placebo. Recent randomized double-blinded, placebo-controlled studies involving patients discharged at home with a patient-controlled never block (PCNB) provided interesting results (42–44). All of these studies involved patients scheduled for orthopedic surgery procedures who underwent placement of an infraclavicular (42), posterior popliteal (43), or interscalene (44) perineural catheter. Patients receiving perineural local anesthetics achieved both clinically and statistically significant lower resting and breakthrough pain scores compared with those using oral opioids for analgesia. Patients who received perineural local anesthetics experienced additional benefits related to improved analgesia. Zero to 30% of patients receiving perineural ropivacaine reported insomnia due to pain, compared with 60% to 70% of patients using only oral opioids. Patients receiving perineural ropivacaine awoke from sleep because of pain an average of zero times on the first postoperative night, compared with two times for patients receiving perineural saline. Lower opioid consumption in patients receiving perineural local anesthetics also resulted in fewer opioid-related side effects. Patients receiving perineural local anesthetics reported satisfaction ratings for their postoperative analgesia of 8.8 to 9.8 compared with 5.5 to 7.7 for patients receiving placebo. Recent prospective studies focusing on outcome benefits concluded that these techniques are not technically challenging and optimized the patient's quality of life and postoperative rehabilitation at home (45–47) (see Chapter 26).

Anticipated Difficult Intubation

Performance of a regional anesthetic in a patient with an anticipated difficult intubation remains controversial (48). For lower limb, forearm, and hand surgery, regional anesthesia is often recommended in the case of anticipated difficult intubation, such as in patients with arthritic conditions. This recommendation is also suitable in the trauma patient. In the case of respiratory risk associated with regional anesthesia, such with the interscalene block, planned fiberoptic intubation is perhaps the better choice, rather than an emergency intubation in a hypoxic patient with a difficult airway, such as in Still disease, ankylosing spondylitis, or rheumatoid arthritis.

Difficult Neuraxial Regional Anesthesia

Rheumatologic patients suffering from spine deformity often require orthopedic lower limb or hip surgery. In some cases, especially in patients with ankylosing spondylitis or severe scoliosis, midline approach for spinal anesthesia may be impossible. Paramedian or lateral approaches may permit neuraxial blockade in these patients, and anesthesiologists working in orthopedic surgery must be familiar with these alternatives (49).

Rehabilitation

As general anesthesia is becoming increasingly safer, it will be more difficult to demonstrate that regional anesthesia and analgesia decreases postoperative mortality. However, evidence suggests that regional anesthesia and analgesia can improve patient rehabilitation after orthopedic surgery (19). In this area, better analgesic control can shorten duration of hospitalization and rehabilitation, improving the global result of surgery (50). In major knee surgery, postoperative analgesia with a continuous femoral nerve catheter increases maximum range of motion of the operated knee, shortens duration of physiotherapy, reduces pain and systemic analgesics, and improves surgical results (50,51).

Economical Aspects

Regional anesthesia is overall less expensive than general anesthesia for orthopedic surgery. Direct and indirect costs of surgery are often reduced with regional anesthesia. For example, Williams and colleagues showed that benchmarking the perioperative processes after having actively incorporated regional anesthesia led to reduced pharmacy and materials cost variability, slightly increased turnover time, improved intraoperative anesthesia and surgical efficiency, improved recovery times, decreased unanticipated admission rates, and a reduction in the number of nursing interventions required for common postoperative symptoms (52). Spinal anesthesia is less expensive than general anesthesia for hip or knee arthroplasty (53). Moreover, spinal anesthesia is often associated with lower postoperative pain in the PACU, leading to reduced administration of analgesics and antiemetics and reduction in PACU length of stay. Intravenous regional anesthesia has been reported as the more cost-effective technique for outpatient hand surgery (54). However, brachial plexus block is more expensive than general anesthesia for upper limb procedures of short duration (55). Shortening postoperative hospital stay and reducing the costs of rehabilitation are other potential economic advantages of regional anesthesia.

REGIONAL ANESTHESIA FOR SPINE SURGERY

Minor Spine Surgery

Minor spine surgery is usually performed under general anesthesia; neuraxial anesthesia is infrequently used for spinal procedures (56). Although complications associated with neurax-

ial anesthesia are rare, spinal or epidural anesthesias have been avoided for spinal surgery as some authors have suggested that neuraxial anesthesia may exacerbate preexisting neurologic disease. However, in selected patients scheduled for intervertebral disk herniation surgery, spinal or epidural anesthesia are efficient alternatives (57). Patient acceptance is higher, and hypotension is less common when surgery is performed with the patient in the lateral position, compared to the standard knee-to-chest position. In the same way, epidural or spinal anesthesia have been compared to general anesthesia for one-level laminectomy (58). A study including 400 patients reported that neuraxial blockade is an intraoperative technique for lumbar laminectomy, and is also associated with several advantages such as a reduction in total operative time and PACU stay, less postoperative nausea and vomiting (PONV), less postoperative pain, and an overall reduction in the postoperative complication rate. Furthermore, bladder dysfunction was less frequent after spinal anesthesia as the total amount of morphine for postoperative pain was reduced.

Postoperative epidural analgesia for lumbar laminectomy results in superior pain control and fewer analgesic requirements than patient-controlled morphine analgesia (59). However, patients poorly accept procedures of long duration, and general anesthesia remains the better choice for spinal surgery of long or uncertain duration. In summary, spinal or epidural anesthesia and analgesia are efficient alternative techniques for nonextensive spine surgery and offer better postoperative pain control than conventional treatments, including patient-controlled morphine analgesia.

Major Spine and Pelvic Surgery

Major spine or pelvic surgery requires general anesthesia. However, evidence suggests that the association of general anesthesia combined with regional anesthesia improves intraoperative conditions and patient outcome.

Spinal Analgesia

Several studies reviewed by Tobias report the intraoperative use of spinal analgesia for extensive anterior or posterior spinal fusion in children (60). Although low doses of intrathecal morphine (2 and 5 μg/kg) are administered (61), most studies report the use of high-dose morphine, ranging from 10 to 20 μg/kg (62–64). These studies have reported better postoperative pain control in the treated groups and a significant decrease in intraoperative blood loss. The decrease in blood loss is postulated to be a result of intraoperative mild and stable hypotension and less hemodynamic reactivity to intraoperative painful stimulation. Furthermore, volatile anesthetic agents, unlike intraoperative spinal opioids (morphine or sufentanil), do not disturb spinal function monitoring (i.e., somatosensory-evoked potentials). No study reports the use of continuous intrathecal analgesia in spinal procedures. Patients receiving high-dose intrathecal opioids required admission to a more intensely monitored unit at least for the first 24 postoperative hours because of the risk of respiratory depression.

Local anesthetics are typically avoided for intraoperative spinal analgesia because of the increased risk of arterial hypotension, the impossibility of monitoring spinal function, and because of the risk of prolonged postoperative motor blockade, which may delay the early diagnosis of neurologic complications.

Epidural Analgesia

Unlike spinal analgesia, the use of perioperative epidural analgesia is more complex, as different options are available (intraoperative versus postoperative use, single-versus double-catheter, continuous infusion versus intermittent dosing, lipophilic versus hydrophilic opioids, additives). Epidural analgesia in extensive spinal surgery provides perioperative analgesia, mild intraoperative hypotension resulting in blood loss reduction, and, potentially, a reduction in postoperative venous thrombosis (65–67). The epidural catheter is usually placed before induction of general anesthesia. If nitrous oxide is used during surgery, the loss-of-resistance technique with air should be carefully considered because of the risk of patchy anesthesia or root compression by neuraxial gas bubbles when their volume is increased by nitrous oxide diffusion (68).

Alternatively, the epidural catheter may be placed under direct vision, by the surgeon at the end of the surgery. This technique allows the placement of two catheters, one directed caudally and the second directed cephalad, to ensure the quality of pain control. The placement of the catheter at the level of surgery results in a significant leak of analgesic solution from the epidural space (69).

UPPER LIMB

Orthopedic surgery of the upper limb may be performed under a large variety of regional anesthetic techniques including brachial plexus block, a combination of individual nerve blocks, or IV regional anesthesia. The choice of a particular technique depends on the need for a tourniquet, the site of surgery, and the anticipated duration of the procedure. Basically, for regional anesthesia, the upper extremity can be divided in four regions: (a) the shoulder and humeral head, (b) the arm and elbow, (c) the forearm, and (d) the wrist and hand. This anatomic division corresponds approximately to the different regional anesthetic techniques described (Table 25-2).

Shoulder and Humeral Head

Shoulder and humeral head surgery can be performed under regional anesthesia alone, but sedation (70) or general anesthesia should be considered for patient comfort, especially for extensive procedures or when surgery is performed in the prone position.

From an anatomic point of view, interscalene block is the paradigm for shoulder surgery as it anesthetizes the roots of the brachial plexus (C5, C6, C7). However, additional blocks may be necessary according to the site of the surgical incision. For example, the superficial nerves of the cervical plexus innervate the anterosuperior aspect of the shoulder. The deltopectoral groove and the axilla are not blocked by an interscalene approach, as extension of the block to the lower roots (C8–T1) is infrequent or unpredictable. Thus, local infiltration for

---

TABLE 25-2

SUGGESTIONS FOR BLOCK TYPE AND NEED FOR CATHETER PLACEMENT FOR UPPER LIMB SURGERY

	Anesthesia	Postoperative analgesia
Surgery	Suggested block	Catheter
Total shoulder arthroplasty	ISB	+++
Rotator cuff repair	ISB	+++
Shoulder arthrolysis	ISB	++
Open acromioplasty	ISB	++
Arthroscopic acromioplasty	ISB	0
Shoulder dislocation (repair)	ISB	±
Clavicular fracture repair	ISB + superficial cervical plexus block	0
Proximal part of humerus fracture repair	ISB or SCB	++
Medial and distal part of humerus	SCB or ICB	±
Elbow arthrolysis	SCB, ICB, AxB	+++
Elbow arthroscopy	SCB	±
Olecranon fracture repair	SCB, ICB, AxB	++
Elbow epicondylitis, neurolysis	ICB, AxB, MHB	0
Forearm and wrist fracture repair	ICB, AxB, MHB	0
Major forearm, wrist or hand trauma or surgery	ICB, AxB	+++
Scheduled surgery for forearm, wrist or hand	AxB, MHB, truncal blocks, IVRA	According to surgery type
Finger surgery	AxB, truncal block(s), IVRA, intrathecal digital block	Selective peripheral truncal blocks

ISB, interscalene block; SCB, supraclavicular block; ICB, infraclavicular block; AxB, axillary block; MHB, midhumeral block; IVRA, intravenous regional anesthesia (Bier block); +++, highly recommended; ++, recommended; ±, may benefit; 0, not recommended.

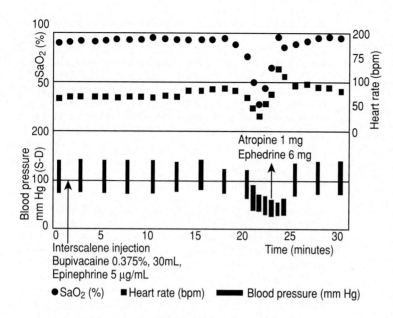

FIGURE 25-1. Record of a hemodynamic event after interscalene block for shoulder surgery in the beach-chair position. Redrawn from the automatic record. From P.J. Zetlaoui, personal data.

cutaneous nerves or paravertebral nerves blocks (T2–T3) may be required.

Several studies have investigated the clinical efficacy of the interscalene block in shoulder surgery. Nearly all report the superiority of this technique for intraoperative and postoperative anesthesia and analgesia compared with other methods (71–73). In a randomized controlled study enrolling patients scheduled for an arthroscopic acromioplasty under general anesthesia, Singelyn and co-workers reported the superiority of the interscalene block for postoperative analgesia when compared with patient-controlled morphine analgesia, suprascapular nerve block, or intra-articular analgesia (74).

The beach-chair position, used to avoid excessive traction on the shoulder (and hence plexus roots), is often required for open or arthroscopic shoulder surgery. The beach-chair position and interscalene block are associated with a high incidence (4%–20%) of significant hemodynamic events involving hypotension and/or bradycardia, sometimes leading to cardiac arrest (75) (Fig. 25-1). This reaction seldom occurs under general anesthesia alone or when interscalene block is combined with general anesthesia. It is more frequent when epinephrine is added in the irrigation solution or to the anesthetic mixture (76). Epinephrine-induced tachycardia and relative hypovolemia due to the beach-chair position are postulated to be major determinants of this hemodynamic compromise. This reaction has been misinterpreted as an activation of the Bezold-Jarisch reflex (75), but the review of Campagna and Carter stated that "the hemodynamic embarrassment seen in shoulder surgery during interscalene block appears not to be related with the Bezold-Jarisch reflex activation" (77), as this reflex is activated by an overfilled left ventricle and never by hypovolemia. Consequently, β-blockers are not required as prophylactic or therapeutic agents, and management of these vasovagal reactions includes fluid loading, ephedrine, atropine, and finally epinephrine use if necessary (78,79).

In emergency cases, such as shoulder dislocation, interscalene block is an effective technique for closed reduction. However, the performance of an interscalene block in such situations should be considered on an individual basis, considering that the nonfasted patient is a relative contraindication for interscalene block because of the risk of recurrent laryngeal nerve paresis with this block (80).

In a review of neurologic complications after shoulder surgery, Boardman and Cofield reported an incidence of 1% to 8%, depending on the specific procedure performed (81). Although traditionally interscalene block was often held responsible for a significant part of these complications, this review reported that surgery and intraoperative position are the major determinants for postoperative neurologic complications, and that the contribution of regional anesthesia is very low. The study of Borgeat and colleagues reports that the incidence of interscalene block–related early or late neurologic complications is about 0.4% (82). These findings are supported by the study of Horlocker and colleagues, who report that the incidence of surgery-related neurologic complications is eight times more frequent than anesthetic-related injuries (83). However, the description by Benumof of four cases of spinal cord damage after interscalene block (17) should be considered and suggests that another approach for the interscalene block, such as that proposed by Borgeat using a lateral modified approach, is considered (84). This approach allows easy catheter placement, less catheter dislodgement, high patient satisfaction, and probably less neurologic risk.

Arthroscopic shoulder surgery overall is reputed to be less painful than open surgery, although the problem of postoperative pain is not resolved. Singelyn and co-workers demonstrated that interscalene block is the superior choice for painful procedures (74). However, for nonextensive or minor interventions, or in the outpatient setting, intra-articular injection of a mixture of local anesthetics with additives (morphine, clonidine, NSAIDs) (85) can provide adequate analgesia with favorable cost-effective and risk-effective ratios. Furthermore, intra-articular analgesia with lidocaine is reported as an effective technique for reduction of acute shoulder dislocation (86).

For surgery to the proximal part of the arm, supraclavicular block is probably preferable to interscalene block because it provides more consistent anesthesia of the posterior aspect of the arm, as blockade of the axillary nerve is more reliable via this approach.

Outpatient Management

Both single-injection and continuous techniques for interscalene block can be used in the outpatient setting. The advantages of continuous infusions of low concentrations/rates of long-acting local anesthetics via portable elastomeric pumps allows early discharge, with less postoperative pain, less PONV, less analgesic consumption, and better patient satisfaction (47,87).

Elbow Surgery

Complete anesthesia of the elbow requires not only effective blockade of three major nerves (radial, musculocutaneous, median) but also blockade of the ulnar nerve and two sensory nerves (medial cutaneous nerves of arm and forearm). In general, anesthesia should always encompass more than the surgical area because of anatomic variations or possible extensions to the surgical procedure. Supraclavicular block is a better choice than interscalene block for elbow surgery, as the ulnar nerve is more consistently blocked, and the incidence of phrenic nerve paresis is very low. However, additional infiltrations in the axilla to block the intercostobrachial nerve and cutaneous medial nerve of the arm are sometimes required. Likewise, infraclavicular and axillary blocks are effective alternatives, with less risk of pneumothorax (88,89).

Forearm and Hand Surgery

Numerous regional anesthetic approaches and techniques have been described to block the forearm and the hand, such as infraclavicular, axillary, midhumeral, and truncal blocks and, finally, IV regional anesthesia (90).

Infraclavicular block is particularly indicated in trauma patients (as it does not require mobilization of the arm) for forearm surgery and for the placement of catheters for postoperative analgesia (because the catheter is placed in glabrous skin and far from the flexion fold of the axilla). The bulk of the pectoralis muscle firmly anchors the catheter, arm movements are not impaired, and hygiene is easily maintained. The rate of failure is low when a distal response is obtained with nerve stimulation. The extrathoracic, infracoracoid technique is preferable to the traditional approaches because of the very low risk of pneumothorax (91).

Axillary and midhumeral blocks exhibit similar efficacy—over 90% success when all nerves are selectively blocked (92). These blocks eliminate the risk of serious adverse effects such as pneumothorax or phrenic nerve paresis. The review by Handoll and Koscielniak-Nielsen concludes that multiple stimulation injection techniques for axillary plexus block provide more effective anesthesia than either double- or single-injection techniques (93). Thus, the main difference between these two techniques is that the axillary approach offers the possibility of placing a catheter, and allows a more proximal tourniquet placement. On the other hand, the midhumeral approach, with discrete blockade of each nerve, allows injection of different anesthetic solutions at each nerve. For example, in patients undergoing outpatient procedures, Bouaziz and co-workers blocked the radial and musculocutaneous nerves with lidocaine (for short-duration blocks to allow elbow movements at the time of discharge) and used bupivacaine for blockade of the ulnar and median nerves (to prolong hand analgesia) (94).

Intravenous regional anesthesia is a basic technique that is almost always effective (even in the hands of nonspecialized anesthesiologists), and it is associated with a very low rate of complications if recognized protocols are followed (95). Nevertheless, two disadvantages to IV regional anesthesia exist. The first is that this technique is only suitable for short or intermediate procedures that last less than 1 hour. The second is the lack

of postoperative analgesia, as anesthesia and analgesia disappear within a few minutes of the tourniquet being removed. Using long-acting, newer local anesthetics, like ropivacaine (2 mg/mL) or levobupivacaine (1.25 mg/mL) instead of lidocaine or prilocaine seems to prolong postoperative analgesia (96,97); however, the real safety of these agents has never been demonstrated with a large series. Using additives like clonidine or ketorolac to prolong postoperative analgesia seems to be safer (98).

Digit Surgery

Anatomically, truncal blocks are feasible for surgery to the digits. The main disadvantage for these distal blocks is use of the tourniquet by the surgeon.

Digital block is a very useful technique for outpatient or emergency finger surgery, particularly in cases of paronychia or acute finger infection (99). Furthermore, this simple and efficient block provides prolonged postoperative analgesia ranging between 18 and 24 hours with low doses of long-acting anesthetics such as bupivacaine or ropivacaine. Epinephrine should be avoided because of the terminal vascularization of fingers. Digital block is suitable for the three long fingers, but is less effective for the thumb. Likewise, for surgery to the fifth finger, truncal ulnar block at the wrist is a better choice. Digital block is preferred to "ring" block, a circular subfascial injection of local anesthetic at the level of the finger injury, as it is an effective, long-lasting, and safe technique (see Chapter 13).

LOWER LIMB SURGERY

Recently, interest has been growing in regional anesthetic techniques for orthopedic lower limb surgery. Investigations have focused on the use of PNBs, particularly continuous technique, to provide anesthesia and postoperative analgesia for major orthopedic surgery. At the same time, spinal anesthesia and the use of epidural analgesia to limit patient morbidity and optimize postoperative rehabilitation have been specifically studied in the outpatient setting (see Chapter 14).

For regional anesthesia, the lower extremity can be divided into four regions: (a) the hip and thigh (femoral bone), (b) the knee, (c) the leg, and (d) the ankle and foot.

Hip and Thigh

Femoral Neck Fractures

Patients presenting with femoral neck fractures are a specific population. Some of these patients previously would not have been considered candidates for surgery because of concomitant disease; for disabled geriatric patients, the 1-year mortality is almost 20%. Several factors influence mortality rates for these older patients: surgical site, emergency surgery, and American Society of Anesthesiologists classification of disease severity. There are potential advantages to anesthetic alternatives. For example, spinal anesthesia is technically easy to administer and has a low failure rate, but can be a dangerous technique in some elderly patients (100). Continuous spinal anesthesia should be considered because of its hemodynamic stability during regional anesthesia induction in comparison with single-injection spinal anesthesia (101,102). Epidural anesthesia may also allow for gradual dosing and titration of local anesthetics to the desired level of anesthesia. In

TABLE 25-3

STUDIES OF NERVE BLOCK USE IN THE PERIOPERATIVE PERIOD

Reference	Patient group	Study type	Outcome	Results
24	30 consecutive patients with neck fractures. Fascia iliaca compartment block. 30 mL 0.5% levobupivacaine	Observational study	Pain levels	VAS 7.2 before to 4.6 after block
			Hip flexion	Mean increase 44°
25	50 patients. 24 femoral nerve blocks and 26 control group. 20 mL 0.5% bupivacaine for three-in-one femoral nerve block and 5–10 mg of morphine in the control group	RCT	Pain levels	Lower pain levels in the block group
			Analgesic consumption	Mean morphine dose/hour: 0.5 mg vs. 1.2 mg
175	36 patients age range 31–95 with fractured neck of femur Femoral nerve block (10 mL 0.5% bupivacaine)	Cohort study	Objective Assessment	29 had reduced sensation; seven failures
			Subjective Assessment	26 patients had reduced pain, four had no pain, six had no change
			Complications	None found
176	50 patients with extracapsular fractures of the femoral neck; age range 68–89 Femoral nerve block (0.3 mL/kg 0.25% bupivacaine) vs. systemic analgesia alone	RCT	Mean pain score using VAS	Greater reduction in nerve block group at 15 mins and 2 hours
			Analgesic requirements	Reduced in the 24 hours from admission in nerve block group
			Incidence of complications	Significantly reduced in nerve block group
177	40 consecutive patients age 67–96 with fractured neck of femur undergoing surgery	RCT	Pain relief (VAS)	Significant difference in psoas block group at 8 and 16 hours preoperatively and 16, 24, and 32 hours postoperatively
	Continuous psoas compartment block (0.8 mL/kg of 0.25% bupivacaine with adrenaline) vs. meperidine analgesia		Complication rate	Three cases of local erythema in psoas group
178	269 patients from seven randomized or quasi-randomized trials with fractured neck of femur; analgesia/anaesthesia given preoperatively in two of these trials Patients given either regional block or intravenous analgesia	Systematic review	Pain levels	Reduction in mean pain score in nerve block groups
			Analgesic requirements	Reduced analgesic requirements in nerve block groups
			Complications	No difference

In part from Mackway-Jones K. Regional nerve block in fractured neck of femur. *Emerg Med J* 2002;19:144–145.
RCT, randomized controlled trial; VAS, visual analog pain scale.

contrast, general anesthesia facilitates control of ventilation, which, in older patients, is more sensitive to the respiratory depressant effects of opioids and sedatives. A number of studies have investigated the impact of neuraxial blocks on the perioperative risk. Meta-analyses show that neuraxial blocks significantly reduce immediate postoperative mortality and morbidity (e.g., deep vein thrombosis, pulmonary embolism, intraoperative blood loss) when compared with general anesthesia (103,104). For hip fracture repair, the results are less consistent (105–109). Urwin and Parkers' meta-analysis reported a nonstatistically significant trend toward lower mortality at 1 month in patients receiving regional anesthesia compared with patients receiving general anesthesia (6.4% versus 9.4%) (109). Compared with conventional analgesia, epidural analgesia with local anesthetics, used in the perioperative period, is associated with a lower incidence of perioperative cardiac ischemic events and significantly reduces death in elderly patients scheduled for femoral neck fracture repair (110,111). In summary, despite the small number of patients studied and substantial weaknesses in study design, some benefit can be obtained with the use of nerve block in fractured femur neck repair in the perioperative setting, most notably in extracapsular fractures (Table 25-3).

For intraoperative anesthesia, de Visme and co-workers showed that psoas compartment block combined with a parasacral block provides similar anesthesia to plain bupivacaine spinal anesthesia for the repair of hip fractures in elderly patients (112). Mannion and colleagues reported that the analgesic duration of single-injection psoas compartment block with levobupivacaine 0.5%, combined with general anesthesia for hip fracture surgery, is increased from a mean of 7.3 hours to 13.6 hours by IV but not perineural clonidine (1 μg/kg), with no differences in hemodynamic or sedation side effects (113).

Although spinal anesthesia is a simple technique with a high success rate, advantages of peripheral blocks include less urinary retention, less hypotension, and the possibility of prolonged postoperative analgesia. Concerning postoperative rehabilitation, Foss and colleagues recently reported that postoperative epidural analgesia provided superior analgesia (attenuating pain as a restricting factor during physiotherapy), but this optimal analgesia regimen did not translate into enhanced rehabilitation (114).

Hip Surgery

Total hip arthroplasty is a major orthopedic procedure associated with significant postoperative pain. Historically, general anesthesia has been the gold standard for surgeons and patients when total hip arthroplasty was performed. However, several regional anesthetic and analgesic techniques are now commonly used. Meta-analyses have reported that the use of epidural or spinal anesthesia during major hip surgery has been linked to a reduced risk of perioperative complications (deep venous thrombosis, less deterioration of cerebral and pulmonary functions in high-risk patients, reduced blood loss) (103,104,115). Modern regional anesthesia/analgesia for major hip surgery includes the use of single-injection and continuous epidural block, single-injection and continuous spinal block, continuous lumbar plexus blockade, and continuous peripheral blockade of the femoral and sciatic nerves. Epidural anesthesia is still widely used. Scharrock and colleagues recently demonstrated that total hip arthroplasty performed under hypotensive epidural anesthesia with propofol sedation enables recovery of cognitive function 2 hours after surgery (116). However, there was no evidence of increased risks, or earlier benefits, with the use of this hypotensive technique (117).

Levobupivacaine 0.5%, bupivacaine 0.5%, or ropivacaine 0.75% produce an epidural block of similar onset, quality, and duration. When prolonging analgesia for the first 12 hours after surgery with a patient-controlled epidural infusion, 0.125% levobupivacaine, 0.125% bupivacaine, and 0.2% ropivacaine provided adequate pain relief with similar recovery of motor function (118). Compared with general anesthesia and postoperative patient-controlled morphine analgesia, epidural anesthesia/analgesia with ropivacaine allowed patients to be discharged earlier from the PACU and provided superior pain relief during the first 24 hours after total hip arthroplasty. A recent placebo-controlled study suggests that continuous spinal anesthesia provides efficient pain relief after total hip arthroplasty (119).

Fournier and co-workers investigated the advantages of single-injection lumbar plexus block via an anterior approach (120). Forty milliliters of 0.5% bupivacaine with epinephrine were compared to a group receiving a sham block. The authors showed that single-injection femoral block for total hip arthroplasty, in association with general anesthesia, improves analgesia for 4 to 5 hours after surgery, but no sparing effect was observed with regard to opioid requirements both intra- and postoperatively for the 48-hour study period. A posterior approach to the lumbar plexus provides blockade of all major branches of the lumbar plexus, in contrast to anterior lumbar plexus block, which is mainly a "femoral" block (121). Stevens and colleagues reported psoas compartment block via the approach of Winnie and co-workers (122) for postoperative analgesia after total hip arthroplasty (123). Single-injection posterior lumbar plexus block was combined with general

anesthesia. A bolus of 0.4 mL/kg of 0.5% bupivacaine with epinephrine was injected. Epidural extension of the block was noted in 11% of patients, but with no adverse effects. Other findings included a decrease in blood loss intraoperatively and also a significant 45% reduction of blood loss 48 hours after the surgery. However, the intraoperative blood-sparing effect was not statistically significant when patients with epidural distribution of the lumbar plexus block were excluded. The proportion of patients requiring supplemental analgesia intraoperatively was significantly greater in the group with general anesthesia alone. In the PACU, VAS scores were significantly lower in the group receiving lumbar plexus block. Pain scores and morphine consumption remained significantly lower in the psoas compartment block group until 6 hours postoperatively.

Although there are a number of approaches to psoas compartment block, for single-injection psoas compartment block combined with spinal anesthesia after total hip arthroplasty or total knee arthroplasty, Mannion and co-workers found no difference between the approach of Capdevila and colleagues (124) and that of Winnie and colleagues (122) in terms of postoperative analgesia, pain scores, extent of lumbar plexus blockade, or bilateral anesthesia (125). Both approaches resulted in median pain scores of 0 at all time periods for the first 24 hours and a mean time to first opioid analgesia of 12 to 13 hours.

Recently, Biboulet and co-workers compared patient-controlled morphine analgesia with single-injection femoral or psoas compartment block for patients undergoing hip surgery (126). They reported an analgesic benefit in patients receiving psoas compartment block for the first 4 hours following surgery (less morphine consumption and lower VAS scores). However, after 4 hours, there was no difference in morphine consumption or pain scores among the three groups, whether at rest or during mobilization. No difference in hip mobility or rehabilitation duration was noted. These data question the need for regional techniques in total hip arthroplasty, especially psoas compartment block, with its potential for serious adverse effects. The authors conclude that patient-controlled morphine analgesia is an efficient and safe analgesic technique for total hip arthroplasty. In another study, Souron and co-workers compared prospectively intrathecal morphine and psoas compartment block techniques after primary total hip arthroplasty (127). They demonstrated that 0.1 mg intrathecal morphine provided better postoperative analgesia than single-injection psoas compartment block but with a greater incidence of urinary retention.

Although, anterior and posterior lumbar plexus blocks have been used for total hip arthroplasty, their contribution to overall outcome remains unclear. Femoral nerve blocks provide an analgesic benefit, but it is of short duration, and no definitive opioid-sparing effect has been noted. Posterior lumbar plexus block provides effective pain relief but its superiority to other analgesic methods remains controversial. The difficulty in establishing the beneficial aspects of regional anesthesia techniques may be in part due to the fact that pain after total hip arthroplasty seems highly variable. However, overall, continuous PNBs provide effective and safe postoperative pain control, reduced opioid consumption, improved and earlier rehabilitation, and high patient satisfaction (see Chapter 14).

Singelyn and Gouverneur have demonstrated that continuous femoral block was efficient in providing comparable analgesia but with fewer side effects and technical problems compared to patient-controlled morphine analgesia or patient-controlled epidural analgesia (128). Visual analog pain scale values at rest were 23 ± 20 min at 24 hours and 11 ± 17 mm at 48 hours. However, during mobilization, VAS scores increased to 46 ± 26 mm at 24 hours and 33 ± 24 mm at

PART III: APPLICATIONS

48 hours. Singelyn and co-workers compared patient-controlled with continuous regimens to evaluate the volume of local anesthetics administered and thereby decrease the potential for toxicity (129). Patient-controlled boluses alone produced analgesia equivalent to a continuous perfusion but with a significantly lower local anesthetics consumption. In this study, two bolus regimens were compared to the continuous infusion: A bolus of 5 mL was possible every 30 minutes and a bolus of 10 mL every 60 minutes; the lowest local anesthetic consumption occurs with a 5 mL bolus and a 30-minute lockout time. Patient satisfaction was also greatest in this group. Capdevila and colleagues also conducted a clinical evaluation of continuous psoas compartment blocks for postoperative analgesia after total hip arthroplasty (124). Only three of the 80 catheters placed were improperly sited. One hour after the block, sensory blockade of the femoral, obturator, and lateral cutaneous femoral nerves was successful in 95%, 90%, and 85%, respec-

tively, of the patients. Postoperative analgesia was adequate; 6.5% of the patients required rescue analgesia. Visual analog pain scale pain scores during the 48-hour study period had a median value of 10 mm at rest and ranged from 18 to 25 mm during physiotherapy. This study proves the efficacy of continuous psoas compartment blocks for pain control after total hip arthroplasty. Few adverse effects were reported, and although 5% exhibited epidural extension, no hemodynamic consequences were observed (see also Chapter 14).

Recently, Fischer and colleagues reported the results of the Procedure-Specific Postoperative Pain Management meta-analysis and recommended the use of epidural local anesthetics and opioids or continuous femoral or posterior lumbar plexus block to decrease postoperative pain and consumption of rescue analgesics after hip replacement (Fig. 25-2) (130). Similarly, Hebl and colleagues combined the effect of minimally invasive surgery and a preemptive multimodal perioperative analgesic

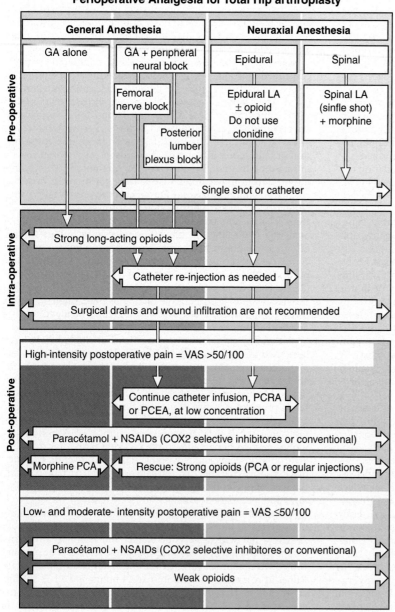

FIGURE 25-2. Perioperative analgesia for total hip arthroplasty. Diagrammatic representation by P.J. Zetlaoui, after Fischer HB, Simanski CJ. A procedure-specific systematic review and consensus recommendations for analgesia after total hip replacement. *Anaesthesia* 2005;60:1189–1202.

regimen featuring PNBs for total arthroplasty and reported that the regional anesthesia group had lower postoperative pain levels at rest and during physiotherapy, met discharge eligibility sooner, and had earlier discharge compared to a historical control group (131). The Mayo Clinic regional anesthesia clinical pathway for hip arthroplasty surgery combines intraoperative and postoperative continuous posterior lumbar plexus block with 0.2% bupivacaine (bolus 10 mL 0.2% bupivacaine on arrival in PACU and 10 mL/hour on day 0, then 12 mL/hour of 0.1% bupivacaine on day 1) and ketorolac, acetaminophen, oxycodone.

Femoral Shaft Fracture

The fascia iliaca compartment block involves a puncture site away from the neurovascular sheath and requires no sophisticated equipment. Lopez and co-workers demonstrated that fascia iliaca block is simple, safe, and efficient in providing prehospital pain relief for femoral fractures at the accident scene (132). Only one block failure was reported out of 27 patients recruited. This technique facilitates transport to a trauma care center and earlier analgesic management at arrival. Even patients with partial block required no further analgesia before going to the operating room (see also Chapter 14).

Knee

Spinal and epidural techniques are obviously widely and traditionally used (see ambulatory surgery section) for knee surgery. However, the enthusiasm for neuraxial technique has decreased in the past 5 years as a result of the routine use of potent anticoagulants by surgeons and the necessity for postoperative rehabilitation. Leading centers now implement continuous peripheral blocks (continuous femoral plus single-injection sciatic and obturator nerve blocks or continuous psoas compartment blocks) as the mainstay of the postoperative multimodal regimen (131) after major knee surgery.

Single-injection Techniques

Single-injection PNBs provide prolonged analgesia and are an alternative to continuous techniques. In a randomized study, Wang and colleagues evaluated the effect of single-injection femoral nerve block (40 mL of 0.25% bupivacaine) on rehabilitation and length of hospital stay following total knee arthroplasty in 30 patients (133). Lower pain scores and morphine consumption in the recovery room for the bupivacaine group were reported, which persisted for 24 hours. Patients receiving bupivacaine performed significantly better in walking distances and knee flexion until discharge. Hospital stay was shorter in the bupivacaine group (3 versus 4 days). Williams and colleagues have retrospectively reviewed 1,200 consecutive cases of outpatient knee surgery (134) to investigate differences in pain associated with surgical complexity and type of blocks used. It was observed, as can be expected, that patients undergoing complex interventions (ligament reconstruction, meniscal reconstruction, and high tibial osteotomy) had a greater risk of experiencing postoperative pain than did patients undergoing less invasive interventions. Results showed that patients who received a femoral and sciatic nerve block for major knee surgery had less pain in the ambulatory unit compared with patients receiving no block or a femoral block alone. Also, fewer unanticipated hospital admissions were noted in patients receiving either femoral block alone or a combination of femoral and sciatic nerve blocks. These findings emphasize

the importance of pain control in the immediate postoperative period, but one cannot conclude on the equivalence of single-injection and continuous femoral block. Based on their findings, Williams and colleagues suggested that there was a greater role for the sciatic nerve in major complex knee surgery. Other investigators have concluded that it appears necessary to combine a sciatic nerve block and/or an obturator nerve block to optimize the results obtained with a femoral block (135,136). Elmas and Atanassoff demonstrated the feasibility of lower limb surgery with the combination of a sciatic and femoral block (137). Only 12% of patients required additional sedation during surgery. Misra and colleagues reported complete analgesia lasting approximately 17 hours in patients receiving combined femoral and sciatic single-injection block before spinal anesthesia for total knee arthroplasty (138). On the other hand, McNamee and colleagues and Macalou and colleagues reported improved analgesia when an obturator nerve block was added to combined sciatic and femoral block after total knee arthroplasty (139,140). Luber and co-workers have reported complete analgesia for about 13 hours following combined lumbar plexus and sciatic block (141). As for the anesthetic efficiency of the block for surgery, 22% of patients required conversion to general anesthesia, despite blockade of all the nerves responsible for innervation of the knee joint.

More recently, regional anesthesia techniques have been compared to the intra-articular administration of local anesthetics following anterior cruciate ligament reconstruction. Iskandar and co-workers showed that analgesia after single-injection femoral block (20 mL of 1% ropivacaine) was better than the same volume of local anesthetics given intra-articularly and also had a significant morphine-sparing effect (142).

Continuous Catheter Techniques

Continuous femoral nerve block provides efficient analgesia after major knee surgery. Ganapathy and colleagues have shown that a continuous femoral perivascular block is efficient in providing pain relief after total knee arthroplasty (143). Although only 40% of catheters reached an ideal location, the use of 0.2% bupivacaine resulted in all patients having a successful block. Singelyn and colleagues evaluated the effect of three analgesic techniques in 45 patients on postoperative pain and rehabilitation after total knee arthroplasty (144). Postoperative analgesia was provided either by patient-controlled morphine analgesia, continuous three-in-one block, or epidural analgesia. Pain scores at rest and during mobilization were significantly lower in patients receiving regional anesthesia techniques. Significantly better knee flexion until discharge was observed in patients with continuous epidural or femoral blocks, compared with the patient-controlled morphine analgesia group. This difference was still present at 6 weeks postoperatively, but not at 3 months. Duration of hospital stay was also significantly longer in patients using patient-controlled analgesia (PCA). Urinary retention and catheter-related problems were significantly more frequent in the epidural group. Similarly, Capdevila and co-workers demonstrated the influence of postoperative analgesic techniques in surgical outcome and convalescence duration after major knee surgery (145). Fifty-six adults scheduled for major knee surgery were randomly assigned to one of three groups: patient-controlled morphine analgesia, continuous femoral block, or continuous epidural infusion. Pain scores at rest and during continuous passive motion were significantly lower in groups receiving continuous femoral or epidural local anesthetic infusion, compared with the PCA group. The duration of stay in the rehabilitation center was significantly shortened in patients receiving regional analgesia techniques.

PART III: APPLICATIONS

Side effects, such as urinary retention, arterial hypotension, and dysesthesias were observed in the epidural group. The authors concluded that continuous femoral nerve block was the better choice for regional analgesia after major knee surgery. Dauri and colleagues compared continuous epidural, continuous femoral block, and intra-articular infusion of ropivacaine for pain relief after anterior cruciate ligament reconstruction (146). The assessment of analgesia for the first 36 hours following surgery showed that patients receiving intra-articular local anesthetic infusion reported significantly higher pain scores compared with the other two groups. Adverse effects were similar in all groups, except for urinary retention, which was significantly more frequent in the epidural group. The authors concluded that a continuous femoral nerve block is the technique of choice for postoperative pain relief after major knee surgery (see Chapter 14 for techniques).

Some authors question the necessity for continuous blocks, alleging that postoperative pain is limited to the immediate postoperative period and therefore could be adequately controlled by single-injection techniques using long-acting local anesthetics. Hirst and colleagues have compared single-injection versus continuous femoral nerve block with 0.5% bupivacaine for analgesia after total knee arthroplasty (147). The continuous block group received an infusion of 0.125% bupivacaine at 6 mL/hour following the surgery. A third group serving as control received a "sham" femoral block. No advantage to continuous femoral block was observed beyond the recovery room period regarding pain scores or morphine consumption. Single-injection femoral nerve block lasted at least 18 hours. The authors concluded that there is no benefit for continuous procedures in postoperative analgesia following total knee arthroplasty. In a study by Mannion and colleagues, single-injection psoas compartment block provided 11 to 14 hours of analgesia post total knee arthroplasty, but there was no increase in analgesic duration with the addition of tramadol (1.5 mg/kg) to levobupivacaine 0.5% (148). Patients receiving either IV or perineural tramadol had median pain scores of 0 for the first 24 hours compared with median pain scores of 2 in the control group. However, this difference was not significant. Salinas and colleagues, in a very similarly designed study, reported that a continuous femoral nerve block allowed a decrease in patient mean maximal VAS values during physical therapy as well as in rescue analgesic consumption compared with a single-injection block (149). However, there was no difference in hospital length of stay and long-term functional recovery.

Watson and co-workers advocated the use of continuous psoas compartment blocks after total knee arthroplasty to reduce postoperative morphine requirements and improve early recovery (150). Williams and colleagues clearly demonstrated the benefits of 0.25% levobupivacaine continuous femoral nerve blocks on VAS scores during movement from day 0 to day 4 after anterior cruciate ligament reconstruction (151). Kaloul and co-workers compared the efficacy of continuous anterior and posterior lumbar plexus blocks with 0.2% ropivacaine for analgesia for the 48 hours following total knee arthroplasty performed under spinal anesthesia (152). Sixty patients were randomly assigned to one of the two regional techniques or to receive patient-controlled morphine analgesia alone. Results showed that continuous femoral block and psoas compartment block reduced total morphine consumption by 48% and 50%, respectively, compared to the PCA group. Pain scores at rest were also significantly lower in patients receiving local anesthetic infusion 6 and 24 hours after surgery. The authors concluded that both continuous femoral and psoas compartment block provided better analgesia than PCA alone after

total knee arthroplasty, but no significant difference was observed between psoas compartment block and femoral block in terms of analgesia.

Ankle and Foot

The optimal anesthetic technique for foot and ankle surgery should provide rapid patient recovery, minimal nursing care requirements in PACU, and reduced hospital discharge times. The postoperative pain that follows can be moderate to severe in intensity and difficult to control with oral analgesics, it and can account for a readmission rate as high as 50% (153). Regional anesthetic techniques have been advocated for such procedures.

Spinal anesthesia is relatively easy to perform. Recently, the use of low doses of local anesthetics and a unilateral spinal block have been recommended in regional anesthesia programs for foot surgery (154–156). However, the risk of hemodynamic instability, urinary dysfunction, TNS, postdural puncture headache, and short postoperative analgesia are significant drawbacks to spinal anesthesia in the ambulatory setting. If adjuvant opioids are used in combination with spinal anesthesia, side effects such as nausea, vomiting, and pruritus may prolong PACU stay, thus increasing costs and decreasing efficiency.

The technical aspects of ankle block are discussed in Chapter 14. Ankle block is a safe and efficient technique indicated in nearly all surgical procedures on the foot, such as Morton neurinoma, bunionectomy, amputation of midfoot or toes, and metatarsal osteotomy. In a large study including more than 1,300 patients requiring foot surgery, general anaesthesia was never required, and patient satisfaction was high (157). Complications included one case (0.07%) of IV injection of local anesthetics with convulsions, and five cases (0.4%) of temporary paresthesias in the area supplied by the posterior tibial nerve. Some authors advocate blocking the posterior tibial nerve systematically and the other nerves (deep peroneal, saphenous, superficial peroneal, and sural) according to the surgical site (157). However, this selective technique is associated with a lower success rate (57% versus 11% of patients felt intraoperative pain and required supplementary anesthesia) than the complete one (blocking all five nerves) (158). Ankle block provides residual analgesia, particularly when long-acting local anesthetics are used. With plain 0.5% bupivacaine, the mean duration of postoperative analgesia is 11.5 hours (159), with a maximal pain-free period of 25 hours in one patient (160). Although of shorter duration, the quality of pain relief was comparable to that obtained with a popliteal sciatic nerve block (159). With 0.75% bupivacaine, analgesia lasted a mean time of 17 hours (161). Ankle block is somewhat time-consuming if five separate injections of local anesthetic agent are required, and the patient may have to assume two separate positions (prone and supine) for the block to be performed. Its performance is relatively painful, particularly when blocking the deep peroneal nerve in the deep planes below the fascia.

Sciatic nerve block with or without a saphenous or femoral nerve block is used for outpatient foot or ankle surgery in many centers. As it preserves hamstring function and thus allows early deambulation with crutches, block at the popliteal level is to be preferred over more proximal approaches. Posterior (162) and lateral (159,163,164) approaches to the popliteal fossa have been described. When performed with a peripheral nerve stimulator, both of these provide efficient and reliable anaesthesia. Ultrasonography is now widely used for the block procedure (165). Less than 5% of blocks failed in experienced hands (166), and a popliteal block can be performed in less than 10 minutes (164). Note that the lateral approach is somewhat more time-consuming than the posterior one. In one study, while most of the patients in the posterior group required only one or two attempts, in the lateral group, most patients required a third or fourth attempt to localize the sciatic nerve (164). One frequently cited disadvantage of the posterior approach is the need to place the patient in the prone position. Combined with a saphenous nerve block, popliteal block provides excellent tolerance of a calf tourniquet, whereas a femoral nerve block allows for the use of a thigh tourniquet (when a more proximal sciatic nerve block is performed) (167). The use of a long-acting local anesthetics provides efficient and prolonged postoperative analgesia. The addition of 1 μg/kg clonidine to 0.75% ropivacaine significantly prolongs the duration of analgesia from 14 hours to 16 to 17 hours without side effects (168). In a recent prospective study of 2,382 outpatient blocks, including 662 patients with a sciatic nerve block, only one patient was identified as having the potential for a neurologic complaint at the 7-day interview (37). In this study by Klein and co-workers, only 5.8% of patients contacted a doctor or nurse to address issues of pain control within the first 24 hours after discharge following sciatic nerve block. No patient required overnight admission. The majority of patients were highly satisfied with their anaesthesia and would choose the same anesthetic again.

Although effective, single-injection block of the sciatic nerve, even with long-lasting local anesthetics, is limited to a period of 10 to 20 hours. For this reason, continuous techniques for sciatic nerve block have been described to improve the analgesia following foot surgery (169–172). Singelyn and colleagues first described a continuous technique for blocking the sciatic nerve at the popliteal fossa (172), and they reported significantly better analgesia in patients receiving continuous sciatic nerve block when compared with patients receiving IV propacetamol and/or intramuscular piritramide and patient-controlled morphine analgesia (Table 25-4). They also noted lower opioid consumption and fewer side effects. Only 6% of patients required conversion to general anesthesia due to inadequate block. No complications were noted. However, in the postoperative period, 25% of catheters presented with technical problems relating to kinks in the catheters.

Patient-controlled analgesia techniques significantly reduce local anesthetic and morphine consumption without compromising pain scores or patient satisfaction (Table 25-5) (171,173). The improvements in equipment and the introduction of new elastomeric pumps for local anesthetic infusion has improved postoperative analgesia and allowed major foot and ankle surgery to be performed as outpatient procedures. Recently, Ilfeld and colleagues have shown, in a randomized, double-blinded study, that local anesthetic infusion via a portable pump through a popliteal sciatic perineural catheter is safe and provides efficient analgesia (170). Eighty percent of their patients receiving perineural ropivacaine did not require any oral opioid analgesics during the 48-hour study period. Average resting pain scores were less than 1 on a scale of 0 to 10. By contrast, in the placebo group, only 7% of patients delayed their first opioid consumption until after infusion discontinuation, and the average resting pain score was 3 to 4. In addition to improved pain control, decreases in opioid consumption, and fewer side effects, they reported a significant decrease in sleep disturbances in the ropivacaine group. These results have been confirmed by another double-blinded placebo-controlled study conducted by White and co-workers, who have also shown a postoperative opioid-sparing effect as well as lower pain scores in the group receiving a local anesthetic infusion in the 48 hours following surgery (174).

TABLE 25-5

PAIN SCORES, MORPHINE, AND LOCAL ANESTHETIC CONSUMPTION IN PATIENTS WITH CONTINUOUS SCIATIC NERVE BLOCKS (SUBGLUTEAL APPROACH) AFTER FOOT SURGERY: PATIENT-CONTROLLED REGIONAL ANALGESIA (PCRA) VERSUS CONTINUOUS INFUSION

	Continuous infusion	PCRA
VAS H6	0.5	0
VAS H12	3	3
VAS H18	3	3
VAS H24	2.5	3
Morphine consumption (mg) at H24 (median)	0 (range: 0–40)	0 (range: 0–20)
Local anesthetic consumption (mg) at H24 (median)	480 (range: 480–480)	280* (range: 240–480)

*P <0.05; VAS (visual analog pain scale) in mm, H, hours, all values are median and range.
From Di Benedetto P, Casati A, Bertini L. Continuous subgluteus sciatic nerve block after orthopedic foot and ankle surgery: Comparison of two infusion techniques. *Reg Anesth Pain Med* 2002;27:168–172, with permission.

TABLE 25-4

COMPARISON BETWEEN CONTINUOUS PERIPHERAL NERVE BLOCK (CPNB) AND INTRAVENOUS MORPHINE PATIENT-CONTROLLED ANALGESIA (PCA) FOR PAIN SCORES AND ADVERSE EVENTS

	CPNB	IV PCA
Highest PPS range (0–3)	0.8 ± 0.1	1.6 ± 0.1
Mean PPS (0–3)	0.3 ± 0.1	0.8 ± 0.1
Nausea/vomiting (%)	5	49*
Urinary retention (%)	0	18*
Sedation (%)	0	11*
Technical problems (%)	25*	0

*p <0.05; PPS, postoperative pain score.
From Eledjam JJ, Cuvillon P, Capdevila X, et al.; French study group. Postoperative analgesia by sciatic nerve block after foot surgery: Continuous versus patient-controlled techniques. *Reg Anesth Pain Med* 2002;27:604–611, with permission.

SUMMARY

Anesthesia for orthopedic surgery encompasses a wide area of anesthetic care, offering anesthesiologists a challenging but rewarding practice, in which neural blockade plays a large and ever-increasing role. The recent developments in regional anesthesia, such as longer-acting, safer local anesthetics and improved techniques, should result in improved outcomes in orthopedic surgery, including reduced postoperative pain and optimized patient rehabilitation.

PART III: APPLICATIONS

References

1. Hebl JR. The importance and implications of aseptic techniques during regional anesthesia. *Reg Anesth Pain Med* 2006;31:311–323.
2. Iohom G, Machmachi A, Diarra DP, et al. The effects of clonidine added to mepivacaine for paronychia surgery under axillary brachial plexus block. *Anesth Analg* 2005;100:1179–1183.
3. Mauermann WJ, Nemergut EC. The anesthesiologist's role in the prevention of surgical site infections. *Anesthesiology* 2006;105:413–421.
4. Capdevila X, Pirat P, Bringuier S, et al. French Study Group on Continuous Peripheral Nerve Blocks. Continuous peripheral nerve blocks in hospital wards after orthopedic surgery: A multicenter prospective analysis of the quality of postoperative analgesia and complications in 1,416 patients. *Anesthesiology* 2005;103:1035–1045.
5. Cuvillon P, Ripart J, Lalourcey L, et al. The continuous femoral nerve block catheter for postoperative analgesia: Bacterial colonization, infectious rate and adverse effects. *Anesth Analg* 2001;93:1045–1049.
6. Phillips JM, Stedeford JC, Hartsilver E, Roberts C. Epidural abscess complicating insertion of epidural catheters. *Br J Anaesth* 2002;89:778–782.
7. Kinirons B, Mimoz O, Lafendi L, et al. Chlorhexidine versus povidone iodine in preventing colonization of continuous epidural catheters in children: A randomized, controlled trial. *Anesthesiology* 2001;94:239–244.
8. Pham-Marcou A, Molina V, Lambert T, et al. Evaluation of continuous femoral nerve block in hemophiliacs after total knee replacement. [Evaluation de l'analgésie continue par cathéter fémoral après prothèse totale de genou chez les hémophiles]. *Ann Fr Anesth Réanin* 2005;24:1173.
9. Horlocker TT, Wedel DJ, Benzon H, et al. Regional anesthesia in the anticoagulated patient: Defining the risks (the second ASRA Consensus Conference on Neuraxial Anesthesia and Anticoagulation). *Reg Anesth Pain Med* 2003;28:172–197.
10. Rowlingson JC, Hanson PB. Neuraxial anesthesia and low-molecular-weight heparin prophylaxis in major orthopedic surgery in the wake of the latest American Society of Regional Anesthesia guidelines. *Anesth Analg* 2005;100:1482–1488.
11. Hebl JR, Horlocker TT, Schroeder DR. Neuraxial anesthesia and analgesia in patients with preexisting central nervous system disorders. *Anesth Analg* 2006;103:223–228.
12. Wiertlewski S, Magot A, Drapier S, et al. Worsening of neurologic symptoms after epidural anesthesia for labor in a Guillain-Barré patient. *Anesth Analg* 2004;98:825–827.
13. Hebl JR, Kopp SL, Schroeder DR, Horlocker TT. Neurologic complications after neuraxial anesthesia or analgesia in patients with preexisting peripheral sensorimotor neuropathy or diabetic polyneuropathy. *Anesth Analg* 2006;103:1294–1299.
14. Mackenzie N. Phantom limb pain during spinal anaesthesia. Recurrence in amputees. *Anaesthesia* 1983;38:886–887.
15. Tessler MJ, Kleiman SJ. Spinal anaesthesia for patients with previous lower limb amputations. *Anaesthesia* 1994;49:439–441.
16. Martin G, Grant SA, Macleod DB, et al. Severe phantom leg pain in an amputee after lumbar plexus block. *Reg Anesth Pain Med* 2003;28:475–478.
17. Benumof JL. Permanent loss of cervical spinal cord function associated with interscalene block performed under general anesthesia. *Anesthesiology* 2000;93:1541–1544.
18. Bogdanov A, Loveland R. Is there a place for interscalene block performed after induction of general anaesthesia? *Eur J Anaesthesiol* 2005;22:107–110.
19. Bonnet F, Marret E. Influence of anaesthetic and analgesic techniques on outcome after surgery. *Br J Anaesth* 2005;95:52–58.
20. Horlocker TT, Abel MD, Messick JM Jr., Schroeder DR. Small risk of serious neurologic complications related to lumbar epidural catheter placement in anesthetized patients. *Anesth Analg* 2003;96:1547–1552.
21. Grady RE, Horlocker TT, Brown RD, et al. Neurologic complications after placement of cerebrospinal fluid drainage catheters and needles in anesthetized patients: Implications for regional anesthesia. Mayo Perioperative Outcomes Group. *Anesth Analg* 1999;88:388–392.
22. Fuzier R, Fourcade O, Fuzier V, et al. The feasibility and efficacy of short axillary catheters for emergency upper limb surgery: A descriptive series of 120 cases. *Anesth Analg* 2006;102:610–614.
23. Minville V, Fourcade O, Idabouk L, et al. Infraclavicular brachial plexus block versus humeral block in trauma patients: A comparison of patient comfort. *Anesth Analg* 2006;102:912–915.
24. Candal-Couto JJ, McVie JL, Haslam N, et al. Pre-operative analgesia for patients with femoral neck fractures using a modified fascia iliaca block technique. *Injury* 2005;36:505–510.
25. Fletcher AK, Rigby AS, Heyes FL. Three-in-one femoral nerve block as analgesia for fractured neck of femur in the emergency department: A randomized, controlled trial. *Ann Emerg Med* 2003;41:227–233.
26. Davis ET, Harris A, Keene D, et al. The use of regional anaesthesia in patients at risk of acute compartment syndrome. *Injury* 2006;37:128–133.
27. Ananthanarayan C, Castro C, McKee N, Sakotic G. Compartment syndrome following intravenous regional anesthesia. *Can J Anaesth* 2000;47:1094–1098.
28. Imarengiaye CO, Song D, Prabhu AJ, Chung F. Spinal anesthesia: Functional balance is impaired after clinical recovery. *Anesthesiology* 2003;98:511–515.
29. Mulroy MF, Salinas FV, Arkin KL, Polissar NL. Ambulatory surgery patients may be discharged before voiding after short-acting spinal and epidural anesthesia. *Anesthesiology* 2002;97:315–319.
30. Freedman JM, Li DK, Drassner K, et al. Transient neurologic symptoms after spinal anesthesia: An epidemiology study of 1.863 patients. *Anesthesiology* 1998;89:633–641.
31. Ben-David B, De Meo PJ, Lucyk C, Solosko D. A comparison of minidose lidocaine-fentanyl spinal anesthesia and local anesthesia/propofol infusion for outpatient knee arthroscopy. *Anesth Analg* 2001;93:319–325.
32. Ben-David B, Maryanovsky M, Gurevitch A. A comparison of minidose lidocaine-fentanyl and conventional-dose lidocaine spinal anesthesia. *Anesth Analg* 2000;91:865–870.
33. Ben-David B, Frankel R, Arzumonov T, et al. Minidose bupivacaine-fentanyl spinal anesthesia for surgical repair of hip fracture in the aged. *Anesthesiology* 2000;92:6–10.
34. Fanelli G, Borghi B, Casati A, et al. Unilateral bupivacaine spinal anesthesia for outpatient knee arthroscopy. *Can J Anaesth* 2000;47:746–751.
35. Buckenmaier CC 3rd, Nielsen KC, Pietrobon R, et al. Small-dose intrathecal lidocaine versus ropivacaine for anorectal surgery in an ambulatory setting. *Anesth Analg* 2002;95:1253–1257.
36. Williams BA, DeRiso BM, Figalloo CM, et al. Benchmarking the perioperative process: III. Effects of regional anesthesia clinical pathway techniques on process efficiency and recovery profiles in ambulatory orthopedic surgery. *J Clin Anesth* 1998;10:570–578.
37. Klein SM, Nielsen KC, Greengrass RA, et al. Ambulatory discharge after long-acting peripheral nerve block 2382 blocks with ropivacaine. *Anesth Analg* 2002;94:65–70.
38. Mulroy MF, Larkin KL, Batra MS, et al. Femoral nerve block with 0.25% or 0.5% bupivacaine improves postoperative analgesia following outpatient arthroscopic ACL repair. *Reg Anesth Pain Med* 2001;26:24–29.
39. Jankowski CJ, Hebl JR, Stuart MJ, et al. A comparison of psoas compartment block and spinal and general anesthesia for outpatient knee arthroscopy. *Anesth Analg* 2003;97:1003–1009.
40. McCartney CJ, Brull R, Chan VW, et al. Early but no long-term benefit of regional compared with general anesthesia for ambulatory hand surgery. *Anesthesiology* 2004;101:461–467.
41. Klein SM, Grant SA, Greengrass RA, et al. Interscalene brachial plexus block with a continuous catheter insertion system and a disposable infusion pump. *Anesth Analg* 2000;91:1473–1478.
42. Ilfeld BM, Morey TE, Enneking FK. Continuous infraclavicular brachial plexus block for postoperative pain control at home: A randomized, double-blinded, placebo-controlled study. *Anesthesiology* 2002;96:1297–1304.
43. Ilfeld BM, Morey TE, Wang RD, Enneking FK. Continuous popliteal sciatic nerve block for postoperative pain control at home: A randomized, double-blinded, placebo-controlled study. *Anesthesiology* 2002;97:959–965.
44. Ilfeld BM, Morey TE, Wright TW, et al. Continuous interscalene brachial plexus block for postoperative pain control at home: A randomized, double-blinded, placebo-controlled study. *Anesth Analg* 2003;96:1089–1095.
45. Ilfeld BM, Vandenborne K, Duncan PW, et al. Ambulatory continuous interscalene nerve blocks decrease the time to discharge readiness after total shoulder arthroplasty: A randomized, triple-masked, placebo-controlled study. *Anesthesiology* 2006;105:999–1007.
46. Ilfeld BM, Gearen PF, Enneking FK, et al. Total knee arthroplasty as an overnight-stay procedure using continuous femoral nerve blocks at home: A prospective feasibility study. *Anesth Analg* 2006;102:87–90.
46a. Ilfeld BM, Gearen PF, Enneking FK, et al. Total hip arthroplasty as an overnight-stay procedure using an ambulatory continuous psoas compartment nerve block: A prospective feasibility study. *Reg Anesth Pain Med* 2006;31:113–118.
47. Capdevila X, Dadure C, Bringuier S, et al. Effect of patient-controlled perineural analgesia on rehabilitation and pain after ambulatory orthopedic surgery: A multicenter randomized trial. *Anesthesiology* 2006;105:566–573.
48. Delgado Tapia JA, Garcia Sanchez MJ, Prieto Cuellar M, et al. Infraclavicular brachial plexus block using a multiple injection technique and an approach in the cranial direction in a patient with anticipated difficulties in tracheal intubation [Spanish]. *Rev Esp Anestesiol Reanim* 2002;49:105–107.
49. Kumar CM, Mehta M. Ankylosing spondylitis: Lateral approach to spinal anaesthesia for lower limb surgery. *Can J Anaesth* 1995;42:73–76.

50. Capdevila X, Barthelet Y, Biboulet P, et al. Effects of perioperative analgesic technique on the surgical outcome and duration of rehabilitation after major knee surgery. *Anesthesiology* 1999;91:8–15.

51. Singelyn FJ, Deyaert M, Joris D, et al. Effects of intravenous patient-controlled analgesia with morphine, continuous epidural analgesia, and continuous three-in-one block on postoperative pain and knee rehabilitation after unilateral total knee arthroplasty. *Anesth Analg* 1998;87:88–92.

52. Williams BA, DeRiso BM, Engel LB, et al. Benchmarking the perioperative process: II. Introducing anesthesia clinical pathways to improve processes and outcomes and to reduce nursing labor intensity in ambulatory orthopedic surgery. *J Clin Anesth* 1998;10:561–569.

53. Gonano C, Leitgeb U, Sitzwohl C, et al. Spinal versus general anesthesia for orthopedic surgery: Anesthesia drug and supply costs. *Anesth Analg* 2006;102:524–529.

54. Chan VW, Peng PW, Kaszas Z, et al. A comparative study of general anesthesia, intravenous regional anesthesia, and axillary block for outpatient hand surgery: Clinical outcome and cost analysis. *Anesth Analg* 2001;93:1181–1184.

55. Schuster M, Gottschalk A, Berger J, Standl T. A retrospective comparison of costs for regional and general anesthesia techniques. *Anesth Analg* 2005;100:786–794.

56. Schenk MR, Putzier M, Kugler B, et al. Postoperative analgesia after major spine surgery: Patient-controlled epidural analgesia versus patient-controlled intravenous analgesia. *Anesth Analg* 2006;103:1311–1317.

57. Silver DJ, Dunsmore RH, Dickson CM. Spinal anesthesia for lumbar disc surgery: Review of 576 operations. *Anesth Analg* 1976;55:550–554.

58. McLain RF, Bell GR, Kalfas I, et al. Complications associated with lumbar anesthesia: A comparison of spinal versus general anesthesia. *Spine* 2004;15(29):2542–2547.

59. Kundra P, Gurnani A, Bhattacharya A. Preemptive epidural morphine for postoperative pain relief after lumbar laminectomy. *Anesth Analg* 1997;85:135–138.

60. Tobias JD. A review of intrathecal and epidural analgesia after spinal surgery in children. *Anesth Analg* 2004;98:956–965.

61. Gall O, Aubineau JV, Berniere J, et al. Analgesic effect of low-dose intrathecal morphine after spinal fusion in children. *Anesthesiology* 2001;94:447–452.

62. Dalens B, Tanguy A. Intrathecal morphine for spinal fusion in children. *Spine* 1988;13:494–498.

63. Blackman RG, Reynolds J, Shively J. Intrathecal morphine: Dosage and efficacy in younger patients for control of postoperative pain following spinal fusion. *Orthopedics* 1991;14:555–557.

64. Goodarzi M. The advantages of intrathecal opioids for spinal fusion in children. *Paediatr Anaesth* 1998;8:131–134.

65. Oshimoto H, Nagashima K, Sato S, et al. A prospective evaluation of anesthesia for posterior lumbar spine fusion: The effectiveness of preoperative epidural anesthesia with morphine. *Spine* 2005;5:863–869.

66. Sekar C, Rajasekaran S, Kannan R, et al. Preemptive analgesia for postoperative pain relief in lumbosacral spine surgeries: A randomized controlled trial. *Spine J* 2004;4:261–264.

67. Blumenthal S, Min K, Nadig M, Borgeat A. Double epidural catheter with ropivacaine versus intravenous morphine: A comparison for postoperative analgesia after scoliosis correction surgery. *Anesthesiology* 2005;102:175–180.

68. Dalens B, Bazin JE, Haberer JP. Epidural bubbles as a cause of incomplete analgesia during epidural anesthesia. *Anesth Analg* 1987;66:679–683.

69. Turner A, Lee J, Mitchell R, et al. The efficacy of surgically placed epidural catheters for analgesia after posterior spinal surgery. *Anaesthesia* 2000;55:370–373.

70. Souron V, Delaunay L, Bonnet F. Sedation with target-controlled propofol infusion during shoulder surgery under interscalene brachial plexus block in the sitting position: Report of a series of 140 patients. *Eur J Anaesthesiol* 2005;22:853–857.

71. Tetzlaff JE, Yoon HJ, Brems J. Interscalene brachial plexus block for shoulder surgery. *Reg Anesth* 1994;19:339–343.

72. Borgeat A, Ekatodramis G. Anaesthesia for shoulder surgery. [Review] *Best Pract Res Clin Anaesthesiol* 2002;16:211–225.

73. Boezaart AP. Continuous interscalene block for ambulatory shoulder surgery. [Review] *Best Pract Res Clin Anaesthesiol* 2002;16:295–310.

74. Singelyn FJ, Lhotel L, Fabre B. Pain relief after arthroscopic shoulder surgery: A comparison of intraarticular analgesia, suprascapular nerve block, and interscalene brachial plexus block. *Anesth Analg* 2004;99:589–592.

75. D'Alessio JG, Weller RS, Rosenblum M. Activation of the Bezold-Jarisch reflex in the sitting position for shoulder arthroscopy using interscalene block. *Anesth Analg* 1995;80:1158–1162.

76. Sia S, Sarro F, Lepri A, Bartoli M. The effect of exogenous epinephrine on the incidence of hypotensive/bradycardic events during shoulder surgery in the sitting position during interscalene block. *Anesth Analg* 2003;97:583–588.

77. Campagna JA, Carter C. Clinical relevance of the Bezold-Jarisch reflex. *Anesthesiology* 2003;98:1250–1260.

78. Liguori GA, Kahn RL, Gordon J, et al. The use of metoprolol and glycopyrrolate to prevent hypotensive/bradycardic events during shoulder arthroscopy in the sitting position under interscalene block. *Anesth Analg* 1998;87:1320–1325.

79. Kahn RL, Hargett MJ. Beta-adrenergic blockers and vasovagal episodes during shoulder surgery in the sitting position under interscalene block. *Anesth Analg* 1999;88:378–381.

80. Blaivas M, Lyon M. Ultrasound-guided interscalene block for shoulder dislocation reduction in the ED. *Am J Emerg Med* 2006;24:293–296.

81. Boardman ND 3rd, Cofield RH. Neurologic complications of shoulder surgery. *Clin Orthop Relat Res* 1999;368:44–53.

82. Borgeat A, Ekatodramis G, Kalberer F, Benz C. Acute and nonacute complications associated with interscalene block and shoulder surgery: A prospective study. *Anesthesiology* 2001;95:875–880.

83. Horlocker TT, Kufner RP, Bishop AT, et al. The risk of persistent paresthesia is not increased with repeated axillary block. *Anesth Analg* 1999;88:382–387.

84. Borgeat A, Dullenkopf A, Ekatodramis G, Nagy L. Evaluation of the lateral modified approach for continuous interscalene block after shoulder surgery. *Anesthesiology* 2003;99:436–442.

85. Tetzlaff JE, Brems J, Dilger J. Intraarticular morphine and bupivacaine reduces postoperative pain after rotator cuff repair. *Reg Anesth Pain Med* 2000;25:611–614.

86. Kosnik J, Shamsa F, Raphael E, et al. Anesthetic methods for reduction of acute shoulder dislocations: A prospective randomized study comparing intraarticular lidocaine with intravenous analgesia and sedation. *Am J Emerg Med* 1999;17:566–570.

87. Ilfeld BM, Enneking FK. Continuous peripheral nerve blocks at home: A review. *Anesth Analg* 2005;100:1822–1833.

88. Ilfeld BM, Wright TW, Enneking FK, Vandenborne K. Total elbow arthroplasty as an outpatient procedure using a continuous infraclavicular nerve block at home: A prospective case report. *Reg Anesth Pain Med* 2006;31:172–176.

89. Schroeder LE, Horlocker TT, Schroeder DR. The efficacy of axillary block for surgical procedures about the elbow. *Anesth Analg* 1996;83:747–751.

90. Dupre LJ. Brachial plexus block through humeral approach. *Cal Anesthesiol* 1994;42:767–769.

91. Chin KJ, Chee VTW, Lee B. Infraclavicular brachial plexus block for regional anaesthesia of the lower arm. [Protocol] *Cochrane Database Sys Rev* 2005;4:CD005487

92. Bouaziz H, Narchi P, Mercier FJ, et al. Comparison between conventional axillary block and a new approach at the midhumeral level. *Anesth Analg* 1997;84:1058–1062.

93. Handoll HH, Koscielniak-Nielsen ZJ. Single, double or multiple injection techniques for axillary brachial plexus block for hand, wrist or forearm surgery. *Cochrane Database Syst Rev* 2006;25:CD003842.

94. Bouaziz H, Narchi P, Mercier FJ, et al. The use of a selective axillary nerve block for outpatient hand surgery. *Anesth Analg* 1998;86:746–748.

95. Henderson CL, Warriner CB, McEwen JA, Merrick PM. A North American survey of intravenous regional anesthesia. *Anesth Analg* 1997;85:858–863.

96. Atanassoff PG, Ocampo CA, Bande MC, et al. Ropivacaine 0.2% and lidocaine 0.5% for intravenous regional anesthesia in outpatient surgery. *Anesthesiology* 2001;95:627–631.

97. Atanassoff PG, Aouad R, Hartmannsgruber MW, Halaszynski T. Levobupivacaine 0.125% and lidocaine 0.5% for intravenous regional anesthesia in volunteers. *Anesthesiology* 2002;97:325–328.

98. Choyce A, Peng P. A systematic review of adjuncts for intravenous regional anesthesia for surgical procedures. [Review] *Can J Anaesth* 2002;49:32–45.

99. Chiu DT. Transthecal digital block: Flexor tendon sheath used for anesthetic infusion. *J Hand Surg [Am]* 1990;15:471–477.

100. Auroy Y, Benhamou D, Bargues L, et al. Major complications of regional anesthesia in France: The SOS Regional Anesthesia Hotline Service. *Anesthesiology* 2002;97:1274–1280.

101. Favarel-Garrigues JF, Sztark F, Petitjean ME, et al. Hemodynamic effects of spinal anesthesia in the elderly: Single dose versus titration through a catheter. *Anesth Analg* 1996;82:312–316.

102. Minville V, Fourcade O, Grousset D, et al. Spinal anesthesia using single injection small-dose bupivacaine versus continuous catheter injection techniques for surgical repair of hip fracture in elderly patients. *Anesth Analg* 2006;102:1559–1563.

103. Rodgers A, Walker N, Schug S, et al. Reduction of postoperative mortality and morbidity with epidural or spinal anaesthesia: Results from overview of randomised trials. *Br Med J* 2000;16(321):1493.

104. Mauermann WJ, Shilling AM, Zuo Z. A comparison of neuraxial block versus general anesthesia for elective total hip replacement: A meta-analysis. *Anesth Analg* 2006;103:1018–1025.

105. O'Hara DA, Duff A, Berlin JA, et al. The effect of anesthetic technique on postoperative outcomes in hip fracture repair. *Anesthesiology* 2000;92:947–957.

106. Gilbert TB, Hawkes WG, Hebel JR, et al. Spinal anesthesia versus general anesthesia for hip fracture repair: A longitudinal observation of 741 elderly patients during 2-year follow-up. *Am J Orthop* 2000;29:25–35.

PART III: APPLICATIONS

107. Sorenson RM, Pace NL. Anesthetic techniques during surgical repair of femoral neck fractures. A meta-analysis. *Anesthesiology* 1992;77:1095–1104.
108. Parker MJ, Handoll HH, Griffiths R. Anaesthesia for hip fracture surgery in adults. *Cochrane Database Syst Rev* 2004;18:CD000521.
109. Urwin SC, Parker MJ, Griffiths R. General versus regional anaesthesia for hip fracture surgery: A meta-analysis of randomized trials. *Br J Anaesth* 2000;84:450–455. Erratum in: *Br J Anaesth* 2002;88:619.
110. Scheini H, Virtanen T, Kentala E, al. Epidural infusion of bupivacaine and fentanyl reduces perioperative myocardial ischaemia in elderly patients with hip fracture: A randomized controlled trial. *Acta Anaesthesiol Scand* 2000;44:1061–1070.
111. Matot I, Oppenheim-Eden A, Ratrot R, et al. Preoperative cardiac events in elderly patients with hip fracture randomized to epidural or conventional analgesia. *Anesthesiology* 2003;98:156–163.
112. de Visme V, Picart F, Le Jouan R, et al. Combined lumbar and sacral plexus block compared with plain bupivacaine spinal anesthesia for hip fractures in the elderly. *Reg Anesth Pain Med* 2000;25:158–162.
113. Mannion S, Hayes I, Loughnane F, et al. Intravenous but not perineural clonidine prolongs postoperative analgesia after psoas compartment block with 0.5% levobupivacaine for hip fracture surgery. *Anesth Analg* 2005;100:873–878.
114. Foss NB, Kristensen MT, Kristensen BB, et al. Effect of postoperative epidural analgesia on rehabilitation and pain after hip fracture surgery: A randomized, double-blind, placebo-controlled trial. *Anesthesiology* 2005;102:1197–1204.
115. Block BM, Liu SS, Rowlingson AJ, et al. Efficacy of postoperative epidural analgesia: A meta-analysis. *JAMA* 2003;12(290):2455–2463.
116. Sharrock NE, Finerty E. Hip replacement, hip seeding, and epidural anaesthesia. *Lancet* 2005;365:1011–1012.
117. Williams-Russo P, Sharrock NE, Mattis S, et al. Randomized trial of hypotensive epidural anesthesia in older adults. *Anesthesiology* 1999;91:926–935.
118. Casati A, Santorsola R, Aldegheri G, et al. Intraoperative epidural anesthesia and postoperative analgesia with levobupivacaine for major orthopedic surgery: A double-blind, randomized comparison of racemic bupivacaine and ropivacaine. *J Clin Anesth* 2003;15:126–131.
119. Standl TG, Horn E, Luckmann M, et al. Subarachnoid sufentanil for early postoperative pain management in orthopedic patients: A placebo-controlled, double-blind study using spinal microcatheters. *Anesthesiology* 2001;94:230–238.
120. Fournier R, Van Gessel E, Gaggero G, et al. Postoperative analgesia with 3-in-1 femoral nerve block after prosthetic hip surgery. *Can J Anesth* 1998;45:34–38.
121. Mannion S, O'Donnell B. Obturator nerve blockade following '3-in-1' block: The role of motor assessment. *Acta Anaesthesiol Scand* 2006;50:645.
122. Winnie AP, Ramamurthy S, Durani Z, Radonjic R. Plexus blocks for lower extremity surgery: New answers to old problems. *Anesthesiol Rev* 1974;1:11–16.
123. Stevens RD, Van Gessel E, Flory N, et al. Lumbar plexus block reduces pain and blood loss associated with total hip arthroplasty. *Anesthesiology* 2000;93:115–121.
124. Capdevila X, Macaire P, Dadure C, et al. Continuous psoas compartment block for postoperative analgesia after total hip arthroplasty: New landmarks, technical guidelines, and clinical evaluation. *Anesth Analg* 2002;94:1606–1613.
125. Mannion S, O'Callaghan S, Walsh M, et al. In with the new, out with the old? Comparison of two approaches for psoas compartment block. *Anesth Analg* 2005;101:259–264.
126. Biboulet P, Morau D, Aubas P, et al. Postoperative analgesia after THA: Comparison of IV PCA with morphine and single injection of femoral nerve or psoas compartment block. A prospective, randomized, double-blind study. *Reg Anesth Pain Med* 2004;29:102–109.
127. Souron V, Delaunay L, Schifrine P. Intrathecal morphine provides better postoperative analgesia than psoas compartment block after primary hip arthroplasty. *Can J Anesth* 2004;51:190–191.
128. Singelyn FJ, Gouverneur JM. Postoperative analgesia after total hip arthroplasty: I.V. PCA with morphine, patient-controlled epidural analgesia, or continuous "3-in-one" block? A prospective evaluation by our acute pain service in more than 1,300 patients. *J Clin Anesth* 1999;11:550–554.
129. Singelyn FJ, Vanderelst PE, Gouverneur JM. Extended femoral nerve sheath block after THA: Continuous vs PCA techniques. *Anesth Analg* 2001;92:455–459.
130. Fischer HB, Simanski CJ. A procedure-specific systematic review and consensus recommendations for analgesia after total hip replacement. *Anaesthesia* 2005;60:1189–1202.
131. Hebl JR, Kopp SL, Ali MH, et al. A comprehensive anesthesia protocol that emphasizes peripheral nerve blockade for total knee and total hip arthroplasty. *J Bone Joint Surg Am* 2005;[87 Suppl 2]:63–70.
132. Lopez S, Gros T, Bernard N, et al. Fascia iliaca compartment block for femoral bone fractures in prehospital care. *Reg Anesth Pain Med* 2003;28:203–207.
133. Wang H, Boctor B, Verner J. The effect of single injection femoral nerve block on rehabilitation and length of hospital stay after TKR. *Reg Anesth Pain Med* 2002;27:139–144.
134. Williams BA, Kentor ML, Vogt MT, et al. Femoral-sciatic nerve blocks for complex outpatient knee surgery are associated with less postoperative pain before same-day discharge. *Anesthesiology* 2003;98:1206–1213.
135. Ben-David B, Schmalenberger K, Chelly JE. Analgesia after total knee arthroplasty: Is continuous sciatic blockade needed in addition to continuous femoral blockade? *Anesth Analg* 2004;98:747–749.
136. Pham Dang C, Gautheron E, Guilley J, et al. The value of adding sciatic block to continuous femoral block for analgesia after total knee replacement. *Reg Anesth Pain Med* 2005;30:128–133.
137. Elmas C, Atanassoff PG. Combined inguinal perivascular and sciatic nerve blocks for lower limb surgery. *Reg Anesth* 1993;18:88–92.
138. Misra U, Pridie AK, McClymont C, Bower S. Plasma concentrations of bupivacaine following combined sciatic and femoral 3 in 1 nerve blocks in open knee surgery. *Br J Anaesth* 1991;66:310–313.
139. McNamee DA, Parks L, Milligan KR. Post-operative analgesia following total knee replacement: An evaluation of the addition of an obturator nerve block to combined femoral and sciatic nerve block. *Acta Anaesthesiol Scand* 2002;46:95–99.
140. Macalou D, Trueck S, Meuret P, et al. Postoperative analgesia after total knee replacement: The effect of an obturator nerve block added to the femoral 3-in-1 nerve block. *Anesth Analg* 2004;99:251–254.
141. Luber MJ, Greengrass R, Vail TP. Patient satisfaction and effectiveness of lumbar plexus and sciatic nerve block for total knee arthroplasty. *Arthroplasty* 2001;16:17–21.
142. Iskandar H, Benard A, Ruel-Raymond J, et al. Femoral block provides superior analgesia compared with intraarticular ropivacaine after ACL reconstruction. *Reg Anesth Pain Med* 2003;28:29–32.
143. Ganapathy S, Wasserman RA, Watson JT, et al. Modified continuous 3-in-1 block for post-operative pain after TKA. *Anesth Analg* 1999;99:1197–1202.
144. Singelyn FJ, Deyaert M, Joris D, et al. Effects of intravenous patient-controlled analgesia with morphine, continuous epidural analgesia, and continuous three-in-one block on postoperative pain and knee rehabilitation after unilateral total knee arthroplasty. *Anesth Analg* 1998;87:88–92.
145. Capdevila X, Barthelet Y, Biboulet P, et al. Effects of perioperative analgesic technique on the surgical outcome and duration of rehabilitation after major knee surgery. *Anesthesiology* 1999;91:8–15.
146. Dauri M, Polzoni M, Fabbi E, et al. Comparison of epidural, continuous femoral block and intraarticular analgesia after ACL reconstruction. *Acta Anesthesiol Scand* 2003;47:20–25.
147. Hirst GC, Lang SA, Dust WN, et al. Femoral nerve block: Single injection vs continuous infusion for TKA. *Reg Anesth* 1996;21:292–297.
148. Mannion S, O'Callaghan S, Murphy DB, Shorten GD. Tramadol as adjunct to psoas compartment block with levobupivacaine 0.5%: A randomized double-blinded study. *Br J Anaesth* 2005;94:352–356.
149. Salinas FV, Liu SS, Mulroy MF. The effect of single-injection femoral nerve block versus continuous femoral nerve block after total knee arthroplasty on hospital length of stay and long-term functional recovery within an established clinical pathway. *Anesth Analg* 2006;102:1234–1239.
150. Watson MW, Mitra D, McLintock TC, Grant SA. Continuous versus single-injection lumbar plexus blocks: Comparison of the effects on morphine use and early recovery after total knee arthroplasty. *Reg Anesth Pain Med* 2005;30:541–547.
151. Williams BA, Kentor ML, Vogt MT, et al. Reduction of verbal pain scores after anterior cruciate ligament reconstruction with 2-day continuous femoral nerve block: A randomized clinical trial. *Anesthesiology* 2006;104:315–327.
152. Kaloul I, Guay J, Cote C, Fallaha M. The posterior lumbar plexus block and the 3-in-1 femoral nerve block provide similar postoperative analgesia after TKR. *Can J Anesth* 2004;51:45–51.
153. Rawal N, Hylander J, Nydahl P, et al. Survey of postoperative analgesia following ambulatory surgery. *Acta Anaesthesiol Scand* 1997;41:1017–1022.
154. Meyer J, Enk D, Penner M. Unilateral spinal anesthesia using low-flow injection through a 29-gauge Quincke needle. *Anesth Analg* 1996;82:1188–1191.
155. Burke D, Kennedy S, Bannister J. Spinal anesthesia with 0.5% S(-)-bupivacaine for elective lower limb surgery. *Reg Anesth Pain Med* 1999;24:519–523.
156. Enk D, Prien T, Van Aken H, et al. Success rate of unilateral spinal anesthesia is dependent on injection flow. *Reg Anesth Pain Med* 2001;26:420–427.
157. Frederic A, Bouchon Y. Analgesia in surgery of the foot: Apropos of 1373 patients. *Cah Anesthesiol* 1996;44:115–118.
158. Delgado-Martinez A, Marchal J, Molina M, Palma A. Forefoot surgery with ankle tourniquet: Complete or selective ankle block? *Reg Anesth Pain Med* 2001;26:184–186.
159. McLeod D, Wong D, Vaghadia H, et al. Lateral popliteal sciatic nerve block compared with ankle block for analgesia following foot surgery. *Can J Anaesth* 1995;42:765–769.
160. Sarrafian S, Ibrahim I, Breihan J. Ankle-foot peripheral nerve block for mid and forefoot surgery. *Foot Ankle* 1983;4:86–90.

161. Mineo R, Sharrock N. Venous levels of lidocaine and bupivacaine after midtarsal ankle block. *Reg Anesth* 1992;17:47–49.
162. Singelyn F, Gouverneur JM. Popliteal sciatic nerve block aided by a nerve stimulator: A reliable technique for foot and ankle surgery. *Reg Anesth* 1991;6:278–281.
163. Zetlaoui P, Bouaziz H. Lateral approach to the sciatic nerve in the popliteal fossa. *Anesth Analg* 1998;87:79–82.
164. Hadzic A, Vloka J. A comparison of the posterior versus lateral approaches to the block of the sciatic nerve in the popliteal fossa. *Anesthesiology* 1988;88:1480–1486.
165. McCartney CJ, Brauner I, Chan VW. Ultrasound guidance for a lateral approach to the sciatic nerve in the popliteal fossa. *Anaesthesia* 2004;59:1023–1025.
166. Hansen E, Eshelmann M, Cracchiolo A. Popliteal fossa neural blockade as the sole anesthetic technique for outpatient foot and ankle surgery. *Foot Ankle Intern* 2000;1:38–44.
167. Fuzier R, Hoffreumont P, Bringuier-Branchereau S, et al. Does the sciatic nerve approach influence thigh tourniquet tolerance during below-knee surgery? *Anesth Analg* 2005;100:1511–1514.
168. Casati A, Magistris L, Fanelli G, et al. Small-dose clonidine prolongs postoperative analgesia after sciatic-femoral nerve block with 0.75% ropivacaine for foot surgery. *Anesth Analg* 2000;91:388–392.
169. Chelly JE, Greger J, Casati A, et al. Continuous lateral sciatic blocks for acute postoperative pain management after major ankle and foot surgery. *Foot Ankle Int* 2002;23:749–752.
170. Ilfeld BM, Morey TE, Wang RD, Enneking FK. Continuous popliteal sciatic nerve block for postoperative pain control at home: A randomized, double-blinded, placebo-controlled study. *Anesthesiology* 2002;97:959–965.
171. Eledjam JJ, Cuvillon P, Capdevila X, et al. Postoperative analgesia by sciatic nerve block after foot surgery: Continuous versus patient-controlled techniques. *Reg Anesth Pain Med* 2002;27:604–611.
172. Singelyn J, Aye F, Gouverneur JM. Continuous popliteal sciatic nerve block: An original technique to provide postoperative analgesia after foot surgery. *Anesth Analg* 1997;84:383–386.
173. Di Benedetto P, Casati A, Bertini L. Continuous subgluteus sciatic nerve block after orthopedic foot and ankle surgery: Comparison of two infusion techniques. *Reg Anesth Pain Med* 2002;27:168–172.
174. White PF, Issioui T, Skrivanek GD, et al. The use of a continuous popliteal sciatic nerve block after surgery involving the foot and ankle: Does it improve the quality of recovery? *Anesth Analg* 2003;97:1303–1309.
175. Finlayson BJ, Underhill TJ. Femoral nerve block for analgesia in fractures of the femoral neck. *Arch Emerg Med* 1988;5:173–176.
176. Haddad FS, Williams RL. Femoral nerve block in extracapsular femoral neck fractures. *J Bone Joint Surg Br* 1995;77:922–923.
177. Chudinov A, Berkenstadt H, Salai M, et al. Continuous psoas compartment block for anesthesia and perioperative analgesia in patients with hip fractures. *Reg Anesth Pain Med* 1999;24:563–568.
178. Parker MJ, Griffiths R, Appadu BN. Nerve blocks (subcostal, lateral cutaneous, femoral, triple, psoas) for hip fractures (Cochrane Review). *Cochrane Database Syst Rev* 2000:CD001159.
179. Singelyn FJ, Felicissimo P, Piovella F, et al. Extended thromboprophylaxis with Fondaparinux (Arixtra®) after major orthopedic lower limb surgery: The EXPERT Study. *J Thromb Haemost* 2005;[3 Suppl 1]:P1102.

PART III: APPLICATIONS

CHAPTER 26 ■ NEURAL BLOCKADE FOR AMBULATORY SURGERY

MICHAEL F. MULROY

Regional anesthesia techniques for surgical patients have grown in popularity because of dramatic advantages in postoperative pain relief, less nausea, and increased alertness. These advantages reduce costs and maximize use of hospital resources. Outpatient surgery has grown to approximately 65% of all surgical procedures performed in the United States, and the use of regional anesthesia in the outpatient setting can also increase efficiency and cost effectiveness, improve recovery, provide postdischarge analgesia, and shorten discharge time.

ADVANTAGES OF REGIONAL ANESTHESIA

The major advantages of regional anesthesia for outpatient procedures center around the superior analgesia obtained with these techniques, without the obtundation and nausea associated with systemic opioids. Pain and nausea are the two major causes of delayed discharge (1) and unplanned admission for outpatients (2,3), and their reduction allows reduced nursing interventions, facilitates bypassing of the postanesthesia care unit (PACU), and ultimately shortens discharge time. Multiple studies have shown these benefits, especially with extremity surgery (4), although faster discharge has been elusive. The potential exists for expanding regional techniques in the outpatient setting, since recent reports have documented a significant problem with postdischarge pain. Apfelbaum and colleagues reported that 85% of surgical patients in the United States still suffer moderate or severe postoperative pain despite modern analgesic drugs (5). Carroll and colleagues showed that, in the outpatient setting, this pain is associated with continued use of oral analgesics for a week after discharge, leading to a high frequency of residual nausea and vomiting at home, even in patients who did not experience nausea in the PACU after outpatient surgery (6). These problems can be reduced by the use of regional techniques, and eliminated even more dramatically by the use of continuous local anesthetic infusions.

The positive aspects of regional techniques must be weighed against the perceived drawbacks, which include the potential need for additional time to perform blocks and the reduced reliability. These challenges also create resistance from some surgeons. Several modifications of regional approaches can overcome each of these drawbacks in the outpatient setting, and make the advantages of this technique available to a larger percentage of outpatients.

MODIFICATIONS FOR REGIONAL ANESTHESIA IN OUTPATIENTS

Selection and Preparation of Patients

The criteria for outpatients receiving regional anesthesia remain the same as for other outpatient procedures, including the level of fitness and fasting status. The advantages of regional analgesia cannot be relied upon to avoid the recognized risks of preexisting medical conditions, such as obstructive sleep apnea. Although regional anesthesia may reduce the need for opioids in such patients, standard guidelines for monitoring and postoperative observation nevertheless must be observed (7). The indications and contraindications for regional techniques also remain the same: the presence of coagulopathy, infection, lack of cooperation, and neurologic disease must be considered. In addition, in the outpatient, significant obesity may increase the potential for block failure and complications (8), although these patients should not necessarily be excluded from consideration.

Patient educations remains a challenge in the outpatient setting. Ambulatory patients are frequently interviewed by the anesthesiologist only on the morning of surgery, and a detailed explanation of a regional technique and acceptance by the patient can consume precious time. Preferably, a preoperative evaluation can be scheduled in advance, or a phone call can at least initiate the educational process. Ideally, the surgeon will be an advocate of regional techniques and start the acceptance process during her preoperative counseling.

Standard American Society of Anesthesiologists (ASA) monitoring guidelines apply. As with all regional techniques, the smallest volume of the local anesthetic drug in a solution of the lowest possible concentration that will give the desired effect should be used. Because of the risk of toxicity, as well as the more common risk of respiratory depression from sedative medications, a dedicated observer trained in advanced life support must be available to monitor mental status, especially with local anesthesia and sedation provided by the surgeon.

Premedication and Sedation

Although rapport, gentleness, and skill in performing the block usually make premedication unnecessary, preoperative sedation for regional anesthesia may be appropriate. Midazolam, 1 to 2 mg, intravenously is an excellent asset to regional anesthesia, often ablating the recall of unpleasant needle insertions or paresthesias. The sedative-amnestic effect can limit its usefulness if the patient becomes confused and can no longer cooperate with the anesthesiologist. Heavy sedation can also prolong time to discharge.

For uncomfortable procedures (which probably includes all multiple needle insertions), analgesia may be provided with a short-acting narcotic such as fentanyl (50 to 100 μg). Again, excessive doses are to be avoided because of the risk of respiratory depression and the potential for increased nausea and vomiting. Supplemental oxygen during the performance of blocks and during surgery is advisable. The short-acting analgesics alfentanil and remifentanil might be appealing, but their duration is too brief to be useful for the performance of most blocks.

If further intraoperative sedation is needed, an intravenous (IV) propofol infusion in doses of 25 to 50 μg/kg/min is useful.

Performance of Blocks: Techniques to Improve Efficiency and Efficacy

In the outpatient setting, speed of room turnover and discharge are important considerations. Although the regional anesthetic techniques described here will allow more rapid discharge and enhanced analgesia, additional time is spent in performing blocks and in allowing adequate onset time of local anesthetic blockade. For the outpatient anesthesiologist, several modifications of choices are helpful.

The selection of rapid-onset blocks and drugs is helpful. In that regard, IV regional and spinal anesthesia techniques are particularly helpful. These can be performed in the operating room itself with little delay in the start of surgery and may be as efficient as general anesthesia itself (9). Selection of rapid-acting drugs, such as 2-chloroprocaine or lidocaine, also provides more rapid onset. Raising the pH of commercial local anesthetic solutions (by adding 1 mEq of sodium bicarbonate to each 10 mL of solution) has also been shown to speed onset of the intermediate duration amino amide local anesthetics for peripheral nerve blocks (10), although this remains controversial.

The optimal time-saver in outpatient surgery is the performance of a block in a location separate from the operating room (9,11). This can be a dedicated anesthesia induction room or a designated corner of the PACU. A separate location, with all of the necessary equipment, drugs, and monitors can allow undisturbed performance of the block and the start of the required "soak time" while the operating room is being prepared. Several investigators have shown that with such an arrangement, the "anesthesia-related time" in the operating room can actually be less than with a general anesthetic technique (12,13). Use of a separate area includes the potential to include additional personnel to aid in block performance. Although an additional anesthesia provider to give sedation and assistance is ideal, PACU nurses or technicians can also help with positioning, preparation of equipment, and manipulation of nerve stimulators or ultrasound devices.

Block technique also impacts efficiency. Selection of simpler techniques with easily identified landmarks (arteries, prominent bones, tendons) will be easier to initiate, and may have higher reliability than techniques that rely on complex geometric measurements and drawings. Similarly, nerve localization technique can improve speed. Electrical neural stimulation identifies nerves at a greater distance than paresthesia techniques, and the use of the more complex ultrasound may prove to be an even faster way to localize nerves and direct injection of the local anesthetic (14,15). The choice of technique must include the level of familiarity and comfort of the operator, since the learning of new approaches is always associated with increased time. All of these considerations should be included when modifying the approach to performing regional anesthesia in the outpatient setting.

Recovery and Discharge

Before discharge, the patient must meet standard discharge criteria for alertness and hemodynamic stability. This does not imply full recovery of a peripheral nerve blockade, since one of the advantages is the potential for discharge with effective residual analgesia. Multiple studies have confirmed the safety of discharging patients with anesthetized extremities (16). Careful instruction must be given in order to avoid injury. In addition, patients must be provided with an appropriate sling for the arm or crutches for the leg, or other protection for the numb extremity or anesthetized area. The usual outpatient precautions about an adult accompaniment home and for the first 24 hours also apply, and are even more essential for the patient with an immobile extremity.

Patients who have received epidural or spinal block must have full recovery of motor function before discharge. If all sensory anesthesia has regressed, particularly with a full return of perineal sensation, then sympathetic blockade and orthostatic hypotension should not be a problem on ambulation. Urinary retention is not a frequent problem with short-acting neuraxial techniques (17), but can occur in older males and in patients who have had operations with groin or perineal incisions. It is most frequently related to overdistention of the bladder during the period of sensory loss. If this overdistention goes beyond the usual cystometric capacity of the bladder, return of function is delayed. This most frequently happens with longer-acting spinal anesthetics such as bupivacaine or higher doses of lidocaine associated with the use of epinephrine. With low doses of lidocaine, very low doses of bupivacaine (5–6 mg), or the use of chloroprocaine, the frequency is similar to that associated with general anesthesia in the outpatient setting. If there is any uncertainty, the bladder volume can be assessed by physical examination or ultrasound, and simple catheter drainage performed if distention is present. Following this (or if no distention is present), most patients can be discharged home with instructions to return to the emergency room should problems develop later.

A delayed complication of spinal anesthesia is the potential for postdural puncture headache. This has occurred as often as 10% in previous reports, but has been significantly reduced by the use of smaller-gauge rounded-bevel needles in the last 15 years. The current literature suggests that the incidence is not greater than 2% in the outpatient setting, and may be considerably lower in patients over 40 years of age. One of the problems is that the symptoms do not usually occur until a day or so following discharge, and thus they may necessitate more complex management in the outpatient setting. Patients should all be advised of the potential symptoms of postdural puncture headache and be given clear instructions for follow-up contacts if these symptoms arise. The diagnosis and treatment are discussed elsewhere in this text, and are generally the same in the outpatient as for the inpatient. It is more problematic to require the outpatient to return to the hospital for therapy, and thus conservative measures are more frequently pursued for a longer period of time. The risk of this complication must be weighed against the definite advantages of the speed of onset of spinal anesthesia, which makes it the most competitive regional anesthetic technique for use in an outpatient environment.

Postoperative and postdischarge analgesia are a challenge in the outpatient. Prolonged regional blockade is ideal, but most patients will also require some supplemental systemic analgesia. To avoid the side effects of opioids, a multimodal postoperative analgesia regimen should be planned for when the regional block resolves. Simple steps such as elevation, immobilization, and cold therapy are appropriate. Nonopioid analgesics should be the first addition. Acetaminophen is underutilized in the United States, but can provide an effective base of analgesia that reduces the need for opioid treatments. Nonsteroidal analgesics are also very effective, and often can be administered preoperatively to provide a preemptive reduction of analgesic needs (18). Intraoperative use of ketorolac has been shown to reduce narcotic requirements without producing nausea or respiratory depression. It is particularly effective in orthopedic and gynecologic procedures, although contraindicated in the presence of significant coagulopathy or renal disease. Doses of 30 mg IV (15 mg in elderly patients) are useful. The use of local infiltration with local anesthetics is another excellent alternative, especially effective in pediatric patients. Instillation of bupivacaine into knee joints following arthroscopy will also reduce narcotic requirements (19).

The most recent addition to the armamentarium of the outpatient anesthesiologist is the use of indwelling peripheral nerve catheters for home infusions after discharge (20). This technique requires more time for insertion, but fortunately is facilitated by the development of new needle/catheter combination sets and the use of stimulating catheters to ensure better localization. Ultrasound had also aided in nerve localization and catheter placement for these techniques. Multiple types of pumps are now available allowing flexibility in dose, patient control, and duration of therapy, and they are generally reliable in delivering the programmed doses (21). Securing the catheters has been a challenge in some locations (especially the neck), but the process of tunneling the catheter and using an occlusive dressing and adhesive has improved the success. Careful patient instruction and close follow-up are required, usually necessitating anesthesiologist availability 24 hours a day by phone. Concern about the potential of local anesthetic toxicity appears to be minimal when dilute concentrations of 0.2% ropivacaine or 0.125% bupivacaine are used. Removal of the catheters can be performed on follow-up visits to the surgeon's office or outpatient center, but most patients are able to remove the catheters safely at home. Arrangements need to be made for recovery of the reusable pumps, or clear instructions about disposal of the disposable model pumps. Despite the added work required for this therapy, extensive experience has shown the reliability and relative safety of these techniques (22). Multiple studies have shown significant advantages in prolonged analgesia, particularly for the more painful orthopedic procedures of the upper and lower extremity, and greatly enhanced patient satisfaction (23).

SPECIFIC PROCEDURES AND TECHNIQUES

The specific details for performing the various nerve blocks are found in other chapters in this text and should be referred to by individuals unfamiliar with a certain technique. This chapter focuses primarily on those surgical procedures commonly performed on an outpatient basis that are appropriate for regional techniques, and comments on the modifications of technique,

drug selection, and recovery aspects that are significant to the outpatient anesthesiologist.

Of the techniques suitable for outpatient application, *local infiltration* of the operative site is the safest and simplest. Intracutaneous and subcutaneous infiltration with a suitable dilute concentration of an intermediate-acting local anesthetic drug is sufficient for removal of superficial scars or lesions. An expansion of this technique is the "field block" by subcutaneous infiltration that blocks minor nerves supplying a particular area. This is most commonly used for hernia blocks or penile blocks for circumcisions. These procedures are usually performed by the surgeon and provide significant postoperative analgesia as well as satisfactory operative anesthesia, if careful infiltration of both deep and superficial layers is performed. The addition of epinephrine to the local anesthetic solution can be helpful in obtaining hemostasis, as well as in reducing plasma levels of drug if a large volume or dose is required.

Head and Neck

Eye Surgery

Retrobulbar or *peribulbar block* for cataract surgery is the ideal example of a peripheral nerve block that provides excellent surgical anesthesia, good postoperative pain relief, and rapid discharge from the hospital (see Chapter 19). In most institutions, these blocks are performed by surgeons, but anesthesiologists can perform them in an adjacent room and reduce turnover time in busy outpatient units. Although sedation often is needed for placement of the block, it is usually not needed intraoperatively, and these patients can leave the operating room in a wheelchair for the second-stage recovery unit and early discharge.

Many other head and neck procedures are relatively superficial, especially removal of skin lesions and cosmetic procedures, and are readily amenable to local infiltration. The two major risks of such procedures are the rapid absorption of local anesthetic from the highly vascular tissues of the face, and the potential for loss of airway related to heavy IV sedation during these procedures.

Upper Extremity

Upper extremity surgery is frequently performed in the outpatient setting. Regional anesthetic techniques are especially suitable for outpatient upper extremity surgery because they have relatively rapid onset and do not limit ambulation at the time of discharge. Many of these blocks can be performed with a single-injection technique, and the nerves are relatively superficial, making it an easy application of regional technique for outpatients.

Surgery to the Forearm and Hand

Hand surgery is a commonly performed outpatient procedure. *Intravenous regional* anesthesia suffices for simple, short operations of the hand (Chapter 15). This is especially true if the surgeon is planning on using a tourniquet to ensure hemostasis. The major hazard of this technique is the accidental or premature release of the tourniquet, or inadequate tourniquet pressure, with resulting excessive blood levels of the local anesthetic drug. Close monitoring is essential, and two-stage release of the tourniquet is suggested if tourniquet time is less than 40 minutes. The use of a wide blood pressure cuff as well as slow injection of the local anesthetic in a peripheral vein, following full exsanguination of the arm, has been shown to reduce the potential for leakage of local anesthetic under the cuff. The technique is relatively simple, although it requires placement of two IV catheters (one for the injection of the drug in the affected limb). Both lidocaine and bupivacaine provide excellent analgesia and anesthesia for hand surgery. Although some analgesia with bupivacaine persists after tourniquet release, it is relatively short-lived and of little clinical significance. Although the use of the double-tourniquet technique has been advocated to allow prolonged tolerance of the tourniquet, in reality this anesthesia technique is generally limited to procedures of less than 45 minutes in duration because of patient discomfort from the tourniquet itself. Fortunately, this includes most outpatient hand surgeries. Although the IV regional technique offers considerable advantages in the rapid return of sensation and function of the arm, the converse is also true—no residual analgesia remains. Nevertheless, it is an extremely useful technique for short, superficial operations such as carpal tunnel release and ganglion excisions. It requires less time than brachial plexus blockade and allows rapid return of arm function, which facilitates rapid discharge (9) and is less expensive than general anesthesia (24).

For lengthy and extensive surgical procedures of the hand and forearm, a deeper and more prolonged blockade of the terminal nerves is more useful (Chapter 15). The *axillary approach* is most commonly preferred because it is easily performed and associated with a lower incidence of complications (specifically pneumothorax) than the other brachial plexus anesthetic techniques. If anesthesia of the hand alone is required, simple blockade of the three terminal nerves surrounding the axillary artery (median, ulnar, radial) is usually sufficient. If surgery will include areas of the forearm or upper arm, or the use of an occlusive tourniquet, then blockade of the supplemental branches of the plexus (musculocutaneous, medial brachial cutaneous, and medial antebrachial cutaneous) is also required. Blockade of all of these branches provides anesthesia for forearm operations such as open reduction and fixation of simple fractures or the creation or revision of arterial venous fistulas. Complete axillary blockade is adequate for elbow surgery. All standard methods of axillary blockade can provide adequate anesthesia (paresthesia, nerve stimulator, ultrasound, transarterial), but the use of the selective mid-humeral approach can allow selective blockade, with the potential for differential motor and sensory blockade of various branches to permit optimal analgesia combined with early return of motor function (25). For most outpatient procedures, the use of an intermediate-duration amino amide, such as lidocaine or mepivacaine, is adequate and allows return of function of the arm within 6 to 8 hours, allowing discharge home. For more painful procedures, the use of the longer-acting amino amides, such as ropivacaine or bupivacaine, may provide 12 to 14 hours or longer of analgesia. With any of these drugs, a protective sling must be provided to the patient to avoid injury to the numb extremity following discharge.

Multiple reports have demonstrated the safety and efficacy of this technique (26,27), with less pain and nausea in the PACU, lower opioid consumption, more frequent phase 1 PACU bypass, and earlier discharge compared to general anesthesia (28). The peripheral nerve block, however, requires longer time for onset of analgesia, ranging from 7 to 20 minutes, depending on the nerve involved and the local anesthetic used (9,27), and the efficiency of this block in an outpatient unit is enhanced by the use of a separate room for block performance (11). Despite the time required, this technique provides superior postoperative analgesia and potential for discharge compared to general anesthesia, although the advantage of analgesia does not persist beyond the first 24 hours (28).

Another alternative for forearm and upper arm anesthesia is anesthesia of the plexus at the level of the cords by use of the *supraclavicular, infraclavicular,* or *subclavian perivascular* technique at the shoulder. Anesthesia of the cords at this level has the advantage of providing dense anesthesia with only two or three injections, rather than the four or five that are required for adequate axillary anesthesia. The disadvantage of these more proximal blocks is that the nerves lie deeper at this level (particularly the infraclavicular), and there may be more discomfort associated with the insertion of the needle, especially as it passes through the pectoralis muscles. Nevertheless, these more proximal blocks can be performed fairly quickly, and they give dense, prolonged anesthesia and analgesia for the entire upper arm, forearm, and hand, so that patients may perceive less discomfort than with the multiple injections required for axillary blockade (29). In comparing the outcome of infraclavicular blocks to general anesthesia, Hadzic has shown less pain in the PACU, more frequent bypass, less analgesic use, earlier ambulation, and faster discharge with infraclavicular anesthesia for hand surgery (30). Ilfeld prolonged these advantages with a continuous infraclavicular catheter home infusion in 30 patients, and found decreased pain, sleep disturbances, narcotic use, and related side effects, and improved overall satisfaction (31).

Arthroscopic Shoulder Surgery

Arthroscopic shoulder surgery is one of the more commonly performed upper extremity surgeries in the outpatient setting. *Interscalene brachial plexus* blockade, with its inherently associated cervical plexus blockade, offers ideal anesthesia for shoulder procedures. Interscalene anesthesia has the advantage of being a single-injection technique, and is thus simple and rapid to perform. Interscalene blockade by itself is sufficient for many of the procedures performed on the shoulder, such as distal clavicle resection, subacromial decompression, and even rotator cuff repair. Insertion of posterior shoulder cannula ports can sometimes be uncomfortable for the patient and may need to be treated with supplemental injections of fentanyl or local anesthesia at the sites. Again, the use of intermediate-duration amino amides provides excellent anesthesia for most of the surgical procedures, as well as 4 to 6 hours of analgesia postoperatively. If longer analgesia is sought with the long-acting amino amides, often a corresponding delay in onset of blockade occurs. For prolonged analgesia, insertion of a continuous catheter is ideal, but again may require more preparation time. Interscalene catheters are especially prone to migration with neck movement, and tunneling and secure dressing is useful. In these situations, an induction room is especially useful (11). Although the interscalene block can be relied on for most surgeries, many practitioners (depending upon the specific traditions of their own operating room) may choose to provide additional supplemental analgesia with a propofol infusion and a laryngeal mask airway to ensure adequate ventilation in a patient who is frequently positioned and draped in a way that makes it difficult for the anesthesiologist to maintain contact with the airway intraoperatively. The use of this technique can also avoid the delay needed for onset of total anesthesia with the regional block, but allow a low dose of propofol and a fully alert and comfortable patient on arrival in PACU. If general anesthesia alone is used, the addition of a suprascapular nerve block at the end of the procedure will add significant analgesia, allowing earlier discharge (32), but this is not useful if an interscalene has been performed (33).

Several investigators have shown significant advantages to the use of the interscalene technique for shoulder surgery, especially in providing early postoperative analgesia, freedom of nausea, increased PACU phase 1 bypass, and reduced overnight admission rates (13,34–37). Several investigators report decreased operating room times when their blocks were performed in an induction area (12,13,36). Most authors have used higher concentrations of long-acting amino amides, such as 0.5% bupivacaine or 0.5% or 0.75% ropivacaine to provide prolonged duration, but lower concentrations can produce less motor blockade, which might be more acceptable to patients (34,35). Unfortunately, with all of these regimens, the duration of analgesia is limited to 12 to 18 hours, and the benefits do not persist long after discharge (38).

This shortcoming can be overcome with continuous infusions. Several reports confirm significant prolonged reductions in postoperative pain (Fig. 26-1), less oral analgesic use, better sleep patterns, and greater patient satisfaction when continuous catheter techniques are used with this block, allowing up to 72 hours of analgesia (39–42). If an interscalene catheter is not used, some advantage is obtained with catheter infiltration of the wound in the subacromial region, but interscalene block is superior (39).

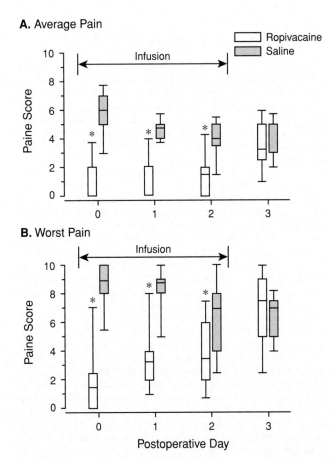

FIGURE 26-1. Pain scores at home with continuous interscalene infusion of ropivacaine. From Ilfeld BM, Morey TE, Wright TW, et al. Continuous interscalene brachial plexus block for postoperative pain control at home: A randomized, double-blinded, placebo-controlled study. *Anesth Analg* 2003;96:1089–1095, with permission.

Trunk and Perineum

Breast Surgery

Breast surgery, excisional biopsies, and even simple mastectomies are often performed on an outpatient basis. Local or general anesthesia is often sufficient, but these can be done with a regional technique, such as a high thoracic epidural or paravertebral blocks, to provide adequate sensory anesthesia. Paravertebral anesthesia requires injection at multiple levels, and a moderate amount of onset time for adequate analgesia. It has been used successfully in the outpatient setting, with prolonged analgesia after discharge and less nausea than with general anesthesia alone (43). There are risks of block failure, epidural spread, and intrapleural injection with this technique (44), and its use may be best restricted to higher-risk patients or situations in which a continuous catheter for prolonged analgesia is desired (45).

Laparoscopy

Laparoscopic procedures for gynecologic diagnosis or therapy are frequent in the outpatient setting. Generally, the prolonged abdominal distension with carbon dioxide makes this procedure uncomfortable for the patient without a general anesthetic, but short procedures with minimal distension are amenable to regional anesthesia. Vaghadia and colleagues have reported the successful use of low-dose hypobaric spinal anesthesia, using 25 mg of lidocaine with 25 μg fentanyl, for laparoscopy with rapid recovery (46). They found discharge and costs were not different from general anesthesia, and that 90% of patients would choose this technique again (24). This may be an acceptable technique if general anesthesia needs to be avoided for specific patient medical or personal reasons.

Extracorporeal Shock Wave Lithotripsy

Extracorporeal shock wave lithotripsy (ESWL) on an outpatient basis can be performed with regional techniques. Although many newer lithotripsy machines employ lower shock energy levels and thus require only sedation and mild analgesia, the older high-energy procedures are painful and merit intervention. Epidural anesthesia with 2-chloroprocaine provides adequate surgical conditions with a competitive discharge in less than 2 hours (47), but the use of longer-duration local anesthetics produces discharge times that are longer than with general anesthesia (Fig. 26-2) (48). Chloroprocaine has had a clouded past because of toxicity associated with previous preservative-containing preparations, but the most common concern with epidural use of the current preparations is postblock back pain. This syndrome presents immediately upon resolution of the blockade and may be related to muscle irritation from the local anesthetic rather than a preservative. It appears to be volume-related, especially with volumes of 40 mL or more (49). Although the back pain responds easily to small doses of opioids, it is best avoided by reserving chloroprocaine for shorter procedures in which reinjection is not needed, or by limiting chloroprocaine use as a "top-up" anesthetic after initial dosing with lidocaine.

Experience with *anorectal surgery* shows a similar pattern of prolonged discharge with longer-acting anesthetics for spinal blockade. One advantage of spinal block is that it can be performed in the operative (jackknife) position if sterile water is added to dilute the local anesthetic to a hypobaric solution. Subarachnoid anesthesia with small doses of hypobaric lidocaine provides good analgesia and the avoidance of

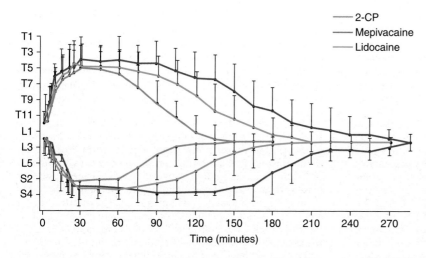

FIGURE 26-2. Duration of epidural anesthesia with chloroprocaine, lidocaine, and mepivacaine, 20 mL volumes with epinephrine added. From Kopacz DJ, Mulroy MF. Chloroprocaine and lidocaine decrease hospital stay and admission rate after outpatient epidural anesthesia. *Reg Anesth* 1990;15:30, with permission.

airway manipulation in the prone position, but requires 2 hours for resolution of blockade (50,51). This can be acceptable in the outpatient setting, but when compared to local anesthesia (52), or when longer-duration bupivacaine is used (53), the discharge times, urinary retention, and PACU costs favor the local infiltration techniques. Chloroprocaine has a potential to provide a shorter-duration hypobaric anesthetic in this situation, but, to date, the drug has not been studied for this application.

Herniorrhaphy

Hernia repair includes inguinal, femoral, umbilical, or incisional herniorrhaphies. Inguinal hernia repair is another excellent opportunity for the use of several regional techniques. *Neuraxial block*, especially spinal anesthesia, is the simplest to perform. Lidocaine spinal anesthesia provides good muscle relaxation and exposure, but with a discharge time slightly longer than general anesthesia (54). The use of longer-acting drugs, such as bupivacaine, is associated with greater variability of block and duration (55), longer discharge, and a higher frequency of urinary retention (56), and may not be competitive in the outpatient setting with local infiltration or general anesthesia (57,58). The evident dilemma is that the use of the higher doses of drug needed for the higher level of anesthesia may also be associated with delayed voiding (17). Thus, the choice of spinal anesthetic for outpatient hernia repair is a challenging one. Epidural anesthesia may offer an acceptable alternative, in which short-acting drugs may be used with a continuous technique, but the longer performance and onset time of epidural blocks limits their use.

Paravertebral blockade has been utilized because it is not associated with urinary retention and does not require resolution before discharge. Compared to general anesthesia, Hadzic found that the paravertebral block took longer to perform, but provided superior analgesia in the PACU, earlier ambulation, and faster discharge (59). Despite the longer time, the potential for failed block, and the potential for epidural spread (60), this technique may have a role in outpatient hernia repair.

Many studies of hernia repair illustrate the advantages of local infiltration for postoperative analgesia in what is otherwise an uncomfortable operation (61). Preincisional blockade of the ilioinguinal and iliohypogastric nerve provides significant pain reduction in the immediate postoperative period (62) and can allow for performance of this procedure under local anesthesia with sedation. This relief is short-lived (58), and the addition of

a multimodal approach, including nonsteroidal analgesics, can reduce narcotic consumption in the first 24 hours after surgery (63).

Lower Extremity

Knee Arthroscopy

Knee arthroscopy is one of the most frequently performed outpatient surgical procedures. It is ideally suited for many forms of regional anesthesia (64). The simplest approach used by many surgeons facile with the procedure, who perform it rapidly, is local infiltration of the arthroscopic portal points complemented by light IV sedation by the anesthesia team. This local sedation is effective for many patients, but not satisfactory for all. In a prospective comparison of local to other modalities, 12% of the patients would have preferred another technique, and 16% of the surgeons found the operating conditions inadequate (65). This may be related to the lack of muscle relaxation around the joint that makes manipulation of the knee difficult under these circumstances. Thus, this technique may be helpful for some patients, but cannot be assumed to be effective and appropriate for all patients coming for knee arthroscopy. It certainly provides rapid discharge (if deep sedation is avoided) because of the intrinsic analgesia associated with this technique.

Virtually all other regional approaches to lower extremity anesthesia have been employed for knee arthroscopy, including psoas compartment block, femoral nerve block, sciatic-femoral block, epidural anesthesia, and spinal anesthesia. Of these, *spinal anesthesia* is the simplest to perform, most rapid in onset, and provides the densest anesthesia. The onset time is competitive with general anesthesia in most situations. The residual analgesia allows for more rapid early recovery, with a high degree of alertness and freedom from nausea (66). The challenge of spinal anesthesia is the selection of the appropriate drug to provide a competitive discharge (67) and to avoid the syndrome of transient neurologic symptoms (TNS). This syndrome usually presents as back pain radiating into the groin or legs, beginning 6 to 24 hours following the resolution of spinal anesthesia and persisting for 3 to 5 days (68). The degree of discomfort is variable, but may be sufficient to preclude return to normal daily activities or to work. There is no simple treatment of the phenomenon, although nonsteroidal anti-inflammatory drugs (NSAIDs) appear to be of some benefit. The phenomenon has been reported with all of the local anesthetics, but most frequently with intrathecal lidocaine. The incidence of the syndrome is generally around 15% with lidocaine, but increases to as high as 30% when knee arthroscopy and lithotomy-position operations are performed using this drug. Many anesthesiologists have abandoned the use of lidocaine for arthroscopy for this reason. Low-dose bupivacaine (5 mg plus fentanyl) has been suggested as an alternative. Ben-David and his colleagues found that a 5-mg dose of plain bupivacaine was inadequate (69), but the addition of fentanyl provided adequate anesthesia for their patients (70). Although the discharge times were acceptable (3 hours from time of injection), the variability of bupivacaine is wide and may result in delayed discharge in some patients. Ben-David and his group have also looked at very-low-dose lidocaine as an alternative to the standard 50-mg lidocaine spinal anesthetic. They reported that 20 mg of lidocaine plus 25 μg of fentanyl produces adequate anesthesia with lower TNS frequency (71). Other investigators have found that a 25-mg dose of lidocaine plus fentanyl does not always produce adequate anesthesia (12% failure rate) and is not associated with a significantly lower risk of TNS (72). Procaine and mepivacaine remain alternatives for knee arthroscopy. Mepivacaine may not have a significantly lower incidence of TNS, and procaine may be associated with more unpleasant side effects when used as a spinal anesthetic (73). The use of 2-chloroprocaine for spinal anesthesia has been reinvestigated lately. Kopacz and colleagues reported that doses of 40 to 50 mg produced adequate spinal anesthesia of approximately 1 hour's duration, with resolution in approximately 2 hours (74) (Fig. 26-3). Casati and colleagues confirmed these volunteer findings in a series of 45 patients undergoing outpatient knee arthroscopy and found no TNS in this small group (75). Further investigation of this is warranted. There remain questions about the history of neurotoxicity with chloroprocaine that also need to be resolved before it can be recommended as a subarachnoid agent (76,77). Nevertheless, spinal anesthesia remains the most reliable and time-effective alternative for regional techniques for outpatient knee arthroscopy, and preservative-free 2-chloroprocaine may be identified as the ideal drug.

Unilateral spinal blockade has been advocated as a technique to reduce the total dosage and duration of spinal anesthesia for arthroscopy. This is usually achieved by placing the patient in a lateral position and injecting a small dose of hyperbaric local anesthetic. If the lateral position is maintained for 10 to 15 minutes, the *majority* of anesthesia is produced in the dependent extremity (78–81). Some spillover inevitably

occurs into the opposite leg, but the blockade there is of short duration. This technique is useful in trying to provide targeted anesthesia of only the involved extremity, but it cannot be relied upon to exclusively anesthetize one side.

A second alternative is the use of *lumbar epidural* anesthesia, which provides an appropriate band of analgesia and anesthesia at the dermatomes needed for the surgical procedure. Again, 2-chloroprocaine is an ideal choice for this procedure because of its rapid onset and predictable 1-hour duration. The block resolves within 2 hours (Fig. 26-2), and thus allows for a discharge time that is competitive with propofol general anesthesia for the same procedure (67,82). The resolution of a 2-chloroprocaine epidural is equivalent to spinal anesthesia with chloroprocaine and is somewhat faster than spinal anesthesia with procaine, lidocaine, or bupivacaine. The disadvantage of epidural injection is the slower onset compared to spinal block, but this can be overcome by the use of an induction area, or by the use of the combined spinal-epidural technique (83). Urmey and colleagues have used this procedure to provide rapid onset, but with the added benefit of the potential for prolonged duration if the procedure becomes prolonged. With both of these neuraxial techniques, patients can generally tolerate the procedure with minimal sedation and thus observe the arthroscopy on the monitor screen and see the anatomy of their own surgical procedure.

With both the neuraxial techniques, block resolution must occur before discharge. One issue is the potential for urinary retention, but, as discussed, this is infrequent with short-acting blocks. More important is the need for postoperative analgesia. In these situations, local infiltration of the wound portals is helpful in reducing postoperative pain. There is also some evidence that installation of bupivacaine and morphine into the knee joint may produce analgesia for several hours or as long as 24 hours following knee arthroscopy. As with the hernia operations, multimodal systemic analgesia is also appropriate, and the use of NSAIDs is especially helpful (18).

Peripheral nerve blockade is also useful for knee arthroscopy. *Psoas compartment block* has been described as an effective single-shot injection for knee surgery (84). The single injection in the back at the lower lumbar level provides blockade of the femoral, lateral femoral cutaneous, and usually the obturator nerves, thus allowing analgesia of the entire anterior medial and lateral portions of the knee joint where the trocar insertion sites are placed. The disadvantage of the psoas block is the somewhat slower onset than spinal anesthesia, but it can certainly be competitive with epidural anesthesia in terms of its onset. It also provides a unilateral block, which may facilitate discharge. Jankowski and colleagues found it provided discharge equivalent to spinal or general anesthesia, with less pain and lower analgesic requirements in PACU (84). As with other nerve block techniques, patients need to be cautioned about the potential for residual blockade of the femoral nerve and the associated quadriceps weakness. If crutches are used to provide discharge ambulation, a prolonged blockade (such as with mepivacaine or even bupivacaine) can provide prolonged analgesia for patients while still providing ambulation.

Femoral nerve block at the inguinal level can be used for the procedure. This is simpler to perform than a psoas compartment block and can be instituted rapidly. Injection of the femoral nerve sheath generally provides reliable blockade of the lateral femoral cutaneous nerve, thus creating sensory analgesia of the anterior portions of the leg where the trocar insertions are usually performed. The muscle relaxation around the knee joint is not as profound as with neuraxial blockade, but the procedure can generally be tolerated with supplemental IV sedation. If total anesthesia for the procedure is desired, a combined

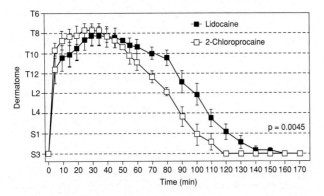

FIGURE 26-3. Extent and duration of subarachnoid anesthesia with 40 mg lidocaine or 2-chloroprocaine in volunteers. From Kouri ME, Kopacz DJ. Spinal 2-chloroprocaine: A comparison with lidocaine in volunteers. *Anesth Analg* 2004;98:75–80.

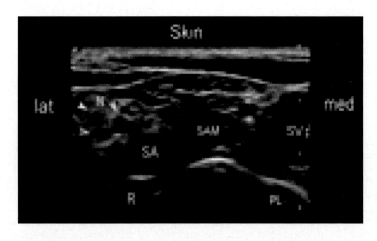

FIGURE 26-4. Pain scores after anterior cruciate ligament repair with placebo, single-shot femoral nerve block, or continuous infusion with levobupivacaine. From Williams BA, Kentor ML, Vogt MT, et al. Reduction of verbal pain scores after anterior cruciate ligament reconstruction with 2-day continuous femoral nerve block: A randomized clinical trial. *Anesthesiology* 2006;104:315–327, with permission.

sciatic and femoral nerve block is more effective (85–88). In experienced hands, the time to surgical readiness is equivalent to spinal anesthesia (87). This technique provides faster recovery than general anesthesia, and can provide faster discharge if a short-acting local anesthetic such as 2-chloroprocaine is used for the blocks (88).

With all of the regional techniques possible for the knee, postoperative analgesia and ambulation must be considered. For routine arthroscopy and meniscectomy, postoperative discomfort is minimal, and can usually be managed with local infiltration of the wound sites and mild systemic analgesics, including NSAIDs, after the neuraxial block or short-acting peripheral block dissipates. With the unilateral peripheral nerve blocks, prolonged analgesia for the more painful procedures of the lower leg, such as anterior cruciate ligament repair with a patellar tendon autograft, can be provided by a longer-acting local anesthetic. A single bupivacaine injection can provide 18 to 24 hours of comfort (89), with decreased pain and analgesic use in the PACU. This technique reduces postoperative pain sufficiently to significantly reduce the chance of overnight admission, potentially by a factor of 10 (90), and to reduce hospital costs dramatically (91). For more complex surgeries, the use of a combined femoral and sciatic block provides additional analgesia (92,93) and also reduces the chance of overnight admission. Discharge with a numb thigh limits ambulation, but can be overcome by the use of crutches and careful patient instruction.

Pain relief can be extended even further by the insertion of a *continuous femoral nerve catheter* (94–96). Williams and colleagues demonstrated that a single-injection femoral nerve block is superior to multimodal systemic analgesia alone, but that continuation of the local anesthetic by a continuous infusion of levobupivacaine provided lower visual analog scale (VAS) scores and lower opioid consumption for 48 hours after surgery (Fig. 26-4) and with continued less analgesic requirements for 7 days after surgery and with a higher degree of patient satisfaction.

Surgery to the Foot and Ankle

Most surgical procedures to the foot and ankle are also performed on an outpatient basis. They vary in intensity and duration from simple bunionectomies to much more complex repairs of the ligaments and bones of the anterior and posterior foot. Many of the less painful procedures can be performed with a simple local anesthetic injection by the surgeon. The more complex operations are amenable to an ankle or popliteal fossa block, particularly if a tourniquet is not to be used (or if

a low calf tourniquet can be employed). For a full ankle block, five separate injections of five nerves are required, and the onset time is somewhat slow. This technique would be ideally performed in a holding area or before the positioning, preparation, and draping in the operating room, to allow adequate time for onset. Anesthesia with bupivacaine will provide up to 12 hours of postoperative pain relief and is useful in allowing patients to go home pain free.

If longer analgesia is required, or for the more extensive and painful operations, more proximal blockade of the nerves can be used. This can most easily be accomplished by a popliteal fossa blockade of the two branches of the sciatic nerve, which must be supplemented by a block of the saphenous branch of the femoral nerve at the level of the tibial head. Popliteal fossa block can be performed either in the traditional posterior approach or in the supine position via a lateral approach between the heads of the biceps femoris and the vastus lateralis. This block is useful for operations performed with the use of a calf tourniquet and when longer analgesia is required, and can be sufficient as the sole anesthetic for the surgery (97). Again, as with the ankle block, the onset is relatively slow, and the block should be placed in a separate area as early as possible before the intended incision.

This approach is also amenable to the use of *continuous catheters*, which can provide superb pain relief for several days after surgery (97,98). White has shown better immediate pain control after extensive foot surgery, facilitating earlier discharge home and lower overnight admission rates (99). Ilfeld and Borgeat have confirmed better analgesia, lower opioid consumption, and better sleep patterns at home with 72 hour continuous popliteal infusions (100,101), Capdevila further evaluated whether this improved analgesia could enhance recovery. Compared to a control group receiving IV morphine, the continuous catheter patients after foot surgery had a faster attainment of minimal activity and return to daily function (102).

For much longer and more complex operations in which a thigh tourniquet is to be used by the surgeon, more central blockade is appropriate, usually through a subarachnoid injection. Although combined blockade of the sciatic and lumbar plexus at the level of the hip could provide adequate analgesia, it would also interfere significantly with ambulation and discharge. The use of a spinal anesthetic combined with more distal block (either popliteal fossa or ankle block) is ideal in this situation for providing adequate surgical anesthesia and excellent residual analgesia to facilitate discharge home. If a spinal anesthetic is used, a unilateral technique can be employed, as described earlier.

As with hand surgery, if regional anesthesia is used on the foot, especially a continuous technique, a generously padded dressing must be placed and specific instructions given to the patient to avoid injury to the extremity while it is still insensate.

Pediatric Regional Techniques

Regional techniques can also be applied to pediatric patients in the outpatient setting to provide the advantages of postoperative analgesia and rapid discharge, as in the adult (see also Chapter 27). The primary applications in this age group for outpatient surgery are aimed at providing pain relief in the healthy child being discharged home the same day. Several techniques have been described. The simplest application is local infiltration, as it is with adults. An alternative for a child is simply to irrigate the wound with local anesthetic; this appears to have efficacy equal to injection techniques for hernia surgery (103).

Ilioinguinal nerve block is simple and useful after hernia repair or scrotal procedures. A 25-gauge needle is introduced into the abdominal wall 1 cm above and medial to the anterior superior iliac spine and a volume of local anesthetic is injected in a fan-wise direction to block the ilioinguinal nerve fibers traveling between the transverse and internal oblique abdominal muscles and the iliohypogastric fibers running superficially to the muscles. A dose of 2 mg/kg of 0.25% to 0.5% bupivacaine is effective (104).

Caudal block is also useful for children. The sacral hiatus is much more easily appreciated in children than in adults, and the cornua on either side can be seen and easily palpated. This block is usually performed with the infant asleep, and it requires very little time in experienced hands (see Chapters 11 and 27).

Another alternative for penile operations is a *penile block*. Two techniques are advocated. The simplest is the subcutaneous ring block, injecting local anesthetic superficial to the fascia of the penile shaft at its base. Alternatively, 1 to 2 mL of local anesthetic can be injected deep to the fascia (Buck fascia) on either side of the dorsal midline. This will provide analgesia for procedures on the distal shaft, although the proximal shaft and the base of the penis are innervated by the genitofemoral and ilioinguinal nerves, which must be blocked by superficial infiltration. In either case, 0.25% bupivacaine provides excellent analgesia; epinephrine is never added to solutions in this area (see Chapter 27).

SUMMARY

At present, about 65% of the surgical procedures in the United States either are being performed or could be performed on an outpatient basis. The principles of anesthetic management for outpatients are the same as those for inpatients, but the added advantages of prolonged analgesia and reduced side effects make neural blockade an excellent anesthetic choice. The customary modifications that have been made for anesthetic management of the outpatient under neural blockade include (a) the selection of patients, surgeons, and anesthetists qualified and motivated toward nerve block anesthesia; (b) written preoperative instructions and information to all patients, because of the short period available for evaluation and rapport; (c) little or no preanesthetic medication; (d) use of regional block anesthetic techniques wherever possible, including infiltration of the wound with a long-acting local anesthetic drug to decrease the need for postoperative narcotics; (e) written postoperative instructions and a method for telephone or return follow-up on discharge; and (f) no limitation as to the ASA physical status of the patients or the techniques of anesthesia. If these considerations are followed, the use of neural blockade in outpatients will be a most satisfying experience.

References

1. Pavlin DJ, Chen C, Penaloza DA, et al. Pain as a factor complicating recovery and discharge after ambulatory surgery. *Anesth Analg* 2002;95:627–634.
2. Fortier J, Chung F, Su J. Unanticipated admission after ambulatory surgery: A prospective study. *Can J Anaesth* 1998;45:612–619.
3. Gold BS, Kitz DS, Lecky JH, Neuhaus JM. Unanticipated admission to the hospital following ambulatory surgery. *JAMA* 1989;262:3008–3010.
4. Liu SS, Strodtbeck WM, Richman JM, Wu CL. A comparison of regional versus general anesthesia for ambulatory anesthesia: A meta-analysis of randomized controlled trials. *Anesth Analg* 2005;101:1634–1642.
5. Apfelbaum JL, Chen C, Mehta SS, Gan TJ. Postoperative pain experience: Results from a national survey suggest postoperative pain continues to be undermanaged. *Anesth Analg* 2003;97:534–540.
6. Carroll NV, Miederhoff P, Cox FM, Hirsch JD. Postoperative nausea and vomiting after discharge from outpatient surgery centers. *Anesth Analg* 1995;80:903–909.
7. Gross JB, Bachenberg KL, Benumof JL, et al. Practice guidelines for the perioperative management of patients with obstructive sleep apnea: A report by the American Society of Anesthesiologists Task Force on perioperative management of patients with obstructive sleep apnea. *Anesthesiology* 2006;104:1081–1093; quiz 117–118.
8. Nielsen KC, Guller U, Steele SM, et al. Influence of obesity on surgical regional anesthesia in the ambulatory setting: An analysis of 9,038 blocks. *Anesthesiology* 2005;102:181–187.
9. Chan VW, Peng PW, Kaszas Z, et al. A comparative study of general anesthesia, intravenous regional anesthesia, and axillary block for outpatient hand surgery: Clinical outcome and cost analysis. *Anesth Analg* 2001;93:1181–1184.
10. Capogna G, Celleno D, Laudano D, Giunta F. Alkalinization of local anesthetics. Which block, which local anesthetic? *Reg Anesth* 1995;20:369–377.
11. Armstrong KP, Cherry RA. Brachial plexus anesthesia compared to general anesthesia when a block room is available. *Can J Anaesth* 2004;51:41–44.
12. Brown AR, Weiss R, Greenberg C, et al. Interscalene block for shoulder arthroscopy: Comparison with general anesthesia. *Arthroscopy* 1993;9:295–300.
13. D'Alessio JG, Rosenblum M, Shea KP, Freitas DG. A retrospective comparison of interscalene block and general anesthesia for ambulatory surgery shoulder arthroscopy. *Reg Anesth* 1995;20:62–68.
14. Sites BD, Gallagher JD, Cravero J, et al. The learning curve associated with a simulated ultrasound-guided interventional task by inexperienced anesthesia residents. *Reg Anesth Pain Med* 2004;29:544–548.
15. Gray AT. Ultrasound-guided regional anesthesia: Current state of the art. *Anesthesiology* 2006;104:368–373, discussion 5A.
16. Klein SM, Nielsen KC, Greengrass RA, et al. Ambulatory discharge after long-acting peripheral nerve blockade: 2382 blocks with ropivacaine. *Anesth Analg* 2002;94:65–70.
17. Mulroy MF, Salinas FV, Larkin KL, Polissar NL. Ambulatory surgery patients may be discharged before voiding after short-acting spinal and epidural anesthesia. *Anesthesiology* 2002;97:315–319.
18. Reuben SS, Bhopatkar S, Maciolek H, et al. The preemptive analgesic effect of rofecoxib after ambulatory arthroscopic knee surgery. *Anesth Analg* 2002;94:55–59.
19. Reuben SS, Sklar J, El-Mansouri M. The preemptive analgesic effect of intraarticular bupivacaine and morphine after ambulatory arthroscopic knee surgery. *Anesth Analg* 2001;92:923–926.
20. Ilfeld BM, Enneking FK. Continuous peripheral nerve blocks at home: A review. *Anesth Analg* 2005;100:1822–1833.
21. Ilfeld BM, Morey TE, Enneking FK. Portable infusion pumps used for continuous regional analgesia: Delivery rate accuracy and consistency. *Reg Anesth Pain Med* 2003;28:424–432.
22. Swenson JD, Bay N, Loose E, et al. Outpatient management of continuous peripheral nerve catheters placed using ultrasound guidance: An experience in 620 patients. *Anesth Analg* 2006;103:1436–1443.

23. Ilfeld BM, Esener DE, Morey TE, Enneking FK. Ambulatory perineural infusion: The patients' perspective. *Reg Anesth Pain Med* 2003;28:418–423.

24. Chilvers CR, Kinahan A, Vaghadia H, Merrick PM. Pharmacoeconomics of intravenous regional anaesthesia vs general anaesthesia for outpatient hand surgery. *Can J Anaesth* 1997;44:1152–1156.

25. Bouaziz H, Narchi P, Mercier FJ, et al. The use of a selective axillary nerve block for outpatient hand surgery. *Anesth Analg* 1998;86:746–748.

26. Davis WJ, Lennon RL, Wedel DJ. Brachial plexus anesthesia for outpatient surgical procedures on an upper extremity. *Mayo Clin Proc* 1991;66:470–473.

27. Gaertner E, Kern O, Mahoudeau G, et al. Block of the brachial plexus branches by the humeral route. A prospective study in 503 ambulatory patients. Proposal of a nerve-blocking sequence. *Acta Anaesthesiol Scand* 1999;43:609–613.

28. McCartney CJ, Brull R, Chan VW, et al. Early but no long-term benefit of regional compared with general anesthesia for ambulatory hand surgery. *Anesthesiology* 2004;101:461–467.

29. Koscielniak-Nielsen ZJ, Rasmussen H, Hesselbjerg L, et al. Infraclavicular block causes less discomfort than axillary block in ambulatory patients. *Acta Anaesthesiol Scand* 2005;49:1030–1034.

30. Hadzic A, Arliss J, Kerimoglu B, et al. A comparison of infraclavicular nerve block versus general anesthesia for hand and wrist day-case surgeries. *Anesthesiology* 2004;101:127–132.

31. Ilfeld BM, Morey TE, Enneking FK. Continuous infraclavicular brachial plexus block for postoperative pain control at home: A randomized, double-blinded, placebo-controlled study. *Anesthesiology* 2002;96:1297–1304.

32. Ritchie ED, Tong D, Chung F, et al. Suprascapular nerve block for postoperative pain relief in arthroscopic shoulder surgery: A new modality? *Anesth Analg* 1997;84:1306–1312.

33. Neal JM, McDonald SB, Larkin KL, Polissar NL. Suprascapular nerve block prolongs analgesia after nonarthroscopic shoulder surgery but does not improve outcome. *Anesth Analg* 2003;96:982–986.

34. Krone SC, Chan VW, Regan J, et al. Analgesic effects of low-dose ropivacaine for interscalene brachial plexus block for outpatient shoulder surgery: A dose-finding study. *Reg Anesth Pain Med* 2001;26:439–443.

35. Al-Kaisy A, McGuire G, Chan VW, et al. Analgesic effect of interscalene block using low-dose bupivacaine for outpatient arthroscopic shoulder surgery. *Reg Anesth Pain Med* 1998;23:469–473.

36. Chelly JE, Greger J, Al Samsam T, et al. Reduction of operating and recovery room times and overnight hospital stays with interscalene blocks as sole anesthetic technique for rotator cuff surgery. *Minerva Anestesiol* 2001;67:613–619.

37. Hadzic A, Williams BA, Karaca PE, et al. For outpatient rotator cuff surgery, nerve block anesthesia provides superior same-day recovery over general anesthesia. *Anesthesiology* 2005;102:1001–1007.

38. Wurm WH, Concepcion M, Sternlicht A, et al. Preoperative interscalene block for elective shoulder surgery: Loss of benefit over early postoperative block after patient discharge to home. *Anesth Analg* 2003;97:1620–1626.

39. Delaunay L, Souron V, Lafosse L, et al. Analgesia after arthroscopic rotator cuff repair: Subacromial versus interscalene continuous infusion of ropivacaine. *Reg Anesth Pain Med* 2005;30:117–122.

40. Klein SM, Grant SA, Greengrass RA, et al. Interscalene brachial plexus block with a continuous catheter insertion system and a disposable infusion pump. *Anesth Analg* 2000;91:1473–1478.

41. Ilfeld BM, Morey TE, Wright TW, et al. Continuous interscalene brachial plexus block for postoperative pain control at home: A randomized, double-blinded, placebo-controlled study. *Anesth Analg* 2003;96:1089–1095.

42. Ilfeld BM, Morey TE, Wright TW, et al. Interscalene perineural ropivacaine infusion: A comparison of two dosing regimens for postoperative analgesia. *Reg Anesth Pain Med* 2004;29:9–16.

43. Klein SM, Bergh A, Steele SM, et al. Thoracic paravertebral block for breast surgery. *Anesth Analg* 2000;90:1402–1405.

44. Terheggen MA, Wille F, Borel Rinkes IH, et al. Paravertebral blockade for minor breast surgery. *Anesth Analg* 2002;94:355–359.

45. Buckenmaier CC 3rd, Klein SM, Nielsen KC, Steele SM. Continuous paravertebral catheter and outpatient infusion for breast surgery. *Anesth Analg* 2003;97:715–717.

46. Vaghadia H, McLeod DH, Mitchell GW, et al. Small-dose hypobaric lidocaine-fentanyl spinal anesthesia for short duration outpatient laparoscopy. I. A randomized comparison with conventional dose hyperbaric lidocaine. *Anesth Analg* 1997;84:59–64.

47. Kopacz DJ, Mulroy MF. Chloroprocaine and lidocaine decrease hospital stay and admission rate after outpatient epidural anesthesia. *Reg Anesth* 1990;15:19–25.

48. Richardson MG, Dooley JW. The effects of general versus epidural anesthesia for outpatient extracorporeal shock wave lithotripsy. *Anesth Analg* 1998;86:1214–1218.

49. Stevens RA, Urmey WF, Urquhart BL, Kao TC. Back pain after epidural anesthesia with chloroprocaine. *Anesthesiology* 1993;78:492–497.

50. Bodily MN, Carpenter RL, Owens BD. Lidocaine 0.5% spinal anaesthesia: A hypobaric solution for short-stay perirectal surgery. *Can J Anaesth* 1992;39:770–773.

51. Waxler B, Mondragon SA, Patel SN, Nedumgottil K. Intrathecal lidocaine and sufentanil shorten postoperative recovery after outpatient rectal surgery. *Can J Anaesth* 2004;51:680–684.

52. Li S, Coloma M, White PF, et al. Comparison of the costs and recovery profiles of three anesthetic techniques for ambulatory anorectal surgery. *Anesthesiology* 2000;93:1225–1230.

53. Sungurtekin H, Sungurtekin U, Erdem E. Local anesthesia and midazolam versus spinal anesthesia in ambulatory pilonidal surgery. *J Clin Anesth* 2003;15:201–205.

54. Burney RE, Prabhu MA, Greenfield ML, et al. Comparison of spinal vs general anesthesia via laryngeal mask airway in inguinal hernia repair. *Arch Surg* 2004;139:183–187.

55. Liu SS, Ware PD, Allen HW, et al. Dose-response characteristics of spinal bupivacaine in volunteers. Clinical implications for ambulatory anesthesia. *Anesthesiology* 1996;85:729–736.

56. Gupta A, Axelsson K, Thorn SE, et al. Low-dose bupivacaine plus fentanyl for spinal anesthesia during ambulatory inguinal herniorrhaphy: A comparison between 6 mg and 7.5 mg of bupivacaine. *Acta Anaesthesiol Scand* 2003;47:13–19.

57. Song D, Greilich NB, White PF, et al. Recovery profiles and costs of anesthesia for outpatient unilateral inguinal herniorrhaphy. *Anesth Analg* 2000;91:876–881.

58. Toivonen J, Permi J, Rosenberg PH. Analgesia and discharge following preincisional ilioinguinal and iliohypogastric nerve block combined with general or spinal anaesthesia for inguinal herniorrhaphy. *Acta Anaesthesiol Scand* 2004;48:480–485.

59. Hadzic A, Kerimoglu B, Loreio D, et al. Paravertebral blocks provide superior same-day recovery over general anesthesia for patients undergoing inguinal hernia repair. *Anesth Analg* 2006;102:1076–1081.

60. Klein SM, Greengrass RA, Weltz C, Warner DS. Paravertebral somatic nerve block for outpatient inguinal herniorrhaphy: An expanded case report of 22 patients. *Reg Anesth Pain Med* 1998;23:306–310.

61. Pavlin DJ, Pavlin EG, Horvath KD, et al. Perioperative rofecoxib plus local anesthetic field block diminishes pain and recovery time after outpatient inguinal hernia repair. *Anesth Analg* 2005;101:83–89.

62. Ding Y, White PF. Post-herniorrhaphy pain in outpatients after pre-incision ilioinguinal-hypogastric nerve block during monitored anaesthetic care. *Can J Anaesth* 1995;42:12–15.

63. Pavlin DJ, Horvath KD, Pavlin EG, Sima K. Preincisional treatment to prevent pain after ambulatory hernia surgery. *Anesth Analg* 2003;97:1627–1632.

64. Horlocker TT, Hebl JR. Anesthesia for outpatient knee arthroscopy: Is there an optimal technique? *Reg Anesth Pain Med* 2003;28:58–63.

65. Jacobson E, Forssblad M, Rosenberg J, et al. Can local anesthesia be recommended for routine use in elective knee arthroscopy? A comparison between local, spinal, and general anesthesia. *Arthroscopy* 2000;16:183–190.

66. Wong J, Marshall S, Chung F, et al. Spinal anesthesia improves the early recovery profile of patients undergoing ambulatory knee arthroscopy. *Can J Anaesth* 2001;48:369–374.

67. Mulroy MF, Larkin KL, Hodgson PS, et al. A comparison of spinal, epidural, and general anesthesia for outpatient knee arthroscopy. *Anesth Analg* 2000;91:860–864.

68. Pollock JE. Transient neurologic symptoms: Etiology, risk factors, and management. *Reg Anesth Pain Med* 2002;27:581–586.

69. Ben-David B, Levin H, Solomon E, et al. Spinal bupivacaine in ambulatory surgery: The effect of saline dilution. *Anesth Analg* 1996;83:716–720.

70. Ben-David B, Solomon E, Levin H, et al. Intrathecal fentanyl with small-dose dilute bupivacaine: Better anesthesia without prolonging recovery. *Anesth Analg* 1997;85:560–565.

71. Ben-David B, Maryanovsky M, Gurevitch A, et al. A comparison of minidose lidocaine-fentanyl and conventional-dose lidocaine spinal anesthesia. *Anesth Analg* 2000;91:865–870.

72. Pollock JE, Mulroy MF, Bent E, Polissar NL. A comparison of two regional anesthetic techniques for outpatient knee arthroscopy. *Anesth Analg* 2003;97:397–401.

73. Hodgson PS, Liu SS, Batra MS, et al. Procaine compared with lidocaine for incidence of transient neurologic symptoms. *Reg Anesth Pain Med* 2000;25:218–222.

74. Kouri ME, Kopacz DJ. Spinal 2-chloroprocaine: A comparison with lidocaine in volunteers. *Anesth Analg* 2004;98:75–80.

75. Casati A, Danelli G, Berti M, et al. Intrathecal 2-chloroprocaine for lower limb outpatient surgery: A prospective, randomized, double-blind, clinical evaluation. *Anesth Analg* 2006;103:234–238.

76. Drasner K. Chloroprocaine spinal anesthesia: Back to the future? *Anesth Analg* 2005;100:549–552.

77. Taniguchi M, Bollen AW, Drasner K. Sodium bisulfite: Scapegoat for chloroprocaine neurotoxicity? *Anesthesiology* 2004;100:85–91.

78. Cappelleri G, Casati A, Fanelli G, et al. Unilateral spinal anesthesia or combined sciatic-femoral nerve block for day-case knee arthroscopy. A prospective, randomized comparison. *Minerva Anestesiol* 2000;66:131–136; discussion 7.

PART III: APPLICATIONS

79. Fanelli G, Borghi B, Casati A, et al. Unilateral bupivacaine spinal anesthesia for outpatient knee arthroscopy. Italian Study Group on Unilateral Spinal Anesthesia. *Can J Anaesth* 2000;47:746–751.
80. Korhonen AM, Valanne JV, Jokela RM, et al. A comparison of selective spinal anesthesia with hyperbaric bupivacaine and general anesthesia with desflurane for outpatient knee arthroscopy. *Anesth Analg* 2004;99:1668–1673.
81. Valanne JV, Korhonen AM, Jokela RM, et al. Selective spinal anesthesia: A comparison of hyperbaric bupivacaine 4 mg versus 6 mg for outpatient knee arthroscopy. *Anesth Analg* 2001;93:1377–1379.
82. Neal JM, Deck JJ, Kopacz DJ, Lewis MA. Hospital discharge after ambulatory knee arthroscopy: A comparison of epidural 2-chloroprocaine versus lidocaine. *Reg Anesth Pain Med* 2001;26:35–40.
83. Urmey WF, Stanton J, Peterson M, Sharrock NE. Combined spinal-epidural anesthesia for outpatient surgery. Dose-response characteristics of intrathecal isobaric lidocaine using a 27-gauge Whitacre spinal needle. *Anesthesiology* 1995;83:528–534.
84. Jankowski CJ, Hebl JR, Stuart MJ, et al. A comparison of psoas compartment block and spinal and general anesthesia for outpatient knee arthroscopy. *Anesth Analg* 2003;97:1003–1009.
85. Casati A, Cappelleri G, Aldegheri G, et al. Total intravenous anesthesia, spinal anesthesia or combined sciatic-femoral nerve block for outpatient knee arthroscopy. *Minerva Anestesiol* 2004;70:493–502.
86. Casati A, Cappelleri G, Berti M, et al. Randomized comparison of remifentanil-propofol with a sciatic-femoral nerve block for out-patient knee arthroscopy. *Eur J Anaesthesiol* 2002;19:109–114.
87. Casati A, Cappelleri G, Fanelli G, et al. Regional anaesthesia for outpatient knee arthroscopy: A randomized clinical comparison of two different anaesthetic techniques. *Acta Anaesthesiol Scand* 2000;44:543–547.
88. Hadzic A, Karaca PE, Hobeika P, et al. Peripheral nerve blocks result in superior recovery profile compared with general anesthesia in outpatient knee arthroscopy. *Anesth Analg* 2005;100:976–981.
89. Mulroy MF, Larkin KL, Batra MS, et al. Femoral nerve block with 0.25% or 0.5% bupivacaine improves postoperative analgesia following outpatient arthroscopic anterior cruciate ligament repair. *Reg Anesth Pain Med* 2001;26:24–29.
90. Williams BA, Kentor ML, Williams JP, et al. Process analysis in outpatient knee surgery: Effects of regional and general anesthesia on anesthesia-controlled time. *Anesthesiology* 2000;93:529–538.
91. Williams BA, Kentor ML, Vogt MT, et al. Economics of nerve block pain management after anterior cruciate ligament reconstruction: Potential hospital cost savings via associated postanesthesia care unit bypass and same-day discharge. *Anesthesiology* 2004;100:697–706.
92. Nakamura SJ, Conte-Hernandez A, Galloway MT. The efficacy of regional anesthesia for outpatient anterior cruciate ligament reconstruction. *Arthroscopy* 1997;13:699–703.
93. Williams BA, Kentor ML, Vogt MT, et al. Femoral-sciatic nerve blocks for complex outpatient knee surgery are associated with less postoperative pain before same-day discharge: A review of 1,200 consecutive cases from the period 1996–1999. *Anesthesiology* 2003;98:1206–1213.
94. Williams BA, Kentor ML, Vogt MT, et al. Reduction of verbal pain scores after anterior cruciate ligament reconstruction with 2-day continuous femoral nerve block: A randomized clinical trial. *Anesthesiology* 2006;104:315–327.
95. Vintar N, Rawal N, Veselko M. Intraarticular patient-controlled regional anesthesia after arthroscopically assisted anterior cruciate ligament reconstruction: Ropivacaine/morphine/ketorolac versus ropivacaine/morphine. *Anesth Analg* 2005;101:573–578.
96. Dauri M, Polzoni M, Fabbi E, et al. Comparison of epidural, continuous femoral block and intraarticular analgesia after anterior cruciate ligament reconstruction. *Acta Anaesthesiol Scand* 2003;47:20–25.
97. Hansen E, Eshelman MR, Cracchiolo A 3rd. Popliteal fossa neural blockade as the sole anesthetic technique for outpatient foot and ankle surgery. *Foot Ankle Int* 2000;21:38–44.
98. Zaric D, Boysen K, Christiansen J, et al. Continuous popliteal sciatic nerve block for outpatient foot surgery: A randomized, controlled trial. *Acta Anaesthesiol Scand* 2004;48:337–341.
99. White PF, Issioui T, Skrivanek GD, et al. The use of a continuous popliteal sciatic nerve block after surgery involving the foot and ankle: Does it improve the quality of recovery? *Anesth Analg* 2003;97:1303–1309.
100. Borgeat A, Blumenthal S, Lambert M, et al. The feasibility and complications of the continuous popliteal nerve block: A 1001-case survey. *Anesth Analg* 2006;103:229–233.
101. Ilfeld BM, Morey TE, Wang RD, Enneking FK. Continuous popliteal sciatic nerve block for postoperative pain control at home: A randomized, double-blinded, placebo-controlled study. *Anesthesiology* 2002;97:959–965.
102. Capdevila X, Dadure C, Bringuier S, et al. Effect of patient-controlled perineural analgesia on rehabilitation and pain after ambulatory orthopedic surgery: A multicenter randomized trial. *Anesthesiology* 2006;105:566–573.
103. Casey WF, Rice LJ, Hannallah RS, et al. A comparison between bupivacaine instillation versus ilioinguinal/iliohypogastric nerve block for postoperative analgesia following inguinal herniorrhaphy in children. *Anesthesiology* 1990;72:637–639.
104. Hannallah RS, Broadman LM, Belman AB, et al. Comparison of caudal and ilioinguinal/iliohypogastric nerve blocks for control of post-orchiopexy pain in pediatric ambulatory surgery. *Anesthesiology* 1987;66:832–834.

CHAPTER 27 ■ NEURAL BLOCKADE FOR PEDIATRIC SURGERY

BERNARD J. DALENS AND RENÉ TRUCHON

Regional anesthetic techniques have become major tools in the management of surgical and nonsurgical pain in pediatric patients. During the last decade, many improvements have occurred, especially regarding technologic aspects such as nerve location, devices specifically designed for pediatric use, and availability of less toxic local anesthetics, but also in terms of the conceptualization of pain management. Currently, ultrasonography is revolutionizing the whole field of regional anesthesia, as nerve stimulation did a few decades ago.

An abundant literature has extensively evaluated the techniques, their indications, the benefits and adverse effects to be expected, and the way to avoid complications. Some anesthesiologists, including pediatric anesthesiologists, are still reluctant to use regional techniques in children, especially in infants, or—worse—they are prone to misuse them. For example, caudal anesthesia is still overused, ignoring the fact that it is a neuraxial block—a major anesthetic procedure, the use of which should be restricted to major surgery only. In this chapter, we summarize the specific factors that differentiate between neonates, infants, children, and adults, and then consider the different block procedures suitable to the pediatric population, focusing on safety aspects. Some indications or therapeutic strategies remain controversial, such as the potential dangers of combined regional and general anesthesia, advantages and hazards of adjuvants, and the risk of masking symptoms of compartment syndromes. These issues will be addressed and, although they will remain controversial, a logical and scientifically founded approach to the individual situations will be proposed, taking also into consideration the relevant medicolegal precautions.

GENERAL CONSIDERATIONS

Differences in Anatomy Between Children and Adults

Overall Influence of Growth Process

The body of a child must be seen as a developing structure that is not anatomically and physiologically completed before the end of puberty and even in the early years of adulthood. The most evident differences pertain to the changes in size, from a length of about 50 cm and a weight of 3 to 3.5 kg at birth to more than 150 cm and 50 kg (often significantly more) at the end of the pediatric period. These considerable increases in size are neither continuous nor proportional; the relative growth of the trunk and limbs is greater than that of

the head. This has marked implications in regional anesthesia because the anatomic landmarks, especially surface landmarks, are constantly changing and must be precisely identified before any block procedure is undertaken. Ultrasound technique may help considerably in locating bony structures and nerve paths (1,2). The use of surface electrolocation techniques, such as surface mapping (3) and percutaneous electrode guidance (4,5), might help in overcoming difficult identification of anatomic landmarks, especially in infants and disabled children with limb and joint malformations.

Another distinctive feature of the pediatric period is the presence of congenital malformations, genetic disorders, and the consequences of fetal/neonatal asphyxia. These conditions impair normal development, and many deformities of bone and joint, as well as neurologic structures, worsen during childhood. These patients usually require repeated orthopedic surgeries; regional block procedures are particularly useful in these indications but anatomic deformities can make the techniques particularly difficult and might expose the patient to complications not usually seen in "normal children," especially in regard to pressure point complications at unusual locations and postoperative monitoring of neurologic functions.

Differences in Growth of Spinal Cord and Spinal Canal

Before birth, during the embryonic period, the spinal cord entirely occupies the spinal canal. During fetal life, the growth of the vertebral column exceeds that of neural structures; thus, the spinal cord and roots are encased within the spinal canal, and the lower end of the spinal cord, as well as that of the dural sac, project at progressively higher levels, L4 and S3/S4, respectively, up to the ninth month of life. By the end of the second year, adult levels are reached, namely T12–L1 and S2, respectively. As a consequence, approaches to the epidural space above L4 should be avoided in small infants to prevent any potential damage to the underlying spinal cord. Also, it should be remembered that, in infancy, the dural sac ending is close to the sacral hiatus; cephalad introduction of the block needle during caudal anesthesia must but limited to 2 to 3 mm to avoid accidental dural puncture.

Delayed Myelinization of Nerve Fibers

Myelinization begins during the fetal period in cervical neuromeres and extends progressively both cephalad and caudad (6,7). This process is not fully completed until the end of the twelfth year of life. This lack of myelin in young patients makes the penetration of local anesthetic easier within the nerve fibers. Diluted solutions of local anesthetic can produce consistent nerve blockade since the nerve fibers are thinner and shorter, which reduces the distance between successive nodes of Ranvier.

Incomplete Ossification of Skeleton

At birth, the skeleton is mostly cartilaginous. This has three practical implications: (a) cartilaginous structures are poorly seen on x-ray films, but ultrasonography can identify cartilage and differentiate it from bone, and visualize underlying neuraxial structures; (b) cartilage offers little resistance to sharp needles; and (c) undamaged ossification nuclei are necessary to allow normal bone growth and ossification. As a consequence, attempts to make boney contact should be avoided as often as possible in children, especially in infants, and use of sharp needles should be avoided; they may severely damage ossification nuclei and adjacent organs or vessels because may not be halted by weak cartilaginous bone.

Development of the spine is not complete at the time of birth. It is gender-related, developing earlier in female than in male fetuses (8). The vertebral arches fuse posteriorly during the first year of life, and their junction with the vertebral body becomes ossified from the third to the sixth year (9,10). This posterior fusion remains incomplete at the level of S5 and also S4 most of the time, demarcating a V-shaped aperture, the sacral hiatus, which is covered by the sacrococcygeal membrane, a continuation of the ligamentum flavum, which is tightly adherent to different sacral ligaments. This strong membrane gives immediate access to the epidural space and can easily be penetrated by a block needle to provide caudal anesthesia.

Another peculiarity of the pediatric spine is that the sacrum is still made up of separate vertebrae, the fusion and ossification of which will not be achieved before adulthood (around the twenty-fifth year of life). Consequently, the epidural space can be approached at sacral levels in the same way as it can be at lumbar levels. On the other hand, since the sacrum is cartilaginous, it can be easily traversed by sharp needles, which can damage ossification nuclei (traumatic and infectious lesions) and pelvic/retroperitoneal organs. It should also be remembered that walking is necessary to the normal fusion of the sacral pieces. Patients confined to bed, especially those suffering from cerebral palsy, keep their intervertebral sacral discs unfused.

Delayed ossification of the iliac crest results in lowering of the crystal line (Tuffier line), which is used to locate the L4–L5 interspace to perform a lumbar epidural. In neonates and infants, this line passes one interspace lower; that is, at the level of the L5–S1 interspace (Fig. 27-1).

Flexures of the Spine

At birth, the spine has a single regular flexure. With the acquisition of head support, the cervical lordosis develops progressively by the sixth month, while the lumbar lordosis appears with the acquisition of stable sitting position between 9 and 12 months of life. This has implications for the performance of an epidural block depending on the spinal level. At birth, the orientation of the epidural needle is the same regardless of the intervertebral space. With the development of the spinal flexures, the orientation of the epidural needle must be adapted accordingly. At age 1, the spine has acquired its definitive shape, and the orientation of epidural needles should be the same as that suitable in adult patients at the same intervertebral space. However, these flexures can be easily emended by forced flexion almost throughout childhood due to the long-lasting persistence of spine flexibility, a major benefit of the pediatric period (in addition to the absence of osteophytes).

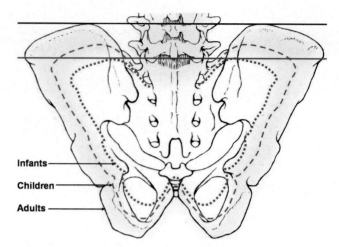

FIGURE 27-1. Variation in size of the pelvic girdle, with subsequent changes in the relative position of the anterior superior iliac crests.

Ability to walk is necessary to acquire normal flexures of the spine. Patients with cerebral palsy usually develop severe deformities of the spine, mainly scoliosis, which often necessitate surgical treatment and make epidural anesthesia particularly challenging, occasionally impossible.

Loose Attachment of Sheaths and Fluidity of Epidural Fat

An important feature of the pediatric period is the loose attachment of fascias and sheaths to nerve trunks and muscles. This allows extended spread of local anesthetic, resulting in high-quality nerve blockade whatever the technique used. This extended diffusion can occasionally result in unwanted or even undesirable distant nerve blocks. This also applies to the sheaths surrounding the spinal roots. The younger the patient, the greater the distal spread of the local anesthetic injected epidurally (caudal or lumbar epidural approach) along the spinal roots. Due to this extended spread, in addition to the incomplete myelination of nerve fibers, the quality of blockade is improved in relevant dermatomes and allows the use of lower concentration of local anesthetics, thus reducing the danger of systemic toxicity. However, leakage along spinal roots has also negative consequences: comparatively larger volumes of local anesthetics are necessary in infants to achieve the same cephalad level as in adults. This may be an incitation to administering potentially toxic amounts of local anesthetics or to attempting hazardous techniques such as distant insertion of epidural catheters (especially via the caudal route) to achieve satisfactory blockade.

Another factor affecting the spread of epidural solution is the consistency of the epidural fat. Up to 6 to 8 years of age, this fat is very fluid. After that age, it becomes more densely packed, with an increased proportion of elastic and collagenous fibers that can significantly impede the distribution of the local anesthetic and the progression of epidural catheters. Caudal anesthesia becomes less reliable after age 6, and the insertion of a distant epidural catheter becomes very hazardous and often impossible.

Not only is the longitudinal spread of local anesthetic increased in children, the diffusion process across nerve sheaths is increased too. In young patients, the structure of the endoneurium is loose, which makes it easily traversed in both directions ("fast in, fast out"). As the child grows, the endoneurium becomes enriched with connective fibers, thus less permeable. The latency and also the duration of nerve blockade increase with age. The most significant characteristics of the pediatric patient that can influence the selection or performance of a regional block procedure are summarized in Table 27-1.

Differences in Pharmacology

Concomitantly with the growth process, the body surface area (BSA) increases throughout childhood; however, when related to patients' weight, the BSA constantly decreases up to the end of adolescence. Drug prescriptions should ideally be related to the BSA, because the doses would be the same as (or in simple ratio with) adult doses, whatever the patient's age (11). However, BSA is not as easy to obtain as body weight and, in practice, dose calculations are usually made according to weight, which requires constant adaptation of doses throughout childhood and could lead to dosage errors.

Local Anesthetics

Although the pharmacodynamics of local anesthetics is similar in children and adults, pharmacokinetic properties differ significantly, especially in neonates and infants (12).

Absorption from the Site of Injection. Nonionized local anesthetics cross almost freely the endothelium of capillaries surrounding the injection site. As the cardiac output and local blood flow of infants are two to three times greater than in adults, systemic absorption of local anesthetics is increased accordingly and vasoactive agents, such as epinephrine, are very effective in slowing down this systemic uptake, especially for short-acting agents.

Mucosal Topical Anesthesia. The absorption of local anesthetics from mucous membranes is increased in infants, and mucosal topical anesthesia has long been contraindicated. However, the technique can be used safely with certain precautions in young children, either by using specific transmucosal patches (13) or sprays of diluted solutions of local anesthetics, mainly lidocaine (14,15). However, it should be remembered that topical lidocaine exaggerates laryngomalacia, thus being a potential cause of increased morbidity in neonates and young infants (16).

Compartment Blocks. Injection of local anesthetics within closed fascial compartments allows easy blockade of nerves running through those compartments. A large compartment requires that a rather large dose be injected to produce satisfactory blockade, and it offers an extended surface of absorption, thus favoring early and high peak plasma concentrations. During intercostal nerve blocks with ropivacaine, the T_{max} is reached 10 (venous blood) and 16 minutes (arterial blood) after injection, with C_{max} values ranging from 0.3 (lowest values with 0.2% ropivacaine) to 5.6 μg/mL (highest values with 1% ropivacaine) (17).

Conduction Blocks (Including Epidural Anesthesia). Amino amides are lipid-soluble and their absorption follows a biphasic curve. Lidocaine undergoes rapid absorption, and its blood concentration increases rapidly following repeat injections. Conversely, bupivacaine and ropivacaine are more efficiently retained at the injection site, and their systemic absorption is slower. In adults, this slow absorption process modifies the

pharmacokinetic profile of long-acting agents after repeat injections or continuous infusion; the decrease in plasma concentration is slower than that expected from single-injection studies, and both the elimination half-life and distribution volume increase.

In children, the pharmacokinetic profiles of bupivacaine, levobupivacaine, and ropivacaine are consistently different. After a single injection in small infants, the T_{max} of bupivacaine is around 30 minutes—the same as in adults—whereas that of levobupivacaine is approximately 50 minutes (18), and that of ropivacaine still longer: 115 minutes in infants and 62 minutes in children ages 3 to 5 years. Only children older than 5 years have T_{max} values similar to those in adults (30 minutes) (19,20). Additionally, several studies also reported a concomitant increase of C_{max} values of ropivacaine in infants and children up to 8 years of age (19), probably due to liver immaturity. This has clinical implications, as the C_{max} of the most recent and supposedly safer local anesthetic could be reached after the infant had left the recovery room following short outpatient surgeries.

Plasma Protein Binding. Two main plasma proteins are involved in local anesthetic binding: human serum albumin (HSA) and α_1-acid glycoprotein (AAG). Human serum albumin has a low affinity for local anesthetic, and many pharmacologic agents can compete at available binding sites. During the first months of life, plasma levels of HSA are low, especially in fasted infants; thus, the protection offered by HSA against systemic local anesthetic toxicity is low and decreases postoperatively (see also Chapter 3).

α_1-Acid glycoprotein has an affinity for local anesthetics of five to 10,000 times greater than that of HSA, thus being very effective in preventing systemic toxicity, as only the nonbound free form is pharmacologically active. However, the plasma concentration of AAG is very low at birth (0.2–0.3 g/L) and does not reach adult levels (0.7–1.0 g/L) until the first year (21–23). Consequently, the free fraction of all local anesthetics is increased in infants. The maximum doses that can be safely administered must be significantly reduced in this age group, even though the plasma concentration of AAG increases postoperatively except in case of liver insufficiency (23).

Red Cell Storage. After their systemic absorption, local anesthetics also distribute in red blood cells, which retain 20% to 30% of the total dose, depending on the specific agent and the hematocrit. Usually, red cell storage does not affect significantly local anesthetic pharmacology except in the following conditions:

- In neonates, due to high hematocrit values (which may exceed 70%) and enlargement of erythrocytes (physiologic macrocytosis), a significantly greater amount of local anesthetic can be entrapped in red blood (decreasing their C_{max} after a single injection) and released secondarily (thus increasing the half-life at this age).
- In infants, red cell storage is decreased due to physiologic anemia, thus increasing the dangers of systemic toxicity when the plasma protein binding sites are saturated (i.e., close to toxic blood concentrations) (24).

Distribution. Distribution of local anesthetics to organs and tissues depends on body fluid content and varies enormously with patient age (Table 27-2): This considerably affects the pharmacokinetics (Table 27-3). During the first 2 years of life, the peak plasma concentration and clearance of all amino amides is decreased after a single injection, while their

TABLE 27-1

CHARACTERISTICS THAT MAY AFFECT SELECTION AND/OR PERFORMANCE OF REGIONAL BLOCK PROCEDURE IN CHILDREN

Pediatric features (infants mainly)	Anatomic/physiologic consequences	Implications for regional anesthesia
Delayed myelinization of nerve fibers	Easier crossing of nerve envelopes by LA	Shortened onset time and increased efficacy of diluted LA.
Cartilaginous structure of bones and vertebrae	Little resistance offered to sharp needles Fragility of ossification nuclei (infection, trauma) which may compromise normal bone/joint growth	Avoid using thin and sharp needles; use short and short-bevel ones instead. Do not apply excessive force on needle: If resistance is felt, stop trying to insert the needle further.
Lower ending of spinal cord	Increased risk of trauma to the spinal cord	Avoid epidural approaches above L3 whenever possible.
Lower ending of dural sac	Increased danger of accidental penetration of the dura mater	Favor low approaches to the epidural space. Check for CSF reflux, including during caudal approaches.
Absence of fusion of sacral vertebrae	Existence of sacral intervertebral spaces	Sacral approaches to epidural spaces are possible.
Delayed curvatures of the spine	Cervical lordosis (3–6 months) Lumbar lordosis (8–9 months)	Adjust needle orientation accordingly when approaching the spinal canal.
Changing orientation of coccyx axis and lack of sacral hiatus growth	Sacral hiatus comparatively smaller with increasing age	Identification of sacral hiatus more difficult above 6–8 years with increased failure rate of caudal anesthesia.
Delayed ossification and growth of iliac crests	Intercristal line (or Tuffier's line) joining the anterior superior iliac spine is lower than in adults	This line passes over L5–S1 interspace instead of L4–L5 interspace.
Increased fluidity of epidural fat	Increased diffusion of LA up to 6–7 years of age	Excellent blockade following caudal anesthesia up to 6–7 years of age.
Loose attachment of sheaths and aponeuroses to underlying structures	Increased diffusion along nerve paths that may reach distant spaces and nerves	Required volume of LA decreases for peripheral blocks but increases for neuraxial (due to leakage along nerve roots).
Enzyme (hepatic) immaturity	Slower metabolism of amino amides (and amino esters) (compensated by other enzyme pathways, not very active in adults)	Increased mean time body residency and half-life, accumulation (especially following repeat injection and continuous infusions of LA).
High heart rate and cardiac output	Increased regional blood flow resulting in increased systemic absorption of LA	Increased systemic absorption of LA: Decreased T_{max}, duration of blockade. Increased efficacy of epinephrine: Vasoconstriction reduces absorption (thus toxicity) and prolongs duration of blockade.
Decrease in extracellular and increase in intracellular body fluid compartment	Increased distribution volume and mean body residency time of LA (and most medications)	Decreased C_{max} after single injection but accumulation with repeat/continuous injections
Low plasma protein content (HSA and AAG)	Competition at nonspecific HSA binding site Limited capacity of specifically binding LA	Increased unbound free fraction of all LAs: Greater danger of toxicity (especially during repeat/continuous injections)
Sympathetic immaturity, diminished autonomic adaptability of the heart, smaller vascular bed in lower extremities	Hemodynamic stability during neuraxial blocks	Fluid preloading and use of vasoactive agents are unnecessary.
Delayed acquisition of body scheme and conceptualization, anxiety	Inability of patients to locate precise body areas, concept of paresthesia not understandable, difficult cooperation	Physical means required to locate nerve and spaces; do not perform a "dangerous" technique while the child is awake (risk of unanticipated panic attack at the wrong time, even in apparently "cooperative" children)

LA, local anesthetic; CSF, cerebrospinal fluid; HSA, human serum albumin; AAG, α_1-acid glycoprotein.

TABLE 27-2

VARIATION OF BODY FLUID DISTRIBUTION ACCORDING TO PATIENT'S AGE

Body fluids	Premature	Full–term	Infant	Children	Adults
Total body water	80%–85%	70%–75%	65%	55%–60%	50%–55%
Intracellular fluids	20%–25%	30%–35%	35%	35%–40%	40%–45%
Extracellular fluids	55%–60%	45%	30%	20%–25%	20%

elimination half-life is consistently prolonged (25,26). During childhood, the clearance increases progressively and becomes higher than that measured in adults before returning to adult levels during adolescence.

If young patients (excluding the neonatal period) are comparatively less prone to develop systemic toxicity after a single local anesthetic injection, the same does not apply in cases of repeat injections or continuous infusion, because of progressive accumulation (26,27). During continuous infusion, the distribution volume and clearance of bupivacaine decrease consistently while the plasma concentration continuously increases, without reaching a plateau. In the same conditions, the distribution volume and clearance of ropivacaine tend to increase while plasma concentration of the unbound (toxic) form reaches a plateau 24 hours following the injection, with no further increase later (28). Little data are yet available on continuous infusion of levobupivacaine but, as for racemic bupivacaine, plasma concentrations do not reach a plateau and continue to increase with time even when a diluted solution (0.0625%) of levobupivacaine is infused (29).

Metabolism

Amino Esters. Amino esters are mainly hydrolyzed by plasma cholinesterases. The activity of these enzymes is low at birth, with no adverse clinical consequences, and gradually increases throughout the first year of life (30) (see also Chapter 3).

Amino amides. Amino amides mainly undergo hepatic microsomal metabolism by the P450 cytochrome enzyme superfamily, the activity of which is reduced during the first months of life (31–33). In adults, bupivacaine is mainly metabolized by the CYP3A4 enzyme (34), the activity of which is low during the first year; however, CYP3A7, a major enzyme in the fetus, is very active at birth and allows bupivacaine metabolism almost as efficiently as CYP3A4 in adults. The metabolism of both ropivacaine (35–37) and levobupivacaine (18) depends mainly on CYP1A2, which is not fully functional before the third year of life, and, to a minor extent, on CYP3A4. This enzyme immaturity is clinically relevant, but to a limited extent (low clearance, delayed T_{max} and, for ropivacaine only, increased C_{max} but within clinically acceptable levels); it does not preclude administering these local anesthetics in neonates and infants.

Clearance

Lidocaine. The hepatic extraction ratio of lidocaine varies from 0.65 to 0.75. The clearance is flow-limited and decreases when cardiac output decreases (12). Continuous infusion of lidocaine also results in considerable decrease in intrinsic clearance, which is further worsened by the fact that lidocaine metabolism is impaired by its own metabolites. Consequently, lidocaine should not be used for continuous infusion, especially in infants (see also Chapter 3).

Bupivacaine and Ropivacaine. The hepatic extraction ratio is low (0.35–0.45), and the clearance is rate-limited for both agents. Protein binding is the key factor influencing clearance. After a single injection, both local anesthetics have a low

TABLE 27-3

INFLUENCE OF AGE ON PHARMACOKINETIC PARAMETERS OF AMINO AMIDES

Local anesthetic	Protein binding (%)	V_{dss} (L/kg)	Clearance (mL/kg/min)
Lidocaine			
Neonate	25	1.4–4.9	5–19
Adult	55–65	0.2–1.0	11–15
Mepivacaine			
Neonate	36	1.2–2.8	1.6–3
Adult	75–80	0.6–1.5	10–13
Bupivacaine			
Neonate	50–70	3.9 ($\pm$ 2.01)	7.1 ($\pm$ 3.2)
Adult	85–95	0.8–1.6	7–9
Ropivacaine			
Infant	94	2.4	6.5
Adult	94	1.1 $\pm$ 0.25	10–13
Levobupivacaine			
Infant	50–70	2.7	13.8
Adult	85–95	0.7–1.4	28–39

clearance at birth, which progressively increases during the first years (38,39). During continuous infusion, the clearance of bupivacaine decreases by more than 40%, whereas that of ropivacaine remains unchanged; ropivacaine therefore represents the safest drug for continuous infusion, especially in infants (23).

Systemic Toxicity. Understanding systemic toxicity is not simple because only total plasma concentration of local anesthetics is easily measurable, whereas only the unbound form is pharmacologically active. Even the dosage of the unbound form in plasma is a poor reflection of the basically unknown concentration at the site of action (intraneuronal concentration of the ionized form, which is the form that blocks sodium channels).

Clinical signs of neurologic toxicity have been reported with plasma concentrations ranging from 7 to 10 μg/mL for lidocaine or mepivacaine, and from 1.5 to 2 μg/mL (intraoperatively) to 2 to 2.5 μg/mL (postoperatively) with bupivacaine. However, plasma concentrations of bupivacaine exceeding 4 μg/mL have been frequently reported without any evidence of clinical toxicity. From studies in adult volunteers (40–42), the following thresholds of toxicity of the unbound form of local anesthetics have been retained: 0.3 μg/mL for unbound bupivacaine; 0.6 μg/mL for unbound levobupivacaine or ropivacaine.

Because of low protein binding, infants are considered at greater risk of systemic toxicity. A noticeable difference with adults is that cardiac toxicity seems to occur concomitantly with central nervous toxicity, instead of being preceded by neurologic symptoms including convulsions (see Chapter 5).

Clinical Implications in Daily Practice. Short-acting agents (lidocaine and mepivacaine) should be restricted to single-injection techniques. For longer duration procedures, bupivacaine, ropivacaine, and levobupivacaine are suitable, either for single-injection blocks or for continuous infusion. In infants, use of ropivacaine or levobupivacaine for single-injection procedures does not represent a significant improvement over racemic bupivacaine in terms of safety; infants given these agents require a longer stay in the recovery room, as their plasma peak concentration is comparatively delayed. Conversely, for continuous infusion, ropivacaine represents a safer choice, as its clearance remains unchanged postoperatively, whereas that of either racemic bupivacaine or levobupivacaine decreases dramatically.

Opioids

The main pharmacokinetic difference between infants and older patients in regard to opioids (mainly morphine) pertains to the elimination half-life, which is consistently increased in infants. After lumbar epidural injection, peak plasma concentration of morphine is reached within 10 minutes. However, following therapeutic epidural or spinal doses, this plasma concentration is far too low to play a significant role in the development of analgesia, which depends only on the drug crossing the dura mater (43,44). The elimination half-life from cerebrospinal fluid (CSF) is similar to that of plasma and follows the same monoexponential elimination curve. As peak CSF concentration of morphine is very high shortly after an epidural injection, it takes 12 to 24 hours before the concentration falls below the minimal effective concentration (10 ng/mL). Therefore, adverse effects, including respiratory depression, can be observed more than 12 hours after an epidural injection, thus requiring close monitoring of vital parameters 24 hours after the last injection. Maximum recommended doses are 30 μg/kg for epidural morphine and 10 μg/kg for intrathecal morphine (Table 27-4). Patients given neuraxial morphine are not eligible for outpatient surgery (see also Chapter 40).

Short-acting lipid-soluble opioids such as fentanyl (1–2 μg/kg) and sufentanil (0.5 μg/kg) can be administered epidurally instead of morphine. They improve the quality of intraoperative analgesia, especially when coadministered with diluted local anesthetic solution. However, they do not prolong significantly the duration of postoperative pain relief unless a continuous infusion or repeat injections are made. Part, if not all, of their action is related to their plasma concentration, which can lead to early and acute respiratory depression (sudden apnea). This condition is very different from the progressive and delayed respiratory depression, preceded by generalized pruritus, sedation, and progressive bradypnea, which is observed following excessive doses of epidural morphine.

TABLE 27-4

COMMONLY USED ADJUVANTS AND RECOMMENDED DOSES

Additive	Recommended doses	Adverse effects
Morphine epidural intrathecal	30 μg/kg 10 μg/kg	Pruritus, nausea and vomiting, urinary retention, delayed respiratory depression, sedation, constipation
Fentanyl (epidural)	1–2 μg/kg	Pruritus, nausea and vomiting, urinary retention, early respiratory depression (apnea), sedation
Sufentanil (epidural)	0.5 μg/kg	Pruritus, nausea and vomiting, urinary retention, early respiratory depression (apnea), sedation
Clonidine (epidural or along peripheral nerves)	1–1.5 μg/kg	Sedation (slight) Hypotension at doses exceeding 2 μg/kg Possible respiratory depression in premature infants and neonates
Ketamine (epidural or occasionally along peripheral nerves)	0.5 mg/kg	Sedation (but no behavioral disturbance)

Another limitation must be considered before prescribing opiates in pediatrics. Experimental administration of a few doses—even a single dose—of opiates can induce tolerance in newly born animals (45–47); this tolerance similarly develops in human neonates and occurs more rapidly in preterm than in term neonates (48,49). Gender plays a consistent role, both in animals (50) and in human (51), with males developing a more intense tolerance than females. The underlying mechanisms of this early tolerance are essentially unknown but should encourage the practitioner to limit exposure of neonates to opiates as often as possible, using alternate medications (continuous local anesthetic infusion and/or other additives).

Other Additives

Epinephrine. Epinephrine is the most commonly used additive (5 mg/L or 1:200,000). Coadministered with local anesthetics (mainly short-acting agents such as lidocaine and mepivacaine), it decreases the plasma peak concentration (52,53) and increases local anesthetic duration of action, especially in children younger than 4 years old (54,55). Its vasoconstrictive properties have raised questions about possible spinal cord ischemia, but this proved to be unfounded (56). Nevertheless, many anesthesiologists prefer using a lower concentration of epinephrine in neonates and infants (2.5 mg/L or 1:400,000). At this concentration, the absorption rate of caudal bupivacaine is decreased by 25% (55), which consistently improves the safety of the technique. Another benefit of using local anesthetics with epinephrine is related to the hypersensitivity of children to IV epinephrine. In most infants and children, an accidental intravascular injection of a solution containing epinephrine would result in early (within 20 seconds) and readily evident ST segment elevation, T wave change (57), and hypertension (58) (see also Chapters 3, 4, 5).

Clonidine. Clonidine is another α_2-adrenergic agonist (like epinephrine) that is extensively used neuraxially (59,60) and peripherally (61) (Table 27-4) at doses of 1 to 2 μg/kg. It increases (by approximately a factor of 2) the duration of blockade with no hemodynamic effects (in children) and decreases peak plasma concentration of the local anesthetic. Clonidine also produces slight sedation for 1 to 3 hours postoperatively, which is more beneficial than detrimental, as it does not preclude hospital discharge provided no more than 2 μg/kg has been administered. The addition of clonidine can often make unnecessary the placement of a catheter and a continuous infusion in many pediatric procedures, thus reducing the overall morbidity and costs of the technique. However, there are some respiratory concerns in neonates (62,63).

Ketamine. Ketamine, especially S-ketamine, has gained considerable interest as a local anesthetic adjuvant due to its blocking effects on N-methyl-D-aspartate (NMDA) receptors and its interaction with sodium channels in a local anesthetic–like fashion (including sharing a binding site with commonly used clinical local anesthetics) (64). Coadministered at a dose of 0.25 to 0.5 mg/kg, ketamine prolongs the duration of analgesia for many hours (65,66) with no significant, especially behavioral, adverse effects (see also Chapter 40).

Other Adjuvants. Many other additives have been occasionally (and questionably from an ethical point of view) administered along with local anesthetics (67). Some may be of interest (corticosteroids, buprenorphine, neostigmine, tramadol, midazolam, and biodegradable bupivacaine/polyester microspheres).

However, many of them produce significant adverse effects. Furthermore, they have no approval for pediatric use.

Immaturity and Perception of Pain

Pain pathways and perception of pain are not mature at birth. They evolve throughout childhood. Furthermore, since the ability of children to communicate is limited both for anatomic (inability to speak, lack of vocabulary) and psychological/emotional reasons, assessment of pain is therefore difficult. The younger is the patient, the more difficult is the evaluation (see Chapters 5, 30, and 47).

Common Applications

Regional techniques are suitable for anesthetic, analgesic, and also a few nonanalgesic purposes.

Anesthetic Indications

Emergency Surgery and Patients at Risk of Severe Complications under General Anesthesia. After halothane had become available, regional anesthetic techniques fell almost completely into disuse. Some regional techniques survived only in a limited number of surgical indications in pediatrics including: (a) emergency procedures on the extremities and lower part of the abdomen and limbs in nonfasted children, and (b) elective surgery in children with severe medical conditions that could be dramatically aggravated either by the general anesthetic itself or the preparation of the patient, such as poor tolerance of fasting in certain metabolic diseases, facial deformities at risk of difficult intubation, malignant hyperthermia–susceptible patients, pulmonary cystic fibrosis, or severe asthma.

Many advances have occurred over the years, including the availability of new anesthetic agents, safer general anesthetic techniques, and new equipment for intra- and postoperative monitoring. Emergency surgery, per se, is no longer an indication for regional anesthesia, even though in many instances, when applicable, it could represent the first choice due to its lower morbidity rate.

Currently, regional blocks are particularly useful in trauma patients with extremity lesions, because they improve the comfort of the child, and allow pain-free clinical and radiologic examinations, wound dressings, even reduction of limb fractures without compromising the vital functions or affecting the evaluation of the status of the central nervous system. In a number of cases, nerve injury (such as median nerve rupture following a supracondylar fracture of the humerus) has resulted from the trauma itself. To avoid irrelevant claims, it is important to make a complete neurologic evaluation before any treatment is undertaken, preferably with the help of an external consultant, and to document the results in the medical files and to the parents. Then, after discussing with the parents and the child the different options for pain relief, a regional block with or without catheter placement will be mutually agreed to or denied.

Patients at risk of compartment syndrome are of special concern (see following discussion), but they should not be deprived of adequate pain relief, including by use of regional procedures (67). Some emergency conditions involving parietal disorders such as torsion of the testis, incarcerated hernia, or paraphimosis in nonfasted patients might benefit greatly from immediate surgery under a regional block procedure (e.g., caudal anesthesia, penile block) without the hazards of either a crash induction or a delayed surgical repair under general anesthesia.

Improvement in the management of diabetic patients and most metabolic disorders does not preclude the performance of a general anesthetic even though regional anesthetic techniques might represent a better choice in many instances. This is especially the case in patients presenting with the following disorders:

- Nonstabilized acute or chronic respiratory insufficiency (status asthmaticus, cystic fibrosis)
- Uncompensated metabolic or endocrine disorders
- Neuromuscular diseases including myopathies, myotonic syndromes, myasthenia, some porphyrias, and some neurologic diseases with demyelinating disorders
- Certain major skeletal deformities and polymalformative syndromes

Instability of the cervical spine is present in patients with Chiari syndrome, and frequent in Down syndrome or achondroplasia. Tracheal intubation in these patients is hazardous and might result in tetraplegia due to mobilization of the cervical spine. Many pediatric syndromes with facial deformities, microstomia, and palatal division are often a cause of difficult or impossible intubation even with the help of a fiberscope (and other devices); using a technique that avoids tracheal intubation is beneficial in these children.

Former preterm infants less than 60 weeks of post gestational age are prone to develop postoperative apnea. Inguinal hernia repair, a common procedure in these patients, is more safely achieved under regional anesthesia alone (spinal, caudal, or sacral/lumbar epidural anesthesia) than with any other technique of anesthesia, provided no sedative agent has been coadministered.

Anesthetic management is extremely difficult to provide to patients suffering from epidermolysis bullosa. Like severely burned patients, these infants are prone to suffer from intense and prolonged pain; regional block procedures may occasionally represent an effective and low-morbidity option, allowing surgery without tracheal intubation and providing long-lasting postoperative pain relief when a catheter is placed.

Elective Surgery

If based on medical indications alone, regional procedures would be extensively used for surgery on the extremities and lower part of the abdomen in children, as it is in adults. This is common practice in a few countries, especially in Northern Europe, where blocks are culturally well established and accepted both by adults and children. However, in the vast majority of countries, children usually fear needle sticks, and regional block procedures have to be performed in anesthetized children, a practice well-established and accepted in this age group (68,69).

Indications for Acute Pain Relief

Analgesia is currently the main indication for regional anesthesia in children, especially in elective surgery involving the extremities, abdomen and, to a lesser extent, the thorax, neck, and head. Intra- and postoperative pain is easily and efficiently prevented by single-injection or continuous techniques depending on the expected duration and intensity of postoperative pain (70–72). All pediatric patients can benefit from these techniques including neonates, preterm infants, and critically ill children (73–75). In some institutions, regional techniques are used in children undergoing cardiac surgery (76–78), but this application remains controversial. Outpatient surgery currently represents a major and cost-effective indication of regional blocks, mainly peripheral nerve blocks, with a very low morbidity provided that appropriate precautions are taken.

In recent years, catheter techniques allowing intermittent, on-demand, or continuous infusion of local anesthetics have become increasingly popular. Originally restricted to neuraxial techniques (28,79,80), catheter placement along a peripheral nerve path or a fascial plane is becoming routine practice in many institutions to provide long-lasting pain relief both in hospitalized and nonhospitalized patients (81–83). Regional blockade is commonly performed to provide analgesia for cancer pain and chronic pain relief. These techniques are detailed in Chapter 47 and are not considered in this chapter.

Nonanalgesic Indications

Occasionally, a regional block procedure may be performed in children for whom analgesia is not the first objective. Examples of these mainly nonanalgesic indications include vasodilation in patients presenting with ischemic disorders (84–86) and maintenance of a motor block throughout the recovery period in the patient with an unstable fracture, fragile nerve suture, or tendon repair.

Contraindications

Contraindications to regional block procedures are basically the same as in adult patients. Regardless of anesthetic technique, the patient's full consent (and parental agreement for children) must be obtained preoperatively. Parent/child refusal should be considered a contraindication. Patients with severe psychoneurotic disorders should also be considered with the greatest attention, and most anesthesiologists would deny regional procedures in these patients.

Contraindications to Neuraxial Blocks

Absolute contraindications to neuraxial blockade include (87,88): infection at the puncture site, septicemia and meningitis; bleeding disorders, either constitutional or secondary to anticoagulant therapy; true allergy to local anesthetic, a very rare event (even with amino esters); uncorrected hypovolemia; and major vertebral anomalies (not spina bifida occulta—for many but not all authors, these include tethered cord syndromes and ventriculoperitoneal shunts).

Patients with mild seizure disorders should not be denied a regional anesthesia if they do not suffer any additional disorder prone to increase the morbidity of the procedure. Preexisting central nervous disorders and degenerative axonal diseases have long been considered as contraindications, at least relatively, even though few data support the hypothesis that a regional block worsens their course. A recent pediatric study involving 139 patients showed that preexisting neurologic disorders were not associated with bad neurologic outcome (the reverse was observed) after central block procedures (89).

Contraindications to Peripheral Nerve Blocks

Peripheral nerve blocks have few contraindications. Although infection close to the insertion site and allergy to local anesthetics are absolute contraindications, bleeding disorders may not contraindicate the performance of most peripheral blocks. Only procedures at risk of damaging large arteries (such as a supraclavicular block) or requiring deep needle insertion in closed muscular compartments (such as psoas compartment blocks or sciatic blocks at the thigh) should be considered with caution.

Patients at Risk of Compartment Syndrome

Compartment syndromes are (very) infrequent but can result in devastating complications. Certain trauma lesions and surgeries are more often concerned, such as displaced humeral supracondylar fractures or tibial shaft and forearm fractures treated by intramedullary nail fixation.

The extremities are divided into distinct muscular compartments by inextensible fascias, within which run nerves and vessels. The intracompartmental pressure must remain low to allow effective venous return. Any expanding lesion or disorder including muscle necrosis, edema, hematoma, injection of a large volume of fluid, or external compression by a cast (90) or a wound dressing inevitably increases the intracompartmental pressure, which may interrupt blood flow. Depending on the local lesions and state of consciousness, this interruption produces "tourniquet" pain, hypoesthesia, or a combination of both, typically summarized by the "5 P's" eponym: pain, pallor, paresthesia, paralysis, and pulselessness. This severe condition must be recognized early, in order to perform extended fasciotomies before irreversible lesions have occurred.

Since pain is one of the cardinal symptoms, any technique aimed at attenuating pain, especially regional blockade, is often claimed to be contraindicated because of the possibility of hiding this presenting symptom and thus delaying the rescuing surgery. However, avoidance of analgesic strategies is not acceptable medically or ethically (91). Intense pain is often associated with bone fractures. Although fractures are very frequent in the pediatric population, compartment syndromes are very rare. Therefore, children should not be deliberately allowed to experience pain because of fear of compartment syndrome, which could be easily and precociously diagnosed using appropriate and easily available monitoring.

Adequate pain management, including continuous epidural analgesia (92), does not preclude early diagnosis but, on the contrary, favors it. In effect, the most sensitive clinical indicator of compartment syndrome is the increase in pain medication requirements, both in dosage and frequency, and this indicator precedes other clinical symptoms of compartment syndrome by an average of 7.3 hours (93). Therefore, adequate pain management, either by the IV route or by using regional procedures with low concentrations of local anesthetics (0.1%–0.15% bupivacaine, levobupivacaine, or ropivacaine) and avoiding motor blockade may considerably facilitate early diagnosis when significant changes happen: (a) because pain is no longer relieved and the child asks for additional analgesia; (b) less often, because the child becomes oversedated with the usual "normal" dose of parenteral narcotics; or (c) because the intensity and distribution of anesthesia is changing (progressive loss of any sensory perception and motor function).

The development of excruciating pain in a child deprived of analgesic medications should no longer be considered the "presenting" symptom of a compartment syndrome. Rather, patients at risk should not have a closed plaster cast and should be monitored by serial clinical evaluation of the distal perfusion and tissue oxygenation of the limb and by noninvasive monitoring of the intracompartmental pressure using, for example, near infrared spectroscopy (94), noninvasive "hardness" measuring devices (95), or ultrasound technique (96), even though these noninvasive techniques are not fully reliable. If the risk is considered high (e.g., displaced humeral fractures, intramedullary nail fixation of tibia or radius, obtunded patients), the intracompartmental pressure close to the fracture site should be invasively monitored because the technique is easy and inexpensive, requiring only a venous cannula, an IV line, and a pressure gauge (as for central venous pressure measurement) (93,97–99).

Selection of the technique, Equipment, and Anesthetic Solution

Selection of the Most Appropriate Block Procedure

Among the pediatric population, regional anesthesia is mostly used for analgesia, rather than anesthesia (as in adults). Therefore, it must offer a risk–benefit ratio superior to alternative analgesic approaches. In making a selection, the following points must be considered:

- The distribution of anesthesia should cover not only the operative field but also the different areas involved in the surgery (e.g., sites of tourniquet placement, skin or bone graft taking).
- The duration of sensory blockade should approximate that of postoperative pain.
- The performance of the block should not aggravate the physical condition of the patient (e.g., risk of bacterial contamination, patient's positioning prone to worsen trauma lesions).
- The anesthetic and surgical techniques should be of the same magnitude (neuraxial blocks should be avoided for minor surgery).
- The anesthesiologist must be familiar with the regional technique planned.

It is recommended that an alternative strategy be selected and explained to patients and family, in case of failure of the primary technique.

Techniques of Nerve Location

As most block procedures are performed on anesthetized children, a reliable technique of nerve localization independent of the patient's cooperation is necessary (nerve stimulation, ultrasound guidance, or both); the overall morbidity of the two combined techniques, regional and general, should be lower than that of any other technique of anesthesia care, meaning usually that general anesthesia should be light (no muscle relaxants and no/minimal narcotics).

Basically, these techniques are the same as in adults; namely, loss-of-resistance technique for epidural anesthesia and compartment blocks, CSF aspiration for spinal anesthesia, and nerve stimulation for peripheral nerves and plexuses.

Ultrasound guidance is opening a new era, one that is particularly exciting in pediatric patients, especially in infants, whose nerves are very superficial and easily identified. However, the size of the probe can be difficult to handle and its application on the skin can change the anatomic landmarks and displace the block needle. The sterility of the procedure can occasionally be difficult to maintain throughout the procedure. Currently, block needles can only be reliably seen and their tip clearly identified when the major axis of the probe is in line with the shaft of the needle. If the probe is perpendicular to the shaft, only a cross-section of the needle can be seen (not always) and no information is obtained regarding the position of the needle tip. Two "tricks" can be helpful (personal data): (a) inject a small amount of 5% dextrose while the ultrasound machine is in Doppler mode—the stream produced at the tip of the needle will give a conical colored signal (dextrose will not compromise

TABLE 27-5

PEDIATRIC DOSES AND CLINICAL CHARACTERISTICS OF COMMONLY USED LOCAL ANESTHETICS

Local anesthetic	Usual concentration (%)	Usual doses (Mg/kg)	Maximum[a] dose (plain) (Mg/kg)	Maximum[a] dose with epinephrine (Mg/kg)	Latency (min)	Duration of effects (h)
Amino esters						
Procaine	1–2	7	10	10	10–15	0.3–1
Chloroprocaine	2–3	7	10	10	7–15	0.5–1
Amino Amides						
Lidocaine	0.5–2	5	7.5	10	5–15	0.75–2
Mepivacaine	0.5–1.5	5–7	8	10	5–15	1–1.25
Bupivacaine	0.25–0.5	2	2.5	3	15–30	2.5–6
Levobupivacaine	0.25–0.5	3	4	4	15–30	2.5–6
Ropivacaine	0.2–10	3	3.5	Not recommended	7–20	2.5–5

[a]Maximum doses are controversial. The doses mentioned in this table are basically safe when given as single injections in children older than 6 months; repeat injections should not be made before half of elimination half-life, and the amount injected should be half that initially injected; a full dose can only be safely injected after two elimination half-lives.
These data are not applicable to spinal anesthesia, intravenous regional anesthesia, and local anesthesia.

further neurostimulation); (b) inject the local anesthetic after dispersing microbubbles in the solution.

Selection of the Anesthetic Solution

Selection of the most appropriate local anesthetic depends on the surgical indication, the expected duration of intense postoperative pain, and the postoperative location of the patient. Commonly administered local anesthetics and their usual doses are displayed in Table 27-5. Short-acting local anesthetics (lidocaine and mepivacaine) are preferred for outpatient surgery. Longer-lasting agents do not preclude hospital discharge, provided motor functions have been restored at least in part and on the condition that the familial environment is competent (i.e., caring and able to make sound judgments). Levobupivacaine and ropivacaine are preferred for continuous infusion or repeat/on-demand injections after a catheter has been inserted along a peripheral nerve or neuraxially to provide long-lasting pain relief. Additives may consistently improve the quality and duration of blockade. Nonopioid additives (clonidine, ketamine) are particularly useful because they have few (and minor) adverse effects, thus not precluding early hospital discharge, and they prolong postoperative pain relief without requiring catheter placement.

For decades, long-lasting postoperative pain relief depended exclusively on continuous epidurals and patient hospitalization. Recently, the development of peripheral catheter techniques has simplified the management of postoperative pain, offering a better risk–benefit ratio than continuous neuraxial blockade, and even allowing hospital discharge and management at home in selected patients. For these techniques, continuous infusion (2–5 mL/h) or on-demand injections (2–5 mL) of low-concentration levobupivacaine or ropivacaine (0.1%–0.2%) represent the best and safest choice.

Equipment

The required equipment to perform regional block in children is basically the same as in adults (see Chapter 8), and this holds particularly true for peripheral nerve blockade (single-injection as well as catheter techniques).

For neuraxial blocks, some notable differences must be considered. For obvious reasons, shorter and thinner needles must be used in infants. For epidural anesthesia, the Tuohy bevel is virtually the only bevel used in children. The recommended medium for the loss-of-resistance technique has elicited many controversies (100). Basically, in children over 6 to 7 years of age, use of normal saline offers the same advantages as in adults. Conversely, in infants and, particularly in neonates, air is the most dependable technique of identification of the epidural space. For spinal blocks, the bevel/tip of the needle does not have the same importance as in adults; the incidence of postdural puncture headache remains (very) low and is not influenced by the design of the needle tip (101,102). Most critical is the distance from the tip of the needle to the distal orifice of the lumen; this distance must be as short as possible to avoid leakage outside the dura mater if the needle is not advanced enough past the dura mater, and to avoid potential damage to the cauda equina if the needle is introduced too deeply. Consequently, pencil-point needles do not improve the overall quality of the procedure and are even suspected of decreasing the success rate by favoring subdural spread of the local anesthetic. The most commonly used devices for regional block procedures in the pediatric patient are listed in Table 27-6.

Technique of Injection

The technique of injection is a critical factor of safety. Meticulous technique must be systematically followed:

1. Perform an aspiration test prior to any injection to verify the absence of blood reflux (or CSF reflux during an epidural).
2. Check cardiac monitoring during and after the injection of a test dose (0.1 mL/kg up to 3 mL) of a solution containing 0.5 to 1 μg/kg of epinephrine for 30 to 60 seconds; any elevation of ST segment or increase in T-wave amplitude (103–107), followed by an increase in blood pressure (108), but only inconstantly by tachycardia, suggests accidental IV injection and requires cessation of the procedure. When epinephrine is contraindicated, isoproterenol (0.05–0.1 μg/kg) should be used instead.
3. Inject the local anesthetic slowly (<10 mL/min) (109) to prevent high peak plasma concentration in case of accidental IV injection.
4. Stop any injection if unusual resistance is felt, to prevent potential intraneural injection.
5. Repeat aspiration tests during injection (every 5 mL) and prior to any catheter reinjection to help verify that the tip of the needle/catheter has not moved into a vessel (or through the dura mater).

TABLE 27-6

RECOMMENDED DEVICES FOR MOST REGIONAL BLOCK PROCEDURES IN PEDIATRIC PATIENTS

Technique	First option	Alternate device
Intradermal wheals	Intradermal needles (25 gauge)	–
Infiltrations and field blocks	Standard IM needles (21–23 gauge)	Intradermal needles (25 gauge)
Compartments blocks (fascia iliaca, ilioinguinal/iliohypogastric nerve, penile, rectus sheath, pudendal nerve blocks)	22- or 20-gauge Tuohy needle	Straight short (25–50 mm) and short bevel (45–55 degree) needles 22-gauge neonatal spinal needle
Peripheral mixed nerve blocks and plexus blocks	Insulated 21–23 gauge short bevel needles of appropriate length connected to a nerve stimulator (0.5–1 mA) Specific catheter (for continuous techniques)	Unsheathed needles with the same characteristics connected to a nerve stimulator (0.5–1 mA) Epidural catheter (for continuous techniques)
Spinal anesthesia	25- or 24-gauge spinal needle (30, 50, or 100 mm long) with Quincke bevel and stylet)	22-gauge neonatal lumbar tap needle (30 mm long) Whitacre spinal needle
Caudal anesthesia	25-gauge short (25–30 mm) and short-bevel (45-degree) needle with stylet	23-gauge short (25–30 mm) and short-bevel (45-degree) needle with stylet Pediatric epidural needle 22- or 20-gauge intravenous cannula
Epidural anesthesia	Tuohy needle (22-, 20-, and 19/18-gauge); LOR[a] syringe and medium; Epidural catheter	Crawford, Whitacre or Sprotte epidural needles appropriately sized; LOR[a] syringe and medium; Epidural catheter

[a]LOR, loss of resistance.

Patient Monitoring during the Block Procedure

Regional anesthesia is an anesthetic procedure. As such, it must be performed by anesthesiologists in an operating room environment with the usual monitoring recommended for any general anesthesia—monitoring of electrocardiogram (ECG), blood pressure, temperature, respiratory rate, oxygen saturation by pulse oximetry and, in patients (especially infants) under assisted ventilation, evaluation of tidal volume and end-tidal CO_2. An IV line must be established prior to any injection of local anesthetic (110), and vitals parameters are to be reported on the anesthesia chart (see Chapter 8).

Assessment of the Block

The quality and distribution of blockade must be evaluated prior to surgery, whatever the patient's age. This evaluation is not easy even in conscious children in the absence of a motor block. It requires that the anesthesiologist has gained the confidence of the child, prevents the child from seeing what he is doing (especially handling of needles), and makes comparative tests in nonblocked areas. Gentle skin pinching is the most dependable technique of sensory testing, especially in lightly anesthetized patients. Electrical stimulation using a nerve stimulator proved to be suitable in healthy volunteers (111,112) but little data are available in children.

Awake versus Asleep Block Placement

Regional blocks can be performed without sedation on cooperative and unpremedicated children (113). However, for elective surgery, children usually should be unconscious during the block procedure. If general anesthesia is not contraindicated for medical reasons, light general anesthesia can be safely used to perform a regional block and is widely accepted in pediatrics (69). In a large multicenter prospective study, only 23 rather minor adverse effects out of 24,000 regional procedures in children were noted, thus confirming the safety of combined regional and general anesthesia (68). A parallel study conducted during the same period in fully awake adult patients reported a similar rate of complications, the severity of which was, however, considerably greater, with several cases of permanent neurologic damage and deaths (114).

Performing a regional block in an anesthetized patient is usually considered unsafe in adults based on case reports (115–117), mainly related to thoracic epidural anesthesia (118). A study involving placement under general anesthesia of a lumbar epidural catheter in 4,298 consecutive adult patients did not report any severe complication (119), thus showing that, in adults too, the combined technique is an acceptable option. However, the real question does not pertain to the safety of the technique but to the benefits expected (relative to the risks) from such a combination (120).

In pediatrics, many reasons make the performance of regional blocks under light general anesthesia mandatory. Young children who have not acquired complete body image cannot grasp the concept of paresthesia. Additionally, whether peripheral nerve trunks and spinal roots have an intrinsic network of sensory innervation, the spinal cord, as well as the brain, does not have sensory nerve supply: Puncturing the spinal cord or the brain is asymptomatic (which allows stereotactic surgery in awake patients) whether or not the child is awake (this applies to adults patients too) (121); conversely, sticking a root or a nerve trunk elicits excruciating pain resulting in an immediate awakening reaction provided the child is lightly anesthetized with no muscle relaxant. Additionally, the background of several decades of placement of epidural catheters and performance of regional blocks under general anesthesia meets the criteria of evidence-based medicine for safe practice.

A further point to be considered is the cooperation of the child, which is not easy to obtain; the occurrence of a panic attack at a critical step of a block procedure can be extremely detrimental. Therefore, all potentially dangerous procedures (interscalene block, thoracic epidural, paravertebral block, etc.) should not be attempted on unanesthetized patients, even if apparently cooperative, because at any time this cooperation may disappear and result in severe damage, as has even been reported in adults (122). In emergency conditions, when it is mandatory to provide pain relief without risking compromising the physical status (especially respiratory and cerebral) of the patient, a regional block offers the best risk–benefit ratio when applicable. In these circumstances, most children experiencing severe pain usually agree to the performance of the block technique while being fully conscious or only lightly sedated.

In conclusion, available data do not show an increase of morbidity when a regional block is performed on an anesthetized child. Conversely, the overall morbidity could be decreased by the combined technique for several reasons: prevention of the potential damages resulting from a loss of behavioral control during the block procedure; and avoidance of the hemodynamic and respiratory complications of deep general anesthesia, provided the associated general anesthetic is light (i.e., without muscle relaxants and with no more than 0.5 MAC of halogenated agents or equivalent IV agents).

The combined technique might also offer psychological benefits, even though difficult to establish, as many children fear needle puncture. In practice, the only pending question pertains to the criteria of "adulthood": At what age a young patient is still managed as a child or as an adult.

Complications

Complications of regional block procedures are basically the same in children as in adults (see Chapters 12 and 20). Schematically, three main categories of complications exist: local, regional, and systemic.

Local Complications

Local complications can result from several conditions: incorrect needle placement and traumatic damage of various anatomic structures; injection of a toxic solution, including epinephrine, which may lead to severe tissue ischemia and gangrene if erroneously injected close to a terminal artery; tissue coring (nonstyletted epidural/spinal needle) that could result in delayed development of an epidermoid tumor in the spinal canal (123); and leakage of the local anesthetic around the insertion point through which a catheter was inserted, which may result in (partial) failure of the technique and bacterial contamination.

All these local complications are considered avoidable by using adequate devices and applying standard precautions (appropriate dressing and bacterial precautions).

Regional Complications

Regional complications are usually a direct consequence of nerve blockade; they develop mainly after neuraxial blocks (e.g., urinary retention, hypoventilation secondary to respiratory muscle paralysis, total spinal anesthesia after unrecognized dural puncture, use of neuraxial narcotics). Occasionally, an asymptomatic or undiagnosed condition (vascular malformation, tumor, tethered cord) can suddenly decompensate during the block procedure (intracranial hypertension, spinal/epidural hematoma, paraplegia).

Systemic Complications

Systemic complications result from an accidental intravascular injection of local anesthetic or, rarely, from a major overdose (12,124). They can be life-threatening and should be managed in the same way as in adults. The major difference between adults and children is that cardiac complications are concomitant with, not preceded by, cerebral signs of toxicity (125).

Postoperative Monitoring and Discharge Criteria

Monitoring in the Recovery Room

After combined regional and general anesthesia, all pediatric patients must be monitored in the recovery room in the same way as following any general anesthetic. The stability of the respiratory and hemodynamic status of the patient must be carefully checked, as well as return to consciousness and adequate responsiveness to nursing care. The quality of analgesia has to be evaluated as precisely as possible using a scoring system, and pain medication should be administered in a timely manner (preferably prior to pain return).

In addition to this standard postanesthetic care, patients under regional blockade require evaluation of the anesthetized area. If motor blockade is present, it should correspond to the expected anatomic distribution according to the block procedure performed. Motor blockade, which is rarely needed by the surgeon, should be avoided as much as possible because it is poorly tolerated by children, making them (and their parents) anxious and agitated. Giving appropriate explanations with a comforting attitude often helps them more than administering sedatives, which may further delay discharge from the recovery room. Patient positioning must be carefully and regularly checked to avoid pressure points, and the anesthetized areas must be protected. This protection, however, should not prevent adequate monitoring, especially in children at risk of compartment syndrome (see earlier discussion).

Urinary retention can be of concern in patients under neuraxial blockade. Although some institutions do not object to discharging children without checking their ability to void, other authors recommend ultrasound bladder monitoring, especially following hypospadias repair (the incidence of urinary retention is greater than usual in this surgery [126]).

Bypassing the recovery room is common practice in adult patients operated on under regional anesthesia only. Even if no sedative or general anesthetic has been administered to the pediatric patient, it is not wise to avoid the benefits of the monitoring provided in a recovery room, both for medical and psychological reasons. Especially in infants who have undergone a short-duration procedure, the plasma peak concentration of the local anesthetic may not be reached yet at the end of the surgery (see the earlier discussion on pharmacology), and the sudden cessation of external stimulation may unmask some compensated adverse effects (hemodynamic and respiratory especially). Adequate monitoring and skilled assistance proved to be critical factors of improvement in immediate postoperative incidents (127).

Discharge from Hospital after Single-injection Procedures

In the absence of motor blockade, discharge from the recovery room relies mainly on the same discharge criteria as following general anesthesia (pediatric adaptation of Aldrete score or specific pediatric score in use in the relevant institution); usually, these patients can be discharged within 15 to 30 minutes.

In case of motor block, discharge should not be permitted before evidence of at least partial motor function restoration. Boisterous children or with a family unable to take appropriate care of them should not be allowed to return home before complete restoration of motor function. On the other hand, reasonable children and those whose family is both responsible and able to understand the limitations and hazards due to the lack of control on some parts of the patient's body are eligible to hospital discharge after partial return of motor function.

Persistence of sensory blockade (without motor blockade) is not a contraindication to early discharge unless the familial environment is inadequate. Systemic analgesics should be systematically prescribed and administered on a regular basis to prevent the return of intense pain at home, when the sensory block is no longer effective (128).

Most additives do not preclude early discharge. However, children given epidural/intrathecal opioids, especially morphine, are not eligible for outpatient surgery and should stay overnight at the hospital.

Continuous Techniques

Catheter techniques have long been considered only in hospitalized patients, either on the ward or even in intensive care units. Typically, only continuous neuraxial blocks must be hospitalized and require close monitoring, especially for respiratory depression. Although selected patients, especially in a context of chronic pain or some forms of cancer pain, can be treated at home but, most of the time, even if no opiates are administered neuraxially, children (especially infants) are maintained hospitalized for the 48 to 72 hours during which they need the epidural, the more so as other treatments and wound dressings are usually necessary.

Continuous peripheral nerve blocks are rather new techniques in the field of pediatric pain management (129). In most institutions, pediatric patients undergoing this technique are maintained hospitalized for safety reasons. A closed and non-modifiable system can be achieved by sterilely connecting a prefilled elastomeric pump to the catheter. If appropriately immobilized and protected, this system is very safe and compatible with early home return, provided both the patient and his family are "adequate."

NEURAXIAL BLOCKS

Caudal Anesthesia

Caudal anesthesia is the oldest and still most commonly used technique of epidural anesthesia via the sacral hiatus in children.

Anatomy

The sacral hiatus is a V-shaped aperture formed by the lack of dorsal fusion of the vertebral arches of the fifth (and fourth, usually) sacral vertebrae. Its lateral borders are formed by two easily palpable bony structures, the sacral cornua. The sacral hiatus is covered by the sacrococcygeal membrane, which is the sacral continuation of the ligamentum flavum. The distance from the skin to the anterior wall of the sacral canal varies from 10 to 39 mm (mean 21 mm) in children ranging in age from 2 months to 7 years (130), which means that the epidural space can usually be entered through the sacrococcygeal membrane at a distance less than 20 mm from the covering skin. The distance from the upper border of the sacral hiatus to the dural sac in children aged 10 months to 18 years equals 30 ± 10.4 mm (range: 13.6 to 54.7 mm) (131). Consequently, caudal blocks should only be performed with short and short-bevel needles to reduce the risks of dural puncture. During infancy and early childhood, the axis of the sacrum changes, making the identification of the sacral hiatus more difficult.

Indications and Contraindications

Indications. Caudal anesthesia is recommended for the intraoperative and postoperative pain relief of many surgical procedures below the umbilicus level, including parietal surgery such as herniorrhaphies, digestive tract surgery (Hirschsprung disease, anorectal malformations, etc.), urinary tract surgery, and orthopedic surgery (pelvic girdle, hip, and lower extremities) (132,133). The technique can be performed on a conscious infant (after local infiltration of the skin), either as a single-injection technique (133–135) or after placement of a caudal catheter that allows reinjection or continuous infusion of local anesthetics (136,137). The technique is especially useful on the preterm baby of less than 60 weeks postconceptual age who is at major risk of postoperative apnea after general anesthesia.

A caudal catheter can be maintained postoperatively for pain relief; it can also be inserted over a long distance, especially in neonates and small infants, to reach higher segmental levels, including thoracic levels (138). Both indications are controversial due to the proximity of the anus and the danger of bacterial complications (139), especially in patients such as infants who have not acquired sphincter control. This technique has also been used for cardiac surgery in pediatric patients (140), but many do not consider it a safe practice in patients under anticoagulant therapy.

Specific Contraindications. Specific contraindications to caudal anesthesia include major malformations of the anorectal area and intracranial hypertension. Patients at risk of compartment syndrome require specific consideration and management (see earlier discussion). Patients presenting with a large intra-abdominal or retroperitoneal tumor usually have severe compression of the inferior vena cava; until the tumor has been completely removed, there is a risk of severe hemodynamic disorders caused by the sympathetic block and an increased risk of injury of engorged epidural veins. Additionally, the spread of local anesthetic in the epidural space is unpredictable due to pressure increase in the epidural veins. Extreme caution is recommended in the selection and volume of the local anesthetic. Some authors recommend delaying the technique until the end of surgery; others suggest placing the catheter, either via the caudal or, preferably, the lumbar route but avoiding administering local anesthetics before completion of the resection.

Technique

Two patient positions are suitable: the lateral decubitus with the patient lying on the side to be operated on, and, less common, the prone position either with a rolled towel slipped under the pelvis or, especially in awake preterm infants, with the patient's legs flexed in the so-called "frog-leg position." The two sacral cornua that delineate the V-shaped sacral hiatus are

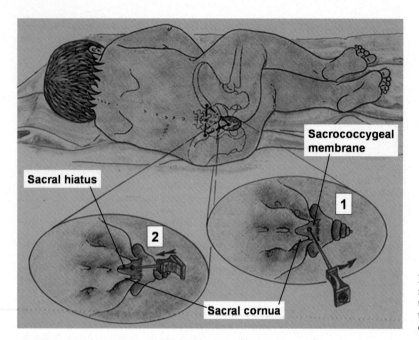

FIGURE 27-2. Caudal anesthesia landmarks and technique: *1*, insertion of the caudal needle at right angles to the sacrococcygeal membrane; *2*, cephalad redirection of the needle (no more than 2–3 mm, to avoid accidental dural mater penetration).

located by palpation of the spinal process line at the level of the sacrococcygeal joint (Fig. 27-2). Classically, the two posterior superior iliac crests and the sacral hiatus delineate an equilateral triangle but, in clinical practice, this assumptive statement does not help in locating the hiatus when palpation is not demonstrative.

Many techniques have been used. The safest approach consists of inserting the caudal needle at a right angle to the skin, close to the upper summit of the sacral hiatus. A resistance is felt as the tip of the needle contacts the sacrococcygeal membrane, then a loss of resistance when the membrane is pierced. Two millimeters of the needle tip should be introduced within the epidural space, either following the same insertion site or after redirecting the needle cephalad, avoiding contacting the anterior wall of the spinal canal before the stylet is removed and the local anesthetic is injected. With such an insertion route, the likelihood of penetrating the dural sac is minimized. The distance from skin to the sacral epidural space is hardly influenced by patient age or weight: It is almost always less than 20 mm (even in adolescents). As mentioned earlier, the distance from skin to the anterior wall of sacral canal (which must not be contacted), ranges from 10 to 39 mm (mean = 21 mm) (130). Years ago, injection of air ("whoosh test") or fluid ("swoosh test") and hearing a characteristic noise along the spine using a stethoscope (141) was recommended by some authors to verify the epidural positioning of the needle. This technique has led to severe complications and should no longer be used.

In experienced hands, especially when placement of a catheter is planned or if an IV cannula is used instead of a caudal epidural needle, the device can be inserted at a 45-degree angle to the skin, close to the summit of the sacral hiatus, until the sacrococcygeal membrane is crossed. Then, the stylet (or introducer needle) is removed and the catheter is introduced without kinking the cannula. In case of catheter placement, as for any epidural, the length of catheter introduced into the epidural space should not exceed 2 to 3 cm. Occasionally, some authors recommend inserting the catheter over a long distance, to reach high lumbar and even thoracic levels. This technique should be considered with extreme caution by experts only; the real position of the tip of the catheter must be controlled

because in 28% of cases it is misplaced (142). Confirmation is usually achieved by performing a radiograph after injecting a contrast medium, but other techniques are effective. Electrical stimulation (at rather high intensities up to 10 mA or above) can be used, but safety of this technique is not established (143,144). A comparison of ECG tracings using a five-lead cardioscope also may be used. An electrode is placed at the desired level of the spinous process line, the metallic wire is connected to the cardioscope, and an ECG tracing corresponding to the position of the tip of the wire that slightly emerges from the catheter ending is obtained. As the epidural catheter progresses upward, this ECG tracing increases in amplitude and becomes identical to that of the "normal" D2 tracing when the catheter tip reaches the level of the dorsal electrode (145). This method is very elegant and noninvasive; however, the "second" ECG tracing is not always easily readable. Ultrasound guidance is the most promising noninvasive technique, but it remains under evaluation.

Tunneling of the caudal catheter (146) theoretically decreases the risks of bacterial contamination but makes the technique more complicated (147).

Volume of Local Anesthetic

The selection of the local anesthetic and additives is made according to the principles detailed earlier. The optimal volume to be administered depends on the size (age and weight) of the patient, and mathematical formulas have been described. These rather complex methods of calculation have little interest in practice due to the considerable interindividual variability of local anesthetic spread within the epidural space. In practice, the prescription scheme of Armitage established many years ago remains the most dependable (148): 0.5 mL/kg constantly produces high sacral blockade; 1 mL/kg ensures high lumbar epidural blockade, and 1.25 mL/kg results at least in mid-thoracic epidural blockade.

Occasionally, the latter dose (1.25 mL/kg) results in excessive rostral spread (above T4) (149). It is therefore preferable to avoid injecting more than 1 mL/kg; if a thoracic level of analgesia is required, it is better to approach the epidural space at high intervertebral lumbar or low thoracic levels; alternatively, some authors recommend inserting a caudothoracic catheter.

Complications

Complications are infrequent, about 1 per 1,000 procedures (68) when a short-bevel needle is used, but the rate of vascular puncture may exceed 10% with a sharp needle (149). These punctures are usually minor, resulting from needle misplacement mainly into soft tissues (failure of the block) but occasionally into a vessel or the anterior wall of the sacral canal (systemic toxicity). If the needle is redirected too cephalad, there is a significant risk of dural penetration and subsequent spinal anesthesia. Penetration into the pelvis has been reported with the use of sharp needles that can easily cross the cartilaginous structure of sacral vertebrae.

Clinically relevant hemodynamic changes are unusual in young children; only patients older than 8 years of age may experience some degree of hypotension. However, epidural anesthesia elicits changes in regional blood flow distribution characterized by (a) an increase in pulmonary arterial resistance and descending aortic blood flow, and (b) a decrease in lower body vascular resistances (150,151). These effects compensate one another in healthy children but may occasionally result in severe hemodynamic disorders in patients with cardiac malformations (aortic stenosis and cardiopathies with intracardiac shunts).

Delayed postoperative voiding was an issue years ago when preoperative fasting was excessively prolonged but with current practices true urinary retention is (very) rare. Other complications include bacterial contamination (although epidural abscesses are rare), development of an inappropriate level of sensory block (too high, lateralized, or too low), and vomiting, which depends more on the general anesthetic given than on the caudal block. Complete failure of the block is not unusual (3 to 5%), especially in children over 7 years of age (108).

Epidural Anesthesia

Anatomy

Apart from obvious differences in size of anatomic structures, few anatomic particularities pertain to the epidural space in children. The most important ones (as previously mentioned) are (a) the progressive development of spinal flexures (as the infant matures, the orientation of the needle must be progressively adjusted up, to the second year of life, when "adult" needle orientation is required); (b) communication of the paravertebral and perineural space surrounding the spinal root, allowing leakage (and thus requiring comparative increases in the injected volume of local anesthetic to obtain an adequate upper limit of analgesia); and (c) the low density of connective fibers in subcutaneous tissues and ligaments—these structures offer little resistance to fluid injection, so that locating the epidural space using the loss-of-resistance technique with saline is unreliable in infants (152,153).

Indications and Contraindications

Indications. Epidural anesthesia is suitable and recommended for all major surgeries of the trunk, including thoracic surgery (154,155), pectus excavatum repair (156), and scoliosis surgery (157,158), but most indications are for surgery below the umbilicus (abdominal, pelvic, retroperitoneal, and lower limb

surgeries). Some authors recommend using the technique for cardiac surgery (159), but this indication is controversial due to the hazards of anticoagulation.

The intervertebral level at which the epidural space should be approached is a matter of debate. Most operations below the umbilicus for which a single-injection procedure is appropriate are performed under caudal anesthesia, especially in infants and children younger than 6 or 7 years of age. When long-lasting postoperative pain relief is required or for surgeries above the umbilicus, depending on local and cultural habits, two strategies are used: either approaching the epidural space below the ending of the dural sac and attempting to insert a long-distance catheter to reach a high lumbar or thoracic levels (caudothoracic catheter for example); or approaching the epidural space 2 to 3 cm below the upper limit of analgesia expected (i.e., including thoracic approaches) and inserting a catheter for no more than 2 to 3 cm.

The simplicity of the first strategy is only apparent, even misleading, because the catheter is misplaced in almost 30% of cases, even in experienced hands (142), and exposes the patient to potentially severe complications (bacterial contamination, traumatic insertion, breakage or nerve injury on removal of the catheter).

Specific Contraindications. In addition to above-mentioned contraindications to caudal anesthesia, specific contraindications to epidural anesthesia include severe malformations of the spine and the spinal cord, such as formerly operated spina bifida (not spina bifida occulta), intraspinal lesions or tumors, and, for most authors, tethered cord syndromes. Patients with a history of hydrocephalus or elevated intracranial pressure, those with reduced intracranial compliance, or with previous operations of the spine (especially with vertebral implants) are not ideal candidates for epidural anesthesia, but these disorders are not absolute contraindications (160).

Techniques

Lumbar Epidural Anesthesia. The epidural space is usually approached on the midline below L3 (i.e., below the conus medullaris), but a paramedian approach is possible and occasionally used in some patients (epidermal lesion on the midline, deformity of the spine). Basically, the procedure is the same as in adults provided an adequately sized epidural needle (typically with a Tuohy bevel) is used. The patient is usually placed in the lateral decubitus position, with the side to be operated lying lowermost and the spine bent to enlarge the interspinous spaces (Fig. 27-3). The sitting position can be used in awake patients (see also Chapter 11).

In infants, the most dependable loss-of-resistance technique is with gas (air or, preferably, CO_2) whereas in children older than 9 to 10 years of age, loss-of-resistance with saline is as reliable as in adults. The distance from the skin to the inner aspect of the ligamentum flavum is correlated with patient's age and weight (Fig. 27-4). The local anesthetic can be injected directly through the needle for single-injection procedures. However, most authors prefer that all injections be made through a catheter, whether or not this catheter is maintained for postoperative pain relief.

The required volume of anesthetic solution depends on the upper level of analgesia required for completion of the surgery, knowing that around 0.1 mL per year of age is necessary to block one neuromere (162). In daily practice, usual volumes of solution range from 0.5 to 1 mL/kg (up to 20 mL), which results in an upper limit of sensory blockade between T9 and T6 in more than 80% of patients. A single epidural injection is

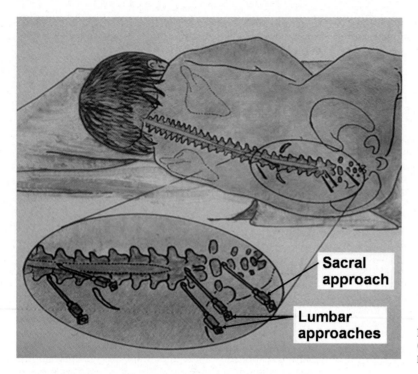

FIGURE 27-3. Epidural anesthesia: Sacral, lumbar (midline and paramedian), and thoracic (midline and paramedian) approaches.

appropriate for many pediatric surgeries, especially when adjuvants such as clonidine (1–2 μg/kg), preservative-free ketamine (0.25–0.5 mg/kg) and, in appropriate indications, morphine (30 μg/kg) are coadministered.

Major surgery and operations resulting in long-lasting postoperative pain are better managed with placement of an epidural catheter with postoperative infusion. The catheter should not be introduced more than 3 cm, to avoid buckling, knotting, lateralization of the block, or migration. Tunneling the catheter decreases the danger of accidental removal and bacterial contamination (161). Catheter insertion over a long distance should be directed using the same techniques as described for caudal catheters. When available, ultrasonographic guidance represents an excellent safety precaution in neonates and infants. As infants are more prone to develop systemic toxicity due to accumulation (see pharmacology section), infusion doses should not exceed 0.25 mg/kg/h in neonates and 0.325 mg/kg/h in infants aged 4 to 12 months. Usual infusion regimens are displayed in Table 27-7.

Sacral Epidural Anesthesia. Sacral epidural interspaces remain unfused at least up to 25 years of age; therefore, intervertebral approaches can be performed at sacral levels in the same way as at lumbar levels in children (Fig. 27-3). Usually, the S2–S3 interspace is identified by palpation 0.5 to 1 cm below the line joining the two posterior superior iliac spines (163). The epidural needle is inserted on the midline, midway between the S2 and S3 spines. As these spines are atrophic, the needle can be oriented upward or, preferably, downward, with the orifice of the Tuohy turned caudally. In this way, the convex part of the needle tip, instead of its cutting edge, faces the dural sac (which ends around this level), thus reducing the hazards of accidental dural penetration. Attention must be paid to the shorter distance from skin to the epidural space at sacral levels as compared to lumbar levels due to the opposite flexures of the spine at these levels.

Indications for sacral epidural blockade are virtually the same as those of caudal anesthesia. In infants, caudal anesthesia is usually preferred, whereas in children over 6 or 7 years of

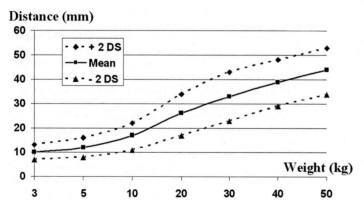

FIGURE 27-4. Distance from skin to the epidural space according to patient's weight.

TABLE 27-7

RECOMMENDED DOSES OF EPIDURAL SOLUTIONS IN CHILDREN

Local anesthetic	Single or first dose	Continuous infusion (maximum doses)	Repeat injections
Bupivacaine Levobupivacaine	Concentration: 0.25% with 5 μg/mL (1:200.000) epinephrine Volume: ■ <20 kg : 0.75 mL/kg ■ 20–40 kg : 8–10 mL or 0.1 mL × age (years) × number of neuromeres ■ >40 kg : As in adults	<4 months: 0.25 mg/kg/h (0.2 mL/kg/h) of a 0.125% (or 0.0625%) solution >4 months: 0.3–0.375 mg/kg/h (0.3 mL/kg/h of a 0.125% (or 0.0625%) solution)	Concentration: 0.25% or 0.125% Volume: 0.1–0.3 mL/kg every 6–12 h according to pain scores
Ropivacaine	Concentration: 0.2% Volume: Same as bupivacaine	Concentration: 0.2% Rate: Same as bupivacaine Stop infusion before the 36th hour in infants <3 months	Concentration: 0.2% 0.1–0.3 mL/kg every 6–12 h according to pain scores
Additives	<6 months: Avoid >6 months: Either ■ fentanyl 1–2 μg/kg ■ sufentanil 0.1–0.6 μg/kg ■ or clonidine 1 μg/kg	Concentration of adjuvant in the local anesthetic: ■ fentanyl 1–2 μg/mL ■ or sufentanil 0.25–0.5 μg/mL ■ or morphine 10 μg/mL ■ or hydromorphone 1–3 μg/mL ■ or clonidine 0.3–1 μg/mL de solution	Morphine: 25–30 μg/kg q8h

age, sacral epidurals are more reliable, require lower doses of local anesthetics and, when required, placement of an epidural catheter is safer than via the caudal route due to the increased distance from the anus.

Thoracic Epidural Anesthesia. As in adults, thoracic epidurals are less commonly performed than lumbar epidurals not only because of limited indications (thoracic and upper abdominal surgery) but also due to the fear of spinal cord damage.

In infants (up to 9 months), the technique is similar to the lumbar approach, with an insertion almost perpendicular to the spinous process line. When the flexures of the spine have developed, the technique is more similar to the midline adult approach, with an upward orientation of the Tuohy needle. The paramedian route can be used instead, but it is rarely necessary in children. The indications and risk–benefit ratio must be precisely evaluated, and the technique should only be performed by experienced pediatric anesthesiologists, typically on anesthetized children (to avoid irrelevant movements at the wrong time) (see also Chapter 11).

Thoracic epidurals are rarely single-injection procedures; a catheter is usually inserted (no more than 3 cm) to allow postoperative infusion of local anesthetic, which requires adequate monitoring by trained pediatric staff. In infants, ultrasonographic guidance is a valuable technique to assist the epidural approach and visualize the dura mater, progression of the needle, and position of the catheter in the epidural space (153).

Cervical Epidural Anesthesia. No indications exist for cervical epidural anesthesia for surgical purposes in pediatric patients. In some chronic pain patients, or in order to prevent phantom limb pain before an amputation of the upper arm at scapular level (osteosarcoma of humerus), a continuous cervical epidural can be considered. These rather rare indications concern mostly adolescents; the block technique and protocols are the same as in adult patients.

Specific Adverse Effects and Complications

Children may experience the same complications as adults (see Chapters 11 and 12). However, the overall rate of severe complications, such as spinal cord trauma, compressive hematoma, spinal ischemia, or severe hemodynamic disorders, is extremely low in children, including those in the neonatal period (68). Only complications related to catheter placement are more frequent than in adults: displacement (difficult draping and taping), leakage around the insertion site (discrepancy between the size of the Tuohy needle and that of the catheter), and occlusion of the infusion pump (high resistance due to the small size of the lumen). These complications usually do not harm the patient but result in a failure of the technique (inadequate pain relief).

Spinal Anesthesia

Anatomy

Apart from the size of the spinal cord and the spine, the main difference between infants and older patients pertains to the ending of the dural sac and the conus medullaris (Table 27-1). Another important feature is that the volume of CSF in infants (4 mL/kg) is twice that of adults (2 mL/kg); furthermore, the proportion of spinal CSF versus cerebral CSF is greater in infants (50%) than in adults (25%). This has a considerable pharmacokinetic impact as, basically, the equivalent dose of spinal local anesthetic is four times greater in infants and partly explains why the duration of a spinal block is much shorter in infants. Also, the hydrostatic CSF pressure in the dorsal recumbent position is significantly lower in neonates than in adults (164). This pressure is further decreased during general anesthesia. Even in conscious infants, this low CSF pressure must be considered while performing a spinal anesthesia. The spinal needle must be inserted slowly, to give enough time for the CSF reflux to become visible at the hub before the needle is further advanced.

TABLE 27-8

CLASSICALLY RECOMMENDED DOSES OF LOCAL ANESTHETIC FOR SPINAL ANESTHESIA IN CHILDREN

Local anesthetic	0–5 kg	5–15 kg	>15 kg
1% plain hyperbaric tetracaine			
dose (mg/kg)	0.5 mg/kg	0.4 mg/kg	0.3 mg/kg
volume (mL/kg)	0.05 ml/kg	0.04 ml/kg	0.03 ml/kg
1% hyperbaric tetracaine with epinephrine			
dose (mg/kg)	0.5 mg/kg	0.4 mg/kg	0.3 mg/kg
volume (mL/kg)	0.05 ml/kg	0.04 ml/kg	0.03 ml/kg
0.5% bupivacaine (hyperbaric or isobaric)			
dose (mg/kg)	0.5 mg/kg	0.4 mg/kg	0.3 mg/kg
volume (mL/kg)	0.1 ml/kg	0.08 ml/kg	0.06 ml/kg

In neonates and infants, most authors give twice the recommended doses (i.e., up to 1 mg/kg of either bupivacaine or tetracaine) to obtain adequate blockade (without adverse effects).

Indications and Contraindications

Indications. Spinal anesthesia is less used in children than in adults. Its main specific indication is for inguinal surgery in awake, preterm infants of less than 60 weeks post gestational age (165,166) because these patients are more prone to develop postoperative apnea following general anesthesia or even mild sedation (167). However, the performance of spinal anesthesia does not guarantee that the baby will not develop a potentially severe postoperative apnea (62,168,169). Therefore, in many institutions, these at-risk patients are maintained hospitalized overnight, although in some they are discharged on the same day (165). The technique is occasionally used in older children (170,171) but the benefits are less evident, even in young infants (172). In some developing countries, the technique is commonly used because it is the only available and safe anesthetic technique. A controversial indication of spinal anesthesia is for cardiac surgery (173) or cardiac catheterization (174).

Intrathecal opioids, especially morphine, provide long-lasting analgesia but may result in postoperative apnea (very rare with recommended doses) and other adverse effects of neuraxial opioids (rather frequent but easily treated with appropriate medications); the technique therefore should be restricted to major and painful operations (scoliosis surgery, upper abdominal and thoracic surgery) (175,176).

Continuous spinal anesthesia has few indications in pediatric patients, and most authors would consider intrathecal catheter placement contraindicated for postoperative acute pain relief even though the technique has been successfully used in open heart surgery (a particularly controversial indication) (177). Some chronic pain patients at terminal stages of fatal diseases (metastatic malignancies especially) may occasionally benefit from the technique (178).

Specific Contraindications. Spinal anesthesia has the same contraindications as epidural anesthesia. Additionally, the short duration of blockade often represents a limitation and even a true contraindication to the technique. The younger the patient, the earlier the restoration of neurologic functions occurs. In neonates, spinal anesthesia with bupivacaine (either hyperbaric or isobaric) rarely exceeds 45 minutes in duration, making the technique inappropriate for longer surgical procedures (bilateral hernia repair often takes more than 45 minutes, even in experienced hands).

Technique

Needle placement is easier when the infant is in the sitting position with an assistant to support the patient's chin to avoid upper airway obstruction. However, as most babies requiring the technique are very small and usually present with several associated disorders, the lateral decubitus is often preferred because it is safer. As mentioned earlier, CSF pressure is low, therefore the progression of the needle should be very slow to detect CSF reflux at the crossing of the dura mater.

Hyperbaric tetracaine and bupivacaine are most often selected, with isobaric bupivacaine as an alternative (170). Ropivacaine (179) and levobupivacaine (180) are not currently approved for spinal administration in pediatric patients. The usual doses of spinal local anesthetics are listed in Table 27-8.

Adverse Effects and Complications

Spinal anesthesia has several drawbacks. The failure rate is rather high, ranging from 10% to more than 25% in infants (167,168). The short duration of blockade is another important limitation that incites many authors to select an alternative procedure (awake caudal anesthesia) or use a complementary block (ilioinguinal/iliohypogastric nerve block); in the latter case, attention must be paid to the total dose of local anesthetic, to avoid hazards of systemic toxicity. A specific complication of the technique is the development of high spinal block (requiring tracheal intubation and assisted ventilation) due to repositioning/moving of the infant's legs (typically to stick a cautery pad on the dorsal aspect of the body). Other complications include those of epidural anesthesia. Postdural puncture headache is less frequent but not exceptional in children than in adults; the incidence might be increased by the use of pencil-point spinal needles (181).

CONDUCTION BLOCKS OF THE UPPER EXTREMITY

Anatomy

Brachial plexus anatomy is basically the same in children as in adults, but two particularities are of critical importance: the size of infants' head is comparatively larger and the neck shorter than in older patients, thus making access to the lateral aspect of the neck and supraclavicular part of the brachial plexus more difficult; and the apical part of the lung overpasses the upper limit of the thorax (plane formed by the first rib and the clavicle). As a result, supraclavicular approaches close to the subclavian artery are contraindicated as they directly threaten the apical pleura.

Indications and Contraindications

Indications

Brachial plexus blocks provide excellent analgesia for all painful procedures on the upper extremity, mainly orthopedic procedures. They can be used as the sole anesthetic technique in compliant children, especially in emergency/trauma conditions, with two provisions: all approaches are not equivalent in terms of safety, especially in younger patients; and several trauma conditions and surgical treatments are at risk for compartment syndrome. Monitoring of these patients is critical, as detailed earlier, and the local anesthetic must be selected to provide "standard" analgesia, not profound sensory or motor blockade.

Axillary block should be considered first due to its low morbidity and high reliability. More proximal approaches are considered only when axillary blocks are not suitable, either due to the distribution of anesthesia or to the required positioning of the arm for the technique when the danger exists of aggravating the lesions or producing intense pain. When a continuous technique is considered, securing and immobilizing the catheter is difficult at axillary levels; the paracoracoid infraclavicular approach or the parascalene supraclavicular represent the best options in this regard. Equally in awake as in anesthetized children, these techniques may benefit greatly from use of ultrasonographic guidance, although large series of pediatric patients have not been studied yet.

Specific Contraindications

Axillary blocks are contraindicated in the presence of local lesions in the axilla, especially lymph node lesions (malignancies, infections) or conditions that could be worsened by moving the arm in order to perform the technique (unstable fractures, extensive wound that could be contaminated, vascular or nerve lesions). Supraclavicular blocks must be avoided in case of respiratory insufficiency.

Techniques

Brachial Plexus Blocks below the Clavicle

At below-the-clavicle level, the brachial plexus consists of three cords surrounding the subclavian, then the axillary artery. Distal to the lower border of the pectoralis minor muscle, the axillary artery becomes the brachial artery, and the brachial plexus ends by giving off its terminal branches.

Axillary Blocks. The child is placed supine, with the relevant upper extremity abducted by 90 degrees, the elbow flexed at 90 degrees, and the forearm and hand supinated (Fig. 27-5). The landmarks are the axillary artery, and the pectoralis major and coracobrachialis muscles. Many insertion sites and routes have been described but, due to loose attachment of perineural fascias in children, the spread of the local anesthetic and the distribution of anesthesia do not differ. The most usual technique consists of inserting the needle at the upper border of the axillary artery, high in the axilla, with a 45-degree cephalad angulation, pointing to the middle of the clavicle. A click is usually felt at the crossing of the neurovascular sheath, and the lateral cord is usually the first to be identified (motor response in muscles of the forearm supplied by the median nerve).

An interesting particularity of the pediatric period is that the circumferential spread of the local anesthetic is excellent: Regardless of which cord the local anesthetic is injected into, the three nerves supplying the limb are almost always blocked (182), therefore multiple nerve localization is unnecessary. However, as in adults, the musculocutaneous nerve remains unchanged when it emerges from the brachial plexus sheath above the axilla, which occurs in 50% of patients approximately.

This limitation can be remedied by performing a transcoracobrachialis approach (183). The insertion site is located at the crossing of the coracobrachialis muscle with the lower border of the pectoralis major muscle (Fig. 27-5); a dimple often marks this crossing. The needle is inserted dorsally in direction of the medial border of the humerus, through the upper and lateral

PART III: APPLICATIONS

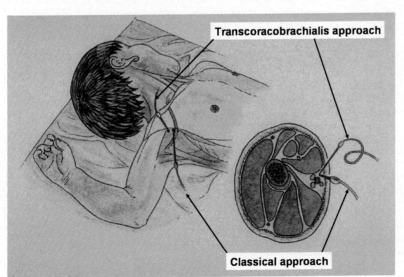

FIGURE 27-5. Axillary approaches to the brachial plexus (cords). *1:* Classical insertion route. *2:* Transcoracobrachialis approach.

TABLE 27-9

RECOMMENDED VOLUMES OF LOCAL ANESTHETIC FOR SINGLE-INJECTION PERIPHERAL NERVE BLOCKS

Block	≤10 kg	11–30 kg	31–60 kg	>60 kg
Brachial plexus block above clavicle	1 mL/kg	10 mL + 0.5 mL/kg above 10 kg	20 mL + 0.25 mL/kg above 30 kg	30 mL
Brachial plexus block below clavicle	0.5 mL/kg	5 mL + 0.25 mL/kg above 10 kg	10 mL + 0.15 mL/kg above 30 kg	15 mL
Lumbar plexus[a]	1 mL/kg	10 mL + 0.5 mL/kg above 10 kg	20 mL	20 mL
Femoral	0.75 mL/kg	7.5 mL + 0.3 mL/kg above 10 kg	14 mL + 0.25 mL/kg above 30 kg	25 mL
Fascia iliaca	1 mL/kg	10 mL + 0.5 mL/kg above 10 kg	20 mL + 0.25 ml/kg above 30 kg	30 mL
Proximal sciatic	1 mL/kg	10 mL + 0.5 mL/kg above 10 kg	20 mL + 0.3 mL/kg above 30 kg	30 mL
Popliteal fossa	0.3 mL/kg	3 mL + 0.15 mL/kg above 10 kg	6 mL + 0.15 mL/kg above 30 kg	12.5 mL

[a]Due to the possibility of epidural spread of the local anesthetic, it is recommended not to inject more than 20 mL of solution. Concentration to be determined in order to provide satisfactory blockade for both surgery and the postoperative course; see text.

part of the coracobrachialis muscle (within which runs the musculocutaneous nerve). The musculocutaneous nerve is usually stimulated first, then, a few millimeters farther, the lateral cord of the plexus. The local anesthetic is injected, then the needle is removed and 1 to 2 mL of local anesthetic is injected within the substance of the coracobrachialis muscle, whether or not the musculocutaneous nerve is identified. This technique can easily be performed with ultrasonographic guidance and does not require any modification, as the probe can be aseptically placed in the axilla with its major axis parallel to the path of the needle (see also Chapter 13).

Commonly used local anesthetic solutions are displayed in Table 27-9 (single-injection techniques) and Table 27-10 (infusion regimen). A catheter can be inserted in the neurovascular sheath for continuous infusion, but its immobilization is difficult and another approach is usually preferred, such as a paracoracoid or parascalene approach.

The morbidity of axillary blocks, whatever the technique used, is extremely low. The most common (albeit very rare) adverse effect is accidental vascular puncture (arterial, then venous). Transient vascular insufficiency, compressive hematoma and, very rarely, pneumothorax (after a very inappropriate insertion route) have been reported.

Infraclavicular Paracoracoid Blocks. Approaches to the brachial plexus cords close to the coracoid process of the scapula are performed with the patient in the dorsal recumbent position, with the ipsilateral arm lying alongside the thorax (183) (Fig. 27-6).

When neurostimulation only is used, the recommended insertion site is located 1 to 2 cm both caudally and medially to the lower border of the coracoid process, within or close to the lower extremity of the deltopectoral groove. The needle is inserted at a right angle to the skin until a motor response is elicited in the upper extremity; if no response is elicited, the needle should be removed and reinserted with a slightly medial insertion route. Either the lateral (motor response in forearm muscles supplied by the median nerve) or the posterior cord (extension of the fingers, usually) is contacted. Although in adults it is preferable to locate the posterior cord, this does not

TABLE 27-10

EFFECTIVE INFUSION RATES WITH OR WITHOUT BOLUS DOSES OF EITHER ROPIVACAINE 0.2%, BUPIVACAINE 0.125%, OR LEVOBUPIVACAINE 0.15–0.2% FOR CONTINUOUS PERIPHERAL NERVE BLOCKS

Techniques	Plexus and proximal conduction nerve blocks[a]	Axillary and popliteal blocks
Infusion rate	0.2 mL/kg/h up to 10 mL/h	0.1 mL/kg/h up to 5 mL/h
Bolus doses	0.2 mL/kg up to 5 mL	0.1 mL/kg/h up to 3 mL
Maximum bolus doses per hour	3	3

[a]Include supraclavicular and coracoid approaches to the brachial plexus, femoral nerve block, fascia iliaca compartment block, proximal approaches to the sciatic nerve. Personal data.

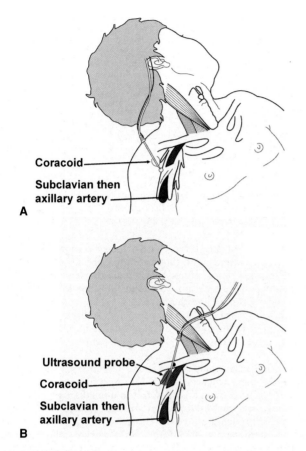

FIGURE 27-6. Infraclavicular approaches to the brachial plexus cords. **A:** Paracoracoid approach. **B:** Midclavicular approach with ultrasound guidance.

matter in children because the excellent circumferential spread of the local anesthetic results in complete blockade of all three cords.

With ultrasound guidance (184), an alternative insertion site just below the midpoint of the lower border of the clavicle is used (185,186) (Fig. 27-6). The subclavian vessels, plexus cords, ribs, and the pleura are first identified at the level of the coracoid process, while the probe is applied with its major axis perpendicular to the deltopectoral groove. Then, the probe is oriented with its major axis aligned with the deltopectoral groove and the neurovascular bundle (i.e., at a 45-degree angle to the lower border of the clavicle), and the block needle is inserted at a 45- to 60-degree angle to the skin and obliquely, toward the axilla, taking care to put in line the major axis of the probe and the shaft of the needle. Once the needle has penetrated the sheath, it is recommended that the nerve stimulator connected to the needle be switched on to verify that motor responses are elicited at appropriate intensities. Then, the (single) injection of the local anesthetic (Table 27-9) is made. A catheter can be inserted and easily secured at this level, allowing continuous infusion of local anesthetic postoperatively when mandatory (Table 27-10). Such infraclavicular approaches are of particular interest when catheter placement is indicated (187,188) because tunneling, draping, immobilizing, and protecting the catheter from accidental removal (especially in boisterous children) is particularly easy. However, these approaches are not as safe as the axillary approach (189–191).

Mid-arm Approach to Brachial Plexus Nerves. Separate blockade of the median, musculocutaneous, radial, and ulnar nerves has limited indications in pediatric patients because the circumferential spread of local anesthetic at the axillary level is excellent.

Brachial Plexus Blocks above the Clavicle

Depending on the level of blockade, different brachial plexus components are approached: roots at the upper part, then primary trunks, then divisions, and, occasionally, cords in the immediate proximity of the upper border of the clavicle. High approaches, such as the interscalene, result in high radicular distribution of anesthesia, meaning that anesthesia of the hand (except the thumb) and the whole medial part of the forearm and arm is often incomplete or absent. On the other hand, primary trunk blockade (as produced by the parascalene approach) results in a distribution of anesthesia more similar to that of peripheral nerve blockade but may miss the fibers deriving from the lower trunk (ulnar nerve and medial cord of the median nerve) or, rarely, the middle trunk (radial nerve).

Parascalene Supraclavicular Block. This approach (192) enters the interscalene space at a consistent distance from other structures such as the apical pleura (193), the carotid artery and superior vena cava, the spinal canal, and the stellate ganglion. It is performed with the child lying supine, his arm extended along the body and his head turned to the nonoperated side. A roll or a pillow is placed under the patient's shoulders to extend the neck, thus stretching and making more superficial the components of the brachial plexus (Fig. 27-7).

The landmarks are the midpoint of the upper border of the clavicle and the transverse process of C6, identified by palpation in the interscalene groove on the circular line passing over the cricoid cartilage. The insertion site is located at the junction of the upper two-thirds with the lower third of the line joining the skin projection of C6 process and the midpoint of the clavicle (Fig. 27-7).

The needle is inserted at right angles to the skin following a strictly anteroposterior insertion route until a motor response is elicited in the upper limb (usually in muscles supplied both by the musculocutaneous and the median nerves). The distance

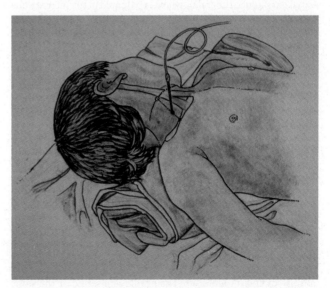

FIGURE 27-7. Parascalene to the brachial plexus (trunks).

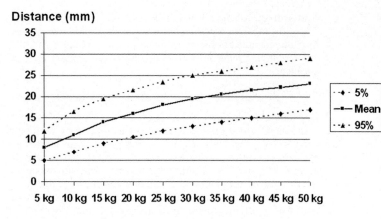

Distance (mm)

FIGURE 27-8. Distance from skin to the brachial plexus trunks via the parascalene approach.

to the primary trunks is correlated with the patient's age and weight, and it is closer than commonly believed, varying from 7 mm (±3 mm) in neonates to 25 mm (±6 mm) in large adolescents (Fig. 27-8).

A single injection of local anesthetic (Table 27-9) is often sufficient but, if needed, a catheter can be inserted in the interscalene space and left in place for repeat injections or continuous infusion (Table 27-10). If judged necessary, the correct positioning of the catheter can be verified either by radiograph, placement of a stimulating catheter, or by ultrasonographic guidance (which additionally allows the progress of the needle to be followed). The success rate of the technique is very high. Occasionally, part of or all the fibers from the lower cord (ulnar nerve and medial branch of the median nerve) remain unblocked.

Interscalene Supraclavicular Block. This approach enters the interscalene space at the junction of its upper and medial parts, close to the transverse process of C6. Ultrasound guidance assists with the overall safety of the technique (184) and allows its performance when nerve stimulation is not possible (194).

The child is placed in the supine position with his arm extended along the body and his head slightly turned opposite to the operated side. The landmarks are (a) the cricoid cartilage, and (b) the anterior ramus of the transverse process of C6 (Chassaignac tubercle), which is palpated in the interscalene groove. The insertion site is the intersection of the semi-circular line, passing over the cricoid cartilage, with the lateral border of the sternocleidomastoid muscle.

Classically, the block needle is inserted at an 80-degree angle (not perpendicularly) to the skin (i.e., dorsally and slightly caudad in direction to the C6 transverse process) until a motor response is elicited in the upper limb (Fig. 27-9). The distance to the roots of the brachial plexus is even less than with the parascalene approach. A catheter can be inserted for long-lasting pain relief. This approach has several drawbacks: It often produces ipsilateral phrenic nerve blockade and carries the risk of vascular damage (especially to the vertebral artery) and accidental cervical epidural/intrathecal penetration/injection. The distribution of anesthesia is radicular, involving C5, C6, and C7 spinal roots, but C8 and T1 often remain unblocked (hand and medial aspect of the arm and forearm remain unchanged). This technique is excellent for shoulder surgery, which is unusual in pediatric patients, but for more distal procedures a distal approach is preferred (see also Chapter 13).

A modified technique has been described in adults (195) and is suitable in children. The needle is inserted at the same site but following a lateral and caudal insertion route toward the midpoint of the clavicle until a motor response is elicited in the upper arm. Using this technique, the tip of the needle localizes the primary trunks at virtually the same place as the parascalene approach and results in the same safety, efficacy, and distribution of anesthesia.

Both interscalene approaches are suitable for single-injection procedure (Table 27-9) as well as for catheter placement (Table 27-10).

Other Supraclavicular Approaches. The interscalene space is quite extensive, thus many needle insertion sites and routes have been used. However, due to the immediate proximity of major vessels, nerves, and vital structures such as the apical pleura, approaches above the clavicle other than the two described here carry a significant risk of severe complications, which is not acceptable when safer options are available.

This limitation, however, may not apply to the posterior approach, as described in adults (196,197). No data are available in children, but the landmarks are easily and precisely identifiable (spinous process of the vertebra prominens and lateral border of the trapezius muscle) and the insertion route (ventral and caudal insertion in direction to a virtual point located 1–2 cm above the midpoint of the clavicle) does not threaten vital structures. Using this technique, the tip of the needle localizes the

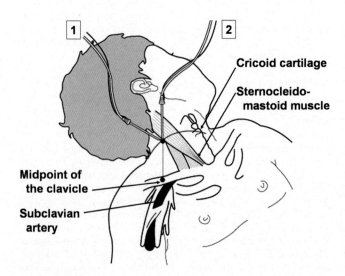

FIGURE 27-9. Interscalene approaches, respectively, to the brachial plexus: *1*, classical approach (roots); *2*, modified approach (primary trunks).

primary trunks at virtually the same place as the parascalene approach and results in a very similar distribution of anesthesia. The distance to the plexus is far greater than that of anterior approaches, and the technique has to be modified in anesthetized children as the sitting position is not suitable, but the lateral decubitus position with the head slightly flexed caudally is appropriate. One of the main interests in this approach (especially in patients undergoing amputation of the arm due to osteosarcoma of the humerus) is that a catheter (198) can easily be inserted at distance from the operative field and securely protected from accidental removal by the child.

Distal Nerve Trunk Blocks

In pediatrics, distal conduction blocks at the elbow or wrist are only complementary blocks of incomplete brachial plexus blocks. Percutaneous nerve location can be very helpful. Ultrasound guidance may be the safest technique, but requires an excellent ultrasound machine and profound knowledge of anatomy, as nerves and tendons look almost the same.

Metacarpal and Transthecal Blocks

Lesions of the finger, especially traumatic lesions, are common in children and often of minor importance. A digital ring block is virtually never used because the technique is very painful, requires several injections, and carries the risk of neurovascular damage, either by direct trauma or by ischemia (compression due to injection of the local anesthetic).

An elegant and easy alternative technique is the so-called "transthecal block" (199–202), which consists of injecting local anesthetic within the space limited by the tendon sheath that surrounds the synovial sheath of the flexor tendon of each digit. As the four digital nerves enter this space, a single injection is sufficient to block them all. Indications include all procedures on the last two phalanxes of any of the fingers.

The block can be performed on nonanesthetized children even though the puncture is somewhat painful, but less so than a digital nerve block. The hand is placed in the supine position and the head of the relevant metacarpal bone is located by palpation. A 25-gauge intradermal needle is inserted perpendicularly to the palm, right in the center of the skin projection of this metacarpal head (Fig. 27-10), until bone contact is made. The needle is then slightly removed to avoid subperiosteal injection, and the local anesthetic (1% or 2% lidocaine without epinephrine) is injected until resistance to injection is felt; at that point, the injection must be immediately ceased.

The size of this "intrathecal" space is very limited at the level of the index, middle, and fourth fingers, and the amount of local anesthetic required to fill it varies from 0.5 to 1 mL in small infants to a maximum of 3 mL in large adolescents. For both the fifth finger and the thumb, this space does not end proximally at the level of the head of the metacarpal bone but up to the wrist, thus requiring larger volumes of anesthetics. The distribution of anesthesia involves the whole ventral aspect of the relevant finger but only the dorsal aspect corresponding to the last two phalanxes. If surgery involves the proximal part of the finger, then a metacarpal block will provide adequate analgesia.

Metacarpal block consists of inserting a 25-gauge needle at right angles to the skin, both laterally then medially to the relevant head of the metacarpal bone, usually with the patient's hand in the prone position, while the anesthesiologist places his

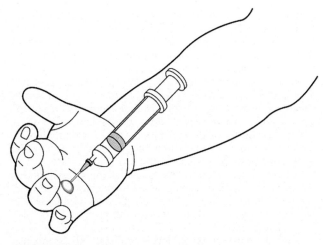

FIGURE 27-10. Digital transthecal block.

finger at the same level on the palmar aspect. When the tissue deformity produced by the tip of the needle is felt on the palmar aspect, the needle is immobilized and 1 mL of solution without epinephrine is injected while the needle is slightly withdrawn. In this way, the two ipsilateral digital nerves are blocked. The procedure is then repeated on the other side of the finger. This two-injection procedure provides quick and excellent analgesia. Although the morbidity is virtually nil, unfortunately, it is as painful as the classical four-injection technique for digital nerve blocks (see also Chapter 13).

CONDUCTION BLOCKS OF THE LOWER EXTREMITY

Anatomy

The main differences of anatomy between adults and children pertain to the size of the patient and the loose attachment of fascia to underlying structures. The major part of the lumbar plexus is located inside the psoas muscle, in the so-called "psoas compartment" that can be percutaneously approached. When they emerge from this compartment, all lumbar plexus nerves run a variable part of their course just below the fascia iliaca, which is the common aponeurosis covering the psoas and iliacus muscles. If a sufficient volume is injected at the inner surface of this fascia, all components of the lumbar plexus can be blocked at once. The sacral plexus cannot be easily approached, but does not have significant considerations unique to children.

Indications and Contraindications

Block of the Lumbar Plexus and Its Branches

Indications of femoral nerve blocks are frequent in pediatric patients. Because of its simplicity, efficacy, and safety, the fascia iliaca compartment block is of major interest in children with a fracture of the femoral shaft (203) as it improves their comfort, especially during transportation; allows pain-free physical and radiologic examinations, wound dressings, and orthopedic procedures; and reduces bleeding. The postoperative course of most elective surgeries on the thigh (soft tissues as well as orthopedic procedures) can be made pain-free with this technique, either after a single injection (with or without additives such as clonidine) or after catheter placement and repeat injections or continuous infusion (204,205).

Psoas compartment blocks have limited indications in children, and are mainly useful when a femoral block cannot be performed because of local lesions. Psoas compartment blocks can represent a valuable alternative to epidural anesthesia for unilateral surgeries on the upper part of the lower limb (hip and thigh), and catheter placement is both easy and very effective in relieving postoperative pain (206).

Saphenous nerve blocks have no indication, per se, but they are an excellent complement to sciatic nerve blocks to provide complete anesthesia below the knee without requiring the large amounts of local anesthetic necessary to produce a complete femoral nerve block.

Lateral cutaneous nerve blocks have few indications; they can be used (as well as femoral blocks) to perform muscle biopsies in conscious children (207). Obturator nerve blocks are occasionally used in children with cerebral palsy suffering from hypertonia of adductor muscles or in cooperative adolescents undergoing knee arthroscopy (as a complement of femoral and sciatic nerve blocks).

There are no specific contraindications to femoral nerve blocks, only general contraindications. Hazards of compartment syndromes require special attention and monitoring (see earlier discussion).

Blockade of Sciatic and Posterior Femoral Nerves

Sciatic nerve blocks are recommended for surgeries involving the leg (except its medial aspect), ankle, and foot. A catheter technique can be used to prolong the duration of pain relief (208); control of the position of this catheter is best achieved when using a stimulating catheter and/or ultrasound guidance (209). There are virtually no indications to specifically block the posterior femoral cutaneous nerve. If the dorsal aspect of the thigh must be anesthetized (tourniquet placement on the thigh, surgery of the posterior aspect of the thigh), a proximal approach to the sciatic nerve is appropriate.

As with lumbar plexus nerve blocks, there are no specific contraindications to sciatic nerve blocks, only general ones, and the hazards of compartment syndromes require special attention and monitoring.

Lumbar Plexus Nerve Blocks

Femoral Nerve Blocks

Femoral nerve blocks are performed with the child in the dorsal recumbent position, preferably with the ipsilateral limb slightly abducted (if possible). The landmarks are the inguinal ligament and the femoral artery. The insertion site is located 0.5 to 1 cm both below the inguinal ligament and lateral to the femoral artery. The block needle is inserted posteriorly, either perpendicularly to the anterior aspect of the thigh or, especially when a catheter has to be inserted, at a 45-degree angle in the cephalad direction, until a motor response is elicited in the quadriceps muscle. Then, local anesthetic is incrementally injected (Table 27-9). A catheter may also be inserted. Usual regimens of repeat injections/continuous infusions are displayed in Table 27-10.

Fascia Iliaca Compartment Block

The fascia iliaca compartment block technique consists of injecting local anesthetic at the inner surface of the fascia iliaca. Depending on the volume injected and the patient's age, the femoral, lateral cutaneous, and often the obturator nerves are blocked with a single injection (210). The technique is performed with the child lying supine. The landmark is the skin projection of the inguinal ligament (extending from the anterior superior iliac spine to the pubic spine), which is divided into three equal parts. The site of needle insertion is 0.5 to 1 cm below the junction of the medial two-thirds and the lateral third of this division (Fig. 27-11). The needle should have a short bevel and is inserted perpendicularly to the skin until a first (fascia lata) then a second (fascia iliaca) loss of resistance is felt. Local anesthetic is subsequently injected (Table 27-9) or a catheter is inserted for continuous infusion or repeat injections (Table 27-10) (211) (see also Chapter 14).

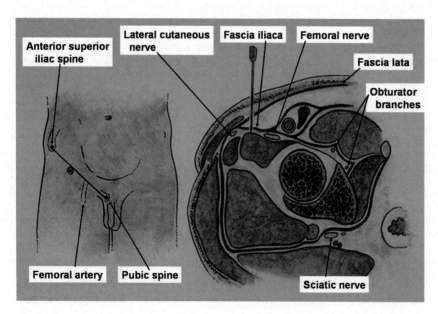

FIGURE 27-11. Fascia iliaca compartment block.

Complete Lumbar Plexus Block (Psoas Compartment Block)

The lumbar plexus can be percutaneously approached within its "psoas compartment" (212) through the quadratus lumborum muscle. The technique is performed with the child placed in the lateral decubitus position. The landmarks are the two iliac crests, ipsilateral posterior superior iliac spine, and L5 spinous process. Two insertion sites can be used: either the midpoint of the line joining the posterior iliac spine to L5 spine (modified Chayen approach) (213), or a point located on the intercristal line, 1 to 2 cm medial to the intersection of this line with the perpendicular line (214) drawn from the posterior iliac spine (Fig. 27-12) (modified Winnie approach). A slight variant consists of locating the puncture point at the union of the lateral third and medial two-thirds of the line extending from the L4 spinous process to the ipsilateral anterior superior iliac spine (215) (see also Chapter 14).

The needle is inserted perpendicularly to the skin until a motor response is elicited in the ipsilateral quadriceps muscle, and the local anesthetic is then injected (Table 27-9). A catheter may be inserted for long-lasting pain relief purposes (Table 27-10).

During the procedure, care must be taken not to direct the needle medially, to avoid damage to great vessels (abdominal aorta, vena cava, iliac vessels) and not to insert it too deeply to avoid damage to the kidney or to other retroperitoneal/intraperitoneal structures. In an attempt to evaluate the distance from skin to the psoas compartment, some authors recommend seeking bone contact (transverse process of L3, L4, or L5 spine), then redirecting the needle slightly below at the same depth or slightly farther. These variations of the technique have not been evaluated in children and appear to be more empiric than scientific (216). It would be safer to use a proper technique and anticipate the distance to the lumbar plexus using age- and weight-related measurements of this distance and an ultrasound-guided technique when possible (which is not always helpful, especially in obese children) (217).

The distribution of anesthesia is usually to those areas supplied by the femoral, lateral cutaneous, and obturator nerves. Occasionally, blockade may spread to the epidural or, very rarely, the subarachnoid space. Because of this potential side effect and the potential threat to intra-abdominal/pelvic organs, indications of this block are usually limited to unilateral operations of significant invasiveness to the hip, femur bone, and knee.

Saphenous Nerve Block

All saphenous nerve block techniques described elsewhere in this textbook (Chapter 14) for use in adults are applicable to children, albeit with the same rather high failure rate (around 30%). With the patient lying supine, the intersection of the upper border of the sartorius muscle and the femoral artery is identified. At this intersection, an insulated block needle is inserted posteriorly at a right angle to the skin, pointing to the lateral border of the artery until a motor response is elicited in the vastus medialis (not the rectus femoris). Injection of 0.1 to 0.2 mL/kg (up to 5 mL) produces a simultaneous block of the vastus medialis (motor) and the saphenous (sensory) nerves since both nerves are contained within a common sheath (Fig. 27-13).

Lateral Cutaneous Nerve Block

The lateral cutaneous nerve is often blocked during fascia iliaca compartment block. Occasionally, this nerve can be individually blocked before performing a muscle biopsy. Two techniques have been specifically evaluated in pediatric patients. The first technique uses the same landmarks and insertion route as for a fascia iliaca compartment block, but only one loss of resistance is sought. At that point, two-thirds of the local anesthetic is injected fan-wise at the inner surface of the fascia lata;

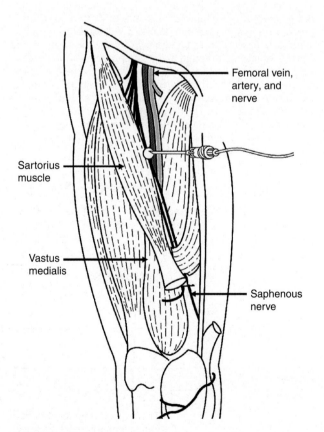

Femoral vein, artery, and nerve

Sartorius muscle

Vastus medialis

Saphenous nerve

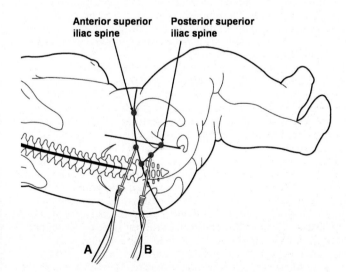

Anterior superior iliac spine   **Posterior superior iliac spine**

A   B

FIGURE 27-12. Direct lumbar plexus blocks. **A:** Modified Winnie approach. **B:** Modified Chayen approach.

FIGURE 27-13. Saphenous nerve block by approaching the vastus medialis motor nerve.

the needle is withdrawn subcutaneously, where the last third is similarly injected (218). Another technique consists of inserting the needle posteriorly, at a right angle to the skin, above the inguinal ligament and immediately medial to the anterior superior iliac spine until a loss of resistance is felt as the needle penetrates the aponeurotic canal containing the nerve (219).

Obturator Nerve Block

Obturator nerve block is infrequently performed in children. The safest technique consists of approaching the two division branches of the nerve below the inguinal ligament and just medial to the lateral border of the adductor longus muscle (220), which is easily palpable on the medial part of the anterior aspect of the thigh, giving the feeling of a groove. The block needle is inserted posteriorly at a right angle to the skin: A first series of motor responses corresponding to the anterior branch of the nerve is elicited in adductor muscles. The needle must be inserted deeper (5–12 mm) until a second series of motor responses corresponding to the stimulation of the posterior branch is elicited (this second branch is important, as it conveys sensory innervation to the knee joint). A 2 to 5 mL volume of local anesthetic is injected close to each of these branches (preferably beginning with the posterior branch, then the anterior branch on removal of the block needle) to anesthetize all obturator nerve fibers (see also Chapter 14).

Sciatic Nerve Blocks

Popliteal Sciatic Nerve Blocks

The sciatic nerve can be easily and safely blocked in the upper portion of the popliteal fossa, where its two constitutive branches separate from one another. All techniques used in adults are applicable to children; however, the simplest one consists of placing the child in the semiprone position (Sim position) with the unblocked side down (221). The landmarks are the tendon of the biceps femoris muscle laterally, and the tendons of the semimembranosus and semitendinosus muscles medially (Fig. 27-14). The needle insertion site lies at the point where the tendons become adjacent at the upper summit of the popliteal fossa. The block needle is inserted into the center of

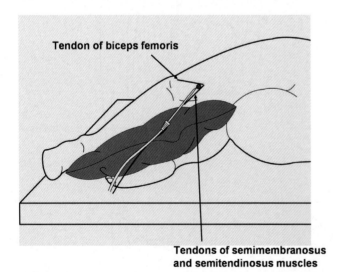

Tendon of biceps femoris

Tendons of semimembranosus and semitendinosus muscles

FIGURE 27-14. Popliteal sciatic nerve block (posterior approach).

this dimple, either at a right angle to the skin or cephalad, at a 45- to 60-degree angle to the skin, until a motor response in the ankle or foot is elicited. A local anesthetic is then injected (Table 27-9), and prolonged pain relief is usually produced (12 hours, occasionally 18 hours with bupivacaine) (222). When needed, especially for club foot or hallux valgus surgery, a catheter can be inserted, which is remarkably easy at this level (Table 27-10).

Proximal Sciatic Nerve Blocks

Proximal approaches to the sciatic nerve are used less commonly than the popliteal fossa in elective surgery but, in emergency procedures, the lateral approach or, occasionally, the anterior approach, are preferred as they do not require mobilization of a patient in pain with a broken leg or other foot, ankle, or leg lesions (223,224). These techniques are performed in children in the same way as they are in adults. Catheter placement allows long-lasting pain relief. Ultrasound guidance may help in locating the nerve (209) (see also Chapter 14).

Metatarsal and Transthecal Blocks

The principles sustaining metacarpal and transthecal blocks are valid for anesthetizing the toes. The landmark is the head of the first metatarsal bone. However, performing a transthecal block is comparatively more difficult than at the level of the hand in small infants. Conversely, metatarsal blocks are easier (but painful in awake children): A standard needle is inserted at the dorsum of the foot, close to the medial then the lateral border of the base of the first metatarsal bone until the tenting produced by the tip of the needle is perceived by palpation at the sole of the foot (225). A volume of 1 to 3 mL of 0.25% to 0.5% plain bupivacaine or ropivacaine is injected while the needle is slowly removed (see also Chapter 14).

BLOCKS OF NERVES SUPPLYING THE TRUNK

Intercostal Nerve Block

Intercostal nerve blocks can be used to provide pain relief for pleural drainage, management of rib fractures, liver transplantation and, in some institutions, for relieving postthoracotomy pain (226), especially via a catheter that allows continuous infusion (see also Chapter 16).

The landmarks are the mid-axillary line and the lower borders of the ribs, corresponding to the intercostal nerves to be blocked. A 22- or 20-gauge (depending on the patient's size) Tuohy needle is connected to a prefilled syringe via a short extension line and is prepared prior to draping. The insertion sites are identified slightly below (2 mm) the crossing of the midaxillary line with the lower border of the relevant ribs. The Tuohy needle is then inserted posteriorly and cephalad at each insertion site, at an 80-degree angle to the chest while continuous pressure is exerted on the barrel of the syringe (as for an epidural). A loss of resistance is felt as the intercostal space is entered: The local anesthetic is then injected slowly (1 mL of 0.125%–0.25% bupivacaine, ropivacaine, or levobupivacaine). Pain relief lasts from 8 to 18 hours. Longer duration of pain relief can be obtained by inserting a catheter into the intercostal space, centering on the area to maintain anesthetized (this catheter can also be installed under visual control by the surgeon at the end of the surgery) (227,228).

The technique has several limitations. It requires several punctures, thus increasing the failure rate and danger of pleural penetration. Absorption from the intercostal space is high, almost equivalent to an IV injection, which means that the hazards of systemic toxicity are significant (229). Only diluted local anesthetic must be injected and, if epinephrine is added, care must be taken not to inject more than 4 μg/kg to avoid significant hemodynamic changes (see Chapter 16).

When a large volume of local anesthetic is injected in a single intercostal space, the solution can spread to adjacent ipsilateral but also contralateral intercostal spaces (via the paravertebral space). The solution may also reach the epidural space. This unpredictable spread of local anesthetic, in addition to the danger of pneumothorax, requires that the child remains hospitalized.

Interpleural/Intrapleural Block

The technique of interpleural (or intrapleural) block consists of injecting a local anesthetic between the two sheaths of the pleura—that is, within the interpleural space—without creating a pneumothorax. This technique elicited some interest a decade ago, in an attempt to provide pain relief following thoracotomy, but contradictory results were reported. For postthoracotomy pain, it proved to be the least effective technique of analgesia, and it cannot be recommended in pediatric patients (230) (see Chapter 16).

Paravertebral Thoracic Space Block

During the last two decades, thoracic paravertebral blocks have elicited a number of applications, including in the pediatric population (231,232). The advantages of this approach are that it avoids thoracic approaches to the epidural space and it provides unilateral analgesia of the chest that can be prolonged for days following catheter placement and infusion of a local anesthetic.

The technique is basically the same in children and in adults (see Chapters 14 and 16). The child is placed in the semiprone position, resting on the nonoperated side. The spinous processes of T4–T6 are identified by palpation. Needle insertion is located 1 to 2 cm lateral to one of these spinous processes. The needle is inserted at right angles to the skin until contact is made with the relevant transverse process. It is then "walked" upward along the surface of this process until the costotransverse ligament is pierced, which gives a loss-of-resistance feeling, and a motor response is elicited in relevant intercostal muscles. A catheter may be inserted for 2 to 3 cm (with some difficulties most of the time), and the local anesthetic is injected (starting dose of 0.5 mL/kg of 0.25% bupivacaine, ropivacaine, or levobupivacaine) followed either by reinjection of half these doses or a 0.25-mL/kg/h continuous infusion of the same local anesthetic.

As in adults, the endothoracic fascia probably plays a major role in the spread of the local anesthetic (233,234). Spread to the lumbar paravertebral space and also to the abdominal cavity (through the medial and lateral arcuate ligaments) (235), the epidural space, and the contralateral thoracic paravertebral space (236) is frequent. In spite of these variations, the failure rate is rather low (237).

Complications include pleural penetration, dural puncture, seizures due to accidental vascular injection, and thoracic epidural spread causing Horner syndrome (238,239). Pharmacokinetic studies show a biphasic absorption of the local anesthetic, the first phase of which is equivalent to an IV injection (240); addition of epinephrine decreases peak plasma concentration.

Rectus Sheath/Periumbilical Block

The rectus sheath/periumbilical block procedure consists of injecting local anesthetic within the substance of the rectus abdominis muscle, where the terminal branch of the tenth intercostal—which supplies sensory innervation to the periumbilical area—courses (241,242). The muscle aponeurosis cannot be traversed by ionized molecules, thus forming a closed compartment within which the local anesthetic distributes easily. The technique is recommended for intra- and postoperative analgesia of periumbilical surgery, especially umbilical hernia repair. It can be adapted by moving the insertion site to the relevant level to provide analgesia to any repair of hernias of the linea alba. An adult study (gynecologic surgery) reported good postoperative analgesia after laparoscopic surgery (243) (see Chapter 16).

The technique is performed with the child in the supine position. The landmarks are the lateral borders of the rectus abdominis muscle on each side of the abdomen or, when they cannot be clearly identified, a parallel line to the midline drawn 2 to 3 cm lateral to the linea alba. Two insertion sites are identified, one per side, at the crossing of these lines with the perpendicular line passing over the center of the umbilicus (Fig. 27-15). A short-bevel needle is inserted medially at a 60-degree angle to the skin, in the direction of the upper border of the umbilical ring, until the rectus sheath is contacted (a strong resistance is felt), then penetrated. A typical "crack" is often perceived at the same time as a loss of resistance is felt.

The local anesthetic (0.5% bupivacaine, ropivacaine, or levobupivacaine) is then injected (0.2 mL/kg per side) in a fan-wise manner. Some authors recommend injecting half the dose at the upper border and half at the lower border of the umbilical ring, then injecting a small amount (1 mL) subcutaneously while the needle is withdrawn (242). The technique is then repeated on the other side. An ultrasound-guided technique was recently reported (244); it allows precise identification of the rectus aponeurosis and visible spread of the local anesthetic, but has no other advantage in terms of reliability or safety as compared to the "blind" technique.

The success rate of the technique is extremely high and, unless a sharp needle is used, the morbidity is minimal because the inner part of the rectus fascia offers the same resistance as the

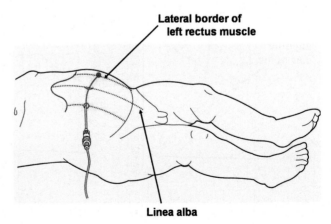

Lateral border of left rectus muscle

Linea alba

FIGURE 27-15. Periumbilical or rectus sheath block.

outer part and cannot be accidentally traversed. Occasionally, especially when the technique is first introduced, the surgeon might complain of "edema" at skin incision but, with experience, will see this as an aid to the identification and dissection of the different fascial planes.

Block of Ilioinguinal, Iliohypogastric Nerves and Genital Branch of Genitofemoral Nerves

Blocking these three nerves provides complete analgesia of the inguinal area including the spermatic cord, thus providing anesthesia and analgesia for virtually all surgeries in this region, especially inguinal hernia, hydrocele of the cord, and undescended testis. The classical technique requires three injections, two at the level of the anterior superior iliac spine and one at the level of the pubic spine. This multi-injection technique can be used in children, but its failure is quite high (245) and there is a potential danger of damaging an intestinal loop (in case of hernia) or an undescended testis at the level of the pubic spine. Use of an ultrasound probe to identify the nerves improves the safety and reliability of the technique close to the iliac crest, but does not prevent the potential injury resulting from the insertion at the level of the pubic spine.

Many pediatric anesthesiologists only perform a two-injection technique near the anterior superior iliac spine, aiming to block the ilioinguinal and the iliohypogastric nerves only. Not surprisingly, the quality of analgesia produced is often unsatisfactory, as sensory supply by the genital branch of the genitofemoral nerve remains unchanged. The contribution of the genitofemoral nerve can be very limited; in these cases, more or less, an ilioinguinal/iliohypogastric nerve block effectively reduces postoperative pain. If this sensory contribution is significant, or if the child has a lower threshold of pain perception, then the technique is not adequate.

A simplified technique takes advantage of the close proximity, in the same fascial plane, of the three nerves close to the subcutaneous inguinal ring formed by the aponeurosis of the external oblique muscle and giving passage to the spermatic cord (round ligament in girls). With the patient in the dorsal decubitus position, the umbilicus and ipsilateral anterior superior iliac spine are localized. The site of insertion lies on the line joining the two landmarks, at the union of the lateral one-

third and the medial two-thirds (Fig. 27-16). A short-beveled needle (a 22- or 20-gauge 50-mm long epidural needle is the best option) is inserted posteriorly and caudally in the direction of the midpoint of the inguinal ligament, until the superficial layer of the aponeurosis of the external oblique muscle (which offers strong resistance) is pierced with a clearly identifiable "crack." The needle is advanced to come close to the midpoint of the inguinal ligament; then the local anesthetic is injected (246). Bupivacaine is more rapidly absorbed from the injection site than ropivacaine (247). A catheter can easily be inserted through the Tuohy needle to provide prolonged analgesia (see also Chapter 16).

The only limitation to this technique is that it does not provide blockade of the sympathetic fibers supplying the spermatic cord. If the surgeon exerts too vigorous a traction on the cord, then autonomic reactions are elicited. These reactions do not appear in case of gentle manipulation of the cord. To avoid these reactions, some authors recommend performing a caudal block. However, inguinal surgery cannot be considered a major surgery; therefore performing a central block procedure in this context is questionable. If gentle manipulation of the cord cannot be guaranteed, it would probably be better to complement the ilioinguinal/iliohypogastric/genitofemoral block with an IV injection of a short-acting narcotic at the time of intraoperative traction.

Pudendal Nerve Block

In recent years, the pudendal nerve block has been increasingly performed in both adults and children undergoing perineal surgery. The technique is particularly indicated to complement an ilioinguinal/iliohypogastric nerve block in case of orchidopexy with scrotal incision. Blocking the pudendal nerves is easy close to the ischial tuberosity, in the ischiorectal fossa, where they give off their terminal branches.

The child is placed supine with knees flexed and soles conjoined (as for bladder catheterization in girls); the gynecologic position as used in adults is suitable too. The landmark is the ischial tuberosity (one per side) (Fig. 27-17). The site of insertion is 0.5 to 1 cm medial to the tuberosity, on the line joining the anal aperture to the tuberosity (248). A short-bevel needle (22- or 20-gauge Tuohy needle especially) connected to a prefilled syringe is inserted posteriorly and laterally, in the direction of

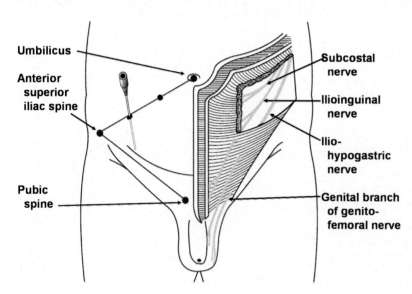

FIGURE 27-16. Combined block of the iliohypogastric nerve, ilioinguinal nerve, and genital branch of the genitofemoral nerve.

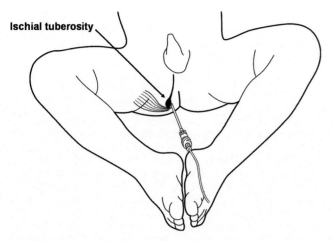

FIGURE 27-17. Pudendal nerve block.

the medial aspect of the ischial tuberosity until a loss of resistance is felt at the crossing of the Colle fascia, indicating that the tip of the needle has entered the ischiorectal fossa. The local anesthetic is then injected or a catheter is introduced to provide prolonged pain relief. Insertion of such a catheter is very easy—even easier than in the epidural space. The technique is then repeated on the other side.

The distribution of anesthesia depends on the volume of local anesthetic injected; with 0.1 mL/kg (up to 5 mL), usually only the perineal nerve, which supplies the posterior part of the scrotum, is blocked. This volume is sufficient to complement an ilioinguinal/iliohypogastric/genitofemoral nerve block to relieve postoperative pain after orchidopexy with a scrotal incision; with 0.3 to 0.4 mL/kg (up to 15 mL), all division branches of the pudendal nerve are blocked, thus providing complete analgesia of the perineum including blockade of the dorsal nerve of the penis.

As the pudendal nerve is a mixed nerve, a nerve stimulator can be used to locate it more precisely if deemed useful. Ultrasound guidance has been described in adults, but identification of the pudendal nerve was only possible in half the cases (249).

As this nerve is accompanied by the pudendal artery, which is a terminal artery, only plain solution of local anesthetics must be injected.

Penile Block via the Subpubic Space

Sensory innervation of the penis depends mainly on the two dorsal nerves of the penis, which are terminal branches of the pudendal nerves. The proximal part of the penis also receives sensory innervation from the ilioinguinal nerve and the genital branch of the genitofemoral nerve; the midline part of the ventral aspect of the penis, including the frenulum, is supplied by the perineal nerve, another terminal branch of the pudendal nerve (250). Within the penis, the dorsal nerves run close to the midline, immediately below the Buck fascia to which they are tightly attached; they cannot be safely approached there. Conversely, after their emergence from the pudendal nerve at the level of the ischiorectal fossa, they pass under the pubic bone and cross the subpubic space within the suspensory ligament of the penis, accompanied by the dorsal arteries, which are terminal arteries (administration of epinephrine must be avoided). In this subpubic space, the nerves can be safely approached.

Penile blocks are indicated for any surface operation on the penis, especially on the foreskin (circumcision, phimosis, and paraphimosis) and glans. These blocks can provide long-lasting analgesia (18 hours) after hypospadias repair but are usually not sufficient intraoperatively, as the midline sensory supply of the posterior aspect of the penis depends on the perineal nerve (a complete pudendal nerve block is preferable, as described earlier).

The child is placed supine and his penis is pulled down either by manual traction or taping (251). The symphysis pubis is identified by palpation and two insertion sites are identified 0.5 cm lateral to the midline on both sides. A short-bevel needle (25-gauge caudal needle, ideally) is then inserted posteriorly and slightly medially until it contacts then crosses with a characteristic loss-of-resistance the Scarpa fascia (the continuation of which is the Buck fascia) (Fig. 27-18). It is important to verify that the Scarpa fascia has been traversed by releasing the needle. If the needle stays in place, the technique is correct; if

Symphysis pubis

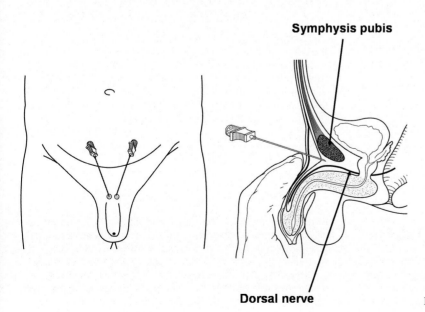

Dorsal nerve

FIGURE 27-18. Penile block via the subpubic space.

the needle spontaneously recoils, the Scarpa fascia has not been traversed but only temporarily displaced. After correct needle insertion, local anesthetic (0.5 mL/kg up to 5 mL) is injected, and the procedure is repeated on the other side. This technique is very easy, and the learning curve is particularly steep (252).

A subcutaneous ring of local anesthetic at the base of the penis can provide satisfactory analgesia but requires relatively large amounts of local anesthetic (2 mg/kg bupivacaine) and fails to provide adequate analgesia in 20% of patients. Topical anesthesia has been recommended for urethral meatotomy and even neonatal circumcision, but the quality of analgesia is less than that obtained from true penile blocks (253).

BLOCK OF NERVES SUPPLYING THE HEAD AND NECK

Blocks of nerves supplying the head and neck are not commonly performed by anesthesiologists in children (see Chapter 17).

Nerve Blocks in the Neck

Cervical Plexus Block

Cervical plexus blocks have very few indications in pediatric surgery; they are occasionally used for cervical lymph node biopsy and excision of thyroid nodules (254). Only the superficial branches are blocked by a subcutaneous infiltration along the lateral border of the sternocleidomastoid muscle.

Stellate Ganglion Block

The stellate ganglion block is a potentially dangerous procedure that has very limited but specific pediatric (nonanalgesic) indications: (a) ventricular tachyarrhythmia due to congenital long QT syndrome (255,256) (a left stellate block is recommended), and (b) severe ipsilateral circulatory disorders of the upper extremity. Some children with herpes zoster ophthalmicus (257) or some unusual forms of chronic pain, such as sympathetically maintained pain syndrome (258,259), may also benefit from the technique (see Chapter 39).

Laryngeal Nerve Block

Laryngeal nerve blocks can be used for short-duration laryngoscopic examinations in conscious patients or to facilitate awake intubation when difficult intubation is suspected. These blocks have also been recommended to prevent or treat laryngospasms (260). The easiest technique consists of subcutaneously injecting local anesthetic just lateral to the extremity of the hyoid horns (on each side) with an intradermal needle inserted perpendicularly to the skin until contact is made with the hyoid cartilage. To obtain an excellent laryngeal nerve block, a rather large volume, 0.1 to 0.2 mL/kg up to a maximum of 8 mL of 1% lidocaine, should be injected subcutaneously after a negative aspiration test (see Chapter 17).

Blocks of Nerves Supplying the Face

Facial innervation depends mainly on terminal branches of the fifth cranial (trigeminal) nerve. These nerves are purely sensory nerves; they are not identifiable by nerve stimulation in anesthetized children. Three infiltration techniques are commonly performed in pediatric patients, either in emergency (skin lacerations) or for elective procedures (superficial procedure, cleft lip/palate repair). Ultrasound guidance has not been described but may be very helpful.

Simultaneous Block of the Supraorbital and Supratrochlear Nerves

These terminal branches of the frontal nerve supply sensory innervation to the upper eyelid, forehead, and scalp and can all be blocked with a single-infiltration technique (on each side). The landmark is the supraorbital foramen, which is palpated at the junction of the lateral two-thirds and the medial one-third of the upper orbital rim. This foramen is located on the same vertical line as the ipsilateral centered pupil and both the infraorbital and mental foramina. An intradermal needle (25-gauge) is inserted posteriorly on this line, 0.5 to 1.5 cm below the supraorbital foramen. When bony contact is obtained, 0.1 mL/kg (up to 3 mL) of local anesthetic is injected to block the supraorbital nerve. The needle is then slightly withdrawn and redirected medially toward the junction of superior orbital rim and the nasal bone. The same volume of local anesthetic is injected while the needle is slowly withdrawn, thus infiltrating the subcutaneous tissues covering the medial side of the upper border of the orbit where the supratrochlear nerve and its division branches are located (see Chapter 17).

Block of the Infraorbital Nerve

The landmark for the infraorbital nerve is the infraorbital foramen, easily palpable on the line joining the ipsilateral centered pupil and supraorbital and mental foramina, below the junction of the medial and the middle third of the lower border of the orbit. The insertion site lies at the crossing of this line, with the perpendicular line passing just below the nostrils. The intradermal needle is directed cephalad toward the lower border of the infraorbital foramen (avoiding penetration inside the foramen) until bony contact is made; then, 0.1 mL/kg (up to 3 mL) of local anesthetic is injected. This block provides excellent analgesia of the lower eyelid, jaw, palate, and ipsilateral nostril. When performed on both sides, it provides excellent intra- and postoperative analgesia for cleft lip repair (261) (see Chapter 17).

Block of the Mental Nerve

The block procedure for the mental nerve is identical to that of the infraorbital nerve but the site of insertion is located 0.5 to 1 cm above the mental foramen on the same line joining the supraorbital, infraorbital, and mental foramina. The main indication of mental nerve block is for surgery involving lower incisor and canine teeth. Bilateral blocks allow pain-free procedures on the lower lip (see Chapter 17).

OTHER PROCEDURES

Intravenous Regional Anesthesia

Intravenous regional anesthesia (Bier block) is becoming outdated in pediatrics even though it is still used in some institutions mainly for fracture repairs (often in emergency departments) (262–264). The technique is the same as in adults (Chapter 15). The inflation pressure of the tourniquet(s) should be two to three times the systolic pressure before the Esmarch bandage is removed and the anesthetic solution is injected.

SUMMARY

The importance of regional anesthetic techniques has considerably and continuously increased during the last three decades. They represent a major therapeutic option for preventing and treating pain both intra- and postoperatively, especially for outpatient surgery (single-injection procedures) and for prolonged postoperative pain relief (with catheter techniques). Over the years, a shift was made from neuraxial techniques toward peripheral nerve blockade. This reduced the overall rate of adverse effects and limitations and allowed patients to be ambulatory and discharged earlier from hospital. These early discharges could take place even with an indwelling catheter, through which local anesthetic is continuously delivered by a nonmodifiable closed system with an elastomeric pump. The expansion of regional anesthesia was favored by the development of devices specifically designed for pediatric use and by techniques that allowed the precise location of nerves trunks without requiring the cooperation of the patient. Nerve stimulation is currently the gold standard for locating nerves and plexuses, but ultrasound guidance is an emerging technique that will probably surpass nerve stimulation in the near future. With increasing accuracy, future scientific studies will evaluate still more precisely the indications, advantages, and limits of the different techniques, as well as the place of regional anesthesia in pediatric care. The use of regional anesthesia in pediatric care will continue to increase, provided that these techniques are extensively and adequately taught to residents in anesthesiology.

References

1. Marhofer P, Bosenberg A, Sitzwohl C, et al. Pilot study of neuraxial imaging by ultrasound in infants and children. *Paediatr Anaesth* 2005;15:671–676.
2. McLeod A, Roche A, Fennelly M. Case series: Ultrasonography may assist epidural insertion in scoliosis patients. *Can J Anaesth* 2005;52:717–720.
3. Bosenberg AT, Raw R, Boezaart AP. Surface mapping of peripheral nerves in children with a nerve stimulator. *Paediatr Anaesth* 2002;12:398–403.
4. Urmey WF, Grossi P. Percutaneous electrode guidance: A noninvasive technique for prelocation of peripheral nerves to facilitate peripheral plexus or nerve block. *Reg Anesth Pain Med* 2002;27:261–267.
5. Capdevila X, Lopez S, Bernard N, et al. Percutaneous electrode guidance using the insulated needle for prelocation of peripheral nerves during axillary plexus blocks. *Reg Anesth Pain Med* 2004;29:206–211.
6. Weidenheim KM, Kress Y, Epshteyn I, et al. Early myelination in the human fetal lumbosacral spinal cord: Characterization by light and electron microscopy. *J Neuropathol Exp Neurol* 1992;51:142–149.
7. Tanaka S, Mito T, Takashima S. Progress of myelination in the human fetal spinal nerve roots, spinal cord and brainstem with myelin basic protein immunohistochemistry. *Early Hum Dev* 1995;41:49–59.
8. Vignolo M, Ginocchio G, Parodi A, et al. Fetal spine ossification: The gender and individual differences illustrated by ultrasonography. *Ultrasound Med Biol* 2005;31:733–738.
9. Verbout AJ. The development of the vertebral column. *Adv Anat Embryol Cell Biol* 1985; 90:1–122.
10. Nolting D, Hansen BF, Keeling J, et al. Prenatal development of the normal human vertebral corpora in different segments of the spine. *Spine* 1998;23:2265–2271.
11. Lack JA, Stuart-Taylor ME. Calculation of drug dosage and body surface area of children. *Br J Anaesth* 1997;78:601–605.
12. Mazoit JX, Dalens BJ. Pharmacokinetics of local anaesthetics in infants and children. *Clin Pharmacokinet* 2004;43:17–32.
13. Leopold A, Wilson S, Weaver JS, et al. Pharmacokinetics of lidocaine delivered from a transmucosal patch in children. *Anesth Prog* 2002;49:82–87.
14. Gjonaj ST, Lowenthal DB, Dozor AJ. Nebulized lidocaine administered to infants and children undergoing flexible bronchoscopy. *Chest* 1997;112:1665.
15. Sitbon P, Laffon M, Lesage V, et al. Lidocaine plasma concentrations in pediatric patients after providing airway topical anesthesia from a calibrated device. *Anesth Analg* 1996;82:1003.
16. Nielson DW, Ku PL, Egger M. Topical lidocaine exaggerates laryngomalacia during flexible bronchoscopy. *Am J Respir Crit Care Med* 2000;161:147–151.
17. Behnke H, Worthmann F, Cornelissen J, et al. Plasma concentration of ropivacaine after intercostal blocks for video-assisted thoracic surgery. *Br J Anaesth* 2002;89:251.
18. Chalkiadis GA, Anderson BJ, Tay M, et al. Pharmacokinetics of levobupivacaine after caudal epidural administration in infants less than 3 months of age. *Br J Anaesth* 2005;95:524–529.
19. Lönnqvist PA, Westrin P, Larsson BA, et al. Ropivacaine pharmacokinetics after caudal block in 1-8 year old children. *Br J Anaesth* 2000;85:506.
20. Karmakar MK, Aun CS, Wong EL, et al. Ropivacaine undergoes slower systemic absorption from the caudal epidural space in children than bupivacaine. *Anesth Analg* 2002;94:259.
21. Mazoit JX, Denson DD, Samii K. Pharmacokinetics of bupivacaine following caudal anesthesia in infants. *Anesthesiology* 1988;68:387–391.
22. Booker PD, Taylor C, Saba G. Perioperative changes in alpha 1-acid glycoprotein concentrations in infants undergoing major surgery. *Br J Anaesth* 1996;76:365–368.
23. Meunier JF, Goujard E, Dubousset AM, et al. Pharmacokinetics of bupivacaine after continuous epidural infusion in infants with and without biliary atresia. *Anesthesiology* 2001;95:87–95.
24. Lönnqvist PA, Herngren L. Effects of pronounced haemodilution on the plasma protein binding of lidocaine. *Perfusion* 1995;10:17.
25. Luz G, Innerhofer P, Bachmann B, et al. Bupivacaine plasma concentrations during continuous epidural anesthesia in infants and children. *Anesth Analg* 1996;82:231–234.
26. Berde C. Local anesthetics in infants and children: An update. *Paediatr Anaesth* 2004;14:387–393.
27. Gunter JB. Benefit and risks of local anesthetics in infants and children. *Paediatr Drugs* 2002;4:649–672.
28. Bosenberg AT, Thomas J, Cronje L, et al. Pharmacokinetics and efficacy of ropivacaine for continuous epidural infusion in neonates and infants. *Paediatr Anaesth* 2005;15:739–749.
29. Lerman J, Nolan J, Eyres R, et al. Efficacy, safety, and pharmacokinetics of levobupivacaine with and without fentanyl after continuous epidural infusion in children: A multicenter trial. *Anesthesiology* 2003;99:1166–1174.
30. Zsigmond EK, Downs JR. Plasma cholinesterase activity in newborns and infants. *Can Anaesth Soc J* 1971;18:278–285.
31. Tateishi T, Nakura H, Asoh M, et al. A comparison of hepatic cytochrome P450 protein expression between infancy and postinfancy. *Life Sci* 1997;61:2567–2574.
32. Tanaka E. In vivo age-related changes in hepatic drug-oxidizing capacity in humans. *J Clin Pharm Ther* 1998;23:247–255.
33. Hines RN, McCarver DG. The ontogeny of human drug-metabolizing enzymes: Phase I oxidative enzymes. *J Pharmacol Exp Ther* 2002;300:355–360.
34. Gantenbein M, Attolini L, Bruguerolle B, et al. Oxidative metabolism of bupivacaine into pipecolylxylidine in humans is mainly catalyzed by CYP3A. *Drug Metab Dispos* 2000;28:383–385.
35. Oda Y, Furuichi K, Tanaka K, et al. Metabolism of a new local anesthetic, ropivacaine, by human hepatic cytochrome P450. *Anesthesiology* 1995;82:214–220.
36. Ekstrom G, Gunnarsson UB. Ropivacaine, a new amide-type local anesthetic agent, is metabolized by cytochromes P450 1A and 3A in human liver microsomes. *Drug Metab Dispos* 1996;24:955–961.
37. Arlander E, Ekstrom G, Alm C, et al. Metabolism of ropivacaine in humans is mediated by CYP1A2 and to a minor extent by CYP3A4: An interaction study with fluvoxamine and ketoconazole as in vivo inhibitors. *Clin Pharmacol Ther* 1998;64:484–491.
38. Hansen TG, Ilett KF, Reid C, et al. Caudal ropivacaine in infants: Population pharmacokinetics and plasma concentrations. *Anesthesiology* 2001;94:579–584.
39. McCann ME, Sethna NF, Mazoit JX, et al. The pharmacokinetics of epidural ropivacaine in infants and young children. *Anesth Analg* 2001;93:893–897.
40. Scott DB, Lee A, Fagan D, et al. Acute toxicity of ropivacaine compared with that of bupivacaine. *Anesth Analg* 1989;69:563–569.
41. Knudsen K, Beckman Suurkula M, et al. Central nervous and cardiovascular effects of i.v. infusions of ropivacaine, bupivacaine and placebo in volunteers. *Br J Anaesth* 1997;78:507–514.
42. Bardsley H, Gristwood R, Baker H, et al. A comparison of the cardiovascular effects of levobupivacaine and rac-bupivacaine following intravenous administration to healthy volunteers. *Br J Clin Pharmacol* 1998;46:245–249.
43. Attia J, Ecoffey C, Sandouk P, et al. Epidural morphine in children: Pharmacokinetics and CO2 sensitivity. *Anesthesiology* 1986;65:590–594.

44. Wolf AR, Hughes D, Hobbs AJ, et al. Combined morphine-bupivacaine caudals for reconstructive penile surgery in children: Systemic absorption of morphine and postoperative analgesia. *Anaesth Intensive Care* 1991;19:17–21.

45. Bardo MT, Hughes RA. Single dose tolerance to morphine induced analgesic and hypoactive effects in infant rats. *Dev Psychobiol* 1981;14:415–423.

46. Thornton SR, Smith FL. Characterization of neonatal rat fentanyl tolerance and dependence. *J Pharmacol Exp Therapeut* 1997;281:514–521.

47. Thornton SR, Smith FL. Long-term alterations in opiate antinociception resulting from infant fentanyl tolerance and dependence. *Eur J Pharmacol* 1998;363:113–119.

48. Anand KJ, Barton BA, McIntosh N, et al. Analgesia and sedation in preterm neonates who require ventilatory support: Results from the NOPAIN trial. Neonatal Outcome and Prolonged Analgesia in Neonates. *Arch Ped Adolesc Med* 1999;153:331–338.

49. Suresh S, Anand KJ. Opioid tolerance in neonates: A state-of-the-art review. *Paediatr Anaesth* 2001;11:511–521.

50. Craft RM, Stratmann JA, Bartok RE, et al. Sex differences in development of morphine tolerance and dependence in the rat. *Psychopharmacology.* 1999;143:1–7.

51. Guinsburg R, de Araujo Peres C, et al. Differences in pain expression between male and female newborn infants. *Pain* 2000;85:127–133.

52. Burm AG, Van Kleef JW, Gladines MP, et al. Epidural anesthesia with lidocaine and bupivacaine: Effects of epinephrine on the plasma concentration profiles. *Anesth Analg* 1986;65:1281–1284.

53. Doyle E, Morton NS, McNicol LR. Plasma bupivacaine levels after fascia iliaca compartment block with and without adrenaline. *Paediatr Anaesth* 1997;7:121–124.

54. Warner MA, Kunkel SE, Offord KO, et al. The effects of age, epinephrine, and operative site on duration of caudal analgesia in pediatric patients. *Anesth Analg* 1987;66:995–998.

55. Hansen TG, Morton NS, Cullen PM, et al. Plasma concentrations and pharmacokinetics of bupivacaine with and without adrenaline following caudal anaesthesia in infants. *Acta Anaesthesiol Scand* 2001;45:42–47.

56. Bouaziz H, Okubo N, Malinovsky JM, et al. The age-related effects of epidural lidocaine, with and without epinephrine, on spinal cord blood flow in anesthetized rabbits. *Anesth Analg* 1999;88:1302–1307.

57. Freid EB, Bailey AG, Valley RD. Electrocardiographic and hemodynamic changes associated with unintentional intravascular injection of bupivacaine with epinephrine in infants. *Anesthesiology* 1993;79:394–398.

58. Liu SS, Carpenter RL. Hemodynamic responses to intravascular injection of epinephrine-containing epidural test-doses in adults during general anesthesia. *Anesthesiology* 1996;84:81–87.

59. Jamali S, Monin S, Begon C, et al. Clonidine in pediatric caudal anesthesia. *Anesth Analg* 1994;78:663–666.

60. De Negri P, Ivani G, Visconti C, et al. The dose-response relationship for clonidine added to a postoperative continuous epidural infusion of ropivacaine in children. *Anesth Analg* 2001;93:71–76.

61. Singelyn FJ, Gouverneur JM, Robert A. A minimum dose of clonidine added to mepivacaine prolongs the duration of anesthesia and analgesia after axillary brachial plexus block. *Anesth Analg* 1996;83:1046–1050.

62. Bouchut JC, Dubois R, Godard J. Clonidine in preterm-infant caudal anesthesia may be responsible for postoperative apnea. *Reg Anesth Pain Med* 2001;26:83–85.

63. Galante D. Preoperative apnea in a preterm infant after caudal block with ropivacaine and clonidine. *Paediatr Anaesth* 2005;15:708–709.

64. Wagner LE 2nd, Gingrich KJ, Kulli JC, et al. Ketamine blockade of voltage-gated sodium channels: Evidence for a shared receptor site with local anesthetics. *Anesthesiology* 2001;95:1406–1413.

65. De Negri P, Ivani G, Visconti C, et al. How to prolong postoperative analgesia after caudal anaesthesia with ropivacaine in children: S-ketamine versus clonidine. *Paediatr Anaesth* 2001;11:679–683.

66. Himmelseher S, Ziegler-Pithamitsis D, Argiriadou H, et al. Small-dose S(+)-ketamine reduces postoperative pain when applied with ropivacaine in epidural anesthesia for total knee arthroplasty. *Anesth Analg* 2001;92:1290–1295.

67. Dalens B. Some controversies in paediatric regional anaesthesia. *Curr Opin Anaesthesiol* 2006;19:301–308.

68. Giaufré E, Dalens B, Gombert A. Epidemiology and morbidity of regional anesthesia in children: A one-year prospective survey of the French-Language Society of Pediatric Anesthesiologists (ADARPEF). *Anesth Analg* 1996;83:904–912.

69. Krane EJ, Dalens BJ, Murat I, et al. The safety of epidurals placed during general anesthesia [Editorial]. *Reg Anesth Pain Med* 1998;23:433–438.

70. Tobias JD. Therapeutic applications of regional anaesthesia in paediatric-aged patients. *Paediatr Anaesth* 2002;12:272–277.

71. Suresh S, Wheeler M. Practical pediatric regional anesthesia. *Anesthesiol Clin North Am* 2002;20:83–113.

72. Zwass MS. Regional anesthesia in children. *Anesthesiol Clin North Am* 2005;23:815–835.

73. Chambliss CR, Anand KJ. Pain management in the pediatric intensive care unit. *Curr Opin Pediatr* 1997;9:246–253.

74. Macfadyen AJ, Buckmaster MA. Pain management in the pediatric intensive care unit. *Crit Care Clin* 1999;15:185–200.

75. Tobias JD. Sedation and analgesia in the pediatric intensive care unit. *Pediatr Ann* 2005;34:636–645.

76. Hammer GB. Regional anesthesia for pediatric cardiac surgery. *J Cardiothorac Vasc Anesth* 1999;13:210–213.

77. Peterson KL, DeCampli WM, Pike NA, et al. A report of two hundred twenty cases of regional anesthesia in pediatric cardiac surgery. *Anesth Analg* 2000;90:1014–1019.

78. Diaz LK. Anesthesia and postoperative analgesia in pediatric patients undergoing cardiac surgery. *Paediatr Drugs* 2006;8:223–233.

79. Hansen TG, Ilett KF, Lim SI, et al. Pharmacokinetics and clinical efficacy of long-term epidural ropivacaine infusion in children. *Br J Anaesth* 2000;85:347–353.

80. Tobias JD. Applications of intrathecal catheters in children. *Paediatr Anaesth* 2000;10:367–375.

81. Dadure C, Pirat P, Raux O, et al. Perioperative continuous peripheral nerve blocks with disposable infusion pumps in children: A prospective descriptive study. *Anesth Analg* 2003;97:687–690.

82. Zaric D, Boysen K, Christiansen J, et al. Continuous popliteal sciatic nerve block for outpatient foot surgery: A randomized, controlled trial. *Acta Anaesthesiol Scand* 2004;48:337–341.

83. Dadure C, Motais F, Ricard C, et al. Continuous peripheral nerve blocks at home for treatment of recurrent complex regional pain syndrome I in children. *Anesthesiology* 2005;102:387–391.

84. Kessell G, Barker I. Leg ischaemia in an infant following accidental intra-arterial administration of atracurium treated with caudal anaesthesia. *Anaesthesia* 1996;51:1154–1156.

85. Elias M. Continuous cervico-thoracic sympathetic ganglion block: Therapeutic modality for arterial insufficiency of the arm of a neonate. *Middle East J Anesthesiol* 2001;16:359–363.

86. Breschan C, Kraschl R, Jost R, et al. Axillary brachial plexus block for treatment of severe forearm ischemia after arterial cannulation in an extremely low birth-weight infant. *Paediatr Anaesth* 2004;14:681–684.

87. Dalens B, Mansoor O. Safe selection and performance of regional anaesthetic techniques in children. *Curr Opin Anaesthesiol* 1994;7:257–261.

88. Mulroy MF. Monitoring opioids. *Reg Anesth* 1996;21[Suppl]:89–93.

89. Hebl JR, Horlocker TT, Schroeder DR. Neuraxial anesthesia and analgesia in patients with preexisting central nervous system disorders. *Anesth Analg* 2006;103(1):223–228.

90. Mubarak SJ, Frick S, Sink E, et al. Volkmann contracture and compartment syndromes after femur fractures in children treated with 90/90 spica casts. *J Pediatr Orthop* 2006;26:567–572.

91. Lejus C. What does analgesia mask? [Editorial]. *Paediatr Anaesth* 2004;14:622–624.

92. Dunwoody JM, Reichert CC, Brown KL. et al. Compartment syndrome associated with bupivacaine and fentanyl epidural analgesia in pediatric orthopaedics. *J Pediatr Orthop* 1997;17:285–288.

93. Battaglia TC, Armstrong DG, Schwend RM. Factors affecting forearm compartment pressures in children with supracondylar fractures of the humerus. *J Pediatr Orthop* 2002;22:431–439.

94. Giannotti G, Cohn SM, Brown M, et al. Utility of near-infrared spectroscopy in the diagnosis of lower extremity compartment syndrome. *J Trauma* 2000;48:396–399.

95. Dickson KF, Sullivan MJ, Steinberg B, et al. Noninvasive measurement of compartment syndrome. *Orthopedics* 2003;26:1215–1218.

96. Wiemann JM, Ueno T, Leek BT, et al. Noninvasive measurements of intramuscular pressure using pulsed phase-locked loop ultrasound for detecting compartment syndromes: A preliminary report. *J Orthop Trauma* 2006;20:458–463.

97. Bibbo C, Lin SS, Cunningham FJ. Acute traumatic compartment syndrome of the foot in children. *Pediatr Emerg Care* 2000;16:244–248.

98. Tiwari A, Haq AI, Myint F, et al. Acute compartment syndromes. *Br J Surg* 2002;89:397–412.

99. Carbonell PG, Prats FL, Fernandez PD, et al. Monitoring antebrachial compartmental pressure in displaced supracondylar elbow fractures in children. *J Pediatr Orthop B* 2004;13:412–416.

100. Evron S, Sessler D, Sadan O, et al. Identification of the epidural space: Loss of resistance with air, lidocaine, or the combination of air and lidocaine. *Anesth Analg* 2004;99:245–250.

101. Kokki H, Heikkinen M, Turunen M, et al. Needle design does not affect the success rate of spinal anaesthesia or the incidence of postpuncture complications in children. *Acta Anaesthesiol Scand* 2000;44:210–213.

102. Kokki H, Turunen M, Heikkinen M, et al. High success rate and low incidence of headache and neurological symptoms with two spinal needle designs in children. *Acta Anaesthesiol Scand* 2005;49:1367–1372.

103. Freid EB, Bailey AG, Valley RD. Electrocardiographic and hemodynamic changes associated with unintentional intravascular injection of bupivacaine with epinephrine in infants. *Anesthesiology* 1993;79:394–398.

104. Fisher QA, Shaffner DH, Yaster M. Detection of intravascular injection of regional anaesthetics in children. *Can J Anaesth* 1997;44:592–596.

105. Tanaka M, Nishikawa T. The efficacy of a simulated intravascular test dose in sevoflurane-anesthetized children: A dose-response study. *Anesth Analg* 1999;89:632–637.
106. Kozek-Langenecker SA, Marhofer P, Jonas K, et al. Cardiovascular criteria for epidural test dosing in sevoflurane- and halothane-anesthetized children. *Anesth Analg* 2000;90:579–583.
107. Guay J. The epidural test dose: A review. *Anesth Analg* 2006;102:921–929.
108. Veyckemans F, Van Obbergh LJ, Gouverneur JM. Lessons from 1100 pediatric caudal blocks in a teaching hospital. *Regional Anesth* 1992;17:119–125.
109. Jiang X, Wen X, Gao B, et al. The plasma concentrations of lidocaine after slow versus rapid administration of an initial dose of epidural anesthesia. *Anesth Analg* 1997;84:570–573.
110. Eyres RL. Local anaesthetic agents in infancy. *Paediatr Anaesth.* 1995;5:213–218.
111. Finkel JC, Yang CI, Yarvitz JL, et al. Neuroselective sensory electrodiagnostic evaluation of 4% liposomal topical lidocaine. *Anesth Analg* 2002;94:1259–1262.
112. Sakai T, Tomiyasu S, Yamada H, et al. Quantitative and selective evaluation of differential sensory nerve block after transdermal lidocaine. *Anesth Analg* 2004;98:248–251.
113. Uguralp S, Mutus M, Koroglu A, et al. Regional anesthesia is a good alternative to general anesthesia in pediatric surgery: Experience in 1,554 children. *J Pediatr Surg* 2002;37:610–613.
114. Auroy Y, Narchi P, Messiah A, et al. Serious complications related to regional anesthesia: Results of a prospective survey in France. *Anesthesiology* 1997;87:479–486.
115. Bromage PR, Benumof JL. Paraplegia following intracord injection during attempted epidural anesthesia under general anesthesia. *Reg Anesth Pain Med* 1998;23:104–107.
116. Benumof JL. Permanent loss of cervical spinal cord function associated with interscalene block performed under general anesthesia. *Anesthesiology* 2000;93:1541–1544.
117. Kao MC, Tsai SK, Tsou MY, et al. Paraplegia after delayed detection of inadvertent spinal cord injury during thoracic epidural catheterization in an anesthetized elderly patient. *Anesth Analg* 2004;99:580–583.
118. Drasner K. Thoracic epidural anesthesia: asleep at the wheal? *Anesth Analg* 2004;99:578–579.
119. Horlocker TT, Abel MD, Messick JM Jr., et al. Small risk of serious neurologic complications related to lumbar epidural catheter placement in anesthetized patients. *Anesth Analg* 2003;96:1547–1552.
120. Rosenquist RW, Birnbach DJ. Epidural insertion in anesthetized adults: Will your patients thank you? [Editorial]. *Anesth Analg* 2003;96:1545–1546.
121. Tsui BC, Armstrong K. Can direct spinal cord injury occur without paresthesia? A report of delayed spinal cord injury after epidural placement in an awake patient. *Anesth Analg* 2005;101:1212–1214.
122. Absalom AR, Martinelli G, Scott NB. Spinal cord injury caused by direct damage by local anaesthetic infiltration needle. *Br J Anaesth* 2001;87:512–515.
123. Krane EJ. Spinal epidermoid tumors: Will a forgotten complication rise again? *Reg Anesth Pain Med* 1999;24:494–496.
124. Dalens BJ, Mazoit JX. Adverse effects of regional anaesthesia in children. *Drug Saf* 1998;19:251–268.
125. Maxwell LG, Martin LD, Yaster M. Bupivacaine-induced cardiac toxicity in neonates: Successful treatment with intravenous phenytoin. *Anesthesiology* 1994;80:682–686.
126. Koomen E, Janssen S, Anderson BJ. Use of ultrasound bladder monitoring in children after caudal anaesthesia. *Paediatr Anaesth* 2002;12:738–741.
127. Kluger MT, Bullock MF. Recovery room incidents: A review of 419 reports from the Anaesthetic Incident Monitoring Study (AIMS). *Anaesthesia* 2002;57:1060–1066.
128. Kokinsky E, Thornberg E, Ostlund AL, et al. Postoperative comfort in paediatric outpatient surgery. *Paediatr Anaesth* 1999;9:243–251.
129. Dadure C, Capdevila X. Continuous peripheral nerve blocks in children. *Best Pract Res Clin Anaesthesiol* 2005;19:309–321.
130. Park JH, Koo BN, Kim JY, et al. Determination of the optimal angle for needle insertion during caudal block in children using ultrasound imaging. *Anaesthesia* 2006;61:946–949.
131. Adewale L, Dearlove O, Wilson B, et al. The caudal canal in children: A study using magnetic resonance imaging. *Paediatr Anaesth* 2000;10:137–141.
132. Dalens BJ. Regional anesthetic techniques. In: Bissonnette B, Dalens B, eds. *Pediatric Anesthesia: Principles and Practice.* New York: McGraw Hill; 2002:528–575.
133. Cucchiaro G, De Lagausie P, El-Ghonemi A, et al. Single-dose caudal anesthesia for major intraabdominal operations in high-risk infants. *Anesth Analg* 2001;92:1439–1441.
134. Gunter JB, Watcha MF, Forestner JE, et al. Caudal epidural anesthesia in conscious premature and high-risk infants. *J Pediatr Surg* 1991;26:9–14.
135. Bouchut JC, Dubois R, Foussat C, et al. Evaluation of caudal anaesthesia performed in conscious ex-premature infants for inguinal herniotomies. *Paediatr Anaesth* 2001;11:55–58.
136. Peutrell JM, Hughes DG. Epidural anaesthesia through caudal catheters for inguinal herniotomies in awake ex-premature babies. *Anaesthesia* 1993;48:128–131.
137. Henderson K, Sethna NF, Berde CB. Continuous caudal anesthesia for inguinal hernia repair in former preterm infants. *J Clin Anesth* 1993;5:129–133.
138. Bosenberg AT. Caudothoracic epidural block. *Techniques Reg Anesth Pain Manage* 1999;3:157–162.
139. Kost-Bierly S, Tobin JR, Greenberg RS, et al. Bacterial colonization and infection rate of continuous epidural catheters in children. *Anesth Analg* 1998;86:712–716.
140. Hammer GH, Wellis V, Boltz G, et al. The use of regional anesthesia in combination with general anesthesia for cardiac surgery in children. *Sem Cardiothor Vascul Anesth* 2001;5:105–112.
141. Orme RM, Berg SJ. The 'swoosh' test: An evaluation of a modified 'whoosh' test in children. *Br J Anaesth* 2003;90:62–65.
142. Valairucha S, Seefelder C, Houck CS. Thoracic epidural catheters placed by the caudal route in infants: The importance of radiographic confirmation. *Paediatr Anaesth* 2002;12:424–428.
143. Tsui BC, Tarkkila P, Gupta S, et al. Confirmation of caudal needle placement using nerve stimulation. *Anesthesiology* 1999;91:374–378.
144. Tsui BC, Wagner A, Cave D, et al. Threshold current for an insulated epidural needle in pediatric patients. *Anesth Analg* 2004;99:694–696.
145. Tsui BC, Seal R, Koller J. Thoracic epidural catheter placement via the caudal approach in infants by using electrocardiographic guidance. *Anesth Analg* 2002;95:326–330.
146. Vas L, Naik V, Patil B, et al. Tunnelling of caudal epidural catheters in infants. *Paediatr Anaesth* 2000;10:149–154.
147. Roberts SA, Galvez I. Ultrasound assessment of caudal catheter position in infants. *Paediatr Anaesth* 2005;15:429–432.
148. Armitage EN. Regional anaesthesia in paediatrics. *Clin Anesthesiol* 1985;3:553–568.
149. Dalens B, Hasnaoui A. Caudal anesthesia in pediatric surgery: Success rate and adverse effects in 750 consecutive patients. *Anesth Analg* 1989;68:83–89.
150. Larousse E, Asehnoune K, Dartayet B, et al. The hemodynamic effects of pediatric caudal anesthesia assessed by esophageal Doppler. *Anesth Analg* 2002;94:1165–1168.
151. Ozasa H, Hashimoto K, Saito Y. Pulmonary Doppler flow velocity pattern during caudal epidural anaesthesia in children. *Paediatr Anaesth* 2002;12:317–321.
152. Marhofer P, Bosenberg A, Sitzwohl C, et al. Pilot study of neuraxial imaging by ultrasound in infants and children. *Paediatr Anaesth* 2005;15:671–676.
153. Willschke H, Marhofer P, Bosenberg A, et al. Epidural catheter placement in children: Comparing a novel approach using ultrasound guidance and a standard loss-of-resistance technique. *Br J Anaesth* 2006;97:200–207.
154. Hammer GB. Pediatric thoracic anesthesia. *Anesthesiol Clin North Am* 2002;20:153–180.
155. Soliman LM, Mossad EB. Thoracic epidural catheter in the management of a child with an anterior mediastinal mass: A case report and literature review. *Paediatr Anaesth* 2006;16:200–205.
156. Futagawa K, Suwa I, Okuda T, et al. Anesthetic management for the minimally invasive Nuss procedure in 21 patients with pectus excavatum. *J Anesth* 2006;20:48–50.
157. Arms DM, Smith JT, Osteyee J, Gartrell A. Postoperative epidural analgesia for pediatric spine surgery. *Orthopedics* 1998;21:539–544.
158. Blumenthal S, Borgeat A, Nadig M, et al. Postoperative analgesia after anterior correction of thoracic scoliosis: A prospective randomized study comparing continuous double epidural catheter technique with intravenous morphine. *Spine* 2006;31:1646–1651.
159. Peterson KL, DeCampli WM, Pike NA, et al. A report of two hundred twenty cases of regional anesthesia in pediatric cardiac surgery. *Anesth Analg* 2000;90:1014–1019.
160. Cooper MG, Sethna NF. Epidural analgesia in patients with congenital lumbosacral spinal abnormalities. *Anesthesiology* 1991;75:370–374.
161. Aram L, Krane EJ, Kozloski LJ, et al. Tunneled epidural catheters for prolonged analgesia in pediatric patients. *Anesth Analg* 2001;92:1432–438.
162. Schulte-Steinberg O. Regional anaesthesia for children. *Ann Chir Gynaecol* 1984;73:158–165.
162. Aram L, Krane EJ, Kozloski LJ, et al. Tunneled epidural catheters for prolonged analgesia in pediatric patients. *Anesth Analg* 2001;92:1432–438.
163. Busoni P, Sarti A. Sacral intervertebral epidural block. *Anesthesiology.* 1987;67:993–995.
164. Kaiser AM, Whitelaw AG. Normal cerebrospinal fluid pressure in the newborn. *Neuropediatrics.* 1986;17:100–102.
165. Frumiento C, Abajian JC, Vane DW. Spinal anesthesia for preterm infants undergoing inguinal hernia repair. *Arch Surg* 2000;135:445–451.
166. Nickel US, Meyer RR, Brambrink AM. Spinal anesthesia in an extremely low birth weight infant. *Paediatr Anaesth* 2005;15:58–62.
167. William JM, Stoddart PA, Williams SA, et al. Post-operative recovery after inguinal herniotomy in ex-premature infants: Comparison between sevoflurane and spinal anaesthesia. *Br J Anaesth* 2001;86:366–371.

PART III: APPLICATIONS

168. Shenkman Z, Hoppenstein D, Litmanowitz I, et al. Spinal anesthesia in 62 premature, former-premature or young infants: Technical aspects and pitfalls. *Can J Anaesth* 2002;49:262–269.

169. Tobias JD, Burd RS, Helikson MA. Apnea following spinal anaesthesia in two former pre-term infants. *Can J Anaesth* 1998;45:985–989.

170. Imbelloni LE, Vieira EM, Sperni F, et al. Spinal anesthesia in children with isobaric local anesthetics: Report on 307 patients under 13 years of age. *Paediatr Anaesth* 2006;16:43–48.

171. Puncuh F, Lampugnani E, Kokki H. Use of spinal anaesthesia in paediatric patients: A single centre experience with 1132 cases. *Paediatr Anaesth* 2004;14:564–567.

172. Koroglu A, Durmus M, Togal T, et al. Spinal anaesthesia in full-term infants of 0-6 months: Are there any differences regarding age? *Eur J Anaesthesiol* 2005;22:111–116.

173. Hammer GB, Ramamoorthy C, Cao H, et al. Postoperative analgesia after spinal blockade in infants and children undergoing cardiac surgery. *Anesth Analg* 2005;100:1283–1288.

174. Katznelson R, Mishaly D, Hegesh T, et al. Spinal anesthesia for diagnostic cardiac catheterization in high-risk infants. *Paediatr Anaesth* 2005;15:50–53.

175. Dalens BJ, Khandwala RS, Tanguy A. Staged segmental scoliosis surgery during regional anesthesia in high risk patients: Report of six cases. *Anesth Analg* 1993;76:434–439.

176. Krechel SW, Helikson MA, Kittle D, et al. Intrathecal morphine (ITM) for postoperative pain control in children: A comparison with nalbuphine patient controlled analgesia (PCA). *Paediatr Anaesth* 1995;5:177–183.

177. Humphreys N, Bays SM, Parry AJ, et al. Spinal anesthesia with an indwelling catheter reduces the stress response in pediatric open heart surgery. *Anesthesiology* 2005;103:1113–1120.

178. Tobias JD. Applications of intrathecal catheters in children. *Paediatr Anaesth* 2000;10:367–375.

179. Kokki H, Ylonen P, Laisalmi M, et al. Isobaric ropivacaine 5 mg/ml for spinal anesthesia in children. *Anesth Analg* 2005;100:66–70.

180. Lee YY, Muchhal K, Chan CK, et al. Levobupivacaine and fentanyl for spinal anaesthesia: A randomized trial. *Eur J Anaesthesiol* 2005;22:899–903.

181. Kokki H, Hendolin H, Turunen M. Postdural puncture headache and transient neurologic symptoms in children after spinal anesthesia using cutting and pencil point paediatric spinal needles. *Acta Anaesthesiol Scand* 1998;42:1076–1082.

182. Carre P, Joly A, Cluzel Field B, et al. Axillary block in children: Single or multiple injection? *Paediatr Anaesth* 2000;10:35–39.

183. Dalens B. Peripheral blocks of the upper extremity. In: Dalens B, ed. *Regional Anesthesia in Infants, Children and Adolescents*. London: Williams & Wilkins; 1995:275–312.

184. Marhofer P, Sitzwohl C, Greher M, et al. Ultrasound guidance for infraclavicular brachial plexus anaesthesia in children. *Anaesthesia* 2004;59:642–646.

185. Borgeat A, Ekatodramis G, Dumont C. An evaluation of the infraclavicular block via a modified approach of the Raj technique. *Anesth Analg* 2001;93:436–441.

186. Sandhu NS, Capan LM. Ultrasound-guided infraclavicular brachial plexus block. *Br J Anaesth* 2002;89:254–259.

187. Dadure C, Raux O, Troncin R, et al. Continuous infraclavicular brachial plexus block for acute pain management in children. *Anesth Analg* 2003;97:691–693.

188. Fisher P, Wilson SE, Brown M, et al. Continuous infraclavicular brachial plexus block in a child. *Paediatr Anaesth* 2006;16:884–886.

189. Salazar CH, Espinosa W. Infraclavicular brachial plexus block: Variation in approach and results in 360 cases. *Reg Anesth Pain Med* 1999;24:411–416.

190. Jandard C, Gentili ME, Girard F, et al. Infraclavicular block with lateral approach and nerve stimulation: Extent of anesthesia and adverse effects. *Reg Anesth Pain Med* 2002;27:37–42.

191. Gentili ME, Deleuze A, Estebe JP, et al. Severe respiratory failure after infraclavicular block with 0.75% ropivacaine. A case report. *J Clin Anesth* 2002;14:459–461.

192. Dalens B, Vanneuville G, Tanguy A. A new parascalene approach to the brachial plexus in children: Comparison with the supraclavicular approach. *Anesth Analg* 1987;66:1264–1271.

193. Vongvises P, Beokhaimook N. Computed tomographic study of parascalene block. *Anesth Analg* 1997;84:379–382.

194. Jan van Geffen G, Tielens L, Gielen M. Ultrasound-guided interscalene brachial plexus block in a child with femur fibula ulna syndrome. *Paediatr Anaesth* 2006;16:330–332.

195. Borgeat A, Ekatodramis G, Kalberer F, et al. Acute and nonacute complications associated with interscalene block and shoulder surgery: A prospective study. *Anesthesiology* 2001;95:875–880.

196. Rucci FS, Pippa P, Barbagli R, et al. How many interscalenic blocks are there? A comparison between the lateral and posterior approach. *Eur J Anaesthesiol* 1993;10:303–307.

197. Rettig HC, Gielen MJ, Jack NT, et al. A comparison of the lateral and posterior approach for brachial plexus block. *Reg Anesth Pain Med* 2006;31:119–126.

198. Boezaart AP, Koorn R, Borene S, et al. Continuous brachial plexus block using the posterior approach. *Reg Anesth Pain Med* 2003;28:70–71.

199. Chiu DT. Transthecal digital block: Flexor tendon sheath used for anesthetic infusion. *J Hand Surg [Am]* 1990;15:471–477.

200. Castellanos J, Ramirez C, De Sena L, et al. Transthecal digital block: Digital anaesthesia through the sheath of the flexor tendon. *J Bone Joint Surg Br* 2000;82:889.

201. Brutus JP, Baeten Y, Chahidi N, et al. Single injection digital block: Comparison between three techniques. *Chir Main* 2002;21:182–187.

202. Cummings AJ, Tisol WB, Meyer LE. Modified transthecal digital block versus traditional digital block for anesthesia of the finger. *J Hand Surg [Am]* 2004;29:44–48.

203. Lopez S, Gros T, Bernard N, et al. Fascia iliaca compartment block for femoral bone fractures in prehospital care. *Reg Anesth Pain Med* 2003;28:203–207.

204. Johnson CM. Continuous femoral nerve blockade for analgesia in children with femoral fractures. *Anaesth Intensive Care* 1994;22:281–283.

205. Tobias JD. Continuous femoral nerve block to provide analgesia following femur fracture in a paediatric ICU population. *Anaesth Intensive Care* 1994;22:616–618.

206. Grant SA, Nielsen KC, Greengrass RA. Continuous peripheral nerve block for ambulatory surgery. *Reg Anesth Pain Med* 2001;26:209–214.

207. Maccani RM, Wedel DJ, Melton A, et al. Femoral and lateral cutaneous nerve block for muscle biopsy in children. *Paediatr Anaesth* 1995;5:223–227.

208. Vas L. Continuous sciatic block for leg and foot surgery in 160 children. *Paediatr Anaesth* 2005;15:971–978.

209. van Geffen GJ, Gielen M. Ultrasound-guided subgluteal sciatic nerve blocks with stimulating catheters in children: a descriptive study. *Anesth Analg* 2006;103:328–333.

210. Dalens B, Vanneuville G, Tanguy A. Comparison of the fascia iliaca compartment block with the 3-in-1 block in children. *Anesth Analg* 1989;69:705–713.

211. Morau D, Lopez S, Biboulet P, et al. Comparison of continuous 3-in-1 and fascia Iliaca compartment blocks for postoperative analgesia: Feasibility, catheter migration, distribution of sensory block, and analgesic efficacy. *Reg Anesth Pain Med* 2003;28:309–314.

212. Chayen D, Nathan H, Chayen M. The psoas compartment block. *Anesthesiology* 1976;45:95–99.

213. Dalens B, Tanguy A, Vanneuville G. Lumbar plexus block in children. A comparison of two procedures in 50 patients. *Anesth Analg* 1988;67:750–758.

214. Winnie AP. Regional anesthesia. *Surg Clin North Am* 1975;55:861–892.

215. Schuepfer G, Johr M. Psoas compartment block in children: Part I: Description of the technique. *Paediatr Anaesth* 2005;15:461–464.

216. Capdevila X, Macaire P, Dadure C, et al. Continuous psoas compartment block for postoperative analgesia after total hip arthroplasty: New landmarks, technical guidelines, and clinical evaluation. *Anesth Analg* 2002;94:1606–1613.

217. Kirchmair L, Entner T, Kapral S, et al. Ultrasound guidance for the psoas compartment block: An imaging study. *Anesth Analg* 2002;94:706–710.

218. McNicol LR. Lower limb blocks for children: Lateral cutaneous and femoral nerve blocks for postoperative pain relief in paediatric practice. *Anaesthesia* 1986;41:27–31.

219. Brown TC, Dickens DR. A new approach to lateral cutaneous nerve of thigh block. *Anaesth Intensive Care* 1986;14:126–1267.

220. Choquet O, Capdevila X, Bennourine K, et al. A new inguinal approach for the obturator nerve block: Anatomical and randomized clinical studies. *Anesthesiology* 2005;103:1238–1245.

221. Konrad C, Johr M. Blockade of the sciatic nerve in the popliteal fossa: A system for standardization in children. *Anesth Analg* 1998;87:1256–1258.

222. Tobias JD, Mencio GA. Popliteal fossa block for postoperative analgesia after foot surgery in infants and children. *J Pediatr Orthop* 1999;19:511–514.

223. Dalens B, Tanguy A, Vanneuville G. Sciatic nerve block in children: Comparison of the posterior, anterior and lateral approaches in 180 pediatric patients. *Anesth Analg* 1990;70:131–137.

224. McNicol LR. Sciatic nerve block for children: Sciatic nerve block by the anterior approach for postoperative pain relief. *Anaesthesia* 1985;40:410–414.

225. Sharrock NE, Waller JF, Fierro LE. Midtarsal block for surgery of the forefoot. *Br J Anaesth* 1986;58:37–40.

226. Matsota P, Livanios S, Marinopoulou E. Intercostal nerve block with Bupivacaine for post-thoracotomy pain relief in children. *Eur J Pediatr Surg* 2001;11:219–222.

227. Downs CS, Cooper MG. Continuous extrapleural intercostal nerve block for post thoracotomy analgesia in children. *Anaesth Intensive Care* 1997;25:390–397.

228. Karmakar MM, Critchley L. Continuous extrapleural intercostal nerve block for post thoracotomy analgesia in children. *Anaesth Intensive Care* 1998;26:115–116.

229. Maurer K, Rentsch KM, Dullenkopf A, et al. Continuous extrapleural infusion of ropivacaine in children: Is it safe? *Can J Anaesth* 2005;52:112–113.

230. Savage C, McQuitty C, Wang D, et al. Postthoracotomy pain management. *Chest Surg Clin North Am* 2002;12:251–263.

231. Lönnqvist PA. Continuous paravertebral block in children. Initial experience. *Anaesthesia* 1992;47:607–609.

232. Karmakar MK. Thoracic paravertebral block. *Anesthesiology* 2001;95:771–780.

233. Lönnqvist PA, Hesser U. Radiological and clinical distribution of thoracic paravertebral blockade in infants and children. *Paediatr Anaesth* 1993;3:83.

234. Naja MZ, Ziade MF, El Rajab M, et al. Varying anatomical injection points within the thoracic paravertebral space: Effect on spread of solution and nerve blockade. *Anaesthesia* 2004;59:459–463.

235. Saito T, Den S, Tanuma K, et al. Anatomical bases for paravertebral anesthetic block: Fluid communication between the thoracic and lumbar paravertebral regions. *Surg Radiol Anat* 1999;21:359–363.

236. Karmakar MK, Kwok WH, Kew J. Thoracic paravertebral block: Radiological evidence of contralateral spread anterior to the vertebral bodies. *Br J Anaesth* 2000;84:263–265.

237. Richardson J, Sabanathan S, Jones J, et al. A prospective, randomized comparison of preoperative and continuous balanced epidural or paravertebral bupivacaine on post-thoracotomy pain, pulmonary function and stress responses. *Br J Anaesth* 1999;83:387–392.

238. Saito T, Tanuma K, Den S, et al. Pathways of anesthetic from the thoracic paravertebral region to the celiac ganglion. *Clin Anat* 2002;15:340–344.

239. Lönnqvist PA, MacKenzie J, Soni AK, et al. Paravertebral blockade: Failure rate and complications. *Anaesthesia* 1995;50:813–815.

240. Karmakar MK, Ho AM, Law BK, et al. Arterial and venous pharmacokinetics of ropivacaine with and without epinephrine after thoracic paravertebral block. *Anesthesiology* 2005;103:704–711.

241. Ferguson S, Thomas V, Lewis I. The rectus sheath block in paediatric anaesthesia: New indications for an old technique? *Paediatr Anaesth* 1996;6:463–466.

242. Courrèges P, Poddevin F, Lecoutre D. Para-umbilical block: A new concept for regional anaesthesia in children. *Paediatr Anaesth* 1997;7:211–214.

243. Azemati S, Khosravi MB. An assessment of the value of rectus sheath block for postlaparoscopic pain in gynecologic surgery. *J Minim Invasive Gynecol* 2005;12:12–15.

244. Willschke H, Bosenberg A, Marhofer P, et al. Ultrasonography-guided rectus sheath block in paediatric anaesthesia: A new approach to an old technique. *Br J Anaesth* 2006;97:244–249.

245. Markham SJ, Tomlinson J, Hain WR. Ilioinguinal nerve block in children: A comparison with caudal block for intra and postoperative analgesia. *Anaesthesia* 1986;41:1098–1103.

246. Dalens B, Ecoffey C, Joly A, et al. Pharmacokinetics and analgesic effect of ropivacaine following ilioinguinal/iliohypogastric nerve block in children. *Paediatr Anaesth* 2001;11:415–420.

247. Ala-Kokko TI, Karinen J, Raiha E, et al. Pharmacokinetics of 0.75% ropivacaine and 0.5% bupivacaine after ilioinguinal-iliohypogastric nerve block in children. *Br J Anaesth* 2002;89:438–441.

248. Dalens B. "Small blocks" in paediatric patients. *Baillières Clin Anaesthesiol* 2001;14:745–758.

249. Kovacs P, Gruber H, Piegger J, et al. New, simple, ultrasound-guided infiltration of the pudendal nerve: Ultrasonographic technique. *Dis Colon Rectum* 2001;44:1381–1385.

250. Yang CC, Bradley WE. Innervation of the human glans penis. *J Urol* 1999;161:97–102.

251. Dalens B, Vanneuville G, Dechelotte P. Penile block via the subpubic space in 100 children. *Anesth Analg* 1989;69:41–45.

252. Schuepfer G, Johr M. Generating a learning curve for penile block in neonates, infants and children: An empirical evaluation of technical skills in novice and experienced anaesthetists. *Paediatr Anaesth* 2004;14:574–578.

253. Butler-O'Hara M, LeMoine C, Guillet R. Analgesia for neonatal circumcision: A randomized controlled trial of EMLA cream versus dorsal penile nerve block. *Pediatrics* 1998;101:E5.

254. Tobias JD. Cervical plexus block in adolescents. *J Clin Anesth* 1999;11:606–608

255. Parris WCV, Reddy BC, White HW, et al. Stellate ganglion blocks in pediatric patients. *Anesth Analg* 1991;72:552–556.

256. Mesa A, Kaplan RF. Dysrhythmias controlled with stellate ganglion block in a child with diabetes and a variant of long QT syndrome. *Reg Anesth* 1993;18:60–62.

257. Elias M, Chakerian MU. Repeated stellate ganglion blockade using a catheter for pediatric herpes zoster ophthalmicus. *Anesthesiology* 1994;80:950–952.

258. Tong HC, Nelson VS. Recurrent and migratory reflex sympathetic dystrophy in children. *Pediatr Rehabil* 2000;4:87–89.

259. Agarwal V, Joseph B. Recurrent migratory sympathetically maintained pain syndrome in a child: A case report. *J Pediatr Orthop B* 2006;15:73–74.

260. Monso A, Riudeubas J, Palanques F, et al. A new application for superior laryngeal nerve block: Treatment or prevention of laryngospasm and stridor. *Reg Anesth Pain Med* 1999;24:186–187.

261. Eipe N, Choudhrie A, Pillai AD, et al. Regional anesthesia for cleft lip repair: A preliminary study. *Cleft Palate Craniofac J* 2006;43:138–141.

262. Bratt HD, Eyres RL, Cole WG. Randomized double-blind trial of low and moderate-dose lidocaine regional anesthesia for forearm fractures in childhood. *J Pediatr Orthop* 1996;16:660–663.

263. Blasier RD, White R. Intravenous regional anesthesia for management of children's extremity fractures in the emergency department. *Pediatr Emerg Care* 1996;12:404–406.

264. Davidson AJ, Eyres RL, Cole WG. A comparison of prilocaine and lidocaine for intravenous regional anaesthesia for forearm fracture reduction in chixsdren. *Paediatr Anaesth* 2002;12:146–150.

PART III: APPLICATIONS

PART IV ■ NEURAL BLOCKADE AND THE MANAGEMENT OF PAIN

CHAPTER 28 ■ PAIN MEDICINE: HISTORY, EMERGENCE AS A MEDICAL SPECIALTY, AND EVOLUTION OF THE MULTIDISCIPLINARY APPROACH

ROLLIN M. GALLAGHER AND SCOTT M. FISHMAN

HISTORY OF PAIN TREATMENT

The treatment of pain reaches back into prehistory. As an alarm system that prompts withdrawal from harm and pursuit of circumstances conducive to healing, pain has an adaptive function. It is ironic that, despite its intrinsic aversive quality, pain commands our attention and is a vital part of life. Although pain is universally avoided, individuals born with a rare condition in which they are unable to perceive pain have a poor quality of life and shortened life expectancy.

The word "pain" can be traced to Poine, the Greek goddess of revenge, which reflects historical appreciation for the emotional complexity of the experience of pain. In ancient times, pain was associated with evil spirits or magic, and its management took place in corresponding domains. Priests or sorcerers might seek relief through sacrificial offerings or dramatic rituals to dispel evil spirits. Ancient cultures employed heat, cold, pressure, trauma, and even primitive operations to relieve pain. Some primitive cultures performed deliberate bleeding or trephination (cutting of holes in the body or skull) to release pain. The ancient Egyptians even employed early neuromodulation by applying electric eels to the body of a person in pain. In the Greek and Roman civilizations, pain was framed as an organized perceptual phenomenon that functioned through discrete organ systems.

During the Renaissance, DaVinci advanced the notion of organ-based physiology and, within this model, posited that the spinal cord and brain subserve transmission and perception of pain. The 17th through 19th centuries saw major advances in the understanding of pain, heralded by Descartes' specificity theory of pain. The 19th century saw the harnessing of the analgesic properties of morphine, aspirin, and cocaine, as well as the discovery of general anesthesia. The rich history of regional anesthesia has in large measure been surveyed by David Brown in Chapter 1.

During the 20th and 21st centuries, enormous advances in understanding and treating pain have revealed a level of complexity that Hippocrates, DaVinci, or Descartes could never have imagined. Much of this information is covered in other chapters of this volume, as synthesized by Allan Basbaum in Chapter 51. Table 28-1 briefly lists selected landmarks in pain control, along with the scientific understanding of nociception and pain, that underpin today's pain medicine practice and the translation of this understanding into clinical practice (1). Yet, despite these gains in the science and art of pain management, translation of this knowledge remains inconsistent. Society at large, while giving greater attention to pain and suffering, even in many respects reaching the threshold of regarding pain relief as a fundamental human right, has struggled with how to value and support pain relief and how best to integrate pain care into modern Westernized biomedicine (2).

Sociobiology of Altruism and the Healing Role

Communication of pain and suffering, and the responses of others who comfort and heal—be it as parent, relative, friend, or even stranger—is closely connected with the human trait of *altruism*. Altruism reflects our species' instinctual response to the perceived suffering of others, a response considered to be a sociobiologically based genetic trait with survival value to our species, one that is shaped and perpetuated by kinship bonds (3). The role of professional healers in social systems can be considered as a behaviorally refined and culturally focused expression of altruism extended to expanded kinship systems. This altruistic motive may be very strong even when it results in no short-term survival benefit for the social group, such as in palliative care of the terminally ill (see Chapter 49). The gradual organization of humans into groups such as tribes, communities, community networks, states, or nations, has promoted the evolution of the healers into defined, intergenerational cultural roles. In Western society, these roles are codified by laws and standards into distinct health professions such as medicine, nursing, and psychology. In many instances, the rules and principles of governance for these professions transcend community and cultural affiliations, as when clinicians are duty-bound to treat sick or injured enemy combatants in times of war. When professional standards of science and ethical practice are engulfed by ideological, political, or economic agendas, the professions suffer—as in the Nazi medical experiments on concentration camp inmates during World War II.

The power of the healing role is evident in the complementary and alternative traditions of healing and caregiving, including the relief of pain. These ubiquitous and ingrained traditions persist despite the ascendance of scientific medicine as the dominant healing profession. Their persistence demands explanations beyond arguments of socioeconomic disparity; that is, that such practices would disappear if every society could afford Western medicine. For example, although Western

TABLE 28-1

A SAMPLING OF MILESTONES IN THE INTELLECTUAL HISTORY OF PAIN MEDICINE

195 A.D.	Cannabis use first documented.
1646	Suarino describes snow and ice for pain relief.
1799	Davy describes the anesthetic properties of nitrous oxide.
1805	Serturner isolates the alkaloid morphine (*Morphium*) and demonstrates its use for sedation and pain control.
1842	Muller postulates the doctrine of specific nerve energies (i.e., afferent sensory neurons are specialized for different sensations), spurring research into pain sensation.
1842	Braid develops hypnosis as an evolution of Mesmer's ideas.
1846	Morton uses ether to allow painless excision of neck tumor at Massachusetts General Hospital.
1861–65	Morphine syringe invented and morphine used extensively in Civil War.
1883	Weir Mitchell describes causalgia in Civil War soldiers and the use of morphine.
1885	Halstead advocates for induction ether anesthesia.
1894	Von Frey initiates research into specific nociceptors in skin and pain pathways in spinal cord and brain.
1894	Goldscheider formulates *Pattern Theory B* (stimulus intensity and central summation determine levels of pain).
1899	Salicylic acid first commercially developed into acetylsalicylic acid (aspirin).
1900	Sherrington postulates physiologic specialization of receptors B.
1901	Frazier performs trigeminal neurectomy for facial pain.
1911	Spillar and Frazier initiate anterolateral cordotomy.
1945	Beecher differentiates intensity of pain from intensity of nociception in describing wounded soldiers in WW II; attributes the disparity to the meaning of the pain (i.e., I will survive and go home versus I have to go back and face battle).
1943	Livingston postulates reverberating spinal cord circuits to account for persistent pain of causalgia.
1953	Bonica introduces the term "pain clinic" to describe the multidisciplinary team that specializes in treating pain, and publishes his seminal textbook, *The Management of Pain*.
1955	White and Sweet describe cingulectomy.
1959	Noordenbos proposes sensory interaction theory: Destruction of the balance of slow small unmyelinated fibres and fast large myelinated fibres leads to pathologic pain.
1961	Gerard proposes loss of spinal pain fiber inhibition.
1965	Melzack and Wall propose the gate theory of pain perception and modulation.
1960s	Carbamazepine first described as effective for trigeminal neuralgia.
1967	Cicely Saunders founds the Saint Christopher's Hospice in Great Britain.
1973	Pert and Snyder (Johns Hopkins), Simon (New York University), and Terenius (Uppsala University) prove the existence of the opiate receptor, demonstrating the existence of the endogenous pain control system.
1973	Bonica (University of Washington) organizes the first scientific meeting devoted solely to pain with support from National Institutes of Health and Industry. This conference (at Issaquah, near Seattle) gives rise to the International Association for the Study of Pain.
1973	Melzack proposes a new conceptual model of pain, with three parallel systems: the gate control system, the motivational-affectivity system, and the sensory-discriminative system.
1973	Fordyce proposes pain as learned behavior and the operant conditioning model of pain.
1973	Sternback proposes pain behavior as an interpersonal identity in the physician–patient relationship.
1974	The International Association for the Study of Pain (IASP) is formed.
1974	The IASP begins its journal, *Pain*, with Patrick Wall as editor-in-chief.
1975	Endogenous opioid peptides—enkephalins—are discovered by Hughes and Kosterlitz (University of Aberdeen).
1978	Biopsychosocial model of medicine articulated by Engel (Rochester) in *Science*.
1982	Blumer describes the reduction of pain in depressed patients taking tricyclic antidepressants.
1986	IASP publishes *Classification of chronic pain: Description of chronic pain syndromes and definition of chronic pain terms*, edited by Mersky and Bogduk. Pain syndromes classified by a multiaxial system: anatomic region, bodily system (e.g., central nervous system), temporal characteristics, subjective intensity, etiology.
1992	Devor, Wall, and Catalan first describe effects of systemic lidocaine (sodium channel blockade) on ectopic firing of injured pain neurons.
1992	U.S. federal government publishes first clinical practice guideline: Topic is acute pain control after surgery or trauma. Multidisciplinary guideline panel, co-chaired by Carr (Boston), establishes a collaborative methodology for developing evidence-based pain guidelines including evidence ratings.
1992	First randomized clinical trial (RCT) demonstrating efficacy of tricyclics over selective serotonin reuptake inhibitors for neuropathic pain, by Max and colleagues (U.S. NIH).
1994	Gabapentin, due to demonstrated safety, begins to be widely used by pain specialists as first-line treatment for neuropathic pain, despite absence of RCTs (which eventually are completed demonstrating efficacy).
1997	Rainville and Bushnell, in *Science*, describe neuroimaging studies demonstrating mediation of affective component of experimental pain by activation of anterior cingulate gyrus and its attenuation with hypnosis.

Dates were obtained from various historical accounts of pain science and pain medicine. The authors are particularly indebted to Isabelle Baszanger's comprehensive treatise, *Inventing Pain Medicine: From the Laboratory to the Clinic*. New Brunswick, NJ: Rutgers University Press, 1998.

scientific medical practice is developing in China alongside, and sometimes blended with, traditional Chinese medical practices, traditional Chinese medical practices have thrived in North America and Europe. Nowhere is the interpenetration of complementary and conventional ("allopathic") therapies better demonstrated than in pain medicine, which combines the most contemporary advances in medical and behavioral neuroscience with ancient Eastern traditions such as acupuncture and meditation. The movement to incorporate complementary and alternative practices into a holistic approach that also offers Western treatments has come not from the medical establishment but to a large extent from consumers seeking relief from pain and suffering. The value of some of these practices no longer mystifies medical science, which has come to recognize efficacy for both acupuncture and meditation and to offer explanatory mechanisms for their beneficial effects. Mechanisms to account for the benefits of needle insertion and stimulation are described by Michael Butler in Chapter 34.

EMERGENCE OF PAIN MEDICINE: A MEDICAL SPECIALTY

It is said that to understand pain is to understand medicine. Pain is a complex phenomenon that encompasses both a neurophysiologic event, explained by a rational biomedical science, and an experience of suffering that mobilizes our human instinct to care. In considering when in the course of our evolution the event of pain became particularly human, one must consider its profoundly personal qualities that reverberate throughout an individuals' consciousness. Suffering is at once profoundly personal and private, but also the most poignant of interpersonal states. The language used to define those interpersonal links is intrinsically human and humane. For example, "empathy" implies a capacity beyond just understanding, that extends to the ability to vicariously experience suffering in others. Altruism and empathy are the instincts that draw us most powerfully to enter medicine and assume the role of healer. Nowhere in medicine is empathy more needed, but more difficult to sustain, than in the care of patients with persistent unrelenting pain (4,5). Although behavioral neuroscientists have made important gains in helping us to understand this encounter and to leverage this understanding to help patients recover from debilitating pain, management of this encounter itself is generally left to instinct, not training, in the traditional medical curriculum.

The problem of understanding the neurophysiology of pain and the pain experience has challenged some of the best minds of medicine. The many new discoveries described in this volume document an explosion of basic and clinical science in this area just in the past few decades. The final chapter of this volume points out that, not only do we possess detailed knowledge of the physiology, molecular biology, and pharmacology of acute pain at the levels of soma, spinal cord, and brain, but we are beginning to glimpse the molecular neurobiology and genetics of chronic pain. As this knowledge becomes more sophisticated, separation of mind and body (e.g., in the concept of "psychogenic pain") no longer is tenable. Brain imaging now enables us to visualize the workings of the mind interacting with the environment through various afferent sensory systems and their modulation, including nociception and analgesia. This knowledge has generated new drug and non-drug treatments at an ever-accelerating pace. When one of the authors (RMG) began his practice of medicine as a family physician in rural Colorado in 1971, outpatient pharmacologic treatment of chronic pain was limited to aspirin, acetaminophen (Tylenol), and occasional brief use of opioid analgesics for acute pain—their use was strongly discouraged for persistent pain, except when due to terminal cancer. The anxiety of acute pain was treated with a new miracle drug called diazepam (Valium). Routine orthopedic treatment for acute low back pain was propoxyphene (Darvon), Valium, and 2 to 3 weeks of bed rest for patients who avoided back surgery—these interventions have since been discredited for most cases of acute low back pain. Today's physician is armed with a myriad of effective pharmacologic, behavioral, and physical therapies; invasive procedures; and cross-cultural complementary and alternative treatments such as acupuncture and meditation. Learning how, when, and in what combination to apply these tools in patients with chronic pain requires physicians to be competently trained in three core clinical skills: to evaluate and formulate the salient biopsychosocial dimensions of chronic pain in each patient; to generate a prioritized, goal-oriented management plan; and to implement that treatment plan effectively within a health care system (6,7). The new specialty of pain medicine comprises this core group of cognitive and behavioral skills (8). Although each traditional medical specialty contributes to this knowledge base and skill set, their respective specialists are not trained to manage the entirety of the spectrum of chronic pain. Table 28-2 outlines the special skills contributed by traditional specialties in pain medicine.

A Climate of Change

Pain medicine is presently practiced as a subspecialty, but has no single most appropriate parent specialty. Its specialized knowledge, education, training, and multidisciplinary nature suggest that pain medicine's evolution as a specialty parallels that of other disciplines, such as emergency medicine or physical medicine and rehabilitation. Knowledge and skills of the latter disciplines, initially fragmented, later coalesced into primary medical specialties because of the inability of multiple specialties to offer an integrated approach that would best serve patients and medical science. Integration of diverse specialties into the formally recognized, differentiated medical specialty of pain medicine benefits the public at a time when society demands improved medical attention to pain (2). This benefit is particularly salient as regulations and standards for pain-related assessment and treatment in all health care facilities proliferate, undergraduate medical and continuing education in pain management are increasingly mandated, and administrative and legal complaints are lodged with increasing frequency against physicians who either overmedicate or undertreat pain.

The knowledge base and skill set of the specialty of pain medicine, as delineated by the American Board of Pain Medicine (9) and more recently by the U.S. Accreditation Council for Graduate Medical Education's Committee on Fellowships (10) comprise the anatomy, physiology, molecular biology, and psychology of the pain experience; the pathophysiology, clinical phenomenology, and epidemiology of conditions leading to chronic pain; the delineation of individual pain problems in a single patient; the appropriate application of relevant treatments (Table 28–2); the administrative aspects of pain treatment within a health system; and goal-oriented treatment planning and chronic disease management. A similar list has been developed by the Faculty of Pain Medicine of the Australia and New Zealand College of Anaesthetists (11).

PART IV: PAIN MANAGEMENT

TABLE 28-2

EXAMPLES OF DISEASE AND TREATMENT CONTRIBUTIONS TO PAIN MEDICINE FROM TRADITIONAL SPECIALTIES

Specialty	Illness/disease knowledge contribution	Medical skill/treatment contribution
Anesthesiology	Acute pain Chronic pain Cancer pain	Regional anesthesia (including neurolytic) Spinal anesthesia Operative anesthesia
Neurology	Peripheral neuropathy Neuropathic pain Central pain Headache	Assessment of neuropathic pain Neuropathic pain analgesia Headache medication
Neurosurgery	Spine disease Central pain	Implantable medication pumps Neurostimulation Spine evaluation and surgery
Orthopedic Surgery	Low back pain Physical disability	Spine evaluation and surgery Joint surgery
Palliative Care	Cancer pain	End of-life symptom management Bioethics
Primary Care	Chronic diseases	Chronic disease management Biopsychosocial medicine
Psychiatry, Behavioral Medicine	Psychiatric comorbidity Somatoform disorders Stress, behavior and emotions Fibromyalgia Personality and coping	Antidepressant analgesia Behavioral rehabilitation Biofeedback and relaxation Biopsychosocial formulation Psychotherapies (Cognitive-behavioral, group, family, hypnosis) Psychiatric diagnosis; psychological and psychometric evaluation Psychopharmacology
Radiological Medicine		Diagnostic imaging Procedure imaging Radiotherapy
Rehabilitation Medicine, Physical Therapy	Musculoskeletal medicine Myofascial pain Physical disability	Physical therapy Physical rehabilitation Transcutaneous electrical nerve stimulation Trigger-point therapy
Rheumatology	Joint diseases Fibromyalgia	Joint injections Peripheral nociceptive analgesia (nonsteroidal anti-inflammatory drugs)
Complementary and Alternative Medicine		Acupuncture Massage Meditation Tai Chi

This constellation of qualifications is not currently contained in any one traditional American Board of Medical Specialties (ABMS) specialty training program. Skillful application of the treatments listed in Table 28–2, often in combination, is required to effectively manage and remediate chronic pain but has not been a goal of previous specialty training. Specialists in pain medicine must be trained to use these tools at a level of evidence-based care that can be standardized and replicated in training programs across the country (12).

The State of Pain Treatment in Medicine

Access to pain treatment is uneven in our society, depending on the race, gender, and socioeconomic status of the patient, as well as on the education and training of the physician (13–19). These socioeconomic factors, which extend into areas such as litigation and reimbursement, are discussed in detail by Professor Loeser in Chapter 29. Despite medicine's traditional mandate "...to relieve often, to comfort always," physicians often harbor mistaken or negative attitudes about treating pain (20). Reimbursement for pain-relieving treatments is often refused by insurance payors, and access to comprehensive pain rehabilitation is almost nonexistent in many areas of the United States. Inadequate access to care takes place despite compelling data to support the effectiveness of comprehensive pain care (in comparison with conventional medical care) in reducing pain, restoring function, and returning injured persons to work (21–26). Access to reimbursement for individualized care related to pain and pain-related drug abuse is also inadequate (27,29). Unnecessary barriers to treatment impose needless suffering on patients and their loved ones, and shift the financial burden of disability from the health insurance sector to businesses and taxpayers (30,31).

Recent actions by regulators, major health care organizations, courts, and legislatures suggest that society is increasingly intolerant of medicine's inattention to pain and suffering (2). The Veteran's Affairs medical system was the first large-scale system to respond to this trend by designating pain as the "fifth vital sign" in all its hospitals (32). The Joint Commission on Accreditation of Healthcare Organizations (JCAHO) followed suit by likewise designating pain as the "fifth vital sign" and by requiring health care institutions to provide organized pain assessment and treatment in order to be accredited (33). Both the American Medical Association (AMA) and the Association of American Medical Colleges (AAMC) recently recommended inclusion of pain and palliative care in every medical school curriculum (34–36).

A recent civil lawsuit finding a physician guilty of elder abuse for undertreating pain led the California State Legislature to require physicians to complete specific pain-related continuing medical education (37). The California State Legislature has also mandated a curriculum in pain and palliative care for all medical schools (38). Nationally, an act of Congress declared 2001–2010 as "The Decade of Pain Control and Research," and The National Institutes of Health has launched a focused initiative in pain research (39–41).

Historically, chronic pain has been treated, at least initially, by primary care physicians. The role of the primary care physician to ease suffering may be eclipsed as the patient with chronic pain is referred to a sequence of specialty physicians, each evaluating the condition from a narrow perspective. Fragmented, costly, and ineffective care often follows, allowing pain to evolve from a symptom to a disease (42). This transformation is characterized by neuropathologic changes such as sensitization, plasticity, and kindling of sensory and affective systems (43). It also shifts the costs of disease burden from insurer to society (30,44,45). The Institute of Medicine recognized the fragmentation of pain care two decades ago, stating: "Such evaluations require expertise in a number of disciplines and in skills such as functional and psychosocial assessment and neurological and musculoskeletal examinations. Currently, few individual clinicians are competent to conduct such multidisciplinary evaluations of pain patients or to recommend and coordinate appropriate therapy. The patient is typically referred to a series of experts, each of whom does part of the assessment and/or part of the treatment. Of course the very problem with this practice is that care is expensive, fragmented, and ineffective" (46).

Treating pain will be—and should always be—part of the clinical responsibility of every physician. Up to 65% of primary care patients report having pain (47,48). The generalist model suffers from diminishing returns when medical and social needs exceed the capacity of the medical care that can be provided by a single generalist. Yet, the number of generalist physicians and allied health practitioners who serve as gatekeepers has grown tremendously (49,50). Although generalist care offers important advantages for the patient in pain, well-designed specialty models are also necessary and feasible within managed care models of health care delivery (51). Evidence suggests that the current focus on having generalists meet the needs of patients must be balanced by maintaining an adequate workforce of pain medicine specialists (52,53) in a collaborative care model in which pain medicine provides workable clinical algorithms that help primary care systems manage pain more effectively but also provides timely clinical back-up (45,54–58).

Specialist care for persistent pain has been associated with improved treatment outcomes, greater patient satisfaction, and lower cost compared with delivery by generalists (52,59–65). For example, Anderson and colleagues found, in a cohort of 398 patients with osteoarthritis or low back pain, that specialist care yielded superior functional outcomes with similar costs compared with care by general internists (52). Mitchell and Carmen compared early intensive treatment by specialists with standard conservative treatments in over 3,000 patients with acute soft-tissue and back injuries (64). Specialist treatment saved $1 to $1.5 million *per month* by preventing lost wages and health care costs. Closer follow-up of a subgroup of 500 patients treated by specialists revealed a lowering of the cost of care by approximately $5,000 per patient.

Formal Recognition as a Specialty: Rationale and Status

The definitive history of the development, recognition, and installment of pain medicine as a distinct specialty has not yet been written because it is a work in progress. The ABMS describes a medical specialty as *"a defined area of medical practice, which connotes special knowledge and ability resulting from specialized effort and training in the special field"* (65). In keeping with this definition, one may trace the evolution of the specialty of pain medicine in three separate but related domains: intellectual (special knowledge), clinical practice (special ability), and clinical training (specialized effort and training).

Pain medicine's *"special knowledge"* has developed relatively recently, on the basis of scientific insights that are integrative in nature. The situation for pain medicine contrasts with that of traditional specialties or subspecialties that organized originally around diseases of specific organ systems (heart, kidney, skin, GI, GU, nervous system) or particular clinical disciplines (surgery, anesthesiology), in many cases before the era of scientific medicine. These traditional specialties marshaled the forces of scientific medicine in the 20th century to develop their intellectual and clinical knowledge base and set standards for training and practice. The explosion of pain medicine's basic and clinical science knowledge base in the past three decades, sparked by a convergence of breakthroughs in biomedical neurosciences such as the gate theory, behavioral medicine research, and methodological refinements in epidemiology, is reflected by a literature search revealing numbers of publications that use pain-related terms (8). Figure 28-1 shows the large increase in publication titles containing the term "pain" from the 1970s to the 1990s. Figure 28-2 shows a much more dramatic rise in the numbers of titles that include the more technical term, *nociception*, which was used rarely before the 1980s.

The key concepts underpinning the "special knowledge" of pain medicine reflect the modern understanding of pain as an experience. Pain is no longer considered merely a symptom

PART IV: PAIN MANAGEMENT

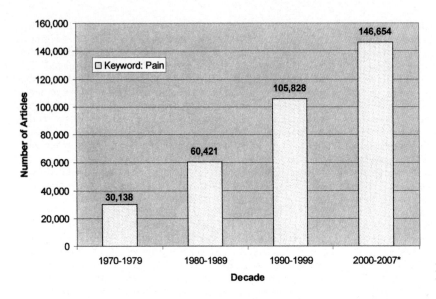

FIGURE 28-1. Articles published, by decade, retrieved using PubMed with keyword "pain."

of tissue injury, one whose empiric treatment necessarily reduces suffering. The appropriate knowledge base for today's practice and teaching of pain medicine now involves an integrated understanding of pain as a multidirectional communication system within the body, spinal cord, and brain, mediated by complex interactions between immunologic, sensorimotor, emotional, and cognitive-behavioral functions, interpreted within a socioeconomic context as described in Chapter 29 by Professor Loeser. Insight into the complex process of pain also involves an understanding of pathophysiologic models of dysfunction and disease, first established in animal studies and now applied to better understand and treat their human disease analogues. Distinct experimental models of neuropathic pain (trauma, vascular compromise, toxic, infection) involve common neural pathways in the peripheral and central nervous system, yet diverse individual neuropathic pain conditions respond differently to interventions in clinical trials. For example, we do not understand why tricyclic antidepressants (TCAs) are effective in treating the neuropathic pain of postherpetic neuralgia and diabetic neuropathy, but not for the neuropathic pain of HIV neuropathy (66).

Pain medicine's "special ability" antedates its "special knowledge." Techniques for treating pain were and still are, in some parts of the world, applied in both prehistoric and prescientific cultures. Some healing practices have evolved into scientifically established, evidence-based enterprises: herbs and plants in folk medicines have evolved to pharmaceuticals, and meditation has evolved to specific, scripted behavioral interventions. The most obvious pharmaceutical examples in pain medicine are aspirin from willow tree bark and morphine from the opium poppy; both purified extracts have routinely been used for over a century in Western medicine (67). Their widespread use prompted the development of two large classes of medications acting through different mechanisms: the nonsteroidal anti-inflammatory drugs (NSAIDs) and the opioid analgesics. Over the last 30 years, pharmacotherapy for pain has expanded well beyond these two mechanisms, often through serendipitous observations of pain relief in persons being treated for other purposes. In the 1970s, pain relief was noted in patients hospitalized for depression and treated with TCAs (68). Although this discovery had the temporarily negative consequence of supporting erroneous arguments for a psychogenic causation of chronic nonmalignant pain, physicians were now provided with a tool that, through well-designed clinical trials, established efficacy specific for types of neuropathic pain in patients without depression, which also suggested a differentiation of efficacy based upon mechanism of action (69). Presently, the analgesic efficacy of TCAs is

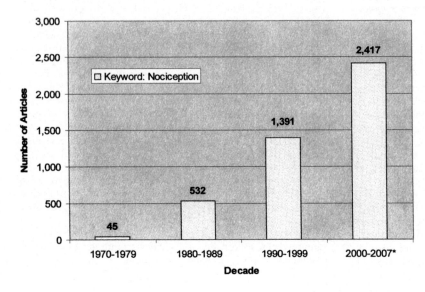

FIGURE 28-2. Articles published, by decade, retrieved using PubMed with keyword "nociception."

thought to be due to several mechanisms, such as the blockade of sodium channels and the inhibition of reuptake of norepinephrine and serotonin leading to activation of descending neuromodulatory pathways (70).

Similar to recognition of the analgesic effect of TCAs independent of their effect upon mood, beginning with carbamazepine in the 1960s, anticonvulsants were observed to ease neuropathic pain independent of their effect upon seizures. By the 1980s, carbamazepine had become a standard treatment for trigeminal neuralgia. In the 1990s, clinicians noted that gabapentin alleviated a variety of neuropathic pain conditions; because of its safety and tolerability profile compared with other anticonvulsants and TCAs (71), it rapidly became the drug of choice for many clinicians treating neuropathic pain well before its efficacy was established by clinical trials (72). Currently, all available antidepressants and anticonvulsants have been tried clinically as analgesics for neuropathic pain, most have been tested for efficacy in randomized clinical trials, and many are recommended in evidence-based clinical pathways, treatment algorithms, and standards (69–73). Important pharmaceutical progress has also been made in developing new methods of delivering analgesic medications, such as through transdermal, transmucosal (e.g., sublingual, buccal, or nasal), and intrathecal routes, as well as in compounding medications for sustained action. Today, numerous medication choices exist for the physician treating a variety of distinct pain disorders and diseases. Their mechanisms of action, interactions, synergies, complications, and indications, as well as training in their use singly, together, or in combination with other therapies, is a fund of knowledge and clinical skills that is large, complex, growing rapidly, and specific to the specialty of pain medicine. As described in Chapters 32 and 33 by Professors Yaksh and Dickenson, respectively, ongoing research in the molecular biology and genetics of pain and the pathophysiology of pain diseases continues to reveal new mechanisms that are targets for new drugs that the biotechnology and specialty pharmaceutical industry will synthesize and deliver.

Other major advances in pain treatment have focused on the elimination or correction of pain-producing pathology caused by disease or trauma. Obvious examples include curative surgical interventions such as for hernias; radiotherapy and chemotherapy to reduce or eliminate cancer metastases; surgery to replace painful arthritic joints; and spinal operations for bony and soft tissue (e.g., disc) disease or injury. Although these interventions promise to eliminate pain generators, we now understand that they themselves have complications (e.g., surgery, radiotherapy, and chemotherapy all may cause nerve damage) including sensitization and centralized pain. Indeed, in the face of preexisting hyperalgesia and chronic pain (e.g., complex regional pain syndrome [CRPS], as described in Chapter 46 by Professor Baron), surgical treatments may aggravate pain.

The development of the specialties of anesthesia and surgery have contributed important advances that are now in the armamentarium of pain treatment, as well-documented in other chapters such as 41 and 42. Morton's demonstration in 1846 of ether anesthesia to control pain during the excision of a jaw tumor revolutionized surgical practice, enabling its evolution over the last 150 years into the complex, life-saving operative procedures that are almost routine today. Now, surgical procedures aim specifically to remediate disabling pain and improve function, either by addressing the underlying pain generator (as in cardiac surgery for painful ischemic heart disease), by implanting neuromodulatory devices, or even in highly selected cases by dividing nociceptive pathways. As described in depth in the first half of this text, regional anesthesia has evolved well beyond the simple procedures commonly used in general

medical and dental practice, such as blocking peripheral nerves for outpatient surgery, dental procedures, suturing in the emergency room, and regional infusions (e.g., Bier blocks) for limb repair. Diverse types of real-time imaging to aid in the precise placement of catheters and needles allow a range of nerve, ganglion, and neuraxial blocks to be applied routinely in operative anesthesia and pain medicine, including widely prevalent spine disorders and palliative care. Identification of pain generators by stimulating specific nerves and testing whether an anesthetic block reduces pain, enables precise thermal ablation or cryoablation and pain relief. Local and general anesthetics introduced to prevent perioperative pain have been found useful for chronic pain conditions; for example, systemic infusions of lidocaine performed periodically to control generalized or regional pain, or ketamine for CRPS. Moreover, local anesthetics and systemic analgesics are now being given preemptively to prevent activation of nociceptive pathways in an effort to reduce the severity of acute postoperative pain, which, if poorly controlled, may predispose to chronic pain. Finally, as described by Drs. Prager and Stanton-Hicks, neurostimulation has evolved beyond the transcutaneous electrical nerve stimulator to include intraspinal, intracranial, transcranial, and peripheral nerve applications.

Rehabilitation medicine has contributed to the expansion of the knowledge base, particularly for musculoskeletal pain, such as myofascial pain and trigger points and their treatment. Specific exercises tailored to individual patients restore muscle function and remediate factors associated with deconditioning. Such factors, including poor posture and disturbed gait, are extremely common comorbidities that perpetuate musculoskeletal pain. Exercise focused on functional gains helps restore the ability to participate in activities across all domains of life that are beneficial physically, psychologically, and socially, and thus enhance the central modulation of pain. Health services research has found that rehabilitation programs integrating the expertise of many disciplines in the service of functional restoration demonstrate both efficacy and cost-effectiveness.

The most recent area of development of the science and practice of pain medicine aims at the interface between mind and brain (43,74–75). Specific treatments aimed at reducing stress and the stress response, such as relaxation training, meditation, biofeedback, and hypnosis have proven to enhance analgesia, well-being, and coping (76). The mechanisms for these positive effects are being elucidated through investigative techniques ranging from neurochemistry to brain imaging. The benefits of these mind–brain therapies can be summarized as threefold. First, they promote self-efficacy by arming patients with the ability to deactivate central and peripheral catecholaminergic arousal (stress response) that stimulates sympathetically maintained neuropathic pain, muscle contraction, and nociceptor activation. Second, they facilitate self-efficacy through the acquisition of new and more effective chronic-disease coping skills (such as avoidance of stress and specific behaviors that activate pain generators) and adherence to regimens of physical, behavioral, and medical treatment. Third, they enhance descending pain modulation. Advances in the neurosciences, specifically neuroimaging, have identified those brain regions that are affected by many of these techniques. Imaging is also being used as a sophisticated form of biofeedback to select optimally scripted exercises aimed at reducing symptoms in CRPS and pain intensity at baseline (76–79).

Outside of traditional medicine, complementary and alternative healing arts have also flourished. The ubiquity of chronic pain, combined with the treatment failures of Western biomedicine, have led to the proliferation of such treatments for pain. Chiropractic focuses on manipulating the spine to relieve pain, although controlled studies are few. The efficacy of acupuncture is supported by well-designed studies of its benefit in reducing pain of several different types, although, as pointed out by Professor Butler in Chapter 34, the nonspecific effects of needle insertion complicate the design and interpretation of such studies. Various other techniques, possibly functioning through psychophysiologic mechanisms such as the placebo effect surveyed in Chapter 36 by Finniss and Benedetti, are used widely, although their efficacy is not established.

The need for "specialized education and training in pain medicine" reflects the poor performance of organized medicine to meet the needs of patients with pain at a time when pain relief is increasingly viewed as a fundamental human right (2). As stated earlier, pain education is lacking at every level of medical education. To date, medicine has been unable to offer effective approaches to pain education that effectively integrate the disparate parts of the field (7,8,12,34–36,80–82). Recent legal and regulatory mandates to teach medical students and physicians about pain reflect a historically fragmented approach to pain education, with many specialties each offering a distinct approach to pain assessment and care, each unable to consolidate the multidisciplinary complexity of pain into a comprehensive curriculum. In light of these deficiencies, change to the current system of patient care and medical education and research must occur. A medical subspecialty is in part defined by the ABMS as "an identifiable component of a specialty to which a practicing physician may devote a significant proportion of time" (10). Unfortunately, no single primary discipline can fully meet this requirement, and multiple specialties can claim to be the appropriate primary specialty for pain medicine. As surveyed earlier, based upon the ABMS's criteria of "special knowledge" and "special ability," pain medicine appears to have rapidly developed as a distinct clinical field (8). Greater recognition of pain medicine as a specialty is needed to translate new knowledge into clinical practice standards, education for students, and training for residents, as well as to attract the support necessary for much-needed translational research.

The circumstances surrounding the historical development of the specialty of emergency medicine are similar to those currently facing pain medicine. It was initially assumed that clinicians from many disciplines could satisfactorily manage patients presenting to the emergency room. Fragmented emergency room activities led to five or six specialists simultaneously addressing a patient, each focusing on her organ system of interest. No single clinician was completely invested in the care of the whole patient. As clinical knowledge expanded, a single specialty was required, comprising those physicians who devoted all their professional activities to the care of the patient with emergent medical needs. This need for a single emergency physician who embodied elements of the various specialties that had traditionally managed patients in this setting led to the creation of the distinct specialty of emergency medicine.

Parallels with pain medicine may be traced with the history of anesthesiology as a primary medical specialty. In North America, the specialty of anesthesiology began with the formation of the Long Island Society of Anesthetists in 1905, the name of which was changed to the New York Society of Anesthetists (NYSA) in 1911 (82,83). In 1936, the word "American" was substituted for "New York," and the Society became the American Society of Anesthesiologists (ASA). Physician anesthesiologists trained as fellows of the NYSA, and later of the ASA. Eventually, leaders in anesthesiology believed that, without immediate action, certification of their specialty would be parsed out to other AMA-sanctioned specialties. The American Board of Anesthesiology (ABA) itself was initially formed as a subordinate board of the American Board of Surgery (ABS), but soon separated to form its own specialty.

Today, in North America, there is no consensus in the medical community as to the duration of additional specialized training and experience required to become a proficient pain specialist. In contrast to the situation for other recognized specialties, disagreements among the several primary disciplines that contribute to the knowledge base and clinical application of pain medicine have, to date, hindered efforts to arrive at such a consensus. The ABA first issued a certificate of added qualification in pain management in 1993 (84). This certificate was followed by applications for subspecialty certificates in pain management from the American Board of Psychiatry and Neurology (ABPN), and the American Board of Physical Medicine and Rehabilitation (ABPMR) in 2000 (84). In an effort to offer board certification to qualifying physicians from all medical specialties, the American Board of Pain Medicine (ABPM) was formed in 1991, as an outgrowth of the American Academy of Pain Medicine (AAPM) (85). Medical licensure boards in three of the largest states, California (1996), Florida (1999), and Texas (2001) found the ABPM board certification to be equivalent to ABMS certification, but the ABPM certificate has not yet been formally recognized by the ABMS.

The recent addition of ABMS-approved certification through the ABPN and the ABPMR indicates that organized medicine is now recognizing the breadth of pain medicine and acknowledging that pain medicine does not currently fit fully under any present single ABMS specialty (82,84). The U.S. Accreditation Council for Graduate Medical Education (ACGME) and ABMS are now tackling the problem of pain specialty training. Proposed solutions range from lengthening current subspecialty-style fellowship programs from 1 year to 2 or more years, to creating specialty residencies in pain medicine (9,12). Residency and fellowship training requirements for the field of pain medicine have been developed conjointly by the AAPM and the ABPM, which have made recommendations to a task force of the ACGME (9). The ACGME task force is also considering recommendations from ABMS member boards to lengthen present fellowship requirements and, starting in 2007, now requires interdisciplinary input for accreditation. To date, however, clarification of standard training in pain medicine has not been achieved in the United States. Of note, the Faculty of Pain Medicine of the Australia New Zealand College of Anaesthetists (FPMANZCA) applied for specialty status for pain medicine and, in 2006, succeeded in being recognized as a separate specialty by the Australian government (85). Among many examples of contributions that can be made when a unified specialty addresses a problem, the FPMANZCA, consisting of about 200 members, provided the first comprehensive, evidence-based review of acute pain management (86) since Carr and colleague's landmark AHCPR clinical practice guideline in 1992, which also established standards for evaluating the strength of the evidence when developing guidelines (87). Today, the momentum to establish standards for pain medicine as a specialty is now global. In 2007, the Section and Board of Anaesthesiology of the European Union of Medical Specialists (EUMS/UEMS) initiated the establishment of the Multidisciplinary Joint Committee on Pain Medicine of the EUMS/UEMS, which has created a certification examination in pain medicine. (88). Also in 2007, the Ministry of Health of the Peoples Republic of China announced the designation of pain medicine as a separate specialty and that departments of pain medicine will be established in major Chinese hospitals (89).

Important events in the organization, education, training, and certification of pain medicine as a specialty are outlined in Table 28-3.

TABLE 28-3	

IMPORTANT EVENTS IN THE ORGANIZATION, EDUCATION, TRAINING, AND CERTIFICATION OF PAIN MEDICINE AS A SPECIALTY

1973	International Association for the Study of Pain (IASP) forms with John Bonica as its first president and Patrick Wall as first editor of *Pain*.
1977	American Pain Society forms as subsidiary of IASP.
1983	American Academy of Pain Medicine (AAPM) forms as a medical specialty society (first called American Academy of Algology).
1991	American Board of Anesthesiology creates an examination for special qualification in pain management for anesthesiologists, and establishes fellowship training in pain management, enabling anesthesiologists to become subspecialty board certified in pain management.
1991	American Board of Pain Medicine (ABPM) is founded (initially incorporated as the American College of Pain Medicine).
1993	ABPM creates specialty board certification in pain medicine: Enables ABMS board-certified anesthesiologists, neurologists, neurosurgeons, psychiatrists, and PM&R specialists who were practicing pain medicine to become board certified in pain medicine following credentialing and examination.
1993	AAPM gains a seat as a separate medical specialty in the American Medical Association.
1993	The European Federation of IASP Chapters (EFIC) forms as a subsidiary of the IASP.
1995	IASP, under its President, Michael Cousins, publishes *Core Curriculum for Professional Education in Pain*. IASP task force publishes Desirable Characteristics for Pain Treatment Facilities.
1998	Faculty of Pain Medicine of the Australia New Zealand College of Anaesthetists (FPMANZCA) founded by specialties of Medicine, Anaesthesia, Surgery, Psychiatry and Rehabilitation Medicine.
1999	FPMANZCA publishes first edition of *Acute Pain Management: Scientific Evidence* (with updated versions in 2004 and 2007).
2000	American Board of Medical Specialties (ABMS) creates subspecialty certification for neurologists, physiatrists, and psychiatrists.
2000	AAPM founds its own journal, *Pain Medicine*, which is indexed by the National Library of Medicine in 2003.
2000–2002	ABPM certification obtains recognition as equivalent to an ABMS certification by the Medical Practice Boards of California, Florida, and Texas.
2001	ABMS proposes to the ACGME Task Force on Fellowship Programs in pain medicine a curriculum for 2- and 3-year primary residencies in pain medicine, the *Essentials of Accredited Training Programs in Graduate Medical Education: Institutional and Program Requirements for Pain Medicine Training Programs*.
2003	The Australian Medical Council (AMC) endorses training and credentialing requirements recommended by the Faculty of Pain Medicine of Australia
2004	FPMANZCA joins AAPM in sponsoring *Pain Medicine* as its official journal.
2004	Ethics Charter published by the AAPM.
2005	The government of Australia formally recognizes pain medicine as a specialty
2005	*Pain Medicine* publishes "The case for pain medicine as a medical specialty."
2006	ACGME approves new standards for pain management fellowships that require multispecialty faculty (anesthesiology, neurology, physiatry, and psychiatry), beginning in 2007.
2007	At the Annual Meeting of the Chinese Association for the Study of Pain, the Ministry of Health of the Peoples Republic of China announces the designation of Pain Medicine as a separate specialty, and that departments of pain medicine will be established in all major hospitals in China.
2008	The Chinese Pain Medicine Association and AAPM hold the East-West Pain Medicine Conference in Shenzhen, China.
2008	The AAPM and ABPM author "Program Requirements for Graduate Medical Education in Pain Medicine", a 4 year residency program, which is published in PAIN MEDICINE.
2008	The first meeting of an international interest group on Pain Medicine Specialty training held at IASP in Glasgow.
2009	FPMANZCA and Chinese Pain Association join the AAPM's first Pacific Pain Medicine Conference in Honolulu, Hawaii.

ORGANIZATIONAL MODELS OF PAIN PRACTICE: THE MULTIDISCIPLINARY APPROACH AND BEYOND

Pain medicine specialty practice initially evolved as clinical innovators and clinical scientists examined specific questions or developed specific techniques for treating pain. As pointed out earlier, this model often leads to sequential referrals without a focus on comprehensive pain control, while risking progression to chronic pain and its psychosocial and economic conse-quences. As health care systems have attempted to address the problems of patients with pain more systematically, new models of organization have emerged based on identified needs. In the 1960s, Dr. John Bonica first organized coordinated care provided by different disciplines in his multidisciplinary pain clinic at the University of Washington (90). Eventually, such multidisciplinary clinics flourished in the United States. Un-fortunately, the dominance of managed care, in which chronic disease management has not been incentivized to achieve improved long-term outcomes (such as return to work) and which carves out multidisciplinary pain treatment, has led to the near-demise of multidisciplinary pain clinics (91). A new model of more efficient collaborative care—the "pain medicine and primary care community rehabilitation model"—combines the efforts of the primary care provider (PCP), other community resources including the patient and their family, and the pain medicine specialist, who embodies the knowledge and skills of the multispecialty team that Bonica envisioned. This model is based on several principles: early, successful intervention with the overriding goal of preventing secondary complications such as nociceptive sensitization, occupational and family stress, and depression; training PCPs to use evidence-based algorithms to guide the management of specific pain disorders and diseases; timely referral to pain medicine specialists for biopsychosocial evaluation and coordination of a goal-oriented management plan; use of other specialists as needed; and shared responsibility for outcomes among patient, PCP, pain medicine center, and community (44,45,54,56).

Table 28-4 outlines four organizational models of pain care and their consequences.

A brief overview of the effectiveness of integrated multidisciplinary pain treatment demonstrates the need for these models, and their value. The evidence is strong (Level 1, i.e., supported by meta-analysis of multiple RCTs) that integrated multidisciplinary pain rehabilitation (IMDR) is effective for reducing pain (92), improving function (93,94), and improving vocational outcomes (95) in chronic low back pain (CLBP), the most common chronic pain condition, and the one that places the greatest economic burden upon society at large. *Pain reduction* ranges from 20% to 40% and tends to be maintained for up to 2 years (92), whereas conventional medical or surgical treatment offers less benefit in long-term pain reduction (96–98). *Function* also improves, with IMDR programs demonstrating a 20% to 40% higher return-to-work rate for CLBP patients compared with conventional treatments (95). A recent systematic review (Level 1 evidence) of RCTs of the effectiveness of IMDR over 5 years in 1,964 patients with CLBP (93) showed strong evidence of improved function, moderate evidence of reduced pain, and mixed evidence regarding vocational outcome. A study of CLBP patients randomized to either lumbar fusion or IMDR showed that the latter improved significantly in muscle strength compared with the former (99). In one study, CLBP patients treated with cognitive behavioral and physical therapies compared with usual medical treatment showed improvement in physical function but not in depression and pain (100). This result demonstrates the importance of analgesic and antidepressant treatment in IMDR programs, and reinforces the

TABLE 28-4

ORGANIZATIONAL MODELS IN PAIN MEDICINE (44, 45)

Model	Description and outcomes
Sequential care model	■ Patients are referred from one expert to another, as each seeks to identify and treat a pain generator according to their specialty training. ■ The process takes many months and accrues high costs. ■ No provider attends to controlling the patients' pain during this process, allowing the progression of the neuropathophysiologic and psychosocial pathologies of chronic pain, such as sensitization, depression, and disability. ■ Outcomes are poor, medical and societal costs are very high.
Multidisciplinary Pain Center Model	■ Patients fail the sequential care model so that the chronic disease of pain and its complications are established. ■ They require a specialized center, usually far from home, where they receive expert treatment from a variety of specialists. ■ Costs are very high, so very few centers exist, and delays of approval worsen clinical conditions. ■ Outcomes are usually good (return to work and function), but patients are sent home without expert follow-up, increasing risk of relapse. ■ Long-term outcomes are determined by availability of expert follow-up treatment.
Managed Care Model	■ Patients are denied referral to specialized pain medicine centers. ■ Behavioral and physical therapies are "carved out" to nonexpert psychologist and physical therapists whose efforts are not coordinated with the pain medicine specialist. ■ Procedures that pay well and take little time are emphasized in clinical practice. ■ Medical management consists of polypharmacy without chronic disease management. ■ Patients often deteriorate, losing jobs and insurance, depending on public assistance for their income and treatment. ■ Collectively, patients increase the tax burden on society and the longitudinal costs of hospitals and clinical care, straining the system.
Pain Medicine and Primary Care Community Rehabilitation Model	■ Evidence-based clinical care algorithms for specific pain diseases/disorders guide evaluation and management for primary care providers (PCPs). ■ Responsibility for outcomes is shared among PCP, patient, family, and pain medicine specialist. ■ Easy, timely access is provided to pain medicine physicians for consultation and referral. ■ Pain medicine specialists support care algorithms and coordinate treatment for complex cases. ■ Early referrals lower the risk of developing chronic pain disease and its complications. ■ System has the capacity to monitor patient outcomes through PCPs. ■ System coordinates longitudinal care among PCP, PT, behavioral, mental health and community supports, and resources. ■ Lower total costs, fewer hidden costs.

need for knowledgeable pain medicine physicians to integrate rehabilitation and analgesic and adjuvant medical treatments (such as antidepressants or anticonvulsants) for the best outcomes.

In a time of rapid evolution of practice models in response to calls for cost-effective and evidence-based practice, examples of studies in which randomization was employed—yet basic flaws in concept and design rendered the results meaningless—should caution readers of the medical literature against assuming that results of an RCT are necessarily superior to those of other study designs (101). For example, in a purported test of different approaches to managing head and neck pain, Canadian researchers randomized a cohort of patients already receiving repeated nerve block therapy for neck and head pain either to continue nerve blocks or to stop them and undergo a course of cognitive behavioral therapy (CBT) (102). Not surprisingly, patients in the latter group wanted to resume nerve blocks, initially having selected and maintained this therapy despite marginal results upon their pain intensity. Despite such obvious evidence for selection bias in this study cohort, the authors did not examine why their patients would choose to continue to undergo nerve blocks despite negative results upon pain intensity. This example illustrates that, although important policy decisions throughout medicine are ostensibly based upon "what the evidence shows," doing so in an uncritical fashion can lead to ignoring a treatment's benefits for important subgroups of responders (103) and overgeneralization or misapplication of trial results, to the detriment of patient care (104). The many examples of bias in systematic reviews of various pain treatments (105) that led to flaws in developing evidence-based guidelines for pain management (106) should caution practitioners and policy-makers to critically review existing literature before developing guidelines and policy from systematic reviews. Clinicians and health services researchers are now reexamining less quantitative forms of clinical evidence, such as narrative and the experience of clinicians, with an eye toward not summarily discarding these sources of potentially worthwhile evidence (107).

Regardless of the clinical practice model employed, an individualized selective combination of diverse treatments to maximize functional outcomes appears to provide the best results (95). The core tenets are: (a) evaluate each patient with chronic pain according to a biopsychosocial perspective that identifies pain generators, pain activators, and pain aggravators, along with psychosocial factors and comorbidities that perpetuate impairment and interfere with treatment response;

(b) provide adequate analgesia to support functional restoration, using medications, regional anesthesia, and neurostimulation as needed; (c) provide physical and occupational therapies focused on functional restoration, without aggravating existing injuries; and (d) provide CBT, supported by psychopharmacology as needed for emotional stability and enhanced coping.

SUMMARY

The need in our health care system has never been greater for the widespread use of timely, selective, cost-effective integrated pain treatment, emphasizing prevention of chronic pain and its consequences and the restoration of function, with a focus on long-term benefit. Pain medicine is a rapidly expanding discipline with an increasingly important role in health care in leading the development of standards for pain treatment and the training of physicians, and setting the clinical research agenda and carrying it out. However, particularly in North America, pain medicine is not optimally positioned within organized medicine for its own growth and the maximal benefit to patients and society. Currently, pain medicine is practiced as a subspecialty of multiple medical specialties without any single one that is clearly most appropriate. The crisis of inadequately treated pain continues to be fueled by fragmentation that is, in part, a result of inadequate acceptance of pain medicine as a distinct medical specialty. Patients in pain require a specialty unencumbered by the boundaries of traditional disciplines, one that is able to assimilate diverse knowledge and treatments in order to provide sound care. Physicians, who are now feeling increasingly vulnerable if they under- or overtreat pain, require a discrete specialty to set standards, produce effective specialty consultants with comprehensive skills and knowledge, and produce role models, teachers, and researchers as the science and practice of pain medicine continue to evolve.

The way in which this new field is positioned for continued development and integration throughout health care will greatly affect the ability of medicine to meet its mission to understand and treat pain. Without leading broad change in the current practices of medical education and clinical care, organized medicine will incur more regulations and laws that will require it to do so. As was true for other recently differentiated specialties, these necessary changes will require unification of the disparate parts of pain medicine that currently reside within multiple specialties.

References

1. Baszanger I. *Inventing Pain Medicine: From the Laboratory to the Clinic.* New Brunswick, New Jersey: Rutgers University Press, 1998.
2. Brennan F, Carr DB, Cousins MJ. Pain management: A fundamental human right. *Anesth Analg* 2007;105:205–221.
3. Wilson EO. *On Human Nature.* Cambridge, MA: Harvard; 1978:149–167.
4. Banja J. Empathy in the physician's pain practice: benefits, barriers, and recommendations. *Pain Med* 2006;7(3):265–275.
5. Gallagher RM. Empathy: A timeless skill for the pain medicine toolbox. *Pain Med* 2006;7(3):213–214.
6. Gallagher RM. Rational polypharmacy in integrated pain treatment. *Am J Phys Med & Reh* 2005;84(3):S64–S76.
7. Gallagher RM. Integrating medical and behavioral treatment in chronic pain management. In: Gallagher RM, ed. Chronic pain. *Med Clin North Am* 1999;83:823–849.
8. Fishman S, Gallagher RM, Carr D, Sullivan L. The case for pain medicine as a medical specialty. *Pain Med* 2004;5(3):281–286.
9. American Board of Pain Medicine. At http://www.abpm.org/what/index.html. Accessed 05 January 2008.
10. Accreditation Council on Graduate Medical Education. At http://www.acgme.org/acWebsite/downloads/RRC_progReq/sh_multiPainPR707.pdf. Accessed 05 January 2008.
11. Australia and New Zealand College of Anaesthetists. At http://www.anzca.edu.au/fpm/trainees/training-program. Accessed 05 January 2008.
12. Gallagher RM. Pain education and training: Progress or paralysis? *Pain Med* 2002;3(3):196–197.
13. Morrison RS, Wallenstein S, Natale DK, et al. "We don't carry that": Failure of pharmacies in predominantly non-white neighborhoods to stock opioid analgesics. *N Engl J Med* 2000;342:1023–1026.
14. Chesterton LS, Barlas P, Foster NE, et al. Gender differences in pressure pain threshold in healthy humans. *Pain* 2003;101:259–266.
15. Katz WA. Musculoskeletal pain and its socioeconomic implications. *Clin Rheumatol* 2002;21[Suppl 1]:S2–S4.
16. Keogh E, Herdenfeldt M. Gender, coping and the perception of pain. *Pain* 2002;97:195–201.
17. Latham J, Davis BD. The socioeconomic impact of chronic pain. *Disabil Rehabil* 1994;16:39–44.

18. Green CR, Wheeler JR, LaPorte F, et al. How well is pain managed? Who does it well? *Pain Med* 2002;3:56–65.
19. Green CR, Wheeler JR. Physician variability in the management of acute postoperative and cancer pain: A quantitative analysis of the Michigan experience. *Pain Med* 2003;4:8–20.
20. Marbach JJ, Lennon MC, Link BG, Dohrenwend BP. Losing face: Sources of stigma as perceived by chronic facial pain patients. *J Behav Med* 1990;13:583–604.
21. Terico A. Perils of payors: A pain center paradigm. In: Cohen MJM, Campbell JN, eds. *Pain Treatment Centers at a Crossroads: A Practical and Conceptual Reappraisal.* The Bristol-Myers Squibb Symposium on Pain Research. Seattle: IASP Press; 1996:109–116.
22. Frederico JV. The cost of pain centers: Where is the return? In: Cohen M, Campbell J, eds. *Pain Treatment at a Crossroads: A Practical and Conceptual Reappraisal.* Progress in pain research and management. Seattle: IASP Press; 1996:257–274.
23. Flor H, Fydrich T, Turk DC. Efficacy of multidisciplinary pain treatment centers: A meta-analytic review. *Pain* 1992;49:221–230.
24. Caudill M, Schnable R, Zuttermeister P, et al. Decreased clinic utilization by chronic pain patients after behavioral medicine intervention. *Pain* 1991;7:305–310.
25. Fishbain DA, Cutler B, Rosomoff H, Steele-Rosomoff R. Pain facilities: A review of their effectiveness and referral selection criteria. *Curr Rev Pain* 1997;1:107–115.
26. Turk DC. Efficacy of multidisciplinary pain centers in the treatment of chronic pain. In: Cohen M, Campbell J, eds. *Pain Treatment at a Crossroads: A Practical and Conceptual Reappraisal.* The Bristol-Myers Squibb Symposium on Pain Research. Seattle: IASP Press; 1996:257–274.
27. Stieg RL, Lippe P, Shepard TA. Roadblocks to effective pain treatment. *Med Clin North Am* 1999;83:809–821, viii.
28. Gammaitoni AR, Gallagher RM, Welz M, et al. Palliative pharmaceutical care: A randomized, prospective study of telephone-based prescription and medication counseling services for treating chronic pain. *Pain Med* 2000;1:317–331.
29. Joranson DE, Gilson AM. Pharmacists' knowledge of and attitudes toward opioid pain medications in relation to federal and state policies. *J Am Pharm Assoc (Wash)* 2001;41:213–220.
30. Burcheil KJ. Social costs of denying access to care. In: Cohen M, Campbell J, eds. *Pain Treatment Centers at a Crossroads: A Practical and Conceptual Reappraisal.* The Bristol-Myers Squibb Symposium on Pain Research. Seattle: IASP Press; 1996:125–142.
31. Gallagher RM, Myers P. Referral delay in back pain patients on worker's compensation. *Psychosomatics* 1996;37:270–284.
32. Pain: The 5th vital sign. *Veterans' Healthy Living* 2001; Winter: 2.
33. Joint Commission on Accreditation of Healthcare Organizations. *Pain Assessment and Management Standards—Health Care Networks. JCAHO Requirement.* Oakbridge Terrace, IL: Joint Commission Resources, 2001.
34. Chang HM. Educating medical students in pain medicine and palliative care. *Pain Med* 2002;3:194–195.
35. Barzansky B, Veloski JJ, Miller R, Jonas HS. Education in end-of-life care during medical school and residency training. *Acad Med* 1999;74[10 Suppl]:S102–S104.
36. Billings JA, Block S. Palliative care in undergraduate medical education. Status report and future directions. *JAMA* 1997;278:733–738.
37. California. Assembly Bill No. 487; 2001.
38. California. Assembly Bill No. 791; 1999.
39. Congress US. H.R. 3244, Title VI, Sec. 1603; 2001.
40. Lippe PM. The decade of pain control and research. *Pain Med* 2000;1:286.
41. Gallagher RM. The pain decade and the public health. *Pain Med* 2000;1:283–285.
42. Babaum AI. Distinct neurochemical features of acute and persistent pain. *Proc Natl Acad Sci USA* 1999;96(14):7739–7743.
43. Rome H, Rome J. Limbically Augmented Pain Syndrome (LAPS): Kindling, corticolimbic sensitization, and the convergence of affective and sensory symptoms in chronic pain disorders. *Pain Med* 2000;1(1):7–23.
44. Gallagher RM. The pain medicine and primary care community rehabilitation model: Monitored care for pain disorders in multiple settings. *Clin J Pain* 1999;15:1–3.
45. Gallagher RM. Primary care and pain medicine. A community solution to the public health problem of chronic pain. *Med Clin North Am* 1999;83:555–583, v.
46. Osterweis M, Kleinman A, Mechanic D. Pain and disability. Clinical, behavioral, and public policy perspectives. In: Institute of Medicine. *Committee on pain, disability, and chronic illness behavior.* Washington, DC: National Academy Press; 1987:280–282.
47. Anderson OW, Morrison EM. The worth of medical care: A critical review. *Med Care Rev* 1989;46:121–155.
48. Kroenke K, Jackson JL. Outcome in general medical patients presenting with common symptoms: A prospective study with a 2-week and 3-month follow-up. *Fam Pract* 1998;15:398–403.
49. Sheldon GF. The health work force, generalism, and the social contract. *Ann Surg* 1995;222:215–228.
50. Sheldon GF. Great expectations: The 21st century health workforce? *Am J Surg* 2003;185:35–41.
51. Grembowski DE, Martin D, Diehr P, et al. Managed care, access to specialists, and outcomes among primary care patients with pain. *Health Serv Res* 2003;38:1–19.
52. Anderson JJ, Ruwe M, Miller DR, et al. Relative costs and effectiveness of specialist and general internist ambulatory care for patients with 2 chronic musculoskeletal conditions. *J Rheumatol* 2002;29:1488–1495.
53. Solomon DH, Katz JN. Generalist, specialist, or both? *J Rheumatol* 2002;29:1345–1347.
54. Bair MJ. Overcoming fears, frustrations, and competing demands: An effective integration of pain medicine and primary care to treat complex pain patients. *Pain Med* 2007;8:544–545.
55. Von Korff M, Moore JC. Stepped care for back pain: Activating approaches for primary care. *Ann Intern Med* 2001;134:911–917.
56. Fishman SM, Mahajan G, Jung SW, Wilsey BL. The trilateral opioid contract bridging the pain clinic and the primary care physician through the opioid contract. *J Pain Symptom Manage* 2002;24(3):335–344.
57. Wiedemer NL, Harden PS, Arndt IO, Gallagher RM. The opioid renewal clinic: A primary care, managed approach to opioid therapy in chronic pain patients at risk for substance abuse. *Pain Med* 2007;8:573–584.
58. Chelminski PR, Ives TJ, Felix KM, et al. A primary care, multi-disciplinary disease management program for opioid-treated patients with chronic noncancer pain and a high burden of psychiatric comorbidity. *BMC Health Serv Res* 2005;5:3.
59. Ward MH, Leigh JP, Fries JF. Progression of functional disability in patients with rheumatoid arthritis. Associations with rheumatology subspecialty care. *Arch Intern Med* 1993;153:2229–2237.
60. Yelin EH, Such CL, Criswell LA, Epstein WV. Outcomes for persons with rheumatoid arthritis with a rheumatologist versus a non-rheumatologist as the main physician for this condition. *Med Care* 1998;36:513–522.
61. Gabriel SE, Wagner JL, Zinsmeister AR, et al. Is rheumatoid arthritis care more costly when provided by rheumatologists compared with generalists? *Arthritis Rheum* 2001;44:1504–1514.
62. Katz JN, Solomon DH, Schaffer JL, et al. Outcomes of care and resource utilization among patients with knee or shoulder disorders treated by general internists, rheumatologists, or orthopedic surgeons. *Am J Med* 2000;108:28–35.
63. Mazzucca SA, Brandt KD, Katz BP, et al. Therapeutic strategies distinguish community based primary care physicians from rheumatologists in the management of osteoarthritis. *J Rheumatol* 1993;20:80–86.
64. Mitchell RI, Carmen GM. Results of a multicenter trial using an intensive active exercise program for the treatment of acute soft tissue and back injuries. *Spine* 1990;15:514–521.
65. *2002 Annual Report and Reference Handbook.* Evanston, IL: American Board of Medical Specialties: Research and Education Foundation; 2002:104.
66. Shlay J, Chaloner K, Max M, et al. Acupuncture and amitriptyline for pain due to HIV-related peripheral neuropathy. *JAMA* 1998;280:1590–1595.
67. Booth M. *Opium: A History.* London, England: Simon & Schuster, Ltd., 1996.
68. Blumer D, Heilbron M. Chronic pain as a variant of depressive disease: The pain-prone disorder. *J Nerv Ment Dis* 1982;170(7):381–406.
69. Max MB, Lynch SA, Muir J, et al. Effects of desipramine, amitriptyline, and fluoxetine on pain in diabetic neuropathy. *N Engl J Med* 1992;326(19):1250–1256.
70. Gallagher RM. Management of neuropathic pain: Translating mechanistic advances and evidence-based research into clinical practice. *Clin J Pain* 2006;22[Suppl 1]:S2–S8.
71. Ramsay RE. Clinical efficacy and safety of gabapentin. *Neurology* 1994;44[Suppl 5]:S23.
72. Backonja M-M, Serra J. Pharmacologic management part 1: Better-studied neuropathic pain diseases. *Pain Med* 2004;5[Suppl 1]:S28–S47.
73. Beydoun A, Backonja M-M. Mechanistic stratification of antineuralgic agents. *J Pain Symptom Manage* 2003;25:S18–S30.
74. Price DD. Psychological and neural mechanisms of the affective dimension of pain. *Science* 2000;288:1769–1772.
75. Rainville P, Duncan GH, Price DD, et al. Pain affect encoded in human anterior cingulate but not somatosensory cortex. *Science* 1997;277(5328):968–971.
76. Hoffman BM, Papas RK, Chatkoff DK, Kerns RD. Meta-analysis of psychological interventions for chronic low back pain. *Health Psychol* 2007;26(1):1–9.
77. Moseley GL. Is successful rehabilitation of complex regional pain syndrome due to sustained attention to the affected limb? A randomised clinical trial. *Pain* 2005;114(1–2):54–61.
78. Moseley GI. Graded motor imagery for pathologic pain: A randomized controlled trial. *Neurology* 2006;97:2129–2134.
79. deCharms RC, Maeda F, Glover GH, et al. Control over brain activation and pain learned by using real-time functional MRI (biofeedback). *Proc Natl Acad Sci USA* 2005;102(51):18626–18631.

80. Bacon DR, Lema MJ. To define a specialty: A brief history of the American Board of Anesthesiology's first written examination. *J Clin Anesthesiol* 1992;4:489–497.

81. Chang HM, Gallagher R, Vaillancourt P, et al. Undergraduate medical education in pain medicine, end-of-life care, and palliative care. *Pain Med* 2000;1:224.

82. Lema MJ. What's the name of the game? *ASA Newsl* 2002:66.

83. New York Society of Anesthetists. At http://www.nyssa-pga.org/society_hist.html. Accessed May 8, 2008.

84. Still AC. Pain medicine: Untangling the web of certification. *ASA Newsletter* 2000;64(11):8–9. At http://www.asahq.org/Newsletters/2000/11_00/still.htm. Accessed May 8, 2008.

85. Cohen M, Goucke R. Pain medicine recognized as a specialty in Australia. *Pain Med* 2006;7(6):473.

86. Walker SM, Macintyre PE, Visser E, Scott D. Acute pain management: Current best evidence provides guide for improved practice. *Pain Med* 2006;7:3–5.

87. Carr DB, Jacox A, et al. Acute Pain Management: Operative or Medical Procedures Clinical Practice Guideline. AHCPR Publication No. 92-0032. Rockville, MD. Agency for Health Care Policy and Research, Public Health Service, U.S. Department of Health and Human Services, Feb. 1992.

88. Cunningham AJ, Knape JT, Adriaensen H, et al. Guidelines for anaesthesiologist specialist training in pain medicine. *Eur J Anaesthesiol* 2007;24(7):568–570.

89. Personal communication from Ji-Sheng Han, MD, President of the Chinese Association for the Study of Pain, December 15, 2007. Public Notice 2007-227. The Ministry of Public Health, People's Republic of China.

90. Bonica JJ. Organization and function of a pain clinic. In: *Advances in Neurology*, Vol. 4. New York: Raven Press, 433–443.

91. Gallagher RM. Selective, tailored, biopsychosocial pain treatment: Our past is our future. *Pain Med* 2007;8(6):471–472.

92. Turk D, Stacey B. Multidisciplinary pain centers in the treatment of chronic pain. In: Fryomoyer J, Ducker T, Hadler N, eds. *The Adult Spine: Principles and Practice*. New York, NY: Raven Press; 1997:253–274.

93. Guzman J, Esmail R, Karjalainen K, et al. Multidisciplinary bio-psychosocial rehabilitation for chronic low back pain. *Cochrane Database Syst Rev* 2002;(1):CD000963.

94. Guzman J, Esmail R, Karjalainen K, et al. Multidisciplinary rehabilitation for chronic low back pain: Systematic review. *Br Med J* 2001;322:1511–1516.

95. Cutler RB, Fishbain DA, Rosomoff HL, et al. Does nonsurgical pain center treatment of chronic pain return patients to work? A review and meta-analysis of the literature. *Spine* 1994;19:643–652.

96. Dvorak J, Gauchat MH, Valach L. The outcome of surgery for lumbar disc herniation. I. A 4–17 years' follow-up with emphasis on somatic aspects. *Spine* 1988;13:1418–1422.

97. Lehmann TR, Spratt KF, Tozzi JE, et al. Long-term follow-up of lower lumbar fusion patients. *Spine* 1987;12:97–104.

98. North RB, Campbell JN, James CS, et al. Failed back surgery syndrome: 5-year follow-up in 102 patients undergoing repeated operation. *Neurosurgery* 1991;28:685–690.

99. Keller A, Brox JI, Gunderson R, et al. Trunk muscle strength, cross-sectional area, and density in patients with chronic low back pain randomized to lumbar fusion or cognitive intervention and exercises. *Spine* 2004;29:3–8.

100. Lang E, Liebig K, Kastner S, et al. Multidisciplinary rehabilitation versus usual care for chronic low back pain in the community: Effects on quality of life. *Spine J* 2003;3:270–276.

101. Jadad AR. Meta-analysis in pain relief: A valuable but easily misused tool. *Curr Opin Anesthesiol* 1996;9:426–429.

102. Gale G, Nussbaum D, Rothbart P, et al. A randomized treatment study to compare the efficacy of repeated nerve blocks with cognitive therapy for control of chronic head and neck pain. *Pain Res Manage* 2002;7:185–189.

103. Witter J, Simon LS, Dionne R. Are means meaningless? The application of individual responder analysis to analgesic drug development. *Aust Prosthodont Soc Bull* 2003;13:1–7.

104. Carr DB. When bad evidence happens to good treatments: Bonica Lecture. *Reg Anesth Pain Med* 2008;33(3):229–240.

105. Chu L. Using evidence in pain practice: Interpreting and applying systematic reviews and clinical practice guidelines. *Pain Med* 2008 (in press).

106. Chu L. Using evidence in pain practice: Assessing quality of systematic reviews and clinical practice guidelines. *Pain Med* 2008 (in press).

107. Carr DB, Loeser JD, Morris DB, eds. Narrative, Pain, and Suffering. (*Progress in Pain Research and Management*, Vol. 34.) Seattle: IASP Press, 2005.

CHAPTER 29 ■ SOCIOECONOMIC FACTORS IN CHRONIC PAIN AND ITS MANAGEMENT

JOHN D. LOESER

In spite of significant advances in the world of medicine and the technology applied to medical problems, chronic pain remains poorly understood and, often, poorly treated. Successful treatment outcomes with both reduction in pain levels and improvement in functional capacities are often not achieved. As described by Gallagher and Fishman in the preceding chapter, one of the reasons for this paradox is the persistence of the biomedical model, in spite of its inadequacies when applied to chronic pain. The biopsychosocial model of pain has much greater utility and offers opportunities for improving outcomes (1) because social factors, most commonly economic, are important contributors to the problems of chronic pain and its treatment (see also Chapters 28, 31, 35, 37).

Socioeconomic factors influence pain, disability, and suffering in all patients, in every culture. They also determine what types, if any, of health care will be available for patients, and the costs to the patient and his society that are associated with an illness (2). Hence, both the health care provider and the patient under his care are influenced by an array of social and economic factors that are not under their own direct control. Social and economic factors are major determinants of the type and quality of health care offered to pain patients. Furthermore, the socioeconomic status of a patient with pain is associated with a wide array of significant health consequences and treatment outcomes. Illness, such as low back pain or headache, has important social and economic consequences for the patient. This chapter reviews studies that have been undertaken to elucidate the role of socioeconomic factors in pain and its management. The literature is immense, and the quality of many studies has been questioned; the inferences to be drawn are of necessity, tentative. On the other hand, the failure of lawmakers, administrators, and health care providers to be cognizant of the ways in which socioeconomic factors can influence both the provider and the patient has led to and will, if not overcome, perpetuate administrative programs and policies that add to the burden of illness, suffering, and disability.

SOCIOECONOMIC INFLUENCES UPON PAIN MANAGEMENT

The extreme examples are quite obvious: If a country is so poor that it has no structured health care system and few providers, no pain management is offered. Folk remedies abound in every such culture, but their efficacy is probably not beyond the placebo effect. When some degree of formal health care exists in a country, governmental regulations may dramatically impact pain management. For example, many governments in

developing countries did not, until recently, allow any opiates to be prescribed for outpatients or inpatients, instead limiting their availability to operating room use. Those who made such rules clearly valued the attempt to prevent drug abuse more than they cared about needless pain and suffering in those with cancer and other serious diseases. Finally, when strenuous international and local efforts successfully made opiates available in some of these countries, the cheapest and most effective standard drug, morphine, was often not on the list of allowable drugs; heavily marketed, patented, more expensive preparations appeared in the local pharmacopoeia. Economic factors (bribes?) were likely influential.

Another example can be seen in a country like Turkey, which has a centrally controlled health care system. Relatively early in the development of pain management, the government established training centers in pain management, established a credentialing board for physicians and treatment facilities, incorporated pain medicine in the curricula of medical schools, and mandated the distribution of accredited pain specialists in major medical centers. Pain management has flourished in this country. Similar examples of governmentally mandated pain management facilities and personnel can be found in the Scandinavian countries and the United Kingdom. As described in the prior chapter, Australia has recently recognized pain management as a specialty and established a reimbursement schedule that will encourage physicians to enter this discipline. These policies will certainly improve the availability of physicians who are willing to undertake the management of complicated chronic pain patients. Social and economic factors are important in the provision of services to pain patients.

There is some experimental data on the influences of socioeconomic factors on pain patients; however, there is very little empirical evidence about how the provision of health care for such patients is influenced by either economic or other social issues. One well-described socioeconomic factor is the economic status and race of the patient. Studies in the United States have documented the unavailability of opiates in pharmacies in New York City that are located in African American and/or poor neighborhoods (3). Other studies have shown that minority patients do not receive the same assessment or treatment as whites (4). Health care for those who suffer is one of the many activities of any culture or state; it tends to be integrated with the concepts of other forms of social support and is not often the subject of scrutiny. In the United States, social and economic events of the past 35 years have led to significant changes in the provision of health care for those who have pain, both chronic and acute. Most of my comments on socioeconomic effects on pain management in this country are based upon first-hand observation (5).

At the dawn of the Pain Movement in the 1960s, there were almost no physicians or psychologists who considered themselves pain specialists. There were few pain clinics, a handful of monographs, no standard texts, no pain journals, few continuing medical education courses, and no professional societies devoted to pain. Pain was usually considered the by-product of a disease and was expected to disappear if the disease was successfully treated. As observed from time immemorial, there certainly were patients suffering with chronic pain, both due to cancer and noncancer diseases, but there were few pain specialists and no guidelines for pain management. Opiates were not widely used, and dosing was minimal when they were. Things evolved in a helter-skelter fashion. Opiate prescriptions increased, and large numbers of patients were referred to the early pain clinics with multiple opiates prescribed by multiple physicians unknown to each other. These patients complained vigorously about their pain despite their heavy medication intake. Pain clinics quickly learned that tapering such painful people off of their opiates, along with physical activation, education, treatment of depression, and focused return-to-work programs reduced their pain and functional disabilities. From these observations arose the dogma that chronic pain patients should not be treated with opiates. The experiences of pain clinics were generalized to the population at large in the absence of any data to indicate that those who came to pain clinics were typical of all who suffered from pain.

Pain clinics proliferated, often with different conceptual underpinnings. The message about inappropriate use of opiates was widely disseminated. Problem patients with high opiate intake became less common. Then the cancer pain movement began, and it was learned that patients with pain due to cancer often required very large doses of opiates to get relief, inexorable dose escalation due to tolerance was not a major problem, and that, with stable disease status, doses of opiates were typically stable. Furthermore, when treatment other than opiates was implemented that alleviated the cause of the pain, such patients rapidly reduced or discontinued their use of opiates without manifesting an abstinence syndrome. With little evidence to support generalization of the experience with cancer pain to noncancer pain, it was loudly advocated by a small number of physicians that every patient should be given whatever dose of opiate was required to obtain pain relief. The physician's life was easier: Just prescribe an opiate in whatever dose the patient wanted and get the patient out of the office. Poor prescribing habits eventually led to inappropriate usage, a rapid increase in emergency room visits and deaths related to prescription opiates, and little reduction in pain and disability in the overall population of patients with chronic pain (6). Public outcry about excessive opiate prescribing and efforts by state and federal officials to discourage opiate usage for medicinal purposes now have made it difficult for appropriately selected patients to obtain chronic opiate prescriptions.

We have seen two revolutions of the opiate-prescribing cycle in the United States. What has been lacking is reliable evidence to support the position of either side in this dispute. Care for patients with chronic pain has fluctuated widely, but certainly not on the basis of scientific evidence. Fortunately, most opiates are inexpensive, and agencies designed to control costs (often labeled as "managed care") have not focused upon their use.

Another example of socioeconomic changes in the provision of care for pain patients is the rapid expansion of pain specialists among anesthesiologists that occurred in the past 20 years both in the United States and in other countries. In the United States, federal agencies determine the charges for services by an arcane process that is not immune to lobbying.

Procedures such as epidural steroids, facet blocks, and nerve blocks are reimbursed far more handsomely than consultation time with the patient. It is no accident, therefore, that proceduralists rapidly increased in number (even in the absence of outcomes-based evidence for efficacy) whereas multidisciplinary pain clinics have rapidly decreased in number, since they do not generate sufficient revenue to satisfy practitioners or hospital administrators. The number of providers is directly related to economic factors such as remuneration for services. This phenomenon is part of the irrational U.S. health care system, and is not seen in countries that have a systematic plan for specialist numbers and distribution.

The advent of managed care in the United States was an attempt to contain costs and in some cases to establish profitable business franchises, disguised as an effort to improve patient management. Although some large managed care organizations persist, this method has not been very successful at either improving management or containing costs. Managed care has dramatically reduced the time that a physician has available to spend with each patient, although successful management of a chronic pain patient requires listening to and understanding the patient's narrative. This cannot occur in a 7-minute visit. Furthermore, managed care organizations often limit access to specialists, tests, drugs, procedures, and surgery; these constraints, too, can be damaging to patients with pain. Chronic pain is often not considered a "real" disease, and sufferers are considered less than deserving of care (7).

As is true for almost every aspect of medical practice, there are wide variations in rates of surgery for low back pain (1,8–11). Economic factors are certainly one of the reasons for this finding. Small area analysis of surgery for low back pain has shown wide variations in the rates of surgery in different states in the United States. These variations are clearly not due to a higher prevalence of patients with defective backs who reside in each high-rate area. Although no satisfactory explanation for all of the variance has been forthcoming, clearly, physician practice style, which is influenced by both peer group pressures and economics, plays a role. Both factors do so in a largely unexamined fashion and lead to increased patient management costs.

When surgeons make a much more handsome living than medical practitioners, it should not surprise anyone that more young doctors choose to go into surgery. The rate of surgery for low back pain is directly proportional to the number of orthopedic and neurologic surgeons in a country, not to the population at risk (10). Within the neurosurgical and orthopedic specialties, it is widely recognized that the most lucrative practice involves spinal fusions using hardware. Hence, the type of care offered to patients with low back pain is largely determined by the availability of providers, which is partially determined by economic factors.

In his fascinating book, *Occupation and Disease*, Dembe documents the socioeconomic factors that have changed the way the Western world looks at low back pain (12). What started out in the 18th and early 19th centuries as a form of rheumatism, whose pathogenesis lay completely within the sufferer, evolved over a 100-year period to be an occupational disorder secondary to trauma. The development of orthopedics as a specialty facilitated this transition and led to increasing surgery to contend with low back pain. The idea that the workplace was the cause of low back pain and that illnesses originating in the workplace should be paid for by the employer completed the change in thinking about how to manage low back pain. Social and economic factors, and not the failure of the working man's back or wrist, are thus responsible for the huge increase in health care costs and disability compensation for conditions such as low back pain and carpal tunnel syndrome.

Despite the remarkable preclinical advances described by Baron, Basbaum, Cousins, Dickenson, Yaksh, and others in this volume, health care is, and always has been determined much more by socioeconomic factors than medical science. Contemporary pain management has not been shaped by evidence of treatment efficacy. If it were, multidisciplinary pain clinics would be flourishing, instead of waning (13).

SOCIOECONOMIC INFLUENCES UPON THE PATIENT WITH CHRONIC PAIN

Influences upon Pain and Pain Behaviors

As we cannot know another's pain, we can only assess the impact of socioeconomic factors upon someone's pain behaviors: the things that are said, done, or not done as a result of pain (14). Whether these external factors alter the perception of a noxious stimulus or alter the response to that stimulus, or both, is not clear. Pain behaviors are influenced by a wide range of socioeconomic factors including culture, gender, family systems, social class, education, employment, and social support systems such as compensation, litigation, and welfare programs (15). As is true for psychological factors in general (see Chapter 35 by Melzack and Katz), the impact of each of these factors varies among individuals, and it is unlikely that any single one determines the experience of or response to pain. The best model would appear to be that, whereas socioeconomic factors do not initiate chronic pain, they do influence pain behaviors and the ensuing disability. It appears heuristically useful to separate effects on pain from those on disability ascribed to pain, even though the things one does or does not do that create disability can also be considered to be pain behaviors.

Culture/Social Support

Over 50 years ago, Zborowski demonstrated in a U.S. population that ethnicity influences beliefs about pain and pain behaviors, but not experimental pain thresholds (16). Thirty years later, Elton and Stanley showed that cultural and ethnic factors strongly influence both the experience of pain and the behaviors associated with it (17). Many papers have alleged that social and cultural factors, typically the family, have strong influences upon the presence of chronic pain, usually based upon the concept of modeling by children of their parents and older relatives. However Turk and colleagues have identified significant methodological flaws in most of these papers, chiefly the lack of control populations, reliance on self-report, and potentially biased recall (2). Chronic widespread pain and fibromyalgia have been found to be associated with weaker social support, a family history positive for chronic pain, and immigrant status (11).

Australian aboriginal culture teaches tolerance of pain and not to display one's distress (18). Cross-cultural studies have often reported differences in prevalence rates of chronic pain, but it is possible that factors biasing responses to questionnaires are the cause of such apparent differences. Being willing to talk about pain is also a cultural trait. A cross-cultural epidemiologic study by Volinn revealed that low back pain was less common in poorer developing countries than in Western Europe, but the author cautioned that study methodologies or other artifacts could account for these conclusions (19).

Musculoskeletal disorders (MSD) are the most common cause of chronic pain and disability in developed countries. Khatun and co-workers found that MSD in Sweden was twice as common in blue-collar workers than white-collar workers at age 30 (20). No such discrepancy was present at ages 16 or 21. It appeared that both early-life and adult-life factors contributed to this finding. A study on the risk factors for temporomandibular pain in Norway found that adverse socioeconomic factors were much more common in those with the condition than in those without it (21). A Finnish study revealed that chronic pain and disability were more frequent with older age, lower education, and lower occupational class (22). Another study of chronic pain in women in Sweden showed that those in a "deprived socioeconomic situation not only run a higher pain risk, but also experience their pain as more severe/disabling than their more privileged counterparts" (23).

The family—parents and siblings for children, spouses for adults—strongly influences one's beliefs and strategies for adapting to life. An extensive literature describes the effects of the family upon the development and persistence of chronic pain (2,24,25). There is little question that the family has substantial effects on individuals' chronic pain behaviors, and that firm social support lessens the burden of chronic pain. There is limited evidence about such influences upon acute pain. Children in Norway were found to be at increased risk of chronic pain if they lived in poorly educated, low-income worker families (26). A body of literature also describes the negative effects of chronic pain upon the patient's spouse and family members (27).

Cultural affiliation has repeatedly been shown to influence the perception of and response to acute and experimental pain. Bates and co-workers, in a series of publications, investigated the relationships between ethnic group, pain perception, and variation in responses to treatment in patients with chronic pain during multidisciplinary pain therapy (28). Cultural differences in attitudes, beliefs, and emotional states predicted pain intensity variation; medications and surgical treatments did not.

In conclusion, socioeconomic status is a significant predictor of prevalence, duration, and severity of almost every type of chronic pain in every country in which studies have been undertaken. Furthermore, this is true even in countries that have a universal health care system, so it is not the deficiency of health care that makes low socioeconomic status an adverse factor in chronic pain patients. The magnitude of the effect varies, and controlled, prospective, random allocation studies are few. Socioeconomic status affects all aspects of health and well-being; there is nothing unique about its effects on pain and disability.

Education

Most, but by no means all, of the reported studies indicate that educational level affects the prevalence and persistence of chronic pain, but it is difficult to separate educational status from social class and type of work performed. Deyo and Tsui-Wu did show that lower levels of education were associated independently of other factors with increased chronic low back pain and duration of disability (29).

Socioeconomic Class

Lower social class is probably a factor in chronic pain in general and low back pain specifically (15), an effect that, in published studies, is larger in males than females. This effect seems to be related primarily to the large number of manual laborers in the lower classes. Whether the recent increase in outside-the-home employment for women will alter this phenomenon is unknown. However, migraine headaches in women are more common in lower-income households in the United States, and women from lower-income households are more likely to use emergency rooms for their health care (30). At the time of the Institute of Medicine review of Pain and Disability in 1987, the available literature strongly suggested that socioeconomic factors were associated with low back pain, lower educational status, low occupational status, and heavy physical demands of the job (31).

Another aspect of the influence of social class on pain was revealed by Richards and colleagues, who studied differences in responses to chest pain between those men who resided in an affluent neighborhood and those who lived in a deprived region in Glasgow (32). Residents of the deprived regions reported greater exposure to ill health, perceived themselves to be more vulnerable to heart disease, yet were less likely to seek cardiology care. The authors concluded that social and cultural factors influenced perceptions of symptoms and illness behavior.

Workmen's Compensation

Considerable evidence supports an important role for worker's compensation in disability due to pain or treatment efficacy for chronic pain. Katz's recent study suggests that onset of back pain and disability in general are related to such socioeconomic factors as job dissatisfaction, strenuous or stressful work, low educational status, and being covered by workers' compensation insurance (33). This same study showed that socioeconomic factors were not related to radiologic findings of disc degeneration. Chronic pain and the disability associated with it were found to be strongly associated with socioeconomic disadvantage, high levels of unemployment, and significant costs to the disabled worker and society in Australia (34). Most pain management physicians agree that a patient who is enmeshed in a compensation system has a potent comorbidity that often intrudes into the rehabilitative process. There is evidence from the review by Rohling (35) that the experience of pain is more intense in those receiving compensation. However, the literature on the effects of compensation upon symptom relief, treatment response, and return to work is not uniformly indicative of the ill effects of compensation. How much of the variance is methodologic and how much is related to different countries and compensation plans is not clear (31,35).

Litigation

Litigation, such as being involved in a compensation system, may alter the disability ascribed to pain, but no evidence supports the idea that pain is caused or perpetuated by litigation. The myth of "cured by a verdict," as promulgated by the English neurologist Henry Miller, in 1961, has never been supported by any research and should be discarded (36,37). Mendelson undertook an extensive review of the relevant literature and showed clearly that Miller's myth was not substantiated by published studies and was often used as a weapon in legal proceedings against injured workers (38). In a separate study, Mendelson found that personal injury litigants did not describe their pain as more severe than nonlitigants, nor were they more psychologically disturbed (39).

A very interesting literature addresses the effects of rear-end auto collisions ("whiplash injury"). First, subjects in a study by Castro and co-workers used bumper cars (as found in an amusement park) to experience collisions at 6 to 9 mph. No one reported neck pain afterward, and there were no abnormalities on magnetic resonance imaging (MRI), electromyography (EMG) or clinical examination (40). This seems odd, as many people involved in rear-end collisions in automobile accidents at similar speeds do ascribe neck pain to their accidents. A report by Schrader suggested that whiplash symptoms were rare in a society that did not offer compensation and litigation for such an injury (41). At the North American Spine Society meeting in 1997, Patheni reported that only 9% of Greeks involved in such an accident had any symptoms, and that none persisted for 6 months (42). There is no tort system for vehicular accidents in that country. Finally, Borchgrevink reported on a sample of 201 whiplash patients who were randomly assigned either to a cervical collar or resumption of normal activities. The group receiving a cervical collar had significantly more symptoms that persisted longer (43). Other studies of whiplash injury report similar findings of a link between litigation and symptom severity.

This sample of the literature shows that socioeconomic factors such as a tort system, expectation of litigation and compensation, and the culture in which an accident occurs, in addition to the physical forces involved, can strongly influence the incidence and persistence of pain. These conclusions are consistent with a recent Australian telephone survey of 484 adults with chronic pain by Blyth, Cousins, and colleagues, in which "litigation . . . was strongly associated with higher levels of pain-related disability, even after taking into account other factors associated with poor functional outcomes." It has also been observed that the presence of litigation or enmeshment in a compensation system can alter treatment outcome (44).

Influences on Disability Ascribed to Pain

Disability ascribed to pain is a major burden in any developed country. The complaint of pain must be discriminated from the disability that is blamed on the existence of pain; it is much easier to measure the disability than the pain itself. In most studies, disability really means failure to be gainfully employed for wages but, particularly in the elderly, disability does not necessarily involve work status. It is wisest to consider disability as the result of an impairment that interferes with activities of daily living, including, but not limited to work.

A study by Thumboo, Chew, and Lewin-Koh in Singapore found that ethnicity, youth, education and employment status, and psychological factors influenced both pain and functioning (45). A Canadian study of whiplash injury victims indicated that longer recovery periods were associated with older age, female sex, having dependents, and not being employed full time. Neurologic findings and the dynamics of the accident also contributed to lengthening recovery time (46). A systematic review, also by Canadian investigators, indicated that workplace factors such as the lack of workplace accommodation and lack of work autonomy predicted chronic pain disability. On the other hand, factors such as lower job satisfaction, perception of difficult work demands, heavy physical demands of the job, private rather than public employment, and lower socioeconomic status were not predictive in that review (21). An interesting study by Peck and colleagues of workers in the state of Washington indicated that having a third-party claim for injury and associated litigation did not increase the duration of disability (47).

Socioeconomic factors are important in the relationships between injury, impairment, and disability (48). An extensive body of literature on wage replacement programs for injured workers and the availability of disability programs for those who do not work has led to the recognition of the moral hazard of these insurance programs: Some people take advantage of such programs to avoid productive employment. In addition, such programs have effects that cannot be part of the injured worker's conscious behaviors. For example, the wage replacement ratio (WRR), which is the ratio of compensation income to preinjury wage, has repeatedly been shown to influence both the likelihood of a compensation claim and the duration of that claim. A synthesis of published data suggested that a 10% increase in workers' compensation benefits led to a 1% to 11% percent increase in the frequency of workers' compensation claims and a 2% to 11% percent increase in duration per claim (49). Twenty years ago, Beals summarized the effects of a compensation system on the recovery from injury and advocated that these systems be changed so as to provide incentives for, rather than impediments to, return to work (50).

Volinn and co-workers, along with the author, studied disability claims for low back pain in the state of Washington (51). We found that socioeconomic factors were strongly implicated in the illness labeled "low back sprain." Among many factors that had a discernible effect, age, monthly wage, family status, and a measure of socioeconomic status were particularly important. A literature review in this paper suggested that male sex, increasing age, heavy labor occupation, transportation occupation, low job satisfaction, low education, single marital status, high wage replacement ratio, the presence of dependent children, and litigation were each likely to increase the risk both of back pain and a claim for disability due to back pain. Not every study, however, provided supported for each of these factors. Another study from the same group investigated the role of socioeconomic factors in the persistence of disability due to low back pain in the state of Washington (52). It was found that three socioeconomic factors—unemployment rate, percentage receiving food stamps, and per capita income—accounted for about one-third of the variance in chronic disability across the 39 counties of this state. The authors proposed that disability was a symptom of social distress and that high levels of job insecurity were predictive that back pain, which is almost a universal complaint, would become disabling.

Influences on Response to Treatment

Van den Hulst and co-workers conducted a comprehensive systematic review of outcome predictors for low back pain patients enrolled in a multidisciplinary rehabilitation treatment program. They found that high job satisfaction, low pain intensity, and less active coping seemed to have some predictive value, but other sociodemographic and physical variables were not predictive. They noted, however, that all of the available studies were descriptive or exploratory, and they called for better studies to accurately assess the role of sociodemographic factors in determining treatment outcomes (53). Michaelson and co-workers found that sociodemographic variables were not reliable predictors of outcome from multidisciplinary pain management (54). In an interesting study based upon emergency room visits in a Level I (i.e., major) trauma center, Gaetz

and colleagues found that only higher income, among a wide array of other socioeconomic variables, predicted pain relief from the emergency room visit (55).

Another facet of the influence of socioeconomic factors on response to treatment was described by Block and colleagues (56). They found that multidisciplinary pain treatment was more effective for patients referred from medical specialties than for those referred by a disability program. The disability referral patients showed less improvement in function, spent more time in hospital, and were less compliant with the treatment program. Block and colleagues advocated an operant model of patient behavior and thought that monetary rewards for disability status were responsible for the treatment outcomes in the two groups. Dworkin and associates suggested that employment status rather than compensation was the determinant of adverse outcomes attributed to compensation by Block and others (57). Patients who were employed at the time of their treatment were much more likely to be at work at follow-up. Carron and colleagues tried to compare patient outcomes from a multidisciplinary pain program in New Zealand with one in the United States (58). Although their study had some methodologic problems, it was highly suggestive that differences in the implementation of compensation systems were responsible for the increased burden of emotional and behavioral disruption found in the U.S. patients. New Zealand had a system that provided wage support whether or not the cause was a work-related injury, in contrast to the adversarial U.S. system. Interestingly, the same magnitude of improvement was seen in both countries: The New Zealanders' lives were less disrupted at the start of treatment and remained so throughout the follow-up period. Of course, other cultural factors could have been influential, but the adversarial nature of the U.S. compensation system and its deleterious effects on patient autonomy and ability to return to work seemed to have a major impact on patient well-being. In sum, the design of a compensation system is a major economic determinant of patient response to a treatment program.

Several studies have concluded that low back pain patients receiving compensation consistently have poorer outcomes from conservative therapies, surgery, and multidisciplinary pain rehabilitation programs (35,59). It appears that compensation delays recovery, by unclear mechanism(s), by up to 30% in published studies. Whether these effects reflect the existence of compensation itself or selection processes that lead to being eligible for compensation (heavier jobs, less education, lower socioeconomic status) is not known. In spite of the potential deleterious effects of compensation upon the results of any form of treatment, we should not exaggerate such adverse influences because three-fourths of injured workers receiving compensation do return to work. To withhold medically indicated therapy because a patient is the recipient of compensation benefits therefore is unjustified and is certainly unethical at a time when pain management is viewed increasingly as a fundamental human right.

SUMMARY

All of the developed nations of the world have significant and increasing costs related to chronic pain and disability. To the prior estimates of the health burden of absenteeism must be added that of "presenteeism," the reduced work performance of employees who remain on their jobs despite chronic pain. Increased understanding of the way in which socioeconomic factors influence individual and group behaviors could lead to immense monetary savings as well as reduced suffering by those who hurt and do not engage in normal daily activities. As many others have stated, higher-quality research will be required to clarify these issues and lead to rational, informed policies. Policy makers and program designers whose work involves the health care and disability management of patients with chronic pain should understand the effects of socioeconomic factors, including health care and wage replacement, that impact upon patients with chronic pain. If it is true that socioeconomic factors can exacerbate both the incidence and duration of pain and disability, then these same factors may potentially be harnessed to improve patient well-being and reduce unnecessary health care costs. Pain behaviors are not solely the product of tissue damage within the patient's body. They represent each individual's response to both internal factors and external influences. Socioeconomic forces are potent modifiers of the experience and report of chronic pain, its associated disability, and its response to treatment.

References

1. Loeser JD. What is chronic pain? *Theor Med* 1991;12(3):213–225.
2. Turk DC, Flor H, Rudy TE. Pain and families. I. Etiology, maintenance, and psychosocial impact. *Pain* 1987;30(1):3–27.
3. Morrison RS, Wallenstein S, Natale DK, et al. "We don't carry that": Failure of pharmacies in predominantly nonwhite neighborhoods to stock opioid analgesics. *N Engl J Med* 2000;342(14):1023–1026.
4. Green CR, Anderson KO, Baker TA, et al. The unequal burden of pain: Confronting racial and ethnic disparities in pain. *Pain Med* 2003;4(3):277–294.
5. Loeser JD. The future. Will pain be abolished or just pain specialists? *Minn Med* 2001;84(7):20–21.
6. Paulozzi LJ, Budnitz DS, Xi Y. Increasing deaths from opioid analgesics in the United States. *Pharmacoepidemiol Drug Saf* 2006;15(9):618–627.
7. Lande SD, Loeser JD. The future of pain management in managed care. *Manag Care Interface* 2001;14(5):69–75.
8. Volinn E, Mayer J, Diehr P, et al. Small area analysis of surgery for low-back pain. *Spine* 1992;17(5):575–581.
9. Volinn E, Turczyn KM, Loeser JD. Patterns in low back pain hospitalizations: Implications for the treatment of low back pain in an era of health care reform. *Clin J Pain* 1994;10(1):64–70.
10. Cherkin DC, Deyo RA, Loeser JD, et al. An international comparison of back surgery rates. *Spine* 1994;19(11):1201–1206.
11. Bergman S. Psychosocial aspects of chronic widespread pain and fibromyalgia. *Disabil Rehabil* 2005;27(12):675–683.
12. Dembe AE. *Occupation and Disease*. New Haven: Yale University Press, 1966.
13. Gatchel RJ, Okifuji A. Evidence-based scientific data documenting the treatment and cost-effectiveness of comprehensive pain programs for chronic nonmalignant pain. *J Pain* 2006;7(11):779–793.
14. Loeser JD. Disability, pain, and suffering. *Clin Neurosurg* 1989;35:398–408.
15. Waddell G, Waddell H. A review of social influences on neck and back pain and disability. In: Nachemson AL, Jonsson E, eds. *Neck and Back Pain*. Philadelphia: Lippincott Williams and Wilkins; 2000:13–55.
16. Zborowski M. Cultural components in responses to pain. *J Soc Issues* 1952;8(1):16–30.
17. Elton D, Stanley G. Cultural expectations and psychological factors in prolonged disability. *Adv Behav Med* 1982;2(2):33–42.
18. Honeyman PT, Jacobs EA. Effects of culture on back pain in Australian aboriginals. *Spine* 1996;21(7):841–843.
19. Volinn E. The epidemiology of low back pain in the rest of the world. A review of surveys in low- and middle-income countries. *Spine* 1997;22(15):1747–1754.
20. Khatun M, Ahlgren C, Hammarstrom A. The influence of factors identified in adolescence and early adulthood on social class inequities of musculoskeletal disorders at age 30: A prospective population-based cohort study. *Int J Epidemiol* 2004;33(6):1353–1360.
21. Teasell RW, Bombardier C. Employment-related factors in chronic pain and chronic pain disability. *Clin J Pain* 2001;17[4 Suppl]:S39–S45.
22. Saastamoinen P, Leino-Arjas P, Laaksonen M, et al. Socio-economic differences in the prevalence of acute, chronic and disabling chronic pain among ageing employees. *Pain* 2005;114(3):364–371.
23. Jablonska B, Soares JJ, Sundin O. Pain among women: Associations with socio-economic and work conditions. *Eur J Pain* 2006;10(5):435–447.
24. Payne B, Norfleet MA. Chronic pain and the family: A review. *Pain* 1986;26(1):1–22.
25. Flor H, Turk DC, Rudy TE. Pain and families. II. Assessment and treatment. *Pain* 1987;30(1):29–45.
26. Groholt EK, Stigum H, Nordhagen R, et al. Recurrent pain in children, socio-economic factors and accumulation in families. *Eur J Epidemiol* 2003;18(10):965–975.
27. Flor H, Turk DC, Scholz OB. Impact of chronic pain on the spouse: Marital, emotional and physical consequences. *J Psychosom Res* 1987;31(1):63–71.

28. Bates MS, Edwards WT, Anderson KO. Ethnocultural influences on variation in chronic pain perception. *Pain* 1993;52(1):101–112.
29. Deyo RA, Tsui-Wu YJ. Functional disability due to back pain. A population-based study indicating the importance of socioeconomic factors. *Arthritis Rheum* 1987;30(11):1247–1253.
30. Stewart WF, Lipton RB, Celentano DD, et al. Prevalence of migraine headache in the United States. Relation to age, income, race, and other sociodemographic factors. *JAMA* 1992;267(1):64–69.
31. Osterweis M, Kleinman A, Mechanic D. *Pain and Disability: Clinical, Behavioral, and Public Policy Perspectives*. Washington, D.C.: National Academy Press, 1987.
32. Richards HM, Reid ME, Watt GC. Socioeconomic variations in responses to chest pain: qualitative study. *Br Med J* 2002;324(7349):1308.
33. Katz JN. Lumbar disc disorders and low-back pain: Socioeconomic factors and consequences. *J Bone Joint Surg Am* 2006;88[Suppl 2]:21–24.
34. Schofield T, ed. *Workplace Health: The Injuries of Neoliberalism: International Journal of Health Sociology: Policy, Promotion, Equity and Practice*. Sydney, Australia: Health Sociology Review, 2005.
35. Rohling ML, Binder LM, Langhinrichsen-Rohling J. Money matters: A meta-analytic review of the association between financial compensation and the experience and treatment of chronic pain. *Health Psychol* 1995;14(6):537–547.
36. Miller H. Accident neurosis. *Br Med J* 1961;1(5231):992–998.
37. Miller H. Accident neurosis. *Br Med J* 1961;1(5230):919–925.
38. Mendelson G. *Psychiatric Aspects of Personal Injury Claims*. Springfield IL: Charles C. Thomas, 1988.
39. Mendelson G. Compensation, pain complaints, and psychological disturbance. *Pain* 1984;20(2):169–177.
40. Castro WH, Schilgen M, Meyer S, et al. Do "whiplash injuries" occur in low-speed rear impacts? *Eur Spine J* 1997;6(6):366–375.
41. Schrader H, Obelieniene D, Bovim G, et al. Natural evolution of late whiplash syndrome outside the medicolegal context. *Lancet* 1996;347(9010):1207–1211.
42. Partheni M, Constantoyannis C, Ferrari R, et al. A prospective cohort study of the outcome of acute whiplash injury in Greece. *Clin Exp Rheumatol* 2000;18(1):67–70.
43. Borchgrevink GE, Kaasa A, McDonagh D, et al. Acute treatment of whiplash neck sprain injuries. A randomized trial of treatment during the first 14 days after a car accident. *Spine* 1998;23(1):25–31.
44. Blyth FM, March L, Nicholas M, et al. Chronic pain, work performance and litigation. *Pain* 2003;103:41–47.
45. Thumboo J, Chew LH, Lewin-Koh SC. Socioeconomic and psychosocial factors influence pain or physical function in Asian patients with knee or hip osteoarthritis. *Ann Rheum Dis* 2002;61(11):1017–1020.
46. Suissa S. Risk factors of poor prognosis after whiplash injury. *Pain Res Manag* 2003;8(2):69–75.
47. Peck CJ, Fordyce WE, Black RG. The effect of pendency of claims for compensation upon behavior indicative of pain. *Wash Law Rev* 1978;53:251–278.
48. Brena SF, Chapman SL, Stegall PG, et al. Chronic pain states: Their relationship to impairment and disability. *Arch Phys Med Rehabil* 1979;60(9):387–389.
49. Loeser JD, Henderlite SE, Conrad DA. Incentive effects of workers' compensation benefits: A literature synthesis. *Med Care Res Rev* 1995;52(1):34–59.
50. Beals RK. Compensation and recovery from injury. *West J Med* 1984;140(2):233–237.
51. Volinn E, Van Koevering D, Loeser JD. Back sprain in industry. The role of socioeconomic factors in chronicity. *Spine* 1991;16(5):542–548.
52. Volinn E, Lai D, McKinney S, et al. When back pain becomes disabling: A regional analysis. *Pain* 1988;33(1):33–39.
53. van der Hulst M, Vollenbroek-Hutten MM, Ijzerman MJ. A systematic review of sociodemographic, physical, and psychological predictors of multidisciplinary rehabilitation: Or, back school treatment outcome in patients with chronic low back pain. *Spine* 2005;30(7):813–825.

54. Michaelson P, Sjolander P, Johansson H. Factors predicting pain reduction in chronic back and neck pain after multimodal treatment. *Clin J Pain* 2004;20(6):447–454.
55. Gaetz A, Miner JR, Schloetter C, et al. The association of socioeconomic status and the physician's perception of socioeconomic status and pain relief in the emergency department. *Acad Emerg Med* 2006;13[Suppl 1]: S123.
56. Block AR, Kremer E, Gaylor M. Behavioral treatment of chronic pain: Variables affecting treatment efficacy. *Pain* 1980;8(3):367–375.
57. Dworkin RH, Handlin DS, Richlin DM, et al. Unraveling the effects of compensation, litigation, and employment on treatment response in chronic pain. *Pain* 1985;23(1):49–59.
58. Carron H, DeGood DE, Tait R. A comparison of low back pain patients in the United States and New Zealand: Psychosocial and economic factors affecting severity of disability. *Pain* 1985;21(1):77–89.
59. Walsh NE, Dumitru D. The influence of compensation on recovery from low back pain. *Occup Med* 1988;3(1):109–121.

CHAPTER 30 ■ DEVELOPMENTAL ASPECTS OF NOCICEPTION

SUELLEN M. WALKER

Although the International Association for the Study of Pain (IASP) definition of pain is based on the individual's report of "a sensory and emotional experience," it is also noted that "the inability to communicate verbally does not negate the possibility that an individual is experiencing pain and is in need of appropriate pain-relieving treatment" (1). This is crucially important in the management of pain in neonates, infants, and young children who are unable to directly describe their experience of pain, although their behavioral and physiologic response to pain may be considered a form of "self-report." The assessment of pain is more difficult at these ages (2), but this does not lessen the need to adequately manage pain, not only for humanitarian reasons, but also because inadequately treated pain can have deleterious short- and long-term effects (3–5).

The immature nervous system responds to pain, injury, and analgesia very differently from the mature one. Activity within sensory pathways is required for normal development, but abnormal or excessive activity related to pain and injury during the neonatal period may alter normal development and produce persistent changes (6–8). Advances in neonatal and pediatric pain management are critically dependent on improved understanding of postnatal changes in: (a) nociceptive processing, (b) effects of different forms of injury, and (c) pharmacokinetic and pharmacodynamic responses to analgesic interventions (9,10).

The rat pup is born at a relatively immature stage and is an established model for investigation of developmental changes. Data collected from human foetal tissue and rat pups show a comparable pattern of progression throughout development, and approximate age correlations can be made across the two species (11). The development of peripheral and spinal cord somatosensory function in the rat from the embryonic day 10 (E10) to birth (E21.5) correlates with the first 24 postconceptional weeks of human gestation, and the first postnatal week in the rat pup corresponds to the later stages of human development from 24 weeks until full-term birth at 40 postconceptional weeks. Rat pups are weaned around the 21st postnatal day (P21) and by this age may be considered developmentally comparable to human adolescents (11,12). Rather than representing absolute correlations, these time lines provide a framework for assessing progressive changes in function throughout development.

This chapter outlines laboratory studies of nociceptive processing throughout postnatal development. More detailed descriptions can be found in recent reviews (13,14) and chapters (15,16). The response to different forms of injury throughout postnatal development will be described and, where possible, findings from laboratory and clinical findings will be compared.

Finally, the developmental pharmacodynamics of common regional analgesics will be outlined.

NOCICEPTIVE PROCESSING

During the first weeks and months of life, significant functional and structural changes in the developing nervous system influence nociceptive transmission. The expression of a number of molecules and channels involved in nociception are developmentally regulated, changes in the distribution and density of many important receptors occur, and the levels and effects of several neurotransmitters alter significantly during the postnatal period (13,14,17).

Peripherally Mediated Responses

The cell bodies of peripheral sensory neurons are located in the dorsal root ganglia (DRG) and send axons both peripherally to innervate target organs such as skin and centrally to synapse within the spinal cord. Large A-fibers innervate the skin before C-fibers, but by birth in the rat and the second trimester in man, sensory fibers are distributed to all body regions (15), and calcitonin gene-related peptide (CGRP) is being expressed in the skin (18). Peripheral cutaneous receptors are capable of responding to a range of stimuli from early development. In the rat pup, recordings from foetal (E16–E20) (19) and neonatal (P0–P14) (20) DRGs identified classes of sensory fibers responding to a similar degree and range of stimuli as adults (i.e., light touch or pressure, noxious pinch, heat, and chemical stimuli). Many different receptors mediate responses to peripheral stimuli, but the developmental profile of relatively few have been investigated. The transient receptor potential vanilloid-1 (TRPV1) receptor is activated by capsaicin, protons and thermal stimuli ($>43°C$), and the TRP ankyrin (TRPA1) receptor responds to pungent compounds such as mustard oil, and possibly noxious cold (21,22). Both TRPA1 and TRPV1 receptors are functional from early development, as primary afferent responses to mustard oil can be observed in fetal (E17–E20) and neonatal rat DRG (19,20), and initial responses to capsaicin are qualitatively similar in cultured DRG cells from neonatal (P0/1) and adult rats (23). TRPV1 nerve terminals are present in cutaneous structures early in development (24), and substance P-IR fibers are present in the skin, sciatic nerve, and dorsal horn at P1 (25). The sensory neuron-specific tetrodotoxin-resistant sodium channels $(Na)_v1.8$ and $Na_v1.9$ are expressed on C-fibers at birth and reach adult levels by P7 (26).

Pain Transmission in the Spinal Cord

Afferent Input

In the adult, C-fiber polymodal nociceptors project to the superficial dorsal horn (lamina I and II), while larger myelinated Aβ-fibers, which subserve light touch and pressure, project to deeper layers of the dorsal horn (lamina III and IV). However, during development, the functional and anatomic relationships between C- and A-fibers change, leading to age-related changes in the processing of sensory inputs. Aβ-fibers enter the cord earlier than C-fibers, initially project throughout lamina I to V of the dorsal horn, and then gradually withdraw to the adult pattern of distribution in lamina III to IV over the first 3 postnatal weeks (18,27–29). A-fibers form synaptic contacts in the superficial laminae in the neonate (30), and A-fiber stimulation evokes postsynaptic spikes and sensitization in dorsal horn cells in the first postnatal week (31,32). As C-fiber function matures with increasing postnatal age, a progressive reduction occurs in A-fiber input and increase in C-fiber input (33,34). Although the intrinsic excitability of superficial dorsal horn neurons is stable throughout development (35), changes in synaptic inputs to these cells result in marked changes in the response to peripheral stimuli throughout development. During the initial period of A- and C-fiber overlap, receptive field sizes of dorsal horn neurons are large, which increases the degree of central activation following stimuli from a given area of peripheral tissue (31,36,37). In addition, the mechanical thresholds of individual dorsal horn sensory neurons are lower at P3 (37), thus increasing the central response to less intense stimuli in early development.

The response of dorsal horn neurons to C-fiber stimulation also varies with postnatal age. Functional synapses between TRPV1-expressing nociceptors and dorsal horn neurons can be identified in spinal cord slice preparations from early development. Initially, these synapses may lack the ability to synchronously release large amounts of transmitter, but a significant enhancement of effect arises from P5 to P10 (38). Extracellular recordings from dorsal horn cells reveal that C-fiber

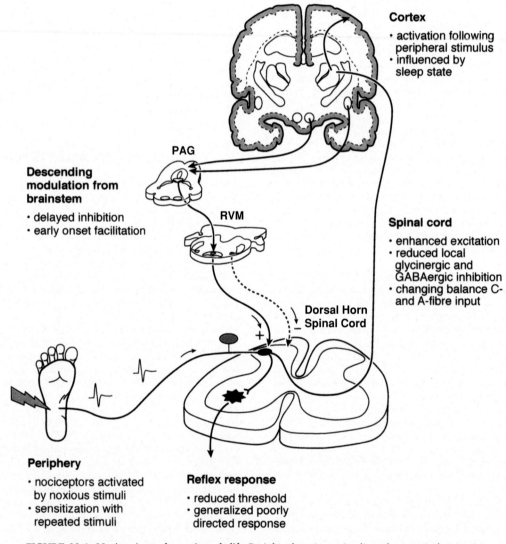

Cortex
- activation following peripheral stimulus
- influenced by sleep state

PAG

Descending modulation from brainstem
- delayed inhibition
- early onset facilitation

RVM

Spinal cord
- enhanced excitation
- reduced local glycinergic and GABAergic inhibition
- changing balance C- and A-fibre input

Dorsal Horn Spinal Cord

Periphery
- nociceptors activated by noxious stimuli
- sensitization with repeated stimuli

Reflex response
- reduced threshold
- generalized poorly directed response

FIGURE 30-1. **Nociceptive pathways in early life.** Peripheral noxious stimuli produce cortical activation following birth even in preterm neonates. Laboratory studies suggest that modulation at the level of the spinal cord, from local and brainstem descending influences, varies throughout postnatal development. PAG, periaqueductal grey; RVM, rostroventral medulla.

electrical stimulation does not evoke postsynaptic responses in the first postnatal week (31,39). However by P10, cells in superficial laminae respond to a C-fiber stimulus, and repetitive C-fiber stimulation produces "wind-up" (31,32,36).

Excitatory Modulation

The balance between excitatory and inhibitory neurotransmission in the dorsal horn alters during postnatal development (14). Enhanced excitatory mechanisms are important for activity-dependent changes during development (6), and there is a tendency for more delayed development of inhibitory mechanisms (40).

Developmental changes in the distribution and subunit composition of glutamate receptors in the spinal cord contribute to the increased excitability of the neonatal spinal dorsal horn (14). α-Amino-3-hydroxy-5-methyl-4-isoxazolepropionic acid (AMPA), kainate, and N-methyl-D-aspartate (NMDA) receptors are activated by glutamate to produce inward cation currents and depolarization of the postsynaptic cell. Binding sites for these receptors are initially higher in density and distributed more widely throughout the dorsal horn (41,42). The AMPA subunits GluR1, -2, and -4 are more highly expressed in the neonate, and increased GluR2 may increase the calcium permeability of the receptor (43–45). The subunits of the NMDA receptor are arranged in a tetrameric fashion, with two NR_1 units and combinations of NR_{2A-D} and/or NR_{3A-B}. Subunit composition changes during development, with the NR_{2D} subunit being highly expressed in neonatal cord (14). The affinity of the receptors for NMDA and the NMDA-induced increase in calcium influx are higher in substantia gelatinosa neurons in the first postnatal week (46). Glutamatergic synapses are functional from birth (38,47), but many synapses present in early development contain NMDA receptors exclusively (approximately 20%) (48). These pure NMDA receptors have been considered to be "silent" as they are not colocalized with AMPA receptors (49), but repetitive stimulation can drive action potential firing and affect neuron excitability in the absence of AMPA (47,50).

Inhibitory Modulation

Inhibitory mechanisms may not be fully mature in early life. Fast inhibitory transmission is mediated by γ-aminobutyric acid (GABA) and glycine receptors, both of which undergo developmental changes in subunit expression that influence channel kinetics (14). In the hippocampus, GABA initially produces depolarizing rather than hyperpolarizing currents, as the intracellular chloride concentration remains high until the potassium-chloride cotransporter KCC2 is upregulated later in development (51,52). However, GABAergic inhibition may mature earlier in the spinal cord. In dorsal horn slices, GABA-produced depolarization in a proportion of cells at P0 to P2, but was insufficient to produce action potentials, and by P6 to P7, only the adult pattern of hyperpolarizing responses was recorded. Glycinergic miniature inhibitory postsynaptic currents (IPSCs) could not be demonstrated at birth, and remained less frequent than GABAergic currents for the first 2 postnatal weeks (40). Application of the $GABA_A$-antagonist gabazine to the spinal cord in vivo produced a similar degree of increased firing at P3 and P21, suggesting that intrinsic spinal GABAergic inhibition is functional during early life (53). Although GABA does not appear to have significant direct excitatory effects in the spinal cord, the overall response is also influenced by descending inputs. When the spinal cord is intact, facilitatory GABA-mediated effects on reflex responses can be identified in pups at P3. Following spinal cord transection, inhibitory GABA effects, as seen in older animals and in isolated spinal cord

preparations, predominate. This suggests that modulation of GABA-mediated transmission by descending nociceptive pathways has important effects on the overall response, and these change throughout early development (54).

The development of interneurons in the superficial dorsal horn, some of which will be inhibitory, lags behind that of projection neurons (55). Descending inhibition of dorsal horn cell responses by stimulation of the dorsolateral funiculus is not present until P10 to P12, and until P22 to P24 is only activated by high-intensity stimulation (56). Diffuse noxious inhibitory controls are not functional in the first 2 postnatal weeks (57), and stimulus-produced analgesia from the periaqueductal gray is not apparent until P21 (58). Therefore, delayed maturation of interneuronal and descending inhibitory mechanisms may further shift the balance toward excitatory responses in the neonatal spinal cord.

The Withdrawal Reflex

Withdrawal reflexes are important models for the investigation of nociceptive processing at all ages, in both laboratory and clinical studies (59,60). Changes in the properties of the withdrawal reflex during development allow assessment of the changing sensitivity and selectivity of the neonatal nervous system to nociceptive stimuli (25,31). Measuring reflex thresholds allows quantification of responses to different forms of injury (61,62) and assessment of analgesic efficacy in preclinical studies (63–66). Similarly, changes in reflex thresholds in infants can provide additional objective evaluation of responses to injury and analgesia in clinical studies (67,68).

In the adult, the withdrawal reflex is selectively elicited by nociceptive stimuli (69). In early life, mechanical and thermal thresholds are lower, and the reflex response has greater amplitude, longer latency, and a higher degree of variability (14,25,70,71). The increase in withdrawal reflex thresholds with age reflects a gradual decrease in the excitability of spinal cord neurons, increased inhibitory input, and reorganization of sensory connections that reduce the size of the receptive field (31). Reflex responses are initially less organized, can be evoked by both noxious and innocuous stimuli, and may result in inappropriate generalized movements. Maturation of sensory and motor inputs, and an activity-dependent process that involves strengthening of appropriate connections and suppression of erroneous movements, leads to tuning of the receptive fields of each withdrawal reflex module. As a result, more specific motor responses develop that selectively move the stimulated area away from the stimulus (72–74).

In clinical studies, changes in reflex thresholds, receptive field size, and specificity of withdrawal responses have been demonstrated that correlate with the developmental pattern seen in laboratory investigations. The mechanical threshold of the hindlimb flexion withdrawal reflex is initially low and increases with postconceptional age (PCA) in preterm neonates, but is still well below adult levels at term (40 weeks PGA) (25,75,76). Electromyographic (EMG) responses of the biceps femoris to mechanical, electrical, and noxious (heel stick for routine blood sampling) stimuli confirmed lower reflex thresholds in infants aged 28 to 42 weeks PGA, and there was good correlation between stimulus intensity and the amplitude of the reflex at all ages (77). Reflex movements are also less synchronized in premature neonates. The receptive field of the hindlimb reflex is large in early development, as withdrawal can be elicited by low-intensity stimuli over the whole limb at 27 weeks PGA. As age increases, withdrawal is more specifically produced by stimuli on the foot, and there occurs a gradient of increasing threshold from distal to proximal sites on the

PART IV: PAIN MANAGEMENT

limb (76). A mechanical stimulus (von Frey hair) applied perpendicular to the abdomen produces a brisk contraction of the ipsilateral abdominal musculature in infants (abdominal skin reflex). In preterm neonates, a more generalized response that includes hip flexion is evoked, but the incidence and degree of hip flexion decreases sharply from 30 to 42 weeks PGA (68). Erroneous reflex movements have also been demonstrated in clinical studies. In an adult, stimulation of the plantar surface of the heel produces plantar flexion of the toes and no response in tibialis anterior (which produces dorsiflexion of toes). However, in neonates aged 30 to 39.5 weeks PGA, low-intensity mechanical (von Frey hairs) or electrical stimuli on the plantar surface of the foot produced an EMG response in tibialis anterior (60). This leads to inappropriate movement toward the stimulus, which resolves with further maturation and tuning of the reflex response.

Cortical Function

The reflex responses and alterations in stress hormones associated with noxious procedures in neonates (and the fetus) are indicators of functional nociceptive and hypothalamo-pituitary-adrenal axis pathways, but do not directly equate with cortical activation or "pain perception" (78). Emphasis has been placed on the presence of thalamocortical fibers as a minimum requirement for pain perception. Although these pathways are anatomically present from 23 to 30 weeks of gestational age in the human (79), functional maturity also needs to be confirmed. Electroencephalographic (EEG) activity can be detected from 24 weeks, and synchronous activity suggesting "wakefulness" from 30 weeks PGA in premature neonates (79). Age- and context-dependent changes in function are particularly pertinent to discussions of fetal "pain." Activity in a premature neonate cannot be directly extrapolated to a fetus at the same gestational age. Differences in environmental factors (constant temperature, amniotic fluid minimizes tactile stimulation) and placental production of inhibitory compounds (such as adenosine and pregnenolone, which suppress cortical activation) are likely to have significant effects on the function of cortical pathways before birth (78,80).

Cortical activation in association with painful procedural interventions has recently been investigated using near-infrared spectroscopy (NIRS) in premature neonates. Heel prick for blood sampling produces changes in cerebral oxygenation over the contralateral somatosensory cortex indicative of cortical activation. These changes could be observed as early as 25 weeks PGA; the magnitude of response increased and latency decreased with age, and greater responses were recorded in awake neonates (81). A later study reported bilateral increases in blood flow over the somatosensory cortex following venipuncture, and a negative correlation was found between cortical activity and gestational age (28 to 36 weeks) (82). Although some results vary due to differing methodology (brief heel lance versus more prolonged venipuncture and squeeze; duration of recordings; time after birth), both studies show that painful interventions produce functional activation of the somatosensory cortex in premature neonates (83).

DEVELOPMENTAL AGE AND RESPONSE TO INJURY

The response to painful tissue injury may vary in degree, duration, and functional consequences in a manner that is critically dependent on the type of injury and the developmental stage at which it occurs. Normal development of the nervous system is activity-dependent, and the formation of synaptic connections and pathways requires appropriate somatosensory input. However, due to the increased plasticity of the developing nervous system, alterations from normal activity may also alter the normal progression of development (6). Reductions in activity due to the destruction of C-fibers (29) or chronic blockade of NMDA receptors in the superficial dorsal horn (84) prevent the normal pattern of C-fiber maturation and A-fiber withdrawal. As a result, an early developmental pattern persists, with large dorsal horn receptive fields and lower mechanical withdrawal thresholds (84). The opposite may also be true—alterations due to *increased* afferent input alter normal development, which may lead to long-term changes in somatosensory function and/or result in effects not seen when the same insult occurs in an adult.

The investigation of long-term consequences of neonatal injury are of considerable importance. There may be effects on nociceptive processing that differ in mechanism and duration from that experienced by older children and adults, and there may be persistent changes in sensory function or an altered response to subsequent stimuli. However, changes are multifactorial, and the following questions need to be considered when interpreting reported long-term effects: (a) Is it specific to early development; (b) is it triggered during a critical period and maintained long after resolution of the initial injury; or (c) is it associated with and maintained by chronic injury?

Primary and Secondary Hyperalgesia

Laboratory Investigations

Primary hyperalgesia is characterized by a decrease in pain threshold and increased response to suprathreshold stimuli due to sensitization of nociceptors within an area of injury (85). Primary hyperalgesia has been demonstrated in a number of early developmental models (62,86). Heating the skin or repeated low-intensity mechanical stimulation produces sensitization of rat foetal DRG afferents and a marked increase in background and evoked activity (19). Similarly, peripheral application of mustard oil, which activates C-fibers via the TRPA1 receptor, enhances the response to subsequent brushing or pinching within the receptive field (11,25). Although hindpaw mustard oil application evokes less immediate reflex activity at P3 than in older pups, the reflex response to mechanical hindpaw stimuli is increased 10 minutes later (i.e., primary hyperalgesia is induced) at all postnatal ages (62). The degree of primary hyperalgesia increases with age, consistent with a developmental increase in the number of TRPV1+ nerve fibers in cutaneous structures (24).

In addition to primary hyperalgesia at the site of injury, noxious C-fiber stimulation produces a surrounding zone of secondary mechanical hyperalgesia (87,88) in adult animals (89,90). Although C-fiber stimuli produce robust primary hyperalgesia in young animals, minimal secondary hyperalgesia is observed in early development (62,91,92), suggesting that the necessary spinal cord and/or supraspinal mechanisms are not mature in the first postnatal week. Recently it has been shown that the distribution and degree of activated extracellular signal-regulated kinase (ERK), which is an important intracellular mediator of increased sensitivity in the dorsal horn following capsaicin injection (93), is significantly reduced in younger pups (62).

Clinical Studies

Primary and secondary hyperalgesia following C-fiber stimulation can be clearly demonstrated and quantified in adult human volunteers (94,95). Tissue injury due to repeated heel-prick blood sampling in neonates results in primary hyperalgesia, as reflected by a reduction in mechanical withdrawal threshold (96,97). Changes in withdrawal threshold in the contralateral limb, suggestive of secondary hyperalgesia, have been reported with more extensive injury (77). The abdominal skin reflex (ASR) has also been used to assess the response to injury in neonates and infants. The mechanical threshold (von Frey hairs) for evoking this reflex is significantly lower for at least 24 hours following abdominal surgery, and can be returned toward baseline values by analgesia (67). Ipsilateral reductions in the ASR threshold have also been shown in infants with unilateral hydronephrosis, suggestive of referred visceral hyperalgesia (68). This suggests that secondary hyperalgesia may be mediated by pathways other than C-fibers in early life, and has implications for the use of analgesics at different ages. Analgesic agents that specifically target C-fiber mechanisms may be advantageous in adults but less so in early development. By contrast, functional opioid receptors are distributed not only on C-fibers but also on a higher proportion of A-fibers in the early postnatal period, and this may contribute to the increased sensitivity to these agents in neonates (98).

Inflammation

Hindpaw inflammation produces hyperalgesia at all postnatal ages in the rat pup, but the degree of acute change varies with age, and long-term changes are critically dependent on the severity of injury (8,65,66). Severe neonatal inflammation produces permanent structural alterations in primary afferent projections in the dorsal horn that are associated with increased behavioral and electrophysiologic responses to subsequent painful stimuli (99,100). As these changes are only seen in association with chronic inflammation, they may have limited clinical significance, but even relatively mild inflammation in neonatal animals produces acute reversible structural changes that are not seen following a similar injury in the adult (8).

Recent rat pup studies have reported a bimodal response following mild neonatal inflammation. A generalized increase in basal sensory thresholds or *hypoalgesia* is seen in all paws when these animals reach adulthood, possibly due to stress-induced alterations in the hypothalamic-pituitary axis (HPA). By contrast, repeated injury in the previously inflamed hindpaw seems to unmask segmental changes of long-term sensitization and produces a greater degree of local *hyperalgesia* (101,102). These changes only occur if inflammation is induced in the first postnatal week and, therefore, a critical period of susceptibility exists for long-term effects following inflammation.

Surgical Incision

Laboratory Investigations

Developmentally regulated responses to surgical incisions are beginning to be investigated in laboratory models. Plantar hindpaw incision produces acute hyperalgesia in 2-week-old rats, which resolves more rapidly than when the same procedure is performed in 4- and 16-week-old animals (103). Effects at earlier stages of development require evaluation. Laparotomy in neonatal mice (P0) produces both acute behavioral responses indicative of pain and distress, as well as long-term changes in sensory function. When these animals reached adulthood, there was a decreased sensitivity to thermal stimuli (increased latency for tail and hindlimb withdrawal) and

a reduced response to a visceral nociceptive stimulus (acetic acid) (104). An increased threshold for hindlimb withdrawal was observed in both the surgery and sham group that had the same degree of stress (anaesthesia, maternal separation, placebo injection) (104). This emphasizes the importance of appropriate control groups, as many factors may influence long-term outcomes, and variable responses may be seen depending on the methodology of individual studies. Maternal separation, maternal behavior, and perinatal stress can all have an impact on subsequent development (105). An initial increase in maternal contact but later neglect was reported after hindpaw inflammation (106), but no change in maternal behavior was seen in mice whose pups had undergone laparotomy (104). Early exposure to an immune challenge can also have long-term effects on nociceptive thresholds in later life (107,108). Increased anxiety but no change in the stress response was reported in adult rats following repeated paw needle prick throughout the first postnatal week (109). In contrast, decreased anxiety and reduced basal and stress-induced release of corticotrophin-releasing factor (CRF) and adrenocorticotropic hormone (ACTH) was reported in adults following hindpaw inflammation at P3 (106). These studies emphasize the complexity of specifically attributing changes in long-term responses to pain in early life. As inflammation, nerve injury, and skin wounding have different developmental profiles (see earlier discussion) but may all contribute to postsurgical pain (110), potential long-term effects of surgical incision are complex and require further investigation.

Clinical Studies

Clinical studies suggest that early pain related to surgery and clinical procedures during intensive care management of premature neonates can have long-term effects upon pain-related behavior and pain perception (7,111). Importantly, analgesia at the time of the initial painful stimulus may modulate long-term effects. Male neonates circumcised without analgesia show an increased behavioral pain response to immunization several months later, but this is partially reduced if local anaesthetic is used prior to surgery (3). Infants who had undergone surgery in the neonatal period with perioperative morphine did not show any increase in later response to immunization when compared with infants without significant previous pain experience (112). Some clinical evidence correlates with the dual pattern of baseline hypoalgesia but increased response to repeated injury that is seen following neonatal inflammation in rat pups (101). Quantitative sensory testing of children 10 years following lateral thoracotomy during the neonatal period found higher mechanical and thermal thresholds both at the site of surgery and at a distant reference point (thenar eminence) compared with an age-matched nonoperated control group (113). Surgery during the first 3 months of life was associated with increased analgesic requirements during subsequent surgery, particularly if performed in the same dermatome (114). Similar studies have not been conducted following surgery performed at different ages, and therefore it remains to be determined if there is a specific age range who are susceptible to long-term changes in sensory function following surgery.

Visceral Injury

Laboratory Investigations

Rat pups subjected to repeated mechanical or chemical (mustard oil) colonic irritation from P8 to P20 had persistent changes in behavior (increased sensitivity to subsequent distension) and central changes (increased firing of dorsal horn neurons) suggestive of persistent hyperalgesia when tested 2 weeks later, despite recovery of peripheral tissues and no detectable changes in bowel histology. Prolonged effects were not seen when the same degree of irritation was performed from P21 to P42, suggesting that this is a specific developmental effect, although older animals were sedated during treatment (115).

Clinical Studies

In infants with unilateral hydronephrosis, the threshold of the abdominal skin reflex was reduced ipsilaterally, reflecting referred visceral hyperalgesia. In addition, the reflex threshold did not follow the normal developmental pattern of increasing threshold with increasing postnatal age and remained lower than in control infants even after corrective surgery (68). This suggests that long-term alterations in sensory processing may occur following early visceral injury.

Full-thickness Skin Wounding

The response to full-thickness skin wounds on the hindpaw differs markedly in neonatal and adult animals. When performed in the first postnatal week, skin wounding results in a reduction in withdrawal threshold that persists well beyond the period of wound healing (116,117), and which is not prevented by a sciatic nerve block at the time of injury (118). Central changes in sensory connections contribute to this persistent sensitivity, as the receptive field size of dorsal horn neurons is significantly greater in wounded compared with control animals 3 and 6 weeks later (119). In addition, marked peripheral hyperinnervation occurs within the wounded area, mediated by local release of neurotrophic factors (120) and changes in short-range inhibitory cues. Ephrins act as contact-mediated guidance molecules during development and repair, and ephrin-A4 inhibits neurite outgrowth. However, following neonatal skin wounding, this inhibition is reduced as ephrin-A4 expression is downregulated, thus allowing an increase in innervation density (121).

Nerve Injury

Laboratory Investigations

In early development, peripheral sensory neurons are dependent on neurotrophins from the target area of innervation (16). Axotomy produces marked cell death within the DRG (122), which is not seen with other forms of injury such as severe inflammation (8). Sciatic nerve axotomy during the first postnatal week leads to a reduction in the central terminal field of these primary afferents, but adjacent saphenous neurons project into the denervated area (123,124) and form functional connections (125). Therefore, despite cell death, central inputs are maintained.

Several different forms of peripheral nerve injury have been used to investigate the pathophysiology of neuropathic pain. Responses during early development differ significantly from those seen when the same injury occurs in adults. Ligation of the spinal nerve roots (L5 and L6) produces significant and prolonged allodynia in adult animals, but changes are of shorter duration if performed at 1 or 2 weeks of age (126,127). Partial sciatic ligation produced minimal difference in threshold from control animals in 2-week-old rat pups, but when performed in 4- or 16-week-old animals, a greater degree and duration of allodynia was observed (127). The spared nerve injury (SNI) model (i.e., division of tibial and common peroneal branches of sciatic nerve while leaving sural nerve intact) produces marked allodynia in adult animals (128). When performed at 3, 7, 10, and 21 days of age, SNI did not produce significant mechanical allodynia at any time in the next 4 weeks, whereas when performed at P33, allodynia occurred but to a lesser degree than in adult animals. Similarly, chronic constriction injury (CCI) at P10 did not produce the prolonged allodynia seen in adults (129). The mechanisms underlying this altered response are currently being investigated.

Clinical Studies

Age-related changes in pain following nerve injury are supported by clinical studies, but further prospective trials with long-term follow-up are required. Traumatic injury to the brachial plexus in adults is frequently followed by severe neuropathic pain (130). By contrast, brachial plexus injury at the time of birth is not associated with chronic neuropathic pain, and restoration of normal sensation and ability to localize stimuli was seen following early surgical repair (131). It has also been postulated that the reduced sensitivity following nerve injury in early life correlates with clinical experience in children with complex regional pain syndrome (CRPS), which is rare before 8 years of age (132). In older children and adolescents, neuropathic pain is recognized. Phantom pain is much more common following surgery or trauma than in children with congenital absence of a limb (133,134) and can be of moderate to severe intensity (6.43 on 0–10 rating scale) (135). Phantom pain also occurs following amputations for burn injury (136) or cancer treatment (137). As 75% of children with phantom pain also had preoperative limb pain (137), it has been suggested that preoperative regional anaesthesia may be beneficial, but no prospective trials have been conducted in children.

DEVELOPMENTAL PHARMACODYNAMICS OF REGIONAL ANALGESICS

Alterations in nociceptive processing and in the distribution and function of receptors may have a significant impact on the efficacy and side-effect profile of regional analgesic agents at different postnatal ages. Laboratory studies allow evaluation of the effect of developmental age on the pharmacodynamic response to analgesics, as effects on baseline sensory function (i.e., antinociceptive effect) and on the hyperalgesia produced by different forms of injury (i.e., antihyperalgesic or analgesic effect) can be tested. Such studies provide information about the effect of developmental stage on the selectivity of drug action and on the sensitivity to analgesic effects and side-effects, and may provide a guide for comparative dose-requirements in subsequent clinical studies.

Local Anaesthetics

Lower concentrations of age-adjusted volumes of epidural bupivacaine reverse inflammatory hyperalgesia in younger pups (P3 <P10 <P21). Selective antihyperalgesic effects were achieved at concentrations that did not affect the sensory threshold of the contralateral paw or produce motor block (65).

Opioids

Opioid receptors and endogenous opioid peptides appear very early in central nervous system (CNS) development, but undergo marked changes in distribution and density throughout the postnatal period. In rat pups, during the first postnatal week, an increased proportion of cells in the DRG express μ opioid receptors (MOR). These receptors are functional and initially distributed on both large ($A\beta$) and small to medium ($A\delta$ and C) DRG cells and, as a result, systemic morphine has a greater effect on the mechanical withdrawal in younger animals (98). By 3 weeks postnatal age, the adult pattern is seen, with fewer cells expressing opioid receptors, and these are predominantly small to medium in size (138). Within the spinal cord, MOR binding sites are relatively diffusely distributed over the dorsal horn at birth (P0). The number of binding sites peaks at P7, and then decreases toward adult levels at P21, with an associated regression of distribution and increased density in the superficial dorsal horn (139).

Epidural morphine has both antinociceptive and antihyperalgesic actions throughout postnatal development. Effects on mechanical withdrawal thresholds occur at lower doses in younger animals (P3 <P10 <P21) (63), and doses required to reverse the mechanical hyperalgesia produced by inflammation are also lower in younger animals (140). It is unlikely that changes in dose requirements relate solely to differences in dural penetration or increased access to the CNS at different ages. The same analgesic effect occurs at lower brain concentrations of opioids in younger pups (141), and the distribution and concentration of [^{3}H]morphine binding sites in the spinal cord did not differ significantly following epidural administration of the same dose at P3, P10, and P21 (63).

α_2-Adrenergic Agonists

The spinal cord has been confirmed as the major site of analgesic action of α_2 agonists, such as clonidine and dexmedetomidine, in adult animals (142). Messenger RNA for the α_{2A}-receptor is present in the dorsal horn both pre- and postnatally (143,144), and binding sites for [^{3}H]dexmedetomidine have been identified in neonatal spinal cord (P1–P2) (145). The analgesic efficacy of subcutaneous dexmedetomidine in the formalin test has been reported to be independent of age from P7 to adult (146), but lower doses suppressed the response in P3 to P5 pups (147). Epidural dexmedetomidine selectively reverses hindpaw inflammatory hyperalgesia throughout postnatal development, and lower doses are effective in the youngest pups (66). Analgesic effects are spinally mediated at all ages, as doses of dexmedetomidine that were effective when administered epidurally had no effect when given systemically. In addition, antihyperalgesic effects were achieved at doses lower than associated with antinociceptive effects or side effects. Dose-dependent sedative effects occur following both epidural and systemic administration, with increased sensitivity in younger pups, but the separation between analgesic and side-effect doses is much greater following epidural administration (66,146).

SUMMARY

Significant advances have been made in our understanding of responses to pain and injury in early life, but effective control of pain remains problematic in many clinical settings. Nociceptive pathways are functional following birth, even in the most premature neonate, but changes in the developing nervous system have a significant impact on the type and degree of response to painful stimuli and the efficacy of analgesic interventions. Alterations in levels of neural activity due to pain and injury have the potential to produce responses not seen in the adult; these may impair normal development and lead to long-term changes in sensory function. Ongoing research will allow further elucidation of the mechanisms underlying developmental changes in nociceptive processing and the response to injury, and will inform translational clinical trials to evaluate developmentally appropriate treatments and enhance effective evidence-based management of pain in patients of all ages.

References

1. Merskey H, Bogduk N. *Classification of Chronic Pain Syndromes and Definitions of Pain Terms*, 2nd ed. Seattle: IASP Press, 1994.
2. Franck LS, Greenberg CS, Stevens B. Pain assessment in infants and children. *Pediatr Clin North Am* 2000;47:487–512.
3. Taddio A, Katz J, Ilersich AL, Koren G. Effect of neonatal circumcision on pain response during subsequent routine vaccination. *Lancet* 1997;349:599–603.
4. Anand KJ, Hickey PR. Halothane-morphine compared with high-dose sufentanil for anesthesia and postoperative analgesia in neonatal cardiac surgery. *N Engl J Med* 1992;326:1–9.
5. Anand KJ. Consensus statement for the prevention and management of pain in the newborn. *Arch Pediatr Adolesc Med* 2001;155:173–180.
6. Fitzgerald M, Walker S. The role of activity in developing pain pathways. In: Dostrovsky J, Carr D, Koltzenburg M, eds. *Proceedings of the 10th World Congress on Pain. Progress in Pain Research and Management*, Vol. 24. Seattle: IASP Press; 2003:185–196.
7. Grunau RE. Long-term consequences of pain in human neonates. In: *Pain Research and Clinical Management*. In: Anand KJS, Stevens BJ, McGrath PJ, eds. Amsterdam: Elsevier; 2000:55–76.
8. Walker SM, Meredith-Middleton J, Cooke-Yarborough C, Fitzgerald M. Neonatal inflammation and primary afferent terminal plasticity in the rat dorsal horn. *Pain* 2003;105:185–195.
9. Fitzgerald M, Howard RF. The neurobiologic basis of pediatric pain. In: Schecter NL, Berde CB, Yaster M, eds. *Pain in Infants Children and Adolescents*. Baltimore: Lippincott Williams and Wilkins; 2002:19–42.
10. Walker S, Howard R. Neonatal pain. *Pain Rev* 2004;9:69–79.
11. Fitzgerald M. The developmental neurobiology of pain. In: Bond M, Charlton JE, Woolf CJ, eds. *Proceedings of the VIth World Congress on Pain. Pain Research and Clinical Management*, Vol. 4. Amsterdam: Elsevier; 1991:253–261.
12. Berde C, Cairns B. Developmental pharmacology across species: Promise and problems. *Anesth Analg* 2000;91:1–5.
13. Fitzgerald M. The development of nociceptive circuits. *Nat Rev Neurosci* 2005;6:507–520.
14. Pattinson D, Fitzgerald M. The neurobiology of infant pain: Development of excitatory and inhibitory neurotransmission in the spinal dorsal horn. *Reg Anesth Pain Med* 2004;29:36–44.
15. Fitzgerald M, MacDermott A. The development of pain systems. In: Hunt S, Koltzenburg M, eds. *The Neurobiology of Pain*. Oxford: Oxford University Press; 2005:207–238.
16. Baccei M, Fitzgerald M. Development of pain pathways and mechanisms. In: McMahon SB, Koltzenburg M, eds. *Wall and Melzack's Textbook of Pain*, 5th ed. New York: Elsevier Churchill Livingstone; 2006:143–158.
17. Alvares D, Fitzgerald M. Building blocks of pain: The regulation of key molecules in spinal sensory neurones during development and following peripheral axotomy. *Pain* 1999;[Suppl 6]:S71–S85.
18. Jackman A, Fitzgerald M. Development of peripheral hindlimb and central spinal cord innervation by subpopulations of dorsal root ganglion cells in the embryonic rat. *J Comp Neurol* 2000;418:281–298.

19. Fitzgerald M. Spontaneous and evoked activity of fetal primary afferents in vivo. *Nature* 1987;326:603–605.
20. Fitzgerald M. Cutaneous primary afferent properties in the hind limb of the neonatal rat. *J Physiol* 1987;383:79–92.
21. Tominaga M, Caterina MJ. Thermosensation and pain. *J Neurobiol* 2004; 61:3–12.
22. Bandell M, Story GM, Hwang SW, et al. Noxious cold ion channel TRPA1 is activated by pungent compounds and bradykinin. *Neuron* 2004;41:849–857.
23. Zhu W, Galoyan SM, Petruska JC, et al. A developmental switch in acute sensitization of small dorsal root ganglion (DRG) neurons to capsaicin or noxious heating by NGF. *J Neurophysiol* 2004;92:3148–3152.
24. Guo A, Simone DA, Stone LS, et al. Developmental shift of vanilloid receptor 1 (VR1) terminals into deeper regions of the superficial dorsal horn: Correlation with a shift from TrkA to Ret expression by dorsal root ganglion neurons. *Eur J Neurosci* 2001;14:293–304.
25. Fitzgerald M, Gibson S. The postnatal physiological and neurochemical development of peripheral sensory C fibers. *Neuroscience* 1984;13:933–944.
26. Benn SC, Costigan M, Tate S, et al. Developmental expression of the TTX-resistant voltage-gated sodium channels Nav1.8 (SNS) and Nav1.9 (SNS2) in primary sensory neurons. *J Neurosci* 2001;21:6077–6085.
27. Fitzgerald M, Butcher T, Shortland P. Developmental changes in the laminar termination of A fiber cutaneous sensory afferents in the rat spinal cord dorsal horn. *J Comp Neurol* 1994;348:225–233.
28. Mirnics K, Koerber HR. Prenatal development of rat primary afferent fibers: II. Central projections. *J Comp Neurol* 1995;355:601–614.
29. Torsney C, Meredith-Middleton J, Fitzgerald M. Neonatal capsaicin treatment prevents the normal postnatal withdrawal of A fibers from lamina II without affecting fos responses to innocuous peripheral stimulation. *Brain Res Dev Brain Res* 2000;121:55–65.
30. Coggeshall RE, Jennings EA, Fitzgerald M. Evidence that large myelinated primary afferent fibers make synaptic contacts in lamina II of neonatal rats. *Brain Res Dev Brain Res* 1996;92:81–90.
31. Fitzgerald M, Jennings E. The postnatal development of spinal sensory processing. *Proc Natl Acad Sci USA* 1999;96:7719–7722.
32. Jennings E, Fitzgerald M. Postnatal changes in responses of rat dorsal horn cells to afferent stimulation: A fiber-induced sensitization. *J Physiol* 1998;509[Pt 3]:859–868.
33. Park JS, Nakatsuka T, Nagata K, et al. Reorganization of the primary afferent termination in the rat spinal dorsal horn during post-natal development. *Brain Res Dev Brain Res* 1999;113:29–36.
34. Nakatsuka T, Ataka T, Kumamoto E, et al. Alteration in synaptic inputs through C-afferent fibers to substantia gelatinosa neurons of the rat spinal dorsal horn during postnatal development. *Neuroscience* 2000;99:549–556.
35. Baccei ML, Fitzgerald M. Intrinsic firing properties of developing rat superficial dorsal horn neurons. *Neuroreport* 2005;16:1325–1328.
36. Fitzgerald M. The post-natal development of cutaneous afferent fiber input and receptive field organization in the rat dorsal horn. *J Physiol* 1985;364:1–18.
37. Torsney C, Fitzgerald M. Age-dependent effects of peripheral inflammation on the electrophysiological properties of neonatal rat dorsal horn neurons. *J Neurophysiol* 2002;87:1311–1317.
38. Baccei ML, Bardoni R, Fitzgerald M. Development of nociceptive synaptic inputs to the neonatal rat dorsal horn: Glutamate release by capsaicin and menthol. *J Physiol* 2003;549:231–242.
39. Fitzgerald M. The development of activity evoked by fine diameter cutaneous fibers in the spinal cord of the newborn rat. *Neurosci Lett* 1988;86:161–166.
40. Baccei ML, Fitzgerald M. Development of GABAergic and glycinergic transmission in the neonatal rat dorsal horn. *J Neurosci* 2004;24:4749–4757.
41. Jakowec MW, Fox AJ, Martin LJ, Kalb RG. Quantitative and qualitative changes in AMPA receptor expression during spinal cord development. *Neuroscience* 1995;67:893–907.
42. Gonzalez DL, Fuchs JL, Droge MH. Distribution of NMDA receptor binding in developing mouse spinal cord. *Neurosci Lett* 1993;151:134–137.
43. Jakowec MW, Yen L, Kalb RG. In situ hybridization analysis of AMPA receptor subunit gene expression in the developing rat spinal cord. *Neuroscience* 1995;67:909–920.
44. Brown KM, Wrathall JR, Yasuda RP, Wolfe BB. Quantitative measurement of glutamate receptor subunit protein expression in the postnatal rat spinal cord. *Brain Res Dev Brain Res* 2002;137:127–133.
45. Engelman HS, Allen TB, MacDermott AB. The distribution of neurons expressing calcium-permeable AMPA receptors in the superficial laminae of the spinal cord dorsal horn. *J Neurosci* 1999;19:2081–2089.
46. Hori Y, Kanda K. Developmental alterations in NMDA receptor-mediated [Ca2+]i elevation in substantia gelatinosa neurons of neonatal rat spinal cord. *Brain Res Dev Brain Res* 1994;80:141–148.
47. Bardoni R. Excitatory synaptic transmission in neonatal dorsal horn: NMDA and ATP receptors. *News Physiol Sci* 2001;16:95–100.
48. Bardoni R, Magherini PC, MacDermott AB. NMDA EPSCs at glutamatergic synapses in the spinal cord dorsal horn of the postnatal rat. *J Neurosci* 1998;18:6558–6567.
49. Li P, Zhuo M. Silent glutamatergic synapses and nociception in mammalian spinal cord. *Nature* 1998;393:695–698.
50. Bardoni R, Magherini PC, MacDermott AB. Activation of NMDA receptors drives action potentials in superficial dorsal horn from neonatal rats. *Neuroreport* 2000;11:1721–1727.
51. Ben-Ari Y. Excitatory actions of GABA during development: The nature of the nurture. *Nat Rev Neurosci* 2002;3:728–739.
52. Rivera C, Voipio J, Payne JA, et al. The K+/Cl− co-transporter KCC2 renders GABA hyperpolarizing during neuronal maturation. *Nature* 1999; 397:251–255.
53. Bremner L, Fitzgerald M, Baccei M. Functional GABA(A)-receptor-mediated inhibition in the neonatal dorsal horn. *J Neurophysiol* 2006; 95:3893–3897.
54. Hathway G, Harrop E, Baccei M, et al. A postnatal switch in GABAergic control of spinal cutaneous reflexes. *Eur J Neurosci* 2006;23:112–118.
55. Bicknell HR Jr., Beal JA. Axonal and dendritic development of substantia gelatinosa neurons in the lumbosacral spinal cord of the rat. *J Comp Neurol* 1984;226:508–522.
56. Fitzgerald M, Koltzenburg M. The functional development of descending inhibitory pathways in the dorsolateral funiculus of the newborn rat spinal cord. *Brain Res* 1986;389:261–270.
57. Boucher T, Jennings E, Fitzgerald M. The onset of diffuse noxious inhibitory controls in postnatal rat pups: A C-Fos study. *Neurosci Lett* 1998;257:9–12.
58. van Praag H, Frenk H. The development of stimulation-produced analgesia (SPA) in the rat. *Brain Res Dev Brain Res* 1991;64:71–76.
59. Woolf CJ. Long term alterations in the excitability of the flexion reflex produced by peripheral tissue injury in the chronic decerebrate rat. *Pain* 1984;18:325–343.
60. Andrews K, Fitzgerald M. Flexion reflex responses in biceps femoris and tibialis anterior in human neonates. *Early Hum Dev* 2000;57:105–110.
61. Fitzgerald M, de Lima J. Hyperalgesia and allodynia in infants. In: Finley G, McGrath P, eds. *Acute and Procedure Pain in Infants and Children. Progress in Pain Research and Management.* Seattle: IASP Press; 2001:1–12.
62. Walker SM, Meredith-Middleton J, Lickiss T, Fitzgerald M. Primary and secondary hyperalgesia can be differentiated by postnatal age and ERK activation in the spinal dorsal horn of the rat pup. *Pain* 2007;128(1–2):157–168.
63. Marsh D, Dickenson A, Hatch D, Fitzgerald M. Epidural opioid analgesia in infant rats I: Mechanical and heat responses. *Pain* 1999;82:23–32.
64. Williams DG, Dickenson A, Fitzgerald M, Howard RF. Developmental regulation of codeine analgesia in the rat. *Anesthesiology* 2004;100: 92–97.
65. Howard RF, Hatch DJ, Cole TJ, Fitzgerald M. Inflammatory pain and hypersensitivity are selectively reversed by epidural bupivacaine and are developmentally regulated. *Anesthesiology* 2001;95:421–427.
66. Walker SM, Howard RF, Keay KA, Fitzgerald M. Developmental age influences the effect of epidural dexmedetomidine on inflammatory hyperalgesia in rat pups. *Anesthesiology* 2005;102:1226–1234.
67. Andrews K, Fitzgerald M. Wound sensitivity as a measure of analgesic effects following surgery in human neonates and infants. *Pain* 2002;99:185–195.
68. Andrews KA, Desai D, Dhillon HK, et al. Abdominal sensitivity in the first year of life: Comparison of infants with and without prenatally diagnosed unilateral hydronephrosis. *Pain* 2002;100:35–46.
69. Woolf CJ. Evidence for a central component of post-injury pain hypersensitivity. *Nature* 1983;306:686–688.
70. Holmberg H, Schouenborg J. Postnatal development of the nociceptive withdrawal reflexes in the rat: A behavioral and electromyographic study. *J Physiol* 1996;493[Pt 1]:239–252.
71. Falcon M, Guendellman D, Stolberg A, et al. Development of thermal nociception in rats. *Pain* 1996;67:203–208.
72. Schouenborg J. Modular organisation and spinal somatosensory imprinting. *Brain Res Brain Res Rev* 2002;40:80–91.
73. Waldenstrom A, Thelin J, Thimansson E, et al. Developmental learning in a pain-related system: Evidence for a cross-modality mechanism. *J Neurosci* 2003;23:7719–7725.
74. Petersson P, Waldenstrom A, Fahraeus C, Schouenborg J. Spontaneous muscle twitches during sleep guide spinal self-organization. *Nature* 2003;424: 72–75.
75. Fitzgerald M, Shaw A, MacIntosh N. Postnatal development of the cutaneous flexor reflex: Comparative study of preterm infants and newborn rat pups. *Dev Med Child Neurol* 1988;30:520–526.
76. Andrews K, Fitzgerald M. The cutaneous withdrawal reflex in human neonates: Sensitization, receptive fields, and the effects of contralateral stimulation. *Pain* 1994;56:95–101.
77. Andrews K, Fitzgerald M. Cutaneous flexion reflex in human neonates: A quantitative study of threshold and stimulus-response characteristics after single and repeated stimuli. *Dev Med Child Neurol* 1999;41:696–703.
78. Derbyshire SW. Can fetuses feel pain? *Br Med J* 2006;332:909–912.
79. Lee SJ, Ralston HJ, Drey EA, et al. Fetal pain: A systematic multidisciplinary review of the evidence. *JAMA* 2005;294:947–954.
80. Mellor DJ, Diesch TJ, Gunn AJ, Bennet L. The importance of 'awareness' for understanding fetal pain. *Brain Res Brain Res Rev* 2005;49:455–471.

81. Slater R, Cantarella A, Gallella S, et al. Cortical pain responses in human infants. *J Neurosci* 2006;26:3662–3666.

82. Bartocci M, Bergqvist LL, Lagercrantz H, Anand KJ. Pain activates cortical areas in the preterm newborn brain. *Pain* 2006;122(1–2):109–117.

83. Slater R, Boyd S, Meek J, Fitzgerald M. Cortical pain responses in the infant brain. *Pain* 2006;123:332; author reply 332–334.

84. Beggs S, Torsney C, Drew LJ, Fitzgerald M. The postnatal reorganization of primary afferent input and dorsal horn cell receptive fields in the rat spinal cord is an activity-dependent process. *Eur J Neurosci* 2002;16:1249–1258.

85. Treede RD, Meyer RA, Raja SN, Campbell JN. Peripheral and central mechanisms of cutaneous hyperalgesia. *Prog Neurobiol* 1992;38:397–421.

86. Koltzenburg M, Lewin GR. Receptive properties of embryonic chick sensory neurons innervating skin. *J Neurophysiol* 1997;78:2560–2568.

87. Treede RD, Magerl W. Multiple mechanisms of secondary hyperalgesia. *Prog Brain Res* 2000;129:331–341.

88. Klede M, Handwerker HO, Schmelz M. Central origin of secondary mechanical hyperalgesia. *J Neurophysiol* 2003;90:353–359.

89. Simone DA, Sorkin LS, Oh U, et al. Neurogenic hyperalgesia: Central neural correlates in responses of spinothalamic tract neurons. *J Neurophysiol* 1991;66:228–246.

90. Reeh PW, Kocher L, Jung S. Does neurogenic inflammation alter the sensitivity of unmyelinated nociceptors in the rat? *Brain Res* 1986;384:42–50.

91. Chen JH, Weng HR, Dougherty PM. Sensitization of dorsal root reflexes in vitro and hyperalgesia in neonatal rats produced by capsaicin. *Neuroscience* 2004;126:743–751.

92. Jiang MC, Gebhart GF. Development of mustard oil-induced hyperalgesia in rats. *Pain* 1998;77:305–313.

93. Ji RR, Baba H, Brenner GJ, Woolf CJ. Nociceptive-specific activation of ERK in spinal neurons contributes to pain hypersensitivity. *Nat Neurosci* 1999;2:1114–1119.

94. LaMotte RH, Lundberg LE, Torebjork HE. Pain, hyperalgesia and activity in nociceptive C units in humans after intradermal injection of capsaicin. *J Physiol* 1992;448:749–764.

95. Koltzenburg M, Lundberg LE, Torebjork HE. Dynamic and static components of mechanical hyperalgesia in human hairy skin. *Pain* 1992;51:207–219.

96. Fitzgerald M, Millard C, MacIntosh N. Hyperalgesia in premature infants. *Lancet* 1988;1:292.

97. Fitzgerald M, Millard C, McIntosh N. Cutaneous hypersensitivity following peripheral tissue damage in newborn infants and its reversal with topical anaesthesia. *Pain* 1989;39:31–36.

98. Nandi R, Beacham D, Middleton J, et al. The functional expression of mu opioid receptors on sensory neurons is developmentally regulated; morphine analgesia is less selective in the neonate. *Pain* 2004;111:38–50.

99. Peng YB, Ling QD, Ruda MA, Kenshalo DR. Electrophysiological changes in adult rat dorsal horn neurons after neonatal peripheral inflammation. *J Neurophysiol* 2003;90:73–80.

100. Ruda MA, Ling QD, Hohmann AG, et al. Altered nociceptive neuronal circuits after neonatal peripheral inflammation. *Science* 2000;289:628–631.

101. Ren K, Anseloni V, Zou SP, et al. Characterization of basal and re-inflammation-associated long-term alteration in pain responsivity following short-lasting neonatal local inflammatory insult. *Pain* 2004;110:588–596.

102. Fitzgerald M. Painful beginnings. *Pain* 2004;110:508–509.

103. Ririe DG, Vernon TL, Tobin JR, Eisenach JC. Age-dependent responses to thermal hyperalgesia and mechanical allodynia in a rat model of acute postoperative pain. *Anesthesiology* 2003;99:443–448.

104. Sternberg WF, Scorr L, Smith LD, et al. Long-term effects of neonatal surgery on adulthood pain behavior. *Pain* 2005;113:347–353.

105. Sternberg WF, Ridgway CG. Effects of gestational stress and neonatal handling on pain, analgesia, and stress behavior of adult mice. *Physiol Behav* 2003;78:375–383.

106. Anseloni VC, He F, Novikova SI, et al. Alterations in stress-associated behaviors and neurochemical markers in adult rats after neonatal short-lasting local inflammatory insult. *Neuroscience* 2005;131:635–645.

107. Boisse L, Spencer SJ, Mouihate A, et al. Neonatal immune challenge alters nociception in the adult rat. *Pain* 2005;119:133–141.

108. Spencer SJ, Boisse L, Mouihate A, Pittman QJ. Long term alterations in neuroimmune responses of female rats after neonatal exposure to lipopolysaccharide. *Brain Behav Immun* 2006;20:325–330.

109. Anand KJ, Coskun V, Thrivikraman KV, et al. Long-term behavioral effects of repetitive pain in neonatal rat pups. *Physiol Behav* 1999;66:627–637.

110. Kehlet H, Jensen TS, Woolf CJ. Persistent postsurgical pain: Risk factors and prevention. *Lancet* 2006;367:1618–1625.

111. Buskila D, Neumann L, Zmora E, et al. Pain sensitivity in prematurely born adolescents. *Arch Pediatr Adolesc Med* 2003;157:1079–1082.

112. Peters JW, Koot HM, de Boer JB, et al. Major surgery within the first 3 months of life and subsequent biobehavioral pain responses to immunization at later age: A case comparison study. *Pediatrics* 2003;111:129–135.

113. Schmelzle-Lubiecki BM, Campbell KA, Howard RF, et al. Long term consequences of early infant injury and trauma upon somatosensory processing. *Eur J Pain* 2007;11(7):799–809.

114. Peters JW, Schouw R, Anand KJ, et al. Does neonatal surgery lead to increased pain sensitivity in later childhood? *Pain* 2005;114:444–454.

115. Al-Chaer ED, Kawasaki M, Pasricha PJ. A new model of chronic visceral hypersensitivity in adult rats induced by colon irritation during postnatal development. *Gastroenterology* 2000;119:1276–1285.

116. Reynolds ML, Fitzgerald M. Long-term sensory hyperinnervation following neonatal skin wounds. *J Comp Neurol* 1995;358:487–498.

117. Alvares D, Torsney C, Beland B, et al. Modelling the prolonged effects of neonatal pain. *Prog Brain Res* 2000;129:365–373.

118. De Lima J, Alvares D, Hatch DJ, Fitzgerald M. Sensory hyperinnervation after neonatal skin wounding: Effect of bupivacaine sciatic nerve block. *Br J Anaesth* 1999;83:662–664.

119. Torsney C, Fitzgerald M. Spinal dorsal horn cell receptive field size is increased in adult rats following neonatal hindpaw skin injury. *J Physiol* 2003;550:255–261.

120. Reynolds M, Alvares D, Middleton J, Fitzgerald M. Neonatally wounded skin induces NGF-independent sensory neurite outgrowth in vitro. *Brain Res Dev Brain Res* 1997;102:275–283.

121. Moss A, Alvares D, Meredith-Middleton J, et al. Ephrin-A4 inhibits sensory neurite outgrowth and is regulated by neonatal skin wounding. *Eur J Neurosci* 2005;22:2413–2421.

122. Himes BT, Tessler A. Death of some dorsal root ganglion neurons and plasticity of others following sciatic nerve section in adult and neonatal rats. *J Comp Neurol* 1989;284:215–230.

123. Fitzgerald M, Woolf CJ, Shortland P. Collateral sprouting of the central terminals of cutaneous primary afferent neurons in the rat spinal cord: Pattern, morphology, and influence of targets. *J Comp Neurol* 1990;300:370–385.

124. Shortland P, Fitzgerald M. Neonatal sciatic nerve section results in a rearrangement of the central terminals of saphenous and axotomized sciatic nerve afferents in the dorsal horn of the spinal cord of the adult rat. *Eur J Neurosci* 1994;6:75–86.

125. Shortland P, Fitzgerald M. Functional connections formed by saphenous nerve terminal sprouts in the dorsal horn following neonatal sciatic nerve section. *Eur J Neurosci* 1991;3:383–396.

126. Lee DH, Chung JM. Neuropathic pain in neonatal rats. *Neurosci Lett* 1996;209:140–142.

127. Ririe DG, Eisenach JC. Age-dependent responses to nerve injury-induced mechanical allodynia. *Anesthesiology* 2006;104:344–350.

128. Decosterd I, Woolf CJ. Spared nerve injury: An animal model of persistent peripheral neuropathic pain. *Pain* 2000;87:149–158.

129. Howard RF, Walker SM, Michael Mota P, Fitzgerald M. The ontogeny of neuropathic pain: Postnatal onset of mechanical allodynia in rat spared nerve injury (SNI) and chronic constriction injury (CCI) models. *Pain* 2005;115:382–389.

130. Kato N, Htut M, Taggart M, et al. The effects of operative delay on the relief of neuropathic pain after injury to the brachial plexus: A review of 148 cases. *J Bone Joint Surg Br* 2006;88:756–759.

131. Anand P, Birch R. Restoration of sensory function and lack of long-term chronic pain syndromes after brachial plexus injury in human neonates. *Brain* 2002;125:113–122.

132. Berde CB, Lebel A. Complex regional pain syndromes in children and adolescents. *Anesthesiology* 2005;102:252–255.

133. Wilkins KL, McGrath PJ, Finley GA, Katz J. Phantom limb sensations and phantom limb pain in child and adolescent amputees. *Pain* 1998;78:7–12.

134. Melzack R, Israel R, Lacroix R, Schultz G. Phantom limbs in people with congenital limb deficiency or amputation in early childhood. *Brain* 1997;120[Pt 9]:1603–1620.

135. Wilkins KL, McGrath PJ, Finley GA, Katz J. Prospective diary study of nonpainful and painful phantom sensations in a preselected sample of child and adolescent amputees reporting phantom limbs. *Clin J Pain* 2004;20:293–301.

136. Thomas CR, Brazeal BA, Rosenberg L, et al. Phantom limb pain in pediatric burn survivors. *Burns* 2003;29:139–142.

137. Krane EJ, Heller LB. The prevalence of phantom sensation and pain in pediatric amputees. *J Pain Symptom Manage* 1995;10:21–29.

138. Beland B, Fitzgerald M. Mu- and delta-opioid receptors are downregulated in the largest diameter primary sensory neurons during postnatal development in rats. *Pain* 2001;90:143–150.

139. Rahman W, Dashwood MR, Fitzgerald M, et al. Postnatal development of multiple opioid receptors in the spinal cord and development of spinal morphine analgesia. *Brain Res Dev Brain Res* 1998;108:239–254.

140. Marsh D, Dickenson A, Hatch D, Fitzgerald M. Epidural opioid analgesia in infant rats II: Responses to carrageenan and capsaicin. *Pain* 1999;82:33–38.

141. Windh RT, Kuhn CM. Increased sensitivity to mu opiate antinociception in the neonatal rat despite weaker receptor-guanyl nucleotide binding protein coupling. *J Pharmacol Exp Ther* 1995;273:1353–1360.

142. Buerkle H, Yaksh TL. Pharmacological evidence for different alpha 2-adrenergic receptor sites mediating analgesia and sedation in the rat. *Br J Anaesth* 1998;81:208–215.

143. Huang Y, Stamer WD, Anthony TL, et al. Expression of alpha(2)-adrenergic receptor subtypes in prenatal rat spinal cord. *Brain Res Dev Brain Res* 2002;133:93–104.

144. Winzer-Serhan UH, Raymon HK, Broide RS, et al. Expression of alpha 2 adrenoceptors during rat brain development: I. Alpha 2A messenger RNA expression. *Neuroscience* 1997;76:241–260.

145. Savola MK, Savola JM. [3H]dexmedetomidine, an alpha 2-adrenoceptor agonist, detects a novel imidazole binding site in adult rat spinal cord. *Eur J Pharmacol* 1996;306:315–323.

146. Sanders RD, Giombini M, Ma D, et al. Dexmedetomidine exerts dose-dependent age-independent antinociception but age-dependent hypnosis in Fischer rats. *Anesth Analg* 2005;100:1295–1302.

147. Otsuguro K, Yasutake S, Ohta T, Ito S. Effects of opioid receptor and alpha2-adrenoceptor agonists on slow ventral root potentials and on capsaicin and formalin tests in neonatal rats. *Brain Res Dev Brain Res* 2005;158:50–58.

CHAPTER 31 ■ INTRODUCTION TO PAIN MECHANISMS: IMPLICATIONS FOR NEURAL BLOCKADE

PHILIP J. SIDDALL AND MICHAEL J. COUSINS

Pain is a complex phenomenon that has additional dimensions that set it apart from other sensations such as vision or hearing. The experience of pain, by nature, has an emotive, aversive component and arises from a multifaceted interaction of biological, psychological, and environmental contributors. In recent years, there has been a huge growth in our understanding of the details in each of these components and how they come together to contribute to the experience of pain. The aim of this chapter is not to provide a comprehensive review of the details of the different mechanisms and contributors to pain. More detailed information on the specific physiologic and pharmacologic processes of nociception, as well as the contribution of psychological factors, can be found in other chapters of this text (Chapters 32–36). Rather, this chapter will seek to provide a broad overview of our current concepts of pain and some of the implications that these concepts have for pain management and neural blockade.

WHAT IS PAIN?

Before looking at some of these concepts, it may be helpful to examine what pain actually is. As mentioned, pain is a sensation that has an aversive quality. The International Association for the Study of Pain (IASP) has defined pain in this way: "Pain is an unpleasant sensory and emotional experience associated with actual or potential tissue damage, or described in terms of such damage" (1). Inherent within this definition is the concept that pain is not only a sensory experience, but a complex interaction that also involves emotional and behavioral factors (Chapter 35).

Nervous System Plasticity

One of the fundamental shifts in our view of pain in the preceding century was the recognition of the adaptations that occur within the nervous system in response to pathophysiologic processes. At the beginning of the 20th century, many regarded pain as a sensation arising from the detection of a noxious stimulus by specific receptors, with transmission of signals along "hard-wired" nerve pathways specifically devoted to this process. However, by the end of the century, it was clear that this view was no longer tenable. Ample evidence now supports that the nervous system responds rapidly and often dramatically to changes in the environment and is in a continual state of flux

that is dependent on the level of inputs arising from the periphery (2–5). For example, trauma to any part of the body, and nerve damage in particular, can lead to changes within other regions of the nervous system that influence subsequent responses to sensory input (6). Not only will an increase in inputs lead to a sensitization of central processing, but loss of inputs also appears to result in changes that are associated with the presence of persistent pain (7).

The *gate theory*, put forward by Melzack and Wall in 1965 (8), also attempted to deal with the problems associated with a hard-wired view of pain. Melzack and Wall proposed that an interaction of inputs occurs within the dorsal horn that can lead to an increase or decrease in the volume of signals transmitted through the dorsal horn to the brain, and that activity in larger primary afferents could inhibit messages traveling from small-diameter fibers. Although some of the details of the gate theory have not been substantiated, the gate theory did much to popularize the concept of modulation of sensory inputs at a spinal level. It also provided a theoretical framework for management approaches, such as stimulation techniques, that appeared to inhibit or "close the gate" on nociceptive inputs (see also Chapter 51).

The extension of the gate theory to include the influence of descending pathways from the brain went even further and helped to provide a framework for the inclusion of emotional and cognitive states in the experience of pain (9). This model set the groundwork for a more comprehensive approach to pain that recognized the contribution of sensory/discriminative, affective/motivational, and cognitive/evaluative components to pain perception and behavior. This model emphasizes the contribution of a person's mood, cognitions and their external environment, and the importance of accurate identification and appropriate management of these contributing factors in the assessment and management of pain. The role and contribution of these psychological aspects to pain is described further in Chapter 35.

Pain in the Clinic

From a clinical point of view, pain is sometimes divided into physiologic and clinical entities (10). This division recognizes that, although many of the processes involved in nociceptive transmission have a role in the perception of acute noxious stimuli, different processes come into play when the stimulus is prolonged or sustained. Physiologic pain describes the situation

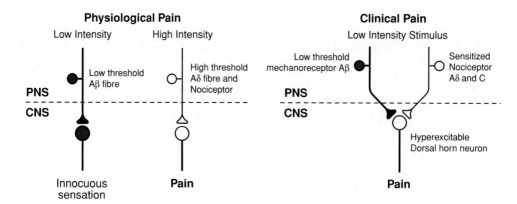

FIGURE 31-1. Right: In the clinical situation, central and peripheral changes lead to abnormal excitability in the nervous system. This means that low-intensity stimuli can produce pain. **Left:** Under "physiologic" conditions, low intensity, non-noxious stimuli activate low-threshold receptors to generate innocuous sensations, and high-intensity, noxious stimuli activate high-threshold nociceptors, which may lead to the sensation of pain. PNS, peripheral nervous system; CNS, central nervous system. From Woolf CJ, Chong MS. Pre-emptive analgesia-treating postoperative pain by preventing the establishment of central sensitization. *Anesth Analg* 1993;77:362, with permission.

in which a noxious stimulus activates peripheral nociceptors, which then transmit sensory information through several relays until it reaches the brain and is recognized as a potentially harmful stimulus (Fig. 31-1, Table 31-1). In the clinical situation, however, this is rarely the situation. More commonly, the insult to the body that produces pain also results in inflammation and tissue injury. The pathophysiologic processes that occur following injury result in a stimulus–response pattern quite different from that seen following physiologic pain, and this phenomenon has therefore been termed *pathophysiologic* or *clinical pain* (Fig. 31-2, Table 31-2). It is the elucidation of these pathophysiological processes that has the most relevance for our understanding and management of pain in the clinical setting. Presentations of visceral pain differ clinically from somatic pain (Table 31-3).

Role of Genetic Factors in Pain

One of the questions raised in the clinical situation is why, in apparently identical situations, some people develop pain and others do not. For example, prevalence studies indicate that around 15% to 50% of people (depending on the condition) will develop neuropathic pain following nervous system trauma (11–14). This may be linked to physical factors, such as the nature of the injury, or to psychological factors that influence the perception and expression of pain. However,

recent findings have also indicated the importance of our innate, genetic makeup in the way that we experience pain. Animal studies indicate that modifications to genetic information, such as occurs in transgenic and knockout mice, result in differences in the prevalence of nociceptive and neuropathic pain and differences in sensitivity to interventions and analgesics (15). Some researchers have suggested a genetic susceptibility to nociceptive and neuropathic pain with excessive and prolonged neuroplastic responses to neuropathic and nociceptive stimuli (16–18).

Some pain disorders have also been shown to have a genetic link. These include hereditary sensory neuropathy type 1 (19), painful congenital myotonia (20), and mutations of CACNL1A4 in people with familial hemiplegic migraine (21) or the neurotrophin receptor tropomyosin receptor kinase A (trkA) in people with congenital insensitivity to pain (22).

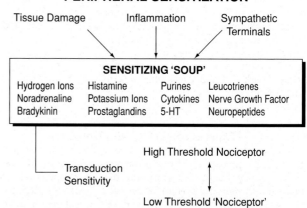

FIGURE 31-2. The sensitivity of high-threshold nociceptors can be modified in the periphery by a combination of chemicals that act as a "sensitizing soup." These chemicals are produced by damaged tissue as part of the inflammatory reaction and by sympathetic terminals. 5-HT, 5-hydroxytryptamine. From Woolf CJ, Chong MS. Pre-emptive analgesia-treating postoperative pain by preventing the establishment of central sensitization. *Anesth Analg* 1993;77:362, with permission.

TABLE 31-1

FEATURES OF PHYSIOLOGICAL PAIN

Pain (Aδ and C fibers) can be differentiated from touch (A*β* fibers)
Pain serves a protective function
Pain acts as a warning of *potential* damage
Pain is transient
Pain is well localized
Stimulus-response pattern is the same as with other sensory modalities, e.g., touch

TABLE 31-2

FEATURES OF CLINICAL PAIN

Pain can be elicited by Aδ and C as well as Aβ fibers
Pain is "pathological," i.e., it is associated with inflammation, neuropathy, etc.
Occurs in the context of peripheral sensitization
Occurs in the context of central sensitization
Pain outlasts the stimulus
Pain spreads to nondamaged areas

μ-Opioid receptor gene polymorphisms (Oprm) (23) cause abnormalities of sensation or changes in response to medication (e.g., differing CYP2D6 phenotype) (24).

An important link between pain and genetic factors has been demonstrated in a study that found that pain responses are modified by alterations in the concentration of an enzyme cofactor, tetrahydrobiopterin (BH4) (25). This study also found that radicular pain in patients following diskectomy was significantly less in people who had a haplotype of the GTP cyclohydrolase gene, which results in reduced production of BH4. This study suggests a strong link between genetic makeup and the development of neuropathic pain. Thus, although the complexity of pain suggests that it is extremely unlikely that a single "pain gene" will be discovered, nevertheless genetic factors are clearly involved in the development of pain under certain conditions and are involved in response to treatment (see also Chapter 33).

Pain as a Disease Entity

Pain has often been regarded merely as a symptom that serves as a passive warning signal of an underlying disease process. Using this model, the goal of treatment has been to identify and address the pathology causing pain in the expectation that this would lead to the resolution of pain. However, it has been suggested that it is more appropriate to consider persistent pain as a disease entity (26,27). As this and the following three chapters demonstrate, accumulating evidence suggests that the transmission of nociceptive signals following injury has a rapid and sustained impact on the physiologic environment at a number of levels (4,6,28–30). In addition, pain has a profound impact on psychological function and social relationships (Chapter 35). These processes, associated with persistent nociceptive inputs, range from changes in receptor function to mood dysfunction, inappropriate cognitions, and social disruption. Therefore, it can be argued that simply regarding pain as a symptom is deficient and fails to recognize the secondary pathophysiologic processes that occur as a result of nociceptive inputs. It also minimizes the impact of pain on the psychological and social milieu of the person in pain. These changes that occur as a consequence of continuing nociceptive inputs and that are described herein argue for the consideration of persistent pain as a disease entity in its own right.

PAIN MECHANISMS

Peripheral Mechanisms

Primary Afferent Nociceptors

The primary afferent nociceptor is generally the initial structure involved in nociceptive processes. Most body structures contain nerve endings that are responsive to mechanical, thermal, and chemical stimuli (see Chapter 30). Nociceptors are primary afferent nerve fibers that are capable of encoding noxious stimuli. Depending on the response characteristics of the nociceptor, stimulation results in propagation of impulses along the primary afferent nerve fiber toward the spinal cord. The receptors associated with transmission of noxious information can be grouped into two main categories: Aδ-fiber mechanothermal and C-fiber polymodal nociceptors (see Chapter 32). Although Aβ-fibers can respond to noxious stimuli, they do not increase their response with increasing stimulus strength and therefore do not encode stimuli in the noxious range.

Receptors

A variety of receptors on primary afferent nociceptors transduce sensory stimuli into nerve activity. These include acid-sensing ion channels (ASIC) (31), P2X receptors (sensitive to adenosine triphosphate [ATP]) (32), and a number of transient receptor potential (TRP) channels such as the cold- and menthol-sensitive transient receptor potential menthol (TRPM8) channel and the heat- and capsaicin-sensitive

TABLE 31-3

VISCERAL PAIN COMPARED WITH SOMATIC PAIN

Site	Somatic well localized	Visceral poorly localized
Radiation	May follow distribution of somatic nerve	Diffuse
Character	Sharp and definite	Dull and vague (may be colicky, cramping, squeezing, etc.)
Relation to stimulus	Hurts where the stimulus is associated with external factors	May be "referred" to another area: associated with internal factors
Time relations	Often constant (sometimes periodic)	Often periodic and builds to peaks (sometimes constant)
Associated symptoms	Nausea usually only with deep somatic pain owing to bone involvement	Often nausea, vomiting, sickening feeling

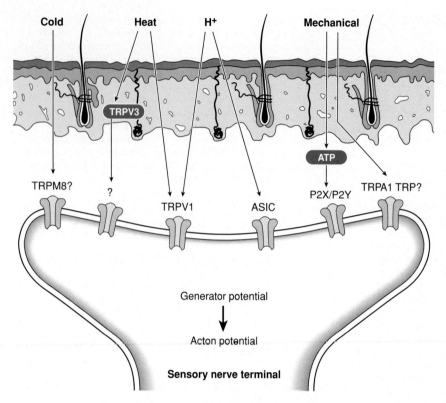

FIGURE 31-3. Peripheral transduction mechanisms. A major advance has resulted from molecular biology studies of nociceptive transduction mechanisms. Noxious mechanical stimuli release adenosine triphosphate, which may act on one or more purine receptors (P_2X and P_2Y). A second mechanism is still uncertain and may involve transient receptor potential (TRP)A_1 or other TRP receptors. Noxious chemical stimuli such as acidity (H^+) act via acid-sensing ion channels (ASICs) or $TRPV_1$ receptors. Noxious heat acts via $TRPV_1$ and $TRPV_2$ (originally called VRL-1) possibly via $TRPV_3$ receptors. Noxious cold acts via TRPM8 receptors (previously called CMR_1). VRL, vanilloid receptor–like; CMR, cold menthol receptor. Modified from Marchand F, Perretti M, McMahon SB. Role of the immune system in chronic pain. *Nat Rev Neurosci* 2005;6: 521–532, with permission.

transient receptor potential vanilloid (TRPV1) channel (33). The TRPV1 receptor responds to heat and lowering of pH and may help mediate the increased pain and hypersensitivity that occurs with inflammation (34) (Fig. 31-3).

Visceral Afferents

Most afferent nerve fibers arising from visceral structures are free nerve endings (35). However, some organs, such as the liver, brain, or lung, do not appear to have sensory innervation and therefore do not respond to traumatic stimuli. The detection of stimuli by visceral structures also appears to be different, and although many structures may be poor in detecting mechanical stimulation such as cutting, they do respond vigorously to other stimuli such as distension. As well as different response properties, visceral afferent pathways are also distinctive from those involved in the transmission of sensory information from somatic structures. Visceral pain is characteristically diffuse and poorly localized (Table 31-3). Like somatic pain, central sensitization may occur in response to an initial insult and result in pain that appears to be out of proportion to the underlying pathology. An example of this is irritable bowel syndrome, which is believed to have a central component leading to a heightened response to relatively minor stimuli. Central sensitization may also be an important component of pain associated with clearly identified pathology, such as ureteric calculi or urinary tract infections, and lead to an exaggeration of response to the underlying pathology.

Referral of visceral pain is also a commonly recognized clinical phenomenon. The mechanism of referral is still a matter of debate but one suggested mechanism is *convergence*. This term refers to the convergence of terminals from visceral and somatic nociceptors onto the same neurons that ascend from the spinal cord to the brain. This makes it difficult for the brain to

distinguish whether signals are arising from somatic or visceral structures (see below Fig. 31-21).

Peripheral Sensitization

Many forms of pain arise from direct activation of primary afferent neurons, especially C-fiber polymodal nociceptors (36). However, the process of nociceptor activation sets in train other processes that modify and enhance responses to further stimuli, a process collectively known as *peripheral sensitization*. For example, a relatively benign noxious stimulus such as a scratch to the skin initiates an inflammatory response in the periphery, which then changes the response properties to subsequent sensory stimuli (Fig. 31-4). After peripheral sensitization, low-intensity mechanical stimuli that would not normally cause pain are now perceived as painful. An increased responsiveness to thermal stimuli also occurs at the site of injury. This zone of primary hyperalgesia surrounding the site of injury is due to peripheral changes and is a feature commonly observed following surgery and other forms of trauma.

Part of the inflammatory response is the release of intracellular contents from damaged cells and inflammatory cells such as macrophages, lymphocytes, and mast cells. Nociceptive stimulation also causes a neurogenic inflammatory response, with the release of substance P, neurokinin A, and calcitonin gene-related peptide (CGRP) from the terminals of nociceptive afferent fibers in the periphery (37). Release of these peptides results in a changed excitability of sensory and sympathetic nerve fibers, vasodilatation, and extravasation of plasma proteins, as well as acting on inflammatory cells to release chemical mediators (38–40). These interactions induce release of a "soup" of inflammatory mediators such as potassium, serotonin, bradykinin, substance P, histamine, cytokines, nitric oxide (NO), and products from the cyclooxygenase and

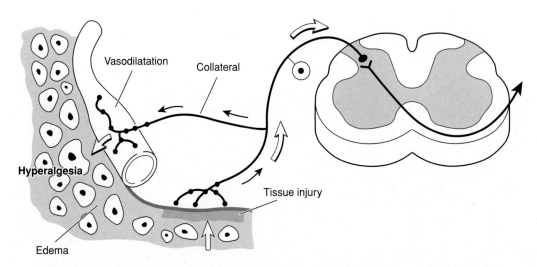

FIGURE 31-4. Effect of antidromic impulses in primary afferents. After tissue injury, antidromic impulses in collaterals of primary afferent fibers results in the release of chemical mediators from the peripheral terminals, which produce vasodilatation (flare), edema (wheal), and hyperalgesia (triple response of Lewis). Modified from Fields HL. *Pain.* New York, McGraw-Hill, 1987, with permission.

lipoxygenase pathways of arachidonic acid metabolism (Fig. 31-5) (39–41).

As well as release of this soup of chemicals, inflammation also results in other changes that may contribute to peripheral sensitization. Neurotrophins act as pain modulators and have an important role in regulating neural function as well as structure (42,43). Nerve growth factor (NGF) and brain-derived neurotrophic factor (BDNF) are two neurotrophins that have received considerable attention. Nerve growth factor acts on the tyrosine kinase A (trkA) receptor and is a peripheral pain mediator that is upregulated in inflammatory conditions. It has numerous actions, which include upregulation of neuropeptides such as CGRP and substance P, receptors such as TRPV1 and P2X3, and ion channels such as tetrodotoxin (TTX)-sensitive or -insensitive sodium channels (33). These actions may all contribute to sensitization of the primary afferent fibers. Modulation of peripheral sensitization may result from peripheral release of opioids from inflammatory cells (Fig. 31-6). Inflammation and peripheral sensitization may also lead to the recruitment of nociceptors that, under normal conditions, are silent. These "silent nociceptors" have been identified in a number of different tissues and species and once again bear testimony to the dynamic nature of sensory function. They are a class of unmyelinated primary afferent neurons that do not respond to excessive mechanical or thermal stimuli under normal circumstances (44). However, in the presence of inflammation and chemical sensitization, they become responsive, discharging vigorously even during ordinary movement and displaying alterations in receptive fields (45).

Peripheral Nerve Injury

Primary afferent nerves are not simply inert conductors of sensory information. Studies have demonstrated that section of, or damage to, a peripheral nerve results in a number of biochemical, physiologic, and morphologic changes that act as a focus of pain in themselves (Fig. 31-7) (30). The damaged end of the nerve fiber sprouts and may produce a spontaneously firing neuroma (Fig. 31-8). It may also demonstrate changed properties in response to various stimuli. These properties include sensitivity to mechanical stimuli, spontaneous firing, and sensitivity to norepinephrine (noradrenaline) (30). Similar changes

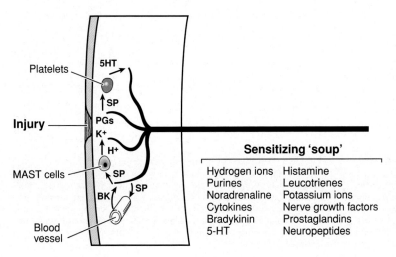

FIGURE 31-5. Peripheral sensitization following injury. Injury results in release of potassium (K^+) from damaged cells, as well as prostaglandins. K^+ strongly activates nociceptive free nerve endings ($A\delta$- and C-fibers). Prostaglandins sensitize nociceptors to activators such as K^+. Antidromic stimuli in collaterals (see Fig. 31-4) activate release of substance P (SP) (and calcitonin-gene-related peptide [CGRP]; not shown), which plays a pivotal role at three sites: SP (and CGRP) increase capillary permeability, thus allowing the peptide bradykinin to cross capillary walls and strongly activate nociceptors, in turn releasing more SP; SP acts on platelets to release 5-hydroxy tryptamine (5HT), which sensitizes nociceptors, again releasing more SP; SP acts also on mast cells to release histamine, sensitizing nociceptors. The foregoing three SP processes set up vicious circles of increasing sensitization. PGs, prostaglandins.

Sensitizing 'soup'

Hydrogen ions	Histamine
Purines	Leucotrienes
Noradrenaline	Potassium ions
Cytokines	Nerve growth factors
Bradykinin	Prostaglandins
5-HT	Neuropeptides

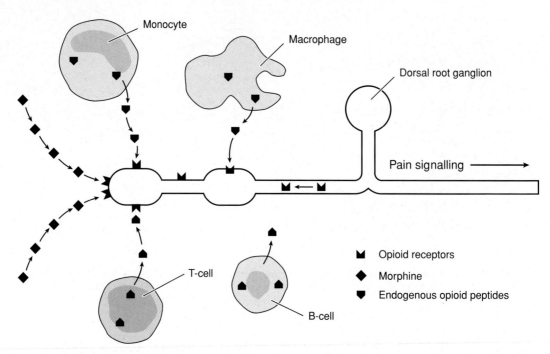

FIGURE 31-6. Peripheral inflammation results in production of opioid receptors by the dorsal root ganglion (*DRG*) and transport of opioid receptors toward the peripheral terminal. Peripheral opioid receptors are activated by exogenous application of morphine and endogenous opioid peptides released by monocytes (*M*), T-cells (*T*), B-cells (*B*), and macrophages (*MP*). Modified from Stein C. Morphine: A local "analgesic." *Pain: Clinical Updates* 1995;3:1, with permission.

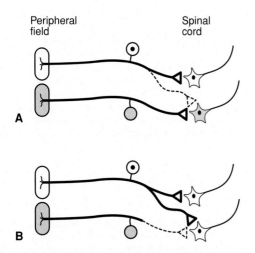

FIGURE 31-7. Neuroplasticity following damage to primary afferent fibers. **A:** Normal connectivity of primary afferent. Primary afferents innervate a defined peripheral region and activate a specific population of spinal cord neurons. In addition, the primary afferent has central connections that are normally ineffective (*dashed line*). In the normal situation, each spinal cord cell responds only to stimulation of its own peripheral field. **B:** When the central process of a primary afferent that innervates an adjacent peripheral field (*stipple*) is interrupted (*dotted line*), the formerly ineffective central connection of the intact primary afferent (*heavy line*) becomes effective. Both spinal cord cells now respond only to stimulation of the innervated peripheral field (*not stippled*). Modified from Fields HL. *Pain.* New York, McGraw-Hill, 1987, with permission.

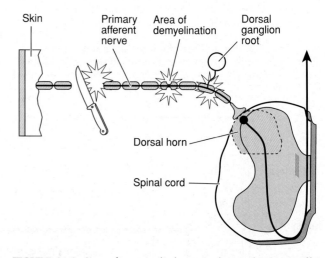

FIGURE 31-8. Sites of ectopic discharge in damaged primary afferent nociceptors. A transected nerve begins to regenerate, sending out sprouts that are mechanically sensitive, sensitive to α-adrenergic agonists, and spontaneously active. In addition, a secondary site of hyperactivity develops near the cell body in the dorsal root ganglion. Ectopic impulses may also arise from a short patch of demyelination on a primary afferent. From Fields HL. *Pain.* New York, McGraw-Hill, 1987, with permission.

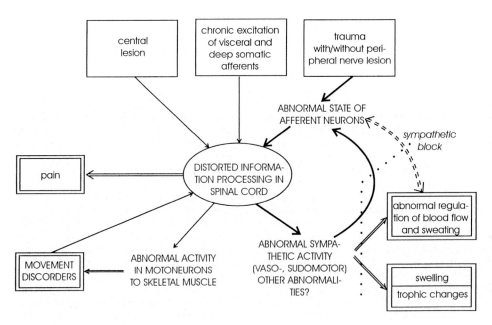

FIGURE 31-9. General hypothesis about the neural mechanisms of the generation of complex regional pain syndrome (CRPS) I and II following peripheral trauma, with and without nerve lesions, chronic stimulation of visceral afferents (e.g., myocardial infarction) and deep somatic afferents and, rarely, central trauma. The clinical observations are double-framed. Note the vicious circle (*arrows in bold black*). An important component of this circle is the excitatory influence of postganglionic sympathetic axons on primary afferent fibers in the periphery. From Jänig W. The puzzle of "reflex sympathetic dystrophy": Mechanisms, hypotheses, open questions. In: Jänig W, Stanton-Hicks M, eds. *Reflex Sympathetic Dystrophy: A Reappraisal.* Seattle, IASP Press, 1996, with permission.

occur within the cell body of the primary afferent nociceptor, the dorsal root ganglion (DRG) (46). Reduction in the blood supply to myelinated fibers ends in demyelination and the production of ectopic impulses.

A number of receptor changes may underlie this increased sensitivity and ectopic activity in primary afferent fibers. Peripheral nerve injury leads to the abnormal expression of receptors such as α_2-adrenergic receptors, calcium channels (47), and novel TTX-sensitive or -insensitive sodium channels (48–50). Novel sodium channel expression may be a source of abnormal ectopic discharges from neuromata and the DRG (51,52) of both injured and uninjured (53) primary afferents. Nerve damage also results in an increased production of neurotrophins such as NGF and BDNF. This upregulation of NGF and BDNF may contribute to the development of pain through both peripheral and central effects (42,43).

Sympathetic Nervous System

The sympathetic nervous system also has an important role in the generation and maintenance of chronic pain states (54,55). Nerve damage and even minor trauma can lead to a disturbance in sympathetic activity (Fig. 31-9), which then leads to a sustained condition now termed a *complex regional pain syndrome* (CRPS), replacing the previously used terms *reflex sympathetic dystrophy* and *causalgia* (1,56). Complex regional pain syndromes are associated with features of sympathetic dysfunction, including vasomotor and sudomotor changes, abnormalities of hair and nail growth, osteoporosis, sensory symptoms of spontaneous burning pain, hyperalgesia and allodynia, and, often, disturbance of motor function (54,56–58).

Basic studies have demonstrated that several changes involving the sympathetic nervous system may be responsible for development of these features (59–61). Inflammation can result in the sensitization of primary nociceptive afferent fibers by prostanoids that are released from sympathetic fibers (62) (Fig. 31-10). Following nerve injury, sympathetic nerve stimulation or administration of norepinephrine can excite primary afferent fibers via an action at α-adrenoceptors (63). There is also innervation of the DRG by sympathetic terminals (59). This means that activity in sympathetic efferent fibers can lead

to abnormal activity or responsiveness of the primary afferent fiber.

Complex regional pain syndromes may be sympathetically maintained or sympathetically independent. Pain problems that are sympathetically maintained may respond to sympathetic blockade by agents administered systemically, epidurally, regionally, or around the sympathetic ganglion (64) (see Chapter 39). Further information on the features, mechanisms, and treatment of CRPS can be found in Chapter 46.

Spinal Mechanisms

Termination Sites of Primary Afferents

The dorsal horn is the site of termination of primary afferents and there is a complex interaction among primary afferent fibers, local intrinsic spinal interneurons, and the endings

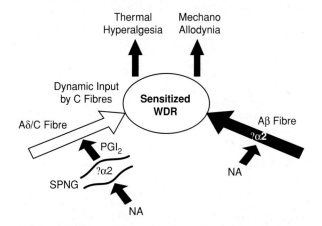

FIGURE 31-10. Inflammation and nerve injury leads to sensitization of wide dynamic range (WDR) neurons in the dorsal horn. This process involves sensitization of nociceptive primary afferents by release of prostanoids (PGI_2) from sympathetic fibers and activation of Aβ-fiber α_2-adrenoceptors by noradrenaline (NA). The effect of these interactions is a resultant thermal hyperalgesia and mechanical allodynia.

of descending fibers from the brain (65) (Chapter 32 and Figure 31-18). Primary afferent nociceptors terminate primarily in laminae I, II (substantia gelatinosa), and V (66), where they connect with several classes of second-order neurons in the dorsal horn of the spinal cord. Large fibers transmitting innocuous inputs primarily terminate in laminae III and IV. Some fibers ascend and descend several segments in the Lissauer tract before terminating on neurons that project to higher centers (see Chapter 32).

Two main classes of second-order dorsal horn neurons are associated with sensory processing. The first class of neurons is termed *nociceptive-specific* or *high-threshold*; the second class is termed *wide dynamic range* or *convergent*. The two classes have different response properties to afferent input and are located in different regions of the dorsal horn. Nociceptive-specific neurons are located within the superficial laminae (I, II) of the dorsal horn and respond selectively to noxious stimuli (67). Wide dynamic range neurons generally are located in deeper laminae (V) and respond to both noxious and non-noxious input (68). Wide dynamic range neurons normally do not signal pain in response to a tactile stimulus at a non-noxious level. However, if they become sensitized and hyperresponsive, they may discharge at a high rate following a tactile stimulus (see Chapter 32). If the activity of the wide dynamic range neuron exceeds a threshold level following this stimulus, then the non-noxious tactile stimulus will be perceived as painful and give rise to the phenomenon of allodynia (69).

Neurotransmitters

Pharmacologic studies have helped to identify the many neurotransmitters and neuromodulators involved in pain processes in the dorsal horn (70) (see Chapter 33). The main neurotransmitter is the excitatory amino acid glutamate. Primary afferent nociceptors are also sometimes divided according to their neurotransmitter content. One group is peptidergic neurons that contain peptides such substance P, neurokinin A, and CGRP. Substance P and neurokinin A act on neurokinin 1 and neurokinin 2 receptors respectively. The other group of nonpeptidergic neurons express the $P2X_3$ purinergic receptor. A number of other receptors are also involved in nociceptive transmission or modulation in the dorsal horn; they include opioid, α-adrenergic, cholinergic, γ-aminobutyric acid (GABAergic), glycinergic, serotonergic (5HT), and tyrosine kinase (trk) receptors (Figs. 31-11 and 31-12).

Excessive neuronal firing may induce prolonged glutamate release and activation of metabotropic glutamate (mgluR)and ionotropic *N*-methyl-*D*-aspartate (NMDA) receptors, with subsequent calcium influx into second-order neurons (71). The excitatory amino acids act at NMDA receptors, non-NMDA receptors (such as α-amino-3-hydroxy-5-methyl-4-isoxazolepropionic acid; AMPA), kainate, and metabotropic glutamate receptors (70,72) (Figs. 31-11 and 31-12).

N-Methyl-D-Aspartate Receptor

A longstanding interest has existed in the role of NMDA receptor in the development of central sensitization, and this receptor appears to be a major contributor to this process. The NMDA receptor channel, in its resting state, is blocked by a magnesium "plug." Priming of the NMDA receptor through the continued release of glutamate and coactivation of neurokinin receptors leads to removal of the magnesium plug and subsequent calcium influx into the cell (Figs. 31-12 and 31-13). Calcium influx, in concert with activation of other receptors on the cell membrane, precipitates activation or production of a number of intracellular messengers or signaling molecules, including phospholipases, polyphosphoinosites (IP_3, DAG), ERK, NO,

cyclic AMP response element-binding protein (CREB), and protein kinases (73–76) (Figs. 31-11 to 31-15). These intracellular messengers then act directly to change the excitability of the cell by feeding back and directly enhancing receptor activation or by feeding forward and inducing gene transcription within the cell nucleus (77). Gene transcription then results in receptor changes that lead to long-term changes in the responsiveness of the cell. All of these processes contribute to the development of central sensitization and some of the medium- and long-term alterations in cellular responsiveness that underlie chronic pain states (78,79) (Figs. 31-11 and 31-15).

The exact role of NO in nociceptive processing is still unclear, and it does not appear to be important in acute nociception (75,80,81). However, production of NO is implicated in the induction and maintenance of chronic pain states (75), and may be one of the factors responsible for the cell death demonstrated to occur under these conditions (Fig. 31-14). The production of arachidonic acid metabolites as part of the cascade that occurs following NMDA receptor activation also raises an interesting potential avenue for intervention that has been explored (82). Although the peripheral effects of nonsteroidal anti-inflammatory drugs (NSAIDs) have been emphasized in the past, it appears that there may be a role for the spinal administration of NSAIDs. Spinal NSAIDs either act directly on receptors, such as the strychnine-insensitive glycine site of the NMDA receptor complex, or influence the production of metabolites within the cell (Figs. 31-11 and 31-13).

Other Receptors

Although much research has focused on the NMDA receptor, as mentioned previously, a number of receptors are involved in nociceptive transmission, such as the metabotropic glutamate, neurokinin, tyrosine kinase (trk), AMPA, and kainate receptors (83,84). These receptors also contribute to the development of central sensitization either as a result of ion influx or activation of intracellular signaling cascades. Neurotrophins also contribute to central sensitization. Brain-derived neurotrophic factor production is upregulated in inflammatory conditions and is released from the central terminations of primary afferents in the dorsal horn, where it acts as a pain modulator. It acts on the tyrosine kinase B (trkB) receptor, which activates signaling cascades within dorsal horn neurons that contribute to the development of central sensitization (42) (Fig. 31-11A).

As well as directly increasing excitability, sensitization may also occur through a reduction in normal inhibitory processes. This may occur as a result of changes in the release of GABA or changes in receptor function. It has been suggested that prolonged stimulation, presumably through sustained and therefore excitotoxic release of glutamate, may result in the death of GABAergic inhibitory neurons and thereby lead to amplification of sensory inputs (85,86). In addition, alterations may occur in GABAergic function. For example, BDNF may act as a signaling molecule that allows communication between glia and neurons and contributes further to central sensitization by reversing the normal inhibitory function of GABA within the dorsal horn (87,88) (Fig. 31-11).

Glia

Glia (microglia and astrocytes) have traditionally been regarded as having a predominantly supportive role in neural signaling, and much of pain research has focused on the function and role of neurons in pain processing. However, abundant evidence now suggests the importance of glia in pain transmission and the development and maintenance of pathologic pain conditions (89,90). Glia are known to be activated by viruses and bacteria, but they also respond to substances released by

A Immediate central sensitization

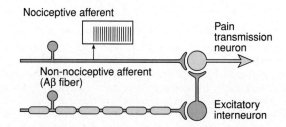

B Delayed central sensitization

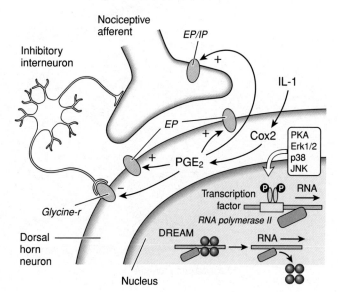

C Changes in synaptic connectivity

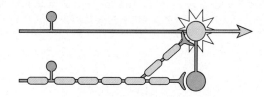

D Loss of inhibition

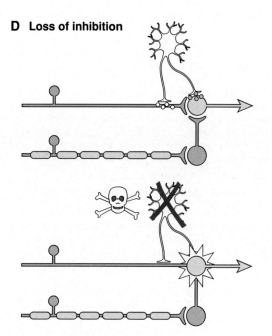

FIGURE 31-11. Non-nociceptor–mediated pain is generated by sensory inputs that would normally produce an innocuous sensation; this reflects a change in the functioning of central neurons. **A:** Activity-
dependent central sensitization. An immediate and relatively short-lasting increase in the excitability and
responsiveness of pain transmission dorsal horn neurons, which is due to phosphorylation of ion channels
and receptors and follows nociceptor-driven transmitter release and activation of intracellular kinases.
Eventually, the response to normally subthreshold inputs is increased. **B:** Transcription-dependent central sensitization. Enhanced gene expression due to the activation of transcription factors, as well as the
removal of repressors like downstream regulatory element antagonist modulator (DREAM), results in
long-lasting changes in the function of dorsal horn neurons. Cyclooxygenase inhibitor (COX2) induction
leads to prostaglandin (PGE₂) production, which acts pre- and postsynaptically to facilitate excitatory
and reduce inhibitory transmission. **C:** After peripheral nerve injury, the central terminals of myelinated
non-nociceptive Aβ-afferents sprout in the dorsal horn and form new connections with nociceptive neurons in laminae I and II. This rewiring of the circuitry of the spinal cord may contribute to persistent pain
hypersensitivity. **D:** Disinhibition. Normal sensory inflow is actively controlled by inhibitory interneurons. Reduced synthesis of the inhibitory neurotransmitters γ-aminobutyric acid (GABA) and glycine
or loss of these inhibitory interneurons after excessive release of the excitotoxic amino acid glutamate
following peripheral nerve injury increases the excitability of pain transmission neurons such that they
begin to respond to normally innocuous inputs. Modified from *Nature Neuroscience* 2002;5:1065, with
permission.

PART IV: PAIN MANAGEMENT

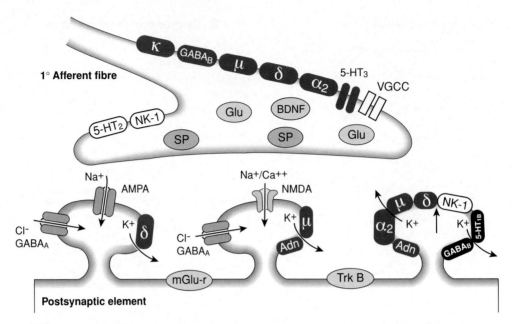

FIGURE 31-12. Possible arrangement of receptors on pre- and postsynaptic structures in the dorsal horn of the spinal cord. *5-HT*, scrotonin; α_2, α_2-adrenoceptor; *Adn*, adenosine; *AMPA*, α-amino-3-hydroxy-5-methyl-4-isoxazolepropionic acid; *GABA*, γ-aminobutyric acid; *Glu*, glutamate; *NMDA*, N-methyl-D-aspartate; *NK-1*, neurokinin 1; μ, δ, κ, opioid receptors; *SP*, substance P. BDNF, brain-derived neurotrophic factor; VGCC, voltage-gated calcium channel; mGlu-r, metabotrophic glutamate receptors; TrK B-tyrosine kinase B receptor.

primary afferent nerve fibers such as substance P, glutamate, and neurotrophins. Activated glia in turn release a variety of neuroactive chemicals such as cytokines, glutamate, NO, and ATP. These substances can then act to enhance release of chemicals from primary afferent terminals or sensitize pain transmission neurons within the dorsal horn (see Chapter 32).

Central Sensitization

As described earlier, it is known that changes occurring in the periphery following trauma lead to an enhanced responsiveness of dorsal horn neurons to further stimuli and a zone of primary hyperalgesia at the site of injury. However, this enhanced responsiveness can only partly be explained by the changes in the

periphery. Following injury, there is an increased responsiveness to normally innocuous mechanical stimuli (allodynia) in a zone of secondary hyperalgesia in uninjured tissue surrounding the site of injury. In contrast to the zone of primary hyperalgesia, no change occurs in the threshold to thermal stimuli. These behavioral changes are believed to be a result of the dorsal horn processes (described earlier) that contribute to the development of central sensitization (Fig. 31-16) (91). Thus, central sensitization refers to the increased responsiveness of neurons in the spinal cord that occurs following strong and sustained inputs from the periphery.

These changes are important in the consideration of clinical pain. A barrage of nociceptive inputs, such as occurs with surgery, results in changes to the response properties of dorsal

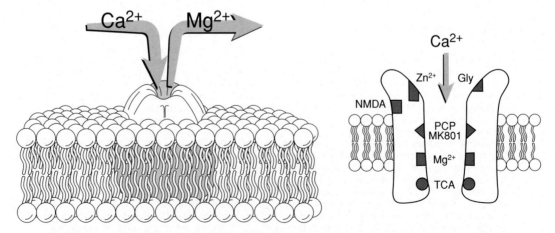

FIGURE 31-13. Representation of the *N*-methyl-*D*-aspartate (NMDA) receptor complex. Removal of the magnesium plug leads to calcium influx. The NMDA receptor complex contains a number of sites, activation of which results in modulation of receptor activity. These sites include: glycine (*GLY*), dizocilpine (*MK-801*), phencyclidine (*PCP*), magnesium (Mg^{2+}), tricyclic antidepressant (*TCA*), and zinc (Zn^{2+}).

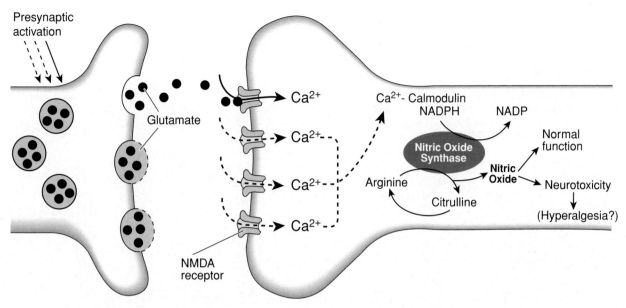

FIGURE 31-14. Diagram illustrating postsynaptic events following release of glutamate from central terminals of primary afferents in the spinal cord. Following priming of the *N*-methyl-*D*-aspartate (NMDA) receptor complex, subsequent glutamate release results in NMDA receptor activation with subsequent calcium influx. Intracellular calcium then acts on a calmodulin-sensitive site to activate the enzyme nitric oxide synthase (NOS). In the presence of a cofactor nicotinamide adenine dinucleotide phosphate (NADPH), NOS uses arginine as a substrate to produce nitric oxide and citrulline. Nitric oxide has a role in normal cellular function, but increased production may be involved in hyperalgesia and may lead to neurotoxicity.

horn neurons (92). It has been demonstrated that a painful stimulus at a level sufficient to activate C-fibers not only activates dorsal horn neurons, but neuronal activity also progressively increases throughout the duration of the stimulus, a phenomenon termed *wind-up* (93). Therefore, with continued nociceptive inputs, a simple stimulus–response relationship does not exist, but rather a gradual increase in spinal cord neuronal activity (see Chapter 32). Wind-up is dependent on activation of the NMDA receptor (71,94) and therefore has

the potential to be modified by agents acting at this site. Thus, wind-up may make these neurons more sensitive to other input and is a component of central sensitization (Figs. 31-16 and 31-17).

Although wind-up is very likely an important underlying mechanism contributing to persistent pain, other processes must be considered as contributors to central sensitization. Long-term potentiation (LTP) refers to the strengthening of the efficacy of synaptic transmission that occurs following

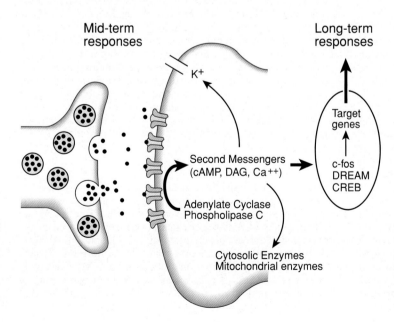

FIGURE 31-15. Neurotransmitter release from the central terminal of peripheral afferents results in activation of receptor sites on the postsynaptic membrane. Activation of phospholipase C and adenylate cyclase leads to the production of the second messengers cyclic adenosine monophosphate (cAMP) and diacylglycerol (DAG). Mobilization of these second messengers may result in a decrease in potassium (K^+) efflux and elevation of intracellular calcium. The increase in intracellular calcium results in the induction of the protooncogene c-fos, production of Fos protein, and a presumed action on target genes to alter long-term responses of the cell to further stimuli. DREAM, downstream regulatory element antagonist modulator; CREB, cyclic adenosine monophosphate (cAMP) response element-binding protein.

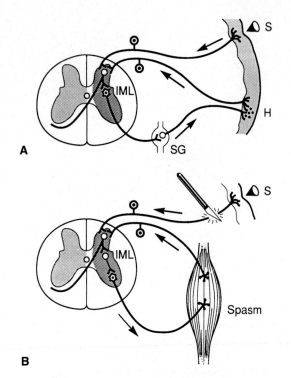

FIGURE 31-16. Depiction of increased spinal neuron activity (hyperactivity) in response to various stimuli. **A:** Nociceptive stimulus delivered at the skin surface (*S*) activates a primary afferent nociceptor that, in turn, activates the sympathetic preganglionic neuron in the intermediolateral column (*IML*). The preganglionic neuron activates the noradrenergic postganglionic neuron in the sympathetic ganglion (*SG*), which sensitizes, and can activate, primary afferent nociceptors (*H*) that feed back to the spinal cord, maintaining the pain. Peripheral injury is associated with an increase in spinal neuron activity, so that there is an enhanced responsiveness to subsequent input. **B:** Section of a peripheral nerve (e.g., following trauma) results in pronounced and long-lasting increases in spinal cord activity. Tissue injury also produces increased activity of spinal neurons, causing activation of ventral horn neurons and muscle spasm. Prolonged muscle spasm activates muscle nociceptors that feed back to the spinal cord to sustain the spasm. From Fields HL. *Pain*. New York, McGraw-Hill, 1987, with permission.

activity across that synapse and is a phenomenon that has long been associated with the hippocampus and memory processes (95). Evidence now suggests that an LTP-like phenomenon may also occur within the dorsal horn (96). In contrast to wind-up, which quickly expires following cessation of the stimulus, LTP may be maintained for hours and possible weeks to months following initiation (96,97). Although some have suggested that LTP only occurs under nonphysiologic conditions and therefore has little clinical relevance, the recent demonstration of a pain amplifier within the spinal cord that is switched on by asynchronous, irregular low-frequency inputs in C-fibers supports the clinical relevance of these findings (98). These changes that occur at a cellular level contribute to the development of behavioral alterations that appear to indicate the presence of central sensitization (38). First, there occurs an expansion in receptive field size (99,100), so that a spinal neuron will respond to stimuli that would normally be outside the region that responds to nociceptive stimuli. Second, there occurs an increase in the magnitude and duration of the response to stimuli that are above threshold in strength (101). Last, there occurs a reduction in threshold, so that stimuli that are not normally noxious activate neurons that normally transmit nociceptive

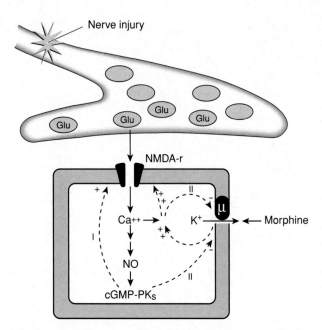

FIGURE 31-17. Nerve injury leads to release of glutamate (*Glu*) from the central terminals of primary nociceptive afferents. Glutamate activates the *N*-methyl-*D*-aspartate (*NMDA*) receptor, which leads to calcium influx and increased production of nitric oxide (*NO*). An increase in NO leads to activation of cyclic guanosine monophosphate (*cGMP*) and various protein kinases (*PK$_s$*). These substances then act as a feedback mechanism at the NMDA receptor (positive feedback) and μ-opioid receptor (negative feedback). This means that subsequent administration of morphine results in a "vicious circle," with further positive feedback at the NMDA receptor.

information. These changes may be important both in acute pain states such as postoperative pain and in the development of chronic pain.

Thus, strong evidence suggests that nociceptive and neuropathic inputs result in an increased responsiveness of central neurons. With increased inputs, as occurs with inflammatory conditions such as osteoarthritis or neuropathic pain associated with a neuroma, central sensitization may be maintained for long periods. However, removal of inputs by neural blockade or approaches that address the underlying pathology, such as joint replacement, in most cases will lead to resolution of pain. There is little evidence that central neurons continue to independently generate nociceptive signals and maintain pain once peripheral inputs are abolished. The notable exception to this rule is neuropathic pain, in which loss of sensory inputs, such as occurs with amputation or spinal cord injury, appears to result in changes within the central nervous system that maintain pain despite the apparent loss of peripheral afferent input.

Nerve Injury

The precise mechanisms that induce pain following nerve injury are uncertain and are undoubtedly complex, with several mechanisms operating even within the same individual (28,102). As well as the peripheral changes described in the previous section of this chapter (Fig. 31-11), peripheral nerve injury can also result in a number of dorsal horn effects such as changes in the distribution and density of AMPA receptors (103,104), release of neurotrophins (105), and sprouting of central terminals (106,107). Disinhibition, either as a result of selective loss of inhibitory GABAergic neurons (85,86,108) or

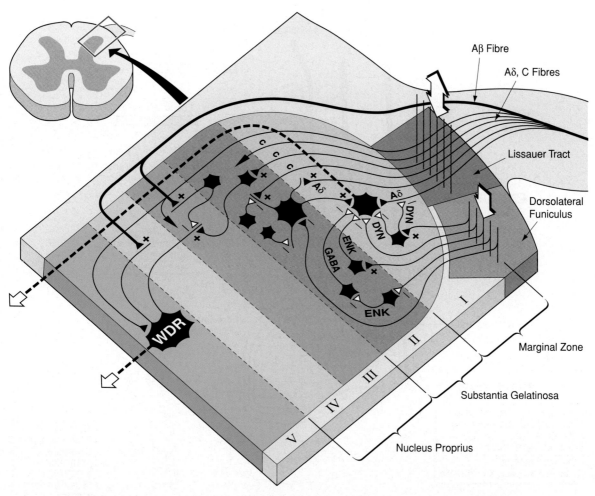

FIGURE 31-18. Diagrammatic representation of primary afferent nociceptor inputs and connections within the dorsal horn of the spinal cord. Large- and small-diameter primary afferent neurons have their cell bodies in the dorsal root ganglia. On entry to the dorsal horn, large-diameter afferent fibers (*thick solid line*) travel medially, and small-diameter afferent fibers (*thin solid lines marked Aδ and C*) travel in the lateral portion of the entry zone. The spinal terminals of the small fibers enter the cord and have collateral branches, which may ascend and descend the spinal cord for several segments, in the Lissauer tract, before synapsing in the dorsal horn. Aβ-fiber afferents terminate in lamina I (marginal zone) and C-fiber afferents terminate in lamina II (substantia gelatinosa). Local interneurons may produce synaptic inhibition of small-diameter afferents and postsynaptic inhibition of projection neurons. Interneurons may have an excitatory action. Modulation also occurs as a result of descending influences arising from fibers in the dorsolateral funiculus. These descending fibers make contact with either projection neurons or interneurons. Neurotransmitters released from interneurons include γ-aminobutyric acid (*GABA*), enkephalin (*ENK*), and dynorphin (*DYN*) in the presence of nerve injury sprouting occurs of axons in laminae III and IV to synapse with neuron cell bodies in laminae I and II.

changes in GABAergic function (87,109,110), may also result in increased responsiveness of central neurons (Fig. 31-11).

Supraspinal Mechanisms

Spinal Pathways

Second-order projection neurons in the dorsal horn, as well as some in the ventral horn and central canal region, project to supraspinal structures through several tracts (see Chapter 32) (111). These include the spinothalamic, spinoreticular, and spinomesencephalic tracts, which ascend the spinal cord in the contralateral anterolateral quadrant (Fig. 31-19). The spinothalamic tract is traditionally regarded as the main pathway involved in nociceptive transmission and contains axons

that have cell bodies in lamina I, II, and V, the regions of the dorsal horn that receive nociceptive inputs. Another pathway ascends from laminae I and V through the dorsolateral funiculus and relays in the parabrachial area of the pons before terminating in the amygdala. This spino-parabrachial-amygdala system may be important in fear and anxiety responses to pain as well as autonomic responses such as vocalization, flight, and cardiorespiratory responses. Although the anterolateral quadrant is viewed as the classical spinal pain pathway, a dorsal column pathway is involved in transmission of nociceptive information (112) (see Chapter 32).

Supraspinal Structures

These ascending tracts terminate in many supraspinal structures throughout the brainstem, thalamus, and cortex

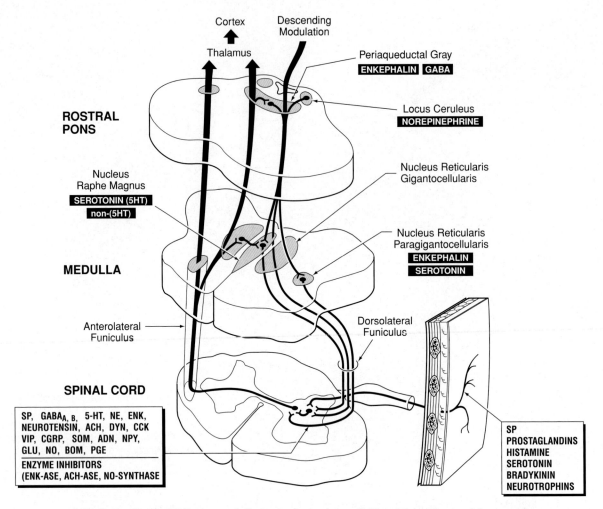

FIGURE 31-19. Simplified schema of afferent sensory pathways (*left*) and descending modulatory pathways (*right*). Stimulation of nociceptors in the skin surface leads to impulse generation in the primary afferent. Concomitant with this impulse generation, increased levels of various endogenous algesic agents (substance P, prostaglandins, histamine, serotonin, bradykinin) are detected near the area of stimulation in the periphery. Primary afferent nociceptors relay to projection neurons in the dorsal horn, which ascend in the anterolateral funiculus to terminate in the thalamus. En route, collaterals of the projection neurons activate multiple higher centers, including the nucleus reticularis gigantocellularis (*NRG*). Neurons from the NRG project to the thalamus and also activate the nucleus raphe magnus (*NRM*) and periaqueductal gray (*PAG*) of the midbrain. Descending fibers from the PAG project to the NRM and reticular formation adjacent to the NRM. These neurons activate descending inhibitory neurons that are located in these regions and travel via the dorsolateral funiculus to terminate in the dorsal horn of the spinal cord. Descending projections also arise from a number of brainstem sites including the locus ceruleus (*LC*). A number of neurotransmitters are released by afferent fibers, descending terminations, or local interneurons in the dorsal horn and modulate peripheral nociceptive input. These include substance P (*SP*), γ-aminobutyric acid (*GABA*), serotonin (*5-HT*), norepinephrine (*NE*), enkephalin (*ENK*), neurotensin, acetylcholine (*ACH*), dynorphin (*DYN*), cholecystokinin (*CCK*), vasoactive intestinal peptide (*VIP*), calcitonin-gene-related peptide (*CGRP*), somatostatin (*SOM*), adenosine (*ADN*), neuropeptide Y (*NPY*), glutamate (*GLU*), nitric oxide (*NO*), bombesin (*BOM*), and prostaglandins (*PGE*). Inhibitors of enzymes such as enkephalinase (*ENK-ASE*), acetylcholinesterase (*ACH-ASE*), and nitric oxide synthase (*NO-SYNTHASE*) may act to modify the action of these neurotransmitters.

(Figs. 31-19 and 31-20; see also Chapter 32). Pain activates regions involved in blood pressure regulation, respiration, vasomotor control, and metabolic homeostasis. Therefore, continuing nociceptive inputs may have deleterious effects on any of these systems (113).

The thalamus is an important relay for the transmission of nociceptive signals. Animal studies indicate that a large spinothalamic projection exists, with terminations within the ventral posterior thalamic nucleus, and that neurons within this region respond preferentially to noxious stimuli (114). The thalamus has traditionally been viewed as a structure organized according to the nature of afferent input with two main divisions: lateral and medial. The lateral region is located within the ventrocaudal or ventroposterior nuclei of the thalamus and is associated with sensory/discriminative processes, such as localization and characterization of the stimulus. The second region is located in the medial nuclei of the thalamus and involved in the affective/motivational processes, which include our emotional responses to nociceptive input (115). A report by Craig and colleagues (116) claims to identify a nucleus within the thalamus that is specific for pain and temperature sensation (for further discussion see Wall [117]). However, it is interesting that stimulation of the ventrocaudal nucleus (analogous to the ventral posterior nucleus in animals and supposedly part of the "pain" pathway) in awake humans rarely results in pain, except in those who have central deafferentation pain (118).

The effect of cortical stimulation and lesions on pain perception is confusing and intriguing but has shed some light on the role of different brain regions in pain perception. It has been known for many years that patients who have had a complete hemispherectomy can have almost normal pain sensation (119). In the awake human, stimulation of primary somatosensory cortex typically evokes nonpainful sensations, with stimulation rarely resulting in pain (115). Neurosurgical lesions of cortical regions produce varying effects, depending on the region ablated (120). Lesions of the frontal lobe and cingulate cortex result in a condition in which pain perception remains. However, the suffering component of pain appears to be reduced. The person reports pain only when queried and spontaneous requests for analgesia are reduced. Functional imaging has added to earlier observations from brain lesioning and stimulation and identified a widely distributed network of cortical and subcortical structures in the brain that are activated by noxious inputs (121–123). Acute painful stimuli fairly consistently result in activation of several key areas, including primary and secondary somatosensory cortices (S1 and S2), anterior cingulate cortex (ACC), and insular cortex (IC) (124–127). Persistent pain, however, is associated with a change in pattern of brain activation that differs from acute pain responses. For example, the prefrontal cortex is activated in many chronic pain studies and, whereas an acute experimental painful stimulus results in an *increase* of activity in the thalamus, (126) people with persistent pain due to cancer (128), fibromyalgia (SPECT) (129), and chronic neuropathic pain (130) demonstrate a *decrease* in activity in the thalamus. Reorganization can also occur with shifts in cortical representation of body structures demonstrated to be associated with persistent pain (7,131). This cortical reorganization may possibly be prevented with the provision of more "normal" afferent inputs following deafferentation (132).

Functional imaging has also contributed to our understanding of the involvement of affective and cognitive factors in our experience of pain. Although it is by no means clear, functional imaging studies (as well as evidence from older reports following brain lesions and stimulation) suggest that those brain regions activated in response to nociceptive inputs have different roles in the perception of pain (133). For example, the somatosensory cortex appears to be primarily involved in the sensory/discriminative aspects of pain such as detecting the locality, intensity, and duration of the stimulus. In contrast, the anterior cingulate cortex may have little discriminative ability but may be part of the affective response to pain and therefore involved in the affective/motivational component of pain. It has also been demonstrated that cognitive influences, such as anticipation (134) and hypnosis (135), modulate activation of brain regions and alter brain responses to nociceptive inputs (136–138).

Modulatory Mechanisms

Descending Inhibition

The observation that cognitions are associated with modulation of activity within specific brain regions that appear to be involved in the experience of pain has given further clarity to our understanding of pain modulatory processes. It has also provided an insight into the physiologic processes involved in the psychological contribution to pain.

Since the beginning of the last century, it was known that powerful descending influences could modulate spinal activity, before the concept was popularized by Melzack and Wall's gate theory (139). It was many years later before it was demonstrated that physical and environmental factors, including stress, could affect the perception of pain, presumably through activation of these descending pathways (140). Subsequent experiments using a variety of approaches identified descending pathways arising from a number of brainstem structures, including periaqueductal gray matter (PAG), locus coeruleus, nucleus raphe magnus, and nucleus paragigantocellularis lateralis (141–143) (Fig. 31-19). The frontal lobes and amygdala also exert a descending influence through projections to the hypothalamus and PAG (144,145) (Fig. 31-20).

Descending inhibition involves the action of a number of endogenous neurotransmitters or neuromodulators, such as opioid peptides, serotonin, norepinephrine (noradrenaline), cannabinoids, GABA, and glycine (146–149). Many of the traditional strategies available in pain management, such as the use of opioids, antidepressants, and anticonvulsants, act at least partially via these inhibitory mechanisms. Elucidation of inhibitory mechanisms has also provided a clearer rationale for techniques already in use and used empirically. These include the use of techniques such as deep brain stimulation, transcutaneous electrical nerve stimulation, acupuncture, and spinal cord stimulation.

Endogenous Opioids

Endogenous opioids include β-endorphin, dynorphins (A and B), enkephalins (met and leu), endomorphins (1 and 2), and nociceptin. These opioids act on a variety of opioid receptors including the μ-, δ-, κ-, and opioid receptor-like receptor (ORL-1) with differing affinities for each receptor (Table 31-4).

Although found both pre- and postsynaptically in the dorsal horn, the majority of opioid receptors (about 75%) are located presynaptically (150). Activation of presynaptic opioid receptors results in a reduction in the release of neurotransmitters from the nociceptive primary afferent (151). However, the changes that occur with inflammation and neuropathy can produce significant changes in opioid sensitivity that involves a number of mechanisms. These include: an interference with opioid analgesia by cholecystokinin (CCK) (152), loss of presynaptic opioid receptors (150), and the formation of the morphine metabolite, morphine-3-glucuronide, which may antagonize the analgesic action normally produced by opioid receptor activation (153).

It has also been demonstrated that the NMDA receptor is involved in the development of tolerance to opioids (154) (Fig. 31-17). Animal studies indicate that administration of an NMDA antagonist reduces the development of tolerance to morphine (155) and prevents the withdrawal syndrome in morphine-tolerant rats (156). Therefore, agents that act as NMDA antagonists, such as dextromethorphan, have the potential to interfere with the development of pain states,

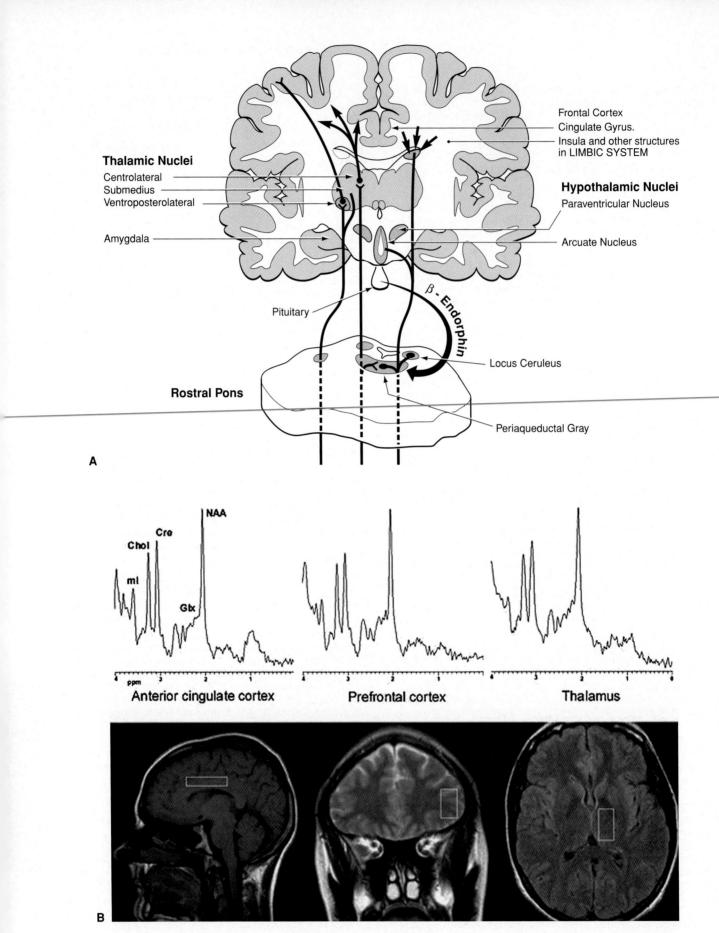

FIGURE 31-20. (See legend next page.)

potentiate the action of opioids (157), and prevent the development of opioid tolerance.

α-Adrenoceptors

Activation of α_2-adrenoceptors in the spinal cord has an analgesic effect either by endogenous release of norepinephrine through descending pathways from the brainstem or by exogenous spinal administration of agents such as clonidine (Fig. 31-12) (158). Furthermore, α-adrenoceptor agonists appear to have a synergistic effect with opioid agonists (159,160). A number of α-adrenoceptor subtypes exist, and the development of selective α-adrenoceptor subtype agonists has the potential to provide effective new analgesic agents with reduced side effects.

γ-Aminobutyric Acid and Glycine

Both GABA and glycine are involved in tonic inhibition of nociceptive input, and loss of their inhibitory action can result in features of neuropathic pain such as allodynia (161). Although $GABA_A$ and $GABA_B$ receptors have been implicated at both pre- and postsynaptic sites, it has been demonstrated that $GABA_A$ receptor–mediated inhibition occurs through largely postsynaptic mechanisms (Fig. 31-12) (162). In contrast, $GABA_B$ mechanisms may be preferentially involved in presynaptic inhibition through suppression of excitatory amino acid release from primary afferent terminals. This finding may help to understand the disparity between laboratory findings that demonstrate that $GABA_B$ receptor agonists such as baclofen have an antinociceptive action (163) and clinical experience, which has found that intrathecal baclofen is of limited use in the management of chronic pain (164). On the other hand, concerns have been expressed about toxicity with long-term administration (165); intrathecal administration of $GABA_A$ agonists may be effective in the management of acute and chronic pain conditions (166).

Modulation at a Spinal Level

Transmission of nociceptive information is subject to modulation at several levels of the neuraxis, including the dorsal horn (see Chapter 32). Afferent impulses arriving in the dorsal horn initiate inhibitory mechanisms that limit the effect of subsequent impulses. Inhibition occurs through the effect of local inhibitory interneurons and descending pathways from the brain. In the dorsal horn, incoming nociceptive messages are modulated by endogenous and exogenous agents that act on opioid

TABLE 31-4

ENDOGENOUS OPIOIDS AND RECEPTORS FOR WHICH THEY HAVE THE HIGHEST AFFINITY

Endogenous opioid	Receptor
β-Endorphin	δ/μ
Dynorphins	κ
Enkephalins	μ/δ
Nociceptin	ORL-1

(167), α-adreno, GABAergic, glycinergic, and cannabinoid receptors located at pre- and postsynaptic sites (Fig. 31-19).

Modulation at a Peripheral Level

Opioids traditionally have been viewed as centrally acting drugs. However, evidence now suggests that endogenous opioids act on peripheral sites following tissue damage (168,169). Opioid receptors are manufactured in the cell body (DRG) and transported toward the central terminal in the dorsal horn and toward the periphery (Fig. 31-6). The peripheral receptors become active following local tissue damage. This occurs with unmasking of opioid receptors and arrival of immunocompetent cells that can synthesize opioid peptides. It is this ability that stimulated interest in peripheral administration of opioids, such as intra-articular administration following knee surgery or arthroscopy (170,171), or topical administration of morphine (172). Despite initial enthusiasm for this technique, some have expressed doubt about the usefulness and cost–benefit of intra-articular morphine, particularly following arthroscopy or minor knee surgery (173).

ASSESSMENT OF PAIN

Identifying Pain Contributors

Pain can be broadly divided into two main types on the basis of the structures affected. Most pain seen clinically falls under the term *nociceptive*. Nociceptive pain is defined as pain due to activation of primary nociceptive nerve endings by nociceptive stimuli. This includes pain arising from pathology in somatic and visceral structures such as fractures, appendicitis,

FIGURE 31-20. A: Rostral projections of nociceptive processing. Ascending projections (*left*) travelling in the anterolateral funiculus, as well as projections from the medulla, pons, and midbrain, terminate in the thalamic nuclear complex. The ventroposterolateral (*VPL*), centrolateral, and submedian nuclei receive nociceptive information. The VPL projects to the somatosensory cortex. The centromedian nucleus projects more diffusely, including projections to regions of the limbic system. The descending fibers (*right*) inhibit the transmission of nociceptive information between primary afferents and projection neurons in the dorsal horn. The periaqueductal gray (*PAG*) receives projections from a number of brain regions including the amygdala, frontal and insular cortex, and the hypothalamus. In addition to direct neural connections, endorphins synthesized in the pituitary are released into the cerebrospinal fluid and blood, where they can exert an inhibitory effect at multiple centers including the PAG. **B:** *Top row:* Typical single-voxel magnetic resonance (MR) spectra collected from anterior cingulate cortex, prefrontal cortex, and thalamus of a patient with low back pain using the STEAM prescription (TE 25-msec, TR 1500 msec, 256 acquisitions). *Bottom row:* Box indicates the placement of each single-voxel measurement on the MR image. Using the anterior cingulate cortex, patients with persistent low back pain could be discriminated from controls with a sensitivity specificity and accuracy of 100%. Reproduced from Siddall et al. *Anesth Analg*, 2006;102:1164–1168 with permission.

and renal calculi. In practice, nociceptive pain is almost invariably accompanied by inflammation. Therefore, this type of pain is also often referred to as *inflammatory pain.*

The other broad category of pain falls under the term *neuropathic* and refers to pain arising from pathology in neural structures. Neuropathic pain has been defined as pain initiated or caused by a primary lesion or dysfunction of the nervous system (1). However, the looseness of the term "dysfunction" has led to some confusion, and it has been argued that this word should be removed from the definition (174). There is now increasing consensus that the term neuropathic pain should be confined to those conditions in which pain is initiated or caused by a primary lesion (due to disease or injury) of the nervous system.

The distinction between nociceptive and neuropathic pain is made because the underlying mechanisms giving rise to pain appear to be different, giving rise to different pain characteristics and responses to treatment. Therefore, despite emerging evidence that considerable overlap exists between nociceptive and neuropathic mechanisms, it is still a useful clinical distinction. Although not diagnostic, neuropathic pain is suggested by descriptors such as burning, electric, and shock-like, with pain present in a region of sensory disturbance. Pain often occurs in the absence of stimulation, and minor stimulation, such as light touch, can lead to exaggerated pain (allodynia).

In addition to dividing pain into two types, depending on the structures giving rise to pain, the contribution of psychological factors must always be considered (Chapter 35). Although it is comparatively rare for people to present with pain arising from psychological causes, psychological factors are invariably involved in the pain experience and are a large determinant of the intensity and quality of the pain experience, as well as the behaviors that arise as a result of nociceptive and neuropathic stimuli. Therefore, the clinician involved in the management of pain needs to be familiar with not only the physical changes that may give rise to the generation of signals in pain pathways but also the emotional, cognitive, and environmental influences that may modify the transmission and processing of these signals and thereby impact on the perception and expression of pain (see also Chapter 37).

Acute and Chronic Pain

Acute Pain

Important differences exist between most types of acute and chronic pain. In *acute pain*, the nervous system usually is intact and the pain is caused by trauma, surgery, acute medical conditions, or a physiologic process such as labor. Facial grimaces and signs of increased autonomic activity and other potentially harmful effects may be evident. For example, hypertension, tachycardia, vasoconstriction, sweating, increased rate and decreased depth of respiration, skeletal muscle spasm, increased gastrointestinal secretions, decreased intestinal motility, increased sphincter tone, urinary retention, venous stasis, potential for thrombosis and possible pulmonary embolism, anxiety, confusion, and delirium all may accompany acute pain. Also, the pain usually ceases when the wound heals or the medical condition improves. Patients are usually aware that the pain will improve as they recover, and that an end to pain is in sight. This may not be so if patients are ill-prepared and poorly informed.

Some severe and prolonged acute pain may become progressively more like chronic pain. Some patients with chronic pain may have superimposed acute pain (e.g., when they require further surgery or develop a bone fracture owing to metastatic cancer) (175). Such patients may not have an intact nervous system and may have marked preexisting psychological problems, opioid tolerance, and other conditions.

Extensive somatic and sympathetic blockade may be required to relieve acute pain associated with some types of major surgery. For example, the following may be involved in pain after thoracoabdominal esophagogastrectomy with cervical anastomosis: C3–C4 and T2–T12 sensory nerves (somatic structures in neck, thorax, and abdomen); cervicothoracic sympathetic chain and celiac plexus (intrathoracic and abdominal viscera); and C3–C4 phrenic nerve sensory afferents (pain from incision in central diaphragm referred to shoulder tip).

Segmental and suprasegmental reflex responses to acute pain result in muscle spasm, immobility, vasospasm, and other adverse effects (see Chapters 6 and 43). This may intensify the pain by way of various vicious cycles (Fig. 31-16), which include increased sensitivity of peripheral nociceptors (see Chapter 32). Acute pain that is unrelieved causes anxiety and sleeplessness, which in turn increase pain; anxiety and feelings of helplessness, both before and after surgery, elevate pain levels. Prevention and relief are valuable adjuncts to other treatments.

After major surgery, severe trauma, or painful medical conditions (e.g., pancreatitis), acute pain can persist for more than 10 days (176). In such situations, the pain and its sequelae become similar to chronic pain. It is not uncommon for such patients to show anger, depression, and other characteristics of chronic pain (176,177). Thus, one should be wary of drawing too sharp a distinction between acute and chronic pain. As acute pain persists, more emphasis may need to be placed on psychological approaches, as well as the traditional physical and pharmacologic approaches to treatment.

Chronic Pain

It has been agreed arbitrarily that chronic pain is pain that persists beyond 3 months (1). However, severe acute pain can become essentially chronic after only about 10 to 14 days. Chronic pain progressively leads to limitation of physical, mental, and social activities, with accompanying anger, depression, and family and socioeconomic disruption. It seems that sympathoadrenal responses habituate, or become exhausted, in chronic pain and then vegetative responses emerge: sleep disturbance, irritability, loss of appetite for food and sex, decreased motor activity, and mental depression (see Chapters 35 and 37). The facial expression of patients with chronic pain may be subdued, sad, or even sleepy, owing to excessive medication. This may give the impression that pain cannot be present. Patients with chronic pain often are exhausted from lack of sleep and from extreme demands on their mental and physical resources. Severe psychoneurosis and other psychological disturbances may result from severe unrelieved chronic pain. These may be rapidly and completely reversed on relief of the pain. Treatment must address these components of chronic pain syndromes (see Chapters 35 and 37).

Cancer Pain

Cancer pain is often regarded as a separate type of pain although, in practice, people with cancer may present with acute or chronic pain, and the factors contributing to cancer pain, (i.e., nociceptive, neuropathic, and psychological) are common to any type of pain. However, cancer pain has a number of characteristics that make it helpful to consider it as a separate category, so that these issues can be addressed satisfactorily. For example, in many situations, people with cancer have an expected lifespan of weeks or months. This will impact choice

TABLE 31-5

TYPES OF PAIN IN PATIENTS WITH CANCER

I. Patients with acute cancer-related pain
  a. Associated with the diagnosis of cancer
  b. Associated with cancer therapy (surgery, chemotherapy, or radiation)
II. Patients with chronic cancer-related pain
  a. Associated with cancer progression
  b. Associated with cancer therapy (surgery, chemotherapy, or radiation)
III. Patients with pre-existing chronic pain and cancer-related pain
IV. Patients with a history of drug addiction and cancer-related pain
  a. Actively involved in illicit drug use
  b. In methadone maintenance programs
  c. With a history of drug abuse
V. Dying patients with cancer-related pain

Incidence of different types of pain is approximately as follows: Directly caused by cancer (78%); caused by treatment (19%); indirectly related or unrelated to cancer (3%). However, many patients have multiple pains (e.g., a high percentage, (30% to 40%) of patients have myofascial syndromes) *in addition* to cancer-related pain. (Data from Foley KM: The treatment of cancer pain. *N Engl J Med* 1985;84:313.)

of treatment, and approaches that may not be considered advisable in those with persistent noncancer pain, such as high-dose opioids, parenteral administration of analgesics or analgesic adjuvants, and neurolytic or surgical procedures, may be considered appropriate for the person with cancer.

Treatment of cancer pain has been helped by clear descriptions of major categories of pain problems that occur commonly in cancer patients, and etiologic factors in cancer pain (175,178,179) (Tables 31-5 to 31-9). Clearly, neural blockade offers an effective means of treatment for only some of these syndromes. Failure to assess *and reassess* cancer pain in the light of these potential etiologies will end in poor results from use of neural blockade. It should be remembered that central neuropathic pain, including deafferentation pain, can occur in patients with cancer (180). This is not responsive, on a continued basis, to neural blockade, except sometimes to stimulation techniques (see Chapter 41). Precise description of the origin and pattern of cancer pain is important. For example, it has been reported that intermittent visceral pain responds poorly to spinal opioids.

Classification of Chronic Pain

In an attempt to standardize the diagnosis and treatment of chronic pain, a pain taxonomy has been developed by the IASP (1). This taxonomy provides definitions of chronic pain syndromes as well as a system of classifying pain types, and it is helpful in improving recognition of various chronic pain syndromes and in providing for the use of a common terminology (see Appendix A).

Several points pertinent to neural blockade can be made:

■ The scheme for coding encourages precise description of region of body, system involved, temporal characteristics of pain, intensity, time since onset, and etiology. This helps to identify pain syndromes that may be responsive to neural blockade and pinpoints anatomic regions involved.

■ The classification refers first to *generalized* syndromes (e.g., peripheral neuropathy) that may have important underlying medical diseases (e.g., amyloid, diabetes). Some of these may be amenable to treatment of the disease as a means of pain treatment, and are frequently, but not invariably, unresponsive to neural blockade. Some may require a good knowledge of the disease process in order to treat the pain effectively *and safely. Regionalized* pain syndromes are described, and some of these are amenable to neural blockade.

■ The use of neural blockade is appropriate and effective only in some of these many syndromes (see Chapters 37–42 and 44–46). Those using neural blockade should be familiar with all of the syndromes in the classification and with the treatments other than neural blockade that are effective for some syndromes. In particular, it should be recognized that, in many well-described pain syndromes, psychological factors play a major role. However, in some of these, neural blockade may be useful as an *adjunct* to psychological measures.

IMPLICATIONS FOR NEURAL BLOCKADE

Peripheral Nerve Blockade

Peripheral nerve blockade is used often as a diagnostic procedure to predict outcome for nerve section or neuroablative procedures. However, it has been demonstrated that isolated, uncontrolled nerve blocks have little diagnostic or predictive value in the assessment of sciatic pain due to lumbosacral disease (181). The recent evidence for physiological and morphologic changes within the nervous system following peripheral pathology, as well as the impact of pain on the whole person, suggests that there are pitfalls in diagnostic neural blockade. First, chronic pain due to peripheral nerve damage may occur independent of peripheral input. For example, a longstanding intercostal neuralgia will not be expected to respond to intercostal neurectomy. Indeed, the pain may increase as a consequence of deafferentation. Second, diagnostic nerve blocks seek to identify a pain source, thereby isolating the person from the disease process thought to be responsible for the pain. Using diagnostic nerve blocks in this way can mean that little recognition is made of the complex psychological issues that can underlie the chronic pain presentation. It may even mean that a psychological diagnosis is made on the basis of the person's response to a diagnostic procedure. For these reasons, diagnostic procedures must be done in the context of a multidisciplinary assessment, with an understanding of the complex biologic and psychological components of chronic pain and placebo response to interventions (see Chapters 7, 28, and 37).

Acute and chronic pain may arise from cutaneous, deep somatic, or visceral structures. Careful mapping of the principal superficial dermatomes is important for effective use of neural blockade techniques. Dermatomes are shown in Chapter 9. Visceral pain is much more vaguely localized than somatic pain and has other unique features (Table 31-3). Convergence of visceral and somatic afferents has been proven, and this helps to explain referred pain (Fig. 31-21).

The relief of visceral pain requires blockade of visceral nociceptive fibers that travel to the spinal cord by way of the sympathetic chain (Fig. 31-21). The viscera and the spinal cord segments associated with their visceral nociceptor afferents are shown in Table 31-10. Visceral pain is referred to the body surface areas, as shown in Figure 31-22. It should be noted that considerable overlap exists for the various organs. Thus,

TABLE 31-6

PAIN SYNDROMES IN PATIENTS WITH CANCER: PAIN DIRECTLY CAUSED BY CANCER[a] (PRIMARY OR METASTATIC)

Mechanism	Common sites and characteristics of pain
Infiltration of bone by tumor	Dull, constant aching; ± muscle spasm
Base of skull (jugular foramen, clivus, sphenoid sinus)	Early onset pain in occiput, vertex, frontal areas, respectively
Vertebral body (subluxation atlas, metastases C7–T1, L1 sacral)	Early onset pain in neck and skull, neck and shoulders, midback, lower back, and coccyx, respectively ± neurologic deficit
Metastatic fracture close to nerves	Acute onset pain + muscle spasm
Hypercalcemia (associated with multiple bone metastases)	Sudden increase in pain ± confusion ± drowsiness
Infiltration or compression of nerve tissue by tumor	
Peripheral nerve (± peripheral and perivascular lymphangitis)	Burning constant pain in area of peripheral sensory loss ± dysesthesia and hyperalgesia ± signs of sympathetic over-activity. See neuropathy definition
Plexus, e.g., lumbar	Radicular pain to anterior thigh and groin (L1–L3) or to leg and foot (L4–S2)
e.g., sacral	Dull aching midline perianal pain + sacral sensory loss and fecal and urinary incontinence
e.g., brachial	Radicular pain in shoulder and arm ± Homer's syndrome (superior pulmonary sulcus or Pancoast syndrome)
Meningeal carcinomatosis	Constant headache ± neck stiffness or low back and buttock pain
Epidural spinal cord compression (± vertebral body infiltration)	Severe neck and back pain locally over involved vertebra, or radicular pain
Obstruction of hollow viscus e.g., gut, genitourinary tract	Poorly localized, dull, sickening pain, typical visceral pain
Occlusion of arteries and veins by tumour	Ischemic pain like rest pain (skin) or claudication (muscle) or pain ± venous engorgement
Stretching of periosteum or fascia, in tissues with tight investment, by tumefaction	Severe localized pain (e.g., periosteum) or typical visceral pain (e.g., ovary)
Inflammation owing to necrosis and infection of tumors (± superficial ulceration)	Severe localized pain (e.g., perineum), visceral pain (e.g., cervix)
Soft tissue infiltration	Localized pain; unsightly and foul-smelling if ulcerated
Raised intracranial pressure	Severe constant headache, behavioral changes, confusion, etc.

[a] A subcategory can be defined as *Pain related to the cancer,* e.g., muscle spasm, constipation, bedsores, lymphedema, candidiasis, herpetic and postherpetic neuralgia, deep venous thrombosis, pulmonary embolism.

it is not surprising that a substantial error rate occurs in the diagnosis of visceral pain. Also, important viscerosomatic and somaticovisceral reflexes may make diagnosis and treatment difficult (Fig. 31-21). Pain pathways for gynecologic pain have been poorly understood; they are shown in Figure 31-23.

Temporary relief of visceral pain by blockade of the somatic referred area poses potential problems of interpretation of diagnostic local anesthetic nerve blocks (see Chapter 38). The processes of peripheral and central sensitization, which have been described previously in this chapter, may be shared by somatic as well as visceral structures. This may account for the heightened response of visceral structures to a relatively benign stimulus following inflammation or tissue damage, termed *visceral hyperalgesia* (see also Chapter 32).

Spinal Administration of Agents

Elucidation of the types of receptors present pre- and post-synaptically around nociceptive transmission neurons in the dorsal horn has led to the use of spinal drug administration as a pain management technique. The application of relatively low doses of agents acting at specific receptor types within the spinal cord, with the relative avoidance of side effects, has been a major advance in the management of some pain problems. Some people who have been unresponsive to administration of oral agents have had greatly improved relief with the use of infusion devices that administer agents such as morphine or clonidine, either alone or in combination, directly into the intrathecal space. In selected cases, intrathecal administration of a combination of morphine and clonidine has been effective in the treatment of some types of neuropathic pain, including pain following spinal cord injury (160) (see Chapter 40).

Although their use is largely experimental at this stage, the availability of spinal drug administration has led to interest in the use of agents not traditionally considered for use by the spinal route. Nonsteroidal anti-inflammatory drugs have an action at the glycine receptor of the NMDA receptor complex, and tricyclic antidepressants (TCAs) also have an action at a receptor within the NMDA complex. Both types of agents have been administered via the spinal route with some success (see Chapter 40).

However, the success that has been achieved by targeting spinal receptors directly has not been without some problems.

TABLE 31-7

PAIN SYNDROMES IN PATIENTS WITH CANCER: PAIN ASSOCIATED WITH CANCER THERAPY

Mechanism	Common sites and characteristics of pain
Following surgery	
Acute postoperative pain	Wound or referred pain; back or other sites (owing to posture during surgery)
Nerve trauma	Neuralgic pain in area of peripheral nerve or spinal nerve
Entrapment of nerves in scar tissue	Superficial wound scar hypersensitivity of area supplied by scarred nerves (e.g., perineum)
Amputation of limb or other area (e.g., breast)	Localized stump pain (neuroma) or phantom pain referred to absent region
Following radiotherapy	
Acute lesions or inflammation of nerves or plexuses	Pain associated with motor and sensory loss (e.g., brachial plexus, lumbar plexus distribution); diffuse limb pain, 6 months to many years after
Radiation fibrosis of nerves or plexuses	radiation ± lymphedema and local skin changes ± sensory loss ± motor loss (difficult to distinguish from tumor recurrence)
Myelopathy of spinal cord	Brown-Sequard syndrome (ipsilateral sensory and contralateral motor loss) with pain at level of spinal cord damage, or referred pain
Peripheral nerve tumors owing to radiation	Painful enlarging mass in area of radiation along line of peripheral nerve or plexus
Following chemotherapy	
Vinca alkaloid (vincristine >vinblastine, taxol)-induced peripheral neuropathy	Burning pain in hands and feet associated with symmetrical polyneuropathy
Steroid pseudorheumatism owing to slow as well as rapid withdrawal of steroid treatment	Diffuse joint and muscle pain with associated tenderness to palpation but no inflammatory signs
	Pain resolves when steroid reinstituted
Aseptic necrosis of bone (femoral or humoral head) with chronic steroid therapy	Pain in knee, leg, or shoulder with limitation of movement; bone scan changes delayed after pain onset
Postherpetic neuralgia, following herpes zoster infection in area of tumor or area of radiotherapy with onset during chemotherapy	Continuous burning pain in area of sensory loss or painful dysesthesias or intermittent, shock-like pain

Many agents, although promising in the laboratory, have severe side effects or are toxic when administered via the spinal route and are therefore unsuitable for this method of administration. Although it was believed early in the use of the technique that dose escalation was not a problem, it has been found that some people using opioids require increasing doses to maintain adequate analgesia. Chronic administration of intrathecal opioids can also result in hormonal changes, and there are reports of paradoxical pain in some people, especially at higher dose levels (182) (see Chapter 40).

Neuroablative Approaches

The location of nociceptive pathways in the anterolateral quadrant would suggest that section of these tracts using an anterolateral cordotomy should be a useful procedure in abolishing or relieving pain. However, results are variable and often transient. A latent ipsilateral pathway progressively takes over from the contralateral spinothalamic pathway following cordotomy, and some nociceptive signals are conveyed through a postsynaptic dorsal column pathway (183). These alternate pathways, or the development of neuropathic pain that follows deafferentation, may account for the eventual failure of analgesia and occasional onset of neuropathic pain following cordotomy (see also Chapters 32 and 42).

Several other procedures are employed to disrupt specific tracts within the spinal cord. These include extralemniscal

TABLE 31-8

PAIN SYNDROMES IN PATIENTS WITH CANCER: PAIN UNRELATED TO CANCER OR CANCER THERAPY

Mechanism	Common sites and characteristics of pain
Neuropathy (e.g., diabetic)	Burning pain in hands, feet
Degenerative disc disease	Back pain ± radicular pain
Rheumatoid arthritis	Joint pain, on movement
Diffuse osteoporosis	Back pain, limb pain (may be like causalgia)
Posture abnormalities after surgery	Back pain and muscle spasm ± radicular pain
Myofascial syndromes owing to anxiety	Local pain in muscle with muscle spasm ± referred pain; trigger areas in muscle
Headache	Typical migraine or tension type

PART IV: PAIN MANAGEMENT

TABLE 31-9

PAIN SYNDROMES IN PATIENTS WITH CANCER: PAIN EXACERBATED OR ENTIRELY CAUSED BY PSYCHOLOGICAL FACTORS

Psychological factor	Possible causes
Anxiety	Sleeplessness
	Fear of death; loss of dignity (loss of self-control)
	Fear of surgical mutilation; uncontrollable pain
	Fear of the future; loss of social position and work
	Confused understanding of disease owing to poor communication
	Family and financial problems
Depression	Sleeplessness
	Loss of physical abilities
	Sense of helplessness
	Disfigurement
	Loss of valued social position, financial problems
Anger	Frustration with therapeutic failures
	Resentment of sickness
	Irritability caused by pain and general discomfort
A vicious circle usually develops:	ANXIETY / SLEEPLESSNESS ← PAIN → ANGER / DEPRESSION

myelotomy and commissural myelotomy (184). Once again, excellent relief can be obtained in the short term, but long-term results are often disappointing, and complications include return of pain, motor weakness, and loss of bladder and bowel function. Therefore, these procedures are usually limited to treatment of cancer pain. Lesioning of the dorsal root entry zone (DREZ) has proven to be effective for neuropathic pain associated with brachial and lumbar plexus avulsion (185). The duration of pain relief of many years seems to be an exception to the rule that neuroplasticity limits the duration after lesions in the nervous system. For example, radiofrequency lesions of the trigeminal ganglion relieve the pain of trigeminal neuralgia for 6 to 12 months, but, inevitably, pain returns (see Chapter 42).

Pharmacologic Approaches

Nonsteroidal Anti-inflammatory Drugs

Nonsteroidal anti-inflammatory drugs are commonly used to reduce the inflammatory response, although they also have a central action (186,187). Agents such as aspirin, paracetamol, and other NSAIDs provide their anti-inflammatory action by blocking the cyclooxygenase pathway and reducing tissue levels of prostaglandins. Nonsteroidal anti-inflammatory drugs are used extensively in treatment of acute postoperative pain (188,189). Although some concern has been raised about the risks of NSAIDs (190), they continue to have a useful role as analgesics in the perioperative period. Nonselective agents such as ibuprofen, naproxen (191), diclofenac (192,193), and ketorolac (194) have been used pre- or postoperatively for some time, with a demonstrated reduction in postoperative pain and reduced opioid requirements (190). The different sites of action

found with NSAIDs and opioids would also suggest additive, or possibly even synergistic, effects and, in clinical practice, they are often used in combination.

With the discovery that cyclooxygenase exists in two forms, COX-1 and COX-2, selective COX-2 inhibitors were developed in the hope that they would confer a clinical advantage by avoiding many of the side effects of nonselective agents (195,196). COX-2 inhibitors such as rofecoxib, meloxicam, celecoxib, etoricoxib, valdecoxib, and parecoxib have been used and appear to have a similar level of efficacy as the nonselective agents (197–199). However, recent evidence of an increased incidence of cardiovascular events in some patients has dampened the initial enthusiasm for these agents.

Antineuropathic Drugs

A number of agents are used with varying degrees of success and levels of evidence in the management of peripheral neuropathic pain (200,201). Treatment of neuropathic pain to a large extent relies on adjuvant medications. These include TCAs; the newer selective serotonin and norepinephrine reuptake inhibitors such as venlafaxine and duloxetine; anticonvulsants such as gabapentin, pregabalin, lamotrigine, carbamazepine, and sodium valproate; clonidine; opioids; local anesthetics, such as lidocaine; and antiarrhythmic agents, such as mexiletine (see Chapter 33).

Systemic administration of local anesthetic agents can culminate in a marked reduction of neuropathic pain (202,203), because relatively low concentrations of local anesthetic can reduce ectopic activity in damaged nerves at levels below the concentration required to produce conduction block (46). A puzzling feature of the response of peripheral neuropathic pain to systemic administration of local anesthetics is the time course of pain relief. Whereas intrathecal or peripheral nerve blockade

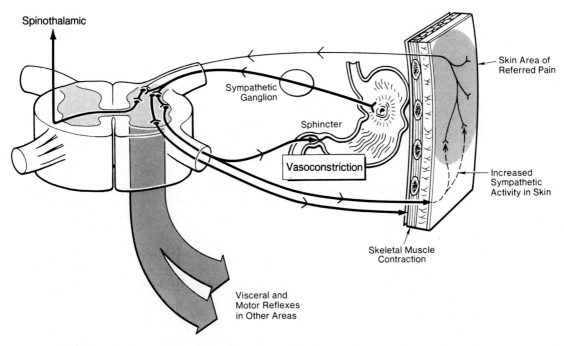

FIGURE 31-21. Visceral pain: Convergence of visceral and somatic nociceptive afferents. Visceral nociceptive afferents converge on the same dorsal horn neuron as do somatic nociceptive afferents. Visceral noxious stimuli are then conveyed, together with somatic noxious stimuli, by means of the spinothalamic pathways to the brain. Note the following: *1.* Referred pain is felt in the cutaneous area corresponding to the dorsal horn neurons upon which visceral afferents converge. This is accompanied by allodynia and hyperalgesia in this skin area. *2.* Reflex somatic motor activity results in muscle spasm, which may stimulate parietal peritoneum and initiate somatic noxious input to dorsal horn. *3.* Reflex sympathetic efferent activity may result in spasm of sphincters of viscera over a wide area, causing pain remote from the original stimulus. *4.* Reflex sympathetic efferent activity may result in visceral ischemia and further noxious stimulation. Also, visceral nociceptors may be sensitized by norepinephrine release and microcirculatory changes. *5.* Increased sympathetic activity may influence cutaneous nociceptors, which may be at least partly responsible for referred pain. *6.* Peripheral visceral afferents branch considerably, causing much overlap in the territory of individual dorsal roots. Only a small number of visceral afferent fibers converge on dorsal horn neurons compared with somatic nociceptor fibers. Also, visceral afferents converge on the dorsal horn over a wide number of segments. Thus, dull, vague, visceral pain is very poorly localized. This is often called *deep visceral pain.*

results in temporary reduction in pain behavior in an animal model of neuropathic pain, systemic administration of lidocaine results in a reduction in mechanical hyperalgesia that persists for 1 week (204). This finding challenges previously accepted explanations for the mechanisms of local anesthetics in reducing neuropathic pain and also suggests possible clinical application (205,206). The broad action of local anesthetics and their resulting side effects has limited their clinical application and use in the treatment of neuropathic pain. The development of novel agents—such as the μO-conotoxin, MrVIB, which is a selective Nav1.8 sodium channel blocker that has excellent analgesic properties and negligible motor effects—offers hope that agents with far more therapeutic usefulness will be available in the near future (207) (see Chapter 33).

The important role of the NMDA receptor in the development of pain is a potential avenue to exploit for treatment. The NMDA antagonists can attenuate alterations in cell responsiveness (71), indicating a role for NMDA antagonists in the relief of some neuropathic pain conditions (208). Several drugs are available, such as ketamine, dextromethorphan, amantadine, and memantine, which appear to block NMDA receptor–mediated changes (71,94,156). Ketamine is the most commonly used NMDA antagonist but can have side effects that are poorly tolerated, and only limited evidence exists for

its efficacy in most chronic pain conditions (209). At present, there is also very limited evidence to support the use of other NMDA antagonists such as memantine and dextromethorphan (210,211). Nevertheless, there still remains a potential for the development of clinically suitable NMDA receptor antagonists, and several agents are being investigated either as analgesics or for use in other medical conditions (208).

Traditional approaches in pain management have focused on classical ligand-receptor blockade as a means to reduce nociceptive or neuropathic input. The rapid progress in our understanding of the molecular and genetic mechanisms involved in nociception provides a new and potentially useful approach to pain management. Using this approach, it may be possible to develop drugs or vectors that regulate gene expression and selectively modify the expression of specific receptors or neuromodulators involved in the transmission of nociceptive and neuropathic messages (212,213).

Preemptive and Preventive Analgesia

Discovery of the changes associated with the phenomenon of central sensitization has led to attempts to prevent these changes (214). It has been demonstrated that early

TABLE 31-10

VISCERA AND THEIR SEGMENTAL NOCICEPTIVE NERVE SUPPLY

Viscus	Spinal segments of visceral nociceptive afferents[a]
Heart	T1–T5
Lungs	T2–T4
Esophagus	T5–T6
Stomach	T6–T10
Liver and gall bladder	T6–T10
Pancreas and spleen	T6–T10
Small intestine	T9–T10
Large intestine	T11–T12
Kidney and ureter	T10–L2
Adrenal glands	T8–L1
Testis, ovary	T10–T11
Urinary bladder	T11–L2
Prostate gland	T11–L1
Uterus	T10–L1

[a]These travel with sympathetic fibers and pass by way of sympathetic ganglia to the spinal cord. However, they are *not* sympathetic (efferent) fibers. They are best referred to as visceral nociceptive afferents. *Note:* Parasympathetic afferent fibers may be important in upper abdominal pain (vagal fibers, celiac plexus).

postoperative pain is a significant predictor of long-term pain (215). It was hoped that steps that would reduce or abolish noxious input to the spinal cord during a painful event such as surgery would reduce or minimize spinal cord changes and thereby lead to reduced pain postoperatively and long-term. However, it is still not known what duration or degree of noxious input is required before these long-term changes occur.

It is also not known how much long-term changes are dependent on the afferent barrage during surgery, and how much they are dependent on *continuing inputs* from the wound after surgery. At both stages, sustained noxious input will occur, and therefore both stages have the capacity to produce central sensitization. However, it would be expected that intervention that preempts central sensitization and seeks to prevent it, rather than attempts to treat it after it has occurred, would be more successful (see Chapter 40 and 43). This implies that treatment must extend before, during, and after surgery.

This concept has led to an increasing interest in the use of preventive analgesia. Local anesthetics, opioids, and NSAIDs have been used alone or in combination, and have been administered locally, epidurally, intrathecally, or systemically. In a preventive approach, they have been administered pre-, intra-, and postoperatively. Many trials have purported to show that preventive analgesia results in reduced pain, decreased analgesic requirements, improved morbidity, and decreased hospital stay (216,217). However, the variability in agents, timing, and method of administration, as well as differences in the type of surgery and anesthetic procedures used, have made it difficult to compare trials that only examine the effectiveness of *preemptive analgesia* (analgesics given before versus after surgery) (218). There have also been several problems with the design of these studies that has made it difficult to draw definite conclusions concerning outcomes. Therefore, despite studies that appear to indicate the advantages of preventive analgesia, the logical appeal of this approach, and its ready application to the clinical arena, there is still lack of evidence to clearly indicate the major clinical benefits of a purely preemptive analgesia (219).

Most studies have focused on the effect of preventive analgesia in reducing pain in the early postoperative period. However, preventive analgesia may also be important in reducing the

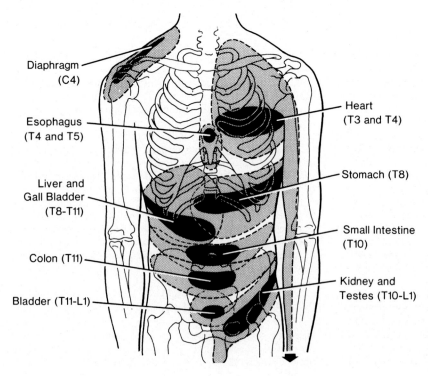

FIGURE 31-22. Viscerotomes. Approximate superficial areas to which visceral pain is referred, with related dermatomes in brackets. The dark areas are those most commonly associated with pain in each viscus. The *gray areas* indicate approximately the larger area that may be associated with pain in the viscus. From Cousins MJ. Visceral pain. In: Andersson S, Bond M, Mehta M, Swerdlow M, eds. *Chronic Non-Cancer Pain: Assessment and Practical Management.* Lancaster, UK: MTP Press, 1987. with permission.

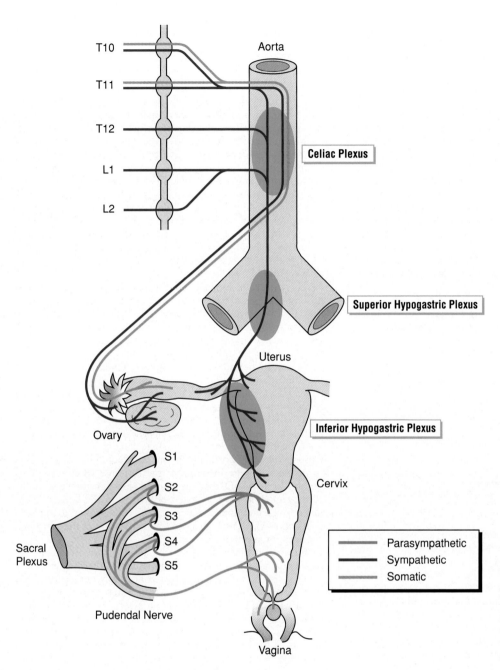

T10

T11

T12

L1

L2

Aorta

Celiac Plexus

Superior Hypogastric Plexus

Uterus

Inferior Hypogastric Plexus

Ovary

S1

S2

S3

S4

S5

Cervix

Sacral
Plexus

Pudendal Nerve

Vagina

	Parasympathetic
	Sympathetic
	Somatic

FIGURE 31-23. Pain pathways in gynecologic pain. Somatic afferents from lower vagina are also shown. From Cousins MJ, Wilson PR. Gynecologic pain. In: Coppleson M, ed. *Gynecologic Oncology*. Edinburgh: Churchill-Livingstone, 1981, with permission.

incidence of chronic pain. An early study that generated interest was the finding by Bach and colleagues (220) that preoperative epidural blockade of patients undergoing lower-limb amputation resulted in a lower incidence of phantom limb pain at 6 and 12 months following surgery, when compared with the control group, which had intraoperative block alone. Although it has been pointed out that there are several inadequacies in the design of this study (216), it does demonstrate that preventive analgesia may have the potential to prevent the development of chronic pain states. In line with this concept, it has been demonstrated that the degree of pain after thoracic surgery predicts long-term postthoracotomy pain (215). However, studies examining prevalence of chronic pain following the use of preventive analgesia have found contradictory results (221,222), and further studies are required to address this important question.

PAIN RELIEF AS A BASIC HUMAN RIGHT

The increasing awareness of the impact of pain at multiple levels has pointed out the need for greater awareness and commitment from the community to providing pain relief for its citizens (223). The problem of persistent pain is now well recognized in our society. Recent studies indicate the high prevalence of persistent pain, the burden of persistent pain on individuals and society as a whole, as well as the limited avenues and resources for appropriate and satisfactory treatment. Therefore, improvements in pain management will not only come from an understanding of the underlying contributors to pain, but from increased accuracy in identifying specific contributors in individuals and the effective application of appropriate interventions. Improvements will also come from a recognition at all levels of society that access to the best pain relief available is a basic human right and that concerted efforts should be made to provide the resources that enable this to be provided to as many people as possible.

SUMMARY

In recent years, substantial progress has been made in our understanding of pain mechanisms. Our understanding of the pharmacology and physiology of nociceptive processes and the identification of neurotransmitters and pathways involved in nociceptive transmission have led to the development of new agents and more effective use of those agents already available. The recognition and characterization of nervous system changes that occur with pain has also had a profound influence on our conceptualization of pain and indicates the potential that exists to modify or prevent the development of chronic pain states by managing acute pain more effectively and in different ways.

APPENDIX A: CLASSIFICATION OF CHRONIC PAIN

Reproduced with permission of the International Association for the Study of Pain (IASP) and IASP Press. The material reproduced is a small portion of the publication "Classification of Chronic Pain: Descriptions of Chronic Pain Syndromes and Definitions of Pain Terms," 2nd edition (1). The reader is strongly encouraged to consult the full document.

Pain Terms

Pain

An unpleasant sensory and emotional experience associated with actual or potential tissue damage, or described in terms of such damage. *Note:* The inability to communicate verbally does not negate the possibility that an individual is experiencing pain and is in need of appropriate pain-relieving treatment. Pain is always subjective. Each individual learns the application of the word through experiences related to injury in early life. Biologists recognize that those stimuli which cause pain are liable to damage tissue. Accordingly, pain is that experience we associate with actual or potential tissue damage. It is unquestionably a sensation in a part or parts of the body, but it is also always unpleasant and therefore also an emotional experience. Experiences which resemble pain but are not unpleasant, e.g., pricking, should not be called pain. Unpleasant abnormal experiences (dysesthesias) may also be pain but are not necessarily so because, subjectively, they may not have the usual sensory qualities of pain.

Many people report pain in the absence of tissue damage or any likely pathophysiological cause; usually this happens for psychological reasons. There is usually no way to distinguish their experience from that due to tissue damage if we take the subjective report. If they regard their experience as pain and if they report it in the same ways as pain caused by tissue damage, it should be accepted as pain. This definition avoids tying pain to the stimulus. Activity induced in the nociceptor and nociceptive pathways by a noxious stimulus is not pain, which is always a psychological state, even though we may well appreciate that pain most often has a proximate physical cause.

Allodynia

Pain due to a stimulus which does not normally provoke pain. *Note:* The term allodynia was originally introduced to separate from hyperalgesia and hyperesthesia, the conditions seen in patients with lesions of the nervous system where touch, light pressure, or moderate cold or warmth evoke pain when applied to apparently normal skin. *Allo* means "other" in Greek and is a common prefix for medical conditions that diverge from the expected. *Odynia* is derived from the Greek word "odune" or "odyne," which is used in "pleurodynia" and "coccydynia" and is similar in meaning to the root from which we derive words with -algia or -algesia in them. Allodynia was suggested following discussions with Professor Paul Potter of the Department of the History of Medicine and Science at The University of Western Ontario.

The words "to normal skin" were used in the original definition but later were omitted in order to remove any suggestion that allodynia applied only to referred pain. Originally, also, the pain-provoking stimulus was described as "non-noxious." However, a stimulus may be noxious at some times and not at others, for example, with intact skin and sunburned skin, and also, the boundaries of noxious stimulation may be hard to delimit. Since the Committee aimed at providing terms for clinical use, it did not wish to define them by reference to the specific physical characteristics of the stimulation, e.g., pressure in kilopascals per square centimeter. Moreover, even in intact skin there is little evidence one way or the other that a strong painful pinch to a normal person does or does not damage tissue. Accordingly, it was considered to be preferable to define allodynia in terms of the response to clinical stimuli and to point out that the normal response to the stimulus could almost always be tested elsewhere in the body, usually in a corresponding part. Further, allodynia is taken to apply to conditions which may give rise to sensitization of the skin, e.g., sunburn, inflammation, trauma.

It is important to recognize that allodynia involves a change in the quality of a sensation, whether tactile, thermal, or of any other sort. The original modality is normally non-painful, but the response is painful. There is thus a loss of specificity of a sensory modality. By contrast, hyperalgesia (q.v.) represents an augmented response in a specific mode, viz., pain. With other cutaneous modalities, hyperesthesia is the term which corresponds to hyperalgesia, and as with hyperalgesia, the quality is not altered. In allodynia the stimulus mode and the response mode differ, unlike the situation with hyperalgesia. This distinction should not be confused by the fact that allodynia and hyperalgesia can be plotted with overlap along the same continuum of physical intensity in certain circumstances, for example, with pressure or temperature.

See also the notes on hyperalgesia and hyperpathia.

Analgesia

Absence of pain in response to stimulation which would normally be painful. *Note:* As with allodynia (q.v.), the stimulus is defined by its usual subjective effects.

Anesthesia Dolorosa

Pain in an area or region which is anesthetic.

Causalgia

A syndrome of sustained burning pain, allodynia, and hyperpathia after a traumatic nerve lesion, often combined with vasomotor and sudomotor dysfunction and later trophic changes.

Central Pain

Pain initiated or caused by a primary lesion or dysfunction in the central nervous system.

Dysesthesia

An unpleasant abnormal sensation, whether spontaneous or evoked. *Note:* Compare with pain and with paresthesia. Special cases of dysesthesia include hyperalgesia and allodynia. A dysesthesia should always be unpleasant and a paresthesia should not be unpleasant, although it is recognized that the borderline may present some difficulties when it comes to deciding as to whether a sensation is pleasant or unpleasant. It should always be specified whether the sensations are spontaneous or evoked.

Hyperalgesia

An increased response to a stimulus which is normally painful. *Note:* Hyperalgesia reflects increased pain on suprathreshold stimulation. For pain evoked by stimuli that usually are not painful, the term allodynia is preferred, while hyperalgesia is more appropriately used for cases with an increased response at a normal threshold, or at an increased threshold, e.g., in patients with neuropathy. It should also be recognized that with allodynia the stimulus and the response are in different modes, whereas with hyperalgesia they are in the same mode. Current evidence suggests that hyperalgesia is a consequence of perturbation of the nociceptive system with peripheral or central sensitization, or both, but it is important to distinguish between the clinical phenomena, which this definition emphasizes, and the interpretation, which may well change as knowledge advances.

Hyperesthesia

Increased sensitivity to stimulation, excluding the special senses. *Note:* The stimulus and locus should be specified. Hyperesthesia may refer to various modes of cutaneous sensibility including touch and thermal sensation without pain, as well as to pain. The word is used to indicate both diminished threshold to any stimulus and an increased response to stimuli that are normally recognized.

Allodynia is suggested for pain after stimulation which is not normally painful. Hyperesthesia includes both allodynia and hyperalgesia, but the more specific terms should be used wherever they are applicable.

Hyperpathia

A painful syndrome characterized by an abnormally painful reaction to a stimulus, especially a repetitive stimulus, as well as an increased threshold. *Note:* It may occur with allodynia, hyperesthesia, hyperalgesia, or dysesthesia. Faulty identification and localization of the stimulus, delay, radiating sensation, and after-sensation may be present, and the pain is often explosive in character. The changes in this note are the specification of allodynia and the inclusion of hyperalgesia explicitly. Previously hyperalgesia was implied, since hyperesthesia was mentioned in the previous note and hyperalgesia is a special case of hyperesthesia.

Hypoalgesia

Diminished pain in response to a normally painful stimulus. *Note:* Hypoalgesia was formerly defined as diminished sensitivity to noxious stimulation, making it a particular case of hypoesthesia (q.v.). However, it now refers only to the occurrence of relatively less pain in response to stimulation that produces pain. Hypoesthesia covers the case of diminished sensitivity to stimulation that is normally painful.

The implications of some of the above definitions may be summarized for convenience as follows:

Allodynia: lowered threshold: stimulus and response mode differ

Hyperalgesia: increased response: stimulus and response mode are the same

Hyperpathia: raised threshold: stimulus and response mode may be the increased response: same or different

Hypoalgesia: raised threshold: stimulus and response mode are the same lowered response.

The above essentials of the definitions do not have to be symmetrical and are not symmetrical at present. Lowered threshold may occur with allodynia but is not required. Also, there is no category for lowered threshold and lowered response—if it ever occurs.

Hypoesthesia

Decreased sensitivity to stimulation, excluding the special senses. *Note:* Stimulation and locus to be specified.

Neuralgia

Pain in the distribution of a nerve or nerves. *Note:* Common usage, especially in Europe, often implies a paroxysmal quality, but neuralgia should not be reserved for paroxysmal pains.

Neuritis

Inflammation of a nerve or nerves. *Note:* Not to be used unless inflammation is thought to be present.

Neurogenic Pain

Pain initiated or caused by a primary lesion, dysfunction, or transitory perturbation in the peripheral or central nervous system.

Neuropathic Pain

Pain initiated or caused by a primary lesion or dysfunction in the nervous system. *Note:* See also Neurogenic Pain and Central Pain. Peripheral neuropathic pain occurs when the lesion or dysfunction affects the peripheral nervous system. Central pain may be retained as the term when the lesion or dysfunction affects the central nervous system.

Neuropathy

A disturbance of function or pathological change in a nerve: in one nerve, mononeuropathy; in several nerves, mononeuropathy multiplex; if diffuse and bilateral, polyneuropathy. *Note:* Neuritis (q.v.) is a special case of neuropathy and is now reserved for inflammatory processes affecting nerves. Neuropathy is not intended to cover cases like neurapraxia, neurotmesis, section of a nerve, or transitory impact like a blow, stretching, or an epileptic discharge. The term neurogenic applies to pain due to such temporary perturbations.

Nociceptor

A receptor preferentially sensitive to a noxious stimulus or to a stimulus which would become noxious if prolonged. *Note:* Avoid use of terms like pain receptor, pain pathway, etc.

Noxious Stimulus

A noxious stimulus is one which is damaging to normal tissues. *Note:* Although the definition of a noxious stimulus has been retained, the term is not used in this list to define other terms.

Pain Threshold

The least experience of pain which a subject can recognize. *Note:* Traditionally the threshold has often been defined, as we defined it formerly, as the least stimulus intensity at which a subject perceives pain. Properly defined, the threshold is really the experience of the patient, whereas the intensity measured is an external event. It has been common usage for most pain research workers to define the threshold in terms of the stimulus, and that should be avoided. However, the threshold stimulus can be recognized as such and measured. In psychophysics, thresholds are defined as the level at which 50% of stimuli are recognized. In that case, the pain threshold would be the level at which 50% of stimuli would be recognized as painful. The stimulus is not pain (q.v.) and cannot be a measure of pain.

Pain Tolerance Level

The greatest level of pain which a subject is prepared to tolerate. *Note:* As with pain threshold, the pain tolerance level is the subjective experience of the individual. The stimuli which are normally measured in relation to its production are the pain tolerance level stimuli and not the level itself. Thus, the same argument applies to pain tolerance level as to pain threshold, and it is not defined in terms of the external stimulation as such.

Paresthesia

An abnormal sensation, whether spontaneous or evoked. *Note:* Compare with dysesthesia. After much discussion, it has been agreed to recommend that paresthesia be used to describe an abnormal sensation that is not unpleasant while dysesthesia be used preferentially for an abnormal sensation that is considered to be unpleasant. The use of one term (paresthesia) to indicate spontaneous sensations and the other to refer to evoked sensations is not favored. There is a sense in which, since paresthesia refers to abnormal sensations in general, it might include dysesthesia, but the reverse is not true. Dysesthesia does not include all abnormal sensations, but only those which are unpleasant.

Peripheral Neurogenic Pain

Pain initiated or caused by a primary lesion or dysfunction or transitory perturbation in the peripheral nervous system.

Peripheral Neuropathic Pain

Pain initiated or caused by a primary lesion or dysfunction in the peripheral nervous system.

References

1. Merskey H, Bogduk N. *Classification of Chronic Pain: Descriptions of Chronic Pain Syndromes and Definitions of Pain Terms.* Seattle: IASP Press, 1994.
2. Calford MB, Tweedale R. Immediate and chronic changes in responses of somatosensory cortex in adult flying-fox after digit amputation. *Nature* 1988;332:446–448.
3. Chen R, Cohen LG, Hallett M. Nervous system reorganization following injury. *Neurosci Biobehav Rev* 2002;111:761–773.
4. Melzack R, Coderre TJ, Vaccarino AL, Katz J. Pain and neuroplasticity. In: Grafman J, Christen Y, eds. *Neuronal Plasticity: Building a Bridge From the Laboratory to the Clinic.* Berlin: Springer-Verlag; 1999:35–52.
5. Melzack R, Coderre TJ, Katz J, Vaccarino AL. Central neuroplasticity and pathological pain. *Ann NY Acad Sci* 2001;933:157–174.
6. Sandkühler J. Learning and memory in pain pathways. *Pain* 2000;88:113–118.
7. Flor H, Elbert T, Knecht S, et al. Phantom-limb pain as a perceptual correlate of cortical reorganization following arm amputation. *Nature* 1995; 375:482–484.
8. Melzack R, Wall PD. Pain mechanisms: A new theory. *Science* 1965;150: 971–979.
9. Melzack R, Casey KL. Sensory, motivational and central determinants of pain: A new conceptual model. In: Kenshalo DR, ed. *The Skin Senses.* Springfield, IL: Thomas; 1968:423–443.
10. Woolf CJ. Recent advances in the pathophysiology of acute pain. *Br J Anaesth* 1989;63:139–146.
11. Callesen T, Bech K, Kehlet H. Prospective study of chronic pain after groin hernia repair. *Br J Surg* 1999;86:1528–1531.
12. Buchanan DC, Mandel AR. The prevalence of phantom limb experience in amputees. *Rehabil Psychol* 1986;31:183–188.
13. Schmader KE. Epidemiology and impact on quality of life of postherpetic neuralgia and painful diabetic neuropathy. *Clin J Pain* 2002;18:350–354.
14. Siddall PJ, McClelland JM, Rutkowski SB, Cousins MJ. A longitudinal study of the prevalence and characteristics of pain in the first 5 years following spinal cord injury. *Pain* 2003;103:249–257.
15. Mogil JS, Wilson SG, Bon K, et al. Heritability of nociception I: Responses of 11 inbred mouse strains on 12 measures of nociception. *Pain* 1999;80:67–82.
16. Inbal R, Devor M, Tuchendler O, Lieblich I. Autotomy following nerve injury: Genetic factors in the development of chronic pain. *Pain* 1980;9:327–337.
17. Mogil JS, Grisel JE. Transgenic studies of pain. *Pain* 1998;77:107–128.
18. Mogil JS, Yu L, Basbaum AI. Pain genes? Natural variation and transgenic mutants. *Annu Rev Neurosci* 2000;23:777–811.
19. Nicholson GA, Dawkins JL, Blair IP, et al. The gene for hereditary sensory neuropathy type I (HSN-I) maps to chromosome 9Q22.1-Q22.3. *Nat Genet* 1996;13:101–104.
20. Rosenfeld J, Sloanbrown K, George AL. A novel muscle sodium channel mutation causes painful congenital myotonia. *Ann Neurol* 1997;42:811–814.
21. Uhl GR, Sora I, Wang ZJ. The mu opiate receptor as a candidate gene for pain: Polymorphisms, variations in expression, nociception, and opiate responses. *Proc Natl Acad Sci USA* 1999;96:7752–7755.
22. Indo Y, Tsuruta M, Hayashida Y, et al. Mutations in the TrkA/NGF receptor gene in patients with congenital insensitivity to pain with anhidrosis. *Nat Genet* 1996;13:485–488.
23. Ophoff RA, Terwindt GM, Vergouwe MN, et al. Familial hemiplegic migraine and episodic ataxia type-2 are caused by mutations in the Ca2+ channel gene CACNL1A4. *Cell* 1996;87:543–552.
24. Meyer UA, Zanger UM. Molecular mechanisms of genetic polymorphisms of drug metabolism. *Annu Rev Pharmacol Toxicol* 1997;37:269–296.
25. Tegeder I, Costigan M, Griffin RS, et al. GTP cyclohydrolase and tetrahydrobiopterin regulate pain sensitivity and persistence. *Nat Med* 2006;12:1269–1277.
26. Siddall PJ, Cousins MJ. Persistent pain as a disease entity: Implications for clinical management. *Anesth Analg* 2004;99:510–520.
27. Loeser JD. Pain as a disease. In: Cervero F, Jensen TS, eds. *Handbook of Clinical Neurology.* Amsterdam: Elsevier B.V.; 2006:11–20.
28. Bridges D, Thompson SWN, Rice ASC. Mechanisms of neuropathic pain. *Br J Anaesth* 2001;87:12–26.

29. Woolf CJ, Mannion RJ. Neuropathic pain: Aetiology, symptoms, mechanisms and management. *Lancet* 1999;353:1959–1964.
30. Devor M. Neuropathic pain and injured nerves: Peripheral mechanisms. *Br Med Bull* 1991;47:619–630.
31. Krishtal O. The ASICs: Signaling molecules? Modulators? *Trends Neurosci* 2003;26:477–483.
32. Burnstock G. Purinergic P2 receptors as targets for novel analgesics. *Pharmacol Ther* 2006;110:433–454.
33. Wang H, Woolf CJ. Pain TRPs. *Neuron* 2005;46:9–12.
34. Caterina MJ, Leffler A, Malmberg AB, et al. Impaired nociception and pain sensation in mice lacking the capsaicin receptor. *Science* 2000;288:306–313.
35. Cousins MJ. Visceral pain. In: Andersson S, Bond M, Mehta M, Swerdlow M, eds. *Chronic Non-Cancer Pain: Assessment and Practical Management.* Lancaster: MTP Press; 1987:119.
36. Meyer RA, Campbell JN, Raja SN, et al. *Peripheral Neural Mechanisms of Nociception. Textbook of Pain.* Edinburgh: Churchill Livingstone; 1994: 13–44.
37. Holzer P, Maggi CA. Dissociation of dorsal root ganglion neurons into afferent and efferent-like neurons. *Neuroscience* 1998;86:389–398.
38. Dubner R, Ren K. Central mechanisms of thermal and mechanical hyperalgesia following tissue inflammation. In: Boivie J, Hansson P, Lindblom U, eds. *Touch, Temperature, and Pain in Health and Disease: Mechanisms and Assessments.* Seattle: IASP Press; 1994:267–277.
39. Forster RW, Ramage AG. The action of some chemical irritants on somatosensory receptors of the cat. *Neuropharmacology* 1981;20:191–198.
40. Perl ER. Sensitization of nociceptors and its relation to sensation. In: Bonica JJ, Albe-Fessard D, eds. *Advances in Pain Research and Therapy.* New York: Raven Press; 1976:17–28.
41. Dray A, Urban L, Dickenson A. Pharmacology of chronic pain. *Trends Pharmacol Sci* 1994;15:190–197.
42. Pezet S, McMahon SB. Neurotrophins: Mediators and modulators of pain. *Annu Rev Neurosci* 2006;29:507–538.
43. Lewin GR, Mendell LM. Nerve growth factor and nociception. *Trends Neurosci* 1993;16:353–359.
44. McMahon S, Koltzenburg M. The changing role of primary afferent neurones in pain. *Pain* 1990;43:269–272.
45. Schaible HG, Schmidt RF. Direct observation of the sensitization of articular afferents during an experimental arthritis. In: Dubner R, Gebhardt G, Bond MR, eds. *Proceedings of the Vth World Congress on Pain,* Vol. 3. Amsterdam: Elsevier; 1988:44–50.
46. Devor M, Wall PD, Catalan N. Systemic lidocaine silences ectopic neuroma and DRG discharge without blocking nerve conduction. *Pain* 1992;48:261–268.
47. Chaplan SR, Pogrel JM, Yaksh TL. Role of voltage-dependent calcium channel subtypes in experimental tactile allodynia. *J Pharmacol Exp Ther* 1994; 269:1117–1123.
48. Devor M, Govrin LR, Angelides K. Na+ channel immunolocalization in peripheral mammalian axons and changes following nerve injury and neuroma formation. *J Neurosci* 1993;13:1976–1992.
49. Chahine M, Ziane R, Vijayaragavan K, Okamura Y. Regulation of Na-v channels in sensory neurons. *Trends Pharmacol Sci* 2005;26:496–502.
50. Rogawski MA, Loscher W. The neurobiology of antiepileptic drugs for the treatment of nonepileptic conditions. *Nat Med* 2004;10:685–692.
51. Devor M. The pathophysiology of damaged peripheral nerves. In: Wall PD, Melzack R, eds. *Textbook of Pain.* London: Churchill-Livingstone; 1994: 79–100.
52. Study RE, Kral MG. Spontaneous action potential activity in isolated dorsal root ganglion neurons from rats with a painful neuropathy. *Pain* 1996;65: 235–242.
53. Gold MS. Spinal nerve ligation: What to blame for the pain and why. *Pain* 2000;84:117–120.
54. Jänig W. The puzzle of "reflex sympathetic dystrophy": Mechanisms, hypotheses, open questions. In: Jänig W, Stanton-Hicks M, eds. *Reflex Sympathetic Dystrophy: A Reappraisal.* Seattle: IASP Press; 1996:1–24.
55. McMahon SB. Mechanisms of sympathetic pain. *Br Med Bull* 1991;47:584–600.
56. Stanton-Hicks M, Jänig W, Hassenbusch S, et al. Reflex sympathetic dystrophy: Changing concepts and taxonomy. *Pain* 1995;63:127–133.
57. Walker SM, Cousins MJ. Complex regional pain syndromes: Including "reflex sympathetic dystrophy" and "causalgia." *Anaesth Intensive Care* 1997; 25:113–125.
58. Wasner G, Schattschneider J, Binder A, Baron R. Complex regional pain syndrome: Diagnostic, mechanisms, CNS involvement and therapy. *Spinal Cord* 2003;41:61–75.
59. McLachlan EM, Jänig W, Devor M, Michaelis M. Peripheral nerve injury triggers noradrenergic sprouting within dorsal root ganglia. *Nature* 1993; 363:543–546.
60. McLachlan EM, Hu P. Axonal sprouts containing calcitonin gene-related peptide and substance p form pericellular baskets around large diameter neurons after sciatic nerve transection in the rat. *Neuroscience* 1998;84:961–965.
61. Lee BH, Yoon YW, Chung KS, Chung JM. Comparison of sympathetic sprouting in sensory ganglia in three animal models of neuropathic pain. *Exp Brain Res* 1998;120:432–438.
62. Levine JD, Fields HL, Basbaum AI. Peptides and the primary afferent nociceptor. *J Neurosci* 1993;13:2273–2286.
63. Satoh J, Perl ER. Adrenergic excitation of cutaneous pain receptors induced by peripheral nerve injury. *Science* 1991;251:1608–1610.
64. Campbell JN, Raja SN, Selig DK, et al. Diagnosis and management of sympathetically maintained pain. In: Fields HL, Liebeskind JC, eds. *Progress in Pain Research and Management.* Seattle: IASP Press; 1994:85–100.
65. Cervero F, Iggo A. The substantia gelatinosa of the spinal cord: A critical review. *Brain* 1980;103:717–772.
66. Light AR, Perl ER. Spinal termination of functionally identified primary afferent neurons with slowly conducting myelinated fibers. *J Comp Neurol* 1979;186:133–150.
67. Christensen BN, Perl ER. Spinal neurons specifically excited by noxious or thermal stimuli: Marginal zone of the dorsal horn. *J Neurophysiol* 1970;33:293–307.
68. Willis WD, Coggeshall RE. *Sensory Mechanisms of the Spinal Cord.* New York: Plenum Press, 1991.
69. Loh L, Nathan PW. Painful peripheral states and sympathetic blocks. *J Neurol Neurosurg Psychiatry* 1978;41:664–671.
70. Dickenson AH, Chapman V, Green GM. The pharmacology of excitatory and inhibitory amino acid-mediated events in the transmission and modulation of pain in the spinal cord. *Gen Pharmacol* 1997;28:633–638.
71. Woolf CJ, Thompson SWN. The induction and maintenance of central sensitization is dependent on N-methyl-D-aspartic acid receptor activation; implications for the treatment of post-injury pain hypersensitivity states. *Pain* 1991;44:293–299.
72. Price DD, Mao JR, Mayer DJ. Central neural mechanisms of normal and abnormal pain states. In: Fields HL, Liebeskind JC, eds. *Progress in Pain Research and Management.* Seattle: IASP Press; 1994:61–84.
73. Martin WJ, Liu H, Wang H, et al. Inflammation-induced up-regulation of protein kinase Cg immunoreactivity in rat spinal cord correlates with enhanced nociceptive processing. *Neuroscience* 1999;88:1267–1274.
74. Malmberg AB, Chen C, Tonegawa S, Basbaum AI. Preserved acute pain and reduced neuropathic pain in mice lacking PKC gamma. *Science* 1997;278: 279–283.
75. Meller ST, Gebhart GF. Nitric oxide (NO) and nociceptive processing in the spinal cord. *Pain* 1993;52:127–136.
76. Ji RR, Baba H, Brenner GJ, Woolf CJ. Nociceptive-specific activation of ERK in spinal neurons contributes to pain hypersensitivity. *Nat Neurosci* 1999;2:1114–1119.
77. Morgan JI, Curran T. Role of ion flux in the control of c-fos expression. *Nature* 1986;322:552–555.
78. Xin W-J, Gong Q-J, Xu J-T, et al. Role of phosphorylation of ERK in induction and maintenance of LTP of the C-fiber evoked field potentials in spinal dorsal horn. *J Neurosci Res* 2006;84:934–943.
79. Dickenson AH. NMDA receptor antagonists as analgesics. In: Fields HL, Liebeskind JC, eds. *Progress in Pain Research and Management.* Seattle: IASP Press; 1996:173–187.
80. Garthwaite J, Charles SL, Chess-Williams R. Endothelium-derived relaxing factor release on activation of NMDA receptors suggests role as intercellular messenger in the brain. *Nature* 1988;336:385–388.
81. Malmberg AB, Yaksh TL. Spinal nitric oxide synthesis inhibition blocks NMDA-induced thermal hyperalgesia and produces antinociception in the formalin test in rats. *Pain* 1993;54:291–300.
82. Eisenach JC. Aspirin, the miracle drug: Spinally, too? *Anesthesiology* 1993; 79:211–213.
83. Ji RR, Kohno T, Moore KA, Woolf CJ. Central sensitization and LTP: Do pain and memory share similar mechanisms? *Trends Neurosci* 2003;26:696–705.
84. Scholz J, Woolf C. Can we conquer pain? *Nat Neurosci* 2002;[Suppl 5]: 1062–1067.
85. Whiteside GT, Munglani R. Cell death in the superficial dorsal horn in a model of neuropathic pain. *J Neurosci Res* 2001;64:168–173.
86. Scholz J, Broom DC, Youn D-H, et al. Blocking caspase activity prevents transsynaptic neuronal apoptosis and the loss of inhibition in lamina II of the dorsal horn after peripheral nerve injury. *J Neurosci* 2005;25:7317–7323.
87. Coull JAM, Boudreau D, Bachand K, et al. Trans-synaptic shift in anion gradient in spinal lamina I neurons as a mechanism of neuropathic pain. *Nature* 2003;424:938–942.
88. Coull JAM, Beggs S, Boudreau D, et al. BDNF from microglia causes the shift in neuronal anion gradient underlying neuropathic pain. *Nature* 2005;438:1017–1021.
89. Watkins LR, Milligan ED, Maier SF. Spinal cord glia: New players in pain. *Pain* 2001;93:201–205.
90. Watkins LR, Milligan ED, Maier SF. Glial activation: A driving force for pathological pain. *Trends Neurosci* 2001;24:450–455.
91. Bennett GJ, Kajander KC, Sahara Y, et al. Neurochemical and anatomical changes in the dorsal horn of rats with an experimental painful peripheral

PART IV: PAIN MANAGEMENT

neuropathy. In: Cervero F, Bennett GJ, Headley PM, eds. *Processing of Sensory Information in the Superficial Dorsal Horn of the Spinal Cord.* Amsterdam: Plenum Press; 1989:463–471.

92. Chi SI, Levine JD, Basbaum AI. Effects of injury discharge on the persistent expression of spinal cord fos-like immunoreactivity produced by sciatic nerve transection in the rat. *Brain Res* 1993;617:220–224.

93. Mendell LM. Physiological properties of unmyelinated fiber projection to the spinal cord. *Exp Neurol* 1966;16:316–332.

94. Dickenson AH, Sullivan AF. Evidence for a role of the NMDA receptor in the frequency dependent potentiation of deep rat dorsal horn nociceptive neurons following C fiber stimulation. *Neuropharmacology* 1987;26:1235–1238.

95. Bliss TV, Lomo T. Long-lasting potentiation of synaptic transmission in the dentate area of the anaesthetized rabbit following stimulation of the perforant path. *J Physiol* 1973;232:331–356.

96. Sandkühler J. Neurobiology of spinal nociception: New concepts. In: Carli G, Zimmerman M, eds. *Progress in Brain Research.* Amsterdam: Elsevier Science; 1996:207–224.

97. Sandkühler J, Liu XG. Induction of long-term potentiation at spinal synapses by noxious stimulation or nerve injury. *Eur J Neurosci* 1998;10:2476–2480.

98. Ikeda H, Stark J, Fischer H, et al. Synaptic amplifier of inflammatory pain in the spinal dorsal horn. *Science* 2006;312:1659–1662.

99. Behbehani MM, Dollberg-Stolik O. Partial sciatic nerve ligation results in an enlargement of the receptive field and enhancement of the response of dorsal horn neurons to noxious stimulation by an adenosine agonist. *Pain* 1994;58:421–428.

100. Takaishi K, Eisele JH Jr., Carstens E. Behavioural and electrophysiological assessment of hyperalgesia and changes in dorsal horn responses following partial sciatic nerve ligation in rats. *Pain* 1996;66:297–306.

101. Laird JMA, Bennett GJ. An electrophysiological study of dorsal horn neurons in the spinal cord of rats with an experimental peripheral neuropathy. *J Neurophysiol* 1993;69:2072–2085.

102. Devor M. Neuropathic pain: What do we do with all these theories? *Acta Anaesthesiol Scand* 2001;45:1121–1127.

103. Carlton SM, Hargett GL, Coggeshall RE. Plasticity in alpha-amino-3-hydroxy-5-methyl-4-isoxazolepropionic acid receptor subunits in the rat dorsal horn following deafferentation. *Neurosci Lett* 1998;242:21–24.

104. Popratiloff A, Weinberg RJ, Rustioni A. AMPA receptors at primary afferent synapses in substantia gelatinosa after sciatic nerve section. *Eur J Neurosci* 1998;10:3220–3230.

105. Walker SM, Mitchell VA, White DM, et al. Release of immunoreactive brain-derived neurotrophic factor in the spinal cord of the rat following sciatic nerve transection. *Brain Res* 2001;899:240–247.

106. Lekan HA, Carlton SM, Coggeshall RE. Sprouting of A-beta fibers into lamina II of the rat dorsal horn in peripheral neuropathy. *Neurosci Lett* 1996;208:147–150.

107. Woolf C, Shortland P, Coggeshall RE. Peripheral nerve injury triggers central sprouting of myelinated afferents. *Nature* 1992;355:75–78.

108. Sugimoto T, Bennett GJ, Kajander KC. Transsynaptic degeneration in the superficial dorsal horn after sciatic nerve injury: Effects of a chronic constriction injury, transection, and strychnine. *Pain* 1990;42:205–213.

109. Drew GM, Siddall PJ, Duggan AW. Mechanical allodynia following contusion injury of the rat spinal cord is associated with loss of GABAergic inhibition in the dorsal horn. *Pain* 2004;109:379–388.

110. Fukuoka T, Tokunaga A, Kondo E, et al. Change in mRNAs for neuropeptides and the GABA(A) receptor in dorsal root ganglion neurons in a rat experimental neuropathic pain model. *Pain* 1998;78:13–26.

111. Willis WD, Westlund KN. Neuroanatomy of the pain system and of the pathways that modulate pain. *J Clin Neurophysiol* 1997;14:2–31.

112. Berkley KJ, Hubscher CH. Are there separate central nervous system pathways for touch and pain? *Nat Med* 1995;1:766–773.

113. Kehlet H. Acute pain control and accelerated postoperative surgical recovery. *Surg Clin North Am* 1999;79:431–443.

114. Kenshalo DR Jr., Giesler GJ Jr., Leaonard RB, Willis WD. Responses of neurons in primate ventral posterior lateral nucleus to noxious stimuli. *J Neurophysiol* 1980;43:1594–1614.

115. Willis WD. *The Pain System. The Neural Basis of Nociceptive Transmission in the Mammalian Nervous System.* Basel: Karger, 1985.

116. Craig AD, Bushnell MC, Zhang ET, Blomqvist A. A thalamic nucleus specific for pain and temperature sensation. *Nature* 1994;372:770–773.

117. Wall PD. Pain in the brain and lower parts of the anatomy. *Pain* 1995;62:389–390.

118. Davis KD, Kiss ZHT, Tasker RR, Dostrovsky JO. Thalamic stimulation-evoked sensations in chronic pain patients and in nonpain (movement disorder) patients. *J Neurophysiol* 1996;75:1026–1037.

119. Barber TX. Toward a new theory of pain: Relief of chronic pain by prefontal leucotomy, opiates, placebos and hypnosis. *Psychol Bull* 1959;56:430–460.

120. Jannetta PJ, Gildenberg PL, Loeser JD, et al. Operations on the brain and brain stem for chronic pain. In: Bonica JJ, ed. *The Management of Pain.* Philadelphia: Lea & Febiger; 1990:2082–2103.

121. Ingvar M. Pain and functional imaging. *Philosophical Transactions of the Royal Society of London: Series B: Biological Sciences (Prog Nucl Energy 6 Biol Sci)* 1999;354:1347–1358.

122. Chen AC. New perspectives in EEG/MEG brain mapping and PET/fMRI neuroimaging of human pain. *Int J Psychophysiol* 2001;42:147–159.

123. Treede RD, Kenshalo DR, Gracely RH, Jones AKP. The cortical representation of pain. *Pain* 1999;79:105–111.

124. Tracey I. Nociceptive processing in the human brain. *Curr Opin Neurobiol* 2005;15:478–487.

125. Davis KD, Wood ML, Crawley AP, Mikulis DJ. fMRI of human somatosensory and cingulate cortex during painful electrical nerve stimulation. *Neuroreport* 1995;7:321–325.

126. Jones AKP, Brown WD, Friston KJ, et al. Cortical and subcortical localization of response to pain in man using positron emission tomography. *Proc R Soc Lond Series B Biol Sci* 1991;244:39–44.

127. Talbot JD, Marrett S, Evans AC, et al. Multiple representations of pain in human cerebral cortex. *Science* 1991;251:1355–1358.

128. Di Piero V, Jones AKP, Ianotti F, et al. Chronic pain: A PET study of the central effects of percutaneous high cervical cordotomy. *Pain* 1991;46:9–12.

129. Kwiatek R, Barnden L, Tedman R, et al. Regional cerebral blood flow in fibromyalgia: Single-photon-emission computed tomography evidence of reduction in the pontine tegmentum and thalami. *Arthritis Rheum* 2000;43:2823–2833.

130. Iadarola MJ, Max MB, Berman KF, et al. Unilateral decrease in thalamic activity observed with positron emission tomography in patients with chronic neuropathic pain. *Pain* 1995;63:55–64.

131. Knecht S, Henningsen H, Hohling C, et al. Plasticity of plasticity: Changes in the pattern of perceptual correlates of reorganization after amputation. *Brain* 1998;121:717–724.

132. Lotze M, Grodd W, Birbaumer N, et al. Does use of a myoelectric prosthesis prevent cortical reorganization and phantom limb pain? *Nat Neurosci* 1999;2:501–502.

133. Price DD. Central neural mechanisms that interrelate sensory and affective dimensions of pain. *Mol Interv* 2002;2:392–402.

134. Wager TD, Rilling JK, Smith EE, et al. Placebo-induced changes in FMRI in the anticipation and experience of pain. *Science* 2004;303:1162–1167.

135. Rainville P, Duncan GH, Price DD, et al. Pain affect encoded in human anterior cingulate but not somatosensory cortex. *Science* 1997;277:968–971.

136. Petrovic P, Ingvar M. Imaging cognitive modulation of pain processing. *Pain* 2002;95:1–5.

137. Villemure C, Bushnell MC. Cognitive modulation of pain: How do attention and emotion influence pain processing? *Pain* 2002;95:195–199.

138. Kupers RC, Faymonville ME, Laureys S. The cognitive modulation of pain: Hypnosis- and placebo-induced analgesia. In: Laureys S, ed. *Progress in Brain Research.* Amsterdam: Elsevier B. V.; 2005:251–269.

139. Frohlich A, Sherrington CS. Path of impulses for inhibition under decerebrate rigidity. *J Physiol* 1902;28:14–19.

140. Watkins LR, Mayer DJ. Organization of endogenous opiate and non-opiate pain control systems. *Science* 1982;216:1185–1192.

141. Reynolds DV. Surgery in the rat during electrical analgesia induced by focal brain stimulation. *Science* 1969;164:444–445.

142. Bandler R, Shipley MT. Columnar organization in the midbrain periaqueductal gray: modules for emotional expression? *Trends Neurosci* 1994;17:379–389.

143. Mayer DJ, Liebeskind JC. Pain reduction by focal electrical stimulation of the brain: an anatomical and behavioral analysis. *Brain Res* 1974;68:73–93.

144. Ongur D, An X, Price JL. Prefrontal cortical projections to the hypothalamus in macaque monkeys. *J Comp Neurol* 1998;401:480–505.

145. An X, Bandler R, Ongur D, Price JL. Prefrontal cortical projections to longitudinal columns in the midbrain periaqueductal gray in macaque monkeys. *J Comp Neurol* 1998;401:455–479.

146. Pert JM, Snyder SH. Opiate receptor: Demonstration in nervous tissue. *Science* 1973;179:1011–1014.

147. Akil H, Richardson DE, Hughes J, Barchas JD. Enkephalin-like material elevated in ventricular cerebrospinal fluid of pain patients after analgetic focal stimulation. *Science* 1978;201:463–465.

148. Mason P. Central mechanisms of pain modulation. *Curr Opin Neurobiol* 1999;9:436–441.

149. Hohmann AG, Suplita RL, Bolton NM, et al. An endocannabinoid mechanism for stress-induced analgesia. *Nature* 2005;435:1108–1112.

150. Besse D, Lombard MC, Zakac JM, et al. Pre- and postsynaptic distribution of mu, delta and kappa opioid receptors in the superficial layers of the cervical dorsal horn of the rat spinal cord. *Brain Res* 1990;521:15–22.

151. Hori Y, Endo K, Takahashi T. Presynaptic inhibitory action of enkephalin on excitatory transmission in superficial dorsal horn of rat spinal cord. *J Physiol* 1992;450:673–685.

152. Xu XJ, Puke MJC, Verge VMK, et al. Up-regulation of cholecystokinin in primary sensory neurons is associated with morphine insensitivity in experimental neuropathic pain in the rat. *Neurosci Lett* 1993;152:129–132.

153. Smith GD, Smith MT. Morphine-3-glucuronide: Evidence to support its putative role in the development of tolerance to the antinociceptive effects of morphine in the rat. *Pain* 1995;62:51–60.

154. Basbaum AI. Mechanisms of substance P-mediated nociception and opioid-mediated antinociception. In: Stanley TH, Ashburn MA, eds. *Anesthesiology and Pain Management*. Dordrecht: Kluwer Academic; 1994:1–17.

155. Wong CS, Cherng CH, Luk HN, et al. Effects of NMDA receptor antagonists on inhibition of morphine tolerance in rats: Binding at mu-opioid receptors. *Eur J Pharmacol* 1996;297:27–33.

156. Trujillo KA, Akil H. Inhibition of morphine tolerance and dependence by the NMDA receptor antagonist MK-801. *Science* 1991;251:85–87.

157. Advokat C, Rhein FQ. Potentiation of morphine-induced antinociception in acute spinal rats by the NMDA antagonist dextrorphan. *Brain Res* 1995; 699:157–160.

158. Yaksh TL, Reddy SVR. Studies in the primate on the analgetic effects associated with intrathecal actions of opiates, alpha-adrenergic agonists and baclofen. *Anesthesiology* 1981;54:451–467.

159. Meert TF, De Kock M. Potentiation of the analgesic properties of fentanyl-like opioids with a2-adrenoceptor agonists in rats. *Anesthesiology* 1994;81:677–688.

160. Siddall PJ, Molloy AR, Walker S, et al. The efficacy of intrathecal morphine and clonidine in the treatment of pain after spinal cord injury. *Anesth Analg* 2000;91:1493–1498.

161. Sivilotti LG, Woolf CJ. The contribution of GABA A and glycine receptors to central sensitization: Disinhibition and touch-evoked allodynia in the spinal cord. *J Neurophysiol* 1994;72:169–179.

162. Lin Q, Peng YB, Willis WD. Role of GABA receptor subtypes in inhibition of primate spinothalamic tract neurons: Difference between spinal and periaqueductal gray inhibition. *J Neurophysiol* 1996;75:109–123.

163. Wilson PR, Yaksh TL. Baclofen is antinociceptive in the spinal intrathecal space of animals. *Eur J Pharmacol* 1995;51:323–330.

164. Fromm GH. Baclofen as an adjuvant analgesic. *J Pain Symptom Manage* 1994;9:500–509.

165. Cousins MJ, Miller RD. Intrathecal midazolam: An ethical editorial dilemma. *Anesth Analg* 2004;98:1507–1508.

166. Tucker AP, Mezzatesta J, Nadeson R, Goodchild CS. Intrathecal Midazolam II: Combination with intrathecal fentanyl for labor pain. *Anesth Analg* 2004;98:1521–1527.

167. Yaksh TL, Rudy TA. Narcotic analgesia produced by a direct action on the spinal cord. *Science* 1976;192:1357.

168. Stein C. Peripheral mechanisms of opioid analgesia. *Anesth Analg* 1993; 76:182–191.

169. Stein C, Millan MJ, Shippenberg TS. Peripheral opioid receptors mediating antinociception in inflammation: Evidence for involvement of mu, delta, and kappa receptors. *J Pharmacol Exp Ther* 1989;248:1269–1275.

170. Haynes TK, Appadurai IR, Power I, et al. Intra-articular morphine and bupivacaine analgesia after arthroscopic knee surgery. *Anaesthesia* 1994;49:54–56.

171. Stein C. Morphine: A local "analgesic." *Pain: Clinical Updates* 1995;3:1–4.

172. Tennant F, Moll D, Depaulo V. Topical morphine for peripheral pain. *Lancet* 1993;342:1047–1048.

173. Aasbo V, Raeder JC, Grogaard B, Roise O. No additional analgesic effect of intra-articular morphine or bupivacaine compared with placebo after elective knee arthroscopy. *Acta Anaesthesiol Scand* 1996;40:585–588.

174. Max MB. Clarifying the definition of neuropathic pain. *Pain* 2002;96:406–407.

175. Foley KM. The treatment of cancer pain. *N Engl J Med* 1985;313:84.

176. Bonica JJ. Biology, pathophysiology and treatment of acute pain. In: Lipton S, Miles J, eds. *Persistent Pain*. Orlando: Grune & Stratton; 1985:1–32.

177. Cousins MJ. Acute Pain Management. In: Phillips GD, ed. *Clinics in Critical Care Medicine*. Edinburgh: Churchill Livingstone, 1986.

178. Bonica JJ. Treatment of cancer pain: Current status and future needs. In: Fields HL, ed. *Advances in Pain Research and Therapy*. New York: Raven Press; 1985:589–616.

179. Bonica JJ. Pain of advanced cancer. In: Ventafridda V, Fields HL, eds. *Advances in Pain Research and Therapy*. New York: Raven Press, 1979.

180. Wall PD. Cancer pain: Neurogenic mechanisms. In: Fields HL, ed. *Advances in Pain Research and Therapy*. New York: Raven Press; 1985:575–587.

181. North RB, Kidd DH, Zahurak M, Piantadosi S. Specificity of diagnostic nerve blocks: A prospective, randomized study of sciatica due to lumbosacral disease. *Pain* 1996;65:77–85.

182. De Conno F, Caraceni A, Martini C, et al. Hyperalgesia and myoclonus with intrathecal infusion of high-dose morphine. *Pain* 1991;47:337–339.

183. Al-Chaer ED, Feng Y, Willis WD. A role for the dorsal column in nociceptive visceral input into the thalamus of primates. *J Neurophysiol* 1998;79:3143–3150.

184. Zeidman SM, North RB. General neurosurgical procedures for management of chronic pain. In: Raj PP, ed. *Current Review of Pain*. Philadelphia: Current Medicine; 1994:103–115.

185. Rath SA, Braun V, Soliman N, et al. Results of DREZ coagulations for pain related to plexus lesions, spinal cord injuries and postherpetic neuralgia. *Acta Neurochir (Wien)* 1996;138:364–369.

186. Urquhart E. Central analgesic activity of nonsteroidal antiinflammatory drugs in animal and human pain models. *Semin Arthritis Rheum* 1993;23:198–205.

187. Walker JS. NSAID: An update on their analgesic effects. *Clin Exp Pharmacol Physiol* 1995;22:855–860.

188. Australian and New Zealand College of Anaesthetists. *Acute Pain Management: Scientific Evidence*, 2nd ed. Sydney: ANZCA, 2005.

189. Merry A, Power I. Perioperative NSAIDs: Towards greater safety. *Pain Rev* 1995;2:268–291.

190. Royal College of Anaesthetists. *Guidelines for the Use of Non-steroidal Anti-inflammatory Drugs in the Perioperative Period*. Oxford, UK: Royal College of Anaesthetists, 1998.

191. Comfort VK, Code WE, Rooney ME, Yip RW. Naproxen premedication reduces postoperative tubal ligation pain. *Can J Anaesth* 1992;39:349–352.

192. Barden J, Edwards J, Moore RA, McQuay HJ. Single dose oral diclofenac for postoperative pain. *Cochrane Database Syst Rev* 2004:CD004768.

193. Laitinen J, Nuutinen L. Intravenous diclofenac coupled with PCA fentanyl for pain relief after total hip replacement. *Anesthesiology* 1992;76:194–198.

194. O'Hara DA, Fragen RJ, Kinzer M, Pemberton D. Ketorolac tromethamine as compared with morphine sulfate for the treatment of postoperative pain. *Clin Pharmacol Ther* 1987;41:556–561.

195. Cannon GW. Cyclooxygenase-2 selective inhibitors. *Drugs Today (Barc)* 1999;35:487–496.

196. Sinatra R. Role of COX-2 Inhibitors in the evolution of acute pain management. *J Pain Symptom Manage* 2002;24:S18–S27.

197. Barden J, Edwards JE, McQuay HJ, Moore RA. Single dose oral celecoxib for postoperative pain. *Cochrane Database Syst Rev* 2003:CD004233.

198. Chavez ML, DeKorte CJ. Valdecoxib: A review. *Clin Ther* 2003;25:817–851.

199. Barden J, Edwards J, Moore RA, McQuay HJ. Single dose oral rofecoxib for postoperative pain. *Cochrane Database Syst Rev* 2005:CD004604.

200. Rice ASC, Hill RG. New treatments for neuropathic pain. *Annu Rev Med* 2006;57:535–551.

201. Finnerup NB, Otto M, McQuay HJ, et al. Algorithm for neuropathic pain treatment: An evidence based proposal. *Pain* 2005;118:289–305.

202. Backonja MM. Local anesthetics as adjuvant analgesics. *J Pain Symptom Manage* 1994;9:491–499.

203. Kalso E, Tramèr MR, McQuay HJ, Moore RA. Systemic local-anaesthetic-type drugs in chronic pain: A systematic review. *Eur J Pain* 1998;2:3–14.

204. Chaplan SR, Bach FW, Shafer SL, Yaksh TL. Prolonged alleviation of tactile allodynia by intravenous lidocaine in neuropathic rats. *Anesthesiology* 1995;83:775–785.

205. Cahana A, Carota A, Montadon ML, Annoni JM. The long-term effect of repeated intravenous lidocaine on central pain and possible correlation in positron emission tomography measurements. *Anesth Analg* 2004;98:1581–1584.

206. Strichartz G. Protracted relief of experimental neuropathic pain by systemic local anesthetics: How, where, and when. *Anesthesiology* 1995;83:654–655.

207. Ekberg J, Jayamanne A, Vaughan CW, et al. muO-conotoxin MrVIB selectively blocks Nav1.8 sensory neuron specific sodium channels and chronic pain behavior without motor deficits. *Proc Natl Acad Sci USA* 2006; 103:17030–17035.

208. Sang CN. NMDA-receptor antagonists in neuropathic pain: Experimental methods to clinical trials. *J Pain Symptom Manage* 2000;19:S21–S25.

209. Hocking G, Cousins MJ. Ketamine in chronic pain management: An evidence-based review. *Anesth Analg* 2003;97:1730–1739.

210. Sang CN, Booher S, Gilron I, et al. Dextromethorphan and memantine in painful diabetic neuropathy and postherpetic neuralgia: Efficacy and dose-response trials. *Anesthesiology* 2002;96:1053–1061.

211. McQuay HJ, Carroll D, Jadad AR, et al. Dextromethorphan for the treatment of neuropathic pain: A double-blind randomised controlled crossover trial with integral n-of-1 design. *Pain* 1994;59:127–133.

212. Akopian AN, Abson NC, Wood JN. Molecular genetic approaches to nociceptor development and function. *Trends Neurosci* 1996;19:240–246.

213. Pezet S, Krzyzanowska A, Wong L-F, et al. Reversal of neurochemical changes and pain-related behavior in a model of neuropathic pain using modified lentiviral vectors expressing GDNF. *Mol Ther* 2006;13:1101–1109.

214. Sandkuhler J, Ruscheweyh R. Opioids and central sensitisation: I. Pre-emptive analgesia. *Eur J Pain* 2005;9:145–148.

215. Katz J, Jackson M, Kavanagh BP, Sandler AN. Acute pain after thoracic surgery predicts long-term post-thoracotomy pain. *Clin J Pain* 1996;12:50–55.

216. Dahl JB, Kehlet H. The value of pre-emptive analgesia in the treatment of postoperative pain. *Br J Anaesth* 1993;70:434–439.

217. Woolf CJ, Chong MS. Preemptive analgesia: Treating postoperative pain by preventing the establishment of central sensitization. *Anesth Analg* 1993;77:362–379.

218. Moiniche S, Kehlet H, Dahl JB. A qualitative and quantitative systematic review of preemptive analgesia for postoperative pain relief: The role of timing of analgesia [Review]. *Anesthesiology* 2002;96:725–741.

219. Dahl JB, Moiniche S. Pre-emptive analgesia. *Br Med Bull* 2004;71:13–27.

220. Bach S, Noreng MF, Tjellden NU. Phantom limb pain in amputees during the first 12 months following limb amputation. *Pain* 1988;33:297–301.

221. Bong CL, Samuel M, Ng JM, Ip-Yam C. Effects of preemptive epidural analgesia on post-thoracotomy pain. *J Cardiothorac Vasc Anesth* 2005;19:786–793.

222. Senturk M, Ozcan PE, Talu GK, et al. The effects of three different analgesia techniques on long-term postthoracotomy pain. *Anesth Analg* 2002;94:11–15.

223. Cousins MJ, Brennan F, Carr DB. Pain relief: A universal human right. *Pain* 2004;112:1–4.

CHAPTER 32 ■ PHYSIOLOGIC AND PHARMACOLOGIC SUBSTRATES OF NOCICEPTION AFTER TISSUE AND NERVE INJURY

TONY L. YAKSH

Certain classes of unconditioned stimuli that interact with visceral, somatic, or muscular sensory receptor systems give rise to a complex syndrome of behavior in the unanesthetized organism that we refer to as pain. This syndrome is frequently characterized by vocalization or efforts to escape. Stimuli able to evoke such behaviors were referred to by Sherrington as being *nociceptive* or painful.[1] An important characteristic is that such "stimuli become adequate as excitants of pain when they are of such intensity as to threaten damage to the skin." To generalize on this phenomenon, we note that other unconditioned stimuli, such as electrical stimuli, that do not produce evident damage will produce the same behavioral syndrome. We would thus conclude that these stimuli have activated portions of the circuitry that mimic the input produced by those stimuli that physically damage the organism. Similarly, instillation of bradykinin onto the cornea, reversible ischemia of cardiac muscle, or gallbladder sphincter contraction, although not necessarily leading to acute and immediate damage, produces similar response syndromes (e.g., vocalization, escape, guarding), which suggest that the organism's response to the input provided by that stimulus is similar to its response to tissue-damaging stimulus. The substrate by which these classes of information gain access to the central nervous system (CNS) and are encoded is the subject of this chapter. The behavior of the organism in context thus provides corollaries that define the "painful" nature of the stimulus. In some instances, the behavioral response reflects a defined pain state (e.g., a pain report, vocalization, guarding), but the stimulus appears inadequate. Thus, a modestly intense stimulus may evoke a response normally associated with a more intense input or a light touch may result in behavior that is normally only associated with tissue injury. In the first case, we might define this behavioral state as reflecting *hyperalgesia*, whereas in the second case, the syndrome may be referred to as *hyperalgesia* or *allodynia*. The apparent alteration of the linkage between stimulus intensity and response constitutes an important example of the dynamic characteristics of those systems that process sensory information. As will be seen, such feedback systems, when activated by repetitive afferent input or by nerve injury, can induce a powerful alteration in the stimulus–response relationship. In some instances, this modulation serves to increase the gain of the system, leading to an exaggerated response (e.g., hyperalgesia); other systems serve to downregulate the system's response and lead to a reduced pain response (analgesia). The

appreciation of this complex relationship between stimulus and response represents one of the major advances in conceptualization of the pain response to have occurred in the past 50 years. It is now apparent that one cannot consider the afferent limb through which "pain" information travels (e.g., the pain pathway) without considering those systems that modulate excitability at every level of that very transmission.

NOCICEPTION: THE BEHAVIORAL CORRELATES

Acute Stimulus

It is commonly appreciated that acute mechanical distortion (pressure), increases in temperature applied to the body surface, or acute distention of a hollow viscus will evoke (a) unlearned but organized escape response with decreasing latency/increasing reliability,[2,3] and (b) the appearance of physiologic reflexes that are evoked by small afferent input (e.g., autonomic responses—blood pressure/heart rate)[4,5] or spinal somatic reflexes (e.g., tail flick, skin twitch).[6,7] In humans, experimental stimuli, such as acute thermal or electrical stimuli, will similarly evoke responses that report pain with increasing rated intensity and increasing certainty as the electrical,[8–11] thermal,[12,13] or mechanical[14,15] stimulus intensity is increased (Fig. 32-1). These acute focal stimulus exposures, both in humans and animals, have several properties:

■ The focus of the behavior and the pain referral is typically limited to the site of stimulus exposure (e.g., it is somatotopically limited).
■ With an intense focal stimulus, it is possible that the observer will frequently report an acute sharp sensation (first pain) followed by a dull throbbing (second pain).[16,17]
■ If the stimulus is limited to a brief exposure, and if the stimulus does not itself produce a local injury, the response measure (latency, pain report) can be shown to be relatively stable over an extended sequence of exposures.
■ If the stimulus is extended, if it results in a persistent state of activity (as with a chemical stimulus that activates small afferents), or if it results in a local injury (e.g., tissue damage or a local burn), the pain report/behavior will show a

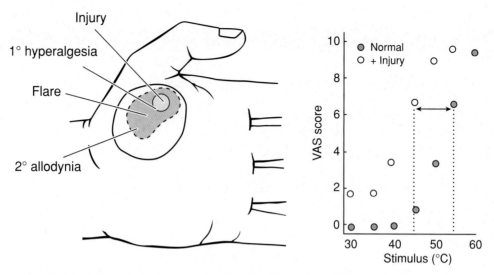

FIGURE 32-1. A thermal stimulus applied to the palm (*left*) will lead to a monotonic increase in the pain report (*right*). Following a focal injury applied to the palm, a mild spontaneous pain report will be referred to the injury site, and the montonic increase in pain report versus intensity of stimulus applied to the injury site will be shifted to the left. This is referred to as *primary hyperalgesia*. Application of a tactile stimulus in areas outside of the original injury will lead to a pain report; this is called *secondary tactile allodynia*. An area of locally increased blood flow and swelling will be noted centering on the injury site ("wheal and flare").

time-dependent enhancement, suggesting an increase in the response generated by the stimulus.[17] This phenomenon will be discussed below.

In general, then, it can be seen that with an acute high-intensity stimulus there is a corresponding faithful representation of the magnitude of the stimulus and its localization on the body surface. The sensation thus induced has great teleogical merit, as it provides an alert that will evoke a tissue-protective reaction.

Persistent Stimulus

If local tissue injury occurs as a result of the stimulus, the magnitude of the response generated by a subsequent test stimulus applied to the injury site is enhanced and a previously innocuous stimulus is reported as aversive. This post-injury state is referred to as *primary hyperalgesia*. In this state, there is (a) a reduction in the threshold needed to produce a pain response, (b) an augmented response to a suprathreshold stimulus, and (c) an ongoing pain report. Importantly, this sensitization is observed for essentially all modalities (e.g., thermal and mechanical) and tends to be localized to the immediate locality of the injury[18,19] (Fig. 32-1).

In contrast, shortly after the induction of a local injury, a region surrounding the local injury appears, substantially larger than the injury, in which low-threshold tactile (but not thermal) stimuli will evoke a significant pain report.[20] Human psychophysical studies have pursued the characteristics of this event systematically by the use of intradermally injected capsaicin. This agent is known to selectively activate C primary afferents.[21] In these studies, it has been shown that intradermal capsaicin will evoke a local primary hyperalgesia that dissipates within the hour and also a large, persistent, secondary hyperalgesia in which low-threshold tactile stimulation (but not thermal) will evoke a pain report.[18,22,23] The mechanism of this sensitization will be considered later; however, it should

be noted here that: (a) the region of secondary hyperalgesia lies considerably beyond the edge of the injury flare (e.g., the axon reflex);[24] (b) the allodynia is mediated by large afferents (e.g., mechanically evoked pain is diminished by a tourniquet that blocks large afferents);[18] and (c) the evolution of the secondary hyperalgesic state is prevented by a local anesthetic block of the region injected with capsaicin prior to the injection of capsaicin, but not after.[25] These latter observations suggest that, in the face of a local injury, there is a locally mediated enhancement of the organism's response to a given stimulus. This primary hyperalgesia is accompanied by the appearance of an extended area of sensitization in which low-intensity mechanical stimuli evoke a pain response. Animal models have similarly been employed in which a local injury, such as that induced by the injection of formalin or carrageenan into the skin,[2,26] the generation of an acute arthritic state,[27,28] a local incision,[29] or a local burn (as with ultraviolet radiation)[30,31] can evoke a prominent facilitation of pain behavior. These observations in humans and animals have striking significance in the treatment of pain states, as they suggest that prior interventions may reduce the magnitude of postinjury stimulus. Accordingly, as will be noted later, the systems activated by such protracted afferent input themselves have unique properties.

NOCICEPTIVE PROCESSING: ROSTRALLY PROJECTING SUBSTRATES

The following sections discuss the substrates through which information generated by high-intensity stimuli gains access to the neuraxis. Anatomically, the substrates may be broadly considered in terms of the primary afferents—the spinal cord, brainstem (medulla, mesencephalon, diencephalon), and cortex. In each case, one must consider the presumptive evidence associating activity in elements of that substrate with the afferent and efferent connections of that substrate and the behavioral sequelae that might be predicted secondary to the physiologic manipulations (lesion, stimulation) of that substrate.

Primary Afferent Systems

Addressed here are the anatomic, physiologic, and pharmacologic characteristics of afferents as they appear to relate to nociceptive transmission.

Primary Afferent Morphology

Myelinated versus Unmyelinated Axons. Afferent fibers can be broadly classified according to whether they are myelinated or unmyelinated. Large-diameter peripheral afferents enveloped in Schwann cell sheets range in diameter from about 6 to 14 μm in the human cutaneous nerve. Nonmyelinated fibers range in diameter from 0.2 to 2.0 μm and, although not possessing the Schwann cell investment, are commonly colocated in proximity with other small fibers within a common Schwann cell sheath (bundles of Remak). Myelinated to unmyelinated fiber ratios in cutaneous nerves are about 1:3 to 1:5 in humans.[32,33] Thus, while although the largest of myelinated fibers represent the largest area in a cross-section of nerve, numerically they are likely to constitute a relatively small proportion of the afferent pathways.

Peripheral Terminals. Afferent axons in the skin ramify profusely,[34] losing their perineural sheath. In this process, some fibers lose their Schwann cell investment and become nonmyelinated. Conduction velocities of myelinated fibers thus decrease and approach that of unmyelinated fibers when measured near their site of termination.[35–37] Large-diameter fibers typically develop specialized terminals with distinctly organized encapsulations constructed of non-neuronal elements.[38–40] However, the vast majority of nerve terminals, and certainly those deriving from unmyelinated fibers, show little morphological specialization.[40] Unmyelinated terminals show extensive branching in a horizontal layer within the superficial dermis. Axon collaterals enter the epidermal layer, with the basement membrane of the nerve terminal becoming contiguous with that of the epidermis. Unmyelinated fiber terminals are directed toward the stratum corneum, and there they lie between the juxtaposed epidermal cells.[41,42] A similar organization is observed in different target tissues such as the cornea. In tooth pulp and knee joint, both myelinated and unmyelinated fibers appear to lose their Schwann cell sheath and show prominent local branching.[20,43] Importantly, these sensory free nerve endings have been typically demonstrated to lie in close anatomic proximity to mast cells and small blood vessels (Fig. 32-2). As will be considered later, injury leads to activation of inflammatory cells and plasma extravasation, which can act upon these free nerve endings; conversely, the products released from the primary afferent terminal can degranulate mast cells and cause vasodilatation and plasma extravasation.

These nonspecialized or so-called *free nerve endings* (e.g. without specialized structures) commonly display agranular vesicles and numerous mitochondria (Fig. 32-3).[41,43–47] As will be discussed in the comments on the peripheral pharmacology of afferents, these vesicle populations provide the substrate for the release of locally active agents at the *distal* terminals of the sensory axon. It appears likely that many "free" nerve endings are characteristically sensitive to physical stimuli that evoke pain behavior. Thus, (a) tissue damage leads to activation of

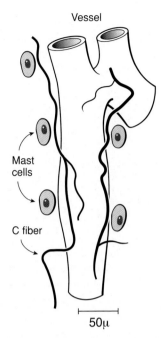

FIGURE 32-2. The fine terminals of small unmyelinated axons innervating bone. These terminals are characterized by free nerve endings that reliably terminate proximal to blood vessels and mast cells. (Derived from Heppelmann B, Messlinger K, Neiss WF, et al. Fine sensory innervation of the knee joint capsule by group III and group IV nerve fibers in the cat. *J Comp Neurol* 1995;351:415–428, with permission.)

small-diameter myelinated and unmyelinated fibers, and most small-diameter fibers end in unencapsulated terminals; and, (b) electrical, mechanical, thermal, or chemical stimuli, applied to certain structures such as the cornea or the tooth pulp, which possess few or no encapsulated endings, will evoke a pain report.[10,48–50]

Primary Afferent Neuron Morphology and Markers

Primary sensory neurons are pseudo-unipolar, with their soma located in the dorsal root ganglion (DRG) or, as in the fifth nerve, in the trigeminal ganglion. The DRG may be divided into two categories[51]: (a) large, lightly staining cells (type A), which give rise to large-diameter myelinated fibers, and (b) small, darkly staining cells (type B) from which derive the small-diameter myelinated or unmyelinated primary afferent axons.[52,53]

Morphologically, type A and type B DRG neurons have been differentiated on the basis of structural components such as relative content of granular and smooth endoplasmic reticulum and of ribosomes, neural filaments and microtubules, Golgi apparatus, and lysosomal bodies.[54]

Primary Afferent Neuron Markers

In addition to morphology, content and cell surface markers have been shown to distinguish subpopulations of afferents (Table 32-1).

Type A cell bodies associated with larger myelinated axons but not type B cells are immunopositive for the neurofilament marker RT97.

Type B DRG cells giving rise to small unmyelinated primary afferents may be subdivided into at least two relatively distinct populations by specific cell surface markers and content. In general, small afferents may contain peptides such as substance

PART IV: PAIN MANAGEMENT

TABLE 32-1

SUMMARY OF MORPHOLOGICAL MARKERS OF PRIMARY AFFERENTS

DRG designation	Type A	Type B	Type B
Morphology			
DRG size	Large	Small	Small
Myelination	Yes	No	No
Spinal projection	Laminae III–V	Lamina I and outer lamina II (IIo)	Inner portion lamina II (IIi)
Histochemistry			
Peptides	No	Yes	No
TRPV1-r (+)	No	Yes	No
IB4 (+)	No	No	Yes
Trk-r(+)	No	No	Yes
FRAP (+)	No	No	Yes
P2X3-r (+)	No	No	Yes

See text for abbreviations, references, and discussion.

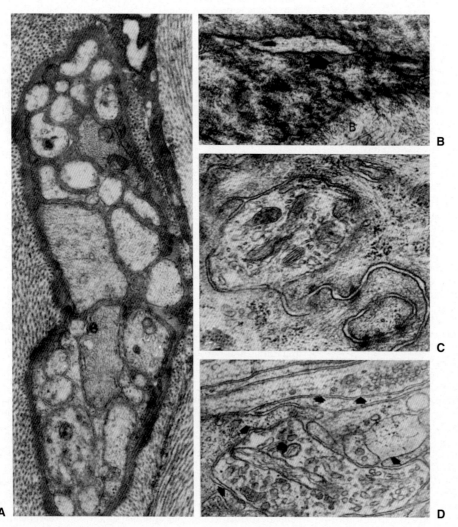

FIGURE 32-3. **A:** A nerve trunk in the stroma of the rat cornea (original magnification ×32,500); electron micrographic image displaying agranular vesicles and numerous mitochondria. **B:** An axon (*arrow*) penetrating between two basal epithelial cells (orignal magnification ×22,000). **C:** An intraepithelial axon profile containing mitochondria and agranular vesicles (original magnification ×59,100). **D:** Two intraepithelial axons (*arrows*) containing agranular vesicles (original magnification ×19,000). From Lervo T, Joo F, Huikuri KT, et al. Fine structure of sensory nerves in the rat cornea: An experimental nerve degeneration study. *Pain* 1979;6:57, with permission.

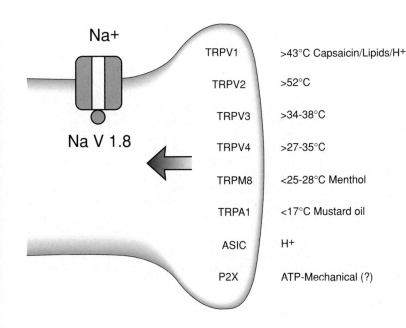

Na+

TRPV1   >43°C Capsaicin/Lipids/H+

TRPV2   >52°C

TRPV3   >34-38°C

Na V 1.8

TRPV4   >27-35°C

TRPM8   <25-28°C Menthol

TRPA1   <17°C Mustard oil

ASIC   H+

P2X   ATP-Mechanical (?)

FIGURE 32-4. Schema showing a variety of transducer channels on an afferent terminal. The range of optimal temperature activation and the various chemicals that also activate these channels are indicated. It is likely that different terminals would express different transducers, which would then define the thermal response properties of that axon. Activation of these channels can lead to a depolarization of voltage sensitive sodium (NaV) channels in the axon. Nav1.8 channels are often found in C-fibers.

P (SP), somatostatin (SST), and calcitonin gene-related peptide (CGRP), and display immunoreactivty for the transient receptor potential vanillin (TRPV1) receptors. Conversely, a second population is not peptidergic, binds to the lectin *Griffonia simplifolia* (IB4) and to the neurotrophin tropomyosin receptor kinase A (TrkA), and displays fluoride-resistant acid phosphatase (FRAP) and P_2X_3 receptors[55-65].

Primary Afferent and Axon Transport. Because axon terminals do not possess ribosomes with which to manufacture peptides and proteins, such materials are synthesized in the soma[66] and transported to the distal terminals of the neuron by means of an energy-dependent axon transport system.[67-69] Differences have not been observed between myelinated and unmyelinated fibers in the velocity or character of axon transport,[70,71] and the ability to conduct an action potential does not depend on the viability of axon transport systems. However, changes in the transport of materials to the distal terminals appear to play several important roles in the maintenance of the axon. Blockade of axon transport (as with certain neuropathy-inducing agents such as colchicine or vinblastine) results in trophic changes in axon structure.[72] Moreover, the likely role of certain peptides in primary afferent neurotransmission and the inability of nerve terminals to synthesize peptides argue for the importance of such a transport system.

Afferent Transduction and Activation Biology

Transduction. As indicated, sensory afferents may be activated by different physical stimuli or a different range of intensities for a given physical modality. This specificity results from the transduction properties of the axon terminal. Transduction is accomplished by specialized structures or receptors at the peripheral terminal. Thus, the myelinated afferent axon displays specialized nerve endings that define the characteristics of the stimulus that initiates axon depolarization (e.g., pacinian corpuscles for rapidly adapting mechanoreceptors), whereas unmyelinated axons typically show "free nerve endings." Although these terminals display no evident morphologic specialization, they will express specific transducer proteins. Thermal, mechanical, or chemical stimuli evoke excitation of the peripheral terminals through an interaction with transduction

proteins. For small sensory afferents, a series of transducing channels (TRPs) sensitive over ranges of hot, warm, cold, have been identified. In addition several channels recognize local pH (TRPV1 and the acid-sensing ion channels [ASIC]). When activated by the appropriate stimulus range, these channels pass sodium (Na+) and/or calcium (Ca2+) ions to depolarize the membrane and activate voltage sensitive sodium (NaV) channels to generate action potentials (Fig. 32-4). In addition to these channels, the terminals of primary afferents are also decorated with a wide variety of receptors for products released from local tissue after injury, inflammation, or plasma extravasation. These are reviewed later.

Action potential frequency is a function of local depolarization and hence stimulus intensity. Some channels also have associated chemical sensitivity. Consistent with the response properties endowed to the sensory axon by the channel activation profile, TRP channels with high temperature threshold profile (such as TRPV1) and with cold threshold profiles (such as TRPM8) are activated respectively by capsaicin and menthol.[73] This selective activation accounts for the psychophysical experience of heat and cold arising from local application of these two chemicals to the skin. Some transducer channel proteins (ASICs) show an enhanced activation in the presence of hydrogen ions (H+), thus accounting for the painful stinging associated with acidic solutions. Interestingly, the wound environment is often acidic. This may directly lead to activation of small afferents. In addition, the acidic environment may shift the stimulus response function of thermal transducing afferents, such that they may be activated by temperatures at or near local skin temperatures, leading to one component of post incision pain

The mechanisms of mechanical transduction are not well defined. Two mechanisms hypothesized to account for such transduction are: (a) mechanical distortion of terminal membranes may yield increased conductance in a nonspecific, large-pore, mechanically gated cation channel, leading to a depolarized membrane;[74] and (b) mechanical distortion of satellite cells releases adenosine triphosphate (ATP), which could then activate purine receptors (P_2X) on the afferent terminal.[75]

In addition to the mechanisms whereby thermal and mechanical transduction can occur, it is appreciated that a variety of chemical stimuli exist in the peri-terminal milieu, particularly

PART IV: PAIN MANAGEMENT

after tissue injury. These can activate small afferents. These chemical entities will be considered further in the discussion of the origins of activation after tissue injury and inflammation.

Action Potential Conduction. Based on conduction velocities, primary afferents have been subdivided into Aβ- (approximately 30–100 m/sec) and Aδ-fibers (approximately 4–30 m/sec). The C component consists of those fibers conducting at less than 2.5 m/sec.[76,77] Conduction velocity of a primary afferent is depdedent upon three factors: (a) axon diameter, (b) myelination, and (c) distribution of Na^+ channels. Based on classical studies, muscle afferents have been divided into the following groups on the basis of axon diameter: group 1, greater than 12 μm; group II, 6 to 12 μm; group III, 1 to 6 μm; and group IV, less than 1 μm.[78] Groups I to III are considered to be myelinated. In myelinated axons, conduction occurs between the nodes formed by adjacent Schwann cells. The larger the axon, the greater is the internodal distance and the greater the rate at which depolarization will travel over a length of axon. Given the close relationship between axon diameter in myelinated/unmyelinated axons and conduction velocities, the following relationships are normally accepted: group I, no sensory homolog; group II, Aβ; group III, Aδ; and group IV, C (Table 32-2).

Action potential conduction in primary afferents is dependent upon several families of voltage-gated sodium channels (VGSC; NaV). These channels consist of tetramers constructed of α and β subunits. Multiple subunits (10 α and three β) define the gating properties of the channel, ion selectivity, and its pharmacology. All VSGC are blocked by agents such as lidocaine, but the channels may be divided into those that are tetrodotoxin-resistant (NaV 1.8 and NaV 1.9) and those that are tetrodotoxin (TTX)-sensitive (the remainder). Molecular techniques have shown that NaV1.6 and NaV1.7 are present in virtually all sensory neurons. NaV1.1 is preferentially expressed in large-diameter sensory neurons; NaV1.8 and NaV1.9, the TTX-resistant channels, are only present in small-diameter neurons. The gating properties of the channels are strongly regulated by phosphorylation at a number of consensus sites. Thus, such phosphorylation can lead to a lowering of depolarization thresholds and an increase in the duration of the channel opening. Such phosphorylation can thus lead to an increase in action potential frequency for any given depolarizing stimulus[79].

Response Properties of the Primary Afferents

The functional characteristics of the primary affferents may be stated in terms of these notable properties:

TABLE 32-2

SUMMARY OF THE SENSORY AFFERENTS AND THEIR CHARACTERISTICS

Receptor type	Effective stimulus	Background activity	Range of conduction velocity (m/sec)	Selected references
Cutaneous mechanoreceptors				
Type I	Indentation of dome	0	30–90	90,199
Type II	Skin deformation	+	30–70	90,199
C mechanoreceptors	Skin indentation	0	<1	866
Meissner corpuscle and Krause end-bulb	Skin indentation	0	40–80	89,867
Pacinian corpuscle	Vibration	0	50–80	89,199
Cutaneous nociceptors				
Aδ mechanical	Damage	0	5–60	198,199
C mechanical	Damage	0	<1	109,198
Aδ heat	Noxious heat or mechanical damage	0	4–40	36,198
C polymodal	Noxious heat; mechanical algesic agents	0	<1	87,122,868
Warm	Increased temperature	+		
Muscle nociceptors				
Group III	Pressure; damage	+/0	60–90	212
Group IV	Pressure; damage	+/0	<2.5	213
Group III	Pressure; damage	+/0	60–90	212
Group IV	Pressure; damage	+/0	<2.5	213
Joint nociceptors				
Aδ	Extreme bending		<30	262
Visceral mechanoreceptors				
Intestine	Distention, tension on mesentry or blood vessels (intestine)	+/0	<1–30	335,869,870
Bladder	Distention or contraction	+/0	<2–20	335,871
Visceral nociceptors				
Intestine	Intense mechanical, thermal, and chemical stimuli	+/0		335

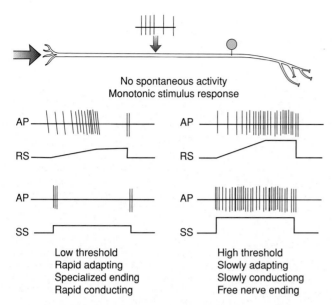

No spontaneous activity
Monotonic stimulus response

AP

RS

AP

SS

Low threshold
Rapid adapting
Specialized ending
Rapid conducting

AP

RS

AP

SS

High threshold
Slowly adapting
Slowly conductiong
Free nerve ending

FIGURE 32-5. Response (action potentials) of a low-threshold primary afferent to a ramped (*RS*) and steady state (*SS*) stimulus. The axon on the left is realtively low-threshold and rapidly adapting, whereas the axon on the right is relatively high-threshold and slowly adapting. Neither axon shows activity in the absence of a stimulus.

▤ Under control conditions, in which little or no stimulus is present, and no injury or inflammation occurs, little or no ongoing activity occurs. Under resting conditions, such spontaneous discharge frequencies may be on the order of 0.1 Hz or less.
▤ In the face of a stimulus of the appropriate modality, the sensory axon will display an increasing frequency of discharge, with the rate of discharge increasing monotonically over a range of stimulus intensities.

The content of the message delivered by a specific axon will depend upon not only the frequency of its discharge, but on its connectivity as well. Thus, a high-threshold and low-threshold A∂ axon may have similar firing rates at two different temperatures, each of which is associated with distinct psychophysical experiences (Fig. 32-5). Although the axons are often functionally subdivided into low- and high-threshold responsiveness (Fig. 32-5), the transduction response profiles of different members of a population of afferents may range relatively continuously between the two extremes.

Correlation of Behavior and Sensory Afferent Activity

Direct Activation of Axons. Electrical stimulation that produced synchronous volleys in high-threshold cutaneous afferents (and therefore slowly conducting and of small diameter) evoked massive sympathetic discharges and pseudo-affective responses even in lightly anesthetized animals,[77] suggesting that the activation was associated with a noxious stimulus. In humans, stimulation that evoked only fast-conducting volleys in cutaneous nerves gave rise to sensations of tickling or light pressure, whereas stimulation that evoked fast and slow components resulted in pain.[80,81] High-intensity stimulation applied during selective blockade of large-diameter fibers by anoxia, leaving Aδ- and or C-fibers active, produces a short-lasting pain of a pricking nature. The sensation appears similar to that often reported as "first" pain. Activation limited to more slowly

conducting fiber populations (C or group IV) gave rise to dull, diffusely localized sensations that were likened to burning or so-called "second pain".[81–87]

Afferent activity evoked by stimuli associated with behavioral signs of pain. Although electrical activation of gross fiber populations may produce pain, it does not necessarily follow that when a high-intensity somatic stimulus is applied, specific afferent populations are activated, or that their specific activation is uniquely correlated with pain sensations. Using single-unit recording in human nerve fascicles in situ, it has been shown that stimuli that produce sensations of light touch or vibration are accompanied by the activation of rapidly conducting afferents.[88–91] Needle pricks associated with verbal reports of marked discomfort evoked rapid firing in C cutaneous afferents (0.5–1.5 m/sec). Chemical (acetic acid or intradermal histamine) or thermal stimuli that produce reports of pain or itch activate populations of slowly conducting fibers.[83–87,92] Such investigations have provided a number of insights:

▤ Activation of only a few C fibers appears not to be sufficient to evoke a pain report.[92,93]
▤ Although the activation of fibers conducting at velocities corresponding to Aδ- and C-fibers is a prerequisite for evoking somatic pain in humans, activity in all slowly conducting fibers is not uniquely associated with a pain event. Populations of slowly conducting afferents communicate information on warmth, cooling, or muscle pressure,[35,39] stimulus conditions that are not normally aversive. This heterogeneity is emphasized in Table 32-2, where the classes of afferents (as defined by conduction velocity) are correlated with the categories of "natural" stimuli that result in their excitation.
▤ Electrical or mechanical stimulation sufficient to activate a slowly conducting component of a compound action potential and evoke a pain event will also evoke activity in rapidly conducting afferent fibers.

Although these observations indicate that the pain report may be obtained in the absence of large fibers, they cannot absolutely exclude them from a role in characterizing the pain event. Thus, prolonged intense mechanical stimuli will give rise to an initial burst of activity in low-threshold afferents which, unlike in the small-diameter fibers, is not sustained. High-frequency stimulation of the sural nerve, at an intensity at which the electrical stimulus was just sufficient to generate a rapidly conducting volley (Aβ), was adequate to provoke reports of pricking pain.[94] Finally, in Fabry disease, in which small-diameter fibers are damaged and the largest fibers remain functional, pain sensations remain.[32,95,96]

Factors Influencing Afferent Activity after Tissue Injury

As noted in the preceding section, mechanical stimuli producing extreme distortion of the skin, or thermal stimuli greater than 42°C to 48°C, will evoke a stimulus-dependent activation of small sensory afferents and a correlated increase in pain behavior. Although such stimuli constitute an important element in the sensory environment of the organism, it is clear that, following tissue injury, there appears a persistent low level of discharge in these small afferents, and, not infrequently, these axons will show an exaggerated response to a subsequent mechanical or thermal stimulus. An example of such an altered stimulus–response relationship is shown in Figure 32-6.[97,98] Of particular interest, systematic studies have revealed that it is often possible to identify slowly conducting afferents with thresholds that exceed the maximum possible mechanical stimulus. In the face of inflammation, however, such axons have

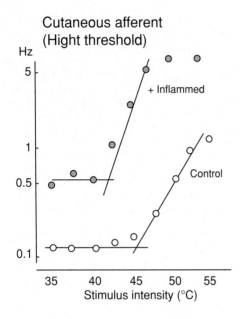

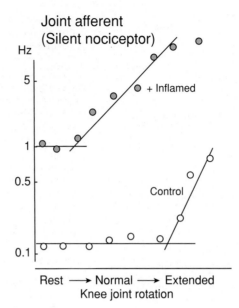

FIGURE 32-6. Firing of small afferent in the skin at increasing temperatures (*left*) or in the articular nerve innervating the knee across degree of joint rotation ranging from normal to hyperextended (*right*). Following the injection of carageenan into the skin or the knee, the afferent shows increasing spontaneous activity, a left shift, and an increase in the slope of the stimulus response curve, indicating a facilitated response to thermal stimuli, such that a modest thermal stimulus or joint rotation yields prominent activity.

been shown to develop spontaneous activity and an exquisite sensitivity to subsequent mechanical stimulation. These axons, frequently found in joint afferents (see following), have been designated as "silent nociceptors."[99] These observations, in conjunction with the observed chemical sensitivity of the small afferent, suggest that the contents of the "inflammatory soup"[100] that has been identified in inflamed tissue may play an important role in the afferent message generated in the post-injury pain state. There are two components to this consideration: (a) the nature of the materials that are elaborated and (b) the effect of these products on afferent activity and pain behavior.

The Post-Injury State. A common result of a high-intensity thermal or mechanical stimulus is tissue damage. This state is defined by Lewis[101] as a "triple response": a flush at the site of the stimulus accompanied by a flare resulting from widespread arterial dilation and a local edema secondary to increased vascular permeability. This state of inflammation is often accompanied by a local decrease in the magnitude of the stimulus required to elicit a pain response, that is, a primary hyperalgesia,[102,103] referred to by Lewis[101] as "nocifensor tenderness." The region of primary hypersensitivity is often surrounded by a much larger region of secondary hypersensitivity[101] (Fig. 32-1). Evidence that at least a fraction of these phenomena were mediated by a peripheral mechanism derives from the following observations: (a) antidromic electrical activation of sensory afferent fibers produces hypersensitivity and flare in the skin region innervated by the nerve, and (b) blockade of the nerve central to the site of antidromic stimulation does not block the hypersensitivity evoked by such nerve stimulation.[104] Because the antidromic volley evokes a primary hyperalgesia and vasodilation in the absence of sympathetic innervation, and the required stimulation intensities evoke discharges in C fibers, it appears likely that the effects are mediated by unmyelinated somatic afferents.[104–106] Lewis[104] presciently suggested that primary hypersensitivity was due to the release of algogenic agents from damaged tissue and from nerve terminals in the skin by means of an axon reflex activated by the proximate tissue damage. In this case, it is suggested that action potentials evoked in the terminals of a sen-

sory fiber located in the damaged regions travel not only back to the spinal cord, but also antidromically into the surrounding vascular bed by means of axon collaterals. This is associated with the release of a vasodilator agent that increases blood flow (thereby producing the flare), increases vascular permeability (producing edema), and, as a result of either a direct effect or a subsequent release of an intermediate agent, activates or facilitates the activation of peripheral sensory afferent terminals (hypersensitivity). The local release of chemical intermediates, as just suggested, may also explain the occurrence of continued sensation after the primary stimulus (e.g., thermal or mechanical) has been removed. Thus, mild heat damage to the receptive fields has been shown to produce significant increases in the excitability of polymodal nociceptors (C-fibers, see following)[107–110] and high-threshold mechanoreceptors.[111] As noted earlier, the parodoxical discharges of cold receptors to noxious heat also display sensitization.[112] A chemical intermediary with a prolonged half-life that alters the environs of the adjacent nerve terminals and facilitates their activity could explain one component of the accompanying hyperalgesia.

Agents Released after Injury and Their Action on Afferents and Behavior. Endogenous agents that may mediate these algogenic and facilitatory effects can be categorized according to their chemical class and their presumed origin, for example: tissue (serotonin, histamine, potassium, H+, members of the arachidonic acid [AA] cascade), plasma (kinins, adenosine), or nerve terminals (SP, CGRP). This listing is meant only to be representative and is neither inclusive nor exclusive.[113] Nevertheless, it provides some sense of the complexity of the chemical milieu that occurs after a local tissue injury (Figs. 32-4 and 32-7).

Potassium/hydrogen. Tissue injury results in prominent release of intracellular potassium (K+) and a lowering of tissue pH. Following intense exercise or burns, for example, extracellular K may reach high mM concentrations.[114,115] Blister base fluid and the pH of the wound environment may display pH values as low as 4 or 5 in cardiac ischemia, fracture-related hematomas, and exercising muscle.[116] The mechanisms of this increase probably reflect failure of cell membrane integrity and

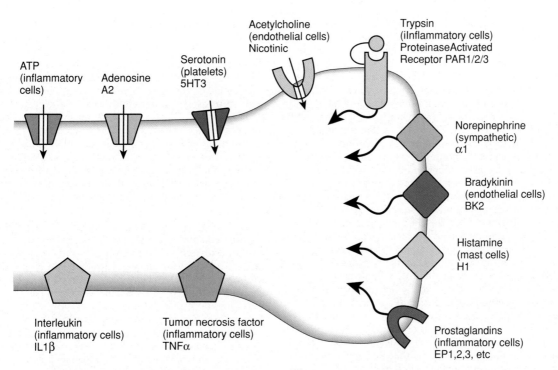

FIGURE 32-7. Schema showing a variety of receptor channels on an afferent terminal. A variety of active products are released in the face of local injury and inflammation. These act upon eponymous ionotrophic (ligand-activated channels indicated by channel/arrow) and metabotrophic (indicated by intracellular tail) receptors to depolarize the terminal and/or act through a variety of kinases to enhance terminal depolarization evoked by a given stimulus.

dysfunction of the Na/K pump function.[114] A population of C-nociceptors sensitive to noxious intensities of mechanical and thermal stimuli also responds in a stimulus-related fashion to solutions of increasing proton concentration injected into their receptive fields. These receptors develop a lower threshold and enhanced response to mechanical stimuli. Similar injections in humans induce a sustained graded pain and hyperalgesia. Increasing evidence suggests that agents such as capsaicin may interact directly with peripheral terminal membranes to increase proton conductance.

Amines. Histamine (granules of mast cells, basophils, and platelets) and serotonin (mast cells and platelets) are released by mechanical trauma, heat, radiation, and certain by-products of tissue damage, most notably neutrophil lysosomal materials, certain immunologic processes, thrombin, collagen, and epinephrine, as well as by lipid acids of the AA cascade, such as the leukotrienes; the prostaglandins (PG),[117–120] histamine, and acetylcholine have all been shown to excite primary afferents. Close intra-arterial injection of serotonin excites populations of cutaneous mechanoreceptive and high-threshold afferents.[121,122] Similar administration of histamine was shown to excite populations of C-fiber/group IV cutaneous mechanoreceptors and nociceptors sensitive to thermal and mechanical stimuli, but not myelinated (presumably non-noxious) mechanoreceptive afferents.[123,124] Administration of the phenethylamine compound 48/80, which releases histamine from mast cells, activated small-diameter fiber nociceptors.[109] A variety of agents (acetylcholine, histamine, serotonin) injected into the ear of a rabbit isolated from the body except for its nerve supply evoked a reflex depressor response indicative of the activation of small-diameter cutaneous nociceptive

afferents.[125] Direct application of histamine or serotonin onto a blister base induced by cantharidin, or the direct injection of these agents into the skin, induced a significant pain response in humans.[126–128] In dogs, the intra-arterial but not the intravenous injection of serotonin and histamine induced pseudo-affective responses (barking, efforts to escape, pupil dilatation)[129] (Fig. 32-1), the most potent agent being brady-kinin.[129]

Kinins. Bradykinin is synthesized by the cascade that is triggered when factor XII is activated by agents such as kallikrein and trypsin. In the course of the cascade, even more kallikrein is produced; this is converted to bradykinin by the enzyme timenogenase.[130,131] Bradykinin is released by noxious insult.[2,132,133] The local injection of bradykinin has been shown to have potent stimulatory effects in small afferents.[122,134–136] After intra-arterial injection in the dog or application in the blister base in humans,[137] bradykinin produces potent pseudo-affective pain behavior. This activity in producing pain behavior and the elaboration of bradykinin during the injury state has led to considerable speculation as to its role in sustaining post-injury evoked activity. Pharmacologic investigations have emphasized the existence of two bradykinin receptors (B_1/B_2^{138}). It appears that, under normal circumstances, pharmacologic studies have indicated a preponderance of B_2 sites, which can activate small afferents, whereas in the face of continued inflammation, an upregulation of B_1 sites appears to occur.[139,140]

Lipidic acids. Prostanoids are synthesized upon the release of cell membrane–derived AA by the activation of phospholipase A.[141] Various agents, including norepinephrine and dopamine, stimulate the synthesis of cellular phospholipids by releasing nonesterified free fatty acid precursors.[142,143] Membrane-bound enzymes, lipoxygenase[144] or cyclooxygenase (COX), act on these substrates to synthesize the leukotrienes and the prostanoids. Agents such as acetylsalicylic acid and indomethacin inhibit COX[145–147] and prevent the synthesis of these agents. Elevated levels of PGs and leukotrienes are found following local injury and inflammation in joints and damaged skin.[133,148,149] Local intra-arterial bradykinin will enhance the formation and release of PGs.[150–153] Prostaglandins injected alone evoked little pain response except in high doses.[154–156] Although these prostanoids commonly have little evocative effect, they readily facilitate the pseudo-affective and autonomic responses produced by intra-arterial administration of bradykinin in dogs and rabbits.[125,155,157] Thus, in the knee joint, PGI_2 will excite and facilitate the responsiveness of slowly conducting joint afferents.[136] In the behaving animal, intradermal injections of PGE_1 augmented the pain evoked by peripheral injections of bradykinin and histamine,[158] the writhing response evoked by intraperitoneal phenylbenzylquinone,[159,160] and the response to pressure in the rat's inflamed paw[161,162] and on the dog's inflamed knee joint.[157] Perfusion of the receptive field of a thermal nociceptive afferent with PGE_2 did not alter its resting discharge. However, PGE_2 produced a dose-dependent increase in the discharge rate of the fiber in response to a stimulus.[163] Similarly, the simultaneous administration of PGE_1 and bradykinin, each in a dose that by itself was ineffective, produced significant activity in afferent fibers.[164] That some or all of bradykinin's algogenic effects may be mediated or potentiated by PGs is suggested by a nociceptive response to the kinin being blocked by prior treatment with a COX inhibitor.[155,157,165] If the PGs produce their sensitizing effects by a common biochemical mechanism in a different species and several organ systems, a common order of potency for the lipidic acids should be observed. Where examined, the following rank order has, in fact, been typically observed: $PGE_1 > PGE_2 > PGF_{2a}, 2\ PGF_{2B}\ 2\ PGA_1 = PGB_2 = PGI_2 = 0$.[125,155,157,162,166]

Adenosine. Adenosine has been shown to be released post-muscle ischemia after exercise, correlating with a reported pain state.[167] Conversely, treatment with a nonselective adenosine receptor antagonist, theophylline, reduced the pain associated with ischemic pain of the forelimb.[168]

Cytokines. Injury and the evolution of the inflammatory state, or local skin injury, will lead to the release into the local extracellular fluid of a number of cytokines such as epidermal growth factor, tumor necrosis factor (TNF)-α, and a number of interleukins (IL), including IL1 and IL8.[169–171] It appears certain that their local interactions can lead to the release of PGs, which can subsequently activate small afferents. This interaction provides mechanisms whereby general immune reactions can be affiliated with activity in small afferents (such as, perhaps, the aching sensation associated with influenza, or the reaction to foreign bodies, as in chimeric antibody therapy for cancer).

Proteinases. Thrombin or trypsin is released from macrophages and mast cells after local injury. These peptidases can cleave tethered peptide ligands that exist on the surface of small primary afferents. These tethered peptides act upon adjacent receptors (proteinase-activated receptors [PARs]) that can serve to depolarize the terminal, causing an orthodromic input and local release of SP and CGRP into the injured tissues.[172,173] These receptors are present on both terminals of the primary afferents modulating the spinal as well as the peripheral sensitivity of the afferent terminal.[174]

Growth factors. Nerve growth factor (NGF) is upregulated in a wide variety of inflammatory conditions in inflammatory cells and Schwann cells and, when released, acts upon TrkA), which is expressed on the terminals of primary afferents. The Trk receptor activates several intracellular signaling cascades, which increase the nociceptor's sensitivity and acts through retrograde transport to initiate delayed and persistent transcriptional processes. This is likely responsible for upregulation of the sensory neuropeptides and neuromodulators (e.g., CGRP, SP, brain-derived neurotrophic factor [BDNF]), receptors (e.g., TRPV1, P_2X), and ion channels (e.g., NaV). With local inflammation, NGF leads to an upregulation of BDNF in TrkA-expressing sensory neuron. Brain-derived neurotrophic factor itself can be released and exert downstream effects.[175]

Afferent peptides. Substance P and CGRP are peptides found in peripheral afferent C-fiber terminals in the skin,[176–178] cortical blood vessels,[179,180] tooth pulp,[181] and eye.[182] Peptide levels in the peripheral tissues are typically elevated in inflamed tissues and joints.[183] Antidromic sensory stimulation has been shown to release SP or CGRP in a variety of peripheral tissues, including tooth pulp,[184] knee joint,[185] skin,[186] and trachea.[187] Importantly, a stimulus that serves to activate the nerve terminal will itself yield the release of the afferent peptide.[187]

With regard to the effects of the afferent peptides, SP has been shown not to be algogenic when administered peripherally,[188] and will not activate peripheral nociceptive afferents.[189] However, it has been shown that conditioning a nerve terminal with SP will result in a facilitation of the response of the terminal to subsequent chemical mediators.[190] Aside from a direct terminal interaction, locally released afferent peptides can serve to alter the local milieu. However, antidromic afferent nerve stimulation will produce flare and sensitization in the region of skin innervated by the stimulated sensory nerve.[191] Exogenously administered SP has been shown to induce plasma extravasation in both normal and denervated skin,[188] and because other peptides, such as vasoactive intestinal peptide (VIP), do not produce such extravasation,[176] SP appears to be a likely mediator for the neurogenically evoked increase in capillary wall permeability. Administration of capsaicin interacts with the TRPV1 receptor present on the terminals of SP- and CGRP-containing C-fibers. This binding will activate and then frequently destroy these terminals. Accordingly, a subsequent depletion of SP/CGRP content occurs in skin.[176] This peptide depletion is accompanied by a loss of the ability of peripheral nerve stimulation to produce extravasation.[192,193] Exogenously administered SP/CGRP or antidromic stimulation of the sensory afferent evokes an increase in local blood flow and capillary permeability. The effects of either manipulation are reversed by these peptide antagonists.[194,195] These observations reflect mechanisms that may be quite common. Thus, the SP/CGRP in plexuses surrounding cerebral vessels and those which originate in the trigeminal ganglion may be released and occasion the vascular component of migraine.[180] Aside from their effects upon the vasculature, the locally released peptides may serve to bring into play a number of systems that may subsequently interact with the afferent terminal. Thus, antidromic stimulation and SP can degranulate mast cells and evoke kinin release.[196] As noted previously, the peptidergic primary afferent terminal in the skin and joint is frequently in close apposition with both blood vessel and mast cells (Fig. 32-2).

Sensory Innervation Excited by Natural Stimuli

Table 32-2 presents a summary of the classes of afferents activated by various physical stimuli capable of evoking pain behavior. In the following section, characteristics of these afferents as a function of their respective innervated organs are discussed.

Cutaneous Stimuli. The cutaneous input is richly innervated by afferents that transduce a variety of stimulus modalities.

Mechanosensitive afferents. High-threshold mechanoreceptive fibers responding only at pressure sufficient to produce damage to innervating glabrous tissue and conducting in the range of Aδ-fibers (15–25 m/sec) have been identified.[39,122,197–199] These afferents tend to respond with a rate of discharge proportional to the magnitude of the pressure applied. Receptive fields for these mechanoreceptors are large in the trunk (1–8 cm[200]) and smaller on the face (1–2 cm[200]); on the limbs, distal receptive fields tend to be smaller than proximal fields. Mechanoreceptors conducting at C-fiber velocities have been shown with thresholds requiring von Frey hair stimuli greater than 2 g and with receptive fields ranging from small (5 mm[200]) to strips covering several square centimeters. These fibers discharge with a frequency that is monotonically proportional to the stimulus intensity.[109,198]

Thermoreceptive afferents. Warm receptors with small peripheral receptive fields (<0.5 mm in diameter) have been observed that respond to temperature increments of less than 1°C within the range of 30°C to 40°C.[201] These fibers have also been shown to respond to thermal stimuli of noxious intensity with an increasing frequency of discharge. High-intensity stimulation within the range of 47°C to 51°C evokes a transient high-frequency discharge. These response characteristics are to be differentiated from those reported for the mechanical–thermal receptive units (see following) in that the response rate commonly is all or none in character.[202,203] Certain afferent cutaneous fibers that respond to decreases in temperature on the order of less than 1°C (i.e., "cold" receptors) may show a paradoxical response to heat. As skin temperature rises to 45°C to 52°C, the fiber's rate of discharge also increases.[112,204–206]

Mechanothermoreceptive nociceptive afferents. Afferents have been reported to respond to high-intensity mechanical and thermal stimulation, conduct within an Aδ range (10–40 m/sec), and exhibit a positively accelerating monotonic stimulus response function.[39,121] The activation threshold may lie between 40°C and 60°C, and a maximum response is commonly observed at 45°C to 53°C.[36,198,202,203] Receptive fields for these units are small (<5 mm[200]) and frequently occur as several spots, suggesting extensive collateralization of the terminals. These afferents may mediate the "first" pain of heat, for example, the pricking sensation reported immediately after the application of a strong thermal stimulus.[207]

Polymodal C-fiber afferents. A major portion of C-fiber afferents that respond to nociceptive stimuli are "polymodal" in character. These fibers may constitute 80% to 90% of the primate nociceptive C-fiber population.[108] These axons are activated equally well by several classes of stimuli, including mechanical (>1 g), thermal (45°–53°C), and frequently chemical stimuli applied to the characteristically small (<3 mm[200]) receptive field. The response to such ongoing stimuli is a sustained, vigorous discharge, in which the frequency is monotonically related to stimuli intensity.[107–109,208]

Recordings in humans from single afferents conducting in the range of 0.5 to 2.0 m/sec have been made from sensory nerves innervating nonglabrous skin. These fibers are activated by strong mechanical stimuli (von Frey hairs of 0.7–13 g; nee-

dle pricks; and local compression) and produce an ongoing discharge that adapts slowly in the presence of the sustained stimulus.[83–87,92,93] Such units are not spontaneously active at temperatures up to 40°C, but temperatures in excess of 45°C evoke activity in an increasing number of units.[83,92,93] Local application of acid, histamine, or potassium chloride evokes a prolonged discharge.[83,92,93] Receptive fields of polymodal C afferents tend to be larger in humans (1 mm–1 cm[200]) but frequently may also display several sites, suggesting extensive collateralization.[83,85,87,92] These slowly conducting fibers, presumably unmyelinated in character, show clear signs of fatigue and failure of conduction upon repeated high-frequency electrical stimulation.[84,86]

Skeletal Muscle. It has been reported that, excluding the stretch receptors, the principal sensory innervation of the skeletal muscle derives from free nerve endings in fascia and the adventitia of blood vessels that arise from myelinated and nonmyelinated fibers.[209] High-threshold groups III and IV mechanoreceptors in muscle activated by intense contraction have been reported.[189,210] Intense thermal stimuli applied to muscle belly evokes monotonically increasing activity in these afferents.[211] Hypertonic solutions of sodium chloride[212] and close intra-arterial injections of a number of algogenic agents (histamine, bradykinin, and serotonin) evoke significant activity in afferent groups III and IV.[124,135,213] However, the terminals are not functionally homogeneous. At least three groups of afferents have been identified: (a) those activated by algogenic agents but not by muscle activity, (b) those activated by muscle activity but not by algogenic agents, and (c) those activated by both sustained muscle activity and algogenic agents.[214] The sensitivity to chemical agents makes it likely that these nociceptive groups III and IV afferents are activated by agents that are released locally during muscle contraction. Extracellular K levels double (5–15 mM) during isometric testing in the cat.[215] Failure of nominal concentrations of phosphate and lactate to alter group IV afferent activity suggests that metabolic by-products alone do not constitute a source of muscle pain.[214] The apparent ability of PGs to sensitize algogenic receptors to otherwise inactive concentrations of chemical stimulants in cardiac muscle (see following), and the likelihood of their release during intense skeletal muscle contraction, could be a significant factor in the activation of groups III and IV skeletal muscle afferents by metabolic by-products.

Cardiac Muscle. The heart receives afferents that travel with both the parasympathetic and the sympathetic tree. In the latter, the cell bodies are in the nodose ganglia, and in the former, the cell bodies are in the respective thoracic dorsal root ganglia. Pain arising from the heart appears to be mediated to a significant degree by activity in the sympathetic afferents, but vagal afferents may play an important, if undefined, role.[216] Occlusion of the coronary artery leading to ischemia of ventricular muscle produces pain in humans[217,218] and pseudo-affective response in animals.[219] Sensory afferents in the inferior cardiac nerve projecting to the T1–T5 segments of the spinal cord mediate the transmission of such information.[220–223] Recording single units from the T2–T3 ramus communicans reveals that, during coronary occlusions, activity in Aδ/C afferents increases.[224–226] The cardiac afferents are activated by moderate- to high-intensity mechanical stimulation,[225,227,228] noxious heating,[229] and several algogenic agents.[229–231] The stimulus for angina may be the release from ischemic muscle of humoral factors that sensitize or activate cardiac afferents. Serotonin and histamine stimulate cardiac afferent fibers,[229,232,233] and blood levels of bradykinin in the coronary sinus after occlusion are sufficient to evoke pseudo-affective responses when administered in dogs.[129,226,234,235] In the heart, reflex cardiovascular changes suggestive of angina discomfort occur following the topical application of several algogenic agents to the wall of the left ventricle, and temporary occlusion of the coronary artery supplying the area of the ventricle under study sensitizes the heart to the algogenic effects of bradykinin.[209] Importantly, coapplication of PGs (PGE$_1$ >PGE$_2$ >PGF$_{2a}$) with bradykinin has significantly potentiated the algogenic effects of bradykinin. Pretreatment with a PG synthesis inhibitor reduced the algogenic effects of bradykinin and the sensitizing effects of prior ischemia. The potentiation of bradykinin's algogenic effects by exogenous PGs was evident for as long as 60 minutes and could not be attenuated by indomethacin. This is consistent with the observation that PGs are formed and released in the heart muscle following hypoxia or ischemia.[236-238] Thus, angina could speculatively result, in part, from the neurohumoral activation of afferent terminals by the joint release of both PGs and bradykinin.

Teeth. Innervation of the teeth occurs both intradentally (within the tooth) and periodontally (within the surrounding connective tissue). Free nerve endings are found within the pulp and the surrounding blood vessels. Fibers that originate in afferent plexuses adjacent to the inner dentinal surface pass through the odontoblasts to the dentinal tubules that run parallel to the odontoblast processes.[239,240] In tooth pulp, the unmyelinated fibers are ensheathed by Schwann cells and interlace with the odontoblast somata. Tooth pulp afferents consist of fibers having diameters and apparent conduction velocities in the Aδ- and C-fiber range.[241-244] The periodontal afferents travel through the maxillary and mandibular branches of the trigeminal nerve to terminate within collagen fibers of the alveolar ligament, with specializations similar to the Meissner corpuscle. Transdentinal electrical stimulation produces a sharp pain of brief duration,[10] which gives rise to jaw opening and closing reflexes and attempts to escape.[245-247] In shock titration paradigms, primates maintain the current intensity of dental stimulation at or immediately above that intensity which, in a single escape paradigm, will support escape behavior.[248] These observations correspond to studies in humans suggesting that the difference between a perceivable threshold stimulus (prepain) and a stimulus sufficient to evoke a pain report is small.[48,49] Conversely, activity in intradentinal sensory nerves has been shown to correlate closely with the sensation of pain.[249] Pressure, touch, or tooth movement is likely to be mediated by afferents from the periodontal and gingival structures in which the tooth is embedded.[250,251]

Thermal stimulation of teeth has been reported to evoke neuronal activity in dental nerves.[252,253] In cats, the frequency of discharge of dental afferents rose when the dentin temperature was elevated from 34°C to 37°C within a 10-second period.[254] Slow heating of the cat tooth surface to 47°C failed to elicit such activity.[255] Repeated intense thermal stimulation of the tooth (60°C), however, did evoke a persistent afferent discharge. Pretreatment, but not posttreatment, with prostaglandin synthesis inhibitors reduced the discharge associated with repetitive heating.[256] The generation of COX products may therefore sensitize nerve endings to stimuli originating in the local pulpal environment. Because nerve endings do not penetrate to the enamel dentin interface, the effective stimulus in tooth sensations has been proposed to be the distortion of odontoblasts or alterations in hydraulic flow produced by changes in temperature.[257] Inflammation or edema associated with thermal damage, as just described, or direct pressure could increase pulpal volume and deform the mechanically sensitive nerve terminals that lie between the odontoblasts. That changes in pulpal pressure can evoke activity in tooth afferents is supported by the observations that (a) bursts of spikes occur in synchrony with the systolic pulse and (b) pulpal pressure changes as much as 5 mm Hg with the systolic pulse pressure in the normal tooth.[254,258] Presumably, where inflammation has occurred, such changes may be augmented because of the increased pulpal volume in a restricted space.

Synovial Joints. Cutaneous afferents and branches of adjacent muscle afferents innervate the joints.[259] Intense deformation or inflammation-induced expansion within the joint will evoke activity in the group III (Aδ) fibers.[260-262] Urate crystals,[263] carrageenan,[157,264] and endotoxin[265] injected into the synovial joint evokes an acute local inflammation, whereas the intradermal injection of killed bacteria suspended in Freund adjuvant results in a chronic polyarthritis.[266] A marked sensitivity to stimulation of the affected limbs is observed in animals so treated. Joint pain associated with gout-induced arthritis in humans probably results from urate crystal deposition.[267] Altered sensitivity to mechanical stimulation may be mediated by the generation of chemical intermediaries such as PGs. The ability of COX or phospholipase A inhibitors to reduce the sensitivity associated with the inflamed joints and to reduce the inflammation is consistent with this hypothesis.[264,268] Other inhibitors of COX are effective against joint pain but exert no effect on arthritic swelling.[269,270] This has led to the speculation that nonsteroidal anti-inflammatory drugs (NSAIDs) may either work by a separate mechanism[271] or be associated with a central action.[272,273]

Visceral Organs. Information regarding the state of the visceral organs projects to the CNS by afferents that travel with both parasympathetic (essentially vagal above the diaphragm and sacral parasympathetics for the abdominal viscera) and sympathetic innervation.[274] For the vagus, the cell body of the afferent lies in the nodose ganglion, whereas for the sympathetic and sacral parasympathetic, the afferent cell body lies in the respective DRG. Many of the axons are small and lightly myelinated or unmyelinated.[216,275,276] Manipulation of a number of healthy visceral organs, such as the liver, kidney, and spleen, does not appear to give rise to reports of pain. However, it appears likely that three conditions associated with visceral stimuli lead to a pain report:

- *Distention of hollow viscus.* Thus, expansion of the gastrointestinal tract (esophagus, stomach duodenum, large and small intestines), smooth muscle organs (gallbladder), and urinary tract (urethra and bladder) will yield short-latency pain behavior in animals and humans.[276,277]
- *Inflammation.* Internal body organs clearly become symptomatic in the presence of mechanical distortion and particularly during inflammation. Based on the ability of some of the inflammatory products outlined earlier, such as bradykinin and PGs, to induce activity in visceral innervation and to induce pain behavior,[209,278-281] such a correlation appears reasonable.
- *Ischemia.* Occlusion of the vasculature is recognized as a potential source of visceral pain. Ischemia induces activity in visceral afferents[282] and results in a septic shock state in which large quantities of active products are released locally and into the circulation (e.g., heart—coronary; viscera—splanchnic). As in the earlier comments on inflammation, the presence of these products can both facilitate and activate the transduction properties of the innervating afferent.

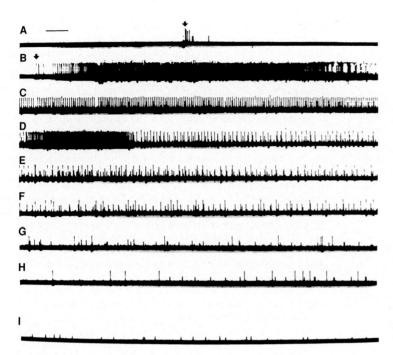

FIGURE 32-8. Effects of dorsal root ganglia (DRG) compression. Multiple-unit recording from a filament of dorsal root. **A:** Compression of dorsal root (*arrow*). **B–H:** Response of same root maintained in dorsal root compression. Each line displays first 3 seconds of recording for each minute after initiation of compression. **I:** Sample taken 25 minutes after start of DRG compression. Time bar: 200 msec. From Howe JF, Loeser JD, Calvin WH. Mechanosensitivity of dorsal root ganglia and chronically injured axons: A physiological basis for the radicular pain of nerve root compression. *Pain* 1977;3:25, with permission.

Origins of Abnormal Activity in Peripheral Afferents. Commonly, orthodromic discharge of a peripheral afferent originates at the distal terminals secondary to generator potentials induced by the appropriate peripheral stimulus. Pressure briskly applied mid-axon evokes only a transient neural activity (Fig. 32-8).[283,284] Acute nerve compression in humans may be reported as transiently painful, if perceived at all.[285,286] Simple, slow distortion of mid-axon regions, however, is ineffective in generating neural activity.[200,284,287–289] Thus, chronic pressure alone, such as that generated by benign tumors, is often not reported as painful.[286] However, mechanical insensitivity of the mid-axon region is altered after nerve injury.

Upon severance of a nerve, a barrage of activity occurs that then disappears. The injured axon undergoes retrograde chromatolysis (dying back). Over an interval of days to weeks, the injured axon initiates sprouting.[290] Collections of these sprouts form a neuroma. Systematic studies in animal models have shown that this neuroma frequently gives rise to ongoing orthodromic activity in the nerve. The activity occurs within fibers having conduction velocities suggestive of large- and small-diameter myelinated and unmyelinated fibers[284,291] and is characerized by patterns of spontaneous and bursting activity in the sprouting axon.[292] Small distortions of the neuroma now produce long periods (30 seconds) of repetitive discharge. These observations suggested that the local injury had transformed that region of the axon and endowed it with properties of excitability similar to those in the terminal region. Importantly, it has been shown that, after such peripheral nerve injury, the DRG cell of the injured nerve also begins to display a spontaneous activity.[291,293]

The origin of the spontaneous activity appears to reflect several mechanisms:[294]

- *Increased expression of NaV channels in the neuroma and DRG of the injured axon.* Following nerve injury, an increased expression of a variety of NaV channels occurs, particularly those that are TTX-resistant.[295,296] Increased ionic conductance of the neuroma may yield the ectopic activity observed in these regenerating axons. Support that this is

indeed the case is provided by the observation that systemic lidocaine at doses that do not block conduction, block ectopic activity in the neuromas and DRG.[293]

- *Potassium channel activity.* An alternate possibility leading to ectopic activity is a reduction in K^+ channel activity. Such a change would similarly contribute to an increased afferent excitability.[297,298]

- *Altered chemosensitivity.* Following nerve injury, application of a variety of amines[299,300] and proinflammatory cytokines (IL-1β, TNFα) to neuromas leads to the initiation of axon activity.[301] An important component of the local milieu after nerve injury is the release from local inflammatory and Schwann cells of cytokine such as I-1β and TNFα. Support for the potential role of such cytokines in nerve injury hyperpathia is provided by the observation that local delivery of IL-1β and TNFα receptor antibodies reduces indices of hyperpathia following nerve injury.[302,303] Growth factors, notably NGF, is also upregulated at the injury site after nerve injury.[175] As reviewed earlier, this neurotrophin may be internalized and transported to the DRG cell body, where it initiates transcription of a wide range of transmitters, receptors, and channels.

Ectopic foci in these injured nerves have been suggested to be the source of the abnormal sensations that occur after amputation.[304,305] Neurotomy in several species, including mice, rats, cats, and rabbits,[284,306,307] gives rise to autotomy of the denervated region, which may result from the abnormal discharges generated by the neuroma formed. The self-mutilation, when and if it does develop, apparently is not due to the anesthetic state, but begins only after several days.[308] Guanethidine, which suppresses the ectopic discharges associated with neuromas in mice, suppresses autotomy in neurectomized rats and mice.[309] Selective spinal tractotomies abolish the autotomy.[306]

Dorsal root ganglion cells are apparent exceptions to the this discussion of nonterminal afferent spike generation. As shown in Figure 32-8, slow, minor distortion of the DRG evokes repetitive firing that lasts minutes. Similar distortion of the dorsal roots was not as effective.[156] It has been proved that this stimulation evoked a pain event by the fact that acute injury to the DRG evokes immediate tachycardia and mass flexion reflexes in the lightly anesthetized animal. These observations support the suggestion that the radicular pain of sciatica might be associated with such a focal distortion of the DRG and not the root or nerve proper. Patients suffering from tic douloureux are often reported to have an artery, small tumor, or plaque impinging upon the trigeminal root.[310–312] Although such mechanical stimulation may not account for the unique sensory barrage associated with tic episodes, the mechanical sensitivity of the dorsal root may provide a background upon which a mechanical stimulus, such as that provided by the adjacent artery, might alter innocuous sensory input and thus generate the pain event.[313–315]

Spinal Terminals of Primary Afferents

Dorsal Root Entry Zone

As the dorsal root approaches the spinal cord, small myelinated and unmyelinated fibers tend to aggregate in the lateral aspect of the dorsal root, and larger myelinated fibers aggregate medially (Fig. 32-9).[316–320] Entering the spinal cord, the primary afferents bifurcate into rostrally and caudally projecting branches. Large fibers proceed along the dorsal columns for varying distances; many terminate in the spinal gray matter.[321,322] Large-diameter afferent collaterals exit from the dorsal column axis perpendicularly and pursue a ballistic trajectory, coursing deeply into the gray matter before turning dorsally to terminate in the upper portions of the gray matter.[323] The smaller-caliber fibers project rostrally and caudally one or two segments into the medial portion of the tract of Lissauer. Small-diameter fibers enter the dorsal gray matter directly and terminate dorsally, as will be discussed. Both large- and small-diameter fibers give rise to collaterals that distribute ventrally in the spinal gray matter (Fig. 32-9).[324]

Although the preponderance of afferents terminate ipsilaterally, evidence suggests that a proportion of the afferents also terminate contralaterally.[317,325–328] These fibers travel dorsal to the central canal to terminate in laminae III and IV of the contralateral dorsal horn, forming a longitudinally oriented plexus one to two segments in length.[329] These contralateral projections occur most commonly at the cervical and sacral levels of the spinal cord, although crossing fibers have been described in the lumbar cord.[317,326] Early work demonstrated the behavioral significance of the medial to lateral distribution of the large and small primary afferents by making discrete lesions in the dorsal root entry zone.[319] Lateral cuts, presumably severing the smaller-caliber myelinated fiber population, produced a significant blockade of the pseudo-affective response of the animal to strong, otherwise aversive, stimuli on the side where the lesions were made. It is likely that such a section also produced local infarcts of the adjacent dorsal gray matter.[330] Discrete surgical lesions directed at the dorsal horn through the dorsal root entry zone have been shown to alleviate pain, particularly that associated with root avulsions.[331,332]

The principal portion of the sensory afferents enters the spinal cord through the dorsal root entry zone, consistent with the "law" of Bell and Magendie. However, a significant number of unmyelinated afferent fibers, which arise from DRG cells, also exist within the ventral roots.[333–337] After the injection of horseradish peroxidase into the spinal gray matter of cats with previously sectioned dorsal roots, reaction products appeared in small DRG cells. Failure to label large DRG neurons is consistent with the observation that the ventral root afferents are largely unmyelinated.[338,339] The relevance of the ventral root afferents in pain transmission remains to be fully defined. This alternate pathway may account for the failure of dorsal rhizotomies to reliably relieve pain.[340] The origin of dorsal and ventral root afferents in DRG neurons would suggest that ganglionectomy would be superior to rhizotomy if afferent input is to be abolished.[341,342]

Afferent Terminals in Dorsal Horn

The dorsal horn was classically recognized from the days of Cajal as being divided into the dorsal root entry zone, superfical dorsal horn (marginal layer), the substantia gelatinosa, the neck of the dorsal horn (nucleus proprius), the ventral horn, and the

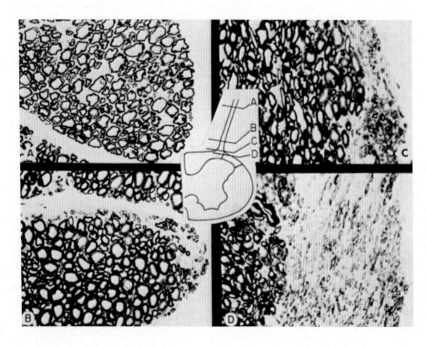

FIGURE 32-9. Distribution of large and small fibers in the L7 dorsal root of the cat at selected distance from root entry zone. **A:** At 5 mm, large- and small-fiber profiles are mixed. **B:** At 1 mm from entry zone, small fibers tend to be arranged in a peripheral ring. **C:** Just before the entry zone, the majority of the small fibers are located in the lateral aspect of the rootlet. **D:** Small fibers have merged with the tract of Lissauer. From Kerr FWL. Pain: A central inhibitory balance theory. *Mayo Clin Proc* 1975;50:685, with permission.

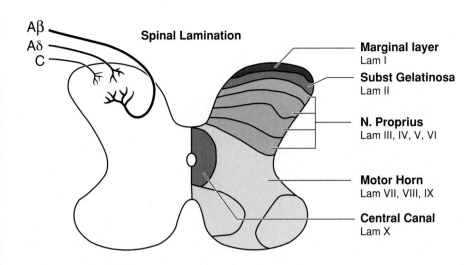

FIGURE 32-10. The Rexed lamination (*right*) and the approximate organization of the approach of the afferents to the spinal cord (*left*) as they enter at the dorsal root entry zone and then penetrate into the dorsal horn to terminate in laminae I and II (A∂/C) or penetrate more deeply to loop upward to terminate as high as the dorsum of lamina III (A*β*).

region around the central canal. The concept that the spinal gray matter of the adult spinal cord may be organized according to a distinctive lamination of cell bodies and terminal regions refines this gross anatomic subdivision to delimit the anatomy of the spinal gray matter (Fig. 32-10).[343,344] The laminations correspond grossly with the classical.

Organization of Terminals by Fiber Type. Retrograde transport of horseradish peroxidase to the distal cut ends of primary afferent fibers after medial section of the dorsal root revealed that the horseradish peroxidase reaction product was located primarily in the most dorsal laminae of the spinal gray matter. Terminals from smaller myelinated fibers were located in the marginal zone, the ventral portion of lamina II, and throughout lamina III.[317] Fine-caliber unmyelinated fibers largely terminated throughout lamina II. In contrast, the large-caliber fibers

passing in the medial portion of the root entry zone terminated largely in the nucleus proprius and in more ventral regions of the dorsal gray matter. These larger fibers made few direct contacts with neurons of the substantia gelatinosa and marginal layer, terminating largely below lamina II. Similar results were obtained in studies in which the distribution of functionally defined afferents was examined after intra-axonal application of horseradish peroxidase.[326] Intermediate- to fine-diameter cutaneous nociceptive mechanoreceptors terminated largely in the marginal zone. Terminals of low-threshold mechanoreceptors activated by low-threhsold mechanical stimuli are distributed in the dorsal portion of laminae IV and V. These comments are summarized schematically in Figure 32-11.[345]

After entry into the dorsal root entry zone, the axons typically display bifurcations or trifurcations. The large afferents send projections rostrally and caudally within the dorsal

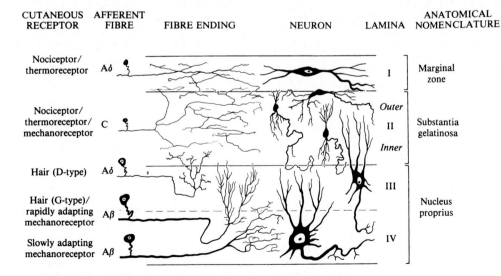

FIGURE 32-11. Schematic diagram of neuronal organization of an afferent input to the superficial dorsal horn. The schematic presents a transverse section illustrating afferent endings and neuronal elements present in the superficial four laminae of the dorsal horn. To the left, the types of afferents and relevant transduction properties are presented. Neurons represent typical morphologic types that have been identified. From top to bottom, these are: a marginal cell, a substantia gelatinosa neuron (outer), two substantia gelatinosa central cells, and two neurons in the nucleus proprius. Note that these nucleus proprius cells have dendrites ascending dorsally into the substantia gelatinosa. From Cervero F, Iggo A. The substantial gelatinosa of the spinal cord. A critical review. *Brain* 1980;103:717, with permission.

PART IV: PAIN MANAGEMENT

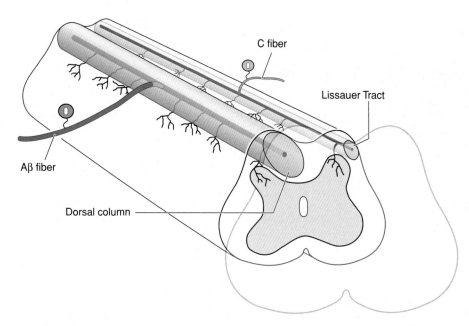

FIGURE 32-12. Schematic diagram displaying the ramification of C fibers (*right*) into the dorsal horn and collateralization into the tract of Lissauer and of Aβ fibers (*left*) into the dorsal columns and into the dorsal horn. Note that the greatest density of terminations is within the segment of entry, and that there are less dense collateralizations into the dorsal horns at the more distal spinal segments. This density of collateralization corresponds to the potency of the excitatory drive into these distal segments.

columns and directly into the dorsal horn (Fig. 32-12). The rostrally projecting collaterals may continue as far forward as the dorsal column nuclei. However, many of the axons send collaterals off into the spinal horn at progressively distal segments. Small axons display a similar collateralization, although the rostrocaudal spread occurs in the lateral tract of Lissauer.[346] Systematic mapping studies have shown that the projections of the "long-ranging afferents" may extend as far as four to 11 segments. Thus, in the rat, labeled terminals from the sural nerve were found in the gray matter up to three to four segments caudal to their root entry, and for the sciatic nerve in S4, four to six segments caudal to the segment of root entry.[347] Importantly, the strength of the excitatory drive is greatest at the segment of entry and diminishes so that inputs from distal dermatomes have a progressively decreasing excitatory influence.[348] The significance of this large- and small-afferent collateralization is that an excitatory drive occurs at spinal segments distal to the segment of entry. Factors that regulate the postsynaptic excitability of the distal cells receiving these projections will serve to define the size of the receptive field of the respective neuron.

PHARMACOLOGY OF PRIMARY AFFERENTS

Spinal Afferent Terminals

The synapse made by primary afferents with neurons of the spinal cord represents the first-order link between the periphery and the CNS. This link has several properties. Classic electrophysiologic studies provided evidence that conducted potentials interact with the second-order neuron by an excitatory synapse. No evidence of a classic monosynaptic inhibitory influence by primary afferents has been hitherto presented.[349] A second property of the neuronal response evoked by afferent excitation is that at least two populations of excitatory postsynaptic potentials are often seen, which are thought to be monosynaptic: (a) fast-onset and short-lasting and (b) delayed and of a relatively extended duration.[350–352] These elec-

trophysiologic findings, in concert with the presence of morphologically distinct vesicle populations in the same terminal, are interpreted as revealing the presence of at least two classes of neurotransmitters released from the same terminal.

Considerable efforts have been directed at establishing the identity of neuroactive substances in the primary afferent. Several criteria are classically accepted as minimum requirements in the establishment of the correspondence between the endogenous material and a given substance: (a) the material must be found in the terminals of the afferent population in question (and it or its precursor in the respective DRG cell), (b) the material must be present in a fraction that is released when the appropriate afferents undergo depolarization, (c) the postsynaptic effects of the exogenously applied materials must mimic the effects that result when the endogenous afferent systems are physiologically activated, and (d) those physiologic effects that result from the actions of the endogenously released and exogenously administered agents must possess an identical pharmacology (i.e., the characteristics of the receptor acted upon by the endogenous and exogenous agents must be indistinguishable) (Fig. 32-13).

Primary Afferent Neurotransmitter Phenotypes

Primary afferent neurotrasmitter phenotypes may be broadly divided according to axon size, state of myelination, and cell surface markers:

- Large primary afferents arising from Type A (large) ganglion cells typically display small, clear-core synaptic vesicles that contain and release excitatory amino acids (glutamate/aspartate).
- The terminals of small afferents arising from type B (small) ganglion cells may display several disitnct phenotypes:
  - *Small clear-core vesicles (containing excitatory amino).* Many of these cells display the IB4 glycoprotein (e.g., IB4+)
  - *Small clear-core vesicles and large dense core vesicles (containing excitatory amino acids and peptides, respectively).* These cells are IB4−. Thus, 90% of the small DRG neurons that are immunopositive for SP, are also glutamate immunopositive.[353]

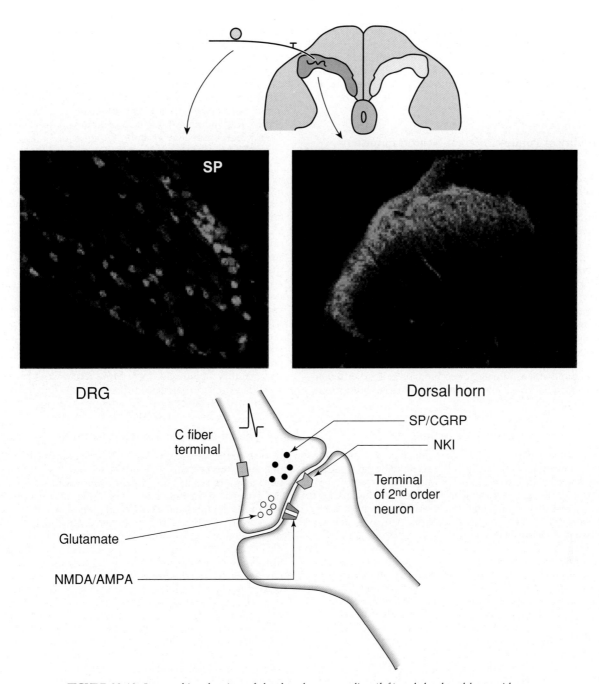

FIGURE 32-13. Immunohistochemisty of the dorsal root ganglion (*left*) and the dorsal horn with an antibody directed at substance P (SP). As indicated, the immunoreactivity in the dorsal root ganglion is present in a small type-B ganglion cell. In the dorsal horn, the immunoreactivity is located in the laminae I and II of the substantia geltaninosa in the region where small primary afferents are known to terminate. Following rhizotomy the dorsal horn immunoreactivity will be abolished (*not shown*). At the electron microscopic level, C-fiber terminals often display small, clear-core vesicles and large, clear-core vesicles that contain glutamate and a peptide (such as SP), respectively (*bottom*). The second-order neurons will typically display receptors for their respective transmitters, such as NMDA and AMPA receptors for glutamate and neurokinin 1 receptors for SP.

■ Peptides identified in the type B ganglion cells and distributed in the superficial (laminae I and II) dorsal horn include SP; CGRP; VIP; SST, a VIP homologue (peptido-histidine-isoleucine [PHI]); cholecystokinin (CCK); angiotensin II; and bombesin.[354,355]

■ The levels of these peptides in the dorsal horn are significantly reduced by rhizotomy or ganglionectomy. These ob-

servations are consistent with findings discussed previously, that unmyelinated afferent fibers course through the dorsal roots but also, to a modest degree, in the ventral roots.

Immunohistochemical studies directed at the dorsal horn have revealed distinguishable differences in the discrete distribution of the several peptides in the dorsal laminae. Substance

P is predominantly located in Rexed lamina I and the outer layer of II; VIP is principally found in lamina I, whereas SST is found in the outer layer of II. Fluoride-resistant acid phosphatase, found in small ganglion cells separate from those containing SP or SST,[63] is distributed primarily in the inner layer of lamina II in regions distinct from those that SP, VIP, or SST project.[356]

Ability of Putative Afferent Neurotransmitters to Be Released

Important considerations are whether the materials present in afferent terminals exist within a releasable fraction and whether the axons from which they derive are relevant to pain transmission. From spinal cord slices, SP and SST levels in the extracellular fluid have been shown to be elevated in a Ca^{2+}-dependent fashion by depolarization.[357–361] In vivo studies using a variety of spinal perfusion models[362] have demonstrated the release of materials from primary afferents, including SP,[363,364] CGRP,[365] VIP, CCK,[366,367] and glutamate.[368–370] Using internalization of the G-protein-coupled neurokinin with these peptides, release was produced by stimulation that activated $A\delta$/C- but not $A\beta$-afferents. The release of SP from the spinal cord has been shown to be antagonized by the local application of μ and δ but not κ opioid agonists and by α_2 agonists.[371] These observations are consistent with the presence of opioid and α-adrenergic receptors on primary afferent terminals and the effects of opiates and adrenergic agonists on afferent terminals.[372–375]

Postsynaptic Actions

Glutamate and aspartate applied onto dorsal horn neurons result in a powerful, reversible depolarization with rapid onset, accompanied by an increase in membrane conductance.[376] Examination of the subclasses of neurons excited by glutamate or aspartate reveals no functional selectivity. Thus, motor horn cells and dorsal horn neurons excited by $A\beta$-, $A\delta$-, and C-fibers show a characteristic excitatory response to glutamate administration.[376,377]

Iontophoretic application onto the dorsal horn of several peptides found in primary afferents has been shown to produce excitatory effects. The focal administration of SP onto spinal neurons results in a slow progressive depolarization of the cell[378–380] mediated in large part though a G-protein-coupled neurokinin 1 (NK1) receptor.[381] Substance P will excite cells that are naturally activated by noxious radiant heat,[378] strong mechanical stimuli,[382] and the intra-arterial injection of bradykinin,[383,384] and it facilitates responses of cells activated by noxious cutaneous stimuli. Other peptides, such as CGRP, SST, CCK, and VIP have been shown to produce excitatory and facilitatory effects on neurons that respond to a wide variety of innocuous stimuli. Calcitonin gene-related peptide may act through two subtypes of receptors.[385] Locally delivered, it facilitates synaptic transmission in dorsal horn neurons, and this effect was exaggerated in spinal slices harvested from rats with inflammatory arthritis.[386] Thus, there appears to be a significant correlation between the ability of SP to evoke a progressive depolarization in a dorsal horn neuron and the existence of an afferent drive from small fibers.[383] Vasoactive intestinal peptide and CCK have been shown to similarly evoke excitation of dorsal horn neurons.[387–389] Somatostatin has been shown to produce an inhibition of the activity of dorsal horn neurons after iontophoretic administration.[382,390] This finding is somewhat surprising, because a monosynaptic inhibition by primary afferents on second-order neurons has not been described, but

reflects the fact that these agents may exist in several systems, not in primary afferents alone.

As noted, populations of afferents, particularly those of a small diameter, have more than one material in their terminals that can be released. Electron microscopy has long indicated the presence of several morphologically distinct vesicle populations in primary afferent terminals, notably those with dense cores and now thought to contain peptides and smaller clear vesicles that may contain amino acids.[391] Intracellular recording in rat spinal cord slices has revealed that repetitive stimulation of the dorsal roots results in an initial burst of monosynaptically driven spikes followed by a prolonged, slow hypopolarization.[351] The slow depolarization of dorsal horn neurons evoked by afferent stimulation or focally applied SP (but not VIP) was blocked by coadministration of a putative SP receptor antagonist or by the prior administration of capsaicin, a neurotoxin that results in the depletion of afferent stores of SP and CCK and destroys small afferents marked by the cytosol enzyme fluoride-resistant acid phosphatase, but has no effect on large-diameter afferents.[392,393] The early depolarization was unaffected by these manipulations. These observations suggest that, for this particular neuronal population in neonatal rat spinal cord, afferent stimulation results in two events: a delayed depolarization likely to be mediated by a population of SP-containing terminals, and an immediate depolarization mediated by a second neuroactive agent, perhaps an excitatory amino acid.[355,394] More recent work has emphasized that the short-latencied primary glutamatergic excitation is mediated by one of several α-amino-3-hydroxy-5-methyl-4-isoxazolepropionic acid (AMPA)-type receptors.[395]

Role of Neurotransmitters in Pain Transmission

In view of the foregoing data, one may tentatively hypothesize that both the excitatory amino acids and one or more peptides may play some role in pain transmission at the level of the primary afferent synapse. The direct application of several of the peptides (SP, CGRP) and glutamate onto the dorsal horn of the spinal cord results in mild scratching behavior and signs of agitation. Importantly, given the co-containment and likely co-release of peptides and glutamate, the effect of the intrathecal agents is translated into a profound increase in behavioral signs of irritation when the peptide is coadministered with glutamate.[396] The potentiating effects are reduced when this is coadministered with low doses of putative SP receptor antagonists. Aside from the direct excitation and behavioral indices of pain, the spinal delivery of several of these peptides and glutamate have been shown to produce a powerful augmentation of the animal's response to an external stimulus. Thus, the iontophoresis of SP and glutamate will increase the size of the receptive field of the cell and enhance its response to light tactile stimulation as well as noxious thermal and mechanical stimuli.[397,398] This increased spinal reactivity after spinal delivery of glutamate is accompanied by behaviorally defined thermal hyperalgesia and tactile allodynia. These effects underlie the prominent states of facilitated processing that will be discussed in the following sections.

NOCICEPTIVE ELEMENTS IN THE SPINAL CORD

The differential distribution in the Rexed laminae[398] of terminals associated with fibers that are activated by specific noxious stimuli is consistent with the existence of populations of second-order neurons relevant to the rostrad transmission of nociceptive information (Fig. 32-14).

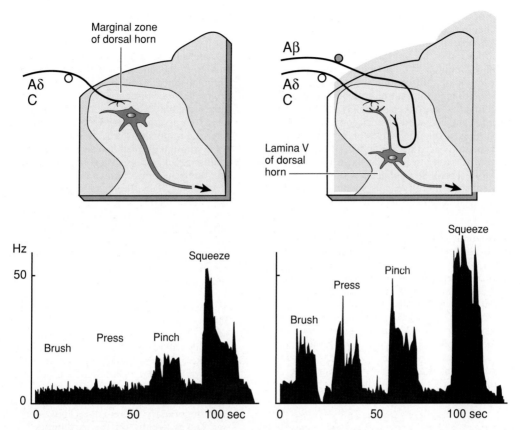

FIGURE 32-14. Firing pattern (frequency of discharge) of a spinal dorsal horn high-threshold (nociceptive-specific marginal) neuron (*left*) and a wide dynamic range (WDR) neuron located primarily in lamina V (*right*) in response to graded intensities of mechanical stimulation (*Brush, Pressure, Pinch, Squeeze*) applied to the receptive fields of each cell. Both cells project supraspinally. Note the relationship between firing patterns and the properties of the afferents with which each cell makes contact.

Marginal Zone (Lamina I)

The superficial layer of the dorsal horn comprises classes of large neurons oriented transversely across the cap of the dorsal gray matter. Some cells project to the brainstem (notably the medullary reticular formation and the mesencephalic parabracheal nucleus thalamus),[316,399–402] while others project intrasegmentally and intersegmentally along the dorsal and dorsolateral white matter.[403–405] The local dendritic plexus of these spinal neurons extends up to several hundred microns along both the transverse and longitudinal axes of the cord, although the dendritic tree is largely confined to the marginal layer.[323,406] As displayed schematically in Figure 32-11, afferent terminals tend to synapse distally in the dendritic tree, whereas nonafferent terminals tend to be proximal on the cell body.[316,407] Lamina I neurons may be divided physiologically into three groups: (a) neurons activated by fibers having Aδ-/C-fiber conduction velocities that respond to intense mechanical stimulation (Fig. 32-14); (b) neurons activated by innocuous skin cooling, with afferents having a conduction velocity akin to those of an Aδ-fiber; and (c) a small percentage of neurons activated by C-fiber polymodal afferents.[399,408–411] Although initial observations suggested that these neurons of lamina I were specifically sensitive to intense stimuli, a significant proportion of these cells also possess a wide dynamic range, that is, a response frequency proportional to the intensity of the stimulus.[408] Importantly, those neurons responding to Aδ- and C-fiber input can also be activated by group III and group IV muscle afferents, indicating a convergence of muscle and cutaneous input.

The role of lamina I neurons in nociception has been directly assessed through spinally delivered neurotoxin (SP; saporin) that destroys neurons that bear the NK1 receptor. In such studies, loss of these cells has been shown to produce a potent reduction in the facilitated nociceptive behavior generated by tissue injury, with little effect upon acute pain thresholds.[412–414]

Substantia Gelatinosa (Lamina II)

The clear band of neural tissue lying ventral to the marginal layer and dorsal to a region of coarser texture known as the nucleus proprius was given the name *substantia gelatinosa* by Rolando.[415] The substantia gelatinosa, defined by gross observation in unfixed or semifixed tissue, corresponds to the laminae II of Rexed. Lamina II is divided into outer and inner layers. The former is characterized by small, densely packed cells and a neuropil made complex by the presence of a larger number of dendrites. The latter zone is similar but has a less coarse texture owing to the relative paucity of terminals. The principal cell type in lamina II is the stalk cell, with cone-shaped dendritic trees arborizing through lamina II into III and axons branching into lamina I.[404,416] The terminals of Aδ-afferents that project to this lamina are a likely source of the numerous axodendritic contacts observed in this region.[55,407,417–420]

A significant proportion of the substantia gelatinosa neurons receive Aδ-/C-fiber input.[421–424] Neurons located in lamina II (the outer portion of the substantia gelatinosa) tend to be excited by activation of thermal receptive or mechanical nociceptive afferents.[423] Neurons retrogradely labeled with horseradish peroxidase and activated by nociceptive input display dendritic branching in the outer layer of the substantia gelatinosa, whereas neurons activated by innocuous mechanical stimuli have dendritic trees in the inner layer of the substantia gelatinosa.[326] Receptive fields of gelatinosa neurons responsive to peripheral stimuli are typically small (<2 cm^{200}). Several properties of gelatinosa neurons have emerged:

■ Unlike those cells lying more deeply (see following), neurons of the substantia gelatinosa commonly exhibit prolonged periods of excitation and inhibition after afferent activation.[424,425]

■ Islet and stalked cells constitute several classes of functionally distinct cells, with variable degrees of background activity, in which afferent input will drive complex "on/off" responses. Significantly, those cells inhibited by non-noxious stimuli were excited by noxious input, whereas cells inhibited by noxious input were excited by non-noxious input.[426,427] Such profiles suggest that the activity of substantia gelatinosa neurons is governed by a convergence of excitation arising from large- and small-fiber input acting either directly on these neurons or by inhibitory interneurons.

Nucleus Proprius (Laminae III, IV, and V)

Lamina III contains fewer neurons and a less dense neuropil than does lamina II. In addition, the islet neuron[428,429] (Golgi type II) appears in high concentration, in contrast to the stalk cells that occur predominantly in the outer layer of lamina II.

Lamina IV, as defined by Rexed, is composed of a broad layer of relatively large neurons (10 to 15 μm in diameter) that endow this region with their characteristic morphology. The dendritic tree of these neurons transversely and dorsally spreads into laminae II and III. The neuropil of lamina II and IV is characterized by axodendritic and axoaxonic synapses,[419,430] originating from afferent input of the large-diameter fibers that contact the apical portion of the dendritic tree,[431] and from local axonal plexuses derived from intrinsic fibers.[316] Lamina V, located along the neck of the dorsal horn, displays a dendritic organization that does not differ prominently from that of neurons in lamina IV.

Neurons in both lamina IV and lamina V project to the ventrobasal thalamus, mesencephalon,[400,401,432–434] and the lateral cervical nucleus,[421,435] and provide propriospinal projections within the spinal cord in various species (see following). Cells in the nucleus proprius may be broadly classed as those that respond to low-threshold (Aβ) input and those that respond at a progressively greater frequency as a function of stimulus intensity. This reflects the convergent input from several classes of functionally defined afferent types (e.g., Aβ, Aδ, and C). These dorsal horn cells are referred to as *wide dynamic range (WDR) neurons*.[436] The latter class of cells responds to transient brush and touch but show no elevation in activity with prolonged pinch; these cells are referred to as lamina IV neurons, whereas the former class of neurons are referred to as lamina V neurons because of the early studies that localized them in that region.[437] Lamina V neurons have several discrete properties

that make them of particular interest to our interpretation of nociceptive mechanisms:

1. In these cells, light innocuous touch evokes activity that increases as the intensity of pressure or pinch is increased. Thermal stimuli applied to the receptive field will similarly evoke a rate of discharge that is proportional to temperature; some units show an exponential increase in discharge rate at temperatures above 45°C.[438–440] Because of this characteristic response profile, these cells are WDR neurons. An acute stimulus applied to a sensory nerve will evoke a characteristic biphasic activation reflecting the excitation evoked first by the rapidly conducting A-fibers and then a second phase mediated by the arrival of the more slowly conducting Aδ- and C-fibers.

2. Repetitive electrical stimulation at a slow rate (<0.1 Hz) results in a stable response. However, at a slightly faster rate (0.5 to 1 Hz), the WDR neurons will show a progressive incrementation in discharge velocity with each subsequent stimulus. This augmentation, referred to as "wind-up," depends upon the activation of C-, but not Aβ-fibers and produces a gradual increase in the frequency discharge until the neuron is in a state of virtually continuous discharge.[436] Many of these cells are indeed projeciton neurons, emphasizing that their exaggerated resposne evoked by a given stimulus will be transmitted to higher centers.[441]

3. Receptive fields for WDR neurons are more extensive than those of the primary afferent neurons that impinge upon them, again indicating a convergence of afferent input onto the dendritic tree of this cell. As with marginal neurons (and the primary afferents), receptive field size decreases as one moves distally on the extremities.[408,442,443] Although somatotopically convergent input is the rule for WDR neurons, and the activity of such neurons can be highly influenced by input from several adjacent spinal cord segments, these neurons are activated most effectively by input arriving from the dermatome in which they lie.[444,445] Importantly, many early investigations were carried out in decerebrate or decerebrate/spinal animals to avoid the use of anesthetics. In experiments using intact anesthetized preparations, receptive fields, sometimes including the whole body, have been found in addition to the more restricted ones observed when the spinal cord has been transected. Moreover, the magnitude of the receptive field is under an ongoing modulation by intrinsic systems that can increase and decrease the size of the complex field (see following).

4. Wide dynamic range neurons commonly demonstrate organ convergence as well as somatic convergence. Thus, neurons in the nucleus proprius have been observed that are activated by (a) stimulation of sympathetic afferents and by coronary artery occlusion, as well as by noxious pinches applied within the dermatomes that coincided with the segmental location of those cells (T1–T5);[221] (b) stimulation of the splanchnic nerve and Aβ/Aδ cutaneous input;[446–449] (c) distention of the hollow viscera (bladder, small intestine, and gallbladder);[450] (d) injection of bradykinin into the mesenteric artery and cutaneous input;[451] and close intra-arterial administration of bradykinin or the injection of hypertonic saline into muscle/tendon or group III afferent stimulation from the gastrocnemius[447,452] and cutaneous input field. Correlation of those areas of the skin (forepaw, hindpaw, hind leg, abdomen, thorax) where stimulation would evoke activity in neurons known to be activated by distention of the gallbladder or the urinary bladder revealed that about one-third of the units examined responded to stimulation of the gallbladder and various cutaneous regions,

with the highest percentage associated with the thorax and perineum.[453] Progressive bladder distention activated cells in widespread dermatomal regions, but most effectively activated neurons responsive to cutaneous stimuli applied to the abdomen. These results indicate that the phenomenon of "referred" visceral pain probably has its substrate in viscerosomatic and musculosomatic convergence onto dorsal horn neurons.[454,455]

Central Canal (Lamina X)

Although the central canal is a parvicellular region, recent studies have demonstrated that branches of small, lightly myelinated fibers were observed to enter the region.[317] Transport studies have further demonstrated that a significant proportion of these neurons projected both ipsilaterally and contralaterally in the ventrolateral tract into the bulbar reticular formation. Electrophysiologic studies in this region have shown that local neurons possess properties similar to those of the marginal cells noted earlier. Thus, cells have been observed that respond primarily to high-threshold temperature and noxious pinch with small receptive fields.[456–458]

ASCENDING SPINAL TRACTS

Spinofugal pathways that originate in the spinal dorsal horn typically ascend into the brainstem and as far rostrally as the diencephalon. Aside from poorly defined intersegmental projection, these ascending pathways synapse in the ventrolateral (anterolateral in bipeds) quadrants. These ascending projection can be divided into those which ascend cotrolaterally and those which remain ipsilateral to the cell of origin. An overview of this pathway is presented in Figure 32-15.

Ventral Funicular Systems

In 1890, William Richard Gower observed in an attempted suicide victim that, prior to death, the patient, who had levelled a pistol through his mouth back to the spinal cord, displayed preserved light touch bilaterally, but loss of pain and temperature on one side. At autopsy, it was found that the bullet had destroyed the ventrolateral aspect of the cord on the side opposite the loss of pain and temperature. This confirmed extensive animal work, which suggested that pain was transmitted via a crossed pathway that ascended in the ventral quadrant, while localizing the epicritic sensation (light touch) to the dorsal columns. That initial observation was confirmed frequently thereafter by the observation that unilateral ventrolateral tractotomies elevate the threshold for visceral and somatic pain reports on the side contralateral to the lesion.[459–462] Conversely, stimulation of the ventrolateral tracts in awake subjects undergoing percutaneous cordotomies has resulted in reports of contralateral warmth and pain.[462,463] The analgesia is characterized by a loss of or reduction in the response to thermal (heat and cold), mechanical (pinprick), itch,[464] and deep somatic (Achilles tendon) stimuli. Midline myelotomies that destroy fibers crossing the midline at the levels of the cut produce bilateral pain deficits.[465,466] These observations suggest that the relevant pathways for nociception are predominantly crossed. It should be stressed that midline myelotomies are not identical to ventrolateral cordotomies. As summarized by Vierck and colleagues,[460] after midline myelotomy there tends to be (a) an increased incidence of paresthesia, (b) no decrease in the magnitude of evoked cutaneous pain, (c) preserved dull–sharp discrimination, and (d) enduring losses of deep pain. The rostrad transmission of nociceptive information, however, is not unique to the ventrolateral funiculus (VLF). This is evidenced by the anomalous recovery of pain 3 months to 1 year after cordotomy, the persistence of contralateral pain sensations after a unilateral lesion (suggestive of bilateral projections), and by the ability of high-intensity stimulation to produce a "breakthrough" of pain resembling the diffuse, burning pain of C-fiber activation.[467]

Cells of Origin

Localization of the cells of origin of the VLF system has been made by examining the chromatolytic reaction after spinal section and antidromic activation of spinal neurons by brainstem electrodes, and by labeling spinal neurons with horseradish peroxidase injected into probable terminal regions of axons

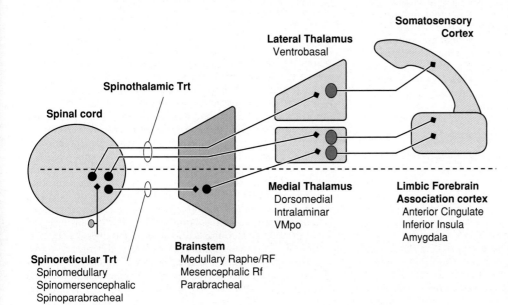

FIGURE 32-15. Schematic organization of principal components of the ascending projection pathways activated by high intensity afferent input. *RF*, reticular formation; *Trt*, tract; *VMpo*, ventral medial nucleus pars oralis.

projecting in the VLF. Retrograde chromatolytic reactions were observed early in neurons of the marginal zone and of the deeper laminae (IV and V) of the dorsal horn of patients with clinically effective lesions of the VLF. Chromatolytic cell bodies lying more deeply in the ventral horn were also found after ventrolateral cordotomy. Injection of horseradish peroxidase into the lateral thalamic nuclei or into the spinothalamic tract itself resulted in labeled neurons in the marginal zone, the substantia gelatinosa,[402] and laminae IV and V.[434] Stimulating electrodes placed in the contralateral VLF at cervical or mesodiencephalic levels will antidromically activate neurons in the marginal zone, the substantia gelatinosa, and laminae IV and V, as well as in laminae VII and VIII in the cat.[432,468–470] Fibers in the ventral funiculi are myelinated with diameters of 1 to 11 μm.[471] Application of the Hurst factor for myelinated fibers estimates conduction velocities that closely correspond to those reported for these fibers by several laboratories (18–58 m/sec in cats[470]; 7–74 m/sec in primates[411]).

Organization

Fibers traveling rostrad in this tract originate in the dorsal horn and cross in the dorsal commissure at levels up to two segments from the point of origin.[402,464] White and associates[472] noted a rostral displacement of the analgesic dermatomes after a ventrolateral cordotomy and suggested that, before crossing, these axons may remain medial for one or two segments. A somatotopic arrangement within the VLF has been so described that the fibers arising from the more caudal segments are located laterally, whereas those entering from the more rostral segments lie medially and ventrally in the funiculi.[473] Although it has been suggested that there may also be an anatomically defined organization by modality in the ventrolateral tract (for example, pain and touch), single-unit recording studies in primates have failed to document such modality segregation.[474]

Rostral Terminals

Because spinofugal tracts do not appear to show major or reliable differences with regard to their point of origin within the spinal gray matter (see later discussion), the tracts projecting rostrally within the VLF are commonly classified according to the brain regions in which they terminate. Long tract systems that may be relevant to the rostrad transmission include the spinoreticular, spinomesencephalic, and spinothalamic tracts. The first two have often been referred to as the paleospinothalamic system, and the last as the neospinothalamic system by virtue of the increasing size of the diencephalic projections in phylogenetically advanced species.[475] It should be remembered, however, that up to half of the fibers in the VLF in humans (which are not destined for the cerebellum) terminate caudal to the rostral aspect of the inferior olive.[476]

Spinoreticular Projections

Spinoreticular axons terminate both ipsilaterally and contralaterally to their site of origin in the spinal cord.[477,478] Entering the medulla, the fibers aggregate laterally, and collaterals of these fibers terminate in the more medially situated brainstem reticular nuclei (the nucleus reticularis gigantocellularis, nucleus reticularis paragigantocellularis, nucleus reticularis pontis caudalis, and nucleus subcoeruleus)[478–482] (Fig. 32-16). Significant terminal fields have also been reported in the nuclei raphe magnus and pallidus,[481,483,484] making both somatic and dendritic contacts.[485] Stimulating electrodes in the reticular formation antidromically activate neurons in laminae V through VIII.[486–488] Discrete injections of horseradish peroxidase into

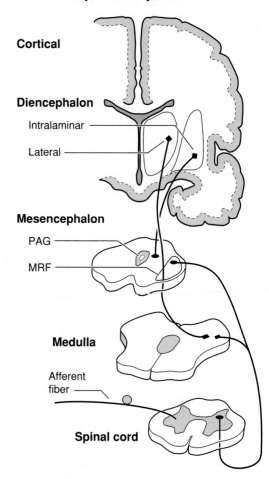

Spinoreticular-Spinomesencephalic Projections Systems

FIGURE 32-16. Schema displaying the connectivity of the spinoreticular/mesencephalic–thalamic projection system. Note the ipsilateral projection of the ventrolateral tract into the medulla and mescenephalon. These cells give rise to prominent rostral projection in the diecephalon. *PAG*, periaqueductal grey; *MRF*, mesencephalic reticular formation.

the nucleus reticularis gigantocellularis and the magnocellular part of the lateral reticular nucleus have labeled neurons situated throughout the contralateral spinal cord in laminae IV, V, and VIII, and in the ipsilateral laminae IV and V.[433,489] It is important to remember that, although many of the projections to the bulbar reticular formation are ipsilateral, a small contingent of fibers may cross at the medullary level. Degeneration in this bulbar region after extensive midline myelotomies has not been observed.[346] Using stimulating electrodes placed at several brainstem levels, it has been shown in cats that axons projecting no further than the brainstem reticular formation do exist and possess cell bodies located throughout the nucleus proprius of the dorsal horn, as well as laminae VI to IX.[486] This suggests that spinoreticular terminals do not represent only the collaterals of fibers in transit to more rostrad sites. Retrograde transport studies have demonstrated, however, that some spinifugal axons do indeed project to both the brainstem and the thalamus.[490,491] With regard to electrophysiologic properties, spinoreticular neurons have been shown to possess receptive fields that may be restricted cutaneous, restricted deep, or complex extensive. Although the receptive fields are predominantly ipsilateral excitatory, bilateral fields and fields with inhibitory components have also been observed. A high proportion of spinoreticular neurons have WDR response characteristics.[486]

Spinoparabrachial Fibers

The parabrachial nucleus located in the pons receives dense projections from contralateral lamina I neurons (Fig. 32-17). Cells in these regions give rise to dense projections into the entrolateral medulla, the periaqueductal gray matter, the ventromedial hypothalamus, VMpo of the thalamus, and the centromedial nucleus of the amygdala.[492,493]

Spinomesencephalic Projections

Fibers originate from neurons located in the spinal gray matter in regions similar to those reported for spinoreticular fibers. Two spinomesencephalic tracts have been reported. The largest tract crosses within the spinal cord; the lesser tract ascends ipsilaterally and crosses in the tegmentum at the level of the intertectal commissure[478,481] (Fig. 32-16). Degenerating terminals

following lesions of the ventrolateral cord have been observed in the midbrain reticular formation; for example, in the nucleus cuneiformis, inferior and superior colliculi, and periaqueductal gray matter of several species.[478–481,494,495] In contrast to the spinoreticular projections, midline myelotomies produce extensive signs of degeneration in the mesencephalon.[346] Using retrograde labeling, cells of origin have been demonstrated in laminae I and V.[496,497] Physiologic properties of identified spinomesencephalic neurons have not been examined extensively. Uniformly shorter response latencies of these neurons in the mesencephalon have been reported for contralateral as compared with ipsilateral somatic stimulation, suggesting a largely crossed afferent input.[498–500] A population of these cells displays a significant response to noxious stimuli.[501]

Spinothalamic Projections

The cells of origin of this tract project monosynaptically to the thalamus. The existence of cell systems lying in the dorsal gray matter is expected, but the density around the neck of the proprius and the central canal emphasizes the possible role of this deep system in nociceptive transmission[458] (Fig. 32-18). The tract ascends predominantly in the contralateral ventral quadrant. Crossed fibers predominate. Retrograde labeling studies revealed that, following unilateral injection of horseradish peroxidase into the thalamus of the monkey, about 25% of the projections from the sacral cord were ipsilateral.[402]

The spinothalamic system ascends in the medulla, dorsolaterally to the pyramid, and inferiorly to the olivary nucleus. In the rostral mesencephalon, fibers are located ventromedially to the inferior colliculus. The spinothalamic fibers differentiate into a lateral and medial component in the posterior portions of the thalamus. The medial component passes through the internal medullary lamina to terminate in the nucleus parafascicularis and intralaminar and paralaminar nuclei.[478,481,502] The majority of fibers pass laterally through the external medullary lamina to terminate in small clusters scattered throughout the nucleus ventralis posterolateralis, the medial aspects of the posterior nuclear complex, and the intralaminar nuclei.[480,481,503–506] In primates, thalamic stimulation evokes antidromic activation of neurons located dorsally in the lateral aspect of the nucleus proprius and in the marginal zone.[400,411,468] From horseradish peroxidase studies, neurons in lamina I project uniquely to the region lying between the rostral, ventrolateral, and caudal ventrolateral thalamic nuclei. Spinothalamic neurons lying in laminae IV and V terminate in the posterior nuclei of the thalamus, whereas neurons in laminae VII and VIII are generally labeled after injections of horseradish peroxidase into the intralaminar thalamic nuclei.[434,507,508]

In the primate, a significant proportion of the neurons projecting laterally in the thalamus (ventral posterior lateral complex) also project to the medial (central lateral nucleus or dorsal medial nucleus) portion. In contrast, a second population of neurons appears to project largely to the medial thalamus. At least four classes of spinothalamic neurons have been identified: (a) narrow dynamic range neurons that respond only to innocuous tactile stimuli (laminae IV and V); (b) neurons situated deep, which are responsive to proprioceptive input (laminae IV and V); (c) WDR neurons that respond in a frequency-dependent fashion to stimuli of increasing intensity, receive convergent input from cutaneous, visceral, and muscle sources, respond to thermal and chemical stimuli in the noxious range, and display a sustained discharge to pressure but a rapid adaptation to light tactile input (lamina V); and (d) neurons that respond uniquely to high-intensity

Spinoparabrachial Projection Systems

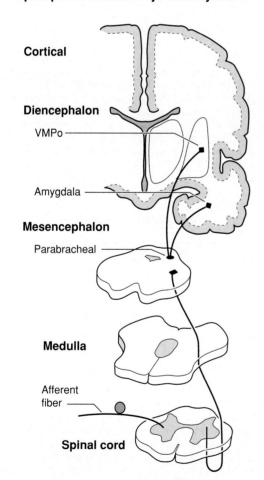

Cortical

Diencephalon

VMPo

Amygdala

Mesencephalon

Parabracheal

Medulla

Afferent fiber

Spinal cord

FIGURE 32-17. Schema displaying the connectivity of the spinoparabrachial–thalamic projection system. Note the crossed pathway into the pons and the projections from the parabrachial to medullary, mesecephalic, and diencephalic targets.

Spinothalamic Projection Systems

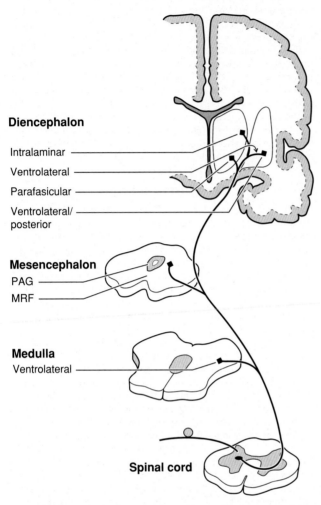

Diencephalon

Intralaminar

Ventrolateral

Parafasicular

Ventrolateral/
posterior

Mesencephalon

PAG

MRF

Medulla

Ventrolateral

Spinal cord

FIGURE 32-18. Schema displaying connectivity of the crossed spinothalamic projection system. Note the collaterals, which are believed to arise from these projection into the medullary and mesecephalic core.

noxious stimuli. These high-threshold units display a slowly adapting response to noxious cutaneous mechanical and thermal stimuli.[509] Lamina I neurons having such properties have been observed.[409,411,422,452,510,511] In the studies noted, neurons that project to *both* the medial and the lateral thalamus display a significant proportion of WDR-type cells. In contrast, medially projecting cells have been largely characterized as high-threshold-selective.[509]

With regard to receptive fields, antidromic activation of spinothalamic neurons from electrodes placed in both the medial thalamus and lateral thalamus reveals three types of spinothalamic neurons: (a) those that project only to the lateral thalamus, (b) those that project only to the medial thalamus, and (c) those that project to both the medial and lateral thalamus. Receptive field properties of those neurons that project to the lateral thalamus are conventional (small fields with larger surrounding regions that require more intense stimulation for activation of the neuron), and many neurons have inhibitory fields extending over broad body areas. Neurons projecting to the medial thalamus display large, often whole-body receptive

fields, although the contralateral field often is most effective in activating the cell. These neurons display discharge patterns that last beyond the stimulus. Severing the cord reduces the receptive field to that observed for spinal animals and abolishes the poststimulus discharge. Thus, somatic stimuli gaining access to supraspinal centers can readdress spinal projection neurons in what appears to be a spino (contralateral)-bulbo (crossed)-spinal (ipsilateral) feedback circuit.[512]

Dorsal Funicular Systems

Transections of the dorsal quadrant of the spinal cord in the cat produce significant increases in the nociceptive threshold.[513] Severance of the dorsal columns or the spinocervical tract, or both, may account for this elevation. In primates and humans, lesions of the dorsolateral quadrant have been reported to produce a hyperalgesia.[514,515] Although large-diameter afferent fibers, sensitive to light touch and vibration, terminate in the dorsal column nuclei after ascending in the dorsal columns, many nonprimary afferent fibers originating in lamina V also ascend in the dorsal column as well.[516,517] These fibers respond to tactile and noxious mechanical and thermal stimuli.[518] Dorsal column lesions in humans do not alter pain threshold,[519] and stimulation of the dorsal columns in humans often gives rise to sensations of vibration, not of pain.[520] In primates, a slight decrease in pain reactivity has been observed.[515] As noted, a postsynaptic pathway originating from lamina V neurons in the dorsal horn has been shown. The role of this system is not known. Axons of spinocervical neurons project ipsilaterally in the dorsolateral quadrant of the spinal cord to terminate in the lateral cervical nucleus.[435,443] These neurons lie predominantly in the nucleus proprius (laminae III and IV).[435,443] Several types of spinocervical neurons have been identified, and they appear to be activated by tactile (hair movement, pressure), noxious thermal (40°–53°C), and noxious mechanical (pinch) stimuli[421,521,522] and close intra-arterial injection of algogenic agents.[523] The spinocervical tract has been well described in cats,[524] but its presence is much reduced in lower primates[525–527] and is practically nonexistent in humans.[528]

Intersegmental Systems

The ability of ventrolateral cordotomies to alter pain illustrates the important role of long tracts in the rostral transmission of nociceptive information. For reasons already stated, the existence of alternate spinal pathways appears certain. Early studies showed that alternating hemisections will abolish neither the behavioral nor the autonomic responses to strong stimuli.[529–531] These observations suggest that systems that project for short distances ipsilaterally may contribute to the rostrad transmission of nociceptive information. Kerr[532,533] proposed that selective destruction of the dorsal gray matter—for example, in spinonucleolysis—might prove to be a possible method of pain management in light of the relevance of nonfunicular pathways traveling in the spinal gray matter. Subsequent work revealed that such lesions could produce significant and prolonged pain relief associated with nerve avulsions and other chronic, otherwise intractable, somatosensory pain syndromes.[331,534] These results offer support for the proposed relevance in pain transmission of systems traveling within the dorsal gray matter. Alternately, the recent role of cell systems in lamina X and the likelihood of local systems traveling in the dorsal columns indicates the possibility that midline myelotomies may act not only by the severance of crossing fibers, but may also be the cause of damage to relevant midline systems. Early studies suggested that visceral pain was dependent upon the central core.[460,535] Several segmental pathways that may be relevant to the rostrad transmission of nociceptive information include the Lissauer tract, the dorsolateral propriospinal system, and the dorsal intracornual tract.

The tract of Lissauer is divided into medial and lateral components. The medial portion of the tract consists largely of collaterals of the unmyelinated or lightly myelinated primary afferent fibers that travel several segments rostrally and caudally before entering the dorsal horn gray matter.[316,318,405,536] The lateral tract lies in the dorsolateral funiculus, immediately lateral to the dorsal root entry zone and consists of myelinated and small myelinated fibers deriving from neurons in the substantia gelatinosa and marginal layers.[344] These fibers may travel only a few millimeters in either direction before disappearing into the dorsal horn.[316,424,485,537] Although the medial and lateral components of the Lissauer tract can be separated at the dorsal root entry zone, they merge at the cervical level and cannot be easily differentiated.[485]

Lesions of the dorsolateral quadrant that destroy the tract of Lissauer have been reported to elevate the nociceptive threshold[513,538] and to enlarge the dermatomal fields associated with a given segment of the spinal cord. Tractotomies of the medial Lissauer tract in primates exert the opposite effect and result in shrinkage of the dermatome associated with a given spinal cord root.[539]

The ipsilateral projections of the dorsolateral propriospinal system travel lateral to the axis of the nucleus proprius and contain axons originating from neurons of the substantia gelatinosa and marginal zone.[323] The role of many marginal neurons in pain transmission and the possibility that these neurons may project into this pathway suggest that a certain proportion of nociceptive information may be transmitted by means of the dorsolateral propriospinal tract. The dorsal intracornual tract consists of small-diameter fibers coursing longitudinally through the medial regions of the nucleus proprius. Because rhizotomies do not reduce the number of these fibers, it appears they arise from intrinsic neurons.[316]

Despite corollary evidence suggesting that intrasegmental systems may transmit nociceptive information, the role of these pathways in pain transmission remains speculative. The results of a ventrolateral cordotomy clearly indicate the importance of crossed pathways; the segmental pathways are largely ipsilaterally organized. Yet evidence suggests that some primary afferent neurons do terminate contralaterally (see previous), and interneurons do cross the midline along the longitudinal axis of the cord, as evidenced by the existence of crossed reflexes. Crossing fibers may serve to transmit the ipsilateral message to a contralateral projection. Moreover, as noted previously, afferent axons collateralize and may project many segments rostrally, where they would initiate an excitation at levels above the spinal long-tract section. The existence of segmental spinal systems might explain the recurrence of pain 3 to 12 months after ventrolateral cordotomy and, particularly, the "breakthrough" mediated by small fibers that occurs when high-intensity stimuli are applied[460] (see previous).

CONSIDERATION OF SPECIAL SENSORY SYSTEMS

In the preceding section, specific interest was directed at general systems whereby sensory information enters the CNS. Although the essential characteristics of the afferent input are rea-

sonably uniform across the sensory systems, two systems have special complexities that engender particular interest. These are the trigeminal system and the systems whereby visceral information enters the CNS.

Trigeminal System

The essential characteristics of afferent input through the trigeminal system are similar to those of the spinal cord. However, certain morphologic and functional considerations make it worth noting this system separately.

Trigeminal Input

The face, head, and buccal regions are innervated by the ophthalmic, mandibular, and maxillary divisions of the trigeminal nerve, the cell bodies of which are located in the ganglion of the fifth nerve (gasserian). The afferents are organized somatotopically in the sensory root in a medial to lateral fashion. The mandibular nerve branch is posterolaterally positioned, the ophthalmic branch anteromedially located, and the maxillary branch situated in an intermediate position.[311,540,541] The more rostral the peripheral terminal fields, the more ventrally and laterally situated are the cell bodies in the ganglia.[311,540,541]

As in the spinal cord, a large proportion of the afferent input enters through the sensory root (the *portio major*), but sensory fibers may enter also by way of the portio minor or the efferent outflow of the trigeminal system. Because visceral efferent fibers are not thought to course in the portio minor, the observation that about 20% of the axons are unmyelinated suggests a situation analogous to that studied in greater detail in the lumbar and sacral cord.[542] The continued presence of these afferent fibers may be a possible reason for the preservation of tactile sensitivity and of various pathologic facial pains following trigeminal nerve rhizotomy.[543,544]

Brainstem Organization

The trigeminal sensory nucleus is divided into the main sensory and the more caudally located spinal nucleus (extending as far caudally as the cervical spinal cord). The spinal nucleus is further divided into three subdivisions: the nucleus oralis, nucleus interpolaris, and nucleus caudalis (rostral–caudal presentation).[545] The central processes of the trigeminal afferent neurons enter the brainstem at the level of the pons to terminate in these nuclei.[546] The somatotopic arrangement of the three branches of the trigeminal nerve observed within the ganglion is maintained in the descending trigeminal tract, in the main sensory nucleus,[311,547] and in the spinal nucleus.[52,311]

Large-diameter afferents bifurcate within the brainstem, giving rise to ascending and descending branches that terminate in the main sensory and spinal nuclei, respectively.[323,548] Horseradish peroxidase injected into axons of physiologically identified afferents of vibrissae has confirmed the bifurcation of these afferents and their coinnervation of the main sensory and spinal nuclei.[549] A population of large-diameter afferents also exists that does not bifurcate but descends in the spinal tract to innervate the entire rostrocaudal extent of the spinal nucleus, a course similar to that followed by smaller-diameter myelinated and unmyelinated fibers. Physiologic studies have supported the anatomic evidence for widespread termination of trigeminal afferents within the nuclear subdivisions. Neurons responsive to tactile stimuli (subserved by activity in large-diameter afferents) are not localized to any one nucleus. Neurons of the nucleus oralis,[550,551] nucleus interpolaris,[550] and nucleus caudalis,[439,550,552,553] and neurons within the main

PART IV: PAIN MANAGEMENT

sensory nucleus[550–552] are activated by the application of tactile stimuli (light touch, hair movement, brush) to their receptive fields. Neurons responsive to thermal or noxious stimuli have been reported in the nucleus caudalis.[207,439,553–556] Significantly, trigeminal neurons may be driven by input from spinal afferent collaterals and other cranial nerves. Thus, stimulation as far caudally as the C2 root will produce an excitatory drive of neurons receiving trigeminal input,[557–560] with the likelihood that unusual pain syndromes, such as those seen in atypical facial neuralgias, might reflect the contribution of these collateral projections. The role of the nucleus caudalis in pain has been emphasized on the basis that trigeminal tractotomy at the level of the medullary obex relieves ipsilateral facial pain with preservation of touch.[464,561] The nociceptive responses of neurons situated in the nucleus caudalis reveal two populations of neurons that are remarkably similar to those reported in the spinal cord.[439] Neurons located in the marginal rim of the nucleus caudalis (corresponding to lamina I of the spinal cord[429]) have been termed "nociceptive specific." The receptive fields of these neurons are predominantly ipsilateral and small in size.[207,439,553,555,556] The second population of nociceptive neurons is of the WDR type and is situated ventrally in the magnocellular portion of the nucleus caudalis. These neurons receive convergent input from large-diameter afferents being activated by stimulation of low-threshold rapidly conducting fibers, as well as by light touch, hair movement, and vibration.[207,439,553]

Ascending Projections

After the injection of horseradish peroxidase into the ventrobasal thalamus of the rat, retrogradely labeled neurons are found throughout the entire trigeminal sensory complex, with the possible exception of the nucleus oralis of the spinal nucleus.[562,563] These trigeminothalamic projections are predominantly contralateral, although a small ipsilateral projection from the main sensory nucleus has been described.[562,563] Neurons in the nucleus caudalis are responsive to noxious or innocuous stimuli, and project to the ventroposterior thalamus[439] and to the adjacent reticular formation.[564] Neurons of the nucleus caudalis also project within the trigeminal tract to the more rostral sensory nuclei.[564–567] This intranuclear projection may serve to modulate the activity of neurons in the more rostral trigeminal sensory nuclei and may explain why neurons responsive to noxious stimuli are not localized to the nucleus caudalis.[551] Neurons of the main sensory nucleus and the nucleus oralis are activated by electrical stimulation of the nucleus caudalis.[551] Activation of nucleus caudalis neurons by topical application of strychnine (a glycine receptor antagonist) potentiates the responses of main sensory and nucleus oralis neurons to both noxious and innocuous stimuli. Conversely, cold block of the nucleus caudalis decreases the responses of neurons in the nucleus oralis and main sensory nucleus to peripheral stimuli.[568] Consistent with these observations, electrical stimulation or strychnine on the nucleus caudalis has been reported to hyperpolarize the preterminal endings of primary afferent neurons in the nucleus oralis.[569] The application of strychnine to the nucleus caudalis potentiates the hyperpolarization induced by dental pulp stimulation of primary afferent terminals located in the rostral sensory nuclei.[570] Thus, neurons of the nucleus caudalis may hyperpolarize primary afferent terminals synapsing on neurons in the more rostral sensory trigeminal nuclei. Behavioral evidence for such a facilitatory action of nucleus caudalis neurons on afferent impulse transmission in the nucleus oralis and main sensory nucleus has been obtained in the cat. After application of strychnine to the nucleus caudalis, strong pseudoaffective responses to stroking of the fur have occurred.[524] Clinical observations of patients with syringomyelia progressing to syringobulbia are not in agreement, however, with the proposed role of ipsilateral projections within trigeminal nuclei in pain. Because this lesion normally does not involve the trigeminal nuclei, the loss of pain coincident with the rostral progression of thermalgesia into the facial region in an onion-skin distribution cannot be attributed to severance of rostrocaudal projections within the trigeminal nuclei. Rather, such observations would suggest that fibers decussating within the brainstem have been interrupted.

Visceral Afferent Organization

Innervation of the visceral organs derives from sensory afferents, the cell bodies of which are in the DRG, and the fibers of which travel with sympathetic and parasympathetic axons. It has been estimated that the visceral afferents account for about 10% of the fibers that run in the dorsal roots. Yet these visceral afferents serve an organ surface area equivalent to about 25% of the body surface, which suggests that visceral sensitivity will be poorly localized. To understand visceral pain, one must recognize that these afferents appear to converge onto somatotopically organized dorsal horn systems, which receive cutaneous input. Gallbladder and urinary bladder stimulation serves to excite cells that have a corresponding cutaneous dermatomal field. Thus, it is not surprising that certain visceral pains are associated predominantly with certain dermatomal segments. Such segments correspond with the cutaneous innervation of that particular spinal segment. With regard to thoracic input, therefore, sensory information from thoracic viscera will serve to activate sensory afferents traveling with sympathetic fibers that terminate in cord segments T1–T4. Similarly, sensory input that results in activity in visceral sympathetic afferents will enter the spinal cord at segments T5–T12/L1, traveling via the splanchnic nerves through the celiac plexus. These afferents enter the dorsal horn of the spinal cord to terminate in the dorsal gray matter. At this point, convergence with somatic afferent input onto common postsynaptic neurons occurs. As noted in previous sections, both spinoreticular and spinothalamic projecting neurons showed such viscerosomatic and muscular somatic convergence as a common property. Such neurons will respond not only to noxious events, that is, cardiac ischemia or smooth muscle spasm, but also to more benign input such as distention of the bladder (see previous).

SUPRASPINAL ELEMENTS IN NOCICEPTIVE TRANSMISSION

Supraspinal nuclear groups participating in the processing of pain-relevant information have been tentatively identified on the basis of their connectivity and their response to a peripheral stimulus adequate to evoke pain behavior. The accessibility of those pathways that project in the VLF has facilitated extensive investigations of the supraspinal connections of these pathways. As noted earlier, there are essentially three major sites of termination: the medulla, the mesencephalon, and the diencephalon (Figs. 32-16 through 32-18).

Medullary Reticular Formation

Given the ipsilateral spinopetal projections and the reticulothalamic projections from the medullary reticular neurons to the intralaminar and ventrobasal nuclei of the thalamus, the medullary reticular formation has been suggested as a "relay" station for the rostrad transmission of nociceptive information. Retrogradely labeled neurons have been localized to neurons in the medullary reticular formation following the injection of horseradish peroxidase into the thalamus.[433] Medullary reticular neurons are activated antidromically by stimulation in the thalamus.[571] Conversely, stimulation of the medullary reticular formation has been reported to activate thalamic neurons.[571–573] Physiologic studies support the anatomic evidence that medullary reticular neurons receive peripheral input by means of spinal systems that travel in the VLF. Neurons of the lateral reticular nucleus,[498] the nucleus gigantocellularis,[574–578] the nuclei raphe magnus and pallidus,[342] and the nucleus locus coeruleus[579] are activated by noxious or innocuous stimuli, or both, applied to their peripheral receptive fields. These receptive fields, both ipsilateral and contralateral, are large, often including an entire limb or extending over the entire body.[342,498,574,580] Because the spinoreticular fibers that project to these regions do not commonly display such broad receptive fields and project predominantly ipsilaterally (see previous), the existence of extensive receptive fields suggests supraspinal convergence. Many of these neurons that are responsive to somatic input are also activated by auditory and visual stimuli.[572]

A significant proportion of neurons of the various medullary reticular nuclei behave as spinal WDR neurons.[342,574,577,579] Neurons of the nucleus gigantocellularis are most effectively activated following electrical stimulation of nerves sufficient to evoke afferent volleys in Aδ- and C-fibers; volleys in larger diameter A-fibers are ineffective or less so.[574,576,578,581] Intraarterial injection of algogenic agents such as bradykinin or intense stimulation of the splanchnic nerve will alter the discharge of nucleus gigantocellularis neurons.[575] Although the number of neurons responding to muscle afferents is small, the most effective input has arisen from group II and III fibers.[278,582]

Several classical lines of evidence have been marshaled to correlate neural activity in the nucleus gigantocellularis with pain behavior in unanesthetized animals:[122,123,126,403]

- In unanesthetized cats, as the intensity of an electrical stimulus applied to the radial nerve is elevated (through chronically implanted electrodes), so too is the discharge frequency of single neurons of the nucleus gigantocellularis. The stimulus intensity that evokes escape behavior is also the minimum intensity that produces a maximum discharge rate in that neuron.
- The discharge frequency of thalamic neurons has been correlated with the intensity of stimuli delivered to the nucleus gigantocellularis and the escape threshold in awake animals.
- Stimulation of the nucleus gigantocellularis may be used to evoke learned escape behavior in rats and cats. Additionally, such stimuli can serve as an unconditioned stimulus in pavlovian conditioning paradigms. In unanesthetized animals, the activity of nucleus gigantocellularis neurons covaries with the intensity of somatic stimulation, and stimuli applied to the nucleus gigantocellularis will drive thalamic neurons, evoke escape behavior, and support pavlovian conditioning.
- Lesions of the nucleus gigantocellularis have been shown to attenuate the response to otherwise aversive stimuli in the absence of any significant signs of motor impairment.

Several cautionary notes should be considered in these and other studies in which the behavioral effects of stimulating and lesioning of supraspinal systems are used to examine the involvement of a given structure in a pain event. Electrical stimulation or lesions of nuclei also affect fibers of passage and so may inhibit or activate ascending or descending pathways relevant to the pain event. Thus, stimulation of spinothalamic fibers could produce a direct drive of thalamic substrates in a manner independent of the system within the nuclei being stimulated. Within the brainstem, particularly the nucleus gigantocellularis, there is a preponderance of connections with autonomic nuclei and sensations related to gastric secretion, nausea, or tachycardia that are likely to be stimulated by activation of efferent/autonomic pathways. These syndromes might be unpleasant, and such sensations themselves might underlie the "aversive" characteristics of local stimulation. It is thus possible that the role played by these nuclei is not related to the "conscious" perception of a pain event, but rather they could serve as the mediators of the autonomic sequelae evoked by high-intensity somatic stimulation.

Parabrachial Nucleus

The parabrachial nucleus is a population of neurons that can be discriminated into a number of subnuclei, each with distinct input–output relationships.[586] Parabrachial neurons project to lateral medulla, the periaqueductal gray, the central nucleus of the amygdala, and to the midline and intralaminar as well as the ventromedial thalamus[493,587] (Fig. 32-17). Single-unit recording has identified nociceptive-responsive cells in the parabrachial region. These cells typically have large receptive fields that include two or more body parts, suggesting that there is significant convergence from spinal lamina I neurons on these cells.[588]

Mesencephalic Reticular Formation and Central Gray Matter

These regions receive crossed and uncrossed projections from spinomesencephalic neurons. Neurons of the central gray project rostrally to terminate in the midline and intralaminar nuclei of the thalamus and the caudal hypothalamus[571,589–592] (Fig. 32-16). Of particular interest are the massive projections that connect the central gray matter with the subjacent tegmentum.[591]

Units in the mesencephalic central gray matter and in the adjacent mesencephalic reticular formation are differentially responsive to innocuous and noxious cutaneous and electrical stimuli, with units phasically excited by innocuous mechanical stimulation but responding to noxious stimuli (i.e., pinching or heating) with sustained discharges.[336,593–596] A close correlation exists between the high-frequency discharge of these neurons evoked by noxious natural stimulation and the ability of electrical C-fiber activation to drive the unit.[594,595,597] As in other brainstem regions, few if any neurons in this region are uniquely nociceptive. Thus, cells that appear to be activated only by noxious tail pinch can be driven by electrical stimulation of the coccygeal nerve at intensities that evoke only a fast-conducting (Aβ) volley.[597] Thus, experiments that examine only "natural" input may fail to observe the presence of weak but clearly present connections. Neurons of the mesencephalic reticular formation display a high degree of convergence with bilateral receptive fields that may include the entire body.[499,593,596,597] Little evidence exists for a specific somatotopic organization of input to these regions, although there may be a distribution.[598,599] Stimulation of the mesencephalic central gray matter and adjacent mesencephalic reticular formation evokes signs of intense discomfort in the cat, as characterized by flattening of the ears, vocalization, pupil dilatation, and attempts to escape. In humans, autonomic responses are elicited along with reports of dysphoria.[600–604]

Although electrolytic lesions of the central gray/mesencephalic reticular nuclei have been reported to alter nociceptive responsiveness,[605,606] a significant portion of the literature suggests little, if any, effects after either lesion or reversible blockade.[607–610] Observation that activation of these areas has an aversive consequence is consistent with the known projections of these nuclei to the medial and intralaminar nuclei of the thalamus. Yet the failure of lesions to elevate the pain threshold indicates that this region is not essential. It might be argued that lesions failed to affect a sufficient volume of tissue and that total destruction of this complex region would leave the animal moribund. The observation that electrical stimulation of the mesencephalic reticular formation would excite spinothalamic cells suggests that pathways either originating in, or passing through, the mesencephalon may exert an excitatory effect on the activity of spinothalamic neurons otherwise evoked by noxious peripheral stimuli.[512] Such a situation might explain why stimulation in the mesencephalon would be aversive, whereas lesions would fail to block the rostrad transmission of information via the diffuse spinothalamic and mesencephalic system and so would not alter the pain threshold (Figs. 32-15 and 32-16).

Diencephalon

As appreciated from the previous sections, sensory information can be broadly considered to reach the thalamic nuclei through monosynaptic or polysynaptic linkages (e.g., spinothalamic versus spinoreticulo, mescephalic, or parabrachial-thalamic connections). Several nuclear groups of the thalamus receive projections primarily from the spinal cord—the posterior nuclear complex, ventrobasal complex, and medial/intralaminar nuclear complex—and are thought to be associated with the transmission of somatic information evoked by noxious stimuli (Fig. 32-19). (For further comments, see previous section on ventrolateral tract projections.)

Posterior Nuclear Complex

The posterior nuclear area comprises the suprageniculate limitants and a heterogeneous region of ill-defined cell groups extending rostrally in the medial geniculate toward the caudal pole of the ventromedial group; the ventral medial nucleus (VMPo).[611] Input into this region is primarily contributed by the spinothalamic system[480,504,612,613] with lemniscal input from the dorsal column nuclei and the parabracheal region. Several projections arise from the posterior complex, but of principal interest are the projections to the posterior portion of the somatosensory area (I–II) of the cortex[611] and the inferior insula.

Populations of neurons in the posterior nuclear complex respond to noxious stimuli.[614–617] These neurons display large bilateral receptive fields. A number of the neurons resemble the WDR neurons in the spinal cord (discharge frequency proportional to the intensity of the applied stimulus). Electrical activation of Aδ afferents from tooth pulp, presumably noxious in nature, also evokes activity in neurons of the posterior thalamic complex.[618] Although these investigations clearly suggest the existence of neurons in the posterior complex that can be activated by nociceptive input, other investigations have failed to observe as large a population of neurons responsive to noxious

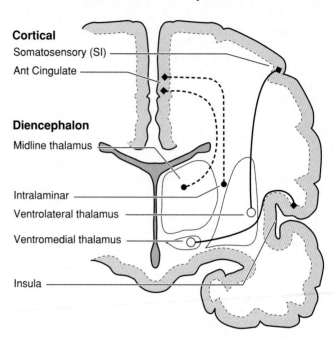

Thalamo-Cortical Projections

FIGURE 32-19. Schema displaying the connectivity of the thalamo-cortical projections. Note the midline and intralaminar projections into the limbic forebrain (anterior cingulate) and inferior insula and the ventrolateral thalamus into the somatosensory cortex.

input.[619–621] Lesions of the monkey posterior nuclear complex reduce the responsiveness of animals to maximum mechanical stimuli,[622] but the literature is generally inconclusive concerning the effects of such lesions in humans; at best, the effects are transient.[623]

Ventrobasal Complex

The lateral thalamus or ventrobasal complex (nucleus ventralis posterior and nucleus ventralis lateralis) is situated in the ventrolateral quadrant of the thalamus. Neurons of this region project in a somatotopic manner to SI and SII of the somatosensory cortex. The projection to SI is greater than to SII. The SII receives no independent input, but rather appears innervated by collaterals of the projection to SI.[624–629]

The ventrobasal nuclei classically have been thought to receive primarily lemniscal input from the dorsal column nuclei.[613,630,631] The spinothalamic tract is a minor source of input.[481,504,632] After sectioning of the dorsal columns, sparing the VLF, only a small number of neurons in the ventrobasal region are activated by either noxious or non-noxious peripheral stimuli.[633] Most neurons in the ventrobasal complex are responsive to innocuous tactile or thermal stimuli, or to joint movement and aversive visceral stimulation.[631,634–638] The number of neurons responsive to noxious stimuli is much smaller, about 6% to 10% of the sample.[618,636,639] In the ventroposterolateral axis, large populations of neurons responsive to noxious input have been identified.[640–642] Lesions in the ventrobasal complex in a variety of species alter somatosensory discrimination. White and Sweet noted in humans that such lesions produce transient analgesia.[464] Similar findings have been reported in cats.[643] Stimulation of the ventrobasal complex in humans commonly produces non-noxious paresthesias and tingling[644] (Fig. 32-19).

Intralaminar and Medial Nuclei

The intralaminar nuclear complex forms a shell around the lateral aspect of the nucleus medialis dorsalis and comprises five nuclear groups: paracentralis, centralis medialis, centromedian, centralis lateralis, and parafascicularis. Input to these nuclei is contributed primarily by the spinothalamic tract[481,504,612,613] and the nucleus reticularis gigantocellularis. These reticulothalamic projections are thought to be a major source of input to the intralaminar complex.[572,645,646] The intralaminar thalamic complex projects diffusely to wide areas of the cerebral cortex, including the frontal, parietal, and limbic regions.[647] Of particular interest are the projections from the intralaminar to the anterior cingulate[648] (Fig. 32-19).

The medial regions receiving ascending input are composed of several nuclear groups, including the centromedian and parafascicular region. The centromedian and parafascicular are said to receive input from the nucleus reticularis gigantocellularis (medulla). The mediodorsal is of particular interest, as it receives input primarily from spinothalamic tract neurons originating in lamina I (high-threshold marginal cells). These regions project heavily to the limbic cortex, notably the anterior cingulate[648] (Fig. 32-19).

Populations of neurons in the medial and intralaminar nuclei respond to noxious stimuli and encode the stimulus intensity in the duration and frequency of patterned discharges.[608] A proportion of neurons in these regions respond exclusively to innocuous stimuli or respond to both innocuous and noxious stimuli.[309,614,633,649-652] Consistent with these observations, volleys in Aδ- and C-fibers produced by electrical stimulation of peripheral nerves evoke activity in neurons of the medial and intralaminar nuclei.[651] The receptive fields of neurons in these regions are large, often bilateral, with little evidence for a somatotopic organization of input.[255,309,649,651,653] Neurons of the medial and intralaminar nuclei receive convergent input from skin, joints, and muscle.[649,651] In humans, neurons in the centromedian–parafascicular region, which possess large receptive fields, occasionally including the contralateral half and ipsilateral upper half of the body, are found to be responsive to noxious stimuli. Two classes of neurons have been described: those activated with a short latency to response and those activated with a long latency. The former category of neurons is found predominantly in the basomedial portions of the parafascicular nucleus, and the latter group is localized to the dorsal centromedian and parafascicular regions.

Although it is argued that intralaminar nuclei, particularly the centromedian–parafascicular region, are involved in nociception, lesion studies conducted in rats, cats, and monkeys have failed to report an alteration in the animals' response to noxious stimuli following large lesions.[654-656] Alternately, such lesions have produced increases in nociceptive threshold as assessed by tooth pulp stimulation in cats[657,658] and operant response to shock in primates.[659,660] In addition, a significant relief of intractable pain arising from neoplastic disease has been reported following lesions of the medial thalamus.[661] In general, the centromedian–parafascicular mediodorsalis complex appears to be a critical compoent of pathways related to affect.[648,662,663]

Cortical Projections

Somatosensory Projection

The somatosensory areas (SI/SII) receive input indirectly from the three major spinal systems through which ascending sensory and noxious information may travel.[38] Investigations have focused attention on the importance of the SII area in the reception and perception of pain information. This area of the cortex may be divided into an anterior and posterior region.[629] The anterior region is thought to receive input primarily from the ventrobasal thalamic nuclei,[624–626,628] and neurons in this region are activated by light tactile stimuli. Input to this region is somatotopically arranged; receptive fields correspond with precise symmetric sites on both sides of the body[629] (Fig. 32-19).

Posterior SII receives input largely from the posterior thalamic complex.[611] Neurons in this region possess receptive fields that encompass large asymmetric areas of the body.[629] These neurons are polysensory, and a number respond to high-intensity mechanical stimuli.[629,664] The responsive properties of these neurons resemble those reported for neurons in the posterior thalamic nuclei.[617,633] Neurons in the posterior thalamic complex are antidromically activated by stimulation of posterior SII, and nociresponsive neurons could still be observed in the cortex of cats having lesions of the dorsal funiculus, suggesting that input eventually arriving at the cortex could, in fact, travel over the ventrolateral quadrants.[665,666] It has been observed that bilateral destruction of that area to which the posterior thalamic nuclei project produces an increase in the nociceptive threshold.

Limbic System

Although these comments document those pathways that are part of the classic somatosensory projection system, it has become increasingly apparent that other regions play an important role. Thus, outflow from the medial thalamic region project into the anterior cingulate cortex (ACC). Other regions, such as the VMPo, produce output that reaches the insula. Regions such as the anterior cingulate, insula, and amygdala are part of the limbic forebrain; they have long been presumed to play an important role in emotionality and are activated by anxiety and stress. These systmes have been shown to play a profound role in modulating the pain response. This will be discussed further in upcoming sections[648,662] (Fig. 32-19).

Correlation of Activation Patterns in Brain Centers with Behavior Evoked by Noxious Input

In the face of increasingly intense stimuli, increasing activation of cortical centers occurs. As shown, such intensity encoding occurs in the primary somatosensory cortex in the human observer as defined using functional magnetic resonance imaging (fMRI) (Fig. 32-20).[667] Specific studies have shown the anticipated localization that has classically defined cortical somatotopic mapping. In addition to the somatosensory cortex, other regions have also been shown to be activated. Of particular interest has been the activation of limbic structures. Thus, it has been found that discrete regions within the anterior cingulate gyrus and the inferior insula of the cortex are activated by noxious stimuli (Fig. 32-20).[662,663,668,669] As noted, these regions are strongly associated with emotionality. As reviewed earlier, these regions receive input from medial aspects of the thalamus (as opposed to the classic relay centers of the lateral thalamus).

PART IV: PAIN MANAGEMENT

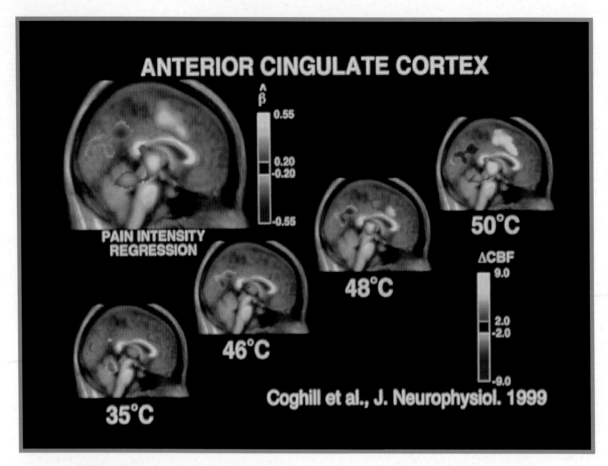

FIGURE 32-20. Functional magnetic resonance imaging showing increasing activation (blood volume/flow) of anterior cingulate (*bottom*) with increasing intensity of thermal stimulus (35°C–50°C) applied to the contralateral forearm in a single human subject. From Coghill RC, Sang CN, Maisog JM, et al. Pain intensity processing within the human brain: a bilateral, distributed mechanism. *J. Neurophysiol* 1999; 82(4):1934–1943.

Functional Relevance of Ascending Limbic and Somatosensory Projections

At present, it is appreciated that the WDR neurons typically project into the lateral thalamus, where their input is mapped precisely onto a sensory homunculus. These cells then project rostrally to the somatosensory cortex, where that input is similarly mapped onto a sensory homunculus. In this system, each site on the body surface is faithfully mapped, and this map is maintained to the cortex. This system is uniquely able to preserve anatomic information as well as information regarding the intensity of the stimulus (as initially provided by the frequency response characteristics of the WDR neuron). This system is able to provide the information necessary for mapping the "sensory-discriminative" dimension of pain.[670]

Although these comments document the pathways relevant to the rostral movement of pain information (i.e., the sensory-discriminative aspects of the stimulus), it is clear that the pain response has an overriding affective–motivational component that is every bit as important to behavior as the initiating stimulus. In the space available, it is not possible to deal with this except to note that a variety of lesion procedures in humans and animals have been shown to psychophysically dissociate the reported stimulus intensity from its affective component. Such disconnection syndromes are produced

by prefrontal lobectomies, cingulotomies, and temporal lobe/amygdala lesions.[671,672] The limbic structures, such as the anterior cingulate and insula, are believed to be associated with emotional content. Preclinical work indicates that the anterior cingulate cortex plays an important role in the processing of affective components of nociception.[673,674] As in humans, fMRI in rats has shown that the ACC is activated by nociceptive stimuli.[675] These limbic circuits thus provide one aspect of a system that appears to be activated by particularly intense stimuli (e.g., receiving strong input from the lamina I nociceptors). Accordingly, such systems might be speculated to underlie the affective–motivational component of the pain pathway.[670]

The potential role of these limbic systems associated with the affective-motivational aspect of the pain response can be suggested by two observations. First, a strong correlation exists between pain and anxiety in the clinical environment.[676,677] Conversely, reduction of anxiety through therapy or drugs can diminish the pain report.[678] Second, it has been shown that the degree of activation of the anterior cingulate covaries with the perceived intensity of the pain stimulus. Rainville and colleagues found that hypnotic suggestions leading to an enhanced pain report in response to a given experimental stimulus resulted in greater activity in the anterior cingulate with no change in the somatosensory cortex[668] (Fig. 32-21).

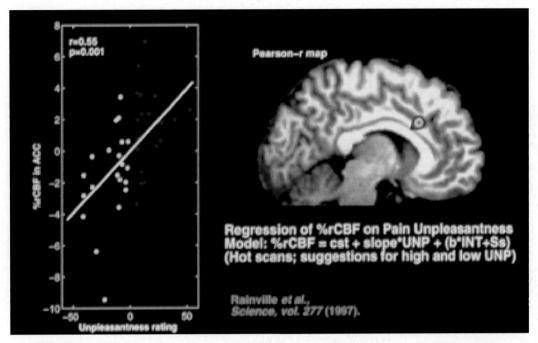

FIGURE 32-21. Subjects were scanned while receiving a fixed thermal noxious stimulus. This typically resulted in the activation of the anterior cingulate gyrus (*right*). The magnitude of the increase in blood flow was plotted against the reported unpleasantness of the stimulus-induced pain state. As noted, a positive covariance occurred between activation and reported pain for the given stimulus. From Rainville P, Duncan GH, Price DD, et al. Pain affect encoded in human anterior cingulate but not somatosensory cortex. *Science.* 1997; 277(5328):968–971.

NOCICEPTIVE PROCESSING: MODULATORY SUBSTRATES

As noted in the introductory sections of this chapter, the consideration of the afferent limb of the ascending pathways through which pain-related information travels may be thought of not only in terms of the elements through which the information travels, but also in terms of the systems that modulate transmission at each level of the synapse. From a historical perspective, the role of modulation has been considered in the context of a suppression of the magnitude of the pain message and the teleology of "endogenous analgesic systems." In the late 1970s and early 1980s, much attention was therefore paid to the role of descending pathways and endogenous, modulatory (endorphinergic) systems. These systems clearly continue to play a role, but of greater interest has been the evolving insight that afferent input can serve to drive a *facilitation* in the response evoked by a given stimulus, that is, tissue injury evokes changes that result in the augmentation of the response evoked by a subsequent stimulus (Fig. 32-1). Further, although it has been appreciated since the early prescient writings of Weir-Mitchell and colleagues[679] that a prominent pain state can be evoked by light touch (allodynia) after nerve injury, the significance of this phenomenon had been poorly incorporated into theoretic mechanisms until recently. As will be discussed, it is clear now that peripheral injury leads to an acute alteration in the response evoked by light touch and to long-term changes in the connectivity of the spinal systems. Accordingly, it is now clear that the encoding of afferent information is much more complex than originally appreciated and that the processing of somatic and visceral information is an extremely dynamic event. Appreciation of these characteristics provides insights into the important principles that define the encoding of information leading to pain behavior.

In the following section, several of the networks that are believed to play an important role in altering the encoding or afferent transmission along the neuraxis will be broadly considered.

Spino-spinal Linkages

Activation of a number of physiologically defined elements has been shown to alter spinal transmission. A number of inhibitory systems have been identified. Dorsal column stimulation activates collaterals of large primary afferents and depresses the C-fiber–evoked discharge of dorsal horn nociceptors.[121] These results fulfilled one prediction of the gate control theory originally proposed by Melzack and Wall,[680] and led to the clinical use of dorsal column stimulation for the relief of pain.[681,682] The neuronal pathways that mediate the mechanisms of inhibition of the cord are believed to involve the activation of inhibitory interneurons that regulate the excitability of the dorsal horn projection neuron (Fig. 32-22). Stimulation of the lateral Lissauer tract (a presumed outflow of gelatinosa neurons) results in the development of segmental dorsal root potentials (DRPs)[683] and a concurrent inhibition of the polysynaptic ventral root reflex, as well as the discharge of WDR neurons evoked by noxious stimulation.[485,684] In contrast, lesion of the Lissauer tract results in an *increased* receptive field size.[539] These observations emhasize the inhibitory role that such gelatinosa neurons play in regulating afferent evoked spinal excitation.

PART IV: PAIN MANAGEMENT

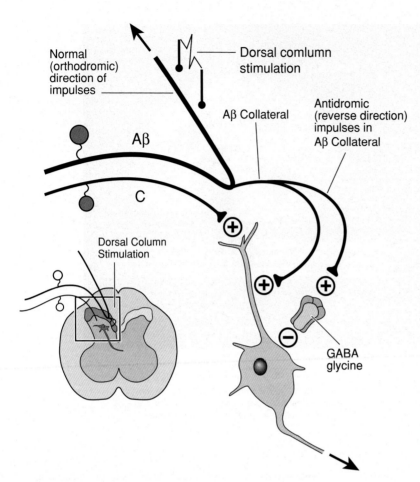

FIGURE 32-22. Schematic displaying small and large afferent drive of dorsal horn neuron. Activation of dorsal column large afferent (Aβ) collateral results in antidromic drive of dorsal horn interneuron, which serves to inhibit through the local release of GABA and/or glycine. This is one mechanism thought to be activated by "dorsal column stimulators" and leading to the antinociceptive effects of this modality.

Brainstem–Spinal Linkages

Classic work by Hagbarth and Kerr[685] demonstrated the ability of descending long-tract systems to modulate spinal-evoked activity. Early on, Takagi and colleagues[686] pointed to a possible role of descending systems in mediating the effects of morphine (Fig. 32-23). It has long been known that activation of the pathways originating in the brainstem and descending to the spinal cord can inhibit activity evoked in flexor reflex afferents.[687–689] Virtually every pathway carrying nociceptive information, including the spinoreticular[690] and spinothalamic,[691] has been shown to be under modulatory control of pathways that originate supraspinally. Bulbospinal projections will diminish the slope of the response (frequency of discharge) versus the stimulus intensity curve of dorsal horn neurons, as well as shift the temperature intercept of the stimulus–response curve to the right, indicating an increase in the threshold stimulus intensity necessary to evoke activity in the cell.[692,693]

The classic observation that microinjections of morphine into the brain stem could inhibit spinal reflex activity,[694] and the subsequent demonstration that stimulation in the mesencephalon and medulla will inhibit the discharge of neurons in the spinal cord and trigeminal nucleus[487,556,691,695,696] evoked by nociceptive stimulation, emphasized the likely role of spinopetal systems in controlling spinal processing. In unanesthetized animals, such stimulation has been shown to alter the response to noxious stimuli and inhibit reflex function.[697,698] The nature of this descending inhibition has been a subject of considerable investigation, and it is increasingly apparent that

a significant proportion of this modulation is mediated by the activation of descending monoaminergic pathways. Evidence for this may be briefly summarized as follows:

- Electrical stimulation or microinjections of opiates at brainstem sites such as the periaqueductal gray or the nucleus gigantocellularis will inhibit nociceptive reflexes, and this effect is antagonized by the intrathecal administration of noradrenergic antagonists.[699–701]
- Microinjections of morphine or focal stimulation in the medulla or periaqueductal gray that alter nociceptive thresholds are associated with an increased release of serotonin or norepinephrine in the spinal cord.[362,702]
- Spinal application of adrenergic or serotonergic agonists either by iontophoresis or by intrathecal administration in the unanesthetized animal will antagonize the Aδ-/C-fiber–evoked activity in dorsal horn neurons and is associated with significant analgesia, respectively.[424,703,704]

As noted, both serotonin and norepinephrine are released in the spinal cord by high- but not low-intensity stimulation of afferent input (sciatic nerve).[705] Importantly, spinal transections inhibit this effect, indicating that the release is mediated by a spinobulbospinal loop. Significantly, stimulation of regions remote from the lumbar spinal cord region from which the release has been measured (infraorbital branch of the trigeminal nerve) also produces release of serotonin and norepinephrine in the lumbar spinal cord region. This suggests that these particular descending systems, the activity of which is manifested by serotonin and norepinephrine release,

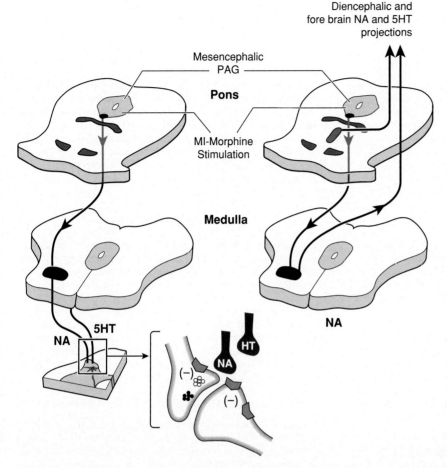

FIGURE 32-23. Several mechanisms whereby opiates in the periaqueductal gray act to alter pain behavior. *Left:* The periaqueductal gray (PAG)–medullary–spinal linkage that regulates dorsal horn excitability. Here, PAG microinjection of a μ-opiate such as morphine will activate PAG–medullary projections. These subsequently lead to activation of bulbospinal monamines that inhibit primary afferent–evoked excitation of dorsal horn wide dynamic range neurons through the spinal release of noradrenaline, acting upon local spinal α_2-receptors present pre- and postsynaptically, on the primary afferent and serotonin (5HT) (see inset). *Right:* Many of the bulbospinal systems activated by opiates have an ascending 5HT and noradrenaline (NA) counterpart arising from the dorsal raphe nucleus and the locus coeruleus, respectively. These ascending monoamine systems project to forebrain regions associated with affect.

are globally activated by afferent input. This is in marked contrast to the enkephalin-evoked release from the spinal cord, in which such distal stimulation has failed to have any influence on spinal release.[705,706] Although the principal interest thus far has focused largely on spinopetal aminergic pathways, other neurotransmitter systems have been shown to project to the spinal cord, including dopamine,[653,707] SP,[653] thyrotropin-releasing hormone,[653] and CCK.[708] The complexity of this system is emphasized further by the fact that a number of these agents may be co-contained, such as SP and serotonin,[709] and enkephalin and serotonin. These several systems clearly provide substrates whereby brainstem systems may interact with spinal cord sensorimotor processing.

Brainstem–Brainstem Linkages

Although most work examining the effects of brainstem manipulations on nociceptive responsiveness has focused on projections to the spinal cord, significant evidence suggests that supraspinal, brainstem, and modulatory influences are exerted by various systems. Thus, the nucleus gigantocellularis, as discussed previously, may represent an important supraspinal link in systems through which nociceptive information may travel en route to higher centers. It has been demonstrated that mesencephalic stimulation will inhibit the discharge of neurons in the nucleus gigantocellularis in response to peripheral stimulation.[710] Thus, although brainstem manipulations that inhibit spinal reflex functions (such as the tail flick) may

indeed alter the rostral transmission of information relevant to pain behavior, it is likely that this is not the only method whereby these supraspinal systems modulate the ascending pain message. Intrathecal administration of aminergic antagonists, therefore, will produce a significant reversal of the effects of these descending systems on spinal reflex function but has a subtotal effect on the supraspinally mediated aspects of the behavior.[699,711,712] This suggests that these supraspinal systems may act at several levels to modulate the animal's processing of nociceptive information.

Brainstem—Forebrain Linkages

Several lines of evidence emphasize the role of ascending systems in the modulation of the organism's response to noxious stimulus. Significant projections exist from the mesencephalic central gray matter into the vicinity of the medial thalamus.[713–715] Although some of these projections may indeed be a part of the ascending sensory projection system, stimulation in the periaqueductal gray matter has been shown to produce a significant inhibition of the response of these medial thalamic neurons.[716,717] The neurotransmitter mediator of this is not known, although ascending serotonergic projections from the raphe have been well described, and the iontophoretic administration of serotonin will reduce the firing of these thalamic neurons.[333,718] Importantly, stimulation of the dorsal raphe will produce similar effects on the firing of parafascicular neurons.[716]

PART IV: PAIN MANAGEMENT

As noted earlier, brainstem stimulation in animals and man is antinociceptive. Although it has been suggested that this brain effect in humans is due to the activation of descending pathways, such stimulation rarely has any effect on human spinal reflex function, even in those cases in which analgesia has been reported and documented.[719-722] These several observations are of particular interest in view of the clinical reports that brainstem stimulation can produce significant changes in the patient's affective response in various chronic pain conditions. Aside from the role played by these pathways in regulating afferent traffic, it should be stressed that all forebrain serotonin and norepinphrine arises from brainstem nuclei such as the dorsal raphe and the locus coreuleus, respectively. There is a general appreciation that the effect of monoamine uptake inhibitors (e.g., tricyclic antidepressants) are likely mediated through effects upon these for brain projections, thus enhancing serotnin and noradrenaline tone by reducing their reuptake.[723]

Early studies have demonstrated that stimulation of the caudate nucleus produces significant interaction of the medial thalamic and interlaminar nuclei and that this interaction is largely inhibitory in character.[724] Electrical stimulation of the caudate nucleus in primates has been reported to reduce the affective response to strong cutaneous stimulation.[725]

Corticospinal systems have long been known to have a significant effect on spinal afferent transmission. Thus, electrical stimulation of the sensory cortex has been reported to affect afferent transmission and reflex pathways.[685,726] Stimulation of the somatosensory SI region of the cortex can result in a significant reduction in the response of spinothalamic neurons to C-fiber activity evoked by high-intensity thermal mechanical stimuli.[727]

DYNAMIC CHARACTERISTICS OF ENCODING SYSTEMS FOR NOCICEPTION

In the preceding section, it was emphasized that a variety of physiologically defined linkages can influence processing at all levels of the neuraxis. In the present section, we focus on several aspects of the afferent processing that emphasize the dynamic and "plastic" nature of the encoding process. These directions of research have provided a rich source for practically defining the mechanisms whereby pain information is encoded.

As noted, principal classes of neurons in the dorsal horn show an excitation evoked by large (low-threshold) and small (high-threshold) primary afferents. We will consider in the following sections that traffic evoked by both large and small afferents is subject to up- and downregulation by a variety of neurochemical systems. In the first section, we will deal with those systems believed to downregulate the response to small and large afferent input.

Inhibitory Systems

As indicated previously, dorsal horn neurons typically display an increasing response in the face of an increasing stimulus intensity. It is likely that this reflects an increased release of afferent excitatory transmitter and the subsequent depolarization of the second-order neuron. Factors that diminish that input–output function would predictably change the magnitude of the pain behavior evoked by a given stimulus. A number of physiologic and pharmacologic mechanisms have been shown to reduce the slope of the stimulus–response relationship at the spinal level. These will be considered in the following sections for input driven by small and large primary afferents.

Modulation of Small-afferent Evoked Excitation

Pharmacologic investigations have revealed that the activation of a variety of spinal receptor systems will depress the discharge of dorsal horn neurons evoked by small high-intensity/small-afferent–mediated input. In contrast, at comparable doses, a minimal effect occurs upon the excitaiton evoked by large low-threshold primary afferents. As indicated in Figure 32-24, some receptor classes, including those for the μ- and δ-opioid, and α_2-adrenergic and γ-aminobutyric acid (GABA)$_B$ receptors, will produce a powerful suppression of the excitation of activated

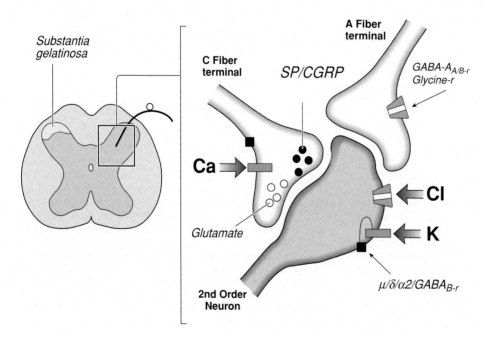

FIGURE 32-24. Organization of several principal modulatory receptors in dorsal horn regulating nociceptive processing. Binding of $\mu/\delta/\alpha_2$ and GABA$_B$ receptor is high in dorsal root ganglia (small, but not large cells) and in the substantia gelatinosa on terminals of small afferents and on second-order neurons. Presynaptic sites reduce release of glutamate/peptides (substance P/calcitonin gene-related peptide) by inhibition of opening of voltage-sensitive calcium channels. Postsynaptic sites hyperpolarize neurons by increasing potassium conductance. GABA$_A$ and glycine sites are present on the terminals of large afferents and second-order neurons.

dorsal horn neurons, produced by the activation of populations of small afferents, and yield an increase in the stimulus intensity required to evoke a given pain response (e.g., analgesia) after spinal delivery. Conversely, in preclinical and clinical models, the response to light touch is unaltered. The mechanisms by which these several modulatory receptor systems exert their surprisingly selective effect upon small, high-threshold afferent-evoked excitation and pain behavior follow a common motif.

Presynaptic Actions. As indicated in Figure 32-24, several of the receptor systems display binding that is presynaptic on primary afferents, and, given the selective effects of capsaicin as a C-fiber neurotoxin in diminishing this binding,[393] this effect appears to occur largely on small fibers.[728,729] Consistent with the presynaptic locus of binding, agonist occupancy of these receptors has been shown to diminish the depolarization-evoked release of spinal excitatory amino acids (glutamate) and peptide (SP and CGRP).[358,364,368,730,731] Given that similar reductions in binding may frequently be produced by treatment with capsaicin and/or rhizotomy suggests that the majority of this primary afferent binding is present on TRPV1 receptor-positive terminals (e.g., C-fibers) and not on large low-threshold primary afferents.

Postsynaptic Actions. Although rhizotomy may diminish significantly the binding for a number of the receptor systems, none has shown a reduction typically greater than 50% to 75%. This suggests that additional binding occurs that is not on the primary afferent. A variety of studies have shown that these receptors exert their effect by increasing K^+ conduction through a $G_{i/o}$-coupled protein. As the equilibrium potential for K^+ is typically lower than the resting membrane potential, increasing K^+ conductance results in membrane hyperpolarization that serves to depress excitability of the respective postafferent neuron.[732]

It is thus considered that agents possessing a joint pre- and postsynaptic action may exert their powerful modulatory influence by a selective effect upon small-fiber input and a coincidental postsynaptic action.[733] The behavioral relevance of these inhibitory receptor systems via pain is emphasized by the observation that the spinal delivery of the appropriate agonists will serve to regulate the animal's response to mechanical, thermal, and chemical stimuli, which would otherwise evoke indices of pain behavior (e.g., escape, vocalization) in animals and humans. Such actions have been substantiated in humans with the spinal actions of μ, δ, and α_2-adrenoceptor agonists on interneurons.[374,375] Such behavioral observations substantiate the powerful role played by these receptor systems in the regulation of afferent traffic evoked by a high-intensity stimulus. The lack of effect of intrathecal opiates on light touch, however, is consistent with the absence of the respective receptors on low-threshold primary afferent terminals.

Endogenous Activity of Small-afferent Inhibitory Systems. The presence of these receptors and the powerful effects of exogenously administered adrenoceptor and opiate agonists on spinal nociceptive functioning lead to the question of what are the *endogenous* systems that normally act on these receptors and what normally activates those systems?

Endogenous Opioids. Several populations of endorphin-containing neurons have been identified throughout the brain and at the spinal level.[734] These neurons contain proteins associated with the pre-/pro-hormones of pro-opiomelanocortin, pre-/pro-enkephalin, and pre-/pro-dynorphin.[735,736] Products of the latter two populations, such as met- and leu-enkephalins, and various extended peptides such as Phe7Arg6-Met5-enkephalin and extended chains of leu-enkephalin (yielding dynorphins), have been identified in dorsal horn neurons. Importantly, these classes of opioids have been shown to possess a differential receptor preference.[735,736] These intrinsic systems have been shown to be activated by a variety of conditions. Release studies have shown that a variety of spinal endorphins are released from the spinal cord in animal models by high-, but not low-intensity, stimulation and irritant stimuli.[705,706,737–740] Ex vivo spinal slice studies have shown that such release is markedly enhanced by a variety of aminopeptidase, dipeptidyl carboxypeptidase, and neutral endopeptidase inhibitors.[741] Interestingly, the role of endogenous opioids should be straightforwardly examined by demonstrating that naloxone blocks the effect of manipulations believed to be modulated by an endogenous opioid.[742–744] It is generally considered that the degree of opioid receptor activation by the endogenous opioid is limited by the amount released and by the rapid metabolism of peptides. As noted, a variety of peptidase inhibitors can increase extracellular opioid peptides, and such treatment has been shown to produce naloxone-reversible analgesia.

Bulbospinal aminergic systems. As noted, bulbospinal pathways containing serotonin and norepinephrine arise from the midline caudal raphe and lateral tegmentum/locus coruleus, respectively, to project into the dorsolateral funiculus to terminate in the dorsal horn.[745,746]

In the dorsal horn, serotonin can act through a variety of excitatory (5HT2/3) and inhibitory (5HT1b) synapses. The receptors are present on membranes that are pre- and postsynaptic to the primary afferent. Given the presence of both excitatory and inhibitory receptors, the antinociceptive effects of spinal serotonin are complex and controversial. The antinociceptive effects of the 5HT3 agonist activity is considered to be mediated in part by the activation of inhibitory interneurons (e.g., GABAergic or opioidergic). As reviewed earlier, in the dorsal horn, norepinephrine acts through local α_2-adrenergic receptors located presynaptically upon dorsal horn neurons and presynaptically on small primary afferents. Activation of bulbospinal projections can accordingly serve to attenuate the release of small-afferent transmitters and reduce the excitability of second-order neurons.

Release studies have shown that both serotonin and norepinephrine are released from the spinal cord by high-, but not low-intensity, stimulation and irritant stimuli.[705,706,737,738,740] It is interesting to note that uptake inhibitors of serotonin and norepinephrine (e.g., tricyclic antidepressants) have been shown to possess analgesic activity after systemic and intrathecal delivery). The mechanisms of this analgesic effect are believed to reflect upon this enhanced spinal extracellular level of norepinephrine. Interestingly, agents selective for serotonin (i.e., serotonin selective reuptake inhibitors; SSRIs) are typically not considered to show comparable preclinical activity,[747] whereas agents selective for norepinephrine uptake inhibition display analgesic efficacy[748] (Fig. 32-25).

It should be stressed that, although these several endogenous systems clearly have the potential of regulating afferent traffic as indicated by the powerful effects of the exogenously delivered receptor agonists, there is surprisingly little support for the thesis that these systems play a significant ongoing role in the regulation of C-fiber–evoked activity. Thus, with few exceptions, antagonists for these systems, such as naloxone (all opiate receptors) or phentolamine (α-adrenoceptor antagonist), fail to produce evident hyperalgesia in a normal animal.[749]

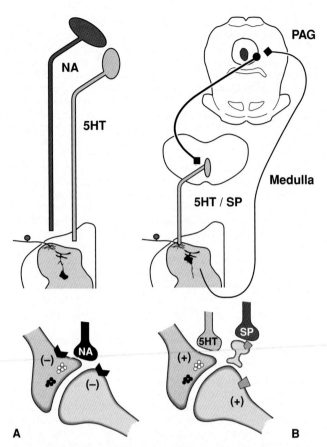

FIGURE 32-25. Complexity of the bulbospinal monamine pathways. **A:** Noradrenaline (NA)-containing cell bodies are present in the brainstem nuclei such as the locus coeruleus. Activation of the bulbospinal NA pathways leads to spinal NA release, which acts through α_2-adrenergic receptors located on the primary afferent and second-order neurons; these serve to inhibit the release of primary afferent transmitter and to hyperpolarize second-order neurons. **B:** Serotonin (5HT)-containing cell bodies are present in the midline raphe nuclei, which give rise to axons that project to the dorsal horn. Here, by an action mediated through excitatory, likely 5HT3 receptors located on second-order neurons, they serve to excite inhibitory interneurons (likely γ-aminobutyric acid), which through their respective receptors inhibit dorsal horn nociceptive neurons. Alternately, these descending pathways may act directly upon dorsal horn nociceptive neurons to facilitate their activation. The indirect connection is thus believed to be antinociceptive, and the second direct projection onto excitatory neurons is pronociceptive.

Modulation of Large-afferent Evoked Excitation

As reviewed earlier, many of the drugs we classify as spinally acting analgesics are present on small, but not large primary afferents. It is clear however that large primary afferent input is subject to powerful regulation by GABA and glycine receptors. As we will see, in contrast to those systems that regulate small-afferent input, large-afferent input is subject to a functionally significant intrinsic regulation by the inhibitory amino acid systems.

γ-Aminobutyric Acid/Glycine Systems

γ-aminotbutyric acid and glycine receptors. γ-Aminobutyric acid and glycine are widely distributed amino acids.

The effects of GABA are mediated not only through a G-protein-coupled receptor (GABA$_B$, see earlier discussion), but by a GABA$_A$, chloride (Cl$^-$) ionophore. γ-Aminobutyric acid effects at the GABA$_A$ site are reversed by bicuculline.[750] Glycine also acts through a ligand-gated Cl$^-$ channel that is blocked by strychnine.[751]

GABA$_A$ and glycine receptors are present throughout the brain. Such neurons are found within the dorsal and ventral horn,[752,753] and glycine[754,755] and GABA[756] binding in the dorsal ventral horn has been demonstrated. These GABA-containing terminals are frequently presynaptic to the large central afferent terminal complexes and may form reciprocal synapses.[757] GABAergic axo-somatic connections on spinothalamic cells have also been identified[752] (Fig. 32-26).

Activation of the GABA$_A$ and glycine receptors results in an increase in Cl$^-$ permeability. Under normal conditions, transmembrane [Cl$^-$] ions at equilibrium are near the resting membrane potential. "Cation-Cl" cotransporters regulate the transmembrane Cl$^-$ gradient by exporting [Cl$^-$]$_i$. Accordingly, it can be seen that, depending upon the membrane potential and the activity of the Cl$^-$ transporter, increasing Cl conductance might lead to an outward or inward current with a net excitatory or inhibitory effect.[758] Typically, in primary afferents, increasing Cl$^-$ permeability is modestly depolarizing. This depolarization induces opening of terminal voltage-sensitive Ca channels, which evokes their inactivation. This effect paradoxically *reduces* transmitter release and is considered to be the mechanism of GABA-mediated primary afferent depolarization (PAD)-induced inhibition. In the second-order neuron, GABA$_A$ activation typically serves to hyperpolarize the membrane, resulting in a net reduction in membrane excitability[759] (Fig. 32-27).

Increasing GABA or glycine tone in the dorsal horn will accordingly serve to reduce net dorsal horn transmission. Perhaps not surprisingly, given the widespread distribution of these ionophores in both the dorsal and ventral horn, their activation by exogenous agonists is frequently associated with motor dysfunction and little evident analgesia.

Endogeneous Activity of Large-afferent Inhibitory Systems. Low-threshold afferents terminate in Rexed lamina below the substantia gelatinosa upon lamina V WDR neurons. As noted in the preceding section, these cells are also activated by small afferents and are believed to play a role in the encoding of the pain message. The afferent barrage evokes activation of GABA/glycinergic interneurons that synapse on adjacent afferent terminals and postsynaptically on second-order neurons. Early studies revealed that the local inhibition of GABA and glycine receptor systems in the vicinity of the primary afferent terminals (using bicuculline or strychnine, respectively) would: (a) significantly enhance the discharge evoked by Aβ-afferents, but only modestly affect the input generated by high-threshold afferents,[551,760] and (b) permit light tactile stroking of the skin to evoke a well-defined pain state as defined by autonomic and behavioral criteria.[761,762] These simple observations suggest that the encoding of low-intensity mechanical stimuli as innocuous depends upon the presence of a tonic activation of intrinsic glycine and/or GABAergic neurons. The relevance of these inhibitory amino acid systems in regulating behavior generated by low-threshold afferent transmission is suggested by: (a) mice[763] and bovines[764] displaying a prominent somatic sensitivity up to a 10-fold decrease in glycine binding; (b) strychnine intoxication in humans, as characterized by a hypersensitivity to light touch;[765] and (c) spinal cord ischemia, known to destroy amino acid–containing interneurons and yield a tactile allodynia.[766–768]

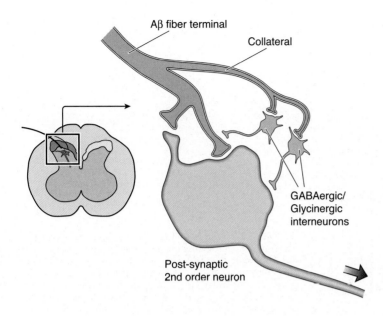

Aβ fiber terminal

Collateral

GABAergic/
Glycinergic
interneurons

Post-synaptic
2nd order neuron

FIGURE 32-26. Connectivity of γ-aminobutryric acid (GABA)/glycinergic interneurons acting presynaptically upon A-fiber afferent terminals and postsynaptically on the second-order neuron through GABA$_A$ and strychnine-sensitive glycine receptors.

An important property of the GABA$_A$ ionophore is that a variety of agents, such as benzodiazepines (e.g., midazolam), will bind to specific populations of GABA$_A$ ionophores that possess the appropriate benzodiazepine recognition site. This binding serves to increase the effects of endogenous GABA in its binding to the ionophore. Midazolam binding is elevated in the dorsal horn, and local delivery has been shown to reduce the postsynaptic discharge. Intrathecal delivery of midazolam can result in a moderate antinociception. These effects thus reflect upon the intrinsic modulatory activity of the spinal GABAergic systems.

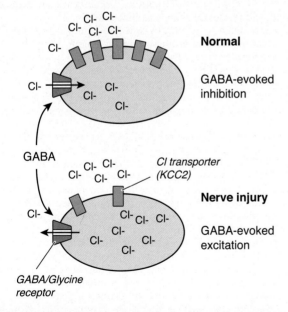

Cl-

Cl- Cl-
Cl- Cl- Cl-

Cl-

Normal

GABA-evoked
inhibition

Cl-

Cl- Cl-

Cl-

GABA

Cl transporter
(KCC2)

Cl- Cl- Cl-
Cl- Cl-

Nerve injury

Cl-

Cl- Cl- Cl-
Cl- Cl-
Cl- Cl-
Cl-

GABA-evoked
excitation

*GABA/Glycine
receptor*

FIGURE 32-27. Following peripheral nerve injury, there is a loss of chloride (Cl) transporter. This leads to an accumulation of intracellular Cl. In these conditions, increasing Cl permeability as by opening the γ-aminobutryric acid (GABA)$_A$ or glycine receptor ionophore may have no inhibitory effect or may lead to an actual excitatory potential. This action may be a mechanism for the enhanced dorsal horn excitability observed after nerve injury.

Facilitatory Systems

The magnitude of the response to a given noxious stimulus may be enhanced in the absence of change in the magnitude of the stimulus. Processes that lead to facilitation of the response to a given input should thus serve to augment the magnitude of the pain behavior. These facilitated states have been well documented in the dorsal horn following repetitive small-afferent input, as occurs with conditions leading to local tissue injury, inflammation, or damage to the nerve. The best example of this was first described by Mendell and Wall.[769] They noted that repetitive activation of C-fibers, but not A-fibers, leads to an augmented response to subsequent C-fiber input (a phenomenon referred to as "wind-up") and to an increase in the size of the receptive field of the respective neuron[436,770] (Fig. 32-28). Behavioral correlates of the event have been observed in a number of animal models in which local injury or inflammation has evoked a prolonged burst of afferent activity followed by an ongoing low level of afferent discharge. One example of this is found in the action of formalin injected into the paw of the rat. In this, recording of saphenous nerve output reveals a prominent burst of activity lasting for approximately 10 minutes, followed by a protracted ongoing barrage of sensory outflow in the small afferent.[771] Examination of the animal's behavior reveals that the injection of the irritant occasions a prominent licking of the paw that lasts for 10 minutes, at which time it subsides. This is followed, approximately 20 minutes later, with a second phase of intense flinching and licking of the injected paw. This second phase occurs in the absence of a significant barrage, and it is believed that this second phase of licking and flinching reflects on a facilitated processing of otherwise modest input (Fig. 32-29). The parallel to this event in the rat has been observed in humans after the intradermal injection of the C-fiber stimulant capsaicin.[23,25]

The following sections reveal a number of process whereby injury and inflammation can increase the local excitability of the dorsal horn projection into the neuronal pool. Thus, synaptic connections that previousy were inadequate to drive a depolarization may now be sufficient to reach threshold. As reviewed in Figure 32-30, dorsal horn neurons receive input from roots at their level of entry, as well as from collaterals

PART IV: PAIN MANAGEMENT

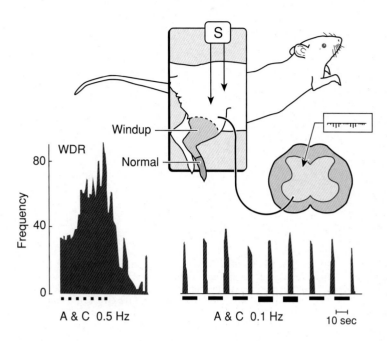

FIGURE 32-28. Single-unit recording from wide dynamic range neuron in response to an electrical stimulus delivered at 0.1 Hz (*right*). A reliable, stimulus-linked response is evoked at this frequency. In contrast, when rate is increased to 0.5 Hz, there is a progressive increase in magnitude of response generated by stimulation (*left*). Facilitation results from the C-fiber input and not an A-fiber input (*middle*) and is called "wind-up."

from distant afferents. These distant (extrasegmental) collaterals possess less excitatory drive than do the local segmental inputs. Increasing the excitability of a given neuron will thus lead to an enhanced resposne from the homosegmental input, but also increase the liklihood that the extrasegmental input can drive activity in that neuron; for example, leading to an increase in the receptive field of that cell. This change likely represents the primary reason why, after local injury, an increase in the apparent receptive field of the cell occurs. This is evident in humans post tissue injury pain states (Fig. 32-1) and during wind-up (Fig. 32-28).

Facilitatory Pharmacology of Spinal Neuronal Systems

Based on the preceding commentary, a reduction in C-fiber–evoked excitation in the dorsal horn occasioned by blocking axonal transmission (local anesthetic, pretreatment with a C-fiber neurotoxin such as capsaicin), by a reduction in the release of small-afferent transmitter (as with intrathecal morphine), or by a blockade of the postafferent receptor (e.g., AMPA receptor for glutamate) will diminish the magnitude of the small-afferent drive arising from tissue injury and, accordingly, diminish the facilitated processing evoked by persistent small-afferent input. However, early work indicated that the wind-up state reflects more than the repetitive activation of a simple excitatory system. In the following sections, we consider the pharmacology of several of these cascades initiated by tissue and nerve injury, which can lead to facilitated states.

Primary Afferent Glutamate and Substance P. The pharmacology of central facilitation suggests that the wind-up state reflects more than simply the repetitive activation of a simple excitatory system. The first real demonstration of this unique pharmacology was presented by showing that the phenomenon of spinal wind-up was prevented by the spinal delivery of antagonists for the *N*-methyl-*D*-aspartate (NMDA) receptor. Several lines of evidence indicate that spinal facilitation evoked by repetitive C-fiber activity (wind-up) is mediated by an SP (NK-1) site and a glutamate receptor of the NMDA subtype: (a) C-fiber–evoked wind-up is blocked or attenuated by the spinal action of NMDA and NK-1 receptor antagonists,[772–774] and (b) direct activation of spinal glutamate and tachykinin receptors with intrathecal agonists will induce an augmented response to a noxious thermal stimulus (i.e., a hyperalgesia[273,775,776]). The relevance of these spinal receptor systems to behavioral indices of a pain state has been well documented. Thus, as described in earlier, injection of an irritant such as formalin into the paw results in a burst of small afferent activity, followed by a prolonged low level of afferent discharge.[777] Behaviorally, the animal displays an initial transient phase of flinching and licking of the injected paw (phase 1), followed, after a brief period of quiescence, by a second prolonged phase of licking and flinching.

Spinal delivery of NMDA and NK-1 antagonists have little effect upon the first phase, but will significantly diminish the magnitude of the second-phase response.[778–780] Physiologic parallels to this behavior have been observed in which NMDA antagonists have little effect on acute excitation of dorsal horn neurons,[781,782] but will significantly reduce the elevated, on-going activity evoked by the induction of a peripheral injury state.[782,783]

As considered earlier, the NMDA receptor does not mediate acute postsynaptic excitation. This reflects upon an important property of this receptor. Under normal resting membrane potentials, the NMDA receptor is in a state referred to as a *magnesium (Mg^{2+}) block*. In this condition, occupancy by glutamate will not activate the ionophore. If a modest depolarization of the membrane occurs (as produced during repetitive stimulation secondary to the activation of AMPA and SP receptors, the Mg^{2+} block is removed, permitting glutamate to now activate the NMDA receptor. When this happens, the NMDA channel permits the passage of Ca (Fig. 32-31). This increase in intracellular calcium ($[Ca^{2+}]_i$) then serves to initiate the downstream components of the excitatory and facilitatory cascade.

Although the NMDA receptor is an important source of increased intracellular calcium, other routes also exist. Work has shown a variant on the AMPA receptors that is also Ca$^-$permeable.[784] Increases in intracellular calcium can also occur through a variety of metabotrophic receptors, such as the NK-1 receptor that acts through inosital triphosphate (IP3) and diacylglycerol pathways (DAG) pathways to release intracellular

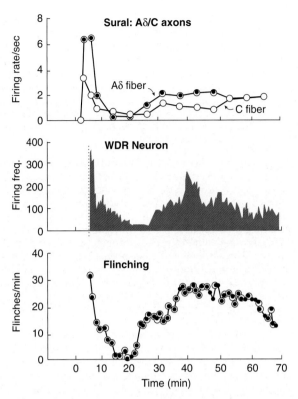

FIGURE 32-29. The injection of formalin into the paw of a rat yields a well-defined series of events representative of spinal facilitation. Schematic displays the afferent activation initiated by paw formalin in sural nerve A∂- and C-fibers (firing rate/sec; *top*), the firing pattern of a wide dynamic range neuron (firing frequency; *middle*), and the incidence of flinching behavior in the unanesthetized rat (Flinches/min; *bottom*); activity measured in the sural nerve of the anesthetized rat; firing of wide-dynamic-range neuron (anesthetized rat, *middle*); and number of flinches in the unanesthetized rat (*bottom*). The subcutaneous injection of formalin into the hind paw occurred at T = 0. Note the low level of input during the second phase, where behavior suggestive of pain is particularly high. Importantly, the second phase of the formalin test persists in spite of the animal being deeply anesthetized during the first.

calcium.[785] The importance of the calcium-permeable AMPA site in initating facilitated states has been demonstrated with intrathecally delivered agents.[786]

Dorsal Horn Facilitatory Cascades. Excitatory input arising from a persistent afferent barrage leads to a marked increase in intracellular Ca^{2+} that induces additional downstream effects that can enhance membrane excitability. Several aspects of these cascades will be discussed as representational of the complexity of these downstream events initiated by persistent small-afferent input.

Protein phosphorylation. Increased $[Ca^{2+}]_i$ can lead to the activation of a number of phosphorylating enzymes including protein kinases A (PKA) and C (PKC) and a variety of mitogen-activated kinases (MAPK) including p38 MAPK, JNK, and ERK.[787,788]

As an example, PKA and PKC are activated by increased intracellular calcium and phosphorylate a variety of proteins (Fig. 32-32). One such protein is the NMDA receptor. Such phosphorylation serves to reduce the threshold for ionophoric activation, leading to an enhanced response of the NMDA ionophore to a given degree of glutamate occupancy.[789,790]

P38 MAPK is activated by increased intracellular calcium. This activation leads to several outcomes. One is to phosphorylate a variety of enzymes, such as members of the family of phospholipase A_2 (PLA$_2$). These enzymes cleave a variety of lipidic acids, such as AA, from the cell membrane and provide the substrate for COX to synthesize PGs.[791] The second is that MAPK activation serves to subsequently activate a variety of transcription factors (such as nuclear factor-κB), which activates the synthesis of a variety of proteins, including nitric oxide synthase (NOS) and COX-2.[792] Thus, MAPK serves not only to mediate acute cellular events that contribute to the facilitated state, but its role as a transcription factor provides a link that, when activated, will promote delayed and persistent changes in cellular function by enhancing the expression of important enzymes, channels, and receptors.

Lipidic acid mediators. Primary afferent stimulation or direct activation of spinal neurons evokes spinal release of prostanoids.[793–795] This synthesis/release arises initially

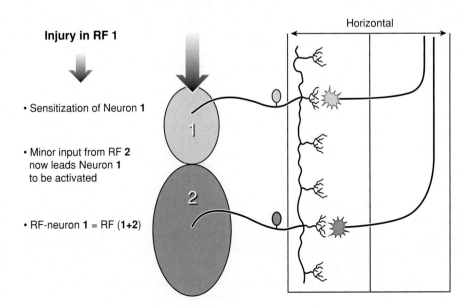

FIGURE 32-30. Receptive field of dorsal horn neuron depends upon its segmental input and the input from other segments that can activate it. After injury in receptive field (*RF*) 1, neuron 1 becomes "sensitized." Collateral input from RF2 normally is unable to initiate sufficient excitatory activity to activate neuron 1, but after sensitization, RF2 input is sufficient. Now the RF of neuron 1 is effectively RF1 + RF2. Thus, local injury can occur through spinal mechanisms and lead acutely to increased receptive fields such that stimuli applied to a noninjured RF can contribute to the post–tissue injury sensation.

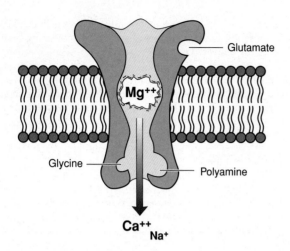

FIGURE 32-31. The *N*-methyl-*D*-aspartate (NMDA) receptor is a ionophore activated by glutamate, resulting in an influx of both calcium (Ca^{2+}) and sodium (Na^{+}). At resting membrane potentials, the channel is inactivated by the presence of magnesium (Mg^{2+}) in the channel. To be activated, the receptor requires the occupancy by glutamate, the removal of the Mg block by a mild membrane depolarization, the occupancy of the "glycine site," along with several allosterically coupled elements, including the "polyamine site." Together, these events permit the ionophore to be activated. Thus, under normal conditions, the NMDA ionophore is inactive even in the presence of glutamate, as with an acute depolarization.

through activation of a variety of PLA_2 isoforms (cytosolic PLA_2, calcium-independent PLA_2, and secreted PLA_2). These lipases cleave lipid chains from the membrane, including AA and lysophospholipids. Each product is acted upon by a variety of downstream enzymes, giving rise to numerous functionally distinct lipid products. Many of these downstream enzymes are constitutively expressed in neuraxial cells. All of these lipid mediators have distinct eponymous receptors that are coupled to membrane excitability. In many cases, lipids within a class may act upon several receptors.

■ *Prostaglandins.* The following provides an example of the complexity of the neuraxial lipid pathways. Thus, AA is acted upon by two COX isoforms (COX-1 and COX-2), which yield a variety of PGs.[796] Isoprostanes are lipid homologs of PGs, but are synthesized through a non-COX pathway. One of these pathways leads to the synthesis of PGE_2. Prostaglandin E_2 can act through four type-E (EP) receptors. The predominant mechanisms behind these effects appear to be largely due to coupling by several prostanoid receptors (EP_1, EP_2, EP_4) to G-proteins.[797] These G-proteins activate PKA, which phosphorylates voltage-sensitive Ca^+ and Na^+ channels in the afferent terminals[798,799] and serves to enhance presynaptic afferent transmitter release.

A postsynaptic effect upon dorsal horn function has been recently described. PGE_2 acting through an EP_2 receptor on the second-order neuron activates PKA and blocks the activation of inhibitory (strychnine-sensitive) glycineric neurotransmission onto superficial dorsal horn neurons.[800] As noted, such a reduction in activation of inhibitory glycine or GABA interneuron regulation can lead to a potent

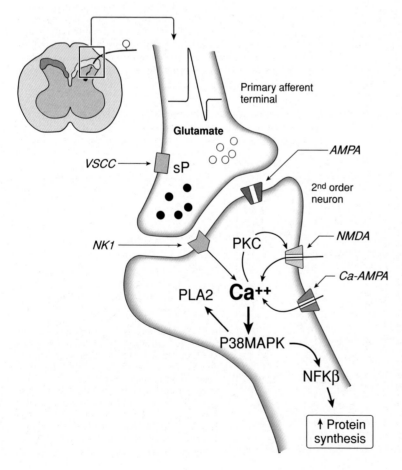

FIGURE 32-32. Activation of second-order neurons by glutamate and substance P released from a primary afferent terminal by activation of a voltage-sensitive calcium channel (VSCC) leads to depolarization of the second-order neurons, which leads to further depolarization of the second-order neuron through the *N*-methyl-*D*-aspartate (NMDA) receptor. This ionophore results in a significant increase in intracellular calcium ($[Ca^{2+}]_i$). Other sources of increased Ca^{2+} include a population of calcium-permeable α-amino-3-hydroxy-5-methyl-4-isoxazolepropionic acid (AMPA) ionophores and metabotrophic receptors such as the neurokinin 1 (NK1) receptor, which works through inositol triphosphate (IP3) and diacylglycerol pathways (DAG) to release intracellular calcium pools. Calcium leads to activation of a number of protein kinases, including protein kinase A and C (PKA and PKC) and several mitogen-activated protein kinases (MAPKs), including P38 MAPK. Protein kinase C can phosphorylate a number of membrane proteins, including the NMDA receptor. This phosphorylation then leads to a facilitation of NMDA ionophore function, increasing Ca influx and further augmenting membrane depolazrization and ($[Ca^{2+}]_i$). P38 MAPK can phosphorylate other protein such as the family of enzymes called phospholipase A_2 (PLA_2). P38 MAPK can also phosphorylate a variety of transcription factors such as nuclear factor κB (NFκB), which can lead to an upregulation in the synthesis of other proteins, such as cyclooxygenase. This increased transcription thus provides an important mechanism whereby an acute input may lead to subsequent persistent changes in system excitability.

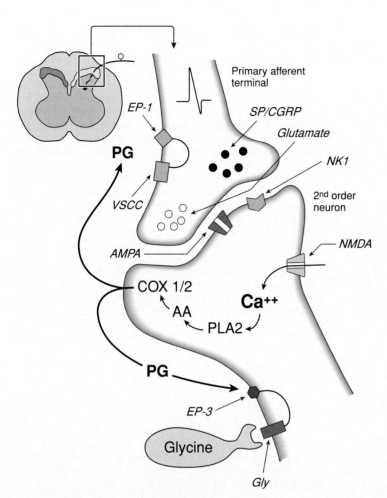

FIGURE 32-33. The phospholipase A_2 (PLA_2)–cyclooxygenase (COX)–prostaglandin (PG) cascade is initiated by the depolarization of the second-order neuron, increased intracellular calcium-and subsequent activation of PLA_2. This leads to an increase in arachidonic acid (AA), which is acted upon by constitutively expressed COX-1 and COX-2 to release PGs into the extracellular space. The PGs acts presynaptically through an E-type PG receptor (EP) upon the primary afferent to enhance transmitter release and upon the second-order neurons through inhibiting activation of a local glycinergic receptor that would otherwise modulate local depolarization. The schematic showing the glycine receptor to be on the same neuron is for presentation purposes only.

facilitation of dorsal horn excitability. Accordingly, this PGE_2-induced "disinhibition" serves to enhance afferent-evoked depolarization of the second-order neuron (Fig. 32-33).

The functional significance of this spinal PLA_2/COX/PG cascade to pain processing is suggested by several observations: (a) PGs facilitate depolarization-evoked increases in Ca^{2+} conductance in DRG cells and increase secretion of primary afferent peptides,[801] (b) intrathecal PGs evoke hyperalgesia after spinal delivery,[802–804] and (c) spinal $cPLA_2$ and COX-2 inhibitors suppress hyperalgesia induced by spinally injected SP or NMDA[273] and the behavioral hyperalgesia resulting from peripheral tissue injury.[500]

■ *Other lipid mediators.* The cascade resulting in central facilitation (i.e., increased activity in the spinal cord) is not uniquely dependent upon downstream products of COX metabolism. Substantial evidence suggests that AA itself may play an important role in facilitating biochemical processes that lead to neuronal excitability.[805–807]

Thus, in the hippocampus, the phenomena of long-term NMDA-mediated potentiation thought to model spinal-facilitated processing in pain appears principally dependent upon AA itself and not its metabolites.

PLA_2-derived AA also serves as a substrate for lipoxygenase, and this lysophospholipid product serves in the formation of platelet activating factor (PAF), both of which alter membrane excitability and activate second-messenger cascades that initiate downstream events leading to enhanced neuronal excitability in a variety of cell systems.[805,808–810]

■ *Nitric oxide synthase.* Nitric oxide (NO) formation is induced by NMDA receptor-mediated increases in Ca^{2+}.[811] The thermal hyperalgesia induced by spinal NMDA[812,813] or the second phase of the formalin test can be blocked by spinal injection of inhibitors of NO synthesis.[812] NO synthase has been found to occur in the dorsal horn[814,815] and in DRG cells (diaphorase-positive type-B ganglion cells[341,816]). Because NO has the ability to readily penetrate cell membranes, it has been proposed as a likely candidate for a retrogradely acting messengers on presynaptic terminals.[817]

Bulbospinal facilitatory systems. Bulbospinal pathways are activated by increases in ascending activity in nociceptive transmission pathways. Although a large component of this descending inhibition mediates local inhibition, considerable evidence suggests that at least one element (the serotonergic pathway) is facilitatory in character, thus contributing to spinal sensitization (Fig. 32-23).

As reviewed, serotonin (5HT) arises from the nucleus raphe magnus, which projects spinally, and the nucleus raphe dorsalis, which provides the principal sources for forebrain serotonin. The former project to the dorsal horn, whereas the latter also to project to the forebrain area. Classic observation has shown that spinopetal serotonin projections can have multiple effects. Activation of bulbospinal pathways can initiate spinal antinociception. The pharmacology of this effect appears to involve inhibitory and excitatory 5HT receptors, the latter of which may activate spinal GABAergic inhibitory interneurons.[818] Alternately, evidence suggests that some of these bulbospinal projections may be facilitatory, directly exciting dorsal horn nociceptive neurons through a 5HT$_3$ receptor[819] (Fig. 32-23). Importantly, this bulbospinal 5HT pathway appears to be activated by high-intensity afferent input through spinobulbar projections arising from the marginal (lamina I) cells in the dorsal horn. These complex effects suggest that, under certain conditions, increasing spinal 5HT tone may facilitate nociceptive processing. Previous work has demonstrated that these bulbospinal 5HT circuits are indeed activated by spinal nociceptive stimuli through the spinobulbospinal loop, as evidenced by in vivo spinal superfusion experiments.[705]

Changes in synaptic function. As noted earlier, GABA$_A$ and glycine receptors are Cl$^-$ ionophores. Under normal conditions, transmembrane [Cl$^-$] are at equilibrium at or just below resting membrane potentials. Increasing Cl$^-$ permeability by GABA$_A$ or glycine receptors yields hyperpolarization and inhibition. "Cation Cl$^-$" cotransporters regulate the Cl$^-$ gradient by exporting [Cl$^-$]$_i$. A recent insight is that, under certain conditions, such as injury to the afferent nerve, a reduction occurs in the expression of the Cl$^-$ transporter protein in dorsal horn neurons. The loss of dorsal horn Cl$^-$ transporter leads to increased intracellular [Cl$^-$]$_i$. Under these conditions, increasing Cl$^-$ permeability may lead to a failure of GABA$_A$/glycine inhibition and in fact turn the GABA/glycine effect into depolarization of the second-order neuron (Fig. 32-24). This change in chloride transporter function may thus represent an important mechanism whereby large-afferent input under reflex inhibitory control by local GABA and glycinergic receptors may thus become pronociceptive, accounting for the paradoxical tactile allodynia that has been shown to accompany nerve injury.

Non-neuronal Cells

Classes of Cells

A variety of non-neuronal cells are present in the CNS, among these being astrocytes and microglia.

Astroctyes perform a variety of important trophic and structural roles, including within in the blood–brain barrier, in mediating capillary glucose transport, by providing a physical support matrix, and by performing phagocytosis. Astrocytes enwrap pre- and postsynaptic structures, forming microdomains to control transmitter dispersion.[820] With neural injury and inflammation, astrocytes undergo hypertrophy (become activated) as shown by markers such as glial fibrillary acidic protein (GFAP).

Microglia derive from macrophages entering the brain during development. Under normal conditions, microglia typically display small cell bodies and long, slender, ramified processes. Upon activation, microglia display hypertrophy-increased expression of major histocompatibility class (MHC) II antigens. Histochemical markers displaying such activation also include epitopes such as Mac-1, ITGAM, TL4R, CD14, and MHC class II (OX-6 marker).[821]

Interaction of Non-neuronal Cells with Neuronal Transmission

Although nonneuronal cells do not establish synaptic contacts, it is evident that several mechanisms serve to influence local terminal excitability (Fig. 32-34).

Neurohumoral Transmission. Ample evidence based on in vitro culture and systems and less directly in vivo have indicated that both astrocytes and microglia have the ability to secrete a variety of products, including ATP, the free radical NO, lipid mediators (PGE$_2$), and a variety of cytokines (IL-1B, TNFα).[822] All of these agents given intrathecally induce a facilitation of neuronal activity, as evidenced by behaviorally defined hyperpathia. Block of their synthesis or their membrane actions by receptor antagonists or binding proteins will attenuate the hyperpathia otherwise induced by tissue or nerve injury. Several examples will be noted. Intracerebrally delivered IL-1B and TNFα yield a dose-dependent hyperpathia,[823] and IL-1B[302] and TNFα[824] binding reduces nerve injury–induced tactile allodynia. Intrathecal delivery of prostanoids will produce hyperalgesia; the hyperalgesia of injury-induced afferent input or caused by the direct activation of dorsal horn NMDA or NK1 receptors is reversed by the spinal delivery of PLA$_2$ or COX-2 inhibitors,[791] reflecting the role of constitutive PLA$_2$ and COX-2 isoforms. Intrathecal ATP agonists potentiate pain behavior, and P$_2$X antagonists reverse some aspects of neuropathic pain. Adenosine triphosphate is released from astrocytes after spinal cord injury,[825] but it is less clear if ATP is specifically released from glia in other neuropathic or inflammatory pain states. As glia as well as neurons express P$_2$X receptors, it is difficult to interpret the mechanism of action of purine receptor antagonists in terms of an effect upon glial activation. Local glutamate concentrations are regulated by their reuptake. Non-neuronal cells, particularly astrocytes, play an important role in the normal economy of extracellular glutamate concentrations. Reduction in uptake or reversal of the transported glutamate will lead to increased extracellular concentrations.[826] The potent effects of intrathecally delivered AMPA and NMDA antagonists emphasize the importance of extracellular glutamate. Importantly, P$_2$X$_7$ receptor activation[827] and local PGs can also stimulate a calcium-dependent release of glutamate from astrocytes.[828]

Electrotonic Activity. It has been appreciated that mechanical/chemical stimulus can initiate a traveling wave of increased [Ca^{2+}]$_i$ in astrocyte populations. This effect is mediated in part by gap junctions. Extracellular glutamate acting through the release of AMPA/NMDARs and mGluRs stimulate ATP and further glutamate release. This traveling wave can serve to modulate local terminal excitability.

Role of Non-neuronal Cells in Nociceptive Processing

Direct support for the potential contribution of non-neuronal cells arises from several perspectives: Do pain states lead to an activation of these non-neuronal cells? And, if one prevents the activation of these cells, will there be corresponding changes in the pain states? We will consider these two questions in the following sections.

Activation of Microglia and Astrocytes after Tissue and Nerve Injury. Following peripheral tissue injury, at intervals of as short as 1 to 2 hours, increases of Mac-1, TLR4, and CD14 mRNA and OX-42 immunoreactivity in homologous spinal dorsal horn has been reported.[829–833]

After nerve injury, markers of neuronal cell activation are increased in the spinal parenchyma.[829,834–839] The temporal pattern of this activation shows parallel with the onset of hyperpathia (allodynia) and spinal microglia/astrocyte activation. After injury, microglial activation typically occurs prior to signs of astrocyte activation.[834,835] Once manifested, neuropathic pain behavior appears to correlate with astrocyte activation.[829,834,836]

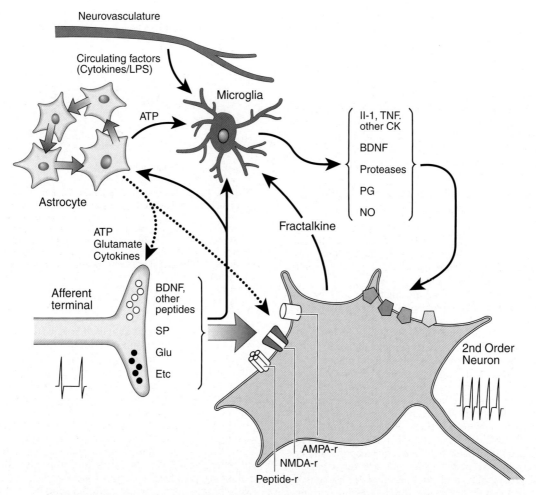

FIGURE 32-34. Synaptic transmission through the dorsal horn of the spinal cord is initiated by afferent input, which activates second-order neurons through the release of several transmitters that activate their eponymous postsynaptic receptors. Synaptic overflow can activate both astrocytes and microglia. Activating local pools of astrocytes can initiate a wave of calcium activation, which can cause spread of the release of a variety of products from astrocytes, including glutamate, adenosine triphosphate, and cytokines; products from neurons, including their transmitters; and a chemokine called fractalkine, which can also stimulate microglia. This in turn leads to the secretion of products from the microglia, which includes cytokines, proteases, growth factors, superoxides, and lipid mediators. These can act upon the neurons and primary afferents to enhance their excitability. Importantly, microglia adjacent to the parenchymal capillaries are able to detect changes in the vascular compartment and initiate secretion in the central nervous system of products that can also alter neuronal excitability.

Defining Non-neuronal Cell Activation. When stimulated, microglia and astrocytes can indeed be shown to display changes in the expression of a variety of membrane proteins on their respective mRNA. Although such degrees of activation when they are noted are of evident importance, those criteria fail to consider that astrocytes and microglia may contribute to the local neurohumoral environment without actually displaying changes in such membrane markers. Although such changes in expression indicate changes in cellular activity, the potential contribution of astrocytes and microglia in otherwise normal nociceptive transmission is also suggested by effects observed after blockade of their function.

Inhibition of the Activation of Astrocyte and Microglial Function. A number of drugs are used in defining the contribution of non-neuronal cells. Fluorocitrate, a glial Krebs cycle inhibitor, will block astrocyte function whereas the substrates isocitrate/2-oxoglutarate, will restore function.[840] Intrathecal flurocitrate reversibly blocks spinal wind-up[841] (the facilitated state produced by local injection of irritants and the pain behavior observed) after a variety of peripheral nerve injuries.[842-845]

Minocycline, a semisynthetic second-generation tetracycline, has potent effects that are independent of its antimicrobial action. This agent reversibly blocks microglial activation under a variety of conditions.[846] Spinal minocycline produces a reversible antihyperpathic effect in models of tissue injury and inflammation, as well as in nerve injury.[847,848] The mechanism of this effect is not certain, but is believed to be mediated by metalloproteinase inhibition.[846] The methylxanthine propentofylline and its homologues are cyclic 3',5'-adenosine monophosphate (cAMP)/cyclic guanosine monophosphate (cGMP) phosphodiesterase inhibitors and serve to increase extracellular adenosine. Adenosine depresses microglial activation, reducing the formation of reactive oxygen radicals and the release of TNFα.[849] Intrathecal propentofylline reduces hyperpathia after nerve injury.[850] Thus, altering the functionality of these non-neuronal cells by a variety of pharmacologic strategies can attenuate the nociceptive behavior generated by tissue and nerve injury. A second important observation is that, although this pharmacology can indeed reduce the expression of those epitopes that we take as signifying activation, the ability of these agents to act upon acute models of tissue injury and inflammation emphasizes that, prior to the expression of an activated phenotype, these cells systems are indeed contributing to the properties of the dorsal horn neuronal processing that leads to the various hyperpathic states after tissue injury.

Linkages between Afferent Input, Microglia, and Astrocytes

Given the potential role for non-neuronal cells in dorsal horn nociceptive processing, it is important to understand the linkages whereby neuronal activity may functionally link to the trophic function of these non-neuronal cells. These principles are presented schematically in Figure 32-34.

First, as discussed, astrocytes and microglia may be activated acutely by a variety of neurotransmitter products, including chemokines such as fractalkine. Second, after tissue injury and inflammation, circulating cytokines (IL-1β/TNFα can activate perivascular astrocytes/microglia. In addition, primary afferent transmitters can overflow to these adjacent non-neuronal cells and lead to their activation. This process is part of a complex cascade referred to broadly as *neuroinflammation*. Upon activation, these non-neuronal cells are then able to contribute to the chemical contents of the extracellular milieu. These glial cells regulate extracellular parenchymal glutamate by their glutamate transporters. This can serve to increase extracellular, activating neuronal glutamate receptors. In addition, these cells may serve as a source for a variety of agents, such as ATP, prostanoids, and cytokines that are upregulated in glia after peripheral injury. Aside from interacting with neurons through the local release of active factors, astrocytes can, as noted above, also exert a spreading excitation through the presence of gap junctions that lead to calcium waves that alter local excitability.

The Injured Axon

In the preceding section, the primary emphasis has been on the transduction of high-intensity, potentially injurious stimuli or in stimuli that arise from the release of active factors that act through transduction mechanisms at the peripheral terminal of the sensory afferent. Injury to the peripheral nerve leads to a variety of pain states that are often characterized by evidently spontaneous painful sensations, and also to the complex facilitated states often associated with tactile allodynia over dermatomes, which exceed the peripheral distribution of the injured nerve. Several limited comments on nerve injury are however appropriate in this section.

"Spontaneous" Pain

Under normal conditions, primary afferents show little if any spontaneous activity. Following an acute injury to the nerve, afferent axons will, however, display an initial burst of afferent firing secondary to the injury, followed by silence for an interval of hours to days, then, over time, the development of a measurable level of spontaneous afferent traffic in both myelinated and unmyelinated axons. This ongoing input is believed to provide

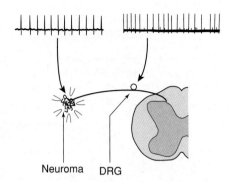

FIGURE 32-35. Following peripheral nerve injury, with failed efforts of regeneration to reach the target, a collection of injured axon sprouts to form a neuroma. These neuromas become ectopic generators of neural activity. In addition, the dorsal root ganglion cells of these injured axons also begin to demonstrate ongoing discharges. These discharges are believed to arise from the overexpression of sodium channels and a variety of receptors that sense the inflammatory products in the injury environment.

the source of the afferent activity that leads to spontaneous ongoing sensation. Single-unit recording from the afferent axon has indicated that the origin of the spontaneous activity in the afferent arises from the neuroma and from DRG of the injured axon. Activity in sensory afferents originates after an interval of days to weeks from the lesioned site (neuroma) and from the DRG of the injured nerve (Fig. 32-35).

The origin of this "spontaneous" activity is a subject of significant interest and several broad concepts can be considered. As reviewed, multiple populations of Na^+ channels exist, differing in their current activation properties and structure. Following peripheral injury, an increase in the expression of Na^+ channels occurs in the neuroma and DRG. This increased ionic conductance may result in the increase in spontaneous activity that develops in a sprouting axon. Systemic lidocaine at concentrations that do not block axon conduction can indeed attenuate the ectopic activity. The sprouted terminals of the injured afferent axon display a characteristic growth cone that possesses transduction properties not possessed by the original axon. These include the expression in neuroma of a variety of receptors and channels that were not normally present, and which can endow the neuroma with significant mechanical and chemical sensitivity. Thus, these spouted endings display a depolarizing response to a variety of humoral factors, such as prostanoids, catecholamines, and cytokines such as TNFα. This evolving sensitivity is of particular importance given that current data suggest that, following local nerve injury, there is the release of a variety of cytokines, particularly TNFα, which can thus directly activate the nerve and neuroma. In addition, following nerve injury, an important sprouting of postganglionic sympathetic efferents occurs, which can lead to the local release of catecholamines. This scenario is consistent with the observation that, following nerve injury, the postganglionic axons can initiate excitation in the injured axon. These events are believed to contribute to the development of spontaneous afferent traffic after peripheral nerve injury.

Facilitated Responses

As regards the evolving enhanced sensitivity of the organism after nerve injury to otherwise innocuous peripheral stimuli, particularly those believed to arise from light touch mediated

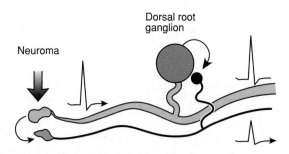

FIGURE 32-36. Functional cross-talk that may occur between injured primary afferent axons (Aβ- and C-fibers) at the site of injury (neuroma) and at the level of the dorsal root ganglia.

by Aβ-afferents, several general mechanisms are believed to be in play.

Peripheral Linkages. Following nerve injury, evidence suggests that "cross-talk" develops between afferents in the DRG and in the neuroma (Fig. 32-36). Here, depolarizing currents in one axon would generate a depolarizing voltage in an adjacent quiescent axon. This depolarization would permit activity arising in one axon to drive activity in a second. In this manner, it is hypothesized that a large low-threshold afferent would drive activity in an adjacent high-threshold afferent.

Afferent Sprouting. Under normal circumstances, large myelinated (Aβ) afferents project into the spinal Rexed lamina III and deeper (Fig. 32-11). Small afferents (C-fibers) tend to project into spinal laminae II and I, a region consisting mostly of nocisponsive neurons. Following peripheral nerve injury, it has been argued that the central terminals of these myelinated afferents (A-fibers) sprout into lamina II of the spinal cord.[851] With this synaptic reorganization, stimulation of low-threshold mechanoreceptors (Aβ fibers) could produce excitation of these neurons and be perceived as painful. The degree to which this sprouting occurs is a point of current discussion and, although it appears to occur, it is less prominent than originally reported.[852]

Sympathetic Sprouting. An additional contributing mechanism may be the increased innervation of the peripheral neuroma by postganglionic sympathetic terminals projecting into the DRG of the injured axons. These postganglionic fibers form baskets of terminals around the ganglion cells.[853] Several properties of this innervation are interesting: (a) It invests all size ganglion cells, but particularly type A (large ganglion cells); (b) the innervation occurs principally in the DRG ipsilateral to the lesion, but in addition, there is innervation of the contralateral ganglion cell; (c) stimulation of the ventral roots of the segments, containing the preganglionic efferents, will produce activity in the sensory axon by an interaction either at the peripheral terminal at the site of injury or by an interaction at the level of the DRG. This excitation is blocked by intravenous phentolamine, emphasizing an adrenergic effect (see Chapter 31).

Dorsal Horn Reorganization. Following peripheral nerve injury, a variety of events occur in the dorsal horn that suggest altered processing, wherein the response to low-threshold afferent traffic can be exaggerated.

Loss of intrinsic GABAergic/glycinergic inhibitory control. As reviewed earlier, large-afferent dorsal horn input is under tonic reflex regulation by GABAergic and glycinergic interneurons. Accordingly, these amino acids normally exert an important tonic or evoked inhibitory control over the activity of Aβ primary afferent terminals and second-order neurons in the spinal dorsal horn. The relevance of this intrinsic inhibition to pain processing is provided by the observation that the simple intrathecal delivery of GABA$_A$ or glycine receptor antagonists will lead to a powerful behaviorally defined tactile allodynia.[749] Similarly, animals genetically lacking glycine-binding sites often display a high level of spinal hyperexcitability.[854,855]

These observations led to the consideration that, following nerve injury, there may be a loss of GABAergic and/or glycinergic neurons. Although some data do support a loss of such GABAergic neurons,[856] the loss appears to be minimal.[857] As reviewed earlier, a second alternative is that excitatory effect is secondary to reduced activity of the membrane Cl$^-$ transporter, which changes the reversal current for the Cl$^-$ conductance. Here, increasing membrane Cl conductance—as occurs with GABA$_A$ receptor activation—results in membrane depolarization.

Spinal glutamate release. There is little doubt that the post–nerve injury pain state is dependent upon the important role of spinal glutamate release. Recent studies have emphasized that, after nerve injury, a significant enhancement occurs in resting spinal glutamate secretion. This release is in accord with an increased spontaneous activity in the primary afferent and with the loss of intrinsic inhibition that may serve to modulate resting glutamate secretion.

Spinal dynorphin. Following peripheral nerve injury, a wide variety of changes take place in the expression of dorsal horn factors. One such example is the increased expression of the peptide dynorphin. Nerve injury leads to a prominent increase in spinal dynorphin expression.[858] Intrathecal delivery of dynorphin can initiate the concurrent release of spinal glutamate and a potent tactile allodynia.[859]

Bulbospinal projections. As noted in previous sections, bulbospinal projections can have a facilitatory effect. Lesion of this projection has been shown to diminish the persistent hyperalgesia noted after nerve injury.[860]

Non-neuronal cells and nerve injury. As reviewed in the preceding section, non-neuronal cells appear to be important contributors to the local neurochemical milieu after nerve injury. Following nerve injury (section or compression), it has been shown that there is a significant increase in activation of spinal microglia and astrocytes in the spinal segments receiving input from the injured nerves.[861,862] Of particular interest is that, in the face of pathology such as bone cancer, such upregulation has been clearly shown. Astrocytes are activated by a variety of neurotransmitters and growth factors. Although the origin of this activation is not clear, it will lead to an increased spinal expression of COX, NOS, glutamate transporters, and proteinases. Such biochemical components have been previously shown to play an important role in the facilitated state.

SUMMARY

In this chapter, an outline has been provided of systems that potentially serve as substrates through which information initiated by high-intensity stimuli may gain access to various regions within the nervous system. The likelihood that "pain-relevant" information passes along a diversity of pathways is clear, even at the level of the spinal cord. Upon reaching the second-order neuron, the most apparent characteristic is that of polymodal convergence. At supraspinal levels, the issue becomes predictably more complex. Although considerable advances have been made in our understanding of the connectivity of these afferent linkages, an equally important component has been the appreciation that the information processing is subject to a variety of modulatory influences that govern the encoding of the afferent message. In the period from 1975 through the early 1980s, the emphasis was on the importance of systems that downregulated the response of the nervous system. The bulbospinal pathways and the endogenous opiates systems were in fact the preeminent part of any consideration of afferent processing. Although these components remain part of the total system, past 10 years has seen a progressive appreciation of the role played by those systems that upregulate the response to a given stimulus. The concept of wind-up and facilitated pain states, and the evolution of changes whereby low-threshold afferent input evokes a pain state, clearly occupy an important place in our current appreciation of pain processing. In the last 5 years, there has been a burgeoning of the experimental literature that considers the contribution of the astrocytes and microglia. Importantly, these lines of research have led to fundamental insights that have practical implications for the management of anomalous pain states. There is indeed a growing appreciation that post–nerve injury pain, far from being a sequelae affecting a small population, may impact on most major pain states such as cancer. Here, tumor compression and the sequelae of chemotherapy and radiation may induce changes that are as florid as those observed after a frank section of the nerve. Accordingly, the pharmacology of nerve injury pain states may have equal significance for chronic pain states, in which tissue injury is the obvious companion to the syndrome. Perhaps the next aspect in the evolution of our understanding of pain is a growth in our understanding of the mechanisms whereby the supraspinal component of the message evoked by a high-intensity stimulus leads to a "consciousness" of the stimulus. It would seem difficult, given the convergence of the many systems, to achieve a selective alteration in that component without altering all components of our psychological status. However, the observation that specific regions of the limbic system and the cortex show a differential response to a strong stimulus provides some support for selective interventions. Moreover, it is widely appreciated that changes in emotional status, such as depression, can significantly alter the pain report in humans and animals.[733] The pharmacology of those states is now beginning to be addressed with respect to pain. The richness of the pharmacology and the complexity of the connections may be daunting, but that very richness and that complexity provide promise that the system is subject to powerful manipulation and control.[863–865]

References

1. Sherrington C. The Integrative Action of the Nervous System. New Haven, Yale University Press, 1947.
2. Hargreaves KM, Troullos ES, Dionne RAea. Bradykinin is increased during acute and chronic inflammation: Therapeutic implications. *Clin Pharmacol* 1988;44:613.
3. Hunskaar S, Berge OG, Hole K. A modified hot-plate test sensitive to mild analgesics. *Behav Brain Res* 1986;21:101–108.
4. Ness TJ, Randich A, Gebhart GF. Further behavioral evidence that colorectal distension is a 'noxious' visceral stimulus in rats. *Neurosci Lett* 1991;131:113.
5. Saeki S, Yaksh TL. Suppression of nociceptive responses by spinal mu opioid agonists: effects of stimulus intensity and agonist efficacy. *Anesth Analg* 1993;77:265–274.
6. Fields HL, Bry J, Hentall I, et al. The activity of neurons in the rostral medulla of the rat during withdrawal from noxious heat. *J Neurosci* 1983;3:2545–2552.
7. Sabbe MB, Grafe MR, Mjanger E, et al. Spinal delivery of sufentanil, alfentanil, and morphine in dogs. Physiologic and toxicologic investigations. *Anesthesiology* 1994;81:899–920.
8. Chapman CR, Casey KL, Dubner R, et al. Pain measurement: an overview. *Pain* 1985;22:1–31.
9. Chapman CR, Schimek F, Colpitts YH, et al. Peak latency differences in evoked potentials elicited by painful dental and cutaneous stimulation. *Int J Neurosci* 1985;27:1–12.
10. Chatrain GE, Canfield RC, Knauss TA, et al. Cerebral responses to electrical tooth pulp stimulation in man: An objective correlate of acute experimental pain. *Neurology* 1975;25:745.
11. Willer JC. Comparative study of perceived pain and nociceptive flexion reflex in man. *Pain* 1977;3:69.
12. Bromm B, Treede RD. Human cerebral potentials evoked by CO2 laser stimuli causing pain. *Exp Brain Res* 1987;67:153–162.
13. Gibson SJ, LeVassEur SA, Helme RD. Cerebral event-related responses induced by CO2 laser stimulation in subjects suffering from cervico-brachial syndrome. *Pain* 1991;47:173–182.
14. Jensen K, Andersen HO, Olesen J, et al. Pressure pain threshold in human temporal region. Evaluation of a new pressure algometer. *Pain* 1986;25:313.
15. Jensen R, Rasmussen BK, Pedersen B, et al. Muscle tenderness and pressure pain thresholds in headache. A population study. *Pain* 1993;52:193.
16. Lewis T, Pochin EE. The double pain response of the human skin to a single stimulus. *Clin Sci* 1937;3:67.
17. Price DD, McHaffie JG. Effects of heterotopic conditioning stimuli on first and second pain: a psychophysical evaluation in humans. *Pain* 1988;34:245–252.
18. La Motte RH, Shain CN, Simone DA, et al. Neurogenic hyperalgesia: Psychophysical studies of underlying mechanisms. *J Neurophysiol* 1991;66:190.
19. Meyer RA, Campbell JN. Myelinated nociceptive afferents account for the hyperalgesia that follows a burn to the hand. *Science* 1981;213:1527.
20. Lewis T. Experiments relating to cutaneous hyperalgesia and its spread through somatic fibers. *Clin Sci* 1935;2:373–423.
21. Bevan S, Szolcsanyi J. Sensory neuron-specific actions of capsaicin: mechanisms and applications. *Trends Pharmacol Sci* 1990;11:330–333.
22. Simone DA, Baumann TK, La Motte RH. Dose-dependent pain and mechanical hyperalgesia in humans after intradermal injection of capsaicin. *Pain* 1989;38:99.
23. Torebjork HE, Lundberg LE, LaMotte RH. Central changes in processing of mechanoreceptive input in capsaicin-induced secondary hyperalgesia in humans. *J Physiol* (Lond) 1992;448:765–780.
24. Koltzenburg M, Lundberg LE, Torebjork HE. Dynamic and static components of mechanical hyperalgesia in human hairy skin. *Pain* 1992;51:207.
25. LaMotte RH, Lundberg LE, Torebjork HE. Pain, hyperalgesia and activity in nociceptive C units in humans after intradermal injection of capsaicin. *J Physiol* (Lond) 1992;448:749–764.
26. Wheeler-Aceto H, Porreca F, Cowan A. The rat paw formalin test: comparison of noxious agents. *Pain* 1990;40:229–238.
27. Nagasaka H, Awad H, Yaksh TL. Peripheral and spinal actions of opioids in the blockade of the autonomic response evoked by compression of the inflamed knee joint *Anesthesiology* 1996;85:808–816.
28. Schott E, Berge OG, Angeby-Moller K, et al. Weight bearing as an objective measure of arthritic pain in the rat. *J Pharmacol Toxicol Methods* 1994;31:79.
29. Zahn PK, Brennan TJ. Primary and secondary hyperalgesia in a rat model for human postoperative pain. *Anesthesiology* 1999;90:863–872.
30. Nozaki-Taguchi N, Yaksh TL. A novel model of primary and secondary hyperalgesia after mild thermal injury in the rat. *Neurosci Lett* 1998;254:25–28.
31. Urban L, Perkins MN, Campbell E, et al. Activity of deep dorsal horn neurons in the anaesthestized rat during hyperalgesia of the hindpaw induced by ultraviolet irradiation. *Neuroscience* 1993;57:167.
32. Dyck PJ, Lambert EH, Nicholas PC. Quantitative measurement of sensation related to compound action potential and number and sizes of myelinated and unmyelinated fibres of the sural nerve in health. Friedrich's ataxia, hereditary sensory neuropathy, and tabes dorsalis Amsterdam, Elsevier/North-Holland, 1971.

33. Ochoa J, Mair WG. The normal sural nerve in man. I. Ultrastructure and numbers of fibers and cells. *Acta Neuropathol* (Berl.) 1967;13:127.
34. Cauna N. The fine morphology of the sensory receptor organs in the article of the rat. *J Comp Neurol* 1969;136:81.
35. Iggo A, Kornhuber HH. A quantitative study of C-mechanoreceptors in hairy skin of the cat. *J Physiol* 1977;271:549–565.
36. Iggo A, Ogawa H. Primate cutaneous thermal nociceptors. *J Physiol* (Lond) 1971;216:77P.
37. MacIver MB, Tanelian DL. Structural and functional specialization of Aδ and C fiber free nerve endings innervating rabbit corneal epithelium. *J Neurosci* 1993;13:4511.
38. Boivie J, Perl ER. Neural substrates of somatic sensation Baltimore, University Press, 1975.
39. Burgess PR, Perl ER. Cutaneous mechanoreceptors and nociceptors. New York, Springer-Verlag, 1973.
40. Winkelmann RK. Sensory receptors of the skin. Spinal Afferent Processing. Edited by Yaksh TL. New York, Plenum Press, 1986, pp. 19–57.
41. Cauna N. Fine structure of the receptor organ and its probable functional significance CIBA Symposium. London, Churchill, 1966.
42. Chouchkov CN. On the fine structure of free nerve endings in human digital skin, oral cavity and rectum. *Z Mikrosk Anat Forsch* 1972;86:273–288.
43. Heppelmann B, Messlinger K, Neiss WF, et al. Ultrastructural three-dimensional reconstruction of group III and group IV sensory nerve endings ("free nerve endings") in the knee joint capsule of the cat: evidence for multiple receptive sites. *J Comp Neurol* 1990;292:103–116.
44. Hoyes AD, Barber P. Ultrastructure of the corneal nerves in the rat. *Cell Tiss Res* 1976;172:133.
45. Tervo T, Joo F, Huikuri KT, et al. Fine structure of sensory nerves in the rat cornea: an experimental nerve degeneration study. *Pain* 1979;6:57–70.
46. Tervo T, Palkama A. Innervation of the rabbit cornea. A histochemical and electronmicroscopic study. *Acta Anat* 1978;102:164.
47. Tervo T, Palkama A. Ultrastructure of the corneal nerves after fixation with potassium permanganate. *Anat Rec* 1978 190:851.
48. Anderson DJ, Curwen MP, Howard LV. The sensitivity of human dentin. *J Dent Res* 1958;37:669.
49. Anderson DJ, Hannam AG, Matthews B. Sensory mechanisms in mammalian teeth and their supporting structures. *Physiol Rev* 1970;50:171.
50. Lele PP, Weddell G. The relationship between neurohistology and corneal sensibility. *Brain* 1956;79:119.
51. Andres KH. Untersuchungen uber den Feinbau von Spinalganglien. *Z Zellforsch* 1961;55:1.
52. Pomepiano O, Swett JE. Actions of graded cutaneous and muscular afferent volleys on brain stem units in the decrebrate, cerebellectomized cat. *Arch Ital Biol* 1963;101:552.
53. Yoshida S, Matsuda Y. Studies on sensory neurons of the mouse with intracellular recording and horseradish peroxidase injection techniques. *J Neurophysiol* 1979;42:1134.
54. Lieberman AR. Sensory ganglia. London, Chapman and Hall, 1976.
55. Coimbra A, Sodre-Borges BP, Magalhaes MM. The substantia gelatinosa Rolandi of the rat. Fine structure, cytochemistry (acid phosphatase) and changes after dorsal root section. *J Neurocytol* 1974;3:199–217.
56. Csilik B, Knyihar E. Biodynamic plasticity in the Rolando substance. Oxford, Pergamon Press, Ltd., 1978.
57. Knyihar E, Cisillik B. Effect of peripheral axotomy on the fine structure and histochemistry of the Rolando substances: Degenerative atrophy of central processes of pseudounipolar cells. *Exp Brian Res* 1976;26:73.
58. Knyihar E, Csillik B. Representation of cutaneous afferents by fluoride-resistant acid phosphatase (FRAP)—active terminals in the rat substantia gelatinosa Rolandi. *Acta Neurol Scand* 1976;53:217.
59. Knyihar E, Gerebtzoff MA. Extra-lysosomal localization of acid phosphatase in the spinal cord of the rat. *Exp Brain Res* 1973;18:383.
60. Kalina M, Bubis JJ. Ultrastructural localization of acetylcholine esterase in neurons of rat trigeminal ganglia. *Experientia* 1967;25:388.
61. Kalina M, Wolman M. Correlative histochemical and morphological study on the maturation of sensory ganglion cells in the rat. *Histochemie* 1970; 22:100.
62. Guo A, Vulchanova L, Wang J, et al. Immunocytochemical localization of the vanilloid receptor 1 (VR1): relationship to neuropeptides, the P2X3 purinoceptor and IB4 binding sites. *Eur J Neurosci* 1999;11:946–958.
63. Nagy JI, Hunt SP. Fluoride-resistant acid phosphatase-containing neurones in dorsal root ganglia are separate from those containing substance P or somatostatin. *Neuroscience* 1982;7:89–97.
64. Braz JM, Nassar MA, Wood JN, et al. Parallel "pain" pathways arise from subpopulations of primary afferent nociceptor. *Neuron* 2005;47:787–793.
65. Molliver DC, Radeke MJ, Feinstein SC, et al. Presence or absence of TrkA protein distinguishes subsets of small sensory neurons with unique cytochemical characteristics and dorsal horn projections. *J Comp Neurol* 1995;361:404–416.
66. Droz B. Renewal of synaptic proteins. *Brain Res* 1973;62:383.
67. Almenar-Queralt A, Goldstein LS. Linkers, packages and pathways: new concepts in axonal transport. *Curr Opin Neurobiol* 2001;11:550–557.
68. Ochs S. Energy metabolism and supply of nerve by axoplasmic transport. *Fed Proc* 1974;33:1049.
69. Ochs S, Hollingsworth D. Dependence of fast axoplasmic transport in nerve on oxidative metabolism. *J Neurochem* 1971;18:107.
70. Byers MR, Fink BR, Kennedy RD, et al. Effects of lidocaine on axonal morphology, microtubules, and rapid transport in rabbit vagus nerve in vitro. *J Neurobiol* 1973;4:125–143.
71. Ochs S, Jersild RA, Jr. Fast axoplasmic transport in umyelinated nerve fibers shown by electron microscopic radioautography. *J Neurobiol* 1974;5:373.
72. Knyihar-Csillik E, Csillik B. FRAP: Histochemistry of the primary nociceptive neuron. *Prog Histochem Cytochem* 1981;14:1.
73. Patapoutian A, Peier AM, Story GM, et al. ThermoTRP channels and beyond: mechanisms of temperature sensation. *Nat Rev Neurosci* 2003;4:529–539.
74. McCarter GC, Levine JD. Ionic basis of a mechanotransduction current in adult rat dorsal root ganglion neurons. *Mol Pain* 2006;2:28.
75. Burnstock G. Purine-mediated signalling in pain and visceral perception. *Trends Pharmacol Sci* 2001;22:182–188.
76. Gasser HS. Unmedullated fibers originating in dorsal root ganglia. *J Gen Physiol* 1950;33:651–690.
77. Zotterman Y. Touch, pain, and tickling: an electrophysiological investigation on cutaneous sensory nerves. *J Physiol* (Lond) 1939;95:1–28.
78. Lloyd DPC. Neuron patterns controlling transmission of ipsilateral hind limb reflexes in cat. *J Neurophysiol* 1943;6:293.
79. Lai J, Porreca F, Hunter J, et al. Voltage-gated sodium channels and hyperalgesia. *Annu Rev Pharmacol Toxicol* 2004;44:371–397.
80. Collins WF, Nulsen FE, Randt CT. Relation of peripheral nerve fiber size and sensation in man. *Arch Neurol* 1960;3:381.
81. Torebjork HE, Hallin RG. Perceptual changes accompanying controlled preferential blocking of A and C fibre responses in intact human skin nerves. *Exp Brain Res* 1973;16:321–332.
82. Heinbecker P, Bishop GH, O'Leary J. Pain and touch fibers in peripheral nerves. *Arch Neurol Psychiatr* (Chic) 1933;29:771.
83. Torebjork HE. Afferent C units responding to mechanical, thermal and chemical stimuli in human non-glabrous skin. *Acta Physiol Scand* 1974; 92:374.
84. Torebjork HE, Hallin RG. Excitation failure in thin nerve fiber structures and accompanying hypalgesia during repetitive electric skin stimulation, Advances in Neurology. Edited by Bonica JJ. New York, Raven Press, 1974, pp. 733–735.
85. Torebjork HE, Hallin RG. Identification of afferent C units in intact human skin nerves. *Brain Res* 1974;67:387.
86. Torebjork HE, Hallin RG. Responses in human A and C fibers to repeated electrical intradermal stimulation. *J Neurol Neurosurg. Psychiatry* 1974;37:653.
87. Van Hees J, Gybels JM. Pain related to single afferent C fibers from human skin. *Brain Res* 1972;48:397.
88. Johansson RS. Tactile sensibility in the human hand: receptive field characteristics of mechanoreceptive units in the glabrous skin area. *J Physiol* 1978;281:101–125.
89. Knibestol M. Stimulus-response functions of rapidly adapting mechanoreceptors in the human glabrous skin area. *J Physiol* (Lond.) 1973;232:427.
90. Knibestol M. Stimulus-response functions of slowly adapting mechanoreceptors in the human glabrous skin area. *J Physiol* (Lond.) 1975;245:63.
91. Knibestol M, Vallbo AB. Single unit analysis of mechanoreceptor activity from the human glabrous skin. *Acta Physiol Scand* 1970;80:178.
92. Torebjork HE, Hallin RG. Skin receptors supplied by unmyelinated (C) fibres in man., Sensory function of the skin in primates. Edited by Zotterman Y. Oxford, Pergamon, 1976, pp. 475–487.
93. Van Hees J. Human C fiber input during painful and nonpainful skin stimulation with radiant heat., Advances in Pain ReseArch and Therapy. Edited by Bonica JJ, Albe-Fessard D. New York, Raven Press, 1976, pp. 35–40.
94. Willer JC, Boureaux F, Albe-Fessard D. Role of large diameter cutaneous afferents in transmission of nociceptive messages: Electrophysiological study in man. *Brain Res* 1978;152:385.
95. Dyck PJ. Detection thresholds of cutaneous sensations in health and disese in man. New York, Raven Press, 1986.
96. Onishi A, Dyck PJ. Loss of small peripheral sensory neurons in Fabry's disease. *Arch Neurol* 1974;31:120.
97. Kocher L, Anton F, Reeh PW, et al. The effect of carrageenan-induced inflammation on the sensitivity of umyelinated skin nociceptors in the rat. *Pain* 1987;29:363.
98. Reeh PW, Kocher L, Jung S. Does neurogenic inflammation alter the sensitivity of umyelinated nociceptors in the rat? *Brain Res* 1986;384:42.
99. Schmidt RF, Schaible HG, Messlinger K, et al. *Prog Pain Res Mgmt* 1994; 2:213.
100. Handwerker HO, Reeh PW. Pain and inflammation. *Pain Res Clin Manage* 1991;4:59–70.
101. Lewis T. Pain. New York, Macmillan, 1942.
102. Bilisaly FN, Goodell H, Wolff HG. Vasodilatation, lowered pain threshold, and increased tissue vulnerability. Effects dependent upon peripheral nerve function. *Arch Intern Med* 1954;94:759.

103. Woolf CJ, Shortland P, Coggeshall RE. Peripheral nerve injury triggers central sprouting of myelinated afferents. *Nature* 1992;355:75–78.
104. Lewis T. Experiments relating to cutaneous hyperalgesia and its spread through somatic nerves. *Clin Sci* 1936;2:373.
105. Chahl LA, Ladd RJ. Local oedema and general excitation of cutaneous sensory receptors produced by electrical stimulation of the saphenous nerve in the rat. *Pain* 1976;2:25–34.
106. Hinsey JC, Gasser HS. The components of the dorsal root mediating vasodilatation and the Sherrington contracture. *Am J Physiol* 1930;92:679.
107. Beitel RE, Dubner R. Fatigue and adaptation in unmyelinated (C) polymodal nociceptors to mechanical and thermal stimuli applied to the monkey face. *Brain Res* 1976;112:402.
108. Beitel RE, Dubner R. Response of unmyelinated (C) polymodal nociceptors to thermal stimuli applied to monkey's face. *J Neurophysiol* 1976;39:1160.
109. Bessou P, Perl ER. Response of cutaneous sensory units with unmyelinated fibers to noxious stimuli. *J Neurophysiol* 1969;32:1025–1043.
110. Perl ER. Sensitization of nociceptors and its relation to sensation., Advances in Pain Research and Therapy. Edited by Bonica JJ, Albe-Fessard D. New York, Raven Press, 1976, pp. 17–28.
111. Fitzgerald M, Lynn B. The sensitization of high threshold mechanoreceptors with myelinated axons by repeated heating. *J Physiol* 1977;265:549–563.
112. Dubner R, Sumino R, Wood WI. A peripheral "cold" fiber population responsive to innocuous and noxious thermal stimuli applied to the monkey's face. *J Neurophysiol* 1975;38:1373.
113. Chahl LA. Pain induced by inflammatory mediators. New York, Raven Press, 1979.
114. Heggers JP, Ko F, Robson MC, et al. Evaluation of burn blister fluid. *Plast Reconstr Surg* 1980;65:798–804.
115. Lindinger MI, Sjogaard G. Potassium regulation during exercise and recovery. *Sports Med* 1991;11:382.
116. Steen KH, Reeh PW, Anton F, et al. Protons selectively induce lasting excitation and sensitization to mechanical stimulation of nociceptors in rat skin, in vitro. *J Neurosci* 1992;12:86–95.
117. Kaliner M, Austen KF. Immunological release of chemical mediators from human tissues. *Ann Rev Pharmacol* 1975;15:177.
118. Morrison DC, Henson PM. Release of mediators from mast cells and basophils induced by different stimuli., Immediate Hypersensitivity: Modern Concepts and Developments. Edited by Bach MK. New York, Marcel Dekker, 1978, pp. 431–502.
119. Sulivan TJ, Parker CW. Possible role of arachidonic acid and its metabolites in mediator release from rat mast cells. *J Immunol* 1979;122:431.
120. Uvnas B. The mechanism of histamine release from mast cell., Handbuch der Experimentallelen Pharmacologie. Edited by Rocha e Silva M. New York, Springer-Verlag, 1978, pp. 75–92.
121. Beck PW, Handwerker HO. Bradykinin and serotonin effects on various types of cutaneous nerve fibers. *Pflugers Arch* 1974;374:209.
122. Beck PW, Handwerker HO, Zimmerman M. Nervous outflow from the cat's foot during noxious radiant heat stimulation. *Brain Res* 1974;67:373.
123. Fjallbrant N, Iggo A. The effect of histamine, 5-hydroxytryptamine and acetylcholine on cutaneous afferent fibres. *J Physiol* 1961;156:578–590.
124. Fock S, Mense S. Excitatory effects of 5-hydroxytryptamine, histamine and potassium ions on muscular group IV afferent units: a comparison with bradykinin. *Brain Res* 1976;105:459–469.
125. Juan H, Lembeck F. Action of peptides and other algesic agents on paravascular pain receptors of the isolated perfused rabbit ear. *Naunyn Schmiedebergs Arch Pharmacol* 1974;283:151–164.
126. Armstrong D, Dry R, Keelee CA, et al. Observations on chemical excitants of cutaneous pain in man. *J Physiol* (Lond.) 1953;120:326.
127. Elliot DE, Horton EW, Lewis GP. Actions of pure bradykinin *J Physiol* (Lond) 1960;153:473.
128. Keele CA, Armstrong D. Substances producing pain and itch London, Edward Arnold, 1964.
129. Guzman F, Braun C, Lim RK. Visceral pain and the pseudaffective response to intra-arterial injection of bradykinin and other algesic agents. *Arch Int Pharmacodyn Ther* 1962;136:353–384.
130. Chan JVC, Burrowes CE, Movat HZ. Surface activation of factor XII (Hageman factor)—Critical role of high molecular weight kininogen and another potentiator. *Agents Actions* 1978;8:65.
131. Cochrane CG. The Hageman factor pathways of kinin formation clotting and fibronylisis. New York, Raven Press, 1976.
132. Roca e Silva M, Antonio A. Release of bradykinin and the mechanism of production of a thermic edema (45Celsius) in the rat's paw. *Med Exp* (Basel) 1960;3:371.
133. Winkelmann RK. Kinins from human skin., The Skin Senses. Edited by Kenshalo DR. Springfield, IL, Charles C. Thomas, 1968, pp. 499–511.
134. He X, Schepelmann K, Schaible HG, et al. Capsaicin inhibits responses of fine afferents from the knee joint of the cat to mechanical and chemical stimuli *Brain Res* 1990;530:147.
135. Mense S, Schmidt RF. Activation of group IV afferent units from muscle by algesic agents. *Brain Res* 1974;72:305.
136. Schepelmann K, Messlinger K, Schaible HG, et al. Inflammatory mediators and nociception in the joint: Excitation and sensitization of slowly

conducting afferent fibers of cat's knee by prostaglandin I2. *Neuroscience* 1992;50:237.
137. Whalley ET, Clegg S, Stewart JM, et al. Antagonism of the algesic action of bradykinin on the human blister base. *Adv Exp Med Biol* 1989;247A: 261.
138. Regoli D, Jukic D, Gobeil F, et al. Receptors for bradykinin and related kinins: A critical analysis. *Can J Physiol Pharmacol* 1993;71:556.
139. Dray A, Perkins M. Bradykinin and inflammatory pain. *Trends Neurosci* 1993;16:99.
140. Perkins MN, Campbell E, Dray A. Antinociceptive acitivity of the bradykinin B1 and B2 receptor antagonists, des-Arg9, [Leu 8]-BK and HOE 140, in two models of persistent hyperalgesia in the rat. *Pain* 1993;53:191.
141. Samuelsson B, Goldyne M, Granström E, et al. Prostaglandins and thromboxanes. *Ann Rev Biochem* 1978;47:997–1029.
142. Flower RJ. Steroidal anti-inflammatory drugs as inhibitors of phospholipase A2 New York, Raven Press, 1978.
143. Marcus AJ. The role of lipids in platelet function with particular reference to the arachidonic acid pathway. *J Lipid Res* 1978;19:793.
144. Nugteren DH. Arachidonate lipoxygenase., Prostaglandins in Hematology. Edited by Silver M, Smith BJ, Kocsis. New York, Spectrum Publications, 1977, pp. 11–25.
145. Flower RJ. Drugs which inhibit prostaglandin biosynthesis. *Pharmacol Rev* 1974;26:33–67.
146. Smith JB, Willis AL. Aspirin selectively inhibits prostaglandin production in human platelets. *Nat New Biol* 1971;231:235–237.
147. Vane JR. Inhibition of prostaglandin synthesis as a mechanism of action for aspirin-like drugs. *Nat New Biol* 1971;231:232–235.
148. Greaves MW, Sondergaard J, McDonald-Gibson W. Recovery of prostaglandins in human cutaneous inflammation. *Br Med J* 1971;2:258–260.
149. Willis AL. Release of histamine, kinin and prostaglandin during carrageenin-induced inflammation in the rat., Prostaglandins, Peptides, and Amines. Edited by Montegazza P, Horton EW. London, Academic Press, 1969, pp. 31–38.
150. Juan H. Mechanism of action of bradykinin-induced release of prostaglandin E. *Naunyn-Schmiedebergs Arch Pharmacol* 1977;300:77.
151. Juan H, Lembeck F. Release of prostaglandins from the isolated perfused rabbit ear by bradykinin and acetylcholine. *Agents Actions* 1976;6:642.
152. Lembeck F, Popper H, Juan H. Release of prostaglandins by bradykinin as an intrinsic mechanism of its algesic effect. *Naunyn Schmiedebergs Arch Pharmacol* 1976;294:69.
153. McGiff JC, Terragno NA, Malik KU, et al. Release of a prostaglandin E-like substance from canine kidney by bradykinin. *Circ Res* 1972;31:36.
154. Crunkchom P, Willis AL. Cutaneous reactions to intradermal prostaglandins. *Br J Pharmacol* 1971;41:49.
155. Ferreira SH, Moncada S, Vane JR. Prostaglandins and the mechanism of analgesia produced by aspirin-like drugs. *Br J Pharmacol* 1973;49:86–97.
156. Horton EW. Acbon of prostaglandin E1 on tissues which respond to bradykinin. *Nature* 1963;200:892.
157. Moncada S, Ferreira SH, Vane JR. Inhibition of prostaglandin biosynthesis as the mechanism of analgesia of aspirin-like drugs in the dog knee joint. *Eur J Pharmacol* 1975;31:250–260
158. Ferreira SH. Prostaglandins, aspirin-like drugs and analgesia. *Nat New Biol* 1972;240:200–203.
159. Collier JG, Karim SMM, Robinson B, et al. Action of prostaglandins A2, B1, E2, F2 on superficial hand veins of man. *Br J Pharmacol* 1972;44:374.
160. James GWL, Church MK. Hyperalgesia after treatment of mice with prostaglandins and arachidonic acid and its antagonism by anti-inflammatory-analgesic compunds. *Arzneimittelforsch* 1978;28:804.
161. Ferreira SH, Lorenzetti BB, Corrêa FM. Central and peripheral antialgesic action of aspirin-like drugs. *Eur J Pharmacol* 1978;53:39–48.
162. Tyers MB, Haywood H. Effect of prostaglandins on peripheral nociceptors in acute inflammation. *Agents Actions* 1979;6 (Suppl.):65.
163. Handwerker HO. Influences of algogenic substances and prostaglandins on the discharges of unmyelinated cutaneous nerve fibers identified as nociceptors, Advances in Pain Research and Therapy. Edited by Bonica JJaA-F, D. New York, Raven Press, 1976, pp. 41–45.
164. Chahl LA, Iggo A. The effects of bradykinin and prostaglandin E1 on rat cutaneous afferent nerve activity. *Br J Pharmacol* 1977;59:343–347.
165. Lembeck F, Juan H. Interaction of prostaglandins and indomethacin with algesic substances. *Naunyn Schmiedebergs Arch Pharmacol* 1974;285:301.
166. Vane JR. The mode of action of aspirin and similar compounds. *J Allergy Clin Immunol* 1976;58:691–712.
167. Sylven C, Jonzon B, Fredholm BB, et al. Adenosine injection into the brachial artery produces ischaemia like pain or discomfort in the forearm. *Cardiovasc Res* 1988;22:674.
168. Jonzon B, Sylven C, Kaijser L. Theophylline decreases pain in the ischaemic forearm test. *Cardiovasc Res* 1989;23:807–809.
169. Ferreira SH. The role of interleukins and nitric oxide in the mediation of inflammatory pain and its control by peripheral analgesics. *Drugs* 1993;46 (Suppl. 1):1.
170. Ferreira SH, Lorenzetti BB, Poole S. Bradykinin initiates cytokine-mediated inflammatory hyperalgesia *Br J Pharmacol* 1993;110:1227.

171. Grayson LS, Hansbrough JF, Zapata-Sirvent RL, et al. Quantitation of cytokine levels in skin graft donor site wound fluid. *Burns* 1993;19:401–405.

172. Vergnolle N, Bunnett NW, Sharkey KA, et al. Proteinase-activated receptor-2 and hyperalgesia: A novel pain pathway. *Nat Med* 2001;7:821–826.

173. Vergnolle N. Modulation of visceral pain and inflammation by protease-activated receptors. *Br J Pharmacol* 2004;141:1264–1274.

174. Koetzner L, Gregory JA, Yaksh TL. Intrathecal protease-activated receptor stimulation produces thermal hyperalgesia through spinal cyclooxygenase activity. *J Pharmacol Exp Ther* 2004;311:356–363.

175. Pezet S, McMahon SB. Neurotrophins: Mediators and Modulators of Pain. *Annu Rev Neurosci* 2006;29:507–538.

176. Gamse R, Holzer P, Lembeck F. Decrease of substance P in primary afferent neurones and impairment of neurogenic plasma extravasation by capsaicin. *Br J Pharmacol* 1980;68:207–213.

177. Hokfelt T, Kellerth JO, Nilsson G, et al. Experimental immunohistochemical studies on the localization and distribution of substance P in cat primary sensory neurones. *Brain Res* 1975;100:235.

178. Hokfelt T, Kellerth JO, Nilsson G, et al. Substance p: localization in the central nervous system and in some primary sensory neurons. *Science* 1975;190:889–890.

179. Mayberg M, Langer RS, Zervas NT, et al. Perivascular meningeal projections from cat trigeminal ganglia: Possible pathway for vascular headaches in man. *Science* 1981;3:228.

180. Moskowitz MA, Reinhard JF, Jr., Romero J, et al. Neurotransmitters and the fifth cranial nerve: Is there a relation to the headache phase of migraine? *Lancet* 1979;1:883.

181. Olgart L, Hokfelt T, Nilsson G, et al. Localization of substance P-like immunoreactivity in nerves in the tooth pulp. *Pain* 1977;4:153.

182. Bill A, Stjernschantz J, Mandahl A, et al. Substance P: release on trigeminal nerve stimulation, effects in the eye. *Acta Physiol Scand* 1979;106:371–373.

183. Larsson J, Ekblom A, Henriksson K, et al. Immunoreactive tachykinins, calcitonin gene-related peptide and neuropeptide Y in human synovial fluid from inflamed knee joints. *Neurosci Lett* 1989;100:326.

184. Brodin E, Gazelius B, Olgart L, et al. Tissue concentration and release of substance P-like immunoreactivity in the dental pulp. *Acta Physiol Scand* 1981;111:141–149.

185. Yaksh TL. Substance P release from knee joint afferent terminals: modulation by opioids. *Brain Res* 1988;458:319–24.

186. Helme RD, Koschorke GM, Zimmermann M. Immunoreactive substance P release from skin nerves in the rat by noxious thermal stimulation. *Neurosci Lett* 1986;63:295.

187. Hua XY, Yaksh TL. Pharmacology of the effects of bradykinin, serotonin, and histamine on the release of calcitonin gene-related peptide from C-fiber terminals in the rat trachea. *J Neurosci* 1993;13:1947–1953.

188. Lembeck F, Gamse R, Juan H. Substance P and sensory nerve endings New York, Raven Press, 1977.

189. Kumazawa T, Mizumura K. Thin-fibre receptors responding to mechanical, chemical, and thermal stimulation in the skeletal muscle of the dog. *J Physiol* (Lond.) 1977;273:179.

190. Kessler W, Kirchhoff C, Reeh PW, et al. Excitation of cutaneous afferent nerve endings in vitro by a combination of inflammatory mediators and conditioning effect of substance P. *Exp Brain Res* 1992;91:467.

191. Szolcsanyi J. Antidromic vasodilatation and neurogenic inflammation. *Agents Actions* 1988;23:4.

192. Jancso N, Jancso-Gabor A, Szolcsanyi J. Direct evidence for neurogenic inflammation and its prevention by denervation and by pretreatment with capsaicin. *Br J Pharmacol Chemother* 1967;31:138–151.

193. Szolcsanyi J, Janeso-Gabor A, Joo F. Functional and fine structural characteristics of the sensory neurone blocking effect of capsaicin. *Naunyn Schmiedebergs Arch Pharmacol* 1975;287:157.

194. Couture R, Cuello AC. Studies on the trigeminal antidromic vasodilatation and plasma extravasation in the rat. *J Physiol* 1984;346:273–285.

195. Rosell S, Olgart L, Gazelius Bea. Inhibition of anhdromic and substance P-induced vasodilatation by a substance P-antagonist. *Acta Physiol Scand* 1981;111:381.

196. Chapman LF, Ramos AO, Goodell H, et al. Neurohumoral features of afferent fibers in man. *Arch Neurol* 1961;4:617.

197. Burgess PR, Perl ER. Myelinated afferent fibers responding specifically to noxious stimulation of the skin. *J Physiol* (Lond.) 1967;190:541.

198. Georgopoulos AP. Functional properties of primary afferent units probably related to pain mechanisms in primate glabrous skin. *J Neurophysiol* 1976;39:71–83.

199. Perl ER. Myelinated afferent fibers innervating the primate skin and their response to noxious stimuli. *J Physiol* (Lond.) 1968;197:593.

200. Adrian ED. The effects of injury on mammalian nerve fibers. *Proc R Soc Lond B* 1930;106:596.

201. Iggo A. Cutaneous thermoreceptors in primates and subprimates. *J Physiol* (Lond) 1969;200:403.

202. Dubner R, Beitel RE. Neural correlates of escape behavior in rhesus monkey to noxious heat applied to the face. New York, Raven Press, 1976.

203. Dubner R, Gobel S, Price DD. Peripheral and central trigeminal "pain" pathways. New York, Raven Press, 1976.

204. Dodt E, Zotterman Y. The discharge of specific cold fibers at high temperatures. *Acta Physiol Scand* 1952;26:358.

205. Hensel H. Cutaneous thermoreceptors Handbook of Sensory Physiology. Edited by Iggo A. New York, Springer-Verlag, 1973, pp. 79–110.

206. La Motte RH, Campbell JN. Comparison of responses of warm and nociceptive C-fiber afferents in monkey with human judgements of thermal pain. *J Neurophysiol* 1978;41:509.

207. Price DD, Hu JW, Dubner R, et al. Peripheral suppression of first pain and central summation of second pain evoked by noxious heat pulses. *Pain* 1977;3:57.

208. Kumazawa T, Perl ER. Primate cutaneous sensory units with umyelinated (C) afferent fibers. *J Neurophysiol* 1977;40:1325.

209. Stacey MJ. Free nerve endings in skeletal muscle of the cat. *J Anat* 1969;105:231.

210. Iggo A. Nonmyelinated afferent fibers from mammalian skeletal muscle. *J Physiol* (Lond) 1961;155:52.

211. Hertel HC, Howaldt B, Mense S. Responses of group IV and group III muscle afferents to thermal stimuli. *Brain Res* 1976;113:201.

212. Paintal AS. Functional analysis of group III afferent fibres of mammalian muscles. *J Physiol* (Lond.) 1960;152:250.

213. Franz M, Mense S. Muscle receptors with group IV afferent fibres responding to application of bradykinin. *Brain Res* 1975;92:369–83.

214. Kniffki KD, Mense S, Schmidt RF. Responses of group IV afferent units from skeletal muscle to stretch, contraction and chemical stimulation. *Exp Brain Res* 1978;31:511.

215. Hnik P, Holas M, Krekvle Iea. Work-induced potassium changes in skeletal muscle and effluent venous blood assessed by liquid ion-exchanger microelectrodes. *Pflugers Arch* 1976;362:85.

216. Meller ST, Gebhart GF. A critical review of the afferent pathways and the potential chemical mediators involved in cardiac pain. *Neuroscience* 1992;48:501.

217. Blumgart HL, Schlesinger MJ, Davis D. Studies on the relation of the clinical manifestations of angina pectoris, coronary thrombosis and myocardial infarction to the pathological findings, with particular reference to the significance of the collateral circulation. *Am Heart J* 1940;19:1.

218. White JC, Bland EF. The surgical relief of severe angina pectoris: Methods employed and end results in 83 patients. *Medicine* (Baltimore) 1948;27:1.

219. Sutton DC, Lueth HC. Experimental production of pain on excitation of the heart and great vessels. *Arch Intern Med* 1930;45:827.

220. Foreman RD. Viscerosomatic convergence onto spinal neurons responding to afferent fibers located in the inferior cardiac nerve. *Brain Res* 1977;137:164.

221. Foreman RD, Ohata CA, Gerhart KD. Neural mechanisms underlying cardiac pain. New York, Raven Press, 1978.

222. Lindgren I, Olivecrona H. Surgical treatment of angina pectoris. *J Neurosurg* 1947;4:19.

223. White JC, Garrey WE, Atkins JA. Cardiac innervation: Experimental and clinical studies. *Arch Surg* 1933;26:765.

224. Brown AM. Excitation of afferent cardiac sympathetic nerve fibres during myocardial ischaemia. *J Physiol* 1967;190:35–53.

225. Brown AM, Malliani A. Spinal sympathetic reflexes initiated by coronary receptors. *J Physiol* 1971;212:685–705.

226. Uchida Y, Murao S. Excitation of afferent cardiac sympathetic nerve fibers during coronary occlusion. *Am J Physiol* 1974;226:1094.

227. Malliani A, Recordati G, Schwartz PJ. Nervous activity of afferent cardiac sympathetic fibres with atrial and ventricular endings. *J Physiol* (Lond.) 1973;229:457.

228. Uchida Y, Kamisaka K, Ueda H. Experimental studies on anginal pain: Mode of excitation of afferent cardiac sympathetic nerve fibers. *Jpn Circulation J* 1971;35:147.

229. Nishi K, Sakanashi M, Takenaka F. Activation of afferent cardiac sympathetic nerve fibers of the cat by pain producing substances and by noxious heat. *Pflugers Arch* 1977;372:53.

230. Burch GE, Depasquale NP. Bradykinin. *Am Heart J* 1963;65:116–123.

231. Uchida Y, Murao S. Bradykinin-induced excitation of afferent cardiac sympathetic nerve fibers. *Jpn Heart J* 1974;25:84.

232. Douglas WW, Ritchie JM. Nonmedullated fibers in the saphenous nerve which signal touch. *J Physiol* 1957;139:385.

233. Nishi K. The action of 5-hydroxytryptamine on chemoreceptor discharges of the cat's carotid body. *Br J Pharmacol* 1975;55:27.

234. Kimura E, Hashimoto K, Furukawa S, et al. Changes in bradykinin level in coronary sinus blood after the experimental occlusion of a coronary artery. *Am Heart J* 1973;85:635.

235. Stazewska-Barczak J, Ferreira SH, Vane JR. An excitatory nociceptive cardiac reflex elicited by bradykinin and potentiated by prostaglandins and myocardial ischemia. *Cardiovasc Res* 1976;10:314.

236. Alexander RW, Kent KM, Pisano JJ. Regulation of canine coronary blood flow by endogenous synthesized prostaglandins. *Circulation* 1973;48 (Suppl. IV).

237. Block AR, Feinberg H, Herbaczynska-Cedra K, et al. Anoxia induced release of prostaglandins in rabbit isolated hearts *Circ Res* 1975;36:34.

238. Wennmalm A, Chanh PH, Junstad M. Hypoxia causes prostaglandin release from perfused rabbit hearts. *Acta Physiol Scand* 1974;91:133.

239. Frank RM. Ultrastructural relationship between the odontoblast, its process and the nerve fiber. London, Livingstone, 1968.

240. Olgart L. Local mechanisms in dental pain., Mechanisms of Pain and Analgesic Compounds. Edited by Beers RF, Bassett EG. New York, Raven Press, 1979, pp. 285–294.

241. Anderson KV, Perl GS. Conduction velocities in afferent fibers from feline tooth pulp. *Exp Neurol* 1974;43:281.

242. Delange A, Hannam AG, Matthews B. The diameters and conduction velocities of fibers in the terminal branches of the inferior dental nerve. *Arch Oral Biol* 1969;14:513.

243. Greenwood LF, Horiuchi H, Matthews B. Electrophysiological evidence on the types of nerve fibers excited by electrical stimulation of teeth with a pulp tester. *Arch Oral Biol* 1972;17:701.

244. Young RF, King RB. Fiber spectrum of the trigeminal sensory root of the baboon determined by electron microscopy. *J Neurosurg* 1973;38:65.

245. Van Hassel HJ, Biedenback MA, Brown AC. Cortical potentials evoked by tooth pulp stimulation in rhesus monkeys. *Arch Oral Biol* 1972;17:1059.

246. Vyklicky L, Keller O. Central projection of tooth pulp primary afferents in the cat. Acta Neurobiol. *Exp* 1973;33:803.

247. Vyklicky L, Keller O, Brozek G, et al. Cortical potentials evoked by stimulation of tooth pulp afferents in the cats. *Brain Res.* 1972;41:211.

248. Oleson TD, Kirkpatrick DB, Goodman SJ. Elevation of pain threshold to tooth shock by brain stimulation in primates. *Brain Res.* 1980;194:79.

249. Edwall L, Olgart L. A new technique for recording of intradental sensory nerve activity in man. *Pain* 1977;3:121–125.

250. Brashear AD. The innervation of the teeth. An analysis of nerve fiber components of the pulp and peridental tissue and their probable significance. *J Comp Neurol* 1936;64:169.

251. Pfaffman C. Afferent impulses from the teeth due to pressure and noxius stimulation. *J Physiol* (Lond.) 1939;97.207.

252. Funakoshi M, Zotterman Y. A study in the excitation of dental pulp nerve fibres. Oxford, Pergamon, 1963.

253. Matthews B. The response of pulpal nerves to thermal stimulation of dentine. *J Dent Res* 1967;46:1279.

254. Scott DJ, Maziarz R. What is the most unique form of stimulus to evoke dental pain?, Advances in Pain Research and Therapy. Edited by Bonica JJ, Albe-Fessard D. New York, Raven Press, 1976, pp. 205–213.

255. Ahlberg KF. Dose-dependent inhibition of sensory nerve activity in the feline dental pulp by anti-inflammatory drugs. *Acta Physiol Scand* 1978;102:434.

256. Ahlberg KF. Influence of local noxious heat stimulation on sensory nerve activity in the feline dental pulp. *Acta Physiol Scand* 1978;103:71.

257. Brannstrom M, Astrom A. The hydrodynamics of the dentine;its possible relationship to dentinal pain. *Int Dent J* 1972;22:219–227.

258. Beveridge EE, Brown A. The measurement of human dental intrapulpal pressure and its response to clinical variables. *Oral Surg* 1965;19:655.

259. Gardner E. The distribution and termination of nerves in the knee joint of the cat. *J Comp Neurol* 1994;80:11.

260. Clark FJ. Central projection of sensory fibers from the cat knee joint. *J Neurobiol* 1972;3:101–110.

261. Clark FJ. Information signaled by sensory fibers in medial articular nerve. *J Neurophysiol* 1975;38:1464–1472.

262. Clark FJ, Burgess PR. Slowly adapting receptors in cat knee joint: can they signal joint angle? *J Neurophysiol* 1975;38:1448–1463.

263. Fitzgerald TJ, Williams B, Uyeki EM. Effects of antimitotic and anti-inflammatory agents on sodium urateinduced pain swelling in mice. *Pharmacology* 1971;6:265.

264. Van Arman CG, Carlson RP, Risley EAea. Inhibitor effects of indomethacin, aspirin and certain other drugs on inflammations induced in rat and dog by carrageenan, sodium urate and ellagic acid. *J Pharmacol Exp Ther* 1970;175:459.

265. Herman AC, Moncada S. Release of prostaglandins and incapacitation after injection of endotoxin in the knee joint of the dog. *Br J Pharmacol* 1975;53:465P.

266. Gouret C, Mocquet G, Raynaud G. Use of Freund's adjuvant arthritis test in anti-flammatory drug screening in the rat: value of animal selection and preparation at the breeding center. *Lab Anim Sci* 1976;26:281–287.

267. McCarty DJ, Gatter RA, Brill JM, et al. Crystal deposition disease-sodium urate (gout) and calcium pyrophate (chondrocalcinosis, pseudogout). *JAMA* 1965;193:129.

268. Brune K, Waltz D, Bucher K. The avian microcrystal arthritis. I. Simultaneous recording of nociceptiona and temperature effect in the inflamed joint. *Agents Actions* 1974;4:21.

269. McCormack K, Brune K. Dissociation between the antinociceptive and anti-inflammatory effects of the nonsteroidal anti-inflammatory drugs. A survey of their analgesic efficacy. *Drugs* 1991;41:533–547.

270. Woodbury DM, Fingl E. Analgesics antipyretics, antiinflammatory agents, and drugs emploed in the therapy of gout., The Pharmacological Basis of Therapeutics., 5th Edition. Edited by Goodman LS, Gilman EA. New York, MacMillan, 1975, pp. 312–344.

271. McCormack K. Non-steroidal anti-inflammatory drugs and spinal nociceptive processing. [published erratum appears in Pain 1995 Mar;60(3):353]. *Pain* 1994;59:9–43.

272. Malmberg AB, Yaksh TL. Antinociceptive actions of spinal nonsteroidal anti-inflammatory agents on the formalin test in the rat. *J Pharmacol Exp Therapeut* 1992;263:136–146.

273. Malmberg AB, Yaksh TL. Hyperalgesia mediated by spinal glutamate or substance P receptor blocked by spinal cyclooxygenase inhibitor. *Science* 1992;257:1276–1279.

274. Bielefeldt K, Christianson JA, Davis BM. Basic and clinical aspects of visceral sensation: transmission in the CNS. *Neurogastroenterol Motil* 2005;17:488–499.

275. Cervero F, Janig W. Visceral nociceptors: a new world order? *Trends Neurosci* 1992;15:374–378.

276. Ness TJ, Gebhart GF. Visceral pain: a review of experimental studies. *Pain* 1990;41:167–234.

277. McMahon SB. Mechanisms of cutaneous, deep and visceral pain. In Melzack, R. and Wall, P.D.: Textbook of Pain. 1994; pp. 129–152.

278. Berkley KJ, Hotta H, Robbins A, et al. Functional properties of afferent fibers supplying the reproductive and other pelvic organs in pelvic nerve of female rat. *J Neurophysiol* 1990;63:256.

279. Berkley KJ, Robbins A, Sato Y. Afferent fibers supplying the uterus in the rat. *J Neurophysiol* 1988;59(110):142.

280. Mizumura K, Sato J, Kumazawa T. Comparison of the effects of prostaglandins E2 and I2 on testicular nociceptor activities studied in vitro. *Naunyn-Schmiedebergs Arch Pharmacol* 1991;344:368.

281. Mizumura K, Sato J, Kumazawa T. Strong heat stimulation sensitizes the heat response as well as the bradykinin response of visceral polymodal receptors. *J Neurophysiol* 1992;68:1209.

282. Haupt P, Janig W, Kohler W. Response pattern of visceral afferent fibres, supplying the colon, upon chemical and mechanical stimuli *Pflugers Archiv Eur J Physiol* 1983;398:41.

283. Howe JF, Loeser JD, Calvin WH. Mechanosensitivity of dorsal root ganglia chronically injured axons: A physiological basis for the radicular pain of nerve root compression. *Pain* 1977;3:25.

284. Wall PD, Gutnick M. Ongoing activity in peripheral nerves: The physiology and pharmacology of impulses originating from a neuroma. *Exp Neurol* 1974;43:580.

285. Dyson C, Brindley GS. Strength-duration curves for the production of cutaneous pain by electrical stimuli. *Clin Sci* 1966;30:237–241.

286. Kelly M. Is pain due to pressure on nerves? Spinal tumors and the intervertebral disk? *Neurology* (Minneap.) 1956;6:32–36.

287. Goldman DE. Responses of nerve fibers to mechanical forces. New York, Springer, 1971.

288. Gray JAB. Effects of stretch on single myelinated fibers. *J Physiol* 1954; 124:84.

289. Julian FJ, Goldman DD. The effects of mechanical stimulation on some electrical properties of axons. *J Gen Physiol* 1962;46:297.

290. Stoll G, Jander S, Myers RR. Degeneration and regeneration of the peripheral nervous system: from Augustus Waller's observations to neuroinflammation. *J Peripher Nerv Syst* 2002;7:13–27.

291. Burchiel KJ, Ochoa JL. Pathophysiology of injured axons. *Neurosurg Clin N Am* 1991;2:105–116.

292. Amir R, Devor M. Spike-evoked suppression and burst patterning in dorsal root ganglion neurons of the rat. *J Physiol* 1997;501 (Pt 1):183–196.

293. Devor M, Wall PD, Catalan N. Systemic lidocaine silences ectopic neuroma and DRG discharge without blocking nerve conduction. *Pain* 1992;48:261–268.

294. Zimmermann M. Pathobiology of neuropathic pain. *Eur J Pharmacol* 2001; 429:23–37.

295. Chahine M, Ziane R, Vijayaragavan K, et al. Regulation of Na v channels in sensory neurons. *Trends Pharmacol Sci* 2005;26:496–502.

296. Kalso E. Sodium channel blockers in neuropathic pain. *Curr Pharm Des* 2005;11:3005–3011.

297. Liu X, Zhou JL, Chung K, et al. Ion channels associated with ectopic discharges generated after segmental spinal nerve injury in the rat. *Brain Res* 2001;900:119–127.

298. Rasband MN, Park EW, Vanderah TW, et al. Distinct potassium channels on pain-sensing neurons. *Proc Natl Acad Sci U S A* 2001;98:13373–13378.

299. Chen Y, Michaelis M, Janig W, et al. Adrenoreceptor subtype mediating sympathetic-sensory coupling in injured sensory neurons. *J Neurophysiol* 1996;76:3721–3730.

300. Shinder V, Govrin-Lippmann R, Cohen S, et al. Structural basis of sympathetic-sensory coupling in rat and human dorsal root ganglia following peripheral nerve injury. *J Neurocytol* 1999;28:743–761.

301. Liu B, Li H, Brull SJ, et al. Increased sensitivity of sensory neurons to tumor necrosis factor alpha in rats with chronic compression of the lumbar ganglia. *J Neurophysiol* 2002;88:1393–1399.

302. Sommer C, Petrausch S, Lindenlaub T, et al. Neutralizing antibodies to interleukin 1-receptor reduce pain associated behavior in mice with experimental neuropathy. *Neurosci Lett* 1999;270:25–8.

303. Sommer C, Schmidt C, George A. Hyperalgesia in experimental neuropathy is dependent on the TNF receptor 1. *Exp Neurol* 1998;151:138–142.

304. Carlen PL, Wall PD, Nadvorna H, et al. Phantom limbs and related phenomena in recent traumatic amputations. *Neurolology* 1978;28:211.

305. Doupe J, Cullen CH, Chance GQ. Post-tramautic pain and the causalgic syndrome. *J Neurol Neurosurg Pyschiatry* 1944;7:33.

306. Basbaum AI. Effects of central lesions on disorders produced by multiple dorsal rhizotomy in rats. *Exp Neurol* 1974;42:490.

307. Devor M, Schonfeld D, Seltzer Z, et al. Two modes of cutaneous reinnervation following peripheral nerve injury. *J Comp Neurol* 1979;185:211–220.

308. Wall PD, Scadding JW, Tomkiewicz MM. The production and prevention of experimental anesthesia dolorosa. *Pain* 1979;6:175–182

309. Pearl GS, Anderson KV. Response of cells in feline nucleus centrum medianum to tooth pulp stimulation. *Brain Res Bull* 1980;5:41.

310. Jannetta PJ. Microsurgical approach to the trigeminal nerve for tic douloureux. *Prog Neurol Surg* 1976;7:180.

311. Kerr FWL. The divisional organization of afferent fibres of the trigeminal nerve. *Brain* 1963;86:721.

312. Kerr FWL. Trigeminal neuralgia, pathogenesis and description of a possible etiology for the cryptogenic variety. *Trans Am Neurol Assoc* 1962;87:118.

313. Baker GS, Kerr FWL. Structural changes in the trigeminal system following compression procedures. *J Neurosurg* 1963;20:181.

314. Calvin WH. Some design features of axons and how neuralgias may defeat them. New York, Raven Press, 1979.

315. Calvin WH, Howe JF, Loeser JD. Ectopic repetitive firing in focally demyelinated axons and some implications for trigeminal neuralgia. Amsterdam, Elsevier/North Holland, 1977.

316. Kerr FW. Neuroanatomical substrates of nociception in the spinal cord. *Pain* 1975;1:325–356.

317. Light AR, Perl ER. Re-examination of the dorsal root projection to the spinal dorsal horn including observations on the differential termination of coarse and fine fibers. *J Comp Neurol* 1979;186:117.

318. Ranson SW. An experimental study of Lissauer's tract and the dorsal roots. *J Comp Neurol* 1914;24:531.

319. Ranson SW, Billingsly PR. The conduction of painful afferent impulses in the spinal nerves. *Am J Physiol* 1916;40:571.

320. Snyder R. The organization of the dorsal root entry zone in cats and monkeys. *J Comp Neurol* 1977;174:47.

321. Carpenter MD, Stein BM, Shriver JE. Central projections of spinal dorsal roots in the monkey. II. Lower thoracic, lumbosacral and coccygeal dorsal roots. *Am J Anat* 1968;123:75.

322. Sterling P, Kuypers HGJM. Anatomical organization of the brachial spinal cord of the cat. I. The distribution of dorsal root fibers. *Brain Res* 1967;4:1.

323. Cajal SR. Histologie du Systeme Nerveux del' Hommes et de Vertebres. Madrid, Instituto Ramon y Cajal, 1909 (1952 reprint).

324. Kerr FWL. Pain: A central inhibitory balance theory. *Mayo Clin Proc* 1975; 50:685.

325. Anderson FD. Distribution of dorsal root fibers in the cat spinal cord. *Anat Rec* 1960;136:154.

326. Light AR, Perl ER. Spinal termination of functionally identified primary afferent neurons with slowly conducting myelinated fibers. *J Comp Neurol* 1979;186:133.

327. Proshansky E, Egger MD. Dendritic spread of dorsal horn neurons in cats. *Exp Brain Res* 1977;28:153.

328. Rethelyi M, Trevino DL, Perl ER. Distribution of primary afferent fibers within the sacrococcygeal dorsal horn: An autoradiographic study. *J Comp Neurol* 1979;185:603.

329. Culberson JL, Haines DE, Kimmel DL, et al. Contralateral projection of primary afferent fibers to mammalian spinal cord. *Exp Neurol* 1979;64:83–97.

330. Heimer L, Wall PD. The dorsal root distribution to the substantia gelatinosa of the rat with a note on distribution in the cat. *Exp Brain Res* 1968;6:89.

331. Nashold B, Urban B, Zorub DS. Phantom pain relief by focal destruction of the substantia gelatinosa of Rolando., Advances in Pain Research and Therapy. Edited by Bonica JJ, Albe-Fessard G. New York, Raven Press, 1976, pp. 959–963.

332. Nashold BJ, Ostdahl RH. Dorsal root entry zone lesions for pain relief. *J Neurosurg* 1979;51:59.

333. Applebaum ML, Clifton GL, Coggeshall REea. Umyelinated fibres in the sacral 3 and caudal 1 ventral roots of the cat. *J Physiol* (Lond.) 1976; 256:557.

334. Clifton GL, Coggeshall RE, Vance WH, et al. Receptive fields of unmyelinated ventral root afferent fibres in the cat. *J Physiol* 1976;256:573–600.

335. Clifton GL, Vance WH, Applebaum ML, et al. Responses of unmyelinated afferents in the mammalian ventral root. *Brain Res* 1974;82:163–167.

336. Coggeshall RE, Applebaum ML, Fazen M, et al. Unmyelinated axons in human ventral roots, a possible explanation for the failure of dorsal rhizotomy to relieve pain. *Brain* 1975;98:157–166.

337. Coggeshall RE, Coulter JD, Willis WD, Jr. Unmyelinated axons in the ventral roots of the cat lumbosacral enlargement. *J Comp Neurol* 1974;153:39–58.

338. MacDermott AB, Mayer ML, Westbrook GL, et al. NMDA-receptor activation increases cytoplasmic calcium concentration in cultured spinal cord neurones. *Nature* 1986;321:519–522.

339. Yamamoto T, Takahashi H, Satomi H, et al. Origins of primary afferent fibers in the spinal ventral roots in the cat as demonstrated by the horseradish peroxidase method. *Brain Res.* 1977;126:350.

340. Onofrio BM, Campa HK. Evaluabon of rhizotomy: Review of 12 years' experience. *J Neurosurg* 1972;36:751.

341. Aimi Y, Fujimura M, Vincent SR, et al. Localization of NADPH-diaphorase-containing neurons in sensory ganglia of the rat. *J Comp Neurol* 1991;306:382–392.

342. Anderson SD, Basbaum AI, Fields HL. Response of medullary raphe neurons to peripheral stimulation and to systemic opiates. *Brain Res* 1977;123:363.

343. Rexed B. A cytoarchitectonic atlas of the spinal cord in the cat. *J Comp Neurol* 1954;100:297.

344. Rexed B. The cytoarchitectonic organization of the spinal cord in the cat. *J Comp Neurol* 1952;96:415–495.

345. Cervero F, Iggo A. The substantia gelatinosa of the spinal cord: a critical review. *Brain* 1980;103:717–772.

346. Kerr FWL, Lippman HH. The primate spinothalamic tract as demonstrated by anterolateral cordotomy and commissural myelotomy. *Adv Neurol* 1974;4:147–156.

347. Wall PD, Shortland P. Long-range afferents in the rat spinal cord. I. Numbers, distances and conduction velocities. Philosophical Transactions of the Royal Society of London. Series B: Biological Sciences 1991;334:85–93.

348. Mendell LM, Sassoon EM, Wall PD. Properties of synaptic linkage from long ranging afferents onto dorsal horn neurones in normal and deafferented cats. *J Physiol* 1978;285:299.

349. Hongo T, Jankowska E, Lundberg A. Post-synaptic excitation and inhibition from primary afferents in neurones of the spinocervical tract. *J Physiol* 1968;199:569–592.

350. King AE, Thompson SW, Urban L, et al. An intracellular analysis of amino acid induced excitations of deep dorsal horn neurones in the rat spinal cord slice. *Neurosci Lett* 1980;89:286.

351. Urban L, Randic M. Slow excitatory transmission in rat dorsal horn: possible mediation by peptides. *Brain ReseArch* 1984;290:336–341.

352. Yoshimura M, Jessell TM. Primary afferent-evoked synaptic responses and slow potential generation in rat substantia gelatinosa neurons in vitro. *J Neurophysiol* 1989;62:96–108.

353. Battaglia G, Rustioni A. Coexistence of glutamate and substance P in dorsal root ganglion neurons of the rat and monkey. *J Comp Neurol* 1988; 277:302–312.

354. Kai-Kai MA. Cytochemistry of the trigeminal and dorsal root ganglia and spinal cord of the rat. *Comp Biochem Physiol A* 1989;93:183–193.

355. Levine JD, Fields HL, Basbaum AI. Peptides and the primary afferent nociceptor. *J Neurosci* 1993;13:2273–2286.

356. Nagy JJ, Hunt SP. The termination of primary afferents within the rat dorsal horn- evidence for rearrangements following capsaicin treatment. *J Comp Neurol* 1983;218:145.

357. Akagi H, Otsuka M, Yanagisawa N. Identification by high-performance liquid chromatography of immunoreactive substance P released from isolated rat spinal cord. *Neurosci Lett* 1980;20:259.

358. Jessell TM, Iversen LL. Opiate analgesics inhibit substance P release from rat trigeminal nucleus. *Nature* 1977;268:549–551.

359. Otsuka M, Konishi S. Release of substances P- like immunoreactivity from isolated spinal cord of newborn rat. *Nature* 1976;264:83.

360. Sawynok J, Kato N, Havlicek V, et al. Lack of effect of baclofen on substance P and somatostatin release from the spinal cord in vitro. *Naunyn Schmiedebergs Arch Pharmacol* 1982;319:78–81.

361. Sheppard M, Kronheim S, Adams C, et al. Immunoreactive somatostatin release from rat spinal cord in vitro. *Neurosci Lett* 1979;15:65.

362. Yaksh TL, Tyce GM. Resting and K+-evoked release of serotonin and norephinephrine in vivo from the rat and cat spinal cord. *Brain Res* 1980; 192:133–146.

363. Go VIW, Yaksh TL. Release of substance P from the cat spinal cord. *J Physiol* 1987;391:141–167.

364. Yaksh TL, Jessell TM, Gamse R, et al. Intrathecal morphine inhibits substance P release from mammalian spinal cord in vivo. *Nature* 1980;286:155–157.

365. Collin E, Mantelet S, Frechilla D, et al. Increased in vivo release of calcitonin gene-related peptide-like material from the spinal cord in arthritic rats. *Pain* 1993;54:203–211.

366. Blank MA, Anard P, Lumb BMea. Release of vasoactive intestinal polypeptide-like immunoreactivity (VIP) from cat urinary bladder in sacal spinal cord during pelvic nerve stimulation. *Dig Dis Sci* 1984;27:115.

367. Yaksh TL, Abay EOd, Go VL. Studies on the location and release of cholecystokinin and vasoactive intestinal peptide in rat and cat spinal cord. *Brain Res* 1982;242:279–290.

368. Malmberg AB, Yaksh TL. Concurrent assessment of formalin-evoked behaviour and spinal release of excitatory amino acids and prostaglandin E2 using micodialysis in awake rats : Effect of systemic morphine. *Br J Pharmacol* 1995;114:1069.

369. Sluka KA, Westlund KN. Spinal cord amino acid release and content in an arthritis model: The effects of pretreatment with non- NMDA,NMDA, and NKI receptor antagonists. *Brain Res* 1993;627:89.

370. Sorkin LS. NMDA evokes an L-NAME sensitive spinal release of glutamate and citrulline. *Neuroreport* 1993;4:479–482.

371. Takano M, Takano Y, Yaksh TL. Release of calcitonin gene-related peptide (CGRP), substance P (SP), and vasoactive intestinal polypeptide (VIP) from rat spinal cord: modulation by alpha 2 agonists. *Peptides* 1993;14:371–378.

372. Jeftinija S, Miletic V, Randic M. Cholecystokinin octapeptide excites dorsal horn neurons both in vivo and in vitro. *Brain Res* 1981;213:231.

373. Yaksh TL. Pharmacology of spinal adrenergic systems which modulate spinal nociceptive processing. *Pharmacol Biochem Behav* 1985;22:845–858.

374. Yaksh TL. The spinal action of opioids. Handbook of Experimental Pharmacology. Edited by Herz A. Berlin, Heidelberg, Springer Verlag, 1993, pp. 53–90.

375. Yaksh TL, Jage J, Takano Y. The spinal actions of a2 adrenergic agonists as analgesics, Bailliere's Clinical Anesthesiology. Edited by Aitkenhead AR, Benard G, Brown BR, Bailliere, 1993.

376. Zieglgansberger W, Phil EA. Actions of glutamic acid on spinal neurons. *Exp Brain Res* 1973;17.

377. Besson JM, Catchlove RFH, Feltz P, et al. Further evidence for postsynaptic inhibitions on lamina V dorsal horn interneurons. *Brain Res* 1974;66:531.

378. Henry JL. Effects of substance P on functionally identified units in cat spinal cord. *Brain Res* 1976;114:439–451.

379. Murase K, Randic M. Actions of substance P on rat spinal dorsal horn neurones. *J Physiol* 1984;346:203.

380. Zieglgansberger W, Tulloch IF. Effects of substance P on neurones in the dorsal horn of the spinal cord of the cat. *Brain Res* 1979;166:273.

381. Page NM. New challenges in the study of the mammalian tachykinins. *Peptides* 2005;26:1356–1368.

382. Randic M, Miletic V. Effects of substance P in cat dorsal horn neurones activated by noxious stimuli. *Brain Res.* 1977;128:164–169.

383. Piercey MF, Einspahr FJ, Dobry PGK, et al. Morphine does not antagonize the substance P mediated excitation of dorsal horn neurons. *Brain Res* 1980;186:421.

384. Wright DM, Roberts MHT. Responses of spinal neurones to a substance P analogue, noxious pinch and bradykinin. *Eur J Pharmacol* 1980;64:165.

385. Poyner DR, Sexton PM, Marshall I, et al. International Union of Pharmacology. XXXII. The mammalian calcitonin gene-related peptides, adrenomedullin, amylin, and calcitonin receptors. *Pharmacol Rev* 2002;54:233–246.

386. Bird GC, Han JS, Fu Y, et al. Pain-related synaptic plasticity in spinal dorsal horn neurons: role of CGRP. *Mol Pain* 2006;2:31.

387. Jeftinija S, Murase K, Nedeljkov V, et al. Vasoactive intestinal polypeptide excites mammalian dorsal horn neurons both in vivo and in vitro. *Brain Res* 1982;243:158–164.

388. Jeftinija S, Semba K, Randic M. Noripinephrine reduces excitability of single cutaneous primary afferent C-fibers in the cat spinal cord. *Brain Res* 1981;219:456.

389. Liu XH, Morris R. Vasoactive intestinal polypeptide produces depolarization and facilitation of C-fibre evoked synaptic responses in superficial dorsal horn neurones (laminae I–IV) of the rat lumbar spinal cord in vitro. *Neurosci Lett* 1999;276:1–4.

390. Jiang N, Furue H, Katafuchi T, et al. Somatostatin directly inhibits substantia gelatinosa neurons in adult rat spinal dorsal horn in vitro. *Neurosci Res* 2003;47:97–107.

391. Hokfelt T. Neuropeptides in perspective: the last ten years. *Neuron* 1991;7:867–879.

392. Buck SH, Burks TF. The neuropharmacology of capsaicin: review of some recent observations. *Pharmacol Rev* 1986;38:179–226.

393. Dray A. Neuropharmocological mechanisms of capsaicin and related substances. *Biochem Pharmacol* 1992;44:611.

394. Jahr CE, Jessell TM. Synaptic transmission between dorsal root ganglion and dorsal horn neurons in culture: antagonism of monosynaptic excitatory postsynaptic potentials and glutamate excitation by kynurenate. *J Neurosci* 1985;5:2281–2289.

395. Tong CK, MacDermott AB. Both Ca2+-permeable and -impermeable AMPA receptors contribute to primary synaptic drive onto rat dorsal horn neurons. *J Physiol* 2006;575:133–144.

396. Mjellem-Joly N, Lund A, Berge OG, et al. Potentiation of a behavioural response in mice by spinal coadministration of substance P and excitatory amino acid agonists. *Neuroscience Letters* 1991;133:121–124.

397. Dougherty PM, Palecek J, Paleckova V, et al. The role of NMDA and non-NMDA excitatory amino acid receptors in the excitation of primate spinothalamic tract neurons by mechanical, chemical, thermal, and electrical stimuli. *J Neurosci* 1992;12:3025–3041.

398. Dougherty PM, Palecek J, Zorn S, et al. Combined application of excitatory amino acids and substance P produces long-lasting changes in responses of primate spinothalamic tract neurons. *Brain Res Rev* 1993;18:227–246.

399. Price DD, Mayer DJ. Neurophysiological characterization of the anterolateral quadrant neurons subserving pain in M. mulatta. *Pain* 1975;1:59.

400. Trevino D, J.D. C, Willis WD. Location of cells of origin of spinothalamic tract in lumbar enlargement of the monkey. *J Neurophysiol* 1973;36:750.

401. Trevino DL, Maunz RA, Bryan RN, et al. Location of cells of origin of the spinothalamic tract in the lumbar enlargement of cat. *Exp Neurol* 1972;34:64.

402. Willis WD, Kenshalo DRJ, Leonard RB. The cells of origin of the primate spinothalamic tract. *J Comp Neurol* 1979;188:543.

403. Burton H, Loewy AD. Descending projections from the marginal cell layer and other regions of the monkey spinal cord. *Brain Res* 1976;116:485–491.

404. Scheibel ME, Scheibel AB. Terminal axonal patternsin the cat spinal cord. II. The dorsal horn. *Brain Res* 1968;9:32.

405. Szentagothai J. Neuronal and synaptic arrangement in the substantia gelatinosa Rolandi. *J Comp Neurol* 1964;122:219–239.

406. Gobel S. Golgi studies of the neurons in layer I of the dorsal horn of the medulla (trigeminal nucleus caudalis). *J Comp Neurol* 1978;180:375–393.

407. Kerr FWL. The fine structure of subnucleus caudalis of the trigeminal: A light and electron microscopic study of degeneration. *Brain Res* 1970;23:147.

408. Cervero F, Iggo A, Ogawa H. Nociceptor-driven dorsal horn neurones in the lumbar spinal cord of the cat. *Pain* 1976;2:5–24.

409. Christensen BN, Perl ER. Spinal neurons specifically excited by noxious or thermal stimuli: marginal zone of the dorsal horn. *J Neurophysiol* 1970;33:293–307.

410. Kumazawa T, Perl ER, Burgess PR, et al. Ascending projections from marginal zone (lamina I) neurons of the spinal dorsal horn. *J Comp Neurol* 1975;162:1–12.

411. Willis WD, Trevino DL, Coulter JD, et al. Responses of primate spinothalamic tract neurons to natural stimulation of hindlimb. *J Neurophysiol* 1974;37:358–372.

412. Suzuki R, Morcuende S, Webber M, et al. Superficial NK1-expressing neurons control spinal excitability through activation of descending pathways. *Nat Neurosci* 2002;5:1319–1326.

413. Yezierski RP, Yu CG, Mantyh PW, et al. Spinal neurons involved in the generation of at-level pain following spinal injury in the rat. *Neurosci Lett* 2004;361:232–236.

414. Mantyh PW, Rogers SD, Honore P, et al. Inhibition of hyperalgesia by ablation of lamina I spinal neurons expressing the substance P receptor. *Science* 1997;278:275–279.

415. Rolando L. Richerche Anatomie Sulla Struttura del Midollo Spinal. Torino, Dalla Stamperia Reale, 1824.

416. Gobel S. Golgi studies of the neurons in layer II of the dorsal horn of the medulla (trigeminal nucleus caudalis). *J Comp Neurol* 1978;180:395–413.

417. Duncan D, Morales R. Relative numbers of several types of synaptic connections in the substantia gelatinosa of the cat spinal cord. *J Comp Neurol* 1978;182:601.

418. Gobel S. Dendroaxonic synapses in the substantia gelatinosa trigeminal nucleus of the cat. *J Comp Neurol* 1976;167:165.

419. Ralston HJ. Dorsal root projection to dorsal horn neurons in the cat spinal cord. *J Comp Neurol* 1968;132:303.

420. Westrum LE, Black RC. Fine structural aspects of the synaptic organization of the spinal trigeminal nucleus (pars interpolaris) of the cat. *Brain Res* 1971;25:265.

421. Cervero F, Iggo A, Molony V. Responses of spinocervical tract neurones to noxious stimulation of the skin. *J Physiol* 1977;267:537–558.

422. Kumazawa T, Perl ER. Differential excitation of dorsal horn and substantia gelatinosa marginal neurons by primary afferent units with fine (A-δ and C) fibers, Sensory Functions of the Skin in Primates, with Special Reference to Man. Edited by Zotterman Y. New York, Pergamon, 1976, pp. 67–88.

423. Light AR, Trevino DL, Perl ER. Morphological features of functionally defined neurons in the marginal zone and substantia gelatinosa of the spinal dorsal horn. *J Comp Neurol* 1979;186:151.

424. Wall PD, Merrill EG, Yaksh TL. Responses of single units in laminae II and III of cat spinal cord. *Brain Res* 1979;160:245–260.

425. Hentall I. A novel class of unit in the substantia gelatinosa of the spinal cat. *Exp Neurol* 1977;57:792.

426. Cervero F. Dorsal horn neurons and their sensory inputs. New York, Plenum Press, 1986.

427. Cervero F, Molony V, Iggo A. Supraspinal linkage of substantia gelatinosa neurones: effects of descending impulses. *Brain Res* 1979;175:351–355.

428. Gobel S. Golgi studies in the substantia gelatinosa neurons in the spinal trigeminal nucleus. *J Comp Neurol* 1975;162:397–415.

429. Gobel S, Hockfield S. An anatomical analysis of the synaptic circuitry of layers I, II and III of trigeminal nucleus caudalis in the cat. Amsterdam, Elsevier/North-Holland, 1977.

430. Kerr FWL. The fine structure of subnucleus caudalis of the trigeminal nerve. *Brain Res* 1970;23:129.

431. Ralston HJ. The organization of the substantia gelatinosa Rolandi in the cat lumbosacral spinal cord. *Z Zellforsch* 1965;67:1.

432. Giesler GJ, Menetrey D, Guilbaud G, et al. Lumbar cord neurons at the origin of the spinothalamic tract in the rat. *Brain Res* 1976;118:320–324.

433. Kerr FWL, Fukushima TF. New observations in the nociceptive pathways in the central nervous system. New York Raven Press, 1980.

434. Trevino DL, Carstens E. Confirmation of the location of spinothalamic neurons in the cat and monkey by the retrograde transport of horseradish peroxidase. *Brain Res* 1975;98:177.

435. Brown AG, Fyffe RE, Noble R, et al. The density, distribution and topographical organization of spinocervical tract neurones in the cat. *J Physiol* 1980;300:409–428.

436. Mendell LM. Physiological properties of unmyelinated fiber projection to the spinal cord. *Exp Neurol* 1966;16:316–332.

437. Wall PD. The laminar organization of dorsal horn and effects of descending impulses. *J Physiol* (Lond) 1967;188:403–423.

438. Le Bars D, Guilbaud G, Turna I, et al. Differential effects of morphine on responses of dorsal horn lamina V type cells elicited by A and C fibre stimulation in the spinal cat. *Brain Res* 1976;115:518.

439. Price DD, Dubner R, Hu JW. Trigeminothalamic neurons in nucleus caudalis responsive to tactile, thermal and nociceptive stimulation of monkey's face. *J Neurophysiol* 1976;39:936.

440. Price DD, Hull CD, Buchwald NA. Intracellular responses of dorsal horn cells to cutaneous and sural nerve A and C fiber stimuli. *Exp Neurol* 1971; 33:291.

441. Willis WD. Long-term potentiation in spinothalamic neurons. *Brain Res Brain Res Rev* 2002;40:202–214.

442. Brown PB, Fuchs JL. Somatotopic representation of hindlimb skin in cat dorsal horn. *J Neurophysiol* 1975;38:1–9.

443. Bryan RN, Trevino DL, Coulter JD, et al. Location and somatotopic organization of the cells of origin of the spino-cervical tract. *Exp Brain Res* 1973;17:177–189.

444. Price DD, Mayer DJ. Physiological laminar organization of the dorsal horn of M. mulatta. *Brain Res* 1974;79:321.

445. Wagman IH, Price DD. Responses of dorsal horn cells of M. mulatta to cutaneous and sural nerve A and C fiber stimuli. *J Neurophysiol* 1969;32:803–817.

446. Hancock MB, Rigamonti DD, Bryan RN. Convergence in the lumbar spinal cord of pathways activated by splanchic nerve and hind limb cutaneous nerve stimulation. *Exp Neurol* 1973;38:337.

447. Pomeranz B, Wall PD, Weber WV. Cord cells responding to fine myelinated afferents from viscera, muscle, and skin. *J Physiol* (Lond.) 1968;199:511.

448. Selzer M, Spencer WA. Convergence of visceral and cutaneous afferent pathways in the lumbar spinal cord. *Brain Res* 1969;14:331.

449. Selzer M, Spencer WA. Interactions between visceral and cutaneous afferents in the spinal cord: Reciprocal primary afferent fiber depolarization. *Brain Res* 1969;14:349.

450. Weber WV. Some actions and interactions of visceral and somatic afferents in the thoracic spinal cord., The Somatosensory System. Thieme Ed. Edited by Kornhuber JJ. Acton, MA, Publishing Sciences Group, 1975, pp. 227–238.

451. Guilbaud G, Benelli G, Besson JM. Responses of thoracic dorsal horn interneurons to cutaneous stimulation and to the administration of algogenic substances into the mesenteric artery in the spinal cat. *Brain Res* 1977;124:437–448.

452. Foreman RD, Schmidt RF, Willis WD. Convergence of muscle and cutaneous input onto primate spinothalamic tract neurons. *Brain Res* 1977;124:555.

453. Fields HL, Partridge LD, Jr., Winter DL. Somatic and visceral receptive field properties of fibers in ventral quadrant white matter of the cat spinal cord. *J Neurophysiol* 1970;33:827–837.

454. Cervero F, Laird JM. Understanding the signaling and transmission of visceral nociceptive events. *J Neurobiol* 2004;61:45–54.

455. Ruch TC. Pathophysiology of pain., Neurophysiology. Edited by Ruch TC, Patton HD, Woodbury JW, Towe AL. Philadelphia, W.B. Saunders, 1961, pp. 350–368.

456. Honda C, Perl ER. Functional and morphological features of neurons in the midline region of the caudal spinal cord of the cat. *Brain Res* 1985;340: 285.

457. Honda CN. Convergence of visceral and somatic afferent conversions onto neurons near the central canal in the sacral spinal cord of the cat. *J Neurophysiol* 1985;53:1059.

458. Nahin RL, Madsen AM, Giesler GI. Anatomical and physiological studies of the grey matter surrounding the spinal cord and central canal. *J Comp Neurol* 1983;220:321.

459. Spiller WG, Martin E. The treatment of persistent pain of organic origin in the lower part of the body by division of anterolateral column of the spinal cord. *JAMA* 1912;58:1489.

460. Vierck CJ, Jr., Greenspan JD, Ritz LA, et al. The spinal pathways contributing to the ascending conduction and the descending modulation of pain sensations and reactions., Spinal Afferent Processing. Edited by Yaksh TL. New York, Plenum, 1986, pp. 275–329.

461. Voris HC. Vanations in the spinothalamic tract in man. *J Neurosurg* 1957; 14:55.

462. White JC, Sweet WH, Hawkins R, et al. Anterolateral cordotomy: Results, complications and causes of failure. *Brain* 1950;73:346.

463. Mayer DJ, Price DD, Becker DP. Neurophysiological characterization of the anterolateral spinal cord neurons contributing to pain perception in man. *Pain* 1975;1:51.

464. White JC, Sweet WH. Pain and the Neurosurgeon. Baltimore, University Park Press, 1969.

465. Hitchcock E. Stereotaxic cervical myelotomy. *J Neurol Neurosurg Pyschiatr* 1970;33:224.

466. Schvarcz JR. Spinal cord stereotactic surgery. Recent Progress in Neurological Surgery. Edited by Sano K, Ishii S, LeVay D. New York, Elsevier, 1974, pp. 234–241.

467. White JC, Sweet WH. Pain, Its Mechanisms and Neurosurgical Control. 1955; Springfield, IL.

468. Albe-Fessard D, Kruger L. Duality of unit discharges from cat centrum medianum in response to natural and electrical stimulation. *J Neurophysiol* 1962;25:3.

469. Albe-Fessard D, Levante A, Lamour Y. Origin of spinothalamic and spinoreticular pathways in cats and monkeys. *Adv Neurol* 1974;4:157.

470. Dilly PN, Wall PD, K.E. W. Cells of origin of the spinothalamic tract in the cat and the rat. *Exp Neurol* 1968;21:550.

471. Lippman HH, Kerr FWL. Light and electron microscopic study of crossed ascending pathways in the anterolateral funiculus in monkey. *Brain Res* 1972;40:496.

472. White JC, Richardson EP, Sweet WH. Upper thoracic cordotomy for relief of pain: Postmortem correlation of spinal incision with analgesic levels in 18 cases. *Ann Surg* 1956;144:407.

473. Hyndman OR, Van Epps C. Possibility of differential section of the spinothalamic tract. *Arch Surg* 1939;38:1036.

474. Willis WD, Coggeshall RE. Sensory Mechanisms of the Spinal Cord. New York, Plenum Press, 1978.

475. Mehler WR. Some neurological species differences- a posteriori. *Ann N Y Acad Sci* 1969;167:89.

476. Bowsher D. Role of the reticular formation in responses to noxious stimulation. *Pain* 1976;2:361–378.

477. Fields HL, Wagner GM, Anderson SD. Some properties of spinal neurons projecting to the medial brain-stem reticular formation. *Exp Neurol* 1975;47:118–134.

478. Zemlan FP, Leonard CM, Kow LM, et al. Ascending tracts of the lateral columns of the rat spinal cord: A study using the silver impregnation and horseradish peroxidase techniques. *Exp Neurol* 1978;62:298.

479. Bowsher D. The subdiencephalic distribution of fibres from the anterolateral quadrant of the spinal cord in man. *Mschr Psychiatr Neurol* 1962;143: 75.

480. Kerr FWL. The ventral spinothalamic tract and other ascending systems of the ventral funiculus of the spinal cord. *J Comp Neurol* 1975;159:335.

481. Mehler WR, Feferman ME, Nauta WJH. Ascending axon degeneration following anterolateral cordotomy. An experimental study in the monkey. *Brain* 1960;83:718.

482. Rossi GF, Brodal A. Terminal distribution of spinoreticular fibers in the cat. *Arch Neurol Pyschiatr* 1957;78:439.

483. Breazile JE, Kitchell RL. Ventrolateral spinal cord afferents to the brain stem in the domestic pig. *J Comp Neurol* 1968;133:363–372.

484. Brodal A, Walberg F, Taber E. The raphe nuclei of the brain stem in cat. II. Afferent connections *J Comp Neurol* 1960;114:261.

485. Wall PD, Yaksh TL. Effect of Lissauer tract stimulation on activity in dorsal roots and in ventral roots. *Exp Neurol* 1978;60:570–583.

486. Fields HL, Basbaum AI, Clanton CH, et al. Nucleus raphe magnus inhibition of spinal cord dorsal horn neurons. *Brain Res* 1977;126:441–453.

487. Fields HL, Clanton CH, Anderson SD. Somatosensory properties of spinoreticular neurons in the cat. *Brain Res* 1977;120:49–66.

488. Levante A, Albe-Fessard D. Localisation dans les couches VII et VIII de Resed de cellules d'origine d'un faisceau spinoreticulaire croise. *CR Acad Sci Hebd Seances Acad Sci D.* 1972;274:3007.

489. Kevetter GA, Haber LH, Yezierski RPea. Cells of the origin of the spinoreticular tract in the monkey *J Comp Neurol* 1982;207:61

490. Kevetter GA, Willis WD. Collaterals of spinothalamic cells in the rat. *J Comp Neurol* 1983;215:453.

491. Kevetter GA, Willis WD. Spinothalamic cells in the rat lumbar cord with collaterals to the medullary reticular formation. *Brain Res* 1982;238:181.

492. Klop EM, Mouton LJ, Hulsebosch R, et al. In cat four times as many lamina I neurons project to the parabrachial nuclei and twice as many to the periaqueductal gray as to the thalamus. *Neuroscience* 2005;134:189–197.

493. Gauriau C, Bernard JF. Pain pathways and parabrachial circuits in the rat. *Exp Physiol* 2002;87:251–258.

494. Antonetty CM, Webster KE. The organization of the spinotectal projection. An experimental study in the rat. *J Comp Neurol* 1975;163:449.

495. Bowsher D. Termination of the central pain pathway in man: the conscious appreciation of pain. *Brain* 1957;80:606–622.

496. Liu RPC. Laminar origins of spinal projection neurons to periaqueductal gray of the rat. *Brain Res.* 1983;264:118.

497. Menetrey D, Chaouch A, Binder D, et al. The origin of the spinomesencephalic tract in the rat: An anatomical study using the retrograde transport of horseradish peroxidase. *J Comp Neurol* 1982;206:193.

498. Amassian VE, Waller HJ. Spatiotemporal patterns of activity in individual reticular neurones, Reticular Formation of the Brain. Edited by Jasper HH, Proctor LD, Knighton RS, Noshay WC. Boston, Little, Brown & Co., 1958.

499. Bell C, Sierra G, Buendia N, et al. Sensory properties of neurons in the mesencephalic reticular formation. *J Neurophysiol* 1964;27:961.

500. Bowsher D, Petit D. Place and modality analysis in nucleus of posterior commissure. *J Physiol* 1970;206:663–675.

501. Yezierski RP, Schwartz RH. Receptive field properties of spinomesencephalic tract (SMT) cells. *Pain* 1984;2:184.
502. Mori F. A new spinal pathway for cutaneous impulses. *Am J Physiol* 1955; 183:245.
503. Berkley KJ. Spatial relationships between the terminations of somatic sensory and motor pathways in the rostral brainstem of cats and monkeys. I. Ascending somatic sensory inputs to lateral diencephalon. *J Comp Neurol* 1980;193:283–317.
504. Boivie J. An anatomical reinvestigation of the termination of the spinothalamic tract in the monkey. *J Comp Neurol* 1979;186:343–369.
505. Craig AD, Jr., Burton H. Spinal and medullary lamina I projection to nucleus submedius in medial thalamus: a possible pain center. *J Neurophysiol* 1981;45:443–466.
506. Peschanski M, Mantyh PW, Besson JM. Spinal afferents to the ventrobasal thalamic complex in the rat: An anatomical study using wheatgerm agglutinin conjugated to horseradish peroxidase. *Brain Res* 1983;278:240.
507. Carstens E, Trevino DL. Laminar origins of spinothalamic projections in the cat as determined by the retrograde transport of horseradish peroxidase. *J Comp Neurol* 1978;182:161–165.
508. Giesler GJ, Jr., Menetrey D, Basbaum AI. Differential origins of spinothalamic tract projections to medial and lateral thalamus in the rat. *J Comp Neurol* 1979;184:107–126.
509. Giesler GJ, Jr., Yezierski RP, Gerhart KD, et al. Spinothalamic tract neurons that project to medial and/or lateral thalamic nuclei: evidence for a physiologically novel population of spinal cord neurons. *J Neurophysiol* 1981;46:1285–1308.
510. Foreman RD, Schmidt RF, Willis WD. Effect of mechanical and chemical stimulation of fine muscle afferents upon primate spinothalamic tract cells. *J Physiol (Lond)* 1979;286:215.
511. Hancock MB, Foreman RD, Willis WD. Convergence of visceral and cutaneous input onto spinothalamic tract cells in the thoracic spinal cord of the cat. *Exp Neurol* 1975;47:240.
512. Willis WD. Ascending somatosensory systems., Spinal Afferent Processing. Edited by Yaksh TL. New York, Plenum Press, 1986, pp. 243–274.
513. Kennard MA. The course of ascending fibers in the spinal cord of the cat essential to the recognition of painful stimuli. *J Comp Neurol* 1954;100:511–525.
514. Nathan PW, Smith MC. Some tracts of the anterior and lateral columns of the spinal cord., Pain. Edited by Knighton RS, Dumke PR. Boston, Little, Brown and Co., 1966, pp. 47–57.
515. Vierck CJ, Jr., Hamilton DM, Thornby JJ. Pain reactivity of monkeys after lesions to the dorsal and lateral columns of the spinal cord. *Exp Brain Res* 1971;13:140.
516. Rustoni A. Nonprimary afferents to the cuneate nucleus in the brachial dorsal funiculus of the cat. *Brain Res* 1974;75:247.
517. Rustoni A. Nonprimary afferents to the nucleic gracilis from the lumbar cord of the cat. *Brain Res* 1973;51:81.
518. Angaut-Petit D. The dorsal column system: Functional properties and bulbar relay of the postsynaptic fibers of the cat's fasciculus gracilis *Exp Brain Res* 1975;22:471.
519. Cook AW, Browder E. Function of posterior columns in man. *Arch Neurol* 1965;22:72.
520. Nashold BS, Jr., Friedman H. Dorsal column stimulation for control of pain. Preliminary report on 30 patients. *J Neurosurg* 1972;36:590–597.
521. Brown AG. Ascending and long spinal pathway: Dorsal columns spinocervical tract and spinothalamic tracting New York, Springer-Verlag, 1973.
522. Brown AG. Organization in the Spinal Cord. New York, Spinger-Verlag, 1981.
523. Kniffki KD, Mense S, Schmidt RF. Activation of neurones of the spinocervical tract by painful stimulation of skeletal muscle. *Proc Int Union Physiol Sci* 1977;13:393.
524. King RB, Barnett JC. Studies of trigeminal nerve potentials. Over-reaction to tactile facial stimulation in acute laboratory preparations. *J Neurosurg* 1957;14:617.
525. Ha H, Kitai ST, Morin F. The Lateral Cervical Nucleus of the Raccoon. *Exp Neurol* 1965;11:441–450.
526. Ha H, Liu CN. Organization of the spino-cervico-thalamic system. *J Comp Neurol* 1966;127:445–470.
527. Nijensohn DE, Kerr FWL. The ascending projections of the dorsolateral funiculus of the spinal cord in the primate. *J Comp Neurol* 1975;161:459.
528. Truex RC, Taylor MJ, Smythe MQ, et al. The lateral cervical nucleus of cat, dog and man. *J Comp Neurol* 1970;139:93.
529. Basbaum AI. Conduction of the effects of noxious stimulation by short-fiber multisynaptic systems of the spinal cord in the rat. *Exp Neurol* 1973;40:699.
530. Breazile JE, Kitchell RL. A study of fiber systems within the spinal cord of the domestic pig that subserve pain. *J Comp Neurol* 1968;133:373–382.
531. Kletzin M, Spiegel EA. Spinal conduction by chains of short neurons. *Fed Proc* 1952;11:83.
532. Kerr FWL. Segmental circuitry and ascending pathways of the nociceptive ssytem. New York, Raven Press, 1979.
533. Kerr FWL. Spinal V nucleolysis and intractable craniofacial pain. *Surg Forum* 1966;17:419.
534. Schvarcz JR. Stereotaxic spinal trigeminal nucleotomy for dysesthetic facial pain. Advances in Pain Research and Therapy. Edited by Bonica JJ, Liebeskind JC, Albe-Fessard D. New York, Raven Press, 1979, pp. 331–336.
535. Davis LE, Hart JT, Crain RC. The pathway for visceral afferent impulses within the spinal cord. II. Experimental dilatation of the biliary ducts. *Surg Gynecol Obstet* 1929;48:647.
536. Ranson SW. The course within the spinal cord of the non-medulated fibers of the dorsal roots: A study of Lissauer's tract in the cat. *J Comp Neurol* 1913;23:259.
537. Cervero F, Molony V, Iggo A. Extracellular and intracellular recordings from neurones in the substantia gelatinosa Rolandi. *Brain Res* 1977;136:565–569.
538. Hyndman OR. Lissauer's tract section. A contribution to chordotomy for the relief of pain (preliminary report). *J Int Coll Surgeons* 1942;5:394.
539. Denny-Brown D, Kirk EJ, Yanagisawa N. The tract of Lissauer in relation to sensory transmission in the dorsal horn of spinal cord in the macaque monkey. *J Comp Neurol* 1973;151:175–200.
540. Beaudreau DE, Jerge CR. Somatotopic representation in the gasserian ganglion of tactile peripheral fields in the cat. *Arch Oral Biol* 1968;13:247.
541. Darian-Smith I, Mutton P, Proctor R. Functional organization of tactile cutaneous afferents within the semilunar ganglion and trigeminal spinal tract in the cat. *J Neurophysiol* 1965;28:682.
542. Young RF. Unmyelinated fibers in the trigeminal motor root. Possible relationship to the results of trigeminal rhizotomy. *J Neurosurg* 1978;49:538.
543. Denny-Brown D, Yanagisawa N. The function of the descending root of the fifth nerve. *Brain* 1973;96:783.
544. Jannetta PJ, Rand RW. Transtentorial retrogasserian rhizotomy in trigeminal neuralgia St. Louis, C.V. Mosby, 1969.
545. Olszewski J. On the anatomical and functional organization of the spinal trigeminal nucleus. *J Comp Neurol* 1950;92:401.
546. Clarke WB, Bowsher D, Terminal distribution of primary afferent trigeminal fibers in the rat. *Exp Neurol* 1962;6:372–383.
547. Kruger L, Michel F. A morphological and somatotopic analysis of single activity in the trigeminal sensory complex of the cat. *Exp Neurol* 1962;5:139.
548. Astrom KE. On the central course of afferent fibers in the trigeminal, facial, glossopharyngeal, and vagal nerves and their nuclei in the mouse. *Acta Physiol Scand* 1953;29 (Suppl. 106):209.
549. Hayashi H. Distribution of vibrissae afferent fiber collaterals in the trigeminal nuclei as revealed by intra-axonal injection of horseradish peroxidase. *Brain Res* 1980;183:442.
550. Kerr FWL, Kruger L, Schwassmann HO, et al. Somatotopic organization of mechanoreceptor units in the trigeminal complex of the macaque. *J Comp Neurol* 1968;34:127.
551. Khayyat GF, Yu UJ, King RB. Response patterns to noxious and non-noxious stimuli in rostral trigeminal relay nuclei. *Brain Res* 1975;97:47–60.
552. Kruger L, Michel F. Reinterpretation of the representation of pain based on physiological excitation of single neurons in the trigeminal sensory complex. *Exp Neurol* 1962;5:157.
553. Mosso JA, Kruger L. Receptor categories represented in spinal trigeminal nucleus caudalis. *J Neurophysiol* 1973;36:472.
554. Dickenson AH, Hellon RF, Taylor DC. Facial thermal input to the trigeminal spinal nucleus of rabbits and rats. *J Comp Neurol* 1979;185:203–209.
555. Mosso JA, Kruger L. Spinal trigeminal neurons excited by noxious and thermal stimuli. *Brain Res* 1972;38:206.
556. Yokota T, Hashimoto S. Periaqueductal gray and tooth pulp afferent interaction on units in caudal medulla oblongata. *Brain Res* 1976;117:508.
557. Kerr FWL. A mechanism to account for frontal headache in cases of posterior-fossa tumors. *J Neurosurg* 1961;18:605.
558. Kerr FWL. Atypical facial neuralgias, their mechanism as inferred from anatomic and physiologic data. *Mayo Clin Proc* 1961;36:254.
559. Kerr FWL. Central relationships of trigeminal and cervical primary afferents in the spinal cord and medulla. *Brain Res* 1972;43:561.
560. Kerr FWL, Olafson RA. Trigeminal and cervical volleys, convergence on single units in the spinal gray at C-1 and C-2. *Arch Neurol* 1961;5:171.
561. Sjoqvist O. Studies on pain conduction of the trigeminal nerve. *Acta Psychiat Neurol Scand* 1938;17(Suppl.):1.
562. Burton H, Craig AD. Distribution of trigeminothalamic projection cells in cat and monkey. *Brain Res* 1976;161:515.
563. Fukushima T, Kerr FW. Organization of trigeminothalamic tracts and other thalamic afferent systems of the brainstem in the rat: presence of gelatinosa neurons with thalamic connections. *J Comp Neurol* 1979;183:169–184.
564. Tiwari RK, King RB. Fiber projections from trigeminal nucleus caudalis in primate (squirrel, monkey and baboon). *J Comp Neurol* 1974;158:191.
565. Gobel S, Purvis MB. Anatomical studies of the organization of the spinal V nucleus: the deep bundles and the spinal V tract. *Brain Res* 1972;48:27–44.
566. Hu JW, Sessle BJ. Trigeminal nociceptive and nonnociceptive neurons: Brain stem intranuclear projections and modulation by orofacial, periaqueductal gray and nucleus raphe magnus stimuli. *Brain Res* 1979;170:547.
567. Stewart W, King RB. Fiber projections from the n. caudalis of the spinal trigeminal nucleus. *J Comp Neurol* 1963;121:271.
568. Greenwood LF, Sessle BJ. Inputs to trigeminal brain stem neurones from facial, oral, tooth pulp and pharyngolaryngeal tissues: II. Role of trigeminal

nucleus caudalis in modulating responses to innocuous and noxious stimuli. *Brain Res* 1976;117:227–238.

569. Scibetta CJ, King RB. Hyperpolarizing influnce of trigeminal nucleus caudalis on primary afferent preterminals in trigeminal nucleus oralis. *J Neurophysiol* 1969;32:229.

570. Young RF, King RB. Excitability changes in the trigeminal primary afferent fibers in response to noxious and nonnoxious stimuli. *J Neurophysiol* 1972;35:87.

571. Mancia M, Marginelli M, Mariotti Mea. Brain stem thalamus reciprocal influences in the cat. *Brain Res* 1974;69:297.

572. Bowsher D, Mallart A, Petit D, et al. A bulbar relay to the centromedian. *J Neurophysiol* 1968;31:288.

573. Keene JJ, Casey KL. Rewarding and aversive brain stimulation: Opposite effects on medial thalamic units. *Physiol Behav* 1973;10:283.

574. Casey KL. Somatic stimuli, spinal pathways, and size of cutaneous fibers influencing unit activity in the medial medullary reticular formation. *Exp Neurol* 1969;25:35–56.

575. Guilbaud G, Besson JM, Oliveras JL, et al. Modifications of the firing rate of bulbar reticular units (nucleus gigantocellularis) after intra-arterial injection of bradykinin into the limbs. *Brain Res* 1973;63:131–140.

576. Le Blanc HJO, Gatipon GB. Medial bulboreticular response to peripherally applied noxious stimuli. *Exp Neurol* 1974;42:264.

577. Pearl GS, Anderson KV. Effects of nociceptive and innocuous stimuli on the firing patterns of single neurons in the feline nucleusreticularis gigantocellularis., Advances in Pain Research and Therapy. Edited by Bonica JJ, Albe-Fessard D. New York, Raven Press, 1976, pp. 498.

578. Pearl GS, Anderson KV. Response patterns of cells in the feline caudal nucleus rebcularis gigantocellularis after noxious trigeminal and spinal stimulation. *Exp Neurol* 1978;58:231.

579. Cedarbaum JM, Aghajanian GK. Activation of locus coeruleus neurons by peripheral stimuli: modulation by a collateral inhibitory mechanism. *Life Sci* 1978;23:1383–1392.

580. Benjamin RM. Single neurons in the rat medulla responsive to nociceptive stimulation. *Brain Res* 1970;24:525.

581. Goldman PL, Collins WF, Taub A, et al. Evoked bulbar reticular unit activity following δ fiber stimulation of peripheral somatosensory nerve in cat. *Exp Neurol* 1972;37:597–606.

582. Limansikyi YP. Response of neurones of the medullary reticular formation to afferent impulses from cutaneous and muscle nerves. *Fiziol Zh* 1965;11:151.

583. Casey KL. Escape elicited by bulboreticular stimulation in the cat. *Int J Neurosci* 1971;2:29–34.

584. Casey KL. Responses of bulboreticular units to somatic stimuli eliciting escape behavior in the cat. *Int J Neurosci* 1971;2:15–28.

585. Casey KL, Keene JJ. Unit analysis of the effects of motivating stimuli in the awake animal: Pain and self stimulation. Springfield, IL, Charles C. Thomas, 1973.

586. Krout KE, Loewy AD. Parabrachial nucleus projections to midline and intralaminar thalamic nuclei of the rat. *J Comp Neurol* 2000;428:475–494.

587. Sarhan M, Freund-Mercier MJ, Veinante P. Branching patterns of parabrachial neurons projecting to the central extended amgydala: single axonal reconstructions. *J Comp Neurol* 2005;491:418–442.

588. Menendez L, Bester H, Besson JM, et al. Parabrachial area: electrophysiological evidence for an involvement in cold nociception. *J Neurophysiol* 1996;75:2099–2116.

589. Bowsher D. Diencephalic projections from the midbrain reticular formation. *Brain Res* 1975;95:211–220.

590. Chi CC. An experimental silver study of the ascending projections of the central gray susbstance and adjacent tegmentum in the rat with observation in the cat. *J Comp Neurol* 1970;139:259.

591. Hamilton BL, Skultety FM. Efferent connections of the periaqueductal gray matter in the cat. *J Comp Neurol* 1970;139:105–114.

592. Robertson RT, Lynch GS, Thompson RF. Diencephalic distributions of ascending reticular systems. 1973.

593. Barnes KL. A quantitative investigation of somatosensory coding in single cells of the cat mesensephalic reticular formation. *Exp Neurol* 1976;50:180.

594. Becker DP, Gluck H, Nuksen FE, et al. An inquiry into the neurophysiological basis for pain. *J Neurosurg* 1969;30:1.

595. Collins WF, Randt CT. Midbrain evoked responses relating to peripheral unmyelinated or 'C' fibers in cat. *J Neurophysiol* 1960;23:47–53.

596. Young DW, Gottschaldt RM. Neurons in the rostral mesencephalic reticular formation of the cat responding specifically to noxious mechanical stimulation. *Exp Neurol* 1976;51:628.

597. Eickhoff R, Handwerker HO, Mc Queen DS, et al. Noxious and tactile input to medial structures of midbrain and pons in the rat. *Pain* 1978;5:99.

598. Groves PM, Miller SW, Parker MV, et al. Organization by sensory modality in the reticular formation of the rat. *Brain Res* 1973;54:207–224.

599. Liebeskind JC, Mayer DJ. Somatosensory evoked responses in the mesencephalic central gray matter of the rat. *Brain Res* 1971;27:133.

600. Delgado JMR, Rosvald HE, Looney E. Evoking conditioned fear by electrical stimulation of subcortical structures in the monkey brain. *J Comp Physiol Psychol* 1956;49:373.

601. Kiser RS, Lebovitz RM, German DC. Anatomic and pharmacologic differences between two types of aversive midbrain stimulation. *Brain Res* 1978;155:331.

602. Nashold BS, Jr., Wilson WP, Slaughter D. Sensation evoked by stimulation in the hindbrain of man. *J Neurosurg* 1969;30:14.

603. Skultety FM. Stimulation of periaqueductal gray and hypothalamus. *Arch Neurol* 1963;8.

604. Spiegel EA, Keltzkin M, Szekely EG. Pain reactions upon stimulation of the lectrum mesencephali. J. Neuropathol. *Exp Neurol* 1954;13:212.

605. Halpern M. Effects of midbrain central gray matter lesions on escape-avoidance behavior in rats. *Physiol Behav* 1968;3:171.

606. Melzack R, Stotler WA, Livingston WK. Effects of discrete brain stem lesions in cats on perception of noxious stimulation. *J Neurophysiol* 1958;21:353.

607. Beven T, Pert A. The effect of midbrain and diencephalic lesions on nociception and morphine induced antinociception in the rat. *Fed Proc* 1975;34:713.

608. Deakin JFW, Dostrovsky JO. Involvement of the periaqueductal grey matter and spinal 5-hydroxytryptaminergic pathways in morphine analgesia. Effects of lesions and 5-hydroxytryptamine. *Br J Pharmacol* 1978;63:159.

609. Lewis VA, Gebhart GF. Evaluation of the periaqueductal central gray (PAG) as a morphine-specific locus of action and examination of morphine-induced and stimulation-produced analgesia at coincident PAG loci. *Brain Res* 1977;124:283–303.

610. Yaksh TL, Yeung JC, Rudy TA. Systematic mapping of the central gray medial thalamic axis of the rat: evidence for a somatotopic distribution of morphine sensitive sites within the penaqueductal gray. *Neuroscience* 1975;1:283.

611. Burton H, Jones EG. The posterior thalamic region and its cortical projection in New World and Old World monkeys. *J Comp Neurol* 1976;168:249–301.

612. Boivie J. The termination of the spinothalamic tract in the cat. An experimental study with silver impregnation methods. *Exp Brain Res* 1971;112:331–353.

613. Lund RD, Webster KE. Thalamic afferents from the spinal cord and trigeminal nuclei. An experimental anatomical study in the rat. *J Comp Neurol* 1967;130:313.

614. Casey KL. Unit analysis of nociceptive mechanisms in the thalamus of the awake squirrel monkey. *J Neurophysiol* 1966;29:727–750.

615. Kenshalo DRJ, Giesler GJ, Leonard RB, et al. Responses of neurons in primate ventral posterior lateral nucleus to noxious stimuli. *J Neurophysiol* 1980;43:1594.

616. Peschanski M, Guilbaud D, Gautron M. Posterior intralaminar region in rat: Neuronal responses to noxious and nonnoxious cutaneous stimuli. *Exp Neurol* 1981;72:226.

617. Poggio GF, Mountcastle VB. A study of the functional contributions of the lemniscal and spinothalamic systems to somatic sensibility. *Bull Johns Hop Hosp* 1960;106:266.

618. Shigenaga Y, Matano S, Okada K, et al. The effects of tooth pulp stimulations in the thalamus and hypothalamus of the rat. *Brain Res* 1973;63:402.

619. Berkley KJ. Response properties of cells in ventrobasal and posterior group nuclei of the cat. *J Neurophysiol* 1973;36:940.

620. Curry MJ. The exteroceptive properties of neurones in the somatic part of the posterior group (PO). *Brain Res* 1972;44:439–462.

621. Nyquist JK, Greenhoot JH. Unit analysis of nonspecific thalamic responses to high-intensity cutaneous input in the cat. *Exp Neurol* 1974;42:609.

622. Schwartzman RJ. Thalamic sensory nuclear ablations in trained monkeys. *Arch Neurol* 1970;23:419.

623. Hassler R. Die Zentralen Systeme des Scmerzes. *Acta Neurochir (Wien)* 1960;8:353.

624. Friedman DP, Jones EG. Focal projection of electrophysiologically defined groupings of thalamic cells on the monkey somatic sensory cortex. *Brain Res* 1980;191:249–252.

625. Jones EG, Powell TP. The cortical projection of the ventroposterior nucleus of the thalamus in the cat. *Brain Res* 1969;13:298–318.

626. Jones EG, Powell TPS. Connexions of the somatic sensory cortex of the rhesus monkey. III. Thalamic connexions. *Brain* 1970;93:37.

627. Manson J. The somatosensory cortical projection of single nerve cells in the thalamus of the cat. *Brain Res* 1969;12:489.

628. Saporta S, Kruger L. The organization of projections to selected points of somatosensory cortex from the cat ventrobasal complex. *Brain Res* 1979;178:275.

629. Whitsel BL, Petrucelli LM, Wemer G. Symmetry and connectively in the map of the body surface in somatosensory area II of primates. *J Neurophysiol* 1969;32:170.

630. Boivie J. Anatomical observations on the dorsal column nuclei, their thalamic projection and the cytoarchitecture of some somatosensory thalamic nuclei in the monkey. *J Comp Neurol* 1978;178:17–48.

631. Poggio GF, Mountcastle VB. The functional properties of ventrobasal thalamic neurons studied in unanesthetized monkeys. *J Neurophysiol* 1963;26:775.

632. Whitlock DG, Perl ER. Thalamic projections of spinothalamic pathways in monkeys. *Exp Neurol* 1961;3:240.

633. Perl ER, Whitlock DC. Somatic stimuli exciting spinothalamic projections to thalamic neurons in cat and monkey. *Exp Neurol* 1961;3:256.

634. Burton H, Forbes DJ, Benjamin RM. Thalamic neurons responsive to temperature changes of glabrous hand and foot skin in squirrel monkey. *Brain Res* 1970;24:179–190.

635. Guilbaud G, Berkley KJ, Benoist JM, et al. Responses of neurons in thalamic ventrobasal complex of rats to graded distension of uterus and vagina and to uterine suprafusion with bradykinin and prostaglandin F2 alpha. *Brain Res* 1993;614:285–290.

636. Harris FA. Wide-field neurons in somatosensory thalamus of domestic cats under barbiturate anesthesia. *Exp Neurol* 1980;68:27.

637. Kruger L, Albe-Fessard D. Distribution of responses to somatic afferent stimuli in the diencephalon of the cat under chloralose anesthesia. *Exp Neurol* 1960;2:442.

638. Poulos DA, Benjamin RM. Response of thalamic neurons to thermal stimulation of the tongue. *J Neurophysiol* 1968;31:28.

639. Nyquist JK. Somatosensory properties of neurons of thalamic nucleus ventralis lateralis. *Exp Neurol* 1975;48:123.

640. Casey KL, Morrow TJ. Ventral posterior thalamic neurons differentially responsive to noxious stimulation of the awake monkey. *Science* 1983;221:675.

641. Honda CN, Mense S, Perl ER. Neurons in ventrobasal region of cat thalamus selectivity responsive to noxious mechanical stimuli. *J Neurophysiol* 1983;49:662.

642. Kniffki KD, Mizumura K. Responses of neurons in VPL and VPL-VL region of the cat to algesic stimulation of muscle and tendon. *J Neurophysiol* 1983;49:649.

643. Glassman RD, Forgus MW, Goodman JE, et al. Somesthetic effects of damage to cat's ventrobasal complex, medial lemniscus or postenor group. *Exp Neurol* 1975;48:460.

644. Talairach J, Hecaen M, David M. Recherches sur la coagulation therapeutique des structures sous-caricates chez l'homme. *Rev Neurol* 1949;81:4.

645. Mancia M, Broggi G, Margnelli M. Brain stem reticular effects on intralaminar thalamic neurons in the cat. *Brain Res* 1971;25:638.

646. Pearl GS, Anderson KV. Interactions between nucleus centrum medianum and gigantocellularis nociceptive neurons. *Brain Res Bull* 1980;5:203.

647. Jones EG, Leavitt RY. Axonal transport and the demonstration of non-specific projections to the cerebral cortex and striatum from thalamic intralaminar nuclei in the rat, cat and monkey. *J Comp Neurol* 1974;154:349.

648. Sewards TV, Sewards MA. The medial pain system: neural representations of the motivational aspect of pain. *Brain Res Bull* 2002;59:163–180.

649. Albe-Fessard D, Levante A, Lamour Y. Origin of spinothalamic tract in monkeys. *Brain Res* 1974;65:503.

650. Angel A. The effect of peripheral stimulation on units located in the thalamic reticular nuclei. *J Physiol* (Lond) 1964;171:42.

651. Dong WK, Ryu H, Wagman IH. Nociceptive responses of neurons in medial thalamus and their relationship to spinothalamic pathways. *J Neurophysiol* 1978;41:1592.

652. Urabe M, Tsubokawa T, Watanabe Y. Alteration of activity of single neurons in the nucleus centrum medianum following stimulation of the peripheral nerve and application of noxious stimuli. *Jpn J Physiol.* 1966;16:421.

653. Bowker RM, Westlund KN, Sullivan MC, et al. Descending serotonergic, peptidergic and cholinergic pathways from the raphe nuclei: a multiple transmitter complex. *Brain Res* 1983;288:33–48.

654. Delacour J, Borst A. Failure to find homology in rat, cat, and monkey for functions of a subcortical structure in avoidance conditioning. *J Comp Physiol Psychol* 1972;80:458–468.

655. Finger S, Frommer GP. Effects of cortical and thalamic lesions on temperature discrimination and responsiveness to foot shock in the rat. *Brain Res* 1970;24:69–89.

656. Yaksh TL, Yeung JC, Rudy TA. Medial thalamic lesions in the rat: effects on the nociceptive threshold and morphine antinociception. *Neuropharmacology* 1977;16:107–114.

657. Kaelber WW, Mitchell CL, Yarmat AJea. Centrum medianum-parafasicularis lesions and reactivity to noxious and non-noxious stimuli. *Exp Neurol* 1975;46:282.

658. Mitchell C, Kaelber W. Effect of medial thalamic lesions on responses elicited by tooth pulp stimulation. *Am J Physiol* 1966;210:263.

659. Marburg DJ. The effect on reaction to painful stimuli of lesions in the centro-median nucleus in the thalamus of the monkey. *Int J Neurosci* 1973;5:153.

660. Tsutsumi H, Mark VH. Experimental local thalamic application of xylocaine through silicone rubber chemode. *J Neurosurg* 1973;38:743.

661. Sano K, Yoshioka M, Ogashiwa Mea. Thalamotominotomy: A new operation for relief of intractable pain. *Confin Neurol* 1966;27:63.

662. Price DD. Central neural mechanisms that interrelate sensory and affective dimensions of pain. *Mol Interv* 2002;2:392–403, 339.

663. Price DD. Psychological and neural mechanisms of the affective dimension of pain. *Science* 2000;288:1769–1772.

664. Carreras M, Andersson SA. Functional properties of neurons of the anterior ectosylvian gyrus of the cat. *J Neurophysiol* 1963;26:100.

665. Andersson SA. Projection of different spinal pathways to the second somatic sensory area in cat. *Acta Physiol Scand* 1962;56 (Suppl. 194):1.

666. Berkley KJ, Palmer R. Somatosensory cortical involvement in response to noxious stimulation in the cat. *Exp Brain Res* 1974;20:363.

667. Coghill RC, McHaffie JG, Yen YF. Neural correlates of interindividual differences in the subjective experience of pain. *Proc Natl Acad Sci U S A* 2003;100:8538–8542.

668. Rainville P, Duncan GH, Price DD, et al. Pain affect encoded in human anterior cingulate but not somatosensory cortex. *Science* 1997;277:968–971.

669. Brooks JC, Tracey I. The insula: a multidimensional integration site for pain. *Pain* 2007;128:1–2.

670. Melzack R, Caesy K. Sensory, motivational and central control determinants of pain: A new conceptual model., The Skin Senses. Edited by Kenshalo D. Springfield, IL, Charles C. Thomas, 1968, pp. 423–443.

671. Foltz EL, White LE, Jr. Pain "relief" by frontal cingulumotomy. *J Neurosurg* 1962;19:89–100.

672. Hassenbusch SJ, Pillay PK, Barnett GH. Radiofrequency cingulotomy for intractable cancer pain using stereotaxis guided by magnetic resonance imaging. *Neurosurgery* 1990;27:220–223.

673. Devinsky O, Morrell MJ, Vogt BA. Contributions of anterior cingulate cortex to behaviour. *Brain* 1995;118(Pt 1):279–306.

674. Johansen JP, Fields HL, Manning BH. The affective component of pain in rodents: direct evidence for a contribution of the anterior cingulate cortex. *Proc Natl Acad Sci U S A* 2001;98:8077–8082.

675. Tuor UI, Malisza K, Foniok T, et al. Functional magnetic resonance imaging in rats subjected to intense electrical and noxious chemical stimulation of the forepaw. *Pain* 2000;87:315–324.

676. Grachev ID, Fredickson BE, Apkarian AV. Dissociating anxiety from pain: mapping the neuronal marker N-acetyl aspartate to perception distinguishes closely interrelated characteristics of chronic pain. *Mol Psychiatry* 2001;6:256–258.

677. Van den Hout JH, Vlaeyen JW, Houben RM, et al. The effects of failure feedback and pain-related fear on pain report, pain tolerance, and pain avoidance in chronic low back pain patients. *Pain* 2001;92:247–257.

678. Dellemijn PL, Fields HL. Do benzodiazepines have a role in chronic pain management? *Pain* 1994;57:137–152.

679. Weir-Mitchell S, Moorhouse GR, Keen WW. Gunshot Wounds and Other Injuries of Nerves. Philadelphia, Lippincott, 1864.

680. Melzack R, Wall PD. Pain mechanisms: a new theory. *Science* 1965;150:971–979.

681. Nielson KP, Adams JE, Hosobuchi Y. Phantom limb pain. Treatment with dorsal column stimulation. *J Neurosurg* 1975;42:301.

682. Shealy CN, Morhmer JT, Hagfors NR. Dorsal column electroanalgesia. *J Neurosurg* 1970;32:560.

683. Wall PD. The origin of a spinal cord slow potential. *J Physiol.* (Lond.) 1962;164:508.

684. Yaksh TL, Wall PD. Activation of a local spinal inhibitory system by focal stimulation of the lateral Lissauer tract in cats. *Fed Proc* (Abstr.) 1978.

685. Hagbarth KE, Kerr DIB. Central influences on spinal afferent conduction. *J Neurophysiol* 1954;17:295–307.

686. Takagi H, Matsurmura M, Yanai A, et al. The effect of analgesics on the spinal reflex activity of the cat. *Jpn J Pharmacol* 1955;4:176–187.

687. Engberg I, Lundberg A, Ryall RW. Reticulospinal inhibition of interneurones. *J Physiol* 1968;194:225–236.

688. Engberg I, Lundberg A, Ryall RW. Reticulospinal inhibition of transmission in reflex pathways. *J Physiol* 1968;194:201–223.

689. Holmqvist B, Lundberg A. On the organization of the supraspinal inhibitory control of interneurones of various spinal reflex arcs. *Arch Ital Biol* 1959;97:340.

690. Holmqvist B, Lundberg A, Oscarsson O. Supraspinal inhibitory control of transmission to three ascending spinal pathways influenced by the flexion reflex afferents. *Arch Ital Biol* 1960;98:60–80.

691. Willis WD, Haber LH, Martin RF. Inhibition of spinothalamic tract cells and interneurons by brain stem stimulation in the monkey. *J Neurophysiol* 1977;40:968–981.

692. Gebhart GF, Sandkuhler J, Thalhammer JG, et al. Inhibition in spinal cord of nociceptive information by electrical stimulation and morphine microinjection at identical sites in midbrain of the cat. *J Neurophysiol* 1984;51:75–89.

693. Gebhart GF, Sandkuhler J, Thalhammer JG, et al. Quantitative comparison of inhibition in spinal cord of nociceptive information by stimulation in periaqueductal gray or nucleus raphe magnus of the cat. *J Neurophysiol* 1983;50:1433–1445.

694. Tsou K. Studies on the site of analgesic action of morphine by intracerebral microinjection. *Acta Physiol Sinica* 1963;26:332–337.

695. Lovick TA, Wolstencroft JH. Inhibitory effects of nucleus raphe magnus in neuronal responses in the spinal trigeminal nucleus to nociceptive compared with nonnociceptive inputs. *Pain* 1979;7:135.

696. Sessle BJ, Dubner R, Greenwood LF, et al. Descending influences of periaqueductal gray matter and somatosensory cerebral cortex on neurones in trigeminal brain stem nuclei. *Can J Physiol Pharmacol* 1975;54:66.

697. Mayer DJ, Liebeskind JC. Pain reduction by focal electrical stimulation of the brain: An anatomical and behavioral analysis. *Brain Res* 1974;68:73.

698. Oliveras JL, Redjemi G, Guilbaud G, et al. Analgesia induced by electrical stimulation of the inferior centralis nucleus of the raphe in the cat. *Pain* 1975;1:139.

699. Camarata PJ, Yaksh TL. Characterization of the spinal adrenergic receptors mediating the spinal effects produced by the microinjection of morphine into the periaqueductal gray. *Brain Res* 1985;336:133–142.

700. Hammond DL, Yaksh TL. Antagonism of stimulation-produced antinociception by intrathecal administration of methysergide or phentolamine. *Brain Res* 1984;298:329–337.

701. Yaksh TL. Inhibition by etorphine of the discharge of dorsal horn neurons: effects on the neuronal response to both high- and low-threshold sensory input in the decerebrate spinal cat. *Exp Neurol* 1978;60:23–40.

702. Hammond DL, Tyce GM, Yaksh TL. Efflux of 5-hydroxytryptamine and noradrenaline into spinal cord superfusates during stimulation of the rat medulla. *J Physiol* (Lond) 1985;359:151–162.

703. Headley PM, Duggan AW, Griersmith BT. Selective reduction by noradrenaline and 5-hydroxytryptamine of nociceptive responses of cat dorsal horn neurones. *Brain Res* 1978;145:185.

704. Reddy SV, Maderdrut JL, Yaksh TL. Spinal cord pharmacology of adrenergic agonist-mediated antinociception. *J Pharmacol Exp Ther* 1980;213:525–533.

705. Tyce GM, Yaksh TL. Monoamine release from cat spinal cord by somatic stimuli: an intrinsic modulatory system. *J Physiol* 1981;314:513–529.

706. Yaksh TL, Elde RP. Factors governing release of methionine enkephalin-like immunoreactivity from mesencephalon and spinal cord of the cat in vivo. *J Neurophysiol* 1981;46:1056–1075.

707. Skagerberg G, Bjorklund A, Lindvall O, et al. Origin and termination of the diencephalo-spinal dopamine system in the rat. *Brain Res Bull* 1982;9:237.

708. Mantyh PW, Hunt SP. Evidence for cholecystokinin-like-immunoreactive neurons in the rat medulla oblongata which project to the spinal cord. *Brain Res* 1984;291:49.

709. Chan-Palay V. Combined immunocytochemistry and autoradiography after in vivo injections of monoclonal antibody to substance P and 3H-serotonin: Coexistence of two putative transmitters in single raphe cells and fiber plexuses. *Anat Embryol* (Berl) 1979;156:241–254.

710. Morrow TJ, Casey KL. Analgesia produced by mesencephalic stimulation: Effect on bulboreticular neurons., Advances in Pain Research and Therapy. Edited by Bonica JJ, Albe-Fessard D. New York, Raven Press, 1976, pp. 503–510.

711. Jensen TS, Yaksh TL. Comparison of antinociceptive action of morphine in the periaqueductal gray, medial and paramedial medulla in rat. *Brain Res* 1986;363:99–113.

712. Jensen TS, Yaksh TL. Examination of spinal monoamine receptors through which brainstem opiate-sensitive systems act in the rat. *Brain Res* 1986;363:114–127.

713. Hamilton BL. Projections of the nuclei of the periaqueductal gray matter in the cat. *J Comp Neurol* 1973;152:45–58.

714. Mantyh PW. Connections of midbrain penaqueductal gray in the monkey. I. Ascending efferent projection. *J Neurophysiol* 1983;49:567.

715. Peschanski M, Besson JM. Diencephalic connections of the raphe nuclei of the rat brainstems: An anatomical study with reference to the somatosensory system. *J Comp Neurol* 1984;224:509.

716. Andersen E, Dafny N. Dorsal raphe stimulation reduces responses of parafasicular neurons to noxious stimulation. *Pain* 1983;15:323.

717. Ishida Y, Kitano K. Raphe induced inhibition of intralaminar thalamic unitary activities and its blockade by para-chlorophenylalanine in cats. *Naunyn Schmiedebergs Arch Pharmacol* 1977;301:1–4.

718. Andersen E, Dafny N. Microiontophoretically applied 5-HT reduces responses to noxious stimuli in the thalamus. *Brain Res* 1982;241:176.

719. Gybels IM. Electrical stimulation of the central gray for pain relief in humans: A critical review. New York, Raven Press, 1979.

720. Hosobuchi Y. The current status of analgesic brain stimulation. *Acta Neurochirur* 1980;30 (Suppl.):219.

721. Meyerson BA, Boethius J, Carlsson AM. Percutaneous central gray stimulation for cancer pain. *App Neurophysiol* 1978;41:57.

722. Richardson DE, Akil H. Pain reduction by electrical brain stimulation in man. *J Neurosurg* 1977;47:178.

723. Delgado PL. Common pathways of depression and pain. *J Clin Psychiatry* 2004;65:16–19.

724. Krauthamer GM, Albe-Fessard D. Inhibition of nonspecific sensory activities following striopallidal and capsular stimulation. *J Neurophysiol* 1965;28:100.

725. Lineberry C, Vierck C. Attenuation of pain reactivity by caudate nucleus stimulation in monkeys. *Brain Res* 1975;98:110.

726. Lloyd DPC. The spinal mechanism of the pyramidal system in cats. *J Neurophysiol* 1941;4:525.

727. Brodin E, Gazelius B, Panopoulos P, et al. Morphine inhibits substance P release from peripheral sensory nerve endings. *Acta Physiol Scand* 1983;117:567–570.

728. Fields HL, Emson PC, Leigh BK, et al. Multiple opiate receptor sites on primary afferent fibres. *Nature* 1980;284:351–353.

729. Ninkovic M, Hunt SP, Kelly JS. Effects of dorsal rhizotomy on the autoradiographic distribution of opiate and neurotensin receptors and neurotensin-like immunoreactivity within the rat spinal cord. *Brain Res* 1981;230:111.

730. Pertovaara A. Noradrenergic pain modulation. *Prog Neurobiol* 2006;80:53–83.

731. Yaksh TL. The effects of intrathecally administered opiod and adrenergic agents on spinal function., Spinal Afferent Processing. Edited by Yaksh TL. New York, Plenum Press, 1986, pp. 505–539.

732. North RA, Williams JT, Suprenant A, et al. μ and α receptors belong to a family of receptors that are coupled to potassium channels. *Proc Natl Acad Sci U S A* 1987;84.

733. Yaksh TL, Malmberg AB. Central pharmacology of nociceptive transmission, Textbook of Pain. Edited by Wall P, Melzack R. New York, Churchill Livingstone, 1994, pp. 165–200.

734. Drolet G, Dumont EC, Gosselin I, et al. Role of endogenous opioid system in the regulation of the stress response. *Prog Neuropsycho Pharmacol Biol Psychiatry* 2001;25:729–741.

735. Yaksh TL. Multiple opioid receptor systems in brain and spinal cord: Part 2. *Eur J Anaesthesiol* 1984;1:201–243.

736. Yaksh TL. Multiple opioid receptor systems in brain and spinal cord: Part I. *Eur J Anaesthesiol* 1984;1:171–199.

737. Cesselin F, Bourgoin S, Artaud F, et al. Basic and regulatory mechanisms of in vitro release of Met-enkephalin from the dorsal zone of the rat spinal cord. *J Neurochem* 1984;43:763–774.

738. Cesselin F, Oliveras JL, Bourgoin S, et al. Increased levels of Met-enkephalin-like material in the CSF of anaesthetized cats after tooth pulp stimulation. *Brain Res* 1982;237:325–38.

739. Yaksh TL, Chipkin RE. Studies on the effect of SCH-34826 and thiorphan on [Met5]enkephalin levels and release in rat spinal cord. *Eur J Pharmacol* 1989;167:367–373.

740. Yaksh TL, Terenius L, Nyberg F, et al. Studies on the release by somatic stimulation from rat and cat spinal cord of active materials which displace dihydromorphine in an opiate-binding assay. *Brain Res* 1983;268:119–128.

741. Song B, Marvizon JC. Peptidases prevent mu-opioid receptor internalization in dorsal horn neurons by endogenously released opioids. *J Neurosci* 2003;23:1847–1858.

742. Zubieta JK, Bueller JA, Jackson LR, et al. Placebo effects mediated by endogenous opioid activity on mu-opioid receptors. *J Neurosci* 2005;25:7754–7762.

743. Julien N, Marchand S. Endogenous pain inhibitory systems activated by spatial summation are opioid-mediated. *Neurosci Lett* 2006;401:256–260.

744. Koppert W, Filitz J, Troster A, et al. Activation of naloxone-sensitive and -insensitive inhibitory systems in a human pain model. *J Pain* 2005;6:757–764.

745. Mason P. Central mechanisms of pain modulation. *Curr Opin Neurobiol* 1999;9:436–441.

746. Yoshimura M, Furue H. Mechanisms for the anti-nociceptive actions of the descending noradrenergic and serotonergic systems in the spinal cord. *J Pharmacol Sci* 2006;101:107–117.

747. Mochizuki D. Serotonin and noradrenaline reuptake inhibitors in animal models of pain. *Hum Psychopharmacol* 2004;19 Suppl 1:S15–S19.

748. Nielsen CK, Lewis RJ, Alewood D, et al. Anti-allodynic efficacy of the chiconopeptide, Xen2174, in rats with neuropathic pain. *Pain* 2005;118:112–124.

749. Yaksh TL. Behavioral and autonomic correlates of the tactile evoked allodynia produced by spinal glycine inhibition: effects of modulatory receptor systems and excitatory amino acid antagonists. *Pain* 1989;37:111–123.

750. Sieghart W. Structure, pharmacology, and function of GABAA receptor subtypes. *Adv Pharmacol* 2006;54:231–263.

751. Betz H, Laube B. Glycine receptors: recent insights into their structural organization and functional diversity. *J Neurochem* 2006;97:1600–1610.

752. Carlton SM, Westlund KN, Zhang D, et al. GABA-immunoreactive terminals synapse on primate spinothalamic tract cells. *J Comp Neurol* 1992;322:528–537.

753. Todd AJ, Sullivan AC. Light microscopic study of the coexistence of GABA-like and glycine-like immunoreactivities in the spinal cord of the rat. *J Comp Neurol* 1990;296:496.

754. Basbaum AI. Distribution of glycine receptor immunoreactivity in the spinal cord of the rat: cytochemical evidence for a differential glycinergic control of lamina I and V nociceptive neurons. *J Comp Neurol* 1988;278:330–336.

755. Zarbin MA, Wamsley JK, Kuhar MJ. Glycine receptor: light microscopic autoradiographic localization with [3H]strychnine. *J Neurosci* 1981;1:532–547.

756. Singer E, Placheta P. Reduction of [3H]muscimol binding sites in rat dorsal spinal cord after neonatal capsaicin treatment. *Brain Res* 1980;202:484–487.

757. Barber RP, Vaughn JE, Saito K, et al. GABAergic terminals are presynaptic to primary afferent terminals in the substantia gelatinosa of the rat spinal cord. *Brain Res* 1978;141:35–55.

758. Price TJ, Cervero F, de Koninck Y. Role of cation-chloride-cotransporters (CCC) in pain and hyperalgesia. *Curr Top Med Chem* 2005;5:547–555.

PART IV: PAIN MANAGEMENT

759. Rudomin P. Selectivity of the central control of sensory information in the mammalian spinal cord. *Adv Exp Med Biol* 2002;508:157–170.

760. Yokota T, Nishikawa N, Nishikawa Y. Effects of strychnine upon different classes of trigeminal subnucleus caudalis neurons. *Brain Res* 1979;168:430–434.

761. Sherman SE, Loomis CW. Morphine insensitive allodynia is produced by intrathecal strychnine in the lightly anesthetized rat. *Pain* 1994;56:17–29.

762. Yaksh TL, Michener SR, Bailey JEea. Survey of distribution of substance P, vasoactive intestinal polypeptide, cholecystokinin, neurotensin, metenkephalin, bombesin and PHI in the spinal cord of cat, dog, sloth and monkey. *Peptides* 1988;9:357.

763. White WF, Heller AH. Glycine receptor alteration in the mutant mouse spastic. *Nature* 1982;298:655–657.

764. Grundlach AL, Dodd PR, Grabara CS, et al. Deficit of spinal cord glycine/strychnine receptors in inherited myoclonus of Poll Hereford calves. *Science* 1988;241:1807–1810.

765. Arena JM. Poisoning Toxicology, Symptoms, Treatments, 4th Edition. Springfield, IL, Charles C. Thomas, 1970.

766. Hao JX, Xu XJ, Aldskogius H, et al. Allodynia-like effects in rat after ischaemic spinal cord injury photochemically induced by laser irradiation. *Pain* 1991;45:175–185.

767. Hao JX, Xu XJ, Yu YX, et al. Baclofen reverses the hypersensitivity of dorsal horn wide dynamic range neurons to mechanical stimulation after transient spinal cord ischemia; implications for a tonic GABAergic inhibitory control of myelinated fiber input. *J Neurophysiol* 1992;68:392–396.

768. Marsala M, Yaksh TL. Reversible aortic occlusion in rats: post-reflow hyperesthesia and motor efects blocked by spinal NMDA antagonism. *Anesthesiology* (Abstr.) 1992;77:A664.

769. Mendell LM, Wall PD. Responses of single dorsal cord cells to peripheral cutaneous unmyelinated fibers. *Nature* 1965;206:97–99.

770. Dickenson AH, Sullivan AF. Evidence for a role of the NMDA receptor in the frequency dependent potentiation of deep rat dorsal horn nociceptive neurones following C fibre stimulation. *Neuropharmacology* 1987;26:1235–1238.

771. Puig S, Sorkin LS. Formalin-evoked activity in identified primary afferent fibers: systemic lidocaine suppresses phase-2 activity. *Pain* 1996;64:345–355.

772. De Koninck Y, Henry JL. Substance P-mediated slow excitatory postsynaptic potential elicited in dorsal horn neurons in vivo by noxious stimulation. *Proc Natl Acad Sci U S A* 1991;88:11344–11348.

773. Dickenson AH, Sullivan AF. Differential effects of excitatory amino acid antagonists on dorsal horn nociceptive neurones in the rat. *Brain Res* 1990;506:31–39.

774. Woolf CJ, Thompson SW. The induction and maintenance of central sensitization is dependent on N-methyl-D-aspartic acid receptor activation; implications for the treatment of post-injury pain hypersensitivity states. *Pain* 1991;44:293–299.

775. Aanonsen LM, Wilcox GL. Nociceptive action of excitatory amino acids in the mouse: effects of spinally administered opioids, phencyclidine and sigma agonists. *J Pharmacol Exp Therapeut* 1987;243:9–19.

776. Cridland RA, Henry JL. Comparison of the effects of substance P, neurokinin A, physalaemin and eledoisin in facilitating a nociceptive reflex in the rat. *Brain Res* 1986;381:93–99.

777. Heapy CG, Jamieson A, Russell NJW. Afferent C-fiber and A-δ activity in models of inflammation. *Br J Pharmacol* 1987;90:164P.

778. Coderre TJ, Melzack R. The contribution of excitatory amino acids to central sensitization and persistent nociception after formalin-induced tissue injury. *J Neuroscience* 1992;12:3665–3670.

779. Yamamoto T, Yaksh TL. Comparison of the antinociceptive effects of pre- and posttreatment with intrathecal morphine and MK801, an NMDA antagonist, on the formalin test in the rat. *Anesthesiology* 1992;77:757–763.

780. Yamamoto T, Yaksh TL. Stereospecific effects of a nonpeptide NK1 selective antagonist, CP-96,345: Antinociception in the absence of motor dysfunction. *Life Sciences* 1991;49:1955–1963.

781. Headley PM, Parsons CG, West DC. The role of N-methylaspartate receptors in mediating responses of rat and cat spinal neurones to defined sensory stimuli. *J Physiol* 1987;385:169–188.

782. Sher GD, Mitchell D. N-methyl-D-aspartate receptors mediate responses of rat dorsal horn neurones to hindlimb ischemia. *Brain Res* 1990;522:55–62.

783. Schaible HG, Grubb BD, Neugebauer V, et al. The effects of nmda antagonists on neuronal activity in cat spinal cord evoked by acute inflammation in the knee joint. *Eur J Neurosci* 1991;3:981–991.

784. Tanaka H, Grooms SY, Bennett MV, et al. The AMPAR subunit GluR2: still front and center-stage. *Brain Res* 2000;886:190–207.

785. Khawaja AM, Rogers DF. Tachykinins: receptor to effector. *Int J Biochem Cell Biol* 1996;28:721–738.

786. Jones TL, Sorkin LS. Calcium-permeable alpha-amino-3-hydroxy-5-methyl-4-isoxazolepropionic acid/kainate receptors mediate development, but not maintenance, of secondary allodynia evoked by first-degree burn in the rat. *J Pharmacol Exp Ther* 2004;310:223–229.

787. Ji RR. Peripheral and central mechanisms of inflammatory pain, with emphasis on MAP kinases. *Curr Drug Targets Inflamm Allergy* 2004;3:299–303.

788. Obata K, Noguchi K. MAPK activation in nociceptive neurons and pain hypersensitivity. *Life Sci* 2004;74:2643–2653.

789. Brenner GJ, Ji RR, Shaffer S, et al. Peripheral noxious stimulation induces phosphorylation of the NMDA receptor NR1 subunit at the PKC-dependent site, serine-896, in spinal cord dorsal horn neurons. *Eur J Neurosci* 2004;20:375–384.

790. Zou X, Lin Q, Willis WD. Effect of protein kinase C blockade on phosphorylation of NR1 in dorsal horn and spinothalamic tract cells caused by intradermal capsaicin injection in rats. *Brain Res* 2004;1020:95–105.

791. Svensson CI, Yaksh TL. The spinal phospholipase-cyclooxygenase-prostanoid cascade in nociceptive processing. *Annu Rev Pharmacol Toxicol* 2002;42:553–583.

792. Karin M. Inflammation-activated protein kinases as targets for drug development. *Proc Am Thorac Soc* 2005;2:386–390; discussion 394–395.

793. Coderre TJ, Gonzales R, Goldyne ME, et al. Noxious stimulus-induced increase in spinal prostaglandin E2 is noradrenergic terminal-dependent. *Neurosci Lett* 1990;115:253–258.

794. Ramwell PW, Shaw JE, Jessup R. Spontaneous and evoked release of prostaglandins from frog spinal cord. *Am Physiol* 1966;211:998.

795. Sorkin LS, Westlund KN, Sluka KA, et al. Neural changes in acute arthritis in monkeys. IV. Time-course of amino acid release into the lumbar dorsal horn. *Brain Res Brain Res Rev* 1992;17:39–50.

796. Leslie JB, Watkins WD. Eicosanoids in the central nervous system. *J Neurosurg* 1985;63:659–668.

797. Narumiya S, Sugimoto Y, Ushikubi F. Prostanoid receptors: structures, properties, and functions. *Physiol Rev* 1999;79:1193–1226.

798. England S, Bevan S, Docherty RJ. PGE2 modulates the tetrodotoxin-resistant sodium current in neonatal rat dorsal root ganglion neurones via the cyclic AMP-protein kinase A cascade. *J Physiol* 1996;495(Pt 2):429–440.

799. Gold MS, Levine JD, Correa AM. Modulation of TTX-R INa by PKC and PKA and their role in PGE2-induced sensitization of rat sensory neurons in vitro. *J Neurosci* 1998;18:10345–10355.

800. Ahmadi S, Lippross S, Neuhuber WL, et al. PGE(2) selectively blocks inhibitory glycinergic neurotransmission onto rat superficial dorsal horn neurons. *Nat Neurosci* 2002;5:34–40.

801. Nicol GD, Klingberg DK, Vasko MR. Prostaglandin E2 increases calcium conductance and stimulates release of substance P in avian sensory neurons. *J Neurosci* 1992;12:1917–1927.

802. Taiwo YO, Levine JD. Indomethacin blocks central nociceptive effects of PGF2 alpha. *Brain Res* 1986;373:81–84.

803. Uda R, Horiguchi S, Ito S, et al. Nociceptive effects induced by intrathecal administration of prostaglandin D2, E2, or F2 alpha to conscious mice. *Brain Res* 1990;510:26–32.

804. Yaksh TL. Central and peripheral mechanisms for the analgesic action of acetylsalicylic acid., Acetylsalicylic acid: New Uses for an Old Drug. Edited by Barett HJM, Hirsh J, Mustard JF. New York, Raven Press, 1982, pp. 137–151.

805. Chen WH, Chen CR, Yang KT, et al. Arachidonic acid-induced H+ and Ca2+ increases in both the cytoplasm and nucleoplasm of rat cerebellar granule cells. *J Physiol* 2001;537:497–510.

806. DeCoster MA, Lambeau G, Lazdunski M, et al. Secreted phospholipase A2 potentiates glutamate-induced calcium increase and cell death in primary neuronal cultures. *J Neurosci Res* 2002;67:634–645.

807. Miller B, Sarantis M, Traynelis SF, et al. Potentiation of NMDA receptor currents by arachidonic acid. *Nature* 1992;355:722–725.

808. Arai A, Lynch G. Antagonists of the Platelet-activating Factor Receptor Block Long-term Potentiation in Hippocampal Slices. *Eur J Neurosci* 1992;4:411–419.

809. Hwang SW, Cho H, Kwak J, et al. Direct activation of capsaicin receptors by products of lipoxygenases: endogenous capsaicin-like substances. *Proc Natl Acad Sci U S A* 2000;97:6155–6160.

810. Bazan NG, Tu B, Rodriguez de Turco EB. What synaptic lipid signaling tells us about seizure-induced damage and epileptogenesis. *Prog Brain Res* 2002;135:175–185.

811. Garthwaite J, Charles SL, Chess-Williams R. Endothelium-derived relaxing factor release on activation of NMDA receptors suggests role as intercellular messenger in the brain. *Nature* 1988;336:385–388.

812. Malmberg AB, Yaksh TL. Spinal nitric oxide synthesis inhibition blocks NMDA-induced thermal hyperalgesia and produces antinociception in the formalin test in rats. *Pain* 1993;54:291–300.

813. Meller ST, Dykstra C, Gebhart GF. Production of endogenous nitric oxide and activation of soluble guanylate cyclase are required for N-methyl-D-aspartate-produced facilitation of the nociceptive tail-flick reflex. *Eur J Pharmacol* 1992;214:93–96.

814. Anderson CR. NADPH diaphorase-positive neurons in the rat spinal cord include a subpopulation of autonomic preganglionic neurons. *Neurosci Lett* 1992;139:280–284.

815. Mizukawa K, Vincent SR, McGeer PL, et al. Distribution of reduced-nicotinamide-adenine-dinucleotide-phosphate diaphorase-positive cells and fibers in the cat central nervous system. *J Comp Neurol* 1989;279:281–311.

816. Morris R, Southam E, Braid DJ, et al. Nitric oxide may act as a messenger between dorsal root ganglion neurones and their satellite cells. *Neurosci Lett* 1992;137:29–32.

817. Schuman EM, Madison DV. A requirement for the intercellular messenger nitric oxide in long-term potentiation. *Science* 1991;254:1503–1506.

818. Alhaider AA, Lei SZ, Wilcox GL. Spinal 5-HT3 receptor-mediated antinociception: possible release of GABA. *J Neurosci* 1991;11:1881–1888.

819. Suzuki R, Rahman W, Hunt SP, et al. Descending facilitatory control of mechanically evoked responses is enhanced in deep dorsal horn neurones following peripheral nerve injury. *Brain Res* 2004;1019:68–76.

820. Grosche J, Matyash V, Moller T, et al. Microdomains for neuron-glia interaction: parallel fiber signaling to Bergmann glial cells. *Nat Neurosci* 1999;2:139–143.

821. Guillemin GJ, Brew BJ. Microglia, macrophages, perivascular macrophages, and pericytes: a review of function and identification. *J Leukoc Biol* 2004;75:388–397.

822. Mrak RE, Griffin WS. Glia and their cytokines in progression of neurodegeneration. *Neurobiol Aging* 2005;26:349–354.

823. Oka T, Wakugawa Y, Hosoi M, et al. Intracerebroventricular injection of tumor necrosis factor-alpha induces thermal hyperalgesia in rats. *Neuroimmunomodulation* 1996;3:135–140.

824. Schafers M, Sorkin LS, Sommer C. Intramuscular injection of tumor necrosis factor-alpha induces muscle hyperalgesia in rats. *Pain* 2003;104:579–588.

825. Zhang JM, Wang HK, Ye CQ, et al. ATP released by astrocytes mediates glutamergic activity-dependent heterosynaptic suppression. *Neuron* 2003;40:971–982.

826. Perea G, Araque A. Synaptic regulation of the astrocyte calcium signal. *J Neural Transm* 2005;112:127–135.

827. Duan S, Anderson CM, Keung EC, et al. P2X7 receptor-mediated release of excitatory amino acids from astrocytes. *J Neurosci* 2003;23:1320–1328.

828. Bezzi P, Carmignoto G, Pasti L, et al. Prostaglandins stimulate calcium-dependent glutamate release in astrocytes. *Nature* 1998;391:281–285.

829. Raghavendra V, Tanga FY, DeLeo JA. Complete Freunds adjuvant-induced peripheral inflammation evokes glial activation and proinflammatory cytokine expression in the CNS. *Eur J Neurosci* 2004;20:467–473.

830. Fu KY, Light AR, Maixner W. Relationship between nociceptor activity, peripheral edema, spinal microglial activation and long-term hyperalgesia induced by formalin. *Neuroscience* 2000;101:1127–1135.

831. Sweitzer SM, Colburn RW, Rutkowski M, et al. Acute peripheral inflammation induces moderate glial activation and spinal IL-1beta expression that correlates with pain behavior in the rat. *Brain Res* 1999;829:209–221.

832. Sweitzer SM, DeLeo JA. The active metabolite of leflunomide, an immunosuppressive agent, reduces mechanical sensitivity in a rat mononeuropathy model. *J Pain* 2002;3:360–368.

833. Wu Y, Wilcockson HH, Maixner W, et al. Suramin inhibits spinal cord microglia activation and long-term hyperalgesia induced by formalin injection. *J Pain* 2004;5:48–55.

834. Colburn RW, DeLeo JA, Rickman AJ, et al. Dissociation of microglial activation and neuropathic pain behaviors following peripheral nerve injury in the rat. *J Neuroimmunol* 1997;79:163–175.

835. Colburn RW, Rickman AJ, DeLeo JA. The effect of site and type of nerve injury on spinal glial activation and neuropathic pain behavior. *Exp Neurol* 1999;157:289–304.

836. Coyle DE. Partial peripheral nerve injury leads to activation of astroglia and microglia which parallels the development of allodynic behavior. *Glia* 1998;23:75–83.

837. Hashizume H, DeLeo JA, Colburn RW, et al. Spinal glial activation and cytokine expression after lumbar root injury in the rat. *Spine* 2000;25:1206–1217.

838. Molander C, Hongpaisan J, Svensson M, et al. Glial cell reactions in the spinal cord after sensory nerve stimulation are associated with axonal injury. *Brain Res* 1997;747:122–129.

839. Winkelstein BA, DeLeo JA. Nerve root injury severity differentially modulates spinal glial activation in a rat lumbar radiculopathy model: considerations for persistent pain. *Brain Res* 2002;956:294–301.

840. Hassel B, Paulsen RE, Johnsen A, et al. Selective inhibition of glial cell metabolism in vivo by fluorocitrate. *Brain Res* 1992;576:120–124.

841. Ma JY, Zhao ZQ. The involvement of glia in long-term plasticity in the spinal dorsal horn of the rat. *Neuroreport* 2002;13:1781–1784.

842. Aumeerally N, Allen G, Sawynok J. Glutamate-evoked release of adenosine and regulation of peripheral nociception. *Neuroscience* 2004;127:1–11.

843. Meller ST, Dykstra C, Grzybycki D, et al. The possible role of glia in nociceptive processing and hyperalgesia in the spinal cord of the rat. *Neuropharmacology* 1994;33:1471–1478.

844. Milligan ED, Mehmert KK, Hinde JL, et al. Thermal hyperalgesia and mechanical allodynia produced by intrathecal administration of the human immunodeficiency virus-1 (HIV-1) envelope glycoprotein, gp120. *Brain Res* 2000;861:105–116.

845. Milligan ED, Twining C, Chacur M, et al. Spinal glia and proinflammatory cytokines mediate mirror-image neuropathic pain in rats. *J Neurosci* 2003;23:1026–1040.

846. Zemke D, Majid A. The potential of minocycline for neuroprotection in human neurologic disease. *Clin Neuropharmacol* 2004;27:293–298.

847. Raghavendra V, Tanga F, DeLeo JA. Inhibition of microglial activation attenuates the development but not existing hypersensitivity in a rat model of neuropathy. *J Pharmacol Exp Ther* 2003;306:624–630.

848. Hua XY, Svensson CI, Matsui T, et al. Intrathecal minocycline attenuates peripheral inflammation-induced hyperalgesia by inhibiting p38 MAPK in spinal microglia. *Eur J Neurosci* 2005;22:2431–2440.

849. Schubert P, Ogata T, Rudolphi K, et al. Support of homeostatic glial cell signaling: a novel therapeutic approach by propentofylline. *Ann N Y Acad Sci* 1997;826:337–347.

850. Raghavendra V, Tanga F, Rutkowski MD, et al. Anti-hyperalgesic and morphine-sparing actions of propentofylline following peripheral nerve injury in rats: mechanistic implications of spinal glia and proinflammatory cytokines. *Pain* 2003;104:655–664.

851. Woolf CJ, Shortland P, Coggeshall RE. Peripheral nerve injury triggers central sprouting of myelinated afferents. *Nature* 1992;355:75–78.

852. Hughes DI, Scott DT, Todd AJ, et al. Lack of evidence for sprouting of Abeta afferents into the superficial laminas of the spinal cord dorsal horn after nerve section. *J Neurosci* 2003;23:9491–9499.

853. McLachlan EM, Jang W, Devor M, et al. Peripheral nerve injury triggers noradrenergic sprouting within dorsal root ganglia. *Nature* 1993;363:543–546.

854. Gundlach AL. Disorder of the inhibitory glycine receptor: inherited myoclonus in Poll Hereford calves. *Faseb J* 1990;4:2761–2766.

855. White WF. The glycine receptor in the mutant mouse spastic (spa): strychnine binding characteristics and pharmacology. *Brain Res* 1985;329:1–6.

856. Moore KA, Kohno T, Karchewski LA, et al. Partial peripheral nerve injury promotes a selective loss of GABAergic inhibition in the superficial dorsal horn of the spinal cord. *J Neurosci* 2002;22:6724–6731.

857. Polgar E, Hughes DI, Riddell JS, et al. Selective loss of spinal GABAergic or glycinergic neurons is not necessary for development of thermal hyperalgesia in the chronic constriction injury model of neuropathic pain. *Pain* 2003;104:229–239.

858. Gardell LR, Ibrahim M, Wang R, et al. Mouse strains that lack spinal dynorphin upregulation after peripheral nerve injury do not develop neuropathic pain. *Neuroscience* 2004;123:43–52.

859. Koetzner L, Hua XY, Lai J, et al. Nonopioid actions of intrathecal dynorphin evoke spinal excitatory amino acid and prostaglandin E2 release mediated by cyclooxygenase-1 and -2. *J Neurosci* 2004;24:1451–1458.

860. Vera-Portocarrero LP, Zhang ET, Ossipov MH, et al. Descending facilitation from the rostral ventromedial medulla maintains nerve injury-induced central sensitization. *Neuroscience* 2006;140:1311–1320.

861. DeLeo JA, Yezierski RP. The role of neuroinflammation and neuroimmune activation in persistent pain. *Pain* 2001;90:1–6.

862. Watkins LR, Maier SF. Immune regulation of central nervous system functions: from sickness responses to pathological pain. *J Intern Med* 2005;257:139–155.

863. Essman WB. Serotonin distribution in tissues and fluids. New York, Spectrum Publications, 1968.

864. Green JP, Johnson CL, Weinstein H. Histamine as a neurotransmitter. New York, Raven Press, 1978.

865. Heppelmann B, Messlinger K, Neiss WF, et al. Fine sensory innervation of the knee joint capsule by group III and group IV nerve fibers in the cat. *J Comp Neurol* 1995;351:415–428.

866. Bessou P, Burgess PR, Perl ER, et al. Dynamic properties of mechanoreceptors with unmyelinated (C) fibers. *J Neurophysiol* 1971;34:116.

867. Talbot WH, Darian-Smith I, Komhuber HH, et al. The sense of flutter-vibration: Comparison of the human capacity with response patterns of mechanoreceptive afferents from the monkey hand. *J Neurophysiol.* 1968;31:301.

868. Croze S, Duclaux R, Kenshalo DR. The thermal sensitivity of the polymodal nociceptors in the monkey. *J Physiol* 1976;263:539–562.

869. Bessou P, Perl ER. A movement receptor of the small intestine. *J Physiol* 1966;182:404.

870. Morrison JFB. The afferent innervation of the gastrointestinal tract, Nerves and the Gut. Edited by Brooks FP, Evers PW. Thorofare, N.J., Slack, 1977, pp. 297–322.

871. Winter DL. Receptor characteristics and conduction velocities in bladder afferents. *J Psychiatr Res* 1971;8:225.

CHAPTER 33 ■ PHARMACOLOGIC SUBSTRATES OF PAIN: PERIPHERAL VOLTAGE GATED ION CHANNELS IN PAIN

LUCINDA C. SEAGROVE AND ANTHONY H. DICKENSON

Peripheral nerves convey external sensory information to the spinal cord. At this first central level, a large amount of convergence and modulation occurs before transmission to the higher centers of the brain where the final perception of the stimulus is established. In addition, descending pathways from the brain to the spinal cord can further shape the output of the dorsal horn by way of inhibitory and facilitatory influences. Thus, processing occurs from both a "bottom-up" and a "top-down" series of events.

However, apart from the poorly understood processes of central pain, activity in peripheral sensory neurons is critical to the genesis of pain. The peripheral terminals of sensory neurons allow the transduction of various modalities such as mechanical, thermal, and chemical stimuli via a number of different proteins, receptors, and ion channels that convert the particular modality into electrical impulses. Critical to this are voltage-gated Na$^+$ channels (VGSCs), which initiate and propagate action potentials that travel the length of the axons, promote neuronal excitability (Fig. 33-1), and lead to the release of transmitters, in the case of sensory neurons, glutamate and peptides. Release of these transmitters into the spinal cord activates receptors on spinal neurons that in turn leads to the activation of projection neurons and interneurons within spinal circuitry.

These mechanisms are fundamental to normal sensation, whether it is signaling innocuous everyday tactile or thermal stimuli or acute painful stimuli, in which case these sensations serve as a warning. However, in pathologic pain states, for example those resulting from peripheral nerve or tissue damage due to disease or trauma, these same mechanisms can become distorted, so that the system (a) becomes hyperexcitable and sensory transmission persists, (b) can be generally not reflective of the magnitude of the evoking stimulus, and (c) can start to generate spontaneous, stimulus-independent activity as well as abnormal evoked activity.

Preclinical experimental studies have been, and continue to be, invaluable in uncovering both physiologic and pathophysiologic mechanisms responsible for sensory signaling and chronic pain conditions, respectively. However it still remains a challenge to translate such findings to clinically observed symptoms and possible therapeutic strategies (1). Blockade of the major drive to activity in cells—the voltage-gated Na$^+$ channel (VGSC)—is a major target in current clinical practice in several therapeutic areas including epilepsy, arrhythmias, and pain, and a number of studies have highlighted Na$^+$ (Na$^+$) channels as important mediators in neuropathic pain. Widely used local anaesthetics, such as lidocaine, act as Na$^+$ channel blockers, and this verifies the potential for targeting these channels as analgesic strategies. In neuropathic pain patients, microneurographic recordings from their peripheral nerves reveals aberrant electrical activity, which interestingly can be reduced by local anaesthetic nerve block in parallel with an attenuation in symptoms (2,3). Further support for the concept that Na$^+$ channels are valid targets comes from the evidence for a therapeutic effect of other drugs with VGSC blocking actions, namely carbamazepine, mexiletine, and lamotrigine (1,4).

Within the nervous system, at least nine subtypes, defined by their pore-forming α-subunit, each with individual functional and expressional characteristics, are expressed (5), with most dorsal root ganglion (DRG) neurons expressing all types (6). Voltage-gated Na$^+$ channels are not restricted to the central nervous system (CNS) and are also found in other excitable tissues, notably, the heart, autonomic neurons, and skeletal muscle. Therefore, without specificity of action or use-dependency, block of Na$^+$ channels per se runs the risk of complete sensory anaesthesia and intolerable side-effects due to potential ubiquitous block of cardiac and brain electrical activity. Although Na$^+$ channel blocking drugs (local anaesthetics, anticonvulsants, antiarrhythmics) used clinically for pain and other indications exhibit some degree of use-dependency in that normal low frequency neuronal firing is not affected, whereas pathologic high-frequency patterns of activity are reduced (7,8), the therapeutic window remains low. Developments in regional blocks can circumvent some of these problems but more selective drugs would be helpful.

Despite many attempts to modify the existing agents and ongoing attempts to identify VGSC subtype-specific ligands, currently no specific agents exist. As a consequence, the roles and potential differential physiologic roles of individual Na$^+$ channel subtypes cannot be studied in vivo by pharmacologic means. Fortunately, in animals, other methodologic approaches can be employed, such as genetic modifications to knock out specific Na$^+$ channel subtypes, a practice which has shed considerable light on the roles of various Na$^+$ channels, as has oligodinucleotide (ODN) antisense knock-down protocols, in which the target protein is temporarily reduced.

Progress in this therapeutic area is therefore dependent on translation of findings from animal studies. For this to be of any use, the animal models, methods of assessment, and inferences drawn need to be carefully established to link the animal biology to the human condition. However, a combination of molecular, genetic, behavioral, and electrophysiologic studies can be highly informative in this respect. The issue with animal

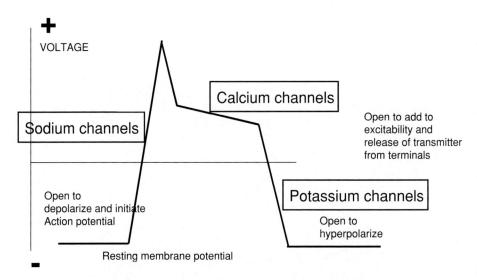

PRODUCTION OF AN ACTION POTENTIAL

FIGURE 33-1. The contribution of ion channels to the action potential and the release of transmitter.

models is that subtle side effects of drugs can be next to impossible to gauge, and so the preclinical approaches will primarily inform on efficacy. Consideration is also needed on what is being measured in animals. A large majority of studies are behavioral, in which the response to a stimulus is defined by the time or force to withdrawal of the animal at a certain intensity of the stimulus. This will be close to the threshold for "pain." Thus, a drug may have reasonable efficacy against a pain of this level but lose or even gain effectiveness at higher intensities, more related to the pains that give rise to clinical problems. This problem can be overcome by recording neuronal activity in vivo (although potentially complicated by general anaesthesia), in which responses of defined sensory neurons, for example in spinal cord, thalamus, or other areas with somatosensory inputs, can be quantified using stimuli that would be above the threshold. Effects on threshold and suprathreshold responses can therefore be revealed. In a similar way, immunohistochemical approaches such as c-fos labeling can also be used (but at a defined time point only) to study responses to suprathreshold stimuli.

Based on discoveries in animals and translation to humans, this chapter gives an account of ion channels in peripheral nerves related to pain as a basis for current and future potentially novel interventions based on the prevention of painful messages from entering the CNS.

VOLTAGE-GATED SODIUM CHANNELS

Primary sensory neurons transmit nociceptive information from the periphery to the spinal cord. Following nerve injury, alterations in the excitability of neurons suggest changes in the expression and density of Na^+ channels within the cell body and neuronal dendrites (9–12). Voltage-gated Na^+ channels are responsible for the inward membrane current in the nervous system, required for the production of the continuously evoked action potentials vital for neuronal transmission of nociceptive and other sensory information (10). They are not only expressed abundantly on primary sensory neurons, but can also be separated into a large family of distinct Na^+ channel sub-

types encoded by a large variety of different genes within the DRG. They are also found to actively alter their expression throughout both development and disease. Some Na^+ channels are specifically confined to sensory neuron populations, as opposed to other neural systems (13).

Voltage-gated Na^+ channels are heteromeric protein complexes, composed of large α- (260 kDa) and smaller β-subunits (33–45 kDa). Each protein complex contains one α-subunit, forming the ion channel pore, and two β-subunits, named $\beta1$, -2, and -3 (12). Originally, there were thought to be eight separate VGSCs within the nervous system, all of which were encoded by eight different genes (9). However, more recent accounts specify nine α-subunit isoforms, named Nav1.1 through 1.9, using modern nomenclature (12) (see Table 33-1). Within the peripheral nervous system, a number of VGSCs have been found, including Nav1.6, 1.7, 1.8, and 1.9. These VGSCs are located on different nerve fiber types and as such, their distribution may alter following neuronal insult (9,12). As interest, both industrially and academically, has risen exponentially over the past few years toward the development of VGSC blockers as neuropathic pain drugs, so has nomenclature changed for a better understanding and a more uniform recognition of the large number of detected VGSCs now cloned (see Table 33-1).

Previously, in situ hybridizations and reverse transcription polymerase chain reaction (PCR) techniques, which reveal the messenger RNAs encoding distinct Na^+ channels, revealed that within the DRG there were only six different Na^+ channel transcripts expressed, namely the Nav1.1 through Nav1.6 channels. These Na^+ channels were found in large quantities, mostly in medium and large DRG cell types. However these Na^+ channels, which elicit Na^+ channel currents, are all found to be expressed at varying levels in other neuronal cell types (9,10,12). The DRG also expresses Na^+ channels that are exclusively or selectively expressed in the primary sensory neurons, as opposed to other neuronal populations; the Nav1.7, Nav1.8, Nav1.9, and NavX channels (9,12,13).

All of these Na^+ channels can be divided based on their pharmacologic sensitivity to the toxin, tetrodotoxin (TTX), a noncompetitive voltage-gated Na^+ channel blocker, into TTX–sensitive and TTX-resistant VGSC categories (9,12).

TABLE 33-1

LOCATION OF VARIOUS SODIUM CHANNEL PROTEINS IN VERTEBRATES

Name	Old name	TTX sensitivity (IC50)	Inactivation	Location
Nav1.1	Brain Type 1	TTSs	Fast	CNS, PC, HPC, SMN, DRG
Nav1.2	Brain Type 2	TTXs (18nm)	Fast	CNS, FB, SN, CML, AT
Nav1.3	Brain Type 3	TTXs (15nm)	Fast	Brain, DRG, CNS
Nav1.4	Skm1	TTXs (5nm)	Fast	Skeletal muscle
Nav1.5	Cardiac	TTXr (1.8μm)	Slow	Heart
Nav1.6	PN4/Nach6	TTXs (1nm)	Fast	DRG, brain, SC, NR-PN
Nav1.7	PN1/hNE	TTXs (2nm)	Fast	DRG (all), brain, SC, NR-PN*
Nav1.8	PN3/SNS	TTXr (>100μm)	Slow	DRG (SDN)
Nav1.9	SNS2/NaN	TTXr (1μm)	Slow	DRG (SDN)
Nax	NaG	?	?	GC, DRG (LDN)

PC, Purkinje cells; HPC, hippocampal pyramidal cells; SMN, spinal motoneurons; DRG, dorsal root ganglia; FB, forebrain; SN, substantia nigra; CML, cerebellum molecular layer; AT, axonal targeting; SC, spinal cord; NR-PN, nodes of Ranvier-peripheral nerve; NR-PN*, rat sciatic nerve only; SDN, small-diameter neurons; GC, glial cells; LN, large neurons.

The TTX–sensitive Na$^+$ channels include Nav1.1, Nav1.2, Nav1.3, Nav1.4, Nav1.6, and Nav1.7, whereas the rest are TTX-resistant Na$^+$ channel types. Nav1.7 Na$^+$ channel transcripts are also located within the terminals of the majority of DRG neurons (12). The Nav1.8 Na$^+$ channel, as well as the Nav1.9 channel, is found in trigeminal neurons as well as small-diameter C-type DRG cells. It has emerged that Nav1.9 is also present in human embryonic kidney (HEK) cells as well. Nav1.8 and Nav1.9, which are TTX-resistant, have caused much interest, as the majority of nociceptive neurons make up small DRG neurons (9–16). Furthermore, it is known from more recent studies that Nav1.8 activates a TTX-resistant current within C-fiber populations, exhibiting slow-activating and inactivating, as well as rapid repriming kinetics (9,12) that would be suggestive of a role in generating abnormal patterns of firing. It is therefore evident that VGSCs are prevalent and participate in the conduction of nociceptive information. Not only is the development of action potentials in small DRG neurons largely diminished in Nav1.8-null mutant mice, but hypoalgesia also develops in response to application of varying forms of noxious stimuli (9,17). Nav1.9 is thought to be active at the resting membrane potential in small DRG cells, and it has therefore been suggested that Nav1.9 regulates the resting membrane potential of nociceptive C-fibers. Recent findings have located Nav1.9 in the hippocampus and therefore lay doubt to the initial hypothesis that Nav1.9 is restricted to the DRG (16).

Much interest has evolved around the concept of Na$^+$ ion channels and their targets as prospective analgesics following nerve injury, because it is now apparent that the type of channels expressed following neuronal insult is altered (9). Recently, development of antisense oligonucleotides that disturb Nav1.8 synthesis have been used to "knock down" Nav1.8 VGSCs, resulting in a 50% reduction in the expression of these VGSCs (12,17). Interestingly, following spinal nerve ligation, "knock-down" has been seen to reduce neuropathic pain and its associated reductions in thermal and mechanical sensory thresholds. The same treatment in normal animals had no such effect on the sensory threshold values to peripherally applied noxious thermal stimuli (12,17). These knock-down studies have not found any effect of downregulation of the channel on thermal or mechanical hypersensitivity in neuropathic animals following attenuation of Nav1.9 synthesis. This is consistent with findings in sham operated animal groups (18).

Following neuronal axotomy, other studies have revealed that both an upregulation of the α-III Na$^+$ channel and a downregulation of Nav1.8 and Nav1.9 gene expression occur within DRG neurons (9,19). Downregulation of Nav1.8 channel proteins in more recent studies following spinal nerve ligation of L5–L6 have specified that Nav1.8 is reduced in the injured DRG cell bodies; thus, Nav1.8 channel functioning is unlikely to occur in damaged nerve fibers (17,20,21). Such downregulation possibly prevents electrical conductivity in damaged C-fiber populations (12,17,22). This is despite original theories that, based on the role of Nav1.8 channels in DRG cell conductance, following nerve injury alterations in the activity of Nav1.8 protein channels could be responsible for spontaneous activity and repetitive firing of DRG cells (6,9). Interestingly, not only does such downregulation result in a reduction of TTX-resistant Na$^+$ currents within the DRG neurons, but also in the development of a rapidly conducting repriming current within the TTX-sensitive Na$^+$ currents in DRG neurons (6,9). This is thought to be due to the upregulation of the previously silent Nav1.3 Na$^+$ channel. This latter channel relates to neuropathic pain and phantom phenomena that are seen after spinal cord injury (SCI), in which any molecular cause based on peripheral fiber ion channel changes cannot be likely due to the central location of the injury. Immunohistochemical investigations demonstrate abnormal expression of the Nav1.3 channel within central spinal cord dorsal horn neurons and also in the projection area of thalamic neurons after SCI. The changed expression of the channel may be a basis for abnormal hyperexcitability whereby denervated neurons start to act as amplifiers and generators (23,24).

Using the spinal nerve ligation (SNL) model of neuropathy, studies have also shown that the levels of Nav1.8 are unaltered in the uninjured L4 ganglia, yet analysis of the sciatic nerve reveals the levels of Nav1.8 are dramatically increased (21). In the neuropathic group, TTX was unable to block the compound action potentials (CAP) at C-fiber latencies, compared to sham operated rats whose CAP remained sensitive (>90%) to TTX (100 μm). These studies strongly emphasize the possible role of Nav1.8 blocking agents in the reversal of neuropathic pain conditions (21). Following Nav1.8 knock-down studies in the sciatic nerve, it has become evident that Nav1.9 channels may be responsible for the observed residual TTXr currents in the C-fiber population (21). However, it is clear that the presence of Nav1.9 channels along the nerve axon is undisturbed by nerve damage, as differences in the density of voltage-gated Na$^+$ channel currents in neuropathic and sham operated animals is minimal. Nav1.8 knockdown in uninjured neurons have also proven to be both antiallodynic and antihyperalgesic in relevant animal models (21). It is feasible that such alterations in Na$^+$ channel expression, as well as changes in Na$^+$ channel densities within DRG neurons, may underlie the spontaneous firing and lower thresholds that are responsible for such abnormal firing after axotomy and nerve damage (25,26). It is also possible that the development of spontaneous activity is a prerequisite of the hypersensitive allodynic and hyperalgesic states that characterize neuropathic conditions, along with the actual insult to the peripheral nerves (4,9,12).

Interestingly, not only does the alteration in Na$^+$ channel expression result in changed conduction properties in neuropathic models, but, in addition, alterations in the production and role of neurotrophins at neuronal sites may influence Na$^+$ channel expression (9). Thus, damage and disruption to the integrity of a nerve and its surrounding tissue may alter the levels and movement of these molecules. Many studies have looked at the role of brain-derived growth factor (BDNF), glial-derived growth factor (GDNF), and nerve growth factor (NGF) in the modulation of Na$^+$ channel expression. Apart from a study that observed a regulatory role of GDNF in the expression of Nav1.9 Na$^+$ channels in small DRG neurons (27), none except for those based on the role of NGF following axotomy has shown any profound function of neurotrophins in Na$^+$ channel expression (9).

Studies have implicated NGF as having a distinct role in the alteration of some Na$^+$ ion channel transcripts, with α-III downregulated upon direct application of NGF to DRG cell bodies (28) and Nav1.8 expression within the DRG increasing following nerve damage (29). These studies are supported by others that reveal an upregulation in TTX-resistant Na$^+$ channel currents in small DRG, as well as Nav1.8 channel currents (mentioned earlier) following direct application of exogenous NGF to the proximal nerve stump. A reduction in the reservoir of neurotrophic factors or a loss of their influence may therefore reveal a valid argument for the contradictory downregulations of such Na$^+$ channel currents following nerve injury (9).

The roles of Nav1.7 have been impossible to judge because the knock-out is lethal in early life, and so the phenotype cannot be ascertained. However, a nociceptor-specific knock-out of the Nav1.7 gene has been generated, and this results in a behavioral phenotype exhibiting dramatic deficits in inflammatory pain models (30). Acutely, Nav1.7 deletion, similar to Nav1.8, produces deficits in mechanosensation, but not to thermal stimuli, although only in the noxious range, as was seen behaviorally using noxious pressure. Marked deficits to noxious von Frey stimulation were observed from electrophysiologic recordings of dorsal horn neuronal activity (30) (Fig. 33-2). Recently, a human heritable pain condition, primary erythromelalgia, in which burning pain is experienced in response to warm stimuli or moderate exercise, has been shown to map to Nav1.7 (31). In contrast to the deficits seen in the nociceptor-specific Nav1.7 knock-out, this is a gain-of-function mutation presented clinically as chronic inflammation and associated pain.

However, Waxman and colleagues have shown that this single mutation can produce hyperexcitability in one neuronal cell type related to pain and yet hypoexcitability in another neuronal cell type. They studied the functional effects of a mutation of Na$^+$ channel Nav1.7 associated with erythromelalgia within sensory and sympathetic ganglion neurons, two cell types in which Nav1.7 is normally expressed. Although this mutation favors depolarization in both neuronal types, the net effect is that sensory neurons become hyperexcitable, yet sympathetic neurons are hypoexcitable. The selective presence of the Nav1.8 channel in sensory, but not autonomic neurons

Deficit in Dorsal Horn Neuronal Response to Mechanical Stimulation in Na$_v$ 1.8 KO mice

(von Frey Hair application over 10s)

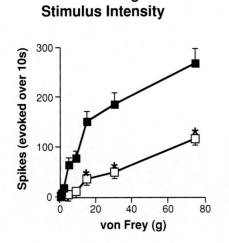

Broad Range Stimulus Intensity

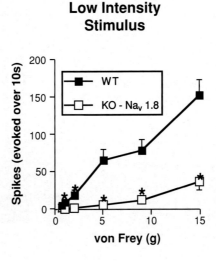

Low Intensity Stimulus

FIGURE 33-2. Data showing the neuronal response of spinal neurons to stimulation of the peripheral receptive field with von Frey hairs. Plotted on the y axis is the mean number of spikes evoked over a 10-second period against increasing von Frey intensity. The first graph shows the entire range; in the second, the lower stimulus range is expanded. Statistically significant over entire range of von Freys. The Nav1.8 knock-out (KO) mice (*open squares*) and the WT mice show graded neuronal responses with increasing mechanical intensity, but the KO mice show a dramatic deficit in the mechanical coding, which is highly significant over the entire range. Data from Matthews EA, Wood JN, Dickenson AH. Nav1.8-null mice show stimulus-dependent deficits in spinal neuronal activity. *Molecul Pain* 2006;2:5, with permission

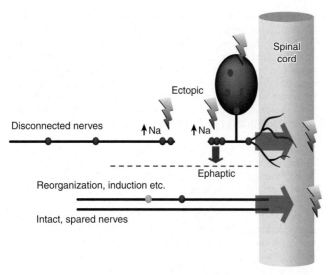

FIGURE 33-3. Altered signalling in damaged and intact nerves leads to some of the initial changes that occur in neuropathic pain. Accumulations of sodium channels at the site injury (e.g., the neuroma) occurs as transport of channels produced in the cell body of the peripheral fiber cannot continue further. Cross-talk or ephaptic activity can occur as a result of demyelination.

(which can be activated at depolarized membrane potentials), is a major determinant of these bidirectional effects. These results provide a molecular basis for the sympathetic dysfunction that has been observed in erythromelalgia (31).

Overall, the findings discussed here have implicated certain distinct Na$^+$ channels in the long search for neuropathic pain treatments, as well as in a firm understanding of the abnormal sensory activities that classify neuropathic pain syndrome and that occur following nerve damage or deafferentation (Fig. 33-3). The widely researched changes in Nav1.8, as well as Nav1.9, protein channel expression, have provided a basis for the development of novel blockers that may prove valuable as analgesic drugs. Specific antisense oligodeoxynucleotides can be used to knock-down DRG PN3/Nav1.8 proteins and have intriguingly been shown to stop the development of injury-induced allodynia and hyperalgesia (9) (Fig. 33-2). Unfortunately, Nav1.9 protein knock-down has failed to replicate such

encouraging results (18). However, this general outcome has led the way for the development of PN3-/Nav1.8-specific Na$^+$ channel blockers, which are ever more attractive due to their restriction on sensory neuron populations. This is important since, although a clear role of Nav1.7 has been revealed (30), the broader distribution of this channel may compromise pharmacologic manipulation unless this could be localized.

Furthermore, recent research using selective antibodies has extended these animals studies to human pain models and found both Nav1.8 and Nav1.9 Na$^+$ channels on peripheral nerves in neurogenic pain patients (32). Immunolocalization enabled the location of such Na$^+$ channels to be discovered within patients who had brachial plexus injury. This study revealed that, following spinal cord root avulsion, Nav1.8 and Nav1.9 Na$^+$ channel expression in neuronal cell bodies is decreased in human models (32).

However, as with previous animal studies, following peripheral axotomy, Na$^+$ channels already synthesized can still be transported to the area of nerve damage and amass at these sites, which may be essential for the development of hypersensitive states (32) (Fig. 33-4). Interestingly, those patients suffering chronic local hyperalgesia had increased levels of Nav1.8 immunoreactivity in neuroma nerve terminal and skin samples, again linking the Nav1.8 Na$^+$ channel with the chronic abnormal and hypersensitive pain symptoms underlying neuropathic pain (32). Also, the majority of patients with brachial plexus injury also had related positive symptoms and demonstrated a positive Tinel sign, fueling belief that blockade of Nav1.8 voltage-gated Na$^+$ channels could aid chronic local hypersensitivity in neuropathic patients (32). Indeed, recent studies looking at the effect of novel Na$^+$ channel blockers in neuropathic and inflammatory pain, as well as their antiallodynic effects, reveal distinct antinociceptive properties (33,34). A summary of the key roles of Nav1.3, –1.7, and –1.8 is given in Table 33-2.

VOLTAGE-GATED POTASSIUM CHANNELS

A great deal of information is available about the importance of Na$^+$ ion channels in peripheral sensory neurons in control of afferent excitability whereas, by comparison, the role(s) of potassium (K$^+$) channels is still not fully characterized. Neuronal hyperexcitability is a feature of epilepsy and both inflammatory

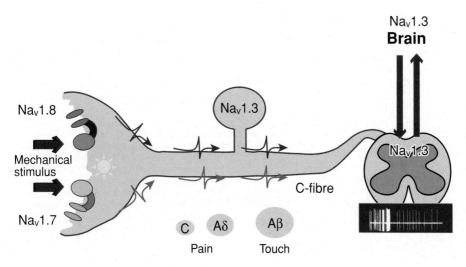

FIGURE 33-4. The two sodium channels Nav1.7 and -1.8 appear to play a key role in the transduction of mechanical stimuli, since genetic deletion of these channels in small afferent fibers markedly reduces the ability of spinal neurons to code this modality. In addition, in cases of nerve injury, the de novo upregulation of Nav1.3 in the cell body, spinal cord, and brain may contribute to peripheral and central neuropathic pains.

TABLE 33-2

SUMMARY OF THE KEY SODIUM CHANNELS IMPLICATED IN PAIN

Na⁺ Channels	
Nav1,7	Expressed in fine fibers Mutations cause sensory and autonomic changes in erythermalgia and others lead to analgesia
Nav1.8	Unique to fine fibers Roles in pain in animals and especially noxious mechanical stimuli Mutations lead to rectal pain
Nav1.5	Mutation implicated in abdominal pain
Nav1.3	Upregulated in DRG, in cord after nerve injury—also in brain after SCI—central pains?

and neuropathic pain. M-currents [IK(M)] play a key role in regulating neuronal excitability, and neuronal KCNQ2/3 subunits—the molecular correlates of IK(M)—are also present in nociceptive sensory systems. Retigabine, an opener of these currents, applied spinally, inhibited C- and Aδ-fiber–mediated responses of dorsal horn neurons evoked by natural or electrical afferent stimulation, as well as "wind-up" after repetitive stimulation, in normal rats and in rats subjected to SNL (35) (Fig. 33-5). This latter result suggests that modulation of this target would remain effective after nerve injury, suggestive of a lack of channel downregulation. Retigabine also inhibited responses to intra-paw application of carrageenan in a rat model of persistent inflammatory pain. It is suggested that IK(M) plays a key role in controlling the excitability of nociceptors and that IK(M) may represent a novel analgesic target (35,36).

Potential roles of other K⁺ channels remain poorly understood, with the exception of calcium-activated K⁺ channels (SK and IK channels). Three mammalian genes (SK1–3/KCNN1–3) produce subunits of small-conductance calcium-activated K⁺ channels. A closely related gene (IK1/SK4/KCNN4) encodes intermediate conductance calcium-activated K⁺ channels (IK channels). SK channels are widely expressed in both the central and peripheral nervous system, and are also found in many other tissues (37). In contrast, IK1 is functionally important for a much more limited range of neurons, although, like the SK channels, IK channels are important in many non-neuronal tissues.

SK and IK channel pharmacology has been extensively studied. The activity of both SK and IK channels can be increased by 1-ethyl-2-benzimidazolinone (1-EBIO) at micromolar concentrations (37). Further, channels formed by either SK2 or SK3 subunits are selectively inhibited at nanomolar or sub nanomolar concentrations by both peptide toxins such as apamin and small-molecule blockers such as UCL 1848 and UCL 1684 (37). IK channels are insensitive to these blockers.

There are conflicting reports about the involvement of SK and IK channels in sensory pathways. In a number of vertebrate species, including man, SK and/or IK channels have been reported in DRG neurons, with suggestions that the channels contribute to calcium-sensitive postspike hyperpolarizations in the cell body (38). The potential functional role of SK and IK channels in the transmission of sensory information remains to be clearly defined, but a recent report strongly supports a role in pain processes (38).

VOLTAGE-DEPENDENT CALCIUM CHANNELS (VDCC)

At present the potential roles of the Na⁺ channel subtypes in peripheral nerves has translated well from animals to humans and the verification of their importance has come not only from the animal studies but from the present use of Na⁺ channel blockers in patients with neuropathic pain (39,40), but the changes in brain expression of Nav1.3 may also provide a future target for a better treatment of central pains (41).

Yet, not only are there alterations in the distribution and number of certain VGSC subtypes expressed following nerve injury and indications for roles in other pain states, but there

Retigabine inhibits electrically evoked dorsal horn responses in vivo

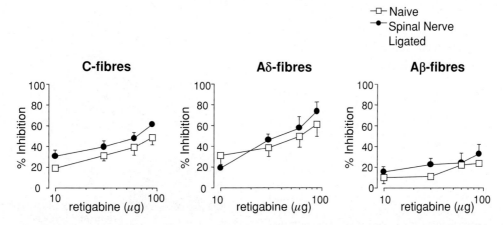

FIGURE 33-5. The effects of the selective potassium channel opener, retigibine, on evoked responses of spinal cord neurons in the anesthetized rat. The drug, which acts on KCNQ channels, causes a selective inhibition of activity evoked by small-fiber stimulation, and this remains after nerve injury. From Passmore GM, Selyanko AA, Mistry M, et al. KCNQ/M-currents in sensory neurons: Significance for pain therapy. *J Neurosci* 2003;23:7227–7236, with permission.

Calcium channels

- Different genes
- Different types
- Different locations
- Different functions

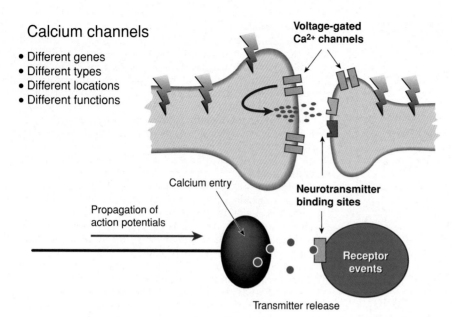

FIGURE 33-6. Transmission from the periphery into the spinal cord where sensory primary afferent fibers terminate is dependent on calcium channel function. The pharmacology of the spine is very complicated, involving a wide range of neurotransmitters, modulators, receptors, and ion channels. What is fundamental to the transmission of sensory information is the release of neurotransmitters from presynaptic terminals, which is under the control of calcium entry into the terminal via voltage-dependent calcium channels.

are also reported changes in the expression and role of calcium (Ca2+) channels (Fig. 33-6). It appears that nerve injury resulting in a neuropathic pain state initiates many changes to the peripheral and central nervous systems that are accountable for the various symptoms that manifest. To summarize, these include changes in spinal cord connectivity, loss of intrinsic modulatory systems, and upregulation of excitatory processes, including the emergence of spontaneous activity and central sensitization. Pivotal to many of these alterations is the concentration of intracellular Ca2+ ions. In addition to release from internal stores heavily implicated in second-messenger systems and gene induction, the major influx route is across the plasma membrane via the N-methyl-D-aspartate (NMDA) receptor/channel complex and voltage-dependent calcium channels (VDCCs), in response to neurotransmitter receptor activation and membrane depolarization. Voltage-dependent calcium channels are critical to the sensory pathway in various aspects, but more specifically, they permit the synaptic transmission of sensory information from the periphery to the brain via the control of depolarization-coupled neurotransmitter release.

Primary Structure of Voltage-dependent Calcium Channels

Voltage-dependent calcium channels can be found in the membrane of many cell types throughout the body, where they mediate Ca2+ entry into the cell in response to membrane depolarization. Originally solubilized and purified from skeletal muscle, VDCCs are hetero-oligomeric complexes consisting of various combinations of an α_1-subunit with auxiliary $\alpha_2\delta$-, β-, and γ-subunits. Hydrophobicity plots, glycosylation, and biochemical analysis of the subunits has revealed their primary structure. The α_1-subunit forms the pore of the channel and is predicted to have four domain repeats (I–IV), each having six transmembrane segments (S1–S6), with a membrane-associated loop between S5 and S6 lining the pore, and the S4 segment forming the voltage-sensor required for activation. The β-subunit is predicted to have no transmembrane regions, and it associates with α_1 intracellularly, in contrast to

the γ-subunit, which has four transmembrane segments. The α_2-subunit is entirely extracellular, with many glycosylation sites, and is anchored to the membrane through a disulfide bond with the δ-subunit. Using in vitro expression systems, generally the α_1-subunit is enough to form functional channels, and the auxiliary subunits serve to modulate its gating and current characteristics via enhancing expression levels, shifting voltage-dependence of activation and inactivation to more negative potentials and increasing the rate of inactivation. In vivo, non-neuronal VDCCs comprise all five subunits, whereas neuronal channels lack the γ-subunit (42) (Fig. 33-7).

Several different classes of VDCCs exist, and these were originally identified by their electrophysiologic and pharmacologic profiles into the L-, N-, P-, Q-, R-, and T–types, each subserving different functional roles relative to their cellular

Voltage-dependent Ca2+ Channel (neuronal)

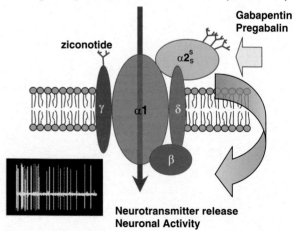

FIGURE 33-7. The structure of calcium channels, whereby the α_1-subunit forms the pore of the channel, the site of action of ziconotide, and the accessory $\alpha_2\delta$-subunit forms the site of action of gabapentin and pregabalin.

TABLE 33-3

CLASSIFICATION, CELLULAR LOCALIZATION, AND FUNCTIONAL SIGNIFICANCE OF VOLTAGE-DEPENDENT CALCIUM CHANNELS

VDCC type	Current type	α_1-Subunit	Tissue localization	Subcellular localization	Spinal cord distribution	Specific blocker	Function
$Ca_v 1.1$	L (HVA)	α_{1S}	Skeletal muscle	T-tubules	×	DHPs	Excitation-contraction coupling
$Ca_v 1.2$	L (HVA)	α_{1C}	Cardiac muscle Smooth muscle Neurons	Membrane surface, t-tubule sarcolemma Cell soma	√ deep dorsal and ventral horns	DHPs	Excitation-contraction coupling, hormone secretion, gene regulation
$Ca_v 1.3$	L (HVA)	α_{1D}	Pancreas Endocrine tissue Neurons	Cell soma and larger dendrites of neurons	√ deep dorsal and ventral horns	DHPs	Hormone secretion, gene regulation
$Ca_v 1.4$	L (HVA)	α_{1F}	Retina		×		Tonic release of neurotransmitters
$Ca_v 2.1$	P/Q (HVA)	α_{1A}	Neurons	Nerve terminals and dendrites	√ throughout	ω-agatoxin IVA	Neurotransmitter release
$Ca_v 2.2$	N (HVA)	α_{1B}	Neurons	Nerve terminals and dendrites	√ mostly concentrated in superficial laminae	ω-conotoxin GVIA	Neurotransmitter release
$Ca_v 2.3$	R (HVA)	α_{1E}	Neurons	Soma, dendrites and terminals	√	None	Neurotransmitter release
$Ca_v 3.1$	T (LVA)	α_{1G}	Neurons Cardiac muscle Skeletal muscle	Soma and dendrites	√ low levels throughout	None	Pacemaking, gradual depolarization for multiple APs and oscillatory behavior, depolarizes cells to threshold for other channels
$Ca_v 3.2$	T (LVA)	α_{1H}	Neurons Cardiac muscle	Soma and dendrites	√ mostly restricted to superficial laminae	None	
$Ca_v 3.3$	T (LVA)	α_{1I}	Neurons	Soma and dendrites	√ throughout, mainly in laminae III–IV	None	

VDCC, voltage-dependent calcium channel; HVA, high-voltage-activated; LVA, low-voltage-activated; DHPs, dihydropiridines; Aps, action potentials.

location. Subsequent advances in molecular biology have identified ten genes encoding the main pore-forming α_1-subunit, termed α_1A to α_1I, and the current nomenclature groups these into three families, Cav1, -2, and -3, based upon structural and functional characteristics. Cav1 and Cav2 comprise the high-voltage-activated (HVA) VDCCs, which allow Ca2+ influx upon substantial membrane depolarization, such as that mediated by an action potential, whereas Cav3 channels are the low-voltage-activated (LVA) VDCCs, such that they permit Ca2+ flux at resting membrane potentials (Table 33-3).

High-voltage-activated Ca2+ channels, activated by large membrane depolarizations, are now thought to be extremely important in pain pathways. A number of different types of high-voltage Ca2+ channels are expressed in the nervous system, which include the four L-, N-, P/Q- and R-type Ca2+ channels (43). These voltage-activated Ca2+ channels (also referred to as VDCCs) are all composed of an α_1-subunit, which forms the Ca2+ channel pore, and related β-, $\alpha_2\delta$-, and γ-subunit proteins (42). Recent studies have now implicated low-voltage T-type channels, found both in and out of the nervous system, in pain processes (44). Using the T-type Ca2+ channel blocker, ethosuximide, it is evident that T-type Ca2+ channels are involved in both noxious electrically, mechanically, and

thermally induced neuronal responses (44). However, following SNL, the role of these T-type Ca2+ channels remains the same.

Following nerve injury, electrophysiologic studies have used intrathecal ω-conotoxin-GVIA, which blocks the N-type VDCC, and results confirm significant reductions in noxious electrically and naturally induced dorsal horn neuronal responses, thus also proving that N-type VDCCs play a distinct role in nociceptive transmission before and after peripheral nerve ligation (43). However, at the lower dose range, block of N-type VDCCs caused a more pronounced inhibition in neuropathic animals, suggesting some upregulation of N-type VDCCs following peripheral nerve ligation (43). Confirming these reports are studies performed on mutant mice lacking the N-type VDCC, which display less neuropathic pain related symptoms compared to control groups (45). The P-type VDCC antagonist ω-agatoxin-IVA did not have as large an effect as the N-type blocker and thus plays a smaller role in electrically and naturally evoked neuronal transmission (43).

Furthermore, monoclonal antibody studies and western blot techniques have also recently suggested an upregulation of $\alpha_2\delta_1$-subunits, an auxiliary protein associated with the channel, and increased gabapentin sensitivity following diabetic-based and mechanical (i.e., sciatic nerve injury and chronic constriction injury [CCI]) neuropathies. This may therefore implicate a role in the development of allodynia in these systems (46). Overall, a variety of studies have signified the involvement of VDCCs, particularly N-type VDCCs, in the development of neuropathic pain–related behaviors and could thus suggest a future role of N-type VDCC antagonists in the treatment of neuropathic pain symptoms.

Indeed, the modified peptide ziconotide is licensed for human pain control. Ziconotide (formerly SNX-111) selectively blocks N-type voltage-sensitive calcium channels and may be effective in patients with pains that are refractory to opioid therapy or those with intolerable opioid-related adverse effects. A double-blind, placebo-controlled, randomized trial conducted on patients with cancer or acquired immune deficiency syndrome (AIDS) using intrathecal ziconotide has been reported. Pain scores improved 53% in the ziconotide group, compared to 18% in the placebo group, without loss of efficacy in a subsequent maintenance phase. The reported pain relief was moderate to complete in just over half the patients in the ziconotide group. However, due to adverse effects by systemic routes, the peptide must be given intrathecally (47).

Interestingly, gabapentin and pregabalin are no longer thought to have any effect on γ-aminobutyric acid (GABA)ergic uptake, metabolism, or receptor action. However, it is believed to block $\alpha_2\delta$–subunits within the Ca2+ channel complex, and therefore exhibit analgesic effects via action at these ion channels (Fig. 33-7) (4,48,49). However, as yet, gabapentin's analgesic effects on neuropathic pain are still not fully elucidated. Numerous studies have confirmed that gabapentin is a good analgesic in patients suffering from painful diabetic neuropathies and postherpetic neuralgia. Interestingly, the side-effect profile of gabapentin is very similar to that of other anticonvulsants (1,48). Electrophysiologic studies using a combination of morphine and gabapentin have illustrated increased effectiveness of morphine when administered with small doses of gabapentin, where morphine previously exerted reduced effectiveness following nerve injury (49). These studies implicate combination treatment as a further choice of therapies in some neuropathic-based pains in which monotherapy is not sufficient.

The target for gabapentin and pregabalin is intriguing. Among the many mechanisms of nerve injury–induced and other pains, the altered expression of genes implicated in neuronal signaling in nociceptive neural circuitry may underlie some of the persistent changes leading to persistent pain (50–55). A growing body of evidence suggests that one of these altered genes may encode the $\alpha_2\delta_1$-subunit (Cav-$\alpha_2\delta_1$ of the VGCC), the binding site for gabapentin and pregabalin. This subunit is markedly upregulated in DRG neurons, suggesting that the subunit is associated with the terminals of afferent fibers but also with spinal dorsal horn neurons following nerve injury (50–55). The time course of the upregulation is highly correlated with the genesis and maintenance of neuropathic pain behavior (46,50). The Cav-$\alpha_2\delta_1$ is a structural subunit that could be involved in the functional assembly of the neuronal Ca2+ channels in the cell membrane (56). Since VGCCs are important in regulating the excitability of sensory and spinal dorsal horn neurons, as well as neurotransmitter release from the presynaptic terminals, altered Cav-$\alpha_2\delta_1$ expression can lead to changes in Ca2+ channel expression and affect sensory information processing. However, the link between upregulation of a particular protein among the many changes that underlie pain behaviors is hard to assess. To investigate the mechanisms underlying the contribution of Cav-$\alpha_2\delta_1$ to neuropathic pain sensations without the influence of other injury factors, Luo and colleagues constructed a transgenic mouse that con-

stitutively overexpresses the Cav-$\alpha_2\delta_1$ in neuronal tissues (57). The study assessed the behavior of the mice, their pharmacology, as well as VGCC properties in DRG neurons and spinal dorsal horn neuron excitability to peripheral stimuli. Cav-$\alpha_2\delta_1$ overexpression resulted in enhanced Ca2+ currents, changes in the properties of VGCC activation in sensory neurons, marked enhancements in both the evoked responses but also prolonged poststimulation firing in dorsal horn neurons, and hypersensitivity to mechanical and thermal stimulation. However, the transgenic mice showed normal dorsal horn responses to wind-up stimulation and normal behavioral responses to tissue injury/inflammatory stimuli. These abnormal pain behaviors in the otherwise normal transgenic mice had a pharmacologic profile similar to that in neuropathic pain and could be reversed by intrathecal gabapentin, even though no nerve injury was present. Thus, elevated neuronal Cav-$\alpha_2\delta_1$ contributes to abnormal sensations through a mechanism mediated by enhanced VGCC activity in sensory neurons and exaggerated dorsal horn neuronal responses to peripheral stimulation (57).

The upregulation of the binding site for the drugs is not the only basis for the ability of $\alpha_2\delta$-ligands to modulate abnormal pain states. Using a substance P-saporin conjugate (SP-SAP), it is possible to selectively ablate neurons in spinal dorsal horn pain pathways that are defined in terms of their location and pharmacologic profiles (58). As substance P binds to its receptor, the neurokinin (NK)1 receptor, it internalizes and thus allows saporin, a neurotoxin, to enter the cell and kill the neuron. This has been done for superficial dorsal horn neurons that express the NK1 receptor for substance P, and this approach may have relevance to the treatment of intractable pain in the future, since it abolished hyperalgesias while leaving acute nociception unaltered (59). These neurons project to the brain and there engage descending brainstem serotonergic influences that enhance spinal excitability via a facilitatory action on serotonin (5HT3) receptors (58). The integrity of this pathway following nerve injury contributes not only to the behavioral allodynia seen, but prevents some of the neuronal plasticity of deep dorsal horn neurons that follows neuropathy (abnormal neuronal coding, including spontaneous activity, increased receptive field size) after SNL. Remarkably, the powerful actions of gabapentin after neuropathy were entirely prevented by either ablation of these specific NK1-expressing neurons or by 5HT3 receptor antagonism using pharmacologic agents (60). By contrast, 5HT3 receptor activation enabled gabapentin to inhibit neuronal activity in normal uninjured animals in a way similar to that observed in animals with overexpression of Cav-$\alpha_2\delta_1$. Thus, activity in this circuit is a key determinant of both the abnormal neuronal and behavioral changes seen after neuropathy and, importantly, the efficacy of gabapentin (60) (Fig. 33-8). Furthermore, since the spino-bulbo-spinal circuit contacts areas of the brain that are implicated in the affective components of pain, this may be one way in which emotional areas of the brain feed back onto the spinal cord to influence the degree of pain in a patient, as well as the effectiveness of the drug treatment (61). The importance of these descending influences on spinal processing is exemplified by a recent study showing their role in models of SCI in which the periphery is unaltered (62,63). Furthermore, Cav-$\alpha_2\delta_1$ has also been shown to play a role in the abnormal pains seen in animal models of cancer-induced bone pain.

One speculation would be that the actions of gabapentin relate to activity in the spinal–brainstem circuits, influenced not only by peripheral and spinal events but by the affective state of the patient (e.g., stress, anxiety, fear) impacting on complex mechanisms relating to attention (60). Only under such

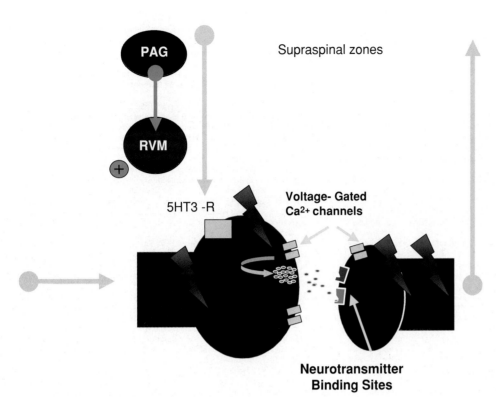

FIGURE 33-8. Ascending messages from spinal cord neurons can contact supraspinal structures that engage descending pathways from the periaqueductal gray (*PAG*) and rostral ventromedial medulla (*RVM*) that further modulate spinal activity. Although descending controls can be excitatory or inhibitory, a descending facilitatory pathway that activates the serotonin (5HT3) receptor at spinal levels appears to not only enhance pain processing but is permissive for the actions of gabapentin and pregabalin, acting through modulation of calcium channels.

circumstances of "heightened excitability" could gabapentin exert its antihyperalgesic effects (i.e., inhibition of stimulus-evoked brainstem activity), thus confirming its state-dependent actions. This state-dependent or permissive interaction may explain why only one in three neuropathic patients achieve more than 50% pain relief following gabapentin in clinical practice (64).

This leads to the idea that the same circuits (spinal and supraspinal) that alter the gain in this sensory system and produce hyperalgesia also permit certain drugs to treat the pain. This appears to be true for both acute experimental pain, such as that induced by capsaicin, and physiopathologic pains, such as that seen after nerve injury. In states of chronic pain, feedback onto this descending modulatory circuitry from higher centers such as the amygdala and anterior cingulate cortex could further amplify spinal nociception, so that the perceived pain is greater.

SUMMARY

Thus, the highest centers of the brain and complex processing at these levels are able to project down to the spinal cord and alter the functional state of ion channels found in terminals of afferent fibers. These key channels, which generate and conduct action potentials, modulate excitability and also are critical for transmitter release, opening and closing in response to membrane voltage changes. But they are also regulated by pathologic states and higher brain functions, showing how the integrated functions of the nervous system and interactions between signaling systems are important for function and, as illustrated by Cav-$\alpha_2\delta_1$, a key to drug action. Future research holds the potential of ion channels as targets for present therapy and also may determine how they may be selectively modulated by future drugs.

References

1. Jensen TS, Baron R. Translation of symptoms and signs into mechanisms in neuropathic pain. *Pain* 2003;102:1–8.
2. Campbell JN, Raja SN, Meyer RA, Mackinnon SE. Myelinated afferents signal the hyperalgesia associated with nerve injury. *Pain* 1988;32:89–94.
3. Nystrom B, Hagbarth KE. Microelectrode recordings from transected nerves in amputees with phantom limb pain. *Neurosci Lett* 1981; 27:211–216.
4. Dickenson AH, Matthews E, Suzuki R. Neurobiology of neuropathic pain: Mode of action of anticonvulsants. *Eur J Pain* 2002;6:51–60.
5. Catterall WA. From ionic currents to molecular mechanisms: The structure and function of voltage-gated sodium channels. *Neuron* 2000;26:13–25.
6. Black JA, Dib-Hajj S, McNabola K, et al. Spinal sensory neurons express multiple sodium channel alpha-subunit mRNAs. *Brain Res Mol Brain Res* 1996;43:117–131.
7. Balser JR, Nuss HB, Orias DW, et al. Local anesthetics as effectors of allosteric gating. Lidocaine effects on inactivation-deficient rat skeletal muscle Na channels. *J Clin Invest* 1996;98:2874–2886.
8. Willow M, Gonoi T, Catterall WA. Voltage clamp analysis of the inhibitory actions of diphenylhydantoin and carbamazepine on voltage-sensitive sodium channels in neuroblastoma cells. *Mol Pharmacol* 1985;27:549–558.
9. Waxman SG. The molecular pathophysiology of pain: Abnormal expression of sodium channel genes and its contributions to hyperexcitability of primary sensory neurons. *Pain* 1999;[Suppl 6]:S133–S140.
10. Waxman SG, Cummins TR, Dib-Hajj SD, et al. Voltage-gated sodium channels and the molecular pathogenesis of pain: A review. *J Rehabil Res Dev* 2000;37:517–528.
11. Waxman SG. Acquired channelopathies in nerve injury and MS. *Neurology* 2001;56:1621–1627.
12. Lai J, Hunter JC, Porreca F. The role of voltage-gated sodium channels in neuropathic pain. *Curr Opin Neurobiol* 2003;13:291–297.
13. Akopian AN, Sivilotti L, Wood JN. A tetrodotoxin-resistant voltage-gated sodium channel expressed by sensory neurons. *Nature* 1966;379:257–262.

14. Sangameswaran L, Fish LM, Koch BD, et al. A novel tetrodotoxin-sensitive, voltage-gated sodium channel expressed in rat and human dorsal root ganglia. *J Biol Chem* 1997;272:14805–14809.
15. Waxman SG, Dib-Hajj S, Cummins TR, et al. Sodium channels and pain. *Proc Natl Acad Sci USA* 1999;96:7635–7639.
16. Blum R, Kafitz KW, Konnerth A. Neurotrophin-evoked depolarization requires the sodium channel Na(V)1.9. *Nature* 2002;419:687–693.
17. Lai J, Gold MS, Kim CS, et al. Inhibition of neuropathic pain by decreased expression of the tetrodotoxin-resistant sodium channel, NaV1.8. *Pain* 2002;95:143–152.
18. Porreca F, Lai J, Bian D, et al. A comparison of the potential role of the tetrodotoxin-insensitive sodium channels, PN3/SNS and NaN/SNS2, in rat models of chronic pain. *Proc Natl Acad Sci USA* 1999;96:7640–7644.
19. Dib-Hajj S, Black JA, Cummins TR, et al. NaN/Nav1.9: A sodium channel with unique properties. *Trends Neurosci* 2002;25:253–259.
20. Decosterd I, Ji RR, Abdi, S, et al. The pattern of expression of the voltage-gated sodium channels Na(v)1.8 and Na(v)1.9 does not change in uninjured primary sensory neurons in experimental neuropathic pain models. *Pain* 2002;96:269–277.
21. Gold MS, Weinreich D, Kim CS, et al. Redistribution of Na(V)1.8 in uninjured axons enables neuropathic pain. *J Neurosci* 2003;23:158–166.
22. Renganathan M, Cummins TR, Waxman SG. Contribution of Na(v)1.8 sodium channels to action potential electrogenesis in DRG neurons. *J Neurophysiol* 2001;86:629–640.
23. Hains BC, Klein JP, Saab CY, et al. Upregulation of sodium channel Nav1.3 and functional involvement in neuronal hyperexcitability associated with central neuropathic pain after spinal cord injury. *J Neurosci* 2003;23:8881–8892.
24. Waxman SG, Kocsis JD, Black JA. Type III sodium channel mRNA is expressed in embryonic but not adult spinal sensory neurons, and is reexpressed following axotomy. *J Neurophysiol* 1994;72:466–470.
25. Matzner O, Devor M. Na+ conductance and the threshold for repetitive neuronal firing. *Brain Res* 1992;597:92–98.
26. Matzner O, Devor M. Hyperexcitability at sites of nerve injury depends on voltage-sensitive Na+ channels. *J Neurophysiol* 1994;72:349–359.
27. Fjell J, Cummins R., Dib-Hajj SD, et al. Differential role of GDNF and NGF in the maintenance of two TTX-resistant sodium channels in adult DRG neurons. *Brain Res Mol Brain Res* 1999;67:267–282.
28. Black JA, Cummins TR, Plumpton C, et al. Upregulation of a silent sodium channel after peripheral, but not central, nerve injury in DRG neurons. *J Neurophysiol* 1999;82:2776–2785.
29. Black JA, Langworthy K, Hinson AW, et al. NGF has opposing effects on Na+ channel III and SNS gene expression in spinal sensory neurons. *Neuroreport* 1997;8:2331–2335.
30. Nassar MA, Stirling LC, Forlani G, et al. Nociceptor-specific gene deletion reveals a major role for Nav1.7 (PN1) in acute and inflammatory pain. *Proc Natl Acad Sci USA* 2004;101:12706–12711.
31. Dib-Hajj SD, Rush AM, Cummins, TR, et al. Gain-of-function mutation in Nav1.7 in familial erythromelalgia induces bursting of sensory neurons. *Brain* 2005;128:1847–1854.
32. Coward K, Plumpton C, Facer P, et al. Immunolocalization of SNS/PN3 and NaN/SNS2 sodium channels in human pain states. *Pain* 2000;85:41–50.
33. Erichsen, HK, Hao JX, Xu XJ, et al. A comparison of the antinociceptive effects of voltage-activated Na+ channel blockers in two rat models of neuropathic pain. *Eur J Pharmacol* 2003;458:275–282.
34. Veneroni O, Maj R, Calabresi M, et al. Anti-allodynic effect of NW-1029, a novel Na(+) channel blocker, in experimental animal models of inflammatory and neuropathic pain. *Pain* 2003;102:17–25.
35. Passmore GM, Selyanko AA, Mistry M, et al. KCNQ/M-currents in sensory neurons: Significance for pain therapy. *J Neurosci* 2003;23:7227–7236.
36. Blackburn-Munro G, Jensen BS. The anticonvulsant retigabine attenuates nociceptive behaviours in rat models of persistent and neuropathic pain. *Eur J Pharmacol* 2003;460:109–116.
37. Stocker M. Ca(2+)-activated K+ channels: Molecular determinants and function of the SK family. *Nat Rev Neurosci* 2004;5:758–770.
38. Bahia PK, Suzuki R, Benton DC, et al. A functional role for small-conductance calcium-activated potassium channels in sensory pathways including nociceptive processes. *J Neurosci* 2005;25:3489–3498.
39. Sindrup SH, Jensen TS. Pharmacotherapy of trigeminal neuralgia. *Clin J Pain* 2002;18:22–27.
40. Hains BC, Saab CY, Waxman SG. Changes in electrophysiological properties and sodium channel Nav1.3 expression in thalamic neurons after spinal cord injury. *Brain* 2005;128:2359–2371.
41. Fields HL, Rowbotham MC, Devor M. *Excitability Blockers: Anticonvulsants and Low Concentration Local Anesthetics in the Treatment of Chronic Pain.* In: Dickenson AH, Besson J-M, eds. London: Springer–Verlag; 1997:93–116.
42. Kochegarov AA. Pharmacological modulators of voltage-gated calcium channels and their therapeutical application. *Cell Calcium* 2003;33:145–162.
43. Matthews EA, Dickenson AH. Effects of spinally delivered N- and P-type voltage-dependent calcium channel antagonists on dorsal horn neuronal responses in a rat model of neuropathy. *Pain* 2001;92:235–246.
44. Matthews EA, Dickenson AH. Effects of ethosuximide, a T-type Ca(2+) channel blocker, on dorsal horn neuronal responses in rats. *Eur J Pharmacol* 2001;415:141–149.
45. Saegusa H, Kurihara T, Zong S, et al. Suppression of inflammatory and neuropathic pain symptoms in mice lacking the N-type Ca2+ channel. *EMBO J* 2001;20:2349–2356.
46. Luo ZD, Calcutt NA, Higuera ES, et al. Injury type-specific calcium channel alpha 2 delta-1 subunit up-regulation in rat neuropathic pain models correlates with antiallodynic effects of gabapentin. *J Pharmacol Exp Ther* 2002;303:1199–1205.
47. Atanassoff PG, Hartmannsgruber MW, Thrasher J, et al. Ziconotide, a new N-type calcium channel blocker, administered intrathecally for acute postoperative pain. *Reg Anesth Pain Med* 2000;25:274–278.
48. Backonja MM. Use of anticonvulsants for treatment of neuropathic pain. *Neurology* 2002;59:S14–S17.
49. Matthews EA, Dickenson AH. A combination of gabapentin and morphine mediates enhanced inhibitory effects on dorsal horn neuronal responses in a rat model of neuropathy. *Anesthesiology* 2002;96:633–640.
50. Luo ZD, Calcutt NA, Higuera ES, et al. Injury type-specific calcium channel alpha 2 delta-1 subunit up-regulation in rat neuropathic pain models correlates with antiallodynic effects of gabapentin. *J Pharmacol Exp Ther* 2002;303:1199–1205.
51. Newton RA, Bingham S, Case PC, et al. Dorsal root ganglion neurons show increased expression of the calcium channel alpha2delta-1 subunit following partial sciatic nerve injury. *Brain Res Mol Brain Res* 2001;95:1–8.
52. Costigan M, Befort K, Karchewski L, et al. Replicate high-density rat genome oligonucleotide microarrays reveal hundreds of regulated genes in the dorsal root ganglion after peripheral nerve injury. *BMC Neurosci* 2002; 3:16–20.
53. Wang H, Sun H, Della Penna K, et al. Chronic neuropathic pain is accompanied by global changes in gene expression and shares pathobiology with neurodegenerative diseases. *Neuroscience* 2002;114:529–546.
54. Xiao HS, Huang QH, Zhang FX, et al. Identification of gene expression profile of dorsal root ganglion in the rat peripheral axotomy model of neuropathic pain. *Proc Natl Acad Sci USA* 2002;99:8360–8365.
55. Valder CR, Liu JJ, Song YH, et al. Coupling gene chip analyses and rat genetic variances in identifying potential target genes that may contribute to neuropathic allodynia development. *J Neurochem* 2003;87:560–573.
56. Williams ME, Brust PF, Feldman DH, et al. Structure and functional expression of an omega-conotoxin-sensitive human N-type calcium channel. *Science* 1992;257:389–395.
57. Li CY, Zhang XL, Matthews EA, et al. Calcium channel $\alpha_2\delta_1$ subunit mediates spinal hyperexcitability in pain modulation. *Pain* 2006;125:20–34.
58. Suzuki R, Morcuende S, Webber M, et al. Superficial NK1-expressing neurons control spinal excitability through activation of descending pathways. *Nat Neurosci* 2002;5:1319–1326.
59. Nichols M, Allen B, Rogers S, et al. Transmission of chronic nociception by spinal neurons expressing the substance P receptor. *Science* 1999;286:1558–1561.
60. Suzuki R, Rahman W, Rygh LJ, et al. Spinal-supraspinal serotonergic circuits regulating neuropathic pain and its treatment with gabapentin. *Pain* 2005;117:292–303.
61. Suzuki R, Rygh LJ, Dickenson AH. Bad news from the brain: Descending 5-HT pathways that control spinal pain processing. *Trends Pharmacol Sci* 2004;25:613–617.
62. Oatway M, Chen Y, Weaver L. The 5-HT3 receptor facilitates at-level mechanical allodynia following spinal cord injury. *Pain* 2004;110:259–268.
63. Donovan-Rodriguez T, Dickenson AH, Urch CE. Gabapentin normalizes spinal neuronal responses that correlate with behavior in a rat model of cancer-induced bone pain. *Anesthesiology* 2005;102:132–140.
64. Rowbotham M, Harden N, Stacey B, et al. Gabapentin for the treatment of postherpetic neuralgia: A randomized controlled trial. *JAMA* 1988;280:1837–1842.

CHAPTER 34 ■ NEUROCHEMICAL AND NEUROPHYSIOLOGIC EFFECTS OF NEEDLE INSERTION: CLINICAL IMPLICATIONS

MICHAEL J. BUTLER AND PHILIP J. SIDDALL

This chapter surveys the effects of needle insertion per se, with an emphasis on controlled animal studies of the neurochemical and neurophysiologic consequences of transdermal needling, particularly analgesia. Human research on the effects of transcutaneous needle insertion, and analgesia in particular, is complicated by the challenge of establishing an appropriate control intervention to isolate the objective effects of needle insertion from other factors such as the placebo response. The placebo response, in turn linked to other factors such as expectation, may play a significant role in the clinical consequences of needling (1,2). Psychological influences upon analgesia, and the placebo effect specifically, are discussed in detail by Katz and Melzack, and Finniss and Benedetti, respectively, in the next two chapters of this volume.

The effects of needle insertion per se during regional anesthetic techniques are difficult if not impossible to ascertain, as active and control groups typically undergo needle insertion at identical skin entry points followed by injection of saline or inactive placebo through the needle (or no solution, in instances of sham injection). Therefore, this chapter emphasizes the substantial basic and clinical evidence amassed during studies of acupuncture. The authors of this chapter were both trained in clinical acupuncture in Beijing, China, then in subsequent years proceeded with initial skepticism to apply this technique to treat a range of disorders. Our practical experience indicated apparently beneficial effects but also noxious side effects that may be of relevance to needle insertion by the regional anesthetist. Controlled animal research on acupuncture analgesia reveals diverse and widespread neurochemical and neurophysiologic effects of needle insertion, beyond simply placebo and nocebo analgesic responses.

Acupuncture is defined as "pricking with a needle, specifically the insertion of needles into living tissues for remedial purposes, other than for the injection of drugs" (3). To *prick* is to "pierce slightly, puncture, or perforate, especially with a fine or sharp point," and to *pierce* is to "penetrate as a sharp pointed instrument does, or to make a hole, opening, or tunnel into or through (something), to bore through or perforate, make (a hole, etc.) by pricking or stabbing with a sharp pointed instrument" (3).

These definitions are important as, too easily, acupuncture is believed to be inseparable from traditional Chinese medical teachings and Oriental medical philosophy that describe presumptive lines of energy (meridians), empirically specifying needle insertion at precise points, and often specifying the type of needle stimulation to be used, either manual or thermal (moxibustion). Yet, one need not practice traditional Chinese medicine to deliver acupuncture treatment.

Most of the animal research summarized below is from Professor Han Ji-Sheng's laboratory at Beijing Medical College. Over many years, this research program elucidated the neurochemical basis of acupuncture analgesia using rigorous experimental and analytical methodology. Although initially these studies were published in Chinese scientific and medical journals in the Chinese language, steadily increasing numbers of publications in this area have appeared in peer-reviewed, English-language scientific and medical journals. We accept that animal research is not devoid of a placebo effect, nor, in relation to pain, is the confounding effect of stress-induced analgesia. Likewise recognizing progressive advances in trial design and experimental rigor of clinical trials in acupuncture, we will adopt a "best available evidence" approach to our survey of relevant clinical trials.

MECHANISMS UNDERLYING NEEDLING EFFECTS

Early Acupuncture Research

The animal research program into acupuncture analgesia (AA) was initiated by Han and colleagues in an effort to understand the results of a human observational study (4,5). The effect of acupuncture on the pain threshold was explored in 66 healthy volunteers and 22 nonstimulated controls, as well as smaller numbers of patients with paraplegia and hemiplegia following strokes ($n = 13$ and 12, respectively). A modified potassium iontophoresis method delivering progressively increasing anodal currents through skin electrodes was employed to produce graded nociceptive stimuli. Eight points, distributed over various sites on the body including the forehead and back, and paired points on the chest, abdomen, and legs, received nociceptive stimuli. Pain thresholds were measured every 10 minutes over 80 minutes, and expressed as a percentage change from baseline in the intensity of electrical current tolerated. Acupuncture (unilateral needle insertion into the thenar eminence at the site of maximal thickness) was given over 15 minutes. A statistically significant increase in pain threshold occurred at all measurement sites, maximal at about 40 minutes and declining rapidly (half-life 16.2 +/- 1.9 minutes) when acupuncture ceased. No significant rise in pain threshold occurred in the unstimulated control group.

The slow increases in pain threshold induced by acupuncture, and the production of a bilateral analgesic effect following unilateral needling, suggested the hypothesis that acupuncture evoked the release of certain chemical substances within the body that in turn produced the analgesic effect. Acupuncture analgesia was blocked by local infiltration of procaine at the site of thenar stimulation, and also was absent when the insensate extremities of paraplegic or hemiplegic patients were stimulated. These observations indicated that afferent impulses to the central nervous system (CNS) were necessary for optimal AA, and led to the decision to focus on the chemistry of the CNS in future planned controlled animal research.

A cerebroventricular perfusion model was developed in rabbits (6) exposed to "finger acupuncture" (i.e., repetitive manual stimulation with the fingers) of the Achilles tendon near its attachment. In fact, either needling of a specific point just distal to the knee or repetitive finger pressure at the Achilles tendon insertion brought about a similar increase in thermal pain threshold of the debristled skin around the nostrils and mouth, indicated by a prolonged latency of head withdrawal. Stainless steel cannulae were stereotactically inserted under general anesthesia with their tips in the lateral cerebral ventricle, thereby allowing withdrawal or infusion of cerebrospinal fluid (CSF). Connection between a donor and recipient rabbit was made with polyethylene tubing between the cannulae, thereby allowing transfer of CSF from donor to recipient rabbits. The tubing was perfused with ice-cold saline to reduce catabolism. In the experimental model, the donor was given finger acupuncture for 30 minutes, and CSF was transferred from donor to the unstimulated recipient. A statistically significant increase in the pain threshold of the recipient occurred, although not as marked as in the donor. This effect was compared with the control experiment of CSF transfer from an unstimulated donor to an unstimulated recipient (Fig. 34-1).

This observation suggested that chemicals with analgesic effect were produced in the brain of the donor rabbit in the course of acupuncture stimulation. Intracerebroventricular (ICV) injection of reserpine enhanced and prolonged the analgesic effect of finger acupuncture. This effect was reversed by ICV replacement of norepinephrine/noradrenaline or dopamine, suggesting that augmentation of finger acupuncture analgesia by reserpine may be related to its effect of depleting monoamines in the brain. Intracerebroventricular injection of atropine significantly reduced the effect of finger acupuncture analgesia, presumably by blocking the muscarinic effect of acetylcholine in the brain. Morphine analgesia and finger acupuncture analgesia were compared: ICV injection of reserpine blocked the analgesic effect of morphine while augmenting that of finger acupuncture analgesia. Intracerebroventricular injection of atropine also blocked morphine analgesia, while substantially reducing finger acupuncture analgesia, suggesting differences between the underlying mechanisms of morphine analgesia and finger acupuncture analgesia.

From 1973, Han and colleagues studied the role of central neurotransmitters in AA, the main questions being: Does needle insertion (acupuncture) bring about any change in the content and turnover rate of central neurotransmitters? Could the effect of AA be modified by selective alteration of these neurotransmitters? For each type of neurotransmitter, the nature of its effect on AA was determined both qualitatively (i.e., facilitatory or inhibitory) and quantitatively (magnitude of effect, dose response, and time course). The site of action in the CNS was also studied.

Animal Models of Acupuncture Analgesia

Two major animal models of AA were studied:

■ The rabbit finger acupuncture model just described, with finger acupuncture to the Achilles tendon attachment and nociceptive (radiant heat) stimuli to the snout or tail, measuring the avoidance response latency (ARL) (7)
■ The rat tail flick model, with radiant heat stimuli either to the lower leg or the tail and tail flick as the response. The nociceptive threshold is measured as tail flick latency (TFL) in seconds between the application of the heat stimulus and withdrawal of the tail (8).

NEUROCHEMICAL BASIS OF ACUPUNCTURE ANALGESIA

A seminal review by Han, co-authored with Terenius of the University of Uppsala, Sweden, was published in 1982 (9). This comprehensive introduction to the complexity of the neurochemical basis of AA emphasized controlled animal research and provided extensive ($n = 193$) references. This large number of references was provided to raise awareness of much of the prior research that had been published in Chinese- and Japanese-language journals not easily accessible to the Western scientific community. The emphasis on research paper selection in this chapter will be on peer-reviewed English-language publications.

Serotonin

To evaluate the effect of ascending serotonergic pathways, 5-6-dihydroxytryptamine (5-6DHT), a chemical depleter of neuronal serotonin (5-hydroxytryptamine, 5HT), was injected into the medial forebrain bundles of rats. A significant reduction in the magnitude of AA occurred, together with selective lowering of forebrain 5HT content, implying that ascending serotonergic fibers may play an important part in mediating the effect of AA (10).

In a study in the rabbit, cinanserin, which blocks the post synaptic 5HT receptor, was injected into the periaqueductal gray (PAG) bilaterally at a dose sufficiently low not to affect basal nociceptive threshold in either electroacupuncture (EA) or morphine analgesia (MA) experiments. The analgesic effect induced by EA and morphine was markedly reduced, suggesting involvement of serotonergic synaptic transmission in the PAG area for EA and morphine analgesia. The site specificity of this effect was also suggested by the observations that bilateral injection was more effective than unilateral injection, and that injection beyond the area of the PAG was ineffective.

In a later study in the rat, an immunocytochemical double-staining technique was used to investigate the effects of EA on the expression of c-fos oncogene in the serotonergic neurons in the nucleus raphe dorsalis (NRD) (11). The number of c-fos positive serotonergic cells in the NRD increased significantly after EA stimulation. Further studies in the rat implicated 5HT receptor subtypes in spinal antinociception (12) and characterized the relevant 5HT receptor subtypes mediating supraspinal μ-opioid–induced analgesia (13).

Repeated or prolonged EA results in a gradual decrease in the analgesic effect in the rat (14). Such EA tolerance and its cross-tolerance to MA can be partially reversed by ICV injection of 5-hydroxytryptophan (5HTP), the precursor of

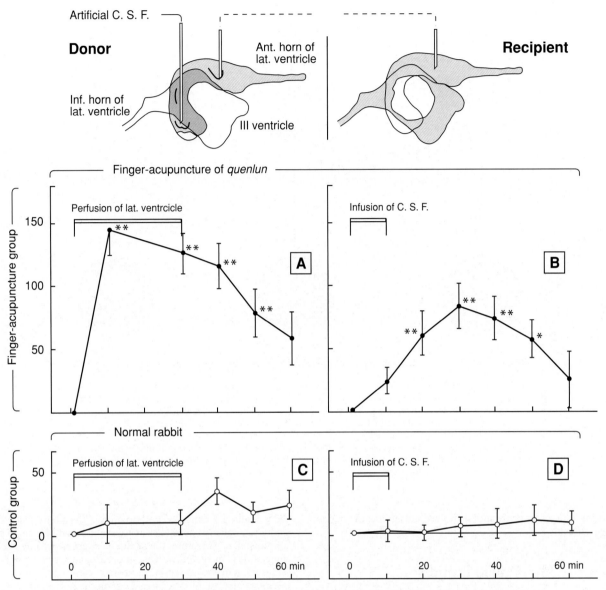

FIGURE 34-1. The effect of finger acupuncture analgesia in cerebrospinal fluid perfusion experiments. From Research Group of Acupuncture Anaesthesia, Peking Medical College, Peking. The role of some neurotransmitters of brain in finger-acupuncture analgesia. *Scientia Sinica* 1974;17:112–130, with permission.

5HT (15). However, no depletion in cerebral 5HT occurred, nor did any decrease in the number of 5HT receptors in the brain of the EA-tolerant animal occur. These negative findings suggest that EA tolerance is likely to be complex and multifactorial. Tolerance to EA analgesia in the rabbit can be reversed by microinjection of 5HT into the nuclei accumbens (16) (Fig. 34-2).

Catecholamines

A series of observations in rat and rabbit suggest that the actions of dopamine and norepinephrine (also called noradrenaline) are antagonistic to AA (17–19). Intracerebroventricular injection of apomorphine, a dopamine receptor agonist, reduced the effect of AA, whereas spiroperidol, a dopamine re-

ceptor antagonist, increased the effect of AA. Selective destruction of ascending noradrenergic fibers by bilateral microinjection of 6-hydroxydopamine (6-OHDA), the chemical depleter of neuronal noradrenaline, into the medial forebrain bundles in rats reduced the cerebral norepinephrine content and significantly increased the effect of AA. Intraperitoneal injection of norepinephrine, which increases the norepinephrine level in the blood but not in the brain, had no significant effect on AA. This implies that intracerebral norepinephrine antagonizes the effect of AA.

In experiments with rabbits, ICV injection of the α_2-adrenergic agonist clonidine antagonized AA, whereas the α_1-adrenergic antagonist phentolamine augmented it. Corresponding results were observed after intraperitoneal injection of these two drugs in rats. Rabbits given ICV injection of the β-adrenergic receptor agonist isoproterenol or the β-adrenergic

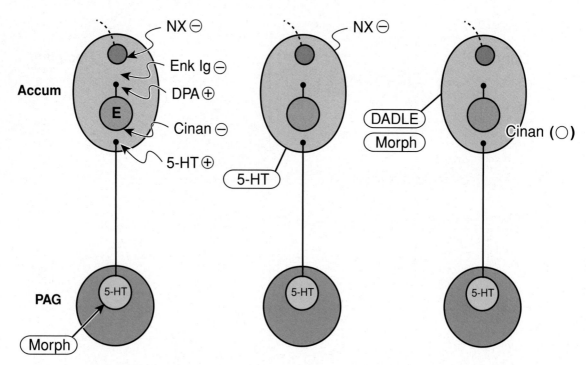

FIGURE 34-2. Diagram summarizing results obtained from studies investigating opioid and serotonin (5HT) involvement. Antinociception induced by injecting morphine (morph) into the periaqueductal gray (PAG) can be modified by drugs administered in the nucleus accumbens (ACCUM): blockade by cinanserin (Cinan), naloxone (NX), or enkephalin IgG (Enk Igg); potentiation by 5HT or D phenylalanine (DPA). Antinociception induced by injecting 5HT into the nucleus accumbens was blocked by naloxone injected into the same site, whereas the antinociceptive effect induced by morphine or [D-Ala2,D-Leu5] enkephalin (DADLE) in the nucleus accumbens was not affected by cinanserin administered in the same site. E, enkephalinergic neuron; ⊕, potentiation; ⊖, blockade; o, no effect. From Xuan YT, Shi YS, Zhou, ZF, Han JS. Studies on the mesolimbic loop of antinociception-II. A serotonin-enkpehalin interaction in the nucleus accumbens. *Neuroscience* 1986;19:403–409, with permission.

receptor antagonist propranolol showed no significant change in AA effect.

Opioid Peptides

The discovery of the opioid peptides in 1975, followed by the progressive definition of families of opioid peptides, was a major advance in the understanding of many forms of analgesia. Han and colleagues studied the effect on AA and morphine analgesia in rabbits of ICV microinjection of naloxone into specific brain sites (20). Localization studies determined that the nuclei accumbens, amygdala, habenula, and PAG are particularly important sites at which endogenous opioids exert their analgesic effects. Electroacupuncture analgesia and morphine analgesia involve both spinal and supraspinal mechanisms, with confirmatory evidence for this from spinally transected rats (21).

The endogenous opioid peptide enkephalin is known to be degraded mainly by two enzymes: the dipeptidyl carboxypeptidase enkephalinase, and aminopeptidase. Microinjection of the enkephalinase inhibitor thiorphan or the aminopeptidase inhibitor bestatin into the nucleus accumbens of the rabbit produced a dose-dependent analgesic effect (22). This analgesic effect was completely reversed by naloxone and by antibodies against met-enkephalin administered at the same site. Antibodies against leu-enkephalin were not effective. Moreover, microinjection of thiorphan or bestatin into the nucleus accum-

bens resulted in a marked potentiation of the after-effect of EA-induced analgesia, as well as analgesia induced by a small dose of morphine. Therefore, the analgesic effect elicited by EA and morphine is mediated, at least in part, by met-enkephalin–like substances in the nucleus accumbens.

Particular attention was focused on the potent analgesic effect of the endogenous analgesic peptide dynorphin injected into the subarachnoid space of the spinal cord of the rat (23–25). Site specificity was shown, in that spinal cord (intrathecal) injection of dynorphin A (1–13) potentiated morphine analgesia whereas brain (ICV) injection antagonized it (26). Intrathecal injection of dynorphin in the rabbit elicited marked analgesia, as measured by TFL, reversible by naloxone, and intrathecal injection of antidynorphin antibody reduced AA by 77%, with the effect lasting for at least 4 hours. No analgesia resulted from dynorphin injection in the PAG, nor was EA analgesia blocked by antidynorphin antibody injected into the PAG. These results suggest that dynorphin reduces nocifensive responses by acting at the spinal cord, and it may play an important role in mediating EA analgesia at the spinal level (27).

Han and colleagues have used highly specific antisera, or the immunoglobulin (Ig)G fractions of such antisera, injected by ICV, intranuclear, or intrathecal routes, to inactivate the target neuropeptides released into the synaptic clefts, leaving the other neuropeptides intact to act on their relevant receptors. The pilot experiments on rats were done "blind": antisera or their IgG fractions against met-enkephalin, β-endorphin, dynorphin, and substance P (SP), together with normal rabbit sera, were sent coded from Terenius at Uppsala University to Beijing Medical College. Injections were given intrathecally or into the PAG of the rabbit to assess their effect upon AA. Similar experiments were performed in collaboration with Goldstein at Stanford University, and Herz and Hollt at the Max Planck Institute of Psychiatry in Munich (28–33). The results indicate that β-endorphin mediates the effect of AA in the PAG, but not in the spinal cord, dynorphin mediates AA in the spinal cord but not in the PAG, and met-enkephalin contributes to AA through actions both in the brain and in the spinal cord.

A later experiment demonstrated involvement of endogenous orphanin FQ (OFQ) in EA analgesia (34). The results suggested that endogenous OFQ exerts a tonic antagonistic effect on EA analgesia, but no such antagonism was observed with intrathecal injection of OFQ. It appeared that spinal OFQ produced a marked analgesic effect and enhanced EA analgesia, consistent with the experimental results in rats, in which morphine analgesia is antagonized by ICV OFQ and potentiated by intrathecal OFQ.

Substance P

Early data in the rat (30), summarized in a review from Han and colleagues (34), indicated that EA releases SP in the PAG, which then accelerates the release of met-enkephalin to produce an antinociceptive effect. In contrast to the actions of SP in the brain, intrathecal injections of SP antiserum augment the effect of AA, consistent with SP's putative role as a neurotransmitter in primary afferent neurons and candidate for nociceptive transmission at the spinal level. Substance P may therefore be regarded as a neurotransmitter playing opposite roles in different parts of the CNS in mediating the effect of AA.

γ-Aminobutyric Acid

Although γ-aminobutyric acid is an important inhibitory neurotransmitter in the CNS, work to date has addressed only its effect on AA (34,35). First, in the rat, intraperitoneal injection of 3-mercaptopropionic acid (3-MP), which blocks both the synthesis and release of GABA, results in a marked potentiation of the effect of AA. The potentiating effect of 3-MP is completely abolished by prior administration of the GABA degrading enzyme inhibitor amino-oxoacetic acid (AOAA). Second, elevation of cerebral GABA content by AOAA is accompanied by a decrease in the effect of AA. This inhibitory effect of AOAA is reversed by the GABA receptor blocker bicuculline methochloride. Third, ICV injection of another GABA-transaminase inhibitor, γ-vinyl-GABA (GVG), produced a fourfold increase in cerebral GABA content and an associated 80% decrease in the effect of AA 12 to 24 hours after ICV GVG administration. A negative correlation was found between the cerebral GABA content and the effectiveness of AA (r = 0.78, p <0.01).

To locate the sites of action for GABA's antagonism of AA, compounds affecting GABA metabolism were injected into the PAG of the rat. Intra-PAG injection of 0.4 μmol of 3-MP produced a 193% increase in the effect of AA, whereas 0.5 to 1.0 nmol of the GABAergic agonist muscimol or 0.1 μmol of GVG reduced the EA effect by more than half. These results suggest that the PAG is one of the target areas for GABA to suppress AA. The GABAergic pathway from habenula to dorsal raphe has been implicated for this effect (36).

Spinal cord GABA does not seem to be involved in the mechanisms of AA; for example, no significant effect on AA was found even when a tenfold dose of 3-MP (5 μmol) was injected intrathecally into the rat (Fig. 34-3).

Cholecystokinin Octapeptide

Considerable experimental evidence from the rat suggests that cholecystokinin octapeptide (CCK-8) provides negative feedback that modulates opioid analgesia (37). Evidence supporting this proposed role of CCK-8 in AA includes:

■ *Suppression of opioid analgesia by CCK-8.*   Rats given EA (15 Hz, 3 V) at specific sites on the hind legs for 10 minutes developed analgesia, as determined by a prolongation of TFL at the end of EA stimulation, an effect that is decreased in a dose-dependent fashion by CCK-8 administered ICV or intrathecally. Antagonism of EA analgesia by CCK-8 was also observed in electrophysiologic and neurochemical studies (38). Electroacupuncture analgesia was shown to inhibit the activity of excitatory nociceptive neurons in the nucleus parafascicularis of the rat and to excite inhibitory nociceptive neurons. These effects of EA were abolished by ICV injection of CCK-8, confirming the results obtained in intact rats that CCK-8 serves as a powerful endogenous modulator antagonizing the antinociceptive effect of EA stimulation (Fig. 34-4).
■ *Potentiation of opioid analgesia by CCK antagonist.* Electroacupuncture stimulation in the rat produced a marked increase of CCK-8 immunoreactivity in spinal cord perfusate (39). The increase was greatest in response to EA of 100 Hz and 15 Hz, and less marked in response to 2 Hz. Since CCK-8 has been shown to possess potent antiopioid activity at the spinal level, blockade of the spinal CCK effect would be expected to potentiate EA-induced analgesia, which is known to be opioid mediated. Intrathecal administration of the CCK-B antagonist L-365,260 did not by itself influence TFL but potentiated EA-induced analgesia in a dose- and frequency-dependent manner. This potentiation was most marked at a dose range of 2.5 to 5.0 ng intrathecally, and at a frequency rank order of 100 Hz >15 Hz >2 Hz. The results suggest that an increased release of CCK-8 following EA may limit the effect of opioid peptides, and that the CCK-B receptor mediates the antiopioid effect of CCK-8 in rat spinal cord.
■ *Reversal of opioid tolerance by CCK-8 antiserum.* As noted, the analgesic effect of EA in the rat was dose-dependently antagonized by ICV or intrathecal injection of CCK-8 (40). This effect had an immediate onset and lasted for at least 4 hours. CCK-8 alone, however, did not affect baseline TFL. Rats subjected to prolonged EA developed tolerance to EA as well as cross-tolerance to morphine. These tolerances could be postponed or reversed by ICV or intrathecal injection of antiserum against CCK-8. Although CCK-8 antagonized opioid analgesia, it did not affect analgesia induced by 5HT or norepinephrine. Moreover, CCK-8 antiserum did not alter the baseline nociceptive responses, nor did it potentiate EA analgesia in naïve rats. It was concluded that prolonged EA stimulation results in a substantial release of endogenous opioids that in turn evoke the release of CCK-8 in the CNS, dampening the opioid component of EA analgesia. This mechanism may mediate, at least in part, the development of EA tolerance. Research in relation to EA tolerance accompanying repeated needle insertion is not reviewed in this chapter, given its focus upon neural blockade.

PART IV: PAIN MANAGEMENT

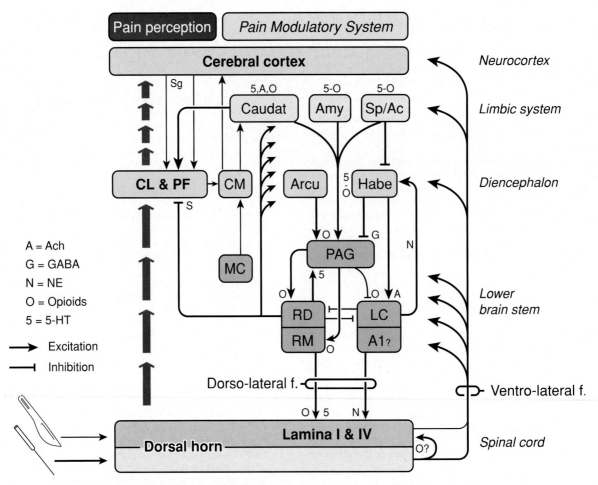

FIGURE 34-3. Possible mechanisms of acupuncture analgesia. *A1*, perikarya of noradrenergic neurons with descending fibers to the spinal cord; *Ac*, nucleus accumbens; *Amy*, amygdala; *Arcu*, arcuate nucleus; *Caudat*, caudate nucleus; CL, controlateralis nucleus of the hypothalamus; *CM*, nucleus centromedianus of the hypothalamus; *Habe*, habenular nucleus; *LC*, locus coeruleus; *MC*, nucleus megalocellularis; *PAG*, periaqueductal gray; *Pf*, nucleus parafascicularis; *RD*, nucleus raphe dorsalis; *RM*, nucleus raphe magnus; *Sp*, septum. From Han JS. Physiologic and neurochemical basis of acupuncture analgesia. In: Cheng TO, ed. *The International Textbook of Cardiology.* New York: Pergamon, 1986:1124–1132, with permission.

■ *Augmentation of CCK-8 released by EA stimulation.* There is evidence both for short-term and prolonged EA that a prompt release of CCK-8 occurs within 30 to 60 minutes. The naloxone reversibility of this CCK-8 release suggests that it is a negative feedback mechanism triggered by opioid receptor activation (41). To determine whether prolonged morphine or EA stimulation augments expression of the gene coding for pre-pro CCK, levels of CCK-mRNA were examined in rats (37,42). The results indicate that continuous EA may induce active transcription of the CCK gene at 8 hours after beginning EA. The concurrent increase of brain CCK content is most probably due to an increase in the enzymatic processing of the preexisting CCK precursor rather than de novo synthesis.

■ *Intracerebral transfer of CCK gene vector decreases the effectiveness EA analgesia.* If CCK-8 in the CNS antagonizes opioid analgesia, one might expect rats with low levels of CCK in the CNS to be highly responsive to EA stimulation. The P77 PMC rat, a breed with audiogenic seizure developed at Beijing Medical College by Pei and colleagues in 1977, has half the content of immunoreactive CCK-8 in

the cerebral cortex and hippocampus compared with derivative Wistar rats (43). P77 PMC rats were demonstrated to be remarkably good responders to AA. Regression analysis showed a positive correlation between the susceptibility to audiogenic seizure and the effectiveness of EA analgesia. The CCK-B antagonist L-365,260, which potentiates EA analgesia in Wistar rats, was not as effective in P77 PMC rats, consistent with reduced CCK-8 in the latter breed (44,45).

If a low CCK-8 content in CNS is the common denominator underlying the high susceptibility of audiogenic seizures and high effectiveness of EA analgesia, normalization of these two parameters would be expected upon reversal by genetic engineering techniques of the congenitally low expression of CCK-8 in the CNS. A p SV2-CCK vector carrying an insertive CCK cDNA in the p SV2 plasmid was constructed and encapsulated within lipofectin (46). An ICV injection of the plasmid–lipofectin complex was given to P77 PMC rats. Using the reporter gene Lacz, instead of CCK cDNA, blue staining of x-Gal appeared in large amounts in the ependymal cells distributed throughout the brain tissue.

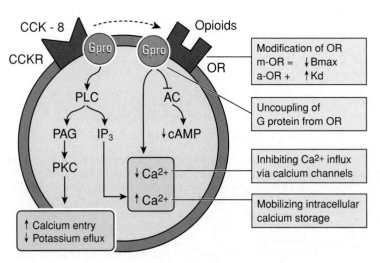

FIGURE 34-4. Possible mechanisms of the antiopioid effect of CCK-8. *AC*, adenyl cyclase; *CCKR*, CCK receptor; *DAG*, diacyl glycerol; *G pro*, G protein; *IP3*, inositol triphosphate; *PKC*, protein kinase C; *PLC*, phospholipases C; $\uparrow$, increase; $\downarrow$, decrease. From Han JS. Molecular events underlying the anti-opioid effect of cholecystokinin octapeptide (CCK-8) in the central nervous system. In: Cuello AC, Collier B, eds. *Pharmacological Sciences: Perspectives for Research and Therapy in the Late 1990s*. Basel: Birkhauser, 1995:199–207, with permission.

The staining was most prominent at days 2 to 4 after ICV injection, and disappeared after 2 to 3 weeks, indicating the time course of expression of the foreign gene in the CNS. Behavioral studies showed concurrent reductions of seizure susceptibility and the effectiveness of EA analgesia in rats receiving p SV2-CCK vector as compared with control rats receiving the empty p SV2 vector (47). The suppressive effects were most marked at days 2 to 4, and returned to normal by days 7 to 12. The implication from this gene transfer experiment is that responders and nonresponders to EA are inter convertible, depending on the balance between the opposing factors influencing these specific behavioral responses.

Taken in total, the evidence indicates that CCK-8 mediates an important negative feedback control mechanism for opioid analgesia. More recent studies have shown that CCK-8 reverses the inhibitory effect induced by EA on C5-evoked discharges in the spinal cord dorsal horn of the rat; that CCK antisense RNA increases the analgesic effect of EA or low-dose morphine, thereby converting low-responder rats into high responders; and that rats with decreased brain CCK levels show increased responsiveness to peripheral EA analgesia (48) (Table 34-1).

FACTORS INFLUENCING THE RESPONSE TO NEEDLING

Frequency-dependent Differential Release of Central Nervous System Opioid Peptides

It was found that 2-Hz EA triggers the release of enkephalins and β-endorphin in the brain and spinal cord, which interacts with the μ- and δ-opioid receptors in the CNS. However, 100-Hz stimulation selectively increases the release of dynorphin in the spinal cord, which interacts with κ-opioid receptors in the spinal cord dorsal horn (49–53) (Fig. 34-5).

More specific studies provide evidence for the differential release of enkephalins in the CNS by low- versus high-frequency EA, attenuation of low- but not high-frequency EA analgesia following microinjection of β-endorphin antiserum into the PAG in rats (54), and tolerance and cross-tolerance to 2-Hz or 100-Hz EA in rats with focal analgesic electrical stimulation of the hypothalamic arcuate nucleus (55,56). The

TABLE 34-1

THE ROLE OF SOME CENTRAL NEUROTRANSMITTERS IN ACUPUNCTURE ANALGESIA

	Brain (PAG)	Spinal cord
5-hydroxytryptamine	+	+
Met-enkephalin	+	+
β-endorphin	+	0
Dynorphin A & B	0	+
Sustance P	+	−
Noradrenaline	−	+
GABA	−	0
CCK-8	−	−

+: potentiation; −: attenuation; 0: no effect.
(from Han 1984).

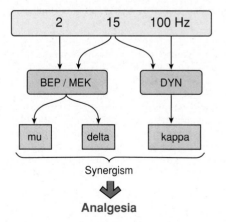

FIGURE 34-5. Activation of different endogenous opioids by different electroacupuncture stimulation frequencies. *BEP*, β-endorphin; *MEK*, met enkephalin; *DYN*, dynorphin. From Han JS, Sun S. Frequency dependence of opioid EA-induced analgesia. *Acupuncture: The Scientific International Journal* 1990;1:19–27, with permission.

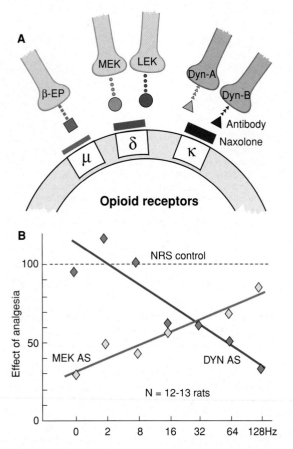

FIGURE 34-6. Diagram of antibody binding to neuropeptides versus blockade of receptor for analysis of synaptic events. **A:** Opioid peptides released from nerve terminals, for example β-endorphin (β-EP); met-enkephalin (MEK); leu-enkephalin (LEK); dynorphin A (Dyn-A); and dynorphin B (Dyn-B) can be selectively bound by specific antibodies recognizing corresponding neuropeptides that prevent receptor activation. Naloxone works through receptor blockade, which does not differentiate the chemical nature of the ligand. **B:** Blockade of analgesic effect of low- and high-frequency electroacupuncture (EA) by intrathecal injection of antiserum against MEK (*MEK AS*) or dynorphin-A (*DYN AS*) respectively. Data were normalized with normal rabbit serum (NRS) control group as 100%. From Han JS, Sun S. Frequency dependence of opioid EA-induced analgesia. *Acupuncture: The Scientific International Journal* 1990;1:19–27, with permission.

diencephalon seems to be a cardinal neural focus for mediating 2-Hz but not 100-Hz EA-induced rat TFL prolongation (57); electrolyte-induced or kainic acid lesions in the ventral PAG of the rat leading to significant attenuation (compared with sham-operated animals) of both low- and high-frequency EA analgesia was measured 4 and 6 days after the lesion in conscious rats (58). A similar experimental procedure relating to the parabrachial nucleus led to significant attenuation of high-frequency EA analgesia but no effect on low-frequency EA analgesia or sham-operated rats (59) (Fig. 34-6).

More recent research showed endomorphin-1 mediates 2-Hz but not 100-Hz EA analgesia in the rat (60) and that endomorphin and μ-opioid receptors in mouse brain mediate the analgesic effect induced by 2-Hz but not 100-Hz EA stimulation (61). Two studies focused on brain substrates activated by EA of different frequencies, the first being a comparative study on the expression of the gene c-fos, a nonspecific marker of

neuronal activation, and different genes coding for three opioid peptides (preproenkephalin [PPE], preprodynorphin [PPD], and proopiomelanocortin [POMC]) (62). The second studied the role of Fos and Jun proteins in EA-induced transcription of PPE and PPD genes (63).

Low versus High Responders for Electroacupuncture Analgesia

Observations in large numbers of rats exposed to EA by Han and colleagues suggest a bimodal distribution of its analgesic effect. Cluster analysis shows two distinct groups: one with an increase of TFL not exceeding 50% (low responders, LR), and the other with an increase of TFL from 50% to 150% (high responders, HR). Rats have stable responses, at least when retested within 2 days. Interestingly, parallelism is seen between LR and HR to EA and sensitivity to systemic morphine analgesia.

Low responsivity to EA reflects several mechanisms at least. First, there may be diminished release of CNS opioid peptides and/or reduced density of CNS opioid receptors. Peets and Pomeranz identified that CXBK mice, known to be deficient in opioid receptors, had low analgesic responsivity to EA (64). Second, there may be enhanced release of CCK-8, which, as already discussed, is a potent antiopioid. An LR rat can be changed into an HR by intracerebral injection of CCK antisense RNA into the brain to block the expression of the gene coding for CCK (65), or by the intracerebral administration of the compound L-365,260, an antagonist to the CCK-B receptor (66).

In the P77 PMC rat, genetically prone to audiogenic seizures, and (as discussed earlier) expressing decreased central levels of CCK, EA had a greater and more prolonged analgesic effect upon TFL than control rats in response to 100-Hz peripheral electrical stimulation. The magnitude of stimulation-produced analgesia correlated with the vulnerability to audiogenic seizures. Radioimmunoassay showed CCK-8 content was significantly lower in cerebral cortex, hippocampus, and PAG in P77 PMC rats than in controls, and parenterally administered CCK-8 blocked EA in the former group, consistent with the already-described role of CCK-8 as an endogenous opioid antagonist (67).

GENETICS AND ACUPUNCTURE ANALGESIA RESPONSE

A recent study of the genetic influence on AA in the mouse examined 10 common inbred strains. The results suggested a role for inherited genetic factors in AA in the mouse, although the low to moderate heritability estimates suggest that environmental factors also modulate the degree of AA response (68). A further study evaluated the characteristics of AA in the mice using three inbred and three outbred strains. Results showed that (a) DBA/Z mice showed the greatest analgesic effect of all strains in response to both 2- and 100-Hz EA; (b) AA increased as the intensity of stimulation increased from 0.5 to 2.0 mA, but it remained at this plateau when the intensity was increased from 2.0 to 3.0 mA; (c) 10 mg/kg naloxone was needed to block the analgesic effect induced by 2.0-Hz EA of 2.0 mA, but to block that from 100-Hz, 25 mg/kg was needed; (d) a positive correlation was observed between analgesia induced by morphine 5 mg/kg and by 100-Hz EA in two tested strains (DBA/2 and C57BL/6J). In conclusion, EA induces reliable, albeit strain-dependent analgesia in mice. The naloxone reversibility of EA, a measure of whether it is opioid or non–opioid mediated, is dependent upon intensity and frequency (69).

OTHER ACUPUNCTURE RESEARCH

Involvement of Different Afferent Fiber Types

It is likely that Aβ- and Aδ-fibers are the most important of the afferent fibers mediating the analgesic response of the CNS to needle insertion. A study in the awake rat using c-fos expression as an indicator of nociceptive processing in the rat dorsal spinal cord showed that formalin-induced c-fos expression can be almost totally abolished by topical application of capsaicin on the sciatic nerve. In the presence of C-fiber dysfunction, EA applied at the leg points of the rat was still able to induce antinociception, using TFL as the measure of nociception (70).

Diffuse Noxious Inhibitory Controls

Diffuse noxious inhibitory controls (DNIC) are triggered by stimulation of peripheral Aδ- and C-fibers; involve brain structures of the lower medulla, including the subnucleus reticularis dorsalis (SRD); and are mediated by descending pathways in the dorsolateral funiculi. Combined measurements of psychophysical and nociceptive reflex responses (RIII) in normal volunteers and patients with spinal cord or brain lesions indicate equivalent, even identical or inhibitory processes in man. Experimental data in both animals and humans support the concept that these mechanisms could be triggered by needle insertion to produce hypoalgesia (71) (Fig. 34-7).

Long-term Potentiation and Depression

Long-term potentiation, the facilitation of neuronal responses to repetitive input, is an important physiologic substrate of memory formation. A form of long-term potentiation within the dorsal horn of the spinal cord has recently been identified as a component of central nociceptive sensitization (72). A reverse phenomenon has also been observed, termed long-term depression; that is, the ability of prior afferent stimulation to attenuate responses to subsequent inputs.

The characteristics of the afferent stimulation determine whether long-term potentiation or long-term depression predominates. Long-term potentiation is a consequence of sustained, high intensity, C-fiber inputs. On the other hand, long-term depression appears to occur after low-frequency, lower intensity, Aδ-fiber inputs (73). Thus, needle insertion per se, by providing a low-intensity input, may reverse or attenuate the central sensitization associated with long-term potentiation evoked by high-intensity inputs. Thus, following trauma and tissue damage, needle insertion may be antihyperalgesic.

Cardiovascular Effects

Since the 1980s, it has been demonstrated that several kinds of experimental hypertension, arrhythmias, and stress-induced pressor responses can be inhibited by needle insertion (EA, 1–3 mA, 2–5 Hz), whereas hypotension and bradycardia can be alleviated by EA (4–6 mA). The neural pathways involved have

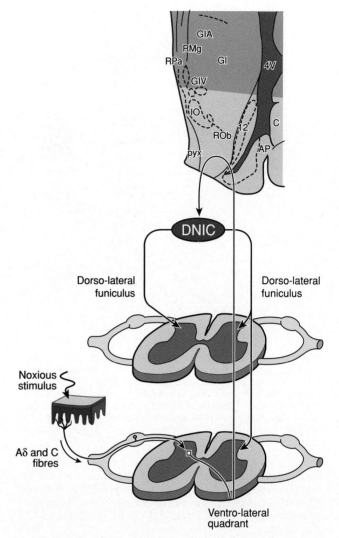

FIGURE 34-7. Triggering of descending inhibitory controls by nociceptive stimulation. *4V*, fourth ventricle; *12*, hypoglossal nucleus; *AP*, area postrema; *C*, cerebellum; *Gi*, gigantocellular nucleus; *GiA*, gigantocellular nucleus pars-α; *GiV*, gigantocellular nucleus ventral; *IO*, inferior olive; *pyx*, pyramidal decussation; *RMg*, nucleus raphe magnus; *RPa*, nucleus raphe pallidus; *Rob*, nucleus raphe obscurus. From LeBars D, Willer J-C. Pain modulation triggered by high-intensity stimulation: Implication for acupuncture analgesia? Acupuncture—is there a physiological basis? Satellite Symposium of the 34th World Congress of the International Union of Physiological Sciences. International Congress Series 2002;1238:11–29, with permission.

been defined (74). For example, central and peripheral neural effects of needle insertion have been studied in a feline model of reversible myocardial ischemia (75). Also, needle insertion and stimulation of the forepaw of anesthetized rats have been shown by laser Doppler measurement to increase cerebral cortical blood flow independent of systemic blood pressure (76) (Fig. 34-8).

Other Autonomic Effects

Other autonomic responses have been examined in anesthetized rats using needle stimulation, such as gastric motility (inhibited by stimulation of the abdominal areas and facilitated

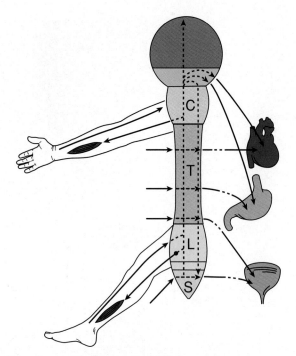

FIGURE 34-8. Reflex pathways for the somato-somatic and somato-autonomic reflexes. From Sato A, Sato Y, Uchida S. Reflex modulation of visceral functions by acupuncture-like stimulation in anaesthetised rats. Acupuncture—is there a physiological basis? Satellite Symposium of the 34th World Congress of the International Union of Physiological Sciences. International Congress Series 2002;1238:111–123, with permission.

by limb stimulation) and rhythmic micturition contractions of the urinary bladder (inhibited by perineal stimulation). The neural pathways involved have been studied (77). An inhibitory effect of cutaneous needle stimulation on L-dopa-induced hyperactivity of the bladder in the rat has been found (78) (Fig. 34-9).

Human Studies

Comprehensive reviews of needle insertion techniques and the clinical effects of needling have been prepared from varying perspectives (79–82). Ongoing studies have applied functional brain imaging to elucidate mechanisms of acupuncture and placebo effects (83,84). Noninvasive clinical brain imaging, using techniques such as functional magnetic resonance imaging (fMRI) and positron emission tomography (PET), have characterized specific brain sites and responses to needle insertion (85–90). Such evidence suggests that the brain sites activated during acupuncture in painful conditions are far more widespread than those seen during acupuncture treatment of nonpainful conditions (91).

CLINICAL EFFICACY AND ADVERSE EFFECTS

The present chapter has briefly surveyed evidence that needle insertion per se modulates nociception and related responses. Basic research on needle insertion effects has deliberately employed animal models for reasons given at the beginning of the chapter. Extrapolating from animal research, it is highly

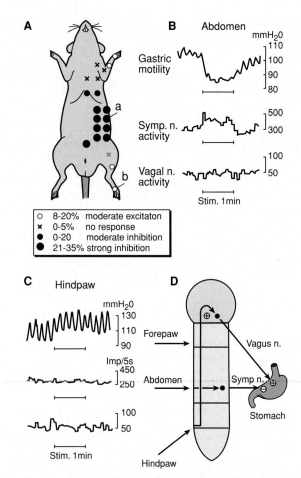

FIGURE 34-9. Effect on gastric motility of acupuncture-like stimulation. **A:** Gastric responses to acupuncture-like stimulation of various segmental areas of the body. Open and filled circles indicate the areas where acupuncture-like stimulation caused excitatory and inhibitory gastric responses, respectively. The size of the circle indicates the magnitude of the response, as shown in the bottom lower inset. **B, C:** Effects on gastric motility (*upper trace*), gastric sympathetic efferent nerve activity (*middle trace*), and vagal efferent nerve activity (*bottom trace*) following acupuncture-like stimulation of the abdomen (**B**) and hind paw (**C**). Nerve activity was counted consecutively every 5 seconds. Stimulation for 1 minute is indicated by the bars. Gastric motility, and sympathetic and vagal efferent nerve activities were recorded in different rats. **D:** Schematic diagram illustrating the proposed reflex responses and their reflex pathways in anesthetized rats. From Sato A, Sato Y, Uchida S. Reflex modulation of visceral functions by acupuncture-like stimulation in anaesthetised rats. Acupuncture—is there a physiological basis? Satellite Symposium of the 34th World Congress of the International Union of Physiological Sciences. International Congress Series 2002;1238:111–123, with permission.

likely that genetic aspects of neurochemical and neurophysiologic responses influence individual human subjects' responses to needle insertion.

Controversy continues in relation to the efficacy of needle insertion in the human to treat acute pain (92,93), based upon the findings of randomized controlled trials. Stronger evidence from randomized controlled trials indicates the efficacy of acupuncture for relief of nausea and vomiting, particularly in postoperative patients (94). Controversy continues as to the efficacy of acupuncture in other conditions related to pain and analgesia, such as opiate addiction (95). However distinction should be made between the acute opiate withdrawal syndrome and the treatment of opiate addiction with its known complex behavioral associations.

Analgesia

The substantial preclinical evidence just summarized concerning the physiologic effects of needle insertion and acupuncture has not translated into unequivocal evidence of clinical efficacy. As mentioned, efficacy studies of needling present a number of methodologic challenges, chiefly the need for a standardized intervention for the control group (96). Despite these challenges, many controlled clinical trials indicate the efficacy of needling and acupuncture for a variety of painful conditions, including acute postoperative pain, low back pain, headache, and osteoarthritis (97–100).

Systematic reviews of these studies have reached varying conclusions (2,101–103). Although many appear pessimistic in their conclusion, the most common conclusion is that insufficient evidence is available to demonstrate efficacy, rather than evidence to demonstrate lack of efficacy. The reviewed studies often enroll small numbers of subjects, employ short durations of follow-up, and lack uniform outcome measures. The most consistent conclusion from systematic reviews of the effects of acupuncture and needle insertion, even those that cite evidence for a positive effect, is the need for funding and accomplishing well-designed trials with larger cohorts of patients (2). A recent attempt to improve the quality and uniformity of trials in this area involves Standards for Reporting Interventions in Controlled Trials of Acupuncture (STRICTA).

Postoperative Nausea and Vomiting

Needling of a specific site on the lower forearm between the tendons of the flexor carpi radialis and the palmaris longus has traditionally been applied to treat nausea and vomiting. An early systematic review of 33 controlled trials studies using this site to relieve nausea and vomiting associated with chemotherapy, pregnancy, or surgery, reached a positive conclusion (104). A subsequent meta-analysis by different authors of needling of this site for postoperative nausea and vomiting included 19 of 24 relevant trials retrieved (105), and was expanded several years later into a Cochrane Collaboration review of 26 studies (106). The positive evidence from the 1999 meta-analysis, which found that nausea but not vomiting was reduced, was challenged by others (107). This is supported by a controlled trial that demonstrated a reduction in postoperative pain, nausea, and opioid consumption with needling of this site (108). A more recent systematic review and meta-analysis of needling to treat chemotherapy-induced nausea and vomiting (109) found efficacy from pooled data from 11 included trials that met quality criteria out of 14 relevant retrieved trials. Given the large number of studies and the overall positive evidence, needling of this site on the forearm appears to have a significant physiologic effect on nausea.

Opiate Addiction

ADVERSE EFFECTS OF NEEDLING

Neurologic complications of regional anesthesia have been described in detail in Chapter 12, and those associated with

pain medicine have been covered in Chapter 50. In the context of acupuncture, the majority of adverse effects are the consequences of poor knowledge of anatomy and inadequate needle sterility (99,110–114). Assuming that nerve damage or other classical pathology (e.g., hematoma) can be excluded when acupuncture increases pain, it is plausible that peripheral needle insertion stimulation may lead to changes in intrinsic CNS pain modulation and result in peripheral nerve sensitization. In that same context, since earlier sections of this chapter have highlighted the neurochemical and neurophysiologic effects of needle insertion, less frequent and perplexing side effects in individual patients may be understood. The authors have themselves observed occasional increases in pain intensity (sometimes accompanied by paresthesias or new hypesthesias); cardiovascular effects such as changes in blood pressure, palpitations, and/or arrhythmias; and neurologic symptoms such as disorientation, mood changes such as euphoria or depression, tremor, or even a seizure (in a patient with a history of epilepsy not on medication at the time). Occasional effects on bowel and/or bladder function are presumed to result from the effects of acupuncture on the autonomic nervous system.

SUMMARY

Acupuncture and other needle insertion techniques have a long history and, despite widespread skepticism, continue to play a significant role in health care. This chapter has emphasized that needle insertion per se has more wide-ranging effects than might be thought. The widespread responses to needle insertion, including acupuncture, are understandable once it is realized that needling produces neurochemical and neurophysiologic effects throughout the CNS, independent of the injection of local anesthetics or active pharmacologic agents. The anesthesiologist using neural blockade techniques should be aware of such nonpharmacologic sequelae of needling.

The traditional practice of acupuncture is reliant on historical philosophical concepts of bodily function. More recently, basic and clinical studies have provided increasing evidence for the physiologic bases by which needle insertion per se may lead to analgesia and alter autonomic function. These effects are mediated through modulation of inputs in the spinal cord, activation of specific brain regions, and alterations in central neurochemistry.

Despite these advances in our understanding of underlying mechanisms, evidence of clinical effectiveness is still limited. Although there is clear evidence for the effectiveness of needle insertion in a number of specific conditions, systematic reviews of efficacy in chronic pain have thus far revealed only moderate treatment effect sizes. This inconclusiveness is due to several factors, such as the number and quality of trials, difficulties in determining a suitable control intervention, and the difficulties of applying a standardized "acupuncture prescription" for the treatment of pain problems. Recent STRICTA guidelines seek to codify the design of trials that examine the sequelae of needle insertion. As such standards become more broadly disseminated and accepted, the quality of trials in this important area may be expected to improve. The scope of such trials should broaden to encompass not only acupuncture according to traditional Chinese practice, but also the regional and systemic effects of needle insertion in the daily practice of regional anesthesia and pain medicine as practiced within a Western, biomedical framework.

PART IV: PAIN MANAGEMENT

References

1. Benedetti F. What do you expect from this treatment? Changing our mind about clinical trials. *Pain* 2007;128(3):193–194.
2. Linde K, Vickers A, Hondras M, et al. Systematic reviews of complementary therapies: An annotated bibliography. Part 1: Acupuncture. *BMC Complement Altern Med* 2001;1(3).
3. Shorter Oxford English Dictionary, 5th ed. 2002.
4. Research Group of Acupuncture Anaesthesia, Peking Medical College, Peking. Effect of acupuncture on pain threshold of human skin. *Chin Med J* 1973;3:35. [English abstract]
5. Research Group of Acupuncture Anaesthesia, Peking Medical College, Peking. The effect of acupuncture on the human skin pain threshold. *Chin Med J* 1973;13:151–157. [Chinese].
6. Research Group of Acupuncture Anaesthesia, Peking Medical College, Peking. The role of some neurotransmitters of brain in finger-acupuncture analgesia. *Sci Sin* 1974;17:112–130.
7. Han JS, Zhou ZF, Xuan YT. Acupuncture has an analgesic effect in rabbits. *Pain* 1983;15:83–91.
8. Ren MF, Han JS. Rat tail flick acupuncture analgesia model. *Chin Med J* 1979;92:576–582.
9. Han JS, Terenius L. Neurochemical basis of acupuncture analgesia. *Ann Rev Pharmacol Toxicol* 1982;22:193–220.
10. Han JS, Chou PH, Chen-Chu L, et al. The role of central 5-hydroxytryptamine in acupuncture analgesia. *Sci Sin* 1979;22:91–104.
11. Ma Q-P, Zhou Y, Yu Y-X, Han JS. Electroacupuncture accelerated the expression of c-fos protooncogene in serotonergic neurons of nucleus raphe dorsalis. *Int J Neurosci* 1992;67:111–117.
12. Xu W, Qiu X, Han JS. Serotonin receptor subtypes in spinal antinociception in the rat. *Neuroreport* 1994;5:2665–2668.
13. Xu W, Cui X, Han JS. Spinal serotonin IA and IC/2 receptors mediate supraspinal mu opioid-induced analgesia. *J Pharmacol Exp Ther* 1994;269:1182–1189.
14. Han JS, Li S-J, Tang J. Tolerance to electroacupuncture and its cross-tolerance to morphine. *Neuropharmacology* 1981;20:593–596.
15. Li S, Tang J, Han JS. The implication of central serotonin in electroacupuncture tolerance in the rat. *Sci Sin [B]* 1982;25:620–629.
16. Xuan YT, Zhou ZF, Han JS. Electroacupuncture analgesia was reversed by microinjection of 5-hydroxytryptophan into nuclei accumbens in the rabbit. *Int J Neurosci* 1982;17:157–161.
17. Han JS, Re MF, Tang J, et al. The role of central catecholamine in acupuncture analgesia. *Chin Med J* 1979;92:793–800.
18. Xie CW, Tang J, Han JS. Central norepinephrine in acupuncture analgesia: Differential effects in brain and spinal cord. In: Advances in Endogenous and Exogenous Opioids, Proceedings of the International Narcotic Research Conference, Kyoto, Japan, July 26–30, 1981, Kodansha Ltd., Tokyo, 288–290.
19. Han JS, Xie CW, Tang J. Central norepinephrine: Its implication in the development of acupuncture tolerance. In: Advances in Endogenous and Exogenous Opioids, Proceedings of the International Narcotic Research Conference, Kyoto, Japan, July 26–30, 1981, Kodansha Ltd., Tokyo, 303–305.
20. Zhou Z, Du M, Wu W, et al. Effect of intracerebral microinjection of naloxone on acupuncture- and morphine-analgesia in the rabbit. *Sci Sin* 1981;24:1166–1178.
21. Han JS. Physiologic and neurochemical basis of acupuncture analgesia. In: Cheng TO, ed. *The International Textbook of Cardiology*. New York: Pergamon; 1986:1124–1132.
22. Jin WQ, Zhou ZF, Han JS. Electroacupuncture and morphine analgesia potentiated by bestatin and thiorphan administered to the nucleus accumbens of the rabbit. *Brain Res* 1986;380:317–324.
23. Han JS, Xie CW. Dynorphin: Potent analgesic effect in spinal cord of the rat. *Life Sci* 1982;31:1781–1783.
24. Han JS, Xie C. Dynorphin: Potent analgesic effect in spinal cord of the rat. *Sci Sin [B]* 1984;27:169–177.
25. Han JS, Xie GX, Goldstein A. Analgesia induced by intrathecal injection of dynorphin B in the rat. *Life Sci* 1984;34:1573–1579.
26. Ren MF, Lu CH, Han JS. Dynorphin-A-(1-13) antagonizes morphine analgesia in the brain and potentiates morphine analgesia in the spinal cord. *Peptides* 1985;6:1015–1020.
27. Han JS, Xie GX. Dynorphin: Important mediator for electroacupuncture analgesia in the spinal cord of the rabbit. *Pain* 1984;18:367–376.
28. Han JS, Xie GX, Zhou ZF, et al. Enkephalin and beta-endorphin as mediators of electroacupuncture analgesia in rabbits: An antiserum microinjection study. In: Costa E, Trabucchi M, eds. *Regulatory Peptides: From Molecular Biology to Function*. New York: Raven Press; 1982:369–377.
29. Xie, GX, Han JS, Hollt V. Electroacupuncture analgesia blocked by microinjection of anti-beta-endorphin antiserum into periaqueductal gray of the rabbit. *Int J Neurosci* 1983;18:287–292.

30. Han JS. Progress in the pharmacological studies of acupuncture analgesia. In: Paton SW, Mitchell J, Turner P, eds. *IUPHAR 9th International Congress of Pharmacology, Proceedings*, Vol. 1. London, 1984:565–572.
31. Han JS, Fei H, Zhou ZF. Met-enkephalin-arg6-phe7-like immunoreactive substances mediate electroacupuncture analgesia in the periaqueductal gray of the rabbit. *Brain Res* 1984;322:289–296.
32. Han JS, Xie GX, Zhou ZF, et al. Acupuncture mechanisms in rabbits studied with microinjection of antibodies against beta- endorphin, enkephalin and substance P. *Neuropharmacology* 1984;23:1–5.
33. Jin WQ, Zhou ZF, Han JS. Substance P in nucleus accumbens of the rabbit mediates acupuncture analgesia. *Kexue Tongbao* 1985;30:464–467.
34. Tian JH, Xu W, Zhang W, et al. Involvement of endogenous orphanin FQ in electroacupuncture-induced analgesia. *Neuroreport* 1997;8:497–500.
35. Fan SG, Qu ZC, Zhe QZ, Han JS. GABA: Antagonistic effect on electroacupuncture analgesia and morphine analgesia in the rat. *Life Sci* 1982;31:1225–1228.
36. Wang RY, Aghajanian GK. Physiological evidence for habenula as major link between forebrain and midbrain raphe. *Science* 1977;1977:89–91.
37. Han JS. Cholecystokinin octapeptide (CCK-8): A negative feedback control mechanism for opioid analgesia. In: Yu ACH, Eng LF, McMahan UJ, et al., eds. *Prog Brain Res* 1995;105(25):263 271.
38. Bian JT, Sun MZ, Han JS. Reversal of electroacupuncture tolerance by CCK-8 antiserum: An electrophysiological study on pain-related neurons in nucleus parafascicularis of the rat. *Int J Neurosci* 1993;72:15–29.
39. Zhou Y, Sun YH, Shen JM, Han JS. Increased release of immunoreactive CCK-8 by electroacupuncture and enhancement of electroacupuncture analgesia by CCK-B antagonist in rat spinal cord. *Neuropeptides* 1993;24:139–144.
40. Han JS, Ding, XZ, Fan SG. Cholecystokinin octapeptide (CCK-8): Antagonism to electroacupuncture analgesia and a possible role in electroacupuncture tolerance. *Pain* 1986a;27:101–115.
41. Shen S, Tian J, Han JS. Electroacupuncture-induced release of cholecystokinin octapeptide mediated by spinal mu- and kappa-opioid receptors. *Chin Sci Bull* 1995;40:1291–1295.
42. Han JS. Molecular events underlying the anti-opioid effect of cholecystokinin octapeptide (CCK-8) in the central nervous system. In: Cuello AC, Collier B, eds. *Pharmacological Sciences: Perspectives for Research and Therapy in the Late 1990s*. Basel: Birkhauser, 1995:199–207.
43. Zhang LX, Zhou Y, Du Y, Han JS. Effect of CCK-8 on audiogenic epileptic seizure in P77PMC rats. *Neuropeptides* 1993;25:73–76.
44. Zhou Y, Sun YH, Zhang ZW, Han JS. Increased release of immunoreactive cholecystokinin octapeptide by morphine and potentiation of mu-opioid analgesia by CCK-B receptor antagonist L-365,260 in rat spinal cord. *Eur J Pharmacol* 1993;234:147–154.
45. Chen XH, Han JS, Huang LT. CCK receptor antagonist L-365,260 potentiated electroacupuncture analgesia in Wistar rats but not in audiogenic epileptic rats. *Chin Med J* 1994;107:113–118.
46. Zhang LX, Wu M, Han JS. Suppression of audiogenic epileptic seizures by intracerebral injection of a CCK gene vector. *Neuroreport* 1992;3:700–702.
47. Zhang LX, Li XL, Smith MA, et al. Lipofectin-facilitated transfer of cholecystokinin gene corrects behavioral abnormalities of rats with audiogenic seizures. *Neuroscience* 1997;77:15–22.
48. Liu NJ, Bao H, Li N, et al. Cholecystokinin octapeptide reverses the inhibitory effect induced by electroacupuncture on C-fiber evoked discharges. *Int J Neurosci* 1996;86:241–247.
49. Han JS, Sun S. Frequency dependence of opioid EA-induced analgesia. *Acupuncture: The Scientific International Journal* 1990;1:19–27.
50. Han JS, Wang Q. Mobilization of specific neuropeptides by peripheral stimulation of identified frequencies. *News in Physiol Sci* 1992;7:176–180.
51. Lin J, Chen XH, Han JS. Antinociception produced by 2 and 5 kHz peripheral stimulation in the rat. *Int J Neurosci* 1992;64:15–22.
52. Chen XH, Han JS. Analgesia induced by electroacupuncture of different frequencies is mediated by different types of opioid receptors: Another cross-tolerance study. *Behav Brain Res* 1992;47:143–149.
53. Han JS. Acupuncture: Neuropeptide release produced by electrical stimulation of different frequencies. *Trends Neurosci* 2003;26:17–22.
54. He C, Han JS. Attenuation of low- rather than high-frequency electroacupuncture analgesia following microinjection of beta-endorphin antiserum into the periaqueductal gray in rats. *Acupuncture: The Scientific International Journal* 1990;1:94–99.
55. Wang Q, Mayo L, Han JS. Analgesic electrical stimulation of the hypothalamic arcuate nucleus: Tolerance and its cross-tolerance to 2 Hz or 100 Hz electroacupuncture. *Brain Res* 1990;518:40–46.

56. Wang Q, Mayo L, Han JS. The arcuate nucleus of hypothalamus mediates low but not high frequency electroacupuncture analgesia in rats. *Brain Res* 1990;513:60–66.
57. Wang Q, Mayo LM, Han JS. Diencephalon as a cardinal neural structure for mediating 2Hz- but not 100Hz-electroacupuncture-induced tail flick reflex suppression. *Behav Brain Res* 1990;37:149–156.
58. Wang Q, Mayo LN, Han JS. The role of periaqueductal gray in mediation of analgesia produced by different frequencies electroacupuncture stimulation in rats. *Int J Neurosci* 1990;53:167–172.
59. Wang Q, Mayo LN, Han JS. The role of parabrachial nucleus in high-frequency electroacupuncture analgesia in rats. *Chin J Physiol Sci* 1991;7:363–367.
60. Han Z, Jiang YH, Wan Y, et al. Endomorphin-I mediates 2Hz but not 100Hz electroacupuncture analgesia in the rat. *Neurosci Lett* 1999;274:75–78.
61. Huang C, Wang Y, Chang JK, Han JS. Endomorphin and mu-opioid receptors in mouse brain mediate the analgesic effect produced by 2Hz but not 100Hz electroacupuncture stimulation. *Neurosci Lett* 2000;294:159–162.
62. Guo HF, Tian JH, Wang X, et al. Brain substrates activated by electroacupuncture of different frequencies (I): Comparative study on the expression of oncogene c-fos and genes coding for three opioid peptides. *Mol Brain Res* 1996;43:157–166.
63. Guo HF, Tian JH, Wang X, et al. Brain substrates activated by electroacupuncture of different frequencies (II): Role of Fos/Jun proteins in EA-induced transcription of preproenkephalin and preprodynorphin genes. *Mol Brain Res* 1996;43:167–173.
64. Peets J, Pomeranz B. CXBK mice deficient in opiate receptors show poor EA analgesia. *Nature* 1978;273:675–676.
65. Tang NM, Dong HW, Wang XM, et al. Cholecystokinin antisense RNA increases the analgesic effect induced by electroacupuncture or low-dose morphine: Conversion of low responder rats into high responders. *Pain* 1997;71:71–80.
66. Tang NM, Dong HW, Zhang LX, et al. Antisense CCK RNA and CCK-B receptor antagonist L-365,260 changed non-responder rat to responder for EA analgesia. *Chin J Pain Med* 1996;2:103–108.
67. Zhang LX, Li XL, Wang L, Han JS. Rats with decreased brain cholecystokinin level show increased responsiveness to peripheral electrical stimulation-induced analgesia. *Brain Res* 1997;745:158–164.
68. Wan Y, Wilson SG, Han JS, Mogil JS. The effect of genotype on sensitivity to electroacupuncture analgesia. *Pain* 2001;91:5–13.
69. Huang C, Wang Y, Han JS, Wan Y. Characteristics of electroacupuncture-induced analgesia in mice: Variation with strain, frequency, intensity and opioid involvement. *Brain Res* 2002;945:20–25.
70. Ji R, Zhang M, Zhang Q, Han JS. Effects of capsaicin on fos expression evoked by formalin and electroacupuncture stimulation in the rat spinal cord. *Pain Res* 1994;9:37–47.
71. LeBars D, Willer J-C. Pain modulation triggered by high-intensity stimulation: Implication for acupuncture analgesia? Acupuncture: Is there a physiological basis? Satellite Symposium of the 34th World Congress of the International Union of Physiological Sciences. *Int Congr Ser* 2002;1238:11–29.
72. Sandkühler J, Liu XG. Induction of long-term potentiation at spinal synapses by noxious stimulation or nerve injury. *Eur J Neurosci* 1998;10:2476–2480.
73. Sandkühler J, Chen JG, Cheng G, Randic M. Low-frequency stimulation of afferent A delta-fibers induces long-term depression at primary afferent synapses with substantia gelatinosa neurons in the rat. *J Neurosci* 1997;17:6483–6491.
74. Li P. Neural mechanisms of the effect of acupuncture on cardiovascular diseases. Acupuncture: Is there a physiological basis? Satellite Symposium of the 34th World Congress of the International Union of Physiological Sciences. *Int Congr Ser* 2002;1238:71–77.
75. Longhurst JC. Central and peripheral neural mechanisms of acupuncture in myocardial ischaemia. Acupuncture: Is there a physiological basis? Satellite Symposium of the 34th World Congress of the International Union of Physiological Sciences. *Int Congr Ser* 2002;1238:79–87.
76. Uchida S, Suzuki A, Kagitani F, Aikawa Y. Effect of acupuncture-like stimulation on cortical cerebral blood flow in anaesthetised rats. Acupuncture: Is there a physiological basis? Satellite Symposium of the 34th World Congress of the International Union of Physiological Sciences. *Int Congr Ser* 2002;1238:89–96.
77. Sato A, Sato Y, Uchida S. Reflex modulation of visceral functions by acupuncture-like stimulation in anaesthetised rats. Acupuncture: Is there a physiological basis? Satellite Symposium of the 34th World Congress of the International Union of Physiological Sciences. *Int Congr Ser* 2002;1238:111–123.
78. Wang S, Wang X. The inhibitory effect of acupuncture on L-dopa-induced hyperactivity of rats' bladder. Acupuncture: Is there a physiological basis? Satellite Symposium of the 34th World Congress of the International Union of Physiological Sciences. *Int Congr Ser* 2002;1238:171–177.
79. Andersson S, Lundeberg T. Acupuncture: From empiricism to science: Functional background to acupuncture effects in pain and disease. *Med Hypotheses* 1995;45:271–281.
80. Mayer DJ. Acupuncture: An evidence-based review of the clinical literature. *Annu Rev Med* 2000;51:49–63.
81. Kaptchuk TJ. Acupuncture: Theory, efficacy, and practice. *Ann Int Med* 2002;136:374–383.
82. Ernst E. Acupuncture: A critical analysis. *J Int Med* 2006;259:125–137.
83. Rainville P, Duncan GH. Functional brain imaging of placebo analgesia: Methodological challenges and recommendations. *Pain* 2006;121:177–180.
84. Dhond RP, Kettner N, Napadow V. Do the neural correlates of acupuncture and placebo effects differ? *Pain* 2007;128:8–12.
85. Wu MT, Hsieh JC, Xiong J, et al. Central nervous pathway for acupuncture stimulation: Localization of processing with functional MR imaging of the brain: Preliminary experience. *Radiology* 1999;212:133–141.
86. Hui KKS, Liu J, Makris N, et al. Acupuncture modulates the limbic system and subcortical gray structures of the human brain: Evidence from fMRI studies in normal subjects. *Hum Brain Mapp* 2000;9:13–25.
87. Hsieh JC, Tu CH, Chen FP, et al. Activation of the hypothalamus characterizes the acupuncture stimulation at the analgesic point in human: A positron emission tomography study. *Neurosci Lett* 2001;307:105–108.
88. Wu MT, Sheen JM, Chuang KH, et al. Neuronal specificity of acupuncture response: A fMRI study with electroacupuncture. *Neuroimage* 2002;16:1028–1037.
89. Zhang WT, Jin Z, Cui GH, et al. Relations between brain network activation and analgesic effect induced by low vs. high frequency electrical acupoint stimulation in different subjects: A functional magnetic resonance imaging study. *Brain Res* 2003;982:168–178.
90. Napadow V, Makris N, Liu J, et al. Effects of electroacupuncture versus manual acupuncture on the human brain as measured by fMRI. *Hum Brain Mapp* 2005;24:193–205.
91. Lewith GT, White PJ, Pariente J. Investigating acupuncture using brain-imaging techniques: The current state of play. *Evid Based Complement Alternat Med* 2005;2(3):315–319.
92. Usichenko TI, Dinse M, Hermsen M, et al. Auricular acupuncture for pain relief after total hip arthroplasty: A randomized controlled study. *Pain* 2005;114:320–327.
93. Lee H, Ernst E. Acupuncture analgesia during surgery: A systematic review. *Pain* 2005;114:511–517.
94. Streitberger K, Ezzo J, Schneider A. Acupuncture for nausea and vomiting: An update of clinical and experimental studies. *Auton Neurosci* 2006;129:107–117.
95. Jordan JB. Acupuncture treatment for opiate addiction: A systematic review. *J Subst Abuse Treat* 2006;30:309–314.
96. Vincent C, Lewith G. Placebo controls for acupuncture studies. *J R Soc Med* 1995;88:199–202.
97. Leibing E, Leonhardt U, Koster G, et al. Acupuncture treatment of chronic low-back pain: A randomized, blinded, placebo-controlled trial with 9-month follow-up. *Pain* 2002;96:189–196.
98. Lin J-G, Lo M-W, Wen Y-R, et al. The effect of high and low frequency electroacupuncture in pain after lower abdominal surgery. *Pain* 2002;99(3):509–514.
99. Melchart D, Weidenhammer W, Streng A, et al. Prospective investigation of adverse effects of acupuncture in 97,733 patients (comments, opinions and brief case reports). *Arch Int Med* 2004;164:104–105.
100. Itoh K, Katsumi Y, Hirota S, Kitakoji H. Effects of trigger point acupuncture on chronic low back pain in elderly patients: A sham-controlled randomised trial. *Acupunct Med* 2006;24(1):5–12.
101. ter Riet G, Kleijnen J, Knipschild P. Acupuncture and chronic pain: A criteria-based meta-analysis. *J Clin Epidemiol* 1990;43:1191–1199.
102. van Tulder MW, Cherkin DC, Berman B, et al. The effectiveness of acupuncture in the management of acute and chronic low back pain: A systematic review within the framework of the Cochrane collaboration back review group. *Spine* 1999;24:1113–1123.
103. Ezzo J, Berman B, Hadhazy VA, et al. Is acupuncture effective for the treatment of chronic pain? A systematic review. *Pain* 2000;86:217–225.
104. Vickers AJ. Can acupuncture have specific effects on health? A systematic review of acupuncture antiemesis trials. *J R Soc Med* 1996;89:303–311.
105. Lee A, Done ML. Stimulation of the wrist acupuncture point P6 for preventing postoperative nausea and vomiting. *Cochrane Database Syst Rev* 2004;3: DOI: 10.1002/14651858.CD003281.pub2.
106. Kimball C, Atwood IV. The P6 acupuncture point and postoperative nausea and vomiting. At The Scientific Review of Alternative Medicine 2004/5; 8(2) http://www.sram.org/current-issue.html. Accessed May 26, 2004.
107. Kotani NMD, Hashimoto HMD, Sato YMD, et al. Preoperative intradermal acupuncture reduces postoperative pain, nausea and vomiting, analgesic requirement, and sympathoadrenal responses. *Anesthesiology* 2001;95(2):349–356.

108. Ezzo J, Richardson MA. Acupuncture-point stimulation for chemotherapy-induced nausea or vomiting. *Cochrane Database Syst Rev* 2006;2: DOI: 10.1002/14651858.CD002285.pub2.

109. White A, Hayhoe S, Hart A, Ernst E. Adverse events following acupuncture: Prospective survey of 32,000 consultations with doctors and physiotherapists. *Brit Med J* 2001;323:485–486.

110. Lao L, Hamilton GR, Fu JP, Berman BM. Is acupuncture safe? A systematic review of case reports. *Altern Ther Health Med* 2003;9:72–83.

111. Chung A, Bui L, Mills E. Adverse effects of acupuncture: Which are clinically significant? *Can Fam Physician* 2003;49:985–989.

112. Ernst E, Strzyz H, Hagmeister H. Incidence of adverse effects during acupuncture therapy: A multicentre survey. *Compl Ther in Med* 2003;11: 93–97.

113. MacPherson H, Scullion A, Thomas KJ, Walters S. Patient reports of adverse events associated with acupuncture treatment: A prospective national survey. *Qual Saf Health Care* 2004;13:349–355.

CHAPTER 35 ■ PSYCHOLOGICAL ASPECTS OF PAIN: IMPLICATIONS FOR NEURAL BLOCKADE

JOEL KATZ AND RONALD MELZACK

Pain is a personal, subjective experience influenced by cultural learning, the meaning of the situation, attention, and other psychological variables. Pain processes do not begin with the stimulation of receptors. Rather, injury or disease produces neural signals that enter an active nervous system that (in the adult organism) is the substrate of past experience, culture, anxiety, and so forth. These brain processes actively participate in the selection, abstraction, and synthesis of information from the total sensory input. Pain, then, is not simply the end product of a linear sensory transmission system; it is a dynamic process that involves continuous interactions among complex ascending and descending systems.

This chapter focuses upon four areas of interest to anesthesiologists and psychologists: (a) the major psychological contributions to pain; (b) theories of pain, which are based on psychological assumptions of the nature of perception, including the gate control and neuromatrix models; (c) the measurement of pain; and (d) labor pain, which is influenced by anesthetic blocks as well as by manipulating psychological variables. Several topics surveyed in this chapter, because of their broad scope and special importance to pain management, are explored in greater detail within dedicated chapters elsewhere in this volume. Examples of the latter include social and cultural influences upon pain and disability (Chapter 29) and the placebo effect (Chapter 36).

PSYCHOLOGICAL CONTRIBUTIONS TO PAIN

When compared with vision or hearing, the perception of pain seems simple, urgent, and primitive. We expect the nerve signals evoked by injury to "get through," unless we are unconscious or anesthetized. But experiments and clinical observations show that pain is much more variable and modifiable than many people have believed in the past. Pain differs from person to person and from culture to culture. Stimuli that produce intolerable pain in one person may be tolerated without a whimper by another. Pain perception, then, cannot be defined simply in terms of particular kinds of stimuli. Rather, it is a highly personal experience that depends in part on psychological factors that are unique to each individual (1).

Cultural Determinants

It is often asserted that variations in pain experience from person to person are due to different "pain thresholds"; however, several thresholds are related to pain, and it is important to distinguish among them. Typically, thresholds are measured by applying a stimulus, such as electric shock or radiant heat, to a small area of skin and gradually increasing the intensity. Four thresholds can be measured by this technique: (a) *sensation threshold* (or lower threshold)—the lowest stimulus value at which a sensation such as tingling or warmth is first reported; (b) *pain perception threshold*—the lowest stimulus value at which the person reports that the stimulation feels painful; (c) *pain tolerance* (or *upper threshold*)—the lowest stimulus level at which the subject withdraws or asks to have the stimulation stopped; and (d) *encouraged pain tolerance*—the same as (c), but the person is encouraged to tolerate higher levels of stimulation.

Evidence now suggests that that all people, regardless of cultural background, have a uniform *sensation threshold*. Sternbach and Tursky (2) made careful measurements of sensation threshold, using electric shock as the stimulus, in American-born women belonging to four different ethnic groups: Italian, Jewish, Irish, and Old American. They found no differences among the groups in the level of shock that was first reported as producing a detectable sensation. The sensory conducting apparatus, in other words, appears to be essentially similar in all people, so that a given critical level of input always elicits a sensation.

Cultural background, however, has a powerful effect on the *pain perception threshold*. For example, levels of radiant heat that are reported as painful by people of Mediterranean origin (such as Italians and Jews) are described merely as warmth by Northern Europeans (3). Similarly, Nepalese porters on a climbing expedition are much more stoic than the Occidental visitors for whom they work. Even though both groups are equally sensitive to changes in electric shock, the Nepalese porters require much higher intensities before they call them painful (4).

The most striking effect of cultural background, however, is on pain tolerance levels. Sternbach and Tursky (2) report that the levels at which subjects refuse to tolerate electric shock, even when they are encouraged by the experimenters, depend in part on the ethnic origin of the subject. Women of Italian descent tolerate less shock than women of Old American or Jewish origin. In a similar experiment (5) in which Jewish and Protestant women served as subjects, the Jewish, but not the Protestant, women increased their tolerance level after they were told that their religious group tolerated pain more poorly than others.

These differences in pain tolerance reflect different ethnic attitudes toward pain. Zborowski (6) found that Old Americans have an accepting, matter-of-fact attitude toward pain and pain expression. They tend to withdraw when the pain is intense, and cry out or moan only when they are alone. Jews and Italians, on the other hand, tend to be vociferous in their complaints and openly seek support and sympathy. The underlying attitudes of the two groups, however, appear to be different. Jews tend to be concerned about the meaning and implications of the pain, whereas Italians usually express a desire for immediate pain relief.

The main findings of these early studies on ethnic and cultural differences have been supported by more recent empirical work using laboratory-induced pain in a variety ethnic groups, including African Americans, White Americans, White British, and South Asians. Pain thresholds do not differ by ethnicity (7). In contrast, heat pain tolerance levels for intensity and unpleasantness ratings show differences between ethnic groups (8–10). Differences in pain tolerance may be partially accounted for by other factors, such as hypervigilance and daily levels of pain (8,9), but even after statistically controlling for these variables, ethnicity remains a significant factor.

Meaning of the Pain-Producing Situation

Considerable evidence shows that people attach variable meaning to pain-producing situations and that the meaning greatly influences the degree and quality of pain they feel. Beecher (11) observed that soldiers wounded in battle rarely complained of pain, whereas civilians with similar surgical wounds usually claimed that they were in severe pain. Beecher (11) concluded the following from his study:

> The common belief that wounds are inevitably associated with pain, and that the more extensive the wound the worse the pain, was not supported by observations made as carefully as possible in the combat zone. . . . The data state in numerical terms what is known to all thoughtful clinical observers: there is no simple direct relationship between the wound per se and the pain experienced. The pain is in very large part determined by other factors, and of great importance here is the significance of the wound. . . . In the wounded soldier [the response to injury] was relief, thankfulness at his escape alive from the battlefield, even euphoria; to the civilian, his major surgery was a depressing, calamitous event.

A similar study (12) of Israeli soldiers with traumatic amputations after the Yom Kippur War provided similar observations. Most of the wounded men spoke of their initial injury as painless and used neutral terms such as "bang," "thump," or "blow" to describe their first sensation. They often volunteered their surprise that the injury did not hurt.

Melzack, Wall, and Ty (13) examined the features of acute pain in patients at an emergency clinic. Patients who had severe, life-threatening injuries or who were agitated, drunk, or "in shock" were excluded from the study. Of 138 patients who were alert, rational, and coherent, 51 (37%) stated that they did not feel pain at the time of injury. The majority of these patients reported onset of pain within an hour of injury, although the delays were as long as 9 hours or more in some patients. The predominant emotions of the patients were embarrassment at appearing careless or worry about loss of wages.

The occurrence of delays in pain onset was related to the nature of the injury. Of 46 patients whose injuries were limited to skin (lacerations, cuts, abrasions, burns), 53% had a pain-free period. Of 86 patients with deep-tissue injuries (fractures, sprains, bruises, amputation of a finger, stabs, and crushes), 28% had a pain-free period. The results indicate that the relation between injury and pain is highly variable and complex.

Attention Diversion and Distraction

If a person's attention is focused on a potentially painful experience, he will tend to perceive pain more intensely than he would normally. Hall and Stride (14) found that the simple appearance of the word "pain" in a set of instructions made anxious subjects more likely to report a given level of electric shock as painful; the same level of shock was rarely reported to be painful when the word was absent from the instructions. Thus, the mere anticipation of pain is sufficient to raise the level of anxiety and thereby the intensity of perceived pain. Similarly, Hill, Kornetsky and associates (15,16) have shown that if anxiety is dispelled (by reassuring the subject that he has control over the pain-producing stimulus), a given level of electric shock or burning heat is perceived as significantly less painful than the same stimulus under conditions of high anxiety.

In contrast to the effects of attention on pain, it is well known that distraction of attention away from pain can diminish or abolish it. Distraction of attention may partly explain why boxers, football players, and other athletes sometimes sustain severe injuries during the excitement of the sport without being aware that they have been hurt.

Distraction of attention, however, is usually effective only when the pain is steady or rises slowly in intensity (17). If radiant heat is focused on the skin, for example, the pain may rise so suddenly and sharply that subjects are unable to control it by distraction. But when the pain rises slowly, people may use various stratagems to distract their attention from it. They often find that the pain actually levels off or decreases *before* it reaches the anticipated intolerable level. Distraction stratagems are used effectively by some people to control pain produced by dental drilling and extraction (18).

Perhaps the simplest method of coping with chronic pain is by means of cognitive and/or behavioral strategies that divert the patient's attention away from pain to some other activity, object, or event (19). The scope of distracting and attention-diverting strategies is extensive, covering direct intentional efforts to reduce pain awareness through techniques such as relaxation and transformational imagery, as well as indirect approaches that accomplish similar goals without distraction being the primary objective (e.g., reading, painting, socializing). Although direct and indirect approaches appear equally effective in reducing awareness of pain, they may result in important differences in patients' attributions and self-efficacy beliefs regarding pain control.

Distraction and attention-diverting strategies are effective for many reasons (20). For example, relaxation and related activities that require sustained, focused attention may actually reduce pain intensity, as well as pain awareness, by decreasing sympathetic nervous system activity (21). Engaging in distracting, social interactions with others may alter the frequency and use of maladaptive strategies, such as catastrophizing and avoidance, in part because of response-incompatibility and in part because of improved mood. At the same time, socializing may also lead to a reduced emphasis on the importance of pain.

The effectiveness of distraction appears to approach a limit as pain intensity increases (20). This is due to an inherent limitation of most distractors; they cannot compete successfully with pain for attentional resources. Simply put, pain may be too intense, unpleasant, and threatening. Recent technological advances have made it possible to employ three-dimensional (3-D) virtual reality (VR) audiovisual devices as adjuncts in the management of painful medical procedures. Virtual reality devices typically consist of a head-mounted display or helmet that provides an immersive 3-D experience. These devices are considered ideal distractors since they create an immersive, interactive experience involving multiple modalities, including vision, proprioception, and audition (22,23).

During invasive medical procedures, VR devices not only distract the patient by redirecting attention to the novel immersive environment, but, by excluding visual and auditory inputs from the surroundings outside the VR device itself, they also distract the patient away from pain and anxiety (24,25). Experimental and clinical studies of VR immersion show significant distraction effects (23). Pain unpleasantness scores and tolerance time to ischemic arm pain were significantly lower among healthy volunteer subjects receiving VR immersion compared with a control group (25).

Hoffman and colleagues have shown significant benefits of VR distraction in children and adults undergoing painful treatment for burn injury (24,26). Not only are pain intensity and unpleasantness reduced significantly by VR distraction, but the duration of time spent thinking about pain during the procedure was reduced by approximately 45% for experimental pain (27) and 75% for clinical pain (26). Moreover, experimental subjects undergoing heat pain stimulation reported an increase in "fun" ratings of 79% when VR and non-VR distraction were compared (27). Virtual reality–induced pain relief is accompanied by reduced activity in five brain regions typically activated by pain, including anterior cingulate cortex, primary and secondary somatosensory cortex, insula, and thalamus (27,28). These results suggest that VR distraction is a promising, new nonpharmacologic therapy for managing pain associated with a variety of painful medical procedures.

Fear of and Avoidance of Pain

Avoidance behavior is usually motivated by fear. Many patients with pain are afraid that movement will cause reinjury and pain (29,30). For example, in the days and weeks after surgery, it is common for pain to be exacerbated by movement. Depending on the location of the incision, deep breathing, coughing, laughing, and getting in and out of bed all may substantially increase pain. Many patients appropriately fear, and therefore avoid, moving about.

Understanding the personal meaning of the fear is important. Patients may fear that in sitting up or walking their stitches will break and the wound will split open. Or, they may fear these activities will cause internal damage. Other patients simply fear the increase in pain associated with activity; they may feel helpless in the presence of intense pain, or they may feel dependent on the nursing staff for pain relief. Apprehension about moving about after surgery is based on first-hand experience that activity causes increased pain. The misinterpretation of activity and pain as harmful engenders avoidance behaviors that may set the stage for decreased activity and increased pain and disability.

Although avoidance by social withdrawal and inactivity may reduce ongoing pain, particularly in the early recovery phase, the long-term consequence of these behaviors is rein-forcement of the belief that avoidance prevents further pain. Such fear-avoidance beliefs are expectations about the consequences of certain actions such as physical activity or work upon pain (31). Avoidance behaviors (e.g., guarding, limping, social withdrawal) may be part of coping with ongoing pain or anticipated increases in pain. However, some of these behaviors may also represent maladaptive ways of coping with concurrent life difficulties. Unpleasant work obligations, aversive household chores, marital strife, and interpersonal difficulties may thus be avoided by the person in pain. Pain behaviors that serve a dual purpose of avoiding not only expected flare-ups in pain, but also other unpleasant life events are at high risk of becoming entrenched because of the multiple sources of negative reinforcement (32).

Patients' fear-avoidance beliefs and negative expectancies about the consequences of activity are meant to reduce anticipated increases in pain through avoidance. Avoidance behaviors tend to increase in frequency as pain becomes chronic, so that pain behaviors and pain intensity become increasingly decoupled (33). This desynchrony sets the stage for reduced self-efficacy beliefs and further avoidance (34). Thus, in attempts to gain control over the pain through avoidant coping, patients report progressively less control over the pain. Self-management programs focused on behavioral exposure and nonavoidance lead to improved self-efficacy and a reduction in preoccupation with pain, because patients acquire increasingly realistic appraisals of the relationship between pain and behavior (34).

Although use of avoidant cognitive coping strategies for pain may be beneficial when pain is acute, long-term use of these strategies is associated with impaired psychosocial functioning, increased pain and disability, and loss of employment. Avoidant coping strategies are adaptive in the early period following an injury because they minimize ongoing pain, reduce the risk of exacerbation through further injury, and thus promote healing. However, once healing has occurred, these strategies are maladaptive because they promote continued isolation, inactivity, and faulty reality testing.

Recent controlled case reports show that pain-related fear can be effectively treated by in vivo exposure, in which patients are exposed to fear-eliciting and hierarchically ordered physical movements. Concomitant reductions in catastrophic thinking, pain intensity, and pain disability were observed (35,36).

Feelings of Control over Pain

It is now clear that the severity of postsurgical pain is significantly reduced when patients are taught how to cope with their pain. In a classic study by Egbert and associates, patients scheduled to undergo major surgery to remove the gallbladder, uterus, or portions of the digestive tract were given detailed information about the pain they would feel after the operation and how they could best cope with it. They were told where they would feel pain, how severe it could be, how long it could last, and that such pain is normal after an operation. They were also shown how to relax by using breathing and relaxation stratagems. Finally, they were told that total relaxation is difficult to achieve and that they should request medication if they were uncomfortable. The results showed that patients who received these instructions reported significantly less pain, asked for much less medication during recovery, and spent less time in hospital than a similar group of patients who received no instructions (37).

It was originally thought that providing information alone is sufficient psychological preparation to reduce the uncertainty and anxiety associated with major surgery. In this case, however, knowledge may increase anxiety because of the certain expectation of pain and other discomforts. It is essential to provide the patient with skills to cope with the pain and anxiety—at the very least, to provide the patient with a sense of control. Recent studies have shown that simply giving patients information about their pain tends to make them focus on the discomforting aspects of the experience, thereby magnifying rather than reducing their pain. However, when patients are taught skills to cope with their pain, such as relaxation or distraction strategies, their pain is less severe (38). Other studies have shown that postsurgical pain intensity is directly proportional to the amount of anxiety perceived by the patient (39). Achieving a sense of control, then, appears to diminish both anxiety and pain.

Suggestion and Placebos

The influence of suggestion on the intensity of perceived pain is clearly demonstrated by studies of the effectiveness of placebos. Chapter 36 by Finniss and Benedetti surveys these studies in detail and discusses their implications for neural blockade, so the present description is deliberately concise. As Beecher carefully documented in the 1950s (11), severe pain, such as postsurgical pain, can be relieved in some patients by giving them a placebo in place of morphine or other analgesic drugs. About 35% of the patients report marked relief of pain after being given a placebo. This is a strikingly high proportion because morphine, even in large doses, relieves severe pain in only about 75% of patients.

Another interesting discovery about placebos is that their effectiveness is of the order of half that of the drug with which they are compared, even in double-blind experiments (40); that is, if the drug is a mild analgesic such as aspirin, the pain relief produced by the placebo is half that of the aspirin. If it is a powerful drug such as morphine, the placebo has greater pain-relieving properties, again about half that of morphine. This indicates that even though the "double-blind" is maintained, the therapist's enthusiasm is conveyed to the patient. However, in a recent analysis of controlled trials, 38% of patients obtained more than 10% of maximum possible pain relief after placebo, whereas 16% obtained greater than 50% relief (50% of maximum with a potent agent). Thus, there was considerable variation among patients in placebo response, within a given study (41).

There are large individual differences in susceptibility to placebos, and studies have been done to determine some of the factors involved (42). These studies have revealed that placebos are more effective for severe pain than for mild pain, and more effective in patients experiencing great stress and anxiety than in those who are not. McGlashan and co-workers (43) have shown that placebo-induced analgesia is not significantly related to suggestibility, hypnotic susceptibility, or anxiety induced specifically by pain or the therapeutic situation (termed *state-anxiety*); however, placebo effects occur more powerfully in people who have chronic, generalized anxiety (*personality-trait anxiety*). Recent work has documented differences in the neurobiology associated with placebo responders and nonresponders. Interestingly, responders and nonresponders differ in the brain areas activated by the ultrashort-acting opioid remifentanil (44). Placebo responders but not nonresponders show activation of the rostral part of the anterior cingulate cortex, a structure associated with attentional processing of pain experience (45), suggesting that placebo responders may have a more effective endogenous opioid system than nonresponders (46).

The placebo response is affected by other fascinating factors. Two placebo capsules, for example, are more effective than one capsule, and large capsules are better than small ones. A placebo is more effective when injected than when given by mouth, and is more potent when accompanied by a strong suggestion that a powerful analgesic has been given. In short, the greater the implicit and explicit suggestion that pain will be relieved, the greater is the relief obtained by the patient. Unfortunately, however, patients tend to get progressively less relief during repeated administration of placebos. We know very little about the extent to which placebo effects actually contribute to pain relief in the clinical setting (47).

The placebo effect is no longer viewed as a nuisance factor or artifact to be controlled, parcelled out, or discounted, but a phenomenon worthy of study in its own right (48). This interest has increased in part because we now know that the opioid antagonist naloxone reverses placebo analgesia, implying that endogenous opioids mediate placebo analgesia (49,50). Moreover, the neurobiology of the placebo response is now better understood as a result of modern imaging techniques (46,51). Using positron emission tomography (PET) scans, Petrovic and co-workers (44) showed that both placebo analgesia and the rapidly acting opioid remifentanil activate the rostral anterior cingulate cortex, suggesting a common underlying neural network. Consistent with this suggestion, a recent functional magnetic resonance imaging study of patients with irritable bowel syndrome found that decreases in the activity of pain-related brain regions, including thalamus, somatosensory cortex, insula, and anterior cingulate cortex accompanied placebo analgesia induced by verbal suggestion (52).

The precise mechanisms underlying the placebo response are not fully understood (47,48), but we know that two non-mutually exclusive factors play important roles in mediating placebo analgesia; namely, expectation and conditioning. *Expectation* usually is generated by verbal suggestions, but may also involve implicit, nonverbal cues. *Conditioning* effects operate by classical or Pavlovian conditioning and typically involve the pairing of an active drug with a specific context or contextual cues. Under most circumstances, placebo responses that arise from expectation induced by verbal suggestions appear to be opioid-mediated, since they are naloxone-reversible. The sensitivity to naloxone of the placebo response following conditioning depends, in part, on the opioidergic status of the unconditioned stimulus (drug). For example, naloxone-reversible placebo responses develop after conditioning with the μ-opioid agonist morphine but not the nonsteroidal anti-inflammatory drug ketorolac (49). The neurobiology of the placebo effect has progressed to the point at which we now know that some drugs act specifically to enhance placebo analgesia. This fascinating finding was first shown by Benedetti and co-workers (53) in a randomized, double-blind controlled trial of patients following posterolateral thoracotomy. After patients had recovered from the general anesthetic, they were randomly assigned to receive a hidden or open injection of saline or proglumide, a cholecystokinin antagonist. Patients in the open injection group received the injection by a physician in full view of the infusion pump and were told that it was a potent analgesic. Patients receiving the hidden injection (by way of an infusion pump that was out of sight) were unaware that an injection had been administered.

Not surprisingly, the results showed that patients who received the hidden injection of saline reported no pain relief whatsoever. In comparison, patients who received the open injection of saline showed significantly more pain relief (i.e., a placebo response due to expectation), and patients who received the open injection of proglumide showed the most pain relief of all (i.e., an apparent analgesic response plus a placebo response due to expectation). These findings appear to be straightforward and suggest that proglumide is an effective analgesic since it produces more pain relief than both a placebo injection and no treatment (i.e., the hidden saline injection). However, this interpretation is clearly incorrect since patients receiving the hidden injection of proglumide showed a total lack of analgesic effect, equal to that of the control group that received the hidden injection of saline. These striking findings suggest that proglumide produces pain relief only in the context of a placebo procedure (i.e., in response to verbal suggestions of pain relief) and that proglumide exerts its effects on an "expectation pathway" to enhance the placebo analgesic response (48).

Context plays an extremely important role in the expression of the placebo response. By context we mean the environmental cues and situations that co-occur with a treatment, along with concurrent words, and past and present meanings attributed to these words. One of the most profound contextual cues known to produce a placebo response consists of the words spoken by a physician to her patient, and in particular, the degree of certainty with which the message is conveyed (54–56). The power of the placebo response generated by a physician's word is best illustrated by Pollo and colleagues (55), who administered a 72-hour continuous intravenous (IV) infusion of saline to three groups of patients after posterolateral thoracotomy. In addition to the background saline infusion, patients in all three groups received 0.15 mg IV buprenorphine on demand for pain relief. Patients in group 1 (natural history) were not told anything about the analgesic action of the saline infusion and believed it was a rehydrating solution. Patients in group 2 (double-blind placebo) were told that the infusion was either buprenorphine or saline and thus were uncertain as to the contents of the infusion. Patients in group 3 (deceptive placebo) were told the infusion contained a powerful painkiller. From their perspective, group 3 patients were certain they were receiving a potent analgesic agent.

The results showed that the number of doses of buprenorphine received by the three groups differed significantly as a function of the instructions they were given and, by implication, the certainty with which patients believed they were receiving an active drug infusion. Patients who were told that the saline was a powerful drug (deceptive placebo) demonstrated the largest placebo effect, a 33.8% reduction in buprenorphine intake compared with the natural history control group. Being less certain about the analgesic properties of the saline infusion (double-blind placebo) produced a 20.8% reduction in buprenorphine use compared with the natural history control group. Since pain scores did not differ significantly among the groups because all were able to self-medicate with buprenorphine upon demand, the magnitude of the placebo effects are indicated by the different doses of buprenorphine taken by the three groups of patients (55).

Not all placebos result in pain reduction. Under certain circumstances, it has been observed that verbal suggestion, conditioning, or expectation can increase pain (57). The term *nocebo hyperalgesia* has been coined to describe the increase in pain that occurs after administration of an inert substance (58). The nocebo response appears to be as robust as the placebo response, but it is not as well researched. Nocebo hyperalgesia is blocked by the cholecystokinin (CCK) antagonist proglumide and is unaffected by naloxone, suggesting that nocebo-induced hyperalgesia is mediated by an opioid independent, CCK-activated increase in anxiety (58). This suggestion is supported by a recent study showing that nocebo hyperalgesia is greatest among individuals high in pain anxiety (59).

Research into the placebo/nocebo effect clearly demonstrates that a physician's choice of words profoundly affects her patients' pain intensity (56) and demand for analgesics after surgery (55,57). Controlled studies designed to better understand the placebo response may require patients to be deceived, providing that backup "rescue" medication is immediately available. However, this clearly is not always feasible in clinical practice. Deceptive administration of a placebo in clinical practice is therefore unethical, since doing so denies patients their legal and ethical rights to informed consent and to refuse treatment (60). Nevertheless, it may be possible to leverage the desirable effects of the placebo response without deception, by emphasizing in a truthfully worded statement the benefits of a procedure or drug whose analgesic efficacy is well documented (47,54).

Hypnosis

The manipulation of attention together with strong suggestion is part of the phenomenon of hypnosis. The hypnotic state eludes precise definition. Loosely speaking, hypnosis is a trance state in which the subject's attention is focused intensely on the hypnotist while attention to other stimuli is markedly diminished. After people are hypnotized they can, with appropriate suggestion, receive normally noxious tactile or thermal stimuli yet report no pain (61,62). They may say that they felt a sharp tactile sensation or strong heat, but they maintain that the sensations never welled up into pain. A small percentage of people can be hypnotized deeply enough to undergo major surgery entirely without anesthesia. For a larger number of people, hypnosis reduces the amount of pain-killing drug required to produce successful analgesia.

Despite the long history of hypnotism, which has been used for hundreds of years under different names such as *animal magnetism* and *mesmerism*, very little is known about its mechanisms. Still worse, most of its major features are highly controversial. For example, there is a vigorous debate about its fundamental nature. Is it a special state of consciousness known as a "trance state," or is it merely a trait of responsiveness to strong suggestion? There is no resolution yet to this question (61).

Nevertheless, anyone who has observed the behavior of people who have been hypnotized realizes that this is an especially interesting phenomenon. Under hypnosis, people tolerate pain, during demonstrations or experiments, from stimuli that would normally cause them to cry out and withdraw. Countless accounts of such observations are supplemented by reports that hypnosis is effective in relieving severe clinical pains, such as phantom limb pain. Although excellent studies of hypnotic analgesia have been carried out with experimentally induced pains (63), there are as yet no convincing studies, using the necessary control groups, of clinical pain. The evidence thus far is observational or "anecdotal."

It is known, however, that not all people can be hypnotized. About 30% of people can reach a state of deep hypnosis, 30% reach a moderate state, 30% achieve a drowsy state, and 10% of people are not susceptible at all. These figures resemble the proportions of placebo reactors and nonreactors. There is, however, strong evidence that hyporesponsiveness to pain in hypnotized subjects is not simply a placebo effect. An elegantly designed experiment (43) has shown that pain perception threshold and pain tolerance level are both strikingly increased during hypnosis but that only pain perception threshold is raised after administration of a placebo. The same study demonstrated that the hypnotic procedure itself has not only a placebo effect, but also an additional effect that raises pain threshold and tolerance still further.

Posttraumatic Stress Disorder and Pain

Posttraumatic stress disorder (PTSD) usually occurs after exposure to a situation or event that is perceived to be threatening to the physical or emotional integrity of an individual. The diagnostic criteria (64) for PTSD comprise three symptom clusters, including (a) reexperiencing the traumatic event (e.g., "flashbacks" and nightmares); (b) emotional numbing (e.g., feeling detached from others) and avoidance of thoughts, feelings, and activities associated with the trauma; and (c) increased arousal (e.g., insomnia, hypervigilance, exaggerated startle reflex). The lifetime prevalence for PTSD ranges from 1% to 14% but may be as high as 58% for at-risk individuals (e.g., soldiers or victims of violent crime) (64). Many more individuals who do not meet all criteria for PTSD may suffer with partial or subthreshold PTSD (65).

Both PTSD and chronic pain are highly prevalent and often difficult to manage effectively. Recent evidence suggests that PTSD and chronic pain occur as comorbidities more frequently than would be expected by chance alone. The prevalence of chronic pain in patients with PTSD ranges from 20% to 80% (66–68). Similarly, the prevalence of PTSD in patients with chronic pain ranges from 10% to 50% (69,70). The high comorbidity has led to a call for routine assessment of both chronic pain and PTSD when either one is diagnosed (71).

Salomons and colleagues (72) present two case reports of patients who developed PTSD following an episode of awareness under anesthesia. In both cases, posttraumatic sequelae persisted for years and included pain symptoms that resembled, in quality and location, the very pain experienced during surgery. In addition to their similarity to the original pain, these persistent pain symptoms were triggered by stimuli associated with the traumatic situation, suggesting that they were flashbacks to the episode of awareness under anesthesia. Both patients received individual, trauma-focused, cognitive-behavioral therapy with resolution of their PTSD.

In an effort to better understand the psychological predictors of excessive use of patient-controlled analgesia (PCA), Katz and associates (73) had 104 women complete measures of mental health and distress 1 week before major gynecologic surgery by laparotomy. Forty-eight hours after surgery, measures of pain and negative affect were obtained. In addition, total opioid consumption and the time of every button press, over the 48 hours, were downloaded from the PCA pump. Multiple regression analyses revealed that intrusive thoughts and avoidant behaviors concerning the upcoming operation in the weeks preceding surgery significantly predicted PCA requests during lock-out periods (i.e., over-frequent attempts at PCA usage), even after controlling for age, preoperative anxiety and depression, postoperative pain, morphine consumption, and negative affect. Furthermore, since pain intensity scores did not significantly predict requests during the lock-out period, a portion of the total morphine patients self-administer may be unnecessary (i.e., not pain-related) and used for purposes other than analgesia. These results suggest that excessive requests for postoperative PCA during lock-out periods reflect poor preoperative adaptation to surgery characterized by the posttraumatic stress symptoms of intrusive thoughts and avoidant behaviors.

The high comorbidity of PTSD and chronic pain may be, in part, a function of the substantial symptom overlap observed in the following domains: anxiety and hyperarousal; attentional biases; avoidant behaviors, emotional lability, and elevated somatic focus (71). This commonality in symptoms suggests the two disorders may be mutually maintaining (71,74). The idea of mutual maintenance may be linked to a common or shared underlying psychological vulnerability that places at-risk individuals at heightened propensity of developing one or both disorders. Anxiety sensitivity has been identified as a likely trait vulnerability factor that predisposes individuals to develop chronic pain, PTSD, or both (71).

The intractability of these two disorders is not surprising when viewed in the context of mutual maintenance and shared vulnerability models. When PTSD and chronic pain co-occur, treatment of one and not the other would be expected to lead only to partial recovery or, if complete recovery occurred in one domain, its duration would be transient (71,72,75). The necessity to detect and treat both conditions concurrently underscores the importance of screening for both disorders when either one is detected.

Medically Unexplained Pain

Pain that does not conform to present-day anatomic and neurophysiologic knowledge is often attributed to psychological dysfunction. Wall has eloquently stated that:

> There are many pains whose cause is not known. If a diligent search has been made in the periphery and no cause is found, we have seen that clinicians act as though there was only one alternative. They blame faulty thinking, which for many classically thinking doctors is the same thing as saying that there is no cause and even no disease. They ignore a century's work on disorders of the spinal cord and brainstem and target the mind.... These are the doctors who repeat again and again to a Second World War amputee in pain that there is nothing wrong with him and that it is all in his head. (76, p. 107)

This view of "psychogenic" pain persists to this day, even in the face of evidence to the contrary. Psychopathology has been proposed to underlie phantom limb pain (77), dyspareunia (78), orofacial pain (79), and a host of other conditions including pelvic pain, abdominal pain, chest pain, and headache (80). However, given the complexity of pain transmission circuitry, many pains that defy our current understanding are likely one day to be explained without having to resort to a psychopathologic etiology. Pain that is "nonanatomical" in distribution, pain that spreads to noninjured territory, pain that is said to be out of proportion to the degree of injury, pain in the absence of injury, pain relief following administration of placebos, have all, at one time or another, been used as evidence to support the idea that psychological disturbance underlies the pain. Yet each of these features of supposed psychopathology can now be explained by neurophysiologic mechanisms that involve an interplay between peripheral and central neural activity (1,79,81).

Recent data linking the immune and central nervous systems have provided an explanation for another heretofore medically unexplained pain problem. Mirror-image pain or *allochiria* has puzzled clinicians and basic scientists ever since it was first documented in the late 1800s (82). Injury to one side of the body is experienced as pain at the site of injury as well as at the contralateral, mirror-image site (83,84). Recent animal studies show that induction of a sciatic inflammatory neuritis by perisciatic microinjection of immune system activators results in hyperalgesia both ipsilaterally and at the mirror-image point on the opposite side, in the territory of the intact contralateral sciatic nerve (85). Moreover, both ipsilateral and contralateral hyperalgesia are prevented or reversed by intrathecal injection of a variety of antagonists to proinflammatory cytokines (86).

Mirror-image pain is likely not a unitary phenomenon and other, nonimmune mechanisms may also be involved (87). Recent human (88) and animal evidence (89) point to a combination of central and peripheral mechanisms. For example, nerve injury to one side of the body results in a 50% reduction in the innervation of the territory of the same nerve on the opposite side of the body in uninjured skin (89). Interestingly, although documented contralateral neurite loss can occur in the absence of contralateral pain or hyperalgesia, the extent of contralateral neurite loss correlates with pain intensity at the site of the injury (88). This observation raises the intriguing possibility that pain at the site of an injury may be prolonged and exacerbated by contralateral neurite loss induced by the original ipsilateral injury (89)—a situation that most clinicians would never have imagined possible.

Taken together, these novel mechanisms that explain some of the most puzzling pain symptoms make us mindful that emotional distress and psychological disturbance in our patients are not at the root of the pain. Attributing pain to a psychological disturbance is damaging to the patient and provider alike, and poisons the patient–provider relationship by introducing an element of mutual distrust and implicit (or even explicit) blame. It is devastating to the patient, who feels at fault, disbelieved, and alone.

The idea that emotional and psychological processes can cause pain traditionally has been tied to the notion of psychopathology. The argument we are making is not that psychological and emotional factors cannot trigger an experience of pain, but that psychopathology per se is not the cause of unexplained pain. There is ample evidence that pain may be triggered by emotional and psychological processes in psychologically healthy individuals (77). However, the presence of comorbid pain and psychopathology does not imply that the pain has its origin in the psychopathology (90).

THEORIES OF PAIN

The Gate Control Theory

The traditional specificity theory of pain, which is still widely taught, proposes that pain is a specific sensation and that the intensity of pain is proportional to the extent of tissue damage. The theory implies a fixed, straight-through transmission system from somatic pain receptors to a pain center in the brain. The evidence just reviewed, however, shows that pain not only is a function of injury, but also is influenced by psychological variables.

In 1965, Melzack and Wall (91) proposed the gate control theory of pain. Basically, the theory proposes that neural mechanisms in the dorsal horns of the spinal cord act as a gate that can facilitate or inhibit the flow of nerve impulses from peripheral fibers to the spinal cord cells that project to the brain. Somatic input is therefore subjected to the modulating influence of the dorsal horn gate before it reaches the brain and evokes pain perception and response. The theory suggests that large-fiber inputs tend to close the gate, whereas small-fiber inputs generally open it, and that the gate is also profoundly influenced by descending influences from the brain. It further proposes that sensory input is modulated at successive synapses throughout its projection from the spinal cord to those brain areas responsible for pain experience and response. Pain occurs

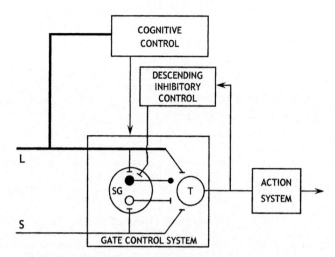

FIGURE 35-1. The gate control theory: Mark II. The new model includes excitatory (*white circle*) and inhibitory (*black circle*) links from the substantia gelatinosa (*SG*) to the transmission (*T*) cells, as well as descending inhibitory control from brainstem systems. The round knob at the end of the inhibitory link implies that its action may be presynaptic, postsynaptic, or both. All connections are excitatory, except the inhibitory link from SG to T cell. Redrawn from Melzack R, Wall PD. *The Challenge of Pain.* New York: Penguin Books, 1982, with permission.

when the number of nerve impulses that arrives at these areas exceeds a critical level.

Melzack and Wall (1) subsequently reassessed the status of the gate-control theory in light of new physiologic research that emerged during the 1990s. Despite considerable controversy and conflicting evidence, the concept of gating (or input modulation) is stronger than ever. A slightly revised model of the gate control theory has been presented (Fig. 35-1). Alternative models are described by Basbaum in the concluding chapter of this volume, on the relevance of gate control theory to regional anesthesia and pain control in the 21st century.

Dimensions of the Pain Experience

Research on pain since the beginning of the 20th century has been dominated by the concept that pain is purely a sensory experience. Yet, pain also has a distinctly unpleasant, affective quality. It becomes overwhelming, demands immediate attention, and disrupts ongoing behavior and thought. It motivates or drives the organism into activity aimed at stopping the pain as quickly as possible. To consider only the sensory features of pain and ignore its motivational–affective properties is to look at only part of the problem. Even the concept of pain as a perception, with full recognition of past experience, attention, and other cognitive influences, still neglects this crucial motivational dimension.

These insights led Melzack and Casey (92) to suggest that pain has three major psychological dimensions: sensory–discriminative, motivational–affective, and cognitive–evaluative. They proposed that these dimensions are subserved by physiologically specialized systems in the brain (Fig. 35-2):

- The sensory–discriminative dimension of pain is influenced primarily by the rapidly conducting spinal systems.
- The powerful motivational drive and unpleasant affect characteristic of pain are subserved by activities in reticular and

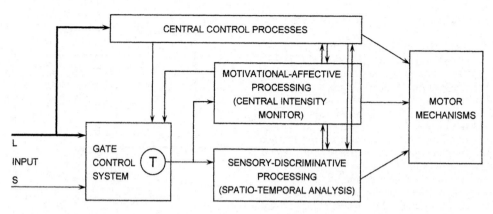

FIGURE 35-2. Conceptual model of the sensory, motivational, and central control determinants of pain. The output of the T cells of the gate control system projects to the sensory–discriminative system (via neospinothalamic fibers) and the motivational–affective system (via the paramedial ascending system). The central control trigger is represented by a line running from the larger fiber system to central control processes; these, in turn, project back to the gate control system and to the sensory–discriminative and motivational–affective systems. All three systems interact with one another and project to the motor system. Redrawn from Melzack R, Casey KL. Sensory, motivational, and central control determinants of pain. In: Kenshalo D, ed. *The Skin Senses*. Springfield, IL: Charles C Thomas, 1968:423–443, with permission.

limbic structures that are influenced primarily by the slowly conducting spinal systems.

■ Discriminative and motivational systems that mediate central nervous system processes, such as evaluation of nociceptive input in terms of past experience, are controlled by neocortical or higher centers.

It is assumed that these three categories of activity interact with one another to provide *perceptual information* on the location, magnitude, and spatiotemporal properties of the noxious stimuli, *motivational tendency* toward escape or attack, *cognitive information* based on past experience, and to predict the likely outcomes of different response strategies. All three forms of activity could then influence motor mechanisms responsible for the complex pattern of overt responses evoked by pain.

Neuromatrix Theory

Melzack (93,94) has recently proposed a new conceptual model, based largely on the properties of phantom limbs and the pain often felt in them (95). He summarized the available data on phantoms in the form of four propositions, which derive from the data:

■ Phantom limbs are experienced as real because their perception is produced by the same brain processes that underlie the experience of the body when it is intact.

■ Neural networks in the brain generate all the qualities of experience that are felt to originate in the body; inputs from the body may trigger or modulate the output of the networks but are not essential for any of the qualities of experience.

■ The experience of the body has a unitary, integrated quality that includes the quality of "self"—that the body is uniquely one's own and not that of any other individual.

■ The neural network that underlies the experience of the body-self is genetically determined but can be modified by sensory experience.

The anatomic substrate of the body-self, Melzack (93,94) proposes, is a network of neurons that extends throughout widespread areas of the brain. He has labeled the network, whose spatial distribution and synaptic links are initially determined genetically and are later sculpted by sensory inputs, as a *neuromatrix*. Thalamocortical and limbic loops that comprise the neuromatrix diverge to permit parallel processing in different components of the neuromatrix and converge repeatedly to permit interactions between the output products of processing. The repeated cyclical processing and synthesis of nerve impulses in the neuromatrix imparts a characteristic pattern or *neurosignature*.

The neurosignature of the neuromatrix is imparted on all nerve impulse patterns that flow through it; the neurosignature is produced by the patterns of synaptic connections, initially innate and later modified by experience, in the entire neuromatrix. All inputs from the body undergo cyclical processing and synthesis, so that characteristic patterns are impressed on them in the neuromatrix. Portions of the neuromatrix are assumed to be specialized to process information related to major sensory events (such as injury) and may be labeled as *neuromodules*, which impress subsignatures on the larger neurosignature.

About 70% of amputees suffer burning, cramping, and other qualities of pain in the first few weeks after amputation. Even 7 years after amputation, 50% still continue to suffer phantom limb pain (96). Why is there so much pain in phantom limbs? Melzack (93) proposes that the active neuromatrix, when deprived of modulating inputs from the limbs or body, produces an abnormal signature pattern that subserves the psychological qualities of hot or burning, the most common qualities of phantom limb pain. Cramping pain, however, may be due to messages from the neuromatrix to produce movement. In the absence of the limbs, the messages to move the muscles may become more frequent and "stronger" in the attempt to move a part of the limb. The end result of the output message may be felt as cramping muscle pain. Shooting pains may have a similar origin, in which the neuromatrix attempts to move the whole limb and sends out abnormal patterns that are felt, for example, as pain shooting down from the groin to the foot. The origins of these pains, then, lie in the brain. Sensory inputs, however, clearly contribute to the phantom; stimulation of the stump or other body sites often produces sensations referred to the phantom limb (97).

Surgical removal of the somatosensory areas of the cortex or thalamus generally fails to relieve phantom limb pain (98). However, the new theory conceives of a neuromatrix that extends throughout selected areas of the whole brain, including the somatic, visual, and limbic systems. Thus, to destroy the neuromatrix for the body-self that generates the neurosignature pattern for pain is impossible. However, if the pattern for pain is generated by cyclical processing and synthesis, it should be possible to block it by injection of a local anesthetic into appropriate discrete areas that are hypothesized to comprise the widespread neuromatrix. Data obtained in rats have shown that localized injections of lidocaine into diverse areas, such as the lateral hypothalamus (99), the cingulum (100), and the dentate gyrus (101), produce striking decreases in experimentally produced pain, including that in an animal model of phantom limb pain (102).

The neuromatrix model has important clinical implications since it searches for brain mechanisms as the causes of pain, rather than focusing exclusively on peripheral factors. The fact that the most common kinds of pain—low back pain and headache (including migraines)—remain a mystery testifies to the extent of our ignorance. The majority of patients who suffer low back pain have no apparent physical signs. A variety of forms of therapy are tried, including disk surgery, trigger-point injections, physical therapy, and behavior modification techniques. Yet a substantial number of people continue to suffer pain in spite of all these efforts. The search for the causes of low back pain is usually focused on the periphery: protruding discs, arthritis, pinched sensory roots, stress on ligaments and joints, spasm in muscles. Given the relatively high frequency of failures in the attempt to rectify possible peripheral causes, it is reasonable to begin considering central mechanisms, such as a neuromatrix responsible for the body's actions.

Because the action neuromatrix maintains specific tensions on all muscles at all times, it is possible that sudden minor accidents (such as a fall) may produce stresses and strains on muscles in a localized part of the body, which then send abnormal messages to the body neuromatrix. The action neuromatrix, in order to maintain posture and balance, may then change the tone in more distant muscles and ultimately produce a vicious cycle of abnormal feedback and output for action.

A brief abnormal message, therefore, may produce a prolonged state of abnormal central outflow. The traditional trigger-point and physical therapies could produce changes in inputs, which sometimes help, but the major cause may be the abnormal messages from the brain that maintain abnormal tensions on a large part of the body musculature. In the attempt to correct the inappropriate feedback, excessive tension may be put on other, distant muscles to maintain balance and readiness for action. In this way, transient minor injury of a shoulder may, for example, lead to pain in the upper back and the other shoulder, and eventually in the lower back and legs. In this case, the therapy that is needed may be far more complex, involving the "re-education" of the musculature of a large part of the body in an attempt to adjust the tone in muscles to a normal, appropriate level.

Myofascial syndromes such as fibromyalgia also remain a mystery and are difficult to understand. It is well known that fibromyalgia (which also has many other names) is associated with a characteristic distribution of trigger spots and sleep disorder, and is usually found in tense, hard-working, younger people. Here again, the initiating cause may be peripheral (muscle tension), but the sustaining cause that maintains abnormal tension is now central. The underlying mechanism is usually sought in long-term activities in the spinal cord, but the cause appears to reside in the brain, and an abnormal output

thus maintains an abnormal pattern of tension on musculature throughout a widespread portion of the body. Once again, therapy may require re-education of the muscles of a large part of the body. Obviously, there are many inputs to the action neuromatrix that may maintain the abnormal activity—such as abnormal muscle feedback, anxiety, depression, and fatigue. All of these provide further avenues for health professionals to attempt to bring about a normal action neuromatrix output.

MEASUREMENT OF PAIN

Psychophysical Approaches

The simplest methods for pain measurement, and, early on, the only available methods, treat pain as though it were a single unique quality that varies only in intensity (11). These methods include the use of verbal rating scales (VRSs), numerical rating scales (NRSs), and visual analogue scales (VASs). These simple methods have all been used effectively in hospital clinics, and have provided valuable information about pain and analgesia. The VRSs, NRSs, and VASs provide simple, efficient, and minimally intrusive measures of pain intensity and have been used widely in clinical and research settings, in which a quick index of pain intensity is required and to which a numerical value can be assigned.

Verbal rating scales typically consist of a series of verbal pain descriptors ordered from least to most intense (e.g., none, mild, moderate, severe) (103). The patient reads the list and chooses the one word that best describes the intensity of his pain at that moment. A score of zero is assigned to the descriptor with the lowest rank, a score of 1 is assigned to the descriptor with the next lowest rank, and so on. Numeric rating scales typically consist of a series of numbers ranging from 0 to 10 (or 0 to 100), with end-points intended to represent the extremes of the possible pain experience and labeled "no pain" and "worst possible pain," respectively. The patient chooses the number that best corresponds to the intensity of his pain at the moment. Although VRSs and NRSs are simple to administer and have demonstrated reliability and validity, the advantages associated with VASs (see later section) make VASs the measurement instrument of choice when a unidimensional measure of pain is required. However, this may not be true when assessing acute and chronic pain in the elderly. Recent evidence suggests that elderly patients with chronic pain make fewer errors on a VRS than on a VAS (104) and that the VAS may not be as sensitive in detecting age differences in postoperative pain as are other measures (105). Moreover, unidimensional measures of pain such as these fail to capture the complexity of the pain experience (106) and, whenever possible, should be coadministered with a multidimensional measure of pain.

The most common VAS consists of a 10-cm horizontal or vertical line with the two end-points labeled "no pain" and "worst pain ever" (or similar verbal descriptors). The patient is required to place a mark on the 10-cm line at a point that corresponds to the level of pain intensity he presently feels. The distance in centimeters from the low end of the VAS to the patient's mark is used as a numerical index of the severity of pain.

Visual analog scales for pain affect have been developed in an effort to include domains of measurable pain experience other than the sensory intensity dimension. The patient is asked to rate the unpleasantness of the pain experience (i.e., how disturbing it is). End-points are labeled "not bad at all" and "the most unpleasant feeling imaginable" (107,108).

Visual analog scales are sensitive to pharmacologic and non-pharmacologic procedures that alter the experience of acute burn pain (109), postoperative pain (110,111), as well as chronic noncancer pain (112,113). Visual analog scales correlate highly with pain measured on verbal and NRSs (114,115). Instructions to patients to rate the amount or percentage of pain relief (e.g., following administration of a treatment designed to reduce pain) may introduce unnecessary bias (e.g., expectancy for change and reliance on memory) that reduces the validity of the measure. It has been suggested, therefore, that a more appropriate measure of change may be obtained by having patients rate the absolute intensity of pain at different points in time, such as before and after an intervention (116). Recent evidence suggests that the relative sensitivity of repeated pain intensity ratings versus measures of pain relief depends upon the characteristics of the sample and not necessarily the psychometric properties of the pain measure used (110). This population-dependent difference in sensitivity highlights the importance of using multiple pain measures in treatment outcome studies.

A major advantage of the VAS as a measure of sensory pain intensity is its ratio scale property (107,113). In contrast to many other pain measurement tools, equality of ratios is implied, making it appropriate to speak meaningfully about percentage differences between VAS measurements obtained either at multiple points in time, or from independent samples of subjects. Other advantages of the VAS include its ease and brevity of administration and scoring, minimal intrusiveness, greater sensitivity to detect the effects of interventions upon pain intensity, and its conceptual simplicity for the patient, providing that adequately clear instructions are given.

Standard VASs have several limitations and disadvantages. These include difficulty with administration in patients who have perceptual–motor problems, cumbersomeness of scoring in a clinical setting where immediate measurement of the patient's response may not be possible, and difficulties for the occasional patient who cannot comprehend the instructions. These limitations and disadvantages of VAS rating scales have been remedied by the development of a visual analogue "thermometer" (VAT), as suggested by Lasagna in 1960, in vertical form (117) and subsequently modified (118). In a currently applied horizontal format (119), the VAT consists of a rigid, plasticized cardboard strip of white color with a horizontal black opening 10 cm long by 2 cm wide. The ends of the opening are labeled "no pain" and "unbearable pain." A red opaque band covers the opening and slides from left to right using a tab operated from the back of the "thermometer." The red strip is moved from left to right across the black opening until the patient stops at a point that corresponds to the intensity of his pain. The back of the VAT also shows a 10-cm ruler to facilitate scoring. The VAT correlates well with a standard paper-and-pencil VAS and a NRS, is sensitive to changes in pain levels, and is preferred over a standard VAS by a substantial number of subjects (120,121).

The main disadvantage of VASs, NRSs, and VRSs is the assumption that pain is a unidimensional experience that can be measured with a single-item scale (122). Although intensity is, without a doubt, a salient dimension of pain, it is clear that the word "pain" refers to a myriad of qualities that are categorized under a single linguistic label, and not to a specific, single sensation that varies only in intensity or affect. The development of rating scales that measure pain affect or pain unpleasantness has partially addressed the problem, but the same shortcoming applies within the affective domain. Each pain has unique qualities. Unpleasantness is only one such quality. The pain of a toothache is obviously different from that of a pin-prick, just as the pain of a coronary occlusion is quite different from the pain of a broken leg. To describe pain solely in terms of intensity or affect is like specifying the visual world only in terms of light flux without regard to pattern, color, texture, and the many other dimensions of visual experience.

The McGill Pain Questionnaire

In the 1970s, Melzack and Torgerson (123,124) made a seminal contribution toward assessing the qualities of pain. In the first part of their study, subjects were asked to classify 102 words, obtained from the clinical literature relating to pain, into smaller groups that describe different aspects of the experience of pain. Based upon these subjects' responses, the words were categorized into three major classes and 16 subclasses. The major classes are (a) words that describe the *sensory qualities* of the experience in terms of temporal, spatial, pressure, thermal, and other properties; (b) words that describe *affective qualities* in terms of tension, fear, and autonomic properties that are part of the pain experience; and (c) *evaluative* words that describe the subjective overall intensity of the total pain experience. Each subclass, which was given a descriptive label, consists of a group of words that were considered by most subjects to be qualitatively similar.

The second part of the study was an attempt to determine the pain intensities implied by the words within each subclass. Groups of doctors, patients, and students were asked to assign an intensity value to each word, using a numeric scale ranging from least (or mild) pain to worst (or excruciating) pain. When this was done, it was apparent that several words within each subclass had the same relative intensity relationships in all three sets. For example, in the spatial subclass, "shooting" was found to represent more pain than "flashing," which in turn implied more pain than "jumping." Although the precise intensity values differed across the three groups of subjects, all three groups provided the same sequence of the words.

Based upon the high degree of agreement on the intensity relationships among pain descriptors by subjects who have different cultural, socioeconomic, and educational backgrounds, it proved possible to develop a questionnaire (Fig. 35-3) for use as a measuring instrument in studies of clinical pain (122,125,126).

One of the most exciting features of the McGill Pain Questionnaire (MPQ) is its value as a diagnostic technique (127). The questionnaire was administered to 95 patients suffering from one of eight known pain syndromes: postherpetic neuralgia, phantom limb pain, metastatic carcinoma, toothache, degenerative disk disease, rheumatoid arthritis or osteoarthritis, labor pain, and menstrual pain. A multiple-group discriminant analysis revealed that each type of pain is characterized by a distinctive constellation of verbal descriptors. Further, when the descriptor set for each patient was classified by computer into one of the eight diagnostic categories, a correct classification was made in 77% of cases.

Further evidence of the discriminative capacity of the MPQ was furnished by Melzack and colleagues (128), who differentiated between the pain of trigeminal neuralgia and atypical facial pain. Fifty-three patients were given a thorough neurologic examination that led to a diagnosis of either trigeminal neuralgia or atypical facial pain. Each patient rated his pain using the MPQ, and the scores were submitted to a discriminant analysis. Ninety-one percent of the patients were correctly classified using seven key descriptors. To determine how well the key descriptors were able to predict either diagnosis, the discriminant function derived from the 53 patients was applied to

McGill Pain Questionnaire

Patient's Name _____   Date _____   Time _____ am/pm

PRI: S _____   A _____   E _____   M _____   PRI(T) _____   PPI_____
     (1-10)   (11-15)   (16)   (17-20)   (1-20)

1 FLICKERING __	11 TIRING __
QUIVERING __	EXHAUSTING __
PULSING __	12 SICKENING __
THROBBING __	SUFFOCATING __
BEATING __	13 FEARFUL __
POUNDING __	FRIGHTFUL __
2 JUMPING __	TERRIFYING __
FLASHING __	14 PUNISHING __
SHOOTING __	GRUELING __
3 PRICKING __	CRUEL __
BORING __	VICIOUS __
DRILLING __	KILLING __
STABBING __	15 WRETCHED __
LANCINATING __	BLINDING __
4 SHARP __	16 ANNOYING __
CUTTING __	TROUBLESOME __
LACERATING __	MISERABLE __
5 PINCHING __	INTENSE __
PRESSING __	UNBEARABLE __
GNAWING __	17 SPREADING __
CRAMPING __	RADIATING __
CRUSHING __	PENETRATING __
6 TUGGING __	PIERCING __
PULLING __	18 TIGHT __
WRENCHING __	NUMB __
7 HOT __	DRAWING __
BURNING __	SQUEEZING __
SCALDING __	TEARING __
SEARING __	19 COOL __
8 TINGLING __	COLD __
ITCHY __	FREEZING __
SMARTING __	20 NAGGING __
STINGING __	NAUSEATING __
9 DULL __	AGONIZING __
SORE __	DREADFUL __
HURTING __	TORTURING __
ACHING __	PPI
HEAVY __	0 NO PAIN __
10 TENDER __	1 MILD __
TAUT __	2 DISCOMFORTING __
RASPING __	3 DISTRESSING __
SPLITTING __	4 HORRIBLE __
	5 EXCRUCIATING __

BRIEF __	RHYTHMIC __	CONTINUOUS __
MOMENTARY __	PERIODIC __	STEADY __
TRANSIENT __	INTERMITTENT __	CONSTANT __

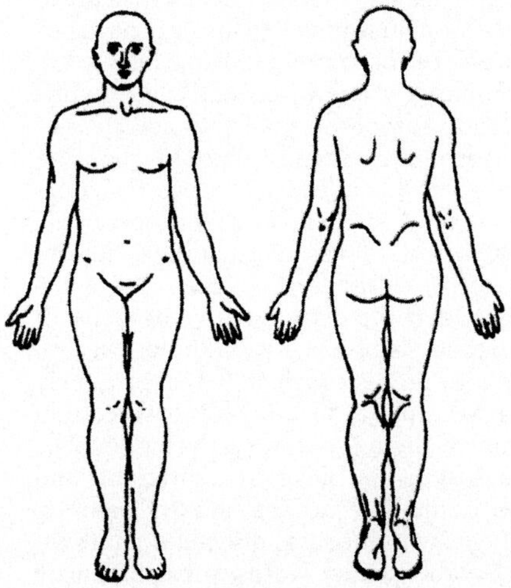

E = EXTERNAL
I = INTERNAL

COMMENTS:

McGill Pain Questionnaire. The descriptors fall into four major groups: sensory, 1-10; affective, 11-15; evaluative, 16; and miscellaneous, 17-20. The rank value for each descriptor is based on its position in the word set. The sum of the rank values is the pain rating index (PRI). The present pain intensity (PPI) is based on a scale of 0 to 5.

FIGURE 35-3. McGill Pain Questionnaire adapted for a study of narcotic drugs. Descriptors fall into four major groups: sensory, 1 to 10; affective, 11 to 15; evaluative, 16; and miscellaneous, 17 to 20. The rank value for each descriptor is based on its position in the word set. The sum of the rank values is the "pain rating index" (PRI). The "present pain intensity" (PPI) is based on a scale of 0 to 5. Redrawn from Melzack R. The McGill Pain Questionnaire: major properties and scoring methods. *Pain* 1975;1:277–299, with permission.

MPQ scores obtained from a second, independent validation sample of patients with trigeminal neuralgia or atypical facial pain. The results showed a correct prediction for 90% of the patients.

Specific verbal descriptors of the MPQ have also been shown to discriminate between reversible and irreversible damage of the nerve fibers in a tooth (129), several facial pain disorders (130,131), and between leg pain caused by diabetic neuropathy and leg pain arising from other causes (132). Mongini and co-workers (133) further showed that the MPQ consistently discriminates between migraine and tension-type headache, confirming an earlier report (134) that cluster headache pain is more intense and distressing than other vascular (migraine and mixed) headache pain and is characterized by a distinct constellation of descriptors. Wilkie and co-workers (135) compared MPQ descriptors chosen by patients with previously classified nociceptive and neuropathic pain sites due to lung cancer. They found that four descriptors (i.e., lacerating, stinging, heavy, suffocating) were used significantly more frequently to describe nociceptive pain sites than neuropathic pain sites and that 11 other descriptors were used more often to describe the latter than the former pain sites. Using a multivariate regression equation, they showed that 78% of the pain sites were accurately identified using 10 MPQ descriptors as nociceptive (81% sensitivity) or neuropathic (59% sensitivity).

It is evident, however, that the discriminative capacity of the MPQ has limits. High levels of anxiety and other psychological disturbance that may produce high affective scores may obscure the discriminative capacity (136). Moreover, certain key words that discriminate among specific syndromes may be absent. Nevertheless, it is clear that there are appreciable and quantifiable differences in the way various types of pain are described, and that patients with the same disease or pain syndrome tend to use remarkably similar words to communicate what they feel.

Worker's Compensation and Pain

Patients who receive worker's compensation or are awaiting litigation after an accident have long been regarded as neurotics or malingerers who are exaggerating their pain for financial gain. There is, however, a growing body of evidence, based on pain measurement, that patients who receive worker's compensation are no different from patients who do not. In particular, a recent study (137) found no differences between compensated and noncompensated patients based on pain scores obtained with the MPQ. A subsequent study of 145 patients suffering low back and musculoskeletal pain also revealed that compensated and noncompensated patients had virtually identical sensory and total pain scores and pain descriptor patterns (138). They were also similar on the Minnesota Multiphase Personality Inventory (MMPI) pain triad (depression, hysteria, hypochondriasis) and on several other personal variables that were examined. The only differences were small but significantly lower affective scores in the low back group and lower evaluative scores in the musculoskeletal group. These results suggest that the financial security provided by compensation decreases anxiety, which is reflected in the lower affective or evaluative ratings but not in the sensory or total MPQ scores. Compensated patients, contrary to traditional opinion, appear not to differ from people who do not receive compensation. Loeser, in Chapter 29, describes the important influence of worker's compensation and litigation upon the outcome of patients with chronic pain. Accidents that produce injury and pain should be considered as potentially psychologically traumatic as well as conducive to the development of subtle physiologic changes, such as trigger points. Patients on compensation or awaiting litigation deserve the same concern and compassion as all other patients who suffer chronic pain. It is prejudice, not evidence, that underlies the old idea of "the compensation neurotic" and adds insult to the patient's injury.

LABOR PAIN

Labor pain provides an excellent model of acute pain. It is associated with obvious sensory stimuli—uterine contractions and cervical dilation—that can be measured in terms of frequency, intensity, spatial extent, and duration. It begins with contractions and ends with the birth of a baby. Labor pain, then, has a specifiable beginning and end, and should reflect all the variables that contribute to other acute pains. As do all pains, labor pain shows an astonishingly high degree of variability among individuals in its intensity and its spatial and temporal distribution (139). This variability allows us to search for the underlying determinants and their contributions to the overall acute pain.

Most women suffer intense pain during labor. In a widely cited study of women in the first stage of labor at the Montreal General Hospital (140), in which one of the authors (RM) employed the MPQ, 60% of primiparas had severe or extremely severe pain, 30% had moderate pain, and only 10% had mild pain. Among multiparas, 45% had severe or extremely severe pain, 30% had moderate pain, and 25% had mild pain. Figure 35-4 shows a comparison of labor pain intensities in relation to different kinds of chronic and acute pain. High pain intensities were also found among Scottish women (141), who are well known for their stoicism; 60% of them reported that labor pain was the most intense pain they had ever experienced.

Although the average labor pain intensity is high, the variability of pain scores is remarkable. Although some women had horrendous pain, others had virtually none. There is some evidence (142) that the latter group of women may generally be less sensitive to all kinds of pain. There is also great individual variability among women in the spatial distribution of pain in the abdomen, sides, and back (143).

Several important variables correlate with labor pain (140, 143). The major determinant is parity; primiparous women have more pain than multiparas. Another determinant is prepared childbirth training, which produces a small (about 10%), statistically significant reduction in both the sensory and affective dimensions of pain. Average pain reductions, depending on the trainer, ranged from 0% to 30%. In addition, older women had less pain than younger women, and women of higher socioeconomic status had less pain than women of lower socioeconomic status. Another determinant is the fact that women who have more painful menstrual periods also have higher levels of labor pain. It is possible that some women produce higher levels of prostaglandins during both menstrual cramps and labor contractions.

Physical factors also play a role (143). Among multiparas, the more the baby weighs, the more pain the mother has, and heavier mothers also tend to have more pain. The pain of primiparas is related to their normal weight-to-height ratio, that is, women who weigh more in relation to their height have more pain.

Yet another determinant is the time of day when the baby is born. Harkness and Gijsbers (144) found that most women tend to give birth at night and, moreover, those who do so have significantly less pain and stress than women who give birth during daylight hours. Previous experience of pain unrelated

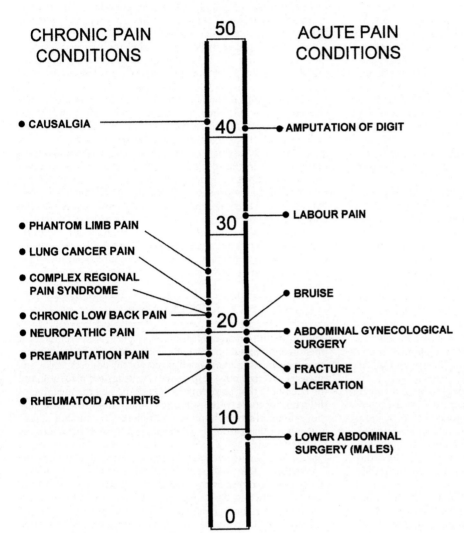

LONG FORM MPQ PAIN SCORES (PRI-T)

CHRONIC PAIN CONDITIONS

ACUTE PAIN CONDITIONS

50

- CAUSALGIA ——————— 40 ——— AMPUTATION OF DIGIT

- LABOUR PAIN

30

- PHANTOM LIMB PAIN
- LUNG CANCER PAIN
- COMPLEX REGIONAL PAIN SYNDROME
- BRUISE
- CHRONIC LOW BACK PAIN 20
- NEUROPATHIC PAIN — ABDOMINAL GYNECOLOGICAL SURGERY
- PREAMPUTATION PAIN
- FRACTURE
- LACERATION
- RHEUMATOID ARTHRITIS

10

- LOWER ABDOMINAL SURGERY (MALES)

0

FIGURE 35-4. Comparison of pain scores, using the McGill Pain Questionnaire, obtained from women during labor (138) and from patients in a general hospital pain clinic (118) and an emergency department (13). The pain score for causalgic pain is reported by Tahmoush (154). Other pain ratings come from studies of patients with chronic pain conditions including lung cancer pain (132), low back pain (155), complex regional pain syndromes (156), neuropathic pain (157), preamputation pain (158), and rheumatoid arthritis (159), as well from patients with acute pain after abdominal gynecological surgery (111) and lower abdominal surgery (160).

to labor also diminishes labor pain (145), presumably due to the opportunity to develop coping strategies.

Low back pain during labor has been the subject of a series of studies. Severe, continuous low back pain is reported by about 33% of women during labor (146). It is described as being qualitatively different from the pains associated with uterine contractions. The pain of contractions felt in the back is often reported as "riding on" the continuous low back pain, so that both together may reach "horrible" or "excruciating" intensities. Continuous low back pain is probably caused by the distention and pressure on adjacent visceral and neural structures in the peritoneum, in contrast to the rhythmic pains that are clearly related to contractions of the uterus. It is possible that each of these major kinds of pain may be controlled by different anesthesiologic and psychological procedures. The former are described at length by Birnbach in Chapter 24.

A further study by Niven and Gijsbers (147) attempted to determine whether episodes of acute low back pain prior to pregnancy are predictive of low back pain during labor. The results show that episodic low back pain before pregnancy is

not correlated with any aspect of labor pain, but is significantly correlated with episodes of low back pain during pregnancy. In contrast, low back pain during menstruation is positively correlated with labor pain scores recorded for back and front contraction pain as well as for continuous back pain. The significant correlation of labor pain with back pain during menstruation suggests that both share a common underlying mechanism. The correlation of low back pain during pregnancy with episodes of acute low back pain before pregnancy suggests that the strain on back muscles during pregnancy may activate the mechanisms that underlie the usual forms of low back pain.

Finally, an experiment (148) carried out by one of the authors (RM) evaluated whether women in labor report less pain when they are in a vertical (sitting or standing) position than in a horizontal (side-lying or supine) position. Pain scores were obtained from 60 women in early labor (dilation 2–5 cm) who alternated between the two positions. The results show that about 35% of women feel less front pain and 50% feel less back pain when they are in a vertical position than in a horizontal position. The amount of decrease in continuous back pain (83%)

was particularly impressive, but the front and back pains associated with contractions were significantly diminished as well. These results, together with earlier observations by Roberts and associates (149), indicate that many women in *early labor* have less pain and are generally more comfortable in a vertical than in a horizontal position. Since early labor comprises a substantial proportion of the entire process of labor and delivery, any simple procedure that alleviates pain without danger to mother or child, such as shifting from a horizontal to a vertical position, should be promoted and employed. During the later stages of labor, however, women prefer to lie down rather than sit because they find the former position more comfortable (149).

Most of the studies described so far are based on data obtained with the MPQ administered during the first stage of labor. When women receive an MPQ after the birth, they report that the second stage is the most painful part of labor and reaches peak intensity at the emergence of the baby's head (149).

Epidural blocks are usually administered during the first stage of labor at the request of the mother when the pain approaches intolerable levels. They are highly effective in about 90% of women (125,140,143). However, the 10% of women who experience a failed epidural block are deeply disappointed. In some of these cases, the epidural appears to be effective for the first hour or so, but then the pain returns at its previously high intensity or higher, sometimes with an unusual spatial distribution (143). In one study (143), the failure rate was about 30%, which is unusually high, and probably was due to the inexperience of incoming residents in anesthesiology. The variability of the effectiveness of anesthesiologists is as distressing as the variability of effectiveness of prepared childbirth trainers to women whose expectations of pain relief are unfulfilled (150).

As a model of acute pain, labor pain highlights individual differences—extraordinary variability occurs in every aspect of pain. Recent studies have revealed a multitude of factors, both psychological and physical, that contribute to the variability of labor pain. Each makes a small contribution, but no single one of them is prepotent in its contribution to pain. Therefore, the relief of labor pain requires multiple convergent approaches (1).

It is clear that prepared childbirth training does not produce the large, dramatic effects promised by many of its proponents and by best-selling books promoting "painless childbirth" (151). The intensity of the feelings of guilt, anger, and failure in some women when they anticipate a "natural, painless birth" and are then confronted with such severe pain or complications that they require an epidural or a cesarean section recently has been documented. Stewart (152) reports that some women may become miserable and depressed (even suicidal), may lose interest in sex and in their marriage, and may require psychotherapy. In some cases, the husbands of women who anticipated "natural" births required psychotherapy after intense feelings of nausea at the sight of blood or seeing their wives in such terrible pain. They experienced a profound sense of guilt and helplessness, and needed therapy for impotence, phobias, and depression.

It is now amply clear that no panaceas exist to abolish labor pain. The Dick-Read (153) and Lamaze (151) procedures have limited effectiveness. The Leboyer method to prevent a "violent birth" has no demonstrable effects (154), and the concept of "early bonding" has fallen by the wayside (155). The recent enthusiasm for birthing chairs has also begun to wane in light of convincing evidence that women in the later stages of labor actually prefer to lie down rather than sit because it is more comfortable (149). Even epidural blocks may fail, forcing women to cope with deep disappointment in addition to pain.

The enormous individual differences in every parameter described lead to the same conclusion reached by Lumley and Astbury: It is absurd to treat all women and all labors in the same way (150). Women should be informed that the "average" labor is a statistical concept, and many women will have patterns of pain that deviate from this concept. In short, any prepared childbirth training course should spend considerable time preparing the prospective mother for possible deviations from the "average"—preparing her for the possibility that she may (or may not) need an epidural block, a forceps delivery, or a cesarean section. Prepared childbirth training and *skillfully* administered epidural analgesia (see Chapter 23) are compatible, complementary procedures that allow recognition of the individuality of each woman.

SUMMARY

Pain, by definition an unpleasant experience, is a psychological phenomenon based upon a complex neurobiological substrate. As surveyed in this chapter, all aspects of the pain response—its intensity, aversiveness, responsivity to drugs (or placebo), and the behaviors that pain evokes—are shaped by the meaning of the pain, its context, the sufferer's beliefs about the pain, and the individual's own, family, vocational, educational, social, and cultural background. All of these factors contribute to the experience and report of pain and must be carefully assessed longitudinally with uniform, validated instruments before the effectiveness or lack thereof of any treatment can be known. Studies of the multiple psychological dimensions of pain have not only refined its assessment, but have also laid the foundation for modern brain imaging studies confirming pain-induced activation of a distributed matrix of brain regions. As reiterated in the final chapter of this book, psychological studies and the models that have sprung from them are crucially relevant not simply to daily practice, but also to the discovery of new drugs and clinical techniques that will carry regional anesthesia and pain medicine well into the 21st century.

ACKNOWLEDGMENTS

Dr. Katz is supported by a Canada Research Chair in Health Psychology at York University. Preparation of this chapter was facilitated by infrastructure support funded by the Canadian Foundation for Innovation and the Ontario Innovation Trust.

References

1. Melzack R, Wall PD. *The Challenge of Pain*, 2nd ed. New York: Basic Books, 1996.
2. Sternbach RA, Tursky B. Ethnic differences among housewives in psychophysical and skin potential responses to electric shock. *Psychophysiology* 1965;148:241–246.
3. Hardy JD, Wolff HG, Goodell H. *Pain Sensations and Reactions*. Baltimore, MD: Williams & Wilkins, 1952.
4. Clark WC, Clark SB. Pain responses in Nepalese porters. *Science* 1980; 209:410–412.

5. Lambert WE, Libman E, Poser EG. Effect of increased salience of membership group on pain tolerance. *J Pers* 1960;28:350.
6. Zborowski M. Cultural components in response to pain. *J Soc Issues* 1952;8:16.
7. Zatzick DF, Dimsdale JE. Cultural variations in response to painful stimuli. *Psychosom Med* 1990;52:544–557.
8. Campbell CM, Edwards RR, Fillingim RB. Ethnic differences in responses to multiple experimental pain stimuli. *Pain* 2005;113:20–26.
9. Edwards RR, Fillingim RB. Ethnic differences in thermal pain responses. *Psychosom Med* 1999;61:346–354.
10. Watson PJ, Latif RK, Rowbotham DJ. Ethnic differences in thermal pain responses: A comparison of South Asian and White British healthy males. *Pain* 2005;118:194–200.
11. Beecher HK. *Measurement of Subjective Responses*. New York, NY: Oxford University Press, 1959.
12. Carlen PL, Wall PD, Nadvorna H, et al. Phantom limbs and related phenomena in recent traumatic amputations. *Neurology* 1978;28:211–217.
13. Melzack R, Wall PD, Ty TC. Acute pain in an emergency clinic: Latency of onset and descriptor patterns related to different injuries. *Pain* 1982;14:33–43.
14. Hall KR, Stride E. The varying response to pain in psychiatric disorders: A study in abnormal psychology. *Br J Med Psychol* 1954;27:48–60.
15. Hill HE, Kornetsky CH, Flanary HG, et al. Effects of anxiety and morphine on discrimination of intensities of painful stimuli. *J Clin Invest* 1952;31:473–480.
16. Hill HE, Kornetsky CH, Flanary HG, et al. Studies on anxiety associated with anticipation of pain. I. Effects of morphine. *AMA Arch Neurol Psychiatry* 1952;67:612–619.
17. Melzack R, Weisz AZ, Sprague LT. Stratagems for controlling pain: Contributions of auditory stimulation and suggestion. *Exp Neurol* 1963;8:239.
18. Gardner WJ, Licklider JC. Auditory analgesia in dental operations. *J Am Dent Assoc* 1959;59:1144–1149.
19. Katz J, Irvine MJ, Ritvo P, et al. Coping with pain. In: Zeidner M, Endler NS, eds. *Handbook of Coping: Theory, Research, Applications*. New York: Wiley; 1996:252–278.
20. McCaul KD, Malott JM. Distraction and coping with pain. *Psychol Bull* 1984;95:516–533.
21. Katz J, Melzack R. Phantom pain. In: Grafman J, Robertson IH, eds. *Handbook of Neuropsychology*. Oxford: Elsevier; 2003:205–230.
22. Slifer KJ, Tucker CL, Dahlquist LM. Helping children and caregivers cope with repeated invasive procedures: How are we doing? *J Clin Psychol Med Settings* 2002;9:131–152.
23. Wismeijer AA, Vingerhoets AJ. The use of virtual reality and audiovisual eyeglass systems as adjunct analgesic techniques: A review of the literature. *Ann Behav Med* 2005;30:268–278.
24. Hoffman HG, Doctor JN, Patterson DR, et al. Virtual reality as an adjunctive pain control during burn wound care in adolescent patients. *Pain* 2000;85:305–309.
25. Magora F, Cohen S, Shochina M, et al. Virtual reality immersion method of distraction to control experimental ischemic pain. *Isr Med Assoc J* 2006;8:261–265.
26. Hoffman HG, Patterson DR, Carrougher GJ. Use of virtual reality for adjunctive treatment of adult burn pain during physical therapy: A controlled study. *Clin J Pain* 2000;16:244–250.
27. Hoffman HG, Richards TL, Coda B, et al. Modulation of thermal pain-related brain activity with virtual reality: Evidence from fMRI. *Neuroreport* 2004;15:1245–1248.
28. Hoffman HG, Richards TL, Bills AR, et al. Using FMRI to study the neural correlates of virtual reality analgesia. *CNS Spectr* 2006;11:45–51.
29. Crombez G, Vlaeyen JW, Heuts PH, et al. Pain-related fear is more disabling than pain itself: Evidence on the role of pain-related fear in chronic back pain disability. *Pain* 1999;80:329–339.
30. Vlaeyen JW, Kole-Snijders AM, Boeren RG, et al. Fear of movement/(re)injury in chronic low back pain and its relation to behavioral performance. *Pain* 1995;62:363–372.
31. Waddell G, Newton M, Henderson I, et al. A Fear-Avoidance Beliefs Questionnaire (FABQ) and the role of fear-avoidance beliefs in chronic low back pain and disability. *Pain* 1993;52:157–168.
32. Fordyce WE. The cognitive/behavioral perspective on clinical pain. In: Loeser JD, Egan KJ, eds. *Managing the Chronic Pain Patient*. New York, NY: Raven Press; 1989:51–64.
33. Philips HC. Avoidance behaviour and its role in sustaining chronic pain. *Behav Res Ther* 1987;25:273–279.
34. Philips HC. The effects of behavioural treatment on chronic pain. *Behav Res Ther* 1987;25:365–377.
35. Boersma K, Linton S, Overmeer T, et al. Lowering fear-avoidance and enhancing function through exposure in vivo. A multiple baseline study across six patients with back pain. *Pain* 2004;108:8–16.
36. Vlaeyen JW, de Jong J, Geilen M, et al. The treatment of fear of movement/(re)injury in chronic low back pain: Further evidence on the effectiveness of exposure in vivo. *Clin J Pain* 2002;18:251–261.
37. Egbert LD, Battit GE, Welch CE, et al. Reduction of postoperative pain by encouragement and instruction of patients. A study of doctor-patient rapport. *N Engl J Med* 1964;270:825–827.
38. Langer EJ, Janis IL, Wolfer J. Reduction of psychological stress in surgical patients. *Exp Soc Psychol* 1975;11:155.
39. Martinez-Urrutia A. Anxiety and pain in surgical patients. *J Consult Clin Psychol* 1975;43:437.
40. McQuay H, Carroll D, Moore A. Variation in the placebo effect in randomised controlled trials of analgesics: All is as blind as it seems. *Pain* 1996;64:331–335.
41. Evans FJ. The placebo response in pain control. *Psychopharmacol Bull* 1981;17:72–76.
42. Wall PD. The placebo and the placebo response. In: Wall PD, Melzack R, eds. *Textbook of Pain*, 3rd ed. Edinburgh: Churchill Livingston, 1994.
43. McGlashan TH, Evans FJ, Orne MT. The nature of hypnotic analgesia and placebo response to experimental pain. *Psychosom Med* 1969;31:227–246.
44. Petrovic P, Kalso E, Petersson KM, et al. Placebo and opioid analgesia: Imaging a shared neuronal network. *Science* 2002;295:1737–1740.
45. Petrovic P, Ingvar M. Imaging cognitive modulation of pain processing. *Pain* 2002;95:1–5.
46. Petrovic P. Opioid and placebo analgesia share the same network. *Semin Pain Med* 2005;3:31–36.
47. Fields HL, Price DD. Placebo analgesia. In: McMahon SB, Koltzenburg M, eds. *Wall and Melzack's Textbook of Pain*, 5th ed. New York, NY: Elsevier Churchill Livingstone; 2006:361–367.
48. Colloca L, Benedetti F. Placebos and painkillers: Is mind as real as matter? *Nat Rev Neurosci* 2005;6:545–552.
49. Amanzio M, Benedetti F. Neuropharmacological dissection of placebo analgesia: Expectation-activated opioid systems versus conditioning-activated specific subsystems. *J Neurosci* 1999;19:484–494.
50. Levine JD, Gordon NC, Fields HL. The mechanism of placebo analgesia. *Lancet* 1978;2:654–657.
51. Benedetti F. Placebo analgesia. *Neurol Sci* 2006;27[Suppl 2]:S100–S102.
52. Price DD, Craggs J, Nicholas Verne G, et al. Placebo analgesia is accompanied by large reductions in pain-related brain activity in irritable bowel syndrome patients. *Pain* 2007;127(1–2):63–72.
53. Benedetti F, Amanzio M, Maggi G. Potentiation of placebo analgesia by proglumide. *Lancet* 1995;346:1231.
54. Benedetti F. How the doctor's words affect the patient's brain. *Eval Health Prof* 2002;25:369–386.
55. Pollo A, Amanzio M, Arslanian A, et al. Response expectancies in placebo analgesia and their clinical relevance. *Pain* 2001;93:77–84.
56. Vase L, Robinson ME, Verne GN, et al. The contributions of suggestion, desire, and expectation to placebo effects in irritable bowel syndrome patients. An empirical investigation. *Pain* 2003;105:17–25.
57. Benedetti F, Amanzio M. The neurobiology of placebo analgesia: From endogenous opioids to cholecystokinin. *Prog Neurobiol* 1997;52:109–125.
58. Benedetti F, Amanzio M, Casadio C, et al. Blockade of nocebo hyperalgesia by the cholecystokinin antagonist proglumide. *Pain* 1997;71:135–140.
59. Staats PS, Staats A, Hekmat H. The additive impact of anxiety and a placebo on pain. *Pain Med* 2001;2:267–279.
60. Sullivan M, Terman GW, Peck B, et al. APS position statement on the use of placebos in pain management. *J Pain* 2005;6:215–217.
61. Spanos NP, Carmanico SJ, Ellis JA. Hypnotic analgesia. In: Wall PD, Melzack R, eds. *Textbook of Pain*. Edinburgh: Churchill Livingston, 1994.
62. Sheehan PW, Perry CW. *Methodologies of Hypnosis: A Critical Appraisal of Contemporary Paradigms of Hypnosis*. Hillsdale, NJ: Erlbaum Associates, 1976.
63. Hilgard ER, Hilgard J. *Hypnosis in the Relief of Pain*. Los Altos, CA: Kaufmann, 1975.
64. American Psychiatric Association, American Psychiatric Association, Task Force on DSM-IV. *Diagnostic and Statistical Manual of Mental Disorders: DSM-IV-TR*, 4th ed. Washington, DC: American Psychiatric Association, 2000.
65. Mylle J, Maes M. Partial posttraumatic stress disorder revisited. *J Affect Disord* 2004;78:37–48.
66. Beckham JC, Crawford AL, Feldman ME, et al. Chronic posttraumatic stress disorder and chronic pain in Vietnam combat veterans. *J Psychosom Res* 1997;43:379–389.
67. McFarlane AC, Atchison M, Rafalowicz E, et al. Physical symptoms in post-traumatic stress disorder. *J Psychosom Res* 1994;38:715–726.
68. White P, Faustman W. Coexisting physical conditions among inpatients with post-traumatic stress disorder. *Mil Med* 1989;154:66–71.
69. Asmundson GJG, Norton GR, Allerdings MD, et al. Posttraumatic stress disorder and work-related injury. *J Anxiety Disord* 1998;12:57–69.
70. Benedikt RA, Kolb LC. Preliminary findings on chronic pain and posttraumatic stress disorder. *Am J Psychiatry* 1986;143:908–910.
71. Asmundson GJG, Coons MJ, Taylor S, et al. PTSD and the experience of pain: Research and clinical implications of shared vulnerability and mutual maintenance models. *Can J Psychiatry* 2002;10:903–937.
72. Salomons TV, Osterman JE, Gagliese L, et al. Pain flashbacks in posttraumatic stress disorder. *Clin J Pain* 2004;20:83–87.

73. Katz J, Buis T, Cohen L. Locked out and still knocking: predictors of excessive demands for postoperative intravenous patient-controlled analgesia. *Can J Anaesth.* 2008;55:88–99.

74. Sharp TJ, Harvey AG. Chronic pain and posttraumatic stress disorder: Mutual maintenance? *Clin Psychol Rev* 2001;21:857–877.

75. Asmundson GJG, Taylor S. PTSD and chronic pain: Cognitive-behavioral perspectives and practical implications. In: Young G, Kane AW, Nicholson K, eds. *Psychological Knowledge in Court. PTSD, Pain, and TBI.* New York, NY: Springer; 2006:225–241.

76. Wall PD. *Pain: The Science of Suffering.* London: Weidenfeld & Nicolson, 1999.

77. Katz J. Individual differences in the consciousness of phantom limbs. In: Kunzendorf RG, Wallace B, eds. *Individual Differences in Conscious Experience: First-person Constraints on Theories of Consciousness, Self-consciousness, and Subconsciousness.* Amsterdam: John Benjamins Publishing Co.; 2000:45–97.

78. Meana M, Binik YM. Painful coitus: A review of female dyspareunia. *J Nerv Ment Dis* 1994;182:264–272.

79. Gagliese L, Katz J. Medically unexplained pain is not caused by psychopathology. *Pain Res Manage* 2000;5:251–257.

80. Stoudemire A, Sandhu J. Psychogenic/idiopathic pain syndromes. *Gen Hosp Psychiatry* 1987;9:79–86.

81. Woolf CJ, Decosterd I. Implications of recent advances in the understanding of pain pathophysiology for the assessment of pain in patients. *Pain* 1999;[Suppl 6]:S141–S147.

82. Basbaum AI. A new way to lose your nerve. *Sci Aging Knowledge Environ* 2004;88:15.

83. Livingston WK. *Pain and Suffering.* Seattle: IASP Press, 1998.

84. Maleki J, LeBel AA, Bennett GJ, et al. Patterns of spread in complex regional pain syndrome, type I (reflex sympathetic dystrophy). *Pain* 2000;88:259–266.

85. Chacur M, Milligan ED, Gazda LS, et al. A new model of sciatic inflammatory neuritis (SIN): Induction of unilateral and bilateral mechanical allodynia following acute unilateral peri-sciatic immune activation in rats. *Pain* 2001;94:231–244.

86. Milligan ED, Twining C, Chacur M, et al. Spinal glia and proinflammatory cytokines mediate mirror-image neuropathic pain in rats. *J Neurosci* 2003;23:1026–1040.

87. Koltzenburg M, Wall PD, McMahon SB. Does the right side know what the left is doing? *Trends Neurosci* 1999;22:122–127.

88. Oaklander AL, Romans K, Horasek S, et al. Unilateral postherpetic neuralgia is associated with bilateral sensory neuron damage. *Ann Neurol* 1998;44:789–795.

89. Oaklander AL, Brown JM. Unilateral nerve injury produces bilateral loss of distal innervation. *Ann Neurol* 2004;55:639–644.

90. Gatchel RJ, Polatin PB, Mayer TG. The dominant role of psychosocial risk factors in the development of chronic low back pain disability. *Spine* 1995;20:2702–2709.

91. Melzack R, Wall PD. Pain mechanisms: A new theory. *Science* 1965;150:971–979.

92. Melzack R, Casey KL. Sensory, motivational, and central control determinants of pain. In: Kenshalo D, ed. *The Skin Senses.* Springfield, IL: Charles C Thomas; 1968:423–443.

93. Melzack R. Labat lecture. Phantom limbs. *Reg Anesth* 1989;14:208–211.

94. Melzack R. The gate control theory 25 years later: New perspectives on phantom limb pain. In: Bond MR, Charlton JE, Woolf CJ, eds. Pain research and therapy: Proceedings of the VIth world congress on pain. Amsterdam: Elsevier; 1991:9–21.

95. Melzack R, Loeser JD. Phantom body pain in paraplegics: Evidence for a central "pattern generating mechanism" for pain. *Pain* 1978;4:195–210.

96. Krebs B, Jensen TS, Kroner K, et al. Phantom limb phenomena in amputees seven years after limb amputation. In: Fields HL, Dubner R, Ceverso F, ed. *Advances in Pain Research and Therapy.* New York, NY: Raven Press; 1985:425–429.

97. Katz J, Melzack R. Referred sensations in chronic pain patients. *Pain* 1987;28:51–59.

98. White JC, Sweet WH. *Pain and the Neurosurgeon.* Springfield, IL: Charles C. Thomas, 1969.

99. Tasker RA, Choiniere M, Libman SM, et al. Analgesia produced by injection of lidocaine into the lateral hypothalamus. *Pain* 1987;31:237–248.

100. Vaccarino AL, Melzack R. Analgesia produced by injection of lidocaine into the anterior cingulum bundle of the rat. *Pain* 1989;39:213–219.

101. McKenna JE, Melzack R. Analgesia produced by lidocaine microinjection into the dentate gyrus. *Pain* 1992;49:105–112.

102. Vaccarino AI, Melzack R. The role of the cingulum bundle in self-mutilation following peripheral neurectomy in the rat. *Exp Neurol* 1991;111:131–134.

103. Jensen MP, Karoly P. Self-report scales and procedures for assessing pain in adults. In: Turk DC, Melzack R, eds. *Handbook of Pain Assessment,* 2nd ed. New York: Guilford Press; 2001:15–34.

104. Gagliese L, Melzack R. Age differences in the quality of chronic pain: A preliminary study. *Pain Res Manage* 1997;2:157–162.

105. Gagliese L, Katz J. Age differences in postoperative pain are scale dependent: A comparison of measures of pain intensity and quality in younger and older surgical patients. *Pain* 2003;103:11–20.

106. de C Williams AC, Davies HT, Chadury Y. Simple pain rating scales hide complex idiosyncratic meanings. *Pain* 2000;85:457–463.

107. Price DD, Harkins SW, Baker C. Sensory-affective relationships among different types of clinical and experimental pain. *Pain* 1987;28:297–307.

108. Price DD, Harkins SW, Rafii A, et al. A simultaneous comparison of fentanyl's analgesic effects on experimental and clinical pain. *Pain* 1986;24:197–203.

109. Choinière M, Melzack R, Girard N, et al. Comparisons between patients' and nurses' assessments of pain and medication efficacy in severe burn injuries. *Pain* 1990;40:143–152.

110. Jensen MP, Chen C, Brugger AM. Postsurgical pain outcome assessment. *Pain* 2002;99:101–109.

111. Katz J, Cohen L, Schmid R, et al. Postoperative morphine use and hyperalgesia are reduced by preoperative but not intraoperative epidural analgesia: Implications for preemptive analgesia and the prevention of central sensitization. *Anesthesiology* 2003;98:1449–1460.

112. Becker N, Sjogren P, Bech P, et al. Treatment outcome of chronic nonmalignant pain patients managed in a Danish multidisciplinary pain centre compared to general practice: A randomised controlled trial. *Pain* 2000;84:203–211.

113. Price DD, McGrath PA, Rafii A, et al. The validation of visual analogue scales as ratio scale measures for chronic and experimental pain. *Pain* 1983;17:45–56.

114. Bijur PE, Latimer CT, Gallagher EJ. Validation of a verbally administered numerical rating scale of acute pain for use in the emergency department. *Acad Emerg Med* 2003;10:390–392.

115. Ekblom A, Hansson P. Pain intensity measurements in patients with acute pain receiving afferent stimulation. *J Neurol Neurosurg Psychiatry* 1988;51:481–486.

116. Carlsson AM. Assessment of chronic pain. I. Aspects of the reliability and validity of the visual analogue scale. *Pain* 1983;16:87–101.

117. Lasagna L. The clinical measurement of pain. *Ann NY Acad Sci* 1960;86:28–37.

118. Szyfelbein SK, Osgood PF, Carr DB. The assessment of pain and plasma beta-endorphin immunoactivity in burned children. *Pain* 1985;22:173–182.

119. Choiniere M, Amsel R. A visual analogue thermometer for measuring pain intensity. *J Pain Symptom Manage* 1996;11:299–311.

120. Melzack R. The McGill Pain Questionnaire: Major properties and scoring methods. *Pain* 1975;1:277–299.

121. Melzack R. The McGill Pain Questionnaire: From description to measurement. *Anesthesiology* 2005;103:199–202.

122. Melzack R, Torgerson WS. On the language of pain. *Anesthesiology* 1971;34:50–59.

123. Melzack R. The short-form McGill Pain Questionnaire. *Pain* 1987;30:191–197.

124. Turk DC, Melzack R. *Handbook of Pain Assessment,* 2nd ed. New York, NY: Guilford Press, 2001.

125. Dubuisson D, Melzack R. Classification of clinical pain descriptions by multiple group discriminant analysis. *Exp Neurol* 1976;51:480–487.

126. Melzack R, Terrence C, Fromm G, et al. Trigeminal neuralgia and atypical facial pain: Use of the McGill Pain Questionnaire for discrimination and diagnosis. *Pain* 1986;27:297–302.

127. Grushka M, Sessle BJ. Applicability of the McGill Pain Questionnaire to the differentiation of "toothache" pain. *Pain* 1984;19:49–57.

128. Mongini F, Italiano M. TMJ disorders and myogenic facial pain: A discriminative analysis using the McGill Pain Questionnaire. *Pain* 2001;91:323–330.

129. Mongini F, Italiano M, Raviola F, et al. The McGill Pain Questionnaire in patients with TMJ pain and with facial pain as a somatoform disorder. *Cranio* 2000;18:249–256.

130. Masson EA, Hunt L, Gem JM, et al. A novel approach to the diagnosis and assessment of symptomatic diabetic neuropathy. *Pain* 1989;38:25–28

131. Mongini F, Deregibus A, Raviola F, et al. Confirmation of the distinction between chronic migraine and chronic tension-type headache by the McGill Pain Questionnaire. *Headache* 2003;43:867–877.

132. Jerome A, Holroyd KA, Theofanous AG, et al. Cluster headache pain vs. other vascular headache pain: Differences revealed with two approaches to the McGill Pain Questionnaire. *Pain* 1988;34:35–42.

133. Wilkie DJ, Huang HY, Reilly N, et al. Nociceptive and neuropathic pain in patients with lung cancer: A comparison of pain quality descriptors. *J Pain Symptom Manage* 2001;22:899–910.

134. Kremer E, Atkinson JH. Pain language as a measure of effect in chronic pain patients. In: Melzack R, ed. *Pain Measurement and Assessment.* New York: Raven Press; 1983:119–127.

135. Mendelson G. Chronic pain and compensation issues. In: Wall PD, Melzack R, eds. *Textbook of Pain,* 3rd ed. Edinburgh: Churchill Livingstone, 1994.

136. Melzack R, Katz J, Jeans ME. The role of compensation in chronic pain: Analysis using a new method of scoring the McGill Pain Questionnaire. *Pain* 1985;23:101–112.

137. Melzack R. The myth of painless childbirth (the John J. Bonica lecture). *Pain* 1984;19:321–337.
138. Melzack R, Taenzer P, Feldman P, et al. Labour is still painful after prepared childbirth training. *Can Med Assoc J* 1981;125:357–363.
139. Niven C, Gijsbers K. Obstetric and non-obstetric factors related to pain. *J Reprod Infant Psychol* 1984;2:61.
140. Niven CA, Gijsbers KJ. Do low levels of labour pain reflect low sensitivity to noxious stimulation? *Soc Sci Med* 1989;29:585–588.
141. Melzack R, Kinch R, Dobkin P, et al. Severity of labour pain: Influence of physical as well as psychologic variables. *Can Med Assoc J* 1984;130:579–584.
142. Harkness J, Gijsbers K. Pain and stress during childbirth and time of day. *Ethol Sociobiol* 1989;10:255.
143. Niven C, Gijsbers K. A study of labour pain using the McGill Pain Questionnaire. *Soc Sci Med* 1984;19:1347–1351.
144. Melzack R, Schaffelberg D. Low-back pain during labor. *Am J Obstet Gynecol* 1987;156:901–905.
145. Melzack R, Belanger E. Labour pain: Correlations with menstrual pain and acute low-back pain before and during pregnancy. *Pain* 1989;36:225–229.
146. Melzack R, Belanger E, Lacroix R. Labor pain: Effect of maternal position on front and back pain. *J Pain Symptom Manage* 1991;6:476–480.
147. Roberts J, Melasanos L, Mendez-Bauer C. Maternal positions in labor. Analysis in relation to comfort and efficiency. *Birth Defects Orig Artic Ser* 1981;17:97.
148. Lumley J, Astbury J. *Birth Rites, Birth Rights*. Melbourne: Sphere Books, 1980.
149. Lamaze F. *Painless Childbirth: Psychoprophylactic Method*. Chicago, IL: Regnery, 1970.
150. Stewart DE. Psychiatric symptoms following attempted natural childbirth. *Can Med Assoc J* 1982;127:713–716.
151. Dick-Read G. *Childbirth Without Fear*. New York, NY: Harper, 1944.
152. Nelson NM, Enkin MW, Saigal S, et al. A randomized clinical trial of the Leboyer approach to childbirth. *N Engl J Med* 1980;302:655–660.
153. Brody JE. Influential theory of "bonding" losing supporters. *New York Times*; reprinted in *The Gazette* [Montreal], April 2, 1983.
154. Tahmoush AJ. Causalgia: Redefinition as a clinical pain syndrome. *Pain* 1981;10:187–197.
155. Scrimshaw SV, Maher CG. Randomized controlled trial of neural mobilization after spinal surgery. *Spine* 2001;26:2647–2652.
156. Birklein F, Riedl B, Sieweke N, et al. Neurological findings in complex regional pain syndromes: Analysis of 145 cases. *Acta Neurol Scand* 2000; 101:262–269.
157. Lynch ME, Clark AJ, Sawynok J. Intravenous adenosine alleviates neuropathic pain: A double blind placebo controlled crossover trial using an enriched enrolment design. *Pain* 2003;103:111–1117.
158. Nikolajsen L, Ilkjaer S, Kroner K, et al. The influence of preamputation pain on postamputation stump and phantom pain. *Pain* 1997;72:393–405.
159. Roche PA, Klestov AC, Heim HM. Description of stable pain in rheumatoid arthritis: a 6 year study. *J Rheumatol* 2003;30:1733–1738.
160. Katz J, Clairoux M, Kavanagh BP, et al. Pre-emptive lumbar epidural anaesthesia reduces postoperative pain and patient-controlled morphine consumption after lower abdominal surgery. *Pain* 1994;59:395–403.

PART IV: PAIN MANAGEMENT

CHAPTER 36 ■ THE PLACEBO RESPONSE: IMPLICATIONS FOR NEURAL BLOCKADE

DAMIEN G. FINNISS AND FABRIZIO BENEDETTI

The placebo response has been a topic of interest for over 200 years and, in recent times, has been gaining more interest in the scientific and clinical communities. Our understanding of the mechanisms of the placebo effect has improved with more rigorous studies using novel research design and technology. This enhanced understanding has led in turn to further questions as to the impact of the placebo effect on clinical practice and clinical trial design (1,2). Much of our knowledge about the mechanisms of the placebo effect has come from the field of pain and analgesia. This chapter surveys the placebo effect per se, as distinct from the well-described physiologic effects of needle insertion that must also be taken into account in evaluating the effects of regional anesthesia. The latter are reviewed in Chapter 34 by Butler and Siddall.

HISTORICAL OVERVIEW

The first documented use of the word *placebo* in medical literature dates back to 1785, and not long after that, the first placebo-controlled trial was apparently conducted (3,4). This trial was conducted between 1799 and 1801 by Haygarth, who experimented with the use of metallic rods ("Perkins tractors") on five patients. It was believed that implantation of these metallic rods would alleviate the symptoms of many diseases, due to the electromagnetic properties of the metal. Haygarth first implanted imitation rods (made from wood) in his five patients, finding that four gained relief. He then repeated the procedure the following day on the same patients, however, this time, he used the metallic rods. Again, four patients gained relief. Possibly the most interesting feature of this trial was one of Haygarth's conclusions. He remarked "an important lesson in physic is here to be learnt, the wonderful and powerful influence of the passions of the mind upon the state and disorder of the body" (3).

Since the trial conducted by Haygarth, a steady if slow increase has occurred in the number of trials using placebo controls, which ultimately resulted in the development of the double-blinded trial (5). The randomized, double-blind, placebo-controlled trial, in which both the clinician and the patient are unaware of whether active treatment or placebo is being given, is now the gold standard in clinical trial design (4,6). Despite placebo use in clinical trials for some years, and the publication over 50 years ago of Beecher's landmark paper analyzing the responses of patients in some of the early placebo-controlled trials (7), the study of the mechanisms of the placebo effect has only recently started to gain more attention in the scientific community.

MECHANISMS OF THE PLACEBO RESPONSE

The mechanisms of the placebo response can be discussed under separate psychological and neurobiologic categories, although it is the integration of these two approaches that provides an opportunity to explore the complexity of the mind–brain–body interaction.

Psychological Mechanisms

The psychological mechanisms of placebo responses studied in greatest detail are those of expectancies and conditioning. Other potential mechanisms that require further investigation include changes in anxiety and desire for pain relief (8,9). The conditioning mechanism is based upon the theory of classical conditioning, whereby a previously neutral stimulus (such as the treatment characteristics or the environment in which treatment is delivered) is paired or "conditioned" with an unconditioned stimulus (the active drug) that is able to elicit a response (conditioned response) (10,11). In the case of injections, the pairing of the context of treatment with an active drug and analgesia may result in a conditioned analgesic response to an injection of a placebo at a later stage (Fig. 36-1). The conditioning mechanism has gained support through a variety of trials both in animals (12,13) and humans (14,15). A recent study demonstrated that placebo analgesic responses were able to be conditioned using both opiate and nonopiate drugs (16). This study also looked at expectancy mechanisms and found that the placebo analgesic response was greatest when both conditioning and expectancy were involved. There is, however, a degree of difficulty in distinguishing the conditioning mechanism from the expectancy mechanism in placebo analgesia, as the conditioning process may influence the expectations of the patient toward the treatment, and thus the placebo analgesic response may in fact be mediated by expectancies (17–19).

One study was able to demonstrate the conditioning mechanism in a clinical population (20). In this study, patients were given standard postoperative analgesia, and ventilatory function was monitored. On the third postoperative day, a placebo was given that resulted in similar changes in ventilatory

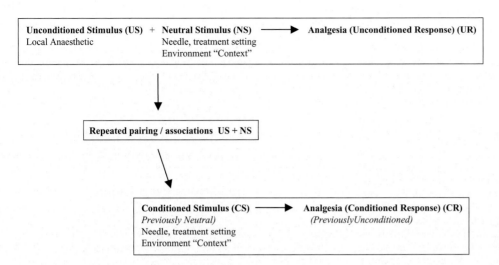

FIGURE 36-1. The classical conditioning mechanism of placebo analgesia.

function (respiratory depression) as had been experienced with the opioids. In this study, the placebo was able to cause a "side effect" similar to that of the active drug. More recent work has also shown that the conditioning mechanism, particularly when involving unconscious processes, such as hormone secretion (18) and immune responses (21,22), may contribute to placebo effects. In the case of placebo analgesia, it would seem that the expectancy mechanism plays a significant role and may be integrated with the conditioning process.

The expectations of the patient regarding the treatment being administered, also termed *response expectancies*, are those held by an individual about his automatic emotional and physiological responses to a particular stimulus (23,24). A variety of studies have investigated the expectancy mechanism using simple verbal cues (suggestibility) (16,25–27), as well as more complicated conditioning protocols aimed at increasing expectations prior to placebo administration (17,28,29). These studies have shown that expectations are powerful contributors to placebo responses, particularly the placebo analgesic response.

Neurobiologic Mechanisms

The neurobiologic mechanisms of the placebo response were highlighted for the first time in 1978, by Levine, Gordon, and Fields, who showed that placebo analgesia was reversed by the administration of naloxone, an endogenous opioid antagonist, suggesting a role of endogenous opioids in the placebo analgesic response (30). The majority of research into the neurobiologic mechanisms of the placebo response has looked at the role of endogenous opioids, although in some studies naloxone has had no effect on placebo analgesia (16,31,32). The occurrence of both positive and negative results for the effects of naloxone suggests that placebo analgesia is mediated by both opioid and nonopioid mechanisms.

One interesting example of the variable role of endogenous opioids is the study by Amanzio and Benedetti in 1999 (16). In this study, both conditioning and expectancy mechanisms were manipulated. Two different types of drugs were used for the conditioning protocol, an opiate analgesic (morphine) and the nonsteroidal anti-inflammatory drug (NSAID) ketorolac. The same drugs were used to explore expectancy manipulations.

Placebo analgesic responses were seen following conditioning with both these drugs, and the responses in the expectancy groups were reversed by naloxone, demonstrating that the expectancy mechanism is mediated by endogenous opioids. Interestingly, in the conditioning groups, only the placebo analgesic response that was conditioned with morphine was able to be reversed by naloxone, whereas the placebo response conditioned with the NSAID was not. This variability demonstrates that different mechanisms (both opioid and nonopioid) are involved in the placebo response and that the drug used to condition the response plays a role in the mechanism of the response.

The role of endogenous opioids has been supported by numerous experiments that have indicated that naloxone can fully (33,34) or partially (35) reverse placebo analgesia, including placebo analgesia elicited through expectation and opioid conditioning (16,25). Interestingly, naloxone is able to reverse spatially or target-specific placebo analgesia in specific parts of the body, suggesting a somatotopic organization of endogenous opioid systems at the level of higher centers in the brain (25). This is a particularly important finding as it demonstrates that the placebo analgesic response acts through release of endogenous opioids at a variety of sites in the nervous system that are involved in the experience of pain. The reversal of placebo-induced respiratory depression (20), decreased heart rate, and decreased β-adrenergic response (36) indicates that the opioid mechanisms of the placebo response also act on other regions and neural circuits, such as the respiratory and cardiovascular centers.

Further interesting examples of the involvement of other neurochemical systems are seen in other recent studies. In one study, preconditioning with a serotonin agonist (sumatriptan) prior to placebo administration resulted in placebo-induced increases in plasma growth hormone and decreases in cortisol (18). Studies of the placebo response in Parkinson disease have added to our understanding of the neurobiology of the placebo response. In Parkinson disease, placebo administration can lead to an increase in dopamine in the ventral (37) and dorsal striatum (38) of sufferers, and this increase in dopamine correlates with improvement in motor function (38). Electrophysiologic evidence has also shown improvements in motor function, along with placebo-induced changes in subthalamic nucleus neuronal activity (39). The relevance of placebo-induced dopamine release for placebo analgesia is that dopamine has been shown to play an important role in reward mechanisms, and placebo administration activates brain areas associated with both reward system and opioid system circuitry (40–43). Parkinson disease has thus emerged as an interesting model to study the placebo response, particularly in light of the increasingly evident anatomic and biochemical relationship between reward and opioid circuitry.

Advances in imaging technology have allowed the investigation of regional brain activation during the experience of pain and during the placebo analgesic response. Positron emission tomography (PET) and functional magnetic resonance imaging (fMRI) studies have shown consistent activation of certain cortical and subcortical areas during the experience of pain compared to control groups who are not experiencing pain (44,45). These areas encompass the neural pathways believed to be responsible for the sensory, affective, and evaluative dimensions of the pain experience. This pattern of activation, termed the *pain matrix*, corresponds to the neuronal substrate of multiple dimensions of pain according to the *neuromatrix model* described by Katz and Melzack in Chapter 35.

Several imaging studies have shown alterations in the pain matrix following placebo administration (42,43,46–48) and expectation of analgesia (49). A recent PET scan study compared activation patterns between injection with a placebo and an opioid (remifentanil), using simple verbal cues and a conditioning protocol to manipulate expectations (42). It was found that the same regions in the brain activated by the opioid injection were also activated by the placebo injection. Of particular interest was the activation of the rostral anterior cingulate cortex (rACC) and orbitofrontal cortex (Obfc), areas that are involved in complex cognitive functions, are rich in opioid receptors, and play a role in descending modulation of pain (50–53). One implication of this study is that expectation-induced placebo analgesia may involve the endogenous opioid–mediated descending pain inhibitory system.

Another study using fMRI investigated pain and reported placebo effects both during the pain experience and in anticipation of pain (43). This study supported the findings of the just described study, showing that activity in the areas involved in the pain matrix decreased upon placebo intervention, again particularly in those areas rich in opioid receptors and involved in the descending pain inhibitory system. Of interest were increases in activation just prior to placebo analgesia, in the dorsolateral prefrontal cortex (DLPFC), Obfc, prefrontal cortex, superior parietal cortex, and periaqueductal gray (PAG), indicating that both cognitive–evaluative and endogenous opioid mechanisms may be involved in the anticipatory phase of the placebo response. Another recent PET imaging study supports the role of endogenous opioids in the placebo analgesic response (54). This study, that captured images using a μ-opioid receptor–selective radiotracer, showed that a placebo can induce the activation of μ-opioid receptors in the dorsolateral prefrontal cortex, pregenual rostral ACC, anterior insular cortex, and nucleus accumbens. These studies offer insights into the role of psychological and neurobiologic mechanisms in altering the processing of pain in the brain, both in sensory, affective, and evaluative dimensions (43).

The study of the mechanisms of the placebo response is still in its infancy. In fact, it is now evident that multiple psychobiologic responses follow administration of a placebo depending upon the drug compared with placebo and other factors, and therefore there exists not one placebo response but many. In the case of placebo analgesia, it is evident that expectations and the endogenous opioid system play a significant

role in altering nociceptive processing. Novel techniques, such as those described earlier, provide important information about the functional neuroanatomy of the placebo response. The integration of imaging and biochemical studies should further enhance our knowledge about the psychobiologic underpinnings of the placebo response.

IMPLICATIONS FOR CLINICAL PRACTICE

Implications from Clinical and Experimental Trials

When discussing the implications of the placebo effect on clinical practice, it is important to look at clinical trial design and interpretation. One important clinical trial design feature relates to the open–hidden paradigm. In this paradigm, the patient can receive a drug in two ways. The first is *hidden administration*, in which the patient is unaware when he receives the drug, and side effects that can provide such cues are minimal. Hidden administration removes the expectation component and other "context effects" from the treatment, implying that the observed response is primarily due to the pharmacologic action of the drug alone. The second is *open administration*, which resembles clinical practice in which an injection is given by the clinician in full view of the patient. Interestingly, many drugs are far less effective when patients do not know they are receiving them (55,56). In other words, removal of the expectation component and the context effects surrounding the injection contributes to a diminution of the response to the drug. In some cases, the drug may actually have little or no effect when given by hidden administration (56,57).

A clinical trial conducted by one of us in 1995 illustrates the importance of open administration. In this trial, a group of patients given a cholecystokinin (CCK) antagonist (proglumide) as an analgesic were compared to a group given a placebo (57). This study was conducted using the gold standard double-blinded, randomized, placebo-controlled trial design (RCT), whereby the efficacy of a drug is defined as the difference between the response to the placebo and the response to the drug (6). The greater the difference between the response to placebo and the response to the active drug, the more efficacious the drug is deemed to be. In this particular trial, the group taking proglumide showed significantly more analgesia compared with the placebo group, indicating that proglumide was an effective analgesic. However, the methodology also included a hidden administration of proglumide, which had no effect on pain (Fig. 36-2). It therefore appeared that proglumide had no specific analgesic properties (contrary to the result of the standard placebo-controlled trial), yet was able to potentiate analgesia through placebo-activated endogenous opioid mechanisms. Several trials have been conducted using the open–hidden paradigm, and each shows differences between the two modalities of drug administration (34,56,58).

Trials using the open–hidden paradigm highlight two significant implications. First, this paradigm may be useful to assess the true pharmacologic action of some drugs (1,55,59). Of note, the open–hidden paradigm provides an ethically attractive alternative to the standard RCT design because this paradigm does not rely upon placebo administration (60). Second, this paradigm offers the opportunity to maximize and quantitate the difference between the open and hidden

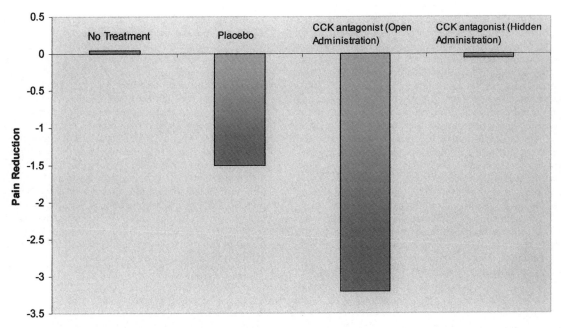

FIGURE 36-2. Adapted from Colloca L, Benedetti F. Placebos and painkillers: Is mind as real as matter? *Nat Rev Neurosci* 2005;6(7):545–552, with permission.

administrations, thereby characterizing the "nonspecific" or placebo-like component of a given treatment. It is clear that a significant proportion of this difference results from the expectation component of the treatment. It is likely, however, that other factors such as the patient–doctor interaction also play a role in this difference. This paradigm therefore allows separation of the effect of a treatment from the context or environment in which the treatment is given.

The power of expectations upon clinical outcomes can be further seen when analyzing the patient's or clinician's perception of which treatment group the patient was allocated to in clinical trials (61,62). A recent double-blinded study addressing human fetal mesencephalic cell transplantation for Parkinson disease assessed the effect of this treatment compared with placebo treatment, according to a standard RCT design (63). They also assessed the patient's perceived assignment to either active or placebo treatment. Amazingly, the perceived assignment of treatment had a more powerful effect upon clinical outcome than did the actual assignment. This perception and concomitant patient expectations had a significant effect on both psychological (quality of life) and physiologic (motor function) outcomes, regardless of whether the patient actually received placebo or active treatment.

The results of the above study have been replicated in a trial of acupuncture analgesia (64). In this study, the perceived assignment to receive sham or true acupuncture better predicted the analgesic response than did the actual assignment, again highlighting the power of expectations in responses both to active and placebo treatments. A recent study has further extended these findings, in that perceived assignment to nicotine replacement or placebo better predicted the outcome (cessation of smoking) than did actual allocation (65).

The power of expectation and potentially exploitable placebo mechanisms is demonstrated in two different studies involving drug administration. One study examined the effects of expectation on regional brain metabolic activity following administration of a stimulant drug (66). This was a controlled study in which the expectations of subjects were manipulated. All patients received the stimulant, but one group expected a dose of the stimulant (similar to an open administration) and the other expected a dose of placebo (similar to a hidden administration). There were significant differences in regional brain glucose metabolism between those patients who expected the stimulant and those who expected a placebo, even though both received the active drug. In this case, despite equal plasma concentrations of the stimulant, manipulation of subjects' expectations was able to change regional brain metabolic activity and the reported perceived "high" in response to the drug, again demonstrating the power of expectations for enhancement of the response to a given treatment.

A second study assessed the effects of placebo administration on opioid intake in patients with postoperative pain (26). In this study, patients were treated with buprenorphine on request for 3 consecutive postoperative days, along with a continuous infusion of saline solution. However, the symbolic meaning of this saline basal infusion was made to differ across three different groups of patients. The first group (natural history or no-treatment group) was told that the infusion was a rehydrating solution, the second (classic double-blind administration) that it could be either a potent analgesic or a placebo, and the third group (deceptive administration) that the infusion was a potent painkiller. It is important to point out that the double-blind group received uncertain verbal instructions (*"It can be either an inert substance or a painkiller"*), whereas the deceptive administration group received certain instructions (*"It is a painkiller"*). The clinical effect of the saline basal infusion (placebo) was measured by recording the amount of buprenorphine requested over the 3-day treatment. A 20.8% decrease in buprenorphine intake, compared with the natural history group, was found with double-blind administration and an even greater reduction (up to 33.8%) occurred with deceptive administration of the saline infusion. It is crucial to point out that pain intensity followed the same time course in the three groups over the 3-day period of treatment; that is, the same analgesic effect was obtained with different doses of buprenorphine. These findings show that patients with strong expectations of analgesia request lower doses of analgesic drugs than those without such expectations.

Ongoing research, particularly involving brain imaging, has highlighted the importance of expectations in modulating brain function (49,67). These emerging findings, along with the prior research on placebo mechanisms mentioned earlier, raise the prospect for opportunities to develop new therapeutic approaches to maximize the benefits of existing treatments. One area of further study is the context or "nonspecific" effects surrounding treatment in pain practice that offer the ability to manipulate the environment surrounding the patient to maximize placebo mechanisms (particularly those mediated by expectations) and thereby enhance the overall efficacy of the intervention. In the case of drug administration, this approach may allow reduction of intake of exogenous, potentially toxic substances by augmenting endogenous placebo mechanisms (68).

The Clinical Interaction, Context Effects and the Placebo Response

A systematic review of context effects on health outcomes concluded that many inconsistencies are present across studies analyzing the emotional and cognitive aspects of different treatments (69). Similarly, attempts at characterizing "placebo responders" have generally been unsuccessful, although it is acknowledged that far more work needs to be done in this area (70). One of the difficulties in identifying placebo responders is the wide variety of psychological, social, and cultural factors that influence the context of a given treatment. For example, a recent meta-analysis comparing oral placebos to subcutaneous placebos for headache showed that injectable placebos are more efficacious than oral ones (71). Interestingly though, this difference was evident in studies conducted in the United States. European studies gave rise to no significant difference between the routes of administration on placebo responses, indicating that cultural factors play a role in placebo responses.

Analyses of the clinical encounter or context of a treatment have focused upon three aspects: the patient, the clinician, and the patient–clinician interaction (or relationship) (72). As just mentioned, further research is required to identify specific patient characteristics that influence the placebo response. Regarding clinician factors, a great deal of inconsistency exists in the literature regarding the specific elements involved in maximizing outcomes to particular treatments (69). However, the power of the clinician to influence outcomes of particular treatments is well recognized (73–76). One interesting study of the clinician's influence upon the outcome of postoperative analgesic drug administration involved manipulation of clinicians rather than patients (77). Patients were divided into two groups. The first received either a placebo or the opioid antagonist naloxone (reduced clinician expectation). The second group received either of these same two drugs or an opiate drug (enhanced clinician expectation). The placebo response was dramatically less for group one (for which the clinician believed that the patient could only receive an opioid antagonist or placebo) than group two (for which clinicians believed that a real analgesic could be delivered). Despite this study's lack of a natural history group, it still revealed a powerful influence by the clinician on the magnitude of patients' placebo responses. Similar results have been seen in a variety of other trials (72), although, as previously mentioned, a great deal of inconsistency exists as to what clinician factors influence the result of treatment (69).

Perhaps the most important way of analyzing nonspecific effects comes through the patient–clinician interaction or relationship, which may comprise a variety of factors such as the environment around the patient, context (78), or meaning (79) of the treatment. There is, however, limited information on which factors play a role and how much of a role they play, not to speak of which particular factors may play differing roles in different contexts. In other words, distinct factors operating in different clinical interactions may activate or modulate distinct placebo mechanisms and responses. Not only will it be important to identify which patient–clinician factors play a role in which particular settings, but it will also be important to better understand placebo mechanisms and their enhancement in a variety of clinical settings.

The Nocebo Effect

When considering the clinical implications of the placebo response, it is worthy to note the potential negative impact of manipulations of expectation on clinical practice. The *nocebo effect* is defined as a negative or undesirable response to an inert treatment. Although our understanding of the nocebo effect is far less than that of the placebo effect, it is believed that the nocebo effect is significantly related to the beliefs and expectations held by the patient about a particular treatment (80–82). Some experimental data support the role of manipulations in expectations in (negatively) mediating responses, highlighting the importance of the clinical encounter (particularly suggestibility) in activating nocebo mechanisms and altering responses (18,83,84). Interestingly, there may be a variety of context effects influencing the nocebo response, such as the information given to the patient along with administration of a particular medication (85). In one recent study of sham acupuncture and placebo antidepressants, a certain percentage of patients in each group reported side effects that mimicked those listed in the informed consent, such as skin irritation at the sham acupuncture site and dry mouth in the placebo amitriptyline. Such findings underscore the importance of the power of the clinical interaction and the context of treatment in potentially activating nocebo mechanisms and eliciting negative responses.

SUMMARY

The placebo response has been a topic of interest for over 200 years and, in recent years, has gained more attention in the scientific and clinical communities. Our understanding of the mechanisms of the placebo effect has improved but is still in its infancy. The placebo response provides an interesting paradigm for researching the complexities of the mind–brain–body interaction and, as Haygarth noted, some two centuries ago, the power of the psychosocial context surrounding a patient on the patient's response to a particular intervention. The challenge for clinicians and researchers is now to further characterize distinct placebo mechanisms active in different contexts and to develop new therapeutic strategies to optimally harness these beneficial mechanisms and improve patient care.

References

1. Finniss DG, Benedetti F. Mechanisms of the placebo response and their impact on clinical trials and clinical practice. *Pain* 2005;114:3–6.
2. Colloca L, Benedetti F. Placebos and painkillers: Is mind as real as matter? *Nat Rev Neurosci* 2005;6(7):545–552.
3. de Craen AJ, Kaptchuk TJ, Tijssen JG, Kleijnen J. Placebos and placebo effects in medicine: Historical overview. *J R Soc Med* 1999;92(10):511–515.
4. Kaptchuk T. Intentional ignorance: A history of blind assessment and placebo controls in medicine. *Bull Hist Med* 1998;72:389–433.
5. Greiner TH, Gold H, Cattell M, et al. A method for the evaluation of effects of drugs on cardiac pain in patients with angina of effort: A study of Khellin (Visammin). *Am J Med* 1950;9:143–155.
6. Kaptchuk TJ. Powerful placebo: The dark side of the randomised controlled trial. *Lancet* 1998;351(9117):1722–1725.
7. Beecher HK. The powerful placebo. *JAMA* 1955;159:1602–1606.
8. Vase L, Robinson ME, Verne GN, Price DD. The contributions of suggestion, desire, and expectation to placebo effects in irritable bowel syndrome patients. An empirical investigation. *Pain* 2003;105(1–2):17–25.
9. Price DD, Chung SK, Robinson ME. Conditioning, expectation and desire for relief in placebo analgesia. *Sem Pain Med* 2005;3:15–21.
10. Siegel S. Explanatory mechanisms for placebo effects: Pavlovian conditioning. In: Guess HA, Kleinman A, Kusek JW, Engel LW, eds. *The Science of the Placebo: Toward an Interdisciplinary Research Agenda.* London: BMJ Books; 2002:133–157.
11. Stewart-Williams S, Podd J. The placebo effect: Dissolving the expectancy versus conditioning debate. *Psychol Bull* 2004;130(2):324–340.
12. Ader R, Cohen N. Behaviourally conditioned immunosuppression. *Psychosom Med* 1975;37:333–340.
13. Herrnstein R. Placebo effect in the rat. *Science* 1962;138:677–678.
14. Voudouris NJ, Peck CL, Coleman G. Conditioned placebo responses. *J Pers Spc Psychol* 1985;48:47–53.
15. Voudouris NJ, Peck CL, Coleman G. Conditioned response models of placebo phenomena: Further support. *Pain* 1989;38:109–116.
16. Amanzio M, Benedetti F. Neuropharmacological dissection of placebo analgesia: Expectation-activated opioid systems versus conditioning-activated specific subsystems. *J Neurosci* 1999;19(1):484–494.
17. Montgomery GH, Kirsch I. Classical conditioning and the placebo effect. *Pain* 1997;72:107–113.
18. Benedetti F, Pollo A, Lopiano L, et al. Conscious expectation and unconscious conditioning in analgesic, motor, and hormonal placebo/nocebo responses. *J Neurosci* 2003;23(10):4315–4323.
19. Colloca L. How prior experience shapes placebo analgesia. *Pain* 2006;124(1–2):126–133.
20. Benedetti F, Amanzio M, Baldi S, et al. Inducing placebo respiratory depressant responses in humans via opioid receptors. *Eur J Neurosci* 1999;11:625–631.
21. Ader R. Conditioned immunomodulation: Research needs and directions. *Brain Behav Immun* 2003;17[Suppl 1]:S51–S57.
22. Pacheco-Lopez G, Engler H, Niemi M, Schedlowski M. Expectations and associations that heal: Immunomodulatory placebo effects and its neurobiology. *Brain Behav Immun* 2006;20(5):430–446.
23. Kirsch I. Response expectancy as a determinant of experience and behavior. *Am Psychol* 1985;40:1189–1202.
24. Caspi O, Bootzin RR. Evaluating how placebos produce change. Logical and causal traps and understanding cognitive explanatory mechanisms. *Eval Health Prof* 2002;25(4):436–464.
25. Benedetti F, Arduino C, Amanzio M. Somatotopic activation of opioid systems by target-directed expectations of analgesia. *J Neurosci* 1999;19(9):3639–3648.
26. Pollo A, Amanzio M, Arslanian A, et al. Response expectancies in placebo analgesia and their clinical relevance. *Pain* 2001;93(1):77–84.
27. De Pascalis V, Chiaradia C, Carotenuto E. The contribution of suggestibility and expectation to placebo analgesia phenomenon in an experimental setting. *Pain* 2002;96(3):393–402.
28. Voudouris NJ, Peck CL, Coleman G. The role of conditioning and verbal expectancy in the placebo response. *Pain* 1990;43:121–128.
29. Price DD, Milling LS, Kirsch I, et al. An analysis of factors that contribute to the magnitude of placebo analgesia in an experimental paradigm. *Pain* 1999;83(2):147–156.
30. Levine JD, Gordon NC, Fields HL. The mechanism of placebo analgesia. *Lancet* 1978;2(8091):654–657.
31. Vase L, Robinson ME, Verne GN, Price DD. Increased placebo analgesia over time in irritable bowel syndrome (IBS) patients is associated with desire and expectation but not endogenous opioid mechanisms. *Pain* 2005;115:338–347.
32. Gracely RH, Dubner R, Wolskee PJ, Deeter WR. Placebo and naloxone can alter post-surgical pain by separate mechanisms. *Nature* 1983;306(5940):264–265.

33. Benedetti F. The opposite effects of the opiate antagonist naloxone and the cholecystokinin antagonist proglumide on placebo analgesia. *Pain* 1996;64(3):535–543.
34. Levine JD, Gordon NC. Influence of the method of drug administration on analgesic response. *Nature* 1984;312(5996):755–756.
35. Grevert P, Albert LH, Goldstein A. Partial antagonism of placebo analgesia by naloxone. *Pain* 1983;16:129–143.
36. Pollo A, Vighetti S, Rainero I, Benedetti F. Placebo analgesia and the heart. *Pain* 2003;102(1–2):125–133.
37. de la Fuente-Fernandez R, Phillips AG, Zamburlini M, et al. Dopamine release in human ventral striatum and expectation of reward. *Behav Brain Res* 2002;136(2):359–363.
38. de la Fuente-Fernandez R, Ruth TJ, Sossi V, et al. Expectation and dopamine release: Mechanism of the placebo effect in Parkinson's disease. *Science* 2001;293(5532):1164–1166.
39. Benedetti F, Colloca L, Torre E, et al. Placebo-responsive Parkinson patients show decreased activity in single neurons of subthalamic nucleus. *Journal* 2004:587–588.
40. de la Fuente-Fernandez R, Schulzer M, Stoessl AJ. Placebo mechanisms and reward circuitry: Clues from Parkinson's disease. *Biol Psychiatry* 2004;56(2):67–71.
41. Mayberg HS, Silva JA, Brannan SK, et al. The functional neuroanatomy of the placebo effect. *Am J Psychiatry* 2002;159(5):728–737.
42. Petrovic P, Kalso E, Petersson KM, Ingvar M. Placebo and opioid analgesia: Imaging a shared neuronal network. *Science* 2002;295(5560):1737–1740.
43. Wager TD, Rilling JK, Smith EE, et al. Placebo-induced changes in fMRI in the anticipation and experience of pain. *Science* 2004;303:1162–1166.
44. Wager TD, Jonides J, Reading S. Neuroimaging studies of shifting attention: A meta-analysis. *Neuroimage* 2004;22(4):1679–1693.
45. Wager TD. The neural bases of placebo effects in anticipation and pain. *Sem Pain Med* 2005;3:22–30.
46. Lieberman MD, Jarcho JM, Berman S, et al. The neural correlates of placebo effects: a disruption account. *Neuroimage* 2004;22:447–455.
47. Kong J, Gollub RL, Rosman IS, et al. Brain activity associated with expectancy-enhanced placebo analgesia as measured by functional magnetic resonance imaging. *Neuroscience* 2006;26(2):381–388.
48. Bingel U, Lorenz J, Schoell E, et al. Mechanisms of placebo analgesia: rACC recruitment of a subcortical antinociceptive network. *Pain* 2006;120(1–2):8–15.
49. Keltner JR, Furst A, Fan C, et al. Isolating the modulatory effect of expectation on pain transmission: A functional magnetic resonance imaging study. *J Neurosci* 2006;26(16):4437–4443.
50. Petrovic P. Opioid and placebo analgesia share the same network. *Sem Pain Med* 2005;3:31–36.
51. Fields HL, Levine JD. Placebo analgesia: A role for endorphins. *Trends Neurosci* 1984;7:271–273.
52. Fields HL, Price DD. Towards a neurobiology of placebo analgesia. In: Harrington A, ed. *The Placebo Effect: An Interdisciplinary Exploration.* Cambridge: Harvard University Press; 1997:93–116.
53. Fields H, Basbaum A. Central nervous system mechanisms of pain modulation. In: Wall PD, Melzack R, eds. *Textbook of Pain,* 4th ed. Edinburgh: Churchill Livingstone; 1999:309–329.
54. Zubieta JK, Bueller JA, Jackson LR, et al. Placebo effects mediated by endogenous opioid neurotransmission and μ-opioid receptors. *J Neurosci* 2005;25(34):7754–7762.
55. Colloca L, Lopiano L, Lanotte M, Benedetti F. Overt versus covert treatment for pain, anxiety, and Parkinson's disease. *Lancet Neurol* 2004;3:679–684.
56. Benedetti F, Giuliano M, Lopiano L. Open versus hidden medical treatments: The patient's knowledge about a therapy affects the therapy outcome. *Prevention & Treatment* 2003;6:Article 1.
57. Benedetti F, Amanzio M, Maggi G. Potentiation of placebo analgesia by proglumide. *Lancet* 1995;346(8984):1231.
58. Amanzio M, Pollo A, Maggi G, Benedetti F. Response variability to analgesics: A role for non-specific activation of endogenous opioids. *Pain* 2001;90(3):205–215.
59. Price DD. Assessing placebo effects without placebo groups: An untapped possibility? *Pain* 2001;90(3):201–203.
60. Kirsch I. Hidden administration as ethical alternatives to the balanced placebo design. *Prevention & Treatment* 2003;6:1–5.
61. Stoessl AJ, de la Fuente-Fernandez R. Willing oneself better on placebo: Effective in its own right. *Lancet* 2004;364:227–228.
62. Benedetti F. The importance of considering the effects of perceived group assignment in placebo-controlled trials. *Eval Health Prof* 2005;28(1):5–6.
63. McRae C, Cherin E, Yamazaki G, et al. Effects of perceived treatment on quality of life and medical outcomes in a double-blind placebo surgery trial. *Arch Gen Psychiatry* 2004;61:412–420.
64. Bausell RB, Lao L, Bergman S, et al. Is acupuncture analgesia an expectancy effect? Preliminary evidence based upon participants' perceived

assignments in two placebo controlled trials. *Eval Health Prof* 2005;28(1): 9–26.

65. Dar R, Stronguin F, Etter JF. Assigned versus perceived placebo effects in nicotine replacement therapy for smoking reduction in Swiss smokers. *J Consult Clin Psychol* 2005;73(2):350–353.

66. Volkow ND, Wang G, Ma Y, et al. Expectation enhances the regional brain metabolic and the reinforcing effects of stimulants in cocaine abusers. *J Neurosci* 2003;23(36):11461–11468.

67. Petrovic P, Dietrich T, Fransson P, et al. Placebo in emotional processing: Induced expectations of anxiety relief activate a generalized modulatory network. *Neuron* 2005;46:957–969.

68. Finniss DG, Benedetti F. The neural matrix of pain processing and placebo analgesia: Implications for clinical practice. *Headache Currents* 2005;2(6):132–138.

69. Di Blasi Z, Harkness E, Ernst E, et al. Influence of context effects on health outcomes: A systematic review. *Lancet* 2001;357(9258):757–762.

70. Moerman D. *Meaning, Medicine and the 'Placebo Effect.'* Cambridge: Cambridge University Press, 2002.

71. de Craen AJ, Tijssen JG, de Gans J, Kleijnen J. Placebo effect in the acute treatment of migraine: Subcutaneous placebos are better than oral placebos. *J Neurol* 2000;247(3):183–188.

72. Kaptchuk TJ. The placebo effect in alternative medicine: Can the performance of a healing ritual have clinical significance? *Ann Intern Med* 2002;136(11):817–825.

73. Benedetti F. How the doctor's words affect the patient's brain. *Eval Health Prof* 2002;25(4):369–386.

74. Brody HB. The symbolic power of the modern personal physician: The placebo response under challenge. *J Drug Issues* 1988;29:149–161.

75. Balint M. The doctor, his patient, and the illness. *Lancet* 1955;1:683–688.

76. Houston WR. The doctor himself as a therapeutic agent. *Ann Intern Med* 1938;11(8):1416–1425.

77. Gracely RH, Dubner R, Deeter WD, Wolskee PJ. Clinicians expectations influence placebo analgesia. *Lancet* 1985;5:43.

78. Di Blasi Z, Kleijnen J. Context effects. Powerful therapies or methodological bias? *Eval Health Prof* 2003;26(2):166–179.

79. Moerman DE, Jonas WB. Deconstructing the placebo effect and finding the meaning response. *Ann Intern Med* 2002;136(6):471–476.

80. Hahn RA. A sociocultural model of illness and healing. In: White L, Tursky B, Schwartz GE, eds. *Placebo: Theory, Research, and Mechanisms.* New York: Guilford; 1985:332–350.

81. Hahn RA. The nocebo phenomenon: Concept, evidence, and implications for public health. *Prev Med* 1997;26[5 Pt 1]:607–611.

82. Hahn RA. The nocebo phenomenon: Scope and foundations. In: Harrington A, ed. *The Placebo Effect: An Interdisciplinary Exploration.* Cambridge: Harvard University Press; 1997:56–77.

83. Staats P, Hekmat H, Staats A. Suggestion/placebo effects on pain: Negative as well as positive. *J Pain Symptom Manage* 1998;15(4):235–243.

84. Johansen O, Brox J, Flaten MA. Placebo and nocebo responses, cortisol, and circulating beta-endorphin. *Psychosom Med* 2003;65(5):786–790.

85. Flaten MA, Simonsen T, Olsen H. Drug-related information generates placebo and nocebo responses that modify the drug response. *Psychosom Med* 1999;61(2):250–255.

CHAPTER 37 ■ ASSESSMENT AND DIAGNOSIS OF CHRONIC PAIN CONDITIONS

CHRISTOPHER VIJE AND MICHAEL A. ASHBURN

The patient with chronic pain comes to the physician with the hope that he can help her find relief from pain and suffering. The initial evaluation starts this process, and what occurs during this evaluation goes a long way toward setting the stage for success or failure. What occurs during the evaluation will impact on the physician's ability to optimize treatment. This interaction plays an important role in establishing the physician–patient relationship, and this relationship is an important contributor to patient outcomes. Therefore, it is reasonable to think of the evaluation process as one that includes several steps, including collection of information, the conduct of a physical examination, the establishment of a physician–patient relationship, the establishment of the initial diagnosis and treatment plan, and the establishment of patient (and family) agreement to the proposed treatment plan.

In this chapter, we review the process of information collection in some detail. However, other chapters in this text also provide valuable information on what data to collect regarding specific disease states. Likewise, this chapter will provide an overview of the physical examination, but other chapters will provide more detailed information regarding the conduct of specific examination techniques related to specific disease states (see Chapters 31, 38, 43–49). We will discuss outcome measurement instruments, as these instruments, when integrated into the care of the pain patient, provide a unique opportunity to track outcomes in a particular patient as well as in populations of patients over time.

OVERVIEW OF THE PROCESS

In as much as possible, the process for the conduct of the initial evaluation, including the documentation of the visit, should be standardized. Although each patient has her own unique story to tell, the use of a standardized process to collect information will improve the likelihood that all necessary information is collected and will lower the chances that valuable information will be overlooked. In addition, as the practice of medicine appropriately moves toward the use of electronic health records, a standardized format will be necessary for data entry. Standardization can include the use of a preprinted initial evaluation form to guide the collection and documentation of information.

The traditional format for the conduct of the patient evaluation, which includes the history of present illness, past medical and surgical history, family history, current medications, drug allergies, review of systems, past radiologic and laboratory studies, physical examination, counseling and coordination of care, impression, and treatment plan, is appropriate. Enhancement can be made, however, to ensure appropriate pain-specific information is collected on the chronic pain patient (detailed history of current pain).

The physician's interactive style has an important impact on the patient's perception of the quality of the care received, and appears to be linked to quality of care (1). An interactive style described as *patient-centered* is associated with better quality (2). Patient-centeredness involves focusing the dialog on the biopsychosocial model of care, rather than a biomedical model of care (3). A patient-centered dialog includes active patient engagement in the medical dialog, with the physician being open and responsive to the patient's agenda and perspective. In this model, the physician also seeks to learn the patient's concerns, expectations, and preferences for treatment, and he makes an effort to establish an emotional rapport with the patient (1).

It is important to note that it is not only what physicians say to their patients, but how they say it that matters (4). A patient extracts meaning from her physician's tone of voice, facial expression, and body cues (5). This nonverbal communication plays an important role in the establishment of trust, liking, and respect, factors deemed by patients to be important parts of the physician–patient relationship (6).

The physician should understand early in the evaluation what the patient hopes to accomplish during the visit. Patients may come to the physician seeking a single, specific therapy. Wasted time and frustration on both the physician and patient's part can be avoided if this expectation is identified and addressed early. Frank, open discussion of whether the physician can meet the patient's expressed goals may avoid frustration later on and allow for education of the patient regarding available treatment options. Such a discussion early may allow patients to make more informed decisions regarding their treatment, thus leading to improved compliance, efficacy, and satisfaction.

At the completion of the visit, treatment goals should be clearly stated and agreed upon. Treatment goals often include improvement in physical and mental function, as well as improvement in pain. Expectations should be reasonable and based on evidence whenever possible. Physicians need to clearly understand what treatment options the patient is willing to consider. For example, medications will not be effective if the patient refuses to take drugs from certain drug classes, or cannot afford to pay for the medications offered. Likewise, physical therapy will not be effective if the patient cannot afford the therapy, or if transportation to the therapist for frequent visits is not possible.

CONDUCT OF THE INITIAL EVALUATION

History of Present Illness

Physicians often form their initial diagnosis from the information collected during this part of the evaluation. As this is usually done first, this also is the part of the evaluation that provides both the physician and the patient with the critical first impression that has a significant impact on the physician–patient relationship going forward. It is important to allow the patient to tell her story as much as possible. Physicians often interrupt the patient very soon after she starts to speak. Such interruptions can be perceived in a negative way by the patient, probably do not allow for more rapid information sharing, and may result in the physician making conclusions based on incomplete information. Therefore, it is important for the physician to develop and practice active listening, especially early in the evaluation.

It is important to collect detailed information regarding the pain experience (Table 37-1). After allowing the patient to "tell her story," gaps in the story should be filled in, so that the physician has complete information regarding the patient's pain. This should include information regarding the circumstances surrounding the onset of the pain, a detailed description of the pain (e.g., site, radiation, character, intensity, precipitating and associated factors; Table 37-1), and past interventions, including the impact of these interventions on the pain experience.

Character of pain refers to the nature of the pain, such as burning, stabbing, dull, aching, tingling, pricking, and many others. The character of the pain can help distinguish the etiology of the pain. A few scales have attempted to assess pain character with numerical scoring, notably the Neuropathic Pain Scale (NPS) (7) and the McGill Pain Questionnaire (MPQ) (8).

The NPS asks respondents to rate their pain based on 10 different characteristics (two global ratings of pain and eight terms common to neuropathic conditions) (9). The advantages of the NPS include its brevity and ability to help discriminate neuropathic pain conditions (10). The main disadvantage of the NPS is that it was developed specifically for neuropathic conditions. Several other neuropathic pain scales are now available, and the two most efficient in detecting neuropathic pain are the PainDetect and S-LANSS (11) (Table 37-2).

The McGill Pain Questionnaire (MPQ), introduced by Melzack and Torgerson, continues to be a standard in assessing pain character. It is more comprehensive than the NPS. The MPQ attempts to score and characterize the character of pain by assigning rank values to different terms used to describe the pain (8). These terms are grouped together and placed in order of intensity. A final score is given to the patient based on different subgroupings of the endorsed terms (sensory, affective, evaluative, and miscellaneous). Although it is difficult to quantify and score an individual's pain experience, the MPQ has been shown to be reproducible, sensitive, and responsive to therapeutic interventions. There is also some evidence that the MPQ can be used to aid in the differential diagnosis of certain pain syndromes. Melzack, largely because of the large amount of time needed to administer the MPQ, developed the short-form MPQ (SF-MPQ) in 1987 (12). It consists of only 15 possible terms to describe the pain, but still correlates well with the pain rating index (PRI) from the original MPQ (13). So, although the quantity of pain is a more common outcome

---

TABLE 37-1

HISTORY TAKING IN PATIENTS WITH PERSISTENT PAIN

- **Presenting Symptoms:** Brief overview of site(s) of pain
- **History of Present Illness:** Includes detailed current pain history (see below)
- **Past & Concurrent Medical/Surgical history:**
  - prior patient submission of "time line"
  - highlight significant issues for current pain/Rx
- **Family history:** Highlight chronic pain problems
- **Medications (Past, Current):**
  - doses/duration, efficacy, side effects
  - include alcohol, substance abuse, smoking etc
- **Other treatments and professionals**
- **Imaging & other investigations**
- **Psychosocial history**
- **Review of systems**

Detailed Current Pain History
- Circumstances associated with pain onset
- Primary site of pain (use of pain diagram)
- Radiation of pain
- Character of pain (using McGill Melzack multidimensional pain inventory [e.g., is pain throbbing, sharp, aching?])
- Intensity of pain (e.g., on visual analogue scale)
  - at rest
  - on movement
  - at present
  - during last week
  - highest level
- Factors altering pain
  - What makes pain worse?
  - What makes it better?
- Associated symptoms (e.g., nausea)
- Temporal factors
  - Is pain present continuously or otherwise? paroxysmal episodes?
- Effect of pain on sleep
- Effect of pain on work and activities of daily living (ADLs)
- Effect of pain on social and recreational activities
- Effect of pain on mood
- Expectations of outcome of pain treatment
- Patient's belief concerning the causes of pain
- Reduction in pain required to resume "reasonable activities"
- Patient's typical coping response for stress or pain
- Family expectations and beliefs about pain, stress and disease
- Ways the patient describes or shows pain
- Patient's knowledge, expectations, and preferences for pain management

---

measurement, assessment of character guides important treatment decisions in neuropathic conditions (14).

Patient report of *pain intensity* can be descriptive ("mild" or "severe") or numerical (on a scale of 0–10). Patient report of pain intensity can be highly variable among patients for a variety of reasons, including differences in perception, demographics, and behavioral patterns (15). Pain intensity can be reported using the Verbal Rating Scales (VRS), Numerical Rating Scales (NRS), or Visual Analogue Scales (VAS), among others (16). The NRS is a commonly used pain intensity measurement

TABLE 37-2

NEUROPATH PAIN SCREENING TOOLS

Items	S-LANSS	painDETECT
Pricking, tingling	+	+
Electric shocks or shooting	+	+
Hot or burning	+	+
Numbness		+
Pain evoked by light touch	+	+
Other symptoms	autonomic changes	temporal & referred patterns
		Pain evoked by hot/ cold
Clinical Examination	brush allodynia raised pin prick threshold	Bennett et al 2007

tool in clinical practice. The NRS is a 11-point categorical scale, where 0 = No Pain, and 10 = Worst Possible Pain. The NRS is easy to administer, and its validity has been well documented (17).

Timing (temporal pattern) refers not only to the duration of the pain, but also time-related qualities (constant versus intermittent) and day or seasonal relationships of the pain. In a patient who has a long history of chronic pain, questioning should attempt to uncover periods of time when pain was absent or much improved. Often, therapy will be less efficacious if the pain is longstanding and progressive in nature (18). Appropriate understanding of timing can help establish realistic treatment goals with the patient. Intermittent, very sudden, spontaneous bursts of pain that may last only seconds to minutes are referred to as *paroxysmal pain*. Such pain is usually of neuropathic origin.

The history of present illness should include an assessment of other key aspects of the patient's life experience that often are altered by the presence of chronic pain. This includes an assessment of the patient's mood, sleep, and functional status.

Patients with chronic pain may suffer from depression, anxiety, or other psychological disturbances (19). These conditions may pre-date the onset of the painful condition or present after the onset of chronic pain. It is important that the pain physician look for and identify psychiatric illness, as these illnesses may have profound impact on outcomes, especially if these illnesses are not properly treated.

Multiple chronic pain conditions have an increased incidence of comorbidity with depressive and anxiety disorders. For example, patients with fibromyalgia have up to a threefold increase risk of developing depression and up to a fivefold increase risk of anxiety disorders (20,21). Increased incidence of mood disorders can also be found in patients with chronic pelvic pain, chronic low back pain, myofascial pain syndrome, and many other conditions seen by the pain specialist. Clearly, mood disturbances can be secondary to chronic impairment from pain, can increase the perception of pain as a somatic condition, and could have developed independently from the primary pain process.

Patients with chronic pain often report disruptions in their sleep (22). Sleep disorders can manifest as insomnia, frequent awakening, early awakening, or restless and disturbed sleep. Sleep disturbances may be due to poorly controlled pain, associated depression, a side effect of the patient's medications, or due to other existing disease. In the United States, the incidence of obstructive sleep apnea appears to be growing as obesity becomes more prevalent (23). It is important for sleep

disturbances and their underlying cause(s) to be identified and treated as part of an integrated pain treatment plan.

Patients with chronic pain often have compromise of their mental and physical functioning (24). Alterations in function may range from an inability to engage in specific activities that are important to the patient to an inability to engage in the activities necessary for daily living. It is important to note that alterations in function include both physical functioning (i.e., inability to raise their arms over their head), and mental functioning (i.e., inability to engage in meaningful conversations with friends and family).

Impairment of function and a diminished ability to perform activities of daily living (ADLs) are often associated with chronic pain conditions (25). This can be related to the pain that causes decreased physical activity and inability to perform social and occupational duties. However, it can also be related to psychosocial and behavioral changes that may impair the mood and motivation of the patient.

An assessment of function begins by establishing baseline lifestyle activities. From this baseline, changes (or percentage changes) in activity can be assessed before and after the pain condition. It is important to include multiple categories in the assessment. Usually, employment status and stability is assessed first. The patient's ability to perform their occupation in a meaningful fashion, perceived job performance, and frequency of job changes can provide insight into the impact of the pain.

Assessment of mental functioning can start with an assessment of the patient's ability to complete family and social responsibilities. If the patient was responsible for dependents, then the patient's ability to provide the usual care for the dependents should be assessed before and after the onset of pain. Social activities in which the patient was involved may also have taken a lesser role in the patient's life coincidental with the onset of pain. In addition, personal recreational activities are often sacrificed secondary to pain.

Basic evaluation of function may include an assessment of physical functioning using a 4-point categorical scale, where 1 = inability to independently complete ADLs, 2 = able to do ADLs, but physical activity severely limited, 3 = unable to independently complete selected tasks important to the patient, and 4 = able to do tasks important to the patient. Detailed assessment of physical functioning can be completed as part of a formal functional capacity evaluation, (FCE) (26). Likewise, a basic assessment of the patient's mental functioning can be completed by questioning the patient regarding any limitations they are experiencing regarding their ability to mentally perform their work (or work equivalent) and interact with their friends and family.

Past Medical History

It is important for the physician to collect complete information regarding past medical and surgical history. Special attention should be paid to medical conditions that can contribute to or be the underlying cause(s) of the painful condition. Prior surgeries can predispose to chronic pain states (for example, the incidence of chronic pain after inguinal herniorrhaphy can range from 10%–54%) (27), and certain medical conditions can either cause pain or mimic a chronic pain state. Important categories include endocrine dysfunction, anatomic abnormalities, cancerous processes, inflammatory conditions, and infectious diseases. Endocrine conditions, such as diabetes, could present with symptoms indicative of peripheral neuropathy. Glycemic control and the presence of other end-organ complications are positively correlated with diabetic neuropathy (28), and this history should be elicited from the patient. Anatomic abnormalities such as cervical syrinx may mimic symptoms of discogenic radicular pain (29), but would require completely different treatment. Clearly, chronic inflammatory conditions, cancer, and chronic infection (e.g., HIV neuropathy) are associated with chronic pain. Treatment of chronic pain in these conditions may be related to success in treating the primary condition (30).

In addition to conditions that may directly affect the patient's pain, the patient's general medical history is important (such as cardiac history, kidney dysfunction, allergies, pulmonary history) because this information will help determine what therapies would be safe and effective in certain population groups.

Past medical history should include documentation of the results of previous evaluations and treatment for the painful condition. This should include all imaging and other tests, as well as response to medical and interventional therapy. It is important to have a clear understanding of what analgesic medications have been tried in the past, and this information should include the dose and duration of therapy, as well as the patient's response to this therapy, including adverse effects and allergies. Because an unlimited number of treatment options does not exist, the physician may miss an opportunity for successful therapy if an assumption is made that a prior attempt at therapy with a particular drug was done appropriately.

It is critical that the physician collect accurate, reliable information regarding the use of all medications, not just what analgesic medications the patient is taking. Often, the patient will be taking medications that can interact with analgesic medications, and an accurate medication history is critical to guiding therapy. Case reports of near fatal interactions of medications with opioids, such as methadone and meperidine, have been reported (31,32). Finally, the physician must obtain information regarding drug allergies, and this information must be clearly documented in the health record.

Collection of what medications the patient is taking should not be limited to prescription medications. Patients often are taking over-the-counter medications, and these medications can clearly impact the pain experience and can adversely interact with prescribed medications. In addition, information regarding dietary supplements and homeopathic therapies should be sought for similar reasons (33). For example, herbal supplements (such as ginkgo, garlic, and ginger) have antiplatelet activity that may interact with nonsteroidal anti-inflammatory

drugs (NSAIDs), and the analgesic effects of opioids may be inhibited by ginseng (34).

Social History

The social history can be critical to guiding chronic pain therapy. Information regarding marital status and living conditions will guide decisions regarding treatment options to optimize physical and social functioning. Education and work history will guide efforts to optimize work-related function, and may provide valuable information that will assist in optimizing patient educational methods. If not already done, the physician should obtain and document information regarding past and ongoing litigation associated with the painful condition. Involvement in worker's compensation or litigation could have an affect on functional outcome in chronic pain states; however, these relationships have not been validated (35). Results of any prior medical disability evaluation should be obtained.

The social history is the point in the evaluation at which the physician collects information regarding alcohol, tobacco, and illicit drug use. Careful attention should be paid to the collection of accurate information on these topics, as past or ongoing substance abuse can have a profound impact on chronic pain therapy (36). The physician should be frank but not judgmental in the collection of this information. In addition, some clinicians are using standardized surveys to standardize and improve the quality of the data collected. Tools such as urine toxicology are being increasingly implemented into the care plan of patients on chronic opioid therapy (37).

Family History

Prior pain experience of members of a patient's family may have a powerful influence on the patient's response. For example, a daughter who nursed her mother with severe cancer pain may have strong fears that her own pain may be due to cancer. A history of oversolicitous behavior in response to pain in a family will likely have a bearing on all family members. An important new dimension is the increasing number of pain conditions that have a genetic basis. The most recent to be characterized is a single-gene, single-ion channel ($NaV_{1.7}$) upregulation causing erythromelalgia (38). Other examples are hereditary hemiplegic migraine and hereditary sensory neuropathy type II. Thus, family history of such conditions is important.

New evidence suggests that a small family of genes controls how much nitric oxide is released in response to nerve injury or inflammation (39). The amount of nitric oxide released is in turn related to the likelihood of the development of persisting pain. This new evidence could lead to a DNA test aimed at identifying patients at risk of developing persistent pain after acute injury or surgery. There may be a family history of such enhanced responses to surgery and/or trauma, although evidence is not yet available for such a linkage.

Review of Systems

The review of systems allows the physician to review a checklist with the patient to ensure that important health information has not been overlooked. This is especially important in patients with a complex medical history. Inquiries within each major body system are made, ensuring that a completed medical history has been obtained. This review commonly unveils additional information that helps to guide diagnosis and therapy.

Physical Examination

Once the history of present illness, past medical and surgical history, review of systems, and medication history has been reviewed, the next step in evaluation is a thorough physical examination. Although the physical examination may be focused on the primary complaint, it is important that the initial examination be comprehensive. The initial physical examination should cover the skin, head and neck, major organs of the thorax and abdomen, and an assessment of the peripheral vascular system. Often, in chronic pain patients, more detail will be spent on the musculoskeletal system and the neurologic system.

Skin examination should search for atypical lesions, signs of trauma, rashes, abnormal patterns of hair and nail growth, changes in temperature, and pressure sores. These signs could clue the physician into possible cancerous processes, drug allergies, or abnormal posturing due to pain conditions. Also, certain changes associated with complex regional pain syndrome (CRPS) can be noted in the skin examination, including abnormal hair growth and nail changes (40) (see Chapter 46).

Head and neck examination should include an examination of the eyes. Exophthalmos could signify thyroid disease, and papilledema could imply some cause of intracranial hypertension or other diagnoses such as brain tumor causing raised intracranial pressure. A sinus examination could illustrate the presence of chronic sinusitis (41). A neck examination should cover palpation of the cervical, submandibular, and supraclavicular lymph nodes. Abnormal adenopathy could be indicative of a cancerous or chronic inflammatory process.

Examination of the thoracic organs involves auscultation of the lungs and heart. Abnormal inspiratory and expiratory sounds, murmurs, and rhythm should be noted. Patterns of breathing and accessory muscle use during respiration could illustrate underlying disease, such as chronic obstructive pulmonary disease or lung cancer.

The abdomen should be examined with palpation, percussion, and auscultation. Palpation in all four quadrants could demonstrate pain or demonstrate organomegaly or other masses. Percussion could illustrate excessive peritoneal fluid, which could signify liver disease or malignancy. Finally, auscultation could reveal abnormal bowel sounds, or diminished activity due to chronic disease or medication use (15).

An examination of the peripheral vascular system entails assessing peripheral pulses, capillary refill, temperature, and sensation in the distal extremities. Calf pain could be associated with peripheral vascular disease. Bruits in the carotid arteries could indicate possible ischemic neurologic dysfunction. Foot examination may reveal sensory dysfunction in diabetic patients and can clue the physician into diabetic neuropathic pain. Vascular examination should also search for deep venous thrombosis, which could be a cause of lower extremity pain or a sign of underlying cancer (present in up to 8% of patients with occult malignancy) (42). Swelling, calf pain with dorsiflexion (Hoffman sign), and lymphedema are all physical examination signs of DVT.

The musculoskeletal examination is often indicated as the area of most complaint; however, it is important to thoroughly examine other areas. Soft-tissue examination of the muscles could illustrate spasm, bands, or trigger points characteristic of myofascial pain syndrome. Active, passive, and resisted range of motion should be tested to detect joint dysfunction and other causes of reduced range of motion. Musculoskeletal examination also includes observation of which positions the patient prefers when unprovoked by the examiner. Upper extremity examination should include assessment for shoulder bursitis, ligamentous inflammation at the elbow joint, and pain in the wrist due to carpal or ulnar tunnel syndrome (if these joints are related to the pain complaint). Examination of the lower extremities should include posture, gait, hip rotation, and assessment of knee and ankle ligaments. The foot can often be affected by plantar fasciitis and other painful conditions.

Examination of the spine is focused on flexion, extension, lateral bend, and rotation. Pain upon palpation of the midline spine may indicate a possible fracture, or paraspinal tenderness may point to muscular causes of pain. Sacroiliac tenderness can often be reproduced upon examination. Radicular symptoms may be elicited with certain movements of the spine in the cervical and lumbar regions. Often, sciatic nerve stretch tests are used (such as the straight leg raise, Patrick test). Radicular pain should further lead to a neurologic examination.

A detailed neurologic examination is necessary, especially when neuropathic pain is considered as a diagnosis. A suspected neuropathic pain complaint should be assessed for motor, sensory, and temperature dysfunction in the distribution of the pain. A nerve root lesion will often be associated with motor and sensory dysfunction in addition to a radicular pain. Abnormal neural functioning can manifest as allodynia (pain reported to a nonpainful stimulus) or hyperalgesia (exaggerated pain response to painful stimuli) (43). Sympathetically maintained pain (or CRPS) are often manifested with changes in skin temperature, color, pattern of vascularity, and hair and nail growth (see also Chapter 46).

The remainder of the neurologic examination should be conducted in standard fashion with regards to mental status, cranial nerve function, motor strength, reflexes, and cerebellar function. Mental status should be assessed for alertness and orientation (Table 37-3). Cranial nerve functions should be grossly documented, or more specific tests should be performed if cranial nerve dysfunction is suspected. Motor strength should be graded on a standard 0–5 scale and should include at least the upper and lower extremities. Reflexes should be rated on briskness to response. Cerebellar function can be assessed with gait examination or Romberg test.

Behavioral and psychological factors are often intertwined with the chronic pain experience and impact the patient's response to therapy. An evaluation of these factors is important to further understand the patient's response to chronic pain and provides important information that can guide therapy. As a result, the pain physician should complete a basic psychiatric evaluation, and should understand the evaluation tools commonly used by our psychology colleagues. Questions should be aimed at uncovering mood and anxiety disorders, and associated functional impairments and presence of suicidal ideation. Evaluation consists of a brief mental status examination (Table 37-3) (44).

Psychological testing can supplement interview data by providing additional information about the patient's response probabilities and biases (Table 37-4). Tests may help discriminate between predominant behavioral or physical factors in the patient's pain (45), help predict success after treatment, or even expose malingering behavior (46). However, the routine use of *personality* testing in chronic pain patients may not be necessary (47). Personality testing may be better used in selected patients to complement the psychological evaluation in understanding of the patient's personality, thus allowing for development of the patient's interdisciplinary pain treatment plan.

TABLE 37-3

COMPONENTS OF MENTAL STATUS EXAMINATION (41)

1. **Appearance:** How does the patient look? Neatly dressed with clear attention to detail? Well groomed?
2. **Level of alertness:** Is the patient conscious? If not, can they be aroused? Can they remain focused on your questions and conversation? What is their attention span?
3. **Speech:** Is it normal in tone, volume and quantity?
4. **Behavior:** Pleasant? Cooperative? Agitated? Appropriate for the particular situation?
5. **Orientation:** Do they know where they are and what they are doing here? Do they know who you are? Can they tell you the day, date and year?
6. **Mood:** How do they feel? You may ask this directly (e.g., "Are you happy, sad, depressed, angry?"). Is it appropriate for their current situation?
7. **Affect:** How do they appear to you? This interpretation is based on your observation of their interactions during the interview. Do they make eye contact? Are they excitable? Does the tone of their voice change? Common assessments include: flat (unchanging throughout), excitable, appropriate.
8. **Thought Process:** This is a description of the way in which they think. Are their comments logical and presented in an organized fashion? If not, how off-base are they? Do they tend to stray quickly to related topics? Are their thoughts appropriately linked or simply all over the map?
9. **Thought Content:** A description of what the patient is thinking about. Are they paranoid? Delusional (i.e., hold beliefs that are untrue)? If so, about what? Phobic? Hallucinating (you need to ask if they see or hear things that others do not)? Fixated on a single idea? If so, about what. Is the thought content consistent with their affect? If there is any concern regarding possible interest in committing suicide or homicide, the patient should be asked this directly, including a search for details (e.g., specific plan, time, etc.). Note: These questions have never been shown to plant the seeds for an otherwise unplanned event and may provide critical information, so they should be asked!
10. **Memory:** Short-term memory is assessed by listing three objects, asking the patient to repeat them to you to ensure that they were heard correctly, and then checking recall at 5 minutes. Long-term memory can be evaluated by asking about the patients job history, where they were born and raised, family history, etc.
11. **Calculations:** Can they perform simple addition, multiplication? Are the responses appropriate for their level of education? Have they noticed any problems balancing their checkbooks or calculating correct change when making purchases? This is also a test of the patient's attention span/ability to focus on a task.
12. **Judgment:** Provide a common scenario and ask what they would do (e.g., "If you found a letter on the ground in front of a mailbox, what would you do with it?").
13. **Reasoning:** Involves interpretation of complex ideas. For example, you may ask them the meaning of the phrase, "People in glass houses should not throw stones." A few common interpretations include: concrete (e.g., "Don't throw stones because it will break the glass"); abstract (e.g., "Don't judge others"); or bizarre.

ASSESSMENT INSTRUMENTS

Several patient assessment instruments can be used during the evaluation process and periodically during treatment to as-

TABLE 37-4

PSYCHOLOGICAL TESTS

Personality tests
1. Minnesota Multiphasic Personality Inventory (MMPI)
2. Rorschach Inkblot Test
3. Thematic Apperception Test
4. Myers-Briggs Type Indicator
5. NEO Personality Inventory
6. Personality Assessment Inventory
7. Sickness Impact Profile
8. Structural Analysis of Social Behavior

Mood tests
1. Beck Depression Inventory
2. Major Depression Inventory
3. Hamilton Rating Scale for Depression
4. Zung Self-Rating Anxiety Scale
5. Spielberger State-Trait Anxiety Inventory

sist in patient evaluation and to document patient response to therapy.

Frequently, attempts are made to document the patient's perception of her quality of life. *Quality of life* is a term that refers to how a person feels and how she functions in daily life (48). Assessment of quality of life may be overly broad and may not allow for precise assessment of the impact of a disease on the patient's life. Therefore, a number of investigators have developed a new term, *health-related quality of life* (HRQL). Health-related quality of life refers to those domains of life that are specifically related to health and that can be potentially influenced by the health care system (49).

Core domains in HRQL assessment include physical and emotional functioning (48). Measures of physical functioning evaluate the ability of the patient to engage in self-care, carry out daily activities such as household chores, walking, work, and travel. In addition, these measures attempt to assess strength and endurance. Emotional functioning refers to an assessment of the level of emotional distress the patient is experiencing, and is not intended to be synonymous with a psychiatric diagnosis or disorder. Emotional functioning is central to a patient's assessment of her overall well-being and satisfaction with life.

Generic measures of health are intended to track health outcomes in large populations of patients. The use of generic measures makes it possible to compare outcomes associated with a given disorder and its treatment with those of different conditions (50). An example of a generic measure

TABLE 37-5

PAIN-SPECIFIC OUTCOME DOMAINS INCLUDED IN THE TOPS (49)

Measure	Explanation
Pain Symptom	The subjective experience of pain without any reference to any consequences of that pain
Functional Limitations	Health-related limitations on the ability to function and do things
Perceived Family Disability	Patient-perceived limitations on the ability to perform family and social roles. These are impressions or feelings of limitation and are specifically attributed to pain in the questions.
Objective Family Disability	The extent to which a person reports physically not engaging in specific family and social activities.
Objective Work Disability	The degree to which a person is classified as disabled in terms of work and receipt of public disability payments
Total Pain Experience	A sum of the above, useful under the biopsychosocial model of pain treatment
Life Control	Patient's perception of control over pain and stress and problem solving abilities.
Passive Coping	The extent to which a person responds to adversity with a passive style as opposed to an active one.
Solicitous Responses	The extent to which a spouse or significant other assists or takes over role function
Upper Body Limitations	Health-related limitations on upper body functions.
Work Limitations	Percentage of time that the patient has difficulty at work.
Fear Avoidance	Patient beliefs that physical activity and work would increase pain.
Patient Satisfaction with Outcomes	The extent to which a patient reports being satisfied with his or her level of pain
Health Care Satisfaction	Satisfaction with the overall care to date.

of health is the Medical Outcomes Study Short Form 36-item Questionnaire, or SF-36 (51). However, generic measures of health are often are not precise enough to track health outcomes over time in an individual patients with chronic pain (52).

Disease-specific measures of health are designed to evaluate the impact of a specific condition on the patient's quality of life. Such measures are more likely to reveal clinically important changes in function that are a result of the condition of interest. In addition, they are precise enough to detect changes in an individual patient over time. One such measure is the Treatment Outcomes in Pain Survey (TOPS) (52,53). The TOPS is a 12-page, 120-item questionnaire that is completed by the patient. The TOPS includes the SF-36, but also includes additional outcome domains specific to the chronic pain population (Table 37-5). The TOPS is precise to document outcomes in individual patients over time.

Recently, The IMMPACT Group identified four core chronic pain domains that should be monitored during the conduct of chronic pain clinical trials (54). These include pain intensity, physical functioning, emotional functioning, and participant rating of overall improvement. They then recommended specific outcome measures to assess these core outcome domains (Table 37-6).

Multidimensional Pain Inventory Scale

The Multidimensional Pain Inventory (MPI) scale is a 60-item patient-completed survey intended to assess the patient's cognitive, behavioral, and affective response to her painful condition (55). The MPI has 12 derived scales that are grouped into three sections (pain and its impact, responses by significant others, activities). The MPI has been used extensively to support pain-related clinical research involving a variety of conditions (56–58). However, there is variability in response by condition, and as a result, the clinical importance of changes in the MPI may vary based on the specific pain condition of the patient.

Brief Pain Inventory Interference Scale

The Brief Pain Inventory Interference (BPI) is a seven-item patient-completed measure intended to assess the extent to which pain interferes with various components of functioning, including physical and emotional functioning, as well as sleep (59,60). The BPI has been used as an outcome measure in multiple pain-related clinical trials.

Beck Depression Inventory

The Beck Depression Inventory consists of 21 groups of four statements that the patient responds to, in order to assess the severity of current symptoms of depressive disorders (61). The Beck Depression Inventory takes 5 to 10 minutes to complete, and has a low (5th or 6th grade) reading level requirement. The

TABLE 37-6

CORE CHRONIC PAIN OUTCOME DOMAINS AND SUGGESTED OUTCOME MEASURES (51)

Chronic pain outcome domain	Outcome measure
Pain Intensity	0–10 numerical rating scale
Physical Functioning	Multidimensional Pain Inventory Scale Brief Pain Inventory Interference Scale
Emotional Functioning	Beck Depression Inventory Profile of Mood States
Overall Improvement	Patient Global Impression of Change Scale

resultant score of between 0 and 63 can be used to identify the intensity of depression. In the general population, a score of below 10 reflects minimal or no depression, 10 to 18 reflects mild to moderate depression, 19 to 29 reflects moderate to severe depression, and 30 or above reflects severe depression. In the chronic pain population, scores of 21 and above identify patients with major depressive disorder (62).

Profile of Mood States

The Profile of Mood States is a 65-item patient-completed survey that provides an evaluation of tension, depression, anger, vigor, fatigue, and confusion (63). This test has been used in a number of clinical trials involving several pain conditions. However, a number of variations of this survey can make it difficult to compare the results of one study with another, and there are limited data to identify what are clinically important changes in the individual Profile of Mood State scales (64).

Patient Global Impression of Change Scale

The Patient Global Impression of Change scale is a single-item patient rating of her response to therapy (Table 37-7) (65). This measure is simple to complete and provides an easily interpretable assessment of the patient's evaluation of the importance of their response to therapy. It is important to note that this measurement scale allows patients to determine not only if they have improved with therapy, but also if they are now worse following therapy.

Assessment of Low Back Pain

Specific measures for low back pain include the North American Spine Society Lumbar Spine Outcome Assessment Instrument, the Oswestry Low Back Disability Questionnaire, and the Roland-Morris Disability Questionnaire (66,67). The Lumbar Spine Outcome Assessment Instrument focuses on lumbar spine pain, disability, and neurogenic symptom subscales. The questionnaire takes about 20 minutes to complete, and has a high test-retest reliability (68). It can be used as a monitoring tool to assess patient's progress with treatment. The Oswestry Low Back Disability Questionnaire is a short, 10-question tool focused on the impact of pain on daily activities. The answers are then scored from 0 to 5. It is a feasible, reliable, and valid tool that can be used as an outcome measure to assess the level of disability caused by low back pain. The Roland-Morris Disability Questionnaire is a 24-item questionnaire that attempts to measure the interference of low back pain in different domains (such as mobility, dressing, and sleeping). It has been proven to be reliable, valid, and easy to use (69).

Assessment of Risk for Substance Abuse

There is increasing interest in the use of assessment tools related to substance abuse, especially in patients in whom administration of opioids is being considered. Several measurement instruments can be used to assist in determining if the patient has an active substance abuse disorder, or is at increased risk of developing problems related to the use of controlled substances. Several assessment tools can provide valuable information regarding the risk for aberrant drug-related behavior associated with the use of opioids for the treatment of pain. These include the Current Opioid Misuse Measure (COMM) (70), Screener and Opioid Assessment for Patient with Pain (SOAPP) (71), and the Opioid Risk Tool (ORT) (72). The inherent drawback to these self reporting measures is that they can be subject to deception by the patient.

The COMM seeks to monitor aberrant medication-related behaviors of chronic pain patients who are being prescribed opioid therapy (70). The COMM is a 40-item self-report measure that has shown consistency and reliability with current aberrant drug-related behavior.

The SOAPP is a self-report measure that seeks to predict aberrant drug behavior in chronic pain patients on opioid therapy (71). The SOAPP has shown reliability, but is susceptible to overt deception. A revised, shortened version (SOAPP-R) has only 18 items and appears to be more resistant to deception (73).

The ORT is a brief, self-administered tool that attempts to document the following risk factors associated with substance abuse: personal and family history of substance abuse, age, and history of preadolescent sexual abuse, as well as certain psychological diseases (72). Completion of the ORT results in scores that categorize the patient as being at low, moderate, or high risk for displaying opioid-related aberrant behaviors.

Normative Data and Automated Records

Instruments that evaluate psychological and physical functioning are valuable in following the progress of patients from baseline through the treatment phase. However, normative data are needed to determine how severely affected by pain patients are when they first present for treatment. Such data are important in evaluating whether various treatment modalities have succeeded in patients with severe problems or mildly affected patients. Thus, it is surprising that the first study to present normative data on a population of patients referred to a pain clinic was published in 2007 (74). This study accumulated data on 6,000 patients over a 10-year period using instruments in all four domains suggested by IMMPACT (Table 37-6) and additionally including a measure of self efficacy, the PSEQ (75). The importance of including psychological instruments as part of the assessment process is accumulating evidence that psychological factors play a key role in the development of chronic pain (76).

The collection and analysis of data from history and instrument is obviously much more consistent and is easier with an automated system. Such systems are now available from a number of different sources.

TABLE 37-7

PATIENT GLOBAL IMPRESSION OF CHANGE SCALE (51)

Value	Response to therapy
7	Very much improved
6	Much improved
5	Minimally improved
4	No change
3	Minimally worse
2	Much worse
1	Very much worse

CONCLUSION

The initial evaluation plays a critical role in the care of the patient with pain. This interaction between the patient and key members of the health care team establishes the cornerstone of what is likely to be a long-term professional relationship. Care should be taken to treat the patient with respect using a patient-centered interactive style. The physician should make every effort to make sure that the patient understands the diagnosis and treatment plan. It is especially important for the physician to understand the patient's treatment goals, and to make sure the patient's goals are taken into account when developing the treatment plan. However, the initial evaluation is only the first of what may be several encounters. The physician should not forget that the evaluation process is ongoing, and careful reassessment is critical to optimizing patient outcomes.

References

1. Bensing JM, Roter DL, Hulsman RL. Communication patterns of primary care physicians in the United States and the Netherlands. *J Gen Intern Med* 2003;18:335–342.
2. Stewart MA. Effective physician-patient communication and health outcomes: A review. *CMAJ* 1995;152:1423–1433.
3. Roter DL. The enduring and evolving nature of the patient-physician relationship. *Patient Educ Couns* 2000;39:5–15.
4. Roter DL. Patient-centered communication. More than a string of words. *BJA* 2004;4:279–281.
5. Roter DL, Frankel RM, Hall JA, Sluyter D. The expression of emotion through nonverbal behavior in medical visits. Mechanisms and outcomes. *J Gen Intern Med* 2006;21: S28–34.
6. Hall JA, Roter DL, Katz NR. Meta-analysis of correlates of provider behavior in medical encounters. *Med Care* 1988;26:657–675.
7. Jensen MP, Friedman M, Bonzo D, Richards P. The validity of the neuropathic pain scale for assessing diabetic neuropathic pain in a clinical trial. *Clin J Pain* 2006;22:97–103.
8. Melzack R. The McGill Pain Questionnaire: Major properties and scoring methods. *Pain* 1975;1:277–299.
9. Galer BS, Jensen MP. Development and preliminary validation of a pain measure specific to neuropathic pain: The Neuropathic Pain Scale. *Neurology* 1997;48:332–338.
10. Carter GT, Jensen MP, Galer BS, et al. Neuropathic pain in Charcot-Marie-Tooth disease. *Arch Phys Med Rehabil* 1998;79:1560–1564.
11. Bennett MI, et al. Using screening tools to identify neuropathic pain. *Pain* 2007;127:199–203.
12. Melzack R. The short-form McGill Pain Questionnaire. *Pain* 1987;30:191–197.
13. Dudgeon D, Raubertas RF, Rosenthal SN. The short-form McGill Pain Questionnaire in chronic cancer pain. *J Pain Symptom Manage* 1993;8:191–195.
14. Jensen MP. Using pain quality assessment measures for selecting analgesic agents. *Clin J Pain* 2006;22:S9–13.
15. Ashburn M, Rice L. *The Management of Pain*. Philadelphia: Church Livingstone, 1998.
16. Turk DC, Dworkin RH, Burke LB, et al. Developing patient-reported outcome measures for pain clinical trials: IMMPACT recommendations. *Pain* 2006;125:208–215.
17. Jensen M, Karoly P, Braver S. The measurement of clinical pain intensity: A comparison of six methods. *Pain* 1986;27:117–126.
18. Abdi S, Datta S, Trescot AM, et al. Epidural steroids in the management of chronic spinal pain: A systematic review. *Pain Physician* 2007;10:185–212.
19. Nicholson B, Verma S. Comorbidities in chronic neuropathic pain. *Pain Med* 2004;5 Suppl 1:S9–S27.
20. Arnold LM, Hudson JI, Keck PE, et al. Comorbidity of fibromyalgia and psychiatric disorders. *J Clin Psychiatry* 2006;67:1219–1225.
21. Fietta P, Manganelli P. Fibromyalgia and psychiatric disorders. *Acta Biomed* 2007;78:88–95.
22. Smith MT, Huang MI, Manber R. Cognitive behavior therapy for chronic insomnia occurring within the context of medical and psychiatric disorders. *Clin Psychol Rev* 2005;25:559–592.
23. Mokhlesi B, Tulaimat A, Faibussowitsch I, et al. Obesity hypoventilation syndrome: Prevalence and predictors in patients with obstructive sleep apnea. *Sleep Breath* 2007;11:117–124.
24. Wittink HM, Rogers WH, Lipman AG, et al. Older and younger adults in pain management programs in the United States: Differences and similarities. *Pain Med* 2006;7:151–163.
25. Gatchel RJ, Peng YB, Peters ML, et al. The biopsychosocial approach to chronic pain: Scientific advances and future directions. *Psychol Bull* 2007; 133:581–624.
26. Gross DP, Battie MC, Asante AK. Evaluation of a short-form functional capacity evaluation: Less may be best. *J Occup Rehabil* 2007;17:422–435.
27. Poobalan AS, Bruce J, Smith WC, et al. A review of chronic pain after inguinal herniorrhaphy. *Clin J Pain* 2003;19:48–54.
28. Ziegler D. Treatment of diabetic neuropathy and neuropathic pain: How far have we come? *Diabetes Care* 2008;31 Suppl 2:S255–61.
29. Porensky P, Muro K, Ganju A. Nontraumatic cervicothoracic syrinx as a cause of progressive neurologic dysfunction. *J Spinal Cord Med* 2007;30: 276–281.
30. Cornblath DR, Hoke A. Recent advances in HIV neuropathy. *Curr Opin Neurol* 2006;19:446–450.
31. Falconer M, Molloy D, Ingerhaug J, Barry M. Methadone induced torsade de pointes in a patient receiving antiretroviral therapy. *Ir Med J* 2007; 100:631–632.
32. Das PK, Warkentin DI, Hewko R, Forrest DL. Serotonin syndrome after concomitant treatment with linezolid and meperidine. *Clin Infect Dis* 2008;46:264–265.
33. Ashar BH, Rowland-Seymour A. Advising patients who use dietary supplements. *Am J Med* 2008;121:91–97.
34. Abebe W. Herbal medication: Potential for adverse interactions with analgesic drugs. *J Clin Pharm Ther* 2002;27:391–401.
35. Landers MR, Cheung W, Miller D, et al. Workers' compensation and litigation status influence the functional outcome of patients with neck pain. *Clin J Pain* 2007;23:676–782.
36. Ballantyne JC, LaForge KS. Opioid dependence and addiction during opioid treatment of chronic pain. *Pain* 2007;129:235–255.
37. Compton P: The role of urine toxicology in chronic opioid analgesic therapy. *Pain Manag Nurs* 2007;8:166–172.
38. Dib-Hajj SD, et al. Gain-of-function mutation in $NaV_{1.7}$ in familial erythromelalgia induces bursting of sensory neurons. *Brain* 2005;128:1847–1854.
39. Tegeder I, et al. GTP cyclohydrolase and tetrahydrobiopterin regulate pain sensitivity and persistence. *Nature Med* 2006;12:1269–1277.
40. Kandi B, Kaya A, Turgut D, et al. Clinical presentation of cutaneous manifestations in complex regional pain syndrome (type 1). *Skinmed* 2007;6:118–121.
41. Clifton NJ, Jones NS. Prevalence of facial pain in 108 consecutive patients with paranasal mucopurulent discharge at endoscopy. *J Laryngol Otol* 2007;121:345–348.
42. Oktar GL, Ergul EG, Kiziltepe U. Occult malignancy in patients with venous thromboembolism: Risk indicators and a diagnostic screening strategy. *Phlebology* 2007;22:75–79.
43. Attal N, Fermanian C, Fermanian J, et al. Neuropathic pain: Are there distinct subtypes depending on the aetiology or anatomical lesion? *Pain* May 4, 2008. Epub ahead of print.
44. Goldberg C. The Mental Status Exam. In: *A Practical Guide to Clinical Medicine*. San Diego: UCSD School of Medicine and VA Medical Center, 2005.
45. Sivik T, Hosterey U. The Thematic Apperception Test as an aid in understanding the psychodynamics of development of chronic idiopathic pain syndrome. *Psychother Psychosom* 1992;57:57–60.
46. Nordin H, Eisemann M, Richter J. MMPI-2 subgroups in a sample of chronic pain patients. *Scand J Psychol* 2005;46:209–216.
47. Turk D, Melzack R. *Handbook of Pain Assessment*, 2nd ed. New York: Guilford Press, 2001.
48. Turk DC, Dworkin RH, Allen RR, et al. Core outcome domains for chronic pain clinical trials: IMMPACT recommendations. *Pain* 2003;106:337–345.
49. Varni JW, Seid M, Rode CA. The PedsQL: Measurement model for the pediatric quality of life inventory. *Med Care* 1999;37:126–139.
50. Dworkin RH, Nagasko EM, Hetzel RD, Farrar JT. Handbook of pain assessment. In Turk DC, Melzack R, *Assessment of Pain and Pain-Related Quality of Life in Clinical Trials*, 2nd ed. New York: Guilford Press, 2001:659–692.
51. Ware JE, Jr., Sherbourne CD. The MOS 36-item short-form health survey (SF-36). I. Conceptual framework and item selection. *Med Care* 1992;30: 473–483.
52. Rogers WH, Wittink H, Wagner A, et al. Assessing individual outcomes during outpatient multidisciplinary chronic pain treatment by means of an augmented SF-36. *Pain Med* 2000;1:44–54.

53. Rogers WH, Wittink HM, Ashburn MA, et al. Using the "TOPS," an outcomes instrument for multidisciplinary outpatient pain treatment. *Pain Med* 2000;1:55–67.

54. Dworkin RH, Turk DC, Wyrwich KW, et al. Interpreting the clinical importance of treatment outcomes in chronic pain clinical trials: IMMPACT recommendations. *J Pain* 2008;9:105–121.

55. Kerns RD, Turk DC, Rudy TE. The West Haven-Yale Multidimensional Pain Inventory (WHYMPI). *Pain* 1985;23:345–356.

56. Scharff L, Turk DC, Marcus DA. Psychosocial and behavioral characteristics in chronic headache patients: Support for a continuum and dual-diagnostic approach. *Cephalalgia* 1995;15:216–223.

57. Turk DC, Okifuji A, Sinclair JD, Starz TW. Pain, disability, and physical functioning in subgroups of patients with fibromyalgia. *J Rheumatol* 1996;23:1255–1262.

58. Turk DC, Rudy TE. The robustness of an empirically derived taxonomy of chronic pain patients. *Pain* 1990;43:27–35.

59. Cleeland CS, Nakamura Y, Mendoza TR, et al. Dimensions of the impact of cancer pain in a four country sample: New information from multidimensional scaling. *Pain* 1996;67:267–273.

60. Cleeland CS, Ryan KM. Pain assessment: Global use of the Brief Pain Inventory. *Ann Acad Med Singapore* 1994;23:129–138.

61. Beck AT, Ward CH, Mendelson M, et al. An inventory for measuring depression. *Arch Gen Psychiatry* 1961;4:561–571.

62. Geisser ME, Roth RS, Robinson ME. Assessing depression among persons with chronic pain using the Center for Epidemiological Studies-Depression Scale and the Beck Depression Inventory: A comparative analysis. *Clin J Pain* 1997;13:163–170.

63. Lin CC, Lai YL, Ward SE. Effect of cancer pain on performance status, mood states, and level of hope among Taiwanese cancer patients. *J Pain Symptom Manage* 2003;25:29–37.

64. Edwards RR, Haythornthwaite J. Mood swings: Variability in the use of the Profile of Mood States. *J Pain Symptom Manage* 2004;28:534.

65. Guy W. *ECDEU assessment manual for psychopharmacology.* (DHEW Publication No. ADM 76–338). Washington, DC: US Government Printing Office, 1976.

66. Rocchi MB, Sisti D, Benedetti P, et al. Critical comparison of nine different self-administered questionnaires for the evaluation of disability caused by low back pain. *Eura Medicophys* 2005;41:275–281.

67. Sigl T, Cieza A, Brockow T, et al. Content comparison of low back pain-specific measures based on the International Classification of Functioning, Disability and Health (ICF). *Clin J Pain* 2006;22:147–153.

68. Bendebba M, Dizerega GS, Long DM. The Lumbar Spine Outcomes Questionnaire: Its development and psychometric properties. *Spine J* 2007;7:118–132.

69. Stroud MW, McKnight PE, Jensen MP. Assessment of self-reported physical activity in patients with chronic pain: Development of an abbreviated Roland-Morris disability scale. *J Pain* 2004;5:257–263.

70. Butler SF, Budman SH, Fernandez KC, et al. Development and validation of the Current Opioid Misuse Measure. *Pain* 2007;130:144–156.

71. Akbik H, Butler SF, Budman SH, et al. Validation and clinical application of the Screener and Opioid Assessment for Patients with Pain (SOAPP). *J Pain Symptom Manage* 2006;32:287–293.

72. Webster LR, Webster RM. Predicting aberrant behaviors in opioid-treated patients: Preliminary validation of the Opioid Risk Tool. *Pain Med* 2005;6:432–442.

73. Butler SF, Fernandez K, Benoit C, et al. Validation of the Revised Screener and Opioid Assessment for Patients With Pain (SOAPP-R). *J Pain* 2008;9:360–372.

74. Nicholas MK, Asghari A, Blyth FM. What do the numbers mean? Normative data in chronic pain measures. *Pain* 2008;134:158–173.

75. Nicholas MK. The pain self-efficacy questionnaire: Taking pain into account. *Eur J Pain* 2007;11:153–163.

76. Blyth FM Macfarlane CJ, Nicholas M. The contribution of psychosocial factors to the development of chronic pain: The key to better outcomes for patients. *Pain* 2007;129:8–11.

CHAPTER 38 ■ DIAGNOSTIC AND PROGNOSTIC NEURAL BLOCKADE

QUINN H. HOGAN AND STEPHEN E. ABRAM

The use of neural blockade to establish the diagnosis or prognosis of painful conditions is motivated by several compelling characteristics of clinical pain treatment: Pain is an entirely subjective phenomenon with limited means of measurement; painful conditions are inexactly delineated, so that a single descriptive label may be applied to a heterogenous group of maladies, and our understanding of the pathophysiology of pain is poorly developed; and, finally, chronic pain is the result of nociception (the stimulation of pain-sensing pathways), sensory modulation (segmental and descending inhibition, descending facilitation, glial and neuronal sensitization), and neuropathy (aberrant neural function), as well as social, emotional, behavioral, financial, and legal influences. The ambiguity caused by these factors argues strongly for the use of neural blockade to gain clear knowledge of the pathophysiology of the pain, specifically the contribution of sympathetic activity, the site of nociception (visceral versus somatic), or the pathway of afferent neural signals (in an extensively injured limb for example). Information gained from neural blockade can be a useful guide toward choice of medicines, therapeutic blocks, or surgical therapy. Also, neural blockade may be used to anticipate response to surgical ablation, which rarely produces a more satisfactory response than does the prognostic block. By means of suitable neural blockade, the patient may experience motor and sensory changes on a temporary basis before committing to a long-term or permanent lesion.

However, the same uncertainties surrounding pain treatment that lead clinicians to seek hard data from neural blockade techniques also cloud the information gained from them. It is rarely simple to interpret even the most meticulously performed procedure. We may unwittingly confirm preconceived expectations or, at worst, respond to the disproportionate remuneration associated with performing procedures. Few blinded and controlled studies exist that test the utility of these alluring methods.

The premise of this chapter is that neural blockade techniques are informative only in proportion to the care with which they are performed and the thoroughness with which the response is evaluated, and that the findings should be interpreted cautiously. Therefore, we emphasize limitations, so that the reader may avoid the pitfalls. Physiologic, anatomic, and psychosocial issues that influence the quality of information from diagnostic blocks are reviewed first, after which the various procedures are discussed.

PAIN PHYSIOLOGY

The rationale for performing diagnostic neural blockade often is based upon the same misconception that prompts sur-

geons to interrupt neural pathways for permanent pain relief, namely the belief that pain is transmitted by a simple and direct "hard-wired" system. This theory, based on the Cartesian model of pain perception conceived in the 17th century, dominated thinking about pain sensation through the mid 20th century and continues to drive much present-day treatment. Use of a nerve block to identify a nerve pathway that is the source of an individual's ongoing pain assumes three potentially false premises: (a) pathology causing pain is located in an exact peripheral location, and impulses from this site travel via a unique and consistent neural route; (b) injection of local anesthetic totally and selectively abolishes sensory function of intended nerves; and (c) relief of pain following local anesthetic block is due solely to blockade of the targeted neural pathway. These assumptions are limited by certain complexities of the anatomy, physiology, and psychology of pain perception, and the effect of local anesthetics on impulse conduction (see Chapters 2 and 31–36).

Nociceptor Activity

Pain that originates in somatic structures is generally associated with activation of nociceptors, sensory receptors that respond to intense, potentially tissue-injuring, stimulation (Table 38-1). There is considerable controversy about the existence of visceral receptors that respond solely to pain, and many researchers argue that visceral pain results from high-frequency discharge of visceral afferents that ordinarily subserve other functions (1,2). In somatic structures, frequency of discharge of nociceptors correlates directly with the intensity of the stimulus. Thermal nociceptors, for instance, increase their discharge frequency in a linear fashion as temperature rises above $43°C$ (3). This schema is compatible with the Cartesian "hard-wired" model.

However, receptor performance is not a fixed function of stimulation, but is also sensitive to tissue factors (see Chapter 31, Figs. 31-2 to 31-4). Bradykinin, histamine, and 5-hydroxytryptamine (5HT; serotonin) are capable of lowering response thresholds of nociceptors (4). Several eicosanoids are important in the sensitization of nociceptors, and at least two of the prostaglandins (PGE_2 and $PGF_{2\alpha}$) increase nociceptor sensitivity, whereas prostacyclin potentiates edema induced by bradykinin and histamine.

The transient receptor potential channel, vanilloid subfamily member 1 (TRPV1) has been identified as an important skin nociceptor, and is well characterized in the basic science literature (5). This receptor is activated extracellularly by heat, acids, and chemicals with a negative electrical charge, and

TABLE 38-1

DIAGNOSTIC BLOCKS—LIMITATIONS FROM VARIABLE 1ry AFFERENT NERVE ACTIVITY

Due to:
- Tissue factors (receptor sensitization)
- Spontaneous discharge (neuroma, dorsal root ganglion)
- Antidromic propagation
- Sympathetic efferent activity (ephapsis, receptor sensitization neuroma stimulation, inflammation)

intracellularly by arachidonic acid products of the lipoxygenase pathway such as anandamide and N-arachadonoyl-dopamine (NADA). Tissue inflammation markedly lowers the TRPV1 threshold to activation by heat (6). Other TRP channels appear to be candidates for cold pain transduction (TRPA1), and TRP channels as well as acid-sensing ion channels (ASICs) may be involved in the initiation of mechanical nociception (6) (see Chapter 32).

Peripheral nerve activity associated with pain perception may arise from injured nerves independent of natural nociceptor activation. It is now well accepted that spontaneous impulses can be initiated from a neuroma or from an injured nerve segment (7,8), and there is evidence that dorsal root ganglia (DRG) proximal to injured or transected nerves participate in abnormal impulse generation (7). Blockade of a nerve proximal to the injured segment may not provide relief of pain if spontaneous activity continues more proximally at the level of the DRG. This may lead to the false assumption that the injured nerve has not initiated the patient's pain (Table 38-1) (see Chapters 31 and 32).

Nerve blocks usually are interpreted in terms of their effect on afferent neural activity, but important efferent traffic must be considered. Impulse generation arising from an injured nerve fiber is likely to be propagated both orthodromically toward the spinal cord and antidromically toward the innervated tissues. For instance, bursts of sural nerve activity are recorded during straight leg-raising in a patient with S1 radiculopathy (9). Antidromic activity from injured sensory nerves (probably only C-fibers) is thought to cause release of substance P and perhaps other substances, such as bradykinin, histamine, 5HT, and prostaglandins, which may produce changes in nociceptor thresholds by direct and indirect means (10). Therefore, nerve block distal to the primary site of nerve pathology may alter pain perception by interrupting antidromic impulses, contrary to the common assumption that axonal function must be interrupted proximal to the area of injury to provide relief. Peripheral blockade of the sciatic nerve has been shown to provide profound relief of pain for patients with documented lumbosacral radiculopathy (11,12), perhaps by blocking those antidromic impulses that arise from the nerve root or DRG and are propagated to the periphery, thus producing changes in nociceptor sensitivity (13) (Table 38-1).

Sympathetic Contributions

Another important type of efferent traffic affected by neural blockade is sympathetic motor activity, which can alter responses in sensory fibers. Receptors at the terminus of C-fibers from an injured nerve become excited during sympathetic stimulation or norepinephrine application and show enhanced responsiveness to irritating stimuli (14). At the site of the nerve in-

jury, sympathetic efferent impulses may depolarize nociceptive afferent fibers, potentially producing both orthodromic and antidromic activity. Increased sympathetic activity or high levels of norepinephrine have been shown to increase discharge rates of spontaneous impulses arising from neuromas (15,16), and the injection of epinephrine in the vicinity of neuromas in pain patients is associated with aggravation of pain (17) (Table 38-1).

In uninjured tissues, it is well accepted that sympathetic supply can modulate sensory responses (18), but the role of the mechanism in producing pain is less certain. Mechanoreceptor sensitivity is heightened by increases in sympathetic discharge rates. Since nociceptors are not excited by sympathetic stimulation, elevated sympathetic efferent activity alone is unlikely to cause pain. However, aberrant central processing of these signals by sensitized wide dynamic range (WDR) neurons in the dorsal horn (see later discussion) may result in the allodynia (18) present in certain cases of complex regional pain syndrome type 1 (CRPS-1) (Fig. 38-1). Following peripheral nerve injury, an increase occurs in the population of sympathetic nerve fibers in the adjacent DRG (19). Sprouting sympathetic fibers arise from the injured spinal nerve and spread into the DRG, creating basket-like structures surrounding cell somata. The functional changes associated with these plasticity changes have not been characterized, but it seems likely that alterations in the activity of these sympathetic efferents may alter the sensitivity of the neurons they contact (see Chapters 31 and 32).

Pain reduction following sympathetic blockade cannot clearly distinguish between several possible pain mechanisms, including irritation of peripheral nociceptor sensitized by sympathetic efferent activity, signal generation in a neuroma induced by normal sympathetic tone, primary pathologic increase in sympathetic activity resulting in abnormally sensitive receptors, and inflammatory or central effects. When local anesthetic blockade of the sympathetic chain produces temporary relief, surgical or neurolytic interruption of the sympathetic pathways can, nonetheless, fail to provide sustained analgesia. Upregulation of adrenergic receptors in the affected limb may lead to such receptor hypersensitivity that circulating catecholamines may be sufficient to reproduce sympathetically maintained pain.

Spinal Processing

Whatever the contribution of receptor, neuropathic, or sympathetic mechanisms, activity in nociceptive afferent fibers is subject to further, variable processing in the spinal cord (Table 38-2). The balance between large- and small-fiber inputs is an important determinant of the response of dorsal horn neurons to noxious stimulation (20). Conceivably, loss of large-fiber activity following peripheral or neuraxial blockade could increase dorsal horn cell activity, particularly if C-fiber input is preserved (see Chapter 35, Fig. 35-1), thus producing a paradoxical increase in pain.

In addition to segmental influences on dorsal horn function, descending pathways modulate the response of spinal cord neurons to sensory stimuli (see Chapter 31, Figs. 31-18 and 31-19). Noradrenergic and serotoninergic fibers originate in the medulla and descend via the dorsolateral funiculus of the spinal cord to terminate in the dorsal horn, where they inhibit nociceptive traffic (21). Since these tracts lie superficially in the cord, they are susceptible to blockade by intrathecally administered local anesthetics, possibly leading to disinhibition of nociceptive transmission. The relative effect of the drug on

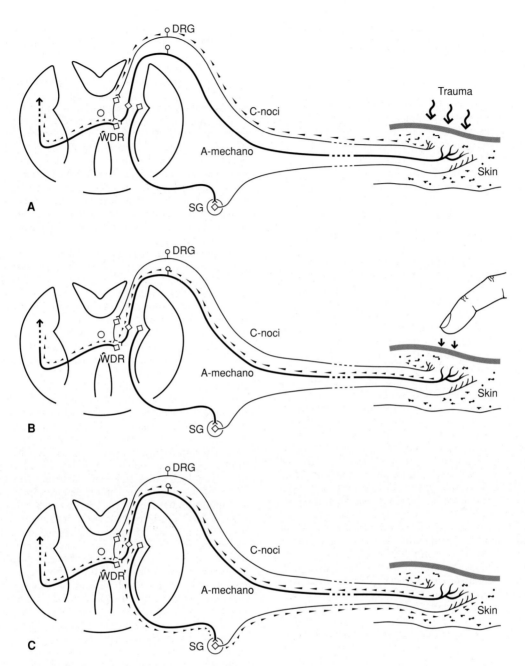

FIGURE 38-1. Robert's hypothesis to explain allodynia and spontaneous pain after tissue trauma, for instance in reflex sympathetic dystrophy. **A:** An initiating injury provides a conditioning stimulus via nociceptive C-fibers, which sensitizes the wide dynamic range (*WDR*) cells in the dorsal horn. **B:** *WDR* cells that transmit to the brain now fire in response to innocuous stimuli conveyed via low-threshold A-mechanoreceptor afferents. **C:** Spontaneous pain is produced by sympathetic efferent actions on A-mechanoreceptor afferents. From Roberts WJ. A hypothesis on the physiological basis for causalgia and related pains. *Pain* 1986;24:297, with permission.

afferent pathways, versus descending inhibitory tracts, would then determine the analgesic effect of a subarachnoid block. Descending cerebral influences may obscure findings during a diagnostic test by producing analgesia in response to stress, independent of the specific nature of the block. Conversely, descending modulation may be stimulatory and produce pain that is independent of sensory input. Dubner and co-workers (22) have demonstrated in primates that nonpainful signals (flashing light) can be associated with nociceptive stimuli (laser heat) by conditioning with repetitive simultaneous presentation. Eventually, the light alone can result in firing of secondary nociceptive neurons and presumably in the sensory experience of pain. The importance of this model is that diagnostic blocks that produce no relief may suggest a diagnosis of malingering or psychiatric disease, when in fact descending influences are generating sensory activity.

DIAGNOSTIC BLOCKS—LIMITATIONS FROM CHANGES IN SPINAL PROCESSING

Via:
- Altered balance between large fiber/small fiber input
- Block of inhibitory descending spinal tracts
- Stress-induced analgesia
- Descending potentiation of nociception
- Convergence (inputs from multiple receptive fields) determine 2° neuron activity

Convergence and Referred Pain

Another feature of pain perception that may confound the application of diagnostic blockade is the phenomenon of convergence (Table 38-2). Many second-order neurons in the spinal cord receive a variety of inputs from primary afferents with either visceral or somatic receptive fields (23) (see Chapter 31, Figs. 31-20 to 31-22). In other instances, convergence is the result of individual C-fiber neurons that have both visceral and cutaneous collaterals (24). When afferent input arises from both somatic and visceral structures, or from separate somatic foci, the perception of pain may be dependent on a summed level of neuronal activity from both components (Chapter 31, Fig. 31-20). Interruption of one limb of the convergent inputs may be enough to provide complete pain relief, leading to false assumptions about the source of the pain. For example, a patient with pain of pancreatic cancer may have inputs from splanchnic nerves, as well as from a focus of myofascial pain in the paravertebral muscles. Infiltration of a painful trigger point in the affected muscle may reduce the combined input to a level insufficient to exceed the pain threshold, and the interpretation would be that the pain is entirely somatic. As a further example, a patient may have combined gluteus medius myofascial pain and S1 radiculopathy, with pain perceived in the distribution of the S1 root. Infiltration of the gluteal trigger point provides blockade of input from muscle afferents to the S1 segment, and may provide sufficient decrease in convergent input to relieve the radicular pain completely on a temporary basis. This could then be interpreted as providing evidence that the patient's pain is entirely myofascial in origin, and the radicular component may be ignored when therapy is proposed.

Plasticity

Sensory processing is not stable but depends on preceding events, a phenomenon called neuronal plasticity (Table 38-3).

DIAGNOSTIC BLOCKS—LIMITATIONS FROM PLASTICITY

- Sensitization (nociceptive potentiation from previous small fiber conditioning stimuli)
- Deafferentation (new receptive fields for nerves after loss of other input)

Small-fiber (nociceptive) activity initiates a series of events in the dorsal horn that lead to heightened responsiveness of neurons activated by noxious stimuli. A brief noxious stimulus produces activation of the α-amino-3-hydroxy-5-methyl-4-isoxazopropionic acid (AMPA) receptor, which in turn produces a brief postsynaptic potential. Repetitive or prolonged firing of small afferent fibers (conditioning stimuli) releases excitatory amino acids, which in turn activates the N-methyl-D-aspartate (NMDA) receptor, causing prolonged postsynaptic potentials. NMDA activation gives rise to a series of intracellular biochemical events (Fig. 38-2) that produce enhanced neurotransmitter release from primary afferents and heightened sensitivity of postsynaptic neurons lasting many minutes to hours (25). In certain instances, more prolonged changes in sensory processing, known as *long-term potentiation* (LTP), may occur (25,26) (see also Chapter 31, Figs. 31-10 to 31-16 and Chapter 32).

In addition to these neuronally mediated mechanisms of central sensitization, activation of glial cells in the central nervous system (CNS), which occurs in response to triggers to neuroimmune activation, such as nerve injury, intense nociceptor activation, inflammation, or infection, can also lead to increased responsiveness of pain projection neurons. The mobilization of microglia, which function as macrophages in the CNS, leads to the increased production and release of proinflammatory cytokines, such as interleukins (IL-1, IL-6) and tumor necrosis factors (TNF-α), which in turn increase the sensitivity of surrounding neurons. Subsequent activation of astrocytes prolongs these responses. The administration of exogenous opioids enhances glial activation, and can in fact directly produce glial activation, cytokine production and hyperalgesia in the absence of tissue or nerve injury (27).

Sensitization in response to noxious stimulation, nerve injury, or chronic opioid administration can affect WDR neurons, which ordinarily respond at very low firing rates to non-noxious (mechanoreceptor, proprioceptor, thermoreceptor) inputs and at high firing rates to nociceptor activity. Following sensitization or LTP, these cells may respond to non-noxious stimuli at sufficiently high firing rates to cause pain perception (allodynia). It is impossible to predict responses to local anesthetic blockade of afferent impulses under conditions of dorsal horn sensitization. Afferent blockade of conditioning stimuli could lead to normalization of dorsal horn responsiveness and profound, prolonged relief. In other circumstances, however, spinal sensitization might persist independently of afferent activity, with little or no change in pain level.

Pain and abnormal sensory responses after injury often are found in a distribution inconsistent with any nerve or root, such as over an entire limb, or in a stocking or glove pattern. This may lead to the diagnosis of psychoneurosis rather than to a neurologic condition. However, injury to a single peripheral nerve may create allodynia in adjacent territories innervated by other nerves, due to altered central processing of afferent signals from the uninjured as well as injured nerve (28). Blockade of the uninjured nerve will relieve pain within the borders of its innervation. The likely but erroneous interpretation would be that the blocked nerve had been injured, which could lead to injection therapy or surgical neurolysis.

Local anesthetic blockade may outlast the duration of local anesthetic effect by hours or days (29), leading to speculation that pain is psychosomatic or factitious. However, it is possible that a period of interruption of nociceptor activity may lead to temporary reversal of the sensitization of spinal cord neurons. Once the peripheral generator recommences, hours or days may go by before sufficient dorsal horn sensitization occurs to cause perception of pain.

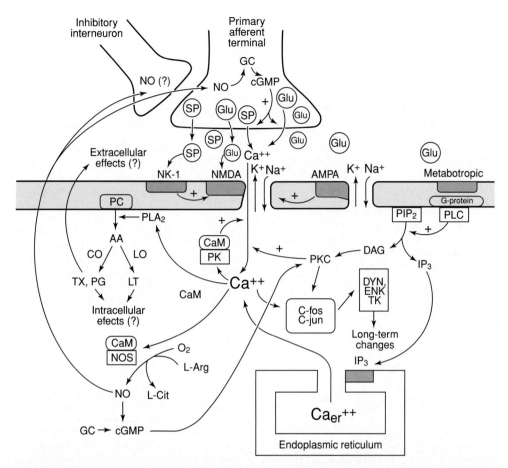

FIGURE 38-2. Sequence of events leading to sensitization of dorsal horn neurons following injury and intense nociceptive stimulation. Intense activation of primary afferent neuron stimulates release of glutamate (*Glu*) and substance P (*SP*). The *N*-methyl-*D*-aspartate (NMDA) receptor, at physiologic magnesium (Mg^{2+}) levels, is initially unresponsive to Glu, but following depolarization of the α-amino-3-hydroxy-5-methyl-4-isoxazopropionic acid (AMPA) receptor by Glu or the neurokinin (NK)-1 receptor by SP, it becomes responsive to Glu, allowing calcium (Ca^{2+}) influx. Action of Glu on the metabotropic receptor stimulates G-protein–mediated activation of phospholipase C (*PLC*), which catalyzes hydrolysis of phosphatidylinositol 4,5-biphosphate (*PIP$_2$*) to produce inositol triphosphate (*IP$_3$*) and diacylglycerol (*DAG*). DAG stimulates production of protein kinase C (*PKC*), which is activated in the presence of high levels of intracellular Ca^{2+} (Ca$_i^{2+}$). IP$_3$ stimulates release of intracellular Ca^{2+} from intracellular stores within the endoplasmic reticulum (Ca$_{er}^{2+}$). Increased PKC induces a sustained increase in membrane permeability and, in conjunction with increased intracellular Ca^{2+}, leads to increased expression of proto-oncogenes such as *c-fos* and *c-jun*. The proteins produced by these proto-oncogenes encode a number of neuropeptides, such as enkephalins (*ENK*), dynorphin (*DYN*), and tachykinins (*TK*). Increased Ca$_i^{2+}$ also leads to activation of calcium-/calmodulin-dependent protein kinase (*CaM PK*), which produces a brief increase in membrane permeability, and to activation of phospholipase A$_2$ (*PLA$_2$*) and to activation of nitric oxide synthase (*NOS*) through a calcium/calmodulin mechanism. PLA$_2$ catalyzes the conversion of phosphatidyl choline (*PC*) to prostaglandins (*PG*) and thromboxanes (*TX*) and by lipoxygenase (*LO*) to produce leukotrienes (*LT*). NOS catalyzes the production of nitric oxide (*NO*) and L-citrulline (*L-Cit*) from L-arginine (*L-Arg*). NO activates soluble guanylate cyclase (*GC*), which increases the intracellular content of cyclic GMP (*cGMP*) and leads to increased production of protein kinases, such as PKC, and alterations in gene expression. NO diffuses out of the cell to the primary afferent terminal, where, through a GC/cGMP mechanism, it increases the release of Glu. It is speculated that NO may interfere with release of inhibitory neurotransmitters from inhibitory neurons.

Conversely, decreases in afferent input can lead to functional changes in the dorsal horn. Following periods of deafferentation, cells that respond to noxious stimulation become hypersensitive to remaining afferent inputs and may develop responsiveness to stimulation of tissues that did not previously produce activation (receptive field expansion) (30). Denervation may also produce sufficient sensitization of WDR neurons so that non-noxious stimulation, including stimuli from out-side the original receptive field, can produce pain (see Chapters 31 and 32). Blockade of such stimulation could cause false indication of the pathology site. Alternatively, blockade of an injured nerve may not provide relief of pain and allodynia if the receptive field of sensitized dorsal horn neurons has spread beyond the distribution of the injured nerve, again leading to the mistaken conclusion that the injured nerve is not involved. Denervation of peripheral afferent fibers has been shown to cause dramatic functional changes in the responses of WDR neurons in the dorsal horn (31).

Summary

These physiologic observations demonstrate that pain is not a process taking place at a single site, is not fixed over time, and is not solely dependent on afferent activity. In addition to the diagnostic implications noted earlier, short-acting local anesthetic blocks often fail to predict beneficial responses to neurodestructive procedures. Nerve regrowth may lead to pain recurrence, but several other factors also cause failure of peripheral neuroablation, despite profound relief from local anesthetic blocks. The nerve injury itself, whether caused by surgical transection, neurolytic block with phenol or alcohol, thermocoagulation, or cryotherapy, may induce spontaneous discharge or increased mechanosensitivity at the site of injury (7,8,15,32). Successful denervation, even in the absence of increased peripheral inputs, may lead to changes in dorsal horn cell function, with sensitization of WDR neurons and expansion of receptive fields.

LOCAL ANESTHETIC PHYSIOLOGY

Intensity of Blockade

Diagnostic and prognostic blocks are accomplished by the action of local anesthetics (and occasionally by neuraxial opioids [33]) upon nerves. It has long been recognized that neural blockade is not an all-or-none response. For instance, analgesia usually is evident earlier and to a greater extent than loss of perception of mechanical stimuli after peripheral neural blockade. This should be recalled when diagnostic sympathetic blocks are performed. The lack of anesthesia to touch in the involved area does not assure that pain relief is accomplished by sympathetic interruption, because a subtle somatic block could produce analgesia without anesthesia, resulting in pain relief independent of a sympathetic mechanism (34). In the opposite sense, apparent intense blockade with complete insensitivity to touch and pain is nonetheless not a complete afferent blockade. Studies of different types of blocks with various agents uniformly demonstrate incomplete elimination of somatosensory potentials evoked by stimulation of the anesthetized region (35). This may be the mechanism behind tourniquet pain and the humoral response to upper abdominal regional anesthesia, both of which occur despite apparently adequate sensory blockade. If pain continues after a diagnostic block, one cannot be certain that the injected pathway is not involved, since neural blockade is rarely complete.

The variable and partial nature of local anesthetic effects is evident also in blockade of efferent sympathetic activity. Skin conduction responses, a manifestation of sympathetic action at sweat glands, often is present in areas of apparently complete somatic blockade (36), and skin cooling has been noted in the center of a truncal band of segmental epidural anesthesia (37). During total thoracolumbar epidural anesthesia, norepinephrine levels decrease by only about 60% (38) or not at all (39), indicating persistent sympathetic synaptic release. These considerations weaken the predictive value of sympathetic blocks, unless monitoring confirms the loss of sympathetic activity concurrent with the onset of relief.

TABLE 38-4

DIAGNOSTIC BLOCKS—LIMITATIONS FROM COMPLEXITY OF LOCAL ANESTHETIC EFFECT

- Blocks rarely complete (afferent sensory, efferent-sympathetic)
- Subtle block without obvious sensory change
- Differential block unpredictable (fiber type, length of exposure)
- Use dependent block (nerve activity influences anesthetic effect)

Differential Block (Table 38-4)

The variable effects of local anesthetics upon fibers performing different functions is termed differential block (Table 38-4). Were it possible to predict and control the neural modalities that are blocked, diagnostic distinctions could be made by selectively interrupting sympathetic or somatic fibers. This goal has proved elusive. The physiologic mechanisms that result in differential effects of local anesthetics are complex and multiple (40) (see also Chapter 2). Most commonly cited is the importance of fiber size. Since fibers of different cross-sectional areas serve different functions (large $A\alpha \rightarrow$ motor, $A\beta$ touch/proprioception; small $A\delta \rightarrow$ cold/hot/pain, B $\rightarrow$ preganglionic sympathetic, C $\rightarrow$ postganglionic sympathetic, pain, temperature), dependence of anesthetic action upon size would explain clinically observed graded blockade of sensory and motor functions by local anesthetics. Erlanger and Gasser formulated this concept in 1929, but despite the appealing simplicity of the model, it has not withstood the test of time. They studied the effects of cocaine upon amphibian nerves, but only examined large myelinated A-fibers at room temperature and not under equilibrium conditions. Further study (41,42) has shown that, contrary to the size principle, the concentrations (C_M) necessary for blockade of A- and B-fibers are less than those for C-fibers. In general, the intrinsic sensitivity of nerve fibers to local anesthetics is probably A <B <C. Problematic for the use of local anesthetics in diagnosis, however, is the great variability of sizes within a fiber type, and the lack of correlation of size and C_M within the group (41,43). The overlap of C_M between different groups "appears to negate any possibility of obtaining steady state differential interruption" by local anesthetics (41).

The size principle fails to explain the differential effects clinically evident during non–steady state conditions, but different diffusion barriers of the various fiber types probably does. The lipid barrier of myelinated A-fibers is a greater impediment to ability of local anesthetics to reach the axonal membrane binding site than it is for C-fibers, which lack the insulating myelin (44). Despite the inherent greater resistance of C-fibers to blockade, they are exposed to higher local anesthetic concentration early in the onset of the block, because of more rapid diffusion, so that the sequence of blockade is usually B first (due to intrinsic sensitivity), then C and Aδ before Aα and Aβ. Using intraneural recording to study conduction in radial nerves of human subjects after injection of 0.25% lidocaine (45), preferential blockade of C-fibers is evident. Full differential block is not possible, however, since completely abolished C-fiber activity is accompanied by partial A-fiber block. Sensory loss progresses in the order of sensibility for warmth, dull ache, cold, prick, and finally touch (46). The combination of

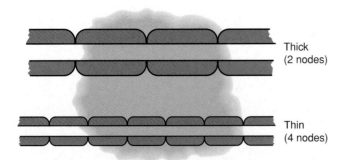

FIGURE 38-3. Effect of exposure length in producing differential block. A large axon with long internodal lengths may continue to conduct despite exposure to local anesthetic at concentrations adequate to block the nodes completely if only two nodes are exposed to local anesthetic. A smaller axon with closer nodes will have more nodes blocked and not be able to conduct. From DeJong RH. *Local Anesthetics*. St. Louis: Mosby–Yearbook, 1994:89, with permission.

high lipid solubility and low pKa (high nonionized fraction) for etidocaine accounts for its thorough penetration into well protected Aα (motor) fibers, and therefore minimal differential block, compared to bupivacaine, which has a weak motor block (see Chapter 2).

Even with concentrations of local anesthetic high enough to eliminate sodium (Na$^+$) conductance completely, an action potential can still "jump" two adjacent totally blocked nodes (about 4 mm for the largest fibers) and excite the nerve beyond the blocked segment. To prevent conduction, at least three nodes in succession must be blocked (47) (see Chapter 2). If local anesthetic is limited in longitudinal extent, large fibers with long internodal distances may lack exposure to three nodes, whereas smaller fibers have the necessary three nodes exposed and are blocked (Fig. 38-3). At concentrations that produce less intense Na$^+$ channel blockade, the influence of exposure length extends even further, so that a concentration of local anesthetic that blocks conduction in 3 cm of exposed nerve may not block conduction when only 2 cm is exposed (48). With low concentrations of local anesthetic, not all Na$^+$ channels are inactivated, so a diminished but present action potential results (i.e., the action potential is not "all-or-none"). Less current reaches the adjacent node, causing it to fire but with an even smaller action potential. During this so-called decremental conduction, the action potential may propagate for many nodes before it finally fails to depolarize the next node. The result is that (a) conduction may fail through a segment of exposed nerve even if none of the nodes have been made completely inexcitable (Fig. 38-4), and (b) C$_M$ is inversely related to exposed nerve length. These phenomena may explain differential blockade that develops with spinal and epidural anesthesia (49), but also dictate that anesthetic potency and the degree of differential effects varies with the length of nerve exposed, an added variable that is hard to control (see also Chapter 2).

Further subtle influences upon local anesthetic action may cloud the interpretation of diagnostic blocks. Sodium channel closure by local anesthetics depends on nerve use; tonic block in an infrequently firing axon is less intense than the phasic block that develops progressively with higher firing rates. Local anesthetic will affect those fibers more completely that are most active. The ongoing activity of B vasomotor fibers may contribute to their preferential blockade, especially since these fibers show the greatest degree of phasic block. Phasic amplification of blockade may play a minor role for C (pain) fibers

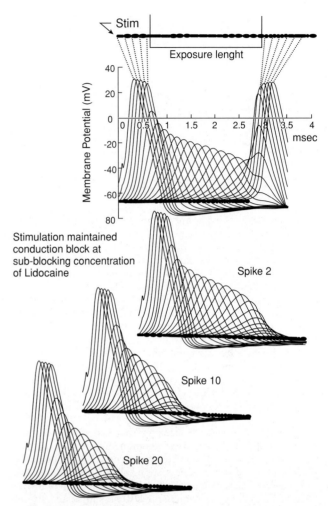

Stimulation maintained conduction block at sub-blocking concentration of Lidocaine

FIGURE 38-4. Modeling of conduction in an axon exposed to local anesthetic concentration below the threshold for complete block at a node. Reduced current from a partially blocked axon provides a diminished stimulus to the next node, so that amplitude declines along the 15-node exposed segment. Intensified block for subsequent impulses causes the signal to perish before it can reach the unexposed node. Signal interruption occurs despite the lack of complete blockade of any node. Response will be highly sensitive to slight changes in signal frequency, exposure length, or anesthetic concentration. From Raymond SA, Strichartz GR. The long and short of differential block. *Anesthesiology* 1989;70:725, with permission.

because their firing rates are too low. The spectrum of anesthetic effects will depend, therefore, upon the pattern of activity of the subject's various neuron types when the diagnostic block is undertaken, and also will depend upon the choice of anesthetic. Bupivacaine, the agent with the greatest degree of phasic block, also shows a high degree of differential blockade. Since the earliest perturbation of nerve function at very low anesthetic concentrations is the prolongation of the latent interval for refiring (43), information encoded with bursts will be transformed into a more continuous signal. By this means, sensations can be made to change without any actual termination of transmission (see Chapter 2).

To summarize, it is now apparent that local anesthetic effects are more subtle, complex, and variable than has been realized in the past. This does not invalidate their use for diagnostic exercises, but does dictate caution in the interpretation of block results.

TABLE 38-5

DIAGNOSTIC BLOCKS—LIMITATIONS FROM LOCAL ANESTHETIC SYSTEMIC EFFECTS

- Suppression of spontaneous neuroma activity
- Depression of spinal nociceptive transmission
- Block of central sensitization (high circulating concentrations)
- Occasional prolonged responses

Systemic Effects

When assessing the response of pain perception to local anesthetic blocks, it is important to consider the systemic effect of the anesthetic as it is absorbed from the site of injection (Table 38-5). Considerable data are available to show that systemic local anesthetic analgesia reduces neuropathic pain, but does relatively little for other painful conditions.

Conventional local anesthetic blood levels that follow blockade even with large volumes of agent (e.g., 1 to 5 μg/mL after 20 mL 1% lidocaine) produce no appreciable effect on impulse conduction in normal peripheral nerves (7,8,32,50) or on cutaneous C-fiber terminal function (50). Local anesthetics also have little or no analgesic effect in animal models of acute nociception (50). Therefore, possible mechanisms for analgesia during neuropathy include effects of the drug on impulse generation in injured nerves or on processing of sensory information in the CNS.

Experimental evidence indicates that systemically administered local anesthetics affect spontaneous impulse generation arising from injured nerves. Intravenous (IV) lidocaine in subconvulsant doses produces suppression of spontaneously active nerve fibers originating from sciatic neuromas in rats (32), and impulse generation in the DRG is suppressed at even lower doses (7). Electrically evoked peripheral nerve activity remains completely intact at these doses. In addition, lidocaine decreases the sensitivity of these neurons to mechanical stimulation. Tanelian and MacIver (8) evaluated the effect of lidocaine on injury-induced discharge of corneal C- and Aδ-fibers. Concentrations ranging from 1 to 20 μg/mL suppress tonic action potential discharge, but do not block electrically evoked nerve conduction until concentrations reach 250 μg/mL.

Nerve injury is associated with significant changes in populations of Na$^+$ channels. The tetrodotoxin (TTX)-sensitive Nav1.3 channel, which is minimally expressed in uninjured nerves except at embryologic stages of development, is upregulated in injured DRG following spinal nerve ligation (SNL) injury. Because this channel subtype recovers rapidly from inactivation, it is able to support rapid firing rates. The TTX-resistant Nav1.8 channel is upregulated in uninjured spinal nerves adjacent to the SNL injury (51). These changes are associated with the development of ectopic discharge and with hyperalgesia and allodynia. Lidocaine is nonspecific in its effect on these channels, but it is effective in blocking the activity of these upregulated channels at blood levels that do not interfere with normal nerve conduction.

Nontoxic doses of systemic local anesthetics also have depressant effects on spinal transmission of nociceptive inputs. Lidocaine significantly suppresses the spinal polysynaptic reflex evoked by stimulation of sural nerve C-fibers (50). An increase in nociceptive flexion reflex thresholds in diabetic patients, and in healthy human subjects, is observed following IV infusion of 5 mg/kg lidocaine (52).

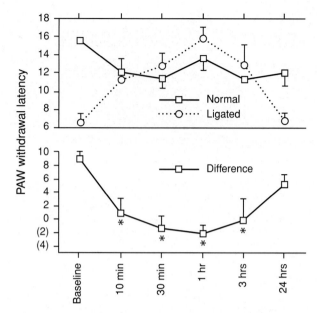

FIGURE 38-5. Effect of systemic lidocaine on hyperalgesia after sciatic nerve ligation in rats. The accelerated paw withdrawal (in seconds) on the side of nerve injury compared with the uninjured normal side, is made normal by lidocaine at a blood level of 1 μg/mL.* Indicate significant difference from baseline. From Abram SE, Yaksh TL. Systemic lidocaine blocks nerve injury-induced hyperalgesia and nociceptor-driven spinal sensitization in the rat. *Anesthesiology* 1994;80:383, with permission.

In an effort to determine the relative potency of local anesthetics on spinal versus peripheral mechanisms, Abram and Yaksh (53) assessed the effects of IV lidocaine on hyperalgesia induced by sciatic nerve ligation and on hyperalgesia due to dorsal horn sensitization following subcutaneous formalin in rats. Intravenous lidocaine at a blood level of 1 μg/mL reversed the thermal hyperalgesia induced by nerve injury (Fig. 38-5). However, spinal sensitization was prevented only when lidocaine blood levels exceeded 6 μg/mL. This indicates that the principal effect of systemic local anesthetics on neuropathic pain is peripheral.

There have been several clinical reports of the efficacy of IV lidocaine in patients with neuropathic pain (8,52,54–57). Although some cite very transient effects (8,57), others indicate analgesic effects lasting several days or more (55,56). Doses of local anesthetic required to relieve neuropathic pain are generally 1 to 3 mg/kg. It would be unlikely, therefore, that a selective nerve root block with 3 mL 1% lidocaine would produce pain relief by a systemic effect. On the other hand, a lumbar sympathetic block, using 15 mL 1% lidocaine, might be capable of relieving neuropathic pain at a location distant from the site of injection.

PSYCHOSOCIAL INFLUENCES

Even though the practitioner uses diagnostic blocks to obtain specific, convincing, "hard" data, she must still be aware that the procedure is also a social interaction (Table 38-6). Although the patient may not seek to deceive the doctor, it is impossible to dissociate the experience of pain from surrounding social and psychological factors (see also Chapters 29 and 35). Important aspects to consider include the following:

TABLE 38-6

DIAGNOSTIC BLOCKS—LIMITATIONS FROM PSYCHOLOGICAL ISSUES

- Communication problems
- Evaluation in an unfamiliar environment
- Divergent patient/physician agendas

- Communication may be incomplete. Answers are reliable only if the physician is able to enter into the same frame of reference as the patient and to use descriptive terms in the same way (58).
- The clinic is not the patient's home (59), and unfamiliarity, stress, and anxiety may create an environment dissimilar to that in which the pain usually exists.
- The patient and physician may not have the same agenda. Whereas the doctor may seek pathophysiologic information, the patient may be looking for reassurance, confirmation of suspicions or proof to persuade doubting family members, certification of disability for legal and financial reasons (see Chapter 29), or may simply wish to please the doctor (see Chapter 36).

Any of these purposes may enter into the patient's reporting.

To diminish the ambiguities created by these psychosocial factors, a physician might choose to inject a placebo (Latin for "I please"), an inert substance with no known pharmacodynamic effect (see Chapter 36). Although desirable in many situations, the use of a placebo is an incomplete means of clarification. Problems include ethical considerations (60) of performing an invasive procedure to inject an inactive substance, and the difficulty of obtaining permission while not revealing that the injected substance is a placebo. This may be circumvented by comparing the duration of response to two local anesthetics with different pharmacokinetics (e.g., lidocaine versus bupivacaine) (61). Comparative durations of relief not in keeping with expected durations of local anesthetic effect could be interpreted as a placebo response, but this unproven method requires more subtle distinctions than the clear case of a response to saline injection, and as noted earlier, relief of pain with local anesthetic may be prolonged long beyond the drug's presence.

A more limiting uncertainty is what to make of a patient who responds favorably to a placebo (Table 38-7). About one-third of patients obtain relief from placebos administered during acute pain (62), and they may be up to twice as likely to obtain relief of chronic pain with a placebo. For example, 82% of patients in a study of chronic arthritis reported definite improvement in pain and function after weekly subcutaneous nor-

mal saline (63). In another study, 59% had relief from a placebo tablet, whereas 57% of those who didn't respond to a pill had relief from a subsequent placebo injection (64). In patients with causalgia, 3 mL of subcutaneous normal saline relieved spontaneous pain in 68% of patients and also relieved mechanically induced pain (allodynia) in 56% and relieved Tinel sign in 67% (65). Probability of analgesia from a placebo is proportionate to the intensity of pain (66). No personality features predict a placebo response (67). Individuals are not consistent in being responders or nonresponders, and most eventually will respond to a placebo if administered repeatedly (68). Thus, it is hard to conclude much from identifying a placebo response. Certainly, this is not a way to determine whether the pain is real.

Psychologic theory explaining placebo response focuses on the subject's expectations (69) and on conditioning (70). In the context of diagnostic blocks, the expectation of a favorable response may make analgesia more likely. By conditioning, a patient's response to an injection is based upon what they experienced after previous similar events. It has been shown that most subjects can be trained to have a placebo response (71) and that a placebo response is more likely if the test with the active agent precedes the placebo administration (72). Other implications are that a patient's previous analgesic experiences will condition the potency of a placebo (73) and that withdrawal of even a pharmacologically inactive therapy may lead to an increase in chronic pain (70). On a physiologic level, the placebo response is a demonstration of the descending modulation of nociception. Evidence of an opioid mechanism includes the antagonism of placebo analgesia with naloxone (74,75) and the documentation of increased cerebrospinal fluid (CSF) endogenous opioid activity after a placebo response, but this is not so if no response occurred (76). In view of this, placebos can be considered active agents in their own right (see also Chapter 36).

When local anesthetic is injected for diagnostic nerve blockade, it is very difficult to be certain that relief has not occurred through a placebo mechanism rather than through neural interruption. In general terms, placebo responses are incomplete, inconsistently repeatable, and may lack the appropriate time course for the onset or duration of the active agent. However, it is difficult to employ these generalizations in any particular clinical case. Placebo action may be as intense as the active agent, usually will mimic the active agent in dose–response and time–effect relationships (77), and may develop over as prolonged an interval as 60 minutes (Fig. 38-6) (78,79). Injections, like surgery, are especially potent placebos (77) (see also Chapter 34).

An important component of the placebo event is the practitioner. It has been demonstrated repeatedly (77,80) that even in carefully blinded protocols, unintended communication from the examiner takes place. When placebo is compared to morphine, the placebo responders have analgesia comparable to that induced by morphine, whereas if aspirin is being tested, the placebo response resembles aspirin. Patients told they might receive either a narcotic analgesic or narcotic antagonist during acute pain developed placebo analgesia (to saline) only if they were in a group that the physician knew would receive fentanyl versus saline, and not if they were in a group which the physician knew would get only naloxone versus saline. This held true even if the physician knew only which group the patient was in and not whether saline or drug was given (Fig. 38-7). The history of new therapies demonstrates the same phenomenon. Initial reports by enthusiasts are commonly contradicted by subsequent blinded and critical trials (81,82). These various observations make it clear that the physician's convictions play a large role in generating placebo responses.

TABLE 38-7

DIAGNOSTIC BLOCKS — LIMITATIONS FROM PLACEBO RESPONSE

- Always possible
- Unpredictable
- Frequent in chronic pain
- Potent with injection
- Based on conditioning, endorphins
- Operator-dependent

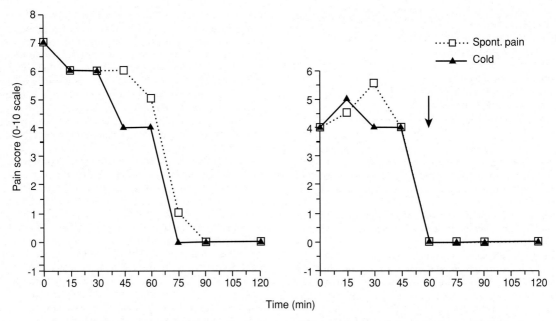

FIGURE 38-6. The time course for development of placebo response in a patient with chronic low back pain. Saline is administered at each 15-minute mark and phentolamine is administered IV at the arrow in the right frame, in a carefully constructed double-blind protocol. Placebo analgesia evolves over 1 hour to both spontaneous and cold-induced pain (*left frame*). From Fine PG, Roberts WJ, Gillette RG, Child TR. Slowly developing placebo responses confound tests of intravenous phentolamine to determine mechanisms underlying idiopathic chronic low back pain. *Pain* 1994;56:235, with permission.

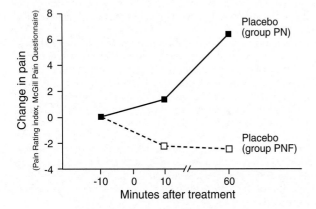

Change in pain rating index between baseline
(10 min before injection) and 10 and 60 min after
administration of placebo.

PN = group that could have either received placebo
or naloxone.
PNF = group that could have received placebo,
naloxone, or lentanyl (PNF)

FIGURE 38-7. The effect of physician awareness on placebo response. No analgesia occurs when placebo is administered to the group *PN* that the physician knew would receive no opioid, only placebo (saline) or Narcan, in a blinded fashion. However, placebo analgesia (downward trend in pain scores) is evident in the group *PNF* that the physician knew might be given fentanyl as one of the blinded choices. From Devor M. Central changes mediating neuropathic pain. In: Dubner R, Gebharrt GF, Bond MR, eds. *Proceedings of the 5th World Congress on Pain.* Amsterdam: Elsevier, 1988:114-128, with permission.

The potency and frequency of the placebo effect is underestimated by the majority of physicians and nurses (83). Far from being a minor inconvenience, this effect is a central concern in the performance of diagnostic blocks. In a sense, each diagnostic block resembles a clinical study of a drug or procedure, but with a study group of only a single subject. Convincing results are elusive without repeated testing with a blinded subject and physician.

What can be done to lessen the confusion introduced by placebo responses? Ironically, when an elaborate protocol is used to control for physician and patient bias, and adequate time is allowed for the full development of placebo response, all subjects have placebo analgesia (78). Our recommendations are to: (a) inform the patient that a placebo injection may be used at some point during diagnostic testing; (b) use more than one trial of a diagnostic block; (c) include a saline injection at least once during a series of blocks, preferably through the same needle that will then be used for the local anesthetic, allowing time between injections for questioning as to relief; (d) if possible, blind the operator performing the block as to the agent injected; (e) recognize relief from a placebo as a normal and expected event; (f) consider a response to local anesthetic more persuasive if it differs in quality, intensity, or timing from the saline injection, or if no placebo response occurred; and (g) bear in mind that relief from local anesthetic injection may still be by a placebo mechanism. A final concern is the negative placebo. From 28% (84) to 34% (85) of subjects given inactive agents will have side effects such as headache, drowsiness, asthenia, dizziness, nausea, and vomiting.

ANATOMICAL CONSIDERATIONS

The use of blocks for diagnosis and prognosis depends on an assumption of anatomic consistency. We expect nerve

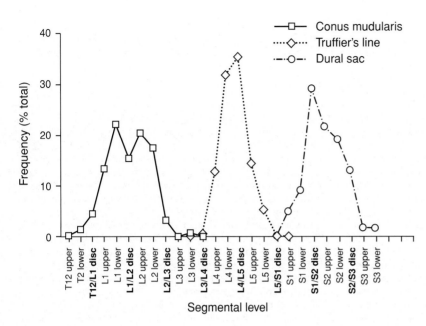

FIGURE 38-8. Bony vertebral levels for conus medullaris, the Tuffier line, and dural sac. Anatomic features such as the termination of the spinal cord and dural sac and the point at which the line between the iliac crests (Tuffier line) crosses the vertebral column are not exact. A normal distribution describes most anatomic measures.

structures to be found in predictable places and to have predictable connections. There are important limitations to these expectations. Like any biologic feature, most anatomic parameters show variability about a norm. For example, the Tuffier line between the iliac crests crosses the vertebral column most often at the L4–L5 disc (perhaps higher on average in men than in women) (86), but the range is from as low as the L5–S1 disc to as high as the L3–L4 disc (86–88). A normal distribution also describes the level of termination of the spinal cord (89) and the termination of the dural sac (Fig. 38-8) (90). This indicates that surface and palpation landmarks are unreliable indicators of deep structures, which is borne out by a 50% accuracy in guessing vertebral level of needle placement without x-ray imaging (91–95).

Anatomic variability is not limited to relative dimensions and positions of structures, but also includes the number and connections of anatomic items, and idealized textbook descriptions hold in only about 50% to 70% of actual subjects (96). For instance, even though patterns of vertebral segmentation are stable in the cervical and thoracic levels, lumbar and sacral regions show a marked variety of segmentation. The last lumbar or first sacral vertebra may be indeterminate in configuration, with fusion of L5 to S1 in 6.2% (sacralization of L5), or incomplete fusion of S1 to S2 in 5.3% (lumbarization of S1), and one or more sacral segments may be absent (97). The distribution of nerve roots to the intervertebral foramina is anomalous in about 8% of subjects (98,99) and includes two root pairs exiting at one level with an adjacent empty foramen (100). These variations occur because the DRG develop from a continuous sheet of neural crest tissue, and separation into segments is imprecise. The clinical consequence of aberrant arrangements is the development of anesthesia in an unexpected distribution following foraminal injection, with resulting diagnostic ambiguity (99).

Separation of somatic input into a discernible segmental pattern is a fundamental concept underlying many diagnostic blocks. No segmentation is evident upon the surface of the spinal cord or by histologic examination of its substance. It is only by the grouping of rootlets into rootlet bundles bound for a common DRG and intervertebral foramen that a pattern of segments is superimposed upon the otherwise seamless connections of the peripheral system with the CNS. There is, however, variability in the formation of segmental spinal nerves and their peripheral distribution. Multiple interconnections of adjacent rootlets and roots are found within the dural sac in all subjects, with between three and nine such intersegmental anastomoses at the upper cervical region and a similar number at the lumbosacral level (101,102). The pattern of spinal nerve contributions to the limb is highly inconsistent. For example, 28% of lumbosacral plexuses have central connections shifted proximally ("prefixed") or distally ("postfixed") along the vertebral column, compared to the usual pattern (103). Seven major configurations of the brachial plexus are possible, with none having more than 57% representation and with 61% of individuals differing in type between right and left (104). The resulting distribution of fibers to the skin has been mapped, using zoster eruptions, residual sensation after sectioning the roots on either side of an intact segment, absent sensation after root section or anesthesia, vasodilatation during stimulation of roots, or pain with nerve root compression and visceral disease (105). The dermatome diagrams these methods produce show considerable disagreement, especially in the extremities. Also, extensive overlap between consecutive peripheral dermatomes is evident, because the division of an individual root rarely produces an appreciable loss of sensibility. As a consequence, the sensory innervation of a particular site cannot be assigned with certainty to any segmental level, and sensory changes after local anesthetic injections about the vertebral column are variable. Segmental inconsistency is also present in the motor innervation of the extremities. Marked departure from the usual distribution of L5 and S1 motor fibers is found in 16% of subjects (106), in whom stimulation of a root produces movement typical of the other root.

Important differences in the peripheral distribution of sympathetic motor fibers are relevant to diagnostic blocks. Preganglionic axons originate only from the T1 through L2 segments. Fibers bound for tissues with cervical or low lumbar and sacral somatic innervation are deployed by the paravertebral chains. Therefore, segmental neuraxial local anesthetic application will block sympathetic innervation to tissues different from those that are somatically denervated. For instance, a low spinal anesthetic may produce intense sensory block to the feet, ankles, calves, and buttocks (low lumbar and sacral segments) without any sympathetic changes in these areas (derived from L1 and L2). Sympathetic outflow is only weakly segmental, due to the crossing of rami communicates (107) and extensive divergence of sympathetic activity in the ganglia. Efferent sympathetic fibers supplying a cutaneous region do not necessarily arrive by the same peripheral nerve as the sensory afferents supplying that area. For example (108), the radial aspect of the dorsum of the hand receives sensory and sudomotor innervation via the radial nerve, but vasomotor innervation from the median nerve. Similarly, the lateral aspect of the foot may receive its sympathetic input from peroneal branches while transmitting sensory information in the sural nerve (109). The extent of sympathetic blockade after regional anesthetic is poorly understood and difficult to predict.

Anatomic variability is also evident in the distribution of injected solutions. Spread is guided by the vagaries of tissue pressures and adherence, and it may be entirely unidirectional, rather than expanding concentrically from the injection site. The vertebral canal is a common pathway for aberrant injectate flow after injections near the vertebral column. As pressure of the solution rises at the injection site, spread to the canal may occur, because pressure in the canal does not rise above CSF pressure (about 15 cm H_2O), since inflow displaces CSF. Epidural anesthetic effect may be an undesired component of various diagnostic blocks (facet, lumbar sympathetic, stellate, nerve root, and plexus blocks).

Less is known about the patterns of visceral sensory connections. Visceral receptive fields are large and overlapping, and extensive convergence of afferent traffic is evident at many CNS levels (24). Most visceral pain travels in sympathetic nerves, but afferents from the thoracic organs, the pancreas, and biliary tree ascend in the phrenic nerve and pass to the thoracic cord via medial branches of the sympathetic chain. From the sigmoid colon, rectum, neck of the bladder, prostate, and cervix of the uterus, most visceral afferent fibers retrace the route of parasympathetic efferent neurons, entering the cord in the posterior roots of S2–S4. A few fibers from these organs ascend in the prevertebral plexuses to enter at L1–L2. Pain that is not relieved by blocks of sympathetic pathways may still be visceral in origin but transmitted by these nonsympathetic routes (see Chapter 31, Figs. 31-20 to 31-22).

The role and even presence of nociceptive fibers from the limbs that travel in sympathetic structures has been debated (110,111). Lumbar sympathetic block prevents the poorly localized dull ache during surgical manipulation of the femoral vein or from lower extremity thrombophlebitis (112,113). Surgical sympathectomy blocks responses to venous distension in canine lower extremities (114) and almost eliminates the aching and stinging pain from cold exposure of human extremities (115). Sympathetic block also interrupts pain from mechanical stimulation of the femoral medullary cavity (116). These observations indicate that interruption of afferent sensory impulses travel from vascular structures in the extremities via sympathetic pathways which, when blocked by diagnostic sympathetic blockade, could be falsely interpreted as an indication of an efferent sympathetic pathogenesis of pain. One recent analysis attributes most "sympathetic dependent" pain to visceral afferent activity (117) (see also Chapter 39 and Chapter 31, Fig. 31-8).

Deep somatic pain from bones, joints, muscles, and fascia shares many features of visceral pain including poor somatotopic localization, referral of pain to distant sites, and a particular ability to generally increase CNS excitability, manifest as elevated motor and autonomic reflexes (110). Additionally, the fibers from many deep somatic elements (costovertebral joint, posterior and anterior longitudinal ligaments, anular ligament

of the intervertebral disc, dura) traverse the sympathetic rami and chain (118–121). It is likely that some pains relieved by sympathetic blocks are unrelated to sympathetic efferent activity (sympathetically maintained pain) and instead are deep somatic pains transmitted by sympathetic pathways (117).

METHODOLOGY

Diagnostic blocks should be performed in a manner that yields the most certain information possible, in order not to add to the inherent ambiguity of clinical pain. In many cases, needle position should be confirmed by radiologic imaging. Determination of the segmental level is unreliable without confirmation by radiography, and studies of a variety of injection procedures have shown inadequate consistency of needle placement without imaging (91,122–124). Since small volumes of local anesthetic need to be used to minimize spread to undesired nerves, meticulous needle placement is required to assure adequate blockade of the desired nerve. Injection of a small amount of radiopaque contrast, prior to the anesthetic, can identify passage into an unwanted space (vascular, subarachnoid) or in an ineffective direction. The usefulness of guiding needle insertion by the nature of provoked pain is limited by the lack of specificity of deep sensations (125,126).

Pain before and after blockade should be evaluated by asking the patient to rate the intensity, between 0 (none) and 10 (worst imaginable), to facilitate communication and documentation. Provocative measures, such as palpation of a tender area or joint movement, may help the patient and clinician discern changes in incident pain, when compared before and after the block. For instance, in a patient who has pain only when ambulating, implantation of a pump for intrathecal opioid treatment is not supported by a prognostic trial during which the patient is kept in bed. Not only may a patient with spontaneous pain respond differently than if he has induced pain, but blocks used may act differently upon pain induced by repetitive dynamic mechanical stimulation (dynamic mechanical allodynia) versus steady pressure (static mechanical allodynia) (127). Careful examination is required to discern these subtle block effects. If the patient is not having the usual pain at the time of a diagnostic block, little can be learned about the pain's mechanism. When pain is relieved by neural blockade, the duration of analgesia should be determined. Relief lasting only the expected duration of the anesthetic effect suggests an ongoing peripheral focus of nociception. If relief obviously outlasts the anesthetic, a central potentiating process may be involved.

Pain relief, however, cannot be the only measured parameter. Direct confirmation of actual neural blockade is necessary, because performing the procedure correctly and with care does not guarantee that the intended nerve will be anesthetized and the desired physiologic change achieved. Detailed sensory and motor testing before and after injection can identify somatic nerve block effects. Meticulous care may be necessary to delineate sensory changes. For instance, vibration transmitted through the skin and soft tissue may stimulate receptors at a considerable distance, creating the misimpression that an area is incompletely insensate (128). Tactile threshold changes can be identified by testing with fibers of different stiffness (von Frey hairs), and fast pain ($A\delta$) sensation can be examined by a scratch, for example using the folded corner of a foil alcohol pad wrapper or a broken tongue blade.

More elaborate methods are necessary for an adequate test of C-fiber (slow pain) sensation. Stimuli should be performed as consistently as possible since a stimulus that is more intense, more frequently repeated, or more broadly distributed may be perceived, whereas weaker stimuli are blocked (129).

Inconsistent stimulation may cause confusion. For instance, subtle somatic blockade may be missed during diagnostic sympathetic block if application of stimuli is more vigorous after the block than during baseline examination.

Many measures have been used to judge the efficacy of sympathetic blockade, although none has become an accepted standard. Horner syndrome documents only blockade of sympathetic fibers to the head. Skin resistance response (sympathogalvanic response) (130,131) and pulse amplitude changes (132,133) are difficult to quantify. Microneurography (131) is invasive and requires elaborate equipment and expertise, as does laser skin blood flow measurement (134). Sweat testing (135) is cumbersome, time-consuming, and not well accepted by patients, and therefore not widely used. Most common is the measurement of skin temperature by thermography or contact thermometry. A temperature increase of $1.0°C$ to $3.0°C$ is typically used (136–138) as a threshold for confirming the onset of sympathetic blockade, but the method is ineffective if skin is warm at the outset of a block. Although local anesthetic blockade of sympathetic activity to the extremities produces vasodilatation, vasoconstriction follows segmental block of sympathetic fibers to the trunk (37), possibly by blockade of sympathetic vasodilator fibers (139). Skin temperature in pathologic conditions is controlled by a balance between sympathetic vasoconstriction and vasodilatation from release of vasoactive peptides from C nociceptors during antidromic activity (140). Temperature change in the field of a blocked peripheral nerve will depend on the relative contribution of these opposing systems.

Pain caused by the procedure may result in a confused diagnosis, because relief following the injection may be due to the termination of the iatrogenic pain and not of the preexisting pain for which the block was done. Also, intense pain from the procedure may diminish the perceived severity of the original pain (noxious counterirritation) (141), creating the illusion that neural blockade effects relieved the pain. For these reasons, the diagnostic blocks should be performed using measures to limit discomfort. Judicious use of local anesthetics in the superficial tissues, small needles, and careful needle guidance limit the pain of the procedure.

SPECIFIC PROCEDURES

In the format adopted below, commonly used diagnostic blocks will be considered individually, first with regard to the rationale behind the procedure, including indications for the block. The discussion of technique that follows also considers methods for monitoring response to the block and for identifying possible complications. (The techniques of blocks discussed more completely elsewhere in this book are covered briefly.) Limitations are reviewed, focusing on sources of error in interpreting results from the injections. If studies of the diagnostic utility of the procedure are available, these are reviewed with emphasis on documentation of success and measures of the diagnostic value. Finally, an evaluation of the utility of the block is offered.

Clinical studies of the blocks vary in quality. Important considerations include entrance criteria (type of patients or normal subjects studied), study size, and the use of controls. The prevalence of placebo responses in pain patients greatly weakens the relevance of studies in which no controls or blinding was used. Where possible, neural blockade tests are evaluated numerically, using standard definitions (see the table immediately following) (142). The importance of the false-positive rate (how often patients without a condition will nonetheless have a positive test) and false-negative rate (how often a patient with

disease will have a negative test for it) is evident, because the rates vary inversely with specificity and sensitivity respectively. (Sensitivity = 1− false negative rate; specificity = 1− false positive rate.) For many painful conditions, however, a credible standard to document the disease for comparison with test results is unavailable, such as when sympathetic involvement is suspected or with cervicogenic headache. At worst, the block under scrutiny may be the defining gold standard. For these blocks, numerical values for diagnostic efficacy are elusive. In many studies, ethical reasons limit operative confirmation of disease to only those patients with positive results from the diagnostic block. The false-negative rate is therefore unknown, and the false-positive rate, which requires knowledge of true disease incidence in the entire group, also cannot be calculated. From these studies, only the positive predictive value (frequency of confirming disease in those with a positive test) can be derived.

	Disease Present	Disease Absent
Test Positive	a	c
Test Negative	b	d
Sensitivity (true positive rate)		a/(a + b)
False-positive Rate		c/(c + d)
Specificity (true negative rate)		d/(c + d)
False-negative Rate		b/(a + b)
Positive Predictive Value		a/(a + c)
Negative Predictive Value		d/(b + d)

The proper interpretation of a positive test must take into consideration the prevalence of the condition. For example, a test with 95% sensitivity will have a positive result in 5% of healthy subjects. If the condition being sought is rare (if, for instance, it occurs in only 2% of the test group), false-positive responses will outnumber true positive tests, and the majority of positive results will occur in subjects who actually are healthy. This issue is especially relevant to the study of painful conditions by diagnostic blocks, since the incidence of most of these maladies is low or unknown.

TISSUE INFILTRATION

Rationale

If nociceptive impulses are thought to arise from a particular site (for example, from a scar, painful structure in a specific muscle, inflamed joint, bursa, or tendon sheath), then the injection of local anesthetic into that site should be of help in establishing the diagnosis. Failure to relieve tenderness by infiltration of superficial tissues, like skin or muscle, focuses attention on a deeper site (bone, joint, nerve root). Painful scars generally are thought to be caused by the development of small neuromas. Although some scars are diffusely tender, most scar pain is associated with very localized areas of tenderness. Some patients who experience relief from local anesthetic will have lasting relief if depot steroids are injected subsequently. When inflammatory processes are the cause of the pain, local anesthetic infiltration may be of prognostic benefit in predicting the response to subsequent steroid injections.

Technique

A skin wheal followed by injection of a small amount of saline in the vicinity of the planned procedure may indicate whether analgesia obtained from local anesthetic injection is due to placebo response. A small amount of local anesthetic is then injected into the affected muscle, joint, tendon sheath, scar, bursa, or like site. It is helpful to determine whether needle placement and local anesthetic injection (as well as the placebo injection) reproduce the clinical pain, and whether local anesthetic injection relieves the pain at rest as well as the pain produced by maneuvers that usually aggravate the pain.

Local infiltration techniques are relatively benign in terms of potential for adverse effects. Infection is always a potential problem in immunocompromised patients, and bleeding may be troublesome if coagulation function is impaired. Extensive infiltration of painful muscles conceivably could result in local anesthetic toxicity or muscle damage (143). In general, the occurrence of complications relates to proximity of the injection to other structures. Injection of the rhomboids or trapezius muscles could cause pneumothorax. Infiltration of muscles or scars near the neuraxis may allow spread of drug epidurally or intrathecally. Infiltration of occipital scars overlying bony cranial defects, following posterior fossa surgery, could mean that drug might be injected into the intracranial CSF, or even into the brain itself. Careful monitoring of blood pressure should be carried out when neuraxial or intracranial injections are possible.

TRIGGER-POINT INJECTION

Rationale

Myofascial pain syndrome is characterized by pain arising from affected muscles, pain associated with movement of those muscles, and reproduction of pain with palpation of well localized "trigger points" in the affected muscle (144). By definition, stimulation or palpation of trigger points causes referred pain, perceived some distance from the site of palpation. Usually, the involved muscle is felt as a tight palpable band. Myofascial syndrome often is found in association with other painful disorders, such as facet arthropathy or radiculopathy, and it is often helpful to determine whether a patient's pain is predominantly myofascial, because appropriate treatment may be very different if such is the case. Other means of documenting myofascial pain, such as electromyelography (EMG), have not proved reliable (145,146), although elevated endplate noise recorded during EMG has recently been proposed as a marker of myofascial trigger points (147). Muscle tenderness also is seen in fibromyalgia, which differs from myofascial pain syndrome in that tender points in the muscle are much more diffuse and numerous, and usually symmetrical, and palpation generally produces local, but not referred pain (148). Trigger-point injections, particularly if repeated several times, may have therapeutic benefit for myofascial pain syndrome but not for fibromyalgia (149).

Technique

The area of maximum tenderness is identified within the affected muscle. It may be helpful to immobilize the muscle between the thumb and forefinger. After antiseptic preparation of the skin, a small-gauge needle is introduced into the trigger point. Often a brief twitch of the affected muscle is noted. The patient should be questioned about the location and intensity of the pain evoked by needle placement. Exacerbation of the pain and the presence of referred pain at this time helps

confirm the diagnosis of myofascial pain syndrome. Following the injection of several milliliters of local anesthetic, the degree of pain relief and the presence or absence of tenderness is reassessed. Pressure algometry may be used to determine the degree of tenderness before and after injection.

A variety of local anesthetics have been used for trigger-point injection. From a diagnostic point of view, there is little reason to choose one over another. Ropivacaine may produce less pain when injected (150). Some clinicians choose to avoid bupivacaine, because accidental blockade of nearby neural structures results in prolonged effects, toxic local anesthetic reactions are potentially more serious, and bupivacaine produces more muscle degeneration than do other anesthetics (151). Ironically, the predictable and selective destruction of mature myocytes by local anesthetic infiltration (143) might be the therapeutic mechanism of long-term response to trigger-point injection, because it encourages the growth of a new generation of myocytes, in which case bupivacaine is a suitable agent. Reproduction of pain during injection and relief of pain after injection suggest that myofascial pain is at least partially responsible for the patient's pain.

The small volume of anesthetic used in trigger-point injection makes this a safe procedure. However, toxicity may result if multiple blocks are performed or if even a small dose reaches the subarachnoid space (152).

Clinical Studies

No studies conclusively demonstrate that trigger-point injection can distinguish myofascial pain from other etiologies, since there is no independent gold standard for identifying myofascial pain other than clinical features. However, utility of this procedure has been shown in studies in which the contribution of myofascial pain is suggested through injection. For instance, pain may be relieved by trigger-point injection in a subset of patients with postthoracotomy pain syndrome (153) or pain following radical neck surgery (154). Myofascial pain presenting as toothache has similarly been identified (155).

Limitations

Pain relief after trigger-point injection does not guarantee that myofascial pain is the principle cause of pain. Placebo effect and systemic uptake of local anesthetic, particularly after multiple injections, may be the cause of the improvement, as may be spread to adjacent nerves. For instance, injection of the piriformis muscle is likely to have some effect on the sciatic nerve, which either penetrates or passes in contact with the muscle. Some doubt about the specificity of the technique is raised by reports showing comparable efficacy from less specific techniques, such as dry needling of trigger points (156) (see also Chapter 34) and jet injection of local anesthetic into the skin overlying trigger points (157).

Evaluation

Reproduction of pain during injection followed by relief of pain is helpful in confirming the tissue site (scar, muscle, etc.) as the focus of nociceptive activity, if the duration of relief is at least as long as the expected duration of local anesthetic. Controlled studies have not confirmed this belief.

SOMATIC NERVE BLOCK

Rationale

A common reason to perform diagnostic peripheral nerve blocks is to determine the likelihood of success after surgical decompression or neurolysis of a peripheral nerve. Diagnostic blocks may be performed before a planned peripheral nerve section, neurolytic block, or cryoanalgesia lesion. Entrapment neuropathies include digital nerve entrapment (Morton neuroma), carpal tunnel entrapment of the median nerve, and tarsal tunnel entrapment of the tibial nerve. Posttraumatic neuropathy of the ilioinguinal and iliohypogastric nerves can occur following herniorrhaphy.

Technique

Techniques for specific peripheral nerve blocks are covered in Chapters 13, 14, and 16 to 19. When performing diagnostic blocks, it is important to use small volumes of anesthetic solution, to document that appropriate sensory blockade is achieved, and to ensure that the block is limited to the intended nerve distribution. In assessing relief of pain, one should determine the duration of the pain relief and the duration of sensory block. If pain returns long before the return of sensory function, the analgesia may be a placebo response. Use of bupivacaine for peripheral diagnostic blocks may be preferable to the use of shorter-acting agents, because it provides a long interval during which placebo responses may subside and a prolonged period for patients to experience the effect of the block. In general, diagnostic blocks are performed with relatively small volumes of local anesthetic (usually 2–3 mL for small nerves, 5 mL for medium-sized nerves, e.g., median nerve at the wrist, and 10 mL for large nerves), and the risk of toxic reactions is small. Intercostal blocks done near the spinal column may be associated with spread of drug to the subarachnoid space, if the needle is placed within the perineurium.

Limitations

It must be kept in mind that relief of pain following blockade of the appropriate nerve does not necessarily confirm the diagnosis of neuropathy at that site. There may be a nociceptive source of pain within the distribution of the blocked nerve, or there may be a neuropathic source of pain proximal to the site of block (e.g., radiculopathy or plexopathy) that may be relieved by the procedure (11–13).

For multiple reasons cited earlier in this chapter, pain relief from local anesthetic block often fails to predict relief of pain from a neuroablative procedure; the local anesthetic block produces profound relief, but the neuroablative procedure fails to provide long-term relief (158).

Study

The diagnostic utility of injection of lidocaine and steroid has been examined in patients suspected to have carpal tunnel syndrome (159). The test identified most patients with the disease demonstrated subsequently at surgery (sensitivity 85%), but it indicated lack of carpal tunnel syndrome in only 38% of those surgically negative (specificity).

Evaluation

Relief of pain from a peripheral nerve block, plus diminished sensation in the distribution of the blocked nerve provides additional, although not conclusive, evidence that the nerve is either the source of neuropathic pain or conveys afferent fibers from a source of nociception. Relief following peripheral block may predict response to neural decompression but has little prognostic value in predicting response to neuroablation, which is often ineffective.

VISCERAL NEURAL BLOCKADE

Rationale

It is often helpful to distinguish whether thoracic, abdominal, or pelvic pain is due to pathology of visceral elements or somatic (body wall) structures. If it can be established that pain is visceral in origin, treatment may be directed toward exploration of abdominal or pelvic organs or toward denervation of visceral structures, if untreatable malignancy is the source of the pain.

In addition to chest pain from pulmonary or cardiac sources, several common painful somatic conditions, such as costal chondritis, myofascial syndrome, and intercostal neuralgia, can cause chest pain. These conditions can be relieved either by intercostal blocks or local infiltration. Sensory innervation to much of the heart can be interrupted by left stellate ganglion block. Information about the origin of a given chest pain may be obtained by comparison of placebo injection, left stellate block, and the appropriate somatic block.

Sensory innervation of the upper abdominal viscera can be interrupted by blocking the celiac plexus or the splanchnic nerves proximal to the site where they join the celiac plexus. Such blocks are useful when it is unclear whether abdominal pain is of visceral origin, such as that which occurs with pancreatitis, distension of the hepatic capsule, or cholecystitis, or of somatic origin, as in the case of entrapment of an intercostal nerve or pain of muscular origin. In such cases, it is helpful to compare the response of celiac or splanchnic block to that of intercostal block or local infiltration of the abdominal wall to that of placebo injection.

It is worthwhile to perform a prognostic celiac or splanchnic block prior to neurolysis for the treatment of pancreatic cancer, since celiac plexus blocks may be relatively ineffective when local tumor spread and resultant inflammation are extensive. In such situations, splanchnic block may still be effective. If tumor spread is extensive enough to involve retroperitoneal somatic structures, both celiac and splanchnic block may be ineffective. This should be tested by the use of local anesthetic blocks. Long-term epidural analgesia may be a preferable technique when cancer is widespread.

Blockade of the afferent innervation of the pelvic viscera can be accomplished by the technique of superior hypogastric plexus block. This technique has been used mainly to predict the response to neurolytic blockade of the superior hypogastric plexus, a technique that has been developed in lieu of surgical presacral neurectomy for treatment of pain due to pelvic cancer (see Chapter 45).

PART IV: PAIN MANAGEMENT

Technique

All patients should have an IV line placed prior to celiac and splanchnic blocks, and possibly before hypogastric plexus block. Patients with a history of congestive failure, or with suspected hypovolemia, may benefit from placement of a central venous line. Frequent monitoring of blood pressure is essential, and continuous verbal contact is helpful to detect signs of local anesthetic toxicity.

Celiac and Splanchnic Blocks

Technique for celiac and splanchnic blocks are described in Chapter 45. Local anesthetic doses of 20 to 30 mL have been advocated for diagnostic celiac blocks (160), although some authors use a total dose of 50 mL (161). A total of 20 mL (10 mL on each side) is adequate for a diagnostic splanchnic block (161). The use of 0.25% bupivacaine or ropivacaine is reasonable in this situation, as this provides fairly prolonged analgesia, allowing the patient to experience the effect on pain of physical activity or eating. Long-acting agents also provide a period of block that is likely to outlast the duration of a placebo response. For example, if pain recurs within 1 hour of the block, it is likely to be a placebo reaction or an effect of absorbed local anesthetics, as opposed to a physiologic response to the block and subsequent recovery from the block.

Diagnostic celiac and splanchnic blocks should be performed using either biplane fluoroscopy or computed tomography (CT) scan. Since subsequent treatment is to be determined by response to the block, and there is no sure way to document its success, it is important to ensure that the anesthetic is placed correctly. The use of small quantities of radiographic dye prior to the anesthetic injection further ensures correct needle placement.

Some clinicians advocate using prognostic blocks at least 24 hours before performance of a neurolytic celiac or splanchnic block, arguing that this gives one time to assess thoroughly the analgesic effects and potential side effects, especially hypotension. Others suggest that if the prognostic local anesthetic block is effective, the neurolytic agent should be injected through the same needles, after a short assessment period to evaluate pain relief, vital signs, and possible presence of somatic block. The rationale for doing the neurolysis immediately is that the local anesthetic injection at that exact site has been shown to provide pain relief and is devoid of somatic blocking effects. In addition, when alcohol is chosen as the neurolytic agent, prior local anesthetic injection will markedly reduce the pain associated with the injection of neurolytic agent.

When the prognostic block is done immediately before neurolysis, a higher concentration of neurolytic agent may be needed. For example, if 30 mL of local anesthetic is injected initially, one may choose to use absolute alcohol rather than 50% alcohol as the neurolytic agent. It may be unwise to choose phenol as the neurolytic agent when such a technique is used because the use of large amounts of local anesthetic plus phenol may produce systemic toxic reactions (seizures).

Serious complications are unusual following local anesthetic celiac or splanchnic blocks. Hypotension, particularly orthostatic hypotension, is fairly common, so that IV fluid loading should be carried out prior to the block, and an attendant should be present if the patient attempts to stand or walk before the block wears off. Toxic reactions to local anesthetic are possible, given the large volumes of local anesthetics used and the proximity of major vessels. Substantial bleeding can occur in patients with coagulopathies. Spread of drug to adjacent nerve roots is possible, particularly with splanchnic blocks. Pneumothorax can occur with either celiac or splanchnic blocks.

Hypogastric Plexus Block

Needles are placed bilaterally at the anterolateral surfaces of the S1 segment of the sacrum (162). As with celiac plexus and splanchnic block, biplane fluoroscopy or CT scan are essential for documentation of proper needle placement. Radiographic dye injection allows documentation of proper spread of the drug. Relatively small volumes, about 6 to 8 mL on each side, are required (see Chapter 45).

Hypotension does not appear to be a common problem. Few complications have been reported. Potential problems include intravascular injection or bleeding following puncture of the iliac vessels, ureteral damage, or somatic nerve (especially L5 nerve root) damage.

Limitations

Given the relatively large volumes of anesthetic often used for these blocks, consideration of systemic local anesthetic effects and possible spread to somatic nerves must be included during interpretation of the response.

Evaluation

Despite the lack of studies documenting prognostic benefits of visceral blocks, it would seem prudent not to pursue neuroablative techniques in the absence of relief from local anesthetics. Information obtained from diagnostic visceral blocks may be helpful in confirming clinical impressions.

SACROILIAC INJECTION

Rationale

It is probable that the sacroiliac joint (SIJ) can be the source of acute or chronic pain, as the joint is well innervated (163). Typically, patients with SIJ pathology demonstrate tenderness over the sacrum just medial to the posterior superior iliac spines. Computed tomography scans of the joint may show erosions, narrowing of the cartilaginous portion of the joint, and bony sclerosis of the adjacent ilium. However, the normal anatomy of the joint shows asymmetry of cartilage thickness (thinner on the iliac side), and cartilage-covered irregularities in the bony surfaces, which interlock with reciprocal depressions on the opposite surface, enhancing joint stability (164). Such changes are more prominent in men, and with age there is a predictable thickening of the capsule, roughening of the cartilage, and growth of marginal osteophytes (165). For these reasons, it is often difficult to identify pathologic changes in SIJs and the extent of the sacroiliac contribution to back pain.

Stimulation by injection of radiographic contrast into the joint, in subjects without complaints of back pain, produces pain in the immediate area, often also in the surrounding gluteal area, and occasionally into the posterior thigh and knee (166).

Diagnostic criteria are uncertain for determining a sacroiliac origin of low back pain. The Gaeslen maneuver, Patrick test, Yeoman test, side-lying iliac compression, or compression of the apex of the sacrum, with the patient prone on a firm surface, may reproduce the pain but the specificity of these tests has been questioned. Other physical examination maneuvers frequently indicate disease in asymptomatic individuals (167) and correlate poorly with diagnoses reached by other means (168). Laslett and co-workers (169) did find some correlation between provocative tests and response to local anesthetic injection into the joint. They found that all patients who had relief from injections demonstrated pain with at least one provocative test. There was 94% sensitivity and 74% specificity when three or more of six provocative tests were positive. Berthelot and colleagues (170) reported discordance between elicitation of pain during contrast injection into the joint and pain relief following injection of local anesthetic. They reported identical response to two consecutive local anesthetic injections in only 60% of patients. They also indicated that injectate spreads outside the joint in the majority of cases and can contact adjacent neural structures.

An alternate source of pain and tenderness in the sacroiliac region is myofascial syndrome involving the sacrospinalis muscle. It is therefore useful to infiltrate the muscle with local anesthetic before SIJ injection. Lack of relief from that procedure rules out placebo response or myofascial pain. It is thought by some clinicians that local anesthetic injections of the joint may have some value in predicting response to intra-articular steroid injections.

Technique

The method for performing sacroiliac injection is more fully discussed in Chapter 44. It is important to recognize that the common method, using palpable landmarks to guide the needle (171), cannot assure passage of the needle tip into the joint space, and anatomic considerations make this unlikely because of the great inter-individual variability in size and contour of SIJs (165) and the inaccessibility of the joint line. Under fluoroscopic or CT control, the inferior extent of the joint can be identified, where the space may be entered more easily, and, thus, success confirmed (166,172). For diagnostic purposes, the patient should be questioned as to whether presence of the needle or injection of the anesthetic reproduces the pain.

Limitations

Without imaging, there is no means to confirm accurate delivery of local anesthetic. When imaging is used to document the intra-articular spread of injectate, intra-articular placement is found to be reliable (166). It is not clear whether intra-articular spread is needed to achieve efficacy. Pain relief after injection actually may be related to infiltration of the sacroiliac ligament or sacrospinalis muscle with anesthetic, and thus gives the incorrect impression that the joint is the pain source. Anesthetic actually injected into the joint may exit the capsule anteriorly and spread along the lumbosacral plexus (173), conceivably relieving pain from sources other than the joint. The character and distribution of pain evoked by needle contact or contrast injection is of uncertain value because exact reproduction of the pain is not significantly more frequent in patients who obtain relief following anesthetic injection compared with those with a negative response to anesthetic (173).

Clinical Studies

A prospective study of radiographically controlled injections (173) indicated that 30% of patients with chronic low back pain below L5 were relieved by local anesthetic sacroiliac injection, most of whom exhibited a tear in the joint capsule. Most subjects with tears, however, did not get relief from block. Groin pain was a distinguishing complaint of subjects who obtained relief from joint injection. Radiation of pain below the knee was as common in patients relieved by sacroiliac injection, as it was in those with no response. Chou and co-workers (174) evaluated the response of intra-articular steroid injections in patients who met stringent criteria, including response to local anesthetic injections, for establishing the SIJ as the source of pain. Eighty-one of 194 patients with sacral pain and more than three positive provocative tests experienced pain relief following fluoroscopically guided, contrast-enhanced SIJ injections. Fifty-four of those patients (67%) achieved at least 80% pain relief after a series of one to four steroid injections. No controlled evaluations of the technique have been published, and no data are available to indicate the sensitivity or specificity of sacroiliac injection as a means of diagnosing the joint as a source of pain.

Evaluation

Analgesia after sacroiliac injection with local anesthetic may be helpful in differentiating sacroiliac arthropathy from facet disease, myofascial pain, or disc disease, although this is unproven.

The majority of patients who experience relief from local anesthetic injection obtain prolonged relief from corticosteroid injections (174). For patients who experience substantial relief from local anesthetic injection of the SIJ, but minimal benefit from corticosteroid injections, radiofrequency denervation of the SIJ may be a reasonable therapeutic option. One-third of patients who obtained pain relief from local anesthetic injection of the joint experienced at least 50% relief for at least 6 months following conventional unipolar radiofrequency denervation procedures (175). With the introduction of bipolar radiofrequency technology, denervation of the nerve supply to the SI joint may be more effective. Multiple lesions up to 6 mm long can be made along the medial aspect of the joint or at the site of the lateral branches of the dorsal primary rami as they exit from the sacral foramina (176) (see Chapter 44).

FACET INJECTION

Rationale

The zygapophyseal (facet) joints are paired diarthrodial articulations between the posterior elements of adjacent vertebrae. The joint surfaces are midway between the axial and coronal plane in the cervical region and are more vertically inclined at the thoracic levels because the inferior articular processes overlap the superior articular processes like shingles on a roof. Lumbar facet joints are complex and formed into a posteriorly concave surface, the posterior portion of the joint almost parallel to the sagittal plane and the anterior portion in a coronal plane (Fig. 38-9). These arrangements determine the relative motions of sections of the vertebral column. The lumbar articulations prevent rotation but allow flexion. Rotation is maximal in the thoracic column, and the cervical vertebrae permit both

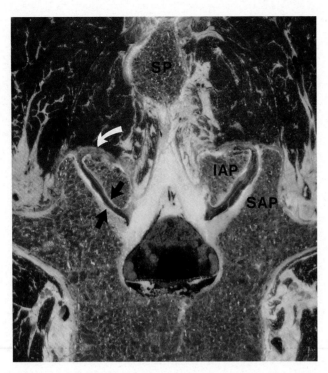

FIGURE 38-9. Unstained axial cryomicrotome section through the third lumbar vertebral body, showing facet joints (*straight arrows*). The medial joint capsule is reinforced by the yellow ligamentum flavum, whereas the posterolateral extent of the joint ends in a redundant pocket (*curved arrows*). Cartilage loss is evident. *IAP*, inferior articular process; *SP*, spinous process; *SAP*, superior articular process.

rotation and extensive movement in the sagittal plane. Rudimentary fibroadipose menisci and synovial folds cushion the superior and inferior poles of the lumbar zygapophyseal joints (177), but with age these typically disappear and the cartilage thins on the joint surfaces (178).

The median branch of the dorsal primary ramus of the spinal nerve supplies the facet joint as well as the supraspinous and intraspinous ligaments. Of these, only the facet joint consistently is found to be well innervated by nociceptive fibers, penetrating the capsule and extending into the synovial folds (179,180). Each facet joint receives branches from the spinal nerve exiting the vertebral canal through the adjacent intervertebral foramen and the nerve, one segment above (181,182). Injection of hypertonic saline into or around the lumbar facet joint capsule produces pain in the back, buttocks, and proximal thigh (125,126). Physiologic recordings in laboratory animals have documented mechanoreceptive sensory fields in facet joints (183,184). Distension of normal cervical facet joint capsules produces unilateral pain ranging from occipital and upper neck from atlanto-occipital, atlanto-axial, and C2–C3 joints, to scapular pain from joint C6–C7 (185,186). Immunohistochemical evidence of substance P in facet capsule neurons (187) also supports the concept of the facet joints as a source of nociception. Rotation and extension between two adjacent vertebrae increases facet stress, as does loss of disc height (188), all of which may be stimuli for facet pain. Facet menisci are innervated by small myelinated nerves (189), in which substance P is present (190) but rare (191). An entrapment syndrome involving the facet menisci has been proposed (177), but no clear evidence implicates this in the production of back pain.

Radicular pain is distinctive (distal radiation and burning, electrical quality), is associated with clear signs of nerve deficit or irritation, correlates fairly well with anatomic defects found on imaging, and usually can be confirmed by electrodiagnostic (EMG, nerve-conduction) studies. In contrast, nonradicular back and neck pain is more ambiguous and almost always poses a diagnostic dilemma. In addition to the facet joints, other structures in the vertebral column also are richly innervated, such as the posterior and anterior longitudinal ligaments, anular ligament of the intervertebral disc, anterior dura mater, and the costovertebral joints (119,120,192–196). Stimulation of these other vertebral elements by injection or during surgery in awake patients with local anesthesia evokes pain in the back, hip, and buttock, indistinguishable from pain produced by facet irritation (194,197–203). Clinical features that suggest a facet joint origin include pain into the proximal but not distal ipsilateral limb, localized paraspinal tenderness, and reproduction of pain with extension and rotation (204). Pain can occur in the absence of changes on plane radiographs of the vertebral column. Computed tomographic imaging is more sensitive, but degenerative facet arthritis is seen in 10.4% of asymptomatic patients (205). Although the value of bone scan is unproven, a positive finding may support the diagnosis of facet arthropathy and may direct attention to a particular joint. Because there is no specific pathognomonic finding or test, the clinical criteria for making the diagnosis of facet pain remain undefined. Therefore, diagnostic injections often are performed to help indicate the contribution of the facet.

Technique

Local anesthetic can be injected either into the joint space or around the nerves innervating the joint. These procedures are described in Chapter 44. For reliable diagnosis, certainty of successful injection requires fluoroscopic imaging at least. With advanced disease and joint changes, CT imaging may be helpful for injection into the joint space (206). When intra-articular injection is used for diagnostic purposes, the patient should be asked to compare the distribution of pain created by needle contact with the joint to his usual pain. No physiologic means exist to test the adequacy of intra-articular anesthesia. When blockade of the posterior primary ramus is performed, two injections are needed to anesthetize a joint because each facet receives terminal fibers from two posterior rami (e.g., the L4–L5 facet is innervated at its upper pole by branches from L3 and at its lower pole by branches from L4). At lumbar levels, there is no cutaneous innervation by these branches, so adequacy of the block cannot be confirmed by superficial examination. Although the medial branches of the third, fourth, and often fifth cervical posterior branches have cutaneous ramifications, they are small areas near the midline and have not been shown to provide accurate evidence of proximal neural blockade. Provocative stimuli of the joint, such as mechanical or chemical irritation, could be performed after the block to check adequacy of denervation, but this has not been investigated. After injection into the joint space or interruption of the sensory nerves to the joint, the patient's pain can be attributed to the facet if pain relief is noted in response to local anesthetic injection, with attention focused on those maneuvers that provoked the pain prior to injection, and if a sensory examination shows no evidence of segmental spinal nerve block.

Limitations

The use of facet or medial branch injections for diagnosis rests upon the assumption that facets are a source of pain. This premise is accepted by most authorities, although the frequency of this as the primary element producing a patient's pain is debated. Disc degeneration is present in all cases of lumbar facet disease evident by CT or magnetic resonance (MR) imaging (207). Disc disease identified by discography was present in 64% of patients with a positive cervical medial branch test for facet joint disease (208). Pathologic changes in facets are a common cause of injury to nerve roots (209), and may irritate afferents on the posterolateral aspect of the disc. These other disease processes could, therefore, be the cause of pain in patients with incidental abnormalities of the facet, or at least could contribute to a condition more complex than a facet origin of pain. Since no histopathologic or imaging standard exists (210), the frequency of pain from the facet per se has been estimated only by relief in response to injections. As is discussed next, this inevitably involves circular logic, but gives a positive indication of cervical facet etiology in unselected patients with posttraumatic neck pain of about 70% (range 63%–100%) (61,208,211–215). In subjects clinically suspected of having lumbar facet pain, confirmation by relief after injection ranges from 16% to 94% (126,204,206,216–221). In a noncontrolled and nonblinded study of patients with chronic low back pain without radiculopathy, 25% of those assigned to receive median branch nerve blockade of a randomly chosen joint had immediate relief, and 38% had relief after injection into the suspected joint (222). These comparable rates are similar to the frequency of placebo response. Total absence of pain after injection of local anesthetic into the lumbar facets is much less common, occurring in only about 7% of back pain patients (216,223). It is reasonable to conclude that in many study groups the facets are an origin of at least part of the patients' pain, but rarely are the unique or major source.

Mechanical irritation of the joint capsule during facet injection may produce discomfort resembling the patient's typical pain. Since cervical (185,224) and lumbar (125,126,224,225) facet stimulation produces broadly overlapping areas of pain distribution, even into the distal extremity (see Chapter 44, Fig. 44-1), this is not a strong indicator of pain origin. Patients whose usual pain is provoked by facet stimulation do not necessarily obtain pain relief by local anesthetic injection in the facet joint (219,226), and a poor correlation exists between pain provocation and relief from local anesthetic injection (227). In one study (220), 31% of patients with a positive response to pain provocation failed to have relief after anesthetic injection into that lumbar facet, and 40% who had relief from injection had not had typical pain during needle stimulation or distension of the facet capsule with contrast.

The specificity of facet denervation depends upon limiting anesthetic spread to the joint or nerves to the joint. Detailed sensory neural testing after these blocks has not been reported. The facet joints are not capacious. Rupture during intra-articular injection has been identified after injection of more than 1 mL into cervical facets (228) and after most lumbar injections (218,229), and has been demonstrated in cadaver facet injections (220). Extravasation from the joint to surrounding tissues or epidural space may uncover a preexisting defect in the capsule. Since this spills local anesthetic into neighboring tissues, pain relieved by facet injection could in fact originate in other structures, such as muscle, periosteum, and ligaments. Passage of anesthetic into the epidural space or intervertebral foramen, which occurs routinely with capsule rupture (see Chapter 44) (218,229), could interrupt nociception from sensitive structures in the vertebral canal, such as anterior dura and posterior longitudinal ligament, or from any distal site through effects on afferent fibers in the spinal roots. Of patients with clinical indications of having lumbar facet

pain, 18% are found to have spondylolysis (230), a defect in the vertebral arch due to chronic stress. With this condition, intra-articular facet injection is followed consistently by spread of solution into the epidural space and to adjacent and contralateral facets, and even laterally along a spinal nerve (230–232), thus limiting the specificity of the test. Injection into the subarachnoid space has been reported (233).

Blockade of medial branches not only denervates the joints they supply, but also muscles, ligaments, and periosteum. Sources of pain in these alternative sites will be relieved by medial branch block. Fluid distribution during cervical medial branch block is variable, with the area of consistent coverage being a small subset of the area into which spread may be observed. Injectate, however, does not travel to anterior primary rami or to medial branches of adjacent posterior rami (212). Since each medial branch supplies parts of two facets, complete denervation of one facet requires partial blockade of the one above and below. Therefore, relief from the blocks cannot distinguish between pain originating at any of the three. Since medial branch blockade more accurately simulates the effect of radiofrequency denervation than does intra-articular injection, it is the appropriate diagnostic test before that procedure.

The reproducibility of the test is uncertain. In one study, facet injections in 176 low back pain patients produced relief in 83 (47%), but a repeat injection was positive in only 26 of those 83 (31%) (234). This indicates either a strong placebo component or subtle technical difficulties that cannot be controlled. (The authors of this study claim that the second injection determines which of the responders to the initial injections were true positives, and not placebo responders. This logic dismisses the explanation that the two time-positive responders were also placebo responders each time.) Even when relief is found during repeated diagnostic injections, no feature of the patients' histories or physical examinations correlates with a positive diagnosis by this more demanding criterion (235), drawing the relevance of blocks into uncertainty.

Studies

Validation of the use of intra-articular and medial branch injections to document facet pain requires demonstration that (a) the injections as described are effective in denervating the joint and (b) such denervation can be used to distinguish between various sources of back pain. No means has been described to test the adequacy of facet denervation, so success rates have not been determined. Relief of pain in patients with presumed facet arthropathy is not a suitable test of physiologic blockade success. Since the diagnosis of a painful facet relies upon injections for confirmation, evidence for either is circular. No block can be assumed to be effective every time, so inability to confirm directly that the block is successful and that the joint is denervated weakens the diagnostic utility of facet and medial branch nerve injections. That is, even though the pain has changed after the injection, to attribute this change securely to the block requires independent evidence to confirm that the block actually happened. Inability to enter the joint during attempted intra-articular injection has been reported in 16% to 38% of lumbar injections (216,236) and 44% of cervical facet injections (215). To a degree, cervical medial branch block has been validated by comparison to intra-articular injection. All of seven patients who were relieved by blockade of the branches innervating a joint had relief after intra-articular injection of that joint on a different occasion, although up to 2 mL of local anesthetic was injected into the joint (213).

Since no standard to confirm facet pain is available for correlation with block findings, the ability of facet blocks to aid in valid diagnosis of the source of back pain has not been established. However, the clinical utility of facet blocks is drawn into question by several findings. In general, a facet etiology is identified infrequently when small intra-articular injectate volumes are used (43,220). This means that either larger volumes (>1.5 mL) are necessary for adequate intra-articular block, or that large-volume injections block pain from sources other than the facet. The only studies done with controls are not optimistic. In one, local anesthetic resulted in relief in 54% of patients with back pain, but 43% of these responders also were relieved by injection of a randomly chosen uninvolved facet joint (219). A controlled trial that examined improvement 1 hour after injection found no difference in groups that had had local anesthetic injected into the joints or outside the joints, or normal saline injected into the joints (237). In a study comparing duration of analgesia following cervical medial branch blocks on two different occasions in order to determine a false-positive rate, 27% either had a duration of analgesia longer for lidocaine than for bupivacaine, or no analgesia at all on the second injection (238). The only study that was controlled and blinded showed no difference in pain relief between intra-articular lidocaine or saline injection (223).

Few data are available on the ability of facet blocks to predict the response to more definitive therapy. Radiofrequency facet denervation failed to benefit 36% of patients who had excellent relief from intra-articular injection (224). In another report (239), the positive predictive value of relief after local anesthetic block of the lumbar medial branch of the posterior primary ramus was 0.45 in anticipating success from radiofrequency denervation (45% of block successes also were radiofrequency successes). Specificity and sensitivity could not be determined because radiofrequency surgery was not performed if blocks provided less than moderate relief. A review of the available literature has not determined what diagnostic block technique is the best predictor of success following medial branch radiofrequency ablation. Several techniques have been advocated, including response to intra-articular local anesthetic, response to a single local anesthetic medial branch block, and comparison of duration of response to lidocaine versus bupivacaine blocks of the medial branches. Because of differences in ablation techniques, outcome measures, and follow-up durations, it is difficult to compare the predictive value of the various diagnostic block techniques (240).

Relief after facet injection has been examined as a prognostic indicator for response to posterolateral lumbosacral fusions (241), but block results did not predict surgical outcome.

Therapeutic responses have been reported following intra-articular zygapophysial joint injection, especially if steroid is included. Steroid injected into the lumbar facet joints results in significant relief, outlasting the local anesthetic in between 30% and 54% of groups of selected patients with back pain (204,206,216,218,236,237,242). Response rates are lower for patients with previous lumbar spine surgery (224) and, after extra-articular injection, are less likely to be therapeutic (236). It is not encouraging to note that the pain returns by 6 months in many of the steroid responders (218) and, in one report, the results for steroid were no different from those for saline injection (237). Beneficial effects of cervical facet injection with steroid have been reported in 91% of patients, but recurrence occurred in half (215). Another study found no benefit from cervical facet steroid injection, even though the same patients had experienced complete relief from local anesthetic (214). A blinded trial of facet steroid injection found that saline in-

jected into lumbar joints produced only slightly less improvement than steroid, and that the completeness of response to local anesthetic did not predict the degree of steroid effect (216). Steroid injection probably is appropriate during a diagnostic injection study, since the additional risk of injecting the steroid after the needle is already in place is minor. However, the efficacy of intra-articular steroid in the facet joint has not been proven. A recent study, however, indicated that positive findings on single photon emission computed tomography (SPECT) identify a population of back pain patients more likely to benefit from injections specifically targeted by this scan (243).

Evaluation

Injections intended to block afferents from facet joints have been found useful by a number of authors. However, the literature on the topic is from relatively few advocates, sometimes with repeated presentation of data (61,238). Also, the inability to confirm success of a block and the lack of convincing evidence for efficacy and diagnostic specificity of these techniques dictates that findings should be interpreted cautiously.

INTERVERTEBRAL DISC INJECTION

Rationale

The annular ligament of the intervertebral disc fuses in the midline with the posterior longitudinal ligament. Both these structures are well innervated by sensory fibers and may provoke pain (95,106,152,242,314,350). Several methods are available to identify pathologic changes, to identify the source of pain in subjects with nonradiating back pain. Because myelography only demonstrates disc abnormalities that deform the dural sac, the injection of radiopaque contrast into the nucleus pulposus of the disc (discography) was developed to reveal the internal details of the disc. More recently, CT and MR have provided sensitive means of identifying changes in disc anatomy. Myelography, CT, and MR imaging all suffer from inadequate specificity, since asymptomatic discs frequently appear abnormal. Myelograms show lumbar nerve root involvement by disc disease in 24% of asymptomatic subjects and cervical involvement in 21% (244). Herniated nucleus pulposus is evident by CT scan in 19.5% of asymptomatic subjects under 40 years old, and in 26.9% of those over 40 (205). Lumbar disc degeneration is documented by MR in one-third to one-half of subjects without clinical evidence of back disease between the ages of 21 and 40 years, and in 90% over the age of 60 years (245–248). By imaging alone, there is no way to tell painful discs from others, especially if abnormal anatomy is evident at multiple levels.

Identifying a particular disc as the source of pain is challenging because of overlapping patterns of pain between various discs, and similar pain from facets. Therefore, discography has been recommended as an objective method for determining a specific disc as the origin of pain and for planning discectomy or vertebral fusion. The premise is that a dynamic test, in which the ability of a disc to produce the patient's typical pain, combined with the sensitivity of detailed intradiscal imaging, can most accurately identify the pathogenic site.

Technique

Since the procedure involves both interpretation of radiographic images, as well as clinical pain phenomena, it is ideally performed by the treating physician in conjunction with a radiologist. Typically, two to three consecutive discs are examined as one procedure. An early method involved passage of a needle in the posterior midline through the dural sac, to enter the disc through the posterior longitudinal ligament (249). Occasionally, this is still necessary for discs that are difficult to enter, especially at L5–S1. A posterolateral approach is used most often (Fig. 38-10) (250). Specially designed needles are available, but a 22-gauge, 5-inch needle is suitable. Sometimes a larger needle is passed first to the disc to guide the needle that actually punctures the anulus. Fluoroscopy is used (251) to determine the disc level and to direct the needle from the skin puncture site about 8 cm from the midline to the posterolateral aspect of the disc, anterior to the spinal nerve. A single needle is placed in each disc, but it must terminate within the nucleus pulposus, which can be assured by placing the tip within the inner one-third of the disc, as seen by both lateral and anteroposterior views. As contrast (water soluble, nonionic, e.g., iopamidol) is injected, the patient is asked to compare the sensation created to his usual pain, in both distribution and quality. The tension in the disc is estimated by the resistance to injection; this has been formally quantified as an indicator of disc condition (252). Injection is stopped when resistance to further injection is noted, when pain is created, or when about 3 mL has entered. Images are recorded with high-quality plane radiographs or CT axial scans.

A discogram is positive for disc degeneration if the image reveals altered texture of the nucleus, clefts in the nucleus and anulus, fissures leading to the perimeter of the anulus, or a radial tear that allows contrast to escape (Fig. 38-11) (253). Discomfort that duplicates the patient's typical pain is also necessary for a completely positive test response.

Reported complications are few and include disc space infection (249,250,254) and allergic response to the contrast.

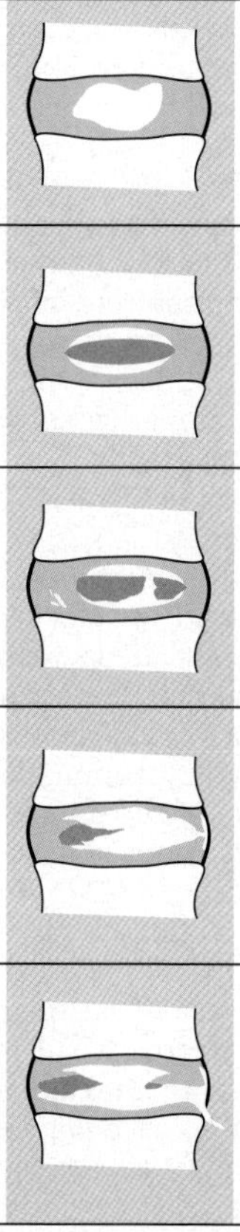

Discogram type		Stage of disc degeneration
1. Cottonball		No signs of degeneration. Soft white amorphous nucleus
2. Lobular		Mature disc with nucleus starting to coalesce into fibrous lumps
3. Irregular		Degenerated disc with fissures and clefts in the nucleus and inner annulus
4. Fissured		Degenerated disc with radial fissure leading to the outer edge of the annulus
5. Ruptured		Disc has a complete radial fissure that allows injected fluid to escape. Can be in any state of degeneration

FIGURE 38-11. The five types of discogram and the stages of disc degeneration they represent. From Neidre A, MacNab I. Anomalies of the lumbosacral nerve roots: Review of 16 cases and classification. *Spine* 1983;8:294, with permission.

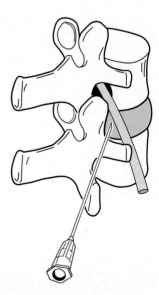

FIGURE 38-10. Needle placement for lumbar discography. From Konings JG, Veldhuizen AG. Topographic anatomical aspects of lumbar disc puncture. *Spine* 1988;13:958, with permission.

Limitations

Authorities report that the quality of testing by discography depends strongly upon the skill and experience of the operator. Proper placement of the needle tip within the nuclear portion of the disc is imperative. Repeated needle insertions or the removal of the needle after injection but prior to imaging may produce artifactual tracks of contrast through the anulus.

Discography is fairly uncomfortable for the subject, but deep sedation should be avoided, so that pain provocation can be evaluated. The value of this invasive test compared to CT and MR imaging is the subject of debate and numerous studies.

Studies

The pathoanatomic validity of discography has been established in cadaver studies by comparison of dissection with plane radiographs (253) and CT or MR imaging (255,256).

Satisfactory discogram testing is impossible to complete in few patients. As with any invasive study, some may find the pain of needle insertion intolerable. Inability to enter the disc and nucleus pulposus occurs in about 4% of discs, often at the L5–S1 level (257,258). Complete disc collapse was reported to preclude discography in 14% of patients (259). Computed tomography imaging after injection probably improves the sensitivity of the test compared to plane radiographs (255).

The false-positive rate determines the practical utility of the test. Early studies of asymptomatic subjects found positive discograms in 93% of cervical injections (260) and in 37% of lumbar injections in 20- to 40-year-olds (261). In part because of these findings, cervical disc injections are performed rarely. A replication of the study of lumbar injections in asymptomatic subjects also found that discograms were falsely positive in 17% of asymptomatic subjects, but if severe and concordant pain is included as a criterion for a positive test, the false-positive rate becomes 0% (262). Others studying patient groups with back pain have found that subjects with pain during injection are a subset of those with abnormal disc anatomy, and that 22% to 40% of discs unresponsive to pain provocation are anatomically abnormal (263,264). These data point to the conclusion that disc degeneration is a predictable age-related process that inconsistently results in pain. Unexplained are the 2% to 24% of back pain patients with induced pain during discography who have normal disc anatomy (263–265).

Since discography is invasive, indications and utility of the test must be compared to MR. Examination of cadaver material shows that radial tears of the annulus were evident by MR in only 67% of the discs with tears shown by discography and documented by dissection (256). In clinical comparison, MR and discography may differ in up to 45% of patients with back pain (254), due to both normal MR with abnormal discography and the reverse. Discography is more prone to operator and interpretation error, which is apparent on reinspection (258). Magnetic resonance images with clear evidence of either present or absent disc pathology usually agree with disc injection testing if provoked pain is included in the evaluation (266), so that discography can be reserved safely for determination of the disease state of discs with intermediate MR patterns.

Although discography with evaluation of induced pain can discern structurally abnormal and sensitive discs, this does not establish whether the test identifies the source of the patient's pain. Using local anesthetic injection to stop disc pain has not been evaluated as an additional phase of the test. However, the pressure-sensitive anulus would not necessarily be affected by anesthetic within the nucleus, and leakage through a disrupted disk would distribute anesthetic to multiple potentially painful elements. The only independent means available for determining the nociceptive source is comparison of the test response to the outcome from surgery, with the assumption that, if surgery at a particular level relieves the pain, then that was the source of the pain. Simmons and colleagues (250) reported the diagnostic accuracy in predicting surgical outcome was 91% at cervical levels and 82% for lumbar discs when discography was used to identify the painful disc. These figures are about twice the accuracy of clinical examination and myelography, but the calculations were not clearly defined. In a prospective study of back pain patients (259) in which all patients subsequently had an operation regardless of discogram result, 88% of patients with pain on injection and an abnormal discogram had a favorable outcome from surgery at the level indicated by testing (positive predictive value = 88%). However, this seemingly persuasive finding is due partly to the very high prevalence of favorable surgical outcomes in the entire group. Regardless of injection test results, 82% of all subjects had a favorable surgical outcome. About equal numbers of surgical nonresponders had positive and negative tests (false-positive rate = 52%), and subjects with a negative discogram image or no pain upon injection (negative test) were equally likely to have surgical success or failure (negative predictive value =

52%). A recent study employing a somewhat different strategy also raises doubt about the predictive value of discography (267). Only 43% of subjects with positive discography had "minimally acceptable outcome" of fusion surgery, whereas spondylolisthesis patients in the same study had 91% success by the same criteria.

The predictive value of discography in determining response to intradiscal thermal annuloplasty (also known as intradiscal electrotherapy, or IDET) is difficult to assess, since nearly all series consider a positive response to provocative discography as an inclusion criterion (268). In addition, the therapeutic benefit of IDET has been questioned. Although a meta-analysis of noncontrolled studies indicated significant improvement in pain scores and physical function following the procedure (268), a randomized controlled trial failed to show a significant advantage of the therapy over placebo (269). A similar technique, radiofrequency thermal annuloplasty (RFA), was shown to be even less effective than IDET in a randomized comparative trial (270).

Evaluation

In settings in which MR imaging is ambiguous, discography is a sensitive although invasive means of obtaining additional anatomic detail about disc structure. Provoking a comparable sensory response to injection is a critical component of the test. Statistical documentation of diagnostic validity has not been achieved.

SELECTIVE SPINAL NERVE INJECTION

Rationale

Radiculopathy is often obvious in its characteristic burning quality and distal radiation of pain. However, patients with more complicated conditions may present in whom the contribution of root inflammation to pain may not be certain or in whom the level of the pathology is unclear. Imaging by CT or MR and electrophysiologic evaluation by EMG may be inconsistent or may not fit with clinical findings. Frequent positive findings in imaging of asymptomatic subjects (205,244,245,247,248) demonstrates the inability of abnormal anatomy to indicate a pain source. A further cause of confusion is the presence of pathology at multiple levels, since the origin of pain may be any one or a combination of sites. This is also true when upper lumbar pathology coexists with hip joint disease. Finally, evaluation is especially difficult after laminectomy, since imaging is impeded by scarring in the epidural space.

In these unclear situations, injection of individual spinal nerves by a paravertebral approach (also termed foraminal injection or nerve root injection, although this latter term is anatomically incorrect), usually at lumbar levels, has been used to elucidate the mechanism and source of pain. The premise is that eliciting the patient's characteristic pain through needle contact will identify the pathologic nerve and that local anesthetic delivered to this nerve will be uniquely analgesic. Advocates point out that selective spinal nerve block, as with facet injection and discography, tests pain production mechanisms dynamically rather than simply displaying anatomic abnormalities that may or may not produce pain. Often this method is

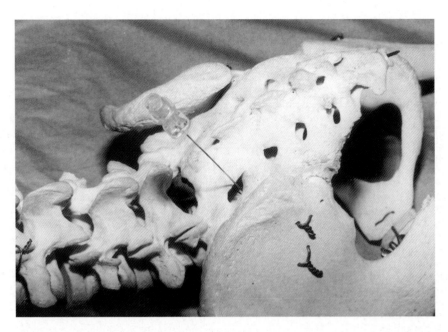

FIGURE 38-12. Trans-sacral approach to the first sacral nerve. The needle is guided by x-ray imaging into the first posterior sacral foramen and advanced to the anterior foramen, either until a paresthesia is evoked or lateral imaging shows the tip flush with the anterior surface of the sacrum.

used for surgical planning, for instance, to determine the site of foraminotomy.

Technique

Technical aspects of this procedure are discussed in detail in Chapter 44.

For diagnostic utility, it is important to obtain a paresthesia by gentle contact with the nerve. At this point, the patient is asked whether the quality and distribution of the provoked sensation is similar to his usual pain. Successful blockade is evident if a segmental sensory deficit develops. This may be subtle, so scratch and cold should be tested as well as touch. Since these patients often have neural dysfunction as part of their pathophysiology, a careful examination is necessary for comparison before injection. Maneuvers that produced pain prior to the block, such as straight leg lift or walking, should be repeated afterwards. A test is considered positive for a given nerve if it produced pain similar to the patient's usual pain, and if relief followed local anesthetic injection. Optimal insight into the origin of the pain is gained by testing two or three adjacent nerves on separate occasions (271).

Block of the first sacral nerve is performed by a transsacral approach with the patient prone (Fig. 38-12). Because of the lumbar lordosis, fluoroscopic guidance is improved when the beam is angled caudally, positioning it perpendicular to the sacrum. With the posterior and anterior sacral foramina superimposed, the needle can be passed to make contact with the spinal nerve in the middle portion of the canal. The rest of the block is done in the same manner as at lumbar levels.

Limitations

The pain provocation portion of the spinal nerve injection test examines pain quality and distribution. Duplication of the typical quality of the pain as a criterion is supported by the demonstration that inflamed nerves are more sensitive to manipulation than are normal nerves (197,202). Whereas mechanical stimulation of normal nerves produces paresthe-

sias, an inflamed nerve reproduces characteristic sciatica when touched. The distribution of the evoked sensation is less certain to be reliable. Since pain with the stimulation of different roots produces overlapping areas of radiation (202), these patterns may not distinguish the involved root from adjacent ones.

Confirmation of successful blockade is a desirable step prior to attributing pain and function changes to the block. It is not clear that anesthetizing a single spinal nerve should produce discernible peripheral sensory changes. Isolated monoradiculopathy commonly is associated with numbness, but this pathologic condition is probably more complex than just segmental nerve dysfunction, including changes in central connections (272). Selective spinal nerve injection reliably produced peripheral sensory changes in dermatome mapping studies, but 2 mL of anesthetic were injected, thus raising the question of spread to adjacent levels (273). Since surgical division of a single root produces no loss of cutaneous sensation (274), it remains uncertain whether cutaneous sensory monitoring can indicate accurately the presence or absence of selective spinal nerve block. No other methods of determining block success, such as thermography or somatosensory-evoked potentials, have been examined.

Pain relief with blockade of a spinal nerve cannot distinguish between pathology of the proximal nerve in the intervertebral foramen or pain transmitted from distal sites by that nerve. Tissue injury in the nerve's distribution and neuropathic pain alike would be relieved by a proximal block of a nerve. The ability of injection to block vertebral pain, without blocking hip pain, has not been demonstrated. The accuracy of spinal nerve block depends upon limiting the spread of anesthetic to the selected nerve alone. Flow into the intervertebral foramen and epidural space is commonly observed (see Chapter 11) and definitely compromises this assumption (275–279). Not only will this block pain transmitted by the sinuvertebral nerve from the dura, posterior longitudinal ligament, and annular ligament of the disc, but spread via the epidural space to other segmental levels could produce misleading results. For instance, injection of a normal S1 with spread to an inflamed L5 could produce relief, with the guilty nerve assumed to be S1. For this reason, this test should not be used outside the context of thorough overall evaluation.

Studies

The frequency of successful spinal nerve blockade has not been determined. In no studies using spinal nerve block for diagnosis were cutaneous sensory changes examined. Satisfactory needle placement could not be achieved in 10% of patients at L4, 15% at L5, and 30% at S1 (277). In another report, 18% of tests failed because of pain that exceeded the patient's tolerance or failure to stimulate the desired root, most often at S1 (280).

Several retrospective studies have investigated the ability of selective spinal nerve blocks to diagnose disease and predict surgical outcome. The positive predictive value (fraction of patients with injections indicating radiculopathy, in whom surgery confirmed radicular pathology at the level indicated by the test), ranged from 87% to 100% (271,276–278). The negative predictive value (percent of patients with a negative injection test and confirmed at surgery to have normal nerve roots) has been poorly studied because few patients had surgery in the negative test groups. Negative predictive values were found in 27% and 38% of the small number of patients operated upon, despite negative tests (276,277). Only one prospective study has appeared, which showed a positive predictive value of 95% and an untested negative predictive value (280). Sensitivity and specificity cannot be determined from these studies because of the unknown disease incidence in the full group. In general, the accuracy of nerve blocks was better than imaging or EMG (277,280). No controls were used in these studies, and the utility of cervical diagnostic spinal nerve injections has not been examined formally.

One retrospective report (275) attempted to predict surgical outcome by evaluating pain relief in response to steroid injection at the spinal nerve. Most subjects were tested with selective spinal nerve blocks, but 20% received epidural injection, and patients who were not relieved by local anesthetic were not included in the steroid test. All patients were operated upon regardless of test outcome, so complete outcome data is available. False-positive rate (percent of patients with failed surgery who had favorable response to injection) was 5%, and false-negative rate (percent of surgical successes who had no response to steroid) was 35%, indicating that patients unlikely to benefit from surgery can be identified reliably by failing to respond to steroid, but some who would benefit from surgery will be missed by this test. In patients with pain lasting longer than 1 year, however, nearly all patients who would benefit from surgery were identified by their response to steroid (false-negative, 15%).

Studies have demonstrated repeatedly that pain relief by paravertebral spinal nerve injection does not predict success by neuroablative surgery either by dorsal rhizotomy (281,282) or dorsal root ganglionectomy (283). Although greater than 50% success has been reported with cervical rhizotomy (282) and ganglionectomy (283) in patients with occipital distribution pain, success rates for these procedures at thoracic and lumbar levels are very low (72,283), and few centers continue to utilize these procedures. Radiofrequency lesioning of cervical (C4, C5, or C6) DRG at relatively low temperatures (67°C) has been shown in a randomized, sham-controlled trial to provide at least 8 weeks of pain reduction (284). All patients had obtained at least 50% relief from local anesthetic nerve root blocks. Evidence for benefit from pulsed radiofrequency lesions of DRG is relatively weak (285).

Selective spinal nerve injections with corticosteroids provide substantial pain relief for some patients with radicular pain. The evidence for benefit from cervical transforaminal steroid injections comes only from uncontrolled studies (285),

and there is substantial concern about spinal cord injury resulting from injection of particulate steroid preparations into a radicular artery. There is evidence from randomized controlled trials that lumbar transforaminal steroid injections are efficacious compared to placebo (286). However, no studies have compared this procedure to lumbar translaminar steroid injections, and there is concern that cord embolization via a radicular artery is a risk, particularly at upper lumbar levels.

Evaluation

Although spinal nerve injection has not been proved to be a valid diagnostic tool by conclusive studies, a broad group of surgical authorities have found benefits in its use for planning decompressive surgery on complicated patients. Controlled and blinded studies are needed to refute or support these beliefs. Its role in evaluating patients for neuroablative procedures is very uncertain.

EPIDURAL STEROID INJECTION

Two studies have used the response to epidural steroids as a prognostic factor. In one (275), subjects receiving epidural injections were mixed with a larger group tested with spinal nerve injections, so that the results cannot be interpreted. In the other report (287), sciatica patients who did not have satisfactory long-term benefit from lumbar epidural steroids had their initial response to epidural steroid injection compared to the outcome of subsequent chemonucleolysis. In a small group, patients who had some relief from steroids uniformly responded to chemonucleolysis, whereas only 46% of steroid nonresponders benefited from chemonucleolysis. No correlation was found between steroid response and surgical outcome. The study was uncontrolled.

GREATER OCCIPITAL NERVE BLOCK

Rationale

The greater occipital nerve is the continuation of the median branch of the posterior primary ramus of the C2 spinal nerve (see Chapter 17, Fig. 17-10), which is the only segmental level in the body at which the posterior primary ramus exceeds the anterior primary ramus in size. It distributes cutaneous sensory fibers to the scalp as far rostral as the vertex, where it abuts the territory of the supraorbital nerve, lateral to the area of the mastoid innervated by the great auricular and lesser occipital nerves of the cervical plexus (anterior primary rami), and inferior to the area of the third occipital nerve in the upper neck. From its origin at the second posterior root ganglion, it emerges between the atlas and axis (C1 and C2 vertebrae), loops under the inferior oblique capitis muscle, ascends medially under the semispinalis capitis muscle, which it penetrates before turning laterally under the trapezius. Emergence to the subcutaneous tissue occurs through the tendinous portion of the trapezius' insertion into the nuchal ridge of the skull adjacent to the occipital artery.

Several theories have proposed involvement of the C2 spinal and greater occipital nerves in production of headache. Initial analysis suggested that the origin of the spinal nerve or the posterior root ganglion may be pinched between the atlas and axis by extension and rotation (288). Further research proved that this is mechanically unlikely (289,290). A more popular theory invokes irritation of the greater occipital nerve as it penetrates the muscle layers. The passage through the muscular portion of the semispinalis capitis rarely is restricted, but the aperture through the trapezius is by a nondistensible channel that typically deforms the nerve (291). Entrapment here may be the origin of nerve irritation that initiates neuralgic pain.

Greater occipital neuralgia and cervical facet arthropathy are putative sources of cervicogenic headache, which is clinically distinguished from migraine and tension-type headaches by unilateral pain, symptoms and signs of neck involvement (ipsilateral neck, shoulder, or arm pain; tenderness or postural pain in the neck; decreased range of neck motion), nonclustering moderate pain that throbs and spreads forward from the neck, and a history of head or neck trauma (292,293). Transient elimination of pain by greater occipital nerve block is used as a key criterion in the work-up of cervicogenic headache (293).

Technique

Although the greater occipital branches to the scalp can be anesthetized by deposition of local anesthetic in a transverse band anywhere rostral to the nuchal ridge (see Chapter 17, Fig. 17-10), selective blockade of the nerve at the proposed pathogenic site requires injection as it penetrates through the trapezius. In two studies, this has been located on average at a point 3.2 cm lateral and 2.2 cm inferior to the external occipital protuberance (291), or 2.4 cm lateral and 1.2 cm inferior (294). There is marked interindividual variability, but 3 to 5 mL of anesthetic (lidocaine 1% or bupivacaine 0.5%) injected at 3 cm lateral and 2 cm inferior to the occipital protuberance (approximately midway between the occipital protuberance and the mastoid process) should spread to block most nerves. Bone should be contacted at a depth of no greater than 1 to 2 cm. A rostral angle and aspiration before injection are important to avoid injection into the CSF of the cisterna magna, with resulting total spinal anesthesia. Injection should be made upon withdrawal a few millimeters from the bone.

Anesthesia should be confirmed by sensory examination of the scalp ipsilateral and rostral to the injection. Determination of changes in headache should follow.

Limitations

Cervicogenic headache is a poorly documented entity (295) with no consistent histopathologic or radiologic findings (296). The typical lack of sensory deficit in the area of distribution of the greater occipital nerve does not support a neuropathic mechanism (289). Alternatively, it is possible that pain radiating in the distribution of the greater occipital nerve represents converging deep somatic input from the lateral atlantoaxial joint, which is innervated by the C2 anterior ramus (289), or from irritation of suboccipital muscles and periosteum, which has been shown to produce ascending headache (297–299).

Since all the proposed pathophysiologies of cervicogenic headache are unproved, the meaning of blockade responses does not rest on a solid mechanistic base. No defined process has been proved when relief follows greater occipital nerve block. Also, the therapeutic plan is not well defined after a favorable response to test injections. There are no data on the use of this block for treatment, and the surgical therapy for

presumed greater occipital neuralgia has not been promising (300,301). Favorable responses to radiofrequency lesions of the greater occipital nerve have been claimed (302). Patients who had pain relief after bilateral greater occipital nerve block, with 10 to 15 mL of local anesthetic on each side, received heat lesions to the nerves during general anesthesia. Although good to excellent relief was reported in 85% of cases, neural interruption was not documented, and no controls were used.

Studies

No information is available regarding rates of successful greater occipital nerve blockade. The ability of the block to identify patients with disease is hampered by inexact definition of cervicogenic headache and no means of certain confirmation. Most studies, as well as the definition of the condition, come from a single group. In one report (303), patients clinically categorized as having migraine, cervicogenic, or tension-type headaches were tested with greater occipital and supraorbital nerve blocks, with the latter as control. Cervicogenic headache patients were most relieved by occipital injection. However, supraorbital block also produced relief (about half as much, and not selective for cervicogenic patients), and the two blocks relieved pain at the other poles of the head. Although this calls into question the basis of relief, a mechanism is offered in which sensory tracts converge on common upper cord and brainstem centers (304,305). In another report (292), the ability of greater occipital nerve block to provide relief (confirmed as successful by sensory examination) was compared to selective blocks of cervical spinal nerves and the C2–C3 facet in patients with symptoms of cervicogenic headache. The patterns of responses were felt to be discriminatory between various origins of pain, but analgesia followed most blocks, to some degree.

Evaluation

The greater occipital nerve is easily blocked and anesthetic efficacy is readily confirmed, but the diagnostic meaning of a favorable analgesic response is clouded by the lack of pathophysiologic understanding of cervicogenic headache.

SELECTIVE SYMPATHETIC BLOCKADE

Rationale

Sympathetic efferent activity is a suspected pathogenic component in a number of conditions. In some, the participation of sympathetic fibers is well documented, such as in hyperhidrosis. In other diseases, such as sudden sensory–neural hearing loss, peripheral vascular disease, dysrhythmia from long-QT syndrome, central pain, pain following plexus injury, and trigeminal or postherpetic neuralgia (306), the diagnosis is clear but the role of sympathetic activity is uncertain and controversial. Finally, in a large category of poorly defined pain states that are grouped under the terms *reflex sympathetic dystrophy* or *causalgia (complex regional pain syndrome types I and II*; see Chapter 46), a sympathetic contribution is suspected, because blood flow and trophic changes are evident, but the pathophysiology is largely obscure. In these settings, selective interruption of sympathetic neural traffic to the involved area may provide diagnostic insight and guidance of future therapy. If sympathetic block relieves pain, indicated therapies might include further local anesthetic blocks, systemic treatment with sympathetically active drugs (e.g., clonidine, prazosin), or destructive therapy with neurolytic injection or surgery. Failure of relief after sympathetic blockade would argue against the use of these treatments.

Peripheral to where the gray rami communicantes deliver postganglionic sympathetic fibers to the spinal nerves, somatic and sympathetic elements are intermixed within nerve trunks, so that both are affected by peripheral neural blockade. (The pathway to a cutaneous destination may not always be the same for sympathetic and sensory fibers, however [108,109].) In contrast to peripheral nerves, the paravertebral sympathetic structures are separate anatomic routes that provide an opportunity for isolated sympathetic blockade (see Chapter 39). Diagnostic block seeks to determine the sympathetic contribution to disease by selective sympathetic interruption, while leaving somatic pathways intact (see Chapter 39). Although epidural or brachial plexus blocks, for example, produce intense sympathetic blockade, changes in disease state during or after these procedures cannot clearly be attributed to somatic or sympathetic effects.

Techniques

The techniques and complications are described in Chapter 39. Several issues are specifically relevant to diagnostic use of these blocks.

Documentation of sympathectomy in the area of disease is essential if diagnostic conclusions are sought regarding sympathetic activity. Block is evident by sudomotor, vasomotor, and ocular changes (see Chapter 39). Since sympathetic activity is most intense in distal portions of the extremity, confirmation of blockade of sympathetic fibers to the arm and leg is best done by examination of sympathetic activity in the glabrous skin, even if the symptomatic site is more proximal. The cervical trunk may be blocked independently of the stellate ganglion or fibers to the brachial plexus, so that the occurrence of ptosis, meiosis, facial anhydrosis, conjunctival hyperemia, or nasal stuffiness does not assure sympathetic block of fibers to the arm. Stellate, thoracic, or lumbar sympathetic injections that produce no measurable evidence of sympathetic blockade reveal nothing about disease pathophysiology, regardless of the pain response.

Careful sensory examination, including the ability to distinguish nociceptive stimuli (e.g., scratch or pin-prick) from touch, should precede and follow diagnostic sympathetic blockade. Otherwise, local anesthetic actions on nociceptive afferents could produce analgesia that is mistakenly viewed as evidence of a sympathetic mechanism.

Limitations

Stellate ganglion injection may fail to produce sympathetic denervation by several causes. Alternative routes allow sympathetic fibers to reach peripheral sites without transit through the stellate ganglion. These include passage in the nerves of Kuntz from the second and third intercostal nerves to the brachial plexus (307,308), distribution via the carotid, subclavian, and vertebral arteries (309–311), and direct entry to the peripheral nerves after entry into synapses outside the sympathetic chain in intermediate ganglia located in spinal nerve roots (312). Sympathetic fibers probably can also bypass the sympathetic chain in the sinuvertebral nerve of Luschka (313). As surgeons learned in previous decades, it is essentially impossible to achieve sympathetic denervation of the upper limb by a single surgical lesion or injection.

The principal reason for failure of injection to produce stellate ganglion blockade is lack of delivery of anesthetic to the ganglion. Whereas the ganglion resides at the lower edge of the head of the first rib (314), solution injected at cervical levels passes anteriorly into the mediastinum (315, 316).

At lumbar levels, multiple pathways of sympathetic fibers include collateral chains (86,317) and cross-over of fibers from the contralateral chain (318–320). These alternative pathways may allow persistent sympathetic innervation to reach the lower extremities, despite a properly performed lumbar sympathetic block. Confusion can result if local anesthetic solution is conveyed to the epidural space through the fibrous tunnel along the waist of the vertebral body (see Chapter 39, Fig. 39-24). The undesired somatic blockade that ensues could produce analgesia, which is then attributed to a sympathetic mechanism.

The diagnostic utility of sympathetic blockade depends upon the ability to interfere selectively with sympathetic activity and to maintain continuity of somatic pathways. The stellate ganglion lies anterior to the anterior primary ramus of the first thoracic spinal nerve at a distance of about 1 cm. Since no fibrous barrier separates these structures, it is likely that local anesthetic delivered to the ganglion would have at least a partial blocking effect on the brachial plexus. Also, injection of solution into the paravertebral space readily enters the epidural space (321). The only study examining detailed somatic sensory changes following sympathetic blocks found that nociceptive block without anesthesia was common (322). A subtle somatic block with analgesia but intact sense of touch would create the impression of analgesia from sympathetic blockade if altered pain sensation is not identified specifically.

Blocks of the paravertebral sympathetic chain inevitably interrupt visceral afferent signals, as well as efferent sympathetic activity (117). This could create a false conclusion about the source and mechanism of pain. For instance, a stellate ganglion block will stop arm pain from myocardial ischemia, but could be credited with identifying a sympathetically dependent pain process.

A fundamental limitation of diagnostic sympathetic blockade is a lack of understanding about the role of the sympathetic nervous system in pain production (323,324). Evidence now indicates that excessive sympathetic activity almost certainly is not the explanation of pain (17,325–328). The enigmatic pathophysiology and ambiguous definitions of reflex sympathetic dystrophy (RSD; CRPS-1; see Chapter 46) and other painful conditions in which the sympathetic nervous system plays a putative role frustrate the interpretation and application of findings from blocks (329), (see Chapter 46, Figs. 46-1 to 46-4).

Studies

Rates of success in actually interrupting sympathetic activity following injections intended for that purpose are incompletely known. After cervical paratracheal injection, Warrick (330) observed that very few patients had warming of the hand. Carron and Litwiller (136) reported that a 3-mL injection produced a temperature increase of 1.5°C in all of more than 700 blocks. Using 15 mL of an equal mix of 1% lidocaine and 0.5% bupivacaine, Ready and co-workers (331) had 100% success in producing a Horner syndrome, but 75% success in warming the ipsilateral hand by 1°C. Malmqvist and colleagues (332) observed an 87% success rate in producing Horner syndrome, but 26 of 54 (48%) subjects with initial ipsilateral hand temperature of 32°C or less failed to warm to 34°C or more within 20 minutes. Only 11.5% of their blocks met five criteria of success: Horner syndrome, increased hand temperature, 50% or greater increase in skin blood flow, increased skin resistance (≥13% baseline), and abolished skin resistance response. In 100 consecutive C6 anterior tubercle blocks in our clinic (138), 84% resulted in a Horner syndrome, indicative of at least some blockade of sympathetic fibers to the head. Only 60% caused the ipsilateral hand to warm by 1.5°C or more, and because the contralateral hand frequently warmed also, in only 27% did the ipsilateral hand warm by 1.5°C more than the contralateral hand. From these studies, it is apparent that sympathetic blockade is a variable result of stellate ganglion injections. There is little difference in the adequacy of sympathetic blockade by paravertebral injection at C7 level, compared with C6 (316,332–334). Injection through a needle placed at the head of the first rib requires CT guidance but assures successful blockade (335).

Success rates for lumbar sympathetic block have not been determined except with use of phenol. With this, success in increasing the skin temperature by more than 1°C was reported in 61% to 68% of patients (336). Diagnostic sympathetic blocks are used most often to evaluate painful conditions (see Chapter 39). No histopathologic or serologic standard exists by which to confirm a sympathetic contribution to pain production, so that few studies exist measuring the ability of blockade to diagnose accurately a sympathetic role. The reports that are available raise doubt as to whether analgesia after sympathetic blockade indicates a sympathetic contribution to pain. For example, the degree of sympathetic dysfunction does not correlate with the response of pain to sympathetic blockade (337), and the timing of changes in pain do not necessarily match the onset of manifestations of sympathetic block. When sympathetic activity is measured with microelectrode neurography in limbs with pain relieved by local anesthetic sympathetic block, sympathetic efferent traffic is normal (17). Response of pain to sympathetic blockade does not predict levels of norepinephrine and its metabolite in the venous effluent from limbs with features of reflex sympathetic dystrophy (327). In fact, catecholamines are consistently fewer on the painful side than on the nonaffected side. These findings make less plausible the belief that sympathetic block analgesia identifies regional sympathetic hyperactivity. The important question of whether the response to sympathetic blockade guides therapy toward a better outcome has not been addressed in any formal way (see also Chapter 39).

Evaluation

Confusion surrounds many aspects of care for patients in whom pain or other dysfunction is suspected to be based in the sympathetic nervous system. Response to a block, therefore, offers an apparently concrete diagnostic insight. The considerations just enumerated, however, suggest that the diagnostic value of sympathetic blockade has been overestimated. Appropriate use calls for care in documenting the desired physiologic response and caution in interpreting the results. One should avoid the circular logic of defining sympathetically maintained pain as those conditions improved by sympathetic blocks, and the blocks defined as successful if they relieve a pain assumed to be sympathetically maintained.

INTRAVENOUS REGIONAL SYMPATHETIC BLOCK

Rationale

Intravenous regional (IVR) injection of both guanethidine (338) and bretylium (339) have been used therapeutically in patients with sympathetically maintained pain (see Chapters 15 and 39). Both drugs inhibit release of norepinephrine from nerve terminals, and guanethidine depletes tissues of norepinephrine. Since a period of regional sympathetic block lasting several hours or more follows these procedures, the patient's response during the postblock period should be an indicator of the extent to which pain is mediated sympathetically.

Technique

With the patient supine, a tourniquet is placed on the upper arm or thigh, and an IV catheter is placed in a vein in the hand or foot. The limb is elevated and exsanguinated by wrapping with an Esmarch bandage. The tourniquet is inflated to at least 100 torr above systolic pressure, the Esmarch is removed, and 20 to 30 mg guanethidine or 2 to 3 mg/kg bretylium in 40 mL normal saline is injected into the venous system. The tourniquet remains inflated for 15 to 30 minutes and is then released. Pain relief may occur while the cuff is still inflated or after deflation. Pain scores and sensory changes are noted before and after the block. Guanethidine often causes severe burning pain in patients with allodynia (226,340), perhaps due to norepinephrine released with the onset of guanethidine action. Itching, piloerection, edema, or engorgement of the tissues in the injected area may also occur. Complications from systemic distribution following release of the cuff have not been observed.

Limitations

The ischemic block produced by the tourniquet may have a profound effect on certain types of pain (see following discussion). It would seem reasonable, therefore, when using this technique diagnostically, to perform the procedure twice: once with guanethidine or bretylium and once with saline alone. A more profound or more prolonged response to the procedure done with the active drug would then indicate a sympathetic component to the pain.

Guanethidine has been demonstrated to affect CNS levels of serotonin and to have anticholinergic effects (341). Local anesthetic effects are not reported, and local anesthetic IVR blockade has produced only brief relief of pain in patients who had prolonged relief following IVR guanethidine (226).

Studies

Intravenous regional guanethidine predictably eliminates allodynia, but has no effects on other sensory function (226,342). Increased peripheral temperature and blood flow follows IVR guanethidine but not IVR saline. Vasodilatation may be delayed by hours after cuff deflation, and complete blockade of vascular control is rare (226). No temporal relationship exists between pain relief and manifestations of sympathetic blockade. This may be due to a vasodilatory action of guanethidine that is independent of effects on norepinephrine release (343).

Bonelli and colleagues (344) found that IVR guanethidine was more effective in patients who exhibited dystrophic changes associated with RSD. Loh and Nathan found that pain and sensory response was congruent in nine of 10 painful limbs when comparing IVR guanethidine and local anesthetic sympathetic chain injections. A high correlation exists between relief of pain from IV phentolamine and from IVR guanethidine (345). These cross-comparisons support the notion that each is producing analgesia by a common sympatholytic mechanism.

There is, so far, no confirmation of the diagnostic value of IVR sympathetic block for identifying patients who can be expected to have long-term therapeutic benefit from systemic or regional sympatholytic measures.

Evaluation

Analgesia following IVR guanethidine or bretylium may in part confirm a sympathetic component of a given patient's pain, particularly if IVR placebo injection fails to do so. Information obtained from the procedure cannot be the sole means of diagnosis, but should be evaluated together with clinical findings and response to other diagnostic interventions, including paravertebral sympathetic blocks, or the phentolamine test.

PRESSURE AND ISCHEMIC DIFFERENTIAL EXTREMITY BLOCK

Rationale

Different fiber types convey a variety of painful sensations that are to a great degree unique to that neuronal category. *First pain*, produced by impulses in small myelinated Aδ-fibers, is prompt, well-localized, and has a pricking and sharp character. *Second pain*, characteristic of nonmyelinated C-fibers, is not felt in an exact location, has gradual onset and offset, and an aching quality. Pain invoked by soft touch of the skin (mechanical allodynia) probably is due to stimulation of fast conducting Aβ-fibers, with subsequent aberrant central processing (see the section on Plasticity). Although the current importance of distinguishing fiber types subserving pain in a particular patient is largely academic, advances in the neuropharmacology of pain may produce therapies suitable only for certain pathophysiologic conditions, making distinctions of fiber types important. For example, it is likely that capsaicin, which depletes substance P from the skin terminals of C-fibers, is effective only in treating pain due to unmyelinated fibers.

Nerve compression is the oldest reported means of producing differential interruption of sensory function, with initial documentation in 1855 (129). Whereas local anesthetics block peripheral nerve C-fibers prior to Aδ and Aβ (45) (see previous discussion), the reverse can be achieved either by direct focal pressure to the nerve or by a tourniquet that produces both compression of the nerve and ischemia of the limb. Both have a preferential effect upon transmission of myelinated fibers. Direct compression of the nerve is limited to sites in which the nerve can be pressed against bone, such as the superficial radial nerve at the wrist (45,46). The psychophysical response to direct compression of a nerve is the same as tourniquet

compression-ischemia (346), which is more generally applicable.

The initial sensory event during compression and ischemia of a nerve is intense paresthesiae (347) due to paralysis of the sodium-potassium (Na$^+$/K$^+$) pump and depolarization of the axon. Fasciculations representing spontaneous activity in motor axons accompany only prolonged periods of nerve compression (348). After about 5 minutes, conduction in ischemic nerves begins to fail in a decremental fashion, in which impulses travel progressively more slowly, and more limited distances, before failing (349). Perception of soft touch fails after 5 to 20 minutes, soon followed by loss of sense of cold and first (sharp) pain. These three sensations may be difficult to separate reliably by compression-ischemia (350). Sense of warmth is inhibited next. Second (aching) pain remains intact after the loss of warmth and may not be completely abolished by compression and ischemia (46,129,351). Efferent sympathetic impulses persist unimpeded (352).

Technique

Meticulous sensory testing should precede the block and be charted during the development of blockade. Direct pressure requires special equipment, and is not generally applicable. For compression-ischemia, an inflatable tourniquet is placed proximal to the site of extremity pain and inflated to a pressure 100 mm Hg above systolic arterial pressure after exsanguination of the limb by elevation. Findings usually are complete within 30 to 45 minutes. Complications are few, although ischemia may be uncomfortable and the tourniquet may not be tolerated on a sensitive extremity. Numbness has persisted for as long as 1 week after blockade (46).

Studies

Persuasive confirmation of the differential specificity of compression and ischemic blockade has been provided by direct microneurographic recording of neuronal impulses (45,46,346). These studies document that susceptibility is greatest for Aβ- and Aδ-fibers, while C-fibers are resistant.

Elimination of sensory potentials recorded proximally from electrical stimulation also confirms that Aβ-afferents are blocked by ischemia while C-fibers remain active (352). Since the timing of electrophysiologically measured conduction block matches the changes of the particular sensory mode transmitted by each fiber type, standard neurologic testing is adequate to detect deactivation of the various fibers.

Compression-ischemic blockade has been used to identify algogenic impulse transmission by myelinated A-fibers (353,354) and nonmyelinated C-fibers (127,346) in painful conditions. In these studies, secondary confirmation by other block techniques and psychophysiologic manipulations has supported the accuracy of differential compression-ischemic block for identifying the fiber type conducting pain.

Evaluation

The physiologic accuracy of differential compression-ischemic block is based on thorough basic research. Practical utility of the test requires further developments in the taxonomy and neuropharmacology of pain.

DIFFERENTIAL NEURAXIAL BLOCK

Rationale

The purpose of differential spinal or epidural block is to provide diagnostic information for patients with lower extremity and/or lower trunk pain (355–357). In the classic approach, a placebo is injected first, followed by a local anesthetic solution capable of selectively blocking sympathetic efferents. If no relief is achieved, a concentration capable of producing sensory blockade is injected. If this produces no pain relief, a solution is then injected that will block motor fibers as well. The changes in pain during the different phases of the block indicate whether the pain is labeled as psychogenic, sympathetic, nociceptive (sensory based), or central.

Technique

A subarachnoid site of injection has been used most extensively. The block is performed with the patient in the lateral decubitus position. A spinal needle is placed in the lumbar subarachnoid space. Blood pressure and pulse are checked at frequent intervals. Prior to the initial injection, and 10 to 15 minutes after each successive injection is performed, the following observations are made in an identical manner:

- A verbal and/or visual analog (VAS) pain score is recorded; if possible, mechanical reproduction of pain (passive movement of legs, pressure over tender points) should be done.
- Skin temperature of the lower extremities is recorded; other measures of sympathetic function, such as galvanic skin response, may be done.
- Sensory and motor testing of the lower extremities is done.

Following placement of the subarachnoid needle, injections are made at 10-minute intervals using the following solutions:

1. Placebo: 5 mL isotonic saline
2. Sympathetic block: 10 mL 0.2% procaine
3. Sensory block: 10 mL 0.5% procaine
4. Motor block: 10 mL 1.0% procaine

If pain relief occurs after placebo injection, this is interpreted as a placebo response. Some authors interpret a placebo response to be evidence of a psychogenic pain mechanism, particularly if relief is prolonged. If the analgesia is brief, it is reasonable to continue on to step 2 (sympathetic blocking anesthetic concentration) and to compare the degree and duration of pain relief to that obtained following saline injection.

Interpretation of response to 0.2% procaine can be made only if there is evidence of sympathetic blockade and no evidence of sensory block (the authors have found this to occur in a relatively small proportion of individuals). If there is indeed pain relief and a differential effect on sympathetic function, this provides evidence of sympathetically maintained pain.

If pain relief occurs following the onset of sensory blockade after injection of 0.5% procaine, this is interpreted as evidence of a somatic mechanism of pain. If pain relief occurs only after the injection of 1% procaine, this again is interpreted as evidence of a somatic mechanism. The higher concentration is thought to be required in some patients because a more complete sensory block is required to relieve the pain, or because motor activity in some way contributes to the clinical pain.

If no relief occurs despite complete motor and sensory blockade, the interpretation is that the pain is of a central mechanism. The possible causes of central pain include:

- A CNS lesion of the upper spinal cord or brain
- Self-sustaining neural activity in the CNS above the level blocked
- Psychogenic pain
- Malingering

A major drawback to the differential spinal block is the prolonged time required to perform and assess the individual steps. In a modified technique (358), only two steps are required. The first is the placebo (saline) injection, as just described. Subsequently, 100 mg procaine (2 mL 5%) is injected intrathecally. Pain relief following placebo response or lack of pain relief from procaine is interpreted as in the classical technique. If the patient experiences pain relief after the procaine injection, the timing of the return of sensation is noted. If the return of pain is coincident with the return of sensation to pin-prick, the interpretation is that the pain is somatic in origin. If pain relief persists until or beyond the return of sympathetic function, the interpretation is that the pain is sympathetically mediated.

An epidural technique also has been used in a fashion similar to the subarachnoid method (33). Following a placebo injection of saline, 0.25% lidocaine is injected to block sympathetic fibers, then 0.5% lidocaine to block sensation as well, and finally 1% lidocaine to produce surgical anesthesia.

A preliminary report has suggested the use of opioid instead of local anesthetic as the analgesic agent (33), arguing that opioid effects are more specific and don't provide a cue of numbness or warmth to trigger placebo or psychogenic responses. Following placebo injections, fentanyl 1 μg/kg in 5 mL normal saline is injected through an epidural catheter. Analgesia indicates a predominantly physical basis for pain, as does reversal of the analgesia by IV injection of naloxone 0.4 mg, unobserved by the subject. Finally, local anesthetic blockade with concentrated lidocaine serves the same purpose as that described in the earlier method.

Limitations

There are a number of possible drawbacks to the traditional differential spinal technique. Even early descriptions of the technique report that either pain fibers or sympathetic fibers may be blocked first (359) and that the injected solutions may fail to provide the desired block (355,356). The entire premise depends on the ability to achieve a steady-state block of certain fiber types while sparing others in the desired order. As discussed, lack of obvious sensory changes does not assure that neural processing has not been altered, and a dense block adequate for surgery does not indicate an absence of afferent sensory traffic or efferent sympathetic impulses. Neurophysiologic study of awake humans and analysis of conduction in various laboratory preparations consistently point to the impossibility of complete block of one fiber type without at least partial block of others.

Further considerations erode the theoretic plausibility of diagnostic differential blockade. When nociceptive afferent fibers are active, as may occur with spontaneous discharge arising from an injured peripheral nerve or from persistent discharge of a nociceptor by a noxious stimulus, they may be subject to use-dependent block and be more affected by low concentrations of anesthetic than normal, quiescent afferents. Additionally, sub-blocking concentrations of local anesthetics are capable of reducing the maximum firing rates of axons (43). Since pain induced by nociceptor activation is proportional to firing frequency, a modest reduction in the firing frequency could result in diminished pain. In both instances, although evidence of sensory block is not detected by sensory testing, pain relief from blockade of nociceptor fibers may be achieved and pain relief may be attributed mistakenly to sympathetic blockade. Although the one-shot technique has the advantage in that it is not dependent upon achieving a critical concentration of anesthetic in the CSF, it does depend on the premise that both A- and C-fibers recover function before B-fibers, which is probably incorrect (see previous discussion).

Even if a true differential block of sympathetic fibers were documented, a number of potential causes exist for uninterpretable responses or misinterpretation:

■ Patients who fail to obtain relief from subarachnoid 0.5% or 1% procaine actually may experience an increase in activity of some spinal cord neurons, because of blockade of certain afferent or spinal cord pathways. For example, A-fibers, including Aβ-fibers, may be blocked by a concentration of anesthetic that spares C-fibers (41), thus reducing the inhibitory effect of large afferent activity on dorsal horn neurons.
■ Intrathecal local anesthetic may block descending inhibitory fibers lying superficially in the dorsolateral funiculus (21), again producing disinhibition.
■ The fact that pain returns after pin-prick sensation does not necessarily imply a sympathetic mechanism. Prolonged pain relief has been described after local anesthetic blocks in conditions other than sympathetic dystrophy (29). Such prolonged effects may be related to changes in central processing. The temporary reduction in sensory input may allow sensitized dorsal horn neurons to return to more normal function, and it may take considerable time before noxious inputs can reestablish spinal cord sensitization.
■ There is no way to assess pain in any position other than lateral recumbent, ruling out any diagnostic benefit for patients whose pain improves when lying down or is activity-dependent.
■ Anatomic consideration makes unlikely a uniform progression of block from sympathetic to sensory. Specifically, complete block of roots caudal to L2 will provide sensory interruption but leave sympathetic fibers unaffected (360), since all white rami communicantes exit the cord between T1 and L2.

Failure of pain to respond to neuraxial opioid does not necessarily indicate that the pain has a psychogenic etiology, since pain with other origins, such as neuropathic and visceral pain or incident pain with movement, may also be resistant to spinal and epidural opioid (361,362). Additionally, systemic naloxone is not likely to reverse completely the analgesic effects of neuraxial opioids (363).

Studies

Despite claims that differential spinal block leads to selection of more effective treatment (357), no outcome studies have documented this belief. Specifically, no data document higher success rates from repeated sympathetic blocks among patients who experienced relief after 0.25% procaine, compared with patients exhibiting other responses. Sanders and co-workers (364). examined the relationship between the presence of psychopathology and the incidence of inappropriate responses to differential spinal. They concluded that psychopathology was no more likely among inappropriate responders.

Evaluation

Minimal evidence supports the ability of differential neuraxial blocks to distinguish the pathophysiologic origin of painful conditions. Current concepts of neurophysiology and local anesthetic action make it unlikely that a predictable and truly selective block can be achieved in a clinical setting.

SYSTEMIC MEDICATIONS

Local Anesthetics

Rationale

A selective action of IV lidocaine has been proposed because it often provides temporary relief of neuropathic pain, but is generally ineffective for nociceptive pain (see the System Effects section under Local Anesthetic Physiology). Therefore, it could be used as a means of distinguishing the pathophysiology of a painful condition. Since lidocaine is structurally analogous with the oral agents tocainide and mexiletine, response to IV lidocaine may be helpful also in predicting which patients with neuropathic pain will gain analgesia from a therapeutic course of these oral Na$^+$ channel blockers.

Technique

When using IV lidocaine to determine possible response to oral mexiletine, a lidocaine infusion is prepared. Initially, pain is assessed using a VAS, and sensory testing is carried out to determine the degree of allodynia. A saline infusion is then begun. After 5 minutes, the VAS and sensory testing is repeated. The placebo testing should be repeated over another 5- to 10-minute interval, then 2 mg/kg lidocaine is infused over a 5-minute period. This is followed by a constant infusion of 50 μg/kg/min, which is continued for 30 minutes. Visual analog scale scores and sensory testing are repeated at the end of the initial bolus dose and several times during the steady-state infusion. If at any time the patient begins to experience symptoms of local anesthetic toxicity (tinnitus, dizziness, tremor, etc.), the infusion is terminated. Blood pressure, heart rate, and electrocardiogram (ECG) are monitored during the infusion. Other authors use as little as 1.5 mg/kg in a single bolus with no infusion (57) or as much as 5 mg/kg over 30 minutes (52,55,56). A computer-controlled infusion pump, using pharmacokinetic parameters, has been reported to result in predictable plasma lidocaine concentration for neuropathic pain (365).

Studies

The effects of systemic lidocaine analgesic on pain with different mechanisms was tested in a study of five patients with a variety of central and peripheral neuropathic pain (54). Ischemic pain of comparable intensity was induced in an uninvolved arm. Both pains responded to the high blood lidocaine concentrations (average 5.6 μg/mL) that immediately followed 3 mg/kg lidocaine IV over 3 minutes, but the clinical pain showed significantly greater analgesia than did the ischemic pain. The lower concentrations of lidocaine (1.5–2.0 μg/mL) that followed infusions of 4 mg/min relieved only the clinical pain. Mild symptoms of toxicity developed during the infusion in two subjects. Another study (366) similarly found that low concentrations of lidocaine achieved during infusions at a rate of 60 μg/kg/min or less fail to alter perception of experimentally produced pain. These results indicate a mild, general, systemic analgesic effect occurs with high blood concentrations of lidocaine, but selective analgesia of central and peripheral neuropathic pain can be expected with lower lidocaine concentrations.

In another placebo-controlled and blinded study (57), 10 patients with chronic neuropathic pain were given saline or lidocaine 1.5 mg/kg IV over 1 minute, and sensory changes were evaluated. There were minimal effects after saline, but pain relief for 15 to 30 minutes was noted in all subjects after lidocaine, including allodynia to cold and mechanical stimuli, as well as the presence of Tinel sign. Four patients felt lightheaded and dizzy. Although this report documents the efficacy of systemic lidocaine in producing analgesia for neuropathic pain, it does not demonstrate a selective effect preferentially upon neuropathic pain, and so does not support a diagnostic use.

Two papers have reported relief from oral mexiletine in patients who previously responded to IV lidocaine (367,368). Randomized and controlled studies, however, have not been done to test the ability of systemic lidocaine to predict the response to mexiletine.

Evaluation

Intravenous lidocaine may be of some diagnostic value in distinguishing between neuropathic and nociceptive pain, although the therapeutic implications of such a distinction may be quite limited. Intravenous lidocaine may be helpful in predicting response to oral Na^+ channel blockers, but this remains to be proved by controlled studies.

Phentolamine

Rationale

The action of endogenous catecholamines upon peripheral sensory afferent neurons has been proposed as a mechanism by which sympathetic efferent activity provokes pain (369). Analgesia that accompanies the IV infusion of phentolamine, an α-adrenergic blocking agent, has been claimed to indicate that a component of a patient's pain is sympathetically mediated. This method has the diagnostic advantage over local anesthetic sympathetic blocks in that it does not interrupt afferent traffic from visceral or somatic structures. Although sudomotor function is mediated by cholinergic transmission and therefore is not affected by adrenergic blockade, sudomotor activity does not play an important role in pain generation (370). Response to IV phentolamine should identify patients who can expect a beneficial response to intermittent or continuous local anesthetic sympathetic blocks, or to oral or transdermal sympatholytic drugs.

Technique

The patient is placed supine and an IV line is placed. Sensory testing is performed to determine the severity and extent of allodynia, and a VAS pain rating is obtained. Sensory testing and VAS ratings are repeated 5 minutes after each placebo or phentolamine injection. Blood pressure and heart rate are monitored throughout the testing period, and skin temperature of the affected and contralateral extremity are recorded continuously. An infusion of normal saline is begun, and 500 mL is infused over a 30-minute period. Some authors recommend administration of propranolol 1 mg IV if the heart rate is greater than 70 min^{-1}. Bolus injections of saline are given at the beginning of the infusion and 15 and 30 minutes later. At 5-minute intervals,

the following doses of phentolamine are administered: 1 mg, 2 mg, 3 mg, 5 mg, 7 mg, and 10 mg. Whenever substantial relief of pain is obtained or significant hypotension occurs, the test is terminated (345,369).

If phentolamine produces evidence of sympathetic block, such as nasal congestion, hypotension, or skin warming, absence of concurrent pain relief indicates no sympathetic contribution. If placebo produces no analgesia but phentolamine does, a sympathetic role is suspected. The appearance of an increase in skin temperature coincident with pain relief provides added assurance of the diagnosis. The procedure is safe, with predictable nasal stuffiness and occasional sinus tachycardia, premature ventricular contractions, dizziness, or wheezing (371). The safety of reduced doses of phentolamine has been confirmed in children (345). Subjects with advanced cardiovascular disease, such as heart block, unstable angina, or congestive heart failure, probably are not suitable for the test.

Limitations

Phentolamine has been shown to have local anesthetic properties (372,373), which raises the question of whether relief could be through pharmacologic mechanisms other than sympathetic block. As with other tests of sympathetic function, a fundamental limitation is the ambiguous role of sympathetic function in pain. The role of α-receptors is uncertain (329). Even though a patient experiences relief from IV phentolamine, oral sympathetic blocking drugs may be ineffective because side effects, particularly orthostatic hypotension, may preclude intense blockade comparable to the potent effect of IV phentolamine.

Studies

Raja and co-workers (369) administered IV phentolamine, 25 to 35 mg in incremental bolus doses, and, on another occasion, local anesthetic sympathetic blocks to 20 patients with suspected sympathetically maintained pain. When comparisons were made of the maximum pain relief from the two procedures, they found a high degree of correlation. Patients generally experienced relief of both spontaneous and evoked pain (allodynia). Only three patients had relief from saline, an extraordinarily low incidence of placebo response (see the discussion of placebo under the section Psychosocial Influences). Arner (345) found that 33% of 48 patients tested with IV phentolamine (5–15 mg) experienced relief of pain. All of the patients who had relief with phentolamine experienced a reduction in pain with IV regional guanethidine, whereas only one of 12 patients who failed the phentolamine test had relief from guanethidine. Overall, they found a false-positive rate of 0% and a false-negative rate of 32% if guanethidine relief is assumed to indicate presence of disease (sympathetically maintained pain).

Shir and colleagues (371) found relief from phentolamine infusion in 25% of pain patients with clinical evidence of a sympathetic contribution. The low response rates in this and the study by Arner and co-workers (345) are at or below typical placebo response rates. Several authors (78,79) caution that placebo responses may require 15 to 60 minutes to become evident. If adequate time is allowed, phentolamine-induced analgesia does not differ from placebo response (79), and placebo analgesia is observed in all subjects, thus making the phentolamine test impossible to administer (78). No studies have been carried out that determine the relationship of response to IV phentolamine with the response to repeated or continuous local anesthetic blocks or to systemic sympathetic blocking agents.

Studies typically report administration of phentolamine to a predetermined dose, rather than until a physiologic effect (nasal congestion, hypotension, skin warming) is achieved. Without such an end-point, it is not possible to distinguish inadequate phentolamine dose from a lack of α-receptor involvement in the pain generation.

Evaluation

Intravenous phentolamine appears to correlate well with responses to local anesthetic paravertebral sympathetic blocks and guanethidine IV regional sympathetic blocks. It is not clear, however, that either of these are an acceptable standard of pure and complete sympathetic interruption (see sections in this chapter on these blocks). Response to phentolamine should be considered in conjunction with clinical findings and other diagnostic tests. Considered alone, it may not be very sensitive or specific. The ability of the phentolamine response to predict outcome of therapy with sympatholytic treatments has not been tested. It is not clear how using a phentolamine trial would improve upon a simple trial of oral therapy in the first place.

Barbiturates

Rationale

Small IV doses of rapidly acting barbiturates have been used in psychiatric practice to promote a state of relaxation to facilitate communication of thoughts (374). In the diagnosis of pain, a light hypnotic state may be used to discern the contribution of cognitive and emotional issues in pain behavior. For example, a limb that relaxes or allodynia that dissipates with sedation may be due to psychological factors such as anxiety, hysterical conversion, or malingering. Non-nociceptive pain, such as pain related to CNS injury, often is relieved by subanesthetic barbiturate doses (375).

Technique

Even if a detailed psychiatric interview is not planned, it probably is wise to perform a barbiturate test with a psychiatrist present who has experience with the technique. Thiopental is injected intravenously in 50-mg increments. The patient is instructed to give a verbal pain score or to relate the degree of pain relief after each dose. Response to provocative stimuli during the hypnotic state are compared to baseline responses. Doses are repeated until either an increase or a decrease in pain occurs, or until the patient becomes too drowsy to cooperate.

Limitations

Because of the complex involvement of cerebral activity and the conscious mind in the production and manifestation of pain, and the resulting behavior, changes during barbiturate administration are very difficult to interpret. Small doses of IV barbiturates are reported to cause an increase in pain that has a nociceptive basis (376). This antianalgesic effect has been demonstrated in pressure algometry studies (377) and may be related to the ability of these drugs to interfere with descending inhibitory mechanisms through a medullary γ-aminobutyric acid (GABA) receptor mechanism (378). The physician should be prepared for the occasional exposure of a distressing, disruptive, and previously unrecognized psychosis during barbiturate administration (379).

Evaluation

The diagnostic utility of this technique has not been tested. Given its purely empirical basis and the inexact nature of the information obtained, it would seem unwise to attach much significance to data collected from this procedure.

References

1. Malliani A. Cardiovascular sympathetic afferent fibers. *Rev Physiol Biochem Pharmacol* 1982;94:11.
2. Perl ER. Is pain a specific sensation? *J Psychiatr Res* 1971;8:273.
3. Zimermann M, Handwerker HO. Total afferent inflow and dorsal horn activity upon radiant heat stimulation of the cat's footpad. In: Bonica JJ, ed. *Advances in Neurology*, Vol. 4. New York: Raven Press; 1974:29–38.
4. Terenius L. Biochemical mediators in pain. *Triangle* 1981;20:19.
5. Cortright DN, Szallasi A. Biochemical pharmacology of the vanilloid receptor TRPV1. *Eur J Biochem* 2004;271:1814.
6. Wang H, Woolf CJ. Pain TRPs. *Neuron* 2005;46:9.
7. Devor M, Wall PD, Catalan N. Systemic lidocaine silences neuroma and DRG discharge without blocking nerve conduction. *Pain* 1992;48:261.
8. Tanelian DL, MacIver MB. Analgesic concentrations of lidocaine suppress tonic A-delta and C-fiber discharges produced by acute injury. *Anesthesiology* 1991;74:934.
9. Nordin M, Nystrom B, Wallin U, Hagbarth K-E. Ectopic sensory discharges and paresthesiae in patients with disorders of peripheral nerves, dorsal roots and dorsal columns. *Pain* 1984;20:231.
10. Cuello AC, Matthews MR. Peptides in the peripheral sensory nerve fibers. In: Melzack R, Wall PD, eds. *Textbook of Pain*. New York: Churchill Livingstone; 1984:65.
11. Kibler RF, Nathan PW. Relief of pain and paraesthesiae by nerve block distal to a lesion. *J Neurol Neurosurg Psychiatry* 1960;23:91.
12. Xavier AV, McDanal J, Kissin I. Relief of sciatic radicular pain by sciatic nerve block. *Anesth Analg* 1988;67:1177.
13. Abram SE. Pain mechanisms in lumbar radiculopathy. *Anesth Analg* 1988;67:1135.
14. Sato J, Perl ER. Adrenergic excitation of cutaneous pain receptors induced by peripheral nerve injury. *Science* 1991;251:1608.
15. Blumberg H, Janig W. Discharge pattern of afferent fibers from a neuroma. *Pain* 1984;20:335.
16. Devor M, Janig W. Activation of myelinated afferents ending in neuroma by stimulation of the sympathetic supply in the rat. *Neurosci Lett* 1981;24:43.
17. Torebjork E. Clinical and neurophysiological observations relating to pathophysiological mechanisms in reflex sympathetic dystrophy. In: Stanton-Hicks M, Janig W, Boas RA, eds. *Reflex Sympathetic Dystrophy*. Boston: Kluwer Academic Publishers; 1990:71–80.
18. Roberts WJ. A hypothesis on the physiological basis for causalgia and related pains. *Pain* 1986;24:297.
19. Chung K, Chung JM. Sympathetic sprouting in the dorsal root ganglion after spinal nerve ligation: Evidence of regenerative collateral sprouting. *Brain Res* 2001;895:204.
20. Melzack R, Wall PD. Pain mechanisms: A new theory. *Science* 1965;150:971.
21. Basbaum AI, Fields HL. Endogenous pain control systems: Brainstem spinal pathways and endorphin circuitry. *Ann Rev Neurosci* 1984;7:309.
22. Dubner R, Hoffman D, Hayes R. Neuronal activity in medullary dorsal horn of awake monkeys trained in a thermal discrimination task. III. Task-related responses and their functional role. *J Neurophysiol* 1981;46:444.
23. Pomeranz B, Wall PD, Weber CV. Cord cells responding to fine myelinated afferents from viscera, muscle, and skin. *J Physiol* 1983;199:511.
24. Ness T, Gebhart GF. Visceral pain: A review of experimental studies. *Pain* 1990;41:167.
25. Wilcox GL. Excitatory neurotransmitters and pain. In: Bond MR, Charlton JE, Woolf CJ, eds. *Proceedings of the 6th World Congress on Pain*. Amsterdam: Elsevier; 1991:97–117.
26. Randic M, Jiang MC, Cerne R. Long-term potentiation and long-term depression of primary afferent neurotransmission in the rat spinal cord. *J Neurosci* 1993;13:5228.
27. DeLeo JA, Tanga FY, Tawfik VL. Neuroimmune activation and neuroinflammation in chronic pain and opioid tolerance/hyperalgesia. *Neuroscientist* 2004;10:40.

28. Tal M, Bennett GJ. Extra-territorial pain in rats with a peripheral mononeuropathy: Mechanohyperalgesia and mechano-allodynia in the territory of an uninjured nerve. *Pain* 1994;57:375.

29. Arner S, Lindblom U, Meyerson BA, Molander C. Prolonged relief of neuralgia after regional anesthetic blocks: A call for further experimental and systematic clinical studies. *Pain* 1990;43:287.

30. Woolf CJ. Central mechanisms of acute pain. In: Bond MR, Charlton JE, Woolf CJ, eds. *Proceedings of the 6th World Congress on Pain.* Amsterdam: Elsevier; 1991:25–34.

31. Devor M. Central changes mediating neuropathic pain. In: Dubner R, Gebharrt GF, Bond MR, eds. *Proceedings of the 5th World Congress on Pain.* Amsterdam: Elsevier; 1988:114–128.

32. Chabal C, Russell LC, Burchiel KJ. The effect of intravenous lidocaine, tocainide, and mexiletine on spontaneously active fibers originating in rat sciatic neuromas. *Pain* 1989;38:333.

33. Cherry DA, Gourlay GK, McLachlan M, Cousins MJ. Diagnostic epidural opioid blockade and chronic pain: Preliminary report. *Pain* 1985;21:143.

34. Dellemijn PLI, Fields HL, Allen RR, et al. The interpretation of pain relief and sensory changes following sympathetic blockade. *Brain* 1994;117:1475.

35. Lund C, Selmer P, Hansen DB, et al. Effects of epidural bupivacaine on somatosensory-evoked potentials after dermatomal stimulation. *Anesth Analg* 1987;66:34.

36. Malmqvist L, Tryggvason B, Bengtsson M. Sympathetic blockade during extradural analgesia with mepivacaine or bupivacaine. *Acta Anaesthesiol Scand* 1989;33:444.

37. Hopf H, Weissbach B, Peters J. High thoracic segmental epidural anesthesia diminishes sympathetic outflow to the legs, despite restriction of sensory blockade to the upper thorax. *Anesthesiology* 1990;73:882.

38. Stevens R, Artuso J, Kao T, et al. Changes in human plasma catecholamine concentrations during epidural anesthesia depend on the level of the block. *Anesthesiology* 1991;74:1029.

39. Stevens R, Beardsley D, White JL, et al. Does the choice of local anesthetic affect the catecholamine response to stress during epidural anesthesia? *Anesthesiology* 1993;79:1219.

40. Raymond S, Gissen AJ. Mechanisms of differential nerve block. In: Strichartz G, ed. *Local Anesthetics.* New York: Springer-Verlag; 1987:95–164.

41. Fink BR, Cairns AM. Lack of size-related differential sensitivity to equilibrium conduction block among mammalian myelinated axons exposed to lidocaine. *Anesth Analg* 1987;66:948.

42. Fink BR, Cairns AM. Differential use-dependent (frequency-dependent) effects in single mammalian axons: Data and clinical considerations. *Anesthesiology* 1987;67:477.

43. Raymond SA. Subblocking concentrations of local anesthetics: Effects on impulse generation and conduction in single myelinated sciatic nerve axons in frog. *Anesth Analg* 1992;75:906.

44. Wildsmith JAW, Gissen AJ, Gregus J, Covino BG. Differential nerve-blocking activity of aminoester local anesthetics. *Br J Anaesth* 1985;57:612.

45. Torebjork HE, Hallin RG. Perceptual changes accompanying controlled preferential blocking of A and C fiber responses in intact human skin nerves. *Exp Brain Res* 1973;16:321.

46. Mackenzie RA, Burke D, Skuse NF, Lethlean AK. Fiber function and perception during cutaneous nerve block. *J Neurol Neurosurg Psychiatry* 1975;38:865.

47. Franz DN, Perry RS. Mechanisms of differential block among single myelinated and nonmyelinated axons by procaine. *J Physiol* 1974;236:193.

48. Raymond S, Steffensen SC, Gugino LD, Strichartz GR. The role of length of nerve exposed to local anesthetics in impulse blocking action. *Anesth Analg* 1989;68:563.

49. Fink BR. Mechanisms of differential blockade in epidural and subarachnoid anesthesia. *Anesthesiology* 1989;70:851.

50. Woolf CJ, Wiesenfeld-Hallin Z. The systemic administration of local anesthetics produces a selective depression of C-afferent fiber-evoked activity in the spinal cord. *Pain* 1985;23:361.

51. Lai J, Porreca F, Hunter JC, Gold MS. Voltage-gated sodium channels and hyperalgesia. *Ann Rev Pharmacol Toxicol* 2004;44:371.

52. Bach FW, Jensen TS, Kastrup J, et al. The effects of intravenous lidocaine on nociceptive processing in diabetic neuropathy. *Pain* 1990;40:29.

53. Abram SE, Yaksh TL. Systemic lidocaine blocks nerve injury-induced hyperalgesia and nociceptor-driven spinal sensitization in the rat. *Anesthesiology* 1994;80:383.

54. Boas RA, Shahnarian A. Analgesic responses to IV lidocaine. *Br J Anaesth* 1982;54:501.

55. Edwards WT, Habib F, Burney RG, Begin G. Intravenous lidocaine in the management of various chronic pain states. *Reg Anesth* 1985;10:1.

56. Kastrup J, Peterson P, Dejgard A, et al. Intravenous lidocaine infusion: A new treatment for chronic painful diabetic neuropathy? *Pain* 1987;28:69.

57. Marchettini P, Lacerenza M, Marangoni C, et al. Lidocaine test in neuralgia. *Pain* 1992;48:377.

58. Smith RC, Hoppe RB. The patient's story: Integrating the patient- and physician-centered approaches to interviewing. *Ann Intern Med* 1991;115:470.

59. Pickering TG, James GD, Boddie C, et al. How common is white coat hypertension? *JAMA* 1988;259:225.

60. Citron ML. Placebos and principles: A trial of ondansetron. *Ann Intern Med* 1993;118:470.

61. Barnsley L, Lord S, Bogduk N. Comparative local anaesthetic blocks in the diagnosis of cervical zygapophysial joint pain. *Pain* 1993;55:99.

62. Beecher HK. The powerful placebo. *JAMA* 1955;159:1602.

63. Sidel N, Abrams MI. Treatment of chronic arthritis: Results of vaccine therapy with saline injections as controls. *JAMA* 1940;114:1740.

64. Traut EF, Passarelli EW. Study in the controlled therapy of degenerative arthritis. *AMA Arch Intern Med* 1956;98:181.

65. Verdugo R, Ochoa JL. High incidence of placebo responders among chronic neuropathic pain patients. *Ann Neurol* 1991;30:294.

66. Levine JD, Gordon NC, Bornstein JC, Fields HL. Role of pain in placebo analgesia. *Proc Natl Acad Sci USA* 1979;76:3528.

67. Liberman R. An experimental study of the placebo response under three different situations of pain. *J Psychiatr Res* 1964;2:233.

68. Houde RW, Wallenstein MS, Rogers A. Clinical pharmacology of analgesics: A method of assaying analgesic effect. *Clin Pharmacol Ther* 1966;1:163.

69. Kirsch I. Response expectancy as a determinant of experience and behavior. *Am Psychol* 1985;40:1189.

70. Voudouris NJ, Peck CL, Coleman G. The role of conditioning and verbal expectancy in the placebo response. *Pain* 1990;43:121.

71. Voudouris NJ, Peck CL, Coleman G. Conditioned placebo responses. *J Per Soc Psychol* 1985;48:47.

72. Kantor TG, Sunshine A, Laska E, et al. Oral analgesic studies: Pentazocine hydrochloride, codeine, aspirin, and placebo and their influence on response to placebo. *Clin Pharmacol Ther* 1966;7:447.

73. Laska E, Sunshine A. Anticipation of analgesia: A placebo effect. *Headache* 1973;13:1.

74. Grevert P, Albert LH, Goldstein A. Partial antagonism of placebo analgesia by naloxone. *Pain* 1983;16:129.

75. Levine JD, Gordon NC, Fields HL. The mechanism of placebo analgesia. *Lancet* 1978;2:654.

76. Lipman JJ, Miller BE, Mays KS, et al. Peak B endorphin concentration in cerebrospinal fluid: Reduced in chronic pain patients and increased during the placebo response. *Psychopharmacology* 1990;102:112.

77. Evans FJ. The placebo response in pain reduction. In: Bonica JJ, ed. *Advances in Neurology,* Vol. 4. New York: Raven Press; 1984;289–300.

78. Fine PG, Roberts WJ, Gillette RG, Child TR. Slowly developing placebo responses confound tests of intravenous phentolamine to determine mechanisms underlying idiopathic chronic low back pain. *Pain* 1994;56:235.

79. Verdugo R, Rosenblum S, Ochoa J. Phentolamine sympathetic blocks mislead diagnosis. *Abstr Soc Neurosci* 1991;17:107.

80. Gracely RH, Dubner R, Deeter WR, Wolskee PJ. Clinical expectations influence placebo analgesia. *Lancet* 1985;1:43.

81. Benson H, McCallie DP. Angina pectoris and the placebo effect. *N Engl J Med* 1979;300:1424.

82. Devor M. What's in a laser beam for pain therapy? *Pain* 1990;43:139.

83. Goodwin JS, Goodwin JM, Vogel AV. Knowledge and use of placebos by house officers and nurses. *Ann Intern Med* 1979;91:106.

84. Rosenzweig P, Brohier S, Zipfel A. The placebo effect in healthy volunteers: Influence of experimental conditions on the adverse events profile during phase I trials. *Clin Pharmacol Ther* 1993;54:578.

85. Dhume VG, Agshikar NV, Diniz RS. Placebo-induced side effects in healthy volunteers. *Clinician* 1975;39:289.

86. Edwards E. Operative anatomy of the lumbar sympathetic chain. *Angiology* 1951;2:184.

87. MacGibbon B, Farfan HF. A radiologic survey of various configurations of the lumbar spine. *Spine* 1979;4:258.

88. Quinnell RC, Stockdale HR. The use of in vivo lumbar discography to assess the clinical significance of the position of the intercrestal line. *Spine* 1983;8:305.

89. Reimann AF, Anson BJ. Vertebral level of termination of the spinal cord with report of a case of sacral cord. *Anat Rec* 1944;88:127.

90. Larsen JL, Olsen KO. Radiographic anatomy of the distal dural sac. *Acta Radiol* 1991;32:214.

91. Ferrer-Brechner T, Brechner VL. Accuracy of needle placement during diagnostic and therapeutic nerve blocks. *Adv Pain Res Ther* 1976;1:679.

92. Gielen MJ, Slappendel R, Merx JL. Asymmetric onset of sympathetic blockade in epidural anesthesia shows no relation to epidural catheter position. *Acta Anaesthesiol Scand* 1991;35:81.

93. Moore DC. Guest discussion. *Anesth Analg* 1970;49:916.

94. Sjogren P, Gefke K, Banning A, et al. Lumbar epidurography and epidural analgesia in cancer patients. *Pain* 1989;36:305.

95. Van Gessel EF, Forster A, Gamulin Z. Continuous spinal anesthesia: Where do spinal catheters go? *Anesth Analg* 1993;76:1004.

96. Bergman RA, Thompson SA, Afifi A, Saadeh FA. *Compendium of Human Anatomic Variation.* Baltimore: Urban and Schwarzenberg, 1988.

97. Willis TA. An analysis of vertebral anomalies. *Am J Surg* 1929;6:163.

98. Kikuchi S, Hasue M, Nishiyama K, Ito T. Anatomic and clinical studies of radicular symptoms. *Spine* 1984;9:23.

PART IV: PAIN MANAGEMENT

99. Nitta H, Tajima T, Sugiyama H, Moriyama A. Study of dermatomes by means of selective lumbar spinal nerve block. *Spine* 1993;13:1782.
100. Neidre A, MacNab I. Anomalies of the lumbosacral nerve roots: Review of 16 cases and classification. *Spine* 1983;8:294.
101. Pallie W. The intersegmental anastomoses of posterior spinal rootlets and their significance. *J Neurosurg* 1959;16:188.
102. Pallie W, Manuel JK. Intersegmental anastomoses between dorsal spinal rootlets in some vertebrates. *Acta Anat* 1968;70:341.
103. Horwitz MT. The anatomy of (A) the lumbosacral nerve plexus: Its relation to variations of vertebral segmentation, and (B), the posterior sacral nerve plexus. *Anat Rec* 1939;74:91.
104. Kerr AT. The brachial plexus of nerves in man, the variations in its formation and branches. *Am J Anat* 1918;23:285.
105. Bonica JJ. *The Management of Pain*, 2nd ed. Philadelphia: Lea and Febiger; 1990:133–146.
106. Young A, Getty J, Jackson A, et al. Variations in the pattern of muscle innervation by the L5 and S1 nerve roots. *Spine* 1983;6:616.
107. Van Rhede van der Kloot E, Drukker J, Lemmens HAJ, Greep JM. The high thoracic sympathetic nerve system: Its anatomic variability. *J Surg Res* 1986;40:112.
108. Campero M, Verdugo RJ, Ochoa JL. Vasomotor innervation of the skin of the hand: A contribution to the study of human anatomy. *J Anat* 1993;182:361.
109. Hoffert MJ, Greenberg RP, Wolskee PJ, et al. Abnormal and collateral innervations of sympathetic and peripheral sensory fields associated with a case of causalgia. *Pain* 1984;20:1.
110. Janig W. Neuronal mechanisms of pain with special emphasis on visceral and deep somatic pain. *Acta Neurochir Suppl* 1987;385:16.
111. Janig W. The sympathetic nervous system in pain: Physiology and pathophysiology. In: Stanton-Hicks M, ed. *Pain and the Sympathetic Nervous System*. Boston: Kluwer Academic Publishers; 1990:17–89.
112. de Sousa PA. The innervation of the veins: Its role in pain, venospasm and collateral circulation. *Surgery* 1946;19:731.
113. Ochsner A, DeBakey M. Treatment of thrombophlebitis by novocaine block of sympathetics. *Surgery* 1939;5:491.
114. Freeman LW, Shumacker HB, Radigan LR. A functional study of afferent fibers in peripheral sympathetic nerves. *Surgery* 1950;28:274.
115. Hyndman OR, Wolkin J. The sympathetic nervous system influence on sensibility to heat and cold and to certain types of pain. *Arch Neurol Psychiatry* 1941;46:1006.
116. Kiaer S. Afferent pain paths in man running from the spongiosa in the femoral head and passing through the lumbar sympathetic ganglia. *Acta Orthop Scand* 1950;19:383.
117. Schott GD. Visceral afferents: Their contribution to "sympathetic dependent" pain. *Brain* 1994;117:397.
118. Bogduk N. The innervation of the lumbar spine. *Spine* 1983;8:286.
119. Groen GJ, Baljet B, Drukker J. Nerves and nerve plexuses of the human vertebral column. *Am J Anat* 1990;188:282.
120. Groen GJ, Baljet B, Drukker J. The innervation of the spinal dura mater: Anatomy and clinical implications. *Acta Neurochir (Wien)* 1988;92:39.
121. Kojima Y, Maeda T, Arai R, Shichicawa K. Nerve supply to the posterior longitudinal ligament and the intervertebral disc of the rat vertebral column as studied by acetylcholinesterase histochemistry. II. Regional differences in the distribution of the nerve fibers and their origins. *Acta Anat* 1990;169:247.
122. Jain S, Shah N, Bedford R. Needle position for paravertebral and sympathetic nerve blocks: Radiologic confirmation is needed. *Anesth Analg* 1991;72:S125.
123. Renfrew D, Moore T, Kathol M, et al. Correct placement of epidural steroid injections: Fluoroscopic guidance and contrast administration. *Am J Neuroradiol* 1991;12:1003.
124. White A, Derby R, Wynne G. Epidural injections for the diagnosis and treatment of low-back pain. *Spine* 1980;5:78.
125. McCall IW, Park WM, O'Brien JP. Induced pain referral from posterior lumbar elements in normal subjects. *Spine* 1979;4:441.
126. Mooney V, Robertson J. The facet syndrome. *Clin Orthop Relat Res* 1976;115:149.
127. Ochoa JL, Yarnitsky D. Mechanical hyperalgesias in neuropathic pain patients: Dynamic and static subtypes. *Ann Neurol* 1993;33:465.
128. Hunt CC. On the nature of vibration receptors in the hind limb of the cat. *J Physiol* 1961;155:175.
129. Sinclair DC, Hinshaw JR. A comparison of the sensory dissociation produced by procaine and by limb compression. *Brain* 1950;73:480.
130. Bengtsson M, Löfström JB, Malmqvist L-Å. Skin conduction changes during spinal analgesia. *Acta Anaesthesiol Scand* 1985;29:67.
131. Lindberg L, Wallin BG. Sympathetic skin nerve discharges in relation to amplitude of skin resistance responses. *Psychophysiology* 1981;18:268.
132. Kim JM, Arakawa K, VonLintel T. Use of pulse-wave monitor as a measurement of diagnostic sympathetic block and of surgical sympathectomy. *Anesth Analg* 1975;54:289.
133. Meijer J, deLange J, Ros H. Skin pulse-wave monitoring during lumbar epidural and spinal anesthesia. *Anesth Analg* 1988;67:356.
134. Bengtsson M, Nilsson GE, Löfström JB. The effect of spinal analgesia on skin blood flow, evaluated by laser Doppler flowmetry. *Acta Anaesthesiol Scand* 1983;17:206.
135. Benzon H, Cheng S, Avram M, Molloy R. Sign of complete sympathetic blockade: Sweat test or sympathogalvanic response. *Anesth Analg* 1985;64:415.
136. Carron H, Litwiller R. Stellate ganglion block. *Anesth Analg* 1975;54:567.
137. Hardy P. Stellate ganglion block with bupivacaine: Minimum effective concentration of bupivacaine and the effect of added potassium. *Anaesthesia* 1989;44:398.
138. Hogan Q, Taylor ML, Goldstein M, et al. Success rates in producing sympathetic blockade by paratracheal injection. *Clin J Pain* 1994;10:139.
139. Kawarai M, Koss MC. Neurogenic cutaneous vasodilation in the cat forepaw. *J Auton Nerv Syst* 1992;37:39.
140. Ochoa JL, Yarnitsky D, Marchettini P, et al. Interactions between sympathetic vasoconstrictor outflow and C nociceptor-induced antidromic vasodilatation. *Pain* 1993;54:191.
141. Sigurdsson A, Maixner W. Effects of experimental and clinical noxious counterirritants on pain perception. *Pain* 1994;57:265.
142. McNeal BJ, Keeler E, Adelstein SJ. Primer on certain elements of medical decision-making. *N Engl J Med* 1975;293:211.
143. Hogan Q, Dotson R, Erickson S, et al. Local anesthetic myotoxicity: A case and review. *Anesthesiology* 1994;80:942.
144. Simons DG, Travell JG. The myofascial genesis of pain. *Postgrad Med* 1952;11:425.
145. Hatch JP, Moore PJ, Cyr-Provost M, et al. The use of electromyography and muscle palpation in the diagnosis of tension-type headache with and without pericranial muscle involvement. *Pain* 1992;49:175.
146. Hubbard DR, Berkoff GM. Myofascial trigger points show spontaneous needle EMG activity. *Spine* 1993;18:1803.
147. Kuan TS, Hsieh YL, Chen SM, et al. The myofascial trigger point region: Correlation between the degree of irritability and the prevalence of endplate noise. *Am J Phys Med Rehabil* 2007;86:183.
148. McCain GA, Scudds RA. The concept of primary fibromyalgia (fibrositis): Clinical value, relation and significance to other musculoskeletal pain syndromes. *Pain* 1988;33:237.
149. Kraus H, Fischer AA. Diagnosis and treatment of myofascial pain. *Mt Sinai J Med* 1991;58:235.
150. Krishnan SK, Benzon HT, Siddiqui T, Canlas B. Pain on intramuscular injection of bupivacaine, ropivacaine, with and without dexamethasone. *Reg Anesth Pain Med* 2000;25:615.
151. Foster AH, Carlson BM. Myotoxicity of local anesthetics and regeneration of the damaged muscle fibers. *Anesth Analg* 1980;59:727.
152. Nelson LS, Hoffman RS. Intrathecal injection: Unusual complication of trigger-point injection therapy. *Ann Emerg Med* 1998;32:506.
153. Hamada H, Moriwaki K, Shiroyama K, et al. Myofascial pain in patients with postthoracotomy pain syndrome. *Reg Anesth Pain Med* 2000;25:302.
154. Sist T, Miner M, Lema M. Characteristics of postradical neck pain syndrome: A report of 25 case. *J Pain Symptom Manage* 1999;18:95.
155. Mascia P, Brown BR, Friedman S. Toothache of nonodontogenic origin: A case report. *J Endod* 2003;29:608.
156. Lewit K. The needle effect in the relief of myofascial pain. *Pain* 1979;6:83.
157. Ready LB, Kozody R, Barsa JE, Murphy TM. Trigger point injections vs. jet injection in the treatment of myofascial pain. *Pain* 1989;15:201.
158. Noordenbos W, Wall PD. Implications of the failure of nerve resection and graft to cure chronic pain produced by nerve lesions. *J Neurol Neurosurg Psychiatry* 1981;44:1068.
159. Green DP. Diagnostic and therapeutic value of carpal tunnel injection. *J Hand Surg* 1984;9A:850.
160. Plancarte R, Velazquez R, Patt RB. Neurolytic blocks of the sympathetic axis. In: Patt RB, ed. *Cancer Pain*. Philadelphia: J. B. Lippincott; 1993:377–425.
161. Abram SE, Boas RA. Sympathetic and visceral nerve blocks. In: Benumof JL, ed. *Clinical Proceedings in Anesthesia Intensive Care*. Philadelphia: J. B. Lippincott; 1992:796–805.
162. Plancarte R, Amescua C, Patt RB, Aldrete JA. Superior hypogastric plexus block for pelvic cancer pain. *Anesthesiology* 1990;73:236.
163. Solonen KA. The sacroiliac joint in light of anatomical, roentgenological, and clinical studies. *Acta Orthop Scand* 1957;27(S):1.
164. Vleeming A, Stoeckart R, Volkers ACW, Snijders CJ. Relation between form and function in the sacroiliac joint. Part I: Clinical anatomic aspects. *Spine* 1990;15:130.
165. Bowen V, Cassidy JD. Macroscopic and microscopic anatomy of the sacroiliac joint from embryonic life until the eighth decade. *Spine* 1981;6:620.
166. Fortin JD, Dwyer AP, West S, Pier J. Sacroiliac joint: Pain referral maps upon applying a new injection/arthrography technique. Part I: Asymptomatic volunteers. *Spine* 1994;19:1475.
167. Dreyfuss P, Dryer S, Griffin J, et al. Positive sacroiliac screening tests in asymptomatic adults. *Spine* 1994;19:1138.
168. Russell AS, Maksymowych W, LeClerq S. Clinical examination of the sacroiliac joints: A prospective study. *Arthritis Rheum* 1981;24:1575.

169. Laslett M, Aprill CN, McDonald B, Youngk SB. Diagnosis of sacroiliac joint pain: Validity of individual provocation tests and composites of tests. *Man Ther* 2005;10:207.

170. Berthelot JM, Labat JJ, Le Goff B, et al. Provocative sacroiliac joint maneuvers and sacroiliac joint block are unreliable for diagnosing sacroiliac joint pain. *Rev Rheum* 2006;73:17.

171. Bonica JJ. *The Management of Pain*. Philadelphia: Lea and Febiger; 1953: 1200.

172. Hendrix RW, Lin PP, Kane WJ. Simplified aspiration or injection technique for the sacroiliac joint. *J Bone Joint Surg* 1982;64A:1249.

173. Schwarzer AC, Aprill CN, Bogduk N. The sacroiliac joint in chronic low back pain. *Spine* 1995;20:31.

174. Chou LH, Slipman CW, Bhagia SM, et al. Inciting events initiating injection-proven sacroiliac joint syndrome. *Pain Med* 2004;5:26.

175. Ferrante FM, King LF, Roche EA, et al. Radiofrequency sacroiliac joint denervation for sacroiliac syndrome. *Reg Anesth Pain Med* 2001;26:137.

176. Pino CA, Hoeft MA, Hofsess C, Rathmell JP. Morphologic analysis of bipolar radiofrequency lesions: Implications for treatment of the sacroiliac joint. *Reg Anesth Pain Med* 2005;30:335.

177. Bogduk N, Engel R. The menisci of the lumbar zygapophyseal joints. *Spine* 1984;9:454.

178. Wang ZL, Yu S, Haughton VM. Age-related changes in the lumbar facet joints. *Clin Anat* 1989;2:55.

179. Giles LGF, Taylor JR. Human zygapophyseal joint capsule and synovial fold innervation. *Br J Rheumatol* 1987;26:93.

180. McLain RF. Mechancoreceptor endings in human cervical facet joints. *Spine* 1994;19:195.

181. Bogduk N, Long DM. The anatomy of the so-called "articular nerves" and their relationship to facet denervation in the treatment of low-back pain. *J Neurosurg* 1979;51:172.

182. Bogduk N. The clinical anatomy of cervical dorsal rami. *Spine* 1982;4:319.

183. Cavanaugh JM, El-Bohy A, Hardy WN, et al. Sensory innervation of soft tissues of the lumbar spine in the rat. *J Orthop Res* 1989;7:378.

184. Yamashita T, Cavanaugh JM, El-Bohy AA, et al. Mechanosensitive afferent units in the lumbar facet joint. *J Bone Joint Surg* 1990;72(A):865.

185. Dwyer A, Aprill C, Bogduk N. Cervical zygapophyseal joint pain patterns I: A study in normal volunteers. *Spine* 1990;15:453.

186. Dreyfuss P, Michaelsen M, Fletcher D. Atlanto-occipital and lateral atlanto-axial joint pain patterns. *Spine* 1994;19:1125.

187. El-Bohy A, Cavanaugh JM, Getchell ML, et al. Localization of substance P and neurofilament immunoreactive fibers in the lumbar facet joint capsule and supraspinous ligament of the rabbit. *Brain Res* 1988;460:379.

188. Dunlop RB, Adams MA, Hutton WS-C. Disc space narrowing and the lumbar facet joints. *J Bone Joint Surg* 1984;66(B):706.

189. Giles LGF, Taylor JR, Cockson A. Human zygapophyseal joint synovial folds. *Acta Anat* 1986;126:110.

190. Giles LGF, Harvey AR. Immunohistochemical demonstration of nociceptors in the capsule and synovial folds of human zygapophyseal joints. *Br J Rheumatol* 1987;26:362.

191. Gronblad M, Korkala O, Konttinen YT, et al. Silver impregnation and immunohistochemical study of nerves in lumbar facet joint plical tissue. *Spine* 1991;16:34.

192. Bogduk N. The innervation of the lumbar spine. *Spine* 1983;8:286.

193. Bogduk N, Tynan W, Wilson AS. The nerve supply to the human lumbar intervertebral discs. *Acta Anat* 1981;132:39.

194. Edgar MA, Ghadially JA. Innervation of the lumbar spine. *Clin Orthop Relat Res* 1976;115:35.

195. Forsythe WB, Ghoshal NG. Innervation of the canine thoracolumbar vertebral column. *Anat Rec* 1984;208:57.

196. Stilwell DL. The nerve supply of the vertebral column and its associated structures in the monkey. *Anat Rec* 1956;125:139.

197. Fernstrom U. A discographical study of ruptured lumbar intervertebral discs. *Acta Chir Scand* 1960;S258:10.

198. Hirsch C, Ingelmark B, Miller M. The anatomical basis for low back pain. *Acta Orthop* 1963;33:1.

199. Kellgren JH. On the distribution of pain arising from deep somatic structures with charts of segmental pain areas. *Clin Sci* 1939;4:35.

200. Kuslich SD, Ulstrom CL. The tissue origin of low back pain and sciatica: A report of pain response to tissue stimulation during operations on the lumbar spine using local anesthesia. *Orthop Clin North Am* 1991;22:181.

201. Murphey F. Sources and patterns of pain in disc disease. *Clin Neurosurg* 1968;15:343.

202. Smyth MJ, Wright V. Sciatica and the intervertebral disc. *J Bone Joint Surg* 1958;40(A):1401.

203. Wiberg G. Back pain in relation to the nerve supply of the intervertebral disc. *Acta Orthop* 1949;19:211.

204. Helbig T, Lee CK. The lumbar facet syndrome. *Spine* 1988;13:61.

205. Wiesel SW, Tsourmas N, Feffer HI, et al. A study of computer-assisted tomography. I. The incidence of positive CAT scans in an asymptomatic group of patients. *Spine* 1984;9:549.

206. Murtagh FR. Computed tomography and fluoroscopy-guided anesthesia and steroid injection in facet syndrome. *Spine* 1988;13:686.

207. Butler D, Trafimow JH, Andersson GBJ, et al. Discs degenerate before facets. *Spine* 1990;15:111.

208. Bogduk N, Aprill C. On the nature of neck pain, discography, and cervical zygapophyseal joint blocks. *Pain* 1993;54:213.

209. Epstein JA, Epstein BS, Lavine LS, et al. Lumbar nerve root compression at the intervertebral foramina caused by arthritis of the posterior facets. *J Neurosurg* 1973;39:362.

210. Murphy WA. The facet syndrome. *Radiology* 1984;151:533.

211. Aprill C, Bogduk N. The prevalence of cervical zygapophyseal joint pain: A first approximation. *Spine* 1992;17:744.

212. Barnsley L, Bogduk N. Medial branch blocks are specific for the diagnosis of cervical zygapophyseal joint pain. *Reg Anesth* 1993;18:242.

213. Bogduk N, Marsland A. The cervical zygapophysial joints as a source of neck pain. *Spine* 1988;13:610.

214. Hove B, Gyldensted C. Cervical analgesic facet joint arthrography. *Neuroradiology* 1990;32:456.

215. Roy DF, Fleury J, Fontaine SB, Dussault R. Clinical evaluation of cervical facet joint infiltration. *J Can Assoc Radiol* 1988;39:118.

216. Carette S, Marcoux S, Truchon R, et al. A controlled trial of corticosteroid injection into facet joints for chronic low back pain. *N Engl J Med* 1991;325:1002.

217. Carrera GF. Lumbar facet joint injection in low back pain and sciatica: Preliminary results. *Radiology* 1980;137:665.

218. Destouet JM, Gilula LA, Murphey WA, Monsees B. Lumbar facet joint injection: Indication, technique, clinical correlation, and preliminary results. *Radiology* 1982;145:321.

219. Fairbank JCT, McCall IW, O'Brian JP. Apophyseal injection of local anesthetic as a diagnostic aid in primary low-back pain syndromes. *Spine* 1981;6:598.

220. Moran R, O'Connell D, Walsh MG. The diagnostic value of facet joint injections. *Spine* 1988;13:1407.

221. Raymond J, Dumas J-M. Intra-articular facet block: Diagnostic test or therapeutic procedure? *Radiology* 1984;151:333.

222. Marks RC, Houston T, Thulbourne T. Facet joint injection and facet nerve block: A randomised comparison in 86 patients with chronic low back pain. *Pain* 1992;49:325.

223. Jackson RP, Jacobs RR, Montesano PX. Facet joint injection in low-back pain: A prospective statistical study. *Spine* 1988;13:966.

224. Lora J, Long D. So-called facet denervation in the management of intractable back pain. *Spine* 1976;2:121.

225. Marks R. Distribution of pain provoked from lumbar facet joints and related structures during diagnostic spinal infiltration. *Pain* 1989;39:37.

226. Loh L, Nathan PW, Schott GD, Wilson PG. Effects of regional guanethidine in certain painful states. *J Neurol Neurosurg Psychiatry* 1980;43:446.

227. Schwarzer AC, Derby R, Aprill CN, et al. The value of the provocation response in lumbar zygapophyseal joint injections. *Clin J Pain* 1994;10:309.

228. Dory MA. Arthrography of the cervical facet joints. *Radiology* 1983;148:379.

229. Dory MA. Arthrography of the lumbar facet joints. *Radiology* 1981;140:23.

230. Maldague B, Mathurin P, Malghem J. Facet joint arthrography in lumbar spondylosis. *Radiology* 1981;140:29.

231. Ghelman B, Doherty JH. Demonstration of spondylolysis by arthrography of the apophyseal joint. *AJR Am J Roentgenol* 1978;130:986.

232. McCormick CC, Taylor JR, Twomey LT. Facet joint arthrography in lumbar spondylolysis: Anatomic basis for spread of contrast medium. *Radiology* 1989;171:193.

233. Goldstone JC, Pennant JH. Spinal anaesthesia following facet joint injection. *Anaesthesia* 1987;42:754.

234. Schwarzer AC, Aprill CN, Derby R, et al. The false-positive rate of uncontrolled diagnostic blocks of the lumbar zygapophysial joints. *Pain* 1994;58:195.

235. Schwarzer AC, Aprill CN, Derby R, et al. Clinical features of patients with pain stemming from the lumbar zygapophyseal joints. *Spine* 1994;19:1132.

236. Lynch MC, Taylor JF. Facet joint injection for low back pain. *J Bone Joint Surg* 1986;68(B):138.

237. Lilius G, Laasonen EM, Myllynen P, et al. Lumbar facet joint syndrome: A randomized clinical trial. *J Bone Joint Surg* 1989;71(B):681.

238. Barnsley L, Lord S, Wallis B, Bogduk N. False-positive rates of cervical zygapophyseal joint blocks. *Clin J Pain* 1993;9:124.

239. North RB, Han M, Zahurak M, Kidd DH. Radiofrequency lumbar facet denervation: Analysis of prognostic factors. *Pain* 1994;57:77.

240. Slipman CW, Bhat AL, Gilchrist FR, et al. A critical review of the evidence for the use of zygapophysial injections and radiofrequency denervation in the treatment of low back pain. *Spine J* 2003;3:310.

241. Jackson RP. The facet syndrome. *Clin OrthopRelat Res* 1992;279:110.

242. Gorbach C, Schmid MR, Elfering A, et al. Therapeutic efficacy of facet joint blocks. *AJR Am J Roentgenol* 2006;186:1228.

243. Pneumaticos SG, Chatziioannou SN, Hipp JA, et al. Low back pain: Prediction of short-term outcome of facet joint injection with bone scintigraphy. *Radiology* 2006;238:693.

244. Hitselberger WE, Witten RM. Abnormal myelograms in asymptomatic patients. *J Neurosurg* 1968;28:204.

PART IV: PAIN MANAGEMENT

245. Boden SD, Davis DO, Dina TS, et al. Abnormal magnetic-resonance scans of the lumbar spine in asymptomatic subjects. *J Bone Joint Surg* 1990;72(A):403.

246. Jensen MC, Brant-Zawadzki MN, Obuchowski N, et al. Magnetic resonance imaging of the lumbar spine in people without back pain. *N Engl J Med* 1994;331:69.

247. Powel MC, Wilson M, Szypryt P, et al. Prevalence of lumbar disc degeneration observed by magnetic resonance in symptomless women. *Lancet* 1986;2:1366.

248. Weinreb JC, Wolbarsht LB, Cohen JM, et al. Prevalence of lumbosacral intervertebral disk abnormalities on MR images in pregnant and asymptomatic nonpregnant women. *Radiology* 1989;170:125.

249. Collis JS, Gardner WJ. Lumbar discography: An analysis of one thousand cases. *J Neurosurg* 1962;19:452.

250. Simmons EH, Segil C. An evaluation of discography in the localization of symptomatic levels in discogenic disease of the spine. *Clin Orthop Relat Res* 1975;108:57.

251. Troisier O. An accurate method for lumbar disc puncture using a single channel intensifier. *Spine* 1990;15:222.

252. Quinnell RC, Stockdale HR, Harmon B. Pressure standardized lumbar discography. *Br J Radiol* 1980;53:1031.

253. Adams MA, Dolan P, Hutton WC. The stages of disc degeneration as revealed by discograms. *J Bone Joint Surg* 1986;68(B):36.

254. Simmons JW, Emery SF, McMillin JN, et al. Awake discography: A comparison with magnetic resonance imaging. *Spine* 1991;16:S216.

255. Videman T, Malmivaara A, Mooney V. The value of the axial view in assessing discograms: An experimental study with cadavers. *Spine* 1987;12:299.

256. Yu S, Haughton VM, Sether LA, Wagner M. Comparison of MR and discography in detecting radial tears of the anulus: A postmortem study. *AJNR Am J Neuroradiol* 1989;10:1077.

257. Friedman J, Goldner MZ. Discography in evaluation of lumbar disk lesions. *Radiology* 1955;65:653.

258. Gibson MJ, Buckley J, Mulholland RC, Worthington BS. Magnetic resonance imaging and discography in the diagnosis of disc degeneration. *J Bone Joint Surg* 1986;68(B):369.

259. Colhoun E, McCall IW, Williams L, Cassar Pullicino VN. Provocation discography as a guide to planning operations on the spine. *J Bone Joint Surg* 1988;70(B):267.

260. Holt EP. Fallacy of cervical discography. *JAMA* 1964;188:799.

261. Holt EP. The question of lumbar discography. *J Bone Joint Surg* 1968;50(A):720.

262. Walsh TR, Weinstein JN, Spratt KF, et al. Lumbar discography in normal subjects. *J Bone Joint Surg* 1990;72(A):1081.

263. Grubb SA, Lipscomb HJ, Guilford WB. The relative value of lumbar roentgenograms, metrizamide myelography, and discography in the assessment of patients with chronic low-back syndrome. *Spine* 1987;12:282.

264. Vanharanta H, Sachs BL, Spivey MA, et al. The relationship of pain provocation to lumbar disc deterioration as seen by CT/discography. *Spine* 1987;12:295.

265. Zucherman J, Derby R, Hsu K, et al. Normal magnetic resonance imaging with abnormal discography. *Spine* 1988;13:1355.

266. Horton WC, Daftari T. Which disc as visualized by magnetic resonance imaging is actually a source of pain? *Spine* 1992;17:S164.

267. Carragee EJ, Lincoln T, Parmar VS, Alamin T. A gold standard evaluation of the "discogenic pain" diagnosis as determined by provocative discography. *Spine* 2006;31: 2115.

268. Appleby D, Andersson G, Totta M. Meta-analysis of the efficacy and safety of intradiscal electrotherapy (IDET). *Pain Med* 2006;7:308.

269. Freeman BJ, Fraser RD, Cain CM, et al. A randomized, double-blind, controlled trial: Intradiscal electrothermal therapy versus placebo for the treatment of chronic discogenic low back pain. *Spine* 2005;30:2369.

270. Kapural L, Hayek S, Malak O, et al. Intradiscal thermal annuloplasty versus intradiscal radiofrequency ablation for the treatment of discogenic pain: A prospective matched control trial. *Pain Med* 2005;6:425.

271. Schutz H, Lougheed WM, Wortzman G, Awerbuck BG. Intervertebral nerve-root in the investigation of chronic lumbar disc disease. *Can J Surg* 1973;16:217.

272. Woolf CJ, Shortland P, Coggeshall RE. Peripheral nerve injury triggers central sprouting of myelinated afferents. *Nature* 1992;355:75.

273. Keegan JJ, Garrett FD. The segmental distribution of the cutaneous nerves in the limbs of man. *Anat Rec* 1948;102:409.

274. Foerster O. The dermatomes in man. *Brain* 1933;56:1.

275. Derby R, Kine G, Saal JA, et al. Response to steroid and duration of radicular pain as predictors of surgical outcome. *Spine* 1992;17:S176.

276. Dooley JF, McBroom RJ, Taguchi T, MacNab I. Nerve root infiltration in the diagnosis of radicular pain. *Spine* 1988;13:79.

277. Haueisen DC, Smith BS, Myers SR, Pryce ML. The diagnostic accuracy of spinal nerve injection studies. *Clin Orthop Relat Res* 1985;198:179.

278. Krempen JS, Smith B, DeFreest LJ. Selective nerve root infiltration for the evaluation of sciatica. *Orthop Clin North Am* 1975;6:311.

279. Tajima T, Furukawa K, Kuramochi E. Selective lumbosacral radiculography and block. *Spine* 1980;5:68.

280. Stanley D, McLaren MI, Euinton HA, Getty CJM. A prospective study of nerve root infiltration in the diagnosis of sciatica. *Spine* 1990;15:540.

281. Loeser JD. Dorsal rhizotomy for the relief of chronic pain. *J Neurosurg* 1972;36:745.

282. Onofrio BM, Campa HK. Evaluation of rhizotomy: Review of 12 years' experience. *J Neurosurg* 1972;36:751.

283. North RB, Kidd DH, Campbell JN, Long DM. Dorsal root ganglionectomy for failed back surgery syndrome: A 5-year follow-up study. *J Neurosurg* 1991;74:236.

284. van Kleef M, Liem L, Lousberg R, et al. Radiofrequency lesion adjacent to the dorsal root ganglion for cervicobrachial pain: A prospective, double blind randomized study. *Neurosurgery* 1996;38:1127.

285. Van Zundert J, Harney D, Joosten EAJ, et al. The role of the dorsal root ganglion in cervical radicular pain: Diagnosis, pathophysiology, and rationale for treatment. *Reg Anesth Pain Med* 2006;31:152.

286. DePalma MJ, Bhargava A, Slipman CW. A critical appraisal of the evidence for selective nerve root injection in the treatment of lumbar radiculopathy. *Arch Phys Med Rehabil* 2005;86:1477.

287. Warfield CA, Crews DA. Epidural steroid injection as a predictor of surgical outcome. *Surg Gynecol Obstet* 1987;164:457.

288. Hunter CR, Mayfield FH. Role of the upper cervical roots in the production of pain in the head. *Am J Surg* 1949;78:743.

289. Bogduk N. The anatomy of occipital neuralgia. *Clin Exp Neurol* 1981;17:167.

290. Weinberger LM. Cervico-occipital pain and its surgical treatment: The myth of the bony millstones. *Am J Surg* 1968;135:243.

291. Vital JM, Dautheribes M, Baspeyre H, et al. An anatomic and dynamic study of the greater occipital nerve (n. of Arnold). *Surg Radiol Anat* 1989;11:205.

292. Bovim G, Berg R, Dale LG. Cervicogenic headache: Anesthetic blockades of cervical nerves (C2-C5) and facet joint (C2-C3). *Pain* 1992;49:315.

293. Sjaastad O, Fredricksen TA, Pfaffenrath V. Cervicogenic headache: Diagnostic criteria. *Headache* 1990;30:725.

294. Bovim G, Bonamico L, Fredriksen TA, et al. Topographic variations in the peripheral course of the greater occipital nerve. *Spine* 1991;16:475.

295. Edmeads J. The cervical spine and headache. *Neurology* 1988;38:1874.

296. Pfaffenrath V, Dandekar R, Pollmann W. Cervicogenic headache: The clinical picture, radiologic findings and hypotheses of its pathophysiology. *Headache* 1987;27:495.

297. Campbell DG, Parsons CM. Referred head pain and its concomitants. *J Nerv Ment Dis* 1944;99:544.

298. Cyriax J. Rheumatic headache. *Br Med J* 1938;2:1367.

299. Feinstein B, Langton JNK, Jameson RM, Schiller F. Experiments on pain referred from deep somatic tissues. *J Bone Joint Surg* 1954;36(A):981.

300. Bovim G, Fredriksen TA, Stolt-Nielsen A, Sjaastad O. Neurolysis of the greater occipital nerve in cervicogenic headache: A follow-up study. *Headache* 1992;32:175.

301. Mayfield FH. Neurosurgical aspects: Symposium on cervical trauma. *Clin Neurosurg* 1955;2:83.

302. Blume H, Kakolewski J, Richardson R, Rojas C. Radiofrequency denaturation in occipital pain: Results in 450 cases. *Appl Neurophysiol* 1982;45:543.

303. Bovim G, Sand T. Cervicogenic headache, migraine without aura and tension-type headache: Diagnostic blockade of greater occipital and supraorbital nerves. *Pain* 1992;51:43.

304. Kerr FWL. Structural relation of the trigeminal spinal tract to upper cervical roots and the solitary nucleus in the cat. *Exp Neurol* 1961;4:134.

305. Kerr FWL, Olafson RA. Trigeminal and cervical volleys. *Arch Neurol* 1961;5:171.

306. Hogan Q. The sympathetic nervous system in postherpetic neuralgia. *Reg Anesth* 1993;18:271.

307. Groen GJ, Baljet B, Boekelaar AB, Drukker J. Branches of the thoracic sympathetic trunk in the human fetus. *Anat Embryol* 1987;176:401.

308. Kirgis H, Kuntz A. Inconstant sympathetic neural pathways. *Arch Surg* 1942;44:95.

309. Hoffman H. An analysis of the sympathetic trunk and rami in the cervical and upper thoracic regions in man. *Ann Surg* 1957;145:94.

310. Kimmel D. Rami communicantes of cervical nerves and the vertebral plexus in the human embryo. *Anat Rec* 1955;121:321.

311. Sheehan D. On the innervation of the blood vessels of the upper extremity: Some anatomical considerations. *Br J Surg* 1932;20:412.

312. Alexander W, Kuntz A, Henderson W, Ehrlich E. Sympathetic ganglion cells in ventral nerve roots: Their relation to sympathectomy. *Science* 1949;109:484.

313. Van Buskirk C. Nerves in the vertebral canal: Their relation to the sympathetic innervation of the upper extremities. *Arch Surg* 1941;43:427.

314. Hogan Q, Erickson S. MR imaging of the stellate ganglion: Normal appearance. *Am J Roentgenol* 1992;158:655.

315. Guntamukkala M, Hardy PAJ. Spread of injectate after stellate ganglion block in man: An anatomical study. *Br J Anaesth* 1991;66:643.

316. Hogan Q, Erickson S, Haddox JD, Abram S. The spread of solutions during "stellate ganglion" blockade. *Reg Anesth* 1992;17:78.

317. Cowley RA, Yeager GH. Anatomic observations on the lumbar sympathetic nervous system. *Surgery* 1949;25:880.

318. Kleiman A. Evidence of the existence of crossed sensory sympathetic fibers. *Am J Surg* 1954;87:839.
319. Weber R. An analysis of the cross-communications between the sympathetic trunks in the lumbar region in man. *Ann Surg* 1957;145:365.
320. Yeager GH, Cowley RA. Anatomical observations on the lumbar sympathetics with evaluation of sympathectomies in organic vascular disease. *Ann Surg* 1948;127:953.
321. Evans J, Dobben G, Gay G. Peridural effusion of drugs following sympathetic blockade. *JAMA* 1967;200:573.
322. Dellemijn PLI, Allen RR, Rowbotham MC, Fields HL. Modulatory influence of the sympathetic nervous system on thermal thresholds and thermal pain as assessed with quantitative sensory testing. *Brain* 1994;117:1475.
323. Bennet G. The role of the sympathetic nervous system in painful peripheral neuropathy. *Pain* 1991;45:221.
324. Schott G. Mechanisms of causalgia and related clinical conditions: The role of the central and of the sympathetic nervous systems. *Brain* 1986;109:717.
325. Casale R, Elam M. Normal sympathetic nerve activity in a reflex sympathetic dystrophy with marked skin vasoconstriction. *Pain* 1992;41:215.
326. Christensen K, Hendriksen O. The reflex sympathetic dystrophy syndrome. *Scand J Rheumatol* 1983;12:263.
327. Drummond PD, Finch PM, Smythe GA. Reflex sympathetic dystrophy: The significance of differing plasma catecholamine concentrations in affected and unaffected limbs. *Brain* 1991;114:2025.
328. Rosen L, Ostergren J, Fagrell BF, Stranden E. Skin microcirculation in the sympathetic dystrophies evaluated by videophotometric capillaroscopy and laser Doppler fluxometry. *Eur J Clin Invest* 1988;18:305.
329. Ochoa J, Verdugo R. Reflex sympathetic dystrophy: Definitions and history of the ideas: A critical review of human studies. In: Low PA, ed. *The Evaluation and Management of Clinical Autonomic Disorders.* Boston: Little, Brown and Co; 1993:473–492.
330. Warrick JW. Stellate ganglion block in the treatment of Ménière's disease and in the symptomatic relief of tinnitus. *Br J Anaesth* 1969;41:699.
331. Ready LB, Kozody R, Barsa JE, Murphy TM. Side-port needles for stellate ganglion block. *Reg Anesth* 1982;7:160.
332. Malmqvist EL, Bengtsson M, Sorensen J. Efficacy of stellate ganglion block: A clinical study with bupivacaine. *Reg Anesth* 1992;17:340.
333. Matsumoto S. Thermographic assessments of the sympathetic blockade by stellate ganglion block: Comparison between C7-SGB and C6-SGB in 40 patients. *Masui* 1991;40:562.
334. Yamamuro M, Kaneko T. The comparison of stellate ganglion block at the transverse process of the 7th and the 6th cervical vertebra. *Masui* 1978;27:376.
335. Erickson SJ, Hogan Q. CT-guided stellate ganglion injection: Description of technique and efficacy of sympathetic blockade. *Radiology* 1993;188:707.
336. Hatangdi V, Boas R. Lumbar sympathectomy: A single-needle technique. *Br J Anaesth* 1985;57:285.
337. Tahmoush AJ, Malley J, Jennings JR. Skin conductance, temperature, and blood flow in causalgia. *Neurology* 1983;33:1483.
338. Hannington-Kiff JG. Intravenous regional sympathetic block with guanethidine. *Lancet* 1974;I:1019.
339. Hannington-Kiff JG. Retrograde intravenous sympathetic target blocks in limbs. In: Stanton Hicks M, ed. *Pain and the Sympathetic Nervous System.* Boston: Klewer Academic Publishers; 1990:191–206.
340. Wahren LK, Torebjork E, Nystrom B. Quantitative sensory testing before and after regional guanethidine block in patients with neuralgia in the hand. *Pain* 199;46:23.
341. Furst CI. The biochemistry of guanethidine. *Adv Drug Res* 1967;4:133.
342. Glynn CJ, Basedow RW, Walsh JA. Pain relief following postganglionic sympathetic blockade with I.V. Guanethidine. *Br J Anaesth* 1981;53:1297.
343. Abboud FM, Eckstein JW. Vasodilator action of guanethidine. *Circ Res* 1962;11:788.
344. Bonelli S, Conoscente F, Movilia BG, et al. Regional intravenous guanethidine vs stellate ganglion block in reflex sympathetic dystrophies. A randomized trial. *Pain* 1983;16:297.
345. Arner S. Intravenous phentolamine test: Diagnostic and prognostic use in reflex sympathetic dystrophy. *Pain* 1991;46:17.
346. Cline MA, Ochoa J, Torebjork HE. Chronic hyperalgesia and skin warming caused by sensitized C-nociceptors. *Brain* 1989;112:621.
347. Merington WR, Nathan PW. A study of post-ischemic paresthesiae. *J Neurol Neurosurg Psychiatry* 1949;12:1.
348. Bostock H, Baker M, Grafe P, Reid G. Changes in excitability and accommodation of human motor axons following brief periods of ischemia. *J Physiol* 1991;441:537.
349. Nielson VK, Kardel T. Decremental conduction in normal human nerves subjected to ischemia? *Acta Physiol Scand* 1974;92:249.
350. Yarnitsky D, Ochoa JL. Sensations conducted by large and small myelinated fibers are lost simultaneously under compression-ischemia block. *Acta Physiol Scand* 1989;137:319.
351. Yarnitsky D, Ochoa JL. Differential effect of compression-ischemia block on warm sensation and heat-induced pain. *Brain* 1991;114:907.
352. Casale R, Glynn C, Buonocore M. The role of ischaemia in the analgesia which follows Bier's block technique. *Pain* 1992;50:169.
353. Campbell JN, Raja SN, Meyer RA, Mackinnon SE. Myelinated afferents signal the hyperalgesia associated with nerve injury. *Pain* 1988;32:89.
354. Gracely RH, Lynch SA, Bennett GJ. Painful neuropathy: Altered central processing maintained dynamically by peripheral input. *Pain* 1992;51:175.
355. Ahlgren EW, Stephen CR, Lloyd EAC, McCollum DE. Diagnosis of pain with a graduated spinal block technique. *JAMA* 1966;195:125.
356. McCollum DE, Stephen CR. The use of graduated spinal anesthesia in the differential diagnosis of pain of the back and lower extremities. *South Med J* 1964;57:410.
357. Ramamurthy S, Winnie AP. Diagnostic maneuvers in painful syndromes. *Int Anesthesiol Clin* 1983;83:47.
358. Akkineni SR, Ramamurthy S. Simplified differential spinal block. *ASA Ann Mtg (Abstr)* 1977;765.
359. Sarnoff SJ, Arrowood JG. Differential spinal block. *Surgery* 1946;20:150.
360. Benzon HT. Caution in interpreting modified differential spinal anesthesia: Does sympathetic block always persist after recovery of motor and sensory modalities? *Reg Anesth* 1983;9:156.
361. Arner S, Arner B. Differential effects of epidural morphine in the treatment of cancer related pain. *Acta Anaesthsiol Scand* 1985;29:32.
362. Hogan Q, Haddox JD, Abram S, et al. Epidural opiates and local anesthetics for the management of cancer pain. *Pain* 1991;46:271.
363. Rawal N, Schott U, Dahlstrom B, et al. Influence of naloxone infusion on analgesia and respiratory depression following epidural morphine. *Anesthesiology* 1986;64:194.
364. Sanders SH, McKeel NL, Hare BD. Relationship between psychopathology and graduated spinal block findings in chronic pain patients. *Pain* 1984;19:367.
365. Schnider TW, Gaeta R, Brose W, et al. Derivation and cross-validation of pharmacokinetic parameters for computer-controlled infusion of lidocaine in pain therapy. *Anesthesiology* 1996;84:1043.
366. Rowlingson JC, DiFazio CA, Foster J, Carron H. Lidocaine as an analgesic for experimental pain. *Anesthesiology* 1980;52:20.
367. Peterson P, Kastrup J. Dercum's disease (adiposa dolorosa): Treatment of the severe pain with intravenous lidocaine. *Pain* 1987;28:77.
368. Scott RM. Mexiletine and vascular headaches. *Aust N Z J Med* 1981;93:92.
369. Raja SN, Treede R-D, Davis KD, Campbell JN. Systemic alpha-adrenergic blockade with phentolamine: A diagnostic test for sympathetically maintained pain. *Anesthesiology* 1991;74:691.
370. Glynn CJ, Stannard C, Collins PA, Casale R. The role of peripheral sudomotor blockade in the treatment of patients with sympathetically maintained pain. *Pain* 1993;53:39.
371. Shir Y, Cameron LB, Raja S, Bourke DL. The safety of intravenous phentolamine administration in patients with neuropathic pain. *Anesth Analg* 1993;76:1008.
372. Northover BJ. A comparison of the electrophysiological actions of phentolamine with those of some other antiarrhythmic drugs on tissues isolated from the rat heart. *Br J Pharmacol* 1983;80:85.
373. Ramirez JM, French AS. Phentolamine selectively affects the fast sodium component of sensory adaptation in an insect mechanoreceptor. *J Neurobiol* 1990;21:893.
374. Kaplan HI, Sadock BJ. *Comprehensive Textbook of Psychiatry*, 4th ed. Baltimore: Williams and Wilkins; 1985:1571.
375. Bonica JJ, Loeser JD. Pain resulting from central nervous system pathology. In: Bonica JJ, ed. *The Management of Pain.* Philadelphia: Lea and Febiger; 1990:271–272.
376. Bonica JJ, Loeser JD. Medical evaluation of the patient with pain. In: Bonica JJ, ed. *The Management of Pain*, 2nd ed. Philadelphia: Lea and Febiger; 1990:570–571.
377. Briggs LP, Dundee JW, Bahar M, Clarke RSJ. Comparison of the effect of diisopropyl phenol (ICI 35868) and thiopentone on response to somatic pain. *Br J Anaesth* 1982;54:307.
378. Drower EJ, Hammond DL. GABAergic modulation of nociceptive threshold: Effects of THIP and bicuculline microinjected in the ventral medulla of the rat. *Brain Res* 1988;450:316.
379. Kidd BL, Cruwys S, Mapp PI, Blake DR. Role of the sympathetic nervous system in chronic joint pain and inflammation. *Ann Rheum Dis* 1992;51:1188.

PART IV: PAIN MANAGEMENT

CHAPTER 39 ■ SYMPATHETIC NEURAL BLOCKADE OF UPPER AND LOWER EXTREMITY

HARALD BREIVIK AND MICHAEL J. COUSINS

The effects of sympathetic nerves in maintaining normal constrictor tone in the blood vessels of the skin have been known since the classic work of Claude Bernard in 1852. The well–known observation of increased skin temperature of the foot after surgical lumbar sympathectomy was first made by Hunter and Royle in 1925 (1). Surgical sympathectomy has been performed at some clinics, as reported by De Bakey in 1950, to promote healing of ischemic cutaneous ulcers and to relieve pain in the foot at rest (*rest pain*) (2); however, in many vascular clinics today more emphasis is placed on vascular grafting and stenting procedures. These refined surgical techniques undoubtedly have greatly improved the prognosis of the patient with occlusive vascular disease. Despite this movement away from sympathetic ablation, there is considerable potential benefit from sympathetic neural blockade as an adjunct to vascular surgery or as primary treatment for patients with rest pain who are not fit for, or not amenable to, vascular reconstruction. The large series of 1,666 patients with neurolytic lumbar sympathetic blocks reported in 1970 by Reid and colleagues bears testimony to this, and it is surprising that many clinics have largely neglected this important option in the treatment of vascular disease (3).

Mandl first described the technique of lumbar sympathetic neural blockade in 1926, and his technique was clearly very similar to that for celiac plexus blockade described by Kappis in 1919 (4,5). A similar neglect of celiac plexus block for analgesia in upper abdominal cancer has been apparent (see Chapter 45). The classic "anterior" approach to stellate ganglion blockade was initiated by Leriche (6) in 1934, and it forms the basis of the technique described in this chapter (7).

Sympathetic blockade is produced together with motor and sensory blockade during regional block for operative surgery (e.g., spinal and epidural anesthesia, brachial plexus block). It has been asserted that "differential" sympathetic blockade without sensory and motor block can be produced using low concentrations of local anesthetic during epidural or spinal subarachnoid block. This selective vulnerability has been applied to clarify the mechanisms of individual patients' chronic pain. We believe that selective sympathetic ganglion block provides more reliable information (see Chapter 38). In the management of acute pain, epidural block at the appropriate segmental level relieves labor pain and the pain of renal colic by blocking visceral (sympathetic afferent) nociceptive and sympathetic efferent nerve fibers (see later discussion and Fig. 39-1). However,

the most specific technique for sympathetic blockade is selective blockade of the sympathetic ganglia.

Because the sympathetic ganglia are, except in the thoracic region, relatively well separated from somatic nerves, it is possible to achieve sympathetic blockade without loss of sensory or motor function. Selective sympathetic blockade offers the possibility of treating a variety of conditions in which reduced sympathetic activity might be beneficial. With careful technique, it is even possible to achieve permanent neurolytic blockade with essentially no loss of somatic sensory and motor function. Thus, sympathetic blockade, at the three major levels indicated in Figure 39-2, is potentially a rewarding series of techniques for the diagnosis and management of acute and chronic pain syndromes and other conditions (Table 39-1). Our clinical experience has been that, of all neural blockade techniques, lumbar sympathetic block for lower extremity rest pain due to vascular insufficiency and celiac plexus block for visceral pain in upper abdominal cancer offer the most benefit at the lowest risk.

Celiac plexus blockade, superior hypogastric plexus block, and ganglion impar block are described in Chapter 45, and cervical, thoracic, and lumbar sympathetic blocks are described in the present chapter, along with intravenous regional sympathetic (IVRS) block. Despite a duration of only up to 2 weeks, repeated IVRS efferent blocks are an attractive alternative to the higher-risk techniques of thoracic sympathetic block and thoracic surgical or thoracoscopic sympathectomy. However, the effects of IVRS blocks differ: Ganglion blocks will intercept efferent as well as afferent nerve fibres, although the latter are in the minority (8), IVRS blocks efferents only.

It may be possible to use either unilateral or bilateral lumbar sympathetic block for some kinds of pelvic pain (particularly urogenital). Doing so poses a much smaller risk than neurolytic subarachnoid block, with its possibility of loss of bladder function (see Chapter 42 and 50), and it is less invasive than subarachnoid opioid plus bupivacaine catheter infusion. To take full advantage of sympathetic neural blockade, it is essential to bear in mind the general features of the anatomy and physiology of the peripheral sympathetic nervous system (as described in the next section) and the regional anatomy, as described in connection with each of the techniques of sympathetic blockade. It is also important to use objective methods to evaluate the completeness of sympathetic blockade and its clinical effects.

SYMPATHETIC PATHWAYS

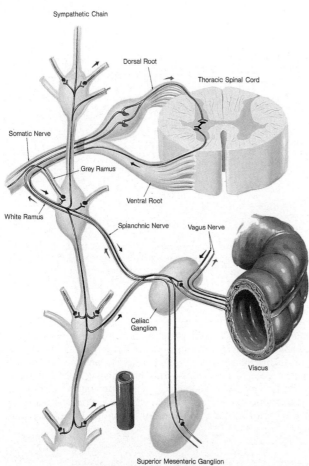

FIGURE 39-1. Peripheral sympathetic nervous system. Cell bodies are located in the intermediolateral cell column of T1–L2 spinal segments. Efferent fibers (cholinergic) pass by way of the ventral root to a white ramus communicans and then to the paravertebral sympathetic ganglia or to more remotely located ganglia, such as the celiac ganglion. From each ganglion, they give rise to adrenergic fibers to supply viscera (e.g., from the celiac ganglion) or to join somatic nerves (from lumbar sympathetic ganglion) to supply efferent fibers to the limbs (sudomotor and vasomotor effects). In the case of lumbar sympathetic ganglia, the adrenergic fibers swing backward by a gray ramus communicans to join the somatic nerve. Afferent fibers travel by way of ganglia, such as the celiac and lumbar sympathetic, without synapsing, and reach somatic nerves and then their cell bodies in the dorsal root ganglia. They then pass to the dorsal root and synapse with interneurons in the intermediolateral area of the spinal cord. These afferent fibers convey pain impulses from the viscera and are similar to nociceptive afferents, except that they pass without synapsing through sympathetic ganglia. Part of the parasympathetic nervous system is indicated by the vagus nerve to and from the gut. These vagal fibers pass through the celiac plexus but do not synapse in the celiac ganglion. Their synapse is at gut wall level (see Fig. 39–5). The submucosal and the myenteric part of the enteric nervous system are indicated in the cross-section of the gut wall.

SYMPATHETIC NERVOUS SYSTEM

Anatomy and Physiology

The peripheral sympathetic nervous system begins as efferent preganglionic fibers from neurons in the intermediolateral column of the spinal cord, passing in the ventral roots from T1 to L2 out of the spinal canal to run separately as white rami communicantes to ganglia in the sympathetic chain, alongside the vertebral bodies (Fig. 39-1). In the lower cervical region, the chain lies at the anterolateral aspect of the vertebral body; in the thorax it is adjacent to the neck of the ribs, still relatively close to somatic roots (Fig. 39-3). In the lumbar region, however, the chain angles forward to lie anterolateral to the vertebral bodies and is separated from somatic roots by psoas muscle and psoas fascia (Fig. 39-4). The preganglionic fibers pass a variable distance in the sympathetic chain to reach neurons in ganglia in the chain, or they may extend to peripherally located ganglia (i.e., in the gut; Fig. 39-1). The inconstant level of relay in the chain itself may be responsible for a number of disappointing results from an apparently technically successful block. Sympathetic ganglia are segmentally located in the chest (T1–T12). There are also three cervical ganglia, four to five lumbar ganglia, four sacral ganglia, and one unpaired coccygeal ganglion (the "ganglion impar"). The postganglionic fibers are widely distributed, partly to join peripheral nerves (via the gray rami communicantes) and partly to join vessels in different organs. The sympathetic chain not only receives efferent preganglionic but also afferent visceral fibers, which conduct pain from head, neck, and upper extremity (cervicothoracic ganglia); abdominal viscera (celiac plexus, hypogastric plexus) (see Chapter 45); and urogenital system and lower extremity (lumbar ganglia; Fig. 39-2).

The sympathetic nervous system is one part of the autonomic nervous system. Most viscera also receive efferent and transmit afferent impulses via the parasympathetic nervous system (Fig. 39-5). The enteric nervous system (the submucosal and myenteric parts) of the gastrointestinal tract interacts with the sympathetic and the parasympathetic systems (Fig. 39-1 and 39-5).

Sympathetic Efferents to Blood Vessels

The great vessels (carotids, aorta, vena cava) receive direct postganglionic filaments from adjacent sympathetic ganglia (Fig. 39-6) and from plexuses (Fig. 39-2). The main outflow of preganglionic fibers through the ventral roots follows four alternative courses: (a) synapse with postganglionic neuron in ganglia at the same level or adjacent ganglia and travel in somatic nerves to the vessels; (b) synapse in ganglia and pass directly to vessels via filaments; (c) pass directly through sympathetic ganglia and synapse in prevertebral plexuses, then reach vessels (Fig. 39-6); or (d) pass through sympathetic ganglia and ascend or descend to synapse in ganglia above (e.g., cervical) or below (e.g., lower lumbar) (Fig. 39-7).

Vascular nerves and filaments from these diverse sources are united around individual vessels in extensive "perivascular adventitial plexuses," which in turn ramify into plexuses between adventitia and media and between media and intima. Plexuses are augmented by branches from nearby cranial or spinal nerves. Thus, there is great overlap of innervation originating from several spinal cord segments. Arteries and arterioles are more richly supplied than veins and venules. Although nerve fibers accompany venules, it is not known whether they serve a vasoconstrictor role.

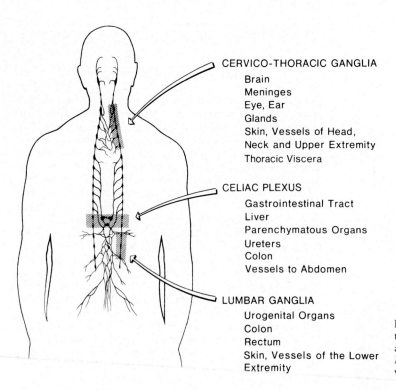

CERVICO-THORACIC GANGLIA
  Brain
  Meninges
  Eye, Ear
  Glands
  Skin, Vessels of Head,
  Neck and Upper Extremity
  Thoracic Viscera

CELIAC PLEXUS
  Gastrointestinal Tract
  Liver
  Parenchymatous Organs
  Ureters
  Colon
  Vessels to Abdomen

LUMBAR GANGLIA
  Urogenital Organs
  Colon
  Rectum
  Skin, Vessels of the Lower
  Extremity

FIGURE 39-2. An outline of the sympathetic nervous system. The three main levels of sympathetic blockade are shown along with major clinical uses. Redrawn from Bonica JJ. *The Management of Pain*. Philadelphia: Lea & Febiger, 1953, with permission.

The complex influences of remote and local factors on vascular tone are illustrated in Figures 39-8 through 39-10.

Sympathetic fibers are generally found in a deep fascial plane and are less accessible than segmental nerves. Interruption of sympathetic nerve fibers by neural blockade can be achieved in the following ways: at the sympathetic chain by anatomically specific sympathetic blockade, at peripheral nerves by a mixed nerve block, at a vessel by perivascular infiltration, or to some extent by intradural or extradural injection of local anesthetic. Sympathetic efferent activity can also be blocked pharmacologically by an α-receptor blocker (phentolamine, Dibenzyline); by a "depleter" of norepinephrine activity in sympathetic nerve ending (guanethidine or reserpine); or by a β-receptor blocker, propranolol (β_1 and β_2) or metoprolol,

TABLE 39-1

CLINICALLY PAINFUL CONDITIONS THAT SYMPATHETIC BLOCKADE MAY BENEFIT

Pain Relief
Acute herpes zoster
Renal colic (lumbar sympathetic block)
Obliterative arterial disease
Acute pancreatitis and pancreatic cancer (celiac plexus block)
Cancer pain from upper abdominal viscera (celiac plexus block; see Chapter 45)
Cardiac pain (thoracic sympathetic or stellate ganglion block)
Paget disease of bone (stellate ganglion or lumbar sympathetic block)
Complex regional pain syndrome (CRPS) type I (11,61) (formerly: reflex sympathetic dystrophy, minor post-traumatic syndrome, post-frostbite syndrome, shoulder/hand syndrome, Sudeck atrophy) (see Chapter 46)
Complex regional pain syndrome (CRPS) type II (11) (formerly: causalgia)
Phantom limb pain
Central pain

To Improve Blood Flow in Vasospastic Disorders (Stellate or Lumbar Sympathetic Block)
Raynaud disease
Accidental intra-arterial injections of thiopentone or other irritants
Early frostbite
Obliterative arterial disease not suitable for vascular surgery (97,98)
Vascular surgery and reimplantation surgery (to improve postoperative blood flow)

To Improve Drainage of Local Edema (Stellate or Lumbar Sympathetic Block)
Upper extremity after mastectomy
Lower extremity after surgery, trauma, thromboembolism

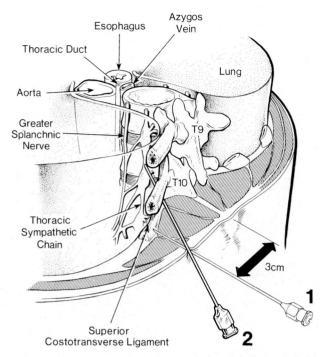

FIGURE 39-3. Thoracic sympathetic (paravertebral) block. Needle insertion is 3 cm from the midline, opposite cephalad aspect of spinous process. Needle is initially inserted perpendicular to skin in all planes to reach rib or transverse process at a depth of about 2.5 to 3.5 cm. Sometimes the needle may need to be angled slightly superiorly or inferiorly to locate rib or transverse process. Needle is then directed cephalad above the rib, and a loss of resistance may be detected as the needle penetrates the costotransverse ligament. At this point, the needle tip lies in the paravertebral space where both sympathetic and somatic thoracic nerves are located. Careful aspiration must be carried out for air (intrapleural), blood (intravascular), or cerebrospinal fluid (intradural).

atenolol, esmolol (mainly β_1-receptor). Norepinephrine released from sympathetic nerve endings acts on both presynaptic and postsynaptic receptors (Fig. 39-11). Phenoxybenzamine and phentolamine are nonspecific α-blockers, acting on both pre- and postsynaptic receptors. Blockade of presynaptic re-

ceptors interrupts the negative feedback that modifies norepinephrine release. More selective postsynaptic blockers (e.g., prazosin) have a much more sustained degree of α-blockade (Fig. 39-11).

Function of α- and β-Blockers

Vasoconstriction by α-Receptors. Arterioles (in the skin and in the splanchnic area), smaller arteries, and, in particular, peripheral veins, are normally under moderate vasoconstrictor influence. Pain, anxiety, and blood loss can provoke a very marked increase in arteriolar vasoconstrictor tone, mediated by the sympathetic nervous system. This increase in resistance, particularly in skin vessels, influences the distribution of blood flow. In addition, the associated increase in venous vascular tone decreases the compliance of the venous system, reducing its blood content and increasing venous pressure. Co-release of neuropeptide-Y from some sympathetic nerve endings increases and prolongs the vasoconstrictive effect of norepinephrine (8).

Heart Muscle Activity (Chronotropic and Inotropic Effect). β_1-Stimulation causes increased heart rate and increased cardiac contractility; thus, high (T1–T4) thoracic sympathetic blockade may cause a marked reduction in cardiac output.

Bronchial Tone. β_2-Stimulation causes bronchodilation, so that it is theoretically possible for thoracic sympathetic blockade to cause bronchoconstriction, although this does not appear to be the case (see Chapter 11).

Vasodilatation. β_2-Stimulation causes vasodilatation in some vascular beds (e.g., muscle); however, this is a minor effect and is overridden by local metabolic effects (see later in this chapter).

Smooth Muscle Tone. In the gut and bladder, β_2-stimulation causes smooth muscle relaxation and sphincter contraction. Thus, sympathetic blockade results in smooth muscle contraction (a small, contracted gut) and sphincter relaxation. These effects provide excellent surgical access during procedures such as abdominoperineal resection. Sudomotor structures (sweat glands) and hair follicles have the same postganglionic efferents as do blood vessels; however, the neurotransmitter in sweat glands is acetylcholine.

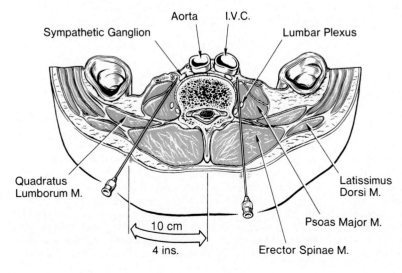

FIGURE 39-4. Lumbar sympathetic block. Note that insertion of needle 10 cm from the midline enables the needle to reach the anterolateral angle of the vertebral body. Insertion of needle closer to the midline takes needle path close to somatic nerve roots and lateral to sympathetic chain. From Cherry DA, Rao DM. Lumbar sympathetic and coeliac plexus blocks: An anatomical study in cadavers. *Br J Anaesth* 1982;54:1037, with permission.

Sympathetic
Nervous System

Parasympathetic
Nervous System

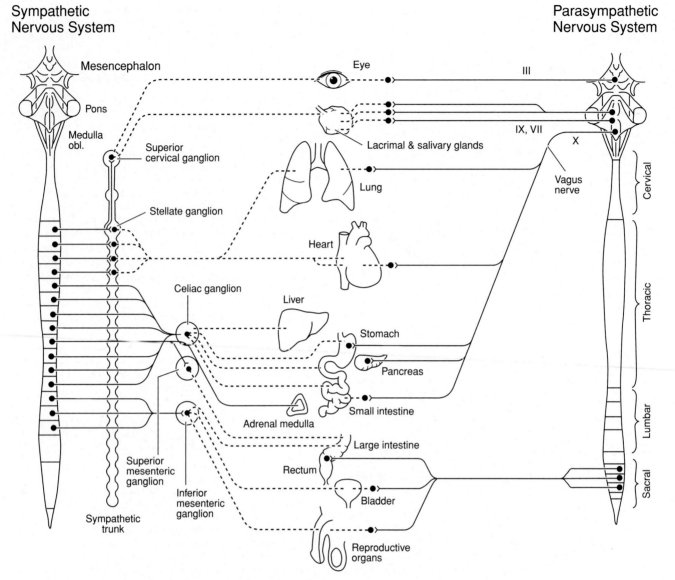

FIGURE 39-5. The sympathetic and parasympathetic parts of the autonomic nervous system. *Continuous lines* are preganglionic axons; *dotted lines* are postganglionic axons. The sympathetic outflow to skin and deep somatic structures of the extremities and trunk are shown in Figure 39-7. *III*, oculomotor nerve; *VII*, facial nerve; *IX*, glossopharyngeal nerve. From Jänig W. The integrative action of the autonomic nervous system. In: *Neurobiology of Homeostasis*. Cambridge: Cambridge University Press, 2006, with permission.

Metabolic. The sympathetic nervous system has a metabolic effect that is said to explain the relaxation of smooth muscle in vessels (β_2) and gut, and its effect on the heart muscle. This metabolic effect is widespread and also affects carbohydrate and lipid distribution and utilization (9).

Nociception is mediated in various ways by the sympathetic nervous system. Uterine nociceptive input, as in labor pain, is transmitted by afferent fibers that traverse the lower thoracic sympathetic ganglia, whereas pain from upper abdominal viscera and the gut, as far distal as the descending colon, can be relieved adequately by celiac ganglion block. Nociceptive input from some pelvic viscera may be transmitted via lumbar sympathetic ganglia (Fig. 39-2). Sympathetic efferents may influence limb pains (10–12). After nerve or tissue trauma,

release of neurotransmitters such as norepinephrine increases discharge from peripheral primary afferent nociceptors. Denervation hypersensitivity from augmented adrenoceptor activity may increase discharge from primary afferent nociceptors in the absence of increased sympathetic efferent nerve activity. (see Chapters 31 and 32). Recently, Jørum and colleagues (13) documented direct stimulation of nociceptive fibers by sympathetic efferent discharge in a patient with sympathetically maintained pain (13). Also, microcirculatory changes caused by intense sympathetic activity may alter the local biochemical environment so as to enhance nociceptor activity (Fig. 39-12). Sympathetic blockade may reverse such effects, provided it is done before abnormal nociceptive activity is permanently established rostral to the spinal cord. Visceral afferent

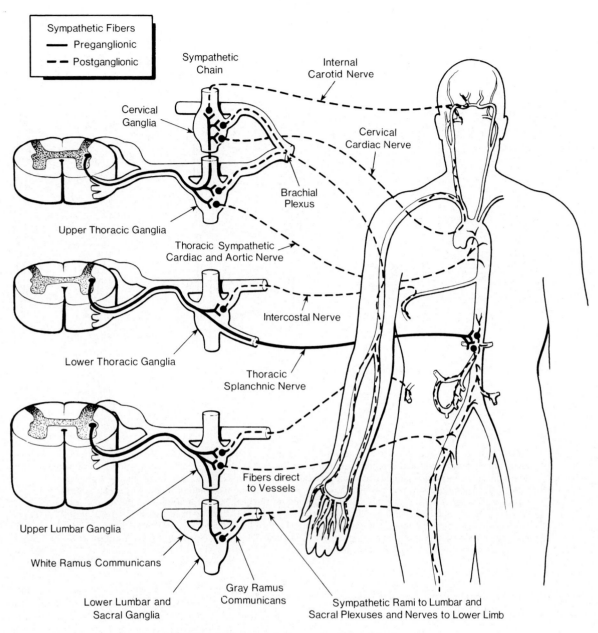

FIGURE 39-6. Sympathetic nerve supply to blood vessels.

inputs can give rise to sensations of pain and discomfort, shape emotions, and produce reflex effects on autonomic target organs.

PHYSIOLOGIC EFFECTS ON PERIPHERAL BLOOD FLOW

A regional sympathetic block has its primary and most obvious effect on vasomotor activity. In a normal subject, this leads to dilatation of veins, promoting an accumulation of blood in the veins, and dilatation of the arterial vessels, leading to a fall in the peripheral resistance and, if the perfusion pressure has not been altered, to an increased capillary blood flow.

In a normal subject, complete sympathetic block will be followed by visibly dilated veins or by increased blood flow, seen clinically in reduced capillary refill time or as measured by plethysmography (Figs. 39-13 and 39-14), laser Doppler flowmetry, (14,15) or ^{133}Xe clearance, all accurate means to measure capillary blood flow. Peripheral pulse waves will be enlarged on oscillometric recordings. Vasoconstrictor responses, as to the "ice response," are abolished (Figs. 39-13 and 39-14). The blood flow increase will, to a large extent, be restricted to the skin, followed by an increase in skin temperature and a marked feeling of warmth in the extremity (Fig. 39-15) (2). Skin capillary oxygen tension and venous oxygen tension and saturation are also increased. A widespread block will cause a peripheral pooling of blood, diminishing the venous return and lowering cardiac output and blood pressure.

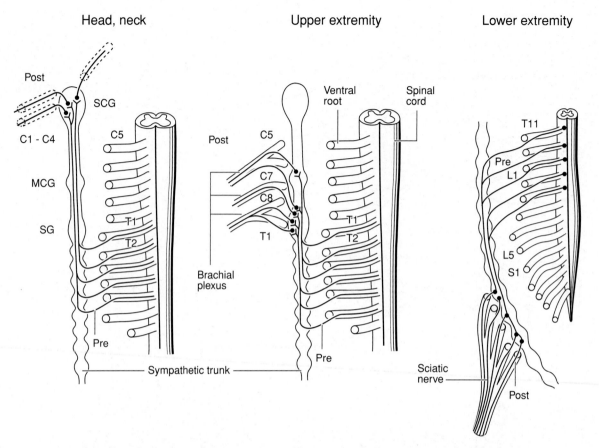

FIGURE 39-7. Sympathetic efferent innervation of head, neck, upper and lower extremities. Preganglionic (*Pre*) neurons in the thoracolumbar spinal cord project through the ventral roots and white rami communicantes to postganglionic neurons in the sympathetic trunk. The postganglionic neurons project with postganglionic fibres (*Post*) through the corresponding gray rami communicantes to the spinal nerves or along the arteries (*i.c.a.*, only internal carotid artery to the head is indicated). *SCG,* superior cervical ganglion; *MCG,* middle cervical ganglion; *SG,* stellate ganglion. Modified from Brodal P. *The Central Nervous System: Structure and Function.* New York. Oxford University Press, 1998; and Jänig W. The integrative action of the autonomic nervous system. In: *Neurobiology of Homeostasis.* Cambridge: Cambridge University Press, 2006, with permission.

Application to Improve Blood Flow in Peripheral Vascular Disease

Muscle blood flow, being automatically regulated according to muscle metabolism, should not be affected by sympathetic blockade at rest, during work, or after ischemia (1). Thus, reduced muscle flow (claudication) may not be helped by sympathetic block (Fig. 35-15). Therefore, it seems logical to use sympathetic blockade to improve the blood flow in a patient with insufficient peripheral superficial blood flow due to vasospasm or arterial disease (i.e., rest pain) (Fig. 39-15) (1,16). It is not possible, however, to predict the effect of sympathetic blockade in a patient with a diseased vascular system, as explained with the aid of the following illustrations. Figure 39-16 shows an artery that divides into two smaller branches. The total flow (Q_A) in the artery is proportional to the perfusion pressure (P) and inversely proportional to the peripheral resistance (PR). In each branch (B and C) the flows (Q_B and Q_C) are affected by the perfusion pressures, almost the same as in the artery (A) and inversely related to the regional resistance (RR_B and RR_C) in each branch. A blockade of the sympathetic fibers to branch B alone will have very little effect on the perfusion pressure (Fig.

39-17). As the regional resistance decreases in branch B, the flow through this vessel will increase. A unilateral sympathetic blockade (in humans) is generally followed by a slight increase in vasomotor tone in the contralateral side, thus increasing the regional resistance and reducing the blood flow through this part of the vascular system.

In Figure 39-18, an arterial obstruction in branch B is shown. Such an obstruction will in itself diminish blood flow by mechanically increasing the regional resistance; however, decreased blood flow across the obstruction might at least be compensated by an increase in the collateral blood flow. A widespread sympathetic blockade, as illustrated in Figure 39-19, will diminish the regional resistance, mainly in branch C with its undamaged vessels. The blood flow will be diverted into this part of the vascular tree, and thus blood will be shunted from the diseased part (branch B). Such "stealing" of blood is known to occur in patients with advanced arterial disease. In theory, stealing can occur at three different levels: a generalized vasodilatation in the body will steal blood from, for instance, one extremity; increased blood flow around the hip and in the pelvis will diminish distal blood flow to the peripheral part of the lower extremity; or increased skin blood flow might steal blood from the muscles (Fig. 39-15) (1,17,18).

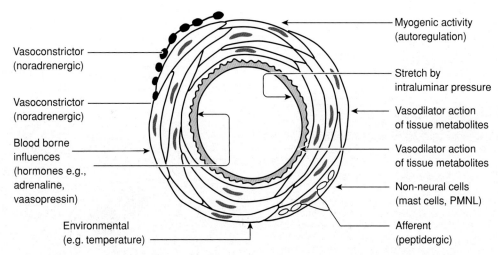

FIGURE 39-8. Blood vessel tone is influenced by remote forces in addition to noradrenergic vasoconstriction, such as nonadrenergic vasodilator, blood-borne adrenaline and vasopressin, and by many local influences: spontaneous myogenic activity, stretch-evoked contractions, endothelium-induced vasodilation via nitric oxide, vasodilation induced by metabolic factors from skeletal muscle, brain (PCO_2 rise), coronary vessels (PO_2 fall). During inflammation, vasodilatory factors from inflammatory cells, calcitonin gene-related peptide, and substance P are released from unmyelinated and thin myelinated fibres. Cold causes enhancement of neuroeffector transmission from vasoconstrictor fibers to skin blood vessels. Modified from Jänig W. The integrative action of the autonomic nervous system. In: *Neurobiology of Homeostasis*. Cambridge: Cambridge University Press, 2006, with permission.

In contrast, a localized vasodilatation that affects the collaterals to branch B and vessels beyond the arterial obstruction should increase blood flow to this region (Fig. 39-20).

If a decrease in vasomotor tone in the collaterals cannot be achieved, the maintenance of a good perfusion pressure is essential, as stressed by Lassen and Larsen (19,20).

From this discussion, it is obvious that the clinical effect of a sympathetic block cannot easily be predicted. Only physiologic studies in patients and clinical experience will identify when a sympathetic block is indicated.

In patients with occlusive vascular disease, the prime indication for surgical or chemical sympathectomy is rest pain in a

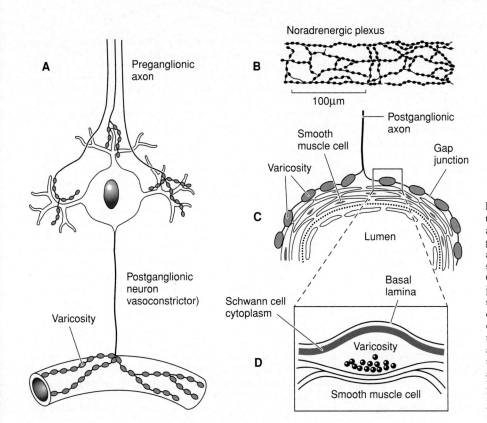

FIGURE 39-9. Neuroeffector synapse of the postganglionic vasoconstrictor neuron and its blood vessel (**A**). The long postganglionic axon forms noradrenergic plexus and many thousand varicosities close to the smooth muscle cells of the blood vessel (**B, C, D**). Smooth muscle cells are coupled by junctional channels forming a functional syncytium (**C**). The varicosity forms close contact with the smooth muscle cells without intervening Schwann cell cytoplasm and the basal laminae of smooth muscle cell and varicosity fuse (**D**). The vesicles contain transmitter. From Jänig W. The integrative action of the autonomic nervous system. In: *Neurobiology of Homeostasis*. Cambridge: Cambridge University Press, 2006, with permission.

PART IV: PAIN MANAGEMENT

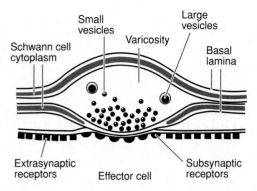

FIGURE 39-10. Neuroeffector transmission to autonomic target cell, such as smooth muscle cells of arterioles or heart. Subsynaptic receptors mediate the effect of transmitter release during physiologic conditions. Norepinephrine from small vesicles causes vasoconstriction of small arterioles via extrasynaptic receptors. Large vesicles contain neuropeptides. From Jänig W. The integrative action of the autonomic nervous system. In: *Neurobiology of Homeostasis.* Cambridge: Cambridge University Press, 2006, with permission.

limb not amenable to direct arterial reconstruction (2). Because of associated coronary artery disease, pulmonary disease, and other physical conditions, many patients in this situation are poor candidates for surgery and are thus better candidates for neurolytic sympathectomy (16). However, the clinical results of both surgical and neurolytic sympathectomy, as reported in the literature, are contradictory. This might be explained by a poor selection of patients or by a lack of use of independent assessment of successful sympathetic ablation and its separate effects on blood flow and pain. This task may be simplified if one of the methods of evaluation in each category depicted in Table 39-2.

The detrimental effects of generalized systemic vasodilation in patients with arteriosclerotic vascular disease that causes rest pain or intermittent claudication have been well described and are generally accepted today. The most important of these effects is the maldistribution of blood flow away from vital organs, such as the myocardium and central nervous system (CNS) (18).

It has been suggested that an increased skin blood flow should always be present in the presence of regional vasodilatation. This finding has also been reported in patients with obliterative arterial disease (21–23).

Although skin blood flow is markedly under the control of sympathetic activity, a decreased blood flow has been demonstrated in patients with severe arteriosclerosis and, in particular, in patients with lower limb vascular disease who have a low ankle blood pressure (less than 60/20 mm Hg) before lumbar sympathetic blockade (23–28). In these patients, the vascular lesions in the periphery are so extreme that, hypothetically, a "proximal stealing" always occurs, and thus a fall in the perfusion pressure peripherally is followed by a vasodilatation in vessels located proximally. Although rare, there are reports of worsening of pain and gangrene (29). Remarkably enough, an increase in skin temperature is not always related to an increase in blood flow through the skin and may merely reflect venous pooling and local inflammatory changes (28). During spinal anesthesia, changes in skin temperature are not closely correlated to changes in skin blood flow, as evaluated by laser Doppler flowmetry (15,30).

The blood flow through muscle is automatically regulated according to local metabolic needs. Thus, in intermittent clau-

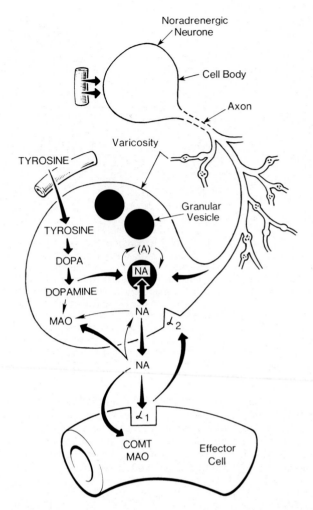

FIGURE 39-11. Sympathetic nerve endings and receptors. Diagram of synapse between a postganglionic sympathetic neuron and postsynaptic receptors on effector cells (e.g., smooth muscle of vessel wall). Stimulation of presynaptic (α_2) receptors by previously released norepinephrine (noradrenaline, NA) results in inhibition of further release of NA from the sympathetic neuron. Stimulation of α_1-receptors results in smooth muscle contraction. *MAO,* monoamine oxidase; *COMT,* catechol-O-methyltransferase.

dication, muscle tissue hypoxia and accumulation of metabolites during exercise should be followed by maximal dilatation of the muscle blood vessels, so that sympathetic blockade should be of no value or may even worsen the symptoms because of "stealing" blood flow to the skin (1,31,32). However, because pain is a primary factor in provoking increased sympathetic activity, its presence could result in vasoconstriction in the collateral vessels that supply the affected muscle (Fig. 39-15). Sympathetic blockade under these circumstances may decrease pain and thereby improve blood flow to muscle, thus explaining why sympathectomy benefits some patients with intermittent claudication (3,21,33). This assumption and the clinical experience of several investigators are supported by a metabolic study in which deep venous blood was drawn before and at the maximum of a one-leg bicycle ergometer test in patients with intermittent claudication (34). In patients with fairly high and segmentally located arterial lesions given sympathetic block (Group I), the rise in femoral venoarterial lactate difference during exercise was not as marked as before

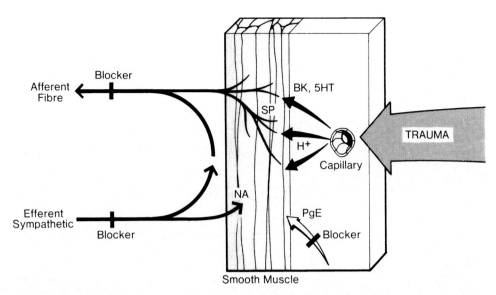

FIGURE 39-12. Peripheral mechanisms of pain, sympathetic activity, and microcirculatory changes. Physical stimuli (e.g., trauma), the chemical environment (e.g., H^+ changes), algesic substance (e.g., serotonin [5HT] and bradykinin [BK]), and microcirculatory changes (e.g., edema) may all modify peripheral nociceptor sensitivity. Increased nociceptor activity increases afferent fiber activity, with resultant increases in efferent sympathetic vasoconstriction, and also norepinephrine (noradrenaline [NA]) release with further increases in nociceptor sensitivity. Thus, a repetitive cycle is set up. Substance P (SP) is probably the peripheral pain transmitter. Prostaglandins (PGE) also increase nociceptor sensitivity. Points of blockade of pain (*shaded and marked "blocker"*) are as follows: 1. Afferent fibers (local anesthetics); 2. efferent sympathetic fibers (local anesthetics); and 3. prostaglandin synthesis (e.g., nonsteroidal anti-inflammatory drugs given orally). All three may relieve pain and produce an associated improvement in microcirculation by breaking the repetitive cycle. New approaches to pain relief include substance P depletion (e.g., by capsaicin). Additional points of blockade to produce vasodilation include the following: *1.* Norepinephrine depletion at sympathetic nerve endings; *2.* norepinephrine receptor blockade (see Fig. 39-33); *3.* selective increase in levels of the prostaglandins PGE and PGE_1 (by intravascular infusion); and *4.* calcium channel blockade (see Fig. 39-33).

their sympathetic block, indicating an improvement in nutrient blood flow. By contrast, in a group of patients with multiple vascular lesions (Group II), no improvement in nutrient blood flow was achieved following sympathetic blockade. In Group I, eight of 10 also experienced less ischemic pain on exercise during the sympathetic blockade. No patients in Group II experienced such pain relief. The most important effect of sympathetic blockade in Group I seemed to be pain relief during exercise, at least partly because of improved blood flow and also enhancement of the development of collateral vessels, which is known to occur over time, providing opportunities for revascularization (Table 39-3). It should be acknowledged that, with respect to pain evaluation, a placebo effect may occur, as has been reported with lumbar sympathetic blockade (35).

Lumbar sympathetic blockade in connection with vascular surgery improves the flow through reconstructed vessels and should be of value in the immediate postoperative period (21,36–39). Although less selective, this effect can also be achieved with epidural sympathetic block. Whether blockade of β-fibers (sympathetic preganglionic fiber) occurs during spinal and epidural blockade has been questioned (15,40–44). Efferent sympathetic change has been studied with the help of skin conductance response (SCR), in which different stimuli (e.g., electrical stimulus, short, deep breath, verbal stimulation) have been used. In spinal analgesia, the sympathetic blockade starts at a level much more caudal than that of analgesia, in contrast to what has historically been stated in the literature (45). Even with T1 blockade (which should block all preganglionic

fibers), an SCR is often seen in the foot, indicating that β-fibers are not blocked as easily as previously thought. In most cases, when a T6 blockade has been achieved, a marked depression of the sympathetic responses is seen mainly in the foot (T12–L1). This partial sympathetic blockade, however, disappears much earlier than the analgesia, in most cases starting 20 to 40 minutes after the injection of the spinal anesthetic. Similar results have been seen when the skin blood flow has been studied with the help of laser Doppler flowmetry (14,15). Also with a high blockade (T4–T6), an increased blood flow was seen only in the foot and in the thigh, at segment levels far below that of analgesia. A very high spinal analgesia is thus needed to make sure that marked depression of sympathetic activity in the lower extremity is produced. Changes in SCR related to the level of epidural blockade are very similar to those seen in spinal analgesia (44).

The increase in limb blood flow resulting from epidural block has been clinically related to a lower incidence of postoperative deep venous thrombosis (see Chapter 11). This effect is most likely correlated with an increase in cardiac output, provoked by the local anesthetic itself (see Chapters 2, 4, and 11). The local anesthetics lidocaine and mepivacaine, when applied directly into the arterial vessels, produce a contraction, in contrast to what is seen during an IV infusion (46).

The limited blocking of sympathetic fibers produced by epidural blockade also explains the fact that a very high epidural blockade is required to ablate stress responses during and after lower abdominal surgery. In upper abdominal surgery, epidural blockade is less effective in blocking the stress

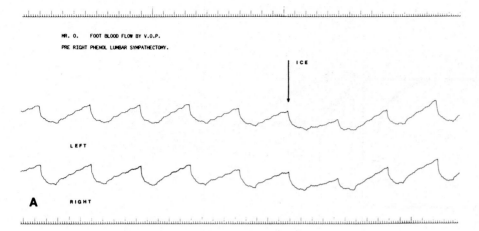

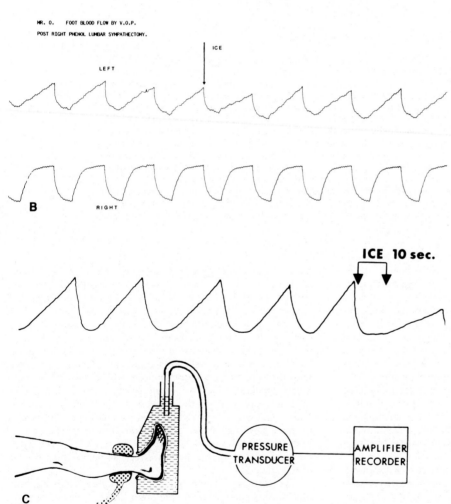

FIGURE 39-13. Skin plethysmography and ice response: Effect of sympathetic block. **A:** Before sympathetic block. Skin blood flow is similar (2 mL/100 mL/min) in both limbs, and the response to ice *(arrow)* is a similar reduction in the height of the pulse wave in both limbs. **B:** After sympathetic block. The blocked limb *(right)* shows a marked increase in the slope of the upward deflection of the pulse wave and an increase in height of the pulse wave; this reflects a tenfold increase of skin blood flow to 22 mL/100 mL/min. There is no change in blood flow in response to ice. In contrast, the unblocked limb *(left)* shows the same shape and height of the pulse wave, and there is a similar marked reduction in blood flow (40% decrease) in response to ice. From Cousins MJ, Reeve TS, Glynn CJ, et al. Neurolytic lumbar sympathetic blockade: Duration of denervation and relief of rest pain. *Anaesth Intensive Care* 1979;7:121, with permission. **C:** Apparatus for venous occlusion skin plethysmography *(VOP)*. The foot is enclosed in a constant-temperature water bath, which surrounds a plethysmograph attached to a pressure transducer. A venous occlusion cuff is placed above the ankle. A typical trace is shown at right. Application of ice to the side of the neck results in a marked increase in sympathetic tone, with a decrease both in the upslope and in the area under the curve. From Walsh JA, Glynn CJ, Cousins MJ, Basedow RW. Blood flow, sympathetic activity, and pain relief following lumbar sympathetic blockade or surgical sympathectomy. *Anaesth Intensive Care* 1984;13:18, with permission.

response. The latter can be rendered much more complete if a splanchnic blockade is added (see Chapter 6).

Proper selection of patients for sympathetic blockade is obviously of great importance. Because the number of patients with vascular disease is very large, complicated and time-consuming physiologic studies are not always feasible. The use of continuous catheter sympathetic blockade that lasts for 5 days is one method of obtaining a clinical evaluation of the

effect of such blockade, which should at least identify patients whose symptoms are exacerbated by blockade (47). A selective alternative is IVRS block, which can eliminate technical failure and is a useful preliminary test for whether surgical sympathectomy or permanent blockade by chemical sympathectomy will be successful (48,49). The often prolonged duration (1–3 weeks) of response to IV sympathetic block can allow adequate time for clinical assessment. A third alternative is to perform

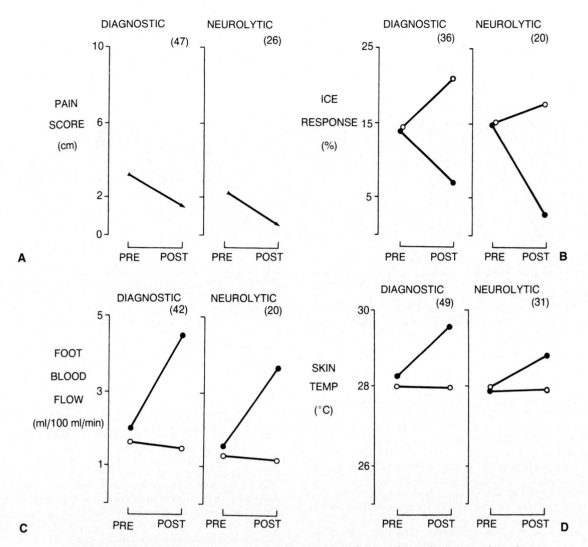

FIGURE 39-14. A: Pain score. Pain score (mean on 10-cm analogue scale) prediagnostic and postdiagnostic local anesthetic (bupivacaine) and neurolytic (phenol) sympathetic blockade in 47 and 26 patients, respectively. Significant decreases in pain score resulted from diagnostic ($p <0.001$) and neurolytic ($p <0.001$) block. **B:** Vasoconstrictor ice response. Effect of diagnostic local anesthetic (bupivacaine, 36 patients) and neurolytic (phenol, 20 patients) sympathetic blockade on vasoconstrictor ice response (%) on treated (•) and control (σ) limb (mean values). Significant decreases in ice response resulted from diagnostic ($p <0.04$) and neurolytic ($p <0.01$) block. **C:** Blood flow. Effect of diagnostic local anesthetic (bupivacaine, 42 patients) and neurolytic (phenol, 20 patients) sympathetic blockade on foot blood flow (mL/100 mL/min) on treated (•) and control (o) limb (mean values). Significant increases in blood flow resulted from diagnostic ($p <0.001$) and neurolytic ($p <0.02$) block. **D:** Skin temperature. Effect of diagnostic local anesthetic (bupivacaine, 49 patients) and neurolytic block (phenol, 31 patients) on foot skin temperature (°C) on treated (•) and control (σ) limbs (mean values). Significant increases in skin temperature resulted from diagnostic ($p <0.001$) and neurolytic ($p <0.01$) block. Parts **A–D** are reproduced from Walsh JA, Glynn CJ, Cousins MJ, Basedow RW. Blood flow, sympathetic activity and pain relief following lumbar sympathetic blockade or surgical sympathectomy. *Anaesth Intensive Care* 1984;13:18, with permission.

diagnostic block with long-acting local anesthetic mixed with contrast medium, and then check the adequacy of sympathetic chain coverage under an image intensifier; however, this has proved the least reliable of the three (16,39).

In a clinical series, Kövamees and Löfström found that the most beneficial effect of sympathetic blockade was relief of rest pain (19 of 23, or 83%), with a somewhat lesser effect of improved healing of ulcers (23 of 55, or 42%) (Table 39-4) (24). Increased walking tolerance (seven of 16, or 44%) was a

significant benefit in a small group of patients with intermittent claudication. Sympathetic blockade was part of a general treatment program that included mobilization and wound treatment, and sometimes infusion of low-molecular-weight dextran. It was not possible to attribute improvement to the sympathetic blockade alone. However, Cousins and colleagues (16) reported that duration of relief of rest pain was similar to duration of lumbar sympathetic blockade, strengthening the link between pain relief and sympathetic denervation. In one study,

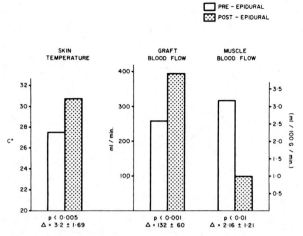

FIGURE 39-15. Blood flow distribution after lumbar sympathetic blockade in arteriosclerotic patients at rest. Blood flow in the femoral artery (electromagnetic flow meter) is increased, as is skin blood flow (skin temperature); however, muscle blood flow (^{133}Xe clearance) is reduced. Note that this is a widespread sympathetic block (both lower limbs), which may sometimes even reduce the skin blood flow through diseased vessels (see Fig. 39-19). From Cousins MJ, Wright CJ. Graft muscle skin blood flow after epidural block in vascular surgical procedures. *Surg Gynecol Obstet* 1971;133:59, with permission.

pain relief was accompanied by increased skin temperature and skin blood flow (venous occlusion plethysmography), whereas regional sweating and vasoconstrictor ice response were decreased (Fig. 39-14) (39). Another study indicated that nutritive blood flow was not increased, but pain was relieved in a high percentage of patients (50). Good results with relief of rest pain in the lower limbs have been reported by others (3,51–52). Very little data are available on upper limb vascular disease, although case reports indicate beneficial results with sympathetic block in vasospastic disorders such as those listed in Table 39-1.

It would appear that the primary benefits that result from sympathetic blockade are pain relief and improved healing of skin lesions; however, controlled studies of efficacy of the sym-

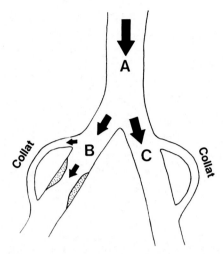

FIGURE 39-17. An arterial obstruction in branch *B* will increase the resistance and thus hamper the blood flow. An increased flow through collaterals (*Collat*) may compensate for a fall in blood flow through the main channel.

pathetic block are required to achieve a better definition of its role in the treatment of vascular disease of the lower and the upper limbs.

Application for Pain Relief other than in Occlusive Vascular Disease

The pain-relieving effect of a sympathetic block in a patient with peripheral arterial disease is said to follow improved blood flow. Good pain relief often occurs, however, when no improvement in peripheral circulation can be noted (50); the possible mechanisms for this are discussed in the next sections (Fig. 39-12). The precise mechanism whereby the nervous system is involved in peripheral pain independent of effects upon blood flow have not yet been fully elucidated (11). It has been suggested that the cutaneous pain threshold, by means of a

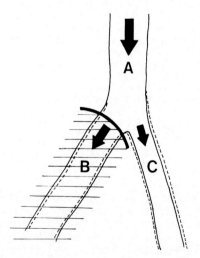

FIGURE 39-16. A limited sympathetic blockade of fibers to branch *B* alone will little affect perfusion pressure. The flow in branch *B* will increase as the regional resistance is diminished. In branch *C*, the flow will be slightly reduced as compensatory vasoconstriction occurs.

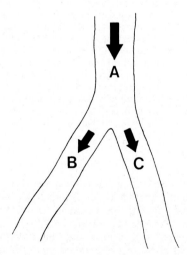

FIGURE 39-18. The blood flows through an artery (*A*) or its branches (*B* and *C*) are proportionate to the perfusion pressures and inversely proportionate to total and regional resistances, respectively.

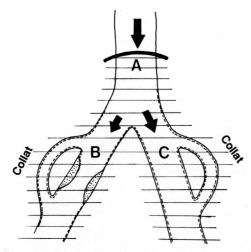

FIGURE 39-19. A widespread sympathetic blockade of fibers to branches *B* and *C* will diminish resistance in undamaged vessels (*C*), thereby potentially stealing blood from a diseased part (*B*) of the vascular tree.

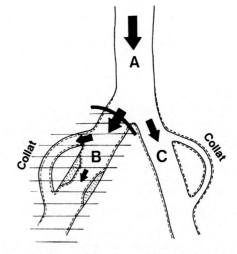

FIGURE 39-20. A vasodilatation restricted to branch *B* and its collaterals (*Collat*) and vessels beyond the arterial obstruction should increase blood flow to this region.

negative feedback loop, is influenced by sympathetic efferents (Fig. 39-12) (53). Interruption of this feedback loop may explain the often remarkable pain relief seen after sympathetic blocks in patients with threatening gangrene, despite a lack of improvement in skin blood flow. It is possible that increased efferent sympathetic activity increases activity in nocireceptors by way of sympathetic fibers in proximity to sensory receptors. This is an explanation for pain relief that may follow stellate

ganglion block in patients with arteriopathy (e.g., associated with scleroderma) in the upper limb, despite the lack of change in blood flow.

Important observations from single-fiber neurography by Jørum's group prove that direct stimulation of nociceptor afferent fibers by sympathetic efferent discharge occurred in a patient with chronic pain in both legs, pain that had repeatedly been eliminated by sympathetic blocks for several weeks

TABLE 39-2
INDEPENDENT TESTS OF SYMPATHETIC FUNCTION, BLOOD FLOW, AND PAIN

Method of Evaluation
Sympathetic function
Skin conductance response (SCR) (41,94,99–101)
Sweat test
Ninhydrin (66)
Cobalt blue (16)
Starch iodine
Skin plethysmography and "ice response" (16)

Blood flow (102)
Plethysmography (muscle and skin) (22,103)
^{133}Xenon clearance (muscle and skin) (32,104,105)
^{24}Sodium clearance (muscle and skin) (106)
Antipyrine clearance (18)
Doppler technique (whole limb) (107,108)
Electromagnetic flow meter (whole limb) (1,21,36,38,109)
Laser Doppler flowmetry (14,15,47,84)
Pulse wave (skin) (102,110–112)
Temperature (skin) (23,25,26,28,34,113)
Size of ulcer (skin) (16)
Distal perfusion pressure (23–28)
Capillary oxygen tension (muscle or skin) (70)
Venous oxygen tension, saturation (muscle) (34)
Metabolism (muscle) (34)

Pain
Pain score (16)
Analgesic requirements
Pain-limited functional activity (e.g., claudication distance)

PART IV: PAIN MANAGEMENT

TABLE 39-3

PERCENTAGE OF PATIENTS WITH OCCLUSIVE VASCULAR DISEASE WHO RESPONDED TO LUMBAR SYMPATHETIC BLOCK

Rest pain (%)	Skin lesions (%)	Claudication (%)	References
	55	13	44, 45
	60	41	106
	64		8
57	45		61
71	55	20	49
62	100 (5/5)		87
63–51	35		105
48 (some)	33		42
57	43		102
	6		41
49 (complete relief)	50	–	24
80 (complete or partial relief)		–	24
–	–	0	43
–	–	0	88

(13). Although such mechanisms have long been suspected, this observation proves that it in fact does occur in patients with chronic pain. Thus, there now exists a solid scientific rationale for why some patients have remarkable pain relief from efferent sympathetic blockade with IV guanethidine or specific sympathetic ganglion blocks with local anesthetic drugs. Such sympathetically maintained pain is not always present in neuropathic pain conditions. Although a history of pain that is aggravated by cold or anxiety may indicate the presence of components of sympathetically maintained pain, only an effective sympathetic blockade can determine the presence of such pain.

Some clinical observations also indicate that early herpes zoster pain and healing of skin vesicles are improved by sym-

pathetic blockade (see Chapter 42) (54,55). That this condition also responds well to a block of the appropriate somatic nerve is well established, so that it is uncertain whether any specific sympathetic involvement is present in this condition. Results of sympathetic block in the treatment of postherpetic neuralgia are uniformly disappointing.

It is well documented that the pain of uterine contraction and cervical dilatation can be abolished by blockade of sympathetic afferents entering the spinal cord at T11–T12 (T10–L1). These fibers are better classified as visceral nociceptive afferents, leaving sympathetic fibers only as efferents. However, interactions between such visceral afferent fibers and the sympathetic efferents are common, as shown in Figures 39-21

TABLE 39-4

RESULTS OF LUMBAR SYMPATHETIC BLOCKADE IN PATIENTS WITH OBLITERATIVE ARTERIAL DISEASE

Primary symptoms	Number of patients		Results of initial continuous local anesthetic and neurolytic block			
			Pain relief 2+	1+	0	–
Gangrene arteriosclerotic	55	L.A.[a]		28	27	0
				∴28 phenol blocks		
			14	9	5	0
Diabetic neuropathic pain	28	L.A.		14	14	
				∴14 phenol blocks		
			8	4	2	0
Severe rest pain	23	L.A.	19	4	0	0
			23			
			∴18 phenol blocks	(5 resolved with L.A.)		
			18	0	0	0
Intermittent claudication	16	L.A.	7	6	2	1
			12			
			∴12 phenol blocks	(1 resolved with L.A.)		
			7	9		

[a]L.A., initial local anesthetic block. (Kövames, A., and Löfström, B.: Continuous lumbar sympathetic block in the treatment of patients with ischemic lower limbs. 10th Congress of Int. Cardiovascular Soc., 1971.)

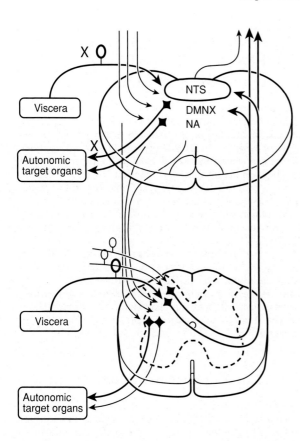

- Sensations:
  non-painful,
  discomfort

- shaping emotions

- Regulations,
  reflexes in
  autonomic
  systems

- Sensations:
  non-painful,
  discomfort,
  painful

- shaping emotions

- Changes in
  referred zones

- Regulations,
  reflexes in
  autonomic
  systems

FIGURE 39-21. Painful and nonpainful stimuli via ("parasympathetic") visceral afferent nerve fibers (about 40,000) via the glossopharyngeal nerve (*IX*) and vagal nerve (*X*) to medulla oblongata (nucleus tractus solitarii [*NTS*]), dorsal motor nucleus of vagus (*DMNX*), and nucleus ambiguus (*NA*). Painful and nonpainful stimuli are also transmitted via ("sympathetic") visceral afferent nerve fibers (about 15,000) in dorsal nerve roots to spinal cord, travelling in the hypogastric, lumbar sympathetic, minor and major splanchnic, and cardiac nerves. Sacral part of the spinal cord also receives visceral afferents ("parasympathetic") from pelvic organs via the sacral nerves and their dorsal root ganglion. General functions of afferent visceral neurons are indicated in the right column; see also the following two figures. Note that the cell bodies of the intrinsic primary afferent neurons of the enteric autonomous nervous system are located in the walls of the intestines. From Jänig W. The integrative action of the autonomic nervous system. In: *Neurobiology of Homeostasis*. Cambridge: Cambridge University Press, 2006, with permission.

through 39-23. The pain of uterine contractions during the first stage of labor is effectively relieved by extradural sympathetic blockade (see Chapter 24).

Also, in a small series of patients with renal colic treated with extradural sympathetic block at L1, nine of 14 patients passed their stones in 10 days and all were pain-free from the start of treatment; this series has now been increased to 32, all of whom obtained complete pain relief (56). This compares favorably with other methods, and it has been suggested that relief of pain and reduction of ureteral spasm is produced by sympathetic blockade of the first lumbar segmental outflow. Chronic pain from the urogenital tract has, in a few cases, been eliminated with chemical lumbar sympathectomy (57).

Cervicothoracic sympathetic blockade is also of value in the treatment of patients with severe angina pectoris, provided that the block extends caudally. The hazards, however, may often outweigh the benefits, except for those with medically intractable angina. Spinal cord stimulation is an alternative method of treating these patients (see Chapter 41).

In posttraumatic complex regional pain syndrome (CRPS), sympathetic blockade is often followed by relief of the burning pain in the injured extremity and a feeling of softening of the tissues, primarily around the joints (7,11,58,59). Symptoms of CRPS may be caused by hyperactivity in the sympathetic nervous system or abnormal supersensitivity of adrenoceptors (11,12), producing vasoconstriction, a decrease in capillary cross-sectional area, redistribution of blood flow, decreased oxygen uptake (tissue hypoxia), increased vascular permeability, and a lack of fluid mobilization (11,60). Clearly, interaction between sympathetic efferent discharge and nociceptive fibers is a possibility (13) (see Chapter 46). A sympathetic blockade

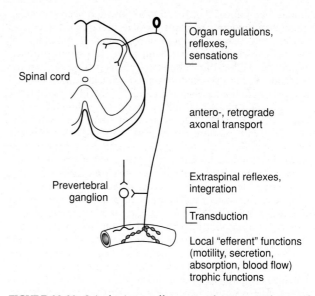

FIGURE 39-22. Spinal primary afferents supplying viscera have multiple functions: They are involved in visceral organ regulations (e.g., motility, secretion, absorption, blood flow), autonomic extraspinal reflexes and conscious sensations from viscera (e.g., pain, nausea, distension/bloating). From Jänig W. The integrative action of the autonomic nervous system. In: *Neurobiology of Homeostasis*. Cambridge: Cambridge University Press, 2006, with permission.

PART IV: PAIN MANAGEMENT

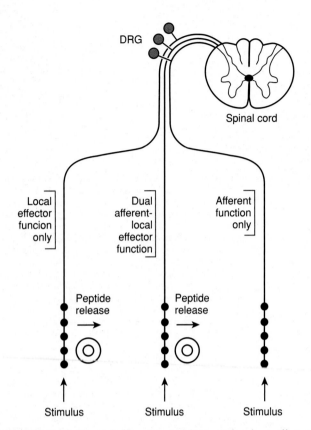

FIGURE 39-23. Visceral afferent neurons having either direct afferent functions to the central nervous system (*right*), local efferent functions to effector organ (*left*), or both (*middle*). From Jänig W. The integrative action of the autonomic nervous system. In: *Neurobiology of Homeostasis*. Cambridge: Cambridge University Press, 2006, with permission.

should then improve nutrient blood flow and decrease the accumulated fluid in the tissue, which explains the increased warmth and the rapid disappearance of tissue edema often seen during this form of treatment. Sympathetic block only produces significant residual clinical improvements if used early in this syndrome. Only two randomized controlled studies ($N = 27$ patients) were found when searching the world literature, and no conclusion of effect could be made (61). Blinding of such studies is not possible, and "evidence of effect" will be difficult to obtain with randomized clinical trials for this treatment. Expert opinion is the best evidence base for recommending sympathetic blocks for CRPS (62) (see also Chapter 46).

Sympathetic block is sometimes not helpful in posttraumatic pain syndromes (10–12). Although reflex hyperactivity of the sympathetic nervous system may be present in sympathetically maintained neuropathic pain, abnormal adrenoceptor hyperactivity, or abnormal interactions between sympathetic efferent and nociceptive afferent fibers, may be more common: Increased or abnormal sensitivity to adrenergic agents in primary afferent nociceptors of damaged nerves may be a result of damaged sympathetic (motor) nerve fibers in mixed peripheral nerves. The resulting denervation hypersensitivity from augmented production of adrenergic receptors means that signs of sympathetic overactivity may be present locally, with a normal (or low) sympathetic nervous system activity (11,63). Also CRPS is associated with pathophysiology at a spinal cord level, which may not be altered by peripheral sympathetic ganglion block (see Chapter 46).

TESTING THE COMPLETENESS OF EFFERENT SYMPATHETIC BLOCKADE

In a patient with a healthy vascular system, a sympathetic blockade produces clear-cut subjective and objective effects on the peripheral circulation, as discussed earlier in this chapter. In a patient with severe arterial disease, however, a complete sympathetic blockade may be achieved with little or no demonstrable effect on the peripheral circulation.

Venous circulation is generally not involved in the disease process, and swelling of the veins can be a valuable indication of a successful block. Table 39-2 lists objective tests that can be used to provide an assessment of completeness of sympathetic block.

The results of all indirect methods that measure blood flow or temperature before and after sympathetic block depend on the initial condition. Low initial temperature (and blood flow) generally implies a large change after the block; a sympathetic block in a patient with high initial temperature (and blood flow) usually will result in only small changes after the block (unless the patient is then exposed to cold after the block) (44).

Skin Conductance Response

Skin conductance response was previously called the sympathogalvanic response (SGR). Skin conduction response tests not only efferent sympathetic activity but also afferent sensory activity and spinal and supraspinal interneurons. Increased sympathetic activity, which in many people can be evoked by a short, deep breath or by pinching the skin, is followed by a change in skin conductance that can be recorded with a simple electrocardiograph (ECG). One ECG electrode is placed on the front and one on the back of the hand or foot (i.e., where sweat glands are abundant). A third grounding electrode is placed anywhere on the body. If necessary, the signal-to-noise ratio of the response may be increased by scrubbing off superficial epithelial cells. In most patients, a slow change will occur in the baseline conductance after such scrubbing, which will stabilize after a few minutes. A short, deep breath or pinching will now, with a 1- to 2-second delay, be followed by a marked deflection that lasts for 4 to 5 seconds. This deflection does not occur if the efferent sympathetic fibers of the extremity are blocked. A partial block of the response will be seen if the patient is atropinized (in clinically used doses). It is preferable to perform separate tests on two limbs simultaneously, thus making it possible to compare the blocked side with the unblocked side. This is essential if the SCR deflections are to be measured in the evaluation of indications for another sympathetic blockade (Fig. 39-24). It is well known that the baseline is far less stable and the deflections much more marked in young than in elderly patients. In elderly patients, it is also more difficult to provoke a sympathetic response, particularly in depressed people and in people who are cold. Also, the SCR undergoes marked habituation; that is, repeated stimuli have a tendency to produce smaller and smaller deflections. Each stimulus should therefore be 2 to 3 minutes apart. When habituation occurs, waiting for a few minutes, putting a warm blanket over the patient, and changing the stimulus from a deep, short breath to pinching or to verbal stimulation or, if available, to a more painful electrical stimulation, usually restores a good response.

Ample experience with SCR has made it clear that it is not always possible to abolish it with sympathetic blockade, even

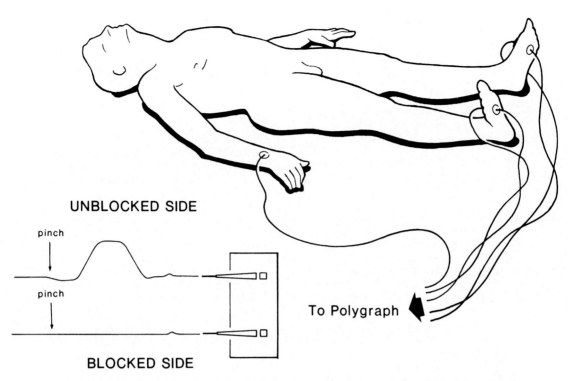

FIGURE 39-24. Skin conductance response (SCR) or sympathogalvanic response. Electrodes are placed on the front and back of hands or feet, and a ground electrode is placed elsewhere on the body. Changes in baseline level on an electrocardiogram (ECG) recorder indicate changes in sweat gland activity.

though the vascular response seems to be maximal. It has been suggested that SCR can be used to predict the value of a sympathetic blockade in patients with arterial disease (30,64). Most patients with a good to moderate deflection on stimulation benefited from a sympathetic block, but not those with little or no deflection. We have also used the SCR to check the completeness of sympathetic denervation following local anesthetic or chemical sympathectomy. When a permanent sympathetic blockade is under consideration and no, or only weak, skin resistance deflections are seen following SCR, a continuous sympathetic blockade is unlikely to be followed by any improvement in the peripheral circulation, although in some cases it may offer pain relief.

Skin Potential Response

The skin potential response (SPR) is an alternative to the SCR (65). The SPR, like the SCR, has a rise time of 1 to 2 seconds and a fall time of 10 to 15 seconds. Skin potential response has an amplitude of 5 mV. Like SCR, SPR is due to an increase in sympathetic activity with subsequent changes in sodium chloride flux in sweat gland ducts and hence, conductance. The benefits claimed for SPR are that electrode size and placement are less critical than for SCR, and no external signal source is required. However, modified ECG recording equipment is needed because (a) most ECG machines have a frequency response of 0.1 to 100 Hz, whereas SPR requires 0.03 to 2 Hz; (b) 50-Hz interference may occur; (c) SPR requires a wider range of input sensitivity than provided by standard ECG machines; (d) ECG recorder paper speed of 25 mm/sec is too fast for SPR; and (e) pre-gelled Ag–Agl electrodes are required (Red Dot; 3M Corp.). A positive electrode is placed over palm or sole and a negative electrode over the dorsum of hand or foot. An indif-

ferent electrode is attached at the contralateral wrist or ankle. Spontaneous changes in sympathetic tone result in negative, then positive, swings on the SPR recording. As with SCR, several factors influence the response: (a) degree of arousal—CNS depression abolishes the response; (b) drugs that alter sympathetic activity, for example, opiates and tranquilizers; (c) anticholinergic drugs abolish the response since acetylcholine is the sudomotor transmitter; and (d) corticosteroids interfere with sodium flux in sweat glands.

Sweat Test

Sweat tests are perhaps the simplest and most sensitive tests of sympathetic activity.

Ninhydrin Photomicrography Method. Fingerprints are taken (at intervals) before and after blockade (66). After suitable preparation, which includes heating, the fingerprints are developed, and each functioning sweat gland can be seen and counted. This test is very accurate and its results reproducible; however, it is time-consuming and does not provide the clinician with an answer at the bedside.

Cobalt Blue Filter Paper Test. Filter papers are soaked in cobalt blue and then dried in an oven, after which they are kept in a desiccator until needed. Two filter papers are removed from the desiccator with forceps and placed on a clean, dry surface, so that the patient can press both feet or hands onto the papers. Sweating is registered on the paper by a change in color from blue to pink. A limb with complete sympathetic block usually produces no color change (Fig. 39-25). Details for preparation of the filter papers are found in Table 39-5.

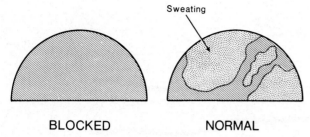

BLOCKED   NORMAL

FIGURE 39-25. Cobalt blue sweat test. The papers are blue (*shaded*) before the test. Sweating from the unblocked limb changes the color to pink (*stippled*).

Starch-Iodine Test. The starch-iodine test works on a principle similar to that of the cobalt blue test. It has the advantage that the material can be spread over a complete limb. It is a messy technique, however, and not well accepted by patients.

Having ensured that sympathetic block is adequate, its effect upon blood flow can then be assessed. If this followed by the ice test (Fig. 39-13), a further evaluation of sympathetic function

can be obtained and, if pain was present before blockade, pain intensity and relief can be independently assessed (Fig. 39-14).

Assessment of Blood Flow Changes

Whole Limb Blood Flow

Indirect

Doppler Ankle/Brachial Index (67). An ultrasound probe is used to facilitate blood pressure measurement with a standard cuff at the brachial artery and also at the ankle. An ankle-to-brachial index is then calculated as follows:

$$Ankle/brachial = (80/50)/(120/80) = 0.65$$

This reading is then repeated after sympathetic block.

Direct

Electromagnetic Flowmeter. This can be applied either directly to a blood vessel during surgery or percutaneously, using a "catheter tip" version.

TABLE 39-5

COBALT BLUE SWEAT TEST

General Requirements
Whatman no. 41 filter papers 5.5 cm (halved) × 100
Cobalt chloride crystals (500 g)
Silica-gel crystals
Thermometer (and antiseptic)
Distilled water
Dressing forceps
Oven and tray
Blankets
Infrared lamps × 2 (or heat cradle)

Filter Paper Preparation
Dissolve 10 g of cobalt chloride in 100 mL of distilled water
Dip and drain halved filter papers, using forceps
Place on tray in oven at approximately 150°C for 20 minutes (avoid excessive drying)
Remove with forceps from oven when pink color changes to bright blue
Seal in airtight jar with silica-gel crystals

Procedure
Record patient's oral temperature
Apply lamp for 30 minutes to trunk and arms (take care not to burn patient or heat face excessively)
Using forceps, place filter paper on firm dry surface, and apply both palms or plantar surfaces of feet, ensuring application is as airtight as possible
Rerecord oral temperature, aiming to increase it by 0.3°F
Cease heat application if the above is recorded or if frank sweating is present

Comments
The procedure should be performed pre- and postblock because some patients have decreased sweating preblock (not including diabetic patients).
Ideally, an area is also needed where the patient may bathe after treatment, because a profuse sweating reaction is desired to ensure that adequate heating has been achieved before adequate denervation exists.

Response	Filter paper
Normal response (profuse sweating)	Blue → pink
Slight reduction (moderate sweating)	Blue → mottled pink/blue small area
Moderate reduction (slight sweating)	Blue → mottled pink/blue large area
Complete reduction (no sweating)	Remains blue

a Available from any large chemical supply house.

Ultrasonic Flowmeter. Very small probes are available that can be placed on the vessel wall at operation and left in situ postoperatively.

Muscle Blood Flow

Venous Occlusion Plethysmography. This has been used in the calf area under the assumption that the calf is mostly muscle with little skin.

Clearance of Radioactive Substances after Direct Injection (e.g., ^{133}Xe). This provides one of the best measurements of nutritive blood flow (Fig. 39-26) (1).

Oxygen Concentration in Blood from Deep Calf Veins. This has also been used as an indirect estimate of oxygen delivery to calf muscle (34). A *mass spectrometer probe* has been developed to measure muscle tissue Po_2 directly.

Skin Blood Flow

Clearance of Radioactive Substances. Radioactive agents, such as ^{133}Xe and ^{124}Na, are injected directly into the skin and their clearance measured.

Laser Doppler Flowmeters. These flowmeters provide a noninvasive assessment of changes in skin blood flow (14,15).

Mass Spectrometer Microprobes and Skin "Cups." These are used to measure changes in skin Po_2 after different forms of treatment.

Skin Occlusion Plethysmography. This method has also been used in the area of the foot, hand, and digits, as described earlier (Fig. 39-13) (16).

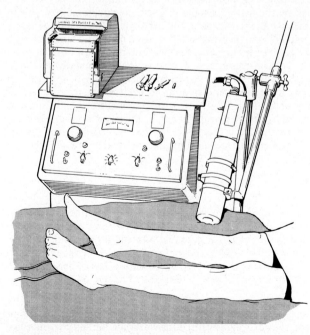

FIGURE 39-26. ^{133}Xenon clearance technique for leg muscle blood flow. ^{133}Xenon is injected into the anterior tibial muscle, and its clearance detected with a portable scintillation detector.

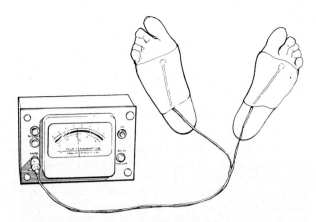

FIGURE 39-27. Skin thermocouple probe and telethermometer. Simultaneous measurements are made on treated and untreated limb.

Skin Temperature Measurements. This technique, using a thermometric camera or contact thermistor or thermocouple skin probes, provides an indirect but easily obtained estimate of changes in skin blood flow (Fig. 39-27). Liquid thermal crystals and heat-sensitive papers are also available.

Optical Density Skin Plethysmography (or Pulse Monitor). Several very sensitive finger "pulse-meters" are available; these use several different wavelengths of light directed into the skin capillary bed. Capillary blood flow results in a cyclical change in optical density, yielding a waveform similar to that shown in Figure 39-13, with an amplitude inversely proportional to sympathetic activity.

Measurement of Size of Skin Ulcers. Progressive documentation of change in ulcer size is a very simple, practical method of checking progress after sympathetic block in patients with ischemic skin lesions.

Pain Assessment

As discussed in Chapters 31, 35, and 37, no objective method of pain assessment exists. Indirect methods such as the pain score (numeric rating scale or visual analogue scale), analgesic requirements, and improved level of activity are used; wherever possible, these should be performed by an independent observer using a double-blind observation (see Chapters 35–37).

Baseline measurement/assessment before sympathetic block should be performed in each case for sympathetic activity, blood flow, and pain score by one of the methods described earlier. After sympathetic blockade, the completeness of sympathetic block, its effect on blood flow, and any effects on pain should be ascertained.

GENERAL CLINICAL APPLICATIONS

The clinical situations in which sympathetic blockade may be considered are summarized in Table 39-1. The present lack of definitive data, and the potential for both short- and long-term morbidity, makes it highly desirable to carry out a diagnostic block before considering permanent blockade. In addition, one or more of the methods of independently assessing blockade, blood flow, and pain relief should be used. When feasible, a sham (placebo) injection should be performed before progressing to irreversible neurolysis or sympathectomy.

General Contraindications

Patients on Heparin

Severe bleeding has been observed, particularly after lumbar sympathetic blockade in a heparinized patient. The bleeding occurs within the psoas fascia, producing minimal symptoms until frank shock occurs. Early symptoms are pain in the groin or pain when the leg is actively lifted and rotated outward. A hematoma may also pass through an intervertebral foramen into the spinal canal after stellate or lumbar sympathetic block, causing pressure on nerves and vessels followed by neurologic symptoms (see also Chapters 11 and 12). Hematoma after stellate block has been reported to interfere with carotid blood flow (see Chapter 12). General considerations related to regional anesthesia in the presence of anticoagulant therapy including newer agents such as low-molecular-weight heparins or antiplatelet agents are discussed in Chapter 12.

Bilateral Injection during One Treatment Session

Bilateral injection during one treatment session should be avoided. Dosage tends to be high, and vascular responses may be a significant problem in this class of patient. Various side effects may pose an increased hazard if both sides are blocked. For example, bilateral recurrent laryngeal block after stellate block may cause stridor (see Chapter 20).

Bilateral Injection in the Lumbar Region for Permanent Blockade

Bilateral injection into the lumbar region may cause loss of ejaculation (68) and should be avoided in young persons; however, impotence does not occur, and the patient does not become sterile.

Agents for Sympathetic Blockade

For short-term block, any of the conventional local anesthetics can be used. The addition of epinephrine to the local anesthetic solution will, to some extent, prolong the duration of action; however, the use of epinephrine in patients with severe vascular disease or vasospasm is questionable. Mepivacaine and bupivacaine, without epinephrine, have durations of 1.5 to 3 and 3 to 10 hours, respectively. These durations are influenced only marginally by the addition of epinephrine, and circulating epinephrine has effects of its own on pain modulation, increasing sensitization of nociceptors to mechanical stimulation and possibly increasing allodynia and hyperalgesia (8, pp. 146–147).

Epinephrine also may produce or worsen subjective feelings of anxiety. Therefore, plain solutions are preferable (69,70). It is useful to add contrast medium (2 mL of iohexol [Omnipaque or Conray-420]), as this allows confirmation of the adequacy of spread of solution (e.g., over L2–L4 ganglia; see Fig. 39-28).

The amount of local anesthetic agent needed in, for example, lumbar sympathetic blockade (1–5 mL, 0.5% mepivacaine or 0.25% bupivacaine at each level), even without epinephrine,

poses a relatively small risk of a toxic systemic reaction from local anesthetic absorption. There is, however, the ever-present risk of acute intravascular injection and the other adverse effects of local anesthetic injection (see Chapter 55). For a permanent block (chemical sympathectomy), 6% to 7% phenol in water, 7% to 10% phenol in water-soluble (e.g., iohexol [Omnipaque/Angiographin]) contrast medium, or 50% to 100% alcohol may be used. The last yields the highest incidence of neuralgia, and most authorities now prefer 7% to 10% phenol in Angiographin because it poses minimal resistance to injection, and its spread can be viewed under radiographic control (16,39,51,71).

TECHNIQUES

Stellate Ganglion Block (Cervicothoracic Sympathetic Block)

Regional Anatomy

The cervical sympathetic chain lies in the prevertebral fascial space, which is limited posteriorly by the fascia over the prevertebral muscles and anteriorly by the carotid sheath (Fig. 39-29).

Although the sympathetic preganglionic fibers for the head, neck, and upper limb leave the spinal cord from segments as widely separated as T1 to T6, pathways converge and pass anteriorly to the neck of the first rib. Here, the first thoracic and inferior cervical ganglion may remain separate or fuse to form the stellate ganglion. In the latter case, the ganglion lies over the neck of the first rib. The ganglion is covered anteriorly in its lower part by the dome of the pleura, and in its upper part by the vertebral artery. Blockade of the stellate ganglion alone may provide disappointing results despite the correct anatomic placement of solution. This failure may be explained by the diverse origin of the sympathetic fibers in the thoracic cord and also by the fact that some thoracic preganglionic fibers lie in other sympathetic ganglia and may bypass the stellate ganglion completely on their way into the head, neck, and upper extremity (72). For best results, the local anesthetic solution has to fill the space in front of the prevertebral fascia caudally to at least T4. This can be achieved by an injection of 15 to 20 mL of weak local anesthetic solution in front of the transverse process of C6 (Fig. 39-30). It is obvious that little advantage is gained by needle placement at C7, and there is a greater risk of pneumothorax at this level. The term *cervicothoracic sympathetic block* thus seems more appropriate than *stellate ganglion block*.

Procedure

A large number of techniques have been described. If the needle is aimed at C7 or the neck of the first rib, the risk of pneumothorax is considerable. On the other hand, the needle may be kept well above the pleura and reliance placed on the spread of a large volume of solution. This is the basis of the anterior approach first described by Leriche (6).

Anterior "Paratracheal" Technique. The patient lies supine with the head slightly lifted forward on a thin pillow and tilted dorsally to stretch the esophagus away from the transverse processes on the left side; a rolled towel under the shoulders helps to increase access to the target area and also stretches

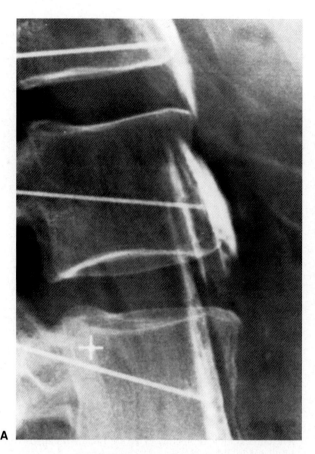 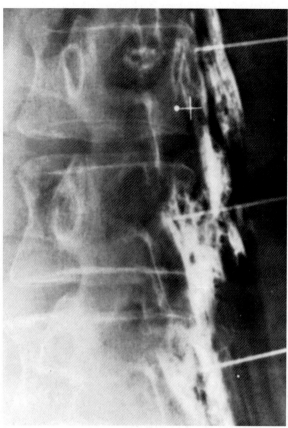

FIGURE 39-28. A: Lateral view. Complete coverage of L2 and L4 vertebral body levels with injection of only 1 mL of 10% phenol on Conray 420 at each level. **B:** Anteroposterior view to show spread of solution following line of psoas muscle. Note limitation of lateral spread to reduce risk of genitofemoral nerve involvement.

the esophagus out of the way. The mouth should be slightly opened to relax the neck muscles.

The trachea and the carotid pulse are gently palpated by inserting two fingers between the sternocleidomastoid muscle and the trachea to find the most prominent cervical transverse process at C6—the Chassaignac tubercle, which lies at the level of the cricoid cartilage (Fig. 39-29). A skin wheal is raised with a fine needle over this transverse process. Two fingers are now gently pressed down to the C6 tubercle, pushing away the carotid artery laterally and the trachea toward the midline with the fingers slightly separated, so that the tubercle lies just in between them (Fig. 39-31).

A 22-gauge, short-bevel, 4- to 5-cm-long needle, with a 20-mL syringe attached, is advanced through the skin and underlying tissues until it hits bone—that is, it rests on the junction of the C6 body and transverse process. The palpating fingers maintain their position; the hand holding the needle is kept braced against the patient, and the needle is withdrawn about 2 mm and fixed (Fig. 39-31).

Aspiration is performed before and after four test doses of 0.5 mL. Injection of even this small dose directly into the vertebral artery can result in a convulsion (see Chapter 5). A high resistance during injection may indicate periosteal injection, and a significant but lesser resistance indicates that the needle is still in prevertebral muscle, whereas radiating pain means the needle is too deep and that it has penetrated a nerve root. While the needle is in situ, it is important that the patient not

talk. If aspiration tests are negative and no sequelae follow the test dose, then the full dose of 15 to 20 mL of local anesthetic is injected in four to five divided doses (Fig. 39-31). In most instances, the patient will quickly feel a lump in the throat and may often be temporarily hoarse; she should be warned beforehand about these events and reassured that they are normal. Because of these effects, patients are more comfortable sitting up after the block is completed. Fluids and food should be withheld while laryngeal reflexes are impaired. As these reflexes return, the initial oral intake should first be sips of water without ice, then clear liquids without ice, such as apple juice.

Continuous Technique. A continuous technique has been described in which a thin radiopaque Teflon catheter is introduced under radiographic control using the paratracheal technique just described. The stylet is withdrawn and the catheter properly fixed (73). It should be recognized, however, that movement of the catheter tip into proximity with vertebral artery, dural cuff, or other structures is possible.

Intravenous Sympathetic Block. This may be a more attractive technique when prolonged effect is required (see Chapter 15 and the following sections).

Signs of a Successful Block

Horner syndrome (Fig. 39-31) results if the cervical sympathetic fibers are blocked successfully: ptosis (drooping upper

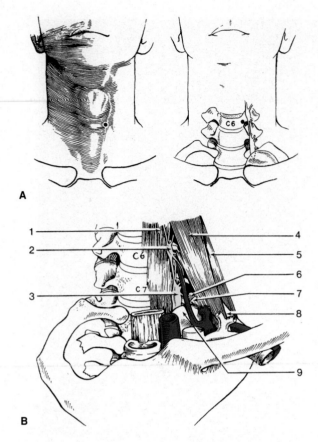

1. Longus Colli Muscle
2. Middle Cervical Ganglion
3. Stellate Ganglion
4. Scalenus Anterior Muscle
5. Scalenus Medius Muscle
6. Transverse Process of First Thoracic Vertebra
7. Tubercle of First Rib
8. Brachial Plexus
9. Dome of Pleura

FIGURE 39-29. Cervicothoracic sympathetic chain: Regional anatomy. **A:** Anterior view. Note stellate ganglion on neck of first rib and extending up to transverse process of C7. At this level, the cervicothoracic sympathetic chain has the vertebral artery on its anterolateral aspect with the pleura covering the lower third of the stellate ganglion. At the level of C6, the vertebral artery has dived posteriorly into the foramen intertransversarium, and the pleura is well below. Note also that even at C6, a large volume of solution may diffuse posteriorly between the slips of origin of scalenus anterior to the roots of the brachial plexus **B:** Cross-section. Note the importance of lateral retraction of the carotid and extension of the neck to draw the esophagus medial to the needle path on the left side. It is necessary to withdraw the needle 2 to 5 mm after contacting the transverse process, in order to clear the anterior aspect of the longus colli muscle. Correct needle direction onto the transverse process is very important, as is the avoidance of force with the risk of penetration of prevertebral fascia and intertransversarium ligaments leading to entry into vertebral artery or dural cuff. Modified from Bryce-Smith R, Macintosh RR. *Local Analgesia: Abdomen.* Edinburgh: Livingstone Press, 1962, with permission.

eyelid), miosis (small pupil), and enophthalmos (sinking in of the eyeball). In addition, other features have been described, such as unilateral nasal congestion (owing to engorgement of nasal mucosa), flushing of conjunctiva and skin, and anhidrosis (lack of sweating). The ptosis and conjunctival engorgement can be relieved by eyedrops of the α-agonist Neo-Synephrine. It should be noted that these signs may be present without com-

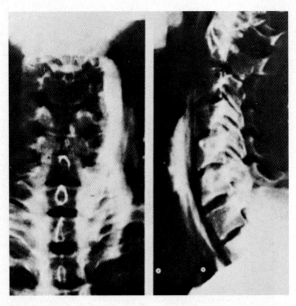

FIGURE 39-30. The spread of 20 mL of local anesthetic solution injected in front of the prevertebral fascia at the sixth transverse process.

plete sympathetic denervation of the upper limb, which may receive sympathetic supply from as far down as T9. The cobalt blue sweat test or SCR is the most useful in this situation.

Indications

The clinical indications for cervicothoracic sympathetic blocks are listed in Table 39-6.

These indications are based largely on anecdotal case reports, so that an initial diagnostic blockade should always be accompanied by a separate assessment, using one of the methods in listed in Table 39-2 for sympathetic ablation, blood flow, and pain.

The most controversial indications are stroke and other conditions in the cranial distribution of the sympathetic chain, such as Ménière disease. At present, no definitive data are available to demonstrate any benefit from sympathetic blockade.

Complications

Intra-arterial and intradural injections are dangerous complications. It should be firmly stated that a negative aspiration test, as described earlier, does not exclude an intra-arterial or an intradural injection owing to a "flap-valve" effect of a vessel wall or dura upon the lumen of the needle tip. To prevent such complications, one must realize that the needle should not meet any resistance after it has passed through the skin, until it rests on what is obviously bone. If the needle is pushed through the prevertebral fascia and the ligaments connecting the transverse processes (this fascia and the ligament can usually be felt), the tip of the needle might be within or adjoining the vertebral artery or the dural sheath enclosing the cervical nerve roots. Spinal analgesia, or even total spinal anesthesia, follows dural sheath injection (see also Chapter 50).

Common complications of cervicothoracic blockade include temporary hoarseness and feeling of a lump in the throat (recurrent laryngeal nerve block), the unpleasant effects of Horner syndrome, hematoma, and neuralgia along chest wall and inner aspect of upper arm. Uncommon complications include brachial plexus injury (rarely), phrenic nerve block, pneumothorax, and osteitis of the transverse process. Severe

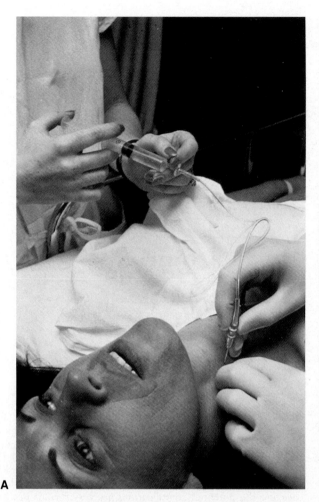
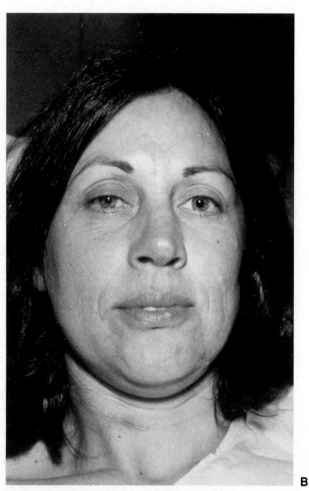

FIGURE 39-31. A: Stellate ganglion block needle correctly placed. Note palpating hand (*left*) retracting carotid sheath laterally and hand holding needle (*right*) braced against clavicle. An extension tubing is used, so that an assistant may aspirate and inject. **B:** Horner syndrome *(right)*. Note ptosis, miosis, anhydrosis, and unilateral conjunctival engorgement. All three of these conditions should be treated at an early stage, for "acute or chronic" episodes.

complications include injection into the vertebral artery, producing immediate CNS effects with grand mal seizures, and intradural injection, with a slower onset of symptoms of spinal anesthesia.

An injection of local anesthetic solution into the paravertebral fascia may also spread along the fascial plane to involve the brachial plexus (74). Bilateral injection is inadvisable since inadvertent bilateral recurrent laryngeal nerve block may result in airway problems (loss of laryngeal reflex). Also, loss of cardioaccelerator activity may result in bradycardia and hypotension.

If a superficial skin hematoma occurs, it might be necessary to inject below C6. This can usually be accomplished because it is possible to feel the prevertebral fascia and the ligaments over C7, after which the needle should be withdrawn several millimeters and the block completed as described; however, the risk of pneumothorax increases.

Osteitis of the transverse process has been described after a stellate ganglion block, possibly because the needle traversed the nonsterile lumen of the esophagus before reaching the transverse process (72).

Chemical Stellate Ganglion Block

An injection of 1 to 2 mL of 6% aqueous phenol or 10% phenol in iohexol (Omnipaque or Conray dye) at C6 will interrupt the cervical chain but will not produce a complete cervicothoracic sympathetic blockade. The arm may escape partially and, in these cases, an injection of the sympathetic chain at T2 and T3 can be used as a supplement; however, this technique is rarely practiced because of the proximity of pleura and somatic nerves (see also Chapter 42). A dural sheath may be entered, and injected solutions may migrate by means of the cerebrospinal fluid (CSF) to the nearby spinal cord with devastating sequelae. A persistent Horner syndrome may also be a problem.

Thoracic Sympathetic Block

Regional Anatomy

The sympathetic chain in the thoracic region lies close to the neck of the ribs, and thus is very close to the somatic roots (Fig. 39-3). In the cervical region, the sympathetic chain is

TABLE 39-6

CLINICAL CONDITIONS THAT CERVICOTHORACIC SYMPATHETIC BLOCKADE MAY BENEFIT

Circulatory Insufficiency in the Arm, due to:
Traumatic or embolic vascular occlusion or impaired circulation (e.g., intra-arterial thiopental)
Postoperatively after reimplantation surgery of fingers/hand (sympathetic and somatic block of brachial plexus are preferable when pain is present)
Postembolectomy vasospasm
Raynaud disease, scleroderma and other arteriopathies, frostbite[a]
Occlusive vascular disease: "acute on chronic" episodes

Pain
Complex regional pain syndromes (CRPS) type I and type II (63) (see Chapter 46)
Causalgia following abdominal injury (114)
Herpes zoster (e.g., ophthalmic herpes zoster)
Phantom limb
Paget disease
Neoplasm
Tropic changes in skin
Pain due to lesions in the CNS (115)

Other
Hyperhidrosis
Miscellaneous conditions in head region: stroke, Ménière disease, tinnitus
Amblyopia due to quinine poisoning (116) (also causes retinal artery spasm and thrombosis)

separated from somatic roots by longus colli and anterior scalene muscles and, in the lumbar region, by the psoas major. In contrast, no such muscle is present in the thoracic region, and the proximity of the pleura to the sympathetic chain adds a second hazard (Fig. 39-3).

Technique

A 10-cm needle is introduced and angled toward the vertebral body two fingerbreadths (3 cm) from the midline opposite the T2 spinous process. As the needle is advanced, it either strikes rib or passes through the intercostal space and continues until it is held up by the body of the vertebra in the true paravertebral space (Fig. 39-3). It is generally easy to decide whether the bone encountered is rib or vertebral body, because the rib is more superficial and transmits through the needle a feeling of smoothness, in contrast to the gritty roughness of the surface of the vertebral body. Because of the anatomic problems outlined earlier, confirmation of position by image intensifier is highly desirable. When the needle reaches the vertebra, it is angled to pass less than 1 cm behind the crest of the vertebral body (Fig. 39-3). At this point, an injection of 2 mL of local anesthetic or, for permanent block, 6% phenol or absolute alcohol, is made, and a successful result is indicated if the patient has a warm dry hand and no evidence of Horner syndrome. The use of image intensifier and injection, under direct vision, of 10% phenol dissolved in iohexol (Omnipaque), Conray-420, or Angiographin greatly increases the safety of this technique.

Indications

Some possible indications for permanent neurolytic sympathectomy for the upper limb syndromes are given in Table 39-1. Many clinics still prefer surgical sympathectomy, although a transaxillary (thoracic) approach is necessary to obtain complete sympathetic denervation of the upper limb; the use of

thoracoscopic technique has been a significant advance. The results and complications of the neurolytic technique using an image intensifier remain to be assessed. Intrathoracic pain, such as status anginosus, has been treated by sympathetic block (by either stellate or thoracic approach); however, the availability of β-blockers has diminished the appeal of sympathetic block, because the potential complications are very serious in a patient with severe myocardial disease. New options for status anginosus are cervical spinal cord stimulation (see Chapter 41) and epidural or intrathecal opioid and nonopioid drugs administration (see Chapter 40).

Complications

The two principal complications of this technique are pneumothorax and intrathecal injection (75) by way of the intervertebral foramen. Because of these two complications, this technique was used only minimally until recent application of image intensifier techniques allowed direct viewing of needle placement and appropriate spread of solution (see Chapter 50).

Lumbar Sympathetic Block

Regional Anatomy

The lumbar part of the sympathetic chain and its ganglia lie in the fascial plane close to the anterolateral side of the vertebral bodies, separated from somatic nerves by the psoas fascia and psoas muscle (Figs. 39-4 and 39-32). An injection of a large volume of fluid (e.g., 25 mL) anywhere in this space will, in most instances, fill the whole space. Theoretically, one injection at L2 or L3 should be enough to achieve adequate longitudinal spread. This single-injection technique is now used by a number of experienced specialists in pain clinics. However, in other clinics, injections are performed at two different levels, particularly with a neurolytic agent such as phenol, to limit

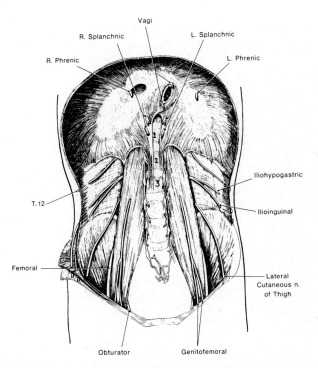

FIGURE 39-32. Posterior abdominal wall, genitofemoral nerve. Note its course anterior to the psoas major, thus being more vulnerable to neurolytic solution spreading laterally from the sympathetic chain. Modified from Bryce-Smith R, Macintosh RR. *Local Analgesia: Abdomen.* Edinburgh: Livingstone Press, 1962, with permission.

lateral spread at any one level. Uncontrolled lateral spread poses a risk of traversing the psoas to reach the genitofemoral nerve, perhaps by a fibrous tunnel to a somatic nerve or, worse still, to a dural cuff region and thence to subarachnoid space (Fig. 39-33) (76). When continuous blockade with catheters is used, it is also preferable to place two catheters because of the tendency for a catheter to slide dorsally out of position.

In an anatomic study, lumbar sympathetic blocks were performed "blind" in cadavers to investigate the frequency of major organ puncture (77). The technique of inserting the needles was based on that of Mandl (see later description). With the cadaver in the lateral position, three 22-gauge, 15-cm needles were inserted about 10 cm from the midline at the approximate levels of L1, L2, and L3. In thin cadavers, the distance of needle insertion from the midline was about 7.5 cm, whereas in obese subjects the distance was greater (up to 12.5 cm). Each needle was advanced onto the vertebral body, gradually positioned more anteriorly until it slipped beyond the anterolateral aspect of the vertebral body (Fig. 39-4), and then advanced to the "hilt" to allow the cadaver to be positioned supine. The cadaver was then rolled over and needle insertion repeated on the other side.

Eighty needles were inserted in the direction of the lumbar sympathetic chain, and 95% passed either through the lumbar sympathetic chain or within 0.5 cm of it. In 90% of those occasions on which the chain was not traversed, the needles were lateral to the chain.

One needle passed through the hilum of the kidney, although in that cadaver there was a large osteophyte over an intervertebral disk that displaced the needle laterally. Two needles were found embedded in grossly osteoporotic vertebral bodies. All three of these placements would, doubtless, have been

prevented by using a C-arm image intensifier like that used routinely in clinical practice. The position of the lumbar sympathetic chain was remarkably consistent on the anterolateral aspect of the vertebral bodies.

Almost all of the needles either passed through the sympathetic chain or lateral to it. As Figure 39-4 shows, the more lateral the insertion of the needle, the closer the tip should be to the lumbar sympathetic chain; there is also a lesser risk of piercing roots of the lumbar plexus or of contacting the transverse process.

Technique (Mandl) with Two Needles

The method of blocking the lumbar sympathetic chain was first introduced by Mandl in 1926, and was similar to that used by Kappis for injecting the celiac plexus (4,5).

The spinous processes of L1 and L4 are marked as reference points. L1 is level with the line between the two points where the lateral margin of the erector spinae muscles meets the twelfth ribs; a line joining the posterior superior iliac crests passes through the lower part of the spine at L4 (Fig. 39-34).

A subcutaneous wheal is raised about 8 to 10 cm laterally to the middle of the spinous processes of L2 and L4. Local anesthetic solution is injected subcutaneously (and with an intramuscular needle, against the transverse process above or below the site of injection by directing the needle 45 degrees cranially or caudally and in between the transverse processes, if these are to be contacted).

A 20- to 22-gauge needle of approximately 12 cm in length (or an 18-gauge needle for continuous blockade) with a rubber marker on its shaft is introduced through the skin until the tip of the needle has reached a transverse process. The marker is pushed down to the skin and the needle withdrawn. The distance from the skin to the transverse process is, in the normal adult, roughly half the distance from the skin to the lateral side of the vertebral body (10 cm). This may be a shorter distance if the patient has thin back muscles, or longer if the muscles are thick. The marker on the needle is moved toward the hub of the needle, so that the distance from the tip to the marker is roughly twice the first marked distance. In general, "hugging" the cephalad edge of the transverse process as the needle is advanced will reduce the likelihood of inadvertent contact with a lumbar root and consequent paresthesia or dural puncture.

The needle is reintroduced and directed slightly medially to pass between the transverse processes. When bone is reached, the marker should be almost flush with the skin, the bevel of the needle being directed toward the lateral side of the vertebral body. A slight change in needle angle will allow the tip of the needle to slide off the vertebra and to reach the sympathetic chain on the ventrolateral aspect of the vertebral body (Fig. 39-34) (78). Correct position can be verified by using a loss-of-resistance test, with a syringe filled with air or saline. Penetration of the psoas fascia gives a resistance change not dissimilar to that of epidural block. Some specialists prefer to avoid the transverse process, so that the needle proceeds directly to the lateral aspect of the vertebral body. A loss of resistance, at a shallower level, is often obtained between psoas and quadratus lumborum in the region of the transverse process (Fig. 39-35). Placement of solution at this level would result in lumbar plexus block—a devastating result if a neurolytic solution is used.

In clinical practice, the anesthesiologist often starts at L2 and, in a second step, introduces the needle at L4. When the needle is correctly placed at L2, that part of the needle outside

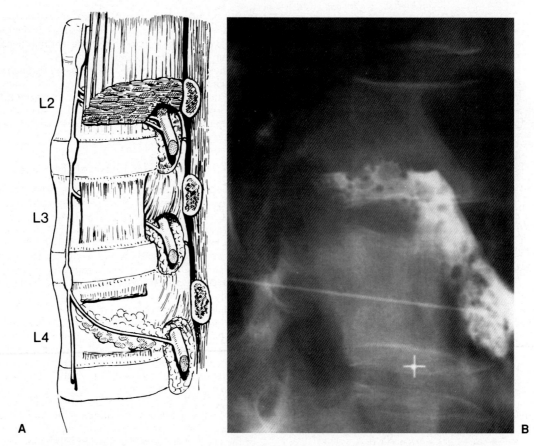

FIGURE 39-33. A: Fibrous arch between paravertebral space and lumbar sympathetic chain. This pathway poses a potential for spread of neurolytic solution to somatic nerve roots, resulting in possible sensory loss or neuralgia. **B:** Contrast medium injected too close to side of vertebral body spreading via fibrous arch. Part **A** is modified from Bryce-Smith R, Macintosh RR. *Local Analgesia: Abdomen.* Edinburgh: Livingstone Press, 1962, with permission.

the skin should be measured, and the marker for L4 properly placed. In most patients, owing to the lumbar lordosis at L4, the distance from the skin to the vertebral body is slightly greater than at L2. It is vitally important to aspirate to ensure that neither blood nor CSF is present, and to check that there is no resistance to injection; resistance could be due to the needle being in the wall of the aorta or vena cava, an abdominal viscus, or an intervertebral disk. Once again, radiographic confirmation (local anesthetic mixed with contrast medium) and injection under direct vision increase safety (16,51,63,71). Placement of the needle on the desired vertebral body can be confirmed on a posteroanterior C-arm view, and proper needle depth confirmed by turning the C-arm to a lateral view. At that point, the tip of the needle should lie along the anterior projection of the vertebral body.

In the most simple cases (e.g., renal colic), one injection of 20 to 30 mL in three to four divided doses, preferably of 0.25% bupivacaine with epinephrine, 1:200,000 (5 μg/mL), at L2 will completely eradicate pain. In patients with obliterative arterial disease, a diagnostic block using 1 to 5 mL of local anesthetic mixed with contrast medium may be made at L2 and L4 under radiographic control. The continuous blockade technique is also very useful; needles are placed at L2 and L4, and, after the proper positioning of each needle, catheters are passed through the needles, which are then withdrawn over the catheters. The catheters are taped to the skin along the erector spinae muscles. The cranial ends of the catheters, each with a needle and a Millipore filter, are placed in a sterile sponge in the supraclavicular fossa. Alternatively, the catheters may be taped laterally, so that their tips lie over the abdomen, in an effort to diminish the effects of the patient bending forward and causing their distal tips to migrate superficially. The time interval between injections may be increased to 6 hours if bupivacaine is used. Continuous blockade is maintained for 5 days, during which its clinical effects should be evaluated. In the case of single-shot diagnostic block, the volume of local anesthetic in contrast medium should be the same as that proposed for neurolytic block. Also, a method of assessment from each category in Table 39-2 should be used immediately after the block. Often, diagnostic blocks are repeated if there is any doubt about results (79).

In most instances, the procedure is short (<30 min) and well tolerated. Heavy premedication or general anesthesia is not necessary and not recommended: Now and then, however, a needle may pass close to a segmental nerve, provoking "electric" pain. The needle should always be advanced slowly and redirected slightly, if paresthesia should occur. The needle should not be directed too much toward the midline. We believe that it is better to be able to detect that the needle is close to a nerve in a lightly medicated patient than to accept the risk of undetected laceration of the nerve with a fairly large needle in a patient under general anesthesia. One case report of severe

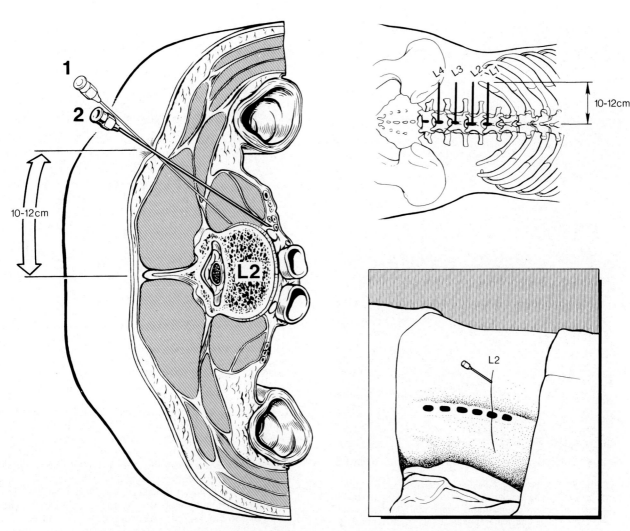

FIGURE 39-34. Technique of lumbar sympathetic block. Note location of skin marks for L1 and L4 spinous processes, which then permit identification of L2 and L3. A line is drawn through the center of the spinous processes; this will lie below the transverse process of that vertebra. Needle insertion (*1*) is at the lateral margin of the erector spinae muscle (approximately 10 to 12 cm from midline). If it is desired to check the depth of the transverse process, the needle must be angled cephalad. Otherwise, the needle is inserted approximately 45 degrees toward the vertebral body until this structure is located. Then, the needle is angled more steeply until it slips just past the vertebral body and through the psoas fascia (*2*). A single needle can be used instead of two or three needles; however, an increased volume must be injected.

segmental neuralgia, most likely the result of a nerve injury, supports this cautious view (16).

Single Injection Technique for Local Anesthetic or Neurolytic Block

Hatangdi and Boas describe the use of the tip of the twelfth rib to act as a marker for needle insertion 2 to 3 cm below and medial to that point (80). This approach allows easy access to the L3 vertebral body, after which placement next to sympathetic chain is verified, as described earlier. Sufficient solution is injected (mixed with contrast medium) to cover L2, L3, and L4 levels. An alternative is to use the twelfth rib to intersect a line drawn through the middle of the L2 spinous process. Needle insertion at this point should be sufficiently lateral to obtain easy access to the L3 level. If desired, the transverse process can be avoided and the needle inserted directly onto the lateral

aspect of the vertebral body. Sufficient solution is then injected to cover the sympathetic chain (Fig. 39-36).

Technique of Bryce-Smith

An alternative approach to local anesthetic lumbar sympathetic blockade has been described by Bryce Smith (in 1951) (81).

Because of the anterolateral position of the ganglia in the lumbar region, the course of the rami communicantes is long and winds around the vertebral body in a fibrous tunnel. This arch forms one of the origins of the psoas muscle and provides indirect access to the lumbar sympathetic chain (Fig. 39-37).

A wheal is raised three fingerbreadths (roughly 6 cm) lateral to the tip of the spinous process of L3, and a 12-cm needle is introduced at a 70-degree angle to the skin and advanced medially toward the body of the vertebra; when the point of the needle reaches the body of the vertebra, it lies within the fibrous

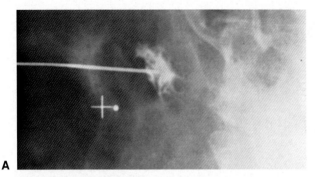

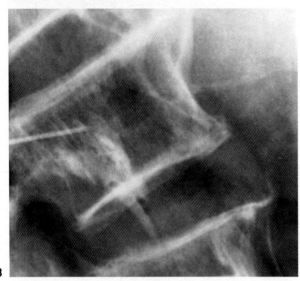

FIGURE 39-35. **A:** Radiograph showing injection of contrast medium into psoas major. **B:** Radiograph showing injection too far posteriorly, probably between psoas and quadratus lumborum aortoiliac (small percentage responding) and femoropopliteal (higher percentage responding).

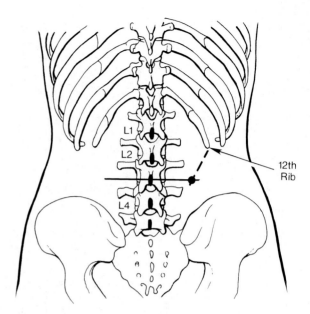

FIGURE 39-36. Single-needle technique of lumbar sympathetic block. Note needle insertion 2 to 3 cm below and medial to the tip of the twelfth rib. This should lie on a line through the center of L3 spinous process. From Hatangdi VS, Boas RV. Lumbar sympathectomy: A single needle technique. *Br J Anaesth* 1985;57:285, with permission.

◼ *Symptoms can be ameliorated without risk of surgery and anesthesia* in a group of patients with a high incidence of severe ischemic heart disease, pulmonary disease, and other problems of old age. In the series reported by Reid and colleagues(3), there was a mortality of 1:1666 injections (less than 0.1%); this compares favorably with surgical sympathectomy, which has a mortality rate of at least 6% (83a) and up to 20% in patients with severe vascular disease. In a series of 386 blocks, only one death occurred within 1 week of blockade, in a patient with severe ischemic heart disease with congestive cardiac failure prior to blockade (16).

tunnel (Fig. 39-37). Fifteen to 20 mL of solution are deposited here, and this tracks forward to reach the sympathetic chain. This approach should not be used when neurolytic solutions are employed, because some of the fluid may backtrack to cause a neuritis of the third lumbar nerve, or it may enter a dural cuff to cause paraplegia.

Because this technique frequently leads to somatic block and does *not* provide a selective sympathetic block, it is also not indicated for diagnosis of pain syndromes.

Lumbar Sympathectomy with Neurolytic Agent

Neurolytic lumbar sympathectomy should be used for the treatment of vascular disease in consultation with a vascular surgeon. It is clear that even a successful sympathetic block in a patient with rest pain may result sometimes in demarcation of a nonviable area, such as a distal phalanx of a toe. This will require appropriate surgical treatment and should not be viewed as a disappointing side effect of the block, but rather as a necessary limitation of a rational treatment regimen (82,83).

The use of lumbar sympathetic block with proper collaboration offers considerable advantages:

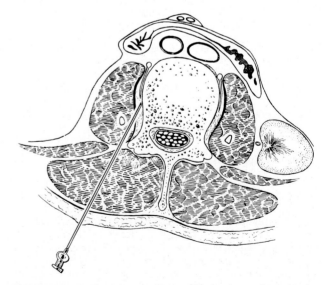

FIGURE 39-37. Alternative technique for local anesthetic lumbar sympathetic block. Modified from Bryce-Smith R, Macintosh RR. *Local Analgesia: Abdomen.* Edinburgh: Livingstone Press, 1962, with permission.

■ *Outpatient treatment.* Treatment may be performed on an outpatient basis, and elderly patients (usually 60–80 years of age) can be released after a short stay. This allows for considerable economy in hospital bed use; surgical sympathectomy often requires several days in the hospital, even when there are no complications.

■ *Fewer postoperative thrombotic phenomena.* Such complications are reduced in the elderly because an operation and bed rest are avoided.

■ *A large turnover of patients* is possible (as many as eight to 10 procedures in a single-day session).

■ *If necessary, a bilateral procedure* can be performed, with the second side blocked 1 week later, also on an outpatient basis.

■ *Duration.* Because the duration of sympathetic ablation is similar with surgical or neurolytic sympathectomy (mean, 6 months), the neurolytic technique offers an advantage. It can be repeated with very minimal morbidity. Nevertheless, the natural history of occlusive vascular disease is such that, in one series, only 5% required repeated blockade (16).

Agents

Absolute alcohol has been used by several groups; however, it has a higher incidence of L1 neuralgia (see Chapter 42) (16). Seven percent phenol in water was used by Reid and colleagues in a very large series because of the low viscosity of the solution and ease of injection (3). Seven percent to 10% phenol in iohexol (Omnipaque), Conray-420 dye, or Angiographin has a similar low resistance to injection and the added advantage of being visible under image intensifier (Fig. 39-38) (16,39,51,71). When the patient is placed on her side under a vertical radiographic beam, it is also of value for the patient to be tilted slightly, ventrally and dorsally, to check that the needle is fairly close to the vertebral column. One report advocates the semi-prone position with vertical x-ray screening to give a more precise view of needle position relative to vertebral body anterolateral aspect, with a single x-ray view (84). If a biplanar image intensifier is available, then both lateral and anteroposterior views should be obtained (Fig. 39-39). A convenient way to determine the spread is to dissolve phenol in an aqueous radiographic contrast medium (Omnipaque, Conray-420, or Angiographin) and inject it under direct radiographic control (Fig. 39-39; Table 39-7). This often allows confirmation of complete coverage of the lumbar sympathetic chain, with as little as 3 to 4 mL of solution (Fig. 39-28).

Technique

The following modifications of local anesthetic blockade are advisable when neurolytic agents are used:

1. A radiopaque marker is placed on the skin (49), and the level of needle insertion is checked under image intensifier. Needle position in the center of the L2 and L4 vertebral bodies is checked with a lateral view (Fig. 39-39). Proximity of the needle to the disk space is avoided.
2. Needle position at the anterolateral angle of the L2 and L4 bodies is also checked in the lateral view (Fig. 39-39). Lack of movement of the needle during deep inspiration and expiration is checked carefully. With correct placement, needle tips should be immobile. Movement on respiration indicates placement lateral to psoas—possibly in the kidney.
3. An anteroposterior view is taken to check that each needle is close to the lateral aspects of the vertebral bodies (Fig. 39-39).

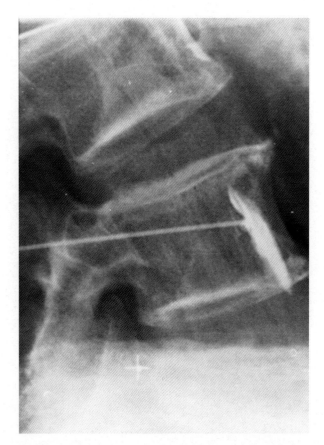

FIGURE 39-38. Injection of 0.5 mL of contrast medium, showing correct linear spread along anterior aspect of psoas fascia.

4. Initially, 0.5 mL of contrast medium is injected and confirmation obtained that a sharp linear spread is occurring (Fig. 39-38). Resistance to injection and the appearance of a "blob" or fuzzy patch of contrast medium indicate injection into muscle or fascia, and injection is ceased pending proper repositioning (Fig. 39-35).
5. As soon as linear spread is obtained, the injection is continued with neurolytic solution until each level has linear coverage. In most instances, this requires no more than 2 mL and often as little as 1 mL of solution (Fig. 39-28).
6. At the completion of the injection, an anteroposterior view is taken to confirm the spread of solution along the lateral aspect of the vertebral body (Fig. 39-28).
7. Finally, 0.5 mL of air is injected immediately before removing each needle to prevent the needle's depositing neurolytic solution on somatic nerve roots during removal.

Patients are kept on their sides for 5 minutes to prevent the solution from spreading laterally toward the genitofemoral nerve or posteriorly between the slips of origin of the psoas major and along the fibrous tunnel occupied by the rami communicates, toward somatic nerve roots (76,81). Patients are then turned supine but instructed not to raise their heads for 30 minutes. Observations of skin temperature, blood pressure, and pulse are continued.

Recovery Procedure

Observations are continued for 1 hour in a recovery room, and, if stable, patients are permitted to sit upright to 45 degrees and

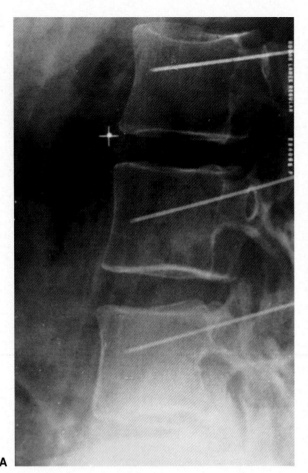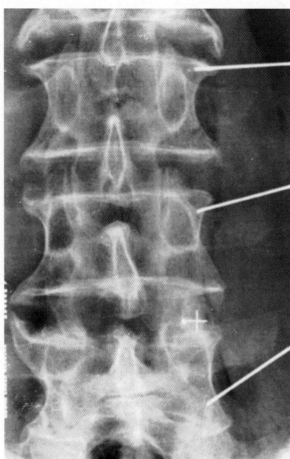

FIGURE 39-39. Radiographs. **A:** Needle placement, lateral view. **B:** Needle placement, anteroposterior view.

resume oral intake. Blood pressure is checked sitting and then standing, and, if unchanged, patients are allowed to ambulate. Most outpatients are then able to go home, accompanied by a friend or relative. Patients with highly unstable cardiovascular disease are to be observed for at least 24 hours postblock prior to discharge.

Indications

The most common clinical indications for lumbar sympathetic blocks are listed in Table 39-8.

Some clinics have stopped using diagnostic blocks for patients with atherosclerotic vascular disease and rest pain, skin ulcers, or gangrene and instead progress directly to neurolytic lumbar sympathetic blockade. Their rationale is that the incidence of adverse effects from neurolytic blockade is extremely low, and many of these patients tolerate multiple procedures poorly. In a series with measurement of pain, blood flow, and sympathetic activity, the results of diagnostic and neurolytic sympathetic blocks were essentially the same in every patient studied (Fig. 39-14) (39). In younger patients whose chronic pain syndromes are less well-defined, however, diagnostic blocks should be performed before neurolytic sympathetic block. As discussed in the section on physiologic effects of sympathectomy, the best rationale for the use of lumbar sympathectomy in arterial disease is to obtain improved skin blood flow; however, pain relief may occur even without improved blood flow. Tables 39-3, 39-4, and 39-9 summarize

clinical data on the use of lumbar sympathectomy for pain and skin ulcers, as well as for other conditions in which its efficacy is more difficult to determine except by diagnostic block in each case.

Complications

Complications of lumbar sympathetic blocks are extremely rare; however, a needle directed too far medially may pass into an intervertebral foramen, causing paraplegia. This may be recognized by the flow of CSF, but it is not always the case. Thus, confirmation of correct placement by radiography is mandatory prior to neurolytic injection (see also Chapter 50).

Common complications of neurolytic lumbar sympathetic blockade[a] include puncture of major vessel or renal pelvis, subarachnoid injection, neuralgia—genitofemoral nerve (5% to 10% pain in the groin), somatic nerve damage—neuralgia (1%), perforation of a disk, stricture of the ureter after phenol or alcohol injection, infection from catheter technique (extremely rare), ejaculatory failure (bilateral block in young males), and chronic back pain.

After surgical and chemical sympathectomies, pain or discomfort in the groin is often seen, hypothetically attributed to a genitofemoral nerve neuralgia. The discomfort may last 2 to 5 weeks (16,51,85,86). This is so-called L1 neuralgia and is

---

[a]See Chapter 30; only useful *early* in these conditions.

TABLE 39-7

PREPARATION OF 10% PHENOL IN IOHEXOL

Name of Preparation
10% phenol in iohexol (Omnipaque), Conray-420 (or Angiographin)

Ingredients
100 g of phenol A.R. (crystals)
IL Conray-420 (or Angiographin)

Equipment
1-liter glass measuring cylinder with stopper
1-liter vacuum flask
Scintered glass filter
Tufryn 0.45 μm 7-mm (Gelmann HT-450) membrane filter mounted in a Millipore Swinnex 47-mm holder
Sterile disposable 50-mL syringe
Connector tube (about 9 inches) for outlet of filter

Identity Number
All washed with pyrogen-free water for injections filtered through a 0.2 μm filter, then dried in hot air oven, with all exposed outlets covered with aluminum foil.

Method of Manufacture
Weigh phenol into 1-L measuring cylinder
Remove outer seals of Conray-420 bottles, leaving stoppers in place
Rinse exterior of these bottles with filtered water for injections
Place bottles in laminar flow cabinet after rinsing, and allow to dry in air stream
Remove stoppers with rinsed forceps
Pour Conray-420 into graduated cylinder containing phenol
Shake to dissolve phenol; make to volume and mix

Container/Closure Description
Container, 20-mL antibiotic vial
Stopper, red merco, lacquered to suit
Crimp cap, gold aluminum, long skirt to suit

Packing—Equipment and Method
Laminar flow cabinet
Filter through sintered glass into 1-L vacuum flask
Pour into Pyrex dish and load 50-mL syringe
Filter from syringe through 47-mm Tufryn filter with connector tube attached to outlet of filter holder and leading to vials.

---

characterized by hyperesthesia in L1 distribution and a burning pain. The patient often says that it is unbearable even to have clothes touch the thigh and may also describe the leg as "feeling as though it will explode." The condition responds well to transcutaneous electrical stimulation. The incidence is much higher with alcohol and appears to occur least when the volume injected at any one level is the minimal amount necessary to achieve coverage of sympathetic ganglia, as checked by image intensifier (16).

After thoracoscopic sympathectomy for hyperhidrosis, very severe discomfort and hyperhidrosis in the neighboring non-sympathectimized regions occurred with alarming frequency and intensity. We are not aware of such complications following lumbar neurolytic sympathetic blocks.

INTRAVENOUS REGIONAL SYMPATHETIC BLOCK

Site of Action and Efficacy

Intravenous regional sympathetic block (87) is based on the "Bier block," a local anesthetic IVR block described in Chapter

15. The sympathetic blocking drug guanethidine (Ismelin) has a high affinity for sympathetic nerve endings, where it displaces norepinephrine from presynaptic vesicles and prevents its reuptake. This causes a brief initial release of norepinephrine, followed by norepinephrine depletion (Fig. 39-11), which results in long-lasting IVRS blocks when the Bier block technique is used. Guanethidine has an advantage over reserpine, which has a similar action, except that reserpine crosses the blood–brain barrier and produces CNS effects, whereas guanethidine does not. Controlled studies have documented the efficacy of IVR guanethidine in increasing blood flow (88,90–95) and skin temperature (88,91) while decreasing the vasoconstrictor ice response (90) and reducing pain (48,88,94) in vascular disease (90) and reflex sympathetic dystrophies (88–90). Sweating is not reduced (90,94) because it is mediated by cholinergic postganglionic sympathetic fibers.

A controlled study in volunteers compared guanethidine and reserpine; it was found that only guanethidine significantly increased temperature after cold challenge and that this effect lasted 3 days (94).

Duration of effect and efficacy of guanethidine was compared with stellate ganglion block in a randomized trial in patients with reflex sympathetic dystrophies (88). In patients treated with stellate ganglion blocks, skin temperature and skin

TABLE 39-8

CLINICAL CONDITIONS THAT LUMBAR SYMPATHETIC BLOCKADE MAY BENEFIT

Circulatory insufficiency in the leg
Arteriosclerotic disease, severe pain gangrene; intermittent claudication in selected cases; diabetic gangrene, Buerger disease
After reconstructive vascular surgery
Arterial embolus

Pain
Renal colic
Complex regional pain syndrome type I and type II (see Chapter 31)
Herpes zoster
Intractable urogenital pain in selected cases
Phantom limb
Amputation stump pain
Chilblains

General
Hyperhidrosis—reduced sympathetic activity to reduce sweating
White leg—phlegmasia alba dolens
Trench foot
Erythromelalgia
Acrocyanosis

Miscellaneous conditions in which reduced sympathetic activity may help to correct an abnormality in nutritive blood flow or venous or lymphatic drainage. Pain in the groin following injection is the most common untoward sequel. Subarachnoid tap is seen occasionally but is easily recognized and should not constitute a hazard. The remaining complications are very rare, when image intensifier control is used.

TABLE 39-9

LUMBAR SYMPATHETIC BLOCK: EXAMPLES OF USES AND RESULTS IN THREE CLINICAL SERIES

Study[a]	Number of cases
After vascular surgery ("continuous" local anesthetic lumbar sympathetic block)	70
Arterial embolism—no surgery	13 (7 improved)
Cytostatic perfusion (melanoma)	4
Frostbite	2
	89
Obliterative arterial disease (local anesthetic block followed by chemical sympathectomy in 72 cases)	122 (see Table 13-2)
Diagnostic local anesthetic followed by neurolytic agent[b]	
Rest pain and ischemic ulcers	386 (80% relieved)
Gangrene of lower extremity (pain relief and speeding up demarcation)	50 (55% relieved)
Reflex sympathetic dysfunction	12 (50% relieved—those treated early)
Claudication	12 (50% relieved; only those with response to local anesthetic block received neurolytic block)
Neurolytic agent over 10-year period[c]	
Rest pain	194 (80% relieved)
Gangrene of lower extremity	40 (50% relieved)
Reflex sympathetic dysfunction (post-traumatic)	42 (45% relieved—those treated early)
Phantom limb	19 (60% relieved)

[a]Data from Löfström B, and Zetterquist S: Lumbar sympathetic blocks in the treatment of patients with obliterative arterial disease of the lower limb. *Int. Anesthesiol. Clin.*, 7:423, 1969.
[b]Data from Cousins MJ, Reeve TS, Glynn CJ, Walsh JA, et al: Neurolytic lumbar sympathetic blockage: Duration of denervation and relief of rest pain. *Anaesth Intensive Care*, 7(2):121, 1979.
[c]Unpublished data from Lloyd JW, et al.

plethysmography measurements were significantly increased at 1 hour but not at later times. In patients treated with guanethidine, skin temperature was increased at 1 hour, 24 hours, and 48 hours postblock. Skin plethysmography measurements were significantly increased at 24 hours and remained so at 48 hours (88).

Stellate blocks every other day (up to a total of eight blocks) produced similar clinical effects to IV guanethidine block every 4 days (up to a total of four blocks) in terms of pain score and clinical signs, when assessed at 1 month and 3 month follow-up (88).

In a within-patient study of IV guanethidine blocks compared to placebo, skin temperature, and hand blood flow were significantly increased at 1 hour postblock (90). At 7 days postblock, hand blood flow, but not skin temperature, was increased. Vasoconstrictor response to ice was decreased at 1 hour and 7 days postblock (90).

Thus, good evidence suggests that an IVRS block offers the following: (a) a less "invasive" and uncomfortable technique for patients; (b) significant diminution of noradrenergic activity, leading to increased blood flow and decreased pain; and (c) effects that are longer-lasting than those of stellate blocks. However, cholinergic activity is *not* modified. Guanethidine blocks only efferent fibers and thus differs from a local anesthetic ganglion block that also affects any afferent fibers passing through the ganglia (8).

A further application of IV sympathetic block is in (upper) limb angiography, where pharmacologic vasodilatation greatly facilitates delineation of the vasculature (95). It is also suggested as an aid to maintaining tissue perfusion in tissue-grafting operations (95). In patients with severe vascular disease, in whom inflation of a tourniquet may be dangerous, guanethidine can be infused slowly into an artery by means of a narrow-gauge needle, with effects similar to those of the IV technique.

Current and Future Options

In some countries, for example, the United States, an IV preparation of guanethidine is no longer available.[b] For this reason, we must examine other potential candidates for use in this valuable technique. Figure 39-40 gives a summary of sympathetic nerve transmission at the adrenergic nerve terminal, sites of action of neurotransmitters, and other factors influencing smooth muscle cells of the vasculature.

Interference with Norepinephrine Synthesis

Methyldopa (Aldomet) was previously thought to have a predominantly peripheral action, leading to formation of a "false transmitter" α-methyl norepinephrine. It now seems, however, that this is metabolized to a powerful agonist, methyl epinephrine. Thus, methyldopa is no longer an attractive choice for IVR block.

Storage Vesicle Depletion and Block of Norepinephrine Reuptake

Guanethidine and reserpine are the only drugs that have been evaluated and remain the only clinical options, where approved. Guanethidine (and also bretylium) block the coupling

of the action potential to norepinephrine release. Bretylium also blocks norepinephrine reuptake.

Reserpine is relatively ineffective and produces many side effects. Bretylium allows only 2 to 7 hours of pain relief after IVRS (93). Many other drugs prevent norepinephrine reuptake, but none have been used for IVRS (e.g., tricyclic antidepressants, cocaine).

Block of Presynaptic (α_2) and Postsynaptic (α_1) Receptors

Phentolamine (Regitine) has been given in a dose of 10 mg IV for IVRS. Precise data on duration of effect are not available. Arnér (94) has shown that IV infusion of phentolamine can predict the therapeutic effect of IVRS with guanethidine ("the IV phentolamine test").

Block of Postsynaptic Receptors (α_1)

Prazosin (Minipress) is a relatively pure α_1-blocker. It does not interfere with the negative feedback on norepinephrine release that is mediated by means of α_2-receptors. No increase in norepinephrine release occurs, and no compensatory tachycardia is seen with phentolamine. Duration of effect with IVRS is not known because an IV preparation has not been approved.

Other α_1-blockers developed and include trimazosin and terazosin. The latter may be of interest because of its reported long duration of effect. All of these drugs pose a potential for postural hypotension and water retention.

Block of Norepinephrine Activity at Level of Vascular Smooth Muscle

This is a complex area, and precise sites of action are not delineated.

Prostaglandins

In most vascular beds, a balance exists between dilatation effects produced by molecules such as PGE_1 and PGI_2 and vasoconstriction effects produced by thromboxanes. PGI_2 is five times more potent than PGE_1 in producing vasodilatation in coronary, renal, mesenteric, and skeletal muscle beds. Effects on arterioles are much greater than on veins. It is possible that the vascular effects are produced by inhibition of norepinephrine release from sympathetic nerve endings. There may also be a direct effect on smooth muscle. Both PGI_2 and PGE_1 inhibit platelet aggregation. It should be noted that PGE_1 causes uterine contraction and is used to produce abortion. Both PGE_1 and PGI_2 have been used by IVRS in patients with severe peripheral vascular disease. Both were reported to give significant and long-lasting improvement in blood flow and tissue oxygenation (95,96). No preparations of these drugs are currently available for IVRS.

Hydralazine (Apresoline) and Diazoxide (Hyperstat IV)

These two drugs have a direct effect on vascular smooth muscle that is as yet poorly defined. Effects on arterioles are greater than on veins. Experimental work has shown a greater effect after intra-arterial than after IV infusion with respect to increased skin temperature and blood flow in limbs.

Neither drug has been evaluated by IVRS. Hydralazine can cause some serious side effects with high-dose and long-term administration, for example, drug-induced lupus erythematosus, peripheral neuropathy, and pancytopenia. Both drugs produce a reflex increase in sympathetic activity as a result of hypotension. This has precipitated angina in susceptible patients.

---

[b]In the United States and some other countries, guanethidine is available for "investigational" use by the IV route.

PART IV: PAIN MANAGEMENT

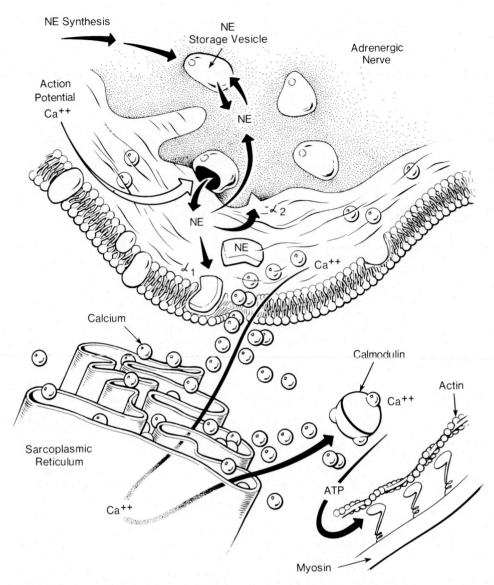

FIGURE 39-40. Peripheral sympathetic neuroeffector synapse and potential sites of action of drugs for intravenous regional sympathetic block. A sympathetic nerve ending (adrenergic nerve terminal), synaptic cleft, cell membrane of smooth muscle of blood vessel wall, calcium (Ca^{2+}) channels, and contractile mechanism are shown. An action potential causes an influx of Ca^{2+} into the nerve terminal, and the norepinephrine (*NE*) storage vesicle fuses with the plasma membrane to release NE. NE then activates α_1-excitatory receptors on smooth muscle (postsynaptic) and α_2-inhibitory receptors on plasma membrane (presynaptic). α_1-Receptor activation in the smooth muscle cell membrane results in an influx of Ca^{2+}, which binds to calmodulin. This regulatory protein molecule then binds to myosin, causing phosphorylation (via adenosine triphosphate [ATP]) and initiation of the actin–myosin contractile process. Potential sites of action for IVRS are as follows: *1.* Norepinephrine synthesis: No drugs currently available for IVRS. *2.* blockade of NE release and reuptake: guanethidine and bretylium block NE reuptake (also block coupling of action potential of NE release), resulting in storage granule depletion. Reserpine also blocks NE reuptake. Note: Tricyclics and cocaine block NE reuptake at plasma membrane of sympathetic nerve ending, which is *not* useful for IVRS. Also, other drugs may inhibit NE release into synaptic cleft: prostaglandin (PGE$_1$) and ATP. *3.* Block of α_2- and α_1-receptors (e.g., phentolamine). *4.* Selective block of α_1-receptors. Prazosin is not available yet as an intravenous preparation. Trimazosin and terazosin (long-acting) are still under development. *5.* Effects on vascular smooth muscle (e.g., diazoxide and hydralazine? action). *6.* Calcium channel blocking drugs: verapamil, nifedipine, diltiazem.

Diazoxide is a relatively weak antagonist to norepinephrine and may have its action mediated by blocking calcium-dependent activation of action potentials in smooth muscle.

Calcium Entry (Calcium Channel) Blocking Drugs

A very large number of drugs of this type are available or under development. In general, they interfere with the flux of Ca^{2+} through smooth muscle cellular membranes, or with the uptake and release of calcium by intracellular membranes. Currently available drugs include verapamil, nifedipine, and diltiazem; however, many more drugs of very diverse structure are being investigated. Nifedipine appears to be more potent as a vasodilator than the other two, but has potent effects on myocardial muscle. It remains to be determined whether any of these drugs will bind firmly enough to vascular smooth muscle with IVRS technique to produce long-lasting vasodilatation, but with minimal cardiac effects. Differences in site of action and physiochemical properties among these drugs may influence their peripheral effects by IVRS technique. For example, nifedipine is a relatively pure slow channel (Ca^{2+}) blocker acting at the "outer gate." Both verapamil and diltiazem appear to act on myosin kinase phosphorylation of myosin at the "inner gate." This prevents myosin–actin cross-bridging, and thus prevents muscle contraction.

Diltiazem may stimulate Ca^{2+} extrusion from the cell, thus lowering sarcoplasmic Ca^{2+}. Because of its deeper site of action and dual action, diltiazem may be more effective for IVRS. However, none of these drugs is approved for IVRS. Because of the role of Ca^{2+} in secretory physiology, endocrine side effects may occur, in addition to cardiovascular side effects resulting from relative overdose.

Technique of Intravenous Regional Sympathetic Block

Guanethidine 10 to 30 mg is dissolved in 25 mL of normal saline for the upper limb and 30 mL for the lower limb. An IV cannula is placed in the nonaffected arm to be used in treatment of side effects. A second cannula is placed in the affected arm. A double cuff, or appropriate equipment, is used to exsanguinate the arm (see Chapter 15). The guanethidine is injected slowly and the cuff kept inflated for a minimum of 20 minutes. The cuff is then slowly deflated while blood pressure is monitored. The patient remains supine until the blood pressure has been stabilized.

Some clinics dilute guanethidine in 20 mL of 0.5% prilocaine to make the injection more comfortable. However, coadministration of a local anaesthetic may interfere with the guanethidine effect on norepinephrine release and reuptake, thus diminishing or abolishing the longer-lasting effect of guanethidine. An alternative technique is to infuse the guanethidine solution slowly into a peripheral artery over 10 to 15 minutes. The results are similar to IVRS, and the technique may be preferable if severe peripheral vascular disease is present.

References

1. Cousins MJ, Wright CJ. Graft muscle skin blood flow after epidural block in vascular surgical procedures. *Surg Gynecol Obstet* 1971;133:59.
2. Wright CJ, Cousins MJ. Blood flow distribution in the human leg following epidural sympathetic blockade. *Arch Surg* 1972;105:334.
3. Reid W, Watt JK, Gray TG. Phenol injection of the sympathetic chain. *Br J Surg* 1970;57:45.
4. Kappis M. Sensibilitat und lokale Anasthesia im chirurginchen Gebiet der Bauchhohle mit besonderer Berucksichtigung der Splanchnicus. *Anasthesie Beitr Z Klin Chir* 1919;115:161.
5. Mandl F. *Die Paravertebrate Injektion*. Vienna: Springer-Verlag, 1926.
6. Lériche R, Fontain R. L'anésthesie isolée du ganglion étoile: Sa technique ses indications ses resultats. *Presse Med* 1934;42:849.
7. Bergan JJ, Conn J Jr. Sympathectomy for pain relief. *Med Clin North Am* 1968;52:147.
8. Jänig W. *The Integrative Action of the Autonomic Nervous System: Neurobiology of Homeostasis*. Cambridge: Cambridge University Press; 2006: 610.
9. Dollery CT, Paterson JW, Conally ME. Clinical pharmacology of beta-receptor-blocking drugs. *Clin Pharmacol Ther* 1969;10:765.
10. Fields HL, Robotham MC. Multiple mechanisms of neuropathic pain: A clinical perspective. In: Fields HL, Liebeskind J, eds. *Progress in Pain Research and Management*. Seattle: IASP Press; 1994:437–445.
11. Jänig W, Stanton-Hicks M, eds. *Reflex Sympathetic Dystrophy: A Reappraisal. Progress in Pain Research and Management*. Seattle: IASP Press; 1996:1–249.
12. Perl ER. A reevaluation of mechanisms leading to sympathetically related pain. In: Fields HL, Liebeskind J, eds. *Progress in Pain Research and Management*. Seattle: IASP Press; 1994:129–150.
13. Jørum E, Ørstabik K, Schmidt R, et al. Catecholamine-induced excitation of nociceptors in sympathetically maintained pain. *Pain* 2006;127:296–301.
14. Bengtsson M. Changes in skin blood flow and temperature during spinal analgesia evaluated by laser Doppler flowmetry and infra-red thermography. *Acta Anaesthesiol Scand* 1984;28:625.
15. Bengtsson M, Nilsson GE, Löfström JB. The effect of spinal analgesia on skin blood flow, evaluated by laser Doppler flowmetry. *Acta Anaesthesiol Scand* 1983;17:206.
16. Cousins MJ, Reeve TS, Glynn CJ, et al. Neurolytic lumbar sympathetic blockade: Duration of denervation and relief of rest pain. *Anaesth Intensive Care* 1979;7(2):121.
17. DeBakey ME, Burch G, Ray T, Ochsner A. The "borrowing-lending" hemodynamic phenomenon (hemometakinesia) and its therapeutic application in peripheral vascular disturbances. *Ann Surg* 1947;126:850.
18. Zetterquist S. Muscle and skin clearance of antipyrine from exercising ischemic legs before and after vasodilating trials. *Acta Med Scand* 1968; 183:487.
19. Larsen OA, Lassen NA. Medical treatment of occlusive arterial disease of the legs: Walking exercise and medically induced hypertension. *Angiologia* 1969;6:288.
20. Lassen NA, Larsen OA, Sorensen AW, et al. Conservative treatment of gangrene using mineralocorticoid-induced moderate hypertension. *Lancet* 1968;1:606.
21. Kovamees A, Löfström B, McCarthy G, Aschberg S. Continuous lumbar sympathetic blocks used to increase regional blood flow after peripheral vascular reconstruction. 18th Congress European Society of Cardiovascular Surgery, 1974.
22. Myers KA, Irvine WT. An objective study of lumbar sympathectomy: II. Skin ischaemia. *Br Med J* 1966;1:943.
23. Thulesius O, Gjores JE, Mandaus L. Distal blood flow and blood pressure in vascular occlusion: Influence of sympathetic nerves on collateral blood flow. *Scand J Clin Lab Invest* 1973;31[Suppl 128]:53.
24. Kovamees A, Löfström B, McCarthy G, Aschberg S. Continuous lumbar sympathetic blocks in the treatment of patients with ischemic lower limbs. 10th Congress of International Cardiovascular Society, 1971.
25. Nielsen PE, Bell G, Augustenborg G, Lassen NA. Reduction in distal blood pressure by sympathetic nerve block in patients with occlusive arterial disease. *Scand J Clin Lab Invest* 1973;31[Suppl 128]:59.
26. Nielsen PE, Bell G, Augustenborg G, et al. Reduction in distal blood pressure by sympathetic block in patients with occlusive arterial disease. *Cardiovasc Res* 1973;7:577.
27. Uhrenholdt A. Relationship between distal blood flow and blood pressure after abolition of the sympathetic vasomotor tone. *Scand J Clin Lab Invest* 1973;31[Suppl 128]:63.
28. Uhrendholdt A, Dam WH, Larsen OA, Lassen NA. Paradoxical effect on peripheral blood flow after sympathetic blockades in patients with gangrene due to arteriosclerosis obliterans. *Vasc Surg* 1971;5:154.
29. Froysaker T. Lumbar sympathectomy in impending gangrene and foot ulcer. *Scand J Clin Lab Invest* 1973;31[Suppl 128]:71.
30. Bengtsson M, Löfström JB, Malmqvist LA. Skin conductance responses during spinal analgesia. *Acta Anaesthesiol Scand* 1985;29:67.

PART IV: PAIN MANAGEMENT

31. Fulton RL, Blakeley WR. Lumbar sympathectomy: A procedure of questionable value in the treatment of arteriosclerosis obliterans of the legs. *Am J Surg* 1968;116:735.

32. Verstraete M. A critical appraisal of lumbar sympathectomy in the treatment of organic arteriopathy. *Angiologia* 1968;5:333.

33. Nielsen J. Thromboangiitis obliterans (Buerger's disease). A study of the prognosis. *Ugeskr Laeger* 1969;131:1740.

34. Löfström B, Zetterquist S. The effect of lumbar sympathetic block upon nutritive blood-flow capacity in intermittent claudication. A metabolic study. *Acta Med Scand* 1967;182:23.

35. Fyfe T, Quin RO. Phenol sympathectomy in the treatment of intermittent claudication: A controlled clinical trial. *Br J Surg* 1975;62:68.

36. Cronestrand R, Juhlin-Dannfeldt A, Wahren J. Simultaneous measurements of external iliac artery and vein blood flow after reconstructive vascular surgery: Evidence of increased collateral circulation during exercise. *Scand J Clin Lab Invest* 1973;31[Suppl 128]:167.

37. Kovamees A. Skin blood flow in obliterative arterial disease of the leg: Effect of vascular reconstruction examined with xenon and iodine antipyrine clearance and skin temperature measurements. *Acta Chir Scand Suppl* 1968;397:1–72.

38. Scheinin TM, Inberg MV. Intraoperative effects of sympathectomy on ipsi- and contralateral blood flow in lower limb arterial reconstruction. *Ann Clin Res* 1969;1:280.

39. Walsh JA, Glynn CJ, Cousins MJ, Basedow RW. Blood flow, sympathetic activity and pain relief following lumbar sympathetic blockade or surgical sympathectomy. *Anaesth Intensive Care* 1984;13:18.

40. Cook PR, Malmqvist L-Å, Bengtsson M, et al. Vagal and sympathetic activity during spinal analgesia. *Acta Anaesthesiol Scand* 1990;34:271.

41. Löfström JB, Malmqvist L-Å, Bengtsson M. Can the "sympatho-galvanic reflex" (skin conductance response) be used to evaluate the extent of sympathetic block in spinal analgesia? *Acta Anaesthesiol Scand* 1984;28:578.

42. Malmqvist L-Å, Bengtsson M, Björnsson G, et al. Sympathetic activity and haemodynamic variables during spinal analgesia in man. *Acta Anaesthesiol Scand* 1987;31:467.

43. Malmqvist L-Å, Trygvasson B, Bengtsson M. Sympathetic blockade during extradural analgesia with mepivacaine or bupivacaine. *Acta Anaesthesiol Scand* 1989;33:444.

44. Malmqvist EL-Å. Sympathetic neural blockade during regional analgesia: Clinical investigation in man. Linköping University medical dissertations, No. 366. Linköping, Sweden, 1992.

45. Greene NM. Preganglionic sympathetic blockade in man: A study of spinal anesthesia. *Acta Anaesthesiol Scand* 1981;25:463.

46. Löfström JB, Thorborg P, Lund N. Direct and indirect effect of some local anesthetics on muscle blood flow-tissue oxygen pressure. *Reg Anaesth* 1985;10:82.

47. Klopfer GT. Neurolytic lumbar sympathetic blockade: A modified technique. *Anaesth Intensive Care* 1983;11:43.

48. Breivik H. Intravenous regional sympathetic blockade with guanethidine. *Tidsskr Nor Lægeforen* 1979;99:935.

49. Hannington-Kiff JG. *Pain Relief*. London: Heinemann Press; 1974:68.

50. Cross FW, Cotton LT. Chemical lumbar sympathectomy for ischemic rest pain. A randomized, prospective controlled clinical trial. *Am J Surg* 1985;150:341.

51. Boas RA, Hatangdi VS, Richards EG. Lumbar sympathectomy: A percutaneous chemical technique. In: Bonica JJ, Albe-Fessard D, eds. *Advances in Pain Research and Therapy*, Vol. 1. New York: Raven Press, 1976:685–689.

52. Hughes-Davies DJ, Redman LR. Chemical lumbar sympathectomy. *Anaesthesia* 1976;31:1068.

53. Procacci P, Francini F, Zoppi M, Maresca M. Cutaneous pain threshold changes after sympathetic block in reflex dystrophies. *Pain* 1975;1:167.

54. Colding A. Treatment of pain. Organization of a pain clinic: Treatment of acute herpes zoster. *Proc R Soc Med* 1973;66:541.

55. Masud KZ, Forster KJ. Sympathetic block in herpes zoster. *Am Fam Physician* 1975;12:142.

56. Lloyd JW, Carrie LES. A method for treating renal colic. *Proc R Soc Med* 1965;58:634.

57. Johansson H. Chemical sympathectomy with phenol for chronic prostatic pain: A case report. *Eur Urol* 1976;2:98.

58. Detakats G. Sympathetic reflex dystrophy. *Med Clin North Am* 1965;49:117.

59. Sternschein MJ, Myers SJ, Frewin DB, Downey JA. Causalgia. *Arch Phys Med Rehabil* 1975;56:58.

60. Linde B. Studies on the vascular exchange function in canine subcutaneous adipose tissue with special reference to effects of sympathetic nerve stimulation. *Acta Physiol Scand Suppl* 1976;433: 1–43.

61. Cepeda MS, Carr DB, Lau J. Local anesthetic sympathetic blockade for complex regional pain syndrome. *Cochrane Database Syst Rev* 2005:CD004598.

62. Livingstone JA, Atkins RM. Intravenous regional guanethidine blockade in the treatment of post-traumatic complex regional pain syndrome type I (algodystrophy) of the hand. *J Bone Joint Surg Br* 2002;84:380–386.

63. Walker SM, Cousins MJ. Complex regional pain syndromes: Including "reflex sympathetic dystrophy" and "causalgia." *Anaesth Intensive Care* 1997;25:113.

64. Boucher JR, Falardeau M, Plante R, et al. Le reflexe sympatho-galvanique (RSG) et la sympathectomie. *Can Anaesth Soc J* 1970;17:504.

65. Cronin KO, Kirsner RL. Assessment of sympathectomy: The skin potential response. *Anaesth Intensive Care* 1979;7:353.

66. Dhuner KG, Edshage S, Wilhelm A. Ninhydrin test: Objective method for testing local anaesthetic drugs. *Acta Anaesthesiol Scand* 1960;4:189.

67. Yao JST, Bergan JJ. Predicting response to sympathetic ablation (quoted in editorial). *Lancet* 1974;1:441.

68. Baxter AD, O'Kafo BA. Ejaculatory failure after chemical sympathectomy. *Anesth Analg* 1984;63:770.

69. Bridenbaugh PO, Moore DC, Bridenbaugh LD. Capillary PO_2 as a measure of sympathetic blockade. *Anesth Analg* 1971;50:26.

70. Nolte H, Ahnefeld FW, Halmagyi M. Die lumbale Grenzstrangblockad zur Beurteilung der Wirkungsdauer von Lokalanaesthetika. *Acta Anaesthesiol Scand* 1966;23[Suppl]:618.

71. Eaton AC, Wright M, Callum KG. The use of the image intensifier in phenol lumbar sympathetic block. *Radiography* 1980;46:298.

72. Moore DC. *Stellate Ganglion Block*. Springfield: Charles C. Thomas, 1954.

73. Linson MA, Leffert R, Todd DP. The treatment of upper extremity reflex sympathetic dystrophy with prolonged continuous stellate ganglion blockade. *J Hand Surg* 1983;8:153.

74. Carron H, Litwiller R. Stellate ganglion block. *Anesth Analg* 1975;54:567.

75. Selander D, Sjostrand J. Longitudinal spread of intraneurally injected local anesthetics. *Acta Anaesthesiol Scand* 1978;22:622.

76. Bryce-Smith R, Macintosh RR. *Local Analgesia: Abdomen*. Edinburgh: Livingstone Press, 1962.

77. Cherry DA, Rao DM. Lumbar sympathetic and coeliac plexus blocks: An anatomical study in cadavers. *Br J Anaesth* 1982;54:1037.

78. Eriksson E. *Illustrated Handbook in Local Anaesthesia*. Copenhagen: Munksgaard, 1969.

79. Bonica JJ. *Clinical Application of Diagnostic and Therapeutic Nerve Blocks*. Oxford: Blackwell Scientific Publications, 1958.

80. Hatangdi VS, Boas RV. Lumbar sympathectomy: A single needle technique. *Br J Anaesth* 1985;57:285.

81. Bryce-Smith R. Injection of the lumbar sympathetic chain. *Anaesthesia* 1951;6:150.

82. Campbell JN, Raja SN, Selig DK, et al. Diagnosis and management of sympathetically maintained pain. In: Fields HL, Liebeskind J, eds. *Progress in Pain Research and Management*. Seattle: IASP Press; 1994:85–100.

83. Ogawa S. Sympathectomy with neurolytics. In: Hyodo M, Oyama T, Swerdlow M, eds. *The Pain Clinic IV*. Utrecht: VSP Publishers; 1992:139–146.

83a. Kim GE, Ibrahim IM, Imparato AM. Lumbar sympathectomy in end stage arterial occlusive disease. *Ann Surg* 1976;183:157–160.

84. Kirnö K. Regional analgesia and sympathetic nerve activity in man. Thesis. University of Göteborg, Sweden, 1992.

85. Dam WH. Therapeutic blockade. *Acta Chir Scand* 1965;33[Suppl]:89.

86. Raskin NH, Levinson SA, Hoffman PM, et al. Postsympathectomy neuralgia amelioration with diphenylhydantoin and carbamazepine. *Am J Surg* 1974;128:75.

87. Hannington-Kiff JG. Sympathetic nerve blocks in painful limb disorders. In: Wall PD, Melzack R, eds. *Textbook of Pain*, 3rd ed. Edinburgh: Churchill Livingstone; 1994:1032–1052.

88. Bonelli S, Conoscente F, Movilia PG, et al. Regional intravenous guanethidine vs. stellate ganglion block in reflex sympathetic dystrophies: A randomized trial. *Pain* 1983;16:297.

89. Driessen JJ, Van Der Werken C, Nicolai JPA, Crul JF. Clinical effects of regional intravenous guanethidine (Ismelin) in reflex sympathetic dystrophy. *Acta Anaesthesiol Scand* 1983;27:505.

90. Glynn CJ, Basedow RW, Walsh JA. Pain relief following post-ganglionic sympathetic blockade with IV guanethidine. *Br J Anaesth* 1981;53:1297.

91. McKain CW, Bruno JU, Goldner JL. The effects of intravenous regional guanethidine and reserpine. *J Bone Joint Surg* 1983;6:808.

92. Vaughan RS, Lawrie BW, Sykes PJ. Use of intravenous regional sympathetic block in upper limb angiography. *Ann R Coll Surg Engl* 1985;67:309.

93. Hanowell LH, Kanefield JK, Soriano SG. A recommendation for reduced lidocaine dosage during intravenous regional bretylium treatment of reflex sympathetic dystrophy. *Anesthesiology* 1989;71:811.

94. Arnér S. Intravenous phentolamine test: Diagnostic and prognostic use in reflex sympathetic dystrophy. *Pain* 1991;46:17.

95. Olsson AG, Carlsson AL. Clinical, hemodynamic and metabolic effects of intra-arterial infusions of prostaglandin E_1 in patients with peripheral vascular disease. *Adv Prostaglandin Thromboxane Res* 1976;1:429.

96. Szczeklik A, Nizankowski R, Splawinski J, et al. Successful therapy of advanced arteriosclerosis obliterans with prostacyclin. *Lancet* 1979;1:1111.

97. Blain A, Zadeh AT, Teves ML, Bing RJ. Lumbar sympathectomy for arteriosclerosis obliterans. *Surgery* 1963;53:164.

98. Gillespie JA. Future place of lumbar sympathectomy in obliterative vascular disease of lower limbs. *Br Med J* 1960;2:1640.

99. Christie MJ. Electrodermal activity in the 1980s: A review. *J R Soc Med* 1981;74:616.

100. Fowles DC, Christie MJ, Edelberg R, et al. Publication recommendations for electrodermal measurements. *Psychophysiology* 1981;18:232.

101. Lewis LW. Evaluation of sympathetic activity following chemical or surgical sympathectomy. *Anesth Analg* 1955;34:334.

102. Gillespie JA. Late effects of lumbar sympathectomy on blood flow in the foot in obliterative vascular disease. *Lancet* 1960;1:891.

103. Myers KA, Irvine WT. An objective study of lumbar sympathectomy. I. Intermittent claudication. *Br Med J* 1966;1:943.

104. Gillespie J. An evaluation of vasodilator drugs in occlusive vascular disease by measurement. *Angiology* 1966;17:280.

105. Hoffman DC, Jepson RP. Muscle blood flow and sympathectomy. *Surg Gynecol Obstet* 1968;127:12.

106. Herman BE, Dworecka F, Wisham L. Increase of dermal blood flow after sympathectomy as measured by radioactive sodium uptake. *Vasc Surg* 1970;4:161.

107. Thulesius O. *Beurteilung des schwergrades arterieller Durchblutungsstorungen mit dem Doppler-Ultraschallgerat.* Angiologie 13. Bern: Hans Huber, 1971.

108. Thulesius O, Gjores JE. Use of Doppler shift detection for determining peripheral arterial blood pressure. *Angiology* 1971;22:594.

109. Weale FE. The hemodynamic assessment of the arterial tree during reconstructive surgery. *Ann Surg* 1969;169:484.

110. Beene TK, Eggers GWN Jr. Use of the pulse monitor for determining sympathetic block of the arm. *Anesthesiology* 1974;40:412.

111. Kim JM, Arakawa K, von Linter T. Use of the pulse-wave monitor as a measurement of diagnostic sympathetic block and of surgical sympathectomy. *Anesth Analg* 1975;54:289.

112. King RD, Kaiser GC, Lempke RE, Shumacker HB. Evaluation of lumbar sympathetic denervation. *Arch Surg* 1964;88:36.

113. Löfström B, Zetterquist S. Lumbar sympathetic blocks in the treatment of patients with obliterative arterial disease of the lower limb. *Int Anesthesiol Clin* 1969;7:423.

114. Szeinfeld M, Saucedo R, Pallares VS. Causalgia of vascular etiology following an abdominal injury. *Anesthesiology* 1982;57:46.

115. Loh L, Nathan PW, Schott GD. Pain due to lesions of central nervous system removed by sympathetic block. *Br Med J* 1981;282:1026.

116. Thomas D. Forced acid diuresis and stellate ganglion block in the treatment of quinine poisoning. *Anaesthesia* 1984;39:257.

PART IV: PAIN MANAGEMENT

CHAPTER 40 ■ SPINAL ROUTE OF ANALGESIA: OPIOIDS AND FUTURE OPTIONS FOR SPINAL ANALGESIC CHEMOTHERAPY

DANIEL B. CARR AND MICHAEL J. COUSINS

Ignored until the late 19th century as a target for anesthesia, and for nearly another hundred years as a substrate for analgesia, the spinal cord has now emerged as a—if not *the*—key target for pain control in clinical anesthesiology. Indeed, the 1984 review of this topic by the senior author (1) has become the mostly frequently cited paper in the 20th century anesthesiology literature (2,3). In successive editions of this text, the topic of spinal analgesia has diffused outward from a small number of chapters, through many others that describe its application in acute pain, cancer pain, obstetrics, orthopedics, and pediatrics, to name but a few. More and more anesthesiologists now give drugs spinally to provide intraoperative (4,5) anesthesia and persistent postoperative analgesia after procedures as diverse as knee arthroscopy (Chapter 25), inguinal hernia repair (Chapter 23), or even (with a "light" general anesthetic) laparoscopic colectomy, thoracoscopy, or coronary artery bypass grafting (Chapter 22) (6). Such operations used to require extensive incisions under general anesthesia, with prolonged and painful hospital stays (7) and the risk of persistent postsurgical pain (8). Today, the combination of minimally invasive surgical techniques and spinal analgesia allows these procedures to be performed on a "fast-track," often outpatient basis (9–11) with demonstrable benefit upon clinical outcome (12–14). Outpatient control of previously refractory cancer pain is now routinely accomplished by implanting pumps for spinal drug delivery (15–18). Intriguing evidence suggests that this approach to pain management may not only improve quality of life but also extend survival (19). These exciting advances harness sophisticated technologies to enhance patient outcomes and quality of life while lowering the cost (20–22) and burden of care. Such progress reflects the continuing translation of new knowledge about spinal analgesia discovered during the decade since the prior edition of this volume. In addition to the preclinical targets described in this chapter in the prior edition (23), newly elucidated mechanisms described by Yaksh in Chapter 32, and Dickenson and Seagrove in Chapter 33, offer promising new targets for spinal analgesia such as ion channels; receptors for a range of ligands, such as cannabinoids and vanilloids; trophic factors; and inflammatory mediators of systemic and local (e.g., glial) origin.

Balanced against these ongoing advances and prospects for spinal analgesia in acute and cancer pain are an emerging series of concerns that have tempered initial enthusiasm for intrathecal (IT) analgesia for chronic noncancer pain. As increasing numbers of patients have been treated for longer durations using implanted IT pumps, long-term risks and adverse effects,

including loss of effectiveness, have become clearer. These negatives include drug-related effects (such as pedal edema or hypogonadism from opioids), possibly catastrophic pump- and catheter-related problems, and other issues such as infection or spinal headache (24). Particular concern has arisen about the inflammatory masses that may develop at the tip of catheters used to infuse opioids (25) and occasionally other drugs such as baclofen (26,27). First described in 1991 (28), such cases now approach 500. As they become more commonplace, new instances are less likely to be reported in the literature and more likely (albeit imperfectly) to be captured in registries. In light of a growing appreciation for the limits of chronic IT infusion, appropriate patient selection is increasingly important (see Appendix). However, the continuing dearth of randomized trials and clinical outcomes studies to inform such selection and subsequent management—a gap well noted in the prior edition published a decade ago—remains disappointingly large (29,30).

The present chapter begins with a brief summary of the history of spinal analgesia, supplementing earlier general historical chapters by Brown, and Gallagher and Fishman. We next survey relevant basic science, although not as comprehensively as Yaksh (Chapter 32), and Dickenson and Seagrove (Chapter 33), and others such as Walker (Chapter 30). The historical development of the modern approach to spinal analgesia has been described elsewhere by the senior author (31). We will then present highlights of the translation of preclinical advances into clinical practice, again in less detail than in other specific clinical chapters. Corresponding to the diffusion of spinal analgesia into many areas of regional anesthesia and pain medicine, it is no longer necessary for this chapter to cover each application of spinal analgesia in depth. Information relevant to pediatric spinal analgesia, for example, is provided in chapters on developmental aspects (Chapter 30), regional anesthesia (Chapter 27), and acute, chronic, and cancer pain (Chapters 43, 45–47). Cancer pain in adults (Chapter 45) is another valuable use of spinal analgesia, as may be complex regional pain syndromes (CRPS) and other forms of neuropathic pain. We will next survey ongoing efforts to translate preclinical insights into improved therapies, with emphasis upon acute pain and cancer pain. It is noteworthy that, in the decade since the prior edition, only one new medication specifically intended for IT use—ziconotide—has cleared all regulatory hurdles to enter the marketplace. Among trends in clinical practice, the use of "combination spinal analgesic chemotherapy," a term introduced in the prior chapter and explored in detail in a subsequent systematic review (32), has burgeoned in the past decade. Combinations of two or more agents coadministered intrathecally are now common, and in some current surveys account for the majority of chronic spinal infusion therapy. We will next discuss current and future prospects for combination therapy, mindful that (as Basbaum has pointed out in Chapter 51) clinical science now has in sight a day when the fundamental neurobiologic disturbances associated with persistent pain may be addressed in a mechanistic fashion, just as in other areas of biomedical science such as oncology or infectious disease. We will conclude with an illustrated approach to the implantation and management of spinal infusion therapy, including adverse events such as device failure or catheter-tip fibromas, whose prevalence has only begun to be fully appreciated. Although in the preparation of this chapter our broad literature search identified hundreds of thousands of publications related in some way to spinal analgesic therapy, the clinical trial literature on chronic spinal drug delivery has not matured sufficiently to support systematic reviews or meta-analyses. The persistent deficiency of high-quality evidence—clearly identified in the prior chapter as well as in the landmark 1984 paper by Cousins and Mather (1)—is a challenge that must urgently be faced, as regulators and third-party payers increasingly withhold support for therapies of unproven efficacy and cost effectiveness. Although lack of evidence does not prove the absence of benefit, particularly on an individual basis (33), failure to meet this challenge may well erode the clinical infrastructure necessary to sustain care and assure progress.

OVERVIEW

Only recently has the spinal cord taken "center stage" in analgesia practice and research. For thousands of years, pain relief could be secured only at the expense of central nervous system (CNS) depression, as with the use of mandragora, wine, and opium in ancient China; mandragora and "poppy" in ancient Egypt, Rome, and Greece; and atropine, opium, cocaine, and hallucinogens by the Incas and ancient Peruvians. Thus, until Koller's daring introduction of local anesthetic blockade in 1884, the major site for pain control was thought to be the brain. In the early 20th century, the visionary surgeon Crile championed intraoperative neural blockade with the recently introduced local anesthetic cocaine used to avert "summation," which we now recognized as *sensitization*, and to diminish the psychological and physiological sequelae of surgery, including persistent pain (34). The brain and axon continued to be the major options for analgesia (35) until the mid-1970s, when preclinical studies proved (36) that the spinal cord can be a target for selective opioid analgesia. By the early 1980s, with speed unprecedented since Koller's time, these basic observations were harnessed in daily clinical practice worldwide (16,37–40). Insight into the chain of events precipitated in the spinal cord by painful peripheral stimuli has spurred novel drug discovery and rekindled interest in the spinal delivery of established drugs alone or in combination (32). This progress, milestones of which are summarized in Table 40-1, has been accelerated by the shared excitement of clinicians and investigators as they participated in a revolution of applied pharmacology. Patient-controlled analgesia (PCA) (41) first applied to the intravenous (IV) route in the 1960s, also was extended to spinal analgesia and, by the 1980s, was in wide use for epidural drug delivery.

Brain, spinal cord, axon, and periphery, once viewed as distinct sites for the actions of different analgesics, are now known to participate jointly as targets for pain control (42–44). Local anesthetics block axons of sensory (superficial) and motor tracts (deep) in the spinal cord (35). Systemically applied opioids and nonopioid compounds such as nonsteroidal anti-inflammatory drugs (NSAIDs) or clonidine have antinociceptive effects at the spinal cord level in animal studies and in humans (45,46). Opioids and NSAIDs also act to reduce pain and inflammation through direct effects upon peripheral tissue (47,48).

Epidural opioids can be absorbed rapidly into the circulation, producing early effects on the brain. Particularly hydrophilic (e.g., morphine) but also lipophilic opioids migrate in cerebrospinal fluid (CSF) to the brain, producing analgesia along with side effects such as sedation, dysphoria, nausea and vomiting, and respiratory depression. Very hydrophilic drugs, such as morphine and glucuronide metabolites, accumulate in the brain, to produce effects such as delayed respiratory depression. It is now clear that the spinal epidural administration of all opioids generates appreciable plasma concentrations that, for many drugs, approach the analgesic range (49–51). Only small amounts of opioid need reach supraspinal sites in order to augment spinal opioid analgesia (52–54). Hence, attempts to isolate the relative contributions of spinal, supraspinal (55,56), and systemic drug (and metabolite) actions during opioid therapy by any route may be irrelevant because all three sites of action are likely involved during treatment using all but the lowest doses and briefest courses.

Understanding of the spinal cord's unique importance as a target for regional and systemic analgesics, reviewed in the prior editions of this text, continues to progress. Interim preclinical and clinical advances allow us to assess the effects of spinal analgesics across many scales of space and time, from interactions of ligand molecules and binding sites on specific receptors in dorsal horn neurons, to clinical outcomes that include patient satisfaction and cost of care. Without exaggeration, one may say that spinal cord sensitization has now replaced pituitary-adrenal activation (57) as the principal undesirable "stress response" whose suppression (or better, preemption) guides the clinical practice of perioperative regional anesthesia and analgesia. In contrast to classical stress responses quantitated as blood hormone levels (58), dorsal horn stress responses are intra- and interneuronal (e.g., remodeling) and manifest as long-term structural and functional changes after noxious input (59,60).

OPIOIDS AND RECEPTORS: TERMINOLOGY

The term *narcotic* ("narco" in Greek is to numb or deaden) is applicable to many drugs and is so vague that it is of little use except as a pejorative term in legal and regulatory contexts. The term *opiate* refers to morphine and related alkaloids derived from the poppy (some reports indicate that opiates are synthesized de novo in mammals, possibly by intestinal flora). *Opioid*, a broader term, includes *exogenous* substances with morphine-like properties as well as *endogenous* peptides (61). Endogenous opioid peptides or *endorphins* all have the aromatic amino acid tyrosine at the initial (i.e., amino or N-terminus) position; all opioids share this tyramine structural motif. Opioid peptides that lack this tyramine moiety do not exert morphine-like effects but still may possess other "non-opioid" biologic actions, such as enhancement of memory or immune modulation.

Full opioid agonists at the morphine or μ receptor include morphine, hydromorphone, meperidine, and fentanyl. These

TABLE 40-1

MILESTONES IN SPINAL ANALGESIC (PARTICULARLY OPIOID) RESEARCH

- Synthesis of naloxone (1961) and other selective opioid antagonists for in vivo and in vitro studies.
- Melzack and Wall's gate theory (1965) suggests nociception is modulated in spinal cord.
- Proposal by Martin (1960s–1970s) of distinct opioid receptors to explain animal and clinical observations of diverse syndromes of addiction and abstinence for different opioids, and predict the possibility of analgesia without respiratory depression.
- Demonstrations that electrical stimulation (1969) or microinjection of morphine into periaqueductal gray elicit naloxone-reversible analgesia mediated by monoaminergic systems descending to the dorsal horn of spinal cord (see Chapters 31 and 32).
- Identification (1973) of saturable, stereoselective receptors for opioids and naloxone independently by Pert and Snyder, Terenius, and Simon and co-workers.
- Isolation and characterization (1975) of endogenous opioids, the enkephalins, by Hughes and others.
- Autoradiographic mapping of opioid receptor distribution (1976 on by Duggan, Yaksh) showing highest densities in substantia gelatinosa of spinal cord, medullary dorsal horn, periaqueductal gray matter, and other brain sites.
- Dose-dependent, stereospecific, naloxone-reversible analgesia demonstrated by Yaksh and Rudy (1977) after intrathecal morphine administration or local, iontophoretic dorsal horn morphine application in the rat (36). Numerous subsequent studies performed by Yaksh and others applying spinal catheterization techniques in animal models to elucidate dose–response relationships, potencies, receptors, and mechanisms of opioid analgesia, toxicity, tolerance, and opioid–nonopioid interactions.
- Synthesis of selective opioid ligands for investigative and therapeutic purposes (Hruby, Porreca, Schiller, Lipkowski, and others).
- Elucidation of antiopioid systems, including hyperalgesic peptides such as substance P or cholecystokinin, excitatory amino acids such as glutamate, and intracellular mediators such as protein kinase C (PKC) and nitric oxide (NO) that act in aggregate to mediate sensitization by nociceptive input, as well as opioid tolerance and latent hyperalgesia during continued opioid use.
- Refinement of animal models for evaluation of analgesics for nociceptive and neuropathic pain (Bennett, Chung).
- Recognition of genes expressed immediately after neuronal activation (e.g., *c-fos*) or in the process of programmed cell death, and their application to elucidate dynamic processes within nociceptive pathways (Basbaum, Besson).
- Clinical application of nonopioid analgesic systems for exploitation singly or in combination with opioids (e.g., α_2, GABAergic).
- Cloning of receptors for the endogenous opioids, synthesis of antisense DNA to evaluate receptor function in vivo, and analysis of subregions' functions by site-specific mutation methods.
- Identification of diverse ion channel types and subtypes as targets for analgesic drug development (TRP, P2X, ASIC, Na, K, Ca).
- Clarification of genetic variants in animals and humans as an important basis for diversity of nociceptive responses and placebo, nocebo, and drug effects
- Clinical outcomes studies of chronic intrathecal analgesia for established drugs and combinations to clarify adverse effects and risks as well as benefits, permitting improved patient selection and management.

TRP, transient receptor potential; P2X, purine receptors; ASIC, acid-sensing ion channel; GABA, γ-aminobutyric acid; Na, sodium; K, potassium; Ca, calcium.

agents bind to μ opioid receptors and activate them to produce dose-dependent analgesia and other effects (62) that are reversed by the opioid antagonist naloxone. As dose increases, there results a maximum or *plateau* of full efficacy. Some opioid agonists have less attraction to (affinity for) the binding site and require higher concentrations to achieve these effects. For other opioids, termed *partial opioid agonists*, this plateau is submaximal; buprenorphine is one example. Opioids that are agonists at one opioid receptor type and antagonists at a different opioid receptor type are termed, somewhat confusingly, *mixed agonist-antagonists*. Nalbuphine or butorphanol fall in this group; both are antagonists at the μ receptor and agonists at the κ receptor. Naloxone, a pure opioid antagonist, has high affinity and zero efficacy. The rate of dissociation of opioids from their receptors influences their duration of action. For example, buprenorphine has a slow rate of dissociation from the μ receptor and a long duration of action. For other drugs with a rapid rate of receptor dissociation, the concentration of opioid in the bloodstream or CSF, and drug redistribution and rate of clearance (e.g., by liver), govern duration of action (61).

The concept that cell membrane *receptors* mediate drug action arose in the 19th century. Descriptions of opioid structure-activity relationships that were presumed to reflect drug–receptor interactions appeared in the 1950s. Different types of opioid receptors were postulated in the 1960s by Martin, who, by the mid-1970s, had painstakingly catalogued heterogeneous profiles of the physiologic effects in dogs exposed to or withdrawn from a variety of opioids (63). Martin discerned three broad patterns of in vivo response to all opioids he evaluated and attributed these three profiles to selective activation of three distinct opioid receptor types. The first he termed "mu (μ)," for morphine; the second, "kappa (κ)," for ketocyclazocine; and the third, "sigma (σ)", for the proprietary drug SKF-10,047. The σ receptor is no longer considered as an opioid receptor; it is activated by phencyclidine. Soon after Martin published his results, Lord (64) and colleagues from the Kosterlitz group in Aberdeen postulated the existence of another opioid receptor type that they termed delta "(δ)" because of its identification in mouse vas deferens. An unusually long interval elapsed between pharmacologic identification of opioid receptor types in vivo and their cloning, reflecting technical obstacles such as the lack of a specific gene product to serve as a marker of opioid receptor activation and the typically inhibitory effect of such activation. All three types of opioid receptors—μ, κ, and δ—were cloned within a relatively short interval in the early 1990s (65).

Cloning of the opioid receptors confirmed and extended much information previously gleaned indirectly from pharmacologic studies (66). All three opioid receptor types are *metabotropic*; that is, coupled to guanyl nucleotide-binding regulatory proteins (G proteins) (67). They share structural features with other G protein-coupled receptors including seven conserved hydrophobic domains that span the cell membrane, disulfide bonds between cysteine residues, glycosylation near the amino terminus, and phosphorylation by protein kinase A (PKA) in the first and third cytoplasmic loops as well as near the carboxy (C) terminus (68). Sequencing of DNA encoding these three receptors in rat and mouse reveals that each contains nearly 400 amino acids, and that all three types share substantial sequence homology not only with each other but also with receptors for somatostatin, angiotensin, and certain chemotactic factors. Messenger RNA for all three types of opioid receptors is present in dorsal root ganglia and superficial layers of the dorsal horn (69). Opioid binding to the μ receptor activates an intracellular G protein, G_i, that inhibits guanyl triphosphate formation (70). Pertussis toxin prevents G_i activation and is useful as a probe of G_i mediation of opioid effects in vivo and in vitro (71).

Perhaps the most exciting consequence of cloning the opioid receptors is the ongoing characterization of the genetic basis for variability of opioid responsiveness (72). Hundreds of reports within the past 5 years associate single nucleotide polymorphisms (SNPs) with individual differences in analgesia following systemic opioid administration. These SNPs affect not only the opioid receptor itself, but related processes including drug transport proteins (73) and enzyme systems such as catechol-O-methyl transferase (74). Gender, being chromosomally based, and race further influence analgesic responses to opioids (75). Principally, studies of the influence of SNPs upon opioid responsivity have involved systemic opioid administration, and the results are not uniform. Thus, much work remains to be done to elucidate the nature of genetic influences upon spinal mechanisms of opioid analgesia. Genetic influences upon non-opioid mechanisms of analgesia, such as sodium (Na) channels such as Na 1.7, are described by Seagrove and Dickenson (Chapter 33), as well as later in this chapter.

The straightforward mechanism of opioid receptor linkage to a G protein, and thence to intracellular effector mechanisms such as ion channels, does not do justice to the complexity of and ongoing controversy about the precise mechanisms by which opioids or other ligands interact with receptors in the cell membrane (76). Several proteins including adenylyl cyclases, G protein receptor kinases, β-arrestins, regulators of G protein signaling, and the scaffold protein spinophilin all play roles in opioid-related cellular signaling (77). These mediators are all involved in varied aspects of tolerance to opioids. Moreover, opioids and other peptides that bind to cell membranes contain helical regions that are *amphipathic*; that is, in which hydrophobic and hydrophilic amino acids are grouped on opposite faces of the helix. This structure positions the ligand, detergent-like, at the surface of the cell membrane (78). Partial immersion of the ligand's amphipathic helical regions within the cell membrane can stabilize or destabilize the membrane independent of any specific ligand–receptor interaction (79). Further relevant to opioid pharmacology is the recognition that activation of G protein-coupled receptors results from a change in conformation from resting to active states, a "two-state" model first developed to describe the opening of transmitter-gated membrane ion channels (80). If a compound has a higher affinity for the conformation of the receptor in its active state, it is an agonist; if its affinity is equal for resting and active states, then it is an antagonist devoid of intrinsic activity; if its affinity is higher for the resting state, then it is an "inverse agonist," capable of producing effects opposite from those of agonists. The relative affinity of a drug for active and resting states of the receptor also determines whether it will behave as a full or partial agonist.

OPIOID RECEPTOR ACTIVATION: ANALGESIC EFFECTS IN VIVO

Martin's definition of opioid receptor types, which employed *in vivo* animal studies to extend and refine clinical observations, has remained the foundation for all subsequent preclinical and clinical studies in this area (81). During this time, efforts to characterize the receptor type selectivity of new opioids have shifted from whole-body pharmacologic studies toward in vitro methods that rely on mathematical analysis of drug–receptor affinity and drug displacement from receptor by highly selective reference opioids. At present, molecular methods to determine the primary sequence of opioid and other receptors, their chemical modification (glycosylation, phosphorylation, disulfide bridging) at specific sites, and the functions of particular subunits are well established. It is likely that the future literature on opioid receptors will continue this progressive shift in focus from bedside, to animal laboratory, to ligand–receptor binding, to molecular analysis of the receptor *per se* down to the level of single amino acid substitutions at ligand binding sites and other functional domains.

Unfortunately for clinicians practicing opioid analgesia, this paradigm shift has taken place unannounced (82). Therefore, the research literature is often confusing because different reports use distinct criteria to determine receptor selectivity of opioids (83,84). These diverse criteria include behavioral observation (e.g., animal performance in a Y-maze or lever-pressing as an index of subjective similarity between a test drug and a reference opioid); relative efficacy against experimental pain of different origins (e.g., heat versus pressure); potency compared with reference drugs in standardized in vitro bioassays (e.g., inhibition of electrical contraction of guinea pig ileum); comparison of dosage of nonselective (pA_2) or selective antagonists to reverse a drug's effects *in vivo* compared to effects of reference drugs; or quantitation of *in vitro* displacement of radiolabeled tracer amounts of test drug from receptor preparations or thin slices of tissue by increasing concentrations of unlabeled drug (Scatchard plot) or selective antagonists. These methods have made it clear that all three major types of opioid receptor—μ, κ, and δ— have subtypes, although information about subtype diversity has not yet had clinical application, and so will not be covered further in this chapter. Currently, preclinical determinations of novel opioids' receptor selectivity rely upon *in vitro* measurements of their binding affinities for purified opioid receptors, concentrations of selective reference opioids necessary to displace them from defined receptors, and the effect of selective receptor alkylating agents in blocking their binding to receptors. On the other hand, the two-state and earlier models of ligand–receptor interaction dictate caution in extrapolating from binding data to inferences about receptor activation. For example, bremazocine binds equally to μ and κ receptors, but is selective in activating κ receptors. Therefore, at present, initial pharmacologic screening and characterization in vitro must be confirmed by testing *in vivo* of potency (e.g., ED_{50} for analgesia) and reversal of effect by selective opioid antagonists (85). This two-stage screening preserves the authenticity of *in vivo* observation yet spares much of its associated imprecision and minimizes animal use. Through this approach, considerable information has emerged on the opioid receptor modulation of analgesia and other clinically important processes such as cardiorespiratory, gastrointestinal, endocrine, and immune function.

Analgesia follows systemic or spinal administration of opioids that act upon μ, δ, or κ receptors (76,86). An important exception to this general rule is the phenomenon of opioid-induced hyperalgesia (87) due to mobilization of excitatory neurotransmitter systems promptly upon opioid exposure (88,89). This phenomenon is described at greater length later. Other causes for hyperalgesia in animal models or case reports include accumulation of algesic metabolites such as morphine-3-glucuronide, opioid inhibition of spinal interneurons that are themselves inhibitory, or stimulation of the excitatory G protein (G_s) in preference to G_i at low opioid concentrations (90). The observation in knock-out mice lacking the μ receptor that high doses of morphine sufficient to activate δ receptors do not produce analgesia on tail flick testing indicates a unique role for the μ receptor in analgesia (91). Enhancement of analgesia (*cooperativity*), and in some reports synergy, occurs when more than one type of opioid receptor is activated simultaneously, such as μ plus δ, that may also form heterodimers. Analgesic enhancement may also be achieved by coadministration of an opioid with other analgesics that act at nonopioid receptors as agonists (adrenergic, cholinergic, etc.) or antagonists (to substance P, cholecystokinin, NMDA, cytokines, etc.) (92–97) that block ion channels (calcium, sodium, etc.), or that inhibit algesic enzyme systems (cyclooxygenase [COX], nitric oxide synthase [NOS], etc.) (98) (see Chapter 32). Cooperativity between opioids active upon distinct receptors, and opioids with nonopioid analgesic molecules, is evident in natural processes of endogenous analgesia. For example, a well-described "mismatch" occurs between receptor selectivity of the opioid molecules released within the spinal cord or into the peripheral circulation, and the opioid receptors that are occupied by these endorphins both adjacent ("paracrine" effect) and distant ("endocrine" effect) to their sites of release. Anatomic sites of opioid analgesic actions are likewise multiple and include supraspinal areas, the spinal cord, and injured tissue in the periphery. Therapeutic benefits therefore follow coadministration not only of different classes of analgesic to the same site (e.g., spinal cord) but also of analgesics to multiple sites at once.

We are not accustomed to viewing the clinical practice of spinal opioid analgesia as involving coadministration of opioids to several sites simultaneously, but this undoubtedly occurs within hours of beginning such therapy. Systemically administered opioids rapidly reach spinal cord, brainstem, and brain. Epidural opioids are distributed into the bloodstream and reach periphery, brainstem, and brain in addition to their spinal target; IT opioids also are carried rostrally in CSF and, to a lesser degree, the peripheral circulation. Brief courses of clinical opioid therapy for routine postoperative pain control by any route last at least a few days, allowing ample time for equilibration and access to multiple anatomic sites rich in opioid receptors. Yet, in contrast to many preclinical reports describing in vivo responses to single doses of spinal or systemic opioids or nonopioid analgesics, relatively few studies detail the analgesic effects of repeated yet short-term opioid administration.

The physiology of nociception and analgesia resulting from actions of spinally (or systemically) administered opioids upon the dorsal horn has been presented in overview in the introductory section and in detail in Chapter 32 by Yaksh. Opioid suppression of excitatory neurotransmitter release (e.g., substance P, calcitonin gene-related peptide, neurokinin A) from C but not A fibers reflects μ, δ, or κ opioid inhibition of calcium channels on the former but not the latter neurons. In particular, opioids act selectively upon small C fibers (99). By contrast, analgesic concentrations of the analgesic peptide somatostatin inhibit calcium channels on large but not small nociceptive afferents. Postsynaptic effects of μ and δ opioids upon wide-dynamic-range (WDR) neurons are both direct, resulting from occupancy of postsynaptic opioid receptors coupled through G_i to potassium channels, and indirect, due to activation of inhibitory pathways that descend from the brainstem to the spinal level. Dual pre- and postsynaptic effects also result from activation of α_2 and γ-aminobutyric acid (GABA) receptors, respectively, by selective agonists such as clonidine or baclofen. Additional opioid analgesic effects at the spinal level include stimulation of adenosine release and activation (i.e., disinhibition) of spinal interneurons, the latter contributing to opioid-induced pruritus. Despite similarities of receptor pharmacology in synapses within distinct nociceptive pathways of the dorsal horn (shown in Fig. 40-1), important preclinical and clinical differences exist between analgesic efficacy of specific drugs applied to treat pain of different origins. By the early 1980s it was clear that μ opioids are more potent than κ opioids against thermal pain, and that the reverse is true for pain of mechanical origin (e.g., pressure) (100). Since then, considerable evidence has accumulated that thermal hyperalgesia at the spinal level is mediated principally by activation of N-methyl-D-aspartate (NMDA) receptors, activation of protein kinase C (PKC), and generation of nitric oxide (NO) and cyclic guanosine monophosphate (cGMP) (101). Mechanical hyperalgesia relies principally on coactivation of spinal α-amino-3-hydroxy-5-methyl-4-isoxazopropionic acid (AMPA) and metabotropic glutamate receptors, activation of phospholipase A_2, and the COX cascade (102). Other models of nociception such as peripheral nerve injury, inflammation from infectious or chemical agents, electrical shock, or application of toxins or irritants to the CNS each produce distinct pathophysiologies and display distinct dose–response profiles in potency testing of various opioid and nonopioid compounds. None of these models exactly duplicates common clinical pain problems such as acute postoperative pain, postcesarean pain, headache, low back pain or cancer pain—syndromes that each involve multiple known and unknown pain mechanisms acting in concert (103).

Tolerance to opioid analgesic effects refers to a decline in analgesic effect and/or the need to escalate opioid dosage during ongoing therapy (104). Opioid tolerance occurs in many preclinical pain models, most reliably in "normal" animals without pain that begin opioid treatment well before challenge with a nociceptive stimulus. This simple yet important phenomenon is complemented by an equally commonplace occurrence that animals or patients who have chronically received an opioid to control pain predictably experience "rebound" hyperalgesia when challenged with an opioid antagonist. Both observations imply that opioid tolerance is not—as believed for years and described in the 2nd edition of this volume—simply a passive consequence of loss of opioid receptors and/or decoupling of opioid–receptor binding from G_i activation (105). If this were all that happened, then challenge with an opioid antagonist might have little effect. Instead, the occurrence of these phenomena implies that opioid tolerance involves mobilization of active processes whose potential to produce latent hyperalgesia is masked so long as opioid dosing is maintained. The presence of these active processes does not mean that downregulation (decreased receptor number) and desensitization (decreased receptor–effector coupling) do not take place: they do (106). However, they cannot by themselves explain the everyday occurrences just mentioned. Thus our view of opioid tolerance has changed during the past 15 years from an analogy with passive muffling of an ongoing signal to one of active cancellation of the signal, followed by rebound of the now-unopposed countersignal when the original signal ceases (107).

Mechanisms of active cancellation of an ongoing opioid analgesic signal involve processes ranging from intracellular

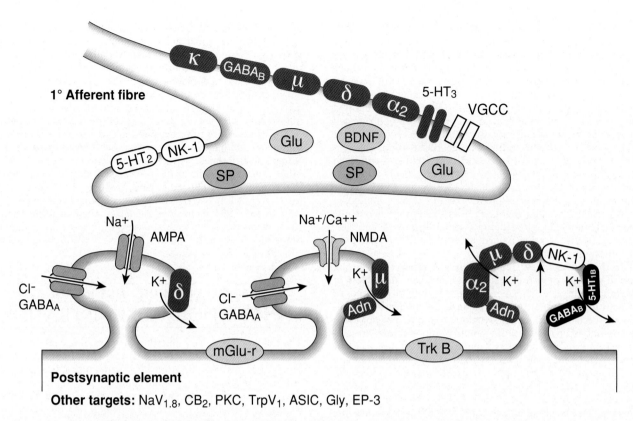

FIGURE 40-1. Schematic of pre and post–synaptic dorsal horn receptors and transmitters (see also Chapter 31, Fig. 31-11 and Chapter 32 Fig. 32-34).

and organ-level metabolic adaptations such as enhanced glucuronidation of morphine, to activation of anti-opioid, hyperalgesic peptide systems and glia. Activation of the μ opioid receptor results in translocation of intracellular PKC and phosphorylation of the calcium channel within the NMDA receptor complex (107). Phosphorylation of this channel removes its magnesium block and allows calcium entry just as after a nociceptive stimulus, even though nociception per se need not have occurred (108). Activation of NOS also mediates NMDA receptor effects, and co-administration of either a NOS inhibitor or an NMDA antagonist along with a μ opioid retards development of tolerance (60). Interestingly, tachyphylaxis to local anesthetic effects is also inhibited in a dose-dependent fashion by a NOS inhibitor or an NMDA antagonist (109). Animal studies have further demonstrated that tolerance develops more slowly when opioids with high intrinsic activity are administered, compared with equianalgesic doses of opioids with low intrinsic activity. Opioids of higher intrinsic activity require fewer receptors to be occupied to produce a response such as analgesia, thereby leaving their target cells with relatively more unoccupied "reserve" or "spare" receptors. Previously, the slower rate of tolerance developed during exposure to opioids of high intrinsic activity was identified with a higher number of remaining spare receptors. Given the connection (104,107) between μ receptor activation and intracellular NO and NMDA effects, a more plausible explanation of the slower development of tolerance during treatment with opioids of high intrinsic activity is that binding and activation of fewer μ receptors yields relatively less stimulation of intracellular NOS and PKC. Phosphorylation of the μ opioid receptor itself during prolonged activation has been proposed as an additional mechanism of opioid tolerance (67,110). In addition to intra-

cellular mechanisms, anti-opioid peptides participate in opioid tolerance. In particular, activation of cholecystokinin and substance P synthesis and release oppose the effect of opioid analgesics, as inferred from augmentation of opioid analgesia after administration of antagonists to either hyperalgesic peptide (111,112).

The contrast between the ease with which profound opioid tolerance can be induced during spinal or systemic infusions in many species of intact animals, and opioids' sustained therapeutic value during chronic use in most clinical settings (113), is still not well understood. In the cat, tolerance to systemic administration of morphine can be demonstrated in dorsal horn neurons after 3 days (114). In the primate, daily IT administration of morphine, β-endorphin, or metkephamid, at doses producing a "just maximum effect" causes a daily reduction in analgesic efficacy. Responsiveness in the primate declines most rapidly for agents having the longest duration of action after each fixed dose. In mice, once-daily doses of opioids of differing intrinsic activity produce tolerance at the same rate, although continuous infusions elicit tolerance more quickly with opioids of low intrinsic activity (115). The latter result is also found during long-term spinal delivery of morphine, sufentanil, and alfentanil in dogs (51). Results from several species indicate that tolerance develops more quickly when a greater proportion of μ receptors is activated by ligand during a greater proportion of each day. Primates made tolerant to IT opioids began to recover opioid responsivity 7 days after the last intrathecal administration, and had near-complete recovery by 2 weeks, indicating that tolerance is reversible (116) and supporting clinicians' common practice of managing tolerance to spinal opioid administration by switching temporarily to an alternative agent, such as spinal local anesthetic. It should be emphasized that tolerance is a greater issue in intact animals or normal volunteers, than during opioid therapy of chronic experimental or clinical pain. Colpaert found that animals exposed to acute pain (mechanical pinch) or chronic pain (intraarticular *Mycobacterium butyricum*) failed to show tolerance to systemically administered opioids when compared with normal controls (117). Similarly, Glynn and Mather (118) reported that tolerance was not an inevitable consequence of prolonged (1 year) treatment of chronic pain in patients receiving systemically administered meperidine. Parallel observations emerged from surveys of IT opioid dose escalation in patients with pain from stable neoplasms by Foley (119), and patients with non-cancer pain by Onofrio and Yaksh (120). In aggregate, observations by practitioners caring for patients with chronic pain from cancer or nonmalignant conditions confirm that systemic or spinal opioid dosage escalation is generally modest and therapeutic effectiveness is sustained, unless the underlying medical condition progresses (120,121).

In the authors' view, rapid dosage escalation early during opioid therapy of chronic pain condition is evidence less of tolerance than of either a behavioral (psychological) issue, or of pain mechanism(s) that are intrinsically insensitive to opioid analgesia. In such cases, switching to a different opioid or nonopioid, or coadministering opioid plus nonopioid, are supported both by preclinical and clinical observations. Animals rendered tolerant to morphine by daily IT injections showed no loss of sensitivity to the δ opioid D-Ala(2),D-Leu(5) enkephalin (DADLE), and only partial loss of effect of the κ opioid ethylketocyclazocine (EKC) (122). Other studies have reported spinal analgesic effects with the κ agonist U-50-488H (123) and a loss of effect of the endogenous κ opioid dynorphin (a κ opioid) in animals made tolerant to EKC. The prospect of maintaining spinal opioid analgesia for prolonged periods by rotating opioid agonists of different receptor selectivity as tolerance develops has clinical potential, and is supported by preclinical and limited clinical studies (124). Some agents that act both at μ and δ receptors, such as metkephamid (125) or biphalin, are effective as analgesics in morphine-tolerant animals, as, too, are hybrid peptides whose structure has one part that functions as an opioid agonist and another that functions (counterintuitively) as a substance P–like agonist (126).

Nonopiate spinal analgesia has been extensively investigated in both animal and human studies and is becoming an increasingly prevalent component of clinical practice. In particular, the α-agonists (e.g., clonidine) have been shown to have powerful antinociceptive effects, which show no cross-tolerance with opioid agonists (116,127,128). Intrathecal and epidural clonidine have been successfully used in humans tolerant to spinal morphine (129), and the combination of clonidine and morphine is associated with sustained analgesic efficacy. In patients with "below level" neuropathic pain after spinal injury, spinal morphine is ineffective (130). However, in a rat model of spinal injury pain coadministration of IT morphine and clonidine does provide analgesia (131), and an initial report supports the clinical value of this drug combination for this purpose (132). Coadministration of catecholamines and enkephalin pentapeptides, secreted together from adrenal chromaffin cells implanted intraspinally, may be a future approach for prolonged analgesia (i.e., to avert tolerance), but early enthusiasm has waned owing to inconsistent results, the possibility of undetected infectious agents in xenotransplanted cells, the expense of this approach, and the potential for this experimental treatment to disqualify spinally injured participants from subsequent trials aimed at restoring spinal cord function per se. Concurrent infusion of spinal local anesthetic plus opioid also retains analgesic effectiveness for prolonged periods

of time. Although the precise explanations for retarding tolerance by pairing opioid and nonopioid analgesic agents may vary, two common factors probably underlie this therapeutic advantage. First, addition of a second class of analgesic to an opioid reduces dorsal horn neuronal responsivity to afferent nociceptive input and hence lessens calcium influx, NOS activation, and PKC translocation. Second, insofar as coadministration of a second agent reduces the fraction of opioid receptors necessary to be activated in order to achieve analgesia, one would likewise expect tolerance to be retarded for the reasons just outlined. Thus, coadministration of opioids and other drugs, or administration of single molecules engineered to act upon opioid plus other pathways (e.g., COX, ion channels, substance P, NMDA, or NOS) is a powerful therapeutic strategy for achieving prolonged analgesia. Spinal antinociceptive systems that are potential targets for nonopioid analgesic molecules are summarized in Chapters 31 through 33. Their clinical relevance is discussed here.

NONANALGESIC EFFECTS OF SPINAL OPIOID ADMINISTRATION

The following summary describes the physiologic effects other than analgesia that directly result from spinal application of opioids. Accordingly, relationships between spinal opioid administration and alterations of respiratory, gastrointestinal, endocrine, cardiovascular, bladder, and sensorimotor function (the latter including pruritus and potential neurotoxicity and granuloma formation) are surveyed herein. Potential side effects of IT and epidural opioid treatment are summarized in Table 40-2 and contrasted with those of local anesthetics.

The present section is intended to complement the earlier discussion of the pharmacology of spinally administered opioid analgesics in preclinical and clinical settings, rather than to provide a comprehensive review of clinical effects, side effects, and outcomes other than analgesia during spinal opioid use. Such outcomes, which involve pulmonary or immune status, morbidity, or length of hospital stay, depend upon multiple processes including many not directly related to spinal opioid actions per se, such as are discussed later in this chapter and also by Liu and Wu in Chapter 7.

Respiratory Depression

Respiratory depression, although infrequent, is always a prime concern after spinal opioid administration, particularly in opioid-naive subjects treated for acute pain. Prompt (less than 2 hours) versus delayed onsets of this side effect have been attributed, respectively, to blood-borne drug quickly reaching the brain (such as after rapid absorption into the circulation of lipophilic opioid given epidurally) versus slow rostral migration of hydrophilic drug (such as morphine deposited within the CSF) (Fig. 40-2).

These two mechanisms are not mutually exclusive, however: sufentanil and meperidine have been detected in cisternal CSF within minutes after epidural or IT administration, respectively. Lipophilic opioids may rapidly cross the dura (Fig. 40-3) and then migrate in CSF to the brainstem (Fig. 40-2). Subacute respiratory depression during chronic use is also a concern. Respiratory depression was not a strong focus of initial animal experiments on opioid receptors or their endogenous ligands that followed the birth of this field in the early to mid 1970s. In large part, this lack of concern reflected the substantially higher

TABLE 40-2

EFFECTS AND SIDE EFFECTS

Effects and side effects	Spinal opioids	Spinal local anesthetics
Respiratory	Early depression[a,b] (0.1–1 h); systemically absorbed drug and? CSF-borne drug Late depression[a,b] (6–24 h); opioid in CSF migrating to brain (see Figs. 40-2 and 40-5)	Usually unimpaired unless cardiovascular collapse
Gastrointestinal	Prolongs intestinal transit time Nausea common postoperatively	Transit time unchanged Nausea less common
Cardiovascular	Minor heart rate changes	Low-block (below T10) sympathetic blockade: postural hypotension
	Usually no postural hypotension	High-block (above T4) sympathetic blockade: postural hypotension
	Vasoconstrictor response intact	Cardio-accelerator block: ↓ HR, ↓ inotropic drive (see Chapter 11)
	Dependent edema with chronic use	
Urinary retention	Yes[a,b]	Yes
CNS		
Sedation	May be marked[a]	Mild or absent, depending on agent
Convulsions	Usually not seen with clinical doses; theoretical possibility at high doses	Expected toxicity from two times overdose or with rapid vascular absorption
Other neurologic abnormalities	Confusion, amnesia, catalepsy, hallucinations (reported with high doses intrathecally)	Not usually seen
Opioid withdrawal	If rapid discontinuation of systemic opioids	
Nausea	Yes[a]	Yes—low incidence
Vomiting	Yes[a]	Yes—low incidence
Pruritis	Yes[a]	No
Miosis	Yes[a,b]	No (unless Homer's syndrome)
Endocrine, harmonal	Feedback loops inhibit pituitary-adrenal and gonadal function	Diminished nociceptive input blunts stress responses and reduces catabolism
Catheter tip **Inflammation, fibromas**	Concentration and dose dependency, especially for morphine	Not observed

[a]Antagonized by naloxone, but repeated doses may be required.
[b]Prevented by naloxone infusion 5–10 μg/kg/h without reversal of analgesic effects.[304,307]

doses (on a mg/kg basis) for opioids to produce respiratory depression in laboratory rats, dogs, and other nonhuman species. The great importance of this and other side effects was soon appreciated once spinal opioid analgesia came into common clinical use in the late 1970s and stimulated detailed animal studies. This concern has, if anything, been strengthened by the increased number of respiratory "near-misses" and catastrophes associated with the concurrent growth in popularity of IV PCA (41,133).

Animal studies provide strong evidence to connect respiratory depression to CSF concentrations of opioids. Data in baboons and in humans after epidural morphine administration indicate peak levels in CSF near the brain at about 3 hours (134–136). Studies in other species of cephalad migration of morphine after IT administration indicate a more rapid time course, with drug reaching the ventral brain after only 15 to 30 minutes and the respiratory center regions by 60 minutes (137). Opioid traveling cephalad in CSF also may stream against the intracranial CSF circulation to gain retrograde access to the fourth ventricle, with subsequent rapid access to respiratory centers. An alternative site of respiratory depression is a group of cells in the ventrolateral medulla, the nucleus ambiguus, and retroambigualis. These loci are involved in control of both inspiratory and expiratory motor output, but are less dense in opioid receptors than the subependymal nuclei in the floor

of the fourth ventricle. In animal studies, direct injection of opioids into the fourth ventricle or into CSF of the ventral brainstem region results in a rapid (3–5 minutes) onset of respiratory depression, which is similar for both sites of injection (138). Thus, diffusion of the drug through the brain tissue to the respiratory centers in the brainstem appears to be rapid once the drug reaches this area in sufficient concentration. Once in the intracranial CSF, opioid removal may occur with great efficiency at the choroid plexus (139), which appears to act as a "cerebral kidney" for these substances (Fig. 40-2). On the other hand, evidence in animals and humans indicates that morphine may be biotransformed within the CNS to active metabolites such as morphine-6-glucuronide, which can have potent and prolonged respiratory depressant as well as analgesic effects (140). It is evident from animal and human studies that μ receptors have a predominant role in opioid-induced respiratory depression, although in some species such as dog, δ receptors are also important in this regard. Central injection of μ-selective opioids in animals reduces ventilation by slowing respiratory rate. Feuerstein and colleagues have attributed the paradoxical effects of a variety of μ-selective opioids, some of which stimulate and others of which depress ventilation, to opposite effects of activation of μ_1 and μ_2 receptor subtypes. Activation of high-affinity μ_1 receptors either by low doses of opioids such as morphine, or by selective μ_1 agonists, appears

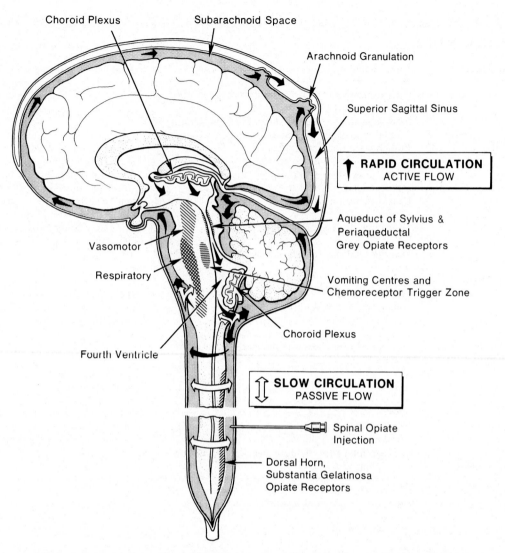

Choroid Plexus
Subarachnoid Space
Arachnoid Granulation
Superior Sagittal Sinus

RAPID CIRCULATION
ACTIVE FLOW

Aqueduct of Sylvius &
Periaqueductal
Grey Opiate Receptors

Vasomotor

Respiratory

Vomiting Centres and
Chemoreceptor Trigger Zone

Choroid Plexus

Fourth Ventricle

SLOW CIRCULATION
PASSIVE FLOW

Spinal Opiate
Injection

Dorsal Horn,
Substantia Gelatinosa
Opiate Receptors

FIGURE 40-2. Model of CSF flow and spread of opioid in CSF. After lumbar intrathecal injection, opioid is carried in the passive flow of CSF to reach peak concentrations in the brain after about 3 hours for morphine and 0.5 to 1 hour for meperidine (Demerol). Rapid spread ensues when the opioid mixes with the active flow of the rapid circulation of intracranial CSF. Spinal and brain stem opioid receptors are shown. The latter are seen to be in proximity to cardiorespiratory and vomiting control centres.

to stimulate ventilation, whereas activation of low-affinity μ_2 receptors by higher opioid doses depresses ventilation. Interestingly, in animal species such as rat, μ_1 receptors develop later than μ_2 receptors, raising the possibility that relatively depressed numbers of μ_1 receptors may underlie neonatal sensitivity to opioid-induced respiratory depression.

Intrathecal opioid, if given clinically as a single excessive dose or supplemented with IV opioid, may result in sudden apnea, necessitating rapid treatment. Onset of respiratory depression after IT morphine administration is variable (137,141–148) but usually is evident within 6 to 10 hours after the opioid injection. Return of normal respiration has required up to 23 hours afterwards. Case reports of respiratory depression when opioids were injected in usual doses intramuscularly within 24 hours of IT opioid (147) therefore, are not unexpected. Usually the progression of respiratory depression and hypercarbia after IT morphine is gradual, allowing time for diagnosis and treatment to avert respiratory arrest. This slow, insidious de-

pression of ventilatory response to carbon dioxide (CO_2) may be followed by sudden apnea, particularly when other risk factors are present, such as concomitant use of CNS depressants. In contrast, local anesthetic–induced convulsions or circulatory depression are usually rapid in onset and mandate urgent treatment.

Delayed respiratory depression after IT morphine for postoperative pain was first reported toward the end of 1979 independently by Glynn and associates (144) and by Liolios and Anderson (146). Glynn and colleagues (144) described two cases of respiratory depression persisting to 18 hours after a single dose of 3 mg and 5 mg of morphine, respectively. The patients were admitted to an intensive care unit and treated with repeated doses of naloxone. High doses of morphine (20 mg) were injected in a hyperbaric solution of dextrose by Samii and co-workers (149) with a similar duration of analgesia to that reported by Wang and others (150). Samii's patients were nursed in a semi-sitting position, and side effects were not noted.

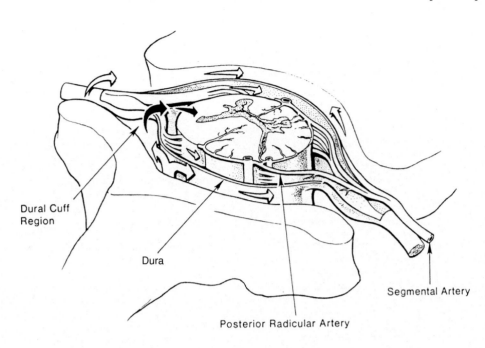

Dural Cuff
Region

Dura

Segmental Artery

Posterior Radicular Artery

FIGURE 40-3. Cross section of spinal cord and epidural space. Opioid spread in epidural space is depicted by *white arrows,* and spread into CSF, and spinal cord, is depicted by *black arrows.* In dural cuff region, posterior radicular spinal artery is readily accessible to opioid, and this artery directly supplies the dorsal horn region of the spinal cord.

However, Liolios and Anderson (146), using a hyperbaric solution of 15 mg of morphine, did observe respiratory depression. Early in 1980, Davies and colleagues reported delayed and prolonged postoperative respiratory depression in three patients who received 1 mg of morphine in an isobaric solution (141,142). All three patients had been premedicated with a long half-life sedative, diazepam, and remained supine postoperatively. In retrospect, it seems likely that the lack of respiratory depression in initial clinical reports by Cousins and others (39,144), Wang and others (150), and Sami and others (149) reflected opioid tolerance, since their patients all had prolonged prior treatment with opioids for cancer pain. In contrast, the cases reported by Glynn and others (144) and Davies and others (141,142) were postoperative and opioid-naive. Lumbar IT injection of radionuclides (151,152) or water-soluble contrast media (153) (metrizamide) is followed by a gradual movement of these substances rostrally to reach the fourth and lateral ventricles after 3 to 6 hours. Contrast media can be demonstrated in the fourth and lateral ventricles 6 hours after lumbar injection, indicating major reflux into the ventricles by way of the foramina of Luschka. Gustafsson and associates found that [^{11}C]-morphine appeared at a high cervical level after 60 to 170 minutes (137). Contrast also appears 6 hours after lumbar injection in the IT space over the entire surface of the brain and shows significant penetration of brain tissue (154,155). In summary, small volumes of opioid injected slowly into the IT space are likely to follow the passive circulation of CSF to reach the cisterns of the brain and then reach the respiratory center by way of the ventral pons (Fig. 40-2).

Risk factors for respiratory depression after IT opioid administration include advanced age (143); poor general condition (156); use of water-soluble opioid (i.e., morphine) (137); high doses (144); marked changes in thoracoabdominal pressure, including artificial ventilation (143); lack of tolerance to opioids (144); and concomitant administration by other routes of opioids or other CNS depressant drugs (142,147). Patients with respiratory disease would be expected to be at risk, as they are with the use of opioids by any route. Age may influence spinal fluid volume and pressure, and the brain in elderly patients may be more susceptible to respiratory depression by opioids (157). The onset and offset of respiratory depression are in agreement with the time courses of minute volume and carbon dioxide response after epidural morphine in volunteers (Fig. 40-4). In many case reports, antagonism of respiratory depression by naloxone has been confirmed, but often several doses or an infusion of naloxone have been required to sustain this antagonism (141,144). Analgesia can be preserved during reversal of spinal opioid-induced respiratory depression by carefully titrating the doses or infusion rate of naloxone (145,156). It has been claimed that the use of the sitting position and a hyperbaric solution of morphine protects against respiratory depression (148). However, respiratory depression has been reported with such maneuvers, and so it seems wiser to limit the dose of drug rather than to rely on the sitting position (156).

Epidural opioid administration may also produce early or delayed respiratory depression. Compared with the IT route, epidural administration is complicated by pharmacokinetic aspects related to dural penetration, fat deposition, and systemic absorption. Pharmacodynamic aspects become complicated, since the larger doses of opioid used result in blood concentrations that cannot be ignored. Simultaneous lumbar epidural injection of morphine and meperidine in patients results in detectable levels of both drugs in cervical CSF at about 30 minutes after injection. Thereafter, CSF meperidine concentrations in the cervical region declines rapidly. The commercial approval of an epidural depot preparation of morphine encapsulated within microspheres of plastic "foam" has introduced another risk factor for prolonged hypoventilation into clinical practice (158).

Most reports of early respiratory depression after epidural meperidine have been in postoperative patients within 1 hour of injection (159,160) and probably reflect vascular absorption by way of epidural veins or possibly rapid redirection to brain by way of the basivertebral venous system (see below and Fig. 40-5A).

Thus, it is plausible that lipid-soluble drugs may cause early respiratory depression at least partly as a result of rapid access to the brain, to achieve peak concentrations near the brainstem at about 30 minutes. This concept is supported by studies of plasma concentrations and respiratory effects of fentanyl: plasma fentanyl concentrations peak after 5 minutes and then

PART IV: PAIN MANAGEMENT

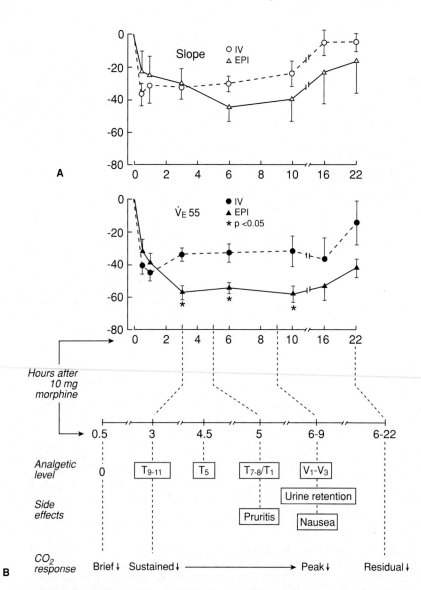

Hours after
10 mg
morphine

	0.5	3	4.5	5	6-9	6-22
Analgetic level	0	T_{9-11}	T_5	T_{7-8}/T_1	V_1-V_3	
Side effects				Pruritis	Urine retention / Nausea	
CO_2 response	Brief ↓	Sustained ↓ ⟶			Peak ↓	Residual ↓

B

FIGURE 40-4. A: Ventilatory response to endogenous carbon dioxide CO_2 after epidural (Epi) and IV morphine 10 mg by separate injection 2 to 4 weeks apart in 6 subjects. Mean ± SEM percentage change in slope and ventilation at end-tidal P_{CO_2} of 55 mm Hg (V_E55). (Reprinted from Neilsen CH, Camporesi EM, Bromage PR et al: CO_2 sensitivity after epidural and IV morphine. *Anesthesiology* 1981;55:A372 with permission of the publisher). B: Respiratory and other side-effects following epidural morphine.

FIGURE 40-5 see next page

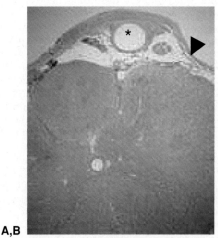
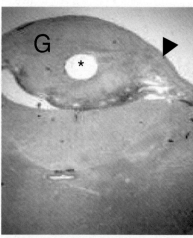
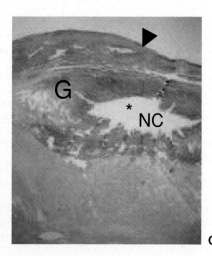

A,B   C

FIGURE 40-6. Spinal catheter-tip fibroma. Histopathology through upper lumbar (A) to caudal lumbar (B, C) spinal cord of a dog receiving intrathecal infusion of morphine (12.5 mg/mL at 40 μL/hr) for 28 days showing the rostrocaudal development of the granuloma from the meninges. Note the necrotic center in the largest area of the mass proximal to the catheter. This pathology is uniformly negative for infectious processes. Abbreviations: **Arrowhead, Dura; G,** granuloma; **NC,** necrotic center;* Catheter lumen. (This figure kindly provided by Prof. T Yaksh) [For radiological camparison see Chapter 50, Fig. 50-19].

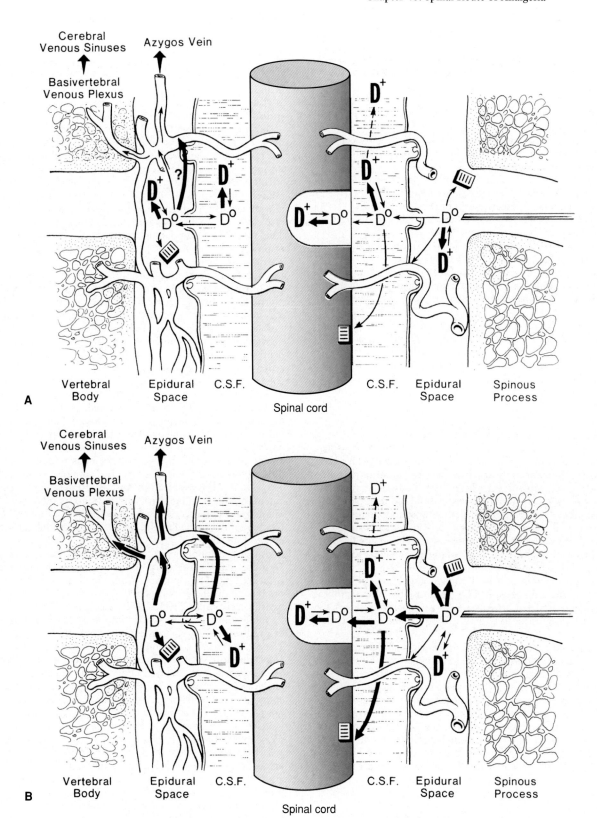

FIGURE 40-5. A: Pharmacokinetic model: Epidural injection of a hydrophilic opioid such as morphine. D^0, Un-Ionized drug; D^+, ionized hydrophilic drug. Major route of clearance is through CSF. Shaded squares are non-specific lipid binding sites. Role of radicular arteries in drug absorption remains unproven. **B:** Epidural injection of a lipophilic opioid such as meperidine or fentanyl. Note rapid passage of un-ionized species (D^0) via CSF into cord and then clearance by epidural veins, leaving less ionized species (D^+) remaining in CSF to migrate to brain.

TABLE 40-3

TABLE 40-3

FACTORS POTENTIALLY CONTRIBUTING TO DELAYED RESPIRATORY DEPRESSION DURING POSTOPERATIVE EPIDURAL OPIOID ANALGESIA

Residual effects of parenteral opioids given before, during, or after surgery. In a number of cases, sizeable doses of intramuscular opioid were given either shortly before or after epidural opioid, when it now is known that significant respiratory interactions are possible.

Residual effects of other CNS-depressant drugs used perioperatively (e.g., benzodiazepines and anti-emetics).

Lack of tolerance to opioid effects or side effects. Most operative patients have not received opioids for prolonged periods before surgery.

Raised intrathoracic pressure, from mechanical ventilation or "grunting" respiration associated with pain.

Raised intra-abdominal pressure and obstruction of inferior vena cava with increased blood flow through azygos system.

Inadvertent dural puncture by needle or delayed catheter penetration.

Large doses (10 mg) of epidural morphine sometimes given for pain relief after major surgery and/or as depot preparations, are associated with a higher incidence of respiratory depression than lower doses of epidural morphine (2–4 mg).

decline rapidly, whereas respiratory depression is seen between 15 and 60 minutes (161,162). These pharmacokinetic considerations are consistent with clinical observations that delayed respiratory depression is most common with epidural morphine (163–167) and absent with epidural fentanyl (161,168). As in the case with IT opioid administration, old age, poor general condition, and respiratory disease probably predispose to respiratory depression (156,163,168,169). Patients subject to Stokes-Adams attacks also require caution (171). Finally, postoperative patients have a number of potential factors that place them at risk for this complication (Table 40-3).

Studies in volunteers by Bromage and others (172–174) suggested that changes in CO_2 responsivity after epidural morphine paralleled its rostral spread, as judged by the cephalad progression of analgesia to ice and pin scratch (Fig. 40-4).

The concurrence of analgesia in the trigeminal distribution, nausea, and peak respiratory depression between 6 to 9 hours after epidural drug administration is strong evidence that significant brain opioid concentrations are reached during this interval. There appears to be a relatively slow progression of analgesia as morphine is carried in the passive flow of the slow circulation of spinal CSF and then merges with the active intracerebral CSF circulation (Figs. 40-2 and 40-3). This time course is in keeping with studies by Gourlay and associates (135), who reported peak morphine concentrations in cervical CSF 3 hours after lumbar epidural administration, as well as animal pharmacokinetic data (137), as described earlier.

Studies by Bromage and others (172–174) and Gourlay and colleagues (135) help in understanding the time delay of approximately 3 to 12 hours in clinical case reports of delayed respiratory depression after epidural morphine (166–167,175). From this work, it may be surmised that further systemic injection of "usual" doses of opioid would be dangerous for up to a day after epidural morphine. Indeed, this risk can be gauged

from the 40% reduction in slope and ventilation after 10 mg of IV morphine, CO_2-response beyond the residual 20% reduction in slope and 40% reduction in ventilation remaining at 22 hours after epidural morphine (173). A similar delay in onset of respiratory depression is seen after IT morphine (141,144,146,156), supporting the importance of the rostral spread of morphine in CSF. In an effort to exploit the effect of posture to inhibit rostral morphine spread, a "between-patient" study found the sitting position to be associated with less respiratory depression than the supine position after epidural morphine (176). However, a controlled study showed no effect of 45-degree elevated posture in protecting against respiratory depression (177). Use of a minimal effective dose of morphine is a more practical approach to achieving safety, since respiratory depression is dose-related (161,178). Doses of 2 to 4 mg morphine result in much milder and briefer depression of respiration than a dose of 10 mg morphine (161,178), which continues to depress respiration for more than 17 hours (178). Depot preparations of morphine present at least as great a duration of ventilatory risk (158). Fortunately, 2 to 4 mg of epidural morphine is often adequate for peripheral surgery, and 4 to 6 mg is adequate for more extensive surgery, provided sufficient time is allowed for onset (161,179,180). A wider therapeutic window can be obtained between analgesia and respiratory depression by using low-dose epidural morphine infusion preceded by a bolus dose in a low volume (1 mL), so that peak concentrations of morphine in brainstem regions are decreased and the incidence of respiratory depression is low (181–183). Respiratory depression can be prevented, or antagonized when it occurs, by naloxone infusion at a dose of 5 μg/kg/hr, without antagonizing analgesia (184). Epidural application of the partial μ agonist buprenorphine, and the mixed κ agonist–μ antagonist butorphanol have both been reported to induce respiratory depression for 12 hours after administration (1,185). *The moral is clear:* respiration must be carefully assessed if parenteral opioid is to be given within 24 hours of any epidural opioid, and parenteral dosage must be kept as low as feasible, preferably through cautious IV titration while an opioid antagonist is nearby.

All of the lipophilic opioids are reported to induce a brief period of early respiratory depression after epidural administration (186–188), possibly from blood-borne access to the brain but more likely as a result of transient peak concentration of drug in cisternal CSF (137,159) (see Fig. 40-2). Because most lipophilic opioids move rapidly into and out of neural tissue, delayed respiratory depression is exceedingly rare (162,189). These theoretical considerations are borne out clinically, provided the dose of fentanyl analogue is kept within the therapeutic margin of about 2, between safe epidural dose and analgesic intramuscular dose. Ventilatory effects of analgesic epidural doses of fentanyl, alfentanil, and sufentanil given to normal volunteers in a dose-ranging study resolved approximately 3 hours after drug administration (50). Also in volunteers, epidural fentanyl did not alter CO_2 response curves over a 24-hour period of study, apart from a brief early depression (167). Low-dose epidural fentanyl infusion (0.5 mcg/kg/h) after a bolus of 1.5 μg/kg was not associated with changes in continuously monitored end-tidal CO_2 or respiratory rate over an 18-hour monitoring period in 21 postoperative patients (161). On the other hand, epidural infusion of 1 μg/kg/hr fentanyl after a bolus dose of 1 μg/kg did depress CO_2 responsivity throughout an 18-hour study period in patients after orthopedic surgery.

Extensive preclinical and clinical attention to spinal opioid–induced respiratory depression is offset by voluminous surveillance data attesting to the low incidence of this complication in tens of thousands of patients treated with IT and epidural opioids. Large-scale surveys in Sweden and elsewhere (57,156,190) have enrolled nearly 30,000 patients and yield incidence estimates of respiratory depression after epidural morphine that range from 0.09% to 0.25%. These estimates compare favorably with published incidence rates for respiratory depression after parenteral morphine, whether given by conventional injection or PCA (39,133). Such surveillance also identified the rarity of respiratory depression occurring more than 12 hours after single doses of epidural morphine, and led the Swedish Society of Anesthesiology and Intensive Care to endorse routine observation for only 12 hours. Although few would question multiple experimental demonstrations of respiratory effects persisting beyond 12 hours in volunteers given epidural morphine, the interpretation of such responses to exogenous CO_2 and their generalizability to patient care is not straightforward. For example, a variety of studies have found benefits of epidural opioid analgesia upon postoperative pulmonary function and oxygenation, presumably derived from enhanced pain control during deep breathing or coughing. Moreover, respiratory depression is recognized to be uncommon in patients who already are opioid tolerant (18,120,191,192), and there have been few reports of such in patients with chronic cancer-related or nonmalignant pain treated with long-term spinal opioids (191,193–196). A heightened risk of epidural opioid use occurs in patients with known or undiagnosed obstructive sleep apnea, in which a small epidural dose of morphine (or even parenteral morphine) can result in severe sedation and respiratory depression (197).

Gastrointestinal Function

Most preclinical studies of the gastrointestinal effects of opioids in vivo have employed transit (propulsion) as an end-point, although some have examined mucosal transport of fluid and ions. These two physiologic effects are clearly separable: in some models, the antidiarrheal effects of opioids result principally from antisecretory rather than antipropulsive effects. The relationship between opioid (or other drug) effects upon gastrointestinal contractions (i.e., motility) versus propulsion (i.e., transit) is not a simple one, nor is it the same at different sites along the gut. For example, opioids delay propulsion in species in which they inhibit contractions; in other species, opioids increase contractions but likewise delay propulsion. Opioids can affect intestinal function (including gastric acid secretion) by actions in the brain, spinal cord, and periphery. Opioid μ agonists given in analgesic doses at any of these three sites inhibit propulsion, gastric acid secretion, and diarrhea. Analgesic doses of κ opioid agonists administered at any of these three sites have little effect upon propulsion or gastric acid secretion, and may even stimulate the latter process when given intravenously. Analgesic doses of δ opioid agonists given intracerebroventricularly or systemically do not affect propulsion or gastric acid secretion, but do inhibit diarrhea. Spinally administered δ opioid agonists, however, inhibit propulsion in preclinical models.

In patients followed postoperatively, gastrointestinal mobility normally decreases, particularly after abdominal surgery. In normal volunteers, opioids given systemically or epidurally delay gastric emptying and decrease gastrointestinal motility. However, one controlled trial in obese patients found a decrease in times to pass flatus and feces postoperatively, and shortened hospital stay, in those given epidural morphine compared with those given systemic (intramuscular) morphine (185). Gastrointestinal effects of postoperative epidural local anesthetics alone are minimal; the benefits of their use postoperatively are described in Chapter 7. Thus, one may provisionally conclude that clinical findings during application of spinal μ opioid agonists are consistent with preclinical effects, in particular that epidural μ opioid administration results in a slowing of postoperative recovery of gastrointestinal function intermediate between systemic opioid administration and spinal analgesia with local anesthetics. A comprehensive picture of the gastrointestinal effects of acute and chronic spinal opioid use in humans, that encompasses non-μ opioids, and coadministration of opioid-sparing analgesics, such as local anesthetics or nonsteroidals (198), has not yet emerged. Recognition of the detrimental effects of opioids upon gut mobility during both acute and chronic administration has prompted the development of peripherally active opioid antagonists (199) such as methylnaltrexone (200,201) and alvimopan (202,203). Nearly all experience with these and other novel agents has been acquired during systemic opioid therapy. As noted earlier, however, there is a significant contribution of central mechanisms to gut hypomotility following spinal opioid administration. Therefore, these and other peripherally active opioid antagonists now under development merit evaluation during spinal opioid analgesia.

Nausea and vomiting occur in approximately one-quarter of postoperative patients treated with spinal opioids, although pain itself has been implicated as a cause of postoperative nausea (180). In a prospective study of 1,085 postoperative patients, Stenseth and associates (180) reported that epidural morphine (dose 4–6 mg) was associated with nausea or vomiting in 34% of patients. In a series of 1,200 postoperative patients, nausea and vomiting were present in 17% of the patients (190), whereas in another series, nausea was present alone in 12%, and with vomiting in 24% (179). In the latter series, the incidence of nausea and vomiting was similar whether morphine was used intramuscularly or epidurally, or saline was injected epidurally. Others, too, have reported a low incidence of nausea and vomiting after epidural morphine in the postoperative period (204). In labor, the incidence of nausea and vomiting has been reported to be low with epidural opioid (186,205) in contrast to a high incidence with IT opioid (206,207). Epidural use of lipid-soluble opioids such as meperidine, fentanyl, and sufentanil (189,208,209) may be associated with the lowest incidence of nausea and vomiting. In a cross-over study in volunteers, Bromage and colleagues (210) observed nausea and vomiting in 50% of subjects approximately 6 hours after epidural morphine, which coincided with other evidence of the rostral spread of morphine in CSF to intracerebral structures, including the vomiting center and the chemoreceptor trigger zone (Fig. 40-4). In contrast, after IV morphine, only one out of ten subjects had nausea lasting 2 hours. Nausea and vomiting in the postoperative setting are antagonized by IV naloxone, without diminishing analgesia, at titrated doses of up to 5 μg/kg/h (211). Fortunately, the incidence of nausea and vomiting seems to be much less with repeated epidural dosing and is low in patients with cancer or nonmalignant pain who require long-term spinal opioid therapy (191,192,196,212).

Cardiovascular Function

Cardiovascular and pain regulatory systems are closely coupled. Activation or inhibition of one system produces changes in the other, often through overlapping anatomic and neurochemical pathways (213). Just as analgesia has multiple components, such as sensory processing or emotion, key aspects of global cardiovascular status—myocardial contractile state,

PART IV: PAIN MANAGEMENT

blood pressure, heart rate, and vascular resistance—although linked, are independently regulated. The bothersome side effect of dependent edema, sometimes observed during chronic spinal opioid therapy (particularly with morphine) likely is mediated through mechanisms unrelated to the just-mentioned parameters. It has been hypothesized, for example, that IT opioid migrating cephalad may stimulate the release of vasopressin (214). Cardiovascular effects of opioids differ between basal, pain-free subjects and those studied perioperatively or while in pain. Also, central injections of receptor-selective opioids in animals may elicit different, even opposite effects upon heart rate and blood pressure if given into nearby sites, or at the same site in low versus high doses. One explanation for dual excitatory and inhibitory effects parallels the explanation for biphasic opioid ventilatory effects, namely, that high-affinity μ_1 receptors mediate excitatory effects and low-affinity μ_2 receptors mediate inhibitory effects (213). Analgesic doses of spinal morphine do not change blood pressure or heart rate in animals and in humans studied under basal conditions in the awake or the anesthetized state (215,216). In halothane-anesthetized or unanesthetized dogs, IT morphine or fentanyl analogues do not change cardiac output or peripheral resistance (127,215). Dose-dependent reductions in heart rate were seen in awake dogs after either epidural or IT administration of boluses of sufentanil, alfentanil, or morphine, with tolerance to these effects during repetitive epidural or IT dosing (51). In resting humans, changes in skin temperature, blood pressure, and heart rate are absent with spinal opioids. Both sudomotor and vasomotor activity (e.g., responses to cold pressor testing or Valsalva maneuver) remain intact (39,173,192,210). The latter is important because of its homeostatic role during upright posture or blood loss.

During noxious stimulation in awake or anesthetized animals and humans, parasympathetic outflow decreases and sympathetic activity increases, as do levels of circulating catecholamines (58,183,217) (see Chapters 6 and 22). Heart rate, blood pressure, myocardial oxygen consumption, systemic vascular resistance, and ventricular vulnerability to fibrillation all increase in this situation. Opioid analgesia by spinal or systemic routes decreases all these parameters (218). One study in dogs reported an increase in cardiac vagal activity after thoracic epidural morphine (219), consistent with previous findings that systemic opioids stimulate both the central baroceptor reflex and vagal afferent activity. Clinical effects of spinal analgesia upon myocardial function have been most evident when local anesthetics, alone or supplemented with opioids, are administered via the thoracic epidural space (220). The greater effect of spinal local anesthetics than opioids upon cardiovascular function during pain or stress probably reflects the more complete sympathetic ablation possible with the former class of agents (221). However, in both experimental and clinical studies, spinal opioid analgesia has not yet been clearly proven to benefit cardiovascular morbidity and mortality beyond what might be attributed to effective analgesia alone (222). Attempts to draw conclusions from published clinical series have been impeded by the small numbers of patients studied, and the likelihood that advances in perioperative monitoring and treatment of myocardial ischemia have advanced sufficiently that it may be necessary to study thousands of patients in order to demonstrate further decrements in cardiovascular complications (222,223). Thus, identification of the impact, if any, of spinal opioid analgesia upon such complications may require pooling of results from studies of high-risk patients undergoing highly invasive procedures—a synthesis that is not yet possible.

Bladder Function

Spinal morphine in humans produces a naloxone-reversible inhibition of the volume-evoked micturition reflex (190) to a greater degree than is seen after systemic administration of equianalgesic doses. This effect seems to be most marked in young males, but demographics are unreliable because many patients treated acutely with spinal opioids are high-risk older patients undergoing major operations, after which they are routinely catheterized (214). It is not yet proven if the incidence varies with the opioid used, the duration of treatment, or between males and females. That these factors may be important is suggested by a series of 40,000 injections of epidural meperidine 50 mg for pain after cesarean section in which catheterization of the bladder was not necessary (208). In this large series, patients routinely had bladder catheterization intraoperatively and for the first 12 hours postoperatively and then did not require recatheterization. The apparently prophylactic effect of this approach is of interest, since another study reported a low incidence of urinary retention using this method compared with a high incidence with "in, out" catheterization intraoperatively followed by epidural morphine (224).

Urinary retention is a more frequently reported complication (37,225–228) of spinal opioids administered to volunteer subjects than spinal opioids administered to patients. Current evidence from volunteer studies indicates that urodynamic effects of epidural morphine are not dose-related within a range of clinically relevant doses but they are reversed by naloxone (225). In a dose–response study of epidural morphine for postoperative pain relief, Martin and associates found that the incidence of urinary retention was the same for doses of morphine of 0.5, 1.0, 2.0, 4.0, and 8.0 mg (185). This was consistent with a urodynamic study in 30 volunteers in whom increased bladder capacity and relaxation of detrusor muscle was similar for epidural doses of morphine of 2, 4, and 10 mg (225). In a study of postoperative patients using CO_2 cystometry, a great variation in bladder response to epidural morphine was found on the day after surgery. Intravenous naloxone reversed bladder effects in those patients who developed urinary retention (229). Naloxone infusion of 5 $\mu g/kg/hr$ in postoperative patients in one study reversed urinary retention with only minimal effects on analgesia (230), but others have reported that naloxone doses large enough to consistently reverse urodynamic changes after epidural morphine (e.g., 10 $\mu g/kg/hr$) may interfere with analgesia. The precise mechanism of spinal opioid interference with bladder function has not been elucidated, although μ opioid receptors are clearly implicated. Anecdotal reports suggest that the incidence of bladder dysfunction may be less with spinal fentanyl (231), meperidine (208,232), and methadone (233) than with morphine but conclusive comparative studies are not available.

Neurotoxic Potential, Inflammatory Mass Formation, and Pruritus

The *neurotoxic potential* of spinally administered opioids has been evaluated extensively in both preclinical and clinical settings (234). High doses of IT morphine in rats may produce two alarming syndromes: (a) convulsive seizures of the hind limbs and hyperreflexia in response to cutaneous stimuli, and (b) intense motor rigidity. Neither of these are antagonized by naloxone, implying mediation by nonopioids such as the algesic metabolite morphine-3-glucuronide or the inhibitory neurotransmitter glycine. This cautionary note is not paralleled by clinical reports: dysesthesia is rare (235) and not clearly distinguishable from pruritus. Similar contrast exists between sobering preclinical evidence (including histopathology) of neurotoxicity and motor paralysis after IT administration of peptides including somatostatin, dynorphin, or δ-selective enkephalin analogs in the rat or dog, and the rarity of corresponding symptoms in clinical trials of these agents. Explanations for this disparity include species differences as well as inclusion criteria in clinical trials that select patients in whom motor effects are undetected because they are already bedridden or inactive.

Apart from the potential neurotoxicity of spinally administered compounds themselves, other factors relevant to the safety of spinal opioid administration are the compatibility of solutions of such agents with CSF and neural tissue, and inflammatory reactions provoked by intraspinal catheters. Solutions of opioids used in spinal injections (morphine, methadone, meperidine, fentanyl, alfentanil, lofentanil, and buprenorphine) and local anesthetics in normal saline have pH values that range from 4.52 to 6.85. When mixed with CSF, all lowered the pH of the CSF by 0.3 or less, but etidocaine lowered pH by 0.82, with clouding of CSF (236). High concentrations of local anesthetics alone, such as 5% lidocaine given intrathecally, are recognized in animal models and clinical reports to have the potential for irreversible neurotoxicity. In fact, clinical adverse events such as cauda equine syndrome led to the withdrawal of spinal microcatheters after otherwise promising use (237). In retrospect, those neurotoxic events were very likely due to the catheters' use to deliver 5% lidocaine rather than the catheters per se. Currently, cautious re-exploration of this potentially valuable technique for perioperative anesthesia and analgesia is proceeding, with reliance upon less problematic solutions such as isobaric (0.5%) bupivacaine (238). Microcatheters are also useful for trials of subacute IT administration of opioids to predict responses to chronic delivery via implanted pump.

Inflammatory mass formation is a problem of increasing concern. Histologic examination of spinal cords of cancer patients who had epidural administration of bupivacaine-morphine mixtures for 3 weeks (239) or morphine for up to 6 months (38) revealed no abnormality attributable to morphine. Two of seven patients had posterior column degeneration consistent with myelopathy of malignancy (240). Animal studies of the potential damage to the spinal cord of epidural catheters and repeated injection of opioids have revealed histologic changes in many but not all models. Yaksh reported that 14 macaque monkeys with epidural catheters in situ for 4 to 16 months and receiving 15 to 122 injections of morphine had no abnormal neurologic signs. Three of the monkeys were sacrificed for autopsy after 6, 8, and 9 months and after 44, 68, and 72 IT injections of a variety of opioids and peptides. No histologic evidence of cord pathology was found (128,241). Similar findings during chronic epidural or IT infusions of sufentanil, alfentanil, morphine, or saline in the dog were later reported by Yaksh and colleagues. In that study, every animal had fibrosis around its infusion catheter whether IT or epidural, and many had histologic evidence of acute and chronic inflammation in the epidural space. Animals with IT catheters, but not epidural catheters, also had acute and chronic inflammation in the meninges. The incidences of all these histologic changes were independent of the dose of opioid used, and were equally likely to occur in animals infused with saline alone. Abouleish and co-workers (239) found no immediate or chronic (42 days) changes in spinal cord histology attributable to a single IT injection of a large dose of morphine (0.07 mg/kg). Coombs and co-workers, however, reported extensive pericatheter reactions in sheep after chronic epidural infusions of high concentrations of hydromorphone and morphine, but not saline. These

reactions were sufficient to produce spinal cord compression, parenchymal damage, and hind limb weakness.

In cats with *intrathecally* implanted catheters receiving only IT saline and killed 19 to 21 days after implantation, an inflammatory response developed, with a thin fibrotic sleeve surrounding the catheter with no obstruction to the tip. Where the catheter lay in contact with the spinal cord, mild deformation and local demyelination were present. Animals that received the ED_{100} for alfentanil or sufentanil daily for 5 days showed spinal cord pathology indistinguishable from those receiving saline. Animals receiving ten times the ED_{100} of either drug showed results similar to controls (127). Chronically implanted epidural catheters in rats resulted in the rapid development of a fibrotic reaction in 36 of 43 rats after only 1 day. After 10 days of catheterization, a thick fibrotic reaction obstructing the catheter tip was observed in 31 of 33 rats. Injection of methylene blue showed no spread into the epidural space; the dye filled the lumen of the catheter and then the sheath, making a blue spot on the skin if the injection was continued. A mild deformation of the dura was observed in all animals (242). Perhaps the most detailed animal studies of catheter-tip inflammatory masses were reported in adjoining papers by Yaksh's group in dogs (243) and Hassenbusch's group in sheep (244), together with an editorial by Follett (245). Figure 40-5 (kindly provided by Professor Yaksh) depicts the rostrocaudal development of a typical inflammatory mass in a dog given an IT infusion of morphine (12.5 mg/mL at 40 μL/hr) for 28 days. No infectious process was detected.

Consideration of these animal studies, and surveillance studies based upon registries of patients who have received implanted spinal drug delivery systems, identify high local concentrations or cumulative doses of opioids, particularly morphine, as risk factors (246). In a "Dear Doctor" letter, however, the manufacturer cautioned that "no dose and/or concentration of morphine sulfate can be considered completely free of risk from inflammatory mass" (247). Intrathecal baclofen, particularly when compounded in nonstandard concentrations or together with opioids, has also been associated with granuloma formation (26,27). The occurrence of catheter tip granuloma formation is estimated at about 1% at 6 years (246), a figure that appears to be rising owing to closer surveillance. Among the tens of thousands of patients worldwide with implanted spinal drug delivery devices, hundreds are known to have developed this problem (245) and more are anticipated, as the average duration of IT infusion therapy increases. A consensus approach endorsed by many leaders in spinal infusion therapy (25) recommends decreasing the risk at the outset of therapy by placing the catheter tip below the conus medullaris and using the lowest doses/concentrations of opioid possible. Because IT clonidine (248,249) and bupivacaine appear much less likely to produce inflammatory masses, either or both of these agents may be coadministered from the outset of therapy with the objective of reducing opioid requirements. Baseline documentation of the patient's neurologic history and physical examination, plus radiologic images of the catheter location, are useful for future comparison. Symptoms that raise the index of suspicion for fibroma formation include an apparent loss of analgesic effectiveness, increased pain intensity, lower extremity weakness, and other neurologic sensorimotor deficits such as bowel or bladder dysfunction (24,247). Magnetic resonance imaging [MRI] with gadolinium enhancement is preferred for diagnostic imaging, but computed tomography [CT] myelography may also be used. The neurologic deficits associated with inflammatory catheter tip masses appear due to a compressive mass effect, rather than the neurotoxic changes described earlier for spinal opioids per se. Treatment should consist of cessation of the infusion (while providing systemic opioids to avert an abstinence syndrome) and expectant observation. Cases in whom this conservative approach does not result in improvement may be considered for surgical excision of the mass, catheter removal, and replacement of the catheter tip two or more levels above or below the mass.

Pruritus is common during spinal opioid therapy but incidence estimates vary widely as its presence (especially if mild) may only be revealed on direct questioning. It seems likely that generalized pruritus associated with spinal opioids is due to widespread alteration in sensory modulation, since it occurs when there is evidence of opioid migration over the entire spinal cord to the brain. Sensory modulatory mechanisms in the upper cervical spinal cord and trigeminal system may be involved, since the onset coincides with the spread of hypalgesia to this region (210). Facial pruritus, which often is reported, may be explained by rapid penetration of opioid to the superficially placed caudal portions of the trigeminal nucleus (137). Pruritus is not due to preservatives, since it occurs with preservative-free opioids, nor is it likely to be due to histamine release (250), since its onset is approximately 3 hours after epidural or spinal opioid administration (172,173,210). Further, it occurs with fentanyl, which does not cause histamine release, as well as with morphine, that does (251). Such benefits as clinicians have observed with antihistamines given for pruritus due to spinal opioid therapy may well derive from their nonspecific sedating actions.

Putative mechanisms of pruritus after spinal opioid therapy include some that involve μ opioid receptor activation, such as stimulation of neuronal G_s (as described earlier) or inhibition of inhibitory interneurons in spinal cord, or stimulation of an itch reflex localized in the trigeminal nucleus. Mechanisms dependent upon μ receptor activation underlie naloxone successful therapy of spinal opioid-induced pruritus (210,230) or other agents with μ-antagonist properties, such as butorphanol or nalbuphine. Indeed, in one obstetric series, the incidence of pruritus was minimal with epidural buprenorphine or butorphanol, but 50% to 60% with epidural morphine or fentanyl (185). In volunteer studies of epidural morphine, 10 mg, pruritus occurred in 100% of subjects in one study (37) and in three of four subjects in another study (227). In postoperative patients, pruritus was present in 28% of patients receiving epidural morphine 10 mg in one study (179) but in only 1% of patients in studies of morphine 5 mg (37) and 2 mg, respectively (166). Pruritus also has been reported with epidural meperidine, fentanyl, alfentanil, sufentanil, and diamorphine, but few comparative data are available. After meperidine 50 mg was given epidurally for postcesarean section pain, Brownridge reported that 50% of 2,000 patients admitted to pruritus (but only on direct questioning), yet only one patient found it troublesome (208). In contrast, in some series, epidural morphine resulted in pruritus in up to 70% of patients, but there was no relationship between incidence of pruritus and dose (250). However, the incidence of severe pruritus that troubles the patient appears to be close to 1% (37). Other putative mechanisms of spinal opioid–induced pruritus that are independent of the μ receptor include the formation of hyperalgesic metabolites such as morphine-3-glucuronide. This metabolite produces scratching behavior and hyperalgesia not reversed by naloxone after injection into monkeys. Further evidence that pruritus need not follow activation of spinal μ opioid receptors is the absence of pruritus after IT administration of β-endorphin (252,253). Hyperesthesia of unclear etiology but not reversible by naloxone, has been observed after high doses of spinal morphine given to patients with cancer pain (254,255). Fortunately, even high doses of sufentanil and alfentanil do not

appear to be associated with this side-effect (255). It has been reported that prior or concomitant use of bupivacaine epidurally reduces the incidence of pruritus with epidural opioids (256). The results of one recent trial suggest that subhypnotic doses of propofol may be an attractive novel means of treating pruritus (257). Pruritus often subsides, as does bladder dysfunction, with continuing doses of opioid.

Endocrine Dysfunction—Hypogonadism

An extensive literature in opioid addicts, patients on methadone maintenance (261,262), and animals has linked opioid administration with impairment of endocrine function. Exogenous opioids mimic an endogenous negative feedback loop (259) in which β-endorphin derived from pituitary proopiomelanocortin inhibits the secretion of hypothalamic corticotrophin-releasing hormone (260,261). However, this phenomenon (the subject of rare case reports) appears to have minimal clinical importance. Yet endogenous opioids do mediate stress-induced hypogonadism through a presumably protective reflex that inhibits male and female reproductive function during acute and chronic illness (including depression) or stressors such as caloric siphoning due to intensive prolonged exercise (263). Therefore it is not surprising that chronic therapy with systemic (264) or spinal opioids (265–268) should give rise to secondary hypogonadism.

The most common endocrine issue related to systemic or central opioid use is hypoandrogenism, both in men and women (265,269). Female hypogonadism is equally likely with chronic opioid use but typically is manifest as loss of libido rather than poor sexual performance. Both male and female opioid-induced hypogonadism may present as accelerated osteoporosis (e.g., hip or vertebral fractures) (270). Estimates of the prevalence of opioid-induced diminished libido and sexual dysfunction vary widely due to different dose ranges employed in the clinical series, different underlying diagnoses and comorbid conditions, varying age ranges reported, and other factors. Patients who note newly decreased libido during chronic opioid therapy regardless of administration route should be evaluated as one would if opioids were not a possible etiologic factor. The clinician should inquire about symptoms frequently associated with hypogonadism: loss of libido; impotence; loss of gender role; depression, anxiety, fatigue; loss of muscle mass and strength; (in females) olio- or amenorrhea (271), galactorrhea; (possibly) worsening of pain; and/or accelerated osteoporosis. The contribution of causes associated with loss of libido and/or erectile dysfunction other than opiotherapy should be assessed, including family stress in chronic pain. Such causes include normal age-related decline, pain during intercourse (e.g., from lumbosacral spine pathology or peripheral nerve dysfunction such as ilioinguinal), weight gain, vascular dysfunction *per se* or related to other intercurrent conditions such as diabetes mellitus or liver disease, nonopioid medications, unrelieved pain, and psychological conditions per se or known to be more likely with chronic pain (anxiety, depression), including marital discord. Physical examination should assess for obesity, peripheral neuropathy, and in men (who are more likely to note symptoms) testicular atrophy, gynecomastia, and decreased beard. Point tenderness upon spine percussion may indicate compression fracture. Laboratory evaluation should include free and total testosterone, keeping in mind that there is a normal age-related decline in testosterone (272). A rule of thumb is that male hypogonadism is excluded if the total (bound + free) testosterone exceeds 300 ng/mL. Low or normal plasma levels of luteinizing hormones and follicle stimulating hormone in the presence of subnormal testosterone levels confirm the diagnosis of secondary hypogonadism due to opioids. A bone densitometry test is useful to disclose bone mineral loss prior to vertebral or long bone fracture.

Therapy for opioid-induced hypoandrogenism may be as simple as rotation of the opioid to permit dose reduction (124). Should that not work, nor opioid doses lowered by the addition of nonopioid adjuvant medication(s), then blood levels of prostate-specific antigen (PSA) should be checked. If the PSA level is normal, testosterone replacement may be started using depot intramuscular injections, oral replacement, or transdermal gel. The goal is to have a total plasma testosterone level of 300–1,200 ng/mL. Monitoring of PSA levels, complete blood count (because of possible erythrocytosis), and lipid profile are recommended. If testosterone therapy is inadvisable, then sildenafil or a similar agent for erectile dysfunction may be used at normal doses, providing there are no contraindications to the latter (e.g., nitrate therapy).

SPINAL OPIOID PHARMACOLOGY

The term *selective spinal analgesia* was suggested by Cousins and associates (39) in 1979 (see later discussion) to emphasize the distinction between spinal opioid analgesia versus analgesia achieved by relatively nonselective blockade of axonal conduction by local anesthetics. From the prior section, it is clear that spinal opioids have many effects other than antinociception. However, animal and human studies have amply validated the concept of "selective spinal analgesia" mediated by multiple opioid and nonopioid spinal antinociceptive systems. Accumulating evidence points to the feasibility of "combination spinal analgesic chemotherapy" (32) to achieve the ideal of analgesia without unwanted side effects by coadministering two or more agents, such as opioids and local anesthetics, that act upon different antinociceptive targets. This section summarizes the preclinical and clinical data that model the pharmacokinetics and pharmacodynamics of IT and epidural opioids given as sole agents or in combination with other opioid and nonopioid compounds.

Physicochemical Properties

Local anesthetics (273) and nonpeptidic opioids have similar molecular weights and pKa values; partition coefficients for individual agents within both drug classes overlap but vary widely (Table 40-4).

Phenylpiperidine derivatives (meperidine, fentanyl, lofentanil) are highly lipid soluble and closest in structure to local anesthetics. In contrast, morphine has low lipid solubility. Morphine's slow onset of action after epidural dosing coincides with delayed peak morphine concentrations in CSF (274,275), and its relative hydrophilicity results in slower efflux from spinal cord and CSF, and greater migration to the brain (135,276). Like lidocaine, meperidine has a rapid onset of analgesia after epidural dosing that coincides with an early peak drug concentration in CSF (39,192,275). High local concentrations of meperidine can produce peripheral nerve block (277), a property that is shared to an extent by other opioids, particularly nonalkaloids, along with many other classes of drugs used in anesthesia. Such high concentrations are unlikely to be infused spinally, and meperidine is the only opioid that has significant local anesthetic actions when applied to individual dorsal root axons or that is effective when used as a sole IT agent for surgery (278,279).

TABLE 40-4

PHYSICOCHEMICAL PROPERTIES OF OPIOIDS AND LOCAL ANESTHETICS

	Molecular weight[a]	pK$_a$ (25°C)	Partition coefficient[b]
Local anesthetics[c]			
Procaine hydrochloride	236	8.9	0.02[c]
Lidocaine hydrochloride	234	7.9	2.9[d]
Bupivacaine hydrochloloride	288	8.1	27.5[d]
Etidocaine hydrochloride	276	7.7	141[c]
Ropivacaine hydrochloride	329	8.1	141[f]
Opioids[e]			
Hydromorphone hydrochloride	322	8.1	1.23[f]
Morphine sulfate	285	7.9[a]	1.42[f]
Meperidine hydrochloride	247	8.5	38.8[f]
Methadone hydrochloride	309	9.3	116[f]
Fentanyl citrate	336	8.4	813[f]
Sufentanil citrate	386	8.0	1,788[f]
(−)Lofentanil cis-oxalate	408	7.8	1,450[f]

[a]Base.
[b]n-Heptane and octanol partition coefficients are strongly correlated for similar compounds in a log–log relationship.
[c]Commonly used forms (see Mather [61]).
[d]n-Heptane/pH 7.4 buffer, partition coefficient.
[e]Tertiary amino group.
[f]Octanol/pH 7.4 buffer partition coefficient.

Onset of analgesia after spinal opioid administration is earlier with more lipid-soluble agents. Other factors such as molecular size and shape also contribute to a degree (280). Morphine, an extreme example of low lipid solubility and high water solubility, has the slowest onset of action. A somewhat quicker onset of clinical analgesia for hydromorphone than morphine after lumbar epidural administration despite comparable lipophilicity and similar blood and CSF pharmacokinetics (281) may reflect more rapid supraspinal action of the former compound (282). Many studies in animals (18,127,241) and humans (157,171,276,283) indicate the importance of lipid solubility for dural transfer (275,284).

Duration of analgesia is inversely related to lipid solubility but also influenced by the rate of dissociation from receptors and accumulation within epidural fat. In rats, the duration of analgesia for fentanyl analogues and morphine in hot plate and tail flick tests is dose-dependent (127). At doses producing an equal magnitude of peak analgesia, the duration of action was lofentanil >morphine >sufentanil >alfentanil ≥fentanyl.

Preclinical Pharmacokinetic Observations

Gustafsson and co-workers performed lumbar IT injections of [14C]-morphine and [3H]-meperidine in rats (285). Whole-body autoradiography revealed that 15 minutes after [14C]-morphine injection, the entire spinal cord and ventral parts of the brain contained high levels of radioactivity. At 60 minutes, parts of the brain, including respiratory and vomiting centers and the trigeminal nucleus, contained radioactivity that remained detectable at 2 but not 4 hours after injection. Only the caudal part of the spinal cord contained radioactivity at 4 hours. Overall, the more lipophilic drug meperidine is rapidly taken up and eliminated from the spinal cord, whereas the hydrophilic drug morphine persists in the spinal cord for much longer. Also, morphine spreads rapidly into basal cisterns and later penetrates into brain.

The same group applied positron emission tomography (PET) to study kinetics of [14C]-labeled morphine and meperidine after lumbar epidural and IT administration in monkeys (137). The technique could differentiate between whole-body versus spinal canal uptake, but not among epidural, IT, or spinal cord uptake. For meperidine, high activity was observed only in the lumbar spinal region. For morphine, radioactivity was fairly constant along the spinal canal up to C4, where it was low. Cervical CSF showed peak radioactivity about 60 minutes after injection of morphine or meperidine. Injection rapidly or in a large volume increased cephalad spread. Peak concentrations of both drugs in blood occurred 5 minutes after spinal injection (137). Strube and associates injected [3H]-morphine in the lumbar epidural space of anesthetized baboons and tracked cisternal CSF radioactivity for 22 hours. Morphine was detected in cisternal CSF 1 hour after administration, reached a peak at 3 hours, then declined, with a half-life of 8 hours (286).

After epidural injection of [3H]-morphine and inulin in dogs, Durant and Yaksh studied distribution in lumbar CSF, azygos venous and femoral arterial blood, and lymph (287). During the first 20 minutes, morphine levels in the azygos blood were three- and tenfold higher, respectively, than in arterial blood and lymph. By 1 hour, half the morphine had passed into the azygos system. The elimination phase from CSF was about 106 minutes. Comparison of blood and lymph values indicated that morphine in lymph was derived from systemic distribution. Morphine appeared to be cleared from CSF through the azygos venous system at a similar rate as inulin. Surprisingly, the fraction of morphine (molecular weight 334) crossing the dura after epidural injection (0.3%) was half that for inulin (0.6%, molecular weight 5,175). A later toxicologic screening study from the same laboratory (51) confirmed rapid systemic redistribution of bolus doses of lumbar epidural or IT sufentanil, alfentanil, and morphine before and after a 15- or 25-day continuous drug infusion.

Colpaert and co-workers studied opiate receptor binding and drug concentrations in plasma and brain after epidural and IV sufentanil in the rat (117). Epidural sufentanil inhibited [3H]-sufentanil binding throughout brain and spinal cord, but more so in thalamus and lumbar spinal cord. Intravenous sufentanil at an analgesic dose inhibited [3H]-sufentanil binding in brain. The epidural route was only half as potent as the IV route in producing detectable levels of sufentanil in plasma and brain. Hence, analgesia with optimal epidural doses of sufentanil probably is due to a spinal action, with a contribution from brain sufentanil action during early stages of analgesia. Increasing epidural doses of sufentanil progressively resemble IV administration as the amount of drug in the brain increases.

The valveless internal vertebral venous plexus communicates with intracranial venous sinuses (see later discussion and Fig. 40-6). Under conditions of increased epidural pressure, venous blood flow may be cephalad, carrying drug absorbed from the epidural space up to the brain. The observation that rapid epidural injection of a small dose of morphine in the cat may provoke retching, yet the same dose given in the femoral vein is without effect (255) suggested that epidural opioids may reach the brain rapidly via a direct vascular channel, in addition to transport in CSF. To test this hypothesis, [3H]-naloxone or [14C]-morphine was injected epidurally and plasma concentrations of tracer measured in the azygos vein (representing epidural venous drainage to superior vena cava) and in internal jugular vein (representing passage of the drug via the internal vertebral venous plexus to intracranial venous sinuses and then to brain). Vena caval compression decreased radioactivity in the azygos outflow but increased radioactivity in jugular blood (127).

Clinical Pharmacokinetics and Pharmacodynamics

In 1979, Wang and others (150) published the first peer-reviewed report of spinal IT opioids in humans conducted as a double-blind, placebo-controlled cross-over study approved by a human studies committee. Eight patients suffering from cancer pain despite chronic systemic opioid therapy received lumbar IT morphine (0.5 or 1.0 mg) or physiologic saline to a total of 17 and 12 injections, respectively. Two patients reported pain relief after both morphine and saline; morphine provided 15 hours of pain relief compared to 7 hours after saline. This incidence (two of eight subjects) and duration of placebo response is consistent with many analgesic trials. In the other six patients, saline injections were ineffective, whereas morphine injections were followed by pain relief in 15 to 45 minutes, lasting 12 to 24 hours. The authors reported no sedation, respiratory depression, or neurologic deterioration (150). Also in 1979, Cousins and colleagues reported that 1 to 2 mg of morphine injected into the thoracic IT space relieved the pain of breast or lung cancer for 24 to 48 hours (39). These patients, who had been treated chronically with systemic opioids, did not experience respiratory depression. Chauvin and associates reported that plasma morphine concentrations were low after 0.02 mg/kg of morphine intrathecally, and thus vascular absorption of morphine was unlikely to contribute to analgesia (288). Following these seminal studies, relief of acute or chronic pain after IT opioid administration has now become an integral part of clinical pain management in many settings, as described throughout this volume.

Epidural opioid therapy was likewise reported in 1979 by Behar and associates (16). The same year, Cousins and colleagues described pharmacokinetic and neurologic findings during epidural meperidine epidural administration (39). Because other neurologic functions, such as sympathetic vasoconstrictor responses were intact, the term *selective spinal analgesia* was advanced to distinguish analgesia achieved with spinal opioids from that accomplished using spinal local anesthetics (39).

Epidural meperidine pharmacokinetics in blood and CSF after epidural or IV drug administration in the same patients were the subject of the earliest studies in this field (289). Blood and CSF meperidine concentrations and analgesic responses varied greatly among patients, but patients having a high CSF-to-blood concentration ratio had complete analgesia. A rapid increase in CSF meperidine concentrations in the first 5 minutes after injection coincided with the onset of analgesia. Analgesia after epidural drug administration lasted well beyond the time when blood concentrations declined below minimally effective levels. These findings have been confirmed by others (1). However, if similar doses of meperidine are given intramuscularly

TABLE 40-5

RELATIVE ANALGESIC POTENCIES

Postoperative intravenous (IV) and epidural (EPID) opioid dose requirements (ODR) over 17 h and relative ODR ratios of various opioids. IV ODR data corrected (corr) for elimination rate are also listed.

	ODR		Relative ODR ratios		
Opioid	(mg) IV	(mg) EPID	IV vs. EPID	EPID MOR vs. EPID opioid	IV corr vs. EPID
Morphine	45.9	5.0	9.2	1.0	35.0
Tramadol	455.0	180.0	2.5	0.03	18.0
Meperidine[a]	442.0	182.0	2.4	0.03	8.1
Methadone	13.0	10.3	1.3	0.5	29.0
Alfentanil	9.1	4.5	2.0	1.1	2.2
Fentanyl	1.2	0.4	3.0	12.5	27.0
Sufentanil	0.152	0.113	1.4	44.0	13.0
Buprenorphine	0.78	0.52	1.5	9.2	3.2

[a]Based upon the "active" R (−)-methadone enantiomer as used in Germany.
Reproduced from Table 29-7 3rd ed *Neural Blockade*.

and epidurally, blood concentrations are similar. Analgesia was significantly greater for epidural compared with intramuscular meperidine between 0.25 and 1 hour in one controlled study (157,159). Also, some patients had evidence of hypalgesia, indicating a weak local anesthetic effect (157). The fact that an effective epidural meperidine dose (e.g., 50 mg) is lower than an effective intramuscular dose (e.g., 100 mg) is consistent with a predominantly spinal action (232,275).

Epidural morphine pharmacokinetics and pharmacodynamics are well characterized and consistent with a spinal site of action after epidural drug administration (167,210,226, 274,280,290–292). Of all opioids studied in the postoperative period, morphine has the greatest dosage-sparing effect for epidural versus IV administration (49). Average postoperative opioid doses and relative dosage requirements for morphine and other opioids given via the IV or epidural routes are shown in Table 40-5. The quality of morphine analgesia is superior when this drug is given epidurally rather than systemically (257), and the analgesic effect of epidural morphine correlates poorly with blood morphine concentration. Consistent with evolving knowledge of genetic heterogeneity in responses to opioid analgesics (see earlier discussion), some patients given epidural morphine report analgesia in the presence of extremely low serum morphine concentrations (290,291), whereas others fail to achieve analgesia in the presence of typically analgesic blood concentrations (167,292–294). Because morphine metabolites appear in plasma shortly after morphine administration, early studies based upon radioimmunoassays that concurrently detect morphine and its metabolites are suspect (e.g., in falsely depicting persistence of morphine or underestimating concentration–analgesia relationships). Nordberg and co-workers (291) used gas chromatography to avoid such analytic pitfalls and found that absorption of epidural morphine into the vascular system occurred rapidly, with peak arterial plasma concentrations occurring within 15 minutes. They reported that the ratio of lumbar CSF-to-plasma morphine concentrations increased with time after injection and ranged from 45:1 to 100:1 at 1 hour to 125:1 to 175:1 at 5 hours. This increase appeared to be caused by dysequilibrium between plasma and tissue concentrations, since elimination half-lives of morphine in plasma and CSF compartments were similar (approximately

4 hours). Gustafsson and colleagues (290) and others (1) confirmed the rapid systemic absorption of epidural morphine and reported that peak plasma morphine concentrations occurred earlier and were also higher (relative to dose) than after intramuscular morphine. Based upon their reevaluation of the octanol-buffer partition coefficient for hydromorphone (281), which revealed it to be closer to that of morphine than previously reported, Cousins and colleagues examined the CSF and blood pharmacokinetics of this drug administered together with morphine and found striking similarity between these two agents (282).

Epidural fentanyl yields a quality of analgesia similar to that produced by epidural morphine and is second only to morphine in the degree of dosage-sparing achieved by epidural versus IV drug delivery (49). Again similar to morphine, postoperative analgesia from epidural fentanyl and sufentanil is evident in patients whose plasma opioid concentrations are below analgesic levels (295,296). Further, analgesia lasted longer and was more profound when the same dose of fentanyl was given epidurally compared with intramuscularly (162,297). A careful experimental study in healthy volunteers by Coda and colleagues (50) demonstrated that lumbar epidural fentanyl, alfentanil, and sufentanil all produced selective lower extremity analgesia. For each of these three agents, low epidural doses yielded plasma levels well below their established minimally effective analgesic concentrations, but higher doses resulted in plasma concentrations that nearly reached minimally effective plasma opioid concentrations. Coda and colleagues concluded that although morphine produces supraspinal effects on the basis of rostral spread in CSF, lipophilic epidural opioids produce supraspinal effects through systemic redistribution. Although one must always be cautious about extrapolating from volunteers (or unstressed animals) to patients because the blood–brain barrier becomes more permeable during environmental stress (298), Coda's conclusion reinforces growing clinical experience that epidural administration of lipophilic opioids alone may offer little advantage over the IV route (49,50,299,300). However, although it is now standard practice to employ opioid–local anesthetic mixtures of drugs for epidural analgesia, it is also appropriate to infuse epidural opioids alone for initial postoperative pain management in unstable patients not yet able

PART IV: PAIN MANAGEMENT

to tolerate epidural local anesthetics. Upon stabilization (e.g., intravascular volume repletion), such patients can be switched to an epidural infusion containing opioid and local anesthetic. When faced with inadequate analgesia cephalad to the epidural catheter tip during a postoperative epidural infusion of fentanyl (with or without local anesthetic), it is helpful first to change the infusate to epidural morphine to increase cephalad coverage and avoid having to reinsert a catheter more cephalad. Such clinical strategies simplify anesthetic and analgesic management by employing the same epidural catheter intra- and postoperatively selecting agent(s) infused and delivery rate according to changing clinical status.

Pharmacokinetic Models of Intrathecal and Epidural Opioids

Pharmacokinetic models of spinal opioid distribution and clearance after IT or epidural injection provide a coherent framework to consolidate preclinical and clinical observations. The just reviewed studies of spinal opioid analgesia have identified dose, delivery mode (bolus versus infusion), injectate volume, lipophilicity, and addition of epinephrine as factors that affect pharmacokinetics and hence analgesic effects of such drugs. Classical compartmental descriptions are somewhat oversimplified, however, as the idealized notion of a solute being cleared with a particular rate constant applies only for a stirred pool.

Intrathecal injection of a highly ionized and hydrophilic drug such as morphine produces extremely high CSF concentrations (274,301–303). The comparable onset times for analgesia after IT and epidural administration of morphine or other opioids has raised the possibility that vascular transport via the posterior radicular artery (304) supplements diffusion from CSF as a mode of drug entry into the cord (Fig. 40-3). Once in the spinal cord, morphine's slow egress produces a long duration of action (284). Cephalad flow carries drug remaining in CSF (305) upwards toward the brain (Fig. 40-2). Spinal CSF flow to the brain may be hastened by Valsalva maneuver or intermittent positive-pressure ventilation. Lazorthes and co-workers (301) measured morphine concentrations in lumbar spinal fluid after IT administration of morphine 5 mg in a hyperbaric solution. They found a distribution half-life of 22 minutes and elimination half-life of 4 hours, the latter value being similar to those reported after IT (274) and epidural (291) administration. By comparison, radiolabeled albumin (which stays in the CSF) passes cephalad, so that 20% to 30% of a lumbar IT dose moves intracranially within 12 hours and almost 100% within 24 hours (151).

Intrathecal injection of an ionized, lipid soluble drug results in low residual concentrations in CSF (192,307) owing to rapid systemic uptake. Hence, less drug is carried in CSF to the brain. High lipid solubility facilitates access via the arterial route into the spinal cord, where drug rapidly enters and binds to opioid receptors and nonspecific binding sites. Unless a particular drug has high affinity for lipid or opioid receptor, however, egress is also rapid.

Pharmacokinetic models of epidural drug injection are identical to those for IT injection, but must in addition take into account drug equilibration and clearance from the epidural space (Fig. 40-6A) (284). After epidural injection of a highly ionized and hydrophilic drug such as morphine, epidural concentrations of nonionized, lipid-soluble drug will be low. Because most of the drug present in CSF is ionized, only a small con-

centration gradient drives diffusion of nonionized drug from CSF into the spinal cord receptors. For the same reason, later egress of drug from spinal cord to spinal fluid will be equally slow. High concentrations of ionized drug in spinal fluid will be carried rostrally with the CSF flow, and will thus extend the level of analgesia as well as migrating to supraspinal structures (Fig. 40-2). For morphine, the foregoing model is consistent with its slow onset and long duration of analgesia, and potential for delayed respiratory depression—effects that correlate well with delayed peak CSF concentrations and prolonged, high levels of morphine in cervical CSF after lumbar administration (Figs. 40-2 and 40-6A) (135,274,275). Epidural injection of a mostly ionized lipophilic drug such as meperidine will produce low concentrations of lipid soluble nonionized drug in the epidural space. Nonionized drug will rapidly be transferred to CSF, spinal radicular arteries, and epidural veins. In the presence of brisk spinal artery blood flow and slow epidural venous flow, transfer of the drug to the spinal cord will predominate while the concentration gradient is high. However, drug absorption into epidural veins will promptly reduce the concentration gradient, and egress from spinal cord receptors will be equally rapid (Fig. 40-6B). Clinical observations confirm that the durations of epidural meperidine and fentanyl do not differ widely (232,297).

Blood concentrations of epidurally administered opioids are greatly influenced by the dynamics of vertebral venous and arterial blood flow. When intrathoracic pressure is high, venous (and drug) flow will be redirected through the basivertebral system up to the brain. Obstruction of the inferior vena cava, as in pregnancy, causes distention of epidural veins and increased flow through the azygos vein, which increases systemic absorption of epidural opioid and leaves less drug available for transfer across the dura to the spinal cord. Meperidine carried in the azygos vein to the superior vena cava is then distributed to the general circulation and cleared rapidly in the liver. Studies during labor confirm more rapid absorption of epidural meperidine than in nonpregnant women (159,306,307). Also in pregnancy, epidural absorption is even more rapid than after intramuscular injection (306).

It seems probable that early respiratory depression (see this section above) after epidural opioid is due to rapid, early vascular absorption together with transient increases in CSF drug concentrations at the base of the brain. For lipid-soluble opioids, such increases are smaller and briefer than for morphine (135,137,276). Late respiratory depression is less likely after lipid-soluble than water-soluble opioids, but both early and late respiratory depression have been described after epidural fentanyl, meperidine, diamorphine, methadone, and sufentanil (185). In such cases, one cannot exclude sudden redirection of blood flow through basivertebral veins to the brain as a result of increased intrathoracic pressure, or inadvertent injection of a portion of the epidural dose into the subarachnoid space. Redistribution, rather than systemic clearance, probably is more important in reducing the risk of respiratory depression from blood-borne drug, since dosing intervals for most epidural opioids will be greater than plasma half-lives.

SPINAL ANALGESIA: CLINICAL OPTIONS

Surveys of clinical practice conducted across the four editions of this text (1980, 1988, 1998, and 2008) leave no doubt that the spinal route of analgesia has evolved to be an integral part of pain management in many settings. In contrast to the growing number of preclinical target candidates for analgesia, however, clinically available agents for spinal analgesia have been few, increasing only at a snail's pace. Only one new application for central administration of a previously marketed systemic drug was approved by the U.S. Food and Drug Administration (FDA) in the 1990s: spinal clonidine in 1997 as an adjunct to morphine (308). Thus far through the 2000s, only one new molecule has been approved for IT analgesia: ziconotide, in 2004 (309). Opioids still predominate in clinical applications, principally morphine but increasingly fentanyl for acute, and sufentanil or hydromorphone for chronic use (the latter selections influenced by the growing problem of morphine-related catheter tip granulomas). These four opioids, together with clonidine, ziconotide, and dilute bupivacaine, account for nearly all chronically, and the great majority of acutely, administered IT analgesics (30,310). Interestingly, early practice guidelines on IT analgesia (311) emphasized morphine and hydromorphone, and noted benefits of adding bupivacaine or clonidine in patients with opioid resistance or tolerance. In 2000, during the first of three Polyanalgesic Consensus Conferences, panelists drew upon their clinical experience and recommended morphine as the first-line agent for IT analgesia. The second line involved addition of either bupivacaine or clonidine, or rotation from morphine to hydromorphone (312). The third line of therapy involved combining morphine, bupivacaine, and clonidine, or rotation of morphine to fentanyl or sufentanil. Miscellaneous agents such as methadone, neostigmine, baclofen, or ketamine were considered fourth-line therapy. The successor conference in 2003 (313) essentially continued this stratification, adding two additional lines of therapy. To those agents recommended in the prior conference were now added adenosine and ketorolac (line five) and ropivacaine, meperidine, gabapentin, buprenorphine, and octreotide (line six). The six lines of therapy were stratified "according to evidence of safety, efficacy, and broad clinical experience." The most recent 2007 Polyanalgesic Conference (30) dropped the "flow chart" structure of the prior summary recommendations, retained six lines of therapy similar to its predecessor, and added the recently FDA-approved ziconotide to each of the top four lines (Table 40-6). A very

similar set of recommendations was issued in mid 2007 by the British Pain Society in collaboration with the Association for Palliative Medicine and the Society for British Neurosurgeons (http://www.britishpainsociety.org/book_ittd_main.pdf). In sum, apart from the addition of ziconotide, little has changed in nearly a decade. On the other hand, a variety of novel spinal analgesics are now in phase 1 and 2 clinical trials around the world (18,314–316). The apparently slow pace of innovation in spinal analgesia may reflect several factors, not all of which are cause for pessimism. First, patient, surgeon, and anesthesiologist satisfaction with currently available agents has remained fairly high since the second edition of this text in 1988 (285), which appeared at the close of the initial decade of clinical spinal analgesia after intense clinical experimentation and refinement around the world. Second, the message that effective analgesia not only improves quality of life but also can reduce short- and long-term cost and burden of care for patients with acute or chronic pain has only recently emerged from basic and clinical research. Third, given the normally long time lag for novel clinical research findings to impact upon practitioners, policy makers, and regulators in any area of medicine (63), delays of a decade or more in translation are not unusual. Fourth, the clinical use of combinations of spinal analgesics, commented upon here and in the prior edition of this text, has dramatically accelerated, so that the handful of primary agents available are now routinely applied in growing numbers of combinations. Finally, increasing public demand for better pain control as a fundamental human right has helped advance medical management of pain, potentially decreasing the need to employ IT analgesia. For these reasons, it is timely to review current and emerging analgesics and combinations as it is likely that the pace of their clinical adoption will quicken during the next decade. Because the preclinical pharmacology of nociception has already been described in Chapter 31 and reviewed in detail in Chapters 32 and 33, the present description will not attempt to be comprehensive, but instead will focus upon agents that practicing anesthesiologists can now (or are likely soon to be able to) obtain (Tables 40-7 and 40-8). We will omit discussion of local anesthetics, whose basic and clinical features have already been described comprehensively in several earlier chapters.

TABLE 40-6

STRATIFIED APPROACH TO DRUG SELECTION FOR CHRONIC INTRATHECAL THERAPY RECOMMENDED BY 2007 POLYANALGESIC CONSENSUS CONFERENCE PANELISTS

Line #1:	morphine	↔	hydromorphone	↔	ziconotide
Line #2:	fentanyl	↔	morphine/hydromorphone + ziconotide	↔	morphine/hydromorphone + bupivacaine/clonidine
Line #3:	clonidine	↔	morphine/hydromorphone/fentanyl (bupivacaine +/or clonidine) + ziconotide		
Line #4:	sufentanil	↔	sufentanil + bupivacaine +/or clonidine + ziconotide		
Line #5:	ropivacaine, buprenophine, midazolam meperidine, ketorolac				
Line #6:	**Experimental Drugs** gabapentin, octreotide, Neostigmine, Adenosine, conpeptides; XEN2174, AM336, ZGX 160				

From Deer T, Krames ES, Hassenbusch SJ, et al. Polyanalgesic Consensus Conference 2007: Recommendations for the management of pain by intrathecal (intraspinal) Drug delivery: Report of an interdisciplinary expert panel. *Neuromodulation* 2007;10:300–328.

TABLE 40-7

CONCENTRATIONS AND DOSES OF CHRONIC INTRATHECAL AGENTS RECOMMENDED BY 2007 POLYANALGESIC CONSENSUS CONFERENCE PANELISTS

Drug	Maximum concentration	Maximum dose/day
Morphine	20 mg/mL	15 mg
Hydromorphone	10 mg/mL	4 mg
Fentanyl	2 mg/mL	No known upper limit
Sufentanil	50 μg/mL, (not available for compounding)	No known upper limit
Bupivacaine	40 mg/mL	30 mg
Clonidine	2 mg/mL	1.0 mg
Ziconotide	100 μg/mL	19.2 μg (Elan recommendations)

From Deer T, Krames ES, Hassenbusch SJ, et al. Polyanalgesic Consensus Conference 2007: Recommendations for the management of pain by intrathecal (intraspinal) drug delivery: Report of an interdisciplinary expert panel. *Neuromodulation* 2007;10:300–328.

Opioids

Postoperative analgesia is the most common indication for spinal opioid use, but long-term spinal opioid infusion has now been applied to tens of thousands of patients for cancer-related and also chronic nonmalignant pain. In the perioperative context, Chapter 43 by Macintyre and Scott, the practical choice between IT versus epidural drug delivery is dictated by the operative procedure and projected duration of the need for optimal postoperative analgesia (317–319). Because of the risk of post–dural puncture headache and CSF leakage when conventional epidural catheters are placed intrathecally, and following with-drawal from the market of microcatheters that allowed continuous perioperative subarachnoid drug delivery, the epidural route remains the choice for all but "one-shot" analgesics (320). As described in Chapters 31 and 32, in preclinical studies, selective opioid agonists possess different selectivity against different types of pain. Thus μ opioid agonists are effective against thermal pain, whereas κ opioid agonists are more effective against pressure or visceral pain models (e.g., formalin). On the other hand, clinically available κ agonists such as butorphanol or nalbuphine are hardly used for spinal application, and buprenorphine, which is used rarely, is a partial μ opioid agonist of low intrinsic efficacy. The reality is at present that virtually all acute and chronic opioid analgesia is accomplished using μ opioid agonists that are phenylpiperidines or alkaloids (Table 40-9). In the largest prospective randomized controlled trial of its type to date, Smith and colleagues (19) randomized 200 patients with cancer pain to receive conventional medical management or IT analgesia using morphine or hydromorphone. About a third had bupivacaine added, and 4% had clonidine added. The group treated with IT analgesia had less pain, and fewer drug-related adverse effects. Most remarkably, the group that received IT analgesia had a 6-month survival rate of 53.9% compared with 37.2% in the conventionally managed group, a result that just missed statistical significance ($p = 0.06$).

In the near term, clinical trials may revisit promising pilot work since the 1970s that suggested a role for δ opioid peptides (321,322) as alternatives to μ agonists, now studying more selective and potent compounds than were earlier available (323–326). Despite the increased potency of the newer δ-selective opioids, they remain relatively costly and require high doses for epidural or systemic use; hence

TABLE 40-8

COMMONLY USED MEDICATIONS IN SIX-MONTH MULTICENTER SURVEY OF IMPLANTED INTRATHECAL INFUSION DEVICES IN PATIENTS WITH CHRONIC NONCANCER LOW BACK PAIN

Medication	Frequency (%)*
Morphine	47.7
Bupivacaine	12.7
Clonidine	10.0
Hydromorphone	7.5
Fentanyl	5.9
Baclofen	5.7
Dilaudid	3.3
Demerol	2.5
Sufentanil	1.8

*Proportion of total medications given.
From Staats P, Whitworth M, Barakat M, et al. The use of implanted programmable infusion pumps in the management of nonmalignant, chronic low-back pain. *Neuromodulation* 2007;10:376–380.

TABLE 40-9

INTRASPINAL OPIOIDS FOR THE TREATMENT OF ACUTE PAIN

Drug	Single dose[a] (mg)	Infusion rate[b] (mg/hr)	Onset (min)	Duration of single dose[c] (hours)
Epidural				
Morphine	1–6	0.1–1.0	30	6–24
Meperidine	20–150	5–20	5	4–8
Methadone	1–10	0.3–0.5	10	6–10
Hydromorphone	1–2	0.1–0.2	15	10–16
Diamorphine	4–6	?	5	12
Fentanyl	0.025–01	0.025–0.10	5	2–4
Sufentanil	0.01–0.06	0.01–0.05	5	2–4
Subarachnoid				
Morphine	0.1–0.3		15	8–24+
Meperidine	10–30		?	10–24+
Diamorphine	1–2		?	20
Fentanyl	0.005–0.25		5	3–6

[a]Low doses may be effective when administered to the elderly or when injected in the cervical or thoracic region.
[b]If combining with a local anesthetic, consider using 0.0625% bupivacaine.
[c]Duration of analgesia varies widely; higher doses produce longer duration.
Modified from the previous edition.

their clinical application will likely be for IT use. Gender differences in the response to systemic κ opioid agonists may reflect estrogen–opioid interactions in the dorsal horn (327).

α_2 and Other Adrenergic Agonists

Spinally applied epinephrine was observed to produce analgesia in animals a century ago and in humans over 50 years ago. Also, for decades, veterinary experience with xylazine and other α_2 adrenergic agonists has provided convincing evidence that systemic administration of these agents produces anesthesia. Unfortunately, these and other veterinary anesthetics that act upon adrenergic pathways are unsuitable for use in humans because they produce unpleasant psychological effects. The present era of integrated preclinical and clinical pharmacologic and toxicologic research dates from the 1980s. Prompted by emerging animal data (116), Tamsen and Gordh administered epidural clonidine to two patients with chronic pain, with encouraging results. Since then, the presence of separate opioid and monoaminergic analgesic systems in the spinal cord has been well defined in a number of basic histologic and pharmacologic studies (328,329). Of the latter, norepinephrine, acetylcholine, and serotonin are the principal, clinically relevant mediators (249). Because of its dose-dependent anxiolytic, sedative, sympatholytic, and anesthetic-sparing actions, clonidine has enjoyed popularity as a premedication, particularly before cardiovascular surgery (330). Its propensity to cause hypotension limits systemic dosing, a side effect that is less prominent with the recently introduced and more potent α_2 agonist dexmedetomidine. Clonidine given systemically has an opioid-sparing effect. Gordh, in his doctoral thesis, further demonstrated in a controlled clinical trial the value of clonidine for epidural analgesia, and others, notably Eisenach (331) and the group of Filos, Goudas, and colleagues (332) carried this work further to show that IT clonidine is nontoxic and can be effective as the sole postoperative spinal analgesic after general or obstetric surgery. As with opioids, clonidine (a lipophilic compound) is active as an analgesic when administered systemically or centrally (333), and in addition has been reported to augment the quality and duration of peripheral neural blockade with local anesthetic. It may be protective against the formation of catheter tip inflammatory masses (246). Several pieces of evidence, parallel to those presented for opioids, indicate that clonidine acts spinally to produce analgesia. Low doses of clonidine infused in the lumbar epidural space produce lower but not upper extremity analgesia, and this analgesia spreads to the upper extremity after prolonged infusion. Clonidine is more potent after epidural than systemic administration, and in volunteers as well as patients, CSF levels of clonidine predict pain relief with much greater accuracy than do blood levels. These promising findings—particularly of clonidine as an adjunct to epidural or IT morphine—have been confirmed in clinical trials for cancer pain (25,334) and in a placebo-controlled, double-blinded study by Siddall and colleagues in chronic pain after spinal cord injury (132). A smaller literature indicates similar promise for other α_2 agents such as tizanidine and dexmedetomidine (335). Xen 2174 is the first conopeptide norepinephrine transporter (NET) blocker, which in animal studies is potent in neuropathic pain models. Its therapeutic index appears to be approximately five times greater than ziconotide. Initial dose-finding studies in cancer patients show promise of efficacy in severe neuropathic pain (M. Cousins, personal communication).

Cholinomimetics and Cholinesterase Inhibitors

Acetylcholine release occurs in response to acute pain in animals and (based upon weaker data) may also occur in clinical settings such as childbirth (4,86,331). These data, along with the observation that α_2 adrenergic analgesia provokes release of acetylcholine from the dorsal horn, suggest that activation of cholinergic receptors is a mechanism of endogenous analgesia. Following the same logic as outlined earlier for α_2 adrenergic spinal analgesia, many of the same preclinical and clinical investigators who advanced clonidine from laboratory into clinical practice also have undertaken studies to clarify and exploit cholinergic mechanisms in clinical spinal analgesia. Preclinical studies employing selective nicotinic and muscarinic agonists reveal a role for the latter, but not the former acetylcholine receptor subtype in mediating spinal analgesic effects. The cholinesterase inhibitor neostigmine also has spinal analgesic properties in preclinical models, an effect that results from augmenting acetylcholine effects upon muscarinic receptors (331). Because preservative-free neostigmine is readily available, phase 1 clinical safety testing began with this agent. Although neurotoxicity of spinal neostigmine was not apparent in animals, in phase 1 clinical testing in volunteers, this agent had a poor effect-to-side effect ratio. Minimal analgesic IT doses (100 μg) produced nausea, vomiting, and transient lower extremity weakness. Initial dose-ranging studies by Lauretti and colleagues (336) in surgical patients confirmed a high incidence of nausea and vomiting at analgesic doses of neostigmine administered as a single IT agent. However, subanalgesic doses of neostigmine had a substantial (30%–70%) dosage-sparing effect upon supplemental analgesia while producing minimal nausea. Further, the epidural administration of neostigmine enhances epidural analgesia from local anesthetics, with apparently fewer gastrointestinal side effects when compared with IT delivery (337). Newer cholinomimetic compounds that enjoy a more favorable effect-to-side effect ratio are reported now to be entering clinical trials.

GABAergic Agonists

Animal studies have demonstrated that muscimol and baclofen, agonists at $GABA_A$ and $GABA_B$ receptors respectively, produce analgesia upon IT administration. Although baclofen is the sole GABAergic agent that has been approved by the FDA for chronic IT use, this approval is limited to therapy of spasticity, for which extensive post-approval clinical data attest to its efficacy and safety. Nonetheless, its analgesic potency in animal models (116,338) led to its adoption for chronic IT administration for patients with spasticity and pain, such as in cerebral palsy, spinal cord injury, or multiple sclerosis (339), or even in dystonia as in CRPS (340). Now, baclofen is at times applied as a component of current multidrug regimens for chronic IT analgesia in patients with chronic pain but without spasticity (310,335). As already noted, although catheter tip granuloma formation does not appear as frequently as with IT morphine, it is still a concern (27), as are multiple clinical observations of the potential lethality both of overdosage and sudden withdrawal of baclofen infusion.

Benzodiazepines such as midazolam, which enhance the effect of endogenous GABA upon $GABA_A$ receptors through a NO-dependent mechanism (341), also produce analgesia when administered into the subarachnoid space in rats (342). This analgesia is reversed by the benzodiazepine antagonist flumazenil as well as the GABA$_A$ antagonist bicuculline. Limited clinical data on IT and epidural administration of midazolam suggest a potential for neurotoxicity based upon prolonged (24 hours) effects after a single dose. However, small case series to date have provided some reassurance in that regard (343–345), including observations in excess of 5 years (346).

Ion Channel Blockers

Because spinal nociception depends upon ion flux to trigger postsynaptic depolarization in dorsal horn neurons, it is not surprising that all clinically useful spinal analgesics inhibit this process either directly or indirectly. The range of specific targets and available agents, as well as the physiologic basis for their action, have been reviewed in detail by Strichartz, Yaksh, Dickenson, and colleagues in Chapters 2, 32, and 33. Mu or δ opioid agonists inhibit potassium flux, κ agonists inhibit calcium flux, and local anesthetics inhibit (principally) sodium flux. The paramount importance of sodium influx in triggering depolarization and calcium influx to initiate the intracellular cascade of genetic and biochemical responses to nociception are indisputable. Over 50 years ago, pioneering electrophysiologists such as Eccles identified alterations in the excitability of spinal neurons following injury to their axons (347). By the 1980s, Wall, Devor, and others recognized that such abnormal action potentials resulted from the accumulation of novel, phenotypically abnormal neuronal voltage-gated sodium channels (348,349). In his essay on "new horizons" in the final chapter of the prior edition of this text, the late Professor Wall commented that the extreme tetrodotoxin sensitivity of uninjured neurons "points to the possibility of a local anesthetic from an entirely new family, which is free of some of the effects of [presently available] local anesthetics" (350). In the decade since Wall's essay, advances in molecular cloning have led to the characterization of at least nine such "Nav" isoforms with distinctive distributions among dorsal root ganglia, peripheral neuromas, and spinal cord, as well as distinctive patterns of response to nerve injury. Of these, a hereditary abnormality leading to loss of function of Nav 1.7 has been recognized as the basis for familial insensitivity to pain (351); another mutation of the same channel (*SCN9A channelopathy*) that leads to increased function is now viewed as the basis for inherited erythermalgia (352). At present, numerous agents are being investigated preclinically for their ability to selectively block specific Nav channels such as 1.7 and 1.8, and we may expect to see clinical trials emerging. MRVIB is the first conopeptide Nav 1.8 blocker (M. Cousins, personal communication). In animal studies, it has a tenfold therapeutic window between Nav 1.8 blockade and blockade of other sodium channels. This compares with a 1.5 therapeutic window of lidocaine; there are no Nav 1.8 sodium channels in myocardium or brain. Thus it is highly likely that MRVIB will be a potent selective IT drug.

Preclinical investigators have also known for decades that calcium channel blockade potentiates opioid analgesia produced by drugs or environmental stress, and suppresses the opioid abstinence syndrome. Clinical studies have not established an important analgesic effect for any of the previously available, L-type voltage-sensitive calcium channel (VSCC) blockers given as sole agents, although many, such as nimodipine, potentiate morphine analgesia (139,353). Recently, however, progress in molecular cloning and electrophysiology has revealed numerous VSCCs with different locations and functional properties (354). N-type VSCCs are located almost ex-

clusively on neurons and are particularly abundant in regions rich in synaptic connections (355). N-type VSCCs function to regulate calcium flux across presynaptic neurons that release neurotransmitters during depolarization. In the mid 1980s, peptide "conotoxins" were isolated from the venom of fish-hunting cone snails that capture their prey by paralyzing them. Some ω-conopeptides, the synthetic analogs of these so-called ω-conotoxins, selectively blocked N-type VSCCs but had little effect upon mammalian neuromuscular transmission. After preclinical testing revealed one of these conopeptides (initially termed SNX-111) to be particularly potent as a spinal analgesic in animal models of acute and chronic pain, clinical development of this agent progressed through initial trials in refractory acquired immunodeficiency syndrome (AIDS) or cancer pain (356) to trials for chronic noncancer pain (309,357). It was approved for IT analgesia by the FDA in 2004 under the name ziconotide (Prialt). The frequent occurrence of side effects such as hypotension or neuropsychiatric symptoms (358) even when dosage increments are cautiously titrated has led to ziconotide's being used more commonly as one of several co-infused medications, rather than as monotherapy. On the other hand, although some in vitro reports indicate substantial stability of a mixture of ziconotide, clonidine, and morphine (359), the manufacturer's current 2008 U.S. product label states that "combination of Prialt with IT opiates has not been studied in placebo-controlled clinical trials and is not recommended."

Gabapentin, a GABA$_A$ analog that produces IT analgesia by several mechanisms, is now believed to have its most important actions at an $\alpha_2\delta$ modulatory (inhibitory) site of N-type VSCCs (360). The high therapeutic index of the oral form of this compound has facilitated its adoption as an opioid adjuvant for acute postoperative pain (11) and as an opioid adjuvant or sole agent for neuropathic pain, including that due to malignancy (361,362). In rats, IT gabapentin prevents delayed hyperalgesia induced by fentanyl exposure (363). Although clinical analgesic trials of its IT use have not yet been reported, this agent is clearly of great interest.

A variety of other ion channels are now being studied as targets for novel selective IT analgesic agents, but have not yet moved beyond the preclinical stage. These include potassium channels such as KCNQ and acid-sensitive ion channels. A particularly interesting story has emerged from studies of the excitatory transient receptor potential vanilloid channel (TRPV1), one of several sensory neuronal TRP channels activated by diverse ligands such as camphor or menthol. TRPV1 is activated by vanilloids such as capsaicin, and is a nonselective (sodium plus calcium) channel that mediates thermal hyperalgesia. In animals, TRPV1 antagonists produce analgesia, in part due to an interaction with spinal cannabinoid receptors (364). However, initial exposure to TRPV1 antagonists in animals and humans has produced hyperthermia, the latter being marked and greater in postsurgical patients than in normal controls (365). Hence, caution has been raised about the prospects for TRPV1 antagonists used alone as clinical analgesics (366). A clever multimodal approach employs the agonist capsaicin to selectively open the TRPV1 channel on nociceptive neurons (367). Opening this channel was hypothesized to allow the normally membrane-impermeant, charged lidocaine derivative QX-314 to enter nociceptive neurons and inactivate them temporarily. In fact, systemic coadministration of capsaicin and QX-314 produced several hours of analgesia without sensory or motor defects. In contrast, administration of lidocaine did produce nonselective neural blockade. Although this strategy employed systemic drug administration, the concept would appear applicable in theory to IT analgesia.

NMDA and AMPA Antagonists

The importance of excitatory amino acids such as glutamate in mediating the transition from immediate to prolonged pain, as well as the development of acute and chronic tolerance to opioids, has been summarized in Chapters 31, 32, and 33. Insight into the role of these mediators is a key advance in understanding pain physiology since the prior edition of this text a decade ago (368,369). Although ketamine has actions at several sites, it is readily available to clinicians and is known to block the open calcium channel on the NMDA receptor complex. Hence, a profusion of studies have been carried out with ketamine in the brief time since its potential clinical value as an NMDA receptor blocker became appreciated (370). Given systemically, ketamine appears to block central summation of experimental second pain and to reduce pain intensity in instances of neurogenic pain, as in postherpetic neuralgia or phantom limb pain (371). Postoperative clinical studies have usually employed it as an adjunctive IV medication, and some have coadministered it in a preemptive fashion at the time of initial epidural analgesia (372). Choe and colleagues, for example, found a greater duration of analgesia and reduction in supplemental postoperative analgesic requirements when ketamine 60 mg was added to morphine 2 mg given epidurally before induction of anesthesia. Cousins and colleagues have found that subcutaneous infusion of ketamine is a valuable adjunct to permit tapering of IT morphine in patients with opioid tolerance after chronic IT infusion (373). In this context, the addition of ketamine prevents rebound hyperalgesia (but not opioid abstinence syndrome) when the IT infusate is switched from morphine to local anesthetic. Ozyalcin and colleagues found that epidural ketamine provided superior analgesia after thoracotomy than intramuscular ketamine (374). Wilson and colleagues (375) described a reduction in perioperative stump and phantom pain following elective lower limb amputation when IT plus epidural bupivacaine were supplemented with epidural ketamine. No long-term effects upon either type of pain were evident, although the investigators noted a long-term benefit upon mood in the patients who received ketamine. Because the incidences for long-term stump and phantom pain were lower than those reported in the literature, they speculated that their combined spinal-epidural local anesthetic improved pain control, so that their study may have been underpowered to detect a ketamine effect. Concerns regarding the potential systemic or spinal neurotoxicity of ketamine have been raised as with other NMDA antagonists, particularly with respect to neonates and infants (376). Consolidation of the relevant literature is difficult owing to species and developmental differences, the influence of the preservative in the particular ketamine formulation used, and the fact that undertreated pain itself produces persistent detrimental effects in the very young (377) as well as in adults (378).

The other NMDA antagonists in common clinical use are dextromethorphan, an inactive opioid isomer long used as an antitussive, and memantine, an antiviral and anti-Parkinson drug. However, neither agent is formulated for spinal use, and clinical trials have administered them orally. Other agents that act upon the open calcium channel of the NMDA receptor complex, such as MK-801 or phencyclidine, produce unacceptable dysphoria and related psychological side effects, and so are unsuitable for systemic administration. Phencyclidine given intrathecally in a pilot clinical study abolished allodynia and hyperpathia due to chronic neurogenic pain. More selective or better tolerated agents that act upon other sites on the NMDA receptor complex, such as its glycine binding site, are now under development. Intriguingly, the venerable antidepressant amitriptyline, used orally for decades to treat neuropathic pain (22), has recently been found to bind with high affinity to the NMDA receptor and to suppress NMDA-induced hyperalgesia after IT administration in animals. As a monoamine uptake inhibitor, amitriptyline also enhances analgesia at the spinal level by augmenting the actions of norepinephrine and serotonin (paralleling the earlier-described effect of IT neostigmine to augment spinal acetylcholine analgesia). Preclinical and phase 1 clinical studies of safety and efficacy of amitriptyline for IT use are now under way, raising the interesting prospect that both old and new drugs may enter clinical use as IT agents targeting NMDA-mediated hyperalgesia.

Glutamate not only activates the NMDA receptor, but it also activates the AMPA/kainate receptor. Preclinical studies demonstrate the efficacy of several AMPA/kainate antagonists in models of acute (379), chronic (380), and neuropathic pain (381) as well as peripheral inflammation (382). Clinical trials of such agents have not yet been reported.

Nonsteroidal Anti-Inflammatory Drugs and Nitric Oxide Synthase Inhibitors

As described earlier, co-release of substance P and glutamate from presynaptic neurons of the dorsal horn evokes prolonged postsynaptic depolarization and intense calcium influx through the NMDA receptor complex (383). Although NMDA receptor antagonism is one promising strategy to develop novel spinal analgesics, an alternative approach is to inhibit key intracellular enzymes activated by calcium entry into the postsynaptic cell (or experimentally by IT application of NMDA). Two such intraneuronal enzymes, both known to play a role in wind-up and hyperalgesia, are NOS and phospholipase A_2 (384). These generate, respectively, NO (385) from arginine and arachidonic acid from membrane phospholipid. Arachidonic acid is a substrate for COX isozymes COX-1 and COX-2 that act upon it to produce a variety of prostanoids. COX-1 is constitutively active in platelets, gastric mucosa, and kidney; inhibition of COX-1 by nonselective NSAIDs correlates with side effects at these sites. COX-2, including spinal COX-2 (386–388) is induced during inflammation and pain. Unfortunately, the increase in cardiovascular risk associated with chronic (389) or even perioperative (390) selective COX-2 inhibition has resulted in a sharp diminution of enthusiasm for this drug class, leaving ketorolac, a "level 5" drug, as the sole NSAID available for consideration for IT use. According to the 2007 Polyanalgesic Consensus Conference, a level 5 drug "is recommended with caution and obvious informed consent regarding the paucity of information regarding the safety and efficacy of their use" (30). Interestingly, NO activates COX-1 and COX-2. Preclinical data (391,392) indicate that spinal administration of the NOS inhibitor nitro-L-arginine methyl ester (L-NAME) blocks thermal hyperalgesia as well as NMDA-induced hyperalgesia, but little work has been done to harness this effect clinically. In contrast, spinal application of NSAIDs dates back to the 1970s, when Devulder administered lysine salicylate intrathecally to provide analgesia for a patient with refractory cancer pain. Other scattered case reports followed, and in the early to mid 1990s were augmented by a number of preclinical observations of spinal cord release of prostanoids along with excitatory amino acids during nociception from peripheral nerve injury or inflammation (393,394). Brune, McCormack (395), Yaksh (396), and others (397) described antinociception and reversal of hyperalgesia by small doses of centrally administered NSAIDs (including acetaminophen) and distinguished between the anti-inflammatory and analgesic mechanisms of NSAIDs (398). A variety of possible mechanisms for the central analgesic effects of NSAIDs are now under preclinical study; prominent among these are inhibition of presynaptic neurotransmitter release in the dorsal horn through inhibition of presynaptic adenylyl cyclase and interference with postsynaptic, NMDA-evoked gene expression.

Adenosine and Nonopioid Peptides

Adenosine receptors are expressed on the surface of nearly all cells. Five adenosine receptors have been identified through pharmacologic and cloning techniques, of which the A_1 receptor appears most closely linked to analgesia, although a delayed analgesic effect mediated through the A_2 receptor has been reported (399). The affinity of a number of adenosine analogs for the A_1 receptor appears to correlate well with their in vivo analgesic potency. Indirect evidence suggests that analgesia from central administration of opioids (400) or serotonin is mediated by spinal cord adenosine release (401). However, although a number of adenosine analogs produce analgesia when given intrathecally in animals (402), and blockade of endogenous adenosine by spinal application of theophylline produces hyperalgesia (403), clinical trials of the possible analgesic effects of spinal adenosine have been few in number. Phase 1 studies of IT adenosine in healthy subjects (404,405) have found it to be generally well tolerated, and it seemed effective in patients with chronic neuropathic pain (406). On the other hand, a postoperative pain trial disclosed no benefit in women undergoing abdominal hysterectomy (407). Not listed at all in the table of IT drug options prepared by the 2007 Polyanalgesia Consensus Conference, its use is likely to remain limited pending detailed assessment of its neurotoxic potential. To date, a single pilot study of IT A_1 antagonism in the human has described touch- or vibration-induced allodynia (408).

A host of peptide systems modulate nociceptive transmission (409) but studies of their value as targets of IT or epidural analgesia have lagged. The inflammatory and nociceptive effects of substance P and related tachykinins are mediated through three receptors termed NK_1, NK_2, and NK_3. Intrathecal injection of NK_1 antagonists blocks hyperalgesia in animal models of formalin injection or sciatic nerve ligature (410). Clinical trials of substance P antagonism have been limited to topical application of a substance P antagonist and have not included spinal administration despite encouraging data from animal studies. Very low doses of substance P itself potentiate opioid analgesia (411), as do peptide hybrids that combine substance P agonism and opioid agonism (126,412). The mechanisms underlying this paradoxical effect may perhaps include presynaptic inhibition of substance P release, but clinical trials have not yet been conducted to exploit the therapeutic potential of this approach. Cholecystokinin (CCK) and neuropeptide FF appear to function as an antiopioid peptides, particularly as active mediators of opioid tolerance at the spinal level (413,414). Given intrathecally along with morphine in animals, antagonists to the CCK_B receptor avert morphine tolerance and augment analgesia but have little effect when used as sole agents (415). Clinical trials of CCK_B receptor antagonists employing the spinal route appear warranted. Of the analgesic peptides employed for spinal administration, the inhibitory peptide somatostatin stands alone in its mixture of success and controversy (416). Initially reported as effective against postoperative as well as refractory cancer pain, its use was clouded by animal data that disclosed substantial neu-

rotoxicity upon IT administration. Hence, its use was abandoned until the stable somatostatin analog octreotide was introduced. Thus far, as with somatostatin itself, there has been no documented clinical neurotoxicity with octreotide despite analgesia for up to 3 months of IT infusion for opioid-resistant cancer pain. It was relegated to level 6 in the Polyanalgesic Consensus Conference (30) recommendations; that is, it "must only be used experimentally and with appropriate Independent Review Board approved protocols." Calcitonin has also been administered epidurally, with favorable if anecdotal results.

COMBINATION ANALGESIC CHEMOTHERAPY

Aggressive treatment of serious medical conditions typically relies upon multiple forms of therapy delivered simultaneously. Examples of this multimodal approach are easy to come by whether one considers infection such as tuberculosis, sepsis, or HIV/AIDS; neoplastic disease; or refractory cases of everyday disorders such as hypertension, cardiac arrhythmias, or depression. The broad power of such an approach no doubt reflects the multivariate nature of these clinical conditions and the utility of attacking as many variables as feasible to decisively bring such disorders under control, particularly in circumstances in which no single agent will suffice. The use of multiple agents for spinal analgesia was already mentioned in earlier reviews of this topic, including the prior edition of this text, where it was termed *combination analgesic chemotherapy* (23). It is now a foundation for acute and chronic spinal analgesia (Table 40-10).

Unfortunately, the standards of rigorous clinical evidence have almost wholly been ignored during this progress, and uncontrolled case series or case reports form by far the largest proportion of this literature. Considering that the number of possible combinations of different analgesics increases as a factorial function of the number of available choices, the optimum choices and relative doses of drugs to apply to different patient populations with different origins of pain require extensive clinical study (417). The corresponding chapter in the prior edition of this volume served as a starting point for a comprehensive systematic review (32) whose findings parallel those of other recent reports (30,310,335). That systematic review, and this portion of the present chapter, assessed whether analgesics available for spinal administration provide a better therapeutic ratio if combined, rather than if either component is administered singly (418,419). We therefore employed a search strategy (Table 40-11) to identify randomized controlled trials that included an experimental group treated with a drug combination and control groups that were each given one component of that combination. Only such trials ($A + B$ versus A versus B) permit comparison of analgesic and safety outcomes resulting from the combination and each of its components (420). We did, however, examine trials in which a second drug, by itself not able to produce analgesia, was added to a known analgesic drug. The possible benefits that we sought were threefold: improvement in analgesic efficacy, reduction in side effects, and slowing of opioid dose escalation.

Opioids and Other Opioids

Combining an opioid with a rapid onset of action and another with a slower onset but longer duration of action may

TABLE 40-10

FREQUENCY OF MULTIPLE INTRATHECAL MEDICATION USE IN 6-MONTH MULTICENTER SURVEY OF IMPLANTED INTRATHECAL INFUSION DEVICES IN PATIENTS WITH CHRONIC NONCANCER LOW BACK PAIN

- One medication: 34.7% (35 out of 101) of patients
- Two medications: 35.6% (36 out of 101)
- Three medications: 19.8% (20 out or 101)
- Four medications: 7.9% (8 out of 101)
- Five medications: 1.0% (1 out of 101)
- Six medications: 1.0% (1 out of 101)

From Staats P, Whitworth M, Barakat M, et al. The use of implanted programmable infusion pumps in the management of nonmalignant, chronic low-back pain. *Neuromodulation* 2007;10:376–380.

improve the quality of early analgesia and prolong its duration. For example, a single epidural injection of morphine plus sufentanil combines the short onset time produced by sufentanil with the long duration of analgesia attributable to morphine, thus providing prolonged analgesia after cesarean delivery (421). Animal studies show that combining opioids with different receptor selectivity has a powerful dosage-sparing effect (128), particularly for μ- plus δ-selective drugs (422,423). The δ opioid receptors in the ventral medial medullary reticular formation may be involved in activation of bulbospinal

TABLE 40-11

SEARCH STRATEGY USED BY THE AUTHORS IN A SYSTEMATIC REVIEW OF CLINICAL TRIALS ON SPINAL DELIVERY OF ANALGESIC DRUG COMBINATIONS

1. Exp narcotics/ or opioid.mp.
2. Exp injections, spinal/or exp spinal cord/or intrathecal.mp.
3. Exp drug combinations/or combinations.mp.
4. 1 and 2 and 3
5. Limit 4 to human
6. Exp analgesia, epidural/or exp epidural space/or exp injections, epidural/or epidural.mp.
7. 2 or 6
8. Exp clonidine/or clonidine.mp.
9. Exp anesthetics, local/or local anesthetics.mp.
10. 1 and 8 and 9
11. 7 and 10
12. 1 or 8 or 9
13. 7 and 12
14. Limit 13 to human and English language
15. Exp morphine/or morphine.mp.
16. 1 and 15
17. 1 or 16
18. Limit 17 to clinical trial
19. Limit 14 to clinical trial
20. 3 and 19

From Walker SM, Goudas LC, Cousins MJ, Carr DB. Combination spinal analgesic chemotherapy: a systematic review. *Anesth Analg* 2002;95:676.

noradrenergic pathways and a descending inhibitory pathway projecting through the dorsolateral funiculus and may thus reinforce other analgesic mechanisms (424,425). Not all opioids induce tolerance at the same rate, and cross-tolerance is incomplete. Tolerance develops more slowly with opioids that have high intrinsic activity than during chronic administration of lower-affinity opioids, such as morphine (23,426). Intrathecal DADLE, a moderately selective δ-receptor agonist, is analgesic in patients tolerant to morphine (427).

Three randomized, controlled trials investigated the combination of epidural fentanyl (428,429) or sufentanil (430) with epidural morphine after abdominal surgery in 289 patients. Early postoperative analgesia was improved by the use of the combination in all three studies, and this benefit for early analgesia was evident even when morphine was given 45 minutes before fentanyl (428,429). A lower dose of morphine (3 mg) was used in the group coadministered sufentanil compared with the group given morphine alone (5 mg). Both the sufentanil-only group and the morphine-sufentanil combination group had larger supplemental opioid requirements than the morphine-only group in the 24 hours after surgery. Not only did the combination not allow a reduction in dosage, but the incidence of side effects was equal between groups (430). In the other two studies, a number of dose combinations of morphine (2–4 mg) and fentanyl (50–100 μg) were investigated with respect to analgesic efficacy. One of these studies reported no augmentation of analgesia when a second drug was added to morphine doses of greater than 2 mg and fentanyl doses of more than 50 μg (428). The other study reported improved late analgesia when a larger dose of 4 mg of morphine (alone or in combination with fentanyl) was compared with 2 mg of morphine (429). A reduction in supplemental opioid requirements in the first 24 hours after surgery was reported by Tanaka and colleagues (428) when combination therapy was compared with either drug as a single therapy. However, in the other studies, combination therapy did not consistently reduce supplemental analgesic requirements when compared with single-drug administration: positive findings were observed with respect to sufentanil alone, but not morphine alone (430), or occurred only with a larger dose of combined drugs (428). The reduction in opioid requirements had little clinical importance because no significant reduction in nausea was reported with the combination compared to single drugs (429,430). In the study by Tanaka and colleagues (428), an additive increase in side effects (vomiting and pruritus) was seen with the largest doses of epidural morphine and fentanyl. In summary, the addition of a relatively rapid onset opioid to morphine improves early analgesia but evidence to support this as a routine practice based upon lowering the incidence of adverse effects during combination regimens of this type is inconclusive.

Opioids and Local Anesthetics

Local anesthetics can produce intense anesthesia, but spinal administration may result in motor weakness and postural hypotension because of sympathetic block. The addition of epidural fentanyl to a local anesthetic improves intraoperative surgical analgesia (meta-analysis of 18 controlled trials) (431), and continued infusion of epidural opioids and local anesthetics is standard practice for management of postoperative pain (432) (Table 40-12). Combinations of an IT opioid and local anesthetic are most often used in the acute setting to prolong the analgesia after single-shot IT anesthesia, and their use for cesarean delivery has recently been reviewed

TABLE 40-12

EPIDURAL OPIOID/BUPIVACAINE COMBINATIONS ADMINISTERED BY CONTINUOUS INFUSION FOR POSTOPERATIVE PAIN

Drug combinations	Solution	Bolus dose of bupivacaine (%)	Basal infusion rate	Rescue doses	Increments in serial rescue doses
Morphine	0.01%		6–8 mL/h	1–2 mL every 10–15 min	1 mL of the solution
+ Bupivacaine	0.05–0.01%	0.5–0.25%			
Hydromorphone	0.0025–0.005%		6–8 mL/h	1–3 mL every 10–15 min	1 mL of the solution
+ Bupivacaine	0.05–0.1%	0.5–0.25%			
Fentanyl	0.001%		0.1–0.15 mL kg^{-1} h^{-1}	1–1.5 mL every 10–15 min	1 mL of the solution
+ Bupivacaine	0.05–0.1%	0.5–0.25%			
Sufentanil	0.0001%		0.1–0.2 mL kg^{-1} h^{-1}	1–1.5 mL every 10–15 min	1 mL of the solution
+ Bupivacaine	0.05–0.1%	0.5–0.25%			

From de Leon-Casasola OA, Lema MJ. Postoperative epidural opioid analgesia: What are the choices? *Anesth Analg.* 1996;83:867.

(433). For chronic pain, clinicians report that opioids are often the first drug of choice for spinal administration, but local anesthetics have long been viewed as the initial supplemental agent when pain is refractory to single-drug administration (434).

Animal studies reveal synergistic antinociception with coadministration of morphine and lidocaine intrathecally (435) or epidurally (436). Dose-dependent development of opioid tolerance was found after IT morphine infusions; this was not affected by the coadministration of lidocaine. However, because an analgesic response was obtained with smaller doses of morphine in the combination group, and because no cross-tolerance was observed, there was an indirect benefit of lidocaine coadministration in that smaller doses of morphine induced less tolerance than larger doses (435). In a prospective clinical study, van Dongen and colleagues (437) reported a less rapid opioid dose escalation between days 10 and 30 of therapy during IT coadministration of morphine and bupivacaine, compared with opioid alone.

Acute Pain

These studies assessed whether a combination of a local anesthetic with an opioid administered spinally produces equal analgesia but fewer side effects, or improved analgesia without increased side effects when compared with either drug administered singly. As indicated earlier, we did not include the large number of postoperative pain trials in which opioids were added to local anesthetics (i.e., *A* versus *A* + *B*). Many such trials have shown that the addition of an opioid reduces local anesthetic requirements or vice versa, but they do not allow conclusions as to the nature of their interaction (432).

Six randomized, controlled trials satisfied our selection criteria. These trials investigated the analgesic effect produced by combinations of opioids (fentanyl in four studies and sufentanil in two studies) with a local anesthetic (bupivacaine in five studies and levobupivacaine in one study) compared with the analgesic effect produced by the opioid and the local anesthetic administered singly through the epidural (four studies) or IT (two studies) route. Five studies investigated analgesic efficacy for the first 24 hours after major lower limb, abdominal, or thoracic surgery, and one study investigated analgesia for 2 hours after a single bolus of study drug during labor (438).

In aggregate, 290 patients were enrolled in six clinical trials. Because of early exclusions (often for unrelated reasons before the administration of study drug), data were able to be evaluated for 262 patients, of whom 239 patients completed the planned study period. The latter withdrawals were predominantly due to inadequate analgesia in two studies (439,440). Two studies investigated analgesia after bolus administration, either a single dose during labor (438) or four doses of different drugs given in a random order at 6-hour intervals during the first 24 hours after surgery (441). The remaining studies investigated spinal analgesic infusions that were either delivered as an investigator-titrated infusion of study drug with an additional supplemental IV PCA opioid (442) or as patient-controlled epidural analgesia (PCEA) (439,440), or IT (443) regimens without supplemental drugs. All studies evaluated self-reported pain intensity at rest either with a visual analog scale (VAS) (0–100) or a 5-point (0–4) verbal rating scale. Four of the six studies also recorded pain intensity upon cough or movement.

Analgesic efficacy of the combination was better than that of local anesthetic alone but was not different from opioid alone in the study by Cooper and colleagues (439), whereas Torda and colleagues (441) found no difference among the effects of boluses of fentanyl alone, local anesthetic alone, or combination therapy. In two studies, overall patient satisfaction was assessed, again with variable results. Cooper and colleagues (439) reported similar levels of satisfaction after either combination therapy or opioid alone, but both were significantly better than local anesthetic alone. Kopacz and co-workers (440) reported similar satisfaction with the combination or local anesthetic alone and found both to be significantly better than with opioid alone. Inadequate analgesia was frequently reported after single-drug therapy, either in both the local anesthetic and opioid single-drug groups (440,442) or in only the local anesthetic group (439).

The ability to evaluate a dosage-sparing effect of combination therapy depends on the study methodology. Similar analgesia was provided by a bolus of 50 mg of bupivacaine alone and by smaller bolus doses of bupivacaine (25 or 12.5 mg) together with fentanyl (441), and therefore the addition of the opioid allowed a reduction in the local anesthetic dose without loss of analgesia. Dosage sparing by combination therapy was assessed in two studies that used an IT PCA regimen (439,443). In both studies, combination therapy reduced opioid and local anesthetic requirements by 50% to 60%, as indicated by a reduction in the number of self-administered spinal boluses (439,443) and use of a less concentrated IT solution in the combination group (439). In a titrated epidural infusion regimen, cumulative epidural medication requirements and supplemental IV PCA morphine requirements were both decreased in the combination group compared with groups that received local anesthetic or opioid alone (442). By contrast, in a study design that used PCEA, there were no significant differences in the number of rescue boluses or cumulative volumes of PCEA solution among groups, despite patients in the single-drug groups reporting increased pain at some time points (440) and having an increased dropout rate.

The ability of combination therapy to reduce analgesic requirements compared with single-drug therapy is clinically useful if there is an associated reduction in opioid-related side effects with combination therapy. In one study, the degree of hypotension after a thoracic epidural bolus was significantly less when a reduced dose of local anesthetic was used in combination with fentanyl (441). In three studies, the incidence of hypotension did not differ significantly among groups (438,440,443). In the study by Kopacz and colleagues (440), hypotension occurred in all treatment groups, including patients receiving opioid alone. Hypotension may have been a residual effect of the large dose of intraoperative local anesthetic, because the timing of the hypotension was not reported. In the remaining studies, hypotension was not observed in any treatment group (439,442). A significant reduction in the degree of motor and sensory block was reported by Cooper and colleagues (439) when the dose of local anesthetic was reduced by combination therapy, but many patients in both the local anesthetic and the combination groups had difficulty mobilizing. In other studies, no significant difference in the degree of motor block was seen in the local anesthetic or combination groups (438,442,443). One study reported a reduction in sedation with combination therapy compared with sufentanil alone (443). These studies provided no evidence for the ability of combination therapy to reduce the side effects of nausea, vomiting, or pruritus compared with opioid alone (438,440), despite reductions in opioid requirements with combination therapy (439,442,443). The overall incidence of a particular side effect is often reported (e.g., the number of patients who vomited) without an indication of the frequency or severity of the adverse event. This failure to discern differences in side effects associated with dosage sparing may in part relate to the relatively small numbers of patients in each treatment arm (10–24 patients) and consequent underpowering. Indeed, power analysis was reported in only two studies. In the study by Kopacz and co-workers (440), the sample size was based on estimates of the primary efficacy end-point (time to first rescue analgesia). The study by Torda and colleagues (441) included calculations based on changes in pain scores, in addition to changes in one selected side effect (hypotension).

In summary, four studies support improved analgesic efficacy with the combination of a local anesthetic and an opioid compared with either drug administered alone. However, in two other studies, no difference in analgesic efficacy was found between the combination and the opioid alone (439) or the combination versus either single drug (441). Most studies indicate that combination therapy reduces dose requirements for either the local anesthetic or the opioid compared to their administration as single drugs. This dose reduction was associated with reduced local anesthetic-related side effects (hypotension and motor block) but little (sedation) or no (vomiting and pruritus) reduction in opioid-related adverse effects.

Chronic and Cancer Pain

Spinal coadministration of a local anesthetic and an opioid has been used extensively for the management of chronic pain. Prolonged use of IT combinations of morphine and bupivacaine has been reported in case series of patients with cancer pain (444), with two series reporting adequate pain control until death in 105 patients (445,446). In 51 patients with cancer pain, 17 proceeded from a morphine-only to a morphine + bupivacaine spinal infusion. Pain intensity subsequently improved in 10 patients, with only moderate improvement in four patients, whereas 11 patients required continuation of oral morphine supplementation (447). In patients with noncancer pain, IT opioid provided satisfactory pain relief in 88% (285 of 323 patients in seven studies), whereas IT opioid plus bupivacaine provided satisfactory pain relief in 93% (96 of 103 patients from two studies) (448). In these case series, bupivacaine was added when pain control was inadequate with the opioid alone. Interpretation of these data is hampered by lack of randomization, variable inclusion criteria (particularly source and type of pain), and variable definitions of satisfactory pain relief. Two prospective studies have shown improvement in analgesia with bupivacaine and morphine combinations compared with opioid alone, although there was neither blinding nor randomization in one study (449) and there was incomplete blinding in the other (437). In both studies, pain intensity at the time of entry varied among patients, who were enrolled for IT therapy when pain was judged refractory to the use of analgesic drugs by other routes (on the basis of the World Health Organization analgesic ladder) or neurolytic techniques. As required clinically, infusions were titrated to effect in each patient, but the resultant variation in dosing makes evaluation of the efficacy and side-effect profile of combination versus single-drug therapy challenging.

Reductions in blood pressure due to sympathetic blockade are often seen in the first 24 hours of IT bupivacaine infusion, but after this initial stabilization, postural hypotension is rarely significant. Side effects of bowel or bladder dysfunction and motor weakness have not been observed at IT bupivacaine doses of less than 30 mg/d (447), but motor weakness may occur with IT doses of more than 25 mg/d (446). These side effects are more likely to be tolerated by patients who are bedridden with terminal disease, and further studies in ambulatory patients are required. A reduction in opioid-related side effects was reported in one study after the initiation of combination therapy (450), but in most series the numbers studied are too few to identify any difference in the incidence of side effects with single or combination therapy.

In summary, only one trial satisfied the selection criteria applied in this systematic review for the use of opioid-local anesthetic combinations in the chronic pain setting. Van Dongen and co-workers (437) reported a diminished progression of IT morphine dose during the coadministration of morphine and bupivacaine when compared with IT morphine alone. However, because infusions were titrated to effect in individual patients who had progressive disease, no assessment of analgesic efficacy with combination therapy was possible. Similarly, many patients had preexisting adverse effects related to analgesic regimens, the underlying disease, or both, thus rendering direct comparison of the incidence of side effects impossible.

PART IV: PAIN MANAGEMENT

Opioids and Clonidine

Opioid–α_2 interactions underlie the dosage-sparing (or analgesia-potentiating) effects of adrenergic agonists upon spinal opioids in preclinical studies that use behavioral or electrophysiologic end-points (248,249,451). Clonidine's analgesic activity is mediated through pre- and postsynaptic α_2 receptors localized in the superficial layers of the spinal dorsal horn (128). In humans, clonidine augments opioid-induced sedation but not respiratory depression; hypotension is not a common side effect of opioids but is frequent with clonidine. In healthy volunteers, the reduction of pain intensity after epidural clonidine correlates with its concentrations in the CSF, but not in serum (451). Much smaller bolus doses of clonidine are needed through the IT route to produce potent and long-lasting analgesia than via the epidural or systemic routes (249). A valuable complementary effect of IT coadministration of opioids with clonidine is the benefit of the latter agent for neuropathic pain, which in general is less sensitive to opioids (452). Clonidine also can benefit sympathetically maintained pain, which is often a component of chronic neuropathic pain due to cancer or nonmalignant causes. The approval in the U.S. of clonidine as an adjunct to epidural opioids for opioid-resistant cancer pain based upon its efficacy in controlled clinical trials has further encouraged spinal coadministration of these two drug classes to treat other refractory pain, such as that from spinal cord injury (130,132). Dexmedetomidine, a second-generation α_2 agonist approved by the FDA in 1999 produces hypotension less frequently than clonidine and is currently used as a preoperative medication for perioperative sympatholysis and analgesia (248). The absence of clinical experience with dexmedetomidine for spinal analgesia leaves clonidine, a "line 2" agent according to the most recent Polyanalgesic Consensus Conference recommendations (30), as the only clinically available α_2 agonist for this purpose.

Seven randomized, controlled trials involving clonidine satisfied our selection criteria. These trials investigated the analgesic effect produced by combinations of opioids (i.e., morphine, fentanyl, and sufentanil) with clonidine, compared with the analgesic effect produced by the opioids or clonidine administered singly through the epidural or IT route for acute postoperative or chronic (cancer or spinal cord injury) pain. In aggregate, 461 patients enrolled in seven clinical trials were randomized to receive an opioid with clonidine, the same opioid alone, or clonidine alone. In five of the seven trials, investigators used the epidural route (334,453–456), whereas the remaining two used IT injections (132,457). Clonidine was combined with morphine in five studies, sufentanil in one study, and fentanyl in one study.

Acute Pain

Pain management after abdominal, orthopedic, or obstetric operations or during labor was investigated in five studies (453–457). In one study, investigators evaluated the analgesic efficacy of the combination of IT sufentanil with clonidine for labor pain (457). Finally, one study compared the combination of epidural fentanyl and clonidine with each drug alone for the management of labor pain (454). This was the only study in this group that evaluated the analgesic interaction by using the isobolographic technique (458). Pooling the outcomes of these studies was not feasible because of differences in a variety of study characteristics; for example, differences in protocols for supplemental opioid consumption and the potential carryover drug effect of the anesthetics (local or general) used for the operation, use of a supplemental IV opioid in the clonidine-only study arm, and the possibility that such an IV drug acts spinally.

Morphine and Clonidine

Carabine and colleagues (453) compared bolus epidural injections of clonidine (150 μg) followed by continuous epidural infusion of clonidine 25 or 50 μg/h, with a bolus injection of morphine (1 mg) followed by epidural infusion of morphine (0.1 mg/mL) and a bolus injection of a mixture of clonidine (150 μg) and morphine (1 mg) followed by continuous epidural infusion of morphine 0.1 mg/h. At both 30 and 60 minutes after the injections, all three groups had significantly lower values for pain intensity compared with the morphine group. Supplemental IV PCA morphine requirements in the combination group were significantly less than in the morphine and clonidine 25 μg groups. Intravenous PCA morphine requirements in the clonidine 50 μg group were also less than in the epidural morphine group. However, the combination and the clonidine 50 μg groups did not differ in IV PCA morphine requirements for supplemental analgesia. Hypotension was significantly more pronounced in the combination group compared with the other groups from 5 until 20 minutes after injection. At 18 and 24 hours after surgery, arterial blood pressure was significantly less in both clonidine groups than in the morphine and combination groups. No differences in other side effects were demonstrated. Collectively, the observations of this trial suggest that there is no demonstrable benefit in the use of the mixture as compared with the 50 μg of clonidine. These results must be interpreted cautiously because all groups received a mixture of clonidine and morphine (the two clonidine groups received supplemental IV PCA morphine). Rockemann and coworkers (455) showed that the combination of a minimally effective epidural morphine dose (2 mg) with a marginally effective clonidine dose ($\sim$280 μg, according to patient weight) produced analgesia that was not significantly different from that produced by morphine alone ($\sim$3.35 mg, according to patient weight). In this study, there were no differences in side effects between study arms. It is noteworthy that the investigators rightly excluded six of 15 patients in the morphine group from data analysis because of requests by these patients for supplemental analgesia. The study demonstrates that the combination of clonidine and morphine is better compared with morphine alone only because of the faster onset of pain relief. Van Essen and colleagues (456) compared clonidine (70 μg), morphine (3 mg), and a combination of the two given as bolus epidural injections 60 minutes after surgery in 28 patients for postoperative pain control. The authors found no difference in pain intensity (verbal analog pain score) in any of the three treatment groups. Statistically significant reductions in blood pressure were observed in the morphine-with-clonidine group but were considered of no clinical importance by the authors. No significant differences were observed in other side effects (urinary retention, nausea, vomiting, and pruritus) after the combination as compared with morphine alone. No supplemental opioid was administered to any of the patients in this study, although it was available.

Fentanyl and Clonidine

Eisenach and colleagues (454) found a slight and insignificant benefit of the combination of epidural clonidine and fentanyl for obstetric pain relief. This was demonstrated as a reduction in the 50% effective dose (ED_{50}) for pain relief of the mixture compared with a theoretical additive ED_{50} calculated from data acquired from the single-drug groups, suggesting an additive interaction between the study drugs. No differences in side effects were demonstrated. The pain outcome was assessed at 10 minutes after epidural injections. Supplemental opioids were used later during the study.

Sufentanil and Clonidine

Gautier and colleagues (457) compared the effects of a single IT bolus of sufentanil (2.5 or 5 μg) and clonidine (15 or 30 μg) with those of their combination (all four possible dose combinations) administered in women in active labor. The combination of 30 μg of clonidine with 2.5 or 5 μg of sufentanil significantly prolonged analgesia compared to 5 μg of sufentanil alone. The dose of 15 μg of clonidine combined with 2.5 or 5 μg of sufentanil produced analgesia of similar duration to that of 5 μg of sufentanil. The mixtures of clonidine and sufentanil did not result in a significant reduction in the incidence of side effects as compared with sufentanil alone. Collectively, there was a significant improvement in the analgesic outcome with use of the mixture of sufentanil and clonidine as compared with sufentanil alone, with no significant difference in side effects.

In summary, these randomized trials in aggregate provide the best available clinical evidence concerning the combination of clonidine and morphine, fentanyl, or sufentanil at the spinal cord for acute pain. Weaknesses of these trials may be the relatively small number of patients enrolled (range, 28–100) and the use of a supplemental opioid in two of the four trials (453,455), with resulting "impure" treatment groups that potentially influence the results. The improved pain outcomes recorded in most cases at single time points include lower pain scores for the combination as compared with the opioid alone, a reduction in supplemental opioid requirement after the combination, or an increase in the duration of analgesia. None of the studies demonstrated a reduction in the incidence or severity of side effects (e.g., hypotension or sedation) after the combination as compared with the single drug. It is also interesting that only one of the studies discussed here used the IT route (452), which is presumed to be in the proximity of the site of interaction between opioids and α_2-adrenergic agonists.

Cancer-related and Other Chronic Pain

We identified two randomized placebo-controlled trials investigating the combination of epidural or IT morphine with clonidine—one for the management of chronic cancer pain (334) and the other for pain after spinal cord injury (132). The Epidural Study Group (334) compared in a blinded fashion the analgesic efficacy of epidural morphine (0.05 mg/kg) plus clonidine (3 μg/ kg) with that of epidural morphine (0.05 mg/kg) plus saline in 85 patients with intractable cancer pain despite large doses of opioids. Success, defined as a reduction of pain intensity or a decrease in morphine use, was significantly increased in the combination group as compared with the morphine-only group. This difference was more pronounced in patients with neuropathic pain. Hypotension was increased in the morphine-plus-clonidine group, whereas nausea was slightly but significantly greater in the morphine-only group. Measurements of quality-of-life indices at baseline and at the end of the study did not differ between groups. These data suggest that the addition of epidural clonidine to morphine for cancer pain management is beneficial, particularly in those patients whose pain has a significant neuropathic component. Siddall and co-workers (132), in a study that used a design especially suitable for combination analgesic drug trials, compared the efficacy of IT administration of saline, morphine (0.2–1 mg), clonidine (50–100 μg), and the combination of clonidine and morphine. The study consisted of two phases.

Each patient received saline, clonidine, and morphine in a random sequence, and one dose per day of each drug was titrated over 3 days toward a positive response (defined as a >50% reduction from baseline pain score) or the occurrence of side effects. The starting doses of IT morphine and clonidine were calculated on the basis of previous use of these drugs. If the patient was regularly taking opioids, then the dose was calculated as 1:100 of the daily IM dose or 1:200 of the daily oral dose. Titration of clonidine and morphine was performed as follows: if there was inadequate pain relief without substantial side effects (sedation or effect on respiratory function), the subject received a 50% larger dose of the same drug on the second day and double the initial dose on the third day. During the second phase of the study, each patient received a combination consisting of 50% of the final dose of morphine combined with 50% of the final dose of clonidine. The authors compared the proportion of those patients who had a positive response at any time during the assessment. Of the 15 patients tested, five had a positive response to saline, three to the largest dose of clonidine alone, four to the largest dose of morphine alone, and seven to the combination of half the largest dose of clonidine plus half the largest dose of morphine. These data suggest that morphine and clonidine are a worthwhile combination but do not permit a distinction between additivity and synergy in their analgesic effect.

Opioids and NMDA Antagonists

A number of animal studies have shown potentiation of opioid analgesia by an NMDA receptor antagonist (459,460) (Fig. 40-7). In clinical practice, spinally administered ketamine has limitations for use as a sole drug, both in terms of efficacy and dose-limiting side effects. On the other hand, low subanesthetic doses of ketamine given systemically are widely used for pain relief (461) and as opioid sparing agents (462–464). Consistent with these observations, the psychological adverse effects of systemically administered ketamine appear to be dose-dependent (465). Intraoperative IT administration of ketamine was inadequate as a sole drug for anesthesia (466), provided minimal benefit when added to bupivacaine (467), and produced significant psychomimetic side effects at higher doses (IT dose range, 25–80 mg). In postoperative studies, limited analgesic efficacy has been reported with epidural bolus doses of up to 30 mg of ketamine (468,469). Although epidural ketamine 30 mg alone produced no significant analgesia, the combination of a smaller dose of 10 mg of ketamine added to 0.5 mg of morphine did provide analgesia (469). The ability of combination therapy to reduce the incidence of side effects varies. Reductions in opioid-related side effects with combination therapy have been reported in a single-bolus epidural study, although the comparison was limited by the much larger dose of morphine being used as a single drug (2 mg of morphine given alone, versus 0.5 mg of morphine and 10 mg of ketamine in combination) (469). Improved analgesia and reduced opioid requirements have been reported with addition of S(+)-ketamine to an IT infusion of morphine in a patient with chronic back and leg pain (470). Further trials are required to establish the efficacy, side-effect profile, and safety of spinally administered ketamine. It is not listed within the 2007 Polyanalgesic Consensus Conference treatment algorithm (30), and assignment of any role will require addressing the latter concern.

The randomized controlled trial literature examining spinally administered ketamine in combination with other agents is limited. Two postoperative randomized, controlled trials have investigated the effect of the addition of ketamine

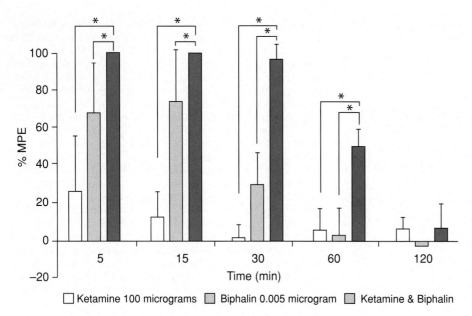

FIGURE 40-7. Combination spinal analgesic therapy. Co-administration of intrathecal (i t) ketamine (100 μg) with biphalin (0.005 μg) significantly (*p <0.05) potentiates and prolongs the antinociceptive effects of biphalin as compared to i t biphalin or ketamine injected alone. (Reproduced with modifications from Kosson D et al. *Europe J Pain* 2008;12:611–616.)

in an infusion-plus-bolus PCEA regimen of morphine (471) or morphine, bupivacaine, and epinephrine (472). The relative concentrations of drugs in the infusions were kept constant, but the size of the bolus dose and the rate of background infusion were adjusted according to the VAS for pain intensity. The interval and duration of pain assessment varied markedly between the two studies. When VAS was assessed daily, the addition of ketamine was reported to significantly reduce VAS at rest on Day 1 and 2 and VAS with coughing for 3 days after surgery (472). When assessed more frequently within the first 24 hour (at 30 minutes and 3, 6, 12, 18, and 24 hours), pain VAS was significantly reduced at 30 minutes and 3 hours only (471). Both studies reported a reduction in PCEA opioid consumption by the addition of ketamine. However, the incidence of nausea and pruritus was not significantly reduced by combination therapy in either study, although a reduction in the incidence of vomiting in the combination group was reported in one study (471).

In patients with terminal cancer pain being treated with epidural morphine 2 mg twice daily, if VAS scores were 4 of 10 or higher, an epidural study drug was added and administered each morning, just after the 2 mg of epidural morphine. The addition of once-daily epidural ketamine 0.2 mg/kg to the regimen of twice-daily epidural morphine administration resulted in improved analgesia when compared with a control group given a third daily bolus of epidural morphine 2 mg. In other treatment groups in this study, the addition of neostigmine 100 μg improved analgesia, but no benefit was reported with epidural midazolam 500 μg (473). Few studies have investigated the analgesic efficacy of IT ketamine. A blinded cross-over trial of twice-daily bolus doses of IT morphine with or without the addition of ketamine 1 mg was conducted in patients with terminal cancer pain. The addition of ketamine resulted in a smaller effective dose of morphine and a reduced requirement for breakthrough analgesia. Although lower VAS pain intensity scores were reported in the combination group, only pre-and posttreatment scores were compared, without a comparison of scores between the medication groups (474). Although combination with IT ketamine reduced IT morphine requirements, no statistical difference in the incidence of side effects was evident, possibly because of the small number of patients studied (474). In summary, current evidence supports the analgesic ef-

ficacy of single-bolus spinal ketamine added to morphine in patients with cancer pain, but there are no controlled data for chronic therapy with this combination and caution must be urged until the neurotoxicity of long-term usage via the spinal route is clarified.

Neostigmine in Combination Therapy

Neostigmine, an acetylcholinesterase inhibitor, produces dose-related analgesia after IT administration through a muscarinic action (475). When administered as a single drug to volunteers, IT neostigmine resulted in a large number of side effects, including nausea, vomiting, and leg weakness at doses greater than 50 μg, and it increased blood pressure and heart rate at doses of 200 μg (476). Therefore, interest has shifted to the potential benefits of small doses of neostigmine coadministered with other IT analgesics.

Neostigmine and Local Anesthetic

The effect of the addition of 25 to100 μg of neostigmine to an IT local anesthetic has been studied in the perioperative period in patients undergoing lower limb orthopedic surgery (477) and vaginal hysterectomy (478). Minor reductions in pain VAS were seen at some time points in the 24 hours after surgery, and postoperative analgesic requirements were reduced. However, a dose-dependent increase in the incidence of nausea occurred in patients receiving neostigmine. In a similar study, prophylactic antiemetics (0.5 mg of IV droperidol, 10 mg of IV metoclopramide, or a 2–4 mg/kg/hr infusion if IV propofol) did not decrease the nausea and vomiting experienced by patients receiving 100 μg of neostigmine added to the IT local anesthetic (478). Because all groups received the same dose of local anesthetic, it is unclear from both studies whether neostigmine has dose-sparing effects when administered with local anesthetic.

Neostigmine and Opioid

Animal studies have shown synergy for neostigmine or other cholinesterase inhibitors and morphine in models of thermal hyperalgesia (176,475) and nerve injury (479). Intrathecal administration of 10 μg of neostigmine had no analgesic action when delivered as a single drug, but reduced the ED_{50} of IT sufentanil for analgesia during labor (481). In a controlled trial, addition of a bolus of epidural neostigmine (100 μg) to epidural morphine increased the duration of analgesia in patients with terminal cancer (473). Current case reports are also limited to effects after single-bolus administration. In two patients with lower limb ischemic pain, single doses of hyperbaric neostigmine 50 μg produced analgesia lasting longer than 6 hours but were associated with nausea and vomiting (482). Two patients with metastatic abdominal cancer achieved relief of pain for approximately 20 hours after single IT injections of neostigmine (100 and 200 μg) (483). In randomized controlled trials, an increased duration of analgesia and reduction in postoperative analgesic requirement has been reported with combinations of neostigmine and opioid when compared with either drug given singly (336,484,485). Initial phases of a study conducted in women during labor by Nelson and co-workers (481) demonstrated a 25% reduction in ED_{50} for sufentanil when combined with neostigmine. The subsequent randomized phase of the study found similar analgesic efficacy when sufentanil 9 μg was compared with a smaller dose of sufentanil (6 μg) in combination with neostigmine, but there was no reduction in side effects. Therefore, although equivalent analgesia has been achieved with smaller doses of opioid when combined with neostigmine, no study has shown clinical advantages of the combination therapy. The number of patients in each treatment group tends to be small in these studies, and evaluation of the relative incidence of side effects is difficult. The incidence of nausea and vomiting is often increased when neostigmine is added, and only one study reported a significant reduction in the incidence of an opioid-related side effect (i.e., pruritus) when IT morphine 50 μg plus neostigmine 12.5 μg was compared with morphine 100 μg (485).

Neostigmine and Clonidine

Because IT clonidine increases CSF acetylcholine levels, supplementation with neostigmine may be expected to enhance spinal analgesia via cholinergic mechanisms. A synergistic antinociceptive interaction has been shown between clonidine and neostigmine in animal studies (475,479,486), including a rat model of neuropathic pain (487). However, an additive, rather than synergistic, interaction between IT neostigmine and epidural clonidine analgesia was found in a volunteer study (488). Because sympathetic nervous system activity is reduced by spinally administered clonidine and is increased by neostigmine, a potential advantage of combination therapy is the inhibition of clonidine-induced hypotension by neostigmine (488). During labor, the incidence of hypotension was less when patients received neostigmine in combination with clonidine, but the number studied was too small to detect a statistically significant difference (489). In randomized controlled trials, the addition of IT neostigmine 50 μg and clonidine 150 μg to bupivacaine spinal anesthesia for cesarean delivery resulted in prolonged postsurgical analgesia compared with neostigmine or clonidine alone plus bupivacaine. However, the dose of drugs was not reduced in the combination group (neostigmine plus clonidine plus bupivacaine), and an increased duration of motor block and an increased incidence of nausea and vomiting were also seen in the combination group (490). Although prolongation of analgesia was maintained with smaller doses of IT clonidine 30 μg and neostigmine 10 μg added to bupivacaine and fentanyl 25 μg during labor, nausea was more common in all patients who received neostigmine (489).

In summary, the relatively frequent incidence of dose-dependent side effects with neostigmine limit its potential role

to that of an adjuvant. Minor improvements in analgesic efficacy have been shown when it is given in combination with a local anesthetic or clonidine, but this is often at the cost of increased side effects. Although the addition of neostigmine allows a reduction in the dose of coadministered opioid, an associated reduction in side effects has not been confirmed. Potential improvements in hemodynamic stability by the combination of neostigmine with clonidine or local anesthetics have not been confirmed in current studies.

Midazolam in Combination Therapy

Animal studies provide evidence of analgesic interactions between $GABA_A$ agonists and morphine (491) after IT coadministration. When administered at a spinal level, midazolam displays additive or synergistic interactions with opioids (492,493), whereas midazolam inhibition of opioid antinociception has been reported at a supraspinal level (494). Synergistic analgesia has also been shown between spinally administered midazolam and glutamate receptor antagonists acting at the NMDA or AMPA receptors. Analgesia was achieved at smaller doses when the drugs were combined, and this was associated with a reduction in the untoward behavioral changes and motor disturbances seen at doses required for single-drug analgesia (495). Investigation of the neurotoxicity of spinally administered midazolam has yielded conflicting results (496–498). In relation to combination therapy, repeated administration of fentanyl 0.005% and midazolam 0.1% was not associated with a more prolonged neurologic effect or greater histologic changes than either drug administered alone, but all animals showed some evidence of cytoplasmic vacuolation in the gray matter on light microscopy examination (499).

An early clinical trial reported prolonged postoperative analgesia after IT midazolam in a small number of patients (500). In chronic low back pain, a single dose of IT midazolam was reported to provide prolonged analgesia comparable to that achieved with epidural steroids (501). A subsequent randomized placebo-controlled trial (although reported only in abstract form) found no analgesic effect and no difference from placebo when IT midazolam 2 mg was administered to patients with chronic mechanical low back pain (502). Infusion of IT midazolam and clonidine improved analgesia in four patients with chronic benign pain (344), and isolated case reports of severe cancer pain have reported improvements with the addition of IT midazolam to IT opioid, local anesthetic, or both (503,504).

A randomized, blinded, controlled study of analgesia after cesarean delivery found little clinical benefit from the addition of midazolam 1 mg to IT bupivacaine. Pain scores were not significantly different and, despite an early reduction in supplemental opioid requirements, there was no reduction in opioid-related side effects. Analgesia was of shorter duration than that achieved with IT diamorphine 0.2 mg, and addition of midazolam 1 mg to diamorphine 0.2 mg provided no appreciable further benefit (505). The addition of midazolam 2 mg to IT bupivacaine in patients undergoing elective knee arthroscopy improved early analgesia, but the duration of follow-up in this study was only 6 hours, and side effects were not well reported (506). In summary, limited data from controlled studies support a clinical benefit of the addition of midazolam to spinal combination therapy, and it is relegated to line 5 of the Polyanalgesic Consensus Conference algorithm. Large controlled clinical trials are required to evaluate its analgesic efficacy and safety as a sole drug or in combination.

PART IV: PAIN MANAGEMENT

Opioids and Droperidol: Evidence from Randomized Controlled Trials

The effect of the addition of droperidol 2.5 mg to epidural morphine 4 mg was studied in an early trial after elective hip replacement (507). No differences in VAS for pain intensity were seen between patients receiving opioid alone and those receiving the combination. The major focus of the study was the incidence of postoperative side effects. Although a reduced incidence of nausea and vomiting, pruritus, and hypotension was reported in patients receiving droperidol, the average number of side effects per patient was significantly reduced at only one time point (8 hours) in the first 24 postoperative hours. A more recent trial examining the effects of adding droperidol 2.5 mg to epidural tramadol 75 mg showed a more rapid onset of analgesia but no differences in pain scores, respiratory rate, or oxygen saturation (508).

Future Agents and Approaches

In the corresponding chapter of the prior edition of this volume, several approaches to prolonging the delivery of then-recognized molecules such as local anesthetic agents or monoamines were surveyed. Unfortunately, such approaches (butamben, depot preparations for chronic use, chromaffin cell implants, or gene therapy) now seem unlikely to advance to clinical application owing to a growing emphasis on the minimization of the risk–benefit ratio for all medical therapies. But an exciting new series of advances in the understanding of pain processing in the spinal cord has taken place in the interim. Rather than becoming a closed field, spinal analgesia has never been more replete with opportunity. In particular, the role of cytokines, neurotrophic factors, and spinal microglial cell proliferation (509) is now clear. Complex interactions between these inflammatory and proliferative processes and recently recognized receptor targets, such as for cannabinoids, are already evident (510). Therefore, future therapies may well be directed more specifically to the underlying pathophysiologic processes that induce and maintain persistent pain. For example, there is increasing evidence for the significant roles played by neurotrophic factors in a number of animal models of acute, inflammatory, and neuropathic pain (511). Two subtypes of dorsal root ganglia (DRG) cells with C-fiber nociceptive axons have been identified: one group synthesizes peptides (substance P and calcitonin gene-related peptide) and expresses the high-affinity nerve growth factor (NGF) receptor tyrosine kinase A (trkA), whereas the second group expresses the purinergic P2X$_3$ receptor, an IB4-lectin binding site, and receptors for glial-derived neurotrophic factor (GDNF) (512). Nerve growth factor is upregulated in peripheral inflamed tissues and increases the firing rate of nociceptors; NGF is also retrogradely transported to the DRG of trkA-expressing C-fiber nociceptors and contributes to upregulation of VR$_1$ and P2X$_3$ purinergic receptors, which further increases excitability. Antagonism of endogenous NGF with trkA/immunoglobulin A reduces inflammatory hyperalgesia (513).

Brain-derived neurotrophic factor (BDNF) is also upregulated in DRG neurons in the presence of NGF and inflammation (514,515). Brain-derived neurotrophic factor transport to the dorsal horn increases (516), leading to modulation of the NMDA receptor (517) and potentiation of C fiber-mediated spinal reflexes (514,515). Brain-derived neurotrophic factor antagonism with trkB/immunoglobulin G attenuates C-fiber evoked responses after NGF pretreatment and inflammation

(519). Brain-derived neurotrophic factor is also upregulated after nerve injury (516,520), and transport to the spinal cord increases, where BDNF becomes demonstrable in deeper laminae of the dorsal horn (521). After nerve injury, antibodies to BDNF administered intraperitoneally (522) or locally to the DRG (523) reduce allodynia and hyperalgesia. Neurotrophin-3 mediates an increase in the neurite outgrowth of DRG cells after nerve injury (524). The IT administration of neurotrophin-3 antisense oligonucleotides attenuates nerve injury–induced sprouting and also behavioral allodynia (525).

Glial-derived neurotrophic factor is a broadly active neurotrophic factor, because both C-and A-fiber DRG cells have the GFR-α receptor for GDNF (526). Intrathecal administration of GDNF reduces ectopic discharges within sensory neurons and reduces mechanical and thermal hyperalgesia after sciatic nerve ligation (527). Although these findings clearly require further investigation and evaluation before clinical application, they hold the potential for novel approaches to pain management in the future. The term *combination analgesic chemotherapy* therefore reinforces not only the concept of targeting multiple analgesic pathways simultaneously, but also the broad therapeutic goal of stopping, if not reversing, a cascade of dysfunctional cellular regulation and growth (528,529).

Therapeutic options available for the future, therefore, are likely to evolve in parallel with other forms of chemotherapy, namely, combinations of several agents aimed at short-term inhibition, together with other agents (including antibodies to trophic factors) aimed at controlling dysfunctional plasticity, both functional and structural—the latter including apoptosis and glial proliferation (530).

SPINAL OPIOID THERAPY IN PRACTICE

In the prior editions of this book, considerable space was devoted to presenting evidence that opioids administered intrathecally or epidurally act primarily upon the spinal cord, rather than simply by systemic absorption and delivery to supraspinal sites. That is no longer necessary. Equal if not more effort was expended to survey emerging clinical experience with spinal opioid analgesia so as to justify its safety and efficacy in the management of severe acute, chronic or cancer-related pain. In the present edition, such justification is no longer necessary and each of these applications is described in depth in specific chapters covering diverse clinical contexts, such as Chapter 43 on acute pain and Chapter 45 on cancer pain. Instead, this section will focus upon the practical approach to provision of spinal (principally IT) analgesia. We will begin by reviewing contraindications for introducing spinal analgesia during the course of chronic pain due to malignancy or nonmalignant conditions, taking care not to duplicate Chapter 12 on neurologic complications of neuraxial blockade and Chapter 50 on complications in pain medicine. Medication options, already surveyed earlier, will not be repeated, although the value of combination drug therapy will be reinforced.

Contraindications

The same contraindications apply to the insertion of a spinal catheter for chronic pain control as for acute pain management, as in obstetrics or general surgery (see Chapters 23 and 24). These include:

■ *Bleeding diathesis.* Hemorrhagic conditions may result in long-term neurologic deficit secondary to the development of an epidural hematoma (531) (see Chapter 12).

■ *Sepsis.* Local superficial infection does not preclude insertion of a spinal catheter at another level because the segmental level chosen is not usually critical, as explained earlier in this chapter. Septicemia is an absolute contraindication because the presence of a foreign body in the epidural space predisposes to formation of an epidural abscess and its sequelae, such as cord compression. If a patient with an implanted epidural catheter subsequently becomes septicemic (e.g., after chemotherapy), then antibiotic therapy combined with prophylactic removal of the catheter is generally indicated (532).

■ *Insulin-dependent diabetics* have proved to be susceptible to infection at the portal site, with potentially serious effects (533), so this condition is regarded by some as a contraindication to spinal catheter placement (193).

■ *Immunosuppression* must be weighed on an individual basis with respect to its magnitude (e.g., CD4 cell count in HIV/AIDS) and likely reversibility.

■ *Epidural metastases* are a relative contraindication. Unless the catheter can be positioned away from such lesions, it is probably wise to avoid spinal catheterization in such cases. The possibility of a needle or catheter penetrating a friable epidural mass, with consequent development of paraplegia, is a risk that must always be considered. The potential for eventual distal loculation of CSF because of pressure on the subarachnoid space by an epidural mass should encourage placement of catheters cephalad to known or suspected spinal metastases (534).

■ *Unmotivated, noncompliant, or cognitively impaired patients* are in general not good candidates for neuraxial opioid therapy, although each case must be approached individually. In some circumstances, placement of an IT catheter for medication infusion via programmable implanted pump offers a simpler and more reliable means to provide analgesia than attempting to follow a complicated oral regimen or maintain a subcutaneous infusion. Indeed, opioid side effects such as cognitive impairment may be dramatically reduced by a switch from systemic to spinal drug administration and the co-infusion of a nonopioid to minimize opioid requirement.

LONG-TERM INTRATHECAL AND EPIDURAL SYSTEMS

Long-term access for the spinal administration of opioids in practice means the use of an IT or epidural catheter system connected to an injection system with or without a reservoir (38,191,194,535,536). Although the dura–arachnoid membrane offers a significant barrier to infection, and therefore the incidence of meningitis should in theory be lower with epidural catheterization, meta-analysis of the relative rates of infection during chronic IT versus epidural catheterization does not support this view. The suggestion from such an analysis that repeated refilling of pump or reservoir may predispose to infectious complications further undermines the intuitive view that the epidural route is the safer of the two. Considering that dosage requirements are lower and hence refilling intervals longer when the IT route is used, one can argue that the IT route may carry a lower infectious risk. The impact of a high standard of specialized care upon complication rates is emphasized by the landmark report of Nitescu, Sjoberg, and colleagues on 200 patients with cancer treated for a total of 14,485 patient days with externalized, tunneled IT catheters for cancer pain control (537). Their protocolized approach involved close follow-up with skilled nursing care to assure sterility during dressing changes, medication refills, and antibacterial filter replacement. Two infections (i.e., rate of 1 per 7,242 treatment days) occurred—an enviable figure but one not likely to be equalled in settings where close follow-up with skilled nursing is not feasible. In this exemplary series, 3.5% of patients had CSF leakage, 1.5% had CSF hygroma, and 15.5% had post–dural puncture headache, although none of the latter persisted. Fibrosis around catheter tips may partly explain dosage escalation, pain with injection, and high failure rate in follow-up studies at about 3 months (191). Also of growing clinical importance is the need for subarachnoid access to deliver drugs such as ziconotide that are ineffective systemically or epidurally. An overview of options for intraspinal drug delivery systems, showing advantages and disadvantages for each, is provided in Table 40-13.

Externalized Catheter Insertion

This method is effective, inexpensive, and potentially available worldwide, although some find it inconvenient to wear, and it interferes to an extent with routine daily activities such as washing, dressing, and sleeping. It is well suited for intermittent spinal drug injection, but opioid infusion can readily be provided by connecting the externalized catheter to one of many available small portable pumps. External infusion can be effective for bedridden as well as ambulatory patients, who can wear the pump in a shoulder holster and use it for many hours to a day or more before refilling.

Figure 40-8 shows a percutaneous epidural catheter tunneled to exit at the lateral chest wall (see Figs. 40-9 and 40-12 for details of tunneling technique).

Three to seven days after a percutaneous catheter is placed, the skin at the catheter exit site can become erythematous or even frankly infected. One means to prevent organisms tracking from skin to the epidural space is to tunnel the catheter laterally from the lumbar interspace, to a percutaneous exit site on the lateral or anterolateral chest wall (Fig. 40-8). A chronic inflammatory response may occur at the skin of the catheter exit site but, in the absence of obstruction, seropurulent material can drain superficially to create a (desirable) sinus. To further minimize opportunistic infection at the exit site, one may apply an airtight, waterproof adhesive dressing, with the epidural catheter running under the dressing to its edge. The safety of this technique is documented in thousands of patient-years, as is a very low incidence of CSF fistula formation (538) or epidural abscess (536,539) despite the immunologically depressed state of many of these patients (196,540,541). Relatively inexpensive, easy-to-insert polyethylene (nylon) catheters are well suited for this application. They do not require a stylet for insertion, nor (contrary to some opinion) do they become excessively brittle and break. Such catheters have been used in patients with cancer pain for periods in excess of 1 year without apparent undue sequelae. Some centers employ softer and more pliable polyurethane and Silastic catheters, as these catheters are believed to induce less tissue reaction in the epidural space and hence to carry a lower likelihood of epidural fibrosis (542). Catheter migration from the epidural space into the subdural or subarachnoid space, or even intravascularly, can occur but is uncommon (543). Allowing for the pressure changes due to cardiovascular and respiratory pulsations, and motion of the catheter tip in response to vertebral column movement by

TABLE 40-13

INTRASPINAL DRUG DELIVERY SYSTEMS

System	Advantages	Disadvantages
Percutaneous temporary catheter	Used extensively both intraoperatively and postoperatively, Useful when prognosis is limited (<1 month).	Mechanical problems include catheter dislodgement, obstruction[a], kinking, or migration. Infection risk with prolonged use.
Permanent silicone-rubber percutaneous epidural catheter	Catheter implantation is a minor procedure. Can deliver bolus injections, continuous infusions, or PCEA (with or without continuous delivery).	Dislodgement, obstruction[a], infection (but less common than with temporary catheters).
Subcutaneous implanted injection port	Increased stability, less risk of dislodgement. Can deliver bolus injections or continuous infusions (with or without PCA). Potentially, reduced infection in comparison to external system.	Implantation more invasive than external catheters. Approved only for epidural catheter in U.S. Potential for infection increases with frequent injections (may obstruct[a]).
Subcutaneous reservoir	Extends duration of therapy without pump implantation.	Difficult to access, and fibrosis may occur after repeated injection.
Implanted pumps (continuous or programmable)	Potentially, decreased risk of infection. Ease of programming. Complex infusion regimens.	Need for more extensive operative procedure. Need for specialized, costly equipment with programmable systems.

[a]A common cause of obstruction is formation of a fibrous sheath around the epidural catheter.
Modified from previous edition.

the patient, one still expects the dura–arachnoid membrane to prevent significant migration. Unrecognized migration into the subarachnoid space may lead to profound respiratory depression (188,208), although patients who have spinal catheters in place are usually tolerant to the respiratory effects of opioids. Hypotension and/or paralysis are theoretical possibilities if the catheter migrates to deliver local anesthetic intrathecally, but this risk is minimal for chronic catheters in which fibrosis is the prime concern. Bacterial filters (Fig. 40-8) can be fitted to the end of the catheter to prevent bacteria from entering the catheter lumen. The need to change filters regularly is a component of cost of this form of therapy.

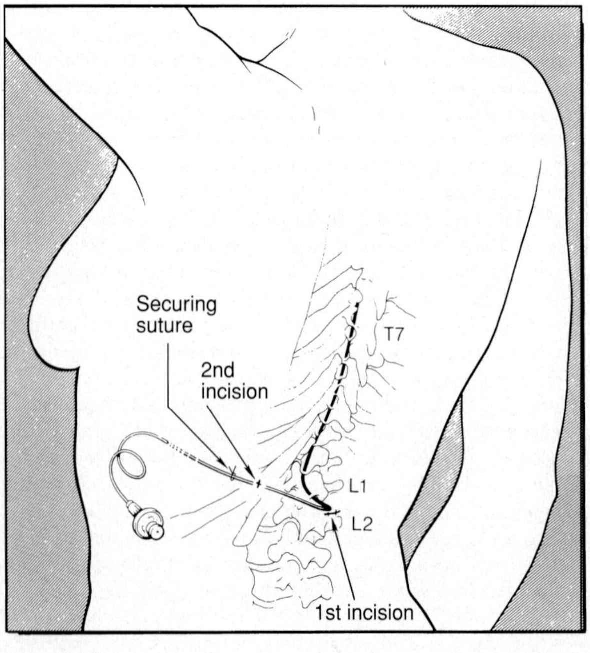

Totally Implanted Systems

Systems that are implanted subcutaneously have obvious advantages in terms of sterility, comfort, and freedom of movement for the patient. Such implanted systems employ either a portal for percutaneous access and bolus injection or an implanted, pump-driven, percutaneously refillable reservoir system. The portal or reservoir is connected to an epidural or IT catheter and positioned on the anterior chest or abdominal wall for convenient access.

Portal systems should have the following characteristics:

- Easily palpable percutaneously
- Self-sealing membrane capable of withstanding 1,000 injections at the pressure required to deliver drug solution through a standard epidural or IT catheter
- Easily discernible endpoint to injection
- Ability to maintain patency
- Injectable by non–medically trained people
- Inexpensive
- Simple to implant under local anesthesia
- Filter to prevent unwanted particulate matter from reaching the epidural or IT space

Implantation of a portal system (Port-A-Cath) is shown in Figure 40-9. Our experience with the insertion of hundreds of these devices for relief of cancer pain previously uncontrolled by oral opioids is that the portal has not been subject to leaking, the membrane has been robust, and staff and patients have found it easy to inject. An early problem of portal outlet

FIGURE 40-8. Percutaneous epidural catheter tunnelled to exit at the lateral chest wall.

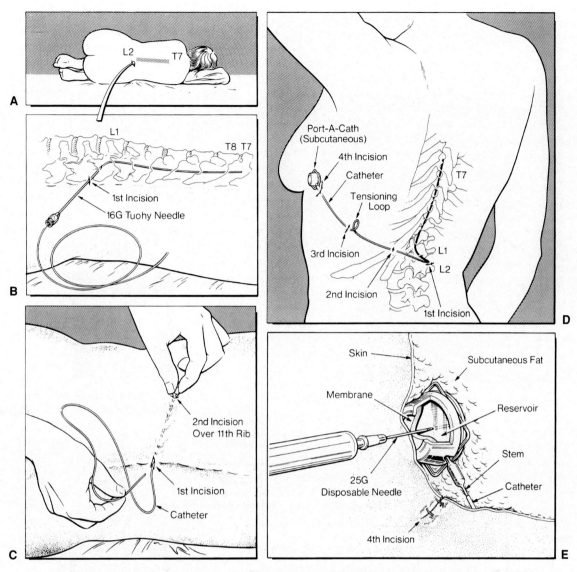

FIGURE 40-9. Implantation of the epidural portal system. **A:** Position of patient before implantation. **B:** Insertion of 16-guage epidural catheter through a Tuohy needle. **C:** Tunneling technique used to relocate the end of the epidural catheter to the anterior chest wall. **D:** Portal attached to the inserted epidural catheter. **E:** Injection technique and exposed view of the epidural portal.

obstruction (193) was overcome by moving the inner end of the outlet tube further into its interior (i.e., so as no longer to be flush with the inner surface of the reservoir), thus avoiding the funneling of debris: bits of silicone released from membrane puncture sites, plugs of dermal layers, and skin-swab fibers. Another early problem of catheter blockage is now prevented by a filter in the port to prevent particulate material from making its way into the catheter.

Implanted Pumps

Pumps designed for subcutaneous implantation must incorporate a drug reservoir as well as some form of powered pump (544). Morphine for intraspinal use should be at concentrations of 20 mg/mL, implying that a patient who requires the highest IT dose, such as 15 mg per 24 hour (see Table 40-7) must receive 0.75 mL per 24 hours. To make the device a practical alternative to the portal/bolus devices, the SynchroMed reservoir capacity was initially 20 mL. This has now been increased

to 40 mL for the same sized pump, allowing over 40 days if morphine alone is used. However, if local anesthetics or other drugs are added, refill times become an issue and can be as frequent as weekly. Together, the reservoir plus pump therefore present a certain minimum volume that in a cachectic patient may impact upon the feasibility of pump implantation. Current systems for this application, such as the IsoMed (Fig. 40-10) (536) and SynchroMed (Fig. 40-11) devices, are compact and the SynchroMed is externally programmable, allowing flexibility in the adjustment of delivered dose (545).

Regardless of the specific choice of implanted pump type or spinal access (IT or epidural), the procedures of catheter placement and tunneling, pump implantation, and linking of catheter and pump follow the same general sequence of steps. Figure 40-12 illustrates these steps for the placement of an IT catheter via the lumbar route for drug delivery through a SynchroMed pump. Figure 40-13 illustrates radiographic confirmation of proper placement of an IT catheter.

Ideally, a pain management unit should work in close harmony with a palliative care team, and this is especially true

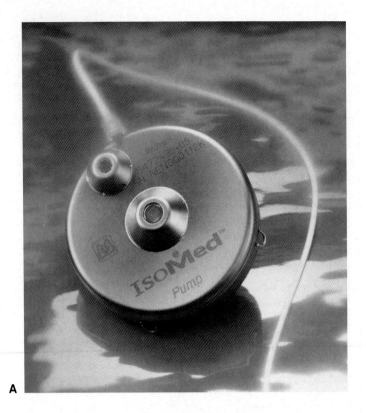

A

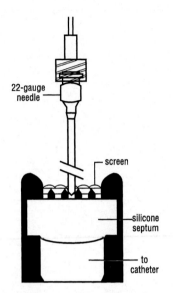

22-gauge needle **cannot** enter
screened catheter access port.   **C (top)**

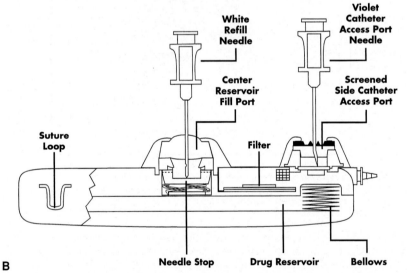

B

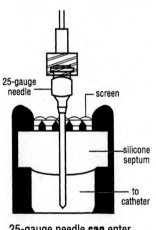

25-gauge needle **can** enter
screened catheter access port.   **C (bottom)**

FIGURE 40-10. "ISOMED" Medtronic Constant Infusion Implantable Pump, for continuous intrathecal (or epidural) administration of opioid and non-opioid drugs. **A:** External appearance of pump: central port and side port serve a similar role to the **SYNCHROMED. B:** Cross-section of pump components. Drug reservoir is driven by an inert gas which compresses the bellows when the reservoir is filled. Note also the different needle for 'central reservoir fill port' and spinal 'catheter access port' which is screened to only accept the 'access port needle'. **C:** Cross section of catheter Access Port. TOP: a 22-gauge needle (as used for central reservoir fill port) is barred entry by the screen. BOTTOM: A 25-gauge needle (supplied in catheter access port kit) can enter. Courtesy of Medtronic Neurological Division, Minneapolis MN, USA. *Caution:* Attempt to refill pump with needle tip still in septum could risk retrograde injection at high pressure driving medication into pump pocket. Aspiration of pump fluid is therefore vital before refill injection is started. (Courtesy of Medtronic Neurological Division, Minneapolis MN, USA.) Note: the high pressure necessary for injection when refilling the pump via the central port poses a potential hazard. If the needle is advertently retracted from the port during high pressure injection, a large bolus of drug may be injected into the pump pocket.

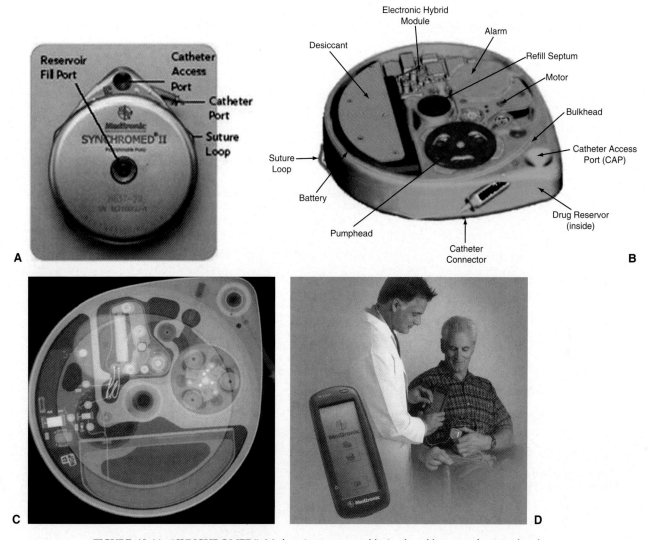

FIGURE 40-11. "SYNCHROMED" Medtronic programmable implantable pump for intrathecal or epidural drug administration. **A: External appearance** of the pump. Central and side ports serve a similar role to the **ISOMED** Pump, however note the tapering orifice of the side port. **B:** Components of the pump consisting of a lithium long life battery an electronic motor; a pumphead which drives drug through the spinal catheter; an electronic hybrid module that receives input from an external programmer and controls the electronic motor; an alarm a drug reservoir which sits on top of all of these components. **C: An x-ray showing the pumphead** at 2 o'clock. Changes in the position of the pumphead after a programmed bolus dose are used to check the functioning of the pump. **D: EXTERNAL PROGRAMMER.** The programmer head is placed over the site of the implanted pump and the programmer module is then used to interrogate the pump and alter the drug infusion as required.

when sophisticated pain treatment technologies are implanted in patients who receive terminal care in the home (see Chapters 45 and 49). This alliance supplies a powerful, hospital-based focus that can then act as a resource for the home care team of home care nurse, volunteers, general practitioners, and other home care professionals. It is essential to conduct a training program for home care nurses and to have a well-organized system for regular communication with them.

Reasons for Lack of Efficacy

Tolerance

Tolerance may reflect a loss of drug effect due to physiologic adaptation, as described earlier; progression of the underly-

ing condition; or catheter tip encasement by fibrous tissue. Drug switching between opioids and addition of or switching to agents from other drug categories are clinically validated strategies involving various drugs described earlier (25). Changing from IT to intraventricular morphine (129) has also been reported to restore morphine responsiveness. The best approach to the problem of tolerance would seem to be based upon proactive, preventive use of drug combinations from the outset, to avoid activating the opioid tolerance/hyperalgesia pathway described above. Such regimens are possible but suitable clinical trials to evaluate whether their use early on could preclude pharmacologic tolerance have not yet been reported.

Catheter Pump Misconnection

Misalignment when connecting the catheter and the pump unit, particularly those with sutureless connectors (546), may be

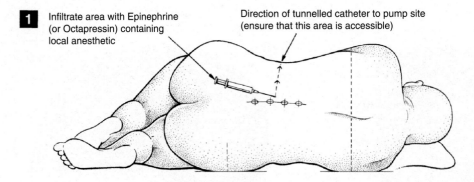

1 Infiltrate area with Epinephrine (or Octapressin) containing local anesthetic

Direction of tunnelled catheter to pump site (ensure that this area is accessible)

Keep hips and shoulders vertical to aid fluoroscopy.
Check spine is not obscured by radio-opaque bars on table

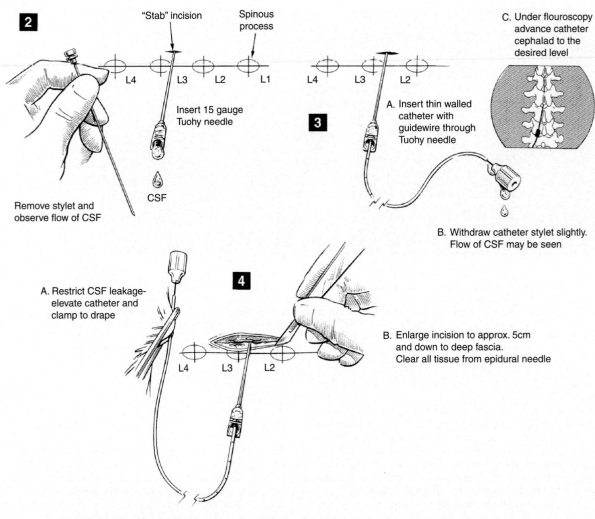

2

"Stab" incision

Spinous process

L4   L3   L2   L1

Insert 15 gauge Tuohy needle

CSF

Remove stylet and observe flow of CSF

C. Under flouroscopy advance catheter cephalad to the desired level

L4   L3   L2

A. Insert thin walled catheter with guidewire through Tuohy needle

3

B. Withdraw catheter stylet slightly. Flow of CSF may be seen

A. Restrict CSF leakage-elevate catheter and clamp to drape

4

L4   L3   L2

B. Enlarge incision to approx. 5cm and down to deep fascia. Clear all tissue from epidural needle

FIGURE 40-12. Intrathecal catheter and pump implantation. (1). Note careful positioning of the spine to allow a true AP and lateral view of the spine during spinal needle insertion. (2). and spinal catheter insertion. (3). The incision is enlarged to the deep fascia level and all tissue is cleared from the epidural needle. (*continued*)

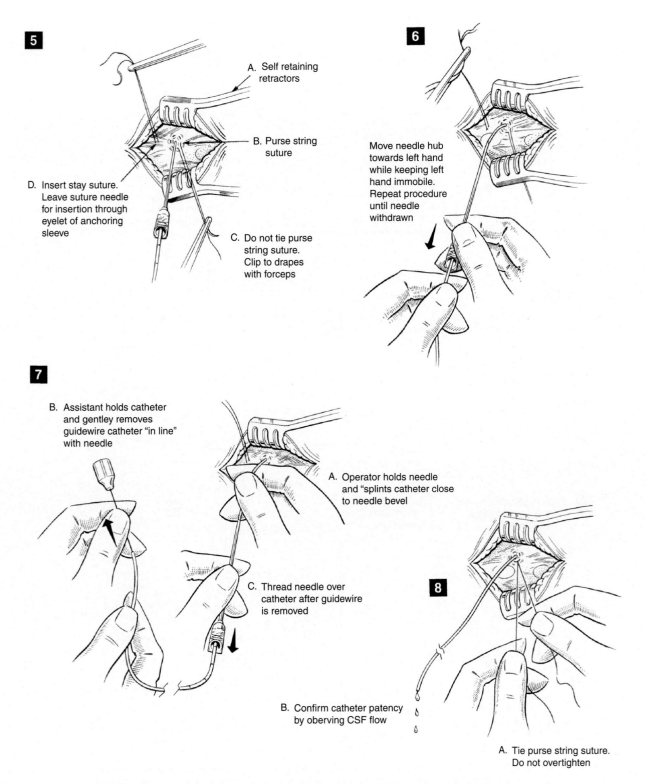

5

A. Self retaining retractors

B. Purse string suture

D. Insert stay suture. Leave suture needle for insertion through eyelet of anchoring sleeve

C. Do not tie purse string suture. Clip to drapes with forceps

6

Move needle hub towards left hand while keeping left hand immobile. Repeat procedure until needle withdrawn

7

B. Assistant holds catheter and gentley removes guidewire catheter "in line" with needle

A. Operator holds needle and "splints catheter close to needle bevel

C. Thread needle over catheter after guidewire is removed

8

B. Confirm catheter patency by oberving CSF flow

A. Tie purse string suture. Do not overtighten

FIGURE 40-12. (*Continued*) **5–8:** Placement of stay suture(s) and purse string suture. Note the use of a self retaining retractor greatly facilitates these steps. (*continued*)

PART IV: PAIN MANAGEMENT

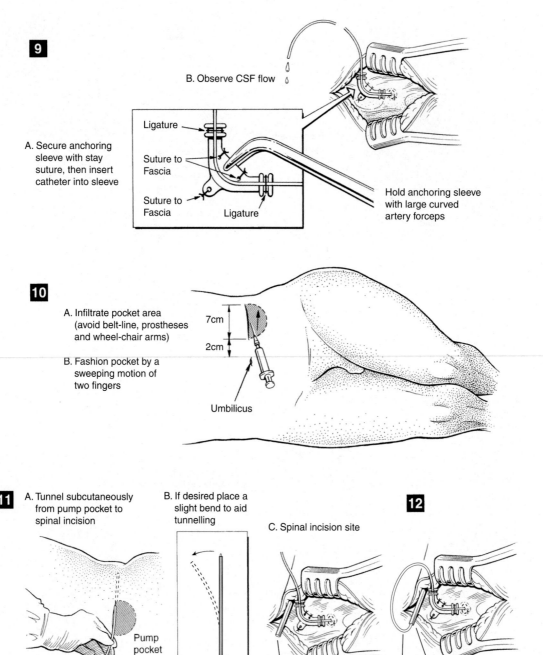

9

B. Observe CSF flow

A. Secure anchoring
sleeve with stay
suture, then insert
catheter into sleeve

Ligature

Suture to
Fascia

Suture to
Fascia

Ligature

Hold anchoring sleeve
with large curved
artery forceps

10

A. Infiltrate pocket area
(avoid belt-line, prostheses
and wheel-chair arms)

7cm

2cm

B. Fashion pocket by a
sweeping motion of
two fingers

Umbilicus

11 A. Tunnel subcutaneously
from pump pocket to
spinal incision

B. If desired place a
slight bend to aid
tunnelling

C. Spinal incision site

12

Pump
pocket

Tunnelling device

Plastic obturator tip

Obturator removed

Feed spinal catheter into
tunnelling device, through to
pump pocket

FIGURE 40-12. (*Continued*) **9:** Securing of anchoring device to fascia or supraspinal ligament, insertion
of spinal catheter in securing device and suturing it into place. Note the use of a large curved artery forcep
to facilitate the process. **10, 11:** Infiltration of site for pump pocket, opening and fashioning of pocket (see
Fig. 41-6–16). **12:** Tunnelling from pump pocket to spinal site, removal of obturator and feeding spinal
catheter to pump pocket. (*continued*)

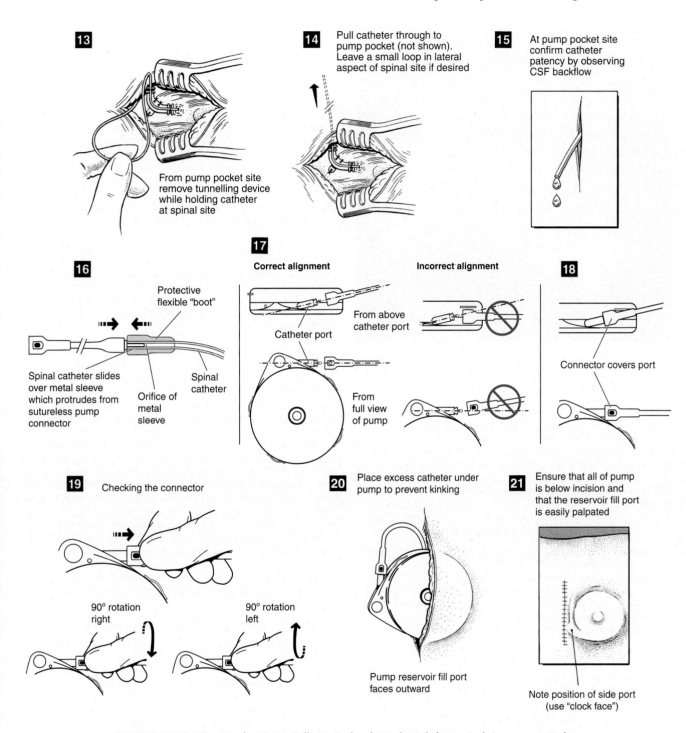

13 From pump pocket site remove tunnelling device while holding catheter at spinal site

14 Pull catheter through to pump pocket (not shown). Leave a small loop in lateral aspect of spinal site if desired

15 At pump pocket site confirm catheter patency by observing CSF backflow

16 Spinal catheter slides over metal sleeve which protrudes from sutureless pump connector

Protective flexible "boot"

Orifice of metal sleeve

Spinal catheter

17 Correct alignment   Incorrect alignment

Catheter port

From above catheter port

From full view of pump

18 Connector covers port

19 Checking the connector

90° rotation right   90° rotation left

20 Place excess catheter under pump to prevent kinking

Pump reservoir fill port faces outward

21 Ensure that all of pump is below incision and that the reservoir fill port is easily palpated

Note position of side port (use "clock face")

FIGURE 40-12. (*Continued*) **13, 14:** Pulling spinal catheter through from spinal site to pump pocket. **15:** Checking CSF flow. **16:** Attachment of spinal catheter to distal end of sutureless pump connector. Note that protective flexible 'boot' must be slid over spinal catheter prior to connection. **17, 18:** Connection of sutureless pump connector to spinal pump. Note correct alignment and firm pressure until a click is felt. **19:** Checking secure and correct connection of the sutureless pump connector by pulling firmly the tapered portion but not the oval marks. Also the connector is rotated 90° to left and to right to check for smooth rotation and maintenance of alignment. **20:** Placement of spinal pump in pocket. Note that redundant spinal catheter should be placed behind the pump and the position of the side-port should be noted. Unless the pocket is very snug, sutures should be placed through the pump 'suture loops' to secure the position of the pump.

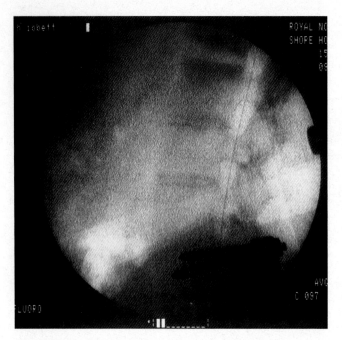

FIGURE 40-13. X-ray showing spinal catheter correctly placed in spinal canal.

followed either by disconnection or occlusion of the catheter lumen. From information provided by one manufacturer, such malfunction need not quickly follow pump placement and catheter connection but may be delayed in onset. In that instance, as of mid 2008 this problem was manifest as disconnection in 34 cases (0.22% of the total implanted) and occlusion in 23 cases (0.15%). This process is illustrated in Figure 40-12, panels 16–19.

Loss of Pump Propellant

A device recall in May 2008 involved instances of missing propellant in SynchroMed II pumps (547). This failure could be manifest either as an excessive rate of drug delivery, or a diminished rate, even to discontinuation, with a corresponding range of symptoms from overdosage to acute abstinence effects. The manufacturer estimated that of the 12,976 pumps at risk for this malfunction, fewer than 21 (0.16%) were so affected.

Gear Shaft Wear and Motor Stall

In a Dear Doctor letter issued in August 2007 (548), the manufacturer (Medtronic) described gear shaft wear and motor stall as the most common cause of failure in SynchroMed EL pumps, accounting for a shaft wear failure rate of 2.2% annually in units manufactured prior to 1999, and 0.5% of those made after 1999. Symptoms are those of drug underinfusion, not always accompanied by an alarm (Fig. 40-11C).

To determine if the pump motor is producing an appropriate response from the pump head (Fig. 40-11C), the pump head position should be checked radiologically, using the image intensifier before and after a programmed bolus dose.

Leakage of Infused Drug

Leakage may occur at the catheter–pump connection, either immediately at the time of implantation or with some delay. A defect may arise in the catheter wall itself, close to the catheter–pump connection (more commonly when using the

SynchroMed EL, with its earlier version of catheter connector). Such a defect may arise anywhere from the level of the side port to the entry of the catheter into the spinal canal. The most immediate cause of such a hole is passage of a needle or instrument through the catheter wall when suturing deep fascia or skin or anchoring the pump unit's "eyelets"; infiltrating additional local anesthetic during closure of the incision; trauma to the catheter by self-retaining retractors or hand-held "cats-paw" retractors; kinking of catheter close to the pump connector, with piercing of the connector by the metal of the connector fastening; or trauma to the catheter by sharp tunneling devices. Because they may be very small, even invisible to the naked eye, the only way to visualize such holes is to carry out a "pumpogram": an injection of radiographic contrast medium under real-time image intensifier observation.

Displacement of Intrathecal Catheter

Rarely, a correctly placed IT catheter becomes displaced. In such instances, often an anchoring device has broken free from the deep fascia and normal movement of the spine incrementally leads to displacement of the catheter tip into the subcutaneous tissues. When that occurs, the open defect in the dura may also allow CSF leakage sufficient to cause a local hygroma. A small seroma may result as fluid accumulates subcutaneously around the dislodged catheter tip. A pumpogram (see previous section) can help diagnose this problem. Less commonly, the catheter tip may migrate into the subdural or epidural space. Again, a pumpogram is needed, complemented by a CT scan with contrast. Such instances of catheter tip migration generally result in a decrease in efficacy.

Hygroma formation due to CSF leakage through the dura or around a displaced catheter is associated with clinical signs of a localized swelling superficial to the spine, that may be transilluminated. Aspiration of this mass yields clear fluid, and laboratory analysis of the fluid is positive for a unique CSF protein, β-transferrin.

Seroma formation may be due to leakage of pump fluid via a hole in the catheter, often with local tissue reaction. Tissue reaction may also occur in response to the securing device or tracking of fluid from the pump site toward the spine. If the rate of fluid leakage is very small, this problem may or may not be manifest as a decrease in clinical effectiveness.

Kinking of Intrathecal Catheter

The IT catheter may become kinked at any level, from the pump itself to the catheter securing device alongside the spine. In such cases, attempts to aspirate CSF or to inject via the pump side port meet unusual resistance or are impossible. If the kinking is intermittent and related to posture, a dynamic pumpogram is required to confirm the diagnosis. Intrathecal catheter kinking, particularly if intermittent, may be difficult to distinguish from pump failure; therefore, it may be necessary to perform both a pumpogram and a pump head check.

Obstruction by Intrathecal Catheter Tip Fibroma or Fibrous Sheath

The likelihood of IT catheter tip fibroinflammatory masses appears to rise with increasing doses and/or concentrations of opioid drugs, particularly morphine. Formation of such masses is usually associated with decreased analgesic effectiveness, new back pain at a different (often higher) level, and possible neurologic deficits along with drug abstinence symptoms. A pumpogram under image intensification will often confirm the diagnosis, but a CT scan or MRI may be a more sensitive diagnostic approach.

Fibrous sheath formation around the intrathecal catheter may extend from the tip to several centimeters proximally, and may even present a septate appearance.

All of the foregoing problems may partially or completely impede flow of infusate into the CSF. In each case, a dynamic pumpogram complemented by CT scan and/or MRI—the latter particularly for catheter tip fibroma—is useful. Such problems tend to be more common if the catheter tip lies at the mid thoracic level, particularly in the anterior IT space where the CSF flow is at its nadir. Withdrawal of the IT catheter so that its tip is in the lumbar thecal sac often restores normal drug delivery and allows spontaneous involution of the fibroma or fibrous sheath. If not, it may be necessary to insert a new catheter with its tip at a different level, to excise the mass, or to cease IT therapy. Estimates of the cumulative incidence of fibroinflammatory mass are still evolving, and currently range from 0.5% to 3% at any time after implantation.

Obstruction to Cerebrospinal Fluid Flow in the Spinal Canal

Numerous case reports describe occlusion of the epidural and subarachnoid spaces, even with compressive symptoms, by large intervertebral discs, abscesses, cancer, or severe spinal stenosis. In such cases, the effective loculation of CSF caudal to the obstruction has prevented spread of opioid within the CSF and resulted in inadequate pain relief (534,542). Diagnosis is by pumpogram confirmed with CT scan or MRI. If not contraindicated, the catheter maybe repositioned cephalad to the mass; however, in practice, such blockage of CSF heralds spinal cord compression, the emergent treatment of which takes priority.

Pain on Injection

Pain is most commonly experienced as a burning, pressure sensation in one or other hip during epidural injection of morphine in saline. This pain is surmised to be an effect of concentrated morphine upon a nerve root but no data prove or disprove this. Such pain can be reduced by administering the injection over 5 to 10 minutes, by pretreating with a small dose of local anesthetic before the morphine injection, or by injecting glucocorticoid through the catheter. Because injection pain may also reflect distension of the fibrous sheath that may form around epidural catheters (287), it is conceivable that glucocorticoid applied locally at this sheath may cause involution, as it does in other fibrous tissue, but this approach remains unproven. Despite these measures, some patients still experience significant pain on injection, in which case the catheter needs to be repositioned. If, despite repositioning of an epidural catheter pain still occurs with injections, the catheter should be resited in the subarachnoid space. In the senior author's experience with hundreds of long-term epidural catheters, this has rarely been found to be necessary (535).

Pumpogram

Pumpograms are usually performed by first turning off the IT pump and then accessing its side port using a side port needle kit. Using this kit, sufficient fluid is aspirated to clear the catheter of drug infusate—if not, an overdosage of drug could be administered upon bolus dosing with contrast medium. After aspiration of drug infusate from the catheter, the patient is placed under a screening x-ray machine and contrast is injected via the previously placed side port needle. Scrutiny of dye must encompass every site from the catheter–pump connection all the way through the IT catheter entry site into the CSF, then to the catheter tip, and finally into the spinal canal above and below the catheter tip. Pressure injection may be necessary, particularly with kinkage or obstruction. Preferably, a video should be saved for later review. Particular attention should be paid to the catheter tip, bearing in mind that such catheters *do not* have end holes but rather side holes close to the tip. Hence, failure to see contrast emerge from the end of the catheter is not diagnostic for catheter tip fibroma. However, uneven spread of contrast from the terminal section of the catheter along its sides, or any defect in the contrast myelogram, may indicate a fibroma. Contrast injected through the IT catheter should flow freely into the spinal canal, and in the lumbar area it should outline the cauda equina. After such studies are complete, an appropriately calculated bolus dose must be given via the pump to ensure that the IT catheter is once again filled with drug infusate solution, and the pump is restarted.

A CT scan immediately after the screening can help to check that the IT catheter is in the IT space. An MRI is the most accurate method of diagnosing a catcher tip fibroma or fibrous sheath and also to check for any myelomalacia in the adjacent spinal cord. Because many radiologists are unfamiliar with pumpograms, direct communication concerning the requirements of the study—if not co-participation or actual performance by the pain physician—is strongly advised.

Pump Head Check

The radiologic appearance of the pump head area differs between the SynchroMed EL and the current SynchroMed II model. Thus, it is essential that the appropriate manufacturer's manual be consulted. With the SynchroMed II, the key area of the pump head is difficult to visualize radiologically. For this reason, at least initially, it may be helpful if the manufacturer's representative is in attendance.

The check itself involves real-time viewing through the image intensifier while the patient is supine on a radiolucent table. Appropriate angulation of the image intensifier must be used to ensure that it gives a true anteroposterior view of the pump head area. Movement of the pump head is observed during a bolus dose (given as per the pump instruction manual) and compared to that expected from the description in the instruction manual. Following the pump head study, the pump programmer is used to check that the pump infusion settings are restored to their prior values.

An additional indicator of the need for a pump head check is a discrepancy between the amount of expected residual volume versus the actual volume of residual fluid aspirated from the pump at the time of a refill. On the other hand, the volume of residual fluid may well exceed that aspirated owing to difficulty in positioning the aspirating needle so as to access all of the residual fluid.

Magnetic Resonance Imaging Scans in Patients with Intrathecal Pumps

Previous concern about carrying out MRI studies in patients with implanted IT pumps has subsided. The catheter itself is nonmagnetic plastic. The IT pump is fabricated of titanium and iridium, neither of which are magnetic. The pump itself may obscure the view of adjacent areas. The SynchroMed II does not have to be turned off prior to MRI, but the pump should be checked after MRI to confirm that it has remained on and its rate has not been altered.

NEED FOR OUTCOMES ASSESSMENT AND IMPROVED CLINICAL EVIDENCE

The techniques for chronic spinal analgesia have remained fairly stable for well over a decade, with only evolutionary advances in their benefits and risks (31). The spinal route of analgesia is now well established as a valuable modality for the control of acute pain and selected cases of cancer pain. Yet, despite tens of thousands of patients having received implanted drug delivery systems, large gaps remain in the fundamental

evidence base regarding the outcomes of such therapy (549). Controversy especially surrounds the use of IT drug delivery for chronic noncancer pain. To this day, as Turner, Sears, and Loeser point out in their recent systematic review of the effectiveness and complications of this modality, "the strongest level of evidence for the efficacy of a pain treatment, at least one systematic review of multiple well-designed randomized controlled trials, is not available for programmable IT drug delivery systems for chronic noncancer pain," nor is "the next strongest level of evidence, a well-designed randomized controlled trial of appropriate size" (29). Their recommendations for future studies are summarized in Table 40-14. However, in the case of cancer pain, a well-designed multicenter study of IT drug therapy compared to comprehensive medical management (CMM) is available (19). In that study, IT drug therapy was associated with better pain control, fewer side effects, improved quality of life, and a trend toward longer survival compared to CMM.

TABLE 40-14

RECOMMENDATIONS FOR FUTURE STUDIES

Study design
- Randomized trial comparing IDDS to alternative treatment (e.g., multidisciplinary pain treatment) and/or "usual care"; if not possible, prospective nonrandomized comparison of IDDS with alternative treatment or usual care with groups matched on important demographic and pain characteristics; if not possible, large prospective cohort study
- Sample size based on a priori statistical power calculations

Assessment
- Timing: Before IDDS trial and at regular, planned follow-ups of at least 1 and preferably 2 years
- Measures: Valid, reliable measures of patient pain, physical functioning, and psychosocial functioning, with treating physician unaware of individual patient responses; systematic, regular assessment of complication types and severity using multiple sources of information (e.g., systematic patient questioning, medical records review, treating physician-completed measures)
- Method: Patient-completed outcome measures administered by someone not part of the treatment team; ideally, supplemented by objective measures (e.g., of physical functioning) completed by someone not part of the treatment team
- Follow-up: Assessment of all patients enrolled in study, regardless of IDDS status

Reporting
- Numbers of patients who (1) were approached for study participation, (2) were ineligible for the study, (3) were eligible but declined to participate, (4) underwent IDDS trial, (5) had a successful trial, (6) had an unsuccessful trial, (7) received permanent IDDS, and (8) provided data at each follow-up
- Sample demographics, pain diagnoses, other relevant clinical characteristics
- Clinical and study-related inclusion and exclusion criteria
- Study enrollment dates
- Surgeon experience with IDDS (as this may affect outcomes and complications)
- Type(s) of pumps and catheters used
- Types of IDDS and other (e.g., oral, transdermal) medications used and dosages initially and at each follow-up
- Separately for patients who were trialed but did not receive permanent IDDS and for those who received permanent IDDS, means and standard deviations of outcome measures before the trial and at 6, 12, and 24 months after the trial
- Statistical tests used (intent-to-treat analysis in RCTs) and results
- Among all patients enrolled, including those who did not receive permanent IDDS, number and proportion with clinically meaningful improvement, as determined by criteria specified before beginning the study (e.g., ≥% pain relief), at 6 month, 1 year, and 2 years; and changes within patients over time in whether they meet the criterion for clinically meaningful improvement (e.g., among patients with ≥50% pain relief at 6 months, how many have this level of pain relief at 1 year).
- For each adverse event mentioned in this review: (1) number and proportion of patients who had the event during the IDDS trial, and (2) number and proportion of patients who had the event during or after permanent IDDS implantation (if no patient had a specific complication, an explicit statement to that effect; if adverse events not mentioned in this review occurred, provision of information about those events). For each adverse event that occurred in the study: (1) length of time between IDDS implantation and the complication, (2) duration of the complication (if a biologic complication such as a drug side effect), and (3) rating of complication severity
- Source(s) of all funding for the study

IDDS, Intrathecal Drug Delivery Systems.
From Turner JA, Sears JM, Loeser JD. Programmable intrathecal opioid delivery systems for chronic noncancer pain: A systematic review of effectiveness and complications. *Clin J Pain* 2007;23:180–195.

Overshadowing the future of the entire field is the fact that very few trials have compared costs, desired and undesired effects, and outcomes during prospective trials of alternative routes of opioid therapy. Instead, nearly all the aggregate data on chronic spinal opioid therapy, including that cited in the series of Polyanalgesic Consensus Conferences (30,312,313), derives from ad hoc case series focused upon the analgesic effects, side effects, and complications during therapy. None of the published Consensus Conference recommendations includes outcomes data for the various techniques and agents surveyed. Abram and Hopwood (550) have questioned whether meta-analysis of invasive techniques for neuraxial opioid therapy can "rescue knowledge from a sea of unintelligible data." Numerous authors have voiced reservations about consolidating weak data from multiple uncontrolled trials enrolling mixed patient populations in diverse contexts (33), and have urged improvement in the design, execution, and reporting of relevant clinical trials (551). As a result, we remain unable to characterize the impact of chronic spinal analgesia upon fundamental dimensions of quality of life such as physical, social, or occupational functioning (552). This missed opportunity to gather outcomes data, combined with growing recognition of adverse events associated with chronic spinal infusion therapy, and an increasing focus on health care cost containment in every industrialized nation, is already endangering the infrastructure needed to safely provide spinal infusion therapy and support clinical research on its impact.

CONCLUSION

Jeanne Stover, a patient who participated in the drafting of U.S. clinical practice guidelines on cancer pain, succumbed to her long-term malignancy while that document was in press. She had written: "My dream is for a medication that can relieve my pain while leaving me alert and with no side effects" (553). Advances in spinal analgesia have brought medical science closer to attaining this vision. Insights into the mechanisms of nociception (Chapters 31–33 and 51) reinforce the importance of acute pain control to enhance postsurgical recovery (Chapter 7) (11,554) and to hinder the development of persistent postsurgical pain (8,14,555). Related insights have led to the use of combination therapies tailored to each person's needs. Combination therapies now form the majority of chronic spinal analgesic infusions in many clinics (310). Researchers are actively assessing the toxicity, stability, compatibility (359,556,557), and efficacy (558) of ever more complicated drug mixtures (559).

Clinical application of new agents for spinal analgesia will certainly continue based upon currently recognized preclinical leads advanced through traditional drug development programs. The experience of the past few decades indicates that the entry of new agents into clinical practice will be slow. At the same time, the theme of individualized analgesia resonates with the promise of personalized care through the application of pharmacogenomics. Advances in the tools of genetics, such as transgenic knock-down mice and microarray-based gene expression profiling ("gene chips"), have deepened our understanding of nociceptive processes shared across individuals and even species (560). The same tools have provided insight into interindividual differences in responses to nociceptive stimuli and analgesic drugs (561,562). As described earlier, genetic "channelopathies" involving sodium channels may lead to pathologically absent (351) or excessive (563) pain,

as may other mutations (564). Polymorphisms for opioid receptors (73) influence the analgesic effectiveness of morphine. Guanosine cyclohydrolase (GCH1), the rate-limiting enzyme for tetrahydrobiopterin (BH4) synthesis, is a key modulator of peripheral neuropathic and inflammatory pain. Inhibiting BH4, an essential cofactor for catecholamine, serotonin, and NO production, appeared analgesic in rat models of inflammation or injury, and administering BH4 was hyperalgesic (565). In the same study, patients with a haplotype of the GCH1 gene had less pain after diskectomy or in response to experimental pain stimuli. GCH1 is thus a promising genetic marker of risk for excessive or persistent pain after acute injury. Intriguingly, one of the earliest proponents of regional anesthesia as a means to avoid persistent postsurgical debility presented his views in 1910 as a visiting lecturer in the "Ether Dome" of the very same department as investigated the GCH1 gene (34). These emerging insights, together with those outlined earlier regarding trophic factors and microglia, offer the therapeutic promise of targeting fundamental processes of "persistent pain as a disease entity" (566).

These exciting scientific advances have been paralleled by a series of societal changes involving medical, ethical, and legal initiatives worldwide that have culminated in pain management being viewed as a fundamental human right (567). This right is explicitly recognized in an increasing number of nations in the form of position papers (http://www.anzca.edu.au/resources/professional-documents/professional-standards/ps45.html) and guidelines (568). This development reflects a megatrend toward patient empowerment in health care systems worldwide, as these systems adopt a more patient-centered focus and shift away from one focused upon pathophysiology (2). Another consequence of society's awakening to the importance of pain control is the quantification of the enormous costs of undertreated pain (569,570). Such costs dwarf the expense of early and aggressive (preemptive when possible) analgesia, especially spinal analgesia, to avert the transition to persistent pain.

Yet, "the best available evidence indicates a major gap between an increasingly sophisticated understanding of the pathophysiology of pain and widespread inadequacy of its treatment" (567). Constant educational efforts targeting health professionals and the public at large, as well as involved regulators, legislators, and third-party payers, are essential to emphasize the importance of pain control. Strengthening the evidence base regarding all aspects of spinal analgesia, particularly its application on a chronic basis, is critical to ensure continued support to provide such care. Such care should be rendered with appropriate training, knowledge of the therapeutic techniques and alternatives as presented in this chapter, and willingness not only to translate research innovations into advances in clinical practice, but also to abandon practices when they simply cannot be shown to be of value (33).

In concluding this chapter in the second edition of this text in 1988, the authors declared that "spinal administration of opioids has proved beyond doubt to produce a powerful antinociceptive action that is substantially due to a spinal action. As with many new techniques, spinal opioids have suffered from too much enthusiasm and too little careful documentation of efficacy, safety, indications, and contraindications in the clinical setting. This is a pity, since the animal studies forming the basis of the technique have been meticulous and clear in their implications for the clinician. Further development of the spinal route of drug administration must continue to be based on relevant pharmacologic and neuropathologic studies in animals before use in humans. Widespread clinical applications of any further agents or techniques should be preceded by controlled clinical studies." These words still ring true today, but the substantial interim advances in preclinical knowledge since they were written, the prospect of new and exciting spinal analgesics based upon novel mechanistic insights, and the elevation of standards for clinical trials and their synthesis make one optimistic for continued progress in and benefits from spinal opioid and nonopioid analgesia well into the future.

ACKNOWLEDGMENTS

Support to D.B.C. during preparation of this chapter was provided by the Saltonstall Fund for Pain Research. Drs. Heinrich Wurm and Michael Entrup, the Chairs of the Department of Anesthesia at Tufts University School of Medicine and Tufts Medical Center during this chapter's preparation, gave ongoing support and encouragement for these and related efforts. Miss Evelyn Hall provided excellent secretarial assistance. Brian Brown and Nicole Dernoski of Lippincott Wolters Kluwer facilitated the preparation of this chapter with grace and forbearance. The section reviewing IT coadministration of two or more analgesic agents was adapted from Walker SM, Goudas LC, Cousins MJ, Carr DB. Combination spinal analgesic chemotherapy: A systematic review. *Anesth Analg* 2002;95:674–715, with permission of the publisher.

APPENDIX

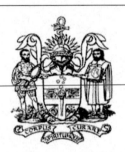

PM6 (2007)

FACULTY OF PAIN MEDICINE

AUSTRALIAN AND NEW ZEALAND COLLEGE OF ANAESTHETISTS
ABN 82 055 042 852

GUIDELINES FOR LONGTERM INTRATHECAL INFUSIONS
(ANALGESICS / ADJUVANTS / ANTISPASMODICS)

To be read in conjunction with Professional Document
PM4 (2005) *Guidelines for Patient Assessment and Implantation of Intrathecal Infusion Devices*

1. INTRODUCTION:

1.1 Persistent pain with associated disability is a common problem.[1]

1.2 In all patients with persistent pain, appropriate evaluation requires assessment of physical, psychological and socio-environmental factors.

1.3 Treatment of only one dimension of the patient's pain may result in less than optimal outcome.

1.4 The long-term intrathecal delivery of drugs is an established method of pain management in a small carefully selected subgroup of patients.

1.5 A range of delivery systems allows for the safe long-term delivery of intrathecal medication.[1]

1.6 Drugs may be administered directly into the intrathecal space, as single or repeated injections or by continuous infusion.

1.7 Non-analgesic drugs may be used for specific indications (e.g. baclofen for spasticity associated with neurological disease of central origin).[17]

2. PRINCIPLES OF USE:

2.1 Intrathecal administration provides direct access into the cerebrospinal fluid for drugs acting at a spinal and/or supra spinal level.

2.2 This invasive form of therapy is generally reserved for patients in whom pain or spasticity is not adequately controlled by less invasive measures and who meet certain criteria.

2.3 Intrathecal drug administration allows the use of relatively small doses of drugs compared with systemic administration.[2]

2.4 Intrathecal drug administration can result in significant undesirable side effects, and has the possibility of morbidity and mortality.[3,4]

2.5 Drugs administered into the intrathecal space need to be carefully assessed in respect of additives and preservatives, which may make them unsuitable for intrathecal use. A small number of medications have been deemed safe for intrathecal use.[2,7]

2.6 Care should be taken when considering off label use of drugs ensuring that additional patient education and consent is obtained.[1]

   2.6.1 In Australia only baclofen is licensed for long-term intrathecal use.

3. METHODS OF ASSESSMENT:

3.1 Effective management of intrathecal therapy requires appropriate patient selection. Education of the patient increases their understanding of the potential benefits, risks and their responsibilities.

3.2 A multidisciplinary assessment must be undertaken. Continuing support by a pain medicine facility is required to provide refills and support with technical problems, but also to allow the patient to gain maximum benefit from the therapy.

3.3 Prior to the consideration of a trial of intrathecal drug therapy, the response to appropriate trials of oral and parenteral therapies should be assessed.

3.4 Prior to the insertion of long term delivery systems, the following should be assessed:

   3.4.1 Intrathecal trials should be undertaken to assess appropriate drugs, doses and efficacy of the drug or drug combinations.

   3.4.2 Testing with temporary catheter systems allows investigation of the potential side effects of the proposed procedure and medication.

   3.4.3 Base line levels of pain, function and Quality of Life should be recorded.

3.5 Treatment requires regular assessment and documentation of efficacy, tailoring therapy to the individual.

3.6 Treatment requires regular assessment, documentation and management of complications of the intervention and side effects of the medication.

   3.6.1 Long-term complications of the intervention include infection, catheter tip masses or failure of the device.

   3.6.2 Long-term side effects of medication include hormonal changes and hyperalgesia.

   3.6.3 If drug combinations are used, interactions with other drugs should be considered, including stability of the mixture.[15]

3.7 Treatment requires ongoing assessment of the patient's pain, function and Quality of Life.

4. PHARMACOLOGICAL THERAPIES:

4.1 Opioids are the most frequently utilised agents for long-term intrathecal therapy. The most common opioid used is Morphine sulphate.[5]

   4.1.1 If good analgesia can be achieved with minimal side effects and risks using alternate routes, there is little evidence for improved outcomes with the intrathecal route.

   4.1.2 Failure to respond to an intrathecal trial or need for a rapidly increasing dose may indicate pain that is poorly responsive to opioids.

   4.1.3 Inadequate analgesia may result in dose escalation of opioid over time. It is important to consider the many factors which may result in inadequate analgesia including:

   - development of tolerance,
   - progression of the underlying disease,
   - emergence of a new source of pain,
   - development of opioid induced hyperalgesia,
   - distress
   - social reinforcers
   - pain which is not opioid responsive

   4.1.4 Increasing analgesic requirements may also result from failure of the infusion device, dislodgement of the intrathecal catheter or other catheter related complications including the development of a catheter tip mass.

4.2 A range of non-opioid spinal analgesic agents are utilised for long-term therapy, some of which are supported by low levels of evidence and for which safety has not been fully established.[2,6,7,8]

    4.2.1 There is level I evidence that intrathecal administration of baclofen is efficacious for the management of muscle spasm of central origin[9,10,17]

    4.2.2 There is level II evidence for efficacy in treating

- neuropathic pain with intrathecal clonidine[11]
- neuropathic pain following spinal cord injury with morphine and clonidine combined[12]
- neuropathic pain with ziconotide[2]

    4.2.3 Intrathecal administration of opioids and local anaesthetics and / or clonidine could be considered as an alternative agent in patients with poorly controlled neuropathic pain in cancer or following spinal cord injury.[8]

    4.2.4 Many of these combinations are "beyond licence" or "off label" and appropriate patient consent must be obtained.[13,14]

4.3 Combinations of intrathecal analgesic agents have potential advantages.[6,8,12]

    4.3.1 Improvement in analgesic efficacy.

    4.3.2 Reduction in side effects if reduced doses of both agents are possible when compared with single agent therapy.

4.4 Combinations of agents may be unstable for long-term use in implantable reservoirs.[15]

4.5 Due to the large number of potential combination therapies, the evidence for the most appropriate agents in different clinical situations is limited.

4.6 Both physician and patient should be aware of current data relating to safety and potential neurotoxicity of proposed intrathecal medications.[7] Toxicological studies to date suggest no long-term adverse effects of baclofen, morphine, bupivacaine or clonidine.[2,15,16]

5. FUTURE DEVELOPMENT:

5.1 Currently, there is limited evidence based data relating to intrathecal therapy for the management of chronic cancer and persistent non-cancer pain.

5.2 Further studies are needed in relation to:

    5.2.1 Inclusion criteria.

    5.2.2 Standardised reporting of the intensity, quality and aetiology of pain.

    5.2.3 Comparison with other routes of administration.

    5.2.4 Long term follow-up of efficacy, side-effects, and technical complications.

    5.2.5 Efficacy of intrathecal agents, both alone and in combination.

    5.2.6 Stability of combination therapies.

    5.2.7 Evaluation of neurotoxicity.

    5.2.8 Development of new agents.

    5.2.9 Assessment of outcome measures from the perspective of analgesia response, function, mood, cognition and quality of life issues (including patient satisfaction).[18]

REFERENCES

1. PM4 2005. Guidelines for Patient Assessment and Implantation of Intrathecal Catheters, Ports and Pumps for Intrathecal Therapy.

2. Schug SA, Saunders D, Kurowski I, Paech MJ. Neuraxial Drug Administration: A Review of Treatment Options. CNS Drugs 2006; 20(11): 917–933.

3. Abs R, Verhelst J, Maeyaert J, et al. Endocrine consequences of long-term intrathecal administration of opioids. J Clin Endocrinol Metab 2000;85:2215–2222.

4. De Conno F, Caraceni A, Martini C, et al. Hyperalgesia and myoclonus with intrathecal infusion of high-dose morphine. Pain 1991;47:337–339.

5. Hassenbusch: Long term intraspinal infusions of opioids: J Pain Symptom Manage: 1995: 10: 527.

6. Bennett G, Serafini M, Burchiel K, et al. Evidence-based review of the literature on intrathecal delivery of pain medication. J Pain Symptom Manage 2001; 20:S12–S36.

7. Hodgson PS, Neal JM, Pollock JE, et al. The neurotoxicity of intrathecal drugs given intrathecally (spinal). Anesth Analg 1999; 88 (4): 797–809.

8. Walker et al: Combination spinal analgesic chemotherapy: A systemic review: Anesth Analg 2002: 95: 674–715.

9. Erickson DL, Blacklock JB, Michaelson M, et al. Control of spasticity by implantable continuous flow morphine pump. Neurosurg 1985; 16:215–216.

10. Penn RD, Kroin JS. Long-term intrathecal baclofen infusion for treatment of spasticity. J Neurosurg 1987;66:181–185.

11. Uhle E-I, Becker R, Gatscher S, et al. Continuous intrathecal clonidine administration for the treatment of neuropathic pain. Stereotact Funct Neurosurg 2000; 75:167–75.

12. Siddall PJ, Molloy AR, Walker S, et al. Efficacy of intrathecal morphine and clonidine in the treatment of neuropathic pain following spinal cord injury. Anesth Analg 2000; 91:1493–1498.

13. British Pain Society: The use of drugs beyond licence in palliative care and pain management (2005): www.britishpainsociety.org.

14. Gazarian M, Kelly M, McPhee JR, Graudins LV, Ward RL and Campbell TJ: Off-label use of medicines: consensus recommendations for evaluating appropriateness: Med J Aust 2006; 185 (10): 544–548.

15. Wulf HW, Gleim M, Mignat C. The stability of mixtures of morphine hydrochloride, bupivacaine hydrochloride, and clonidine hydrochloride in portable pump reservoirs for the management of chronic pain syndromes. J Pain Symptom Manage 1994;9:308–311.

16. Yaksh TL, Allen JW. The use of intrathecal midazolam in humans: a case study of process. Anesth Analg 2004; 98: 1536–45, PMID: 15155302.

17. Ochs GA. Intrathecal baclofen. Baillieres Clin Neurol 1993; 2 (1):73–86.

18. Dworkin RH, Turk DC et al. Core outcome measures for chronic pain trials: IMMPACT recommendations. Pain 2005: 113:9–19.

FACULTY OF PAIN MEDICINE PROFESSIONAL DOCUMENTS

POLICY – defined as 'a course of action adopted and pursued by the Faculty. These are matters coming within the authority and control of the Faculty.

RECOMMENDATIONS – defined as 'advisable courses of action'.

GUIDELINES – defined as 'a document offering advice'. These may be clinical (in which case they will eventually be evidence-based), or non-clinical.

STATEMENTS – defined as 'a communication setting out information'.

This document has been prepared having regard to general circumstances, and it is the responsibility of the practitioner to have express regard to the particular circumstances of each case, and the application of this policy document in each case.

Professional documents are reviewed from time to time, and it is the responsibility of the practitioner to ensure that the practitioner has obtained the current version. Professional documents have been prepared having regard to the information available at the time of their preparation, and the practitioner should therefore have regard to any information, research or material which may have been published or become available subsequently.

Whilst the College and Faculty endeavours to ensure that documents are as current as possible at the time of their preparation, they take no responsibility for matters arising from changed circumstances or information or material which may have become available subsequently.

Promulgated: 2007
Date of current document: Feb 2007

Faculty Website: http://www.fpm.anzca.edu.au

References

1. Cousins MJ, Mather LE. Intrathecal and epidural administration of opioids. *Anesthesiology* 1984;61:276–310.

2. Strassels SA, Carr DB, Meldrum M, et al. Toward a canon of the pain and analgesia literature: A citation analysis. *Anesth Analg* 1999;89:1528–1533.

3. Baltussen A, Kindler CH. Citation classics in anesthetic journals. *Anesth Analg* 2004;98:443–451.

4. Abram SE. Alternative neuraxial pain management techniques. *Reg Anesth* 1996;21:129–34.

5. Carpenter, RL. Future epidural or subarachnoid analgesics: Local anesthetics. *Reg Anesth* 1996;21(6S):75–80.

6. Carpenter RL, Abram SE, Bromage PR, et al. Consensus statement on acute pain management. *Reg Anesth* 1996;21:152–156.

7. Carpenter RL. Future directions for outcome research in acute pain management: Design of clinical trials. *Reg Anesth* 1996;21:137–138.

8. Cousins MJ, Power I, Smith G. 1996 Labat lecture: Pain—A persistent problem. *Reg Anesth Pain Med* 2000;25:6–21.

9. Carr DB. The evolving practice of regional anesthesia. *Curr Opin Anesth* 1994;7:427.

10. Kehlet H. Organizing postoperative accelerated recovery programs. *Reg Anesth* 1996;21(6S):149–151.

11. White PF, Kehlet H, Neal JM, et al., and the Fast-Track Surgery Study Group. The role of the anesthesiologist in fast-track surgery: From multimodal analgesia to perioperative medical care. *Anesth Analg* 2007;104:1380–1396.

12. Block BM, Liu SS, Rowlingson AJ, et al. Efficacy of postoperative epidural analgesia: A meta-analysis. *JAMA* 2003;290:2455–2463.

13. Carli F, Mayo N, Klubien K, et al. epidural analgesia enhances functional exercise capacity and health-related quality of life after colonic surgery: Results of a randomized trial. *Anesthesiology* 2002;97:540–549.

14. Reuben SS, Buvanendran A. Preventing the development of chronic pain after orthopaedic surgery with preventive multimodal analgesic techniques. *J Bone Joint Surg Am* 1997;89:1343–1358.

15. Ballantyne JC, Carr DB, Berkey CS, et al. Comparative efficacy of epidural, subarachnoid, and intracerebroventricular opioids in patients with pain due to cancer. *Reg Anesth* 1996;21:542–546.

16. Behar M, Olshwang D, Magora F, et al. Epidural morphine in treatment of pain. *Lancet* 1979;1:527–529.

17. Chrubasik J, Chrubasik S. Meta-analysis in the efficacy of intrathecal and epidural opiates. In: Parris W, ed., *Cancer pain management*. Boston: Butterworth-Heinemann, 1997:207–214.

18. Yaksh TL. Intrathecal and epidural opiates: A review. In: Campbell JN, ed., *Pain 1996 – An updated review*. Seattle: IASP Press, 1996:381–393.

19. Smith TJ, Staats PS, Deer T, et al. Randomized clinical trial of an implantable drug delivery system compared with comprehensive medical management for refractory cancer pain: Impact on pain, drug-related toxicity, and survival. *J Clin Oncol* 2002;20:4040–4049.

20. Carr DB, Goudas LC. Postoperative pain control: A survey of promising drugs and pharmacoeconomic criteria for purchasing them. In: Campbell, JN, ed., *Pain 1996 – An Updated Review*. Seattle, IASP press, 1996:189–194.

21. Fisher DM, Macario A. Economics of anesthesia care: A call to arms! *Anesthesiology* 1997;86:1018–1022.

22. Jadad AR. Opioids in the treatment of neuropathic pain: A systematic review of controlled clinical trials. In: Portenoy RK, Bruera E, eds., *Supportive care medicine*. Oxford: Oxford University Press, 1996.

23. Carr DB, Cousins MJ. Spinal route of analgesia. Opioids and future options. In: Cousins MJ, Bridenbaugh PO, eds. *Neural blockade in clinical anesthesia and management of pain*, 3rd ed. Philadelphia: Lippincott-Raven Publishers; 1998:915–983.

24. Staats PS. Complications of intrathecal therapy. *Pain Med* 2008;9[Suppl 1]: S102–S107.

25. Hassenbusch S, Burchiel K, Coffey RJ, et al. Management of intrathecal catheter-tip inflammatory masses: A consensus statement. *Pain Med* 2002; 3:313–323.

26. Murphy PM, Skouvaklis DE, Amadeo RJJ, et al. Intrathecal catheter granuloma associated with Isolated baclofen infusion. *Anesth Analg* 2006; 102:848–852.

27. Deer TR, Raso LJ, Coffey RJ, et al. Intrathecal baclofen and catheter tip inflammatory mass lesions (granulomas): A reevaluation of case reports and imaging findings in light of experimental, clinicopathological, and radiological evidence. *Pain Med* 2008;9:391–395.

28. North RB, Cutchis PN, Epstein JA, et al. Spinal cord compression complicating subarachnoid infusion of morphine: Case report and laboratory experience. *Neurosurgery* 1991;29:778–784.

29. Turner JA, Sears JM, Loeser JD. Programmable intrathecal opioid delivery systems for chronic noncancer pain: A systematic review of effectiveness and complications. *Clin J Pain* 2007;23:180–195.

30. Deer T, Krames ES, Hassenbusch SJ, et al. Polyanalgesic Consensus Conference 2007: Recommendations for the management of pain by intrathecal (intraspinal) drug delivery: Report of an interdisciplinary expert panel. *Neuromodulation* 2007;10:300–328.

31. Cousins MJ. History of the development of pain management with spinal opioid and non-opioid drugs. In: Meldrum ML, ed., *Opioids and pain relief: A historical perspective. (Progress in pain research and management*, Vol. 25). Seattle: IASP Press; 2003:141–155.

32. Walker SM, Goudas LC, Cousins MJ, Carr DB. Combination spinal analgesic chemotherapy: A systematic review. *Anesth Analg* 2002;95:674–715.

33. Carr DB. When bad evidence happens to good treatments. *Reg Anesth Pain Med* 2008;33;229–240.

34. Crile GW. Phylogenetic association in relation to certain medical problems. Address delivered at the Massachusetts General Hospital on the sixty-fourth anniversary of Ether Day, Oct. 15, 1910. *Boston Med Surg J* 1910;163:893–904.

35. Cousins MJ, Mather LE, Gourlay GK. Axon, spinal cord and brain: Targets for acute pain control. In: Scott DB, McClure J, Wildsmith, JA, eds. *Regional anaesthesia 1884–1984*. Denmark: J.H. Schultz, 1984.

36. Yaksh TL, Rudy TA. Studies on the direct spinal action of narcotics in the production of spinal analgesia in the rat. *J Pharmacol Exp Ther* 1977;202: 411–428.

37. Bromage PR, Camporesi E, Chestnut, D. Epidural narcotics for postoperative analgesia. *Anesth Analg* 1980;59:473–480.

38. Coombs DW, Saunders RL, Harbaugh, R, et al. Relief of continuous chronic pain by intraspinal narcotics infusion via an implanted reservoir. *JAMA* 1983;250:2336–9.

39. Cousins MJ, Mather LE, Glynn CJ, et al. Selective spinal analgesia. *Lancet* 1979;1:1141–1142.

40. Poletti CE, Cohen AM, Todd DP, et al. Cancer pain relieved by long-term epidural morphine with permanent indwelling systems for self-administration. *J Neurosurg* 1981;55:581–584.

41. Hudcova J, McNicol E, Quah C, et al. Patient controlled opioid analgesia versus conventional opioid analgesia for postoperative pain. *Cochrane Database Syst Rev* 2006;(4):CD003348. DOI: 10.1002/14651858. CD003348.pub2.

42. Jones AKP, Derbyshire SWG. Positron emission tomography as a tool of understanding the cerebral processing of pain. In: Boivie J, Hansson P, Lindblom U, eds., *Touch, temperature, and pain in health and disease: Mechanisms and assessments*. Seattle: IASP Press, 1993;491–520.

43. Proudfit HK, Yeomans DC. The modulation of nociception by enkephalin-containing neurons in the brainstem. In: Tseng LF, ed., *The pharmacology of opioid peptides*. Langhorn, PA: Harwood Academic Press, 1995:197–218.

44. Tseng LF, Tsai JHH, Collins KA, et al. Spinal delta2-, but not delta1-, μ-, or k-opioid receptors are involved in the tail-flick inhibition induced by β-endorphin from nucleus raphe obscurus in the pentobarbital-anesthetized rat. *Eur J Pharmacol* 1995;277:251–256.

45. Johnson SM, Duggan AW. Evidence that opiate receptors of the substantia gelatinosa contribute to the depression by intravenous morphine of the spinal transmission of impulses in the unmyelinated primary afferents. *Brain Res* 1981;207:223–228.

46. Kitahata LM, Collins JG. Spinal action of narcotic analgesics. *Anesthesiology* 1981;54:153–163.

47. Stein C. Peripheral and non-neuronal opioid effects. *Curr Op Anesth* 1994; 7:347.

48. Stein C. The control of pain in peripheral tissue by opioids. *N Engl J Med* 1995;332:1685–1690.

49. Chrubasik J, Chrubasik S, Mather L, eds. *Postoperative epidural opioids*. Berlin: Springer-Verlag, 1993.

50. Coda BA, Brown MC, Schaffer R, et al. Pharmacology of epidural fentanyl, alfentanil, and sufentanil in volunteers. *Anesthesiology* 1994;81:1149–1161.

51. Sabbe MB, Grafe MR, Mjanger E, et al. Spinal delivery of sufentanil, alfentanil, and morphine in dogs. Physiologic and toxicologic investigations. *Anesthesiology* 1994;81:899–920.

52. Le Bars D, Bouhassira D, Villanueva L. Opioids and diffuse noxious inhibitory control (DNIC) in the rat. In: Bromm B, Desmedt JE, eds., *Advances in pain research and therapy*. New York: Raven Press 1995;22:517–539.

53. Ossipov M, Kovelowski C, Nichols M, et al. Characterization of supraspinal antinociceptive actions of opioid delta agonists in the rat. *Pain* 1995;62:287–293.

54. Stamford JA. Descending control of pain. *Br J Anaesth* 1995;75:217–227.

55. DeLander GE, Wahl JJ. Morphine (intracerebroventricular) activates spinal systems to inhibit behavior induced by putative pain neurotransmitters. *J Pharmacol Exp Ther* 1989;251:1090–1095.

56. Gogas KR, Presley RW, Levine JD, Basbaum AI. The antinociceptive action of supraspinal opioids results from an increase in descending inhibitory control: Correlation of nociceptive behavior and c-fos expression. *Neuroscience* 1991;42:617–628.

57. Pechnick RN. Effects of opioids on the hypothalamo-pituitary-adrenal axis. *Annu Rev Pharmacol Toxicol* 1993;32:353–382.

58. Kehlet H. The modifying effect of general and regional anaesthesia on the endocrine metabolic response to surgery. *Reg Anaesth* 1982;7[Suppl]:538–548.

59. Cepeda, MS, Carr DB. The stress response and regional anesthesia. In: Brown DL. ed., *Regional anesthesia and analgesia*. Philadelphia: W.B. Saunders Company, 1996.

60. Dubner R, Ren K. Central mechanisms of thermal and mechanical hyperalgesia following tissue inflammation. In: Boivie J, Hansson P, Lindblom U, eds. *Touch, temperature, and pain in health and disease: Mechanisms and assessments*. Seattle: IASP Press, 1993;267–277.

61. Mather LE, Cousins MJ. Pharmacology of opioids. Part 1. Basic aspects. *Med J Aust* 1986;144:424–7

62. Zieglgansberger W, Tolle TR, Zimprich A, et al. Endorphins, pain relief, and euphoria. In: Bromm B, Desmedt JE, eds., *Advances in pain research and therapy*, Vol. 22. New York: Raven Press, 1995:439–457.

63. Carr DB, Lipkowski AW. Today's versus tomorrow's opioids for cancer pain: Who will close the gap? *Analgesia* 1996;2:1:227–235.

64. Lord JA, Waterfield AA, Hughes J, et al. Endogenous opioid peptides: Multiple agonists and receptors. *Nature* 1977;267:495–499.

65. Miotto K, Magendzo K, Evans CJ. Molecular characterization of opioid receptors. In: Tseng, LF, ed., *The pharmacology of opioid peptides*. Langhorn, PA: Harwood Academic Publishers GmbH, 1995:57–71.

66. Dickenson AH. Where and how do opioids act? In: Gebhart GF, Hammond DL, Jensen TS eds., *Proceedings of the 7th World Congress on Pain*. Seattle: IASP Press, 1994;525–552.

67. Garzon J. Cellular transduction regulated by μ and δ-opioid receptors in supraspinal analgesia: GTP binding regulatory proteins as pharmacological targets. *Analgesia* 1995;1:131–8.

68. Pennypacker KR. Pharmacological regulation of opioid peptide gene expression: Second and third messenger systems. In: Tseng LF, ed., *The pharmacology of opioid peptides*. Langhorn, PA: Harwood Academic Press, 1995:73–86.

69. Mansour A, Fox CA, Akil H, Watson SJ. Opioid-receptor mRNA expression in the rat CNS: Anatomical and functional implications. *TINS* 1995;18:22–29.

70. Law P. G-proteins and opioid receptors' functions. In: Tseng LF, ed., *The pharmacology of opioid peptides*. Langhorn, PA: Harwood Academic Press, 1995;109–130.

71. Coleman DE, Berghuis AM, Lee E, et al. Structures of active conformations of G1α1 and the mechanism of GTP Hydrolysis. *Science* 1994;265:1405–1412.

72. Mogil JS. The genetics of pain. *Progress in pain research and management*, Vol. 28. Seattle: IASP Press, 2004.

73. Campa D, Gioia A, Tomei A, et al. Association of ABCB1/MDR1 and OPRM1 gene polymorphisms with morphine pain relief. *Clin Pharmacol Ther* 2008;83:559–566.

74. Zubieta J-K, Heitzeg MM, Smith YR, et al. COMT val158met Genotype Affects μ-Opioid Neurotransmitter Responses to a Pain Stressor. *Science* 2003;299:1240–1243.

75. Cepeda MS, Farrar JT, Baumgarten M, et al. Side effects of opioids after short term administration: Effect of age, gender, race, and type of opioid on side effects after opioid administration. *Clin Pharmacol Ther* 2003;74:102–112.

76. Dickenson AH. Spinal cord pharmacology of pain. *Br J Anaesth* 1995;75:193–200.

77. Charlton JJ, Allen PB, Psifogeorgou K, et al. Multiple actions of spinophilin regulate mu opioid receptor function. *Neuron* 2008;58:238–247.

78. Epand RM, Shai Y, Segrest JP, et al. Mechanisms for the modulation of membrane bilayer properties by amphipathic helical peptides. *Biopolymers (Peptide Science)* 1995;37:319–338.

79. Deber CM, Li S. Peptides in membranes: Helicity and hydrophobicity. *Biopolymers (Peptide Science)* 1995;37:295–318.

80. Leff P. The two-state model of receptor activation. *Trends Pharmacol Sci* 1995;16:89–97.

81. Carr DB, Lipkowski AW. Mechanisms of opioid analgetic actions. In: Rogers M, Tinker JH, Covino BG, Longnecker DE, eds., *Principles and practice of anesthesiology*. Vol. 1. St. Louis: Mosby Year Book, 1993:1105–1130.

82. Carr DB. Opioids. *Int Anesthesiol Clin* 1988;26:283.

83. Nock B. Kappa and ∈ opioid receptor binding. In: Tseng LF, ed., *The pharmacology of opioid peptides*. Langhorn, PA: Harwood Academic Press, 1995:29.

84. Porreca F, Bilsky EJ, Lai J. Pharmacological characterization of opioid δ- and κ-receptors. In: Tseng LF, ed., *The pharmacology of opioid peptides*. Langhorn, PA: Harwood Academic Publishers GmbH, 1995.

85. Knapp RJ, Vaughn LK, Yamamura HI. Selective ligands for μ and δ opioid receptors. In: Tseng LF, ed. *The pharmacology of opioid peptides*. Langhorn, PA: Harwood Academic Publishers GmbH, 1995.

86. Dohi S. Spinal antinociception. *Curr Op Anesth* 1996;9:404–409.

87. DeConno F, Caraceni A, Martini C, et al. Hyperalgesia and myoclonus with intrathecal infusion of high-dose morphine. *Pain* 1991;47:337–339.

88. Simonnet G. Preemptive antihyperalgesia to improve preemptive analgesia. *Anesthesiology* 2008;108:352–354.

89. Angst MS, Clark JD. Opioid-induced hyperalgesia: A qualitative systematic review. *Anesthesiology* 2006;104:570–587.

90. Huang LM. Cellular mechanisms of excitatory and inhibitory actions of opioids. In: Tseng LF, ed., *The pharmacology of opioid peptides*. Langhorn, PA: Harwood Academic Press, 1995;131–150.

91. Matthes HW, Maldonado R, Simonin F, et al. Loss of morphine-induced analgesia, reward effect and withdrawal symptoms in mice lacking the mu-opioid-receptor gene. *Nature* 1996;383:819–823.

92. Kellstein DE, Mayer DJ. Chronic administration of cholecystokinin antagonists reverses the enhancement of spinal morphine analgesia induced by acute pretreatment. *Brain Res* 1990;516:263–270.

93. Kellstein DE, Mayer DJ. Spinal co-administration of cholecystokinin antagonists with morphine prevents the development of opioid tolerance. *Pain* 1991;47:221–229.

94. Kellstein DE, Price DD, Mayer DJ. Cholecystokinin and its antagonist lorglumide respectively attenuate and facilitate morphine-induced inhibition of C-fiber evoked discharges of dorsal horn nociceptive neurons. *Brain Res* 1991;540:302–306.

95. Poggioli R, Vergoni AV, Sandrini M, et al. Influence of the selective cholecystokinin antagonist L-364,718 on pain threshold and morphine analgesia. *Pharmacology* 1991;42:197–201.

96. Wiertelak EP, Maier SF, Watkins LR. Cholecystokinin antianalgesia: Safety cues abolish morphine analgesia. *Science* 1992;256:830–833.

97. Wiesenfeld-Hallin Z, Xu X, Hughes J, et al. PD134308, a selective antagonist of cholecystokinin type B receptor, enhances the analgesic effect of morphine and synergistically interacts with intrathecal galanin to depress spinal nociceptive reflexes. *Proc Natl Acad Sci* 1990;87:7105–7109.

98. Salvemini D, Misko TP, Maferrer JL, et al. Nitric oxide, an inhibitor of lipid oxidation by lipoxygenase, cyclooxygenase and hemoglobin. *Lipids* 1992;27:46.

99. Swenson JD, Hullander RM, Bready RJ, et al. A comparison of patient controlled analgesia by the lumbar versus thoracic route after thoracotomy. *Anesth Analg* 1994;78:215–218.

100. Price DD. Psychophysical measurement of normal and abnormal pain processing. In: Boivie J, Hansson P, Lindblom U, eds. *Touch, temperature, and pain in health and disease: Mechanisms and assessments*. Seattle: IASP Press, 1993:3–26.

101. Henry JL, Radhakrishnan V. Hyperalgesia following noxious thermal, mechanical, or chemical stimulation involves overlapping spinal mechanisms and interactive participation of excitatory amino acids and neuropeptides. *APS Journal* 1994;3:249–256.

102. Meller ST. Thermal and mechanical hyperalgesia. A distinct role for different excitatory amino acid receptors and signal transduction pathways? *APS Journal* 1994;3:215.

103. Abram SE. Necessity for an animal model of postoperative pain. *Anesthesiology* 1997;86:1015–1017.

104. Basbaum A. Insights into the development of opioid tolerance. *Pain* 1995;61:349–352.

105. Cox BM. Molecular and cellular mechanisms in opioid tolerance. In: Basbaum AI, Besson JM, eds., *Towards a new pharmacotherapy of pain*. New York: Wiley Interscience, 1991;137–156.

106. Fleming WW, Taylor DA. Cellular mechanisms of opioid tolerance and dependence. In: Tseng LF, ed., *The pharmacology of opioid peptides*. Langhorn, PA: Harwood Academic Press, 1995;463.

107. Mao J, Price DD, Mayer DJ. Mechanisms of hyperalgesia and morphine tolerance: A current view of their possible interactions. *Pain* 1995;62:259–274.

108. Mayer D, Mao J, Price D. The development of morphine tolerance and dependence is associated with translocation of protein kinase C. *Pain* 1995;61:365–374.

109. Wilder RT, Shoales MG, Berde CB. NG-Nitro-L-arginine Methyl Ester (L-NAME) prevents tachyphylaxis to local anesthetics in a dose-dependent manner. *Anesth Analg* 1996;83:1251–1255.

110. Sadee W, Wang Z, Arden, JR, et al. Constitutive activation of the μ-opioid receptor: A novel paradigm of receptor regulation in narcotic analgesia, tolerance, and dependence. *Analgesia* 1994;1:11–14.

111. Gericke M, Morgenstern R, Ott T. The influence of tifluadom on cholecystokinin-induced antinociception. *Eur J Pharmacol* 1990;180:187–190.

112. Goodman CB, Elmer GI, Yang HT, et al. Modulation of opioid receptors by anti-opioid peptides. In: Tseng LF, ed., *The pharmacology of opioid peptides*. Langhorn PA: Harwood Academic Press, 1995;303–320.

113. Portenoy RK. Opioid tolerance and responsiveness: Research findings and clinical observations. In: Gebhart GF, Hammond DL, Jensen TS, eds., *Proceedings of the 7th World Congress on Pain*. Seattle: IASP Press, 1994:595–619.

114. Johnson SM, Duggan AW. Tolerance and dependence of dorsal horn neurones of the cat: The role of the opiate receptors of the substantia gelatinosa. *Neuropharmacology* 1981;20:1033–1038.

115. Duttaroy A, Pharm BS, Byron MS, et al. The effect of intrinsic efficacy on opioid tolerance. *Anesthesiology* 1995;82:1226–1236.

116. Yaksh TL, Reddy SV. Studies on the primate on the analgetic effects associated with intrathecal actions of opiate alpha-adrenergic agonists and baclofen. *Anesthesiology* 1981;54:451–467.

117. Colpaert FC, Leysen LE, Michiels M, et al. Epidural and intravenous sufentanil in the rat: Analgesia, opiate receptor binding, and drug concentrations in plasma and brain. *Anesthesiology* 1986;65:41–49.

118. Glynn CJ, Mather LE. Clinical pharmacokinetics applied to patients with intractable pain: Studies with pethidine. *Pain* 1982;13:237–246.

119. Foley KM. Clinical tolerance to opioids. In: Basbaum AI, Besson JM, eds. *Towards a new pharmacotherapy of pain: Dahlem Konfrenzen (The Dahlem Conference)*. Chichester, England: John Wiley & Sons; 1991:181–204.

120. Onofrio BM, Yaksh TL. Long-term pain relief produced by intrathecal morphine infusion in 53 patients. *J Neurosurg* 1990;72:200–209.

121. Plummer JL, Cherry DA, Cousins MJ, et al. Long-term spinal administration of morphine in cancer and non-cancer pain: A retrospective study. *Pain* 1991;44:215–220.

122. Tung AS, Yaksh TL. In vivo evidence for multiple opiate receptors mediating analgesia in the rat spinal cord. *Brain Res* 1982;247:75–83.

123. Cardan E. Spinal morphine in enuresis. *Br J Anaesth* 1985;57:354.

124. McNicol E, Horowicz-Mehler N, Fisk RA, et al. Management of opioid side effects in cancer-related and chronic noncancer pain – a systematic review. *J Pain* 2003;4:231–256.

125. Yaksh TL, Huang SP, Rudy RT, et al. The direct and specific opiate-like effect of met5–enkephalin and analogues on the spinal cord. *Neuroscience* 1977;2:593–596.

126. Foran SE, Carr DB, Lipkowski AW, et al. A substance P-opioid chimeric peptide as a unique nontolerance-forming analgesic. *Proc Natl Acad Sci USA* 2000;97:7621–7626.

127. Yaksh TL, Noueihed RY, Durant AC. Studies of the pharmacology and pathology of intrathecally administered 4-aminopiperidine analogues and morphine in the rat and cat. *Anesthesiology* 1986;64:54–66.

128. Yaksh TL, Malmberg AB. Interaction of spinal modulatory receptor systems. In: Fields HL, Liebeskind JC, eds., *Pharmacological Approaches to*

the treatment of chronic pain: New concepts and critical issues. Seattle: IASP Press, 1994:151–171.

129. Coombs DW, Saunders RL, LaChance D, et al. Intrathecal morphine tolerance: Use of intrathecal clonidine, DADLE, and intraventricular morphine. *Anesthesiology* 1985;62:358–363.

130. Siddall PJ, Grat M, Rutkowski S, et al. Intrathecal morphine and clonidine in the management of spinal cord injury pain: A case report. *Pain* 1994;59: 147–148.

131. Siddall PJ, Xu CL, Cousins, MJ. Allodynia following traumatic spinal injury in the rat. *Neuroreport* 1995;6:1241–4.

132. Siddall PJ, Molloy AR, Walker S, et al. Efficacy of intrathecal morphine and clonidine in the treatment of neuropathic pain following spinal cord injury. *Anesth Analg* 2000;91:1493–1498.

133. Overdyk FJ, Carter R, Maddox RR, et al. Continuous oximetry/capnometry monitoring reveals frequent desaturation and bradypnea during patient-controlled analgesia. *Anesth Analg* 2007;105:412–418.

134. Chrubasik J, Scholler K, Bammert J. Epidural morphine injection and cisternal cerebellomedullary CSF bioavailability of morphine in dogs. In: Erdmann W, Oyama T, Pernak M, eds., *The pain clinic*. Utrecht: UNU Science Press, 1985:47–49.

135. Gourlay GK, Cherry DA, Cousins MJ. Cephalad migration of morphine in CSF following lumbar epidural administration in patients with cancer pain. *Pain* 1985;23:317–326.

136. Strichartz G. Protracted relief of experimental neuropathic pain by systemic local anesthetics. *Anesthesiology* 1995;83:654–655.

137. Gustafsson LL, Hartvig P, Bergstrom K, et al. Distribution of 11C-labelled morphine and pethidine after spinal administration to Rhesus monkey. *Acta Anaesthesiologica Scandinavica* 1989;33:105–111.

138. Florez J, McCarty LE, Borison HL. A comparative study in the cat of the respiratory effects of morphine injected intravenously and into the cerebrospinal fluid. *J Pharmacol Exp Ther* 1968;163:448–455.

139. Filos KS, Goudas LC, Patroni O, et al. Analgesia with epidural nimodipine. *Lancet* 1993;342:1047.

140. Goudas LC, Langlade A, Serrie A, et al. Acute decreases in cerebrospinal fluid glutathione levels after intracerebroventricular morphine for cancer pain. *Anesth Analg* 1999;89:1209–1215.

141. Davies GK, Tolhurst-Cleaver CL, James TL. CNS depression from intrathecal morphine. *Anesthesiology* 1980;52:280.

142. Davies GK, Tolhurst-Cleaver CL, James TL. Respiratory depression after intrathecal narcotics. *Anaesthesia* 1980.35:1080–1083.

143. Gjessing J, Tomlin, PJ. Postoperative pain control with intrathecal morphine. *Anaesthesia* 1981;36:268–276.

144. Glynn CJ, Mather LE, Cousins MJ, et al. Spinal narcotics and respiratory depression. *Lancet* 1979;2:356–357.

145. Jones RDM, Jones JG. Intrathecal morphine: Naloxone reverses respiratory depression but not analgesia. *Br Med J* 1980;281:645–646.

146. Liolios A, Anderson FH. Selective spinal analgesia. *Lancet* 1979;2: 357–362.

147. Odoom JA. Respiratory depression after intrathecal morphine. *Anesth Analg* 1982;61:70.

148. Paulus DA, Paul W, Munson ES. Neurologic depression after intrathecal morphine. *Anesthesiology* 1981;54:517–518.

149. Samii K, Feret J, Haran A, et al. Selective spinal analgesia. *Lancet* 1979;1: 1142.

150. Wang JK, Nauss LE, Thomas JE. Pain relief by intrathecally applied morphine in man. *Anesthesiology* 1979;50:149–151.

151. DiChiro G. Movement of the cerebrospinal fluid in human beings. *Nature* 1964;204:290–291.

152. DiChiro G. Observations on the circulation of the cerebrospinal fluid. *Acta Radiol [Diagn] (Stockh)* 1966;5:988–1002.

153. Drayer BP, Rosenbaum AE. Studies of the third circulation. Amipaque CT cisternography and ventriculography. *J Neurosurg* 1978;48:946–956.

154. Sage M. Kinetics of water-soluble contrast media in the central nervous system. *Am J Neuroradiol* 1983;4:897–906.

155. Sage M, Kilatrick C, Fon GT, et al. Brain parenchyma penetration by metrizamide following lumbar myelography. *Aust Radiol* 1984;28: 90–96.

156. Rawal N, Arner S, Gustaffson LL, et al. Present state of extradural and intrathecal opioid analgesia in Sweden. A nationwide follow-up survey. *Br J Anaesth* 1987;59:791–799.

157. Gustafsson LL, Johannisson J, Garle M. Extradural and parenteral pethidine as analgesia after total hip replacement: Effects and kinetics. A controlled clinical study. *Eur J Clin Pharmacol* 1986;29:529–534.

158. Gambling D, Hughes T, Martin G, et al., for the Single-Dose EREM Study Group. A comparison of DepoDurTM, a novel, single-dose extended-release epidural morphine, with standard epidural morphine for pain relief after lower abdominal surgery. *Anesth Analg* 2005;100:1065–1074.

159. Gustafsson, L.L, Garle, M, Johannisson, J, et al. Regional epidural analgesia: Kinetics of pethidine. *Acta Anaesthesiol Scand* 1982;74[Suppl]:165–8.

160. Scott DB, McClure J. Selective epidural analgesia. *Lancet* 1979;1:1410–1411.

161. Ahuja BR, Strunin L. Respiratory effects of epidural fentanyl. *Anaesthesia* 1985;40:949–955.

162. Lomessy A, Magnin C, Viale J-P, et al. Clinical advantages of fentanyl given epidurally for post-operative analgesia. *Anesthesiology* 1984;61:466–469.

163. Bilsback P, Rolly G, Tampubolon O. Efficacy of the extradural administration of lofentanil, buprenorphine or saline in the management of postoperative pain. A double-blind study. *Br J Anaesth* 1985;57:943–948.

164. Christensen V. Respiratory depression after extradural morphine. *Br J Anaesth* 1980;52:841.

165. Muller H, Borner U, Stoyanov M, and Hempelmann G. Intraoperative peridural opiate analgesia. *Anaesthesist* 1980;12:656–657.

166. Reiz S, Ahlin J, Ahrenfeld B, et al. Epidural morphine for postoperative pain relief. *Acta Anaesthesiol Scand* 1981;25:111–114.

167. Wedel SJ, Ritter RR. Serum levels following epidural administration of morphine and correlation with relief of post surgical pain. *Anesthesiology* 1981;54:210–214.

168. Lam AM, Knill RL, Thompson WR, et al. Epidural fentanyl does not cause delayed respiratory depression. *Can Anaesth Soc J* 1983;30:578–579.

169. Boas RA. Hazards of epidural morphine. *Anaesth Intens Care* 1980;8:377–378.

170. Klinck JR, Lindop MJ. Epidural morphine in the elderly. A controlled trial after upper abdominal surgery. *Anaesthesia* 1982;37:907–912.

171. Christensen P, Brandt MR. Extradural morphine and Stokes-Adams attacks. *Br J Anaesth* 1982;54:363.

172. Bromage PR, Camporesi EM, Durant PAC, et al. Rostral spread of epidural morphine. *Anesthesiology* 1982;56:431–436.

173. Bromage PR, Camporesi E, Leslie J. Epidural narcotics in volunteers: Sensitivity to pain and to carbon dioxide. *Pain* 1980;9:145–160.

174. Camporesi EM, Nielsen CH, Bromage PR, et al. Ventilatory CO2 sensitivity after intravenous and epidural morphine in volunteers. *Anesth Analg* 1983;62:633–640.

175. Knill RL, Clement JL, Thompson WR. Epidural morphine causes delayed and prolonged ventilatory depression. *Can Anaesth Soc J* 1981;28:537–543.

176. McCaughey W, Graham JL. The respiratory depression of epidural morphine. Time course and effect of posture. *Anaesthesia* 1982;37:990–995.

177. Molke JF, Madsen JB, Guldager H, et al. Respiratory depression after epidural morphine in the postoperative period. Influence of posture. *Acta Anaesthesiol Scand* 1984;28:600–602.

178. Rawal N, Wattwil M. Respiratory depression following epidural morphine. An experimental and clinical study. *Anesth Analg* 1984;63:8–14.

179. Lanz E, Kehrberger E, Theiss D. Epidural morphine: A clinical double-blind study of dosage. *Anesth Analg* 1985;64:786–791.

180. Stenseth R, Sellevold O, Breivik H. Epidural morphine for postoperative pain: Experience with 1095 patients. *Acta Anaesthesiol Scand* 1985;29:148–156.

181. Chrubasik J, Meynadier J, Blond S, et al. Somatostatin, a potent analgesic. *Lancet* 1984;2:1208–1209.

182. Chrubasik J, Wiebers K. Continuous-plus-on-demand epidural infusions of morphine for postoperative pain relief by means of a small, externally worn infusion device. *Anesthesiology* 1985;62:263–267.

183. El-Baz NM, Faber LP, Jensik RJ. Continuous epidural infusion of morphine for treatment of pain after thoracic surgery: A new technique. *Anesth Analg* 1984;63:757–764.

184. Rawal N, Schott U, Dahlstrom B, et al. Influence of naloxone on analgesia and respiratory depression following epidural morphine. *Anesthesiology* 1986;64:194–201.

185. Rawal N. Neuraxial administration of opioids and nonopioids. In: Brown DL, ed., *Regional anesthesia and analgesia*. Philadelphia: WB Saunders Company, 1996:208–231.

186. Brownridge P, Wrobel J, Watt-Smith J. Respiratory depression following accidental subarachnoid pethidine. *Anaesth Intens Care* 1983;11:237–240.

187. Chauvin M, Salbaing J, Perrin, D, et al. Clinical assessment and plasma pharmacokinetics associated with intramuscular or extradural alfentanil. *Br J Anaesth* 1985;57:886–891.

188. Watson J, Moore A, McQuay H, et al. Plasma morphine concentrations and analgesic effects of lumbar extradural morphine and heroin. *Anesth Analg* 1984;63:629–634.

189. Donadoni, R, Rolly, G, Noorduin, H, et al. Epidural sufentanil for postoperative pain relief. *Anaesthesia* 1985;40:634–638.

190. Reiz S, Westberg M. Side effects of epidural morphine. *Lancet* 1980;2:203–204.

191. Coombs DW, Maurer LH, Saunders RL, et al. Outcomes and complications of continuous intraspinal narcotic analgesia for cancer pain control. *J Clin Oncol* 1984;2:1414–1420.

192. Glynn CJ, Mather LE, Cousins MJ, et al. Peridural meperidine in humans: Analgesic response, pharmacokinetics and transmission into CSF. *Anesthesiology* 1981;55:520–526.

193. Cherry DA, Gourlay GK, Cousins MJ, et al. A technique for the insertion of an implantable portal system for the long term epidural administration of opioids in the treatment of cancer pain. *Anaesth Intens Care* 1985;13:145–152.

194. Coombs DW, Sanders RL, Gaylor M, et al. Epidural narcotic infusion reservoir: Implantation technique and efficacy. *Anesthesiology* 1981;55:469–473.

195. Crawford ME, Andersen HB, Augustenborg G, et al. Pain treatment on outpatient basis utilizing extradural opiates: A Danish multicentre study comprising 105 patients. *Pain* 1983;16:41–47.

196. Zenz M. Epidural opiates: Long term experiences in cancer pain. *Klin Wochenschr* 1985;63:225–229.

197. Lamarche, Y, Martin, R, Reiher, Y, et al. The sleep apnea syndrome and epidural morphine. *Can Anaesth Soc J* 1986;33:231–233.

198. Petring OU, Dawson PJ, Blake DW, et al. Normal postoperative gastric emptying after orthopaedic surgery with spinal anesthesia and i.m. ketorolac as the first postoperative analgesic. *Br J Anaesth* 1995;74:257–260.

199. McNicol ED, Boyce D, Schumann R, Carr DB. Efficacy and safety of mu opioid antagonists in the treatment of opioid induced bowel dysfunction: Systematic review and meta-analysis of randomized controlled trials. *Cochrane Database Syst Rev* 2008 Apr 16;(2):CD006332.

200. Yuan CS, Foss JF, O'Connor M, et al. Methylnaltrexone for reversal of constipation due to chronic methadone use: A randomized controlled trial. *JAMA* 2000:283:367–372.

201. Yuan CS, Israel RJ. Methylnaltrexone, a novel peripheral opioid receptor antagonist for the treatment of opioid side effects. *Expert Opin Investig Drugs* 2006;15:541–552.

202. Camilleri M. Alvimopan, a selective peripherally acting mu-opioid antagonist. *Neurogastroenterol Motil* 2005;17:157–165.

203. Webster L, Jansen JP, Peppin J, et al. Alvimopan, a peripherally acting mu-opioid receptor (PAM-OR) antagonist for the treatment of opioid-induced bowel dysfunction: Results from a randomized, double-blind, placebo-controlled, dose-finding study in subjects taking opioids for chronic non-cancer pain. *Pain* 2008;137:428–440.

204. Torda TA, Pybus DA. Clinical experience with epidural morphine. *Anaesth Intensive Care* 1981;9:129–134.

205. Perriss BW, Malins AF. Pain relief in labour using epidural pethidine with adrenaline. *Anaesthesia* 1981;36:631–633.

206. Baraka A, Noueihed R, Hajj S. Intrathecal injection of morphine for obstetric analgesia. *Anesthesiology* 1981;54: 136–140.

207. Scott PV, Bowen FE, Cartwright P, et al. Intrathecal morphine as sole analgesic during labour. *Br Med J* 1980;281:351–355.

208. Brownridge P. Epidural and intrathecal opiates for postoperative pain relief. *Anaesthesia* 1983;38:74–76.

209. Welchew EA. The optimum concentration for epidural fentanyl. *Anaesthesia* 1983;38:1037–1041.

210. Bromage, PR, Camporesi EM, Durant PAC, et al. Nonrespiratory side effects of epidural morphine. *Anesth Analg* 1982;61:490–495.

211. Rawal N, Sjostrand U, Christoffersson E, et al. Comparison of intramuscular and epidural morphine for postoperative analgesia in the grossly obese: Influence on postoperative ambulation and pulmonary function. *Anesth Analg* 1984;63:583–592.

212. Howard RP, Milne LA, Williams NE. Epidural morphine in terminal care. *Anaesthesia* 1981;36:51–53.

213. Paakkari P, Feuerstein G. Opioid peptides in cardiovascular and respiratory regulation. In: Tseng LF, ed., *The pharmacology of opioid peptides*. Langhorn, PA: Harwood Academic Press, 1995:425–444.

214. Chaney MA. Side effects of intrathecal and epidural opioids. *Can J Anaesth* 1995;42:891–903.

215. Atchison SR, Durant P, Yaksh TL. Cardiorespiratory effects and kinetics of intrathecally injected DADLE and morphine in unanesthetized dogs. *Anesthesiology* 1986;65:609.

216. Duggan AW, Morton CR, Johnson SM, et al. Opioid antagonists and spinal reflexes in the anaesthetized cat. *Brain Res* 1984;297:33–40.

217. Cowen MJ, Bullingham RES, Paterson GMC, et al. A controlled comparison of the effects of extradural diamorphine and bupivacaine on plasma glucose and plasma cortisol in postoperative patients. *Anesth Analg* 1982;61:15–18.

218. Cozian A, Pinaud M, Lepage JY, et al. Effects of meperidine spinal anesthesia on hemodynamics, plasma catecholamines, angiotensin I, aldosterone, and histamine concentrations in elderly men. *Anesthesiology* 1986;64:815–819.

219. Hotvedt R, Refsum H. Cardiac effects of thoracic epidural morphine caused by increased vagal activity in the dog. *Acta Anaesthesiol Scand* 1986;30:76–83.

220. Reiz S, Bennett S. Cardiovascular effects of epidural anaesthesia. *Curr Op Anesth* 1993;6:813.

221. Chaney MA. Intrathecal and epidural anesthesia for cardiac surgery. *Anesth Analg* 2006;102:45–64.

222. Bode RH, Lewis KP, Zarich SW, et al. Cardiac outcome after peripheral vascular surgery: Comparison of general and regional anesthesia. *Anesthesiology* 1996;84:3–13.

223. Go AS, Browner WS. Cardiac outcomes after regional or general anesthesia: Do we have the answer? *Anesthesiology* 1996;84:1–2.

224. Kerr-Wilson RH, McNally S. Bladder drainage for caesarean section under epidural analgesia. *Br J Obstet Gynaecol* 1986;93:28–30.

225. Rawal N, Mollefors K, Axelsson K, et al. An experimental study of urodynamic effects of epidural morphine and of naloxone reversal. *Anesth Analg* 1983;62:641–647.

226. Thompson WR, Smith PT, Hirst M, et al. Regional analgesic effect of epidural morphine in volunteers. *Can Anaesth Soc J* 1981;28:530–536.

227. Torda TA, Pybus DA, Liberman H, et al. Experimental comparison of extradural and I.M. morphine. *Br J Anaesth* 1980;52:939–943.

228. Walts LF, Kaufman RD, Moreland JR, et al. Total hip arthroplasty. An investigation of factors related to postoperative urinary retention. *Clin Orthop* 1985;194:280–282.

229. Husted S, Djurhuus JC, Husegaard HC, et al. Effect of postoperative extradural morphine on lower urinary tract function. *Acta Anaesthesiol Scand* 1985;29:183–185.

230. Rawal N, Schott U, Tandon B, et al. Influence of intravenous naloxone infusion on analgesia and untoward effects of epidural morphine. *Anesth Analg* 1985;64:270.

231. Naulty JS, Johnson M, Burger GA, et al. Epidural fentanyl for post cesarean delivery pain management. *Anesthesiology* 1983;59:A415.

232. Brownridge P, Frewin DB. A comparative study of techniques of postoperative analgesia following caesarean section and lower abdominal surgery. *Anaesth Intensive Care* 1985;13:123–130.

233. Evron S, Samueloff A, Simon A, et al. Urinary function during epidural analgesia with methadone and morphine in post-cesarean section patients. *Pain* 1985;23:135–144.

234. Abram SE. Spinal cord toxicity of epidural and subarachnoid analgesics. *Reg Anesth* 1996;21:84–88.

235. Rozan JP, Kahn CH, Warfield CA. Epidural and intravenous opioid-induced neuroexcitation. *Anesthesiology* 1995;83:860–863.

236. Borner U, Muller H, Stoyanov M, et al. Epidural opiate analgesia. Compatibility of opiates with tissue and CSF. *Anaesthesist* 1980;29:570–571.

237. Hurley RJ, Lambert DH. Continuous spinal anesthesia with a micro-catheter technique: The experience in obstetrics and general surgery. *Reg Anesth* 1989;14:3–8.

238. Kumar CM, Corbett WA, Wilson RG. Spinal anaesthesia with a micro-catheter in high-risk patients undergoing colorectal cancer and other major abdominal surgery. *Surg Oncol* 2008;17:73–79.

239. Abouleish E, Barmada MA, Nemoto EM, et al. Acute and chronic effects of intrathecal morphine in monkeys. *Br J Anaesth* 1981;53:1027–1032.

240. Coombs DW, Fratkin JD, Meier FA, et al. Neuropathologic lesions and CSF morphine concentrations during chronic continuous intraspinal morphine infusion. *Pain* 1985;22:337–351.

241. Yaksh TL. In vivo studies on spinal opiate receptor systems mediating antinociception. I. Mu and delta receptor profiles in the primate. *J Pharmacol Exp Ther* 1983;226:303–316.

242. Durant PA, Yaksh TL. Epidural injections of bupivacaine, morphine, fentanyl, lofentanil and DADL in chronically implanted rats: A pharmacologic and pathologic study. *Anesthesiology* 1986;64:43–53.

243. Yaksh TL, Horais KA, Tozier NA, et al. Chronically infused intrathecal morphine in dogs. *Anesthesiology* 2003;99:174–187.

244. Gradert TL, Baze WB, Satterfield WC, et al. Safety of chronic intrathecal morphine infusion in a sheep model. *Anesthesiology*, 2003;99:188–198.

245. Follett KA. Intrathecal analgesia and catheter-tip inflammatory masses. *Anesthesiology* 2003;99:5–6.

246. Yaksh TL, Hassenbusch S, Burchiel K, et al. Inflammatory masses associated with intrathecal drug infusion: A review of preclinical evidence and human data. *Pain Med* 2002;3:300–313.

247. Medtronic January 2008. Letter. Updated Information—Inflammatory mass (granuloma) at or near the distal tip of intrathecal catheters. Retrieved August 14, 2008 from: http://www.medtronic.com/neuro/spasticity/itbtherapy/downloads/Inflammatory_Mass_Letter.pdf.

248. Goudas LC. Clonidine. *Curr Op Anesth* 1995;8:455–460.

249. Goudas LC, Carr DB, Filos KS, et al. The spinal clonidine-opioid analgesic interaction: From laboratory animals to the postoperative ward. A literature review of preclinical and clinical evidence. *Analgesia* 1998;3:277–290.

250. Ballantyne JC, Loach AB, Carr DB. Itching after epidural and spinal opiates. *Pain* 1988;33:149–160.

251. Rosow CE, Moss J, Philbin DM, et al. Histamine release during morphine and fentanyl anesthesia. *Anesthesiology* 1982;56:93–96.

252. Oyama T, Matsuki A, Taneichi T, et al. Beta-endorphin in obstetric analgesia. *Am J Obst Gynecol* 1980;137:613–616.

253. Oyama T, Jin T, Yamaya R, et al. Profound analgesic effects of beta-endorphin in man. *Lancet* 1980;1:122–124.

254. Mathews E. Epidural morphine. *Lancet* 1979;1:673.

255. Yaksh TL, Harty GJ, Onofrio BM. High doses of spinal morphine produce a non-opiate receptor mediated hyperesthesia. Practical and theoretical implications. *Anesthesiology* 1986;64:590–597.

256. Scott PV, Fisher HB. Intraspinal opiates and itching: A new reflex? *Br Med J* 1982;284:1015–1016.

257. Brown DV, McCarthy RJ. Epidural and spinal opioids. *Curr Opin Anesth* 1995;8:337.

258. Cicero TJ, Bell RD, Wiest WG, et al. Function of the male sex organs in heroin and methadone users. *N Engl J Med* 1975;292:882–887.

259. Mendelson JH, Mendelson JE, Patch VD. Plasma testosterone levels in heroin addiction and during methadone maintenance. *J Pharmacol Exp Ther* 1975;192:211–217.

PART IV: PAIN MANAGEMENT

260. Taylor T, Dluhy RG, Williams GH. Beta-endorphin suppresses adrenocorticotropin and cortisol levels in normal human subjects. *J Clin Endocrinol Metabol* 1983;57(3):592–596.

261. Cepeda MS, Carr DB. The stress response and regional anesthesia. In: Brown DL, ed., *Regional anesthesia and analgesia*. Philadelphia: Saunders; 1996:108–123.

262. Carr DB. Caveats in the evaluation of stress hormone responses in analgesic trials. In: Max MB, Portenoy RK, Laska EM, eds., *The design of analgesic clinical trials*. (*Advances in pain research and therapy*, Vol. 18). New York: Raven Press; 1991:599–605.

263. Carr DB, Bullen BA, Skrinar GS, et al. Physical conditioning facilitates the exercise-induced secretion of beta-endorphin and beta-lipotropin in women. *N Engl J Med* 1981;305:560–563.

264. Daniell HW. Opioid-induced androgen deficiency. *Curr Opin Endocrinol Diabetes* 2006;13(3):262–266.

265. Abs R, et al. Endocrine consequences of long-term intrathecal administration of opioids. *J Clin Endocrinol Metab* 2000;85(6):2215–2222.

266. Doleys DM, Dinoff BL, Page L, et al. Sexual dysfunction and other side effects of intraspinal opiate use in the management of chronic noncancer pain. *AJPM* 1998;8:5–11.

267. Finch PM, Roberts LJ, Price L, et al. Hypogonadism in patients treated with intrathecal morphine. *Clin J Pain* 2000;16(3):251–254.

268. Paice JA, Penn RD, Ryan WG. Altered sexual function and decreased testosterone in patients receiving intraspinal opioids. *J Pain Symptom Manage* 1994;9:126–131.

269. Katz N. The Impact of opioids on the endocrine system. *Pain Management Rounds (Massachusetts General Hospital)* 2005;1(9). Retrieved August 14, 2008 from: www.painmanagementrounds.com.

270. Jackson J, Riggs MW, Spiekerman AM. Testosterone deficiency as a risk factor for hip fractures in men: A case-control study. *Am J Med Sci* 1992; 304(1):4–8.

271. Paice JA, Penn RD. Amenorrhea associated with intraspinal morphine. *J Pain Symptom Manage* 1995;10:582–583.

272. Kaufman JM, Vermeulen A. The decline of androgen levels in elderly men and its clinical and therapeutic implications. *Endocrine Rev* 2005;26: 833–876.

273. McClure JH. Ropivacaine. *Br J Anaesth* 1996;76:300–307.

274. Nordberg G. Pharmacokinetic aspects of spinal morphine analgesia. *Acta Anaesthesiol Scand* 1984;79:1–38.

275. Sjostrom S, Hartvig P, Persson P, et al. Pharmacokinetics of epidural morphine and meperidine in man. *Anesthesiology* 1987;67:877–888.

276. Max MB, Inturrisi CE, Kaiko RF, et al. Epidural and intrathecal opiates: Cerebrospinal fluid and plasma profiles in patients with chronic cancer pain. *Clin Pharmacol Ther* 1985;38:631–641.

277. Way EL. Studies on the local anaesthetic properties of isonipecaine. *J Am Pharm Assoc* 1946;35:44–47.

278. Mirceau N, Constaninescu C, Jianu C, et al. Anesthesie sous-arachnoidienne par la pethidine. *Ann Fr Anesth Reanim* 1982;1:167.

279. Sangarlangkarn S, Klaewtanong V, Jonglerttrakool P, et al. Meperidine as a spinal anesthetic agent: A comparison with lidocaine-glucose. *Anesth Analg* 1987;666:235–240.

280. Moore RA, Bullingham RSJ, McQuay HJ, et al. Spinal fluid kinetics of morphine and heroin in man. *Clin Pharmacol Ther* 1984;35:40–45.

281. Plummer JL, Cmielewski PL, Reynolds GD, et al. Influence of polarity on dose-response relationships of intrathecal opioids in rats. *Pain* 1990;40:339–347.

282. Brose WG, Tanelian DL, Brodsky JB, et al. CSF and blood pharmacokinetics of hydromorphone and morphine following lumbar epidural administration. *Pain* 1991;45:11–15.

283. Max M, Inturrisi CE, Grabrinsh P, et al. Epidural opiates: Plasma and cerebrospinal fluid (CSF) pharmacokinetics of morphine, methadone and beta-endorphin. *Pain* 1981;11[Suppl 1]:S123.

284. Sjostrom S, Tamsen A, Persson P, et al. Pharmacokinetics of intrathecal morphine and meperidine in man. *Anesthesiology* 1987;67:889–895.

285. Cousins MJ, Cherry DA, Gourlay GK. Acute and chronic pain: Use of spinal opioids. In: Cousins MJ, Bridenbaugh PO, eds., *Neural blockade*. Philadelphia: Lippincott, 1988:955–1029.

286. Strube PJ, Downing JW, Brock-Utne JG. CSF pharmacokinetics of extradural morphine. *Br J Anaesth* 1984;56:921–922.

287. Durant PA, Yaksh TL. Distribution in cerebrospinal fluid, blood and lymph of epidurally injected morphine and inulin in dogs. *Anesth Analg* 1986;65:583–592.

288. Chauvin M, Samii K, Schermann JM, et al. Plasma morphine concentration after intrathecal administration of low doses of morphine. *Br J Anaesth* 1981;53:1065–1067.

289. Yarnell RW, Polis T, Reid GN, et al. Patient-controlled analgesia with epidural meperidine after elective cesarean section. *Reg Anesth* 1992;17:329–333.

290. Gustafsson LL, Friberg-Nielsen S, Garle M. Extradural and parenteral morphine: Kinetics and effects in postoperative pain. A controlled clinical study. *Br J Anaesth* 1982;54:1167–1174.

291. Nordberg G, Hedner T, Mellstrand T, et al. Pharmacokinetic aspects of epidural morphine analgesia. *Anesthesiology* 1983;58:545–551.

292. Rawal N, Sjostrand UH, Dahlstrom B. Postoperative pain relief by epidural morphine. *Anesth Analg* 1981;60:726–731.

293. Chauvin M, Samii K, Schermann JM, et al. Plasma pharmacokinetics of morphine after I.M. extradural and intrathecal administration. *Br J Anaesth* 1981;54:843–847.

294. Dailey PA, Brookshire GL, Shnider SM, et al. The effects of naloxone associated with the intrathecal use of morphine in labor. *Anesth Analg* 1985;64:658–666.

295. Tan S, Cohen SE, White PF. Sufentanil for analgesia after cesarean section: Intravenous versus epidural administration. *Anesth Analg* 1986;65 [Suppl1]:1.

296. Wolfe MJ, Davies GK. Analgesic action of extradural fentanyl. *Br J Anaesth* 1980;52:357–358.

297. Justins DM, Knott C, Luthman J, et al. Epidural versus intramuscular fentanyl: Analgesia and pharmacokinetics in labor. *Anaesthesia* 1983;38:937–942.

298. Freidman A, Kaufer D, Shemer J, et al. Pyridostigmine brain penetration under stress enhances neuronal excitability and induces early immediate transcriptional response. *Nature Med* 1996;12:1382–1385.

299. Cheam EWS, Morgan M. The superiority of epidural opioids for postoperative analgesia – fact or fallacy? *Anaesthesia* 1994;49:1019–1021.

300. Delvecchio L, Bettinelli S, Klersy C, et al. Comparing the efficacy and safety of continuous epidural analgesia in abdominal and urological surgery between two opioids with different kinetic properties: Morphine and sufentanil. *Minerva Anestesiol* 2008;74:69–76.

301. Lazorthes Y, Gouarderes CH, Verdie JC, et al. Analgesie par injection intrathecale de morphine. Etude pharmacocinetique et application aux douleurs irreducibles. *Neurochirurgie* 1980;26:159–164.

302. Moore RA, Bullingham RSJ, McQuay HJ, et al. Dural permeability to narcotics: In vitro determination and application to extra-dural administration. *Br J Anaesth* 1982;54:1117–1128.

303. Tung A, Maliniak K, Tenicela R, et al. Intrathecal morphine for intraoperative and postoperative analgesia. *JAMA* 1980;244:2637–2638.

304. Cousins MJ, Bridenbaugh PO. Spinal opioids and pain relief in acute care. In: Cousins MJ, Phillips GD, eds., *Acute pain management*. New York: Churchill Livingstone, 1986:151–185.

305. Sato O, Asai T, Amaro Y, et al. Formation of cerebrospinal fluid in spinal sub-arachnoid space. *Nature* 1971;233:129–130.

306. Husemeyer RP, Cummings AJ, Rosankiewicz JR, et al. A study of pethidine kinetics and analgesia in women in labour following intravenous, intramuscular and epidural administration. *Br J Clin Pharmacol* 1982;13:171–176.

307. Husemeyer RP, Davenport HT, Cummings AJ, et al. Comparison of epidural and intramuscular pethidine for analgesia in labour. *Br J Obstet Gynecol* 1981;88:711–717.

308. Carr DB. Economics of patient-controlled analgesia: An annotated bibliography. In: Campbell JN, ed., *Pain 1996 – an updated review*. Seattle, IASP Press 1996:437–439.

309. Rauck RL, Wallace MS, Leong MS, et al. A randomized, double-blind, placebo-controlled study of intrathecal ziconotide in adults with severe chronic pain. *J Pain Symptom Manage* 2006;31(5):393–406.

310. Staats P, Whitworth M, Barakat M, et al. The use of implanted programmable infusion pumps in the management of nonmalignant, chronic low-back pain. *Neuromodulation* 2007;10:376–380.

311. Krames ES. Intraspinal opioid therapy for chronic nonmalignant pain: Current practice and clinical guidelines. *J Pain Symptom Manage* 1996;11:333–352.

312. Bennett G, Burchiel K, Buchser E, et al. Clinical guidelines for intraspinal infusion: Report of an expert panel. *J Pain Symptom Manage* 2000;20:S37–S43.

313. Hassenbusch SJ, Portenoy RK, Cousins M, et al. Polyanalgesic consensus conference 2003: An update on the management of pain by intraspinal drug delivery— report of an expert panel. *J Pain Symptom Manage* 2004;27:540–563.

314. Carr DB. Preemptive analgesia implies prevention. *Anesthesiology* 1996;85:1498–1499.

315. Schmidt WK. Survey of current and investigational drugs for the treatment of acute and chronic pain. American Pain Society Annual Meeting, 1995.

316. U.S. Food and Drug Administration (FDA). *Guidelines for the clinical evaluation of analgesic drugs*. Docket Number 91D-0425. Group for analgesic drugs pilot drug evaluation staff (HFD-007). Washington DC: Author, December, 1992.

317. Ferrante FM, VadeBoncouer TR. Epidural analgesia with combinations of local anesthetics and opioids. In: Ferrante FN, VadeBoncouer TR, eds., *Postoperative pain management*. New York: Churchill-Livingstone, 1993;305–333.

318. Fields HL, ed. *Core curriculum for professional education in pain*, 2nd ed. Seattle: IASP Press, 1995.

319. Ready LB, Ashburn M, Caplan M, et al. Practice guidelines for acute pain management in the perioperative setting. *Anesthesiology* 1995;82:1071–1081.

320. Glass PS, Grichnik KP. The role of opioids for epidural analgesia. *Curr Opin Anaesthesiol* 1995;8:283–286.

321. Anderson HB, Jorgensen BC, Engquist A. Epidural met-enkephalin (FK 33–824). A dose-effect study. *Acta Anaesthesiol Scand* 1982;26:69–71.
322. Moulin DE, Max MB, Kaiko RF, et al. The analgesic efficacy of intrathecal D-Ala2–D-Leu5–enkephalin in cancer patients with chronic pain. *Pain* 1985;23:213–221.
323. Dooley CT, Chung NN, Wilkes BC, et al. An all D-amino acid opioid peptide with central analgesic activity from a combinatorial library. *Science* 1994;266:2019–2022.
324. Malmberg AB, Grafe MR, Haaseth RC, et al. Spinal toxicology of [D-Pen2, D-Pen5]Enkephalin (DPDPE) after multiple lumbar intrathecal injections in the rat. *Neurotoxicology* 1995 (submitted).
325. Schmauss C, Shimohigashi Y, Jensen TS, et al. Studies on spinal opiate receptor pharmacology. III. Analgetic effects of enkephalin dimers as measured by cutaneous-thermal and visceral-chemical evoked responses. *Brain Res* 1985;337:209–215.
326. Siegel JE, Weinstein MC, Russell LB, et al. Recommendations for reporting cost-effective analyses. *JAMA* 1996;276:1339–1341.
327. Amandusson A, Hermanson O, Blomquist A. Estrogen receptor-like immunoreactivity in the medullary and spinal dorsal horn of the female rat. *Neurosci Lett* 1995;196:25–28.
328. Yaksh TL. Direct evidence that spinal serotonin and noradrenaline terminals mediate the spinal antinociceptive effects of morphine in the periaqueductal gray. *Brain Res* 1979;160:180–185.
329. Yaksh TL, ed. *Spinal afferent processing.* New York: Plenum Press, 1986.
330. De Kock M. Alpha-2 adrenoceptor agonists: Clonidine, dexmedetomidine, mivazerol. *Curr Opin Anesth* 1996;9:295–299.
331. Eisenach JC. Three novel spinal analgesics: Clonidine, neostigmine, amitriptyline. *Reg Anesth* 1996;21:81–83.
332. Filos KS, Goudas LC, Patroni O, et al. Intrathecal clonidine as a sole analgesic for pain relief after cesarean section. *Anesthesiology* 1992;77:267–274.
333. Bernard J, Kick O, Bonnet F. Comparison of intravenous and epidural clonidine for postoperative patient-controlled analgesia. *Anesth Analg* 1995; 81:706–712.
334. Eisenach JC, DuPen S, Dubois M, et al. Epidural clonidine analgesia for intractable cancer pain. *Pain* 1995;61:391–399.
335. Schug SA, Saunders D, Kurowski I, Paech MJ. Neuraxial drug administration: A review of treatment options for anaesthesia and analgesia.[Erratum appears in *CNS Drugs* 2007;21(7):579]. *CNS Drugs* 2006;20(11):917–933.
336. Lauretti GR, Reis MP, Prado WA, et al. Dose response study of intrathecal morphine versus intrathecal neostigmine, their combination, or placebo for postoperative analgesia in patients undergoing anterior and posterior vaginoplasty. *Anesth Analg* 1996;82:1182–1187.
337. Roelants F, Lavand'homme P, Mercier-Fuzier V. Epidural administration of neostigmine and clonidine to induce labor analgesia: Evaluation of efficacy, and local anesthetic-sparing effect. *Anesthesiology* 2005;102:1205–1210.
338. Wilson PR, Yaksh TL. Baclofen is antinociceptive in the spinal intrathecal space of animals. *Eur J Pharmacol* 1978;51:323–330.
339. Slonimski M, Abram SE, Zuniga RE. Intrathecal baclofen in pain management. *Reg Anesth Pain Med* 2004;29:269–276.
340. Zuniga RE, Perera S, Abram SE. Intrathecal baclofen: A useful agent in the treatment of well-established complex regional pain syndrome. *Reg Anesth Pain Med* 2002;27:90–93.
341. Cao JL, Ding HL, He JH, et al. The spinal nitric oxide involved in the inhibitory effect of midazolam on morphine-induced analgesia tolerance. *Pharmacol Biochem Behav* 2005;80:493–503.
342. Whitwam JG. Benzodiazepine receptors. *Anaesthesia* 1983;38:93–95.
343. Yaksh TL, Allen JW. The use of intrathecal midazolam in humans: A case study of process. *Anesth Analg* 2004;98:1536–1545.
344. Borg PA, Krijnen HJ. Long-term intrathecal administration of midazolam and clonidine. *Clin J Pain* 1996;12:63–68.
345. Rainov NG, Heidecke V, Burkert W. Long-term intrathecal infusion of drug combinations for chronic back and leg pain. *J Pain Symptom Manage* 2001;22:862–871.
346. Canavero S, Bonicalzi V, Clemente M. No neurotoxicity from long-term (>5 years) intrathecal infusion of midazolam in humans. *J Pain Symptom Manage* 2006;32:1–3.
347. Eccles JC, Libet B, Young RR. The behavior of chromatolysed motoneurons studied by intracellular recording. *J Physiol (Land)* 1958;143:l–40.
348. Wall PD, Devor M. The effect of peripheral nerve injury on dorsal root potentials and on transmission of afferent signals into the spinal cord. *Brain Res* 1981;209:95–l11.
349. Devor M, Keller CH, Deerinck TJ, Ellisman MH. Na+ channel accumulation on axolemma of afferent endings in nerve end neuromas in Apteronotus. *Neuroscience Lett* 1989;102:149–154.
350. Wall PD. New horizons: An essay. Chapter 34 in third edition, pp 1135–43.
351. Cox JJ, Reimann F, Nicholas AK, et al. An SCN9A channelopathy causes congenital inability to experience pain. [See comment]. *Nature* 2006;444:894–898.
352. Yang Y, Wang Y, Li S, et al. Mutations in SCN9A, encoding a sodium channel alpha subunit, in patients with primary erythermalgia. *J Med Genetics* 2004;41:171–174.

353. Santillan R, Maestre JM, Hurle MA, et al. Nimodipine, a calcium channel blocker, enhances opiate analgesia in patients with cancer pain tolerant to morphine. In: Gebhart GF, Hammond DL, Jensen TS, eds., *Proceedings of the 7th World Congress on Pain.* Seattle: IASP Press, 1994:587–594.
354. Bowersox SS, Miljanich GP, Sugiura Y, et al. Differential blockade of voltage-sensitive calcium channels at the mouse neuromuscular junction by novel w-concopeptides and w-agatoxin-IVA. *J Pharmacol Exp Ther* 1995;273:248–256.
355. Valentino K, Newcomb R, Gadbois T, et al. A selective N-type calcium channel antagonist protects against neuronal loss after global cerebral ischemia. *Proc Natl Acad Sci USA* 1993;90:7894–7897.
356. Staats PS, Yearwood T, Charapata SG, et al. Intrathecal ziconotide in the treatment of refractory pain in patients with cancer or AIDS: A randomized controlled trial. *JAMA* 2004;291: 63–70.
357. Wallace MS, Charapata SG, Fisher R, et al. Intrathecal ziconotide in the treatment of chronic nonmalignant pain: A randomized, double-blind, placebo-controlled clinical trial. *Neuromodulation* 2006;9(2): 75–86.
358. Thompson JC, Dunbar E, Laye RR. Treatment challenges and complications with ziconotide monotherapy in established pump patients. *Pain Physician* 2006;9:147–152.
359. Shields D, Montenegro R. Chemical stability of ziconotide-clonidine hydrochloride admixtures with and without morphine sulfate during simulated intrathecal administration. *Neuromodulation* 2007;10[Suppl 1]:6–11.
360. Cheng JK, Chiou LC. Mechanisms of the antinociceptive action of gabapentin. *J Pharmacological Sci* 2006;100:471–486.
361. Dworkin RH, Backonja M, Rowbotham MC, et al. Advances in neuropathic pain: Diagnosis, mechanisms, and treatment recommendations. *Arch Neurology* 2003;60:1524–1534.
362. Attal N, Cruccu G, Haanpää M, et al. EFNS guidelines on pharmacological treatment of neuropathic pain. *Eur J Neurol* 2006;13:1153–1169.
363. Van Elstraete AC, Sitbon P, Mazoit J-X, et al. Gabapentin prevents delayed and long-lasting hyperalgesia induced by fentanyl in rats. *Anesthesiology* 2008;108:484–494.
364. Horvath G, Kekesi G, Nagy E, et al. The role of TRPV1 receptors in the antinociceptive effect of anandamide at spinal level. *Pain* 2008;134:277–284.
365. Gavva NR, James JS, Treanor AS, et al. Pharmacological blockade of the vanilloid receptor TRPV1 elicits marked hyperthermia in humans. *Pain* 2008;136(1–2):202–210.
366. Caterina MJ. On the thermoregulatory perils of TRPV1 antagonism. *Pain* 2008;136:3–4.
367. Binshtock AM, Bean BP, Woolf CJ. Inhibition of nociceptors by TRPV1-mediated entry of impermeant sodium channel blockers. *Nature* 2007;449: 607–610.
368. Dickenson AH. NMDA receptor antagonists as analgesics. In: Fields HL, Liebeskind JC, eds., *Pharmacological approaches to the treatment of chronic pain: New concepts and critical issues.* Seattle: IASP Press, 1994;173–187.
369. Woolf CJ, Thompson SWN. The induction and maintenance of central sensitization is dependent on N-methyl-D-aspartic acid receptor activation: Implications for the treatment of post-injury pain hypersensitivity states. *Pain* 1991;44:293–299.
370. Yaksh TL. Epidural ketamine: A useful, mechanistically novel adjuvant for epidural morphine? *Reg Anesth* 1996;21:508–513.
371. Knox DJ, McLeod BJ, Goucke CR. Acute phantom limb pain controlled by ketamine. *Anaesth Intensive Care* 1995;23:620–622.
372. Choe H, Choi Y-S, Kim Y-H, et al. Preemptive analgesia with epidural morphine and ketamine in upper abdominal surgery. *Anesth Analg* (in press).
373. Walker SM, Cousins MJ. Reduction in hyperalgesia and intrathecal morphine requirements by low-dose ketamine infusion. *J Pain Symptom Manage.* 1997;14:129–133.
374. Ozyalcin NS, Yucel A, Camlica H, et al. Effect of pre-emptive ketamine on sensory changes and postoperative pain after thoracotomy: Comparison of epidural and intramuscular routes. *Br J Anaesth* 2004;93:356–361.
375. Wilson JA, Alastair F, Nimmo SM, et al. A randomised double blind trial of the effect of pre-emptive epidural ketamine on persistent pain after lower limb amputation. *Pain* 2008;135(1–2):108–118.
376. Degos V, Loron G, Mantz J, Gressens P. Neuroprotective strategies for the neonatal brain. *Anesth Analg* 2008;106:1670–1680.
377. Anand KJ, Soriano SC. Anesthetic agents and the immature brain: Are these toxic or therapeutic? *Anesthesiology* 2004;101(2):527–530.
378. May A. Chronic pain may change the structure of the brain. *Pain* 2008; 137:7–15.
379. Jin HC, Keller AJ, Jung JK, et al. Epidural tezampanel, an AMPA/kainate receptor antagonist, produces postoperative analgesia in rats. *Anesth Analg* 2007;105:1152–1159.
380. Coderre TJ, Van Empel I. The utility of excitatory amino acid (EAA) antagonists as analgesic agents. I. Comparison of the antinociceptive activity of various classes of EAA antagonists in mechanical, thermal and chemical nociceptive tests. *Pain* 1994;59:345–352.

381. Chaplan SR, Malmberg AB, Yaksh TL. Efficacy of spinal NMDA receptor antagonism in formalin hyperalgesia and nerve injury evoked allodynia in the rat. *J Pharmacol Exp Ther* 1997;280:829–838.

382. Sluka KA, Westlund KN. Centrally administered non-NMDA but not NMDA receptor antagonists block peripheral knee joint inflammation. *Pain* 1993;55:217–225.

383. Sukiennik AW, Kream RM. N-methyl-D-aspartate receptors and pain. *Curr Op Anesth* 1995;8:445.

384. Ballantyne JC, Dershwitz M. The pharmacology of non-steroidal anti-inflammatory drugs for acute pain. *Curr Opin Anesth* 1995;8:461–468.

385. Kitto KF, Haley JE, Wilcox GL. Involvement of nitric oxide in spinally mediated hyperalgesia in the mouse. *Neuroscience Lett* 1992;148:1–5.

386. Samad TA, Moore KA, Sapirstein A, et al. Interleukin-1beta-mediated induction of Cox-2 in the CNS contributes to inflammatory pain hypersensitivity. *Nature* 2001;22;410(6827):471–475.

387. Broom DC, Samad TA, Kohno T, et al. Cyclooxygenase 2 expression in the spared nerve injury model of neuropathic pain. *Neuroscience* 2004; 124(4):891–900.

388. Lee IO, Seo Y. The effects of intrathecal cyclooxygenase-1, cyclooxygenase-2, or nonselective inhibitors on pain behavior and spinal fos-like immunoreactivity. *Anesth Analg* 2008;106:972–977.

389. Antman EM, Bennett JS, Daugherty A, et al. Use of nonsteroidal antiinflammatory drugs: An update for clinicians: A scientific statement from the American Heart Association. *Circulation* 2007;115:1634–1642.

390. Nussmeier NA, Whelton AA, Brown MT, et al. Complications of the COX-2 inhibitors parecoxib and valdecoxib after cardiac surgery. *N Engl J Med* 2005;352:1081–1091.

391. Malmberg AB, Yaksh TL. Spinal nitric oxide synthase inhibition blocks NMDA induced thermal hyperalgesia and produces antinociception in the formalin test in rats. *Pain* 1993;54:291–300.

392. Yamamoto T, Shimoyama N. Role of nitric oxide in the development of thermal hyperesthesia induced by sciatic nerve constriction injury in the rat. *Anesthesiology* 1995;82:1266–1273.

393. Minami T, Uda R, Horiguchi S, et al. Allodynia evoked by intrathecal administration of prostaglandin F2a to conscious mice. *Pain* 1992;50:223–229.

394. Sorkin LS, Moore JH. Evoked release of amino acids and prostanoids in spinal cords of anesthetized rats: Changes during peripheral inflammation and hyperalgesia. *Am J Ther* 1996;3:268–275.

395. McCormack K. Non-steroidal anti-inflammatory drugs and spinal nociceptive processing. *Pain* 1994;59:9–43.

396. Malmberg AB, Yaksh TL. Antinociceptive actions of spinal non-steroidal anti-inflammatory agents on the formalin test in the rat. *J Pharmacol Exp Ther* 1992;163:136–146.

397. Uda R, Horiguchi S, Ito S, et al. Nociceptive effects induced by intrathecal administration of prostaglandin D2, E2, or F2alpha to conscious mice. *Brain Res* 1990;510:26–32.

398. Chapman V, Dickensen AH. The spinal and peripheral roles of bradykinin and prostaglandins in nociceptive processing in the rat. *Eur J Pharmacol* 1992;219:427–433.

399. DeLander GE, Hopkins CJ. Involvement of A2 adenosine receptors in spinal mechanisms of antinociception. *Eur J Pharmacol* 1987;139:215–223.

400. DeLander GE, Hopkins CJ. Spinal adenosine modulates descending antinociceptive pathways stimulated by morphine. *J Pharmacol Exp Ther* 1986;239:88–93.

401. DeLander GE, Hopkins CJ. Interdependence of spinal adenosinergic, serotonergic and noradrenergic systems mediating antinociception. *Neuropharmacology* 1987;26:1791–1794.

402. DeLander GE, Keil GJ, II. Antinociception induced by intrathecal coadministration of selective adenosine receptor and selective opioid receptor agonists in mice. *J Pharmacol Exp Ther* 1993;268:943–951.

403. DeLander GE, Wahl JJ. Behavior induced by putative nociceptive neurotransmitters is inhibited by adenosine or adenosine analogs coadministered intrathecally. *J Pharmacol Exp Ther* 1988;246:565–570.

404. Eisenach JD, Hood DD, Curry R. Phase I safety assessment of intrathecal injection of an American formulation of adenosine in humans. *Anesthesiology* 2002;96(1):24–28.

405. Rane K, Segerdahl M, Goiny M, et al. Intrathecal adenosine administration: A phase 1 clinical safety study in healthy volunteers, with additional evaluation of its influence on sensory thresholds and experimental pain. *Anesthesiology* 1998;89(5):1108–1115.

406. Måns B, Segerdahl M, Arnér S, Sollevi A. The safety and efficacy of intrathecal adenosine in patients with chronic neuropathic pain. *Anesth Analg* 1999;89:136.

407. Sharma M, Mohta M, Chawla R. Efficacy of intrathecal adenosine for postoperative pain relief. *Eur J Anaesthesiol* 2006;23(6):449–453.

408. Lipkowski AW, Maszczynska I. Peptide, N-methyl-D-aspartate and adenosine receptors as analgesic targets. *Curr Op Anesth* 1996;9:443–448.

409. Lipkowski A, Carr DB. Neuropeptides: Peptide and non-peptide analogs. In: Gutte B., ed., *Peptides: Synthesis, structures and applications*. San Diego: Academic Press, 1995;287–320.

410. Bernstein JE. Substance P and substance P antagonists. *Curr Opin Anesth* 1994;7:462.

411. Kream RM, Kato T, Shimonaka H, et al. Substance P markedly potentiates the antinociceptive effects of morphine sulfate administered at the spinal level. *Proc Natl Acad Sci* 1993;90:3564–3568.

412. Foran SE, Carr DB, Lipkowski AW, et al. Inhibition of morphine tolerance development by a substance P-opioid peptide chimera. *J Pharmacol Exp Ther* 2000;295:1142–1148.

413. Melton PM, Riley AL. An assessment of the interaction between cholecystokinin and the opiates within a drug discrimination procedure. *Pharmacol Biochem Behav* 1993;46:237–242.

414. Stanfa LC, Dickenson, AH. Descending control of pain in the enhanced potency of spinal morphine following carrageen in inflammation. *Br J Pharmacol* 1993;180:967–973.

415. Dourish CT, O'Neill MF, Schaffer LW, et al. The cholecystokinin receptor antagonist devazepide enhances morphine-induced analgesia but not morphine-induced respiratory depression in the squirrel monkey. *J Pharmacol Exp Ther* 1990;255:1158–1169.

416. Yaksh TL. Spinal somatostatin for patients with cancer. Risk-benefit assessment of an analgesic. *Anesthesiology* 1994;81:531–533.

417. Lasagna L, ed. *Combination drugs: Their use and regulation*. New York: Stratton, 1975.

418. Eisenach JC. Drug combination studies. In: Max M, ed., *Pain 1999: An updated review—refresher course syllabus*. Seattle: IASP Press, 1999:309–313.

419. Max M. Methodological issues in the design of analgesic clinical trials. In: Max M, ed., *Pain 1999: An updated review—refresher course syllabus*. Seattle: IASP Press, 1999: 299–308.

420. Goldstein D, Brunelle RL. Commentary: Dose-response model for combination analgesic drugs. In: Max M, Portenoy RK, Laska E, eds., *The design of analgesic clinical trials*. New York: Raven Press, 1991:125–136.

421. Dottrens M, Rifat K, Morel DR. Comparison of extradural administration of sufentanil, morphine and sufentanil-morphine combination after caesarean section. *Br J Anaesth* 1992;69:9–12.

422. Adams JU, Tallarida RJ, Geller EB, et al. Isobolographic superadditivity between delta and mu opioid agonists in the rat depends on the ratio of compounds, the mu agonist and the analgesic assay used. *J Pharmacol Exp Ther* 1993;266:1261–1267.

423. Traynor JR, Elliott J. Delta-opioid receptor subtypes and crosstalk with mu-receptors. *Trends Pharmacol Sci* 1993;14:84–86.

424. Kovelowski CJ, Ossipov MH, Hruby VJ, et al. Lesions of the dorsolateral funiculus block supraspinal opioid delta receptor mediated antinociception in the rat. *Pain* 1999;83:115–122.

425. Grabow TS, Hurley RW, Banfor PN, et al. Supraspinal and spinal delta(2) opioid receptor-mediated antinociceptive synergy is mediated by spinal alpha(2) adrenoceptors. *Pain* 1999;83:47–55.

426. Dirig DM, Yaksh TL. Differential right shifts in the dose-response curve for intrathecal morphine and sufentanil as a function of stimulus intensity. *Pain* 1995;62:321–328.

427. Krames ES, Wilkie DJ, Gershow J. Intrathecal D-Ala2–D-Leu5enkephalin (DADL) restores analgesia in a patient analgetically tolerant to intrathecal morphine sulfate. *Pain* 1986;24:205–209.

428. Tanaka M, Watanabe S, Ashimura H, et al. Minimum effective combination dose of epidural morphine and fentanyl for post-hysterectomy analgesia: A randomized, prospective, double-blind study. *Anesth Analg* 1993;77:942–946.

429. Tanaka M, Watanabe S, Matsumiya N, et al. Enhanced pain management for postgastrectomy patients with combined epidural morphine and fentanyl. *Can J Anaesth* 1997;44:1047–1052.

430. Sinatra RS, Sevarino FB, Chung JH, et al. Comparison of epidurally administered sufentanil, morphine, and sufentanil-morphine combination for postoperative analgesia. *Anesth Analg* 1991;72:522–527.

431. Curatolo M, Petersen-Felix S, Scaramozzino P, Zbinden AM. Epidural fentanyl, adrenaline and clonidine as adjuvants to local anaesthetics for surgical analgesia: Meta-analyses of analgesia and side-effects. *Acta Anaesthesiol Scand* 1998;42:910–920.

432. Wheatley RG, Schug SA, Watson D. Safety and efficacy of postoperative epidural analgesia. *Br J Anaesth* 2001;87:47–61.

433. Dahl JB, Jeppesen IS, Jorgensen H, et al. Intraoperative and postoperative analgesic efficacy and adverse effects of intrathecal opioids in patients undergoing cesarean section with spinal anesthesia: A qualitative and quantitative systematic review of randomized controlled trials. *Anesthesiology* 1999;91:1919–1927.

434. Hassenbusch SJ, Portenoy RK. Current practices in intraspinal therapy: A survey of clinical trends and decision making. *J Pain Symptom Manage* 2000;20:S4 –S11.

435. Saito Y, Kaneko M, Kirihara Y, et al. Interaction of intrathecally infused morphine and lidocaine in rats. I. Synergistic antinociceptive effects. *Anesthesiology* 1998;89:1455–1463.

436. Maves TJ, Gebhart GF. Antinociceptive synergy between intrathecal morphine and lidocaine during visceral and somatic nociception in the rat. *Anesthesiology* 1992;76:91–99.

437. van Dongen RT, Crul BJ, van Egmond J. Intrathecal coadministration of bupivacaine diminishes morphine dose progression during long-term intrathecal infusion in cancer patients. *Clin J Pain* 1999;15:166–172.

438. Campbell DC, Camann WR, Datta S. The addition of bupivacaine to intrathecal sufentanil for labor analgesia. *Anesth Analg* 1995;81:305–309.

439. Cooper DW, Ryall DM, McHardy FE, et al. Patient-controlled extradural analgesia with bupivacaine, fentanyl, or a mixture of both, after Caesarean section. *Br J Anaesth* 1996;76:611–615.

440. Kopacz DJ, Sharrock NE, Allen HW. A comparison of levobupivacaine 0.125%, fentanyl 4 microg/mL, or their combination for patient-controlled epidural analgesia after major orthopedic surgery. *Anesth Analg* 1999;89:1497–1503.

441. Torda TA, Hann P, Mills G, et al. Comparison of extradural fentanyl, bupivacaine and two fentanyl-bupivacaine mixtures of pain relief after abdominal surgery. *Br J Anaesth* 1995;74:35–40.

442. George KA, Chisakuta AM, Gamble JA, et al. Thoracic epidural infusion for postoperative pain relief following abdominal aortic surgery: Bupivacaine, fentanyl or a mixture of both? *Anaesthesia* 1992;47:388–394.

443. Vercauteren MP, Geernaert K, Hoffmann VL, et al. Postoperative intrathecal patient-controlled analgesia with bupivacaine, sufentanil or a mixture of both. *Anaesthesia* 1998;53:1022–1027.

444. Mercadante S. Intrathecal morphine and bupivacaine in advanced cancer pain patients implanted at home. *J Pain Symptom Manage* 1994;9:201–207.

445. Sjoberg M, Appelgren L, Einarsson S, et al. Long-term intrathecal morphine and bupivacaine in "refractory" cancer pain. I. Results from the first series of 52 patients. *Acta Anaesthesiol Scand* 1991;35:30–43.

446. Sjoberg M, Nitescu P, Appelgren L, et al. Long-term intrathecal morphine and bupivacaine in patients with refractory cancer pain: Results from a morphine:bupivacaine dose regimen of 0.5:4.75 mg/ml. *Anesthesiology* 1994;80:284–297.

447. van Dongen RT, Crul BJ, De Bock M. Long-term intrathecal infusion of morphine and morphine/bupivacaine mixtures in the treatment of cancer pain: A retrospective analysis of 51 cases. *Pain* 1993;55:119–123.

448. Dahm P, Nitescu P, Appelgren L, et al. Efficacy and technical complications of long-term continuous intraspinal infusions of opioid and/or bupivacaine in refractory nonmalignant pain: A comparison between the epidural and the intrathecal approach with externalized or implanted catheters and infusion pumps. *Clin J Pain* 1998;14:4–16.

449. Nitescu P, Dahm P, Appelgren L, et al. Continuous infusion of opioid and bupivacaine by externalized intrathecal catheters in long-term treatment of "refractory" nonmalignant pain. *Clin J Pain* 1998;14:17–28.

450. Krames ES. Intrathecal infusional therapies for intractable pain: Patient management guidelines. *J Pain Symptom Manage* 1993;8:36–46.

451. Eisenach JC, De Kock M, Klimscha W. Alpha(2)-adrenergic agonists for regional anesthesia: A clinical review of clonidine (1984–1995). *Anesthesiology* 1996;85:655–674.

452. Ossipov MH, Lopez Y, Bian D, et al. Synergistic antinociceptive interactions of morphine and clonidine in rats with nerve ligation injury. *Anesthesiology* 1997;86:196–204.

453. Carabine UA, Milligan KR, Mulholland D, et al. Extradural clonidine infusions for analgesia after total hip replacement. *Br J Anaesth* 1992;68:338–343.

454. Eisenach JC, D'Angelo R, Taylor C, et al. An isobolographic study of epidural clonidine and fentanyl after cesarean section. *Anesth Analg* 1994;79:285–290.

455. Rockemann MG, Seeling W, Brinkmann A, et al. Analgesic and hemodynamic effects of epidural clonidine, clonidine/ morphine, and morphine after pancreatic surgery: A double-blind study. *Anesth Analg* 1995;80:869–874.

456. van Essen EJ, Bovill JG, Ploeger EJ. Extradural clonidine does not potentiate analgesia produced by extradural morphine after meniscectomy. *Br J Anaesth* 1991;66:237–241.

457. Gautier PE, De Kock M, Fanard L, et al. Intrathecal clonidine combined with sufentanil for labor analgesia. *Anesthesiology* 1998;88:651–656.

458. Tallarida RJ. *Drug synergism and dose-effect data analysis.* Boca Raton, FL: Chapman & Hall/CRC, 2000.

459. Yamamoto T, Yaksh TL. Studies on the spinal interaction of morphine and the NMDA antagonist MK-801 on the hyperesthesia observed in a rat model of sciatic mononeuropathy. *Neurosci Lett* 1992;135:67–70.

460. Kosson D, Klinowiecka A, Kosson P, et al. Intrathecal antinociceptive interaction between the NMDA antagonist ketamine and the opioids, morphine and biphalin. *Eur J Pain* 2008;12:611–616.

461. Visser E, Schug SA. The role of ketamine in pain management. *Biomed Pharmacother* 2006;60(7):341–348.

462. Liu SS, Wu CL. Effect of postoperative analgesia on major postoperative complications: A systematic update of the evidence. *Anesth Analg* 2007;104:689–702.

463. Weinbroum AA. A single small dose of postoperative ketamine provides rapid and sustained improvement in morphine analgesia in the presence of morphine-resistant pain. *Anesth Analg* 2003;96:789–795.

464. Subramaniam B, Subramaniam K, Dilip K, et al. Preoperative epidural ketamine in combination with morphine does not have a clinically relevant intra- and postoperative opioid-sparing effect. *Anesth Analg* 2001;93 1321–1326.

465. Tucker AP, Kim YI, Nadeson R, Goodchild CS. Investigation of the potentiation of the analgesic effects of fentanyl by ketamine in humans: A double-blinded, randomised, placebo controlled, crossover study of experimental pain. *Anesthesiology* 2005;5:2.

466. Hawksworth C, Serpell M. Intrathecal anesthesia with ketamine. *Reg Anesth Pain Med* 1998;23:283–288.

467. Kathirvel S, Sadhasivam S, Saxena A, et al. Effects of intrathecal ketamine added to bupivacaine for spinal anaesthesia. *Anaesthesia* 2000;55:899–904.

468. Kawana Y, Sato H, Shimada H, et al. Epidural ketamine for postoperative pain relief after gynecologic operations: A double-blind study and comparison with epidural morphine. *Anesth Analg* 1987;66:735–738.

469. Wong CS, Liaw WJ, Tung CS, et al. Ketamine potentiates analgesic effect of morphine in postoperative epidural pain control. *Reg Anesth* 1996;21:534–541.

470. Sator-Katzenschlager S, Deusch E, Maier P, et al. The long-term antinociceptive effect of intrathecal S(+)-ketamine in a patient with established morphine tolerance. *Anesth Analg* 2001;93:1032–1034.

471. Tan PH, Kuo MC, Kao PF, et al. Patient-controlled epidural analgesia with morphine or morphine plus ketamine for postoperative pain relief. *Eur J Anaesthesiol* 1999;16:820–825.

472. Chia YY, Liu K, Liu YC, et al. Adding ketamine in a multimodal patient-controlled epidural regimen reduces postoperative pain and analgesic consumption. *Anesth Analg* 1998;86:1245–1249.

473. Lauretti GR, Gomes JM, Reis MP, et al. Low doses of epidural ketamine or neostigmine, but not midazolam, improve morphine analgesia in epidural terminal cancer pain therapy. *J Clin Anesth* 1999;11:663–668.

474. Yang CY, Wong CS, Chang JY, et al. Intrathecal ketamine reduces morphine requirements in patients with terminal cancer pain. *Can J Anaesth* 1996;43:379–383.

475. Naguib M, Yaksh TL. Antinociceptive effects of spinal cholinesterase inhibition and isobolographic analysis of the interaction with mu and alpha 2 receptor systems. *Anesthesiology* 1994;80:1338–1348.

476. Hood DD, Eisenach JC, Tuttle R. Phase I safety assessment of intrathecal neostigmine methylsulfate in humans. *Anesthesiology* 1995;82:331–343.

477. Lauretti GR, Mattos AL, Reis MP, et al. Intrathecal neostigmine for postoperative analgesia after orthopedic surgery. *J Clin Anesth* 1997;9:473–477.

478. Lauretti GR, Hood DD, Eisenach JC, et al. A multi-center study of intrathecal neostigmine for analgesia following vaginal hysterectomy. *Anesthesiology* 1998;89:913–918.

479. Abram SE, Winne RP. Intrathecal acetyl cholinesterase inhibitors produce analgesia that is synergistic with morphine and clonidine in rats. *Anesth Analg* 1995;81:501–507.

480. Hwang JH, Hwang KS, Choi Y, et al. An analysis of drug interaction between morphine and neostigmine in rats with nerve-ligation injury. *Anesth Analg* 2000;90:421–426.

481. Nelson KE, D'Angelo R, Foss ML, et al. Intrathecal neostigmine and sufentanil for early labor analgesia. *Anesthesiology* 1999;91:1293–1298.

482. Klamt JG, Garcia LV, Prado WA. Analgesic and adverse effects of a low dose of intrathecally administered hyperbaric neostigmine alone or combined with morphine in patients submitted to spinal anaesthesia: Pilot studies. *Anaesthesia* 1999;54:27–31.

483. Klamt JG, Dos RM, Barbieri NJ, et al. Analgesic effect of subarachnoid neostigmine in two patients with cancer pain. *Pain* 1996;66:389–391.

484. Lauretti GR, Mattos AL, Reis MP, et al. Combined intrathecal fentanyl and neostigmine: Therapy for postoperative abdominal hysterectomy pain relief. *J Clin Anesth* 1998;10:291–296.

485. Chung CJ, Kim JS, Park HS, et al. The efficacy of intrathecal neostigmine, intrathecal morphine, and their combination for post-cesarean section analgesia. *Anesth Analg* 1998;87:341–346.

486. Bouaziz H, Tong C, Eisenach JC. Postoperative analgesia from intrathecal neostigmine in sheep. *Anesth Analg* 1995;80:1140–1144.

487. Lavand'homme P, Pan HL, Eisenach JC. Intrathecal neostigmine, but not sympathectomy, relieves mechanical allodynia in a rat model of neuropathic pain. *Anesthesiology* 1998;89:493–499.

488. Hood DD, Mallak KA, Eisenach JC, et al. Interaction between intrathecal neostigmine and epidural clonidine in human volunteers. *Anesthesiology* 1996;85:315–325.

489. Owen MD, Ozsarac O, Sahin S, et al. Low-dose clonidine and neostigmine prolong the duration of intrathecal bupivacaine-fentanyl for labor analgesia. *Anesthesiology* 2000;92:361–366.

490. Pan PM, Huang CT, Wei TT, et al. Enhancement of analgesic effect of intrathecal neostigmine and clonidine on bupivacaine spinal anesthesia. *Reg Anesth Pain Med* 1998;23:49–56.

491. Hara K, Saito Y, Kirihara Y, et al. The interaction of antinociceptive effects of morphine and GABA receptor agonists within the rat spinal cord. *Anesth Analg* 1999;89:422–427.

492. Wang C, Chakrabarti MK, Whitwam JG. Synergism between the antinociceptive effects of intrathecal midazolam and fentanyl on both A delta and C somatosympathetic reflexes. *Neuropharmacology* 1993;32:303–305.

493. Plummer JL, Cmielewski PL, Gourlay GK, et al. Antinociceptive and motor effects of intrathecal morphine combined with intrathecal clonidine, noradrenaline, carbachol or midazolam in rats. *Pain* 1992;49:145–152.

494. Luger TJ, Hayashi T, Lorenz IH, et al. Mechanisms of the influence of midazolam on morphine antinociception at spinal and supraspinal levels in rats. *Eur J Pharmacol* 1994;271:421–431.

495. Nishiyama T, Gyermek L, Lee C, et al. Analgesic interaction between intrathecal midazolam and glutamate receptor antagonists on thermal-induced pain in rats. *Anesthesiology* 1999;91:531–537.

496. Hodgson PS, Neal JM, Pollock JE, et al. The neurotoxicity of drugs given intrathecally (spinal). *Anesth Analg* 1999;88:797–809.

497. Nishiyama T, Matsukawa T, Hanaoka K. Acute phase histopathological study of spinally administered midazolam in cats. *Anesth Analg* 1999;89:717–720.

498. Erdine S, Yucel A, Ozyalcin S, et al. Neurotoxicity of midazolam in the rabbit. *Pain* 1999;80:419–423.

499. Bahar M, Cohen ML, Grinshpoon Y, et al. An investigation of the possible neurotoxic effects of intrathecal midazolam combined with fentanyl in the rat. *Eur J Anaesthesiol* 1998;15:695–701.

500. Goodchild CS, Noble J. The effects of intrathecal midazolam on sympathetic nervous system reflexes in man: A pilot study. *Br J Clin Pharmacol* 1987;23:279–285.

501. Serrao JM, Marks RL, Morley SJ, et al. Intrathecal midazolam for the treatment of chronic mechanical low back pain: A controlled comparison with epidural steroid in a pilot study. *Pain* 1992;48:5–12.

502. Baaijens PFJ, van Dongen RTM, Crul BJP. Intrathecal midazolam for the treatment of chronic mechanical low back pain: A randomized double-blind placebo-controlled study. *Br J Anaesth* 1995;74;[Suppl 1]:A470.

503. Aguilar JL, Espachs P, Roca G, et al. Difficult management of pain following sacrococcygeal chordoma: 13 months of subarachnoid infusion. *Pain* 1994;59:317–320.

504. Barnes RK, Rosenfeld JV, Fennessy SS, et al. Continuous subarachnoid infusion to control severe cancer pain in an ambulant patient. *Med J Aust* 1994;161:549–551.

505. Valentine JM, Lyons G, Bellamy MC. The effect of intrathecal midazolam on post-operative pain. *Eur J Anaesthesiol* 1996;13:589–593.

506. Batra YK, Jain K, Chari P, et al. Addition of intrathecal midazolam to bupivacaine produces better post-operative analgesia without prolonging recovery. *Int J Clin Pharmacol Ther* 1999;37:519–523.

507. Naji P, Farschtschian M, Wilder-Smith OH, et al. Epidural droperidol and morphine for postoperative pain. *Anesth Analg* 1990;70:583–488.

508. Gurses E, Sungurtekin H, Tomatir E, et al. The addition of droperidol or clonidine to epidural tramadol shortens onset time and increases duration of postoperative analgesia. *Can J Anaesth* 2003;50(2):147–152.

509. Watkins LR, Milligan ED, Maier SF. Glial proinflammatory cytokines mediate exaggerated pain states: Implications for clinical pain. *Adv Exp Biol Med* 2003;521:1–21.

510. Romero-Sandoval A, Nutile-McMenemy N, DeLeo JA. Spinal microglial and perivascular cell cannabinoid receptor type 2 activation reduces behavioral hypersensitivity without tolerance after peripheral nerve injury. *Anesthesiology* 2008;108:722–734.

511. McMahon SB, Bennett DL. Trophic factors and pain. In: Wall PD, Melzack R, eds., *Textbook of pain.* New York: Churchill Livingstone, 1999:105–127.

512. Hunt SP, Mantyh PW. The molecular dynamics of pain control. *Nat Rev Neurosci* 2001;2:83–91.

513. McMahon SB, Bennett DL, Priestley JV, et al. The biological effects of endogenous nerve growth factor on adult sensory neurons revealed by a trkA-IgG fusion molecule. *Nat Med* 1995;1:774–780.

514. Kerr BJ, Bradbury EJ, Bennett DL, et al. Brain-derived neurotrophic factor modulates nociceptive sensory inputs and NMDA-evoked responses in the rat spinal cord. *J Neurosci* 1999;19:5138–5148.

515. Michael GJ, Averill S, Nitkunan A, et al. Nerve growth factor treatment increases brain-derived neurotrophic factor selectively in TrkA-expressing dorsal root ganglion cells and in their central terminations within the spinal cord. *J Neurosci* 1997;17:8476–8490.

516. Cho HJ, Kim JK, Zhou XF, et al. Increased brain-derived neurotrophic factor immunoreactivity in rat dorsal root ganglia and spinal cord following peripheral inflammation. *Brain Res* 1997;764:269–272.

517. Levine ES, Crozier RA, Black IB, et al. Brain-derived neurotrophic factor modulates hippocampal synaptic transmission by increasing N-methyl-d-aspartic acid receptor activity. *Proc Natl Acad Sci USA* 1998;95:10235–10239.

518. Mannion RJ, Costigan M, Decosterd I, et al. Neurotrophins: Peripherally and centrally acting modulators of tactile stimulus-induced inflammatory pain hypersensitivity. *Proc Natl Acad Sci USA* 1999;96:9385–9390.

519. Thompson SW, Bennett DL, Kerr BJ, et al. Brain-derived neurotrophic factor is an endogenous modulator of nociceptive responses in the spinal cord. *Proc Natl Acad Sci USA* 1999;96:7714–7718.

520. Michael GJ, Averill S, Shortland PJ, et al. Axotomy results in major changes in BDNF expression by dorsal root ganglion cells: BDNF expression in large trkB and trkC cells, in pericellular baskets, and in projections to deep dorsal horn and dorsal column nuclei. *Eur J Neurosci* 1999;11:3539–3551.

521. Walker SM, Mitchell VA, White DM, et al. Release of immunoreactive brain-derived neurotrophic factor in the spinal cord of the rat following sciatic nerve transection. *Brain Res* 2001;890:240–247.

522. Theodosiou M, Rush RA, Zhou XF, et al. Hyperalgesia due to nerve damage: Role of nerve growth factor. *Pain* 1999;81:245–255.

523. Zhou XF, Deng YS, Xian CJ, et al. Neurotrophins from dorsal root ganglia trigger allodynia after spinal nerve injury in rats. *Eur J Neurosci* 2000;12:100–105.

524. White DM. Contribution of neurotrophin-3 to the neuropeptide Y-induced increase in neurite outgrowth of rat dorsal root ganglion cells. *Neuroscience* 1998;86:257–263.

525. White DM. Neurotrophin-3 antisense oligonucleotide attenuates nerve injury-induced Abeta-fibre sprouting. *Brain Res* 2000;885:79–86.

526. Bennett DL, Boucher TJ, Armanini MP, et al. The glial cell line-derived neurotrophic factor family receptor components are differentially regulated within sensory neurons after nerve injury. *J Neurosci* 2000;20:427–437.

527. Boucher TJ, Okuse K, Bennett DL, et al. Potent analgesic effects of GDNF in neuropathic pain states. *Science* 2000;290:124–127.

528. Carr DB, Goudas LC. Acute pain. *Lancet* 1999;353:2051–2058.

529. Echeverry S, Shi XQ, Zhang J. Characterization of cell proliferation in rat spinal cord following peripheral nerve injury and the relationship with chronic pain. *Pain* 2008;135:37–47.

530. Okuse K. Pain signaling pathways: From cytokines to ion channels. *Int J Biochem Cell Biol* 2007;39:490–496.

531. Horlocker TT, Wedel DJ, Benzon H, et al. Regional anesthesia in the anticoagulated patient: Defining the risks (the second ASRA Consensus Conference on Neuraxial Anesthesia and Anticoagulation). *Reg Anesth Pain Med* 2003;28,172–197.

532. Schneider MC, Hampl KF. Complications of epidural and spinal anesthesia in adults. *Curr Op Anesth* 1995;8:414.

533. Kamei J, Kasuya, Y. The effects of diabetes on opioid-induced antinociception. In: Tseng LF, ed., *The pharmacology of opioid peptides.* Langhorn, PA: Harwood Academic Press, 1995;271.

534. Cherry DA, Gourlay GK, Cousins MJ. Extradural mass associated with lack of efficacy of epidural morphine, and undetectable CSF morphine concentrations. *Pain* 1986;25:69.

535. Cherry DA. Drug delivery systems for epidural administration of opioids. *Acta Anaesthesiol Scand* 1987;[Suppl]:54–59.

536. Coombs DW. Management of chronic pain by epidural and intrathecal opioids. Newer drugs and delivery systems. In: Sjostrand UH, Rawal N, eds., Regional opioids in anesthesiology and pain management. *Int Anesthesiol Clin* 1986;24:59–74.

537. Nitescu P, Sjoberg M, Appelgren L, Curelaru, I, et al. Complications of intrathecal opioids and bupivacaine in the treatment of "refractory" cancer pain. *Clin J Pain* 1995;11:45–62.

538. Wanscher M, Riishede L, Krogh, B. Fistula formation following epidural catheter: A case report. *Acta Anaesthesiol Scand* 1985;29:552–553.

539. Nielson TH, Husegaard HC, Joensen F. Tunnel-leret spiduralkateter og infektion. *Ugeskr Laeger* 1985;147:1548–1549.

540. Muller H, Borner U, Stoyanov M, et al. Pendurale opiatapplikation bie malignombedingten chronischen schmerzen. *Anaesth Intensivther Notfallmed* 1981;16:251–257.

541. Zenz M, Schappler-Scheele B, Neuhans R, et al. Long term peridural morphine analgesia in cancer pain. *Lancet* 1981;1:91.

542. Rodan BA, Cohen FL, Bean WJ, et al. Fibrous mass complicating epidural morphine infusion. *Neurosurgery* 1985;16:68–70.

543. Crul B, Delhass E. Technical complications during long-term subarachnoid or epidural administration of morphine in terminally ill cancer patients: A review of 140 cases. *Reg Anesth* 1991;16:209–213.

544. Laffer U, Brachman-Mettler I, Metzger U, eds. *Implantable drug delivery systems.* Switzerland: S Karger AG, 1991.

545. Penn RD, Paice JA, Gottschalk W, et al. Cancer pain relief using chronic morphine infusion. Early experience with a programmable implanted drug pump. *J Neurosurg* 1984;61:302–306.

546. Medtronic. Letter from Archana Sabananthan (June 27, 2008). Proper Connection of Sutureless Connector Intrathecal Catheters. Retrieved August 14, 2008 from: http://www.medtronic.com/restoreultra/product-advisories.html.

547. Medtronic. Letter from George Aram (May 2008). Medical Device Recall. SynchroMed® II Missing Propellant. Retrieved August 14, 2008 from: http://www.medtronic.com/restoreultra/product-advisories.html.

548. Medtronic. Letter (August 2007). SynchroMed® EL Pump Motor Stall Due To Gear Shaft Wear. Retrieved August 15, 2008 from: http://www.medtronic.com/restoreultra/product-advisories.html.

549. Carr DB, Eidelman A. Clinical study design. In: Krames E, Peckham PH, Rezai AR, eds., *Textbook of neuromodulation.* Oxford: Blackwell Publishing, in press.

550. Abram SE, Hopwood M. Can meta-analysis rescue knowledge from a sea of unintelligible data? *Reg Anesth* 1996;21:514–516.
551. Jadad AR. Meta-analysis in pain relief: A valuable but easily misused tool. *Curr Op Anesth* 1996;9:426–429.
552. Wittink HM, Carr DB, eds. *Pain management: Evidence, outcomes and quality of life*. St. Louis: Elsevier, 2008.
553. Jacox AK, Carr DB, Payne R, et al. Management of Cancer Pain. Clinical Practice Guideline No. 9. Rockville, MD: Agency for Health Care Policy and Research, Public Health Service, U.S. Department of Health & Human Services; 1994. AHCPR Pub. No. 94-0592.
554. Rathmell JP, Wu CL, Sinatra RS, et al. Acute post-surgical pain management: A critical appraisal of current practice. *Reg Anesth Pain Med* 2006;31[Suppl 1]:1–42.
555. Perkins FM, Kehlet H. Chronic pain as an outcome of surgery: A review of predictive factors. *Anesthesiology* 2000;93:1123–1133.
556. Shields D, Montenegro R, Aclan J. Chemical stability of admixtures combining ziconotide with baclofen during simulated intrathecal administration. *Neuromodulation* 2007;10[Suppl 1]:12–17.
557. Shields D, Montenegro R, Aclan J. Chemical stability of an admixture combining ziconotide and bupivacaine during simulated intrathecal administration. *Neuromodulation* 2007;10[Suppl 1]:1–5.
558. Curatolo M, Schnider TW, Petersen-Felix S, et al. A direct search procedure to optimize combinations of epidural bupivacaine, fentanyl, and clonidine for postoperative analgesia. *Anesthesiology* 2000;92:325–337.
559. Eastman M, Johnson S. Ziconotide combination intrathecal therapy. *Practical Pain Manage* 2007;30–38.
560. Mogil JS, McCarson KE. Finding pain genes: Bottom-up and top-down approaches. *J Pain* 2000;1[Suppl1]:66–80.
561. Mogil JS. The genetic mediation of individual differences in sensitivity to pain and its inhibition. *Proc Natl Acad Sci USA* 1999;96:7744–7751.
562. Coghill RC, McHaffie JG, Yen Y. Neural correlates of interindividual differences in the subjective experience of pain. *Proc Natl Acad Sci USA* 2003; 100:8538–8542.
563. Dib-Hajj SD, Rush AM, Cummins TR, et al. Gain of function mutation in NaV1.7 in familial erythromelalgia induces bursting of sensory neurons. *Brain* 2005;128:1847–1854.
564. Nagasako EM, Oaklander AL, Dworkin RH. Congenital insensitivity to pain: An update. *Pain* 2003;101:213–219.
565. Tegeder I, Costigan M, Griffin RS, et al. GTP cyclohydrolase and tetrahydrobiopterin regulate pain sensitivity and persistence. *Nature Med* 2006;12:1269–1277.
566. Siddall PJ, Cousins MJ. Persistent pain as a disease entity: Implications for clinical management. *Anesth Analg* 2004 99:510–520.
567. Brennan F, Carr DB, Cousins MJ. Pain management: A fundamental human right. *Anesth Analg.* 2007;105:205–221.
568. Carr DB. The development of national guidelines for pain control: Synopsis and commentary. *Eur J Pain* 2001;5[Suppl A]:91–98.
569. Stewart WF, Ricci JA, Chee E, et al. Lost productive time and cost due to common pain conditions in the US workforce. *JAMA* 2003;290:2443–2454.
570. Van Leeuwen MT, Blyth FM, March LM, et al. Chronic pain and reduced work effectiveness: The hidden cost to Australian employers. *Eur J Pain* 2006;2:161–166.

CHAPTER 41 ■ NEUROSTIMULATION

JOSHUA P. PRAGER AND MICHAEL STANTON-HICKS

For more than 30 years, interventional pain specialists have used spinal cord stimulation (SCS) to treat a variety of pain syndromes. Unlike neuroablation, SCS offers the opportunity to evaluate efficacy during a preimplantation screening trial, spares nerve tissue, and can later be reversed if necessary. In 1967, Shealy and colleagues reported on the first clinical application of SCS for pain management using electrodes placed surgically within the subarachnoid space (1). Building on the gate control theory of pain postulated only a few years earlier by Melzack and Wall (2), they sought to activate large-diameter nerve fibers selectively, thereby closing the gate for transmission of pain via small-diameter fibers in the dorsal horn of the spinal cord. Early enthusiasm for the procedure waned due to mixed clinical results (3,4). Two developments spurred renewed interest in SCS—consistent definitions of pain types by the International Association for the Study of Pain (IASP), which allowed the indications for SCS to be refined and standardized, and technologic advances in stimulation equipment, including multichannel implanted pulse generators (IPGs) and a variety of implantable or percutaneous electrodes placed through a needle without need for incision. The percutaneous technique permitted a prognostic trial of stimulation, to demonstrate potential efficacy before committing to an open surgical procedure. As the specific indications for SCS were defined and new stimulation systems became available, outcomes improved (5). Ample clinical evidence now supports the value of SCS in relieving chronic neuropathic pain resulting from failed back surgery syndrome (FBSS), complex regional pain syndrome (CRPS) I and II, and a variety of other pain conditions (6). Equipment also continues to evolve, with rechargeable miniaturized devices, robust programming capabilities, variation of lead design for specific applications, and greater patient control of devices being among the most recent improvements.

DORSAL COLUMN STIMULATION

Historical Overview

Electrotherapy boasts an ancient although not always distinguished history. In 46 A.D., the Roman physician Scribonius Largus, who first wrote about the medical application of electricity, mentions using the electrical discharge of torpedo fish to treat gout and headache (7). The invention of the Leyden jar in 1745 allowed manmade electricity to be applied to the treatment of pain (8). By the late 18th century, the English surgeon, John Birch, reported treating cases of low back pain and gout with electrostatic machines. The Galvani–Volta controversy, which led to the invention of the electrochemical battery in 1800, introduced "galvanism," the application of galvanic cur-

rent to the human body. This therapeutic "contact electricity" eliminated the painful sparks that often accompanied earlier static electrical treatments. In 1823, Chevalier Sarlandiére proposed delivering electric current through acupuncture needles, and he began using electroacupuncture to treat patients suffering from gout, arthritis, and sciatic and lumbo-sacral neuralgias (9). The Danish scientist Hans Christian Oersted launched modern electrotherapy in 1891, by demonstrating that a magnetic field surrounds an electric current. Numerous European scientists and physicians began studying electromagnetic induction and applying "localized electrization," "catalytic action," and "interrupted" current clinically. In his *Treatise on Medical Electricity*, Julius Althaus became the first to report using transcutaneous current applied to peripheral nerves as a method of pain relief (10,11).

In North America, electrotherapy was championed by the medical profession as well as exploited by quacks. In 1891, Drs. Beard and Rockwell (12) published a popular and influential treatise on electrotherapy that contained a chapter on neuralgia and low back pain. By the turn of the 19th century, the majority of American physicians were employing electrical machines in their practices, often without any scientific basis. Release of the Flexner Report in 1910 triggered major reforms in medical education and effectively ended the era of pseudoscientific therapies, including electrotherapy. In addition, conditions previously treated with electrotherapy increasingly seemed amenable to diagnosis with radiography and treatment with analgesics. Yet electrophysiologic experiments continued, most notably using induction coil techniques for cardiac pacing (13) The gate theory of pain, proposed by Melzack and Wall in 1965 (2), furnished a credible anatomic and physiologic explanation for the efficacy of analgesic electrotherapy that could be tested experimentally. Their theory—that nonpainful stimuli can inhibit pain—formed the original basis for contemporary neurostimulation. As the gate theory continues to be refined and expanded, and simultaneously as the mechanism of neurostimulation is better understood, there is now controversy as to how well the gate theory explains how SCS actually produces pain relief.

Shealy and his neurosurgeon colleagues (1), noting that Wall had demonstrated pain reduction by peripheral nerve stimulation (14), viewed dorsal column stimulation as a natural extension. They applied advances in cardiac pacemaker technology to the electrical inhibition of neuropathic pain due to cancer by directly delivering current through electrodes implanted subdurally using externally powered stimulators. First reports of their experimental results were so controversial that they were refused publication in the *Journal of Neurosurgery* (15). Although Shealy made remarkable gains and enjoyed early success, he eventually abandoned dorsal column stimulation because of technical problems, surgical complications,

TABLE 41-1

DEFINITIONS OF KEY TERMS ASSOCIATED WITH SPINAL CORD STIMULATION

Array	A two-dimensional arrangement of stimulating contacts either prefabricated on insulated backing as a paddle or plate, or created by insertion of percutaneous electrodes in parallel. Most commonly, and of necessity if placed percutaneously, the contacts are arranged longitudinally in columns; an array may have any number of columns. A prefabricated paddle or plate may have contacts in a diamond pattern or in rows.
Channel	A pulse generator or radiofrequency (RF) receiver output, which is independent of other outputs, in particular as to amplitude (voltage or current). A true multichannel stimulator will allow simultaneous delivery of different amplitudes to different contacts. (A programmable multicontact stimulator which allows rapid sequential delivery of pulses to different contacts approaches this, but it is not, strictly speaking, a multichannel device.)
Contact	An electrically conductive point or surface from which current passes into tissue. Contemporary electrode arrays have multiple contacts.
Electrode	An assembly of electrically conductive contacts and wires, along with insulating spacers, catheters, and backing material. Most often used to refer to the "business end" of the assembly, where contacts deliver stimulation current to tissue. (Sometimes used to refer simply to a stimulating contact; but electrodes include insulation and other materials.)
Implantable pulse generator (IPG)	A battery-driven power source for electrically activating a contact array(s); designed to be implanted in a subcutaneous location not requiring an external apparatus to activate but may have an external control for off-on, amplitude, and rate control.
Lead	A linear arrangement of conductors and insulations—wires and their circumferential insulation, between stimulating contacts and connectors. (Sometimes used to refer to the entire electrode, particularly if it is a percutaneous, catheter design.)
Paddle	A flat, essentially two-dimensional insulated electrode or array. As it cannot be inserted percutaneously (through a needle) it is implanted in the spinal canal by laminotomy or laminectomy. Also termed a plate electrode.
Receiver	With regard to SCS, a device that is implanted in a subcutaneous location and designed to receive AM radio frequency transmissions from an external source. These transmissions are converted to an electrical signal, which activates an implanted contact array(s).

North American Neuromodulation Society. Definitions.

the difficulty of selecting appropriate patients, and high failure rates among patients in the hands of inexperienced implanters. Subsequent progress in all of these areas has established neurostimulation as an effective therapy for carefully selected and screened patients in expert hands. Today the North American Neuromodulation Society and the International Neuromodulation Society act as interdisciplinary forums for continuing improvements.

Practitioners adopted the broader term "spinal cord stimulation" to describe the procedure more accurately, as the complex mechanisms of electrical stimulation became clearer. The clinical goals of SCS have always been to relieve pain and to reduce the use of medication, with patients potentially benefitting from better quality of life (QOL), renewed ability to perform activities of daily living (ADL), and return to work in some cases (6). Achieving these goals depends, in turn, on the technical goal of producing "stimulation paresthesia at a subjectively tolerable (comfortable) level, overlapping (covering) a patient's topography of pain" (6). Yet, technical success does not necessarily guarantee clinical success. Thus, the development of SCS has relied heavily on clinical observations, continuing elucidation of the anatomy, physiology, and psychology of pain, and successive technical improvements. Two clinical observations stand out—SCS more effectively curbs neuropathic or sympathetically mediated pain than nociceptive pain, and stimulation appears to suppress chronic but not acute pain. Today, the most common indication for SCS in North America is chronic neuropathic pain (6,16). Europeans use SCS most often to treat ischemic pain associated with intractable angina pectoris (17) and peripheral vascular disease (18).

As SCS has become more standardized, so too have the definitions for key terms. This chapter uses the terminology and

definitions developed by the North American Neuromodulation Society (Table 41-1) (19).

MECHANISM OF ACTION

The first application of SCS for chronic pain was based on the gate theory of pain (2), which postulated that a gate existed in the dorsal horn of the spinal cord that governed the central transmission of neural activity signaling pain. This gate was opened when small afferent fiber activity exceeded large afferent fiber activity in the peripheral nervous system; conversely, the gate was closed when large fiber activity predominated. To its early proponents, SCS represented a means of electively closing the gate, thereby reducing or eliminating painful inputs to the spinal cord and brain. Although the general mechanism of pain relief produced by SCS is still understood in these gating terms, the truth is considerably more complex. How can we explain, for example, that closing the gate works effectively to manage chronic, neuropathic pain but not acute, nociceptive pain? Researchers at the Karolinska Institute in Sweden (20) and the University of Oklahoma (21) have published in-depth reviews of current experimental and clinical studies of the mechanisms operating in SCS.

Understanding the mechanism of action that underlies SCS begins with a knowledge of the anatomy of the peripheral nervous system (PNS) and central nervous system (CNS). Figure 41-1 depicts the peripheral nerve fibers and their relationship to the spinal cord tract. Electrical impulses (action potentials) generated by sensory stimuli travel along afferent nerve fibers of the PNS to the spinal cord, which is part of the CNS. These sensory impulses ascend three orders of neurons

PART IV: PAIN MANAGEMENT

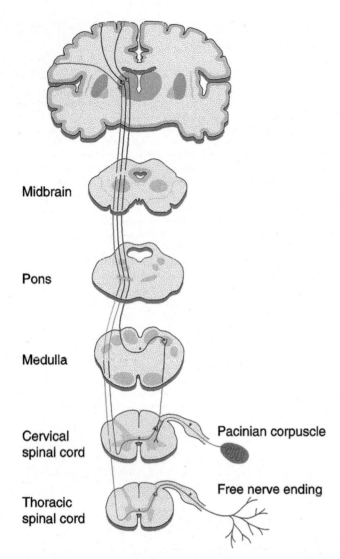

Midbrain

Pons

Medulla

Cervical
spinal cord

Pacinian corpuscle

Free nerve ending

Thoracic
spinal cord

FIGURE 41-1. The spinal cord tract and peripheral fibers. From Oakley JC, Prager JP. Spinal cord stimulation: Mechanisms of action. *Spine* 2002;27(22):2574–2583, with permission.

as they move from the PNS to the CNS. First-order neurons are the primary afferent fibers. Second-order neurons exist in the dorsal horn of the spinal cord, where excitatory and inhibitory signals are processed and modulated. Projection to higher brain structures involves third-order neurons. The brain receives, interprets, and responds to incoming nociceptive signals projected from the spinal cord to the thalamus, which processes input before relaying it to the cerebral cortex. The cerebral cortex identifies, modulates, and interprets sensations, and then oversees behavioral responses. Initially, the brain may suppress incoming impulses through antinociception or a descending analgesic pathway, thereby reducing pain perception. However, intense, prolonged noxious stimuli eventually cause tissue damage, which sensitizes peripheral nerves. In the presence of persistent and prolonged pain, signals in the spinal cord switch from inhibition to amplification, and damaged nerves undergo physiologic changes resulting from intracellular enzyme cascades, receptor modifications, and novel gene expression. These changes characterize the progression of pain as a symptom of acute injury to pain itself as a chronic disease (see Chapters 31 and 32).

TABLE 41-2

RELATIVE CONDUCTIVITY OF INTRASPINAL ELEMENTS

Tissue	Relative conductivity
Gray matter	0.23
White matter	
Longitudinal	0.6
Transverse	0.08
Cerebrospinal fluid	1.7
Epidural fat	0.04
Dura mater	0.03
Vertebral bone	0.02
Electrode insulation	0.002

Electrical Effects

Electrical stimulation depends on the conductivity of the intraspinal elements in relation to the electrical lead position. A depolarized neuron that is electrically positive (+) produces an action potential, allowing painful signals to proceed. A hyperpolarized, negatively charged (–) neuron loses the ability to propagate an action potential or raises the threshold for propagation. Careful placement of external electrodes allows SCS to produce the same effects. The negatively charged cathode is the active electrode in SCS; the positively charged anode shields neuronal structures from the effects of stimulation. The relative position of electrodes and their distance from the spinal cord are major determinants of axonal activation and paresthesia distribution (22).

Cerebrospinal fluid (CSF) is the most conductive intraspinal element, so any electrical field that encompasses the CSF has the greatest potential to be conducted to nearby structures (Table 41-2). Of the intraspinal structures, the longitudinal white matter demonstrates the greatest conductivity, transverse white matter is much less conductive, and gray matter falls in between (Fig. 41-2). Epidural fat demonstrates high impedance; thus, a lead placed in the most posterior region of the epidural space, in a part of the spine with large epidural spaces such as in the thoracic region, demonstrates low conductivity. Thus, paresthesia thresholds are highest in the mid thoracic region and lowest in the cervical area, where the posterior epidural space is smallest. Dura mater, which also has low conductivity, presents no significant resistance because it is so thin. Vertebral bone is least conductive, insulating thoracic (the heart) and pelvic organs from the electrical field produced by SCS.

Large-diameter nerve fibers have relatively low thresholds for recruitment by external cathodes. In the spinal cord, particularly near the dorsal column, the primary afferent fibers are conveniently segregated from motor fibers, which may possess a similar activation threshold. These afferent neurons can be selectively activated and may close the gate through their respective collateral processes to the dorsal horn. The original term "dorsal column stimulation" came from the position of the stimulating electrodes over the dorsal columns of the spinal cord. Although topographically accurate, the term proved physiologically simplistic and "spinal cord stimulation" is now preferred (see also Chapter 32).

The clinical goal of SCS is to produce an electrical field that stimulates the relevant spinal cord structures without stimulating the nearby nerve root. The threshold current necessary

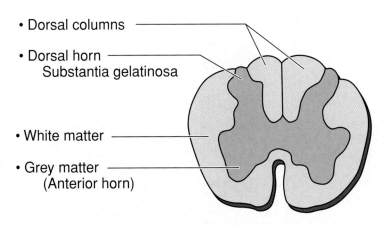

- Dorsal columns
- Dorsal horn
  Substantia gelatinosa
- White matter
- Grey matter
  (Anterior horn)

FIGURE 41-2. Cross-section of the spinal cord. Dorsal root sensory fibers are curved and their large diameter significantly reduces the threshold required for their activation. Dorsal column fibers are straight and carry nonpainful sensation (Aβ). They have collateral branches for reflexes and decrease in size as they ascend. From Oakley JC, Prager JP. Spinal cord stimulation: Mechanisms of action. *Spine* 2002;27(22):2574–2583, with permission.

to stimulate a nerve fiber increases with the distance between the fiber and the cathode, and is inversely related to the fiber diameter (23). This information allows predictions regarding the recruitment order of fibers, whether in a peripheral nerve, spinal root, or central pathway. Short pulses favor stimulation of large nerve fibers; wide pulses favor stimulation of smaller fibers. In SCS, improved paresthesia coverage may be achieved with pulses of 0.5 to 1 ms.

Barolat described the placement of the active electrode (cathode) in relation to the area in which paresthesia is produced (24). He and his colleagues mapped sensory responses to epidural stimulation, as demonstrated in Figure 41-3. The lead contact typically rests several levels above the intended area for concordant paresthesia. If the lead is close to the midline, the electrical field will reach the spinal cord before reaching the nerve root at the level of the lead. The low threshold of the dorsal root sensory fibers makes it imperative that lead position be sufficiently midline to avoid recruitment of the root. Stimulation of the low-threshold nerve root produces the sensation of paresthesia along the nerve root and, although it is neurostimulation, it is not SCS.

The goal of SCS is to create paresthesia that completely and consistently covers the painful areas, yet does not cause uncomfortable sensations in other areas (25). This paresthesia production is accomplished by stimulating Aβ fibers in the dorsal column (DC) and/or the dorsal roots (DR). Dorsal column stimulation typically causes paresthesia in several dermatomes at and below the level of the cathode. In contrast, DR stimulation activates fibers in a limited number of rootlets in close proximity to the cathode and causes paresthesia in only a few dermatomes. Because of these factors, DR stimulation may not produce sufficient pain relief. Another potential drawback to DR stimulation is that the roots also contain large proprioceptive fibers which, when stimulated, can cause uncomfortable sensations and motor responses (26). These side effects can occur at pulse amplitudes that are below the value needed for full paresthesia coverage.

Because the perception of pain is subjective, the appropriate usage level must be individually defined. The usage range is the interval between the perception threshold, the amplitude necessary to produce paresthesia, and the discomfort threshold, the point at which the patient can no longer tolerate the paresthesia. The maximum therapeutic amplitude rarely exceeds 170% of the perception threshold (23). During screening, a lead activated in the mid usage range can be physically moved to the position that produces the best pain relief coverage for the patient (22). This technique is described as active electrode screening, commonly referred to as "trolling." More

advanced systems now allow trolling to be performed electronically, minimizing the need to physically move the lead. At amplitudes used clinically for pain relief, SCS produces peripheral, antidromically activated compound action potentials over major peripheral nerves (see Chapter 32, Fig. 32-32). Peripheral nerve stimulation reduces primary afferent conduction velocity, the conduction safety factor, and neuroma discharge (14,27), and these effects are selective according to fiber size. Thus, stimulation peripherally likely blocks normal afferent activity, suggesting that SCS relieves pain partially through peripheral effects.

Clinical observations have also demonstrated that therapeutic response only occurs in a limited range of frequencies. For example, nerve fibers fail to conduct action potentials when stimulated at higher frequencies (≥300–500 pps) (23) due to a depolarization block or neurotransmitter depletion, an effect known as frequency dependent conduction. Others describe clinically useful higher-frequency stimulation (28), which may produce phase cancellation. When the pulse frequency becomes smaller than the refractory period, the largest fibers will continue to activate regularly whereas smaller fibers will not. This effect is most pronounced at junctures where larger fibers branch into smaller ones, such as where primary afferent neurons to the dorsal column branch to the dorsal horn (29). Similarly, frequencies lower than 25 to 30 Hz may exacerbate pain in patients undergoing SCS.

Evoked activity occurs in the dorsal and ventral spinal cord at the level of the dorsal horn (30). In patients who experience pain relief, inhibition of the RIII flexor reflex suggests a local dorsal horn contribution (31). Recordings from the human thalamus have also shown CNS effects during SCS, perhaps representing an evoked potential effect related to pain relief. In animals, SCS activates the anterior pretectal nucleus, which controls descending pain inhibitory action. The period of inhibitory influence noted in animals is consistent with the pain relief reported by humans after stimulation.

Neurochemical Effects

Neurochemically, SCS may act to restore normal γ-aminobutyric acid (GABA) levels in the dorsal horn and possibly to effect the release of the central neuromodulator adenosine (32), thus reducing neuropathic pain. In rats, SCS induces GABA release (33), which apparently attenuates the release of excitatory amino acids, such as glutamate and aspartate (34). Spinal cord stimulation clearly does not work through the endogenous opioid system. However, work with neurotransmitters suggests that the infusion of adenosine or

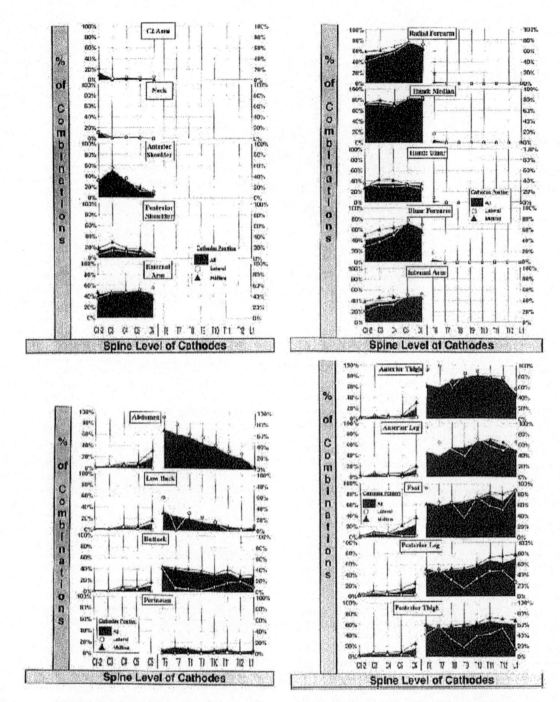

FIGURE 41-3. Distribution of paresthesias induced by epidural stimulation of neural structures. From Oakley JC, Prager JP. Spinal cord stimulation: Mechanisms of action. *Spine* 2002;27(22):2574–2583, with permission.

GABA$_B$ agonist baclofen may be helpful in potentiating the effects of stimulation (30,33,35).

Sympathetic Nervous System Effects

The use of SCS in treating angina pectoris suggests that dorsal column stimulation can produce both anti-anginal and anti-ischemic activity in an organ. Canine studies have documented modulated intrinsic cardiac neuronal activity when the dorsal aspect of the thoracic cord is stimulated electrically (36). Both sympathetic afferent and efferent fibers likely contribute to suppression of intrinsic cardiac activity during SCS. Anti-anginal effects decrease noxious inputs to pain pathways in the spinal cord, and the anti-ischemic effects are mediated by release of vasoactive substances. Linderoth and colleagues (37) and Croom and colleagues (38) demonstrated that stimulation increased blood flow at two-thirds and 90% of motor stimulation threshold, respectively. The vasodilative effect requires intact

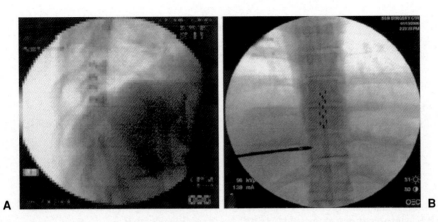

FIGURE 41-4. Transverse tripolar spinal cord stimulation using three Pisces Quad leads and a Synergy internal pulse generator (AP view). Programming with the Synergy system allows two separate simultaneous programs and multiple permutations of contact combinations. The marker is on T_{10}. The cathodes are in the middle, anodes guard laterally. From Oakley JC, Prager JP. Spinal cord stimulation: Mechanisms of action. *Spine* 2002;27(22):2574–2583, with permission.

dorsal roots. Release of calcitonin gene-related peptide (CGRP) at the synaptic terminal sites also causes vasodilation, mediated through antidromic activation of interneurons (38). At high stimulation thresholds (80%), antidromic effects are seen; at low stimulation thresholds (63%), orthodromic effects are seen. The anti-ischemic and analgesic benefits of SCS noted in patients with angina may also apply to those with peripheral ischemia, and possibly to those with CRPS.

Neurophysiologic Effects

Spinal cord stimulation appears to mainly affect pain related to Aβ fiber functions but not C fibers (31). Sciatic nerve injury, for example, increases the spontaneous firing of wide-dynamic-range (WDR) neurons responsive to sensory input from mechanical, chemical, and thermal receptors in the deeper lamina of the rat dorsal horn. Spinal cord stimulation suppresses these effects (24,39). Dorsal column lesions substantially lessen the effect of SCS, suggesting a dorsal column contribution to the SCS effect. Transecting the spinal cord above the level of SCS further reduces the effect of stimulation, indicating both supraspinal and segmental mechanisms. In animals, SCS modifies brainstem activity in the anterior pretectal nucleus, which is associated with descending pain inhibitory pathways (40).

Computer Modeling

A finite-element computer model has been used to study the distribution of electrical fields in spinal tissues of varying densities, to design electrodes, and to select targets for stimulation (41). The model predicts that the DR and DC fiber thresholds for stimulation are dependent on the dorsal CSF space, the position of the stimulating cathode with respect to the physiologic midline of the spinal cord, and the arrangement of negative and positive electrodes within a stimulating array (26). Modeling predicts the clinically confirmed observation that stimulation of the dorsal column is most efficient with closely spaced longitudinal bipolar (+/−) or tripolar (+/−/+) configurations centered on the spinal cord, where the main delivered current corresponds to the orientation of the nerve fibers (42). The model also predicts that narrower electrode spacing produces a more centralized stimulation with improved stimulation selectivity, although at the expense of power consumption (43). The model suggests that a transverse tripolar arrangement across

the spinal cord can be used to steer the paresthesias electrically into an area of pain, rather than moving an electrode mechanically until pain control is achieved (44).

Better DC versus DR recruitment, higher usage ranges, and preferential avoidance of dorsal roots have been modeled successfully with a 4-8-4 array and transverse tripoles (45,46).

Most predictions of the model have been confirmed clinically. Figure 41-4 illustrates transverse tripolar SCS in a patient with failed back syndrome (47). Spinal cord stimulation has been traditionally recognized as an effective therapy in the treatment of radicular pain; its use to achieve pain relief in the axial low back has been more difficult (24,48). A small, theoretical region found between the T8 and T9 vertebral level junction (i.e., corresponding to the L1 and L2 spinal nerves innervating the low back) has been identified as an optimal SCS target for low back pain (49,50).

INDICATIONS FOR SPINAL CORD STIMULATION

The clinical results of SCS demonstrate that it controls the neuropathic component of pain more effectively than the nociceptive component, and treats pain associated with the sympathetic nervous system more effectively than that caused by the somatic nervous system. Neuropathic pain results from injury to the nervous system and commonly coexists with nociceptive or ischemic pain (see also Chapter 46). Anxiety and depression can also add to the perception of pain, complicating the clinical presentation. Results of SCS reported in the clinical literature support its use, in order of effectiveness, for the following indications: intractable angina (90% effective) (17), ischemic pain due to peripheral vascular disease (18), CRPS types I and II (formerly called reflex sympathetic dystrophy or causalgia) (16), and persistent neuropathic pain after spinal surgery (50% effective) (51). Recently North, Shipley, and members of The Neuromodulation Therapy Access Coalition (NTAC) published *Practice Parameters for the Use of Spinal Cord Stimulation in the Treatment of Chronic Neuropathic Pain,* a comprehensive, evidence-based literature review and consensus statement regarding SCS (6). Their detailed analyses represent the most extensive examination to date of

TABLE 41-3

INDICATIONS FOR SPINAL CORD STIMULATION SUPPORTED BY AN
EVIDENCE-BASED LITERATURE REVIEW AND CONSENSUS STATEMENT

Indication	Grade and evidence sources
Failed back surgery syndrome or lumbosacral root injury pain (arachnoiditis)	A ■ Well-designed randomized controlled trial (RCT) ■ Well-designed clinical studies ■ Weighing risk vs. potential benefit and expert consensus reveals a high likelihood of a favorable outcome
Complex regional pain syndrome (CRPS) I (reflex sympathetic dystrophy) and CRPS II (causalgia)	A ■ Well-designed RCT ■ Well-designed clinical studies ■ Weighing risk vs. potential benefit and expert consensus reveals a high likelihood of a favorable outcome
Other indications: peripheral neuropathic pain, phantom limb/postamputation syndrome, postherpetic neuralgia, root injury pain, spinal cord injury/lesion	B ■ Well-designed clinical studies ■ Case reports ■ Weighing risk vs. potential benefit and expert consensus reveals a good likelihood of a favorable outcome

From North RB, Shipley J. The Neuromodulation Therapy Access Coalition. Practice parameters for the use of spinal cord stimulation in the treatment of chronic neuropathic pain. *Pain Med* 2007;8:S200–S275, with permission.

the likelihood of success with SCS for specific indications and of the associated risks and benefits.

Failed Back Surgery Syndrome

Failed back surgery syndrome euphemistically describes a varied group of conditions suffered by patients who continue to experience debilitating nociceptive-neuropathic pain after lumbar spine surgery. Cases of FBSS described in the literature include lumbosacral pain, buttock pain, and sometimes diffuse lower extremity pain, which are attributed to incorrect diagnosis, wrong level of surgery, psychological illness, arachnoiditis, lumbosacral epidural fibrosis, radiculitis, vertebral instability, and recurrent disk herniations (52).

The lifetime prevalence of lumbar surgery in the United States is higher than in any other industrialized country, ranging from one to three surgeries per 100 Americans (53,54). Of the 200,000 Americans who undergo lumbosacral surgery to relieve chronic low back pain annually, 20% to 40% will experience continuing pain (55). As the population ages, the number of surgeries for degenerative lumbar conditions is expected to increase, as is the risk of FBSS. Unfortunately, many patients with FBSS who were referred to one multidisciplinary pain treatment center did not meet the criteria customarily accepted by neurosurgeons for surgical intervention at the time of their first surgery (56). This fact, coupled with persistent postoperative pain and sometimes by maladaptive behavior, complicates their subsequent medical management. However, some patients with FBSS are candidates for SCS, provided they meet patient selection criteria and successfully complete a screening trial.

In developing their practice parameters for the use of SCS, NTAC analyzed one randomized controlled trial (RCT) (57), 17 long-term follow-up studies, 12 short-term follow-up studies, four case or miscellaneous studies, and 31 studies of mixed indications for FBSS (6). The group also examined 16 studies of low back/leg pain or mixed indications that were not necessarily FBSS. From these sources, they concluded that there was excellent evidence (A = recommended or required; valid, useful, or non-negotiable) to support the use of SCS in treating FBSS (Table 41-3). Results of another RCT have since been published (58). These two RCTs offer compelling evidence of the efficacy of SCS in treating FBSS while also clarifying the necessary conditions for success. Both were well-controlled, randomized, crossover studies, one comparing SCS with repeat spine surgery and the other with conventional medical management (CMM). Compared with repeat spine surgery, SCS was significantly more successful ($p < 0.01$), patients initially randomized to SCS were significantly less likely to cross over than those initially randomized to surgery ($p = 0.02$), and patients randomized to reoperation required increased doses of analgesics significantly more often than those randomized to SCS ($p < 0.025$) (57). Compared with CMM, significantly more SCS patients had greater than 50% pain relief in their legs ($p < 0.001$) 6 months after the start of the study (58). The SCS group experienced significantly improved ($p < 0.05$) leg and back pain relief, QOL, functional capacity, and treatment satisfaction. Between 6 and 12 months, five SCS patients crossed to CMM and 32 CMM patients crossed to SCS.

The remaining body of evidence helps clarify the conditions necessary for successful treatment of FBSS with SCS. Numerous investigators have emphasized the importance of proper patient selection, a subject examined later in this chapter. It should be noted, however, that specific pain syndromes, such as angina, peripheral vascular disease, and CRPS are beginning to include SCS as a treatment option, rather than as a last resort, for patients meeting well-defined diagnostic criteria (59). In FBSS, SCS has demonstrated efficacy for managing intractable leg pain, and to a lesser extent, low back pain (52). Yet most experienced implanters have found that SCS is far more effective in relieving radicular pain than in treating axial low back pain. Thus, FBSS patients with predominant low back pain, or mixed nociceptive-neuropathic pain may be difficult to treat with SCS. Some success in treating low back pain has been achieved using paddle electrodes and high-voltage radio-frequency coupled systems, especially those with sophisticated programming options (52). However, extensive reprogramming and long-term follow-up are probably necessary to maintain effective paresthesia coverage.

Patients with FBSS who are considering SCS should have had chronic, intractable back and leg(s) pain for more than 6 months, the radicular component should be more severe than the axial component, and there should be no indication for additional spine surgery (such as progressive deformity, a lesion, or progressive motor deficit) (59). Contraindications to SCS for FBSS include an inadequate course of optimum nonsurgical care and previous failure of an SCS screening trial performed properly using current technology.

Several studies have considered the cost utility of SCS in treating FBSS. Bell and colleagues (60) compared the costs of SCS with surgeries and other treatments and reported that, in patients who responded favorably to SCS, the therapy paid for itself within 2.1 years. Devulder and colleagues (61) calculated an average annual cost of $3,660 per patient for SCS, which may be cost-effective if other therapies for FBSS have failed. In 2007, North and co-workers (62) reported on the difference in cost (cost effectiveness) and cost utility (quality adjusted life years) of SCS versus reoperation using data collected in a crossover RCT. The mean per-patient costs were US$48,357 for SCS versus $38,160 for reoperation (intention to treat), $48,357 for SCS versus $105,928 for reoperation (treated as intended), and $34,371 for SCS versus $36,341 for reoperation (final treatment). Thus, SCS was less expensive and more effective than reoperation in selected FBSS patients.

Complex Regional Pain Syndrome

In 1864, Mitchell first described causalgia (later called "reflex sympathetic dystrophy"), but the condition's many variations and puzzling pathophysiology created a formidable diagnostic challenge. In 1994, the International Association for the Study of Pain (IASP) replaced the name "reflex sympathetic dystrophy" with "complex regional pain syndrome" (63). The change acknowledged the unclear role of the sympathetic nervous system in the disorder, and the fact that dystrophy does not occur in all patients. Instead, two forms of CRPS were defined: type I, in which all the features of reflex sympathetic dystrophy are present but with no definable nerve injury; and type II (formerly called causalgia), in which the nerve injury is definable (64). See Chapter 46, by Binder and Baron, for a much more detailed review of CRPS.

Traditionally CRPS has been treated with physical therapy in an attempt to prevent contractures, minimize atrophy, and facilitate return to function. Several pain-relieving therapies have been offered to enhance the patient's ability to participate in physical therapy. Sympathetic nerve blocks can be used if they provide a sufficient duration of analgesia, or if the period of postprocedure analgesia increases with each block. Nu-

merous systemic medications have been administered to provide "balanced" analgesia during physical therapy, including serotonin/norepinephrine reuptake blockers, nonsteroidal anti-inflammatory drugs, steroids, opioids, α-adrenergic blocking agents, membrane stabilizers, N-methyl-D-aspartate (NMDA) antagonists (28) and gabenoids, gabapentin, and pregabalin. Continuous epidural infusion of anesthetics, clonidine, or opioids can also provide analgesia during rehabilitation, although the technique is labor intensive, expensive, and prone to complications such as infection or catheter occlusion. Neuroablation of the sympathetic chain provides longer-lasting analgesia but is fraught with complications, irreversible, and not uniformly effective (65). In light of the emerging understanding of peripheral–cord–brainstem interactions, neurodestructive techniques should be considered a last resort (28), if at all (66).

The NTAC found excellent evidence supporting the use of SCS to treat CRPS (Table 41-3) (6). They identified three RCTs, six long-term follow-up studies, six short-term follow-up studies, 10 case studies, and numerous studies of CRPS in mixed indications. Kemler and colleagues reported results of the first RCT in 2000 (67). Enrolled patients met the diagnostic criteria for CRPS type I established by the IASP, and all of the patients had experienced severe pain that was unresponsive to conventional treatment for at least 6 months. Patients were randomly assigned to receive SCS plus physical therapy ($n = 36$) or physical therapy alone ($n = 18$). The stimulator was implanted only if trial stimulation was successful. Intention-to-treat analysis demonstrated a significant reduction in pain for patients in the SCS group compared with patients in the physical therapy group ($p < 0.001$). Thirty-nine percent of patients in the SCS group had a much improved global perceived effect score compared with 6% in the other group ($p = 0.01$). None of the patients had clinical improvement in functional status. The QOL improved by 11% overall, but only in the 24 patients who actually underwent stimulator implantation. Six of these patients required additional procedures due to complications, including removal of one device.

The same researchers reported on their original patients after 2-year follow-up (68). The SCS plus physical therapy group still had significantly improved pain relief and global perceived effect compared with the physical therapy-only group ($p \leq 0.001$). There was no clinically important improvement in functional status for either group. The investigators concluded that SCS provided long-term pain reduction and improved the health-related QOL in these patients treated for CRPS. At 5-year follow-up, the effects of SCS or physical therapy only were equivalent with regard to all measured variables (69). Global perceived effect for SCS patients ($n = 20$) was still significantly better ($p = 0.02$) than for physical therapy patients ($n = 13$), but there was no difference in pain relief ($p = 0.06$). Despite the diminishing effect of SCS over time, the overwhelming majority (95%) of SCS-treated patients said they would repeat the treatment for the same result. The statistical artifact that SCS provides short-term relief without demonstrating long-term pain relief is produced by the study design of intent-to-treat analysis, with patients having the ability to cross over to SCS if more conservative therapy failed (70).

The third RCT compared the analgesic effects of carbamazepine (600 mg/day) or sustained-release morphine (90 mg/day) in patients with CRPS who were pretreated with SCS (71). Forty-three patients had SCS switched off before receiving the pain medications or placebo. They could reactivate SCS if the pain became intolerable. Compared with placebo, carbamazepine significantly delayed a pain increase, but morphine did not, perhaps because the dose was too low. Two patients taking carbamazepine and one taking morphine preferred to continue the medication. Thirty-five returned to SCS.

Most of the published studies describing treatment of CRPS with SCS have been retrospective. In reviewing 10 of these, Bennett and Cameron (28) found an overall success rate of 82% (148/180) for patients with CRPS I and 79% (23/29) for patients with CRPS II. These results are encouraging, considering that many physicians reserve SCS until all other conservative therapies have failed. These results were also obtained with relatively limited stimulation systems having few electrode contacts and limited output capabilities. More sophisticated stimulation systems, although not yet tested in RCTs, have demonstrated statistically significant improvements in pain scores and overall patient satisfaction compared with baseline (72). For example, Bennett and co-workers (72) found greater improvement in patients with dual octapolar leads versus a single quadripolar lead, probably because octapolar leads can safely deliver higher frequencies and be carefully programmed to maximize paresthesia coverage. They believe that the more flexibility afforded by a stimulation system—through numbers or arrays of electrodes; range of pulse width, frequency, and amplitude; dual-channel capabilities; and programming options—the more attractive the system is for treating CRPS.

Current thinking regarding CRPS suggests that early intervention provides a higher probability of complete reversal of symptoms or a greater degree of symptom resolution (73). Given the demonstrated efficacy of SCS in treating longer-standing cases, Prager and Chang reported on the temporary use of SCS to provide adjuvant analgesia while patients underwent interdisciplinary treatment that commenced within 8 weeks of their injury (47). Eight patients had an external pulse generator system connected to an implanted lead to facilitate physical therapy. The lead was to remain for 4 weeks, with permanent pulse generator implantation performed if stimulation was required for a longer time. After that time, if the patient desired explantation, the lead was removed. Five of the eight patients (62.5%) had sufficient symptom resolution to remove the lead. Temporary SCS is relatively inexpensive compared to multiple serial sympathetic blocks or maintenance of an epidural infusion. In addition, an implanted SCS lead without an internal pulse generator can be converted to a permanent, totally implanted system, if necessary, after functional rehabilitation is completed.

A retrospective analysis was performed of 16 consecutive patients who had permanent SCS systems implanted to treat CRPS (74); two (12.5%) had their systems explanted (at 5 and 18 months) and were relatively symptom free 2 years later. Ample evidence in the current literature supports the efficacy of SCS in treating pain due to CRPS I and II compared to other modalities, such as physical therapy and medication. Its greatest utility, however, may be in combination with other therapies early in the course of CRPS, when therapeutic interventions may prevent or moderate disability. In a preliminary report of patients receiving treatment for various types of neuropathic pain, SCS or intrathecal drug therapy was used in combination with cognitive behavioral therapy (CBT), given before or after CBT. Improvements in mental and physical function occurred only when SCS was combined with CBT (76a).

Spinal Cord Stimulation and CRPS in Children

Complex regional pain syndrome type I is not uncommon in children. Early treatment is often effective provided it com-

prises CBT, including reprogramming of motor function, sometimes supported by a short course of "neuropathic drugs." However, some children are referred very late or the condition escalates rapidly, so that all conservative treatments fail. In this situation, a short course of epidural clonidine may be helpful but requires hospitalization. A better option is the placement of a percutaneous SCS lead, which may be sufficient, over a week or so, to allow CBT to proceed. Severely affected children may be markedly improved by implantation of an SCS system (76b). This should only be carried out by highly experienced SCS implanters.

Peripheral Vascular Disease

Critical limb ischemia (CLI) is the most common vascular indication for SCS (75). In nondiabetic patients, CLI is defined as "the presence of rest pain or tissue necrosis (ulceration or gangrene) with an ankle systolic pressure of 50 mm Hg or less, or a toe pressure of 30 mm Hg or less (76). Vascular surgeons have proposed adding a microcirculatory measure to the definition, perhaps a combination of toe blood pressure (<30–50 mm Hg) and transcutaneous oxygen tension ($TcpO_2$, <30–50 mm Hg) (77).

Intermittent pain (vascular claudication) is the earliest symptom of ischemia and probably includes both nociceptive and neuropathic elements. The analgesic effect of SCS on CLI may be due to modulation of neuropathic pain, antinociception, and primary or secondary anti-ischemic effects (78). Decades ago, Cook noticed that SCS generated autonomic changes and pain relief in patients with spinal cord lesions or multiple sclerosis (79). About the same time, Dooley observed increased peripheral blood flow in patients treated with SCS for CNS disorders (80). More recently, Ghajar and Miles (81) found that SCS increased blood flow and skin temperature in the legs if the stimulating electrode was positioned below the T10 vertebral level, preferably at T12. Exactly how SCS influences blood flow remains a matter for further study, although sustained vasodilation has been demonstrated in humans and animals during antidromic stimulation of dorsal root afferents (82). Tallis and co-workers proposed that conventional pain relief might reverse the sympathetic vasoconstriction that accompanies pain, or that SCS induces an electrical sympathetic paralysis (82).

Beginning in Europe during the 1990s, epidural SCS was used to treat peripheral vascular disease in patients who could not undergo vascular reconstruction. In these diverse patients with severe limb ischemia, SCS relieved pain, permitted greater mobility, and promoted ulcer healing due to enhanced blood flow (75). Clinicians were encouraged by these results, because the alternative was generally amputation. The Second European Consensus Document on Critical Limb Ischaemia (76) added microcirculatory criteria to the Fontaine staging system previously used to grade peripheral arterial disease. The randomized studies that have since been conducted demonstrated no statistically significant advantage for SCS in limb preservation over medical management, but have documented pain relief, greater mobility, and improved QOL for patients treated with SCS (83,84). In a study of 120 patients randomly assigned to SCS or standard treatment, limb survival was 60% in the SCS group and 46% in the standard treatment group after 2 years (84). Further refinement of the patient selection criteria, especially with regard to microcirculatory measurements, may more accurately identify CLI patients who would respond optimally to SCS.

Intractable Angina Pectoris

Angina pectoris, a reversible myocardial ischemia, represents an imbalance between oxygen demand and supply that is caused by blood vessel obstruction or vasospasm. Angina can be triggered by exercise, blood redistribution to digestion after eating, cold, or mental stress. Patients with ischemic heart disease now enjoy increased QOL and longer life expectancy due to surgical and pharmacologic therapies. In a subset of patients, however, angina pectoris proves refractory to all treatments (85,86). The European Study Group on the Treatment of Refractory Angina Pectoris offers this definition for refractory angina pectoris: "A chronic condition characterized by the presence of angina, caused by coronary insufficiency in the presence of coronary artery disease, which cannot be adequately controlled by a combination of medical therapy, angioplasty, and coronary artery bypass surgery. The presence of reversible myocardial ischemia should be clinically established to be the cause of symptoms" (87).

Approximately 100,000 patients in Europe and the United States meet this definition, most of them male, relatively young (in their early sixties), and previously treated with multiple revascularization procedures (88,89). Of all the available adjunct therapies, from medications such as amiodarone to experimental angiogenesis, SCS is considered one of the most successful and safest (90,91). For this reason, the European Study Group on the Treatment of Refractory Angina Pectoris recommends SCS as a treatment of choice (along with transcutaneous electrical nerve stimulation or TENS) for refractory angina (87). Relief of angina is most pronounced when SCS is applied in the epidural space at levels T1 to T2 (17).

Randomized and observational studies of SCS for refractory angina have demonstrated fewer anginal episodes, less use of short-acting nitrates, improved exercise capacity, and more favorable perceived QOL (92). The benefits of SCS persist for at least a year in 80% of patients, and almost 60% experience improved exercise capacity and QOL for up to 5 years (89,93, 94). Separate from its pain-relieving effects, SCS therapy reduces myocardial ischemia as gauged by exercise stress testing and ambulatory ECG monitoring (95,96). Fears that SCS might obliterate the warning signs of angina, thus putting patients at risk of adverse myocardial events, are not borne out by the evidence. Spinal cord stimulation elevates the pain threshold but does not completely eliminate anginal pain, and pain perception reportedly remains intact during myocardial infarction (97,98). Nor is mortality adversely affected, according to prospective and retrospective studies of SCS for refractory angina pectoris (92). For example, in a retrospective follow-up study of 517 patients who had refractory angina and were treated with SCS, there was no negative effect on mortality (89). In a prospective study that compared SCS with bypass surgery, there was no difference between SCS and surgery regarding symptom relief at 6 months (95). The SCS group had lower mortality and cerebrovascular morbidity than the bypass group. Two-year follow-up showed that SCS was more cost effective than bypass (99) and 5-year follow-up that there was no difference in mortality (94).

Other Pain Conditions

When considering the scientific and clinical evidence for using SCS, members of the NTAC (6) analyzed well-controlled clinical studies and case reports describing other pain conditions, such as phantom limb/postamputation syndrome, pos-

therpetic neuralgia (PHN), root injury pain, and spinal cord injury/lesion (Table 41-3). Weighing risk versus benefit and expert consensus, they concluded that SCS offers a good likelihood of a favorable outcome in treating these conditions (B = recommended; uncertain validity, apparently useful). In the absence of RCTs comparing SCS with other treatments for these pain syndromes, some individuals and groups have expressed skepticism or counseled extreme caution (100). A number of retrospective studies, however, do demonstrate long-term (5 to 20 years) successful outcomes for patients with these conditions (51,101–105). Many of the studies included mixed indications, with chronic, refractory pain the common denominator. This fact underscores the importance of patient selection (105,106) and the necessity of demonstrating SCS efficacy during a preimplantation trial (101,106). These factors are discussed in more detail later in this chapter.

Phantom Limb/Postamputation Syndrome

The IASP defines phantom limb pain as "pain referred to a surgically or traumatically removed limb or portion thereof" (107). Severe phantom pain affects 0.5% to 5% of amputees (108) for up to 71% of the time (109). Stump pain may arise from skin changes, circulatory problems, and infection or bone abnormalities, and may not always be neuropathic (108). Most reports of treating phantom limb pain with SCS are embedded in retrospective reviews of all types of chronic pain. Krainick and colleagues (110) followed 84 patients treated with dorsal column stimulation between 1972 and 1974, including 64 amputees. Good results were obtained in 52.4% after 2 years and 39% after 5 years. Tasker and Dostrovsky (111) reported 56% of 16 patients treated with SCS responded favorably. In a series of 15 patients, Oakley found that the five with neuropathic stump pain experienced improvement of more than 50% (112). In the same series, four of the 10 patients with painful phantom said they no longer experienced phantom discomfort, although phantom awareness persisted. Pain relief was related to subjective reports of paresthesia in the phantom. These results demonstrate that SCS can provide pain relief in some cases of phantom limb/postamputation syndrome, while also pointing to the need for further study of this application.

Postherpetic Neuralgia

Two studies offer evidence of efficacy for SCS in treating PHN. The first examined outcomes for 109 patients who underwent SCS between 1978 and 1986, 10 of whom had PHN (104). Six of the 10 experienced 52.5% mean analgesia and reported long-term implant success. In a more recent study, Harke and colleagues (113) reported on 28 patients with PHN of more than 2 years duration. Long-term pain relief was achieved in 23 patients (82%), eight of whom became completely pain free. Four patients with acute PHN noted immediate improvement, although perhaps as a result of the natural resolution of PHN.

Spinal Cord Injury or Lesion

In patients with brachial plexus damage or complete avulsion of the nerve roots from the spinal cord, SCS will not relieve pain because the relevant neurons have been destroyed or severed (114). These patients can be identified through radiography and neurologic examination. In patients with less severe injuries, the extent and location of damage helps determine whether SCS will be efficacious. Still, patients with the same diagnosis may experience widely varying responses to SCS. This truth highlights our incomplete understanding of the etiology and pathophysiology of neuropathic conditions and underscores the importance of trial stimulation before permanent implantation. However, even trial stimulation cannot guarantee longer-term success, as proven by the 60% to 70% success rate obtained after successful trial. The literature contains a number of case studies and reports from several groups on SCS for the treatment of spinal cord injury or lesion.

In a series of 109 patients followed between 1978 and 1986, 15 with an incomplete spinal cord lesion, Meglio and colleagues (104) found no clinical usefulness for SCS in treating pain associated with central deafferentation. Cioni and colleagues (115) instituted trial stimulation in 25 paraplegic patients suffering from intractable pain due to a spinal cord lesion. Fewer than half (40.9%) reported pain relief and underwent permanent implantation. Just over 3 years later, only 18.2% had a greater than 50% reduction in their pain.

Lazorthes and co-workers (116) followed 692 patients with neurogenic pain, 17 with brachial plexus lesions and 101 with spinal cord lesions, for 20 years. Their patients were enrolled as two study groups: one a series of 279 patients and the other of 413 patients. Percutaneous SCS trials lasting 3 to 14 days were used to screen candidates. One month after implantation, the success rates were 86% and 85% for the two groups, respectively. At a mean of 10 years follow-up, the success rates were 54% and 52%. For the period from 1984 to 1990, the success rate in 301 patients was higher, 68% and 60%, respectively. The researchers concluded that SCS had therapeutic value in treating neurogenic pain secondary to partial deafferentation. For upper limb pain, they recommended ipsilateral radicular stimulation, and in cases of brachial plexus avulsion, herpes zoster, and pain of spinal or cerebral origin, they recommended thalamic stimulation if SCS failed. Their recommendations illustrate the evolution of electrical stimulation, and the newly emerging techniques of motor cortex and deep brain stimulation. In reviewing 25 years of experience with 1,336 cases of motor disorders, including 303 spinal cord injuries, Waltz (103) cited numerous technical advances, as well as our progressive understanding of neurophysiologic mechanisms, as the keys to improving the efficacy of SCS.

WEIGHING POTENTIAL RISK VERSUS BENEFIT

Any pain treatment plan must balance benefit against risk. Consequently, the classic chronic pain treatment continuum begins with less invasive and costly options and progresses if they fail (117). In this context, SCS has usually been relegated to the status of last resort. The decision to choose SCS ultimately falls to the patient and physician, who together can discuss individual circumstances. The potential benefits of SCS are listed in Table 41-4. It should be noted that the NTAC, in drawing up its practice parameters for SCS, classified its reported benefits as useful for information, in part because there are no generally accepted standards for measuring many of the benefits and only two RCTs available for consideration.

The most obvious potential benefit of SCS is pain relief. The criterion of 50% pain reduction has been used as a definition of success for decades (139) but lacks standardization because pain itself fluctuates, and the perception of pain is highly subjective and idiosyncratic. The commonly used visual analog scale (VAS) creates an individual framework for the assessment of pain over time, with a reduction in score considered a measure of success. Yet, patients reporting relatively modest reductions in VAS may have disproportionately greater gains in function or decreases in pain medication. For example, in one

prospective study, only 26% of patients said SCS conferred 50% or greater reduction in pain, yet 70% said the therapy helped them and they would recommend it (130). Two years post implantation, two-thirds of these patients had reduced or stopped their narcotic medications. In another study, 55% of patients met the pain reduction criterion, but 90% had reduced or stopped their medication (140). Given the intractable nature of the chronic pain syndromes treated with SCS, patients may view any reduction in pain as advantageous, particularly if it allows functional improvement and less reliance on pain medications. Both RCTs (of treatment for FBSS) found significantly greater pain relief with SCS than with alternative treatments (reoperation or CMM) (57,58).

Numerous studies, including one RCT, have documented pain relief (or reduced need for medication) due to SCS for a variety of indications (see North et al., (6) for a comprehensive bibliography). The RCT compared SCS to lumbosacral spine surgery for chronic pain. Patients randomly assigned to reoperation required significantly more opiate medication than those assigned to SCS ($p < 0.025$) (57). One prospective, multicenter study of SCS for chronic back and extremity pain found no reduction in medication among patients treated with SCS (118). However, all pain and quality-of-life measures showed statistically significant improvement during the year after implantation. This included improvements measured by the average pain VAS, the McGill Pain Questionnaire, the Oswestry Disability Questionnaire, the Sickness Impact Profile, and the Beck Depression Inventory. Using 50% pain relief as the definition of success, SCS managed pain in 55% of the patients.

In their review, the NTAC (6) found 13 long-term and 12 short-term follow-up studies that demonstrated increased ability to undertake ADLs or improved QOL for patients treated with SCS. Seven years after SCS implantation, a majority of patients in one retrospective, consecutive series of 205 patients had maintained improvements in ADLs (51). In a retrospective long-term (mean 37.5 months) follow-up of 81 patients with SCS, 80% reported an improvement in QOL (123). They experienced significant reductions in the Oswestry Disability Index ($p < 0.01$), the Hospital Anxiety and Depression (HAD) Index ($p < 0.01$), and VAS scores ($p < 0.001$). In the same study, patients in two "control" groups, who had no trial of SCS or a failed trial of SCS, deteriorated over time. Spinal cord stimulation reduced the frequency of awakenings during the night in 20 patients treated for FBSS (124). Ten of these patients, (59%) said SCS had increased their ability to participate in social activities or pursue a hobby. Budd noted improvements in sleep, mood, and mobility in a retrospective study of 20 patients treated for FBSS (120).

No standard measure of patient satisfaction with treatment exists. In one study of SCS for FBSS, 53% of patients expressed satisfaction with the procedure at 2.2 years follow-up and 47% at 5 years postoperatively (5). A nationwide survey by the health insurer in Belgium found that among 70 patients with a mean follow-up of 3.5 years, the effect of SCS was judged good or very good by 52% of the patients (134). Among 153 patients followed for 4 years after implantation in Belgium, 68% rated their result as excellent to good (125). One convincing measure of patient satisfaction with SCS is the fact that in the two RCTs, patients were significantly less likely to cross over to reoperation or CMM than to stay with SCS (57,58).

Several studies have noted fewer symptoms of depression in patients successfully treated with SCS (6,16,101,118,123,137). Burchiel and colleagues (137), using the depression subscale of the Minnesota Multiphasic Personality Inventory (MMPI), noted that increased depression scores correlated negatively with post-treatment pain status as measured by VAS. However,

TABLE 41-4

POTENTIAL BENEFITS OF SPINAL CORD STIMULATION (SCS)

Benefit	Comments
Pain relief (5,42,51,57,58,118)	The primary outcome measure of SCS success is patient-reported pain relief, generally using a standard pain scale such as the Visual Analog Scale (VAS), Functional Rating Index, McGill Pain Questionnaire (6) A majority of patients may experience at least 50% reduction in pain
Increased activity levels or function (5,42,51,101,118–128)	As demonstrated by activities of daily living, such as walking, climbing stairs, sleeping, engaging in sex, driving a car and sitting at a table (6) Measured by the Oswestry Disability Index (specific for low back pain), the Sickness Impact Profile (for general health), Functional Rating Index, Pain Disability Index
Reduced use of pain medications (5,51,57,119–120,124,125,129,130)	Patients in whom SCS is successful should be able to reduce or eliminate their intake of pain medication (6)
Improvement in quality of life (6,120–125,131)	
Patient satisfaction with treatment (5,6,42,57,72,101, 121,123,125,132–136)	Would repeat treatment to achieve the same result (6)
Fewer symptoms of depression (6,16,101,123,137)	Measured by the Beck Depression Inventory
Improved neurologic/physical function (6)	Better lower extremity strength and coordination, sensation, bladder/bowel function might be indirect benefits of pain control or discontinuation of other treatments (opioids, for example) Measured by patient self-report, neurologic examination, or a validated scale such as exists for spinal cord injury
Return to work in patients whose uncontrolled chronic pain was the only impediment to gainful employment (5,6,61,120,121,122,131,135,138)	Employment status depends on many factors beyond pain control, including the patient's education, field of employment, work history, overall physical condition, and age. Many patients were disabled by pain and unable to work for long periods of time while they were unsuccessfully treated with other therapies before SCS. Long periods of unemployment decrease the likelihood of returning to work, even after successful treatment. However, some SCS patients do return to work (6).
Reduced consumption of health care resources (6)	Measured by patient self-report, medical records, tracking of patient cross over to an alternative treatment, or an instrument, such as the Medication Quantification Scale

Consult the *Practice Parameters for the Use of Spinal Cord Stimulation in the Treatment of Chronic Neuropathic Pain* (6) for a comprehensive bibliography of studies that support the benefits of spinal cord stimulation. Selected long-term or seminal studies are cited here, including two randomized controlled trials; short-term studies and case reports are not.

May and co-workers (123) did not find any correlation between initial depression scores and subsequent levels of pain relief. Two prospective studies offer additional evidence. Oakley and Weiner (16) observed a trend toward improvement ($p < 0.06$) in the Beck Depression Inventory scores, which dropped from 13.18 pre-implant to 5.18 post-implant, at an average follow-up of 7.9 months in patients being treated for CRPS. Burchiel et al., (118) measured a significant ($p = 0.02$) decline in the Beck Depression Inventory score 1 year after implantation in 70 patients being treated for chronic back and extremity pain.

Improved physical or neurologic function has been documented in a variety of long-term follow-up studies of SCS in treating intractable leg pain (130), FBSS (120), axial low back pain (135), mixed indications (101), and spinal cord injury (126,127). Isometric lower extremity function was significantly improved ($p < 0.01$) 12 and 24 months after implantation in 40 patients treated for intractable leg pain (130). In a cost–benefit study with 5-year follow-up, physical functioning improved by a mean of 30% postimplantation (120). A prospective study of epidural spinal cord stimulation in 48 patients with spinal cord injury showed a statistically significant reduction in the severity of spasms at 6, 12, and 24 months after SCS implantation (126). The number of spasms continued to decrease over time, and no patient experienced neurologic deterioration. A more recent case report documents the recovery of functional walking after SCS in a patient with incomplete spinal cord injury (127). Even modest gains in neurologic or physical function can have disproportionate impact for patients with extensive injuries, and for their care givers.

For employers and health care payers, return to work for previously employed patients represents a desired goal of SCS therapy. The NTAC (6) found 13 long-term and nine short-term follow-up studies demonstrating that some patients treated with SCS return to work. They also identified five studies that documented no improvement in work status. The discrepancy points to the complex and sometimes competing motivations of patients, payers, physicians, employers, and societies. Obviously, successful pain control by itself does not guarantee a person's ability or willingness to return to work. Many patients disabled by pain were unable to work for long periods of time before failing conservative therapies and becoming eligible for SCS. Long periods of unemployment decrease the chances of finding work again, even if SCS treatment is successful. The fact remains, however, that some SCS patients do return to work.

A retrospective analysis of 235 patients over 15 years found 47 of 111 successfully implanted patients (42%) were gainfully employed, compared with only 22 patients employed before implantation (122). In a 5-year retrospective analysis of 49 patients with FBSS, eight of 21 patients who received SCS had returned to work, and 13 (four retired and nine unemployed) had resumed daily activities (138). In a prospective well-controlled study of 20 patients with FBSS or axial low back pain, eight of 17 (40%) employed before their illness were working immediately before SCS implantation, and seven (35%) at 2.3 year follow-up (57). Two cost–benefit studies included work status among the examined outcomes. In the first, of 20 patients who had undergone SCS for FBSS, four remained at work but functioned more efficiently after treatment, four returned to work, 10 not employed remained so, and one patient returned to work but retired 2 years later due to age (120). The authors observed, "There was a suspicion that, in a time of relatively high unemployment, the likelihood of obtaining suitable work was unlikely and that remaining 'disabled' offered at least a tolerable life style. Consequently, rehabilitation was not always pursued with enthusiasm on the part of the patient and the outcome was not always as successful as anticipated following what appeared to be a satisfactory procedure from a clinical point of view." In the second study, 15% (9/60) of SCS-treated patients returned to work because of superior pain control or lower drug intake (121). By contrast, none of the 44 patients receiving best medical treatment or conventional pain therapy returned to work.

The NTAC (6) also compiled five studies that showed no improvement in work status (57,118,124,133,141). All included patients with FBSS or chronic back and leg pain. In the one RCT, 52% ($n = 45$) of the study population was retired or permanently disabled at the study's start (57). Patients receiving workman's compensation agreed to randomization as often as other patients but were treated significantly less often ($p < 0.01$) because third-party authorization was denied to nine of 10 such candidates for SCS. There was no significant treatment difference in patients' ability to return to work whether they were treated with SCS or reoperation. Of those who were employed before the study began, all but one remained employed at 3-year follow-up, and one went from part-time to full-time employment.

Reduced consumption of health care resources will be considered later in this chapter in the cost-effectiveness section. Suffice it to say that the high cost of equipment has often been cited as a justification for delaying SCS until all other therapies have failed. However, increasing evidence suggests that neurostimulation is cost effective when treating chronic conditions (142).

One newly emerging and intriguing benefit of SCS is the possibility of favorably altering the pathogenesis of pain by early application of SCS (142). The chance of salvaging limbs in CLI, producing a cardioprotective effect in cardiac ischemia, and halting the debilitating effects of CRPS should spur additional research in the future.

The Risks of Spinal Cord Stimulation

The risks of SCS can be categorized as related to surgery, to the implanted devices, or to stimulation itself (Table 41-5). Infection ranks as the primary surgery-related risk. In a survey

---

TABLE 41-5

POTENTIAL RISKS OF SPINAL CORD STIMULATION

Surgical complications: hematoma, epidural hemorrhage, paralysis, seroma, cerebrospinal fluid leakage, infection, erosion

Device-related complications: hardware malfunction or migration, pain at implant site, allergic response, reoperation

Stimulation-induced complications: undesirable change in stimulation (discomfort, jolting, shocking), loss of pain relief, chest wall stimulation

Precautions
Patients should:
▓ Be detoxified from narcotics before lead placement.
▓ Avoid activities that may put undue stress on the implanted components.
▓ Should not scuba dive below 10 meters of water or enter hyperbaric chambers >2.0 atmosphere absolute.
▓ Disable the stimulator system before entering magnetic fields (metal detectors, security screening systems, etc.).
Contraindications: diathermy or therapeutic ultrasound

---

of 31 studies, perioperative infections were reported in 5% of cases (0% to 12%) (143). Two decades of experience with SCS turned up a similar 5% incidence of infections, but no spinal cord injury, meningitis, or life-threatening infection (51). Surgical risks exclusive of infections include spinal fluid leaks, hemorrhage, or neurologic injury, which reportedly occur in approximately 9% of cases (0% to 42%) (59). Many practitioners administer antibiotic prophylaxis intravenously 1 hour before a procedure to minimize the chance of infection.

Device-related complications present the greatest challenge to successful implantation, occurring in as many as 30% of cases in a review of 13 studies published in 1995 (143). Electrode migration posed the biggest difficulty, accounting for 24% of device-related complications and frequently resulting in loss of paresthesia coverage. Surgical revision or replacement of a system component was necessary for 12 of 219 (5%) patients tracked by Burchiel and colleagues (118). Multichannel systems have proven significantly more reliable than single-channel laminectomy or percutaneous leads (51). Remarkable technological advances in the past decade promise to further decrease the number of complications attributable to equipment.

Patients occasionally report that stimulation has become uncomfortable or increases underlying pain. Stimulation-related complications vary widely, and few studies have examined the precise reasons for failure. Five of 219 patients (3%) in one series (118) reported discomfort or loss of pain relief. Posture-induced changes in paresthesia are sometimes cited. Oakley reviewed 126 patients with 2-year follow-up, 26 (20%) of whom had discontinued stimulation or requested removal of the system (59). He found three reasons for failure: disease progression in 12 patients (55% of failures), appropriate paresthesia with loss of pain relief in nine patients (41% of failures), and painful hardware at the implant site in one patient. Four patients (3%) enjoyed such successful pain resolution that they no longer required SCS.

On balance, the risks of SCS must also be judged against those of other possible therapies or the option of doing nothing. In this calculus, the patient should be told of the deleterious side effects of systemic medications, such as mental impairment, sedation, nausea, constipation, weight gain (142), and endocrine suppression (144). In the United States, medical therapies are often favored over surgical ones by physicians, payers, and patients. Yet the most frequent and serious complications of SCS are not related to stimulation itself or to its long-term use. Thus, a preimplantation screening trial (to determine efficacy) combined with careful immediate postimplant management offers the potential to resolve side effects early in the course of treatment. The side effects of pain medications, however, can persist as long as their use endures.

Every patient contemplating SCS should be engaged in a detailed discussion of the risks and benefits that might be experienced personally. It is desirable to engage family members when appropriate. A well-informed patient with a good support system becomes an active partner in the treatment plan. Patients should be aware that they have responsibilities, and their committed participation in preoperative, postoperative, and maintenance therapy will influence outcome.

PROGNOSTIC FACTORS

Clearly, SCS works well in some cases and not in others. Even with a definitive diagnosis and a successful preimplantation trial of SCS, some patients fail to achieve the expected benefits of therapy. Thus, the search for prognostic factors continues. The NTAC found excellent evidence for age and gender as prognostic factors (Table 41-6) and inadequate information to make a judgment regarding life expectancy or worker's compensation status. Regarding age, the safety and effectiveness of SCS in children has not been established. One study found that advanced age might reduce the chances of a good outcome

(137), but four studies found no age difference in outcome (101,122,123,131). The Coalition recommends assessing each patient individually, not solely on the basis of age.

Eight studies identified by the NTAC found differences between the genders in response to SCS. However, the advantages to one gender or the other did not hold across studies. For example, the nationwide survey of SCS treatment in Belgium documented an advantage for men (134), whereas a 5-year follow-up study of patients with FBSS documented a significant advantage for women (5). Four additional studies found no difference in response between the genders (6). Coalition members concluded that there was no reason to exclude patients based on their gender. The one exception is pregnancy, during which the safety of SCS remains to be established and must be balanced against the known or potential adverse effects of pain medications or other treatments. Use of fluoroscopy to facilitate lead placement during pregnancy is contraindicated for the fetus and therefore renders new implantation during pregnancy impractical. There are no data suggesting that a previously implanted SCS system has any undesirable effects on pregnancy.

The NTAC could recommend the pain states likely to be treated successfully with SCS, on the basis of seven well-controlled studies (Table 41-7) (6). Numerous retrospective series of SCS patients have examined heterogeneous groups of patients. It is more difficult to determine specific outcomes without stratifying according to diagnosis. Among patients treated for FBSS, for instance, many had no clear indication for their first surgery (56). Unless objective pathology resulting from that surgery exists, such as scarring or arachnoid fibrosis, further treatment with SCS has little chance of yielding better results than the previous intervention(s) (145). For this reason, several groups have been working to develop patient-selection

TABLE 41-6

PROGNOSTIC FACTORS FOR SPINAL CORD STIMULATION (SCS) SUPPORTED BY AN EVIDENCE-BASED LITERATURE REVIEW AND CONSENSUS STATEMENT

Factor	Grade and recommendations
Does patient age affect the potential benefit from SCS?	A
	▪ The safety and effectiveness of SCS in children has not been established
	▪ Advanced age might reduce the chances of a good outcome, but each patient must be assessed on an individual basis
	▪ Weighing risk vs. potential benefit and expert consensus reveals a high likelihood of a favorable outcome
	▪ Only option (in some cases)
Does patient sex affect the potential benefit from SCS?	A
	▪ The safety of SCS during pregnancy remains to be established (and must be balanced against the known or potential adverse effects of medication and other treatments for pain)
	▪ Weighing risk vs. potential benefit and expert consensus reveals a high likelihood of a favorable outcome
What pain states are likely to be treated successfully with SCS?	B
	▪ Weighing risk vs. potential benefit and expert consensus reveals a high likelihood of a good outcome
Does life expectancy dictate how SCS is used?	Inadequate information to determine
Does worker's compensation status have an effect on SCS outcome?	Inadequate information to determine

Consult the *Practice Parameters for the Use of Spinal Cord Stimulation in the Treatment of Chronic Neuropathic Pain* (6) for a comprehensive bibliography of studies regarding prognostic factors associated with successful spinal cord stimulation.

TABLE 41-7

PAIN STATES MOST LIKELY TO BE TREATED SUCCESSFULLY WITH SPINAL CORD STIMULATION (SCS)

- Radicular or radiating pain rather than axial in distribution (predominant low back pain is more difficult to treat) and neuropathic rather than nociceptive pain
- Pain with an objective basis and a distribution consistent with the results of the physical examination and diagnostic imaging studies
- Painful condition linked to a specific diagnosis
- Objective findings predominate, as opposed to functional, nonphysiologic signs
- Pain is adequately relieved during an SCS screening trial

criteria for SCS that would maximize the opportunity for therapeutic success.

For patients with a very short life expectancy, such as those with terminal cancer, using an SCS system with an external stimulator is the most cost-effective method of neurostimulation (146). The longer-term use of an external pulse generator connected to an implanted lead must be weighed against the increased risk of infection associated with systems that are contiguous with the outside of the body. Inadequate information exists to determine if worker's compensation status exerts any influence on SCS outcome.

Three additional studies of prognostic factors deserve mention. Burchiel and co-workers (137) retrospectively analyzed a variety of demographic, physical, psychosocial, and functional variables for 40 patients treated with SCS for FBSS in search of factors that might have predicted their pain outcome 3 months after implantation. Three prognostic factors—age, the MMPI depression scale, and McGill Pain Questionnaire scores—correctly predicted the postoperative change in VAS for 85% of the patients. Younger patients who were less depressed were more likely to report good pain relief, and patients who considered their overall pain as intense preoperatively were more likely to report larger improvements at 3 months.

Investigators at the University of Birmingham conducted two systematic literature reviews designed to assess prognostic factors: one for patients with chronic back and leg pain and FBSS (147) the other for patients with CRPS (148). In the first, the chief prognostic factors for increased pain relief were poor study quality, short follow-up, multicenter (versus single-site) studies, and inclusion of patients with FBSS (versus chronic back and leg pain). The other review, of patients with CRPS, identified no statistically significant predictors of pain relief with SCS. Since the first of these reviews was published in 2004, considerable effort has been expended to improve the quality of case studies and series, including using better methodology and controls, defining diagnoses, and conducting RCTs that compare SCS with alternative therapies.

PATIENT SELECTION FOR A SCREENING TRIAL

The literature is virtually unanimous in emphasizing the importance of appropriate patient selection if SCS is to be successful (149). Pain treatment algorithms rely on a stepwise approach that begins with therapies that are less invasive, likely to have few side effects, and reversible. Spinal cord stimulation is a minimally invasive procedure and should, therefore, follow appropriate noninvasive therapies. By the same reasoning, a screening trial of SCS should precede ablative therapies (e.g., sympathectomies, dorsal root entry zone [DREZ] lesions, or dorsal root ganglionectomy) and major surgical procedures (reoperation in FBSS patients). There is good evidence that the tests listed in Table 41-8 will reveal information about a patient's suitability to proceed to a screening trial (6).

Most candidates for SCS have a long medical history, and reviewing it is a crucial first step in the selection process. Specific criteria exist for making a diagnosis of the pain syndromes for which SCS is indicated, including FBSS, CRPS types I and II, peripheral vascular disease, and intractable angina pectoris. Patient questionnaires can cover pain history, current medication and other therapies, disability status, and a VAS for rating current pain (149). An initial clinical interview can also elicit the patient's subjective experience of pain by saying, "Tell me what your pain feels like to you." The resulting narrative can contextualize the patient's experience. Issues such as timely medical treatment, response to conservative and aggressive interventions, past involvement with implantable devices, and ancillary treatments may predict how the proposed implantation will be received. Information provided by the patient should be carefully reviewed against records from the referring physician to provide corroborative evidence and supply results from earlier diagnostic studies. The physical examination, including complete neurologic assessment, will document the patient's current pain symptoms. In some cases, a complete diagnostic workup may be necessary to identify treatable causes of pain.

Magnetic resonance imaging (MRI) should be performed in any suspected case of stenosis, disk herniation, or other anatomic abnormality that might increase the procedural risk of SCS (6). Some clinicians rely on an MRI to gain information about the depth of dorsal cerebrospinal fluid (CSF) and the position of the spinal cord, dimensions that vary among individuals and affect electrode selection, placement, and adjustment. Others forgo a routine, pre-trial MRI because of the cost.

Table 41-9 lists patient inclusion and exclusion criteria (59) and relative and absolute contraindications for SCS (6). These should be considered carefully, as inappropriate patient selection undoubtedly accounts for some of the disparate results of SCS reported in the literature. In general, if neurostimulation can be used for a given pain syndrome, it is preferred and attempted initially (149). That is because when neurostimulation is effective, it requires less ongoing maintenance and expense than drug administration systems. The valuable and continuing work performed by the North American Neuromodulation Society, the IASP, and other groups has contributed to a more precise understanding of the patient selection criteria associated with successful neurostimulation, and their insights should not be overlooked. Where controversies exist, with the necessity for psychological testing, for example, clinical judgment comes to the fore.

Medicare and many health insurers already require psychological screening as a condition for SCS (150). Information from a psychological assessment can expose psychological factors that should be treated, guide specific treatments that can help resolve psychological risk factors, facilitate patient selection, and provide clues as to the patient's possible response to treatment. On the other hand, no psychological assessment can confirm the cause of pain or the relative contribution of organic versus psychological factors. Doleys and Olson (150) recommend looking for an accumulation of risk factors or an overall level of distress when conducting psychological testing. Severe

TABLE 41-8

EVIDENCE FOR PATIENT SELECTION CRITERIA

Criteria	Grade and recommendations
What tests reveal information about a patient's suitability to proceed to spinal cord stimulation (SCS) trial?	B ▨ History; pain location and intensity; physical examination; MRI as appropriate, and flexion-extension radiographs, computed tomography, myelography, or discography to reveal abnormalities concordant with the pain complaint and surgically remediable causes of neurologic deficit ▨ Weighing risk vs. potential benefit and expert consensus reveals a high likelihood of a good outcome
What are the psychological characteristics of patients most likely to benefit from SCS?	B ▨ Interventional pain treatments should be reserved for patients with no evident unresolved major psychiatric comorbidity ▨ Medicare requires a psychological evaluation before SCS implantation and many private insurers follow suit ▨ Weighing risk vs. potential benefit and expert consensus reveals a high likelihood of a good outcome
What are the relative contraindications to SCS?	A ▨ Weighing risk vs. potential benefit and expert consensus reveals a high likelihood of a favorable outcome
What are the absolute contraindications to SCS?	A ▨ Weighing risk vs. potential benefit and expert consensus reveals a high likelihood of a favorable outcome

Consult the *Practice Parameters for the Use of Spinal Cord Stimulation in the Treatment of Chronic Neuropathic Pain* (6) for a comprehensive bibliography of studies regarding patient selection criteria.

---

pain by itself can cause psychological disturbances, and cognitive behavioral therapy can help patients control pain (151). Thus, a psychological assessment could uncover treatable psychological factors that would improve the chances for success. In this context, a psychological assessment is designed to ensure that no significant psychological dysfunction precludes a screening trial. After psychological evaluation, we categorize a patient's suitability for implantation as: (a) no contraindicated; (b) contraindicated due to behavioral issues; (c) contraindicated due to behavioral issues, implantation trial acceptable; or (d) patient unsuitable (149).

CONDUCTING A SCREENING TRIAL

Screening trials provide valid patient selection information (Table 41-10) (6). They offer both the physician and patient an opportunity to evaluate SCS before committing to it. Approximating the conditions of long-term therapy during the trial seems to offer the best chance for assessing efficacy and tolerance. The trial should answer two fundamental questions:

Is the patient's pain responsive to SCS therapy, and can the patient tolerate the treatment (149)? The physician and patient should agree in advance on the goals of the trial and on the measures used to assess those goals. For example, if returning to work is a goal of treatment, then a rehabilitation specialist should evaluate the patient during the screening trial. In general, candidates should proceed to implantation if their pain can be reduced by at least 50% (70% optimally) (152), the area of paresthesia is tolerable and concordant with the area of pain (59), analgesic medication intake remains stable or can be decreased, and functional improvement has been assessed (different clinics employ different tools for physical evaluation). As many as a third of potential SCS candidates will be eliminated during the screening trial (59).

Numerous screening protocols exist, and none can be considered superior or definitive based on the current literature (153). Multiple factors influence the choice of protocol, including the patient's overall condition, the physician's preference and experience, available facilities and resources, practice environment, and payer coverage. Table 41-11 compares trial techniques. Medicare requires a screening trial before reimbursing for SCS therapy and may dictate some trial conditions. Generally, trials last for 1 week or longer and use externalized

TABLE 41-9

PATIENT SELECTION CRITERIA AND RELATIVE AND ABSOLUTE CONTRAINDICATIONS FOR SPINAL CORD STIMULATION (SCS)

Inclusion criteria (59)
- Established diagnosis of specific pain syndrome (peripheral neuropathic pain, peripheral vascular disease, complex regional pain syndrome, or angina pectoris)
- Appendicular pain following at least one previous spine surgery
- Leg pain which radiates below the knee greater than back pain
- Informed consent
- Clearance after psychological evaluation

Exclusion criteria (59)
- Surgical procedure within 6 months of screening trial
- Evidence of active, disruptive psychiatric disorder; active drug abuse; personality disorders that might affect pain perception, compliance with intervention, or ability to evaluate therapy
- Patients <18 years old
- Patients who have not received an adequate course of nonsurgical care
- Patients who have failed a previous SCS trial

Relative contraindications (6)
- An unresolved major psychiatric comorbidity
- The unresolved possibility of secondary gain
- An inappropriate dependency on pharmaceuticals (especially controlled substances)
- Inconsistency among the patient's history, pain description, physical examination, and diagnostic studies
- Abnormal or inconsistent pain ratings
- Predominance of nonorganic signs (e.g., Waddell signs)
- Alternative therapies with a risk/benefit ratio comparable to that of SCS remain to be tried
- Pregnancy
- Occupational risk (e.g., employment requires climbing ladders or operating certain machinery)
- Local or systemic infection
- Presence of a demand pacemaker or cardiac defibrillator
- Foreseeable need for an MRI
- Presence of a major comorbid chronic pain syndrome
- Anticoagulant or antiplatelet therapy

Absolute contraindications (6)
- Inability to control the device
- For patients with failed back surgery syndrome
  - Nerve compression amenable to surgery and causing a serious neurologic deficit
  - Gross spinal instability at risk for progression
- Coagulopathy, immunosuppression, or other condition associated with an unacceptable surgical risk
- Need for therapeutic diathermy (a contraindication for implantable devices)

lead wires and a temporary external transmitter. Most screening trials use percutaneous electrodes placed under fluoroscopy (Fig. 41-5), because they provide access to many levels of the spine with the use of a single epidural needle (6). A surgical plate/paddle can be used in the minority of patients in whom the epidural space is otherwise inaccessible. Whenever possible, electrodes should be placed under local anesthetic, so that the patient can describe paresthesia coverage, react to changes in stimulation, and report any unusual intraoperative events.

Cogent arguments exist for and against anchoring the screening electrode for later use if the screening trial is successful. Anchoring the electrode reduces the cost of hardware in patients who have a successful trial but increases the cost of the screening procedure because it must then be performed in an operating room. An anchored electrode also increases incisional pain, which may be a factor in judging the extent of pain relief during the trial. Yet, pain relief with an anchored

electrode eliminates the possibility that a replacement electrode will not produce the same paresthesia. If the trial fails, the anchored electrode must also be removed in an operating room. However, a temporary percutaneous electrode is less expensive than an implantable electrode, and is easily removed if the trial fails. The parameters of neurostimulation may need to be adjusted during the screening trial and after SCS implantation. A diagrammatic summary of the procedural steps for permanent implantation of spine electrodes and pulse generator is shown in Figure 41-6.

MANAGING PROCEDURAL RISK

Although the risks of SCS are real (Table 41-5), proactive risk management can pay dividends (Table 41-12) (6). Manufacturers offer detailed instructions for implantation of their

TABLE 41-10

VALUE OF A SCREENING TRIAL

Criteria	Grade and recommendations
Does a screening trial provide valid patient-selection information?	A ▪ Medicare requirement ▪ Weighing risk vs. potential benefit and expert consensus reveals a high likelihood of a favorable outcome
Does the length of a screening trial affects its ability to provide valid information?	B ▪ Weighing risk vs. potential benefit and expert consensus reveals a good likelihood of a favorable outcome
What is the optimum length of a screening trial?	B ▪ Weighing risk vs. potential benefit and expert consensus reveals a good likelihood of a favorable outcome
What type of electrode should be used for the screening trial?	A ▪ Weighing risk vs. potential benefit and expert consensus reveals a high likelihood of a favorable outcome
What is the impact of anchoring the screening electrode at the time of implantation for chronic use if the screening trial is successful?	B ▪ Weighing risk vs. potential benefit and expert consensus reveals a good likelihood of a favorable outcome
What should be done to control procedural pain during trial electrode placement?	A ▪ Only option (in some cases) ▪ Weighing risk vs. potential benefit and expert consensus reveals a high likelihood of a favorable outcome
What constitutes a successful screening trial?	Information only
When should a screening trial be repeated?	Information only

Consult the *Practice Parameters for the Use of Spinal Cord Stimulation in the Treatment of Chronic Neuropathic Pain* (6) for a comprehensive bibliography of studies regarding screening trials of SCS.

products as well as troubleshooting tips. Any physician offering SCS should have completed residency, fellowship training, or a preceptorship in SCS in a setting with adequate patient volume to include a full range of candidates for SCS and a complete continuum of pain management strategies. The literature provides no evidence regarding the impact that physician experience with SCS may have on outcome. However, retrospective studies of other therapies demonstrate that high patient volume and relevant physician experience correlate positively with improved outcomes. Finally, never underestimate the importance of enlisting patient and family cooperation in SCS therapy. Thorough discussion of the risks and benefits of therapy, of realistic expectations for pain relief, and of the pa-

tient's responsibilities sets the stage for a successful therapeutic intervention. Discharge instructions must include information about when and how to contact the implanting physician, the device manufacturer, and emergency care providers.

DEVICE SELECTION

Lead wires contain the electrodes used for spinal cord stimulation and are available in a variety of configurations (Fig. 41-7) designed for implantation percutaneously or through laminotomy (59). The simplest leads allow bipolar stimulation with two electrodes, but lead wires with four, eight, or 16 contacts

TABLE 41-11

PURE PERCUTANEOUS TRIAL VS. IMPLANTED SPINAL CORD STIMULATOR TRIAL

Pure percutaneous trial	Implanted trial
▪ Less O.R. time initially ▪ Incisionless removal ▪ Less post op pain to complicate the trial	▪ Same lead(s) used (decreased cost for full implantation) ▪ No need to find the position at second stage (May save O.R. time) ▪ Facilitates longer trial ▪ Requires second open surgery to remove lead if trial is unsuccessful.

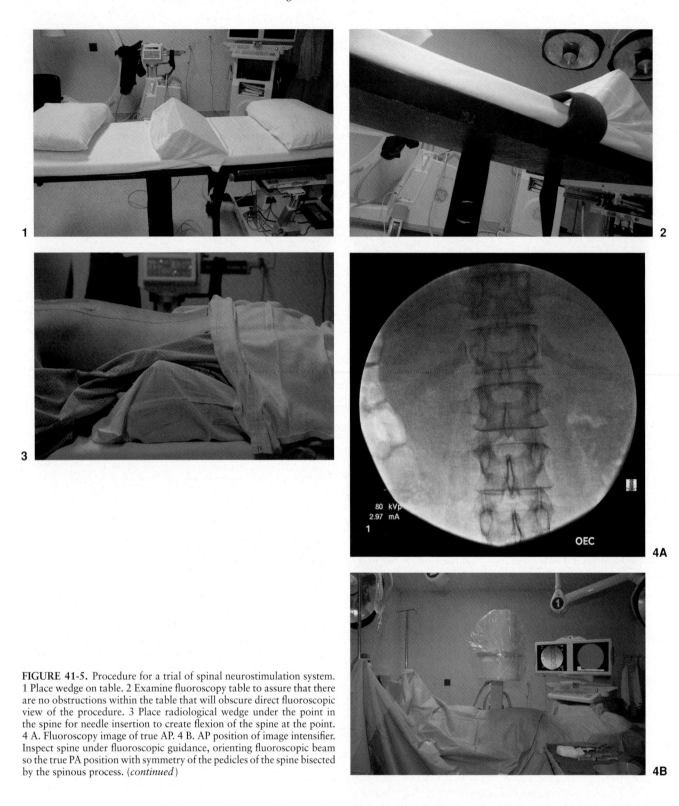

FIGURE 41-5. Procedure for a trial of spinal neurostimulation system. 1 Place wedge on table. 2 Examine fluoroscopy table to assure that there are no obstructions within the table that will obscure direct fluoroscopic view of the procedure. 3 Place radiological wedge under the point in the spine for needle insertion to create flexion of the spine at the point. 4 A. Fluoroscopy image of true AP. 4 B. AP position of image intensifier. Inspect spine under fluoroscopic guidance, orienting fluoroscopic beam so the true PA position with symmetry of the pedicles of the spine bisected by the spinous process. (*continued*)

are also available. Arrays consist of one or two columns of contacts in paddle or plate styles. A newer transverse tripolar configuration enables programming of current across the spinal cord and requires a special transmitter. There is no inherent difference in fracture rates for the various electrodes (6). Systems are powered by internal batteries or by external radiofrequency

(RF) devices. Totally implantable, battery-powered devices resemble cardiac pacemakers (Fig. 41-8) and have a battery life of 2 to 5 years, depending on power demands; rechargeable devices are now available (Fig. 41-9). An implantable pulse generator (IPG) is programmed transcutaneously using a wand attached to a computer. A handheld controller can be used to turn

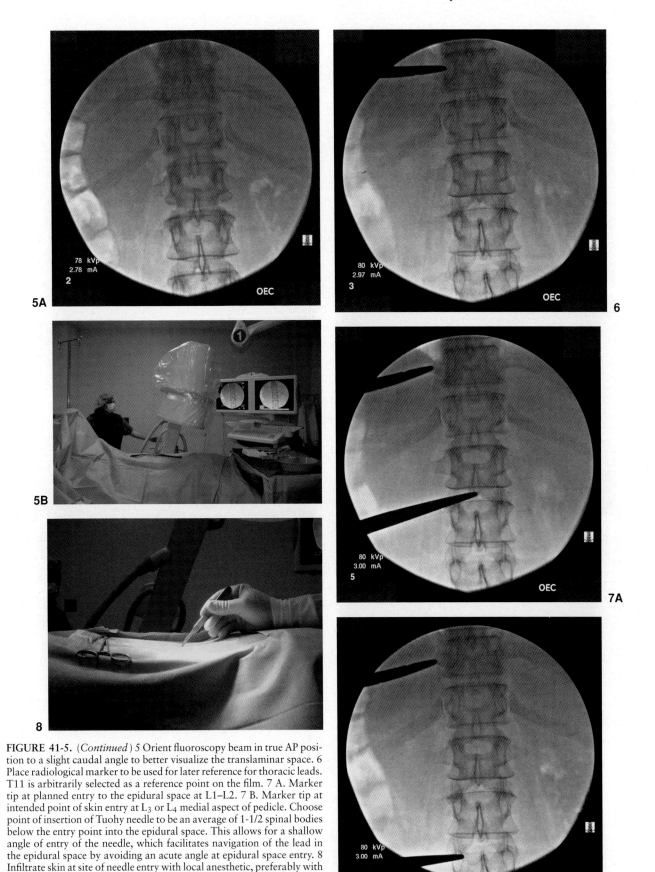

FIGURE 41-5. (*Continued*) 5 Orient fluoroscopy beam in true AP position to a slight caudal angle to better visualize the translaminar space. 6 Place radiological marker to be used for later reference for thoracic leads. T11 is arbitrarily selected as a reference point on the film. 7 A. Marker tip at planned entry to the epidural space at L1–L2. 7 B. Marker tip at intended point of skin entry at L$_3$ or L$_4$ medial aspect of pedicle. Choose point of insertion of Tuohy needle to be an average of 1-1/2 spinal bodies below the entry point into the epidural space. This allows for a shallow angle of entry of the needle, which facilitates navigation of the lead in the epidural space by avoiding an acute angle at epidural space entry. 8 Infiltrate skin at site of needle entry with local anesthetic, preferably with bicarbonate to enhance rapid action and without epinephrine to avoid excess discomfort at time of injection. Make a small skin nick with a scalpel to avoid dulling needle tip. (*continued*)

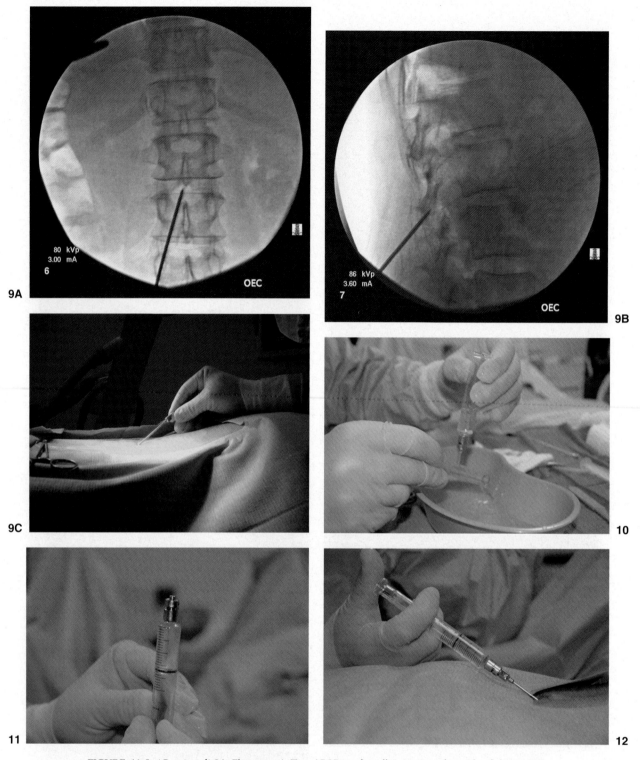

FIGURE 41-5. (*Continued*) 9A. Fluoroscopic True AP View of needle entry into the epidural space at L1-L2. 9 B. Fluoroscopic lateral view of needle engaged in ligamentum flavum prior to entry into the epidural space by loss of resistance technique. 9 C. Needle photograph. Notice angles produced by paramedian approach and the obliqueness of the needle. Advance needle with a paramedian approach, entering at the medial aspect of the pedicle 1-1/2 interspaces below the entry point directed toward the midline toward the point below the inferior aspect of the spinous process at the entry point in the epidural space. Advance needle initially with PA image to assure proper direction of the needle. Convert fluoroscopic beam to lateral view to determine depth of needle at the time of entry into the epidural space. Advance the needle utilizing loss-of-resistance technique while viewing laterally. 10 Prelubricate the loss of resistance syringe with saline. As part of preparation for loss-of-resistance technique, assure that the syringe is properly lubricated with saline. Luer lock syringe assures that high pressure can be developed during the loss-of resistance technique process without dislodging the syringe from the needle. 11 Luer lock syringe, assembled. Note dark ring where the plunger of syringe forms a glass-fluid lock with the barrel wall. 12 Loss-of-resistance technique with constant pressure. Note that the thumb is engaged as the needle advances. (*continued*)

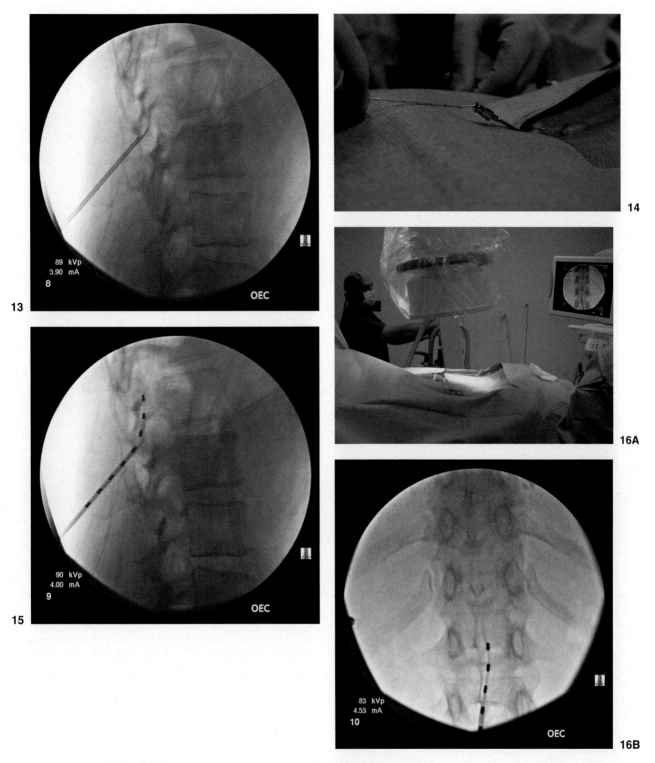

FIGURE 41-5. (*Continued*) 13 Loss of resistance has been achieved. Note, the needle bevel is now rotated to face posteriorly after loss of resistance to facilitate navigation of the lead posteriorly. 14 Insert spinal cord stimulator lead into the needle with the bend of the stylette in the lead oriented toward the ceiling and advance the lead in lateral view to determine that the lead is advancing in the posterior epidural space. 15 In lateral position observe that the lead is directed in the posterior epidural space. 16 A. Rotate the fluoroscopic beam to PA position. Orient the beam with a slight cephalad tilt from the true PA position. This permits real time navigation of the lead without having the operator's hand directly in the fluoroscopy beam. 16 B. the needle tip at 6 o'clock on the fluoroscopy screen. A magnified image at this point enhances the ability to determine small movements of the lead as it advances in the cephalad direction, If difficulties in navigation are encountered, consider changing the acuity of the angle of the stylette at the lead tip to facilitate navigation. (*continued*)

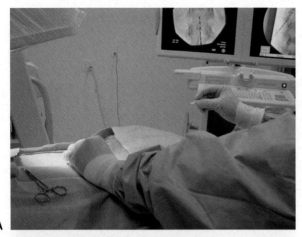

17A

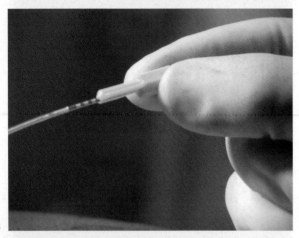

17B

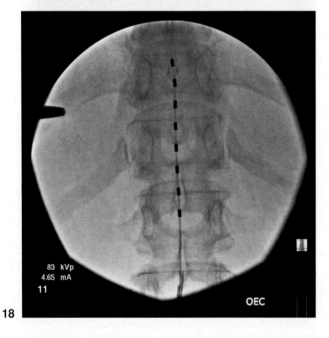

18

FIGURE 41-5. (*Continued*) If the lead is oriented properly but not advancing due to small adhesions, consider changing to a straight stylet to advance in the desired direction. While advancing the lead, it is important to steer the lead in the proper direction and then advance whenever the lead is moving with the appropriate trajectory. When adhesions are present in the epidural space that prevent advancing the lead, mild adhesions can often be avoided by bolusing small amounts of saline immediately prior to reinserting the lead within the needle. Alternatively, contrast can be injected to help delineate any obstruction to lead passage. However, once contrast is injected, the entire procedure becomes encumbered by the stickiness of the contrast solution about the lead. For coverage of an extremity, the lead is usually best placed just off the midline with the lead obscuring the PA view of the fluoroscopy image of the lateral cortex of the ipsilateral spinous process. Obviously, midline leads are placed bisecting the lateral margins of the cortex of the spinous process. Entry points for thoracic leads are usually placed at L1-2 because this entry point is the most stable in the spine. This usually allows for enough placement of the lead in the posterior epidural space without a need for excess lead in the lumbar spine. For cervical lead placement, leads can enter at T1-2 or T2-3 where the posterior epidural space is considerably larger than in the cervical region where it is far more dangerous and ill advised to enter. This allows for sufficient lead in the epidural space prior to reaching the target. 17 A. The lead is advanced with the non-dominant hand close to the hub of the needle and steered with the dominant hand. 17 B Notice steering with the fingers of the dominant hand. The handle at the proximal aspect of the lead provides leverage for steering and its angles provide visual-tactile feedback. 18 Final position of the lead in true AP with the lead centered. Note the marker at T11 for later reference. A reference marker is imperative to identify the site in the thoracic spine in which the lead is placed because often it is not possible to be oriented to exact position if the first lumbar vertebra is absent from the field to identify the lower border of the thoracic spine. It is imperative to have a true AP film for later reference and also to center the beam over the midpoint of the lead contacts to avoid parallax errors that can confuse later viewing of the film when attempting to replace the lead. A true AP without any parallax with good identification with radiological markers can allow for reproduction of the placement of the lead at a later time. A confirmatory lateral view provides data to demonstrate the posterior position of the lead at the time of placement.

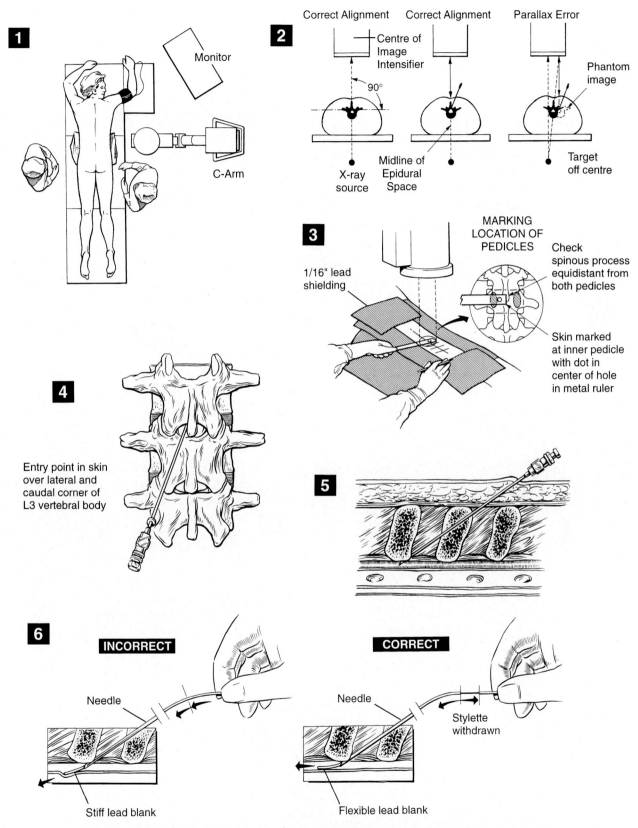

FIGURE 41-6. Diagrammatic summary of procedure for implantation of spinal cord stimulation electrodes and pulse generator (IPG). (*1, 2*) Positioning patient and image intensifier to eliminate parallax errors. (*3*) Marking location of pedicles and checking that spinous processes are equidistant from both pedicles. (*4*) Needle entry through skin at L3 pedicle level and entry into epidural space at L1 spinous process. (*5*) Note shallow angle of needle. (*6*) Electrode stylet withdrawn 1 cm to prevent indentation of dura. (*continued*)

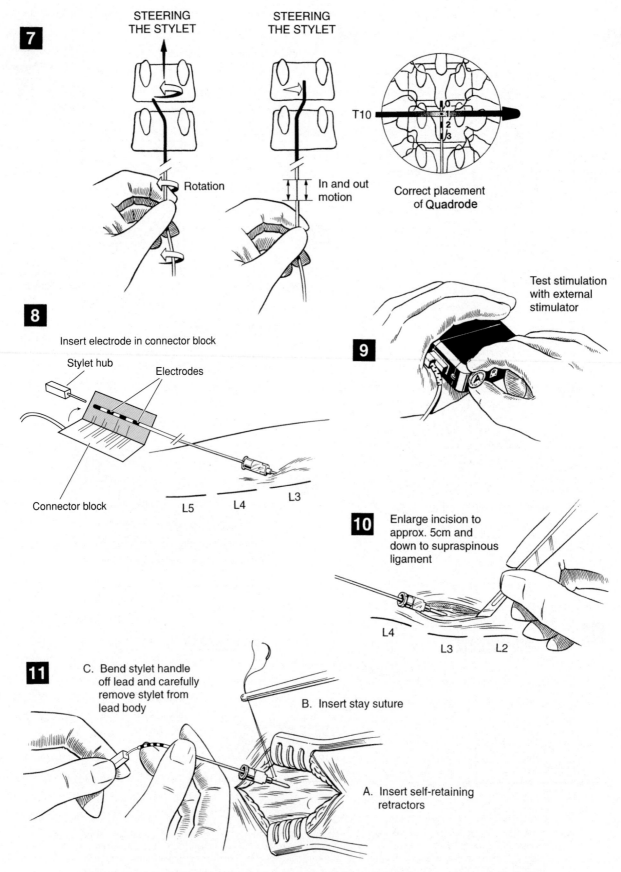

FIGURE 41-6. (*Continued*) (7) Steering of the stylet to final position desired e.g., T10 level. (8, 9) Connection of electrode for trial stimulation. (10) Enlarging incision. (11) Insertion of stay suture. (*continued*)

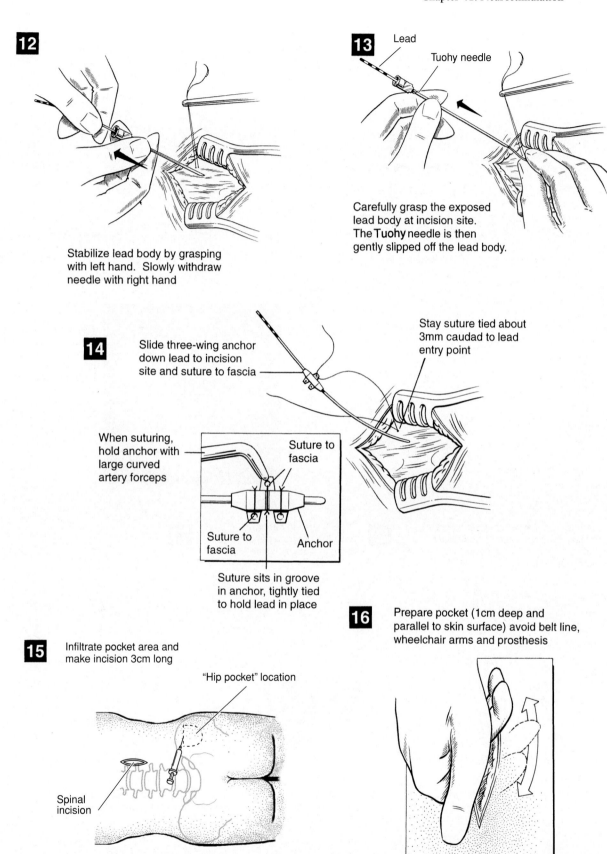

12 Stabilize lead body by grasping with left hand. Slowly withdraw needle with right hand

13 Lead

Tuohy needle

Carefully grasp the exposed lead body at incision site. The Tuohy needle is then gently slipped off the lead body.

14 Slide three-wing anchor down lead to incision site and suture to fascia

Stay suture tied about 3mm caudad to lead entry point

When suturing, hold anchor with large curved artery forceps

Suture to fascia

Suture to fascia

Anchor

Suture sits in groove in anchor, tightly tied to hold lead in place

15 Infiltrate pocket area and make incision 3cm long

"Hip pocket" location

Spinal incision

16 Prepare pocket (1cm deep and parallel to skin surface) avoid belt line, wheelchair arms and prosthesis

FIGURE 41-6. (*Continued*) (*12, 13*) Removal of Tuohy needle. (*14*) Anchoring spinal electrode. (*15, 16*) Marking pulse generator pocket. (*continued*)

PART IV: PAIN MANAGEMENT

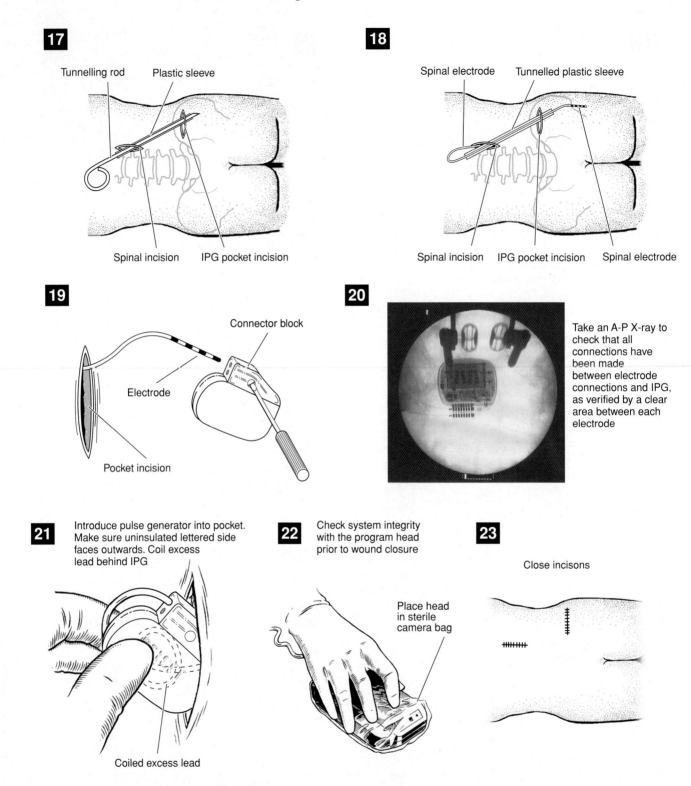

17

Tunnelling rod   Plastic sleeve

Spinal incision   IPG pocket incision

18

Spinal electrode   Tunnelled plastic sleeve

Spinal incision   IPG pocket incision   Spinal electrode

19

Connector block

Electrode

Pocket incision

20

Take an A-P X-ray to check that all connections have been made between electrode connections and IPG, as verified by a clear area between each electrode

21   Introduce pulse generator into pocket. Make sure uninsulated lettered side faces outwards. Coil excess lead behind IPG

Coiled excess lead

22   Check system integrity with the program head prior to wound closure

Place head in sterile camera bag

23

Close incisons

FIGURE 41-6. (*Continued*) (*17, 18*) Tunneling spinal electrode to hip pocket. (*19*) Connecting electrode to pulse generator. (*20*) Check x-ray to confirm electrode connection. (*21*) Insertion of IPG into pocket. (*22*) Checking function of entire system. (*23*) Closure of all incisions.

TABLE 41-12

PROACTIVE RISK MANAGEMENT

Surgical complications
- Obtain an MRI of the target spinal site to identify suspected stenosis or anatomic conditions that might increase risk
- Use an anesthetic technique that allows the patient to provide feedback during insertion or implantation of the electrodes
- Avoid needle placement in areas of pre-existing scarring
- Review the patient's coagulation history, medications, and preoperative blood studies if epidural hematoma is a concern
- Use normal sterile techniques, maintain sterile dressing during the trial, and administer prophylactic intravenous antibiotics before permanent implantation to reduce infection risk

Device-related complications
- Prevent electrode migration by applying silicone elastomer adhesive when anchoring electrodes
- During implantation, avoid putting mechanical stress on leads
- Avoid crossing a mobile joint with subcutaneous lead wire or extension cable
- Use absorbable sutures to eliminate focal stress after the electrode becomes encapsulated
- Avoid using extra connectors, or locate them near existing points of fixation
- Create service loops from redundant cable or lead wire and place them where they can provide strain relief (behind the implantable generator, for example)

Stimulation-induced complications
- Avoid crossing a mobile area of the body with subcutaneous lead wire or extension cable to reduce motion stress from postural changes

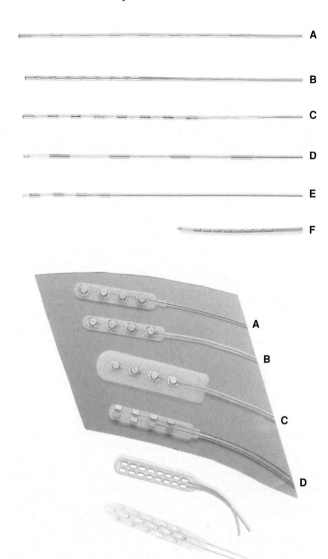

FIGURE 41-7-1. Examples of lead electrodes: **A:** standard eight electrode. **B:** subcompact, eight electrode. **C:** compact, eight electrodes. **D:** pisces quad plus electrodes **E:** Pisces Z quadr, four electrodes **F:** Super compact eight electrodes (Boston). **FIGURE 41-7-2** Examples of paddle electrodes.

the IPG on and off, and set amplitude and rate parameters. The newest IPGs permit independent control of two, four-contact leads. The RF devices rely on an external power pack that broadcasts a radio signal to the implanted receiver and lead wire(s) or to periodically recharged internal batteries (Fig. 41-9). These devices are programmed at the transmitter, which may allow several programs to be stored, so that the patient exerts some control over the stimulation (154).

The choice of stimulator device depends on many factors, including the patient's pain condition, the implanter's experience with various systems, the necessity for postimplantation adjustments, and the patient's ability to control the device. There exists excellent evidence (grade A) from an RCT, well-designed clinical studies, and consensus regarding the respective advantages of percutaneous catheter electrodes versus surgical plate/paddle electrodes (6). Obviously, insertion and removal of a percutaneous electrode is less invasive than the same procedures for plate or paddle electrodes, which require laminectomy or laminotomy. However, surgical plates and paddles are less likely to migrate, once encased in fibrous tissue, than are single or paired electrodes. Targeting of certain sites may be facilitated with specific electrode arrays designed to maximize pain/paresthesia overlap, clinically useful patterns of stimulation, and battery life (42). In the treatment of low back and leg pain, for example, use of an insulated surgical plate or paddle electrode improved paresthesia coverage, pain relief,

and clinical outcome (155). In axial low back pain, a single-column electrode of contacts placed on the midline produces superior results compared with a plate or paddle with dual-column contacts (135,156). Finally, computer modeling studies and short-term clinical results indicate that using transverse tripole electrodes with three columns, which reduce segmental side effects, may be advantageous (46,47,157). The dorsal insulation on plate or paddle electrodes prevents uncomfortable stimulation of nerve fibers in the ligamentum flavum (6).

PATIENT MANAGEMENT

Typically, candidates for SCS have suffered unresolved pain for lengthy periods of time, and they may approach the procedure with fears, skepticism, or wildly unrealistic expectations.

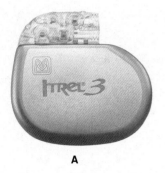
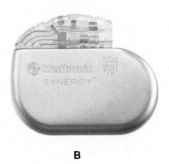
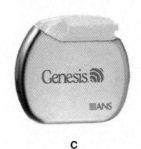

A   B   C

FIGURE 41-8. Examples of non-rechargeable implanted pulse generators.

These should be addressed when reviewing the new patient's history and through continuing patient education. Patients should know that SCS reduces but does not eliminate pain. They should also know that SCS can be used with other pain treatments, as there is no indication of cross-tolerance (6). Adjunct treatments may be especially helpful if a patient's pain has a nociceptive component, which is not likely to be managed by SCS. Patient participation in SCS involves all of the items listed in Table 41-13. Follow-up is mandatory, especially in the first 6 to 8 weeks, when most system adjustments are made. On postoperative day 7 to 14, staples or sutures will be removed and any necessary SCS adjustments made. After that, follow-up visits should be scheduled as necessary to ensure safe and effective operation of the SCS system. Initially, this may mean monthly visits, which can be gradually tapered to yearly visits. Patients with SCS units implanted elsewhere should be followed up as new patients, so that the physician can become familiar with the patient's pain condition and response. Every patient should know how to contact the implanting physician and device manufacturer in case of emergency.

COST EFFECTIVENESS

Payers generally view SCS as a costly therapy because of the initial investment necessary to pay for the screening trial and equipment. Yet there is excellent evidence, including RCTs, to support the cost effectiveness of SCS in treating FBSS and CRPS (6). In the case of FBSS, the per patient costs were U.S. $31,530 for SCS vs. $38,160 for reoperation (using intention-to-treat analyses), $48,357 for SCS vs. $105,928 for reoperation (treated as intended), and $34,371 for SCS vs. $36,341 for reoperation (final treatment) (62). SCS proved consistently superior in the incremental cost-effectiveness and cost-utility ratios compared with reoperation. Budd et al., (120) concluded in their analyses that cost neutrality could be reached with SCS in 5 years or less, even given the high initial cost of the device,

screening trial and necessary follow-up adjustments. Bell et al., (60) reported that successful SCS therapy would pay for itself in 2.1 years. These calculations fall within the break-even or payback range reported by Kumar et al. (121) in their economic analysis of SCS vs. conventional medical therapy. In some centers the time to cost neutrality (payback) was as short as 15 months but ranged up to 5 years at other centers. The payback period is influenced by several variables, including SCS efficacy, battery and electrode life, and the SCS usage (148).

As for CRPS, in an RCT in Holland, the per-patient cost of treatment in the first year after implantation was $4000 higher for SCS than for physical therapy (control) (158). Most of the additional cost (83%) was associated with the implantation procedure. However, after initial treatment the costs in the SCS group were significantly ($p < 0.003$) less than in the control group, primarily due to less need for medical care. After 3 years, the cost differences were permanently reversed in favor of SCS. Thus, in the lifetime analyses, SCS was $60,000 less expensive per patient than the control therapy. In addition, at 1 year follow-up, pain relief ($p < 0.001$) and health-related QOL ($p = 0.004$) were both significantly better for the SCS patients. The authors concluded that the clinical benefits of SCS plus physical therapy were greater than for the control therapy, and because the lifetime costs of SCS plus physical therapy were less, it should be considered the "dominant" therapy.

A British RCT of patients treated for CRPS I found a lifetime cost saving of approximately U.S. $60,800 for the SCS group compared with the physical therapy group (148). The mean cost per quality-adjusted life-year was $23,480 at 12-month follow-up. Another cost-benefit study in Canada compared the cost of SCS with conventional pain therapy for a consecutive series of 104 patients treated in a constant health care delivery environment (121). Over a 5-year period, the mean cumulative cost was Canadian $29,123 for SCS compared with $38,029 for conventional pain management. Costs for the SCS group exceeded those for the conventional management group during the first 2.5 years, but dipped below for the rest of the

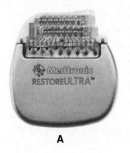
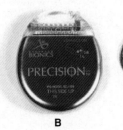

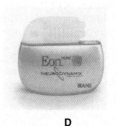

A   B   C   D

FIGURE 41-9. Examples of rechargeable implanted pulse generators.

TABLE 41-13

PATIENT PARTICIPATION IN SPINAL CORD STIMULATION (SCS)

- Understand the goals, benefits and risks of SCS therapy
- List the alternatives to neurostimulation
- Explore the relative merits of various SCS systems and know why a specific system has been selected
- Know what to expect during the trial screening period
- Prepare for the immediate postoperative recovery period
- Work closely with the physician to achieve optimal pain relief after implantation
- Communicate openly with the health care team about response to therapy and report problems immediately
- Commit to regular follow-up appointments

follow-up period. A number of strategies, such as those listed in Table 41-14, can be employed to optimize the cost-effectiveness of SCS.

SACRAL STIMULATION FOR PELVIC PAIN AND INTERSTITIAL CYSTITIS

Recent progress in understanding the pathophysiology of several pain syndromes suggests that neurostimulation could be effective in their treatment. One such syndrome is interstitial cystitis (IC), sometimes described as "reflex sympathetic dystrophy of the bladder." Up to 100 million people in the United States are afflicted with IC. The condition has been recognized for more than 150 years, and is characterized by dysuria, dyspareunia, pelvic pain, urinary frequency and urgency, hematuria, and glomerulation or ulcers. Patients often suffer with worsening symptoms for years before a diagnosis is made (159). Early explanations for the pathogenesis of IC focused on the bladder itself, specifically bladder mucosal defects. However, more than 20 years ago Dr. Stephen McMahon created an animal model of visceral hyperalgesia that tied repeated irritation of the bladder (with turpentine oil) to neurogenic inflammation, in which repeated peripheral nerve stimulation induces vasodilation, edema, and other inflammatory changes (160). In fact, the histologic features of neurogenic inflammation look remarkably similar to the cystoscopic and pathological findings of IC. Persistent irritation may first lead to sensitization of the

nociceptor, and eventually to neural remodeling and hypersensitivity. Thus, normally quiescent sacral dorsal root ganglion neurons could be activated, providing new receptors for pain mediators, such as substance P and neurokinin (NK)-1 (161). If neurogenic inflammation alters central processing of pain signals at the dorsal root, then therapy for IC, which traditionally relied on neurodestruction, can instead be aimed at inhibiting C-fiber nociceptors with neurostimulation.

Several small clinical studies have evaluated sacral stimulation to treat refractory IC, and one device (Interstim, Medtronic, Minneapolis, MN) has been approved by the U.S. Food and Drug Administration (FDA) to stimulate sacral nerve roots in patients with urge incontinence. A prospective, multicenter study using this device followed patients with urinary urge incontinence, urgency-frequency, or retention for up to 3 years (162). Some of these patients likely had urgency-frequency due to IC. After 3 years, 59% of the urge incontinent patients had greater than 50% reduction in leaking and 46% were completely dry.

In a prospective study of 15 women with refractory IC, Maher and co-workers (163) succeeded in significantly increasing mean voiding volume ($p <0.001$), and in decreasing mean daytime ($p <0.012$) and nighttime ($p = 0.007$) frequency, and mean pain score ($p <0.001$) using percutaneous sacral nerve stimulation. During stimulation, the women reported significantly improved QOL measured by social functioning, bodily pain, and general health. Seventy-three percent of the women subsequently asked for complete sacral nerve root implantation. Feler and colleagues (164) used a retrograde lumbar approach to stimulate S2 and S3 nerve roots in patients with IC in whom pain therapy has failed and cystectomy was being considered. By using relatively high frequencies (200–1,000 Hz), they achieved a 75% success rate in more than 100 patients. These outcomes are encouraging, given the generally poor results associated with other current treatments for IC.

The transsacral route is well described and is an approved treatment for IC. The retrograde approach for sacral stimulation employs electrodes directed to the S2, S3, and S4 sacral nerves by a percutaneous retrograde, oblique, extradural approach at either L5–S1 or L4–L5 interlaminar spaces. Usually, two electrodes on each side, as shown in Figure 41-10 are

TABLE 41-14

STRATEGIES FOR OPTIMIZING COST-EFFECTIVENESS

- Adjust stimulation parameters to prolong battery life
- Minimize complications, especially those related to system explantation and replacement
- Improve equipment design and performance
- Select patients carefully
- Offer spinal cord stimulation before ablative therapies, such as sympathectomy, dorsal root gangliectomy, or reoperation

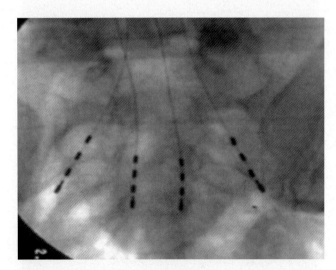

FIGURE 41-10. Sacral nerve root stimulation, retrograde approach. Fluoroscopic image of four electrodes placed via a retrograde epidural approach. (Image courtesy of Michael Stanton-Hicks.)

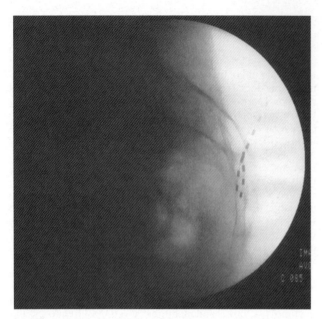

FIGURE 41-11. Sacral nerve root stimulation, trans-sacral approach. Fluoroscopic image, lateral view of transsacral electrode insertion. Note octrode traversing sacral foramen to presacral location.

sufficient to achieve stimulation paresthesia in the pelvis or pelvic floor. Intraoperative testing for paresthesiae in the appropriate region is always performed to assure satisfactory location of the electrodes. Motor fiber stimulation in S2 results in buttock muscle contraction. Stimulation of S3 or S4 supply to external anal sphincter results in contraction of the anus. Any electrode instability with changing paresthesiae that is experienced by the patient during the trial may make it necessary to consider a transsacral percutaneous technique (Figs. 41-11 and 41-12) or a laminectomy at L5–S1, with direct placement

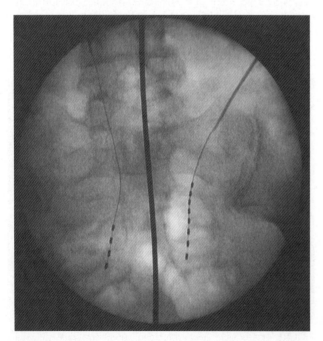

FIGURE 41-12. Sacral nerve root stimulation, trans-sacral approach. Anteroposterior view of two electrodes in situ.

of a laminectomy paddle electrode in the same position as that found to provide therapeutic paresthesiae during the trial. A trial is necessary before implantation of these electrodes. As with other peripheral nerves, the stimulation parameters used for sacral nerve stimulation are very small. After a week's successful trial, the electrodes are removed and a new set is introduced to the same position. These are tunneled to the buttock, where a pocket for a dual-channel IPG is made.

PERIPHERAL NERVE STIMULATION

The use of peripheral nerve stimulation (PNS) can be traced back through millennia. Various species of fish were used in Asia by the Chinese and, undoubtedly, contemporaneously by the Greeks, Romans, and ancient Egyptians for the treatment of a number of medical conditions including headache and gout. The clinical demonstration of pain relief and anesthesia during stimulation of major nerve trunks was included in a treatise describing the use of medical electricity by Althaus (10). With the publication of the gate control theory by Melzack and Wall (2), research in animals and later in humans demonstrated the tremendous potential of neurostimulation to control a number of painful neuropathic conditions (27,165–167).

Early experiments in animals by Shealy and colleagues (168) showed that both SCS and stimulation of peripheral nerves could produce behavioral changes to painful stimuli. In fact, the very first implant of a spinal cord stimulator by Shealy, a neurosurgeon, resulted from his work with a colleague, Mortimer, who was at the time a predoctoral student of biomedical engineering at Case Western Reserve University in Cleveland (169). Stimulation-produced analgesia (SPA), a term introduced by Reynolds (165), applies to all forms of neurostimulation, of which PNS is but one modality.

The development of PNS in parallel with SCS in the early 1970s opened an era of managing pain that was poorly addressed by pharmacologic means. Unfortunately, the early success of these two modalities was overshadowed by technical problems related to the devices that were implanted in the spine and on peripheral nerves. Although the development of SCS devices continued to improve with the advent of percutaneous leads (79,170–172), similar developments in the design and application of peripheral nerve stimulators was lacking. By the late 1970s, the morbidity associated with many PNS surgeries had driven away all but a dedicated minority of surgeons, who recognized the peculiar advantages conferred by PNS. The revival of PNS relates to its special attributes in modulating neuropathic pain and to the technical developments that are now defining the application of PNS as a valuable tool for neurostimulation.

Functional Neuroanatomy

Peripheral Nerve Trunks

Peripheral nerves contain afferent and efferent axons, which, with their Schwann cells, are enclosed in a delicate layer of endoneurial tissue (endoneurium). (See Chapter 2, Figure 2-4.) This connective tissue allows the diffusion of fluids to and from neural structures. The perineurium encloses each bundle of axons (e.g., the *gaine lamelleuse* forms the perineurium)

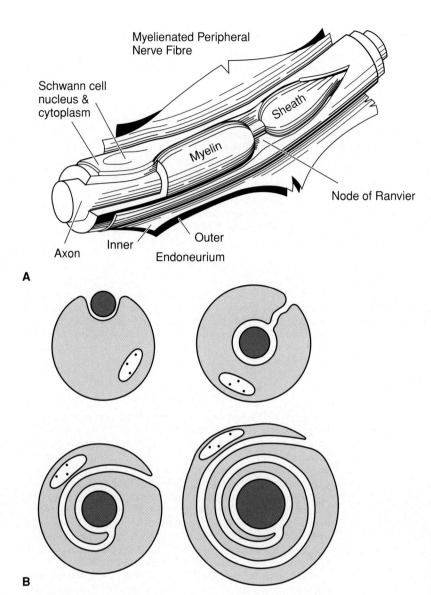

Myelienated Peripheral
Nerve Fibre

Schwann cell
nucleus &
cytoplasm

Sheath

Myelin

Node of Ranvier

Axon   Inner   Outer
              Endoneurium

A

B

FIGURE 41-13. A: Peripheral nerve trunk structure. Morphology of a myelinated axon. Note delicate layer of endoneural tissue (after Sunderland). **B:** Changing axon–Schwann cell relationship, with development of concentric lamellae.

(Fig. 41-13). Each sensory cell body has only one process, an axon with a long branch that extends from its functional source and a shorter branch that extends from the cell body to the spinal cord. Otherwise, the axon is unipolar. Axons transmit sensory information from receptors in the periphery to the second-order neurons in the spinal cord. In contrast, motor neurons with cell bodies in the ventral horn of the spinal cord are multipolar, having many dendrites that channel impulses to the periphery in order to activate particular effector organs. The dendrites and cell bodies of these neurons are specialized to integrate postsynaptic currents that modulate effector organs (see Chapter 2, Fig. 2-1).

Myelinated nerve fibers are made up of many laminae that arise from a single Schwann cell (Fig. 41-13B). The fibers are interrupted at intervals by nodes of Ranvier (see Chapter 2, Fig. 2-2). The diameter of an axon can vary along its length from as little as 2 microns to 11.75 microns (173,174). To preserve regional distribution, nerve fibers must divide into many branches. This architecture allows for the innervation of a significant tissue mass by a single neuron. As a result, referred

pain that may originate within a single neuron is transferred by branches to other tissues in the same region. Axon reflex represents another mechanism responsible for pain being felt in undisturbed adjacent tissue. Antidromic and orthodromic transmission also causes expansion of the painful area. Table 41-15 lists the diameters of nerve fibers, their conduction velocities, and functions.

Morphology of Nerve Trunks

We owe an accurate picture of the fascicular nerve supply to Sunderland (Figs. 41-14 and 41-15) (175–177). Fascicles vary in size from 0.04 to 4 mm. Most fall within the range of 0.04 to 2 mm. As fascicles approach a joint, they tend to divide into smaller and more numerous fibers, which become more topographically discrete as the nerve fibers proceed distally. In addition, the orientation of fascicles moves radially as they prepare to distribute into the nerve branches arising from sensory receptors, or supplying motor units (motor fibers), or both—mixed sensory and motor nerves. The ulnar nerve behind the medial

TABLE 41-15

NERVE FIBERS, CONDUCTION VELOCITIES, AND FUNCTION

Nerve fiber	Diameter Nm	Conduction velocity m/s	Function
A alpha	12–20	70–120	Motor, Extrafusal Muscle Fibers, Proprioceptors
Beta	5–12	30–70	Touch, Pressure
Gamma	3–6	15–30	Motor, Intrafusal Muscle Fibers
Delta	2–5	10–30	Nociceptors, Touch, Temperature
B	1.5–3	3–15	Pre-Ganglionic Sympathetic Fibers
C	<2	0.5–2	Post-Ganglionic Sympathetic Fibers

epicondyle illustrates fascicular variability, as many nerve fibers are grouped into a single fascicle in this location. Other examples of this intraneural arrangement are the radial nerve in the spiral groove, the axillary nerve behind the humerus, and the common peroneal nerve in the lower thigh.

The epineurium also influences the effect of neurostimulation. The epineurial tissue as a percentage of nerve tissue may vary between 30% and almost 78% in the sciatic nerve, for example. The greater the thickness, the more attenuated the electrical field. The thickness of the epineurium and the electrical attenuation also influence the amount of local anesthetic necessary to diffuse through an axon and determine the resulting analgesic effect (see Chapter 2, Fig. 2-4).

Nerve Blood Supply

Collateral veins and arteries to peripheral nerves are derived from adjacent blood vessels (Fig. 41-16). These vasa nervorum are generally tortuous, in order to accommodate transitional movement of the nerve. The extent of the movement increases with proximity to a joint. Also, the variability with which blood vessels provide additional flow to a nerve is considerable throughout the length of each nerve. This has the effect of creating a "natural water shed" zone in each nerve between each collateral source. However, it has been shown that while the loss of collateral flow at a given site (from surgical resection, for example) reduces the interneural flow, this flow is generally reestablished within 3 days (178–180).

Many past therapeutic failures of PNS can be attributed to induced morbidity at the time of electrode placement. Anything that induces sclerosing pathology or materially occludes

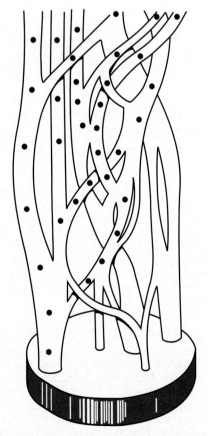

FIGURE 41-14. Arrangement of nerve fascicles. Representation of fascicular dispersal with branching fibers in the fascicular plexuses.

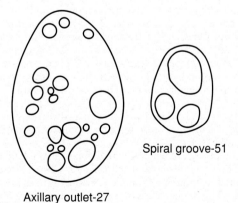

Spiral groove-51

Axillary outlet-27

FIGURE 41-15. Transverse section of radial nerve showing distribution of fascicles at the axillary outlet and in the spiral groove.

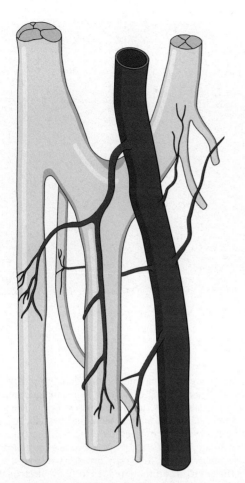

FIGURE 41-16. Collateral blood supply to two separate nerves.

nutrient arteries of nerves can cause neural ischemia. Intraepineural sclerosis is an insidious cause of neural morbidity. Even given the forgoing observations, however, loss of the collateral blood supply for peripheral nerve trunks is not so critical in most cases because of the extensive longitudinal vascular plexus within each nerve. Compression or contusional injury to a nerve is a far greater potential factor of neural morbidity.

Indications for Peripheral Nerve Stimulation

An extensive bibliography, mostly anecdotal, and case reports have identified a wide range of conditions that are amenable to PNS (Table 41-16). That PNS is an effective modality for the treatment of neuropathic pain in one or two nerves is well described by surgeons who have persisted with the technique, in spite of the many reports describing associated complications and morbidity (181–189). Although the use of large surface-contact metal electrodes became very popular, their use has certainly not been concordant with the underlying neuroarchitecture or function of peripheral nerves. Small-diameter electrodes, which can be placed through a needle subcutaneously, were used by Wall and Sweet (1967) to demonstrate the effects of neurostimulation on each other's infraorbital nerves, and temporary subcutaneous placement of electrodes on peripheral

TABLE 41-16

POTENTIAL SITES FOR PNS

Cranial Nerves
    Trigeminal and Branches
    Supra Orbital
    Infraorbital

Occipital Nerve

Segmental Nerves
    Nerve Root
    Intercostal
    Ilioinguinal
    Iliohypogastric
    Genitofemoral

Upper and Lower Extremity
    Ulnar
    Median
    Radial
    Lateral Cutaneous
    Sciatic
        Peroneal
        Tibial
        Posterior tibial

Brachial Plexus

Lumbosacral Plexus

nerves has also been advocated by Campbell and Long (182) to predict the efficacy of PNS. A surgical trial of PNS, using either an electrode adjacent to a nerve or inserting a microelectrode under the epineurium, can be undertaken before implantation of the power source (an IPG or RF receiver). A successful outcome of PNS can be improved by incorporating the measures shown in Table 41-17.

During electrode placement, investigators (190,191,184) determined that the amplitude required to stimulate sensory fibers almost reached the minimum threshold for stimulation of motor fibers, thereby reducing the efficacy of the technique. Goldner and colleagues (192), Waisbrod and colleagues (193), and Gybels and Kupers (194) demonstrated that paddle-type electrodes, previously developed for SCS, improved the therapeutic success of the procedure, and these electrodes were subsequently approved for PNS. Racz and co-workers (195,196) reported on the use of fascia, either as a free graft or from adjacent tissue, to separate the electrode contacts from the nerve in the belief that foreign-body reaction and scarring would be reduced. This technique was later adopted by other implanters with improved results (186,187,197–199).

TABLE 41-17

CRITERIA FOR PERIPHERAL NERVE STIMULATION

Neuropathic pain arising in the distribution of a single nerve.
EMG and NCS evidence of axonal damage.
Demonstration by nerve block of pain relief.
Psychological clearance excluding adverse behavioral or
    psychiatric pathology.

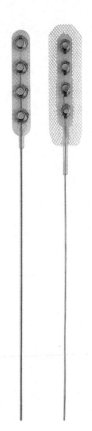

FIGURE 41-17. Electrodes approved for peripheral nerve stimulation in the United States.

In the United States, only two electrodes are approved by the FDA: the Resume or On-Point electrodes (Medtronic Corporation, Minneapolis, MN; see Fig. 41-17).

These electrodes were originally approved for use with an RF transmitter. Recently, this approval has been extended to cover a fully implanted pulse generator. The stability of paddle electrodes will be inversely affected by the dynamic nature of the tissues within which they are implanted and the nature of scarring resulting from their surgical placement. Any separation from the nerve by distraction, loss of longitudinal orientation, or tipping will degrade the efficiency of the electrical field supplied to the nerve, resulting in either partial or complete loss of therapeutic neurostimulation and, therefore, of analgesia.

Although most peripheral nerves are ovoid or oval in shape, many different electrode designs have been suggested. Buschmann and Oppel (200) described one type of microelectrode that has been used extensively for functional electrical stimulation (FES) (201–203).

Surgical Technique

Five sites for access to peripheral nerves will be described: (1) the median and ulnar nerves, at the mid humerus level; (2) the radial nerve in the spiral grove, also mid humerus; (3) the sciatic and (4) common peroneal nerves, easily reached behind the iliotibial band at the lateral aspect of the mid thigh;

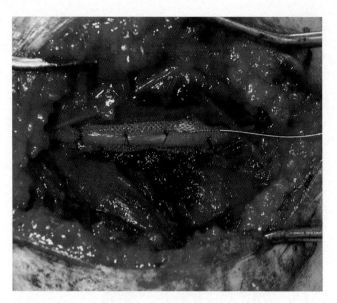

FIGURE 41-18. On-point electrode sutured via Gortex skirt to ulnar nerve.

and (5) the posterior tibial nerve immediately proximal to the medial malleolus. During dissection to reach each nerve, care is taken to preserve any cutaneous nerve and, in the arm, the medial antebrachial cutaneous nerve and vessels. A length of each target nerve is then carefully dissected free from its surrounding tissue, taking care to preserve any motor branches or collateral circulation. It is only necessary to free a length of nerve sufficient to accommodate the On-point electrode, which is then secured by use of its Gortex "skirt" with 4.0 monofilament nylon sutures. Because of their size, two On-point electrodes are placed on the sciatic nerve, taking care to position them adjacent to the peroneal and tibial divisions (Figs. 41-18 and 41-19). For a two-stage surgical procedure, usually a short 48-hour trial suffices. An extension attached to the electrode

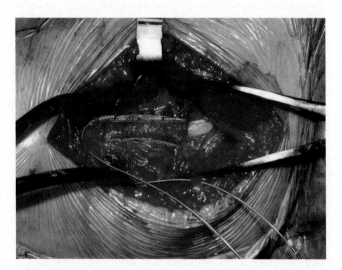

FIGURE 41-19. Two On-point electrodes attached to the sciatic nerve.

lead is passed through the skin some distance from the main incision, and then attached to the externalized pulse generator. After a successful trial, the wound is reopened. For an upper extremity implant, the pocket for the RF receiver or IPG is generally made beneath the clavicle, either under the fascia of the pectoris major muscle or, in thin individuals, beneath the muscle itself on the chest wall. For PNS procedures in the leg, the IPG can be placed behind the iliotibial band in the thigh, thereby reducing the length of the extension and eliminating the need for it to pass the hip joint, as would be necessary for a buttock site.

Stimulation Characteristics

Most nerves that are currently amenable to neurostimulation are mixed nerves. For this reason, the plexus-like fascicular morphology will influence the sensory threshold, making it more difficult to separate sensory from motor sensation.

As can be seen in Figure 41-19, an ideal situation would be to achieve a bipole on several sensory fascicles, using the smallest possible current to achieve sensory thresholds for topographical paresthesiae while remaining well below the threshold for motor stimulation. Arguably, this situation should provide optimal inhibition of pain pathways and therefore analgesia. Stimulation currents required for PNS are markedly lower than those required for SCS. Typically, the amplitude to achieve therapeutic stimulation is 0.1 to 1 volt, with pulse widths of 120 to 180 ms being optimal, and frequencies typically varying between 50 and 90 Hz. Given the contemporary electrode technology, it is not necessary to undertake intraoperative programming similar to that used during SCS in an awake patient. With the future development of electrodes that have multiple small contacts that conform to the shape of peripheral nerves, routine fascicular mapping will be possible, thereby allowing optimal analgesia to be achieved with the least current required in each affected nerve.

Current Outcomes

The clinical outcome of eight studies published during the past 17 years will be described. All these studies report uniform improvement and agreement regarding outcome measures, yet none of the studies are prospective. Cooney and Strege (197,198) reported their combined results in 60 patients over a 2-year period. Pain relief occurred in 80% of these patients, with analgesia being maintained at 2 years. Half of the patients studied had good pain relief and either returned to their full-time occupation or changed from no employment to part-time employment.

Schetter and colleagues (204) described 70% and 80% pain relief in 117 males and females, respectively. Sixty-five percent of these patients increased their ADLs, and 75% said that they were happy with the therapy.

In 1999, Buschman and Oppel described 52 patients in whom micro-, subepineurial electrodes were implanted for a variety of neuropathic pain conditions (200). They reported good results in 80% of their patients; 22 patients returned to either full- or part-time work, and two patients changed their occupations.

Novak and MacKinnon (199) reported their experience with 17 patients. Sixty percent described good to excellent

pain relief, four had fair relief, and three had poor relief at 21 months. Six of their patients returned to work.

A review of results from three centers was undertaken by Eisenberg and co-workers (205) in 46 patients with neuropathic pain treated between 1993 and 1995. Their review is especially compelling because they examined earlier data that had been published at one of the centers (Mainz) covering cases from 1985 to 1986. Four patients had failed previous therapies, and all had a good response with relief of their neuropathic pain after a diagnostic local anesthetic block of the affected nerve. The results were classified as good in 26 patients (78%) and poor in 10 (22%). Overall pain intensity, before and after surgery, was a mean of 69 and 24 using the VAS scale of 0 to 100 mm ($p <0.001$).

Johnson and Burchiel (206) reported on the successful implantation of PNS in 11 patients who had postherpetic neuralgia affecting the supraorbital (eight patients) and infraorbital nerves (three patients). The one patient who had sustained a traumatic injury to the infraorbital nerve did not respond to PNS. After 26 months, at least 50% pain relief was sustained in 70% of all patients. Medication use declined by 70%. In two patients, PNS failed to address their neuropathic symptoms, most likely a reflection of the degree of axon loss. Mobbs and colleagues (207) described a reduction in neuropathic pain in almost half of their patients. Sixty-three percent of the patients reduced or eliminated their use of oral analgesics. Activity levels were improved in 47%, unchanged in 37%, and worse in 16%.

Occipital Nerve Stimulation

Weiner and colleagues (208) were the first to publish their experience with greater occipital nerve stimulation (GONS). A second publication elaborated on the original procedure (209). This technique was introduced primarily to address pain arising in the occipital nerve distribution, and is recommended for its management when all other headache-relief techniques have failed. Like many other "diagnostic nerve" blocks (see Chapter 38), response to local anaesthetic greater occipital nerve block does not predict the success of GONS (210). However some advocate demonstrating symptomatic relief by two local anesthetic blocks of the occipital nerve prior to considering GONS. Then a trial of neurostimulation is undertaken using a percutaneous approach with either a quadripolar or octapolar SCS lead. After a successful trial, a permanent percutaneous type of SCS lead, similar to that used for the trial or a quadripolar laminectomy (paddle) electrode is introduced in the subcutaneous tissue at the C1–C2 level (Figs. 41-20 to 41-22). Percutaneous leads are increasingly preferred because of the tendency for paddle electrodes to erode the skin and lead to infection. It is important to undertake electronic testing intraoperatively to determine that topical paresthesiae are perceived in the distribution of the occipital nerve. Surgical access is gained through a small midline incision, allowing either unilateral or bilateral electrodes to be positioned if the headache is on both sides. The electrodes are retained in situ by braided nylon or silk sutures, making a generous strain-relief loop that will accommodate extension and flexion of the neck. This procedure is particularly important to prevent dislodgement when a longer extension is used for connection to the IPG in the buttock. The IPG can also be placed in a pocket inferior to the clavicle. Although initially occipital stimulation was mainly used for occipital neuralgia, other applications are

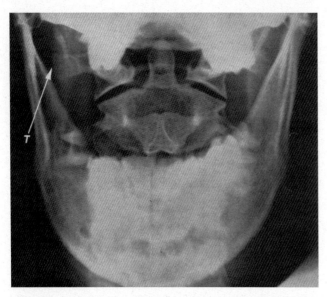

FIGURE 41-20. Suboccipital nerve stimulation. Anteroposterior radiograph of cervical spine. The transverse process of C1 (the atlas) is marked (*T*). The large upward projecting "peg" of C2 (the axis) clearly identifies C2. The large articular processes of C2–C2 are seen sloping laterally and slightly inferiorly above the body of C2. Most clinicians target the body of C2, whereas others advocate the C1–C2 articulation as a more reliable target for occipital nerve stimulation.

emerging. Patients with severe intractable migraine (211,210) have emerged as good candidates. Some respond to GONS and some do not, thus trial stimulation is the only method of determining which patients are suitable for implantation. Controlled trials are now underway in migraine patients (the PRISM trial [212]).

Initial reports indicate that cluster headache and hemicrania continua may also respond to G0NS. Thirteen patients with intractable cluster headache were followed up for 19 months after GONS: three improved by 90%; two by 40% to 60%; five by 20% to 30% and three had no improvement. Ten of the study group said they would recommend the treatment to other patients (213,214). Other reports with long-term follow-up also indicate positive outcomes in about 50% of patients with migraine, cluster headache, and hemicrania continua (215–217).

Possible Mechanisms of Occipital Nerve Stimulation

Greater occipital nerve (see Chapter 17) has been used for many years to provide short-term relief of severe headache, including migraine (218). Usually both local anesthetic and corticosteroid were employed. The mechanism of relief beyond the duration of the local anesthetic (sometimes of the order of 1 month) was unknown. A neurosurgeon and pain research pioneer, Fred Kerr of the Mayo Clinic, suggested many years ago that there was a major anatomical overlap of the nucleus caudalis of the trigeminal system and the C2 segment of the cervical spinal cord—the so-called *trigeminocervical complex* (TCC) (219).

However, only recently, direct connections have been described in the TCC of afferents from the brain meninges and cervical afferents. A population of neurons in the C2 dorsal horn was identified that received convergent input from supratentorial dura mater and the GON (220,221). Furthermore, the TCC has ascending and descending connections with brainstem structures such as the periaqueductal gray (PAG), nucleus raphe magnus, and rostroventral medulla (see Chapters 31 and 32).

Stimulation of the foregoing brain areas produces profound antinociception (47). In chronic migraine patients, PET brain scanning reveals that ONS alters thalamic activation in parallel with improvement in head pain (51). A review of current thinking on mechanisms of GONS has been provided by Goadsby and colleagues (220).

Supraorbital and Supratrochlear Neuralgia

Dunteman (222) published a description of supraorbital and supratrochlear nerve stimulation in 2002. The procedure is undertaken for cases of refractory postherpetic or trigeminal neuralgia after all conservative or regional anesthetic measures have failed. Supraorbital and supratrochlear blocks must first demonstrate complete symptomatic relief before the trial stimulation is undertaken with a percutaneous electrode (Fig. 41-23). The most suitable electrode for this purpose is a closely spaced quadripolar or octipolar SCS electrode.

Entry through the skin is by means of an SCS needle, curved to conform to the curvature of the skull, which is introduced above and anterior to the tragus of the ear. During insertion of the needle, care must be taken to avoid disturbing the su-

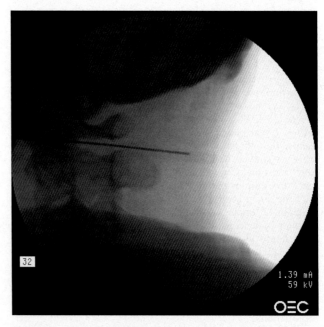

FIGURE 41-21. Suboccipital nerve stimulation. Lateral fluoroscopic image with marker for target site placed just below C1.

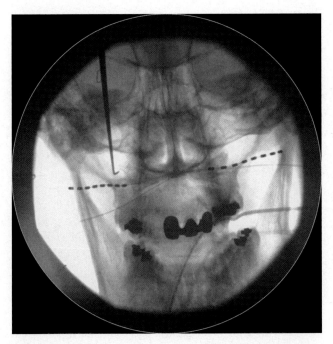

FIGURE 41-22. Suboccipital Stimulation A-P view. Electrodes have been placed bilaterally across the superior aspect of the articulation of C_1–C_2, at the base of the dens ("peg") of C_2 which is seen projecting superiorly. Superimposed on the peg is the midline septum of the symmetrically placed ethmoid air cells. The peg has been aligned midway between the two orbits (at the top of the x-ray). The octrode on the reader's right of the image is correctly placed to cover both greater and lesser occipital nerves. The marker on the reader's left has been placed to indicate the intended lateral extent of the three electrodes that will be used to stimulate the greater occipital nerve. On the right side, the electrodes are in place. Final correction is being made on the left side, with the electrode being moved medially. Note the lateral extent of both electrode arrays about 1 cm below the mastoid processes.

perficial temporal artery, nerve, and the superficial temporal branches of the auriculotemporal nerve. After a successful trial of stimulation, another subcutaneous quadripolar SCS electrode is passed to the same site through a tiny incision that will allow retention using braided nylon or silk sutures. After connecting the lead wire to an extension, this is passed through a subcutaneous tunnel over the ear and down the neck, posterior to the sternomastoid muscle to a site where a pocket for the IPG is made just below the clavicle. The lead and IPG are connected, and the IPG retained in its pocket using braided nylon or silk sutures.

Trigeminal Nerve Stimulation

The treatment of trigeminal neuralgia and postherpetic neuralgia in the second or third divisions of the trigeminal nerve is difficult to achieve. The use of neurostimulation can be considered after other conservative or surgical techniques have failed. Although PNS is still regarded as a technique of last resort, because of its nondestructive nature a strong argument can be made for earlier use of neurostimulation. The approach originally described by Meglio (223), Meyerson and Håkansson (224), and more recently Taub and colleagues (225) uses the percutaneous approach originally described by Härtel. A 5 to

7 mm electrode length is passed through the foramen ovale. Accurate positioning of the electrode can be achieved using stimulation paresthesiae in the appropriate nerve distribution. A trial will allow the patient to appreciate whether PNS is likely to be successful in obtaining pain relief.

Percutaneous Field Stimulation

Field stimulation, a potential alternative to direct nerve stimulation, offers promise of pain relief in a number of applications. This approach may be used in conjunction with either PNS or SCS. In principle, the percutaneous insertion of an SCS lead into the subcutaneous tissue where pain is experienced presumably influences small nerve fibers, thereby inhibiting the expression of pain in this distribution. The following situations exemplify percutaneous filed stimulation.

Facial Pain

Pain occurring on the forehead might be addressed by passing a percutaneous SCS lead to the site of pain. The lead wire is then connected to an external pulse generator for a period of trial stimulation. One week should be sufficient to determine if there is symptomatic relief. If the technique succeeds, an electrode can be implanted at the same site and tunneled to a site beneath the clavicle where a pocket for the IPG is made.

Residual Pain after Spinal Surgery

Another example is residual low back pain after spinal surgery that is unrelieved by SCS. Back pain may represent as much as 70% of a patient's total pain. The residual pain may be addressed by placing two percutaneous octapolar SCS leads

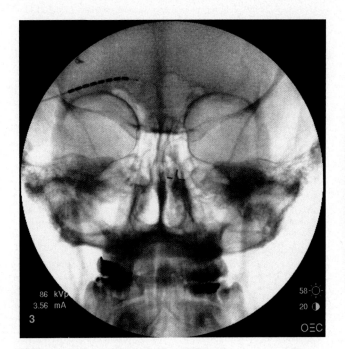

FIGURE 41-23. Supraorbital electrode in situ.

subcutaneously, parallel to the lumbar spine. A trial of 1 week is generally sufficient to determine whether percutaneous field stimulation will provide any additional symptomatic relief. Although lacking any rigorous supportive studies, this technique may offer another means of treating an otherwise difficult pain problem.

Post Inguinal Herniorrhaphy Neuralgia

It has now become apparent that approximately 10% of patients continue to experience neuropathic pain, at the operative site in the inguinal region, more than a year after surgery (see Chapter 31). Some of these patients fail to obtain relief with maximum medical treatment and become candidates for neuromodulation. An Octrode lead is inserted via a Tuohy needle into the center of the painful inguinal area. A trial stimulation is performed using an external pulse generator. If successful, a permanent lead and generator are implanted. The inguinal region is conveniently located very close to an often used lower abdominal site for pulse generator implantation. Initial results are encouraging but consist only of case series (226).

References

1. Shealy CN, Mortimer JT, Reswick J. Electrical inhibition of pain by stimulation of the dorsal column: Preliminary clinical reports. *Anesth Analg* 1967;46:489–491.
2. Melzack R, Wall PD. Pain mechanisms: A new theory. *Science* 1965;150: 971–979.
3. Siegfried J, Lazothes Y. Long-term follow-up of dorsal column stimulation for chronic pain syndrome after multiple lumbar operations. *Appl Neurophysiol* 1982;45:201–204.
4. Erickson DL, Long DM. Ten-year follow-up of dorsal column stimulation. In: Bonica JJ, Lindblom U, Iggo A, eds. *Advances in Pain Research and Therapy*, Vol. 5. New York: Raven; 1983:583–589.
5. North RB, Ewend MG, Lawton MT, et al. Failed back surgery syndrome: 5-year follow-up after spinal cord stimulator implantation. *Neurosurgery* 1991;28(5):692–699.
6. North RB, Shipley J, The Neuromodulation Therapy Access Coalition. Practice parameters for the use of spinal cord stimulation in the treatment of chronic neuropathic pain. *Pain Med* 2007;8:S200–S275.
7. Kellaway D. The William Osler Medal Essay. The part played by electric fish in the early history of bioelectricity and electrotherapy. *Bull Hist Med* 1946;20:112–137.
8. Hoff HE. An account of stimulation of tissue by electricity before Galvani. *Arm Sci* 1963;1:157.
9. Sarlandiére JB, ed. *Memoires sur l'électro-puncture*. Paris: Delaunay, 1825.
10. Althaus J. *Treatise on Medical Electricity, Theoretical and Practical and Its Use in the Treatment of Paralysis Neuralgia and Other Diseases*. London: Trubner, 1859.
11. Kane K, Taub A. A history of local electrical analgesia. *Pain* 1975;1(2):125–138.
12. Beard G, Rockwell A, eds. *Medical and Surgical Uses of Electricity*. New York: W. Wood Co., 1891.
13. Glenn WWL, Mauro A, Longo P, et al. Remote stimulation of the heart by radiofrequency transmission. *N Engl J Med* 1959;261:948.
14. Wall PD. The past and future of local nerve and brain stimulation. *Abstracts of the International Congress of the International Neuromodulation Society*, Rome, 1992:1–4.
15. Rossi U. The history of electrical stimulation of the nervous system for the control of pain. In: Simpson BA, ed. *Electrical stimulation and the relief of pain. Pain Research and Clinical Management*, Vol. 15. Amsterdam: Elsevier; 2003:5–16.
16. Oakley JC, Weiner RL. Spinal cord stimulation of complex regional pain syndrome: A prospective study of 19 patients at two centers. *Neuromodulation* 1999;2:47–50.
17. DeJongste MJL. Spinal cord stimulation for ischemic heart disease. *Neurol Res* 2000;22:293–298.
18. Huber SJ, Vaglienti RM, Huber JS. Spinal cord stimulation in severe, inoperable, peripheral vascular disease. *Neuromodulation* 2000;3:131–143.
19. North American Neuromodulation Society. Definitions.
20. Meyerson BA, Linderoth B. Mechanisms of spinal cord stimulation in neuropathic pain. *Neurol Res* 2000;22:285–292.
21. Linderoth B, Foreman RD. Physiology of spinal cord stimulation: Review and update. *Neuromodulation* 1999;2:150–164.
22. Oakley JC, Prager JP. Spinal cord stimulation: Mechanisms of action. *Spine* 2002;27(22):2574–2583.
23. Holsheimer J. Principles of neurostimulation. In: Simpson BA, ed. *Electrical stimulation and the relief of pain. Pain Research and Clinical Management*, Vol. 15. Amsterdam: Elsevier; 2003:17–36.
24. Barolat G, Massaro F, He J, et al. Mapping of sensory responses to epidural stimulation of the intraspinal neural structures in man. *J Neurosurg* 1993;78:233–239.
25. Law, 1983

26. Holsheimer J. Which neuronal elements are activated directly by spinal cord stimulation. *Neuromodulation* 2002;5:25–31.
27. Wall PD, Sweet WH. Temporary abolition of pain in man. *Science* 1967;155:108–109.
28. Bennett DS, Cameron TL. Spinal cord stimulation for complex regional pain syndromes. In: Simpson BA, ed. *Electrical stimulation and the relief of pain. Pain Research and Clinical Management*, Vol. 15. Amsterdam: Elsevier; 2003:111–129.
29. Yakhnitsa V, Linderoth B, Meyerson BA. Spinal cord stimulation attenuates dorsal horn neuronal hyperexcitability in a rat model of mononeuropathy. *Pain* 1999;79:223–233.
30. Meyerson BA, Cui J-G, Yakhnitsa V, et al. Modulation of spinal pain mechanisms by spinal cord stimulation and the potential role of adjuvant pharmacotherapy. *Stereotact Funct Neurosurg* 1997;68:129–140.
31. Ren B, Linderoth B, Meyerson BA. Effects of spinal cord stimulation on the flexor reflex and involvement of supraspinal mechanisms: An experimental study in mononeuropathic rats. *J Neurosurg* 1996;84:244–249.
32. Cui JG, Sollevi A, Linderoth B, et al. Adenosine receptor activation suppresses tactile hypersensitivity and potentiates effect of spinal cord in mononeuropathic rats. *Neurosci Lett* 1997;223:171–176.
33. Linderoth B, Stiller CO, Gunasekera L, et al. Gamma-aminobutyric acid is released in the dorsal horn by electrical spinal cord stimulation: An in vivo microdialysis study in the rat. *Neurosurgery* 1994;34:484–489.
34. Cui JG, O'Connor WT, Ungerstedt U, et al. Spinal cord stimulation attenuates augmented dorsal horn release of excitatory amino acids in mononeuropathy via a GABAergic mechanism. *Pain* 1997;73:87–95.
35. Cui JG, Meyerson BA, Sollevi A, et al. Effects of spinal cord stimulation on tactile hypersensitivity in mononeuropathic rats is potentiated by GABA$_B$ and adenosine receptor activation. *Neurosci Lett* 1998;247:183–186.
36. Foreman RD, Linderoth B, Ardell JL, et al. Modulation of intrinsic cardiac neurons by spinal cord stimulation: Implications for its therapeutic use in angina pectoris. *Cardiovasc Res* 2000;47:367–375.
37. Linderoth B, Fedoresak I, Meyerson BA. Peripheral vasodilatation after spinal cord stimulation: Animal studies of putative effector mechanisms. *Neurosurgery* 1991;28:187–195.
38. Croom JE, Foreman RD, Chandler MJ, et al. Cutaneous vasodilation during dorsal column stimulation is mediated by dorsal roots and CGRP. *Am J Physiol* 1997;272:H950–H957.
39. Dubuisson D. Effect of dorsal column stimulation on gelatinosa and marginal neurons of the cat spinal cord. *J Neurosurg* 1989;70:257–265.
40. Roberts MHT, Rees H. Physiological basis of spinal cord stimulation. *Pain Rev* 1994;1:184–198.
41. Holsheimer J, Wesselink WA. Effect of anode-cathode configuration on paresthesia coverage in spinal cord stimulation. *Neurosurgery* 1997;41:654–660.
42. North RB, Ewend MG, Lawton MT, Piantadosi S. Spinal cord stimulation for chronic, intractable pain: Superiority of "multichannel" devices. *Pain* 1991;44:119–130.
43. Holsheimer J. Wesselink WA. Optimum electrode geometry for spinal cord stimulation. The narrow bipole and tripole. *Med Biol Eng Comput* 1997;35:493–497.
44. Holsheimer J, Nuttin B, King GW, et al. Clinical evaluation of paresthesias steering with a new system for spinal cord stimulation. *Neurosurgery* 1998;42:541–549.
45. Miyazawa G, Greenberg J, King G, et al. Guarded cathode arrays allow differential spinal cord stimulation effects. Poster presented at _____;_____.
46. Prager JP, Ross EL, Wesselink W. Spinal cord stimulation using a midline cathode had a better dorsal column recruitment ratio. Presented at the 2006 Annual Meeting of the American Society of Anesthesiologists, Chicago, IL, 2006.

47. Prager JP, Chang JH. Transverse tripolar spinal cord stimulation produced by a percutaneously placed triple lead system. Paper presented at: Worldwide Pain Conference, Meeting of the International Neuromodulation, North American Neuromodulation Society, and World Institute of Pain; July 15–21, 2000.

48. Stojanovic & Abdi 2002.

49. Schade CM. Active electrode screening for low back pain. Paper presented at: Worldwide Pain Conference, Meeting of the International Neuromodulation, North American Neuromodulation Society, and World Institute of Pain; July 15–21, 2000.

50. Stojanovic & Abdi in Boswell and Cole 2006.

51. North RB, Kidd DH, Zahurak M, et al. Spinal cord stimulation for chronic, intractable pain: Two decades' experience. J Neurosurg 1993;32:384–395.

52. Barolat G, Sharan A, Ong J. Spinal cord stimulation for back pain. In: Simpson BA, ed. Electrical stimulation and the relief of pain. Pain Research and Clinical Management, Vol. 15. Amsterdam: Elsevier; 2003:79–86.

53. Annunziata CC, Lauerman WC. When back surgery fails: What's the next step? J Musculoskeletal Med 1999;16(6):342.

54. Frymoyar JW, Cats-Baril WL. An overview of the incidences and costs of low back pain. Orthop Clin North Am 1991;22:263–271.

55. Wilkinson HA. The Failed Back Syndrome: Etiology and Therapy, 2nd ed. Philadelphia: Harper and Row, 1991.

56. Long DM, Filtzer DL, BenDebba M, Hendler NH. Clinical features of the failed-back syndrome. J Neurosurgery 1988;69:61–71.

57. North RB, Kidd DH, Farrokhi F, Piantadosi S. Spinal cord stimulation versus repeated lumbosacral spine surgery for chronic pain: A randomized, controlled trial. Neurosurgery 2005;56(1):98–106.

58. Kumar K, Taylor RS, Jacques L, et al. Spinal cord stimulation versus conventional medical management for neuropathic pain: A multicentre randomised controlled trial in patients with failed back surgery syndrome. Pain 2007;132(1–2):179–188.

59. Oakley JC. Spinal cord stimulation for the treatment of chronic pain. In: Follett KA, ed. Neurosurgical Pain Management. Philadelphia: Saunders; 2004:131–144.

60. Bell GKK, Kidd DH, North RB. Cost-effectiveness analysis of spinal cord stimulation in treatment of failed back surgery syndrome. J Pain Symptom Manage 1997;13(5):286–295.

61. Devulder J, de Laat M, van Bastelaere M, Rolly G. Spinal cord stimulation: A valuable treatment for chronic failed back surgery patients. J Pain Symptom Manage 1997;13(5):296–301.

62. North RB, Kidd DH, Shipley J, Taylor RS. Spinal cord stimulation versus reoperation for failed back surgery syndrome: A cost effectiveness and cost utility analysis based on a randomized, controlled trial. Neurosurgery 2007;61(2):361–368.

63. Stanton-Hicks M, Janig W, Hassenbusch SJ, et al. Reflex sympathetic dystrophy: Changing concepts and taxonomy. Pain 1995;3:127–133.

64. Schwartzman RJ. New treatments for reflex sympathetic dystrophy. New Engl J Med 2000;343:654–656.

65. Furlan AD, Lui PW, Mailis A. Chemical sympathectomy for neuropathic pain: Does it work? Case report and systematic literature review. Clin J Pain 2001;17(4):327–336.

66. Prager JP. Invasive modalities for the diagnosis and treatment of pain in the elderly. Clin Geriatr Med 1996;(3):549–561.

67. Kemler MA, Barendse GAM, van Kleef M, et al. Spinal cord stimulation in patients with chronic reflex sympathetic dystrophy. New Engl J Med 2000;343:618–624.

68. Kemler MA, De Vet HC, Barendse GA, et al. The effect of spinal cord stimulation in patients with chronic reflex sympathetic dystrophy: Two years' follow-up of the randomized controlled trial. Ann Neurol 2004;55(1):13–18.

69. Kemler MA, De Vet HC, Barendse GA, et al. Effect of spinal cord stimulation for chronic complex regional pain syndrome Type I: Five-year final follow-up of patients in a randomized controlled trial. J Neurosurg 2008;108:292–298.

70. North __, Prager JP, Stanton-Hicks __. N Engl J Med ____;__:___

71. Harke H, Gretenkort P, Ladleif HU, et al. The response of neuropathic pain and pain in complex regional pain syndrome I to carbamazepine and sustained-release morphine in patients pretreated with spinal cord stimulation: A double-blinded randomized study. Anesth Analg 2001;92(2):488–495.

72. Bennett DS, Alo KM, Oakley J, Feler C. Spinal cord stimulation for complex regional pain syndrome (RSD): A retrospective multicenter experience from 1995–1998 of 101 patients. Neuromodulation 1999;2:202–210.

73. Boas RA. Complex regional pain syndromes: Symptoms, signs and differential diagnosis. In: Janig W, Stanton-Hicks MD, eds. Reflex Sympathetic Dystrophy: A Reappraisal. Progress in Pain Research and Management. Seattle, WA: IASP Press; 1996:79–92.

74. Prager JP. Spinal cord stimulation as a temporary treatment for complex regional pain syndrome. Paper presented at: Worldwide Pain Conference, Meeting of the International Neuromodulation, North American Neuromodulation Society, and World Institute of Pain; July 15–21, 2000.

75. Spincemaille GH. Spinal cord stimulation in peripheral vascular disease. Simpson BA, ed. Electrical Stimulation and the Relief of Pain. Pain Research and Clinical Management, Vol. 15. Amsterdam: Elsevier; 2003:131–142.

76. European Working Group on critical leg ischemia. Second European consensus document on chronic critical leg ischemia. Eur J Vasc Surg 1992;6(Suppl. A):1–32.

76a. Molloy AR, Nicholas MK, Asghari A. Does a combination of intensive cognitive-behavioural pain management and a spinal implantable device confer any advantage? A preliminary examination. Pain Pract 2006;6:96–103.

76b. Olsson GL, Meyerson BA, Linderoth B. Spinal cord stimulation in adolescents with complex regional pain syndrome type I (CRPS-I). Eur J Pain 2008;12:53–59.

77. Definition and nomenclature for chronic critical limb ischemia. J Vasc Surg 2000;31(1):__-__.

78. Petrakis IE, Sciacca V. Does autonomic neuropathy influence spinal cord stimulation therapy success in diabetic patients with critical lower limb ischemia? Surg Neurol 2000;53:182–188.

79. Cook AW, Oygar A, Baggenstos P, et al. Vascular disease of extremities: Electrical stimulation of spinal cord and posterior roots. NY State J Med 1976;76:366–378.

80. Dooley D, Kasprak M. Modifications of blood flow to the extremities by electrical stimulation of the nervous system. South Med J 1976;69:1309–1311.

81. Ghajar AW, Miles JB. The differential effect of the level of spinal cord stimulation on patients with advanced peripheral vascular disease in the lower limbs. Br J Neurosurg 1998;12:402–408.

82. Tallis R, Jacobs M, Miles J. Spinal cord stimulation in peripheral vascular disease (editorial). Br J Neurosurg 1992;6:101–106.

83. Suy R, Gybels J, Van Damme H, et al. Spinal cord stimulation for ischemic rest pain. The Belgian randomised study. In: Horsch S, Claeys L, eds. Spinal Cord Stimulation: An Innovative Method in the Treatment of PVD. Darmstadt: Steinkoph-Verlag; 1994:197–202.

84. Klomp HM, Spincemaille GH, Steyerberg EW, et al. Efficacy of spinal cord stimulation in critical limb ischaemia. Lancet 1999;353:1040–1044.

85. Parmley WW. Optimal treatment of stable angina. Cardiology 1997;88(Suppl. 3):27–31.

86. Zanger DR, Solomon AJ, Gersh BJ. Contemporary management of angina: Part II. Medical management of chronic stable angina. Am Fam Physician 2000;61:129–138.

87. Mannheimer C, Camici P, Chester, MR, et al. The problem of chronic refractory angina: Report from the ESC Joint Study Group on the Treatment of Refractory Angina. Eur Heart J 2002;23:355–370.

88. Mukherjee D, Bhatt D, Roe MT. Direct myocardial revascularization and angiogenesis: How many patients might be eligible? Am J Cardiol 1999;84:598–600.

89. TenVaarwerk I, Jessuran G, DeJongste M, et al. Clinical outcome of patients treated with spinal cord stimulation for therapeutically refractory angina pectoris. Heart 1999;82:82–88.

90. Fallen EL. Commentary on spinal cord stimulation was effective in the treatment of chronic intractable angina pectoris. Evid Based Cardiovasc Med 1999;3:20.

91. Mulcahy D, Knight C, Stables R, Fox K. Lasers, burns, cuts, tingles and pumps: A consideration of alternative treatments for intractable angina. Br Heart J 1994;71:406–407.

92. Eliasson T, DeJongste MJL, Mannheimer C. Neuromodulation for refractory angina pectoris. In: Simpson BA, ed. Electrical Stimulation and the Relief of Pain. Pain Research and Clinical Management, Vol. 15. Amsterdam: Elsevier; 2003:141–159.

93. Bagger JP, Jensen BS, Johannsen G. Long-term outcome of spinal cord electrical stimulation in patients with refractory chest pain. Clin Cardiol 1998;21:286–288.

94. Ekre O, Eliasson T, Norrsell H, et al. Long-term effects of spinal cord stimulation and coronary artery bypass grafting on quality of life and survival in the ESBY study. Eur Heart J 2002;23:1938–1945.

95. Mannheimer C, Eliasson T, Augustinsson L-E, et al. Electrical stimulation versus coronary artery bypass grafting in severe angina pectoris. Circulation 1998;97:1157–1163.

96. Hautvast R, Brouwer J, DeJongsteM, Lie K. Effect of spinal cord stimulation on heart rate variability and myocardial ischemia in patients with chronic intractable angina pectoris: A prospective ambulatory electrocardiographic study. Clin Cardiol 1998;21:33–38.

97. Andersen C, Hole P, Oxhøj H. Does pain relief with spinal cord stimulation conceal myocardial infarction? Br Heart J 1994;71:419–421.

98. Jessurun G, Ten Vaarwerk I, DeJongste M, et al. Sequelae of spinal cord stimulation for refractory angina pectoris. Reliability and safety profile of long-term clinical application. Coron Artery Dis 1997;8:33–37.

99. Andrell P, Ekre O, Eliasson T, et al. Cost-effectiveness of spinal cord stimulation vs. coronary artery bypass grafting in patients with severe angina pectoris: Long-term results from the ESBY study. Cardiology 2003;99:20–24.

100. Mailis-Gagnon A, Furlan AD, Sandoval JA, Taylor R. Spinal cord stimulation for chronic pain. *Cochrane Database Syst Rev* 2007;4:abstr.

101. Kumar K, Hunter G, Demeria D. Spinal cord stimulation in treatment of chronic benign pain: Challenges in treatment planning and present status, a 22-year experience. *Neurosurgery* 2006;58(3):481–496.

102. Kay AD, McIntyre MD, Macrae WA, Varma TR. Spinal cord stimulation: A long-term evaluation in patients with chronic pain. *Br J Neurosurg* 2001;15(4):355–341.

103. Waltz JM. Spinal cord stimulation: A quarter century of development and investigation. A review of the development and effectiveness in 1,336 cases. *Stereotact Funct Neurosurg* 1997;69(1–4 Pt. 2):288–299.

104. Meglio M, Cioni B, Rossi GF. Spinal cord stimulation in management of chronic pain. A 9-year experience. *J Neurosurg* 1989;70(4):519–524.

105. Van de Kelft E, De La Porte C. Long-term pain relief during spinal cord stimulation. The effect of patient selection. *Qual Life Res* 1994;3(1):21–27.

106. Kumar K, Wilson JR. Factors affecting spinal cord stimulation outcome in chronic benign pain with suggestions to improve success rate. *Acta Neurochir Suppl* 2007;97(Pt. 1):91–99.

107. International Association for the Study of Pain. Subcommittee on Taxonomy. Classification of chronic pain. Description of chronic pain syndromes and definitions of pain terms. *Pain* 1986:(Suppl. 3).

108. Jensen TS, Rasmussen P. Phantom pain and other phenomena after amputation. In: Wall PD, Melzack R, eds. *Textbook of Pain*, 3rd ed. Edinburgh: Churchill Livingstone; 1994:651–665.

109. Loeser JD. Pain after amputation: Phantom limb and stump pain. In: Bonica JJ, ed. *The Management of Pain*, 2nd ed. Philadelphia: Lea and Febiger; 1990:255–256.

110. Krainick JU, Thoden U, Riechert T. Pain reduction in amputees by long-term spinal cord stimulation. Long-term follow-up study over 5 years. *J Neurosurg* 1980;52(3):346–350.

111. Tasker RR, Dostrovsky JO. Deafferentation and central pain. In: Wall PD, Melzack R, eds. *Textbook of Pain*, 2nd ed. Edinburgh: Churchill Livingstone; 1989:154–180.

112. Oakley JC. Spinal cord stimulation for neuropathic pain. In: Simpson BA, ed. *Electrical stimulation and the relief of pain. Pain Research and Clinical Management*, Vol. 15. Amsterdam: Elsevier; 2003:79–86.

113. Harke H, Gretenkort P, Ladleif HU. Spinal cord stimulation in postherpetic neuralgia and in acute herpes zoster pain. *Anesth Analg* 2002;94:694–700.

114. Simpson BA. Selection of patients and assessment of outcome. In: Simpson BA, ed. *Electrical stimulation and the relief of pain. Pain Research and Clinical Management*, Vol. 15. Amsterdam: Elsevier; 2003:237–249.

115. Cioni B, Meglio M, Pentimalli L, Visocchi M. Spinal cord stimulation in the treatment of paraplegic pain. *J Neurosurg* 1995;82(1):35–39.

116. Lazorthes Y, Siegfried J, Verdie JC, Casaux J. Chronic spinal cord stimulation in the treatment of neurogenic pain. Cooperative and retrospective study on 20 years of follow-up. *Neurochirurgie* 1995;42(2):73–86.

117. Krames E. Implantable technologies: Spinal cord stimulation and implantable drug delivery systems. Accessed January 18, 2008 at: http://www.nationalpainfoundation.org/My Treatment/news_implantab.

118. Burchiel K, Anderson VC, Brown FD, et al. Prospective, multicenter study of spinal cord stimulation for relief of chronic back and extremity pain. *Spine* 1996;21(23):2786–2794.

119. Racz G, McCarron RF, Talboys P. Percutaneous dorsal column stimulator for chronic pain control. *Spine* 1989;14(1):1–4.

120. Budd K. Spinal cord stimulation: Cost-benefit study. *Neuromodulation* 2002;5(2):75–78.

121. Kumar K, Malik S, Demeria D. Treatment of chronic pain with spinal cord stimulation versus alternative therapies: Cost-effectiveness analysis. *Neurosurgery* 2002;51(1):106–115.

122. Kumar K, Toth C, Nath RK, Laing P. Epidural spinal cord stimulation for treatment of chronic pain: Some predictors of success. A 15-year experience. *Surg Neurol* 1998;50(2):110–120.

123. May MS, Banks C, Thomson SJ. A retrospective, long-term, third-party follow-up of patients considered for spinal cord stimulation. *Neuromodulation* 2002;5(3):137–144.

124. Van Buyten J-P, van Zundert JV, Milbouw G. Treatment of failed back surgery syndrome patients with low back and leg pain: A pilot study of a new dual lead spinal cord stimulation system. *Neuromodulation* 1999;2(3):258–265.

125. Van Buyten J-P, van Zundert J, Vueghs P, Vanduffel L. Efficacy of spinal cord stimulation: 10 years of experience in a pain centre in Belgium. *Eur J Pain* 2001;5(3):299–307.

126. Barolat G, Singh-Sahni K, Staas WE, et al. Epidural spinal cord stimulation in the management of spasms in spinal cord injury: A prospective study. *Stereotact Funct Neurosurg* 1995;64(3):153–164.

127. Carhart MR, He J, Herman R, et al. Epidural spinal-cord stimulation facilitates recovery of functional walking following incomplete spinal-cord injury. *IEEE Trans Neural Syst Rehabil Eng* 2004;12(1):32–42.

128. Kiwerski J. Stimulation of the spinal cord in the treatment of traumatic injuries of cervical spine. *Appl Neurophysiol* 1986;49(3):166–171.

129. Harke H, Gretenkort P, Ladleif HU, Rahman S. Spinal cord stimulation in sympathetically maintained complex regional pain syndrome type I with severe disability. A prospective clinical trial. *Eur J Pain* 2005;9(4):363–373.

130. Ohnmeiss DD, Rashbaum RF, Bogdanffy GM. Prospective outcome evaluation of spinal cord stimulation in patients with intractable leg pain. *Spine* 1996;21(11):1344–1350.

131. Kumar K, Toth C. The role of spinal cord stimulation in the treatment of chronic pain postlaminectomy. *Curr Pain Headache Rep* 1998;2:85–92.

132. Aló KM, Yland MJ, Charnov JH, Redko V. Multiple program spinal cord stimulation in the treatment of chronic pain: Follow-up of multiple program SCS. *Neuromodulation* 1999;2(4):266–272.

133. De Mulder PA, te Rijdt B, Veeckmans G, Belmans L. Evaluation of a dual quadripolar surgically implanted spinal cord stimulation lead for failed back surgery patients with chronic low back and leg pain. *Neuromodulation* 2005;8(4):219–224.

134. Kupers RC, Van den Oever R, Van Houdenhove B, et al. Spinal cord stimulation in Belgium: A nation-wide survey on the incidence, indications and therapeutic efficacy by the health insurer. *Pain* 1994;56(2):211–216.

135. North RB, Kidd DH, Olin J, et al. Spinal cord stimulation for axial low back pain: A prospective, controlled trial comparing dual with single percutaneous electrodes. *Spine* 2005;30(12):1412–1418.

136. Ohnmeiss DD, Rashbaum RF. Patient satisfaction with spinal cord stimulation for predominant complaints of chronic, intractable low back pain. *Spine J* 2001;1(5):358–363.

137. Burchiel KJ, Anderson VC, Wilson BJ, et al. Prognostic factors of spinal cord stimulation for chronic back and leg pain. *Neurosurgery* 1995;36(6):1101–1110.

138. Dario A, Fortini G, Bertollo D, et al. Treatment of failed back surgery syndrome. *Neuromodulation* 2001;4(3):105–110.

139. Long DM, Erickson DE. Stimulation of the posterior columns of the spinal cord for relief of intractable pain. *Surg Neurol* 1975;4:134–141.

140. De La Porte C, Van De Kelft E. Spinal cord stimulation in failed back surgery syndrome. *Pain* 1993;52:55–61.

141. Spiegelmann R, Friedman WA. Spinal cord stimulation: A contemporary series. *Neurosurgery* 1991;28(1):65–70.

142. Simpson BA. The role of neurostimulation: The neurosurgical perspective. *J Pain Symptom Manage* 2006;31[4Supp]:S3–S5.

143. Turner JA, Loeser JD, Bell KG. Spinal cord stimulation for chronic low back pain: A systematic synthesis. *Neurosurgery* 1995;37:1088–1096.

144. Katz N. The impact of opioids on the endocrine system. *Pain Management Rounds* 2005;1(9).

145. North RB, Guarino AH. Spinal cord stimulation for failed back surgery syndrome: Technical advances, patient selection and outcome. *Neuromodulation* 1999;2(3):171–178.

146. Hassenbusch SJ, Paice JA, Patt RB, et al. Clinical realities and economic considerations: Economics of intrathecal therapy. *J Pain Symptom Manage* 1997;14(3 Suppl):S36–S48.

147. Taylor RS, Taylor RJ, Van Buyten J-P, et al. The cost effectiveness of spinal cord stimulation in the treatment of pain: A systematic review of the literature. *J Pain Symptom Manage* 2004;27:370–378.

148. Taylor RS, Van Buyten J-P, Buchser E. Spinal cord stimulation for complex regional pain syndrome: A systematic review of the clinical and cost-effectiveness literature and assessment of prognostic factors. *Eur J Pain* 2006;10(2):91–101.

149. Prager JP, Jacobs M. Evaluation of patients for implantable pain modalities: Medical and behavioral assessment. *Clin J Pain* 2001;(3):206–214.

150. Doleys DM, Olson K. *Psychological Assessment and Intervention in Implantable Pain Therapies*. Minneapolis: Medtronic Neurologic, 1997.

151. Turk DC, Gatchel R, eds. *Psychological Approaches to Pain Management: A Practitioner's Handbook*, 2nd ed. New York: Guilford Publications, 2002.

152. Caudill MA, Holman GH, Turk D. Effective ways to manage chronic pain. *Patient Care* 1996;31(11):154–166.

153. Prager JP. Neuraxial medication delivery: The development and maturity of a concept for treating chronic pain of spinal origin. *Spine* 2002;27(22):2593–2605.

154. Aló KM, Yland MJ, Kramer DL, et al. Computer assisted and patient interactive programming of dual octrode spinal cord stimulation in the treatment of chronic pain. *Neuromodulation* 1998;1:30–40.

155. North RB, Kidd DH, Olin J, Sieracki JN. Spinal cord stimulation electrode design: Prospective, controlled trial comparing percutaneous and laminectomy electrodes: Part I: Technical outcomes. *Neurosurgery* 2002;51(2):381–390.

156. North RB, Kidd DH, Olin J, et al. Spinal cord stimulation for axial low back pain: A prospective controlled trial comparing 16-contact insulated electrode arrays with 4-contact percutaneous electrodes. *Neuromodulation* 2006;9(1):56–67.

157. Struijk JJ, Holsheimer J, Spincemaille GHJ, et al. Theoretical performance and clinical evaluation of transverse tripolar spinal cord stimulation. *IEEE Trans Rehabil Eng* 1998;6(3):277–285.

158. Kemler MA, Furnee CA. Economic evaluation of spinal cord stimulation for chronic reflex sympathetic dystrophy. *Neurology* 2002;59:1203–1209.
159. Koziol JK, Clark DC, Gittes RF, Tan EM. The natural history of interstitial cystitis: A survey of 374 patients. *J Urol* 1993;149:465–469.
160. McMahon SB, Abel C. A model for the study of visceral pain states: Chronic inflammation of the chronic decerebrate rat urinary bladder by irritant chemicals. *Pain* 1987;28(1):109–127.
161. Lecci A, Guiliani S, Santicioli P, Maggi CA. Involvement of spinal tachykinin NK1 and NK2 receptors in detrusor hyperreflexia during chemical cystitis in anesthetized rats. *Eur J Pharmacol* 1994;259:129–135.
162. Siegel SW, Catanzaro F, Dijkema HE. Long-term results of a multicenter study on sacral nerve stimulation for treatment of urinary urge incontinence, urgency, frequency, and retention. *Urology* 2000;56(Suppl. 6A):87–91.
163. Maher CF, Carey MP, Dwyer PL, Schlucter PL. Percutaneous sacral nerve root neuromodulation for intractable interstitial cystitis. *J Urol* 2001;165:884–886.
164. Feler CA, Whitworth LA, Brookhoff D, Powell R. Recent advances: Sacral nerve root stimulation using retrograde method of lead insertion for the treatment of pelvic pain due to interstitial cystitis. *Neuromodulation* 1999;2:211–216.
165. Reynolds DB. Surgery in the rat during electrical analgesia induced by central brain stimulation. *Science* 1969;164:444–445.
166. Mayer DJ, Liebeskind JC. Pain reduction by focal electrical stimulation of the brain: an anatomical and behavioral analysis. *Brain Res* 1974;68:73–93.
167. Long BM, Hagfors N. Electrical stimulation in the nervous system: The current status of electrical stimulation of the nervous system for relief of pain. *Pain* 1975;1:109–123.
168. Shealy CN, Mortimer JT, Reswick JB. Electrical inhibition of pain by stimulation of the dorsal columns: Preliminary clinical report. *Anesth Analg* 1967;46:489.
169. Shealy CM, Mortimer JT, Hagfors NR. Dorsal column electroanalgesia. *J Neurosurg* 1970;32:560–564.
170. Shimoji K, Higashi H, Kano T. Electrical management of intractable pain. *Jpn J Anesthesiol* 1971;20:444–447.
171. Dooley DM. Percutaneous electrical stimulation of the spinal cord. Association of Neurological Surgeons. Bal Harbour, Florida; 1975.
172. Zumpano BJ, Saunders RL. Percutaneous epidural dorsal column stimulation. *J Neurosurg* 1976;45:459–460.
173. Peters A, Palay SL, Webster HF. *Defined Structure of the Nervous System: The Neuron and Supporting Cells.* Philadelphia: Saunders, 1976.
174. Hubbard JJ. *The Peripheral Nervous System.* New York: Premium Press, 1976.
175. Sunderland S. The intraneural topography of the radial, median and ulnar nerves. *Brain* 1945;68:242–299.
176. Sunderland S. *Nerves and Nerve Injuries,* 2nd ed. Edinburgh: Churchill-Livingston, 1978.
177. DiRosa F, Giuzzi P, Battistone B. Radial nerve anatomy and fascicular arrangement. In: Brunelli G, ed. *Textbook of Microsurgery.* Milan: Masson; 1988:571.
178. Ogata K, Naito M. Blood flow of peripheral nerves: Effects of dissection, stretching and compression. *J Hand Surg* 1986;11b:10.
179. Smith JW. Factors influencing nerve repair. I. Blood supply of peripheral nerves. *Arch Surg* 1966;93:335.
180. Smith JW. Factors influencing nerve repair. II. Collateral circulation of peripheral nerves. *Arch Surg* 1966;93:433.
181. Nashold BS, Mellen JB, Avry R. Peripheral nerve stimulation for pain relief using a multi-contact electrode system. *J Neurosurg* 1979;51:872–873.
182. Campbell N, Long DM. Peripheral nerve stimulation in the treatment of intractable pain. *J Neurosurg* 1976;45:692–699.
183. Kirsch WN, Lewis JA, Simon RH. Experience with electrical stimulation devices for the control of chronic pain. *Med Instr* 1975;9:217–220.
184. Law JT, Sweet J, Kirsch W. Retrospective analysis of 22 patients with chronic pain treated by peripheral nerve stimulation. *J Neurosurg* 1981;52:482–485.
185. Sweet WH, Wepsic JG. Stimulation of the posterior columns of the spinal cord for pain control: Indications, techniques and results. *Clin Neurosurg* 1974;21:278–310.
186. Cooney WP. Electrical stimulation in the treatment of complex regional pain syndrome of the upper extremities. Hand Clinics, Upper extremity pain dysfunction: Somatic and sympathethic disorders 1997;14:519–526.
187. Hassenbusch SJ, Stanton-Hicks M, Schoppa AD, et al. Long-term peripheral nerve stimulation for reflex sympathetic dystrophy. *J Neurosurg* 1996;84:415–423.
188. Stanton Hicks M, Salamon R. Stimulation of the central and peripheral nervous system for the control of pain. *J Clin Neurophysiol* 1997:46–62.
189. Stanton Hicks M. Transcutaneous and peripheral nerve stimulation. In: Simpson B, ed. *Electrical stimulation and relief of pain. Pain Research and Clinical Management,* Vol. 15. Amsterdam: Elseview; 2003:37–55.
190. Nashold BS, Goldner L, Mullen JB, Bright DS. Long-term pain control by direct peripheral nerve stimulation. *J Bone Joint Surg Am* 1975;64:1–10.
191. Nashold BS, Goldner L, Mellen JB, Bright DS. Long-term pain control by direct peripheral nerve stimulation. *J Bone Joint Surg Am* 1982;64:1–10.
192. Goldner JL, Nashold BS, Hendrix PC. Peripheral nerve stimulation. *Clin Orthop* 1982;163:33–41.
193. Waisbrod H, Banhan SC, Hansen D, et al. Direct nerve stimulation for painful peripheral neuropathies. *J Bone Joint Surg* 1985;67:420–422.
194. Gybels J, Kupers R. *Acta Neurochirurgica* 1987;38(Suppl.):64–75.
195. Racz GB, Brown NT, Lewis R. Peripheral stimulator implant for treatment of causalgia caused by electrical burns. *Text Med* 1988;84:45–50.
196. Racz GB, Lewis R, Heavner JE, et al. Peripheral nerve stimulator implant for treatment of causalgia. In: Stanton-Hicks M, ed. *Pain and the Sympathetic Nervous System.* Norwell, Massachusetts: Kluwer Academic Publishers; 1990:225–239.
197. Cooney WP. Chronic pain treatment of direct electrical nerve stimulation. In: Geberman RH, ed. *Operative Nerve Repair and Reconstruction.* Philadelphia: JB Lippincott; 1991:1551–1561.
198. Strege W, Cooney WG, Wood MB, et al. Chronic peripheral nerve pain treated with direct electrical neurostimulation. *J Hand Surg Am* 1994;19:931–939.
199. Novak CV, MacKinnon SE. Outcome following implantation of a peripheral nerve stimulator in patients with chronic nerve pain. *Plast Reconstr Surg* 1999;105:1967–1972.
200. Buschmann N, Oppel F. Peripheral nerve stimulation. *Schmerz* 1999;13:113–120.
201. Brummer SB, Turner MJ. Electrical stimulation with Pt electrodes. I. A. Method for determination of "real" electrode areas. *IEEE Trans Biomed Eng* 1977;34:436–438.
202. Brummer SB, Turner MJ. Electrical stimulation with Pt electrodes. II. Estimation of maximum service redux (theoretical non-gassing) limits. *IEEE Trans Biomed Eng* 1977;34:440.
203. Brummer SB, Turner MJ. Electric chemical considerations for safe electrical stimulation of the nervous system with platinum electrodes. *IEEE Trans Biomed Eng* 1977;24:69.
204. Schetter AG, Racz GB, Lewis R, Heavner JE. Peripheral nerve stimulation. In: North RB, Levy RN, eds. *Management of Pain.* New York, NY: Springer Verlag; 1997:261–270.
205. Eisenberg E, Waisbrod H, Gerbershagen HU. Long-term peripheral nerve stimulation for painful nerve injuries. *Clin J Pain* 2004;20:143–146.
206. Johnson MD, Birchiel KJ. Peripheral stimulation for the treatment of trigeminal post herpetic neuralgia and trigeminal post traumatic neuropathic pain: A pilot study. *Neurosurgery* 2004;55:135–142.
207. Mobbs RJ, Nair S, Blum NP. Peripheral nerve stimulation for the treatment of chronic pain. *J Clin Neuroscience* 2007;14:216–221.
208. Weiner RL, Reed KL. Peripheral neurostimulation for control of intractable occipital neuralgia. *Neuromodulation* 1999;2:217–221.
209. Weiner L. The future of peripheral nerve stimulation. *Neurol Res* 2000;22:299–303.
210. Goadsby PJ, Bartsch T, Dodick DW. Occipital nerve stimulation for headache: Mechanisms and efficacy. *Headache* 2008;48(2):313–318.
211. Matharu MS, Bartsch, T, Ward N, et al. Central neuromodulation in chronic migraine patients with suboccipital stimulators: A PET study. *Brain* 2004;127:220–230.
212. Goadsby PJ, Dodick D, Mitsias P, et al. ONSTIM: Occipital nerve stimulation for the treatment of chronic migraine. *Eur J Neurol* 2005;12(2):198.
213. Burns B, Watkins L, Goadsby PJ. Treatment of medically intractable cluster headache by occipital nerve stimulation: Long term follow up 13 patients. *Cephalalgia* 2007;27:1197–1198.
214. Burns B, Watkins L, Goadsby PJ. Successful treatment of medically intractable cluster headache using occipital nerve stimulation (ONS). *Lancet* 2007;369:1099–1106.
215. Schwedt T, Dodick D, Trentman T, Zimmerman R. Occipital nerve stimulation for chronic cluster headache and hemicrania continua: Pain relief and persistence of autonomic features. *Cephalalgia* 1006;26:1025–1027.
216. Schwedt TJ, Dodick DW, Hentz J, et al. Occipital nerve stimulation for chronic headache: Long term safety and efficacy. *Cephalalgia* 2007;27:153–157.
217. Dodick DW, Schwedt TJ, Trentman TL, et al. Trigeminal autonomic cephalalgias: Current and future treatments. *Headache* 2007;47:981–986.
218. Anthony M. Arrest of attacks of cluster headache by local steroid injection of the occipital nerve. In: Rose FC, ed. *Migraine: Clinical and Research Advances.* London: Karger; 1985;169–174.
219. Kerr FW, Olafsen RA. Trigeminal and cervical volleys. *Arch Neurol* 1961;5:69–76.
220. Goadsby PJ, Hoskin KL, Knight YE. Stimulation of the greater occipital nerve increases metabolic activity in the trigeminal nucleus caudalis and cervical dorsal horn of the cat. *Pain* 1997;73:23–28.
221. Bartsch T, Goadsby PJ. Stimulation of the greater occipital nerve induces increased central excitability of dural afferent input. *Brain* 2002;125:1496–1509.
222. Dunteman E. Peripheral nerve stimulation for unremitting ophthalmic post-herpetic neuralgia. *Neuromodulation* 2002;5:32–37.

223. Meglio M. Percutaneously implantable chronic electrode for radiofrequency stimulation of Gasserian ganglion: A perspective in the management of trigeminal pain. *Acta Neurochir (Wein)* 1984;33[Suppl]:521–525.

224. Meyerson B, Håkansson S. Alleviation of atypical trigeminal pain by stimulation of the Gasserian ganglion via an implanted electrode. *Acta Neurosurg* 1980;30:303–309.

225. Taub E, Munz M, Taskar R. Chronic electrical stimulation of the Gasserian ganglion for the relief of pain in a series of 34 patients. *J Neurosurg* 1997; 86:197–202.

226. Stinson LW, Rodever GT, Cross NE, Davis BE. Peripheral subcutaneous electrostimulation for control of intractable postoperative inguinal pain: A case report series. *Neuromodulation* 2001;4:99–104.

CHAPTER 42 ■ PERCUTANEOUS NEURAL DESTRUCTIVE TECHNIQUES

DAVID NIV AND MICHAEL GOFELD

HISTORY

The idea of relieving intractable pain by severing a nerve as if it were a rope connecting an injured part with the brain probably originated in Descartes' mechanical model of sensations; however, it took another 300 years to put this concept into practice. In his pioneering work *La Chirurgie de la douleur*, René Leriche proclaimed the term "pain surgery," which eventually became a synonym of interventional pain management (1). He invented principles for operations on either sensory or autonomic parts of the nervous system to fight intractable pain. His most important contribution was probably the assertion of the concept of a "pain disorder." Leriche wrote in his manuscript: "The disorder and its expression are confined within the nervous system. Localized in appearance, it affects virtually the whole individual" (1). Many years later, chronic pain would be defined as a disease in its own right (2). Even before surgical approaches emerged, descriptions of percutaneous methods of chemical ablation started to appear in the literature. Trigeminal ganglion ablation with absolute alcohol was first described by Härtel in 1912 (3). In 1926, Swetlow injected 85% alcohol paravertebrally in the upper thoracic level for the treatment of angina pectoris (4). Dogliotti described a technique of subarachnoid alcohol neurolysis for the treatment of sciatic pain in 1931 (5). Alcohol splanchnic nerve block was first described in 1957 (6), and several years later Brindenbaugh published the technique of neurolytic celiac plexus block for the management of cancer-related abdominal pain (7).

Interestingly, chemical neurodestructive procedures were mainly invented initially for the treatment of nonmalignant pain. The potential for devastating complications (8,9), the discovery of the sequelae of deafferentation pain (10), and especially the publication and overwhelming recognition of the gate control theory (11) diverted clinicians toward neuromodulation rather than neuroablation (see Chapters 40 and 41). Chemical neuroablation has fallen into disfavor and currently, with few exceptions, pertains to cancer pain management, where the limited life expectancy "protects" the patient from the development of deafferentation syndrome, and the loss of motor and sensory functions is perceived as an unfortunate but less important event (see Chapter 45).

The search for more predictable and localized neural destruction and fading interest in chemical ablation resulted in the invention of two physical approaches in the 1960s: radiofrequency (RF) neurotomy and cryoablation. Radiofrequency ablation of the Gasserian ganglion was described by Sweet and Wepsic and quickly became a well-accepted procedure, successfully concurring with results of alcohol and retrogasserian glyc-erol injections, but with fewer complications (12). Rapidly, several RF techniques were developed to treat various chronic pain conditions: spinal facet joint denervation, dorsal root ganglion lesion, percutaneous cordotomy, and sympathectomy (13–17).

At the same time, cryoanalgesia was introduced, initially to treat parkinsonism (18) and then to treat chronic pain. The idea of limiting lesion size within the boundaries of the target nerve, thus avoiding complications associated with inadvertent spread of the neurolytic solution, was so attractive that clinical applications of this method often preceded scientific knowledge. In fact, only a few randomized controlled studies were published on RF neurotomy of cervical and lumbar facet joints (19–23). The history of lumbar facet denervation merely mirrors the battle between clinicians' desire to implement a new and virtually complications-free procedure and the lack of compelling knowledge of applied anatomy and physics. Positive results from randomized controlled trials (RCTs), in which selection criteria and surgical techniques were flawed, suggest another problem: namely, the difficulty of producing high-quality clinical trials in the field of neurodestructive procedures. Cervical facet neurotomy ran a more favorable course since its use was preceded by anatomic studies and only then followed by a carefully performed randomized controlled study by Lord and colleagues (23) that provided compelling evidence of efficacy. This study unequivocally demonstrated the benefit of an RF procedure performed using an anatomically correct approach. Therefore, any other technique should be considered as a nonvalidated method.

Obviously, clinical trials of interventional procedures have technical, methodological, and ethical restraints, especially in cancer pain management. Only neurolytic celiac block has shown a sufficient level of evidence (24) in comparison with conservative treatment. Evidence of efficacy is restricted to case series and case reports for other neurolytic procedures. Only one randomized trial was published comparing cryoanalgesia with phenol block of peripheral nerves, reporting slightly better results after phenol injection (25).

CURRENT SITUATION

Notwithstanding the limited evidence of efficacy for many procedures, several percutaneous neural destructive techniques have earned a reputation as being reliable and effective. This chapter concentrates on describing techniques that can be recommended in routine clinical practice. Other procedures will be mentioned as a matter of curiosity and for the sake of comprehensiveness.

TABLE 42-1

CLASSIFICATION OF PERCUTANEOUS NEURAL
DESTRUCTIVE PROCEDURES

Applications
1. Cancer-related pain
2. Nonmalignant chronic pain
3. Spasticity

Methodology
1. Chemical neurolysis: alcohol, phenol, glycerol
2. Cryoablation
3. Radiofrequency lesion

Anatomy
1. Peripheral neurotomy (such as destruction of intercostal, ilioinguinal nerves)
2. Rhizotomy (spinal dorsal root rhizotomy, trigeminal rhizotomy)
3. Destruction of sensory pathways in the spinal cord (midline punctuate myelotomy, cordotomy)
4. Destruction of brain sensory centers (hypophysectomy)
5. Sympathectomy

The era of "blind" injections belonging to a small group of "experts" has passed. Neurolytic procedures must be performed under imaging guidance. This approach ultimately eliminates any question of technical error or misplacement of the needle or cannula and greatly reduces the rate of complications. In addition, visualization of the spread of radiopaque contrast before an ablation procedure or injection of a chemical agent can help predict anticipated effects and further decrease adverse outcomes associated with intravascular injection or a misplaced neuroablation device. Computed tomography (CT) and fluoroscopy are invaluable tools for cranial and spinal procedures, and ultrasonography has emerged as the standard tool for peripheral soft-tissue procedures.

CLASSIFICATION AND BASIC PRINCIPLES OF PERCUTANEOUS TECHNIQUES

Percutaneous neural destructive techniques can be classified according to application, methodology, and anatomy (Table 42-1). This chapter will be concerned with procedures for the relief of intractable pain by means of RF and cryoablation. Chemical neurolysis in nonmalignant pain will be highlighted as well. Injection of neurolytic agents for palliation of cancer pain is discussed in Chapter 45.

Percutaneous neurolytic techniques can be used in several ways to treat intractable pain (Table 42-1). Most obvious are the destructive techniques that interrupt transmission in pain pathways, such as neurectomy, rhizotomy, and destructive lesions in the spinal cord. However, percutaneous destructive techniques of autonomic pathways also have been developed. They target either sympathetic ganglion (thoracic sympathectomy) or preganglionic sympathetic fibers (splanchnic neurolysis). Thus, neurolytic procedures are divided into the destruction of nociceptive conduction or the destruction of autonomic pathways.

Methods are classified according to modality: chemical (alcohol, phenol, and glycerol) or thermal (heating, cooling).

Logically, the division of neurolytic approaches may be based on anatomic site: peripheral, central, and, separately, autonomic. This classification system allows stepwise neurolysis and also produces cessation of nerve conduction in that part of the nervous system that anatomically corresponds to the painful site.

SELECTION OF PATIENTS FOR DESTRUCTIVE PROCEDURES

The selection of patients for procedures for the relief of pain is a complex, multidimensional process. First, all simpler methods of treatment must have been tried and found ineffective. Second, the proposed invasive procedure should have a reasonable chance of relieving the problem for which it is proposed, commensurate with the severity of the symptoms it is intended to relieve, the impact of the procedure, and the likely complications. Third, the patient and family should understand that the procedure is intended to control specific symptoms, not the underlying disease and other problems related to it. For instance, a procedure for pain caused by spinal cord injury does not affect the paraplegia. Fourth, it should be clearly recognized that procedures for pain relief seldom give permanent relief. Pain usually recurs in time no matter what operation is done (26), quite apart from early failure that may reflect waning of an initial placebo effect, which is usually more transient than a procedure-specific effect (27). Finally, destructive procedures for pain relief may give rise in themselves to iatrogenic neuropathic or deafferentation pain syndromes (28).

Prior to a neurodestructive procedure, a diagnostic trial of local anesthetic to block the nerve target must be carried out. Anesthesia of the potential source of the patient's pain should provide almost complete pain relief for the duration of action of the specific analgesic or for longer than expected. Placebo-controlled blocks, considered as the gold standard in research applications, have been disproved for clinical practice because of both logistic and ethical concerns (see also Chapter 38). Deceptive use of a placebo is unethical, and a set of three diagnostic tests is probably overzealous and costly in a busy clinical practice. Comparative medial branches blocks recommended before RF zygapophysial neurotomy should be considered as an acceptable and validated method for any diagnostic spinal nerve injection (29,30). The main idea behind this strategy is to produce an unbiased response due to a patient's unawareness of the type of local anesthetic injected. For instance, diagnostic workup of lumbar zygapophysial pain includes fluoroscopy-guided low-volume injections of the medial branches of the dorsal rami at the suspected levels. In the first block, 0.5 mL of 0.5% bupivacaine without epinephrine is injected at each target level. The patient has to complete a self-administered pain score diary and use a telephone answering system to report the degree and duration of pain relief according to a numeric pain score (from 0–10) before the procedure and every 30 minutes for up to 6 hours afterward. The response is considered positive if the patient experiences a decrease in numeric pain score of at least 80% for more than 3 hours.

Patients with a positive result after the first block undergo a second block on a separate occasion with 0.5 mL of 2% lidocaine. The same method is used to determine pain before and after the procedure. The block is determined successful if greater than 80% pain relief is obtained for more than 1 hour.

Radiofrequency facet denervation is proposed for patients who experience pain relief (according to the stated definitions) in both diagnostic studies. Concordant response, in which the patient reports relief of pain for a shorter duration following lidocaine injection and for a longer duration after bupivacaine use, confirms the diagnosis with a confidence level of 85% (31). If the patient reports more than 80% pain reduction but with no appropriate differential response, this result should be interpreted as "discordant." Nevertheless, discordant response provides a 65% level of confidence (31). Discrepant or negative response exists when the patient fails to obtain pain relief on a second confirmative block (see also Chapter 38).

NEURAL DESTRUCTIVE PROCEDURES: PHYSICAL PRINCIPLES AND BIOLOGIC EFFECT

Wherever possible, RF lesion-making is the preferred procedure because of the ease of making a graded lesion of planned reproducible size (14,32,33) (Fig. 42-1). This is accomplished by controlling the diameter and length of the active tip of the cannula, the duration of current flow, and the tip's temperature during lesion-making. Radiofrequency electrical current is a high-frequency (500-KHz) signal. A large positive electrode, a *ground pad*, is applied on the skin. Electric flow concentrates on a very limited area of the negative pole, the *active tip*. Oscillations of electrical current produce molecular friction and, therefore, elevation of temperature. If the active tip is equipped with a thermocouple, the temperature can be recorded. In addition, impedance of the tissue is usually monitored. A temperature of 45°C to 50°C is considered as a "minimal lethal margin" for biologic tissue. Obviously, higher temperature creates a bigger lesion; however, no further extension of lesion is found with the temperature higher than 80°C (33). Moreover,

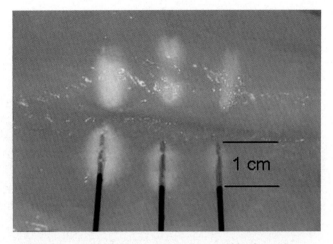

FIGURE 42-2. Radiofrequency lesion is increased by the temperature elevation. From left to right: 80°C, 70°C, and 60°C. Duration of lesion is 75 seconds. Courtesy of Baylis Medical Inc.

higher temperature can lead to charcoaling and boiling. Therefore, the routine temperature recommended is 80°C (Fig. 42-2). Similarly, lesion size depends on the size and shape of the active tip (Fig. 42-3). The maximal useful diameter is thought to be 15-gauge, since no further increase in lesion size occurs with a cannula bigger than that (33). Last, but not least, it is mandatory to place the cannula parallel to the target nerve, because the RF lesion is created from the sides of the cannula, not from the tip (34). The maximal lesion size is roughly two cannula diameters circumferentially (35).

An RF lesion-making generator usually includes other features, such as data recording, a nerve stimulator, and an impedance monitor, to facilitate control of the procedure (Fig. 42-4).

The technique of RF lesion-making is similar wherever applied, and details will be given here only for selected procedures. Most RF procedures are performed under local anesthesia with intravenous (IV) sedation. Care is taken to provide the necessary analgesia for the patient's ongoing pain, but

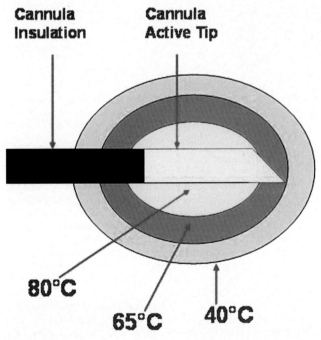

FIGURE 42-1. Diagram of a typical radiofrequency cannula with 80°C temperature setting.

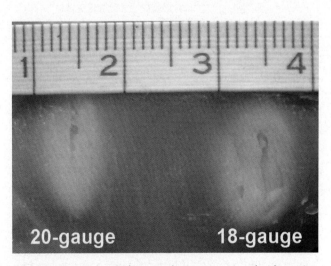

FIGURE 42-3. Two radiofrequency lesions were created with rotation of active tip in opposite directions. The maximal diameter of the lesion was measured: 18-gauge cannula produces 9-mm width burn, whereas 20-gauge creates only a 5.5-mm width lesion.

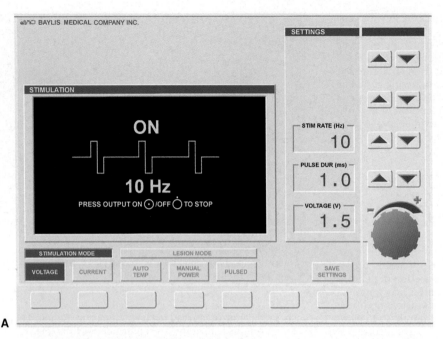

A

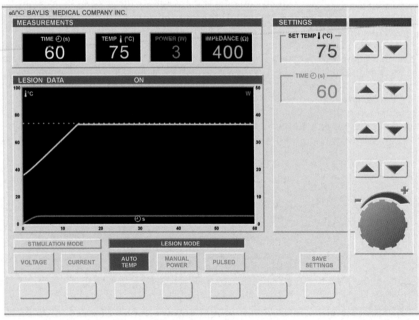

B

FIGURE 42-4. Radiofrequency generator monitor shows (A) stimulation mode and (B) lesion mode. Courtesy of Baylis Medical Inc.

not sufficient sedation to cloud the patient's ability to cooperate with physiologic testing. The RF cannula is introduced toward the intended target under fluoroscopy or computed tomography (CT) guidance. When it appears to be in the correct anatomic location, this fact can be further corroborated in a number of ways. Contrast medium can be injected, then monitored under image intensification. Impedance monitoring is helpful, with levels of 400 Ohms being typical of cerebrospinal fluid (CSF), 800 to 1,200 Ohms typical of the spinal cord, and 100 to 400 Ohms being normally recorded during rhizotomies and neurotomies. If high resistance is encountered for the conventional musculoskeletal procedure, it can and must be reduced by injecting a small volume of normal saline or local anesthetic. Recording is also useful; microelectrode recording

is probably limited to lesion-making in the brain or perhaps the spinal cord, but recording of evoked potentials is much more generally applicable. However, macro stimulation is most often applied for physiologic corroboration. Usually, threshold stimulation is applied at low (2 Hz for motor) and high (50 Hz for sensory) frequencies, and the responses are compared with ideal findings expected for the specific target. Once localization is deemed satisfactory, an RF lesion is made with parameters appropriate to the procedure.

Cryoablation, the second physical modality for the treatment of pain, was implemented by Lloyd in 1976 (36). The cryoprobe consists of a hollow tube with a smaller inner tube (Fig. 42-5). Pressurized gas (usually nitrogen dioxide or carbon dioxide) at 600 to 800 PSI flows through the inner tube and

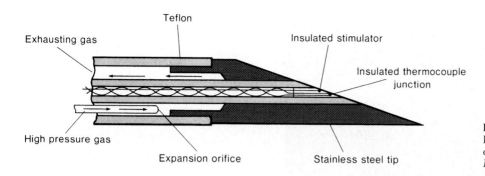

FIGURE 42-5. Details of cryoprobe tip. From Lloyd J, Barnard J, Glynn C. Cryoanalgesia, a new approach to pain relief. *Lancet* 1976;2:932–934.

is released into the larger outer tube through a very fine aperture (0.002 mm). This process extracts heat from the tip of the probe, resulting in a temperature drop (Joule-Thompson effect) and formation of an ice ball, with temperatures in the range of $-70°C$ (37). The gas is then scavenged through an outer tube. A 2.0-mm probe forms a 5.5-mm ice ball, and a 1.4-mm probe forms a 3.5-mm ice ball (Fig. 42-6). A cryoablation machine also includes a nerve stimulator, which allows precise localization of the target nerve, and some models include a thermostat for the temperature monitor (Fig. 42-7).

The application of cold to tissues creates a conduction block, similar to the effect of local anesthetics. At $10°C$, larger myelinated fibers stop conducting, and at $-20°C$, all nerve fibers stop conducting. Long-term pain relief from nerve freezing occurs because ice crystals create vascular damage to the vasa nervorum, which produces severe endoneural edema and creates Wallerian degeneration, but leaves the myelin sheath and endoneurium intact (38). The Schwann cell basal lamina is spared and ultimately provides the structure for regeneration. Although demyelination and degeneration of the axon occurs, the intact endoneurium prevents neuroma formation, and the nerve is typically able to regenerate at a rate of 1.0 to 1.5 mm per week (39).

In comparison with RF, cryodestruction also provides satisfactory lesion-making, but it requires a rather larger probe that is easily damaged, a supply of liquid nitrogen, and a delivery system that is prone to blockage and other problems. Furthermore, cryosurgery is more time-consuming, requiring two to three freezing cycles of 3 minutes each at each target. Unlike the RF cannula, which usually does not require attention during the procedure, the cryoprobe must be kept steady by the operator, which may lead to fatigue and subsequent dislodgement.

Multiple potential indications for cryodestruction have been reviewed recently, including treatment of craniofacial pain, thoracic and abdominal wall pain, pelvic pain, and spinal problems, as well as destruction of a peripheral nerve and neuroma (40). Unfortunately, cryoneurolysis usually fails to provide the lasting pain relief, usually fading within about 3 months. Furthermore, the level of evidence of efficacy of cryoablation may be defined as indeterminate to limited (level V to IV) (41) since the vast majority of available publications are nonexperimental descriptive studies and case reports. Only one randomized trial assessed the efficacy of cryoablation versus phenol block, and it showed better results in the phenol group (25). Nevertheless, because a thermal heat lesion is perceived to have high potential for nerve injury pain, cryoneurolysis could be recommended for the treatment of chronic pain wherever lesion of a peripheral nerve or neuroma is warranted.

Destructive chemicals also have been used extensively (42–46) in neurodestructive procedures. Absolute alcohol, phenol, and glycerol are most commonly used (Chapter 45); hypertonic and cold saline also have been used intrathecally (47). The introduction of chemicals has the advantage of applying a destructive agent that diffuses widely beyond the tip of the introductory needle, which is particularly useful when introduced into the CSF, say, in the Meckel cave or spinal canal. However, all these techniques have the disadvantage of erratic, unpredictable spread and variable degrees of penetration of nervous tissue; none is selective for pain fibers. They tend to produce incomplete and nonpermanent lesions. The danger of tracking is also significant; for example, alcohol injected into the infraorbital nerve may leak into the orbit and cause oculomotor palsy or blindness.

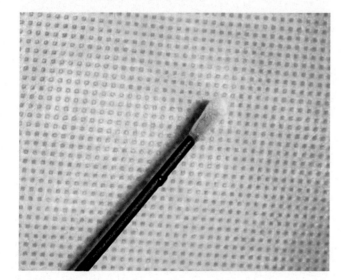

FIGURE 42-6. Ice-ball around the active tip of 12-gauge Lloyd cryoprobe.

Percutaneous Neurectomy and Rhizotomy

Conceptually, percutaneous neurectomy or rhizotomy provide the simplest technique for treating pain syndromes that depend on pain transmission. Unfortunately, such procedures often are not useful either because pain is seldom restricted to the domain of one or a few nerves or roots, or because the inevitable concomitant sensory loss and/or motor impairment is not acceptable (48). Ineffectiveness of surgery on peripheral structures suggests that the source of the pain is to be found in central structures (49).

PART IV: PAIN MANAGEMENT

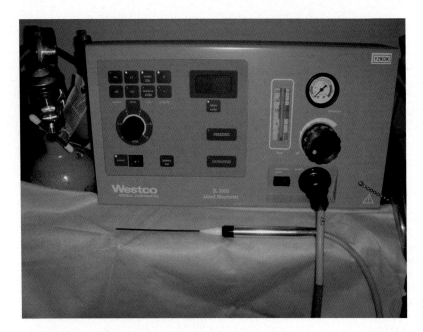

FIGURE 42-7. Cryoanalgesia machine. (Manufactured by Westco Medical Corporation.)

Occipital Neurotomy

For pain syndromes amenable to treatment by denervation in the occipital nerve distribution, occipital neurectomy is commonly advocated. It can be accomplished using either RF or cryoablation. There is poor consensus on indications for occipital neurectomy, the procedure being advocated for diverse pain syndromes in occipital territory including occipital neuralgia, postherpetic neuralgia, and cervicogenic headaches (CH). The procedure should not be expected to relieve steady neuropathic pain, and conceptually it would not seem useful for the relief of pain caused by lesions proximal to the site of the denervation. It may be, however, that denervation of the projected field of the pain would prove to be effective treatment regardless of the site of the causative lesion, although it appears that no study of this issue has been undertaken. In a study of C2 ganglionectomy, microsurgical decompression of the C2 root and ganglion has some utility in treating CH. The accepted diagnostic criteria and success of anesthetic blockade of C2 should identify the subset of patients with CH predominantly caused by C2 root or ganglion effect at this level, which may favor surgical treatment (50). Although occipital neurectomy should eliminate the allodynia and hyperpathia of postherpetic neuralgia in C2–C3 territory by denervating the responsible receptors, this strategy is seldom worthwhile, since the steady element of the pain persists or may become worse as a result of deafferentation neuropathic pain.

Another condition in which occipital neurectomy has been recommended is occipital headache. Patients with recurrent attacks of headache located consistently in the same territory sometimes gain temporary relief from division of the peripheral nerves that supply the region of the head involved in the pain, including the occipital region.

The technique of percutaneous RF occipital neurectomy consists of introducing an RF cannula with an active tip 2 to 4 mm in length (Fig. 42-8) through the scalp to the expected location of the greater and/or lesser occipital nerves on the affected side at the base of the skull, using surface landmarks. Then 50-Hz stimulation is applied, and the needle is moved until paresthesia is produced in occipital nerve territory at the

lowest threshold; an RF lesion is made and the degree of sensory loss is verified. Usually, a maximal lesion is required, achieved by several cycles of 80°C for 90 seconds.

It is difficult to present outcome data because these depend on the syndrome treated and the nature of the pain; reports fail to distinguish these matters. Published data suggest that 75%

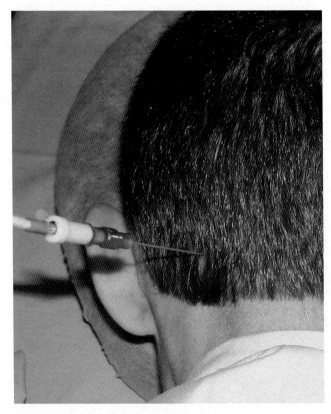

FIGURE 42-8. Greater occipital radiofrequency neurotomy of the left greater occipital nerve. 21-gauge 4-mm active tip cannula in place.

of patients enjoy amelioration of occipital pain generally over a 1- to 4-year follow-up (51).

Complications are few, with neuropathic pain in the denervated area being an ever-present concern. Recurrence after nerve regeneration is to be expected. Thus, the technique of suboccipital peripheral nerve stimulation has emerged as a preferable neuromodulatory technique (see Chapter 41).

Intercostal Neurotomy

Various pain syndromes, such as postherpetic neuralgia, postthoracotomy pain, intercostal neuralgia, and the pain of cancer, affect the chest wall. For these conditions, percutaneous RF intercostal neurectomy, first used by Tasker in 1972, may seem a promising procedure because it is not followed by significant functional deficit (52). However, comments made regarding occipital postherpetic neuralgia also apply to intercostal postherpetic neuralgia; and, for obscure reasons, intercostal neurectomy is practically useless in treating postthoracotomy syndrome, with only 25% of 44 patients reporting useful relief (52). Intercostal neuralgia usually results from compression of a thoracic root by a thoracic disk or foraminal stenosis, although sometimes no cause can be found. Because intercostal nerve section distal to a site of irritation is all that can be accomplished in treating intercostal neuralgia caused by disk compression or stenosis, this procedure appears to be ineffective. Destruction of the dorsal root proximal to the lesion site usually is necessary. Intercostal neurectomy is useful chiefly to treat pain caused by cancer of the chest wall; all of Tasker's eight patients experienced relief when denervation of the painful area was possible and when the pain did not incorporate an old thoracotomy incision.

Chemical destruction is accomplished by injection of 1 to 2 mL of 10% phenol, using the same technique as that used for intercostal block with local anesthetic. Fluoroscopic guidance or ultrasonography is generally recommended to prevent inadvertent spread of the neurolytic solution into the epidural space.

Radiofrequency lesioning is usually performed under local anesthesia with fluoroscopy or ultrasound guidance. An 18-gauge RF cannula with a curved 10-mm active tip is "walked down" and slid under the inferior margin of the rib related to the nerve to be sectioned, proximal to the expected site of nerve involvement, until it enters or lies alongside the neurovascular bundle (see Chapter 16). Then, 2-Hz stimulation is performed as the needle tip is moved about, and contractions in the appropriate intercostal muscles are monitored until a site is found where the these contractions occur at 0.3 to 0.8 V. Two cycles of RF lesion are then made for 90 seconds, using a temperature of 80°C. It is wise to make a second lesion adjacent to the first to ensure adequate denervation. Efficacy is checked by ensuring that appropriate anesthesia has been achieved and/or by demonstrating increased threshold for motor response. An upright chest radiograph is performed immediately postoperatively to exclude pneumothorax, which occurred in approximately 3% to 6% of patients and required chest drainage in 2% (52).

Cryodenervation is also a feasible option. Local anesthesia of skin and intercostal space is performed with 1% to 2% lidocaine with 1:200 000 epinephrine. Epinephrine solution is useful for any cryoablation because it diminishes to some degree the bleeding associated with inserting a 12-gauge cryoprobe, and a spasm of blood vessels prevents the dissipation of cold. A Lloyd cryoprobe (12-gauge) is inserted so as to place the tip parallel to and under the corresponding rib (Fig. 42-9). Flu-

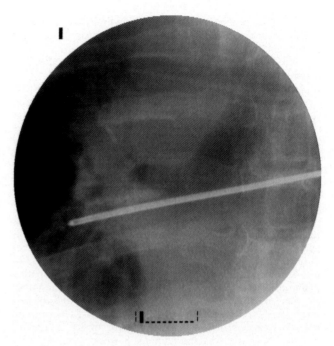

FIGURE 42-9. Intercostal neurotomy. Lloyd 12-gauge cryoprobe is placed in the medial-lateral direction and positioned below the rib.

oroscopy may greatly help to place the probe accurately and avoid pneumothorax. Three cycles of freezing for 3 minutes each are executed, followed by slight advancement or retraction of the probe and duplication of the same process of freezing. Three consecutive lesions are sufficient for the ablation of the nerve. Spinal cord stimulation is often a better option in patients with neuropathic thoracic chronic noncancer pain (see Chapter 41).

Miscellaneous Neurotomies

Several miscellaneous applications for peripheral nerve destruction have been published. Phenol neurolytic block of the suprascapular nerve and articular branches of the circumflex nerve was claimed to be effective in palliation of arthritic shoulder pain (53). Four patients obtained sustained pain relief after RF neurotomy of sensory branches of the obturator and femoral nerves for the treatment of nonoperable hip pain (54). Cryoanalgesia has been attempted in the treatment of painful peripheral nerve lesions (55). However, the risk of neuropathic pain is ever present.

Peripheral nerve destruction is occasionally recommended for the treatment of cancer pain (see Chapter 45) and spasticity. Discussion of the interventional treatment of spasticity is beyond the objectives of this chapter.

Dorsal Rhizotomy

According to Gybels and Sweet (56), Uematsu and his colleagues (15,57) were the first to report percutaneous RF dorsal rhizotomy. Although percutaneous RF dorsal rhizotomy has the advantage over neurectomy of not inducing motor deficits unless electrode positioning is faulty, and of usually denervating a larger area of the body, it still results in proprioceptive loss, a serious problem if roots supplying limbs are sectioned. The fact that the radicular arteries that accompany roots may be end-arteries for the spinal cord—especially at the C1, T1–T4, and T11–L1 levels—means that their accidental occlusion may result in cord infarction and paraplegia.

Although experience with open rhizotomy has been extensively published, outcome data for the percutaneous technique are limited. In general, the pain syndromes for which dorsal rhizotomy should be considered are nociceptive pain caused by cancer or by spinal pathology that compresses nerve roots and the evoked or neuralgic elements of neuropathic pain. Control of malignant pain is limited to cases in which the entire area involved can be denervated by rhizotomy lesions that lie proximal to the tumor site. In practice, this is rarely practicable.

Radiofrequency dorsal rhizotomy for radicular pain is currently an ill-defined procedure, with the results of clinical trials mixed. Several observational studies found the procedure effective in the long term for about 50% of patients (58–60). Surprisingly, the complication rates of a new neuropathic pain, sensory loss, and motor loss were low. Painful dysesthesia was observed in 4% of patients (10), but it disappeared after 6 weeks. One RCT of cervical dorsal root RF rhizotomy showed clearly beneficial results in favor of RF treatment, but the follow-up was shorter than 8 weeks (61). Another RCT failed to prove the efficacy of RF posterior rhizotomy in treating lumbosacral radicular pain (62); however, this study contained several methodological and statistical biases (63). Currently, the procedure should only be considered for those patients suffering severe radicular pain when alternative nondestructive methods (multimodal medical treatment, fluoroscopy-guided epidural injection, spinal cord stimulation, and rehabilitation strategies) have failed and the patients are not candidates for neurosurgical correction of underlying pathology. Patients must understand the temporal nature of the treatment and its potential complications, including sensory and motor loss and dysesthetic pain.

Even when a single root can be incriminated by careful selective local anesthetic root blocks, the permanent rhizotomy may fail because the lesion cannot be made proximal to the site of entrapment or irritation. Also, because of innervation overlap within somatic areas, lesioning of a single nerve root may produce only temporary denervation. In patients with neuropathic pain in whom allodynia or hyperpathia are prominent features, rhizotomy may also be useful, as in cases of spinal cord injury with a radicular distribution of allodynia at the level of the cord lesion. If a limb is to be denervated, even with a single-level rhizotomy, the accompanying loss of position sense must be considered, and this is best assessed at the time of the essential diagnostic root blockade. However, such diagnostic blocks do not correlate precisely with the outcome of rhizotomy (see Chapter 38). Multiple consecutive rhizotomies are even riskier.

Notwithstanding the discretion needed in administering RF posterior rhizotomy for radicular pain, the procedure seems to be highly effective for the treatment of spasticity (64,65), producing an improvement in 94% of patients, with excellent results in 73%.

The technique consists of identifying the correct root(s) to be denervated by clinical means and diagnostic local blocks. Then, with the patient either under neuroleptic analgesia or local anesthesia or both, a 20-gauge RF cannula with a 5-mm active tip is introduced into the dorsal portion of the appropriate intervertebral foramen, under intermittent fluoroscopic guidance. Sensory stimulation, first at 50 Hz, should elicit tingling sensation at the corresponding dermatome, with a threshold

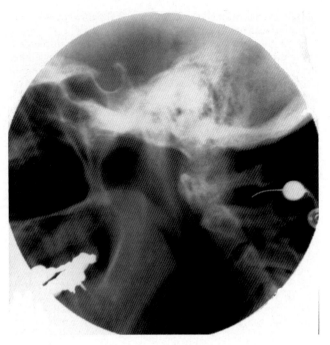

FIGURE 42-10. C2 dorsal root ganglion rhizotomy. Radiofrequency cannula is introduced at the border of the anterior third, within the posterior two-thirds of the atlanto-axial arch.

of 0.3 to 0.5 V. Motor stimulation at 2 Hz must not produce muscle twitching below the level of the double sensory response current (i.e., if the patient experienced paresthesia at 0.5 V, one should avoid starting RF lesion if the motor response obtained was below 1 V). This strategy prevents inadvertent damage of the ventral motor portion of the nerve root. Traditionally, a temperature of 67°C, applied for 60 to 120 seconds, has been recommended for the RF dorsal rhizotomy.

Cervical Dorsal Rhizotomy

At the C2 level, the cannula should be introduced at the border of the anterior third with the posterior two-thirds of the atlanto-axial arch seen on the lateral view (Fig. 42-10). On the anteroposterior (AP) view, the tip should be seen at the middle of the atlanto-axial joint shadow (Fig. 42-11). Further insertion may result in dural puncture and spinal cord injury.

Placement of the cannula at any other cervical level is accomplished by using the oblique position of the image intensifier to "open up" the intervertebral foramina. Under tunnel vision, the cannula is aimed toward the posterior border of the foramen at its inferior third. After bone contact is made, the AP view is obtained and the cannula further introduced until positioned at the middle of the facet joint shadow. Often, the correct cannula position is heralded by paresthesia. Caution has to be taken not to introduce the cannula into the anterior portion of the foramen lest the vertebral artery be damaged.

Thoracic Dorsal Rhizotomy

At the thoracic levels, the cannula should be introduced into the superior portion of the intervertebral foramina in tunnel view. The AP image should confirm the position of the tip at the level of the facet joint line (Fig. 42-12).

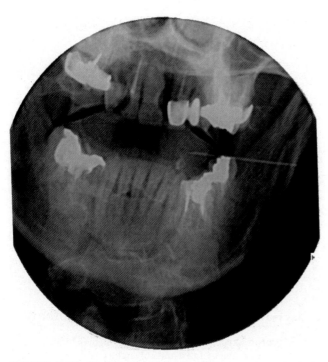

FIGURE 42-11. C2 dorsal root ganglion rhizotomy. Cannula tip is seen at the middle of the atlanto-axial joint shadow.

Lumbar Dorsal Rhizotomy

In the lumbar area, the cannula is introduced into the dorsal third of the foramen using a tunnel view with approximately 30 to 40 degrees of lateral rotation. As a rule of thumb, the shadow of the spinous process should superimpose the con-

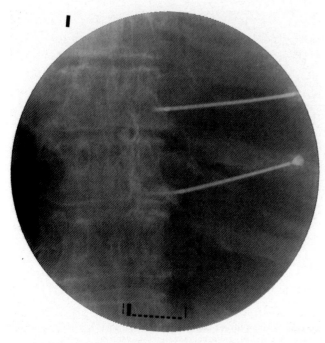

FIGURE 42-12. Thoracic dorsal root ganglions radiofrequency rhizotomy. Two 20-gauge 10-mm curved active tip cannulae are positioned (anteroposterior view).

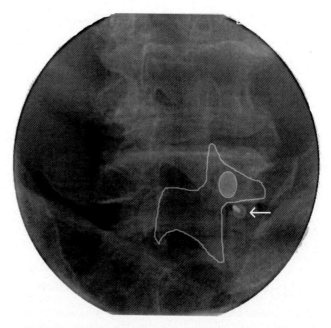

FIGURE 42-13. Radiofrequency rhizotomy of the fifth lumbar dorsal root ganglion. The cannula is positioned under "tunnel vision" fluoroscopy immediately laterally to the apex of the S1 superior articular process (under the "chin of the Scotty dog").

tralateral facet joint. In this position, the cannula is aimed under the "chin on the Scotty-dog" (Fig. 42-13). In the AP view, similar to the thoracic levels, the tip of the cannula should be seen at the facet joint line. If, at the L5 level, a tunnel view often cannot be achieved because of the superimposed iliac crest, the cannula is introduced laterally and inferiorly into the space between the transverse process of L5 and the ala of the sacrum, aimed at the neck of the L5 transverse process. Progress is often impeded here by "sacralization" of L5 and/or osteophytes. Sacral ventral roots are reached through appropriate posterior sacral foramina, bringing the electrode tip to the anterior foramina. Here, one must be alert to the risks of causing bladder and sexual dysfunction.

Uematsu and colleagues (15,57) reported seven excellent and two good results out of 17 patients operated upon for various pain syndromes. Pagura (66) reported 76% pain relief in 50 patients, 13 suffering from cancer and 37 from intervertebral disk disease, with a 4% incidence of temporary postoperative paresis.

Dubuisson (67) lists the data quoted in Table 42-2. Of the patients reported by van Kleef and colleagues (68), 13 suffered from degenerative disk disease in the C4–C6 region; of these, 75% enjoyed pain relief after 3 months and 50% after 6 months. Not unexpectedly, dysesthetic burning from iatrogenic deafferentation occurred in 12 patients (60%) but did not persist past 3 weeks; decreased sensation was seen in seven (35%) but disappeared after 6 weeks; no motor or reflex deficits were seen.

In the published data collected by Gybels and Sweet (56), of 192 patients with nonmalignant pain, 69% were enjoying useful pain relief; of six with pain caused by cancer, all were relieved. Follow-ups for these patients were short.

The complications of rhizotomy, other than failure and pain recurrence, include sensory and motor loss, iatrogenic neuropathic pain, and the risk of direct spinal cord damage or ischemic infarction due to injury of the radicular artery. These complications explain why few patients undergo rhizotomy,

TABLE 42-2

RESULTS OF PERCUTANEOUS RF DORSAL RHIZOTOMY

Authors	Levels treated	Initial relief	Late relief	Mortality	No. of cases
Uematsu et al. (1974)[332]	Spinal roots	39%	?	0	13
Lazorthes et al. (1976)[135]	Spinal roots	65%	?	0	20
Nash (1986)[206]	Spinal ganglia	58%	50%	0	26
van Kleef et al. (1993)[334]	Spinal ganglia	75%	39%	0	20

RF, radiofrequency.
From Dubuisson, D.: Root surgery. In Wall PD, and Melzack R. (eds.): *Textbook of Pain*, 3rd Ed. pp. 1055. Edinburgh, Churchill Livingstone, 1994.

but rather are treated with less-invasive methods including spinal cord stimulation (see Chapter 41).

Spinal Zygapophysial Joint Neurotomy

This category of percutaneous nerve destruction is probably the most extensively published and clinically applied. Prevalence of zygapophysial joint pain is high, estimated as the source of pain in 15% to 45% of a heterogeneous group of patients with chronic low back pain, 42% to 48% of patients with thoracic pain, and 54% to 67% of patients with chronic neck pain. Individuals younger than 65 have lower incidence of facet joint pain (30%), whereas those older than 65 have higher prevalence (52%); males are slightly less affected (38%) as compared with females (43%) (69).

Prior to zygapophysial nerve destruction, the diagnosis must be confirmed by double comparative local anesthetic blocks, as described earlier. Multiple potential pain generators could be involved in spinal pain, including intervertebral disks, spinal nerves, and adjacent structures, and nonorganic components may play a significant role; therefore, establishing the correct diagnosis of the facet pain is imperative.

Cervical Zygapophysial Joint Neurotomy

The neurotomy technique for C3 to C7 medial branches was originally described by Lord and colleagues, and this is the only time it was validated in a RCT (23). More recently, an acceptable method of third occipital neurotomy was also described, but it has not been validated in a RCT (70). Medial branches of C3 to C6 take off from dorsal rami and are uniformly found at the waist of corresponding articular pillars. The third occipital nerve (TON) is in fact the posterior ramus of the third cervical root, much thicker than the ventral ramus. It usually lies on the line of C2–C3 facet joint or, alternatively, may be located slightly above or below the joint (Fig. 42-14).

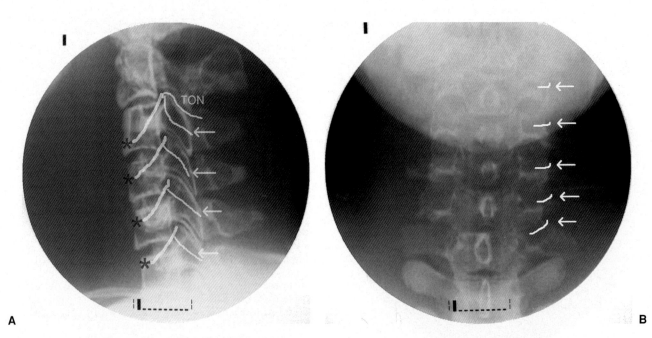

FIGURE 42-14. A: Lateral radiograph with diagram of surgical anatomy of cervical medial branches and the third occipital nerve. *TON,* the third occipital nerve; *arrows,* medial branches; *asterisks,* ventral cervical rami. **B:** Posteroanterior radiograph with drawing of the medial branches of C3–C7 at the middle of corresponding articular pillars (*arrows*). TON cannot be drawn on this figure because of mandible shadow.

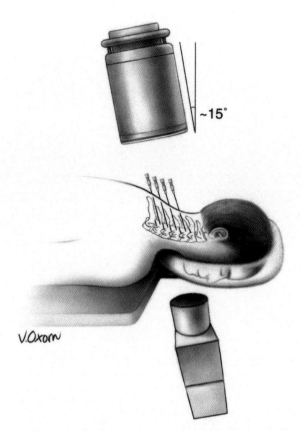

FIGURE 42-15. Cervical medial branch neurotomy (prone position). Patient placed prone with face on a padded ring. Image intensifier positioned anteroposteriorly and tilted 15 degrees caudad. *Note:* If the neck remains somewhat extended on a flat table, the caudad angulation must increase to 25 to 35 degrees (see Chapter 44, Fig. 44-28). Reprinted from Faclier G, Kay J. Cervical facet radiofrequency neurotomy. *Tech Reg Anesth Pain Manage* 2000;4:120–125, with permission.

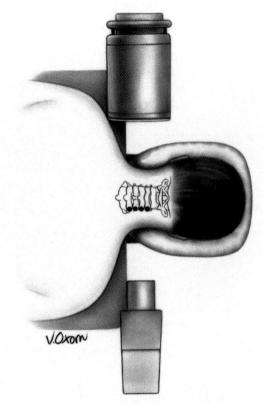

FIGURE 42-16. Cervical medial branch neurotomy (prone position). Patient placed prone with face on padded ring. Image intensifier rotated to the lateral position. Reprinted from Faclier G, Kay J. Cervical facet radiofrequency neurotomy. *Tech Reg Anesth Pain Manage* 2000;4:120–125, with permission.

Here, we describe the method used for cervical facet neurotomy from the TON to the C7 medial branch (71). The most important recommendation is to place the cannula parallel to the target nerve at the anatomically correct area of the cervical spine.

The patient is positioned prone on the fluoroscopy table, with the head flexed 5 to 10 degrees in a soft frame (Figs. 42-15 and 42-16). Arms are positioned alongside the patient's body, and shoulders are pulled on a caudad direction. Application of adhesive tape on the trapezius areas facilitates shoulder traction and helps to maximize the operator's comfort and fluoroscopic visualization of the lower cervical vertebrae at the lateral view. Conscious sedation and local anesthesia with 2% lidocaine are sufficient to alleviate discomfort and to allow operator–patient communication. Under AP fluoroscopic view, the lateral masses of facet joints are seen. Recognition of the target level can be facilitated by either cephalo-caudad or caudo-cephalad tilt of the image intensifier. At the C1–C2 levels, the dens of C2 and the line of the atlanto-axial joint are useful landmarks. At the C2–C3 levels, the line caudad to the atlanto-axial joint is the C2–C3 facet joint, which is the target for the third occipital neurotomy. The waist of each lateral mass is the landmark for medial branch neurotomy (Fig. 42-14B). Alternatively, the C7 vertebra, with its wide transverse process, is used as the starting point to count more cephalad cervical vertebrae. At times, the mandible and the dentition may obscure the view.

On such occasions, the patient's head should be gently and slightly rotated contralaterally, and the patient asked to open the mouth.

Universally, the skin entry point is chosen somewhat laterally to the bone at the level of a facet joint below the target (i.e., if the C4 medial branch has to be coagulated, the entry point should be 1.0–1.5 cm lateral to the C5–C6 facet joint). This routine allows cannula placement parallel to the nerve. A 22-gauge 5-mm RF cannula is inserted in a mesiad and cephalad direction to contact the facet nerve at the waist of each articular pillar (Fig. 42-17). For the third occipital neurotomy, the cannula is inserted to contact the midpoint of the C2–C3 facet joint line.

An alternative approach is to obtain a sublaminar AP view at a position that allows radiographic separation of facet joints. Since the sagittal line of the facet joints is parallel to the medial branch at the corresponding waist of the pillar, this fluoroscopy view secures insertion of the cannula parallel to the nerve. With a slight oblique rotation of 5 to 10 degrees, the skin entry point is superimposed on the midpoint of the pillar waist edge, and the cannula is positioned using "tunnel vision" technique until it makes contact with bone (Fig. 42-18).

The lateral view then confirms that the cannulae are in proper position and do not project anteriorly to the pillar (Fig. 42-19). A thermocouple electrode is inserted into the lumen of each cannula and stimulated with frequencies of 50 Hz (sensory) and 2 Hz (motor) (Fig. 42-20). The patient should experience a tingling sensation covering the painful area, but no radicular distribution. Usually, contractions of multifidus

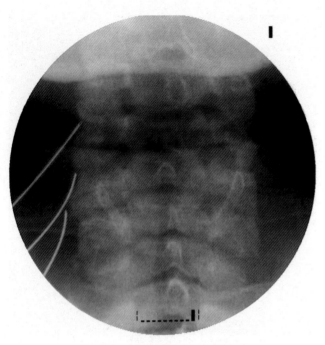

FIGURE 42-17. Cervical medial branch neurotomy (prone position). Anteroposterior view shows cannulae positioned at the waist of left cervical facet pillars C3, C4, and C5. The lower cannula seemed to be displaced, however this radiographic picture is misleading due to severe deformation of the articular pillar of C5.

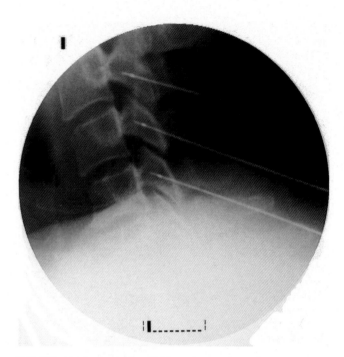

FIGURE 42-19. Cervical medial branch neurotomy (prone position). The lateral view confirms the proper cannulae position at the middle of the waists of C3, C4, and C5 articular pillars. The cannulae are positioned parallel to the target nerves and do not project anterior to the pillar. Radiopaque bead highlights the proximal end of active tip.

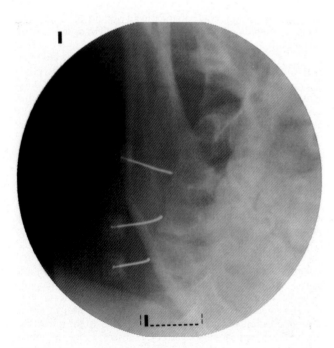

FIGURE 42-18. Cervical medial branch neurotomy (prone position). Anteroposterior view with caudo-cephalad tilt. The entry point is superimposed on the middle of the pillar waist edge, and the cannulae are positioned using the "tunnel vision" technique.

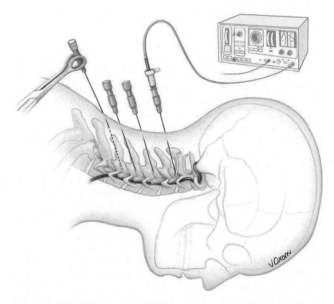

FIGURE 42-20. Cervical medial branch neurotomy (prone position). Lateral view shows ideal positioning of radiofrequency cannulae adjacent to the target nerves at the C2–C3 joint and C4 and C5 pillars. A cannula is being inserted to contact the C6 pillar. A thermocouple electrode has been inserted into the C2–C3 cannula in preparation for stimulation and radiofrequency neurotomy. Reprinted from Faclier G, Kay J. Cervical facet radiofrequency neurotomy. *Tech Reg Anesth Pain Manage* 2000;4:120–125, with permission.

muscles are seen during the motor stimulation. Another approach, with the patient positioned on the side, is discussed in Chapter 44 (see Fig. 44-30 and 44-31).

Following appropriate responses to stimulation, 0.5 mL of 2% lidocaine or 0.5% ropivacaine is injected through each cannula to abolish pain during the RF lesion, which is made at 80°C for 60 seconds. With proper anatomic position and concordant stimulation, two cycles of lesion are sufficient for the medial branch neurotomy at C3 to C7. However, two or three consecutive lesions, made by repositioning the cannula cephalad and caudad, were recommended in the original article published on this technique (23). At the level of C2–C3 (TON), three lesions are executed: at the level of the joint, immediately above it, and then below the joint line on the lateral view. The TON is the thickest, and its pathway is variable. Depending on the electrical stimulation, occasionally a lesion at the level of the joint and two additional burns above or below the joint are required.

Usually, RF neurotomy is performed at a minimum of three levels that correspond to the patient's pain. Suboccipital pain and headaches require third occipital neurotomy and C3 and C4 medial branch neurotomies. Neck pain with radiation to the upper trapezius needs to be addressed by C4 to C6 neurotomies, whereas pain referred to the shoulder and scapula requires C5 to C7 neurotomies.

Fluoroscopic control, proper cannula placement, and the use of stimulation before nerve destruction make complication rates fairly low. However, if RF inadvertently damages the posterior ramus and/or its lateral branch, cutaneous dysesthesia and sometimes anesthesia can result, but this usually resolves within 3 to 4 months. In Lord's study, five of 12 patients had numbness or dysesthesia in the cutaneous territory of the coagulated nerves, but they did not rate it as a troublesome or requiring treatment (23). The TON supplies cutaneous sensation over a small area of the occiput. Thus, numbness and neuritic pain may occur in the area around the suboccipital region and usually resolves within weeks to months. Rarely, if the procedure fails to provide pain relief, some patients may report transient escalation of their pain. Failure of the procedure may be a result of poor patient selection, missing the target nerve, proximity of blood vessels close to the tip of the cannula producing a heat sink, a relatively small burn area compared with the local anesthetic coverage, or alternate afferent pathways.

Median pain relief after cervical zygapophysial neurotomy is 7 to 14 months, and repeated procedures reliably reinstitute the initial analgesic effect (23,72).

Thoracic Zygapophysial Joint Neurotomy

The anatomic basis for this procedure has been investigated in a cadaveric study (73). At the upper (T1–T3) and lower (T9–T10) levels, the medial branch consistently passes across the intertransverse space, making contact with the lateral end of the superior border of the transverse process (Fig. 42-21). The T11 medial branch passes across the base of the superior articular process (SAP) of T12. The T12 medial branch runs similarly to the lumbar levels (see next section). At midthoracic levels (T4–T8), the course of a medial branch is less constant. Usually, at these levels, the nerve passes somewhere in the intertransverse space without making contact with bone.

Prior to neurotomy, double comparative local anesthetic block should establish the diagnosis of thoracic facet pain. Although medial branch anesthetic block is a simple and straight-forward technique, the situation is completely different for the performance of RF neurotomy. No validated technique has

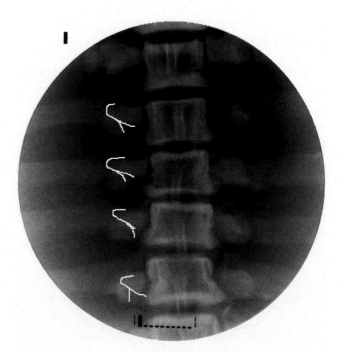

FIGURE 42-21. Thoracic medial branch neurotomy (prone position). Drawing (*white lines*) on the radiographic image shows upper thoracic medial branches emerge through intertransverse space, make contact with the lateral end of the superior border of the transverse process, and continue in mesiad-caudad direction.

been published yet. Only one published prospective observational study of 40 patients claimed some benefit, reporting good to excellent pain relief for an average duration of 31 months, but the method used cannot be considered as anatomic (74).

In theory, contralateral cannula insertion should align the position of the active tip parallel to the target nerve. The authors follow this principle in clinical practice in the neurotomy of T1 to T3 and T9 to T10 (Fig. 42-22); however, we refrain from recommending it before a formal validation study is performed. T11 and T12 neurotomies are performed similarly to those at the lumbar levels (see next section).

Lumbar Zygapophysial Joint Neurotomy

The anatomy of lumbar zygapophysial nerves and the position of RF cannulae are illustrated in Figure 42-23. Each facet joint is innervated by two nerves: the medial branch of the dorsal ramus at the same level and from the level above, excluding the L5–S1 facet joint, which is thought to be innervated by the L4 medial branch and the L5–S1 dorsal rami. All lumbar medial branches and the L5 dorsal ramus pass the base of the superior articular process (SAP) between the intervertebral foramen and the mamillo-accessory ligament (75,76). The S1 posterior ramus leaves the S1 posterior foramen at 12 o'clock, sending the ascending branches to innervate the L5–S1 facet joint (77).

The principle of lumbar zygapophysial joint neurectomy is the same as for the other areas: placement of the RF cannula parallel and adjacent to the target nerve.

Facet neurotomy is performed under local analgesia and light neuroleptic anesthesia. The patient is placed in the prone position on a fluoroscopy table with a pillow under the abdomen to alleviate lumbar lordosis (Fig. 42-24). The AP

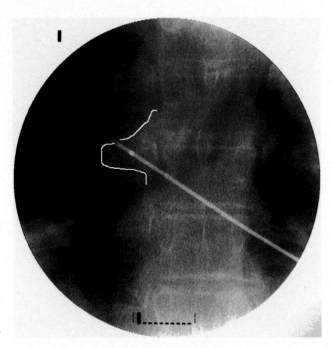

FIGURE 42-22. Thoracic medial branch neurotomy (prone position). A 18-gauge 10-mm curved active tip radiofrequency cannula is inserted from the level of the spinous process and directed toward costo-transverse junction. Active tip is parallel to thoracic medial branch nerve. White drawing delineates the transverse and superior articular processes of thoracic vertebra.

fluoroscopic view is obtained with maximal exposure of the target points. Lidocaine 2% or ropivacaine 0.5% is used for the local anesthesia. The selected skin entry point is somewhat lateral to the pedicle, one level caudal for every lumbar level, excluding L5 and S1. For the L5 dorsal ramus, the entry point

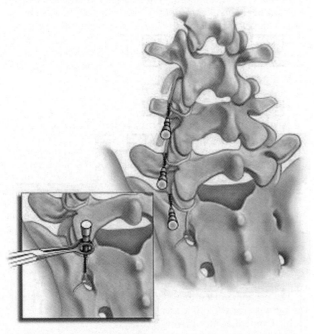

FIGURE 42-23. Lumbar medial branch neurotomy (prone position). The medial branches of L3 and L4 and the posterior primary rami of L5 and the first sacral vertebra (S1), with cannulae placed parallel to the nerves (S1 inset).

is approximately at the level of the S1 posterior foramen, but less laterally than for the upper levels, so as not to superimpose the iliac crest on the sacral ala. For the S1 level, a tunnel view of the posterior neural foramen is obtained. The entry point is situated at the 12 o'clock position of the foramen (Fig. 42-25; see also Chapter 44, Figs. 44-34 to 44-37).

An 18-gauge cannula with a curved 10-mm active tip is probably the best suited disposable device for this application. Although the best published results (78) were reached when a 15-gauge solid Ray electrode was used, the lack of available supply of that device and the fact that it is not disposable make an 18-gauge single-use cannula a suitable alternative. A 10-mm active tip completely corresponds to 1 cm of exposed nerve before it disappears under the mamillo-accessory ligament.

Standard Technique

The cannula is inserted and advanced toward the target using intermittent AP fluoroscopy. Several steps are taken to ensure placement of the cannula at the correct final position at the base of the corresponding SAP. First, the contact with bone is made just caudal to the superior edge of the transverse process (or the sacral ala for L5), immediately lateral to the base of the SAP (Fig. 42-26A; see also Chapter 44 Figs. 44-37 and 38).

The image intensifier is then rotated to the lateral view. The cannulae are advanced until loss of bony contact is felt and seen on fluoroscopy. Lateral views are used to ensure that the tip of the cannula did not pass the posterior boundary of the intervertebral foramen but is situated close to the anterior border of the SAP (Fig. 42-26B).

The 10- to 20-degree oblique view is used to demonstrate correct cannula placement parallel to the base of the SAP. The cannula tip is obliquely crossing the shadow of corresponding pedicle in this projection (Fig. 42-27).

At the S1 level, the cannula is introduced at the 12 o'clock position while constant bony contact is maintained. A lateral view is used to verify the position of the cannula tip outside the sacral canal (Fig. 42-28).

Finally, electrical stimulation at 50 Hz is performed for sensory testing; a dermatomal pattern is considered unacceptable. A frequency of 2 Hz is then applied for motor stimulation. Any motor response other than twitching of the multifidus muscles must be interpreted as stimulation of the ventral ramus. In this situation, the cannula must be repositioned, usually by slight withdrawal, until no dermatomal or motor response is obtained.

A small volume (0.5–1.0 mL) of local anesthetic is injected before activation of the RF generator. The first lesion is created with the cannula tip rotated caudally, following the curvature of the bone (7 o'clock for the right and 5 o'clock for the left side). The duration of the cycle is 90 seconds with 80°C temperature. The second lesion is generated after dorsal rotation (11 o'clock for the right and 1 o'clock for the left side), moving up on the SAP, to increase the size of the lesion. This rotation is warranted because variations in the path of the medial branch occur in the caudo-cephalad direction on the surface of SAP.

S1 dorsal ramus RF neurotomy is performed with the same parameters. The cannula's active tip, initially faced cephalad (12 o'clock), is rotated to 2 o'clock and the first lesion created. The second lesion is performed at the 10 o'clock position.

Tunnel Vision Technique

The principle of this technique is to insert RF cannulae under fluoroscopic tunnel vision guidance, avoiding the difficulties of

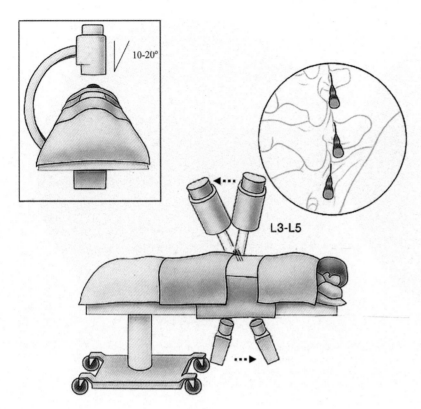

FIGURE 42-24. Lumbar medial branch neurotomy (prone position). Diagram showing patient's position and cannulae placement at the L3–L4, L4–L5, and L5–S1 levels. If image intensifier is tilted caudo-cephalad (*arrows*), the radiographic anteroposterior view becomes sublaminar "tunnel vision" view.

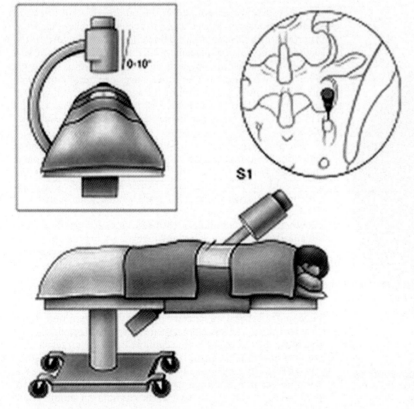

FIGURE 42-25. S1 medial branch neurotomy (prone position). Position of patient, fluoroscopic image intensifier, and site of the cannula placed at the foramen for S1 dorsal ramus neurotomy.

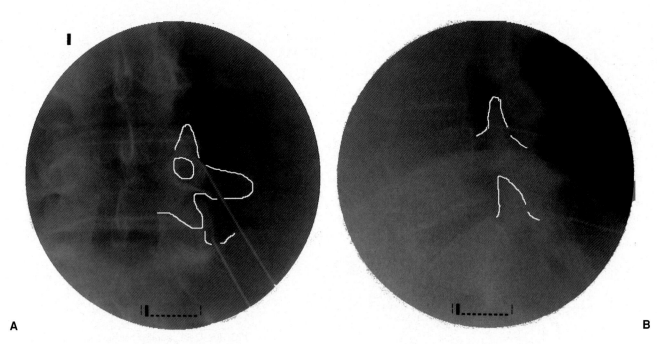

A   **B**

FIGURE 42-26. Lumbar medial branch neurotomy (prone position). **A:** Anteroposterior view shows cannulae at the L4–L5 and L5–S1 levels. The tip of the cannula is positioned at the junction of the superior articular process and the transverse process/sacral ala. **B:** Lateral view shows that the cannula tip remains within the shadow of the base of the superior articular process, parallel to the medial branch and L5 dorsal ramus.

two-dimensional vision inevitably encountered with the technique described earlier for the L1 to L5 levels.

First, a lateral image of the lumbar spine is obtained. The scout image of the target segment is printed, and the angles between the upper border of the vertebra and the base of the SAP

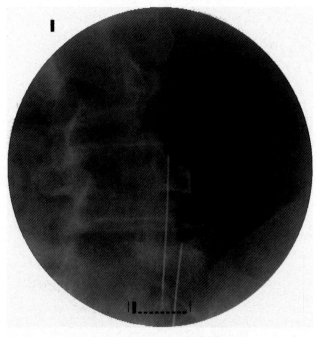

FIGURE 42-27. Lumbar medial branch neurotomy (prone position). Oblique view of the radiofrequency cannulae positioned parallel to the base of corresponding superior articular processes.

are measured (Fig. 42-29). This measurement will give the exact angle of caudo-cephalad axial rotation needed to correctly position the cannula in the sagittal plane. This angle is typically 20 to 40 degrees, depending on individual lordotic curvature.

Next, the AP view of the lumbar spine is obtained. The image intensifier is then rotated in the caudo-cephalad direction to the previously measured angle to achieve a sublaminar view. Insertion of the cannula parallel to the base of the SAP in the sagittal plane ensures placement analogous to that of the target nerve. The last alignment is an oblique rotation. Dynamic fluoroscopy is used to rotate the image ipsilaterally by 10 to 20 degrees until the junction of the superior proximal edge of the transverse process and the SAP is visualized (Fig. 42-30). This fluoroscopic view can be termed the "sublaminar oblique view."

The final position at the L5 level may be different because of individual anatomic variations of iliac crest height. The image intensifier is rotated until the S1 SAP is clearly seen. The degree of obliquity depends on the extent to which the iliac crest obscures the target point. This angle will vary between 5 and 10 degrees.

When the target point is identified, skin marks are made. Local anesthetic is administered through a 25-gauge spinal needle to diminish pain from insertion of the large-bore RF cannula. Cannulae are inserted using the tunnel view technique (i.e., the target point, the tip, and the hub of the cannula should appear as a dot). The cannula, with the tip facing caudad, is inserted until contact is made with bone. The tip of the cannula is rotated cephalad and advanced a further 3 to 5 mm until bony contact is lost. The cannula is then rotated caudad and mesiad to expose the full length of the cannula tip to the target site. To confirm proper placement, lateral fluoroscopy is performed. A true lateral view is obtained when the bony landmarks are superimposed, thus eliminating the double contour appearance of vertebral bodies. In that view, the cannula tip should reach

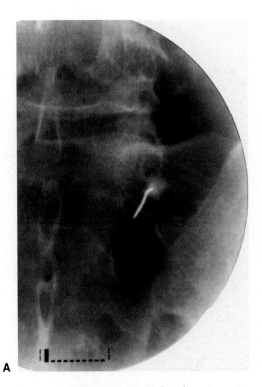
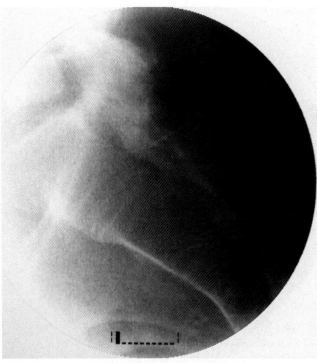

FIGURE 42-28. S1 dorsal ramus neurotomy (prone position). **A:** Anteroposterior view shows cannula at the 12 o'clock position of the superior border of the S1 posterior foramen. **B:** Lateral view shows cannula situated within dorsal sacral foramen.

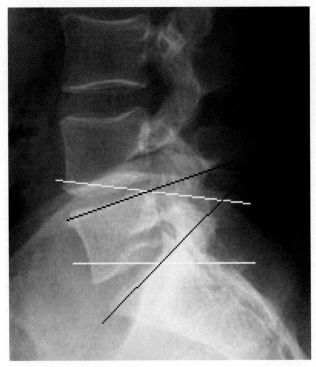

FIGURE 42-29. Radiographic lateral view of lumbar spine in natural vertical position. Prone positioning with a pillow usually partially eliminates lumbar lordosis. *Black lines* represent the sagittal plane of the superior endplate of the vertebrae. *White lines* are plotted through the bases of the superior articular processes.

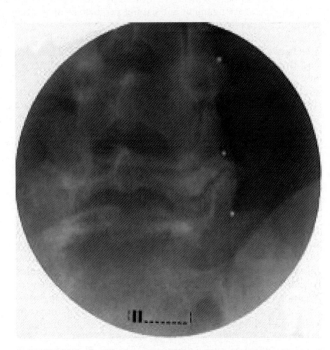

FIGURE 42-30. Lumbar medial branch neurotomy. Sublaminar and slightly oblique view clearly shows the junction of the superior articular processes with the corresponding transverse processes of L3, L4, and the sacral ala (*white dots*).

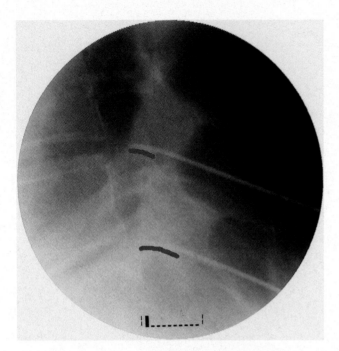

FIGURE 42-31. Lumbar medial branch neurotomy. Lateral view of two cannulae positioned at the base of the L5 and S1 superior articular processes. *Red lines* represent the medial branch of L4 and the posterior primary ramus of L5.

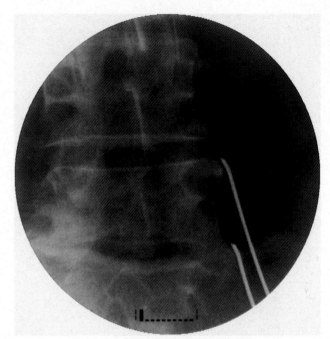

FIGURE 42-32. Lumbar medial branch neurotomy. Anteroposterior view of two cannulae positioned at the base of the L5 and S1 superior articular processes.

the anterior two-thirds of the base of the SAP. This position ensures maximal contact between the active tip of the cannula and the target nerve. Deeper positioning may cause inadvertent contact with an exiting dorsal root ganglion or ventral ramus. A more posterior position means that the active tip is lying on the mamillo-accessory ligament and cannot produce a substantial lesion of the nerve (Fig. 42-31).

If the procedure is to be successful, the lesion should be created between the posterior border of the intervertebral foramen and the mamillo-accessory ligament, where the target nerves hug the base of the SAP.

The cannula position should be confirmed in the AP view. The active tip should make contact with the bone to ensure maximal exposure to the target nerve. The cannula must be positioned snugly against the base of the SAP (Fig. 42-32).

The technique of S1 dorsal ramus lesioning is the same. The RF lesions are made as in the previously described technique.

Outcome

Numerous small studies of RF neurotomy have been done, with widely varying, but mostly positive results. The plethora of small observational studies prompted several RCTs to confirm the efficacy of the procedure, and four such studies have been published to date (19–22). Unfortunately, they all contained methodologic and technical flaws and, therefore, failed to clarify the efficacy of RF neurotomy for the treatment of zygapophysial pain. None of these studies used comparative or placebo-controlled blocks, nor did they use an anatomically validated technique (i.e., placement of the electrode parallel to the target nerve) (79).

Only Dreyfuss and colleagues (78) applied strict patient selection criteria, conducted comparative double diagnostic blocks, and performed the RF procedure according to the anatomy of the target nerves. These authors also used mul-

tiple outcome tools and had a follow-up period of appropriately long duration. About 60% of the patients in their study experienced at least 90% pain relief at 12 months, and 87% experienced at least 60% relief at that time point. The only major limitation of this study was the small number of patients followed (15 patients).

Nevertheless, because of this work, practitioners are now called upon to use validated and anatomically correct techniques.

A large clinical audit suggested that anatomic RF denervation of lumbar zygapophysial joints provides long-term pain relief. In this study, 68.4% of patients obtained more than 50% pain relief for a median duration of 9 months (80). Notably, most patients were able to decrease their analgesic medication intake and increase physical activities.

Cryoablation of lumbar medial branches is technically feasible as well. However, the data are limited to only two prospective observational trials with questionable methodology. In the first study, patients with postlaminectomy syndrome were not excluded, and those patients (not surprisingly) obtained good (more than 50%) pain relief in 46% of cases, whereas the success rate was 85% in patients without previous surgery (81). The second study was flawed because the diagnostic protocol included only a single block. The authors reported success (pain reduction of 50% or more) in 59% of patients at 6 months' follow-up, and in 45.6% at 12 months (82).

Sacroiliac Joint Neurotomy

The surgical anatomy of the sacroiliac joint (SIJ) innervation is not completely clear. Several anatomic studies provide differing descriptions of the various combinations of dorsal and ventral rami of the L4 to S3 branches that contribute to the SIJ nerve supply (83). A recent anatomic study, however, has

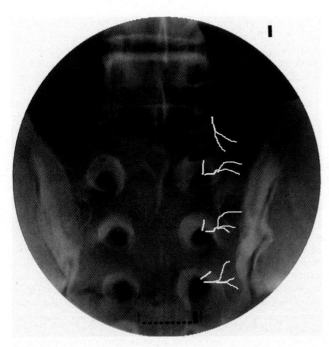

FIGURE 42-33. Lumbo-sacral lateral branch neurotomy (prone position). L5–S3 lateral branches topographic fluoroscopic anatomy (*white lines*).

demonstrated predominant dorsal innervation of the SIJ in humans by sensory fiber types from the L5 dorsal ramus and the lateral branches of the S1–S3 dorsal rami (84) (Fig. 42-33). Thus, either RF or cryoablation of the nerves is theoretically feasible.

The diagnosis of SIJ pain must be confirmed by diagnostic blockade. However, comparative block has not been validated in the context of intra-articular injections. Because the duration of action of local anesthetics is not well defined when they are administered into a joint, a method of anatomical control has been proposed (85). A positive response to the SIJ block is more compelling if the patient had a negative response to the zygapophysial nerve block and/or to lumbar provocation discography. The fact that the patient has not exhibited a placebo response following previous injection might increase the credibility of the response to the SIJ block.

As for RF or cryoablation of SIJ nerves, both procedures share the inconsistencies published for the nerve supply and diagnostic algorithm. The technique of cryoablation has been briefly outlined without data on outcome (40). Two essentially different techniques of RF treatment have been described. The first, called nonstimulation-guided bipolar RF lesioning along the posterior joint line, has yielded mediocre results, with only 36.4% of patients having obtained more than 50% pain relief for more than 6 months (86). The second method, selective lesioning of symptomatic lateral branches, is more theoretically attractive. Using this method, 64% of patients reported more than 50% pain relief, and 36% were pain-free after 6 months of follow-up (87). In another study, Cohen and Abdi evaluated RF lesioning of the L4 medial branch, the L5 dorsal ramus, and lateral branches of S1 to S3 in nine patients, reporting that 89% obtained more than 50% pain relief from this procedure that persisted at the 9-month follow-up (88).

Unfortunately, both studies were retrospective and small, consisting of 14 and nine patients, respectively. Furthermore,

radiograms of the procedure are not convincing enough to conclude that cannulae were placed parallel to the nerves. Therefore, the current level of evidence for RF neurotomy in the treatment of SIJ pain should be considered as indeterminate.

Technique

A curved 100-mm, 20-gauge RF cannula with a 10-mm active tip is suitable for this procedure. Under fluoroscopic imaging, the cannula is placed at the base of the S1 SAP, as described earlier, to perform the lesion of the L5 dorsal ramus. Separately, the RF cannulae are directed to the lateral edge of the dorsal sacral foraminal apertures of S1 to S3 (sacral dorsal rami lateral branch nerves). At each location, 50-Hz, 1-ms stimulation is applied at 0.4 to 0.7 V ("searching" voltage). The RF cannulae are finely manipulated under fluoroscopic imaging around the target structures until either a reproduction of concordant/usual pain or paresthetic cutaneous sensation is elicited. Stimulation has to be performed through the 2 o'clock to 6 o'clock zone on the right or the 6 o'clock to 10 o'clock zone on the left (if the dorsal sacral foramen is viewed as a clock face). Stimulation voltage must be as low as 0.1 to 0.2 V to ensure the contact with the target nerve. Absolutely consistent and reproducible elicitation of specific and concordant pain is interpreted as successful localization of the symptomatic lateral branch, whereas the elicitation of cutaneous paresthesiae without pain is interpreted as localization of asymptomatic nerves.

Once a symptomatic branch is identified, an RF lesion is created. Before RF lesion, 0.5 to 1.0 mL of preservative-free 2% lidocaine is injected to anesthetize the target nerve. Radiofrequency lesions are created at 80°C for a period of 60 seconds (87).

Radiofrequency Neurotomy of Rami Communicans

Interventional management of discogenic pain is comprehensively discussed in Chapter 44.

The method of RF lesioning of rami communicans in the treatment of discogenic pain has been described in two studies. The first was small, with only five patients, and the RF lesion was performed on the L2 ramus communicans. Four of the patients reduced their pain medication, and all reported improvement in sitting tolerance and functioning (89). The second study was a randomized single blind trial of rami communicans neurotomy in patients who failed to obtain pain relief by previously performed, ineffective interventional treatment. In comparison with the sham group, the RF group's Visual Analog Score pain scores decreased by 2.5 points (p <0.05). The outcome scores of the RF lesion group improved by a mean increase of 11.3 points (p <0.05) on the SF-36 bodily pain subscale, and by a mean increase of 12.4 points on the physical function subscale (p <0.05) (90). The weaknesses of this work were the short follow-up (4 months) and the selection bias associated with including patients after previous ineffective interventional treatment.

CRANIAL NERVE PROCEDURES

Table 42-3 summarizes the percutaneous destructive procedures available for treatment of pain in the distribution of the cranial nerves, of which tic douloureux is the most prevalent.

Tic Douloureux

Tic douloureux is a unique pain syndrome nearly always affecting cranial nerve V and rarely, nerves IX and X or VII. The diagnosis is based solely on the patient's description of the pain. In trigeminal territory, this pain affects the genders approximately equally (45% in males) and the right side possibly more frequently; the incidence increases with age. It can affect any or all portions of the territory supplied by nerve V, but the lower face is preferentially affected; with tic being most common in V2 and V3 together, next most common in V3 and then in V2, and rarest in V1. In 3% of cases, the disease becomes bilateral. The typical diagnostic features of the pain include abrupt onset of severe intermittent lancinating pain consistently affecting a particular portion of the trigeminal territory, interrupted by periods of remission, with the pain gradually becoming more severe and frequent with time and often slowly spreading to adjacent trigeminal territory. Triggering always arises from ipsilateral stimulation, most commonly in the nose and mouth region, not necessarily in the field of pain; occasionally, triggering occurs from outside trigeminal territory, including the C2 and C3 dermatomes. The pain can be triggered by touching the face, talking, swallowing, brushing the teeth, washing the face, or feeling drafts of wind (91–94). Usually, no abnormality is detectable on neurologic examination or by imaging. In a small number of patients, typical tic accompanies multiple sclerosis. Occasionally, an underlying lesion appears to be responsible, particularly a schwannoma, rarely an arteriovenous malformation, and exceptionally rarely, hydrocephalus (95). Although many processes, both central and peripheral, have been advocated as the underlying cause of tic, especially compression of the nerve's dorsal root entry zone by an arterial or, less often, venous loop (96), the etiology remains uncertain. With the availability of magnetic resonance angiography (MRA), vascular compression of the trigeminal system is more commonly demonstrated.

Treatment of Tic Douloureux

When treatment with anticonvulsants and adjuvants (baclofen, opioids) fails, an interventional approach is often required, with most of the currently practiced surgical modalities being accomplished percutaneously except for microvascular decompression of the root in the posterior fossa. Tic is unique in that denervation of the field to which the pain is referred always stops the pain, although recurrence is common because of regeneration; thus, several of the surgical techniques advocated for its treatment involve trigeminal denervation by various means at various levels.

Various compression and/or decompression procedures also can result in relief of the pain without accompanying sensory loss, including (a) the Taarnhöj (97) and Sheldon (98) procedures, which are now probably of historical interest, in which the roots of the nerve are either lightly traumatized (compressed) or freed of arachnoid adhesions (decompressed) in the middle fossa; (b) the Mullan microcompression (99) technique; and (c) Jannetta microvascular decompression (100,101). The mechanism of action of these procedures relevant to the underlying pathophysiology of tic is highly debated. It is important to reiterate that these procedures, so successful for tic, are inappropriate in most other types of craniofacial pain.

Furthermore, despite the fact that tic douloureux is a unique type of chronic intractable pain, there exists for it, by far, the most successful medical and surgical treatment of any chronic pain syndrome. Two of the most popular surgical modalities are percutaneous RF coagulation of the Gasserian ganglion and/or its roots and microvascular decompression in the posterior fossa, which yield about 50% (after 10 years) and 20% (after 15 years) long-term relief, respectively (92). Radiofrequency thermocoagulation offers higher rates of complete pain relief, as compared with glycerol rhizolysis and stereotactic radiosurgery, although it demonstrates the greatest number of complications (102).

Although tic is one of the most common pain syndromes for which surgery is performed, outcome data are seldom published because the procedures used have been known for a long time.

Percutaneous Denervation of the Supraorbital or Infraorbital Nerves

The simplest percutaneous technique for treating tic is percutaneous denervation of the supraorbital or infraorbital nerves by the injection of absolute alcohol. Although simple and perhaps indicated in the very elderly or very ill with well-defined tic in the appropriate territory, any benefit is reversed within a few months to a year by nerve regeneration; also, there is a risk of blindness and oculomotor palsy. Such peripheral denervation may also result in neuropathic pain; it is worthy of note that traumatic damage to the infraorbital nerve in facial fracturing is a common cause of deafferentation pain.

Radiofrequency Coagulation of the Trigeminal Nerve

Conventional Procedure. The conventional technique will be discussed first. Based on the original work of Härtel (3) and Kirshner (103), the technique underwent certain refinements, including RF lesion-making as described by Sweet and Wepsic (12), before precision became satisfactory and risks low enough for general acceptance.

Technique. The patient is placed supine, head precisely in the anatomic position, monitors applied, and supplemental oxygen given by nasal prongs. Light neuroleptic analgesia provides for the patient's comfort during the procedure. The image intensifier is positioned in a submandibular view with slight ipsilateral oblique rotation. The foramen ovale is typically identified just medially to the mandibular ramus (Fig. 42-34A). To facilitate the correct position of the image intensifier, a radiopaque bead can be attached to the skin 2 cm lateral to the lateral angle of the mouth. This hint may improve the orientation of fluoroscopy because the bead should be approximately superimposed on the shadow of the foramen ovale at the final position. The RF cannula should be directed into the medial third of the foramen

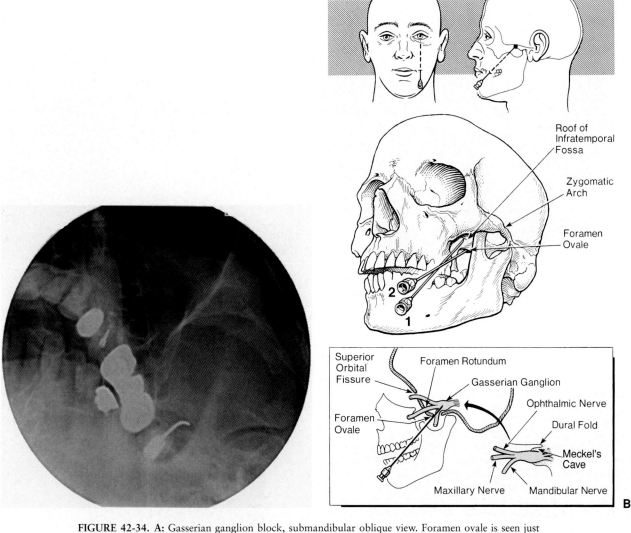

FIGURE 42-34. A: Gasserian ganglion block, submandibular oblique view. Foramen ovale is seen just medially to the mandibular ramus with the radiofrequency cannula in situ. **B:** Gasserian ganglion block. *Top panel*: Note that the needle is inserted in the cheek about 2 cm lateral to the angle of the mouth as shown and directed toward the pupil in the anterior view and the midpoint of the zygoma in the lateral view. In patients with teeth, needle insertion in the cheek is superficial to the teeth of the upper jaw. In edentulous patients, this may lie a variable distance between the angle of the mouth and a line midway between upper lip and nose. A palpating finger in the mouth helps to prevent needle penetration into the mouth. *Middle panel*: As the needle is advanced into the infratemporal fossa, it will usually strike the roof of the infratemporal fossa initially (*1*); this is the correct depth to seek the foramen ovale. The needle is then directed slightly posteriorly (*2*) to obtain a mandibular nerve (V3) paresthesia. *Lower panel*: The needle can then be advanced through the foramen ovale into the middle cranial fossa, where it will be adjacent to the Gasserian ganglion, as shown. Note the relationships of the dural fold and Meckel cave, containing cerebrospinal fluid. A needle advanced too far through the foramen ovale can enter the Meckel cave, and subsequent injections could enter the cranial CSF and produce total spinal anesthesia.

ovale, the center, or the lateral third to reach the V1, V2, or V3 root, respectively (Fig. 42-34B).

Several types of cannulae can be used. The simplest tool is a 22-gauge RF cannula with a 2-mm active tip; however, the Tew kit, designed by Tew and Cosman, enables off-axis or straight electrode tip extensions for greater flexibility in lesion size and positioning in the ganglion. A curved Tew electrode may greatly help to reach difficult positions, such as the V1 ganglion division (Fig. 42-35).

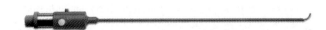

FIGURE 42-35. Gasserian ganglion radiofrequency lesioning. Tew curved TC electrode and cannula. Manufactured by Cosman® Medical, Inc. Reprinted with permission of Cosman Medical, Inc.

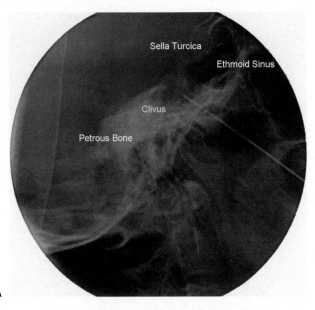

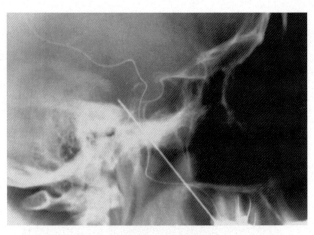

A

B

FIGURE 42-36. **A:** Gasserian ganglion radiofrequency lesioning. Lateral fluoroscopic view showing 21-gauge radiofrequency cannula inserted though the foramen ovale. Anatomic landmarks are marked. **B:** Gasserian ganglion radiofrequency lesioning. Lateral fluoroscopic view showing radiofrequency cannula inserted though the foramen ovale, where stimulation produced paresthesia in the forehead.

A cannula is inserted through the skin and advanced under tunnel vision fluoroscopic view into the desired part of the foramen ovale (Fig. 42-34). Entrance into the oral cavity must be avoided, and, if it occurs, the cannula is replaced. When a cannula "walks off" the pterygoid plate or the base of the skull into the foramen ovale, a sudden contraction of jaw muscles or an exacerbation of pain may occur. When a cannula attains perfect direction and remains steady in the soft tissue, the image intensifier is rotated to the lateral view (Fig. 42-36A). Two major landmarks help to obtain the true lateral view: shadows of the angles of the mandible and the external acoustic meatuses must be superimposed. The cannula tip should not rise above the line connecting the crest of the petrous ridge and the posterior clinoid as its progress is followed on the image intensifier. For third-division (V3) tic, the tip should lie relatively low on this trajectory, as shown in Figure 42-36A; for first-division tic (V1), relatively high, as shown in Figure 42-36B. If CSF flow occurs, a more permanent and often more complete denervation is likely, since the cannula is positioned among preganglionic rootlets. In V3 tic, this situation need not be sought, as the procedure is easily repeated in the event of recurrence, when a postganglionic lesion is made.

It may not be radiographically apparent when the cannula lies in alternate adjacent foraminae except for the jugular, as shown in Figure 42-37, hence the importance of physiologic localization. If arterial blood is encountered in the foramen lacerum, the cannula need only be withdrawn and reinserted. In proper position, stimulation at 2 Hz may elicit ipsilateral masticatory muscle contractions at thresholds under 1 to 2 V. There is no need to reposition the cannula to try to avoid these; any masseter weakness induced is likely to be transient, and unilateral permanent weakness is seldom apparent. However, bilateral RF coagulation should be approached with caution. The level of sedation is lowered now and stimulation performed at 50 Hz. This action should induce paresthesias in the area where the pain occurs, preferably at less than 0.3 V, certainly at no more than 0.8 V. Under repeated IV sedation, an RF lesion is now

made, with progressively increasing current flow and the temperature at 50°C to 90°C, over 30 to 90 seconds. A visible flush will often appear in the denervated part of the face. Between cycles, pin-prick analgesia and the corneal reflex are checked. Lesion cycles are repeated to the point of inducing analgesia

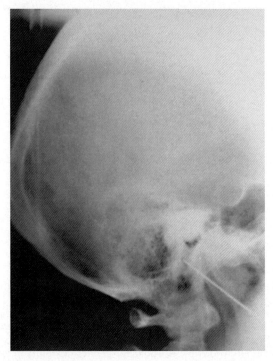

FIGURE 42-37. Glossopharyngeal nerve radiofrequency lesioning. Lateral fluoroscopic view showing radiofrequency cannula for thermocoagulation of glossopharyngeal nerve in jugular foramen.

without loss of appreciation of touch in the painful area of the face. Unexpected, massive sensory loss, even spreading beyond the confines of the patient's pain, may still occur despite all attempts to avoid it. Alternatively, and when deep sedation is not a suitable option, 0.2 to 0.5 mL of preservative-free lidocaine is injected after successful sensory stimulation. The RF lesion is then performed for two to three cycles of maximal temperature (80°C–90°C). This practice, however, makes sensory testing impractical and, theoretically, may lead to an extensive sensory loss. Injection of depo-steroids (betamethasone, triamcinolone) also has been advocated to reduce postprocedural neuritis, but this practice has limited validity.

Selective Procedure. A modification of the just-described technique is referred to as the "selective technique" (104,105), in which a specially designed Tew kit is used. When the introductory 19-gauge needle is positioned into the foramen ovale, the stylet is removed and a curved electrode is inserted. Gentle rotation of the electrode during sensory stimulation brings it into the closest contact with a root. This has two advantages over the conventional technique: (a) since the electrode and its tip are smaller, a smaller and more selective lesion can be made, which is better tailored to selectively induce analgesia in the area of pain; and (b) the electrode tip can be withdrawn into the introductory needle and rotated, like the hands of a clock, then readvanced to test a large area of adjacent nerve fibers with a single needle position until the ideal lesion site is found. Using this technique, Tew and his colleagues (105,106) found their results to be better than with the conventional technique. Complications consisted of a 9% incidence of masseter weakness, 11% unpleasant paresthesias, and 2% keratitis. Tasker suggested that recurrence is more likely when the selective method is used (107).

Results. Tew and colleagues (108) reported 93% excellent-to-good results in 400 patients with tic after using the conventional technique. Fourteen percent complained of unpleasant sensory effects; in 1%, these were so severe as to lead to excoriation of the face, nostril, or scalp. Only 2% developed keratitis, although 30% had corneal analgesia. Two percent exhibited transient diplopia, and 22% paresis in the distribution of the motor root, which was usually transient. The latter was occasionally associated with complaints referred to the ear because of paralysis of the tensor veli palatini or tensor tympani. Over 1 to 8 years, tic recurred in 14%, and 9% underwent a second operation. In a subsequent review (105), Tew and associates reported 76% excellent, 17% good, 6% fair, and 1% poor results with 700 procedures, also performed in the conventional way, over a 10-year period; of the 24% with recurrence, 9% underwent reoperation. Complications in this larger series using the conventional method consisted of a 24% incidence of masseter weakness, 27% unpleasant paresthesias, 2% diplopia, and 4% keratitis.

Latchaw and co-workers (109) reported 52% good results with the conventional method, without recurrence in 96 patients with tic, particularly if the patient had not been previously exposed to open surgery and particularly if dense sensory loss was achieved. All patients without persistent sensory loss suffered recurrence; 26% had depressed and 13% absent corneal reflexes, 2% keratitis, 5% masseter paresis, 42% unintended sensory loss, 26% unpleasant sensory effects, and 1% anesthesia dolorosa. The severity of the latter was related to the degree of sensory loss. Latchaw's useful literature review suggests a 7% to 22% incidence of corneal anesthesia, 0 to 5% keratitis, 1% to 19% dysesthesia, and 15% to 50% unintended sensory loss. Recurrences were reported in these series

in 6% to 46% over 2 to 2.5 years, 9% to 53% over 4 to 5 years, 18% to 22% over 7 to 8 years, and 80% in longer follow-ups.

Turnbull (94) reported his experience in 41 patients in a graphic and particularly interesting way. Anesthesia in at least part of the face occurred in the only patient with V1 tic, four of nine with V1–V2 tic, six of 14 with V2 tic, three of nine with V2–V3 tic, and two of 11 with V3 tic. Pain was relieved in all, but recurred in five patients over the first 4 years. Motor weakness occurred in nine, keratitis in two, and corneal areflexia in eight, six of whom did not have V1 tic to start with. Five developed dysesthesia and one, anesthesia dolorosa. Anesthesia occurred in facial areas not afflicted with tic in one of nine with V1–V2 tic, five of 14 with V2 tic, one of nine with V2–V3 tic; no anesthesia was recorded among patients with pure V1 and V3 tic. Analgesia occurred in unafflicted areas in one of one, two of nine, nine of 14, two of nine, and two of 11 patients with V1, V1–V2, V2, V2–V3, and V3 tic, respectively.

Whatever the technique, the chief disadvantages of RF thermocoagulation of nerve V are that it deliberately produces sensory loss with an unavoidable incidence of neuropathic pain and, if the patient is followed long enough, recurrence of tic (80% in 10 years) (92). "Anesthesia dolorosa" is more likely to occur in relation to patient age, degree of sensory loss induced, and height of sensory loss on the face. Sweet (32) noted that, after RF coagulation of trigeminal nerve, early relief was reported in 96% to 100% of cases, with reoperation being needed after 1 to 13 years in 7% to 31%. In larger series, the most significant complication was deafferentation pain occurring in 0.2% to 7.9% of patients. Corneal anesthesia affected 1% to 35%; keratitis, 0.4% to 20%; motor weakness, 13% to 40%; and oculomotor palsy, 0.2% to 6.5% in large series. Complications were somewhat different in smaller series. Epilepsy from temporal lobe damage, dry eye (3%), nasal wetness (23%), and increased (17%) or decreased (3%) salivation also occur (Tables 42-4 and 42-5).

Sweet (32) advised abandoning the procedure until another day should the carotid artery be punctured, although Tasker has uneventfully completed the procedure after needle replacement at the same sitting in numerous cases; serious sequelae occur, however, if an RF lesion is made in the foramen lacerum. Sweet mentions that the foramina of Vesalius and Arnold, as well as anomalous ones, may also be entered, paying careful attention to essential physiologic monitoring lest complications occur. Finally, damage to the trochlear nerve may occur, even with a correctly placed lesion, due to heat spread, but it usually recovers after 3 months; damage to the temporal lobe can occur similarly. X-ray monitoring should prevent entry into the supraorbital fissure or jugular foramen.

Bilateral RF lesions in bilateral tic should be undertaken with caution for fear of the devastating complication of bilateral trigeminal motor root paralysis. Since the motor root also supplies the tensor tympani and tensor veli palatini, RF tic damage to the motor root can produce aberrations of function of the middle ear musculature or eustachian tube, resulting in various, fortunately usually temporary, auditory aberrations or ear pain.

Although percutaneous thermocoagulation of the trigeminal nerve is still a procedure with low morbidity and mortality, Tasker (107) reported on the following problems: (a) two incidences of fatal hemorrhage unrelated to the lesion, one in a personal case, possibly caused by acute hypertension induced by needle introduction and preventable by appropriate premedication; (b) one case of bacterial meningitis; (c) one case of temporal lobe abscess; and (d) a stroke following puncture of the carotid artery and carotid cavernous fistula. Sweet (32) reviews these problems in some detail (Table 42-6).

TABLE 42-4

TRIGEMINAL THERMAL RHIZOTOMY: 31 SERVICES WITH LESS THAN 600 PROCEDURES

Author[a]	No. of pts.	No. of RF ops[b]	Early complete relief[b]	Follow-up period range-average	% Recurrence not requiring reoperation	% Recurrence requiring reoperation	Anesthesia, analgesia hypalgesia dolorosa	Dysesthesias controlled with drugs	Keratitis	Corneal anesthesia	Masticator paralysis	Oculomotor paresis temp.
Apfelbaum	48	51	88%	0–36 mo — 19 mo	10%	12%	12%				14%	2%	
Brandt	229	–325		1–13 yr	23%	28%	3.5%				8%	3%	1%
Browne	106	121	100%	0–4 yr		14%				5% in 50% of pts with V1 pain			1 pt 1%
Burchiel	78	92	77%	56 mo	41%	23%	4%		3%	20%	25%	1 pt
Campos	72	79	93%	6 mo–3 yr	6%	12%	3–3.5%	10%	2.5%	6%	0%	0%
Eiras	36	?40	98%	3–23 mo		6%	0%		0%	7%	30%	0%
Ferguson	55	58		1–50 mo — 30 mo	31%	11%	2%	0%				
Fraioli	481			4.2 yr		9%	0%	11%				
Galbraith	102	120	92%	1–7 yr — 3 yr		20%						0%
Graziussl	205	219	93%	6 mo–5 yr — 3 yr		20% { 65% 1st yr; 23% 2nd yr; 6% 3rd & 4th yr }	6%	62%	4%	4%	15%	0.4%
Guidetti	167	173	99.4%	2 yr			0.6%		0%	4%	3.4%	0.6%
Hitchcock	47	70	98%	Up to 40 mo	13%	28%	4%		2%	2%	8%	0%
Kanpolat	256	290	94% of 240 pts (final)			12% of 256	1.8%			5%		
Lahuerta	30	35	97%	15–26 mo			10%	7%	3%	19%		2 pts = 6%
Latchaw	96	135	100%	2–8 yr — 5 yr	8%	48% at 5 yr	2%	32%	3%	19%	5%	
Mittal	216	267	91%	3 mo–8 yr — 3.8 yr		21%	9%	6%	4%			3 pts = 1%
Onofrio	135	140	97%	Up to several yr	6%	6% (16 pts slight sensory loss—recurrence 2 wk–14 mo)	1.5%		1.5%	8%	15%	0.8%
Penzhoiz	232	57	85%	1–9 yr	7%	24%	1.3%	5%				2%
Perez Calvo	50	113	100%	0.5–5 yr — 11 mo		6% in <1 yr; 13%	2%					1%
Pertruiset	100	60	100%	Longest 3 yr — 11 mo				5%	0%	3%	2%	1 pt
Philippon	50			2–6 yr — 3 yr		>40% after 3 yr	0	4%	2%	17%	2.5% Gone in 6 mo	
Salar	46	?50	100%	More than 1 yr		7%	1 pt	10%	0%	0%	0%	0%
Schiirmann	282	351; 413	100%	1963–1975		22% or 193 pts >3-yr follow-up			0%		12%	0%
Schvarcz	400	411		1–6 yr in 75% — 4 yr	6%	9%	0%			3%		0%
Sengupta	39		92%	2–20 mo		3%			5%	15%	0%	
Silverberg	38		95%	2–36 mo		14%	0%		0%	0%		0%
Spincemaille	53		85%	6–42 mo — 2 yr		5%	0	8%	0%			
Steude	194		100%	10–50 mo		11%	0.5%		0%		0%	0%
Thiry	225	(1950–1960)	100%	Up to 23 yr		17%			3%	9%		3%
Thiry	140	(1960–1970)	98%	Up to 13 yr		27%			1%	4%		3%
Turnbull	41		100%	6 mo–3 yr		7%	2.5%	10%	5%	22%	22%	0%
Turner	51	64	92%		5%	26%	2%		2%	6%		0%

[a] For complete References, see source of Table (Sweet[284]).
[b] Includes those relieved after early operation.
RF, radiofrequency.
From Sweet WH: Treatment of trigeminal neuralgia by percutaneous rhizotomy. In Youmans JR (ed.): *Neurological Surgery. A Comprehensive Reference Guide to the Diagnosis and Management of Neurosurgical Problems*, 3rd ed. Philadelphia, Saunders, 1990, p. 3888.

TABLE 42-5
TRIGEMINAL THERMAL RHIZOTOMY: 11 SERVICES WITH 600 OR MORE PROCEDURES

Author[a]	No. of pts.	No. of RF ops	Early complete relief	Follow-up period range-average	No. of recurrences not requiring reoperation	No. of recurrences requiring reoperation	Anesthesia, analgesia hypalgesia doiorosa	Dysesthesias controlled with drugs	Keratitis	Corneal anesthesia	Masticator paralysis	Oculomotor paresis temp.	Oculomotor paresis temp.
Broggi	1000		100%	1–10 yr		13%	7.9% "often unbearable"		Tarsorr. 0.4%	Reduced or absent 21%	10%		0.3%
Frank	939	>600	100%	6 mo–5 yr		21%		11.6%					
Maxwell	unstated	~800					0.6%		1%	1%	1%		
Nugent	643	~1500		4.7 yrs		23%	2%	5%	0.5%	2% last 600 ops 1 loss of eye		10%	0.25%
Rhoton	unstated						1%			4%			
Rovit	550	600				19%	0.2%	0.7%					0.2%
Siegfried	1000		100%	135 pts followed 5½–8 yr	4%	21% at 5½–8 yr	3%	24% at 5½–8 yr	0.8%	2.8%	15%	25%	4%
Sindou	609		100%	1–13 yr		7%		25% "painful"	20%	35%	Lasting 2% Temp. 25%		6.5%
Sweet	702	1119	99%	1–33 yr avg 5.6 yr	6%	31%	2.1%	6%	3% Tarsorr. 1.5%	9%	25%	40%	0.4%
Tew	1100	1150	98%	1–18 yr avg 8 yr	9%	8%	1%	9%	3%			13% (curved electrode)	1.5%
Thurel	890		96%			23%	0.6%	7%	2%	6%		25%	0.7%

[a]For complete References, see source of Table (Sweet[284]).
[b]Includes relief after early reoperation.
RF, radiofrequency.
From Sweet WH: Treatment of trigeminal neuralgia by percutaneous rhizotomy. In Youmans JR (ed.): *Neurological Surgery. A Comprehensive Reference Guide to the Diagnosis and Management of Neurosurgical Problems*, 3rd ed. pp. 3888. Philadelphia, Saunders, 1990.

TABLE 42-6

COMPLICATIONS OF PERCUTANEOUS RADIOFREQUENCY TRIGEMINAL RHIZOTOMY[a]

	Number of cases
Central retinal artery occlusion	1
Optic nerve lesion	
Blindness, ipsilateral, permanent	2
Amblyopia, ipsilateral, transient	1
Blindness, complete, permanent	4
Myocardial infarction	
Death (91-year-old patient)	1
Recovery	1
Intracerebral abscess	
Death	3
Mental impairment, permanent	1
Recovery	3
Meningitis	
Death	1
Recovery	21
Hemorrhages	
Related to needle puncture	
Subdural, infratemporal	
Recovered	1
Intracerebral	
Death	2
Recovered	1
Disabled, permanent	1
Not related to needle puncture	
Intracerebral	
Death	8
Disabled, permanent	4
Hemiplegia, transient	3
Hemiparesis	
Transient	1
Permanent	1
Subarachnoid hemorrhage	
Death	3
Recovered	2
Neuroparalytic keratitis	18
Carotid cavemous fistulas	5
Meningeal reaction	
Negative cultures	8
Oculomotor palsy	
Temporary	16
Permanent	2
Seizure, intraoperative	2
Psychosis, postoperative	
Transient	1

[a] Reported from 92 service with over 7000 patients. Not all services gave the number of patients, and as a result not all are included in the figure of 7000 patients; however, the complications they reported are included in this Table.
From Sweet WH: Treatment of trigeminal neuralgia by percutaneous rhizotomy. In Youmans JR (ed.): *Neurological Surgery*. A Comprehensive Reference Guide to the Diagnosis and Management of Neurosurgical Problems. 3rd Ed. pp. 3888. Philadelphia, Saunders, 1990.

Alcohol Injection. Although probably of historical interest today, the injection of absolute alcohol into the CSF of the Meckel cave was popular well past the middle of the 20th century (110) but has probably been replaced by other procedures.

Percutaneous Injection of Glycerol. Håkansson (111) introduced the treatment of tic by the injection, through a 22-gauge needle, of 0.2 to 0.4 mL of glycerol into the CSF of the Meckel cave under local anesthesia, using a technique similar to that used for RF coagulation. The CSF is drained, and metrizamide slowly injected in 0.2- to 0.4-mL increments until the cistern is filled and dye starts to empty into the posterior fossa. Cisternal metrizamide is emptied by head positioning to uncover those parts of the root intended to be affected by glycerol (Fig. 42-38). The calculated volume of the cistern is used to estimate the volume of glycerol needed. If the entire cistern is exposed to glycerol, all three divisions will be affected; leaving metrizamide in place to cover rootlets uninvolved with tic will protect them from the injection. In 15% of Håkansson's cases, the first attempt failed, pain recurred in 18% over a period of 2 to 48 months, and 60% noted slight facial numbness for the first postoperative week. None suffered from dysesthesia, and alteration of facial sensation was barely detectable in "the majority." Eighty-six percent of 75 patients were totally free of their pain, half immediately and half within 4 to 6 days. One patient died of pulmonary embolism.

Sweet and Poletti (112) note that Håkansson's recurrence rate was 31% over 1 to 6 years in 100 patients. They themselves treated 31 patients, 27 suffering from tic, three from atypical facial pain, and one from posttraumatic pain. Pain was relieved in 24 of the 27 with tic. The only failures were in patients who did not develop analgesia during or after the injection, and 16 of their patients had persistent sensory loss, including nine who developed dysesthesia and five with reduced corneal reflexes.

Lunsford and Bennett (113) reported 67% complete and 23% partial control of tic in 112 patients followed from 4 to 28 months. Seventy-three percent had no sensory loss, 3% developed aseptic meningitis, and 3.6% had severe postoperative dysesthesia. None of their patients developed motor weakness, oculomotor disturbance, or keratitis.

Sweet (32,112) and Gybels and Sweet (56) have exhaustively studied the published results with glycerol injection (Table 42-7). They note that initial failure ranges from 4% to 18%, that early relief is often delayed up to 1 week, and that the first attempt yields 69% to 96% relief, with 9% to 30% of patients requiring reoperation. They also note that corneal anesthesia, although rare, does occur.

It appears that the technique exposes patients to the same risks, including neuropathic pain, as RF coagulation, that it requires more attention to detail to perform (extreme head positioning after the needle has been inserted), and that its somatotopic selectivity is not established. Its great advantage is that it can be used to treat V1 tic without the need to produce significant sensory loss in V1 territory, with the ensuing risk of keratitis and the greater chance of neuropathic pain than that seen after denervation of the lower face.

Percutaneous Compression of Trigeminal Nerve. Harking back to the technique of open compression or decompression of the Meckel cave advocated by Taarnhoj (97) and by Sheldon and associates (98) for the treatment of tic, Mullan and Lichtor (99) have introduced a method for percutaneous compression of the nerve. Under endotracheal general anesthesia and using biplanar imaging, a No. 4 (0.75- to 1.0-mL capacity) Fogarty balloon catheter is inserted through a liver biopsy needle and passed through the foramen ovale after slightly filling its space with a radiopaque contrast dye (Conray). The catheter is now advanced 1 cm and slowly inflated with Conray diluted to a manageable viscosity until the balloon fills the Meckel cave and begins to assume a pear shape by slowly expanding into the posterior fossa. The balloon is held inflated for 3 to 10 minutes

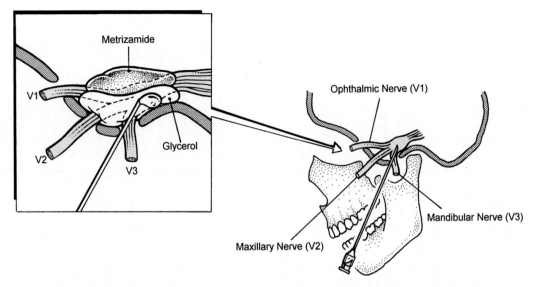

FIGURE 42-38. Gasserian ganglion neurolytic blockade with glycerol. A needle is inserted via the foramen ovale as described in Figure 42-34B. However, in this technique, the needle tip must penetrate the dural fold and then lie in the gasserian cistern of the Meckel cave (inset). Cerebrospinal fluid is aspirated to confirm placement in the Gasserian cistern and then water-soluble contrast medium, such as metrizamide, is injected to confirm correct placement, to outline the Meckel cave, and to indicate the volume required to bathe part or whole of the Gasserian ganglion. In one approach to blocking V3, or V2 and V3, the metrizamide is removed and the injection made. In an alternative approach, the metrizamide is removed only to the extent that a residue covers V1 in the supine position with the head extended; then the glycerol is injected while maintaining the same position; glycerol will sit on top of the metrizamide (*inset panel*). In the unusual situation in which V1 and V2 need to be blocked while sparing V3, metrizamide is removed until only enough for one division remains and then glycerol is injected while the patient is in the sitting position, so that V3 will be covered with the metrizamide while the glycerol will sit on top of the metrizamide, thus blocking V1 and V2.

with 0.5 to 1.0 mL of Conray, then collapsed and withdrawn. Difficulties may be encountered in patients with a scarred cave, including rupture of the balloon (not a dangerous occurrence). In 50 patients with tic, 49 obtained immediate relief, six experienced recurrence in 6 to 31 months, three suffered from dysesthesia, four from analgesia, and one from trochlear nerve palsy. All patients experienced subjective numbness and ipsilateral motor paralysis; some experienced sensory loss persisting 4 to 6 months.

Bricolo and Dalle Ore (114) reported results of the procedure in 51 patients, all of whom experienced pain relief; few had mild to moderate changes in sensation. None of them had impaired corneal reflexes, although in a small group a mild objective deficit of the ipsilateral masseter muscle was present. Recurrent pain was observed in 10 cases, but only six of them required reoperation. Lobato and colleagues (115) reported three recurrences in 100 patients in 7 to 11 months; 29% still had sensory loss after 1 year, while 18% had minor dysesthesia and 3%, significant dysesthesia. Belber and Rak (116) recorded 100% initial pain relief in 33 patients, with 24% experiencing recurrence over 7 years; one patient had mild dysesthesia.

It has been suggested that recurrence is likely to occur if pressure in the balloon was low (0.9 Bar); conversely the highest values of pressure (1.9–2.4 Bars) were observed in most of the patients suffering from untoward side effects (117).

Radiofrequency Coagulation of Trigeminal Nerve for Pain Other Than Tic. The conventional percutaneous thermocoagulation technique also can be used to treat trigeminal pain caused by cancer as well as migrainous pain that consistently afflicts one part of the trigeminal territory, although it should be avoided in atypical facial pain, deafferentation pain, and postherpetic neuralgia unless intended for the control of allodynia or hyperpathia alone.

In cancer, pain is rarely confined to the trigeminal territory, so that trigeminal denervation alone is nearly always unsuccessful, and cancerous destruction of the base of the skull may prevent needle positioning. In those few selected suitable candidates, denervation for the relief of cancer pain should be as complete as possible. Siegfried and Broggi (118) relieved pain in ten of their 20 patients who had pain caused by cancer. Maxwell (119) relieved all eight of his patients with migrainous neuralgia, although pain eventually recurred in three. Watson and colleagues (120) reported pain relief in eight of 13 patients with cluster headache treated by percutaneous thermocoagulation. One developed anesthesia dolorosa, and five suffered from recurrence, one of whom did not respond to repeated coagulation. Pain relief required sensory loss in the area of pain.

Gybels and Sweet (56) note that denervation in migrainous face pain results in a greater incidence of dysesthetic pain than in tic and that a greater degree of sensory loss is necessary than in tic to achieve pain relief; however, in six of their own patients, pain relief did not accompany any sensory loss in the painful area. They quote the results of Onofrio and Campbell (121), who experienced 11 early failures and one recurrence after 6 months in 22 patients.

Few data have been recorded for glycerol injection in migrainous pain.

Cluster Headache

Cluster headache, unlike migraine, affects predominantly males in a ratio of 3:1 or 4:1. The prevalence is 0.1% to 0.3% of

TABLE 42-7

TRIGEMINAL GLYCEROL RHIZOTOMY: 16 SERVICES

Author[a]	No. of patients	Initial failure	Days to relief	Relief 1st op	Relief 2nd op	Average follow-up	Recurrence: reoperation not needed	Recurrence: reoperation needed	Corneal anesthesia	Sensory status
Arias	100	5%	2–4 days in 6%			6–36 mo			0	Never more than 30% loss in any division
Beck	58	17%		69%	72%	2–40 mo Avg 18 mo	16%	9%	1%	17%–? intraganglion inj. in 1; 1 lasting total analgesia
Burchlel	48	12%				Mean time to recurrence 5 mo in 43% of 46 ops			7%	Sensory loss >1 mo in 72%
Dieckmann	51	4%				78% relief at 1 yr				40% anesthesia dolorosa 2%
Hakansson	100		4–6 days in 50%	96%	90%	1–6 yr	16%	15%	0	Never more than mild No dysesthesias
Igarashi	27		Up to 1 wk						Decreased with more than 0.4 ml	Hypalgesia at 8 wk 30% 3 high-grade dysesthesias
Lunsford	73	14%	Avg 5 days up to 21 days	86%	90%	Up to 3 yrs Avg 15 mo	10% of 73 19% of 62 pts	13% of 73 15% of 62 pts		6% dysesthesias 0 anesthesia dolorosa
Lunsford Rappaport	225 43		Relief at once 54%; 46% relief in avg 3 days—max 14 days	81%	97%		Pain-free at follow-up Recurrence rate 25% at 1 yr	65%	0	Hypalgesia 38%; of 7 recurrences 6 did not have sensory deficit
Saini	412		Relief in 2–42 hr							3.4% anesthesia dolorosa 13% dysesthesias
Shetter	64	14%		86%		2–45 mo Avg 18 mo	61% pain-free at avg 18 mo	28%	3%	Analgesia 1 of 64; dysesthesia bothers about 5%
Slettebo	60	10%		90%		Avg 24 mo	11%	30% at avg 2 yr		Higher proportion sensory deficits than in earlier articles
Sweet	88	18%	Up to 1 wk in 24%	82%		Avg 2.9 yr 1–8½ yr		22%	14% 50% of 14 V1 trigger zones	27 hyp; 49 analg, 4 anesth (2 anesth dol; 1 hyp dol; 0 hyp dol since 1983; 0 analg dol since 1980; 0 anesth dol since 1983)
Takusagawa	122	10%		79%		1–3 yr	58% pain-free; 17% improved; 25% in pain			Anesth dol 2 pts 1.5%; hypesthesia 80%; dysesthesias 35%
Thurel	50	18%		75%		Avg 15 mo		15%	2%	1 anesthesia complete V1, V2 at 5 mo but no major dysesthesias
Waltz	184	18%		70%	81%	1–52 mo	12%	17%		Hypesthesia 67%; "sensory deficit mild with one exception"
Young	157	6%					Pain-free 79%		5%	67% significant sensory loss 0% anesthesia dolorosa 2% dysesthesias

[a]For complete References, see source of Table (Sweet[284]).
From Sweet WH: Treatment of trigominal neuralgia by percutaneous rhizotomy. In Youmans JR (ed.): *Neurological Surgery. A Comprehensive Reference Guide to the Diagnosis and Management of Neurosurgical Problems.* 3rd Ed. pp. 3888. Philadelphia, Saunders, 1990.

the population. Most patients have a history of smoking and alcohol consumption. In the majority of cases, attacks begin between the ages of 20 and 40. The pathophysiology of cluster headache is unknown, however a typical picture is of severe pain that wakes a patient from sleep and is accompanied by lacrimation, conjunctival injection, nasal congestion, ptosis, and myosis, which suggests involvement of autonomic nervous system (122). When conservative treatment by ergotamine tartrate, isometheptene, triptans, and oxygen inhalation fails, a trial of diagnostic sphenopalatine ganglion block during the attack is warranted. Responders may benefit from radiofrequency rhizotomy. The procedure was proposed by Salar in 1987 (123). The evidence of efficacy of the method is limited so far. Apart from a few case reports and reviews, only one large observational study was published (124). Radiofrequency lesions of the sphenopalatine ganglion were made in 66 patients suffering from either episodic (56 patients) or chronic (10 patients) cluster headache. Authors reported complete relief of pain in 34 (60.7%) among patients with episodic headache, but only in three (30%) who suffered from the chronic form of cluster headache. The mean time of follow up was 29.1 +/− 10.6 months.

As to side effects and complications, temporary postoperative epistaxis was observed in eight patients and a cheek hematoma in 11 patients; a partial RF lesion of the maxillary nerve was inadvertently made in four patients. Nine patients complained of hypesthesia of the palate, which disappeared in all cases within 3 months (124).

Glossopharyngeal Neuralgia

Radiofrequency lesioning of glossopharyngeal ganglion seems to be appropriate for the treatment of throat pain due to cancer or idiopathic glossopharyngeal neuralgia (125).

Glossopharyngeal neuralgia, first recognized by Sicard and Robineau in 1920, requires special attention, not because it is common (its incidence is 1:40 to 1:250 that of trigeminal tic) but because it is so rare and unfamiliar to many that it can be confused with other craniofacial pain syndromes. Inappropriate treatment may be *disastrous*. The peak age incidence is 40 to 60 years, incidence is equal for the two genders, and it is more common on the left side; 10% to 30% of cases coexist with trigeminal tic, and in up to 25% of cases, it occurs bilaterally. The same etiologies have been suggested as for trigeminal tic, except that it apparently has not been recognized in multiple sclerosis. It tends to be less severe than trigeminal tic, with 67% of patients suffering a single episode (29% in trigeminal tic) and 42% requiring no treatment (9% in trigeminal tic) (124–130).

Like trigeminal tic, the condition can be diagnosed only on the basis of the history of the pain with the absence of neurologic or imaging abnormalities, a difficult exercise since the symptomatology is complex. Apart from rare purely syncopal attacks, most patients complain of pain, although syncopal attacks, first described in 1942 by Riley, may accompany the pain (127,131). The pain may be of two main types, typical (tic-like lancinating) and atypical. Atypical pain can be dull, aching, burning, pressure-like, or swelling. Even typical pain may be preceded by itching, tickling, tingling, or a feeling of sticking, choking, or scratching from a foreign body and, as in trigeminal tic, may be followed by an after-pain.

Both types of pain begin either (a) in the ear, mandibular angle, eustachian tube, or front of the ear or (b) in the pharynx, tonsil, or posterior tongue, and may project from either to the other site. Rarely, pain spreads over the mastoid and adjacent occipital area. Triggering is sometimes seen, induced by swallowing (especially of cold fluids), yawning, chewing, coughing, sneezing, clearing the throat, blowing the nose, talking, or turning the head, or by touching the gingivae, external canal of the ear, tongue, periauricular skin, tonsillar pillars, or pharynx; sometimes triggering occurs from outside glossopharyngeal-vagal territory. It may be accompanied by tinnitus, by soreness in the cheek or mandible, and, like trigeminal tic, occasionally by sensory loss. There are several more bizarre symptoms: uncontrolled gestures, involuntary coughing, dyspnea, hoarseness, sweating, dryness of the mouth, salivation, choking, hiccups, flushing, mydriasis, and tearing. In 10% of patients, bradycardia, hypotension, asystole, syncopal fits accompany the pain, sometimes resulting in sudden death.

When surgical therapy becomes necessary, the chief options are open section of cranial nerve IX and the upper one-quarter to one-third of the roots of cranial nerve X, microvascular decompression of these nerves, or percutaneous RF thermocoagulation. In this condition, open surgery may be preferable to avoid the indiscriminate damage to other lower cranial nerves that may follow the percutaneous technique, causing hoarseness and cardiovascular instability (105,125,132–135).

The percutaneous technique consists of introducing a needle into the external pars nervosa portion of the jugular canal in which the vein lies laterally. The foramen is located in line with, but posterior to, the foramen ovale, behind the temporomandibular joint and anterior to the occipital condyle, medial to the carotid artery. The needle is passed 20 degrees posterior and 5 to 10 degrees medial to the course used to enter the foramen ovale, being in a more posterior position (Fig. 42-37). Electrocardiogram (ECG) and blood pressure should be monitored to avoid problems associated with alterations in vagus nerve function; correct positioning is indicated when 0.1- to 0.3-V stimulation produces paresthesias, some say pain, in the external auditory meatus or the ipsilateral side of the pharynx. Trapezius contractions should be avoided, and alterations in blood pressure and ECG pattern monitored. After a test lesion to avoid untoward effects, a 60- to 90-second RF lesion is made starting at 60°C, with 5°C increments, watching for alterations in pulse or blood pressure; if these occur, repositioning of the electrode is necessary. The lesion is enlarged until the tonsillar pharynx is analgesic and the gag reflex is lessened. Since vocal cord paralysis may occur, the percutaneous technique is better suited to cases of cancer than to those of tic.

Isamat and associates (125) used this procedure in four patients with glossopharyngeal tic. No complications occurred, although pain recurred in two. The procedure was successfully repeated in one. Tew and co-workers (105) and Lazorthes and Verdie (133) relieved pain in three patients, but dysarthria and dysphasia were observed postoperatively. Tew and associates (105) treated nine patients with cancer in glossopharyngeal distribution, eight of whom were relieved. Broggi (135) used the procedure in five patients with cancer, with two excellent results and two recurrences successfully managed by reoperation. Dubuisson (67) summarized reported experience, as shown in Table 42-8.

Pagura treated 15 patients with pain secondary to cancer using RF glossopharyngeal rhizotomy by the percutaneous approach. Eleven patients had complete relief, whereas four patients had partial relief. All patients presented after surgery with some impairment in glossopharyngeal function (136).

Sindou and colleagues (130) reviewed 15 cases from the literature and three of their own treated by thermocoagulation, finding complications greater than in cases treated by open means. In 18 patients operated upon, one procedure was not completed because of coronary ischemia and one that was

RESULTS OF PERCUTANEOUS RF COAGULATION OF IX NERVE

Authors	Levels treated	Initial relief	Late relief	Mortality	No. of cases
Lazorthes and Verdie (1979)[136]	Ninth/tenth cranial (cancer) (glossopharyngeal neuralgia)	?	73%	0	11
Isamat et al. (1980)[104]	Ninth/tenth cranial (glossopharyngeal neuralgia)	? 100%	100% 75%	0 0	1 4
Tew (1982)[322]	Ninth/tenth cranial (cancer) (glossopharyngeal neuralgia)	56% 100%	? ?	0 0	9 2
Giorgi and Broggi (1984)[76]	Ninth/tenth cranial (cancer) (glossopharyngeal neuralgia)	100% 100%	100% 60%	0 0	5 5

RF, radiofrequency.
From Dubuisson D: Root surgery. *In* Wall PD and Melzack R (eds.): *Textbook of Pain.* 3rd Ed. pp. 1055. Edinburgh, Churchill Livingstone, 1994.

completed led to the cardiac arrest; 14 (78%) enjoyed excellent and two (11%) partial pain relief. Complications affected 10 (56%) patients; in addition to the above-mentioned cardiac complications, seven patients suffered sensory loss; six, suppression of gag reflex; five, transient dysphagia; one, persistent dysphagia; and one, deafness. Ori and colleagues (134) reported thermocoagulation in nine patients, in one of whom two repetitions were required; six of 11 procedures caused cardiac dysrhythmia or over a 50% fall in blood pressure or heart rate, causing syncope in two cases and seizures in one.

A lateral cervical approach is also available, as described by Salar and co-workers (137). The needle is introduced anterior to the mastoid process, below the external auditory meatus, perpendicular to the skin and is advanced until the styloid process is reached at a depth of 1.5 to 2.0 cm. The needle is pulled back and pushed across the styloid posteriorly for 2 cm, until the tip lies tangential to and below the lateral part of the jugular foramen. After x-ray confirmation of the needle's location pointing toward the medial pars nervosa, stimulation induces slightly painful paresthesias in the retropharyngeal-tonsillar area, as well as in the external meatus. Suprathreshold stimulation may cause laryngeal muscle contraction. Vagal hyperactivity may also be seen with a fall in blood pressure and heart rate, in which case the needle must be repositioned. Then a thermal lesion is made as before.

SYMPATHECTOMY

Sympathectomy has a long and varied history, having been used to treat a vast array of problems from epilepsy through pain to vascular disease. Currently, the indications appear to include hyperhydrosis, vascular insufficiency, and pain. Under the latter indication, it is used in patients with visceral pain, including that from cancer of the pancreas, pain associated with vascular insufficiency in the limbs, and sympathetically maintained pain. In general, sympathectomy is less useful in controlling intractable "nonmalignant" pain than that of cancer pain, although the sympathetic dystrophic changes that sometimes accompany deafferentation pain may be relieved (138–140) without affecting the underlying pain.

Institution of sympathetic blocks in the treatment of complex regional pain syndrome (CRPS) is controversial (141). The compelling evidence of efficacy as either a diagnostic or ther-

apeutic tool has not been published. The role of sympathetic blockade in the treatment of CRPS was reviewed by Cepeda and colleagues (142). Their analysis suggests that less than one-third of CRPS patients are likely to respond to sympathetic blockade. Most likely, those who exhibit a pattern of mechanical and especially cold allodynia may benefit from a sympatholysis (143) (see also Chapter 46).

Anatomy

Cervical Level

Preganglionic fibers to the head and neck leave the spinal canal with the ventral roots of T1 and T2, and then continue as white rami communicans before joining the sympathetic chain and passing cephalad to synapse at the inferior, middle, or superior cervical ganglion. All preganglionic nerves either synapse or pass through the inferior (stellate) ganglion; therefore, the stellate ganglion should be targeted to achieve sympathetic block of the head and neck (see Chapter 39).

Thoracic Level

Sympathetic fibers to the upper extremity exit with T2 to T8 ventral roots and travel as white rami communicans to the sympathetic chain before they synapse the second and, possibly, the third thoracic ganglion. Thus, a T2 and/or T3 lesion will reliably deprive the upper extremity from the sympathetic innervation (144) (see Chapter 39).

Abdomen

Innervation of the viscera originates in T5 to T11, with occasional T4 and T12 preganglionic fibers. They do not synapse in the sympathetic chain, but rather pass through the chain to synapse at distal locations (i.e., the celiac, renal, and superior mesenteric ganglia). T5 to T9 preganglionic fibers coalesce to build the greater splanchnic nerve; T10 and T11 constitute the lesser and T12, the least splanchnic nerves (145).

Lumbar Level

Each lumbar sympathetic chain lies at the anterolateral aspect of the vertebral bodies L1 to L4, whereas the L5 ganglion is situated more dorsally at the level of the L5–S1 intervertebral disk. The sympathetic ganglia of the lumbar sympathetic chain are variable in both numbers and position. In most cases, only four are found. There tends to be fusion of L1 and L2 ganglia in most patients, and ganglia are aggregated at the L2–L3 and L4–L5 disks. Also, there is considerable variability in the size of the ganglia, some being fusiform and as long as 10 to 15 mm, and others being round and approximately 5 mm long (146) (see also Chapter 39).

Pelvis and Perineum

The most caudal domain of the sympathetic chain includes the superior hypogastric plexus and the impar (Walter) ganglion. The superior hypogastric plexus is the extension of the aortic plexus below the level of aortic bifurcation. It is situated at the anterior aspect of the promontorium, with somewhat of a left side shift. The impar ganglion is the most caudal part of the sympathetic chain, located just ventrally to the sacrococcygeal junction.

Stellate Gangliotomy

There is only indeterminate to limited evidence of efficacy (V–IV) (41) of the stellate ganglion lesion in the management of postherpetic neuralgia in the distribution of the trigeminal nerve and in the management of upper extremity CRPS. Moreover, phenol injection in the vicinity of the spinal cord and vertebral artery may result in direct neural damage, vascular injury, and neural infarcts (147). Evidence of efficacy of the RF technique is confined to a small prospective study with only short-term success (148) and to a retrospective study in which only 40.7% reported pain reduction of more than 50% (149).

Upper Thoracic Percutaneous Sympathectomy

Thoracic sympathectomy has been used to manage various painful conditions and vascular insufficiency of the upper extremities. There are numerous potential indications for thoracic sympathetic blockade and sympathectomy, including CRPS, ischemic and vasospastic painful conditions, frostbite, hyperhidrosis, and malignant and nonmalignant thoracic visceral pain. Acute vascular occlusive events, such as Raynaud syndrome, are often accompanied by excruciating pain refractory to systemic analgesics. Sympathetic block and sympathectomy can have major roles for both nutritional blood flow restoration and pain control (150) (see also Chapter 39). Despite the high rate of recurrence, when used in Raynaud syndrome, thoracic sympathectomy clearly produced a high success rate and showed potential for reducing the severity of refractory symptoms (151).

Although chemical thoracic sympathectomy was one of the first described neural destructive procedures (4), it was eventually abandoned. Proximity of the thoracic sympathetic ganglia to the intercostal nerves and neuroforamina resulted in high rates of neurologic complications (152). A large volume of injectate and use of a "blind" technique was likely the cause of the complications. More recently, the technique has been reintroduced. Small-volume phenol injection under fluoroscopic guidance has been reported to be successful, with only minor side effects (153).

To maximize the probability of success of the RF procedure, the RF electrode must be located precisely, as close to the sympathetic ganglion as possible. According to the anatomic study of Wilkinson, the T2 ganglion is situated roughly in the middle of the vertebra rostro-caudally and one-third dorso-ventrally (154) (Fig. 42-39A,B). Others have found that approximately

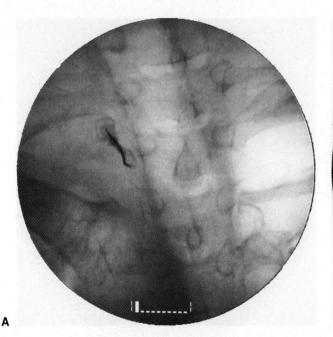

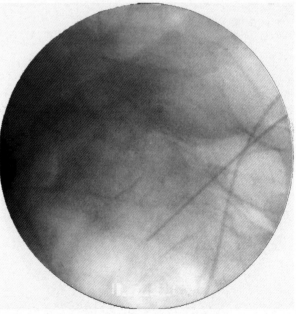

A

B

FIGURE 42-39. Upper thoracic sympathetic ganglion radiofrequency lesioning. **A:** Anteroposterior view: an 18-gauge curved active tip radiofrequency cannula is inserted beneath the head of T2 rib. **B:** Lateral view: an 18-gauge curved active tip radiofrequency cannula is positioned in the middle of the T2 vertebra. To ensure ablation of the T2 ganglion, sequential lesions have to be made with the cannula withdrawal dorsally.

90% of the T2 or T3 sympathetic trunks are located on the head of the corresponding rib (155). A recent study found that the second thoracic ganglion is usually located (in 92.5% of patients) in the second intercostal space at the level of the intervertebral disk, between the second and third thoracic vertebrae (156). Although a variation of 1.0 to 1.5 cm is not of great importance during a surgical sympathectomy, it is crucial for RF electrode placement; therefore, addition of 1 to 2 mL of radiopaque phenol 10% has been recommended (157).

Wilkinson (158) has described a percutaneous RF technique for upper thoracic sympathectomy. A modified technique using a curved-tip cannula probably simplifies cannula positioning and lessens the risk of pneumothorax. With the patient prone under local anesthesia, using fluoroscopy guidance, an RF cannula is introduced 4 to 5 cm from the midline and directed toward three sites. An 18-gauge electrode with a 10-mm curved active tip is inserted between the third and fourth ribs medial to the scapular margin and aimed at a point 2 to 5 mm lateral and rostral to the midpoint of the T3 vertebra. The electrode tip is positioned at the ventral edge of T3 in the lateral x-ray image under the head of the third rib. The next lesion is made by passing the electrode between the second and third ribs just lateral to the T2–T3 interspace. The third lesion is made through the same rib space, but the tip is rotated to the rostral portion of the T2 body beneath the head of the second rib (Fig. 42-39A,B). When each electrode is properly positioned, stimulation is carried out and positioning effected so as to avoid a somatic motor or sensory response below 0.5 V. This avoids damage to the somatic roots. A test lesion at 60°C for 60 seconds is made to guard against Horner syndrome, while plethysmography and hand temperature monitoring indicate whether sympathetic interruption is occurring. When all criteria have been satisfied, a 90°C 180-second lesion is made and enlarged by withdrawing the tip 8 to 10 mm.

In Wilkinson's study (158), 20 procedures on 27 sides produced 24 instances of sympathetic denervation. Two patients suffered from pneumothorax, three from brachial neuralgia, and one from unwanted Horner syndrome.

Gybels and Sweet (56) collected 65 cases treated by upper thoracic percutaneous RF sympathectomy; postoperatively, eight suffered initial and one delayed failure (14%), one developed pneumonia, and four developed new pain syndromes.

In a recent series of 1,742 cases of hyperhidrosis, the authors concluded that the modified technique was associated with very good long-term results and a low complication rate. Similar outcomes were obtained when the sympathectomy was performed at the T2 and T3 levels, or at the T2 level only (159).

Splanchnic Neurolysis

Splanchnic and celiac plexus neurolysis pertains almost completely to the pain management of abdominal malignancies (see Chapter 45). Nevertheless, several observational studies suggest that the procedure can be effective in the treatment of chronic pancreatic pain (160,161).

To create a lesion of the splanchnic nerve, the RF cannula has to be positioned at the mid-third portion of the lateral side of the T11 or T12 vertebral body. A curved 10-cm long cannula with a 10-mm active tip is recommended. The cannula should remain retrocrural and posterior to the descending aorta. To achieve this position, a 10- to 20-degree fluoroscopic view of the T11 or T12 vertebra is obtained. The cannula is introduced under tunnel fluoroscopic view under the 11th or 12th rib (Fig. 42-40A,B). The image intensifier is rotated to the lateral view, and the cannula is advanced with the tip rotated medially until reaching the anterior third of the vertebral body (see Chapter 45). The bony contact has to be consistently maintained. Once the cannula is in place, sensory stimulation at 50 Hz is conducted up to 1 V. The patient may report a vague stimulation in the epigastric region. This is typical and satisfactory. If the stimulation is in a girdle-like fashion around the intercostal

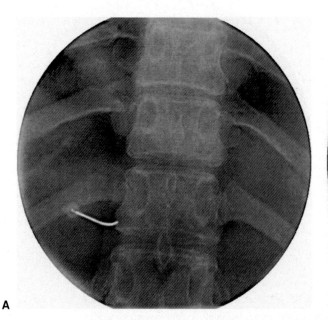

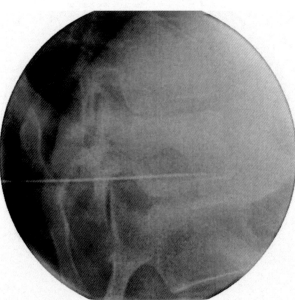

A   **B**

FIGURE 42-40. Splanchnic radiofrequency lesioning. A: Anteroposterior view: an 18-gauge radiofrequency cannula with curved active tip rotated medially is positioned adjacent to the T12 vertebra. B: Lateral view: an 18-gauge curved active tip radiofrequency cannula is seen at the lateral surface of the T12 vertebral body reaching the anterior third of the vertebral shadow.

spaces, the cannula must be advanced anteriorly. At 2 Hz, motor stimulation is increased to 3 V. The intercostal muscle contraction should not be seen or perceived. Prior to the RF lesion, 2 mL of local anesthetic is injected. The active tip is rotated upward or downward. A 90-second 80°C lesion is performed. The cannula is rotated 180 degrees, and the second lesion is performed at the same setting. If the procedure is for bilateral neurolysis, then the same procedure of testing and lesioning should be completed on the opposite site.

Lumbar Sympathectomy

Gybels and Sweet (56) reviewed the development of percutaneous lumbar sympathectomy with phenol usually for relief of symptoms of peripheral vascular disease, quoting results from Reid and co-workers (162) of 77% initial and 60% longer-term relief of ischemic rest pain in 189 men. Dondelinger and Kurdziel (163) suppressed pain in 60% of patients, but vascular improvement occurred in only 33%. Cross and Cotton (164) recorded a 67% reduction in rest pain persisting for 6 months. Gybels and Sweet note the confusion as to whether the procedure achieved its results in patients with peripheral vascular disease by virtue of vasodilation or of pain fiber interruption. Cousins and colleagues (165) reported that 80% of 386 patients with rest pain had complete or partial pain relief, with a mean duration of 6 months, regardless of changes in blood flow (see Chapter 39).

Because of the anatomic variability of the lumbar sympathetic ganglia, RF ablation has not yet gained popularity, and its efficacy still needs to be confirmed. In one publication, 89% of patients in the phenol group showed signs of sympathetic blockade after 8 weeks, as compared with 12% in the RF group (166). Another small study reported success in only five patients for 5 months to 3 years after the RF sympatholysis. Fifteen patients had temporary or no relief at all. The procedure was temporarily complicated by an excessively hot, swollen foot, and by postsympathectomy (genitofemoral) neuralgia in a few cases (167).

Superior Hypogastric Plexus and Impar Ganglion Destruction

Superior hypogastric plexus is not amenable to RF ablation because this structure is a network of nerve fibers rather than a ganglionic formation. Apart from an application for the treatment of cancer pain (168) (see Chapter 45), neurolytic superior hypogastric block has been proposed in the management of chronic pelvic pain associated with endometriosis and pelvic inflammatory disease (169,170).

Radiofrequency lesioning of the impar ganglion has been described in the treatment of chronic perineal nonmalignant pain in a small study, demonstrating that it can decrease pain severity by at least 35% (171).

PERCUTANEOUS DESTRUCTIVE PROCEDURES ON THE SPINAL CORD

Percutaneous procedures aimed at the spinal cord for the control of intractable pain are listed in Table 42-9; of these, percutaneous cordotomy is most often used since the spinal cord

---

TABLE 42-9

PERCUTANEOUS PROCEDURES FOR PAIN RELIEF IN THE SPINAL CORD

Percutaneous cordotomy:
  Lateral high approach
  Dorsal high approach
  Low anterior approach

Percutaneous cervical myelotomy

Percutaneous trigeminal nucleotomy/tractotomy

Percutaneous punctate midline myelotomy

---

can readily be approached percutaneously only at the occipital C1 and the C1–C2 interspaces.

Open versus Percutaneous Cordotomy

Although there are still advocates of open cordotomy, a careful review of the situation reveals few indications for the open procedure. Pathologic and anatomic abnormalities virtually never interfere with the percutaneous approach, so the lesser impact and increased precision of this approach should give it priority, except when a surgeon capable of performing the procedure is not readily available to a sick patient who cannot travel. If a patient's inability to cooperate precludes local anesthesia, percutaneous cordotomy can be performed under general anesthesia without muscle paralysis (172–175). Percutaneous cordotomy is the operative cordotomy procedure of choice in cancer pain, whenever it is not contraindicated (176,177).

There is minimal evidence of efficacy and safety of the percutaneous cordotomy in the management of nonmalignant pain (178) (see also Chapter 31).

Percutaneous Cordotomy

Percutaneous cordotomy, modeled after the open operation of Spiller and Martin (179), was first employed by Mullan and colleagues (180) using the lateral approach between C1 and C2, and using a radiostrontium source to make the lesion. In a short time, the procedure was perfected by the addition of myelography (181) to guide electrode position, electrical impedance monitoring (182) to guide cord penetration, RF lesion-making (13,14) to replace the radioactive source, physiologic corroboration (183–185), and CT guidance (186). Meanwhile, Hitchcock (187,188) and others (189) developed a dorsal approach in the occiput–C1 space requiring the use of a stereotactic frame, whereas Lin and colleagues (190) introduced a low anterior cervical approach to avoid potential damage to the pathways responsible for respiratory control. Of these, the lateral high cervical method has been the most popular.

Indications

Percutaneous cordotomy by the lateral high cervical approach is indicated in cases of nociceptive cancer pain below the C5 dermatome; above this level lasting analgesia cannot be achieved. The usual cause of the pain is malignant involvement of the lumbosacral plexus, for which it is the procedure of choice, although it may be indicated rarely for nociceptive

TABLE 42-10

DIFFERENTIAL EFFECT OF SURGICAL PROCEDURES ON DIFFERENT ELEMENTS OF CENTRAL PAIN OF SPINAL CORD ORIGIN

Pain element	% of Patients significantly relieved	
	Destructive surgery[a]	Chronic stimulation[b]
Steady, causalgic dysesthetic, aching	26	36
Intermittent shooting	89	0
Allodynia and hyperpathia	84	16

[a]Cordotomy, cordectomy, dorsal root entry zone (DREZ).
[b]Dorsal column, deep brain stimulation producing paraesthesias in pain area.

pain caused by nonmalignant disease (however, see Chapter 31). The lancinating element of central spinal cord pain, that is common with thoracolumbar injuries, and allodynia or hyperpathia associated with neuropathic pain in the lower extremities are also indications (191,192) (Table 42-10).

In general, severe pain in a single lower extremity is the best indication; bilateral lower limb pain requiring bilateral cordotomy exposes the patient to the risk of bladder dysfunction and respiratory complications. Bilateral lower truncal-pelvic-perineal pain is a poor indication (193), partly because it responds poorly, possibly due to elements of neuropathic pain caused by previous surgery and/or radiation—and partly because it requires bilateral operation. Neuroaxial drug delivery may be superior here.

Respiratory contraindications require special comment (194–200). Voluntary respiration, in response to the command "take a deep breath," is controlled by the corticospinal tract, rarely damaged during percutaneous cordotomy. On the other hand, unconscious respiration, as in sleep, is mediated by the strictly ipsilaterally distributed reticulospinal tracts. Since these lie adjacent to the cervical dermatomes of the spinothalamic tract, they are easily damaged by a cordotomy lesion that achieves high levels of cervical analgesia. This is of no concern if both lungs and their innervation are functioning normally. However, if, for example, an apical carcinoma has destroyed the phrenic nerve on one side and a cordotomy is being contemplated on the other to produce analgesia into the upper cervical dermatomes, the remaining reticulospinal tract will be interrupted and unconscious respiration abolished, with fatal results. In such situations, cordotomy is either contraindicated or fraught with much risk. The same issues apply if a previous cordotomy has interrupted the tract and a new cordotomy is now being considered on the second side. Lema and Hitchcock (200) found that respiratory function (measured as the forced expiratory volume in 1 second) was interfered with to a greater degree by high dorsal percutaneous cordotomy than by percutaneous myelotomy or trigeminal tractotomy.

Other contraindications, such as anomalies or disease in the C1–C2 area, virtually never interfere, and in children or confused patients who cannot cooperate, general anesthesia may be used.

The choice of percutaneous technique depends upon the surgeon's experience and preferences. The dorsal (13,183,189)

approaches requiring a stereotactic frame can achieve a slightly higher level of analgesia than the lateral high cervical approaches, but these appear to have been little exploited. The low anterior approach (190) has two disadvantages: it achieves a low level of analgesia, and it requires first traversing the cervical disk and part of the cord with the electrode before the spinothalamic tract is reached. Thus, small changes of electrode position require withdrawal of the electrode through the disk first and then reinsertion.

Technique: Lateral High Cervical Cordotomy

The lateral high cervical procedure is usually carried out under local anesthesia with IV sedation, but, as mentioned, it can be performed under general anesthesia without paralysis, and without stereotactic subjective backup of proper electrode position (173). With the patient positioned supine, a spinal needle is introduced into the middle of the C1–C2 space under lateral image intensification (Fig. 42-41). Imaging of the dentate ligament is obtained by rapid injection of a small volume of a mixture of CSF, air, and contrast medium when the subarachnoid space is entered. Oil-based contrast medium, which is superior to the evanescent water-soluble types, although associated with aseptic arachnoiditis (201), is now difficult to obtain. Water-soluble contrast can also be used (202). The cordotomy electrode (Fig. 42-42) is now introduced into the spinal needle. This is a monopolar insulated sharpened wire with a 2-mm active tip, which locks into the spinal needle so that 2 mm of insulated part, in addition to the active tip, projects beyond the tip of the spinal needle (Fig. 42-42). It is grounded against an indifferent electrode in the ipsilateral upper arm. These dimensions ensure the optimum 2-mm penetration of the cord for lesioning the spinothalamic tract and provide standard impedance measurements. The electrode/needle assembly is directed toward the image of the dentate ligament and advanced so as to penetrate the cord at that site, penetration being signaled by an impedance rise from the 400 watts characteristic of CSF to the 800–1,200 watts of cord (Fig. 42-43). Stimulation is now carried out. If the electrode is correctly positioned, 2-Hz stimulation should produce muscle contractions in the ipsilateral neck and sometimes in the upper limb, whereas 50-Hz stimulation should produce contralateral warm/cold or "wind" sensations. If these contractions are felt in the lower limb, the electrode tip lies in the distal dermatomes of the spinothalamic tract; if felt in the hand, it lies in the proximal dermatomes. When all parameters are satisfactory, the first low-temperature (50°C) lesion is performed for 60 seconds. If it produces at least partial pain relief in the corresponding pain area and muscle power hasn't changed at the ipsilateral side, subsequent 90°C RF lesions are made until the desired level and degree of analgesia are achieved. Otherwise, the electrode must be repositioned and the previous steps repeated.

If cordotomy is to be performed on the second side, an interval of at least a week should be taken. Extreme caution must be observed to avoid respiratory complications; persisting unconscious respiration on the first side should be radiologically confirmed preoperatively, and the patient should be observed in an intensive care unit postoperatively, with monitoring of blood gases to detect a rising arterial carbon dioxide level forewarning of respiratory arrest. A significant risk of bladder dysfunction must be anticipated after bilateral cordotomy.

Results

The results of percutaneous cordotomy are perhaps best displayed in tabular form. Table 42-11 summarizes published results of unilateral procedures, Table 42-12 summarizes those

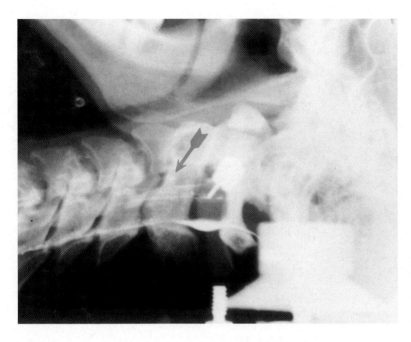

FIGURE 42-41. Percutaneous cordotomy. Lateral radiograph of neck during percutaneous cordotomy. A contrast medium (*arrow*) lies on the anterior cord margin. The ventral root line and dorsal dura are well outlined. The electrode tip is impaling the cord at the level of the dentate ligament, where a lesion produced analgesia up to T6 without complications.

of bilateral cordotomy, and Table 42-13 summarizes complications.

In a series of 244 cases (173), the procedure was completed in 99% of patients, achieving spinothalamic interruption in 92.4%. In unilateral cases, effective pain relief was obtained in 94.4% at the time of discharge from hospital and in 82.3% in longer-term follow-up. Incidence of pain relief after bilateral cordotomy obeys the P-squared rule and is therefore lower than for unilateral cordotomy (82.3% × 82.3% = 67.7%). Recurrence of the nociceptive pain for which the procedure was performed virtually never occurs in an area of persisting analgesia. Nevertheless, persistent or recurrent pain after cordotomy can result from various causes: (a) technical failure of the procedure; (b) spread of cancer beyond the site involved at the time of the cordotomy (6% of 244 cases developed pain above their cordotomy level); (c) presence or development of neuropathic pain from plexus destruction (203); and (d) development of, or intensification of, ipsilateral or "mirror" pain (41% of 244 cases) (173). The last development is particularly interesting. Once thought to be the result of unmasking of lesser pain on the other side of the body, it now seems more likely to be the result of opening up of previously inactive ipsilateral spinothalamic cord synapses after successful cordotomy, allowing painful

stimuli applied to the now analgesic site to be appreciated in the mirror position on the other side of the body (204–207). In those patients in whom cordotomy was performed for other than malignant disease (191), levels of analgesia tended to fade with time and pain recurred. In six of 24 paraplegics undergoing cordotomy, this happened after 1, 1.5, 4, 5, 13, and 21 years; pain relief has been restored in two patients after 5 and 21 years, respectively, by repetition of the cordotomy (191).

It is unfortunate that percutaneous cordotomy has been so nearly supplanted in many centers by subcutaneous infusion of opioids using an external pump or by intrathecal/epidural administration of opioids and local anesthetics (see Chapter 40). Because of tolerance, the former therapy may result in enormous daily dosages of morphine, with their inevitable secondary effects; and the latter, neuroaxial delivery, requires continual attendance at a medical facility. In selected patients, particularly those with lower limb pain, cordotomy—a once-only procedure—may achieve sufficient lasting pain relief so that the patient may require only small doses of oral analgesics postoperatively until the terminal stages of the illness.

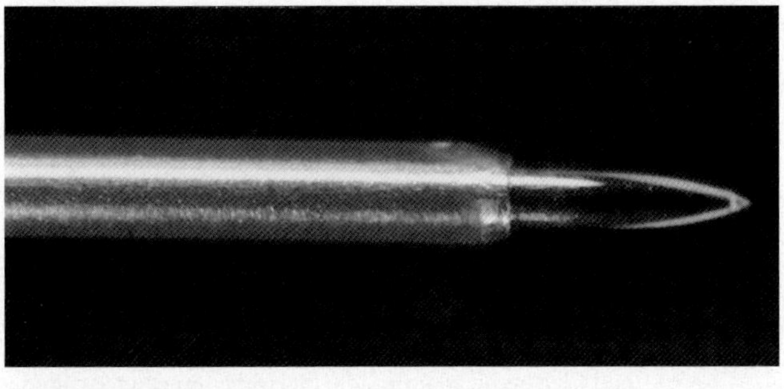

Other Spinal Cord Procedures

Hitchcock (208) has evolved a high cervical dorsal percutaneous technique in the occipital–C1 space for central myelotomy, a substitute for longitudinal myelotomy done by open laminectomy. This latter curious procedure, introduced by Armour (209), was originally intended to interrupt decussating spinothalamic fibers in the anterior commissure and thus to raise the analgesic level achieved by a cordotomy at the same level. The open operation also achieved the same effect as cordotomy if performed over many levels; when performed in the cervical area, it avoided the risk of respiratory complications. Hitchcock's percutaneous operation, however, performed in the upper cervical spine, can relieve pain at any level in the cord, and any analgesia induced bears no somatotopographic relationship to the level of the pain relieved. Thus, it is thought to interrupt an extralemniscal pain pathway whose

FIGURE 42-42. Percutaneous cordotomy. Tip of cordotomy electrode (×15 magnification).

TABLE 42-11

PUBLISHED SUCCESS AFTER UNILATERAL PERCUTANEOUS CORDOTOMY
(% PATIENTS)

Pain relief (% of patients)		References
Complete	Significant	
63		O'Connell (1969)[220]
75	96	Lorenz (1976)[166]
77	89	Grote and Roosen (1976)[a79]
75	83	von Schröttner (1978)[a340]
79	—	Meglio and Cioni (1981)[178]
—	68	Kühner (1981)[123]
75	—	Lipton (1981)[153]
—	79.1	Ventafridda, DeConno and Fochi (1982) (literature review)[335]
	50% after 3 mos.	
71	82.3	Tasker (1982)[298]
—	75	Siegfried Kühner and Sturm (1984)[269]
	80	Lipton (1984)[154]
—	71	Ischia et al. (1984)[109]
64	87	Lahuerta Lipton and Wells (1985)[126]
76	92.5	Ischia et al. (1985)[106]
—	89	Farcot et al. (1988)[62]
74.5	87.8	Tasker (1988)[304]
90—immediately		Rosomoff et al. (1990)[249]
84—@ 3 months		
61—@ 1 year		
43—1–5 years		
37—5–10 years		
64	82	Amano et al. (1991)[1]
	59–96	Tasker (1993) (literature review)[308]
72	84	Tasker (1995)[309]
	81.1	Ischia et al. (1984)[108]

[a]Mostly cancer pain and unilateral cordotomy.

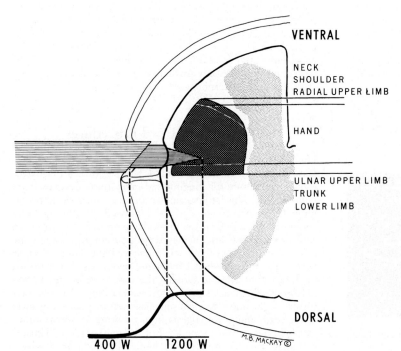

FIGURE 42-43. Percutaneous cordotomy. Diagram illustrating technique of percutaneous cordotomy by the lateral high cervical approach, including impedance changes on cord impilation and anatomic organization of the region.

TABLE 42-12

PUBLISHED SUCCESS AFTER BILATERAL PERCUTANEOUS CORDOTOMY (% PATIENTS)

Relief		
Complete	Significant	Reference
58	77	Rosomoff (1969)[245]
—	71.4	Tasker (1982)[298]
47	59.5	Ischia et al. (1984)[107]
76	95	Amano et al. (1991)[1]
	47	Tasker (1993) (literature review)[308]

nature is unclear and which is distinct from the spinothalamic tract (210). The procedure is an option in patients with pain caused by cancer, whereas its role in those with deafferentation pain needs further observation. It is a useful alternative to intrathecal or epidural opiate instillation in patients with midline or bilateral trunk pain in the lower body.

High cervical commissurotomy is performed percutaneously under local anesthesia through the occipital–C1 interspace with the patient sitting, using a suitable frame. A cisternal myelogram outlines the dorsal and ventral aspects of the medulla and cord. A sharpened 0.5-mm electrode is introduced under impedance control with stimulation for physiologic localization. It is passed toward a point 5 mm anterior to the dorsal cord margin in the midsagittal plane. As the electrode enters the cord, stimulation of dorsal columns produces paresthesias in both feet. More deeply near the central canal, stimulation effects are referred to more dorsal aspects of the lower limbs. At the central canal region, paresthesiae occur in the soles, spreading to the dorsal aspects of the legs as the current is increased. Sometimes paresthesiae affect the whole face, crossed limbs, or bilateral upper limbs, or else burning in the trunk occurs. Lesions are made as in cordotomy, just anterior to or at the sites of distal lower limb responses. Lesions produce subjective analgesia without clinically demonstrable sensory loss unrelated in location to areas of pain relief.

Results

Hitchcock (208) reported ten excellent and two good results in 14 patients with cancer pain and excellent results in three with deafferentation pain associated with unpredictable bilateral alterations in the appreciation of pin-prick. Eiras and co-workers (211) reported good initial results in patients with cancer pain, with recurrence in some patients. Papo (212) found the pain relief from the procedure to be short-lived. Gybels and Sweet (56) compiled outcome data in 260 cases of percutaneous cervical RF myelotomy in patients with noncancerous pain syndromes; 66% derived useful relief. In 141 patients with pain caused by cancer, 63% were relieved.

Percutaneous Tractotomy of Caudal Nucleus and Descending Tract of Trigeminal Nerve

Percutaneous tractotomy of the trigeminal nerve has been performed at both the lower medullary (213–217) and the upper cervical (187,188,208,218) levels. Unlike the previously discussed destructive techniques aimed at interrupting pain transmission in the management of nociceptive pain, this procedure at the cord level has been directed toward the management of

deafferentation pain in the face, although the mechanism of this relief is unknown. Possibly it is similar to that in the so-called dorsal root entry zone introduced by Hyndman (219) and elaborated by Sindou and co-workers (130) in the treatment of cancer pain, by Nashold and Ostdahl (220) for deafferentation pain at the cord level, and by Bernard and colleagues (221) for deafferentation pain affecting the trigeminal nerve. Crue and colleagues (213,222) first performed trigeminal medullary tractotomy primarily for the treatment of nociceptive pain; Fox (214,215) introduced radiographic localization.

Technique

Medullary. The patient is positioned prone under local anesthesia. A 18-gauge lumbar puncture needle is introduced between occiput and C1 into the midline of the cisterna magna, and 1 mL of a contrast dye emulsified with 1 mL of CSF is injected under lateral image intensification, outlining the floor of the fourth ventricle, the dorsum of the brainstem, and the obex, the latter appearing as a step in the shadow of the contrast medium. Four centimeters lateral to the midline, a second 18-gauge thin-wall lumbar puncture needle is passed over C1 lamina and aimed toward cisterna magna, terminating 12 mm from the midline as measured uncorrected on the posteroanterior film and 8 mm caudal to obex at the level of the dorsum of the brainstem on the lateral film (also uncorrected). These x-rays are achieved with a 30-inch tube-to-target and a 40-inch tube-to-film distance so as to afford reproducible measurements. A second electrode, such as the stylet of a 22-gauge, 4.5-inch lumbar puncture needle insulated with vinyl tubing (except for a 3-mm bare tip), is passed through the laterally placed guide needle into the brainstem under impedance control at a site 0 to 10 mm from the midline of the odontoid on the uncorrected posteroanterior film and at, or just caudal to, the obex and 4 mm anterior to the level of the floor of the fourth ventricle on the lateral film. In proper position, 50-Hz stimulation should cause ipsilateral facial sensation, whereupon a graded RF lesion up to 50 mA for 10 to 60 seconds is made with serial sensory testing.

Cervical. Hitchcock and Schvarcz (218) performed the procedure with the patient in the sitting position under local anesthesia using a stereotactic frame. A needle is passed through the occipital–C1 interspace in the midsagittal plane, and a contrast dye is injected to outline the anterior/posterior aspects of the cord and the cisterna magna. The caudal dermatomes of the spinal tract of the fifth nerve at this location are said to lie 3 to 4 mm anterior to the posterior aspect of the cord and 6 mm lateral. Rostral dermatomes lie more laterally and anteriorly, and intermedius, ninth, and tenth dermatomes more posteriorly and medially. A 0.5-mm sharpened insulated electrode with a 2-mm bare tip enclosed in a nylon tube is advanced under radiologic and impedance control using monopolar stimulation until stimulation induces sensation in the face, said to be paresthetic (216) or painful (218). Stimulation of the dorsal columns or their nuclei may induce ipsilateral sensory effects; stimulation of the spinothalamic tract, contralateral sensory effects; the trigeminal effects are ipsilateral. At the level of C1, all of the trigeminal fibers, including those for the circumoral dermatomes, are present, the latter not being represented more distally. As soon as satisfactory positioning is achieved, a graded RF lesion is made.

Results. Fox (214) operated on eight patients with cancer, two with postherpetic neuralgia, one with tic, and one with questionable iatrogenic deafferentation facial pain. Analgesia of the

TABLE 42-13

REPORTED COMPLICATIONS OF PERCUTANEOUS CORDOTOMY (% OF PATIENTS)

Complication References	Unilateral																Bilateral							
	220	79	152	180	123	335	269	109	154	126	106	62	226	249	308	309	283	245	123	121	107	1	308	309
Death (most respiratory)	1.5	1.5			4.5			1.4	6.2	5	4.2		0.6		0–6	0.3	3.3	2	9.9	27.2		0	→27	1.6
Severe respiratory failure	2		6.2	9		5–20							0.6	1	2.6–27	0.8	0.8	2		292		0	→36	
Mild respiratory problems					5.7						3.9			3		1.2			27.0	4.5				1.6
Transient respiratory problems		3.2		7.9		1–15							2.4	2	0.3	0.3			18.1					3.2
Significant paresis or ataxia	5.5	2	2.5	10.5	6	2–100	8	10.1	8–20	4	3.9	18		6	1–2	1.0	1.5	5		13.6	2.8	0		1.6
Mild or transient paresis or ataxia	11	2.9	20		48.5		100		100	69	31	47	4.3	25	→100	17.9		39		67.8	36.1		→67	29.5
Significant worsening micturition	13	3.2	5.3		4	2–35	7.2			3	8.7		2	2	→19	3.5	1.1	2	9.9	18.1	58	6.7		21.3
Mild, transient worsening micturition	18				8					19		10.5	6.1	10	0–8.7	7.0		15	36.3				→100	9.8
Transient bowel incontinence																2.1								9.8
Transient hypotension					2.6											1.8		4	54.5		36.1		40	8.1
Contralateral limb weakness										6						0								0
Postcordotomy dysesthesia		14.1 / 0.7 severe			3	1–50	8.7	8.7		6	6.8	16		1	→20	8.3	0.7							
Horner's syndrome					75			94	100	100	most	42	most		→100	23.0 $1/2$ persist				59	100	common		23% $1/4$ persist
Neck pain					50				100	26		58				2.4								1.6
Other significant																0.3								1.6
Other transient, minor																0.6								1.6

fifth, seventh, ninth, and tenth nerves occurred in seven, V2–V3 analgesia in the rest. Complications included transient ipsilateral ataxia (common), three instances of contralateral body analgesia, and nearly all patients suffered from postoperative hyperpyrexia of 38°C to 39°C.

Schvarcz (215,217) reported 53 procedures in 52 patients with 87.5% relief of postherpetic neuralgia, 56% of anesthesia dolorosa, and 74% of "dysesthetic pain." He reported 83.8% relief of pain in 31 cancer patients. Complications consisted of contralateral hypalgesia and ipsilateral ataxia. Full evaluation of this interesting technique requires further studies.

Percutaneous Punctate Midline Myelotomy

Spinal visceral pain transmission can be successfully interrupted by lesion of the most anterior and medial part of the dorsal column. Nauta and colleagues targeted this pathway through an open T8 punctate midline myelotomy and reported excellent results (223). Since this report, a percutaneous CT-guided method has been described (224). The patient is positioned prone on the CT table. Under local anesthesia, a 16-gauge venous catheter pierces the skin strictly in the midline and directed toward the posterior margin of the vertebral canal, as confirmed by lateral scanograms. The catheter is carefully advanced until CSF is obtained, and up to 5 mL of air is injected to delineate the posterior surface of the cord. The needle is then carefully introduced in the posterior midline of the cord to a depth of 4 to 5 mm. Another axial slice is performed to confirm proper placement and depth (all other slices are performed without the needle to avoid metal artifact). The needle, with a length 4 mm longer than the catheter, is introduced with its bevel upwards, downwards, to the right, to the left, rotated twice, and then withdrawn.

Pituitary Ablation

Pituitary ablation (neuroadenolysis of the pituitary, chemical hypophysectomy) is performed in a limited number of centers to treat intractable pain due to disseminated bone metastases, especially in patients with primary breast or prostate cancer.

Surgical hypophysectomy was first advocated to reduce tumor spread in 1952 (225). The observation that some patients experienced postsurgical pain relief led Greco (226) and later Moricca (227) and others to suggest pituitary destruction by percutaneous injection of absolute alcohol as a primary treatment for oncogenic pain. When indicated, a needle-based technique with alcohol, and less commonly performed cryogenic lesions (228) and even electrical stimulation (229), is preferred to surgical extirpation because the former approaches are comparatively simple, safe, and inexpensive, and entail only a brief hospitalization. It is curious that pituitary ablation has not secured a more uniform place in the cancer pain specialist's armamentarium since, although its conduct is technically demanding, considerable published experience reflects favorably on its efficacy and safety (228–233). Although experience is greatest in patients with breast and prostate cancer, recent reports suggest efficacy in patients with other malignant neoplasms, especially if the presenting complaint is head or neck pain (230,231,233). Major advantage of pituitary ablation is its applicability for bilateral and disseminated pain. Onset of relief is typically rapid and often complete, but like most ablative procedures, efficacy tends to deteriorate beyond 6 to 12 months.

Mechanism

The mechanism underlying the action of pituitary ablation remains obscure (234), although authorities favor theories that involve activation of a pituitary inhibitory system (229), alterations in hormonal feedback, and suppression of the hypothalamic axis (235). It has been further postulated that the capacity for pituitary procedures to relieve pain may involve a stress response similar to that which is observed in animal models, after battle injuries, and in athletes (231). Although there are some conflicting data, activation of endogenous opioids seems unlikely based on reports that analgesia is not reliably reversed by naloxone administration (236). Although observations of the spread of contrast medium near the third ventricle led to theories of hypothalamic injury, this mechanism is inconsistent with reports of pain relief after more discrete procedures (cryolesioning and electrical stimulation). Evidence suggests that pituitary destruction, in and of itself, is unlikely to be causal: primate research has demonstrated that neither complete destruction of the gland nor even significant injury is required to achieve pain relief (237). Similar outcomes in humans treated with alcohol injection and stimulation (229), and an absence of correlation between the degree of injury observed at autopsy and clinical outcomes, further argue against such a mechanism. Neither is tumor regression a likely explanation, since pituitary injections, oophorectomy, adrenalectomy, and orchidectomy all may produce almost immediate pain relief in appropriate patients. Finally, there is little evidence that hypofunction of the pituitary or the anterior hypothalamus, or straightforward hormonal changes underlie pain relief, in that outcome does not correlate with measurable changes in circulating levels of hormones. In addition, the presence and severity of diabetes insipidus, one marker for glandular injury, does not correlate with pain relief (231).

Technique

Pituitary ablation has been carried out variously by neurosurgical or anesthesiology teams, or in collaboration, with apparently similar results (238,239). Both radiologically guided "freehand" and stereotactic techniques have been advocated (235). Plain radiographs of the skull are reviewed to survey the size and position of the sella turcica, as well as to identify any bony abnormalities. Typically, light general endotracheal anesthesia is induced, and a topical vasoconstrictive anesthetic (4% cocaine paste or 7.5% to 20% cocaine-impregnated packs) is applied to the nasal mucosa of the most patent nostril, which is then cleansed with an organic iodine solution.

Modified Moricca ("Freehand") Technique. For the "freehand" or (modified) Moricca approach, with the patient positioned supine and the head semiflexed, a specially designed "Moricca" needle or 17-gauge styletted spinal needle is passed through one nostril toward the pituitary fossa by the transsphenoidal route (Fig. 42-44). Under fluoroscopic guidance, the needle is directed posteriorly, superiorly, and slightly medially toward the glabella (from the frontal plane) and zygomatic arch (viewed laterally). The needle is passed through the posterior nasal mucosa until resistance is encountered, which correlates to the skull base, and it is then advanced incrementally by means of gently tapping its hub with a small metal hammer. The position of the needle tip within the anterior bony margins of the pituitary fossa is confirmed with anterior and posterior radiographs (Figs. 42-45 and 42-46), and the Queckenstedt maneuver is performed to exclude extrusion of CSF or blood. A smaller (20-gauge) needle may be introduced through the original needle and advanced a few millimeters into the substance

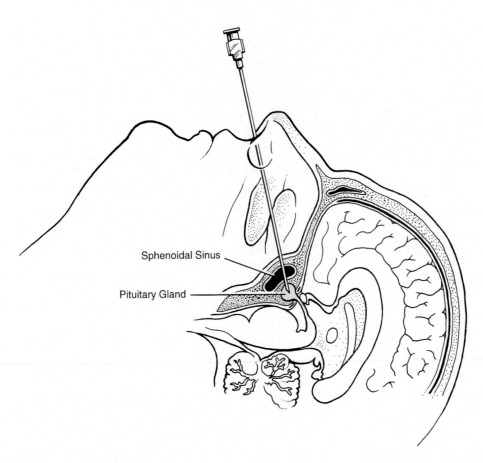

FIGURE 42-44. Pituitary ablation. Technique for pituitary ablation.

of the gland, after which the spread of the injection of a minute quantity of contrast medium is monitored. Moricca's original technique, which employed the administration 2 to 6 mL of absolute alcohol, has yielded to protocols that call for the injection of a total of 0.8 to 1.0 mL of absolute alcohol in 0.1-mL increments over 10 to 15 minutes. During the injection, anesthesia is lightened to facilitate detection of pupillary movement or dilation that may signal damage to the optic chiasm. If pupillary changes occur, some clinicians advocate discontinuing the injection, turning the patient laterally, and administering corticosteroids intracisternally. When the injection is complete, after withdrawing the needle to the sella's anterior border, many advocate the injection of 0.5 mL of cyanomethacralate resin as a sealant to prevent CSF leakage (240).

Stereotactic Technique. A stereotactic approach, pioneered by Levin (231), differs in just a few important ways from Moricca's technique. It involves positioning the patient in a Todd-Wells head holder equipped with a transverse quadrant assembly (Fig. 42-47). The unit's needle holder is advanced through the

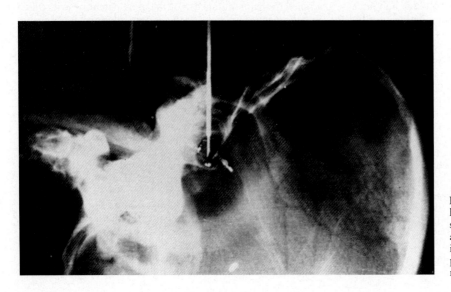

FIGURE 42-45. Pituitary ablation. Chemical hypophysectomy. Radiograph, lateral view, showing needle passing through sphenoid sinus and floor of sella turcica. Tip of needle is immediately below level of posterior clinoid processes. Some injected Myodil can be seen moving up the pituitary stalk.

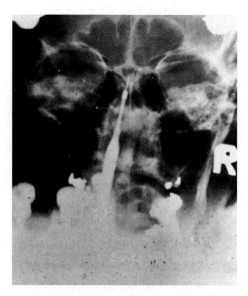

FIGURE 42-46. Pituitary ablation. Anteroposterior view showing needle in midline at target. From Levin AB, Ramidel LL. Treatment of cancer pain with hypophysectomy: Surgical and chemical. In: Benedetti C eds., *Advances in pain research and therapy.* New York: Raven Press, 1984;7:631–646, with permission.

prepared nostril and, with fluoroscopic guidance, the posterosuperior aspect of the sella, just below the posterior clinoid processes in the midline, is targeted using a trajectory that maximizes glandular penetration. After additional infiltration, a 6-inch 18-gauge spinal needle is used to penetrate the floor of the sphenoid sinus, where bacitracin is administered. The 18-gauge needle is replaced with a 6-inch 20-gauge spinal needle, which is gently inserted until its tip is radiographically confirmed to have reached the target region. One to 2 mL of absolute alcohol is slowly injected, following which the needle is withdrawn to a point halfway between the target and the sella's floor, where a second 1- to 2-mL injection is made, and finally, after further withdrawal, a third 1 to 2-mL injec-

tion is performed distally. Anesthesia is lightened and the eyes are monitored during injections, so that the procedure can be discontinued should pupillary changes occur.

In addition to visual impairment, postoperative problems may include CSF leak and diabetes or Addisonism, which may require hormone replacement. Monitoring of blood sugar and urine volume is instituted to detect hormonal insufficiency and diabetes insipidus. Typically, patients are given oral hydrocortisone and, if necessary, vasopressin and/or thyroid supplementation.

Results

Results vary among studies owing in part to differences in patient selection and technique. Bonica and colleagues (238) reviewed the results of 15 clinical series that reported good or complete pain relief in 39% to 87% of patients, and calculated a mean incidence of 86% fair-good results (63% complete or good, 23% fair). In at least one case, analgesia was so profound as to allow a patient previously immobile from pain to return to work for an extended period. Some patients remained free of pain for up to 2 years, and a significant number of patients died painlessly. Pain relief usually develops gradually over the first 24 to 48 hours following the procedure, but in some cases it is immediate and in others accrues over more prolonged periods.

Miles reported six procedure-related deaths in an early series of 250 patients (239), but in recent, more representative studies there is typically no mortality attributed to the procedure (233). The most frequent complications in a large series were self-limited headache (17%), diabetes insipidus (17%), and nausea (9%) (228). Visual disturbance, a potentially serious complication, occurs infrequently.

CONCLUSION

The treatment of intractable pain by means of neural destructive procedures first requires that the pain problem be dissected into its various components, such as somatic, neuropathic, and visceral domains. Feasibility of a procedure should be weighted against projected quality of life, psychological state, and

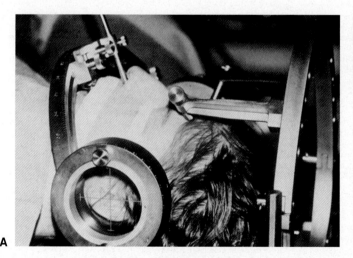

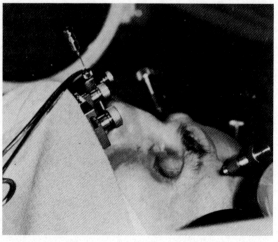

FIGURE 42-47. Pituitary ablation. Chemical hypophysectomy. **A:** Stereotaxic apparatus in place on patient's head. Note needle guide inserted into the nostril. **B:** Spinal needle (20-gauge) inserted into needle guide and then passed into sella turcica. From Levin AB, Ramidel LL. Treatment of cancer pain with hypophysectomy: Surgical and chemical. In: Benedetti C eds., *Advances in pain research and therapy.* New York: Raven Press, 1984;7:631–646, with permission.

social and family dynamics. Treatment techniques must then be selected starting with the simplest percutaneous techniques whenever possible. Progression to more complex techniques is pursued in parallel with the disability caused by the pain, not the underlying disease. The risk-to-benefit ratio is always assessed, bearing in mind the stage of disease and pain in each patient and other factors (physical, psychological, and environmental).

ACKNOWLEDGMENTS

David Niv died suddenly while this chapter was underway. This untimely death was a great loss to the pain community. The preparation of the manuscript was supported by research grant of Department of Anesthesia, Sunnybrook Health Sciences Centre.

References

1. *La Chirurgie de la Douleur.* Paris: Masson, 1937.
2. Siddall P, Cousins MJ. Persistent pain as a disease entity: Implications for clinical management. *Anesth Analg* 2004;99:510–520.
3. Härtel F. Die Leitungsanesthesie und injektions behandlung des ganglion Gasseri und der trigeminusaste. *Arch Klin Chir* 1912;100:193–292.
4. Swetlow G. Paravertebral alcohol block in cardiac pain. *Am Heart J* 1926;1: 393–412.
5. Dogilotti AM. Traitement des syndromes douloreaux de la peripherie par l'alcoholisation subarachnoidienne des racines posterieures à leur émergence de la moelle epineri. *Presse Med* 1931;39:1249–1252.
6. Jones RR. A technique of injection of the splanchnic nerves with alcohol. *Anesth Analg* 1957;36:75–77.
7. Bridenbaugh LD, Moore DC, Campbell DD. Management of upper abdominal cancer pain: Treatment with celiac plexus block with alcohol. *JAMA* 1964;190:877.
8. Mandl F. *Die paravertebral injektion.* Vienna, J Springer, 1926.
9. Totoki T, Kato T, Nomoto Y, et al. Anterior spinal artery syndrome-a complication of cervical intrathecal phenol injection. *Pain* 1979;6:99–104.
10. Sweet WH. Deafferentation pain after posterior rhizotomy, trauma to a limb, and herpes zoster. *Neurosurgery* 1984;15:928–932.
11. Melzack R, Wall PD. Pain mechanisms: A new theory. *Science* 1965;150: 971–979.
12. Sweet WH, Wepsic JC. Controlled thermocoagulation of trigeminal ganglion and rootlets for differential destruction of pain fibers. Trigeminal neuralgia. *J Neurosurgery* 1974;40:143–156.
13. Sweet WH, Mark VH, Hamlin H. Radiofrequency lesions in the central nervous system of man and cat: Including case reports of eight bulbar pain-tract interruptions. *J Neurosurg* 1960;17:213–225.
14. Rosomoff HL, Brown CJ, Sheptak P. Percutaneous radiofrequency cervical cordotomy: technique. *J Neurosurg* 1965;23:639–644.
15. Uematsu S, Udvarhelyi GB, Benson DW, et al. Percutaneous radiofrequency rhizotomy. *Surg Neurol* 1974;2:319–325.
16. Shealy CN. Percutaneous radiofrequency denervation of spinal facets. Treatment for chronic back pain and sciatica. *J Neurosurg* 1975;43:448–451.
17. Wilkinson HA. Radiofrequency percutaneous upper-thoracic sympathectomy. Technique and review of indications. *N Engl J Med* 1984;311:34–36.
18. Cooper IS, Riklan M. Cryothalamectomy for abnormal movement disorders. *St Barnabas Hosp Med Bull* 1962;1:17–23.
19. van Kleef M, Barendse GA, Kessels A, et al. Randomized trial of radiofrequency lumbar facet denervation for chronic low back pain. *Spine* 1999;24: 1937–1942.
20. Gallagher J, Petriccione Di Vadi PL, Wedley JR, et al. Radiofrequency facet joint denervation in the treatment of low back pain: A prospective controlled double-blind study to assess its efficacy. *Pain Clin* 1994;7:193–198.
21. Leclaire R, Fortin L, Lambert R, et al. Radiofrequency facet joint denervation in the treatment of low back pain: A placebo-controlled clinical trial to assess efficacy. *Spine* 2001;26:1411–1416.
22. van Wijk RM, Geurts JW, Wynne HJ, et al. Radiofrequency denervation of lumbar facet joints in the treatment of chronic low back pain: A randomized, double-blind, sham lesion-controlled trial. *Clin J Pain* 2005;21:335–344.
23. Lord SM, Barnsley L, Wallis BJ, et al. Percutaneous radio-frequency neurotomy for chronic cervical zygapophyseal-joint pain. *N Engl J Med* 1996;335: 1721–1726.
24. Eisenberg E, Carr DB, Chalmers TC. Neurolytic celiac plexus block for treatment of cancer pain: A meta-analysis. *Anesth Analg* 1995;80:290–295.
25. Ramamurthy S, Walsh NE, Schoenfeld LS, et al. Evaluation of neurolytic blocks using phenol and cryogenic block in the management of chronic pain. *J Pain Symptom Manage* 1989;4:72–75.
26. Tasker RR. The recurrence of pain after neurosurgical procedures. *Qual Life Res* 1994;3:S43–S49.
27. Wall PD. The placebo effect: An unpopular topic. *Pain* 1992, 51:1–3.
28. Cassinari V, Pagni CA. *Central pain: A neurosurgical survey.* Cambridge, Harvard, 1969.
29. Barnsley L, Lord S, Bogduk N. Comparative local anesthetic blocks in the diagnosis of cervical zygapophysial joints pain. *Pain* 1993;55:99–106.
30. Bogduk N. Diagnosing lumbar zygapophysial joint pain. *Pain Med* 2005;6: 139–142.
31. Lord S, Barnsley L, Bogduk N. The utility of comparative local anesthetic blocks versus placebo-controlled blocks for the diagnosis of cervical zygapophysial joint pain. *Clin J Pain* 1995;11:208–213.
32. Sweet WH. Treatment of trigeminal neuralgia by percutaneous rhizotomy. In: Youmans JR, ed. *Neurological surgery: A comprehensive reference guide to the diagnosis and management of neurosurgical problems,* 3rd ed. Philadelphia: WB Saunders, 1990:3888–3921.
33. Goldberg SN, Gazelle GS, Dawson SL, et al. Tissue ablation with radiofrequency: Effect of probe size, gauge, duration, and temperature on lesion volume. *Acad Radiol* 1995;2:399–404.
34. Bogduk N, Macintosh J, Marsland A. Technical limitations to the efficacy of radiofrequency neurotomy for spinal pain. *Neurosurgery* 1987;20:529–534.
35. Lord SM, McDonald GJ, Bogduk N. Percutaneous radiofrequency neurotomy of the cervical medial branches: A validated treatment for cervical zygapophysial joint pain. *Neurosurgery Quarterly* 1998;8:288–308.
36. Lloyd J, Barnard J, Glynn C. Cryoanalgesia, a new approach to pain relief. *Lancet* 1976;2:932–934.
37. Garamy G. Engineering aspects of cryosurgery. In: Rand RW, Rinfret AP, von Leden H, eds., *Cryosurgery.* IL: Springfield, Charles C. Thomas, 1968:92–132.
38. Myers RR, Powell HC, Heckman HM, et al. Biophysical and pathological effects of cryogenic nerve lesion. *Ann Neurol* 1981;10:478–485.
39. Sunderland S. *Nerves and nerve injuries.* Edinburgh & London: Livingstone, 1968.
40. Trescot A. Cryoanalgesia in interventional pain management. *Pain Physician* 2003;6:345–360.
41. Manchikanti L, Abdi S, Lucas L. Evidence synthesis and development of guidelines in interventional pain management. *Pain Physician* 2005;8:73–86.
42. Katz J. The current role of neurolytic agents. *Adv Neurol* 1974;4:471–476.
43. Moore DC. Role of nerve block in neurolytic solutions for pelvic visceral cancer pain. In: Bonica JJ, Ventafridda V, eds., *Advances in pain research and therapy.* New York: Raven Press, 1979;2:593–596.
44. Papo I, Visca A. Phenol subarachnoid rhizotomy for the treatment of cancer pain: A personal account on 290 cases. In: Bonica JJ, Ventafridda V, eds., *Advances in pain research and therapy.* New York: Raven Press, 1979;2:339–346.
45. Robertson DH. Transsacral neurolytic nerve block. An alternative approach to intractable perineal pain. *Br J Anaesth* 1983;55:873–875.
46. Swerdlow M. Subarachnoid and extradural neurolytic blocks. In: Bonica JJ, Ventafridda V, eds., *Advances in pain research and therapy.* New York: Raven Press, 1979;2:325–337.
47. Ventafridda V, Spreafico R. Subarachnoid saline perfusion. In: Bonica JJ, ed. *Advances in neurology.* New York: Raven Press, 1974;4:477–484.
48. Meyerson BA. Neurosurgical approaches to pain treatment. *Acta Anaesthesiol Scand* 2001;45:1108–1113.
49. Carlsson CA, Persson K, Pelletieri L. Painful scars after thoracic and abdominal surgery. *Acta Chir Scand* 1985;151:309–311.
50. Pikus HJ, Phillips JM. Outcome of surgical decompression of the second cervical root for cervicogenic headache. *Neurosurgery* 1996;39:63–70.
51. Blume HG. Radiofrequency denervation in occipital pain: A new approach in 114 cases. In: Bonica JJ, Albe-Fessard DG, eds., *Advances in pain research and therapy.* New York: Raven Press, 1976;1:691–698.
52. Tasker RR. Deafferentation. In: Wall PD, Melzack RM, eds., *Textbook of pain.* Edinburgh: Churchill Livingstone, 1984:119–132.
53. Lewis RN. The use of combined suprascapular and circumflex (articular branches) nerve blocks in the management of chronic arthritis of the shoulder joint. *Eur J Anaesthesiol* 1999;16:37–41.

54. Malik A, Simopolous T, Elkersh M, et al. Percutaneous radiofrequency lesioning of sensory branches of the obturator and femoral nerves for the treatment of non-operable hip pain. *Pain Physician* 2003;6:499–502.

55. Wang JK. Cryoanalgesia for painful peripheral nerve lesions. *Pain* 1985:22:191–194.

56. Gybels JM, Sweet WH. Neurosurgical treatment of persistent pain; physiological and pathological mechanisms of human pain. In: Gildenberg PL, ed. *Pain and headache*. Basel: Karger, 1989:1–402.

57. Uematsu S. Percutaneous electrothermocoagulation of spinal nerve trunk. ganglion and rootlets. In: Schmidek HH, Sweet W, eds., *Operative neurosurgical techniques: Indications that method, and results*. New York: Grune & Stratton,1982:1177–1198.

58. Nash TP. Percutaneous radiofrequency lesioning of dorsal root ganglia for intractable pain. *Pain* 1986;24:67–73.

59. van Kleef M, Barendse GA, Dingemans WA, et al. Effects of producing a radiofrequency lesion adjacent to the dorsal root ganglion in patients with thoracic segmental pain. *Clin J Pain* 1995;11:325–332.

60. van Wijk RM, Geurts JW, Wynne HJ. Long-lasting analgesic effect of radiofrequency treatment of the lumbosacral dorsal root ganglion. *J Neurosurg* 2001;94:227–231.

61. van Kleef M, Liem L, Lousberg R, et al. Radiofrequency lesion adjacent to the dorsal root ganglion for cervicobrachial pain: A prospective double blind randomized study. *Neurosurgery* 1996;38:1127–1131.

62. Geurts JW, van Wijk RM, Wynne HJ, et al. Radiofrequency lesioning of dorsal root ganglia for chronic lumbosacral radicular pain: A randomised, double-blind, controlled trial. *Lancet* 2003;361:21–26.

63. Carr DB, Goudas LC. Burning questions, randomized controlled trials, and the pain doctor's dilemma. *Reg Anesth Pain Med* 2003;28:360–361.

64. Herz DA, Parsons KC, Pearl L. Percutaneous radiofrequency foraminal rhizotomies. *Spine* 1983;8:729–732.

65. Kasdon DL, Lathi ES. A prospective study of radiofrequency rhizotomy in the treatment of posttraumatic spasticity. *Neurosurgery* 1984;15:526–529.

66. Pagura JR. Percutaneous radiofrequency spinal rhizotomy. *Appl Neurophysiol* 1983;46:138–148.

67. Dubuisson D. Root surgery. In: Wall PD, Melzack R, eds., *Textbook of pain*, 3rd ed. Edinburgh: Churchill Livingstone, 1994:1055–1065.

68. van Kleef M, Spaans F, Dingemans W, et al. Effects and side effects of a percutaneous thermal lesion of the dorsal root ganglion in patients with cervical pain syndrome. *Pain* 1993;52:49–53.

69. Sehgal N, Shah RV, McKenzie-Brown A, et al. Diagnostic utility of facet (zygapophysial) joint injections in chronic spinal pain: A systematic review of evidence. *Pain Physician* 2005;8:211–224.

70. Govind J, King W, Bailey B, et al. Radiofrequency neurotomy for the treatment of third occipital headache. *J Neurol Neurosurg Psychiatry* 2003;74:88–93.

71. Faclier G, Kay J. Cervical facet radiofrequency neurotomy. *Tech Reg Anesth Pain Manage* 2000;4:120–125.

72. McDonald GJ, Lord SM, Bogduk N. Long-term follow-up of patients treated with cervical radiofrequency neurotomy for chronic neck pain. *Neurosurgery* 1999;45:61–67.

73. Chua WH, Bogduk N. The surgical anatomy of thoracic facet denervation. *Acta Neurochir* 1995;136:140–144.

74. Stolker RJ, Vervest AC, Groen GJ. Percutaneous facet denervation in chronic thoracic spinal pain. *Acta Neurochir (Wien)* 1993;122:82–90.

75. Bogduk N, Long DM. The anatomy of the so-called "articular nerves" and their relationship to facet denervation in the treatment of low-back pain. *J Neurosurg* 1979;51:172–177.

76. Lau P, Mercer S, Govind J, et al. The surgical anatomy of lumbar medial branch neurotomy (facet denervation). *Pain Med* 2004;5:289–298.

77. Paris S. Anatomy as related to function and pain. *Orthop Clin North Am* 1983;14:475–489.

78. Dreyfuss P, Halbrook B, Pauza K, et al. Efficacy and validity of radiofrequency neurotomy for chronic lumbar zygapophysial joint pain. *Spine* 2000;25:1270–1277.

79. Gofeld M. Radiofrequency facet denervation: A randomized control placebo versus sham procedure. *Clin J Pain* 2006;22:410–411.

80. Gofeld M, Jain J, Faclier G. Radiofrequency denervation of the lumbar zygapophysial joints: 10-year prospective clinical audit. *Pain Physician* 2007;10:291–300.

81. Barlocher CB, Krauss JK, Seiler RW. Kryorhizotomy: An alternative technique for lumbar medial branch rhizotomy in lumbar facet syndrome. *J Neurosurg* 2003;98:14–20.

82. Birkenmaier C, Veihelmann A, Trouillier H, et al. Percutaneous cryodenervation of lumbar facet joints: A prospective clinical trial. *Int Orthop* 2006 Aug 23; [Epub ahead of print].

83. Forst SL, Wheeler MT, Fortin JD, et al. The sacroiliac joint: Anatomy, physiology and clinical significance. *Pain Physician* 2006;9:61–67.

84. Grob K, Neuhuber W, Kissling R. Innervation of the sacroiliac joint of the human. *Z Rheumatol* 1995;54:117–122.

85. Bogduk N, ed. ISIS guidelines. Practice guidelines for spinal diagnostic and treatment procedures. San Francisco, CA: International Spine Intervention Society; 2004.

86. Ferrante FM, King LF, Roche EA, et al. Radiofrequency sacroiliac joint denervation for sacroiliac syndrome. *Reg Anesth Pain Med* 2001;26:137–142.

87. Yin W, Willard F, Carreiro J, et al. Sensory stimulation-guided sacroiliac joint radiofrequency neurotomy: Technique based on neuroanatomy of the dorsal sacral plexus. *Spine* 2003;28:2419–2425.

88. Cohen SP, Abdi S. Lateral branch blocks as a treatment for sacroiliac joint pain: A pilot study. *Reg Anesth Pain Med* 2003;28:113–119.

89. Simopoulos TT, Malik AB, Sial KA, et al. Radiofrequency lesioning of the L2 ramus communicans in managing discogenic low back pain. *Pain Physician* 2005;8:61–65.

90. Oh WS, Shim JC. A randomized controlled trial of radiofrequency denervation of the ramus communicans nerve for chronic discogenic low back pain. *Clin J Pain* 2004;20:55–60.

91. Katusic S, Williams DB, Beard CM, et al. Epidemiology and clinical features of idiopathic trigeminal neuralgia and glossopharyngeal neuralgia: Similarities and differences, Rochester, Minnesota, 1945–1984. *Neuroepidemiology* 1991;10:276–281.

92. Loeser JD. Tic douloureux and atypical face pain. In: Wall PD, Melzack R. eds., *Textbook of pain*, 3rd ed. Edinburgh: Churchill Livingstone, 1994:669–710.

93. Loeser JD. Herpes zoster and postherpetic neuralgia. *Pain* 1986;25:149–164.

94. Turnbull IM. Percutaneous rhizotomy for trigeminal neuralgia. *Surg Neurol* 1974;2:385–389.

95. Tucker WS, Fleming R, Taylor FA, et al. Trigeminal neuralgia in aqueduct stenosis. *Can J Neurol Sci* 1978;5:331–333.

96. Jannetta PJ. Arterial compression of the trigeminal nerve at the pons in patients with trigeminal neuralgia. *J Neurosurg* 1967;26 Suppl:159–162.

97. Taarnhöj P. Decompression of the trigeminal root and the posterior part of the ganglion as treatment in trigeminal neuralgia. Preliminary communication. *J Neurosurg* 1952:9:288–290.

98. Sheldon CH, Pudenz RH, Freshwater DB, et al. Compression rather than decompression for trigeminal neuralgia. *J Neurosurg* 1955;12:123–126.

99. Mullan S, Lichtor T. Percutaneous microcompression of the trigeminal ganglion for trigeminal neuralgia. *J Neurosurg* 1983;59:1007–1012.

100. Jannetta PJ. Observation on the etiology of trigeminal neuralgia, hemifacial spasm, acoustic nerve dysfunction, and glossopharyngeal neuralgia: Definitive microsurgical treatment and results in 117 patients. *Neurochirurgia* 1977;20:145–154.

101. Apfelbaum RI. Surgical management of disorders of the lower cranial nerves. In: Schmidek HH, Sweet WH, eds., *Current techniques in operative neurosurgery*, 2nd ed. New York: Grune & Stratton, Inc., 1988:1097–1109.

102. Lopez BC, Hamlyn PJ, Zakrzewska JM. Systematic review of ablative neurosurgical techniques for the treatment of trigeminal neuralgia. *Neurosurgery* 2004;54:973–982.

103. Kirschner M. Elektrokoagulation des Ganglion Gasseri. *Zentralbl Chir* 1932;47:2841.

104. Nugent GR, Berry B. Trigeminal neuralgia treated by differential percutaneous radiofrequency coagulation of the Gasserian ganglion. *J Neurosurg.* 1974;40:517–523.

105. Tew JM Jr., Taha JM. Percutaneous rhizotomy in the treatment of intractable facial pain (trigeminal, glossopharyngeal, and vagal nerves). In: Schmidek HH, Sweet WH, eds., *Operative neurosurgical techniques: Indications, methods, and results*. Philadelphia: WB Saunders, 1995:1469–1484.

106. Tobler WD, Tew JM Jr., Cosman E, et al. Improved outcome in the treatment of trigeminal neuralgia by percutaneous stereotactic rhizotomy with a new, curved tip electrode. *Neurosurgery* 1983;12:313–317.

107. Tasker R. Neurostimulation and percutaneous neural destructive techniques. In: Cousins MJ, Bridenbaugh PO, eds., *Neural blockade in clinical anesthesia and management of pain*, 3rd ed. Philadelphia: Lippincott-Raven, 1998:1063–1112.

108. Tew JM Jr., Keller JT. The treatment of trigeminal neuralgia by percutaneous radiofrequency technique. *Clin Neurosurg* 1977;24:557–578.

109. Latchaw JP Jr., Hardy RW Jr., Forsythe SB, et al. Trigeminal neuralgia treated by radiofrequency coagulation. *J Neurosurg* 1983;59:479–484.

110. Ecker A, Perl T. Alcoholic gasserian injection for relief of tic douloureux; preliminary report of a modification of Penman's method. *Neurology* 1958;8:461–468.

111. Hakanson S. Trigeminal neuralgia treated by the injection of glycerol into the trigeminal cistern. *Neurosurgery* 1981;9:638–646.

112. Sweet WH, Poletti CE, Macon JB. Treatment of trigeminal neuralgia and other facial pains by the retrogasserian injection of glycerol. *Neurosurgery* 1981;9:647–653.

113. Lunsford LD, Bennett MH. Percutaneous retrogasserian glycerol rhizotomy for tic douloureux: Part 1. Technique and results in 112 patients. *Neurosurgery* 1984;14:424–430.

114. Bricolo A, Dalle Ore G. Percutaneous microcompression of the gasserian ganglion for trigeminal neuralgia; preliminary results. *Acta Neurochir* 1983;69:102.

115. Lobato RD, Rivas JJ, Sarabia R, et al. Percutaneous microcompression of the gasserian ganglion for trigeminal neuralgia. *J Neurosurg* 1990;72:546–553.

PART IV: PAIN MANAGEMENT

116. Belber CJ, Rak RA. Balloon compression rhizolysis in the surgical management of trigeminal neuralgia. *Neurosurgery* 1987;20:908–913.
117. Zanusso M, Curri D, Landi A, et al. Pressure monitoring inside Meckel's cave during percutaneous microcompression of gasserian ganglion. *Stereotact Funct Neurosurg* 1991;56:37–43.
118. Siegfried J, Broggi G. Percutaneous thermocoagulation of the gasserian ganglion in the treatment of pain in advanced cancer. In: Bonica JJ, Ventafridda V, eds., *Advances in pain research and therapy*. New York: Raven Press, 1979;2:463–469.
119. Maxwell RE. Surgical control of chronic migrainous neuralgia by trigeminal ganglio-rhizolysis. *J Neurosurg* 1982;57:459–466.
120. Watson CP, Morley TP, Richardson JC, et al. The surgical treatment of chronic cluster headache. *Headache* 1983 Nov;23(6):289–295.
121. Onofrio BM, Campbell JK. Surgical treatment of chronic cluster headache. *Mayo Clin Proc* 1986;61:537–544.
122. Rozenal JM. Cluster headache. In: Benzon HT, Raja SN, Borsook D, Molloy RE, Stricharz G, eds., *Essentials of pain medicine and regional anesthesia*. Philadelphia: Churchill Livingstone, 1999:191–193.
123. Salar G, Ori C, Iob I, et al. Percutaneous thermocoagulation for sphenopalatine ganglion neuralgia. *Acta Neurochir (Wien)* 1987;84:24–28.
124. Sanders M, Zuurmond WW. Efficacy of sphenopalatine ganglion blockade in 66 patients suffering from cluster headache: A 12- to 70-month follow-up evaluation. *J Neurosurg* 1997;87:876–880.
125. Isamat F, Ferran E, Acebes JJ. Selective percutaneous thermocoagulation rhizotomy in essential glossopharyngeal neuralgia. *J Neurosurg* 1981;55:575–580.
126. Bruyn GW. Superior laryngeal neuralgia. *Cephalalgia* 1983;3:235–240.
127. Katusic S, Williams DB, Beard CM, et al. Incidence and clinical features of glossopharyngeal neuralgia, Rochester, Minnesota, 1945–1984. *Neuroepidemiology* 1991;10:266–275.
128. King J. Glossopharyngeal neuralgia. *Clin Exp Neurol* 1987;24:113–121.
129. Rushton JG, Stevens JC, Miller RH. Glossopharyngeal (vagoglossopharyngeal) neuralgia: A study of 217 cases. *Arch Neurol* 1981;38:201–205.
130. Sindou M, Fischer G, Goutelle A, et al. La radicellotomie postérieure sélective. Premiers résultats dans la chirurgie de la douleur. *Neurochirurgie* 1974;20:391–408.
131. Reddy K, Hobson DE, Gomori A, et al. Painless glossopharyngeal "neuralgia" with syncope: A case report and literature review. *Neurosurgery* 1987;21:916–919.
132. Giorgi C, Broggi G. Surgical treatment of glossopharyngeal neuralgia and pain from cancer of the nasopharynx. A 20-year experience. *J Neurosurg* 1984;61:952–955.
133. Lazorthes Y, Verdie JC. Radiofrequency coagulation of the petrous ganglion in glossopharyngeal neuralgia. *Neurosurgery* 1979;4:512–516.
134. Ori C, Salar G, Giron GP. Cardiovascular and cerebral complications during glossopharyngeal nerve thermocoagulation. *Anaesthesia* 1985;40:433–437.
135. Broggi G, Siegfried J. Percutaneous differential radiofrequency rhizotomy of glossopharyngeal nerve in facial pain due to cancer. In Bonica JJ, Ventafridda V, eds., *Advances in pain research and therapy*. New York: Raven Press, 1979;2:469–473.
136. Pagura JR, Schnapp M, Passarelli P. Percutaneous radiofrequency glossopharyngeal rhizotomy for cancer pain. *Appl Neurophysiol* 1983;46:154–159.
137. Salar G, Ori C, Baratto V, et al. Selective percutaneous thermolesions of the ninth cranial nerve by lateral cervical approach: Report of eight cases. *Surg Neurol* 1983;20:276–279.
138. Tasker RR, Dostrovsky JO. Deafferentation and central pain. In: Wall PD, Melzack R, eds., *Textbook of pain,* 2nd ed. Edinburgh: Churchill Livingstone, 1988:154–180.
139. Loh L, Nathan PW, Schott GD. Pain due to lesions of central nervous system removed by sympathetic block. *Br Med J (Clin Res Ed)* 1981;282:1026–1028.
140. Kim SH, Chung JM. Sympathectomy alleviates mechanical allodynia in an experimental animal model for neuropathy in the rat. *Neurosci Lett* 1991; 134:131–134.
141. Schott GD. Interrupting the sympathetic outflow in causalgia and reflex sympathetic dystrophy. *Br Med J* 1998;316:791–793.
142. Cepeda MS, Lau J, Carr DB. Defining the therapeutic role of local anesthetic sympathetic blockade in complex regional pain syndrome: A narrative and systematic review. *Clin J Pain* 2002;18:216–233.
143. Hartrick CT, Kovan JP, Naismith P. Outcome prediction following sympathetic block for complex regional pain syndrome. *Pain Practice* 2004;4:222–228.
144. Kuntz A. Distribution of the sympathetic nerve to the brachial plexus. *Arch Surg* 1927;15:871–877.
145. Abram SE, Boas RA. Sympathetic and visceral nerve blocks. In: Benumof JL, ed., *Clinical procedures in anesthesia and intensive care*. Philadelphia: JB Lippincott, 1993:787–805.
146. Rocco AG, Palomgi D, Raeke D. Anatomy of the lumbar sympathetic chain. *Reg Anesth* 1995;20:13–19.
147. Superville-Sovak B, Rasminsky M, Finlayson MH. Complications of phenol neurolysis. *Arch Neurol* 1975;32:226–228.
148. Kastler B, Michalakis D, Clair CH, et al. Stellate ganglion radiofrequency neurolysis under CT guidance. Preliminary study. *BR-BTR* 2001;84:191–194.
149. Forouzanfar T, van Kleef M, Weber WE. Radiofrequency lesions of the stellate ganglion in chronic pain syndromes: Retrospective analysis of clinical efficacy in 86 patients. *Clin J Pain* 2000;16:164–168.
150. Koman LA, Smith BP, Pollock FE Jr., et al. The microcirculatory effects of peripheral sympathectomy. *J Hand Surg [Am]* 1995;20:709–717.
151. Matsumoto Y, Ueyama T, Endo M, et al. Endoscopic thoracic sympathectomy for Raynaud's phenomenon. *J Vasc Surg* 2002;36:57–61.
152. Raj PP, Lou L, Erdine S, et al, eds., T2 and T3 Sympathetic Nerve Block and Neurolysis. *Radiographic imaging for regional anesthesia and pain management*. Philadelphia: Churchill Livingstone, 2003:132–137.
153. Wang YC, Wei SH, Sun MH, et al. A new mode of percutaneous upper thoracic phenol sympatholysis: Report of 50 cases. *Neurosurgery* 2001;49:628–634.
154. Yarzebski JL, Wilkinson HA. T2 and T3 sympathetic ganglia in the adult human: A cadaver and clinical-radiographic study and its clinical application. *Neurosurgery* 1987;21:339–342.
155. Wang YC, Sun MH, Lin CW, et al. Anatomical location of T2–3 sympathetic trunk and Kuntz nerve determined by transthoracic endoscopy. *J Neurosurg* 2002;96:68–72.
156. Singh B, Ramsaroop L, Partab P, et al. Anatomical variations of the second thoracic ganglion. *Surg Radiol Anat* 2005;27:119–122.
157. Gofeld M, Faclier G. Bilateral pain relief after unilateral thoracic percutaneous sympathectomy. *Can J Anaesth* 2006;53:258–262.
158. Wilkinson HA. Percutaneous radiofrequency upper thoracic sympathectomy: A new technique. *Neurosurgery* 1984;15:811–814.
159. Chuang KS, Liu JC. Long-term assessment of percutaneous stereotactic thermocoagulation of upper thoracic ganglionectomy and sympathectomy for palmar and craniofacial hyperhidrosis in 1742 cases. *Neurosurgery* 2002;51:963–969.
160. Malfertheiner P, Dominquez-Munoz JE, Buchler MW. Chronic pancreatitis: Management of pain. *Digestion* 1994;55(Suppl 1):29–34.
161. Garcea G, Thomasset S, Berry DP, et al. Percutaneous splanchnic nerve radiofrequency ablation for chronic abdominal pain. *ANZ J Surg* 2005;75:640–644.
162. Reid W, Watt JK, Gray TG. Phenol injection of the sympathetic chain. *Br J Surg* 1970;57:45–50.
163. Dondelinger R, Kurdziel JC. Percutaneous phenol neurolysis of the lumbar sympathetic chain with computed tomography control. *Ann Radiol* 1984; 27:376–379.
164. Cross FW, Cotton LT. Chemical lumbar sympathectomy for ischemic rest pain. A randomized, prospective controlled clinical trial. *Am J Surg* 1985; 150:341–345.
165. Cousins MJ, Reeve TS, Glynn CJ, et al. Neurolytic lumbar sympathetic blockade: Duration of denervation and relief of rest pain. *Anaesth Intensive Care* 1979;7:121–35.
166. Haynsworth RF Jr., Noe CE. Percutaneous lumbar sympathectomy: A comparison of radiofrequency denervation versus phenol neurolysis. *Anesthesiology* 1991;74:459–463.
167. Rocco AG. Radiofrequency lumbar sympatholysis. The evolution of a technique for managing sympathetically maintained pain. *Reg Anesth* 1995; 20:3–12.
168. Plancarte R, Amescua C, Patt RB, et al. Superior hypogastric plexus block for pelvic cancer pain. *Anesthesiology* 1990;73:236–239.
169. Wechsler RJ, Maurer PM, Halpern EJ, et al. Superior hypogastric plexus block for chronic pelvic pain in the presence of endometriosis: CT techniques and results. *Radiology* 1995;196:103–106.
170. McDonald JS. Management of chronic pelvic pain. *Obstet Gynecol Clin North Am* 1993;20:817–838.
171. Reig E, Abejón D, del Pozo C, et al. Thermocoagulation of the ganglion impar or ganglion of Walther: Description of a modified approach. Preliminary results in chronic, nononcological pain. *Pain Practice* 2005;5:103–110.
172. Izumi J, Hirose Y, Yazaki T. Percutaneous trigeminal rhizotomy and percutaneous cordotomy under general anesthesia. *Stereotact Funct Neurosurg* 1992;59:62–68.
173. Tasker RR. Percutaneous cordotomy: The lateral high cervical technique. In: Schmidek HH, Sweet WH, eds., *Operative neurosurgical techniques indications, methods, and results,* 2nd ed. Philadelphia: WB Saunders, 1988:1191–1205.
174. Tasker RR. Percutaneous cordotomy. In: Youmans JR, ed. *Neurological surgery. A comprehensive reference guide to the diagnosis and management of neurosurgical problems,* 3rd ed. Philadelphia: Saunders, 1990:4045–4069.
175. Tasker RR. Percutaneous cordotomy. In: Schmidek HH, Sweet WH, eds., *Operative neurosurgical techniques,* 3rd ed. Philadelphia: Saunders, 1995: 1595–1611.
176. Poletti CE. Open cordotomy and medullary tractotomy. In: Schmidek HH, Sweet WH. *Operative neurosurgical techniques,* 3rd ed. Philadelphia: Saunders, 1995:1557–1572.

177. Siegfried J, Kuhner A, Sturm V. Neurosurgical treatment of cancer pain. *Recent Results Cancer Res* 1984;89:148–156.
178. Probst CL. Microsurgical cordotomy in 20 patients with epi/intradural fibrosis following operation for lumbar disc herniation. *Acta Neurochir* 1990;107:30–36.
179. Spiller WG, Martin E. The treatment of persistent pain of organic origin in the lower part of the body by division of the anterolateral column of the spinal cord. *JAMA* 1912;58:1489–1490.
180. Mullan S, Harper PV, Hekmatpanah J, et al. Percutaneous interruption of spinal pain tracts by means of a strontium-90 needle. *J Neurosurg* 1963;20:931–939.
181. Onofrio BM. Cervical spinal cord and dentate delineation in percutaneous radiofrequency cordotomy at the level of the first to second cervical vertebrae. *Surg Gynecol Obstet* 1971;133:30–34.
182. Gildenberg PL, Zanes C, Flitter M, et al. Impedance monitoring device for detection of penetration of the spinal cord in anterior percutaneous cervical cordotomy. Technical note. *J Neurosurg* 1969;30:87– 92.
183. Hitchcock ER, Tsukamoto Y. Distal and proximal sensory responses during stereotactic spinal tractotomy in man. *Ann Clin Res* 1973;5:68–73.
184. Taren JA, Davis R, Crosby EC. Target physiologic corroboration in stereotactic cervical cordotomy. *J Neurosurg* 1969;30:569–584.
185. Tasker RR, Organ LW, Smith KC. Physiological guidelines for the localization of lesions by percutaneous cordotomy. *Acta Neurochir* 1974;Suppl 21:111–117.
186. Kanpolat Y, Deda H, Akyar S, et al. CT-guided percutaneous cordotomy. *Acta Neurochir* 1989;46:67–68.
187. Hitchcock ER. An apparatus for stereotactic spinal surgery. *Lancet* 1969;1:705–706.
188. Hitchcock ER. Stereotactic spinal surgery. A preliminary report. *J Neurosurg* 1969;31:386–392.
189. Crue BL, Todd EM, Carregal EJA. Posterior approach for high cervical percutaneous radiofrequency cordotomy. *Confin Neurol* 1968;30:41–52.
190. Lin PM, Gildenberg PL, Polakoff PP. An anterior approach to percutaneous lower cervical cordotomy. *J Neurosurg* 1966;25:553–560.
191. Tasker R. Pain resulting from central nervous system pathology (central pain). In: Bonica JJ, ed., *The management of pain*, 2nd ed. Philadelphia: Lea & Febiger, 1990:264–283.
192. Tasker RR, de Carvalho GT, Dolan EJ. Intractable pain of spinal cord origin: Clinical features and implications for surgery. *J Neurosurg* 1992;77:373–378.
193. Jones B, Finlay I, Ray A, et al. Is there still a role for open cordotomy in cancer pain management? *J Pain Symptom Manage* 2003;25:179–184.
194. Fox JL. Localization of the respiratory pathway in the upper cervical spinal cord following percutaneous cordotomy. *Neurology* 1969;19:1115–1118.
195. Hitchcock ER, Leece B. Somatotopic representation of the respiratory pathways in the cervical cord of man. *J Neurosurg* 1969;27:320–329.
196. Mullan S, Hosobuchi Y. Respiratory hazards of high cervical percutaneous cordotomy. *J Neurosurg* 1968;28:291–297.
197. Nathan PW. The descending respiratory pathway in man. *J Neurol Neurosurg Psychiatry* 1963;26:487–499.
198. Rosomoff HL, Krieger AJ, Kuperman AS. Effects of percutaneous cervical cordotomy on pulmonary function. *J Neurosurg* 1969;31:620–627.
199. Tenicela R, Rosomoff HL, Feist J, et al. Pulmonary function following percutaneous cervical cordotomy. *Anesthesiology* 1968;29:7–16.
200. Lema JA, Hitchcock E. Respiratory changes after stereotactic high cervical cord lesions for pain. *Appl Neurophysiol* 1986;49:62–68.
201. Navani A, Dominguez CL, Hald JK, et al. An injection from the past: Fluoroscopic evidence of remote injections of radiopaque substances. *Reg Anesth Pain Med* 2006;31:82–85.
202. Krol G, Arbit E. Percutaneous lateral cervical cordotomy: Target localization with water-soluble contrast medium. *J Neurosurg* 1993;79:390–392.
203. Tasker RR. The problem of deafferentation pain in the management of the patient with cancer. *J Palliat Care* 1987;2:8–12.
204. Bowsher D. Contralateral mirror-image pain following anterolateral cordotomy. *Pain* 1988;33:63–65.
205. Ischia S, Ischia A. A mechanism of new pain following cordotomy (letter). *Pain* 1988;32:383–384.
206. Nagara T, Kimura S, Arai T. A mechanism of new pain following cordotomy: Reference of sensation. *Pain* 1988;30:89–91.
207. Nagara T, Amakawa K, Arai T, et al. Ipsilateral referral of pain following cordotomy. *Pain* 1993;55:275–276.
208. Hitchcock ER. Stereotactic cervical myelotomy. *J Neurol Neurosurg Psychiatry* 1970;33:224–230.
209. Armour D. Surgery of the spinal cord and its membranes. *Lancet* 1927;i:691–697.
210. Cook AW, Nathan PW, Smith MC. Sensory consequences of commissural myelotomy. A challenge to traditional anatomical concepts. *Brain* 1984;107:547–568.
211. Eiras J, Garcia J, Gomez J, et al. First results with extralemniscal myelotomy. *Acta Neurochir Suppl (Wien)* 1980;30:377–381.
212. Papo I. Commissural posterior spinal rhizotomy and myelotomy in the treatment of cancer pain. In: Bonica JJ, Ventafrida V, eds., *Advances in pain research and therapy*. New York: Raven Press, 1979;2:439–448.
213. Crue BL, Todd EM, Carregal EJ, et al. Percutaneous trigeminal tractotomy— case report utilizing stereotactic radiofrequency lesion. *Bull Los Angeles Neurol Soc* 1967;32:86–92.
214. Fox JL. Delineation of the obex by contrast radiography during percutaneous trigeminal tractotomy. Technical note. *J Neurosurg* 1972;36:107–112.
215. Fox JL. Percutaneous trigeminal tractotomy. Variations in delineation of the obex using emulsified Pantopaque. *Confin Neurol* 1974;36:97–100.
216. Schvarcz JR. Spinal cord stereotactic techniques re trigeminal nucleotomy and extralemniscal myelotomy. *Appl Neurophysiol* 1978;41:99–112.
217. Schvarcz JR. Stereotactic spinal trigeminal nucleotomy for dysesthetic facial pain. In: Bonica JJ, Liebeskind JC, Albe-Fessard DG, eds., *Advances in pain research and therapy*. New York: Raven Press, 1979;3:331–336.
218. Hitchcock ER, Schvarcz JR. Stereotaxic trigeminal tractotomy for postherpetic facial pain. *J Neurosurg* 1972;37:412–417.
219. Hyndman O R. Lissauer's tract section. Contribution to chordotomy for the relief of pain (preliminary report). *J Internat Coll Surgeons* 1942;5:394–400.
220. Nashold BS, Ostdahl RH. Dorsal root entry zone lesions for pain relief. *J Neurosurg* 1979;51:59–69.
221. Bernard EJ Jr., Nashold BS Jr., Caputi F, et al. Nucleus caudalis DREZ lesions for facial pain. *Br J Neurosurg* 1987;1:81–91.
222. Todd EM, Crue BL, Carregal EJ. Posterior percutaneous tractotomy and cordotomy. *Confin Neurol* 1969;31:106–115.
223. Nauta HJ, Soukup VM, Fabian RH, et al. Punctate midline myelotomy for the relief of visceral cancer pain. *J Neurosurg.* 2000;92:125–30.
224. Vilela Filho O, Araujo MR, Florencio RS, et al. CT-guided percutaneous punctate midline myelotomy for the treatment of intractable visceral pain: A technical note. *Stereotact Funct Neurosurg* 2001;77:177–182.
225. Luft R, Olivecrona H, Sjogren B. Hypophysectomy in man. *Nord Med* 1952;47:351–354.
226. Greco T. [Alcoholization of the pituitary gland. Advantages of this method in the treatment of malignant tumors ond of their recurrence.] *Urol Int* 1965;19:54–57.
227. Moricca G. Chemical hypophysectomy for cancer pain. In: Bonica JJ, ed., *Advances in neurology*. New York: Raven Press, 1974;4:707–714.
228. Duthie AM, Ingham V, Dell AE, et al. Pituitary cryoablation. The results of treatment using a transsphenoidal cryoprobe. *Anaesthesia* 1983;38:448–451.
229. Yanagida H, Corssen G, Trouwborst A, et al. Relief of cancer pain in man: Alcohol-induced neuroadenolysis vs electrical stimulation of the pituitary gland. *Pain* 1984;19:133–141.
230. Katz J, Levin AB. Treatment of diffuse metastatic cancer pain by instillation of alcohol into the sella turcica. *Anesthesiology* 1977;46:115–121.
231. Levin AB, Ramirez LL. Treatment of cancer pain with hypophysectomy: Surgical and chemical. In: Benedetti C ed., *Advances in pain research and therapy*. New York: Raven Press, 1984;7:631–646.
232. Lloyd JW, Rawlinson WA, Evans PJ. Selective hypophysectomy for metastatic pain: A review of ethyl alcohol ablation of the anterior pituitary in a regional pain relief unit. *Br J Anaesth* 1981;53:1129–1233.
233. Lahuerta A, Lipton S, Miles J, et al. Update on percutaneous cervical cordotomy and pituitary alcohol neuroadenolysis: An audit of our recent results and complications. In: Lipton S, Miles J, eds., *Persistent pain: Modern methods of treatment*. Orlando FL: Grune & Stratton, 1985;5:197–223.
234. Levin AB, Katz J, Benson RC, et al. Treatment of pain of diffuse metastatic cancer by stereotactic chemical hypophysectomy: Long term results and observations on mechanism of action. *Neurosurgery* 1980;6:258–262.
235. Cousins MJ, Dwyer B, Gibb D. Chronic pain and neurolytic neural blockade. In: Cousins MJ, Bridenbaugh PO, eds., *Neural blockade*, 2nd ed. Philadelphia: JB Lippincott, 1988:1053–1084.
236. Misfeldt DS, Goldstein A. Hypophysectomy relieves pain not via endorphins. *N Engl J Med* 1977;297:1236–1237.
237. Yanagida H, Corssen G, Ceballos R, et al. Alcohol-induced pituitary adenolysis: How does it control intractable cancer pain? An experimental study using tooth pulp-evoked potentials in rhesus monkeys. *Anesth Analg* 1979;58:279–287.
238. Bonica JJ, Buckley FP, Moricca G, et al. Neurolytic blockade and hypophysectomy. In: Bonica JJ, ed., *The management of pain*, 2nd ed. Philadelphia: Lea & Febiger, 1990:2039–2059.
239. Miles J. Pituitary destruction. In: Wall PD, Melzack R, eds., *Textbook of pain*. New York: Churchill Livingstone, 1984:656–665.
240. Waldman SD, Feldstein GS, Allen ML. Neuroadenolysis of the pituitary: Description of a modified technique. *J Pain Symptom Manage* 1987;2:45–49.

CHAPTER 43 ■ ACUTE PAIN MANAGEMENT AND ACUTE PAIN SERVICES

PAMELA E. MACINTYRE AND DAVID A. SCOTT

The International Association for the Study of Pain (IASP) defines pain in general as "an unpleasant sensory and emotional experience associated with actual or potential tissue damage, or described in terms of such damage" (1). This highlights the influence of a variety of factors (affective and subjective) on the pain experience and the need to consider all relevant biopsychosocial (pathophysiologic, psychological, and social) factors when assessing and managing pain, whether that pain is acute or chronic.

Ready and Edwards (2) defined acute pain as "pain of recent onset and probably limited duration" and said that "it usually has an identifiable temporal and causal relationship to injury." They characterized chronic pain as that which "commonly persists beyond the time of healing of an injury and frequently there may not be any clearly identifiable cause." However, it is realized that acute pain and chronic pain are not separate entities but part of a pain continuum. This is reflected in the increasing overlap of therapies used in both acute and chronic pain settings.

Earlier chapters have already reviewed in detail the various drugs and techniques used for neuraxial and peripheral neural blockade in acute pain management (efficacy, side effects, complications, clinical applications, etc.). Therefore, this chapter only briefly mentions these topics, and instead concentrates on other aspects of acute pain management.

Analgesic techniques and drugs will be discussed briefly, especially those used for systemic rather than regional analgesia, and the importance of multimodal analgesia will be emphasized. However, the main focus will be on the consequences of and reasons for the continued undertreatment of acute pain, the very important issue of transition of acute to chronic (persistent) pain, preemptive and preventive analgesia, the organizational requirements needed to deliver safe and effective acute pain management (especially assessment and monitoring of patients), and the influence that patient variables (e.g., patient age, gender, and psychological factors) may have on some of the drugs and techniques used.

UNDERTREATMENT OF ACUTE PAIN

Evidence for Undertreatment

It is an unfortunate fact that 25% to 67% of patients (surgical and medical) in hospitals experience at least one episode of moderate to severe pain during their stay (3–6). Although these figures depend on the population surveyed, inadequate pain relief has been a consistent observation over the last 20 years, despite the significant improvements in the understanding of acute pain and advances in the sophistication of acute pain management options that have occurred over this time. This failure stems from a number of causes, as has been investigated by many professional organizations in addition to the Joint Council of American Hospital Organizations (JCAHO), the United States Department of Veteran Affairs (VA), and the Australian National Institute for Clinical Studies (NICS).

Consequences of Undertreatment

"Nobody ever died from pain after surgery" is an aphorism that is unfortunately frequently cited as a justification for avoiding the perceived complexities of acute pain management. In particular, this sort of statement reflects an attitude that acute pain is usually expected, short-lived, and, therefore, not a high priority. Yet, from a basic humanitarian point of view, the relief of pain and suffering is clearly important (7). It has also been believed for many years that the relief of acute pain would result in improved outcomes. Although this has been difficult to demonstrate until recently, these potential benefits formed one of the bases for the establishment of the first organized acute pain services (APS) in the 1980s.

In a retrospective review of esophagectomy patients, a lower incidence of cardiorespiratory complications and decreased mortality was associated with patients managed by an APS using epidural or parenteral opioid analgesia, compared with those receiving traditional as-required (p.r.n.) intramuscular opioids (8). Although such uncontrolled studies may be criticized on methodological grounds, an established body of evidence now supports the conclusion that effective pain relief can lead to improved clinical outcomes (see later and also Chapters 6 and 7). The effective management of acute postoperative pain has benefits relating to the facilitation of rehabilitation, and, therefore, recovery, by reducing stress responses that may impact the body in a number of ways and by reducing the incidence and intensity of long-term complications such as chronic pain.

It is not ethically possible to design studies to investigate the effects of inadequately treated pain, and, therefore, outcome data generally relate to comparisons of one analgesic technique with another. Often not detailed, however, are the outcomes in trials in which the primary analgesic technique has failed and, as a result, the patient may have experienced inadequate pain relief for a significant period of time. One such set of outcomes was reported in a trial by Bode et al. (9) in a study investigating the effect of regional anesthesia and analgesia versus general anesthesia on cardiovascular outcomes in high-risk vascular patients. Although no differences in cardiac outcomes were observed between the two study groups, there were 32 failed regional anesthetics in 235 patients; these patients had non-significantly higher cardiac morbidity (failed regional, regional, general anesthesia: myocardial infarction 6.3%, 3.6%, 4.9%, respectively; cardiac failure 15.6%, 7.1%, 8.9%, respectively) and significantly higher mortality (9.4%, 2.7%, 1.5%, respectively; $p = .03$). In a case report describing a fatal postoperative in-stent thrombosis in a patient with coronary artery stents having a thoracotomy and lobectomy, inadequate postoperative pain relief was associated with severe tachycardia and hypertension prior to the event (10). The temporal association of the hemodynamic responses to the undertreated pain and subsequent fatal myocardial infarction highlights the importance of maintaining effective pain control and promptly intervening when necessary. In a retrospective review of a small number of patients ($n = 43$) following lung reduction surgery, an association was seen between inadequate analgesia and complications such as atrial fibrillation and respiratory failure (11).

Long-term effects on the central nervous system (CNS) also need to be considered in the context of undertreated pain. A number of investigations now show evidence of an association between the intensity of acute pain with the development of persistent pain. For example, in a survey of 265 mastectomy patients, chronic pain in the breast area was significantly associated with intensity of postoperative pain (multivariate odds ratio [OR] 1.65; range, 1.16–2.35) (12). Similar studies in thoracic surgical patients support the link between acute pain intensity and persistent pain (13–15). Further examples are given later in the section discussing the transition of acute to chronic pain.

Overall, the increasing evidence that undertreated pain is associated with adverse clinical outcomes is supported by the wide range of clinical investigations comparing alternative analgesic techniques and associated improved clinical outcomes with improved quality of analgesia.

Reasons for Undertreatment

A number of reasons have been put forward in an attempt to explain the failure to provide consistently effective acute pain management in the hospital setting (16). This failure is despite the improvements gained by the now widespread adoption of some form of APS in most large hospitals. Many of these reasons parallel those barriers that are described for the provision of effective care for chronic pain sufferers, and can be divided into institutionally, clinician-, and patient-based factors (17).

At an institutional level, a key factor limiting the effectiveness of acute pain management is a lack of resource provision. Such resources include adequate and appropriate staffing, time and personnel to educate staff and patients and to carry out appropriate assessment and monitoring of patients, and the provision and use of proper guidelines and protocols for analgesic drugs and methods of drug administration. In addition, although APSs may be established, their structure may vary (e.g., anesthesiologist-based or nurse-based). Despite evidence for improved pain outcomes associated with an APS (18–21), the cost-effectiveness of the various APS structures is still not clear (8,19,22).

The diffuse nature of the problem is yet another factor limiting institutional awareness of the problem of undermanaged pain. Acute pain management is an element of care in all hospital settings, but particularly in the emergency department and postsurgical areas, including intensive care. As such, it crosses the boundaries of clinical specialty practice, as well as affecting clinicians at different levels (nurse aid, nurse, resident doctor,

consultant, etc.). Without a clear focus for attention or an obvious economic driver, it falls upon clinicians to recognize the value of integrated pain management, to make a case for such integration, and to draw together the necessary resources. It was from these concerns that APSs were initially developed in the mid-1980s; however, the nature of the implementation of such services is still inconsistent and leaves room for improvement (19).

Cultural changes within institutions are necessary to overcome some of these administrative and organizational barriers. Clear lines of responsibility need to be established while remaining cognizant of the significant professional boundaries that exist.

Institution-wide changes cannot be implemented without appropriate audit and review, which surveys suggest is not consistently undertaken even by APSs (23). A salutatory example of the benefits of review, and the risks of an unbalanced strategy for pain management, was documented by Vila et al. (24). In response to the JCAHO call for improved pain assessment and intervention, an institution-wide algorithm-based strategy for titration of analgesia according to numerical pain scores was adopted. This resulted in lower pain scores but also an increased incidence of respiratory depression. The recommendations from this experience were to improve the awareness of increasing sedation as a predictor of opioid-induced CNS and respiratory depression, and promote the routine use of sedation scoring. This example emphasizes the need for an integrated approach to pain management, including the full cycle of implementation of carefully thought out strategies with appropriate education and training, followed by assessment and reporting of outcomes. Such reporting also has the advantage of raising the profile of pain management with the organization.

At a clinician level, there also exist many barriers to be overcome before a patient's pain can be effectively managed. Over the years, a number of surveys have been done documenting the beliefs and attitudes of nurses and doctors regarding pain assessment and prescription of analgesic drugs. These consistently find that pain assessment is infrequent (16) and that it often underestimates pain compared with the patient's own perceptions (25). With regard to prescribing, one of the most commonly held misconceptions is still that short-term opioid use in the treatment of acute pain poses an increased risk of addiction. This may be reinforced by "pseudo-addiction" (26) or pain behaviors that appear to be inappropriately drug-seeking when in fact they are an appropriate response to undertreated pain. No evidence supports these concerns (27). Another key reason for undertreatment of acute pain is the fear of overtreatment, leading to drug-related side effects and complications.

Drug administration practices are often outdated, both in the prescription of drug orders and their implementation. The factors just mentioned, relating to fear of overuse and addiction, often result in the prescription of doses that are inadequate or given too infrequently. In addition, p.r.n. drug orders must be used carefully to avoid reactive rather than proactive pain management. Conventional, intramuscular p.r.n. administration is known to be ineffective in controlling acute postoperative pain, with incidences of moderate to severe pain of 67% and severe pain of 29% reported in one review (5).

Clearly, circumstances arise in which breakthrough or incident pain may trigger an unexpected need for supplementation. In these cases, the cycle from need to response must be short, but this may not always be achievable in a busy ward environment. This situation is an example in which patient-controlled analgesia (PCA) provides more effective care than traditional p.r.n. approaches (5,28,29). Strategies for using p.r.n. or PCA

PART IV: PAIN MANAGEMENT

opioid analgesia proactively (i.e., in anticipation of mobilization, physiotherapy, etc.), coupled with appropriate regular (time-based) analgesic prescriptions are likely to be the most effective in providing acute pain relief.

Education programs for medical and nursing staff are essential and should include the need for frequent and regular assessment of pain, the appropriate use of prescribed drugs, and the need to titrate pain relief for each patient. Clinicians also must be more aware of the options available for multimodal analgesic therapy. This includes a wide range of pharmacologic options, but also includes consideration of physical therapies and other strategies that may improve patient comfort. The use of multimodal analgesia, appropriate education and policies, frequent patient assessment, and appropriate titration, are all necessary components in preventing inadequate analgesia.

Finally, many patient factors may limit effective acute pain management. In chronic pain, as in acute pain settings, patients may be reluctant to report pain for fear of being judged a "complainer" or a "bad patient" (30). In addition, without appropriate education, patients often feel that they are "supposed" to have significant pain and that it is, therefore, inevitable. These attitudes are strongly affected by individual cultural and social characteristics, and may be aggravated by communication difficulties posed by language or cognitive barriers. Fear of addiction to opioids is also a concern for some patients. Wherever possible, preoperative education regarding the importance of pain reporting and providing an explanation of ways this can be achieved is an important first step in improving the effectiveness of pain assessment and hence pain treatment (31). Finally, specific characteristics of the patients themselves (discussed in more detail later) may affect their management, such as prior pain experience, adverse drug reactions, opioid tolerance, age, culture, gender, and genetics, as well as psychological factors.

The implementation of some sort of APS structure is not enough on its own to address the problems of undertreatment of acute pain. Overall, to overcome the barriers described and to improve the management of acute pain, education strategies need to be developed and underpinned by widespread institutional support with respect to both principles and also practice, in terms of resources. Quality improvement and risk management strategies also need to be implemented (32). It is only through a unified approach throughout the hospital system that the goals of effective pain management will be achieved (33). The Australian and New Zealand College of Anaesthetists (ANZCA) Faculty of Pain Medicine has developed a Statement of Rights to Pain Management (34) that is directed at these issues. These patient rights include (in abbreviated form):

- Education about effective pain management options
- Appropriate assessment and management of pain
- Regular recording of assessment results to facilitate ongoing care
- Care from health professionals with appropriate training and experience
- Appropriate effective pain management strategies supported by appropriate policies and procedures

TRANSITION FROM ACUTE TO CHRONIC PAIN

Persistent Pain Syndromes

Chronic or persistent pain (pain lasting more than 3 months after the expected resolution of the cause) has long been regarded as a separate entity from acute pain, with significantly different clinical characteristics. Acute pain may be described by patients as sharp, localized, and often triggered by movement if it is somatic in origin, or dull, aching, and nauseating if it is visceral in origin. Persistent pain, especially if neuropathic in origin, may be described as stabbing, burning, and not clearly associated with a trigger action. Other characteristics of neuropathic pain include sensory deficits, paresthesiae, hyperalgesia, and allodynia.

Neuropathic pain—pain resulting from injury to or disorder of the nervous system—has traditionally been placed in the "chronic pain" category of pain syndromes, and often clinicians involved in the management of postoperative pain have ignored or overlooked the possibility of neuropathic pain being a significant component of acute pain. Yet, by simply observing most surgical procedures, it is clear that damage to peripheral nerves is unavoidable although usually inadvertent. It is now known from laboratory research that behavioral signs of neuropathic pain may appear within hours of nerve injury and persist for weeks to months thereafter.

This has several implications for the clinician. The first and most obvious is that the acute pain experienced by patients postoperatively or after an injury may comprise elements of both nociceptive ("normal" acute pain) and neuropathic pain, and that these pain types may respond to different treatment strategies. The second is that there may be different surgical techniques or analgesic approaches that can be implemented during surgery to minimize the risk of neuropathic pain postoperatively. Finally, the incidence of long-term chronic or persistent pain disorders following surgical procedures may be reduced by perioperative interventions designed to avoid or treat acute neuropathic pain.

The association between surgical procedures and persistent pain was highlighted in the early 1990s by a survey of pain clinics in northern Britain (35) and by studies investigating postthoracotomy pain (13,15). In the survey of chronic pain clinics (35), over 20% of patients associated the onset of their persistent pain with a surgical procedure. This has been confirmed by other authors, especially with respect to neuropathic pain (36–38). The incidence of persistent pain as a long-term consequence following surgery is especially high after certain procedures, such as surgery involving the chest wall (thoracotomy, mastectomy, and midline sternotomy for cardiac surgery). This may be related to the likelihood of surgical trauma to one or more branches of the intercostal nerves supplying sensation to these regions.

Other procedures with a strong association include herniorrhaphy, knee joint procedures, and limb amputation (37,39,40) (Table 43-1).

Factors Associated with an Increased Risk of Persistent Pain

Some of the risk factors shown to be associated with an increased incidence of persistent pain are listed in Table 43-2. It is important to note that not all patients develop persistent pain syndromes despite having technically similar surgical procedures. This implies that other factors are involved that increase the likelihood of developing a long-term problem. Although not exhaustive, these factors include preexisting pain, postoperative pain intensity, psychological factors, concurrent neurologic injury, genetic factors, and gender. Some of these factors may impact on the intensity of postoperative pain (e.g., female gender) (41) and the incidence of chronic pain (e.g., depression)

TABLE 43-1

ESTIMATED INCIDENCE OF CHRONIC POSTOPERATIVE PAIN AND DISABILITY AFTER SELECTED SURGICAL PROCEDURES

Type of operation	Incidence of chronic Pain (%)
Amputation	30–85
Thoracotomy	5–67
Mastectomy	11–57
Cholecystectomy	3–56
Inguinal hernia	0–63
Vasectomy	0–37
Dental surgery	5–13

From Australian and New Zealand College of Anaesthetists and Faculty of Pain Medicine. *Acute Pain Management: Scientific Evidence*, 2nd ed. Melbourne: Australia and New Zealand College of Anaesthetists, 2005, with permission.

(12), whereas others may increase the likelihood of nerve injury or impaired healing (e.g., radiotherapy or chemotherapy).

Preexisting Pain

Preexisting pain has been recognized as a factor associated with postoperative phantom pain since the publication by Bach (42) citing the beneficial effects of preoperative pain control before lower limb amputation. In a small trial of 25 patients with painful lower limbs, 11 patients received epidural analgesia for 3 days prior to amputation. The incidence of phantom limb pain at 6 months was significantly reduced (none in the pretreatment group and five in the control group), and this continued as a trend to 1 year. Although criticized for its size and other uncontrolled factors, this study has been widely cited as

TABLE 43-2

FACTORS CONTRIBUTING TO THE DEVELOPMENT OF PERSISTENT POSTSURGICAL PAIN

Preexisting pain
   Central nervous system hyperexcitability
   Opioid tolerance

Physical nerve injury
   Location of surgical procedure (e.g., chest wall)
   Surgical technique

Postoperative pain severity
   Inadequate analgesia techniques
   Extent of tissue injury
   Psychological factors (e.g., depression)
   Gender
   Genetics including pharmacogenetics

Impaired nerve repair (or aggravated injury)
   Radiotherapy
   Chemotherapy

Other factors
   Genetic
   Psychological

being a clinical example of the effectiveness of "preemptive analgesia." However, preemptive analgesia (discussed later) is more specifically the prevention of central sensitization by using an analgesic technique prior to and during the time of nociceptive input. Nonetheless, the presence of preexisting pain induces some degree of CNS hyperexcitability or sensitization, and this certainly contributes to postsurgical pain (43).

A further example is provided in a prospective study of 346 patients undergoing abdominal surgery, in whom moderate to severe preoperative pain was significantly associated with an increased severity of postoperative pain (OR 2.96; 95% confidence interval [CI]; 1.32–6.60) (41). In the same study, the presence of a chronic pain condition was also linked to an increase in postoperative pain (OR 1.75; 95% CI; 1.03–2.98).

The risk does not just apply to patients having surgery. For example, higher levels of pain in patients with acute herpes zoster are associated with a higher incidence and severity of postherpetic neuralgia (44).

Nerve Injury

Nerve injury resulting from the site and extent of surgery is an important factor in the development of neuropathic pain (40) and may present in the early perioperative period (37). This has clinical implications for acute pain management because neuropathic pain is often less responsive to opioid analgesics, thus reinforcing the need for a multimodal analgesic strategy.

At the site of nerve injury, an inflammatory response is initiated by local factors and also by mediators that are conducted down the injured axon. The local neuronal membrane characteristics alter, so that there is a lowered threshold for depolarization with the expression of low-threshold sodium (Na^+) channels at the site of injury (45,46). In normal nerve regrowth, this may be seen in the Tinel sign, in which the progress of the axon down the peripheral nerve sheath can be determined by tapping on the course of the nerve until the patient reports a tingling sensation. Unsuccessful attempts at nerve regrowth may result in local neuroma formation with local hypersensitivity. Neuropathic pain results from a constant stream of afferent discharge to the CNS, coupled with central neural responses to axonal injury, causing nerve growth factor and other cytokines to be expressed in the dorsal root ganglion and the dorsal horn of the spinal cord. New, nonconventional connections form that do not have the same presynaptic inhibitory opioid receptor responses as the conventional nociceptive pathways (47). This impacts on possible therapeutic options.

Postoperative Pain

Evidence for the role of neuropathic pain and altered neuronal excitability in early postoperative pain comes from the clinical characteristics of patients' pain and clinical trials (48). The characteristics of neuropathic pain, including sensory changes, dysesthesia, and allodynia, can be elicited by asking patients about the character of their pain and not simply relying on unidimensional pain scores.

Studies using low doses of intravenous (IV) lidocaine have shown a reduction in postoperative analgesic requirements well beyond the expected pharmacologic effect of the drug (49). The plasma levels attained with these regimens have been demonstrated to be effective in blocking low-threshold Na^+ channels, such as those occurring at the site of nerve injury (46,50). Acting at a central site, the antineuropathic drug gabapentin is effective in reducing perioperative analgesic requirements

PART IV: PAIN MANAGEMENT

(51,52), also reinforcing the role of neuropathic pain as a component of acute postoperative pain.

As noted earlier, the intensity of postoperative pain is associated with the development of persistent pain. Although this could be attributed solely to the extent of tissue trauma, a number of studies have shown that, for identical surgical procedures, the severity of postoperative pain is a factor in influencing chronic pain outcomes. In a retrospective study of 509 breast surgery patients, both the type of operation (e.g., with or without axillary dissection) and the severity of postoperative pain were associated with the presence of chronic breast pain (53). In both retrospective and prospective surveys of thoracotomy patients, early postoperative pain has been significantly associated with persistent pain (13,15). Two studies comparing different types of analgesia following thoracotomy also demonstrated this effect (14,54). Taken together, convincing evidence suggests that the modification of pain intensity in the immediate postoperative period can influence the incidence of longer-term persistent pain syndromes.

Phantom pain is a characteristic form of postamputation pain that can vary in intensity from mild discomfort to excruciating pain. Although most frequently associated with limb amputation, it may also occur with resection of other parts of the body, including breast and teeth. Phantom limb sensation occurs in a majority of amputees and diminishes over months to years. Phantom pain occurs in up to 80% of patients, and 1 year later, may still persist in up to two-thirds of these (55). Phantom pain is probably a form of "pain memory," and is likely to be a manifestation of central sensitization prior to or during the amputation, and cortical reorganization following the event (56). It has many similarities with other forms of neuropathic pain.

Radiotherapy and Chemotherapy

Radiotherapy has been identified as an independent risk factor in the development of chronic postmastectomy pain (53) and the intensity of that pain (57), possibly because of the effect on the healing of injured chest wall nerves or the development of fibrotic scar tissue. Chemotherapeutic agents such as vincristine have long been known to be associated with painful peripheral neuropathies, and recent laboratory evidence suggests that this mechanism is different from that of traumatic neuropathic pain (58). Thus, it is likely that the combination of the neurologic insults of chemotherapy with surgical nerve trauma may have at least an additive effect on neuropathic pain outcomes.

Prevention Strategies

The key objectives in preventing or reducing the transition from acute to chronic pain are to (a) modify risk factors wherever possible and (b) provide the current best practice as far as preventive therapies are concerned. As already noted, the etiologic mechanisms of postsurgical neuropathic pain remain incompletely characterized, and it is unclear why the same injury will cause neuropathic pain in some individuals but not others. This finding even extends to the laboratory where, despite carefully controlled circumstances, some animals will manifest allodynia following nerve injury and others will not. Thus, it is not surprising that evidence for precise recommendations is still limited.

Surgical strategies that minimize nerve injury and decrease the extent of tissue damage should result in an improvement in outcomes. Perioperative pain is decreased by the use of minimally invasive surgical techniques such as video-assisted thoracic surgery (VATS) and laparoscopic cholecystectomy. Although this would be expected to translate into reduced persistent pain problems, the results have been modest. A retrospective review of 343 patients reported a 30% incidence of persistent pain in the months following VATS thoracotomy, compared with a 44% incidence in those having open procedures (59). There was no difference at 12 months. This may reflect the difficulty in avoiding injury to intercostal nerves even after minimal-access procedures. Laparoscopic cholecystectomy has also been associated with mixed long-term outcomes compared with open surgery. This may be due in part to more complex issues relating to the source of pain being from the gallbladder bed or biliary tract (60). Nonetheless, on the basis of reduced acute pain intensity alone, modification of surgical techniques should be encouraged.

Optimizing postoperative analgesia using multimodal techniques remains the most significant contribution that clinicians can make. Recognition of the potentially opioid-resistant components of neuropathic pain in postoperative patients justifies consideration of drugs that have been shown to be effective in treating neuropathic pain, in addition to conventional analgesics in high-risk patients (40). A number of potentially useful drugs are already being used, such as nonsteroidal anti-inflammatory drugs (NSAIDs). In addition to their peripheral anti-inflammatory effect, which may also reduce inflammation at sites of nerve injury, there is evidence for cyclooxygenase (COX)-2–mediated mechanisms involved in central hypersensitivity at a spinal cord level. Tramadol may also be of benefit in neuropathic pain, possibly because of its nonopioid effects (61). Ketamine should be considered in the perioperative setting for high-risk patients because it is well tolerated in low doses, is morphine sparing (62), and is effective in the treatment of certain types of neuropathic pain (63).

Regional analgesic techniques should be encouraged. Epidural local anesthetics and/or opioids result in better analgesia after abdominal surgery than do parenteral opioids (64). Evidence from thoracic surgery and lower limb amputation suggests that regional techniques are associated with lower incidences of persistent pain (14) and severe phantom pain (65).

Obata et al. (54) compared 28 patients in whom epidural analgesia was commenced before surgery with 30 patients in whom epidural analgesia was started immediately postoperatively; both regimens were continued for 72 hours after surgery. Pain relief was significantly better in the preoperative epidural group; the incidence of chronic pain at 6 months was 33%, compared with 67% in the postoperative group. Similarly, Senturk et al. (14) allocated 86 thoracotomy patients to receive preoperative epidural analgesia lasting 48 hours, postoperative epidural analgesia lasting 48 hours, or IV PCA morphine only. The incidence of chronic pain at 6 months was 45%, 63%, and 78%, respectively, and chronic pain was associated with postoperative pain on day 2.

A number of investigations have attempted to identify factors that could be modified to reduce or prevent phantom pain. The early series published by Bach (referred to earlier [42]), suggested that strategies that allow the CNS to "unwind" or desensitize prior to amputation may result in a lower incidence and severity of phantom or neuropathic pain (47). Over the succeeding decades, many approaches have been tried to prevent the onset of phantom pain, including regional analgesia (66), sympathetic interruption (67), ketamine (63,68,69), and anticonvulsants (e.g., gabapentin) (70,71). Evidence to guide therapy is limited, despite the large number of reports published, because many are uncontrolled case series or clinical trials that were small or poorly controlled (72).

However, perioperative regional anesthesia and analgesia may offer some advantage. Gehling et al. (65) conducted a closer examination of published studies, looking at regional anesthesia and phantom limb pain after amputation using more graded end-points. It was concluded that a definite benefit accrues when regional techniques are used in these patients, particularly in diminishing the intensity of phantom limb pain.

Cyclooxygenase (COX)-2 inhibitors may also reduce the incidence of chronic pain after surgery. Celecoxib given perioperatively reduced pain scores and the incidence of chronic donor site pain after spinal fusion (73).

The decision to use other drugs with known efficacy in the treatment of established neuropathic pain, such as amitriptyline, venlafaxine, gabapentin, pregabalin, and lidocaine, in an attempt to reduce the risk of chronic pain, must be based on individual clinical assessment of the likely benefit versus tolerability and side effects (46,47,74,75).

Amitriptyline, given in the early stages of acute herpes zoster, has been shown to reduce the risk of chronic postherpetic neuralgia (76). It has also been reported that venlafaxine, given prior to surgery, reduced the incidence of chronic pain after breast surgery (77), although other investigators have not shown the same result (78). However, although antidepressants may have a role, their side effects may not always be well tolerated (79).

Gabapentinoids are being increasingly used for neuropathic pain and have recently been recommended as second- or third-line therapy (80). The mechanism of action of gabapentin is, despite its name, unrelated to γ-aminobutyric acid (GABA) receptors or metabolism, and is more likely to be a direct modulator of neuronal calcium channels. A meta-analysis of placebo-controlled randomized studies showed a positive effect of gabapentin in diabetic neuropathy and postherpetic neuralgia, and uncontrolled studies also suggest a benefit in other painful neuropathic conditions (81). The role of gabapentin in acute pain is not well defined, although it has been shown to be opioid-sparing, and may have long-term benefits. In a study of mastectomy patients, 66 patients received mexiletine (a Na$^+$ channel blocker), gabapentin, or placebo for 10 days, starting preoperatively (78). Pain scores were reduced from day 2 to 6 in both active treatment groups. At 6 months, analgesic use was lower, and there was no difference in throbbing or aching nociceptive pain, although the incidence of neuropathic (burning) pain was significantly lower (5% in each of mexiletine and gabapentin groups versus 25% in the placebo group). However, in a study involving lower limb amputation, gabapentin given immediately postoperatively and continued for 30 days did not reduce the intensity or incidence of postamputation stump or phantom pain (71).

It is clear that acute pain management and chronic pain issues are interlinked. It is, therefore, important that all clinicians know about the potential benefits of effective analgesia in reducing the incidence and intensity of persistent pain, including phantom pain and other neuropathic pain. Although not all techniques have an established evidence base, the use of regional anesthesia and analgesic techniques, ketamine, and possibly antidepressants and anticonvulsants should be considered in selected patients.

Preemptive and Preventive Analgesia

The concept of preemptive analgesia was first proposed by Crile in 1913, a surgeon who advocated the use of nerve blocks to supplement general anesthesia to prevent painful wound scars (82). This was an important conceptual step, because it integrated both the notion of preventing pain before it occurred, and the possibility that acute events could influence long-term pain. Identification of neurophysiologic mechanisms stimulated modern clinical interest when laboratory research demonstrated a reduction in central hypersensitivity and plasticity ("wind-up") when analgesic drugs were administered prior to the imposition of a nociceptive stimulus (83).

This appeared to be confirmed by small-scale clinical studies such as that by Bach (42), showing a reduction in postamputation phantom limb pain with preoperative epidural analgesia. However, over the following two decades, clinical studies in acute surgical pain have frequently failed to show a significant or sustained reduction in postoperative analgesic requirements or postoperative pain, despite preincisional analgesia (84). In addition, until recently, there have been relatively few studies of chronic pain. This failure to confirm the neurophysiologic evidence is due to a number of factors, including the definition of preemptive analgesia, but it does not invalidate the underlying principles (85,86). In support of this perspective, a recent meta-analysis of a large number of clinical studies (87) has concluded that preemptive analgesia is effective in certain clinical circumstances.

The terminology relating to preemptive analgesia is frequently misunderstood. Common use of the concept is that the commencement of an analgesic strategy prior to surgery will result in profoundly decreased pain or analgesic requirements following the procedure, in comparison with initiation of pain relief once the stimulus has begun. Although this is to some extent true, preemptive analgesia actually refers to a process initiated prior to an acute nociceptive stimulus (the surgery or injury) that prevents CNS sensitization (central hypersensitivity).

To be most effective, preemptive analgesia strategies must interact at all sites of nociceptive input into the spinal cord: Thus, wound infiltration with local anesthetics will not block inputs from deeper structures, and epidural analgesia may not block all relevant dermatomes or autonomic nociceptive pathways. Importantly, the period of intense nociceptive input may continue well into the postprocedural period and be heightened by peripheral hypersensitivity (including inflammatory processes). Thus, the treatment used should extend in time to cover this stimulus as well (86). To achieve this level of control of central sensitization is very difficult in clinical practice, which explains why the treatment effect seen in many studies is small or absent despite encouraging laboratory work.

Seeking out strategies for preemptive analgesia has a broader justification because of the significant growth in recognition of persistent or chronic pain following surgical procedures (40). Central sensitization at the time of surgery may contribute to both the degree of acute postoperative pain and the likelihood of chronic neuropathic pain. Because the terminology associated with preemptive analgesia has often been confused, many investigators were not assessing changes in central hypersensitivity itself but rather looking for surrogate end-points such as analgesic requirements. In support of this approach, more recent studies have shown evidence that preemptive analgesia reduces acute and chronic pain after thoracotomy (14) and major abdominal surgery (88).

There are many studies, which by design, have potentially modified the sensitization process without demonstrating true "preemptive" analgesia. In these situations, the administration of a treatment strategy (drug/nerve block/wound infiltration) could be deemed to have had a "preventive" analgesic effect if the outcome outlasted the known effect-site activity. Thus, preventive analgesia (86) is demonstrated when a treatment or agent results in a reduction in analgesic consumption or pain scores beyond the expected pharmacotherapeutic duration of action of the treatment. Preventive analgesic effects relating to acute pain outcomes have been demonstrated in a recent meta-analysis by Ong et al. (87).

Thus, the impact of both preemptive analgesia and preventive analgesia can be ascertained from properly designed clinical investigations. For preemptive analgesic strategies to show benefits in hypersensitivity reduction and decreased chronic pain, they must attenuate a significant degree of nociceptive afferent input, and they must be maintained for sufficient duration—that is, into the postoperative period. Preventive analgesia is also a valuable concept, because even if hyperalgesia is not fully attenuated, the outcomes of reduced opioid requirements and decreased pain intensity are beneficial in themselves.

ASSESSMENT AND MONITORING

Patients with acute pain must be assessed at frequent intervals to optimize analgesia and detect and manage side effects or complications at an early stage (89). Infrequent or inadequate assessment may contribute to the undertreatment of pain and poor clinical outcomes. Such assessments need to be undertaken using clearly described criteria and tools and need to include a pain history, measurement of pain intensity and functional impact of the pain, and monitoring of relevant vital signs, including sedation scoring for those receiving opioids. The results should be documented in a standardized fashion.

Wherever possible, a proper pain history and patient education should be done prior to elective surgery (90). At this time, the opportunity also exists to develop a pain management plan with the patient, advise on expectations and concerns, and discuss pain measurement tools and the importance of communicating pain experiences openly with his or her clinical caregivers (90).

Strategies should be in place to manage deviations from expected parameters. Although a deterioration in pain scores may indicate a need for increasing or modifying analgesic therapy, a significant unexpected increase in pain may be due to the onset of a new clinical condition (e.g., perforated viscus or compartment syndrome) and should be evaluated accordingly. Likewise, aggressive pain management without appropriate clinical monitoring may lead to an increase in adverse outcomes (24).

All of this must be undertaken within the context of the patient's situation; that is, within the history of the acute pain event, history of past and ongoing long-term pain experiences, and with full knowledge of current analgesic and medical history. This may not be achievable in some circumstances (e.g., severe trauma) or in patients with poor communication abilities, including those with dementia.

Pain History

In acute pain, the pain history is important even if the clinical situation is clearly defined and the expectations are for a relatively rapid recovery. Although in some circumstances clinical priorities may dictate a need for a rapid pain control (e.g., in the emergency department), an exploration of the patient's pain history, both acute and chronic, is important for the provision of effective and safe pain relief.

The key objectives of the pain history in patients with acute pain are:

■ Establish communication and rapport with the patient.

■ Understand the context of the current condition.
■ Learn the location, character, and intensity of the pain being experienced.
■ Establish the functional impact of the pain on the patient's activity.
■ Identify all current drug therapies and the indications for their use.
■ Identify drug contraindications, adverse reactions, or "allergies" that might affect analgesic options.
■ Determine underlying chronic pain issues and treatments.
■ Learn about previous relevant acute pain episodes and how they responded to treatment.

The last two items are important in maximizing the effectiveness of treatment and also in interpreting pain intensity measurements.

The pain description provides the most valuable information used to guide treatment. Whenever possible, a detailed description of the patient's pain should be made, guided by descriptors similar to those used in assessing chronic pain. These descriptors can be obtained reasonably quickly and include:

■ Site
■ Intensity: The subjective pain score or rating, measured at rest and with movement/activity
■ Character: Stabbing, burning, shooting, aching, etc.
■ Radiation
■ Aggravating or relieving factors
■ Associated symptoms: Nausea/vomiting, light headedness, etc.

For example, patients following thoracic surgery often have significant pain, but there may be multiple components. The wound itself may be acutely painful, especially if there has been surgical rib resection; there may be muscle spasm and pain in the chest wall as a reflex response to the pain or secondary to rib retraction or costochondral pain; and there may be referred pain from diaphragmatic irritation by the chest drains. The therapeutic strategies and expected time course for resolution of each of these components differs significantly, and management of any one element only will lead to incomplete treatment of the patient's pain.

Pain Intensity Measurement

The IASP definition of pain emphasizes that it is a subjective experience; that it can be affected profoundly by other factors in the environment, such as anxiety and depression; and that its expression is related to the social and cultural background of the individual. Importantly, acute pain, like chronic pain, is not unidimensional and may not be effectively categorized by one measurable index. Many scales have been developed in an attempt to record the perceived level of pain (pain intensity scores) or to assess the degree of pain relief (analgesia scores). A number of these have direct application in a controlled research environment, whereas others have less reliability or are less complex but are simpler to apply and hence more useful on a day-to-day clinical basis.

Intensity is the subjective component of pain and is measured and recorded using one or more scales or tools. Tools for measuring pain intensity should be meaningful to the patient and clinician. A ranked scale is important to assess the response over time and to changes in therapy. It is most helpful if all scales can be recorded in a similar way on the patient's observation chart, the most commonly used system for documentation being a numeric index from 0 to 10 (which is, therefore, an 11-point scale). This index can be used to describe the result from a range of pain intensity tools.

A summary of the types of tools and scales used is shown in Table 43-3 (91–105). The optimal measurement tool or scale may change from time to time because of the circumstances of the patient (e.g., sedation, confusion, etc.). Pain intensity should be assessed and recorded both at rest, and with movement that is relevant to the patient's condition. However, these measures do not necessarily give the clinician a clear idea of the impact that the pain is having on limiting physical activity or rehabilitation. For this to be done, a functional activity assessment must be made.

Many scales are available for pain assessment in children (106). Children at different ages and with differing abilities will need appropriate tools for assessment, including parent's or caregiver's opinion and the response to analgesia. In the absence of demonstrated superiority of any one tool, it is important for an institution to adopt a consistent multidimensional approach to pain measurement and reporting. Refer to Chapter 47 for more details.

Pain assessment in patients with dementia presents a challenge because of the limited communication abilities of the sufferers. As with children, behavioral tools have proved effective, as has the use of reports from family members or personal caregivers. A number of projects have evaluated systems for use in dementia including the PAINAD (107) and Abbey scales (108). Although many of these are too time-consuming for frequent use (they lend themselves to the assessment of persistent pain), elements are applicable to acute pain, such as the modified FLACC scale (Table 43-3).

A limited and consistent set of tools should be established throughout the institution. This will improve care, because clinical staff moving from one area to another will have immediate familiarity with assessments and will know what responses might be necessary. In addition, patients can be educated about how to report their pain and even choose those tools they feel suit them best. An appropriate selection for an adult hospital might be a visual analog scale (VAS; with slide rulers provided), a numerical rating scale (NRS; with consistent wording used), a faces scale, and a behavioral tool (such as FLACC) when needed. All scores should be graded on a 0 to 10 scale for charting, and all patient observation charts throughout the institution should have a specific entry line for pain scoring. Clearly, if a patient does not have a painful condition then pain scoring need only be done once per shift, but otherwise assessments may need to be hourly or as required.

Functional Assessment

The functional impact of the patient's pain can be assessed by history and if possible, direct observation. Pain management can only be considered to be fully effective if it both relieves the patient's suffering and enables appropriate physical function. Without being able to undertake relevant activities, which in most cases involve rehabilitation, recovery from an underlying injury or surgery may be impaired (109). Pain also impacts on other aspects of function, such as the ability to sleep, and this should also be assessed.

One method for scoring functional impact is the Functional Activity Scale (FAS), which was developed as part of a pain management toolkit project in Australia (110). The activity to be used for assessing the FAS score must be determined on an individual basis: Coughing may be an appropriate activity target following abdominal surgery, whereas tolerance of physiotherapy and joint mobilization may be appropriate fol-

lowing knee surgery, or the ability to tolerate a lighted room for patients with migraine headaches. The FAS score is a simple three-level ranked categorical score designed to be applied at the bedside. Its fundamental purpose is to assess whether the patient can undertake appropriate activity at his or her current level of pain control, and to act as a trigger for intervention should this not be the case. This differs from, but is related to, pain intensity scoring with movement. It comprises both objective and subjective components in that the clinician asks the patient if he is able to perform the activity and gains the pain intensity score at the time. The patient is asked to perform the activity, or is taken through the activity in the case of structured physiotherapy (joint mobilization) or nurse-assisted care (e.g., ambulation, turning in bed). The ability to complete the activity is then assessed using the FAS, as detailed in Table 43-4.

A FAS score of A represents optimal pain control; B represents an adequate functional outcome, but further pain relief is required for comfort; and C represents inadequate pain control or unacceptable complications of pain control (motor block from neuraxial analgesia, nausea or sedation from opioids, etc.). The score of A needs to be determined relative to the patient's pre-acute baseline function (which may already have limitations, as from severe arthritis). The FAS score is simple and flexible but requires staff education to be consistently applied; it has not yet been validated in large clinical trials (in part because there exists no "gold standard" for reference).

Overall, it is well recognized that clinical recovery depends on effective rehabilitation. This can be best achieved by careful patient questioning, combined with the use of selected tools to measure pain intensity and functional capacity, linked to appropriate guidelines for intervention should pain relief be inadequate (see example in Table 43-5). Finally, when reassessing patients during treatment for acute pain, it is important to remember that the patient's current condition may well have altered since the last visit, even if only recent. Ambulation or physiotherapy, changes in drug therapy, side effects of drug treatment (e.g., nausea), the effects of altered sleep patterns, and even relationships with caregivers may all impact on the current situation.

Monitoring for Side Effects and Complications

Provision of safe and effective acute pain management includes regular evaluation of the patient to detect and limit any side effects or complications. Although the regular assessment of heart rate, blood pressure, and respiratory rate is well-established practice, the widespread use of parenteral opioids requires routine and frequent assessment of sedation, as this almost always precedes respiratory depression (24,111). All assessments should be documented, and patient observation charts throughout the institution should contain a specific place for recording sedation scores as well as the "routine" observations in addition to pain scoring.

Little benefit is provided to the patient if the regular assessments for pain and side effects are not coupled with clearly defined trigger levels for intervention (Table 43-5). Such interventions may be as straightforward as the alteration of analgesia dosing, ranging through consultation with senior or more experienced clinicians, to resuscitation (e.g., oxygen, naloxone etc.).

The side effects and complications that are most common or important for consideration are listed in Table 43-6. This list has been drawn from a number of sources (112,113).

UNIDIMENSIONAL PAIN INTENSITY MEASURES

Measure	Description	Merits	Comments
Verbal Rating Scales (VRS) or Verbal Descriptor Scales (VDS)	A list of words describing pain of increasing intensity; e.g., the four-level VRS-4 (91): (0 – No Pain; 1 – Mild Pain; 2- Moderate pain; 3- Severe Pain)	Pro: Simple; word choice important; some correlation with VAS. Con: Limited set of responses; subjective; not readily convertible to an 11-point score	Used in McGill Pain Questionnaire; emergency triage systems (92)
Numerical Rating Scale (NRS)	Verbal (VNRS) or visual grading of pain by patient using a 0–10 (NRS-11) (or 0–5) scale. *"On a scale of 0 to 10 with 0 being no pain at all and 10 being the worst pain imaginable, how would you rate the pain you are experiencing now?"*	Pro: Conceptually simple; visual alternatives useful (93); results easy to record; well validated Con: Anchor terms important; some people have trouble using numbers to grade a subjective sensation	Most widely used in clinical practice; gradings comparable to VAS (94); emergency triage systems (92)
Visual Analogue Scale (VAS)	An unmarked horizontal or vertical line typically 100 mm in length, anchored by textual descriptors and/or pictures at each end. Labels (only at ends) "no pain" (equals a score of 0) at the left end, "worst pain imaginable" or "worst possible pain" (a score of 10 or 100) is placed at the right end. The patient is asked to indicate a point along the line using a pencil, finger, or slider.	Pro: Reliable and validated; anchor terms easily translated; easy to use in research; does not need language or numeracy skills once taught Con: Anchor terms/pictures important; physical tool required; requires some dexterity	Widely used in research; results easy to record; orientation does not matter (95); linearity validated (96,97)
Pictorial Face Scales	A row of face pictures indicating increasing pain intensity, usually cartoon-like. Usually 6 faces e.g. Wong-Baker FACES Pain Rating Scale (99); (suitable for 3 years and older); Faces Pain Scale – Revised (98) Oucher scale (photographs) (100)	Pro: Suitable for children 3 years and older and cognitively or linguistically limited adults; faces can be converted to numeric scale for recording Con: Physical tool required; actual imagery may overlay some nonpain emotional content (101)	Widely used in pediatrics; well-validated
Pain Drawings	A graphical image of the body on which the patient can shade or label character and location of pain (102)	Pro: Useful for recording of longer-term pain conditions; can be used in situations where speech is not possible (e.g., ICU); potentially multidimensional Con: Requires alertness and dexterity; time-consuming	Used mostly in chronic pain; may be suitable in intensive care and similar environments (103)
Behavioral Assessment Tools and Scales	A set of behavioral criteria that can be observed and scored to achieve a "pain score": e.g., for children the FLACC index (facial expression, leg movement, activity, cry, and consolability [104]) or modified for adults (105)	Pro: Provides a structured set of criteria instead of relying on a global subjective evaluation; may be recorded numerically Con: Items are still subjective; time-consuming; need to have the guide available	Suitable for children and adults who are unable to communicate effectively; difficult to validate

TABLE 43-4

FUNCTIONAL ACTIVITY SCORES

A: No limitation	The patient is able to undertake the activity without limitation due to pain (pain intensity score typically 0–3).
B: Mild limitation	The patient is able to undertake the activity but experiences moderate to severe pain (pain intensity score typically 4–10).
C: Significant limitation	The patient is unable to complete the activity due to pain (or pain treatment-related side effects); independent of pain intensity scores.

Nausea and Vomiting

Nausea and vomiting, although usually a minor adverse effect, is a significant source of patient dissatisfaction (114). In some circumstances, it can compromise surgical outcome (e.g., abdominal or chest wall flap reconstruction). An evidence-based strategy should be in place to manage perioperative nausea and vomiting (115).

Opioid exposure is a common cause of nausea and vomiting, and there is a known correlation between the risk of nausea and vomiting and increasing opioid dose (116–118). Risk factors other than opioids have been identified (119); nausea and vomiting may also occur without any postoperative opioid use (120). Intrathecal opioids are associated with a high incidence of nausea and vomiting, but this may not be dose-related (121).

The use of multimodal analgesia results in a decreased need for opioids, which is associated with a decreased incidence of nausea and vomiting as well as sedation (62,117).

In the review by Dolin and Cashman, the incidence of nausea was reported to be higher with PCA than following intramuscular/subcutaneous opioid analgesia (Table 43-6), but there was no difference in the incidence of vomiting (112). It is possible that this difference could be related to opioid dose. The much higher number of patients reporting moderate to severe or severe pain with intramuscular analgesia (5) would suggest that lower opioid doses were used in these patients.

Three meta-analysis have shown no difference in the incidence of nausea and vomiting with PCA compared with conventional methods of opioid delivery (29,122,123).

Pruritus

Pruritus is a common opioid-related side effect, but its mechanism is not yet fully understood. The role of histamine remains unclear, as pruritus may occur after the administration of opioids that do not release histamine. The fact that drugs such as naloxone (a μ-receptor antagonist) can reverse opioid-related pruritus suggests that a μ-receptor–mediated mechanism may be in play (123).

The incidence of pruritus is significantly higher in patients given PCA opioids compared with those receiving systemic opioids by other routes (29,112).

Sedation

The importance of monitoring for opioid-induced CNS depression cannot be overstated. Significant sedation or respiratory depression occurring in patients receiving parenteral

TABLE 43-5

REPORTABLE OBSERVATION GUIDE

Notify APS or Unit responsible for patient if any of the following parameters occur:

PAIN

Pain Intensity Score (0–10)	Persistent severe pain-Consecutive scores >7
Functional Activity Score (A-C)	Severe Limitation – 2 Consecutive FAS of C

SEDATION

Sedation Score (0–3)	Sedation Score >1 or 1s
	Sedation Score >0 and Respiratory Rate <8

MOTOR (Epidural)

Bromage Score	Motor Block >1 for prolonged period (>4h)
	Unexpected increase in motor block post (including after epidural catheter removal)

BACK PAIN (Epidural)

	Potential Emergency must assess within 1 hour
	Unexpected or new back pain
	Pain, Inflammation or Swelling at the epidural catheter site plus Fever >38.5°C
	Altered sensation or power in lower limbs
	New urinary or fecal incontinence

HIGH BLOCK (Epidural)

T4 or above Nipple line	Tingling/numbness in fingers
	Weakness in arm(s)
	Respiratory Difficulty

HYPOTENSION (Epidural)

	Systolic Blood Pressure <90 mmHg
	Pulse Rate <55 with Blood Pressure <100 mmHg

PRURITUS

	If patient requests treatment

NAUSEA/VOMITING

	Unresponsive to prescribed treatment

URINARY RETENTION

	Patient unable to void

TABLE 43-6

ADVERSE OUTCOMES ASSOCIATED WITH ACUTE PAIN MANAGEMENT

	Pooled frequency (%) (95% CI)	IM/SC opioids	IV PCA opioids	Epidural analgesia
Nausea	25.2 (19.3–32.1)	17.0 (6.6–37.4)	32.0 (26.8–37.6)	18.8 (14.0–24.8)
Vomiting	20.2 (17.5–23.2)	21.9 (17.1–27.6)	20.7 (17.1–24.8)	16.2 (12.5–20.7)
Pruritus	14.7 (11.9–18.1)	3.4 (1.6–6.9)	13.8 (10.7–17.5)	16.1 (12.8–20.0)
Urinary Retention	23.0 (17.3–29.9)	15.2 (9.3–23.8)	13.4 (6.6–25.0)	29.1 (21.5–38.1)
Hypotension	4.9 (2.7–8.8)	3.8 (1.9–7.5)	0.4 (0.1–1.9)	5.6 (3.0–10.2)
Sedation*	2.6 (2.3–2.8)	5.2 (4.1–6.4)	5.3 (4.6–6.4)	1.2 (0.9–1.4)
Respiratory Depression**	0.3 (0.1–1.3)	1.4[†] (0.1–12.7)	1.9 (1.9–2.0)	0.1 (01.–0.2)

Percentage (95% CI). IM, intramuscular; SC, subcutaneous; *, excessive sedation/extreme somnolence/hard to rouse; **, based on naloxone requirement.
†, low patient numbers (112,113). Data from studies including but not limited to randomized-controlled trials.

opioids may lead to significant morbidity. The assumption that respiratory rate monitoring will effectively detect opioid-induced respiratory depression is flawed (24,111), and sedation scoring should be employed on a routine basis in addition to the other core clinical observations.

The need to use sedation as an indicator of respiratory depression rather than rely on a decrease in respiratory rate is unfortunately commonly still not recognized. Cashman and Dolin (112,113) reported the incidences of sedation and respiratory depression (Table 43-6) in different papers; respiratory depression was defined in a number of ways by the authors of the various studies included in these reviews, none of which included an assessment of sedation.

The biggest weakness of sedation scoring is for patients who are assumed to be asleep, and who, therefore, may not be disturbed by clinical staff. At these times, patients should

be noted to rouse slightly when clinical observations are made (e.g., pulse or blood pressure), and if they do not do so, then the stimulus should be increased until they respond. A suitable sedation scoring system is based on a scale from 0 to 3 (Table 43-7). The aim is for a sedation score of 0 or 1. A higher sedation score should require clinical intervention (reassessment, escalation of care, etc.).

Complications Associated with Neuraxial Analgesia

A list of potential complications associated with neuraxial analgesia is listed in Table 43-8 (124–132), but more detail is given in other chapters of this book.

Patients receiving neuraxial infusions (i.e., epidural or subarachnoid) need regular assessment of motor and sensory block and body temperature, and inspection of the catheter insertion

TABLE 43-7

EXAMPLE OF A SEDATION SCORING SYSTEM

0 = Awake, alert	The patient is awake, alert, and responds appropriately to verbal command.
1 = Mild sedation, easy to rouse	The patient rouses easily from sleep/rest, is able to stay awake and is alert and cooperative.
1s = Asleep, easy to rouse	This sedation scoring option is to be used at night when the patient would normally be expected to be asleep. The patient must be assessed if he or she is on any opioid or sedative agents to ensure he or she is not deteriorating in his sedation level despite having a normal respiratory rate. When doing the normal BP and pulse observations at night, the patient should stir or move at this time. If this does not occur, then an attempt to wake the patient should be made to ensure they are arousable.
2 = Moderate sedation, unable to remain awake	The patient is frequently asleep or drowsy when observed. Usually drowsy on waking. He or she is able to follow commands but unable to remain awake.
3 = Difficult to rouse	The patient is difficult to rouse or unarousable. He or she has difficulty with, or inability to follow commands.

TABLE 43-8

ADVERSE OUTCOMES ASSOCIATED WITH
PERINEURAL AND EPIDURAL INFUSIONS

	Perineural infusion	Epidural infusion
Catheter insertion site infection	0.25–3.0	0.8–2.8
Hematoma	0.25	0.01–0.02
Epidural abscess	n/a	0.015–0.05
Residual neurological deficit (>3 months)	0.016–1.0	0.01

Incidence Range or Incidence (Percent and 95% CI) (124–132).

site. Any unexpected progression of motor block, or the failure of it to resolve, should be considered suspicious and justifies an escalation of clinical care and thorough assessment of the patient. Ideally, low doses of local anesthetic should be used in epidural infusions, so that even if the catheter is placed at a lumbar spinal levels, the likelihood of motor block is low. Motor block is most frequently evaluated using the Bromage score (133). This scale is widely used and validated, and it is easy to train clinical staff in its use. It does not replace formal neurologic assessment should neurologic deficit be suspected.

Although the onset of new backache or neurologic signs should be a trigger for prompt neurologic consultation and/or magnetic resonance image (MRI) scanning, investigation should not be delayed if clinical suspicion is high (134). Suggestive features include systemic pyrexia in association with purulence or cellulitis at the catheter insertion site (128). Delay in decompression of an epidural hematoma or abscess increases the risk of poor recovery of function (132).

The use of anticoagulants during epidural infusions needs to be identified and carefully monitored. Guidelines should be established for hospital use to ensure appropriate timing and size of dosing (132). Good coordination with surgical or medical treating teams will help to avoid unnecessarily increasing a patient's risk of complications should full systemic anticoagulation be required (e.g., following myocardial ischemia or pulmonary thromboembolism). This also applies to patients receiving perineural infusions (e.g., brachial plexus or femoral), although these are generally more straightforward to manage.

One approach to guiding clinical interventions is shown in Table 43-5. An institution's guidelines are summarized and placed in an accessible location (e.g., reverse side of the observation chart or nursing procedure manual). This can provide a consistent response to abnormal or undesirable observations throughout the institution.

DELIVERY OF EFFECTIVE ACUTE PAIN MANAGEMENT

Regardless of the drugs and techniques available to treat acute pain, the best patient outcomes can only be achieved if these are used as effectively and safely as possible. In general, this requires the provision of appropriate educational programs and suitable organizational structures. When more advanced methods of pain relief are used, or when acute pain management is needed in more complex patients, treatment may be supervised by an APS in some institutions.

General Requirements

Central to the ability to deliver safe and effective pain relief, regardless of the drug or technique used, are education (staff and patients), appropriate assessment and monitoring of patients (see earlier discussion), and the provision of proper guidelines and protocols for analgesic drugs and methods of drug administration.

Education

Patients. The need to provide appropriate education for patients seems to be well accepted. However, the best way in which to do this (e.g., verbally, by leaflet or video) has yet to be identified, and any evidence of benefit in terms of better pain relief remains inconsistent.

Most of the studies involve patients undergoing surgery. Although preoperative education will increase both patient and caregiver knowledge and understanding about pain and pain management (135–138), it may not always lead to improvements in postoperative pain relief.

Some studies have suggested that patient education improves pain relief (138–142); others have not been able to show any benefit either generally (135–137,143–147) or after specific types of surgery, such as total hip or knee arthroplasty (144), cardiac surgery (145,146), or gynecological surgery (147). In addition, patient satisfaction may (142,147) or may not (143) be increased, and anxiety may (140,142) or may not be reduced (136,137,145).

Nursing and Medical Staff. Education of staff (medical, nursing, and allied health) is usually seen as a requirement for effective and safe pain relief. The effect of staff education on pain management in general, as well as specific pain management techniques and prescribing practices, has been studied.

Improvements in the assessment of pain, prescribing practices, and the effectiveness of traditional methods of opioid analgesia have followed the implementation of education programs and introduction of guidelines (89,148). Others have also shown benefits both in general terms (149,150) and for specific medications, such as meperidine (pethidine) (151), acetaminophen (paracetamol) (152), and NSAIDs (153,154).

Education of staff can also affect the efficacy of more advanced methods of pain relief such as epidural analgesia and PCA. For example, the introduction of an APS nurse, whose role included routine education of ward staff, was followed by marked improvements in pain relief with PCA and significantly fewer side effects associated with epidural analgesia (155). Improvements in knowledge about epidural analgesia also followed the reintroduction of an epidural education program (156), and pain relief and patient evaluation of treatment in an emergency department was significantly improved after education of the junior medical staff (157).

Guidelines and Protocols

Institutional guidelines and protocols that cover drug prescription, assessment, and monitoring of patients, and recognition and treatment of any adverse effects of pain relief, can lead to improvements in the efficacy and safety of acute pain management techniques—using both the more advanced methods of pain relief such as PCA and epidural analgesia (see the later section on acute pain services) and simple methods of pain relief.

The introduction of a simple algorithm for intermittent intramuscular opioid administration in 15 hospitals in the United

Kingdom, accompanied by an education program and a requirement for formal assessment and monitoring of pain and pain relief, resulted in significant reductions in the number of patients with moderate to severe pain, and in the incidence of nausea and vomiting (148).

Professional bodies in a number of countries have issued guidelines for the management of acute pain. These include the ANZCA (111) and the American Society of Anesthesiology (90). Operative site-specific guidelines for acute pain management have been developed by the Veterans Health Administration and Department of Defense in the United States (158) and the European-based PROSPECT group (159).

However, the benefit or otherwise of any guidelines, whether developed by institutions or professional bodies, will depend on their relevance, effective dissemination and implementation, whether they accurately reflect current knowledge, and degree of compliance. Compliance with guidelines is known to be variable, although it may be better in larger institutions (160) and where staff with pain management expertise and formal quality assurance programs that monitor pain management are available (161).

Acute Pain Services

Variations in Terminology

The term *acute pain service* is used to cover a variety of different types of service. These can range from those that are a low-cost nursed-based service (162,163) to those that are led by an anesthesiologist but depend on acute pain nurses and are without daily input from an anesthesiologist (164–166), through to those that are comprehensive services with acute pain nurses and sometimes other staff such as pharmacists, and which have daily input from and 24-hour cover by anesthesiologists (167–169). In addition, although some APS restrict their activities essentially to supervision of the more sophisticated methods of acute pain management, others will also assist in optimizing all forms of acute pain therapies to all patient within an institution (170,171).

Effectiveness

Given the variety of services provided under the one title and the quality of the studies (often audits or before–after studies) looking at APS, it has not been possible to perform a proper meta-analysis of their benefits or otherwise (172). However, individual studies have suggested that an APS, whether nurse- or anesthesiologist-based, can improve pain relief and reduce the incidence of side effects after surgery, and that this benefit can be seen using the simpler forms of opioid analgesia as well as more sophisticated methods of pain relief.

When conventional intramuscular analgesia was supervised by an APS, pain scores were significantly lower (89), both at rest and with movement (148), and there were significantly fewer side effects (148). In a survey of 23 U.S. hospitals, of which 49% had an anesthesiologist-based APS, patients in the hospitals with an APS reported significantly lower pain scores, fewer side effects, and higher satisfaction ratings (21). Similar results were reported after the inception of nurse-based (18) and nurse-based, anesthesiologist-led APS (20), which resulted in significant improvements in pain scores. Stadler et al. (22) assessed pain relief and costs after the introduction of a nurse-based APS and showed that, once again, pain relief was improved, although it was associated with a small increase in cost.

Provision of a dedicated APS nurse led to a marked decrease in moderate to severe pain with PCA and epidural analgesia, significantly fewer side effects, increased patient satisfaction,

and increased use of oral analgesia (155). A comparison of the effectiveness of PCA and epidural analgesia before and after the introduction of an APS showed that resting and dynamic pain scores were significantly lower with both techniques when supervised by an APS (173). Similarly, when PCA was supervised by an APS, compared with the primary clinic a year earlier, patients used significantly more opioids but the incidence of side effects was almost halved (174). The APS was more likely to ensure that patients were comfortable before starting PCA, PCA bolus doses were altered more often to suit the individual patient, and patients were more likely to be given oral analgesia after PCA was ceased (174).

Werner et al. (19), in a review of publications looking at APS effectiveness, concluded that pain relief was significantly improved. However, they also noted that it was not possible to measure the role that other factors (e.g., regular visits by an APS, use of more effective analgesia techniques, and a general increased awareness of the need for better postoperative pain management) might have played in this improvement.

All APSs rely on APS nurses and, regardless of the model chosen, an organized team approach is important. However, regular scheduled input from anesthesiologists and the provision of 24-hour cover may offer additional advantages (170). As well as availability of advice about pain management problems, the anesthesiologist will have expert knowledge about the pharmacology of all analgesic agents, as well as the different delivery techniques available and their risks and benefits.

The anesthesiologist will also have a good understanding of the disease processes of the patients they are seeing, and may, if called on, be able to assist with acute postoperative and other medical problems. When an APS also performed a critical care "outreach" role and systematically reviewed high-risk postoperative patients for the first 3 days after surgery, the incidence of serious adverse events decreased from 23 to 16 events per 100 patients, and 30-day mortality was reduced from 9% to 3% ($p = 0.004$) (175).

Role

The role of an APS may differ according to APS type and the institution involved. The APS must provide resources ranging from defining policies and procedures to bedside consultation and the provision of clinical advice and management strategies. These must always be done within a cooperative and team-based approach with the primary clinicians caring for the patient.

In general, the role of an APS includes (170):

- Organization and standardization of initial and ongoing education of staff and patients (see earlier)
- Introduction and supervision of more advanced analgesic techniques
- Assistance in improving traditional opioid and nonopioid analgesic treatment regimens
- Assistance to standardize a number of aspects of acute pain care, including equipment, preprinted orders for advanced analgesic techniques, drugs used (including doses and concentrations), recognition and management of side effects and complications, monitoring requirements, nursing procedure protocols, and nondrug treatment orders (e.g., use of oxygen)
- Regular audit of activity and continuous quality improvement

Guidelines incorporating these aspects of care will help lead to consistent practices and may potentially improve analgesic efficacy and patient safety (176).

In addition, and in view of the complexity of patients often seen by an APS, collaboration and communication with other medical and nursing services including chronic pain, drug and alcohol, palliative care, and surgical services, is essential (170).

ANALGESIC DRUGS AND TECHNIQUES

In this section, most of the information will relate to analgesic drugs and techniques used for other than regional analgesia, as the latter subject is covered in depth in other chapters of this book.

As noted earlier, suboptimal acute pain management may, in some circumstances, result in potential harm to some patients. This information, as well as the data from many surveys published since the 1950s showing that acute pain (both postoperative and in medical wards) was often undertreated, encouraged many of the advances in both acute pain management techniques and drugs made over the last two to three decades. However, these advances have not always led to the anticipated improvements in pain relief. Factors other than just the efficacy of the many techniques and drugs now available for the treatment of acute pain play a part in determining overall patient outcome and include safety (side effects and complications), cost, and any influence on patient outcome, including morbidity and recovery. Therefore, factors affecting efficacy and safety are often inextricably linked.

Efficacy and Outcomes

Information about the efficacy of various analgesic drugs and techniques comes from a variety of sources. Although the best evidence is commonly assumed to result from meta-analyses of randomized controlled trials (RCTs), it is possible, when studies are undertaken to look at various techniques and drugs, that efficacy improves because of the study environment. For example, the close interest shown by investigators could lead to greater nursing attention paid to conventional methods of pain relief, with a consequent improvement in pain relief using these techniques—the "Hawthorn effect" (177). Therefore, data from other sources such as cohort studies, case-controlled studies, and audits, in addition to RCTs can provide a "real-life" perspective, even though the quality of evidence is less.

Patient-controlled Analgesia (Systemic Opioids)

Two meta-analyses (28,29), examining 15 and 55 RCTs respectively, have shown that PCA results in significantly better analgesia than conventional methods of opioid administration, although the magnitude of the improvement was only small. Other findings included significantly greater patient satisfaction, but no difference in length of hospital stay or the incidence of opioid-related side effects (except for an increased incidence of pruritus in the second analysis (29). A third meta-analysis (122) that looked at 32 RCTs found no difference in pain scores or side effects; PCA was only better if all pain outcomes (pain relief, pain intensity, and need for rescue analgesia) were considered; patients preferred PCA; and the risk of pulmonary complications was reduced.

The lack of a marked difference between PCA and conventional methods of opioid analgesia is a little surprising, given the results from a paper by Dolin and Cashman (5). These authors reviewed information obtained from published cohort studies, case-controlled studies, and audit reports as well as RCTs and looked at the percentage of patients who experienced moderate to severe pain and severe pain associated with as-needed intramuscular opioid analgesia, IV PCA, and epidural analgesia during the first 24 hours after surgery. For intramuscular analgesia, the mean (95% CI) percentage of patients with moderate to severe pain was 67.2% (58.1%–76.2%); for IV PCA, 35.8% (31.4%–40.2%); and for epidural analgesia, 20.9% (17.8%–24.0%). The results for severe pain were 29.1% (18.8%–39.4%), 10.4% (8.0%–12.8%), and 7.8% (6.1%–9.5%), respectively. Thus, in this review, PCA was significantly more effective than intermittent intramuscular opioid analgesia, although there was considerable room for improvement with all techniques.

Although studies other than RCTs provide a lower quality of evidence, it may be that they give a better view of "real life" effectiveness in a clinical setting, as noted earlier. As well as the advantageous influences of study conditions, it is possible that the way in which PCA was used in most of these studies did not adequately allow for interpatient variations (e.g., fixed program parameters) and significantly limited the flexibility of the technique (178).

A fourth meta-analysis (179) that specifically looked at the effectiveness of PCA after cardiac surgery found that PCA was no better than nurse-administered analgesia during the first 24 hours after surgery, but resulted in better pain relief during the second 24 hours. It is possible that where high nurse-to-patient ratios exist—when it may be possible to give any analgesia truly "on demand"—there is little difference between the techniques. This lack of difference has been noted by other authors comparing PCA with nurse-administered analgesia in areas likely to have higher nurse-to-patient ratios, such as the emergency department (180) and after cardiac surgery (181–183).

Three recent meta-analyses have shown that IV PCA is less effective than continuous epidural analgesia (64,184,185) and patient-controlled epidural analgesia (185), except when compared with hydrophilic opioid-only epidural regimens (185). Patient-controlled analgesia had higher incidences of nausea and sedation but was less likely to cause pruritus or urinary retention (64).

Although the term *patient-controlled analgesia* more commonly refers to IV PCA, PCA opioids may also be administered via other routes. Intranasal PCA (PCINA), using metered dose devices that allow the intranasal administration of a fixed dose of opioid, can provide analgesia that is as effective as IV PCA (186,187). Use of the subcutaneous route for PCA administration is also effective, although opioid dose requirements may be higher (188,189).

Recent developments in PCA have centered on the iontophoretic transdermal PCA fentanyl system, which uses a low-intensity electric current to drive the drug from the reservoir through the skin and into the systemic circulation (190). The PCA device, which is applied to the chest or upper outer arm, delivers a fixed dose of 40 μg fentanyl over a 10-minute period following a patient demand (190,191). The device allows delivery of up to six doses each hour, up to a maximum of 80 doses in 24 hours (191,192). It must be replaced every 24 hours, is not yet available in all countries, and is designed for in-hospital use only. Unlike fentanyl patches used for chronic pain management, no reservoir of drug is left in the skin once the device is removed (193).

Transdermal fentanyl PCA has been shown to be as effective as IV PCA using bolus doses of 1 mg morphine (194). Although the system is easy to use, does not require IV access, enables easier patient mobility, and avoids the programming errors that can occur with the use of electronic PCA devices, the cost and lack of dose flexibility may limit its widespread use.

PART IV: PAIN MANAGEMENT

Use in Patients with Obstructive Sleep Apnea. Patients with obstructive sleep apnea (OSA) are a group for whom concerns are often raised about the risks of opioid administration, including via PCA. The prevalence of OSA in the adult population is surprisingly high, with up to 20% estimated to have mild OSA, approximately 7% to have moderate to severe OSA, and up to 5% of adults estimated to have undiagnosed OSA that could benefit from treatment (195).

In the acute pain setting, there is concern that the patient with OSA is at increased risk of respiratory depression and hypoxia if given opioid or sedative drugs. This concern is not unreasonable given that, in any patient, it is known that opioid administration can lead to recurrent episodes of upper airway obstruction when the patient is asleep (i.e., not unlike OSA) and that hypoxemic episodes are more likely to be associated with upper airway obstruction rather than decreases in respiratory rate (196–198).

Case reports of life-threatening respiratory depression have been published following opioid administration via a number of routes (but especially using IV PCA) and are often used to "demonstrate" the potential danger of opioid administration in patients with OSA.

Four of these reports involved the use of PCA in patients with OSA: one patient given PCA set to deliver (inappropriately) a background infusion of morphine of 2 mg/hr was found unconscious with a PaCo$_2$ of 94 mm Hg (199); another was "found to be unarousable" with a PaCo$_2$ of 76 mm Hg (200); yet another was "heavily sedated and hypercapnic" (201); and a final composite case derived from reported claims cases was "found in respiratory arrest" 1 hour after "his last normal vital signs" (202).

However, complications have also been documented in patients given opioids via other routes. Respiratory arrest and the death of three patients receiving postoperative bupivacaine and fentanyl epidural infusions have also been reported (203). The usual sign of respiratory depression described was a decrease in ventilatory frequency. In another report, a patient died after being given intramuscular morphine; during the 2 hours after the injection, he was noted to be "sleeping" and then "unresponsive," and an order was given to continue monitoring of vital signs (204).

It would seem, from these reports, that the significance of increasing sedation as the best early clinical indicator of respiratory depression was not recognized, and inappropriate reliance was placed on monitoring of the patient's respiratory rate.

There remains a paucity of good evidence to guide the best choice of technique or drug in patients with OSA. In addition, many patients with undiagnosed OSA are likely to present for surgery or in other situations that require treatment of their acute pain. Therefore, it is important to provide adequate and appropriate analgesic regimens, including monitoring—and in particular monitoring of sedation level—for all patients given opioids, not just those with diagnosed OSA.

The use of PCA with appropriate bolus doses and monitoring in patients who were morbidly obese, and, therefore, more likely to have OSA (195), has been reported to be safe (205), and as safe as intramuscular opioids (206) and epidural analgesia (207), although patient numbers were small and, therefore, the studies were unlikely to be able to show any difference in the incidence of respiratory depression.

In addition, supplemental oxygen given to patients with OSA (not in a perioperative setting) has been shown to be as effective as continuous positive airway pressure (CPAP) ventilation in reducing the risk of significant hypoxemia (208,209). Despite concerns about reducing respiratory drive during apneic periods (202), the routine use of supplemental oxygen would seem appropriate in all patients with OSA, or suspected of having OSA, and receiving opioids for the treatment of their pain.

Epidural Analgesia

Because detailed information relating to efficacy and outcomes of epidural is given in Chapter 7, a short summary only of the beneficial effects of epidural analgesia is given in this section.

As outlined earlier, epidural analgesia provides better pain relief compared with parenteral opioids including IV PCA opioids. Compared with systemic and epidural opioid analgesia, epidural analgesia with a local anesthetic agent leads to earlier recovery of bowel function after abdominal surgery; the effects are more likely to be seen with thoracic rather than lumbar epidural pain relief (210–212). Thoracic epidural analgesia has also been shown to reduce the risk of pneumonia and ventilator days in patients with fractured ribs (213) and reduce the incidence of postoperative myocardial infarction (214).

In patients having elective open abdominal aortic surgery, the use of postoperative epidural analgesia (especially thoracic epidural analgesia) resulted in better pain relief for up to 3 days after surgery, a reduction in duration of mechanical ventilation of 20%, and a lower risk of cardiovascular and renal complications compared with systemic opioid administration (215). Also compared with systemic opioids, epidural local anesthetics led to a reduction in the incidence of pulmonary complications and improved oxygenation (216).

Continuous Peripheral Nerve Block Analgesia

The use of continuous peripheral nerve blockade (CPNB) is becoming increasingly common and is described in more detail in other chapters in this book.

A recent meta-analysis (217) of 19 RCTs that looked at the effectiveness of CPNB concluded that CPNB, regardless of anatomic location, results in better pain relief, decreases opioid use, and reduces the incidence of opioid-related side effects compared with opioid-only analgesia. Similar results were reported in a review of lower extremity CPNB (218), which concluded that the technique provides effective analgesia in the postoperative period, reduces opioid requirements, and improves rehabilitation.

The risk of major neurologic and infectious complications seems to be rare. Capdevila et al. (131) performed a prospective analysis of CPNB after orthopedic surgery in 1,416 patients. They found that effective analgesia was obtained in over 96% of patients. The following incidences were also noted: hypoesthesia 3%, numbness 2.2%, femoral nerve lesions (all resolved between 3 days and 10 weeks) 0.21%, local inflammation 3%, and psoas abscess 0.07% (131). Other complications associated with the use of various types of CPNB include diaphragmatic paralysis (interscalene block) and drug toxicity.

Multimodal Analgesia

Multiple mechanisms, often coexisting, are involved in pain perception (219). It is, therefore, not surprising that treatment of pain may require multimodal strategies. Indeed, the use of multimodal analgesia in the treatment of acute pain should be the rule rather than the exception for most patients.

The term *multimodal* refers to the use of a combination of drugs from more than one class of analgesic agent (e.g., opioid, local anesthetic, and acetaminophen) having different mechanisms and/or sites of action; these drugs may be delivered using a variety of techniques. The aim is to maximize the pain relief achieved, particularly dynamic pain, while minimizing the incidence of analgesia-related side effects (220). Multimodal analgesia should also be combined with multimodal and multidisciplinary rehabilitation programs to assist and speed patient recovery (220).

Options for multimodal analgesia, therefore, include a variety of systemically and regionally administered analgesic agents. Only the systemic administration of analgesic drugs is covered in this chapter, as their use in regional analgesia is discussed in detail elsewhere in the book.

Analgesic Drugs

Acetaminophen (Paracetamol)

Acetaminophen is an effective analgesic agent (221), but its exact mechanisms of action are yet to be clearly defined. It has no known endogenous binding sites; it does not appear to inhibit peripheral COX activity; inhibition of COX-2 activity in the CNS is possible; and there may be selective inhibition of putative COX-3 activity by acetaminophen (222–224). It has also been suggested that part of the analgesic action of acetaminophen results from modulation of descending inhibitory serotonergic pathways (225).

Acetaminophen can be given intravenously. The preparation first introduced into clinical practice for IV use was propacetamol, a prodrug that was rapidly metabolized to acetaminophen; an IV preparation of acetaminophen itself is now available. These two preparations have comparable efficacy but a higher incidence of local pain occurs at the infusion site with propacetamol (226,227).

The onset of analgesia after propacetamol is shorter than after oral acetaminophen (228); compared with propacetamol, oral administration of acetaminophen results in a large and unpredictable variation in plasma concentration (229). Loading doses of 2 g acetaminophen IV have been suggested, as this has been shown to be significantly better than 1 g IV in terms of magnitude and duration of analgesia effect (230), but further studies are probably needed before this can be recommended.

Acetaminophen given as a regularly administered adjunct to opioid analgesia leads to significant opioid-sparing, but this may or may not improve pain relief, and does not reduce the incidence of opioid-related adverse effects. Romsing et al. (231) showed that the combination using oral or rectal acetaminophen resulted in significantly better pain relief and a reduction in opioid requirements of 20% to 30%. A later meta-analysis by Remy et al. (232) looked at the morphine-sparing effect of acetaminophen when given orally or intravenously in conjunction with morphine PCA. Again, a morphine-sparing effect of 20% was noted, but this was not associated with a reduction in morphine-related side effects. Similarly, another meta-analysis by Elia et al. (233) found significant opioid-sparing with acetaminophen but no benefit in terms of pain relief or adverse effects.

The analgesic efficacy of acetaminophen is improved by the addition of an NSAID (231,234).

Acetaminophen is well-tolerated by most patients, giving rise to few adverse effects (221,235), and it is an important component of multimodal analgesia. Compared with NSAIDs and COX inhibitors, it has a more favorable cardiovascular and gastrointestinal safety profile (236) and is the preferred choice in high-risk patients (234).

Concerns about the risks of cardiovascular events associated with the use of NSAIDs are discussed later. Chan et al. (237) have suggested that the use of high-frequency or high doses of acetaminophen, but not more moderate use, is also associated with an increase in the risk of major cardiovascular events. However, a case control study of acetaminophen in relation to myocardial infarction found no such increased risk (238).

Acetaminophen is often avoided in patients with chronic liver disease. However, evidence for this practice is not strong. A review by Benson et al. (239) concluded that acetaminophen can be used safely in patients with liver disease and would be the preferred analgesic/antipyretic in these patients. In addition, it would seem that therapeutic doses of acetaminophen are unlikely to result in hepatotoxicity in patients who take moderate to large amounts of alcohol (235,240).

Nonsteroidal Anti-inflammatory Drugs and COX-2 Inhibitors

Prostaglandins, produced by the COX enzyme, play a key role in the maintenance of many normal physiologic functions. They are also released in response to tissue damage. This enzyme has two isoforms, COX-1 and COX-2 (and possibly COX-3, as noted earlier). The physiologic roles of prostaglandins are mainly regulated by COX-1, which is said to be "constitutive"; tissue damage results in COX-2 production (i.e., it is "inducible") and synthesis of prostaglandins, resulting in pain and inflammation, although COX-2 is also constitutive in some tissues (e.g., the kidney). Inhibition of the COX enzyme leads to a reduction in prostaglandin synthesis, with analgesic and anti-inflammatory effects. This mechanism is also responsible for many of the adverse effects of COX inhibition.

Nonsteroidal anti-inflammatory drugs are nonselective inhibitors of both the COX-1 and COX-2 isoenzymes. They are effective analgesics (111,241). Although drugs that selectively inhibit COX-2 do not result in better pain relief than nonselective NSAIDs (242,243), they have a significantly lower incidence of gastrointestinal complications (242,244–247). Other benefits of COX-2 inhibitors include a lack of platelet inhibition, less impairment of bone healing, and safety of use in patients with aspirin-exacerbated respiratory disease (245,248). However, the risk of other adverse effects, including effects on renal function and exacerbation of cardiac failure, is similar to nonselective NSAIDs (242,244,245,249).

The use of both nonselective, nonaspirin NSAIDs and COX inhibitors may increase the risk of cardiovascular and cerebrovascular events (237,250–253), although most information is gained from studies of other than short-term use (days) for the treatment of acute pain. Short-term use may not have the same associated risks (254). In addition, regular use of NSAIDs may interfere with the clinical benefits of low-dose aspirin (255,256).

Two recent meta-analyses (117,233) have shown that NSAIDs have a 30% to 55% sparing effect on morphine consumption and a resultant decrease in the incidence of nausea, vomiting, and sedation; however, the risk of severe bleeding was increased (233). A similar opioid-sparing effect has been reported in meta-analyses looking at COX-2 inhibitors, but an associated reduction in opioid-related adverse events was not seen (233,257,258). Pain relief is also improved (233). Selective COX-2 inhibitors did increase the risk of renal failure in cardiac surgical patients (233).

Opioids and Tramadol

In general and at equianalgesic doses, no one particular opioid administered by a systemic route appears to be better than any other, either in terms of efficacy, patient satisfaction, or incidence of adverse effects (111). Individual patients may gain benefit from one opioid over another. In a cross-over three-way double-blinded RCT comparing morphine, fentanyl, and pethidine (that is, all three opioids were studied in each patient), Woodhouse et al. (259) showed that, whereas overall analgesia was equivalent for all three drugs, some patients were able to tolerate one or more of the opioids better than another.

Side effects of opioid analgesia have been discussed earlier (see section on Assessment and Monitoring). As noted previously, the importance of monitoring a patient's level of sedation to detect early respiratory depression cannot be overemphasized (111).

The key to effective analgesia with opioids is titration to effect for each patient. Considerable inter- and intra-patient variability is possible in the pharmacodynamics and pharmacokinetics of opioids (260), and the effective minimal analgesic concentrations (MEAC) of opioids vary four- to fivefold between patients (261–264). Therefore, to obtain good pain relief in individual patients, doses must be altered according to regular assessments of pain and adverse effects (particularly sedation), as discussed earlier.

Differences may be seen between different opioids when given in conjunction with neuraxial analgesia (see Chapter 11).

Tramadol is an effective analgesia agent and an effective treatment for neuropathic pain (61). In general, tramadol is less likely to cause respiratory depression (265,266), constipation (267), or delayed gastric emptying (268) than pure agonist opioids.

Local Anesthetic Agents

Local anesthetic drugs are discussed in detail in Chapters 1 to 5.

Adjuvant Analgesic Drugs

A number of other drugs are often given as adjuvant medications in the management of acute pain.

A recent meta-analysis (62) of low-dose ketamine given in conjunction with opioid therapy has shown that it is opioid sparing and results in less nausea and vomiting, and adverse effects are either mild or absent. The issue of optimal dose remains unresolved.

Although there is little evidence of any benefit of most antidepressant drugs on nociceptive acute pain (111), they may reduce the risk of development of persistent pain after surgery (see earlier discussion under Prevention Strategies). However, perioperative use of gabapentin can lead to significant reductions in postoperative pain intensity and analgesic use.

Three recent meta-analyses have looked at the use of gabapentin for postoperative analgesia (269–271). All reported that gabapentin resulted in better pain relief and a reduction in opioid requirements; increased sedation was noted in two of the studies (270,271).

Systemic administration of clonidine is also opioid-sparing (272) and improves pain relief (273). However, side effects such as sedation and hypotension can limit its usefulness in the clinical setting (111). Magnesium also improves pain relief and reduces postoperative opioid requirements (274).

The use of adjuvant drugs with regional analgesia is discussed in other chapters in this book.

Regional Analgesia

The efficacy, management, and complications of techniques used in regional analgesia (including central neuraxial, plexus, and peripheral nerve block) are covered in detail in other chapters in this book. A brief summary of side effects of epidural analgesia has been included earlier in this chapter.

Regional Analgesia after Ambulatory Surgery

The use of continuous peripheral nerve blocks for pain relief at home after ambulatory surgery was first described in 1998 (275) and followed the introduction of lightweight and portable infusion pumps. The technique has rapidly gained acceptance, and the literature pertaining to its use has grown markedly over just the last few years. The types of continuous peripheral nerve infusion that have been used include paravertebral, interscalene, infraclavicular, axillary, psoas compartment, femoral, sciatic, and tibial.

A recent detailed review by Ilfeld and Enneking (276) summarized this relatively new information and highlighted some of the important issues to be considered when using these methods of pain relief at home. The benefits reported included improved pain relief, better sleep, lower opioid consumption, a decreased incidence of opioid-related side effects, and increased patient satisfaction (276). These authors also highlighted the need for appropriate patient selection, accurate catheter placement, firm fixation of the catheter, selection of a suitable infusion solution and infusion regimen (this will vary according to the anatomic site), and use of a reliable pump. Most importantly, they stress the need for verbal and written patient and caregiver information and education, and organization of patient contact and follow-up, as well as catheter removal.

Patient-controlled Analgesia

As noted earlier, PCA, whether administered by IV or other routes is a very effective analgesic technique. The topic is covered in detail in recent reviews (177,178,277), so a brief summary only will be included in this chapter.

The PCA concept dates back to 1968, when Sechzer (278) allowed patients to choose the timing of administration of 1 mL IV doses of opioid given to them by a nurse according to their level of pain. Later, in 1971, he described a machine that allowed patients to self-administer these bolus doses as needed (279). He found that this analgesic demand system provided better pain relief than fixed-dose, nurse-administered regimens.

There are two main types of PCA devices, electronic and disposable. The latter includes the transdermal PCA system just described. With the use of some disposable devices, the drug and drug concentration may be varied, but the volume of the bolus dose cannot be changed; in others, neither the drug administered nor the bolus dose delivered can be altered. Thus, dose regimens are much less flexible compared with electronic devices. The drug reservoirs for these devices are also more readily accessible, raising security issues.

Electronic PCA pumps allow flexibility in use through variations in programmed parameter settings, which can help maximize both the efficacy and safety of the technique. The various parameters must be specified as part of the PCA prescription, and this should be done in a way that takes into account the evidence (where it exists) for choosing a particular setting. The variable PCA parameters and any evidence for choosing a particular setting are summarized in Table 43-9 (177,178,280–287).

Little evidence suggests that any one opioid is better than any other when used with IV PCA in terms of side effects (111). Possible opioid-related side effects have been covered in an earlier section of this chapter.

TABLE 43-9

PROGRAMMABLE PATIENT-CONTROLLED ANALGESIA (PCA) VARIABLES

Variable	Comment
Bolus dose	■ "Optimal" dose that provides consistent, satisfactory analgesia without producing excessive or dangerous side effects ■ Optimal doses may be 1 mg for morphine (280) and 30 μg fentanyl delivered over 5 minutes (281) or 40 μg for fentanyl, delivered over 10 minutes (282). ■ The size of the bolus dose will need to be increased or decreased as needed according to subsequent reports of pain or the onset of any side effects (178). ■ PCA is neither a "one size fits all" nor a "set and forget" therapy (283).
Lockout interval	■ No difference in analgesia was shown with lockout intervals (for IV PCA) of 7 to 11 minutes for morphine and 5 to 8 minutes for fentanyl (284).
Loading dose	■ Enormous interpatient differences in loading dose requirements mean that individual titration of the loading dose is usually required prior to starting PCA (177).
Background infusions (in opioid naive patients)	■ Do not improve analgesia (285) or sleep (286) ■ Increase the risk of respiratory depression (287)
Dose limit	■ No good evidence shows benefit (or otherwise) from the use of a dose limit (177). ■ For PCA to be used effectively in all patients, a wide range of opioid doses may be required.

PATIENT VARIABLES THAT MAY INFLUENCE TREATMENT

As noted earlier, operative site-specific guidelines for acute pain management have been developed by the U.S. Veterans Health Administration and Department of Defense (158) and by the European-based PROSPECT group (159). The PROSPECT group in particular has developed excellent and very detailed evidence-based guidelines for a number of procedures to date, and work on other procedures is ongoing. The reader is referred to the organization's Web site.

However, occasions will arise when these guidelines may not be as applicable to some patients as they will be to others, as a number of patient factors may also influence treatment. These include the age of the patient, the culture from which the patient comes, the patient gender, differences in genetic and psychological makeup, and if the patient is opioid-tolerant or has a substance abuse disorder (SAD).

Patient Age

Effect on Opioids

Age, rather than patient weight, appears to be a better determinant of the amount of opioid an adult is likely to require for effective management of acute pain. Clinical and experimental evidence suggests a two- to fourfold decrease in opioid requirements as patient age increases (288–294). The decrease in opioid requirement is not associated with reports of increased pain (288,290).

Although interpatient variability in pharmacokinetics and MEAC is well-documented, it would seem that this age-related decrease in opioid requirement is due mainly to pharmacodynamic rather than pharmacokinetic factors (292,293). The reasons for the pharmacodynamic differences are not yet clear but could be due to changes in the number or function of opioid receptors in the CNS, or an increased penetration of opioids into the CNS (295). It is known that aging is associated with changes, such as reductions in the density of neurons, neurotransmitters, and receptors in the CNS (296,297), that may predispose the elderly to increased drug sensitivity (298,299).

As renal function inevitably declines with age, the elderly patient may also be at risk of accumulation of any active metabolites of opioids such as morphine, normeperidine, and dextropropoxyphene, and tramadol. For this reason, meperidine (300) and dextropropoxyphene (244) should be avoided in the elderly, and lower daily maximum dose limits of tramadol are suggested for patients older than 75 years (301).

As noted earlier, there appears to be little difference in the side-effect profiles of different opioids at equianalgesic doses in most patients. However, in the elderly, fentanyl may cause less depression of postoperative cognitive function (302) and confusion (303). No difference in cognitive effects was seen in a comparison of fentanyl and tramadol in patients groups with average ages of 61 and 63 years, respectively (304). The elderly patient seems less likely to suffer from opioid-related nausea and vomiting (305) or pruritus (306).

The range of techniques available for opioid administration in the elderly patients is the same as for their younger counterparts. Patient-controlled analgesia can be a safe and very effective method of pain relief in elderly patients, providing they have reasonably normal cognitive function (289,307,308). As

PART IV: PAIN MANAGEMENT

with younger patients, PCA is more effective than conventional methods of opioid administration in older patients (309,310).

Like parenteral opioids, epidural opioid requirements also decrease as patient age increases (311).

Effect on Local Anesthetics

The half-lives of local anesthetics such as bupivacaine (312) and ropivacaine (313) are significantly increased, and clearances significantly decreased, in older patients. These patients are also more sensitive to the effects of local anesthetics because of age-related physiologic changes that include an increase in sensory neuron degeneration, decreases in the densities of peripheral nerve fibers and CNS neurons, and a slowing of nerve fiber conduction velocities (296,297,314).

Age is also a factor determining the spread of local anesthetic in the epidural space and degree of motor blockade. It has been shown that, in older patients, epidural doses of levobupivacaine (315) and ropivacaine (316) result in a higher block level, thus smaller volumes will be needed to cover the same number of dermatomes. In addition, when the same volume of local anesthetic is given, the same concentration results in more intense motor blockade (316,317).

As with younger patients, epidural analgesia results in lower pain scores at rest and movement, higher satisfaction scores, and more rapid recovery of bowel function compared with IV PCA (308). However, older patients may be more susceptible to some of the side effects of epidural analgesia, including hypotension (316,318,319).

Age-related changes have also been reported with other forms of regional analgesia. For example, the duration of action of sciatic nerve (320) and brachial plexus blocks (321) may be prolonged.

Gender

The effect of patient gender on reported pain scores and opioid use in the acute pain setting remains poorly understood (322). Evidence suggests that opioids may be more effective in females but that this can depend on the opioid used, with the main differences being reported with κ-agonist opioids (322).

Evidence for any difference in opioid requirements varies. For example, higher morphine requirements in the immediate postoperative period have been reported for female patients (323,324), whereas no difference was seen in adolescent patients using PCA (325). In Chinese patients using PCA morphine in the postoperative period, female patients consumed significantly less morphine than their male counterparts (326). After knee ligament reconstruction, no difference in morphine consumption was seen (327).

In comparisons of reported pain scores after surgery, it has been found that female patients report higher scores than male patients. Higher VAS scores have been seen in the immediate postoperative period after a variety of surgical procedures (323,324) in adolescent patients using PCA after their surgery (325) and after specific types of surgery, for example after intraoral implants (328), knee ligament reconstruction (327), and arthroscopy (329).

Psychological Factors

Psychological factors may play a significant role in the pain experience, whether acute or chronic, or during the transition from acute to chronic pain (330,331).

Preoperative anxiety (41,332–335), high Pain Catastrophizing Scale (PCS) scores (336–338), preoperative depression (41,335,339), and neuroticism (340) have all been associated with higher intensities of postoperative pain. As noted earlier, depression may also be associated with an increased incidence of persistent postsurgical pain (12).

Locus of control has been investigated and found not to be associated with postoperative pain intensity in patients using PCA (334). Others have noted lower pain ratings with perceived control (341) or no change (342).

Genetics

Genetic variability may also affect a patient's response to opioids. A recent review by Klepstad et al. (343) looked at the effects on morphine pharmacology by variability in genes coding μ-opioid receptors, blood–brain barrier transport of morphine by multidrug resistance transporters, and morphine metabolism.

The μ-opioid receptor gene plays a role in mediating the endogenous and exogenous effects of opioids. The effects on morphine consumption of single nucleotide polymorphism at nucleotide position 118 on the μ-opioid receptor gene have been studied after two different types of surgery. To reach adequate levels of analgesia after total abdominal hysterectomy, Chou et al. (344) found that patients homozygous for G118 required more morphine than did patients who were homozygous for A118; that is, they had a poorer response to morphine, although the difference in total morphine dose was small and of minimal clinical significance. The same group also reported similar results in patients after total knee arthroplasty (345). A different group looked at the differences in patients undergoing colorectal surgery and were unable to find a statistically significant difference, although there was a trend toward higher morphine use in patients carrying the G118 allele, but the proportion of patients with this allele was low (291). The correlation of G118 and higher opioid requirements has also been noted in patients with cancer pain (346).

Patient genotype can also influence the efficacy of tramadol. Genetic polymorphism can result in absent enzyme activity of CYP2D6 in patients who are "poor metabolizers" (about 10% of the Caucasian population); these patients have a reduced analgesic response to tramadol compared with patients who are "extensive" (normal) metabolizers (347,348). Poor metabolizers are also known to get no pain relief from codeine (348).

Opioid Tolerance

Tolerance has been defined as "the phenomenon whereby chronic exposure to a drug diminishes its antinociceptive or analgesic effect, or creates the need for a higher dose to maintain this effect" (349).

The mechanisms underlying the development of tolerance are still not fully understood, but they appear to overlap with those mechanisms that are thought to produce and maintain persistent pain states, and include desensitization and downregulation (i.e., a decrease in responsiveness) of μ-opioid receptors and involvement of the N-methyl-D-aspartate (NMDA) receptor (349). These mechanisms may also overlap with those underlying opioid-induced hyperalgesia (OIH), a term used to indicate that, in some circumstances, opioids can, paradoxically, lead to increased pain sensitivity (hyperalgesia) rather than analgesia.

In the acute pain setting, when opioid requirements are known to be markedly increased in opioid-tolerant patients (350), it may be difficult to differentiate between this mix of tolerance to opioids and OIH. However, with OIH and unlike tolerance, increasing opioid doses will not improve analgesia. It is possible that those interventions outlined in the following section that may help to attenuate tolerance may also be effective for OIH.

Management of Acute Pain in Opioid-tolerant Patients

The main aims of treatment in opioid-tolerant patients are to provide adequate analgesia and to prevent the onset of withdrawal signs and symptoms. Therapies aimed at attenuating tolerance may also be useful.

Analgesia. In general, multimodal analgesic regimens that include opioids, regional analgesia (where indicated), NSAIDs or COX-2 inhibitors, ketamine, and clonidine will be of most benefit in these patients (351).

The doses of opioid that are required by opioid-tolerant patients for the management of their acute pain are usually significantly greater than those needed by their opioid-naïve counterparts. Rapp et al. (350) found that postoperative PCA opioid doses were three times higher in patients who were taking opioids prior to admission for treatment of cancer or chronic pain, or because the patient was taking illicit opioids, than in matched opioid-naïve patients. Interestingly, although the incidence of nausea and vomiting was less in the opioid-tolerant group, the risk of excessive sedation (used as an indicator of early respiratory depression) was higher.

However, determination of the appropriate starting dose of opioid can be difficult, and limited data are available on which to base this decision. Davis et al. (352) developed a technique whereby they can establish individualized doses in opioid-tolerant patients. Using a preoperative high-dose fentanyl infusion and pharmacokinetic simulation, they were able to determine the fentanyl effect site concentration associated with a respiratory rate of less than 5 breaths/minute for individual patients. This was used to predict a postoperative hourly infusion rate that would result in analgesic effect site concentrations, half of which was then delivered as a basal infusion and the other half as patient-demand bolus doses.

An alternative suggestion is to convert the patient's normal preadmission opioid requirement to the equivalent amount of the opioid to be used in PCA and calculate the hourly rate (mg/hr); if the patient cannot take his usual opioid, then this rate can be used as a background infusion. The bolus dose will usually need to be increased as well, and a reasonable initial bolus dose in mg would be the same as the background infusion in mg/hr (170). These doses can then be adjusted as required.

Prevention of Withdrawal. Continuation of the patient's normal preadmission opioid requirements (the doses of which should be verified where possible, especially if a patient is taking high doses or is part of a drug-dependence program) or the equivalent using an alternative opioid or route of administration will prevent withdrawal. Tramadol given as the sole analgesic will not prevent withdrawal; the use of partial agonist and agonist-antagonist opioid drugs may precipitate withdrawal, and the doses of opioids administered by the epidural or intrathecal routes may not be enough to prevent withdrawal (351).

In patients with a substance abuse disorder, dependence on other drugs such as benzodiazepines or alcohol is common. Treatment must also aim to prevent withdrawal from these drugs. It is also worth noting that withdrawal from amphetamines can result in severe sedation, which can impact on the safety of giving adequate doses of opioid.

Attenuation of Tolerance. A number of strategies may help attenuate opioid tolerance to a certain degree and improve analgesia. Those that might be of some use in the acute pain setting include:

- *Addition of nonopioids, including paracetamol and NSAIDs/COX-2 inhibitors.* In rats, it has been shown that COX may be involved in the development of opioid tolerance (353).
- *Opioid rotation.* A change to another opioid, in smaller than equivalent doses, may result in better analgesia and an improved side-effect profile (354).
- *Use of regional analgesic techniques.*
- *Use of NMDA receptor antagonists such as ketamine or drugs such as clonidine (354).* Some limited evidence suggests that ketamine may reduce opioid requirements and improve pain relief in opioid-tolerant patients (355–358).
- *Use of naloxone and nalbuphine.* Animal evidence shows that ultra-low-dose naloxone infusions attenuate opioid-tolerance (359,360) and that coadministration of nalbuphine has a similar effect (361).

Patients with a Substance Abuse Disorder

Patients with a substance abuse disorder who are dependent on opioids can present additional concerns. In addition to being opioid-tolerant, management may be complicated by associated psychological and behavioral factors, by the presence of other drugs of abuse (polyabuse is common) or medications that assist with drug withdrawal and/or rehabilitation, and by possible complications related to drug abuse, including infectious diseases. In some patients, concerns may arise because of the difficulty in balancing anxieties about undertreatment of pain against safety and possible diversion of the drug (351). Close liaison with drug and alcohol services and other treating clinicians is recommended.

A number of papers have been published recently reviewing the management of acute pain in these patients (351,362–365). To date, however, most information is based on experience and little, if any, good quality evidence is available to guide treatment (111).

In general, management of a patients with a SAD involving opioids is similar to that of any patients who is opioid-tolerant, except that it must also take into account the factors just noted (psychological and behavioral factors, presence of other drugs of abuse, medications used in the treatment of drug dependence). No evidence exists for concerns that the use of opioids may lead to a relapse of the SAD; in fact, unrelieved pain may be more likely to be a trigger for relapse (365). Unrelieved pain may also be a more common cause of these patients asking for ("seeking") more opioid (a term that has been coined "pseudo-addiction" [26]), rather than an occasion of the patient exhibiting true aberrant drug-seeking behaviors (365). Patients may also "seek" opioids if they are concerned about the risk of withdrawal (365).

Drugs Used in the Treatment of Substance Abuse Disorders. Methadone is a long-acting pure opioid agonist often used in the management of patients with an opioid SAD. In the acute pain setting, if the patient cannot take their usual oral methadone, substitution with parenteral methadone or another pure opioid agonist will be needed (351,363).

Naltrexone is a pure opioid antagonist with a similar structure to naloxone, but it is much more effective when given orally and it has a longer duration of action (362). It is used in the treatment of both opioid and alcohol addiction. It has been suggested, where possible and in view of its prolonged action, that it be ceased at least 24 hours prior to surgery (351,363); others have suggested 48 to 72 hours (362). Some experimental evidence exists of opioid receptor upregulation following cessation of naltrexone, and patients may, therefore, be more sensitive to opioids (366), so that lower than expected opioid requirements may be seen once the effect of naltrexone has faded. Although naltrexone is more commonly administered orally, long-acting implantable pellets are also available in some countries, which can make adequate pain relief in the acute setting more difficult.

Buprenorphine is a partial μ-agonist and κ-antagonist (367) that is increasingly being used in the treatment of opioid SADs. There is no good evidence on which to base treatment of these patients as yet. The main choice is whether to cease or continue buprenorphine; if the latter course is chosen, a change to another opioid (e.g., methadone) will be required to prevent withdrawal (365). Otherwise management is similar to that of the opioid-tolerant patient described earlier.

SUMMARY

Significant advances in acute pain management continue to develop at a rapid rate. In the future, it is likely that there will be a better understanding of the reasons behind the inter-individual variation in response to opioids and that the major advances in the treatment of pain using opioids will involve the concurrent use of adjuvants rather than new pure agonist opioids. Peripheral regional analgesia is likely to increase in popularity now that more surgery is done on an ambulatory basis, and pain relief techniques will need to evolve to suit "fast-track" surgery. Importantly, the link between acute pain and persistent pain will be further explored and, hopefully, strategies will be developed that may reduce the burden of chronic postsurgical pain.

References

1. Merskey H. Pain terms: A list with definitions and notes on usage. Recommended by the Subcommittee on Taxonomy. *Pain* 1979;6:249–252.
2. Ready LB, Edwards WT. *Management of Acute Pain: A Practical Guide.* Taskforce on Acute Pain. Seattle: IASP Publications, 1992.
3. Apfelbaum JL, Chen C, Mehta SS, et al. Postoperative pain experience: Results from a national survey suggest postoperative pain continues to be undermanaged. *Anesth Analg* 2003;97:534–540.
4. Dix P, Sandhar B, Murdoch J, et al. Pain on medical wards in a district general hospital. *Br J Anaesth* 2004;92:235–237.
5. Dolin SJ, Cashman JN, Bland JM. Effectiveness of acute postoperative pain management: I. Evidence from published data. *Br J Anaesth* 2002;89:409–423.
6. Yates P, Dewar A, Edwards H, et al. The prevalence and perception of pain amongst hospital in-patients. *J Clin Nurs* 1998;7:521–530.
7. Cousins MJ, Brennan F, Carr DB. Pain relief: A universal human right. *Pain* 2004;112:1–4.
8. Tsui SL, Law S, Fok M, et al. Postoperative analgesia reduces mortality and morbidity after esophagectomy. *Am J Surg* 1997;173:472–478.
9. Bode RH Jr., Lewis KP, Zarich SW, et al. Cardiac outcome after peripheral vascular surgery. Comparison of general and regional anesthesia. *Anesthesiology* 1996;84:3–13.
10. Marcucci C, Chassot PG, Gardaz JP, et al. Fatal myocardial infarction after lung resection in a patient with prophylactic preoperative coronary stenting. *Br J Anaesth* 2004;92:743–747.
11. Hooten WM, Karanikolas M, Swarm R, et al. Postoperative pain management following bilateral lung volume reduction surgery for severe emphysema. *Anaesth Intensive Care* 2005;33:591–596.
12. Tasmuth T, Blomqvist C, Kalso E. Chronic post-treatment symptoms in patients with breast cancer operated in different surgical units. *Eur J Surg Oncol* 1999;25:38–43.
13. Katz J, Jackson M, Kavanagh BP, et al. Acute pain after thoracic surgery predicts long-term post-thoracotomy pain. *Clin J Pain* 1996;12:50–55.
14. Senturk M, Ozcan PE, Talu GK, et al. The effects of three different analgesia techniques on long-term postthoracotomy pain. *Anesth Analg* 2002;94:11–15.
15. Kalso E, Perttunen K, Kaasinen S. Pain after thoracic surgery. *Acta Anaesthesiol Scand* 1992;36:96–100.
16. Schafheutle EI, Cantrill JA, Noyce PR. Why is pain management suboptimal on surgical wards? *J Adv Nurs* 2001;33:728–737.
17. Dahl JL. Pain: Impediments and suggestions for solutions. *J Natl Cancer Inst Monogr* 2004:124–126.
18. Salomaki TE, Hokajarvi TM, Ranta P, et al. Improving the quality of postoperative pain relief. *Eur J Pain* 2000;4:367–372.
19. Werner MU, Soholm L, Rotboll-Nielsen P, et al. Does an acute pain service improve postoperative outcome? *Anesth Analg* 2002;95:1361–1372.
20. Bardiau FM, Taviaux NF, Albert A, et al. An intervention study to enhance postoperative pain management. *Anesth Analg* 2003;96:179–185.
21. Miaskowski C, Crews J, Ready LB, et al. Anesthesia-based pain services improve the quality of postoperative pain management. *Pain* 1999;80:23–29.
22. Stadler M, Schlander M, Braeckman M, et al. A cost-utility and cost-effectiveness analysis of an acute pain service. *J Clin Anesth* 2004;16:159–167.
23. Stamer UM, Mpasios N, Stuber F, et al. A survey of acute pain services in Germany and a discussion of international survey data. *Reg Anesth Pain Med* 2002;27:125–131.
24. Vila H Jr., Smith RA, Augustyniak MJ, et al. The efficacy and safety of pain management before and after implementation of hospital-wide pain management standards: Is patient safety compromised by treatment based solely on numerical pain ratings? *Anesth Analg* 2005;101:474–480.
25. Maciocia PM, Strachan EM, Akram AR, et al. Pain assessment in the paediatric Emergency Department: Whose view counts? *Eur J Emerg Med* 2003;10:264–267.
26. Weissman DE, Haddox JD. Opioid pseudoaddiction: An iatrogenic syndrome. *Pain* 1989;36:363–366.
27. Porter J, Jick H. Addiction rare in patients treated with narcotics. *N Engl J Med* 1980;302:123.
28. Ballantyne JC, Carr DB, Chalmers TC, et al. Postoperative patient-controlled analgesia: Meta-analyses of initial randomized control trials. *J Clin Anesth* 1993;5:182–193.
29. Hudcova J, McNicol E, Quah C, et al. Patient controlled intravenous opioid analgesia versus conventional opioid analgesia for postoperative pain control: A quantitative systematic review. *Acute Pain* 2005;7:115–132.
30. Patrick DL, Ferketich SL, Frame PS, et al. National Institutes of Health State-of-the-Science Conference Statement: Symptom Management in Cancer: Pain, Depression, and Fatigue, July 15–17, 2002. *J Natl Cancer Inst* 2003;95:1110–1117.
31. Scott DA, McDonald W. *Measuring Pain Management.* Melbourne: Victorian Quality Council, 2004.
32. Gordon DB, Pellino TA, Miaskowski C, et al. A 10-year review of quality improvement monitoring in pain management: Recommendations for standardized outcome measures. *Pain Manag Nurs* 2002;3:116–130.
33. Ready LB. Acute pain: Lessons learned from 25,000 patients. *Reg Anesth Pain Med* 1999;24:499–505.
34. Australian and New Zealand Collage of Anaesthesiologists, Faculty of Pain Medicine. Statement on patients' rights to pain management, 2001.
35. Davies H, Crombie I. Pain clinic patients in northern Britain. *The Pain Clinic* 1992;5:127–198.
36. Hayes C, Browne S. Neuropathic pain in the Acute Pain Service. *Acute Pain* 2002;4:45–48.
37. Hayes C, Molloy AR. Neuropathic pain in the perioperative period. *Int Anesthesiol Clin* 1997;35:67–81.
38. Crombie IK, Davies HT, Macrae WA. Cut and thrust: Antecedent surgery and trauma among patients attending a chronic pain clinic. *Pain* 1998;76:167–171.
39. Perkins FM, Kehlet H. Chronic pain as an outcome of surgery. A review of predictive factors. *Anesthesiology* 2000;93:1123–1133.
40. Kehlet H, Jensen TS, Woolf CJ. Persistent postsurgical pain: Risk factors and prevention. *Lancet* 2006;367:1618–1625.

41. Caumo W, Schmidt AP, Schneider CN, et al. Preoperative predictors of moderate to intense acute postoperative pain in patients undergoing abdominal surgery. *Acta Anaesthesiol Scand* 2002;46:1265–1271.
42. Bach S, Noreng MF, Tjellden NU. Phantom limb pain in amputees during the first 12 months following limb amputation, after preoperative lumbar epidural blockade. *Pain* 1988;33:297–301.
43. Nikolajsen L, Ilkjaer S, Kroner K, et al. The influence of preamputation pain on postamputation stump and phantom pain. *Pain* 1997;72:393–405.
44. Jung BF, Johnson RW, Griffin DR, et al. Risk factors for postherpetic neuralgia in patients with herpes zoster. *Neurology* 2004;62:1545–1551.
45. Birch PJ, Dekker LV, James IF, et al. Strategies to identify ion channel modulators: Current and novel approaches to target neuropathic pain. *Drug Discov Today* 2004;9:410–418.
46. Mao J, Chen LL. Systemic lidocaine for neuropathic pain relief. *Pain* 2000;87:7–17.
47. Woolf CJ. Dissecting out mechanisms responsible for peripheral neuropathic pain: Implications for diagnosis and therapy. *Life Sci* 2004;74:2605–2610.
48. Eisenberg E. Post-surgical neuralgia. *Pain* 2004;111:3–7.
49. Koppert W, Weigand M, Neumann F, et al. Perioperative intravenous lidocaine has preventive effects on postoperative pain and morphine consumption after major abdominal surgery. *Anesth Analg* 2004;98:1050–1055.
50. Strichartz GR, Zhou Z, Sinnott C, et al. Therapeutic concentrations of local anaesthetics unveil the potential role of sodium channels in neuropathic pain. *Novartis Found Symp* 2002;241:189–201.
51. Dirks J, Fredensborg BB, Christensen D, et al. A randomized study of the effects of single-dose gabapentin versus placebo on postoperative pain and morphine consumption after mastectomy. *Anesthesiology* 2002;97:560–564.
52. Rorarius MG, Mennander S, Suominen P, et al. Gabapentin for the prevention of postoperative pain after vaginal hysterectomy. *Pain* 2004;110:175–181.
53. Tasmuth T, Kataja M, Blomqvist C, et al. Treatment-related factors predisposing to chronic pain in patients with breast cancer: A multivariate approach. *Acta Oncol* 1997;36:625–630.
54. Obata H, Saito S, Fujita N, et al. Epidural block with mepivacaine before surgery reduces long-term post-thoracotomy pain. *Can J Anaesth* 1999;46:1127–1132.
55. Manchikanti L, Singh V. Managing phantom pain. *Pain Physician* 2004;7:365–375.
56. Woodhouse A. Phantom limb sensation. *Clin Exp Pharmacol Physiol* 2005;32:132–134.
57. Poleshuck EL, Katz J, Andrus CH, et al. Risk factors for chronic pain following breast cancer surgery: A prospective study. *J Pain* 2006;7:626–634.
58. Siau C, Bennett GJ. Dysregulation of cellular calcium homeostasis in chemotherapy-evoked painful peripheral neuropathy. *Anesth Analg* 2006;102:1485–1490.
59. Landreneau RJ, Mack MJ, Hazelrigg SR, et al. Prevalence of chronic pain after pulmonary resection by thoracotomy or video-assisted thoracic surgery. *J Thorac Cardiovasc Surg* 1994;107:1079–1085.
60. Macrae WA. Chronic pain after surgery. *Br J Anaesth* 2001;87:88–98.
61. Duhmke RM, Cornblath DD, Hollingshead JR. Tramadol for neuropathic pain. *Cochrane Database Syst Rev* 2004:CD003726.
62. Bell RF, Dahl JB, Moore RA, et al. Perioperative ketamine for acute postoperative pain. *Cochrane Database Syst Rev* 2006:CD004603.
63. Hocking G, Cousins MJ. Ketamine in chronic pain management: An evidence-based review. *Anesth Analg* 2003;97:1730–1739.
64. Block BM, Liu SS, Rowlingson AJ, et al. Efficacy of postoperative epidural analgesia: A meta-analysis. *JAMA* 2003;290:2455–2463.
65. Gehling M, Tryba M. Prophylaxis of phantom pain: Is regional analgesia ineffective? *Schmerz* 2003;17:11–19.
66. Flor H. Phantom-limb pain: Characteristics, causes, and treatment. *Lancet Neurol* 2002;1:182–189.
67. Mailis A, Furlan A. Sympathectomy for neuropathic pain. *Cochrane Database Syst Rev* 2003:CD002918.
68. Dertwinkel R, Heinrichs C, Senne I, et al. Prevention of severe phantom limb pain by perioperative administration of ketamine: An observational study. *Acute Pain* 2002;4:12–16.
69. Hayes C, Armstrong-Brown A, Burstal R. Perioperative intravenous ketamine infusion for the prevention of persistent post-amputation pain: A randomized, controlled trial. *Anaesth Intensive Care* 2004;32:330–338.
70. Bone M, Critchley P, Buggy DJ. Gabapentin in postamputation phantom limb pain: A randomized, double-blind, placebo-controlled, cross-over study. *Reg Anesth Pain Med* 2002;27:481–486.
71. Nikolajsen L, Finnerup NB, Kramp S, et al. A randomized study of the effects of gabapentin on postamputation pain. *Anesthesiology* 2006;105:1008–1015.
72. Halbert J, Crotty M, Cameron ID. Evidence for the optimal management of acute and chronic phantom pain: A systematic review. *Clin J Pain* 2002;18:84–92.
73. Reuben SS, Ekman EF, Raghunathan K, et al. The effect of cyclooxygenase-2 inhibition on acute and chronic donor-site pain after spinal-fusion surgery. *Reg Anesth Pain Med* 2006;31:6–13.
74. Sindrup SH, Jensen TS. Efficacy of pharmacological treatments of neuropathic pain: An update and effect related to mechanism of drug action. *Pain* 1999;83:389–400.
75. Hempenstall K, Nurmikko TJ, Johnson RW, et al. Analgesic therapy in postherpetic neuralgia: A quantitative systematic review. *PLoS Med* 2005;2:E164.
76. Bowsher D. The effects of pre-emptive treatment of postherpetic neuralgia with amitriptyline: A randomized, double-blind, placebo-controlled trial. *J Pain Symptom Manage* 1997;13:327–331.
77. Reuben SS, Makari-Judson G, Lurie SD. Evaluation of efficacy of the perioperative administration of venlafaxine XR in the prevention of postmastectomy pain syndrome. *J Pain Symptom Manage* 2004;27:133–139.
78. Fassoulaki A, Patris K, Sarantopoulos C, et al. The analgesic effect of gabapentin and mexiletine after breast surgery for cancer. *Anesth Analg* 2002;95:985–991.
79. Sindrup SH, Otto M, Finnerup NB, et al. Antidepressants in the treatment of neuropathic pain. *Basic Clin Pharmacol Toxicol* 2005;96:399–409.
80. Finnerup NB, Otto M, McQuay HJ, et al. Algorithm for neuropathic pain treatment: An evidence based proposal. *Pain* 2005;118:289–305.
81. Mellegers MA, Furlan AD, Mailis A. Gabapentin for neuropathic pain: Systematic review of controlled and uncontrolled literature. *Clin J Pain* 2001;17:284–295.
82. Crile GW. The kinetic theory of shock and its prevention through anociassociation. *Lancet* 1913;185:7–16.
83. Woolf CJ, Chong MS. Preemptive analgesia: Treating postoperative pain by preventing the establishment of central sensitization. *Anesth Analg* 1993;77:362–379.
84. Moiniche S, Kehlet H, Dahl JB. A qualitative and quantitative systematic review of preemptive analgesia for postoperative pain relief: The role of timing of analgesia. *Anesthesiology* 2002;96:725–741.
85. Kissin I. Preemptive analgesia. *Anesthesiology* 2000;93:1138–1143.
86. Kissin I. Preemptive analgesia at the crossroad. *Anesth Analg* 2005;100:754–756.
87. Ong CK, Lirk P, Seymour RA, et al. The efficacy of preemptive analgesia for acute postoperative pain management: A meta-analysis. *Anesth Analg* 2005;100:757–773.
88. Lavand'homme P, De Kock M, Waterloos H. Intraoperative epidural analgesia combined with ketamine provides effective preventive analgesia in patients undergoing major digestive surgery. *Anesthesiology* 2005;103:813–820.
89. Gould TH, Crosby DL, Harmer M, et al. Policy for controlling pain after surgery: Effect of sequential changes in management. *BMJ* 1992;305:1187–1193.
90. ASA. Practice guidelines for acute pain management in the perioperative setting: An updated report by the American Society of Anesthesiologists Task Force on Acute Pain Management. *Anesthesiology* 2004;100:1573–1581.
91. Breivik EK, Bjornsson GA, Skovlund E. A comparison of pain rating scales by sampling from clinical trial data. *Clin J Pain* 2000;16:22–28.
92. Bible D. Pain assessment at nurse triage: A literature review. *Emerg Nurse* 2006;14:26–29.
93. Department of Veterans' Affairs. *VHA Pain Outcomes Toolkit*, 2003.
94. Moore A, Edwards J, Barden J, McQuay H. An evidence-based guide to treatments. *Bandolier's Little Book of Pain*. Oxford, U.K.: Oxford University Press, 2003.
95. Breivik EK, Skoglund LA. Comparison of present pain intensity assessments on horizontally and vertically oriented visual analogue scales. *Methods Find Exp Clin Pharmacol* 1998;20:719–724.
96. Myles PS, Troedel S, Boquest M, et al. The pain visual analog scale: Is it linear or nonlinear? *Anesth Analg* 1999;89:1517–1520.
97. Myles PS, Urquhart N. The linearity of the visual analogue scale in patients with severe acute pain. *Anaesth Intensive Care* 2005;33:54–58.
98. Hicks CL, von Baeyer CL, Spafford PA, et al. The Faces Pain Scale-Revised: Toward a common metric in pediatric pain measurement. *Pain* 2001;93:173–183.
99. Wong DL, Baker CM. Pain in children: Comparison of assessment scales. *Pediatr Nurs* 1988;14:9–17.
100. Beyer JE, Denyes MJ, Villarruel AM. The creation, validation, and continuing development of the Oucher: A measure of pain intensity in children. *J Pediatr Nurs* 1992;7:335–346.
101. Chambers CT, Craig KD. An intrusive impact of anchors in children's faces pain scales. *Pain* 1998;78:27–37.
102. Margolis RB, Tait RC, Krause SJ. A rating system for use with patient pain drawings. *Pain* 1986;24:57–65.
103. Puntillo KA. Dimensions of procedural pain and its analgesic management in critically ill surgical patients. *Am J Crit Care* 1994;3:116–122.
104. Merkel SI, Voepel-Lewis T, Shayevitz JR, et al. The FLACC: A behavioral scale for scoring postoperative pain in young children. *Pediatr Nurs* 1997;23:293–297.
105. Erdek MA, Pronovost PJ. Improving assessment and treatment of pain in the critically ill. *Int J Qual Health Care* 2004;16:59–64.
106. Franck LS, Greenberg CS, Stevens B. Pain assessment in infants and children. *Pediatr Clin North Am* 2000;47:487–512.

PART IV: PAIN MANAGEMENT

107. Lane P, Kuntupis M, MacDonald S, et al. A pain assessment tool for people with advanced Alzheimer's and other progressive dementias. *Home Healthc Nurse* 2003;21:32–37.

108. Abbey J, Piller N, De Bellis A, et al. The Abbey pain scale: A 1-minute numerical indicator for people with end-stage dementia. *Int J Palliat Nurs* 2004;10:6–13.

109. Kehlet H. Effect of postoperative pain treatment on outcome-current status and future strategies. *Langenbecks Arch Surg* 2004;389:244–249.

110. Scott DA, McDonald W. Acute pain management performance measurement toolkit. Melbourne: Victorian Quality Council, Department of Human Services, 2005.

111. Australian and New Zealand College of Anaesthesiologists. *Acute Pain Management: Scientific Evidence*, 2nd ed. Melbourne: ANZCA, 2005.

112. Dolin SJ, Cashman JN. Tolerability of acute postoperative pain management: Nausea, vomiting, sedation, pruritus, and urinary retention. Evidence from published data. *Br J Anaesth* 2005;95:584–591.

113. Cashman JN, Dolin SJ. Respiratory and haemodynamic effects of acute postoperative pain management: evidence from published data. *Br J Anaesth* 2004;93:212–223.

114. Myles PS, Williams DL, Hendrata M, et al. Patient satisfaction after anaesthesia and surgery: Results of a prospective survey of 10,811 patients. [See comments] *Br J Anaesth* 2000;84:6–10.

115. Habib AS, Gan TJ. Evidence-based management of postoperative nausea and vomiting: A review. *Can J Anaesth* 2004;51:326–341.

116. Roberts GW, Bekker TB, Carlsen HH, et al. Postoperative nausea and vomiting are strongly influenced by postoperative opioid use in a dose-related manner. *Anesth Analg* 2005;101:1343–1348.

117. Marret E, Kurdi O, Zufferey P, et al. Effects of nonsteroidal antiinflammatory drugs on patient-controlled analgesia morphine side effects: Meta-analysis of randomized controlled trials. *Anesthesiology* 2005;102:1249–1260.

118. Zhao SZ, Chung F, Hanna DB, et al. Dose-response relationship between opioid use and adverse effects after ambulatory surgery. *J Pain Symptom Manage* 2004;28:35–46.

119. Gan TJ. Risk factors for postoperative nausea and vomiting. *Anesth Analg* 2006;102:1884–1898.

120. Scott D, Chamley D, Mooney P, et al. Epidural ropivacaine infusion for postoperative analgesia after major lower abdominal surgery: A dose finding study. *Anesth Analg* 1995;81:982–986.

121. Raffaeli W, Marconi G, Fanelli G, et al. Opioid-related side-effects after intrathecal morphine: A prospective, randomized, double-blind dose-response study. *Eur J Anaesthesiol* 2006;23:605–610.

122. Walder B, Schafer M, Henzi I, et al. Efficacy and safety of patient-controlled opioid analgesia for acute postoperative pain. A quantitative systematic review. *Acta Anaesthesiol Scand* 2001;45:795–804.

123. Kjellberg F, Tramer MR. Pharmacological control of opioid-induced pruritus: A quantitative systematic review of randomized trials. *Eur J Anaesthesiol* 2001;18:346–357.

124. Rygnestad T, Borchgrevink PC, Eide E. Postoperative epidural infusion of morphine and bupivacaine is safe on surgical wards. Organisation of the treatment, effects and side-effects in 2000 consecutive patients. [See comments] *Acta Anaesthesiol Scand* 1997;41:868–876.

125. Auroy Y, Narchi P, Messiah A, et al. Serious complications related to regional anesthesia: Results of a prospective survey in France. *Anesthesiology* 1997;87:479–486.

126. Barrington MJ, Olive D, Low K, et al. Continuous femoral nerve blockade or epidural analgesia after total knee replacement: A prospective randomized controlled trial. *Anesth Analg* 2005;101:1824–1829.

127. Bergman BD, Hebl JR, Kent J, et al. Neurologic complications of 405 consecutive continuous axillary catheters. *Anesth Analg* 2003;96:247–252.

128. Cameron CM, Scott DA, McDonald WM, Davies MJ. A review of neuraxial epidural morbidity: Experience of over 8000 cases at a single teaching hospital. *Anesthesiology* 2007;107(6):1034–1035.

129. Scott DA, Beilby DS, McClymont C. Postoperative analgesia using epidural infusions of fentanyl with bupivacaine. A prospective analysis of 1,014 patients. *Anesthesiology* 1995;83:727–737.

130. Wang LP, Hauerberg J, Schmidt JF. Incidence of spinal epidural abscess after epidural analgesia: A national 1-year survey. *Anesthesiology* 1999;91:1928–1936.

131. Capdevila X, Pirat P, Bringuier S, et al. Continuous peripheral nerve blocks in hospital wards after orthopedic surgery: A multicenter prospective analysis of the quality of postoperative analgesia and complications in 1,416 patients. *Anesthesiology* 2005;103:1035–1045.

132. Horlocker TT, Wedel DJ, Benzon H, et al. Regional anesthesia in the anticoagulated patient: Defining the risks (the second ASRA Consensus Conference on Neuraxial Anesthesia and Anticoagulation). *Reg Anesth Pain Med* 2003;28:172–197.

133. Lanz E, Theiss D, Kellner G, et al. Assessment of motor blockade during epidural anesthesia. *Anesth Analg* 1983;62:889–893.

134. Royakkers AA, Willigers H, van der Ven AJ, et al. Catheter-related epidural abscesses: Don't wait for neurological deficits. *Acta Anaesthesiol Scand* 2002;46:611–615.

135. Greenberg RS, Billett C, Zahurak M, et al. Videotape increases parental knowledge about pediatric pain management. *Anesth Analg* 1999;89:899–903.

136. Chumbley GM, Ward L, Hall GM, et al. Pre-operative information and patient-controlled analgesia: Much ado about nothing. *Anaesthesia* 2004;59:354–358.

137. Chumbley GM, Hall GM, Salmon P. Patient-controlled analgesia: What information does the patient want? *J Adv Nurs* 2002;39:459–471.

138. Chen HH, Yeh ML, Yang HJ. Testing the impact of a multimedia video CD of patient-controlled analgesia on pain knowledge and pain relief in patients receiving surgery. *Int J Med Inform* 2005;74:437–445.

139. Devine EC. Effects of psychoeducational care for adult surgical patients: A meta-analysis of 191 studies. *Patient Educ Couns* 1992;19:129–142.

140. Giraudet-Le Quintrec JS, Coste J, Vastel L, et al. Positive effect of patient education for hip surgery: A randomized trial. *Clin Orthop Relat Res* 2003:112–120.

141. Guruge S, Sidani S. Effects of demographic characteristics on preoperative teaching outcomes: A meta-analysis. *Can J Nurs Res* 2002;34:25–33.

142. Sjoling M, Nordahl G, Olofsson N, et al. The impact of preoperative information on state anxiety, postoperative pain and satisfaction with pain management. *Patient Educ Couns* 2003;51:169–176.

143. Griffin MJ, Brennan L, McShane AJ. Preoperative education and outcome of patient controlled analgesia. *Can J Anaesth* 1998;45:943–948.

144. McDonald S, Hetrick S, Green S. Pre-operative education for hip or knee replacement. *Cochrane Database Syst Rev* 2004:CD003526.

145. Shuldham CM, Fleming S, Goodman H. The impact of pre-operative education on recovery following coronary artery bypass surgery. A randomized controlled clinical trial. *Eur Heart J* 2002;23:666–674.

146. Watt-Watson J, Stevens B, Katz J, et al. Impact of preoperative education on pain outcomes after coronary artery bypass graft surgery. *Pain* 2004;109:73–85.

147. Lam KK, Chan MT, Chen PP, et al. Structured preoperative patient education for patient-controlled analgesia. *J Clin Anesth* 2001;13:465–469.

148. Harmer M, Davies KA. The effect of education, assessment and a standardised prescription on postoperative pain management. The value of clinical audit in the establishment of acute pain services. *Anaesthesia* 1998;53:424–430.

149. Humphries CA, Counsell DJ, Pediani RC, et al. Audit of opioid prescribing: The effect of hospital guidelines. *Anaesthesia* 1997;52:745–749.

150. Ury WA, Rahn M, Tolentino V, et al. Can a pain management and palliative care curriculum improve the opioid prescribing practices of medical residents? *J Gen Intern Med* 2002;17:625–631.

151. Gordon DB, Jones HD, Goshman LM, et al. A quality improvement approach to reducing use of meperidine. *Jt Comm J Qual Improv* 2000;26:686–699.

152. Ripouteau C, Conort O, Lamas JP, et al. Effect of multifaceted intervention promoting early switch from intravenous to oral acetaminophen for postoperative pain: Controlled, prospective, before and after study. *BMJ* 2000;321:1460–1463.

153. Figueiras A, Sastre I, Tato F, et al. One-to-one versus group sessions to improve prescription in primary care: A pragmatic randomized controlled trial. *Med Care* 2001;39:158–167.

154. May FW, Rowett DS, Gilbert AL, et al. Outcomes of an educational-outreach service for community medical practitioners: Non-steroidal anti-inflammatory drugs. *Med J Aust* 1999;170:471–474.

155. Coleman SA, Booker-Milburn J. Audit of postoperative pain control. Influence of a dedicated acute pain nurse. *Anaesthesia* 1996;51:1093–1096.

156. Richardson J. Post-operative epidural analgesia: Introducing evidence-based guidelines through an education and assessment process. *J Clin Nurs* 2001;10:238–245.

157. Jones JB. Assessment of pain management skills in emergency medicine residents: The role of a pain education program. *J Emerg Med* 1999;17:349–354.

158. Office of Veterans' Affairs/Department of Defense. *Clinical Practice Guidelines for the Management of Postoperative Pain*, 2002.

159. Kehlet H, Wilkinson RC, Fischer HB, et al. PROSPECT: Evidence-based, procedure-specific postoperative pain management. *Best Pract Res Clin Anaesthesiol* 2007;21(1):149–159.

160. Carr DB, Miaskowski C, Dedrick SC, et al. Management of perioperative pain in hospitalized patients: A national survey. *J Clin Anesth* 1998;10:77–85.

161. Jiang HJ, Lagasse RS, Ciccone K, et al. Factors influencing hospital implementation of acute pain management practice guidelines. *J Clin Anesth* 2001;13:268–276.

162. Rawal N. Organization of acute pain services: A low-cost model. *Acta Anaesthesiol Scand Suppl* 1997;111:188–190.

163. Shapiro A, Zohar E, Kantor M, et al. Establishing a nurse-based, anesthesiologist-supervised inpatient acute pain service: Experience of 4,617 patients. *J Clin Anesth* 2004;16:415–420.

164. Powell AE, Davies HT, Bannister J, et al. Rhetoric and reality on acute pain services in the UK: A national postal questionnaire survey. *Br J Anaesth* 2004;92:689–693.

165. Harmer M. When is a standard, not a standard? When it is a recommendation. *Anaesthesia* 2001;56:611–612.

166. Nagi H. Acute pain services in the United Kingdom. *Acute Pain* 2004;5:89–107.

167. Ready LB, Oden R, Chadwick HS, et al. Development of an anesthesiology-based postoperative pain management service. *Anesthesiology* 1988;68:100–106.

168. Schug SA, Haridas RP. Development and organizational structure of an acute pain service in a major teaching hospital. *Aust N Z J Surg* 1993;63:8–13.

169. Macintyre PE, Runciman WB, Webb RK. An acute pain service in an Australian teaching hospital: The first year. *Med J Aust* 1990;153:417–421.

170. Macintyre PE, Schug SA. *Acute Pain Management: A Practical Guide*, 3rd ed. London: Elsevier, 2007.

171. Breivik H. How to implement an acute pain service. *Best Pract Res Clin Anaesthesiol* 2002;16:527–547.

172. McDonnell A, Nicholl J, Read SM. Acute pain teams and the management of postoperative pain: A systematic review and meta-analysis. *J Adv Nurs* 2003;41:261–273.

173. Sartain JB, Barry JJ. The impact of an acute pain service on postoperative pain management. *Anaesth Intensive Care* 1999;27:375–380.

174. Stacey BR, Rudy TE, Nellhaus D. Management of patient-controlled analgesia: A comparison of primary surgeons and a dedicated pain service. *Anesth Analg* 1997;85:130–134.

175. Story DA, Shelton AC, Poustie SJ, et al. Effect of an anaesthesia department led critical care outreach and acute pain service on postoperative serious adverse events. *Anaesthesia* 2006;61:24–28.

176. Wheatley RG, Madej TH. Organization of an acute pain service. In: Rowbotham DJ, Macintyre PE, eds. *Clinical Pain Management: Acute Pain.* London: Arnold Publishers, 2003.

177. Macintyre PE. Safety and efficacy of patient-controlled analgesia. *Br J Anaesth* 2001;87:36–46.

178. Macintyre PE. Intravenous patient-controlled analgesia: One size does not fit all. *Anesthesiol Clin North America* 2005;23:109–123.

179. Bainbridge D, Martin JE, Cheng DC. Patient-controlled versus nurse-controlled analgesia after cardiac surgery: A meta-analysis. *Can J Anaesth* 2006;53:492–499.

180. Evans E, Turley N, Robinson N. Randomised controlled trial of patient controlled analgesia compared with nurse delivered analgesia in an emergency department. *Emerg Med J* 2005;22:25–29.

181. Munro AJ, Long GT, Sleigh JW. Nurse-administered subcutaneous morphine is a satisfactory alternative to intravenous patient-controlled analgesia morphine after cardiac surgery. *Anesth Analg* 1998;87:11–15.

182. Myles PS, Buckland MR, Cannon GB, et al. Comparison of patient-controlled analgesia and nurse-controlled infusion analgesia after cardiac surgery. *Anaesth Intensive Care* 1994;22:672–678.

183. Tsang J, Brush B. Patient-controlled analgesia in postoperative cardiac surgery. *Anaesth Intensive Care* 1999;27:464–470.

184. Werawatganon T, Charuluxanun S. Patient controlled intravenous opioid analgesia versus continuous epidural analgesia for pain after intra-abdominal surgery. *Cochrane Database Syst Rev* 2005:CD004088.

185. Wu CL, Cohen SR, Richman JM, et al. Efficacy of postoperative patient-controlled and continuous infusion epidural analgesia versus intravenous patient-controlled analgesia with opioids: A meta-analysis. *Anesthesiology* 2005;103:1079–1088.

186. Toussaint S, Maidl J, Schwagmeier R, et al. Patient-controlled intranasal analgesia: Effective alternative to intravenous PCA for postoperative pain relief. *Can J Anaesth* 2000;47:299–302.

187. Paech MJ, Lim CB, Banks SL, et al. A new formulation of nasal fentanyl spray for postoperative analgesia: A pilot study. *Anaesthesia* 2003;58:740–744.

188. Dawson L, Brockbank K, Carr EC, et al. Improving patients' postoperative sleep: A randomized control study comparing subcutaneous with intravenous patient-controlled analgesia. *J Adv Nurs* 1999;30:875–881.

189. Urquhart ML, Klapp K, White PF. Patient-controlled analgesia: A comparison of intravenous versus subcutaneous hydromorphone. *Anesthesiology* 1988;69:428–432.

190. Banga AK. Iontophoretic topical and transdermal drug delivery. *Drug Delivery Report* 2005;Autumn/Winter:51–53.

191. Koo PJ. Postoperative pain management with a patient-controlled transdermal delivery system for fentanyl. *Am J Health Syst Pharm* 2005;62:1171–1176.

192. Chelly JE. An iontophoretic, fentanyl HCl patient-controlled transdermal system for acute postoperative pain management. *Expert Opin Pharmacother* 2005;6:1205–1214.

193. Sathyan G, Jaskowiak J, Evashenk M, et al. Characterisation of the pharmacokinetics of the fentanyl HCl patient-controlled transdermal system (PCTS): Effect of current magnitude and multiple-day dosing and comparison with IV fentanyl administration. *Clin Pharmacokinet* 2005;44[Suppl]1:7–15.

194. Viscusi ER, Reynolds L, Chung F, et al. Patient-controlled transdermal fentanyl hydrochloride vs intravenous morphine pump for postoperative pain: A randomized controlled trial. *JAMA* 2004;291:1333–1341.

195. Young T, Skatrud J, Peppard PE. Risk factors for obstructive sleep apnea in adults. *JAMA* 2004;291:2013–2016.

196. Catley DM, Thornton C, Jordan C, et al. Pronounced, episodic oxygen desaturation in the postoperative period: Its association with ventilatory pattern and analgesic regimen. *Anesthesiology* 1985;63:20–28.

197. Jones JG, Sapsford DJ, Wheatley RG. Postoperative hypoxaemia: Mechanisms and time course. *Anaesthesia* 1990;45:566–573.

198. Wheatley RG, Somerville DJ, Sapsford DJ, et al. Postoperative hypoxaemia: Comparison of extradural, IM and patient-controlled opioid analgesia. *Br J Anaesth* 1990;64:267–275.

199. VanDercar DH, Martinez AP, De Lisser EA. Sleep apnea syndromes: A potential contraindication for patient-controlled analgesia. *Anesthesiology* 1991;74:623–624.

200. Etches RC. Respiratory depression associated with patient-controlled analgesia: A review of eight cases. *Can J Anaesth* 1994;41:125–132.

201. Parikh SN, Stuchin SA, Maca C, et al. Sleep apnea syndrome in patients undergoing total joint arthroplasty. *J Arthroplasty* 2002;17:635–642.

202. Lofsky A. Sleep apnea and narcotic postoperative pain medication: Morbidity and mortality risk. *Anesthesia Patient Safety Foundation Newsletter* 2002;17:24.

203. Ostermeier AM, Roizen MF, Hautkappe M, et al. Three sudden postoperative respiratory arrests associated with epidural opioids in patients with sleep apnea. *Anesth Analg* 1997;85:452–460.

204. Cullen DJ. Obstructive sleep apnea and postoperative analgesia: A potentially dangerous combination. *J Clin Anesth* 2001;13:83–85.

205. Choi YK, Brolin RE, Wagner BK, et al. Efficacy and safety of patient-controlled analgesia for morbidly obese patients following gastric bypass surgery. *Obes Surg* 2000;10:154–159.

206. Kyzer S, Ramadan E, Gersch M, et al. Patient-controlled analgesia following vertical gastroplasty: A comparison with intramuscular narcotics. *Obes Surg* 1995;5:18–21.

207. Charghi R, Backman S, Christou N, et al. Patient controlled i.v. analgesia is an acceptable pain management strategy in morbidly obese patients undergoing gastric bypass surgery. A retrospective comparison with epidural analgesia. *Can J Anaesth* 2003;50:672–678.

208. Landsberg R, Friedman M, Ascher-Landsberg J. Treatment of hypoxemia in obstructive sleep apnea. *Am J Rhinol* 2001;15:311–313.

209. Phillips BA, Schmitt FA, Berry DT, et al. Treatment of obstructive sleep apnea. A preliminary report comparing nasal CPAP to nasal oxygen in patients with mild OSA. *Chest* 1990;98:325–330.

210. Jorgensen H, Wetterslev J, Moiniche S, et al. Epidural local anaesthetics versus opioid-based analgesic regimens on postoperative gastrointestinal paralysis, PONV and pain after abdominal surgery. *Cochrane Database Syst Rev* 2000:CD001893.

211. Steinbrook RA. Epidural anesthesia and gastrointestinal motility. *Anesth Analg* 1998;86:837–844.

212. Liu S, Carpenter RL, Neal JM. Epidural anesthesia and analgesia. Their role in postoperative outcome. *Anesthesiology* 1995;82:1474–1506.

213. Bulger EM, Edwards T, Klotz P, et al. Epidural analgesia improves outcome after multiple rib fractures. *Surgery* 2004;136:426–430.

214. Beattie WS, Badner NH, Choi P. Epidural analgesia reduces postoperative myocardial infarction: A meta-analysis. *Anesth Analg* 2001;93:853–858.

215. Nishimori M, Ballantyne JC, Low JH. Epidural pain relief versus systemic opioid-based pain relief for abdominal aortic surgery. *Cochrane Database Syst Rev* 2006;3:CD005059.

216. Ballantyne JC, Carr DB, DeFerranti S, et al. The comparative effects of postoperative analgesic therapies on pulmonary outcome: Cumulative meta-analyses of randomized, controlled trials. *Anesth Analg* 1998;86:598–612.

217. Richman JM, Liu SS, Courpas G, et al. Does continuous peripheral nerve block provide superior pain control to opioids? A meta-analysis. *Anesth Analg* 2006;102:248–257.

218. Navas AM, Gutierrez TV, Moreno ME. Continuous peripheral nerve blockade in lower extremity surgery. *Acta Anaesthesiol Scand* 2005;49:1048–1055.

219. Woolf CJ. Pain: Moving from symptom control toward mechanism-specific pharmacologic management. *Ann Intern Med* 2004;140:441–451.

220. Joshi GP. Multimodal analgesia techniques and postoperative rehabilitation. *Anesthesiol Clin North America* 2005;23:185–202.

221. Barden J, Edwards J, Moore A, et al. Single dose oral paracetamol (acetaminophen) for postoperative pain. *Cochrane Database Syst Rev* 2004:CD004602.

222. Bonnefont J, Courade JP, Alloui A, et al. Antinociceptive mechanism of action of paracetamol. *Drugs* 2003;63(2):1–4.

223. Botting R. COX-1 and COX-3 inhibitors. *Thromb Res* 2003;110:269–272.

224. Schwab JM, Schluesener HJ, Meyermann R, et al. COX-3 the enzyme and the concept: Steps towards highly specialized pathways and precision therapeutics? *Prostaglandins Leukot Essent Fatty Acids* 2003;69:339–343.

PART IV: PAIN MANAGEMENT

225. Pickering G, Loriot MA, Libert F, et al. Analgesic effect of acetaminophen in humans: First evidence of a central serotonergic mechanism. *Clin Pharmacol Ther* 2006;79:371–378.

226. Moller PL, Juhl GI, Payen-Champenois C, et al. Intravenous acetaminophen (paracetamol): Comparable analgesic efficacy, but better local safety than its prodrug, Propacetamol, for postoperative pain after third molar surgery. *Anesth Analg* 2005;101:90–96.

227. Flouvat B, Leneveu A, Fitoussi S, et al. Bioequivalence study comparing a new paracetamol solution for injection and Propacetamol after single intravenous infusion in healthy subjects. *Int J Clin Pharmacol Ther* 2004;42:50–57.

228. Moller PL, Sindet-Pedersen S, Petersen CT, et al. Onset of acetaminophen analgesia: Comparison of oral and intravenous routes after third molar surgery. *Br J Anaesth* 2005;94:642–648.

229. Holmer Pettersson P, Owall A, Jakobsson J. Early bioavailability of paracetamol after oral or intravenous administration. *Acta Anaesthesiol Scand* 2004;48:867–870.

230. Juhl GI, Norholt SE, Tonnesen E, et al. Analgesic efficacy and safety of intravenous paracetamol (acetaminophen) administered as a 2 g starting dose following third molar surgery. *Eur J Pain* 2006;10:371–377.

231. Romsing J, Moiniche S, Dahl JB. Rectal and parenteral paracetamol, and paracetamol in combination with NSAIDs, for postoperative analgesia. *Br J Anaesth* 2002;88:215–226.

232. Remy C, Marret E, Bonnet F. Effects of acetaminophen on morphine side-effects and consumption after major surgery: Meta-analysis of randomized controlled trials. *Br J Anaesth* 2005;94:505–513.

233. Elia N, Lysakowski C, Tramer MR. Does multimodal analgesia with acetaminophen, nonsteroidal antiinflammatory drugs, or selective cyclooxygenase-2 inhibitors and patient-controlled analgesia morphine offer advantages over morphine alone? Meta-analyses of randomized trials. *Anesthesiology* 2005;103.1296–1304.

234. Hyllested M, Jones S, Pedersen JL, et al. Comparative effect of paracetamol, NSAIDs or their combination in postoperative pain management: A qualitative review. *Br J Anaesth* 2002;88:199–214.

235. Graham GG, Scott KF, Day RO. Tolerability of paracetamol. *Drug Saf* 2005;28:227–240.

236. Whelton A. Clinical implications of nonopioid analgesia for relief of mild-to-moderate pain in patients with or at risk for cardiovascular disease. *Am J Cardiol* 2006;97:3–9.

237. Chan AT, Manson JE, Albert CM, et al. Nonsteroidal antiinflammatory drugs, acetaminophen, and the risk of cardiovascular events. *Circulation* 2006;113:1578–1587.

238. Rosenberg L, Rao RS, Palmer JR. A case-control study of acetaminophen use in relation to the risk of first myocardial infarction in men. *Pharmacoepidemiol Drug Saf* 2003;12:459–465.

239. Benson GD, Koff RS, Tolman KG. The therapeutic use of acetaminophen in patients with liver disease. *Am J Ther* 2005;12:133–141.

240. Rumack BH. Acetaminophen misconceptions. *Hepatology* 2004;40:10–15.

241. Royal College of Anaesthetists. *Guidelines for the Use of Nonsteroidal Antiinflammatory Drugs in the Perioperative Period.* London: Royal College of Anaesthetists, 1998.

242. Savage R. Cyclo-oxygenase-2 inhibitors: When should they be used in the elderly? *Drugs Aging* 2005;22:185–200.

243. Romsing J, Moiniche S. A systematic review of COX-2 inhibitors compared with traditional NSAIDs, or different COX-2 inhibitors for post-operative pain. *Acta Anaesthesiol Scand* 2004;48:525–546.

244. Argoff CE. Pharmacotherapeutic options in pain management. *Geriatrics* 2005;[Suppl]:3–9.

245. Schug SA. The role of COX-2 inhibitors in the treatment of postoperative pain. *J Cardiovasc Pharmacol* 2006;47[Suppl 1]:S82–S86.

246. Bombardier C, Laine L, Reicin A, et al. Comparison of upper gastrointestinal toxicity of rofecoxib and naproxen in patients with rheumatoid arthritis. VIGOR Study Group. *N Engl J Med* 2000;343:1520–1528.

247. Silverstein FE, Faich G, Goldstein JL, et al. Gastrointestinal toxicity with celecoxib vs nonsteroidal anti-inflammatory drugs for osteoarthritis and rheumatoid arthritis: The CLASS study: A randomized controlled trial. Celecoxib Long-term Arthritis Safety Study. *JAMA* 2000;284:1247–1255.

248. West PM, Fernandez C. Safety of COX-2 inhibitors in asthma patients with aspirin hypersensitivity. *Ann Pharmacother* 2003;37:1497–1501.

249. Curtis SP, Ng J, Yu Q. Renal effects of etoricoxib and comparator nonsteroidal anti-inflammatory drugs in controlled clinical trials. *Clin Ther* 2004;26:70–83.

250. Kearney PM, Baigent C, Godwin J, et al. Do selective cyclo-oxygenase-2 inhibitors and traditional non-steroidal anti-inflammatory drugs increase the risk of atherothrombosis? Meta-analysis of randomised trials. *BMJ* 2006;332:1302–1308.

251. Johnsen SP, Larsson H, Tarone RE, et al. Risk of hospitalization for myocardial infarction among users of rofecoxib, celecoxib, and other NSAIDs: A population-based case-control study. *Arch Intern Med* 2005;165:978–984.

252. McGettigan P, Henry D. Cardiovascular risk and inhibition of cyclooxygenase: A systematic review of the observational studies of selective and nonselective inhibitors of cyclooxygenase 2. *JAMA* 2006;296:1633–1644.

253. Zhang J, Ding EL, Song Y. Adverse effects of cyclooxygenase 2 inhibitors on renal and arrhythmia events: Meta-analysis of randomized trials. *JAMA* 2006;296:1619–1632.

254. Nussmeier NA, Whelton AA, Brown MT, et al. Safety and efficacy of the cyclooxygenase-2 inhibitors parecoxib and valdecoxib after noncardiac surgery. *Anesthesiology* 2006;104:518–526.

255. Kurth T, Glynn RJ, Walker AM, et al. Inhibition of clinical benefits of aspirin on first myocardial infarction by nonsteroidal antiinflammatory drugs. *Circulation* 2003;108:1191–1195.

256. MacDonald TM, Wei L. Effect of ibuprofen on cardioprotective effect of aspirin. *Lancet* 2003;361:573–574.

257. Romsing J, Moiniche S, Mathiesen O, et al. Reduction of opioid-related adverse events using opioid-sparing analgesia with COX-2 inhibitors lacks documentation: A systematic review. *Acta Anaesthesiol Scand* 2005;49:133–142.

258. Straube S, Derry S, McQuay HJ, et al. Effect of preoperative Cox-II-selective NSAIDs (coxibs) on postoperative outcomes: A systematic review of randomized studies. *Acta Anaesthesiol Scand* 2005;49:601–613.

259. Woodhouse A, Ward M, Mather L. Inter-subject variability in post-operative patient-controlled analgesia (PCA): Is the patient equally satisfied with morphine, pethidine and fentanyl? *Pain* 1999;80:545–553.

260. Upton RN, Semple TJ, Macintyre PE, et al. Population pharmacokinetic modelling of subcutaneous morphine in the elderly. *Acute Pain* 2006;8:109–116.

261. Austin KL, Stapleton JV, Mather LE. Multiple intramuscular injections: A major source of variability in analgesic response to meperidine. *Pain* 1980;8:47–62.

262. Austin KL, Stapleton JV, Mather LE. Relationship between blood meperidine concentrations and analgesic response: A preliminary report. *Anesthesiology* 1980;53:460–466.

263. Woodhouse A, Mather LE. The minimum effective concentration of opioids: A revisitation with patient controlled analgesia fentanyl. *Reg Anesth Pain Med* 2000;25:259–267.

264. Baumann TJ, Smythe MA, Marikis B, et al. Meperidine serum concentrations and analgesic response in postsurgical patients. *DICP* 1991;25:724–727.

265. Tarkkila P, Tuominen M, Lindgren L. Comparison of respiratory effects of tramadol and oxycodone. *J Clin Anesth* 1997;9:582–585.

266. Tarkkila P, Tuominen M, Lindgren L. Comparison of respiratory effects of tramadol and pethidine. *Eur J Anaesthesiol* 1998;15:64–68.

267. Wilder-Smith CH, Hill L, Osler W, et al. Effect of tramadol and morphine on pain and gastrointestinal motor function in patients with chronic pancreatitis. *Dig Dis Sci* 1999;44:1107–1116.

268. Wilder-Smith CH, Hill L, Wilkins J, et al. Effects of morphine and tramadol on somatic and visceral sensory function and gastrointestinal motility after abdominal surgery. *Anesthesiology* 1999;91:639–647.

269. Seib RK, Paul JE. Preoperative gabapentin for postoperative analgesia: A meta-analysis. *Can J Anaesth* 2006;53:461–469.

270. Hurley RW, Cohen SP, Williams KA, et al. The analgesic effects of perioperative gabapentin on postoperative pain: a meta-analysis. *Reg Anesth Pain Med* 2006;31:237–247.

271. Ho KY, Gan TJ, Habib AS. Gabapentin and postoperative pain: A systematic review of randomized controlled trials. *Pain* 2006;126:91–101.

272. Park J, Forrest J, Kolesar R, et al. Oral clonidine reduces postoperative PCA morphine requirements. *Can J Anaesth* 1996;43:900–906.

273. Jeffs SA, Hall JE, Morris S. Comparison of morphine alone with morphine plus clonidine for postoperative patient-controlled analgesia. *Br J Anaesth* 2002;89:424–427.

274. Unlugenc H, Ozalevli M, Guler T, et al. Postoperative pain management with intravenous patient-controlled morphine: Comparison of the effect of adding magnesium or ketamine. *Eur J Anaesthesiol* 2003;20:416–421.

275. Rawal N, Axelsson K, Hylander J, et al. Postoperative patient-controlled local anesthetic administration at home. *Anesth Analg* 1998;86:86–89.

276. Ilfeld BM, Enneking FK. Continuous peripheral nerve blocks at home: A review. *Anesth Analg* 2005;100:1822–1833.

277. Lehmann KA. Recent developments in patient-controlled analgesia. *J Pain Symptom Manage* 2005;29:S72–S89.

278. Sechzer PH. Objective measurement of pain. *Anesthesiology* 1968;29:209–213.

279. Sechzer PH. Studies in pain with the analgesic-demand system. *Anesth Analg* 1971;50:1–10.

280. Owen H, Plummer JL, Armstrong I, et al. Variables of patient-controlled analgesia: 1. Bolus size. *Anaesthesia* 1989;44:7–10.

281. Prakash S, Fatima T, Pawar M. Patient-controlled analgesia with fentanyl for burn dressing changes. *Anesth Analg* 2004;99:552–555.

282. Camu F, Van Aken H, Bovill JG. Postoperative analgesic effects of three demand-dose sizes of fentanyl administered by patient-controlled analgesia. *Anesth Analg* 1998;87:890–895.

283. Etches RC. Patient-controlled analgesia. *Surg Clin North Am* 1999;79:297–312.

284. Ginsberg B, Gil KM, Muir M, et al. The influence of lockout intervals and drug selection on patient-controlled analgesia following gynecological surgery. *Pain* 1995;62:95–100.

285. Dal D, Kanbak M, Caglar M, et al. A background infusion of morphine does not enhance postoperative analgesia after cardiac surgery. *Can J Anaesth* 2003;50:476–479.

286. Parker RK, Holtmann B, White PF. Effects of a nighttime opioid infusion with PCA therapy on patient comfort and analgesic requirements after abdominal hysterectomy. *Anesthesiology* 1992;76:362–367.

287. Sidebotham D, Dijkhuizen MRJ, Schug SA. The safety and utilization of patient-controlled analgesia. *J Pain Symptom Manage* 1997;14:202–209.

288. Burns JW, Hodsman NBA, McLintock TTC, et al. The influence of patient characteristics on the requirements for postoperative analgesia. *Anaesthesia* 1989;44:2–6.

289. Gagliese L, Jackson M, Ritvo P, et al. Age is not an impediment to effective use of patient-controlled analgesia by surgical patients. *Anesthesiology* 2000;93:601–610.

290. Macintyre PE, Jarvis DA. Age is the best predictor of postoperative morphine requirements. *Pain* 1996;64:357–364.

291. Coulbault L, Beaussier M, Verstuyft C, et al. Environmental and genetic factors associated with morphine response in the postoperative period. *Clin Pharmacol Ther* 2006;79:316–324.

292. Scott JC, Stanski DR. Decreased fentanyl and alfentanil dose requirements with age. A simultaneous pharmacokinetic and pharmacodynamic evaluation. *J Pharmacol Exp Ther* 1987;240:159–166.

293. Minto CF, Schnider TW, Egan TD, et al. Influence of age and gender on the pharmacokinetics and pharmacodynamics of remifentanil. I. Model development. *Anesthesiology* 1997;86:10–23.

294. Shafer SL. Pharmacokinetics and pharmacodynamics of the elderly. In: McKleskey C, ed. *Geriatric Anesthesiology*. Baltimore: Williams and Wilkins, 1997.

295. Macintyre PE, Upton RN, Ludbrook GL. Acute pain in the elderly. In: Rowbotham DJ, Macintyre PE, eds. *Clinical Pain Management: Acute Pain*. London: Arnold, 2007.

296. Gibson SJ, Farrell M. A review of age differences in the neurophysiology of nociception and the perceptual experience of pain. *Clin J Pain* 2004;20:227–239.

297. Gibson SJ. Pain and aging: The pain experience over the adult life span. In: Dostrovsky JO, Carr DB, Koltzenburg M, eds. *Proceedings of the 10th World Congress on Pain*. Seattle: IASP Press, 2003.

298. Aubrun F. Management of postoperative analgesia in elderly patients. *Reg Anesth Pain Med* 2005;30:363–379.

299. Ginsberg G, Hattis D, Russ A, et al. Pharmacokinetic and pharmacodynamic factors that can affect sensitivity to neurotoxic sequelae in elderly individuals. *Environ Health Perspect* 2005;113:1243–1249.

300. Davis MP, Srivastava M. Demographics, assessment and management of pain in the elderly. *Drugs Aging* 2003;20:23–57.

301. Barkin RL, Barkin SJ, Barkin DS. Perception, assessment, treatment, and management of pain in the elderly. *Clin Geriatr Med* 2005;21:465–490, v.

302. Herrick IA, Ganapathy S, Komar W, et al. Postoperative cognitive impairment in the elderly. Choice of patient-controlled analgesia opioid. *Anaesthesia* 1996;51:356–360.

303. Narayanaswamy M, Smith J, Spralja A. Choice of opiate and incidence of confusion in elderly postoperative patients. In: Annual Scientific Meeting of the Australian and New Zealand Society of Anaesthetists. Adelaide, Australia, 2006.

304. Ng KF, Yuen TS, Ng VM. A comparison of postoperative cognitive function and pain relief with fentanyl or tramadol patient-controlled analgesia. *J Clin Anesth* 2006;18:205–210.

305. Quinn AC, Brown JH, Wallace PG, et al. Studies in postoperative sequelae. Nausea and vomiting: Still a problem. *Anaesthesia* 1994;49:62–65.

306. Macintyre PE. Nine years experience in an acute pain service. In: J. Keneally and M. Jones, eds. *Australasian Anesthesia*. Melbourne: Australian and New Zealand College of Anaesthetists, 1998.

307. Mann C, Pouzeratte Y, Eledjam JJ. Postoperative patient-controlled analgesia in the elderly: Risks and benefits of epidural versus intravenous administration. *Drugs Aging* 2003;20:337–345.

308. Mann C, Pouzeratte Y, Boccara G, et al. Comparison of intravenous or epidural patient-controlled analgesia in the elderly after major abdominal surgery. *Anesthesiology* 2000;92:433–441.

309. Keita H, Geachan N, Dahmani S, et al. Comparison between patient-controlled analgesia and subcutaneous morphine in elderly patients after total hip replacement. *Br J Anaesth* 2003;90:53–57.

310. Egbert AM, Parks LH, Short LM, et al. Randomized trial of postoperative patient-controlled analgesia vs intramuscular narcotics in frail elderly men. *Arch Intern Med* 1990;150:1897–1903.

311. Ready LB, Chadwick HS, Ross B. Age predicts effective epidural morphine dose after abdominal hysterectomy. *Anesth Analg* 1987;66:1215–1218.

312. Veering BT, Burm AG, van Kleef JW, et al. Epidural anesthesia with bupivacaine: Effects of age on neural blockade and pharmacokinetics. *Anesth Analg* 1987;66:589–593.

313. Simon MJ, Veering BT, Vletter AA, et al. The effect of age on the systemic absorption and systemic disposition of ropivacaine after epidural administration. *Anesth Analg* 2006;102:276–282.

314. Sadean MR, Glass PS. Pharmacokinetics in the elderly. *Best Pract Res Clin Anaesthesiol* 2003;17:191–205.

315. Simon MJ, Veering BT, Stienstra R, et al. Effect of age on the clinical profile and systemic absorption and disposition of levobupivacaine after epidural administration. *Br J Anaesth* 2004;93:512–520.

316. Simon MJ, Veering BT, Stienstra R, et al. The effects of age on neural blockade and hemodynamic changes after epidural anesthesia with ropivacaine. *Anesth Analg* 2002;94:1325–1330.

317. Li Y, Zhu S, Bao F, et al. The effects of age on the median effective concentration of ropivacaine for motor blockade after epidural anesthesia with ropivacaine. *Anesth Analg* 2006;102:1847–1850.

318. Crawford ME, Moiniche S, Orbaek J, et al. Orthostatic hypotension during postoperative continuous thoracic epidural bupivacaine-morphine in patients undergoing abdominal surgery. *Anesth Analg* 1996;83:1028–1032.

319. Veering BT. Hemodynamic effects of central neural blockade in elderly patients. *Can J Anaesth* 2006;53:117–121.

320. Hanks RK, Pietrobon R, Nielsen KC, et al. The effect of age on sciatic nerve block duration. *Anesth Analg* 2006;102:588–592.

321. Paqueron X, Boccara G, Bendahou M, et al. Brachial plexus nerve block exhibits prolonged duration in the elderly. *Anesthesiology* 2002;97:1245–1249.

322. Kest B, Sarton E, Dahan A. Gender differences in opioid-mediated analgesia: Animal and human studies. *Anesthesiology* 2000;93:539–547.

323. Aubrun F, Salvi N, Coriat P, et al. Sex- and age-related differences in morphine requirements for postoperative pain relief. *Anesthesiology* 2005;103:156–160.

324. Cepeda MS, Carr DB. Women experience more pain and require more morphine than men to achieve a similar degree of analgesia. *Anesth Analg* 2003;97:1464–1468.

325. Logan DE, Rose JB. Gender differences in post-operative pain and patient controlled analgesia use among adolescent surgical patients. *Pain* 2004;109:481–487.

326. Chia YY, Chow LH, Hung CC, et al. Gender and pain upon movement are associated with the requirements for postoperative patient-controlled iv analgesia: A prospective survey of 2,298 Chinese patients. *Can J Anaesth* 2002;49:249–255.

327. Taenzer AH, Clark C, Curry CS. Gender affects report of pain and function after arthroscopic anterior cruciate ligament reconstruction. *Anesthesiology* 2000;93:670–675.

328. Morin C, Lund JP, Villarroel T, et al. Differences between the sexes in post-surgical pain. *Pain* 2000;85:79–85.

329. Rosseland LA, Stubhaug A. Gender is a confounding factor in pain trials: Women report more pain than men after arthroscopic surgery. *Pain* 2004;112:248–253.

330. Linton SJ. A review of psychological risk factors in back and neck pain. *Spine* 2000;25:1148–1156.

331. Pincus T, Vlaeyen JW, Kendall NA, et al. Cognitive-behavioral therapy and psychosocial factors in low back pain: Directions for the future. *Spine* 2002;27:E133–E138.

332. Nelson FV, Zimmerman L, Barnason S, et al. The relationship and influence of anxiety on postoperative pain in the coronary artery bypass graft patient. *J Pain Symptom Manage* 1998;15:102–109.

333. Kalkman CJ, Visser K, Moen J, et al. Preoperative prediction of severe postoperative pain. *Pain* 2003;105:415–423.

334. Brandner B, Bromley L, Blagrove M. Influence of psychological factors in the use of patient controlled analgesia. *Acute Pain* 2002;4:53–56.

335. Ozalp G, Sarioglu R, Tuncel G, et al. Preoperative emotional states in patients with breast cancer and postoperative pain. *Acta Anaesthesiol Scand* 2003;47:26–29.

336. Pavlin DJ, Sullivan MJ, Freund PR, et al. Catastrophizing: A risk factor for postsurgical pain. *Clin J Pain* 2005;21:83–90.

337. Jacobsen PB, Butler RW. Relation of cognitive coping and catastrophizing to acute pain and analgesic use following breast cancer surgery. *J Behav Med* 1996;19:17–29.

338. Ferber SG, Granot M, Zimmer EZ. Catastrophizing labor pain compromises later maternity adjustments. *Am J Obstet Gynecol* 2005;192:826–831.

339. Kudoh A, Katagai H, Takazawa T. Increased postoperative pain scores in chronic depression patients who take antidepressants. *J Clin Anesth* 2002;14:421–425.

340. Bisgaard T, Klarskov B, Rosenberg J, et al. Characteristics and prediction of early pain after laparoscopic cholecystectomy. *Pain* 2001;90:261–269.

341. Pellino TA, Ward SE. Perceived control mediates the relationship between pain severity and patient satisfaction. *J Pain Symptom Manage* 1998;15:110–116.

342. Taylor NM, Hall GM, Salmon P. Patients' experiences of patient-controlled analgesia. *Anaesthesia* 1996;51:525–528.

PART IV: PAIN MANAGEMENT

343. Klepstad P, Dale O, Skorpen F, et al. Genetic variability and clinical efficacy of morphine. *Acta Anaesthesiol Scand* 2005;49:902–908.

344. Chou WY, Wang CH, Liu PH, et al. Human opioid receptor A118G polymorphism affects intravenous patient-controlled analgesia morphine consumption after total abdominal hysterectomy. *Anesthesiology* 2006; 105:334–337.

345. Chou WY, Yang LC, Lu HF, et al. Association of mu-opioid receptor gene polymorphism (A118G) with variations in morphine consumption for analgesia after total knee arthroplasty. *Acta Anaesthesiol Scand* 2006;50:787–792.

346. Klepstad P, Rakvag TT, Kaasa S, et al. The 118 A >G polymorphism in the human micro-opioid receptor gene may increase morphine requirements in patients with pain caused by malignant disease. *Acta Anaesthesiol Scand* 2004;48:1232–1239.

347. Stamer UM, Lehnen K, Hothker F, et al. Impact of CYP2D6 genotype on postoperative tramadol analgesia. *Pain* 2003;105:231–238.

348. Stamer UM, Bayerer B, Stuber F. Genetics and variability in opioid response. *Eur J Pain* 2005;9:101–104.

349. South SM, Smith MT. Analgesia tolerance to opioids. *Pain – Clinical Updates (IASP)* 2001;5:104.

350. Rapp SE, Ready LB, Nessly ML. Acute pain management in patients with prior opioid consumption: A case-controlled retrospective review. *Pain* 1995;61:195–201.

351. Mitra S, Sinatra RS. Perioperative management of acute pain in the opioid-dependent patient. *Anesthesiology* 2004;101:212–227.

352. Davis JJ, Swenson JD, Hall RH, et al. Preoperative "fentanyl challenge" as a tool to estimate postoperative opioid dosing in chronic opioid-consuming patients. *Anesth Analg* 2005;101:389–395.

353. Wong CS, Hsu MM, Chou R, et al. Intrathecal cyclooxygenase inhibitor administration attenuates morphine antinociceptive tolerance in rats. *Br J Anaesth* 2000;85:747–751.

354. Mercadante S, Portenoy RK. Opioid poorly-responsive cancer pain. Part 3. Clinical strategies to improve opioid responsiveness. *J Pain Symptom Manage* 2001;21:338–354.

355. Sator-Katzenschlager S, Deusch E, Maier P, et al. The long-term antinoci-

356. Bell RF. Low-dose subcutaneous ketamine infusion and morphine tolerance. *Pain* 1999;83:101–103.

357. Eilers H, Philip LA, Bickler PE, et al. The reversal of fentanyl-induced tolerance by administration of "small-dose" ketamine. *Anesth Analg* 2001; 93:213–214.

358. Haller G, Waeber JL, Infante NK, et al. Ketamine combined with morphine for the management of pain in an opioid addict. *Anesthesiology* 2002; 96:1265–1266.

359. Crain SM, Shen KF. Ultra-low concentrations of naloxone selectively antagonize excitatory effects of morphine on sensory neurons, thereby increasing its antinociceptive potency and attenuating tolerance/dependence during chronic cotreatment. *Proc Natl Acad Sci USA* 1995;92:10540–10544.

360. Wang HY, Friedman E, Olmstead MC, et al. Ultra-low-dose naloxone suppresses opioid tolerance, dependence and associated changes in mu opioid receptor-G protein coupling and Gbetagamma signaling. *Neuroscience* 2005;135:247–261.

361. Jang S, Kim H, Kim D, et al. Attenuation of morphine tolerance and withdrawal syndrome by coadmistration of nalbuphine. *Arch Pharm Res* 2006;29:677–684.

362. Vickers AP, Jolly A. Naltrexone and problems in pain management. *Br Med J* 2006;332:132–133.

363. Jage J, Bey T. Postoperative analgesia in patients with substance use disorders: Part 1. *Acute Pain* 2000;3:141–156.

364. Mehta V, Langford RM. Acute pain management for opioid dependent patients. *Anaesthesia* 2006;61:269–276.

365. Alford DP, Compton P, Samet JH. Acute pain management for patients receiving maintenance methadone or buprenorphine therapy. *Ann Intern Med* 2006;144:127–134.

366. Lee MC, Wagner HN, Jr., Tanada S, et al. Duration of occupancy of opiate receptors by naltrexone. *J Nucl Med* 1988;29:1207–1211.

367. Johnson RE, Fudala PJ, Payne R. Buprenorphine: Considerations for pain management. *J Pain Symptom Manage* 2005;29:297–326.

CHAPTER 44 ■ SPINAL PAIN AND THE ROLE OF NEURAL BLOCKADE

JAMES P. RATHMELL, CARLOS A. PINO, AND SHIHAB AHMED

Low back pain is a nonspecific term, typically used to refer to pain that is centered over the lumbosacral junction. To be more precise in our approach to diagnosis and treatment, it is important to differentiate pain that is primarily over the axis of the spinal column from pain that is primarily referred to the leg (Fig. 44-1). *Lumbar spinal pain* is pain inferior to the inferior aspect of the 12th thoracic spinous process and superior aspect of the 1st sacral spinous process (1). *Sacral spinal* pain is pain inferior to the first sacral spinous process and superior to the sacrococcygeal joint (1). *Lumbosacral spinal pain* is pain in either or both of these regions and constitutes what is commonly referred to as "low back pain." A subset of patients will present with pain that is predominantly localized within the leg and is commonly called "sciatica," because of its distribution in the area innervated by the sciatic nerve; the proper term for this type of pain is *radicular pain*, and this pain is evoked by stimulation of the nerve roots or the dorsal root ganglion of a spinal nerve.

Pain in the thoracic and cervical regions is less common than low back pain, and our understanding of treatment is less well developed. Nonetheless, cervical and thoracic pain are common. *Cervical spinal pain* is pain inferior to the occiput, extending inferiorly to the inferior aspect of the 7th cervical spinous process. *Thoracic spinal pain* is pain anywhere between the 1st and 12th thoracic spinous processes. As described for lumbosacral pain, when approaching patients with spinal pain in the cervical or thoracic areas, one of the most important issues is to distinguish between pain that occurs predominantly along the axis of the spine and radicular pain that is referred along the course of one or more spinal nerves.

EPIDEMIOLOGY

Low back pain is the second most common problem that leads patients to seek medical attention (2). The majority of episodes of acute low back pain with or without radicular pain will resolve without specific treatment. Overall, 60% to 70% of those who experience a first episode of acute low back pain will recover by 6 weeks, and 80% to 90% will do so by 12 weeks (Fig. 44-2) (3). For those with new onset of radicular pain due to an acute disc herniation, recovery with or without surgical discectomy occurs in nearly all individuals within the first 12 months (4); however, recovery is slow and uncertain. Fewer than 50% of those individuals disabled for longer than 6 months will return to work. The return-to-work rate for those absent from work for 2 years is near zero (5). There is a high lifetime recurrence rate, with the vast majority of those who have a single episode of back pain experiencing a second episode at

some point during their lives (3). Both biologic and psychosocial factors lead some individuals to have a higher probability of developing chronic low back pain. Biologic factors predicting chronicity include longer duration of back pain, a past history of back pain, presence of leg pain, and obesity (3,6). Among the most predictive psychosocial factors are job dissatisfaction, depression, poor coping skills, and fear of reinjury. Chronic back pain is ubiquitous and a leading cause for medical intervention, disability, and long-term suffering among our patients.

PATHOPHYSIOLOGY

The basic functional unit of the spine is termed the *functional spinal unit* and is comprised of two adjacent vertebral bodies with two posterior facet joints, an intervertebral disc, and the surrounding ligamentous structures (Fig. 44-3). The intervertebral disc distributes the load evenly from one spinal segment to the next while allowing movement of the protective bony elements; it also serves to absorb energy (7). Mechanical stressors such as lifting, bending, twisting, or whole-body vibration have the potential to injure elements of the spine. With injury and aging, progressive degenerative changes appear in each element of the functional spinal unit, along with the onset of characteristic symptoms associated with specific degenerative changes (Fig. 44-3). The earliest change in the lumbar facet joints is synovitis, which progresses to degradation of the articular surfaces of the facet joints, capsular laxity and subluxation, and finally enlargement of the articular processes (facet hypertrophy). Progressive degeneration also occurs within the intervertebral discs, starting with the loss of hydration of the nucleus pulposus, followed by the appearance of circumferential or radial tears within the annulus fibrosis (internal disc disruption). Lumbosacral pain can arise from the degenerating facet joints or the annulus fibrosis, a structure that is richly innervated in the outer one-third of its circumference (8). With this internal disruption of the intervertebral disc, a localized protrusion of the disc called a *disc herniation* can appear (herniated nucleus pulposus or HNP). When disc material reaches the epidural space adjacent to the spinal nerve, this incites an intense inflammatory reaction (9). Those with HNP typically present with acute radicular pain. Hypertrophy of the facet joints and calcification of the ligamentous structures within the spinal canal can lead to a critical reduction in the dimensions of the intervertebral foramina and/or the central spinal canal (spinal stenosis), with the onset of radicular pain or neurogenic claudication.

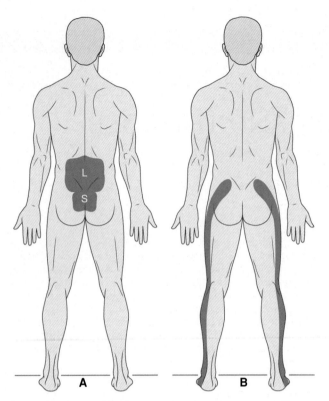

FIGURE 44-1. The definition of low back pain. **A:** "Low back pain" is more precisely termed *lumbosacral spinal pain,* and encompasses *both lumbar spinal pain (L)* and *sacral spinal pain (S).* **B:** *Radicular pain* refers to pain that is referred to the lower extremity and is caused by stimulation of a spinal nerve.

An increasing number of patients present with prior lumbar surgery and either recurrent or persistent low back pain. This group, often termed *failed back surgery syndrome,* require special attention (10). All patients who have pain after prior lumbar surgery are not the same: Understanding what type of surgery was done, why the surgery was done, and the initial results of the surgery, as well as the time course and characteristics of any changes in the pattern and severity of symptoms is essential. Recurrent pain or progressive symptoms signal the need for further diagnostic evaluation in efforts to determine if a new and treatable cause for the pain can be identified.

APPROACH TO EVALUATION AND TREATMENT

In the initial approach to evaluating any patient with low back pain, several key principles apply (Table 44-1). Features in the history that point to the need for prompt and detailed investigation include patients with new-onset or worsening back pain in the face of any history of trauma, infection, or previous cancer (Table 44-2). Those with progressive neurologic deficits (typically worsening numbness or weakness) or the appearance of bowel or bladder dysfunction also warrant immediate imaging to rule out a compressive lesion.

Because the lines of treatment available follow fairly discrete paths, it is reasonable to divide patients into four discrete categories, then proceed with diagnosis and treatment accordingly. First, determine if the pain is primarily along the axis of the cervical or lumbosacral spine or primarily radicular; then,

establish the duration of the pain. *Acute* pain is often defined as pain that has been present less than 3 months, and *chronic* pain as pain that has been present for at least 3 months (1).

Acute Radicular Pain

A herniated intervertebral disc typically causes acute radicular pain, with or without radiculopathy (signs of dysfunction including numbness, weakness, or loss of deep tendon reflexes referable to a specific spinal nerve). In the elderly or those with extensive spondylosis, it is not uncommon to have the onset of acute radicular symptoms caused by narrowing of one or more intervertebral foramina. Initial treatment is symptomatic, and the symptoms will resolve without specific treatment in the majority of patients.

Chronic Radicular Pain

Persistent arm or leg pain in the distribution of a spinal nerve is not uncommon in those who have had a disc herniation, with or without subsequent surgery. In those with persistent pain, a search for a reversible cause for ongoing nerve root compression is warranted. In many individuals, extensive scarring surrounding the nerve root at the operative site can be seen on magnetic resonance imaging (MRI) (11), and electrodiagnostic studies will suggest typical patterns suggestive of chronic radiculopathy. This group is similar in characteristic to those who suffer from other chronic nerve injuries and have ongoing pain due to abnormal function of the nervous system, termed *neuropathic pain.* Like those with painful diabetic neuropathy and postherpetic neuralgia, this group is best approached initially with pharmacologic treatment for neuropathic pain.

Acute Cervical or Lumbosacral Pain

Most patients presenting with acute-onset axial cervical or lumbosacral pain without radicular symptoms will have no obvious signs of abnormality on physical examination, and imaging is unlikely to be of significant benefit in the acute setting. Traumatic sprain of the muscles and ligaments of the spine or the zygapophyseal joints, as well as early internal disc disruption, are all significant causes of acute cervical or lumbosacral pain. Like those with acute radicular pain, this group is best managed symptomatically with mild oral analgesics with or without muscle relaxants and prompt return to full activity.

Chronic Lumbosacral Pain

Perhaps the most challenging is the patient with persistent axial cervical or lumbosacral pain, particularly those with significant and ongoing disability. Chronic cervical and lumbosacral pain has many causes, and there is no means to identify the "pain generator" in any given individual with absolute certainty. The structures that have been most commonly implicated in causing chronic cervical or lumbosacral pain include the sacroiliac joint, the lumbar facets, and the intervertebral discs. The incidence of symptomatic conditions in these areas in patients presenting with chronic low back pain has been estimated to be 39% for internal disc disruption (range, 29%–49%), 15% for facet joint pain (10%–20%), and 15% for sacroiliac joint pain (7%–23%) (12). The gold standard for diagnosing sacroiliac and facet joint pain has been injection of local anesthetic

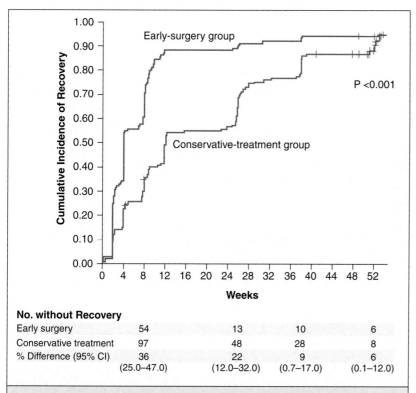

No. without Recovery

Early surgery	54	13	10	6
Conservative treatment	97	48	28	8
% Difference (95% CI)	36	22	9	6
	(25.0–47.0)	(12.0–32.0)	(0.7–17.0)	(0.1–12.0)

Inverse Kaplan–Meier Estimating the Cumulative Incidence of Recovery

The median time to recovery was 4.0 weeks (95% CI, 3.7 to 4.3) in the early-surgery group and 12.1 weeks (95% CI, 9.5 to 14.8) in the conservative-treatment group. The number of patients who had not yet recovered at each examination is shown, as are the absolute percent difference between the conservative-treatment group and the early-surgery group is patients who had recovered (95% confidence interval). Recovery was defined as complete or nearly complete according to the Likert 7-point scale (higher scores indicate worse outcome). The hazard ratio, estimated with the unadjusted Cox model with recovery as an end point, was 1.97 (95% CI, 1.72 to 2.22) in favor of early surgery.

FIGURE 44-2. Cumulative incidence of recovery. From Peul WC, van Houwelingen HC, van den Hout WB, et al. Leiden-The Hague Spine Intervention Prognostic Study Group. Surgery versus prolonged conservative treatment for sciatica. *N Engl J Med* 2007;356: 2245–2256, with permission.

into the joint (13).However, the use of uncontrolled local anesthetic blocks for diagnostic purposes is plagued by a frequent placebo response and other factors (see Chapter 36). For those attaining significant pain relief with diagnostic blocks, radiofrequency treatment offers a simple, minimally invasive treatment that is modestly effective for treating facet-related pain. Finally, pain arising from degenerating intervertebral discs is also a common source of chronic axial neck or back pain. Diagnostic provocative discography has been used to identify symptomatic discs prior to intradiscal treatment with emerging therapies such as intradiscal electrothermal therapy (IDET) or surgical fusion; however, again, interpretation of response to provocative discography is not as straightforward as often claimed (see Chapter 38).

MEDICAL THERAPIES

Neuropathic Pain Medications

Treatment of neuropathic pain in the form of chronic lumbar radicular pain is extrapolated from randomized trials examining the treatment of the more common forms of neuropathic

pain, diabetic neuropathy and postherpetic neuralgia. Discrete characteristics suggest neuropathic pain and, in the presence of these abnormal sensations (Table 44-3), beginning treatment with oral neuropathic pain medications is warranted, even in the absence of an identifiable neurologic deficit. Anticonvulsants and antidepressants have shown significant efficacy in treating neuropathic pain. Tricyclic antidepressants (e.g., amitriptyline, nortriptyline, desipramine) and certain other antidepressants (i.e., bupropion, venlafaxine, duloxetine) are effective in the treatment of neuropathic pain (14). First-generation antiepileptic drugs (i.e., carbamazepine, phenytoin) and second-generation antiepileptic drugs (e.g., gabapentin, pregabalin) are also effective in the treatment of neuropathic pain (14).

Chronic Opioid Therapy

The use of chronic opioid therapy for the long-term treatment of noncancer pain remains a topic of significant controversy (15–17). Advocates point toward the significant long-term efficacy and improvement in function in patients with chronic painful conditions, including chronic low back pain. Opponents point to the difficulties with using these drugs over

PART IV: PAIN MANAGEMENT

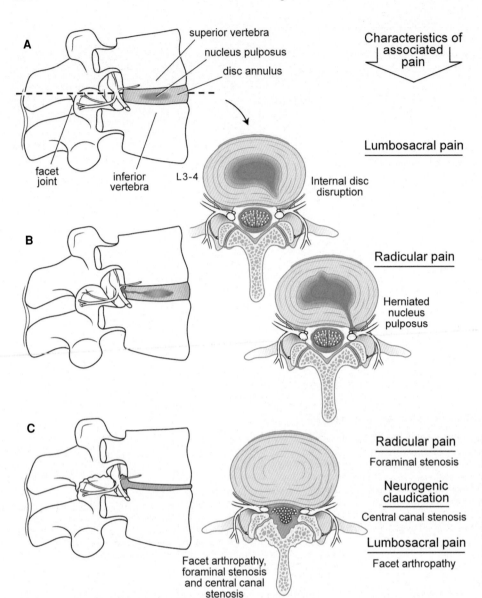

FIGURE 44-3. The functional spinal unit and the degenerative changes that lead to lumbosacral and radicular pain. **A:** The normal functional spinal unit. **B:** The degenerative changes of internal disc disruption and facet arthropathy leading to lumbosacral (discogenic pain, facet joint pain) and radicular pain (herniated nucleus pulposus). **C:** The degenerative changes of lumbar spondylosis leading to lumbosacral (facet joint pain), radicular pain (foraminal stenosis causing radicular pain), and neurogenic claudication (central canal stenosis).

the long-term (18). Although aberrant drug-related behavior (e.g., losing prescriptions, escalating drug dose beyond the prescriber's recommendations) are relatively common in those receiving the medications for the treatment of chronic pain (19), overt addiction is uncommon (20). However, treating acute pain in the opioid-tolerant patient is a difficult proposition (21,22), and there is emerging recognition that chronic opioid use can actually worsen pain in the form of opioid-induced hyperalgesia (23). The current prevailing opinion seems to be that the use of modest doses of opioids can help to reduce pain and improve function in a select group of patients with chronic noncancer pain (24). However, the selection process is empiric, and there is no standard approach to choosing those who will do well.

When opting to treat a patient with long-term opioids, a wide array of opioid analgesics is available to choose from. The traditional paradigm for treating pain with opioids arose from the treatment of cancer pain (25). Using this approach, those with significant ongoing pain are given a long-acting opioid to provide continuous pain relief without the fluctuations in pain control associated with short-acting opioids. In addition, a small, intermittent dose of a short-acting agent is made available to treat pain that occurs with activity and "breaks through" the control provided by the long-acting agent alone. Nearly every available opioid has been used successfully in treating chronic low back pain, including short-acting agents alone or in combination formulations with ibuprofen or acetaminophen (e.g., hydrocodone, oxycodone) and long-acting agents (e.g., methadone, transdermal fentanyl, controlled-release oxycodone). Recently, a new type of opioid, termed *ultra-fast onset,* has emerged (e.g., oral transmucosal fentanyl citrate, fentanyl buccal tablet) for the rapid treatment of break-through pain (26). Like the patient selection process, choosing the best agent and the appropriate dose of opioid remains empiric. The choice between using short- or long-acting agents alone or in combination is best tailored to each patient and their individual pattern of pain. Ample evidence suggests that opioids significantly reduce pain during the first several months after initiating treatment, but studies of long-term treatment are just starting to appear (27).

TABLE 44-1

KEY PRINCIPLES IN THE EVALUATION OF PATIENTS WITH LOW BACK PAIN

- Serious causes of neck and back pain (e.g., infection, tumor, trauma, acute spinal canal, or foraminal stenosis) are rare, but must be excluded.
- The etiology of pain in a significant number of patients with back and neck pain may remain unknown. Nonspecific back or neck pain is a legitimate diagnosis.
- History and physical examination have a limited role in the diagnosis of back and neck pain but are important in ruling out serious pathology.
- It is important to distinguish pain limited to the axis of the spine from radicular pain and radiculopathy.
- It is important to reassure patients with acute back and neck pain that the vast majority of patients recover within weeks, without specific treatment.
- Discogenic pain is the single most common cause for axial low back pain.
- Cervical facet joints are among the most common causes of axial neck pain.
- Diagnostic local anesthetic blocks can be helpful in establishing an anatomic diagnosis.

Physical Therapy

Physical therapy, generally consisting of stretching, strengthening, and aerobic exercise in conjunction with patient education, is widely used and has shown benefit in treating patients with low back pain persisting beyond 6 weeks (28). Following acute lumbar strain with or without radicular pain, exercise therapy is no more effective than other conservative treatments, includ-

ing no intervention (29). Even brief patient education through one-on-one, group, or video instruction can lead to significantly less disability and less worry about reinjury (30). Physical therapy can include the use of various modalities, including heat, ultrasound, and transcutaneous electrical stimulation (TENS); these modalities may provide short-term symptomatic relief, but evidence that they alter the long-term course of acute or chronic low back pain is lacking (29,31).

Behavioral Therapy

Persistent pain is recognized as a problem that often has psychological and social/occupational dimensions, as well as biologic or physical components. Two main types of behavioral therapy have been used for back pain, operant conditioning and cognitive therapy. *Operant conditioning* aims to eliminate maladaptive pain behaviors. *Cognitive therapy* addresses how patients cope with their pain: what they actually do as a result of their pain and how their thoughts and feelings influence their behavior. Behavioral therapy significantly reduces pain intensity and behavioral outcomes (e.g., pain behavior, cognitive errors, perceived or observed levels of tension, anxiety, depression) compared with no treatment (32).

Multidisciplinary Pain Treatment Programs

The typical multidisciplinary treatment program includes a medical manager, usually a physician, who oversees all aspects of the treatment program, working together with other health care professionals who deliver behavioral therapy and physical therapy. In recent years, declining reimbursement has forced many inpatient programs to evolve to outpatient day treatment programs. Intensive (>100 hours of therapy) multidisciplinary biopsychosocial rehabilitation with functional

TABLE 44-2

RED FLAG FOR POTENTIALLY SERIOUS CONDITIONS

Possible fracture	Possible tumor or infection	Possible cauda equina syndrome
From medical history - Major trauma, such as a motor vehicle accident or a fall from a height - Minor trauma or even strenuous lifting in an older or potentially osteoporotic patient	- Age over 50 or under 20 - History of cancer - Risk factors for spinal infection: recent bacterial infection, IV drug abuse, immune suppression (steroid therapy, transplant, HIV) - Pain that worsens when supine; severe nighttime pain	- Saddle anesthesia - Recent onset of bladder dysfunction, such as urinary retention, increased frequency, or overflow incontinence - Severe or progressive neurologic deficit in the lower extremity
From physical examination —	—	- Unexpected laxity of the anal sphincter - Perianal/perineal sensory loss - Major motor weakness: quadriceps (knee extension); ankle plantar flexors, evertors, or dorsiflexors (foot drop)

IV, intravenous; HIV, human immunodeficiency virus.
From Bigos S, Bowyer O, Braen G, at al. Acute low back problems in adults. *Clinical Practice Guideline, Quick Reference Guide Number 14.* Rockville, MD: U.S. Department of Health and Human Services, Agency for Health Care Policy and Research, AHCPR Pub. No. 95-0643. December 1994.

TABLE 44-3

THE ABNORMAL SENSATIONS OF NEUROPATHIC PAIN

Pain is a normal physiologic process and serves as a signal that tissue injury has occurred and that the injured region should be protected while healing ensues. As the tissue heals, the pain diminishes and usually resolves completely. Pain associated with tissue injury is usually well-localized and associated with sensitivity in the region. Pain signals are carried toward the central nervous system via the peripheral sensory nerves. This type of pain is termed *nociceptive pain.*

In contrast, pain associated with many nerve injuries, termed *neuropathic pain*, includes chronic pain states in which pain signals are carried through the sympathetic nervous system. These types of pain share a number of characteristics. The diagnosis of neuropathic pain is made largely on the basis of the patient's description of one or more of the following characteristics:

- *Spontaneous pain.* Pain that occurs without a specific sensory stimulus (e.g., the sudden lancinating pain described by those with postherpetic neuralgia).
- *Paresthesias/dysesthesias.* Abnormal pain distant from the site of actual tissue injury that may be spontaneous or evoked (e.g., the radiating pain associated with lumbar nerve root compression).
- *Hyperalgesia.* An exaggerated painful response to a normally noxious stimulus (e.g., light pin-prick leads to extreme and prolonged pain).
- *Allodynia.* A painful response to a normally non-noxious stimulus (e.g., light touch causes pain).

restoration significantly reduces pain and improves function compared with inpatient or outpatient non-multidisciplinary treatments or usual care; some improvements in physical function are sustained over long-term follow-up (33). Multidisciplinary pain treatment programs remain a viable and important treatment option for those with chronic pain accompanied by significant impairment in function.

OTHER THERAPIES

Acupuncture

Determining the efficacy of acupuncture has been hindered by the lack of well-controlled trials (34). A recent meta-analysis analyzed 33 randomized clinical trials (RCTs) comparing acupuncture with sham intervention for the treatment of back pain (35). The investigators found that acupuncture effectively relieves chronic low back pain, but the data regarding the effectiveness of acupuncture for treating acute low back pain remains inconclusive. The effectiveness of acupuncture when compared to other available treatments has not been studied; the frequency and duration of treatment required to produce ongoing pain reduction also remain in question.

Spinal Manipulation

No universally accepted definition of spinal manipulation exists. In general terms, spinal manipulation involves the use of hands applied to the patient to deliver a forceful load to specific body tissues, typically with the intent of reducing pain and/or improving range of movement (36). Postulated mechanisms include increase of joint movement, changes in joint kinematics, increase of pain threshold, increase of muscle strength, and release of endogenous analgesic peptides (37). The available data are conflicting, but on balance show that spinal manipulation brings about a more rapid recovery in some patients if applied within 3 weeks of onset of acute low back pain (38). The outcomes regarding treatment of chronic low back pain are less clear, and the conclusions of systematic reviews are at odds. One recent systematic review concluded that spinal manipulation for chronic low back pain has an effect similar to an efficacious prescription of nonsteroidal anti-inflammatory drug; it is effective in the short-term when compared to placebo and general practitioner care, and in the long-term when compared to physical therapy (38). In contrast, another group systematically reviewed a series of 16 different systematic reviews regarding spinal manipulation and concluded that spinal manipulation was not effective for treating any condition, including low back pain (36). Nonetheless, they pointed to the paucity of data and called for additional clinical trials.

THE ROLE FOR NEURAL BLOCKADE: INTERVENTIONAL PAIN THERAPY

Interventional pain therapy refers to a group of targeted treatments used for specific spine disorders; many of these treatments evolved through modification of traditional techniques used for neural blockade for surgical anesthesia. These interventions range from epidural injection of steroids to percutaneous intradiscal techniques. Some of these interventional pain therapies have undergone extensive validation through RCTs, whereas others have progressed into widespread use without critical evaluation. When these treatment techniques are applied logically to the disorders that they have the most likelihood to benefit, they are a good addition to the armamentarium used to treat low back pain; when used haphazardly, they are unlikely to help patients and may be associated with significant risk of harm.

Despite the paucity of scientific evidence to guide pain practitioners, particularly evidence to support the use of many interventional modalities, a number of techniques appear to have efficacy based on limited observational data; these have been adopted into widespread use. Practitioners are left to choose among many available modalities, often with only anecdotal and personal experience to guide them, to treat a group of desperate patients with intractable pain who are willing to accept almost any intervention, even those which remain unproved. No single practice pattern exists that any pain specialist can point to as the correct way to treat patients with chronic pain. The best pain medicine practitioners strike a reasonable balance between interventional and noninterventional management. This practice pattern is sustainable, and those adopting a balanced style of practice will be able to adapt to evolving scientific evidence that appears in support of any particular pain treatment, regardless of its type. A balance between treatment modalities also allows practitioners to switch from one mode to another, or to incorporate multiple treatment approaches simultaneously.

Use of Image-guided Techniques in Pain Medicine

Little more than a decade ago, radiographic guidance was used infrequently by pain practitioners, being reserved for major procedures like neurolytic celiac plexus block. During the last several years, however, two forces have been at work. First, pain practitioners are now being called upon to serve as diagnosticians. Patients and referring practitioners expect pain physicians to have familiarity with imaging modalities and their usefulness in diagnosing pain conditions. At the same time, pain practitioners have come to realize the usefulness of radiographic guidance in achieving precise anatomic placement of needles and catheters. Although the evidence supporting the need for routine radiographic guidance is still evolving, the intuitive appeal of this more precise approach has caught firm hold, to the point where the majority of practitioners now perform at least a portion of their injections using fluoroscopic guidance (39). In some cases—as in patients with intractable pain associated with metastatic cancer—radiographic guidance has proven invaluable in the planning and implementation of therapy directed toward pain relief.

We have examined the distribution of injectate in a series of patients who received epidural steroid injections for radicular pain associated with a new herniated disc (40). We found that the injectate often spread to the side opposite the disc herniation. This is not at all surprising; if a disc herniation is present on one side, this might well obstruct the flow of fluid through the relatively confined epidural space. The fluid follows the path of least resistance, spreading preferentially to the contralateral, unaffected side and exiting the contralateral intervertebral foramina. This study and others (41,42) have challenged the conventional wisdom that suspending the steroid in a modest volume was sufficient to consistently produce spread of the injectate to the affected levels, regardless of where the solution was placed within the epidural space. Perhaps the blind loss-of-resistance technique is not the best way to deliver steroid to the site of inflammation.

Using radiographic guidance, bony structures can be visualized directly and in real time. The needle can be seen within the radiographic field, and simple geometry can be used to guide the needle directly from the skin's surface to its destination. However, the field of pain medicine suffers from a lack of well-controlled studies to guide the choice of the most effective therapies. Indeed, many of the techniques described in this chapter lack clear evidence to support their efficacy. Even so, the techniques described here are in widespread clinical use. In the sections that follow, a clear summary of the current evidence available supporting the use of each technique has been given, but all too often these data are scant. With more consistent methodology, we can begin the much-needed work of assembling RCTs to determine which of these techniques are most useful in aiding those with intractable pain.

Specific Interventional Techniques

In the following sections, we provide an overview of the most common techniques used in interventional pain medicine. The section begins with a discussion of the anatomy relevant to image-guided interventions for treating chronic pain. Thereafter, we briefly describe the clinical utility of each technique and the technical aspects of conducting each intervention. We provide illustrations for the most common techniques, but detailed illustration of less common techniques is beyond the scope of this chapter. Many books have been published with detailed technical descriptions of these techniques, and we refer the interested reader to one of these texts (43).

Anatomy Relevant to Image-guided Intervention for Spinal Pain

The key to success in any interventional pain technique is a clear understanding of the normal anatomy. The procedures described in this text require understanding of the normal anatomy of the spine, including the epidural and subarachnoid spaces, the zygapophyseal joints, intervertebral discs and, most importantly, the spinal cord with its somatic and sympathetic components (see Chapter 9). In this section, we review the basic anatomy relevant to common interventions used in the treatment of chronic pain.

Anatomy of the Spine. The anatomy of the bony spine, individual vertebrae, meninges, spinal cord, spinal nerves, spinal vasculature, and cerebrospinal fluid (CSF) is described in detail in Chapter 9 (see Figs. 9-1 to 9-41).

Normally, the vertebral canal is nearly triangular, surrounded by the bony components of the vertebrae. There are 33 vertebrae: 7 cervical, 12 thoracic, 5 lumbar, 5 fused elements that make up the sacrum, and 4 to 5 fused ossicles that form the coccyx (Fig. 44-4) (44). A typical vertebra consists of a vertebral body and two pedicles that extend posteriorly, surrounding the spinal canal and epidural space to join a pair of arched laminae (Fig. 44-5). The laminae fuse in the midline to form a dorsal projection called the *spinous process*. Near the junction of the pedicles and the laminae are found the lateral transverse processes, and the superior and the inferior articular processes (zygapophyses or facets). The pedicles and their articulating processes form the superior and inferior vertebral notches. In the articulated spine, these notches form the intervertebral foramina (44).

The zygapophyseal or "facet" joints are paired structures that lie posterolaterally on the bony vertebrae at the junction of the lamina and pedicle, medially, and on the base of the transverse process, laterally. The facet joints are true joints, with opposing cartilaginous surfaces and a true synovial lining, and they are subject to the same inflammatory and degenerative processes that affect other synovial joints throughout the body (44). Two opposing articular surfaces comprise each facet joint. The facet joint articular processes are named for the vertebra to which they belong. Thus, each vertebra has a superior articular process and an inferior articular process. This nomenclature can be confusing, as the superior articular process of a given vertebra actually forms the inferior portion of each facet joint.

The intervertebral disc is comprised of glucosaminoglycans with a relatively fluid inner nucleus pulposus surrounded by a stiff, lamellar outer annulus fibrosis (44). With aging, the hydration of the intervertebral discs declines, leading to loss of disc height and fissure formation in the annulus fibrosis. These fissures begin centrally, near the border between the nucleus pulposus and the annulus fibrosis and can extend to the periphery of the disc space (Fig. 44-3B). This process of degradation is called *internal disc disruption* and is believed responsible for producing discogenic pain. The annulus contains neural elements from the sinuvertebral nerve, which is believed to be responsible for pain transmission (Figs. 44-6 and 44-7) (45). These same radial fissures within the annulus represent paths through which nuclear material can pass and extrude as a herniated nucleus pulposus. When this extruded material is adjacent

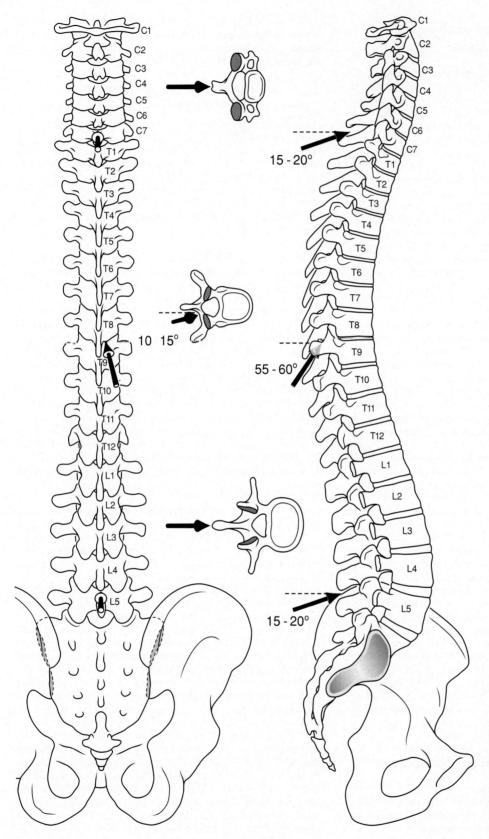

FIGURE 44-4. Anatomy of vertebral column. The most prominent spinous process at the base of the neck is C7 in most humans (the vertebrae prominens). Note that the angle of the spinous processes changes dramatically from cervical to lumbar levels, with the steepest angle in the mid thoracic region. The approximate plane of midline needle entry for interlaminar epidural injection is shown for cervical, thoracic, and lumbar levels. From Rathmell JP. *Atlas of Image-guided Intervention in Regional Anesthesia and Pain Medicine.* Philadelphia: Lippincott Williams & Wilkins, 2006, with permission.

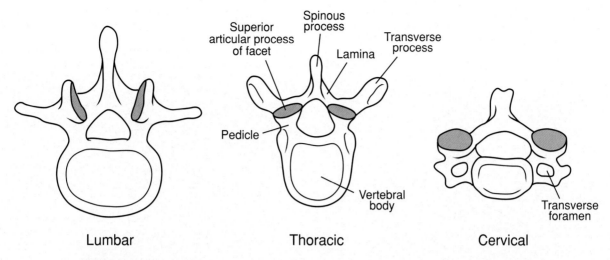

FIGURE 44-5. Anatomy of the cervical, thoracic, and lumbar vertebrae. From Rathmell JP. *Atlas of Image-guided Intervention in Regional Anesthesia and Pain Medicine*. Philadelphia: Lippincott Williams & Wilkins, 2006, with permission.

to an exiting spinal nerve root, it can lead to intense inflammation, nerve root compression, and radicular pain with or without radiculopathy (nerve root dysfunction in the form of numbness, weakness, and/or loss of deep tendon reflexes; Fig. 44-3B). The paired facet joints, along with the vertebral bodies and intervertebral discs, form the three weight-bearing support columns that distribute the axial load on the vertebral column while allowing for movement in various planes. The structure of the vertebrae varies from cephalad to caudad and should be thoroughly reviewed by the practitioner, especially when utilizing imaging (Figs. 44-4 and 44-5). Of importance when performing injections, the spinous processes of the cervical and lumbar regions approach the lamina in a nearly perpendicular fashion, which facilitates a midline approach when performing epidural or subarachnoid injections. The cervical facet joints are oriented nearly parallel to the axial plane, where the atlas (C1) articulates with the occiput, and become gradually more steeply angulated in a cephalad to caudad direction at lower cervical levels. The orientation of the cervical facet joints in a plane close to the axial plane allows for a great degree of rotation of the neck as well as flexion and extension.

The mid thoracic (T5–T9) spinous processes are acutely angled caudad, making the midline approach to the epidural space more difficult than the paramedian approach (see Chapter 11). The thoracic facet joints are so steeply angulated that they approach the frontal plane, which makes intra-articular injection difficult or impossible. At mid thoracic levels, the inferior articular process of the vertebra forming the superior portion of each thoracic facet joint lies directly posterior to the superior articular process forming the inferior portion of each joint. This allows for some degree of flexion and extension, but limited rotation of the spinal column in the thorax.

The spinous processes of the lumbar vertebrae approach the lamina in a nearly perpendicular fashion. The lumbar facet joints are angled with a somewhat oblique orientation, allowing for flexion, extension, and rotation that is greater than that in the thorax, but less than in the cervical region. The sacral hiatus is the area where the 5th sacral vertebra lacks both the laminae and the spinous process posteriorly (Fig. 44-8). The two sacral cornua lie on either side of the sacral hiatus and cephalad to the coccyx, and provide useful landmarks when performing an epidural from a caudal approach (see Chapter 11).

The midline distance from the ligamentum flavum to the dural sac varies considerably depending on the level of entry, increasing from 2 mm at C3–6 to 5 to 6 mm in the midlumbar region (46). The epidural space narrows posterior and laterally toward the intervertebral foramina. The anterior boundary of the epidural space is provided by the posterior longitudinal ligament covering the vertebral bodies and the intervertebral discs. Posteriorly, the epidural space is limited by the periosteum of the anterior surfaces of the laminae, the articulating facet processes (zygapophyses), and the ligamentum flavum. Laterally, the pedicles and the intervertebral foramina limit the epidural space (see Chapter 9, Figs. 9-5 to 9-30).

Knowledge of surface anatomy enhances safety when performing procedures under imaging and is of absolute necessity when imaging is not available. Important surface landmarks include the spinous process at C7 (*vertebra prominens*), which is the most prominent cervical spinous process palpable when the neck is flexed. The spinous process at T7 lies opposite the inferior angle of the scapula when the arm is at the side. A line joining the superior aspects of the iliac crests will pass through the spinous process of the fourth lumbar vertebrae. The spinal cord generally terminates at the L2 level, and the dural sac ends at S2, which corresponds to the level of the posterior superior iliac spines (see also Fig. 9-3). The tip of an equilateral triangle drawn between the posterior superior iliac spines and directed caudally overlies the sacral cornua and sacral hiatus.

Additionally, the articulated spine is supported by the anterior and posterior longitudinal ligaments, the supraspinous and interspinous ligaments, and ligamentum flavum (see Fig. 9-8) (46). Many of the pain management procedures discussed later will make reference to the ligamentum flavum. The ligamentum flavum or "yellow ligament" is a structure of variable thickness and completeness, composed of elastic fibers, that defines the posterolateral soft tissue boundaries of the epidural space. Because its leather-like consistency resists active expulsion of fluid from a syringe, loss of this resistance is valuable in signaling entry into the epidural space. The ligament's structure is steeply arched and tent-like, so much so that the lateral reflection may be up to 1 cm deeper than at the midline. In the cervical and thoracic epidural spaces, the ligamentum flavum often does not fuse in the midline, which can become problematic during loss-of-resistance techniques. When the dense ligamentum flavum

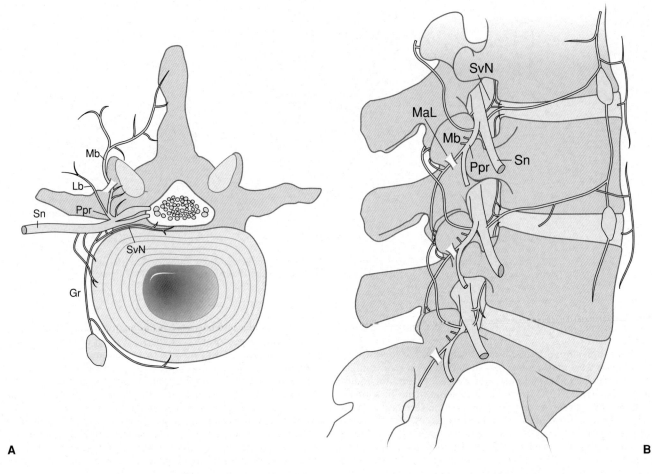

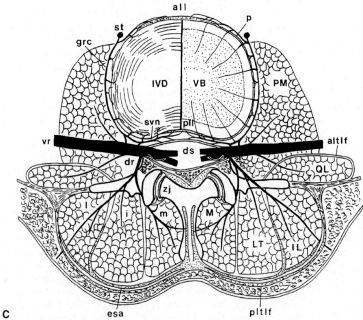

FIGURE 44-6. Lumbar spine innervation. Sketch of the innervation of the lumbar spinal structures in transverse (**A**) and lateral (**B**) views. **A:** Note the posterior primary ramus *(Ppr)* leaving the spinal nerve *(Sn)* and splitting into a lateral branch *(Lb)* and a medial branch *(Mb)*. The medial branch passes under the mamilla-accessory ligament *(mal)* to innervate the facet joint and capsule, the spinous process, and the multifidus muscles. Sensory fibers traveling with the gray rami *(Gr)* from the sinuvertebral nerve *(SvN)* provide sensory function to the disc annulus. **C:** A cross-sectional view incorporating the level of the vertebral body (*B*) and its periosteum (*p*) on the right of the intervertebral disc *(IVD)* on the left. *PM*, psoas muscle; *QL*, quadratus lumborum; *IL*, iliocostalis lumborum; *LT*, longissimus thoracicus; *M*, multifidus; *altf*, anterior layer of thoracolumbar fascia; *pltf*, posterior layer of thoracolumbar fascia; *esa*, erector spinae aponeurosis; *ds*, dural sac; *zj*, zygapophyseal joint; *pll*, posterior longitudinal ligament; *vr*, ventral ramus; *dr*, dorsal ramus; *de*, dorsal sac; *m*, medial nerve; *grc*, gray ramus communicans; *st*, sympathetic trunk. From Boguk N, Twomey LT. Nerves of the lumbar spine. In: *Clinical Anatomy of the Lumbar Spine*, 2nd ed. Melbourne: Churchill Livingstone, 1996, with permission.

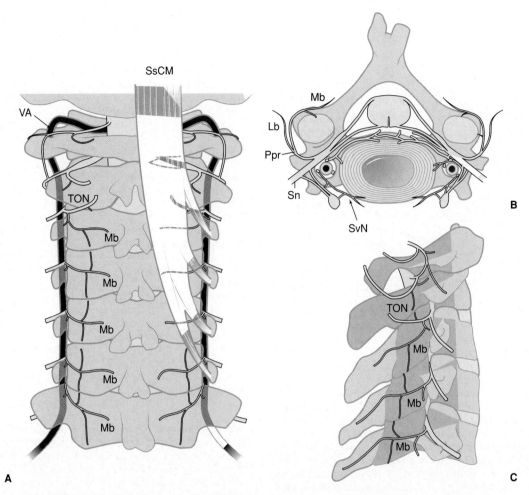

FIGURE 44-7. Cervical spine innervation. Sketch of the innervation of the cervical spine in posterior (**A**), transverse (**B**), and lateral (**C**) projections. Note the posterior primary ramus (*Ppr*) leaving the spinal nerve (*Sn*) in **B** and splitting into a lateral branch (*Lb*) and a medial branch (*b*). Note the covering for the medial branch provided by the insertion of the splenius capitis muscles (*ScCM*). The innervation of the C2 facet is provided by the large myelinated third occipital nerve (*TON*). Note the proximity of the medial branches in relation to the vertebral artery (*VA*). As in the lumbar spine, sensory fibers traveling in the gray rami from the sinuvertebral nerve (*SvN*) provide innervation to the disc annulus.

is absent in the midline, it is possible to enter the epidural space without ever sensing significant resistance to injection. The ligamentum flavum is thickest at the lumbar and thoracic levels, and thinnest at the cervical level. Its thickness also diminishes at the cephalad aspect of each interlaminar space, and as the ligamentum flavum tapers off laterally (see Chapter 9, Figs. 9-5 to 9-30). In patients who have undergone previous spinal surgery, scarring of the posterior epidural space is common, such that the loss-of-resistance and the flow of injected solutions are less predictable.

The spinal cord is a cylindrical structure comprised of an external white matter and internal gray matter, protected by the bony vertebral column. White matter represents the myelinated ascending and descending tracts of the spinal cord, which conduct information to and from the brain. The gray matter contains axons, dendrites, and synaptic terminals arranged grossly in the shape butterfly wings. The spinal cord receives its vascular supply from arteries of the brain and from segmental spinal arteries of the subclavian artery, aorta, and iliac arteries (44). The posterior spinal cord receives its blood sup-

ply from a paired system of arteries arising from the posterior inferior cerebellar arteries. The anterior spinal artery (ASA) is a single, discontinuous vessel formed by the union of a terminal branch from each vertebral artery that descends along the anterior midline of the spinal cord. In all regions of the cord, the ASA provides the nutrition to approximately 75% of the cord tissue, including all of the gray matter (46), which makes this territory most vulnerable to ischemia (see Chapter 9).

The spinal nerve at each level traverses the intervertebral foramen and divides into anterior and posterior primary rami. The anterior ramus contains the majority of sensory and motor fibers at each vertebral level. Of importance, a small branch of the anterior ramus, the sinuvertebral nerve, provides neural branches to the posterior outer layers of the annulus of the disc (see Chapter 9, Fig. 9-39) (45). The posterior primary ramus, in turn, divides into a lateral branch that provides innervation to the paraspinous musculature and a small, variable sensory distribution to the skin overlying the spinous processes, whereas the medial branch courses over the base of the transverse process, where it joins with the superior articular process of the

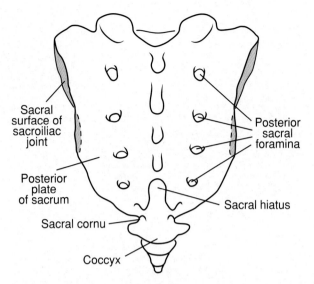

FIGURE 44-8. Anatomy of the posterior sacrum and coccyx. From Rathmell JP. *Atlas of Image-guided Intervention in Regional Anesthesia and Pain Medicine.* Philadelphia: Lippincott Williams & Wilkins, 2006, with permission.

facet joint and courses along the articular process to supply sensation to the joint. Each facet joint receives sensory innervation from the medial branch nerve at the same vertebral level, as well as from a descending branch from the vertebral level above; thus, two medial branch nerves must be blocked to anesthetize each facet joint (e.g., medial branch blocks at the base of the L4 and L5 transverse processes are needed to anesthetize the L4–L5 facet joint). The specific course of the medial branch nerves and cannula position for radiofrequency treatment at specific spinal levels is discussed in the sections that follow.

Epidural Injection of Steroids: Interlaminar and Transforaminal Approaches

Numerous randomized trials have examined the efficacy of epidural injection of steroids for treating acute radicular pain. The rationale behind injecting glucocorticoid into the epidural space is to combat the inflammatory response associated with acute disc herniation (47). In acute radicular pain associated with herniated nucleolus pulposus, the evidence in systematic reviews (47), as well as more recent RCTs (48,49), demonstrates that epidural steroids reduce the severity and duration of pain between 3 and 6 weeks after onset. There do not appear to be any long-term reductions in pain or disability that stem from long-term epidural steroid use (47,50). Use of this therapy for lumbosacral pain without radicular symptoms has never been proven to be of benefit.

The theoretical background supporting the use of epidural steroids is based on the existence of inflammation as the basic pathophysiologic process. Nerve root edema has been demonstrated surgically and with computed tomography (CT) in patients with herniated discs (51). Inflammation of nerves in the presence of a herniated disc has further been confirmed during surgery (52), myelography (53), and histologic examinations (54,55). More recently, phospholipase A2 (PLA2), the rate-limiting enzyme in the conversion of arachidonic acid to prostaglandins and leukotrienes, has been found in high levels in patients undergoing discectomy for herniated disc (56). Other inflammatory mediators such as prostaglandins have

also been shown to produce hyperalgesia (57). Clinically, improvement of pain has been shown to coincide with resolution or decrease in nerve root edema, despite a persistent herniated disc (45).

In laboratory animals, PLA2 has been implicated as a primary inflammatory mediator, and its administration in lumbar nerve roots produces motor weakness and decreased mechanical withdrawal thresholds (58). Histologic examination shows reversible demyelination, vacuolar degeneration in the nerve roots, and unclear axonal margins (54). In another animal model of radiculopathy, Hayashi et al. (59) ligated the left L4 and L5 nerve roots while surgically placing an epidural catheter with the tip between the ligated nerve roots. All rats demonstrated reversible motor weakness, which completely resolved in 4 weeks, and all of the animals exhibited thermal hyperalgesia. The rats were separated into groups receiving either epidural betamethasone alone, normal saline, or epidural betamethasone plus bupivacaine. All treatment groups demonstrated a transient reduction in thermal hyperalgesia, but both betamethasone groups showed prolonged benefit lasting 3 to 4 weeks.

Steroids decrease inflammation by inducing the biosynthesis of a PLA2 inhibitor and preventing prostaglandin generation (60,61). Steroids have also been shown to suppress ongoing discharge in chronic neuromas and prevent the development of ectopic neural discharges from experimental neuromas, which has been attributed to direct membrane action (62). Steroids may also block nociceptive input. Local application of methylprednisolone was found to reversibly block transmission in the unmyelinated C-fibers, but not in Aβ-fibers (63).

Patient Selection. Recent reviews of epidural steroid injection have yielded contradictory results, although considerable overlap occurred between the trials included in these reviews (64,65). Koes et al. (64) reviewed 12 RCTs on the efficacy of epidural steroid injections for low back pain and sciatica. One-half of the trials reported positive outcomes of epidural steroid injections, and the other half reported negative outcomes. There were significant flaws in the design of most studies included in this analysis, although there appeared to be no relationship between the methodologic quality of the trials and the reported outcomes. Koes et al. concluded that the efficacy of epidural injections has not yet been established.

Watts et al. (65) performed a meta-analysis of 11 placebo-controlled trials on the efficacy of epidural steroid injections in the treatment of sciatica (9 of the same trials were considered by Koes). The quality of the trials was generally good. A clinically relevant response to treatment was at least 75% improvement or reduction in pain. With respect to short-term pain relief (1–60 days), the pooled odds ratio (OR; based on 10 trials) was 2.61 (95% confidence interval [CI], 1.80–3.77); with respect to long-term pain relief (12 weeks to 1 year), the pooled OR (based on 5 trials) was 1.87 (95% CI, 1.31–2.68). Watts et al. concluded that epidural steroid injections are effective in the management of patients with sciatica.

In 1999, Nelemans et al. (66) performed another systematic review of RCTs on the efficacy of injection therapy in patients with low back pain. This review differed from the previous reviews because it was not restricted to epidural steroid injections, and it also considered epidural injections with anesthetics and other injection sites, such as facet joint and local injections. The Nelemans group's review was restricted to RCTs that included patients with duration of low back pain of longer than 1 month; twenty-one RCTs met this criterion. Eleven studies compared injection therapy with placebo injections. The methodologic quality of many studies was low. There were only three well-designed explanatory clinical trials: one on injections into the facet joints with a short-term OR of 0.89 (95% CI, 0.65–1.21) and a long-term OR of 0.90 (95% CI, 0.69–1.17); one on epidural injections with a short-term OR of 0.94 (95% CI, 0.76–1.15) and a long-term OR of 1.00 (95% CI, 0.71–1.41); and one on local injections with a long-term OR of 0.79 (95% CI, 0.65–0.96).

Within the six subcategories of explanatory studies, the pooled OR with 95% confidence intervals were: facet joint, short-term, 0.89 (0.65–1.21); facet joint, long-term, 0.90 (0.69–1.17); epidural, short-term, 0.93 (0.79–1.09); epidural, long-term, 0.92 (0.76–1.11); local, short-term, 0.80 (0.40–1.59); and local, long-term, 0.79 (0.65–0.96).

Nelemans et al. concluded that convincing evidence is lacking on the effects of injection therapies for low back pain, pointing toward the need for more well-designed explanatory trials in this field.

All three systematic reviews are now significantly outdated, and the Cochrane database review performed by Nelemans in 1999 was withdrawn in January 2005, citing the need for an update. It is worth noting that a 80% to 90% probability exists that patients with low back pain will recover within 3 months.

Newer Studies. Several more recent RCTs have been performed that point toward a limited role for epidural corticosteroid injections in reducing the duration of acute pain. The efficacy of epidural corticosteroid injection in the conservative management of sciatica was examined by Buchner et al. (67). Thirty-six patients with lumbar radicular pain due to herniated nucleolus pulposus were randomized to receive epidural steroid injections or no injection. At 2 weeks after injection, those receiving epidural steroid injections had superior improvement in straight-leg raise. There were no differences in pain reduction or functional status at 6 weeks or 6 months after injection. The authors concluded that epidural steroid injections can be recommended only in the acute phase for the conservative management of lumbosciatic pain.

Wilson-Macdonald et al. (68) conducted a prospective randomized trial of epidural steroid injection compared with intramuscular steroid injection in 93 patients with pain due to lumbar nerve root compression. All patients had been categorized as potential candidates for surgical nerve root decompression before treatment. A significant reduction of pain occurred early (35 days) in those having an epidural steroid injection, but no difference was noted in the longer-term effects (2-year follow-up). Eighteen percent of patients in the epidural group and 15% of those in the control group underwent operative decompression during the 2-year follow-up (p = NS).

In 2005, a large multicenter trial of epidural corticosteroid injections for sciatica appeared, the Wessex Epidural Steroid Trial (WEST) study (69). Two-hundred-twenty-eight patients with unilateral sciatica of 1 to 18 months' duration were randomized to receive either three epidural steroid injections or three interligamentous injections over a 3-week period. At 3 weeks, those receiving epidural steroids demonstrated a significantly greater reduction in pain, but no difference between groups was seen from 6 to 52 weeks of follow-up. The authors concluded that epidural steroid injections afforded patients earlier relief of pain, but no long-term benefit in pain or need for surgery.

When earlier studies are reexamined, a similar early reduction in pain can be seen despite the lack of long-term benefit from epidural steroid injections. Indeed, the much-cited trial performed by Carrette et al. (70) examined the effectiveness of epidural steroid injections as compared with saline for the treatment of acute radicular pain due to disc herniation and concluded there were no long-term benefits of epidural steroid injection. In this RCT of 158 patients, although there were no demonstrable differences between epidural steroid and placebo treatment groups at 3 months following injection, there was significant earlier reduction in pain and improvement in sensory deficits (3 weeks after treatment) in those receiving epidural steroid injections.

The route of injection has also been the subject of much debate in recent years. The transforaminal approach to placing epidural steroids has been advocated as a means of delivering the steroid in high concentration directly to the site of inflammation near the spinal nerve within the lateral epidural space. A recent randomized trial (71) compared the efficacy of transforaminal versus interspinous corticosteroid injection in treating radicular pain in 31 patients. They demonstrated significantly better pain reduction in the transforaminal group at 30-day follow-up. A mailed questionnaire also revealed significantly better pain relief and daily activity levels at 6 months after injection. This small study warrants further validation in a larger controlled trial. We are still lacking studies that compare the transforaminal route to the interlaminar route.

Two additional recent reviews reinforce the conclusions of earlier publications regarding the use of epidural steroids. Young et al. (72) published a comprehensive review of epidural steroid injections for treating spinal disease and concluded that "lumbar epidural steroid injections are a reasonable nonsurgical option in select patients," particularly for providing earlier resolution of pain in patients with lumbar radicular pain. In addition, The American Academy of Neurology's Technology Assessment Subcommittee published a focused assessment of the use of epidural steroid injections to treat radicular lumbosacral pain (73). This group concluded that, "1) Epidural steroid injections may result in some improvement in radicular lumbosacral pain when assessed between 2 and 6 weeks following the injection, compared to control treatments (Level C, Class I–III evidence). The average magnitude of effect is small and generalizability of the observation is limited by the small number of studies, highly selected patient populations, few techniques and doses, and variable comparison treatments; 2) in general, epidural steroid injection for radicular lumbosacral pain does not impact average impairment of function, need for surgery, or provide long-term pain relief beyond 3 months."

Collectively, the numerous studies and reviews that have been carried out examining the usefulness of epidural steroids for the treatment of acute radicular pain due to herniated nucleolus pulposus fail to show any long-term benefit in pain reduction nor do these injections obviate the need for surgical intervention. However, the bulk of the studies do demonstrate more rapid resolution of pain in those receiving epidural steroid injections. Thus, the role for epidural steroid injections in the conservative management of radicular pain is simply to facilitate earlier pain relief and return to full function.

Drug Selection for Epidural Steroid Injection. Most studies in the literature have used either a mixture of local anesthetics and steroid, saline with steroid, or steroid alone. The steroids most commonly used are either methylprednisolone acetate (Depo-Medrol) or triamcinolone diacetate (Aristocort). The doses of methylprednisolone most widely used in the literature vary from 80 mg to 120 mg, and the doses of triamcinolone most commonly used vary from 50 to 75 mg (31,74–76).

Methylprednisolone acetate has been approved for intramuscular, intrasynovial, soft-tissue, or intralesional injection. It is a glucocorticoid with an elimination half-life of 139 hours, with a range of 58 to 866 hours (77). Triamcinolone diacetate, with an elimination half-life of 18 to 36 hours, possesses glucocorticoid properties while being essentially devoid of mineralocorticoid activity, thus causing little or no sodium retention. It has been approved for administration by intramuscular, intraarticular, or intrasynovial routes (78).

In a review of the literature, Kepes et al. found that methylprednisolone was the least irritating, most beneficial, and longest acting (79), whereas Delaney et al. prefer triamcinolone because of its excellent anti-inflammatory effect and low potential for sodium retention (80). No study has compared the effectiveness of triamcinolone and methylprednisolone, and they are probably equally effective. Both of these preparations contain polyethylene glycol, which has been found to impair nerve transmission in rabbit's vagus nerve and cause degenerative lesions in rat sciatic nerves (81,82). Also, both preparations contain benzyl alcohol, which is potentially toxic when administered locally to neural tissue (83). Neither of these preparations should be used intrathecally.

Most practitioners dilute the steroid with local anesthetic or sterile saline, and the results are apparently comparable with either diluent (84). Some authors have recommended the use of local anesthetics "in the presence of muscle spasms" (85,86). However small the dose, the use of local anesthetic carries some risks, including hypotension, arrhythmias, and seizures from intravascular injections. Benzon (31) suggests that, since the results are comparable, the use of saline is probably sufficient. Some investigators have combined epidural methylprednisolone with morphine. In an initial study, Cohn et al. (87) showed encouraging results in postlaminectomy patients; however, a subsequent study was unable to confirm such beneficial effects (88).

Traditionally, the volume of diluent has depended on the site of injection, whether lumbar, caudal, or transforaminal. When using a caudal approach, 20 to 25 mL of a solution has been recommended to assure epidural spread cephalad to the desired level (89,94). When using a lumbar interlaminar approach, a volume of 5 to 10 mL has been recommended to reach those areas most commonly involved in the lumbar region (90). Other practitioners use smaller volumes (2–3 mL), especially when using the transforaminal approach. Some authors (91) have suggested that several nerve roots may also be inflamed in addition to those adjacent to the herniated or bulging disc, and recommend against the use of small volumes of diluent. Additionally, Wood et al. suggested diluting the steroid, after their study showed degenerative lesions in rat sciatic nerves attributed to the polyethylene glycol vehicle in the steroid preparation (82). The optimal volume of injectate and site of epidural placement remain unresolved.

Epidural steroids have been associated with glucose intolerance and pituitary-adrenal axis suppression for up to 3 weeks after repeated administration (92–94). Ward et al. (95) measured insulin sensitivity, fasting blood glucose, fasting plasma insulin, and fasting serum cortisol in 10 healthy individuals 24 hours before and 1 week after an epidural administration of 80 mg of triamcinolone via a caudal route. They found that at 24 hours after the epidural steroid injection, insulin sensitivity had decreased to nearly half the baseline, fasting insulin levels increased 1.4-fold, and fasting glucose had increased 1.1-fold. All of these values had normalized by 1 week after injection, and they demonstrate marked changes in insulin sensitivity in nondiabetic healthy individuals after an epidural steroid injection.

Technique. The epidural space can be approached through the interlaminar space (median or paramedian), the intervertebral foramen (transforaminal), or the sacral hiatus (caudal). The approach selected will depend on patient selection, indication for the injection, the practitioner's experience, and availability of imaging. The patient can be positioned in the lateral decubitus position, sitting or prone, depending on the technique to be used.

Interlaminar Technique for Epidural Steroid Injection. The term *interlaminar* has been used to describe the traditional posterior approach to the epidural space, to easily differentiate it from the transforaminal or caudal approach. The interlaminar approach can be either midline or paramedian, and correct epidural placement with this technique does not require the use of imaging guidance (see Chapter 11). As reported by Sharrock et al., anesthesiologists have a success rate of epidural anesthesia that approaches 99% (96). However, more recent reports have demonstrated that reliance on loss of resistance leads to a high rate (25.7%) of inaccurate needle-tip placement in the posterior soft tissues of the back during lumbar epidural steroid administration employing a 20-gauge Tuohy needle (97). This high rate of inaccurate needle placement during interlaminar epidural injection has led some experts to call for a mandate to use fluoroscopy to confirm needle placement. When using the midline approach, the point of insertion will depend on the level of entry and angle of the corresponding spinous processes. For cervical and lumbar midline approach, the needle should be almost perpendicular to the neuraxis, in line with the corresponding spinous process. This is also true with low thoracic approach below T9 (see Chapter 11). In the mid thoracic region, the spinous processes are sharply angled caudad, such that the tip of the spinous processes lies opposite the lamina of the inferior vertebral body. In this region, the midline approach requires that the needle be inserted with a steep cephalad angle, often approaching 130 degrees. Many practitioners prefer the paramedian approach in the mid thoracic region. The choice of needles when using the interlaminar approach is similar to those available for anesthesia, the most common type being the 18- or 20-gauge Tuohy needle (see Chapter 11).

For cervical interlaminar epidural injections, most practitioners will place the patient in a sitting or prone position. In the sitting position, the patient is asked to sit comfortably and flex the neck anteriorly. The forehead may be supported against a sturdy, but padded, horizontal surface to minimize involuntary movement. This position will avoid rotation of the spine and widen the lower cervical epidural space. When the prone position is utilized for the cervical interlaminar approach, most practitioners prefer to use image guidance. This allows for good visualization of the interlaminar space and needle advancement between adjacent spinous processes.

Cervical Epidural Steroid Injection Technique. Classically, the epidural space has been identified using three modalities: hanging-drop technique, loss-of-resistance to saline, or loss-of-resistance to air. Regardless of the approach, sterile technique must be strictly observed. The skin and subcutaneous tissues overlying the interspace where the block is to be carried out are anesthetized with local anesthetic. The cervical interspaces with the largest interlaminar distance are typically found at C6–7 and C7–T1. The long spinous process of C7 (vertebra prominens) serves as a surface landmark. Because of the ease of entry, many practitioners will place the needle via one of these larger interspaces, regardless of the level of pathology, and rely on the flow of steroid in the epidural space to reach the level of pathology. The same technique can be utilized in all cervical interspaces below C3–4. Interlaminar injection above the C2–3 level has not been described.

An 18- or 20-gauge Tuohy needle is placed through the skin and advanced several centimeters until it is firmly seated in the interspinous ligament. An anteroposterior (AP) image is then taken, and the needle is redirected toward midline. We use the loss-of-resistance technique with saline to find the epidural space. Repeat images taken after every 1- to 1.5-mm of needle advancement will assure that the needle direction does not stray from midline. A firm grasp of the anatomy of adjacent structures and the spinal meninges and spinal cord is essential during cervical interlaminar epidural injection. After the needle tip enters the epidural space, the position is confirmed by injecting nonionic radiographic contrast, and adequate spread is verified in the AP and lateral planes. If lateral imaging of the cervicothoracic junction and low cervical spine is hindered by the adjacent structures of the torso and arms, a second lateral image taken just above the shoulders can often be much simpler to interpret when trying to confirm epidural contrast flow. Once epidural needle position has been confirmed, a solution containing steroid diluted in preservative-free saline is injected. In our practice, we routinely use 80 mg of methyl prednisolone acetate or the equivalent diluted in 5 mL total volume.

Mid Thoracic Epidural Steroid Injection. Because of the steep angulation of the spinous processes at this level, image guidance is often used. The patient lies prone, with the head turned to one side. The C-arm is rotated 40 to 50 degrees caudally from the axial plane without any oblique angulation. This allows for good visualization of the interlaminar space and needle advancement between adjacent spinous processes.

The skin and subcutaneous tissues approximately 1 cm lateral and 2 to 3 cm caudad to the interspace where the block is to be carried out are anesthetized. An 18- or 20-gauge Tuohy needle is placed through the skin and advanced several centimeters until it is firmly seated in tissue. An AP image is then taken, and the needle is directed toward the superior margin of the lamina below the interspace that is to be entered, near the junction of the spinous process and the lamina. Although a midline approach can be used at low thoracic levels, the spinous processes are angled too steeply to allow for true coaxial needle placement at the mid thoracic levels. Thus, the needle is best directed toward the superior margin of the lamina. While advancing, repeat images are taken; care must be taken to keep the needle tip over the lamina until bone is gently contacted. The periosteum is then anesthetized, and the needle is slowly advanced over the superior margin of the lamina until loss-of-resistance occurs. Because the needle is unlikely to lie within the interspinous ligament when using a paramedian approach, there will be little resistance to injection until the needle enters the interlaminar space and traverses the ligamentum flavum (see Chapter 11, Fig. 11-12). A firm understanding of the adjacent structures and the proximity of the spinal cord is essential during thoracic interlaminar epidural injection. After the needle tip enters the epidural space, the position is confirmed by injecting nonionic radiographic contrast, and spread is verified in the AP and lateral planes. Lateral imaging of the thoracic spine is hindered by the overlying structures of the thorax. Once epidural needle position has been confirmed, a solution containing steroid diluted in preservative-free saline is injected and the needle is removed.

Lumbar Epidural Steroid Injection. Epidural injection at the lumbar level can be administered with the patient in a sitting or prone position. The patient is asked to sit comfortably with his back to the anesthesiologist, curving the spine posteriorly and pushing the lumbar region against the examiners fingers in an attempt to separate the spinous processes. If the procedure

is to be done in the prone position under fluoroscopic imaging, a pillow is placed under the mid and lower abdomen to reduce the lumbar lordosis and increase the separation between adjacent spinous processes. The C-arm is rotated 15 to 20 degrees caudally from the axial plane without any oblique angulation. This allows for good visualization of the interlaminar space and needle advancement between adjacent spinous processes.

The skin and subcutaneous tissues overlying the interspace where the block is to be carried out are anesthetized. An 18- or 20-gauge Tuohy needle is placed through the skin and advanced 1 to 2 cm until it is firmly seated in the interspinous ligament. If the patient is prone, an AP image should be taken as the needle is advanced, until loss-of-resistance occurs. If the patient is sitting, adequate positioning will allow a proper midline approach. A firm knowledge of the adjacent structures and the proximity of the thecal sac and cauda equina is essential during lumbar interlaminar epidural injection (Fig. 44-9). After the needle tip enters the epidural space, and aspiration is negative for CSF or blood, the position is confirmed by injecting nonionic radiographic contrast, and spread is verified in the AP and lateral planes. Lateral imaging of the lower lumbar spine is hindered by the overlying iliac crests, and visualization can also be quite difficult in the obese patient. Once epidural needle position has been confirmed, a solution containing steroid diluted in preservative-free saline is injected, and the needle is removed. In the lumbar region, we usually use 80 mg of methyl prednisolone acetate or the equivalent diluted in 5 to 10 mL total volume. When larger injectate volumes are used, the solution spreads extensively in both the anterior and posterior aspects of the epidural space. In patients with significant lumbar pathology, the injectate will tend to follow the path of least resistance, often flowing toward the side opposite to the pathology (40).

Caudal Epidural Steroid Injection. Anesthesiologists will be familiar with caudal injections administered to pediatric patients in the operating room. Because of difficulty identifying the sacral hiatus clinically in adults (see Chapter 9, Figs. 9-6 and 9-7 and Chapter 11, Figs. 11-18 and 11-19), these procedures are usually done under fluoroscopy. The patient lies prone with the head turned to one side. The C-arm is rotated 20 to 30 degrees caudally from the axial plane without any oblique angulation. This allows for good visualization of the sacrum, sacral hiatus, and coccyx.

Once the sacral hiatus is identified radiographically, the overlying skin and subcutaneous tissues are anesthetized. However, the sacral hiatus can be quite difficult to visualize radiographically. The approximate location can be identified by palpating the paired sacral cornua in the midline, near the superior extent of the gluteal cleft. An 18- or 20-gauge Tuohy needle can be used, but a smaller 22-gauge, 3.5-inch spinal needle is adequate. The needle is placed through the skin and advanced directly through the sacrococcygeal ligament (see Chapter 11, Figs. 11-18 and 11-19). Once the needle has passed through the sacrococcygeal ligament and is within the caudal spinal canal, the angle of the needle is decreased to lie closer to the plane of the sacrum, and the needle is advanced into the spinal canal an additional 1 to 2 cm. A firm grasp of the anatomy of the sacral hiatus and the caudal epidural space is essential during caudal epidural injection. AP and lateral imaging confirm the needle's position within the caudal epidural space. The caudal epidural space is generously supplied with veins, and intravascular needle placement is ruled out by injecting nonionic radiographic contrast under live fluoroscopy. Once caudal epidural needle position has been confirmed, a solution containing steroid diluted in preservative-free saline is injected and the needle is

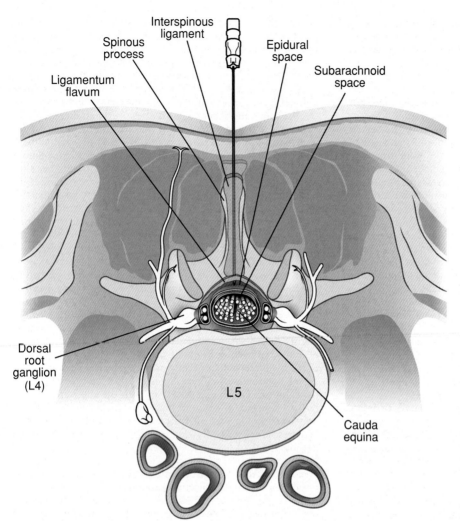

Interspinous ligament

Spinous process

Ligamentum flavum

Epidural space

Subarachnoid space

Dorsal root ganglion (L4)

L5

Cauda equina

FIGURE 44-9. Axial diagram of interlaminar lumbar epidural injection. The epidural needle is advanced in the midline between adjacent spinous processes to traverse the ligamentum flavum and enter the dorsal epidural space in the midline. The normal epidural space is approximately 4- to 6-mm wide (from the ligamentum flavum to the dura mater in the axial plane). Note the proximity of the underlying cauda equina during lumbar epidural injection. From Rathmell JP. *Atlas of Image-guided Intervention in Regional Anesthesia and Pain Medicine*. Philadelphia: Lippincott Williams & Wilkins, 2006, with permission.

removed. The caudal epidural space is distant from the usual sites of nerve root inflammation near the lumbosacral junction, thus a significant volume of injectate is usually required to affect spread to the level of the lumbosacral junction. For this approach, we use 80 mg of methyl prednisolone acetate or the equivalent diluted in at least 10 mL total volume.

Complications of the interlaminar approach include dural puncture with subsequent post–dural puncture headache (PDPH), which can occur when this technique is used at any level of the spine. Although in a different patient population, the incidence of dural puncture in parturients undergoing lumbar epidurals ranges between 0% and 2.6% (98). Post dural puncture headaches are very frequent after unintended dural puncture with large epidural needles. The incidence of headache following cervical dural puncture is lower than that following lumbar puncture, likely due to the diminished column of CSF cephalad to the point of dural puncture.

Although cervical and thoracic epidural blood patches using small volumes of autologous blood have been described, most practitioners will manage PDPH following cervical or thoracic epidural injection conservatively with fluids and oral analgesics. Dural puncture can also occur during caudal epidural injection, but usually this occurs only if the needle is advanced several centimeters cephalad within the caudal spinal canal. The thecal sac extends to the level of approximately S2, and the position can be approximated by palpating the adjacent posterior superior iliac spines, which lie at the same

level. Epidural blood patch using autologous blood is a safe and effective treatment that relieves the headache symptoms promptly in 70% to 98% of those who fail to improve after 24 to 48 hours of conservative treatment and oral analgesics (99). The incidence of unintentional dural puncture may be higher in those with previous lumbar surgery, due to scarring within the epidural space and adhesion of the dura to the posterior elements.

Although direct neurologic needle trauma is rare (<0.6%) (100), injury to the spinal cord with catastrophic consequences including quadriplegia, has been described, particularly if epidural injections are performed in heavily sedated patients (101–103). The level of sedation during this procedure should allow for direct conversation between the practitioner and the patient to assure that the patient can report contact with neural elements before significant traumatic injury occurs. Caution should also be taken to avoid interlaminar epidural injection at any level where there is effacement of the epidural space (104). Complete effacement of the epidural space, as well as the CSF column surrounding the spinal cord within the thecal sac, occurs in high-grade spinal stenosis, particularly that due to a large central or paramedian disc herniation. Direct trauma to the cauda equina or exiting nerve roots is unlikely during lumbar epidural injection when disciplined use of radiographic guidance is employed to assure that the needle tip does not stray from the midline. Direct trauma to the cauda equina or the exiting nerve roots is unlikely with the caudal approach.

Regardless of the level of injection, epidural bleeding or infection can occur. Epidural hematoma or abscess can lead to significant compression of the spinal cord or cauda equina. Interlaminar epidural injection should be avoided or postponed in those receiving anticoagulants (105).

Transforaminal Technique for Epidural Steroid Injection. Transforaminal epidural steroid injection and selective nerve root injection can be performed using similar techniques. Indeed, the distinction between the two techniques is questionable, as the fascial sheath surrounding the spinal nerves is contiguous with the dura mater within the epidural space. A solution injected around a spinal nerve may well enter the epidural space, whether or not the needle tip is advanced through the intervertebral foramen prior to injection. Nonetheless, many practitioners reserve the term "selective nerve root injection" for injections that are performed with the needle tip adjacent to the spinal nerve, *outside* of the intervertebral foramen and the term "transforaminal injection" for injections that are performed with the needle tip within the intervertebral foramen. Unlike the interlaminar technique, the transforaminal approach *requires* the use of radiographic imaging if it is to proceed with safety (106).

Several important anatomical aspects are unique to transforaminal epidural and selective nerve root injections (Figs. 44-10 to 44-13). At *cervical levels*, the ventral and dorsal roots of the spinal nerves descend in the vertebral canal to form the spinal nerve in the intervertebral foramen. The foramen faces

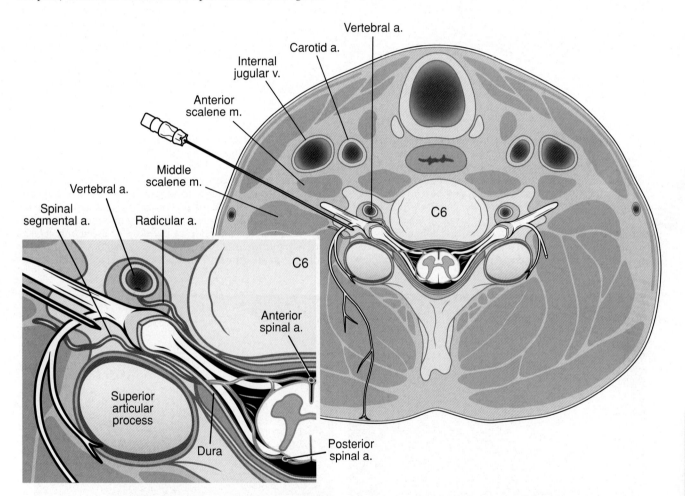

FIGURE 44-10. Axial view of cervical transforaminal injection at the level of C6. The needle has been inserted along the axis of the foramen and is illustrated in final position within the posterior aspect of the foramen. Insertion along this axis avoids the vertebral artery, which lies anterior to the foramen, and the exiting nerve root. Spinal segmental arteries arise from the deep or ascending cervical artery, enter the foramen at variable locations, and often course through the foramen, penetrate the dura, and join the anterior or posterior spinal arteries that supply the spinal cord (*inset*). An arterial branch that joins the anterior spinal artery is a segmental "medullary" artery. Likewise, arterial branches arise variably from the vertebral artery to supply the nerve root itself (here a branch to the nerve root or "radicular" artery is illustrated); similar branches from the vertebral artery often penetrate the dura to join the anterior or posterior spinal artery. Great anatomic variation occurs in the vascular supply in this region. The anatomic variant illustrated is shown to demonstrate how a small artery that provides critical reinforcing blood supply to the spinal cord can be entered during cervical transforaminal injection. Injection of particulate steroid directly into one of these vessels can lead to catastrophic spinal cord injury. Anatomic descriptions are based on cadaveric dissections carried out in our laboratory. Preliminary data appear in Hoeft MA, Rathmell JP, Monsey RD, et al. *Anatomy of the Cervical Radicular Arteries: Implications for Cervical Transforaminal Injection.* Presented at the annual fall meeting of the American Society of Regional Anesthesia and Pain Medicine, Phoenix, AZ, November 11–14, 2004, with permission.

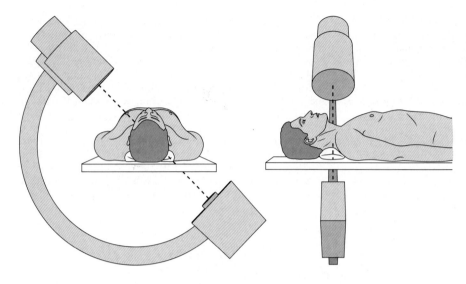

FIGURE 44-11. Patient position for cervical transforaminal injection. The patient is positioned supine with the C-arm axis rotated obliquely 45 to 65 degrees until the intervertebral foramina are clearly visualized. Most C-arms are limited in their ability to rotate obliquely to the side opposite the mobile base (the limit is typically 45–55 degrees). When performing cervical transforaminal injection on the side opposite the base unit, the limits of oblique angulation can be overcome by placing a foam wedge beneath the patient to angle him toward the side of the base unit, thereby gaining an additional degree of oblique angulation toward the opposite side. The limits of oblique angulation can also be overcome by inverting the C-arm, so that the x-ray source is above the patient and the image intensifier below; however, this results in a dramatic increase in radiation exposure to both the patient and the operator. From Rathmell JP. *Atlas of Image-guided Intervention in Regional Anesthesia and Pain Medicine*. Philadelphia: Lippincott Williams & Wilkins, 2006, with permission.

obliquely anterior and laterally. Its roof and floor are formed by the pedicles of the articulated vertebrae. Its posterolateral wall is formed largely by the superior articular process of the lower vertebra, and in part by the inferior articular process of the upper vertebra and the capsule of the zygapophysial joint. The anteromedial wall is formed by the lower end of the upper vertebral body, the uncinate process of the lower vertebra, and the posterolateral corner of the intervertebral disc. Immediately lateral to the external opening of the foramen, the vertebral artery ascends within the *foramen transversarium* in close proximity

to the spinal nerve and anterior to the articular pillars of the zygapophysial joint (Fig. 44-10). The spinal nerve, in its dural sleeve, lies in the lower half of the foramen, whereas the upper half is occupied by periradicular veins. Arterial branches arise from the vertebral arteries to supply the nerve roots (radicular arteries) or the spinal cord via the anterior and posterior spinal arteries (medullary arteries). Medullary and radicular arterial branches may also arise from the deep or ascending cervical arteries and traverse through the entire length of the foramen adjacent to the spinal nerve. It is these spinal segmental arteries

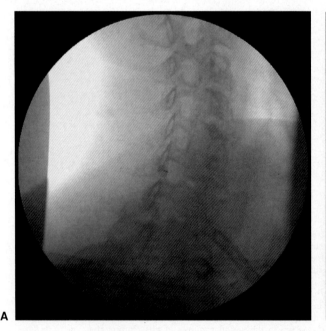

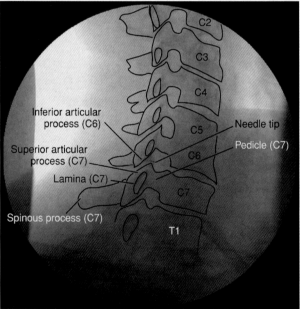

FIGURE 44-12. Right oblique view of the cervical spine during right C6–7 transforaminal injection. **A:** The needle is in proper position in the posterior aspect of the foramen for right C6–7 transforaminal injection (C7 nerve root). Note that this patient has had a prior C5–6 interbody fusion, and no discernible disc space exists between these two vertebrae. **B:** Labeled image. From Rathmell JP. *Atlas of Image-guided Intervention in Regional Anesthesia and Pain Medicine*. Philadelphia: Lippincott Williams & Wilkins, 2006, with permission.

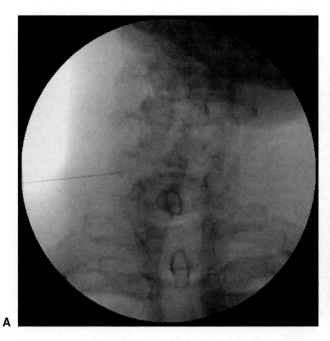
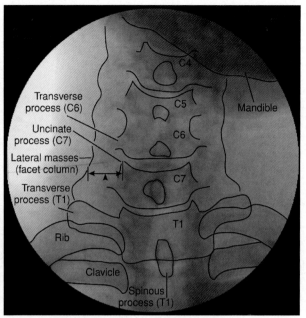

A

B

FIGURE 44-13. Posterior–anterior view of the cervical spine during C6–7 transforaminal injection. **A:** The needle is in proper position within the right C6–7 intervertebral foramen (C7 nerve root). Note that this patient has had a prior C5–6 interbody fusion, and no discernible disc space exists between these two vertebrae. **B:** Labeled image. From Rathmell JP. *Atlas of Image-guided Intervention in Regional Anesthesia and Pain Medicine.* Philadelphia: Lippincott Williams & Wilkins, 2006, with permission.

that are at risk for penetration during cervical transforaminal injection (Fig. 44-10).

At the *lumbar levels*, the ventral and dorsal roots of the spinal nerves descend within the vertebral canal to form the spinal nerve in the intervertebral foramen. Its roof and floor are formed by the pedicles of consecutive vertebrae. Its posterior wall is formed largely by the superior articular process of the lower vertebra, and in part by the inferior articular process of the upper vertebra and the capsule of the zygapophysial joint. The anterior wall is formed by the vertebral body and the intervertebral disc. The spinal nerve, in its dural sleeve, lies in the anterior and superior portion of the foramen, just inferior to the pedicle (Figs. 44-14 and 44-15).

The most common indication for a transforaminal approach or selective nerve root injection is to place the corticosteroid immediately adjacent to the inflamed nerve root causing the radicular symptoms. Nerve root inflammation may stem from an acutely herniated intervertebral disc, causing nerve root irritation or other causes of nerve root impingement such as isolated foraminal stenosis due to spondylitic spurring of the bony margins of the foramen. However, it should be noted that currently no evidence shows better clinical outcome with the transforaminal approach versus the interlaminar approach (106). Selective nerve root injection with local anesthetic has also been employed diagnostically to determine which nerve root is causing symptoms when pathology exists at multiple vertebral levels. This information can prove invaluable in planning surgical intervention.

Cervical Transforaminal Steroid Injection. The patient lies supine, facing directly forward. The C-arm is rotated 45 to 55 degrees lateral oblique until the neural foramina are clearly visualized (Figs. 44-11 and 44-12). The patient may also be asked to rotate his head away from the side of injection. Al-

though this facilitates access to the side of the neck, the neural foramina and bony elements of the cervical spine will no longer be aligned. This may prove confusing to the inexperienced practitioner.

A 25-gauge 1.5-inch blunt-tipped needle is sufficient in length for all but the most obese patients. To avoid the vertebral artery and the spinal nerve, the needle is advanced toward the posterior and middle aspect of the intervertebral foramen (Fig. 44-12). Care is taken to be sure that the needle tip remains superimposed on the bone of the facet column during advancement. In this way, the superior articular process of the facet just posterior to the foramen is first contacted, preventing needle advancement through the foramen and into the spinal canal. Once the needle contacts the facet, it is then walked anteriorly into the foramen and advanced no more than an additional 2 to 3 mm (Figs. 44-12 and 44-13). The depth is then assessed by obtaining an image in the direct AP plane. To avoid direct trauma to the spinal cord and intrathecal injection, the needle should be advanced no further than halfway across the facet column. Nonionic radiographic contrast is then injected under "live" or real-time fluoroscopy (or digital subtraction cineradiography) to assure that the needle tip lies in close proximity to the nerve root, without any intravascular or intrathecal spread. The solution containing the steroid can then be injected safely. In our practice, we typically use 40 mg of triamcinolone acetonide or the equivalent diluted in 0.5 to 1 mL of 1% lidocaine.

Lumbar Transforaminal Steroid Injection. The patient lies prone on the fluoroscopy table. The C-arm is rotated 20 to 30 degrees lateral oblique (Fig. 44-16) to allow direction of the needle toward the superolateral aspect of the intervertebral foramen (Figs. 44-14 and 44-15). A somewhat less oblique approach will result in a final needle position slightly lateral to the intervertebral foramen and has been advocated by some

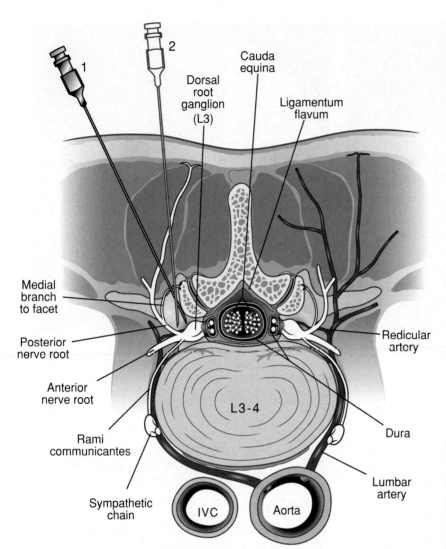

FIGURE 44-14. Axial view of lumbar transforaminal and selective nerve root injection. The anatomy and proper needle position (axial view) for right (*1*) L3–4 transforaminal injection and (*2*) L3 selective nerve root injection. From Rathmell JP. *Atlas of Image-guided Intervention in Regional Anesthesia and Pain Medicine.* Philadelphia: Lippincott Williams & Wilkins, 2006, with permission.

practitioners as a means of limiting spread of the injectate to a single nerve root. However, even small volumes of injectate will often be seen to track along the exiting nerve root to enter the lateral epidural space. A 22- or 25- gauge 3.5-inch spinal needle is sufficient in length for patients of average build, whereas a 5-inch needle may be needed in obese patients. To avoid the spinal nerve, the needle is advanced coaxially (Fig. 44-17) toward the superior aspect of the intervertebral foramen, just inferior to the pedicle and inferolateral to the pars interarticularis (Fig. 44-17). This serves as an effective depth marker. Once this bony margin is contacted, the C-arm is rotated to a lateral view, and the needle is slowly advanced toward the anterior and superior aspect of the foramen (Fig. 44-18A,B). If a paresthesia is reported by the patient at any time during needle advancement, the needle should be withdrawn slightly, and the position confirmed with radiographic contrast. With the needle in final position, nonionic radiographic contrast is injected under real-time fluoroscopy (or digital subtraction cineradiography) in the AP position to assure that the needle tip lies in close proximity to the nerve root, without any intravascular or intrathecal spread (Fig. 44-18C). Obtaining a final AP image will allow assessment of the extent of spread of the injectate.

Complications of the transforaminal technique can be catastrophic. A firm grasp of the anatomy of adjacent vascular and neural structures is essential to avoid complications during cervical and lumbar approaches (Fig. 44-14). Direct intravascular injection into the vertebral artery may produce generalized seizures when local anesthetic is utilized or cerebral ischemia when particulate steroid solutions are used (106,107). Direct injection of particulate steroid into a medullary or radicular artery supplying the spinal cord at the cervical or lumbar level, respectively, can lead to catastrophic spinal cord infarction. Needle positioning toward the posterior aspect of the foramen and advancing the needle in a plane parallel to the nerve root reduces the risk of entering a vascular structure. Again, particular care should be taken when performing transforaminal injection on the left between T8 and L3, as the artery of Adamkiewicz lies between these levels. However, the use of radiographic contrast injected during live or real-time fluoroscopy (or digital subtraction cineradiography) to visualize final needle position and detect any hint of intravascular injection is the only means to accurately verify that injectate is not injected within an artery.

Subarachnoid injection may also occur if the needle is advanced too far medially and pierces the dural cuff as it extends laterally onto the exiting nerve root. Direct trauma to the

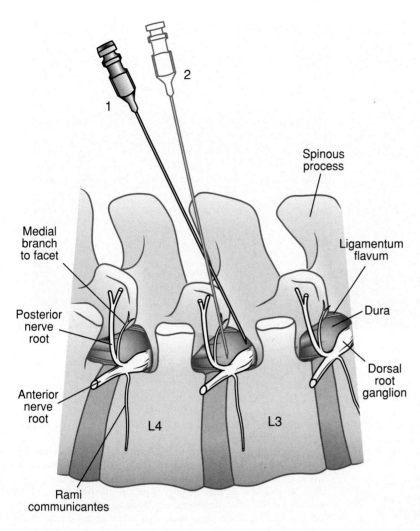

Spinous
process

Medial
branch
to facet

Ligamentum
flavum

Posterior
nerve
root

Dura

Dorsal
root
ganglion

Anterior
nerve
root

L4   L3

Rami
communicantes

FIGURE 44-15. Lateral view of lumbar transforaminal and selective nerve root injection. Anatomy and proper needle position (lateral view) for right (*1*) L3–4 transforaminal injection and (*2*) L3 selective nerve root injection. From Rathmell JP. *Atlas of Image-guided Intervention in Regional Anesthesia and Pain Medicine.* Philadelphia: Lippincott Williams & Wilkins, 2006, with permission.

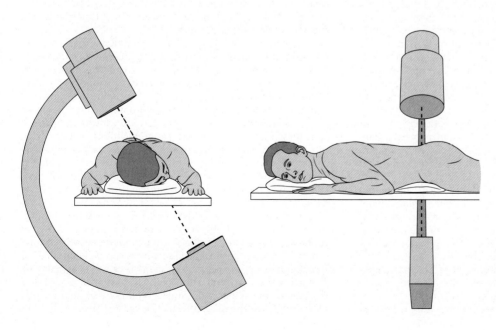

FIGURE 44-16. Patient position for lumbar transforaminal and selective nerve root injection. The patient is positioned prone, with the C-arm axis rotated obliquely 20 to 30 degrees until the facet joint and pars interarticularis are clearly visualized. From Rathmell JP. *Atlas of Image-guided Intervention in Regional Anesthesia and Pain Medicine.* Philadelphia: Lippincott Williams & Wilkins, 2006, with permission.

PART IV: PAIN MANAGEMENT

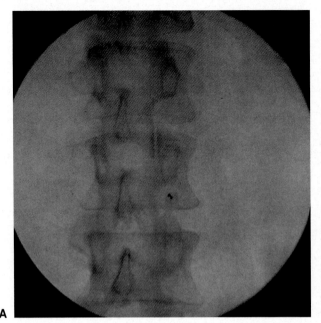
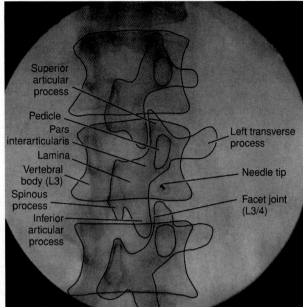

FIGURE 44-17. Left oblique radiograph with needle in final position for right L3–L4 transforaminal injection. **A:** The needle tip lies directly inferior to the pedicle and inferolateral to the pars interarticularis. **B:** Labeled image. From Rathmell JP. *Atlas of Image-guided Intervention in Regional Anesthesia and Pain Medicine.* Philadelphia: Lippincott Williams & Wilkins, 2006, with permission.

exiting nerve root or the spinal cord itself may also occur. Intradiscal placement of the needle during attempted transforaminal epidural steroid injection has also been reported, and is usually without sequelae (108).

Facet Joint Injections: Intra-articular Injections, Medial Branch Blocks, and Radiofrequency Treatment

Facet Blocks and Radiofrequency Treatment. Pain arising from the lumbar facet joints affects up to 15% of patients with chronic low back pain (109). Clinical experience and a limited number of published observational studies suggest that the intra-articular injection of local anesthetic and steroid leads to intermediate term (1–3 months) pain relief in a small subset of patients with pain accompanied by an active inflammatory process (109). Radiofrequency denervation delivers energy through a small-diameter insulated needle that is positioned adjacent to the sensory nerve of the facet joint; this creates a small burn that denervates the facet joint. A recent systematic review examining a total of six RCTs concluded that there is moderate evidence that radiofrequency denervation provides better pain relief than sham intervention (110). Approximately 50% of patients treated will report at least 50% pain reduction. Pain typically returns between 6 and 12 months after treatment, and denervation can be repeated without apparent diminution in efficacy (111).

Intra-articular facet injection has been largely supplanted by radiofrequency treatment techniques for facet-related pain. Clinical experience and a limited number of published observational studies suggest that the intra-articular injection of local anesthetic and steroid leads to relief of facet-related pain that is limited in duration (112,113). In contrast, radiofrequency treatment is safe and modestly effective in producing longer-term pain relief in the same group of patients. Nonetheless, an understanding of facet-related pain syndromes and the methods for placing medication directly within the facet joint may

still prove useful for those practitioners who are unable to provide radiofrequency treatment.

Osteoarthritis of the spine is ubiquitous and an inevitable part of aging. The degenerative cascade that leads to degeneration of the intervertebral discs causes progressive disc dehydration and loss of disc height. Typically starting in the third decade of life, disc degeneration leads to increased mobility of adjacent vertebrae, and increased shear forces on the facet joints themselves. This can lead to a pattern of pain over the axis of the spine that increases with movement, particularly with flexion and extension, but produces little or no pain radiating toward the extremities. In the past, the only available treatment for those with debilitating facet-related pain was segmental fusion of the spine to completely arrest motion within the painful portion of the spine (114).

The majority of patients will have pain that is gradual in onset and can be localized only to a general region of the spinal axis (115). However, a subgroup of patients will present with sudden onset of pain, often associated with trauma in the form of sudden flexion or hyperextension of the spine in the affected region. In those with pain of sudden onset, it may be possible to isolate one or more facets that are causing the pain. It is in these instances of sudden-onset, well-localized pain that intra-articular facet injection with local anesthetic and steroid can prove most beneficial. Patients with facet-related pain are difficult to distinguish from those with other causes of axial spinal pain. Some patients will present with sudden onset of pain following a significant flexion-extension (whiplash) injury, but more commonly the onset is insidious, over months to years. Patients with myofascial or discogenic pain, as well as those suffering from sacroiliac dysfunction present with similar symptoms. Nonetheless, certain features can be helpful in differentiating facet-related pain from other causes of spinal pain. The pain caused by facet arthropathy is most pronounced over the axis of the spine itself, and is typically maximal directly in the region of the most affected joints. The pain tends to be

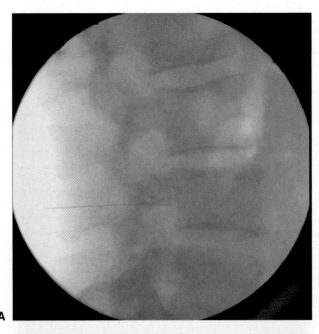

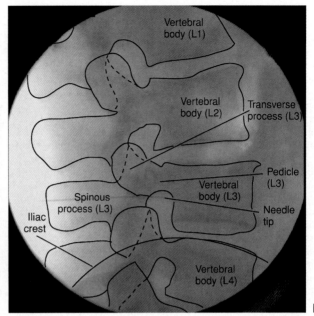

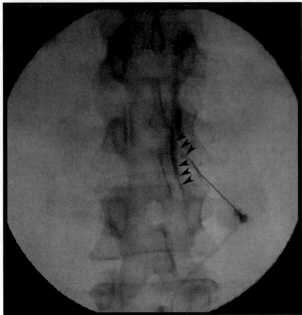

FIGURE 44-18. Lateral radiograph with needle in final position for right L3–4 transforaminal injection. **A:** The needle tip lies directly inferior to the pedicle within the anterior and superior aspect of the L3–4 intervertebral foramen. **B:** Labeled image. **C:** Anterior–posterior radiograph of the lumbar spine following lumbar transforaminal injection (after contrast injection). The needle is in final position for right L3–4 transforaminal injection following injection of 1 mL of radiographic contrast. The needle tip lies directly inferior to the pedicle, and contrast extends to the right lateral epidural space beneath the pedicle (*upper group of arrowheads*). Contrast also extends along the right lateral aspect of the epidural space to outline the L4 nerve root as it exits through the right L4–5 intervertebral foramen (*lower group of arrowheads*). From Rathmell JP. *Atlas of Image-guided Intervention in Regional Anesthesia and Pain Medicine.* Philadelphia: Lippincott Williams & Wilkins, 2006, with permission.

exacerbated by movement, particularly extension of the spine, which forces the inflamed articular surfaces of the facet joints together. However, axial spinal pain at rest or worsening with forward flexion or rotation of the spine is also a common feature. The most important historical feature is a predominance of axial spinal pain; those patients who report that the predominance of their pain is in the extremities are more likely to have acute or chronic radicular pain, rather than facet-related pain. In axial spinal pain, the quality of the pain is typically deep and aching, which waxes and wanes with activity. Burning or stabbing qualities suggest neuropathic pain rather than facet arthropathy.

Diagnostic studies are often unrevealing. Patients with significant facet-related pain may have unremarkable plain radiographs and/or imaging studies of the spine, or they may show

facet arthropathy at multiple levels. Patient selection for facet injection or radiofrequency treatment is empiric, and relies on excluding other causes of pain and a pattern of pain that corresponds to facet-related pain.

The patterns of pain caused by abnormalities in specific facet joints has been established by injecting a mild irritant into a specific facet joints in healthy volunteers and then recording the pattern of pain produced (116–118). The levels treated are chosen by correlating the patient's report of pain to these pain diagrams. Occasionally, a patient will present with evidence of facet arthropathy and a pattern of pain that corresponds to a single level, but this is uncommon. Most patients will have more diffuse pain that can only be narrowed to a specific region. Treatment should be directed to the joint or joints that most closely matches the pattern of referred pain that has been established for each joint, and that typically requires treatment at more than one level.

Intra-articular Facet Joint Injections versus Radiofrequency Treatment. Choosing between intra-articular facet injection and diagnostic medial branch blocks followed by radiofrequency treatment is a frequent clinical scenario. Limited outcome studies of intra-articular injection, particularly at the cervical level, have demonstrated only transient pain relief lasting from days to weeks in most patients (112,113,119). In a randomized trial, Marks et al. (120) showed equal pain relief in patients receiving facet joint injections and medial branch blocks. Those patients who obtain significant pain relief from diagnostic blocks of the medial branch nerves may attain significant and longer-lasting pain reduction from radiofrequency treatment. Two RCTs have shown that radiofrequency ablation provides prolonged pain relief, up to 6 months (121,122). Based on this improved efficacy and a long track record of safety, more and more practitioners are beginning immediately with radiofrequency treatment rather than intra-articular injection. Intra-articular injection remains valuable in those patients who have recent-onset, discrete location pain that suggests involvement of a single facet joint. Intra-articular injection is also a reasonable alternative when the expertise or equipment for radiofrequency treatment is not available, but it will provide only transient symptomatic relief in those with facet-related pain who have failed conservative treatment.

Intra-articular Facet Injection. Key anatomic features are illustrated in Figures 44-6 and 44-7.

Cervical Intra-articular Facet Injection. The patient lies prone, facing directly toward the table with a small headrest under the forehead to allow for air flow between the table and the patient's nose and mouth. The C-arm is rotated 25 to 35 degrees caudally from the axial plane without oblique angulation (Fig. 44-19). This brings the axis of the x-rays in line with the axis of the facet joints and allows for good visualization of the joints (Fig. 44-20). Although the cervical facet joints can also be entered from a lateral approach with the patient lying on his side, advancing a needle using radiographic guidance in the AP plane allows the operator to directly see the position of the spinal canal at all times and avoid medial needle direction that could lead to spinal cord injury (Figs. 44-20 and 44-21).

The skin and subcutaneous tissues overlying the facet joint where the block is to be carried out are anesthetized. The cervical level is easily identified by counting upward from the T1 level, where the T1 vertebra is easily distinguished by the presence of a large transverse process that articulates with the first rib. A 22-gauge, 3.5-inch spinal needle is placed through the skin and advanced until it is seated in the tissues in a plane that is coaxial with the axis of the x-ray path (Fig. 44-19). The needle is then advanced in 0.5- to 1-cm increments, using repeat images to redirect the needle toward the facet joint. Once the surface of the joint space is contacted, a lateral radiograph is obtained, and the needle is advanced slightly to penetrate the posterior joint capsule (Fig. 44-21). The needle should not be advanced into the joint between articular surfaces; this serves no purpose and is likely to abrade the articular surfaces and lead to worsened pain once the local anesthetic block subsides. Although intra-articular location of the needle tip can be confirmed with radiographic contrast, this is unnecessary if the needle location is correct in both AP and lateral planes.

Thoracic Intra-articular Facet Injection. Thoracic intra-articular facet injection is not commonly employed. The plane of the thoracic facet joints is steeply angled, nearing the frontal plane (Fig. 44-22). Even with steep angulation of the C-arm, the joint space cannot be visualized directly, but must be inferred from the position of adjacent structures. The patient is positioned prone, with the head turned to one side. The C-arm is angled 50 to 60 degrees in a caudad direction from the axial plane. The plane of the mid and lower thoracic facet joints lies at an angle of 60 to 70 degrees from the axial plane, but further angulation of the C-arm is impractical without the image intensifier resting against the patient's back. This angle allows visualization of structures adjacent to the facet joint, from which the position of the joint can be inferred (Fig. 44-23). The inferior articular process (superior aspect of the joint) lies posteriorly, directly over the superior articular process (inferior aspect of the joint). The needle tip is advanced toward the inferior aspect of the joint.

The thoracic level is easily identified by counting upward from the T12 level where the twelfth and lowest rib joins

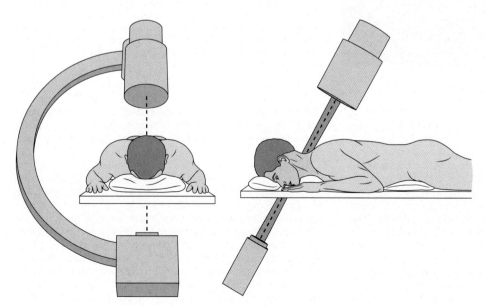

FIGURE 44-19. Position for intra-articular cervical facet joint injection. The patient is placed prone with a small headrest under the forehead to allow for air flow between the table and the patient's nose and mouth. The C-arm is angled 25 to 35 degrees caudally from the axial plane. From Rathmell JP. *Atlas of Image-guided Intervention in Regional Anesthesia and Pain Medicine.* Philadelphia: Lippincott Williams & Wilkins, 2006, with permission.

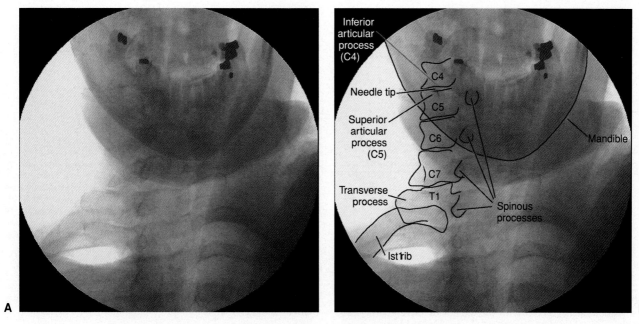

FIGURE 44-20. Anterior–posterior radiograph of the cervical spine during intra-articular cervical facet injection. **A:** A 22-gauge spinal needle is in position in the left C4–5 facet joint. The needle tip is angled slightly to the left. **B:** Labeled image. From Rathmell JP. *Atlas of Image-guided Intervention in Regional Anesthesia and Pain Medicine*. Philadelphia: Lippincott Williams & Wilkins, 2006, with permission.

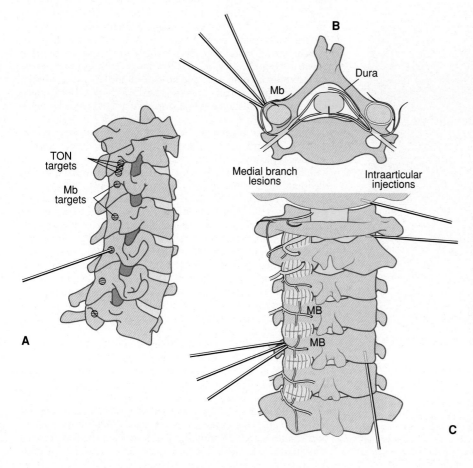

FIGURE 44-21. Diagram of cervical zygapophysial joint blocks (medial branch and intra-articular). Diagram of needle placements for cervical medial branch (*Mb;* **B** and **C,** *left*) and intra-articular (**B** and **C,** *right*) injections. The joint capsule has been removed on the right to demonstrate the intra-articular entry. Note the proximity of the anterior joint capsule wall and the epidural space. Although medial branch blocks can be performed with a single injection, the denervation procedures often require multiple lesions as indicated by the multiple projections on the left. **A** indicates the targets for local anesthetic block in an oblique projection. In **A,** note the multiple injection sites required for adequate blockade of the third occipital nerve—a larger myelinated nerve. For comparison to lower cervical blocks, the needle placements for atlanto-occipital and atlanto-axial intra-articular blocks are indicated.

PART IV: PAIN MANAGEMENT

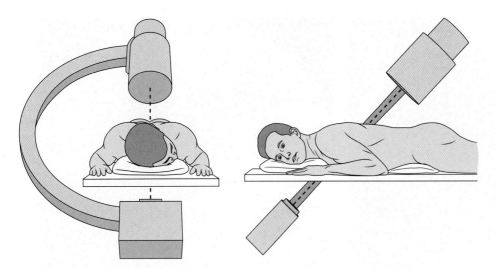

FIGURE 44-22. Position for intra-articular thoracic facet joint injection. The patient is placed prone with the head turned to one side. The C-arm is angled 50 to 60 degrees caudally from the axial plane. From Rathmell JP. *Atlas of Image-guided Intervention in Regional Anesthesia and Pain Medicine.* Philadelphia: Lippincott Williams & Wilkins, 2006, with permission.

the T12 vertebra. A 22-gauge, 1.5-inch spinal needle is placed through the skin and advanced until it is seated in the tissues in a plane that is coaxial with the axis of the x-ray path. The needle is adjusted to remain coaxial and advanced toward the inferior margin of the joint space. Because of the joint's steep angle, the needle can be advanced only into the inferior- and

posterior-most extent of the joint (Fig. 44-24). Lateral radiography is difficult to interpret because of the overlying structures of the thorax.

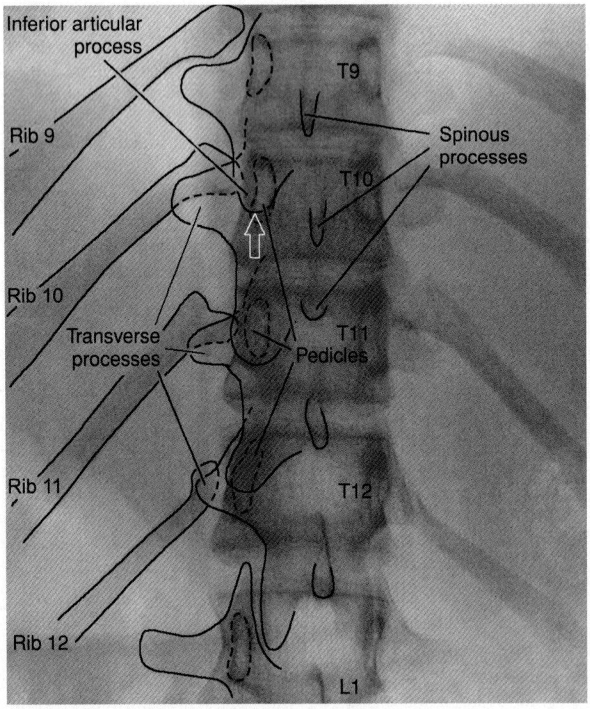

Lumbar Intra-articular Facet Injection. The anatomy of the lumbar facet joint and surrounding structures is illustrated in Figure 44-25. The patient is positioned prone, with the head turned to one side. The C-arm is angled obliquely 25 to 35 degrees from the sagittal plane and without caudal angulation (Fig. 44-26). This angle allows direct visualization of the facet joint (Fig. 44-27). The skin and subcutaneous tissues overlying the facet joint where the block is to be carried out are anesthetized. The lumbar level is easily identified by counting upward from the sacrum. A 22-gauge, 3.5-inch spinal needle is placed through the skin and advanced until it is seated in the tissues, in a plane that is coaxial with the axis of the x-ray path. The needle is adjusted to remain coaxial and advanced toward the joint space.

Whether the intra-articular injection is done at the cervical, thoracic, or lumbar level, the facet joint itself holds only limited volume, typically less than 1.5 mL. Placing contrast in the joint will limit the ability to place local anesthetic and steroid within the joint. Intra-articular injections are commonly carried out at the lumbar levels. At this level, the articular space is Z-shaped, with the superior recess extending slightly lateral to the axis of the articular surfaces, and the inferior recess extending slightly medial to the axis of the articular surfaces. Once needle position has been confirmed, a solution containing steroid and local anesthetic is placed. A total dose of 80 mg of methylprednisolone acetate or the equivalent should be divided over all of the joints to be injected, but more than 40 mg per joint is probably unnecessary. Using concentrated steroid (40 or 80 mg/mL) allows a 1:1 mixture with local anesthetic (0.5% bupivacaine) to provide some immediate pain relief.

Complications associated with intra-articular facet injection are uncommon. The most likely adverse effect is an exacerbation of pain. This is frequent when intra-articular cervical facet injection is carried out and the needle is advanced within the joint space. The joint space is narrow, and advancing the needle within the joint can abrade the articular surfaces, causing increased pain. This exacerbation is usually self-limited. Infection can also occur, leading to abscess within the paraspinous musculature, but the incidence is exceedingly low (123). Bleeding complications have not been associated with intra-articular facet injection.

FIGURE 44-23. Anterior–posterior radiograph of the low thoracic spine. Because of their steep angle, the thoracic facet joints cannot be seen directly but must be inferred from the position of adjacent structures. The superior aspect of each joint (inferior articular process) lies posteriorly (*arrow*), directly over the inferior aspect of the joint (superior articular process). This position can be inferred by following the inferior margin of the lamina from the spinous process laterally (*arrow*). From Rathmell JP. *Atlas of Image-guided Intervention in Regional Anesthesia and Pain Medicine.* Philadelphia: Lippincott Williams & Wilkins, 2006, with permission.

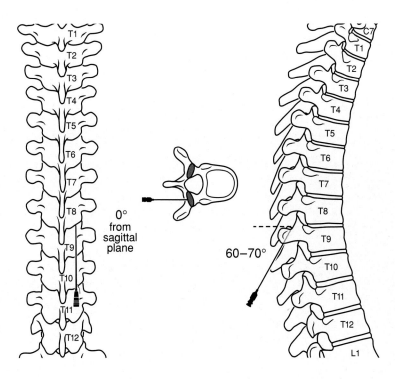

0°
from
sagittal
plane

60–70°

FIGURE 44-24. Position and angle of needle entry for intra-articular thoracic facet injection. A 22-gauge spinal needle is advanced in the sagittal plane overlying the facet joint with 60 to 70 degrees of caudad angulation from the axial plane. From Rathmell JP. *Atlas of Image-guided Intervention in Regional Anesthesia and Pain Medicine.* Philadelphia: Lippincott Williams & Wilkins, 2006, with permission.

Facet Medial Branch Blocks and Radiofrequency Treatment.
In those patients who receive only temporary relief from therapeutic intra-articular facet injections, or who have pain that is more diffuse and requires treatment at numerous levels, radiofrequency treatment can produce significant, enduring pain relief. Many investigators have pointed to the need for controlled diagnostic injections to determine who will respond to radiofrequency treatment. Despite the value of placebo-controlled injections, this is impractical in most clinical settings. Most practitioners rely on a single set of diagnostic local anesthetic blocks to the medial branch nerves at the levels of suspected pathology to determine who should receive radiofrequency treatment. Those who report significant pain relief, usually defined as 50% or greater pain reduction lasting the average duration of the local anesthetic, go on to radiofrequency treatment. Similar, transient pain relief with intra-articular injection of local anesthetic can also be used as a reasonable prognostic test before proceeding with radiofrequency treatment.

Conventional radiofrequency treatment produces a small area of tissue coagulation surrounding the active tip of an insulated cannula. When the tip of the radiofrequency cannula is placed in close proximity to a neural structure, the lesion encompasses the nerve, causing denervation. The most commonly used cannulae for facet treatment are 22-gauge Sluijter-Mehta cannulae (SMK) and come in 5-, 10-, and 15-cm lengths. These radiofrequency cannulae have a noninsulated area where coagulation occurs, called the *active tip*, which may be 4, 5, or 10 mm in length. Conventional radiofrequency damages neural tissue by creating an electrical field between the active tip of the needle connected to a voltage generator and an inactive or dispersion electrode at a distance. This induces the movement of a tissue ionic current that follows the alternating current, generating friction, and, therefore, creating heat surrounding the needle tip. Radiofrequency power produces heat by current flow and not through heat transfer from the tip (124). The lesion, although variable, is well circumscribed and reproducible when the physical parameters are properly controlled. The size is mostly dependent on needle diameter, length of the active tip, tissue vascularization, tip temperature, and time of exposure. Lesions are characterized by a central core filled with blood, related to the electrode placement, surrounded by an area of coagulation necrosis and separated by a wall of neuroglial proliferation from a zone of liquefaction necrosis. The lesion is then surrounded by an area of demyelination (125,126). For all but the most obese patients, the 10-cm cannulae with 5-mm active tips are used (see also Chapter 42, Figs. 42-1 to 42-5).

In recent years, pulsed radiofrequency treatment has come into frequent use. Studies that looked into the effects of tissues exposed to the typical electromagnetic field generated during radiofrequency treatment without tissue heating showed that the so-called isothermal (42°C–45°C) radiofrequency procedure induced physiologic changes in tissues (127). Recently, Van Zundert et al. showed increased expression of c-fos in the dorsal horn of experimental animals up to 7 days after pulsed radiofrequency treatment, which suggests sustained activation of a pain-inhibiting process (128). Although the concept of long-lasting pain reduction without neural destruction is appealing, as yet little clinical evidence supports the efficacy of this new technique (129).

The key concept when using conventional versus pulsed radiofrequency is to understand where the lesion or pulse radiofrequency energy will occur relative to the active tip. The lesion produced by conventional radiofrequency is along the shaft of the needle surrounding the active tip. Scant tissue destruction occurs at the tip of the needle, thus the active tip of the cannula must be placed along the course of the nerve. In contrast, the highest density of voltage change during pulsed radiofrequency emanates directly from the tip of the radiofrequency cannula; thus, the tip of the needle should be directed along the course of the nerve to be treated. Techniques for both conventional and pulsed radiofrequency treatment will be discussed in the next sections.

PART IV: PAIN MANAGEMENT

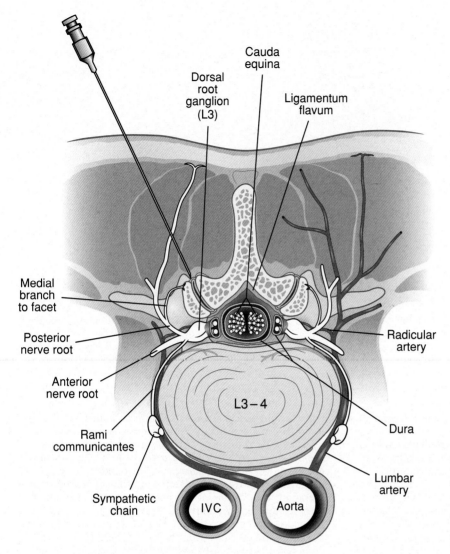

FIGURE 44-25. Axial diagram of intra-articular lumbar facet injection. The axis of the facet joint lies 25 to 35 degrees from the sagittal plane. Note the innervation to the facet joint. From Rathmell JP. *Atlas of Image-guided Intervention in Regional Anesthesia and Pain Medicine.* Philadelphia: Lippincott Williams & Wilkins, 2006, with permission.

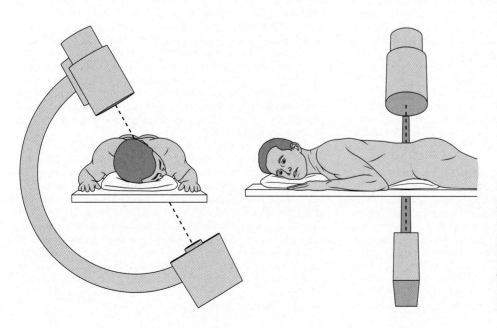

FIGURE 44-26. Position for intra-articular lumbar facet joint injection. The patient is placed prone with the head turned to one side. The C-arm is angled 25 to 35 degrees from the sagittal plane parallel to the axial plane. From Rathmell JP. *Atlas of Image-guided Intervention in Regional Anesthesia and Pain Medicine.* Philadelphia: Lippincott Williams & Wilkins, 2006, with permission.

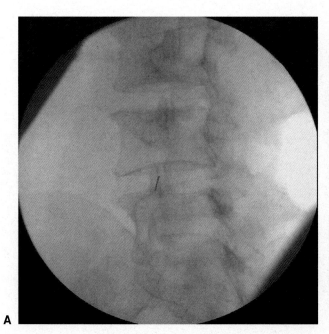
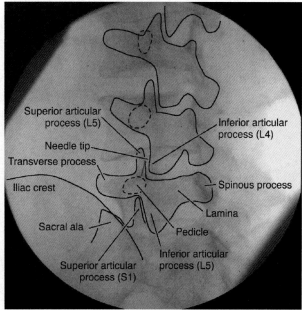

FIGURE 44-27. Oblique radiograph of the lumbar spine during lumbar intra-articular facet injection. **A:** The needle is in place in the left L4–L5 facet joint. The needle travels from inferior to slightly superior. **B:** Labeled image. From Rathmell JP. *Atlas of Image-guided Intervention in Regional Anesthesia and Pain Medicine*. Philadelphia: Lippincott Williams & Wilkins, 2006, with permission.

Cervical Facet Medial Branch Block and Radiofrequency Treatment. The medial branch nerves to the cervical facets course across the articular pillar, midway between the superior and inferior articular processes (Fig. 44-7, and also see Chapter 42, Fig. 42-14). The nerves can be anesthetized by placing a needle from a posterior or lateral approach (Fig. 44-21). For the patient, the lateral approach is more comfortable, as he can lie on one side rather than face down, and the needle must traverse less tissue en route to the target. However, when the needles are inserted from a lateral approach, they are directed toward the spinal cord; even slight rotation of the neck can confuse identification of the left and right articular pillars and result in needle entry into the spinal canal. For performing diagnostic medial branch blocks, either approach is adequate, as the local anesthetic will be deposited in the same location with both approaches. For conventional radiofrequency treatment, the cannulae should be placed using a posterior approach, as this will allow the entire length of the 5-mm active tip to be placed along the course of the nerve on the articular pillar. For pulsed radiofrequency treatment, the cannulae can be placed from a lateral approach, as the voltage fluctuations are maximal at the tip of the cannula.

POSTERIOR APPROACH. The patient lies prone, facing directly toward the table, with a small headrest under the forehead to allow for air flow between the table and the patient's nose and mouth. The C-arm is rotated 25 to 35 degrees caudally from the axial plane without any oblique angulation. This brings the axis of the x-rays in line with axis of the facet joints and allows for good visualization of the articular pillars. (Figs. 44-28 and 44-29). If the neck can be flexed, using a special attachment at the end of the table, the C-arm needs to be angled caudally only 15 degrees (see Chapter 42, Fig. 42-15).

LATERAL APPROACH. The patient lies in the lateral decubitus position with a pillow under the head to keep the neck hori-zontal and minimize lateral flexion of the neck to either side. The C-arm is placed directly over the patient's neck without rotation or angulation (Fig. 44-30). Care must be taken to assure that the left and right articular pillars are aligned directly over one another (Fig. 44-31). This is a point of great confusion among practitioners who are inexperienced with radiographic anatomy of the cervical spine. Even a small degree of rotation can place the left and right facet joints in significantly different locations on lateral radiographs. It is difficult to discern the left side from the right, and if a needle is advanced toward the contralateral facet target in error, the needle can easily penetrate into the spinal canal.

DIAGNOSTIC MEDIAL BRANCH BLOCKS. The cervical level can be identified by counting upward from T1 or downward from C2. Radiographically, T1 is identified in the AP view by its large transverse process that articulates with the head of the first rib, and C2 can be identified by its odontoid process in the AP view and its large spinous process in the lateral view (Fig. 44-29). The skin and subcutaneous tissues overlying the facet target where the block is to be carried out are anesthetized and a 22-gauge, 3.5-inch spinal needle is placed through the skin and advanced just until it is seated in the tissues, in a plane that is coaxial with the axis of the x-ray path. The needle is adjusted to remain coaxial and advanced toward the medial branch target in the middle of the articular pillar, midway between superior and inferior articular surfaces of the vertebra. This appears as an invagination or "waist" on AP radiographs, and as a trapezoid on lateral radiographs (Fig. 44-29). From the posterior approach, the needle is gently seated on the lateral margin of the facet column in the middle of the "waist" (Fig. 44-29, and also see Chapter 42, Fig. 42-14B); from a lateral approach, the needle tip is seated in the middle of the trapezoid (Fig. 44-32). Needle position is confirmed with AP and lateral radiographs. Once needle position has been confirmed, a small

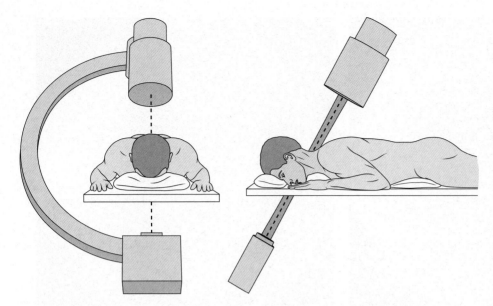

FIGURE 44-28. Position for cervical medial branch blocks and radiofrequency treatment (posterior approach). The patient is placed prone with a small headrest under the forehead to allow for air flow between the table and the patient's nose and mouth. The C-arm is angled 25 to 35 degrees caudally from the axial plane. From Rathmell JP. *Atlas of Image-guided Intervention in Regional Anesthesia and Pain Medicine.* Philadelphia: Lippincott Williams & Wilkins, 2006, with permission.

volume of local anesthetic is placed at each level, and the needles are removed. The patient is instructed to assess his degree of pain relief in the hours immediately following the diagnostic blocks.

RADIOFREQUENCY TREATMENT. Radiofrequency cannulae are placed using a technique identical to that described for medial branch blocks. For *conventional* radiofrequency treatment, 5-cm SMK cannulae with 5-mm active tips are used and placed from a posterior approach. Once the lateral margin of the facet column is contacted, the needle is walked laterally off

the facet and advanced 2 to 3 mm to position the active tip along the course of the medial branch nerve (see Chapter 42, Figs. 42-17 to 42-20). Proper testing for sensory–motor dissociation is conducted. For sensory testing, the patient is asked to report pain or tingling during stimulation at 50 Hz at less than 0.5 V. Motor testing is carried out at 2 Hz, slowly increasing the output to three times the sensory threshold. No motor stimulation should be made to the affected myotome throughout the testing period. We routinely increase the output to 3 V to rule out stimulation of the nerve root, before we proceed

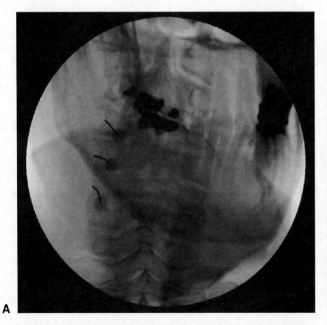

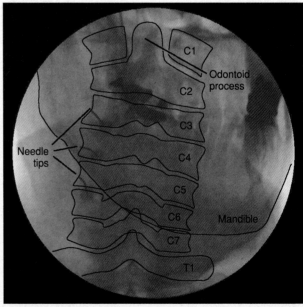

A   **B**

FIGURE 44-29. Anterior–posterior radiograph of the cervical spine during cervical medial branch block or radiofrequency treatment (posterior approach). **A:** Three radiofrequency cannulae are in place in the middle of the facet pillar at C3, C4, and C5 on the left. The caudad angulation of 25 to 35 degrees brings the facet joints into clear view and allows placement of the cannulae along the course of the medial branch nerves. **B:** Labeled image. From Rathmell JP. *Atlas of Image-guided Intervention in Regional Anesthesia and Pain Medicine.* Philadelphia: Lippincott Williams & Wilkins, 2006, with permission.

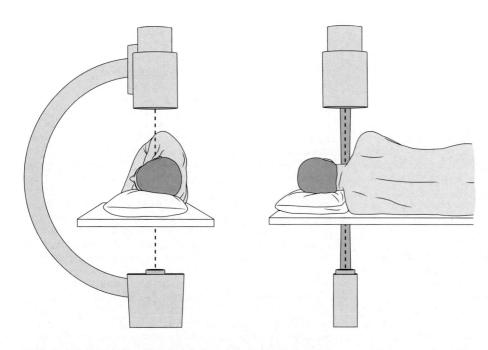

FIGURE 44-30. Position for cervical medial branch blocks and radiofrequency treatment (lateral approach). The patient is placed on his side with a pillow under the head. The pillow should keep the cervical spine in alignment without lateral flexion to either side. The C-arm is placed directly over the patient's neck in the axial plane without angulation. From Rathmell JP. *Atlas of Image-guided Intervention in Regional Anesthesia and Pain Medicine*. Philadelphia: Lippincott Williams & Wilkins, 2006, with permission.

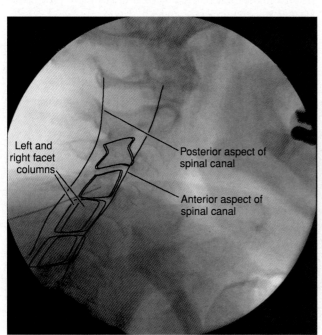

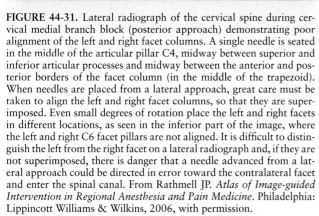

FIGURE 44-31. Lateral radiograph of the cervical spine during cervical medial branch block (posterior approach) demonstrating poor alignment of the left and right facet columns. A single needle is seated in the middle of the articular pillar C4, midway between superior and inferior articular processes and midway between the anterior and posterior borders of the facet column (in the middle of the trapezoid). When needles are placed from a lateral approach, great care must be taken to align the left and right facet columns, so that they are superimposed. Even small degrees of rotation place the left and right facets in different locations, as seen in the inferior part of the image, where the left and right C6 facet pillars are not aligned. It is difficult to distinguish the left from the right facet on a lateral radiograph and, if they are not superimposed, there is danger that a needle advanced from a lateral approach could be directed in error toward the contralateral facet and enter the spinal canal. From Rathmell JP. *Atlas of Image-guided Intervention in Regional Anesthesia and Pain Medicine*. Philadelphia: Lippincott Williams & Wilkins, 2006, with permission.

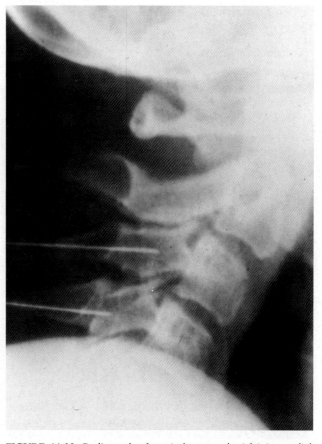

FIGURE 44-32. Radiograph of cervical zygapophysial joint medial branch nerve block at the C3 and C4 level. Lateral radiograph demonstrating the position of needle tips at the center of the trapezoid-shaped articular process in the cervical spine. Injection here would allow minimal diffusion because of insertion of the splenius capitis muscle groups.

with radiofrequency procedure. Thereafter, great care must be taken to prevent any movement of the cannulae. Each level is anesthetized prior to ablation, and lesions are created at 80°C for 60 to 90 seconds.

For pulsed radiofrequency treatment, 5-cm cannulae with 5-mm active tips are inserted from a lateral approach. The tip is placed in the center of the trapezoid of the target facet, midway between articular surfaces and midway between the anterior and posterior extent of the facet column. Proper testing for sensory thresholds is conducted as in conventional radiofrequency. Each level is then treated with *pulsed* radiofrequency adequate to maintain voltage fluctuations of 40 to 45 V for 120 seconds, without exceeding a tip temperature of 42°C centigrade. Local anesthesia is not needed for pulsed radiofrequency treatment, but may be placed before the cannulae are removed.

Thoracic Facet Medial Branch Block and Radiofrequency Treatment. The medial branch nerves to the thoracic facets course over the base of the transverse processes, where they join with the superior articular processes. The patient lies prone, with the head turned to one side. The C-arm is positioned over the thoracic spine, in a direct anterior–posterior plane without any angulation. The transverse processes of the thoracic vertebrae are best seen from this angle at both high and low thoracic levels (Fig. 44-33).

DIAGNOSTIC MEDIAL BRANCH BLOCKS. The thoracic level can be identified by counting downward from T1 or upward from T12. The skin and subcutaneous tissues overlying the facet target where the block is to be carried out are anesthetized

and a 22-gauge, 3.5-inch spinal needle is placed through the skin and advanced just until it is seated in the tissues in a plane that is coaxial with the axis of the x-ray path. The needle is adjusted to remain coaxial and advanced toward the base of the transverse process where it joins the superior articular process, and is seated just on the bony margin (Fig. 44-34). Once the needle is in position, a small volume of local anesthetic is placed at each level, and the needles are removed. The patient is instructed to assess his degree of pain relief in the hours immediately following the diagnostic blocks.

RADIOFREQUENCY TREATMENT. Radiofrequency cannulae are placed using a technique identical to that described for medial branch blocks (Fig. 44-34). For conventional radiofrequency treatment, 5- or 10-cm SMK cannulae with 5-mm active tips are used. Once the needle is seated against the superior margin of the transverse process where it joins the superior articular process of the facet, the cannula is walked superolaterally off of the transverse process and advanced 2 to 3 mm to position the active tip along the course of the medial branch nerve. Proper testing for sensory–motor dissociation is conducted as previously described. Thereafter, great care must be taken to prevent any movement of the cannulae. Each level is anesthetized, and lesions are created at 80°C for 60 to 90 seconds. Cannula placement for thoracic pulsed radiofrequency treatment is carried out in the same manner. Further discussion is provided in Chapter 42, Figures 42-21 and 42-22.

Lumbar Facet Medial Branch Blocks and Radiofrequency Treatment. The medial branch nerves to the lumbar facets

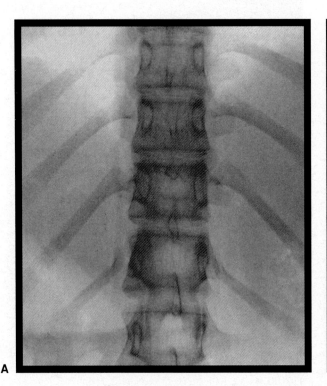
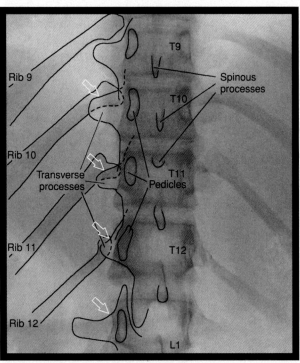

FIGURE 44-33. Anterior–posterior radiograph of the low thoracic spine. **A:** The transverse processes are less prominent at low thoracic levels and are often difficult to see at all at T12. The base of the transverse process joins the superior articular process just superolateral to the pedicle, and the pedicle is used as a landmark to locate the target for injection. **B:** Labeled image. The arrows indicate the targets for medial branch nerve blocks or radiofrequency treatment at T10–L1 levels on the left. From Rathmell JP. *Atlas of Image-guided Intervention in Regional Anesthesia and Pain Medicine.* Philadelphia: Lippincott Williams & Wilkins, 2006, with permission.

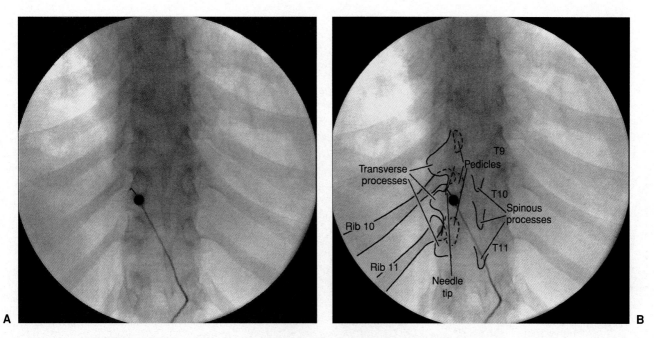

FIGURE 44-34. Anterior–posterior radiograph of the thoracic spine during radiofrequency treatment of the thoracic facets. **A:** A single radiofrequency cannulae is in place along the superolateral margin of the left T10 transverse process, where it joins the superior articular process. **B:** Labeled image. From Rathmell JP. *Atlas of Image-guided Intervention in Regional Anesthesia and Pain Medicine.* Philadelphia: Lippincott Williams & Wilkins, 2006, with permission.

course over the base of the transverse process where they join with the superior articular processes (Figs. 44-6 and 44-35). The medial branch nerve lays in the groove between the transverse process and the superior articular process, which slopes inferolaterally (see also Chapter 42, Fig. 42-23). The patient lies prone, with the head turned to one side (Fig. 44-35). A pillow is placed under the lower abdomen in an effort to tilt the pelvis backward and swing the iliac crests posteriorly away from the lumbosacral junction. The C-arm is positioned over the lumbar spine with 25 to 35 degrees of *oblique* angulation (Fig. 44-36), so that the facet joints themselves and the junction between the transverse process and the superior articular process are clearly seen. For medial branch blocks, the needle can be advanced in the axial plane without caudal angulation. However, for radiofrequency treatment, the C-arm should be angled 25 to 30 degrees caudal to the axial plane, so that the active tip of the radiofrequency cannulae will be parallel to the medial branch nerve within the groove between the transverse process and the superior articular process as it slopes inferomedially. A variation of this approach is described in Chapter 42, Figures 42-24 to 42-28.

DIAGNOSTIC MEDIAL BRANCH BLOCKS. The lumbar level can be identified by counting upward from the sacrum. The skin and subcutaneous tissues overlying the facet target where the block is to be carried out are anesthetized, and a 22-gauge, 3.5-inch spinal needle is placed through the skin and advanced until it is gently seated in the tissues in a plane that is coaxial with the axis of the x-ray path. The needle is adjusted to remain coaxial and advanced toward the base of the transverse process where it joins the superior articular process, and is seated just on the bony margin, just superolateral to the "eye of the scotty dog" (Fig. 44-37). Once the needle is in position, a small volume of local anesthetic is placed at each level, and the needles are removed. The patient is instructed to assess his degree of

pain relief in the hours immediately following the diagnostic blocks.

RADIOFREQUENCY TREATMENT. Radiofrequency cannulae are placed using a technique identical to that described for medial branch blocks, however the C-arm is angled 25 to 30 degrees caudal to the axial plane, so that the active tip of the radiofrequency cannulae will be parallel to the medial branch. Some clinicians prefer to position the C-arm in an anterior–posterior plane, with 25 degrees caudad angulation but no oblique angulation (Fig. 44-38). For conventional radiofrequency treatment, 10-cm SMK cannulae with 5-mm active tips are used. Once the needle is seated against the superior margin of the transverse process where it joins the superior articular process of the facet, the cannula is walked off the superior margin of the transverse process and advanced 2 to 3 mm to position the active tip along the course of the medial branch nerve (see also Chapter 42, Figs. 42-26 and 42-27). Proper testing for sensory–motor dissociation is conducted as previously described, assuring no stimulation of the motor nerves to the lower extremities occurs. Thereafter, great care must be taken to prevent any movement of the cannulae. Each level is anesthetized, and lesions are created at 80°C for 60 to 90 seconds. Cannula placement for lumbar pulsed radiofrequency treatment is carried out in the same manner, with the exception that the active tip does not need to be parallel to the medial branch nerve. A "tunnel view" technique is described in Chapter 42, Figures 42-29 to 42-32.

Complications of Medial Branch Block and Radiofrequency Treatment. Complications associated with diagnostic medial branch nerve blocks are uncommon and similar to those following intra-articular facet injections. Unlike intra-articular injection, it is unusual for medial branch blocks to cause an exacerbation of pain. Patients should be warned to expect mild pain

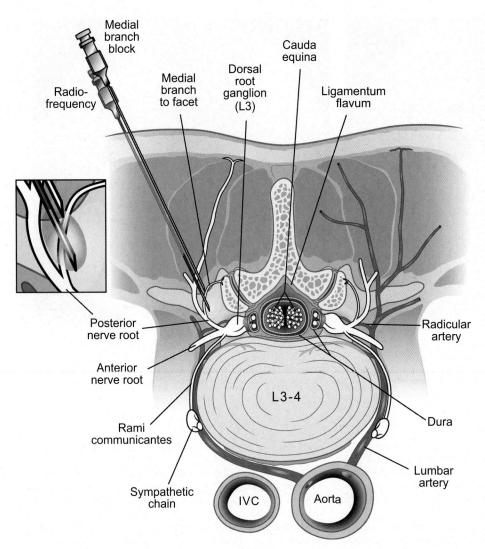

FIGURE 44-35. Axial diagram of lumbar medial branch nerve blocks and radiofrequency treatment. A 22-gauge, 3.5-inch spinal needle (or 22-gauge, 10-cm SMK radiofrequency cannula with a 5-mm active tip) is advanced toward the base of the transverse process where it joins with the superior articular process. Cannulae placement for conventional radiofrequency treatment should be carried out with 25 to 30 degrees of caudal angulation of the C-arm to bring the axis of the active tip parallel to the course of the medial branch nerve in the groove between the transverse process and the superior articular process. From Rathmell JP. *Atlas of Image-guided Intervention in Regional Anesthesia and Pain Medicine.* Philadelphia: Lippincott Williams & Wilkins, 2006, with permission.

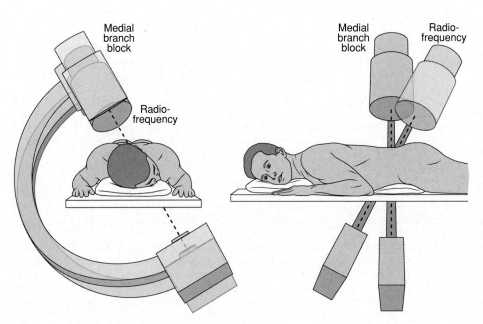

FIGURE 44-36. Position for lumbar medial branch blocks and radiofrequency treatment. The patient is placed prone with the head turned to one side. The C-arm is positioned over the lumbar spine with 25 to 35 degrees of oblique angulation, so that the facet joints themselves and the junction between the transverse process and the superior articular process are clearly seen. For medial branch blocks, the needle can be advanced in the axial plane without caudal angulation. However, for radiofrequency treatment, the C-arm should be angled 25 to 30 degrees caudal to the axial plane, so that the active tip of the radiofrequency cannulae will be parallel to the medial branch nerve in the groove between the transverse process and the superior articular process. From Rathmell JP. *Atlas of Image-guided Intervention in Regional Anesthesia and Pain Medicine.* Philadelphia: Lippincott Williams & Wilkins, 2006, with permission.

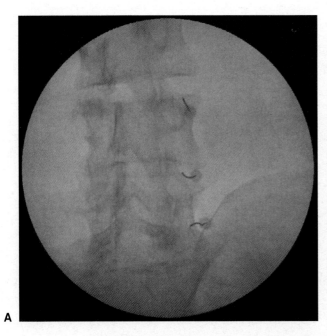
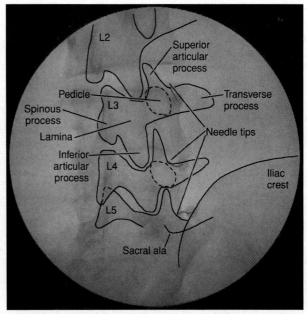

FIGURE 44-37. Oblique radiograph of the lumbar spine during lumbar radiofrequency treatment of the lumbar facet joints. **A:** Three radiofrequency cannulae are in place at the base of the transverse processes and superior articular processes at the L3, L4, and L5 levels on the right. **B:** Labeled image. From Rathmell JP. *Atlas of Image-guided Intervention in Regional Anesthesia and Pain Medicine.* Philadelphia: Lippincott Williams & Wilkins, 2006, with permission.

at the injection site, lasting a day or two after the procedure. Radiofrequency treatment of the facets is also associated with few complications. Despite the fact that conventional radiofrequency produces actual tissue destruction, injury to the spinal nerve roots is uncommon, perhaps because of sensory and mo-

tor testing. Injury to the spinal nerve root has been reported following radiofrequency treatment, and this could present with new-onset radicular pain, with or without radiculopathy. The importance of physiologic testing before each lesion should be emphasized, since this will reduce the chance that the active tip

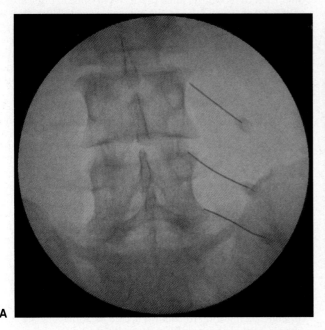
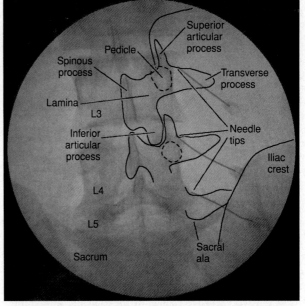

FIGURE 44-38. Anterior–posterior radiograph of the lumbar spine during lumbar radiofrequency treatment of the lumbar facet joints. **A:** Three radiofrequency cannulae are in place at the base of the transverse processes and superior articular processes at the L3, L4, and L5 levels on the right. Note the angle of the entering cannulae. **B:** Labeled image. From Rathmell JP. *Atlas of Image-guided Intervention in Regional Anesthesia and Pain Medicine.* Philadelphia: Lippincott Williams & Wilkins, 2006, with permission.

of the cannula will be close enough to the anterior nerve root to cause injury.

Exacerbation of pain following conventional radiofrequency treatment is common, and patients should be instructed to expect an increase in pain, similar in character to their usual pain, that will last from several days to a week or more. A smaller group of patients will report uncomfortable dysesthesia, usually in the form of a sunburn-like feeling of the skin overlying the spinous processes and often accompanied by allodynia. This adverse effect is more common following cervical radiofrequency treatment and usually subsides over several weeks. These dysesthesia likely stem from partial denervation of the lateral branch of the posterior primary ramus, which supplies a variable region of cutaneous innervation overlying the spinous processes. Likewise, some patients will report a small patch of complete sensory loss in this same region.

Pulsed radiofrequency treatment does not produce tissue destruction, thus it is not surprising that most patients will have no worsening of their pain following treatment, or only a transient, mild, short-lived exacerbation. Painful dysesthesia and other consequences of nerve injury do not occur with pulsed radiofrequency treatment. It is precisely this lack of neural destruction and associated adverse effects that has made pulsed radiofrequency treatment so popular among practitioners; if controlled trials emerge to support the efficacy of pulsed radiofrequency treatment, it may rapidly replace conventional radiofrequency ablation (129).

Sacroiliac Joint Injection

Pain arising from the sacroiliac joints (SIJ) is common and difficult to distinguish from other causes of pain in the area of the lumbosacral junction. Sacroiliac joint dysfunction typically presents with localized pain in the lower back or upper buttock overlying the SIJ (130). Pain may be referred to the posterior thigh, but pain extending below the knee is unusual. In most cases, the etiology is unclear, and the onset is gradual over months to years. Sacroiliac joint pain has been estimated to comprise 15% to 25% of patients with lumbosacral pain (130). Trauma, infection, and tumor are uncommon causes of SIJ pain. The inflammatory arthropathies associated with ankylosing spondylitis, Reiter syndrome, and inflammatory bowel diseases are also infrequent but well-established causes of sacroiliac-related pain. Intra-articular injection of the SIJ with local anesthetic and steroid can provide short-term pain relief and assist diagnostically in establishing the source of low back pain (131). Radiofrequency treatments for SIJ-related pain have been devised, but are only modestly effective in a fraction of treated patients (132). A long-term solution to SIJ-related pain is one of the unmet needs of our current armamentarium.

Patients with facet-related pain are difficult to distinguish from those with other causes of axial spinal pain, tending to report pain location over the SIJs to either side of midline near the lumbosacral junction (Fig. 44.1). Physical examination may reveal localized tenderness over the joint, and tests aimed at evoking SIJ-related pain (Table 44.4), including the Patrick (or FABER) test are positive in up to 20% of asymptomatic patients (133). Degenerative change of the joint on radiograph is uncommon and nonspecific; most patients with SIJ-related pain have normal SIJ appearance on radiography. Resolution of pain following intra-articular injection of local anesthetic under fluoroscopic or CT guidance is the best diagnostic tool available for SIJ pain; like facet joint pain, definitive diagno-

TABLE 44-4

PROVOCATIVE TESTS FOR SACROILIAC PAIN

The Patrick or flexion, abduction, external rotation (FABER) test. The knee is flexed and the lateral malleolus of the ankle placed on the contralateral patella. The knee is then slowly lowered toward the examination table in external rotation. Pain caused by hip disease (e.g., osteoarthritis of the hip) is produced by this maneuver and is reported radiating to the groin along the inguinal ligament. During the same maneuver, the examiner presses over the flexed knee while stabilizing the contralateral side of the pelvis over the anterior, superior iliac spine. This stresses the sacroiliac joint (SIJ), and report of pain over the SIJ should raise the suspicion of SIJ etiology.

The Gaenslen test. An alternate test for pain arising from the SIJ, the Gaenslen test is performed by placing the patient supine along the edge of the examination table. One leg is placed over the edge of the examination table and lowered toward the floor in hyperextension, while the pelvis is held stable. Pain related to the SIJ is reproduced by this maneuver.

sis is hindered by the significant placebo and other effects of diagnostic injection (see Chapter 38).

Intra-articular Sacroiliac Joint Injection. The patient lies prone, with the head turned to one side. The C-arm is rotated 25 to 35 degrees caudally from the axial plane to place the posterior superior iliac spine and the iliac crest cephalad along the line of the SIJ. The C-arm is then rotated (Figs. 44-39 and 44-40) obliquely 0 to 30 degrees until the posterior, inferior aspect of the SIJ is clearly visible. Two features of the SIJ are important to recognize. First, the SIJ is curvilinear, often arcing somewhat laterally toward the anterior aspect. This can lead to confusing overlying shadows of the anterior and posterior portion of the joint. The second important feature is the overlying iliac crest, which can block entry to the SIJ. Using caudal angulation of the C-arm and limiting injection to the inferior aspect of the joint are used to avoid placing a needle on the iliac crest rather than in the SIJ itself.

The skin and subcutaneous tissues overlying the SIJ where the block is to be carried out are anesthetized with 1 to 2 mL of 1% lidocaine. A 22-gauge, 3.5-inch spinal needle is placed through the skin and advanced just until it is seated in the tissues in a plane that is coaxial with the axis of the x-ray path. The needle is adjusted to remain coaxial or angled in a slightly cephalad direction toward the inferior aspect of the joint and advanced toward the joint space using repeat AP images after every 2- to 4-mm of needle advancement. Once the surface of the joint space is contacted, the needle is advanced just slightly to penetrate the posterior joint capsule. As the needle enters the joint space, the tip often curves slightly, following the contour of the surface of the ilium. In older patients and those with significant osteoarthritis, it may be difficult or impossible to penetrate into the joint space, and only periarticular infiltration can be carried out. In most instances, there is no need for contrast injection to confirm needle location. The SIJ itself often holds only limited volume (typically <2 mL), and placing contrast in the joint limits the ability to place local anesthetic and steroid. A total dose of 80 mg of methylprednisolone acetate or the equivalent can be administered, or divided between both SIJs if bilateral injection is necessary. Using concentrated

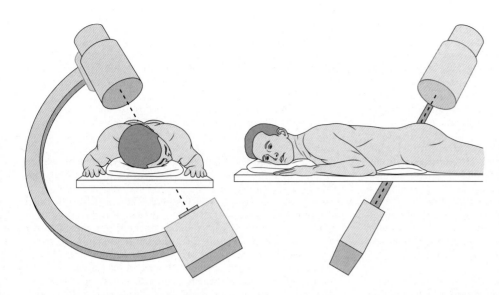

FIGURE 44-39. Position for intra-articular sacroiliac joint injection. The patient is placed prone with the head turned to one side. The C-arm is angled 25 to 35 degrees caudally from the axial plane and 0 to 30 degrees obliquely until the posterior-inferior aspect of the joint is clearly visible. From Rathmell JP. *Atlas of Image-guided Intervention in Regional Anesthesia and Pain Medicine.* Philadelphia: Lippincott Williams & Wilkins, 2006, with permission.

steroid (40 or 80 mg/mL) allows a 1:1 mixture with local anesthetic (0.5% bupivacaine) to provide immediate pain relief. An alternative technique is to carry out radiofrequency lesioning of lateral branches as they emerge from the sacral foramina at the midpoint of the lateral border of the foramen (133) (see Chapter 42, Fig. 42-33).

Complications associated with intra-articular SIJ injection are uncommon. The most likely adverse effect is an exacerbation of pain in the days following resolution of the local anesthetic effect, likely owing to distention of the SIJ during the injection procedure. This exacerbation is usually mild and self-limited. Infection can also occur, leading to abscess within the presacral musculature, but the incidence is exceedingly low.

Bleeding complications have not been associated with intra-articular sacroiliac injection.

Treatment for SIJ pain remains inadequate and controversial. Currently, periodic intra-articular injection of steroid with local anesthetics is the most common therapy for SIJ pain, but this typically provides only transient relief (130).

Lumbar Discography and Intradiscal Treatments

Discography is a diagnostic test in which radiographic contrast is injected into the nucleus pulposus of the intervertebral disc. Although originally developed for the study of disc herniation, discography is now used most commonly to identify

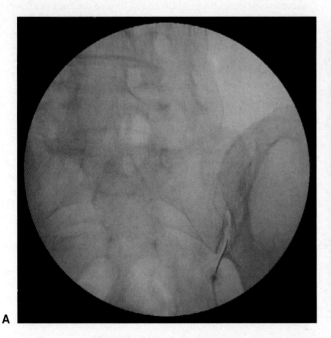

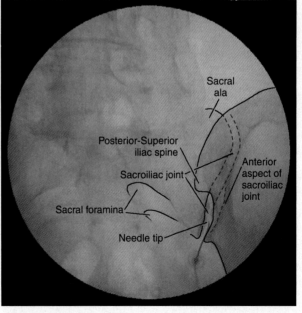

Sacral ala

Posterior-Superior iliac spine

Sacroiliac joint

Sacral foramina

Anterior aspect of sacroiliac joint

Needle tip

A   B

FIGURE 44-40. Anterior–posterior radiograph of the sacroiliac (S1) joint during intra-articular S1 joint injection. **A:** A 22-guage spinal needle is in position in the posterior-inferior aspect of the right S1 joint. Note the medial deflection of the needle tip along the medial aspect of the ilium where the needle enters the joint space. **B:** Labeled image. From Rathmell JP. *Atlas of Image-guided Intervention in Regional Anesthesia and Pain Medicine.* Philadelphia: Lippincott Williams & Wilkins, 2006, with permission.

PART IV: PAIN MANAGEMENT

symptomatic disc degeneration. Discography has two components: the anatomic appearance of contrast spread within the disc (using plane radiographs and/or CT), and the presence or absence of typical pain during contrast injection within the disc (pain provocation). The usefulness of discography remains controversial. Some clinicians routinely use discography to identify symptomatic discs prior to surgical fusion or intradiscal thermal annuloplasty, whereas others believe the test is of unproved benefit in identifying symptomatic discs (134,135). Discography remains the only test available that attempts to correlate pain response from the patient during provocation, with abnormal discs discovered on imaging studies. Improved surgical outcomes following lumbar fusion have been reported when guided by the use of discography (135–138). Intradiscal electrothermal therapy is a minimally invasive procedure that offers an alternative treatment to a subset of those patients with discogenic low back pain. Much like its use prior to fusion, discography is used to identify symptomatic intervertebral discs prior to IDET (139).

The patient with low back or neck pain originating from the vertebral disc often presents with deep, aching, axial midline pain. Pain can be referred to the buttocks and posterior thigh from lumbar discs, but does not extend to the distal extremities. Patients with discogenic pain are often young and otherwise healthy; discogenic pain is common in those with jobs that require repetitive motion of the affected spine segment (such as package handlers) or which expose the spine to excessive vibration (such as long-distance truck drivers, helicopter pilots, and jack-hammer operators). Onset of symptoms is usually gradual. Pain is experienced with prolonged sitting (sitting intolerance), standing, and bending forward. The referred pain usually remains in the proximal part of the extremity. Results of physical examination are usually nonspecific, with limited range of motion at the affected segment, or pain with movement, particularly on flexion.

Proponents of discography argue that MRI and CT reveal only nonspecific findings, such as loss of disc height and/or hydration. Jensen et al. showed that over 50% of asymptomatic patients have abnormal findings on MRI scans, in at least one intervertebral disc (140). The presence of a high-intensity zone on MRI at the posterior aspect of the disc indicates that a radial tear or fissure may be present in the annulus fibrosis, again a nonspecific finding common in those without back pain.

Treatment for discogenic pain starts with conservative therapy, including physical therapy and oral nonsteroidal anti-inflammatories (NSAIDs). In those with prolonged or disabling pain that is suspected to be of discogenic origin, provocative discography can help to identify the affected level and guide targeted therapy.

Diagnostic Lumbar Discography. Lumbar discography is a painful procedure, even when performed by the most skilled practitioners. Intravenous sedation can facilitate the procedure; however, caution must be used to avoid oversedation, which could impede ongoing communication with the patient. The patient must be able to report paresthesiae before neural injury occurs. Discography relies on the patient to report the location and severity of symptoms during provocation, thus excessive sedation can make interpretation of the results difficult (141).

The patient lies prone, with the head turned to one side. A pillow is placed under the lower abdomen, above the iliac crest, in an effort to reduce the lumbar lordosis. Asking the patient to rotate the inferior aspect of the pelvis anteriorly toward the table will tip the iliac crest posteriorly and is often key to successfully performing discography at the L5–S1 level. The C-arm is rotated 25 to 35 degrees obliquely, centered on the disc space

to be studied. The C-arm is then angled in a caudad-cephalad direction, the degree of which will vary from patient to patient, depending on the disc to be studied and each patient's degree of lumbar lordosis. In general, the L3–L4 disc lies close to the axial plane and requires no cephalad angulation to align the vertebral end plates; the L4–5 disc requires 0 to 15 degrees of cephalad angulation; and the L5–S1 disc requires 25 to 35 degrees of cephalad angulation (Figs. 44-41 and 44-42). Proper alignment of the C-arm is critical to the safety and success of discography.

The skin and subcutaneous tissues overlying the disc space where discography is to be carried out are anesthetized, and additional local anesthetic is instilled liberally as the needle is advanced. A 22-gauge, 5-inch spinal needle is placed through the skin and advanced just until it is seated in the tissues in a plane that is coaxial with the axis of the x-ray path. A 7- or 8-inch spinal needle is often required in obese patients, and is often needed at the L5–S1 level due to the long and oblique trajectory to the disc space. Without careful use of a coaxial technique throughout the entire course of needle advancement, discography will require multiple repositioning of the needle, if it can be done successfully at all. The direction of the needle should be rechecked after every 1 to 1.5 cm of needle advancement and adjusted to remain coaxial. The position of the exiting nerve root beneath the pedicle should be kept in mind at all times, and efforts to assure that the needle does not stray cephalad or lateral to the intended point over the middle of the disc will reduce the likelihood of striking the nerve root en route to the disc (Fig. 44-43).

Once the needle is in contact with the surface of the disc, a notable increase in resistance to needle placement will occur. At this point, the C-arm should be rotated to a lateral position, and the needles advanced halfway from the anterior to the posterior margin of the disc (Fig. 44-44). Proper final placement is then checked in the AP plane, where again the needle should be in the midportion of the disc space. The nucleus pulposus occupies the central one-third of the disc space, and placement of the needle tip anywhere within the nucleus should suffice. The final needle path lies just inferior to the exiting nerve root and, in many patients, it is difficult or impossible to position the needle exactly in the center of the disc.

Once the needles are in final position at all levels to be tested, provocative testing is carried out. A small volume of radiographic contrast containing antibiotic is placed at each level (<1.5 mL of iohexol 180 mg/mL containing 1 mg/mL of cefazolin). The contrast material is injected under live fluoroscopy to observe the pattern of contrast spread within the disc. As the contrast is injected, the resistance to injection is noted, and the patient is questioned about his symptoms. Some practitioners use an in-line pressure monitoring device to assure that excess pressure is not delivered during the provocative test. There is some evidence that pain reproduction using small volumes without excessive pressure during injection correlates most closely with symptomatic discogenic pain; injection under high pressure or with large volumes may well produce pain even in normal discs (142).

A concordant discogram result occurs when the patient reports his typical pattern of severe pain during injection at the level of suspected pathology and the same patient reports no pain on injection of an adjacent disc that is normal in appearance (141,143). After injection of all levels, final AP and lateral radiographs should be obtained to document the levels tested and the patterns of contrast spread during injection. Some practitioners advocate for subsequent CT scans to assess the patterns of disc disruption using axial imaging, but the usefulness of CT-discography in planning subsequent therapy is unclear.

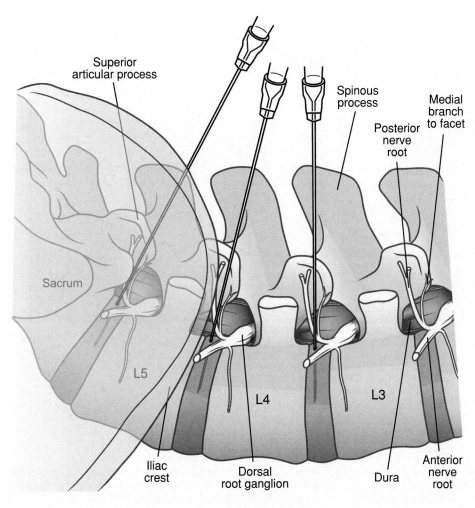

FIGURE 44-41. Anatomy of the lumbar intervertebral discs. In general, the L3–4 disc lies close to the axial plane, the L4–5 disc is angled caudally 0 to 15 degrees, and the L5–S1 disc is angled caudally 25 to 35 degrees. Needles can be safely inserted into each disc through the posterolateral aspect of the annulus fibrosis, just caudal to the exiting nerve root. From Rathmell JP. *Atlas of Image-guided Intervention in Regional Anesthesia and Pain Medicine.* Philadelphia: Lippincott Williams & Wilkins, 2006, with permission.

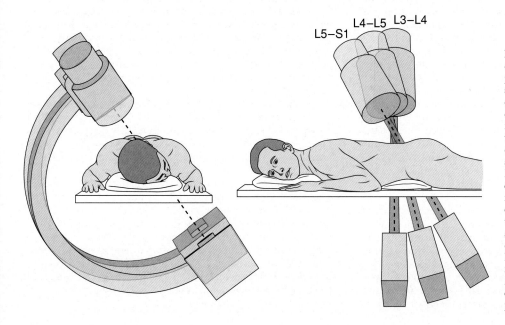

FIGURE 44-42. Position for lumbar discography. The patient is placed prone, with the head turned to one side. The C-arm is rotated 25 to 35 degrees obliquely and centered on the disc space to be studied. The C-arm is then angled in a cephalad direction that will vary from patient to patient, depending on the disc to be studied and each patient's degree of lumbar lordosis. In general, the L3–4 disc lies close to the axial plane and requires no angulation to align the vertebral end plates, the L4–5 disc requires 0 to 15 degrees of cephalad angulation, and the L5–S1 disc requires 25 to 35 degrees of cephalad angulation. From Rathmell JP. *Atlas of Image-guided Intervention in Regional Anesthesia and Pain Medicine.* Philadelphia: Lippincott Williams & Wilkins, 2006, with permission.

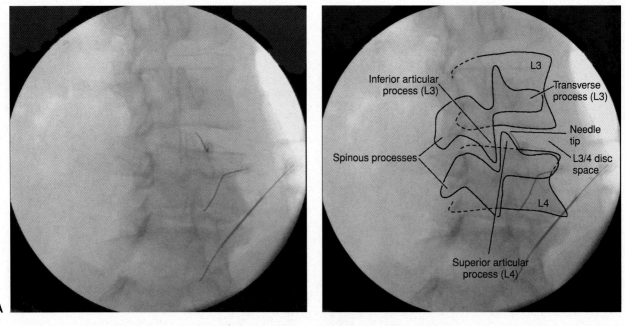

FIGURE 44-43. Oblique radiograph during lumbar discography (L3–4). **A:** The superior endplate of the L4 vertebral body is aligned with the inferior endplate of the L3 vertebral body. The junction of the L4 transverse process with the superior articular process lies just caudal to the L3–4 disc space. A needle is directed slightly superior and posterior toward the L3–4 disc space. The exiting L3 nerve root transverses inferior to the L3 pedicle and courses laterally, well superolateral to the path of the needle as it enters the disc space. **B:** Labeled figure. From Rathmell JP. *Atlas of Image-guided Intervention in Regional Anesthesia and Pain Medicine.* Philadelphia: Lippincott Williams & Wilkins, 2006, with permission.

Complications of Lumbar Discography. The majority of patients will experience a marked exacerbation of their typical back pain in the days following discography. They should be warned to expect this and given a short course of oral analgesics for treatment of the exacerbation. Less commonly, injury to the exiting nerve roots can occur. The position of the nerve roots is in close proximity to the needle's path. Care must be taken to advance the needle slowly as it passes over the transverse process en route to the posterolateral margin of the disc. If the patient reports a paresthesia to the lower extremity, the needle should be withdrawn and redirected. Paresthesia will occur in a small proportion of patients, even with good technique. Persistent paresthesiae are uncommon and typically ensue only after repeated paresthesiae occur during the procedure.

Infection can also occur, leading to abscess within the presacral musculature, but the incidence is exceedingly low. Infection within the disc space (discitis) is the most feared complication of discography and occurs with an incidence of less than 1 in 1,000 cases. Treatment of discitis may require long-term administration of IV antibiotics and/or the need for surgical removal of the infection. There have been no cases of discitis reported to date in patients who have received intradiscal antibiotics during discography. Bleeding complications have not been associated with intradiscal injection.

Intradiscal Electrothermal Therapy. The intervertebral disc is thought to contribute to pain in between 29% and 49% of patients with chronic low back pain (12). Discography has been used to select patients for surgical fusion, although the ability of discography to predict surgical outcome remains in question (144). Discography has also been used to select patients for a newer procedure called IDET, aimed at treating discogenic pain. Intradiscal electrothermal therapy employs a

steerable thermal resistance wire placed along the posterior annulus fibrosus. Thermal energy is then applied to destroy penetrating nociceptive fibers and to change the cross-linking of glucosaminoglycans, thereby stiffening the intervertebral disc (145). Clinical studies have been mixed, with two recent, high-quality RCTs: one demonstrating significant efficacy in pain reduction and improved function in about one-third of treated patients (146), while the other demonstrated no effect (147). On balance, the available literature suggests a modest overall reduction in pain and improvement in function in less than half of patients receiving IDET at a single level who have concordant discography and well-preserved disc height (148); IDET cannot be used in those with more advanced disc degeneration and significant loss of disc height. The usefulness of IDET has only been demonstrated for treating symptomatic degenerative disc disease causing chronic lumbosacral pain.

Spinal fusion has been reserved for patients with advanced disc degeneration, with clinical results varying between 46% and 82% (114,137). Patients who have early degenerative disc disease with preservation of near normal disc height (>75% of normal disc height remaining), but severe ongoing back pain that does not improve with conservative therapy, may be adequate candidates for intradiscal thermal coagulation (149). The mechanism of action of IDET is unclear, but thermal energy has been shown to coagulate neural tissue (150) and induce collagen denaturation (151), thereby addressing both nociceptive and mechanical aspects of discogenic pain (152). Early prospective studies demonstrated significant pain reduction and improvement in physical function in 30% to 50% of patients treated with IDET (149,152). However, two recent RCTs have reached conflicting conclusions when comparing IDET to placebo (153,154).

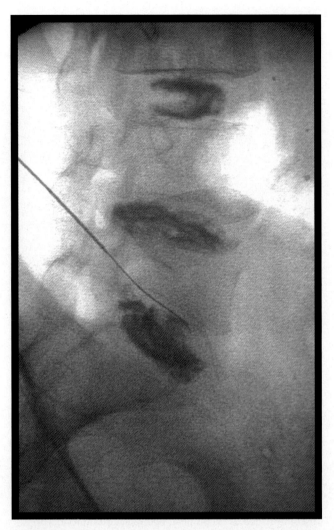

FIGURE 44-44. Lateral radiograph of the lumbar spine following lumbar discography at the L3–4, L4–5, and L5–S1 levels. Disc height is normal at the L3–4 level, markedly reduced at the L4–5 level, and minimally reduced at the L5–S1 level. The L3–4 discogram has the characteristic bilobed appearance of normal contrast spread within the nucleus pulposus, without any contrast extension into the annulus fibrosus. The L4–5 discogram has diffuse linear spread of the dye to the limits of the annulus, with posterior extension of contrast into the epidural space. The L5–S1 discogram has a small extension of contrast into the epidural space. From Tarver JM, Rathmell JP, Alsofrom GF. Lumbar discography. *Reg Anesth Pain Med* 2001;26:264, with permission.

Patients suitable for IDET present with concordant pain on discography at one or two spinal levels, and no pain during provocation of an adjacent control disc. Intradiscal electrothermal therapy makes use of a navigable thermal resistance wire that is placed percutaneously and positioned along the posterior aspect of the annulus fibrosis. Once in position, the disc is heated using a standardized protocol. Like discography, IDET is a painful procedure, even when performed by the most skilled practitioners. Intravenous sedation can facilitate the procedure, but a level of sedation that allows for ongoing communication with the patient is essential. The patient must be able to report paresthesiae or excess discomfort during the intradiscal treatment before neural injury occurs. Placement of the cannulae for

IDET is identical to that for needle placement during discography. The patient lies prone, with the head turned to one side. A pillow is placed under the lower abdomen, above the iliac crest, in an effort to reduce the lumbar lordosis. The C-arm is rotated 25 to 35 degrees obliquely, centered on the disc space to be studied. The C-arm is then angled in a caudad-cephalad direction that will vary from patient to patient, depending on the disc to be studied and their degree of lumbar lordosis.

As in discography, the L3–4 disc lies close to the axial plane and requires no cephalad angulation to align the vertebral end plates, the L4–5 disc requires 0 to 15 degrees of cephalad angulation, and the L5–S1 disc requires 25 to 35 degrees of cephalad angulation (Fig. 44-41). Proper alignment of the C-arm is critical to the safety and success of IDET. The technique for placing the cannulae through which the IDET catheter is introduced into the disc is similar to that for needle placement for discography. However, the final position of the introducer is best placed in the anterolateral aspect of the nucleus, rather than the central portion of the nucleus. This allows for a more gradual angle as the IDET catheter exits the introducer and curves around the inner aspect of the annulus (Fig. 44-45). The skin and subcutaneous tissues overlying the disc space where IDET is to be carried out are anesthetized, and additional local anesthetic is instilled liberally as the cannulae are advanced. A 17-gauge introducer supplied by the manufacturer is placed through the skin and advanced just until it is seated in the tissues in a plane that is coaxial with the axis of the x-ray path. The IDET introducer is stiff and easy to redirect and advance. The direction of the cannula should be rechecked after ever 1 to 1.5 cm of needle advancement and adjusted to remain coaxial. The position of the exiting nerve root beneath the pedicle should be kept in mind at all times, and efforts to assure that the needle does not stray cephalad or lateral to the intended point over the middle of the disc will reduce the likelihood of striking the nerve root en route to the disc.

Once the needle is in contact with the surface of the disc, a notable increase in resistance to needle placement will occur. At this point, the C-arm should be rotated to a lateral position, and the needles advanced halfway from the anterior to the posterior margin of the disc (Fig. 44-46). Proper final placement is then checked in the AP plane, where again the needle should be in the midportion of the disc space (Fig. 44-47).

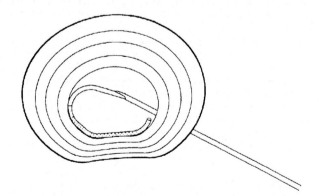

FIGURE 44-45. Axial diagram of intradiscal electrothermal therapy introducer and catheter in proper position for treatment. The introducer is placed in the anterolateral portion of the nucleus pulposus. The catheter is then threaded through the introducer and steered along the inner circumference of the annulus fibrosis until the catheter is in place along the entire posterior annular wall. From Smith & Nephew Orthopaedics, Memphis, TN, with permission.

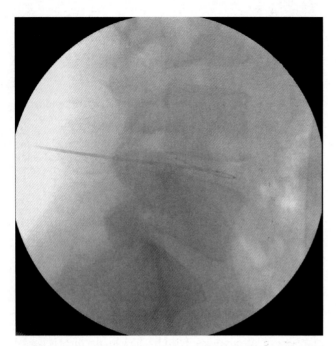

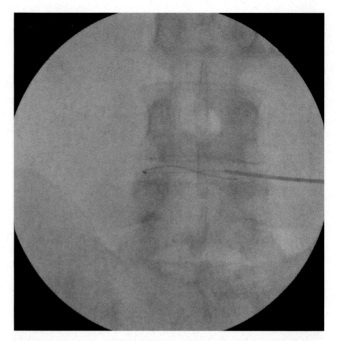

FIGURE 44-46. Lateral radiograph of the lumbar spine during initial placement of the catheter for intradiscal electrothermal therapy (IDET). After the introducer is in position, the IDET catheter is threaded initially using radiographic guidance in the lateral view. In this plane, the IDET catheter can be followed as it hugs the contralateral inner annular wall and travels toward the posterior annular wall. When the tip of the cannula reaches the posterior annular wall, it should turn toward the ipsilateral side and hug the posterior annular wall. Great care should be taken to observe the position of the catheter along the posterior annular wall because, in the presence of a significant posterior annular tear, the catheter can easily exit the disc space and enter the epidural space. From Rathmell JP. *Atlas of Image-guided Intervention in Regional Anesthesia and Pain Medicine.* Philadelphia: Lippincott Williams & Wilkins, 2006, with permission.

FIGURE 44-47. Anterior–posterior radiograph of the lumbar spine during final placement of the catheter for intradiscal electrothermal therapy (IDET). When the IDET catheter tip reaches the posterior annular wall in the lateral radiograph, the view is changed to the anterior–posterior plane before the catheter is advanced further. The catheter is then guided across the posterior annular wall until the radiographic markers extend across the entire posterior annulus. From Rathmell JP. *Atlas of Image-guided Intervention in Regional Anesthesia and Pain Medicine.* Philadelphia: Lippincott Williams & Wilkins, 2006, with permission.

Once the IDET introducer is satisfactorily positioned, the navigable thermal resistance wire (SpineCATH, Smith and Nephew) is introduced. The tip of the wire slides along the medial circumference of the annulus and can be guided by gently rotating the proximal end of the catheter. The catheter is first advanced beyond the tip of the introducer and into the disc space using lateral radiography. When the tip of the catheter passes to the posterior aspect of the annulus and begins to traverse along the posterior annulus, the C-arm is then rotated to the AP view, and the catheter is advanced into final position across the entire posterior annulus (Fig. 44-47). The catheter has two radiopaque guides that indicate the active treatment portion of the catheter, and these markers should be positioned to either side of the disc to indicate that the entire posterior annulus will be treated.

This brief description is overly simplistic; guiding the IDET catheter into final position can be quite challenging and requires delicate manipulation of the catheter to keep the tip from advancing into radial tears within the annulus. Overly aggressive handling of the catheter will cause it to kink and, once kinked, it will be difficult or impossible to steer.

Once the catheter is in final position, heat is introduced using a specific protocol designed to gradually raise the temperature within the disc to 80°C to 90°C and maintain that temperature for a minimum treatment period, typically 14 to 16 minutes. It is important that the patient is not overly se-

dated during the actual heat treatment, so that they can report discomfort due to excess heat, before neural injury occurs.

Complications of IDET. Patients should be warned of the typical postprocedural flare-up in pain symptoms that occurs after IDET. This results in an exacerbation of their typical axial back pain, often lasting several days to weeks. Less commonly, injury to the exiting nerve roots can occur. The position of the nerve roots is in close proximity to the needle's path. Care must be taken to advance the needle slowly as it passes over the transverse process en route to the posterolateral margin of the disc. If the patient reports a paresthesia to the lower extremity, the needle should be withdrawn and redirected. Paresthesia will occur in a small proportion of patients, even with good technique. Persistent paresthesiae are uncommon and typically ensue only after repeated paresthesiae occur during the procedure.

Cauda equina syndrome, with severe neuropathic pain in the lower extremities, as well as bowel and bladder dysfunction, has been reported to occur from IDET (155,156). Injury to the cauda equina is more likely to occur when there is an insufficient posterior annulus and the thermal catheter lies in close proximity to the thecal sac. The catheter can also exit the disc space to enter the epidural space; however, this should be evident on lateral radiographs before treatment. Assuring that the patient is awake enough to report excessive discomfort during the IDET treatment should reduce the chances of significant neural injury. Finally, overly aggressive handling of the IDET catheter leads to kinking of the catheter near the point where it exits the tip of the introducer within the intervertebral disc. Repeated attempts to reposition the catheter once it is kinked can lead to shearing of the catheter tip. Catheter breakage and migration of the tip has also been described (157).

A key to successful outcome following IDET is strict adherence to a structured rehabilitation program that guides the patient through gradual increases in physical activity over a 6-week to 3-month period. The rehabilitation following IDET is similar to those programs used following lumbar fusion.

Spinal Cord Simulation

Based on the theory that non-noxious input can interfere with the perception of pain, investigators developed the concept of direct activation of those ascending fibers within the dorsal columns of the spinal cord that transmit nonpainful stimuli as a means of treating chronic pain. Moderate evidence from observational trials alone suggests that spinal cord stimulation is effective, particularly in patients with chronic lumbosacral or radicular pain following prior lumbar surgery (158–160). Spinal cord stimulation appears to be most effective in patients with chronic radicular pain isolated to a single extremity, with or without radiculopathy. The majority of patients will continue to report at least 50% pain relief with ongoing use of the device 5 years after implant (160). Use of spinal cord stimulation to treat chronic, axial low back pain has been less satisfactory, but results have improved with the advent of dual-lead systems and electrode arrays that allow for a broad area of stimulation (161). Spinal cord stimulation is more effective than reoperation as a treatment for persistent radicular pain, and it can obviate the need for repeat surgery (162). Spinal cord stimulation is discussed in more detail in Chapter 41.

Intrathecal Drug Delivery

Evidence that direct application of morphine to the spinal cord could produce spinally mediated analgesia first appeared in 1976 (163). Intrathecal opioids are now widely used as useful adjuncts in the treatment of acute and chronic pain, and a number of nonopioid agents show promise as analgesic agents with spinal selectivity. The advent of small, programmable pumps that can be implanted within the subcutaneous tissues of the abdominal wall to deliver precise, continuous drug infusions via a catheter tunneled to the intrathecal space has allowed application of this technology to treat patients with chronic noncancer pain. The nondestructive nature and reversibility of intrathecal drug delivery makes this method an attractive alternative to neuroablative procedures for refractory pain. Continued improvement of catheter and pump technologies, along with physicians' willingness to combine opioids with adjuvants, contributes to the steady rise in use of this treatment modality (164). Intrathecal drug delivery is discussed in detail in Chapter 40; the purpose of this section is to briefly review the role of intrathecal drug delivery in the treatment of spinal pain.

In general, intrathecal drug delivery is reserved for patients with severe pain that does not respond to conservative treatment. An RCT comparing maximal medical therapy with intrathecal drug delivery for cancer-related pain has demonstrated improved pain control and reduction in opioid-related side effects in those who received intrathecal pain therapy (165). Although morphine is currently the only opioid approved by the U.S. Food and Drug Administration for intrathecal use, the use of other agents and combinations of agents is common and largely untested. A recent randomized trial of the novel neuron-specific calcium-channel blocker ziconotide demonstrated significant pain reduction in adults with severe chronic pain, although adverse drug-related effects were common (166). Ziconotide has now been approved.

Use of intrathecal drug delivery in noncancer pain has not been subject to controlled trials and remains controversial, but numerous observational trials suggest significant efficacy in patients with chronic pain that fails to respond to more conservative treatment (167,168). Recently, Turner et al. published a systematic review of the effectiveness and complications of intrathecal drug delivery for chronic noncancer pain (169). The majority of the patients included in this review had chronic spine-related pain, including failed back surgery syndrome. The authors concluded that the majority of patients treated with intrathecal drug delivery do achieve pain relief after initial device implantation. However, the available trials lacked any control treatment, thus the superiority of intrathecal drug delivery over any other form of treatment, including no treatment at all, cannot yet be established with certainty. In addition, the long-term efficacy of the intrathecal drug delivery therapy in improving pain and function remains unclear. Complications were common, with 27% of the patients requiring repeat surgery to revise the device, most often for replacement of a dislodged intrathecal catheter. Other cited limitations of intrathecal drug delivery include side effects from the drugs used, including endocrine dysfunction and urinary retention; catheter tip granuloma formation; the high initial cost of equipment and surgery; and failure of the therapy to show meaningful functional improvement, such as the ability to return to work (170–172).

Appropriate patient selection for intrathecal drug delivery remains critical and almost entirely empirical. Experts point to the importance of a successful trial using epidural or intrathecal administration of morphine or another agent or agents before implantation. Further controlled studies are desperately needed to define the role of intrathecal drug delivery in treating patients with chronic noncancer pain.

Epiduroscopy and Epidural Adhesiolysis

Fewer than 5% of people who experience an episode of acute back pain will go on to develop chronic low back pain (3).°Chronic low back pain can take one of several forms, the most common being chronic lumbosacral pain with or without radicular pain extending into the lower extremity (Fig. 44-1). Chronic low back pain can occur without prior lumbar surgery, take the form of persistent pain following surgery, or appear as new onset of pain following surgery. Many patients with chronic lumbosacral or radicular pain will have undergone numerous diagnostic studies, and no specific cause for the pain can be identified. In a subset of this group, MRI will reveal extensive epidural and/or periradicular scarring in the form of regions that enhance on images taken following infusion of gadolinium contrast. For this group of patients with chronic lumbosacral pain with or without radicular pain, the approach to treatment is not well established. As described earlier, the use of spinal cord stimulation has proven beneficial for many of these patients. However, a direct approach to treating epidural adhesions using a treatment termed *epidural lysis of adhesions* or *epidural adhesiolysis* has emerged in recent years.

The normal process of healing following surgical trespass of the epidural space is the ingrowth of fibrous tissue (173,174). Epidural and periradicular fibrosis can also occur in the absence of prior spinal surgery, particularly following intervertebral disc herniation (174,175). Kulisch et al. (176) performed a series of routine spinal surgeries under local anesthesia, allowing them to directly expose and stimulate various spinal structures in this group of awake patients who could then report the resulting symptoms. In many of these patients, they found one or more hyperemic spinal nerves with extensive surrounding fibrotic tissue, and direct stimulation reproduced the typical radicular pain of many of these individuals. Many investigators believe that mechanical tethering caused by epidural fibrosis may contribute to chronic lumbosacral and radicular pain in a significant subset of patients (177), and epidural adhesiolysis has been developed in an effort to directly alleviate chronic pain associated with epidural adhesions.

Epidural adhesiolysis relies on *epidurography* to identify and treat epidural adhesions. Epidurography refers to the introduction of radiographic contrast into the epidural space and the subsequent analysis of contrast flow within the epidural space on radiographs taken in multiple planes (178). Prior to the advent of CT and MRI, epidurography was used as a method to identify disc herniations, which appeared as filling defects within the ventral epidural space adjacent to the nerve root and intervertebral foramen. Epidurography is used during adhesiolysis to identify regions of epidural scarring, which appear as filling defects or barriers to free flow of contrast within the epidural space (179,180). Once epidural adhesions are identified using epidurography, the adhesions are removed by single or serial injections of solution into the epidural space. Various protocols have been tested, and there appears to be no single, best approach to performing epidural adhesiolysis. Protocols that have been subjected to RCTs have been carried out over from 1 to 3 days of treatment using solutions of normal saline or hypertonic saline with or without hyaluronidase, a common proteolytic enzyme aimed at facilitating the breakdown of fibrotic tissue. Many of the treatment protocols also place corticosteroid within the epidural space at the conclusion of treatment. The steroid solution is often directed to one or more affected spinal nerves using an epidural catheter directed to the site under fluoroscopic guidance. Alternately, *epiduroscopy* using a flexible fiberoptic scope that can be introduced directly into the epidural space, allows direct visualization and treatment of the inflamed spinal nerves following epidural adhesiolysis (179,180).

Trescott et al. (177) recently conducted a systematic review of the effectiveness and complications of epidural adhesiolysis in the management of chronic spinal pain. Currently four RCTs are available that have examined the effectiveness of this treatment. The studies are technically heterogeneous, precluding any direct comparisons, with variation in the duration of treatment between 1 and 3 days, differences in the lytic solution employed, and varying control groups (181–184). All of these studies demonstrated significant short-term (<6 months) and long-term (>6 months) improvements, with benefit typically to about half of treated patients. All studies demonstrated significant reduction in pain, and several studies showed improvements in other outcomes, including reductions in analgesic use, improvements in physical function, and higher return-to-work rates. Complications associated with epidural adhesiolysis are uncommon, but include transient sensory deficits, dural puncture with resultant subarachnoid block and/or PDPH, and infection at the skin entry site or within the epidural or subarachnoid space (177). In their systematic review, Trescott et al. (177) concluded that, in this subset of patients with chronic lumbosacral or radicular pain associated with identifiable epidural adhesions, epidural adhesiolysis may be an effective intervention.

Epiduroscopy has been used to deliver corticosteroid directly to the site of spinal nerve inflammation. Studies of epiduroscopy have been conducted in patients following epidural adhesiolysis (185), as well as in patients with acute radicular pain and no prior surgery or evidence of epidural adhesions (186). This single available RCT of endoscopic corti-

costeroid placement versus caudal epidural injection of steroid revealed no significant differences in outcome using the endoscopic technique. The single RCT of endoscopic adhesiolysis demonstrated significant improvement in both short- and long-term pain relief, as well as return-to-work rate (187). Complications specific to epiduroscopy have not been detailed separately from those associated with epidural adhesiolysis, but some investigators have hypothesized that high hydrostatic pressure within the epidural space, which may arise when excessive volumes of saline are infused, can lead to direct neural injury by compressing neural elements (188).

Mounting evidence suggests that percutaneous adhesiolysis with or without epiduroscopy may be valuable in treating a subset of patients with persistent lumbosacral and/or lumbar radicular pain associated with epidural adhesions. However, the available evidence provides little guidance on the best approach to selecting optimal patients, or the optimal technique for carrying out this treatment.

Emerging Treatments

Cytokine Inhibition and Radicular Pain Due to Herniated Nucleus Pulposus

Tumor necrosis factor (TNF)-α has been shown to be an important mediator of sciatica in animal models of disc herniation (189). Initial, uncontrolled trials of the systemic administration of the anti-TNFα agents infliximab (190) and etanercept (191) showed a beneficial effect on speeding resolution of pain and lowering the incidence of recurrent pain. However, a subsequent RCT showed no benefit of infliximab over placebo (192). Although systemic administration of anti-TNFα agents has proven disappointing, trials examining the direct periradicular infiltration of similar agents are currently under way.

Gene Therapy and Lumbosacral Pain Due to Degenerative Disc Disease

Although no single factor that leads to degenerative disc disease has been identified, progressive loss of proteoglycan within the nucleus pulposus has proven to be a characteristic factor. A number of growth factors (human transforming growth factor [TGF-β1]; tissue inhibitor of matrix metalloproteinase-1 [TIMP-1]) have been identified that are capable of upregulating the anabolism or inhibiting the catabolism of proteoglycans within isolated intervertebral disc cells (193,194). Because these factors have short elimination half-lives, direct delivery is impractical. Gene therapy using the adenoviral-mediated delivery of growth factors has proven successful in increasing proteoglycan synthesis (195,196). The idea that direct intradiscal injection of genes that encode the protein in question might be used to regenerate a more normal disc or slow the process of disc degeneration is enticing. Clinical trials in humans will undoubtedly emerge soon.

TRAINING IN INTERVENTIONAL PAIN MEDICINE

In our rapidly changing world of modern health care, new technologies are appearing at a dizzying rate. Many of these new treatments require physicians to acquire detailed new knowledge and technical skills. Interventional pain medicine is evolving as a distinct discipline that requires detailed new knowledge and expertise. Familiarity with radiographic anatomy for the conduct of image-guided injection and the minor surgical skills needed to place implanted devices such as spinal cord stimulators and implanted drug delivery systems are just a few of the techniques that practitioners must master. As we set out to introduce new interventional techniques to our own pain practices, we must assure that we have been properly trained to conduct these techniques to assure safety and success.

SUMMARY

The field of evidence-based medicine (EBM) has emerged as a new paradigm to guide practicing physicians (197). This field endeavors to educate practitioners about how to frame specific questions based on the clinical problems they are faced with every day. They then access the published scientific literature with focused questions about prevention, treatment, and diagnosis of a specific clinical condition. Many EBM centers offer concise and periodically updated summaries about specific clinical conditions. The idea is to get the best information available to the practicing clinician; EBM describes the best available evidence and, if no good evidence is available, it says so. In pain medicine, we are faced with an expanding array of treatment options that strike us as logical developments that *should* provide pain relief for our patients. However, there is a dearth of clinical evidence to guide the rational choice and application of the majority of these emerging treatments.

Merrill (198) recently presented a detailed analysis of the current state of evidence guiding the use of interventional treatments in the field of pain medicine. He points out the frequent flaws in existing studies, including the lack of valid comparators (such as no treatment) and concludes that "the practice of invasive pain medicine teeters at a particularly critical juncture . . . crippled by a lack of vigorous self-evaluation of its role in the treatment of chronic pain." Merrill goes on to detail the means by which we, as scientists and clinicians, can proceed to build a better body of evidence for the treatments we are using.

The field of pain medicine is young and in its early stage of development, and it is perhaps unreasonable to expect an accumulation of RCTs just yet. The EBM movement gives little guidance to practitioners whose tools are still under development. It simply reminds us that no evidence exists regarding many of our techniques. As individual practitioners, we must monitor our own outcomes using valid measures, be more reflective and systematic in studying our own outcomes and patterns of care, and provide this information to our patients as part of the decision-making process. As pain practitioners, we have an expanding range of treatment options available to us, few with convincing evidence of efficacy superior to alternate treatments. We must evaluate each patient and use the limited evidence available to us to guide compassionate and rational, if not evidence-based, use of therapy for our patients.

References

1. Merskey H, Bogduk N, eds. *Classification of Chronic Pain. Descriptions of Chronic Pain Syndromes and Definitions of Pain Terms*, 3rd ed. Seattle: IASP Press, 1994.
2. Hart LG, Deyo RA, Cherkin DC. Physician office visits for low back pain. *Spine* 1995;20:11–19.
3. Andersson GBJ. Epidemiological features of chronic low-back pain. *Lancet* 1999;354:581–585.
4. Peul WC, van Houwelingen HC, van den Hout WB, et al. Surgery versus prolonged conservative treatment for sciatica. *N Engl J Med* 2007;356:2245–2256.
5. Spitzer WO, LeBlanc FE, Dupuis M, et al. Scientific approach to the assessment and management of activity-related spinal disorders: A monograph for clinicians. Report of the Quebec Task Force on Spinal Disorders. *Spine* 1987;12:S1–S59.
6. Bogduk N, McGuirk B. *Pain Research and Clinical Management, Vol. 13. Medical Management of Acute and Chronic Low Back Pain: An Evidence-based Approach*. Amsterdam: Elsevier Science B.V.; 2002:19–25.
7. Pope MH, DeVocht JW. The clinical relevance of biomechanics. *Neur Clin N Amer* 1999;17:17–41.
8. Schwarzer AC, Aprill CN, Derby R, et al. The prevalence and clinical features of internal disc disruption in patients with chronic low back pain. *Spine* 1995;20:1878–1883.
9. Olmarker K. Radicular pain: Recent pathophysiologic concepts and therapeutic implications. *Schmerz* 2001;15:425–429.
10. Onesti ST. Failed back syndrome. *Neurologist* 2004;10:259–264.
11. BenDebba M, Augustus van Alphen H, Long DM. Association between peridural scar and activity-related pain after lumbar discectomy. *Neurol Res* 1999;21[Suppl 1]:S37–S42.
12. Bogduk N, McGuirk B. *Pain Research and Clinical Management, Vol. 13. Medical Management of Acute and Chronic Low Back Pain: An Evidence-based Approach*. Amsterdam: Elsevier Science; 2002:123.
13. Schwarzer AC, Aprill CN, Bogduk N. The sacroiliac joint in chronic low back pain. *Spine* 1995;20:31–37.
14. Maizels M, McCarberg B. Antidepressants and antiepileptic drugs for chronic non-cancer pain. *Am Fam Physician* 2005;71:483–490.
15. Furlan AD, Sandoval JA, Mailis-Gagnon A, Tunks E. Opioids for chronic noncancer pain: A meta-analysis of effectiveness and side effects. *Can Med Assoc J* 2006;174:1589–1594.
16. Morley-Forster PK, Clark AJ, Speechley M, Moulin DE. Attitudes toward opioid use for chronic pain: A Canadian physician survey. *Pain Res Manag* 2003;8:189–194.
17. Kalso E, Edwards JE, Moore RA, McQuay HJ. Opioids in chronic non-cancer pain: Systematic review of efficacy and safety. *Pain* 2004;112:372–380.
18. Ballantyne JC, Mao J. Opioid therapy for chronic pain. *N Engl J Med* 2003;349:1943–1953.
19. Martell BA, O'Connor PG, Kerns RD, et al. Systematic review: Opioid treatment for chronic back pain: Prevalence, efficacy, and association with addiction. *Ann Intern Med* 2007;146:116–127.
20. Michna E, Ross EL, Hynes WL, et al. Predicting aberrant drug behavior in patients treated for chronic pain: Importance of abuse history. *J Pain Symptom Manage* 2004;28:250–258.
21. Mackenzie JW. Acute pain management for opioid dependent patients. *Anaesthesia* 2006;61:907–908.
22. Mitra S, Sinatra RS. Perioperative management of acute pain in the opioid-dependent patient. *Anesthesiology* 2004;101:212–227.
23. Pud D, Cohen D, Lawental E, Eisenberg E. Opioids and abnormal pain perception: New evidence from a study of chronic opioid addicts and healthy subjects. *Drug Alcohol Depend* 2006;82:218–223.
24. Trescot AM, Boswell MV, Atluri SL, et al. Opioid guidelines in the management of chronic non-cancer pain. *Pain Physician* 2006;9:1–39.
25. Mercadante S. Opioid titration in cancer pain: A critical review. *Eur J Pain* 2007;11(8):823–830.
26. Portenoy RK, Messina J, Xie F, Peppin J. Fentanyl buccal tablet (FBT) for relief of breakthrough pain in opioid-treated patients with chronic low back pain: A randomized, placebo-controlled study. *Curr Med Res Opin* 2007;23:223–233.
27. Rauck RL, Bookbinder SA, Bunker TR, et al. A randomized, open-label study of once-a-day AVINZA (morphine sulfate extended-release capsules) versus twice-a-day OxyContin (oxycodone hydrochloride controlled-release tablets) for chronic low back pain: The extension phase of the ACTION trial. *J Opioid Manag* 2006;2:325–328, 331–333.
28. Foye PM, Sullivan WJ, Sable AW, et al. Industrial medicine and acute musculoskeletal rehabilitation. 3. Work-related musculoskeletal conditions: The role for physical therapy, occupational therapy, bracing, and modalities. *Arch Phys Med Rehabil* 2007;88[3 Suppl 1]:S147.
29. Koes B, Van Tulder M. Acute low back pain. *Am Fam Physician* 2006;74:803–805.
30. Von Korff M, Moore JE, Lorig K, et al. A randomized trial of a lay person-led self-management group intervention for back pain patients in primary care. *Spine* 1998;23:2608–2615.

31. van Tulder M, Koes B. Chronic low back pain. *Am Fam Physician* 2006; 74:1577–1579.

32. van Tulder MW, Ostelo R, Vlaeyen JWS, et al. Behavioural treatment for chronic low back pain. In: *The Cochrane Library*, Issue 4. Chichester, UK: John Wiley & Sons, Ltd., 2004.

33. Guzman J, Esmail R, Karjalainen K, et al. Multidisciplinary rehabilitation for chronic low back pain: Systematic review. *Br Med J* 2001;322:1511–1516.

34. NIH Consensus Development Panel on Acupuncture. Acupuncture. *JAMA* 1998;280:1518–1524.

35. Manheimer E, White A, Berman B, et al. Meta-analysis: Acupuncture for low back pain. *Ann Intern Med* 2005;142:651–663.

36. Ernst E, Canter PH. A systematic review of systematic reviews of spinal manipulation. *J R Soc Med* 2006;99:192–196.

37. Meeker WC, Haldeman S. Chiropractic: A profession at the crossroads of mainstream and alternative medicine. *Ann Intern Med* 2002;136:216–227.

38. Bronfort G, Haas M, Evans RL, Bouter LM. Efficacy of spinal manipulation and mobilization for low back pain and neck pain: A systematic review and best evidence synthesis. *Spine J* 2004;4:335–356.

39. Cluff R, Mehio AK, Cohen SP, et al. The technical aspects of epidural steroid injections: A national survey. *Anesth Analg* 2002;95:403–408.

40. Rathmell JP, Torian D, Song T. Lumbar epidurography. *Reg Anesth Pain Med* 2000;25:540–545.

41. Stojanovic MP, Vu TN, Caneris O, et al. The role of fluoroscopy in cervical epidural steroid injections: An analysis of contrast dispersal patterns. *Spine* 2002;27:509–514.

42. Kim KM, Kim HS, Choi KH, Ahn WS. Cephalic spreading levels after volumetric caudal epidural injections in chronic low back pain. *J Korean Med Sci* 2001;16:193–197.

43. Rathmell JP. *Atlas of Image-guided Intervention in Regional Anesthesia and Pain Medicine*. Philadelphia: Lippincott Williams and Wilkins, 2006.

44. Parke WW. Applied anatomy of the spine. In: Rothman RH, Simeone FA, eds. *The Spine*, 3rd ed. Vol. I. New York: W.B. Saunders; 1992:35–87.

45. Williams KD, Park AL. In: Canale ST, ed. *Campbell's Operative Orthopaedics*, 10th ed. St. Louis: Mosby, 2003:1955–2028.

46. Cousins MJ, Bromage PR. Epidural neural blockade. In: Cousins MJ, Bridengaugh PO, eds. *Neural Blockade*, 2nd ed. Philadelphia: Lippincott, 1988:253–360.

47. McLain RF, Kapural L, Mekhail NA. Epidural steroid therapy for back and leg pain: Mechanisms of action and efficacy. *Spine J* 2005;5:191–201.

48. Wilson-MacDonald J, Burt G, Griffin D, Glynn C. Epidural steroid injection for nerve root compression. A randomised, controlled trial. *J Bone Joint Surg Br* 2005;87:352–355.

49. Arden NK, Price C, Reading I, et al. A multicentre RCT of epidural corticosteroid injections for sciatica: The WEST study. *Rheumatology* 2005; 44:1399–1406.

50. Koes BW, Scholten RJPM, Mens JMA, et al. Epidural steroid injections for low back pain and sciatica: An updated systematic review of randomized clinical trials. *Pain Digest* 1999;9:241–247.

51. Takata K, Inoue S, Takahashi K, Ohtsuka Y. Swelling of the cauda equina in patients who have herniation of a lumbar disc: A possible pathogenesis of sciatica. *J Bone Joint Surg Am* 1988;70:36.

52. Murphy RW. Nerve roots and spinal nerves in degenerated disc disease. *Clin Orthop Related Res* 1977;129:46–60.

53. Berg A. Clinical and myelographic studies of conservatively treated cases of lumbar intervertebral disc protrusion. *Acta Chir Scand* 1953;104:124–129.

54. Lindahl O, Rexed B. Histologic changes in spinal nerve roots of operated cases of sciatica. *Acta Orthop Scand* 1950;20:215–225.

55. Marshall LL, Trethwie ER. Chemical irritation of nerve root in disc prolapse. *Lancet* 1973;2:230.

56. Saal JS, Franson R, Dobrow R, et al. High levels of inflammatory phospholipase A2 activity in lumbar disc herniation. *Spine* 1990;15:674–678.

57. Ferreira SH. Prostaglandins: Peripheral and central analgesia. In: Bonica JJ, Lindblom U, Iggo A, et al., eds. *Advances in Pain Research and Therapy*, Vol. 5. New York: Raven Press, 1983.

58. Chen C, Cavanaugh JM, Ozaktay AC, et al. Effects of phospholipase A2 on lumbar nerve root structure and function. *Spine* 1997;22:1057–1064.

59. Hayashi N, Weinstein JN, Meller ST, et al. The effect of epidural injection of betamethasone or bupivacaine in a rat model of lumbar radiculopathy. *Spine* 1998;23:877–885.

60. Fowler RJ, Blackwell GJ. Anti-inflammatory steroids induce biosynthesis of a phospholipase A2 inhibitor which prevents prostaglandin generation. *Nature* 1979;278:456–459.

61. Granstrom E. Biochemistry of the prostaglandins, thromboxanes, and leukotrienes. In: Bonica JJ, Lindblom U, Iggo A, eds. *Advances in Pain Research and Therapy*, Vol. 5. New York: Raven Press, 1983.

62. Devor M, Govrin-Lippmann R, Raber P. Corticosteroids suppress ectopic neural discharge originating in experimental neuromas. *Pain* 1985;22:127.

63. Johansson A, Hao J, Sjölund B. Local corticosteroid application blocks transmission in normal nociceptive C fibers. *Acta Anaesthesiol Scand* 1990;34:335.

64. Koes BW, Scholten RJPM, Mens JMA, Bouter LM. Efficacy of epidural steroid injections for low-back pain and sciatica: A systematic review of randomized clinical trials. *Pain* 1995;63:279–288.

65. Watts RW, Silagy CA. A meta-analysis on the efficacy of epidural corticosteroids in the treatment of sciatica. *Anaesth Intensive Care* 1995;23:564–569.

66. Nelemans PJ, de RA Bie, de HCW Vet, Sturmans F. Injection therapy for subacute and chronic benign low-back pain. *Cochrane Database Syst Rev* 1999, Issue 4. Art No.:CD001824.

67. Buchner M, Zeifang F, Brocai DRC, Schiltenwolf M. Epidural corticosteroid injection in the conservative management of sciatica. *Clin Orthop Relat Res* 2000;375:149–156.

68. Wilson-MasDinald J, Burt J, Griffin D, Glynn C. Epidural steroid injection for nerve root compression. A randomized, controlled trial. *J Bone Joint Surg Br* 2005;87B:352–355.

69. Arden NK, Proce C, Reading I, et al. A multicentre randomized controlled trial of epidural corticosteroid injections for sciatica: The WEST study. *Rheumatology* 2005;44:1399–1406.

70. Carrette S, Leclaire R, Marcoux S, et al. Epidural corticosteroid injections for sciatica due to herniated nucleus pulposus. *New Engl J Med* 1997;336:1634–1640.

71. Thomas E, Cyteval C, Abiad L, et al. Efficacy of transforaminal versus interspinous corticosteroid injection in discal radiculalgia: A prospective, randomised, double-blind study. *Clin Rheumatol* 2003;22:299–304.

72. Young IA, Hyman GS, Packia-Raj LN, Cole AJ. The use of lumbar epidural/transforaminal steroids for managing spinal disease. *J Am Acad Orthop Surg* 2007;15(4):228–238.

73. Armon C, Argoff CE, Samuels J, Backonja MM. Therapeutics and Technology Assessment Subcommittee of the American Academy of Neurology. Assessment: Use of epidural steroid injections to treat radicular lumbosacral pain: Report of the Therapeutics and Technology Assessment Subcommittee of the American Academy of Neurology. *Neurology* 2007;68(10):723–729.

74. Green PW, Burke AJ, Weiss CA, Langan P. The role of epidural cortisone injection in the treatment of diskogenic low back pain. *Clin Orthop Relat Res* 1980;153:121–125.

75. Arnhoff FN, Triplett HB, Pokorney B. Follow up status of patients treated with nerve blocks for low back pain. *Anesthesiology* 1977;46:170–178.

76. Yates DW. A comparison of the types of epidural injection commonly used in the treatment of low back pain and sciatica. *Rheumatol Rehab* 1978;17:181–186.

77. *Physicians' Desk Reference*, 57th ed. 2003;2733–2735.

78. *Physicians' Desk Reference*, 57th ed. 2003;1367–1368.

79. Kepes ER, Duncalf D. Treatment of backache with spinal injections of local anesthetics, spinal and systemic steroids. A review. *Pain* 1985;22:33–47.

80. Delaney TJ, Rowlingson JC, Carron H, et al. Epidural steroid effects on nerves and meninges. *Anesth Analg* 1980;59:610–614.

81. Benzon HT, Gissen AJ, Strichartz GR, et al. The effect of polyethylene glycol on mammalian nerve impulses. *Anesth Analg* 1987;66:553–559.

82. Wood KM, Arguelles J, Noremberg MD. Degenerative lesions in rat sciatic nerves after local injections of methylprednisolone in aqueous solution. *Reg Anesth* 1980;5:13–15.

83. Brown FW. Management of diskogenic pain using epidural and intrathecal steroids. *Clin Orthop Relat Res* 1977;129:72–78.

84. Heyse-Moore GH. A rational approach to the use of epidural medication in the treatment of sciatic pain. *Acta Orthop Scand* 1978;49:366–370.

85. Buchner M, Zeifang F, Brocai DR, Schiltenwolf M. Epidural corticosteroid injection in the conservative management of sciatica. *Clin Orthop Relat Res* 2000;375:149–156.

86. Kelman H. Epidural injection therapy for sciatic pain. *Am J Surg* 1944; 64:183–190.

87. Cohn ML, Huntington CT, Byrd SE, et al. Epidural morphine and methylprednisolone. New therapy for recurrent low back pain. *Spine* 1986;11:960–963.

88. Dallas TI, Lin RL, Wu WH, et al. Epidural morphine and methylprednisolone for low-back pain. *Anesthesiology* 1987;67:408–411.

89. Dilke TF, Burry HC, Grahame R. Extradural corticosteroid injection in management of lumbar nerve root compression. *Br Med J* 1973;2:635–637.

90. White AH, Derby R, Wynne G. Epidural injections for the diagnosis and treatment of low back pain. *Spine* 1980;5:78–86.

91. Benzon HT, Braunschweig R, Molloy RE. Delayed onset of epidural anesthesia in patients with back pain. *Anesth Analg* 1981;60:874–877.

92. Jacobs S, Pullan PT, Potter JM, Shenfield GM. Adrenal suppression following extradural steroids. *Anaesthesia* 1983;38:953–956.

93. McMahon M, Gerich J, Rizza R. Effects of glucocorticoids on carbohydrate metabolism. *Diabetes Metab Rev* 1988;4:17–30.

94. Kay J. Epidural triamcinolone suppresses the pituitary-adrenal axis in human subjects. [Abstract]. *Anesth Analg* 1994;79(3):501–505.

95. Ward A, Watson P, Wood C, et al. Glucocorticoid epidural for sciatica: Metabolic and endocrine sequelae. *Rheumatology* 2002;41:68–71.

96. Sharrock NE, Urquhart B, Mineo R. Extradural anaesthesia in patients with previous lumbar spine surgery. *Br J Anaesth* 1990;65:237–239.

97. Bartynski WS, Grahovac SZ, Rothfus WE. Incorrect needle position during lumbar epidural steroid administration: Inaccuracy of loss of air pressure resistance and requirement of fluoroscopy and epidurography during needle insertion. *AJNR Am J Neuroradiol* 2005;26:502–505.

98. Reynolds F. Dural puncture and headache. *Br Med J* 1993;306:874–876.

99. Abouleish E, Vega S, Blendinger I, Tio TO. Long-term follow-up of epidural blood patch. *Anesth Analg* 1975;54:459–463.

100. Neal, Joseph M. Neurologic complications. In: Rathmell JP, Neal JM, Viscomi CM, eds. *Regional Anesthesia: The Requisites in Anesthesiology.* Philadelphia, PA: Elsevier Mosby, 2004.

101. Hodges SD, Castleberg RL, Miller T, et al. Cervical epidural steroid injection with intrinsic spinal cord damage: Two case reports. *Spine* 1998;23:2137–2142.

102. Bromage, PR, Benumof JL. Paraplegia following intracord injection during attempted epidural anesthesia under general anesthesia. *Reg Anesth Pain Med* 1998;23:104–107.

103. Abram SE, O'Connor TC. Complications associated with epidural steroid injection. *Reg Anesth* 1996;21:149–162.

104. Field J, Rathmell JP, Stephenson JH, Katz NP. Neuropathic pain following cervical epidural steroid injection. *Anesthesiology* 2000;93(3):885–888.

105. Horlocker TT, Wedel DJ, Benzon H, et al. Regional anesthesia in the anticoagulated patient: Defining the risks. (The second ASRA consensus conference on neuraxial anesthesia and anticoagulation). *Reg Anesth Pain Med* 2003;28(3):172–197.

106. Rathmell JP, Benzon HT. Transforaminal injections of steroids: Should we continue? *Reg Anesth Pain Med* 2004;29(5):397–399.

107. Kozody R, Ready LB, Barsa JE, Murphy TM. Dose requirement of local anaesthetic to produce grand mal seizure during stellate ganglion block. *Can Anaesth Soc J* 1982;29(5):489–491.

108. Finn KP, Case JL. Disk entry: A complication of transforaminal epidural injection: A case report. *Arch Phys Med Rehabil* 2005;86(7):1489–1491.

109. Cohen SP, Raja SN. Pathogenesis, diagnosis, and treatment of lumbar zygapophysial (facet) joint pain. *Anesthesiology* 2007;106:1–21.

110. Guerts JW, van Wijk RM, Stolker RJ, Groen GJ. Efficacy of radiofrequency procedures for the treatment of spinal pain: A systematic review of randomized clinical trials. *Reg Anesth Pain Med* 2001;26:394–400.

111. Schofferman J, Kine G. Effectiveness of repeated radiofrequency neurotomy for lumbar facet pain. *Spine* 2004;29:2471–2473.

112. Carette S, Marcoux S, Truchon R, et al. A controlled trial of corticosteroid injections into facet joints for chronic low back pain. *N Engl J Med* 1991;325:1002–1007.

113. Lilius G, Harilainen A, Laasonen EM, et al. Chronic unilateral low back pain: Predictors of outcome of facet joint injection. *Spine* 1990;15:780–782.

114. Thomsen K, Christensen FB, Eiskjaer SP, et al. 1997 Volvo award winner in clinical studies. The effect of pedicle screw instrumentation on functional outcome and fusion rates on posterolateral spinal fusion: A prospective, randomized clinical study. *Spine* 1997;22(24):2813–2822.

115. Nelemans PJ, deBie RA, deVet HC, Sturmans F. Injection therapy for subacute and chronic benign low back pain. *Spine* 2001;26(5):501–515.

116. Dreyfuss P, Tibiletti C, Dreyer S. Thoracic zygapophyseal joint pain patterns. *Spine* 1994;19:807–811.

117. Boas RA. Facet joint injections. In: Stanton-Hicks MA, Boas RA, eds. *Chronic Low Back Pain.* New York: Raven Press, 1982.

118. Bogduk N, Marsland A. The cervical zygapophysial joints as a source of neck pain. *Spine* 1988;13:610–617.

119. Resnick DK, Choudhri TF, Dailey AT, et al. Guidelines for the performance of fusion procedures for degenerative disease of the lumbar spine. Part 13: Injection therapies, low-back pain, and lumbar fusion. *J Neurosurg Spine* 2005;2(6):707–715.

120. Marks RC, Houston T, Thulbourne T. Facet joint injection and facet nerve block: A randomised comparison in 86 patients with chronic low back pain. *Pain* 1992;49:325–328.

121. Gallagher J, Petriccione di Vadi PL, Wedley JR, et al. Radiofrequency facet joint denervation in the treatment of low back pain: A prospective controlled double-blind study to assess its efficacy. *Pain Clin* 1994;7:193–198.

122. Van Kleef M, Barendse GAM, Kessels A, et al. Randomized trial of radiofrequency lumbar facet denervation for chronic low back pain. *Spine* 1999;24:1937–1942.

123. Orpen NM, Birch NC. Delayed presentation of septic arthritis of a lumbar facet joint after diagnostic facet joint injection. *J Spinal Disord Tech* 2003;16(3):285–287.

124. Alberts W, Wright E, Feinstein B, von Bonin G. Experimental radiofrequency brain lesion size as a function of physical parameters. *J Neurosurg* 1966;25:421–423.

125. Vinas FC, Zamorano L, Dujovny M, et al. Vivo and in vitro study of lesions produced with a computerized radiofrequency system. *Stereotactic Funct Neurosurg* 1992;58:121–133.

126. Dieckman G, Gabriel E, Hassler R. Size, form and structural peculiarities of experimental brain lesions obtained by thermocontrolled radiofrequency. *Confin Neurol* 1965;26:134–142.

127. Sluijter ME, Cosmas ER, Ritman WB 3rd. Characteristics and mode of action of pulsed radiofrequency fields applied to the dorsal root ganglion: A preliminary report. *Pain Clin* 1998;11:109–117.

128. Van Zundert J, de Louw AJA, Joosten EA, et al. Pulsed and continuous radiofrequency current adjacent to the cervical dorsal root ganglion of the rat induces late cellular activity in the dorsal horn. *Anesthesiology* 2005;102:125–131.

129. Richebe P, Rathmell JP, Brennan TJ. Immediate early genes after pulsed radiofrequency treatment: Neurobiology in need of clinical trials. *Anesthesiology* 2005;102(1):1–3.

130. Cohen SP. Sacroiliac joint pain: A comprehensive review of anatomy, diagnosis, and treatment. *Anesth Analg* 2005;101:1440–1453.

131. Maigne JY, Aivaliklis A, Pfefer F. Results of sacroiliac joint double block and value of sacroiliac pain provocation tests in 54 patients with low back pain. *Spine* 1996;21:1889–1892.

132. Hansen HC, McKenzie-Brown AM, Cohen SP, et al. Sacroiliac joint interventions: A systematic review. *Pain Physician* 2007;10:165–184.

133. Dreyfuss P, Dryer S, Griffin J, et al. Positive sacroiliac screening tests in asymptomatic adults. *Spine* 1994;19:1138–1143.

134. Tehranzadeh J. Discography 2000. *Radiol Cllin North Am* 1998;36:463–495.

135. Whitecloud TS 3rd, Seago RA. Cervical discogenic syndrome. Results of operative intervention in patients with positive discography. *Spine* 1987;12:313–316.

136. Colhoun E, McCall IW, Williams L, et al. Provocation discography as a guide to planning operations on the spine. *J Bone Joint Surg* 1988;70:267–271.

137. Wetzel FT, LaRocca SH, Lowery GL, Aprill CN. The treatment of lumbar spinal pain syndromes diagnosed by discography. Lumbar arthrodesis. *Spine* 1994;19:792–800.

138. Derby R, Howard MW, Grant JM, et al. The ability of pressure-controlled discography to predict surgical and non-surgical outcomes. *Spine* 1999;24:364–372.

139. Cohen SP, Larkin TM, Barna SA, et al. Lumbar discography: A comprehensive review of outcome studies, diagnostic accuracy and principles. *Reg Anesth Pain Med* 2005;30(2):163–183.

140. Jensen MC, BrantZawadzki MN, Obuchowski N, et al. Magnetic resonance imaging of the lumbar spine in people without back pain. *N Engl J Med* 1994;331:69–73.

141. Tarver JM, Rathmell JP, Alsofrom GF. Lumbar discography. *Reg Anesth Pain Med* 2001;26(3):263–266.

142. Cohen SP, Larkin TM, Barna SA, et al. Lumbar discography: A comprehensive review of outcome studies, diagnostic accuracy, and principles. *Reg Anesth Pain Med* 2005;30:163–183.

143. Anderson MW. Lumbar discography: An update. *Semin Roentgenol* 2004;39(1):52–67.

144. Carragee EJ, Lincoln T, Parmar VS, Alamin T. A gold standard evaluation of the "discogenic pain" diagnosis as determined by provocative discography. *Spine* 2006;31:2115–2123.

145. Freeman BJ, Walters RM, Moore RJ, Fraser RD. Does intradiscal electrothermal therapy denervate and repair experimentally induced annular tears in an animal model? *Spine* 2003;28:2602–2608.

146. Pauza KJ, Howell S, Dreyfuss P, et al. A randomized, placebo-controlled trial of intradiscal electrothermal therapy for the treatment of discogenic low back pain. *Spine J* 2004;4:27–35.

147. Freeman BJ, Fraser RD, Cain CM, et al. A randomized, double-blind, controlled trial: Intradiscal electrothermal therapy versus placebo for the treatment of chronic discogenic low back pain. *Spine* 2005;30:2369–2377.

148. Appleby D, Andersson G, Totta M. Meta-analysis of the efficacy and safety of intradiscal electrothermal therapy (IDET). *Pain Med* 2006;7:308–316.

149. Saal JS, Saal JA. Management of chronic discogenic low back pain with a thermal intradiscal catheter: A preliminary report. *Spine* 2000;25:382–388.

150. Letcher F, Foldring S. The effect of radiofrequency current and heat on peripheral nerve action potential in the cat. *J Neurosurg* 1968;29:42–47.

151. Shah RV, Lutz GE, Lee J, et al. Intradiscal electrothermal therapy: A preliminary histological study. *Arch Phys Med Rehabil* 2001;82:1230–1237.

152. Saal JA, Saal JS. Intradiscal electrothermal therapy for the treatment of chronic discogenic low back pain. *Operative Tech Orthop* 2000;10:271–281.

153. Freeman BJ, Fraser RD, Cain CM, et al. A randomized, double blind controlled trial: Intradiscal electrothermal therapy (IDET) versus placebo for the treatment of chronic discogenic low back pain. *Spine* 2005;30(21):2369–2377.

154. Pauza KJ, Howell S, Dreyfuss P, et al. A randomized, placebo controlled trial of intradiscal electrothermal therapy for the treatment of discogenic low back pain. *Spine J* 2004;4(1):27–35.

155. Hsui A, Isaac K, Katz J. Cauda equine syndrome from intradiscal electrothermal therapy. *Neurology* 2000;55:320.

156. Wetzel FT. Cauda equine syndrome from intradiscal electrothermal therapy. *Neurology* 2001;56:1607.

157. Orr RD, Thomas SA. Intradural migration of broken IDET catheter causing a radiculopathy. *J Spinal Disord Tech* 2005;18(2):185–187.

158. Taylor RS, Van Buyten JP, Buchser E. Spinal cord stimulation for chronic back and leg pain and failed back surgery syndrome: A systematic review and analysis of prognostic factors. *Spine* 2005;30:152–160.

159. Mailis-Gagnon A, Furlan AD, Sandoval JA, Taylor R. Spinal cord stimulation for chronic pain. *Cochrane Database Syst Rev* 2004;3:CD003783.

160. Turner JA, Loeser JD, Deyo RA, Sanders SB. Spinal cord stimulation for patients with failed back surgery syndrome or complex regional pain syndrome: a systematic review of effectiveness and complications. *Pain* 2004;108:137–147.

161. North RB, Kidd DH, Olin J, et al. Spinal cord stimulation for axial low back pain: A prospective, controlled trial comparing dual with single percutaneous electrodes. *Spine* 2005;30:1412–1418.

162. North RB, Kidd DH, Farrokhi F, Piantadosi SA. Spinal cord stimulation versus repeated lumbosacral spine surgery for chronic pain: A randomized, controlled trial. *Neurosurgery* 2005;56:98–106.

163. Yaksh TL, Rudy TA. Analgesia mediated by a direct spinal action of narcotics. *Science* 1976;192:1357–1358.

164. Hassenbusch SJ, Portenoy RK, Cousins M, Buchser E, et al. Polyanalgesic consensus conference 2003: An update on the management of pain by intraspinal drug delivery: Report of an expert panel. *J Pain Symptom Manage* 2004;27:540–563.

165. Smith TJ, Coyne PJ, Staats PS, et al. An implantable drug delivery system (IDDS) for refractory cancer pain provides sustained pain control, less drug-related toxicity, and possibly better survival compared with comprehensive medical management (CMM). *Ann Oncol* 2005;16:825–833.

166. Rauck RL, Wallace MS, Leong MS, et al. Ziconotide 301 Study Group. A randomized, double-blind, placebo-controlled study of intrathecal ziconotide in adults with severe chronic pain. *J Pain Symptom Manage* 2006;31:393–406.

167. Prager JP. Neuraxial medication delivery: The development and maturity of a concept for treating chronic pain of spinal origin. *Spine* 2002;27:2593–2605.

168. Turner JA, Sears JM, Loeser JD. Programmable intrathecal opioid delivery systems for chronic noncancer pain: A systematic review of effectiveness and complications. *Clin J Pain* 2007;23:180–195.

169. Turner JA, Sears JM, Loeser JD. Programable intrathecal opioid delivery systems for chronic noncancer pain: A systemic review of effectiveness and complications. *Clin J Pain* 2007;23:180–195.

170. Anderson VC, Burchiel KJ. A prospective study of long-term intrathecal morphine in the management of chronic nonmalignant pain. *Neurosurgery* 1999;44:289–300.

171. Winkelmuller M, Winkelmuller W. Long-term effects of continuous intrathecal opioid treatment in chronic pain of nonmalignant etiology. *J Neurosurg* 1996;85:458–467.

172. Miele VJ, Price KO, Bloomfield S, et al. A review of intrathecal morphine therapy related granulomas. *Eur J Pain* 2006;10:251–261.

173. LaRocca H, McNab I. The laminectomy membrane. Studies in its evolution, characteristics, effects and prophylaxis in dogs. *J Bone Joint Surg Br* 1974;56B:545–550.

174. McCarron RF, Wimpee MW, Hudkins PG, Laros GS. The inflammatory effect of nucleus pulposus. A possible element in the pathogenesis of low-back pain. *Spine* 1987;12:760–764.

175. Cooper RG, Freemont AJ, Hoyland JA, et al. Herniated intervertebral disc-associated periradicular fibrosis and vascular abnormalities occur without inflammatory cell infiltration. *Spine* 1995;20:591–598.

176. Kuslich SD, Ulstrom CL, Michael CJ. The tissue origin of low back pain and sciatica: A report of pain response to tissue stimulation during operations on the lumbar spine using local anesthesia. *Orthop Clin North Am* 1991;22:181–187.

177. Trescot AM, Chopra P, Abdi S, et al. Systematic review of effectiveness and complications of adhesiolysis in the management of chronic spinal pain: An update. *Pain Physician* 2007;10:129–146.

178. Rathmell JP, Song T, Torian D, Alsofrom GF. Lumbar epidurography. *Reg Anesth Pain Med* 2000;25:540–545.

179. Manchikanti L, Bakhit CE. Percutaneous lysis of epidural adhesions. *Pain Physician* 2000;3:46–64.

180. Viesca CO, Racz GB, Day MR. Special techniques in pain management: Lysis of adhesions. *Anesthesiol Clin North America* 2003;21:745–766.

181. Veihelmann A, Devens C, Trouillier H, et al. Epidural neuroplasty versus physiotherapy to relieve pain in patients with sciatica: A prospective randomized blinded clinical trial. *J Orthop Sci* 2006;11:365–369.

182. Heavner JE, Racz GB, Raj P. Percutaneous epidural neuroplasty: Prospective evaluation of 0.9% NaCl versus 10% NaCl with or without hyaluronidase. *Reg Anesth Pain Med* 1999;24:202–207.

183. Manchikanti L, Pampati V, Fellows B, et al. Role of one day epidural adhesiolysis in management of chronic low back pain: A randomized clinical trial. *Pain Physician* 2001;4:153–166.

184. Manchikanti L, Rivera JJ, Pampati V, et al. One day lumbar epidural adhesiolysis and hypertonic saline neurolysis in treatment of chronic low back pain: A randomized, double-blind trial. *Pain Physician* 2004;7:177–186.

185. Manchikanti L, Pampati V, Bakhit CE, Pakanati RR. Non-endoscopic and endoscopic adhesiolysis in post-lumbar laminectomy syndrome: A one-year outcome study and cost effectiveness analysis. *Pain Physician* 1999;2:52–58.

186. Dashfield AK, Taylor MB, Cleaver JS, Farrow D. Comparison of caudal steroid epidural with targeted steroid placement during spinal endoscopy for chronic sciatica: A prospective, randomized, double-blind trial. *Br J Anaesth* 2005;94:514–519.

187. Manchikanti L, Boswell MV, Rivera JJ, et al. A randomized, controlled trial of spinal endoscopic adhesiolysis in chronic refractory low back and lower extremity pain. *BMC Anesthesiol* 2005;5:10.

188. Racz GB, Haevner JE. Complications associated with lysis of epidural adhesions and epiduroscopy. In: Neal JM, Rathmell JP, eds. *Complications in Regional Anesthesia and Pain Medicine*. Philadelphia: Saunders Elsevier; 2007:301–312.

189. Igarashi T, Kikuchi S, Shubayev V, et al. Exogenous tumor necrosis factor alpha mimics nucleus pulposus-induced neuropathology: Molecular, histologic, and behavioral comparisons in rats. *Spine* 2000;5:2975–2980.

190. Karppinen J, Korhonen T, Malmivaara A, et al. Tumor necrosis factor-alpha monoclonal antibody, infliximab, used to manage severe sciatica. *Spine* 2003;28:750–753.

191. Genevay S, Stingelin S, Gabay C. Efficacy of etanercept in the treatment of acute and severe sciatica: A pilot study. *Ann Rheum Dis* 2004;63:1120–1123.

192. Korhonen T, Karppinen J, Paimela L, et al. The treatment of disc-herniation-induced sciatica with infliximab: One-year follow-up results of FIRST II, a RCT. *Spine* 2006;31:2759–2766.

193. Thompson JP, Oegema TR Jr., Bradford DS. Stimulation of mature canine intervertebral disc by growth factors. *Spine* 1991;16:253–260.

194. Nagase H, Woessner JF Jr. Matrix metalloproteinases. *J Biol Chem* 1999;274:21491–21494.

195. Nishida K, Kang JD, Gilbertson LG, et al. Modulation of the biologic activity of the rabbit intervertebral disc by gene therapy: An in vivo study of adenovirus-mediated transfer of the human transforming growth factor beta 1 encoding gene. *Spine* 1999;24:2419–2425.

196. Wallach CJ, Sobajima S, Watanabe Y, et al. Gene transfer of the catabolic inhibitor TIMP-1 increases measured proteoglycans in cells from degenerated human intervertebral discs. *Spine* 2003;28:2331–2337.

197. Rathmell JP, Carr DB. The scientific method, evidence-based medicine, and rational use of interventional pain treatments. *Reg Anesth Pain Med* 2003;28:498–501.

198. Merrill DG. Hoffman's glasses: Evidence-based medicine and the search for quality in the literature of interventional pain medicine. *Reg Anesth Pain Med* 2003;28:547–560.

CHAPTER 45 ■ TREATMENT OF CANCER PAIN: ROLE OF NEURAL BLOCKADE AND NEUROMODULATION

ALLEN W. BURTON, PHILLIP C. PHAN, AND MICHAEL J. COUSINS

EPIDEMIOLOGY

Cancer

Almost 1.4 million Americans were newly diagnosed with cancer in 2004, approximately 4,000 per day (1). In the same year, 564,000 U.S. deaths were attributed to cancer, about 22% of all deaths. It is estimated that over 10 million people in the United States are living with cancer at present, around 3% of the population. The demographic of cancer continues to slowly evolve with the overall number of cases slowly trending upward, and the number of long-term survivors, including those with chronic pain issues, continuing to grow (2).

Cancer Pain and Related Symptom Burden

The diagnosis of cancer is distressing to the patient in many ways. First, the patient fears that cancer will shorten his life. Second, the patient is apprehensive that the cancer will bring with its progression significant pain and suffering. Indeed, pain is already experienced by 20% to 50% of cancer patients initially at time of diagnosis. With cancer progression, 75% of patients with advanced cancer will experience pain (3). Up to 80% of cancer patients described their pain as having moderate to severe intensity.

According to the World Health Organization (WHO), an estimated 6.6 million people worldwide die from cancer every year (4). Recent WHO studies pointed out that cancer-related pain continued to be a significant source of global health concern. With advances in therapeutic modalities, about 80% of cancer pain can be controlled easily (5). Unfortunately, even with these advances, cancer pain remains widely undertreated even in developed countries (6). In the United States, the reasons for undertreatment of cancer pain are complex and encompasses many barriers, as outlined in Table 45-1.

Recently, there is a growing awareness that pain control is an essential part of comprehensive cancer care. Some studies have showed a direct correlation between good pain control and cancer patient's length of survival, as well as responsiveness to timely oncologic treatment (7,8). In addition to problems stemming from immobility (deep venous thrombosis, pneumonia), uncontrolled pain has also proven to be major risk factor in cancer-related suicides (9,10). Further, issues of long-term survival with increasing treatment options prolonging survival add to the complexity of care required. The landscape of "cancer pain" is shifting quickly into a chronic pain situation in many instances, thereby blurring previous lines of distinction in treatment strategies most suited for "noncancer" versus "cancer" pain (2).

ASSESSMENT

Pain is always subjective and is experienced only by the patient. Because of the subjective nature of pain, versus an objectively measurable parameter such as blood pressure or tumor size, much research has been directed toward accurate measurement of pain *and* correlation with interference in activities. Over the past 20 years, the assessment of pain has been the subject of much research and refinement of techniques and instruments (see Chapters 37–38 and 46–49). A cursory review is presented in this section; the reader is directed to the references cited for more details on the assessment of cancer pain. In addition to evaluating the pain symptom, the physician has to focus on a myriad of related symptoms. The cancer patient often experiences fatigue, insomnia, depression, anxiety, somnolence, and even cognitive impairment. Increasingly, certain symptoms are thought to cluster, perhaps related to alterations in cytokine levels, and new research is focused in this area. The psychological symptoms, such as anxiety and depression, are deeply intertwined with, and can often have a large impact on, the patient's perception and expression of pain. Furthermore, the patient can develop symptoms such as nausea, vomiting, and headaches as side effects of therapeutic intervention. The cancer patient thus commonly presents with a constellation of symptoms that have profound impact on the patient's psychological well-being, functional status, and quality of life.

Screening Instruments

Many pain clinics utilize a questionnaire to aid in and standardize assessment.

Brief Pain Inventory

The Wisconsin Brief Pain Inventory (BPI) and Memorial pain assessment card are well-accepted and standard tools for evaluating cancer pain (11,12). At The University of Texas MD Anderson Cancer Center, an institutionally approved MD Anderson questionnaire (modified BPI) is used for initial and follow-up assessment of patients (Fig. 45-1).

TABLE 45-1

BARRIERS TO EFFECTIVE CANCER PAIN CONTROL

I. Barriers by health care providers
 A. Inadequate assessment by physicians
 B. Lack of knowledge regarding current treatments by providers
 C. Outdated beliefs by practitioners
  1. Cancer pain expected with disease progression
  2. Opioids prescribed only for dying patients
  3. Patient's pain complaints unreliable
 D. Reluctance to prescribe opioids by physicians
  1. Fear of regulatory controls
  2. Fear of increasing liability for over-prescribing
  3. Increased work and effort for opioid management
II. Patient and family-related barriers
 A. Fear of developing addiction to "narcotics"
 B. Reluctance to discuss pain with physician
 C. Fear of acknowledging pain as disease progression
III. Barriers from health care system
 A. Lack of coordination for effective treatment of pain
 B. Inadequate resources for dedicated pain treatment

Advantages to the Wisconsin Brief Pain Inventory (BPI) include the following:

■ 15-minute questionnaire, which can be self-administered
■ Includes several questions about the characteristics of the pain and associated symptoms, including its origin and the effects of prior treatments
■ It incorporates two valuable features of the McGill Pain Questionnaire, a graphic representation of the location of pain and groups of qualitative descriptors. Severity of pain is assessed by a series of 0 to 10 scales (11-point numerical rating scales or NRS) that score pain at its best, worst, and on average. The perceived level of interference with normal function (on several measures including fatigue, nausea, depression, anxiety, drowsiness, difficulty thinking clearly, shortness of breath, poor appetite, insomnia, and overall feeling of well-being) is quantified with a NRS also.
■ Consistent evidence suggests that the BPI is cross-culturally valid and is useful, particularly when patients are not fit to complete a more thorough or comprehensive questionnaire (13,14). Further evidence shows its validity and usefulness in documenting outcomes and health status of noncancer pain patients (15).

Pediatric Cancer Pain Assessment

This complex topic is beyond the scope of this chapter, but pain assessment in the child should be undertaken in an age-appropriate manner, using the proper tool. Examples of pediatric assessment tools include Beyer's The Oucher, Eland's color scale-body outline, Hester's poker chip tool, McGrath's faces scale, and others (16) (see Chapter 47).

Pain History

Objective observations of grimacing, limping, and vital signs (tachycardia) may be useful in assessing the patient, but these signs are often absent in patients with chronic pain (see Chapter 37). Pain evaluation should be integrated with a detailed oncologic, medical, and psychological history. The initial eval-

uation should include evaluation of the patient's feelings and attitudes about the pain and disease, family concerns, and the premorbid psychological history. A comprehensive but objective approach to assessment instills confidence in the patient and family that will be valuable throughout treatment.

A comprehensive evaluation of the patients with cancer pain includes the following:

■ *Primary complaint.* The chief complaint is obtained to ensure appropriate triage (i.e., a patient with severe pain due to a bowel obstruction may need to be sent to the emergency center for urgent treatment).
■ *Oncologic history.* Next, the oncologic history is obtained to gain the context of the pain problem. The oncologic history includes diagnosis and stage of disease; therapy and outcome, including side effects; and the patient's understanding of the disease process and prognosis.
■ *Pain history.* The pain history should include any premorbid chronic pain. For each new pain site, record onset and evolution, site and radiation, pattern (constant, intermittent, or unpredictable), and intensity (best, worst, average, current) using numeric rating 0 to 10 scales, character of pain, exacerbating and relieving factors, pain interference with usual activities, neurologic and motor abnormalities (including bowel and bladder continence), vasomotor changes, and current and past analgesics (use, efficacy, side effects). Prior treatments for pain should also be noted (radiotherapy, nerve blocks, physiotherapy, etc.).
■ *Medical record and radiologic studies review.* Many of the treatments for cancer can cause pain (e.g., chemotherapy- and radiotherapy-induced neuropathies or postoperative pain syndromes; Table 45-2) (17). Many specific cancers can cause well-established pain patterns due to known likely sites of metastasis, for example, breast to long bones, spine, chest wall, brachial plexus, and spinal cord; colon to pelvis, hips, lumbar plexus, sacral plexus, and spine; and prostate to long bones, pelvis, hips, lung, and spine (18). (See Chapter 31, Tables 31-5 to 31-9.)
■ *Psychological history.* This should include marital and residential status, employment history and status, educational background, functional status, activities of daily living, recreational activities, support systems, health and capabilities of spouse or significant other, and past (or current) history of drug or alcohol abuse (19,20).
■ *Medical history (independent of oncologic history).* This includes coexisting systemic disease, exercise intolerance, allergies to medications and medication use, prior illness and surgery, and a thorough review of systems, including the following:
  ■ General (including anorexia, weight loss, cachexia, fatigue, weakness, insomnia)
  ■ Neurologic (including sedation, confusion, hallucination, headache, motor weakness, altered sensation, incontinence)
  ■ Respiratory (including dyspnea, cough, pneumonia)
  ■ Gastrointestinal (including dysphagia, nausea, vomiting, dehydration, constipation, diarrhea)
  ■ Psychological (including irritability, anxiety, depression, dementia, suicidal ideation)
  ■ Genitourinary (including urgency, hesitancy, or hematuria)

Physical Examination

The physical examination must be thorough, although at times it is appropriate to perform a focused examination. In patients

THE UNIVERSITY OF TEXAS
MD ANDERSON
CANCER CENTER

**Follow-Up And
Progress Notes**

Pain Management Center-Follow-Up Visit
Page 1 Of 2

Burton (Pump)

Patient
MDA #   Date 01/05/2005
DOB 12/15/1937 FC M   SEX M

DATE
1/5/05
10-
$10/50
R

Temp: 97   Pulse: 65   Resp: 14   BP: 137/78   Wt: 110.6   Ambulatory: (Yes) No   Assistive Devices:

Pain / Chief Complaint: Fore-head, entire head, too, right eye

How long have you had this pain? Very long time, about 1996

Has pain changed in intensity and/or character since last visit? If yes, describe. Not much change
Was in emergency Room New years eve for pain

Where is it located: (Shade diagram, mark worst spot(s) with an X)

hurts to touch
constant pain

Pain Pain

Mark Location

PAIN SCALE: 0 1 2 3 4 5 6 7 8 9 (10)
None   Worst

Over the last week, rate:

Worst Pain: 0 1 2 3 4 5 6 7 8 9 (10)

Least Pain: 0 1 2 3 (4 5) 6 (7) 8 9 10

Usually: 0 1 2 3 4 5 6 7 8 (9 10)

Right Now: 0 1 2 3 4 5 6 7 (8 9) 10

Acceptable Level: 0 1 2 3 4 5 6 7 8 9 10
                        Low as possible

Current Medications: Allergies: Tetanus (swelling)
I.—Medications

Name	Dose	Frequency	Side Effects	% Pain Relieved
R 10/day Loratab. 10/500	1 every 4 hrs		none	0
Liscol	1 per day		none	
topral 100	1 per day		none	
furosimide	1 per day		none	
methadone twice daily	(given in ER) 5d		none	15%
dilaudid in pump			none	10%
Xanax 1-3 times daily			none	

II. Physical Therapy: (no) yes
III. TENS Unit: (no) yes
IV. Nerve Blocks: (no) yes   Dilaudid
V. Other: (no) yes. Specify Zoloft 50mg qday
                                Fiorcet

Follow-Up and Progress Notes
File Under: Progress Notes/Dictated Reports

SCP483010

FIGURE 45-1. MD Anderson modified brief pain inventory (BPI) assessment form. (*Continued*)

with spinal pain and known or suspected metastatic disease, a complete neurologic examination is mandatory. When cognitive impairment is suspected, a mini-mental status examination will clarify the level of impairment and allow tracking over time (see Chapter 37). Gonzales et al. found new evidence of metastatic disease in 64% of patients, and this finding resulted in new antitumor therapy for 18% of patients evaluated by their pain service (21).

Clinical Plan of Care

The clinical plan of care is developed after all items of the history are evaluated.

■ *Formulate clinical impression (diagnosis).* Multiple diagnoses usually apply, and it is optimal to use the most specific

TABLE 45-2

INCIDENCE OF DEVELOPING CHRONIC POSTOPERATIVE PAIN BY TYPE OF SURGERY

Type of surgery	Reported incidence of chronic pain
Limb amputation	30%–80%
Thoracotomy	22%–70%
Cholecystectomy	3%–56%
Inguinal hernia	0%–37%

Modified from Perkins FM and Kehlet H. Chronic pain as an outcome of surgery. *Anesthesiology* 2000;93:1123–1133, with permission.

PART IV: PAIN MANAGEMENT

**Follow-Up And
Progress Notes**

Pain Management Center-Follow-up Visit

Page 2 Of 2

	Patient MDA #	Date 01/05/2005
	DOB 12/15/1937 FC M	SEX M

DATE

Other Symptoms:

Bowel Patterns: Usual Frequency: _2-3 days_   Consistency: _med_

Last B M: _2 days ago_   Bowel Regimen: ✓ No ____ Yes

Sexual Disfunction: No _____   Yes ✓

Other Symptoms:

	NONE (Best)										Worst
Fatigue	0	1	2	3	4	5	⑥	7	8	9	10
Nausea	⓪	1	2	3	4	5	6	7	8	9	10
Depression	0	1	2	3	4	5	6	⑦	8	9	10
Anxiety	0	1	2	3	4	5	6	7	⑧	9	10
Drowsiness	0	1	2	3	4	⑤	6	7	8	9	10
Difficulty Thinking Clearly	0	1	2	3	4	⑤	6	7	8	9	10
Shortness of Breathe	0	1	2	3	4	5	6	7	⑧	9	10
Poor Appetite	0	1	2	3	4	⑤	6	7	8	9	10
Insomnia	0	1	2	3	4	5	⑥	7	8	9	10
Feeling of Well-Being	0	1	2	3	4	5	6	7	⑧	9	10

Anything Else We Can Help You With Today?

Needs refill on Zoloft & Lortab

IT pump refill done in clinic

Plan Of Care:

Teaching: see ITPR _____→ _see IPOCTR_____

Treatment Plan of Care: see IPTP _____

Other: _RTC- 6/6/05 for IT pump refill_

Signature: _____   R.N.

Follow-Up and Progress Notes
File Under: Progress Notes/Dictated Reports

SCP483010

FIGURE 45-1. (*Continued*)

known diagnosis. For example, T11 compression fracture (pathologic versus osteoporotic) with severe incidental pain; metastatic breast carcinoma (with known bony metastasis; nausea with dehydration; and constipation).

▨ *Formulate recommendations (plan) and alternatives for each problem.* For example (related to the above problem list), magnetic resonance imaging (MRI) of the thoracic and lumbar spine with consideration of vertebroplasty if appropriate; oxycodone slow-release 10 mg twice daily, with oral transmucosal fentanyl citrate for breakthrough pain; management including further chemotherapy, radiotherapy, or bisphosphonates as deemed appropriate by the patient's oncologist; metoclopramide 10 mg orally 30 minutes prior to meals and as needed for nausea; and addition of Senokot-S twice daily for constipation.

▨ *Coordinate care.* A call to the referring oncologist and/or primary care provider (and copying them on any clinical notes) helps to ensure good communication and coordination of care between all of a patient's physicians.

▨ *Exit interview.* The exit interview with the patient is ideally performed by the physician, but any trained professional can be designated for this important duty. Items to be addressed include:

▨ Explain the probable cause of symptoms in terms the patient can understand.

▨ Discuss prognosis for symptom relief, management options, and specific recommendations. In addition to writing prescriptions, oral and written instructions should be provided. Educational material regarding medications, pain management strategies, procedures, or other issues should be provided. Potential side effects should be discussed.

▨ Arrange for follow-up with clinic contact information, including an "after-hours" contact number, which is imperative because of the dynamic nature of cancer pain.

▨ A dictated summary (in addition to the phone call) should be sent to referring and consulting physicians to keep them apprised of the patient's present status and treatment offered.

ETIOLOGY AND CLASSIFICATION OF CANCER PAIN SYNDROMES

Pain in cancer patients can have many causes. Most cancer pain syndromes are tumor-related, but an increasing array of more chronic treatment-related painful syndromes are seen with increasing life expectancy (see Chapter 31, Tables 31-5 to 31-9). Numerous schemas for classification of cancer pain syndromes have been explored. This chapter explores time course and pathophysiology as relevant classifications in relation to treatment strategies.

Pain Syndrome Time Course: Acute

The large majority of acute cancer pain is due to tumor invasion of pain-sensitive structures. This invasion causes a derangement of physiologic processes including inflammation, edema, acidosis, and necrosis of pain-sensitive tissues. Further pathologic processes may include invasion of bone or soft tissues, obstruction of lymphatic or vascular vessels, distention of hollow organs, distortion of solid organs, and compression of nervous system structures (22). All of these cause typical acute cancer pain syndromes, most of which are diagnosable during the oncologic workup (see also Chapter 31, Tables 31-5 through 31-9). Many of these same pains improve with successful treatment of the tumor, thus reassessment is important because of the dynamic nature of tumor-related pain.

Pain Syndrome Time Course: Chronic

A significant source of pain can also be related to the cancer treatments. Most of the time, this pain is more chronic, with a gradual onset and often delayed diagnosis and treatment. Certain types of chemotherapy often cause painful peripheral neuropathy including the taxanes, platinum compounds, vincristine and its analogs, and some newer agents such as bortezomib (23). Often, this neuropathy is dose-related and resolves with a lowering of the dose of the offending agent in subsequent courses of chemotherapy. However, in some patients, the painful neuropathy is permanent, severe, and very disabling. It can lead to problems with gait or fine motor tasks of the hands. Radiation treatment may also cause neural injury in the form of plexopathy, chronic radiation myelopathy, and chronic radiation enteritis and proctitis, as well as nonspecific postradiation head and neck pain, most likely a myofascial pain syndrome (24). Other postradiation problems include an increase in long-term pelvic fractures (25).

Surgical treatment also can lead to chronic postoperative pain syndromes. For example, the post–radical mastectomy patient often has pain in the posterior upper arm, axilla, and anterior chest wall secondary to damage of the intercostobrachial nerve (26). Similarly, nerve damages during thoracotomy and radical neck dissection can cause pain in the distribution of the affected nerves (27). Phantom limb pain is especially common after amputation procedures, with burning and cramping sensation in the area of the amputated limb (28) (see also Chapter 31 and Tables 31-5 to 31-9).

The increasing use of combination treatments in numerous cancers, such as combined chemoradiation prior to surgical re-

section of head and neck or breast tumors for example, have increased cure rates. However, they may also increase the toxicity and long-term sequelae of treatment. In such cases, chronic pain may not be attributable to one or another of the therapies, and the term *treatment–related toxicity* has been coined to describe this new phenomenon (29).

As the pain syndromes become chronic—defined as lasting beyond the expected healing time course—the treatment algorithms become similar to those used for noncancer chronic pain. Many confusing issues may develop within this patient population, such as those patients with very slowly progressive cancer and associated pain that may last many years. In many cases the lines between treating cancer pain versus noncancer pain syndromes are blurring (2,30).

Cancer Pain Pathophysiologic Classification

In any assessment of cancer pain, an understanding of pain classification is helpful in delineating both the mechanism of pain and its responsiveness to therapeutic interventions. Pain can be broadly classified into *nociceptive* and *neuropathic* pain; however, in many patients, both mechanisms may be operating, and in all patients, psychological and environmental factors contribute to pain.

Nociceptive Pain

Somatic. Nociceptive pain occurs when non-neurologic tissues suffer insult or injury. The associated neurologic structures, however, are not injured and remain functional. Consequently, the injuries of the damaged tissues are detected as noxious stimuli, and these noxious signals are transmitted along the various pain pathways (see Chapters 31 and 32). The pain perceived by the patient is only very broadly proportional to the degree of tissue damage caused by the cancer, and this is also strongly influenced by psychologic and environmental factors. This pain experienced by the patient may be responsive to nonsteroidal anti-inflammatory drugs (NSAIDs) because tissue damage from cancer inevitably initiates activation of cellular phospholipase A2 to release arachidonic acids (AA) from cell lipid membrane. Cyclooxygenase (COX) enzymes then act on AA to produce potent inflammatory mediators such as thromboxanes, prostaglandins, and leukotrienes. Nonsteroidal anti-inflammatories, including the COX inhibitors, attenuate this initial inflammatory reaction at the site of the tissue damaged by cancer and thus reduce the initial pain signals. One must be aware of the growing concerns about cardiovascular side effects associated this group of compounds (31).

Opiate therapy is also effective in helping to control nociceptive pain. Opioid analgesics act on pain receptors at the level of spinal cord and in the brain to modulate pain pathways in the central nervous system (CNS). Nociceptive pain responds to opioids in a scaled manner, such that pain control is generally proportional to opioid dosage (32).

Nociceptive pain can further be categorized into nociceptive *somatic pain* and nociceptive *visceral pain*. Nociceptive somatic pain results from activation of nociceptive receptors in somatic tissues. These nociceptors are sensitive to mechanical, chemical, and thermal stimuli. They are located in skin, bone, muscle, tendon, joint, and connective tissues. The pain signals from these nociceptors are carried along sensory nerve fibers. The patient's perception of nociceptive somatic pain is characterized typically as aching, dull, sharp, throbbing, and is well localized to the injured tissue site.

Visceral Pain

Nociceptive visceral pain, in contrast, is poorly localized. It originates typically from solid organs of the chest, abdomen, and pelvis. The nociceptive receptors in these solid organs typically do not respond to cutting or burning stimuli. They are, however, extremely sensitive to any mechanical stress or torsion of organs, as well as to tension or traction on mesenteric or vascular attachments to organs. The visceral nociceptive pain signals are carried by autonomic sympathetic fibers. The pain is often described as a vague, dull, aching, or pressure-like (33). The patient often perceives this nociceptive visceral pain as a referred pain that is falsely localized to a distant site. For example, pancreatic cancer pain often presents as a referred mid-back pain, and cancer involvement of diaphragm causes pain in the shoulder (see also Chapter 31 and Figs. 31-21 and 31-22).

Neuropathic Pain

The second major class of cancer pain is neuropathic pain. This pain differs from nociceptive pain in that the cancer causes direct injury to the neural tissues. Tumor destruction of peripheral nerves will cause abnormal and exaggerated pain signal transmission. Tumor invasion of peripheral or central nervous systems results in abnormal pain signal processing, integration, and perception. The cancer patient often reports extraordinary pain perception, with pain feeling different from the usual pain sensation (34). Neuropathic pain is often described as diffuse with superficial areas, is excessively sensitive to noxious stimuli (hyperalgesia/hyperesthesia), occurs even with non-noxious stimuli (allodynia), and includes abnormal painful sensations (dysesthesias). Neuropathic pain is thought to be slightly less responsive to opioid analgesics, and also requires adjuvant medications and, at times, interventional therapy for effective control (35) (see also Chapters 31, 32, 37, and 46).

TREATMENT MODALITIES

Pharmacologic Therapy

World Health Organization Guidelines

As discussed earlier, the barriers to effective pain control are multifold. As a result, clinicians have traditionally undertreated cancer pain. A growing recognition of this health issue has led to the development of numerous guidelines for treating cancer pain, including, most famously, the World Health Organization (WHO) step-ladder approach to treating cancer pain. Although too simple to serve as a comprehensive treatment algorithm, the principle of treating more resistant cancer-related pain with stronger/higher doses of opioids is generally sound (Table 45-3). (The treatment of chronic noncancer pain syndromes with chronic opioids remains controversial.)

Nonopioid Analgesics

The nonopioid class of analgesics includes both acetaminophen, NSAIDs, and perhaps tramadol. Nonopioids are commonly used for mild cancer pain, as directed by the WHO analgesic ladder. Even in the patient with advanced cancer, nonopioid analgesics are often used as co-analgesics combined with opioid (see also Chapter 33). Nonopioids help to reduce the dosage requirement of opioids, thus decreasing the opioid-associated side effects of nausea, constipation, somnolence, and cognitive impairment. However, both acetaminophen and

TABLE 45-3

THE WORLD HEALTH ORGANIZATION (WHO) THREE-STEP ANALGESIC LADDER FOR CANCER PAIN

Step 1: Mild cancer pain $\longrightarrow$ Nonopioid analgesics $\pm$ Adjuvant medications

Step 2: Moderate cancer pain $\longrightarrow$ "Weak" opioids $\pm$ Nonopioid analgesics $\pm$ Adjuvant medications

Step 3: Severe cancer pain $\longrightarrow$ "Strong" opioids $\pm$ Nonopioid analgesics $\pm$ Adjuvant medications

NSAIDs can suppress a fever response, indicative of a mounting infection in the immunocompromised patient who is undergoing immunosuppressive chemotherapy.

Adjuvant Medications

The heterogeneous class of adjuvant medications has a defined role in the WHO three-step analgesic ladder. These agents fall into five general categories: antidepressants, anticonvulsants, oral local anesthetics, corticosteroids, and miscellaneous (Table 45-4).

These adjuvant medications act to promote certain desirable effects (or prevent opioid-related side effects) in the cancer patient. Tricyclic antidepressants are useful in certain types of neuropathic pain, especially burning dysesthetic pain. They produce significant sedation as a side effect at high dose. Consequently, they can be helpful in the cancer pain patient with insomnia and depression. Anticonvulsants and local anesthetics have a membrane-stabilizing effect and are extremely effective in neuropathic pain secondary to nerve injury in both peripheral and central nervous systems. Corticosteroids have potent anti-inflammatory effects and thus are helpful in cancer patients with spinal cord compression, intracranial tumors, organ capsule distention, and bone infiltration. Steroids also have CNS effects, improving mood and a sense of well-being in the cancer patient. Antiemetics and stool softeners should routinely be prescribed along with opioids. The other miscellaneous adjuvant medications have variable effects and are tailored to the patient's individual pain and associated symptoms.

Opioid Analgesics

Opioid analgesics are a mainstay of treatment for cancer pain. In the WHO three-step analgesic ladder, "weak" opioids are recommended for treatment of moderate cancer pain, whereas "strong" opioids are prescribed for severe cancer pain. The weak opioids have slightly less potency and also fewer side effects. Some common oral weak opioids are listed in Table 45-5.

These weak opioids are produced in combination with acetaminophen or aspirin, thus they are "weak" because of the limitation imposed by acetaminophen or aspirin ceiling doses, above which the patient is at higher risk of renal and liver toxicity.

The "strong" opioids are more potent because they are made in pure form, without addition of aspirin or acetaminophen. These opioids do not have a maximum ceiling dose, but at higher dosages, the patient tends to experience more frequent and significant side effects of nausea and vomiting, constipation, pruritus, somnolence, and cognitive impairment. Some common strong opioids are listed in Table 45-6.

TABLE 45-4

ADJUVANT DRUGS FOR TREATMENT OF CANCER PAIN

I.	Antidepressants:	
	Amitriptyline	Doxepin
	Nortriptyline	Paroxetine
	Desipramine	Venlafaxine
	Duloxetine	
II.	Anticonvulsants:	
	Gabapentin	Valproic Acid
	Carbamazepine	Clonazepam
	Pregabalin	Topiramate
III.	Local Anesthetics:	
	Mexiletine	Topical & systemic (IV, SCI) lidocaine
IV.	Corticosteroids:	
	Dexamethasone	Prednisolone
	Methylprednisolone	Cortisone
V.	Miscellaneous:	
	Psychostimulants- Dextroamphetamine, methylphenidate	
	γ-Aminobutyric acid (GABA) agonist: Baclofen	
	α_2-Antagonist: Clonidine	
	N-methyl-D-aspartate (NMDA) antagonist: Ketamine	
	Antiemetics*: Metoclopramide, ondansetron, corticosteroids	
	Laxatives/stool softeners*: Senna, docusate, polyethylene glycol powder	

*Recommended in all patients receiving opioids.

Failure of Noninterventional Therapies

It has been claimed that 70% to 90% of patients with cancer pain have satisfactory pain relief from pharmacologic therapies alone, following the WHO guidelines (36). This means, however, that 10% to 30% of these patients have pain that cannot be effectively managed with medications alone. Additionally, it must be pointed out that the standard 70% to 90% success rates using the WHO step-ladder include patients with mild, moderate, and severe pain grouped together, with higher success rates in the mild pain group. Thus, the 70% to 90% adequate cancer pain treatment almost certainly overestimates WHO approach success in the most severe cancer pain syndromes. The reasons for this failure of pharmacologic treatment are variable (37), varying from physician- to patient-related factors. The physician-related reasons for pharmacologic failure include inaccurate assessment of pain and deficiency in knowledge of current analgesics and adjuvant medications. Patient-related reasons range from fear of addiction to appearance of adverse side effects (38,39). Failure of pharmacologic control of cancer pain due to lack of efficacy of existing drugs in some patients is also commonly seen with cancer progression. Patients with advanced disease can present with intractable pain from multiple metastases and multiple pain sites (see Chapter 31, Tables 31-5 to 31-9).

INTERVENTIONAL PAIN THERAPIES

Goal of Intervention

Patients who fail to respond to conservative pharmacologic treatments may be candidates for interventional therapies. A large armamentarium of invasive procedures is available to achieve better control of cancer pain. However, the role of interventional therapies must be placed in the proper context. Usually, these procedures cannot be employed as the sole

TABLE 45-5

"WEAK" OPIOIDS FOR TREATMENT OF MODERATE CANCER PAIN

Generic name	Examples of U.S. trade names
Hydrocodone	Lortab, Vicoden, Lorcet, Norco
Codeine	Tylenol #3, #4
Propoxyphene	Darvon, Darvocet

TABLE 45-6

"STRONG" OPIOIDS FOR TREATMENT OF SEVERE CANCER PAIN

Generic Name	Examples of U.S. trade names
Morphine/MS-CR	MSIR, MS Contin, Oramorph, Kadian, Avinza
Oxycodone/ oxycodone-CR	Roxicodone, OxyContin
Fentanyl	Duragesic (time release transdermal), Actiq (oral immediate release)
Hydromorphone	Dilaudid
Methadone	Methadose, Dolophine
Oxymorphone/ Oxymorphone-CR	Numorphan, Opana, Opana-CR

treatment for cancer pain, especially for advanced cancer patients. Rather, they should be used as part of a multimodality approach in the treatment of cancer pain (40,41). However, in cases in which the risk–benefit ratio is favorable and outcome evidence is strong (i.e., celiac plexus block), the patient need not "fail" WHO ladder therapy to be a candidate for interventional pain therapy. As discussed previously, the etiologies of cancer pain are diverse, and pain is interrelated with the constellation of symptoms experienced by the cancer patient. Consequently, a global, multimodal approach to treatment of cancer pain is necessary. It includes the appropriate antineoplastic therapy, management of analgesics and adjuvant pain medications, behavioral and psychiatric support, and finally interventional therapies. Most often, interventional pain procedures will not completely eliminate the need for pain medications. The therapeutic goal of such procedures is to help alleviate cancer pain, reduce the overall analgesic need, and thereby minimize associated opioid-related side effects, with the overall aim of enhancing quality of life.

Communication

Prior to proceeding with any invasive pain procedure, communication between the pain physician and the relevant parties is absolutely essential. The patient must first be educated about the risks and benefits of the interventional procedure. He must be allowed an opportunity to have questions about the procedure extensively and satisfactorily answered. He must, at the same time, be grounded in realistic expectations in terms of outcomes and possible complications from the chosen procedure. The patient should be made aware of the efficacy of the procedure, duration of effectiveness, and possibility of failure of the procedure to provide complete or even partial pain relief. He must understand that the interventional procedure is part of a multimodal approach to pain control.

With cancer patients, especially those critically ill or preterminal, family members and caregivers are often involved in the decision-making process. Family support helps the patient cope emotionally with cancer disease and with procedural interventions. Like the patient, the family must also be educated and have realistic expectations about the procedure.

Effective communication with other professional members of the care team is also important. These include the patient's oncologists, primary care providers, and all the relevant consultants. Treatment of cancer is a multidisciplinary effort. The interventional procedure should be planned in coordination with the overall cancer treatment. For example, the cancer patient may undergo chemotherapy with resultant thrombocytopenia. In such case, the interventional procedure must be carried out prior to or following chemoinduction, when the patient's platelet count is normalized. Typically, other members of the patient's care team are informed about the planned interventional procedure and given a chance to voice any input or concern.

Detailed Physical Examination

A thorough physical examination of the patient prior to the procedure is also critical. This entails a complete neurologic evaluation. Interventional procedures for pain control involve neurologically sensitive tissues such as nerves and CNS structures. The objective of intervention is to disrupt or modulate pain pathways involved in nociception. Interventional procedures like neurolysis of peripheral nerves will not only block pain transmission but also block sensory and motor innervations as well. Consequently, it is important to document before and after the procedure a complete and thorough physical examination, with focus especially on pain and neurologic changes. Changes such as sensory and motor blockade are closely monitored after procedures.

Categories of Interventional Techniques

Interventional therapies can be categorized into three groups: neurolytic techniques, neuromodulatory techniques, and surgical techniques. Neurolytic or neuroablative techniques are procedures that target the destruction of those nerves or neural structures that are involved in the generation or transmission of pain signals. Neurolytic lesions can be created using a variety of agents. Lysis is achieved with chemicals (glycerol, alcohol, or phenol), heat (radiofrequency coagulation), or cold (cryotherapy) (see also Chapters 39, 42, and 44).

Neuromodulatory techniques have as their basis Wall and Melzack's gate control theory of pain (42) (see Chapters 40 and 41), which is also discussed in light of current knowledge in Chapter 51. Regardless of the exact locus of such a gate, the concept is accurate in describing how afferent input of all types is heavily modulated along the route of transmission into the brain. All of these modulation sites become therapeutic targets when discussing the treatment of pain (43). Neuromodulative techniques aim to modulate pain signals along the transmission pathway. These techniques include local anesthetic blockade or regional infusion of drugs at epidural, intrathecal, intraventricular, or perineural sites, and the electrical stimulation of the CNS and peripheral nervous system (PNS).

Surgical techniques are another class of interventional pain procedures, ranging from minimally invasive percutaneous vertebroplasty to highly invasive neurosurgical destructive techniques, including percutaneous cordotomy, dorsal root entry zone (DREZ) lesions, thalamotomy, cingulotomy, hypophysectomy, and trigeminal tractomy. Most of these procedures are done stereotactically under monitored anesthesia care (MAC) and fluoroscopic or computed tomography (CT) guidance. Nondestructive neurosurgical techniques include deep brain stimulation and motor cortex stimulation; both of these are currently experimental.

NEUROLYTIC PROCEDURES

Over the past century, many chemical and physical ablative techniques have been developed with the goal of disrupting the transmission of pain signals along the neural pathways. Chemical neurolysis is achieved with alcohol (50%–100%), phenol (5%–15%), and glycerol (100%). These agents produce nerve injury that results in degeneration of nerve fiber distal to the lysis lesion (Wallerian degeneration) (44). This disrupts the nerve cell transmission of pain and results in a nociceptive block. However, after Wallerian degeneration, the nerve axon can regenerate within 3 months. Thus, chemical neurolysis provides a temporary block of nociception lasting about 3 to 6 months (44,45).

In the past, alcohol has been classically used in neurolysis (46). Many clinicians today favor the use of phenol for peripheral neurolysis because it is less neurotoxic than alcohol (47). Alcohol is used in concentrations up to 100%. It causes nonselective destruction of all nerves, as well as surrounding soft tissues. Alcohol is rapidly soluble in blood and is hypobaric relative to cerebrospinal fluid (CSF). If injected into the intraspinal space, it will rise rapidly against gravity, diffusing away from the initial injection site. Specifically, it damages nerves by extracting fatty substances and precipitating proteins in the nerve axon, resulting in Wallerian degeneration (48). The lesion is proportional to both the concentration and volume of alcohol used. There may be a higher risk of neuritis associated with alcohol injection versus other techniques (49). Also, patients usually experience intense burning pain initially with alcohol injection. However, after intrathecal injection, patients experience a warm numb feeling.

Phenol, now more commonly used, is thought to be associated with lower risk of postablation neuritis (49). Phenol 5% is equivalent to alcohol 40% concentration in neurolytic potency (50). Phenol is less water-soluble than alcohol and thus tends to concentrate more around the injection site. It acts by diffusing into the axon and denaturing proteins, causing Wallerian degeneration. Many clinicians prefer phenol because the intensity (or "density") and duration of neural blockade are less with phenol and thus provide a wider margin of safety.

Less commonly used is glycerol in peripheral neural blockade. It is used primarily for treatment of trigeminal neuralgia. It is injected directly into the trigeminal cistern (cave of Meckel) with good efficacy in treating trigeminal neuralgia. Other neurolytic chemicals that have been tried include ammonium salt compounds and hypertonic and hypotonic saline solutions, with variable results (44). Radiofrequency thermocoagulation (RFTC) or radiofrequency ablation (RFA) is also employed to produce a physical nociceptive block (51). As opposed to chemical neurolysis, the lesion created by radiofrequency heating is discrete, and the size of the lesion is controlled by the temperature of the probe and duration of application. Some studies have shown that radiofrequency ablation can produce a longer-lasting block versus chemical neurolytic techniques (52) (see Chapters 42 and 44).

Cryotherapy can also be used to achieve neurolytic lesioning. Applying extreme cold to the nerve will result in long-lasting nerve blockade (44). Intraoperative cryoneurolysis of intercostal nerves has been reported with good efficacy in controlling postthoracotomy pain (53). Wide application of cryoablation has been hindered by the large size of the probe (14 g), relative complexity of the equipment involved (requires a compressed nitrogen source), and the relatively short duration of the lesion versus the aforementioned techniques (see Chapter 42).

Patient selection for chemical neurolysis, radiofrequency ablation, and cryoneurolysis techniques is extremely important in achieving the desired outcome. In most cases, the patient should have an advanced, progressive cancer with a limited life expectancy (6–12 months). The pain should be severe, persistent, refractory to conservative treatment, and amenable to neural blockade (discrete and localized to a region served by one or two nerves, i.e., the chest wall or jaw line). Potential risks are associated with neuroablation, as outlined in Table 45-7. Despite the inherent risks of neuroablation however, patients with advanced cancer and well-localized nociceptive pain can benefit greatly from neurolytic blockade. Peripheral, central, and sympathetic neurolysis has been used for many decades to alleviate suffering in cancer patients with intractable pain (54).

Neural Blockade in Head and Neck

Over 40,000 patients are diagnosed with head and neck cancer each year in the United States, and over 500,000 are diagnosed worldwide (55). Cancer of the head and neck constitutes about 5% of all malignant diseases in the United States, and affects

TABLE 45-7

POTENTIAL RISKS WITH NEUROABLATION TECHNIQUES

Dysesthetic pain: Painful neuralgia due to deafferentation, neuritis, or neuroma formation
Tissue damage: Accidental injury to nontargeted neurologic and non-neurologic tissues
Motor paralysis: Especially with intrathecal neurolysis
Sensory deficit: Areas of paresthesia or numbness
Failure to relieve pain: Due to incomplete ablation or incorrect nerve target
Short-term pain relief: Due to central nervous system plasticity, axonal regrowth, or tumor progression

about 6.6 million worldwide (56). Because of dense facial and neck innervations, cancer commonly causes not only disfiguring facial lesions but also disabling pain in face and neck. The incidence of pain following treatment for head and neck cancer may be as high as 50%, with more than 50% disabled 1 year after diagnosis, highly correlated to pain scores (57–59). Blocking relevant trigeminal or cervical nerve branches can control such pain. Efficacy of interventional nerve block, however, can be affected by tumor distortion of anatomy, radiation-induced fibrosis of local tissues, and possible overlapping sensory innervations of neighboring cranial nerves V, VII, IX, X, and upper cervical nerves (see Chapter 17). Careful anatomic evaluation of facial pain and proper selection of nerve block with a local anesthetic test block is indicated prior to consideration of neurolytic blockade in these patients.

Trigeminal Nerve Block

Indications. Blockade of trigeminal ganglion or specific branches of trigeminal nerves will alleviate somatic and neuropathic pain from cancer. Trigeminal neuralgia (tic douloureux) is discussed in Chapter 42.

Anatomy. The trigeminal or Gasserian ganglion is formed from two nerve roots that arise from the ventral pons of the brainstem. These roots fuse anteriorly and enter the Meckel cave, a recess in the middle cranial fossa. Three sensory divisions then exit anteriorly as the ophthalmic nerve (V1), maxillary nerve (V2), and the mandibular nerve (V3). Destruction of the Gasserian ganglion may be useful in alleviating intractable pain from invasive tumors of the orbit, maxillary sinus, and mandible (60). Conversely, each individual sensory nerve can be blocked separately, if selective blockade is desired.

Techniques. Local anesthetic, neurolytic, and radiofrequency lesioning techniques for Gasserian ganglion blockade are described in Chapter 42 (see Figs. 42-34 to 42-38). Radiographs showing the position of the needle are presented in Figure 45-2.

Complications. After local anesthetic or neurolytic agent injection, inadvertent vascular puncture can lead to neurotoxicity, including seizure and death. When the needle is directed through the pterygopalatine fossa, injury to blood vessels can result in facial hematoma or ocular subscleral hematoma. Postprocedure neuritis can cause significant dysesthetic pain in trigeminal sensory areas. Ocular dryness and masticator weakness are also possible after neurolytic trigeminal block (see also Chapter 20).

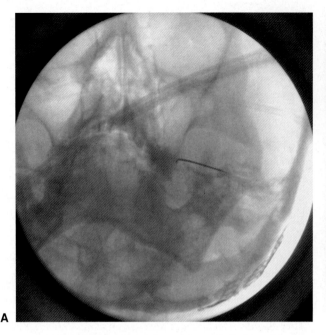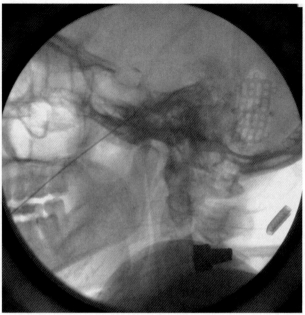

FIGURE 45-2. Trigeminal nerve block showing radiographic appearance. **A:** Anteroposterior view. **B:** Lateral view.

Occipital Nerve Block

Indications. Occipital nerve block is effective in treating oncologic pain in the posterior scalp and occipital region.

Anatomy. Most of the posterior scalp is innervated by the greater occipital nerve, which arises from the dorsal rami of the C2 nerve root (see Chapter 17, Fig. 17-2). It emerges subcutaneously in the posterior scalp just slightly inferior to the superior nuchal line and 2 to 3 cm lateral to the greater occipital protuberance. At this point of emergence, it is just medial to the occipital artery (61) (see Chapter 17, Fig. 17-10).

Techniques. The occipital nerve block technique is described in Chapter 17 (see Fig. 17-10). In the case of occipital neuralgia, the patient may be a candidate for suboccipital peripheral nerve stimulation (see Chapter 41). Radiographs showing the final position of suboccipital electrodes are presented in Figure 45-3.

Complications. Because of the superficial location of the greater occipital nerve and relative ease of this block, complications are minimal. The close proximity of the greater occipital artery may increase risk of intravascular injection, which can be avoided by frequent aspiration while slowly injecting the neurolytic solution. Neuritis can also occur with neurolytic agents, especially with alcohol (see also Chapter 20).

Superficial Cervical Plexus Block

Indications. Superficial cervical plexus block is often used to treat cancer pain in the dermatome of the neck innervated by the cervical plexus.

Anatomy. The superficial and deep cervical plexus arise from the first four cervical nerves. The cervical plexus lies just lateral to the first cervical vertebrae. It is located anterior to the levator scapulae and middle scalene muscles, and posterior to the sternocleidomastoid (SCM) muscle. The plexus gives off both superficial sensory branches and deep motor branches. This anatomic division of sensory and motor nerves allows for selective sensory blockade of the superficial sensory branches of the cervical plexus without compromising the motor function of the neck muscles.

These superficial branches arise from the plexus and pierce the deep fascia of the neck at the posterior border of the SCM muscle (see Chapter 17, Fig. 17-9). It is at this point, where the bundle of the superficial cervical plexus emerges, that sensory innervation to the plexus can be blocked easily (62). The superficial cervical plexus gives rise to the sensory nerves that supply sensation to the skin and superficial fascia of the head, neck, and shoulder. These include the lesser occipital, greater auricular, accessory, anterior cervical, and suprascapular nerves (63).

Techniques. The technique for this block is described in Chapter 17 (see Fig. 17-9). If local anesthetic block is successful, it can be followed with neurolytic agents to achieve a longer blockade. In this region, the authors use a dilute (3%) phenol solution because of the vascular structures and muscles in the area. A note of caution is that the external jugular vein crosses the midpoint of the lateral border of the SCM. Careful aspiration prior to infiltration is helpful to avoid intravascular injection (64).

Complications. There are few complications with this superficial cervical block. The most common complication is intravascular injection into the external or internal jugular vein, with resulting systemic toxicity. Also, placement of needle into the jugular vein may result in hematoma or even air embolism (see also Chapter 20).

Neural Blockade of Upper Extremity

Brachial Plexus Block

Indications. Malignancy involving the upper extremity includes sarcoma of bone as well as soft tissue sarcoma. In the

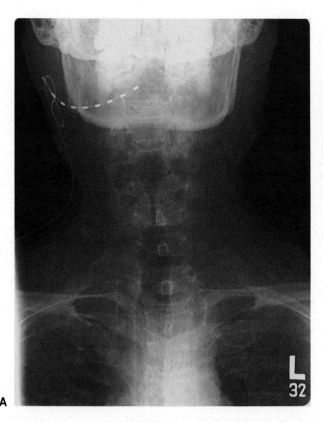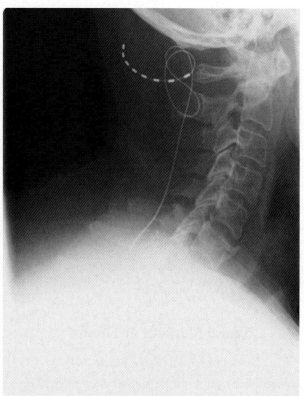

A   **B**

FIGURE 45-3. Suboccipital electrodes in situ. **A:** Anteroposterior view. **B:** Lateral view.

United States, almost 13,000 new cases of bony sarcoma and 7,000 new cases of soft tissue sarcomas are diagnosed each year (65). In most cases, surgical resections of sarcomas with limb-sparing procedures are performed with good result. These patients, however, often have severe pain from direct tumor invasion of the neurovascular bundle or as a consequence of surgical tumor resection. Neural blockade of the brachial plexus is effective in controlling somatic nociceptive pain in upper extremity cancer.

For short-term palliation of cancer pain, brachial plexus block can also be performed with a catheter left in place for continuous infusion of local anesthetic. In cases of severe intractable pain from invasive tumors of the brachial plexus or soft tissues and bone of the shoulder and upper extremity, destruction of the brachial plexus may be indicated. The patient should be made aware of the full consequences of neurolysis of the brachial plexus, including paralysis of the upper extremity. Many patients who are candidates for this block will already have significant motor deficits in the extremity (66).

Anatomy. The brachial plexus is formed from fusion of the ventral rami of C5–T1 nerve roots. These nerve roots, with possible contribution from C4 and T2, emerge from the lateral aspect of the vertebral bodies and run laterally and inferiorly, in the interscalene compartment. These nerves of the brachial plexus run down the interscalene compartment to pass behind the clavicle and above the top of the first rib, then into the axilla (see Chapter 13, Figs. 13-1 to 13-5).

Techniques. There are multiple approaches to the brachial plexus blockade, including interscalene block, supraclavicular block, and axillary block. In cancer pain from tumor involve-

ment of the shoulder, interscalene block is preferred (67). The techniques are described and illustrated in Chapter 13, Figures 13-6 to 13-15.

Once efficacy of local anesthetic blockade in relieving cancer pain has been proven, the patient may wish to proceed with a longer-lasting neurolytic block using phenol. A volume of 20 mL of 6% phenol is slowly injected into the intrascalene compartment of the brachial plexus. The neurolytic block is done under fluoroscopic guidance in our facility. Again, motor paralysis of the upper extremity can be expected with this neurolysis of the brachial plexus. Another method of neurolysis of the brachial plexus produces a radiofrequency lesion of the cervical nerve roots (see Chapter 42), which we have done in our institution in some cases of pain refractory to brachial plexus neurolysis.

If a less prolonged blockade of the brachial plexus is desired, a continuous local anesthetic infusion of the brachial plexus can be performed. The infraclavicular approach for brachial plexus block is preferred here, because the catheter can remain in the same position for up to 3 weeks (68). The infraclavicular entry site permits easy catheter threading into the plexus, and catheter position is not affected by the patient's movement. The technique for infraclavicular block and insertion of a catheter for infusion is described in Chapter 13, Figures 13-20 to 13-21. Once the infraclavicular catheter has been inserted and the catheter is sutured well in place, infusion of 0.125% or 0.25% bupivacaine is used to provide continuous brachial plexus analgesia. It is effective in controlling somatic pain for several days and sympathetically mediated pain for up to a few weeks.

The patient will lose protective reflexes in the extremity and should be counseled to periodically examine his extremity for

PART IV: PAIN MANAGEMENT

lesions and/or infection for the duration of the block. Further, the patient should be fitted with a sling for the duration of the block.

Complications. Complications from interscalene block are possible because of its proximity to many sensitive structures in the neck. Intravascular injection, as mentioned earlier, will lead to systemic toxicity including seizure. Subarachnoid injection can cause sensory, motor, total spinal anesthesia, and even death. Phrenic nerve block is an expected condition that accompanies a successful interscalene block. In patients with respiratory compromise, the patient's ability to tolerate a local anesthetic phrenic nerve block with hemidiaphragm paralysis should be considered before neurolytic blockade.

Complications for infraclavicular brachial plexus block are similar to interscalene block. Proximity to the subclavian artery and vein increases the potential for intravascular injection. The apex of the lung is also close, so pneumothorax risk is higher also. Although the probability of phrenic nerve block is less with the infraclavicular approach, the risk of recurrent laryngeal nerve blockade and consequent vocal cord paralysis is higher (see also Chapters 20 and 50).

Neural Blockade in Thorax

Intercostal Nerve Block

Indications. Lung cancer is the number-one cancer killer in both males and females. It accounts for 15% of malignant disease in males and 13% in females. Patients diagnosed with lung cancer often require thoracotomy, with surgical biopsy or resection of tumor mass. Many such patients experience chest wall pain from either direct tumor involvement or from surgical trauma to intercostal nerves (69). In addition to lung cancer, aggressive breast cancer may also invade ribs and intercostal nerve bundles to cause pain (70).

Tumor invasion of lung parenchyma and visceral pleura is not thought to cause pain because these are nociceptive-insensitive structures. However, cancer involvement of the parietal pleura will elicit a pain response. Pain is transmitted from parietal pleura along somatic nerves, including the intercostal nerves from T1 to T12. Intercostal nerve blockade is effective in blocking this somatic pain (71).

Anatomy. The intercostal nerves are formed from the ventral rami of thoracic nerves from T1 to T12. Each nerve, joined by an intercostal vein and artery, runs in a neurovascular bundle in the subcostal groove. It gives off four branches as it runs anteriorly in the intercostal space. The first is the gray rami communicantes, which joins the sympathetic ganglion. The second branch is the posterior cutaneous nerve, which innervates the paravertebral region. The third branch is the lateral cutaneous nerve, which innervates the axilla and lateral chest wall. The fourth is the anterior cutaneous nerve, which innervates the anterior thorax (see Chapter 16, Fig. 16-4). Considerable sensory overlap occurs between those branches as well as between the intercostal nerves themselves. Thus, pain from one area may require blockade of multiple adjacent intercostal nerves (72).

Techniques. For neurolytic block, the procedure should be performed under fluoroscopic or ultrasound guidance. Also, some new data support increased efficacy with proximal radiofrequency lesioning of the dorsal root ganglion (DRG) (see also Chapter 42). The details of this technique are described in Chapter 16, Figures 16-6 to 16-12. Once the needle is in place, water-soluble contrast dye injected into this groove should show a nice spread along the inferior border of rib. A neurolytic solution of 10% phenol can be injected, using 3 to 5 mL for each intercostal block. The proximal approach to the DRG is generally done under fluoroscopic guidance, using an oblique approach and a curved needle. Sensory testing with radiofrequency allows the operator to manipulate the needle tip in the foramen to optimal position (i.e., until the paresthesia reproduces the patient's pain; see Chapter 42).

Complications. Some common complications with intercostal nerve blockade include pneumothorax and systemic toxicity. Pneumothorax results from needle puncture through parietal and visceral pleura. This will create an air leak from lung into pleural space. A simple pneumothorax may progress into a tension pneumothorax with its life-threatening implications. The patient should be closely monitored after the procedure, and a postprocedure chest radiograph is recommended.

Another complication is systemic toxicity from absorption of anesthetic or neurolytic solution into the intercostal neurovascular bundle. Because of the close proximity of the intercostal artery and vein to nerve, absorption of injected solution into the intercostal space is likely. However, considering the small volume used for neurolysis, systemic toxicity is less likely. Another less likely complication is neuraxial spread of the anesthetic or neurolytic solution. A clear risk is the development or worsening of preexisting neuropathic pain as a result of neuroplastic changes in response to the intercostal denervation.

Instead of chemical neurolysis, cryoanalgesia and radiofrequency ablation have also been used in intercostal nerve blockade (see Chapter 42). Cryoanalgesia or freezing of intercostal nerves has been shown to control pain in postthoracotomy patients if done under direct visualization of the intercostal bundle at termination of surgery (72).

Intercostal nerve radiofrequency ablation of the DRG can also be used for long-lasting blockade. A blunt-tipped 100-mm 22-gauge radiofrequency electrode with a 5-mm active tip is inserted into the subcostal space (see Chapter 42). One mL of 2% lidocaine is injected into the electrode cannula. Lesioning is then accomplished by coagulation at 80°C for 60 seconds or using other similar lesioning parameters. We use a curved-tip probe to optimally locate the DRG in the proximal neural foramen (Figs. 45-4 and 45-5).

Sympathetic Blockade for Cancer Pain

Visceral pain arises from cancer involvement of sympathetically innervated organs. Innervation of viscera is best described as being through "visceral nociceptive afferents," since such fibers utilize sympathetic plexuses and ganglia as an anatomic route to the DRG. Insults to these organs can be from abnormal distention of organ wall or viscus, tension or torsion on mesenteric vessels, and ischemia. Such visceral pain is commonly seen with gastrointestinal malignancies such as hepatic metastases, intestinal tract tumor, and pancreatic cancer. Sympathetically mediated pain (SMP) can be part of a neuropathic pain problem (most commonly complex regional pain syndrome or CRPS), as when there is direct injury to nervous tissue such as occurs in brachial and lumbosacral plexopathies (73,74) (see Chapter 46). No evidence suggests that sympathetic blockade provides long-term relief of SMP, despite some patients obtaining short- to medium-term relief. Studies have shown that sympathetic blockade may provide short-term relief of SMP (74,75) (see Chapters 39 and 46).

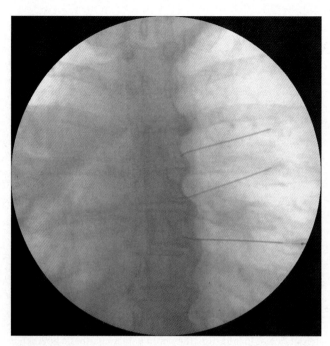

FIGURE 45-4. Intercostal nerve radiofrequency ablation at level of dorsal root ganglion (DRG). Fluoroscopy image showing needle in final position. Anteroposterior view.

Anatomy. The sympathetic axis is made up primarily of a pair of ganglionated paravertebral chains that run from the base of the skull to the tip of the coccyx. It also consists of several major vertebral plexuses, including the celiac, cardiac, and hypogastric plexuses (see Chapter 39). Table 45-8 lists major sympathetic structures and the corresponding tissues innervated (75).

These sympathetic structures are attractive targets for blockade of visceral pain (75–86) and ischemic limb pain (82,83) (see

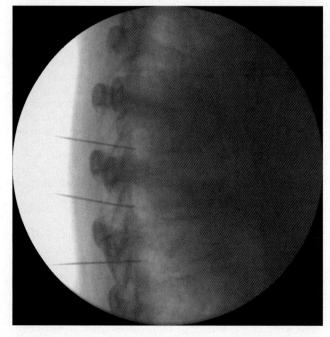

FIGURE 45-5. Thoracic dorsal root ganglion ablation. Lateral view.

TABLE 45-8

SYMPATHETIC STRUCTURES

Sympathetic ganglia/ plexuses	Innervated tissues
Stellate ganglia	Brain, ear, tongue, pharynx, larynx, skin of neck, head, and upper extremity
Thoracic ganglia	Mediastinal contents, esophagus, trachea, bronchus, pericardium, heart, lung
Celiac plexus	GI tract (from distal esophagus to mid transverse colon), pancreas, stomach, liver, adrenals, ureters, abdominal vessels
Lumbar ganglia	Skin and vessels of lower extremity, kidneys, ureters, transverse colon, testes
Hypogastric plexus	Descending and sigmoid colon, rectum, vaginal fundus, bladder, prostate, prostatic urethra, testes, seminal vesicles, uterus, and ovaries
Ganglion impar	Perineum, distal rectum and anus, distal urethra, vulva and distal third of vagina

Chapter 39), as well as SMP (see Chapter 46). Interruption of pain pathways at these discrete sites has been demonstrated to have a useful role in controlling oncologic pain (76,77). Sympathetically mediated pain associated with CRPS is much more difficult to manage, probably because of the central neuroplastic changes associated with CRPS (see Chapter 46).

Stellate Ganglion Block

Indications. Stellate ganglion block helps control SMP in the head, neck, and upper extremity. Sympathically mediated pain is commonly seen in tumor invasion of brachial plexopathy or in Pancoast tumor (78).

Anatomy. The stellate or cervicothoracic ganglion is formed from fusion of the inferior cervical and the first thoracic sympathetic ganglia. A detailed description of the efferent sympathetic nerves and cervicothoracic sympathetic ganglia is given in Chapter 39.

Techniques. Because of many sensitive structures in the neck adjacent to the stellate ganglion, fluoroscopic imaging is recommended. The patient is placed in the supine position with neck slightly extended. The classic technique is to identify the Chassaignac tubercle at C6 and enter the needle at this site (see Chapter 39, Figs. 39-26 to 39-28). However, many clinicians recommend Racz's technique at the C7 level for its improved safety margin (79). The patient's neck is prepared in a sterile manner with Betadine, and the skin over the body of the C7 vertebral body is anesthetized with local 1% lidocaine. The proceduralist's nondominant hand is used to palpate the carotid artery at the level of C7 and retract it laterally. The dominant hand introduces a 1.5-inch, 22-gauge needle just medial to the palpated carotid artery and directs that needle in a medial direction. The target of the needle tip is the ventrolateral aspect of the C7 vertebral body, not the transverse process, as seen in

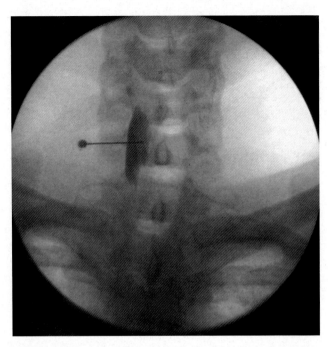

FIGURE 45-6. Stellate ganglion block at C7 level. Fluoroscopy image after injection of contrast media.

the classic approach. Once the needle tip contacts the C7 vertebral body, it is slightly withdrawn about 1 mm. The needle is then carefully aspirated for CSF or blood. A contrast dye, 1 to 2 mL, is injected to confirm the caudocephalad spread in front of the prevertebral facia (Fig. 45-6). For gangliolysis, a mixture of 3% phenol, local anesthetic, and steroid is used (i.e., 5 mL of 6% phenol in saline, 5 mL of 0.5% bupivacaine, and 80 mg of methylprednisone).

The volume of this mixture injected is dependent on the blockade desired. A volume of 10 mL of neurolytic mixture is adequate for stellate ganglion blockade of SMP to the head and upper extremity. If blockade of pain from thoracic viscera is desired, a volume of 15 to 20 mL of neurolytic mixture is necessary. During injection, the clinician must exercise caution to prevent intravascular injection. Even 1 mL of local anesthetic injected into carotid or vertebral artery can cause loss of consciousness and seizure. An initial test dose, frequent aspiration, and slow injection are good safety measures.

Efficacy. Evidence of sympathetic blockade in the head can include a myriad of symptoms characteristic of Horner syndrome such as miosis, ptosis, enophthalmos, facial anhidrosis, and nasal congestion. Sympathetic blockade to the upper extremity results in visible engorgement of veins in the hands and forearm. Resolution of prior pain suggests that such pain is sympathetically mediated. (However, see Chapter 38 describing diagnostic and prognostic neural blockade.)

Complications. Because of anatomic proximity to critical structures, serious complications of stellate ganglion block can include pneumothorax, anesthetic-induced seizure from intravascular injection, and total spinal anesthesia from subarachnoid injection. Other less serious problems include localized hematoma, infection, or neck muscle tenderness. Many clinicians fear a permanent Horner syndrome with neurolysis. Anecdotally, Racz et al., however, have not reported any long-

term Horner syndrome using their modified technique just discussed (79).

Celiac Plexus Blockade

Indications. Celiac plexus blockade continues to be an extremely effective intervention for pain from pancreatic cancer and malignancies involving the upper and mid abdomen (80). Pancreatic cancer carries such a poor diagnosis that palliation of pain symptoms is a priority in these patients, who have a survival rate of typically less than 6 months. These patients often present initially with upper abdominal pain with referred pain to back (81). The pain is described as severe, increasing with disease progression, and poorly relieved by opioids or other medications. Celiac plexus block is the interventional treatment of choice for pain control in pancreatic cancer patients.

Anatomy. The celiac plexus is the largest of the great plexuses of the sympathetic nervous system. The cardiac plexus innervates structures that are primarily thoracic, the celiac plexus innervates abdominal organs, and the hypogastric plexus supplies pelvic organs. All three contain visceral afferent and efferent fibers. In addition, they hold parasympathetic fibers that pass through these ganglia after originating in cranial or sacral areas of the nervous system. Although the latter fibers may be found in these plexuses, all are primarily sympathetic nervous system structures. They contain no somatic fibers, but do innervate most of the abdominal viscera, to include stomach, liver, biliary tract, pancreas, spleen, kidneys, adrenals, omentum, and small and large bowel. (Although the terms *plexus* and *ganglion* often are used interchangeably, it is important to realize that plexus is the more inclusive term. A plexus is composed of a number of ganglia and nerve fibers that converge in a fairly well-defined anatomic location.)

According to most standard anatomic textbooks, there are three splanchnic nerves—great, lesser, and least. The great splanchnic nerve arises from the roots of T5 or T6 to T9 or T10. It runs paravertebrally in the thorax, through the crus of the diaphragm to enter the abdominal cavity, and ends in the celiac (or semilunar) ganglion on that side. The lesser splanchnic nerve arises from the T10 to T11 segments and passes lateral to, or with, the great nerve to the celiac ganglion. It sends postganglionic fibers to the celiac and renal plexuses. The least splanchnic nerve arises from T11–T12 segments and passes through the diaphragm to the celiac ganglion. It is worth remembering that all three splanchnic nerves are preganglionic and that the paired celiac (or semilunar) ganglia are where they synapse. The postganglionic fibers radiate to the abdominal viscera (Fig. 45-7).

Of more importance to performance of celiac plexus block is an understanding of the anatomy of the surrounding structures that will be subjected to the potential trauma of needles and drug. The celiac ganglia are situated in close relation to the first lumbar vertebra. On the right side and anterior is the vena cava, and, on the left, anteriorly, is the aorta. The kidneys are lateral on either side. The paired ganglia are close to the midline on each side between the adrenal glands and are immediately above the pancreas. The postganglionic nerves are flat, and rest against the crus of the diaphragm. Covered partially by the vena cava on the right and the pancreas on the left, they become interconnected to form the plexus. The plexus anterior to the aorta, around the base of the celiac artery and superior mesenteric artery, is referred to as the solar (or celiac) plexus (Fig. 45-8).

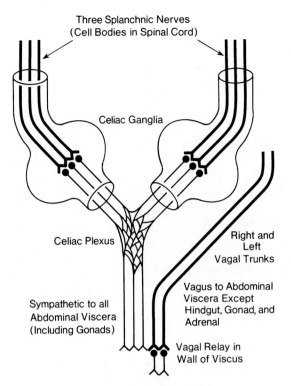

FIGURE 45-7. Constituents of celiac plexus. Redrawn from Last RJ. *Anatomy, Regional and Applied*, 6th ed. Edinburgh: Churchill Livingstone, 1978, with permission.

The celiac ganglia vary in number, size, and location. On either side, the number vary from one to five and the size from 0.5 to 4.5 cm in diameter. Ganglia on the left are uniformly lower than on the right by an average of less than one vertebral level; the extreme is 1.5 vertebral levels. On both sides, the ganglia are 0.6 to 0.9 cm below the celiac artery. The most consistent relationship of the ganglia is to the anterior vertebral margin, most frequently less than 1.5 cm anterior to this margin. Moore et al. (80) verified needle placement and spread of injected solution by radiograph and by CT scan in 20 cancer patients. They noted that spread of the solution tended to be confined to the sides of the injection. They also noted that the anterior portion of the aortic plexus was 2 to 2.5 cm anterior to the anterior vertebral margin (see Fig. 45-10).

Technique. Multiple techniques have been described (up to 13 approaches) for sympathetic blockade at the level of the celiac plexus (76,80–82). Posteriorly, clinicians can employ the classic retrocrural, transcrural, or transaortic techniques using fluoroscopy, CT, or ultrasound guidance. Anteriorly, one can use percutaneous gangliolysis with CT guidance or direct intraoperative celiac gangliolysis.

Celiac plexus nerve block is of special interest in that both bony and vascular landmarks can be used to good advantage in the performance of this block. As with any nerve block, it is advisable to mark out a diagram on the skin that, projected mentally, can yield a three-dimensional perspective for the ultimate placement of the needles. The easiest and most useful avenue of approach to the well-guarded celiac plexus is posterolateral. The patient is placed in a prone position, with a pillow under the abdomen, head turned flat to the table or cart, and arms dangling down at each side. The primary external

topographic features are the 12th ribs and the inferior aspects of the T12 and L1 spinous processes (Fig. 45-8). The figure formed by connecting the spine of T12 and L1 with points 7 to 8 cm lateral at the lower edges of the 12th ribs is that of a flattened isosceles triangle. The equal sides of this triangle serve as directional guides for the two needles. They are passed under the edge of each of the 12th ribs to approach the midline anterior to the body of L1. A 10- to 15-cm, 20-gauge needle is used, dictated by either the frailty or obesity of the patient. Skin wheals are raised 7 to 8 cm from the midline at the inferior edge of the 12th rib. Infiltration with a small amount of local anesthetic solution can be carried deeper for 1 to 3 cm. An awake patient should be warned about brief twinges of pain, which result from the advancing needle coming in contact with the periosteum or lumbar nerves.

At first insertion, the needle is tilted about 45 degrees from the horizontal, so that contact can be made with the lateral body of L1 at an average depth of 7 to 9 cm (Fig. 45-8). Bony contact at a more superficial level indicates that a vertebral transverse process has been encountered, requiring a slightly more caudal redirection of the needle. This must be recognized for what it is, because an incorrect judgment might lead to a superficial injection of anesthetic solution just 2 to 3 cm deep to the transverse process. An ensuing epidural, spinal, or psoas muscle injection could result in a widespread somatic nerve paralysis. This point is of special importance when neurolytic solutions are to be used. The depth of L1 will depend on the patient's size and on the location on the vertebral body at which contact is made (i.e., posterolateral or anterolateral). Once the vertebral body is identified at a usual depth of 8 to 10 cm, the needle is withdrawn to a subcutaneous level and its angle increased to allow the tip of the needle to pass 2 to 3 cm deeper than the previous point of bony contact. The needle's angle may have to be readjusted two or three times until it slides off the anterolateral side of the vertebral body. Determining the precise depth to which the needle should be advanced is of major importance. The simplest method is to advance the left-sided needle slowly to about 2-cm depth, until sensitive fingertips feel aortic pulsations transmitted up the shaft (Fig. 45-8). Once this aortic depth is discovered, the right-sided needle can be inserted and readily advanced to a depth of 3 to 4 cm past the vertebral body. Problems caused by bleeding from penetration of either the aorta or inferior vena cava are extremely rare. The goal is for the tip of the left needle to be just posterior to the aorta, and the right needle anterolateral to the aorta. When neurolytic solutions are to be injected, use of a test dose should be meticulously performed, and the use of contrast media and an image intensifier (fluoroscopy or CT scan) is highly desirable (Fig. 45-9). Diagnostic (local anesthetic) and therapeutic (neurolytic agent) blockade can be performed at the same time, if the patient is kept lucid enough that it can be determined that relief is from the block and not the sedation. In this scenario, it is probably better to give a smaller volume initially (e.g., 6–10 mL local anesthetic through each needle), so that, once the block proves efficacious, the later injection of neurolytic agent does not spread excessively. Neurolytic agent (10–12 mL 50% alcohol or 6% phenol) is injected on each side, preferably mixed with contrast medium for a total dose of 50 mL (Fig. 45-10).

There have been reports of a number of other techniques for celiac plexus nerve block. Although the transaortic method of Ischia (87) would seem to have the theoretical advantage of spreading solution anterior to the aorta, this has yet to be demonstrated. Using a combination of fluoroscopy and fingertip feel, a 22-gauge needle is advanced to penetrate both walls of the aorta and to rest directly in the preaortic nerve network

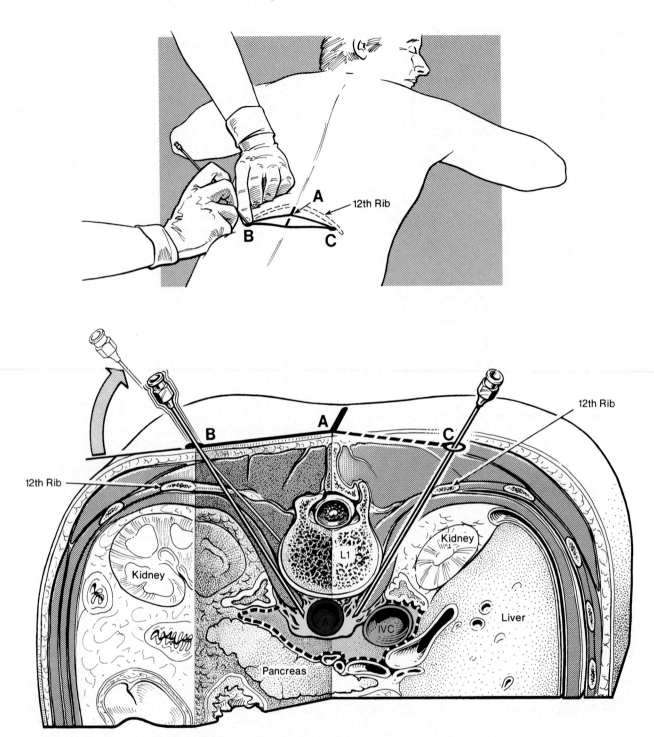

FIGURE 45-8. *Upper panel*: Celiac plexus block. Skin markings, position of patient, and initial insertion of needle. *Note:* Triangle formed by skin marks on lower border of twelfth ribs (*B* and *C*) in line with inferior border of L1 spinous process and joined to inferior border of T12 (*A*). *Lower panel*: Needle insertion and deep anatomy. Skin markings and triangle (*A, B, C*) are still shown. Needle initially is directed in the plane of the line *BA* or *CA*, and at 45 degrees to the horizontal axis of the body, to contact the lateral aspect of the L1 vertebral body. It passes inferior to the twelfth rib and medial to the kidney. The angle of insertion to the *horizontal axis* of the body is then increased until the needle slips past the lateral aspect of the vertebral body, still in the line *BA* or *CA*, to reach the anterolateral aspect. On the left side, the aortic pulsations will be detected at the needle hub before puncturing the artery. Spread of a test dose of contrast medium (in the approximate area indicated by the light blue color) is a valuable guide to correct placement prior to diagnostic or therapeutic celiac block.

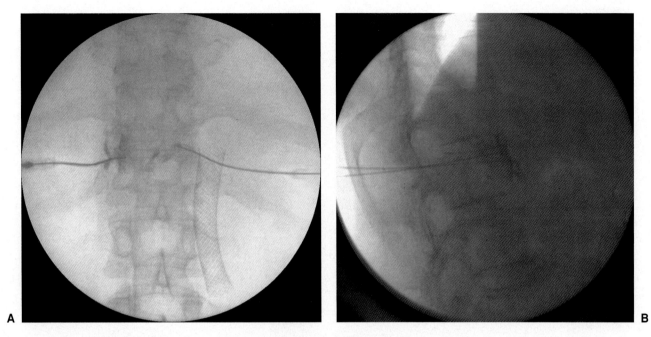

FIGURE 45-9. Retrocrural celiac plexus block. Fluoroscopy images. **A:** Anteroposterior view. **B:** Lateral view with contrast.

of the celiac plexus (Fig. 45-11). A loss-of-resistance technique as the needle passes through the anterior aortic wall can also be employed (88). Although this would seem to guarantee correct placement of local anesthetic or neurolytic solutions, these solutions may be diluted with extravasated blood, and there is also the theoretical concern of dislodging atherosclerotic plaque in elderly patients. Postblock CT scans showed

no retroperitoneal hematoma in six patients. Other authors have described variations of needle placement that emphasize the differences between transcrural celiac block and retrocrural splanchnic nerve block (89). Perhaps the boldest is the ultrasound-guided (percutaneous) anterior approach, which does not seem to have any higher risk of complications and may be of value in patients who cannot tolerate the prone

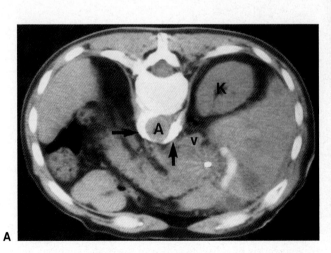

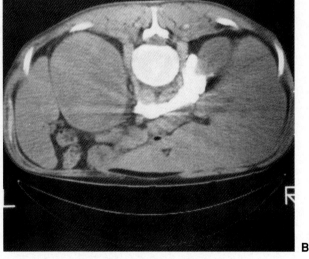

FIGURE 45-10. Computed tomography (CT) scan of contrast media injection during celiac plexus block. **A:** Needles have been inserted through the crus of the diaphragm (on right and left) and contrast medium injected. (In this case, 25 mL of a solution of 50% alcohol containing iothalamate was injected through each needle.) Note contrast almost surrounding aorta in a similar distribution to that shown in Figure 45-8. *A*, aorta; *V*, vena cava; *K*, kidney; *arrows*, spread of contrast media. *B.* Patient with large metastasis in left adrenal gland, seen as large mass to the left of vertebral body. The kidney and liver are seen on the right. *L*, left; *R*, right. In this situation, only one needle through the diaphragm on the left side would have a high chance of piercing the aorta. From Moore DC. *Intercostal Nerve Block and Celiac Plexus Block for Pain Therapy*, Vol. 7. New York: Raven Press, 1984, with permission.

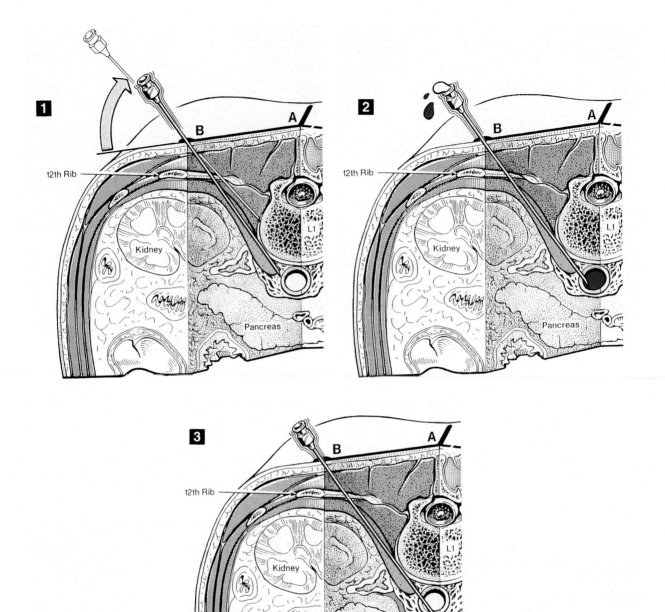

FIGURE 45-11. Transaortic coeliac plexus block.

position, or who are having radiologic biopsies performed simultaneously (90). Anatomic variations make precise needle placement a difficult matter, even though fluoroscopy, standard radiographs, or CT guidance may be used (Fig. 45-10). It is possible that the block may actually occur at nerve, ganglion, or plexus sites with any of the described techniques, and the reported results are quite similar for any of these various combinations.

Efficacy. Celiac plexus block can be used alone or in various combinations with intercostal nerve block to help in the dif-

ferential diagnosis of visceral versus abdominal wall pain (see Chapter 38). The block can be of therapeutic value in acute pancreatitis by relieving spasm of ducts and sphincters in the pancreatic system (91). When used in this regard, methylprednisolone may be mixed and injected along with the local anesthetic solution. The pains of hepatic artery embolization for metastatic malignancies, and of percutaneous interventional biliary manipulations, have been controlled with celiac plexus blockade (92–94). Although the efficacy of neurolytic celiac plexus block in pancreatic cancer pain management has been questioned, when compared to aggressive opiate regimens,

TABLE 45-9

RATIONALE FOR EARLY INTERVENTION WITH CELIAC PLEXUS BLOCK IN ABDOMINAL CANCER

Overall favorable risk:benefit ratio

Better efficacy before extensive perineural infiltration shelters targeted nerves

Increased ease and safety prior to development of massive organomegaly and anatomic distortion

Interventions generally better tolerated in less medically ill patients

May forestall development of chronic pain behavior

Improvements in performance status more likely to meaningfully increase activity and function

May improve compliance with antitumor therapy

Improved performance status may enhance candidacy for investigational therapy

Collateral effects may result in improved gastrointestinal motility

Preliminary evidence of improved survival

TABLE 45-10

FACTORS LIMITING PHAMACOTHERAPY FOR NEOPLASTIC ABDOMINAL PAIN

Modality	Limitations
NSAIDs	Gastropathy, renal dysfunction, bone marrow depletion, or concerns of masking fever
Oral analgesics	Xerostomia, dysphagia, malabsorption, obstruction, nausea, vomiting, coma
Transdermal analgesics	Dose requirements for opioids that exceed limitations of dose form
Parenteral analgesics	Inadequate household or community support to manage infusions
Opioids	Ileus, partial obstruction, intractable constipation
Opioids	Reduced responsivity due to neuropathic component of pain
Opioids	Dose-limiting side effects due to asthenia and cachexia

NSAIDs, nonsteroidal anti-inflammatory drugs.

alcohol celiac plexus block appears to have fewer side effects (95,96). It is the most effective of all therapeutic endeavors commonly used in the treatment of pancreatic cancer pain (97). A comparison of the three posterior approaches (transaortic, classic retrocrural, and bilateral splanchnicectomy) appears to show no significant differences in the results obtained; 70% to 94% of patients report good and immediate relief, which lasts until death in approximately 75% of these patients (99). Recent studies have higher success rates, due to better patient selection, improved technique, and use of imaging. In contrast, alcohol celiac block does not lead to good, prolonged pain relief in patients with chronic pancreatitis or other chronic benign abdominal pain syndromes (98,99).

Rationale for Early Intervention. Table 45-9 summarizes the rationale for this approach. Systemic agents all have limitations for treatment of abdominal cancer pain (Table 45-10). Two studies suggest that early celiac block increases survival in pancreatic cancer (100,101).

Complications. Although not strictly a complication, sympatholysis with its side effects should be considered in celiac blockade. Significant hypotension, especially orthostatic, may occur and should be anticipated (102). Unopposed parasympathetic activity will lead to gastrointestinal hypermotility. The consequent diarrhea is usually transient and does not last more than 2 days (103), but may be severe and continuing. Possible complications of celiac plexus block include subarachnoid, epidural, intraosseous, or intra psoas injection; intravascular injection; retroperitoneal hematoma secondary to bleeding from aorta or vena cava; and puncture of viscera (most often kidney), the lymphatic duct, abscesses, or cysts. Other complications reported after neurolytic blocks include paralysis, lower extremity dysesthesias, and sexual dysfunction. In such cases, the solution obviously had spread to contaminate the lumbar plexus or central neuraxis. Another, more remote possibility is the impairment of blood supply due to hematoma, radicular artery spasm, or perivascular pressure of injected solution. Some drop in blood pressure will occur in 30% to 60% of patients, depending on blood volume and physical status. It is usu-

ally not abrupt in onset. Misplaced injections are best prevented by experience, drawing the proper skin markings, and having the patient fully prone for the injection. Although celiac block can be performed on patients who are in a lateral or semiprone position, these positions make it more difficult to ensure proper orientation to anatomic details. Initial aspiration and the use of a test dose of local anesthetic solution are other precautionary measures against the complications of misplaced injections.

Neurologic Complications. The most common neurologic complication of celiac neurolysis is somatic nerve injury, which was documented as numbness and/or weakness in the T10–L2 dermatomes in 8% of patients in one large series (104). Even after confirmation of accurate needle placement, drug may conceivably track backward between the attachments of the psoas muscle or defects in the crura (105), resulting in deposition near somatic nerves and consequent neurologic injury, most commonly manifest as numbness or dysesthetic pain over the anterior thigh and lower abdominal wall and/or quadriceps weakness (106). This outcome has been postulated to be more likely when retrocrural techniques are utilized (107).

Of over 3,000 cases (most without radiographic guidance), Moore (108) reported 18 episodes of dural puncture (0.006%) which, in all but one case, was heralded by the spontaneous appearance of CSF. Other possible anomalous modes of entry to the spinal canal include retrograde spread via an elongated dural cuff near a nerve root, and through annular tears after accidental disk penetration (109–110). Although well-controlled comparisons between guided and blind procedures are unavailable, radiographic assistance is likely to help one avoid and detect subarachnoid and epidural placement. A case of unilateral paraplegia (111), presumably due to accidental psoas compartment block, was reported after a celiac block was performed without radiologic guidance in a patient positioned laterally because of obesity and ascites.

An important mechanism of potential neurologic injury is spasm of, disruption in, or accidental injection into one of the spinal cord's small nutrient vessels, which may result in ischemic injury, typically to the pyramidal and spinothalamic tracts, with relative sparing of proprioception. The artery of Adamkiewicz (arteria radicularis magna), the largest of the cord's ventral radicular arteries, provides nutrient blood flow to the lower two-thirds of the spinal cord. After leaving the aorta, it runs laterally, about 80% of the time on the left, and typically reaches the cord between T8 and L4, making it vulnerable to injury during celiac block (see Chapter 9, Figs. 9-40, 9-41). This mechanism has been postulated to be responsible for at least five episodes of serious neurologic morbidity after celiac block. De Conno et al. (111) reported a case of flaccid paraplegia, after an otherwise uneventful fluoroscopically guided celiac plexus block undertaken using Moore's technique. Despite clinical demonstration of a T8 sensory-motor deficit that persisted despite corticosteroids, MRI examinations were normal 1 day and 1 week after the block. However, the patient did achieve complete pain relief, which was maintained for 5 months until death. In another case, which utilized neither radiologic guidance nor test doses of local anesthetic, rapid onset of persistent paraplegia followed celiac neurolysis with 6 mL of 6% aqueous phenol in a patient with pancreatic carcinoma (112). The onset of paraplegia was delayed for 2 hours in a third case, which was performed under general anesthesia with the patient in the lateral position, using a single needle and 25 mL of absolute alcohol (113). Arterial blood had been obtained prior to repositioning the needle for subsequent neurolysis.

A survey of pain clinics performing celiac neurolysis in England and Wales during the 5-year interval between 1986 and 1990 elicited 160 responses (73% response rate) and disclosed four instances of permanent paraplegia, accompanied in three cases by urinary and fecal incontinence (114). An aggregate of 2,730 neurolytic blocks had been performed, representing an unsettling one in 683 incidence of serious neurologic morbidity. Only one of the cases had previously been reported in the literature, and results were verified by a survey of three medical defense societies. The techniques used were not detailed, although it was reported that alcohol was used in varied concentrations (50%, 66%, 90%, 100%), and the blocks were performed for cancer (n = 1), pancreatitis (n = 2), and an unknown indication. Radiologic imaging was utilized in all cases, making direct neuraxial injection a less likely explanation than indirect ischemic medullary injury. Two of the four cases were performed under general anesthesia, a fact that eliminates the opportunity to detect potential difficulties with test doses of local anesthetic. A third, performed for pancreatic pain, represented the eighth in a series of blocks, suggesting that repeated neurolysis might produce anatomic abnormalities that predispose to a poor outcome.

Vascular Complications. Although it is an essential safeguard, intermittent aspiration may be inadequate to identify intravascular placement and should be augmented by the preliminary injection of a local anesthetic, coupled with a neurologic examination and the use of fluoroscopy to detect "vascular run-off." The use of general anesthesia, which limits the value of test doses, should be discouraged except when specifically indicated (e.g., in pediatric patients) (115). Large vessels may be punctured accidentally (116) or intentionally (117,118) but, if recognized, the puncture is usually innocuous. Although clinically significant bleeding and hematoma have not been reported, even after transaortic blocks, pretreatment coagulation status should be investigated and, if necessary, optimized.

A generalized seizure accompanied by transient loss of consciousness was reported following an apparent accidental intravascular injection of phenol (119). French investigators (120) described a case of severe cardiac dysrhythmia followed by circulatory arrest after celiac neurolysis performed under general anesthesia with 30 mL of 6.6% phenol. These cases underscore the need for concern related to the potential for systemic toxicity with large volumes of phenol.

Visceral Injury. Perforation of adjacent viscera, especially the kidney, probably occurs more frequently than is appreciated clinically (106) and is a more significant risk in patients who are obese or have altered anatomy due to tumor compression, organomegaly, or surgery (121). Although renal puncture and attendant hematuria are characteristically self-limited, the accidental injection of an appreciable volume of neurolytic drug may produce injury and infarction. Based on cadaver studies, Moore (121) states that renal puncture is more likely when needles are inserted more than 7.5 cm lateral to the midline, when needle tips lie excessively lateral to the vertebral body, and when a higher vertebral body (T11) is targeted. With careful attention to technique, perforation of the viscera should not occur; an obvious advantage of CT guidance, however, is direct visualization of viscera, particularly in patients in whom normal anatomy is distorted by the presence of massive tumor.

Pneumothorax has been reported in a patient treated without radiologic guidance, and in another after a block that relied on just plain films for guidance (102). Based on this experience, chest tube drainage may not be required. Two cases of self-limited pleural effusion were reported after posterior block with 90% alcohol despite CT confirmation of accurate placement (122). Diaphragmatic irritation from overflow of alcohol into the left subdiaphragmatic space was proposed to explain these complications. Chylothorax, an occasional complication of high translumbar aortography (123), has been reported after fluoroscopically guided phenol celiac plexus block (124). In a study of nonradiologically guided paravertebral celiac block (10 cm from the midline) on 20 cadavers, the only cases of visceral injury documented were three instances of pleural puncture (125). Ejaculatory failure occurred in 2% of one large series (104) but is otherwise rarely reported, presumably because patients needing treatment are rarely sexually active. This complication should be borne in mind when treating nonmalignant pain, but is rarely of concern in medically ill cancer patients.

Wilson (109) documented two instances of accidental intervertebral disk penetration, in one case with epidural spread through an annular defect, during attempted celiac block. Disk penetration is usually heralded by increased resistance to needle passage and pain, especially on injection, both of which were absent in these cases, presumably due to disk degeneration. Disk penetration per se is usually innocuous and is even deliberately undertaken with modified transdiscal approaches to splanchnic (126) and celiac (127) block, but if unrecognized may produce disastrous complications.

Metabolic and Chemical Complications

ALCOHOL INTOXICATION. Serum ethanol levels after celiac block have been documented to range between 21 and 54 mg/dL, values well below legal levels of intoxication, and thus ordinarily insufficient to produce systemic effects (128–130). One study demonstrated significantly higher serum alcohol levels in patients with gastric as opposed to pancreatic cancer, due presumably to surgical changes (130). Consideration should still be given to the potential interactions of even low serum alcohol levels and the effects of other concurrently administered CNS depressants. Accidental intravascular injection of large volumes of alcohol may induce intoxication, seizures, and unconsciousness.

ACETALDEHYDE SYNDROME. Occasional systemic reactions consisting of facial flushing, palpitations, and diaphoresis observed after alcohol celiac plexus block have been suggested to represent acetaldehyde syndrome (131). This phenomenon has been postulated to be due to abnormal metabolism of alcohol and high levels of acetaldehyde in individuals with an atypical phenotype for the enzyme aldehyde dehydrogenase (ALDH-1 deficiency). Up to 38% of Japanese possess this phenotype (131). In addition, susceptible patients may give a history of facial flushing after social consumption of small amounts of alcohol. In one study, blood levels of acetaldehyde were 20 times normal in "flushers" (131). This syndrome is probably underdiagnosed because it is relatively innocuous. A similar but more serious reaction—consisting of flushing, diaphoresis, dizziness, nausea, vomiting, hypotension, and tachycardia—which resolved only after 4 to 8 hours, was observed in a patient taking a *b*-lactam antibiotic, moxalactam (132). Alcohol neurolysis should be undertaken only cautiously in patients on disulfiram (Antabuse) therapy for alcohol abuse, and who provide a history of taking other drugs with the capacity to inhibit ALDH such as *b*-lactam antibiotics (including moxalactam), metronidazole (Flagyl), chloramphenicol (Chloromycetin), tolbutamide (Orinase), and chlorpropamide (Diabinese) (133).

OTHER METABOLIC COMPLICATIONS. Unchanged levels of serum amylase in 20 patients who underwent celiac plexus neurolysis suggested that pancreatic injury is unusual (134). Alterations in serum creatinine phosphokinase (CPK) levels occasionally occur, but typically are minimal, suggesting that skeletal muscle injury is infrequent. Interestingly, in one series (129), the two of 20 patients with significantly elevated CPKs (4,242 and 1,640 IU/L) experienced side effects consistent with muscle injury (bilateral L1 neuritis and back pain).

Phenol Complications. Intravascular injection or absorption of phenol may produce transient tinnitus and flushing. Higher doses may produce CNS stimulation, myoclonus, seizures (119), unconsciousness, hypotension, cardiac arrhythmias, and hepatic and renal insufficiency (135). Patients may experience malaise for 24 hours after the administration of doses near the upper recommended limits (600–2,000 mg) (136,137). Owing to the potential for systemic toxicity, especially given trends toward the use of higher concentrations, Boas recommends that phenol be avoided for celiac block and reserved for splanchnic block, which is usually accomplished with lower volumes (139). In an unrandomized trial of alcohol and phenol blocks, Jain (138) demonstrated a higher incidence of untoward effects in the latter group.

Splanchnic Nerve Block

Technique. The splanchnic nerves can be blocked above the diaphragm, at the upper border of T12, using a technique similar to celiac plexus block. The needle is directed, however, to the anterolateral angle of the vertebral body of T12 (139), to the same point on the vertebral body as in the lumbar sympathetic block (see Chapter 39). This block is not recommended for surgical application. For diagnosis and treatment of chronic abdominal pain, it is possible to obtain pain relief with a much smaller volume of solution than is the case with celiac block. Needle insertion is carried out under image intensifier control (Fig. 45-12). A small volume (1 mL) of contrast media (e.g., Angiographin) is injected to check that a linear spread is obtained, in anteroposterior and lateral views, along the anterolateral aspects of vertebral bodies immediately above the diaphragm (Fig. 45-13). Either local anesthetic or neurolytic solution may

be injected for diagnostic or therapeutic block, respectively. The neurolytic solution of choice is phenol in contrast media (e.g., 10% phenol in Angiographin), which can be viewed directly as it spreads. Usually only 3 to 7 mL is required on each side (139).

Complications. Complications of this technique are similar to those of celiac block. Postural hypotension is less, however, because lumbar sympathetic ganglia are not blocked. The risk of pneumothorax is considerable, and it is important to keep the needle as close as possible to the vertebral body. The thoracic duct may be damaged, leading to chylothorax, or it may become obstructed, leading to lymphedema. Vascular puncture and hematoma formation may occur as in celiac block.

Radiologic Guidance for Various Techniques. Although radiographic guidance does not prevent complications, some form of radiographic guidance would seem to be indicated whenever neurolytic block is undertaken because of the serious nature of potential complications. A 1993 survey (140) completed by 130 U.S. pain programs determined that only 3.4% of neurolytic celiac blocks were performed without radiologic guidance, and that 75% and 21.5% were performed with the aid of fluoroscopy and CT, respectively. Thirty-six percent of respondents used CT occasionally, and an additional 25% would if facilities were available.

Although inexpensive and usually accessible, plain radiography is least preferred because it is time-consuming and cannot provide real-time information. The obvious advantage of CT scanning relates to its capacity to directly demonstrate tumor spread and details of visceral and vascular anatomy, thus minimizing the likelihood of injury to these structures. These advantages are, to some extent, offset by the limited availability of CT, its cost, the requirement for cooperation from a knowledgeable radiologist, time required, and limited acceptance in claustrophobic patients. Fluoroscopy is an adequate alternative (134), especially when anatomy is not grossly abnormal and when special techniques are not undertaken. Computed tomography is advisable after failed attempts at fluoroscopically guided neurolysis, when prior studies have demonstrated distortion of normal anatomy (e.g., massive ascites, large pleural effusions, hepato- or splenomegaly, displaced kidneys), and when a transcrural or anterior approach is undertaken (141). Ultrasonography appears to be a reasonable alternative when an anterior approach is planned. Regardless of which anatomic approach or type of guidance is selected, the routine application of fundamental precautions (attention to topographic landmarks, observation for paresthesias, serial aspiration, and the use of a local anesthetic test dose) and contrast media injection are essential.

Choice of Technique. The bulk of experience is with the classic retrocrural approach, and thus it can be regarded as being an extremely reliable and overall acceptable approach. Its main advantages are that it is familiar to clinicians and that, except when anatomy is distorted, it can be performed safely under fluoroscopic guidance. Its theoretic disadvantages relate to the requirement for large volumes of neurolytics administered in the retroaortic region. The thrust of most newer techniques involves ensuring maximal spread of drug to the preaortic space, where the celiac plexus tends to be most concentrated. The classic retrocrural technique has been demonstrated to actually block the splanchnic nerves directly and less reliably to block the celiac plexus, since, in order to do so, drug must traverse the diaphragm through the aortic hiatus or through crural defects (105). Although preaortic spread often occurs with

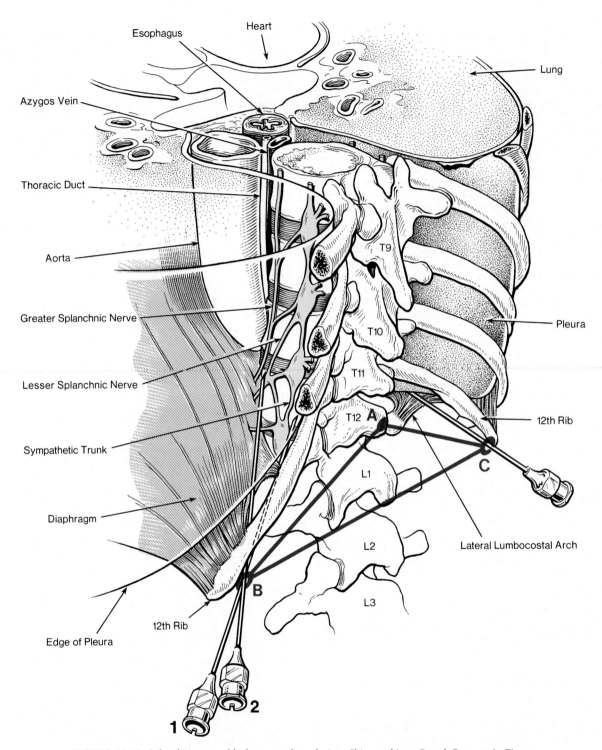

FIGURE 45-12. Splanchnic nerve block, posterolateral view. Skin markings *B* and *C* are as in Figure 45-10, but aimed along *BA* and *CA* to the superior aspect of T12. Note the proximity of pleura and also the thoracic duct on left side.

retrocrural approaches, it is inconstant and seems to depend on the administration of large volumes of drug. Although the retrocrural approach is preferred by some (142), advocates of alternate approaches cite the theoretic advantages of depositing drug more directly into the preaortic region, which may result in more profound analgesia, despite the routine use of lower volumes, and may reduce complications because drug is deposited farther from the spinal axis (142).

Each variant has features that recommend its use, as well as potential drawbacks. Although it is often combined with a classic right-sided block, the transaortic approach requires only a single needle. The aorta serves as a reliable landmark,

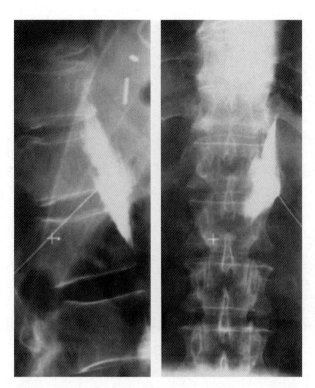

FIGURE 45-13. Splanchnic nerve block. Fluoroscopy image of spread of contrast medium. Anteroposterior (*right*) and lateral (*left*) view.

ensuring anterior deposition of drug. Although it has been described alternately using fluoroscopic and CT guidance, with the former, the aorta will not always be encountered. It should probably be avoided in the presence of recent coagulopathy, significant aneurysm, and mural thrombus. Although they have not emerged as clinically significant problems, hemorrhage, hematoma, and aortic dissection are possible. Although CT or sonographic guidance and attendant expertise are required, the anterior approach has several practical advantages. It, too, requires only a single needle and maximizes preaortic spread and, in addition, is quick and relatively painless. Anterior approaches are unique in that they are extremely well tolerated in patients who cannot lie prone, and thus general anesthesia or deep sedation may be avoided. Although they have not been reported, hemorrhage, infection, and visceral injury are conceivable risks. The posterior transcrural approach resembles the classic approach, but with the aid of CT scanning, preaortic spread is enhanced and a lower volume of drug can be utilized. High splanchnic block is relatively simple to perform since needles do not need to be advanced beyond the vertebral body, and CT scanning is not ordinarily required. The incidence of pneumothorax is low, and this approach is particularly advantageous in the presence of extensive subdiaphragmatic tumor and lymphadenopathy, which may inhibit the spread of drug with other techniques. Despite the potential that neurologic injury might be masked by general anesthesia, intraoperative therapeutic or prophylactic neurolysis is a reasonable option for patients with pancreatic cancer undergoing laparotomy. No particular advantage seems to be associated with transdiscal and transcatheter approaches, although they may emerge as experience accrues.

Choice of Drug and Needle. Diagnostic blockade is typically achieved using a total of 20 to 50 mL of 0.25% bupivacaine or a similar agent injected through one or two needles. Smaller volumes are often used for local anesthetic as opposed to neurolytic block based on the view that the former spreads more readily in tissue. For therapeutic blockade, 25 mL of 50% alcohol and 0.125% bupivacaine or saline is most often administered bilaterally. Moore's experience and anatomic investigations have led him to advocate the use of a total 50-mL volume administered through two needles for retrocrural block. Phenol and other strengths of alcohol (25% to 100%) have been utilized in volumes ranging from 20 to 80 mL without apparent differences.

Although controlled trials of alcohol versus phenol are lacking, alcohol (50% to 100%) would seem to be the agent of choice based on global experience. Alcohol, however, has the disadvantage of producing severe, although transient, pain on injection and is less miscible with contrast medium than is phenol. Phenol (6% to 10%) mixes readily with contrast medium, but must be prepared by a compounding pharmacist (143,144). The apparently greater affinity of phenol for vascular tissue (145) has been cited as a theoretic disadvantage (146), since this might be predicted to correlate with higher incidences of injury to the spinal cord's nutrient vessels, but the actual clinical significance is unknown. Large volumes of phenol may be associated with systemic and cardiac toxicity (120), and accidental intravascular injection has been reported to produce seizures (119). Phenol may be best reserved for (lower volume) splanchnic block, especially if high concentrations are used, because of its potential systemic toxicity (136).

Both 20- and 22-gauge needles are advocated. Although it is more difficult to maintain a straight trajectory with a 22-gauge needle, and higher intraluminal pressures interfere with the manual appreciation of differences in tissue compliance, it is reasonable to utilize 22-gauge needles to minimize pain and tissue trauma (102) as long as radiologic guidance is employed to offset disadvantages. The use of a 22-gauge needle is recommended for anterior (147) and transaortic approaches (148).

Lumbar Sympathetic Block

Indications. Lumbar sympathetic blockade has been used to treat sympathetically mediated cancer pain due to tumor invasion or metastases to the lumbosacral region, chemotherapy or radiation therapy–induced lumbar plexopathy, phantom limb pain, and lower extremity neuropathy secondary to malignancy (82). Unfortunately, it is rarely the case that sympathetic blockade alone is sufficient when somatic nerve roots and/or lumbosacral plexus are involved. The main indication remains lower limb vascular ischemia and pain (see Chapter 39).

Anatomy. The lumbar sympathetic chain is quite variable in size and location. The sympathetic ganglia are usually located between the L2 to L4 vertebral bodies. Classically, the sympathetic chain lies in the fascial plane, anterolateral to lumbar vertebral bodies, just anterior and medial to psoas major muscles. Details of anatomy are provided in Chapter 39, Figures 39-32 to 39-39.

Techniques. Techniques of lumbar sympathetic block are described in Chapter 39, Figs. 39-32 to 39-39. Fluoroscopic images of needle placement and contrast injection are shown in Figure 45-14.

Complications. Side effects of lumbar sympatholysis include hypotension and diarrhea, although both are rare. Intestinal

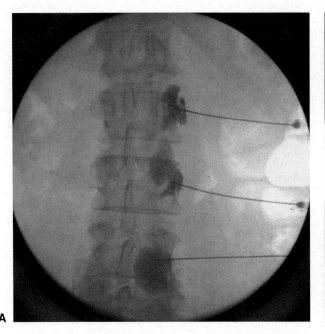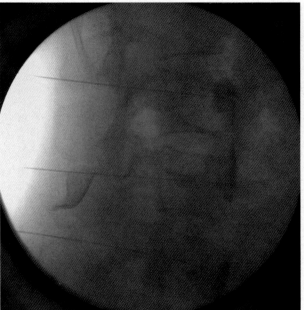

A   B

FIGURE 45-14. Lumbar sympathetic neurolytic block. Fluoroscopic images of needle placement and injection of contrast with A: anterior-posterior and B: lateral views.

hypermotility is self-limited to a few days (83). Other complications include psoas muscle necrosis, kidney or visceral damage, and, rarely, paraplegia. The most common complication with lumbar sympatholysis is genitofemoral neuralgia. Most cases are transient and resolve in a few weeks, although some can be severe and "permanent," particularly if alcohol is used rather than phenol.

Superior Hypogastric Plexus Block

Indications. Pelvic malignancies can affect multiple organs in the pelvis. Such cancers include the gynecologic, rectal, and prostate. Each year in the United States, 18,400 new cases of gynecologic cancer of the uterine cervix, vulva, and vagina are diagnosed; and about 6,300 deaths occur from these cancers. The patient with pelvic malignancy often experiences pain described as vague, poorly localized in the pelvic region, and colicky in character (see Chapter 31, Figs. 31-22 and 31-23). Surgical destruction of the hypogastric plexus (presacral neurectomy) has been shown to relieve pelvic pain (84,85). Subsequently, Plancarte et al. reported a technique for hypogastric blockade with good results for controlling pelvic pain secondary to cancer (86). In this anecdotal report, all 28 patients with intractable pelvic cancer pain reported good pain relief after the procedure. There were no reported complications. No confirmatory studies have been reported. Unfortunately, many patients with pelvic visceral cancer also have somatic structures involved, thus limiting the usefulness of this technique.

Because of the ease of applying epidural, caudal, or spinal anesthesia for surgery in the pelvic region, and because hypogastric plexus block is exclusively an autonomic blockade, it is likely that it will remain within the realm of pain management.

Anatomy. The (superior) hypogastric plexus constitutes the most caudal of the great plexus of the sympathetic nervous system. It is formed from pelvic visceral afferent and efferent sympathetic nerves from branches of the aortic plexus and fibers from the L2 and L3 splanchnic nerves. These pass through the plexus en route to and from all pelvic viscera (bladder, uterus, vagina, prostate, rectum) via the hypogastric nerves. The superior hypogastric plexus is retroperitoneal and distinctly situated at the sacral promontory, between the lower third of the fifth lumbar vertebrae and the upper third of the first sacral vertebral body, where it is accessible to blockade by a percutaneous needle. In this area, it is in close proximity to the bifurcation of the common iliac vessels (Fig. 45-15). The inferior hypogastric plexus (right and left) are intertwined with the viscera of the pelvis, and, for this reason, they cannot be isolated and separately blocked. However, as all of the sympathetic fibers must have passed first through the superior plexus, this is not a concern. Neither the superior nor the inferior hypogastric plexus contain somatic nerve fibers, however, they do receive parasympathetic fibers from S2–S4.

Technique. The patient is placed in the prone position, the same as for intercostal or celiac plexus blockade. In many respects, needle placement for hypogastric plexus block is identical to that for the celiac plexus block, but in the reverse direction (Fig. 45-15). The target for a hypogastric plexus block is just anterior to the caudal end of the lumbar lordosis (L5–S1) instead of anterior to the cephalad end of the lordosis (L1), as in celiac plexus blockade. After the patient is adequately sedated, the skin is prepped with topical antiseptic, and the lumbosacral region is draped in a sterile manner. Bilateral skin wheals are raised 5 to 7 cm lateral to the L4–L5 interspace (intercristal line). A 10- to 15-cm, 20-gauge needle, with its bevel oriented in the medial direction, is introduced toward the midline at a 45-degree angle, and in the caudal direction at a 30-degree angle. Should the transverse process of L5 or iliac crest be encountered, first redirection slightly cephalad or caudad, then movement of insertion points 1 cm laterally or medially may be necessary. The needle is advanced until the body of L5 is contacted. The needle is then removed to the subcutaneous tissue and, maintaining the same caudal angle, redirected with

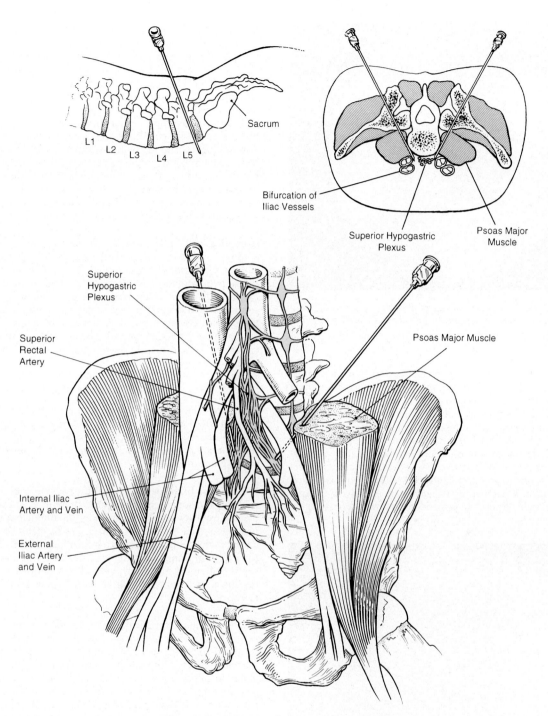

FIGURE 45-15. Superior hypogastric plexus block.

slightly less medial angle and readvanced until it is felt to slide off the vertebral body. A slight loss of resistance from the psoas muscle fascia may be felt as the needle is advanced 1 cm more to reach its eventual position just anterior to the L5–S1 interspace (Fig. 45-15). The second needle is placed in a similar manner on the opposite side. Fluoroscopic guidance is useful to facilitate passage of the needles and to demonstrate final positioning by injection of contrast (Fig. 45-16). Computed tomography scan guidance may be beneficial in visualizing the common iliac vessels, or in determining whether exceptional anatomic alter-

ations exist in the region, due to disease involvement. Contrast material (3 to 4 mL) should remain anterior to the vertebral bodies (Fig. 45-17) with relatively smooth anterior (retroperitoneal space) and posterior (psoas muscle) borders on lateral images, and should meet but be confined to midline region on anteroposterior (AP) projections (Figs. 45-16 and 45-17). A single-needle technique has been described, which may be useful for evaluation of nonmalignant conditions. For malignant conditions in which disease may prohibit adequate spread, the two-needle approach just described is recommended.

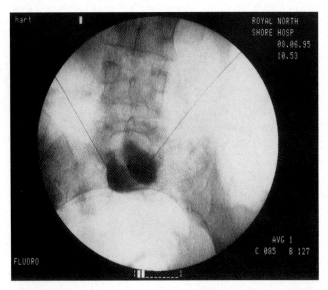

FIGURE 45-16. Fluoroscopic image of needle placement and contrast injection for superior hypogastric plexus block (anterior-posterior view).

Gentle aspiration should be performed in four quadrants, and, if negative, a 3-mL test dose of epinephrine, containing local anesthetic, is injected to rule out intravascular or subarachnoid malpositioning. Substantial resistance to injection suggests improper positioning in the psoas muscle or the L5–S1 intervertebral disc. To confine solution to the plexus region, and to avoid spillage onto the nearby sacral somatic roots, injected volumes should be limited to 6 to 8 mL through each needle. For diagnostic/prognostic purposes, 0.25% bupivacaine is recommended. When neurolytic agents are employed, use of a test dose should be performed meticulously, with repeated gen-

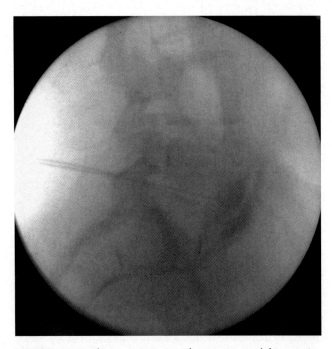

FIGURE 45-17. Fluoroscopic image of contrast spread for superior hypogastric plexus block. Lateral view.

tle aspiration through the remainder of injection. Neurolytic blockade has been described using 10% phenol in water, although 10% phenol in contrast medium seems preferable.

Applications. Hypogastric block may be useful in the differential diagnosis and treatment of chronic pelvic pain, particularly of neoplastic origin. Patients with pain due to cervical, endometrial, prostatic, testicular, and colorectal cancers have been treated with superior hypogastric blockade. Success (visual analogue scale for pain assessment [VAS] <4 and significant reductions in opioid usage) appears to occur in 70%, with a duration until patient demise (3–12 months) in most reported patients. In three patients with pain felt to be secondary to complications of radiotherapy (enteritis, cystitis, proctitis), symptoms had not recurred after 2 years of follow-up.

Complications. Intramuscular, intravascular, subarachnoid, epidural, and intraperitoneal injection are all theoretically possible complications. Vascular puncture could lead to retroperitoneal hematoma formation, and neurologic damage could occur through direct needle trauma or with spillage of neurolytic solutions onto somatic nerves. Visceral puncture (ureter, bowel, uterus, and kidney) is possible. None of these possible complications have yet been reported. The incidence of these complications is, therefore, unknown, but should be minimized with strict adherence to technique.

Ganglion Impar Block

Anatomy. The ganglion impar is a solitary retroperitoneal structure located at the level of the sacrococcygeal junction. The two parallel sympathetic chains fuse together anterior to the superior border of the coccyx to form the ganglion impar or ganglion of Walther.

Indications. In the perineum, a diffuse network of mixed sympathetic and somatic innervation is present. Perineal pain thus usually involves both somatic and sympathetic pathways. Perineal pain can be due to cancer involvement of the lower colon, rectum, bladder, cervix, and endometrium. Blockade of the ganglion impar with the goal of disrupting visceral nociceptive afferents has been reported to be effective in managing intractable perineal cancer pain in anecdotal case series (149,150).

Anatomy. Characteristically, sympathetic pain in the perineal region has distinct qualities—it tends to be vague and poorly localized and is frequently accompanied by sensations of burning and urgency. Although the anatomic interconnections of the ganglion impar are rarely described in any detail in even the anatomic literature, it is probable that the sympathetic component of these pain syndromes derives, at least in part, from this structure. The ganglion impar is a solitary retroperitoneal structure located at the level of the sacrococcygeal junction that marks the termination of the paired paravertebral sympathetic chains (Fig. 45-18).

Technique. The patient is positioned in the lateral decubitus position, and a skin wheal is raised in the midline at the superior aspect of the intergluteal crease, over the anococcygeal ligament, and just above the anus. The stylet is removed from a standard 22-gauge, 3.5-inch spinal needle, which is then manually bent about 1 inch from its hub to form a 25- to 30-degree angle. This maneuver facilitates positioning of the needle tip anterior to the concave curvature of the sacrum and coccyx. The needle is inserted through the skin wheal with its concavity

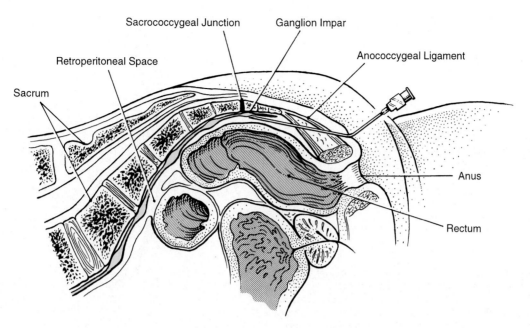

FIGURE 45-18. Ganglion impar block.

oriented posteriorly and, under fluoroscopic guidance, is directed anterior to the coccyx, closely approximating the anterior surface of the bone, until its tip is observed to have reached the sacrococcygeal junction (Fig. 45-18). Retroperitoneal location of the needle is verified by observation of the spread of 2 mL of water-soluble contrast medium, which typically assumes a smooth-margined configuration resembling an apostrophe. Four milliliters of 1% lidocaine or 0.25% bupivacaine is injected for diagnostic and prognostic purposes, or alternatively, 4 to 6 mL of 10% phenol is injected for therapeutic neurolytic blockade.

Under most circumstances, needle placement is relatively straightforward. Local tumor invasion, particularly from rectal cancer, may prohibit the spread of injected solutions.

Efficacy. The first report of interruption of the ganglion impar for relief of perineal pain appeared in 1990 (149). Sixteen patients were studied (13 women, 3 men), ranging in age from 24 to 87 (median = 48). All patients had advanced cancer (cervix, nine; colon, two; bladder, two; rectum, one; endometrium, two), and pain had persisted in all cases despite surgery and/or chemotherapy and radiation, analgesics, and psychological support. Localized perineal pain was present in all cases, and was characterized as burning and urgent in eight patients and of a mixed character in eight patients. Pain was referred to the rectum (seven cases), perineum (six cases), or vagina (three cases). Following preliminary local anesthetic blockade and subsequent neurolytic block, eight patients experienced complete (100%) relief of pain, and the remainder experienced significant reduction in pain (one, 90%; two, 80%; one, 70%; four, 60%) as determined with a VAS. Blocks were repeated in two patients, with further improvement. Follow-up depended on survival and was carried out for 14 to 120 days. In patients with incomplete relief of pain, residual somatic symptoms were treated with either epidural injections of steroid or sacral nerve blocks. A modified version of ganglion impar block was reported in 1995 (150).

Complications. Observation that the spread of contrast material is restricted to the retroperitoneum is essential, as we have had experience with one case in which epidural spread within the caudal canal was evident. Also, unless care is taken to confirm the needle's posteroanterior orientation, perforation of the rectum or periosteal injection is possible. In addition, anatomic abnormalities of the sacrococcygeal vertebral column, specifically exaggerated anterior curvature, may inhibit access, in which case the needle may be further modified with an additional bend.

Subarachnoid Neurolysis

Indications. Although indications are limited, subarachnoid neurolysis is a valuable technique in carefully selected patients with refractory cancer pain and life expectancy that is unlikely to exceed 1 year. The most suitable pain problems involve only a few dermatomes, and are ideally unilateral. Intrathecal neurolysis is intended to produce discrete lesions at the level of the cord's posterior roots within the dural sac (chemical rhizolysis). Rather than the extensive anesthesia that accompanies perioperative local anesthetic spinal anesthesia, subarachnoid neurolysis endeavors to produce a band of analgesia that corresponds to or slightly overlaps the boundaries of the patient's pain. Coupled with prudent patient selection, complications are few, and favorable results are common. Difficulties, however, are more likely to arise when its use is extended for pain that is bilateral or diffuse, and in the presence of neurologic or undiagnosed disease (151,152).

Although chlorocresol, cold or hypertonic saline, and ammonium salts are occasionally used, concentrated solutions of alcohol or phenol are preferred. Since the neurolytic effects of these agents are not selective, patients are exposed to risks that include motor weakness and incontinence. These risks can be minimized (although not entirely eliminated) by careful patient selection and by combining the use of hyperbaric or hypobaric solutions with careful positioning of the patient and strict attention to protocol.

TABLE 45-11

CONSIDERATIONS FOR SUBARACHNOID NEUROLYSIS

Patient education and consent
Consideration of periprocedural sedation
Selection of neurolytic agent (alcohol or phenol)
Selection of concentration (absolute alcohol, 5%–15% phenol in glycerine)
Determination of targeted dermatomes and roots
Determination of injection site
Need for single-versus-multiple needles
Upper and lower volume limits
Positioning of patient
Adjustment of opioid dose and follow-up

Considerations Common to Subarachnoid Alcohol and Phenol Neurolysis. A number of factors must be considered prior to commencing treatment (Table 45-11). An absence of controlled studies compares outcomes for alcohol versus phenol, so these agents are used almost interchangeably. Despite early suggestions that phenol was associated with preferential effects on small fibers subserving pain (153,154), subsequent animal and autopsy studies have confirmed that the effects of alcohol and phenol are nonselective, resulting in indiscriminate damage to nerve fibers, the extent of which is dependent on volume and concentration (132,155). Pathologic findings and mechanisms have been amply reviewed by Papo and Visca (156). Expert opinion suggests that hyperbaric phenol may be more controllable than hypobaric alcohol, but that the neurolytic effects of alcohol may be more potent and lasting (157,158). Alcohol is preferred to phenol when the patient cannot lie on his painful side. In addition, failed neurolysis with one agent may be best followed with a trial of treatment using another.

In general, subarachnoid neurolysis should not be undertaken if more than six spinal segments are involved, especially since treatment usually aims to block one dermatome above and below the boundaries of the painful region. Some controversy surrounds the treatment of bilateral symptoms. Some authorities recommend unilateral neurolysis of the more painful side first, followed a few days later by treatment of the contralateral side (159). However, intrathecal and epidural opioid and nonopioid drugs are better alternatives (see Chapter 40). The patient's overall condition is an important factor in making such decisions. Epidural neurolysis may also be considered for pain that is bilateral or more widely distributed.

Anatomy. The topographic distribution of pain is determined through a careful history, following which anatomic charts are consulted to confirm which spinal nerve roots innervate the painful region. Owing to differential growth, the length of the adult vertebral column exceeds that of the spinal cord; along the caudal half of the axis, nerve roots emerge from the cord a variable number of spinal segments above the level from which they exit the vertebral column through their intervertebral foramen. The targeted roots may be approached either at the interspace where they arise from the cord or somewhat lower, where they exit the bony canal. This controversy relates only to lumbar and low thoracic blocks, since more proximal roots have a shorter, more horizontal intradural course. Based on the view that the effects of alcohol are most profound at the level at which the fine rootlets (fila radicularia) arise from the cord, most authorities (152,160) recommend that the roots be

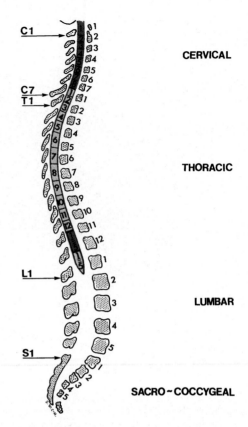

FIGURE 45-19. Drawing of vertebral column and spinal cord, indicating segmental relationships. Significant difference between the vertebral and cord levels occurs only in the lower thoracic and lumbosacral regions.

targeted at the level at which they arise from the cord. A chart depicting the relationship between the spinal nerve roots and the vertebral column is consulted to determine the appropriate interspace for needle placement (Fig. 45-19).

In general, both therapeutic and toxic effects correlate with the volume and concentration of neurolytic used. Owing to the absence of controlled comparative studies among treatment protocols, arbitrary, although reasonable, upper limits have been proposed by various authors based on their clinical experience. Although limits customarily regarded as safe are exceeded at the peril of increased risk of serious neurologic morbidity, the treatment protocol that is ultimately applied must, to a degree, be individualized. For example, upper volume limits may be reasonably amplified in the mid thoracic region, which is distant from the outflow to the brachial and lumbosacral plexus; likewise, volume limits are less critical in preterminal patients who are already confined to bed and in whom continence is not an issue.

The administration of small volumes of drug through multiple needles placed in neighboring interspaces is preferable to using larger volumes through a single needle (156,161). All aspects of the injection technique should be designed to minimize turbulence that might produce aberrant flow and untoward neurologic changes.

Techniques

Patient Preparation. The need to remain immobile during and immediately after the injection must be explained. Patients should be led to expect little discomfort during needle placement, but must be warned of the necessity for assuming an uncomfortable position during and just after the injection. They are coached regarding the need to provide real-time feedback regarding the development of new sensations, especially burning, tingling, warmth, numbness, or pain relief. Ideally, premedication is omitted or used sparingly to preserve patient cooperation. The blood pressure cuff is placed on the uppermost arm and used infrequently during the procedure to avoid artifactual numbness from decreased circulation. Finally, it is essential that a careful preprocedural neurologic assessment be performed to familiarize patients with the intraprocedural routine and document preexisting deficits.

Subarachnoid Alcohol Neurolysis. For alcohol injection, the patient lies with the painful side uppermost on an adjustable bed, of the type typically used for surgery. The patient is positioned so that, after needle placement, the injection site can be elevated above the neighboring spinal segments by means of table adjustments and support provided by padding. A firm bolster comprised of folded sheets is preferable to bulky pillows.

The theca can be accessed through a midline or paravertebral approach, although ideally the needle tip should ultimately rest at the superior (uppermost) aspect of the subarachnoid space near the targeted roots. A 22-gauge needle should be utilized to facilitate placement, ensure easy detection of CSF, and minimize any jet effects during injection. The bevel is oriented toward the ceiling to maximize the migration of hypobaric alcohol toward the targeted roots. Free flow of CSF is obtained, following which a 1-mL syringe is firmly connected to the needle's hub, taking care not to alter the needle's depth. The table is adjusted to ensure that the injection site is the least dependent (highest) portion of the vertebral column, and the patient is rolled 45 degrees forward to direct the hypobaric alcohol toward the posterior (sensory) roots (Fig. 45-20). Alcohol is instilled slowly and steadily in aliquots of 0.1 to 0.2 mL/min. The patient is coached to report new sensations, espe-

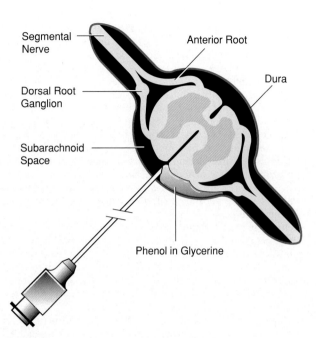

FIGURE 45-21. Lateral supine position used for subarachnoid injection of phenol.

cially burning, tingling, warmth, or pain relief. Between injections, a brief neurologic examination is serially performed. If paresthesias or numbness are encountered just above or below the targeted dermatomes, the table's tilt is modified away from the direction in which further spread is desired. If altered sensation occurs distant from the targeted dermatomes, treatment should be halted and the needle repositioned in an alternate interspace.

Subarachnoid Phenol Neurolysis. The technique for subarachnoid neurolysis with phenol is similar to that which has been described for alcohol except, insofar as the use of a hyperbaric as opposed to hypobaric solution mandates different positioning of the patient. The patient is positioned laterally, with the painful side dependent, and provisions are made for adjusting the table and inserting pads, so that the injection site is rendered lower than the adjacent vertebral segments. Because the patient will ultimately be tilted 45 degrees posteriorly (toward the operator) to maximize the spread of hyperbaric phenol to the posterior roots (Fig. 45-21), he must initially be positioned near the edge of the bed to avoid contact between the bed and needle/syringe. A 20- to 22-gauge spinal needle is required because of the viscosity of phenol and glycerine formulations. The needle bevel is directed downward, and whether introduced in a midline or paramedian trajectory, its tip should ultimately lie near the lower portion of the spinal axis.

When using hyperbaric phenol, it is critical that utmost care be exercised in creating a firm seal between the syringe and the needle's hub. Phenol in glycerine is so viscous that, even when injected through a 1-mL syringe, the pressure required to advance the plunger often breaks the seal, introducing the risk that the neurolytic solution will spill onto the patient's skin or injure the clinician's eyes. Ease of injection can be facilitated by immersing the ampule containing the phenol solution in hot water before aspirating it into the syringe.

In contrast to the transient or burning pain that may immediately follow subarachnoid alcohol injection, intrathecal

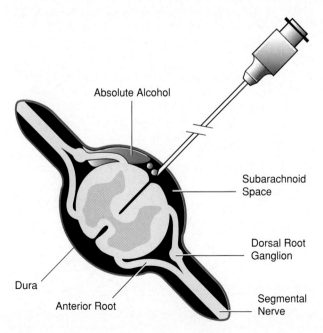

FIGURE 45-20. Lateral prone position used for subarachnoid injection of alcohol.

phenol characteristically produces relatively mild feelings of warmth, tingling, or prickling in affected dermatomes, presumably owing to its initial local anesthetic effects.

Other Considerations Common to Subarachnoid Alcohol and Phenol Neurolysis. Brief but careful serial neurologic examinations are performed throughout the procedure to determine the extent of ongoing neural blockade and to detect early signs of motor weakness. Documentation of baseline neurologic function is essential, and patients should be cautioned to move as little as possible during motor and sensory testing. Prolonged maintenance of the lateral decubitus position and frequent blood pressure checks occasionally produce artifactual numbness of the dependent limb(s), which may be mistaken for denervation.

Once the predetermined volume of neurolytic has been injected, the needle(s) stylet should be replaced and the needle tip is allowed to be washed by CSF, to minimize the potential for sinus formation and backache due to the escape of residual drug from the needle as it is withdrawn. The patient's position should be maintained for about 15 minutes following the injection.

Matsuki et al. carried out a series of investigations in humans and dogs to determine the rapidity at which CSF concentrations of absolute alcohol (162) and 7% phenol in glycerine (163) decline following therapeutic neurolysis. They determined that the neurolytic solution is rapidly diluted by CSF, which is a reasonable explanation for the inadequate results often observed clinically. Immediately after the completion of incremental injections of 1.0 mL of each agent, the CSF alcohol concentration was only 25.6%, and phenol and glycerine concentrations were, respectively, 30% and 40% of their original concentrations. Ten minutes following the completion of injection, CSF alcohol concentrations had fallen to 3.1%, and 15 minutes after phenol injection, the mean CSF concentrations of phenol and glycerine were 0.1% and 3%, respectively.

Several important conclusions can be drawn from these experiments. Rapid decline in CSF levels of the agents studied suggest that patients can be safely repositioned 15 minutes after the spinal injection is complete. In addition, the nearly immediate reduction in concentrations support the need for carefully positioning needles near the targeted roots, rather than relying on modifications of the table to affect precise localization of effect. Finally, rapid decline of CSF levels of both phenol and glycerine argues against Maher's (154) contention that glycerine acts as a mordant or carrying agent, releasing phenol slowly.

Cervical Subarachnoid Neurolysis. Typically, only a moderate proportion of patients experience lasting pain relief after cervical subarachnoid neurolysis (146), as exemplified by a large series that reported excellent to good results in 77% of patients overall, but in only 50% of patients treated with cervical block. This has been suggested to be due to anatomic factors that limit contact between the neurolytic and the targeted roots, including the relatively short intradural course of the cervical roots, the narrower caliber of the cervical canal, and rapid dissipation of the lytic agent due to brisk CSF flow. Subdural block, although once advocated as an alternative to cervical subarachnoid neurolysis, is not now commonly used, and experience with cervical epidural neurolysis is meager.

Puncturing the dura at the cervical level is not technically difficult. The cervical column's spinous processes are relatively blunt, and when the neck is flexed, they usually do not overlap. The cervical interspaces can usually be easily palpated, and the theca accessed in the midline from a nearly perpendicular trajectory (see Chapter 9, Figs. 9-1 and 9-2). Obviously,

the needle needs initially to be advanced cautiously to avoid spinal cord injury. Notwithstanding this important consideration, the cord is routinely penetrated during cordotomy (164), and workers have reported accidentally piercing the cord with no complications other than transient pain (165,166). Cervical CSF pressure may be low in the patient in the prone position. If free flow of CSF is not easily established, localization can be aided by gentle aspiration, or, alternatively, the puncture can be performed with the patient sitting, provided that the return to the decubitus position is undertaken carefully.

The most important potential complications of cervical subarachnoid neurolysis are cranial nerve dysfunction and upper extremity weakness. Cranial nerve palsy is unlikely when proper technique is followed, and few reports are encountered in the literature. Perese (165) described one patient with diplopia of 2 months' duration after C1–C2 alcohol block. Careful positioning, scrupulous attention to technique, and serial neurologic assessment are employed to minimize the risk of limb paresis, except when the limb has already been rendered useless, in which case ipsilateral motor weakness is not a concern and slightly more liberal volumes can be used. When performing high cervical blocks or attempting to block pain distributed over more than one or two dermatomes, one should consider inserting multiple spinal needles into the two or three neighboring, relevant interspaces and injecting smaller increments of absolute alcohol through each needle. It may be best to initially exaggerate the head-up and head-down position for hyperbaric and hypobaric techniques, respectively, after which the table can be gently readjusted (Fig. 45-22).

Thoracic Subarachnoid Neurolysis. The approaches to high and low thoracic intraspinal injections are relatively straightforward and are similar to those employed for cervical and lumbar puncture, respectively. The architecture of the mid thoracic spine's posterior elements often renders access to the theca difficult at this level. The thoracic spinous processes are elongated and project from the column at an acute angle (see Chapter 11, Fig. 11-12) and, as a result, overlapping adjacent processes may render it difficult to introduce a needle into the subarachnoid space. This difficulty may be obviated by adopting a paramedian approach (see Chapter 11, Fig. 11-12). If the desired

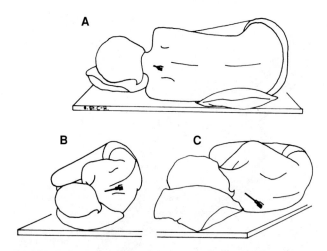

FIGURE 45-22. Positioning of the patient for cervical subarachnoid injection. **A:** Posterior view. **B:** Lateral-prone position used for the injection of absolute alcohol. **C:** Lateral-supine position used for the injection of hyperbaric solutions.

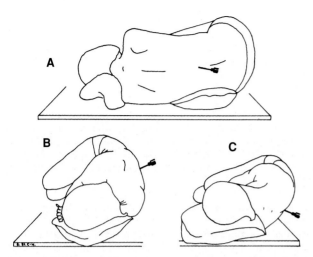

FIGURE 45-23. Positioning of the patient for subarachnoid injection in the thoracolumbar region. **A:** Posterior view. **B:** Lateral-prone position used for the injection of absolute alcohol. **C:** Lateral-supine position used for the injection of hyperbaric solutions.

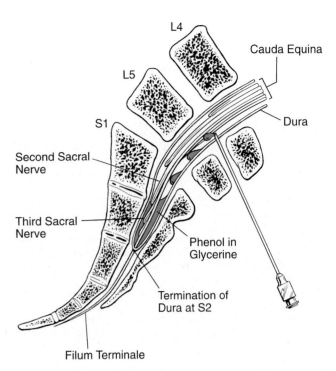

FIGURE 45-24. Saddle block with phenol and other hyperbaric solutions is used in the treatment of midline perineal pain of malignant origin.

interspace still cannot be accessed, an attempt may be made one to two segments above or below. If successful, the table is tilted to direct the injectate toward the roots subserving the painful region, and neurolysis can be cautiously initiated (Figs. 45-20 through 45-23).

Relative to the rest of the cord, the mid thoracic region is relatively distant from the fibers that subserve limb, bowel, and bladder function and, as a result, neurolysis is, overall, safest in this region (Fig. 45-19). Although selective sensory effects are never guaranteed owing to the potential for drug spilling onto anterior motor roots, if segmental unilateral paresis of the intercostal muscles occurs, it rarely embarrasses ventilation. Occasionally, a functional hernia develops which, although inconvenient, can be managed with an abdominal binder. Greater caution should be exercised when the upper or lower thoracic roots are targeted.

Lumbar Subarachnoid Neurolysis. Because of the proximity of fibers subserving pain and lower limb, bowel, and bladder function, lumbar subarachnoid neurolysis is ill-advised except in carefully selected circumstances. In patients with unilateral limb pain, normal strength, and intact bowel and bladder function, percutaneous cordotomy is preferred. If cordotomy is not feasible and lower extremity strength is already compromised, lumbar neurolysis may be carried out cautiously, albeit with a risk of increased weakness of the affected extremity, contralateral weakness, and sphincter disturbances. Incontinence usually, although not consistently, can be avoided by combining careful positioning and modest volumes. In patients with normal strength but impaired ambulation secondary to intractable pain, function may improve even if motor weakness ensues, although this outcome cannot be predicted with certainty. In patients already confined to bed owing to neurologic or systemic effects of cancer, lumbar neurolysis can be performed more freely. The bedbound patient with a urinary diversion and colostomy is subject to insignificant risks. Bedbound patients with intact sphincter function are more likely to accept the modest risk of incontinence than their ambulatory counterparts. In most series, urinary difficulties occur infrequently, and usually are transient, whereas incontinence of stool is even more rare.

Lumbosacral Neurolysis (Saddle Block). Perineal analgesia can be produced reliably and easily with phenol saddle block, making it an excellent option for midline pain due to rectal and pelvic malignancies in selected patients. Incontinence is relatively common, and, as is the case after lumbar block, the incidence of urinary dysfunction exceeds bowel problems, with effects that are usually but not always transient. Nevertheless, saddle block is usually avoided in patients with normal sphincters. Superior hypogastric plexus or ganglion impar blocks can be considered when pain is of sympathetic origin; these procedures block the individual sacral nerve roots as they emerge from their foramina and are preferred for somatic pain.

Lumbosacral Subarachnoid Phenol Injection (Saddle Block). The technique is fairly simple, but can be made even more so with adequate preparation. The block is performed with the patient seated and simply requires lumbar puncture at the L5–S1 (or L4–L5) interspace (Fig. 45-24). The bevel of the needle is directed downward, and the needle's caliber (20- or 22-gauge) must be sufficient to allow easy passage of hyperbaric phenol. Ultimately, before commencing phenol administration, the patient is inclined 45 degrees backward, a position that is nearly impossible to maintain without support. This difficulty can be overcome by positioning the patient backward on a chair, so that its back rest can be held by the patient with both arms. Once the needle is in place, the chair can be moved toward a wall equipped with a safety railing; the railing supports the upper part of the patient's back, while the space between the railing and wall leaves room to connect a syringe and perform the injection. This position is intended to ensure that the hyperbaric phenol is deposited preferentially on the posterior (sensory) roots, and must be maintained for about 15 minutes after the injection is complete. Patients usually begin to experience pain relief after the first drops of drug are administered.

PART IV: PAIN MANAGEMENT

Sensory testing of the perineum is somewhat difficult because of the patient's seated position, but still must be performed serially, along with tests of lower extremity strength. Administering up to 1.2 mL of 5% phenol, Stovner and Endressen (167) encountered six cases of urinary incontinence and two of bowel incontinence, none of which persisted beyond 10 days. In another series that used 1 mL of 10% phenol (168), urinary incontinence occurred after 22% of 133 blocks, but resolved within 3 to 7 days in all but two patients. Using 0.8 mL of 5%, 10%, or 15% phenol, Ischia et al. (169) observed both progressively better pain relief and higher incidences of incontinence using stronger solutions. In a subsequent series (170), utilizing 0.6 to 1 mL of 7.5%, 10%, and 15% phenol, better efficacy was again observed using more concentrated formulations, and one-third of patients with intact urinary function experienced incontinence. Urinary incontinence was observed only in males in the latter series, and neither fecal incontinence nor leg weakness occurred in either series. Their recommendation is to use stronger concentrations, especially when urinary diversion is already present.

In patients with normal bladder and bowel function in whom alternate procedures are inappropriate, the position may be modified by placing padding beneath the buttock that corresponds to the least painful side. Although perineal pain usually crosses the midline, it is often vague, and "bilateral" pain is sometimes eliminated with a predominantly unilateral block on the most affected side. If pain persists, the alternate side can be blocked after an interval of a few days.

Lumbosacral Subarachnoid Alcohol Injection. Because it is so straightforward, phenol saddle block is preferred for perineal pain, although alcohol can be used for the rare patient who cannot sit because of severe pain. The considerations for using alcohol are similar to those described for phenol. Because patients must assume a "jackknife position" (buttocks elevated), difficulty in obtaining a free flow of CSF sometimes arises. Bilateral pain can be treated by having the patient adopt a prone position or, if sphincter function is a concern, padding can be placed beneath the most painful side, and a contralateral injection can be performed on another occasion, if it is still indicated.

Chemical Cordectomy. In their classic treatises on regional block, Moore (171) and Bonica (172) refer to so-called alcohol "cordectomy," induced by injecting large volumes (10 mL) of absolute alcohol intrathecally, but little detail or outcome data are provided. This technique has been used mostly to treat refractory severe muscle spasm after spinal cord injury, but occasionally to treat pain of malignant origin. Autopsies performed on patients treated with 4 to 8 mL of intrathecal alcohol for spasticity, however, suggest that results are due to lesions involving the spinal roots rather than the cord (173). Posterior nerve root degeneration, which was present in all cases, exceeded more limited effects observed on the anterior roots. Evidence of myelitis was limited to a characteristic zone of myelination and gliosis rimming the cord's periphery. Leptomeningeal changes were manifest as fibrosis of the pia and arachnoid, but the dura and major blood vessels were unaffected. Their observation that pathology was similar in patients administered 4 and 8 mL of alcohol led them to conclude that further benefit was unlikely to accompany the administration of larger volumes.

Bruno (174) administered 10 to 12 mL of absolute alcohol intrathecally to 42 paraplegic patients with good results, overall. He injected 2 mL/min at or below the L1 level in patients positioned with the targeted roots uppermost, but tilted backward to maximize motor effects. He reported considerable functional improvement, with easier positioning, mobilization, facilitation of physical therapy, and decreased bladder spasm. Complications were limited to three cases of immediate flushing, dizziness and nausea, and occasional postural headache. The authors have utilized injections of large volumes of subarachnoid alcohol (so-called "cordectomy") on six occasions with excellent results (unpublished data). Each patient was already bedbound and incontinent, and suffered from extensive lower extremity and back pain due to malignancy. The administration of 10 mL of alcohol was well tolerated in all cases, and it reduced pain and spasm considerably without affecting upper extremity function.

Overall Results for Subarachnoid Neurolysis. Interpretation of the results of the clinical series published over the last few decades is difficult because of variations in investigators' techniques, a lack of uniformity in methods of reporting outcome, and highly varied provision of detail. Studies have not thoroughly evaluated the influence of mechanistic or pathologic factors on efficacy, although a few general statements may be made. Investigators have reported inadequate results in pain due to herpes zoster, lymphedema, and phantom limb (167). Some early investigators reported that patients with long-standing pain were less likely to achieve favorable results, postulating failure due to sheltering of the targeted roots by tumor or inflammation (154,167,175). This finding has not been uniformly recognized (176), suggesting that these outcomes may also be due to "central sensitization" or to a failure to address prolonged suffering or to recognize physical dependency on opioids. Papo and Visca (177) noted early recurrences to be more common in patients treated for upper limb pain, high rates of failure for abdominal visceral pain, and especially favorable results for pelvic and saddle pain. In a careful review of the published experience with nonmalignant pain, Papo and Visca (156) conclude "the results are not encouraging, and the indications, if any, for the method in this area are extremely limited."

Pain Relief. Although subarachnoid neurolysis is not technically difficult, attention to detail and experience undoubtedly influence outcome. In the hands of experts, results for alcohol and phenol neurolysis seem to be similar (178), with excellent to good results typically reported in one-half to two-thirds of patients (142,160,167–170,175,177,179). In a literature review of over 2,000 cases of subarachnoid alcohol neurolysis, Gerbershagen (180) reported good results in 60%, fair results in 21%, and poor results in 19%. Similarly, in a review of 2,500 cases from 13 published series of intrathecal phenol neurolysis, Swerdlow noted good relief in 58%, fair relief in 21%, and little or no relief in 20% (181).

Duration. Unfortunately, although not well characterized by all investigators, duration of relief is highly variable. Although no evidence from controlled trials shows that duration of relief differs for alcohol or phenol, clinical experience suggests that the effects of the former are often more lasting. Using alcohol, Perese (165) reported greater than 6 months' duration in half of 57 patients who obtained initial relief. Using phenol, Lifschitz (185) documented 1 to 2 months' relief in 52%, greater than 2 months' duration in 27%, and less than 2 weeks in 14%. Based on their review of large numbers of reports, Hay (160) and Gerbershagen (180) suggest that, overall, the average duration of relief is 4 months.

Most studies report a moderate proportion of patients who experience excellent relief of just a few days duration, a phenomenon that is most likely due to technical failure from either blockade of too few segments or the use of a neurolytic agent of insufficient strength. The preliminary local anesthetic effect of phenol, which quickly fades, may initially suggest a slightly more ample extension of effect than ultimately encountered. If clinically indicated, it is reasonable, especially when using phenol, to treat initially with the intent of extending the upper and lower limits of hypalgesia one segment beyond the targeted dermatomes. In a comparison of the results of subarachnoid neurolysis with 5% to 15% phenol, Ischia et al. (169,170) noted better outcomes and longer durations of relief in patients treated with more concentrated solutions. It is reasonable to consider repetition in cases of early failure, with consideration for modifying the agent, its concentration, and/or its volume. Although atypical, most studies also report a small proportion of patients who experience relief of greater than 1 year's duration (177,180).

Complications. Complications vary according to a variety of factors, but especially patient selection, the site that is blocked, and technical aspects. Although some older literature reports high rates, in more recent series significant complications present at 1-month follow-up can be found in about 2% of patients (180). In a review of 1,478 subarachnoid alcohol blocks, Gerbeshagen (180) reported transient complications in 12% of patients and permanent complications in 2%. In 2,125 alcohol blocks performed in 1,478 patients, of 232 complications, the duration was as follows: 28% resolved within 3 days, 23% within 1 week, 21% within 1 month, 9% within 4 months, and only 18% lasted longer than 4 months (180).

Other than self-limited back pain, the most significant minor complication is postdural puncture headache, which seems to occur less frequently than with local anesthetic blocks, despite the use of large-bore needles (182). Major complications are mostly neurologic and, depending on their severity and duration and the patient's overall condition, these can range from annoying to devastating in effect.

Unanticipated Complications. When providing informed consent, it is perhaps most useful to refer to significant complications as either expected or unexpected. A modest incidence of regional neurologic complications that varies with the site of injection is anticipated, but in addition, in a minute proportion of patients, devastating neurologic deterioration may occur from unexpected complications due to spinal artery injury, herniation, or injection near a metastasis (133,152). Citing two cases of paraparesis after cervicothoracic subarachnoid neurolysis, Lipton recommends ensuring free flow of CSF before commencing neurolysis, and warns of increased risks in patients with superior sulcus (Pancoast) tumor, which often extends into the contiguous epidural space (133). Patients with complete obstruction of the subarachnoid space are at risk for neurologic deterioration if dural puncture and removal of CSF is undertaken distal to the obstruction, because of downward traction on the medulla. The phenomenon is reflected in a review of 100 patients with complete spinal block: No morbidity occurred in 50 patients undergoing C1–C2 myelography, whereas seven of 50 patients deteriorated after a lumbar approach was undertaken (151).

Anticipated Complications. All patients should be warned of the potential for numbness in the painful dermatomes, although this is usually gratefully accepted in exchange for relief of pain. Most often, however, pain relief is accompanied by a mildly dull sensation (hypalgesia) and only rarely, complete anesthesia or anesthesia dolorosa (painful dysesthesia)

ensues. Although attention to careful positioning, titration to effect, and respect for upper dose limits reduces spread of the neurolytic agent to anterior motor roots, a small proportion of patients will experience regional, usually unilateral, motor weakness. The true incidence of weakness is often difficult to determine since pretreatment pain often interferes with the accuracy of neurologic testing. Even in the presence of weakness, patients may report increased functional capacity, since muscle guarding due to pain may diminish.

Thoracic subarachnoid neurolysis is associated with a low incidence of complications, since the site of injection is distant from the outflow of motor fibers to the limbs and sphincters, and intercostal weakness, should it occur, is usually well tolerated. A single case of a severe pneumothorax has been reported (183).

Subarachnoid neurolysis undertaken in the cervical and lumbar regions is associated with moderate risks of limb paresis. The risk seems to be greater in the lumbar region, perhaps because nerve roots are grouped closely between the levels of the T11 and L1 spinous processes (Fig. 45-19). Lumbar neurolysis should be carried out cautiously, if at all, in patients with intact lower extremity strength, but it is generally well tolerated in patients who are bedbound. Bowel and bladder complications are infrequent when leg pain is being treated, especially if the injection is undertaken at the low thoracic level, where the lumbar roots exit the cord. Lumbosacral neurolysis, whether performed as a saddle block or in the jackknife position, is associated with significant risks of bowel and bladder difficulties. Bladder function is more commonly affected (167), and although incontinence is usually transient it is often demoralizing; thus, normal urinary function is usually regarded as a relative contraindication to lumbosacral neurolysis.

Hypertonic and Isotonic Saline

Subarachnoid Saline. This technique, which was introduced in the 1960s by Hitchcock, enjoyed transient popularity and subsequently has been almost entirely abandoned. The original technique involved the removal of large volumes of CSF, which were replaced by similar volumes of iced isotonic saline (184). Observations that thawing isotonic saline produced a hypertonic supernatant led to the development of a more accepted modification that substituted normothermic hypertonic (12%–15%) saline and did not involve removal of significant volumes of CSF (185). Although the mechanisms of pain relief are unclear, postmortem studies after iced saline infusion have demonstrated areas of peripheral demyelination in the cord and brainstem (186).

General anesthesia is required to ameliorate the severe pain that follows injection and to facilitate safe recovery. Treatment is frequently followed by fasciculations, piloerection, venostasis, and cyanosis of the lower limbs. Tachypnea and hypertension are common responses, and the use of potent antihypertensives has been advocated to limit morbidity (184). Although Hitchcock (185) and others have reported favorable results, morbidity is significant (187,188). A survey reporting on 2,105 patients treated with normothermic hypertonic saline or iced isotonic saline injection revealed a 10.6% incidence of adverse outcomes, of which muscle spasm, blood pressure changes, and seizure were most prominent, but which also included para- or quadriplegia in 22 patients and two deaths from myocardial infarction (187).

Epidural Hypertonic Saline

The epidural administration of hypertonic saline is used as a component of a procedure advocated by Racz and others for the relief of back and radicular pain due to epidural fibrosis and scarring (189). The procedure involves placement of a specialized epidural catheter (Racz catheter) near the site of scarring and serial injections of contrast dye, local anesthetic, corticosteroid, and 10% saline, often on a daily basis. Although widespread trials have not been carried out, treatment seems to be relatively safe and effective. In this setting, hypertonic saline is postulated to act not as a neurolytic agent, but as an osmotic means to reduce local swelling and pressure by driving water out of cells (see Chapter 44).

Epidural Neurolysis

Given that the epidural route is in such wide use by contemporary anesthesiologists, it is surprising that there have been relatively few reports on epidural neurolysis. After numerous anecdotal reports, early investigators became disenchanted with epidural neurolysis owing either to pain on injection (alcohol) or to disappointing results (phenol) (181). Lack of efficacy of early single-shot techniques relative to subarachnoid injections presumably relates to reduced contact of the neurolytic with the targeted nerves because of the barrier to diffusion presented by the dura.

Some resurgence of interest in epidural neurolysis has occurred, primarily related to technical modifications that appear to be associated with improved results. The main change has been the use of serial instillations of dilute phenol through a percutaneous catheter and monitoring of spread of injectate by image intensifier. Although treatment has been associated with few adverse neurologic sequelae, a study of 6% to 12% epidural phenol in monkeys suggests the potential for considerable damage to the posterior and anterior roots, as well as parts of the cord (190). In light of these findings, repeated treatments with dilute concentrations would seem to be most prudent.

Brechner (191) reported on 12 cancer patients treated with single-shot epidural injections of 10% phenol. Volumes were based on the volume requirement for analgesia with epidural lidocaine to a maximum of 8 mL. Results were good and fair in one-third and one-half of patients, respectively, and one case each of urinary incontinence and leg weakness occurred. These disappointing results emphasize the rationale for consideration of serial injections of low volumes of dilute phenol. Korevaar (192) administered alcohol to 36 patients on 3 successive days via an indwelling catheter and reported an 89% incidence of greater than 70% relief, averaging a mean of 3.3 months and until death in 20 patients. Few serious side effects were reported. Racz (193,194) employs a specially designed catheter formulated from spiraled stainless steel coils coated with fluoropolymers designed to facilitate radiologic localization, aspiration, and repositioning. The catheter is advanced through a specially designed nonshearing needle under fluoroscopy until the desired spinal level is reached, and doses of 2.5 to 5.0 mL of 5.5% phenol in saline are injected daily until complete or nearly complete relief is obtained for 24 hours. The procedure is halted if signs of motor involvement appear at any stage. He reported significant benefit in 70% (of a mixed population of 60 patients) that lasted less than 1 month in about 50% and 2 to 6 months in the remainder. Best results were achieved in patients with cancer pain or spasticity, and no complications were reported. Using a similar technique (two to six daily injections of 2–4 mL 5% phenol and glycerine), Salmon et al. (195) obtained good relief in 93% of 16 patients (duration unspecified) with no serious complications. Jain et al. (196) employed three daily 5-mL transcatheter injections of 5% epidural phenol in water to relieve extensive neoplastic chest wall pain and, in a preliminary report, three of seven patients experienced complete relief and four moderate relief. As an alternative to daily injec-

tions, others have successfully performed serial epidural neurolysis after allowing an interval of hours to elapse (Plancarte, R., personal communication, 1994). A special use of epidural neurolysis has been recommended by Doughty. He administers 10% phenol in glycerine epidurally at the level of T12–L1 to relieve attacks of tenesmus and burning pain in rectal cancer (personal communication).

Technique. The patient is positioned on the painful side in a 45-degree posterior tilt, as for intrathecal phenol block. After antiseptic skin preparation and infiltration of the skin and pertinent interspace with local anesthesia, an epidural needle is introduced into the epidural space and an epidural catheter is threaded under image-intensifier control to the level of the middle of the painful dermatomes. Because of the relatively large volume of solution employed, accidental intrathecal injection must be carefully excluded, ideally with the injection of a small amount of nonionic contrast medium to confirm appropriate spread in the epidural space. Some workers recommend use of a small volume of local anesthetic as a test dose, such as 2.0 mL 1% lidocaine, in which case a period of 2 hours or more should be allowed for its effects to dissipate before administering phenol. On the basis of nuclear medicine studies (195) that suggest that the spread of epidural phenol and glycerine may be extensive and variable (mean of 13 segments/3 mL with a range of 6–23), volumes larger than 3.0 mL should probably be avoided. This study suggested that distribution was unaffected by position, and that the extent of spread was less robust with repeat injections. Volumes of up to 5 mL of phenol in water (196) or saline (181) have, however, been used safely.

If a standard catheter is being used, difficulties may be encountered if a standard viscous glycerine-phenol preparation is employed, even when warmed and administered through a 1-mL syringe. This problem may be overcome by using phenol dissolved in a contrast medium such as Angiographin. Because of the vascularity of the epidural space, intravascular placement or migration of the catheter tip should be excluded before each neurolytic injection. Although the influence of gravity is uncertain, if a unilateral block is desired, the patient should be kept on his side for about 40 minutes following completion of the injection. In contrast to subarachnoid injection, the patient usually cannot immediately verify the anatomic localization of the neurolytic solution relative to the affected nerve roots. Pain usually disappears about 10 to 15 minutes after each administration.

Complications. Epidural neurolysis is rarely followed by complications other than backache and, after the administration of alcohol, occasionally neuritis. However, both urinary incontinence (191,197) and muscle paresis (191) have been reported. In addition, animal studies (190) suggest the potential for anterior root and cord injury with concentrations of 6% and greater. It is inadvisable to administer epidural injections to patients who are anticoagulated because of the risk of epidural hemorrhage if a vein is injured. Cousins (198) recommends that CT or MRI scan be carried out before performing epidural block to exclude local tumor invasion and the potential for hemorrhage, spinal cord compression, and neurologic injury. Furthermore, distortion of the epidural space by tumor may cause the neurolytic solution to spread unpredictably.

As noted, radiographic confirmation of both the integrity of the catheter, which may be chemically or physically damaged (199), and the position of its tip in the epidural space is recommended before each neurolytic injection. In addition, owing to anecdotal reports of transient widespread anesthesia when neurolytic injection immediately follows a local anesthetic test dose (192), it is suggested that a reasonable interval be allowed to elapse between injections, and that the neurolytic agent should be injected slowly.

Advantages Vis-a-Vis Subarachnoid Neurolysis. Theoretically, epidural neurolytic injection has potential advantages over subarachnoid block, particularly for pain with an extensive anatomic/topographic distribution. Risks of spread to the cranial cavity and meningeal irritation are fewer, and the incidence of sphincter dysfunction, motor weakness, and headache may be less, especially when incremental treatment using dilute phenol is administered serially.

Disadvantages Vis-a-Vis Subarachnoid Neurolysis. These advantages are offset by historical impressions of inferior results for single-shot injections. Although further work is needed to characterize the efficacy of serial epidural neurolysis, certain technical aspects favor subarachnoid neurolysis, at least in certain settings.

The main advantage of subarachnoid neurolysis is that it is a relatively simple procedure that can usually be performed on an outpatient basis. Although subarachnoid puncture is easily verified by the return of CSF, localization of the epidural space must be inferred from the results of epidurograms or test doses of local anesthetic. Although serial epidural neurolysis appears to be efficacious, it is time-consuming, mandates inpatient hospitalization, and requires serial epidurograms. Also, although reports suggest that gravity and position can be partially relied on to control the spread of epidural hyperbaric phenol (191), these factors can be utilized to exert more precise control for subarachnoid injection. A graded intensity of lesioning may perhaps be accomplished with repeat epidural phenol injections, but localization is better assured with subarachnoid administration.

Further trials of serial epidural neurolysis are indicated before it can be determined that it is reliably associated with actual advantages over intrathecal neurolysis. Meanwhile, it is reasonable to employ these methods in suitable cases of malignant pain arising from several dermatomes, particularly if other relevant therapies have been unsuccessful.

Subdural (Interarachnoid) Block

Subdural block, usually regarded as a complication of attempted subarachnoid or epidural block, in which case it is usually manifest as diffuse, spotty anesthesia, is occasionally intentionally sought to relieve cancer pain (154). Subdural block has been proposed as an alternative to cervical subarachnoid neurolysis, because access is purportedly easier in the cervical region and because it prevents dilution from rapidly circulating cranial CSF. As a consequence of its disposition between the dura and arachnoid membranes, subdural injection is undertaken deep to the epidural space, after dural puncture has occurred, but before the return of CSF is noted. The subdural space differs from the epidural space in that anatomic studies suggest that it is not a true potential space and only exists as a consequence of iatrogenic cleaving by injection or bleeding, hence the suggestion that it be referred to as the *interarachnoid space* (200,201). This, combined with its small caliber, makes intentional subdural injection difficult and sometimes impossible, and has probably contributed to the infrequent use of blocks in this region. The dura and arachnoid appear to be separated by a thin fluid film and, once injection occurs, by strands of connective tissue, which are responsible for the "honeycombed" appearance of AP contrast studies (Figs. 45-25 and 41-26).

Mehta and Maher (202) advocated locating the cervical epidural space with a short-beveled needle introduced through

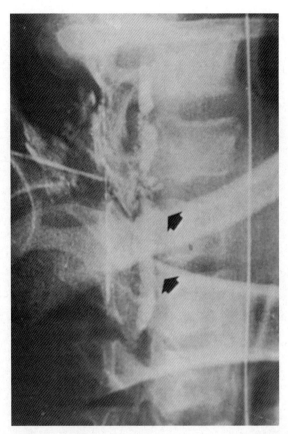

FIGURE 45-25. Subdural block. Radiograph showing lateral view. Needle tip has been placed in the subdural space and 0.5 mL of iophendylate (Myodil) has been injected. Note the fine line extending up and down from needle tip. Also, there is a second broader line *(arrows)* in which contrast medium tends to arrange itself like a "rosary." From Ischia S, Maffezzoli GF, Luzzani A, Pacini L. Subdural extra-arachnoid neurolytic block in cervical pain. *Pain* 1982;14 :347, with permission.

the midline using a loss-of-resistance technique. The needle is then slightly advanced and rotated 180 degrees until a sudden increase in resistance heralds subdural placement, which is subsequently confirmed radiologically. Swerdlow recommended the instillation of no more than 3 mL of 5% phenol in glycerine, but noted that relief is usually short-lived (178). Although the older literature proposes subdural neurolysis as a reasonable option for cervicothoracic pain, its viability in contemporary practice is questionable.

Chlorocresol

Chlorocresol (parachlormetacresol), a phenol derivative, was introduced by Maher (203) in an effort to identify an agent that would selectively damage pain fibers and would more effectively penetrate nerve roots sheltered by tumor or inflammation. Neither property has been confirmed.

NEUROMODULATION TECHNIQUES

Intraspinal Drug Delivery

Administration of neuraxial or spinal analgesics offers many advantages over irreversible neurodestructive procedures to

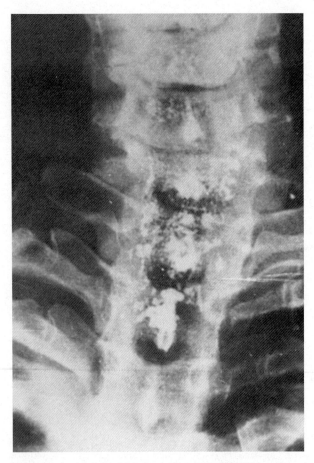

FIGURE 45-26. Subdural block. Radiograph showing anteroposterior view after injection of 0.5 mL of Myodil. Note the bilateral spread confined to the interior of the canal, over several segments. The appearance of the contrast medium is like a "nail scratch" shape. From Ischia S, Maffezzoli GF, Luzzani A, Pacini L. Subdural extra-arachnoid neurolytic block in cervical pain. *Pain* 1982;14:347, with permission.

control pain, such as neurolytic blockade. It is very effective in patients with multiple pain sites, such as those with advanced cancer with multiple sites of metastases. An indwelling neuraxial catheter allows for titration of opioid dosage and rotation of analgesic agents, if necessary. The use of intraspinal opioids is selective for the pain transmission pathway at the spinal level, without any discernible effect on the motor, sensory, or sympathetic system (see Chapter 40).

As discussed earlier, intraspinal analgesics are effective in modulating pain pathways at the spinal level. The significant side effects from systemic high-dose opioid administration (including nausea, constipation, confusion, increased somnolence, or lethargy) can be minimized with intraspinal delivery of opioids. Deposition of opioids into close proximity to spinal cord receptors provides for potent analgesia with fewer side effects. If the opioid is delivered via the epidural route, only 20% to 40% of the systemic dose is required to achieve equianalgesia. The intrathecal route is even more potent, requiring only 1% of the systemic dose for equianalgesia (204–208). This therapy is effective in two broad groups of patients: those with refractory pain syndromes and those with intolerable opioid-related side effects (209). The ability to treat pain effectively while minimizing these side effects has a significant impact on quality of life (210). One advantage of intraspinal analgesia is that a trial of therapy can be undertaken with minimal risk to

the patient. The main benefit of the trial is to determine which drugs can be tolerated by the patient at various dose levels and whether intolerable side effects are experienced. Deciding on which cancer patients will benefit from implantation of an intrathecal pump is complex and involves multiple factors.

Intraspinal delivery of opioids and other agents can be achieved using a variety of approaches, including epidural bolus, intermittent intrathecal injection, and continuous epidural and intrathecal infusions. Continuous infusion via either the epidural or intrathecal route requires the use of catheter system and either external or implantable infusion pumps to deliver the analgesic medications. There is little consensus on when to use the intrathecal versus the epidural route of administration and when to use an implantable versus external pump. With prolonged epidural infusions of greater than 6 to 9 months, complications with catheter obstruction, fibrosis, and loss of analgesic efficacy have been observed, leading most clinicians to favor the intrathecal route for long-term intraspinal analgesic infusions (211) (see Chapter 40).

Many factors are considered in the decision for an external pump system versus an implantable pump. Factors supporting use of an external system include a short life expectancy (<3 months), the need for frequent patient-controlled doses (such as with severe incident pain), the need for an epidural infusion (which generally requires infusion volumes too great for the implanted pump), a lack of reprogramming/refilling capabilities near the patient's home, and payor constraints, as well as the ability of the patient and family to take care of an externalized catheter system (212–214). We use a variety of catheters for our external systems including a tunneled Arrow Flex-Tip catheter (Arrow Inc., Reading, PA), the Du Pen epidural catheter (Bard Access Systems Inc., Salt Lake City, UT), and the Sims Epidural Portacath (Sims-Deltech, St. Paul, MN).

Factors that influence the selection of an implantable intrathecal pump include a longer life expectancy (>3 months), access to pump refill/reprogramming capabilities, diffuse pain (e.g., widespread metastasis), and favorable response to an intrathecal trial (214–215). The cost of an implanted intrathecal pump plays a role in the decision for implantation in cancer patients. We recently published our decision-making algorithm (214).

Implanted infusion pump systems utilize either fixed (factory preset at 0.5 or 1.0 mL/day) or programmable flow rate. All implantable pumps come with a refillable drug reservoir. In addition, they all have an access port and a side port system that allows for direct injection of a drug into the implanted catheter system (see Chapter 40, Figs. 40-10 and 40-11). Changing the dose in a fixed-rate pump requires the medication concentration be changed, mandating a pump refill each time the dose is adjusted. These implantable pumps come in a variety of reservoir volumes (up to 60 mL), allowing selection based on a patient's needs and body habitus.

Medtronic Inc. (Minneapolis, MN) has the only programmable pump on the market today. Medtronic's Synchromed I and II pumps can hold up to 20 and 40 mL of medication, respectively. They can be programmed to deliver a single bolus, time-specific boluses, or a complex regimen of continuous infusion of intrathecal analgesic. A function exists for a patient-controlled "demand dose" via a remote control, the so-called "patient therapy manager" or PTM device from Medtronic. Although these fixed-rate and programmable pumps can be used to deliver either epidural or intrathecal medications, they are more suited to intrathecal delivery. Epidural infusions usually require a significantly higher daily volume and thus are typically managed with an external pump system (211) (see Figs. 40-8 and 40-9).

Intraspinal Analgesic Trial

Once intraspinal analgesia has been considered as an option, first an intrathecal trial must be accomplished. This trial is to evaluate efficacy and side effects of the intraspinal medication in improving pain control, level of functioning, and overall quality of life. There is no standard for neuraxial trials, although numerous approaches have been advocated (214–220). We do not trial patients undergoing catheter-external pump systems, as the trial procedure and catheter "implant" procedure are virtually identical. For consideration of intrathecal catheter-pump implantation, our preference is a single-shot (one subarachnoid opioid or opioid/local anesthetic injection) trial in most cases. If the analgesia is equivocal, or the patient has a severe incidental pain syndrome, a tunneled intrathecal catheter trial is done, usually with an opioid/local anesthetic or opioid/clonidine combination. Also, in those cases in which we anticipate the need for local anesthetic combination therapy, an intrathecal catheter trial is helpful in adjusting and achieving the right opioid and local anesthetic mix prior to pump implantation. Criteria for successful intraspinal opioid trial are variable, with some effective indicators being reduction in pain scores, improvement in function, and decreased opioid requirement, as well as reduction in opioid-related side effects.

Efficacy of Intraspinal Opioids in Cancer Pain

Intrathecal delivery of opioids has been shown to reduce pain levels in patients with intractable cancer pain (214,216,218,219–221). The results of three recent studies of intrathecal therapy demonstrate the effectiveness of this therapy in management of severe pain from cancer (214,218–219). Our group at MD Anderson reported our results utilizing intraspinal analgesia in 87 of 4,107 evaluated patients using our previously mentioned algorithm (214). Retrospective evaluation of 8-week follow-up revealed improved pain control, decreased oral opioid intake, and decreased drowsiness and mental clouding. This study analyzed the effectiveness of intraspinal analgesia by comparing pain scores, oral opioid intake, and self-reported symptoms before and after the intraspinal intervention. After administration of intraspinal analgesia either via epidural or intrathecal route, a significant reduction occurred in the proportion of patients in severe pain (with pain score 7–10, NRS) from 86% to 17% (p <0.001). The patient numerical pain scores decreased significantly from 7.9 ± 1.6 to 4.1 ± 2.3 (p <0.001). Oral opioid intake decreased from 588 mg/day morphine-equivalent daily dose (MEDD) to 294 mg/day (p <0.001). Self-reported drowsiness and mental clouding (0–10) also significantly decreased from 6.2 ± 3.0 and 5.4 ± 3.4 to 3.2 ± 3.0 and 3.1 ± 3.0 respectively (p <0.001).

In a prospective, randomized, multicenter clinical trial, the use of an implanted intrathecal drug delivery system was shown to improve pain control, reduce side effects, and improve survival in cancer patients with refractory pain (218). At study entry, all patients ($n = 202$) had unrelieved cancer pain, as indicated by their visual analog pain scores of 5 or greater on a 0 to 10 scale. Patients were randomized to receive either morphine via intrathecal delivery and comprehensive medical management per the 1994 Agency for Health Care Policy and Research (AHCPR) Cancer Pain Relief guidelines, or comprehensive medical management alone. At week 4 of follow-up, 60 (84.5%) of the 71 patients in the intrathecal delivery arm achieved clinical success, as indicated by a 20% or greater reduction in VAS pain scores or a 20% or greater reduction in toxicity. By contrast, in the comprehensive medical management arm, only 51 (70.8%) of 72 patients achieved clinical

success. Mean toxicity scores declined in the intrathecal delivery and comprehensive medical management-only arm by 50% and 17%, respectively ($p = 0.004$). Further, the intrathecal delivery group had significant reduction in fatigue and depressed level of consciousness (p <0.05). Moreover, slightly greater improvement in 6-month survival was seen in the intrathecal delivery group compared to medical management-only group (53.9% versus 37.2%, $p = 0.06$).

In a third study, Rauck et al. evaluated intrathecal drug delivery systems in the management of episodic or breakthrough pain in a prospective, open-label study (219). In this study of 119 cancer patients with refractory cancer pain and/or uncontrollable side effects, better analgesia was achieved when the patients managed their pain with an implantable, patient-controlled intrathecal drug delivery system. Such a system allowed patients to self-administer a bolus dose of morphine sulfate on demand. Results of the study showed that the mean numerical analog pain score significantly decreased from 6.1 to 4.2 at month 1 (p <0.01, $n = 99$), and was maintained through month 7 (p <0.01, $n = 14$) and month 13 (p <0.05, $n = 10$). In addition, the MEDD use of systemic opioids was significantly reduced throughout the study (p <0.01). Overall success (50% or greater reduction in numeric analog pain score, systemic opioid use, or severity of opioid side effects) was reported at month 1 in 83% and at month 4 in 91% of patients.

Clearly, in these three and many other studies, intraspinal administration of opioids and analgesics has been shown to play a significant role in controlling cancer pain, reducing opioid-related toxicities, and even improving survival outcomes (214–221). Intraspinal analgesic therapy is an effective mode of pain control in cancer patients with difficult to control, refractory pain (see also Chapter 40).

Complications

Complications fall into two broad categories: device-related or drug-related. Device-related complications include wound infection, catheter breakage/migration, and catheter tip granuloma. A growing body of literature documents sterile granuloma at the catheter tip, which is being increasingly reported. The consensus is that this is related to highly concentrated medications, especially morphine, and the index of suspicion should be high in patients with new-onset back pain, prompting MRI evaluation and appropriate management as outlined elsewhere (222,225) (see Chapter 50).

Drug-related complications include dosing/programming errors, misfilling, and the spectrum of opioid-related side effects including nausea, sedation, urinary retention, pruritus, and respiratory depression. These side effects are minimized through patient monitoring and careful dose adjustments, and by double-checking pump programming prior to the patient's departure to the clinic. In general, in a stable patient who begins to have side effects shortly after pump refill, the programming should be promptly double-checked and the drug changed only if needed (see Chapter 40).

In cases of suspected pump malfunction, a plain radiograph should be ordered to check catheter patency. Next, a dye study with injection of contrast via the side port may be revealing of catheter malposition or disruption. Pump battery life is around 5 years, with the more recent devices lasting longer than older devices. Algorithms for device assessment have been published and, if the practitioner is in doubt, the pump manufacturer should be consulted. The possibility of opioid abuse via the pump should be considered (223). Implanted pumps have a wound infection rate of less than 5%; although an infection may lead to pump explant, local treatment and leaving the pump in place has been advocated in some cases (224). Rare, but serious infections reinforce the need for strict asepsis both at implant and with pump refill (see Chapter 40).

Neurostimulation

Because many cancer patients now live much longer, and some of these develop neuropathic pain due to their cancer, treatment, or other causes, neurostimulation is an important treatment option. The major targets are the peripheral nerves, spinal cord, and brain. These treatment options are considered in Chapter 41. Brain stimulation techniques are still at a developmental level, but one technique already stands out from others: Motor cortex stimulation is emerging as a promising option for very severe intractable neuropathic pain, such as CRPS (see Chapter 41).

Neurosurgical Neurodestructive Techniques

As a result of much improved use of systemic multimodal analgesia, spinal drug administration, and other methods described in this chapter, more invasive neurodestructive techniques are much less commonly used today. However, some important additional options remain clinically valuable, and these are described in Chapter 42. These methods include percutaneous cordotomy (see Figs. 42-41 to 42-43 and Tables 42-11 to 42-13), percutaneous tractotomy of the caudal nucleus and descending tract of the trigeminal nerve, percutaneous punctuate midline myelotomy, pituitary ablation, and dorsal root entry zone (DREZ) lesions for plexus avulsion.

Other Techniques

Vertebroplasty/Kyphoplasty

As mentioned earlier, neurosurgical procedures can be employed to treat intractable pain. Percutaneous vertebroplasty (PV) (Figs. 45-27 and 45-28) and kyphoplasty (PK) (Figs. 45-29 and 45-30) are minimally invasive approaches to treating painful compression fractures due to osteoporosis or malignancy. Such malignant tumors include solid tumor with spinal metastasis, lymphomas, myeloma, and others. These techniques involve injection of polymethylmethacrylate (PMMA) cement into the diseased vertebral body (226,227).

Outcomes in Cancer. Fourney et al. reported a retrospective review of 56 patients undergoing 65 PV (vertebroplasty) and/or 32 PK (kyphoplasty) procedures for cancer-associated vertebral compression fractures (VCFs) (228). Twenty-one patients had myeloma, whereas 35 had other primary and metastatic neoplasms. Mean age was 62, with a mean duration of symptoms of 3.2 months; 84% of patients reported marked or complete pain relief post procedure, with a mean follow-up of 4.5 months. No treatment-related complications were seen. Asymptomatic PMMA leakage was noted in 9.2% of 65 levels treated with PV, whereas there was no PMMA leakage in the PK group. These authors presented an algorithm for choosing PV, PK, surgery, or radiotherapy in the cancer patient.

Dudeney et al. prospectively evaluated a series of patients with multiple myeloma undergoing PK for painful VCFs (229). Eighteen patients underwent 55 PK procedures due to multiple myeloma. Short Form (SF-36) pain scales showed postproce-

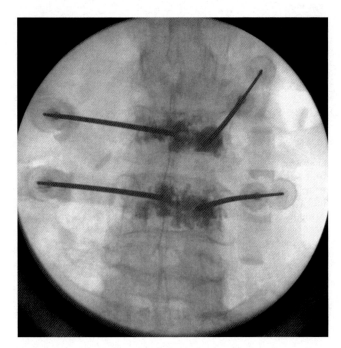

FIGURE 45-27. Vertebroplasty. Fluoroscopy image PA view.

dure improvement for the bodily pain, physical function, vitality, and social functioning scales. On average, 34% of lost vertebral height was restored. No major complications were seen, and asymptomatic PMMA leakage was seen in 4% of treated levels.

Wang et al. in our institution reported in abstract form our experience with myeloma patients (230). Retrospective analysis

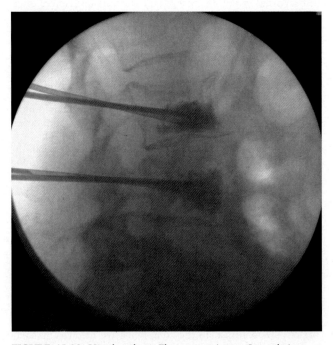

FIGURE 45-28. Vertebroplasty. Fluoroscopy image. Lateral view.

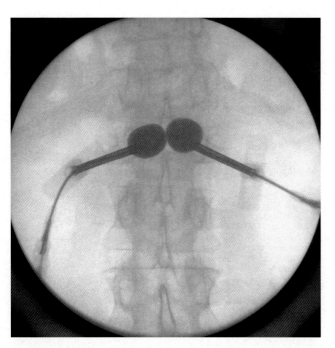

FIGURE 45-29. Kyphoplasty. Fluoroscopy image posterior–anterior view.

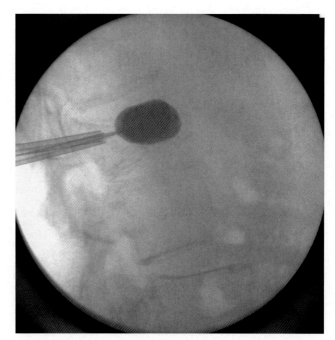

FIGURE 45-30. Kyphoplasty. Fluoroscopy image. Lateral view.

of 32 patients undergoing 43 PV and 24 PK procedures was undertaken; 91% of patients reported marked or complete pain relief post procedure. Mean preprocedure pain score was 7 of 10, and the postoperative mean pain score was 2 of 10, which was durable to a 12-month follow-up period. No major complications were seen, but asymptomatic PMMA extravasation was noted in 4% of the patients undergoing PV. Our group has reported value in this procedure in selected patients even in the very end stages of advanced metastatic disease (231).

ratio is favorable and more conservative therapies are failing, interventional pain techniques may be helpful—even extremely helpful. It is wise in treating the advanced cancer patient to keep some tenets of palliative medicine in mind; these are adopted from Field et al. (232) and Foley et al. (233). Symptom control is a paramount concern. It is critical to discuss openly and compassionately the patient's goals of care and tailor your treatments in accordance with the patient's wishes. The patient's overall well-being directly impacts on the caregiver's quality of life. Be honest with patients and family members while being cautious not to extinguish hope (see Chapter 49).

PALLIATIVE CARE

Palliative care is defined as comprehensive care of the terminally ill patient (see Chapter 49). In overall oncologic care, much effort and treatment is utilized in the palliative treatment mode. Many patients have meaningful, life-extending and life-enhancing palliative (as distinct from "curative") treatments. These treatments include chemotherapy, radiotherapy, tumor ablative procedures, surgery, and the interventional treatments outlined earlier in this chapter.

Effective palliation in the patient with advanced cancer always starts with a complete assessment and aggressive pharmacologic management. In some cases in which the risk–benefit

SUMMARY

Cancer pain management is a complicated challenge. It requires a thorough understanding of the cancer disease process, the pain diagnosis, and the treatment modalities available to treat the pain condition. In addition to pain, the patient often presents with a constellation of symptoms arising from their cancer and oncologic treatment. Both pharmacologic and interventional modalities of treatment are necessary to help the patient control pain and reach a satisfactory quality of life. In carefully selected patients, the diverse interventional techniques help the physician and patient to achieve effective control of cancer pain, thereby optimizing quality of life.

References

1. American Cancer Society. Cancer Facts and Figures 2004. At http://www.cancer.org/downloads/STT/CAFF_finalPWSecured.pdf. Accessed 25 October 2005.
2. Burton AW, Fanciullo GJ, Beasley RD, Fisch MJ. Chronic pain in the cancer survivor: A new frontier. *Pain Med* 2007;8(2):189–198.
3. Von Roenn JH, Cleeland CS, Gonin R. Physician attitudes and practice in cancer pain management. A survey from the Eastern Cooperative Oncology Group. *Ann Int Med* 1993;119:121–126.
4. World Health Organization. *Cancer Pain Relief and Palliative Care*, 2nd ed. Geneva: World Health Organization; 1996:12–15.

5. Zech DF, Grond S, Lynch J, et al. Validation of World Health Organization Guidelines for cancer pain relief: A 10-year prospective study. *Pain* 1995;63(1):65–76.
6. Ventafridda V, DeConno FD. Status of cancer pain and palliative care worldwide. *J Pain Symptom Manage* 1996;12:79.
7. Lillemoe KD, Cameron JL, Kaufman HS, et al. Chemical splanchnicectomy in patients with unresectable pancreatic cancer. *Ann Surg* 1993;217:447–457.
8. Smith TJ, Coyne PJ, Staats PS, et al. An implantable drug delivery system (IDDS) for refractory cancer pain provides sustained pain control, less drug-related toxicity, and possibly better survival compared with comprehensive medical management (CMM). *Ann Oncol* 2005;16(5):825–833.
9. Breitbart W. Suicide in the cancer patient. *Oncology* 1987;1:49–54.
10. Bolund C. Medical and care factors in suicides by cancer patients in Sweden. *J Psychosomat Oncology* 1985;3:31–52.
11. Daut RL, Cleeland CS, Flannery RC. Development of the Wisconsin brief pain questionnaire to access pain in cancer and other diseases. *Pain* 1983;17:197–210.
12. Fishman B, Pasternak S, Wallenstein SL, et al. The Memorial pain assessment card: A valid instrument for the evaluation of cancer pain. *Cancer* 1987;60:1151–1158.
13. Ger LP, Ho ST, Sun WZ, et al. Validation of the Brief Pain inventory in a Taiwanese population. *J Pain Symptom Manage* 1999;18:316–322.
14. Yun YH, Mendoza TR, Heo DS, et al. Development of a cancer pain assessment tool in Korea: A validation study of a Korean version of the brief pain inventory. *Oncology* 2004;66:439–444.
15. Validity of the brief pain inventory for use in documenting the outcomes of patients with noncancer pain. *Clin J Pain* 2004;20:308–318.
16. Stanford EA, Chambers CT, Craig KD. The role of developmental factors in predicting young children's use of a self-report scale for pain. *Pain* 2006;120:16–23.
17. Perkins FM and Kehlet H. Chronic pain as an outcome of surgery. *Anesthesiology* 2000;93:1123–1133.
18. Cleeland CS, Gonin R, Hatfield AK, et al. Pain and its treatment in outpatients with metastatic cancer. *N Engl J Med* 1994;330:592–596.
19. Novy D, Berry MP, Palmer JL, et al. Somatic symptoms in patients with chronic non-cancer related and cancer-related pain. *J Pain Symptom Manage* 2005;29:603–612.
20. Passik SD, Kirsh KL. Managing pain in patients with aberrant drug-taking behaviors. *J Support Oncol* 2005;3:83–86.
21. Gonzales GR, Elliott KJ, Portenoy RK, Foley KM. The impact of a comprehensive evaluation in the management of cancer pain. *Pain* 1991;47:141–144.
22. Lindsay TH, Jonas BM, Sevcik MA, et al. Pancreatic cancer pain and its correlation with changes in tumor vasculature, macrophage infiltration, neuronal innervation, body weight and disease progression. *Pain* 2005;119(1–3):233–246.
23. Cata JP, Weng HR, Lee BN, et al. Clinical and experimental findings in humans and animals with chemotherapy-induced peripheral neuropathy. *Minerva Anestesiol* 2006;72:151–169.
24. van Wilgen CP, Dijkstra PU, van der Laan BF, et al. Morbidity of the neck after head and neck cancer therapy. *Head Neck* 2004;26:785–791.
25. Baxter NN, Habermann EB, Tepper JE, et al. Risk of pelvic fractures in older women following pelvic irradiation. *JAMA* 2005;294:2587–2593.
26. Tasmuth T, von Smitten K, Hietanen P, et al. Pain and other symptoms after different treatment modalities of breast cancer. *Ann Oncol* 1995;6:453–459.
27. Rogers ML, Duffy JP. Surgical aspects of chronic post-thoracotomy pain. *Eur J Cardiothorac Surg* 2000;18:711–716.
28. Borsje S, Bosmans JC, Van Der Schans CP, et al. Phantom pain: A sensitivity analysis. *Disabil Rehabil* 2004;26:905–910.
29. Small W Jr., Kachnic L. Postradiotherapy pelvic fractures: Cause for concern or opportunity for future research? *JAMA* 2005;294:2635–2637.
30. Robb KA, Williams JE, Duvivier V, Newham DJ. A pain management program for chronic cancer-treatment-related pain: A preliminary study. *J Pain* 2006;7(2):82–90.
31. Hermann M, Krum H, Ruschitzka F. To the heart of the matter: Coxibs, smoking, and cardiovascular risk. *Circulation* 2005;112:1024–1029.
32. Zech DFG, Grong S, Lynch J, et al. Validation of the World Health Organization guidelines for cancer pain relief: A 10-year prospective study. *Pain* 1996;63:65–76.
33. Rigor BM. Pelvic cancer pain. *J Surg Oncol* 2000;75:280–300.
34. Kori SH, Foley KM, Posner JB. Brachial plexus lesions in patients with cancer: 100 cases. *Neurology* 1981;31:45–50.
35. Paice JA. Mechanisms and management of neuropathic pain in cancer. *J Support Oncol* 2003;1:107–120.
36. Zech DF, Grond S, Lynch J, et al. Validation of the World Health Organization guidelines for cancer pain relief: A 10-year prospective study. *Pain* 1995;63:65–76.
37. Portnoy RK. Inadequate outcome of opioid therapy for cancer pain: Influences on practitioners and patients. In: Patt RB, ed. *Cancer Pain*. Philadelphia: JB Lippincott;1993:119–128.
38. Colleau S, Toranson DE. Fear of addiction: Confronting a barrier to cancer pain relief. *Cancer Pain Release* 1998;113:1–3.
39. Lyss AP, Portenoy RK. Strategies for limiting the side effects of cancer pain therapy. *Semin Oncol* 1997;24:S128–S123.
40. Ferrante FM, Bedder M, Caplan KA, et al. Practice guidelines for cancer pain management. *Anesthesiology* 1996;94:1243–1257.
41. Patt RB, Jain S. Therapeutic decision-making for invasive procedures. In: Patt RB, ed. *Cancer Pain*. Philadelphia: Lippincott; 1993:275–283.
42. Melzak R, Wall P. Pain mechanisms: A new theory. *Science* 1965;150:971–979.
43. Oakley J, Prager J. Spinal cord stimulation: Mechanism of action. *Spine* 2002;(27)22:2574–2583.
44. Patt RB, Cousins MJ. Neurolytic blockade techniques for chronic and cancer pain. In: Cousins MJ, ed. *Neural Blockade*, 3rd ed. Philadelphia: JB Lippincott, 1998:1007–1061.
45. Ramamurthy S, Wash NE, Scholenfeld LS, et al. Evaluation of neurolytic block using phenol and cryogenic block in management of chronic pain. *J Pain Symptom Manage* 1989;4:72–75.
46. Swetlow GI, Weingarten B. Alcohol nerve block for pain in malignant disease. *Med J Rec* 1926;123:728.
47. Politis MJ, Schaumburg HA, Spence PS. Neurotoxicity of selected chemicals. In: Spense PS, ed. *Experimental and Chemical Neurotoxicity*. Baltimore: William and Wilkins; 1980:613.
48. Rumbsy MG, Finean JB. The action of organic solvents in the myelin sheath of peripheral nerve tissue. *J Neurochem* 1966;12:1509.
49. Lipton S. Neurolysis: Pharmacology and drug selection. In: Patt RB, ed. *Cancer Pain*. Philadelphia: Lippincott; 1993:343–358.
50. Molles JE, Helweg-Larson J, Jacobson E. Histopathological lesions in the sciatic nerve of the rat following perineural application of phenol and alcohol solutions. *Dan Med Bull* 1969;16:116–119.
51. Kline MT. Radiofrequency techniques in clinical practice. In: Waldman SD, ed. *Interventional Pain Management*. Philadelphia: WB Saunders, 1996.
52. Cheng TM, Cascino TL, Onofrom BM. Comprehensive study of diagnosis and treatment of trigeminal neuralgia secondary to tumors. *Neurology* 1993;43:2298–2302.
53. Glynn CJ, Lloyd JW, Barnard JD. Cryoanalgesia in management of pain after thoracotomy. *Thorax* 1980;35:325–327.
54. Bonica JJ, Buckley FP, Morrica G, et al. Neurolytic blockade and hypophysectomy. *The Management of Pain*. Philadelphia: Lea and Febriger; 1990:1980–2040.
55. Landis S, Murray J, Bolden S. Cancer statistics. *CA Cancer J Clin* 1999;49:8–10.
56. Vokes EE, Weickselbaum RR, Lippman SM. Medical progress: Head and neck cancer. *N Engl J Med* 1993;328:184–186.
57. Taylor JC, Terrell JE, Ronis DL, et al. Disability in patients with head and neck cancer. *Arch Otolaryngol Head Neck Surg* 2004;130:764–769.
58. van Wilgen CP, Dijkstra PU, van der Laan BF, et al. Morbidity of the neck after head and neck cancer therapy. *Head Neck* 2004;26:785–791.
59. Evensen JF, Bjordal K, Knutsen BH, et al. Side effects and quality of life after inadvertent radiation overdosage in brachytherapy of head-and-neck cancer. *Int J Radiat Oncol Biol Phys* 2002;52:944–952.
60. Waldman SD. Blockade of Gasserian ganglion. In: Waldman SD, ed. *Interventional Pain Management*. New York: WB Saunders; 2001:316–320.
61. Vital JM, Grenier F, Dautheribes M, et al. An anatomic and dynamic study of the greater occipital nerve. *Surg Radiol Anat* 1989;11:205–210.
62. Pai U, Raj PP. Peripheral nerve blocks: Cervical plexus. In: Raj PP, ed. *Handbook of Regional Anesthesia*. New York: Churchhill Livingstone; 1985:163–167.
63. Wertheim HM, Rovenstine EA. Cervical plexus block. *NY State J Med* 1939;1311–1315.
64. Master RD, Castresana FJ, Castresana MR. Superficial and deep cervical plexus block: Technical considerations. *AANA J* 1995;63:235–243.
65. Landis S, Murray J, Bolden S. Cancer statistics. *CA Cancer J Clin* 1998;48:6–11.
66. Kori SH, Foley KM, Posner JB. Brachial plexus lesions in patients with cancer: 100 cases. *Neurology* 1981;31:45–50.
67. Bonica JJ. Musculoskeletal disorders of the upper limb. In: Bonica JJ, ed. *The Management of Pain*, 2nd ed. Philadelphia: Lea & Febriger; 1990:891–893.
68. Raj PP. Continuous regional analgesia. In: Raj PP, ed. *Practical Management of Pain*, 3rd ed. St. Louis: Mosby; 2000:710–722.
69. Rogers ML, Duffy JP. Surgical aspects of chronic post-thoracotomy pain. *Eur J Cardiothorac Surg* 2000;18:711–716.
70. Wallace MS, Wallace AM, Lee J. Pain after breast surgery: A survey of 282 women. *Pain* 1996;66:195–205.
71. Moore DC. Intercostal nerve block in 4333 patients: Indications, techniques, and complications. *Anesth Analg* 1962;41:1–10.
72. Conacher ID. Percutaneous cryotherapy for post thoracotomy neuralgia. *Pain* 1986;25:227–230.
73. Debacker LJ, Kienzle WK, Keasley HH. A study of stellate ganglion block for pain relief. *Anesthesiology* 1959;20:618–625.
74. Bonica JJ. Autonomic innervation of viscera in relation to nerve block. *Anesthesiology* 1968;29:793–795.

75. Plancarte R, Velaquez R, Patt RB. Neurolytic blocks of the sympathetic axis. In: Patt RB, ed. *Cancer Pain*. Philadelphia: JB Lippincott; 1993:377–3425.
76. Brown DL, Bulley CK, Quiel EL. Neurolytic celiac plexus block for pancreatic cancer pain. *Anesth Analg* 1987;66:869–873.
77. Plancarte R, Amescua C, Patt RB et al. Superior hypogastric block for pelvic cancer pain. *Anesthesiology* 1990;73:236–240.
78. Warfield CA, Crews DA. Use of stellate ganglion blocks in treatment of intractable limb pain in lung cancer. *Clin J Pain* 1987;3:13–15.
79. Racz GB, Holubec JT. Stellate ganglioin phenol lysis. In: Racz GB, ed. *Techniques of Neurolysis*. Boston: Kluwer Academic; 1989:133–140.
80. Thompson GE, Moore DC, Bridenbaugh PO, et al. Abdominal pain and celiac plexus nerve block. *Anesth Analg* 1977;56:1–3.
81. Reber HA, Foley KM. Pancreatic cancer pain: Presentation, pathogenesis, and management. *J Pain Symptom Manage* 1988;3:163–176.
82. Boas RA. Sympathetic blocks in clinical practice. *Int Anesthesiol Clin* 1978;16:149–155.
83. Reid W, Watt JK, Gray TG. Phenol injection of sympathetic chain. *Br J Surg* 1970;57:45–50.
84. Moore DC, Bush WH, Burnett LL. Plexus block: a roentgenographic anatomic study of technique and spread of solutions. *Anesth Analg* 1981; 60(6):369–379.
85. Lee RB, Stone K, Magelssen D, et al. Presacral neurotomy for chronic pelvic pain. *Obstet Gynecol* 1986;68:517–521.
86. Plancarte R, de Leon-Casasola OA, El-Helaly M, et al. Neurolytic superior hypogastric plexus block for chronic pelvic pain associated with cancer. *Reg Anesth* 1997;22:562–568.
87. Ischia S, Luzzan A, Ischia A, Faggion S. A new approach to the neurolytic block of the celiac plexus: The transaortic technique. *Pain* 1983;16:333.
88. Feldstein GS, Waldman SD, Allen ML. Loss-of-resistance technique for transaortic celiac plexus block. *Anesth Analg* 1986;65:1092.
89. Singler R. An improved technique for alcohol celiac plexus nerve block. *Anesthesiology* 1982;56:137.
90. Montero MA, Vidal LF, Aguilar SJ, Donoso BL. Percutaneous anterior approach to the coeliac plexus, using ultrasound. *Br J Anaesth* 1989;62:637.
91. Kune G, Cole R, Bell S. Observations on the relief of pancreatic pain. *Med J. Aust* 1975;2:789.
92. Lieberman RP, Nance PN, Cuka DJ. Anterior approach to celiac plexus block during interventional biliary procedures. *Radiology* 1988;167:562.
93. Loper KA, Coldwell DM, Lecky J, Dowling C. Celiac plexus block for hepatic arterial embolization: A comparison with intravenous morphine. *Anesth Analg* 1989;69:398.
94. Whiteman MS, Rosenberg H, Haskin PH, Teplick SK. Celiac plexus block for interventional radiology. *Radiology* 1986;161:836.
95. Sharfman WH, Walsh TD. Has the analgesic efficacy of neurolytic celiac plexus block been demonstrated in pancreatic cancer pain? *Pain* 1990;41: 267.
96. Mercadante S. Celiac plexus block versus analgesics in pancreatic cancer pain. *Pain* 1993;52:187.
97. Eisenberg E, Carr D, Chalmers TC. Neurolytic celiac plexus block for cancer pain: A meta-analysis. 1995;80:290–295.
98. Brown DL, Bulley CK, Quiel EL. Neurolytic celiac plexus block for pancreatic cancer pain. *Anesth Analg* 1987;66:869.
99. Ischia S, Ischia A, Polati E, Finco G. Three posterior percutaneous celiac plexus block techniques: A prospective, randomized study in 61 patients with pancreatic cancer pain. *Anesthesiology* 1992;76:534.
100. Lillemoe KD, Cameron JL, Kaufman HS, et al. Chemical splanchnicectomy in patients with unresectable pancreatic cancer: A prospective randomized trial. *Ann Surg* 1993;217:447.
101. Staats PS et al. the effects of alcohol celiac plexus block on pain, mood, longevity in patients with unresectable pancreatic cancer: A double blinded randomized, placebo controlled study. *Pain Med* 2002;2:28–34.
102. Brown BL, Bulley CK, Quiel EC. Neurolytic celiac plexus block for pancreatic cancer pain. *Anesth Analg* 1987;66:869.
103. Teeple E, Ghia JN. Problems with neurolytic blocks for cancer pain in patients receiving narcotics and psychoactive drugs. *Reg Anesth* 1981;6: 152.
104. Black A, Dwyer B. Coeliac plexus block. *Anaesth Intens Care* 1973;1:315.
105. Naidich DP, Megibow AJ, Ross CR, et al. Computed tomography of the diaphragm: Normal anatomy and variants. *J Comput Assist Tomogr* 1983;7:633.
106. Haaga JR., Reich NE, Havrilla TR, Alfidi RJ. Interventional CT scanning. *Radiol Clin North Am* 1977;15:456.
107. Singler RC. An improved technique for alcohol neurolysis of the celiac plexus. *Anesthesiology* 1982;56:137.
108. Moore DC. Celiac (splanchnic) plexus block with alcohol for cancer pain of the upper intra-abdominal viscera. *Adv Pain Res Ther* 1979;2:357.
109. Wilson PR. Incidental discography during celiac plexus block. *Anesthesiology* 1992;76:314.
110. Thompson GE, Moore DC, Bridenbaugh PO, et al. Abdominal pain and celiac plexus nerve block. *Anesth Analg* 1977;56:1.
111. De Conno F, Caraceni A, Aldrighetti L, et al. Paraplegia following coeliac plexus block. *Pain* 1993;55:383.

112. Galizia EJ, Lahiri SK. Paraplegia following coeliac plexus block with phenol. *Br J Anaesth* 1974;46:539.
113. Cherry DA, Lamberty J. Paraplegia following coeliac plexus block. *Anaesth Intens Car* 1984;12:59.
114. Davies DD. Incidence of major complications of neurolytic coeliac plexus block. *J R Soc Med* 1993;86:264.
115. Tanelian D, Cousins MJ. Celiac plexus block following high dose opiates in a four-year-old child. *J Pain Symptom Manage* 1989;4:82.
116. Hilgier M, Rykowski J. One needle transcrural celiac plexus block. *Reg Anesth* 1994;19:277.
117. Jackson SH, Jacobs JB, Epstein RA. A radiographic approach to celiac plexus block. *Anesthesiology* 1969;31:373.
118. Lieberman RP, Waldman SD. Celiac plexus neurolysis with modified transaortic approach. *Radiology* 1990;175:274.
119. Benzon HT. Convulsions secondary to intravascular phenol: A hazard of celiac plexus block. *Anesth Analg* 1979;58:150.
120. Gaudy JH, Tricot C, Sezeur A. Troubles du rhythme cardiaque graves apres phénolisation splanchnique peroperatoire. *Can J Anaesth* 1993;40:357.
121. Moore DC, Bush WH, Burnett LL. Celiac plexus block: A roentgenographic, anatomic study of technique and spread of solution in patients and corpses. *Anesth Analg* 1981;60:369.
122. Fujita Y, Takaori M. Pleural effusion after CT-guided alcohol celiac plexus block. *Anesth Analg* 1987;66:911.
123. Cook EE, Flaherty RA, Willmarth CL, et al. Chylothorax: A complication of translumbar aortography. *Radiology* 1960;75:251.
124. Fine PG, Bubela C. Chylothorax following celiac plexus block. *Anesthesiology* 1985;63:454.
125. Cherry DA, Rao DM. Lumbar sympathetic and coeliac plexus blocks: An anatomical study in cadavers. *Br J Anaesth* 1982;54:1037.
126. Masadu R, Yokoyama K. Study of needle placement for sympathetic blocks under computed tomography (paravertebral approach in thoracic sympathetic block and transdisc approach in splanchnic nerve block. Abstracts; pp. 342. 7th World Congress on Pain, Paris, 1993.
127. Koboyashi M, Ina H, Imai S, et al. Under CT guided celiac plexus block: Trans-intravertebral disc approach. *Reg Anesth* 1992;17[Suppl]:122.
128. Jain S, Hirsh R, Shah N, et al. Blood ethanol levels following celiac plexus block with 50% ethanol. *Anesth Analg* 68:S 1989;35.
129. Lubenow TR, Ivankovich AD. Serum alcohol, CPK and amylase levels following celiac plexus block with alcohol. *Reg Anesth* 1988;13[Suppl]: 64.
130. Sato S, Okubu N, Tajima K, et al. Plasma alcohol concentrations after celiac plexus block in gastric and pancreatic cancer. *Reg Anesth* 1993;18:366.
131. Noda J, Umeda S, Mori K, et al. Acetaldehyde syndrome after celiac plexus block. *Anesth Analg* 1986;65:1300.
132. Umeda S. Disulfiram-like reaction to moxalactam after celiac plexus block. *Anesth Analg* 1985;64:377.
133. Lipton S. Neurolysis: Pharmacology and drug selection. In: Patt RB, ed. *Cancer Pain*. Philadelphia: JB Lippincott;1993:343–358.
134. Lu G, Frost EAM, Goldiner PL. Another aspect of celiac plexus block. *Anesthesiology* 1987;67:1017.
135. Churcher M. Peripheral nerve blocks in the relief of intractable pain. In: Swerdlow M, Charlton, JE, eds. *Relief of Intractable Pain*, 4th ed. Amsterdam: Elsevier; 1989:195.
136. Abram SE, Boas RA. Sympathetic and visceral nerve blocks. In: Benumof JL, ed. *Clinical Procedures in Anesthesia and Intensive Care*. Philadelphia: JB Lippincott; 1993:787–805.
137. Smith JL. Care of people who are dying. The hospice approach. In: Patt RB, ed. *Cancer Pain*. Philadelphia: JB Lippincott; 1993:543–552.
138. Jain S, Kestenbaum A, Khan Y. Ethanol or phenol for peripheral neurolysis? Does it make a difference? *Pain* 1990;5[Suppl]:2.
139. Boas RA Sympathetic blocks in clinical practice. *Int Anesthesiol Clin* 1978; 16:149.
140. Honet JE, Shea KL, Seltzer JL. Celiac plexus neurolytic block: Survey of pain programs. *Reg Anesth* 1993;18[Suppl]:45.
141. Fujita Y, Oshumi A, Takaori M. CT scan and celiac plexus block. *Anesthesiology* 1988;68:968.
142. Moore DC, Bush WH, Burnett LL. An improved technique for celiac plexus block may be more theoretical than real. *Anesthesiology* 1982;57:347.
143. Raj PP. *Practical Management of Pain*, 2nd ed. St. Louis: Mosby Year Book 1992:1021–1022.
144. Swenson C, Patt RB. Manufacturing processes. In: Patt RB, ed. *Cancer Pain*. Philadelphia: JB Lippincott; 1993:612–615.
145. Nour-Eldin F. Preliminary report: Uptake of phenol by vascular and brain tissue. *Microvasc Res* 1970;2:224.
146. Swerdlow M. Spinal and peripheral neurolysis for managing Pancoast syndrome. *Adv Pain Res Ther* 1982;4:135.
147. Matamala AM, Lopez FV, Martinez I. Percutaneous approach to the celiac plexus using CT guidance. *Pain* 1988;34:285.
148. Ischia S, Luzzani A, Ischia A, et al. A new approach to neurolytic block of the celiac plexus: The transaortic technique. *Pain* 1983;16:333.
149. Plancarte R, Amescua C, Patt RB. Presacral blockade of the ganglion impar (ganglion of Walther). *Anesthesiology* 73:A 1990;51.

150. Wemm K, Saberski L. Modified approach to block ganglion impar (ganglion of Walther) *Reg Anesth* 1995;20:544–5.
151. Hollis PH, Malis L, Zappulla RA. Neurological deterioration after lumbar puncture below complete spinal subarachnoid block. *J Neurosurg* 1986; 64:253.
152. Swerdlow M, ed. *Relief of Intractable Pain*, 3rd ed. Amsterdam: Excerpta Medica, 1983.
153. Iggo A, Walsh EG. Selective block of small fibers in the spinal roots by phenol. *Brain* 1960;83:701.
154. Maher RM. Relief of pain in incurable cancer. *Lancet* 1955;18.
155. Nathan PW, Sears TA, Smith MC. Effects of phenol solutions on the nerve roots of the cat: An electrophysiological and histological study. *J Neurol Sci* 1965;2:7.
156. Papo I, Visca A. Intrathecal phenol in the treatment of pain and spasticity. *Proc Neurol Surg* 1976;7:56.
157. Stern EL. Chronic painful conditions amenable to relief by intraspinal (subarachnoid) injection of alcohol. *Am J Sur* 1937;36:509.
158. Stewart WA, Lourie H. An experimental evaluation of the effects of subarachnoid injections of phenol-Pantopaque in cats: A histological study. *J Neurosurg* 1963;20:64.
159. Katz J. Current role of neurolytic agents. *Adv Neurol* 1974;4:471.
160. Hay RC. Subarachnoid alcohol block in the control of intractable pain: Report of results in 252 patients. *Anesth Analg* 1962;41:12.
161. Bonica JJ, Buckley FP, Moricca G, et al. Neurolytic blockade and hypophysectomy. In: Bonica JJ, ed. *Management of Pain*, 2nd ed. Philadelphia: Lea & Febiger; 1990:1980.
162. Matsuki M, Kato Y, Ichiyanagi K. Progressive changes in the concentration of ethyl alcohol in the human and canine subarachnoid spaces. *Anesthesiology* 1972;36:617.
163. Ichiyanagi K, Matsuki M, Kinefuchi S, Kato Y. Progressive changes in the concentrations of phenol and glycerine in the human subarachnoid space. *Anesthesiology* 1975;42:622.
164. Lipton S. Neurodestructive procedures in the management of cancer pain. *J Pain Symptom Manage* 1987;2:219.
165. Perese DM. Subarachnoid alcohol block in the management of pain of malignant disease. *Arch Surg* 1958;76:347.
166. Rauck R. Sympathetic nerve blocks. In: Raj PP, ed. *Practical Management of Pain*, 2nd ed. St. Louis: Mosby–Year Book;1992:778–812.
167. Stovner J, Endressen R. Intrathecal phenol for cancer pain. *Acta Anaesth Scand* 1972;16:17.
168. Lifshitz S, Debacker LJ, Buchsbaum HJ. Subarachnoid phenol block for pain relief in gynecologic malignancy. *Obstet Gynecol* 1976;48:316.
169. Ischia S, Luzzani A, Pacini L, Maffezzoli GF. Lytic saddle block: Clinical comparison of the results, using phenol at 5, 10, and 15 percent. *Adv Pain Res Ther* 1984;7:339.
170. Ischia S, Luzzani A, Ischia A, et al. Subarachnoid neurolytic block (L5–S1) and unilateral percutaneous cervical cordotomy in the treatment of pain secondary to pelvic malignant disease. *Pain* 1984;20:139.
171. Moore DC. *Regional Block*, 4th ed. Springfield, IL: Charles C. Thomas 1965.
172. Bonica JJ. Introduction: semantic, epidemiologic, and educational issues. In: Casey KL (ed.) *Pain and the Central Nervous System: the Central Pain Syndromes*. New York: Raven Press, 1991, pp 13–29.
173. Hughes JT. Pathological findings following the intrathecal injection of ethyl alcohol in man. *Paraplegia* 1988;26:71–82.
174. Bruno G. Intrathecal alcohol block: Experiences on 41 cases. *Paraplegia* 1975;12:305.
175. Maher RM. Neurone selection in relief of pain: Further experiences with intrathecal injections. *Lancet* 1957;16.
176. Evans RJ, MacKay IM. Subarachnoid phenol blocks for relief of pain in advanced malignancy. *Can J Surg* 1972;15:50.
177. Papo I, Visca A. Phenol subarachnoid rhizotomy for the treatment of cancer pain: A personal account on 290 cases. *Adv Pain Res Ther* 1979;2: 339.
178. Swerdlow M. Neurolytic blocks of the neuroaxis. In: Patt, RB, ed. *Cancer Pain*. Philadelphia: JB Lippincott; 1993:427–442.
179. Mark VH, White JC, Zervas NT, et al. Intrathecal use of phenol for the relief of chronic severe pain. *N Engl J Med* 1962;267:589.
180. Gerbershagen HU. Neurolysis: Subarachnoid neurolytic blockade. *Acta Anœsth Belg* 1981;1:45.
181. Swerdlow M. Subarachnoid and extradural blocks. *Adv Pain Res Ther* 1979;2:325.
182. Patt RB, Wu CL, Reddy S, et al. Incidence of postdural puncture headache following intrathecal neurolysis with large caliber needles. *Reg Anesth* 1994;19[Suppl 2]:86.
183. Patt RB, Reddy S, Wu CL, Catania JA. Pneumothorax as a consequence of thoracic subarachnoid block. *Anesth Analg* 1994;78:160.
184. Hitchcock E. Hypothermic subarachnoid irrigation for intractable pain. *Lancet* 1967;1133.
185. Hitchcock E. Subarachnoid saline infusion. In: Morley TP, ed. *Current Controversies in Neurosurgery*. Philadelphia: WB Saunders; 1976: 515.
186. Lloyd JW. Treatment of intractable pain with cerebrospinal fluid barbotage. In: Morley TP, ed. *Current Controversies in Neurosurgery*. Philadelphia: W.B. Saunders; 1976:520.
187. Lucas JT, Ducker TB, Perot PL Jr. Adverse reactions to intrathecal saline injection for control of pain. *J Neurosurg* 1975;42:557.
188. Thompson GE. Pulmonary edema complicating intrathecal hypertonic saline injection for intractable pain. *Anesthesiology* 1971;35:425.
189. Racz GB, Heavner JE, Singleton W, Carline M. Hypertonic saline and corticosteroid injected epidurally for pain control. In: Racz GB, ed. *Techniques of Neurolysis*. Boston: Kluwer Academic Publishers; 1989:73–86.
190. Gregg RV, Sehlhorst CS, Liwnicz BH. Histopathology of epidural phenol in the monkey. Abstracts; p. 93. 7th World Congress on Pain, Paris, 1993.
191. Ferrer-Brechner T. Epidural and intrathecal phenol neurolysis for cancer pain. *Anesthesiol Rev* 1981;8:14.
192. Korevaar WC. Transcatheter thoracic epidural neurolysis using ethyl alcohol. *Anesthesiology* 1988;69:989.
193. Racz GB, Heavner J, Haynsworth R. Repeat epidural phenol injections in chronic pain and spasticity. In: Lipton S, Miles J, eds. *Persistent Pain*, Vol. 5. Orlando FL: Grune & Stratton; 1985:157.
194. Racz GB, Sabonghy M, Gintautas J, Kline WM. Intractable pain therapy using a new epidural catheter. *JAMA* 1982;248:579.
195. Salmon JB, Finch PM, Lovegrove FTA, Warwick A. Mapping the spread of epidural phenol in cancer pain patients by radionuclide admixture and epidural scintigraphy. *Clin J Pain* 1992;8:18.
196. Jain S, Foley K, Thomas J, et al. Factors influencing efficacy of epidural neurolysis therapy for intractable cancer pain. Suppl. 4. Proc 5th World Congress I.A.S.P, 1987.
197. Grunwald I. Neurlise com fenol: Uso de via peridural no tratomento da dolor de cancer. *Rev Brasil de Anest* 1976;26:628.
198. Cousins MJ, Dwyer B, Gibb D. Chronic pain and neurolytic neural blockade. In: Cousins MJ, Bridenbaugh PO. *Neural Blockade*, 2nd ed. Philadelphia: JB Lippincott; 1988:1053–1084.
199. Coombs DW. Potential hazards of transcatheter serial epidural phenol neurolysis. *Anesth Analg* 1985;64:1205.
200. Haines DE. On the question of a subdural space. *Anat Rec* 1991;230:3.
201. Shantha TR. Subdural space: What is it? Does it exist? *Reg Anesth* 1992; 17[Suppl]:85.
202. Mehta M, Maher R. Injection into the extra-arachnoid subdural space. *Anaesthesia* 1977;32:76.
203. Maher RM. Intrathecal chlorocresol in the treatment of pain in cancer. *Lancet* 1963;965.
204. Hassenbusch SJ, Portenoy RK, Cousins M, et al. Polyanalgesic Consensus Conference 2003: An update on the management of pain by intraspinal drug delivery- report of an expert panel. *J Pain Symptom Manage* 2004;27:540– 563.
205. Max MB, Inturrisi CE, Kaido RF, et al. Epidural and intrathecal opiates: CSF and plasma profiles in patients with chronic cancer pain. *Clin Pharmacol The* 1985;38:631.
206. Gourlay RF, Cherry BA, Cousins MJ. Cephalad migration of morphine in CSF following lumbar epidural administration in patients with cancer pain. *Pain* 1985;23:317.
207. Walker SM, Goudas LC, Cousins MJ, Carr DB. Combination spinal analgesic chemotherapy: A systematic review. *Anesth Analg* 2002;95:674– 715.
208. Smith TJ, Coyne PJ. How to use implantable intrathecal drug delivery systems for refractory chronic pain. *J Support Oncol* 2003;1:73–76.
209. Kedlaya D, Reynolds L, Waldman S. Epidural and intrathecal analgesia for cancer pain. *Best Pract Res Clin Anaesthesiol* 2002;16:651–655.
210. Gallagher RM. Epidural and intrathecal cancer pain management: Prescriptive care for quality of life. *Pain Med* 5(3);235, 2004.
211. Crul BJ, Delhaas EM. Technical complications during long-term subarachnoid or epidural administration of morphine in terminally ill cancer patients: A review of 140 cases. *Reg Anest* 1991;16:209–213.
212. Hans JE, Peters J, Eikermann M. Epidural analgesia at the end of life: Facing empirical contraindications. *Anesth Analg* 2003;97:1740–1742.
213. Mercadante S. Epidural treatment in advanced cancer patients (letter). *Anesth Analg* 2004;98:1503.
214. Burton AW, Rajagopal A, Shah HN, et al. Epidural and intrathecal analgesia is effective in treating refractory cancer pain. *Pain Med* 2004;5:238–246.
215. Burton AW and Hassenbusch SJ. The double catheter technique for intrathecal medication trial: A brief clinical note and report of five cases. *Pain Med* 2(4):352–354, 2001.
216. Hassenbusch SJ, Pillay PK, Magdinec M, et al. Constant infusion of morphine for intractable cancer pain using implanted pump. *J Neurosur* 1990;73:405–409.
217. Krames ES. Intraspinal opioid therapy for chronic nonmalignant pain: Current practice and clinical guidelines. *J Pain Symptom Manag* 1996;11:333– 352.
218. Smith TJ, Staats P, Deer T, et al. Randomized clinical trial of an implantable drug delivery system compared with comprehensive medical management for refractory cancer pain: impact on pain, drug-related toxicity, and survival. *J Clin Oncol* 2002;20:4040–4049.

219. Rauck RL, Cherry D, Boyer MF, et al. Long-term intrathecal opioid therapy with a patient-activated implanted delivery system for the treatment of refractory cancer pain. *J Pain* 2003;4:441–447.
220. Krames ES. Continuous infusion of spinally administered narcotics for the relief of pain due to malignant disorders. *Cancer* 1985;Aug 1;56:696–702.
221. Gilmer-Hill HS, Boggan JE, Smith KA, et al. Intrathecal morphine delivered via subcutaneous pump for intractable cancer pain: A review of the literature. *Surg Neuro* 1999;51:12–15.
222. Follett KA. Intrathecal analgesia and catheter-tip inflammatory masses. *Anesthesiology* 2003;99:5–6.
223. Borton AW, Conroy B, Garcia E, et al. Illicit substance abuse via implanted intrathecal pump. *Anesthesiology* 1998;89(5):1264–1267.
224. Boviatsis EJ, Kouyialis AT, Boutsikakis I, et al. Infected CNS infusion pumps. Is there a chance for treatment without removal? *Acta Neurochir (Wien)* 2004;146:463–467.
225. Hassenbusch S, Burchiel K, Coffey RJ, Cousins MJ, et al. Management of intrathecal catheter tip inflammatory masses: a consensus statement. *Pain Med* 2002;2:313–323
226. Burton AW, Rhines LD, Mendel E. Vertebroplasty and kyphoplasty: A comprehensive review. *Neurosurg Focus* 2005;18(3):E1:1–9.
227. Cotton A. Percutaneous vertebroplasty for osteolytic metastases and myeloma: effects of the percentage of lesion filling and the leakage of methylmethacrylate at clinical followup. *Radiolog* 1996;200:525–530.
228. Fourney DR, Schomer DF, Nader R, et al. Percutaneous vertebroplasty and kyphoplasty for painful vertebral body fractures in cancer patients. *J Neurosurgery (Spine 1)* 2003;98:21–30.
229. Dudeney S, Lieberman IH, Reinhardt MK, Hussein M. Kyphoplasty in the treatment of osteolytic vertebral compression fractures as a result of multiple myeloma. *J Clin Oncol* 2002;20(9):2382–2387.
230. Wang M, Weber D, Fourney D, et al. Value of vertebroplasty and kyphoplasty for painful vertebral compression fractures in multiple myeloma [Abstract No. 1565]. *Blood* 1002;100(11):403a.
231. Burton AW, Reddy SK, Shah HN, et al. Percutaneous vertebroplasty-a technique to treat refractory spinal pain in the setting of advanced metastatic cancer: A case series. *J Pain Sympt Manage* 30(1):87–95, 2005.
232. Field MJ, Behrman RE, eds. *When Children Die: Improving Palliative and End-of-Life Care for Children and Their Families.* Washington DC: The National Academy Press, 2003.
233. Foley KM, Gelband H, eds. *Improving Palliative Care for Cancer.* Washington DC: The National Academy Press, 2001.

CHAPTER 46 ■ COMPLEX REGIONAL PAIN SYNDROME, INCLUDING APPLICATIONS OF NEURAL BLOCKADE

ANDREAS BINDER AND RALF BARON

The term *complex regional pain syndrome* (CRPS) describes a variety of painful conditions following injury that appears regionally with a distal predominance of abnormal findings. The symptoms exceed in both magnitude and duration the expected clinical course of the inciting event and often result in significant impairment of motor function. The disorder shows a variable progression over time. These chronic pain syndromes comprise different additional clinical features including spontaneous pain, allodynia, hyperalgesia, edema, autonomic abnormalities, and trophic signs. In CRPS type I (reflex sympathetic dystrophy) minor injuries or limb fractures precede the onset of symptoms; CRPS type II (causalgia) develops after injury to a major peripheral nerve (1–3).

COMPLEX REGIONAL PAIN SYNDROME TYPE I (REFLEX SYMPATHETIC DYSTROPHY)

The most common precipitating event is a trauma affecting the distal part of an extremity (65%), especially fractures, postsurgical conditions, contusions, and strain or sprain. Less common occasions are central nervous system (CNS) lesions, such as spinal cord injuries and cerebrovascular accidents, as well as cardiac ischemia (4).

CRPS I patients develop asymmetrical distal extremity pain and edema without presenting an overt nerve lesion (Fig. 46-1). These patients often report a *burning, spontaneous pain* felt in the distal part of the affected extremity. Characteristically, the pain is disproportionate in intensity to the inciting event. The pain usually increases when the extremity is in a dependent position. Stimulus-evoked pains are a striking clinical feature. These sensory abnormalities often appear early, are most pronounced distally, and have no consistent spatial relationship to individual nerve territories or to the site of the inciting lesion. Typically pain can be elicited by movement of and pressure on the joints (deep somatic allodynia), even if these are not directly affected by the inciting lesion.

Autonomic abnormalities include swelling and changes in sweating and skin blood flow. In the acute stages of CRPS I, the affected limb is often warmer than the contralateral limb (5,6). In chronic phases, vasoconstriction and cold skin is induced by endothelial damage (7). Sweating abnormalities, either hypohidrosis or, more frequently, hyperhidrosis, are present in nearly all CRPS I patients. The acute distal swelling of the affected limb depends very critically on aggravating stimuli.

Since it diminishes after sympathetic blocks, it is likely that this swelling is maintained by sympathetic activity.

Trophic changes, such as abnormal nail growth, increased or decreased hair growth, fibrosis, thin glossy skin, and osteoporosis may be present, particularly in chronic stages. Restrictions of passive movement are often present in long-standing cases and may be related to both functional motor disturbances and trophic changes of joints and tendons.

Weakness of all muscles of the affected distal extremity is often present. Small, accurate movements are characteristically impaired. Nerve conduction and electromyography studies are normal, except in patients in very chronic and advanced stages. About half of the patients have a postural or action tremor representing an increased physiologic tremor. In about 10% of cases, dystonia of the affected hand or foot develops.

COMPLEX REGIONAL PAIN SYNDROME TYPE II (CAUSALGIA)

The symptoms of CRPS II are similar to those of CRPS I. The only exception is that a lesion of peripheral nerve structures and subsequent focal deficits are mandatory for the diagnosis. The symptoms and signs spread beyond the innervation territory of the injured peripheral nerve and often occur *remote* from the site of injury, although a restriction to the territory is not in conflict with the current definition.

EPIDEMIOLOGY

A population-based study in the United States on CRPS I calculated an incidence of about 5.5 per 100,000 person years at-risk and a prevalence of about 21 per 100,000 (8). An incidence of 0.8 per 100,000 person years at-risk and a prevalence of about 4 per 100,000 was reported for CRPS II. In contrast, a European population-based study determined a much higher incidence of 26.2 for CRPS in general when using a different diagnostic approach (9). However, CRPS I develops more often than CRPS II. The incidence of CRPS II in peripheral nerve injury varies from 2% to 14% in different series, with a mean of around 4% (10). Estimations suggest an incidence of CRPS I of 1% to 2% after fractures, 12% after brain lesions, and 5% after myocardial infarction. However, the latter data for brain lesions and myocardial infarctions are relatively high and must be interpreted with some caution because of the lack of

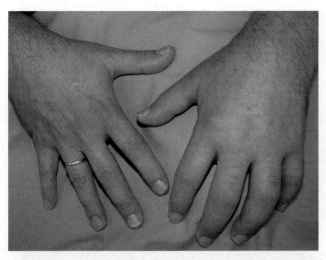

FIGURE 46-1. Clinical picture of patient with complex regional pain syndrome type I of the upper left extremity following distortion of the left wrist.

uniform diagnostic criteria. Females are more often affected than males, with a female-to-male ratio ranging from 2:1 to 4:1. CRPS shows a distribution over all ages, with a mean age peak at diagnosis of 40 to 50 years and highest incidence rates at 61 to 70 years. Differences in ethnicity, socioeconomic status, and different diagnostic criteria used may contribute to epidemiologic differences (9).

Predominantly, CRPS occurs in one extremity. Retrospective studies in large cohorts showed a distribution in the upper and lower extremity from 1:1 to 2:1. In 113 retrospectively reviewed cases, the symptoms occurred in 47% on the right, in 51% on the left side, and in 2% bilaterally. Multiple extremities were affected in up to 7% (10).

ARE STAGES APPROPRIATE?

A sequential progression of untreated CRPS has been repeatedly described, each stage of which (usually three are proposed) differing in patterns of signs and symptoms. Nevertheless, this concept has come into question in the last few years. In 2002, the clinical validity of this concept was tested by Bruehl et al. in 113 patients (11). Using a cluster analysis, three subgroups were identified that could be differentiated by their symptoms and signs regardless of disease duration. The sequential concept relies on the course of untreated CRPS; however, to date, all studies performed to test its clinical validity investigated patients already under treatment. Furthermore, vascular disturbances and skin temperature measurements indicated different thermoregulatory types, depending on time.

In conclusion, it is questionable whether staging of CRPS is appropriate. It is much more practical, with direct implication to therapy, that patients with CRPS be graded according to the intensity of their sensory, autonomic, motor, and trophic changes as having mild, moderate, or severe impairment.

PSYCHOLOGY

Most patients with CRPS exhibit significant psychological distress, most commonly depression and anxiety. Many patients become overwhelmed by the pain and associated symptoms and, without adequate psychosocial support, may develop maladaptive coping skills. Based on these symptoms, there is a tendency to ascribe the etiology of CRPS to emotional causes, and it has been proposed that CRPS is a psychiatric illness. In fact, it is sometimes difficult to recognize the organic nature of the symptoms. However, when describing the clinical picture, Livingston was convinced: "The ultimate source of this dysfunction is not known but its organic nature is obvious and no one seems to doubt that these classical pain syndromes are real." Covington (12) drew several conclusions on psychological factors in CRPS: (a) No evidence was found to support that CRPS is a psychogenic condition; (b) because anxiety and stress increases nociception, relaxation and antidepressive treatment is helpful; (c) the pain in CRPS is the cause of psychiatric problems, and not the converse; (d) maladaptive behavior by the patients, such as volitional or inadvertent actions, are mostly due to fear, regression, or misinformation and do not indicate psychopathology; and (e) some patients with conversion disorders and factitious diseases have been diagnosed incorrectly with CRPS. In summary, the author concludes that the widely proposed "CRPS personality" is clearly unsubstantiated. This assumption was further strengthened when no differences in psychological patterns were found in those patients with radius fracture who developed CRPS I in comparison to patients who recovered without developing CRPS (13).

According to this view, an even distribution of childhood trauma, pain intensity, and psychological distress was confirmed in patients with CRPS in comparison to patients with other neuropathic pain syndromes and chronic back pain (14). Further studies demonstrated a high psychiatric comorbidity, especially depression, anxiety, and personality disorders in CRPS patients. These findings are also present in other chronic pain patients and are more likely a result of the long and severe pain disease (15). In comparison with patients with low back pain, CRPS patients showed a higher tendency to somatization but did not show any other psychological differences (16). In 145 patients, 42% reported stressful life events in close relationship to the onset of CRPS, and 41% had a history of chronic pain before CRPS (17). Thus, stressful life events could be risk factors for the development of CRPS.

IMPORTANT ISSUES UNIQUE TO COMPLEX REGIONAL PAIN SYNDROME

Motor Abnormalities

About 50% of the patients with CRPS show motor abnormalities (18,19). It is unlikely that these motor changes are related to a peripheral process (e.g., influence of the sympathetic nervous system on neuromuscular transmission and/or contractility of skeletal muscle). These somatomotor changes are more likely generated by central changes of activity in the motoneurons. In a recent study, the motor dysfunction in CRPS patients was analyzed using kinematic analysis and functional imaging investigations to study the cerebral representation of finger movements. First, patients were investigated in a kinematic analysis assessing possible changes of movement patterns during target reaching and grasping. Compared with controls, CRPS patients particularly showed a significant prolongation of the target phase in this paradigm. The pattern of motor

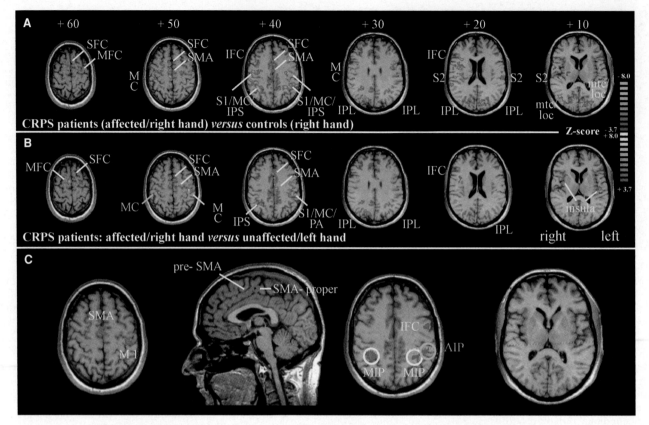

FIGURE 46-2. Contrast map of the GLM model calculated by subtracting the tapping condition of controls (right hand) from the tapping condition in patients (complex regional pain syndrome [CRPS]-affected side; i.e., right hand). Brain slices are referred to by the superior–inferior level in millimeters relative to a line through the anterior and posterior commissure (AC–PC line). Z score indicates level of significance. **B:** Contrast map of the GLM model calculated by subtracting the tapping condition on the unaffected side (i.e., left hand) from the affected side (i.e., right hand) in CRPS patients. Brain slices are referred to by the superior–inferior level in millimeters relative to a line through the anterior and posterior commissure (AC–PC line). Z score indicates level of significance. **C:** Implementation of the individual degrees of motor impairment (Z values of tapping frequencies; i.e., values of the individual maximum tapping frequencies are normalized to the mean maximum tapping frequencies of controls, see methods) as regressors in the GLM model for the condition "tapping on the CRPS-affected side." In this approach, we sought to isolate brain areas correlating with the degree of motor impairment. The statistical map was thresholded at $p < 0.0001$. Maihofner C, et al. The motor system shows adaptive changes in complex regional pain syndrome. *Brain* 2007;130[Pt 10]:2671–2687, with permission.

impairment was consistent with a disturbed integration of visual and proprioceptive inputs in the posterior parietal cortex. Second, functional magnetic resonance imaging (fMRI) was used to investigate cortical activations during tapping movements of the CRPS-affected hand. During finger tapping of the affected extremity, CRPS patients showed a significant reorganization of central motor circuits, with an increased activation of primary motor and supplementary motor cortices (SMA) (Fig. 46-2). Furthermore, the ipsilateral motor cortex showed a markedly increased activation. When the individual amount of motor impairment was introduced as regressor in the fMRI analysis, we were able to demonstrate that activations of the posterior parietal cortices (i.e., areas within the intraparietal sulcus), SMA, and primary motor cortex were correlated with the extent of motor dysfunction. Thus, substantial adaptive changes within the CNS may contribute to motor symptoms in CRPS (20). According to the bilateral cortical changes, the motor performance was also slightly impaired on the contralateral unaffected side (21).

Moreover, a neglect-like syndrome was clinically described to be involved in the disuse of the extremity (22). Recent controlled studies also support an incongruence between central motor output and sensory input as underlying mechanism in CRPS. Using the method of mirror visual feedback, the visual input from a moving unaffected limb to the brain was able to reestablish the pain-free relationship between sensory feedback and motor execution. After 6 weeks of therapy, pain and function were improved, as compared with the control group (23,24). Furthermore, a sustained inhibition of the motor cortex was found in CRPS patients on the contralateral as well as ipsilateral hemisphere (25,26).

Immune Cell–mediated Inflammation and Cytokine Release

Several studies in CRPS patients address the question to what extent an immune cell–mediated inflammation is involved

(Fig. 46-3). Skin biopsies in these patients showed a striking increase in the number of Langerhans cells, which can release immune cell chemoattractants and proinflammatory cytokines (27). In accordance, in the fluid of artificially produced skin blisters, significantly higher levels of interleukin (IL)-6 and tumor necrosis factor (TNF)-α, as well as tryptase (a measure of mast cell activity), were observed in the involved extremity as compared with the uninvolved extremity (28,29). In CRPS patients with hyperalgesia, higher levels of the soluble TNFα receptor type I were found (30). Accordingly, significant increases in IL-1β and IL-6, but not TNF-α, were demonstrated in the cerebrospinal fluid of individuals afflicted with CRPS as compared with controls (31).

In this context, it is of particular interest that cutaneous denervation can cause rapid activation and proliferation of Langerhans cells that continues until reinnervation occurs. Thus, one might speculate that such cell proliferation may reflect also a functional denervation of cutaneous sympathetic outflow that occurs in CRPS (5,32).

The patchy osteoporosis that is found in more advanced CRPS cases may also be consistent with a regional inflammatory process in deep somatic tissues. Both, IL-1 and IL-6 cause proliferation and activation of osteoclasts and suppress the activity of osteoblasts.

Changes in hair growth can also be created by proinflammatory cytokines. TNF and IL-1 directly inhibit hair growth. Keratocyte-derived TNF and IL-6 cause retarded hair growth, signs of fibrosis, and, in turn, immune infiltration of the dermis, all present in CRPS patients.

Autoimmune Etiology

Several studies focus on an autoimmune response in patients with CRPS. Autoantibodies against rat sympathetic neurons were detected in 40% of CRPS patients, whereas only 5% of other neuropathy patients showed these autoantibodies (33,34). Immunoreactivity to *Campylobacter* was found in many early CRPS patients, in particular associated with minimal trauma, thus indicating a postinfectious autoimmune basis in some patients (35).

Sensitization to Adrenergic Stimuli: Sympathetically Maintained Pain

Sympathetically Maintained Pain

On the basis of experience and clinical studies, the term *sympathetically maintained pain* (SMP) was redefined: Neuropathic pain patients presenting with similar clinical signs and symptoms can clearly be divided into two groups by the negative or positive effect of selective sympathetic blockade or blockade of α-adrenoceptors (36,37). The pain component that is relieved by specific sympatholytic procedures is considered "sympathetically maintained pain." Thus, SMP is now defined to be a symptom in a subset of patients with neuropathic disorders and not a clinical entity. The positive or negative effect of a sympathetic blockade is not essential for the diagnosis of CRPS I. On the other hand, the only possibility to differentiate between SMP and *sympathetically independent pain* (SIP) is the efficacy of a correctly applied sympatholytic intervention (38,39).

Influence of Sympathetic Activity and Catecholamines on Primary Afferents

Clinical studies in humans support the idea that cutaneous nociceptors develop catecholamine sensitivity after partial nerve lesions (CRPS II). Intracutaneous application of norepinephrine into a symptomatic area rekindles spontaneous pain and dynamic mechanical hyperalgesia/allodynia that had been relieved by sympathetic blockade (40,41). Intracutaneous injection of norepinephrine in control subjects does not elicit pain.

The question arises whether, in CRPS I, similar mechanisms of SMP exist, although no major nerve lesion is present. To address this issue, we performed a study in patients with CRPS I using physiologic stimuli to excite sympathetic neurons (42). Cutaneous sympathetic vasoconstrictor outflow to the painful extremity was experimentally activated to the highest possible physiologic degree by whole-body cooling. During the thermal challenge, the affected extremity was clamped to 35°C to avoid thermal effects at the nociceptor level. The intensity of spontaneous pain and mechanical hyperalgesia (dynamic and punctate) increased significantly in patients who had been classified as having SMP by positive sympathetic blocks but not in SIP patients (Fig. 46-4).

The experimental intervention used in the present study selectively alters sympathetic cutaneous vasoconstrictor activity without influencing other sympathetic systems innervating the deep somatic tissues (e.g., muscle vasoconstrictor neurons [43,44]). Therefore, the interaction of sympathetic and afferent neurons measured here is likely to be located within the skin, as predicted by the pain-enhancing effect of intracutaneous norepinephrine injections in CRPS II. Interestingly, the relief of spontaneous and evoked pain after sympathetic blockade was more pronounced than changes in spontaneous and evoked pain that could be induced experimentally by sympathetic activation. One explanation for this discrepancy might be that a complete sympathetic block affects *all* sympathetic outflow channels projecting to the affected extremity. It is very likely that, in addition to a coupling in the skin, a sympathetic–afferent interaction may also occur in other tissues, in particular in the deep somatic domain such as bone, muscle, or joint. Supporting this view, these structures are in particular extremely painful in some patients with CRPS (45). Furthermore, patients may exist who are characterized by a selective or predominant sympathetic–afferent interaction in deep somatic tissues, sparing the skin (32) (Fig. 46-5).

Mechanisms Involved in Sympathetically Maintained Pain

The quantitative measurements shown in Figure 46-6 on patients with CRPS I and with SMP clearly demonstrate that the underlying mechanism of SMP must be a coupling between sympathetic noradrenergic neurons and primary afferent neurons in the periphery of the body. The mechanisms of these couplings are not revealed by the experiments performed on human patients. However, it must be inferred from experiments on human patients that these are different for SMP in CRPS II compared with SMP in CRPS I.

Following nerve lesions, afferent nociceptive and nonnociceptive neurons, as well as sympathetic postganglionic neurons, undergo dramatic changes leading to sprouting, shrinkage, and eventually even death of the lesioned neurons, as well as to up- or downregulation of transmitters (including neuropeptides), ionic channels, transduction molecules, and other entities, one such change being upregulation of

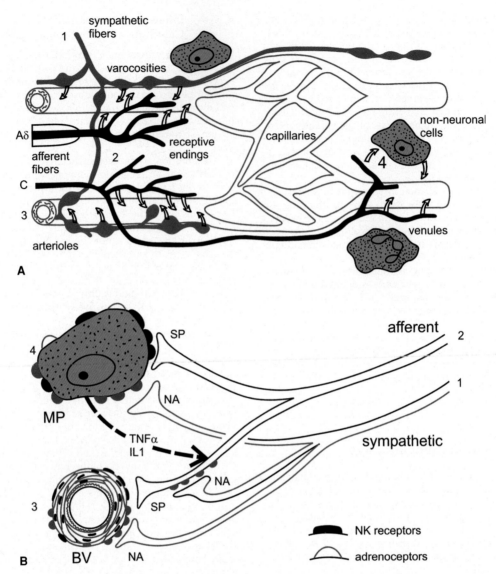

FIGURE 46-3. A: The micro milieu of nociceptors. The microenvironment of primary afferents is thought to affect the properties of the receptive endings of myelinated (*A*) and unmyelinated (*C*) afferent fibers. This has been particularly documented for inflammatory processes, but one may speculate that pathologic changes in the direct surroundings of primary afferents may contribute to other pain states as well. The vascular bed consists of arterioles (directly innervated by sympathetic and afferent fibers), capillaries (not innervated and not influenced by nerve fibers), and venules (not directly innervated but influenced by nerve fibers). The micro milieu depends on several interacting components: Neural activity in postganglionic noradrenergic fibers (*1*) supplying blood vessels (*3*, BV) causes release of noradrenaline (NA) and possibly other substances and vasoconstriction. Excitation of primary afferents (Aδ- and C-fibers) (*2*) causes vasodilation in precapillary arterioles and plasma extravasation in postcapillary venules (C-fibers only) by the release of substance P (SP) and other vasoactive compounds (e.g., calcitonin gene-related peptide, CGRP). Some of these effects may be mediated by non-neuronal cells, such as mast cells and macrophages (*4*). Other factors that affect the control of the microcirculation are the myogenic properties of arterioles (*3*) and more global environmental influences, such as a change of the temperature and the metabolic state of the tissue. **B:** Hypothetical relation between sympathetic noradrenergic nerve fibers (*1*), peptidergic afferent nerve fibers (*2*), blood vessels (*3*), and macrophages (*4*). The activated and sensitized afferent nerve fibers activate macrophages (MP), possibly via substance P release. The immune cells start to release cytokines, such as tumour necrosis factor (TNF)-α and interleukin (IL)-1, which further activate afferent fibers. Substance P (and CGRP) released from the afferent nerve fibers reacts with neurokinin (NK)-1 receptors in the blood vessels (arteriolar vasodilation, venular plasma extravasation; neurogenic inflammation). The sympathetic nerve fibers interact with this system on three levels: (*1*) via adrenoceptors (mainly α) on the blood vessels (vasoconstriction); (*2*) via adrenoceptors (mainly β) on macrophages (further release of cytokines), and (*3*) via adrenoceptors (mainly α) on afferents (further sensitization of these fibers). Modified from 1. Jänig W, Baron R. Complex regional pain syndrome: Mystery explained? *Lancet Neurol* 2003;2(11):687–697, with permission.

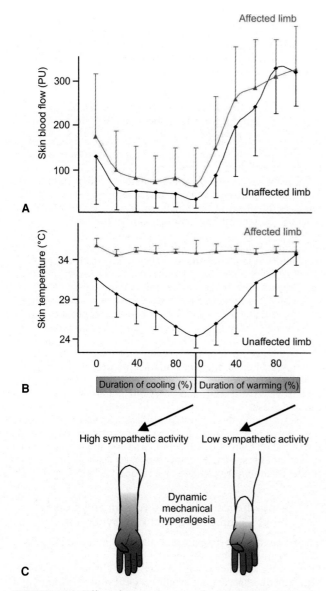

A

B

C

High sympathetic activity   Low sympathetic activity

Dynamic mechanical hyperalgesia

FIGURE 46-4. Effect of cutaneous sympathetic vasoconstrictor activity on skin blood flow, skin temperature, and mechanical hyperalgesia in one patient with complex regional pain syndrome (CRPS). Online recording of skin blood flow and skin temperature during whole-body cooling and warming. High sympathetic vasoconstrictor activity during cooling induces considerable drop in skin blood flow on the affected and unaffected extremity (laser Doppler flowmetry, *A*). On the unaffected side, the decrease of skin temperature secondary to vasoconstriction is shown. On the affected side, the forearm temperature was clamped at 35°C. Activation of sympathetic neurons leads to a considerable increase of the area of dynamic mechanical allodynia indicating that, in CRPS, a pathologic coupling between sympathetic and nociceptive neurons does exist. Modified from Baron R, Jänig W. Complex regional pain syndromes: How do we escape the diagnostic trap? *Lancet* 2004;364(9447):1739–1741, with permission.

α-adrenoceptors (46,47). Noradrenaline released by the sympathetic nerve fibers may activate and/or sensitize the afferent neurons. The sympathetic–afferent coupling may occur at the lesion site, along the lesioned nerve, or even in the dorsal root ganglion, although the latter, as attractive as it may be, appears to be unlikely. Overall animal models clearly support these

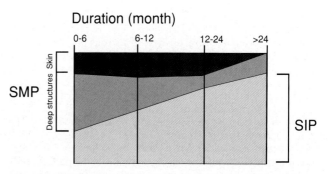

FIGURE 46-5. Different components of sympathetic maintained pain (SMP). The component of pain that depends on the cutaneous sympathetic innervation (skin SMP), on the deep somatic sympathetic innervation (deep SMP), and the pain component that is not maintained by sympathetic activity (sympathetically independent pain [SIP]) during the course of the disease. Modified from Schattschneider J, Binder A, Siebrecht D, et al. Complex regional pain syndromes: The influence of cutaneous and deep somatic sympathetic innervation on pain. *Clin J Pain* 2006;22(3):240–244, with permission.

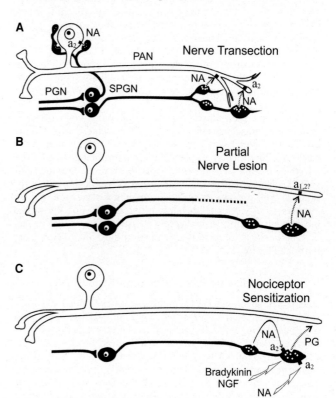

FIGURE 46-6. Influence of sympathetic activity and catecholamines on primary afferent neurons. **A:** Complete nerve lesion. The sympathetic–afferent interaction is located in the neuroma and in the dorsal root ganglion. It is mediated by norepinephrine (NA) released from postganglionic neurons (SPGN) and α-adrenoreceptors expressed at the plasma membrane of afferent fibers. PGN, preganglionic neuron. **B:** Partial nerve lesion. Partial nerve injury is followed by a decrease of the sympathetic innervation density (stippled postganglionic neuron). This induces an upregulation of functional α_2-adrenoceptors at the membrane of intact nociceptive fibers. **C:** After tissue inflammation, intact but sensitized primary afferents acquire norepinephrine sensitivity. Norepinephrine is not acting directly on afferents but induces the release of prostaglandins (PG) from sympathetic terminals that sensitize the afferents. In accordance, bradykinin- and nerve growth factor (NGF)-induced nociceptor sensitization is also mediated by the release of prostaglandins from postganglionic fibers.

peripheral mechanisms of SMP occurring in CRPS II (48–52). It should be kept in mind that not only coupling of sympathetic neurons to nociceptive afferent neurons but also to non-nociceptive afferent (e.g., mechanosensitive, cold) neurons may emerge as important. Sympathetic activation of these afferent neurons may excite sensitized or hyperexcitable central neurons of the somatosensory system (e.g., in the dorsal horn) and contribute to mechanical or cold allodynia in CRPS II patients.

Unfortunately, we have no animal models for SMP in CRPS I. It is unlikely that mechanisms of SMP occurring in CRPS II (i.e., after trauma with nerve lesion) can explain SMP in CRPS I. For the mechanisms underlying SMP in CRPS I patients only a minor component of the coupling occurs in the skin. We suggest that an important sympathetic–afferent coupling also occurs in the deep somatic tissues, and that the mechanism of this coupling is indirect, involving the vascular bed and possibly other non-neural components. This mode of coupling has been repeatedly postulated (48,50–52). However, it has never been explored experimentally using animal models.

Other potential ways of coupling may exist between sympathetic neurons and afferent nociceptive neurons, which have been developed from experiments using animals but which have not been explored in patients. These modes of coupling do not involve activity in the sympathetic nerve fibers, but the sympathetic fibers may mediate the effects of inflammatory (e.g., bradykinin) or other compounds (e.g., nerve growth factor) to nociceptive fibers in the peripheral tissue. This sympathetic–afferent coupling may emerge as important in inflammatory pain and in CRPS I (51,53–55).

Finally, the sympathetic nervous system may be involved in coupling to nociceptive neurons via the adrenal medulla. This mechanism, which has been shown to exist in rats (using behavioral experiments), implies that epinephrine released by the adrenal medulla (during its activation by preganglionic neurons) leads to sensitization of nociceptors for mechanical stimulation. The process of sensitization has a slow time course of days to 2 weeks to develop fully. We do not know the mechanism leading to nociceptor sensitization in this model or whether it is important in understanding SMP in patients with CRPS I (51,56–58).

Pain-relieving Effect of Sympathetic Blocks

The pain-relieving effect of sympathetic blocks using local anesthetics applied to the sympathetic chain in CRPS patients with SMP, as documented by quantitative measurements (59), is puzzling. Pain relief outlasts the conduction block of sympathetic neurons by at least one order of magnitude. Sometimes only a few (in the extreme, only one!) temporary sympathetic blocks are necessary to produce permanent pain relief. The long-lasting pain-relieving effects of sympathetic blocks clearly argue that activity in sympathetic neurons, which is of central origin, maintains a positive feedback circuit via the primary afferent neurons. Animal models for positive feedback circuits are absent. We postulate that activity in sympathetic neurons maintains a central state of hyperexcitability (e.g., of neurons in the spinal dorsal horn), via excitation of afferent neurons initiated by an intense noxious event. The persistent afferent activity necessary to maintain such a central state of hyperexcitability is probably low in rate. This central state of hyperexcitability is switched off during a temporary block of conduction in the sympathetic chain lasting only for a few hours, and it cannot be switched on again when the block wears off and the sympathetic activity (and therefore also the sympathetically induced activity in afferent neurons) returns. Finally, the tacit assumption made is that cutaneous (sympa-

thetic and afferent) systems are primarily involved. However, whether sympathetic systems and afferent systems innervating deep somatic tissues are more important in this hypothetical positive feedback circuit has never been tested and needs to be investigated experimentally (42).

Possible Link between Inflammation and Sympathetic Nervous System

In some patients, sympatholytic procedures can ameliorate pain as well as inflammation and edema. Accordingly, animal studies have demonstrated that the sympathetic nervous system can influence the intensity of an inflammatory process (48,60–63). The question arises whether the sympathetic nervous system might be involved in the inflammatory process in CRPS and whether it might interact with immune cells.

Under normal conditions, catecholamines act via β_2-adrenoceptors on immune cells to inhibit the production and release of proinflammatory cytokines. These cells do not express α-adrenoceptors under basal conditions. However, the situation can dramatically change in chronic inflammation. Here, immune cells downregulate their expression of β_2-adrenoceptors and upregulate their expression of α_1-adrenoceptors over time (64). In contrast to β_2-adrenoceptors, α_1-adrenoceptors stimulate the production and release of proinflammatory cytokines. If α_1-adrenoceptors were to become expressed by the resident and/or recruited immune or immunocompetent cells of the affected CRPS extremity, then sympathetic activation would be predicted to cause pain and other inflammatory signs via cytokine release.

Summarizing the hypothetical ideas just described, Figure 46-3 illustrates the possible interactions between sympathetic fibers, afferent fibers, blood vessels, and non-neural cells related to the immune system (e.g., macrophages) leading theoretically to the inflammatory changes observed in CRPS patients.

Sympathetically Maintained Pain and Course of Complex Regional Pain Syndrome

The percentage of the pain that depends on sympathetic activity steadily declines during the course of the disease (Fig. 46-5). After 24 months, only a very small chance remains that sympathetic interventions might be successful. This finding is supported by studies that analyzed the effect of sympathetic blockade as well as cutaneous injections of norepinephrine in a group of acute patients and in the same patients after up to 10 years (41). Most of the chronic patients did not respond to sympathetic blockade, and the pain did not change after norepinephrine injection although this subgroup demonstrated favorable effects in the acute phase.

From these data it should be concluded that patients with acute CRPS should be assigned to diagnostic and, if applicable, to therapeutic sympathetic interventions as soon as possible to achieve the highest degree of pain relief in order to facilitate physiotherapy and have a better chance at full rehabilitation.

DIAGNOSTIC PROCEDURES

For the present, the lack of universally valid diagnostic criteria results in inherent difficulties in distinguishing CRPS from other pain syndromes in extremities. The diagnosis is predominantly based upon clinical criteria. There is no gold standard to compare with, nor is there an objective diagnostic test procedure.

The definition of standardized diagnostic criteria for CRPS in 1995 was a major advance (38). However, these criteria were derived based upon the consensus opinion of a small group of expert clinicians. Although this was an appropriate first step, it is important to continuously improve the criteria, to validate and, if necessary, modify these initial consensus-based criteria based upon results of systematic validation research. The 1995 CRPS diagnostic criteria were adequately sensitive (i.e., rarely miss a case of actual CRPS). However, both internal and external validation research suggests that CRPS was over-diagnosed (65,66). For example, an external validation of the International Association for the Study of Pain (IASP) criteria in 117 patients with CRPS and 43 patients with neuropathic pain without CRPS etiology demonstrated a sensitivity of 0.98 and a specificity 0.36. For example, the inclusion of a category "motor and trophic signs and symptoms" improves specificity considerably without losing sensitivity (11).

Based on this validation research, a novel diagnostic algorithm was recently proposed (Table 46-1) (67,68). In addition to the improved clinical categories, it became possible to distinguish between criteria for clinical use and a classification for research purposes. For the clinician, and particularly for the patient, it is important to have a high sensitivity value combined with a fair specificity (e.g., 0.85 versus 0.60, Table 46-1). For research purposes, however, it is much more important to have

TABLE 46-1

REVISED DIAGNOSTIC CRITERIA FOR COMPLEX REGIONAL PAIN SYNDROME

Categories of clinical signs/symptoms
1. Positive sensory abnormalities:
   - Spontaneous pain
   - Mechanical hyperalgesia
   - Thermal hyperalgesia
   - Deep somatic hyperalgesia
2. Vascular abnormalities:
   - Vasodilation
   - Vasoconstriction
   - Skin temperature asymmetries
   - Skin color changes
3. Edema, sweating abnormalities:
   - Swelling
   - Hyperhidrosis
   - Hypohidrosis
4. Motor, trophic changes:
   - Motor weakness
   - Tremor
   - Dystonia
   - Coordination deficits
   - Nail, hair changes
   - Skin atrophy
   - Joint stiffness
   - Soft tissue

Interpretation
Clinical use:
≥1 symptoms of ≥3 categories each AND ≥1 signs of ≥2 categories each:
Sensitivity 0.85   Specificity 0.60
Research use:
≥1 symptoms of = 4 categories each AND ≥1 signs of ≥2 categories each:
Sensitivity 0.70   Specificity 0.96

TABLE 46-2

DIAGNOSTIC TESTS IN COMPLEX REGIONAL PAIN SYNDROME

	Sensitivity	Specificity
Plain radiograph (only chronic stages)	73	57
Bone scan (only acute stages)	97	86
Quantitative sensory testing (QST)	High	Low
Temperature differences (during sympathetic stimulation)	76	93
Magnetic resonance imaging (skin, joint, etc.)	91	17

a high specificity to perform studies in a precisely diagnosed population (e.g., 0.7 versus 0.96, Table 46-1).

Tests Aiding in Diagnosis

Several diagnostic procedures have been evaluated in recent years (Table 46-2). New techniques to assess specific signs objectively are in the experimental testing phase. Cortical reorganization underlying somatosensory and motor abnormalities can be visualized using magnetoencephalography and fMRI. Video-assisted kinematic and tremor analyses are used to quantify and qualify motor abnormalities such as weakness, coordination deficits, and tremor. The acute inflammatory component of the disorder, in particular the role of specific inflammatory mediators, is explored using microdialysis techniques and analyzing the content of suction blister fluid. These and other investigations will pave the way for a quantitative and objective analysis of these abnormalities. Furthermore, genetic patterns of patients at risk to develop CRPS have already been revealed, and the discovery of more genes determining the susceptible patient is to come.

In summary, we must encourage researchers from various fields to unravel the diagnostic puzzle of the CRPS mystery using an interdisciplinary research approach.

THERAPY

Lack of understanding of the underlying pathophysiologic abnormalities and lack of objective diagnostic criteria result in inherent difficulties in conducting clinical trials of various therapeutic modalities. Therefore, only few evidence-based treatment regimens exist for CRPS. In fact, three literature reviews of outcome studies find discouragingly little consistent information regarding pharmacologic agents and methods for treatment of CRPS (69–71). Moreover, within the only 30 studies available, the methodology is often of low quality. In the absence of more specific information about pathophysiologic mechanisms and treatment of CRPS, one has to rely on outcomes from treatment studies for other neuropathic pain syndromes.

Pharmacologic Therapy

- *Nonsteroidal anti-inflammatory drugs.* Nonsteroidal anti-inflammatory drugs (NSAIDs) have not been investigated in the treatment of CRPS so far. However, from clinical experience, they can control mild to moderate pain.

- *Opioids.* Opioids are clearly effective in postoperative, inflammatory, and cancer pain. The use of opioids in CRPS has not been studied. In other neuropathic pain syndromes, compounds such as tramadol, morphine, oxycodone, and levorphanol are clearly analgesic when compared to placebo. However, there are no long-term studies of oral opioids use for treatment of neuropathic pain, CRPS included. Even without solid scientific evidence, the expert opinion of pain clinicians is that opioids could and should be used as a part of a comprehensive pain treatment program. Given that some patients with neuropathic pain may obtain considerable pain relief from opioids, they should be prescribed immediately if other agents do not achieve sufficient analgesia.

- *Antidepressants.* Tricyclic antidepressants (TCAs) have been intensely studied in different neuropathic pain conditions, but not in CRPS. Solid evidence suggests that reuptake blockers of serotonin and noradrenaline, such as amitriptyline, and selective noradrenaline blockers, such as desipramine, produce pain relief in diabetic or postherpetic neuropathy. The effectiveness of selective serotonin reuptake inhibitors in neuropathic pain states is still being investigated. Only one of four studies performed so far showed a significant pain reduction in painful diabetic neuropathy. None has been performed on CRPS patients.

- *Sodium channel–blocking agents.* Lidocaine administered intravenously is effective in CRPS I and II regarding spontaneous and evoked pain (72). Carbamazepine has not been tested in CRPS.

- *γ-Aminobutyric acid (GABA) agonists.* Intrathecally administered baclofen is effective in the treatment of dystonia in CRPS (73). Oral baclofen has been effective in the treatment of trigeminal neuralgia. No further trials in CRPS are available, and there is no evidence for an analgesic effect of baclofen, valproic acid, vigabatrin, and benzodiazepines in CRPS or other neuropathic pain conditions.

- *Gabapentin.* A randomized, double-blind, placebo-controlled trial demonstrated a mild effect of gabapentin on pain and a good effect on sensory deficit symptoms in CRPS I (74). Gabapentin is effective in painful diabetic neuropathy and postherpetic neuralgia.

- *Steroids.* Orally administered prednisone, 10 mg three times daily, has clearly demonstrated efficacy in the improvement of the entire clinical status (up to 75%) in acute CRPS patients (<13 weeks) (75). In CRPS I following stroke, 40 mg prednisolone for 14 days followed by tapering improved significantly the signs and symptoms compared to piroxicam 20 mg daily (76). No evidence has been obtained with other immune-modulating therapies, such as immunoglobulins or immunosuppressive drugs. A cytokine modulator, lenalidomide, showed efficacy in an open-label trial.

- *N-methyl-D-aspartate (NMDA) receptor blockers.* Clinically available compounds that are demonstrated to have NMDA receptor-blocking properties include ketamine, dextromethorphan, and memantine. Dextromethorphan, for example, is effective in the treatment of painful diabetic neuropathy, but not effective in postherpetic neuralgia and central pain. NMDA blockers may offer new options for treatment of CRPS pain, but studies that will help clinicians to fully utilize these agents are not available.

- *Calcium-regulating drugs.* Calcitonin administered three times daily intranasally demonstrated a significant pain reduction in CRPS patients (77). Intravenous (IV) clodronate 300 mg daily and IV alendronate 7.5 mg daily showed a significant improvement in pain, swelling, and movement range in acute CRPS (78,79). A non–placebo-controlled trial showed the same efficacy for calcitonin 200 I/U/day together with physiotherapy when compared to the combination of paracetamol 1,500 mg/day and physiotherapy (80). The mode of action of these compounds in CRPS is unknown.

- *Free radical scavengers.* Recently, a placebo-controlled trial was performed using the free radical scavengers dimethylsulfoxide (DMSO) 50% topically or N-acetylcysteine (NAC) orally for the treatment of CRPS I (81). Both drugs were found to be equally effective; DMSO seemed more favorable for "warm" and NAC for "cold" CRPS I. The results were negatively influenced by a longer disease duration. A previous trial with DMSO failed to show a positive result in CRPS (82), whereas DMSO has been more effective than regional blocks using guanethidine in a small population of CRPS patients (83).

- *Clonidine.* Transdermal application of the α2-adrenoceptor agonist clonidine, which is thought to prevent the release of catecholamines by a presynaptic action, may be helpful when small areas of hyperalgesia are present (84).

Interventional Therapy

Sympathetic Blockade

Currently, two therapeutic techniques to block sympathetic nerves are used: injections of a local anaesthetic around sympathetic paravertebral ganglia that project to the affected body part (sympathetic ganglion blocks) and regional IV application of guanethidine, bretylium, or reserpine (which all deplete noradrenaline in the postganglionic axon) to an isolated extremity blocked with a tourniquet (IV regional sympatholysis, IVRS).

Many uncontrolled surveys in the literature review the effect of sympathetic interventions in CRPS. In acute CRPS, about 85% of the patients report a positive effect. The efficacy of these procedures is, however, still discussed controversially and has been questioned in the past (69,85–90). In fact, the specific and long-term results, as well as the techniques used have been rarely adequately evaluated.

One controlled study in patients with CRPS I has shown that sympathetic ganglion blocks with local anaesthetic have the same immediate effect on pain as a control injection with saline (91). However, after 24 hours, patients in the local anaesthetic group were much better, indicating that nonspecific effects are important initially and that evaluating the efficacy of sympatholytic interventions is best done after 24 hours. With these data in mind, the uncontrolled studies here mentioned must be interpreted cautiously. Only 10 out of the 24 studies we reviewed assessed long-term effects.

Neither IV phentolamine nor guanethidine used for sympathetic blocks was effective in CRPS (89). No improvement was found following reserpine given together with guanethidine or guanethidine-only (IVRS) (92,93). However, stellate blocks with bupivacaine and regional blocks with IVRS guanethidine demonstrated a significant improvement of pain compared to baseline, but showed no differences between these two drugs (94). The cross-over study performed by Hord (95) showed a significant pain reduction due to the sympathetic blockade using lidocaine and bretylium. No differences were obtained between sympathetic blocks with IVRS guanethidine or lidocaine (96). No effect was obtained by IVRS droperidol (97). Hanna et al. (98) demonstrated a significant improvement of pain due to a single IVRS bolus of ketanserin. Bounameaux (99) failed to show any significant effect using the same procedure.

In summary-controlled studies using IVRS guanethidine, all but one (94) did not show a beneficial effect (92,93,96, 100,101). One study demonstrated that IVRS bretylium and lidocaine produce significantly longer pain relief than does lidocaine alone (95). Two studies showed that IVRS reserpine was ineffective (92,101).

In our view, there is a desperate need for controlled studies that assess the acute as well as the long-term effect of sympathetic blockade on pain and other CRPS symptoms, in particular motor function. Well-performed sympathetic ganglion blocks should be preferred over IVRS.

Surgical Sympathectomy

Only limited evidence exists regarding the efficacy of thoracoscopic or surgical sympathectomy. Four studies report on partly long-lasting benefits in CRPS I and II (102–105). The most important independent factor in determining a positive outcome of sympathectomy is time of less than 12 months between injury and intervention (104,105). The videoscopic lumbar sympathectomy is equally effective as the open surgical intervention (106).

We investigated skin blood flow, sympathetic vasoconstrictor reflexes, and pain after surgical sympathectomy in a small cohort of CRPS patients (107). Postoperatively, no vasoconstriction due to deep inspiration (vasoconstrictor reflex) could be elicited at the affected extremity, indicating complete sympathetic denervation. Additionally, the skin temperature at the affected hand increased. After 4 weeks, skin temperature decreased without signs of reinnervation. This denervation supersensitivity was associated with the recurrence of pain and is thought to rely on a vascular supersensitivity to cold and circulating catecholamines. Only two of 12 patients experienced long-term pain relief.

The irreversible sympathectomy may be effective in selected cases. Because of the risk of development of adaptive supersensitivity even on nociceptive neurons and consecutive pain increase and prolongation, these procedures should not be recommended on a broad indication basis.

Stimulation Techniques

Transcutaneous electrical nerve stimulation (TENS) may be effective in some cases and has minimal side effects.

Epidural spinal cord stimulation (SCS) has shown efficacy in one randomized study in selected chronic CRPS patients (108). It improved pain and health-related quality of life, but not functional outcome assessed 2 years later. Interestingly, these patients had previously undergone unsuccessful surgical sympathectomy. The pain-relieving effect was not associated with peripheral vasodilatation, suggesting that central disinhibition processes are involved. Sensory detection thresholds were not affected by the stimulation (109). A meta-analysis showed that, in selected patients, SCS can relieve pain and allodynia and improve quality of life (110) with an adverse event rate of 34% (111) but further studies are still warranted. Cervical and lumbar devices seem to be equally effective (112). SCS was also effective in selected CRPS patients with SMP (113), but further predicting factors in addition to test stimulations are still under investigation (114). A health economics study revealed that the use of SCS in combination with physiotherapy compared with physiotherapy alone is associated with a lifetime cost saving of 58,000 Euro per patient (115).

Other stimulation techniques, such as peripheral nerve stimulation using implanted electrodes, repetitive transcranial magnetic stimulation, and deep brain stimulation (sensory thalamus and medial lemniscus, motor cortex) have been reported to be effective in selected cases of CRPS (116–118).

Spinal Drug Application

In selected patients with severe refractory CRPS, the epidural application of clonidine showed a greater pain reduction in higher dosages (700 μg) than in lower dosages (300 μg) (119). However, the drug was associated with marked side effects (e.g., sedation and hypotension). Intrathecally administered baclofen is effective in the treatment of dystonia in CRPS (73).

Physical and Occupational Therapy

It should be stressed that clinical experience clearly indicates that physiotherapy is of utmost importance in achieving the recovery of function and rehabilitation. Standardized physiotherapy has shown long-term relief in pain and physical dysfunction in children (120). Recent developments of mirror and limb recognition techniques have advanced this field.

Physical and, to a lesser extent, occupational therapy are able to reduce pain and improve active mobility in CRPS I (121). Lymph drainage provides no benefit when applied together with physiotherapy in comparison with physiotherapy alone (122). Patients with initially less pain and better motor function are predicted to benefit to a greater degree than others (123). Physical therapy in CRPS is both more effective and less costly than either occupational therapy or control treatment (124).

Mirror visual feedback treatment in CRPS type I (i.e., observing the mirror image of the unaffected limb mimicking painless movement of the affected limb) reduces pain and improves function (23).

Recent studies have demonstrated that the combination of hand laterality recognition training, imagination of movements, and mirror movements reduces pain and disability in CRPS patients (125,126). It is important to recognize that only the order of training—laterality recognition, movement imagination, followed by mirror movements—is effective. If used, a numbers needed to treat (NNT) rate of 3 for a 6-month period can be achieved and is therefore more effective than physiotherapy without these techniques. Thus, physical and occupational therapy and attentional training have become an important part of successful therapy in CRPS patients.

Psychological Therapy

Although some evidence suggests a psychological impact on CRPS patients, only one study has addressed the efficacy of psychological treatment. A prospective, randomized, single-blind trial of cognitive-behavioral therapy (CBT) was conducted together with physical therapy of different intensities in children and adults and showed a long-lasting reduction of all symptoms in both arms (127). Fear of injury or reinjury by moving the affected limb is thought to be a possible predictor of chronic disability. Thus, in a small group of patients, graded exposure therapy was successful in decreasing pain-related fear, pain intensity, and consecutively disability. In addition to the lack of well-controlled studies, a sequenced protocol for psychological treatment has been proposed recently:

1. Education regarding the nature of the disease for all patients and their families

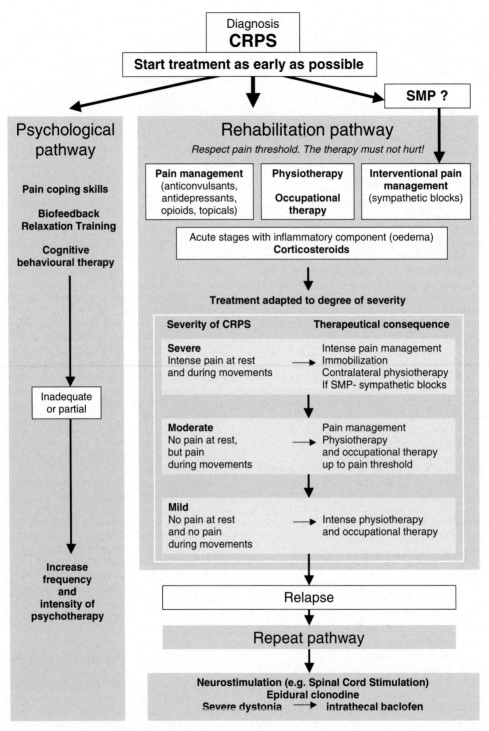

FIGURE 46-7. Treatment algorithm. Treatment must be directed toward restoration of full function of the extremity. The severity of the disease determines a stepwise therapeutic regime. The reduction of pain is the precondition for all other approaches. (*1*) At the acute stage of complex regional pain syndrome (CPRS) with severe pain at rest, immobilization and careful contralateral physical therapy should be the treatment of choice. Sympatholytic procedures, preferably sympathetic ganglion blocks, should identify that component of the pain maintained by the sympathetic nervous system. (*2*) If resting pain subsides, physical therapy should be performed in combination with sensory desensitization programs and pain therapy. (*3*) If movement-induced pain subsides, then physio- and occupational should be intensified.

Psychological treatment must flank the regime to strengthen coping strategies and discover contributing factors. In refractory cases, spinal cord stimulation and epidural clonidine could be considered. If refractory dystonia develops, intrathecal baclofen application is worth considering. Modified from Stanton-Hicks M, et al. An updated interdisciplinary clinical pathway for CRPS: Report of an expert panel. *Pain Pract* 2002;2(1):1–16; and Baron R, et al. Complex regional pain syndrome. Reflex sympathetic dystrophy and causalgia. *Nervenarzt* 2002;73(4):305–318, with permission.

2. If disease duration exceeds 6 to 8 weeks, patients should be evaluated psychologically and treated with CBT
3. In case of psychiatric comorbidities and major ongoing life stressors, these issues should be addressed in conjunction with the use of general CBT (128).

THERAPY GUIDELINES

Treatment should be immediate and, most importantly, directed toward restoration of full function of the extremity. This objective is best attained in a comprehensive interdisciplinary setting, with particular emphasis on pain management and functional restoration (129,130). The pain specialists should include neurologists, anesthesiologists, orthopedic surgeons, physiotherapists, psychologists, and the general practitioner.

The severity of the disease determines the therapeutic regime (Fig. 46-7). The reduction of pain is the precondition with which all other interventions have to comply. Interestingly, relative pain reduction of at least 50% and 30 mm on the 100 mm VAS are judged to be the result of a "successful" therapy (71). No therapeutic approaches must hurt; at the acute stage of CRPS, when the patient still suffers from severe pain at rest and during movements, it is nearly impossible to carry out intensive active therapy. Painful interventions, and in particular aggressive physical therapy, at this stage often lead to deterioration. Therefore, immobilization and careful contralateral physical therapy should be the acute treatment of choice, and intense pain treatment should be initiated immediately. First-line analgesics and co-analgesics are opioids, tricyclic antidepressants, gabapentin, and carbamazepine. Additionally, corticosteroids should be considered if inflammatory signs and symptoms are predominant. Sympatholytic procedures, preferably sympathetic ganglion blocks, should identify that component of the pain maintained by the sympathetic nervous system.

For efficacy, a serial regime of treatment should be undertaken. Calcium-regulating agents should be used in cases of refractory pain. If resting pain subsides, first passive physical therapy, then later active isometric followed by active isotonic training should be performed in combination with sensory desensitization programs until restitution of complete motor function. Psychological treatment must flank the regime to strengthen coping strategies and discover contributing factors. In refractory cases, spinal cord stimulation and epidural clonidine could be considered. If refractory dystonia develops, intrathecal baclofen application is worth considering.

PREVENTION

Zollinger (131) proved a significantly reduced incidence of CRPS following Colles fracture using vitamin C (500 mg/day) treatment. Reuben et al. demonstrated a significantly lower occurrence rate using axillary block or IVRA with lidocaine and clonidine, compared to general anesthesia or IVRA with lidocaine for Dupuytren contracture (132).

The recurrence rate in patients with a history of CRPS undergoing surgery of the formerly affected extremity was significantly reduced by a perioperative stellate ganglion block (133). Preoperatively administered guanethidine did not prevent CRPS in patients undergoing fasciectomy for Dupuytren disease (134). In patients with a history of CRPS, IVRA with lidocaine and clonidine, but not lidocaine alone, reduced significantly the recurrence rate (135).

PROGNOSIS

The disease duration is variable and may persist over decades (10). In rare cases, a causal therapy, such as the decompression of an entrapment syndrome, may lead to complete recovery (136,137).

A 5.5-year follow-up study showed that 62% of the patients were still limited in their activities of daily living, with pain and motor impairment listed as the most important factors (83,137,138). In more than 60% of patients with CRPS II, the complaints remained unchanged even after 1 year of intensive therapy (139). In contrast, a retrospective population-based study reported a resolution of symptoms in 74% of the patients with CRPS I (8). In a 13-month follow-up study in a small cohort, nearly all patients still suffered from a functional impairment of the affected extremity, although most of the other clinical features of CRPS had resolved (140).

Severity, not etiology, seems to determine the disease course (141,142), and age, gender, and affected side are not associated with the outcome (8). Fractures may be associated with a higher resolution rate (91%) than sprain (78%) and other inciting event (55%) (8). In 1,183 patients, the incidence of recurrence was 1.8% per year. Those patients with a recurrent CRPS were significantly younger but did not differ in gender or primary localization. The symptoms and signs were few in case of recurrence, in half of the patient's of spontaneous origin and affected the symmetrical limb.

A low skin temperature at the onset of the disease may predict an unfavorable course and outcome (10). This study hypothesis is weakened by a possible discrepancy between the patients' retrospective assessment and the missing objective assessment of the skin temperature (143).

A retrospective analysis of 1,006 CRPS cases showed an incidence of severe complications in about 7%. These comprised infection, ulceration, chronic edema, dystonia, and/or myoclonus. Mostly female and younger patients with CRPS of the lower limb were affected (144).

ACKNOWLEDGMENTS

This work was supported by the Deutsche Forschungsgemeinschaft (DFG Ba 1921/1-2), the German Ministry of Research and Education within the German Research Network on Neuropathic Pain (BMBF, 01EM05/04), and an unrestricted educational grant of Pfizer (Germany).

PART IV: PAIN MANAGEMENT

References

1. Jänig W, Baron R. Complex regional pain syndrome: Mystery explained? *Lancet Neurol* 2003;2(11):687–697.
2. Baron R, Fields HL, Jänig W, et al. National Institutes of Health Workshop: Reflex sympathetic dystrophy/complex regional pain syndromes: State-of-the-science. *Anesth Analg* 2002;95(6):1812–1816.
3. Baron R. Mechanistic and clinical aspects of complex regional pain syndrome (CRPS). *Novartis Found Symp* 2004;261:220–233; discussion 233–238, 256–261.
4. Wasner G, Schattschneider J, Binder A, Baron R. Complex regional pain syndrome: Diagnostic, mechanisms, CNS involvement and therapy. *Spinal Cord* 2003;41(2):61–75.
5. Wasner G, Schattschnedier J, Heckmann K, et al. Vascular abnormalities in

reflex sympathetic dystrophy (CRPS I): Mechanisms and diagnostic value. *Brain* 2001;124[Pt 3]:587–599.

6. Wasner G, Heckmann K, Maier C, Baron R. Vascular abnormalities in acute reflex sympathetic dystrophy (CRPS I): Complete inhibition of sympathetic nerve activity with recovery. *Arch Neurol* 1999;56(5):613–620.

7. Schattschneider J, Hartung K, Stengel M, et al. Endothelial dysfunction in cold type complex regional pain syndrome. *Neurology* 2006;67(4):673–675.

8. Sandroni P, Benrud-Larson LM, McClelland RL, Low PA. Complex regional pain syndrome type I: Incidence and prevalence in Olmsted county, a population-based study. *Pain* 2003;103(1–2):199–207.

9. de Mos M, de Bruijn AG, Huygen FJ, et al. The incidence of complex regional pain syndrome: A population-based study. *Pain* 2007;129(1–2):12–20.

10. Veldman PH, Reynen HM, Arntz IF, Goris RJ. Signs and symptoms of reflex sympathetic dystrophy: Prospective study of 829 patients. *Lancet* 1993;342(8878):1012–1016.

11. Bruehl S, Harden RN, Galer BS, et al. Complex regional pain syndrome: Are there distinct subtypes and sequential stages of the syndrome? *Pain* 2002;95(1–2):119–124.

12. Covington EC. Psychological issues in reflex sympathetic dystrophy. In: Jänig W, Stanton-Hicks M, eds. *Reflex Sympathetic Dystrophy: A Reappraisal. Progress in Pain Research and Management.* Seattle: IASP Press; 1996:192–216.

13. Puchalski P, Zyluk A. Complex regional pain syndrome type 1 after fractures of the distal radius: A prospective study of the role of psychological factors. *J Hand Surg [Br]* 2005;30(6):574–580.

14. Ciccone DS, Bandilla E, Wu W. Psychological dysfunction in patients with reflex sympathetic dystrophy. *Pain* 1997;71(3):323–333.

15. Monti DA, Herring CL, Schwartzman RJ, Marchese M. Personality assessment of patients with complex regional pain syndrome type I. *Clin J Pain* 1998;14(4):295–302.

16. Bruehl S, Husfeldt B, Lubenow TR, et al. Psychological differences between reflex sympathetic dystrophy and non-RSD chronic pain patients. *Pain* 1996;67(1):107–114.

17. Birklein F, Riedl B, Sieweke N, et al. Neurological findings in complex regional pain syndromes: Analysis of 145 cases. *Acta Neurol Scand* 2000;101(4):262–269.

18. Deuschl G, Blumberg H, Lücking CH. Tremor in reflex sympathetic dystrophy. *Arch Neurol* 1991;48(12):1247–1252.

19. Bhatia KP, Bhatt MH, Marsden CD. The causalgia-dystonia syndrome. *Brain* 1993;116[Pt 4]:843–851.

20. Maihofner C, Baron R, DeCol R, et al. The motor system shows adaptive changes in complex regional pain syndrome. *Brain* 2007;130[Pt 10]:2671–2687.

21. Ribbers GM, Mulder T, Geurts AC, den Otter RA. Reflex sympathetic dystrophy of the left hand and motor impairments of the unaffected right hand: Impaired central motor processing? *Arch Phys Med Rehabil* 2002;83(1):81–85.

22. Galer BS, Butler S, Jensen MP. Case reports and hypothesis: A neglect-like syndrome may be responsible for the motor disturbance in reflex sympathetic dystrophy (Complex Regional Pain Syndrome-1). *J Pain Symptom Manage* 1995;10(5):385–391.

23. McCabe CS, Haigh RC, Ring EF, et al. A controlled pilot study of the utility of mirror visual feedback in the treatment of complex regional pain syndrome (type 1). *Rheumatology (Oxford)* 2003;42(1):97–101.

24. Moseley GL. Graded motor imagery is effective for long-standing complex regional pain syndrome: A randomised controlled trial. *Pain* 2004;108(1–2):192–198.

25. Juottonen K, Gockel M, Silén T, et al. Altered central sensorimotor processing in patients with complex regional pain syndrome. *Pain* 2002;98(3):315–323.

26. Schwenkreis P, Janssen F, Rommel O, et al. Bilateral motor cortex disinhibition in complex regional pain syndrome (CRPS) type I of the hand. *Neurology* 2003;61(4):515–519.

27. Calder JS, Holten I, McAllister RM. Evidence for immune system involvement in reflex sympathetic dystrophy. *J Hand Surg [Br]* 1998;23(2):147–150.

28. Huygen FJ, de Bruijn AG, Klein J, Zijlstra FJ. Neuroimmune alterations in the complex regional pain syndrome. *Eur J Pharmacol* 2001;429(1–3):101–113.

29. Huygen FJ, de Bruijn AG, De Bruin MT, et al. Evidence for local inflammation in complex regional pain syndrome type 1. *Mediators Inflamm* 2002;11(1):47–51.

30. Maihofner C, Handwerker HO, Neundörfer B, Birklein F. Mechanical hyperalgesia in complex regional pain syndrome: A role for TNF-alpha? *Neurology* 2005;65(2):311–313.

31. Alexander GM, van Rijn MA, van Hilten JJ, et al. Changes in cerebrospinal fluid levels of pro-inflammatory cytokines in CRPS. *Pain* 2005;116(3):213–219.

32. Wasner G, Heckmann K, Maier C, Baron R. Vascular abnormalities in acute reflex sympathetic dystrophy (CRPS I): Complete inhibition of sympathetic nerve activity with recovery. *Arch Neurol* 1999;56:613–620.

33. Blaes F, Schmitz K, Tschernatsch M, et al. Autoimmune etiology of complex regional pain syndrome (M Sudeck). *Neurology* 2004;63(9):1734–1736.

34. Blaes F, Tschernatsch M, Braeu ME, et al. Autoimmunity in complex-regional pain syndrome. *Ann NY Acad Sci* 2007;1107:168–173.

35. Goebel A, Vogel H, Caneris O, et al. Immune responses to Campylobacter and serum autoantibodies in patients with complex regional pain syndrome. *J Neuroimmunol* 2005;162(1–2):184–189.

36. Arnér S. Intravenous phentolamine test: Diagnostic and prognostic use in reflex sympathetic dystrophy. *Pain* 1991;46(1):17–22.

37. Raja SN, Treede RD, Davis KD, Campbell JN. Systemic alpha-adrenergic blockade with phentolamine: A diagnostic test for sympathetically maintained pain. *Anesthesiology* 1991;74(4):691–698.

38. Stanton-Hicks M, Jänig W, Hassenbusch S, et al. Reflex sympathetic dystrophy: Changing concepts and taxonomy. *Pain* 1995;63(1):127–133.

39. Schurmann M, Gradl G, Wizgal I, et al. Clinical and physiologic evaluation of stellate ganglion blockade for complex regional pain syndrome type I. *Clin J Pain* 2001;17(1):94–100.

40. Ali Z, Raja SN, Wesselmann U, et al. Intradermal injection of norepinephrine evokes pain in patients with sympathetically maintained pain. *Pain* 2000;88:161–168.

41. Torebjörk E, Wahren L, Wallin G, et al. Noradrenaline-evoked pain in neuralgia [see comments]. *Pain* 1995;63(1):11–20.

42. Baron R, Schattschneider J, Binder A, et al. Relation between sympathetic vasoconstrictor activity and pain and hyperalgesia in complex regional pain syndromes: A case-control study. *Lancet* 2002;359(9318):1655–1660.

43. Jänig W, McLachlan EM. Characteristics of function-specific pathways in the sympathetic nervous system. *Trends Neurosci* 1992;15(12):475–481.

44. Jänig W, McLachlan EM. Neurobiology of the autonomic nervous system. In: Mathias CJ, Bannister R, eds. *Autonomic Failure.* Oxford: Oxford University Press; 1999:3–15.

45. Baron R, Wasner G. Complex regional pain syndromes. *Curr Pain Headache Rep* 2001;5(2):114–123.

46. Baron R. Mechanisms of disease: Neuropathic pain: A clinical perspective. *Nat Clin Pract Neurol* 2006;2(2):95–106.

47. Shi TS, Winzer-Serhan U, Leslie F, Hokfelt T. Distribution and regulation of alpha(2)-adrenoceptors in rat dorsal root ganglia. *Pain* 2000;84(2–3):319–330.

48. Jänig W, Levine JD, Michaelis M. Interactions of sympathetic and primary afferent neurons following nerve injury and tissue trauma. *Prog Brain Res* 1996;113:161–184.

49. Jänig W, Baron R. Complex regional pain syndrome is a disease of the central nervous system. *Clin Auton Res* 2002;12(3):150–164.

50. Jänig W, Koltzenburg M. Plasticity of sympathetic reflex organization following cross-union of inappropriate nerves in the adult cat. *J Physiol* 1991;436:309–323.

51. Jänig W, Habler HJ. Sympathetic nervous system: Contribution to chronic pain. *Prog Brain Res* 2000;129:451–468.

52. Jänig W, Koltzenburg M. What is the interaction between the sympathetic terminal and the primary afferent fiber? In: Basbaum AI, Besson J-M, eds. *Towards a New Pharmacotherapy of Pain, Dahlem Workshop Reports.* Chichester: John Wiley and Sons; 1991:331–352.

53. Jänig W, Levine JD, Michaelis M. Interactions of sympathetic and primary afferent neurons following nerve injury and tissue trauma. *Prog Brain Res* 1996;113:161–184.

54. Woolf CJ, Ma QP, Allchorne A, Poole S. Peripheral cell types contributing to the hyperalgesic action of nerve growth factor in inflammation. *J Neurosci* 1996;16(8):2716–2723.

55. McMahon SB. NGF as a mediator of inflammatory pain. *Philos Trans R Soc Lond B Biol Sci* 1996;351(1338):431–440.

56. Khasar SG, Miao FJ, Jänig W, Levine JD. Vagotomy-induced enhancement of mechanical hyperalgesia in the rat is sympathoadrenal-mediated. *J Neurosci* 1998;18(8):3043–3049.

57. Khasar SG, Miao FJ, Jänig W, Levine JD. Modulation of bradykinin-induced mechanical hyperalgesia in the rat skin by activity in the abdominal vagal afferents. *Eur J Neurosci* 1998;10:435–444.

58. Jänig W, Khasar SG, Levine JD, Miao FJ. The role of vagal visceral afferents in the control of nociception. *Prog Brain Res* 2000;122:273–287.

59. Price DD, Long S, Wilsey B, Rafii A. Analysis of peak magnitude and duration of analgesia produced by local anesthetics injected into sympathetic ganglia of complex regional syndrome patients. *Clin J Pain* 1998;14:216–226.

60. Perl ER. Cutaneous polymodal receptors: Characteristics and plasticity. *Prog Brain Res* 1996;113:21–37.

61. Miao FJ, Green PG, Coderre TJ, et al. Sympathetic-dependence in bradykinin-induced synovial plasma extravasation is dose-related. *Neurosci Lett* 1996;205(3):165–168.

62. Miao FJ, Jänig W, Green PG, Levine JD. Inhibition of bradykinin-induced synovial plasma extravasation produced by intrathecal nicotine is mediated by the hypothalamopituitary adrenal axis. *J Neurophysiol* 1996;76(5):2813–2821.

63. Levine JD, Dardick SJ, Basbaum AI, Scipio E. Reflex neurogenic inflammation. I. Contribution of the peripheral nervous system to spatially remote

inflammatory responses that follow injury. *J Neurosci* 1985;5(5):1380–1386.

64. Gazda LS, Milligan ED, Hansen MK, et al. Sciatic inflammatory neuritis (SIN): Behavioral allodynia is paralleled by peri-sciatic proinflammatory cytokine and superoxide production. *J Peripher Nerv Syst* 2001;6(3):111–129.

65. Harden RN, Bruehl S, Galer BS, et al. Complex regional pain syndrome: Are the IASP diagnostic criteria valid and sufficiently comprehensive? *Pain* 1999;83(2):211–219.

66. Bruehl S, Harden RN, Galer BS, et al. External validation of IASP diagnostic criteria for Complex Regional Pain Syndrome and proposed research diagnostic criteria. *Pain* 1999;81(1–2):147–154.

67. Burton AW, Bruehl S, Harden RN. Current diagnosis and therapy of complex regional pain syndrome: Refining diagnostic criteria and therapeutic options. *Expert Rev Neurother* 2005;5(5):643–651.

68. Baron R, Jänig W. Complex regional pain syndromes: How do we escape the diagnostic trap? *Lancet* 2004;364(9447):1739–1741.

69. Kingery WS. A critical review of controlled clinical trials for peripheral neuropathic pain and complex regional pain syndromes. *Pain* 1997;73(2):123–139.

70. Perez RS, Kwakkel G, Zuurmond WW, de Lange JJ. Treatment of reflex sympathetic dystrophy (CRPS type 1): A research synthesis of 21 randomized clinical trials. *J Pain Symptom Manage* 2001;21(6):511–526.

71. Forouzanfar T, Köke AJ, van Kleef M, Weber WE. Treatment of complex regional pain syndrome type I. *Eur J Pain* 2002;6(2):105–122.

72. Wallace MS, Ridgeway BM, Leung AY, et al. Concentration-effect relationship of intravenous lidocaine on the allodynia of complex regional pain syndrome types I and II. *Anesthesiology* 2000;92(1):75–83.

73. van Hilten BJ, van de Beek WJ, Hoff JI, et al. Intrathecal baclofen for the treatment of dystonia in patients with reflex sympathetic dystrophy. *N Engl J Med* 2000;343(9):625–630.

74. van de Vusse AC, Stomp-van den Berg SG, Kessels AH, Weber WE. Randomised controlled trial of gabapentin in Complex Regional Pain Syndrome type 1 [ISRCTN84121379]. *BMC Neurol* 2004;4:13.

75. Christensen K, Jensen EM, Noer I. The reflex dystrophy syndrome response to treatment with systemic corticosteroids. *Acta Chir Scand* 1982;148(8):653–655.

76. Kalita J, Vajpayee A, Misra UK. Comparison of prednisolone with piroxicam in complex regional pain syndrome following stroke: A randomized controlled trial. *QJM* 2006;99(2):89–95.

77. Gobelet C, Waldburger M, Meier JL. The effect of adding calcitonin to physical treatment on reflex sympathetic dystrophy. *Pain* 1992;48(2):171–175.

78. Adami S, et al. Bisphosphonate therapy of reflex sympathetic dystrophy syndrome. *Ann Rheum Dis* 1997;56(3):201–204.

79. Varenna M, Zucchi F, Ghiringhelli D, et al. Intravenous clodronate in the treatment of reflex sympathetic dystrophy syndrome. A randomized, double blind, placebo controlled study. *J Rheumatol* 2000;27(6):1477–1483.

80. Sahin F, Yilmaz F, Kotevoglu N, Kuran B. Efficacy of salmon calcitonin in complex regional pain syndrome (type 1) in addition to physical therapy. *Clin Rheumatol* 2006;25(2):143–148.

81. Perez RS, Zuurmond WW, Bezemer PD, et al. The treatment of complex regional pain syndrome type I with free radical scavengers: A randomized controlled study. *Pain* 2003;102(3):297–307.

82. Zuurmond WW, Langendijk PN, Bezemer PD, et al. Treatment of acute reflex sympathetic dystrophy with DMSO 50% in a fatty cream. *Acta Anaesthesiol Scand* 1996;40(3):364–367.

83. Geertzen JH, de Bruijn H, de Bruijn-Kofman AT, Arendzen JH. Reflex sympathetic dystrophy: Early treatment and psychological aspects. *Arch Phys Med Rehabil* 1994;75(4):442–446.

84. Davis KD, Treede RD, Raja SN, et al. Topical application of clonidine relieves hyperalgesia in patients with sympathetically maintained pain [see comments]. *Pain* 1991;47(3):309–317.

85. Schott G. Clinical features of algodystrophy: Is the sympathetic nervous system involved? *Funct Neurol* 1989;4(2):131–134.

86. Schott GD. Visceral afferents: Their contribution to "sympathetic dependent" pain. *Brain* 1994;117[Pt 2]:397–413.

87. Schott GD. Interrupting the sympathetic outflow in causalgia and reflex sympathetic dystrophy [editorial]. *BMJ* 1998;316(7134):792–793.

88. Ochoa JL. Truths, errors, and lies around "reflex sympathetic dystrophy" and "complex regional pain syndrome." *J Neurol* 1999;246(10):875–879.

89. Verdugo RJ, Ochoa JL. "Sympathetically maintained pain." I. Phentolamine block questions the concept [see comments]. *Neurology* 1994;44(6):1003–1010.

90. Verdugo RJ, Campero M, Ochoa JL. Phentolamine sympathetic block in painful polyneuropathies. II. Further questioning of the concept of "sympathetically maintained pain." *Neurology* 1994;44(6):1010–1014.

91. Price DD, Long S, Wilsey B, Rafii A. Analysis of peak magnitude and duration of analgesia produced by local anesthetics injected into sympathetic ganglia of complex regional pain syndrome patients. *Clin J Pain* 1998;14(3):216–226.

92. Blanchard J, Ramamurthy S, Walsh N, et al. Intravenous regional sympatholysis: A double-blind comparison of guanethidine, reserpine, and normal saline. *J Pain Symptom Manage* 1990;5(6):357–361.

93. Jadad AR, Carroll D, Glynn CJ, McQuary HJ. Intravenous regional sympathetic blockade for pain relief in reflex sympathetic dystrophy: A systematic review and a randomized, double-blind crossover study. *J Pain Symptom Manage* 1995;10(1):13–20.

94. Bonelli S, Conoscente F, Movilia PG, et al. Regional intravenous guanethidine vs. stellate ganglion block in reflex sympathetic dystrophies: A randomized trial. *Pain* 1983;16(3):297–307.

95. Hord AH, Rooks MD, Stephens BO, et al. Intravenous regional bretylium and lidocaine for treatment of reflex sympathetic dystrophy: A randomized, double-blind study. *Anesth Analg* 1992;74(6):818–821.

96. Ramamurthy S, Hoffman J. Intravenous regional guanethidine in the treatment of reflex sympathetic dystrophy/causalgia: A randomized, double-blind study. Guanethidine Study Group. *Anesth Analg* 1995;81(4):718–723.

97. Kettler RE, Abram SE. Intravenous regional droperidol in the management of reflex sympathetic dystrophy: A double-blind, placebo-controlled, crossover study. *Anesthesiology* 1988;69(6):933–936.

98. Hanna MH, Peat SJ. Ketanserin in reflex sympathetic dystrophy. A double-blind placebo controlled cross-over trial. *Pain* 1989;38(2):145–150.

99. Bounameaux HM, Hellemans H, Verhaeghe R. Ketanserin in chronic sympathetic dystrophy. An acute controlled trial. *Clin Rheumatol* 1984;3(4):556–557.

100. Glynn CJ, Basedow RW, Walsh JA. Pain relief following post-ganglionic sympathetic blockade with I.V. guanethidine. *Br J Anaesth* 1981;53(12):1297–1302.

101. Rocco AG, Kaul AF, Reisman RM, et al. A comparison of regional intravenous guanethidine and reserpine in reflex sympathetic dystrophy. A controlled, randomized, double-blind crossover study. *Clin J Pain* 1989;5(3):205–209.

102. Singh B, Moodley J, Shaik AS, Robbs JV. Sympathectomy for complex regional pain syndrome. *J Vasc Surg* 2003;37(3):508–511.

103. Bandyk DF, Johnson BL, Kirkpatrick AF, et al. Surgical sympathectomy for reflex sympathetic dystrophy syndromes. *J Vasc Surg* 2002;35(2):269–277.

104. Schwartzman RJ, Liu JE, Smullens SN, et al. Long-term outcome following sympathectomy for complex regional pain syndrome type 1 (RSD). *J Neurol Sci* 1997;150(2):149–152.

105. AbuRahma AF, Robinson PA, Powell M, et al. Sympathectomy for reflex sympathetic dystrophy: Factors affecting outcome. *Ann Vasc Surg* 1994;8(4):372–379.

106. Lacroix H, Vander Velpen G, Peninckx F, et al. Technique and early results of videoscopic lumbar sympathectomy. *Acta Chir Belg* 1996;96(1):11–14.

107. Baron R, Maier C. Reflex sympathetic dystrophy: Skin blood flow, sympathetic vasoconstrictor reflexes and pain before and after surgical sympathectomy. *Pain* 1996;67(2–3):317–326.

108. Kemler MA, Barendse GA, van Kleef M, et al. Spinal cord stimulation in patients with chronic reflex sympathetic dystrophy. *N Engl J Med* 2000;343(9):618–624.

109. Kemler MA, Barendse GA, van Kleef M, Egbrink MG. Pain relief in complex regional pain syndrome due to spinal cord stimulation does not depend on vasodilation. *Anesthesiology* 2000;92(6):1653–1660.

110. Taylor RS. Spinal cord stimulation in complex regional pain syndrome and refractory neuropathic back and leg pain/failed back surgery syndrome: Results of a systematic review and meta-analysis. *J Pain Symptom Manage* 2006;31[4 Suppl]:S13–S19.

111. Turner JA, Loeser JD, Deyo RA, Sanders SB. Spinal cord stimulation for patients with failed back surgery syndrome or complex regional pain syndrome: A systematic review of effectiveness and complications. *Pain* 2004;108(1–2):137–147.

112. Forouzanfar T, Kemler MA, Weber WE, et al. Spinal cord stimulation in complex regional pain syndrome: Cervical and lumbar devices are comparably effective. *Br J Anaesth* 2004;92(3):348–353.

113. Harke H, Gretenkort P, Ladleif HU, Rahman S. Spinal cord stimulation in sympathetically maintained complex regional pain syndrome type I with severe disability. A prospective clinical study. *Eur J Pain* 2005;9(4):363–373.

114. Eisenberg E, Backonja MM, Fillingim RB, et al. Quantitative sensory testing for spinal cord stimulation in patients with chronic neuropathic pain. *Pain Pract* 2006;6(3):161–165.

115. Kemler MA, Furnee CA. Economic evaluation of spinal cord stimulation for chronic reflex sympathetic dystrophy. *Neurology* 2002;59(8):1203–1209.

116. Hassenbusch SJ, Stanton-Hicks M, Schoppa D, et al. Long-term results of peripheral nerve stimulation for reflex sympathetic dystrophy. *J Neurosurg* 1996;84(3):415–423.

117. Pleger B, Janssen F, Schwenkreis P, et al. Repetitive transcranial magnetic stimulation of the motor cortex attenuates pain perception in complex regional pain syndrome type I. *Neurosci Lett* 2004;356(2):87–90.

118. Son UC, Kim MC, Moon DE, Kang JK. Motor cortex stimulation in a patient with intractable complex regional pain syndrome type II with hemibody involvement. Case report. *J Neurosurg* 2003;98(1):175–179.

119. Rauck RL, Eisenach JC, Jackson K, et al. Epidural clonidine treatment for refractory reflex sympathetic dystrophy. *Anesthesiology* 1993;79(6):1163–1169; discussion 27A.

120. Sherry DD, Wallace CA, Kelley C, et al. Short- and long-term outcomes of children with complex regional pain syndrome type I treated with exercise therapy. *Clin J Pain* 1999;15(3):218–223.

121. Oerlemans HM, Oostendorp RA, de Boo T, et al. Adjuvant physical therapy versus occupational therapy in patients with reflex sympathetic dystrophy/complex regional pain syndrome type I. *Arch Phys Med Rehabil* 2000;81(1):49–56.

122. Uher EM, Vacariu G, Schneider B, Fialka V. Comparison of manual lymph drainage with physical therapy in complex regional pain syndrome, type I. A comparative randomized controlled therapy study. *Wien Klin Wochenschr* 2000;112(3):133–137.

123. Kemler MA, Rijks CP, de Vet HC. Which patients with chronic reflex sympathetic dystrophy are most likely to benefit from physical therapy? *J Manipulative Physiol Ther* 2001;24(4):272–278.

124. Severens JL, Oerlemans HM, Weegels AJ, et al. Cost-effectiveness analysis of adjuvant physical or occupational therapy for patients with reflex sympathetic dystrophy. *Arch Phys Med Rehabil* 1999;80(9):1038–1043.

125. Moseley GL. Is successful rehabilitation of complex regional pain syndrome due to sustained attention to the affected limb? A randomised clinical trial. *Pain* 2005;114(1–2):54–61.

126. Moseley GL. Graded motor imagery for pathologic pain: A randomized controlled trial. *Neurology* 2006;67(12):2129–2134.

127. Lee BH, Scharff L, Sethna NF, et al. Physical therapy and cognitive-behavioral treatment for complex regional pain syndromes. *J Pediatr* 2002; 141(1):135–140.

128. Bruehl S, Chung OY. Psychological and behavioral aspects of complex regional pain syndrome management. *Clin J Pain* 2006;22(5):430–437.

129. Stanton-Hicks M, Baron R, Boas R, et al. Complex regional pain syndromes: Guidelines for therapy. *Clin J Pain* 1998;14(2):155–166.

130. Stanton-Hicks M, Burton AW, Bruehl SP, et al. An updated interdisciplinary clinical pathway for CRPS: Report of an expert panel. *Pain Pract* 2002;2(1):1–16.

131. Zollinger PE, Tuinebreijer WE, Kreis RW, Breederveld RS. Effect of vitamin C on frequency of reflex sympathetic dystrophy in wrist fractures: A randomised trial. *Lancet* 1999;354(9195):2025–2028.

132. Reuben SS, Pristas R, Dixon D, et al. The incidence of complex regional pain syndrome after fasciectomy for Dupuytren's contracture: A prospective observational study of four anesthetic techniques. *Anesth Analg* 2006;102(2):499–503.

133. Reuben SS, Rosenthal EA, Steinberg RB. Surgery on the affected upper extremity of patients with a history of complex regional pain syndrome: A retrospective study of 100 patients. *J Hand Surg [Am]* 2000;25(6):1147–1151.

134. Gschwind C, Fricker R, Lacher G, Jung M. Does peri-operative guanethidine prevent reflex sympathetic dystrophy? *J Hand Surg [Br]* 1995;20(6):773–775.

135. Reuben SS, Rosenthal EA, Steinberg RB, et al. Surgery on the affected upper extremity of patients with a history of complex regional pain syndrome: The use of intravenous regional anesthesia with clonidine. *J Clin Anesth* 2004; 16(7):517–522.

136. Wilhelm A, Suden R. Proximal radial nerve compression syndrome. Treatment and results. *Handchir Mikrochir Plast Chir* 1985;17(4):219–224.

137. Maier C. Sympathische Reflexdystrophie - M Sudeck. In: Diener HC, Maier C, eds. *Das Schmerz-Therapiebuch*. Baltimore: Urban und Schwarzenberg; 1996:170–180.

138. Atkins RM, Duckworth T, Kanis JA. Features of algodystrophy after Colles' fracture. *J Bone Joint Surg Br* 1990;72(1):105–110.

139. Karstetter K, Sherman RA. Use of thermography for initial detection of early reflex sympathetic dystrophy. *J Am Podiatr Med Assoc* 1991;81:437–443.

140. Zyluk A. The natural history of post-traumatic reflex sympathetic dystrophy. *J Hand Surg [Br]* 1998;23(1):20–23.

141. Gold B, Brickner D, Sukenik S. Reflex sympathetic dystrophy syndrome following minor trauma. *Isr J Med Sci* 1989;25(2):107–109.

142. Bonica JJ. Causalgia and other reflex sympathetic dystrophies. In: Bonica JJ, ed. *The Management of Pain*, Vol. 2. Philadelphia: Lea & Febiger; 1990: 220–243.

143. Oerlemans HM, Oostendorp RA, de Boo T, et al. Signs and symptoms in complex regional pain syndrome type I/reflex sympathetic dystrophy: Judgment of the physician versus objective measurement. *Clin J Pain* 1999; 15(3):224–232.

144. van der Laan L, Veldman PH, Goris RJ. Severe complications of reflex sympathetic dystrophy: Infection, ulcers, chronic edema, dystonia, and myoclonus. *Arch Phys Med Rehabil* 1998;79(4):424–429.

145. Schattschneider J, Binder A, Siebrecht D, et al. Complex regional pain syndromes: The influence of cutaneous and deep somatic sympathetic innervation on pain. *Clin J Pain* 2006;22(3):240–244.

146. Baron R, Binder A, Ulrich W, Maier C. Complex regional pain syndrome. Reflex sympathetic dystrophy and causalgia. *Nervenarzt* 2002;73(4):305–318.

CHAPTER 47 ■ THE TREATMENT OF PAIN IN NEONATAL AND PEDIATRIC PATIENTS

CONSTANCE S. HOUCK, JOSEPH D. TOBIAS, MARY ELLEN TRESGALLO, K. J. S. ANAND, AND WILLIAM S. SCHECHTER

During the preceding 50 years, numerous changes, refinements, and advancements have occurred in the understanding and treatment of acute and chronic pain in neonates, infants, and children. This revolution in pediatric pain management began with the rejection of misconceptions and unfounded beliefs that neonates, infants, and children do not perceive and re-act to painful stimuli because of the immaturity of their peripheral and central nervous system (CNS). These false tenets, compounded by fears of addiction and adverse effects, led to the historical undertreatment of acute and chronic (including cancer-related) pain in children. This chapter focuses on the practical management of pediatric pain whether it be acute, chronic, or cancer-related—categories whose distinctiveness is useful from a didactic perspective, but that frequently overlap in clinical practice (e.g., acute pain associated with diagnostic and therapeutic procedures contributes substantially to cancer-related pain in children).

This chapter begins with an overview of the anatomy and development of the nociceptive system. It does not provide the detail given by Walker in Chapter 30 on developmental aspects of nociception, nor that by Dickenson and Yaksh in Chapters 32 and 33 on pharmacology and neuroanatomy, but aims simply to present a preclinical basis for the clinical approach presented later in the chapter. Next, we outline commonly used techniques for the assessment of pain in infants and children. Because many of the interventions used to treat acute pain are fundamental to the armamentarium for treatment of chronic pain and cancer-related pain, we next describe pharmacotherapy for acute pain along with relevant regional anesthetic techniques. Readers interested to learn more about the latter are referred to the comprehensive account by Dalens in Chapter 27.

Clinical studies have demonstrated that infants and children experience a similar severity of postoperative pain as adults and that even preterm infants demonstrate alterations in physiologic and biochemical markers of stress following painful stimuli (1–8). In fact, increases in biochemical measures of perioperative stress are frequently well in excess of those seen in the adult population (1,8). Inadequate treatment of pain during infancy may have long-lasting consequences including the development of chronic pain syndromes or a heightened sensitivity to subsequent painful stimuli, both of which may persist throughout childhood (2,5,9). The latter portion of the chapter addresses the spectrum of chronic and cancer-related pain in infants and children of all ages.

THE ANATOMY OF PAIN AND DEVELOPMENT OF NOCICEPTION

Nociceptive systems develop during the second and third trimesters of gestation and continue to mature during the first 2 years of life. Part of the traditional reluctance to aggressively treat pain during the neonatal period and infancy arose from the belief that the pain system was immature during these times. Given the nonverbal state of neonates and infants, they are incapable of reporting and describing the subjective phenomenon of pain. Therefore, it was erroneously concluded that these age groups were also incapable of nociception.

Normal nociception begins in the peripheral nervous system (PNS). In contrast to touch, pressure, heat or cold, there are no specific pain sensors. Rather, pain is sensed by free nerve endings. Cutaneous sensory receptors appear in the perioral area at 7 weeks of gestation, spread to the hands and feet by 11 weeks, and are present throughout all cutaneous and mucous surfaces by 20 weeks of gestation. The sensation of pain is mediated via free nerve endings of $A\delta$ and C fibers. These fibers do not demonstrate fatigue: repeated or continuous stimulation increases the ease of transmission of the impulse. Histologic studies show that the density of nociceptive nerve endings in newborn skin is similar to that in adult skin. More importantly, the neurophysiologic properties of the earliest nociceptors are also similar to those of adult skin. Rapidly adapting pressure receptors are the first to appear during fetal life, followed by the development of slowly adapting pressure receptors, and then rapidly adapting mechanoceptors. The depolarization responses of these receptors to mechanical injury, chemical irritants, and inflammatory mediators are similar to those of adult receptors.

Fetal sensory receptors are located on or close to the skin surface soon after development. As the stratum corneum develops, fetal sensory receptors gradually become subepidermal. Reflex movements to cutaneous perioral sensory stimulation occur as early as the seventh week of gestation; for the rest of the face, palms of the hands, and the soles of the feet by the eleventh week; for the trunk and proximal parts of the arms and legs by the fifteenth week; and for all cutaneous and mucosal surfaces by the twentieth week. The development of these sensory reflexes is preceded by synaptogenesis between afferent fibers and sensory neurons in the dorsal horn of the spinal cord. Myelinated fibers are the first to grow into the developing spinal cord and form connections with deeper layers of the dorsal horn, with collaterals to neurons in the substantia gelatinosa. Following the ingrowth of C fibers (unmyelinated fibers) and synaptogenesis with superficial dorsal horn neurons, these collaterals undergo developmental degeneration. Nociceptive stimuli in fetal life (and in the extremely premature neonate) are transmitted by myelinated A fibers until the maturation of C-fiber connections.

In the first trimester of pregnancy, the development of the spinal cord and CNS begins with the closure of the neural canal. At this time, the dorsal horn begins to appear. Electron microscopic and immunochemical studies demonstrate development of the various neuronal cell types in the dorsal horn with their laminar arrangement, interneuronal connections, and the expression of their specific neurotransmitters and receptors, before 13 weeks of gestation and completion by 30 to 32 weeks of gestation. Initially, the receptive fields of dorsal horn neurons are very large, with extensive overlap between receptive fields of adjacent neurons. As maturation occurs, receptive fields of individual dorsal horn cells progressively shrink to become more precisely defined.

On a cellular level, the transmission of nociceptive impulses through the dorsal horn of the spinal cord is mediated via the release of multiple neurotransmitters, such as substance P, glutamate, calcitonin gene-related peptide (CGRP), vasoactive intestinal polypeptide (VIP), neuropeptide Y, and somatostatin. Modulation of this nociceptive transmission occurs by the release of met-enkephalin from local interneurons and norepinephrine, dopamine, and serotonin (5-HT) from descending inhibitory axons. These descending inhibitory axons originate in supraspinal centers and terminate at all levels of the spinal cord and brainstem. During the first and second trimesters up until the latter half of the third trimester, an imbalance exists between the mechanisms that facilitate and inhibit nociceptive input with the former being favored. Of the nociceptive neurotransmitters, substance P, CGRP, and somatostatin are expressed in the dorsal horn of 8- to 10-week-old human fetuses. Glutamate, VIP, and neuropeptide Y appear at 12 to 16 weeks of human gestation. Modulation of incoming noxious stimuli in extremely premature infants may occur through the local release of met-enkephalin, which is first expressed at 12 to 16 weeks of gestation. However, this mechanism is unlikely to be effective in diminishing the transmission of intensive painful stimuli. In the latter half of the third trimester, with the maturation of the descending inhibitory pathways from supraspinal centers, inhibition of incoming sensory stimuli can occur with the release of dopamine and norepinephrine in the dorsal horn of the spinal cord. These neurotransmitters are first expressed at 34 to 38 weeks of human gestation followed in the postneonatal period by 5-HT.

Conduction of nociceptive impulses to the supraspinal centers occurs via the spinothalamic, spinoreticular, and spinomesencephalic tracts located primarily in the anterolateral and lateral white matter tracts of the spinal cord. Delayed myelination in these tracts was proposed as an index of immaturity of the neonatal CNS and used to support the argument that neonates cannot feel pain or fail to react to nociception as do adults. This argument was widely supported despite the common knowledge that incomplete myelination does not imply lack of function, but merely slows conduction velocity. Additionally, any slowing of central conduction velocity would be completely offset by shorter interneuronal distances that must be traversed in infants, compared to much larger (and longer) adult axons. Nociceptive tracts to the brainstem and thalamus are completely myelinated by 30 weeks of human gestation, and thalamocortical pain fibers are fully myelinated by

37 weeks. The emergence of the thalamocortical connection is of crucial importance for cortical perception, since most sensory pathways to the neocortex have synapses in the thalamus. In the primate fetus, thalamic neurons produce axons that arrive in the cerebrum before midgestation. These fibers remain just below the neocortex until migration and dendritic arborization of cortical neurons are complete and finally establish synaptic connections at 20 to 24 weeks of gestation.

The functional maturity of the cerebral cortex is suggested by the presence of fetal and neonatal electroencephalographic (EEG) patterns and by the behavioral development of neonates. Intermittent EEG bursts in both cerebral hemispheres first seen at 20 weeks of gestation, become sustained at 22 weeks, and are bilaterally synchronous at 26 to 27 weeks of gestation. By 30 weeks, the distinction between wakefulness and sleep can be made on the basis of EEG patterns. Cortical components of somatosensory, auditory, and visually evoked potentials have been recorded in preterm babies before 26 weeks of gestation. Several forms of behavior imply cortical function during fetal life. Well-defined periods of quiet sleep, active sleep, and wakefulness occur even in utero, beginning at 28 weeks of gestation. In addition to specific behavioral responses to pain, neonates have various cognitive, coordinative, and associative capabilities in response to visual and auditory stimuli, attesting to the presence of cortical function. Several lines of evidence suggest that the nervous system as a whole is active during prenatal development and that detrimental or developmental changes in any part can affect the whole.

Recent evidence indicates that selective cortical activation occurs after painful stimuli in preterm neonates (10). Bartocci and colleagues (11), using near-infrared spectroscopy in preterm infants aged 28 to 36 weeks gestation, demonstrated increased blood flow in the somatosensory cortex but not the occipital cortex after venipuncture. In a similar study, Slater and colleagues recorded cortical activation after heel sticks in 18 infants between 25 and 45 weeks gestation (12). No cortical response was noted after tactile stimulation even when this stimulation was accompanied by reflex limb withdrawal. Taken together, these studies imply conscious sensory perception of painful stimuli in preterm newborns.

Thus, it is now well established that even premature human newborns have the functional components of a pain system and are capable of pain perception. In fact, the slow development of the pain inhibitory system suggests that the pain threshold may be lower in preterm neonates than term neonates or older infants. The cutaneous flexor reflex has a lower threshold in preterm neonates than in term neonates or adults (8). Thresholds for the flexor withdrawal reflex are decreased after repeated stimulation or local tissue injury in preterm neonates. Sensitization of this reflex may result from immature segmental or descending inhibition in the spinal cord, the immaturity of other spinal or supraspinal mechanisms, or factors associated with the intensive care environment (e.g., noise) and critical illness. Such sensitization is prevented by topical analgesia applied before local tissue injury (13).

Opioid receptor labeling in the fetal brainstem demonstrates very high densities in multiple supraspinal centers associated with sensory perception. These inhibitory opioid receptors may protect developing neuronal systems from constant overstimulation in the presence of the underdeveloped inhibitory gate-control mechanisms in the dorsal horn of the spinal cord. Brain development in neonatal rats can be significantly altered by exposure to naloxone, but is relatively unaltered after treatment with exogenous opioids.

The magnitude of endocrine-metabolic and other stress responses to invasive procedures or surgical operations is much greater in neonates than in adults. Neonatal catecholamine and metabolic responses are three to five times those of adult patients undergoing similar types of surgery (2). Pharmacokinetic studies of anesthetic drugs show that higher plasma concentrations are required to maintain effective surgical anesthesia in preterm neonates than in older age groups (2). An additional manifestation of the decrease in pain threshold, known as the *wind-up phenomenon*, occurs in neonates after exposure to a painful stimulus (1,11,14,15). The wind-up phenomenon results from prolonged responses of neurons in the dorsal horn of the spinal cord (3). The temporal summation of these responses produces a condition of prolonged or recurrent hypersensitivity that is disproportionate to the extent of the original injury (5). During these prolonged periods of hypersensitivity, even non-noxious stimuli (such as those produced by handling, physical examination, checking vital signs, etc.) are perceived as noxious, evoking stress and stimulating the systemic neuroendocrine stress responses (see Chapters 31, 32).

PAIN ASSESSMENT

As with any type of treatment or therapy, a method of assessing response is the first step in achieving success. For pain management in infants and children, a means of assessing pain helps not only to determine the severity of pain, but also the child's response to therapy. Tools for this purpose range from simple, bedside checklists with four to five components that require only 5 to 10 seconds to complete, to complex lengthy surveys that are too cumbersome and time-consuming for use in a busy office practice or hospital setting. Tools initially applied to assess pain in adult patients, which relied on self-reporting, are difficult if not impossible to apply to preverbal patients such as neonates and infants, or cognitively impaired children and adolescents. Although tools have been developed to assess pain in nonverbal or cognitively impaired populations (16–18), clinical practice that involves the routine assessment of pain in pediatric patients in a standardized fashion cannot do so in a consistent fashion in the majority of clinical scenarios. Nonetheless, the development and use of broadly applicable scales for pediatric use has recently been encouraged by the mandate of various hospital credentialing boards and regulatory agencies to use the presence of pain management protocols as a benchmark criterion for quality assessment.

Pain assessment tools can be categorized into five broad categories including self-report, observational, physiologic, neurophysiologic, and hormonal-metabolic (changes in stress hormones such as epinephrine, norepinephrine, or cortisol). Pain assessment in the verbal child most commonly relies on self-report of pain intensity by means of a visual analogue score (VAS), as is routinely done in adults. Such scales ask patients to indicate where their pain intensity falls on a straight line from 0 (no pain) to 10 (worst imaginable pain). These techniques rely on the patients' ability to assess and report their own pain. Variations aimed at being more user friendly and usable in younger children (down to 3–5 years of age) include the use of poker chips, a ladder, colored crayons, or pictures of children in varying degrees of distress. With the poker chip scale, the child expresses pain as a number of red poker chips on a pile (1 to 4). Mild pain would be one poker chip, whereas four poker chips are "the most hurt" the child could have. The pain ladder is a picture of a ladder with nine steps or rungs. At the bottom of the ladder is "no hurt" and at the top of the ladder is "hurt as bad as it could be." The child is asked to point at the place on the ladder that indicates the amount of pain he is experiencing. The severity of pain can also be expressed by selecting a crayon from a spectrum of colors, with red indicating severe pain and blue indicating little or no pain. However, the use of colors to express pain may have some variability among various ethnic groups, as the association of blue with calm or no pain and red with pain does not cross all ethnic groups. Alternatively, the child can use a Faces scale first described by Bieri and co-workers (17). The scale uses photographs of a child in various degrees of distress. One advantage of the Faces scale is that it is available in various versions for different ethnic groups. Although the Faces scale is meant to be used as a self-report type of scoring system, some centers have modified its use and used the Faces scale as an observational tool. In this application, the health care provider assesses the child and selects the face corresponding to the intensity of pain that they believe the patient is manifesting. A revised version of the Bieri Faces Scale (FPS-R) that has six computer-generated face drawings rather than the original seven (allowing an easier comparison with the most commonly used 0–10 VAS scale) was subsequently found to correlate very closely with VAS for acute pain in hospitalized children from 4 to 12 years of age (19) (Fig. 47-1).

In the pediatric population acute illnesses, cognitive states, or very young age may preclude the use of self-report scales. Assessment tools have been described and validated for various patient populations including neonates (20,21), preterm infants (22–25), and patients with cognitive impairment. The latter group of patients, a growing subgroup of the pediatric patient population, has received significant attention in the past 5 to 10 years and now benefits from a number of options for pain assessment. The noncommunicative children's pain checklist (NCCPC-PV) was developed specifically for use in this population (23). It includes the grading of several specific behaviors such as vocalization, socialization, facial expression, activity, body and limb positioning, and physiologic signs that have been shown to be indicative of pain in children with cognitive impairment. Alternatively, scales such as the Face Legs Activity Cry and Consolability (FLACC) scoring system, which is used for preverbal children, can be modified for cognitively impaired children by the addition of specific descriptors and parent-identified behaviors for each individual patient (24). These tools have been shown to have excellent interobserver reliability and are quick and easy to use even in a busy clinical practice (Table 47-1).

Physiologic parameters applied in pain assessment include heart rate, blood pressure, respiratory rate, oxygen saturation, palmar sweating, or changes in pupillary size. However, factors other than pain may alter these physiologic parameters or their responses to the painful stimulus. For example, the use of

  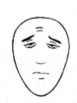 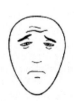 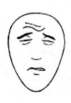 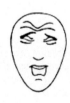

FIGURE 47-1. The Faces Pain Scale–Revised. From Hicks CL, von Baeyer CL, Spafford PA, et al. The Faces Pain Scale-Revised: Toward a common metric in pediatric pain measurement. *Pain* 2001;93:173–183.

TABLE 47-1

FLACC BEHAVIORAL SCALE

Categories	Scoring*		
	0	1	2
Face	No particular expression or smile	Occasional grimace or frown, withdrawn, disinterested	Frequent to constant frown, quivering chin, clenched jaw
Legs	Normal position or relaxed	Uneasy, restless, tense	Kicking or legs drawn up
Activity	Lying, quietly, normal position, moves easily	Squirming, shifting back and forth, tense	Arched, rigid, or jerking
Cry	No cry (awake or asleep)	Moans or whimpers; occasional complaint	Crying steadily, screams or sobs, frequent complaints
Consolability	Content, relaxed	Reassured by occasional touching, hugging, or being talked to; distractible	Difficult to console or comfort

Note: *Each of the five categories Face (F), Legs (L), Activity (A), Cry (C), and Consolability (C) is scored from 0–2, which results in a total score between 0 and 10.
From Merkel SI, Voepel-Lewis T, Shayevitz JR, Malviya S. The FLACC: A behavioral scale for scoring postoperative pain in young children. *Pediatric Nursing* 1997;23:293–297.

blood pressure elevation as an indicator of pain in a critically ill infant or child in an intensive care unit (ICU) is precluded when blood pressure is low due to a comorbid disease process. Observational tools rely upon assessment of stereotypic behaviors that suggest pain: facial expression, body positioning, and the presence or absence of crying. One such tool is the Children's Hospital of Eastern Ontario Pain Score (CHEOPS) developed by McGrath and colleagues (18). This scale assigns a score of 0 to 2 for six categories including cry, facial expression, verbal complaints of pain, position of the torso, whether the child is touching the painful site, and position of the legs.

The last category of pain assessment tools use neurophysiologic and metabolic-hormonal changes. Both are generally restricted to research protocols and have limited applicability for everyday pediatric pain management. Neurophysiologic monitoring is the least well known and least well studied of pain assessment tools. Potential neurophysiologic measures include ECG monitoring and waveform analysis, pupillary responses, brainstem evoked responses, galvanic skin changes, and perhaps even metabolic changes in the subcortical areas of the brain and brainstem. Hormonal-metabolic changes such as alterations in plasma levels of stress hormones including epinephrine and cortisol have been used to study pain management regimens for patients with acute illnesses or those undergoing major surgical procedures (1,4,8). However, blood cortisol levels may decline acutely in patients given opioids, regardless of whether analgesia is achieved. Such a decline is simply the manifestation of a well-defined endocrine feedback loop in which exogenous opioids inhibit pituitary-adrenal activation just as they inhibit pituitary-gonadal function (see Chapter 40).

THE PHARMACOLOGIC MANAGEMENT OF ACUTE PAIN

Factors that influence the choice of regimens for pain management in infants and children include the health care provider's assessment of the severity of pain, the patient's age, the setting in which the pain will be managed (outpatient versus inpatient), and the presence of comorbid disease. Pain treatment regimens should incorporate a graded, stepwise approach similar to that applied for cancer-related pain (26). This graded or ladder approach includes the use of a nonsteroidal anti-inflammatory agent (NSAID), acetaminophen, or salicylate for the treatment of mild pain; addition of an opioid commonly used for moderate pain (oxycodone, hydrocodone, codeine) to one of the above agents; and the use of intravenous (IV) opioids or regional anesthesia for acute moderate to severe pain. An initial assessment of the severity of pain (mild, moderate, or severe) is made to guide initial therapy and the treatment escalated as needed. A second consideration in the treatment of acute pain must be the setting in which the pain is treated. Non-IV routes (e.g., oral) are needed for outpatient management, whereas the inpatient setting offers an infrastructure appropriate for administration of parenteral opioids.

An example of this graded approach to the treatment of pain includes treatment with a nonopioid analgesic agent (acetaminophen, acetylsalicylic acid, or an NSAID such as ibuprofen) for mild pain such as that following a surgical procedure on soft tissue or mild pain from a medical illness such as pharyngitis or otitis media. Moderate pain such as that following a fracture or an orthopedic procedure on bone can usually be controlled in the outpatient using a combination of acetaminophen, acetylsalicylic acid, or an NSAID such as ibuprofen together with a weak opioid (e.g., an acetaminophen with codeine preparation). Severe pain such as that accompanying a sickle cell vaso-occlusive crisis, major burns, or after a major surgical procedure (e.g., thoracotomy or an exploratory laparotomy), generally requires either a regional anesthetic technique and/or parenteral opioids.

Mild to Moderate Pain in the Outpatient

With tissue disruption and lysis of cell membranes, fatty acids are released and metabolized to prostaglandins, which results in local inflammation and pain through the stimulation of the free nerve endings of $A\delta$ and C fibers. NSAIDs, acetaminophen, and salicylates inhibit the enzyme cyclooxygenase (COX), blocking prostaglandin formation. In contrast to opioids, prostaglandin synthesis inhibitors demonstrate a

TABLE 47-2

ORAL DOSING GUIDELINES FOR COMMONLY USED NONOPIOID ANALGESICS

Drug	Dose (mg/kg) (<60 kg)	Dose (mg) (>60 kg)	Interval (hours)	Daily maximum dose (mg/kg) (<60 kg)	Daily maximum dose (mg) (>60 kg)
Acetaminophen	10–15	650–1,000	4	90[1]	4,000
Ibuprofen	6–10	400–600[3]	6	40[2,3]	2,400[3]
Naproxen	5–6[3]	250–375[3]	12	24[2,3]	1,000[3]
Aspirin[4]	10–15[3,4]	650–1,000[3]	4	80[2,3,4]	3,600[3]

[1] Maximum daily doses for acetaminophen in term neonates and infants, should be reduced to 60 mg/kg and to 40 mg/kg in preterm neonates]. [2] Dosing guidelines for neonates and infants have not been established. [3] Higher doses may be used in selected cases for treatment of rheumatologic conditions in children. [4] Aspirin carries a risk of precipitating Reye syndrome in infants and children. If other analgesics are available, aspirin use should be restricted to indications where antiplatelet or anti-inflammatory effect is required, rather than as a routine analgesic or antipyretic in neonates, infants, or children. Dosing guidelines for aspirin in neonates have not been established. Adapted from Berde CB, Sethna NF. Analgesics for the treatment of pain in children. *N Engl J Med* 2002;347(14):1094–1103.

ceiling effect, so that once a therapeutic plasma concentration is achieved, increasing the dose does not improve analgesia but may increase the incidence of adverse effects. The majority of such agents are available as over-the-counter medications and represent an effective and relatively safe means of controlling mild to moderate pain. When evaluated in a cohort of pediatric patients with recent musculoskeletal injury, ibuprofen (10 mg/kg) was shown to be superior to either acetaminophen (15 mg/kg) or codeine (1 mg/kg) in reducing pain scores from baseline and in providing effective analgesia, defined as a VAS less than 30 (0–100 scale) (27).

Recent pharmacokinetic and pharmacodynamic data have provided the clinician with ample information to suggest appropriate dosing guidelines for the pediatric population (Table 47-2). Although salicylate use in pediatrics has declined following recognition of its association with Reye syndrome, choline magnesium trisalicylate combines the analgesic properties of a salicylate with limited effects on platelet function, thereby allowing its use in patients with qualitative and quantitative platelet issues.

Given acetaminophen's safety profile and potential concerns with both salicylates and the NSAIDs in the pediatric population, it is the most frequently used medication from this group. Recent studies in preterm neonates and infants have provided useful guidelines for treatment with acetaminophen in neonates as young as 28 weeks of gestational age (Table 47-3) (28).

Several potential concerns with the NSAIDs, in particular ibuprofen, have recently been raised but the supporting evidence is conflicting. Although NSAID use has been reported to result in an increased incidence of invasive group A streptococcal disease (necrotizing fasciitis) with varicella infections, other investigations have failed to support this association (29,30). Additional concerns with the NSAIDs include alterations in renal blood flow resulting in acute renal failure in the setting of dehydration (29), as well as the longstanding concern that NSAIDs are hazardous in patients with asthma. In a prospective, randomized trial, the need for an outpatient visit for asthma was less frequent with ibuprofen than acetaminophen when used to treat fever in children with underlying asthma who had no known sensitivity to salicylates (31). Further evidence for the safety of ibuprofen is provided by Lesko and colleagues in a prospective, randomized trial of 27,065 febrile children younger than 2 years of age. The children were randomized to receive acetaminophen (12 mg/kg), ibuprofen (5 mg/kg), or ibuprofen (10 mg/kg) for the treatment of fever. The authors reported no statistical difference in adverse effects,

including acute GI bleeding, acute renal failure, anaphylaxis, Reye syndrome, asthma, bronchiolitis, and vomiting/gastritis among the three groups. Although not statistically significantly different from acetaminophen, three patients in the ibuprofen group were hospitalized for GI bleeding, giving a risk of 17 per 100,000. The authors caution that although they noted no difference in the adverse effect profile of these two agents, the study did not evaluate long-term administration nor examine the use of both agents simultaneously. (See below for an expanded discussion of the adverse effect profile of the NSAIDs.)

The role of COX inhibitors in the treatment of acute pain includes their use as the sole agent for mild pain, their combination with opioids for oral administration in moderate pain, and their addition to parenteral opioids and regional anesthetic

TABLE 47-3

RECOMMENDATIONS FOR ADMINISTRATION OF ACETAMINOPHEN TO PRETERM AND FULL-TERM INFANTS*

Preterm infants 28–32 weeks[†]
 ORAL 10–12 mg/kg q6–8h
 RECTAL 20 mg q12h

MAXIMUM DOSE 40 mg/kg/day

Preterm infants 32–36 weeks and full-term infants <10 days of age
 ORAL 10–15 mg/kg q6h
 RECTAL 30 mg/kg loading dose and 15 mg/kg q8h[‡]

MAXIMUM DOSE 60 mg/kg/day

Full-term infants >10 days of age
 ORAL 10–15 mg/kg q4–6h
 RECTAL 30 mg/kg loading dose and 20 mg/kg q6–8h

MAXIMUM DOSE 90 mg/kg/day

Of note: *Caution should always be observed in administering acetaminophen to infants who have evidence of severe systemic illness (i.e. sepsis, bowel obstruction, dehydration) or who have evidence of liver dysfunction.
[†] There is currently no pharmacokinetic data for preterm infants younger than 28 weeks, so no recommendation is made for these infants.
[‡] Loading doses are not included in maximal daily dose calculations

techniques for severe pain. In the latter situation, their use does not eliminate the need for opioids, but rather provides adjunctive analgesia and a reduction of opioid requirement. As the majority of opioid-related adverse effects are dose-related, modalities that decrease total opioid consumption significantly may decrease or prevent opioid-associated adverse effects.

Although oral administration is used most frequently, this route of administration can be difficult in young children, who may refuse or spit out medication whose taste they find objectionable. Oral administration also has a slower onset and lower bioavailability than parenteral administration, nor can it be used effectively in children with gastrointestinal symptoms such as vomiting, ileus, or abdominal pain. Because they are available in several preparations suitable for use in pediatric patients of all ages including tablets, capsules, chewable tablets, elixirs, and infant drops, acetaminophen and ibuprofen are the most commonly prescribed medications of this group. Acetaminophen is also available in suppository form and sustained-release tablets. Intravenous acetaminophen products (the prodrug, Propacetamol which is metabolized to acetaminophen and recently released pure acetaminophen form) are available outside of the United States.

Recent studies in children older than 1 year have demonstrated that the initial dose for rectal administration of acetaminophen should be 40 mg/kg to achieve an analgesic plasma concentration of 10 to 20 μg/mL (32). Anderson and colleagues published recommendations for dosing of acetaminophen in neonates and infants by analyzing individual data from six pediatric acetaminophen dosing studies (28). Based on these studies, the route of administration, and the type of product (oral elixir, suppository, etc.), the authors formulated a helpful table that provides suggested initial doses, subsequent doses, and a dosing interval based on the infant's gestational and chronological age (Table 47-3).

Several options are available for the timing of the administration of these agents. In the perioperative setting, acetaminophen (15 mg/kg) or ibuprofen elixir (10 mg/kg) can be combined with the oral premedication midazolam (33). This technique allows the medication to achieve a plasma concentration that will provide effective analgesia by the time of awakening, and also masks the unpleasant taste of the IV preparation of midazolam when it is given orally. An alternative to preoperative administration is placement of an acetaminophen suppository (40 mg/kg) following anesthetic induction. A third option is postoperative administration of either ibuprofen or acetaminophen once the child complains of pain in the recovery room. This combination technique can also be used for outpatients with acute pain. This latter option is less desirable in the perioperative setting, since the onset of activity of any of these agents following oral or rectal administration is 20 to 30 minutes. Acetaminophen remains a cornerstone in the perioperative setting due to its lack of platelet effects, raising no additional concerns of increased intraoperative or postoperative bleeding.

When administering or prescribing acetaminophen, the health care provider must ensure that the infant or child is not receiving acetaminophen in other forms, such as in over-the-counter cold medicines. Additionally, given that several different acetaminophen preparations are available from numerous manufacturers, it is equally important to ensure that parents and health care providers know the amount of acetaminophen or ibuprofen in the specific product. The most common cause of acetaminophen toxicity in patients younger than 10 years of age remains inadvertent parental overdosing (34).

For outpatient treatment of moderate pain or when the first step of the pharmacotherapy ladder fails to control mild

pain, the NSAIDs, aspirin or acetaminophen can be combined with an opioid (codeine, oxycodone, or hydrocodone). Several such combination preparations are available in both liquid and tablet formulations, offering a wide range of choices for the pediatric patient of all ages. For younger patients, acetaminophen with codeine elixir containing 120 mg of acetaminophen and 12 mg of codeine per 5 mL is a frequently chosen option, with dosing based on the codeine component (0.5–1.0 mg/kg every 4–6 hours). Tablet preparations are also available that contain 325 mg of acetaminophen with 15 mg of codeine (Tylenol #2, Ortho-McNeil Pharmaceutical, Raritan, NJ), 30 mg of codeine (Tylenol #3, Ortho-McNeil Pharmaceutical, Raritan, NJ), or 60 mg of codeine (Tylenol #4, Ortho-McNeil Pharmaceutical, Raritan, NJ).

Recent investigations have questioned the efficacy of codeine for analgesia, as codeine is dependent on hepatic metabolism to morphine for a significant part of its analgesic effect. Williams and colleagues reported that 47% of pediatric patients had genotypes associated with a reduction of the activity of the enzymes necessary for the conversion of codeine to morphine (35). In 36% of the patients, neither morphine nor its metabolites could be detected after codeine administration. The authors concluded that diminished ability to metabolize codeine may be more common than previously reported and result in inadequate analgesia. Codeine is also available as a parenteral formulation, which although marketed for subcutaneous administration, has also been used for IV administration—a practice that is not recommended due to the potential for allergic and anaphylactoid reactions. Although health care practitioners may choose codeine over other opioids because of a misconception that it has less sedative and/or respiratory depressant effects, opioids, when used in equipotent doses, produce equivalent degrees of sedation and respiratory depression.

Alternatives to codeine for oral administration include oxycodone or hydrocodone preparations. As these agents are not dependent on hepatic microsomal enzyme activity for metabolism to active moieties, there should be less genetic contribution to variation in their pharmacokinetics. These opioids are also available in both liquid and tablet forms in combination with either acetaminophen or acetylsalicylic acid. Newer products include a tablet preparation including ibuprofen with either hydrocodone or oxycodone. The dose of these preparations should be based on their oxycodone or hydrocodone component, starting at 0.1 to 0.15 mg/kg (maximum starting dose 5 mg) every 4 to 6 hours. Regardless of the preparation used, with dose escalations, the amount of acetaminophen may exceed the maximum recommended daily dose of 60 to 90 mg/kg. Therefore, if higher doses of the opioid component are needed, preparations that contain codeine, oxycodone, or hydrocodone without the acetaminophen or aspirin should be used to avoid toxicity. A sustained-release formulation of oxycodone (OxyContin, Purdue Pharma LP, Stamford, CT) is also available. Its sustained release maintains an analgesic plasma concentration during a dosing interval of 8 to 12 hours. Although used occasionally to achieve a baseline steady-state plasma concentration of opioid to provide analgesia following major operative procedures, the inability to titrate a long-acting medication to match fluctuating analgesic requirements, and a lack of data regarding its pharmacokinetics in pediatric-aged patients, the risk–benefit ratio of such regimens must be considered (36).

Another option to control mild to moderate pain in the outpatient setting is Tramadol (Ultram, Ortho-McNeil, Raritan, NJ) (37–40). Tramadol's analgesic effect results from several potential mechanisms including opioid agonism at the μ opioid receptor, antagonism of the N-methyl-D-aspartate (NMDA) receptor, and inhibition of norepinephrine and 5-HT reuptake in the dorsal horn of the spinal cord. Despite the initial suggestion that there was limited abuse potential, clinical experience has demonstrated an abuse potential that may be similar to that of other "weak opioids." Tramadol's potency is roughly equivalent to that of meperidine. Worldwide, it is available as an injectable solution, suppository, liquid, and tablet. Tablets containing 50 mg of tramadol or the combination of 37.5 mg of tramadol with 325 mg of acetaminophen (Ultracet) are the only two preparations available in the United States. The 50-mg tablet is scored and can be cut in half, thus allowing its administration to smaller pediatric patients. The manufacturer's recommendations for dosing include 0.5 to 1.0 mg/kg (initial maximum dose of 50 mg) every 3 to 4 hours as needed. However, doses up to 2 mg/kg have been used in some pediatric trials. To date, there have been a limited number of reported clinical trials of tramadol in the pediatric population. Viitanen and Annila compared the analgesic efficacy of an IV intraoperative dose of tramadol (2 mg/kg) with placebo in 80 children following outpatient surgery (adenoidectomy) (40). There was a decrease in the need for rescue opioid analgesia in the recovery room in patients receiving tramadol. Forty-five percent of children receiving tramadol required no supplemental postoperative analgesia, compared with 15% of children receiving placebo ($p = 0.003$). There were no differences in adverse effects and recovery times. Rose and co-workers evaluated the efficacy of oral tramadol in a cohort of 113 children, ranging in age from 7 to 16 years (38). The study was limited to patients who weighed at least 20 kg and were expected to require analgesia for 7 to 30 days. Dosing was initiated with 1 mg/kg and increased up to 2 mg/kg as needed. Tramadol analgesia was rated as very good or excellent by 69% of parents and 70% of patients. The authors concluded that tramadol was well tolerated and provided effective pain relief. Adverse events were rated as mild or moderate, and similar in incidence to that seen with other oral opioids.

Tramadol has a longer half-life (6–7 hours) than other previously discussed oral opioids agents, and its active metabolite has a half-life of 10 to 11 hours. The active metabolite is renally excreted and can accumulate in patients with renal insufficiency or failure, thereby making it a poor choice in that setting. Despite tramadol's longer half-life, Viitanen and Annila did not observe a decrease in analgesic needs after discharge when tramadol was compared with placebo. The adverse effect profile of tramadol is similar to that of other opioids; however, as with meperidine, seizures may occur with large doses or in patients with renal failure (41).

One advantage of tramadol over other "weak opioids" suggested by preliminary data is that there may be less respiratory depression with equipotent doses of tramadol (42). In a randomized double-blind, placebo-controlled study, Bosenberg and Ratcliffe evaluated the respiratory effects of IV tramadol (1 or 2 mg/kg) with 1 mg/kg of pethidine (meperidine) during halothane anesthesia in children, ranging in age from 2 to 10 years. Respiratory rate decreased by 1.7 ± 1.8 breaths/minute in the placebo group, by 7.3 ± 3.6 breaths/minute after 1 mg/kg of tramadol, and by 11.4 ± 4.9 breaths/minute after 1 mg/kg of pethidine. The decreases in respiratory rate were accompanied by an increase in end-tidal carbon dioxide (CO_2) concentration. Thirteen episodes of apnea occurred with pethidine, 11 of which required naloxone, whereas none were noted after either dose of tramadol. In addition to its limited effect upon respiratory function, there appeared to be an analgesic advantage for the larger dose of tramadol during the first 6 postoperative hours, as the proportion of patients requiring

supplemental analgesia was greater for pethidine than 2 mg/kg of tramadol.

Moderate to Severe Pain in the Inpatient

In the inpatient setting, the options for acute pain management expand to include the use of parenteral prostaglandin synthesis inhibitors and the strong opioids. Even when the choice is made to escalate pain therapy to include parenteral opioids, the prostaglandin synthesis inhibitors can be used to lower postoperative opioid requirements and thereby decrease opioid-related adverse effects. Although there has been a significant amount of favorable literature regarding the use of the parenteral NSAID, ketorolac, it may be that less expensive alternatives including oral ibuprofen and acetaminophen may provide equal benefit. These potential benefits were demonstrated by Maunuksela and co-workers following inpatient surgery in a cohort of pediatric patients (43). Children who received rectal ibuprofen (40 mg/kg/day) had lower pain scores; decreased opioid requirements in the recovery room, during the day of operation, and 72 hours following the procedure; and a decreased incidence of opioid-related adverse effects. Although rectal preparations of ibuprofen are not available in the United States, similar results have been reported in both children and adults for the use of rectal indomethacin or acetaminophen (44).

When oral or rectal administration is not feasible, IV administration using the parenteral NSAID ketorolac should be considered. Although initial clinical trails suggested that ketorolac was as effective as opioids in treating acute pain, its practical clinical role is similar that of other NSAIDs as an adjunct to opioid analgesia, as demonstrated by Vetter and Heiner (45). A single IV dose of ketorolac was administered just prior to the completion of a surgical procedure as a supplement to morphine patient-controlled analgesia (PCA). Patients receiving ketorolac had decreased morphine requirements, lower pain scores, and a decreased incidence of adverse effects during the initial 12 postoperative hours.

Dsida and colleagues evaluated the pharmacokinetics of a single dose of ketorolac (0.5 mg/kg) in 36 children, stratified into four age groups (1–3 years, 4–7 years, 8–11 years, and 12–16 years) (46). No differences in pharmacokinetics were noted among the various age groups. The authors concluded that in patients ranging in age from 1 to 16 years, the pharmacokinetic properties of ketorolac were similar to those reported in adults, and a plasma concentration in the adult therapeutic range can be maintained for 6 hours in the majority of patients. Although Dsida and colleagues recommended a dosing regimen of 0.5 mg/kg every 6 hours, recent information from the adult literature has suggested the need to reevaluate these practices. In the adult population, a ceiling effect upon opioid sparing was noted following lumbar spine surgery for doses greater than 7.5 mg (47).

To date, there are limited data regarding ketorolac use in patients younger than 1 year of age (48,49). In a retrospective analysis of ketorolac use in infants younger than 6 months of age, daily morphine requirements (0.04 ± 0.05 versus 0.15 ± 0.06 mg/kg/day, $p < 0.01$) were significantly decreased in 10 infants who received ketorolac (1–1.5 mg/kg/day for up to 48 hours) when compared with eight control patients who did not receive ketorolac (48). No difference in pain scores were noted between the two groups, and no adverse effects related to ketorolac were noted. Moffett and colleagues reported no adverse renal or hematologic effects in their retrospective review of ketorolac use in 53 children younger than 6 months of age who received at least one dose of ketorolac following surgery for congenital heart disease (49). The greatest increase in serum creatinine from baseline was 0.3 mg/dL. Four patients had minor episodes of bleeding while receiving ketorolac.

A major issue with any of the NSAIDs is their effect on platelet function and the potential for bleeding, particularly given ketorolac's relative selectivity in inhibiting COX-1. These concerns are illustrated by the study of Rusy and co-workers, who randomized 50 children undergoing tonsilloadenoidectomy to receive either ketorolac (1 mg/kg) or acetaminophen (35 mg/kg rectally) following anesthetic induction. Patients receiving ketorolac had significantly more blood loss (2.67 versus 1.44 mL/kg) and required more surgical interventions to control bleeding. Despite the concerns illustrated by the study of Rusy and co-workers, increased bleeding with the use of ketorolac has not been demonstrated in two other types of potentially high-blood loss procedures including surgery for congenital heart surgery and spinal fusion (50–53). In a retrospective analysis, there was no difference in the need for surgical reexploration in infants and children following surgery for congenital heart disease who received ketorolac compared to case-matched controls (50). In a prospective, randomized trial in the same population, there was no difference in median chest tube output (13.3 versus 16.5 mL/kg/day) when comparing patients randomized to ketorolac or placebo (53).

The adverse effects of NSAIDs and acetylsalicylic acid result from the inhibition of homeostatic prostaglandins that regulate normal physiologic processes, including renal blood flow and the protection of the gastric mucosa. Alterations in glomerular filtration and the development of renal insufficiency or failure is uncommon except in patients with preexisting renal dysfunction, during concomitant administration of other nephrotoxic agents, in the presence of hypovolemia, or with prolonged administration. A review of the short-term use (48 hours) of IV ketorolac in over 1,700 children at Children's Hospital Boston demonstrated a low rate of complications. Four children (0.2%) demonstrated hypersensitivity reactions (urticaria and/or bronchospasm), two children (0.1%) had evidence of renal impairment (although both had other underlying problems that could account for the renal insufficiency) and one child (0.05%) had melena at the completion of a 48-hour course of the drug (54).

A concern with ketorolac or other NSAIDs is the potential for inhibition of new bone formation. In an adult population, a retrospective review of 288 patients revealed the incidence of nonunion to be five of 121 in patients who received no NSAIDs compared to 29 of 167 in patients receiving ketorolac following lumbar spinal fusion (55). Therefore, some health care providers avoid the use of ketorolac in patients undergoing spinal fusion and other procedures in which bone grafts are used. An anecdotal report also describes the temporal association of the intraoperative administration of ketorolac with the development of bradycardia in two children whose heart rates decreased from 98 to 48 beats/minute and from 138 to 32 beats/minute (56). Although no physiologic explanation was provided in this report, the authors cautioned against the use of ketorolac without electrocardiogram (EKG) monitoring and suggested premedication with an anticholinergic agent.

Efforts to provide analgesia while diminishing the incidence of adverse effects of NSAIDs have focused on the use of specific isomers of the NSAIDs or agents that selectively inhibit COX-2 versus COX-1. Although NSAID isomers are still in the investigational phase, experience with other medications has demonstrated the potential for decreasing adverse effects while maintaining efficacy by separation of the two enantiomers of a chiral compound. Ibuprofen is a chiral mixture of its two optical iso-

mers and animal data suggest that the $S(+)$ isomer may provide analgesia while having limited effects on the homeostatic COX, thereby limiting its adverse effect profile (57). COX-1, referred to as the *homeostatic COX*, controls renal blood flow, protects the gastric mucosa, and maintains normal platelet function. COX-2, referred to as *inducible COX*, is responsible for the inflammatory process. Celecoxib and rofecoxib were the first selective COX-2 inhibitors introduced into clinical use. Like nonspecific NSAIDs and acetaminophen, when used as an adjunct to opioid analgesia, they decrease opioid requirements and opioid-related adverse effects (58). However, the enthusiasm for these agents and their clinical use has decreased dramatically following several investigations demonstrating their association with an increased risk of cardiovascular events including myocardial infarctions (59–61). Currently, celecoxib is the only COX-2 inhibitor marketed in the United States, and it is only available in tablet form, limiting its use to older children.

In the inpatient setting, management strategies to control severe pain generally include the use of the strong opioids. The clinically relevant differences between the opioids are their potency, duration of action, and their metabolic fate, including the presence or absence of active metabolites (Table 47-4). Opioids interact with specific opioid receptors (μ or κ) in the PNS and CNS. They may act as either pure agonists (binding to and activating μ and κ receptors) or agonist/antagonists (binding to and activating κ receptors while binding to, but not activating, or even antagonizing, μ receptors). The agonist/antagonists in common clinical use include nalbuphine, butorphanol, and pentazocine (Table 47-4). The major caveat with the use of these agents in patients of any age is that they should not be administered to patients chronically receiving opioids, as their μ-antagonism can precipitate withdrawal. One of the cited potential clinical advantages of these agents is a decreased potential to cause respiratory depression. Given this property, these agents may be chosen to provide analgesia in patients with comorbid disease processes that place them at risk for opioid-related adverse effects. The potency and efficacy of agonists/antagonists for severe pain is less than that of pure agonists, and a ceiling dose exists for their analgesic effects, above which dose escalations do not augment analgesia. Given these restrictions, they may also be useful for mild to moderate pain when oral administration of other agents, such

TABLE 47-4

POTENCY AND HALF-LIFE OF PARENTERAL OPIOIDS

Opioid agonists	Potency	Half-life	Active metabolites
Morphine	1	2–3 hours	Yes
Meperidine	0.1	2–3 hours	Yes
Hydromorphone	5–8	2–3 hours	No
Oxymorphone	10	1–4 hours	No
Methadone	1	12–24 hours	No
Fentanyl	100	20–30 minutes	No
Sufentanil	1000	20–30 minutes	No
Alfentanil	20	10–15 minutes	No
Remifentanil	100	5–8 minutes	No
Agonist/antagonists			
Butorphanol	5	2–4 hours	No
Nalbuphine	1	4–5 hours	No
Pentazocine	0.3–0.4	2–3 hours	No

as acetaminophen with codeine, is not feasible or when the IV route is preferred to provide a more rapid onset of action. An additional benefit of a drug such as nalbuphine is that it clinically provides more sedation than other opioids because of its effects on the κ opioid receptor. Therefore, in addition to providing analgesia, it may also provide sedation for the agitated postoperative patient. Nalbuphine has also been shown to be effective in the treatment of emergence agitation following inhalational anesthesia in children (62). The agonist/antagonists should also be considered when supplemental IV analgesia is required in patients who are receiving or have received neuraxial (epidural or intrathecal) opioids within the last 24 hours. There may be a diminished risk of respiratory depression if an agonist/antagonist is used intravenously to supplement analgesia after neuraxial morphine rather than a pure agonist such as morphine. Additionally, these agents may effectively control adverse effects such as pruritus following neuraxial opioids.

When potent opioids are chosen for postoperative analgesia, three choices must be made: the type of opioid, the mode of administration, and the route of administration. There is limited data concerning the optimal opioid for postoperative analgesia in the pediatric patient. Several acceptable alternatives are available, any of which will provide equivalent analgesia provided that equipotent doses are administered. In the critically ill ICU patient, in the presence of comorbid diseases such as a compromised cardiovascular status or when there is a risk for pulmonary hypertension, the synthetic phenylpiperidine opioids (fentanyl, sufentanil, alfentanil, remifentanil) offer cardiovascular stability, the ability to modulate pulmonary vascular resistance, and the ability to blunt the sympathetic stress response. As the synthetic opioids have short plasma half-lives (<30 minutes), they need to be administered by a continuous infusion to maintain a plasma concentration adequate to provide analgesia. Anecdotal experience has also described the use of fentanyl-PCA in the pediatric patient (63,64). However, this practice remains the exception rather than the rule and is indicated only in selected clinical scenarios when other opioids fail or are associated with debilitating adverse effects.

There seems to be no inherent advantage to one synthetic opioid over the others except that fentanyl is the least expensive. Remifentanil, metabolized by plasma esterases, has the shortest half-life of any of the synthetic opioids (approximately 10 minutes) and, unlike the other opioids that undergo hepatic metabolism, there is no difference in its half-life across age ranges beginning with neonates. Kinder-Ross and colleagues evaluated the pharmacokinetics of remifentanil (bolus dose of 5 μg/kg) in 42 pediatric patients undergoing elective surgical procedures (65). The patients were divided into six groups according to age, including young infants (younger than 2 months), older infants (2 months to 2 years), young children (2–7 years), older children (7–13 years), adolescents (13–16 years), and young adults (16–18 years). The volume of distribution was largest in infants who were 2 months of age or younger (452 mL/kg) and decreased to 223 and 308 mL/kg in the two oldest groups of patients. There was a more rapid clearance in the infants younger than 2 months of age (90 mL/kg/min) and infants 2 months to 2 years of age (92 mL/kg/min) than in the older groups (46 to 76 mL/kg/min). The authors concluded that remifentanil, as in adults, is eliminated extremely rapidly in all pediatric age groups. The fast clearance rates observed in neonates and infants, as well as the lack of age-related changes in half-life, are in sharp contrast to the pharmacokinetic profile of other opioids. Given these properties, it has become a popular agent for intraoperative use. Unlike the other synthetic opioids, remifentanil does not demonstrate changes in its context-sensitive half-life, so that prolonged infusions do not result in increases in the plasma half-life (66). Given this property, it may be used to transition from other sedatives/analgesics prior to extubation to allow for elimination of other medications or to allow for periods of deep sedation/analgesia during mechanical ventilation in the pediatric ICU while providing a rapid wake-up following its discontinuation (67).

Aside from its cost, an issue with remifentanil that may preclude its long-term use in the ICU setting is the rapid development of tolerance, an effect attributed to the avidity with which it binds to the μ opioid receptor. The potential impact of this effect can be illustrated by the study of Crawford and co-workers, who randomized adolescents (12–17 years of age) undergoing posterior spinal fusion to an anesthetic regimen that included either intermittent doses of morphine or a remifentanil infusion (68). Postoperative pain scores were similar between the two groups, but patients given remifentanil required 30% more morphine during the initial 24 postoperative hours (1.65 ± 0.41 versus 1.27 ± 0.32 mg/kg, $p < 0.001$).

Although the synthetic opioids maintain stable hemodynamics and are frequently used in patients with compromised cardiovascular function, alternative agents such as morphine are acceptable to treat most other types of acute severe pain in the pediatric population. In a cohort of 44 children following surgery for congenital heart disease, Lynn and co-workers demonstrated that morphine in doses of 10 to 30 μg/kg/hr provided effective analgesia without impeding weaning from mechanical ventilation (69). This morphine infusion resulted in plasma concentrations of less than 30 ng/mL and was not associated with elevated $Paco_2$. Five extubated patients breathed spontaneously and 35 patients were weaned from assisted to spontaneous ventilation with normal $Paco_2$ values while receiving morphine. In the 12 patients who were old enough to provide verbal pain scores, pain was relieved when serum morphine levels exceeded 12 ng/mL. The same group of investigators have shown that there is no difference in morphine clearance or its effects on ventilation when comparing infants with cyanotic and acyanotic congenital heart disease (70). However, they did note significant interpatient variability (two- to threefold) in morphine clearance in infants of similar ages.

In addition to its efficacy, outcome studies of patients treated with morphine during the neonatal period have not demonstrated adverse effects on neurocognitive development (71). MacGregor and colleagues assessed 87 children who had been enrolled into neonatal sedation studies. The authors reported no effect from exposure to morphine given in the neonatal period to facilitate mechanical ventilation upon measures of intelligence, motor function, or behavior when these children are assessed at 5 to 6 years of age. When compared with fentanyl, morphine offers the advantage of the less rapid development of tolerance and less withdrawal issues following prolonged administration. Franck and co-workers reported that infants sedated with morphine during extracorporeal membrane oxygenation (ECMO) required fewer supplemental doses, had a lower incidence of withdrawal (1 of 11 versus 13 of 27, $p < 0.01$), and had a shorter hospital stay (31.1 ± 14 versus 21.5 ± 7.0 days, $p = 0.01$) when compared to patients receiving fentanyl (72). Given these findings and the vast clinical experience with its use, morphine is generally the opioid of choice for the treatment of acute severe pain. As with any medication that is dependent on hepatic metabolism, the pharmacokinetics of morphine are significantly different in neonates and infants compared to older children and adults. Additionally, significant interpatient variability occurs when comparing patients of comparable gestational and chronological ages (69,70). Lynn and Slattery provided preliminary data regarding morphine

PART IV: PAIN MANAGEMENT

TABLE 47-5

MORPHINE DOSING GUIDELINES*

Initial IV titration for acute, moderate to severe pain:
   10–20 μg/kg every 10 minutes, titrated to effective analgesia

P.r.n. or fixed interval dosing:
   50 μg/kg q2–3h

Continuous infusion:
   10–30 μg/kg/hour

Patient-controlled analgesia:
   Bolus: 20 μg/kg every 7–10 minutes
   Basal infusion: 4–5 μg/kg/hour

*The doses listed are guidelines for starting doses in patients who have not previously been receiving opioids. These doses should be adjusted up or down as necessary to achieve the desired level of analgesia while limiting adverse effects. When opioids are used in infants younger than 3 months of age, or in patients with severe systemic illnesses or other comorbid diseases that place them at risk for opioid-related adverse effects, the starting dose should be half of the listed doses, and monitoring of cardiorespiratory function is suggested.

pharmacokinetics in 10 infants born at a gestational age of 36 to 41 weeks who were less than 10 weeks of age (73). Infants younger than 10 days of age showed longer morphine elimination half lives than older infants (6.8 versus 3.9 hours), and morphine clearance in these younger infants was less than one-half that found in older infants (6.3 versus 23.8 mL/min/kg). The authors also suggested that the half-life of morphine approaches adult values at about 1 month of age, although they cautioned that this conclusion was based on findings in only 3 infants. Due to decreased hepatic metabolism and a suggestion that differences in the permeability of the blood–brain barrier in infants may lead to an increased risk of respiratory depression (74), dosing for the control of acute pain is started at 50% of the usual doses for infants younger than 3 months of age (Table 47-5). Furthermore, monitoring of respiratory function with continuous pulse oximetry is recommended when opioids are used in this age group or in patients with compromised cardiorespiratory status. Morphine's predominant hemodynamic effect is peripheral vasodilatation, which may decrease preload and result in hypotension. Clinically significant hemodynamic effects are uncommon in patients with normal cardiovascular function, but may be accentuated with comorbid cardiac disease or in the setting of hypovolemia. Preterm neonates may be especially susceptible to these effects. A recent review of a large group of ventilated preterm infants ($n = 898$) who received morphine boluses and infusions as preemptive treatment in the neonatal ICU found that morphine can cause significant hypotension in preterm neonates between 23 and 26 weeks of gestational age (75). The authors of this study suggest close monitoring and cautious use in these particularly vulnerable infants.

Histamine release from morphine may lead to pruritus, an adverse effect that tends to be particularly common in adolescents and young adults or patients with skin symptoms from other disease processes. Morphine is metabolized in the liver to morphine-6-glucuronide (M6G), which is significantly more potent that the parent compound. As it is water soluble, M6G penetrates the CNS poorly and, in most circumstances, is of little consequence. However, M6G is cleared by the kidneys and can accumulate in patients with renal failure or insufficiency

and lead to respiratory depression. In such patients, alternative opioids such as hydromorphone, which has no comparably active metabolites, should be considered.

Other opioids used in the treatment of acute pain include hydromorphone (Dilaudid), meperidine (Demerol), and methadone (Dolobid). Hydromorphone may be advantageous when adverse effects related to histamine release, such as pruritus, occur with morphine. Hydromorphone's potency is five to eight times that of morphine and therefore one-fifth to one-eighth of the morphine dose is used. Pediatric PCA solutions can be prepared so that an equipotent amount of the opioid is present in each milliliter of the solution (1 mg/mL for morphine, 1 mg/mL for nalbuphine, 0.15 mg/mL for hydromorphone, and 10 mg/mL for meperidine).

Meperidine (pethidine in Europe and the United Kingdom) is approximately one-tenth as potent as morphine. It is associated with a relatively high incidence of adverse CNS effects, including dysphoria, agitation, and seizures. Meperidine's CNS toxicity, including its epileptogenic potential, results from the accumulation of normeperidine, a metabolite produced by the hepatic N-methylation of the parent compound. Normeperidine has a long half-life (15–20 hours) and is dependent on renal clearance. High or toxic levels occur more commonly in the setting of renal failure/insufficiency, with the coadministration of drugs such as phenobarbital that stimulate hepatic microsomal enzymes, and with large doses (greater than 2 g/day in an adult). Since meperidine offers no particular advantage over other opioids and, in fact, may be less efficacious than morphine in controlling acute pain (76), its use is discouraged in favor of morphine or hydromorphone.

Methadone has a potency similar to that of morphine; however, its serum half-life is 12 to 24 hours, thereby providing a prolonged therapeutic serum concentration following a single bolus dose. This effect can be used to provide prolonged postoperative analgesia without the need for a continuous infusion or the use of a PCA device. Intraoperatively, a single IV methadone dose of 0.2 mg/kg resulted in lower pain scores and a decreased need for supplemental opioid analgesic agents during the initial 36 postoperative hours (77). Although effective, the use of IV methadone in the acute pain setting remains investigational and is therefore limited to institutions involved in ongoing clinical trials or in the hands of investigators with significant experience with its use. The IV preparation may not be readily available in many institutions.

Once the specific drug is selected, the second decision to be made regarding opioid analgesia for infants and children is the mode of administration. Options include on demand ("as needed" or "p.r.n." dosing), fixed interval administration, continuous infusion, or nurse-controlled analgesia (NCA). To provide optimal analgesia, opioids should be administered in a manner that maintains a steady-state serum concentration. For moderate to severe pain, "on demand" administration generally does not provide adequate analgesia, as a significant delay can occur from the time that it is recognized that the child is in pain until the medication is drawn up, administered, and has time to take effect. Patient-controlled analgesia minimizes such delays by allowing the patient to administer a pre-set amount of opioid at specific intervals. These devices may be used in children as young as 5 or 6 years of age (78).

Appropriate education for the patient, family, nurse, pharmacist and the entire care team is required prior to instituting a pediatric PCA program to minimize potential adverse effects and ineffective use of this technique. Decisions regarding PCA include the opioid to be used, the bolus dose, the lockout interval (the minimum time that must elapse between doses), whether a continuous or basal infusion will be used in addition to the intermittent bolus doses, and the maximum total hourly dose. Although any opioid can be used with PCA, the majority of experience is with morphine. A common starting pointing for the bolus dose is 20 μg/kg every 7–10 minutes as needed. Dose adjustments may be needed based on the patient's previous exposure to opioids, comorbid disease processes, and interpatient variability. Prior to starting PCA for acute pain, titration of opioid to achieve an effective plasma concentration to provide analgesia must be achieved. To accomplish this, sequential bolus doses of morphine (20 μg/kg every 5–10 minutes) are titrated until the desired level of analgesia is obtained. Once this is accomplished, the PCA device is started. A frequent problem is that patients are provided adequate analgesia in the recovery room, the emergency department, or the inpatient ward, followed by a delay until the PCA pump arrives, is programmed, and hooked up. By that time, patients may need to repeatedly push the PCA button to reestablish an analgesic plasma concentration of the opioid.

One controversial issue regarding PCA is whether to include a low basal infusion rate in addition to patient-administered bolus doses. The use of a basal infusion rate is thought by some to oppose the inherent safety factor of PCA that patients who are somnolent cannot push the button and administer additional opioid. With a basal infusion rate, opioid is infused regardless of the patient's demands. Different outcomes have been reported in pediatric patients depending on the dose used for the basal infusion rate. Doyle and co-workers compared PCA (morphine 20 μg/kg every 5 minutes as needed) with and without a basal infusion rate of 20 μg/kg/hour (79). Although there was no difference in the pain scores, there were more adverse effects including nausea, sedation, and hypoxemia in the patients who received the basal infusion. In a follow-up study, the same investigators compared three different regimens of PCA that included morphine 20 μg/kg every 5 minutes as needed with no basal infusion rate (group 1), a basal infusion of 10 μg/kg/hour (group 2), or a basal infusion rate of 4 μg/kg/hour (group 3) (80). Although pain scores were equivalent in all three groups, there was increased time spent asleep during the first two postoperative nights in groups 2 and 3 with no difference in time asleep during the day. There was an increased incidence of nausea and vomiting in the group 2. The authors concluded that a low basal infusion of 4 μg/kg/hour improved the sleep pattern when compared with no basal infusion.

When used in classic fashion, PCA requires an awake, cooperative patient who is able to comprehend its purpose and push the button to initiate delivery of the medication. Therefore, its use may be limited in certain patient populations due to age, underlying illness, or cognitive capabilities. A second controversy regarding PCA is whether to allow the use of nurse and/or family controlled PCA (PCA by proxy) in these patient populations. When used in this fashion, the PCA device eliminates the delay in opioid administration that may occur with traditional as-needed dosing when the nurse signs out the medication and draws it up. Murphy and colleagues demonstrated equivalent levels of analgesia and equivalent opioid consumption when comparing PCA with NCA in an adult population (81). They noted no difference in the incidence of adverse effects or level of analgesia achieved in their study cohort. Recent studies in infants and children have established NCA, provided according to a standardized protocol, to be a generally safe and effective alternative to intermittent dosing or continuous infusions of opioids. Closer monitoring of respiratory status (i.e., cardiorespiratory monitoring and/or pulse oximetry) is essential during NCA, since younger children remain at somewhat higher risk of respiratory depression whenever opioids are administered.

Monitto and colleagues recently reviewed their experience with NCA in 212 infants and children from newborn to 6 years of age (82). They noted a 1.7% incidence of respiratory depression requiring treatment with naloxone and a need for supplemental oxygen in 25% of patients to maintain oxygen saturation greater than 95% in the first 24 hours after surgery. This incidence of respiratory depression is significantly higher than the 0.2% to 0.7% reported for PCA in adults. As with other studies of opioids in children, the youngest children appeared to be at the highest risk. All of the episodes of respiratory depression occurred in children 3 years of age or younger, and most (56%) were in infants under 1 year of age. This increased risk in younger patients during NCA was also found in the review of Lloyd-Thomas and Howard (83). They reported a 1% incidence of respiratory depression in pediatric patients receiving NCA and no significant respiratory depression in the older children who self-administered their own doses. Although practices vary, many pediatric institutions currently use NCA in patients who are unable to activate the device, but for safety purposes most do not permit family members to activate the PCA device for acute postoperative pain.

The Nonintravenous Administration of Opioids for Acute Pain

In the majority of clinical scenarios, moderate to severe acute pain is treated with IV opioids. However, certain situations may arise in which venous access is limited, drug incompatibilities are present, or other factors preclude the use of the IV route. In these situations, non-IV routes of administration may become necessary to ensure adequate analgesia. Non-IV routes employed to deliver opioids include subcutaneous, oral, transdermal, and transmucosal (sublingual, buccal, intranasal, rectal, inhaled) administration (84). Some of these techniques are considered investigational and therefore likely to have a limited role in the day-to-day management of acute pain in children. The intramuscular route is strictly avoided as variability in uptake and absorption leads to erratic serum levels and ineffective analgesia. Additionally, children will deny pain to avoid a "shot."

The simplest and cheapest of the non-IV routes remains oral administration. Although this route is frequently chosen for outpatients, its use remains limited in hospitalized patients. Oral administration of the "weak opioids," including codeine and oxycodone has been previously discussed in this chapter. This technique is a viable option even in hospitalized patients, provided their pain is mild to moderate, or when transitioning from IV opioids or regional anesthetic techniques. When compared with IV administration, issues with oral administration include a delay in onset of action, the need for larger doses due to decreased bioavailability and first-pass hepatic metabolism, and underlying medical/surgical problems that preclude the use of the gastrointestinal tract. Litman and Shapiro reported their experience with a novel technique that they termed "oral PCA" using either hydromorphone or morphine to treat acute pain related to medical illnesses in a cohort of four pediatric patients (85). When no IV access is available, oral methadone can also be used for acute postoperative pain. Methadone is available in an elixir form and has excellent bioavailability via the oral route, ranging from 60 to 90% (86). A sliding scale regimen has been used at Children's Hospital, Boston for many years utilizing "reverse p.r.n." dosing. Patients are assessed by the nursing staff at intervals no less frequent than every 4 hours. A "sliding scale" adjusts the methadone dose according to the nurse's assessment of the child's pain as severe (0.07 mg/kg), moderate (0.05 mg/kg), or mild (0.03 mg/kg). This method is convenient, inexpensive, and permits easy adjustment of dosing to patients' variable requirements. Subcutaneous administration has generally been reserved for the terminal cancer patient. However, preliminary experiences outside of the cancer population suggest its efficacy for controlling acute pain of various etiologies. Doyle and colleagues investigated the efficacy of PCA by the subcutaneous route in children following appendectomy (87). Patients were randomized to either IV or subcutaneous administration with a standard PCA regimen that included morphine (bolus doses of 20 μg/kg every 5 minutes as needed, plus a basal infusion of 5 μg/kg/hour). The subcutaneous PCA was delivered through a 22-gauge IV cannula that was placed into the subcutaneous tissue over the deltoid muscle during the operative procedure. There was no difference in the pain scores at rest or with activity between the two groups. There were significantly more hypoxemic events, defined as an oxygen saturation less than 90%, with IV compared with subcutaneous administration. Additional experience with use of subcutaneous opioids for the management of acute pain in children was reported by Lamacraft and colleagues in a cohort of 220 pediatric patients (88). Morphine was administered via an indwelling catheter that was placed into the subcutaneous tissue after the induction of anesthesia. No patient complained of infusion site pain during subcutaneous administration of morphine. When compared with the intermittent intramuscular administration of opioids, 95% of the nurses preferred the subcutaneous route, and 74% of them stated that they would give morphine more readily via the subcutaneous route compared to the intramuscular route. Dietrich and co-workers reported similarly encouraging efficacy with the use subcutaneous fentanyl in a cohort of 24 children (89). Unlike the two previous reports, their cohort included a more heterogeneous population. Opioid administration was required for the gradual weaning of opioid administration following prolonged ICU care, for acute pain problems, and during terminal care. Reasons for using subcutaneous administration included either lack of venous access or drug incompatibilities that precluded IV administration.

Although the number of reports in the pediatric population regarding subcutaneous opioid administration is small, they have been uniformly favorable in documenting it as an effective alternative to IV administration. For subcutaneous administration, a butterfly needle or a standard IV catheter is inserted into the subcutaneous tissue of the thigh, abdominal wall, subclavicular area, or above the deltoid. Dosing regimens, including basal infusions, continuous infusions, and boluses, are the same as for IV administration. Although the steady-state plasma concentration of the opioid during subcutaneous administration is equivalent to those achieved with IV administration, peak plasma concentrations are lower with subcutaneous versus IV administration. In our practice, we suggest that the fluid volume used to deliver the opioid be restricted to a maximum of 1 to 3 mL/hour. The site should be changed at 7-day intervals or sooner if erythema or local tissue reaction are noted. Several different opioids, including morphine, hydromorphone, and fentanyl are suitable for subcutaneous administration. Methadone is not recommended for subcutaneous administration because it can cause significant tissue reaction with erythema.

Adverse Effects of Opioids

Adverse effects of opioids frequently interfere with the delivery of effective analgesia (Table 47-6). Respiratory depression is

TABLE 47-6

ADVERSE EFFECTS OF OPIOIDS AND TREATMENT STRATEGIES*

Adverse effect	Treatment strategy
Respiratory depression	Stop opioid Airway management as needed Naloxone 1 μg/kg every 3 minutes up to 10 μg/kg; consider use of infusion for longer acting opioids
Constipation or ileus	Stool softeners Cathartic agents Motility agent (metoclopramide) Osmotic agents (70% sorbitol)
Nausea or vomiting	Phenothiazine (promethazine 0.25 mg/kg up to 12.5 mg)* 5–HT$_3$ antagonist: ondansetron (0.1 mg/kg up to 4 mg)
Pruritus	Diphenhydramine (0.5 mg/kg up to 12.5 mg)* Low-dose nalbuphine (0.01 mg/kg) Change opioid

*Monitoring of respiratory status is suggested when opioids are used in patients with comorbid disease processes, in infants, or conjunction with other medications that may potentiate opioid-induced respiratory depression.

directly related to potency: equianalgesic doses of all opioids produce equivalent degrees of respiratory depression. Respiratory depression may be more likely to occur at the extremes of age, in patients with severe underlying systemic diseases or preexisting altered mental status, and with the addition of other medications known to potentiate the central respiratory depressant effects of opioids including benzodiazepines, barbiturates, chloral hydrate, and phenothiazines (Table 47-7). The

TABLE 47-7

PATIENTS AT RISK FOR OPIOID-RELATED ADVERSE EFFECTS*

1. Extremes of age (infants <6 months of age)

2. Patients with severe underlying systemic illness:
   Cardiorespiratory dysfunction
   Hepatic insufficiency
   Renal insufficiency
   Altered mental status
   Airway obstruction
   Central or obstructive sleep apnea

3. Concomitant use of other medications:
   Barbiturates
   Phenothiazines
   Benzodiazepines

*The presence of these problems does not preclude opioid administration. When opioids are used in these patients, half the usual dose is recommended, with continuous monitoring of cardiorespiratory function.

presence of such risk factors does not preclude the use of opioids in children; however, initial doses in such cases should start at approximately 50% of the usual regimen, with aggressive monitoring of cardiorespiratory function to facilitate early identification of cardiovascular and, particularly respiratory compromise. Respiratory depression may also occur in the setting of renal insufficiency or failure in patients receiving morphine. Although the parent compound (morphine) undergoes primarily hepatic metabolism, the metabolite (M6G) is dependent on renal excretion. M6G possess respiratory depressant and analgesic activity several-fold higher on a per-weight basis than the parent compound. In the setting of altered renal function, an opioid such as hydromorphone, which does not have comparably active metabolites, may be a safer alternative. A recent study in patients undergoing adenotonsillectomy also revealed that children with severe obstructive sleep apnea and chronic hypoxemia may be at increased risk for opioid-induced postoperative respiratory depression (90).

In patients who develop respiratory depression, the first priority is airway management with provision of supplemental oxygen or bag-mask ventilation as needed. Airway control is then followed by the incremental administration of naloxone. When administering naloxone, the concentration should be noted, as different strengths are commercially available. Standard pediatric ampules contain either 0.4 or 1.0 mg/mL. For the reversal of respiratory depression, naloxone is administered in incremental doses of 1 to 2 μg/kg, repeated every 3 minutes as needed up to a total dose of 10 μg/kg. Titration using small incremental doses of naloxone can reverse opioid-induced respiratory depression without reversing analgesia. The naloxone dose of 10 to 15 μg/kg that is sometimes recommended in reference texts is meant to be used only in the emergency department setting to reverse opioid overdose in the absence of any underlying pain. Using such large doses in a patient with underlying pain can precipitously reverse analgesia, leading to agonizing consequences for the patient. As incremental naloxone doses are cautiously administered, ongoing respiratory support is provided as needed until the respiratory depression has been treated. Once the respiratory depression is reversed, continued monitoring of the patient is necessary since the half-life of naloxone is 20 to 30 minutes, compared to 2 to 3 hours or longer for many opioids such as morphine, meperidine, or hydromorphone. Although two longer-acting opioid antagonists (naltrexone and nalmefene) are available, there is limited information regarding their use in children (91).

The non–life-threatening adverse effects of opioids may also interfere with the delivery of effective analgesia. Inadequate analgesia may occur in pediatric patients of all ages because of unfounded fears of addiction. Although drug-seeking behaviors may occur in patients of any age, addiction in patients receiving opioids for acute pain management is rare and should not limit the delivery of effective analgesia. Additionally, a long history of morphine analgesia in the neonatal population of all gestational ages has demonstrated its safety without fears of adverse effects on subsequent neurocognitive development. However, physical dependence is common following the prolonged administration of opioids and sedative agents. This potential should not limit the use of opioids, but rather emphasizes the need to have protocols in place to prevent and treat such problems in the at-risk population (92).

Additional adverse effects of opioids include sedation, constipation, pruritus, and nausea/vomiting. Careful attention to the patient's bowel habits and the use of stool softeners and stimulant laxatives concurrently with opioid therapy may help to avoid constipation. Although tolerance to some of the other adverse effects of opioids such as sedation may develop, opioid effects on gastrointestinal motility generally persist during chronic therapy. Osmotic agents (70% sorbitol) may be needed for refractory cases or when constipation has already developed. Preventing constipation with a daily dose of magnesium sulfate and/or a stool softener during opioid therapy is easier than treating the problem once it is established. Infants and children receiving opioids for acute pain are frequently inactive and may have subnormal fluid intake, which exacerbates constipation. Although pediatric experience with new opioid antagonists such as methylnaltrexone, which do not cross the blood–brain barrier is limited, they offer an attractive approach to eliminating opioid constipation while preserving analgesia.

Nausea and vomiting are probably the most debilitating of the acute non–life-threatening adverse effects of opioids. Mechanisms involved include the direct stimulation of the central chemoreceptor trigger zone of the medulla, decreased gastrointestinal motility with increased pyloric tone, and sensitization of the vestibular apparatus. Regardless of the mechanisms involved, treatment is primarily symptomatic and may include phenothiazines, metoclopramide, and 5-HT$_3$ antagonists. A new class of drug, the neurokinin (NK)-1 receptor antagonists, has recently been introduced for clinical use to supplement the armamentarium for treatment of opioid-related nausea and vomiting. These latter agents are available in only a tablet formulation, which may limit their use in smaller pediatric patients and infants. To date, reports regarding this new agent are limited to the adult population. Phenothiazines, such as promethazine, are available in preparations for both rectal and IV administration and the 5-HT$_3$ antagonist, ondansetron, is available in oral and IV formulations in addition to a wafer that dissolves in the mouth. Although there is extensive clinical experience with the use of the phenothiazines for the treatment of vomiting, their adverse-effect profile includes dystonic reactions, lowering of the seizure threshold, alteration of cardiac repolarization, and potentiation of opioid-induced respiratory depression.

Pruritus may occur as an isolated symptom or in association with urticaria. The mechanisms of opioid-induced pruritus are multifactorial and include a direct central effect as well as histamine release. Strategies to control pruritus include the administration of antihistamines such as diphenhydramine (0.5 mg/kg up to 12.5 mg) or changing to another opioid. The sedative properties of diphenhydramine may also potentiate opioid-induced sedation. When pruritus is not controlled with antihistamines, changing to another opioid, with less histamine release such as hydromorphone or fentanyl, may be helpful. Clinical experience has suggested that pruritus may be more common in specific pediatric populations including adolescents, sickle cell patients, and patients with severe skin diseases such as cutaneous involvement of graft-versus-host disease.

REGIONAL ANESTHETIC TECHNIQUES

Regional anesthetic techniques such as neuraxial blockade (epidural or spinal/intrathecal analgesia) or peripheral nerve blockade can provide profound analgesia for infants and children undergoing surgery. These techniques are generally performed under general anesthesia and can be continued into the postoperative period by the placement of indwelling catheters. Single-shot injections of local anesthetic agents combined with adjuvants such as clonidine are frequently performed in children undergoing minor or short-stay surgical procedures. Detailed information about the performance of single-shot neuraxial and peripheral blocks in children can be found in Chapter 27. Most infants and children undergoing major surgery, however, benefit from the placement of a catheter to provide continuous analgesia for several days postoperatively.

CONTINUOUS EPIDURAL ANALGESIA

Continuous epidural analgesia can provide excellent postoperative analgesia in children undergoing thoracic, abdominal, perineal, and lower extremity surgery. With the availability of shorter and smaller epidural needles and catheters, epidural analgesia can be easily administered even to very young infants. The safety and efficacy of epidural infusions in children has been demonstrated in several studies (93–95). In 1983, Meignier first showed that children with severe pulmonary disease recover rapidly following thoracic epidural anesthesia combined with light general anesthesia (96). Two retrospective studies (97,98) suggest that ICU and hospital stays can be shortened when regional anesthesia is combined with general anesthesia and continued in the postoperative period for thoracic and upper abdominal surgical procedures. McNeely and colleagues found significantly lower oxygen requirements and days of hospitalization after Nissen fundoplication when epidural anesthesia was used (98). In addition, Bosenberg found a significant difference in the requirement for postoperative mechanical ventilation when a caudal epidural catheter was placed and threaded cephalad to the thoracic area during repair of tracheo-esophageal fistula (19). Prospective studies are needed to confirm these reports.

Continuous Epidural Anesthesia via the Caudal Route

Bosenberg and colleagues first demonstrated in the late 1980s that a catheter could be reliably threaded to the thoracic region from a caudal approach in neonates and young infants (99). This would allow neonates to have thoracic-level epidural analgesia using the simpler caudal approach. This technique tends to be quite reliable in infants of less than 5 kg, but may be unreliable in older children (100). Since placement of the tip of the catheter at or near the spinal levels innervating the surgical site is crucial for the success of this technique, confirmation of tip position should be routinely verified by radiography (101). This may be done with a simple radiograph if a radiopaque (Arrow) catheter is used or by the injection of radiopaque dye through the catheter. For the latter, 0.5 mL of Omnipaque 180 or Isovue 200 can be used to assure placement in the epidural space as well as optimal location of the catheter tip (Fig. 47-2).

Technique of Lumbar Epidural Placement in Children

The epidural space may be approached at any level, but is most frequently approached via the lumbar route in children. For upper abdominal or thoracic procedures, a thoracic epidural approach may used, but this is commonly reserved for older children who can cooperate with the procedure under light sedation. Performance of thoracic puncture under general anesthesia should only be performed by personnel experienced with this approach in younger children. Although placement of

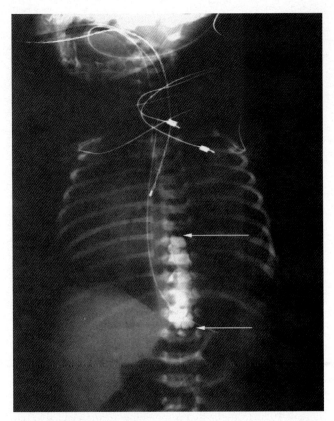

FIGURE 47-2. Epidurogram in patient with indwelling epidural catheter advanced from the caudal approach.

epidural catheters in the lumbar region is not much different in children than adults, there are some notable distinctions:

1. Catheters are generally placed in children after induction of general anesthesia and often after the administration of muscle relaxants, therefore removing many of the usual indicators of improper placement, such as paresthesias or motor block.
2. Heart rate responses to intravascular epinephrine are blunted by general anesthesia and therefore intravascular placement may be harder to detect. Higher doses of epinephrine after pretreatment with atropine are generally required in order to detect intravascular placement (i.e., 0.75 μg/kg rather than the usual 0.5 μg/kg) (102,103).
3. Distance from the skin to the epidural space is much less in infants and young children, generally no more than 1 to 2 cm, depending on size and age. The simple rule of thumb of allowing 1 millimeter of depth for each kilogram of body weight can be used for infants and children between 6 months and 10 years to estimate the distance from the skin to the epidural space (104).
4. Shorter needles (i.e., 2-inch rather than 3.5-inch) are generally used in children younger than 8 to 10 years of age to make placement easier.
5. Saline loss of resistance is used rather than air, in order to avoid the accumulation of air bubbles within the epidural space and the associated "patchy" block (105). A case report of air embolism has also been reported when loss of resistance was obtained with air in a small infant (106).
6. Since young children tend to be more prone to skin irritation, the less irritating adhesive Mastisol is often preferred to

TABLE 47-8

SUGGESTED DOSING FOR PEDIATRIC EPIDURAL INFUSIONS

Solution	Suggested rates in mL/kg/hr	Comments
Infants and children >2 months		
Bupivacaine 0.1%	0.2–0.3 Max = 0.4	
Bupivacaine 0.1% with fentanyl 2 μg/mL	0.2–0.3 Max = 0.4	
Bupivacaine 0.1% with clonidine 0.4 μg/mL	0.2–0.3 Max = 0.4	Not recommended for infants <4 months
Bupivacaine 0.1% with fentanyl 2 μg/mL and clonidine 0.4 μg/mL	0.2–0.3	Not recommended for infants <4 months
Bupivacaine 0.1% with hydromorphone 10 μg/mL	0.1–0.2 Max = 0.2	Not recommended for infants <4 months cardiovascular monitoring required
Bupivacaine 0.1% with hydromorphone 10 μg/mL and clonidine 0.4 μg/mL	0.1–0.25 Max = 0.2	Not recommended for infants <4 months cardiovascular monitoring required
Neonatal Solutions		
1.5% 2-chloroprocaine	0.2–0.45	
1.5% 2-chloroprocaine with Fentanyl 0.2 μg/mL	0.2–0.45	
Bupivacaine 0.05% with Fentanyl 1 μg/mL	0.2–0.3 Max = 0.4	

tincture of benzoin to secure the epidural catheter. Since replacing the catheter postoperatively in small children can be extremely difficult, it is important to reinforce the Tegaderm dressing with some sort of adhesive to prevent inadvertent dislodgement. It has recently been suggested that Mastisol is actually more effective than tincture of benzoin for securing catheters used for anesthesia (107).

7. Because of the higher pressures noted within the epidural space in young children, it is not unusual for epidural catheters to "leak" postoperatively (108). This can be anxiety provoking for nurses and parents caring for these children but generally does not lead to a significant reduction in postoperative analgesia. Even a significant amount of leakage under the dressing does not generally indicate catheter dislodgement, so decisions regarding the effectiveness of epidural analgesia are made on pain assessment only.

8. In patients younger than 8 years of age, clinically significant blood pressure changes associated with neuraxial sympathectomy are unusual. Children have reduced resting sympathetic tone and an increased ability to compensate for decreased systemic vascular resistance (109).

9. Infants younger than 6 months of age are at higher risk of respiratory depression with epidural opioids and local anesthetic toxicity due to decreased metabolism and clearance. Hydrophilic opioids are generally avoided in young infants, and reductions in bupivacaine infusion rates are required.

Epidural Infusions

When the tip of the epidural catheter is placed at spinal levels innervating the operative site, excellent analgesia can generally be provided with local anesthetic-based solutions. Dilute solutions (0.1%–0.125%) of bupivacaine or ropivacaine are generally used either alone or in combination with the lipophilic opioid, fentanyl and/or the α_2 agonist, clonidine. The standard infusions used at Children's Hospital Boston are shown in Table 47-8. After lower abdominal and lower extremity procedures, between 0.2 and 0.3 mL/kg/hour of this solution is generally required in the first postoperative day, with a maximum rate of 0.4 mL/kg/hour.

When the surgery is extensive and involves many dermatomes or when the catheter is placed in the lumbar region for upper abdominal or thoracic surgery, hydrophilic opioid-based solutions are generally necessary to provide adequate analgesia. In the mid 1980s, bolus doses of epidural morphine in the range of 30 to 50 μg/kg were shown to be both efficacious and safe in children (110,111). Respiratory depression was noted in infants when higher doses (70–100 μg/kg) were administered (112,113). Pruritus was also a significant problem, leading some children to literally excoriate their skin (114). For this reason, many pediatric institutions prefer to use hydromorphone as a bolus or infusion when hydrophilic opioids are indicated. Studies in adult patients suggest that the analgesic efficacy is similar but the incidence of moderate to severe pruritus is much less with hydromorphone than with morphine (115). Hydromorphone is roughly three to five times as potent as morphine via the epidural route and is preservative free. Because the cost compared to preservative-free morphine is similar milligram to milligram, it is also significantly less expensive to use. A preliminary study suggested that doses in the range of 2 to 8 μg/kg could provide pain relief for an average duration of 9 hours with significantly less respiratory depression and pruritus than higher doses (116). Further studies are needed to determine the optimal dosing for continuous infusions of hydromorphone in children.

Clonidine is rapidly becoming one of the preferred adjuncts to provide enhanced analgesia for both peripheral and neuraxial blocks. Clonidine is a selective partial agonist for α_2 adrenergic receptors with an α_2 to α_1 ratio of approximately 200:1.

Its hemodynamic effects appear at the level of the medullary vasomotor center, reducing norepinephrine turnover and decreasing sympathetic outflow from the CNS (117). It also centrally stimulates parasympathetic outflow, thereby slowing the heart rate. Children, possibly due to the differences in parasympathetic tone noted in early life, generally demonstrate more of a heart rate response and rarely demonstrate significant hypotension when clonidine is administered perioperatively.

Clonidine has proven to be an excellent adjunct for regional anesthesia in children due to the ability of this drug to significantly prolong the duration of single-shot caudal blockade. The exact mechanism for this effect is unknown, but clonidine has been demonstrated to activate α-adrenoreceptors in the dorsal horn gray matter of the spinal cord (118–120). Clinical effects when given via the neuraxial route are more closely correlated with concentrations of clonidine in the cerebrospinal fluid (CSF) than in the plasma, suggesting a direct effect at the spinal cord level (121,122). A recent study suggests that its effects on α_2 receptors in the PNS may be even more profound than that in the CNS (123). The introduction of a preservative-free preparation of clonidine (Duraclon) in 1999 has made this drug widely available for regional anesthesia in the United States. The addition of clonidine 1 to 2 μg/kg has been shown to prolong single-shot caudal blockade with bupivacaine by 46% to 114% in several pediatric studies (124–127) and significantly reduce subsequent analgesic requirements over the next 24 hours. Side effects have generally been mild with short-lived (<3 hours) clinically relevant hypotension and bradycardia only observed when larger doses (i.e., 5 μg/kg) are used (128).

Clonidine enhances postoperative analgesia when given by continuous infusion via the epidural route. De Negri and colleagues found that clonidine dosages in the range of 0.08 to 0.12 μg/kg/hr combined with ropivacaine 0.08% provided improved postoperative analgesia for infants undergoing hypospadias repair compared to either plain ropivacaine 0.1% or ropivacaine + clonidine 0.04 μg/kg/hr (129). Although there was a tendency toward more sedation with the highest dose of clonidine, no clinically significant side effects were noted during the 48-hour study period. One of the clearest advantages of the addition of clonidine to continuous infusions of local anesthetics for postoperative pain relief is the decrease in side effects. Comparisons between infusions of local anesthetic with clonidine and local anesthetic with morphine have shown a profound decrease in pruritus and vomiting (130). Clonidine in the range of 0.12 mg/kg/hr is often added to infusions of bupivacaine + fentanyl or bupivacaine + hydromorphone when postoperative analgesia is inadequate, but few studies have compared these combined infusions with those containing clonidine or epidural opioids alone.

Beyond the neonatal period, clonidine appears to have minimal respiratory side effects in children. Dupeyrat demonstrated no difference in transcutaneous CO_2 between infants who received 1 μg/kg of clonidine for regional analgesia compared to those who had not received clonidine (131). A study of healthy adults found no changes in the CO_2 response curve when clonidine was administered orally (132). In addition, no increase in respiratory depression was noted when morphine and clonidine were administered simultaneously, beyond that found with morphine administration alone.

In contrast, most likely due to the immaturity of the central respiratory drive, neonates and premature infants appear to have an increased risk of apnea when clonidine is administered as a part of neuraxial anesthesia. Several case reports have demonstrated an increased risk of apnea when clonidine was added to either epidural or spinal local anesthetics in neonates and preterm infants (133,134). Increased binding of α_2 agonists

---

TABLE 47-9

PAIN SERVICE GUIDELINES FOR EPIDURAL INFUSIONS

1. A representative of the pediatric pain service or the anesthesia department is available in the hospital 24 hours a day to rapidly deal with any complication that may arise.
2. Respiratory rates and quality along with level of sedation are monitored and recorded every hour for at least the first 24 hours postoperatively.
3. Heart rate, blood pressure, and pain scales are recorded at least every 4 hours.
4. The patient is evaluated by a member of the pain service at least once a day.
5. Any changes in respiratory rate, quality, or level of sedation must be promptly reported to a member of the pain service.
6. Any patient under the age of 6 months, having severe neurologic deficits, receiving hydrophilic opioids, or at an otherwise increased risk for respiratory depression should be placed on a cardiorespiratory monitor.
7. Heels should be padded to prevent pressure necrosis.

No systemic opioids are given concurrent with epidural opioids.

Adapted from Protocols for Pain Management. Report of an ad hoc committee, Children's Hospital, Boston, Massachusetts.

---

in the locus coeruleus has been demonstrated in tissues from the brainstems of fetuses and newborns compared to older children (135). For this reason, the use of neuraxial clonidine is not recommended in children under 3 months of age.

Continuous epidural anesthesia/analgesia can be safely administered on the surgical and medical wards if proper observation is maintained and a management protocol is in place. The nursing staff must be educated about the potential complications that may arise with these infusions and the appropriate measures to take if such complications arise. A sample of such a protocol used at Children's Hospital, Boston can be found in Table 47-9.

Two case reports and an analysis of retrospective data from 13 pediatric institutions have identified risk factors for systemic toxicity (primarily seizures) with the use of continuous epidural infusions of local anesthetics (136,137). Based on the available data, it has been recommended that the initial epidural bolus of bupivacaine (caudal or lumbar) not exceed 2 to 2.5 mg/kg for children older than 6 months of age and that subsequent infusions of bupivacaine be maintained no greater than 0.4 mg/kg/hour.

Particular caution must be exercised when local anesthetics are administered to neonates and young children. Neonates have low concentrations of albumin and α_1–acid glycoprotein, which can lead to decreased protein binding of local anesthetics and increases in the plasma concentrations of the unbound drug (138). As well, amide local anesthetics are metabolized by the microsomal P450 enzyme system in the liver, which does not exhibit full activity for weeks after birth. This combined with a decrease in liver blood flow found with respiratory diseases and cardiac insufficiency can lead to a significantly prolonged terminal half-life of these agents in sick newborns. Recent pharmacokinetic studies of bupivacaine infusions in newborns have suggested that infusion rates in neonates should not exceed 0.2 mg/kg/hr and may need to be adjusted downward if the epidural infusion is continued beyond 72 hours (139,140).

More recently, due to these concerns regarding bupivacaine toxicity, some pediatric institutions have begun using 2-chloroprocaine for postoperative epidural infusions in neonates. Since 2-chloroprocaine is an ester local anesthetic and, therefore broken down by plasma cholinesterases, it is rapidly metabolized and cleared from the circulation. Theoretically then, higher infusion rates can be administered with less likelihood of accumulation. A study by Henderson and colleagues supported this and showed rapid clearance in neonates even at high infusion rates (1 mL/kg/hour) (141). The activity of the plasma cholinesterase enzymes is diminished in the first 6 months of life, however, suggesting that clearance of the ester local anesthetics may be prolonged in certain circumstances. Further studies are needed to assess the efficacy and safety of long-term infusions of 2-chloroprocaine, since limited data are currently available in adults.

Although bupivacaine is still the standard amide local anesthetic used in many pediatric institutions for continuous epidural and peripheral block infusions, several of the newer, potentially less cardiotoxic amide local anesthetics have been studied for use in infants and children. Their use is steadily increasing as more pediatric pharmacokinetic and pharmacodynamic information becomes available.

Ropivacaine

Ropivacaine, most likely due to its intrinsic vasoconstrictive properties, is absorbed more slowly from the epidural space and provides a less neuro- and cardiotoxic alternative to bupivacaine. In volunteer studies in adults, ropivacaine exhibited less CNS and cardiac toxicity than bupivacaine, with adults tolerating an average of 25% more ropivacaine infused intravenously than bupivacaine before the onset of signs of CNS toxicity (142). Since studies to compare local anesthetic toxicity in infants and children cannot be performed, the toxicity and therapeutic index for ropivacaine and bupivacaine was compared using infant, adolescent, and adult rats (143). Using this model, ropivacaine was less toxic (larger dose per kilogram to produce respiratory distress and larger lethal dose per kilogram) than bupivacaine at all ages. For both bupivacaine and ropivacaine, infant rats had larger lethal doses per kilogram than adults.

Several recent studies in infants and children have suggested that ropivacaine may also result in less motor block while inducing a sensory block of similar quality to bupivacaine. Breschan and colleagues demonstrated significantly less motor blockade for the first 2 hours postoperatively when an equivalent volume (1 mL/kg) of 0.2% ropivacaine and 0.2% bupivacaine were compared for single-shot caudal blockade in children (144). This same difference was noted when continuous infusions of 0.125% bupivacaine were compared to equivalent concentrations of ropivacaine and levobupivacaine for 48 hours postoperatively (145). No motor block was noted throughout the study period in the ropivacaine or levobupivacaine groups, whereas 21% of patients in the bupivacaine infusion group had evidence of motor block beginning 12 hours after the onset of the infusion. Khalil and colleagues recently compared 1 mL/kg of different concentrations of ropivacaine (0.1%, 0.15%, 0.175%, and 0.2%) in infants of 1 to 12 months of age undergoing outpatient urologic surgery (primarily circumcision and hypospadias repair) and found significant differences in duration of analgesia and return of motor function (146). Infants receiving the lower concentrations (0.1% and 0.15%) required more pain medicine in the immediate postoperative period and had a shorter duration of motor block.

Infants in the 0.175% and 0.2% groups had median caudal durations (defined as time to first analgesic) of 454 minutes and more than 974 minutes, respectively.

Pharmacokinetic studies in school age children have shown that clearance is somewhat slower for epidural infusions of ropivacaine than bupivacaine (147). However, a recent pharmacokinetic study of continuous epidural infusions of ropivacaine in neonates and infants demonstrated that levels of both total and unbound ropivacaine did not increase after 48 hours of continuous infusion (148). Epidural infusions in this study were maintained at 0.2 mg/kg/hour in infants younger than 180 days and 0.4 mg/kg/hour in older infants. Although the levels of unbound ropivacaine were higher in neonates, all levels were below threshold concentrations for CNS toxicity in adults (<0.35 mg/L).

Levobupivacaine

Levobupivacaine (Chirocaine) is an isomeric form of bupivacaine ($S-$) with less affinity for cardiac and brain tissue. It has lower cardiac and neurotoxicity, with a similar clinical analgesia profile. Although used extensively in Europe, levobupivacaine is not currently available commercially in the United States. Dose response studies in pediatric patients have suggested that caudal blockade with 1 mL/kg of 0.2% levobupivacaine provides better analgesia than 0.15% and less motor blockade than 0.25% after outpatient subumbilical surgery (149). As with other local anesthetics, recent pharmacokinetic studies during epidural infusion in infants and children indicate that the drug is absorbed more slowly, and clearance is reduced in neonates and young infants (150).

CHRONIC PAIN IN PEDIATRICS: OVERVIEW AND PREVALENCE

Methods for the assessment and treatment of acute pain in infants and children overlap to a degree with those encountered during chronic pain treatment. However, the International Association for the Study of Pain definition of chronic pain as "pain lasting several months in duration" is rooted in the adult literature and is based upon the natural course of acute tissue injury, inflammation and repair. Chronicity is presumed when pain lasts beyond normal tissue healing time, presumed to be approximately 3 months (151). Understanding when to term pain in infants and children as "chronic" is more of a challenge. Some authors have attempted to extend the definition of chronicity to the very young by classifying chronic pain as either subacute (<1 month duration), recurrent with pain-free intervals, or persistent (>6 months duration) (152,153). Thus, a 2-week-old neonate with a diagnosis of epidermolysis bullosa and severe pain associated with skin sloughing would properly be categorized as having chronic pain.

In pediatrics, an indistinct time frame for the definition of chronicity reinforces the concept that pain is a dynamic process that must be conceptually viewed within biopsychosocial, neurodevelopmental, and cultural domains (154,155). A premature infant may rightfully be said to suffer from both chronic and recurrent pain if, during neonatal intensive care, the infant endures multiple, untreated painful interventions such as heel lancing, dressing changes, catheter insertions, and other daily procedures. Similarly, the teenager with sickle cell disease, whose pain began with dactylitis in infancy and who has had multiple hospital admissions because of vaso-occlusive crisis, also suffers from both chronic and recurrent acute pain even although there may be some pain-free intervals. Many chronically ill children also fall into a category of almost daily pain or discomfort punctuated by episodes of exacerbation. As is amply illustrated in Chapter 30, abundant research demonstrates that the pediatric nervous system is highly plastic. As summarized earlier in this chapter, ample data also suggests that changes in nervous system structure and function may be induced by repetitive painful experiences (156). Intense or excessive pain experiences early in life may have long-term consequences in terms of pain processing (157). Paradoxically, such experiences may result in either hyper- or hypoalgesia to painful stimuli that may last through childhood and even into adulthood (158–161). Plasticity may be assessed behaviorally or measured utilizing quantitative sensory testing (162). The long-term consequences of pain early in life appear to be dependent upon the type of painful stimulus, its intensity and duration, and the point at which it takes place in relation to postnatal development (157,163,164). Objective signs of pain, such as increased adrenergic tone as manifested by increases in heart rate or blood pressure, or changes in facial expression, may be lacking in the patient with chronic daily pain, making it easier for the inexperienced physician to disbelieve the patient's pain complaint and therefore confound both diagnosis and treatment. The patient's stage of cognitive development, underlying temperament, and parental and cultural influences all affect the degree of suffering and probability of therapeutic success following an intervention.

Chronic pain in childhood, whatever the underlying etiology, may have significant consequences besides physical suffering (165). Emotional sequelae and a loss of function may convert a minor or temporary disability into a true handicap with lifelong repercussions. The financial consequences of increased health care utilization place a stress on society as a whole, since children with chronic pain utilize greater medical services and medications than their peers (166–171). In addition, chronic pain also imposes an enormous psychosocial and financial burden on the family (172–174). Pain in childhood may result in poor coping patterns and contribute to the development of chronic adult pain. Therefore, aggressively pursuing treatment strategies in the psychosocial domain becomes paramount.

Bursch, Walco, and Zeltzer have coined the term *pain-associated disability syndrome* (PADS) to describe a subset of patients with chronic pain. This syndrome can arise from any diagnosis and may result in withdrawal from school and progressive social isolation (175,176). Table 47-10 illustrates several diagnoses at very high risk of PADS. This list is by no means exhaustive. One could also include children with any chronic medical illness such as cancer, cystic fibrosis, and a myriad of other disorders associated with pain. The disorders listed in Table 47-10 remain diagnostically vague and incompletely understood. In addition, these syndromes may overlap; for example, the child with chronic abdominal pain may also complain of chronic headache.

Treatment of PADS generally requires referral to a pediatric pain management center for intensive multimodal therapy that addresses contextual issues (177). Occasionally, intensive inpatient treatment may be helpful (178).

The general approach to chronic pain in children usually consists of a detailed patient and family narrative, physical therapy, and psychological supportive care. Medications and, in some cases, neural blockade may also be indicated. Certain invasive approaches, validated as treatment in adults with chronic pain symptomatology, when provided without the necessary developmental and family focus may be inappropriate or potentially harmful when applied to children.

Various investigators have attempted to estimate the prevalence of chronic pain in children. Many of these studies are flawed because they are retrospective and subject to historical differences in diagnostic criteria and sampling error, since they often reference only patients who come to the attention of pain consultants or who are hospitalized. Early epidemiologic studies have attempted to comprehensively define the broad categories of chronic pain problems that beset children, their prevalence, and demographics in both the hospital and community setting (179). Goodman and McGrath's review of the literature suggests that chronic pain is experienced by at least 15% to 20% of children. More recent studies have confirmed initial observations that chronic pain in children is indeed a common entity, in all age ranges, and is independent of geography, socioeconomic status or cultural milieu. Often the pain is recurrent, rather than the persistent pain that is more common in adults (180–184). Scharff and co-workers have noted that common, yet poorly understood pain syndromes in childhood follow a predictable pattern at each age range: colic in infancy, lower limb pain ("growing pains") in the preschool child, followed by abdominal pain later in childhood, then headache during adolescence (185).

Perquin and colleagues randomly surveyed over 6,600 Dutch children using a structured pain questionnaire (186). Of the 82% who responded, 54% had experienced some form of pain within the previous 3 months, and 25% of the respondents reported having chronic pain. The prevalence of chronic pain was greater for girls as their age increased, peaking in early adolescence. The most common categories of pain were limb pain, headache, and abdominal pain. Half of the respondents reported multiple sites of pain, and one-third reported their pain as frequent and severe. A similar study was conducted by Roth-Isigkeit and colleagues in Germany (187). The most common complaints, in descending order 'were headache, abdominal pain, limb pain and back pain. Pain duration of greater than 3 months was reported by 45% of children, and 35% of children reported a duration of greater than 6 months. Pain occurring at least once a week was reported by a third of the children surveyed Table 47-11.

TABLE 47-10

SOME DIAGNOSES AT HIGH RISK FOR DEVELOPMENT OF PAIN ASSOCIATED DISABILITY SYNDROME (PADS)

Chronic regional pain syndrome 1
Juvenile primary fibromyalgia
Recurrent abdominal pain
Chronic headache

Chronic Noncancer Pain

Unfortunately, children are subject to many of the numerous painful conditions that affect adults. The contributing role of psychological and environmental stressors is even more important in children than in adults. Thus, the biopsychosocial framework for assessment and treatment is vital.

TABLE 47-11

MEAN PAIN INTENSITIES FOR CHILDREN WITH CHRONIC PAIN VERSUS NON-CHRONIC PAIN BY GENDER, AGE GROUPS, LOCATION OF PAIN AND SINGLE/MULTIPLE PAIN[a]

	Chronic pain			Non-chronic pain		
	Mean intensity	SD	P value	Mean intensity	SD	P value
Total	54.4	24.2		41.2	24.4	
Gender			<0.001			NS
Boys	50.7	25.0		40.2	24.5	
Girls	56.6	23.5		42.1	24.4	
Age (years)			<0.001			<0.001
0–3	54.7	27.7		36.6	27.7	
4–7	45.9	23.5		32.7	24.1	
8–11	58.3	24.7		43.7	25.6	
12–15	54.9	23.5		42.1	22.4	
16–18	54.4	21.8		37.5	20.8	
Location of pain			<0.001			<0.001
Head	53.1	22.1		34.7	22.7	
Abdomen	49.5	24.7		39.0	24.0	
Limb	51.2	24.1		42.0	24.0	
Back	57.6	23.5		40.5	22.3	
Ear	58.9	23.8		42.4	25.1	
Throat	57.1	24.4		40.4	24.2	
Unknown	59.1	23.9		67.3	24.8	
Other site	59.5	24.2		45.3	26.5	
Single/multiple pain			<0.001			<0.001
Single pain	51.0	24.5		38.0	23.7	
Multiple pain	57.6	23.4		44.2	24.7	

[a]The intensity of pain, measured with the Visual Analogue Scale, ranged from 0 (no pain) to 100 mm (worst pain). Data were based on one pain report per child. Differences were tested by Student's *t*-tests or analysis of variance.
From Perquin CW, Hazebroek-Kampschreur AAJM, Hunfeld JAM. Pain in children and adolescents: A common experience. *Pain* 2000;87:51–58, with permission.

Back Pain

Back and neck pain, so common in adults, are less so in children, in whom school avoidance issues replace the work avoidance issues seen in working adults. The presentation of back pain in children differs from that of adults. *Back or neck pain in a child without a clear history of antecedent trauma requires thorough evaluation for neoplasia or congenital malformation.* In adolescents, discogenic pain has been reported in 11% of patients, and muscle or tendon strain in 6% of patients who presented to a pediatric sports medicine clinic (188). Forty-seven percent of patients in this population had pain associated with spondylolysis stress fractures of the pars interarticularis, whereas only 5% of adults presenting with back pain had such an etiology. In the pain clinic settings, the presentation of discogenic and spondylolysis-related pain may be even more common in adolescents. For spondylosis pain, the use of NSAIDs and bracing is often sufficient, although some patients benefit from the use of a tricyclic such as nortriptyline. Neuropathic radicular pain associated with disc protrusion frequently resolves with time, but if severe, may respond to epidural steroid injection with similar results to those seen in adults (see Chapter 44). Transforaminal injection in older children is theoretically another option if computed tomography (CT) guidance is used and all appropriate precautions are taken (see Chapter 44). These interventions are very seldom needed in children, and currently no studies in the literature assess long-term outcomes following such interventional approaches in children.

Complex Regional Pain Syndromes and Other Neuropathic Pain

Complex regional pain syndrome (CRPS) type 1 is discussed in detail in Chapter 46. Its exact incidence in children is not known. The outcome is highly variable, but with proper therapy may be more benign in terms of disability than in the adult presentation (189). It is both a gender- and age-related syndrome demonstrating a female (6:1) and pubertal predominance, with a mean age at onset of 12.5 years and a range of 5 to 17 years (190). Most patients seek medical help within 2 weeks of symptom onset; however, the time to an accurate diagnosis may be quite prolonged, sometimes ranging to months. Most children present with high pain scores and many immobilize the affected extremity. Concurrent complaints of other pains, such as muscle aches, headache, or abdominal pain are common. Signs and symptoms may occasionally show generalized spread from a distal location to a more proximal distribution or even to the contralateral extremity. Often these children are engaged in competitive sports, dance, or gymnastics prior to the onset of symptoms.

Diagnosis requires a detailed history and physical examination. Often there is antecedent history of minor trauma. The neurologic examination, especially the motor examination, may be limited by pain requiring patience and multiple evaluations over time. A hallmark of diagnosis is mechanical allodynia and hyperalgesia; ambient cold temperatures typically are poorly tolerated. Bone scans may be useful to rule out other conditions. Plain films may demonstrate osteopenia, which can be a sign of disuse. A temperature difference between the affected and unaffected limb of greater than 3°C where the affected limb is at least 3°C cooler is another criterion suggested for diagnosis. Staying of the syndrome is similar to that described for adults. Some children may also demonstrate a movement disorder characterized either by weakness, dystonia, tremor, or choreoathetosis; bizarre contractures may also be present with progressive disease (191–195).

In Wilder's series of 70 patients, high-risk indicators for treatment failure included prolonged duration of symptoms and time to correct diagnosis; older age at the time of injury; female gender; the presence of vegetative or sympathetic signs such as trophic skin changes, mottling, cyanosis or edema; immobilization; number of school days missed; and high pain scores in the presence of functional disability. In general, younger patients (<11 years) had milder disease. In terms of outcome, two-thirds of children improved with physical therapy alone, and 50% percent of children believed that cognitive-behavioral interventions are of benefit. Two-thirds of children did not benefit from the administration of either corticosteroids or NSAIDs, although half described benefit from tricyclic antidepressants (TCADs). Two-thirds of patients appeared to benefit from sympathetic or somatic block (190).

The essential elements of treatment are physical therapy and psychological intervention (196,197). Medications, such as gabapentin, TCADs, and NMDA antagonists such as ketamine and the opioid methadone, have been utilized for treatment of symptoms. Opioids such as oxycodone, hydromorphone, or morphine, may provide some limited benefit, especially when administered around the initiation of physical therapy.

Tricyclic antidepressants may be helpful, especially with respect to the well-described sleep disturbance associated with this illness. Although TCADs have been shown to decrease pain in diabetic neuropathy, postherpetic neuralgia, and central poststroke pain syndromes, efficacy data specifically for CRPS is largely empirical. The mechanism of action is believed to be related to both sodium channel blockade (local anesthetic effect) as well as to decreased reuptake of 5-HT and norepinephrine (NE). Nortriptyline is the least sedating and has relatively fewer anticholinergic effects than other drugs in this class. Amitriptyline has also been used with success. Both medications are usually given at bedtime. Since TCADs may prolong the PR, QRS, and QTc intervals, a baseline EKG with a rhythm strip is warranted prior to initiating therapy. Tricyclics should not be administered to children with an unresolved history of syncope, palpitations, thyroid disease, or family history of dysrhythmia. Serum levels may be helpful to assure that the drug is being taken appropriately or if higher than anticipated doses are being administered. Serial EKGs should be performed if the daily dose is greater than 1 mg/kg/day.

Gabapentin has also been utilized for treatment of neuropathic pain in children. Its pharmacology and safety profile is well understood in pediatrics, however the U.S. Food and Drug Administration (FDA) has recently issued a warning about an increase in neuropsychiatric events and possible increase in suicidality with this drug (198). Initially, it is usually administered at night to limit the effect of potentially disturbing side effects, especially sedation. The dosage may then be increased gradually to minimize adverse effects during the daytime. Dosing every 8 hours is usually required for full therapeutic efficacy. Gabapentin may be associated with the adverse effects of light-headedness, sleepiness, double vision, or fluid retention. Nystagmus and ataxia are signs of gabapentin overdose. It is eliminated unchanged by the kidneys.

Pregabalin, another calcium channel g-subunit blocker similar to gabapentin, has high bioavailability that is independent of the dose. It has been used for the treatment of neuropathic conditions and fibromyalgia in adults but has not been well studied in pediatrics (Table 47-12).

Other classes of drugs that have been utilized for neuropathic pain in children include sympathetically active agents, other classes of anticonvulsants, and some topical agents. They have all demonstrated limited empirical efficacy and, in some cases, their use has been limited by adverse effects.

The major role for neural blockade in CRPS is to facilitate physical therapy, particularly weightbearing and speedy return to normal activities, including school. Options that may be part of a "therapeutic trial," if conservative treatment is unsuccessful, include sympathetic blocks (see Chapter 39), epidural analgesia with local anesthetic with or without epidural clonidine (see Chapters 27 and 40), transcutaneous electrical nerve stimulation (TENS), acupuncture, or variations of an IV block (Bier block). Dadure has reported efficacy in treating refractory or recurrent CRPS 1 with a combination of peripheral local anesthetic nerve block combined with an IV regional block using a mixture that included lidocaine, hydroxyethyl starch, and buflomedil (an α_1 and α_2 adrenergic blocker) followed by a continuous infusion of local anesthetic using a disposable elastomeric pump on an ambulatory basis (199).

Imaging guidance is essential when performing a stellate ganglion block or lumbar paravertebral sympathetic block in children. Precise placement of the needle or catheter minimizes the dose of agent administered and the likelihood of catastrophic adverse events. Ketamine administered either intravenously, topically, or perineurally has occasionally been described as being helpful (200–202). Intravenous block with a combination of ketamine and lidocaine has been utilized with some success (203). Temporary spinal cord stimulation with tunnelled electrodes (see Chapter 41) or peripheral nerve stimulation by using implanted electrodes is rarely advocated for use in children or adolescents. Similarly, teenagers who are diagnosed with severe CRPS that remains refractory to conservative multimodal treatment may, under exceptional circumstances, be offered a trial of spinal cord stimulation (SCS) via a tunnelled electrode, which would then possibly be followed by implantation of a spinal electrode and an implanted pulse generator (IPG) (204) (see Chapter 41). Alternatively, a tunnelled epidural catheter may be used to deliver epidural clonidine, with or without local anesthetic, for a limited period of time to facilitate physical therapy (see Chapter 40).

Psychological interventions include counseling and creating realistic expectations for improvement as well as avoidance of the "sick role." Elimination of reinforcement for dysfunctional behavior as well as facilitation of a return to school and other social activities are critical for recovery. Formal psychotherapy (to diagnose and treat comorbid psychiatric conditions) as well as cognitive behavioral techniques such as relaxation, distraction, imagery, focused breathing, hypnosis, and biofeedback, and the teaching of coping skills are essential elements in the armamentarium. Stressful family dynamics and abuse must also be explored as contributing factors.

Physical therapy including gentle reactivation, tactile desensitization, and passive and active range of motion, followed by weightbearing and muscle strengthening is often helpful.

TABLE 47-12

SAMPLE TITRATION PROCEDURES FOR MEDICATIONS COMMONLY USED FOR NEUROPATHIC PAIN

1. Slow titration (e.g., ambulatory outpatients who are attending school or work)		
	<50 kg	>50 kg
a. Nortriptytine or amitriptyline	obtain baseline ECG	
Days 1–4	0.2 mg/kg q.h.s.	10 mg q.h.s.
Days 5–8	0.4 mg/kg q.h.s	20 mg q.h.s.
increase as tolerated every 4 to 6 days until		
i. good analgesia or		
ii. limiting side effects or		
iii. dosing reaches 1 mg/kg/d (<50 kg) or 50 mg (>50 mg)		
iv. if condition iii, consider measuring plasma concentration and ECG before further dose escalation. Consider twice-daily dosing (25% in morning, 75% in evening).		
b. Gabapentin		
	<50 kg	>50 kg
Days 1–2	2 mg/kg q.h.s	100 mg q.h.s.
Days 3–4	2 mg/kg b.i.d.	100 mg b.i.d.
Days 4–6	2 mg/kg t.i.d.	100 mg t.i.d.
Days 7–9	2, 2, 4 mg/kg (t.i.d. schedule)	100, 100, 200 mg
increase as tolerated every 3 days (with 50% of daily dose in the evening) until		
i. good analgesia		
ii. limiting side effects		
iii. dosing reaches 60 mg/kg daily (<50 kg) or 3 g daily (>50 kg)		
2. Rapid Titration (e.g., nonambulatory patients with widely metastatic cancer)		
a. Tricyclics; begin at 0.2 mg/kg (10 mg for >50 kg) and titrate up every 1 to 2 days in steps according to the slow titration regimen		
b. Gabapentin: begin at 6 mg/kg b.i.d. (300 mg b.i.d. for >50 kg) for 1 to 2 days, 6 mg/kg t.i.d. (300 mg t.i.d. for >50 kg) for 1 to 2 days, 6 mg/kg morning and midday, 12 mg/kg q.h.s. (300, 300, 600 mg for >50 kg) for 1 to 2 days, and increase as tolerated to 60 mg/kg daily (3 g/d for >50 kg) over 5 to 10 days.		

ECG, electrocardiogram; q.h.s., once daily at bedtime; b.i.d., twice daily; t.i.d., three times daily.
From Schechter NL, Berde CB, Yaster M, eds. *Pain in infants, children and adolescents*, 2nd ed. Philadelphia: Lippincott, Williams & Wilkins, 2003;851.

Aqua-therapy, swimming, and aerobic conditioning are also frequently utilized. Finniss and colleagues demonstrated that children often respond to cognitive behavioral therapy with motor function reprogramming, combined with a brief course of neuropathic drugs such as gabapentin (205).

Neural blockade may be particularly beneficial for children with postamputation pain or other neuropathic pain following traumatic injury (206–208). It is the opinion of many anesthesiologists that presurgical blockade offers the greatest likelihood of modulating and potentially eliminating phantom limb pains or sensations.

Diagnosis and Treatment of Common Chronic Pain Syndromes in Children

Headache

Headache and facial pain are common in children and may have complex presentations and differential diagnostic considerations. Interdisciplinary consultation is essential. Bruxism and temporomandibular joint (TMJ) disease may contribute to chronic orofacial pain that may often benefit from physical therapy and splint therapy. Suboccipital neurostimulation has been reported to be valuable in adults with headaches but is yet to be assessed in children (see Chapter 41). It may be an option for some teenagers with severe intractable migraine that can have a devastating effect on school, family, and personal life. Neural blockade has been utilized diagnostically and therapeutically in the treatment of headache (209,210). Commonly utilized blocks (described in Chapter 17) include sphenopalatine nerve block for aborting the pain of refractory migraine, and greater and lesser occipital nerve blocks, which can provide benefit for the treatment of occipital neuralgia and cervicogenic headache.

Pelvic Pain

Pelvic pain in adolescent females is an increasingly recognized problem and is often due to endometriosis diagnosed laparoscopically. Pelvic inflammatory disease is another common problem, requiring specialized gynecological management. Neural blockade is rarely indicated in these patients, however severe intractable pelvic pain from interstitial cystitis may benefit from treatment with retrograde spinal cord stimulation (see Chapter 41).

Abdominal Pain

Abdominal pain is common in children, but unlike in adults, it tends to be recurrent rather than constant. It is the subject of two recent Cochrane evidence-based reviews that discuss pharmacologic and psychosocial interventions for this group of patients (211,212). The Rome II Multinational Working Teams have provided guidance on nosology, diagnosis, and treatment of the "functional" gastrointestinal disorders including recurrent abdominal pain (RAP) (213). Apley's definition of RAP requires that pain must occur at least once monthly, be accompanied by pain-free intervals, and be severe enough to interfere with normal activities (214). Recurrent abdominal pain is estimated to have a population prevalence of 9% to 25%, and is more common in girls than boys. It is frequently associated with chronic headaches and migraine headaches. The pain is rarely if ever related to physiologic events such as eating, menses, urination, or defecation. Usually the pain is difficult to describe and may be periumbilical in location. Severe pain episodes rarely last more than several hours. The pain usually does not awaken the patient from sleep, and often no intervention can be found to help. Abdominal pain symptoms may be associated with diaphoresis, pallor, nausea, or vomiting.

Signs and symptoms that would lead one away from the diagnosis of RAP include weight loss, pain that awakens the child from sleep, fevers, pain far from the umbilicus, dysuria, guaiac positive stools, anemia, elevated white blood cell count, elevated erythrocyte sedimentation rate (ESR) or c-reactive protein (CRP), or a positive urine analysis and urine culture. Evaluation of weight and growth curves are essential elements of diagnosis. Other laboratory testing such as serum amylase, lipase, imaging studies, and stool examinations for infectious or neoplastic etiologies may be warranted. In the absence of a "red flag" for pathology, common, easily treated entities such as lactose intolerance, malabsorption syndromes, *Helicobacter pylori* infection, and inflammatory bowel syndrome should be ruled out as well. Constipation and food intolerance are increasingly recognized as causes of RAP. *The extent of the workup must be guided by clinical acumen; an unhurried history and physical examination is the best guide to the need for further studies.* Only 10% of children will have a diagnosable etiology for their abdominal pain. Visceral hyperalgesia, often associated with enteroparesis, is a vaguely described entity of the neuroenteric system. It may be associated with hormonal abnormalities or follow nonspecific infection (215).

Once potentially dangerous pathology has been ruled out by a carefully directed workup, one must explore the psychological and/or environmental factors that are commonly causal. Anxiety, depression, other stressors, secondary gain, family and peer issues, school pressure, school avoidance and phobias, and parental discord. Physical and sexual abuse are as important to investigate as are the pathologic tissue diagnoses. Neural blockade has no role for treatment, but on occasion can be exceedingly helpful for diagnostic purposes (see Chapter 38). If pain persists despite a dense subarachnoid block, central or psychological causes of the pain must be pursued.

Treatment is often based upon the stress management and cognitive behavioral techniques described earlier in this chapter. Selective serotonin reuptake inhibitors (SSRIs) or selective norepinephrine reuptake inhibitors (SNRIs) may be particularly helpful pharmacologic adjuvants.

Juvenile Primary Fibromyalgia

Juvenile primary fibromyalgia syndrome (JPFS) is characterized by diffuse muscle pain and tender points on digital examination. It is usually accompanied by fatigue without objective signs of systemic disease. Criteria for JPFS have been proposed (216). The etiology of this entity is idiopathic, but there appears to be a familial predisposition. Juvenile primary fibromyalgia is more commonly described in girls than boys and usually presents in adolescence. It is frequently associated with headaches, fatigue and sleep disturbances, morning stiffness, abdominal pain, depression, and subjective swelling (217,218). The sleep disturbance is characterized by long sleep latency and shortened sleep duration (219,220). The prognosis in children is generally better than that for adults (221).

Treatment consists of psychosocial support and a cognitive behavioral approach along with exercise, particularly aerobic exercise (222,223). SSRIs, SNRIs pregabalin, gabapentin, and TCADs have also been utilized for treatment of JPFS. Occasional trigger point injections and acupuncture may also be helpful.

Pain Associated with Chronic Illness in Childhood

Cystic Fibrosis

Cystic fibrosis is the most common lethal childhood disease in the United States (224). Although tremendous strides have been made in the care of these children, many older patients with cystic fibrosis suffer from chronic or recurrent pain. According to Ravilly and colleagues, cystic fibrosis may be associated with muscular pain from coughing; pain associated with rib fractures, pleuritis, and pneumothorax; chronic sinusitis; and headache, as well as abdominal pain associated principally with gastroesophageal reflux, episodes of pancreatitis, and meconium ileus equivalent. Back and limb pain is also common in children with cystic fibrosis because of the muscle strain associated with coughing and increased respiratory effort. Osteopenia may contribute to fractures of vertebrae and ribs. Prolonged postthoracotomy pain has also been reported in this population. Chronic pain increases dramatically in the last 6 months of life. Headache may be associated with increasing degrees of hypercarbia or hypoxia (225,226). Nonpharmacologic approaches may be particularly helpful, especially relaxation techniques. NSAIDs can also be used, although concerns about bleeding, especially in patients with pulmonary hypertension, should be taken into consideration. Exacerbation of bronchospasm may also be a consequence of NSAID administration. Opioids may be administered systemically for pain control, as well as for treatment of air hunger and may also be used as a cough suppressant, if needed, in the final stages of disease. Anxiolytics, such as the benzodiazepines may also be helpful in the terminal phases of illness to treat the fear associated with breathlessness. Meticulous enforcement of a bowel regimen, including softeners, lubricants, and osmotic agents is essential if opioid therapy is employed. Epidural blockade (thoracic), including tunnelled catheters, may be particularly helpful in this group of patients, particularly those with refractory chest pain. Intercostal nerve blocks may also be helpful, although the risk of pneumothorax may be catastrophic.

Sickle Cell Disease

Chronic and recurrent pain is the hallmark of the sickle hemoglobinopathies (hemoglobin SS, SC, and Sβ-thalassemia). Vaso-occlusive crisis and ensuing ischemia or tissue infarction account for the pain. Central pain syndromes associated with stroke are rare but may also occur. Treatment consists of hydration, systemic administration of opioid, paracetamol, and NSAIDs. Maintenance of adequate oxygenation is achieved by administering supplemental oxygen and, if required, transfusion therapy (either a simple transfusion or exchange transfusion). The latter treatment strategy may also serve to temporarily suspend reticulocytosis and hence sickle cell production. Treating acidosis and maintaining the patient in a warm, comfortable environment will also decrease vasoconstriction and improve rheology and tissue perfusion.

Opioid therapy for sickle cell crisis usually involves a combination of strategies. For an acute crisis, an immediate-acting opioid such as morphine, oxycodone, or hydromorphone can be administered orally. If around-the-clock dosing is required, and dosing requirements have been ascertained, consideration should be given to utilizing a sustained-release preparation of morphine or oxycodone. Sustained-release preparations should not be used in patients with rare crises who are opioid naive. Opioid requirements must be clearly established before any sustained release formulation is prescribed. Sustained-release tablets cannot be chewed, thus limiting their usefulness to the younger patient. They may, however, play a critically important role in the older patient who has frequent, recurrent crises. If oral opioids fail, administration of parenteral opioids by a demand-dose PCA is the next logical step. If the patient is not on a sustained release oral preparation, a continuous infusion delivered by PCA should be considered. Nurse-administered boluses may be utilized with proper monitoring for breakthrough pain. If the patient is on a sustained-release preparation of opioid, it may be continued in lieu of a continuous infusion. NSAIDS are utilized as co-analgesics. Once pain is under control, the patient is transitioned to an oral regimen utilizing one of two approaches. The patient can be placed either on an immediate-release opioid that is continued around-the-clock for 24 hours (doses are not administered if the patient is comfortable, asleep, sedated, or bradypneic) followed by as-needed dosing or, if the patient's total daily opioid dose requirement is high enough, the patient is placed on a sustained-release preparation and immediate-release opioid is given as needed for mild breakthrough pain. Once symptoms are completely resolved, the sustained-release opioid preparation is gradually weaned. Oral methadone is the only long-acting opioid preparation available in liquid formulation.

Methadone has also been shown to be remarkably effective in patients who may have refractory pain symptoms from diseases such as sickle cell disease and cancer. Methadone should be prescribed with great care since it has a large volume of distribution and long $t_{1/2\beta}$, which can lead to delayed sedation and possible respiratory depression. This may occur within 24 to 72 hours after initiation of treatment. It may also affect cardiac repolarization by blocking the slow inward potassium current, possibly leading to dysrhythmias (227,228). Methadone also interacts pharmacodynamically with a wide variety of other drugs, such as the macrolide antibiotics. Its metabolism is also known to be affected by retrovirals and antifungals, among other drugs (229). It can be used as an adjuvant for the treatment of refractory pain at very low dose; that is, 0.1 mg/kg either intravenously or orally every 8 to 12 hours for 24 to 72 hours and then slowly weaned.

Epidural analgesia utilizing local anesthetic alone or in combination with opioid has been infrequently used in the management of vaso-occlusive crisis (230,231). It may be useful for refractory cases.

Since sickle cell patients are on intensive opioid protocols for prolonged periods of time, a rigorous bowel hygiene regimen is necessary to prevent constipation. 5-HT$_3$ agents are frequently needed for treatment of nausea, although over time this symptom usually resolves. Pruritus may be problematic as well (232). Antihistamines may have limited efficacy for the treatment of pruritus. Low doses of naloxone in the range of 0.25 μg/kg/hour may decrease pruritus, nausea, and vomiting while not interfering with opioid analgesia. Some evidence suggests that at this low dose, naloxone may paradoxically enhance analgesia (233).

Often sickle-cell patients may report high pain scores yet appear nonchalant. This "affective-sensory disconnect" that many clinicians have observed may lead to underestimation or skepticism as to the severity of the patient's pain and consequent undertreatment. Close, long-term follow-up and a therapeutic alliance between the medical provider and the patient are therefore essential for good care.

Pain in Children with Cognitive Impairment

Cognitively impaired children constitute a challenging group of patients. Assessment of acute or chronic pain can be difficult in this population. For many of these children, the causes of their suffering remain occult, even after careful investigation. Potential reasons for chronic pain may include contractures, gastroesophageal reflux, decubitus ulcers, and spasticity. These children commonly undergo surgical procedures such as shunt placement and revision, gastrostomy tube placement, contracture releases, and osteotomies. Some are said to suffer "neural agony" for no discrete cause. Comfort measures (swaddling, feeding, assuring warmth and dryness) may be helpful in eliminating causes of general discomfort. Judicious use of analgesics including opioids, with appropriate monitoring, may be necessary and humane. Botulinum toxin injections may be helpful for treatment of spasticity, and baclofen has been utilized either systemically or via intrathecal pump, particularly in children with spastic cerebral palsy (234–236). Dorsal rhizotomy has also been advocated in a select group of patients (237).

Finally, it should be remembered that children occasionally suffer from chronic pain of unexplained or uncertain etiology. Somatization, conversion disorders, or malingering, and, in rare, cases Munchausen syndrome by proxy must be considered.

MANAGEMENT OF CANCER PAIN IN CHILDREN

The incidence of cancer in children has remained stable over the past 25 years, but overall survival has increased as therapies have become more effective. As a consequence, pain is one of the most common symptoms reported in childhood cancer (238,239). Two-thirds of pediatric patients who are diagnosed with cancer report pain as a presenting symptom and more than 80% of inpatients with cancer report pain during hospitalization and rate its intensity as moderate to severe (240–242).

Management of cancer pain in children is particularly challenging because of its emotional impact on the child, family, and medical staff. Many of the principles outlined by Burton and Phan in the chapter on cancer pain in adults (Chapter 45) can be applied in children, although neurolytic procedures are much less commonly used. The general framework of palliative care in adults described by Fine (Chapter 49) is also applicable in children, except that children tend to be more commonly managed in the hospital or, whenever possible, at home (243). In contradistinction to adult palliative care, pediatric palliative care is viewed as a continuum that may coexist with curative intent. The World Health Organization (WHO) analgesic ladder provides a broad pharmacologic approach to the management of cancer pain. However, as in adults, multimodal treatment is usually tailored to the type and severity of the child's pain, with the stage of cancer being a secondary but still significant consideration (244–246). As is the case in adults and children with chronic pain in general, the biopsychosocial framework outlined by Katz and Melzack in Chapter 35 is used to assess physical, psychological, and environmental factors in the child's pain and thereby guiding therapy. The methods for assessment of pain described earlier in this chapter are applicable to cancer pain in children.

It is worth noting that most pain in cancer patients is *not* tumor-related (242). Procedure-related pain from lumbar punctures, bone marrow aspiration and biopsy, IV catheter placement, chest tube placement, and surgical pain account for a significant proportion of recurrent pain. Procedural pain in children with cancer requires special attention, with treatment plans that are individualized for each child. The full range of options for procedural analgesia should always be considered, including general anesthesia (154). Topically applied local anesthetics may also be of benefit.

The adverse effects of chemotherapy or radiation may result in the development of mucositis or neuropathies. Stem cell transplantation can be associated with the skin and visceral consequences of graft-versus-host disease, which can be both painful and distressing. Pain late in the course of cancer may be related to both tumor invasion and metastasis. Plexopathies and bone pain can be particularly difficult treatment challenges, often requiring a variety of adjuvants and techniques. The severity and quality of cancer pain is related to tumor type, size, and location. In general, blood dyscrasias, such as leukemia, are intrinsically less painful than solid tumors. Central nervous system tumors may be associated with unremitting headache. It is also worth noting that overall patient distress may be related to poor control of symptoms other than pain. Attention should be given to the management of fatigue, anxiety, depression, insomnia, delirium, constipation, pruritus, nausea and vomiting as well as existential or spiritual concerns. Guidelines have been published by the American Pain Society and the WHO that can help guide therapy.

In general, management begins with a detailed assessment of the pain. Likely cancer pain syndromes associated with the particular tumor type and its location should be considered. Rapid titration of opioids for the treatment of a "pain emergency" has immediate priority. Adverse affects of pain treatment must be anticipated and proactively addressed. Adjuvants and co-analgesics may be helpful in improving pain control and limiting opioid related adverse effects. Pain must be temporally anticipated, based upon the type of chemotherapy or radiation administered and the likely time course of the neutropenic nadir. The need for long-acting medications is frequently warranted.

Pharmacologic treatment of cancer pain in children utilizes the range of opioid and nonopioid drugs described earlier in this chapter, with some additional agents and strategies (247). Opioids are often effective in children with cancer pain and, if the gastrointestinal tract is intact and vomiting is not an issue, the majority can be treated via the oral route (248). If a child can reliably swallow a pill or capsule whole, sustained-release preparations can be employed once dose requirements have been firmly determined. In the case of sustained-release morphine, it may be necessary to dose three times daily, rather than

the twice daily regimen of adults because of different morphine pharmacokinetics in children (249). As in adults, methadone is often utilized. Dosing strategies for methadone depend upon whether it is used as a co-analgesic (along with a short-acting oral opioid) or as the sole opioid. Some authors have advocated the use of methadone as a "poor man's PCA" administering a sliding scale of medication at regular intervals based upon the level of reported pain and withholding the drug if the patient is comfortable (250–252).

Unfortunately, opioids may cause frequent side effects in children with cancer, including sedation, confusion, dysphoria, and constipation, even when systematic anticipatory treatment of side effects is used (253). Tolerance to the constipating effects of opioids does not develop and requires prophylactic therapy.

It is sobering to note the high level of suffering that persists despite best efforts today in dying children (253). In her research, Wolfe and colleagues identified that suffering from pain was not relieved in 30% of patients and that other distressing symptoms were frequently inadequately controlled. Contributing to this failure was the parental perception that providers were not adequately aware of the degree of their child's suffering. To manage opioid side effects, patients at risk should be identified (Table 47-7) and medical orders should be ready for staff to utilize if such side effects occur (Table 47-6).

It may occasionally be necessary to use psychostimulants in children with cancer who require opioid treatment. Stimulants such as dextroamphetamine or methylphenidate should be considered if opioid rotation or dose adjustment, in combination with the use of nonopioid analgesics, does not reduce unwanted sedative side effects. Children receiving both methylphenidate and clonidine (to enhance local anesthetic effects of epidural blockade or for neuropathic symptoms) are at some increased risk of dysrhythmias, particularly bradyrhythmias (254). Modafinil has also been used to treat unwanted sedation and fatigue but has not been studied rigorously in children (255–257).

Sometimes changing to a different opioid or different route of administration may solve the problem of excessive side effects. For example, subcutaneous opioid infusions may permit the use of smaller hourly dose rates, but with improved analgesia and reduced side effects compared to some other routes of administration (244). Hydromorphone, oxycodone, or transdermal fentanyl may be associated with improved analgesia if oral morphine has failed to provide analgesia without unacceptable side effects. A small percentage of children tolerate fentanyl better than morphine (258).

Like any long-acting preparation, transdermal fentanyl should never be used in the opioid-naive patient, nor should it be used for the acute relief of pain since it takes approximately 12 to 24 hours to achieve stable serum levels. Its greatest utility is for patients who cannot utilize the enteral route of administration. The 12.5 µg/hour patch is approved for use in children older than 2 years of age. Upon removal of the patch, the serum concentration decreases to 50% by about 17 hours. Other options for opioid analgesia in cancer pain include sustained-release preparations of oxycodone or morphine; often hydromorphone is a better choice orally or by subcutaneous infusion but it is no longer available in the United States as a sustained-release preparation. Fentanyl is an attractive option for breakthrough pain, either via the transmucosal "lozenge" or the very rapidly absorbed transbuccal tablet, and may be suitable in older adolescents. Adverse effects of the fentanyl Oralet that have been reported in children include excessive sedation and oxygen desaturation (259). Therefore, if employed, it should initially be used in a monitored setting. In Europe, a "transdermal PCA," the IONSYS system is available. This consists of a special patch containing a microchip and current-regulated delivery system to provide precise amounts of fentanyl across the skin. The transdermal or subcutaneous route can be valuable in children who cannot tolerate the oral route for various reasons, or who are being cared for in a nonhospitalized setting.

Intravenous or subcutaneous PCA is valuable for severe pain that is acute, often varying in intensity, and not amenable to the oral route. It is the "gold standard" for treatment of most forms of moderate to severe cancer pain encountered in the hospital setting (260). Ketamine in subanesthetic doses is occasionally employed in cases of severe cancer pain, especially when opioid adverse effects may be limiting (261,262).

Caution should be exercised in prescribing NSAIDs for children with cancer. Underlying hepatopathy, nephropathy, gastropathy, or coagulopathy may contraindicate their use. Choline magnesium trisalicylate may be a useful co-analgesic, since it does not irreversibly inactivate platelet function. It is, however, associated with the other adverse effects ascribed to salicylates including the risk of Reye syndrome.

Mucositis pain is a classic example of treatment-associated pain in children undergoing radiation therapy or chemotherapy (263), and is the principle reason for PCA initiation in this population. Hydromorphone may be better tolerated than morphine for PCA in children and has about five times the potency of morphine (263). As described earlier in this chapter, demand-dosing by PCA device can be utilized in the child who is cognitively able to understand the concept. Most children with mucositis will require a continuous infusion and should be monitored accordingly. In addition to demand doses, clinician-administered boluses may be given for breakthrough pain following appropriate evaluation. Clinician bolus doses may be between 25% and 200% of the hourly infused dose, and may be repeated at appropriate intervals, usually no more frequent than every 15 to 30 minutes up to a preset limit. The admonition to "start low and go slow" should be heeded. Parent-controlled analgesia or "PCA by proxy" is controversial and not without serious risk, as described earlier in this chapter. It can be utilized, with careful selection of both patient and proxy in certain circumstances, only once institutional guidelines and specific training programs have been established (264–267). Children with mucositis also benefit from a variety of local "magic mouthwashes" that coat and soothe raw surfaces.

Sudden severe pain, often described as a "pain emergency," requires prompt attention. Often, patients with such pain are already receiving chronic opioid therapy. It is essential that treatable causes of pain be immediately assessed and addressed. Analgesic treatment in this circumstance must be swift and aggressive (268). Medication may be rapidly titrated every 15 minutes until relief is achieved or further dosing becomes limited by sedation or hypoventilation. Pain score, level of consciousness, vital signs, and oxygen saturation must be monitored. Titration requires a clinician at the bedside until the pain is reduced to a satisfactory level. Bioavailability issues (when changing the route of administration of medication from enteral to parenteral) and issues of incomplete cross-tolerance (when changing the specific type of opioid) must be taken into consideration when deciding upon the appropriate dosage of IV medication for use in such an emergency. Anecdotally, some patients benefit from opioid rotation (269).

Despite optimization of opioids, NSAIDs, acetaminophen (paracetamol), and other appropriately prescribed adjuvants, some children's pain is poorly responsive. One reason for this failure is that some children with cancer have neuropathic pain (occasionally consistent with a diagnosis of CRPS-2) that is poorly responsive to opioids and NSAIDs. The diagnosis of neuropathic pain has now become more precise with the availability of validated instruments such as Pain-detect and S-LANSS (see Chapter 46). Neuropathic pain is best treated by the addition of "neuropathic drugs" such as antidepressants and anticonvulsants. These have been discussed earlier in the chapter. Nortriptyline is a noradrenergic TCAD that has proven efficacy for neuropathic pain and is well tolerated by children; a titration regimen is given in Table 47-12. Gabapentin and pregabalin are the most common anticonvulsants prescribed at present, with a greater experience available for gabapentin.

As is the case for treatment of acute pain, neural blockade techniques are highly effective and well tolerated for relief of cancer pain (270). The main indication for neural blockade is failure of multimodal pharmacotherapy or intolerable side effects. However, even when this indication is adhered to, too few children with cancer are afforded the superior pain relief and reduction of side effects that clinicians commonly observe with this modality of treatment. Unfortunately, there is no randomized, prospective controlled study of "optimized medical management" compared to, for example, intrathecal infusion of opioids as reported in adults (271).

The most commonly used neural blockade technique in children with cancer pain is epidural infusion of preservative-free local anesthetic, opioid, clonidine, and sometimes other drugs such as (S)–ketamine. This technique is described in detail for pediatric application in Chapter 27. Additional relevant discussion on epidural analgesia is offered in Chapter 11 by Cousins and Veering, among other places in this volume. However, nearly all of the techniques described in Chapter 27 on neural blockade for pediatric surgery can be utilized with appropriate application in children with cancer.

It is not uncommon for a child who has been on high-dose opioids to become somnolent and hypopneic immediately after receiving an effective block. These children require careful monitoring for a decrease in respiratory drive due to unopposed opioid effect following sudden cessation of severe pain. As is the case for surgery, such techniques will be mostly initiated in the operating room, under general anesthesia. Usually the technique employed utilizes a catheter to permit a continuous infusion. Thus, confirmation of correct placement of the catheter is essential, and image intensifier control as well as contrast injection is highly recommended. For peripheral nerve and plexus blocks, the use of ultrasound guidance provides added precision and probable improvement in efficacy and safety.

Children with diffuse pain and a short life expectancy are best managed with a tunnelled intrathecal catheter, placed according to the technique described for adults by Carr and Cousins in Chapter 40, with appropriate modification. Those few children with severe pain and a life expectancy of more than 3 to 6 months may benefit from an intrathecal catheter connected to a programmable implanted intrathecal pump (e.g., SynchroMed, Medtronic). Because of the size of such pumps, children younger than 5 to 7 years of age are generally too small for their use, and are best managed with a tunnelled catheter and portable external pump.

Children with a more defined area of pain such as pelvic, lower limbs, abdomen, or thoracic region may be managed with an epidural catheter; the tip of the catheter should be located close to the segmental distribution of the pain, as described earlier. Since the doses required for epidural infusion are much greater than for intrathecal infusion, almost invariably a tunnelled epidural catheter will be used with an external portable pump. However, in some situations a "port" may be used to provide access to the epidural catheter. Initially, twice-daily injections via the port may be sufficient; however, when the pain becomes more severe a "right-angled" needle may be inserted into the port and an infusion pump utilized (see Chapter 40). The main advantage of the port is the initial freedom from an attached pump and probably a lower incidence of infection. Infection at the exit site of a tunnelled catheter is usually a minor problem treated locally. Infection of a port can require removal of the port and epidural catheter, as well as treatment with systemic antibiotics.

Neurolytic blockade is rarely used in children; however, celiac plexus block remains a valuable option for severe upper abdominal visceral pain. Computed tomography guidance and IV contrast injection to identify the aorta and celiac artery greatly increases the safety and efficacy (272) (see also Chapter 45 on adult cancer pain relief). In the presence of lower limb ischemia and pain, neurolytic lumbar sympathetic block, as described in Chapter 39, may be very valuable.

In children with cancer of one limb requiring amputation or extensive surgery, a continuous catheter technique for upper or lower extremity blockade may be of enormous assistance in relieving acute pain and possibly preventing development of neuropathic pain or phantom limb pain (see Chapter 27). Less commonly, cancer affecting other regions, such as the head and neck, may be amenable to use of specific neural blockade techniques with catheter placement for continuous infusion (see Chapter 27).

It is important to remember that children with cancer may develop neuropathic pain including CRPS (see Chapter 46) as a result of the cancer, its progression, radiotherapy, chemotherapy, or surgery, and that early diagnosis and appropriate treatment are vital to prevent loss of function. Even more rarely, teenage children may require radiofrequency lesioning (RF) techniques. For example, a teenager who has become very deconditioned during cancer treatment may develop mechanical facet-related spinal pain. Diagnostic medial branch blocks may confirm the foregoing diagnosis, leading to possible use of RF lesioning (see Chapters 42 and 44).

Corticosteroids, radiation, and chemotherapy may prove to be useful for palliation when all else has failed. Hormonal therapies such as medroxyprogesterone acetate to improve weight gain and sense of well-being have been reported as beneficial in the adult literature, but the literature on their use in pediatrics is anecdotal. The value of bisphosphonates or calcitonin in treating bone metastasis is of undetermined value in pediatrics. Octreotide infusions have been anecdotally helpful in cases of severe abdominal cramping and diarrhea, such as may be seen in graft-versus-host disease and may also be helpful in the palliation of malignant bowel obstruction (273,274). Children with cancer pain or other cancer-related symptoms such as nausea are also potential candidates for treatment with acupressure or acupuncture in its various forms (see Chapter 34).

SUMMARY

Ongoing evidence continues to demonstrate the deleterious physiologic effects of pain and the beneficial effects of effective analgesia upon recovery after surgical procedures and maintenance or recovery of function during chronic illness, including cancer. Even without positive impacts upon secondary outcomes, relief of pain and suffering per se—particularly in society's most vulnerable members—must be a goal of any humane society. Indeed, the growing body of clinical evidence on the influence of pain control upon function has coincided with the growing awareness by professionals and the public of the importance of pain management to the well-being of infants and children. The American Academy of Pediatrics has published position statements advocating the proper assessment and treatment of pain in infants and children. Regulatory bodies and professional organizations are vocal advocates for the adequate treatment of pain in children. The Joint Commission on Accreditation of Healthcare Organizations (JCAHO) has focused on the issue of pain assessment and treatment in its standards and on-site surveys. The JCAHO standards require all hospitals to establish institution-wide methods to deal with pain management, including procedural sedation in patients, including infants and children. Compliance with these guidelines has become a major area of focus of JCAHO site visits.

Pharmacotherapy of acute, chronic, and cancer-related pain in children, as in adults, relies upon the basic three-step, graded WHO ladder based upon assessment of the severity of pain. This strategy utilizes a combination of NSAIDs or acetaminophen, so-called "weak" opioids (codeine, oxycodone, hydrocodone), and strong opioids. Parenteral opioids or neuraxial regional anesthetic techniques may be applied according to the nature of the pain being addressed, its anticipated severity, and the resources of the setting in which care is provided. Even in the setting of moderate to severe pain, acetaminophen or an NSAID can be used on a fixed-interval basis as a means of decreasing total opioid consumption and thereby opioid-related adverse effects. Decisions regarding opioid use include the choice of opioid, its route of administration, and its mode of administration. For the treatment of severe pain in the hospitalized patient, PCA is the preferred mode of administration. Although the IV administration of opioids remains the primary route of administration for the control of moderate and severe pain in the hospital setting, future formulations and developments may allow for the increased use of other routes. Anecdotal experience has demonstrated the effective use of subcutaneous opioids when IV administration is not feasible. Regional anesthetic techniques are frequently used to control acute postoperative pain, although these techniques may also be applicable to moderate or severe pain of other etiologies such as CRPS or cancer. Although used initially in the adult population, there is now extensive experience with all techniques of regional anesthesia, including neurolytic blocks, in even our youngest pediatric patients. Advances in technology and the availability of appropriately sized equipment has facilitated the migration of such techniques from adult practice to the care of infants and children. In addition to the choice of appropriate medications and regional anesthetic techniques, an integral aspect of pediatric pain management is the assessment of the patient's pain, its meaning for the patient and family, and its biopsychosocial context.

Given the persistent impact that pain in infants and children may have throughout much of the patient's lifetime, early and aggressive treatment (and preemption when possible) is mandatory. For chronic and cancer pain, such treatment includes comprehensive rehabilitation to address the nearly universal disruptions of psychological and social well-being, and physical functioning, that emerge when pain persists—and that involve the family as well as the patient. After millennia of neglect, the importance of appropriate pain control is now recognized, particularly in children. Basic and clinical knowledge is emerging at an accelerated pace to fill gaps in our knowledge. With translation of this knowledge, the goal of providing appropriate analgesia to children of all ages is in sight.

References

1. Anand KJ. Effects of perinatal pain and stress. *Prog Brain Res* 2000;122:117–129.
2. Anand KJ, Hickey PR. Halothane-morphine compared with high-dose sufentanil for anesthesia and postoperative analgesia in neonatal cardiac surgery. *N Engl J Med* 1992;326:1–9.
3. Arendt-Nielsen L, Petersen-Felix S. Wind-up and neuroplasticity: Is there a correlation to clinical pain? *Eur J Anaesthesiol Suppl* 1995;10:1–7.
4. Fitzgerald M, Beggs S. The neurobiology of pain: Developmental aspects. *Neuroscientist* 2001;7:246–257.
5. Melzack R, Coderre TJ, Katz J, et al. Central neuroplasticity and pathological pain. *Ann N Y Acad Sci* 2001;933:157–174.
6. Rose SA, Schmidt K, Riese ML, et al. Effects of prematurity and early intervention on responsivity to tactual stimuli: A comparison of preterm and full-term infants. *Child Dev* 1980;51:416–425.
7. Schechter NL, Allen DA, Hanson K. Status of pediatric pain control: A comparison of hospital analgesic usage in children and adults. *Pediatrics* 1986;77:11–15.
8. Whitfield MF, Grunau RE. Behavior, pain perception, and the extremely low-birth weight survivor. *Clin Perinatol* 2000;27:363–379.
9. Porter FL, Grunau RE, Anand KJ. Long-term effects of pain in infants. *J Dev Behav Pediatr* 1999;20:253–261.
10. Anand KJ. Pain assessment in preterm neonates. *Pediatrics* 2007;119:605–607.
11. Bartocci M, Bergqvist LL, Lagercrantz H, et al. Pain activates cortical areas in the preterm newborn brain. *Pain* 2006;122:109–117.
12. Slater R, Cantarella A, Gallella S, et al. Cortical pain responses in human infants. *J Neurosci* 2006;26:3662–3666.
13. Fitzgerald M, Millard C, McIntosh N. Cutaneous hypersensitivity following peripheral tissue damage in newborn infants and its reversal with topical anaesthesia. *Pain* 1989;39:31–36.
14. Anand KJ, Runeson B, Jacobson B. Gastric suction at birth associated with long-term risk for functional intestinal disorders in later life. *J Pediatr* 2004;144:449–454.
15. Peters JW, Schouw R, Anand KJ, et al. Does neonatal surgery lead to increased pain sensitivity in later childhood? *Pain* 2005;114:444–454.
16. Beyer JE, Wells N. The assessment of pain in children. *Pediatr Clin North Am* 1989;36:837–854.
17. Bieri D, Reeve RA, Champion GD, et al. The Faces Pain Scale for the self-assessment of the severity of pain experienced by children: Development, initial validation, and preliminary investigation for ratio scale properties. *Pain* 1990;41:139–150.
18. McGrath PJ, Johnson G, Goodman JT, et al. CHEOPS: A behavioral scale for rating postoperative pain in children. In: Fields HL, ed., *Advances in pain research & therapy*, Vol. 9. New York: Raven Press; 1985:395–402.
19. Hicks CL, von Baeyer CL, Spafford PA, et al. The Faces Pain Scale-Revised: Toward a common metric in pediatric pain measurement. *Pain* 2001;93:173–183.
20. Krechel SW, Bildner J. CRIES: A new neonatal postoperative pain measurement score. Initial testing of validity and reliability. *Paediatr Anaesth* 1995;5:53–61.
21. Taddio A, Nulman I, Koren BS, et al. A revised measure of acute pain in infants. *J Pain Symptom Manage* 1995;10:456–463.
22. Stevens B, Johnston C, Petryshen P, et al. Premature Infant Pain Profile: Development and initial validation. *Clin J Pain* 1996;12:13–22.
23. Breau LM, Finley GA, McGrath PJ, et al. Validation of the Non-communicating Children's Pain Checklist-Postoperative Version. *Anesthesiology* 2002;96:528–535.
24. Malviya S, Voepel-Lewis T, Burke C, et al. The revised FLACC observational pain tool: Improved reliability and validity for pain assessment in children with cognitive impairment. *Paediatr Anaesth* 2006;16:258–265.
25. McGrath PJ, Rosmus C, Canfield C, et al. Behaviours caregivers use to determine pain in non-verbal, cognitively impaired individuals. *Dev Med Child Neurol* 1998;40:340–343.
26. Schug SA, Zech D, Dorr U. Cancer pain management according to WHO analgesic guidelines. *J Pain Symptom Manage* 1990;5:27–32.
27. Clark E, Plint AC, Correll R, et al. A randomized, controlled trial of acetaminophen, ibuprofen, and codeine for acute pain relief in children with musculoskeletal trauma. *Pediatrics* 2007;119:460–467.
28. Anderson BJ, van Lingen RA, Hansen TG, et al. Acetaminophen developmental pharmacokinetics in premature neonates and infants: A pooled population analysis. *Anesthesiology* 2002;96:1336–1345.
29. Leroy S, Mosca A, Landre-Peigne C, et al. [Ibuprofen in childhood: evidence-based review of efficacy and safety]. *Arch Pediatr* 2007;14:477–484.
30. Lesko SM, O'Brien KL, Schwartz B, et al. Invasive group A streptococcal infection and nonsteroidal antiinflammatory drug use among children with primary varicella. *Pediatrics* 2001;107:1108–1115.
31. Lesko SM, Louik C, Vezina RM, et al. Asthma morbidity after the short-term use of ibuprofen in children. *Pediatrics* 2002;109:E20.
32. Birmingham PK, Tobin MJ, Henthorn TK, et al. Twenty-four-hour pharmacokinetics of rectal acetaminophen in children: An old drug with new recommendations. *Anesthesiology* 1997;87:244–252.
33. Tobias JD, Lowe S, Hersey S, et al. Analgesia after bilateral myringotomy and placement of pressure equalization tubes in children: Acetaminophen versus acetaminophen with codeine. *Anesth Analg* 1995;81:496–500.
34. Rivera-Penera T, Gugig R, Davis J, et al. Outcome of acetaminophen overdose in pediatric patients and factors contributing to hepatotoxicity. *J Pediatr* 1997;130:300–304.
35. Williams DG, Patel A, Howard RF. Pharmacogenetics of codeine metabolism in an urban population of children and its implications for analgesic reliability. *Br J Anaesth* 2002;89:839–845.
36. Cicero TJ, Inciardi JA, Munoz A. Trends in abuse of OxyContin and other opioid analgesics in the United States: 2002–2004. *J Pain* 2005;6:662–672.
37. Finkel JC, Rose JB, Schmitz ML, et al. An evaluation of the efficacy and tolerability of oral tramadol hydrochloride tablets for the treatment of postsurgical pain in children. *Anesth Analg* 2002;94:1469–1473.
38. Rose JB, Finkel JC, Arquedas-Mohs A, et al. Oral tramadol for the treatment of pain of 7–30 days' duration in children. *Anesth Analg* 2003;96:78–81.
39. Tobias JD. Tramadol for postoperative analgesia in adolescents following orthopedic surgery in a third world country. *Amer J Pain Manage* 1996;6:51–53.
40. Viitanen H, Annila P. Analgesic efficacy of tramadol 2 mg kg(−1) for paediatric day-case adenoidectomy. *Br J Anaesth* 2001;86:572–575.
41. Tobias JD. Seizure after overdose of tramadol. *South Med J* 1997;90:826–827.
42. Bosenberg AT, Ratcliffe S. The respiratory effects of tramadol in children under halothane an anaesthesia. *Anaesthesia* 1998;53:960–964.
43. Maunuksela EL, Ryhanen P, Janhunen L. Efficacy of rectal ibuprofen in controlling postoperative pain in children. *Can J Anaesth* 1992;39:226–230.
44. Sims C, Johnson CM, Bergesio R, et al. Rectal indomethacin for analgesia after appendicectomy in children. *Anaesth Intensive Care* 1994;22:272–275.
45. Vetter TR, Heiner EJ. Intravenous ketorolac as an adjuvant to pediatric patient-controlled analgesia with morphine. *J Clin Anesth* 1994;6:110–113.
46. Dsida RM, Wheeler M, Birmingham PK, et al. Age-stratified pharmacokinetics of ketorolac tromethamine in pediatric surgical patients. *Anesth Analg* 2002;94:266–270.
47. Reuben SS, Connelly NR, Lurie S, et al. Dose-response of ketorolac as an adjunct to patient-controlled analgesia morphine in patients after spinal fusion surgery. *Anesth Analg* 1998;87:98–102.
48. Burd RS, Tobias JD. Ketorolac for pain management after abdominal surgical procedures in infants. *South Med J* 2002;95:331–333.
49. Moffett BS, Wann TI, Carberry KE, et al. Safety of ketorolac in neonates and infants after cardiac surgery. *Paediatr Anaesth* 2006;16:424–428.
50. Gupta A, Daggett C, Drant S, et al. Prospective randomized trial of ketorolac after congenital heart surgery. *J Cardiothorac Vasc Anesth* 2004;18:454–457.
51. Gupta A, Daggett C, Ludwick J, et al. Ketorolac after congenital heart surgery: Does it increase the risk of significant bleeding complications? *Paediatr Anaesth* 2005;15:139–142.
52. Munro HM, Walton SR, Malviya S, et al. Low-dose ketorolac improves analgesia and reduces morphine requirements following posterior spinal fusion in adolescents. *Can J Anaesth* 2002;49:461–466.
53. Vitale MG, Choe JC, Hwang MW, et al. Use of ketorolac tromethamine in children undergoing scoliosis surgery. an analysis of complications. *Spine J* 2003;3:55–62.
54. Houck CS, Wilder RT, McDermott JS, et al. Safety of IV ketorolac therapy in children and cost savings with a unit dosing system. *J Pediatr* 1996;129:292–296.
55. Glassman SD, Rose SM, Dimar JR, et al. The effect of postoperative non-steroidal anti-inflammatory drug administration on spinal fusion. *Spine* 1998;23:834–838.
56. Foster PN, Williams JG. Bradycardia following IV ketorolac in children. *Eur J Anaesthesiol* 1997;14:307–309.
57. Bonabello A, Galmozzi MR, Canaparo R, et al. Dexibuprofen (S+-isomer ibuprofen) reduces gastric damage and improves analgesic and antiinflammatory effects in rodents. *Anesth Analg* 2003;97:402–408.
58. Joshi W, Connelly NR, Reuben SS, et al. An evaluation of the safety and efficacy of administering rofecoxib for postoperative pain management. *Anesth Analg* 2003;97:35–38.
59. Howard PA, Delafontaine P. Nonsteroidal anti-Inflammatory drugs and cardiovascular risk. *J Am Coll Cardiol* 2004;43:519–525.
60. Konstam MA, Weir MR, Reicin A, et al. Cardiovascular thrombotic events in controlled, clinical trials of rofecoxib. *Circulation* 2001;104:2280–2288.
61. Solomon DH, Glynn RJ, Levin R, et al. Nonsteroidal anti-inflammatory drug use and acute myocardial infarction. *Arch Intern Med* 2002;162:1099–1104.

62. Dalens BJ, Pinard AM, Letourneau DR, et al. Prevention of emergence agitation after sevoflurane anesthesia for pediatric cerebral magnetic resonance imaging by small doses of ketamine or nalbuphine administered just before discontinuing anesthesia. *Anesth Analg* 2006;102:1056–1061.

63. Tobias JD. Patient-controlled analgesia using fentanyl in pediatric patients with sickle-cell vaso-occlusive crisis. *Amer J Pain Manage* 2000;10:149–153.

64. Tobias JD, Baker DK. Patient-controlled analgesia with fentanyl in children. *Clin Pediatr (Phila)* 1992;31:177–179.

65. Ross AK, Davis PJ, Dear GD, et al. Pharmacokinetics of remifentanil in anesthetized pediatric patients undergoing elective surgery or diagnostic procedures. *Anesth Analg* 2001;93:1393–1401.

66. Egan TD, Lemmens HJ, Fiset P, et al. The pharmacokinetics of the new short-acting opioid remifentanil (GI87084B) in healthy adult male volunteers. *Anesthesiology* 1993;79:881–892.

67. Tobias JD. Remifentanil: Applications in the pediatric ICU population. *Amer J Pain Manage* 1998;8:114–117.

68. Crawford MW, Hickey C, Zaarour C, et al. Development of acute opioid tolerance during infusion of remifentanil for pediatric scoliosis surgery. *Anesth Analg* 2006;102:1662–1667.

69. Lynn AM, Opheim KE, Tyler DC. Morphine infusion after pediatric cardiac surgery. *Crit Care Med* 1984;12:863–866.

70. Lynn AM, Nespeca MK, Bratton SL, et al. Ventilatory effects of morphine infusions in cyanotic versus acyanotic infants after thoracotomy. *Paediatr Anaesth* 2003;13:12–17.

71. MacGregor R, Evans D, Sugden D, et al. Outcome at 5–6 years of prematurely born children who received morphine as neonates. *Arch Dis Child Fetal Neonatal Ed* 1998;79:F40–43.

72. Franck LS, Vilardi J, Durand D, et al. Opioid withdrawal in neonates after continuous infusions of morphine or fentanyl during extracorporeal membrane oxygenation. *Am J Crit Care* 1998;7:364–369.

73. Lynn AM, Slattery JT. Morphine pharmacokinetics in early infancy. *Anesthesiology* 1987;66:136–139.

74. Vandeberghe H, MacLeod S, Chinyangra H, et al. Pharmacokinetics of IV morphine in balanced anesthesia studies in children. *Drug Metabol Rev* 1983;14:887–903.

75. Hall RW, Kronsberg SS, Barton BA, et al. Morphine, hypotension, and adverse outcomes among preterm neonates: who's to blame? Secondary results from the NEOPAIN trial. *Pediatrics* 2005;115:1351–1359.

76. Vetter TR. Pediatric patient-controlled analgesia with morphine versus meperidine. *J Pain Symptom Manage* 1992;7:204–208.

77. Berde CB, Beyer JE, Bournaki MC, et al. Comparison of morphine and methadone for prevention of postoperative pain in 3- to 7-year-old children. *J Pediatr* 1991;119:136–141.

78. Berde CB, Lehn BM, Yee JD, et al. Patient-controlled analgesia in children and adolescents: A randomized, prospective comparison with intramuscular administration of morphine for postoperative analgesia. *J Pediatr* 1991;118:460–466.

79. Doyle E, Robinson D, Morton NS. Comparison of patient-controlled analgesia with and without a background infusion after lower abdominal surgery in children. *Br J Anaesth* 1993;71:670–673.

80. Doyle E, Harper I, Morton NS. Patient-controlled analgesia with low dose background infusions after lower abdominal surgery in children. *Br J Anaesth* 1993;71:818–822.

81. Murphy DF, Graziotti P, Chalkiadis G, et al. Patient-controlled analgesia: A comparison with nurse-controlled IV opioid infusions. *Anaesth Intensive Care* 1994;22:589–592.

82. Monitto CL, Greenberg RS, Kost-Byerly S, et al. The safety and efficacy of parent-/nurse-controlled analgesia in patients less than six years of age. *Anesth Analg* 2000;91:573–579.

83. Lloyd TD, Orr S, Skett P, et al. Cryopreservation of hepatocytes: A review of current methods for banking. *Cell Tissue Bank* 2003;4:3–15.

84. Tobias JD. The non-IV administration of opioids in children. *Am J Anesthesiol* 1997;24:254–263.

85. Litman RS, Shapiro BS. Oral patient-controlled analgesia in adolescents. *J Pain Symptom Manage* 1992;7:78–81.

86. Gourlay GK, Cherry DA, Cousins MJ. A comparative study of the efficacy and pharmacokinetics of oral methadone and morphine in the treatment of severe pain in patients with cancer. *Pain* 1986;25:297–312.

87. Doyle E, Morton NS, McNicol LR. Comparison of patient-controlled analgesia in children by i.v. and s.c. routes of administration. *Br J Anaesth* 1994;72:533–536.

88. Lamacraft G, Cooper MG, Cavalletto BP. Subcutaneous cannulae for morphine boluses in children: Assessment of a technique. *J Pain Symptom Manage* 1997;13:43–49.

89. Dietrich CC, Tobias JD. Subcutaneous fentanyl infusions in the pediatric population. *Amer J Pain Manage* 2003;13:146–150.

90. Brown KA, Laferriere A, Lakheeram I, et al. Recurrent hypoxemia in children is associated with increased analgesic sensitivity to opiates. *Anesthesiology* 2006;105:665–669.

91. Chumpa A, Kaplan RL, Burns MM, et al. Nalmefene for elective reversal of procedural sedation in children. *Am J Emerg Med* 2001;19:545–548.

92. Tobias JD. Tolerance, withdrawal, and physical dependency after long-term sedation and analgesia of children in the pediatric intensive care unit. *Crit Care Med* 2000;28:2122–2132.

93. Berde CB, Sethna NF, Yemen TA. Continuous epidural bupivacaine-fentanyl infusions in children following ureteral reimplantation. *Anesth Analg* 1990;73:A1128.

94. Desparmet J, Meistelman C, Barre J, et al. Continuous epidural infusion of bupivacaine for postoperative pain relief in children. *Anesthesiology* 1987;67:108–110.

95. Ecoffey C, Dubousset AM, Samii K. Lumbar and thoracic epidural anesthesia for urologic and upper abdominal surgery in infants and children. *Anesthesiology* 1986;65:87–90.

96. Meignier M, Souron R, Le Neel JC. Postoperative dorsal epidural analgesia in the child with respiratory disabilities. *Anesthesiology* 1983;59:473–475.

97. Bosenberg AT, Hadley GP, Murray WB. Postoperative ventilation requirements following esophageal atresia repair. *J Pain Symptom Manage* 1991;6:209.

98. McNeely JK, Farber NE, Rusy LM, et al. Epidural analgesia improves outcome following pediatric fundoplication. A retrospective analysis. *Reg Anesth* 1997;22:16–23.

99. Bosenberg AT, Bland BA, Schulte-Steinberg O, et al. Thoracic epidural anesthesia via caudal route in infants. *Anesthesiology* 1988;69:265–269.

100. Blank JW, Houck CS, McClain BC, et al. Cephalad advancement of epidural catheters: radiographic correlation. *Anesthesiology* 1994;81:A1345.

101. Valairucha S, Seefelder C, Houck CS. Thoracic epidural catheters placed by the caudal route in infants: The importance of radiographic confirmation. *Paediatr Anaesth* 2002;12:424–428.

102. Desparmet J, Mateo J, Ecoffey C, et al. Efficacy of an epidural test dose in children anesthetized with halothane. *Anesthesiology* 1990;72:249–251.

103. Sethna NF, Sullivan L, Retik A, et al. Efficacy of simulated epinephrine-containing epidural test dose after IV atropine during isoflurane anesthesia in children. *Reg Anesth Pain Med* 2000;25:566–572.

104. Bosenberg AT. Lower limb nerve blocks in children using unsheathed needles and a nerve stimulator. *Anaesthesia* 1995;50:206–210.

105. Dalens B, Bazin JE, Haberer JP. Epidural bubbles as a cause of incomplete analgesia during epidural anesthesia. *Anesth Analg* 1987;66:679–683.

106. Sethna NF, Berde CB. Venous air embolism during identification of the epidural space in children. *Anesth Analg* 1993;76:925–927.

107. Patel N, Smith CE, Pinchak AC, et al. The influence of tape type and of skin preparation on the force required to dislodge angiocatheters. *Can J Anaesth* 1994;41:738–741.

108. Vas L, Raghavendran S, Hosalkar H, et al. A study of epidural pressures in infants. *Paediatr Anaesth* 2001;11:575–583.

109. Oberlander TF, Berde CB, Lam KH, et al. Infants tolerate spinal anesthesia with minimal overall autonomic changes: Analysis of heart rate variability in former premature infants undergoing hernia repair. *Anesth Analg* 1995;80:20–27.

110. Attia J, Ecoffey C, Sandouk P, et al. Epidural morphine in children: pharmacokinetics and CO$_2$ sensitivity. *Anesthesiology* 1986;65:590–594.

111. Krane EJ, Jacobson LE, Lynn AM, et al. Caudal morphine for postoperative analgesia in children: A comparison with caudal bupivacaine and IV morphine. *Anesth Analg* 1987;66:647–653.

112. Krane EJ. Delayed respiratory depression in a child after caudal epidural morphine. *Anesth Analg* 1988;67:79–82.

113. Valley RD, Bailey AG. Caudal morphine for postoperative analgesia in infants and children: A report of 138 cases. *Anesth Analg* 1991;72:120–124.

114. Krane EJ, Tyler DC, Jacobson LE. The dose response of caudal morphine in children. *Anesthesiology* 1989;71:48–52.

115. Chaplan SR, Duncan SR, Brodsky JB, et al. Morphine and hydromorphone epidural analgesia. A prospective, randomized comparison. *Anesthesiology* 1992;77:1090–1094.

116. Houck CS, McClain BC, Wilder RT, et al. The dose response of epidural hydromorphone in children. *Anesthesiology* 1994;81:A1346.

117. Aantaa R, Scheinin M. Alpha 2-adrenergic agents in anaesthesia. *Acta Anaesthesiol Scand* 1993;37:433–448.

118. Eisenach J, Detweiler D, Hood D. Hemodynamic and analgesic actions of epidurally administered clonidine. *Anesthesiology* 1993;78:277–287.

119. Maze M. ASA Refresher Course Lectures. 1992;274:1–7.

120. Maze M, Tranquilli W. Alpha-2 adrenoceptor agonists: Defining the role in clinical anesthesia. *Anesthesiology* 1991;74:581–605.

121. De Kock M, Crochet B, Morimont C, et al. Intravenous or epidural clonidine for intra- and postoperative analgesia. *Anesthesiology* 1993;79:525–531.

122. Ivani G, Bergendahl HT, Lampugnani E, et al. Plasma levels of clonidine following epidural bolus injection in children. *Acta Anaesthesiol Scand* 1998;42:306–311.

123. Ivani G, Conio A, De Negri P, et al. Spinal versus peripheral effects of adjunct clonidine: Comparison of the analgesic effect of a ropivacaine-clonidine mixture when administered as a caudal or ilioinguinal-iliohypogastric nerve blockade for inguinal surgery in children. *Paediatr Anaesth* 2002;12:680–684.

124. Ivani G, Mattioli G, Rega M, et al. Clonidine-mepivacaine mixture vs plain mepivacaine in paediatric surgery. *Paediatr Anaesth* 1996;6:111–114.

125. Jamali S, Monin S, Begon C, et al. Clonidine in pediatric caudal anesthesia. *Anesth Analg* 1994;78:663–666.
126. Klimscha W, Chiari A, Michalek-Sauberer A, et al. The efficacy and safety of a clonidine/bupivacaine combination in caudal blockade for pediatric hernia repair. *Anesth Analg* 1998;86:54–61.
127. Lee JJ, Rubin AP. Comparison of a bupivacaine-clonidine mixture with plain bupivacaine for caudal analgesia in children. *Br J Anaesth* 1994;72:258–262.
128. Motsch J, Bottiger BW, Bach A, et al. Caudal clonidine and bupivacaine for combined epidural and general anaesthesia in children. *Acta Anaesthesiol Scand* 1997;41:877–883.
129. De Negri P, Ivani G, Visconti C, et al. The dose-response relationship for clonidine added to a postoperative continuous epidural infusion of ropivacaine in children. *Anesth Analg* 2001;93:71–76.
130. Cucchiaro G, Dagher C, Baujard C, et al. Side-effects of postoperative epidural analgesia in children: A randomized study comparing morphine and clonidine. *Paediatr Anaesth* 2003;13:318–323.
131. Dupeyrat A, Goujard E, Muret J, et al. Transcutaneous CO2 tension effects of clonidine in paediatric caudal analgesia. *Paediatr Anaesth* 1998;8:145–148.
132. Bailey PL, Sperry RJ, Johnson GK, et al. Respiratory effects of clonidine alone and combined with morphine, in humans. *Anesthesiology* 1991;74:43–48.
133. Bouchut JC, Dubois R, Godard J. Clonidine in preterm-infant caudal anesthesia may be responsible for postoperative apnea. *Reg Anesth Pain Med* 2001;26:83–85.
134. Breschan C, Krumpholz R, Likar R, et al. Can a dose of 2 microg.kg(−1) caudal clonidine cause respiratory depression in neonates? *Paediatr Anaesth* 1999;9:81–83.
135. Mansouri J, Panigrahy A, Assmann SF, et al. Distribution of alpha 2–adrenergic receptor binding in the developing human brainstem. *Pediatr Dev Pathol* 2001;4:222–236.
136. Agarwal R, Gutlove DP, Lockhart CH. Seizures occurring in pediatric patients receiving continuous infusion of bupivacaine. *Anesth Analg* 1992;75:284–286.
137. McCloskey JJ, Haun SE, Deshpande JK. Bupivacaine toxicity secondary to continuous caudal epidural infusion in children. *Anesth Analg* 1992;75:287–290.
138. Mazoit JX, Denson DD, Samii K. Pharmacokinetics of bupivacaine following caudal anesthesia in infants. *Anesthesiology* 1988;68:387–391.
139. Larsson BA, Lonnqvist PA, Olsson GL. Plasma concentrations of bupivacaine in neonates after continuous epidural infusion. *Anesth Analg* 1997;84:501–505.
140. Luz G, Innerhofer P, Bachmann B, et al. Bupivacaine plasma concentrations during continuous epidural anesthesia in infants and children. *Anesth Analg* 1996;82:231–234.
141. Henderson K, Sethna NF, Berde CB. Continuous caudal anesthesia for inguinal hernia repair in former preterm infants. *J Clin Anesth* 1993;5:129–133.
142. Scott DB, Lee A, Fagan D, et al. Acute toxicity of ropivacaine compared with that of bupivacaine. *Anesth Analg* 1989;69:563–569.
143. Kohane DS, Sankar WN, Shubina M, et al. Sciatic nerve blockade in infant, adolescent, and adult rats: A comparison of ropivacaine with bupivacaine. *Anesthesiology* 1998;89:1199–1208; discussion 1110A.
144. Breschan C, Jost R, Krumpholz R, et al. A prospective study comparing the analgesic efficacy of levobupivacaine, ropivacaine and bupivacaine in pediatric patients undergoing caudal blockade. *Paediatr Anaesth* 2005;15:301–306.
145. De Negri P, Ivani G, Tirri T, et al. A comparison of epidural bupivacaine, levobupivacaine, and ropivacaine on postoperative analgesia and motor blockade. *Anesth Analg* 2004;99:45–48.
146. Khalil S, Lingadevaru H, Bolos M, et al. Caudal regional anesthesia, ropivacaine concentration, postoperative analgesia, and infants. *Anesth Analg* 2006;102:395–399.
147. McCann ME, Sethna NF, Mazoit JX, et al. The pharmacokinetics of epidural ropivacaine in infants and young children. *Anesth Analg* 2001;93:893–897.
148. Bosenberg AT, Thomas J, Cronje L, et al. Pharmacokinetics and efficacy of ropivacaine for continuous epidural infusion in neonates and infants. *Paediatr Anaesth* 2005;15:739–749.
149. Ivani G, De Negri P, Lonnqvist PA, et al. A comparison of three different concentrations of levobupivacaine for caudal block in children. *Anesth Analg* 2003;97:368–371, table of contents.
150. Chalkiadis GA, Anderson BJ. Age and size are the major covariates for prediction of levobupivacaine clearance in children. *Paediatr Anaesth* 2006;16:275–282.
151. Elliott AM, Smith BH, Penny KI et al. The epidemiology of chronic pain in the community. *Lancet* 1999;354:1248–1252.
152. Wong CM, McIntosh N, Menon G, et al. The pain (and stress) in infants in a neonatal intensive care unit. In: Schechter NL, Berde CB, Yaster M, eds. *Pain in Infants, Children and Adolescents*, 2nd ed. Philadelphia: Lippincott, Williams and Wilkins, 2003;669–692.
153. Schechter NL, Berde CB, Yaster M. Pain in infants, children and adolescents: An overview. In: Schechter NL, Berde CB, Yaster M, eds. *Pain in infants, children and adolescents*, 2nd ed. Philadelphia: Lippincott, Williams & Wilkins, 2003;3–18.
154. Schechter NL, Berde CB, Yaster M, eds. *Pain in infants, children and adolescents,* 1st ed. Philadelphia: Lippincott, Williams & Wilkins, 1993.
155. McGrath PJ, Unruh A. *Pain in children and adolescents.* Amsterdam: Elsevier Science, 1987.
156. Fitzgerald M. Developmental biology of inflammatory pain. *Br J Anaesth* 1995;75:177–185.
157. Fitzgerald M. Painful beginnings. *Pain* 2004;110:508–509.
158. Taddio A, Goldbach M, Ipp M, et al. Effect of neonatal circumcision on pain responses during vaccination in boys. *Lancet* 1995;345: 291–292.
159. Taddio A, Stevens E, Craig K, et al. Efficacy and safety of lidocaine-prilocaine cream for pain during circumcision. *N Engl J Med* 1997;336:1197–201.
160. Andrews KA, Desai D, Dhillon HK, et al. Abdominal sensitivity in the first year of life: Comparison of infants with and without prenatally diagnosed unilateral hydronephrosis. *Pain* 2002;100:35–46.
161. Schmelzle-Lubiecki BM, Campbell KA, Howard RH, et al. Long-term consequences of early infant injury and trauma upon somatosensory processing. *Eur J Pain* 2007;11:799–809.
162. McGrath PA, Brown SC. Quantitative Sensory Testing in children: Practical considerations for research and clinical practice. *Pain* 2006;123:1–2.
163. Alvares D, Torsney C, Beland B, et al. Modelling the prolonged effects of neonatal pain. *Prog Brain Res* 2000;129:365–373.
164. Ren K, Anseloni V, Zou SP, et al. Characterization of basal and re-inflammation-associated long-term alteration in pain responsivity following short-lasting neonatal local inflammatory insult. *Pain* 2004;110:588–596.
165. Eccleston C, Jordan A, McCracken LM, et al. The Bath Adolescent Pain Questionnaire (BAPQ): Development and preliminary psychometric evaluation of an instrument to assess the impact of chronic pain on adolescents. *Pain* 2005;118:263–270.
166. Vetter TR. A primer on health-related quality of life in chronic pain medicine. *Anesth Analg* 2007;104:703–718.
167. Vetter TR. The application of economic evaluation methods in the chronic pain medicine literature. *Anesth Analg* 2007;105:114–118.
168. Vetter TR. A clinical profile of a cohort of patients referred to an anesthesiology-based pediatric chronic pain medicine program. *Anesth Analg* 2008;106:786–794.
169. Geist R. Psychosocial care in the pediatric hospital. The need for scientific validation of clinical and cost effectiveness. *Gen Hosp Psychiatry* 1995; 17:228–234.
170. Keren R, Pati S, Feudtner C. The generation gap: Differences between children and adults pertinent to economic evaluations of health interventions. *Pharmacoeconomics* 2004;22:71–81.
171. Sleed M, Eccleston C, Beecham J, et al. The economic impact of chronic pain in adolescence: Methodological considerations and a preliminary costs-of-illness study. *Pain* 2005;119:183–190.
172. Palermo TM. Impact of recurrent and chronic pain on child and family daily functioning: A critical review of the literature. *J Dev Behav Pediatr* 2000;21: 58–69.
173. Hunfeld JA, Perquin CW, Hazebroek-Kampschreur AA, et al. Physically unexplained chronic pain and its impact on children and their families: The mother's perception. *Psychol Psychother Theory Res Pract* 2002;75:251–260.
174. Scharff L, Langan N, Rotter N, et al. Psychological, behavioral, and family characteristics of pediatric patients with chronic pain: A 1-year retrospective study and cluster analysis. *Clin J Pain* 2005;21:432–438.
175. Bursch B, Walco GA, Zeltzer L. Clinical assessment and management of chronic pain and pain-associated disability syndrome. *J Dev Behav Pediatr* 1998;19:45–53.
176. Zeltzer L, Bursch B, Walco G. Pain responsiveness and chronic pain: A psychobiological perspective." *J Dev Behav Pediatr* 1997;18:413–422.
177. Bursch B, Joseph MH, Zeltzer LK. Pain-associated disability syndrome. In: Schechter NL, Berde CB, Yaster M, eds., *Pain in infants, children and adolescents*, 2nd ed. Philadelphia: Lippincott, Williams and Wilkins, 2003;841–848.
178. Zeltzer LK, Bush JP, Chen E, et al. A psychobiologic approach to pediatric pain: Part 1. History, physiology, and assessment strategies. *Curr Probl Pediatr* 1997;27:225–253.
179. Goodman JE, McGrath PJ. The epidemiology of pain in children and adolescents: A review. *Pain* 1991;46:247–264.
180. Apley J, Naish N. Recurrent abdominal pain: A field survey of 1,000 school children. *Arch Dis Child* 1958;33:165–170.
181. Oster J. Recurrent abdominal pain, headache and limb pain in children and adolescents. *Pediatrics* 1972;50:429–436.
182. Bille B. A 40 year follow up of school children with migraine. *Cephalalgia* 1997;17:488–491.
183. Coleman WL. Recurrent chest pain in children. *Pediatr Clin North Am* 1984;31:1007–1026.
184. Oster J, Nielson A. Growing pains: A clinical investigation of a school population. *Acta Paediatr Scand* 1972;61:329–334.

185. Scharff L, Leichtner AM, Rappaport LA. Recurrent abdominal pain. In: Schechter N, Berde CB, Yaster M, eds. *Pain in infants, children and adolescents,* 2nd ed. Philadelphia: Lippincott, Williams and Wilkins, 2003:719–731.

186. Perquin CW, Hazebroek-Kampschreur AA, Hunfeld JA, et al. Pain in children and adolescents: A common experience. *Pain* 2000;87:51–58.

187. Roth-Isigkeit A, Thyen U, Raspe HH, et al. Reports of pain among German children and adolescents: An epidemiological study. *Acta Paediatr* 2004;93:258–263.

188. Micheli LJ. Back pain in young athletes. Significant differences from adults in causes and patterns. *Arch Pediatr Adolesc Med* 1995;149:15–18.

189. Berde CB, Lebel A. Complex regional pain syndromes in children and adolescents. *Anesthesiology* 2005;102:252–255.

190. Wilder RT, Berde CB, Wolohan M, et al. Reflex sympathetic dystrophy in children. Clinical characteristics and follow-up of seventy patients. *J Bone Joint Surg* 1992;74:910–919.

191. Schwartzman RJ, Kerrigan J. The movement disorder of reflex sympathetic dystrophy. *Neurology* 1990;40:57–61.

192. Birklein F, Riedl B, Sieweke N, et al. Neurological findings in complex regional pain syndromes–analysis of 145 cases. *Acta Neurol Scand* 2000;101:262–269.

193. Verdugo RJ, Ochoa JL. Abnormal movements in complex regional pain syndrome: Assessment of their nature. *Muscle Nerve* 2000;23:198–205.

194. Ribbers GM, Mulder T, Geurts AC, et al. Reflex sympathetic dystrophy of the left hand and motor impairments of the unaffected right hand: Impaired central motor processing? *Arch Phys Med Rehabil* 2002;83:81–85.

195. Oaklander AL. Progression of dystonia in complex regional pain syndrome. *Neurology* 2004;63:751.

196. Lee BH, Scharff L, Sethna NF, et al. Physical therapy and cognitive-behavioral treatment for complex regional pain syndromes. *J Pediatr* 2002;141:135–140.

197. Sherry DD, Wallace CA, Kelley C, et al. Short- and long-term outcomes of children with complex regional pain syndrome type I treated with exercise therapy. *Clin J Pain* 1999;15:218–223.

198. www.fda.gov/cder/drug/InfoSheets/HCP/antiepilepticsHCP.htm.

199. Dadure C, Motais F, Ricard C, et al. Continuous peripheral nerve blocks at home for treatment of recurrent complex regional pain syndrome I in children. *Anesthesiology* 2005;102:387–391.

200. Kishimoto N, Kato J, Suzuki T, et al. [A case of RSD with complete disappearance of symptoms following IV ketamine infusion combined with stellate ganglion block and continuous epidural block]. *Masui - Jpn J Anesthesiol* 1995;44:1680–1684.

201. Lin TC, Wong CS, Chen FC, et al. Long-term epidural ketamine, morphine and bupivacaine attenuate reflex sympathetic dystrophy neuralgia. *Can J Anaesth* 1998;45:175–177.

202. Ushida T, Tani T, Kanbara T, et al. Analgesic effects of ketamine ointment in patients with complex regional pain syndrome type 1. *Reg Anesth Pain Med* 2002;27:524–528.

203. Suresh S, Wheeler M, Patel A. Case series: IV regional anesthesia with ketorolac and lidocaine: Is it effective for the management of complex regional pain syndrome 1 in children and adolescents? *Anesth Analg* 2003;96:694–695.

204. Olsson GL, Meyerson BA, Linderoth B, et al. Spinal cord stimulation in adolescents with complex regional pain syndrome type 1 (CRPS-I). *Eur J Pain* 2008;12:53–59.

205. Finniss DG, Murphy PM, Brooker C, et al. Complex regional pain syndrome in children and adolescents. *Eur J Pain* 2006;10:767–770.

206. Krane EJ, Heller LB, Pomietto ML. Incidence of phantom sensation and pain in pediatric amputees. *Anesthesiology* 1991;75:A691.

207. Berde CB, Lebel AA, Olsson G. Neuropathic pain in children. In: Schechter NL, Berde CB, Yaster M, eds., *Pain in infants, children and adolescents,* 2nd ed. Philadelphia: Lippincott Williams & Wilkins, 2003:620–638.

208. Wilkins KL, McGrath PJ, Finley GA, et al. Phantom limb sensations and phantom limb pain in child and adolescent amputees. *Pain* 1998;78:7–12.

209. Suresh S, Wheeler M. Practical pediatric regional anesthesia. *Anesthesiol Clin North Am* 2002;20:83–113.

210. Suresh S, Voronov P. Head and neck blocks in children: An anatomical and procedural review. *Paediatr Anaesth* 2006;16:910–918.

211. Huertas-Ceballos A, Logan S, Bennett C, et al. Pharmacological interventions for recurrent abdominal pain (RAP) and irritable bowel syndrome (IBS) in childhood. *Cochrane Database Syst Rev* 2008; Issue 1. Art.No.:CD003017. DOI:10.102/14651858.CD003017.pub2.

212. Huertas-Ceballos A, Logan S, Bennett C, et al. Psychosocial interventions for recurrent abdominal pain (RAP) and irritable bowel syndrome (IBS) in childhood. *Cochrane Database Syst Rev* 2008, Issue 1. Art.No.:CD003014. DOI:10.1002/14651858.CD003014.pub2.

213. Drossman DA, Corazziari E, Talley NJ, et al. *The functional gastrointestinal disorders.* Lawrence: Allen Press, Inc, 2000.

214. Apley J. Psychosomatic aspects of gastrointestinal problems in children. *Clin Gastroenterol* 1977;6:311–320.

215. American Academy of *Pediatrics* Subcommittee on Chronic Abdominal Pain. Chronic abdominal pain in children. *Pediatrics* 2005;115:812–815.

216. Yunus MB, Masi AT. Juvenile primary fibromyalgia syndrome. A clinical study of thirty-three patients and matched normal controls. *Arthritis Rheum* 1985;28:138–145.

217. Gedalia A, Garcia CO, Molina JF, et al. Fibromyalgia syndrome: Experience in a pediatric rheumatology clinic. *Clin Exp Rheumatol* 2000;18:415–419.

218. Siegel DM, Janeway D, Baum J. Fibromyalgia syndrome in children and adolescents: Clinical features at presentation and status at follow-up. *Pediatrics* 1998;101:377–382.

219. Roizenblatt S, Tufik S, Goldenberg J, et al. Juvenile fibromyalgia: Clinical and polysomnographic aspects. *J Rheumatol* 1997;24:579–585.

220. Tayag-Kier CE, Keenan GF, Scalzi LV, et al. Sleep and periodic limb movement in sleep in juvenile fibromyalgia. *Pediatrics* 2000;106:E70.

221. Buskila D, Neumann L, Hershman E, et al. Fibromyalgia syndrome in children–an outcome study. *J Rheumatol* 1995;22:525–528.

222. Walco GA, Ilowite NT. Cognitive-behavioral intervention for juvenile primary fibromyalgia syndrome. *J Rheumatol* 1992;19:1617–1619.

223. Degotardi PJ, Klass ES, Rosenberg BS, et al. Development and evaluation of a cognitive-behavioral intervention for juvenile fibromyalgia. *J Pediatr Psychol* 2006;31:714–723.

224. Robinson WM, Ravilly S, Berde C, et al. End-of-life care in cystic fibrosis. *Pediatrics* 1997;100:205–209.

225. Ravilly S, Robinson W, Suresh S, et al. Chronic pain in cystic fibrosis. *Pediatrics* 1996;98:741–747.

226. Koh JL, Harrison D, Palermo TM, et al. Assessment of acute and chronic pain symptoms in children with cystic fibrosis. *Pediatr Pulmonol* 2005;40:330–335.

227. Lugo RA, Satterfield KL, Kern SE. Pharmacokinetics of methadone. *J Pain Palliat Care Pharmacother* 2005;19:13–24.

228. Byrne A, Stimmel B. Methadone and QTc prolongation. *Lancet* 2007;369:366; author reply 366–367.

229. Ferrari A, Coccia CPR, Bertolini A, et al. Methadone—Metabolism, pharmacokinetics and interactions. *Pharmacol Res* 2004;50:551–559.

230. Yaster M, Kost-Byerly S, Maxwell LG. The management of pain in sickle cell disease. *Pediatr Clin North Am* 2000;47:699–710.

231. Yaster M, Tobin JR, Billett C, et al. Epidural analgesia in the management of severe vaso-occlusive sickle cell crisis. *Pediatrics* 1994;93:310–315.

232. Ganesh A, Maxwell LG. Pathophysiology and management of opioid-induced pruritus. *Drugs* 2007;67:2323–2333.

233. Maxwell LG, Kaufmann SC, Pitzer S, et al. The effects of a small-dose naloxone infusion on opioid-induced side effects and analgesia in children and adolescents treated with IV patient-controlled analgesia: A double-blind, prospective, randomized, controlled study. *Anesth Analg* 2005;100:953–958.

234. Gibson N, Graham HK, Love S. Botulinum toxin A in the management of focal muscle overactivity in children with cerebral palsy. *Disabil Rehabil* 2007;29:1813–1822.

235. Hoving MA, van Raak EPM, Spincemaille GHJJ, et al. Intrathecal baclofen in children with spastic cerebral palsy: A double-blind, randomized, placebo-controlled, dose-finding study. *Dev Med Child Neurol* 2007;49:654–659.

236. Kolaski K, Logan LR. A review of the complications of intrathecal baclofen in patients with cerebral palsy. *Neurorehabilitation* 2007;22:383–395.

237. Sgouros S. Surgical management of spasticity of cerebral origin in children. *Acta Neurochir* 2007;97:193–203.

238. Collins JJ. Cancer pain management in children. *Eur J Pain* 2001;5:37–41.

239. Collins JJ, Weisman SJ. Management of pain in childhood cancer. In: Schechter N, Berde CB, Yaster M, eds., *Pain in infants children and adolescents,* 2nd ed. Philadelphia: Lippincott, Williams and Wilkens, 2003:517–538.

240. Miser AW, McCalla J, Dothage JA, et al. Pain as a presenting symptom in children and young adults with newly diagnosed malignancy. *Pain* 1987;29:85–90.

241. Collins JJ, Byrnes ME, Dunkel IJ, et al. The measurement of symptoms in children with cancer. *J Pain Symptom Manage* 2000;19:363–377.

242. Ljungman G, Gordh T, Sorensen S, et al. Pain variations during cancer treatment in children: A descriptive survey. *Pediatr Hematol Oncol* 2000;17:211–221.

243. Goldman A, Hain R, Liben S, eds. *Oxford Textbook of Palliative Care for Children.* New York: Oxford University Press, 2006.

244. Miser AW, Davis DM, Hughes CS, et al. Continuous subcutaneous infusion of morphine in children with cancer. *Am J Dis Child* 1983;137:383–385.

245. Collins JJ, Grier HE, Kinney HC et al. Control of severe pain in children with terminal malignancy. *J Pediatr* 1995;126:653–657.

246. Stevens M, Dalla Pozza L, Cavalletto B, et al. Pain and symptom control in paediatric palliative care. *Cancer Surv* 1994;21:211–231.

247. Zernikow B, Smale H, Michel E, et al. Paediatric cancer pain management using the WHO analgesic ladder—results of a prospective analysis from 2265 treatment days during a quality improvement study. *Eur J Pain* 2006;10:587–595.

248. Goldman A. Home care of the dying child. *J Palliat Care* 1996;12:16–19.

249. Hunt A, Joel S, Dick G, et al. Population pharmacokinetics of oral morphine and its glucuronides in children receiving morphine as immediate-release

liquid or sustained-release tablets for cancer pain. *J Pediatr* 1999;135: 47–55.

250. Yaster M, Kost-Byerly S, Maxwell LG. Opioid agonists and antagonists. In: Schechter N, Berde CB, Yaster M, eds., *Pain in infants, children and adolescents*, 2nd ed. Philadelphia: Lippincott, Williams and Wilkins: 181–224.

251. Berde CB. Pediatric postoperative pain management. *Pediatr Clin North Am* 1989;36:921–940.

252. Shannon M, Berde CB. Pharmacologic management of pain in children and adolescents. *Pediatr Clin North Am* 1989;36:855–871.

253. Wolfe J, Grier HE, Klar N, et al. Symptoms and suffering at the end of life in children with cancer. *N Engl J Med* 2000;342:326–333.

254. Daviss WB, Patel NC, Robb AS, et al. Clonidine for attention-deficit/hyperactivity disorder: II. ECG changes and adverse events analysis. *J Am Acad Child Adolesc Psychiatry* 2008;47:189–198.

255. Reineke-Bracke H, Radbruch L, Elsner F. Treatment of fatigue: Modafinil, methylphenidate, and goals of care. *J Palliative Med* 2006;9:1210–1214.

256. Breitbart W, Alici-Evcimen Y. Update on psychotropic medications for cancer-related fatigue. *J Nat Comp Canc Net* 2007;5:1081–1091.

257. Carroll JK, Kohli S, Mustian KM, et al. Pharmacologic treatment of cancer-related fatigue. *Oncologist* 2007;12:43–51.

258. Collins JJ, Dunket IJ, Gupta SK, et al. Transdermal fentanyl in children with cancer pain: feasibility, tolerability, and pharmacokinetic correlates. *J Pediatr* 1999;134:319–323.

259. Malviya S, Voepel-Lewis T, Huntington J, et al. Effects of anesthetic technique on side effects associated with fentanyl Oralet premedication. *J Clin Anesth* 1997;9:374–378.

260. Friedrichsdorf SJ, Finney D, Bergin M, et al. Breakthrough pain in children with cancer. *J Pain Symptom Manage* 2007;34:209–216.

261. Bell RF, Eccleston C, Calso E. Ketamine as an adjuvant to opioids for cancer pain. *Cochrane Database Syst Rev* 2003;1: CD003351.DOI: 10.1002/14651858.CD003351.

262. Finkel JC, Pestieau SR, Quezado ZMN. Ketamine as an adjuvant for treatment of cancer pain in children and adolescents. *J Pain* 2007;8:515–521.

263. Collins JJ, Geake J, Grier HE, et al. Patient-controlled analgesia for mucositis pain in children: A three-period crossover study comparing morphine and hydromorphone. *J Pediatr* 1996;129:722–728.

264. Voepel-Lewis T, Marinkovic A, Kostrzewa A, et al. The prevalence of and risk factors for adverse events in children receiving patient-controlled analgesia by proxy or patient-controlled analgesia after surgery. *Anesth Analg* 2008;107:70–75.

265. Joint Commission on Accreditation of Healthcare Organizations. Patient controlled analgesia by proxy. *Jt Comm Perspect* 2005;25:10–11.

266. Kenagy A, Turner H. Pediatric patient-controlled analgesia by proxy. *AACN Adv Crit Care* 2007;18:361–365.

267. Wuhrman E, Cooney MF, Dunwoody CJ, et al. Authorized and unauthorized ("PCA by proxy") dosing of analgesic infusion pumps: Position statement with clinical practice recommendations. *Pain Manag Nursing* 2007;8:4–11.

268. Moryl N, Coyle N, Foley KM. Managing an acute pain crisis in a patient with advanced cancer: This is as much of a crisis as a code. *JAMA* 2008;299:1457–1467.

269. McNicol E, Horowicz-Mehler N, Fisk RA, et al. Management of opioid side effects in cancer-related and chronic noncancer pain: A systematic review. *J Pain* 2003;4:231–256.

270. Saroyan JM, Schechter WS, Tresgallo ME, et al. Role of intraspinal analgesia in terminal pediatric malignancy. *J Clin Oncol* 2005;23:1318–1321.

271. Smith TJ, Staats PS, Deer T et al. Randomized clinical trial of an implantable drug delivery system compared with comprehensive medical management for refractory cancer pain: Impact on pain, drug related toxicity, and survival. *J Clin Oncol* 2002;20:4040–4049.

272. Tanelian D, Cousins MJ. Celiac plexus block following high dose opiates for chronic non-cancer pain in a four-year-old child. *J Pain Symptom Manage* 1989;4:82–85.

273. Heikenen JB, Pohl JF, Werlin SL, et al. Octreotide in pediatric patients. *J Pediatr Gastroenterol Nutr* 2002;35:600–609.

274. Watanabe H, Inoue Y, Uchida K, et al. Octreotide improved the quality of life in a child with malignant bowel obstruction caused by peritoneal dissemination of colon cancer. *J Pediatr Surg* 2007;42:259–260.

CHAPTER 48 ■ THE TREATMENT OF PAIN IN OLDER PATIENTS

ROBERT D. HELME AND JULIA A. FLEMING

This chapter summarizes strategies applicable to the pain management, including neural blockade, in older patients. Whereas acute pain has a prevalence within the community of approximately 5% at all ages, chronic pain affects approximately 55% of the population older than 65 years (1). Within hospitals, a significant proportion of older people undergo surgical procedures requiring postoperative pain management. Undertreatment of pain is common and may relate to misperceptions regarding pain intensity experienced in the aging population, difficulties assessing pain, concerns regarding adverse effects of analgesic medications, and older patient barriers to expressing pain and requesting treatment. Strategies to manage acute and cancer-related pain are similar across all age groups, although some specific management principles do apply to older patients.

Chronic pain is defined as pain persisting beyond the period of normal recovery after injury. By consensus, this has been taken to be 3 months in the absence of an ongoing cause for the pain. The term *chronic pain* is usually used in the context of persistent pain accompanied by functional disability and adverse psychosocial consequences. Chronic pain is best assessed from a multidisciplinary perspective. Optimal outcomes are likely to be achieved with a seamless blend of anaesthetic interventions, together with pharmacologic, physical, and psychological therapies in a multidisciplinary environment (see Chapter 28 on the multidisciplinary approach). There is a tendency, however, to "medicalize" chronic pain management in older people and insist on prolonged investigations and treatments, often with excessive emphasis on an external controlling approach, whether it be with medication or interventions. When curative approaches are determined not to be feasible or acceptable to the older patient, a symptom management approach should be adopted, aiming to reduce pain to tolerable levels, enhance the individual's coping strategies, and minimize any pain-related handicap.

Although the pathophysiology of experimental pain in older individuals is reasonably well understood, understanding the development and management of chronic pain in older persons remains limited. This chapter summarizes pertinent data in this field and presents a model for the assessment and management of chronic pain in older people.

EPIDEMIOLOGY OF PAIN IN OLDER PEOPLE

We live in an aging world (2). This fact is most apparent in Western countries, notably Europe; for example, in the United Kingdom, the population over 65 years of age will increase from 16% at present to 19% by 2020, and plateau around 23% by 2050. In younger Western societies, such as Australia and the United States, with more postwar immigration and higher birth rates, those over 65 years are projected to increase from 13%, currently, to approximately 17% in 2020, then catch up to the older countries by 2050. In the United States, the population over 85 years is increasing faster than any other age group. Even developing countries are aware of aging in their societies, albeit from a lower starting point. With time, an increasing number of older patients will experience pain after surgery, and develop malignancies, degenerative diseases, or other painful medical conditions. In general, pain is poorly recognized and undertreated in this group. Thus, substantial increases in the numbers of health professionals with the motivation, knowledge, skill, and understanding of the special needs of older persons will be required.

The prevalence of pain in different age groups has been examined in a number of studies. Crook et al. published one of the most widely cited prevalence studies of the effect of age upon pain (3). This telephone survey of a random sample obtained from a group general practitioner list was one of the first studies to clearly demonstrate increased pain complaints with increasing age, and highlighted the importance of pain as a frequent problem for a large number of older people. However, very few respondents were over the age of 80, a problem common to most community-based studies that seek to explore issues relevant to older people. The questions asked in this study regarding the temporal nature of pain were not framed according to the usual definitions of acute and chronic pain, which means their classification of pain as "temporary" or "persistent" is not easily compared with other studies. An intriguing finding was that "temporary" pain had the same prevalence at all ages. This remains the only study in the literature that has reported age-related prevalence figures for acute pain of any type in community practice.

Other studies have not uniformly replicated these results (4,5). Collectively, however, the literature suggests a peak or plateau in the prevalence of pain by age 65 years, at around 55%, and a later decline in reported pain in those over 80 years of age. This is surprising, given that age-related increases in disease prevalence continue into the seventh, eighth, and ninth decades of life. When age-related, progressive severity of disease is taken into account, it appears that the very old do report disproportionately lower levels of pain intensity (6–8).

The most likely reason for the interstudy variation in absolute prevalence figures is the heterogeneity of the survey questions: the pain recall interval, the time in pain within this interval, the severity or interference of the pain in daily life (often recorded as whether the pain is "troubling" or "bothersome"), and the effect of prompting or cueing (for instance, specifically asking about back pain, neck pain, headache, etc.) (1).

Certain trends have emerged from the number of studies that have examined pain at particular body sites. The prevalence of articular joint pain more than doubles in adults over 65 years when compared to young adult samples (9–12). Conversely, the prevalence of headache shows a progressive decrease with increasing age after a peak prevalence at 45 to 50 years of age (9,11). The frequency of facial/dental pain and abdominal/stomach pain also appears to diminish beyond middle age (13). Chest pain probably peaks during late middle age, concurrent with the peak of ischemic heart disease presentation, but declines thereafter despite continuing high mortality from this disease (9). The findings are equivocal with respect to back pain (14), with reports of both an increase (9,10) and decrease (11) in back pain with advancing age. A summary view is that aging to 65 years is associated with an increasing prevalence of chronic pain but not acute pain. Pain in the head, abdomen, and chest is reduced among older people, and joint pain is increased.

Cancer Pain

The incidence of cancer increases with age. In the United States, the rate of malignancy in the older population is nearly 10-fold that in the young, being 2,183 per 100,000 population for people over 65 versus 224 per 100,000 for those under 65 (15). However, cancer-related pain is less well recognized and treated in older persons, and the need for clinicians to facilitate symptom control for elderly patients with cancer is anticipated to steadily increase. As described in Chapter 45 by Burton and Phan, people with cancer may have multiple causes of pain, resulting in deterioration in function, nutrition, and mood. Older individuals may be reticent to seek treatment for pain, and may be reluctant to take medications for pain (16); many other barriers to effective pain management have been highlighted, as discussed later. A study of 1,308 outpatients with metastatic cancer revealed higher reporting of poor pain control in older patients; age over 70 years was predictive of inadequate pain management, with an odds ratio (OR) of 2.4 (17). Data from more than 13,000 aging patients with cancer discharged from hospital to nursing homes revealed that one-third had ongoing daily pain, and, of these, one in four did not receive any analgesic medication (18). Despite ongoing pain, patients older than 85 years were half as likely to receive morphine as those aged 65 to 74 years.

Educational programs targeting clinicians, patients, and caregivers have been identified as a means to improve inadequate cancer pain management in older persons.

Acute Postoperative Pain

In parallel with the occurrence of cancer, the rate of surgical and anesthetic interventions increases with age, with a concomitant increase in numbers of aging patients requiring postoperative analgesia. A survey of anesthetic practice in France during 1996 indicated that the annual rate of anesthetic procedures had increased since 1980, particularly in older age groups, to 25% to 30% of men and 19% to 24% of women over 65 years, compared to an overall rate of 14% (19). Notably, the rate of regional anesthesia rose markedly, to 23% of anesthetic procedures in 1996. As expected, the American Society of Anesthesi-

ologists (ASA) status generally increased with age, reflecting increased comorbidity, although the largest group had ASA II status, indicating the variability of health in the aged. Surgery for ophthalmic, urologic, vascular, cardiac, and pulmonary procedures was more frequent in older patients. It is anticipated that the rate of surgery will continue to increase proportionally in older age groups, relative to the young. Regional anesthetic techniques are frequently used in these older individuals, notably for orthopedic, genito-urologic, abdominal, and gynecologic surgery, and for postoperative pain control that optimizes cognitive function.

Postoperative pain management, surveyed in general terms in Chapter 43 by Macintyre and Scott, is often poorly addressed in the older patient. An analysis of the impact of pain on morbidity after hip fracture in 411 cognitively intact patients with a median age of 82 years indicated that 50% of patients experienced moderate to severe postoperative pain, and 87% received no regular analgesia (20). Increased postoperative pain, but not total opioid dose, was associated with longer hospital stay, delayed ambulation, reduction in rehabilitation, and function impairment at 6 months. Analgesia prescribed only on an as-needed (p.r.n.) basis was associated with increased length of stay and time to ambulation. Some studies indicate that older patients receive less postoperative analgesia (21,22).

THE CONCEPT OF AGING AS APPLIED TO PAIN

Prior to simple assessment of pain, we should have a framework for the management of illness that applies to all older people. Aging involves a progressive generalized impairment of function resulting in a loss of adaptive responses to stress and a growing risk of age-related disease (23). Even more succinctly, aging can be defined as a loss of functional reserve with increasing chronologic age, although functional reserve may also be limited in children. The reasons for functional decline with aging include biological aging, disease, environmental effects on cohorts, and disuse. Biological aging is universal and progressive, and also characterized by degenerative structural change. Theories of the mechanism of biological aging include concepts of ongoing random errors of gene transcription and translation resulting in progressive deterioration of multiple biologic functions, especially immunologic and endocrine, and of a nonrandom species-specific programmed "biological clock" (24).

Biological Aging and Pain

One way of examining the effects of biological aging on pain perception is to use psychophysical measures, most of which have examined pain threshold. A meta-analysis undertaken on age differences in pain threshold has clearly demonstrated an increase in threshold with age, when measured using brief thermal stimuli (25). This increase in pain threshold is attenuated somewhat by increasing the duration of the thermal stimulus, but the difference still persists (26). The central nervous system is also involved in aging processes, and the effects of descending nociceptive inhibitory pathways in the brainstem have also been examined for age-related differences (27). Using a cold immersion technique, it has been shown that young people recruit a descending inhibitory system. In older people, recruitment of these inhibitory pathways was less effective, and increases in pain thresholds were limited in comparison to younger persons. This difference suggests that older people are less able to tolerate a persistent painful stimulus; other literature also supports this concept (25). Overall, therefore, with aging there appears to be diminished function of those descending spinal pathways that modulate the perception of noxious stimuli in the cerebral cortex. The precise nature of these effects remains unexplained; they may be structural or functional in nature. Age-related changes in the pharmacodynamics of central endogenous opioid actions are likely to contribute to these findings (28).

There also appears to be age-related impairment in pain perception mediated differentially by Aδ and C-fibers (29), and in the effectiveness of temporal summation at a spinal cord level (30). Older people rely less upon well-localized Aδ activation and more upon poorly localized C-fiber activation, before reporting the presence of pain (29).

Disease-related Pain

Many age-related diseases are associated with pain. Conversely, many clinical studies of pain and aging suggest there may be reduced pain with increasing age in conditions such as myocardial ischaemia, postoperative and procedural pain, inflammatory disease in the abdomen, and pain associated with malignancy (31). However, these latter findings, generally derived from clinical audit studies, may be misleading because of difficulties in controlling for severity of pathology and uniform application of measurement tools.

Environmental Influences on Pain

Functional declines with age that are the result of environmental effects on cohorts are often difficult to detect. Nevertheless, scrutiny of the literature on prevalence of chronic pain with age by body site reveals distinct differences. Hip, knee, and foot pain increase in prevalence with age as opposed to visceral causes of pain; these joint pains are considered often to be related to physical work in men and ill-fitting shoes in women.

Comorbidity, Beliefs, and Attitudes

The presence of multiple pathologies in older people must be considered in planning an approach to pain management. Both active and inactive comorbidities, in addition to physical and cognitive impairments such as visual impairment, deafness, loss of dexterity, gait impairment, and memory loss need to be taken into account. One also has to ask the question: Is the treatment appropriate for the older person? Specific objectives and treatment goals may vary as a function of age. It is likely that the goals of care will be symptom control and, wherever possible, functional independence rather than cure. The empowerment of patients and caregivers is very important in this age group. It must also be remembered that older cohorts often are unfamiliar with psychological approaches. Some older adults have low self-efficacy for psychological treatment objectives. There are also age-related differences in beliefs and attitudes toward pain. Older people often consider pain to be a normal companion to aging, rather than attributing pain to disease, and they are often focused on past regrets instead of future prospects. The social reinforcers of pain behavior often differ from those seen at younger ages. Litigation and avoidance of work re-

sponsibility are much less evident, whereas the need for social contact, the effects of widowhood, and the solicitous spouse may influence behaviors in response to pain.

An interesting but unanswered question is whether disuse affects the pain experience. Over the last several years, the question of stoicism as it relates to age has been studied (32,33). One attribute of stoicism includes reluctance to label a noxious stimulus as being painful. Older pain-free subjects subjected to an experimental pain stimulus may be reluctant to describe the stimulus as painful. However, when such stoicism is assessed across a wide age range in patients with pain, no age effect is observed. This suggests that reluctance to label may be a consequence of disuse in this age group, due to limited recent experience of pain.

THE BIOPSYCHOSOCIAL CONCEPT OF CHRONIC PAIN IN OLDER PEOPLE

Pain is never a consequence of age alone, and very rarely does it have an entirely psychological genesis in older people. Although maladaptive attitudes or beliefs and inappropriate behaviors often accompany chronic pain in the older population, evidence of either nociceptive or neuropathic activity is found in nearly all situations where chronic pain occurs. The current concept of chronic pain is that cognitions (appraisal of the situation and beliefs about pain and its treatment) are interposed between stimulus and outcome. For all age groups, some beliefs can be particularly counterproductive to effective pain management. These harmful beliefs include the ideas that the pain is due to ongoing damage from disease, that physical activity will make the underlying condition worse, that the individual has no control over the pain, that only medical interventions can relieve the pain, and that the situation is catastrophic. Conversely, other beliefs, including that the individual is able to cope despite pain, often lead to better psychological and functional outcomes. Thus, an approach that targets only the pain stimulus and its nociceptive pathway, without taking into consideration the individual's appraisal of the situation, may lead to suboptimal outcomes.

Chronic pain is frequently associated with mood disturbance (34). Community-based epidemiologic data indicates that mild symptomatic depression affecting quality of life in older people ranges up to 40%. The prevalence of anxiety is less well defined, as the instruments used to determine affective disturbance overlap on these domains. However, in pain clinic samples, older patients generally express less anxiety than their younger counterparts. Other mood states that are rarely pursued during clinical assessment include frustration, anger and demoralization. Validated psychometric instruments that explore these other facets of mood disturbance in older people, such as the Profile of Mood States (35), have not been applied to date in large-scale epidemiologic studies. The physical impact of chronic pain alone is often difficult to differentiate from the physical disability associated with other comorbid medical conditions common in the older population. In a recent epidemiologic survey among community-dwelling Australians, about 60% of the sample aged 65 years and above expressed that pain interfered with their daily activities (1).

The belief systems that modulate the effects of nociceptive inputs are diverse, as indicated in the psychological literature and surveyed in Chapter 35 by Melzack and Katz. The commonest approach is to consider coping strategies, or their converse, catastrophizing behaviors, which may be associated with feelings of despair, fear, or helplessness (34). Other concepts, however, such as stoicism and fear avoidance may also be explored.

A relationship between pain and gender has not been clearly identified in the elderly, although certain conditions are diagnosed more commonly in elderly females, such as joint pain, chronic widespread myofascial pain, and fibromyalgia. Chronic pain is more prevalent in widows living alone than in married women. The effect of ethnicity on pain in older people is not known.

ASSESSMENT

Supplementing the general overview of pain assessment provided in Chapter 35 by Katz and Melzack, a comprehensive detailed approach to the assessment of the older person with pain has recently been prepared and published as an interdisciplinary expert consensus statement (36). This statement contains advice on measurement tools applicable to clinical situations and for research.

Persistent pain may be only one of many factors that modulates the well-being of an older patient. The aging process is associated with multiple social, personal, and health-related losses. Establishing the impact of persistent pain upon overall quality of life is important in planning treatment, and may necessitate a multidisciplinary approach when the patient's pain is resistant to conventional treatment modalities. In practice, the skills of a pain medicine specialist, psychologist, and physiotherapist, all experienced in the care of older people, are com-

plementary and allow a broad multidimensional picture of the impact of pain in the older patient to be assembled. Important contributions to assessment and development of a management plan may be made by a nurse clinician, occupational therapist, and pharmacist. The total time commitment to assessment of a complex patient may be several hours if multidisciplinary assessment is coordinated; full assessment may take several days if personnel are not immediately available. Special attention is required to differentiate the impact of pain on the individual, her social interactions and functional ability, from the impact of other factors.

Domains of Assessment

Any assessment of the older patient in pain should lead to a formulation that includes medical, functional, social, cognitive and mood-related domains (Table 48-1).

The Medical/Physical Assessment

The initial screen should exclude organic causes of pain that require urgent or specific interventions. If the exact pathology cannot be accurately ascertained, however, a diagnosis should not be relentlessly pursued in the absence of features to suggest a deleterious outcome. The lack of a progression of symptoms, or alternately, underlying pathology becoming apparent, may be reassuring. "Red flags" indicative of severe underlying disease include weight loss, chronic ill health, and a history of other systemic illness such as malignancy, progressive neurologic deficit, progressively worsening pain, and increased

---

TABLE 48-1

FORMULATION OF THE PAIN PROBLEM IN OLDER PATIENTS

1. Medical:
   - What is the pathologic process that resulted in the present pain syndrome, and are other pathologies maintaining the pain?
   - Is the pain primarily nociceptive in origin, neuropathic, a combination of both, or unexplained?
   - How many medical comorbidities coexist, and do any comorbidities or their treatment affect the management of pain?
   - Is specific disease management or a symptom management approach required, or both?
   - Are features present that suggest a more sinister pathology?
   - Is polypharmacy an issue complicating the management of the pain problem?
   - What factors are likely to limit compliance?
2. Functional:
   - What are the functional implications of pain? Consider activities of daily living, including instrumental activities for self-care, discretionary and vocational activities, and the ability to attend to health care strategies.
3. Social:
   - What impact does the pain have on social relationships?
   - Are aspects of the relationship maintaining the chronic pain syndrome?
4. Cognition:
   - What beliefs does the patient hold regarding the cause, prognosis, and treatment options of the pain?
   - How do these beliefs interact with her pain?
   - What is the level of cognitive function?
   - Is pain or the consequences of pain influencing cognitive function?
   - Is general cognitive failure, delirium, and/or dementia interfering with assessment, coping, or management?
5. Mood:
   - Is pain associated with depression, anxiety, anger, or other mood disturbance?

intensity of pain at rest. The recurrence of severe pain in an older individual with previously well-controlled pain warrants close reassessment. If a good correlation exists between clinical findings and radiologic studies, specific management of the underlying pathology may be considered, for example, knee joint replacement. Age per se is no excuse to withhold beneficial surgical management. Where curative treatment is not feasible or is declined by the patient, the focus should be on symptom control.

The prevalence and number of medical comorbidities affects treatment outcomes in older persons with pain (37). Drug–illness interactions are also important considerations. Some medications exacerbate common geriatric syndromes; for example, opioids can increase constipation, delirium, or somnolence, and tricyclic antidepressants (TCAs) can worsen obstructive lower urinary tract symptoms, glaucoma, constipation, and postural hypotension. As noted in the following chapter on palliative care, the selection of pharmacologic agent is often based more on suitability and tolerability for the aging individual being treated than on the efficacy of the particular agent for the condition being treated.

Psychological Assessment

Psychological assessment should take into account the affect, pain-related cognitions, and pain-related behaviors of the patient.

Common symptoms in the aging population, such as altered sleep and poor appetite, overlap with those observed in depressed patients. Therefore, the Geriatric Depression Scale (38) was developed with the purpose of focusing on attitudes rather than somatic symptoms. Similarly, the Profile of Mood States gives an overall view of mood and has been validated in older people (35). Establishing any temporal relationship between the pain problem and the mood disorder is important, as treatment of a primary affective disorder requires a different approach from management of pain-related mood disturbance.

Adaptive and maladaptive pain-related cognitions, in the form of beliefs, thoughts, and appraisals, must be identified. Beliefs relating to the meaning of pain and any associated illness, the available modes of treatment, the amount of self-control over pain, and the type of strategies that one can use to cope with pain are important to ascertain. Maladaptive beliefs that can lead to poor outcomes include (a) the intensity of pain correlates with the severity of the underlying illness; (b) severe ongoing pain might represent an undiagnosed cancer or severe ongoing damage; (c) only medications or an operation will resolve the pain; and (d) all physical activity should be limited until pain resolves. Pain-associated behaviors include grimacing, rubbing the affected area, lying down in the presence of company, and avoidance of activity. Avoidance of activity because of a pain-related fear of movement (kinesophobia) may comprise avoidance of all everyday activities or a simple reduction in the frequency or intensity of these activities. An undue emphasis on passive strategies (such as massage, traction, and heat) and overreliance on others to bring the pain under control are maladaptive in the context of chronic pain, because these strategies reinforce one's daily focus on pain. Some individuals have unrealistic beliefs regarding the efficacy of doctors or of prayer.

Catastrophizing about pain, and associated fear and helplessness, is a maladaptive behavior that inhibits independence and the adoption of pain coping strategies. Conversely, cognitive factors that can lead to better outcomes include high self-efficacy (a person's positive appraisal of her ability to undertake coping behaviors), a belief that active strategies (relaxation,

exercise) are helpful, and the patient feeling able to control her own pain. The first and last factors represent an internal locus of control as opposed to an external locus of control, which is also generally maladaptive.

Social Assessment

The support of concerned relatives is often helpful in the rehabilitation of chronic pain sufferers. However, excessively solicitous behavior by relatives and caregivers can result in a worsening of chronic pain and pain behaviors. For example, if a spouse insists on undertaking activities for the patient, deconditioning may occur, resulting in exacerbation of musculoskeletal pain. An expectation of solicitous behavior on the part of the patient can also result in social conflicts. The evaluation should also consider the possibility of caregiver stress, which may adversely impact on the patient's pain severity or cognitions. Social (including economic) factors in pain management are covered in greater detail by Loeser in Chapter 29.

Assessment of Pain in Patients with Delirium and Dementia

Available measurement tools for delirium and dementia do not provide the specificity to differentiate between these conditions nor assign to each a percentage contribution when both are present with enough reliability to enable their use in clinical situations. The clinician relies on clinical acumen to determine the time course of onset of cognitive impairment and the ancillary factors of variability in attention and change in conscious state. Asterixis, or metabolic flap, may be helpful, if present in the examination of the patient with suspected delirium, in raising awareness of an organic mental syndrome.

Given the high prevalence of chronic pain and delirium/dementia among older people, these two problems often coincide. There are many causes of delirium and dementia, and even within a single diagnostic group individuals differ in regard to their cognitive and communication abilities. Dementia is usually associated with impairment of memory, thus compromising the ability to give a pain history. Cognitive impairment is often associated with language impairment; for example, aphasia in vascular dementia and increasing paucity of vocabulary in advanced Alzheimer's disease. Multiple observations may be required for accurate and reliable diagnosis, and a separate history should be sought. The inability of an individual to recall or report pain does not exclude the possibility that her pain is sufficiently severe to warrant treatment.

In patients with delirium and dementia, pain is poorly recognized, difficult to document, and undertreated (36,39–41). The inability of some older people to express their pain and the perception of some clinicians and caregivers that pain is less severe in individuals with cognitive impairment are important barriers to effective pain management in patients with dementia (41). Pain in older people with communication difficulties may present as either silent withdrawal or aggressive agitation, often alternating in the same individual. The first step is adequate assessment for the presence and impact of pain. The problem of severity assessment increases as dementia worsens. For patients who are communicative, the pain intensity scales used in cognitively normal older people are still relevant. There is no consensus as to which scale is the most appropriate in older individuals. There is some suggestion that word descriptor scales are able to be completed more frequently than numerical rating scales in communicative individuals with moderate to severe dementia. It is best to try a number of different scales, and select the instrument the person appears to manage best. In this way, most people with significant cognitive impairment or moderate to severe dementia are still able to have their pain assessed with some degree of accuracy and less observer bias.

In noncommunicative older individuals, as in infants, observer interpretation of pain behavior is used. Some features include facial expressions, such as brow lowering, orbit tightening, raised upper eyelids or eyelid closure; others relate to vocalizations, guarding, or protective posturing, and altered motor activity. Measures and audit tools for these behaviors continue to be developed (36,40–42).

Impact and Assessment of Postoperative Pain

In the older patient, poor postoperative analgesia can increase morbidity, yet pain management may be inadequate because of perceived or actual treatment constraints due to concurrent medical morbidity, polypharmacy, and debility. Suboptimal postoperative analgesia in the aging patient, just as in younger patients (see Chapter 43), is associated with delayed recovery, heightened sympathetic activation, increased cardiopulmonary morbidity, immobility, anxiety, impaired cognition, prolonged hospital stay, and impaired rehabilitation with reduced functional status months after surgery (21). In older patients, chronic musculoskeletal and other pain may be exacerbated in the perioperative period, related to the stress of surgery, operative positioning, and immobility. Optimal outcomes in the older surgical patient require attention to detail in pain management, ongoing assessment, and a coordinated approach to reducing functional disability related to acute postoperative and chronic pain states.

Studies of postoperative pain in the older population echo those of chronic pain in the same population. Acute postoperative pain may be difficult to assess in older patients, particularly in the presence of cognitive impairment. Postoperative pain management after surgery for hip fracture has been extensively studied and serves as a model to inform the principles of postoperative analgesia in older patients. A prospective study of older patients with hip fracture highlighted that pain was undertreated, both before and after surgery, with over 40% of cognitively intact older patients describing their *average* pain intensity as severe or very severe (44). Analgesia was inadequate given the high intensity of pain, with the mean postoperative opioid dose equivalent to 4.1 mg/day morphine in cognitively intact patients and significantly less in patients with advanced dementia, with doses 1.5 mg/day. Analgesics were prescribed at regular intervals for a minority (25%) of patients, despite the predictable nature of pain after hip fracture. Notably a subsequent multicenter prospective cohort study of over 400 older patients after hip fracture indicated a higher, but suboptimal, mean daily morphine dose (12 mg), and a persistent trend for a lack of standing analgesic orders (21). This prospective study also demonstrated the hidden costs of poor postoperative analgesia after hip fracture in terms of longer length of hospital admission, delayed ambulation, and ongoing impairment of mobility at 6 months. Persistent pain was a frequent outcome in the frail older patient (45).

Postoperative cognitive impairment is common in the older patient. Acute delirium, characterized by alterations of consciousness, attention, memory, perception, and sleep, may also occur in older patients after surgery, and this is associated with significantly increased morbidity and mortality (46). Many perioperative events can trigger postoperative delirium, including hypoxemia, medications, fluid and electrolyte imbalance,

metabolic and endocrine derangements, sepsis, sleep deprivation, and physical restraint (47). The impact of anesthetic technique has also been investigated: Regional anesthesia for hip fracture surgery was associated with a reduction in acute postoperative confusion (48). Anticholinergics, TCAs, opioids, and benzodiazepines may precipitate delirium in older patients. The use of the opioid meperidine and benzodiazepines were independently associated with the development of postoperative delirium in elderly patients after orthopedic surgery (49).

The concern that opioids impact adversely on cognition in older patients is a major barrier to effective analgesia. However, pain itself may impair cognition and increase the rate of postoperative delirium (50–54). A systematic review by Fong et al. indicated limited (level II–III) evidence for the impact of postoperative opioids on cognition in older patients (53). In a randomized controlled trial of older patients after knee or hip arthroplasty, sample size was inadequate, and no significant difference in postoperative confusion after morphine or fentanyl patient-controlled analgesia could be determined; confusion was observed in 14% and 4% patients after morphine and fentanyl, respectively, with no difference in pain scores between groups (55). All other studies indicated that meperidine was associated with increased postoperative delirium relative to morphine and other opioids, although analgesic efficacy was not assessed (21,48,56). Subsequent investigations indicated that pain intensity correlated with cognitive decline (50), higher resting pain intensity scores were associated with increased rates of delirium after non–cardiac surgery (51), and suboptimal analgesia was an independent risk factor for postoperative delirium after hip fracture (57).

Because cognitive impairment, delirium, and dementia all impact adversely on pain assessment, their presence must be considered when determining appropriate pain management strategies. Patients with dementia may be unable to clearly express pain, recall episodes of pain, or request analgesia. Patient-controlled analgesia techniques are inappropriate in patients unable to comprehend or recall instructions for their use. Indicators of pain may be subtle, including excessive sleep due to exhaustion from pain, groaning, grimacing, and reluctance to move or be moved (58). Pain-induced behavior may seem irrational and be attributed to dementia (41). Although medical and nursing staff may be concerned that analgesic medications could cause sedation, further deterioration in cognitive state and delirium due to undertreatment of pain must be considered.

MANAGEMENT STRATEGIES

General Strategy

In most cases, the cause of acute pain is apparent following assessment, and the pain is self-limited. When possible, the underlying cause of the pain should be identified and, if possible, rectified. In practice, a short course of symptomatic treatment with analgesia, modified activity, and physical rehabilitation is often adequate. A more comprehensive management approach is required if initial measures fail and pain has become chronic. The aim is to promote self-management by the patient, in active collaboration with the health care team and caregivers. The focus is upon maintaining functional independence. A multidisciplinary approach to the management of chronic pain is recommended if a good response is not achieved by a single clinician. For ease of description, the subsequent discussion divides management into individual conditions and modalities, although frequently the management program is multidimensional from the beginning.

Procedural Modalities of Management

Ongoing pain may warrant consideration of anesthetic or surgical interventions. Hip or knee arthoplasty are good examples of interventions that improve pain and function in appropriately selected older individuals. Interventional procedures (discussed in detail across Chapters 39–44) offer the possibility of rapid-onset (albeit often transitory) analgesia and improvement in mobility that, in aggregate, may defuse an acute pain crisis, restore confidence, and prevent a cycle of disuse, weakness, and further injury. However, due consideration should be given to: potential for harm in the older patient; inadequate comprehension of the procedure; poor comprehension of the related risk–benefit ratio as this relates to informed consent, associated medical comorbidities, and treatments; ability to cooperate during any procedure; monitoring; and necessity for aftercare. Assessment must take place on an individual basis. Referral to a multidisciplinary pain clinic or pain specialist should be considered when planning interventional procedures in frail patients.

Specific interventions may be more commonly utilized in the older population. The place of vertebroplasty in vertebral compression fractures due to either osteoporosis or malignancy is not yet fully established and is discussed later. Other interventions, such as epidural injections of local anaesthetics and corticosteroids, may provide short-term relief; to date, however, there is no clear evidence of any long-term benefit. Most studies of anaesthetic interventions for chronic pain have not included older subjects, particularly those in residential care, so that outcomes for most interventions in the aged are based on low levels of evidence. Although neural blockade and invasive procedures have a specific role in selected patients, many older patients with chronic pain benefit from thoughtfully applied pharmacologic management.

Vertebral Compression Fractures

Vertebral compression fracture presents particular pain management issues in the older patient with osteoporosis. Vertebral fracture may cause localized pain, loss of height or kyphosis, and potential spinal instability. Patients are often frail, and conservative treatments, including bed rest, bracing and analgesics may fail, with concomitant adverse drug reactions, increasing disability, loss of independence, and increased morbidity. There has been increasing interest in minimally invasive procedures, such as vertebroplasty and kyphoplasty, that offer the prospect of analgesia and early mobilization after fracture stabilization with bone cement.

Performed under radiologic guidance, percutaneous vertebroplasty with polymethylmethacrylate bone cement was originally described for treatment of hemangiomata in 1987 (59). Subsequently, this technique has been used to manage pain and increase bone strength after vertebral compression fractures due to osteoporosis, spinal metastasis and multiple myeloma. Cement leakage is relatively common, with spread reported into paravertebral, venous, intradiscal intraforaminal, epidural, and even intradural spaces (60); serious neurologic sequelae are uncommon, but if they occur they may lead to permanent incapacity. Risk of cement leakage is higher in metastatic vertebral disease. In a more recently introduced percutaneous technique, kyphoplasty, a balloon is first placed within the collapsed vertebral body and then inflated to restore vertebral height and reduce spinal deformity prior to injection of bone cement (61). Both procedures require considerable experience and expertise, have the potential for major adverse events, and should be carried out only in major centers with appropriately trained personnel and resources.

Current outcome data, derived from nonrandomized trials and case series, indicate that a considerable proportion of patients derive substantial analgesia and improved mobility from these procedures. A systematic literature review of nonrandomized, peer-reviewed trials (37 retrospective, 25 prospective, and 7 unspecified) by Hulme et al. included 2,958 vertebroplasty and 1,288 kyphoplasty subjects (61). The authors concluded that standardized methodology and reporting would assist validity and applicability of future studies. Apparent findings were that 90% patients derived some analgesic benefit, bone cement leakage rates were higher with vertebroplasty (41%) than kyphoplasty (9%), vertebral height restoration occurs in about two-thirds of patients after kyphoplasty and in a subset of vertebroplasty patients, and that new fractures of uncertain etiology were found in adjacent vertebrae after both procedures. Issues to be resolved include mechanisms of analgesia, strategies to minimize cement leak, appropriate selection criteria, outcome differences after the two procedures, and methods to prevent new fractures.

In a prospective nonrandomized study of outcomes after kyphoplasty with conservative management versus conservative medical management alone (bisphosphonate, calcium, vitamin D_3, analgesics, physiotherapy), a number of benefits were identified (62). Vertebral height was significantly greater early after kyphoplasty, and at 6 and 12 months. New vertebral fractures were less frequent after kyphoplasty at 12 months, although the rate of fracture of an adjacent vertebra was similar between groups. Relative to conservative medical management, pain scores were significantly lower early, and at 6 and 12 months, after kypholasty. At 12 months, individual pain scores were lower in 31 of 40 patients who underwent kyphoplasty and 11 of 20 patients who elected for conservative management only, the difference in numbers was not significant. A functional benefit was noted at 6 months, but not at 12 months, after kyphoplasty.

As indicated earlier, additional, often adjacent, vertebral fractures have been reported after these procedures. A causal relationship between the increased frequency of osteoporotic fractures and vertebroplasty is debated and remains controversial (63). Further fractures might simply reflect the underlying bone structural abnormality or clustering of fractures around the thoracolumbar region. Alternately, the pressure required to inject bone cement potentially increases mechanical forces on adjacent vertebrae.

Postherpetic Neuralgia

The incidence and duration of postherpetic neuralgia both increase with age and are a significant cause of debilitating and unremitting pain in older populations. The increased incidence is believed to reflect a normal age-related decrease in cell-mediated immunity. Other medical conditions that cause immune compromise, in addition to corticosteroids, chemotherapy, and radiotherapy, also predispose to reactivation of the varicella zoster virus (64).

Early treatment of herpes zoster (shingles) is important, not only to relieve acute pain and treat the virus, but to decrease the incidence of postherpetic neuralgia. Antiviral treatment within 3 days of the development of rash has been shown to decrease the duration of the rash and associated acute pain. Where not contraindicated, concomitant oral corticosteroids decrease acute pain, but evidence for any reduction in incidence or severity of postherpetic neuralgia is controversial; any benefits must be balanced by the consideration of effects on co-morbidities such as diabetic control, and the theoretical risk of immunosuppression and herpes dissemination.

A systematic review of treatments for postherpetic neuralgia indicated that there was good evidence for moderate efficacy of TCAs, gabapentin, pregabalin, opioids, and lignocaine patches (65). A randomized placebo-controlled trial in older patients indicated that early treatment with amitriptyline 25 mg/day significantly reduced the incidence of pain due to postherpetic neuralgia at 6 months (66). There was less efficacy, or lower levels of evidence, for topical aspirin or capsaicin formulations. No adverse effects were reported in a clinical trial that compared a series of four intrathecal or epidural injections of 80 mg preservative-free methylprednisolone; this trial concluded that intrathecal, but not epidural, steroid reduced pain at up to 2 years follow-up, with an NNT of 1.4 (95% confidence interval [CI], 1.0–2.1) (67). However, specific cautions have been published, indicating the lack of regulatory approval for intrathecal corticosteroid administration and potential neurotoxicity, including arachnoiditis, transverse myelitis and chemical meningitis potentially related to sensitivity to local anesthetic, the corticosteroid, hyperbaric formulations, or preservatives in the corticosteroid such as benzyl alcohol, benzalkonium chloride, and polyethylene glycol (68). The use of intrathecal methylprednisolone should thus be considered experimental at this time.

Various other interventions to relieve neuralgic pain have been trialed, with a low level of evidence for any benefit. A recent randomized controlled trial of 598 patients over 50 years of age with acute herpes zoster, comparing numbers with zoster-associated pain after standard therapy (antivirals and analgesics) combined with a single epidural injection of local anaesthetic (bupivacaine 10 mg) and steroid (methylprednisolone 80 mg), or standard therapy alone, demonstrated a significant reduction in the number of patients with pain at 1 month after epidural injection (48%, versus 58% after standard treatment alone; RR 0.83, 90% CI, 0.71–0.97). However, there was no difference in outcome at 3 and 6 months (69). The use of repeated subcutaneous infiltration of local anaesthetic, triamcinolone, or a combination during the acute phase may provide short-term relief, but clear evidence of long-term benefit is lacking (70) and comparison with oral corticosteroids is not available.

A comprehensive review by Wu et al. of the role of local anaesthetic sympathetic block concluded that the intervention may provide a benefit in acute herpes zoster, but has no demonstrable long-term efficacy in postherpetic neuralgia (71). Although sympathetic block may reduce the pain of acute zoster, most studies were observational and unable to demonstrate a reduction in the incidence of postherpetic neuralgia, or were uninterpretable due to methodologic flaws. A short-term benefit was found in 30% to 50% of patients in some studies, indicating that sympathetic block may have a limited role in this context. Adequately controlled prospective studies in the field are needed.

Opstelten et al. reviewed a number of retrospective or observational studies of local anaesthetic epidural block, with or without corticosteroids, that suggested a short-term benefit but again, long-term improvement was unclear (70). However, a longer-term benefit of epidural management was indicated by a large prospective study of 600 patients aged over 55 years (range 55–94) with severe acute zoster pain, recruited within 7 days of developing rash (72). Treatment was randomized to either antiviral therapy (treatment period 9 days) plus prednisolone (21 days), or epidural bupi-

vacaine and methylprednisolone (7–21 days). Analysis was based on the intention-to-treat population; 485 patients completed the 12-month study period, at which time the incidence of pain was significantly less in the group that had received epidural management (1.6%) than the group receiving antiviral and prednisolone therapy (22%); superior pain control in the epidural group was noted at 1 month. The reduced incidence of postherpetic neuralgia after epidural intervention was consistent with previous uncontrolled studies. The authors indicated that the anti-inflammatory actions and antilysosomal protection afforded by corticosteroids may diminish neuronal damage by virus, and they also speculated that local anaesthetics act by blocking intra-axonal transport of virus toward the spinal cord dorsal horn. The importance of early therapy was emphasized. Adverse effects after epidural treatment were all reversible and included inadvertent dural puncture resulting in 48-hour treatment delay, post–dural puncture headache, and failure to complete the course of treatment (leg paresis and oliguria in one patient, diaphoresis and fainting in two, and neck pain after one cervical epidural). Temporary ocular complications were equivalent in both groups. An editorial accompanying this study questioned the widespread feasibility and projected health care costs of such treatment and reiterated concerns relating to epidural corticosteroid use, including the lack of use of bacterial filters and potential hazards of inadvertent subarachnoid administration, as well as lack of evidence for the corticosteroid component of treatment (73).

In the future, the burden of disease in the aged due to the herpes zoster virus will hopefully decrease. Recent regulatory approval of a live attenuated varicella zoster vaccine has been supported by a large randomized, controlled, double-blind trial in over 38,546 patients older than 60 years. This study found a 60% reduction in the burden of illness from the zoster virus, and a 67% decrease in the incidence of postherpetic neuralgia (74).

Degenerative Spinal Disease

Spinal canal stenosis involving the lumbar spine is a leading cause of pain and disability in the older person and is believed to now be the most common reason for spinal surgery in adults over 65 years of age (75). There is ongoing debate as to the most effective treatments for canal stenosis, which may depend upon the extent, symptoms, and complications of the degenerative condition, in addition to the responses to conservative management and the medical condition of the individual. A recent Cochrane review of the role of surgery for degenerative lumbar spondylosis concluded that insufficient scientific evidence is available for any firm conclusions to be made regarding the clinical outcomes and cost-effectiveness of spinal surgeries, including newer procedures for degenerative diseases of the spine such as intradiscal electrothermal treatment (IDET) and disc arthroplasty and that well-designed randomized clinical trials are required (75). A comprehensive review of spinal pain and the role of neural blockade in its treatment is provided by Rathmell in Chapter 44.

In the older person, degenerative central canal and lateral recess stenosis may be consequent to hypertrophy of the ligamentum flavum or zygapophyseal (facet) joints, vertebral body osteophytes or disc protrusion, or spondylolisthesis. The impact of degenerative changes may be compounded in a congenitally narrow canal or when associated with acquired conditions resulting from trauma, previous surgery, or medical comorbidities such as malignant neoplasia, Paget disease of bone, ankylosing spondylitis and vertebral compression fracture.

Central canal stenosis may result in neurogenic claudication and, ultimately, cauda equina syndrome. Lateral recess or intraforaminal stenosis may result in radicular nerve root pain, due to compression of the exiting nerve root or the lower nerve root descending within the lateral recess. Degenerative spinal stenosis most commonly affects the L3–L4 and L4–L5 spinal segments. A review of foraminal stenosis indicated that the incidence of nerve root involvement was L5 (75%), L4 (15%), L3 (5%), and L2 (4%), relating to larger size of the L5 nerve root and its associated dorsal root ganglion relative to the exit foramen and increased frequency of disc degeneration and spondylosis at L4 and L5 (76). Foraminal stenosis may be static or dynamic, with lumbar flexion increasing (12%) and extension decreasing (15%) the size of the foramen. Hence, nerve root compression may be intermittent, depending on posture and activity. In one study, the incidence of foraminal nerve root compression was 21% in neutral, 15% in flexed, and 33% in extended positions (77). Exacerbation of leg pain during spine extension should therefore prompt consideration of foraminal stenosis.

Imaging findings should always be correlated with clinical symptoms and examination. Jenis and An (76) suggest that plain radiographic dynamic flexion and extension studies may be misleading because of the oblique orientation of the lower lumbar intervertebral foramina. Myelography may not detect lateral pathology because of termination of the dural sheath, which prevents contrast medium from reaching the lateral nerve root sheath. Combined computed tomography (CT) and magnetic resonance imaging (MRI) studies will delineate bone encroachment on the foramen and enable a full assessment of lumbar foramina and vertebral disc changes. Magnetic resonance changes suggestive of foraminal stenosis are reduction in foramen dimensions and loss of perineural fat in T1-weighted images. Important conditions, including malignant neoplasia and infection, should be considered and excluded and the patient carefully evaluated for evidence of any neurologic deficit, in order to enable timely referral and treatment that may prevent permanent or progressive impairment.

However, a prospective 10-year study of the outcomes of spinal decompressive surgery (78) by Amundsen et al. in 100 patients with a median age of 59 years, concluded that outcomes were generally better with surgery than conservative care in patients with sciatica, radiologic signs of stenosis and nerve root compression, and no previous back surgery. Conservative care was an alternative for patients with mild to moderate symptoms, resulting in 50% achieving a reduction in symptoms after 3 months; good results could still be obtained from surgery after failure of a trial of conservative care. However, patient and physician agreement on outcomes was low (κ coefficient of 0.41 at 4 years). Also, there was no difference in claudication at 4 years between surgical and conservatively treated groups, and more patients reported back pain at 4 years after operative intervention. There was an overall decrease in claudication symptoms from 90% at baseline to 20% after 10 years.

medications used for general and regional anaesthesia and postoperative pain management (79,80). As aging progresses, responses become less predictable, with wide variability in response to medications and interventions being the result of the overlay of purely age-based changes on those related to evolving medical comorbidities.

Age-related changes in the impact of neuraxial block relate to altered function of cardiovascular, respiratory, and nervous systems, and also to increase in upper height of block. Following neuraxial block, hypotension and bradycardia are more frequent in the older patient, related to higher dermatomal levels of analgesia and sympathetic block after dose-equivalent spinal and epidural procedures; these cardiovascular changes pose greater risk to older individuals with reduced cardiac reserve (81–88). Increased hypotension may be attributable to an increase in the upper level of analgesia with age, seen after epidural bupivacaine 0.5%, levobupivacaine 0.5%, and ropivacaine 0.5% to 1%; some studies have noted an increased speed of onset and intensity of motor block. With neuraxial block, the older patient is less able to compensate for hypovolemia or the redistribution of blood flow to the lower limbs and splanchnic circulation, due to decreased cardiac reserve and reduced sensitivity of the β-adrenergic system and baroreceptor reflexes. Bradycardia may occur as a consequence of neuraxial cardiac sympathetic block at T1–T4, age-related reduction in baroreceptor reflex mediated heart rate responses to hypotension or reflex slowing of heart rate in response to decreased venous return that relates to decreased atrial and pacemaker stretch and decreased ventricular mechanoreceptor reflex response. These factors all contribute to cardiovascular instability with increasing age. Judicious administration of intravenous fluids and vasopressors is required, taking care to avoid the fluid overload that may emerge as the neuraxial block regresses and the intravascular space contracts.

Both local anesthetic dose and solution volume influence the upper epidural block height in the older patient, as in younger patients (see Chapter 11 on epidural blockade by Veering and Cousins). The age-related increase in upper block height after a fixed dose of local anesthetic may be the consequence of a number of factors (88). There may be decreased loss of epidural solution related to sclerosis and calcification of intervertebral foramina, or reduced epidural fat and decreased resistance to flow within the epidural space. In addition, greater flux of epidural solutions across the dura may be due to increased size of arachnoid villi and changes in the connective tissue matrix with age. Variability in age-related response with changes in solution volume may result in considerable interindividual variability in epidural block height in the older person. Thus, it may be preferable to consider transforaminal fluoroscopic or CT-guided "mini-dose" neural blockade using local anaesthetic and corticosteroid when pain arises mainly from a single nerve root. However, significant complications can arise even with small doses of drugs administered transforaminally (see Chapter 50).

NEURAL BLOCKADE IN THE ELDERLY

Anatomic and pathophysiologic changes with aging alter the responses to neuraxial and peripheral neural blockade and impact on the pharmacokinetics and pharmacodynamics of individual agents used. Recent reviews provide a more comprehensive overview of those changes in pharmacokinetics and pharmacodynamics in older patients that result in an increased sensitivity to both the therapeutic and adverse effects of many

Neural Blockade Options in the Older Age Group

Neural blockade and neuromodulatory techniques are potentially helpful in the management of pain associated with many of the most common conditions affecting the older age group. The subsections immediately following touch upon the value of these techniques in specific contexts such as low back pain, angina, peripheral vascular disease, and peripheral nerve injury. Comprehensive surveys of interventions related to musculoskeletal pain are described by Prager et al., and Rathmell, respectively, in Chapters 41 and 44. Percutaneous neurolytic blocks (e.g., for trigeminal neuralgia) are described by Gofeld and Niv and Gofeld in Chapter 42, and interventions for cancer pain control are covered by Burton and Phan in Chapter 45.

Low Back Pain

Low back pain has many causes, as discussed above and in Chapter 44. In the older age group, degenerative changes associated with osteoarthritis, spondylosis, and osteoporosis are common causes of back pain. Low back pain due to facet joint disease can be diagnosed by means of medial branch blocks and, if appropriate, radiofrequency lesions can be performed. This is a simple day case procedure that is well tolerated in the older age group. Further details on this and other spinal procedures are provided in Chapter 42 on percutaneous neurodestructive techniques by Niv and Gofeld, and Chapter 44 on spine pain by Rathmell.

Back and leg pain associated with foraminal stenosis may be treated with epidural or transforaminal steroid and local anaesthetic injection. Central canal stenosis may sometimes be relieved by translaminar epidural steroid injection; however, the evidence for efficacy in the older age group is weak. Patients with lower limb neuropathic pain may be candidates for spinal cord stimulation (see Chapter 41 on neurostimulation by Prager et al.). Back pain due to internal disc disruption is difficult to treat. Currently only two procedural options are available: fusion or IDET. The results of IDET, although initially encouraging, now indicate that only a small subgroup of patients may benefit.

Back pain due to osteoporotic, or other, crush fractures may be treated by vertebroplasty or kyphoplasty (see earlier section on Vertebral Compression Fractures). For safety and logistical reasons, usually only a single level is treated. Not all patients respond with long-term pain relief. An alternative option is to place a tunneled epidural catheter, with the catheter tip at the level of the fracture. Very low doses of local anaesthetic and opioid can be used safely and effectively (see Chapter 40 on spinal analgesia by Cousins and Carr).

Peripheral Vascular Disease

Severe lower limb pain (rest pain and vascular claudication) may be relieved in a substantial percentage of patients by using neurolytic lumbar sympathetic blockade (see Chapter 39 on sympathetic block by Breivik and Cousins). Through the use of local anesthetic stellate ganglion blockade, patients with severe "acute on chronic" episodes of vascular ischemia in the upper limbs may obtain pain relief and the breaking of a vicious cycle of ischaemia. Another option is sympathetic block by means of intra-arterial infusion of a vasodilator.

In patients unsuitable for vascular reconstruction, spinal cord stimulation (SCS) has a high success rate for relief of rest pain and claudication, as well as healing of ischemic ulcers (see Chapter 41 on neurostimulation by Prager et al.).

Intractable Angina

Patients who have exhausted the options for coronary artery stent placement or bypass procedures can be difficult to manage using available systemic cardiovascular medications. A suitable alternative may be cervicothoracic SCS. Angina, together with the pain of peripheral vascular disease, has the highest likelihood of success of all indications for SCS. Indeed, a randomized prospective controlled study of SCS compared to coronary artery bypass grafting reported comparable symptomatic control of pain with the two methods.

Pain Associated with Peripheral Nerve Damage

Older patients may suffer from persistent neuropathic pain after operations or trauma, cancer-related "peripheral neuropathic pain," or other neuropathic pain conditions such as occipital neuralgia. An important emerging option for such conditions is peripheral nerve stimulation involving the placement of SCS or similar electrodes percutaneously across the course of the affected peripheral nerve or nerves. This technique has been particularly effective in occipital neuralgia and postoperative neuropathic pain, such as post–inguinal herniorrhaphy pain.

PHARMACOLOGIC MANAGEMENT

Despite the fact that pharmacologic management has become the mainstay of pain management in older people, limited data are available regarding the pharmacologic treatment of chronic pain specifically in this age group. Principles of management are based on clinical practice, which is often extrapolated from data available from the young and from patients with malignant pain. These data should be interpreted with caution. Published studies tend to be based on highly selected populations quite atypical of patients seen on a day-to-day basis. Positive trial outcomes are often achieved over short time frames, at doses much higher than those tolerated by frail older individuals.

Analgesia may be administered as pain-contingent (as required), time-contingent, or prophylactic (just prior to an activity known to exacerbate pain). Efforts to ensure good compliance are often as important as the selection of the medication itself. Side effects are common in this age group and in many instances predictable. Tolerance to side effects may be achieved by commencement at a low dose with slow titration, as tolerated; that is, *start low and go slow*. The benefits and disadvantages of treatments need to be openly explained and discussed with patients and caregivers, particularly in managing chronic pain when the goal is to optimize pain relief without causing intolerable side effects. Attempts to eradicate pain entirely will often result in drug side effects that are as troublesome as the pain itself. Side effects can usually be managed effectively by dose adjustment or the addition of an adjuvant medication that does not compromise analgesic benefits (e.g., a senna laxative used preemptively to avert constipation during long-term opioid analgesia). Of equal note, the use of a neural blockade technique to remove one component of pain may permit dose reduction of a systemic analgesic to a level at which the medication can be tolerated.

Simple Analgesics

Paracetamol (called acetaminophen or APAP in North America) remains the first line of treatment for mild to moderate, chronic, nonmalignant pain. Full dosing can begin immediately at 1 g four times a day if necessary. Efficacy is not significantly different from ibuprofen. Paracetamol is a relatively safe drug. The risk of liver failure with paracetamol toxicity is increased in alcoholics and malnourished individuals; frail older patients following major surgery may fall into the latter group. Paracetamol is still probably a safer option than opioids and anti-inflammatory agents in the older population, provided that the maximum daily dose of 4 g/day is not exceeded.

Nonsteroidal anti-inflammatory drugs are effective analgesics and represent one of the most widely used classes of medication. There is concern, however, about the safety of both cyclooxygenase (COX)-1 and COX-2 inhibitors in older individuals (89). Particular caution is required in patients with renal impairment or those prescribed diuretics and angiotensin-converting enzyme inhibitors. Cardiovascular risk may be increased by specific and nonspecific COX-2 inhibitors. Anti-inflammatory agents should be reserved for use in transient or subacute musculoskeletal pain that is believed to have an inflammatory pathogenesis. Prolonged use of NSAIDs should be avoided.

Other Analgesics

For patients with pain not adequately controlled with simple analgesics, an intermediate step can be taken before embarking on treatment with conventional (i.e., strong) opioids. The medications in this intermediate group include codeine, tramadol, and dextropropoxyphene. These medications are often used in combination with paracetamol (acetaminophen). As a group, their efficacy is not always predictable and side effects are common; their use remains under scrutiny because of their adverse event profile in older patients.

Codeine (also called methylmorphine) is an opioid analgesic with a short half-life. Codeine is frequently administered in fixed combination tablets with paracetamol (acetaminophen) or with aspirin. The analgesic effects of codeine require biotransformation to morphine within the liver by the microsomal enzyme CYP2D6. Congenital absence of this enzyme occurs in about 8% of Caucasians and 2% of Asians, rendering these subgroups resistant to the analgesic effect of codeine. Codeine may be used for incident, predictable, short-lasting, and infrequent pain in older patients; however, a role for codeine use in chronic pain management is less clearly defined. The maximum dose in older people should be limited to 60 mg four times a day; frail individuals will only tolerate 30 mg. Codeine can easily cause constipation, nausea and confusion in older people.

Tramadol is an atypical, centrally acting analgesic with weak action on the μ-opioid receptor. Additional pharmacologic actions, including inhibition of neuronal noradrenaline and serotonin reuptake, lead to tramadol's being classified separately from the opioid analgesics. Immediate-release and sustained-release oral preparations are available. Dose reduction is usually required in older people, to a daily maximum dose of 300 mg/day. The starting dose is 50 mg of the short-acting preparation. Once a daily maintenance dose has been determined, tramadol can be prescribed in a twice daily, controlled-release preparation. Up to one-third of patients are unable to tolerate tramadol; common adverse symptoms include nausea, vomiting, sweating, dizziness, tremors, and headaches. More serious side effects include delirium and hallucinations, and also serotonergic syndrome, precipitated when other serotonergic medications, including selective serotonin reuptake inhibitors and TCAs, or herbal remedies such as St. John's wort, are used concurrently.

Dextropropoxyphene should only be used with extreme caution in the elderly (90). The usual dose is 32.5 mg to 65 mg, up to four times a day. Dextropropoxyphene use for chronic pain is controversial; a recent review of efficacy and safety data in older patients suggested that better-quality outcome data were required to evaluate its role in this population. Dextropropoxyphene and the major metabolite nordextropropoxyphene both have long half-lives; which are increased in the elderly to 36 hours (range 24–51 hours) and 53 hours (25–76 hours), respectively. Fixed-dose combinations with paracetamol (acetaminophen) are inappropriate, as the opioid and its major metabolite can accumulate with chronic use. Also, first-pass metabolism decreases with chronic use, thus increasing the risk of gastrointestinal and central nervous system side effects, including psychosis, hallucinations, and seizures. Nordextropropoxyphene is cardiotoxic.

The analgesic properties of codeine, tramadol, and dextropropoxyphene are limited by ceiling effects. Dose escalation may cause toxicity without conferring additional analgesia. Our general preference, if additional analgesia is required, is to switch to a low dose of a strong opioid, rather than escalating the dosage of any of these agents.

Opioid Analgesia

Opioids have an established role in the treatment of severe cancer pain in the elderly. Opioids are increasingly gaining acceptance for the management of severe nonmalignant pain in this age group as well. This trend is seen as positive, in the sense that individuals should not be left to suffer uncontrolled pain. The potency of this class means that additional precautions are required. It is possible to mask the symptoms of pathology in cases in which specific treatment is more appropriate. Care is needed to select the most appropriate opioid analgesic and to manage opioid dosing and side effects. All opioids have the tendency to produce constipation, nausea, sedation, cognitive impairment, gait instability, and respiratory depression, thus necessitating a low starting dose with gentle titration. Tolerance to many side effects occurs over time, apart from constipation, which tends to persist. Prophylactic treatment of constipation is generally required.

Initiation of opioid analgesia for chronic noncancer pain usually involves a low dose of a immediate-release (IR) opioid administered orally, for example 5 mg of oxycodone or 10 mg of morphine. The dose is titrated according to response, as limited by side effects. Once the maintenance dose has been determined, a sustained-release oral preparation can be supplemented by an immediate-release preparation for breakthrough pain. Each breakthrough dose is usually on the order of one-sixth to one-tenth of the daily maintenance dose, depending on the selected opioid half-life.

Sustained-release preparations of morphine and oxycodone are available in a large range of doses and are appropriate for use in the elderly, provided appropriate cautions are given regarding the use of sustained-release medications. Methadone has a very long half-life, with a potential to accumulate, and should only be used with caution in this age group and under the supervision of clinicians experienced in methadone use. Methadone accumulation may cause sedation and confusion. Methadone has no active metabolites. Alternate routes of administration of opioids may be considered for patients who cannot tolerate oral preparations. Recently introduced formulations have assisted opioid-rotation from low doses of oral opioids to transdermal controlled-release opioids in older patients. Transdermal fentanyl patches offer the advantage of infrequent application every 72 hours (fentanyl patches) or 7 days (buprenorphine patches). However, the 25 μg/hr strength transdermal fentanyl patch is often too high a dose for many older patients and the recent availability of a 12 μg/hr "matrix" fentanyl patch has proven useful. Likewise, the partial agonist buprenorphine is available as a 7-day transdermal patch starting at a very low dose of 5 μg/hr; this dose is often well tolerated even in the elderly. However, even the smallest transdermal opioid dose may prove too potent for opioid naïve patients, and initial use should be cautiously monitored, particularly because of slow onset and offset.

The use of opioid analgesia in nonmalignant pain raises other issues. Maier et al. (91) demonstrated that only approximately one-third of patients responded well to opioid analgesia, one-third respond partially, and one-third did not respond. Of the responders, only half continued to benefit in the long term. This compares poorly with the use of opioids in malignant pain, in which 90% of patients will have opioid-responsive pain. The risk–benefit ratio in older patients is currently unknown. In general, older patients respond to lower doses of opioids, at which level fewer side effects would be expected to occur, but they have a greater tendency toward adverse effects.

Adjuvant Analgesics

Commonly used agents for neuropathic pain include TCAs and antiepileptic drugs. Some antiarrhythmic are used, but they generally have a limited therapeutic window in older people that precludes their use.

Amitriptyline remains the most commonly used antidepressant for neuropathic pain. No other antidepressant drug has been shown to be superior to amitriptyline, although other TCAs including nortriptyline have fewer side effects (92). The TCAs can be used for any form of neuropathic pain. As with any other medication used in older people, the clinician is advised to initiate therapy at a low dose and titrate slowly according to response. Amitriptyline and nortriptyline are usually commenced at 5 to 10 mg taken an hour before retiring and increased every few days by a similar dose until a benefit is achieved or side effects preclude further use. A dose of 50 mg to 75 mg is usually considered to be enough to achieve an analgesic effect if one is going to occur. Common side effects include dry mouth, postural hypotension, drowsiness, and urinary retention. Newer selective noradrenaline or serotonin reuptake inhibitors have not been shown to be effective for pain relief outside their antidepressant effects.

The widespread use of antiepileptic drugs for neuropathic pain is based on clinical experience rather than large numbers of placebo-controlled trials. Carbamazepine is a frequent choice for trigeminal neuralgia. A starting dose of 50 mg is suggested, as some older people are very sensitive to the adverse effects of this medication. The best-studied antiepileptic drugs at present are gabapentin and pregabalin (92). They have been proved to be useful in the management of postherpetic neuralgia and diabetic neuropathy, with use in other syndromes by extrapolation and clinical experience. They can produce somnolence, giddiness, and ataxia in the elderly at therapeutic doses, which can increase the risk of falls. In the frail elderly, the dose of gabapentin can begin at 100 mg at night, increasing every few days to a target of 300 mg three times a day; pregabalin can be commenced at a dose of 75 mg at night, increasing to 300 mg twice a day as tolerated. The dose must be reduced if renal impairment is present. Other antiepileptic agents may occasionally be of benefit in neuropathic pain.

In summary, good evidence confirms the benefit of TCAs, antiepileptic agents, and opioids for the management of chronic neuropathic pain, but that evidence is limited in older people. In the absence of head-to-head comparative studies, the choice of initial medication is based on the likely tolerability of the medication for the individual being treated, its availability, and its cost.

PSYCHOLOGICAL MODALITIES

As described in Chapters 28 and 35, most modern chronic pain management programs are based on the cognitive behavioral therapy (CBT) model. Such programs consist of patient and family education, contingency management, relaxation training, training in goal-setting and problem-solving skills, training in effective communication, behavioral reactivation, and cognitive restructuring. The last requires attention to specific constructs identified in individual patients. These might include a fear of increased damage from activity or increased pain levels, or excessive reliance on "powerful others" such as doctors and medications.

In the general population, CBT has been shown to have unequivocal benefit. However, only limited studies have been undertaken in older people. Cook demonstrated that 10 weekly sessions of CBT were effective in the institutionalized elderly (93). Puder has also shown that age was not a factor in determining the success of a CBT program (94). CBT is also useful in the treatment of depression in the elderly.

PHYSICAL MODALITIES

Exercise therapy is an integral part of CBT programmes. It is most effective if it has a specific goal orientation. Exercise therapy should include stretching, strengthening, aerobic exercise, and postural correction where feasible. Weight loss can help in painful conditions involving the weight-bearing joints and can assist in slowing the progression of degenerative arthritis. Other techniques, such as bracing, trigger point deactivation, massage therapy, acupuncture, transcutaneous electrical stimulation (TENS), heat, and cold have also been used. Hydrotherapy and use of an exercise bike may promote range of movement and confidence. TENS is useful in subacute injury and postherpetic neuralgia. Controlled trials of TENS using experimental pain models are usually only effective at high intensities of stimulation. TENS has the advantage of being able to be used for long periods at a time, but post stimulus effects are short-lived. The clinician should be aware of the dangers of overreliance on passive therapies, especially in patients who have an external locus of control. Advice on simple maneuvers for lifting and walking may be of great functional benefit, for instance leaning on the supermarket trolley/cart in patients with vertebral canal stenosis as a means to increase their walking distance.

Assistive devices, such as canes/walking sticks and walkers, can be useful to improve function and reduce pain. However, such measures should be applied judiciously, so as not to risk overreliance or promote deconditioning. Physiotherapists can also counsel patients in approaches to avoid exacerbations of musculoskeletal pains.

PART IV: PAIN MANAGEMENT

MANAGEMENT OF SOCIAL CIRCUMSTANCES

The importance of social (and economic) factors in pain management has been emphasized in Chapter 29 by Loeser. The patient's family must be educated about the nature of chronic pain. First, they must be assured that the problem is real, and the patient is not in any way trying to "fake the pain" to obtain some advantage. Second, they must be educated that the aim is to decrease pain and maintain function. The risk that solicitous behavior can impair a patient's function should be explained to caregivers. The family should also be educated about the need to maintain a paced level of physical activity and be taught the same methods of nonpharmacologic pain management as the patient. Such measures may increase the sense of mastery for both patient and family. The family may play an important role in the management of patients with dementia, who may not be able to maintain a therapeutic approach without on-going prompting and supervision. Frequently, loneliness and a loss of meaning can present as somatic complaints, including pain. Pain management in these instances may best address the source by encouraging or arranging for social or other meaningful activities.

SUMMARY

Any patient with chronic pain requires meticulous multidimensional assessment and properly planned and monitored interventions. Empowerment is a key factor in ensuring satisfying and durable outcomes; the patient and her caregivers must be active participants in therapy at all times. Although limited high-quality published information is available about the management of chronic pain in older people, this scarcity of evidence is likely to be rectified in coming years as chronic pain is increasingly recognized as a highly prevalent, major health burden in the geriatric population.

References

1. Helme RD, Gibson SJ. Pain in the elderly. In: Jensen TS, Turner JA, Wiesenfeld-Hallin Z, eds. *Proceedings of the 8th World Congress on Pain.* Seattle: IASP Press; 1999:919–944.
2. http://www.census.gov/ipc/www.idbpyr.html
3. Crook J, Rideout E, Browne G. The prevalence of pain complaints in a general population. *Pain* 1984;18:299–314.
4. Gibson SJ, Helme RD. Age differences in pain perception and report: A review of physiological, psychological, laboratory and clinical studies. *Pain Rev* 1995;2:111–137.
5. Helme RD, Gibson SJ. Pain in older people. In: Crombie IK, Croft PR, Linton SJ, et al., eds. *Epidemiology of Pain.* Seattle: IASP Press; 1999:103–111.
6. Miller PF, Sheps DS, Bragdon EE, et al. Ageing and pain perception in ischaemic heart disease. *Am Heart J* 1990;120:22–31.
7. Moss MS, Lawton MP, Glicksman A. The role of pain in the last year of life of older persons. *J Gerontol* 1991;46:51–57.
8. Lasch H, Castell DO, Castell JA. Evidence for diminished visceral pain with ageing: Studies using graded intraoesophageal balloon distension. *Am J Physiol* 1997;272:G1–G3.
9. Harkins SW, Price DD, Bush FM, Small RE. Geriatric pain. In: Wall PD, Melzack R, eds. *Textbook of Pain.* New York: Churchill Livingstone; 1994: 769–784.
10. Von Korff M, Dworkin SF, LeResche L. Graded chronic pain status: An epidemiologic study. *Pain* 1990;40:279–291.
11. Sternback RA. Survey of pain in the United States: The Nuprin Pain Report. *Clin J Pain* 1986;2:49–53.
12. Barberger-Gateau P, Chaslerie A, Dartigues J, et al. Health measure correlates in a French elderly community population: The PAQUID study. *J Gerontol* 1992;472:S88–S95.
13. Kay L, Jorgensen T, Schult-Larsen K. Abdominal pain in a 70 year old Danish population. *J Clin Epidemiol* 1992;45:1377–1382.
14. Dionne CE, Dunn KM, Croft PR. Does back pain prevalence really decrease with increasing age? A systematic review. *Age Ageing* 2006;35:229–234.
15. Ries LAG, Harkins D, Krapcho M, et al. SEER Cancer Statistics Review, 1975–2003. Bethesda, MD: National Cancer Institute. Available at http://seer.cancer.gov/csr/1975_2003/, based on November 2005 SEER data submission.
16. Ward SE, Goldberg N, Miller-McCauley V, et al. Patient-related barriers to management of cancer pain. *Pain* 1993;52:319–324.
17. Cleeland CS, Gonin R, Hatfield AK, et al. Pain and its treatment in outpatients with metastatic cancer. *N Engl J Med* 1994;330:592–596.
18. Bernabei R, Gambassi G, Lapane K, et al. Management of pain in elderly patients with cancer. *JAMA* 1998;279(23):1877–1882.
19. Clergue F, Auroy Y, Pequignot F, et al. French survey of anesthesia in 1996. *Anesthesiology* 1999;91:1509–1520.
20. Morrison RS, Magaziner J, McLaughlin MA, et al. The impact of postoperative pain on outcomes following hip fracture. *Pain* 2003;103:303–311.
21. Closs SJ. An exploratory analysis of nurses' provision of postoperative analgesic drugs. *J Adv Nurs* 1990;15:42–49.
22. Faherty B, Grier M. Analgesic medication for elderly people post-surgery. *Nurs Res* 1984;33:369–372.
23. Kirkwood T. Evolution theory and mechanics of ageing. In: Tallis R, Fillit H, Brocklehurst JC, eds. *Brocklehurst's Textbook of Geriatric Medicine and Gerontology,* 5th ed. Edinburgh: Churchill, Livingstone; 1998:45–49.
24. Kirkwood T. *Time of Our Lives: The Science of Aging.* Oxford: Oxford University Press, 1999.
25. Gibson SJ. Pain and aging: The pain experience over the adult lifespan. In: Dostrovsky JO, Carr DB, Koltzenburg M, eds. *Proceedings of the 10th World Congress on Pain.* Seattle: IASP Press; 2003:767–790.
26. Helme RD, Meliala A, Gibson SJ. Methodologic factors which contribute to variations in experimental pain threshold reported for older people. *Neurosci Lett* 2004;361:144–146.
27. Washington LL, Gibson SJ, Helme RD. Age-related differences in the endogenous analgesic response to repeated cold water immersion in human volunteers. *Pain* 2000;89:89–96.
28. Washington LL, Gibson SJ. Application of the R111 reflex and naxolone to monitor the spinal action of age-dependant endogenous analgesia. *11th World Congress on Pain.* Sydney, 2005;827–P69.
29. Chakour MC, Gibson SJ, Bradbeer M, Helme RD. Effect of age on A-Delta fibre modulation of thermal pain perception. *Pain* 1996;64:143–152.
30. Chang WC, Helme RD, Farrell MJ, Gibson SJ. Age interacts with frequency in the temporal summation of painful electrical stimuli. *10th World Congress on Pain.* San Diego, 2002;906-P176.
31. Gibson SJ, Helme RD. Age related differences in pain perception and report. *Clin Geriatr Med* 2001;17:433–456.
32. Yong H-H, Gibson SJ, de La Horne DJ, Helme RD. Development of a pain attitudes questionnaire to assess stoicism and cautiousness for possible age differences. *J Gerontol B Psychol Sci Soc Sci* 2001;56B:279–284.
33. Yong H-H, Bell R, Workman B, Gibson SJ. Psychometric properties of the Pain Attitudes Questionnaire (revised) in adult patients with chronic pain. *Pain* 2003;104:673–681.
34. Gibson SJ. Age differences in psychosocial aspects of pain. In: Gibson SJ, Weiner DK, eds. *Pain in Older Persons.* Seattle: IASP Press; 2005: 87–107.
35. Gibson SJ. The measurement of mood states in older adults. *J Gerontol B Psychol Sci Soc Sci* 1997;52:167–174.
36. Hadjistavropoulos T, Herr K, Turk DC, et al. An interdisciplinary expert consensus statement on assessment of pain in older persons. *Clin J Pain* 2007;23[1 Suppl]:S1–S43.
37. Leong IY, Farrell MJ, Helme RD, Gibson SJ. The relationship between medical comorbidity and self-rated pain, mood disturbance and function in older people with chronic pain. *J Gerontol A Biol Sci Med Sci* 2007;62(5):550–555.
38. Yesavage JA, Brink TL, Rose TL, et al. Development and validation of a geriatric depression screening scale: A preliminary report. *J Psychiatr Res* 1983;17:37–49.
39. Ferrell BA, Ferrell BR, Rivera L. Pain in cognitively impaired nursing home patients. *J Pain Symptom Manage* 1995;10:591–598.
40. Zwakhalen SMG, Jamers JPH, Abu-Saad HH, Berger MPF. Pain in elderly people with severe dementia: A systematic review of behavioural pain assessment tools. *BMC Geriatr* 2006;3:1–15.

41. Herr K, Bjoro K, Decker S. Tools for assessment of pain in nonverbal older adults with dementia: A state-of-the-science review. *J Pain Symptom Manage* 2006;31:170–192.

42. Morello R, Jean A, Alix M, et al. A scale to measure pain in non-verbally communicating older patients: the EPCA-2 Study of its psychometric properties. *Pain.* 2007;133:87–98.

43. Shea RA, Brooks JA, Dayhoff NE, et al. Pain intensity and postoperative pulmonary complications among the elderly after abdominal surgery. *Heart Lung* 2002;31:440–449.

44. Morrison RS, Siu AL. A comparison of pain and its treatment in advanced dementia and cognitively intact patients with hip fracture. *J Pain Symptom Manage* 2000;19:240–248.

45. Herrick C, Steger-May K, Sinacore DR, et al. Persistent pain in frail older adults after hip fracture repair. *J Am Geriatr Soc* 2004;52:2062–2068.

46. Inouye SK, Schlesinger MJ, Lydon TJ. Delirium: A symptom of how hospital care is failing older persons and a window to improve quality of hospital care. *Am J Med* 1999;106:565–573.

47. Inouye SK, Charpentier PA. Precipitating factors for delirium in hospitalized elderly persons: Predictive model and interrelationship with baseline vulnerability. *JAMA* 1996;275:852–857.

48. Parker MJ, Handoll HH, Griffiths R. Anaesthesia for hip fracture surgery in adults. *Cochrane Database Syst Rev* 2004;18:CD000521.

49. Marcantonio ER, Juarez G, Goldman L, et al. The relationship of postoperative delirium with psychoactive medications. *JAMA* 1994;272:1518–1522.

50. Duggleby W, Lander J. Cognitive status and postoperative pain: Older adults. *J Pain Symptom Manage* 1994;9:19–27.

51. Lynch EP, Lazor MA, Gellis JE, et al. The impact of postoperative pain on the development of postoperative delirium. *Anesth Analg* 1998;86:781–785.

52. Marcantonio ER, Goldman L, Mangione CM, et al. A clinical prediction rule for delirium after elective noncardiac surgery. *JAMA* 1994;271:134–139.

53. Fong HK, Sands LP, Leung JM. The role of postoperative analgesia in delirium and cognitive decline in elderly patients: A systematic review. *Anesth Analg* 2006;102:1255–1266.

54. Vaurio LE, Sands LP, Wang Y, et al. Postoperative delirium: The importance of pain and pain management. *Anesth Analg* 2006;102:1267–1273.

55. Herrick IA, Ganapathy S, Komar W, et al. Postoperative cognitive impairment in the elderly: Choice of patient-controlled analgesia opioid. *Anaesthesia* 1996;51:356–60.

56. Adunsky A, Levy R, Heim M, et al. Meperidine analgesia and delirium in aged hip fracture patients. *Arch Gerontol Geriatr* 2002;35:253–259.

57. Morrison RS, Magaziner J, Gilbert M, et al. Relationship between pain and opioid analgesics on the development of delirium following hip fracture. *J Gerontol A Biol Sci Med Sci* 2003;58:76–81.

58. Pasero C, McCaffery M. Postoperative pain management in the elderly. In: Ferrell BR, Ferrell BA, eds. *Pain in the Elderly.* Seattle: IASP Press; 1996:45–68.

59. Galibert P, Deramond H, Rosat P, et al. Preliminary note on the treatment of vertebral angioma by percutaneous acrylic vertebroplasty [in French]. *Neurochirurgie* 1987;33:166–168.

60. Chen Y-J, Tan T-S, Chen W-H, et al. Intradural cement leakage: A devastatingly rare complication of vertebroplasty. *Spine* 2006;31:E379–E382.

61. Hulme PA, Krebs J, Ferguson SJ, Berlemann U. Vertebroplasty and kyphoplasty: A systematic review of 69 clinical studies. *Spine* 2006;31:1983–2001.

62. Grafe IA, Da Fonseca K, Hillmeier J, et al. Reduction of pain and fracture incidence after kyphoplasty: 1-year outcomes of a prospective controlled trial of patients with primary osteoporosis. *Osteoporos Int* 2005;16:2005–2012.

63. Trout AT, Kallmes DF. Does vertebroplasty cause incident vertebral fractures? A review of available data. *AJNR AM J Neuroradiol* 2006;27:1397–1403.

64. Stankus SJ, Dlugopolski M, Packer D. Management of herpes zoster (shingles) and postherpetic neuralgia. *Am Fam Physician* 2000;61:2437–2444, 2447–2448.

65. Dubinsky RM, Kabbani H, El-Chami Z, et al. Practice parameter: Treatment of postherpetic neuralgia. An evidence-based report of the Quality Standards Subcommittee of the American Academy of Neurology. *Neurology* 2004;63:959–965.

66. Bowsher D. The effects of pre-emptive treatment of postherpetic neuralgia with amitriptyline: A randomized, double blind, placebo-controlled trial. *J Pain Symptom Manage* 1997;13:327–331.

67. Kotani N, Kushikata T, Hashimoto H, et al. Intrathecal methylprednisolone for intractable postherpetic neuralgia. *N Engl J Med* 2000;343:1514–1519.

68. Nelson DA, Landau WM. Intraspinal steroids: History, efficacy, accidentality, and controversy with review of United States Food and Drug Administration reports. *J Neurol Neurosurg Psychiatry* 2001;70:433–443.

69. van Wijck AJ, Opstelten W, Moons KG, et al. The PINE study of epidural steroids and local anaesthetics to prevent postherpetic neuralgia: A randomised controlled trial. *Lancet* 2006;367:219–224.

70. Opstelten W, van Wijck AJ, Stolker RJ. Interventions to prevent postherpetic neuralgia: Cutaneous and percutaneous techniques. *Pain* 2004;107:202–206.

71. Wu CL, Marsh A, Dworkin RH. The role of sympathetic nerve blocks in herpes zoster and postherpetic neuralgia. *Pain* 2000;87:121–129.

72. Pasqualucci A, Pasqualucci V, Galla F, et al. Prevention of post-herpetic neuralgia: Acyclovir and prednisolone versus epidural local anesthetic and methylprednisolone. *Acta Anaesthesiol Scand* 2000;44:910–918.

73. Johnson RW. Prevention of post-herpetic neuralgia: Can it be achieved? Editorial. *Acta Anaesthesiol Scand* 2000;44:903–905.

74. Oxman MN, Levin MJ, Johnson GR, et al. A vaccine to prevent herpes zoster and postherpetic neuralgia in older adults. *New Engl J Med* 2005;352:2271–2284.

75. Gibson JNA, Waddell G. Surgery for degenerative lumbar spondylosis: Updated Cochrane review. *Spine* 2005;30:2312–2320.

76. Jenis LG, An HS. Spine update. Lumbar foraminal stenosis. *Spine* 2000;25:389–394.

77. Infusa A, An HS, Lim TH, et al. Anatomic changes of the spinal canal and intervertebral foramen associated with flexion-extension movement. *Spine* 1996;21:2412–2420.

78. Amundsen T, Weber H, Nordal HJ, et al. Lumbar spinal stenosis: Conservative or surgical management? A prospective 10-year study. *Spine* 2000;25:1425–1435.

79. Sadean MR, Glass PSA. Pharmacokinetics in the elderly. *Best Pract Res Clin Anaesthesiol* 2003;17:191–205.

80. Vuyk J. Pharmacodynamics in the elderly. *Best Pract Res Clin Anaesthesiol* 2003;17:206–218.

81. Veering BT, Burm AG, van Kleef JW, et al. Spinal anesthesia with glucose-free bupivacaine: Effects of age on neural blockade and pharmacokinetics. *Anesth Analg* 1987;66:965–970.

82. Veering BT, Burm AG, Spierdijk J. Spinal anesthesia with hyperbaric bupivacaine. Effects of age on neural blockade and pharmacokinetics. *Br J Anaesth* 1988;60:187–194.

83. Veering BT, Burm AG, van Kleef JW, et al. Epidural anesthesia with bupivacaine: Effects of age on neural blockade and pharmacokinetics. *Anesth Analg* 1987;66:589–593.

84. Hirabayashi Y, Shimizu R. Effect of age on extradural dose requirement in thoracic extradural anaesthesia. *Br J Anaesth* 1993;71:445–456.

85. Wolff AP, Hasselström L, Kerkkamp HE, Gielen MJ. Extradural ropivacaine and bupivacaine in hip surgery. *Br J Anaesth* 1995;74:458–460.

86. Simon MJ, Veering BT, Stienstra R, et al. The effects of age on neural blockade and hemodynamic changes after epidural anesthesia with ropivacaine. *Anesth Analg* 2002;94:1325–1330.

87. Simon MJ, Veering BT, Stienstra R, et al. Effect of age on the clinical profile and systemic absorption and disposition of levobupivacaine after epidural administration. *Br J Anaesth* 2004;93:512–520.

88. Veering BT. Hemodynamic effects of central blockade in elderly patients. Editorial. *Can J Anesth* 2006;53:117–121.

89. Juni P, Dieppe P. Older people should not be prescribed "coxibs" in place of conventional NSAIDs. *Age Ageing* 2004;33:100–104.

90. Goldstein DJ, Turk DC. Dextropropoxyphene: Safety and efficacy in older patients. *Drugs Aging* 2005;22:419–432.

91. Maier C, Hildebrandt J, Klinger R, et al. Morphine responsiveness, efficacy and tolerability in patients with chronic non-tumour associated pain-results of a double-blind placebo-controlled trial (MONTAS). *Pain* 2002;97:223–233.

92. Finnerup NB, Otto M, McQuay HJ, et al. Algorithm for neuropathic pain treatment: An evidence based proposal. *Pain* 2005;118:289–305.

93. Cook AJ. Cognitive-behavioural pain management for elderly nursing home residents. *J Gerontol B Psychol Sci Soc Sci* 1998;53:P51–P59.

94. Puder RS. Age analysis of cognitive-behavioural group therapy for chronic pain outpatients. *Psychol Aging* 1998;3:3204–3207.

CHAPTER 49 ■ PALLIATIVE CARE AND PAIN CONTROL IN OLDER PERSONS AND THOSE WITH TERMINAL ILLNESS

PERRY G. FINE

The recent and rapidly growing emphasis on optimizing quality of life throughout the course of chronic progressive illness reflects a rededication to humanistic principles in the health care professions. This modern movement can be traced to several converging initiatives in the latter decades of the 20th century that recognized that "good medicine" requires attention to the burden of disease for the patient and family in addition to disease-specific, biomedically focused treatments. The global hospice movement, the World Health Organization (WHO) cancer pain relief program, and the worldwide emergence of pain medicine as a differentiated specialty that recognizes the importance of interdisciplinary care for complex pain-related disorders all contributed to this still-evolving shift in thinking. In economically developed nations, a major force driving this paradigm change is the substantial economic impact of contemporary medical and public health efforts. Such efforts have increased not only life expectancy but also costs of care to the point where such costs consume a significant and rising portion of the gross domestic product. For example, advancing rates of hospitalization during progressive illness result in almost a third of the total $100 billion U.S. Medicare budget spent on health care costs in the last year of life, and one-sixth of the total spent in the last 2 months of life, even though significant deficiencies continue to be documented for outcomes such as pain control or adherence to advance directives (1,2). These topics are described in greater detail in other chapters of this volume, such as Chapter 28 by Gallagher and Fishman on the emergence of pain medicine as a specialty, and Chapter 29 by Loeser on socioeconomic factors in pain management.

Hygiene and medical technology have together not only prolonged life, but extended the process of dying. In the face of accumulated comorbid conditions, the burdens of illness are numerous and, without due attention and skillful intervention, these can lead to tremendous unnecessary suffering and despair, and financial hardship. These burdens increase with advancing age, as described by Helme and Fleming in the preceding chapter on the treatment of pain in older people. Optimizing quality of life for the patient and family throughout the entire disease trajectory, including bereavement, has become the province of the current palliative care movement. Notwithstanding the limited curative and disease-modifying therapies available at the time, in retrospect, Sir William Osler was uncannily prescient when he stated a century ago, "Care more particularly for the individual patient than for the special features of the disease. To accept a great group of maladies, against which we have never had and can scarcely ever hope to have curative measures, makes some men as sensitive as though we were ourselves responsible for their existence. These very cases are 'rocks of offence' to many good fellows whose moral decline dates from the rash promise to cure. We work by wit and not by witchcraft, and while patients have our tenderest care, and we must do what is best for the relief of their sufferings, we should not bring the art of medicine into disrepute by quack-like promises to heal, or by wire-drawn attempts at cure, adding 'continuate and inexorable maladies'" (3).

Although the substance of the present chapter is relevant across medical disciplines and specialties, it is intended to capture the collective wisdom and imagination of anesthesiologists in particular. Anesthesiologists—especially those with additional training and credentials in pain management—may be called upon as consultants to help relieve pain and related forms of suffering. Far too few anesthesiologists, however, have entered palliative care practice (including hospice as an end-of-life domain of palliative care) as integrated members of a palliative care or hospice team. This gap is unfortunate because the knowledge and skills acquired during anesthesiology postgraduate training and clinical practice well prepare anesthesiologists to relieve many of the burdens associated with advanced illness. The unique combination of expertise in neural blockade, analgesic pharmacology, and sedation (based on experience and skill in safe, effective, goal-directed drug titration that is a hallmark of anesthesiology) and the carefully cultivated ability to create an environment of calm among seriously ill, anxious, and agitated patients and their families, together create an invaluable foundation from which to contribute to palliative care teams (4).

SOCIAL CHANGE AND RECENT DEVELOPMENTS

Palliative care has long been a recognized field in British Commonwealth nations, but it has been slower to develop in the United States and in many other nations. From the author's North American perspective, an inflection point occurred in the United States 25 years ago, upon legislative passage of the Medicare Hospice Benefit in 1982. Since then, access and utilization of hospice services have increased dramatically to an annual level of over one million patients served by hospice programs (5). Moreover, the 1995 SUPPORT study (6), which showed egregious deficiencies in end-of-life care, and the 1997 report from the U.S. Institute of Medicine (2), which provided a comprehensive assessment and elaboration of needs, prompted influential philanthropic foundations such as the Robert Wood Johnson and Mayday Funds to foster improvement in end-of-life care. As a result, there is now a burgeoning academic discipline of palliative medicine, including fellowship training programs for physicians and approval in 2006 by the American Board of Medical Specialties of a medical subspecialty in palliative medicine. Largely through the efforts of the Center to Advance Palliative Care (CAPC) at Mount Sinai School of Medicine in New York City, a sizeable proportion of U.S. hospitals currently have some form of organized palliative care consultation service. This was accomplished by philanthropic funding of regional training courses around the nation, led by CAPC faculty. Participants were instructed in ways to engender support for program development and operations in their parent institutions.

On a global basis, the initial 2004 IASP-EFIC-WHO Global Day Against Pain clearly enunciated the concept that pain relief should be a universal human right, as encapsulated in an accompanying editorial statement and subsequently reviewed in detail (7). Key elements of that message included that satisfactory palliation of pain in patients with substantial life expectancy, as well as in the terminally ill hospice population, should be achievable in most circumstances, and patients should be educated to expect that reasonable measures will be taken to achieve pain relief and support quality of life. Efforts are now being made by the National Hospice and Palliative Care Organization and the Foundation for Hospice in Sub-Saharan Africa, among others, to translate and export the lessons learned through these experiences to economically developing and underdeveloped nations, in order to mitigate the overwhelming consequences of the acquired immune deficiency syndrome (AIDS) epidemic and other life-limiting diseases that produce great suffering and high mortality rates.

In recent years, several evidence-based and consensus guidelines and supporting documents in the somewhat overlapping areas of geriatric pain management (Chapter 48) and palliative care address what "good care" can and should be. The first guideline that specifically addressed pain care for older patients was developed by a committee under the auspices of the American Geriatrics Society in 1998, with a revision in 2002 (8). Subsequently, the American Medical Directors Association created a similar document, to direct attention to appreciable deficiencies in pain assessment and management in nursing homes (institutional long-term care settings) (9). Most recently, the Canadian and U.S. governments have funded an interdisciplinary panel of experts to create a consensus document on the assessment of pain in older patients experiencing pain (10). The results of these efforts on patient outcomes have yet to be determined, but adherence to pain assessment and management processes and procedures is now required for U.S. nursing homes to pass regulatory surveys.

The late 2000s witnessed a convergence of extraordinary efforts to create systematic change in end-of-life care in North America. In 2004, the National Consensus Project for Quality Palliative Care, a consortium of professional organizations including the American Academy of Hospice and Palliative Care (AAHPM), the Center to Advance Palliative Care (CAPC), the Hospice and Palliative Nurses Association (HPNA), the National Hospice and Palliative Care Organization (NHPCO), and the Last Acts Partnership (subsequently merged into NHPCO), produced a monograph entitled "Clinical Practice Guidelines for Quality Palliative Care" (http:www.nationalconsensusproject.org). This document expands upon domains drawn from the work of previous efforts to produce standards of care in this field (Australia, New Zealand, Canada, Children's Hospice International, and the NHPCO) (Table 49-1). More recently, a framework for preferred practices in palliative and hospice care has been embraced by the National Quality Forum (NQF), a private consortium of not-for-profit organizations created to develop and implement a national strategy for health care quality measurement and reporting (http://www.qualityforum.org/txpalliative1pager+RCpublic4-05-05.pdf).

The National Hospice and Palliative Care Organization convened an expert panel to create and publish a research agenda for palliative care, a field that historically has had sparse funding for research and, for this and other reasons such as a culture that emphasized bedside care over clinical research, a very limited evidence base (11). Growing awareness of this problem led the U.S. National Institutes of Health (NIH) to host a State-of-the-Science conference in December, 2004, the recommendations from which have been published (12). In a similar vein, the NIH also hosted an expert task force to create guidelines for ethical research in end-of-life care, and these findings, too, have been published in the peer-reviewed medical literature (13). Together, these guidelines, policy statements, and consensus documents provide a roadmap to direct improvements in all aspects of palliative care and templates for the creation of standards and outcome measures.

DEFINITIONS

The WHO has defined palliative care as: *The active and total care of patients whose disease is not responsive to curative treatment. Control of pain, of other symptoms, and of psychological, social, and spiritual problems is paramount. The goal of palliative care is achievement of the best quality of life for patients and their families.* (14). This definition has been modified by the NQF in its recently approved consensus document entitled "National Framework and Preferred Practices for Palliative and Hospice Care" to read: *Palliative care means patient- and family-centered care that optimizes quality of life by anticipating, preventing, and treating suffering. Palliative care throughout the continuum of illness involves addressing physical, intellectual, emotional, social, and spiritual needs and to facilitate patient autonomy, access to information, and choice* (15). Note how this latter definition broadens care. That is, the time frame to begin palliative care has been moved "upstream" to include patients for whom curative and disease-modifying interventions may add years of life.

Because of the expansion of the time frame of palliative care, hospice care is now viewed as a "subset" of palliative care. Hospice care is therefore now defined by the NQF consensus group as: *A service delivery system that provides palliative care for patients that have a limited life expectancy and require comprehensive biomedical, psychosocial, and spiritual support as they enter the terminal stage of an illness or condition. It also supports family members coping with the complex consequences of illness, disability, and aging as death nears. Hospice care further addresses bereavement needs of the family following the death of the patient* (15). An integrated model of these concepts, which ties them together as a system of care that addresses the needs of patients throughout the continuum of care, is shown in Figure 49-1.

THE ETHICAL IMPERATIVE TO RELIEVE PAIN AT LIFE'S END

In patients with far-advanced disease, beyond the subjective nature of suffering, unrelieved persistent pain negatively impacts

TABLE 49-1

DOMAINS AND GUIDELINES FOR QUALITY PALLIATIVE CARE

Domain 1: Structure and Processes of Care
Guideline 1.1. The plan of care is based on a comprehensive interdisciplinary assessment of the patient and family.
Guideline 1.2. The care plan is based on the identified and expressed values, goals, and needs of patient and family, and is developed with professional guidance and support for decision-making.
Guideline 1.3. An interdisciplinary team provides services to the patient and family, consistent with the care plan.
Guideline 1.4. The interdisciplinary team may include appropriately trained and supervised volunteers.
Guideline 1.5. Support for education and training is available to the interdisciplinary team.
Guideline 1.6. The palliative care program is committed to quality improvement in clinical and management practices.
Guideline 1.7. The palliative care program recognizes the emotional impact on the palliative care team of providing care to patients with life-threatening illnesses and their families.
Guideline 1.8. Palliative care programs should have a relationship with one or more hospices and other community resources to ensure continuity of the highest-quality palliative care across the illness trajectory.
Guideline 1.9. The physical environment in which care is provided should meet the preferences, needs, and circumstances of the patient and family to the extent possible.

Domain 2: Physical Aspects of Care
Guideline 2.1. Pain, other symptoms, and side effects are managed based on the best available evidence, which is skillfully and systematically applied.

Domain 3: Psychological and Psychiatric Aspects of Care
Guideline 3.1. Psychological and psychiatric issues are assessed and managed based on the best available evidence, which is skillfully and systematically applied.
Guideline 3.2. A grief and bereavement program is available to patients and families, based on the assessed need for services.

Domain 4: Social Aspects of Care
Guideline 4.1. Comprehensive interdisciplinary assessment identifies the social needs of patients and their families, and a care plan is developed to respond to these needs as effectively as possible.

Domain 5: Spiritual, Religious, and Existential Aspects of Care
Guideline 5.1. Spiritual and existential dimensions are assessed and responded to based on the best available evidence, which is skillfully and systematically applied.

Domain 6: Cultural Aspects of Care
Guideline 6.1. The palliative care program assesses and attempts to meet the culture-specific needs of the patient and family.

Domain 7: Care of the Imminently Dying Patient
Guideline 7.1. Signs and symptoms of impending death are recognized and communicated, and care appropriate for this phase of illness is provided to patient and family.

Domain 8: Ethical and Legal Aspects of Care
Guideline 8.1. The patient's goals, preferences, and choices are respected within the limits of applicable state and federal law, and form the basis for the plan of care.
Guideline 8.2. The palliative care program is aware of and addresses the complex ethical issues arising in the care of persons with life-threatening debilitating illness.
Guideline 8.3. The palliative care program is knowledgeable about legal and regulatory aspects of palliative care.

Extracted from National Consensus Project for Quality Palliative Care Clinical Practice Guidelines for Quality Palliative Care, http://wwwnationalconsensusproject.org/GuidelinesDownload.asp. Accessed 6 August, 2006.

functional capacities, cognitive and emotional states, and, perhaps, survival. Yet, despite recent strong evidence to the contrary (16,17), aggressive pain control has in the past sometimes been erroneously assumed and taught to contribute to reduced life expectancy. Less quantifiable, but of tremendous significance to patients and their families, is the suffering, erosion of the sense of self, and loss of will to live caused by incessant, unrelieved severe pain (18,19). Furthermore, poorly managed pain is a frequent cause of readmission to the acute care hospital, which adds significantly to patient care costs (20).

The ethical imperatives that compel us to attend to these consequences of disease are core values of the health care professions: to relieve suffering and limit pathology caused by it, including premature death caused by suffering itself (21). These values should serve as a consistent and unifying tie that binds all clinicians, regardless of specialty or discipline (22). Virtually all medical interventions have a possible although unin-

tended downside. The conventional *doctrine of double effect* states that a foreseeable but unintended adverse outcome of a therapeutic intervention is ethically justified (under conditions specified). This principle allows care providers to proceed with therapeutic intent without being paralyzed by the ethical dread of causing unintentional harm. The doctrine of double effect applies across all medical practice. Application of this doctrine to justify any treatment implies that the following conditions are met: (a) the intervention must not be intrinsically wrong; (b) the motivation for the intervention is to provide a therapeutic effect, not an adverse one; (c) the potential adverse effect must not be the means of achieving the desired effect; (d) the value of the therapeutic intervention must outweigh the unintended but possible harms (23).

The doctrine of double effect has been given greater weight in terminal care than in other clinical settings because of the perceived risks of hastening death with aggressive symptom

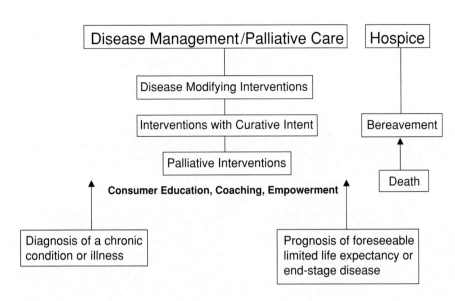

FIGURE 49-1. Conceptual model of comprehensive system of palliative care throughout the life continuum. Modified from Fine PG, Davis M. Hospice: Comprehensive care at the end of life. *Anesthesiol Clin* 2006;24(1):181–204, with permission.

management (e.g., using opioids). Yet, techniques of symptom control have become more refined, practitioners have become more skilled, and quality of life and reduced burden of illness have become increasingly accepted as priorities for mainstream medicine. Therefore, it is anticipated that patient autonomy, in the form of informed consent (by patient or legal proxy) will emerge as the leading ethical principle, as it has in other domains of medical care. In other words, special moral justification *should not* (and predictably *will not*) be required to attend to the dire needs of patients with incurable illness experiencing onerous symptoms, such as excruciating pain (24).

PAIN ASSESSMENT AND MANAGEMENT IN OLDER PATIENTS WITH TERMINAL ILLNESS

Pain is common in older individuals as they approach the end of life. The reported prevalence of persistent pain lies between 20% and 50% in community-dwelling adults, and reaches 84% in nursing home patients (25,26). As described in Chapter 48, pain in older patients is undertreated (27). This population—especially the cognitively impaired—is at greater risk of undertreatment than younger patients with comparable pain-producing diagnoses (28). Older patients are also at risk of complications from pain therapies, largely because of adverse drug reactions, drug interactions, and medical comorbidities (e.g., anticoagulation) that complicate invasive therapies (29). Notwithstanding these sobering facts, pain can be safely and effectively managed in terminally ill older persons by applying well-described multimodal approaches, incorporating nonpharmacologic, pharmacologic, and interventional therapies when indicated (30–33). Thus, it is very important to seek underlying causes that are amenable to specific pain relief strategies; for example, a vertebral crush fracture that may possibly be suitable for percutaneous vertebroplasty or the low-dose epidural infusion of suitable agents.

The key to pain control in palliative care of older patients, as in all age groups, depends upon assessment sufficient to determine etiology and indications for a range of available interven-

tions. Two important added and often confounding dimensions in older patients, particularly those with far-advanced illness, are the inherent difficulties of assessment in those with cognitive impairment (e.g., dementing illness, expressive aphasia, etc.) and limited anticipated life expectancy (short prognosis).

Pain assessment in patients with cognitive impairment who are unable to self-report using standardized pain intensity assessment tools and verbal descriptors requires interpretation of behaviors. An ongoing problem in this context is to validate proposed instruments, since purported pain behaviors and behavioral responses to analgesics may be ambiguous. There has been a proliferation of new pain assessment tools for older patients with dementing illness, varying in length, content, and complexity of interpretation. Purely from the standpoint of decreasing assessor burden, in most clinical settings (in contrast to psychometric research or clinical trials), the Pain Assessment in Advanced Dementia (PAINAD) tool is recommended (34). This scale consists of five items, each of which is scored on a three-point, 0 to 2 scale corresponding to specific descriptors with regard to breathing, vocalization, facial expression, body language, and consolability. Analgesic protocols applied to patients with dementing illness have been shown to reduce these scores (35).

In patients with a relatively short life expectancy (e.g., weeks to months), certain therapies (e.g., implanted intrathecal pump) that might otherwise be highly appropriate for a longer-lived patient (>3 months) may be less applicable due to an excessive opportunity cost-to-benefit ratio (36). Nevertheless, even in patients with limited prognoses, regional anesthetic interventions that can provide definitive relief (e.g., neurolytic celiac plexus block, as described in Chapter 45 by Burton and Phan) should be considered as early as possible to reduce pain and suffering and optimize physical and functional outcomes by reducing adverse effects associated with systemic analgesic therapy (37). "Low-tech," minimally invasive methods of spinal drug delivery can offer a high benefit-to-cost ratio in this setting. These methods include tunneled epidural and intrathecal catheters that are exteriorized and connected to portable infusion pumps, or intrathecal or epidural port systems (e.g., Port-A-Cath) as described in Chapter 40.

Conversely, in the terminal phase of a disease, when comfort—rather than maximizing cognitive and functional capacities—may be the patient's highest priority, prior concerns

TABLE 49-2

MECHANISM-SPECIFIC PAIN THERAPIES FOR PATIENTS RECEIVING PALLIATIVE CARE

Pain type	Underlying pain mechanism	Examples	Treatment approach
Nociceptive	Activation of pain receptors resulting from inflammation, mechanical deformation, ongoing injury, tissue destruction, ischemia, visceral obstruction, or dilatation	▪ Arthritis ▪ Ischemic disease ▪ Mechanical low back pain ▪ Pathologic fractures ▪ Surgery ▪ Myofascial pain ▪ Procedural pain	Responds well to traditional interventions: ▪ Nonpharmacologic ▪ Cognitive-behavioral ▪ Systemic and topical analgesics ▪ Regional anesthetics
Neuropathic	Pathology involving peripheral or central nervous system. Upregulation of receptors, central sensitization and neuroplastic changes, N-methyl-D-aspartate receptor involvement are among current theories of underlying mechanisms for neuropathic pain.	▪ Diabetic neuropathy ▪ Neuropathic back pain ▪ Postherpetic neuralgia ▪ Post-stroke pain ▪ Phantom limb pain ▪ Postoperative neuropathic pain syndromes (e.g., post-mastectomy, post-thoracotomy) ▪ Trigeminal neuralgia ▪ Radiation neuritis ▪ Chemotherapy neuritis ▪ HIV neuropathy ▪ Complex regional pain syndromes (CRPS I, II)	Does not predictably or fully respond to traditional analgesics; interpatient variability of response to adjuvant analgesics, opioids, oral/topical/peripheral/ regional local anesthetics, spinal pharmacotherapy, neurostimulation (e.g., peripheral or dorsal column stimulation; transcutaneous or percutaneous nerve stimulation). Commonly requires multimodal therapy and combinations of treatments. Parenteral local anesthetic infusion and/or subanesthetic ketamine may be required in intractable cases, especially in end-of-life care.
Mixed or unknown	Mixed or unknown mechanisms	▪ Chronic low back pain ▪ Recurrent headache ▪ Vasculitis	May require combinations of traditional and nontraditional approaches.
Psychological disorders	Psychiatric conditions and personality disorders that predispose to or exacerbate pain perception and experiences that are refractory to conventional pain treatment	▪ Anxiety disorders ▪ Bipolar disorders ▪ Borderline personality disorder ▪ Major depressive illness ▪ Dementing illness ▪ Schizo-affective disorders	Traditional pain therapies should only be applied to target specifically defined pathology. Absent or paradoxical treatment responses should be anticipated and managed with psychiatric strategies.

about mental clouding, sedation, ataxia, and other dose-limiting adverse effects of analgesic drugs may become less important. Similarly, drugs whose long-term use should be avoided whenever possible in older patients, such as NSAIDs and corticosteroids, may provide great benefit during the last days to weeks of a patient's life. In older patients in general, knowledge of concurrent medication use and medical history, laboratory assessment of hepatic and renal function, and the patient's report of prior experience with analgesics best prepares the clinician to anticipate and mitigate against treatment complications (38).

It is sensible to direct therapies at the pathophysiologic mechanism(s) of pain whenever possible, using disease-modifying approaches, but also to palliate distressing symptoms while medical, surgical, or (in cancer care) radiotherapeutic management is optimized. In some cases, palliative therapies may be temporizing (e.g., epidural analgesia during acute herpes zoster in an immunocompromised elderly patient), whereas in other cases, palliation may be the dominant theme of treatment during a course of years (e.g., for chronic severe neuropathic pain due to long-standing diabetes mellitus). Regardless, mechanism-specific treatments offering the least likelihood of added complications should guide treatment decisions. A sum-

mary of pain mechanisms and treatment approaches is outlined in Table 49-2.

A generic method for the treatment of pain was developed by the WHO 20 years ago in an effort to provide a simple, worldwide, easily explained means of relieving cancer pain. The WHO three-step analgesic ladder has been shown to be highly effective in controlling cancer pain in most patients most of the time (39). However, an appreciable number of patients with persistent pain syndromes have insufficient responses or intolerable drug- and dose-related side effects. A modification of the WHO model, shown in Figure 49-2, has therefore been proposed that draws upon additional pain-relieving modalities to provide a better therapeutic index for pain control, both in cancer and noncancer conditions (4).

THE MANY BURDENS OF CHRONIC PROGRESSIVE ILLNESS

It is important to remember that pain is but one of a panoply of symptoms associated with aging, chronic progressive disease, and terminal illness. Pain and other highly prevalent

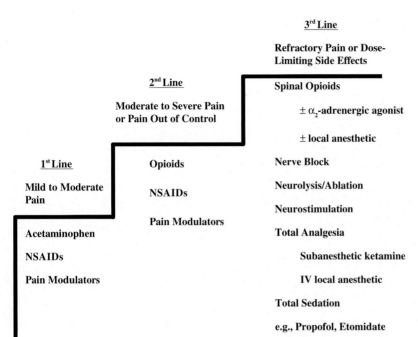

FIGURE 49-2. Modification of World Health Organization Step Ladder Approach to Pain Control. Adapted from Fine PG. The evolving and important role of anesthesiology in palliative care. *Anesth Analg* 2005;100:183–188, with permission.

symptoms such as dyspnea, gastrointestinal disturbances, fatigue and weakness, cognitive impairment, and mood disturbances often amplify each other, as do treatment effects (e.g., opioid adverse effects) (40). Therefore, comprehensive palliative therapy and the role of the pain specialist within palliative care teams require knowledge of evaluation, prevention, and treatment of all burdensome and distressing symptoms, consistent with the patient's goals of care. Specific to the domain of pain management, and the currently irreplaceable role of opioid analgesics, it is appearing hopeful that the advent of peripherally acting opioid receptor antagonists (e.g., alvimopan, methylnaltrexone) (41) will obviate one of the most commonly caused complications of opioid therapy that significantly impacts quality of life in older patients: opioid-induced bowel dysfunction, including constipation, bloating, reflux, and nausea, among others (42).

Finally, the complexities of pain syndromes must be continually recalled. Once a patient's baseline pain is controlled, as discussed in Chapter 45 on cancer pain control, breakthrough pain (BTP) is very common in patients with far-advanced disease (43). Breakthrough pain must be assessed and treated to optimize quality of life at the end of life in all patients with persistent pain problems. Noninvasive, but rapid-onset, transmucosal delivery formulations of fentanyl have been found to be highly effective for the treatment of BTP. In many cases, the speed of onset is preferred to more conventional oral opioid formulations (pills, capsules, liquids), but demonstrated tolerance to opioid effects at the start of BTP therapy mandates cautious titration to prevent toxicity (44).

SUMMARY

Pain and other emotionally distressing and physically disabling symptoms are very common during chronic progressive illnesses, and these problems become intensified with end-stage disease. Palliative care programs that meet physical, emotional, and spiritual needs effectively address the principal concerns voiced by those facing life-limiting illness (45,46). There is a subset of patients for whom conventional approaches to pain and symptom management do not provide adequate comfort or facilitate optimal functioning. In these persons, immediate consultation with an expert in the management of refractory symptoms is required. Anesthesiologists, by virtue of their unique training, should logically serve in this capacity. Expertise in determining indications for and providing interventional therapies, the ability to weigh lost opportunities to enhance quality of life when such therapies are delayed, and the ability to consider the myriad of contextual nuances of patients and their clinical and social circumstances, are required skills. Guiding principles for interventional therapies, when they are indicated, have been proposed (47), and are reviewed in detail in earlier chapters on cancer pain, interventional and neurolytic therapies, and spinal analgesia. In the author's view, these include:

- *Know the patient.* This should not be confused with knowing the disease. A deep understanding of what might constitute a "mortal blow" to the individual's sense of personhood—that is, what is really at stake and what has meaning to the patient—is required to adequately ascertain acceptable risk.
- *Know all available therapeutic options.* This includes full knowledge of likely risks and benefits, within the context of each patient's unique set of circumstances. Informed consent implies a fully informed clinician to advise the patient.
- *Precede permanent interventions with temporary (diagnostic) maneuvers,* whenever time and circumstances allow, to better gauge the likely long-term benefits and risks.

To meet the growing challenge of maximizing quality of life in our aging societies, with an increasing proportion of individuals with protracted, chronic illnesses, grounding in both the pragmatic and ethical issues of geriatric and end-of-life care is necessary (Table 49-3). In providing this expertise, we can assure all patients and their families that the last phases of life need not be met with a sense of trepidation or despair. With sufficient preparation and application of available knowledge and clinical tools, it is now possible—ethically, legally, and safely—to realize the long-heralded admonition to "provide comfort always."

TABLE 49-3

KEY ELEMENTS FOR PHYSICIANS IN OPTIMIZING PAIN MANAGEMENT IN OLDER PATIENTS WITH FAR-ADVANCED DISEASE

Goals of Care

1. Determine and review the patient's priorities with regard to goals of pain management and trade-offs from potential or likely pain treatment–related adverse effects:
   - Activity and functional capacities
   - Improved sleep
   - Interpersonal/social interactions
   - Reduction in pain-related mood disorders (anxiety, depression)
   - Comfort
2. Reconcile goals and range of available treatment options with opportunity costs:
   - Potential reduction in mental clarity for optimum comfort during final weeks, days, hours of life
   - Time and effort to access certain types of treatment (e.g., palliative radiation therapy)
   - Benefits and burdens associated with interventional (invasive) therapies (e.g., intraspinal drug delivery, nerve blocks, parenteral infusions)

Differential Diagnosis: Assessment of Pain Etiology

1. Comprehensive assessment: also consider information provided by other professionals (e.g., RN's comprehensive assessment, other test reports, etc.).
2. Common causes of tumor-related pain:
   - Nociceptive pain:
     - Visceral pain (obstruction, tumor invasion, abscess/necrosis/ischemia)
     - Somatic pain (tumor infiltration of soft tissues, bone lesions)
   - Neuropathic pain:
     - Infiltration of peripheral nerves, nerve roots/plexus, spinal cord compression
3. Treatment-related pain:
   - Chemotherapy-induced neuropathy
   - Postradiation pain
   - Postsurgical pain (e.g., postmastectomy pain; postthoracotomy pain)
4. Nonmalignant pain disorders:
   - Osteoarthritis, headache, postherpetic neuralgia, diabetic neuropathy, etc.

Rapid Response to Pain Crisis (Severe/excruciating pain not responsive to existing therapeutic approaches as designated under the plan of care)

1. Determine whether this is a new pain or recurrence/exacerbation of preexisting pain.
2. Rapid formulation of differential diagnosis by history and exam findings, to the extent possible:
   - Institute disease-modifying therapies if pertinent (e.g., antimicrobials for infection, octreotide for bowel obstruction; high-dose corticosteroids for refractory inflammation or tumor-encroachment symptoms) only if consistent with patient's goals of care.
   - Institute pain crisis protocols (e.g., rapid titration of opioids [APS Guideline, page 43]; trial of ketamine [APS Guideline, page 98, 102]).
   - Consult with established pain expert if pain remains out of control or intolerable treatment-related adverse effects prevail.

Routine Pain Management

1. Assure that nonpharmacologic therapies are being applied appropriately (e.g., positioning, heat, cold).
2. Assure adequate management of pain-amplifying cognitive/mood disorders (e.g., anxiety, depression, boredom, agitation) through milieu and cognitive-behavioral therapies or pharmacotherapy.
3. Identify temporal patterns of persistent continuous pain and break-through pain (severe episodic pains occurring against a background of otherwise well-controlled pain) and provide treatment for both.
4. Choose route of administration that is least invasive and a function of patient preference, considering route that provides access and is therapeutically effective.
5. Prescribe pharmacotherapy based on sufficient understanding of pain etiology to address pain mechanisms when possible; combine lowest effective doses of mechanistically different drugs to optimize therapeutic effects and minimize adverse effects:
   - Nonsteroidal anti-inflammatory drugs (NSAIDs) for nociceptive inflammatory disease processes (e.g., pain associated with bone metastasis)
     - Use nonselective NSAIDs very cautiously in patients with compromised platelet function or those who are at risk of bleeding.
     - Use all NSAIDs very cautiously in patients at risk for congestive heart failure and those with renal insufficiency
   - Opioid therapy for moderate to severe pain of any cause where opioids are not absolutely contraindicated
   - Adjuvant analgesics (e.g., low-dose secondary amine tricyclic antidepressants [desipramine, nortriptyline], anticonvulsants [gabapentin, pregabalin], norepinephrine serotonin reuptake inhibitors (NSRIs) [venlafaxine, duloxetine] for neuropathic pain
   - Additional adjuvant agents (e.g., corticosteroids, bisphosphonates, calcitonin) for bone pain
   - See attached drug tables with dosing and drug selection recommendations for older adults.

(continued)

TABLE 49-3

(CONTINUED)

6. Refer to equianalgesic tables for initial opioid dosing, drug conversion and opioid rotation.
7. Titrate opioid analgesics and adjuvants according to the pharmacokinetic profile of the drug, the patient's response to therapy, and the impact of the patient's pain on quality of life.
   - An acceptable outcome is pain that is controlled to a patient's defined level of comfort within 48 hours of admission to hospice and on an ongoing basis through the time of death.
   - Initiate opioid therapy for older adults at a 25%–50% lower dose than that recommended for younger adults and slowly titrate dosage by 25% on an individual basis until there is either a 50% reduction in the patient's pain rating or the patient reports satisfactory pain relief.
8. Use long-acting opioid formulations for continuous moderate to severe pain and immediate-release or rapid onset opioids for break-through pain.
   - Break-through (rescue) doses may be made available every 1–2 hours during oral opioid therapy and every 30–60 minutes during parenteral or intraspinal therapy.
   - Break-through doses may be taken at any time, even at the same time as the ATC opioid.
   - Recommended dosing for break-through pain is 10%–15% of the total daily dose of ATC oral opioid analgesic and 25%–50% of the hourly parenteral or intraspinal dose.
9. Morphine, oxycodone, hydromorphone, fentanyl, oxymorphone, methadone, and hydrocodone are the opioids of choice for moderate to severe pain.
   - *Morphine* has active metabolites (M-3-G, M-6-G) that are cleared via the kidney. Excessive sedation, agitation, myoclonus, or hyperalgesia should be considered possible consequences of morphine metabolite toxicity and an indication for conversion to an alternative opioid.
   - *Methadone* must be used with great caution due to its highly variable half-life and nonlinear relative analgesic equivalents. Follow dose-conversion guidelines carefully when switching to methadone from another opioid (APS Guideline, page 56). Titrate slowly and monitor drug effects frequently.
   - *Hydrocodone* safety and efficacy in patients with severe pain is limited by acetaminophen content, which should not exceed 4 g in patients with normal renal and hepatic function.
10. Follow-up by clinical staff (monitoring) should include evaluation of both therapeutic effects and common adverse effects.
    - Lack of sufficient efficacy but tolerable side effects: titrate to a higher dose or consider an alternative and/or additional "synergistic" agent from a different pharmacologic class (e.g., combine low-dose anticonvulsant therapy with low-dose opioid therapy for the treatment of neuropathic pain).
    - The best strategy for opioid-induced side effect management is decreasing the dose of the opioid by 25%–50%, depending on severity of side effects.
    - Opioid-induced bowel dysfunction (constipation): institute a bowel regimen at the onset of opioid use. Assure that there is no symptomatology consistent with fecal impaction prior to prescribing motility agents (APS Guideline, page 67–68).
    - Excessive sedation or mental clouding: allow ample time for patient to habituate to this common effect. Temporize with central nervous system stimulants (APS Guideline, page 69) as indicated and desired by the patient.
    - Nausea: if temporally connected to initiation of opioid therapy or dose escalation, allow ample time for patient to habituate to this common opioid effect. Temporize with antiemetics; if no resolution within a few days, consider other causes and switching to a different opioid or nonenteral delivery system (e.g., transdermal patch).

Intractable Pain and Implementing Palliative Sedation
1. Review patient's Advance Directives and goals of care.
2. Assure that all usual therapies have been appropriately applied.
3. Assure that staff and family understand the gravity of the situation and benefits/risks associated with palliative sedation protocols.
4. Consider relative merits of General Inpatient versus Continuous Care level of hospice care.
5. Seek additional expert consultation and rapid resolution of issues if unsure of indications, ethical circumstances, family member or staff conflicts, concerns with clinical protocols.
6. Review pharmacologic options: opioids, benzodiazepines, barbiturates, ketamine, propofol.
7. Ensure that neuroleptic agents (e.g., chlorpromazine, haloperidol), if indicated, are properly used and not merely masking emotional or physical distress. These drugs should be used only highly selectively for the treatment of agitation, delirium, or psychosis that is not remedied by more etiology-specific therapies. They should not be used for palliative sedation.

Data from Herr K, Bjoro K, Steffensmeier J, Rakel B. Guideline for the Management of Cancer Pain in Adults and Children. *American Pain Society,* 2005; Clinical Practice Guidelines for Quality Palliative Care. *National Consensus Project for Quality Palliative Care,* 2004; Evidence-Based Practice Guideline: Acute Pain Management in Older Adults, 2006.

References

1. Dartmouth Medical School Center for the Evaluative Clinical Sciences. *The Dartmouth Atlas of Healthcare*, 3rd ed. Chicago: American Hospital Association Services, 1999.
2. Field M, Cassell C. *Approaching Death: Improving Care at the End of Life*. Washington, DC: Institute of Medicine, National Academy Press, 1997.
3. Osler W. Address to students of the Albany Medical College. *Albany Med Ann* 1899;20:307–309.
4. Fine PG. The evolving and important role of anesthesiology in palliative care. *Anesth Analg* 2005;100:183–188.
5. Center for the Evaluative Clinical Sciences, Dartmouth College. *Dartmouth Atlas of Healthcare*. The care of patients with severe chronic illness. A report on the Medicare Program by the Dartmouth Atlas Project, 2006.
6. The SUPPORT Principal Investigators. A controlled trial to improve care for seriously ill hospitalized patients: The Study to Understand Prognoses and Preferences for Outcomes and Risks of Treatment (SUPPORT). *JAMA* 1995;274:1591–1598.
7. Brennan F, Carr DB, Cousins MJ. Pain management: A fundamental human right. *Anesth Analg* 2007;105:205–221.
8. AGS Panel on Persistent Pain in Older Persons. The management of persistent pain in older persons. *J Am Geriatr Soc* 2002;50:S205–S224.
9. American Medical Directors Association (AMDA). Pain management in the long-term care setting. Columbia MD: American Medical Directors Association (AMDA), 2003:1–36.
10. Hadjistavropoulos T, Fine PG, Herr KA, et al. An interdisciplinary expert consensus statement on assessment of older persons experiencing pain. *Clin J Pain* 2007;23:S1–S43.
11. National Hospice and Palliative Care Organization. Development of the NHPCO research agenda. *J Pain Symptom Manage* 2004;28(5):488–496.
12. NIH Select Panel. National Institutes of Health State of the Science Conference to Improve Care at the End of Life. *J Palliat Med* 2005;8[Suppl 1]:S1–S115.
13. Fine PG. Maximizing benefits and minimizing risks in palliative care research that involves patients near the end of life. *J Pain Symptom Manage* 2003;25(4):S53–S62.
14. World Health Organization. *Cancer Pain Relief and Palliative Care*. Report of a WHO expert committee (World Health Organization Technical Report Series, 804). Geneva: World Health Organization; 1990:1–75.
15. National Quality Forum. *National Framework and Preferred Practices for Palliative and Hospice Care*. Washington, DC: National Quality Forum, Washington; 2006:vi.
16. Morita T, Tsunoda J, Inoue S, Chihara S. Effects of high dose opioids and sedatives on survival in terminally ill cancer patients. *J Pain Symptom Manage* 2001;21:282–289.
17. Portenoy RK, Sibirceva BA, Smout MS, et al. Opioid use and survival at the end of life: A survey of a hospice population. *J Pain Symptom Manage* 2006;32(6):532–540.
18. Chochinov HM, Krisjanson LJ, Hack TF, et al. Dignity in the terminally ill: Revisited. *J Palliat Med* 2006;9(3):666–672.
19. Fine PG. Discussing assisted suicide. American College of Physicians, Physicians' Information and Education Resource. Available at http://pier.acponline.org/physicians/ethical_legal/el025.html. Accessed 5 Aug, 2006.
20. Grant M, Ferrell B, Rivera L, Lee J. Unscheduled readmissions for uncontrolled symptoms. *Nurs Clin North Am* 1995;30:673–682.
21. Connor S, Pyenson B, Fitch K, et al. Comparing hospice and nonhospice patient survival among patients who die within a three-year window. *J Pain Symptom Manage* 2007;33(3):238–246.
22. Fine PG. The ethical imperative to relieve pain at life's end. *J Pain Symptom Manage* 2002;23(4):273–277.
23. Kamm F. The doctrine of double effect: Reflections on theoretical and practical issues. *J Med Philos* 1991;16:571–585.
24. Quill TE, Dresser R, Brock D. The rule of double effect: A critique of its role in end-of-life decision making. *New Engl J Med* 1997;337:1768–1771.
25. Blyth FM, March LM, Brnabic AJ, et al. Chronic pain in Australia: A prevalence study. *Pain* 2001;89:127–134.
26. Hartikainen SA, Mantyselka PT, Louhivouri-Laako KA, Sulkava RO. Balancing pain and analgesic treatment in the home-dwelling elderly. *Ann Pharmacother* 2005;39:11–16.
27. Teno JM, Weitzen S, Wetle T, Mor V. Persistent pain in nursing home residents. *JAMA* 2001;285:2081.
28. Morrison RS, Siu AL. A comparison of pain and its treatment in advanced dementia and cognitively intact patients with hip fracture. *J Pain Symptom Manage* 2000;19:240–248.
29. Weiner DK, Hanlon JT. Pain in nursing home residents: Management strategies. *Drugs Aging* 2001;18:13–29.
30. Fine PG. Benefits of pain management in the elderly. *Manag Care* 2005;30[12 Suppl]:46–55.
31. Paice J, Fine PG. Pain management at end of life. In: Ferrell B, Coyle N, eds. *Oxford Textbook of Palliative Nursing*, 2nd ed. New York: Oxford University Press, 2005.
32. Bernstein C, Lateef B, Fine PG. Interventional pain management procedures in older patients. In: Gibson S, Weiner D, eds. *Pain in Older Persons*. Seattle: IASP Press, 2005.
33. Fine PG, Davis M. Hospice: Comprehensive care at the end of life. *Anesthesiol Clin* 2006;24(1):181–204.
34. Warden V, Hurley AC, Volicer L. Development and psychometric evaluation of the Pain Assessment in Advanced Dementia (PAINAD) scale. *J Am Med Dir Assoc* 2003;4:9–15.
35. Cohen-Mansfield J, Lipson S. The utility of pain assessment for analgesic use in persons with dementia. *Pain* 2008;134:16–23.
36. Smith TJ, Staats PS, Deer T, et al. Randomized clinical trial of an implantable drug delivery system compared with comprehensive medical management for refractory cancer pain: Impact on pain, drug-related toxicity, and survival. *J Clin Oncol* 2002;20(19):4040–4049.
37. Wong GY, Schroeder DR, Carns PE, et al. Effect of neurolytic celiac plexus block on pain relief, quality of life, and survival in patients with unresectable pancreatic cancer. *JAMA* 2004; 291(9):1092–1099.
38. Fine PG, Herr KA. Efficacy, safety, and tolerability of pharmacotherapy for management of persistent pain in older persons. *Annals of Long-Term Care* 2006;14(3):25–33.
39. Zech DF, Grond S, Lynch J, et al. Validation of World Health Organization Guidelines for cancer pain relief: A 10-year prospective study. *Pain* 1995;63:65–76.
40. Schonwetter R, Roscoe LA, Nwosu M, et al. Quality of life and symptom control in hospice patients with cancer receiving chemotherapy. *J Palliat Med* 2006;9(3):638–645.
41. Paulson DM, Kennedy DT, Donovick RA, et al. Alvimopan: An oral, peripherally acting μ-opioid receptor antagonist for the treatment of opioid-induced bowel dysfunction: A 21-day treatment-randomized clinical trial. *J Pain* 2005;6(3):184–192.
42. McNicol E, Boyce DB, Schumann R, Carr D. Efficacy and safety of mu opioid antagonists in the treatment of opioid induced bowel dysfunction: Systematic review and meta-analysis of randomized controlled trials. *Pain Med* 2007;Epub.
43. Fine PG, Busch M. Characterization of breakthrough pain by hospice patients and their caregivers. *J Pain Symptom Manage* 1998;16:179–183.
44. Fine PG. Oral transmucosal opioid analgesics. In: Fine PG. *The Diagnosis and Treatment of Breakthrough Pain*. New York, Oxford University Press, 2008.
45. Steinhauser KE, Christakis NA, Clipp EC, et al. Factors considered important at the end of life by patients, family, physicians, and other care providers. *JAMA* 2000;284:2476–2482.
46. Emanuel L, Alpert HR, Baldwin DC, Emanuel EJ. What terminally ill patients care about: Toward a validated construct of patients' perspective. *J Palliat Med* 2000;3:419–431.
47. Fine PG. Response to a complication of midline myelotomy. *J Cancer Pain Symptom Pall* 2005;1(2):51–53.

CHAPTER 50 ■ COMPLICATIONS IN PAIN MEDICINE

JAMES P. RATHMELL

Complications arise in the course of any type of medical treatment, and the common interventions used to treat acute and chronic pain are no exception. The best approach to preventing adverse outcomes during the majority of these treatments is to have detailed knowledge of the patient's medical condition and of the pharmacology/physiology of the intervention. Also required are a detailed knowledge of the anatomy of the adjacent structures that lie near the target site for each intended treatment and a clear understanding of how the technique has been devised to minimize the risk of harm to these structures. Many pain procedures are now best carried out with the use of radiographic guidance, and the widespread availability of fluoroscopy has increased both the precision and safety of many techniques. When complications do arise, prompt recognition and treatment can often prevent serious sequelae. This chapter reviews complications associated with many of the treatments used in the practice of pain medicine.

COMPLICATIONS ASSOCIATED WITH EPIDURAL, FACET JOINT, AND SACROILIAC INJECTION

Direct injection of local anesthetic with or without long-acting corticosteroid suspensions has been used in the diagnosis and treatment of pain arising from spinal structures. Among the most common applications is the injection of corticosteroid into the epidural space in efforts to reduce the pain associated with acute lumbar disc herniation and spinal stenosis (1,2). In those with acute radicular pain caused by herniation of an intervertebral disc, epidural steroid injection appears to speed the resolution of acute pain. The degenerative cascade that leads to loss of intervertebral disc height with ageing can cause increased stress on the zygapophyseal (facet) joints, and these facet joints are well recognized as a source of chronic axial back pain. Injection of the local anesthetic and corticosteroid within the facet joints has been used with limited success to treat axial back pain (3). Injection of local anesthetic along the course of the medial branch nerve to the facet joints is often used as a diagnostic test before proceeding with radiofrequency ablation. The sacroiliac joint (SIJ) is a less common cause for axial low back pain, and injection of local anesthetic into the joint has been used as a diagnostic test for SIJ-related pain, whereas injection of corticosteroid has been used with limited success to afford longer-term pain resolution (4).

Few reports of serious complications are associated with epidural, facet joint, and sacroiliac joint injection of corticosteroids. However, it is difficult to estimate the actual incidence of complications with any certainty, as no mandatory reporting system exists for such adverse events in the United States. The American Society of Anesthesiologists (ASA) maintains an ongoing surveillance of malpractice claims that have been settled through the ASA Closed Claims study, and a recent report stemming from this project detailed 114 complications associated with chronic pain treatment (Table 50-1) (5). In addition, there remain significant concerns regarding the neurotoxic potential of the available corticosteroid preparations (6). Neurotoxicity, neurologic injury, and the pharmacologic effects of corticosteroids have all been reported as complications following epidural, facet joint, and sacroiliac corticosteroid injections.

Neurotoxicity

The intrathecal injection of neurotoxic substances can result in inflammation of the meninges with or without direct neural injury in the form of arachnoiditis or cauda equina syndrome. Arachnoiditis is an inflammatory condition of the meninges that can extend to the underlying neural structures. This inflammation usually follows significant spinal infection, often following tertiary syphilis or advanced tuberculosis (7). However, arachnoiditis can also arise following the intrathecal injection of radiographic contrast or following surgical breach of the spinal canal during spinal surgery. Cauda equina syndrome is a broad descriptive term that refers to neurologic signs and symptoms that arise from direct compression of the cauda equina. The syndrome is characterized by bilateral sciatica, saddle hyperesthesia, lower extremity weakness; and bowel, bladder, and sexual dysfunction. Although cauda equina syndrome is most often seen in association with a compressive lesion (e.g., epidural extension of a metastatic tumor or a large central disc herniation), similar symptoms can also arise in association with severe arachnoiditis. The typical signs and symptoms of arachnoiditis are shown in Table 50-2 (see also Fig. 50-30).

Concern regarding the potential for neurotoxicity associated with epidural steroid injections stems from reports of arachnoiditis that arose during the course of repeated intrathecal injections administered for the treatment of multiple sclerosis (8–10). Two cases of arachnoiditis were reported among a series of 23 patients receiving repeated injections of intrathecal methylprednisolone acetate (MPA), and concern was raised about the drug vehicle, polyethylene glycol, as the possible causative agent (8). Only one case of documented arachnoiditis has been reported following epidural steroid injection for sciatica due to lumbar disc disease complicated by a traumatic tap; the symptoms resolved following subsequent discectomy (11).

TABLE 50-1

PRIMARY OUTCOME FOR CLAIMS RELATED TO EPIDURAL STEROID INJECTIONS

Nerve injury	28
Infection	24
Death/brain damage	9
Headache	20
Increased pain/no relief	10

Data from Fitzgibbon DR, Posner KL, Caplan RA, et al. Chronic pain management: American Society of Anesthesiologists Closed Claims Project. *Anesthesiology* 2004;100:98–105.

Aseptic meningitis has also been reported following intrathecal injection of MPA (12,13). This condition can arise after the intrathecal injection of nearly any substance, including normal saline (14). Aseptic meningitis is generally a benign and self-limited condition that produces signs of neurologic irritation, including burning pain in the legs, headache, meningismus, and, in severe cases, seizures. Fever and nausea are often reported. Cerebrospinal fluid (CSF) examination reveals pleocytosis, elevated protein, and decreased glucose. Several cases of aseptic meningitis have been reported after intrathecal corticosteroid injection (12,15,16) and one case has been reported after epidural (17) corticosteroid injection. In at least one case (17), the symptoms were severe and prolonged, resolving over a period of more than 3 weeks.

Limited evidence suggests that any component of the available long-acting corticosteroid preparations may be neurotoxic. Following the appearance of arachnoiditis during the intrathecal injection of MPA, propylene glycol was suggested as the offending agent (6). The polyethylene glycol preparation used in steroid suspensions has a molecular weight of 3,350 and is present in concentrations of 2.8% to 3%. However, propylene glycol has no acute effects on either sheathed or unsheathed neurons in concentrations up to 10%, with mild slowing appearing at 20% to 30%, and complete abolishment of conduction at 40% (18). This effect was reversible following washout in both sheathed and unsheathed nerves. Benzyl alcohol 0.9% is present as a preservative in several steroid suspension preparations, including multidose vials of Depo-Medrol brand MPA (Pharmacia & Upjohn, Kalamazoo, MI) and Aristocort Intralesional brand triamcinolone diacetate (American Cyanamid, Madison, NJ). Mild, transient inflammatory changes appear in the nerve roots, cord root entry zone, and meninges after epidural injections of triamcinolone diacetate plus lidocaine in cats (19); however, no discernible effects on neurologic function or histology were seen in a separate study examining repeated intrathecal injections of triamcinolone diacetate (20). Direct intrathecal injection of up to 9% benzyl alcohol (10 times the concentration used as a preser-

TABLE 50-2

SYMPTOMS OF ADHESIVE ARACHNOIDITIS

Constant, burning pain in low back, legs
Urinary frequency, incontinence
Muscle spasm, back and legs
Variable sensory loss
Variable motor dysfunction

vative) in dogs produced transient neurologic dysfunction related to the local anesthetic effect of this agent without the appearance of any discernible long-term sequelae or histologic changes (21).

Much public controversy surrounded the risk of arachnoiditis following epidural MPA administration in Australia during the 1990s. This led some practitioners to adopt the use of Celestone Chronodose (betamethasone 5.7 mg, as betamethasone sodium phosphate 3.9 mg [in solution] and betamethasone acetate 3 mg/mL [in suspension] in an aqueous vehicle; Schering-Plough, Kenilworth, NJ) for epidural injection. This product contains sodium phosphate monobasic, disodium edetate, benzalkonium chloride, and water. However, a study in sheep demonstrated arachnoiditis in animals receiving 2 mL or more of this preparation intrathecally (22). More recently, practitioners have moved to the use of the potent, soluble steroid dexamethasone for epidural use; a recent study in rodents found no evidence of arachnoiditis or neural injury following intrathecal administration of this agent (23).

It is not clear that a single intrathecal injection of any of the available corticosteroid preparations will cause any harm. Indeed, a recent study of repeated intrathecal administration of MPA for postherpetic neuralgia failed to find any evidence of either aseptic meningitis or arachnoiditis among 89 patients treated with four 60-mg injections (24). However, it is important for practitioners to realize that, despite their widespread use for epidural injection, the U.S. Food and Drug Administration nor any other regulatory agency labels these steroid preparations for epidural use. The concern regarding arachnoiditis appears to be limited to intrathecal administration (e.g., following inadvertent dural puncture in the course of attempted epidural placement); large case series and randomized trials of epidural injections of long-acting particulate steroids are devoid of reports of arachnoiditis. Thus, the most prudent approach is to use all means available to avoid intrathecal injection of corticosteroid. A local anesthetic test dose administered prior to steroid injection can effectively rule out intrathecal placement. Use of radiographic guidance and injection of a small amount of radiographic contrast can also be used to accurately confirm epidural localization of the injectate. In those patients in whom a dural puncture occurs during needle placement, it is prudent to consider abandoning the procedure; placement of the corticosteroid at an adjacent interspace will reduce, but not completely eliminate the chance of the steroid reaching the intrathecal space.

Neurologic Injury

Direct injury to the spinal nerves or the spinal cord itself can occur during needle placement for epidural injection. The most common form of nerve injury is persistent paresthesia. More severe injury to the spinal cord can occur when the advancing needle enters the substance of the spinal cord. Surprisingly, needle penetration into the cord is not in itself always catastrophic and may even occur without the patient reporting symptoms (25). More significant injury occurs if bleeding into the spinal cord occurs or if injectate of any kind is placed through the needle into the substance of the spinal cord (26,27). Neural injury occurred in 14 patients following epidural steroid injection reported in the Closed Claims Study (5). Six of these resulted in paraplegia, one in quadriplegia. Another mechanism of injury is injection of steroid suspension into a radicular artery, with embolization of end arteries in the spinal cord or cerebellum; this complication will be discussed in detail in the section later in this chapter on transforaminal injection of steroids.

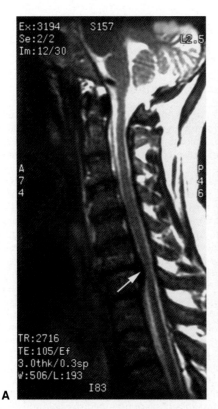
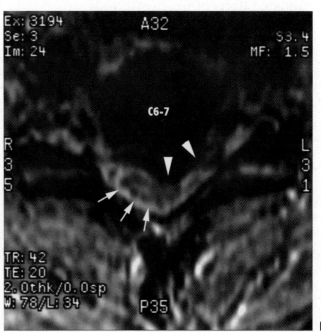

A   **B**

FIGURE 50-1. Cervical magnetic resonance imaging (MRI) of large disc herniation causing effacement of the epidural fat and cerebrospinal fluid (CSF) surrounding the spinal cord. Field et al. (29) reported three cases of transient neurologic injury that followed otherwise uneventful cervical epidural steroid injections in awake patients. All three patients had large disc herniations causing effacement of the epidural fat and spinal fluid surrounding the spinal cord at the level of injection. **A:** Midline sagittal, T2-weighted MRI showing large disc herniation at the C6–7 level (*arrow*) that effaces the epidural fat and CSF signal both anterior and posterior to the spinal cord. **B:** Axial, T1-weighted MRI, showing a large central and left-sided disc herniation (*arrow heads*) displacing the spinal cord (*arrows*) to the right posterolateral limits of the spinal canal. Reproduced from Field J, Rathmell JP, Stephenson JH, Katz NP. Neuropathic pain following cervical epidural steroid injection. *Anesthesiology* 2000;93:885–888, with permission.

The risk of direct injury to the spinal cord is greatest when epidural injection is carried out at the high lumbar, thoracic, or cervical levels, where the spinal cord lies directly anterior to the path of the advancing needle. Two cases of spinal cord injury following cervical epidural steroid injections conducted with fluoroscopic guidance were reported (28). The details of use of fluoroscopy were not given, and it is not clear if the final needle position was confirmed using both anteroposterior (AP) and lateral images and/or with use of radiographic contrast. In both cases, the patients received sedation with midazolam and propofol. The authors postulate that these patients failed to report any symptoms associated with needle contact with the cord because of the level of sedation. Both patients developed persistent upper extremity pain and lower extremity paresthesias. A more recent report details three cases of transient neurologic injury that followed otherwise uneventful cervical epidural steroid injections in awake patients (29). All three patients had large disc herniations that caused effacement of the epidural fat and spinal fluid surrounding the spinal cord at the level of injection (Fig. 50-1). The authors hypothesized that direct injury to the spinal cord or dorsal nerve root could occur even without dural puncture when narrowing or obliteration of the epidural space, caused by a large disc herniation, displaces the spinal cord posteriorly.

The use of fluoroscopy offers some protection against neural injury. The position of the needle tip in the AP view can be kept midline as it is advanced, eliminating the risk of lateral deviation and injury to the nerve roots or the spinal nerve. Although the primary means of detecting penetration of the epidural space remains the loss of resistance to injection as the needle is advanced, a lateral view on fluoroscopy can be used to assure that the needle tip is at the level of the posterior border of the bony spinal canal. Once the tip of the needle appears to be in good positron in both AP and lateral views, injection of a small volume of radiographic contrast can be used to assure that the injectate is within the epidural space. Most reports describe the immediate onset of severe pain in one or both lower extremities reported by awake patients receiving epidural injections who went on to develop spinal cord injuries (26,27,29). Thus, minimizing sedation is an important measure—the patient should be alert enough to respond to paresthesias induced by needle contact with neural structures. In the majority of cases, probably little more than supportive care can be offered to those patients who do suffer neural injury in the course of epidural injection. Immediate neurosurgical consultation and diagnostic imaging is warranted in those cases in which injury to the spinal cord is suspected; consideration should be given to administration of a course of high-dose intravenous (IV) corticosteroids, as this approach has proven beneficial in reducing neuronal injury following traumatic spinal cord injury (30).

Pharmacologic Effects of Corticosteroids

The administration of exogenous corticosteroids can lead to both hypercortisolism and suppression of the adrenal cortex's normal production of endogenous glucocorticoids. Cushing's syndrome occurs as the result of excessive endogenous cortisol production by the adrenal cortex and results in a characteristic pattern of obesity associated with hypertension. Prolonged administration of exogenous glucocorticoids can result in similar manifestations and is termed *cushingoid syndrome*. The long-acting corticosteroid preparations used for epidural steroid injection slowly release the active steroid over 1 to 3 weeks. Fluid retention and weight gain, increased blood pressure, and congestive heart failure have been reported after epidural steroid injections (31,32), and may be more likely in those with a history of previous congestive heart failure or chronic diuretic use. Cushingoid side effects have been reported even after a single epidural administration of corticosteroid (33).

Epidural administration of long-acting corticosteroid preparations leads to prompt, marked, and prolonged suppression of serum cortisol levels. In 12 patients who received 80 mg of epidural methylprednisolone acetate, adrenocorticotropic hormone (ACTH) and plasma cortisol levels were depressed from 1 to 21 days after treatment, and the ability of exogenous ACTH to raise plasma cortisol levels was reduced over the same interval (34). Three epidural injections of 80 mg of triamcinolone acetate given at weekly intervals also reduced ACTH and serum cortisol levels, starting within 45 minutes of the first injection; levels were nearly normal 30 days following the last injection (35). Steroid-induced myopathy, characterized by progressive proximal muscle weakness, increased serum creatinine kinase levels, and a myopathic electromyelogram (EMG) and muscle biopsy specimen has been reported following a single epidural dose of triamcinolone (36). Severe cases of cushingoid syndrome and steroid myopathy are rare, and these have been reported after a single epidural injection of corticosteroid, thus it is unlikely that these complications can be completely avoided. However, the use of systemic corticosteroids in any form is not without risk, thus making it essential to judge the response from each treatment before administering additional corticosteroid. No specific treatment is available for the adrenal suppression that follows epidural injection of corticosteroid; however, it seems prudent to consider coverage with an additional dose of exogenous steroid in those undergoing major surgery in the weeks following epidural steroid injection.

Glucocorticoid administration reduces the effect of insulin and results in increased blood glucose levels and insulin requirements in diabetics for 48 to 72 hours. A single caudal epidural injection of triamcinolone acetonide resulted in an increase in serum insulin levels and a suppression of serum glucose response to insulin within 24 hours, and a return to normal after 1 week (37). There is little published information about the effects of epidural injection of steroids on glucose control in diabetic patients. Glucose levels in diabetic patients should be monitored closely during the week following administration of any type of long-acting steroid. Patients must be informed that adjustment of insulin dose may be required. Brittle diabetics should consult their internist or endocrinologist prior to initiating steroid treatment.

Although rare, allergic reaction to systemic administration of corticosteroid has been documented (38,39). Signs and symptoms of a delayed allergic reaction appeared in one pa-

tient a week after epidural injection of triamcinolone diacetate, and subsequent skin testing resulted in recurrence of symptoms (40).

Bleeding Complications

Similar to single-shot epidural placement for surgical anesthesia, epidural injection for pain treatment carries the risk of intraspinal bleeding. Significant bleeding within the epidural space can cause compression of neural elements and potentially result in paraplegia or quadriplegia. Both epidural (41) and subdural (42) hematomas have been reported following epidural steroid injections in patients without any apparent coagulopathy. The patient with the epidural hematoma regained normal neurologic function following emergent surgical decompression. The patient with the subdural hematoma initially developed quadriplegia; although neurologic function recovered after surgery, the patient subsequently developed meningitis and died. A case of quadriplegia following cervical epidural steroid injection in a patient receiving clopidogrel and diclofenac has also been reported; this patient regained upper extremity function after surgical decompression (43). In the Closed Claims Study (5), two epidural hematomas occurred following epidural steroid injections; both patients had been receiving anticoagulants.

The risks and considerations regarding neuraxial blockade in patients receiving anticoagulation are similar in those receiving the injections for treatment of pain to those who are receiving epidural anesthesia or perioperative epidural analgesia (44). Epidural injection of steroids should be avoided in patients receiving systemic anticoagulants (e.g., Coumadin or heparin) or potent antiplatelet agents (e.g., clopidogrel or ticlopidine). However, nonsteroidal anti-inflammatory drugs (NSAIDs), including aspirin, do not appear to increase the risk of epidural hematoma formation associated with epidural injection. In a series of 1,035 patients who received a total of 1,214 epidural steroid injections, no bleeding complications were seen; one-third of these patients had been taking NSAIDs at the time of treatment (134 on aspirin, 249 on other NSAIDs, 34 on multiple NSAIDs) (45).

Infectious Complications

Injection therapy for pain treatment carries a small risk of both superficial and deep infection, including neuraxial infection such as epidural abscess (46) (see also Fig. 50-22). Both superficial and deep infections have been reported after injection therapies for pain including epidural steroid injections (47–49), facet injections (50), and trigger point injections (51). It is not possible to discern the actual incidence of infection from the available published data.

The most worrisome and potentially devastating infectious complication is epidural abscess. Abscess formation within the epidural space can occur without injection or instrumentation of the spinal canal. In a series of 46 cases of spontaneous epidural abscess, 46% occurred in diabetic patients (52). Common presenting symptoms included paralysis (80%), localized spinal pain (89%), radicular pain (57%), and chills and fever (67%). The erythrocyte sedimentation rate (ESR) was always elevated. *Staphylococcus aureus* was the most common organism isolated. A recent review detailed 14 cases of epidural abscess following epidural steroid injection that have been reported in the literature (53). Patient characteristics and outcomes for those cases and one additional reported case (48)

TABLE 50-3

DATA REGARDING CASES OF EPIDURAL ABSCESS FOLLOWING EPIDURAL STEROID INJECTIONS

Total number of cases	15
Onset ≤1 week	9
Onset >1 week	6
Patients with diabetes	5
Caudal epidural injection	1
Lumbar epidural injection	10
Thoracic epidural injection	1
Cervical epidural injection	3
Required laminectomy	11
Deaths	2
Residual motor dysfunction	5

Data from Huang RC, Shapiro GS, Lim M, et al. Cervical epidural abscess after epidural steroid injection. *Spine* 2004;29:E7–E9; and Hooten WM, Kinney MO, Huntoon MA. Epidural abscess and meningitis after epidural corticosteroid injection. *Mayo Clin Proc* 2004;79:682–686.

are shown in Table 50-3. Infection was listed in the Closed Claims Study (5) as a cause for litigation in 24 cases involving epidural steroid injections. Twelve cases of meningitis and three cases of osteomyelitis occurred. Seven cases of epidural abscess were noted, six requiring surgical decompression and one resulting in permanent lower extremity motor dysfunction. In one claim, both meningitis and epidural abscess occurred, and in one a combination of meningitis, abscess, and osteomyelitis.

Similar to epidural infections, the majority of cases of septic arthritis of the facet and sacroiliac joints occur in the absence of injection or instrumentation. Systematic reviews have reported 27 cases of facet joint infection (54) and 166 cases of bacterial sacroiliitis (55). Following intraarticular facet injection, septic arthritis in the facet joints can extend to involve the paraspinous muscles (56) and the epidural space (57).

No well-tested guidelines for the prevention of infection during injection treatment for chronic pain are available. Considerations regarding sterile technique and use of disinfectant solutions are similar to those recommended for single-shot regional anesthetic techniques performed in the perioperative period (58,59). Most experts recommend the use of an iodine-based skin preparation solution, routine use of sterile drapes and gloves, and strong consideration of routine use of face masks and hats. Routine use of preprocedure antibiotics does not appear to be warranted in the majority of single-shot spinal and perispinal injections (46). Pain practitioners should establish written postprocedural guidelines for their patients that include a clear description of the signs and symptoms of evolving infection and a clear process for contacting pain clinic personnel to report the appearance of any worrisome signs or symptoms (46). Although some isolated paraspinous infections have been treated with needle aspiration, most will require open surgical incision and drainage along with the administration of systemic antibiotics.

COMPLICATIONS ASSOCIATED WITH TRANSFORAMINAL INJECTIONS

Transforaminal injections are those delivered onto a spinal nerve within the intervertebral foramen. The rationale for in-

jecting steroids is that they suppress inflammation of the nerve, which, in many instances, is believed to be the basis for radicular pain (60,61). The rationale for using a transforaminal route of injection rather than an interlaminar route is that the injectate is delivered directly onto the target nerve. This ensures that the medication reaches the site of the suspected pathology in maximum concentration. When used for diagnostic purposes, transforaminal blocks can be used to pinpoint the particular spinal nerve responsible for radicular pain when imaging studies are ambiguous; the drug injected is a local anesthetic agent. When used as a therapeutic intervention, a combination of a local anesthetic and a corticosteroid preparation is injected. Most practitioners use lidocaine (in concentrations of 0.5%, 1%, or 2%) but some use small volumes of bupivacaine (0.5%). The steroid preparation depends on practitioner preference, and available choices include betamethasone, dexamethasone, and methylprednisolone. Numerous reports document complications associated with both the cervical and lumbar transforaminal injection of steroids.

Cervical Transforaminal Injections

The most concerning risk of transforaminal injection involves unintentional vascular injection of the steroid solution. The incidence of intravascular injection was 19% in a series of 504 cervical transforaminal injections (62). Although the authors do not differentiate intra-arterial and IV injections, the observed vascular injections seem to have been IV, and no adverse outcomes occurred. Intravenous injection is an innocuous event during transforaminal injection; particulate steroid injected intravenously will simply be carried away from the site of inflammation, thus reducing any local anti-inflammatory effect. In contrast, intra-arterial injection is far less common, but the effects may lead to catastrophic neurologic injury (63).

In the cervical spine, the vertebral artery, the ascending cervical artery, and the deep cervical artery each furnish spinal branches that enter the intervertebral foramina. These spinal branches supply the vertebral column but also give rise to radicular arteries that accompany the dorsal and ventral roots of the spinal nerves (Fig. 50-2). Not infrequently, anterior radicular arteries are of significant caliber and reinforce the anterior spinal artery. Such reinforcing arteries can occur at any cervical level, but appear to be more common at lower cervical levels (64). If particulate steroid is injected within a reinforcing radicular artery during transforaminal injection, infarction of the cervical spinal cord could ensue. The vertebral artery lies anterior to the cervical intervertebral foramina, and should not be encountered in a carefully executed transforaminal injection. However, radicular arterial branches arising from the vertebral artery can also join the arterial supply that reaches the anterior spinal artery; it is feasible that injectate placed within a radicular artery during transforaminal injection could reach the vertebral artery via retrograde flow through an arterial anastomosis (64). If particulate steroid reaches the vertebral artery during transforaminal injection, infarction of the posterior circulation of the brain, including the cerebellum, could ensue.

The first report of a complication attributed to cervical transforaminal injection of steroids described a patient who died from a spinal cord infarction (65). The location of the infarction implied that a radicular artery that reinforced the anterior spinal artery had been compromised, but no evidence was offered about the mechanism by which the artery had been compromised. Images of the placement of the needle were not published. A subsequent case report did describe a possible mechanism by which the spinal cord could be compromised

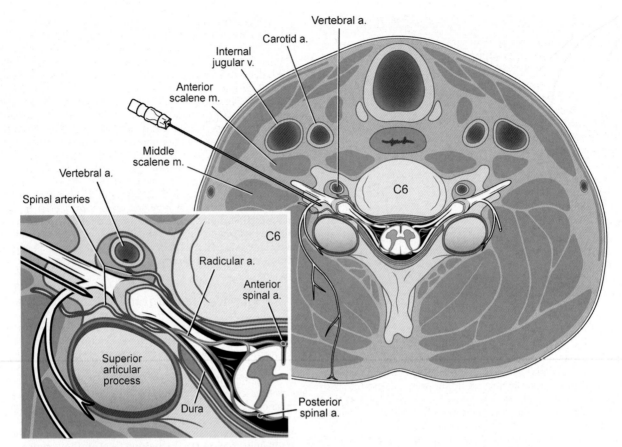

FIGURE 50-2. Axial view of cervical transforaminal injection at the level of C6. The needle has been inserted along the axis of the foramen and is in final position against the posterior aspect of the intervertebral foramen. Insertion along this axis places the needle behind the spinal nerve, and behind the vertebral artery, which lies anterior to the foramen. *Inset:* A spinal artery arises from the vertebral artery. It supplies the vertebral column. Another spinal artery enters the intervertebral foramen from the ascending cervical artery or deep cervical artery. It furnishes radicular branches that accompany the nerve roots and ultimately reach the anterior and posterior spinal arteries of the spinal cord. Modified from Rathmell JP. *Atlas of Image-guided Intervention in Regional Anesthesia and Pain Medicine*, 1st ed. Philadelphia: Lippincott Williams & Wilkins, 2005, with permission.

(66). During a C5–C6 transforaminal injection, the operator injected a test dose of contrast medium to ensure that the injectate properly dispersed along the course of the spinal nerve and its root sleeve. At that time, filling of a transversely running vessel that satisfied the features of a radicular artery was observed (Fig. 50-3). The procedure was terminated and the patient suffered no ill effects. The authors postulated that unintentional injection of an anterior radicular artery could occur during transforaminal injection. If particulate steroids were to be injected into a reinforcing artery, they could act as an embolus to infarct the spinal cord. This view was reiterated in a later review article (63), which described another case of radicular artery filling during cervical transforaminal injection. Further circumstantial evidence of this mechanism was provided in another case report (67). Upon injecting contrast medium, the operator found no evidence of intra-arterial injection during a C6–C7 transforaminal injection. He next injected local anesthetic. The patient developed neurologic features consistent with anesthetization of the anterior and anterolateral columns of the cervical spinal cord. The posterior columns were spared. These features indicate that injection was made into a radicular artery, which reinforced the anterior spinal artery. The

procedure was terminated and the patient recovered within 20 minutes.

Several reports have now appeared implicating vertebral artery injection as the mechanism of injury during cervical transforaminal injection. After attempted C5–C6 and C4–C5 transforaminal injections, a patient developed bilateral blindness, and magnetic resonance imaging (MRI) revealed bilateral parenchymal enhancement of the occipital lobes (68). The clinical features and the imaging results implicated unintentional injection into the vertebral artery. The offending agent was not apparent, as only contrast medium and air were used during the procedure. The authors argued that either the contrast medium or air embolism could have caused the cerebral injury. In a second report implicating vertebral artery injection, a patient developed respiratory and cardiovascular collapse shortly after a C6–C7 transforaminal injection of steroids and died in a coma 1 day later (69). A computed tomography (CT) scan revealed a large hemorrhage around the brainstem. A postmortem examination revealed cerebral edema, extensive hemorrhage in the brainstem and left cerebellum, and a thrombus in the left vertebral artery. A third patient developed quadriparesis after a right C5–C6 transforaminal injection and expired the

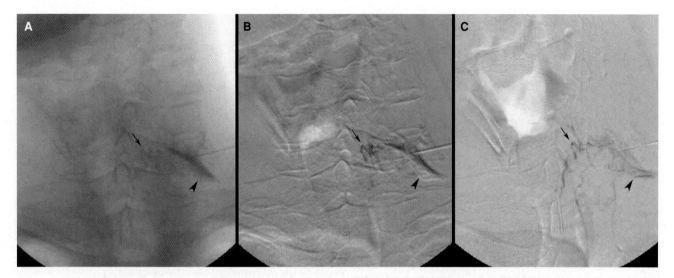

FIGURE 50-3. Anteroposterior view of the cervical spine during C7–T1 transforaminal injection (digital subtraction sequence after contrast injection). An anteroposterior view of an angiogram obtained after injection of contrast medium, prior to planned transforaminal injection of corticosteroids. **A:** Image as seen on fluoroscopy. The needle lies in the left C7–T1 intervertebral foramen no further medially than its mediolateral point. Contrast medium outlines the exiting nerve root (*arrowhead*). The radicular artery appears as a thin thread passing medially from the site of injection (*small arrow*). **B:** Digital subtraction angiogram more clearly reveals the radicular artery extending medially (*small arrow*). **C:** Digital subtraction angiogram after pixel-shift re-registration reveals that the radicular artery (*small arrow*) extends to the midline to join the anterior spinal artery. Reproduced from Rathmell JP, Aprill C, Bogduk N. Cervical transforaminal injection of steroids. *Anesthesiology* 2004;100:1595–1600, with permission.

following day (70). No imaging or postmortem findings were provided.

These case reports indicate that serious complications can occur as a result of unintentional intra-arterial injection in the course of cervical transforaminal injections. Either a radicular artery or the vertebral artery can be involved.

Published guidelines for the conduct of cervical transforaminal injections (63,71) are designed to guard against these complications (Table 50-4). The needle must be accurately and correctly placed against the posterior wall of the intervertebral foramen. In securing this position, it is essential that the needle be introduced along a correctly obtained oblique view of the target foramen (Fig. 50-2). Needle advancement using less than oblique or lateral views risks penetration of the vertebral artery en route to the foramen. Once the needle has been placed, a test dose of contrast medium should be injected and its flow carefully monitored during injection, using "live" or "real-time" fluoroscopy with or without digital subtraction. Under normal circumstances, the injectate should flow around the target nerve and into the lateral epidural space. Simultaneously, but more critically, this test dose of contrast shows if intravascular injection occurs. Close attention is required to notice if the injection is intra-arterial. The rapid flow through arteries means that intra-arterial contrast medium will appear only fleetingly. This event is unlikely to be captured by postinjection spot films. The flow of contrast medium must be monitored using continuous fluoroscopy throughout the injection.

TABLE 50-4

PREVENTING COMPLICATIONS DURING CERVICAL TRANSFORAMINAL INJECTION

- Advance the needle using fluoroscopic guidance from an anterior oblique approach.
- Ensure that the needle remains over the superior articular process along the posterior aspect of the intervertebral foramen. The vertebral artery lies anterior to the foramen. Keeping the needle posterior avoids risk of penetrating the vertebral artery.
- Use anterior-posterior radiography to adjust final needle depth. Do not advance the needle more than 50% across the medial-lateral dimension of the foramen to avoid penetrating the dural sleeve.
- Once the needle is in final position, inject a small volume of radiographic contrast under live or real-time fluoroscopy to ensure that injection into an artery does not occur. Digital subtraction angiography is a fluoroscopic technique that offers advantages over conventional fluoroscopy by subtracting out the overlying radiodense structures and improving visualization of contrast spread.

Lumbar Transforaminal Injections

Minor complications occurred in about 9% of a series of 322 lumbar transforaminal injections (72). Transient headaches (3%), increased back pain (2%), facial flushing (1%), increased leg pain (0.6%), and vasovagal reaction (0.3%) were the most frequently reported (Table 50-5). These complications are similar to those associated with lumbar interlaminar and caudal injections.

Similar to the major complications seen with cervical transforaminal injections, the major complications associated with lumbar transforaminal injections involve the reinforcing radicular artery, known as the artery of Adamkiewicz. Although this artery typically arises at thoracic levels, in 1% of individuals, this artery arises as low as L2, and more rarely as low as the

TABLE 50-5
ADVERSE EFFECTS ASSOCIATED WITH LUMBAR TRANSFORAMINAL INJECTION
■ Overall incidence of minor adverse effects: 9% of cases (72)
■ Transient headaches (3%)
■ Increased back pain (2%)
■ Facial flushing (1%)
■ Increased leg pain (0.6%)
■ Vasovagal reaction (0.3%)

sacral levels (73). In those with a low-lying radicular artery, the artery can be entered during lumbar transforaminal injections (Fig. 50-4). There have been two reports of complications that likely resulted from direct injection into this vessel.

In one report, three patients developed paraplegia after lumbar transforaminal injections. In two cases the injections were performed at L3–L4 and in the third, the injection was at S1 (74). In all cases, MRI demonstrated increased signal intensity of the low thoracic spinal cord. A second report described one patient who developed paraplegia after an injection at L2–L3 (75). MRI showed increased signal intensity in the lower thoracic spinal cord and conus medullaris. The injection had been

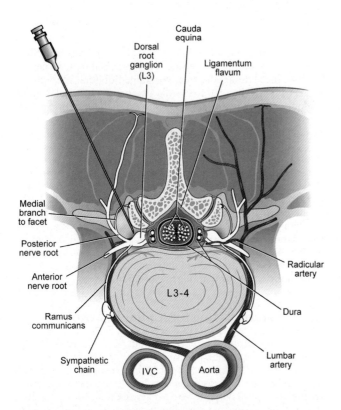

FIGURE 50-4. Axial view of lumbar transforaminal selective nerve root injection. On the right of the specimen, a needle has been placed in the intervertebral foramen, aiming at the nerve root complex. On the left, a radicular artery is accompanying the nerve roots. Such a vessel could be susceptible to penetration during a transforaminal injection. Modified from Rathmell JP. *Atlas of Image-guided Intervention in Regional Anesthesia and Pain Medicine*, 1st ed. Philadelphia: Lippincott Williams & Wilkins, 2005, with permission.

performed under CT guidance without a test dose of contrast medium.

The exact mechanism of spinal cord injury following lumbar transforaminal injections has not been determined. The pattern of injury seen on subsequent MRI strongly suggests occlusion of a reinforcing radicular artery. Both spasm of the artery or embolism of particulate steroids could account for these outcomes, but spasm seems less likely in light of the permanent and catastrophic outcomes. However, direct evidence is still lacking.

Published guidelines for lumbar transforaminal injections emphasize a technique similar to that used for cervical transforaminal injections (76). A test dose of contrast medium with real-time fluoroscopic monitoring is essential. Furthermore, during this test, a view of the lumbar spine that includes several segments cephalad of the level of injection should be used to assure that flow of contrast medium to the thoracic levels can be detected.

Neurologic complications of transforaminal injections are typically catastrophic. They are immediately obvious, with the onset of spinal weakness and numbness. Their recognition requires no special investigations. Magnetic resonance imaging of the spinal cord and hindbrain serves only to identify the location and extent of the neurologic damage. Immediate treatment is with ventilatory and cardiovascular support as needed, and subsequent management and rehabilitation follow standard protocols for spinal cord injury or stroke.

COMPLICATIONS ASSOCIATED WITH SYMPATHETIC BLOCKS

A number of acute, posttraumatic, and chronic neuropathic pain conditions are maintained through nociceptive impulses that travel through the sympathetic nervous system; these conditions often improve with sympathetic blockade. A recent evidence-based review (77) suggests that appropriate applications for sympathetic blocks include diagnosis of pain that is responsive to sympathetic blockade (e.g., complex regional pain syndrome or CRPS) and the treatment of ischemic pain. Pain arising from the viscera and sympathetically maintained pain (SMP) that arises after injury in the periphery can be effectively relieved in many instances by using local anesthetic or neurolytic blockade of the sympathetic nervous system at one of three main levels: the cervicothoracic ganglia (including the stellate ganglion); the celiac plexus; or the lumbar ganglia.

Sympathetic blocks including stellate ganglion, celiac plexus, and lumbar sympathetic blocks have been used for more than half a century. Practitioners have developed a relatively good understanding of the risks and complications of performing these procedures. Some newer techniques, such as hypogastric plexus block, and newer approaches to the sympathetic nerves, such as transdiscal approaches, have been described, but little is known about the risks of these approaches.

Stellate Ganglion Block

Complications from stellate ganglion block arise from vascular, epidural, and intrathecal injection (Table 50-6). Needle trauma can result in injuries to vessels or nervous tissue in the neck. Pneumothorax can also occur following a stellate ganglion block. Infections are uncommon. No published reports are available that offer an estimate of the frequency of complications associated with stellate ganglion block. In a recent

TABLE 50-6

COMPLICATIONS ASSOCIATED WITH STELLATE GANGLION BLOCK

Common
- Recurrent laryngeal and phrenic nerve block
- Brachial plexus block

Uncommon
- Pneumothorax
- Generalized seizure
- Total spinal anesthesia
- Severe hypertension

Rare
- Transient locked-in syndrome
- Paratracheal hematoma
- Soft-tissue infection/osteomyelitis

survey of members of the Canadian Anesthesiologists' Society, approximately one-third of the anesthesiologists surveyed reported that they incorporate chronic pain treatment into their practice, and the most commonly practiced interventions included stellate ganglion block (61%) and lumbar sympathetic block (50%), suggesting that these techniques are commonly practiced. Most complications described, however, appear only in the form of sporadic case reports (see Chapter 39).

Several arteries and veins lie in close proximity to the intended injection site, the anterior tubercle of C6 or C7 (Fig. 50-5). Injections into the vein do not commonly result in sequelae since the volume and concentration of local anesthetic should not produce a toxic effect. The risk of local anesthetic toxicity can further be reduced by the use of dilute local anesthetic concentrations, such as 0.25% bupivacaine. Arterial injections do not offer the same measure of safety. As little as 2.5 mg of bupivacaine or a mixture of bupivacaine 1.25 mg and lidocaine 5 mg injected into the vertebral or internal carotid artery has been reported to produce seizures (78). Vertebral injections occur when the needle is inserted too medially and posteriorly. The practitioner often contacts bone but mistakes

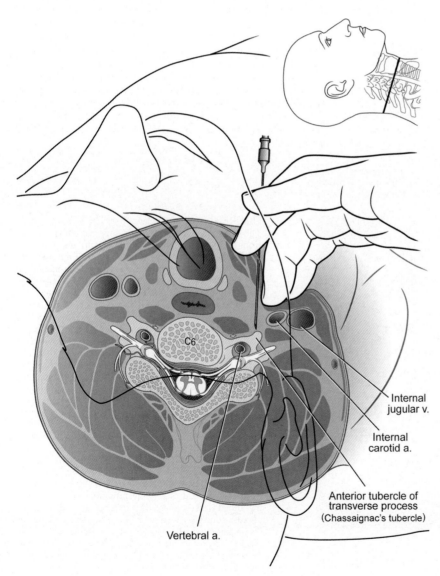

Internal
jugular v.

Internal
carotid a.

Anterior tubercle of
transverse process
(Chassaignac's tubercle)

Vertebral a.

FIGURE 50-5. Axial diagram of stellate ganglion block. The great vessels of the neck are gently retracted laterally, and the needle is seated on the anterior tubercle of the transverse process of C6 (Chassaignac tubercle). Note the position of the vertebral artery within the foramen transversarium, the spinal nerve root and dural cuff, and the carotid artery and jugular vein. Reproduced from Neal JM, Rathmell JP. *Complications in Regional Anesthesia and Pain Medicine*. Philadelphia: Saunders Elsevier, 2007, with permission.

the posterior tubercle for the anterior tubercle. Slight withdrawal of the needle from the posterior tubercle, particularly if in a medial position, can produce a vertebral artery injection. The carotid artery also lies near the site of entry for a stellate ganglion block. It is advisable to feel for the carotid pulse, then retract the vessel laterally prior to inserting the needle. This should prevent insertion into the carotid artery in most cases. Injection into the carotid artery can be expected to produce similar effects as vertebral artery injection.

Rarely is this procedure performed secondary to direct inflammation of the ganglion. Sympathetic blocks (e.g., stellate ganglion block) are performed diagnostically and therapeutically to denervate the sympathetic nerves. Local anesthetics effectively block these nerves temporarily. Long-term benefits have been reported following local anesthetic blocks. The addition of corticosteroids has not been demonstrated to enhance the effect of the local anesthetic. If there has been trauma at the site of the ganglion (e.g., a gunshot wound) then injection of corticosteroid with local anesthetic would seem reasonable. Routine administration of corticosteroid in these injections might be questioned because of the risk of intra-arterial injection into either the vertebral, carotid, or spinal radicular artery. Specifically, particulate corticosteroids (suspensions such as MPA) can cause an embolic stroke if unintentionally injected into any of these arteries.

Careful aspiration prior to injection helps to prevent intravascular injection but is not 100% effective. Slight movement of the needle can change the position from extravascular to intravascular. Attaching tubing to the needle and having a second person perform the aspirations and injections may further decrease the chance of intravascular injections, although no studies have been performed to confirm this. Incremental injections of local anesthetic injection are also advocated to minimize the chance of a large intravascular injection. If an intravascular (arterial) injection occurs, a grand mal seizure often results. Fortunately, these are transient and usually resolve prior to initiation of any therapy. Therapy is directed at maintaining an airway and preventing oral (teeth or tongue) trauma. Oxygen should be administered as soon as possible, although the seizure often ends before therapy can be initiated. The most serious risk from a grand mal seizure is aspiration of vomitus. For this reason, it is advisable to have a patient adhere to an "n.p.o." status prior to the procedure. An IV line should be considered, particularly in patients with potentially difficult airways or larger than average necks (see also Chapter 39).

The cervical spinal nerves traverse the intervertebral foramen near the location for a stellate ganglion block (Fig. 50-6). If the needle is positioned posterior to the anterior tubercle, it can be positioned into either the epidural compartment or into a dural sleeve that accompanies the exiting nerve. Although CSF would be expected on aspiration if the needle were inside the subarachnoid space, this may be overlooked as the practitioner focuses on the more likely risk of vascular aspiration and injection. Paresthesias in the distribution of the brachial plexus may or may not occur. If present, one should consider repositioning the needle more anteriorly. Epidural injection of 10 mL of local anesthetic at the C6 or C7 level produces variable effects and is dependent on the concentration of local anesthetic and whether or not the entire volume of drug is injected. In our experience, epidural injection (with high concentrations of local anesthetic) can produce a profound sensory and motor block but often spares the phrenic nerve. Subjective respiratory distress is common secondary to block of the intercostal nerves. If airway reflexes are intact, continuous oxygen saturation monitoring and cardiac monitoring will allow the patient to be cared

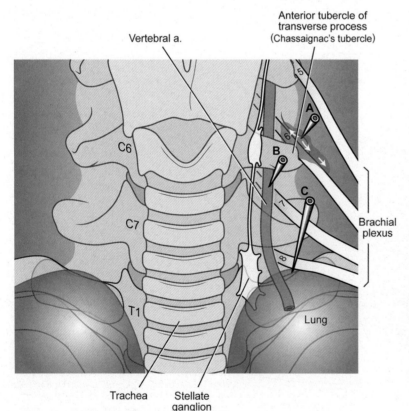

FIGURE 50-6. Frontal view of stellate ganglion block. The stellate ganglion conveys sympathetic fibers to and from the upper extremities and the head and neck. The ganglion is comprised of the fused superior thoracic ganglion and the inferior cervical ganglion and is named for its fusiform shape (in many individuals, the two ganglia remain separate). The stellate ganglion lies over the head of the first rib at the junction of the transverse process and uncinate process of T1. The ganglion is just posteromedial to the cupola of the lung and medial to the vertebral artery, and these are the two structures most vulnerable. Stellate ganglion block is typically carried out at the C6 or C7 level to avoid pneumothorax, and a volume of solution that will spread along the prevertebral fascia inferiorly to the stellate ganglion is employed (usually 10 mL). When radiographic guidance is not used, the operator palpates the anterior tubercle of the transverse process of C6 (Chassaignac tubercle), and a needle is seated in the location. With radiographic guidance, it is simpler and safer to place a needle over the vertebral body just inferior the uncinate process of C6 or C7. Incorrect needle placement can lead to pneumothorax, damage to the vertebral artery or intra-arterial injection, or spread of the injectate adjacent to the exiting spinal nerves where they join to form the brachial plexus; contrast can also course proximally along the spinal nerves to the epidural space. Reproduced from Neal JM, Rathmell JP. *Complications in Regional Anesthesia and Pain Medicine*. Philadelphia: Saunders Elsevier, 2007, with permission.

for supportively (oxygen and IV fluids) and not require intubation. Small doses of benzodiazepines can be administered to allay the patient's fears while the block subsides.

Intrathecal injection of local anesthetic at this site commonly produces a total spinal block. Loss of airway reflexes and phrenic nerve function often occurs. Patients often describe difficulty breathing or an inability to move their arms as initial symptoms. Contralateral motor block develops as further confirmation, along with block of the lower extremities. Intubation and assisted ventilation will be required until the block abates. Blood pressure, cardiac, and oxygen-saturation monitoring should be performed until the block resolves. The duration of the block depends on the drug and the total dose injected. The patient will commonly remain awake during the event. Once the airway is protected and vital signs stabilized, some sedation to keep the patient comfortable is advised. Verbal reassurance of the patient can further calm fears and assure her that the effects she is experiencing are temporary.

Horner syndrome is often observed following a stellate ganglion block. In fact, many practitioners look for Horner syndrome as evidence of sympathetic denervation following the stellate ganglion injection of local anesthetic. Horner syndrome is, theoretically, a side effect, since a stellate ganglion block is most commonly performed for patients with upper extremity pain (diagnostically to rule in SMP or therapeutically for CRPS type I or II). Horner syndrome consists of miosis (papillary constriction), ptosis (drooping of the upper eyelid), and enophthalmos (recession of the globe within the orbit). The presence of Horner syndrome does not necessarily equate to sympathetic denervation of the upper extremity. A study by Malmqvist et al. used five measures of sympathetic denervation (including the presence of Horner syndrome, increased temperature of the blocked extremity, and sympathogalvanic skin response) to evaluate the effectiveness of a stellate ganglion block (79). The authors found only 15 of 54 blocks had four of five positive measures following stellate ganglion block. A study by Hogan et al. examined the distribution and spread of contrast following stellate ganglion block using MRI (80). They found that injectate was not delivered to the stellate ganglion but rather passed anterior to it (with or without caudad extension to the stellate ganglion). This could produce Horner syndrome but not sympathetic denervation to the extremity. Other sites of spread included the brachial plexus, the subclavian plexus, and the epidural or subarachnoid spaces. Horner syndrome following stellate ganglion injection with local anesthetic resolves when the local anesthetic effect ends. Ideally, the analgesic effect outlives the Horner syndrome. Use of neurolytic solutions can produce permanent Horner syndrome when injected near the stellate ganglion. Use of dilute neurolytic solutions has been reported by Racz et al. as safe, in that they may not produce permanent Horner syndrome (personal communication). However, the use of neurolytic solutions near the stellate ganglion cannot be advocated for routine cases and should be used only in special situations following clear discussions of risks and benefits with the patient.

Recurrent laryngeal and phrenic nerve blocks are frequent side effects of a stellate ganglion block. They occur from local anesthetic injection that spills from the area of the ganglion. Since diffusion of drug is required to obtain a satisfactory block, it can be expected that these nerves will often be temporarily blocked. Symptoms of a recurrent laryngeal nerve block include hoarseness and, occasionally, respiratory stridor. Patients often complain of difficulty in getting their breath and the sensation of a lump in their throats. Symptomatic treatment is sufficient along with reassurance that these sensations will resolve as the local anesthetic dissipates. Pa-

tients should be cautioned to drink clear liquids initially after a stellate ganglion block to make sure that their upper airway function is not compromised. Once they feel comfortable swallowing liquids, they can progress to regular food. Phrenic nerve block rarely presents a problem for patients unless they have preexisting severe respiratory compromise. The potential for producing phrenic nerve block is one reason that bilateral stellate ganglion blocks are rarely performed at the same time. Most practitioners wait several days or a week between injections.

The pleural dome of the lung extends variably above the first rib. Most commonly, this dome passes laterally to the intended C6 injection site for the stellate ganglion block (Fig. 50-6). Using the anterior C7 approach to the stellate ganglion, the pleural dome is closer and may be entered in unusual cases. This can be accentuated in patients with pulmonary disease and hyperinflated lungs, such as patients with chronic obstructive pulmonary disease (COPD). The posterior approach to the upper thoracic sympathetic chain is extremely close to the parietal pleura. Anyone using this approach should be cautious and guided by fluoroscopy or CT techniques. Pneumothorax can result despite careful attention to detail, and patients should be warned of this potential complication prior to a posterior approach of the sympathetic chain or stellate ganglion.

If air is aspirated during placement of the needle, the clinician should decide if the trachea or pulmonary parenchyma has been entered. Breath sounds should be examined following the procedure if one suspects a pulmonary problem. Any abnormalities should be followed up with a chest radiograph. Inspiration and expiration films should be considered. Delayed presentation of a pneumothorax is always possible. If a pneumothorax is suspected but unconfirmed, patients should be warned to call or go to an emergency facility if they become symptomatic. Patients who develop a pneumothorax should be hospitalized and watched closely, with appropriate consultation with a respiratory physician or a cardiothoracic surgeon, if indicated.

Brachial plexus block can occur following a stellate ganglion injection. The majority of sympathetic nerves that travel to the upper extremity leave the sympathetic chain to accompany the somatic nerves of the brachial plexus. A few sympathetic nerves of the upper extremity, often referred to as the anomalous Kuntz nerves, may not pass through the stellate ganglion but later join the brachial plexus (81). These upper extremity sympathetic fibers can only be blocked by either a brachial plexus block or a posterior approach to the upper thoracic sympathetic chain. In a standard, anterior (C6) approach to the stellate ganglion, the brachial plexus will not be blocked. However, partial block of the nerve roots that form the brachial plexus is commonly seen after a stellate ganglion block. This occurs most commonly when the needle has been inserted too deeply, bypasses the anterior tubercle, and rests on the posterior tubercle. After retraction from the posterior tubercle, the injection of local anesthetic is likely to block one or more of the exiting nerve roots of the brachial plexus.

There are no long-term sequelae of a block of the brachial plexus with local anesthetic. An intraneural injection is almost impossible, but extreme radiating pain during injection should be avoided in the unlikely event that the needle has pierced the epineurial layer of a nerve. Outpatients who develop a partial brachial plexus motor block should be warned about being insensate for possibly 24 hours or more (dependent on the volume and concentration of local anesthetic used) and should avoid putting the extremity in an unsafe position, such as one in which a burn could occur. Use of a sling may help diminish any risk associated with a motor block.

Partial brachial plexus block may make interpretation of the stellate ganglion block difficult. Complete sympathetic denervation may not coexist if the stellate ganglion is not equally blocked or if the entire brachial plexus denervated. Patients can also be distracted by the motor block and experience dysesthesias, anesthesia dolorosa, and the like. Although complete brachial plexus denervation can be an excellent therapeutic modality for patients with severe dystonia and CRPS, partial block following stellate ganglion block should be viewed as an undesired, although most frequently harmless, side effect.

Paratracheal hematoma causing airway obstruction and death has been reported after stellate ganglion block (82). This may occur if the vertebral artery or carotid artery has been entered. In the event of a hematoma, direct pressure should be held. Communication with the patient should continue to make sure that there is no compromise of arterial blood flow to the cerebral cortex while pressure is maintained. A more serious, although very rare, situation develops if a plaque is dislodged following unintentional arterial puncture of either the carotid or vertebral artery. Presentation would be expected to mimic an evolving stroke. Similarly, unintentional puncture can also produce an arterial wall dissection. This is more likely in the rare situation in which the needle rests in the wall of the artery, negative aspiration is noted, and subsequent injection of the local anesthetic produces the dissections. This should be viewed as a medical emergency, with life care support and direct transport to an emergency facility indicated.

Infections are very uncommon following stellate ganglion injections, but case reports of cervical vertebral osteomyelitis do exist (83,84). Risk of infection is minimized by use of alcohol preparation of the site and good technique with sterile surgical gloves. More formal surgical preparation using Betadine or a similar solution and sterile drapes can also be recommended. Many clinicians believe it is important, however, to watch the patient during the injection for immediate feedback if an intravascular injection occurs and therefore recommend avoiding the use of drapes over the patient's face. If an infection occurs, the most likely organism would be a strain of *Staphylococcus* unless the esophagus was inadvertently entered. Since the needle can contact bone during the procedure, any infection should be treated with antibiotics and followed closely. An infectious disease consult should be considered in patients who do not respond to a course of oral antibiotics.

Two separate case reports have reported a transient locked-in syndrome following stellate ganglion block (85,86). In both cases, the patients remained conscious but were unable to breathe or move, with sparing of eye movement. The authors of both reports believed these cases were the result of intra-arterial injections of the vertebral artery. In our practice, we have seen two cases of a similar presentation in 20 years. However, we attributed both cases to a total spinal injection. Whether these cases represent a different phenomenon or a misdiagnosis is unclear. Fortunately, in all four cases (ours and the published cases), the patients recovered uneventfully. Care should be taken to provide sedation and frequent reassurance to these patients, as they are conscious but unable to move or breathe.

Wallace and Milholland have reported a case of contralateral and bilateral Horner syndrome following stellate ganglion injection (87). They also reported a bilateral recurrent laryngeal nerve block, which can potentially produce life-threatening airway compromise and must be monitored closely.

Intubation may be required if patients cannot sustain acceptable oxygen saturation.

Kimura et al. have reported severe hypertension following stellate ganglion block (88). They reported seven patients who developed a systolic blood pressures of greater than 200 mm Hg after a stellate ganglion block. They postulated that local anesthetic diffused along the carotid sheath, resulting in block of the vagus nerve, attenuation of the baroreceptor reflex, and subsequent unopposed sympathetic activity.

Lumbar Sympathetic Block

Lumbar sympathetic block is commonly performed for either diagnostic or therapeutic purposes in patients with suspected SMP in the lower extremities and for vascular ischemia (see Chapter 39). No published data present any estimate of the frequency of complications associated with this block, and the complications described here are derived from case reports. Complications that have been reported with lumbar sympathetic block include intravascular injection, intraspinal injection, infection (including discitis), postdural puncture headache (PDPH), and hematoma formation (Table 50-7).

On the left side of the spine, the aorta lies close to the needle placement site for a lumbar sympathetic block, and the inferior vena cava is near the placement site for needles placed on the right side (Fig. 50-7). Large volumes of local anesthetic, particularly bupivacaine, injected into either vessel can cause seizures and/or cardiovascular collapse if injected into either vessel. Resuscitation can be prolonged and difficult if bupivacaine is injected. Careful, frequent aspiration and intermittent injection is recommended. If the solution contains epinephrine, changes in heart rate may serve as a signal of intravascular injection.

It is possible for the needle to come to rest in a nerve root sleeve, with final placement in either the epidural or intrathecal space, although this occurs less frequently now that fluoroscopy is commonly used during these procedures. Entry into the spinal canal when using the "blind" technique (i.e., using surface landmarks alone to guide needle placement) occurs when the angle of needle placement is too shallow and aims directly toward the intervertebral foramen rather than the anterolateral surface of the vertebral body. Intraspinal injection should occur rarely, if ever, with the proper use of radiographic guidance during LSB. If a local anesthetic is the only drug used, side effects should resolve over time. Supportive care and vasopressors may be required.

Neurolytic lumbar sympathetic block has been advocated in efforts to produce long-lasting pain relief in those patients who receive temporary relief following local anesthetic injection. Fluoroscopic use should decrease the incidence of complications from LSB injections. A comparison of alcohol and phenol demonstrated that alcohol blocks were more likely to produce an L2 neuralgia than was phenol. However, either agent can produce an L2 neuralgia, and this complication can occur with good spread of contrast (see Chapter 39). For this reason, some

---

TABLE 50-7

COMPLICATIONS OF LUMBAR SYMPATHETIC BLOCK

- Intravascular injection (generalized seizure, cardiovascular collapse)
- Intraspinal injection (spinal or epidural block)
- Infection (retroperitoneal abscess, discitis)
- Postdural puncture headache
- Hematoma (superficial, retroperitoneal)
- L1 neuralgia (neurolytic block)

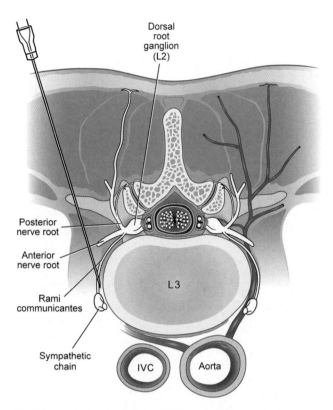

FIGURE 50-7. Axial diagram of lumbar sympathetic block. A single needle passes over the transverse process, and the tip is in position adjacent to the lumbar sympathetic ganglion over the anteromedial surface of the L3 vertebral body. Reproduced from Rathmell JP. *Atlas of Image-guided Intervention in Regional Anesthesia and Pain Medicine*, 1st ed. Philadelphia: Lippincott Williams & Wilkins, 2006, with permission.

practitioners advocate the use of radiofrequency denervation. Multiple lesions are required using radiofrequency to achieve adequate denervation (89). There is insufficient published information on the radiofrequency technique to understand if it will reduce the incidence of neuralgia; however, neuralgia has been reported in several cases following neurolytic LSB using radiofrequency (89).

The intervertebral disc lies near the path of a LSB needle (Fig. 50-7). It is not uncommon for the needle to unintentionally pass through part of the disc. Normally, this does not result in a complication, but discitis can occur. Historically, complete surgical drape, gown, and other precautions are not used for a LSB (as one might for a discogram). Whether this increases the risk of discitis is unclear. In modern practice, sterile technique should be used for LSB. Also, it would seem prudent to avoid the intervertebral disc whenever possible, given the potentially serious consequences of discitis. Our practice has seen one serious discitis from a "blind" LSB that was done before fluoroscopy was in common use. The patient ultimately required surgery and partial vertebrectomy to resolve the infection.

Severe bleeding following LSB was reported in two patients: a large subcutaneous hematoma in one case, and a massive retroperitoneal hematoma in the second (90). Both patients were receiving irreversible platelet aggregation inhibitors (ticlopidine or clopidogrel). The considerations for performing sympathetic blocks in patients receiving these agents are similar to those proposed for neuraxial blockade (44). Discontinuing use of anticoagulants or other drugs used to inhibit platelet aggregation carries its own set of risks. Patients have suffered

embolic strokes when appropriately stopped from their anticoagulant medications prior to interventional procedures. The risk–benefit ratio of stopping or continuing any of these drugs should be carefully considered. Alternative therapies may be appropriate. Consulting the patient's primary care physician or the specialist who is prescribing the anticoagulant is indicated.

Post–dural puncture headache after LSB has been reported in two cases (91). The cases most likely occurred as a result of the needle passing near a nerve root sleeve that contained spinal fluid. One patient underwent an unsuccessful attempt at an epidural blood patch. Needles that are placed too laterally and posteriorly will come to rest in the psoas sheath or muscle. A striated appearance on fluoroscopy is indicative of needle placement into the muscle. If local anesthetic is injected, patients will develop a motor block of the femoral plexus, with resultant lower extremity weakness. Renal trauma or puncture of a ureter can occur with needles that begin too far laterally. Most practitioners avoid inserting the needle more than 7 to 8 cm from the midline. Fortunately, sequelae are minimal unless a neurolytic agent is injected, resulting in possible ureteral stricture or extravasation of urine.

Celiac Plexus Block

Neurolytic celiac plexus block (NCPB) has been shown to be an effective analgesic technique for management of pain in patients with intra-abdominal malignancies, especially pancreatic cancer (92–95). The technique of NCPB involves injection of neurolytic solutions in the area of the celiac plexus or splanchnic nerves, which are neural structures that transmit the majority of visceral pain from the upper abdomen (96). The celiac plexus is comprised of a diffuse network of nerve fibers and individual ganglia that lie over the anterolateral surface of the aorta, primarily at the T12–L1 vertebral level. Sympathetic innervation to the abdominal viscera arises from the anterolateral horn of the spinal cord between the T5 and T12 levels. Nociceptive information from the abdominal viscera is carried by afferents that accompany the sympathetic nerves. Presynaptic sympathetic fibers travel from the thoracic sympathetic chain toward the ganglia, traversing over the anterolateral aspect of the inferior thoracic vertebrae as the greater (T5–T9), lesser (T10–T11), and least (T12) splanchnic nerves (Fig. 50-8). Presynaptic fibers traveling via the splanchnic nerves synapse within the celiac ganglia, over the anterolateral surface of the aorta surrounding the origin of the celiac and superior mesenteric arteries at approximately the L1 vertebral level. Postsynaptic fibers from the celiac ganglia innervate the upper abdominal viscera, with the exception of the descending colon, sigmoid colon, rectum, and pelvic viscera.

Celiac plexus block using a transcrural approach places the local anesthetic or neurolytic solution in direct contact with the celiac ganglion anterolateral to the aorta (Fig. 50-8). The needles pass directly through the crura of the diaphragm en route to the celiac plexus. Because of the diaphragm, spread of the solution toward the posterior surface of the aorta may be more limited, perhaps reducing the chance of nerve root or spinal segmental artery involvement. In contrast, splanchnic nerve block (Fig. 50-8) avoids the risk of penetrating the aorta, uses smaller volumes of solution, and is unlikely to be affected by anatomic distortion caused by extensive tumor of the pancreas or metastatic lymphadenopathy. Because the needles remain posterior to the diaphragmatic crura in close apposition to the T12 vertebral body, this has been termed the *retrocrural technique*. Splanchnic nerve block is a minor modification

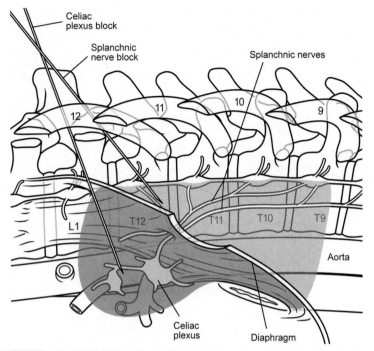

FIGURE 50-8. Anatomy of the celiac plexus and splanchnic nerves. The celiac plexus is comprised of a diffuse network of nerve fibers and individual ganglia located in close proximity to the anterolateral surface of the aorta at the T12–L1 vertebral level. Presynaptic sympathetic fibers travel from the thoracic sympathetic chain toward the celiac ganglia, traversing over the anterolateral aspect of the inferior thoracic vertebrae as the greater (T5–T9), lesser (T10–T11), and least (T12) splanchnic nerves. Celiac plexus block using a transcrural approach places the local anesthetic or neurolytic solution in direct contact with the celiac ganglion anterolateral to the aorta. The needles pass through the crura of the diaphragm en route to the celiac plexus. In contrast, for splanchnic nerve block, the needles remain posterior to the diaphragmatic crura in close apposition to the T12 vertebral body. Shading indicates the pattern of solution spread for each technique. Reproduced with permission from Rathmell JP. *Atlas of Image-guided Intervention in Regional Anesthesia and Pain Medicine*, 1st ed. Philadelphia: Lippincott Williams & Wilkins, 2006, with permission.

of the classic retrocrural celiac plexus block, the only difference being that, for splanchnic block, the needles are placed over the midportion of the T12 vertebral body rather than the cephalad portion of L1. Retrocrural celiac plexus block at the superior aspect of the L1 vertebral body and splanchnic nerve block at the mid T12 vertebral body have both been described, and they are essentially the same technique, both relying on cephalad spread of solution to block the splanchnic nerves in a retrocrural location. In most cases, celiac plexus (transcrural or retrocrural) and splanchnic nerve block can be used interchangeably to produce the same results. Although there are those who strongly advocate one approach or the other, there is no evidence that either results in superior clinical outcomes (95). From the perspective of complications in this chapter, NCPB may refer to neurolytic blockade of either celiac plexus or splanchnic nerves (see also Chapter 45).

Overall, the NCPB is considered to be a relatively safe procedure in clinical practice. Despite the infrequency of significant complications, there is still a range of potential complications associated with NCPB that must be considered, including cardiovascular, gastrointestinal, genitourinary, pulmonary, systemic, and neurologic (Table 50-8).

Many of the minor complications of NCPB are the result of effective sympathetic block due to neurolysis of the celiac ganglia. These side effects can usually be treated in a symptomatic manner without a significant effect on the patient. For example, orthostatic hypotension typically improves shortly after equilibration of the intravascular volume. Another example, bowel hypermotility, is usually transient, and may actually be desirable in many patients with opioid-induced constipation.

Major complications are often related to significant neurologic deficits or vascular events, but are extremely uncommon. Neurologic complications, such as loss of sensation or motor function of the lower extremities, are very uncommon, but can have significant clinical impact and lasting duration (97). In patients with intra-abdominal malignancies, these resultant

neurologic deficits often continue for the remainder of their lives. Serious vascular events may involve uncontrolled arterial bleeding or aortic dissection (98,99), which may be life-threatening.

Most cases of complications and derived frequencies of complications are based on patients receiving NCPB from a posterior approach. The celiac plexus and splanchnic nerves are primarily sympathetic nervous system structures. Neurolytic blockade of these sympathetic structures results in a relative increase in parasympathetic tone to the splanchnic region. Therefore, vasodilation of the splanchnic vasculature can result in orthostatic hypotension, and relative increase in parasympathetic tone may cause bowel hypermobility (see Chapter 45).

Meta-analysis of the literature regarding patients undergoing NCPB found that hypotension occurred in 38% of cases and bowel hypermotility occurred in 44% of cases (100). A case series of 136 patients who had NCPB reported that eight patients (6%) with symptomatic orthostatic hypotension required treatment (101). Another study (61 patients), prospectively comparing different CPB techniques, reported a 38% incidence of transient decreases in systolic blood pressure of more than 33% compared to baseline measurements (95). Bowel hypermotility also occurred in 31% of these patients. In the largest series (2,730 patients) evaluating neurologic complications associated with NCPB, four cases (0.15%) of permanent paraplegia were identified (97). In three of these cases, loss of anal and bladder sphincter function also occurred. Radiographic guidance with radiocontrast dye was used for CPB in all four cases. In a case series by Brown et al., there were no cases of permanent paraplegia in 136 patients with NCPB (101). Meta-analysis of the literature revealed a 1% incidence of neurologic complications, including lower extremity weakness, paresthesia, epidural anesthesia, and lumbar puncture, after NCPB (100).

Complications of celiac plexus and splanchnic nerve block include hematuria, intravascular injection, and pneumothorax.

TABLE 50-8

SUMMARY OF COMPLICATIONS ASSOCIATED WITH CELIAC PLEXUS BLOCK, THEIR CLINICAL SIGNS AND SYMPTOMS, DIAGNOSTIC EVALUATION, TREATMENT, AND MANAGEMENT

Organ system	Complication	Clinical signs and symptoms	Diagnostic evaluation	Treatment and management
Cardiovascular				
	Vascular bleeding	Hypotension, pain	Radiographic image	Ranging from self-limited to surgery or interventional radiology
	Aortic dissection	Hypotension, pain	Radiographic image	Emergent surgery or interventional radiology
	Orthostatic hypotension	Postural hypotension; lightheadedness and dizziness while upright	Blood pressure assessment in supine and sitting position	Ranging from self-limited to fluid resuscitation, leg wraps, α_1-agonist (midodrine)
Gastrointestinal				
	Bowel hypermotility	Diarrhea	Clinical assessment	Lomotil, self limited
	Loss of anal control	Stool incontinence	Neurologic evaluation	Limited treatment available
Genitourinary				
	Kidney puncture	Hematuria; hypotension	Radiographic imaging	Urology consult
	Loss of bladder control	Urinary incontinence	Neurologic evaluation	Limited treatment available
	Impotence (males)	Sexual and/or erectile dysfunction	Neurologic and Urologic evaluation	Limited treatment available
Pulmonary				
	Lung puncture	Dyspnea; tachypnea; hypotension	Radiographic image	Ranging from self-limited to chest tube
Systemic				
	Drug sensitivity	Rash; hives; urticaria; dyspnea; nausea/vomiting	Clinical history and examination	Ranging from self-limited to antihistamine; corticosteroid; epinephrine; airway management
Nervous system				
	Sensory/motor deficits of trunk/lower extremities	Paraplegia; paraparesis; numbness; paresthesia; weakness	Neurologic examination; radiographic imaging	Emergent neurology evaluation and possibly interventional radiology to vasodilate, if vascular spasm

Reproduced from Wong G. Complications associated with neurolytic celiac plexus block. In: Neal JM, Rathmell JP. *Complications in Regional Anesthesia and Pain Medicine.* Philadelphia: Saunders Elsevier, 2007, with permission.

Computed tomography (CT) allows visualization of the structures located adjacent to the celiac ganglia as the block is being performed (Fig. 50-9). The kidneys extend from between T12 and L3, with the left kidney slightly more cephalad than the right. The aorta lies over the left anterolateral border of the vertebral column. Cardiovascular-related complications may include needle puncture injury resulting in aortic or major arterial bleeding (98,99). The inferior vena cava lies just to the right of the aorta, over the anterolateral surface of the vertebral column. The medial pleural reflection extends inferomedially as low as the T12–L1 level.

Gastrointestinal-related complications such as bowel hypermotility (100) can occur frequently from effective sympathetic block due to neurolysis of the celiac plexus. The blockade of sympathetic outflow to the viscera during continued parasympathetic outflow to the viscera is likely to result in increased peristalsis and bowel hypermotility. Another complication, the loss of anal sphincter control, could result from the inadvertent neurolysis of relevant central and/or peripheral nerves (97). The mechanism of injury in this report is unclear; one can only speculate that neurolytic solution might have tracked either centrally (epidural or intrathecal) to a minor extent or contacted one of the sacral roots. Genitourinary-related complications can occur due to needle puncture of the kidney (102). Separately, contact of neurolytic solution with relevant central and/or peripheral nerves can result in loss of bladder control (97) and impotence in males (103). Pulmonary-related complications are infrequent but are related to pneumothorax resulting from needle puncture traversing from the back passing excessively anteriorly (101).

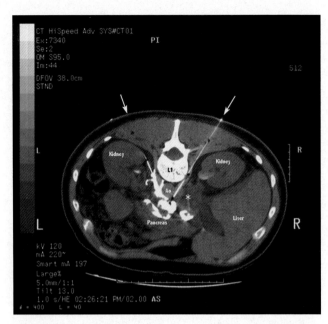

FIGURE 50-9. Computed tomography during neurolytic celiac plexus block. Cross-sectional view after placement of two transcrural needles for neurolytic celiac plexus block. Neurolytic solution (10% phenol in iohexol 100 mg/mL) has been injected through both needles (10 mL on each side). The arrows indicate the approximate needle trajectory on each side. Contrast extends over the left anterolateral surface of the aorta and anteriorly along the posterior surface of the pancreas. A large soft-tissue mass is adjacent to the right-sided needle (*asterisk*), consistent with lymphadenopathy or metastatic tumor. Reproduced from Rathmell JP, Gallant JM, Brown DL. Computed tomography and the anatomy of celiac plexus block. *Reg Anesth Pain Med* 2000;25:411–416, with permission.

sensitivities, and vascular spasm of the major anterior radicular artery (artery of Adamkiewicz).

Radiographic guidance, such as fluoroscopy or CT, is commonly used in contemporary practice to recognize grossly inaccurate needle placement. The use of radiographic guidance may provide improved visualization of anatomic structures relevant to the NCPB. Improved sense of the anatomy may lower the risk of some complications due to incorrect needle direction or placement. Radiocontrast dye can confirm appropriate needle position based on appropriate spread of injected solution. Despite its apparent usefulness, it is important to consider that radiographic guidance cannot provide complete prevention of neurologic complications. In the large case series of 2,730 patients with NCPB, four cases of permanent paraplegia occurred. All four cases of paraplegia involved the use of radiography and radiocontrast dye to confirm final needle placement. Nonetheless, there seems to be consensus in the specialty for the use of radiographic guidance for NCPB in the contemporary practice of interventional pain medicine.

Minor complications, such as orthostatic hypotension and bowel hypermotility, are common and typically self-limited. Orthostatic hypotension, if symptomatic, can be treated by increasing oral fluid intake or by IV fluids. Leg wrappings with elastic bandages or support stockings can also decrease venous capacitance and improve hypotension. Short-term use of oral ephedrine tablets 15 to 30 mg/q8h may be useful at times to allow patients to ambulate.

In the event of a major vascular complication such as significant arterial bleeding or aortic dissection, immediate radiographic imaging coupled with emergent surgical evaluation is recommended. If neurologic deficits occur during the NCPB, emergent consultation with a neurologist is recommended. There are no known remedies for relieving arterial spasm once it has occurred, but at least one case of transient paraplegia following neurolytic celiac plexus block has been reported and attributed to arterial spasm (106).

Superior Hypogastric Block

The sympathetic nervous system is involved in the pathophysiology of pain arising from the bladder, uterus, rectum, vagina, and prostate. Block of the superior hypogastric plexus has been described as a technique for treating pain arising from the pelvic viscera, but only limited observational data point to the usefulness of these techniques (108,109). Few complications have been reported, therefore much of the following discussion will focus on potential complications (see Chapter 45).

The superior hypogastric plexus is situated in the retroperitoneum, bilaterally extending from the lower third of the fifth lumbar vertebral body to the upper third of the first sacral vertebral body (Fig. 50-11). It receives fibers from the inferior hypogastric plexus, which in turn receives all the afferent fibers from the pelvic organs.

The combined experience of more than 200 cases indicates that neurologic complications have not occured as a result of this block (110) (Table 50-9). However, incorrect needle placement may lead to catastrophic results. If the needle tips are placed too posteriorly, they will lie adjacent to the intervertebral foramina at the L5–S1 level, and injectate may easily spread to surround the spinal nerve and extend into the epidural space. Thus, the tip of needle must be placed adjacent to the inferior third of L5 to avoid this potential problem. Because of the close proximity of the iliac vessels, intravascular injection can easily occur. Careful evaluation of images taken

Acetaldehyde dehydrogenase deficiency results in sensitivity to ethanol, which is frequently used for neurolysis (104). Following ethanol injection, individuals with aldehyde dehydrogenase deficiency have increased systemic levels of acetaldehyde, causing skin flushing, nausea, headache, tachycardia, hypotension, and drowsiness (105) (see also Chapter 45).

Neurologic complications involve sensory and/or motor deficits of the lower extremities. Although the incidence is extremely infrequent, these neurologic deficits often represent the most worrisome complications associated with NCPB. Different mechanisms are possible, with the most likely cause involving the injection or contact of neurolytic solutions with neural structures other than the celiac ganglia or splanchnic nerves. Possible routes could include inadvertent needle placement or injection into the intrathecal or epidural space, thoracic or lumbar nerve roots, or lumbar plexus within the psoas muscle compartment. Another separate mechanism involves the interruption of blood flow due to injury or spasm of the major anterior radicular artery, also known as the artery of Adamkiewicz, which provides blood flow to the anterior spinal artery (106,107) (Fig. 50-10). Interruption of blood flow to the spinal cord can result in permanent sensory and motor deficits of the lower trunk and/or extremities.

Some of the complications associated with NCPB may be difficult to prevent even in the care of an experienced pain medicine specialist. These complications include needle puncture injuries, complications related to sympatholysis from an effective block (e.g., bowel hypermotility), unexpected drug

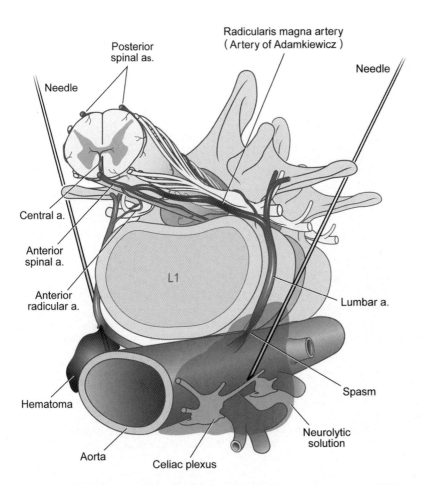

Posterior spinal as.

Radicularis magna artery (Artery of Adamkiewicz)

Needle

Needle

Central a.

Anterior spinal a.

Anterior radicular a.

L1

Lumbar a.

Hematoma

Aorta

Celiac plexus

Spasm

Neurolytic solution

FIGURE 50-10. Arterial supply of the spinal cord at the level of low thoracic and high lumbar vertebral levels. The largest feeding artery to the spinal cord is the artery of Adamkiewicz (anterior radicular artery), which branches from the lumbar artery (in this figure). Reproduced from Neal JM, Rathmell JP. *Complications in Regional Anesthesia and Pain Medicine.* Philadelphia: Saunders Elsevier, 2007, with permission.

after injection of radiographic contrast must be done to rule out abnormal spread or intravascular injection.

COMPLICATIONS ASSOCIATED WITH NEUROLYTIC BLOCKADE

Chemical Neurolysis and the Pharmacology of Neurolytic Agents

Neurolytic blocks are performed in patients with severe pain secondary to advanced cancer or occlusive vascular disease. Their use in chronic nonmalignant pain (e.g., chronic relapsing pancreatitis) is controversial. Neurolytic blocks are best suited for patients suffering from severe pain despite aggressive attempts to control the pain using more conservative means and a short life expectancy. The results of neurolytic blockade can be devastating to the patient and must be carefully weighed against the anticipated benefits. For instance, neuraxial neurolysis can provide profound pain relief for patients with pain related to invasive tumors involving the pelvis, but this approach often leads to loss of bowel and/or bladder function and may well also produce weakness in the lower extremities. Neurolytic blocks can be peripheral, neuraxial, or visceral. Peripheral neurolytic blocks are rarely performed because the block can cause motor deficit when mixed nerves are blocked, neuritis and deafferentation pain are consequences, and the block is not predictably permanent (111). The risks and complications

associated with neurolytic celiac plexus block have been covered in detail earlier in this chapter; here we will discuss the pharmacology and pathophysiology of chemical neurolysis of other structures (see also Chapter 45).

The neurolytic agents that are commonly employed include ethyl alcohol and phenol. Occasionally, glycerol is used. Ethyl alcohol causes neurolysis by extracting cholesterol, phospholipids, and cerebrosides from the nervous tissue and precipitating lipoproteins and mucoproteins. Its injection into a peripheral nerve results in Wallerian degeneration, wherein the axon and the Schwann cell are both damaged (112). When neurolytic agents are injected into the subarachnoid space, the changes occur in the dorsal roots, posterior portion of the spinal cord, and the Lissauer tract (113). Alcohol is commercially available as a 95% concentration. Studies showed that a concentration of 33% or greater is necessary to produce neurolysis (114). Alcohol is commonly used for visceral sympathetic blocks (celiac plexus, superior hypogastric plexus) and injections into the subarachnoid space. Because of the risk of neuralgia, it is now rarely used for neurolytic blocks of the lumbar sympathetic ganglia and the trigeminal ganglia. It is an irritant and causes burning pain on injection. Alcohol is injected undiluted when used for peripheral injections. In celiac plexus blocks, the alcohol is usually diluted with a local anesthetic to a concentration of 50% to diminish the pain on injection. Alcohol is hypobaric with respect to the CSF, and the patient must be positioned with the painful side up when intrathecal injection is performed. Denervation and relief of pain usually occurs over a few days after injection and is complete after 1 week (111). Intravascular injection of 30 mL of 100% ethanol will result in a blood

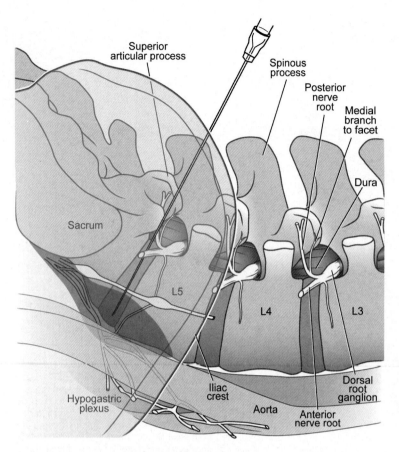

FIGURE 50-11. Anatomy of the superior hypogastric plexus. The superior hypogastric plexus is comprised of a loose, web-like group of interlacing nerve fibers that lie over the anterolateral surface of the L5 vertebral body and extend inferiorly over the sacrum. Needles are positioned over the anterolateral surface of the L5–S1 intervertebral disc of the inferior aspect of the L5 vertebral bodies to block the superior hypogastric plexus. Reproduced from Rathmell JP. *Atlas of Image-guided Intervention in Regional Anesthesia and Pain Medicine*, 1st ed. Philadelphia: Lippincott Williams & Wilkins, 2006, with permission.

ethanol level well above the legal limit for intoxication, but below the danger of severe alcohol toxicity; IV injection is usually uneventful but may cause thrombosis of the vessel (115).

Phenol causes neurolysis by precipitating proteins in the nervous tissue. At lower concentrations, it acts as a local anesthetic. As a result, minimal discomfort occurs on injection of the drug. It has a strong affinity for vascular tissue, and injury to the blood vessels at or near nervous tissues may contribute to its neurotoxicity (116). Five percent phenol is equivalent to 40% alcohol in neurolytic potency (117). The intrathecal injection of phenol causes changes similar to that of alcohol. Degeneration of fibers occurs in the posterior columns and posterior nerve roots. The concentrations of phenol that are used for neurolysis range from 3% to 15%. Phenol is relatively insoluble in water and, at concentrations above 6%, has to be prepared with the addition of glycerin or contrast medium. At these concentrations, it is fairly viscous. Phenol has a clinical biphasic action,

with the initial relief secondary to its local anesthetic effect. This relief fades within the first 24 hours, and lasting analgesia occurs 3 to 7 days after the injection secondary to the neurolytic action of the drug. Phenol is hyperbaric with respect to CSF, and the patient must be positioned with the painful side down when subarachnoid injection is performed. The intravascular injection of phenol results in convulsions secondary to an increase in the excitatory transmitter acetylcholine in the central nervous system (118). Large systemic doses of phenol (>8.5 g) cause effects similar to those seen with local anesthetic overdose: generalized seizures and cardiovascular collapse; renal damage due to nephrotoxicity is also possible. Clinical doses up to 1,000 mg are unlikely to cause serious toxicity.

Intercostal and Thoracic Paravertebral Neurolysis

Intercostal blocks are used in the treatment of thoracic or abdominal wall pain. Prior to the widespread use of continuous thoracic epidural analgesia, the use of intercostal blocks was common. Complications include pneumothorax, intravascular injection, intrapulmonary injection with consequent bronchospasm, and neuraxial spread (Fig. 50-12). When multiple intercostal nerve blocks are administered to provide analgesia following thoracotomy, the incidence of pneumothorax detected by radiograph is 0.082% to 2% (119,120). Clinically significant pneumothorax occurs at a low rate, and chest tube insertion is rarely required. Paravertebral somatic block is an alternative to intercostal or epidural blockade, and involves placing local anesthetic or neurolytic solution in the space just

---

TABLE 50-9

PREVENTING COMPLICATIONS DURING SUPERIOR HYPOGASTRIC PLEXUS BLOCK

- Pay strict attention to needle placement using radiographic guidance. The tip of the needle must be at the junction of L5–S1.
- Avoid the use of the traditional approach in patients with evidence of atherosclerotic disease of the iliac vessels. Under these circumstances, the transdiscal approach at the L5–S1 would be a better choice.

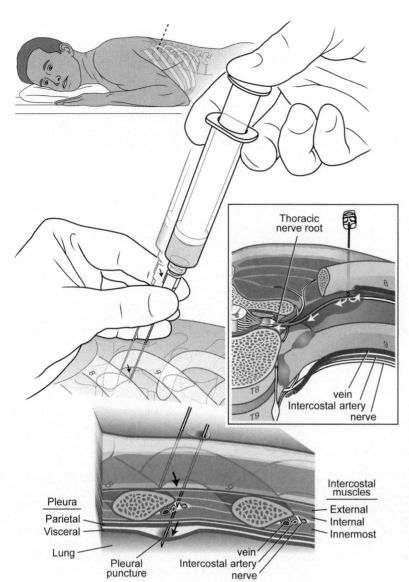

FIGURE 50-12. Complications of intercostal neurolysis. The thoracic nerve roots exit the spinal canal through the intervertebral foramina and divide into anterior and posterior primary rami. The anterior rami course laterally to enter a groove beneath the inferior margin of each rib, where they traverse laterally inferior to the intercostal vein and artery. Intercostal nerve block is carried out by inserting a needle just inferior to the rib margin. When the needle tip is directly adjacent to the intercostal nerve, the intercostal vessels lie in close proximity, thus intravascular injection often occurs. Advancing the needle deep beyond the rib margin may result in pneumothorax. Proximal spread of injectate along the course of the intercostal nerve can result in epidural spread. Reproduced from Neal JM, Rathmell JP. *Complications in Regional Anesthesia and Pain Medicine*. Philadelphia: Saunders Elsevier, 2007, with permission.

outside of the intervertebral foramen. Although most of the studies looked at the utility of paravertebral block for surgery, it may also be useful to treat metastatic breast cancer pain from the chest wall or ribs (121,122). No data are available to guide use of this technique. The short-term consequences are likely similar to those encountered with local anesthetic intercostal blocks. In the author's hands, the use of intercostal or paravertebral neurolysis using 6% to 10% phenol can produce nearly immediate and profound analgesia limited to one or two adjacent dermatomes on one side of the chest wall. However, incomplete neurolysis, likely due to limited spread of the neurolytic solution, can cause severe neuralgic-type pain requiring repeat neurolysis. This technique is rarely if ever indicated in noncancer patients because of the high risk of neuralgia.

Neuraxial Neurolysis

With the advent of intrathecal drug delivery, neuraxial neurolytic blocks are now used very infrequently. Indeed, much of the following information can be found only in old textbooks, with little appearing even in the older peer-reviewed literature. Subarachnoid neurolytic (Fig. 50-13) blocks are utilized in patients with short life expectancy, whose pain is somatic in origin, is limited to two or three dermatomes, is not completely relieved by analgesic and adjunctive medications, and is completely relieved by prognostic local anesthetic blocks (123). The recommended dose of subarachnoid alcohol and phenol is very small; 0.1 mL increments are injected up to a total of 0.8 mL. Subarachnoid alcohol is injected with the painful side up, while phenol is injected with the painful side down, positioning with respect to the baricity of the alcohol or phenol. The patient must remain in position for at least 30 minutes after the injection, and air is injected to clear the needle before it is withdrawn. Complications include PDPH, aseptic meningitis, bowel and bladder dysfunction, numbness, muscle weakness, and dysesthesia (Table 50-10) (123,124). The incidences of these complications ranged from 1% to 26% for rectal and urinary dysfunction, 1% to 14% for lower extremity paresis, 1% to 21% for sensory loss, and 0.3% to 4% for paresthesia/neuritis (125). The nature of the complication depends on

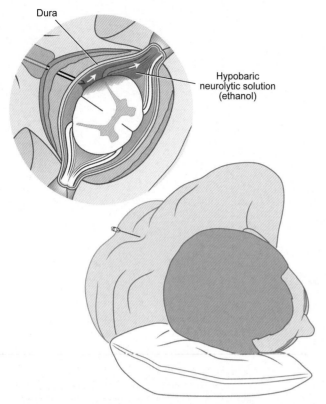

FIGURE 50-13. Anatomy of intrathecal neurolysis. Intrathecal neurolysis is performed infrequently for those who have intractable pain of the trunk or lower extremities associated with locally invasive cancer. When the block is performed using alcohol, a hypobaric solution, the patient is placed in the lateral position with the painful region upward or nondependent and the torso rotated 45 degrees anteriorly to bring the dorsal roots to the highest point within the cerebrospinal fluid. The alcohol solution is then administered in small increments, and the hypobaric solution rises to bathe the dorsal roots. The neurolytic solution is placed directly adjacent to the spinal cord, and damage to the cord is a distinct possibility during intrathecal neurolysis. Reproduced from Neal JM, Rathmell JP. *Complications in Regional Anesthesia and Pain Medicine.* Philadelphia: Saunders Elsevier, 2007, with permission.

the site of injection. Motor weakness is noted when the injection is at the lumbar or cervicothoracic area, whereas bladder complications usually occur when the level of injection is below the thoracic nerve roots. Because of the severity of the complications, it is important that patients are properly selected and informed of the complications; patients should be properly positioned and the needle be inserted at the proper interspace (see Chapter 42).

TABLE 50-10

COMPLICATIONS OF SUBARACHNOID NEUROLYTIC BLOCKS

Dural puncture headache
Bowel paralysis
Bladder paralysis
Numbness
Muscle weakness
Dysesthesia

The epidural approach to chemical neurolysis has been advocated for improved efficacy at the thoracic and cervicothoracic junction, increased safety, ease of repeated injections, and relief of bilateral pain (126,127). Although no serious complications were noted in previous publications, the safety of epidural neurolysis has been questioned. In primates, lower extremity weakness has been noted clinically, and posterior nerve root damage was demonstrated histologically (128). Autopsy studies in a patient showed destruction at the outer third of the dura with no abnormality of the spinal cord or the nerve roots (129).

Radiofrequency Neurolysis

Experimental attempts to use electricity to produce discrete tissue lesions were reported as early as the 1870s in animals and introduced into clinical practice in the 1930s (130). Sweet and Mark attempted to use direct current (DC), but found that this led to unpredictable and irregular lesions that varied in size by a factor of four (131). Sweet and subsequent investigators suggested that use of a high-frequency current might produce more predictable lesions. From their experimental work on hemostasis, Aranow and Cosman adapted a radiofrequency technique for producing neural lesions in the 1950s (132). Radiofrequency generators utilize high-frequency waves in the range of 300 to 500 kHz to produce tissue lesions via ionic means; since high frequencies in this range were also used in radio transmitters, the current was named *radiofrequency* current. Conventional radiofrequency treatment uses a constant output of high-frequency electric current, produces controllable tissue destruction surrounding the tip of the treatment cannula and, when placed at precise anatomic locations, has demonstrated success in reducing pain in a number of different chronic pain states, including chronic neck pain after whiplash injury (133) and trigeminal neuralgia (134).

Pulsed radiofrequency uses brief "pulses" of high-voltage, radiofrequency-range (~300 kHz) electrical current that produces the same voltage fluctuations in the region of treatment that occur during conventional radiofrequency treatment but without heating to a temperature at which tissue coagulates. The conceptual appeal of a minimally invasive, nondestructive technique that is useful in treating chronic pain of any sort is compelling. In clinical practice, a mass migration has occurred to the use of pulsed radiofrequency despite few data to support the efficacy of this new technique. The modality has great appeal, specifically because it is not neurodestructive. With conventional radiofrequency, the thermal lesion occasionally leads to worsening pain and even new onset of neuropathic pain (135). A small retrospective case series (136) and extensive clinical experience among practitioners suggest that pulsed radiofrequency results in neither increased pain nor any risk of neuropathic pain, and that it is very well tolerated by patients from treatment through recovery. Not a single randomized trial compares the efficacy of pulsed radiofrequency to any type of control treatment or to conventional radiofrequency treatment; this technique is in need of further study to validate its usefulness.

Conventional wisdom holds that the usefulness of radiofrequency stems from the ability to produce a small lesion of precise dimensions in a specific anatomic location (137). Pulsed radiofrequency produces the same voltage fluctuations in the region of treatment as conventional radiofrequency but without tissue coagulation. Complications associated with radiofrequency treatment fall into two broad categories: those that arise during placement of the radiofrequency cannula and those that result from neural destruction during conventional radiofrequency neurotomy. As may occur with any technique that requires needle placement, direct injury to neural or vascular structures in the vicinity of treatment can occur. Both conventional and pulsed radiofrequency treatment are associated with a similar risk of injury during needle placement. Conventional radiofrequency neurotomy using a heat lesion that produces neural destruction is also associated with the sequelae of neural injury that follow placement of lesions. Even with proper technique, conventional radiofrequency lesions are associated with sensory loss and onset of neuropathic pain in a subset of patients; the frequency and severity of these neural changes vary with the specific site of treatment and are most common after intracranial radiofrequency lesioning of the trigeminal ganglion. Injury to adjacent nerves can also occur, and the frequency of these complications is minimized by the proper use of sensory and motor stimulation before lesioning.

Radiofrequency Treatment for Trigeminal Neuralgia

Trigeminal neuralgia (tic douloureux) is a common, idiopathic form of neuropathic pain that presents with paroxysms of pain involving one or more divisions of the trigeminal nerve (cranial nerve V). The disorder typically strikes those in the sixth decade of life, is of sudden onset without a precipitating event, and has a 2:1 predominance in females (138). Patients report episodic and severe pain involving one or more branches of the trigeminal nerve. The most commonly affected branches are the second and third divisions together, followed closely by involvement of either the second or third division alone. Those affected often describe a small area that "triggers" paroxysms of pain—perhaps pressure on an incisor or slight touch to the margins of the lip precipitates lancinating pains along the entire course of the involved division of the trigeminal nerve. The pain typically occurs in brief paroxysms lasting just seconds at a time, but may escalate to a frequency of many episodes daily (139). The underlying etiology remains unknown, but experts have hypothesized that second-order neurons within the trigeminal ganglion become sensitized and, following sensory input from the trigger area, seizure-like hyperactivity is triggered in adjacent sensory neurons and is manifested as pain. Recurrent trauma due to pulsatile compression of the ganglion caused by the small branch vessels from the adjacent carotid siphon has been postulated as the underlying cause of neural injury that leads to trigeminal neuralgia (140,141), and from this hypothesis, treatment via posterior craniotomy and microvascular decompression has evolved as a successful method to alleviate the pain (142) (see also Chapter 42).

Invariably, a proportion of patients will continue to experience debilitating pain despite drug treatment, or their pain will recur and become refractory to pharmacologic management, and this group will seek further treatment. A wide range of neuroablative techniques have been developed, all aimed at destroying a small number of cells within the affected area of the trigeminal ganglion and thereby eliminating the neuronal excitability (143). Available techniques range from chemical destruction with glycerol to focused external-beam radiotherapy (radiosurgery). Among these neuroablative techniques, the most widely used has been percutaneous radiofrequency ablation of the trigeminal ganglion (144). All of the available neuroablative techniques will produce some degree of sensory and/or motor loss.

Radiofrequency ablation of the trigeminal ganglion has been in use for decades, and there are large retrospective series conducted in a similar fashion to guide our understanding of the usefulness and complications associated with this approach. Currently, its use has declined and is now limited to those patients who have failed pharmacologic therapy and are not deemed medically fit or decline to undergo microvascular decompression (144). The initial success rates for all surgical interventions ranges from 92% to 98%. The rate of pain recurrence among percutaneous techniques is lowest with radiofrequency rhizotomy (20% in 9 years) when compared with glycerol rhizotomy (54% in 4 years) and balloon compression (21% in 2 years) (144). The most common complications and adverse effects (some of which are an expected part of the treatment) include facial numbness (98%), dysesthesia (24%), anesthesia dolorosa (1.5%), corneal anesthesia (7%), keratitis (1%), and trigeminal motor dysfunction (24%). Recent reviews detail the range of incidence of complications from the published literature (Table 50-11) (145).

The mechanism of injury during radiofreqency rhizotomy for trigeminal neuralgia may be related to injury caused during placement of the cannula or injury that results from the thermal destruction during radiofrequency treatment. The radiofrequency cannula is inserted through the skin just adjacent to the lateral margin of the mouth and cephalad via the foramen ovale in the base of the skull until the active tip lies adjacent to or within the trigeminal ganglion. Placement of the cannula generally requires brief intervals of heavy sedation. En route to the trigeminal ganglion, the cannula courses medial to the body of the mandible, just beneath the oral mucosa, and there is significant risk of piercing the oral mucosa

TABLE 50-11

COMPLICATIONS OF RADIOFREQUENCY RHIZOTOMY FOR TRIGEMINAL NEURALGIA. (ADAPTED FROM REFERENCE)

Complication	Estimated incidence (%)
Attributable to lesions of the trigeminal nerve	
Numbness	71–98
Dysesthesia	11–27
Anesthesia dolorosa	0.2–7.9
Corneal anesthesia	1–21
Keratitis	0.2–20
Masseter weakness (motor root)	1–25
Due to inclusion/injury of adjacent nerves	
Optic nerve lesion	0.001
Diplopia (CN III, IV, or VI)	0.5–2
Hearing problems	0.01–2
Due to injury of other adjacent structures	
Carotid-cavernous fistula	0.1
Subdural, infratemporal hemorrhage	0.0002
Intracerebral hemorrhage (needle puncture)	0.0006
Other	
Intracerebral hemorrhage (not due to needle)	0.002
Subdural hemorrhage	0.0007
Seizure	0.0002
Hemiparesis	0.0003
Perioperative mortality (all causes)	0.0006–0.0026

Adapted from Mikeladze G, Espinal R, Finnegan R, et al. Pulsed radiofrequency application in treatment of chronic zygapophyseal joint pain. *Spine J* 2003;3:360–362, with permission.

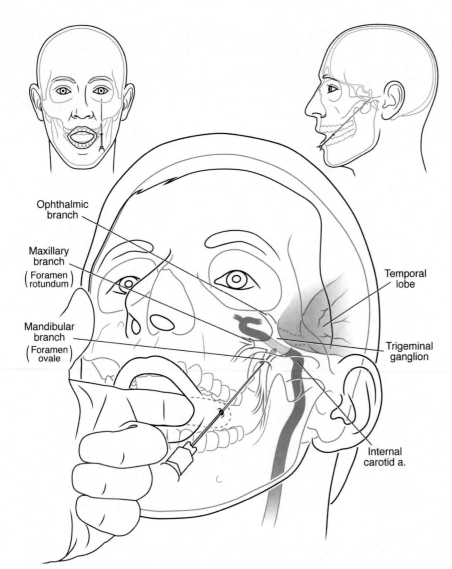

Ophthalmic branch

Maxillary branch
(Foramen)
(rotundum)

Mandibular branch
(Foramen)
(ovale)

Temporal lobe

Trigeminal ganglion

Internal carotid a.

FIGURE 50-14. Mechanism of complications that arise during radiofrequency treatment for trigeminal neuralgia. The radiofrequency cannula is inserted just lateral to the lateral margin of the lips and advanced medial to the mandible and lateral to the oral mucosa. The index finger of the operator is placed in the patient's mouth to ensure that the tip of the cannula does not penetrate the oral mucosa en route to the foramen ovale. Note the close proximity of the carotid artery, the temporal lobe, and the brainstem to the final position of the cannula. *Insets:* The proper trajectory of the needle and final needle position are shown in the frontal and axial planes. Reproduced from Neal JM, Rathmell JP. *Complications in Regional Anesthesia and Pain Medicine.* Philadelphia: Saunders Elsevier, 2007, with permission.

and dragging bacteria into the cranium. Meningitis is a rare complication, and the exact portal of bacterial entry is usually uncertain (146,147). Within the skull, the trigeminal ganglion lies lateral to the posterior clinoid process of the sella turcica, just lateral to the internal carotid artery, anterior to the pons, and medial to the inferomedial aspect of the temporal lobe of the brain (Fig. 50-14). Excessive advancement of the needle risks injury to these structures. Indeed, case reports of brainstem injury have appeared (148). Excessive anterior angulation of the advancing cannula can lead it through the pterygopalatine fossa up through the inferior orbital fissure and into the optic canal, where optic nerve injury and monocular blindness have occurred (149). In addition, toward its posterior aspect, the trigeminal ganglion is enveloped closely within dural reflections, and even proper placement of the cannula often results in the appearance of CSF flowing freely from the cannula. This rarely creates any long-term sequelae, but may lead to reports of CSF rhinorrhea (150), believed to be retrograde flow of CSF through the foramen ovale and into the auditory (eustachian) tube through an opening in the canal created during needle placement.

Neural injury during radiofrequency ablation of the trigeminal ganglion is universal and indeed the goal of this treatment

modality. Direct destruction of a small area of neurons within the distal portion of the ganglion or the nerve rootlets is believed to be the mechanism that interrupts the episodic pain. To target the radiofrequency treatment area, the cannula is advanced until a low-voltage, high-frequency current produces a paresthesia within the area where the patient typically experiences pain. Thereafter, heat lesioning is begun for 60-second intervals at 60°C under brief periods of general anesthesia. Between treatments, the patient is allowed to recover enough to allow sensory testing within the cutaneous distribution where the pain is localized. Repeated lesions are created at gradually increasing temperatures (typically 2°C increments) to increase the degree of neural destruction until the patient reports the appearance of slight hypesthesia in the affected region. The most common adverse effects of this approach are related to the size and location of the thermal lesion (Table 50-11). Judging the extent of the sensory change following each lesion can be quite difficult and is often clouded by effects of the anesthetic. If the extent of the lesion is excessive, the area of sensory loss can extend to the ophthalmic division of the trigeminal nerve (V1), and can result in loss of the corneal reflex, corneal anesthesia, and keratitis may ensue. The majority of patients (98%) (143) will report some detectable degree of sensory loss within the region treated, and this loss of sensation can be bothersome to some. Others have reported dense sensory anesthesia and ongoing neuropathic pain in the region of treatment (anesthesia dolorosa). Treatment of the mandibular division of the trigeminal nerve (V3) involves motor fibers to the masseter muscle, and weakness during mastication is common. Finally, direct heating of the trigeminal rootlets can lead to dramatic rises in blood pressure and intracranial bleeding (151). In a recent large review examining 6,205 patients treated with radiofrequency rhizotomy for trigeminal neuralgia, the latter complication has not been reported (144), perhaps due to the advent of more rapidly acting sedative hypnotics and meticulous intraoperative monitoring. Diagnosis of adverse effects and complications associated with radiofrequency treatment for trigeminal neuralgia is usually self-evident. Masticatory weakness, variable degrees of hypesthesia, and anesthesia dolorosa occur with sufficient frequency that they should be expected, and patients should be counseled regarding each as a part of the informed consent process prior to treatment. CSF rhinorrhea is typically painless and self-limited. New onset of a focal neurologic deficit or headache after treatment warrants immediate imaging of the brain using MRI to rule out hematoma formation with reversible compression of neural elements. Although direct neural injury is by far the more common cause leading to new focal deficits, a reversible cause should be ruled out. Indeed, this technique has been largely performed by neurosurgeons; ongoing and close collaboration with a neurosurgeon is warranted for anesthesiologists and others who perform the technique independently, and immediate neurosurgical consultation should be readily available whenever the technique is used. For those patients who develop corneal anesthesia following the procedure, consultation with an ophthalmologist is required.

Treatment of the most common adverse effects associated with radiofrequency ablation for trigeminal neuralgia is symptomatic. Most problems are self-limited. Like other forms of neuropathic pain stemming from neural injury, anesthesia dolorosa is difficult to treat. The use of antiepileptic and antidepressant drugs is the cornerstone of management for this problem. In the immediate time interval following radiofrequency treatment, the pain can be extreme, and use of opioid analgesics, often in high doses, is the only available means of temporizing. Onset of a new focal neurologic deficit may herald significant, direct neural trauma. Therapy is guided by diagnostic imaging. In the event that significant intracranial bleeding occurs, immediate surgical decompression may be warranted.

Central to successful application of radiofrequency treatment for trigeminal neuralgia is the use of meticulous image-guided placement of the radiofrequency cannula and creation of the smallest anatomically correct lesion that will produce mild hypesthesia in the region affected. Correct needle placement begins with advancing the needle over the medial aspect of the mandible beneath the oral mucosa. Penetration of the oral mucosa and further advancing the needle risks seeding the intracranial vault with oral bacteria. This can be avoided by placing a gloved hand in the patient's mouth and palpating the needle beneath the oral mucosa as it is advanced. Once the needle has been advanced beyond the posterior extent of the mandible toward the base of the skull, there is no further risk of penetrating the oral mucosa. Trauma to extracranial vascular structures near the skull base, including the carotid artery as it enters the carotid canal, is minimized by use of fluoroscopic guidance. The foramen ovale should be identified near the base of the lateral pterygoid plate, and excessive deviation from this location should be avoided. Once the needle has entered the foramen ovale, fluoroscopic images in the AP

and lateral planes should be used to avoid excessive cranial advancement. The needle tip should not be inserted beyond a line drawn between the superior aspects of the anterior and posterior clinoid processes in a lateral radiograph to avoid direct trauma to the temporal lobe and brainstem. Sensory stimulation should then be carried out just after traversing the foramen. Repeated sensory stimulation after each small (2–3 mm) advance of the needle will ensure that the needle reaches the proper position without excessive advancement within the cranium.

For those patients with involvement of the ophthalmic division of the trigeminal nerve (V1), many experts question the usefulness of radiofrequency treatment (144). Since thermal injury to the ganglion to the point of sensory loss is required for successful treatment, some degree of corneal anesthesia is to be expected if the lesion is targeted to this region of the ganglion. Nonetheless, when other treatment options are not available, even those with involvement of V1 have been successfully treated, albeit at a heightened risk of corneal anesthesia and subsequent keratitis.

Radiofrequency Treatment for Facet-related Pain

Neck and low back pain are ubiquitous and have many causes. Each element of the spine can give rise to distinct pain syndromes. Facet-related pain has been recognized as a common cause of axial neck and low back pain (i.e., pain that is primarily along the spinal axis as opposed to radicular pain that extends into the extremities and suggests neural compression) (152). The diagnosis of facet-related pain is made on the basis of symptoms. No definitive diagnostic studies are possible, thus the diagnosis is imprecise at best. Patients with facet-related pain typically report deep aching pain that predominantly overlies the spinal axis. The pain may be unilateral or bilateral. The most common causes of facet-related pain appear to be degenerative changes within the facet joints, most often osteoarthritis ("spondylosis"). There may be some history of trauma, particularly in facet-related neck pain. The most common injuries are sudden twisting or flexion–extension injuries (e.g., "whiplash"). Symptoms are usually exacerbated by extension. Well-documented patterns of referred pain arising from various facet joints help with deciding where treatment should be focused (153–155). Imaging studies (CT, MRI) may be completely normal, even though facet arthropathy of varying degrees is quite common. Most clinicians rely on diagnostic injections to guide patient selection for radiofrequency facet denervation. Intra-articular facet injections or blocks of the medial branch nerves to the facet using local anesthetic should produce transient relief of the symptoms before proceeding with radiofrequency treatment.

Despite widespread use of radiofrequency thermoablation for facet-related pain, limited data are available regarding the safety of this technique and its associated complications. No formal safety assessment has been performed (156). In the absence of such formal assessment, knowledge must be gleaned from a review of published studies. Attempts to evaluate incidence and severity of complications are frustrated by variability in the published literature. Authors have differed widely regarding the detail with which complications have been reported, and some authors have neither reported complications nor remarked on their absence. Nonetheless, numerous reports have confirmed the safety of radiofrequency facet denervation. Several large series of patients treated with lumbar radiofrequency denervation have been reported without major complications (157). Notably, there have been few reports of major neurologic injury resulting from this technique, and it is rare to see anything more than transient exacerbation of symptoms following radiofrequency facet denervation. The primary limitations of this technique are the rate of failure and return of pain after treatment.

It is clear that fewer than half of reported patients who undergo diagnostic blocks proceed to neurolysis. Of those undergoing lumbar facet denervation, about half of patients obtain good to excellent pain relief. In a summary report of numerous uncontrolled studies, the proportion of patients achieving greater than 50% pain relief varied from 17% to 82%, with a mean success rate of 48%; however, the proportion of patients obtaining complete relief was unstated, and the duration of follow-up was often less than a year (158). In contrast, more recent studies have incorporated rigorous patient selection criteria and sham controls; among the best designed and conducted of trials was a recent prospective, randomized, placebo-controlled (sham) study of patients with cervical pain (whiplash) that demonstrated 50% pain reduction for a median of 9 months after facet denervation versus 8 days in the sham-treated group (159). A recent systematic review concluded that percutaneous radiofrequency neurolysis of the sensory nerves to the facet joints is a safe and modestly effective treatment for facet-related pain (160).

A recent review details the adverse effects and complications associated with cervical radiofrequency neurotomy (Table 50-12) (145). In a series of 28 patients who received cervical radiofrequency treatment, McDonald et al. reported no complications (161). In a comment on this article, Burchiel asserted the importance of warning patients about the possibility of both cutaneous dysesthesia and postoperative pain and numbness that could last between 2 and 34 months (162), both of which are common sequelae of cervical radiofrequency neurotomy and are often considered expected outcomes rather than complications. The most common complications associated with cervical medial branch neurotomy include postoperative pain (97%); ataxia, unsteadiness, and spatial disorientation (23%); and vasovagal syncope (2%) (Table 50-12). Lord found that brief postoperative pain was the only side effect of lower cervical procedures, but ataxia occurred when the third occipital nerve was treated (163). Because the third occipital nerve carries a large proportion of fibers involved in cutaneous innervation, numbness routinely accompanies lesioning of this nerve. In patients whose treatment was successful, this numb patch regressed over 1 to 3 weeks and was replaced by dysesthesia and pruritus, followed by the return of normal cutaneous sensation and pain. Unsuccessful treatment was characterized by the loss of numbness and return of pain within 1 week.

The incidence of expected treatment-related adverse effects and complications associated with lumbar radiofrequency medial branch neurotomy is markedly lower than that observed following treatment at cervical levels. Postoperative pain has emerged as the most prevalent complication of radiofrequency medial branch neurotomy. This pain is usually transient, although neuritic pain may occasionally last for months to years. Information related to radiofrequency complications was contained mainly in anecdotal reports, with most large series reporting no complications (157,164–166). In a contemporary retrospective study designed to assess that frequency of complications, Kornick et al. found that 92 patients who received 616 lumbar radiofrequency lesions in 116 procedures performed over a 5-year period, had a 1% incidence of postoperative pain (167). Only one-half of those affected experienced pain for more than 2 weeks. There were no major complications, such as infection or new neurologic deficit. In 122 patients who received lumbar, cervical, or thoracic radiofrequency treatment with a minimum follow-up of 1 year, 22% reported transient discomfort and burning pain; universally, resolution occurred within 1 month (168).

Major complications have been acknowledged mainly in the form of case reports. Serious complications appear to be rare, and the available data prevent meaningful systematic analysis. Kornick et al. noted minor burns due to insulation breaks in electrodes, improper function of grounding pads, or unexplained reasons (136). There is no evidence of any significant risk of infection or hemorrhage. Radiofrequency ablation is also used as a minimally invasive means for local treatment of several types of solid malignancies (169). Three cases of lumbosacral radiculopathy were reported following radiofrequency ablation of intra-abdominal metastases, suggesting that when radiofrequency thermocoagulation is applied directly to a lumbosacral nerve root, thermal injury is likely (170).

Separate consideration should be given to the emerging use of *pulsed radiofrequency* techniques that do not cause neurodestruction. Munglani noted that this technique produces no clinical evidence of neural damage and minimal postoperative soreness (171). Manchikanti asserted that this technique "may be used in neuropathic pain without adverse sequelae and safely in CRPS" (172). Despite the enthusiasm for pulsed radiofrequency, precisely because it does not appear to be neurodestructive, the nature and extent of lesions made by these methods have not been described, and no evidence has been published to demonstrate their efficacy.

Similar to radiofrequency treatment of trigeminal neuralgia, complications during radiofrequency ablation of the medial branch nerves may be related to injury caused during placement of the cannula and injury that results from the thermal destruction during radiofrequency treatment. The anatomic configuration of the sensory nerves to the facet joints allows safe destruction without damage to the sensory and motor nerves to the extremities. The spinal nerve roots exit the spinal canal via the intervertebral foramina and divide into anterior and

TABLE 50-12

OBSERVED COMPLICATIONS OF CERVICAL MEDIAL BRANCH NEUROTOMY

Complication	Observed frequency (%)	95% CI (%)
Vasovagal syncope	2	0–6
Postoperative pain	97	94–100
Ataxia, unsteadiness, spatial disorientation	23	14–32
Cutaneous numbness		
TON procedures	88	75–100
C3–C4 procedures	80	55–100
Lower levels	19	8–30
Dysesthesias		
TON procedures	56	37–75
C3–C4 procedures	30	2–58
Lower levels	17	6–27
Dermoid cyst	1	0–4
Transient neuritis	2	0–6

CI, confidence interval; TON, third occipital nerve
Modified from McDonald GJ, Lord SM, Bogduk N. Long-term follow-up of patients treated with cervical radiofrequency neurotomy for chronic neck pain. *Neurosurgery* 1999;45:61–67, with permission.

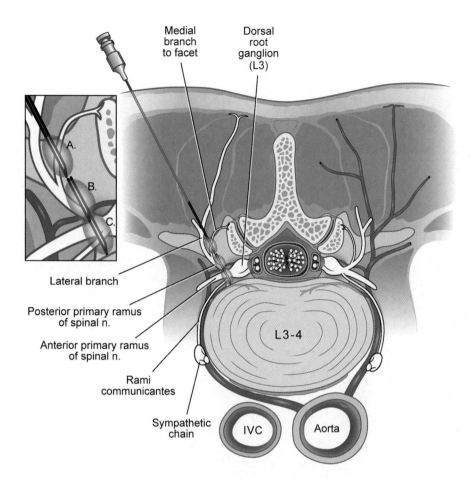

Medial
branch
to facet

Dorsal
root
ganglion
(L3)

Lateral branch

Posterior primary ramus
of spinal n.

Anterior primary ramus
of spinal n.

Rami
communicantes

Sympathetic
chain

IVC

Aorta

L3-4

A.

B.

C.

FIGURE 50-15. Mechanism of complications that arise during lumbar radiofrequency medial branch neurotomy. Axial diagram of lumbar radiofrequency medial branch neurotomy. A 22-gauge, 10-cm radiofrequency cannula with a 5-mm active tip is advanced just anterior to the base of the transverse process where it joins with the superior articular process (see insert). **A:** A radiofrequency cannula in correct position for lumbar radiofrequency medial branch neurotomy. The point of bifurcation of the posterior primary ramus of the spinal nerve into medial and lateral branches is variable, and conventional radiofrequency treatment commonly destroys both nerves. The medial branch supplies sensation to the facet joint, and the lateral branch provides motor innervation to the paraspinous musculature and a small and variable patch of sensory innervation to the skin overlying the spinous processes. **B:** Neurolysis of the lateral branch does not have any demonstrable effect on strength of the paraspinous muscles; however, cutaneous hyperesthesia and/or hypoesthesia do occur infrequently. **C:** Placement of the radiofrequency lesion directly on the anterior primary ramus of the spinal nerve can cause severe and persistent radicular pain. Reproduced from Neal JM, Rathmell JP. *Complications in Regional Anesthesia and Pain Medicine.* Philadelphia: Saunders Elsevier, 2007, with permission.

posterior primary rami (Fig. 50-15). The anterior ramus supplies sensory and motor innervation to the trunk and extremities according to the spinal level of the nerve root. The posterior primary ramus divides again into medial and lateral branches. The lateral branch of the posterior primary ramus provides motor innervation to the spinal erector muscles and a small, variable area of cutaneous sensory innervation to the area directly overlying the spinous processes. The medial branch of the posterior primary ramus supplies sensory innervation to the facet joints. The medial branch, or nerve to the facet, travels along the base of the superior articular process of the facet joint of each vertebra, where it joins with the medial-most portion of the transverse process. In this location, radiographic guidance allows precise placement of the radiofrequency cannula, and lesions can be produced without affecting the anterior primary ramus (i.e., without risk of unwanted damage to the sensory or motor nerves to the trunk and extremities).

Direct injury to soft tissues and periosteum during traumatic needle placement can lead to transient local pain for several days following treatment. The needle can also be advanced anteriorly and cause direct injury to the exiting spinal nerve. More likely is that the patient will report a transient paresthesia extending to the peripheral distribution of the nerve as the needle contacts the spinal nerve. Paresthesia are not uncommon and typically resolve immediately with needle repositioning; however, persistent paresthesia may occur.

Thermal injury caused by incorrect position of the radiofrequency cannula has also been reported (170). The precise anatomic location of the bifurcation of the posterior primary

ramus of the spinal nerve into medial and lateral branches is variable, and often the cannula cannot be positioned at a point that allows close enough proximity to the medial branch without the lesion also engulfing the lateral branch (Figs. 50-15 and 50-16). The lateral branch supplies some motor innervation to the lumbar paraspinous musculature; EMG studies of these muscle groups following radiofrequency medial branch neurotomy at a single level yields denervation potentials (positive sharp waves and fibrillation potentials) in adjacent muscle segments have demonstrated polysegmental innervation from each spinal level (173). This polysegmental innervation likely accounts for the lack of significant clinically detectable weakness following radiofrequency medial branch neurotomy. Indeed, many practitioners view motor stimulation in the paraspinous muscle groups without motor stimulation in the lower extremities as a reliable sign of good cannula positioning. The lateral branch also carries a small and variable number of sensory fibers that supply sensation to a small area overlying the spinous processes. Transient hyperesthesia manifested as a sunburn-like sensation has been reported after lumbar radiofrequency treatment and, more commonly, after cervical radiofrequency treatment. The large sensory distribution of the cervical medial branch nerves is responsible for the high incidence of cutaneous sensory loss and dysesthesias, particularly with treatment of the third occipital nerve and the medial branch nerves at C3 and C4.

More concerning is a cannula position that is so far anterior to the transverse process that the active tip lies in contact with the spinal nerve (Figs. 50-15 and 50-16). This position should

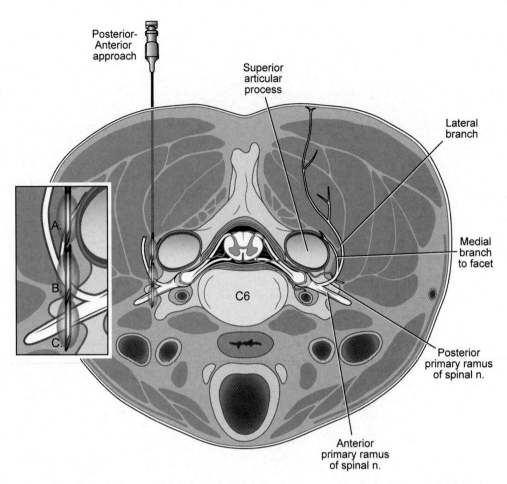

FIGURE 50-16. Mechanism of complications that arise during cervical radiofrequency medial branch neurotomy. Axial diagram of cervical radiofrequency medial branch neurotomy. When a posterior approach is used, the needle is first seated on the lateral margin of the facet column and then walked off the lateral margin of the facet column and advanced 2 to 3 mm to place the active tip along the course of the medial branch nerve (see insert). **A:** A radiofrequency cannula in correct position for cervical radiofrequency medial branch neurotomy. The point of bifurcation of the posterior primary ramus of the spinal nerve into medial and lateral branches is variable, and conventional radiofrequency treatment commonly destroys both nerves. The medial branch supplies sensation to the facet joint, and the lateral branch provides motor innervation to the paraspinous musculature and a small and variable patch of sensory innervation to the skin overlying the spinous processes. **B:** Neurolysis of the lateral branch does not have any demonstrable effect on strength of the paraspinous muscles; however, cutaneous hyperesthesia and/or hypoesthesia do occur infrequently. This is particularly frequent following conventional radiofrequency treatment of the third occipital nerve and the C3 and C4 medial branch nerves, owing to their large cutaneous sensory components. **C:** Placement of the radiofrequency lesion directly on the anterior primary ramus of the spinal nerve can cause severe and persistent radicular pain. Reproduced from Neal JM, Rathmell JP. *Complications in Regional Anesthesia and Pain Medicine.* Philadelphia: Saunders Elsevier, 2007, with permission.

be easily detected during sensory and motor stimulation prior to lesion creation (see further discussion under Prevention). However, once local anesthetic has been placed through the cannula prior to lesion creation, if the cannula is moved anteriorly, spinal nerve injury can occur without any warning signs. Despite this theoretic concern, not even a single case report of persisting new-onset radicular pain following radiofrequency treatment has appeared.

Reports of new-onset radicular pain following radiofrequency medial branch neurotomy are typically self-limited. Physical examination is likely to reveal a limited area of sensory loss or allodynia without any motor deficit. Large fibers within

the spinal nerve are resistant to destruction during radiofrequency treatment. Thus, diagnosis relies on familiarity with the technical aspects of cannula placement during a particular treatment and physical examination alone. If a large sensory deficit is present or discernible focal weakness is apparent, neurologic consultation and consideration of diagnostic imaging to rule out other causes of nerve compression (e.g., herniated nucleus pulposus or localized hematoma) is warranted.

Most sequelae following radiofrequency medial branch neurotomy are self-limited and require nothing more than reassurance and time to resolve. Patients should be warned to expect a transient increase in back pain for several days to weeks following treatment. Providing a brief course of oral analgesics can obviate unnecessary return visits. If new-onset radicular pain with or without allodynia appears, spinal nerve injury should be suspected, and oral neuropathic pain treatment with a tricyclic antidepressant or anticonvulsant should be started. Localized allodynia described as a "sunburn" sensation is common, particularly following radiofrequency treatment of the high cervical medial branch nerves (TON, C3, and C4). A topical 5% lidocaine patch (Lidoderm, Endo Pharmaceuticals, Chadds Ford, PA) can prove invaluable for symptomatic management in these cases, which also tend to resolve within days to weeks of treatment. Persistent numbness is also common and rarely requires specific treatment.

Injury to the spinal nerves during lumbar radiofrequency medial branch neurotomy is best avoided by precise anatomic placement of the radiofrequency cannula using fluoroscopic guidance. The cannula should be gently advanced to contact the superior margin of the transverse process precisely where it joins the superior articular process of the facet, then advanced no more than 2 to 3 mm further over the superior margin of the transverse process to lie along the course of the medial branch nerve. By contacting the transverse process, the depth of the advancing cannula is assured before it approaches the more anterior spinal nerve within the intervertebral foramen.

Similarly, the spinal cord and great vessels of the neck can be avoided during cervical radiofrequency medial branch neurotomy by careful patient positioning and use of radiographic guidance. The medial branch nerves to the facets course across the articular pillar, midway between the superior and inferior articular processes. The nerves can be anesthetized by placing a needle from either a posterior or lateral approach. The lateral approach is more comfortable for the patient, as she can lie on one side rather than face down, and the needle must traverse less tissue en route to the target. However, when the needles are inserted from a lateral approach, they are directed toward the spinal cord; even slight rotation of the neck can lead to confusing the left and right articular pillars and lead to cannula entry into the spinal canal or anteriorly toward the vertebral artery within the foramen transversarium.

The physiologic testing conducted after placement of radiofrequency cannulae and prior to lesion generation is likely the factor that makes complications so uncommon and has assured clinicians that this neuroablative technique is safe. Once the cannulae have been positioned using radiographic guidance, their proper position is confirmed with electrical stimulation similar to that used for nerve localization, using a nerve stimulator to conduct peripheral nerve blocks. Proper testing for sensory–motor dissociation is conducted (the patient should report pain or tingling during stimulation at 50 Hz at less than 0.5 V, and have no motor stimulation to the affected myotome at 2 Hz at no less than three times the sensory threshold or 3 V). Thereafter, great care must be taken to prevent any movement of the cannulae. Each level is anesthetized with 0.5 mL of 2% lidocaine, and lesions are created at 80°C for 60 to 90 seconds. Radiofrequency medial branch neurotomy is safe and modestly effective for treatment of facet-related pain. The most common adverse effect is a transient increase in pain following treatment. Consultation should be sought whenever unexpected sequelae ensue. These sequelae include the appearance of a previously undetected focal neurologic deficit following radiofrequency treatment. Although most will be in the form of a transient radicular pain or area of cutaneous hyperesthesia, the appearance of a previously undetected motor deficit or a progressive deficit warrants immediate neurologic consultation. Direct injury to the spinal cord or vertebral artery may prove catastrophic, indicating immediate neurosurgical con-

sultation, with diagnostic evaluation guided by the presenting signs and symptoms and the suspected injury.

Lumbar Discography

The ability to access the intervertebral disc percutaneously using image guidance has proven to be a safe approach that allows for diagnostic and therapeutic interventions within the nucleus pulposus. Lumbar discography is a controversial diagnostic test that has seen a resurgence in popularity in recent years. Recent modifications incorporating measures of intradiscal pressure into the diagnostic algorithm appear to offer some promise of improving the diagnostic accuracy of discography for identifying symptomatic discs (174). Until the last several years, the role of discography was solely to identify the intervertebral disc or discs that were causing a given patient's pain, thereby allowing the surgeon to rationally plan surgical fusion. In recent years, discography has been used to identify symptomatic discs prior to minimally invasive intradiscal procedures for treating discogenic low back pain and contained disc herniations.

Intradiscal electrothermal therapy (IDET) is a recently introduced technique that employs a steerable thermal resistance wire inserted into the intervertebral disc through a rigid cannula (SpineCATH, Smith & Nephew, Andover, MA). Using radiographic guidance, the catheter is placed along the posterior border of the posterior annulus fibrosus. Thermal energy is then applied using a standardized heating protocol. In experimental animals, this approach has been shown to destroy penetrating nociceptive fibers and to change the cross-linking of glucosaminoglycans, thereby stiffening the intervertebral disc (175). Clinical studies have been mixed, with two recent, high-quality randomized controlled trials (RCTs): one demonstrating significant efficacy in pain reduction and improved function in about one-third of treated patients (176), whereas the other demonstrated no effect (177). On balance, the available literature suggests a modest overall reduction in pain and improvement in function in less than half of patients receiving IDET at a single level who have concordant discography and well-preserved disc height (178). The usefulness of IDET has only been demonstrated for the treatment of symptomatic degenerative disc disease causing axial low back pain.

The use of percutaneous techniques for treatment of radicular pain associated with contained disc herniations has also developed rapidly in recent years. A range of different techniques has been developed that all rely on the same principle. For treatment of radicular pain (primarily leg pain) associated with a disc bulge or contained disc herniation, a cannula is introduced into the nucleus pulposus, and one of several techniques is used to remove a fraction of the central portion of the intervertebral disc (179). The idea is that, by removing a fraction of the central disc, the pressure within the disc can be reduced, thereby allowing the protruding disc to fall away from the spinal nerve. A number of techniques have been developed to allow for percutaneous discectomy, including chemonucleolysis with chymopapain, laser discectomy, automated percutaneous lumbar discectomy (mechanical removal of a portion of the disc using a cutting and/or suction device), and nucleoplasty using a technique called *Coblation* to vaporize a portion of the disc. Chemonucleolysis using chymopapain has undergone extensive testing; a recent meta-analysis demonstrated that chemonucleolysis is superior to placebo for treating radicular pain associated with disc herniations; however, treatment outcomes were inferior to those who received microsurgical discectomy (180). A significant proportion of patients undergoing chemonucleolysis required repeat discectomy within

2 years, and the results of subsequent discectomy were inferior to those who received primary microsurgical discectomy. A number of other techniques for performing percutaneous discectomy are available. One such technique is called *nucleoplasty* and employs a technology called Coblation (Arthrocare Corporation, Austin, Texas) (181). Coblation uses radiofrequency energy to excite the electrolytes in tissue, creating a precisely focused plasma. The plasma's energized particles have sufficient energy to break the molecular bond within tissue, causing tissue to dissolve at relatively low temperatures (typically 40°C–70°C). The result is volumetric removal of target tissue with minimal damage to surrounding tissue. When Coblation is applied to remove tissue within the nucleus pulposus (nucleoplasty), intradiscal pressure is reduced in experimental animals (182). Although nucleoplasty is in widespread clinical use, validation of the efficacy of this approach to percutaneous discectomy is still emerging.

Complications associated with discography, IDET, and nucleoplasty have been described, but are uncommon. All of these techniques share the common element of introducing a cannula into the nucleus pulposus using a percutaneous approach (Fig. 50-17), and direct trauma to the spinal nerve can occur. Likewise, bleeding and infection can follow the introduction of the cannula. With any of these intradiscal techniques, discitis is an inherent risk—a delayed and insidious infection within the disc space that can be difficult to diagnose and treat. The thermal

wire used to perform IDET is subject to mechanical breakage, and the thermal energy delivered during both IDET and nucleoplasty can cause direct thermal injury to neural elements when incorrectly positioned.

Complications associated with lumbar discography range from exacerbation of pain to spondylodiscitis (Table 50-13). All complications associated with discography can also be expected with any of the other intradiscal treatments, as placement of a needle or cannula into the nucleus pulposus of an intervertebral disc is common to all of these procedures (Fig. 50-17). En route from the skin's surface to the intervertebral disc, the needle or cannula must pass inferior and medial to the spinal nerve, just inferior to where the nerve root traverses the intervertebral foramen. Although direct trauma to the spinal nerve typically produces only a transient paresthesia, persistent neuropathic pain can result. Bleeding within the subcutaneous tissues or paraspinous musculature can result in significant hematoma, which is typically self-limiting. Likewise, infection within the superficial and deep paraspinous tissues can occur as the result of needle placement for discography or cannula placement for intradiscal procedures.

Spondylodiscitis, infection within the disc space, is a well-recognized complication of diagnostic discography, with an overall incidence of less than 0.15% per patient and less than 0.08% per disc injected (183). Discitis appears to result from infection introduced by the needle tip (184). The most common

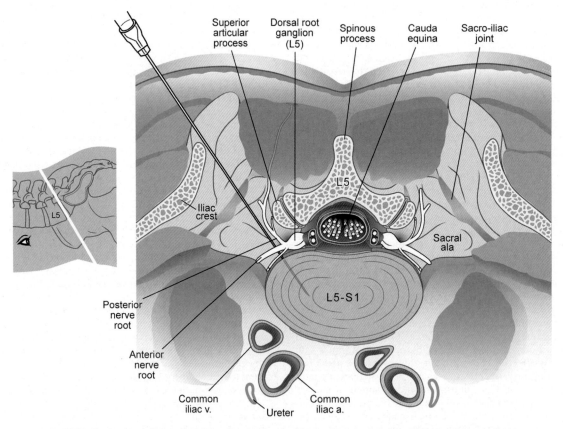

FIGURE 50-17. Axial diagram of L5–S1 discography. The needle enters the posterolateral aspect of the intervertebral disc, just inferomedial to the exiting L5 nerve root. The inset indicates the approximate plane of the L5–S1 disc and needle. All intradiscal treatments share the common element of introducing a hollow needle or introducer cannula percutaneously into the nucleus pulposus of the intervertebral disc. Reproduced from Rathmell JP. *Atlas of Image-guided Intervention in Regional Anesthesia and Pain Medicine.* Philadelphia: Lippincott Williams & Wilkins, 2006, with permission.

TABLE 50-13

COMPLICATIONS ASSOCIATED WITH INTRADISCAL PROCEDURES

Complications associated with intradiscal needle or cannula placement
  Hematoma
  Superficial abscess
  Deep abscess (paraspinous)
  Allergic reaction to radiographic contrast or antibiotic
  Direct needle trauma to a spinal nerve with transient or persistent paresthesia
  Spondylodiscitis
Complications associated with electrothermal treatment
  Thermal injury to a spinal nerve
  Epidural placement of IDET catheter resulting in thermal injury to the cauda equina
  Fracture of the IDET catheter resulting in retained intradiscal catheter fragment
  Vertebral osteonecrosis
  Disc herniation

TABLE 50-14

ANTIMICROBIAL DRUGS OF CHOICE FOR PROPHYLAXIS DURING DISCOGRAPHY AND OTHER INTRADISCAL TREATMENT TECHNIQUES

Drug	Dose	Comments
Cefazolin	1–2 g IV 30 minutes prior to discography OR cefazolin 1–10 mg/mL with intradiscal contrast	
Clindamycin	600 mg IV 30 minutes prior to discography OR clindamycin 7.5 mg/mL with intradiscal contrast	In patients with β-lactam allergy
Vancomycin	1 g IV over 60 minutes prior to discography	In patients who are documented carriers of methicillin-resistant *Staphylococcus aureus* (MRSA)

organisms identified are *Staphylococcus aureus* and *S. epidermidis* (184).

Discitis is an insidious infection that presents initially with worsening back pain. The clinical presentation and time course are highly variable. A detailed discussion of the diagnosis and management of discitis is beyond the scope of this manuscript, but is available in several recent review articles (185,186). Early in the course of discitis, few systemic symptoms are present, as the disc space is poorly vascularized, and systemic bacteremia is uncommon. In a series of 29 consecutive patients with spontaneous disc space infections, 10 patients (34%) had elevated serum leukocyte count and 21 patients (72%) had an elevated ESR (186). Diagnosis is dependent on maintaining a high index of suspicion and is confirmed by characteristic changes seen within the disc space on MRI (187). Practitioners should suspect discitis in patients who report worsening back pain during the weeks following discography, particularly a change in the pattern of long-standing back pain. Successful conservative treatment of discitis relies on early detection (186). Pain practitioners should establish written postprocedural guidelines for their patients that include a clear description of the signs and symptoms of evolving infection and a clear process for contacting pain clinic personnel to report the appearance of any worrisome signs or symptoms. Practitioners performing discography should be familiar with the principles of diagnostic evaluation and management of the patient with discitis.

Animal studies suggest that both IV and intradiscal administration of antibiotic prophylaxis can prevent the development of discitis even when bacteria are directly introduced into the disc (188,189). Because discitis can be classified as potentially catastrophic, the 1999 Centers for Disease Control (CDC) Guideline for Prevention of Surgical Site Infection supports the use of routine antimicrobial prophylaxis during discography and other intradiscal treatment techniques (190). Only limited animal data are available to guide the selection of antimicrobial agent and the route of administration for prophylaxis during discography and intradiscal treatments. Discography is commonly carried out with use of radiographic contrast material injected into the intervertebral disc; cefazolin and clindamycin both remain active in vitro when mixed with radiographic contrast (iohexol) (188). Extrapolation from animal

data (188,189) and the CDC recommendations (189) support the routine use of intradiscal or IV antibiotics prior to discography and other intradiscal techniques (Table 50-14); the advantage of one route of administration over another is not clear.

Intradiscal Electrothermal Therapy

Similar to any intradiscal technique, transient paresthesia, and exacerbation of back pain in the first several days following treatment are a common and expected part of IDET. Indeed, back pain may increase, requiring treatment with oral analgesics. This increase in pain level typically returns to the preoperative or better level of pain within several days to weeks following treatment.

Published cohort trials have indicated that the studied patients had experienced no IDET-related complications (191–196). Nonetheless, sporadic case reports have appeared of thermal injury to the cauda equina, disc herniation, and osteonecrosis of the vertebral endplates following IDET (Table 50-14).

Transient spinal nerve injury appears to be the most common complication associated with IDET. In most of these circumstances, the operator has reported nerve contact at the time of intradiscal needle placement with the affected nerve. Thermal injury to the nerve root may be possible, particularly if catheter placement is not entirely within the disc. To date, there are no reported cases of thermal nerve root injury that remained permanent in cases where the catheter was within the confines of the disc.

A recent analysis of the U.S. Food and Drug Administration (FDA) Medical Device Reports found 21 cases of IDET catheter breakage (197). Two were removed percutaneously and one was excised at time of disc excision. In the 18 cases in which a small piece of catheter remained in the disc, there were no reports of patient morbidity. It has been estimated

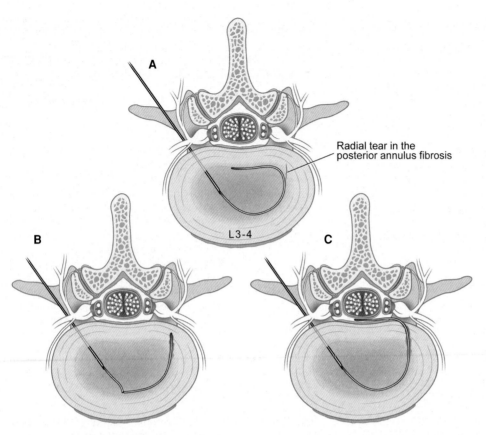

Radial tear in the posterior annulus fibrosis

L3-4

FIGURE 50-18. Mechanisms that lead to catheter breakage and thermal injury to the cauda equine during intradiscal electrothermal therapy (IDET). **A:** Catheter in good position for IDET treatment with the thermally active portion of the catheter (*shaded*) along the inner aspect of the posterior annulus fibrosis. **B:** Radial tears that extend from the nucleus pulposus into the annulus fibrosis are common in patients with degenerative disc disease. The IDET catheter often extends into one or more of these radial tears during placement. Repeated attempts to forcibly advance the IDET catheter can lead to kinking of the catheter and catheter breakage. **C:** Radial tears can extend from the nucleus pulposus all the way to the outer limit of the annulus fibrosis. The IDET catheter can advance through a radial tear in the annulus and out into the anterior epidural space, where the catheter will lie in close proximity to the cauda equina. IDET treatment with the catheter in this position can cause direct thermal injury to the cauda equina. Reproduced from Neal JM, Rathmell JP. *Complications in Regional Anesthesia and Pain Medicine.* Philadelphia: Saunders Elsevier, 2007, with permission.

that 35,000 catheters had been used during that time period. Currently, there appears to be no indication that surgical removal of a sheared catheter that is left in the disc is required. Long-term observation of these patients should be undertaken to determine the long-term consequences of this occurrence. Catheter breakage can be minimized or eliminated if the operator performs the procedure carefully, avoids catheter kinking, and does not make repeated attempts at forceful removal of a kinked catheter back through the introducer needle (Fig. 50-18).

The single case of cauda equina injury following IDET that was reported occurred in a patient who was oversedated and unresponsive. As the IDET catheter was advanced, the tip extended beyond the posterior margin of the annulus fibrosis and into the anterior epidural space, immediately adjacent to the thecal sac (Fig. 50-18). The catheter's location went unnoticed because the practitioners did not examine a lateral radiograph to determine the final position of the catheter. Treatment with a standard heating protocol commenced. Normally, as the temperature of the catheter is slowly raised, a patient who is awake would report progressively worsening discomfort in the back and extending to the lower extremities, signaling that excessive heat was reaching the nerves of the cauda equina within the thecal sac. The absolute temperature of the catheter and/or the rate at which the temperature was increased would normally be reduced in the face of such reports in the patient. However, this patient was heavily sedated and unable to report the discomfort that would have heralded dangerous excessive heating before irreparable injury ensued.

There is one published report of a disc herniation following IDET (198). This may represent weakening of the annular wall due to thermal modification of collagen. It appears to be an infrequent finding, but practitioners must be aware of it and inform their patients of this possibility. All of the post-IDET disc herniations reported here were successfully treated without residual symptoms. One required disc excision, and the remainder were treated with nonoperative care. Disc herniation following IDET could be due to accelerated natural history of that particular disc, secondary weakening of a disrupted annulus, or change in character of the nucleus following exposure to thermal energy. The significance of individual case reports of disc herniation must be placed in clinical perspective. Lumbar disc herniations are part of the natural history of lumbar degenerative disc disease. Large case series are needed to develop an accurate analysis of the frequency of disc herniation following IDET. Of incidental note was the occurrence of a disc herniation at a nontreated disc level in a patient in a recent randomized, controlled trial examining the efficacy of IDET (199).

One case of vertebral osteonecrosis was discussed in a published report (200). The authors of the report did not perform the IDET, discogram, or any of the spinal injections that the patient may have undergone prior to the IDET. It is unclear whether antibiotics were used for the IDET or discogram, or if the patient underwent any intradiscal injections prior to or after the IDET. The report did not present objective evidence of catheter positions during the procedure, nor was there detailed information regarding the heating protocol that was used. It has been hypothesized that placing the IDET catheter in close proximity to the vertebral endplate and conducting treatment using standard heating protocols may induce osteonecrosis.

Saal and Saal (197) carried out a survey of five centers that performed IDET. These centers were selected on the basis of their high case volumes and operator type. Each center represented a different specialty performing the IDETs. In one center, the procedures were performed by orthopedic spine surgeons, at one center by an anesthesiologist/pain physician, at two centers by an interventional radiologist, and at one center by physiatrists (physical medicine and rehabilitation). Each center was sent a detailed questionnaire asking them to list the total number of IDET cases performed during the survey period, and all the complications that followed IDET procedures. In addition, they were asked to detail the outcome and follow-up care required to resolve any complications. The survey documented 1,675 consecutive IDET cases performed at the five centers between July 1997 and February 2001. Six cases of transient spinal nerve injuries were reported; five cases were believed by the operator to be due to needle placement, and one was believed to be thermally mediated. All neurologic symptoms resolved, and no persisting lesions remained. One disc space infection was noted, which was treated with antibiotics. It occurred in an immunosuppressed patient who was undergoing chemotherapy for metastatic cancer. There were no cases of catheter breakage or cases of severe pain that required hospitalization. There were five cases of post-IDET disc herniation; three were noted at the IDET-treated disc level and two at adjacent levels. The composite complication rate was 10 of 1,675. It is interesting to note that these centers reflect a multidisciplinary spectrum of practitioners that perform IDET and includes spine surgeons, anesthesiologists, interventional radiologists, and physiatrists.

Cohen noted eight patients out of a cohort group of 79 that had increasing symptoms following IDET (201). One was a case of foot drop that completely resolved in 6 weeks, one was a case of burning sensation in the leg that resolved in 2 weeks, another was a case of leg paresthesias that resolved in 4 weeks, and there occurred one case of increased thigh pain that persisted after IDET and one case of increased back and thigh pain in a patient who demonstrated a new disc abnormality at an adjacent untreated level.

Disc space infection (discitis) has been reported with other intradiscal techniques, particularly diagnostic discography; however, there have been no reports of discitis associated with IDET.

It is clear that complications related to IDET do occur. Practitioners must be aware of these potential problems and appropriately inform patients who are considering IDET. The complication rates appear to be low, and most may be avoided with careful technique. Expertise in intradiscal needle placement is required, along with an accurate understanding of radiologic spinal anatomy and multiplanar fluoroscopic technique. IDET certainly has a risk profile that is far below that of fusion surgery (202).

The most severe complications associated with IDET stem from situations in which the catheter is placed outside the confines of the disc space. It is critical that the operator be certain of the intradiscal location of the catheter before heating is initiated. Clearly, the knowledge of three-dimensional fluoroscopic anatomy on the part of the treating physician is essential. This requires familiarity with accurate interpretation of anteroposterior, lateral, and oblique radiographs of the lumbar spine using fluoroscopy. Symptoms must be monitored by the operator to ensure that no undue lower extremity or perineal symptoms develop. These would warrant halting the procedure and reconfirming the location of the catheter. Excessive sedation during IDET can reduce or eliminate the ability of the patient to report dangerous symptoms during treatment, and must be avoided.

Theoretically, paravertebral soft tissue or disc space infection could occur following IDET despite close attention to aseptic technique. Most practitioners routinely administer in-

tradiscal and/or IV antibiotics during IDET. Guidelines for prophylactic antibiotic use during IDET are similar to those for discography (Table 50-15).

Nucleoplasty

Nucleoplasty is the term given to a novel approach to percutaneous discectomy that uses a patented technology called Coblation to remove a portion of the nucleus pulposus and thereby reduce intradiscal pressure for the treatment of radicular pain due to contained disc herniations. Similar to other percutaneous discectomy techniques, the treatment probe is placed into the nucleus pulposus of an intervertebral disc through an introducer cannula. The probe is then advanced while energy is applied, and the active tip of the treatment probe creates a series of small channels within the nucleus pulposus. This treatment effectively reduces intradiscal pressure in experimental models (182). Like other approaches to percutaneous discectomy, the concept is to reduce intradiscal pressure, thereby allowing a bulging disc or contained disc herniation to fall away from the spinal nerve, thus relieving radicular pain. This technique is simple, and few adverse events are reported in the literature despite widespread application of the new technology, suggesting that the technique is safe. However, to date, few clinical trials are available to confirm the safety or demonstrate the effectiveness of nucleoplasty.

Similar to other intradiscal techniques, the primary complications associated with nucleoplasty are associated with the placement of the intradiscal introducer cannula (Table 50-16); this group of complications has been discussed earlier, in the section on discography. Although the introducer cannula used for nucleoplasty is larger in diameter than the typical 22-gauge spinal needle used to perform discography, no evidence suggests that a higher complication rate is associated with the use of this large-bore introducer. Nonetheless, it stands to reason that use of a larger needle may well lead to greater neural injury in the event of contact with a neural structure.

Early cohort studies reported favorable outcomes following nucleoplasty without any reported complications (203,204). Bhagia et al. (205) recently detailed the side effects and complications associated with nucleoplasty. In a series of 53 patients, the most common side effects at 24 hours after treatment were soreness at the needle insertion site (76%), new numbness and tingling (26%), increased intensity of preprocedure back pain (15%), and new areas of back pain (15%). At 2 weeks after nucleoplasty, no patient had soreness at the needle insertion site or new areas of back pain; however, new numbness and tingling was present in 15% of patients. Two patients (4%) had increased intensity of preprocedure back pain and opted for surgical discectomy.

A number of theoretical risks that have not been reported during clinical use are possible. The technology results in marked temperature elevation and tissue destruction that is limited to the area immediately adjacent to the treatment tip of the probe (206). If the treatment tip is withdrawn too far, and the active tip is pulled back into the metal introducer, this can theoretically cause heating of the entire length of the introducer cannula. In this way, it is possible to produce thermal injury to any structure along the course of cannula. Excessive extension of the treatment probe can lead to penetration of the anterior annulus fibrosis and extension into the retroperitoneal space, with potential damage to vascular structures in this area.

Prevention of complications associated with placement of the intradiscal cannula during nucleoplasty is similar to prevention during any other intradiscal technique and has been

TABLE 50-15

RECOMMENDED ANTIBIOTIC PROPHYLAXIS PRIOR TO IMPLANTATION OF AN INTRATHECAL DRUG DELIVERY SYSTEM OR SPINAL CORD STIMULATION SYSTEM. (ADAPTED FROM REFERENCE)

Antibiotic	Dose and administration
Cefazolin	1–2 g IV 30 minutes prior to incision
Clindamycin (β-lactam allergic patients)	600 mg IV 30 minutes prior to incision
Vancomycin (methicillin-resistant *Staphylococcus aureus* [MRSA] carriers)	1 g IV over 60 minutes prior to incision

Adapted from The Centers for Disease Control and Prevention Guideline for Prevention of Surgical Site Infection. *Infect Control Hosp Epidemiol* 1999;20:217–278, with permission.

described in the prior section on discography. Prevention of complications associated with the Coblation treatment used to perform nucleoplasty relies on the disciplined use of radiographic guidance during insertion of the intradiscal cannula to assure that the extent of treatment is contained within the limits of the nucleus pulposus. Thus, the extent of anterior advancement, as well as retraction, of the treatment probe during treatment must be guided radiographically in the lateral view. Like IDET, excess sedation during the active treatment removes

a potential early warning from the patient that thermal injury to neural structures is occurring.

COMPLICATIONS ASSOCIATED WITH INTRATHECAL DRUG DELIVERY

Surgically implantable intrathecal drug delivery systems with subcutaneous drug reservoirs and programmable pump mechanisms are now widely available for the treatment of chronic and cancer-related pain that is unresponsive to more conservative treatments (see Chapter 40). The use of intrathecal drug delivery pumps is associated with complications that can be classified as surgical, device-related, or drug-related. Initially, pumps were used primarily for cancer patients and those with spasticity. Over the past 15 years, use of these devices has grown to include more patients with pain of noncancer origin. Long-term intrathecal drug delivery has been associated with a number of complications related to drug infusion via an intrathecal catheter (ITC) or pump failure.

The reported incidence of adverse events ranges from 3% to 24%, most of which are minor and related to the infused drug (206). Recently, it has been found that long-term intrathecal drug delivery can lead to formation of an inflammatory mass at the tip of the catheter, within the thecal, posing significant risk of neurologic injury (207). Most device-related complications occur at the time of implantation, and many of these surgical complications can be avoided with careful surgical technique and recent improvements in technology. Drug-related

TABLE 50-16

COMPLICATIONS ASSOCIATED WITH SPINAL CORD STIMULATION, THEIR DIAGNOSIS, AND TREATMENT

Complication	Diagnosis	Treatment
Complication involving the neuraxis		
Nerve injury	CT or MRI, EMG/NCS/physical examination	Anticonvulsants, neurosurgery consult
Epidural fibrosis	Increased stimulation amplitude	Lead reprogramming, lead revision
Epidural hematoma	Physical examination, CT, or MRI	Surgical evacuation
Epidural abscess	Physical examination, CT or MRI, CBC, blood work	Surgical evacuation, IV antibiotics, infectious disease consult
Postdural puncture headache	Positional headache, blurred vision, nausea	IV fluids, rest, blood patch
Complications outside of the neuraxis		
Seroma	Serosanguineous fluid in pocket	Aspiration; if no response, surgical drainage
Hematoma	Blood in pocket	Pressure dressing and aspiration, surgical revision
Pain at generator	Pain on palpation	Topical local anesthetic, local injection, revision
Wound infection	Fever, rubor, drainage	Antibiotics, incision and drainage, removal
Device-related complications		
Unacceptable programming	Lack of stimulation in area of pain	Reprogramming of device, revision of leads
Lead migration	Inability to program, x-rays	Reprogramming, surgical revision
Current leak	High electrode impedance, pain at site of current leak	Revision of connectors, generator, or leads
Generator failure	Inability to read device	Replacement of generator

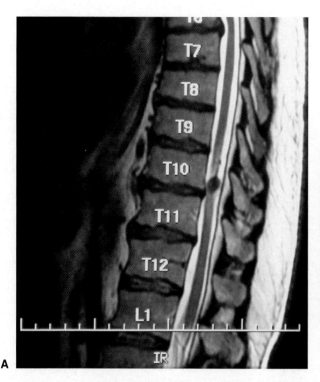

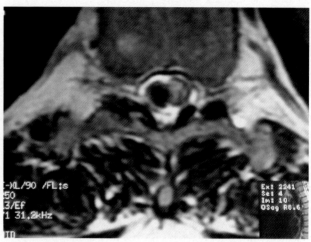

FIGURE 50-19. Magnetic resonance imaging study of a patient with an inflammatory mass surrounding the tip of an implanted intrathecal drug delivery catheter. **A:** Midline, sagittal, T2-weighted image. The inflammatory mass involves the dorsal aspect of the spinal cord at the level of the inferior end plate of T10. **B:** Axial, T2-weighted image through the inflammatory mass. The mass displaces the spinal cord toward the left. Reproduced from Neal JM, Rathmell JP. *Complications in Regional Anesthesia and Pain Medicine*. Philadelphia: Saunders Elsevier, 2007, with permission.

complications are common and typically evolve over several months following implantation (209).

Complications Involving the Neuraxis

During initial implantation of an ITC, direct trauma to the spinal cord, spinal nerve roots, or spinal nerves can result from needle or catheter placement. Traumatic syrinx (210) and direct intraparenchymal placement of the ITC (211) have been described. Other complications that may occur at or soon after the initial surgical period include CSF leak, hygroma formation, and chronic PDPH. Neuraxial infectious complications are uncommon and include meningitis and direct infection of the spinal cord near the catheter tip, resulting in transverse myelitis (212).

The occurrence of inflammatory masses surrounding the tip of ITCs during long-term intrathecal infusion of morphine was first reported in 1999 and, in more recent years, the number of reports and agents associated with inflammatory masses has grown. The inflammatory mass appears to be a chronic, fibrotic, noninfectious mass that develops at the tip of the ITC over the course of months or years. As the inflammatory mass grows larger, patients often present with neurologic signs and symptoms that reflect direct compression of the spinal cord or other neural elements by the expanding mass (208). These inflammatory masses are characterized by dense collections of lymphocytes, monocytes, macrophages, and plasma cells that formed well-defined masses in the intrathecal space. The cellular constitution of the mass typically reflects a chronic or

chronic–active inflammation (213). The cause of this chronic inflammation is uncertain. Reported cases have been linked to high concentrations of morphine or hydromorphone at the catheter tip (214). A consensus statement by a panel of experts recommended that the concentration of morphine be limited to 30 mg/mL and that the concentration of hydromorphone be limited to 20 mg/mL (215) (see Chapter 40).

The typical clinical course of a patient with an inflammatory mass begins with loss of pain relief followed by the appearance of variable, but progressive sensory and motor deficits. Signs and symptoms include loss of proprioception, pain in the dermatomal distribution of the catheter tip, change in sensation or strength, and eventually bladder and bowel symptoms (urinary retention followed by loss of urinary and anal sphincter control). Left untreated, progressive expansion of the inflammatory mass can lead to complete paraplegia. Diagnosis is reliant on maintaining a high index of suspicion in patients receiving intrathecal drug therapy. Diagnosis is confirmed using MRI with and without gadolinium contrast enhancement (Fig. 50-19). If the patient cannot undergo an MRI, diagnosis can also be established using CT combined with myelography to delineate the intrathecal mass (216). The FDA issued a Medwatch Safety Alert in March 2008 with updated information regarding granuloma formation at or near the distal tip of ITCs. In this communication, the FDA cited an overall incidence of 0.49% for granuloma formation in all patients ever implanted (217). The following specific recommendations were offered to clinicians: (a) the lowest effective dose and concentration of intrathecal opioid should be used, (b) patients should be closely monitored for the prodromal signs of a developing inflammatory mass, and (c) in patients with new neurologic symptoms, prompt imaging and neurosurgical consultation should be considered.

Direct trauma to the cord or nerve roots can result in paralysis, pain, and traumatic radiculitis. Treatment is initiated as soon as the diagnosis is confirmed by MRI or CT. Immediate neurosurgical consultation and initiation of high-dose IV steroids should be considered. If the injury involves a catheter, removal of the catheter should be urgently performed. CSF leak is treated conservatively by fluid intake, bed rest, and caffeine. If that should fail, some would consider an epidural blood patch. If the clinician chooses to perform a blood patch, care must be taken to avoid impaling the catheter with the needle.

In the event of neuraxial infection, rapid intervention is required. Meningitis is seen in less than 0.1% of all cases of infection associated with implanted intrathecal drug delivery devices (218), and it is treated in a manner consistent with other patients with meningitis. There is no consensus in the literature on the need to remove the device in the setting of meningitis. Epidural abscess is a much more serious event in most situations, and can result in paralysis if rapid action is delayed. This problem is identified by pain in the back outside of the intensity and character of typical postoperative pain, accompanied by fever and malaise. Diagnosis is confirmed by MRI or CT, and treatment is often surgical, requiring drainage and removal of the catheter. Since the catheter is intrathecal, the incidence of epidural abscess is extremely low. Transverse myelitis is a rare complication. Treatment consists of a high-dose IV steroid administration and consultation with an infectious disease specialist to rule out and treat any identifiable viral or bacterial causes of this disorder (212).

Inflammatory mass varies in its presentation. Deer showed in a series of consecutive patients examined by MRI that patients can have these lesions but show no symptoms (216). Coffey and Burchiel presented a series of patients with much more serious outcomes, including paraplegia (208). In asymptomatic patients, treatment may consist of repeat MRI and observation, a change of drug, or removal of the ITC. Animal studies have shown that persistent exposure to the inciting drug leads to advancement of the lesion. The infusion of saline may lead to lesion regression, but results in cessation of the therapy. As a result, many clinicians opt for removing the catheter. If a catheter revision is carried out, the patient should be kept responsive. The incision is made and the catheter is exposed. Once the catheter is located, it should be gently removed. If resistance develops or unexpected pain occurs, the catheter should be left in place. Options at this point include occluding the catheter at the level of the ligamentum flavum with suture or surgical clips and leaving it in place, or surgical resection to remove the inflammatory mass. In cases in which no obvious neurologic compromise is present, surgical resection is not usually warranted. Once the catheter has been corrected, the offending agent should be avoided in the future and alternative drugs should be used (219).

Complications Involving Nonspinal Tissues

Infection involving the implanted pump or catheter can result in the need to remove the device. The incidence of wound infection ranges from 0% to 4.5%, although higher rates of infection have been reported (218). In those with superficial infections involving the subcutaneous pocket in the abdominal wall, the diagnosis of infection can be confused with that of noninfectious fluid accumulation (seroma). Both can involve redness and edema of the pocket. The presence of a fever, el-

evated white blood count, elevated C-reactive protein, or elevated ESR raises the level of suspicion of an infectious process. Gram stain and culture of fluid aspirated from the pump pocket are helpful in verifying the presence of infection and identifying the causative organism. The noninfectious build-up of serosanguineous fluid in the pocket surrounding an implanted pump (seroma formation) can impede wound healing and cause pain and wound breakdown. Seroma is usually diagnosed by the appearance of a painful, erythematous, fluctuant mass surrounding the implanted device, accompanied by normal laboratory values and lack of fever. Diagnosis is confirmed by aspirate that does not show bacteria on microscopic analysis or subsequent culture.

Bleeding within the pocket can lead to hematoma, wound dehiscence, and the need to re-explore the pump pocket. Diagnosis is typically straightforward, and heralded by postoperative pain and swelling at the pocket site. Breakdown of the skin overlying the implanted device can occur over the long term. This often occurs in patients who experience a significant weight loss.

Because implanted devices used for chronic pain therapy extend to the neuraxis, and infection can prove catastrophic, routine antimicrobial prophylaxis is warranted in all patients (Table 50-15). The CDC published an extensive Guideline for Prevention of Surgical Site Infection (219) in 1999 that discuss all aspects of prevention. Rathmell has reviewed infectious complications associated with chronic pain therapies (220). When infection occurs, treatment options vary with the severity of tissue involvement. In superficial infections, treatment options include oral antibiotics and observation or open incision and drainage. Once infection has spread to the deeper tissues, the pump and catheter must be removed and antibiotics administered by either an oral or IV route. Consultation from an infectious disease specialist can be helpful in determining the optimal antibiotic regimen and guiding the duration of treatment. Culture results are used to guide therapy. If the device is removed and replaced in the future, an infectious disease specialist can be helpful in identifying preoperative precautions to reduce the risk of recurrent infection. In removing an implanted device because of tissue infection, wound dehiscence, or seroma, the clinician must be extremely vigilant to avoid overdose or withdrawal symptoms of opioid, clonidine, or baclofen (209).

To minimize the risk of seroma formation, trauma to tissues should be minimized and close attention paid to achieving hemostasis before wound closure. Once a seroma occurs, treatment involves sterile aspiration and analysis of the fluid to rule out infection. If aspiration is performed repeatedly without resolution of the seroma, surgical incision and drainage is warranted. A drain may be used postoperatively to avoid reaccumulation of fluid, but is controversial because of the perceived increased risk of infection. Recurrent seroma may lead to the need to move the pump pocket to a new location. Postoperative bleeding is treated with a pressure dressing and observation. If the hematoma is rapidly expanding, immediate surgical re-exploration is needed; treatment is evacuation of the hematoma, irrigation of the wound, identification of the bleeding source, and hemostasis. The considerations regarding management of anticoagulant agents prior to surgery are similar to those for neuraxial blockade (see Chapter 12). The risk of discontinuing antiplatelet agents prior to surgery should be discussed with each patient's primary care physician, so that an appropriate analysis of the risk of recurrent thromboembolic event can be weighed against the risk of perioperative bleeding.

Long-term skin breakdown can occur and lead to cellulitis and exposure of the device, mandating removal. If pain develops around the pump, a careful examination should be performed to rule out the need for surgical revision, before skin breakdown occurs.

Complications Involving the Implanted Intrathecal Catheter

The ITC is the most common cause of complications related to the implanted device itself. In a prospective observational study, Follet and Naumann reported a complication rate of 4.5% due to the ITC over the first 9 months of therapy (221). Complications include migration, kinking, or dislodgement of the catheter. Migration of the ITC most often leads to movement into the epidural space or completely out of the spinal canal. Catheter migration can also occur into the intervertebral foramen toward a spinal nerve, causing radicular pain or sciatica (222). Migration into the substance of the spinal cord itself has also been reported; this can occur without pain and can go undiagnosed until significant neurologic injury develops (223). Placement of the catheter into the spinal cord at the time of implantation has also been reported (224). To minimize the risk of direct trauma to the spinal cord, some authors advise that ITCs should be placed with a level of sedation that allows for verbal communication with the patient throughout catheter placement (210). Migration of the catheter into the subdural space has also been described (225). Subdural migration leads to decreased efficacy, because the drug no longer mixes freely with the CSF. It has been hypothesized that subdural catheter migration can also create a loculated region containing high concentrations of the infused drug between the dura mater and the arachnoid mater; this pocket is contained only by the fragile arachnoid membrane, and sudden rupture and release of the loculated drug into the intrathecal space could cause a sudden overdose.

Progressive myelopathy, presumably caused by direct trauma as the catheter tip repeatedly contacts the spinal cord, has been described even in the absence of an inflammatory mass. The presentation in one case mimicked transverse myelitis, and it remains uncertain if this complication was directly related to the catheter or to the infused drug (210).

Catheters can become blocked by fibrosis, resulting in difficulty aspirating or injecting through the catheter. The extent of fibrosis ranges from a minor problem to the dangerous inflammatory masses described earlier. Catheter kinking, leak, or fracture is identified by injecting radiographic contrast through the side port of the infusion pump under fluoroscopy. In the event that the plain film does not show leakage of contrast, and no fluid can be aspirated from the side port of the infusion pump, some experts recommend surgical exploration and revision of the entire catheter. Catheter fracture leads to a disconnection between the distal and proximal ends of the catheter. In some cases, the distal end may be floating in the CSF.

Catheter malfunction is the most common problem seen with implanted pumps. This problem can lead to symptoms of opioid or other drug withdrawal, increased pain, and the need for surgical correction. Diagnosis of the catheter malfunction is often made by x-ray screening, side port contrast study (as described earlier), or MRI. Treatment involves correction of the identified problem. If the catheter has migrated out of the subarachnoid space, the entire catheter may need to be replaced. An alternative is to replace the intrathecal portion and then to use a splice to connect it to the catheter remnant leading to the pump. Catheter migration into the cord is extremely rare and requires consultation with a neurosurgeon and removal of the system.

Catheter kinking or fracture can necessitate replacing the entire catheter. If the kink is at the level of the anchor or near the midline incision, a splice kit can be used, so that only the posterior wound needs to be explored. If the catheter fractures at a more proximal location, the entire catheter should be replaced.

Development of a fibrous tissue tube around the catheter can lead to decreased drug effect, and is apparent when painful injection occurs during a side port study. This complication can be treated by either withdrawing the catheter to the desired level or revising the distal portion of the catheter. Some experts suggest a revision of the intrathecal portion of the catheter and insertion at a different vertebral level in this situation.

In the event of catheter fracture within the subarachnoid space, a new catheter is required. There is no consensus regarding the need to remove the retained catheter fragment; removal requires laminectomy and durotomy. Experience with fractured ventriculo-peritoneal shunts offers good evidence that the presence of a retained catheter in the intrathecal space presents little risk over time, and that the risk of surgical exploration and removal may well be greater than leaving the catheter fragment in place.

Complications Involving the Implanted Drug Delivery Pump

In patients with implanted pumps, a refill is required at intervals ranging from 14 to 120 days. During each refill, the pump reservoir must be accessed percutaneously, and there is a risk of error during the refill procedure, as well as a risk of infection, as the device is accessed percutaneously for each refill. Errors that can occur during periodic refill of the pump drug reservoir include: pharmacy errors leading to over- or underdosing; injection of part or all of refill volume into subcutaneous tissue with subsequent systemic absorption, causing overdose (226); and contamination of refill solution with toxic (e.g., alcohol prep solution), infective, or particulate material. The risk of infection is minimized by use of appropriate sterile technique and employing an in-line bacterial filter. Despite the need to frequently perform this procedure, the infection rates appear to be low and should occur in less than 1% of all refills (227).

Currently available programmable pumps are driven by a rotor coupled to a motor with gears. Mechanical failure, including jamming of the gears or rotor failure can occur and results in sudden cessation of the intrathecal drug infusion. Examination of the pump under fluoroscopy at timed intervals will reveal that there is no movement of the pump's rotor. Sudden pump failure may result in signs of opioid withdrawal. The side port of the pump allows for injection and aspiration (Fig. 50-20). This side port communicates with tubing within the pump that carries drug from the reservoir to the ITC (see Chapter 40). A leak in either the side port tubing or the access port can lead to pump failure. The access port to the pump is accessed by a noncoring needle. Despite the specialized needle, the access port can be damaged over time, and drug may leak from the reservoir into the surrounding tissue; if such leakage occurs at the time of pump refill, systemic absorption of a large amount of drug could result in opioid or nonopioid overdose, a potentially dangerous complication. Finally, drug overdose and device infection have been reported after attempts to access the port and remove the drug by unauthorized persons. In one case, the patient was trying to gain access to and sell the drug in the pump, and IV injection of the drug resulted in overdose (228).

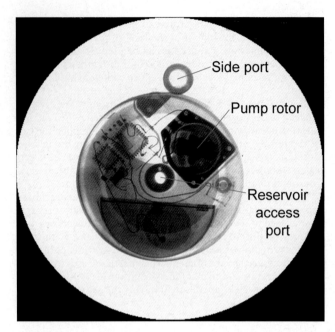

FIGURE 50-20. Plain radiograph of the Medtronic SynchroMed programmable intrathecal drug delivery pump. Used with permission from the manufacturer. The pump shown is the most common pump in use worldwide in 2008, the SynchroMed pump manufactured by Medtronic Neurological, Minneapolis, MN.

The most common reason to revise or remove a pump is the battery reaching end of life. Battery exhaustion is expected, and available devices will need replacement every 5.5 years, on average. Significant overdosing can occur at the time of pump replacement, and vigilance must be maintained to correctly identify the drug dose, catheter length, and bridge bolus. This can usually be accomplished in the outpatient setting with a minimal risk, but when uncertainties about the bridge dosing arise during pump replacement, the patient should be admitted for careful observation until the entire bridge bolus has been completed and significant time from the new baseline infusion has elapsed.

The pump can turn over within the pocket after implantation, so that the access port is facing toward the abdominal wall. If technically feasible, the problem can be avoided by securing the pump in position by inserting sutures at the pump securing points. Pump turn-over can occur due to change in body habitus that leads to laxity in the tissue of the abdominal wall; the pump can also turn over if the patient repeatedly attempts to move it within the pocket. In these instances, the pump may be repositioned and an abdominal binder can be used to hold it in position. Eventually, a surgical correction may be required. This process involves removing some of the surrounding adipose tissue to anchor the pump to the fascia. In the morbidly obese, this may be impossible since it may lead to the pump being so far from the surface that it can no longer communicate with the telemetry device used in programming. In these cases, a Dacron pouch may be used to anchor to the surrounding tissue in the hope that development of fibrosis will help to avoid further movement of the pump.

Mechanical failure, including a stalled rotor or jammed gear in a programmable pump, requires replacement of the entire device. Pump replacement is also required if the side port develops a leak or if the access port develops a loss of integrity.

Complications Involving Specific Intrathecal Agents

The reported frequency of complications associated with long-term infusion of opioids is shown in Table 50-17. Penn and Paice demonstrated in a multicenter review that complications can be common and can affect several body systems (229). Winkelmuller and Winkelmuller showed a similarly high rate of adverse effects with intrathecal opioids (230).

Peripheral edema of the lower extremities has been reported with opioids, most commonly morphine. The incidence of this complication appears to vary from 1% to 20%, depending on the vascular status of patients prior to implantation. The mechanism appears to be related to a direct effect on the hypothalamic-pituitary-adrenal axis by intrathecal opioids (231). The appearance of inflammatory catheter-tip masses has been described in detail earlier.

Several other drugs are commonly delivered as chronic intrathecal infusions. Clonidine is an α_2-receptor agonist and can cause hypotension and somnolence. Clonidine is also associated with severe rebound hypertension upon sudden withdrawal or reduction (232). Ziconotide (SNX-111) is a synthetic analogue of an N-type voltage-dependent calcium channel blocker that was first isolated from the marine snail, *Conus magnus*. Ziconotide was approved for intrathecal use by the FDA in late 2004, and has shown some promise in treating refractory pain associated with cancer and acquired immunodeficiency syndrome (AIDS) (233). However, the high frequency of side effects (Table 50-18) mandates slow dose escalation over a prolonged time period and has led to limited use of this new agent.

In the event that a sudden change in analgesia, increased somnolence, or other effects appear soon after the reservoir has been refilled, a drug error should by suspected. In these circumstances, the drug must be sent for analysis. Possible causes include giving the wrong patient the intended drug, mislabeling by the pharmacist, or improper calculation when preparing or ordering the drug. The first sign of the placement of an inaccurate drug may be patient distress or respiratory depression. Because of this troubling diagnostic dilemma, it is critical to

TABLE 50-17

COMPLICATIONS REPORTED WITH LONG-TERM INTRATHECAL INFUSION OF OPIOIDS

Complication	Reported frequency
Constipation	50%
Difficulty urinating	42.7%
Nausea and vomiting	24.4%–36.6%
Impotence	26.8%
Nightmares	23.2%
Pruritus	13.3%–14.6%
Edema	6.1%–11.7%
Diaphoresis	7.2%–8.5%
Weakness	7.2%
Weight gain	5.4%
Diminished libido	4.9%

Data derived from Burton AW, Conroy B, Garcia E, et al. Illicit substance abuse via an implanted intrathecal pump. *Anesthesiology* 2005;89:1264–1267; and Paice JA, Penn RD, Shott S. Intraspinal morphine for chronic pain: A retrospective, multicenter study. *J Pain Symptom Manage* 1996;11:71–80, with permission.

TABLE 50-18

COMPLICATIONS REPORTED WITH SHORT-TERM INTRATHECAL INFUSION OF ZICONOTIDE (SNX-111).

	No. of patients (%)	
Complication	Ziconotide ($n = 72$)	Placebo ($n = 40$)
Patients with any adverse event	70 (97.2)	29 (72.5)
Patients with any serious adverse event	22 (30.6)	4 (10.0)
Cardiovascular system	24 (33.3)	4 (10.0)
Postural hypotension	17 (23.6)	2 (5.0)
Hypotension	6 (8.3)	2 (5.0)
Nervous system	60 (83.3)	14 (35.0)
Dizziness	36 (50.0)	4 (10.0)
Nystagmus	33 (45.8)	4 (10.0)
Somnolence	17 (23.6)	3 (7.5)
Confusion	15 (20.8)	2 (5.0)
Abnormal gait	9 (12.5)	0
Urogenital system	23 (31.9)	0
Urinary retention	13 (18.1)	0
Urinary tract infection	7 (9.7)	0

Adapted from Rauck RL, Wallace MS, Leong MS, et al., Ziconotide 301 Study Group. A randomized, double-blind, placebo-controlled study of intrathecal ziconotide in adults with severe chronic pain. *J Pain Symptom Manage* 2006;31:393–406, with permission.

double-check each refill solution at the pharmacy and in the pain center to assure accuracy. Additional testing is needed to determine accuracy of concentration, stability, and lack of bacterial contamination.

Complications from opioids, such as nausea and vomiting, pruritus, dysuria, constipation, edema, diaphoresis, weakness, weight gain, and diminished libido generally dissipate over time with no specific treatment. Of these problems, edema can be persistent and troubling. Treatment consists of conservative measures including diuretics and support stockings. Maximizing control of preexisting edema prior to implant may also help in reducing the subsequent incidence of this problem in such patients. If these options are not successful, then a change of drug is required. Constipation can be problematic, although it is less common than with other routes of opioid administration. Similar to those receiving long-term oral opioid analgesics, options are to place the patient on a good bowel regimen to increase activity and increase fiber in the diet.

Some drugs have complications specific to their receptor-mediated actions. Clonidine is active at the α_2-receptors. To prevent somnolence or hypotension, the dose of this drug should be increased with caution. Side effects are more likely to occur if the catheter tip is in the high thoracic or cervical region. Bupivacaine has also been shown to cause specific problems with loss of sensation. This can be avoided by starting at a low dose of 1 to 2 mg/day and increasing the dose with caution. At higher doses (20–30 mg/day), motor deficits and bladder/bowel incontinence may occur.

Ziconotide has specific problems related to its infusion (Table 50-18). These problems include dizziness, confusion, hallucination, somnolence, and nausea. Recent work in follow-up studies (233) shows that a slow titration can reduce the incidence of these problems and improve the ability of patients to tolerate the drug.

Potential complications of drug mislabeling or the presence of contaminates must be under surveillance at the pharmacy level. The physician should have discussions with the pharmacy that is employed to provide the pump drugs and confirm that they are using international standards to make compounds and create admixtures. The pharmacist should also be well versed in the concentrations of drugs that are safe to administer in the device.

Arachnoiditis

Spinal injection of incorrect solutions may result in inflammation and subsequent fibrosis of the meninges (arachnoiditis). Arachnoiditis results in adhesion of the spinal nerve roots to the arachnoid membranes (Fig. 50-20) and progressive fibrosis resulting in areas of spinal nerve root demyelination, leading to severe neuropathic pain and possible neurologic deficit. It is unlikely that approved spinal formulations of local anesthetics, opioids, and other drugs cause arachnoiditis. However, a high degree of care and vigilance is required to ensure the use of only approved drugs and to prevent the contamination of "spinal drug solutions" with alcoholic preparation solutions or similar materials.

COMPLICATIONS ASSOCIATED WITH SPINAL CORD STIMULATION

Spinal cord stimulation (SCS) refers to the use of an epidural electrode connected with an energy source called an *implantable pulse generator* (IPG) that directly stimulates the dorsal columns of the spinal cord and offers significant long-term pain reduction for a number of painful conditions. The history, rationale, indications, contraindications, and outcomes of SCS are discussed in Chapter 41. Complications associated with SCS are those relating to the neuraxis, those that arise in other tissues outside the neuraxis, and those relating to the device itself (Table 15-16). To successfully manage complications, the physician must understand the surgical approach to SCS and corrective measures for each problem that may arise during the use of these systems.

The incidence of complications associated with spinal cord stimulator placement has been reported as ranging from 0% to 81%, depending on the study and the specific adverse event. A recent systematic review showed that, in evidence-based studies, the mean complication rate was 34%. Surgical revision was necessary to correct the problem in 23% of patients. Life-threatening or serious complications occurred less than 1% of the time (235). In another long-term analysis of 102 patients with implanted SCS devices, the surgical revision rate was 32% over 10 years of follow-up (236). Burchiel et al. reported a 17% revision rate in a group of patients implanted for 1 year or more (237). Kumar found lead complication rates of 5.3%, epidural fibrosis rates of 19%, and infection rates of 2.7% (238). It is important to recognize that SCS technology and techniques have improved markedly and thus results of earlier studies may not equate with current practice.

Complications Involving the Neuraxis

Complications involving the spinal canal and its contents are most likely to occur during the initial placement of the SCS

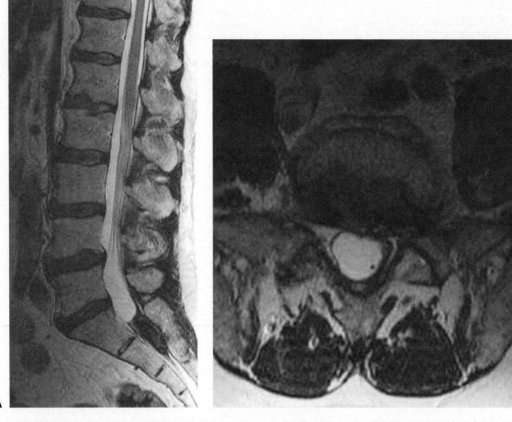

A   **B**

FIGURE 50-21. Arachnoiditis. **A:** Lumber magnetic resonance image scan, midline sagittal T₂-weighted. Cauda equina is clearly visible down to L₄-L₅ level, but it is completely "cut off" at this level. **B:** Axial view at L₅ level. Thecal sac appears empty because the roots of the cauda equina are adherent to the meninges at the periphery of the dural sac. One nerve root can be seen peripherally at about the 3:30 on the clock face position. Images courtesy of Dr. David Brazier.

lead in the dorsal epidural space. These complications are largely similar to those that can follow placement of an epidural catheter to provide continuous epidural analgesia and include hematoma and abscess formation, injury to the spinal cord or spinal nerves, and PDPH.

Epidural Hematoma and Abscess

Among the most feared complications of SCS is the development of an epidural hematoma, which can lead to paralysis if not treated urgently (239). No epidural hematomas appear in published series, thus the incidence of this complication is low, although an exact estimate of the incidence cannot be derived from the existing SCS literature. Because SCS involves placing a large introducer needle into the epidural space and threading an electrode many levels cephalad within the spinal canal, it seems likely that the incidence of epidural hematoma formation would be somewhat higher than that during single-shot or continuous epidural analgesia (see Chapter 12). The patient may complain of numbness accompanied by severe and often increasing back or leg pain developing in the immediate postoperative period. Weakness in the postoperative period should immediately raise suspicion of an epidural hematoma. Use of anticoagulants or drugs affecting platelet adherence may increase the risk (see Chapter 12). Some authors have postulated other risks specific to SCS that might increase the risk of epidural hematoma formation, including difficult lead placement with

multiple lead passes, the need to place a surgical lead requiring laminectomy, and reoperation in a previously implanted area. This complication is more commonly seen with surgical instrumentation requiring extensive bony insult (235). Diagnosis of an epidural hematoma in this setting requires CT. To date, because of concerns regarding inductive heating of the epidural electrode during MRI, MRI imaging has not been approved by the FDA for use in patients with spinal cord stimulator leads in place.

Infections of the spinal structures can also be potentially life-threatening complications. Possible infections include epidural abscess, discitis, and meningitis. The incidence of these critical events is small, and no data exist for SCS on the exact incidence, but most authors have speculated that the incidence is <0.1% (240). Epidural abscess is the most common of these complications, and considerations are similar to those discussed for epidural analgesia (see Chapters 11 and 40). Diagnosis of an epidural abscess (Fig. 50-21) is best accomplished using CT. Diagnosis of meningitis is best made through CSF analysis (241).

Treatment of epidural hematoma usually involves urgent surgical evacuation. In some instances, when the hematoma is small, careful observation alone is warranted. When epidural abscess is diagnosed, treatment involves surgical decompression, infectious disease consultation, and proper antibiotic coverage. Minor injury to nerves or the spinal cord is sometimes difficult to differentiate from nerve root irritation. Prolonged or difficult lead placement or significant patient report of pain

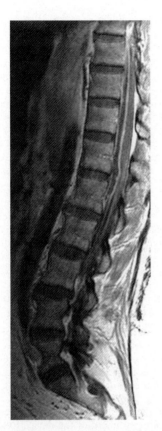

FIGURE 50-22. Epidural abscess. Lumbar magnetic resonance image scan, midline saggital T$_2$-weighted. An extensive mass is present in the anterior epidural space from L$_1$–T$_{10}$. Following epidural infusion, the patient presented with new severe upper lumbar pain and fever. Subsequently lower limb weakness developed bilateral. Image courtesy of Dr. David Brazier.

during lead placement should signal the possibility of neurologic injury. In the absence of hematoma or abscess, usually little can be done surgically to correct the problem (239,240), apart from ongoing review by a neurologist and appropriate arrangements for neurologic rehabilitation.

Nerve Injury

Injury to the spinal cord or nerve roots are potential risks of SCS. Direct trauma to neural structures caused by the epidural needle used to introduce the electrode is the most common suspected mechanism for this complication, with other mechanisms involving injury by lead placement, lead removal, and traction on the nerve while placing a surgical laminectomy lead. In many reported cases of nerve injury, the patient was under general anesthesia or deep sedation at the time of injury and could not respond with complaints of pain or paresthesia at the time of neural insult. Thus, many experts advocate for lead placement under local anesthesia and light sedation rather than heavy sedation or general anesthesia. Evaluation should be guided by the symptoms. Imaging studies are unlikely to reveal abnormalities following isolated injury to a single nerve root, even in the patient reporting ongoing painful dysesthesia. In contrast, any patient who develops signs or symptoms suggesting injury to the spinal cord should undergo immediate imaging with CT (in the event the epidural electrode remains in place) or MRI (if the lead was removed). MRI is far more sensitive in delineating subtle injury to the substance of the spinal

cord itself. Electromyograms and nerve conduction studies can also be helpful in defining the location and extent of nerve injury, but may not show an abnormality for several weeks following injury (see Chapter 20) (241).

Post–Dural Puncture Headache

A more frequent but less worrisome neuraxial complication of SCS is that of unintentional dural puncture. In a study involving patients with CRPS reported by Kemler, 11% of 36 patients in the randomized clinical trial had evidence of PDPH (242). Other authors have noted similar rates of this complication. Factors that may predispose to this complication are previous surgery in the area of needle placement, calcified ligaments, obesity, and patient movement during SCS epidural needle placement. Technique may also play a role, with a higher rate of dural puncture occurring with the midline approach, a steep angle of needle placement (above 60 degrees), and the use of a needle to introduce a retrograde lead (i.e., a lead extending caudally from the interspace of entry). An extremely rare but more severe complication is a longitudinal dural tear with subsequent chronic CSF leak. This can lead to chronic positional headache, nausea, tinnitus, and malaise.

When an accidental puncture of the dura occurs, the initial treatment is to increase perioperative fluids and provide perioperative antiemetics. Symptoms of PDPH can also be improved by use of an abdominal binder. The use of prophylactic blood patches has not been shown to prevent the occurrence of PDPH (see Chapters 11 and 12). The decision to perform a therapeutic blood patch in the presence of an epidural SCS lead is complicated, because of the worry of introducing blood into the epidural space in the presence of a foreign body and theoretically increasing the risk of epidural infection. No data are available to suggest the best course of action if the symptoms do not abate with conservative measures. Blood patch should be performed only as the last resort in cases where headache persists after conservative therapy.

Other Neuraxial Complications

The introduction of a foreign body into the epidural space can result in a reaction creating scarring of the epidural tissues. This problem is more common with surgical leads, but can occur with the smaller percutaneous leads. There is no evidence that midline dorsal epidural scarring at the thoracic or cervical level results in any specific problems or leads to any type of new pain syndrome. Patients who require SCS often have significant pathologic changes of the bony spine, and these abnormalities can progress in the years following placement of an implanted system. In cases in which a lead is successfully placed, the development or worsening of spinal stenosis may result in a compression of the spinal structures, and the presence of an electrode in the epidural space may well contribute to the degree of central canal stenosis, resulting in new radicular symptoms or signs of myelopathy (243). In the event of critical stenosis that becomes symptomatic after lead placement, surgical consultation should be sought; treatment is likely surgical decompression and revision or removal of the lead. In patients who have not been implanted, the decompression of the stenotic area should be addressed prior to consideration of lead placement.

Complications Outside the Neuraxis

Complications involving structures outside the neuraxis vary in severity and can be as simple as pain at the incision site or as complicated as serious wound infection leading to sepsis (244–247). Infections may occur in the pocket, lead placement incision, or tunneled subcutaneous tissue. Infections may involve only the superficial tissues or may extend from the pocket to the epidural space.

Infection in Tissues Outside the Neuraxis

Diagnosis and treatment of infections at the site of the subcutaneous pocket where the IPG for SCS is placed is the same as for intrathecal pump pocket infection (248). Seroma can occur at the pocket site and must be borne in mind in the differential diagnosis (see the section Complications Involving Nonspinal Tissues). Prevention, diagnosis, and treatment of infection at the site of SCS lead insertion and along the course of the lead follows the same principles as for intrathecal catheter infections (see earlier discussion).

Bleeding in Tissues Outside The Neuraxis

Bleeding can occur in the wound of the IPG or lead placement area. The bleeding can range from superficial bruising to a large hematoma requiring evacuation. Initial treatment includes compression of the wound, discontinuation of any anticoagulants, and assessment for and correction of any abnormalities in coagulation status. If these conservative measures fail, surgical exploration and evacuation of the hematoma may be necessary to halt any ongoing bleeding and remove the hematoma to reduce pain and allow for normal wound healing.

Device-related Complications

Device-related complications are those that are directly due to malfunction or incorrect use of the implanted components of the SCS device. SCS devices are comprised of multiple components, including an energy source (IPG), one or more electrodes, and a lead extension that joins the lead to the IPG when they are separated by a distance that does not allow the lead to be connected directly to the IPG. The IPG is typically programmable, allowing for delivery of electrical energy through different combinations of stimulating electrodes at varying amplitudes, pulse widths, and frequencies. Epidural leads come in many shapes and sizes. The two large groups of leads are those that can be placed percutaneously and those that must be placed through a surgical laminotomy incision. The epidural leads are comprised of several electrodes and wires that transmit the electrical impulses from the IPG to the electrodes. Device-related complications can arise due to incorrect positioning of the electrode or a change in position of the electrode that occurs after implantation, malfunction of the IPG, or fracture of a lead or lead extension. Device-related complications are often difficult to distinguish from overall adverse events in published reports. Taylor et al. reported a 43% device complication rate. The actual events are not broken down by category, but many of these events were minor and not felt to be clinically significant (249). Alo et al. reported problems with the SCS device requiring revision in 6% of patients and device removal in a similar number of patients (250). In a recent RCT comparing SCS with conventional medical management for failed back surgery syndrome, one or more complication occurred in 32% of patients, with lead displacement requiring reoperation in 10% and infection or wound breakdown in 8% (238).

TABLE 50-19

DIAGNOSING THE CAUSE FOR LOSS OF STIMULATION IN THE PATIENT WITH AN IMPLANTED SPINAL CORD STIMULATOR (SCS)

Perform an analysis using the SCS device programmer to:
- Ensure that the implanted pulse generator is functional and that sufficient battery life remains
- Check lead impedance (excessive impedance or no impedance reading may indicate lead fracture)
- Reprogram the lead configuration in attempts to regain stimulation

Obtain a plain anterior-posterior and lateral radiograph of the region where the epidural SCS lead was placed and compare to films obtained at the time of initial placement to assure that the lead position has not changed

Loss of Stimulation, Painful Stimulation, and Positional Stimulation

The most common complication during use of SCS is the loss of adequate stimulation covering the painful region. In many cases, this results from lead migration or changes in the patient's pain pattern. Regions may exist within the epidural space in some patients that do not result in perceived stimulation even at high amplitudes and wide pulse widths.

Determining the cause for loss of stimulation begins with analysis and reprogramming of the device followed by radiographs to assess lead integrity and position (Table 50-19). Simple reprogramming of the stimulation parameters and stimulating electrode combinations will often restore successful stimulation. Plain radiographs can reveal lead disconnection, fractures, or migration. Comparing current films with the initial postoperative films will readily establish lead migration. Electronic analysis of the IPG can also detect high impedance in one or more electrodes caused by fluid within the lead connector or a break in the lead. Fluid can leak in at the point of connection between the lead extension and the epidural lead or at the point where the lead or extension join the IPG, resulting in loss of stimulation and high impedance readings on analysis. In the case of either fluid leak or lead fracture, repair requires surgical exploration with testing of the lead, connectors, and generator, and replacement of any malfunctioning components.

After an SCS system has been in place for some years, the patient may experience a loss of stimulation that is not explained by reprogramming, x-ray analysis, or impedance abnormalities. This may signal progression of disease (e.g., spinal stenosis), but making this diagnosis is difficult. All other parameters may be normal, yet the pattern of stimulation has significantly changed or stimulation has been lost altogether. Particularly in those patients with preexisting spinal stenosis, progression in narrowing of the central spinal canal should be suspected; CT myelography may be necessary to determine the level and degree of stenosis.

Painful stimulation can occur as a result of a current leak in the system, change in programming, lead migration, or change in disease state. Painful stimulation accompanied by high impedance suggests a lead fracture, with current leak from the lead as a cause for pain. Sudden change in the position of the perceived stimulation signals lead migration. Lateral lead migration may result in painful stimulation of the spinal nerve roots sensed over the dermatomal distribution of the corresponding spinal nerve (typically in the anterior chest or

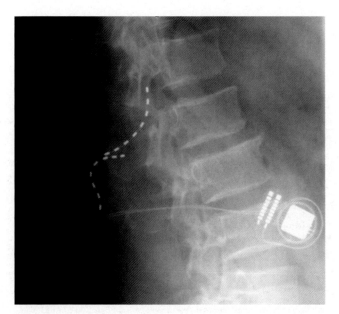

FIGURE 50-23. Spinal cord stimulator lead migration. This patient presented with sudden loss of stimulation. Both leads have migrated, with one of the two located completely outside of the epidural space. The cause for this loss of stimulation was easily detected using plain radiographs. Reproduced from Neal JM, Rathmell JP. *Complications in Regional Anesthesia and Pain Medicine.* Philadelphia: Saunders Elsevier, 2007, with permission.

abdominal wall). Positional stimulation often occurs because the spinal cord itself moves within the thecal sac during normal activity; thus, the distance between the epidural electrode and the dorsal columns changes, causing increases or decreases in the perceived intensity of stimulation.

When stimulation is lost because of migration of the lead (Fig. 50-22) that cannot be corrected by reprogramming, surgical revision is required. The incidence of lead migration can be reduced by careful postoperative instructions to the patient to limit movement during the first 4 to 6 weeks after surgery. Migration may also be reduced by careful attention to surgical technique when anchoring the lead. In the event that a percutaneous lead migrates on more than one occasion, the use of a surgical lead should be considered.

Pain at the Site of the Implanted Device

Persistent pain associated with the implanted SCS system is uncommon, occurring most commonly at the IPG site or the point where the lead is anchored to the paraspinous fascia. Pain at the implant site can be caused by the hardness of the lead anchoring device itself, irritation at connection sites that rub against overlying clothing or an underlying bony prominence,

pain from the generator, or neuroma formation. Pain leading to removal of the system occurs in 6% of patients across numerous trials and is more common in patients who gain significant weight after implantation (235).

SUMMARY

Few serious complications are associated with the majority of interventional techniques currently in use for the treatment of chronic pain. Careful history and physical examination will help identify risk factors such as diabetes, immunosuppression, coagulopathy, and occult infection. Having a thorough familiarity with the anatomy relevant to each treatment technique and coupling this knowledge with meticulous use of radiographic guidance can minimize complications. The use of IV sedation during these procedures remains controversial. Although modest levels of sedation that allow the patient to communicate verbally with the operator throughout the procedure seem reasonable, the use of heavy sedation or general anesthesia that prevents any verbal communication with the patient is unwise. Patients should be informed of the most serious complications, as well as of common minor complications like accidental dural puncture and PDPH. They should be instructed to promptly report neurologic changes, new or increasing pain, headache, and fever. Several complications arise in the course of pain treatment that, when recognized and treated early in their course, may well result in less catastrophic outcomes, foremost among them are evolving epidural abscess or hematoma. A system of night and weekend coverage should be available, and patients should know how to contact the on-call physician, such that any adverse sequelae of these treatment techniques can be promptly recognized and treated.

ACKNOWLEDGMENTS

Much of this chapter has been distilled from contributions to a textbook that I edited together with Joseph Neal, M.D. (Neal JM, Rathmell JP. *Complications in Regional Anesthesia and Pain Medicine.* Philadelphia: Saunders Elsevier, 2007). I am indebted to the following authors for their contributions to the original textbook and the additional textbook chapters and monographs I have written together with many of them. These earlier published works served as an invaluable guide as I distilled the present book chapter from their detailed analyses: Stephen E. Abram, M.D. (epidural, facet joint, and sacroiliac joint injections), Honorio T. Benzon, M.D. (neurolytic blocks), Nikolai Bogduk, M.D. (transforaminal injection), Oscar A. de Leon-Casasola, M.D. (superior hypogastric and ganglion impar blocks), Timothy Deer, M.D. (intrathecal drug delivery and spinal cord stimulation), Richard L. Rauck, M.D. (sympathetic blocks), and Joel S. Saal, M.D. and Jeffrey Saal, M.D. (IDET).

References

1. Abram SE. The use of epidural steroid injections for the treatment of lumbar radiculopathy. *Anesthesiology* 1999;91:1937–1941.
2. Delport EG, Cucuzzella AR, Marley JK, et al. Treatment of lumbar spinal stenosis with epidural steroid injections: A retrospective outcome study. *Arch Phys Med Rehabil* 2004;85:479–484.
3. Carrera GF. Lumbar facet joint injection in low back pain and sciatica: Preliminary results. *Radiology* 1980;137:665–667.
4. Slipman CW, Lipetz JS, Plastaras CT, et al. Fluoroscopically guided therapeutic sacroiliac joint injections for sacroiliac joint syndrome. *Am J Phys Med Rehabil* 2001;80:425–432.
5. Fitzgibbon DR, Posner KL, Caplan RA, et al. Chronic pain management: American Society of Anesthesiologists Closed Claims Project. *Anesthesiology* 2004;100:98–105.
6. Nelson DA. Dangers from methylprednisolone acetate therapy by intraspinal injection. *Arch Neurol* 1988;45:804–806.
7. Wright MN, Denney LC. A comprehensive review of spinal arachnoiditis. *Orthop Nurs* 2003;22:215–219.
8. Nelson DA, Vates TS, Thompson RB. Complications from intrathecal steroid therapy in patients with multiple sclerosis. *Acta Neurol Scand* 1973;49:176–188.

9. Bernat JL, Sadowski CH, Vincent FM, et al. Sclerosing spinal pachymeningitis. *J Neurol Neurosurg Psychiatry* 1976;39:1124–1128.

10. Carta F, Canu C, Datti R, et al. Calcification and ossification of the spinal arachnoid after intrathecal injection of Depo Medrol. *Zentralbl Neurochir* 1987;48:256–261.

11. Ryan MD, Taylor TKF. Management of lumbar nerve root pain by intrathecal and epidural injection of depot methylprednisolone acetate. *Med J Aust* 1981;2:532–534.

12. Plumb VJ, Dismukes WE. Chemical meningitis related to intrathecal corticosteroid therapy. *South Med J* 1977;70:1241.

13. Seghal AD, Tweed DC, Gardner WH, et al. Laboratory studies after intrathecal corticosteroids. *Arch Neurol* 1963;9:74–78.

14. Bedford THB. The effect of injected solutions on the cell count of the cerebrospinal fluid. *Br J Pharmacol* 1948;3:80–83.

15. Gutknecht DR. Chemical meningitis following epidural injections of corticosteroids. *Am J Med* 1987;82:570.

16. Abram SE. Subarachnoid corticosteroid injection following inadequate response to epidural steroids for sciatica. *Anesth Analg* 1978;57:313–315.

17. Morris JT, Konkol KA, Longfield RN. Chemical meningitis following epidural methylprednisolone injection. *Infect Med* 1994;11:439–440.

18. Benzon HT, Gissen AJ, Strichartz GR, et al. The effect of polyethylene glycol on mammalian nerve impulses. *Anesth Analg* 1987;66:553–559.

19. Delaney TJ, Rowlingson JC, Carron H, et al. Epidural steroid effects on nerves and meninges. *Anesth Analg* 1980;59:610–614.

20. Abram SE. Subarachnoid corticosteroid injection following inadequate response to epidural steroids for sciatica. *Anesth Analg* 1978;57:313–316.

21. Deland FH. Intrathecal toxicity studies with benzyl alcohol. *Toxicol Appl Pharmacol* 1973;25:153–156.

22. Latham JM, Fraser RD, Moore RJ, et al. The pathologic effects of intrathecal betamethasone. *Spine* 1997;22:1558–1562.

23. Hoeft MA, Rathmell JP. Acute intrathecal administration of dexamethasone sodium phosphate: Neurotoxicity in an animal model. American Society of Regional Anesthesia and Pain Medicine Annual Fall Pain Meeting, San Francisco, CA, 2006.

24. Kotani N, Kushikata T, Hashimoto H, et al. Intrathecal methylprednisolone for intractable postherpetic neuralgia. *N Engl J Med* 2000;343:1514–1519.

25. Simon SL, Abrahams JM, Sean Grady M, et al. Intramedullary injection of contrast into the cervical spinal cord during cervical myelography: A case report. *Spine* 2002;27:E274–E277.

26. Pradhan S, Yadav R, Maurya PK, Mishra VN. Focal myelomalacia and syrinx formation after accidental intramedullary lidocaine injection during lumbar anesthesia: A report of 3 cases. *J Neurol Sci* 2006;251:70–72.

27. Wilkinson PA, Valentine A, Gibbs JM. Intrinsic spinal cord lesions complicating epidural anaesthesia and analgesia: Report of three cases. *J Neurol Neurosurg Psychiatry* 2002;72:537–539.

28. Hodges SD, Castleberg RL, Miller T, et al. Cervical epidural steroid injection with intrinsic spinal cord damage: Two case reports. *Spine* 1998;23:2137–2140.

29. Field J, Rathmell JP, Stephenson JH, Katz NP. Neuropathic pain following cervical epidural steroid injection. *Anesthesiology* 2000;93:885–888.

30. Hall ED, Springer JE. Neuroprotection and acute spinal cord injury: A reappraisal. *Neuro Rx* 2004;1:80–100.

31. Knight CL, Burnell JC. Systemic side effects of extradural steroids. *Anaesthesia* 1980;35:593–594.

32. Stambough JL, Booth RE, Rothman RH. Transient hypercorticism after epidural steroid injection. *J Bone Joint Surg* 1984;66A:1115–1116.

33. Tuel SM, Meythaler JM, Cross LL. Cushing's syndrome from methylprednisolone. *Pain* 1990;40:81–84.

34. Jacobs S, Pullan PT, Potter JM, et al. Adrenal suppression following extradural steroids. *Anaesthesia* 1983;38:953–956.

35. Kay J, Findling JW, Raff H. Epidural triamcinolone suppresses the pituitary-adrenal axis in human subjects. *Anesth Analg* 1994;79:501–505.

36. Boonen S, Van Distel G, Westhovens R, et al. Steroid myopathy induced by epidural triamcinolone injection. *Br J Rheumatol* 1995;34:385–386.

37. Ward A, Watson J, Wood P, et al. Glucocorticoid epidural for sciatica: Metabolic and endocrine sequelae. *Rheumatology* 2002;41:68–71.

38. Nakamura H, Matsuse H, Obase Y, et al. Clinical evaluation of anaphylactic reactions to intravenous corticosteroids in adult asthmatics. *Respiration* 2002;69:309–313.

39. Saito R, Moroi S, Okuno H, Ogawa O. Anaphylaxis following administration of intravenous methylprednisolone sodium succinate in a renal transplant recipient. *Int J Urol* 2004;11:171–174.

40. Simon DL, Kunz RD, German JD, et al. Allergic or pseudoallergic reaction following epidural steroid deposition and skin testing. *Reg Anesth* 1989;14:253–255.

41. Williams KN, Jackowski A, Evans PJD. Epidural hematoma requiring surgical decompression following repeated epidural steroid injections for chronic pain. *Pain* 1990;42:197–199.

42. Reitman CA, Watters W. Subdural hematoma after cervical epidural steroid injection. *Spine* 2002;27:E174–E176.

43. Benzon HT, Wong HY, Siddiqui T, et al. Caution in performing epidural injections in patients on several antiplatelet drugs. *Anesthesiology* 1999;91:1558.

44. Horlocker TT, Wedel DJ, Benzon H, et al. Regional anesthesia in the anticoagulated patient: Defining the risks (the second ASRA Consensus Conference on Neuraxial Anesthesia and Anticoagulation). *Reg Anesth Pain Med* 2003;28(3):172–197.

45. Horlocker T, Bajwa ZH, Zubaira A, et al. Risk assessment of hemorrhagic complications associated with nonsteroidal anti-inflammatory medications in ambulatory pain clinic patients undergoing epidural steroid injection. *Anesth Analg* 2002;95:1691–1697.

46. Rathmell JP, Lake T, Ramundo MB. Infectious risks of chronic pain treatments: Injection therapy, surgical implants, and intradiscal techniques. *Reg Anesth Pain Med* 2006;31:346–352.

47. Cooper AB, Sharpe MD. Bacterial meningitis and cauda equina syndrome after epidural steroid injections. *Can J Anesth* 1996;43:471–474.

48. Huang RC, Shapiro GS, Lim M, et al. Cervical epidural abscess after epidural steroid injection. *Spine* 2004;29:E7–E9.

49. Knight JW, Cordingley JJ, Palazzo MG. Epidural abscess following epidural steroid and local anaesthetic injection. *Anaesthesia* 1997;52:576–578.

50. Okazaki K, Sasaki K, Matsuda S, et al. Pyogenic arthritis of a lumbar facet joint. *Am J Orthop* 2000;29:222–224.

51. Elias M. Cervical epidural abscess following trigger point injection. *J Pain Symptom Manage* 1994;9:71–72.

52. Tang HJ, Lin HJ, Liu YC, et al. Spinal epidural abscess: Experience with 46 patients and evaluation of prognostic factors. *J Infection* 2002;45:76–81.

53. Hooten WM, Kinney MO, Huntoon MA. Epidural abscess and meningitis after epidural corticosteroid injection. *Mayo Clin Proc* 2004;79:682–686.

54. Muffoletto AJ, Ketonen LM, Mader JT, et al. Hematogenous pyogenic facet joint infection. *Spine* 2001;26:1570–1576.

55. Vyskocil JJ, McIlroy MA, Brennan TA, et al. Pyogenic infection of the sacroiliac joint. Case reports and review of the literature. *Medicine* 1991;70:188–197.

56. Cook NJ, Hanrahan P, Song S. Paraspinal abscess following facet joint injection. *Clin Rheumatol* 1999;18:52–53.

57. Alcock E, Regaard A, Browne J. Facet joint injection: A rare cause of epidural abscess formation. *Pain* 2003;103:209–210.

58. Birnbach DJ, Meadows W, Stein DJ, et al. Comparison of povidone iodine and DuraPrep, an iodophor-in-isopropyl alcohol solution, for skin disinfection prior to epidural catheter insertion in parturients. *Anesthesiology* 2003;98:164–169.

59. Yentur EA, Luleci N, Topcu I, et al. Is skin disinfection with 10% povidone iodine sufficient to prevent epidural needle and catheter contamination? *Reg Anesth Pain Med* 2003;28:389–393.

60. Kang JD, Georgescu HI, McIntyre-Larkin L, et al. Herniated cervical intervertebral discs spontaneously produce matrix metalloproteinases, nitric oxide, interleukin-6 and prostaglandin E2. *Spine* 1995;22:2373–2378.

61. Furusawa N, Baba H, Miyoshi N, et al. Herniation of cervical intervertebral disc. Immunohistochemical examination and measurement of nitric oxide production. *Spine* 2001;26:1110–1116.

62. Furman MB, Giovanniello MT, O'Brien EM. Incidence of intravascular penetration in transforaminal cervical epidural steroid injections. *Spine* 2003;28:21–25.

63. Rathmell JP, Aprill C, Bogduk N. Cervical transforaminal injection of steroids. *Anesthesiology* 2004;100(6):1595–1600.

64. Huntoon MA. Anatomy of the cervical intervertebral foramina: Vulnerable arteries and ischemic neurologic injuries after transforaminal epidural injections. *Pain* 2005;117(1–2):104–111.

65. Brouwers PJAM, Kottnik EJBL, Simon MAM, et al. A cervical anterior spinal artery syndrome after diagnostic blockade of the right C6-nerve root. *Pain* 2001;91:397–399.

66. Baker R, Dreyfuss P, Mercer S, et al. Cervical transforaminal injection of corticosteroids into a radicular artery: A possible mechanism for spinal cord injury. *Pain* 2002;103:211–215.

67. Karasek M, Bogduk N. Temporary neurologic deficit after cervical transforaminal injection of local anesthetic. *Pain Med* 2004;5:202–205.

68. McMillan MR, Crumpton C. Cortical blindness and neurologic injury complicating cervical transforaminal injection for cervical radiculopathy. *Anesthesiology* 2003;99:509–511.

69. Rozin L, Rozin R, Koehler SA, et al. Death during a transforaminal epidural steroid nerve root block (C7) due to perforation of the left vertebral artery. *Am J Forensic Med Path* 2003;24:351–355.

70. Tiso RL, Cutler T, Catania JA, et al. Adverse central nervous system sequelae after selective transforaminal block: The role of corticosteroids. *Spine J* 2004;4:468–474.

71. Standards Committee of the International Spine Intervention Society. Cervical transforaminal injection of corticosteroids. In: Bogduk N, ed. *Practice Guidelines for Spinal Diagnostic and Treatment Procedures*. San Francisco: International Spine Intervention Society, 2004:237–248.

72. Botwin KP, Gruber RD, Bouchlas CG, et al. Complications of fluoroscopically guided transforaminal lumbar epidural injections. *Arch Phys Med Rehabil* 2000;81:1045–1050.

73. Lo D, Vallee JN, Spelle L, et al. Unusual origin of the artery of Adamkiewicz from the fourth lumbar artery. *Neuroradiology* 2002;44:153–157.

74. Houten JK, Errico TJ. Paraplegia after lumbosacral nerve root block: Report of three cases. *Spine J* 2002;2:70–75.

75. Somyaji HS, Saifuddin A, Casey ATH, et al. Spinal cord infarction following therapeutic compute tomography-guided left L2 nerve root injection. *Spine* 2005;30:E106–E108.

76. Standards Committee of the International Spine Intervention Society. Lumbar transforaminal injection of corticosteroids. In: Bogduk N, ed. *Practice Guidelines for Spinal Diagnostic and Treatment Procedures*. San Francisco: International Spine Intervention Society, 2004:163–287.

77. Boas RA. Sympathetic nerve blocks: In search of a role. *Reg Anesth Pain Med* 1998;23:292–305.

78. Kozody R, Ready LB, Barsa JE, et al. Dose requirement of local anaesthetic to produce grand mal seizure during stellate ganglion block. *Can Anaesth Soc J* 1982;29:489–491.

79. Malmqvist EL, Bengtsson M, Sorensen J. Efficacy of stellate ganglion block: A clinical study with bupivacaine. *Reg Anesth* 1992;17:340–347.

80. Hogan QH, Erickson SJ, Haddox JD, et al. The spread of solutions during stellate ganglion block. *Reg Anesth* 1992;17:78–83.

81. Cho HM, Lee DY, Sung SW. Anatomical variations of rami communicantes in the upper thoracic sympathetic trunk. *Eur J Cardiothorac Surg* 2005;27:320–324.

82. Kashiwagi M, Ikeda N, Tsuji A, et al. Sudden unexpected death following stellate ganglion block. *Leg Med (Tokyo)* 1999;1:262–265.

83. Shimada Y, Marumo H, Kinoshita T, et al. A case of cervical spondylitis during stellate ganglion block. *J Nippon Med Sch* 2005;72:295–299.

84. Maeda S, Murakawa K, Fu K, et al. A case of pyogenic osteomyelitis of the cervical spine following stellate ganglion block. *Masui* 2004;53:664–667.

85. Dukes RR, Alexander LA. Transient locked-in syndrome after vascular injection during stellate ganglion block. *Reg Anesth* 1993;18:378–380.

86. Tuz M, Erodlu F, Dodru H, et al. Transient locked-in syndrome resulting from stellate ganglion block in the treatment of patients with sudden hearing loss. *Acta Anaesthesiol Scand* 2003;47:485–487.

87. Wallace MS, Milholland AV. Contralateral spread of local anesthetic with stellate ganglion block. *Reg Anesth* 1993;18:55–59.

88. Kimura T, Nishiwaki K, Yokota S, et al. Severe hypertension after stellate ganglion block. *Br J Anaesth* 2005;94:840–842.

89. Rocco AG. Radiofrequency lumbar sympatholysis. The evolution of a technique for managing sympathetically maintained pain. *Reg Anesth* 1995;20:3–12.

90. Maier C, Gleim M, Weiss T, et al. Severe bleeding following lumbar sympathetic blockade in two patients under medication with irreversible platelet aggregation inhibitors. *Anesthesiology* 2002;97:740–743.

91. Artuso JD, Stevens RA, Lineberry PJ. Post dural puncture headache after lumbar sympathetic block: A report of two cases. *Reg Anesth* 1991;16:288–291.

92. Wong GY, Schroeder DR, Carns PE, et al. Effect of neurolytic celiac plexus block on pain relief, quality of life, and survival in patients with unresectable pancreatic cancer. *JAMA* 2004;291:1092–1099.

93. Goudas L, Carr DB, Bloch R, et al. Management of Cancer Pain. Evidence Report/Technology Assessment No. 35. Rockville, MD: Agency for Healthcare Research and Quality (Prepared by the New England Medical Center Evidence-based Practice Center under Contract No 290-97-0019). AHCPR Publication No. 02-E002, 2001.

94. Lillemoe KD, Cameron JL, Kaufman HS, et al. Chemical splanchnicectomy in patients with unresectable pancreatic cancer. A prospective randomized trial. *Ann Surg* 1993;217:447–457.

95. Ischia S, Ischia A, Polati E, et al. Three posterior percutaneous celiac plexus block techniques. A prospective randomized study in 61 patients with pancreatic cancer pain. *Anesthesiology* 1992;76:534–540.

96. Moore DC. Intercostal nerve block combined with celiac plexus (splanchnic) block. In: Moore DC, ed. *Regional Block*, 4th ed. Springfield: Charles C Thomas Publisher, 1981.

97. Davies DD. Incidence of major complications of neurolytic coeliac plexus block. *J R Soc Med* 1993;86:264–266.

98. Kaplan R, Schiff-Keren B, Alt E. Aortic dissection as a complication of celiac plexus block. *Anesthesiology* 1995;83:632–635.

99. Sett SS, Taylor DC. Aortic pseudoaneurysm secondary to celiac plexus block. *Ann Vasc Surg* 1991;5:88–91.

100. Eisenberg E, Carr DB, Chalmers TC. Neurolytic celiac plexus block for treatment of cancer pain: A meta-analysis. *Anesth Analg* 1995;80:290–295.

101. Brown DL, Bulley CK, Quiel EL. Neurolytic celiac plexus block for pancreatic cancer pain. *Anesth Analg* 1987;66:869–873.

102. Weber JG, Brown DL, Stephens DH, et al. Retrocrural computed tomographic anatomy in patients with and without pancreatic cancer. *Reg Anesth* 1996;21:407–413.

103. Black A, Dwyer B. Coeliac plexus block. *Anaesth Intensive Care* 1973;1:315–318.

104. Noda J, Umeda S, Mori K, et al. Acetaldehyde syndrome after celiac plexus alcohol block. *Anesth Analg* 1986;65:1300–1302.

105. Noda J, Umeda S, Mori K, et al. Acetaldehyde syndrome after celiac plexus alcohol block. *Anesth Analg* 1986;65:1300–1302.

106. Thomasson HR, Crabb DW, Edenberg HJ, et al. Alcohol and aldehyde dehydrogenase polymorphisms and alcoholism. *Behav Genet* 1993;23:131–136.

107. Wong GY, Brown DL. Transient paraplegia following alcohol celiac plexus block. *Reg Anesth* 1995;20:352–355.

108. Brown DL, Rorie DK. Altered reactivity of isolated segmental lumbar arteries of dogs following exposure to ethanol and phenol. *Pain* 1994;56:139–143.

109. Plancarte R, Amescua C, Patt RB, et al. Superior hypogastric plexus block for pelvic cancer pain. *Anesthesiology* 1990;73:236–239.

110. de Leon-Casasola OA, Kent E, Lema MJ. Neurolytic superior hypogastric plexus block for chronic pelvic pain associated with cancer. *Pain* 1993;54:145–151.

111. Rosenberg SK, Tewari R, Boswell MV, et al. Superior hypogastric plexus block successfully treats severe penile pain after transurethral resection of the prostate. *Reg Anesth Pain Med* 1998;23:618–620.

112. Raj PP. Peripheral neurolysis in the management of pain. In: Waldman SD, Winnie AP, eds. *Interventional Pain Management*. Philadelphia: WB Saunders;1996:392–400.

113. Myers RR, Katz J. Neurolytic agents. In: Raj PP, ed. *Practical Management of Pain*, 2nd ed. St. Louis: Mosby-Year Book; 1992:701–712.

114. Gallagher HS, Yonezawa T, Hoy RC, et al. Subarachnoid alcohol block. II: Histological changes in the central nervous system. *Am J Pathol* 1961;35:679.

115. Labat G. The action of alcohol on the living nerve. Experimental and clinical considerations. *Anesth Analg Curr Res* 1933;12:190–196.

116. Swerdlow M. Complications of neurolytic neural blockade. In: Cousins MJ, Bridenbaugh PO, eds. *Neural Blockade in Clinical Anesthesia and Management of Pain*, 2nd ed. Philadelphia: JB Lippincott; 1988:719–735.

117. Wood KM. The use of phenol as a neurolytic agent. *Pain* 1978;5:205–229.

118. Moller JE, Helweg-Larson J, Jacobson E. Histopathological lesions in the sciatic nerve of the rat following perineural application of phenol and alcohol solutions. *Dan Med Bull* 1969;16:116–119.

119. Benzon HT. Convulsions secondary to intravascular phenol: A hazard of celiac plexus block. *Anesth Analg* 1979;58:150–151.

120. Bridenbaugh PO, Dupen SL, Moore DC, et al. Postoperative intercostals nerve block analgesia versus narcotic analgesia. *Anesth Analg* 1973;52:81.

121. Benumof JF, Semenza J. Total spinal anesthesia following intrathoracic intercostal nerve blocks. *Anesthesiology* 1975;43:124–125.

122. Purcell-Jones G, Pither CE, Justins DM. Paravertebral somatic nerve block: A clinical radiographic, and computed tomographic study in chronic pain patients. *Anesth Analg* 1989;68:32–39.

123. Perttunen K, Nilsson E, Heinonen J, et al. Extradural, paravertebral and intercostal nerve blocks for post-thoracotomy pain. *Br J Anaesth* 1995;75:541–547.

124. Winnie AP. Subarachnoid neurolytic blocks. In: Waldman SD, Winnie AP, eds. *Interventional Pain Management*. Philadelphia: WB Saunders; 1996:401–405.

125. Gerbershagen HY. Neurolysis: Subarachnoid neurolytic blockade. *Acta Anaesthesiol Belg* 1982;1:45.

126. Cousins MJ. Chronic pain and neurolytic neural blockade. In: Cousins MJ, Bridenbaugh PO, eds. *Neural Blockade in Clinical Anesthesia and Management of Pain*, 2nd ed. Philadelphia: JB Lippincott; 1988:1053–1084.

127. Korevaar WC. Transcatheter thoracic epidural neurolysis using ethyl alcohol. *Anesthesiology* 1988;69:989–993.

128. Racz GB, Sabongy M, Gintautas J, et al. Intractable pain therapy using a new epidural catheter. *JAMA* 1982;248:579–581.

129. Katz JA, Selhorst S, Blisard KS. Histopathological changes in primate spinal cord after single and repeated epidural phenol administration. *Reg Anesth* 1995;20:283–290.

130. Hayashi I, Odashiro M, Sasaki Y. Two cases of epidural neurolysis using ethyl alcohol and histopathologic changes in the spinal cord. *Masui* 2000;49:877–880.

131. Kirschner M. Zur Elektrochirurgie. *Arch Klin Chir* 1931;167:761.

132. Sweet WH, Mark VH. Unipolar anodal electrolyte lesions in the brain of man and rat: Report of five human cases with electrically produced bulbar or mesencephalic tractotomies. *AMA Arch Neurol Psychiatry* 1953;70:224–234.

133. Aranow S. The use of radiofrequency power in making lesions in the brain. *J Neurosurg* 1960;17:431–438.

134. Lord SM, Barnsley L, Wallis BJ, et al. Percutaneous radio-frequency neurotomy for chronic cervical zygapophyseal-joint pain. *N Engl J Med* 1996;335:1721–1726.

135. Kanpolat Y, Savas A, Bekar A, Berk C. Percutaneous controlled radiofrequency trigeminal rhizotomy for the treatment of idiopathic trigeminal neuralgia: 25-year experience with 1,600 patients. *Neurosurgery* 2001;48:524–532.

136. Kornick C, Kramarich SS, Lamer TJ, Sitzman B. Complications of lumbar facet radiofrequency denervation. *Spine* 2004;29:1352–1354.

PART IV: PAIN MANAGEMENT

137. Mikeladze G, Espinal R, Finnegan R, et al. Pulsed radiofrequency application in treatment of chronic zygapophyseal joint pain. *Spine J* 2003;3:360–362.

138. Lord SM, Bogduk N. Radiofrequency procedures in chronic pain. *Best Pract Res Clin Anesthesiol* 2002;16:597–617.

139. Taha JM, Tew JM Jr., Buncher CR. A prospective 15-year follow up of 154 consecutive patients with trigeminal neuralgia treated by percutaneous stereotactic radiofrequency thermal rhizotomy. *J Neurosurg* 1995;83:989–993.

140. Eller JL, Raslan AM, Burchiel KJ. Trigeminal neuralgia: Definition and classification. *Neurosurg Focus* 2005;18:E3.

141. Dandy WE. Concerning the cause of trigeminal neuralgia. *Am J Surg* 1934;24:447–455.

142. Gardner WJ, Sava GA. Hemifacial spasm: Reversible pathophysiologic state. *J Neurosurg* 1962;21:240–247.

143. Janetta P. Treatment of trigeminal neuralgia by micro-operative decompression. In: Youmans J, ed. *Neurological Surgery*. Philadelphia: WB Saunders; 1990:3928–3942.

144. Taha JM, Tew JM. Comparison of surgical treatments for trigeminal neuralgia reevaluation of radiofrequency rhizotomy. *Neurosurgery* 1996;38:865–871.

145. Lord SM, Bogduk N. Radiofrequency procedures in chronic pain. *Best Pract Res Clin Anesthesiol* 2002;16:597–617.

146. Mitchell RG, Teddy PJ. Meningitis due to Gemella Hoaemolysans after radiofrequency trigeminal rhizotomy. *J Clin Pathol* 1985;38:558–560.

147. Göçer AI, Çetinalp E, Tuna M, et al. Fatal complication of the radiofrequency trigeminal rhizotomy. *Acta Neurochir (Wein)* 1997;139:373–374.

148. Berk C, Honey CR. Brain stem injury after radiofrequency trigeminal rhizotomy. *Acta Neurochir (Wein)* 2004;146:635–636.

149. Egan RA, Pless M, Shults WT. Monocular blindness as a complication of trigeminal radiofrequency rhizotomy. *Ophthalmology* 2001;131:237–240.

150. Ugur HC, Savas A, Elhan A, Kanpolat Y. Unanticipated complication of percutaneous radiofrequency trigeminal rhizotomy rhinorrhea report of three cases and a cadaver study. *Neurosurgery* 2004;54:1522–1526.

151. Sweet WH, Poletti CE, Roberts JT. Dangerous rises in blood pressure upon heating of the trigeminal rootlets: Increased bleeding times in patients with trigeminal neuralgia. *Neurosurgery* 1985;17:843–844.

152. Cavanaugh JM, Lu Y, Chen C, Kallakuri S. Pain generation in lumbar and cervical facet joints. *J Bone Joint Surg Am* 2006;88[Suppl 2]:63–67.

153. Bogduk N, Marsland A. The cervical zygapophyseal joints as a source of pain. *Spine* 1988;13:610–617.

154. Boas RA. Facet joint injections. In: Stanton-Hicks MA, Boas RA, eds. *Chronic Low Back Pain*. New York: Raven Press, 1982.

155. Dreyfuss P, Tibiletti C, Dreyer SJ. Thoracic zygapophyseal joint pain patterns. *Spine* 1994;19:807–811.

156. Kornick C, Kramarich SS, Lamer TJ, Sitzman BT. Complications of lumbar facet radiofrequency denervation. *Spine* 2004;29:1352–1354.

157. North RB, Han M, Zahurak M, Kidd DH. Radiofrequency lumbar facet denervation: Analysis of prognostic factors. *Pain* 1994;57:77–83.

158. North RB, Misop H, Zahurak M, Kidd DH. Radiofrequency lumbar denervation: Analysis of prognostic factors. *Pain* 1994;57:77–83.

159. Lord SM, Barnsley L, Wallis BJ, et al. Percutaneous radiofrequency neurotomy in the treatment of cervical zygapophyseal joint pain. *N Engl J Med* 1996;335:1721–1726.

160. Guerts JW, van Wijk RM, Stolker RJ, Groen GJ. Efficacy of radiofrequency procedures for the treatment of spinal pain: A systematic review of randomized clinical trials. *Reg Anesth Pain Med* 2001;26:394–400.

161. McDonald GJ, Lord SM, Bogduk N. Long-term follow-up of patients treated with cervical radiofrequency neurotomy for chronic neck pain. *Neurosurgery* 1999;45:61–67.

162. Burchiel KJ. Comments. *Neurosurgery* 1999;45:67–68.

163. Lord SM, Barnsley L, Bogduk N. Percutaneous radiofrequency neurotomy in the treatment of cervical zygapophysial joint pain: A caution. *Neurosurgery* 1995;36:732–739.

164. Dreyfuss P, Halbrook B, Pauza K, et al. Efficacy and validity of radiofrequency neurotomy for chronic lumbar zygapophysial joint pain. *Spine* 2000;25:1270–1277.

165. van Kleef M, Barendse GA, Kessels A, et al. Randomized trial of radiofrequency lumbar facet denervation for chronic low back pain. *Spine* 1999;24:1937–1942.

166. Leclaire R, Fortin L, Lambert R, et al. Radiofrequency facet joint denervation in the treatment of low back pain: A placebo-controlled clinical trial to assess efficacy. *Spine* 2001;26:1411–1416.

167. Kornick C, Kramarich SS, Lamer TJ, Sitzman BT. Complications of lumbar facet radiofrequency denervation. *Spine* 2004;29:1352–1354.

168. Pevsner Y, Shabat S, Catz A, et al. The role of radiofrequency in the treatment of mechanical pain of spinal origin. *Eur Spine J* 2003;12:602–605.

169. Dupuy DA, Goldberg SN. Image-guided radiofrequency tumor ablation challenges and opportunities. *J Vasc Interv Radiol* 2001;12:1135–1148.

170. Coskun DM, Gilchrist J, Dupuy D. Lumbosacral radiculopathy following radiofrequency ablation therapy. *Muscle Nerve* 2003;28:754–756.

171. Mungliani R. The longer term effect of pulsed radiofrequency for neuropathic pain. *Pain* 1999;80:437–439.

172. Manchikanti L. The role of radiofrequency in the management of complex regional pain syndrome. *Curr Rev Pain* 2000;4:437–444.

173. Wu PB, Date ES, Kingery WS. The lumbar multifidus muscle in polysegmentally innervated. *Electromyogr Clin Neurophysiol* 2000;40:483–485.

174. Derby R, Lee SH, Kim BJ, et al. Pressure-controlled lumbar discography in volunteers without low back symptoms. *Pain Med* 2005;6:213–221.

175. Freeman BJ, Walters RM, Moore RJ, Fraser RD. Does intradiscal electrothermal therapy denervate and repair experimentally induced annular tears in an animal model? *Spine* 2003;28:2602–2608.

176. Pauza KJ, Howell S, Dreyfuss P, et al. A randomized, placebo-controlled trial of intradiscal electrothermal therapy for the treatment of discogenic low back pain. *Spine J* 2004;4:27–35.

177. Freeman BJ, Fraser RD, Cain CM, et al. A randomized, double-blind, controlled trial: Intradiscal electrothermal therapy versus placebo for the treatment of chronic discogenic low back pain. *Spine* 2005;30:2369–2377.

178. Appleby D, Andersson G, Totta M. Meta-analysis of the efficacy and safety of intradiscal electrothermal therapy (IDET). *Pain Med* 2006;7:308–316.

179. Singh K, Ledet E, Carl A. Intradiscal therapy: A review of current treatment modalities. *Spine* 2005;30[17 Suppl]:S20–S60.

180. Gibson JN, Grant IC, Wadell G. The Cochrane review of surgery for lumbar disc prolapse and degenerative lumbar spondylosis. *Spine* 1999;24:1820–1832.

181. Pomerantz SR, Hirsch JA. Intradiscal therapies for discogenic pain. *Semin Musculoskelet Radiol* 2006;10:125–135.

182. Chen YC, Lee SH, Saenz Y, Lehman NL. Histologic findings of disc, end plate and neural elements after coblation of nucleus pulposus: An experimental nucleoplasty study. *Spine J* 2003;3:466–470.

183. North American Spine Society. Position statement on discography. *Spine* 1988;20:2048–2059.

184. Fraser RD, Osti OL, Vernon-Roberts B. Discitis after discography. *J Bone Joint Surg Br* 1987;69:26–35.

185. Tay BK, Deckey J, Hu SS. Spinal infections. *J Am Acad Orthop Surg* 2002;10:188–197.

186. Friedman JA, Maher CO, Quast LM, et al. Spontaneous disc space infections in adults. *Surg Neurol* 2002;57:81–86.

187. Maiuri F, Iaconetta G, Gallicchio B, et al. Spondylodiscitis: Clinical and magnetic resonance diagnosis. *Spine* 1997;22:1741–1746.

188. Osti OL, Fraser RD, Vernon-Roberts B. Discitis after discography. The role of prophylactic antibiotics. *J Bone Joint Surg Br* 1990;72:271–274.

189. Klessig H, Showsh SA, Sekorski A. The use of intradiscal antibiotics for discography: An in vitro study of gentamicin, cefazolin, and clindamycin. *Spine* 2003;28:1735–1738.

190. Mangram AJ, Horan TC, Pearson ML, et al. Guideline for prevention of surgical site infection, 1999. Hospital Infection Control Practices Advisory Committee. *Infect Control Hosp Epidemiol* 1999;20:250–278.

191. Karasek M, Bogduk N. Twelve-month follow-up of a controlled trial of intradiscal thermal annuloplasty for back pain due to internal disc disruption. *Spine* 2000;25:2601–2607.

192. Saal JS, Saal JA. Management of chronic discogenic low back pain with a thermal intradiscal catheter: A preliminary report. *Spine* 2000;25:382–388.

193. Saal, JA Saal JS. Intradiscal electrothermal treatment for chronic discogenic low back pain: A prospective outcome study with minimum one year follow-up. *Spine* 2000;25:2622–2627.

194. Saal JA, Saal JS. Intradiscal electrothermal treatment for chronic discogenic low back pain: A prospective outcome study with minimum two-year follow-up. *Spine* 2002;27:966–974.

195. Derby R, Eck B, Chen Y, et al. Intradiscal electrothermal annuloplasty (IDET): A novel approach for treating chronic discogenic back pain. *Neuromodulation* 2000;3:69–75.

196. Lutz C, Lutz GE, Cooke PM. Treatment of chronic lumbar diskogenic pain with intradiskal electrothermal therapy: A prospective outcome study. *Arch Phys Med Rehab* 2003;84:23–28.

197. Saal JS, Saal JS. Complications associated with intradiscal electrothermal therapy. In: Neal JM, Rathmell JP, eds. *Complications in Regional Anesthesia and Pain Medicine*. Philadelphia: Saunders Elsevier; 2007:267–272.

198. Cohen S, Larkin T, Polly D. A giant herniated disc following intradiscal electrothermal therapy. *J Spine Disord Tech* 2002;15:537–541.

199. Pauza KS, Howell P, Dreyfuss P, et al. A randomized placebo-controlled trial of intradiscal electrothermal therapy (IDET) for treatment of discogenic low back pain. *Spine J* 2004;4:27–35.

200. Scholl BM, Theiss SM, Lopez-Ben R, et al. Vertebral osteonecrosis related to intradiscal electrothermal therapy: A case report. *Spine* 2003;28:E161–E164.

201. Cohen SP, Larkin T, Abdi S, et al. Risk factors for failure and complications of intradiscal electrothermal therapy: A pilot study. *Spine* 2003;28:1142–1147.

202. Lonstein JE, Denis F, Perra J, et al. Complications associated with pedicle screws. *J Bone Joint Surg* 1999;81A:1519–1528.

203. Sharps LS, Isaac Z. Percutaneous disc decompression using nucleoplasty. *Pain Physician* 2002;5:121–126.

204. Singh V, Piryani C, Liao K. Role of percutaneous disc decompression using Coblation in managing chronic discogenic low back pain: A prospective, observational study. *Pain Physician* 2004;7:419–425.
205. Bhagia SM, Slipman CW, Nirschl M, et al. Side effects and complications after percutaneous disc decompression using coblation technology. *Am J Phys Rehabil* 2006;85:6–13.
206. Nau WH, Diedrich CJ. Evaluation of temperature distributions in cadaveris spine during nucleoplasty. *Phys Med Biol* 2004;49:1583–1594.
207. Winkelmuller M, Winkelmuller W. Long-term effects of continuous intrathecal opioid treatment in chronic pain of nonmalignant etiology. *J Neurosurg* 1996;85:458–467.
208. Coffey RJ, Burchiel KJ. Inflammatory mass lesions associated with intrathecal drug infusion catheters: Report and observations on 41 patients. *Neurosurgery* 2002;50:78–86.
209. Thimineur MA, Kravitz E, Vodapally MS. Intrathecal opioid treatment for chronic non-malignant pain: A 3-year prospective study. *Pain* 2004;109:242–249.
210. Harney D, Victor R. Traumatic syrinx after implantation of an intrathecal catheter. *Reg Anesth Pain Med* 2004;29:606–609.
211. Huntoon MA, Hurdle MF, Marsh RW, et al. Intrinsic spinal cord catheter placement: Implications of new intractable pain in a patient with a spinal cord injury. *Anesth Analg* 2004;99:1763–1765.
212. Ubogu EE, Lindenberg JR, Werz MA, et al. Transverse myelitis associated with *Acinetobacter baumanii* intrathecal pump catheter-related infection. *Reg Anesth Pain Med* 2003;28:470–474.
213. Yaksh TL, Horais KA, Tozier NA, et al. Chronically infused intrathecal morphine in dogs. *Anesthesiology* 2003;99:174–187.
214. Allen JW, Horais KA, Tozier NA, Yaksh TL. Opiate pharmacology of intrathecal granulomas. *Anesthesiology* 2006;105:590–598.
215. Hassenbusch SJ, Portenoy RK, Cousins M, et al. Polyanalgesic Consensus Conference 2003: An update on the management of pain by intraspinal drug delivery: Report of an expert panel. *J Pain Symptom Manage* 2004;27:540–563.
216. Deer T. A prospective analysis of intrathecal granuloma in chronic pain patients. A review of the literature and report of a surveillance study. *Pain Physician* 2004;7:225–228.
217. At www.fda.gov/medwatch/safety/2008/Medtronic_Neuromod_DHCP.pdf. Accessed 26 March 26.
218. Follett KA, Boortz-Marx RL, Drake JM, et al. Prevention and management of intrathecal drug delivery and spinal cord stimulation system infections. *Anesthesiology* 2004;100:1582–1594.
219. The Centers for Disease Control and Prevention Guideline for Prevention of Surgical Site Infection. *Infect Control Hosp Epidemiol* 1999;20:217–278.
220. Rathmell JP, Lake T, Ramundo MB. Infectious risks of chronic pain treatments: Injection therapy, surgical implants, and intradiscal techniques. *Reg Anesth Pain Med* 2006;31:346–352.
221. Follett KA, Naumann CP. A prospective study of catheter-related complications of intrathecal drug delivery systems. *J Pain Symptom Manage* 2000;19:209–215.
222. Milbouw G. An unusual sign of catheter migration: Sciatica. *Neuromodulation* 2005;8:233.
223. Albrecht E, Durrer A, Chedel D, et al. Intraparenchymal migration of an intrathecal catheter three years after implantation. *Pain* 2005;118:274–278.
224. Levin GZ, Tabor DR. Paraplegia secondary to progressive necrotic myelopathy in a patient with an implanted morphine pump. *Am J Phys Med Rehabil* 2005;84:193–196.
225. Lew S, Psaty E, Abbott R. An unusual cause of overdose after baclofen pump implantation: Case report. *Neurosurgery* 2005;56:E624.
226. Coyne PJ, Hansen LA, Laird J, et al. Massive hydromorphone dose delivered subcutaneously instead of intrathecally: Guidelines for prevention and management of opioid, local anesthetic, and clonidine overdose. *J Pain Symptom Manage* 2004;28:273–276.
227. Dario A, Scamoni C, Picano M. The infection risk of intrathecal drug infusion pumps after multiple refill procedures. *Neuromodulation* 2005;8:36.
228. Burton AW, Conroy B, Garcia E, et al. Illicit substance abuse via an implanted intrathecal pump. *Anesthesiology* 2005;89:1264–1267.
229. Paice JA, Penn RD, Shott S. Intraspinal morphine for chronic pain: A retrospective, multicenter study. *J Pain Symptom Manage* 1996;11:71–80.
230. Winkelmuller M, Winkelmuller W. Long-term effects of continuous intrathecal opioid treatment in chronic pain of nonmalignant etiology. *J Neurosurg* 1996;85:458–467.
231. Aldrete JA, Couto da Silva JM. Leg edema from intrathecal opiate infusions. *Eur J Pain* 2000;4:361–365.
232. Hassenbusch SJ, Gunes S, Wachsman S, et al. Intrathecal clonidine in the treatment of intractable pain: A phase I/II study. *Pain Med* 2002;3:85–91.
233. Staats PS, Yearwood T, Charapata SG, et al. Intrathecal ziconotide in the treatment of refractory pain in patients with cancer and AIDS. *JAMA* 2003;291:62–70.
234. Rauck RL, Wallace MS, Leong MS, et al., Ziconotide 301 Study Group. A randomized, double-blind, placebo-controlled study of intrathecal ziconotide in adults with severe chronic pain. *J Pain Symptom Manage* 2006;31:393–406.
235. Turner JA, Loeser JD, Deyo RA, et al. Spinal cord stimulation for patients with failed back surgery syndrome or complex regional pain syndrome: A systematic review of effectiveness and complications. *Pain* 2004;108:137–147.
236. Quigley DG, Arnold J, Eldridge PR, et al. Long-term outcome of spinal cord stimulation and hardware complications. *Stereotact Funct Neurosurg* 2003;81:50–56.
237. Burchiel KJ, Anderson VC, Brown FD, et al. Prospective, multicenter study of spinal cord stimulation for relief of chronic back and extremity pain. *Spine* 1996;21:2786–2794.
238. Kumar K, Taylor RS, Jacques L, et al. Spinal cord stimulation versus conventional medical management for neuropathic pain: A multicentre randomised controlled trial in patients with failed back surgery syndrome. *Pain* 2007;132:179–188.
239. Franzini A, Ferroli P, Marras C, Broggi G. Huge epidural hematoma after surgery for spinal cord stimulation. *Acta Neurochir (Wien)* 2005;147:565–567.
240. Martin RJ, Yuan HA. Neurosurgical care of spinal epidural, subdural, and intramedullary abscesses and arachnoiditis. *Orthop Clin North Am* 1996;27:125–136.
241. Mailis-Gagnon A, Furlan AD, Sandoval JA, et al. Spinal cord stimulation for chronic pain. *Cochrane Database Syst Rev* 2004;(3):CD003783.
242. Kemler MA, Barendse GA, van Kleef M, et al. Spinal cord stimulation in patients with chronic reflex sympathetic dystrophy. *N Engl J Med* 2000;343:618–624.
243. Barolat G. Spinal cord stimulation for chronic pain management. *Arch Med Res* 2000;31:258–262.
244. North RB, Ewend MG, Lawton MT, et al. Failed back surgery syndrome: 5-year follow-up after spinal cord stimulator implantation. *Neurosurgery* 1991;28:692–699.
245. Krames E. Spinal cord stimulation: Indications, mechanism of action, and efficacy. *Curr Rev Pain* 1999;3:419–426.
246. North RB, Wetzel FT. Spinal cord stimulation for chronic pain of spinal origin: A valuable long-term solution. *Spine* 2002;27:2584–2591.
247. Heidecke V, Rainov NG, Burkert W. Hardware failures in spinal cord stimulation for failed back surgery syndrome. *Neuromodulation* 2000;3:27–30.
248. Torrens JK, Stanley PJ, Ragunathan PL, et al. Risk of infection with electrical spinal-cord stimulation. *Lancet* 1997;349:729.
249. Taylor RS, Van Buyten JP, Buchser E. Spinal cord stimulation for chronic back and leg pain and failed back surgery syndrome: A systematic review and analysis of prognostic factors. *Spine* 2005;30:152–160.
250. Alo KM, Holsheimer J. New trends in neuromodulation for the management of neuropathic pain. *Neurosurgery* 2002;50:690–703.

CHAPTER 51 ■ NEW HORIZONS

ALLAN I. BASBAUM

This chapter occupies the same concluding position as the late Pat Wall's essay on "new horizons" in the prior edition. Although it is now more than 40 years since Melzack and Wall's publication of the gate control theory of pain (1), and much has been written about the impact of this theory on pain research and management, I fear that practitioners of regional anesthesia and pain management need to be reminded of its relevance—its increasing relevance—to the development of new treatments that will advance their practice in the near term. Certainly, the rationale for many current pain treatments is based on the view that they "close the gate." Unfortunately, endless discussions with both clinicians and basic scientists have convinced me that the great majority of pain researchers and clinicians have an incomplete understanding of the underlying principles of gate control theory. They appreciate that gate control theory argues strongly against the Cartesian view of pain as having a single labeled line for transmission, with pain afferents, pathways, and cortical areas, but overlook or do not understand many critical elements of this theory.

In formulating the gate control theory of pain, Melzack and Wall recognized the variability of the clinical condition of pain. The word *allodynia* had yet to be coined, but they understood that pain was not merely a consequence of the individual being exposed to a noxious stimulus. Gate control theory, of course, postulated that the activity of small-diameter afferents that respond to noxious stimulation—*nociceptors* in today's parlance—is not the sole determinant of the magnitude of pain experienced. Rather, pain is a consequence of the balance of activity in small- and large-diameter afferents and the central nervous system (CNS) circuits engaged by these afferents. Later elaborations of gate control theory incorporated the important contribution of the affective/emotional impact of the particular noxious stimulus, and the importance of the context in which the stimulus is experienced; that is, the critical contribution of experiential and cognitive factors (2). Together, these ideas underscore the view that pain is a complex perception, not simply the registering of a stimulus. Although it is highly likely that an intense noxious stimulus will be experienced as painful by most individuals, and indeed in the majority of medical and surgical settings in which the stimulus is generated, this type of acute pain is very different from chronic pain conditions that pain physicians generally face. We must explain why innocuous stimuli produce pain (allodynia) after tissue or nerve injury or why pain can persist after the injury resolves.

This marvelous book covers many aspects of the pathophysiologic basis of persistent pain and illustrates the many ways that blockade or inhibition of nerve conduction can influence pain processing. It seemed redundant, therefore, merely to summarize the field in the present concluding essay. I decided instead to look back at the gate control theory, to emphasize its major features—not all of which relate to "closing the gate"—

and perhaps most importantly, to ask if it is still relevant today. I believe that it is, but not for the reasons that one might expect!

GATE CONTROL THEORY: A PRIMER

In Figure 51.1, I have broken down the major components of the spinal cord network that constitute the elements of gate control theory of pain. The classic Melzack and Wall paper appeared soon after Patrick Wall published his seminal electrophysiologic studies on the laminar organization of the spinal cord dorsal horn (3). At that time, the focus on neurons that are responsive to noxious stimulation was in the neck of the dorsal horn, specifically lamina V. Of particular interest was the wide dynamic range (WDR) neuron, which receives convergent inputs from small- and large-diameter primary afferents. Many of these neurons send projections to supraspinal regions (reticular formation and thalamus). Gate control theory referred to this neuron as the "T cell", for transmission neuron. Today, it would likely be identified with the lamina V WDR neuron and almost certainly as well to the lamina I nociresponsive neurons (4). Interestingly, many of the latter receive no direct monosynaptic input from large-diameter myelinated ($A\beta$) afferents, which partly accounts for their nociceptive-specific properties. On the other hand, it is almost certain that, in the setting of injury, many of the lamina I neurons are transformed into WDR cells, so that we can safely include laminae I and V neurons in the output that is regulated by the gate of the original gate control theory. Note that gate control theory did not equate the output of the T cell with "pain." Rather, Melzack and Wall depicted an arrow pointing to an "action system," a more generic term that emphasizes the motivational dimension of stimuli and circuits that produce pain. "Action system" also connotes that noxious stimuli not only evoke pain, but also generate a behavioral repertoire through which the organism responds to noxious stimuli.

Gate control theory begins with the simple view that C-fibers (i.e., nociceptors) directly activate spinal cord projection neurons that transmit a nociceptive message to higher centers (Fig. 51.1A). It is of interest that this conclusion was based on electrophysiologic grounds and on mistaken anatomy. Thus, in 1965 it was argued, based on remarkably insensitive anatomic tracing techniques, that C-fibers do not project to the superficial dorsal horn (i.e., to laminae I or II), but only to the deep dorsal horn, where they could monosynaptically activate the WDR neurons in this region. This conclusion was consistent with electrophysiologic recordings that unequivocally established that increasing the current to activate C-fibers in a peripheral nerve excited WDR neurons over and above

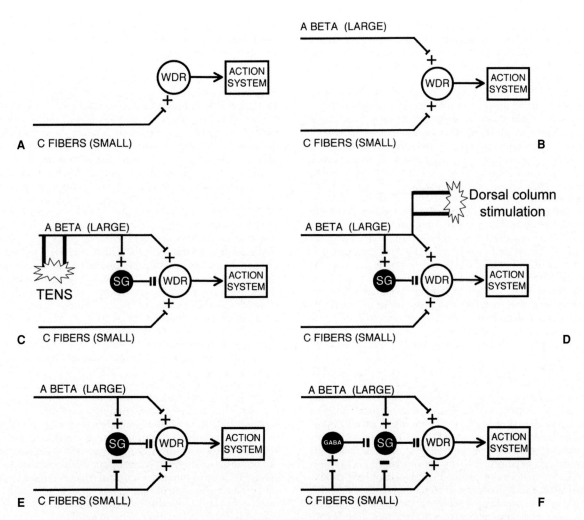

FIGURE 51-1. The essential circuit elements described in the gate control theory of pain. The major output cell controlled by the gate corresponds to the wide dynamic range (WDR) neuron of the dorsal horn of the spinal cord. The WDR neurons, in turn, activate an *action system*, which corresponds to the complex matrix of responses associated with the experience of pain. There are two major excitatory drives to the WDR neuron, from small-diameter, unmyelinated C-fiber primary afferents, most of which are nociceptors (**A**) and from large-diameter, myelinated Aβ primary afferents (**B**), most of which respond to innocuous stimuli. Through a feed-forward inhibitory circuit involving interneurons of the substantia gelatinosa (SG), large-diameter non-nociceptive primary afferents also inhibit the firing of the WDR neurons, thus "closing" the gate (**C**). **C:** Activation of large-diameter primary afferents, as by transcutaneous electrical nerve stimulation (TENS), will predominantly bring into play the inhibitory controls exerted via inhibitory interneurons in the SG. To activate larger numbers of large-diameter primary afferents, electrodes can be placed on the dorsal columns of the spinal cord (**D**). Although the mechanism of inhibitory control exerted by dorsal column stimulation is not known, antidromic activation of the afferents, and ensuing activation of the SG interneurons is a reasonable possibility.

Critical to gate control theory is the mechanism through which the gate is opened. **E:** Unmyelinated afferents not only directly activate WDR neurons, but also hold the gate in an open state by blocking the inhibitory controls exerted by SG interneurons. As the latter inhibitory controls are presumed to be tonically active (from tonic activation of large-diameter afferents), noxious stimulation effectively counters the closing of the gate, which is initiated and maintained by large-diameter primary afferents. **F:** One simple circuit through which excitatory nociceptors may regulate (inhibit) the firing of SG interneurons. In this case, the nociceptor is proposed to activate a normally silent γ-aminobutyric acid (GABA)ergic inhibitory interneuron. When activated, the GABAergic interneuron decreases the firing of the SG interneuron, thereby decreasing inhibitory controls exerted upon WDR neurons. This disinhibitory circuit maintains the gate in an open position and contributes to persistent pain.

that produced by electrical stimulation of large myelinated afferents. In fact, modern anatomic techniques have established not only that primary afferent C-fibers massively project to laminae I and II, but also that few if any project directly to lamina V. Of course, C-fibers can directly activate some deep dorsal horn WDR neurons because the dendrites of some of these neurons extend dorsally into the superficial dorsal horn.

If pain is purely a function of the activity of nociceptors, then the direct activation of WDR neurons by "pain-responsive" C-fibers is the modern equivalent of the Cartesian, specificity view of "pain" transmission. But Melzack and Wall emphasized that the output of the WDR neuron is under incredibly complex controls. Based on other studies from Wall's laboratory, they incorporated the contribution of the circuits engaged by large-diameter primary afferents, which generally do not respond to noxious stimulation, and which, on that basis, would be excluded from the Cartesian view of pain processing. As illustrated in Figure 51.1B, large-diameter primary afferent fibers regulate the firing of the WDR neurons by two very different mechanisms. First, they *excite* the neurons, something that is often forgotten. Presumably this results from direct monosynaptic excitatory input to the WDR cell or via a chain of excitatory interneurons. Second, and perhaps more importantly, large-diameter, rapidly conducting afferents also *inhibit* the WDR cell, via a feed-forward inhibitory mechanism.

Some of Pat Wall's most elegant electrophysiologic studies identified the site and mechanisms through which feed-forward inhibitory control is exerted (4). The then-prevailing view was that inhibitory controls, including the circuitry that underlies presynaptic inhibition of primary afferent fibers, involve interneurons in the deep dorsal horn. Pat Wall's studies turned attention to what at the time were completely enigmatic interneurons of the substantia gelatinosa (SG) of the superficial dorsal horn (lamina II). Space does not permit a discussion of how the SG was implicated. But it is of interest to remind readers that this postulate was formulated well before extracellular or intracellular recordings had been made from SG neurons, even before it was known that C-fibers directly project to the SG, and well before the incredibly complex neurochemistry of the SG had been characterized (see later discussion). Pat Wall's inferences were drawn from studies of cord dorsum potentials, which led to the view that large-diameter afferents excite some SG interneurons. These interneurons, in turn, via both pre- and direct postsynaptic inhibitory controls, were proposed to regulate/inhibit the output of the dorsal horn WDR neuron. This critical feature of gate control theory is illustrated in Figure 51.1C.

It did not take long for this simple circuit to be cited as the explanation for many common clinical findings and, for that matter, for the anecdotal experiences of almost everyone. Rub your hand when it hurts, and it gets better. Shake it, and it gets better. Rubbing and shaking, of course, activate large-diameter afferents, which should "close the gate." Interestingly, if you burn the tip of your finger, you would not just rub the tip. This is reasonable, as it will hurt even more, presumably because you have not only activated sensitized C-fibers, whose threshold has now dropped, but almost certainly the large-diameter afferents innervating the injury site. These are the large-diameter afferents that directly excite the "pain" transmission "T cell" of gate control theory. However, when you rub the area that *surrounds* the zone of injury, it causes profound inhibition of the WDR neuron. This inhibition is almost certainly mediated by γ-aminobutyric acid (GABA)ergic and glycinergic interneurons in the SG.

Clinically, the consequence of engaging the circuits that are activated via large-diameter primary afferents is a reduction of ongoing pain. Not surprisingly, from the moment gate control theory was published, many physicians tried to develop new and better methods to "close the gate." Vibration is effective for some types of pain, but transcutaneous nerve stimulation (TENS) is probably the most dramatic offshoot, albeit a somewhat more expensive approach to closing the gate (Figure 51.1C). Transcutaneous stimulation does work for some conditions. Why its effects are so limited is of interest in and of itself. The explanation may teach us much about the limits that the surround inhibitory circuitry in the dorsal horn can exert upon the output of "pain" transmission neurons.

Among the most significant clinical successes that emanated from the publication of gate control theory was the development of dorsal column stimulation for the treatment of pain. The idea was to activate populations of large-diameter afferents that not only collateralize into the spinal cord, but that also send major branches via the dorsal columns to the dorsal column nuclei of the medulla (Figure 51.1D). Describing the development of dorsal column stimulation for pain control, Pat Wall wrote, in a 1996 retrospective on gate control theory (5), "to activate more large fibers we next inserted the stimulating electrodes in the cauda equina . . . . William Sweet's resident, Norman Shealey advanced the electrodes rostrally, and placed them directly on the dorsal columns. . . ." The paper describing this procedure was published in *Science* (6) and provided a dramatic and remarkably rapid example of translating basic science observations to the clinic. It is not clear whether the mechanism of inhibition involves antidromic activation of large-diameter afferents and their collaterals that enter the dorsal horn, thus activating local inhibitory circuits, or involves a loop through the brainstem. Interestingly, the original gate control theory included a "central control trigger" through which spinocorticospinal loops were hypothesized to regulate the output of the gate. Although Melzack and Wall postulated that the ascending loop of the central control trigger coursed in the dorsal columns, the control that it was thought to subserve is in many respects comparable to the controls exerted by descending inhibitory circuits that arise in midbrain periaqueductal gray and medullary raphe (7,8), which are generally considered to be activated by "painful" inputs. It is of interest that recent studies of Porreca and colleagues (9) have provided significant evidence for a contribution of ascending axons in the dorsal columns to the activation of spinal-bulbospinal loops that influence the transmission of nociceptive signals by dorsal horn neurons.

That large-diameter fibers, which do not respond to noxious stimulation, engage circuits that "close the gate" is the part of gate control theory that most people remember. And when gate control theory is taught in medical and graduate schools, often only its closing is mentioned. Indeed clinicians and other pain management specialists often argue, incorrectly, that this or that treatment for pain is effective because the treatment "closes the gate." The problem is that everyone forgets, or completely ignores, why the word "gate" was chosen in the first place. Gates do not just close, they also open; and the opening part of gate control theory is not merely a monosynaptic excitatory input of C-fibers to the WDR projection neurons.

THE KEY TO OPENING THE GATE

What, then, is the key that opens the gate and ultimately enhances transmission of injury messages to the brain? The key resides in the circuitry of the SG. As Figure 51.1E illustrates, gate control theory postulated that small fibers "open" the gate by blocking the closing mechanisms; that is, by shutting off the inhibitory controls exerted by the large-diameter afferents. This hypothesis derived directly from Patrick Wall's studies of spinal cord dorsum potentials that identified a special contribution of activity from unmyelinated C-fibers, and that postulated that this effect of C-fibers was exerted via circuits in the SG (10).

The Neurochemistry of the Substantia Gelatinosa in 1965

In 1965, almost nothing was known about the complex circuitry of the SG. At that time, only five neurotransmitters had been identified in the dorsal horn. Glutamate was known to be the major excitatory neurotransmitter of nerve fibers, and certainly of the primary afferent fiber. Inhibitory GABAergic and glycinergic interneurons had also been described and implicated in local inhibitory mechanisms in the dorsal horn. And, in 1965, Dahlström and Fuxe published their pioneering studies on the monoamines, serotonin and norepinephrine, and demonstrated that the spinal cord content of these neurotransmitters arises from projection neurons in the brainstem (11).

So, how might the C-fiber "opening" mechanism postulated by gate control theory operate according to 1965 neurochemistry? Figure 51.1F illustrates one simple possibility. This circuit is based upon several assumptions, but the overall circuit is entirely plausible. The first assumption is that there is a tonic inhibition of the WDR cell by the same SG interneuron that is engaged by the large-diameter afferents. The second assumption is that this SG interneuron can be regulated by a population of GABAergic inhibitory interneurons. Third, it must be assumed that the GABAergic interneuron is normally not spontaneously active. The final assumption is that injury-induced excitation of C-fibers not only directly activates the WDR neuron, but also enhances WDR activity by activating the GABAergic inhibitory interneuron, resulting in inhibition of the tonic SG inhibitory controls. To the extent that the SG inhibition is generated by tonic activity of large-diameter afferent activity, this opening mechanism clearly results from a circuit that counteracts the tonic inhibitory controls exerted by large-diameter afferents. In other words, opening the gate and keeping it open involve inhibition of the circuit through which large-diameter fibers normally keep the gate tonically closed.

This is a relatively simple feed-forward disinhibitory circuit, which likely exists in the superficial dorsal horn, even according to 1965 neurochemistry. Note that the gate control theory publication did not outline plausible circuits. To the contrary, the formulation was very much black box. Single lines did not represent single neurons, and plus and minus signs were not meant to illustrate whether a particular neuron was excitatory or inhibitory. Rather these elements of the gate represented the integrated sum of the output of populations of neurons. But amidst this apparent simplicity, the authors of gate control theory made a prediction based on creative examination and a keen insight into the basic anatomy and physiology of the spinal cord. For reasons of which I am completely ignorant, Melzack and Wall suggested that there was something "special" about the interneurons of the SG. They pointed out that the SG seemed to be relatively resistant to normal stains, although they didn't specify which stains. And the confusion about the extent to which there was a direct C-fiber input to these neurons, not to mention whether there was a direct descending inhibitory input, contributed to their conclusion that this was a particularly unusual population of interneurons.

How true that observation was! Almost every month, a new paper appears identifying yet another molecule that is enriched in interneurons of the SG, from neuropeptides, to growth factors, to protein kinases, and so on. It may be impossible to draw the wiring diagram of the SG, but it is not difficult to imagine a chemical circuit in the superficial dorsal horn that could overcome the tonic inhibition generated by large-diameter afferents. There are numerous routes through which C-fibers could generate disinhibition and thus enhance transmission of nociceptive messages; in other words, there are numerous means by which the gate may not only be opened, but also held open.

To me, holding the gate open is critical, as it bears on the problem of persistent pain and, in this regard, answers the question of whether gate control theory is relevant today. In my opinion, gate control theory is remarkably relevant, not because of the nature of the circuits that it postulates, but because of the underlying principle at its heart. Chronic or persistent pain is not merely long-lasting acute pain. Nor is it merely a result of maintained C-fiber activity. Rather, the development of chronic pain also depends on the evolution of an altered dorsal horn, one that amplifies and prolongs "pain" signals, and indeed one that can alter the perception of non-noxious as well as noxious stimuli. In the following section, I argue that central *sensitization*, a CNS process by which injury signals induce an amplified nociceptive message, is the modern version of gate control theory, not so much in terms of the circuit described, but rather in terms of the message that gate control theory conveys and the impact that it has for understanding the genesis of persistent pain.

CENTRAL SENSITIZATION

Central sensitization refers to the incredible plasticity and malleability of information flow in the "pain" transmission system (12). Dozens of molecules have been implicated in the sensitization of dorsal horn circuits, any of which can amplify the effects of the afferent signal, establish long-lasting sensitization, and enhance nociceptive processing (13–19). Central sensitization connotes a pathophysiologic process through which the gate of gate control theory can be held open. Because the mechanisms through which central sensitization occurs do not exclusively involve disinhibitory circuits that counter the effects of large-diameter afferents, central sensitization is not merely a restatement of gate control theory. On the other hand, there is no question that the process of central sensitization highlights the great differences between the Cartesian and the Melzack and Wall view of pain processing, particularly as it relates to the generation of persistent pain, which is clearly a profoundly important clinical problem.

Interesting Modes of Central Sensitization

In additional to the more traditional and better-studied N-methyl-D-aspartate (NMDA) receptor-mediated long-term facilitatory changes in the spinal cord, there are other changes that result from loss of inhibitory control, either through downregulation of receptors that are targeted by GABAergic inhibitory interneurons or because of frank loss of the inhibitory neurons themselves. Dysregulation of glycinergic inhibitory controls is of particular interest, as the evidence for its occurrence points to a mechanism through which cyclooxygenase (COX) inhibition at the level of the spinal cord could regulate central sensitization and nociceptive processing. In these studies, Ahmadi and colleagues (20) demonstrated that prostaglandin E_2 (PGE_2), by blocking action at a strychnine-sensitive subunit of the glycine receptor, reduces glycinergic inhibitory tone in the cord. As injury and the ensuing activity of nociceptors evokes the release of PGE_2 in the dorsal horn (perhaps from non-neuronal cells), this is conceivably one of the mechanisms through which the gate can be held open and through which inhibitory tone may be countered. Most importantly, of course, this mechanism is amenable to clinical manipulation with COX inhibitors. And, it is of particular interest that by using an intrathecal rather than systemic route, it may be possible to avoid some of the unfortunate adverse side effects of systemically administered COX-2 inhibitors.

Targeting Central Sensitization for Treatment

Of course, the list of possible ways to regulate central sensitization is long, and indeed some of these approaches are being developed within evolving clinical practice, as the anesthesiologist deals with the problem of persistent pain. Many of these methods are beautifully described throughout this textbook, and thus it is not my intention in this essay to provide a detailed discussion of targets or approaches that modern molecular genetic and behavioral studies have identified. The good news is that so many possible targets exist. I am not a betting man, however, so if asked which molecule to put my money on, I will pass. But I will emphasize my optimism, not only because I believe that the relatively near future will see the development of therapies that target molecules critical to central sensitization, but also that the methodology for producing long-term downregulation of these processes is on the horizon. I am particularly optimistic about the development of molecular approaches to regulating the genes that are at the heart of the problem. Antisense technology has been disappointing, for reasons of specificity and difficulties in relevant drug delivery. But the excitement surrounding the use of small interfering RNAs to disrupt mRNAs is not only palpable, but to me justified. The approach is already in the clinic (for example, for the treatment of age-dependent macular degeneration). Intrathecal application of these molecules provides a convenient route of therapy, which adds to my optimism.

THERAPEUTIC TARGETS: CENTRAL SENSITIZATION OR AFFERENT DRIVE OF THE NOCICEPTORS

Unfortunately, the downside to the identification of so many molecules as candidate mediators of central sensitization is that one wonders whether it will ever be sufficient to target a single site. A further problem is that many, if not the majority, of molecules implicated in central sensitization have been implicated in the process of long-term potentiation (21), which is critical to the establishment of memories. Thus, a high likelihood exists for producing significant adverse side effects upon memory when trying to interfere with central sensitization. The alternative, of course, is not to target the underlying mechanisms of central sensitization, which may or may not correspond to the circuit through which the gate is held open, but rather to target the input that activates the sensitization process.

A recent satellite meeting of the International Association for the Study of Pain (IASP) triennial World Congress on the topic of central pain was instructive in this regard. Not sur-prisingly, discussion focused on pains associated with multiple sclerosis, stroke, and spinal cord injury. Of particular interest to me was the make-up of the audience. Despite the fact that the IASP membership has a preponderance of anesthesiologists, very few attended the central pain meeting. The major clinical representation was from neurologists and a few neurosurgeons. Presumably, this attendance reflects the fact that anesthesiologists do not generally treat pains that arise from injury to the CNS. Rather, these patients end up in the hands of the neurologist. I am not certain that the neurologists have better solutions, other than the traditional anticonvulsants and other drugs that are used for a variety of neuropathic pain conditions, but they were there and took part in what was a lively discussion.

There is a lesson here, of course. The majority of anesthesiologists who specialize in the treatment of chronic pain employ techniques of regional anesthesia, particularly neural blockade. Such therapies are primarily directed at blocking ongoing activity of peripheral afferent fibers. Some anesthesiologists implant pumps and other neuromodulatory devices in the spinal column, perhaps with benefit for some patients with central pain, but these patients constitute a small part of the chronic pain population. It is not surprising, therefore, that any look to the future of pain therapy as it is likely to affect the regional anesthesiologist must concentrate on local anesthetic–responsive pathophysiologic conditions that contribute to persistent pain, and to the development of novel drugs that can block voltage-gated sodium (Na^+) channels with fewer adverse effects compared to presently available agents.

Importance of Ongoing Peripheral Input for Perpetuating Chronic Pain

I am, in fact, a very strong advocate of the view that the vast majority, if not all, of chronic pain conditions are maintained, to a great extent, by ongoing activity of peripheral afferents (see also Devor [22] for review). This is certainly true for evoked pain (e.g., the mechanical allodynia associated with a variety of peripheral nerve injury conditions), and I believe it is also true for ongoing pain. Indeed, the great majority of ongoing pains (both nociceptive/inflammatory and neuropathic) can be blocked, at least transiently, by peripheral local anesthetic injection. The block will, of course, wear off and the pain will return, but in some fortunate patients the relief significantly outlasts the anesthetic duration. Almost inevitably, however, the pain will return. One can speculate that the prolonged relief results from a transient quieting of the central sensitization that is driven by ongoing peripheral nerve activity. Regardless, the fact that peripheral block almost always yields some benefit (something that I observed repeatedly while working under the direction of the late Peter Nathan at the National Hospital in London) illustrates the importance of peripheral afferent input, and more importantly, the utility of peripheral nerve block.

Without question, therefore, local anesthetics will remain the mainstay of the regional anesthesiologist. On the horizon, however, are local anesthetics that will be far more efficacious for pain, as they will target Na^+ channels that are uniquely or at least much more selectively expressed by primary afferent nociceptors. To the extent that the distribution of these channels is anatomically limited, the therapeutic window for pain therapy will be enlarged, so that adverse side effects are dramatically reduced. The discovery of novel Na^+ channel blockers and their local delivery via innovative techniques will revolutionize the approaches taken by the regional anesthesiologist. Therefore, I believe that the future of regional techniques in pain management is very bright.

Regulation of Nociceptor Drive: NaV1.7, 1.8, 1.9, and More

Of particular interest is the development of drugs that selectively target the tetrodotoxin (TTX)-resistant, voltage-gated Na$^+$ channels, which many view as the Holy Grail for pain therapy, if one exists (23). NaV1.8 and 1.9 are only expressed by primary afferents, and the majority of these are small-diameter nociceptors. Considerable evidence also exists for a critical contribution of this class of voltage-gated Na$^+$ channels to injury-induced persistent pain. Whether it will be possible to selectively block the NaV1.8 subtype of Na$^+$ channel remains to be seen, but industry is making strides in that direction. We should soon learn whether this Na$^+$ channel subtype is indeed a worthwhile site to target clinically.

There is perhaps even more exciting news concerning the possible contribution of the NaV1.7 subtype of voltage-gated Na channel, which until very recently received attention because a gain of function mutation in the channel is the cause of erythromelalgia (24). Cox et al reported on a Pakistani firewalker who has a loss of function mutation in the gene that encodes NaV1.7 (25). This individual never experiences pain and apparently has no adverse side-effects associated with the loss of pain sensibility, a phenotype that to me was quite unexpected. This is because, unlike the TTX-resistant channels, which are exclusively located in primary afferents, the NaV1.7 subtype is likely also found, at least to some extent, in brain and spinal cord. Furthermore, although mice with a deletion of the gene that encodes NaV1.7 show abnormalities of pain sensation, including a dramatic reduction in the production of inflammatory pain, the mice are not "pain free" (26). Indeed, these mice still develop nerve injury-associated pain conditions in models of neuropathic pain. In fact, even double deletion mutants of 1.8 and 1.7 are not as pain free as the firewalker (27). Exactly what this means for understanding mechanism is not clear, but it certainly suggests caution in drawing conclusions about human correlates from results in which mice with single gene deletions are studied. One thing that can be predicted with high confidence, however, is that the number one target on the analgesic radar screen of the pharmaceutical industry is now 1.7, rather than 1.8.

There are, of course, other approaches to regulating afferent drive, and many of these are already in use. Chief among these are therapies directed at decreasing calcium (Ca^{2+}) entry into the presynaptic terminal of the primary afferent nociceptor. In this group are the opioids, which inhibit Ca^{2+} influx into nociceptive neurons, and also hyperpolarize postsynaptic neurons by increasing their potassium (K$^+$) conductance. The precise mechanisms through which gabapentin and related compounds that interact with the $\alpha_2\delta$-subunit of Ca^{2+} channels (28) produce analgesia is not certain, but also likely involves regulation of transmitter release from primary afferents. Ziconotide, an N-type Ca^{2+} channel blocker also acts directly to decrease neurotransmitter release (29). As more and more molecules unique to the nociceptor are identified, and as the functional significance of subsets of nociceptors is better characterized, it may be possible for the regional anesthesiologist to achieve even more selective blockade of relevant afferent input.

SUMMARY

The major message of the gate control theory of pain is still relevant today. Pain is not simply the consequence of inputs transmitted by primary afferent nociceptors, but rather depends on activity in populations of afferents, not all of which are nociceptors, and in circuits in the spinal cord and brain that modify these inputs. Of particular importance are circuits that amplify the signals generated by nociceptors. Recognizing that the gate may be opened as well as closed is critical to understanding the important contribution of gate control theory. For this reason, it is essential to understand the many processes that open the gate and maintain it in an open position if we are to develop novel therapies for persistent pain.

Central sensitization is, in some respects, a metaphor for the process that maintains the gate in an open state, altering the central consequences of nociceptor activity. Treating pain, therefore, can involve regulation of central sensitization processes, but more simply, it can involve selective blockade of afferent input, because doing so should reduce the duration of central sensitization. The latter approach assumes that central sensitization is more tractable in the absence of the afferent drive, a principle that is not universally accepted and clearly needs to be tested. Taken together with recent breakthroughs in understanding the complexity of voltage-gated Na$^+$ channels, the potential for the pharmaceutical industry to develop drugs that selectively target those channels, and ongoing insights into the myriad other ways that afferent drive can be regulated, we can optimistically expect that remarkable new therapies will soon be available for the regional anesthesiologist who treats chronic pain.

ACKNOWLEDGMENTS

This work was supported by NIH grants NS14627 and NS48499.

References

1. Melzack R, Wall PD. Pain mechanisms: A new theory. *Science* 1965;150:971–979.
2. Melzack R, Casey KL. Sensory motivational and central control determinants of pain: A new conceptual model. In: Kenshalo DR, ed. *The Skin Senses.* Springfield, IL: Charles C. Thomas; 1968:423–439.
3. Wall PD. Cord cells responding to touch, damage, and temperature of skin. *J Neurophysiol* 1960;23:197–210.
4. Christensen BN, Perl ER. Spinal neurons specifically excited by noxious or thermal stimuli: Marginal zone of the dorsal horn. *J Neurophysiol* 1970;33:293–307.
5. Wall PD. Comments after 30 years of the Gate Control Theory. *Pain Forum* 1996;5:12–22.
6. Wall PD, Sweet WH. Temporary abolition of pain in man. *Science* 1967;155:108–109.
7. Basbaum AI, Fields HL. Endogenous pain control mechanisms: Review and hypothesis. *Ann Neurol* 1978;4:451–462.
8. Fields HL, Basbaum AI. Brainstem control of spinal pain-transmission neurons. *Annu Rev Physiol* 1978;40:217–248.
9. Sun H, Ren K, Zhong CM, et al. Nerve injury-induced tactile allodynia is mediated via ascending spinal dorsal column projections. *Pain* 2001;90:105–111.
10. Mendell LM, Wall PD. Presynaptic hyperpolarization: A role for fine afferent fibres. *J Physiol* 1964;172:274–294.
11. Dahlström A, Fuxe K. Evidence for the existence of monoamine neurons in the central nervous system. II. Experimentally induced changes in the intraneuronal amine levels of bulbospinal neuron systems. *Acta Physiol Scand* 1965;[Suppl S247]:1–36.
12. Woolf CJ. Evidence for a central component of post-injury pain hypersensitivity. *Nature* 1983;306:686–688.

13. Woolf CJ, Salter MW. Neuronal plasticity: Increasing the gain in pain. *Science* 2000;288:1765–1769.
14. Suzuki R, Dickenson A. Spinal and supraspinal contributions to central sensitization in peripheral neuropathy. *Neurosignals* 2005;14:175–181.
15. Petersen-Zeitz KR, Basbaum AI. Second messengers, the substantia gelatinosa and injury-induced persistent pain. *Pain* 1999;[Suppl 6]:S5–S12.
16. McMahon SB, Cafferty WB, Marchand F. Immune and glial cell factors as pain mediators and modulators. *Exp Neurol* 2005;192:444–4462.
17. Julius D, Basbaum AI. Molecular mechanisms of nociception. *Nature* 2001;413:203–210.
18. Ji RR. Peripheral and central mechanisms of inflammatory pain, with emphasis on MAP kinases. *Curr Drug Targets Inflamm Allergy* 2004;3:299–303.
19. Basbaum AI, Woolf CJ. Pain. *Curr Biol* 1999;9:R429–R431.
20. Ahmadi S, Lippross S, Neuhuber WL, et al. PGE$_2$ selectively blocks inhibitory glycinergic neurotransmission onto rat superficial dorsal horn neurons. *Nat Neurosci* 2002;5:34–40.
21. Sanes JR, Lichtman JW. Can molecules explain long-term potentiation? *Nat Neurosci* 1999;2:597–604.
22. Devor M. Sodium channels and mechanisms of neuropathic pain. *J Pain* 2006;7:S3–S12.
23. Amir R, Argoff CE, Bennett GJ, et al. The role of sodium channels in chronic inflammatory and neuropathic pain. *J Pain* 2006;7:S1–29.
24. Waxman SG, Dib-Hajj S. Erythermalgia: Molecular basis for an inherited pain syndrome. *Trends Mol Med* 2005;11:555–562.
25. Cox JJ, Reimann F, Nicholas AK, et al. An SCN9A channelopathy causes congenital inability to experience pain. *Nature* 2006;444:894–898.
26. Nassar MA, Stirling LC, Forlani G, et al. Nociceptor-specific gene deletion reveals a major role for Nav1.7 (PN1) in acute and inflammatory pain. *Proc Natl Acad Sci USA* 2004;101:12706–12711.
27. Nassar MA, Levato A, Stirling LC, et al. Neuropathic pain develops normally in mice lacking both Nav1.7 and Nav1.8. *Mol Pain* 2005;1:24.
28. Field MJ, Cox PJ, Stott E, et al. Identification of the alpha2-delta-1 subunit of voltage-dependent calcium channels as a molecular target for pain mediating the analgesic actions of pregabalin. *Proc Natl Acad Sci USA* 2006;103:17537–17542.
29. McGivern JG. Targeting N-type and T-type calcium channels for the treatment of pain. *Drug Discov Today* 2006;11:245–253.

Note: Page numbers followed by *f* and *t* denote figure and table, respectively.